ENDOCRINOLOGY

ENDOCRINOLOGY

FOURTH EDITION

Edited by

LESLIE J. DeGROOT

J. LARRY JAMESON

Henry G. Burger

D. Lynn Loriaux

John C. Marshall

Shlomo Melmed

William D. Odell

John T. Potts, Jr.

Arthur H. Rubenstein

Volume

2

W.B. SAUNDERS COMPANY

A Harcourt Health Sciences Company

Philadelphia London New York St. Louis Toronto Sydney

W.B. SAUNDERS COMPANY
A Harcourt Health Sciences Company

The Curtis Center
Independence Square West
Philadelphia, Pennsylvania 19106

Library of Congress Cataloging-in-Publication Data

Endocrinology/edited by Leslie J. DeGroot, J. Larry Jameson [and] Henry Burger . . . [et al.]—4th ed.

p. cm.

Includes bibliographical references and index.

ISBN 0–7216–7840–8 (set)

1. Endocrine glands—Diseases. 2. Endocrinology. I. DeGroot, Leslie J. II. Jameson, J. Larry.

[DNLM: 1. Endocrine Diseases. 2. Endocrine Glands. 3. Hormones. WK 140 E5585 2001]

RC648.E458 2001 616.4—dc21

DNLM/DLC 00-030134

Acquisitions Editor: Richard Zorab
Developmental Editor: Hazel N. Hacker
Manuscript Editor: Deborah Thorp, Marjory Fraser
Production Manager: Norman Stellander
Illustration Specialist: Walter Verbitski
Book Designer: Steven Stave

ISBN 0–7216–7841–6 (vol. 1)
ISBN 0–7216–7842–4 (vol. 2)
ISBN 0–7216–7843–2 (vol. 3)
ISBN 0–7216–7840–8 (set)

ENDOCRINOLOGY

Printed in the United States of America.

Last digit is the print number: 9 8 7 6 5 4 3 2 1

Contributors

Rexford S. Ahima, MD, PhD
Assistant Professor of Medicine, Division of Endocrinology/Diabetes and Metabolism, Department of Medicine, University of Pennsylvania School of Medicine; Attending Endocrinologist, Hospital of the University of Pennsylvania; Director, Physiology Core Laboratory, Penn Diabetes Center, Philadelphia, Pennsylvania
Leptin

Nobuyuki Amino, MD
Professor of Medicine, Department of Laboratory Medicine, Osaka University Medical School, Osaka, Japan
Chronic (Hashimoto's) Thyroiditis

Marianne S. Anderson, MD
Assistant Professor, Department of Pediatrics, University of Colorado School of Medicine, Denver, Colorado
Fuel Homeostasis in the Fetus and Neonate

Josephine Arendt, BSc, PhD, FRCPath
Professor of Endocrinology, School of Biological Sciences, University of Surrey; Director, Centre for Chronobiology, Surrey, England
The Pineal Gland: Basic Physiology and Clinical Implications

Lora Armstrong, RPh, PharmD, BCPS
Clinical Pharmacist, Clinical Services Department, Caremark, Northbrook, Illinois
Drugs and Hormones Used in Endocrinology

David C. Aron, MD, MS
Professor of Medicine and Professor of Epidemiology and Biostatistics, Case Western Reserve University School of Medicine; Senior Scholar and Associate Chief of Staff for Education, Louis Stokes Cleveland Veterans Affairs Medical Center, Cleveland, Ohio
Diagnostic Implications of Adrenal Physiology and Clinical Epidemiology for Evaluation of Glucocorticoid Excess and Deficiency

Sylvia L. Asa, MD, PhD
Professor, Department of Laboratory Medicine and Pathobiology, University of Toronto; Consultant in Endocrine Pathology, Department of Pathology and Laboratory Medicine, Mount Sinai Hospital, Toronto, Ontario, Canada
Functional Pituitary Anatomy and Histology

Richard J. Auchus, MD, PhD
Assistant Professor, Division of Endocrinology and Metabolism, Department of Internal Medicine, University of Texas Southwestern Medical Center; Attending Physician, Parkland Memorial Hospital, VANTHCS, Dallas, Texas
The Principles, Pathways, and Enzymes of Human Steroidogenesis

Louis V. Avioli, MD
Schoenberg Professor of Medicine and Director, Division of Bone and Mineral Diseases, Washington University School of Medicine; Director, Division of Endocrinology and Metabolism, The Jewish Hospital of St. Louis, St. Louis, Missouri
Disorders of Calcification: Osteomalacia and Rickets

Joseph Avruch, MD
Professor of Medicine, Harvard Medical School; Physician and Chief, Diabetes Unit, Medical Services, and Member, Department of Molecular Biology, Massachusetts General Hospital, Boston, Massachusetts
Receptor Tyrosine Kinases

Lloyd Axelrod, MD
Associate Professor of Medicine, Harvard Medical School; Physician and Chief, James Howard Means Firm, Massachusetts General Hospital, Boston, Massachusetts
Glucocorticoid Therapy

Sami T. Azar, MD
Assistant Professor in Medicine, American University in Beirut, Beirut, Lebanon
Hypoaldosteronism and Mineralocorticoid Resistance

David T. Baird, MB, DSc
MCR Clinical Research Professor, Faculty of Medicine, University of Edinburgh; Director, Reproductive Medicine, Royal Infirmary, Edinburgh, Scotland
Amenorrhea, Anovulation, and Dysfunctional Uterine Bleeding

H. W. Gordon Baker, MD, PhD, FRACP
Principal Research Fellow, Department of Obstetrics and Gynaecology, University of Melbourne, Melbourne; Andrologist, The Royal Women's Hospital, Clayton, Victoria, Australia
Male Infertility

Giuseppe Barbesino, MD
Assistant Professor, Department of Endocrinology, University of Pisa Medical School, Pisa, Italy
Graves' Disease

Randall B. Barnes, MD
Associate Professor, Department of Obstetrics and Gynecology, University of Chicago Pritzker School of Medicine; Attending Physician, Chicago Lying-in Hospital, Chicago, Illinois
Hyperandrogenism, Hirsutism, and the Polycystic Ovary Syndrome

George B. Bartley, MD
Associate Professor of Ophthalmology, Mayo Medical School; Chair, Department of Ophthalmology, Mayo Clinic, Rochester, Minnesota
Ophthalmopathy

Etienne-Emile Baulieu, MD, PhD
Professor, Collège de France; Chef de Service de Biochimie Hormonale, Hôpital de Bicêtre, Bicêtre, France
Nuclear Receptor Superfamily

Peter H. Baylis, BSc, MD, FRCP
Dean of Medicine and Professor of Experimental Medicine, University of Newcastle Upon Tyne Medical School; Consultant Endocrinologist, Royal Victoria Infirmary, Newcastle Upon Tyne, England
Vasopressin, Diabetes Insipidus, and Syndrome of Inappropriate Antidiuresis

Paolo Beck-Peccoz
Professor of Endocrinology, Institute of Endocrine Sciences, University of Milan; Chief, Endocrine Unit, Ospedale Maggiore IRCCS, Milan, Italy
TSH-Producing Adenomas; Resistance to Thyroid Hormone

Graeme I. Bell, PhD
Professor of Biochemistry and Molecular Biology, Medicine, and Human Genetics, University of Chicago Pritzker School of Medicine; Investigator, Howard Hughes Medical Institute, Chicago, Illinois
Chemistry and Biosynthesis of the Islet Hormones: Insulin, Islet Amyloid Polypeptide (Amylin), Glucagon, Somatostatin, and Pancreatic Polypeptide

Eren Berber, MD
Fellow, Department of General Surgery, Cleveland Clinic Foundation, Cleveland, Ohio
Adrenal Surgery

Richard M. Bergenstal, MD
Executive Director and Chief Medical Officer, International Diabetes Center; Consultant in Endocrinology, Park Nicollet Clinic, Minneapolis, Minnesota
Management of Type 2 Diabetes: A Systematic Approach to Meeting the Standards of Care, I: Self-Management Education, Medical Nutrition Therapy, and Exercise; II: Oral Agents, Insulin, and Management of Complications

John P. Bilezikian, MD
Professor of Medicine and Pharmacology, Department of Medicine, Columbia University College of Physicians and Surgeons; Attending Physician, New York–Presbyterian Hospital, New York, New York
Primary Hyperparathyroidism

Richard E. Blackwell, PhD, MD
Professor, Department of Obstetrics and Gynecology, University of Alabama School of Medicine, Birmingham, Alabama
Female Infertility: Evaluation and Treatment

Stephen R. Bloom, MD, DSc, FRCP, FRCPath
Professor of Medicine, Imperial College School of Medicine; Chief, Investigative Sciences, The Hammersmith Hospital, London, England
Gastrointestinal Hormones and Tumor Syndromes

Jeffrey A. Bluestone, PhD
Daniel K. Ludwig Professor, University of Chicago Pritzker School of Medicine; Director, Ben May Institute for Cancer Research, Chicago, Illinois
Immunologic Mechanisms Causing Autoimmune Endocrine Disease

Manfred Blum, MD
Professor of Clinical Medicine and Radiology, New York University School of Medicine; Attending Physician and Director, Nuclear Endocrine Laboratory, Tisch Hospital, New York, New York
Thyroid Imaging

Roger Bouillon, MD, PhD
Professor of Endocrinology, Faculty of Medicine, Katholieke Universiteit Leuven; Chairman, Department of Endocrinology, University Hospitals, Gasthuisberg, Leuven, Belgium
Vitamin D: From Photosynthesis, Metabolism, and Action to Clinical Applications

Andrew J. M. Boulton, MD, FRCP
Professor of Medicine, Faculty of Medicine, University of Manchester; Consultant Physician, Manchester Royal Infirmary, Manchester, England
Diabetes Mellitus: Neuropathy

Glenn D. Braunstein, MD
Professor and Vice Chair, Department of Medicine, University of California, Los Angeles, UCLA School of Medicine; Chairman, Department of Medicine, Cedars-Sinai Medical Center, Los Angeles, California
Hypothalamic Syndromes

F. Richard Bringhurst, MD
Associate Professor of Medicine, Harvard Medical School; Physician and Chief of Staff, Medical Services, Massachusetts General Hospital, Boston, Massachusetts
Regulation of Calcium and Phosphate Homeostasis

Arthur E. Broadus, MD, PhD
Professor of Medicine, Yale University School of Medicine; Chief of Endocrinology, Yale–New Haven Hospital, New Haven, Connecticut
Malignancy-Associated Hypercalcemia

Edward M. Brown, MD
Professor of Medicine, Harvard Medical School; Senior Physician, Brigham and Women's Hospital, Boston, Massachusetts
Parathyroid Hormone and Parathyroid Hormone–Related Peptide in the Regulation of Calcium Homeostasis and Bone Development; Familial Hypocalciuric Hypercalcemia and Other Disorders Due to Calcium-Sensing Receptor Mutations

Henry B. Burch, MD
Associate Professor of Medicine, Uniformed Services University of the Health Sciences, Bethesda, Maryland; Assistant Chief, Endocrine–Metabolic Service, Walter Reed Army Medical Center, Washington, D.C.
Ophthalmopathy

Henry G. Burger, MD, FRACP
Honorary Professor of Medicine, Faculty of Medicine, Monash University; *formerly* Director, Prince Henry's Institute of Medical Research, Monash Medical Centre, Clayton, Victoria, Australia
Gonadal Peptides: Inhibins, Activins, Follistatin, Müllerian-Inhibiting Substance (Antimüllerian Hormone); Menopause and Hormone Replacement

Gerard N. Burrow, MD
David Paige Smith Professor of Medicine and Professor of Obstetrics and Gynecology, Yale University School of Medicine, New Haven, Connecticut
Diagnosis and Treatment of Thyroid Disease During Pregnancy

Jose F. Caro, MD
Professor of Medicine, Indiana University School of Medicine, Indianapolis, Indiana
Obesity

Don H. Catlin, MD
Associate Professor, Department of Medicine and Department of Molecular and Medical Pharmacology, University of California, Los Angeles, UCLA School of Medicine, Los Angeles, California
Use and Abuse of Anabolic Steroids

Ralph R. Cavalieri, MD
Professor Emeritus, Department of Medicine and Department of Radiology, University of California, San Francisco, School of Medicine; Consultant in Endocrinology and Nuclear Medicine, Veterans Administration Medical Center, San Francisco, California
Thyroid Imaging

Alan Chait, MD
Professor of Medicine and Head, Division of Metabolism, Endocrinology, and Nutrition, Department of Medicine, University of Washington School of Medicine, Seattle, Washington
Diabetes, Lipids, and Atherosclerosis

John R. G. Challis, PhD, DSc, FIBiol, FRCOG, FRSC
Ernest B. and Leonard B. Smith Professor and Chair, Department of Physiology, and Professor of Obstetrics and Gynecology, MRC Group in Fetal and Neonatal Health and Development, Faculty of Medicine, University of Toronto, Toronto; Affiliate Scientist, Samuel Lunenfeld Research Institute, Mount Sinai Hospital; Toronto Affiliate, Lawson Research Institute, London, Ontario, Canada
Endocrinology of Parturition

Shu J. Chan, PhD
Associate Professor of Biochemistry and Molecular Biology, University of Chicago Pritzker School of Medicine; Senior Research Associate, Howard Hughes Medical Institute, Chicago, Illinois
Chemistry and Biosynthesis of the Islet Hormones: Insulin, Islet Amyloid Polypeptide (Amylin), Glucagon, Somatostatin, and Pancreatic Polypeptide

Roland D. Chapurlat, MD
Assistant Professor, Department of Rheumatology and Bone Diseases and INSERM U403, Hôpital E. Herriot, Lyon, France
Osteoporosis

V. Krishna Chatterjee, MBChB, FRCP
Professor of Endocrinology, Department of Medicine, Faculty of Medicine, University of Cambridge; Honorary Consultant Physician, Addenbrooke's Hospital, Cambridge, England
Resistance to Thyroid Hormone

Qiao-Yi Chen, MD, PhD
Assistant Professor, Department of Pediatrics Louisiana State University School of Medicine in New Orleans, New Orleans; Research Institute for Children, Harahan, Louisiana
The Autoimmune Polyglandular Syndromes

Luca Chiovato, MD
Assistant Professor, Department of Endocrinology, University of Pisa Medical School, Pisa, Italy
Graves' Disease

George P. Chrousos, MD
Chief, Pediatric and Reproductive Endocrinology Branch, National Institute of Child Health and Human Development, National Institutes of Health, Bethesda, Maryland
Interactions of the Endocrine and Immune Systems

David R. Clemmons, MD
Chief, Division of Endocrinology, and Kenan Professor of Medicine, University of North Carolina at Chapel Hill School of Medicine; Attending Physician, UNC Hospitals, Chapel Hill, North Carolina
Insulin-Like Growth Factor-I and Its Binding Proteins

Jack W. Coburn, MD
Adjunct Professor of Medicine, University of California, Los Angeles, UCLA School of Medicine; Staff Physician, VA West Los Angeles Medical Center, Los Angeles, California
The Renal Osteodystrophies

Georges Copinschi, MD, PhD
Professor of Endocrinology, Free University of Brussels Medical School; Consultant in Endocrinology, Erasme University Hospital, Brussels, Belgium
Endocrine and Other Biologic Rhythms

Gerald R. Cunha, PhD
Professor, Department of Anatomy, University of California, San Francisco, School of Medicine, San Francisco, California
Endocrinology of the Prostate and Benign Prostatic Hyperplasia

Leona Cuttler, MD
Professor of Pediatrics, Case Western Reserve University School of Medicine; Endocrinologist, Rainbow Babies and Children's Hospital, Cleveland, Ohio
Somatic Growth and Maturation

Jamie Dananberg, MD
Senior Physician-Scientist and Senior Clinical Research Physician, Lilly Research Laboratories, Eli Lilly and Company, Indianapolis, Indiana
Obesity

David L. Daniels, MD
Professor of Radiology, Medical College of Wisconsin; Froedtert Memorial Lutheran Hospital, Milwaukee, Wisconsin
Radiographic Evaluation of the Pituitary and Anterior Hypothalamus

Mario De Felice, MD
Associate Professor of Immunology, University of Messina Medical School, Messina; Scientist, Stazione Zoologica Anton Dohrn, Naples, Italy
Anatomy and Development

Ralph A. DeFronzo, MD
Professor of Medicine, University of Texas Health Sciences Center School of Medicine; Chief, Diabetes Division, South Texas Veterans' Health Care System, Audie Murphy Division, San Antonio, Texas
Regulation of Intermediary Metabolism During Fasting and Feeding

Leslie J. DeGroot, MD
Professor of Medicine, Thyroid Study Unit, University of Chicago Pritzker School of Medicine; Attending Physician, University of Chicago Hospitals, Chicago, Illinois
Nonthyroidal Illness Syndrome; Thyroid Neoplasia

David M. de Kretser
Professor and Director, Institute of Reproduction and Development, Monash University; Consultant, Reproductive Biology Unit, Monash Medical Centre, Clayton, Victoria, Australia
Functional Morphology

Pierre D. Delmas, MD, PhD
Professor of Medicine and Director, INSERM U403, Department of Rheumatology and Bone Diseases, Hôpital E. Herriot, Lyon, France
Osteoporosis

Ruben Diaz, MD, PhD
Instructor in Pediatrics, Harvard Medical School; Assistant in Medicine, Children's Hospital, Boston, Massachusetts
Familial Hypocalciuric Hypercalcemia and Other Disorders Due to Calcium-Sensing Receptor Mutations

Roberto Di Lauro, MD
Full Professor of Human Genetics, University of Naples Federico II Medical School; Head, Laboratory of Biochemistry and Molecular Biology, Stazione Zoologica Anton Dohrn, Naples, Italy
Anatomy and Development

Sean F. Dinneen, MD, FACP, FRCPI
Consultant Diabetologist, Addenbrooke's Hospital, Cambridge, England
Classification and Diagnosis of Diabetes Mellitus

Annemarie A. Donjacour, PhD
Assistant Researcher, Department of Anatomy, University of California, San Francisco, School of Medicine, San Francisco, California
Endocrinology of the Prostate and Benign Prostatic Hyperplasia

John L. Doppman, MD
Staff Radiologist, Department of Radiology, The Clinical Center, National Institutes of Health, Bethesda, Maryland
Adrenal Imaging

Daniel J. Drucker, MD
Professor, Department of Medicine, University of Toronto Faculty of Medicine; Staff Physician and University Division Director, Endocrinology, Toronto General Hospital, Toronto, Ontario, Canada
Glucagon Secretion, α Cell Metabolism, and Glucagon Action

Jacques E. Dumont, MD, PhD
Professor of Biochemistry, Free University of Brussels Medical School, Brussels, Belgium
Thyroid Regulatory Factors

John T. Dunn, MD
Professor, Division of Endocrinology, Department of Medicine, University of Virginia School of Medicine; Attending Physician, University of Virginia Hospital, Charlottesville, Virginia
Biosynthesis and Secretion of Thyroid Hormones

Christopher R. W. Edwards, MD
Professor of Clinical Medicine, Department of Medicine, University of Edinburgh; Honorary Consultant Physician, Western General Hospital, Edinburgh, Scotland
Primary Mineralocorticoid Excess Syndromes

David A. Ehrmann, MD
Associate Professor, Section of Endocrinology, Department of Medicine, University of Chicago Pritzker School of Medicine; Attending Physician, University of Chicago Hospitals, Chicago, Illinois
Hyperandrogenism, Hirsutism, and the Polycystic Ovary Syndrome

Ilia J. Elenkov, MD, PhD
Guest Researcher, Pediatric Endocrinology Section, Pediatric and Reproductive Endocrinology Branch, National Institute of Child Health and Human Development, and Inflammatory Joint Diseases Section, Arthritis and Rheumatism Branch, National Institute of Arthritis and Musculoskeletal and Skin Diseases, National Institutes of Health, Bethesda, Maryland
Interactions of the Endocrine and Immune Systems

Gregory F. Erickson, PhD
Professor, Department of Reproductive Medicine, University of California, San Diego, School of Medicine, La Jolla, California
Folliculogenesis, Ovulation, and Luteogenesis

Eric A. Espiner, MD, FRACP, FRS(NZ)
Professor in Medicine, Christchurch School of Medicine; Department of Endocrinology, Christchurch Hospital, Christchurch, New Zealand
Hormones of the Cardiovascular System

Erica A. Eugster, MD
Clinical Assistant Professor, Department of Pediatrics, Division of Endocrinology and Diabetes, Indiana University School of Medicine; Staff, James Whitcomb Riley Hospital for Children, Indianapolis, Indiana
Precocious Puberty; Delayed Puberty

Giovanni Faglia, MD
Professor of Endocrinology, School of Medicine, Faculty of Medicine, and Postgraduate School of Endocrinology and Metabolism, University of Milan; Chief, Division of Endocrinology, Ospedale Maggiore IRCCS, Milan, Italy
Prolactinomas and Hyperprolactinemic Syndrome

Lisa A. Farah, MD
Courtesy Assistant Clinical Professor, University of Florida Medical Center (Jacksonville); Physician, North Florida Gynecologic Specialists, Jacksonville, Florida
Female Infertility: Evaluation and Treatment

Murray J. Favus, MD
Professor of Medicine, University of Chicago Pritzker School of Medicine; Director, Bone Program, and Director, Clinical Research Center, University of Chicago Hospitals, Chicago, Illinois
Clinical Approach to Metabolic Bone Disease

Eleuterio Ferrannini, MD
Professor of Internal Medicine, Department of Internal Medicine and CNR Institute of Clinical Physiology, University of Pisa School of Medicine, Pisa, Italy
Regulation of Intermediary Metabolism During Fasting and Feeding

Joel S. Finkelstein, MD
Associate Professor of Medicine, Harvard Medical School; Associate Physician, Endocrine Unit, Massachusetts General Hospital, Boston, Massachusetts
Medical Management of Hypercalcemia

Delbert A. Fisher, MD
Professor Emeritus, Department of Pediatrics and Department of Medicine, University of California, Los Angeles, UCLA School of Medicine, Los Angeles; Vice President, Science and Innovation, Quest Diagnostics, Nichols Institute, San Juan Capistrano, California
Fetal and Neonatal Endocrinology; Endocrine Testing

Susan J. Fisher, PhD
Departments of Stomatology, Obstetrics and Gynecology and Reproductive Sciences, Pharmaceutical Chemistry and Anatomy, University of California at San Francisco, San Francisco, California
Implantation and Placental Physiology in Early Human Pregnancy: The Role of the Maternal Decidua and the Trophoblast

Jeffrey S. Flier, MD
George C. Reisman Professor of Medicine, Harvard Medical School; Vice Chair for Research, Department of Medicine, and Chief, Division of Endocrinology, Beth Israel Deaconess Medical Center, Boston, Massachusetts
Leptin; Syndromes of Insulin Resistance and Mutant Insulin

Maguelone G. Forest, MD, PhD
Hôpital Debrousse, Lyon, France
Diagnosis and Treatment of Disorders of Sexual Development

Daniel W. Foster, MD
Donald W. Seldin Distinguished Chair in Internal Medicine and Chairman, Department of Internal Medicine, University of Texas Southwestern Medical School, Dallas, Texas
Acute Complications of Diabetes Mellitus: Ketoacidosis, Hyperosmolar Coma, and Lactic Acidosis

Jayne A. Franklyn, MBChB, MD, PhD, FRCP
Professor of Medicine, Division of Medical Sciences, University of Birmingham; Consultant Physician, Queen Elizabeth Hospital, Birmingham, England
Thyroid Function Tests

Marion J. Franz, MS, RD, CDE
Director of Nutrition and Professional Education, International Diabetes Center, Minneapolis, Minnesota
Management of Type 2 Diabetes: A Systematic Approach to Meeting the Standards of Care, I: Self-Management Education, Medical Nutrition Therapy, and Exercise; II: Oral Agents, Insulin, and Management of Complications

Aaron L. Friedman, MD
Professor and Chair, Department of Pediatrics, University of Wisconsin School of Medicine, Madison, Wisconsin
Hormonal Regulation of Electrolyte and Water Metabolism

Eli A. Friedman, MD
Distinguished Teaching Professor and Chief, Renal Disease Division, State University of New York Downstate Medical Center College of Medicine, Brooklyn, New York
Nephropathy: A Major Diabetic Complication

Peter J. Fuller, MBBS, BMedSc, PhD, FRACP
Associate Professor, Monash University Department of Medicine; NH&MRL Principal Research Fellow, Prince Henry's Institute of Medical Research, Clayton, Victoria, Australia
Biochemistry of Mineralocorticoids

John W. Funder, BA, MDBS, PhD, FRACP
Professor, Monash University, Department of Medicine, Alfred Hospital; Director, Baker Medical Research Institute, Victoria, Australia
Biochemistry of Mineralocorticoids

Dana Gaddy-Kurten, MD
Associate Professor, Department of Medicine and Endocrinology, University of Arkansas for Medical Sciences, Little Rock, Arkansas
Hormone Signaling via Cytokine Receptors and Receptor Serine Kinases

Robert F. Gagel, MD
Professor of Medicine and Chairman, Department of Internal Medicine Specialties, University of Texas–Houston Medical School; Chief, Section of Endocrine Neoplasia and Hormonal Disorders, M. D. Anderson Cancer Center, Houston, Texas
Multiple Endocrine Neoplasia Type 2

Thomas J. Gardella, PhD
Assistant Professor in Medicine, Harvard Medical School; Assistant Professor in Biochemistry, Massachusetts General Hospital, Boston, Massachusetts
Parathyroid Hormone and Parathyroid Hormone–Related Peptide in the Regulation of Calcium Homeostasis and Bone Development

Bruce D. Gaylinn, PhD
Research Assistant Professor, Department of Internal Medicine, University of Virginia School of Medicine, Charlottesville, Virginia
Growth Hormone–Releasing Hormone and Growth Hormone Secretagogues: Basic Physiology and Clinical Implications

Harry K. Genant, MD
Professor of Radiology, Medicine, Epidemiology, and Orthopaedic Surgery, University of California, San Francisco, School of Medicine, San Francisco, California
Bone Density and Imaging of Osteoporosis

Hans Gerber, MD
Privatdozent, University of Bern School of Medicine; Head of Division, Department of Clinical Chemistry, University Hospital, Inselspital, Bern, Switzerland
Multinodular Goiter

John E. Gerich, MD
Professor of Medicine, University of Rochester School of Medicine, Rochester, New York
Hypoglycemia

Marvin C. Gershengorn, MD
Abby Rockefeller Mauze Distinguished Professor of Endocrinology in Medicine, Weill Medical College and Graduate School of Medical Sciences of Cornell University, New York, New York
Second Messenger Signaling Pathways: Phospholipids and Calcium

Mohammad A. Ghatei, PhD
Reader in Regulatory Peptides, Imperial College School of Medicine, London, England
Gastrointestinal Hormones and Tumor Syndromes

Gary W. Gibbons, MD
Professor of Surgery, Boston University School of Medicine; Executive Director, Foot Care Specialists of Boston Medical Center, Boston, Massachusetts
Management of the Diabetic Foot Complication

Neil J. L. Gittoes, BSc, MBChB, MRCP, PhD
Lecturer in Medicine, Division of Medical Sciences, University of Birmingham; Specialist Registrar in Endocrinology and Diabetes, Queen Elizabeth Hospital, Birmingham, England
Thyroid Function Tests

Linda C. Giudice, MD, PhD
Department of Obstetrics and Gynecology, Division of Reproductive Endocrinology, Stanford University Medical Center, Stanford, California
Endometriosis; Implantation and Placental Physiology in Early Human Pregnancy: The Role of the Maternal Decidua and the Trophoblast

Francis H. Glorieux, MD, PhD
Professor of Surgery and Pediatrics, McGill University Faculty of Medicine; Director of Research and Head, Genetics Unit, Shriners Hospital for Children, Montreal, Quebec, Canada
Hereditary Defects in Vitamin D Metabolism and Action

Steven R. Goldring, MD
Associate Professor of Medicine, Harvard Medical School; Chief of Rheumatology, New England Deaconess Hospital; Clinical Associate, Massachusetts General Hospital, Boston, Massachusetts
Disorders of Calcification: Osteomalacia and Rickets

Theodore L. Goodfriend, MD
Professor of Internal Medicine and Pharmacology, University of Wisconsin Medical School; Associate Chief of Staff, Research, Veterans Hospital, Madison, Wisconsin
Hormonal Regulation of Electrolyte and Water Metabolism

William G. Goodman, MD
Professor of Medicine, University of California, Los Angeles, UCLA School of Medicine; UCLA Medical Center, Los Angeles, California
The Renal Osteodystrophies

Louis J. G. Gooren, MD, PhD
Professor of Endocrinology, Hospital of the Vrije Universiteit, Amsterdam, The Netherlands
Gender Identity and Sexual Behavior

Colum A. Gorman, MB, BCh, PhD
Professor of Medicine, Mayo Medical School; Consultant, Mayo Clinic, Rochester, Minnesota
Ophthalmopathy

William J. Gradishar, MD
Associate Professor of Medicine, Department of Medicine, Northwestern University Medical School; Director, Breast Medical Oncology, Robert H. Lurie Comprehensive Cancer Center, Chicago, Illinois
Breast Cancer and Hormonal Management

Mathis Grossmann, MD
Research Officer, The Walter and Eliza Hall Institute of Medical Research, Parkville, Victoria, Australia
Thyroid-Stimulating Hormone and Regulation of the Thyroid Axis

Joel F. Habener, MD
Professor of Medicine, Harvard Medical School; Associate Physician, Massachusetts General Hospital; Investigator, Howard Hughes Medical Institute, Boston, Massachusetts
The Cyclic AMP Second Messenger Signaling Pathway

Steven Haffner, MD
Professor of Medicine, University of Texas Health Science Center, San Antonio, Texas
Diabetes, Lipids, and Atherosclerosis

Charles B. Hammond, MD
E. C. Hamblen Professor and Chairman, Department of Obstetrics and Gynecology, Duke University School of Medicine, Durham, North Carolina
Gestational Trophoblastic Neoplasms

David J. Handelsman, MBBS, FRACP, PhD
Professor of Reproductive Endocrinology and Andrology, University of Sydney Faculty of Medicine; Director, ANZAC Research Institute and Department of Andrology, Concord Hospital, Sydney, New South Wales, Australia
Androgen Action and Pharmacologic Uses; Male Contraception

Victor M. Haughton, MD
Professor of Radiology and Director of MRI Research, Medical College of Wisconsin; Radiologist, Milwaukee County Medical Complex, Froedtert Memorial Lutheran Hospital; Consultant in Radiology, Veterans Affairs Medical Center, Milwaukee, Wisconsin
Radiographic Evaluation of the Pituitary and Anterior Hypothalamus

William W. Hay, Jr., MD
Professor, Department of Pediatrics, University of Colorado School of Medicine; Scientific Director, Perinatal Research Center; Director, Training Program in Neonatal Perinatal Medicine, University of Colorado Health Sciences Center, Denver, Colorado
Fuel Homeostasis in the Fetus and Neonate

Simon W. Hayward, PhD
Assistant Adjunct Professor, Department of Urology, University of California, San Francisco, School of Medicine, San Francisco, California
Endocrinology of the Prostate and Benign Prostatic Hyperplasia

David Heber, MD, PhD
Professor of Medicine and Chief, Division of Clinical Nutrition, Department of Medicine, University of California, Los Angeles, UCLA School of Medicine; Director, Clinical Nutrition Research Unit, UCLA Medical Center, Los Angeles, California
Starvation and Nutritional Therapy

Laszlo Hegedüs, MD
Department of Endocrinology, Odense University Hospital, Odense, Denmark
Multinodular Goiter

Georg Hennemann, MD, PhD, FRCP, FRCP(E)
Professor of Medicine and Endocrinology, Medical Faculty, Erasmus University, Rotterdam, The Netherlands
Autonomously Functioning Thyroid Nodules and Other Causes of Thyrotoxicosis

Kevan C. Herold, MD
Associate Professor of Clinical Medicine, Columbia University College of Physicians and Surgeons; Associate Attending Physician, New York Presbyterian Hospital, New York, New York
Immunologic Mechanisms Causing Autoimmune Endocrine Disease

Yoh Hidaka, MD
Associate Professor, Department of Laboratory Medicine, Osaka University Medical School, Osaka, Japan
Chronic (Hashimoto's) Thyroiditis

Patricia M. Hinkle, PhD
Department of Pharmacology and Physiology, University of Rochester Medical Center, Rochester, New York
Second Messenger Signaling Pathways: Phospholipids and Calcium

Ken K. Y. Ho, MD, FRACP
Professor of Medicine, University of New South Wales Faculty of Medicine; Head, Pituitary Research Unit, The Garvan Institute of Medical Research, St. Vincent's Hospital, Sydney, New South Wales, Australia
Growth Hormone Deficiency in Adults

Joseph J. Hoet, MD*
Anatomy, Developmental Biology, and Pathology of the Pancreatic Islets

*Deceased.

Nelson D. Horseman, MS, PhD
Professor, Department of Molecular and Cellular Physiology and Department of Medicine, University of Cincinnati College of Medicine, Cincinnati, Ohio
Prolactin

Eva Horvath, PhD
Associate Professor, Department of Laboratory Medicine and Pathobiology, University of Toronto, Faculty of Medicine; Research Associate, Department of Laboratory Medicine, St. Michael's Hospital, Toronto, Ontario, Canada
Functional Pituitary Anatomy and Histology

Aaron J. W. Hsueh, PhD
Professor, Division of Reproductive Biology, Stanford University Medical School, Stanford, California
Ovarian Hormone Synthesis

John M. Hutson, MD(Monash), MD(Melb), FRACS
Professor and Director of Paediatric Surgery, Department of Paediatrics, Faculty of Medicine, University of Melbourne; Director of General Surgery, Royal Children's Hospital; Associate Director (Clinical Sciences), Murdoch Children's Research Institute, Melbourne, Victoria, Australia
Cryptorchidism and Hypospadias

J. Larry Jameson, MD, PhD
Irving S. Cutter Professor of Medicine and Chairman, Department of Medicine, Northwestern University Medical School; Physician-in-Chief, Northwestern Memorial Hospital, Chicago, Illinois
Applications of Molecular Biology and Genetics in Endocrinology; Mechanisms of Thyroid Hormone Action

Reza Jarrahy, MD
Resident, Department of Surgery, New York University Medical Center, New York, New York; Fellow, Division of Skull Base Surgery, Cedars-Sinai Medical Center, Los Angeles, California
Surgical Management of Pituitary Tumors

Michael Jergas, MD
Assistant Professor of Radiology, Teaching Hospital of the University of Cologne; Director, Department of Radiology, St. Katharinen-Hospital, Frechen, Germany
Bone Density and Imaging of Osteoporosis

V. Craig Jordan, PhD, DSc
Diana, Princess of Wales Professor of Cancer Research, Northwestern University Medical School; Director, Lyn Sage Breast Cancer Research Program, Robert H. Lurie Comprehensive Cancer Center, Chicago, Illinois
Breast Cancer and Hormonal Management

Nathalie Josso, MD
Research Director, École Normale Supérieure; Physician (Consultant), Hôpital St. Vincent de Paul, Paris, France
Anatomy and Endocrinology of Fetal Sex Differentiation

Harald W. Jüppner, MD
Associate Professor of Pediatrics, Harvard Medical School; Associate Biologist and Associate Pediatrician, Endocrine Unit, Department of Medicine and Pediatrics, Massachusetts General Hospital, Boston, Massachusetts
Parathyroid Hormone and Parathyroid Hormone–Related Peptide in the Regulation of Calcium Homeostasis and Bone Development; Genetic Disorders of Calcium Homeostasis Caused by Abnormal Regulation of Parathyroid Hormone Secretion or Responsiveness

Edwin L. Kaplan, MD
Professor of Surgery, University of Chicago Pritzker School of Medicine; University of Chicago Hospitals, Chicago, Illinois
Surgery of the Thyroid

Walter H. Kaye, MD
Professor of Psychiatry, University of Pittsburgh School of Medicine; Director, Center for Overcoming Problem Eating, Department of Psychiatry, Western Psychiatric Institute and Clinic, Pittsburgh, Pennsylvania
Anorexia Nervosa and Other Eating Disorders

Rasa Kazlauskaite, MD
Fellow, Division of Endocrinology, Diabetes and Nutrition, Department of Medicine, University of Maryland School of Medicine, Baltimore, Maryland
Thyroid-Stimulating Hormone and Regulation of the Thyroid Axis

Gary L. Keeney, MD
Assistant Professor, Mayo Medical School; Consultant, Department of Laboratory Medicine and Pathology, Division of Anatomic Pathology, Mayo Clinic, Rochester, Minnesota
Ovarian Tumors with Endocrine Manifestations

Harry R. Keiser, MD
Scientist Emeritus; Attending Physician, The Clinical Center, National Institutes of Health, Bethesda, Maryland
Pheochromocytoma and Related Tumors

David M. Kendall, MD
Medical Director, Adult Diabetes Services and Affiliate Program, International Diabetes Center; Consultant in Endocrinology, Park Nicollet Clinic, Minneapolis, Minnesota
Management of Type 2 Diabetes: A Systematic Approach to Meeting the Standards of Care, I: Self-Management Education, Medical Nutrition Therapy, and Exercise; II: Oral Agents, Insulin, and Management of Complications

Jeffrey B. Kerr, PhD
Associate Professor, Department of Anatomy, Monash University, Clayton, Victoria, Australia
Functional Morphology

Ronald Klein, MD, MPH
Professor, Department of Ophthalmology and Visual Sciences, University of Wisconsin Medical School, Madison, Wisconsin
Diabetes Mellitus: Oculopathy

David L. Kleinberg, MD
Professor of Medicine, New York University School of Medicine; Chief of Endocrinology, Department of Veterans Affairs, New York Harbor Health Care System, New York, New York
Endocrinology of Mammary Development, Lactation, and Galactorrhea

Christian A. Koch, MD
Senior Fellow, National Institutes of Health, National Institute of Child Health and Human Development, Bethesda, Maryland
Aging, Endocrinology, and the Elderly Patient

John J. Kopchick, MS, PhD
Department of Biomedical Sciences, College of Osteopathic Medicine, Ohio University; Edison Biotechnology Institute, Athens, Ohio
Growth Hormone

Stanley G. Korenman, MD
Professor of Medicine (Endocrinology) and Associate Dean, Ethics and Medical Sciences Training Program, University of California, Los Angeles, UCLA School of Medicine, Los Angeles, California
Erectile Dysfunction

Kenneth S. Korach, PhD
Professor of Endocrinology, University of North Carolina at Chapel Hill School of Medicine, Chapel Hill; Duke University School of Medicine, Durham; North Carolina State University, Raleigh; Program Director, Environmental Disease and Medicine Program, and Chief, Laboratory of Reproductive and Developmental Toxicology, National Institute of Environmental Health Science, National Institutes of Health, Research Triangle Park, North Carolina
Environmental Agents and the Reproductive System

Kalman Thomas Kovacs, MD, PhD
Professor, Department of Laboratory Medicine and Pathobiology, University of Toronto Faculty of Medicine; Pathologist, Department of Laboratory Medicine, St. Michael's Hospital, Toronto, Ontario, Canada
Functional Pituitary Anatomy and Histology

James M. Kozlowski, MD
Associate Professor, Department of Urology, Northwestern University Medical School, Chicago, Illinois
Prostate Cancer

Stephen M. Krane, MD
Persis, Cyrus and Marlow B. Harrison Professor of Medicine, Harvard Medical School; Physician and Chief of Arthritis Unit, Massachusetts General Hospital, Boston, Massachusetts
Disorders of Calcification: Osteomalacia and Rickets

Henry M. Kronenberg, MD
Professor of Medicine, Harvard Medical School; Chief, Endocrine Unit, Massachusetts General Hospital, Boston, Massachusetts
Parathyroid Hormone and Parathyroid Hormone–Related Peptide in the Regulation of Calcium Homeostasis and Bone Development

Yolanta T. Kruszynska, PhD, MRCP
Associate Professor of Medicine, University of California, San Diego, School of Medicine, La Jolla, California
Type 2 Diabetes Mellitus: Etiology, Pathogenesis, and Natural History

Anjli Kukreja, PhD
Research Associate, Department of Pediatrics, Weill Medical College of Cornell University, New York, New York
The Autoimmune Polyglandular Syndromes

Sandeep Kunwar, MD
Assistant Professor, Department of Neurological Surgery, University of California, San Francisco, School of Medicine; Principal Investigator, Brain Tumor Research Center, University of California at San Francisco, San Francisco, California
Sellar and Parasellar Tumors in Children

John M. Kyriakis, PhD
Associate Professor of Medicine, Department of Medicine, Harvard Medical School; Assistant Biochemist, Diabetes Unit, Department of Medicine, Massachusetts General Hospital, Boston, Massachusetts
Mitogen-Activated Protein Kinase and Growth Factor Signaling Pathways

Hop N. Le, MD
Research Fellow, Department of Surgery, University of California, San Francisco, School of Medicine, San Francisco, California
Surgical Management of Hyperparathyroidism

Harold E. Lebovitz, MD
State University of New York Downstate Medical Center College of Medicine, Brooklyn, New York
Hyperglycemia Secondary to Nondiabetic Conditions and Therapies

Chung Lee, PhD
Professor, Northwestern University Medical School, Chicago, Illinois
Prostate Cancer

Åke Lernmark, MD
Professor, Department of Medicine, University of Washington School of Medicine, Seattle, Washington
Type 1 (Insulin-Dependent) Diabetes Mellitus: Etiology, Pathogenesis, and Natural History

Michael A. Levine, MD
Professor of Pediatrics, Medicine, and Pathology, and Director, Division of Pediatric Endocrinology, Johns Hopkins University School of Medicine; Physician, Johns Hopkins Hospital, Baltimore, Maryland
Hypoparathyroidism and Pseudohypoparathyroidism

Stephen L. Lin, MD
Fellow in Endocrinology, Diabetes, and Nutrition and Assistant Clinical Instructor, Department of Medicine, University of Maryland School of Medicine, Baltimore, Maryland
Appetite Regulation

Jill S. Lindberg, MD
Evanston–Northwestern Hospital, Evanston, Illinois
Nephrolithiasis

Jonathan Lindzey, PhD
Assistant Professor, Department of Biology, University of South Florida, Tampa, Florida
Environmental Agents and the Reproductive System

Catherine Ann Lissett, MBChB, MRCP
Clinical Research Fellow, Department of Endocrinology, Christie Hospital, Manchester, England
Hypopituitarism

D. Lynn Loriaux, MD, PhD
Professor of Medicine and Head, Division of Endocrinology, Diabetes and Clinical Nutrition, Department of Medicine, Oregon Health Sciences University School of Medicine, Portland, Oregon
An Introduction to Endocrinology; Adrenal Insufficiency

Noel K. Maclaren, MD
Professor of Pediatrics, Weill College of Medicine of Cornell University; Director, Cornell Juvenile Diabetes Center, New York Hospitals, New York, New York
The Autoimmune Polyglandular Syndromes

Carl D. Malchoff, MD, PhD
Associate Professor, Department of Medicine, University of Connecticut School of Medicine, Farmington, Connecticut
Generalized Glucocorticoid Resistance

Diana M. Malchoff, PhD
Assistant Professor, Department of Medicine, University of Connecticut School of Medicine, Farmington, Connecticut
Generalized Glucocorticoid Resistance

Rayaz A. Malik, MD, PhD
Clinical Lecturer, Faculty of Medicine, University of Manchester; Senior Registrar, Manchester Royal Infirmary, Manchester, England
Diabetes Mellitus: Neuropathy

Susan J. Mandel, MD, MPH
Assistant Professor, Department of Medicine, University of Pennsylvania School of Medicine; Associate Chief for Clinical Affairs, Division of Endocrinology, Diabetes, and Metabolism, Hospital of the University of Pennsylvania, Philadelphia, Pennsylvania
Diagnosis and Treatment of Thyroid Disease During Pregnancy

Christos Mantzoros, MD, DSc
Assistant Professor, Department of Medicine, Division of Endocrinology, Harvard Medical School; Attending Endocrinologist, Beth Israel Deaconess Medical Center, Boston, Massachusetts
Syndromes of Insulin Resistance and Mutant Insulin

Leighton P. Mark, MD
Professor of Radiology, Medical College of Wisconsin; Froedtert Memorial Lutheran Hospital, Milwaukee, Wisconsin
Radiographic Evaluation of the Pituitary and Anterior Hypothalamus

John C. Marshall, MD, PhD
Arthur and Margaret Ebbert Professor of Medical Science Professor of Internal Medicine, University of Virginia School of Medicine; Director, Center for Research in Reproduction, University of Virginia Health Sciences Center, Charlottesville, Virginia
Regulation of Gonadotropin Synthesis and Secretion; Hormonal Regulation of the Menstrual Cycle and Mechanisms of Ovulation

T. John Martin, MD, DSc, FRACP
Director, St. Vincent's Institute of Medical Research, Melbourne, Victoria, Australia
Calcitonin

Thomas F. J. Martin, PhD
Department of Biochemistry, University of Wisconsin Medical School, Madison, Wisconsin
Control of Hormone Secretion

Lawrence S. Mathews, PhD
Department of Biochemistry, University of Michigan, Ann Arbor, Michigan
Hormone Signaling via Cytokine Receptors and Receptor Serine Kinases

Walter J. McDonald, MD
Associate Dean for Education, Oregon Health Sciences University; Active Staff, University Hospital, Portland, Oregon
Adrenal Insufficiency

Samy I. McFarlane, MD, FACE, CCD
Assistant Professor, Department of Medicine, Division of Endocrinology, Diabetes, and Hypertension, State University of New York, Health Science Center at Brooklyn, Brooklyn, New York
Hyperglycemia Secondary to Nondiabetic Conditions and Therapies

J. Denis McGarry, PhD
Clifton and Betsy Robinson Chair in Biomedical Research and Professor of Internal Medicine and Biochemistry, University of Texas Southwestern Medical School, Dallas, Texas
Acute Complications of Diabetes Mellitus: Ketoacidosis, Hyperosmolar Coma, and Lactic Acidosis

Michael J. McPhaul, MD
Professor of Internal Medicine, Division of Endocrinology and Metabolism, University of Texas Southwestern Medical Center, Dallas, Texas
Mutations That Alter Androgen Receptor Function

Geraldo Medeiros-Neto, MD, PhD
Professor of Endocrinology, Department of Clinical Medicine, University of São Paulo Medical School; Chief, Thyroid Unit, Hospital Das Clinicas FMUSP, São Paulo, Brazil
Iodine Deficiency Disorders

James C. Melby, MD
Professor of Medicine, Boston University School of Medicine, Boston, Massachusetts
Hypoaldosteronism and Mineralocorticoid Resistance

Shlomo Melmed, MD, FACP
Professor of Medicine and Associate Dean, University of California, Los Angeles, UCLA School of Medicine; Director, Research Institute, Cedars-Sinai Medical Center, Los Angeles, California
Evaluation of Pituitary Masses; Acromegaly

Jan Mester
Signalisation et Fonctions Cellulaires: Application au Diabete et aux Cancers Digestifs, INSERM, Paris, France
Nuclear Receptor Superfamily

Boyd E. Metzger, MD
Professor of Medicine, Northwestern University Medical School; Attending Physician, Northwestern Memorial Hospital, Chicago, Illinois
Diabetes Mellitus and Pregnancy

Roger L. Miesfeld, PhD
Professor of Biochemistry, University of Arizona College of Medicine, Tucson, Arizona
Glucocorticoid Action: Biochemistry

Robert Peter Millar BSc(Hons), MSc, PhD, FRCPath(Chem)
Professor, University of Edinburgh; Director, MRC Human Reproductive Sciences Unit, and Department of Medical Biochemistry, University of Cape Town, Cape Town, South Africa
Gonadotropin-Releasing Hormone (GnRH) and GnRH Receptors

Walter L. Miller, MD
Professor of Pediatrics, Chief of Endocrinology, and Director, Child Health Research Center, University of California, San Francisco; Director, Pediatric Endocrine Services, Moffit/Long Hospitals, San Francisco, California
The Principles, Pathways, and Enzymes of Human Steroidogenesis

Daniel R. Mishell, Jr., MD
Lyle G. McNeil Professor and Chairman, Department of Obstetrics-Gynecology, Keck School of Medicine, University of Southern California; Chief, Professional Services, Los Angeles County–University of Southern California Medical Center, Women's and Children's Hospital, Los Angeles, California
Contraception

Mark E. Molitch, MD
Professor of Medicine, Center for Endocrinology, Metabolism and Molecular Medicine, Northwestern University Medical School; Attending Physician, Northwestern Memorial Hospital, Chicago, Illinois
Hormonal Changes and Endocrine Testing in Pregnancy

Richard M. Mortensen, MD, PhD
Assistant Professor of Medicine, Harvard Medical School; Associate Physician, Brigham and Women's Hospital, Boston, Massachusetts
Aldosterone Action

Jane M. Moseley, PhD
Associate Professor of Medicine, University of Melbourne; Principal Research Fellow (NHMRC), St. Vincent's Institute of Medical Research, Melbourne, Victoria, Australia
Calcitonin

William R. Moyle, PhD
Professor of Obstetrics and Gynecology, University of Medicine and Dentistry of New Jersey–Robert Wood Johnson (Rutgers) Medical School, Piscataway, New Jersey
Gonadotropins

Allan Munck, PhD
Professor of Physiology, Dartmouth Medical School, Lebanon, New Hampshire
Glucocorticoid Action: Physiology

Martin G. Myers, Jr., MD, PhD
Assistant Professor in Medicine, Harvard Medical School; Assistant Investigator, Joslin Diabetes Center, Boston, Massachusetts
The Molecular Basis of Insulin Action

Anikó Náray-Fejes-Tóth, MD
Professor of Physiology, Dartmouth Medical School, Lebanon, New Hampshire
Glucocorticoid Action: Physiology

Ralf Nass, MD
Research Associate, University of Virginia School of Medicine, Charlottesville, Virginia
Growth Hormone–Releasing Hormone and Growth Hormone Secretagogues: Basic Physiology and Clinical Implications

Jerald C. Nelson, MD
Professor of Medicine and Pathology, Loma Linda University, School of Medicine, Loma Linda; Senior Medical Director, Quest Diagnostics, Nichols Institute, San Juan Capistrano, California
Endocrine Testing

Maria I. New, MD
Harold and Percy Uris Professor of Pediatric Endocrinology and Metabolism and Professor, Department of Pediatrics, Weill Medical College of Cornell University; Chairman, Department of Pediatrics, and Chief, Pediatric Endocrinology, New York–Presbyterian Hospital, New York, New York
Defects of Adrenal Steroidogenesis

Lynnette K. Nieman, MD
Chief, Unit on Reproductive Medicine, Developmental Endocrinology Branch, and Senior Staff Physician, National Institute of Child Health and Human Development, National Institutes of Health, Bethesda, Maryland
Cushing's Syndrome

John H. Nilson, PhD
John H. Hord Professor and Chair, Department of Pharmacology, and Director, Medical Scientist Training Program, Case Western Reserve University School of Medicine, Cleveland, Ohio; Editor-in-Chief, *Molecular Endocrinology*
Hormones and Gene Expression: Basic Principles

Christopher F. Njeh, BSc, MSc, PhD, CPhys
Assistant Adjunct Professor, Department of Radiology, University of California, San Francisco, School of Medicine, San Francisco, California
Bone Density and Imaging of Osteoporosis

Jeffrey A. Norton, MD, FACS
Vice Chairman, Department of Surgery, University of California, San Francisco, School of Medicine; Chief, Department of Surgery, San Francisco Veterans Affairs Medical Center, San Francisco, California
Surgical Management of Hyperparathyroidism

William D. Odell, MD, PhD, MACP
Emeritus Professor of Medicine and Physiology, University of Utah School of Medicine, Salt Lake City, Utah
Endocrinology of Sexual Maturation; Menopause and Hormone Replacement

Jerrold M. Olefsky, MD
Professor of Medicine and Chief, Endocrinology and Metabolism Division, University of California, San Diego, School of Medicine, La Jolla, California
Type 2 Diabetes Mellitus: Etiology, Pathogenesis, and Natural History

Niall M. O'Meara, MD
Consultant Physician/Endocrinologist, Department of Diabetes and Endocrinology, Mater Misericordiae Hospital, Dublin, Ireland
Secretion and Metabolism of Insulin, Proinsulin, and C Peptide

Furio Pacini, MD
Associate Professor, Department of Endocrinology, University of Pisa Medical School, Pisa, Italy
Thyroid Neoplasia

Lawrence N. Parker, MD
Professor of Medicine, Division of Endocrinology, University of California, Irvine, College of Medicine; Assistant Chief, Endocrinology Section, Veterans Affairs Medical Center, Long Beach, California
Adrenarche

Samuel Parry, MD
Assistant Professor, University of Pennsylvania School of Medicine, Philadelphia, Pennsylvania
Placental Hormones

Yogesh C. Patel, MD, PhD, FACP, FRCP(C), FRSC
Professor, Department of Medicine, Department of Neurology and Neurosurgery, and Department of Pharmacology and Therapeutics, McGill University Faculty of Medicine; Director, Division of Endocrinology and Metabolism, McGill University Health Center, Montreal, Quebec, Canada
Neurotransmitters and Hypothalamic Control of Anterior Pituitary Function

Luca Persani, MD, PhD
Senior Research Fellow, Institute of Endocrine Sciences, University of Milan; Senior Research Fellow, Istituto Auxilogico Italiano IRCCS, Milan, Italy
TSH-Producing Adenomas

Ora Hirsch Pescovitz, MD
Edwin Letzter Professor of Pediatrics and Professor of Physiology and Biophysics, Indiana University School of Medicine; Director of Pediatric Endocrinology and Diabetology, James Whitcomb Riley Hospital for Children, Indianapolis, Indiana
Precocious Puberty; Delayed Puberty

Richard L. Phelps, MD
Assistant Clinical Professor of Medicine, Northwestern University Medical School; Attending Physician, Northwestern Memorial Hospital, Chicago, Illinois
Diabetes Mellitus and Pregnancy

Aldo Pinchera, MD
Professor and Chairman, Department of Endocrinology, University of Pisa Medical School, Pisa, Italy
Graves' Disease

JoAnn Pinkerton, MD
Associate Professor, Department of Obstetrics and Gynecology; Director, Midlife Health University of Virginia Health Sciences Center, Charlottesville, Virginia
Benign Breast Disorders

Kenneth S. Polonsky, MD
Chairman, Department of Medicine, Washington University School of Medicine, St. Louis, Missouri
Secretion and Metabolism of Insulin, Proinsulin, and C Peptide

John T. Potts, Jr., MD
Jackson Distinguished Professor of Clinical Medicine, Harvard Medical School, Boston; Director of Research, Massachusetts General Hospital, Charlestown, Massachusetts
Parathyroid Hormone and Parathyroid Hormone–Related Peptide in the Regulation of Calcium Homeostasis and Bone Development

Lisa P. Purdy, MD, CM, MPH
Assistant Professor of Medicine, University of Rochester School of Medicine and Dentistry; Attending Physician, Genesee Hospital, Rochester General Hospital, and Strong Memorial Hospital, Rochester, New York
Diabetes Mellitus and Pregnancy

Charmian A. Quigley, MBBS
Assistant Professor, Indiana University School of Medicine; Clinical Research Physician, Department of Endocrinology, Lilly Research Laboratories, US Medical Division, Eli Lilly and Company, Indianapolis, Indiana
Genetic Basis of Sex Determination and Sex Differentiation

Christine Campion Quirk, PhD
NRSA Post-Doctoral Fellow, Department of Pharmacology, Case Western Reserve University School of Medicine, Cleveland, Ohio
Hormones and Gene Expression: Basic Principles

Miriam T. Rademaker, BSc, PhD
Research Fellow, Department of Medicine, Christchurch School of Medicine, Christchurch, New Zealand
Hormones of the Cardiovascular System

Ewa Rajpert-De Meyts, MD, PhD
Senior Scientist, Department of Growth and Reproduction, Copenhagen University Hospital (Rigshospitalet), Copenhagen, Denmark
Testicular Tumors with Endocrine Manifestations

Valerie Anne Randall, BSc, PhD
Senior Lecturer in Biomedical Sciences, Department of Biomedical Sciences, University of Bradford, Bradford, England
Physiology and Pathophysiology of Androgenetic Alopecia

David W. Ray, MD, PhD
Endocrine Science Research Group, School of Biological Sciences, University of Manchester, Manchester, England
Adrenocorticotropic Hormone

Nancy E. Reame, MSN, PhD
Professor, Center for Nursing Research, and Research Scientist, Reproductive Sciences Program, University of Michigan, Ann Arbor, Michigan
Premenstrual Syndrome

Gerald M. Reaven, MD
Professor of Medicine (Active Emeritus), Stanford University School of Medicine, Stanford, California
Syndrome X

Gézard Redeuilh
Signalisation et Fonctions Cellulaires: Application au Diabete et aux Cancers Digestifs, INSERM, Paris, France
Nuclear Receptor Superfamily

Samuel Refetoff, MD
Professor of Medicine and Pediatrics, University of Chicago Pritzker School of Medicine; Attending Physician, University of Chicago Hospitals, Chicago, Illinois
Thyroid Function Tests

Claude Remacle
Professor, Université Catholique de Louvain, Faculté des Sciences, Louvain-la-Neuve, Belgium
Anatomy, Developmental Biology, and Pathology of the Pancreatic Islets

Brigitte Reusens, DSc
Université Catholique de Louvain, Faculté des Sciences, Louvain-la-Neuve, Belgium
Anatomy, Developmental Biology, and Pathology of the Pancreatic Islets

Gail P. Risbridger, PhD
NH and MRC Senior Research Fellow, Institute of Reproduction and Development, Monash University, Melbourne, Australia
Functional Morphology

Robert A. Rizza, MD
Professor of Medicine, Mayo Medical School; Chair, Division of Endocrinology, Diabetes and Metabolism, Mayo Clinic, Rochester, Minnesota
Classification and Diagnosis of Diabetes Mellitus

R. Paul Robertson, MD
Affiliate Professor of Pharmacology, University of Washington School of Medicine; University of Washington Medical Center; CEO/Scientific Director, Pacific Northwest Research Institute, Seattle, Washington
Pancreas and Islet Transplantation

Gideon A. Rodan, MD, PhD
Adjunct Professor of Pathology, University of Pennsylvania School of Medicine, Philadelphia; Research Vice President, Bone Biology and Osteoporosis, Merck Research Laboratories, West Point, Pennsylvania
Bone Development and Remodeling

Ron G. Rosenfeld, MD
Professor and Chair, Department of Pediatrics, and Professor, Department of Cell and Developmental Biology, Oregon Health Sciences University School of Medicine; Physician-in-Chief, Doernbecher Memorial Hospital for Children, Portland, Oregon
Growth Hormone Deficiency in Children

Robert L. Rosenfield, MD
Professor of Pediatrics and Medicine, University of Chicago Pritzker School of Medicine; Head, Section of Pediatric Endocrinology, University of Chicago Children's Hospital, Chicago, Illinois
Somatic Growth and Maturation; Hyperandrogenism, Hirsutism, and the Polycystic Ovary Syndrome

Jesse Roth, MD
Raymond and Anna Lublin Professor of Medicine, Division of Geriatric Medicine and Gerontology, Johns Hopkins University School of Medicine, Baltimore, Maryland
Aging, Endocrinology, and the Elderly Patient

Kristina I. Rother, MD
Clinical Investigator, Diabetes Branch, NIDDK, National Institutes of Health, Bethesda, Maryland
Aging, Endocrinology, and the Elderly Patient

Peter S. Rotwein, MD
Professor of Medicine, Molecular Medicine Division, Department of Medicine, Oregon Health Sciences University School of Medicine, Portland, Oregon
Peptide Growth Factors Other Than Insulin-Like Growth Factors or Cytokines

Brian G. Rowan, PhD
Postdoctoral Fellow, Department of Molecular and Cellular Biology, Baylor College of Medicine, Houston, Texas
Estrogen and Progesterone Action

Arthur H. Rubenstein, MB, BCh
Dean and Gustave L. Levy Distinguished Professor, Mount Sinai School of Medicine of New York University, New York, New York
Chemistry and Biosynthesis of the Islet Hormones: Insulin, Islet Amyloid Polypeptide (Amylin), Glucagon, Somatostatin, and Pancreatic Polypeptide; Management of Type 2 Diabetes: A Systematic Approach to Meeting the Standards of Care, I: Self-Management Education, Medical Nutrition Therapy, and Exercise; II: Oral Agents, Insulin, and Management of Complications

Robert T. Rubin, MD, PhD
Professor of Neurosciences and Psychiatry, MCP Hahnemann University School of Medicine; Director, Center for Neurosciences Research, Allegheny General Hospital, Pittsburgh, Pennsylvania
Anorexia Nervosa and Other Eating Disorders

Irma M. Russo, MD
Professor, Jefferson Medical College of Thomas Jefferson University; Director, Molecular Endocrinology, Breast Cancer Research, Fox Chase Cancer Center, Philadelphia, Pennsylvania
Hormonal Control of Breast Development

Jose Russo, MD
Professor, Jefferson Medical College of Thomas Jefferson University; Director, Breast Cancer Research, Fox Chase Cancer Center, Philadelphia, Pennsylvania
Hormonal Control of Breast Development

Isidro B. Salusky, MD
Professor of Pediatrics, University of California, Los Angeles, UCLA School of Medicine; Director, Pediatric Dialysis Program, and Director, General Clinical Research Center, UCLA Medical Center, Los Angeles, California
The Renal Osteodystrophies

Richard J. Santen, MD
Professor of Medicine, University of Virginia School of Medicine, Charlottesville, Virginia
Hormonal Control of Breast Development; Benign Breast Disorders; Gynecomastia

David H. Sarne, MRCP, PhD
Associate Professor of Medicine and Director, Endocrine Clinic, Department of Medicine, University of Illinois, Chicago, Illinois
Thyroid Function Tests

Maurice F. Scanlon, BSc, MD, FRCP
Professor of Endocrinology, University of Wales College of Medicine; Honorary Consultant Physician, University Hospital of Wales, Cardiff, Wales
Thyrotropin-Releasing Hormone and Thyroid-Stimulating Hormone

Agnes Schonbrunn, PhD
Professor, Department of Integrative Biology and Pharmacology, University of Texas–Houston School of Medicine, Houston, Texas
Somatostatin

David E. Schteingart, MD
Professor of Internal Medicine and Associate Division Chief for Faculty Affairs, University of Michigan Medical School, Ann Arbor, Michigan
Adrenal Cancer

Machelle M. Seibel
Medical Director, Faulkner Center for Reproductive Medicine, Boston, Massachusetts
Ovulation Induction and Assisted Reproduction

Patrick M. Sexton, PhD
National Health and Medical Research Council Fellow, Molecular Pharmacology Laboratory, Department of Pharmacology, University of Melbourne, Melbourne, Victoria, Australia
Calcitonin

Hrayr K. Shahinian, MD
Director, Division of Skull Base Surgery, Department of Surgery, Cedars-Sinai Medical Center, Los Angeles, California
Surgical Management of Pituitary Tumors

Stephen Michael Shalet, MD, FRCP
Professor of Medicine (Endocrinology), Faculty of Medicine, University of Manchester; Attending Physician, Christie Hospital, Manchester, England
Hypopituitarism

Andrew Shenker, MD, PhD
Assistant Professor of Pediatrics, Molecular Pharmacology and Biological Chemistry, Northwestern University Medical School; Crown Family Young Investigator in Developmental Systems Biology, Children's Memorial Institute for Education and Research, Children's Memorial Hospital, Chicago, Illinois
Hormone Signaling via G Protein–Coupled Receptors

Yoram Shenker, MD
Associate Professor of Medicine and Interim Section Head, Endocrinology, Diabetes, and Metabolism, Department of Medicine, University of Wisconsin Medical School; Chief, Section of Endocrinology, William S. Middleton Memorial VA Hospital, Madison, Wisconsin
Hormonal Regulation of Electrolyte and Water Metabolism

Michael C. Sheppard, MBChB, PhD, FRCP
Professor of Medicine and Head, Division of Medical Sciences, University of Birmingham; Consultant Physician, Queen Elizabeth Hospital, Birmingham, England
Thyroid Function Tests

Shonni J. Silverberg, MD
Associate Professor, Department of Medicine, Columbia University College of Physicians and Surgeons; Associate Attending Physician, New York–Presbyterian Hospital, New York, New York
Primary Hyperparathyroidism

Frederick R. Singer, MD
Clinical Professor of Medicine, University of California, Los Angeles, UCLA School of Medicine, Los Angeles; Director, Endocrine/Bone Disease Program, John Wayne Cancer Institute, St. John's Health Center, Santa Monica, California
Paget's Disease of Bone

Allan E. Siperstein, MD
Staff Surgeon and Head, Section of Endocrine Surgery, Cleveland Clinic Foundation, Cleveland, Ohio
Adrenal Surgery

Niels E. Skakkebaek, MD, DSc
Professor, University of Copenhagen; Head, Department of Growth and Reproduction, Copenhagen University Hospital (Rigshospitalet), Copenhagen, Denmark
Testicular Tumors with Endocrine Manifestations

Peter J. Snyder, MD
Professor of Medicine, University of Pennsylvania School of Medicine, Philadelphia, Pennsylvania
Gonadotroph Adenomas

John T. Soper, MD
Professor, Department of Obstetrics and Gynecology, Duke University School of Medicine, Durham, North Carolina
Gestational Trophoblastic Neoplasms

Stuart M. Sprague, DO
Associate Professor of Medicine, Northwestern University Medical School, Chicago; Director, Metabolic Bone and Stone Disease Program, Evanston Northwestern Healthcare, Evanston, Illinois
Nephrolithiasis

René St-Arnaud, PhD
Associate Professor of Surgery and Human Genetics, McGill University Faculty of Medicine; Senior Staff Scientist, Genetics Unit, Shriners Hospital for Children, Montreal, Quebec, Canada
Hereditary Defects in Vitamin D Metabolism and Action

Donald L. St. Germain, MD
Professor of Medicine and Physiology, Dartmouth Medical School, Lebanon, New Hampshire
Thyroid Hormone Binding and Metabolism: Thyroid Hormone Metabolism

Donald F. Steiner, MD
Professor of Biochemistry and Molecular Biology and Medicine, University of Chicago Pritzker School of Medicine; Senior Investigator, Howard Hughes Medical Institute, Chicago, Illinois
Chemistry and Biosynthesis of the Islet Hormones: Insulin, Islet Amyloid Polypeptide (Amylin), Glucagon, Somatostatin, and Pancreatic Polypeptide

Andrew F. Stewart, MD
Professor of Medicine, University of Pittsburgh School of Medicine; Chief of Endocrinology, University of Pittsburgh Medical Center, Pittsburgh, Pennsylvania
Malignancy-Associated Hypercalcemia

Jan R. Stockigt, MD, FRACP, FRCPA
Professor of Medicine, Monash University; Senior Endocrinologist, Ewen Downie Metabolic Unit, Alfred Hospital, Melbourne, Victoria, Australia
Thyroid Hormone Binding and Metabolism: Thyroid Hormone Binding; Transport Protein Variants

Jerome F. Strauss III, MD, PhD
Luigi Mastroianni, Jr. Professor and Director, Center for Research and Reproduction and Women's Health, and Associate Chairman, Department of Obstetrics and Gynecology, University of Pennsylvania School of Medicine; Staff Physician, Hospital of the University of Pennsylvania, Philadelphia, Pennsylvania
Ovarian Hormone Synthesis; Placental Hormones

David H.P. Streeten, MBBCh, DPhil, FRCP, FACP
Professor Emeritus of Medicine and *former* Head, Section of Endocrinology, State University of New York Upstate Medical University, Syracuse, New York
Orthostatic Hypotension

Sonia L. Sugg, MD
Assistant Professor of Surgery, University of Chicago Medical Center, Chicago, Illinois
Surgery of the Thyroid

Mariusz W. Szkudlinski, MD, PhD
Assistant Professor, Division of Endocrinology, Diabetes and Nutrition, Department of Medicine, University of Maryland School of Medicine; Chief, Section of Protein Engineering, Laboratory of Molecular Endocrinology, Institute of Human Virology, University of Maryland Biotechnology Institute, Baltimore, Maryland
Thyroid-Stimulating Hormone and Regulation of the Thyroid Axis

Hisato Tada, MD
Assistant Professor, Department of Laboratory Medicine, Osaka University Medical School, Osaka, Japan
Chronic (Hashimoto's) Thyroiditis

Shahrad Taheri, BSc, MSc, MBBS, MRCP
Wellcome Trust Research Fellow, Imperial College School of Medicine and The Hammersmith Hospital, London, England
Gastrointestinal Hormones and Tumor Syndromes

Robert B. Tattersall, MD, FRCP
Retired; former Professor of Clinical Diabetes, University of Nottingham, Nottingham, England
The Relationship of Diabetic Control to Complications

Rajesh V. Thakker, MD, FRCP, FRCPath, FMedSc
May Professor of Medicine, University of Oxford; Consultant Physician and Endocrinologist, Nuffield Department of Medicine, John Radcliffe Hospital, Oxford, England
Genetic Disorders of Calcium Homeostasis Caused by Abnormal Regulation of Parathyroid Hormone Secretion or Responsiveness; Multiple Endocrine Neoplasia Type 1

Axel A. Thomson, PhD
Group Leader, MRC Reproductive Biology Unit, Edinburgh, England
Endocrinology of the Prostate and Benign Prostatic Hyperplasia

Michael O. Thorner, MB, BS, DSc
Henry B. Mulholland Professor of Medicine and Chair, Department of Medicine, University of Virginia School of Medicine, Charlottesville, Virginia
Growth Hormone–Releasing Hormone and Growth Hormone Secretagogues: Basic Physiology and Clinical Implications

Andrew A. Toogood, MB, ChB, MRCP
Lecturer in Medicine, Department of Medicine, Division of Medical Sciences, Queen Elizabeth Hospital, Birmingham, England
Growth Hormone–Releasing Hormone and Growth Hormone Secretagogues: Basic Physiology and Clinical Implications

Jorma Toppari, MD, PhD
Senior Scientist of the Academy of Finland, Department of Pediatrics and Department of Physiology, University of Turku, Turku, Finland
Testicular Tumors with Endocrine Manifestations

Fred W. Turek, PhD
Charles E. and Emma H. Morrison Professor of Biology and Director, Center for Circadian Biology and Medicine, Professor of Neurobiology and Physiology, Northwestern University, Evanston, Illinois
Endocrine and Other Biologic Rhythms

Helen E. Turner, MA, MBChB, MRCP
Senior Registrar, Department of Endocrinology, Radcliffe Infirmary, Oxford, England
Ectopic Hormone Syndromes

Eve Van Cauter, PhD
Professor of Medicine, University of Chicago Pritzker School of Medicine, Chicago, Illinois
Endocrine and Other Biologic Rhythms

Gilbert Vassart, MD, PhD
Professor of Genetics, Faculty of Medicine, Institute of Interdisciplinary Research, University of Brussels; Head, Medical Genetics, Erasme Hospital, Brussels, Belgium
Thyroid Regulatory Factors; Thyroid-Stimulating Hormone Receptor Mutations

Jan J. M. de Vijlder, MSc, PhD
Professor of Biochemistry, University of Amsterdam; Emma Children's Hospital, Academic Medical Center, Amsterdam, The Netherlands
Genetic Defects in Thyroid Hormone Synthesis and Action: Defects in Thyroid Hormone Synthesis

Aaron I. Vinik, MD
Professor of Internal Medicine and Anatomy/Neurobiology and Director, Diabetes Research Institute, Eastern Virginia Medical School, Norfolk, Virginia
Carcinoid Tumors

Robert Volpé, MD, FRCP(C), MACP, FRCP(Edin and Lond)
Professor Emeritus, Division of Endocrinology and Metabolism, Department of Medicine, University of Toronto Faculty of Medicine; Active Staff, Division of Endocrinology and Metabolism, Wellesley Division, St. Michael's Hospital, Toronto, Ontario, Canada
Infectious, Subacute, and Sclerosing Thyroiditis

Thomas Vulsma, MD, PhD, MSc
Associate Professor of Pediatric Endocrinology, University of Amsterdam; Pediatric Endocrinologist, Emma Children's Hospital, Academic Medical Center, Amsterdam, The Netherlands
Genetic Defects in Thyroid Hormone Synthesis and Action: Defects in Thyroid Hormone Synthesis

Michael P. Wajnrajch, MD
Assistant Professor of Pediatrics, Department of Pediatrics, Division of Pediatric Endocrinology, Weill Medical College of Cornell University; Visiting Associate Research Scientist, Department of Pediatrics, Division of Molecular Genetics, Columbia University College of Physicians and Surgeons, New York, New York
Defects of Adrenal Steroidogenesis

John A. H. Wass, MA, MD, FRCP
Professor of Endocrinology, University of Oxford; Consultant Physician, Department of Endocrinology, Radcliffe Infirmary, Oxford, England
Ectopic Hormone Syndromes

Anthony P. Weetman, MD, DSc
Professor of Medicine and Dean, Medical School, University of Sheffield; Honorary Consultant Physician, Northern General Hospital, Sheffield, England
Autoimmune Thyroid Disease

Nancy L. Weigel, PhD
Associate Professor, Department of Molecular and Cellular Biology, Baylor College of Medicine, Houston, Texas
Estrogen and Progesterone Action

Bruce D. Weintraub, MD
Professor, Department of Medicine, University of Maryland School of Medicine; Chief, Laboratory of Molecular Endocrinology, Institute of Human Virology, University of Maryland Biotechnology Institute, Baltimore, Maryland
Thyroid-Stimulating Hormone and Regulation of the Thyroid Axis

Anne White, PhD
Professor of Endocrine Sciences, School of Biological Sciences and Faculty of Medicine, University of Manchester, Manchester, England
Adrenocorticotropic Hormone

Morris F. White, PhD
Harvard Medical School; Principal Investigator, Joslin Diabetes Center, Boston, Massachusetts
The Molecular Basis of Insulin Action

Wilmar M. Wiersinga, MD, PhD
Professor of Endocrinology, Department of Medicine, University of Amsterdam; Chief, Department of Endocrinology and Metabolism, Academic Medical Center, Amsterdam, The Netherlands
Hypothyroidism and Myxedema Coma

John F. Wilber, MD
Professor, Department of Medicine, University of Maryland School of Medicine, Baltimore, Maryland
Appetite Regulation

Gordon H. Williams, MD
Professor of Medicine, Harvard Medical School; Senior Physician and Chief, Endocrine-Hypertension Service, Brigham and Women's Hospital, Boston, Massachusetts
Aldosterone Action

Charles B. Wilson, MD, MSHA, DSc
Professor, Department of Neurological Surgery, University of California, San Francisco, School of Medicine; Principal Investigator, Brain Tumor Research Center, University of California at San Francisco, San Francisco, California
Sellar and Parasellar Tumors in Children

Stephen J. Winters, MD
Professor of Medicine and Chief, Division of Endocrinology and Metabolism, University of Louisville School of Medicine, Louisville, Kentucky
Clinical Disorders of the Testis

Robert J. Witte, MD
Assistant Professor of Radiology, Mayo Medical School, Rochester, Minnesota; Consultant, Mayo Clinic, Diagnostic Radiology, Jacksonville, Florida
Radiographic Evaluation of the Pituitary and Anterior Hypothalamus

Hans H. Zingg, MD, PhD
Professor, Department of Medicine, McGill University Faculty of Medicine; Director, Laboratory of Molecular Endocrinology, Royal Victoria Hospital, Montreal, Quebec, Canada
Oxytocin

Preface

The changes buffeting endocrinology have accelerated in the 5 years between the third edition and this, the fourth edition of *Endocrinology.* New hormones and factors abound. The discovery of leptin and agouti protein, along with their receptors, provides just one example. Whole groups of factors—interleukins, chemokines, and others—have been characterized but are yet to be fully integrated into the structure of endocrinology as it is generally conceived. Genetic approaches to endocrine diseases bring new discoveries almost weekly, and several hundred endocrine diseases are now understood at the genetic level. These include disorders such as the multiple endocrine neoplasia syndromes, the various forms of "maturity-onset diabetes of the young," numerous hormone resistance syndromes, and myriad defects in transcription factors and enzymes that control glandular development and hormone synthesis. The instrumentation available for bone density measurements, imaging techniques, minimally invasive surgery, and noninvasive continuous monitoring glucose is changing the way in which we practice endocrinology. Development of specialization in assisted fertility, breast disease, and prostate disease has wrested out of our hands certain illnesses that were long considered to be part of endocrinology. The care of diabetic patients is shifting to teams of doctors, nutritionists, and educators; increasingly, daily management is transferred to the patient, while we attempt to attain a level of glycemic control that was previously thought impossible. Paperwork engulfs us and detracts from patient care, while we attempt to survive economically.

However, despite all of this, the practice of endocrinology remains the same cottage industry that it has always been. One patient pours out his or her troubles and his or her heart to one physician, who does his or her best to provide scientifically based care in a humanistic manner. The physician must often be wise enough to do this in a setting complicated by rampant "anti-scientism," much poorly digested information gleaned from the Internet, and a host of practitioners who offer cures by diet therapy, holistic medicine, acupuncture, and the numerous "natural" herbal remedies.

Perhaps the newly board-certified endocrinologist can get by on the material that he or she learned in training for a few months or a year. But beyond that time, the endocrinologist must again become a student, seeking continuing education at meetings and in journals and textbooks, if he or she is to remain abreast of this field. The reality of our rapidly changing field is that we are students for life—a role that is challenging but rewarding. It is these students of endocrinology who want to, and must, continuously refresh their knowledge to whom we dedicate *Endocrinology.* We believe that this book can serve as an invaluable resource for the busy practitioner who encounters an unfamiliar endocrine problem, as well as the investigator who wishes to find an updated and scholarly review of a topic. It is our intention to provide a complete, current review and analysis of all aspects of endocrinology, both basic and clinical. We hope to provide a source that will answer any endocrine question, which is perhaps at least a laudable goal, even if it is not always reached. We strive to integrate the lessons learned from basic research into the practice of clinical endocrinology. We have provided both the traditional gland-by-gland analysis of disease processes and sections that integrate the hormonal systems and the immune and hormonal systems.

The current edition consists of 194 chapters. About one third of these are completely new, and the remainder have been completely rewritten and brought up to date. There are new sections on Growth and Maturation, Immunology and Endocrinology, Obesity and Nutrition, and Endocrinology of the Breast and two additional "minibooks" on Endocrine Testing and Drugs and Hormones used in Endocrinology. Some readers describe our book as the "Bible of Endocrinology." Whether that is appropriate or not, we are certain that readers will find many of the chapters to be absolutely the best presentation of the topic that has ever been put together. We are very proud of the scholarship that is evident throughout.

With more than 300 authors, it is not possible to give individual credit for outstanding contributions. But here the Editors offer their thanks and appreciation to all of the authors who have contributed such outstanding chapters. Their erudition and ability to make science and practice readable make *Endocrinology* a special book. We also owe thanks to Hazel Hacker and Richard Zorab at W.B. Saunders for their commitment to quality publishing and for expeditiously preparing this book to keep the information current.

We are very pleased that Shlomo Melmed has joined our group as the editor of the neuroendocrine section, and we wish to acknowledge the important contributions of Michael Besser to this section in previous editions. The wisdom, hard work, and friendship of our co-editors—Henry G. Burger, D. Lynn Loriaux, John C. Marshall, Shlomo Melmed, William D. Odell, John T. Potts, Jr., and Arthur H. Rubenstein—have made this experience pleasurable, as well as enlightening. Last, we note with special pleasure the contribution of Dr. J. Larry Jameson as co-editor in chief.

Leslie J. DeGroot, MD
J. Larry Jameson, MD, PhD

NOTICE

Endocrinology is an ever-changing field. Standard safety precautions must be followed, but as new research and clinical experience broaden our knowledge, changes in treatment and drug therapy may become necessary or appropriate. Readers are advised to check the most current product information provided by the manufacturer of each drug to be administered to verify the recommended dose, the method and duration of administration, and the contraindications. It is the responsibility of the treating physician, relying on experience and knowledge of the patient, to determine dosages and the best treatment for each individual patient. Neither the publisher nor the editor assumes any liability for any injury and/or damage to persons or property arising from this publication.

THE PUBLISHER

Contents

Color Plates follow frontmatter.

Volume 1

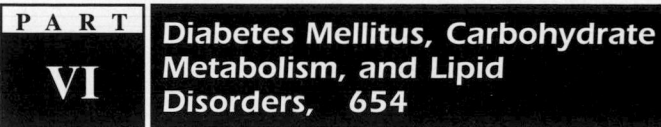

Editor: Arthur H. Rubenstein

Volume 2

PART VII Parathyroid Gland, Calciotropic Hormones, and Bone Metabolism, 969

Editor: John T. Potts, Jr.

BASIC PHYSIOLOGY, 969

CLINICAL DISORDERS, 1062

PART VIII Thyroid Gland, 1268

Editor: Leslie J. DeGroot

BASIC PHYSIOLOGY, 1268

Volume 3

PART X Endocrine Hypertension and Mineralocorticoids, 1777

Editor: D. Lynn Loriaux

BASIC PHYSIOLOGY, 1777

CLINICAL DISORDERS, 1820

PART XI Reproductive Endocrinology and Sexual Development, 1885

Editor: William D. Odell

BASIC PHYSIOLOGY, 1885

CLINICAL DISORDERS, 1974

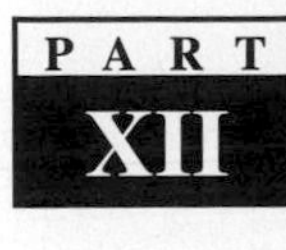

PART XII Female Reproduction, 2043

Editor: John C. Marshall

BASIC PHYSIOLOGY, 2043

CLINICAL DISORDERS, 2086

PART XIII Endocrinology of the Breast, 2181

Editor: John C. Marshall

PART XIV Male Reproduction, 2209

Editor: Henry G. Burger

BASIC PHYSIOLOGY, 2209

CLINICAL DISORDERS, 2243

ENDOCRINOLOGY

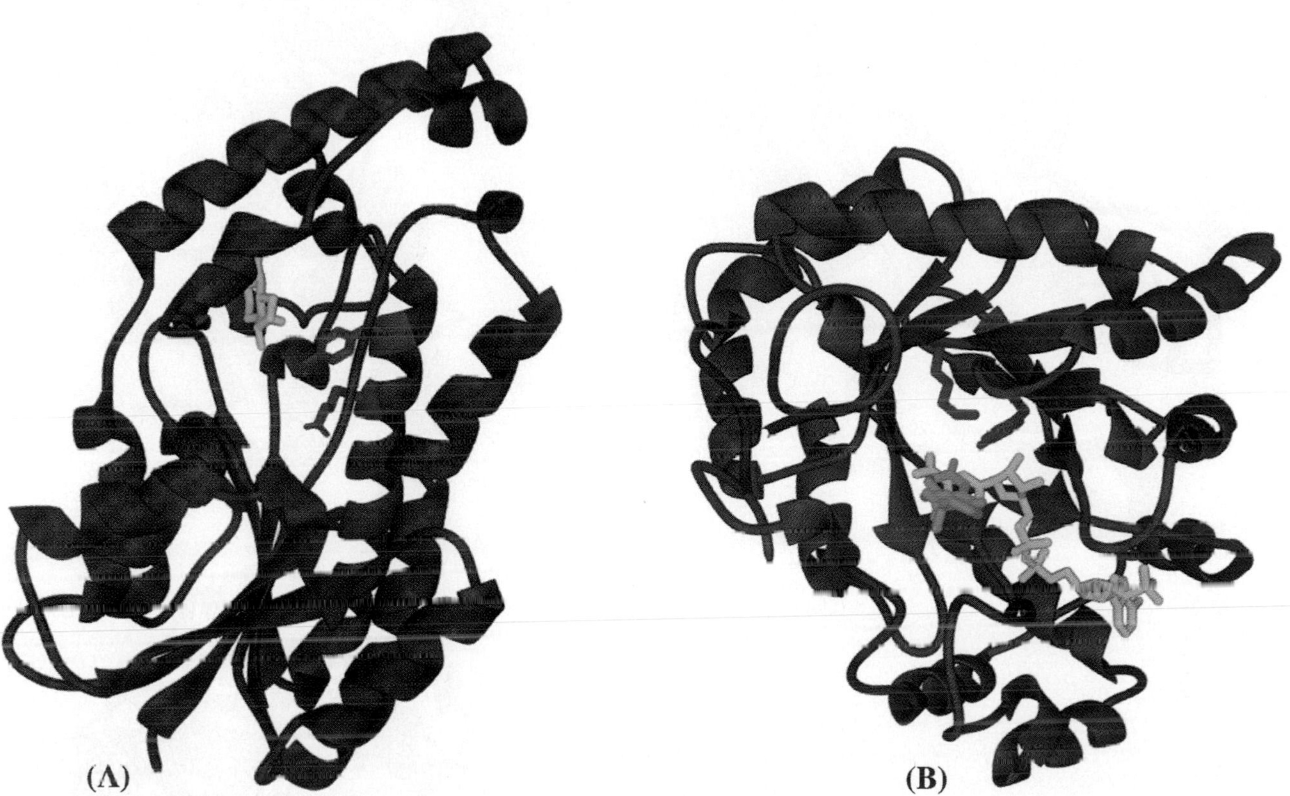

FIGURE 115–5. The two types of hydroxysteroid dehydrogenase (HSD) structures. The representative structure for the short-chain dehydrogenase reductase (SDR) class is human 17β-HSDI (research collaboratory for structural bioinformatics [rcsb, website http://www.rcsb.org] PDB ID No. 1IOL, panel A), with bound estradiol in yellow, and the Tyr and Lys residues critical for catalysis are shown in magenta and blue, respectively. The basic SDR structure contains the strands of a β-sheet core (upward *arrows* at the bottom of the figure) plus helices on the top and sides of the molecule. The representative structure for the aldo-keto reductase (AKR) class is rat liver 3α-HSD (rcsb PDB ID No. 1AFS, panel B). The bound substrate testosterone is in green; cofactor $NADP^+$ is in yellow; and the Tyr and Lys residues that are critical for catalysis are shown in magenta and blue, respectively. The TIM barrel structure of the AKR enzymes is the circular array of β-sheets *(arrows)* with the active site at the "hole" in the barrel and helices at the periphery of the molecule. Note that the Tyr and Lys occupy similar juxtaposition in three-dimensional space in both structures, although the two residues lie on adjacent turns of the same helix in 17β-HSDI but on adjacent β-sheet strands in 3α-HSD.

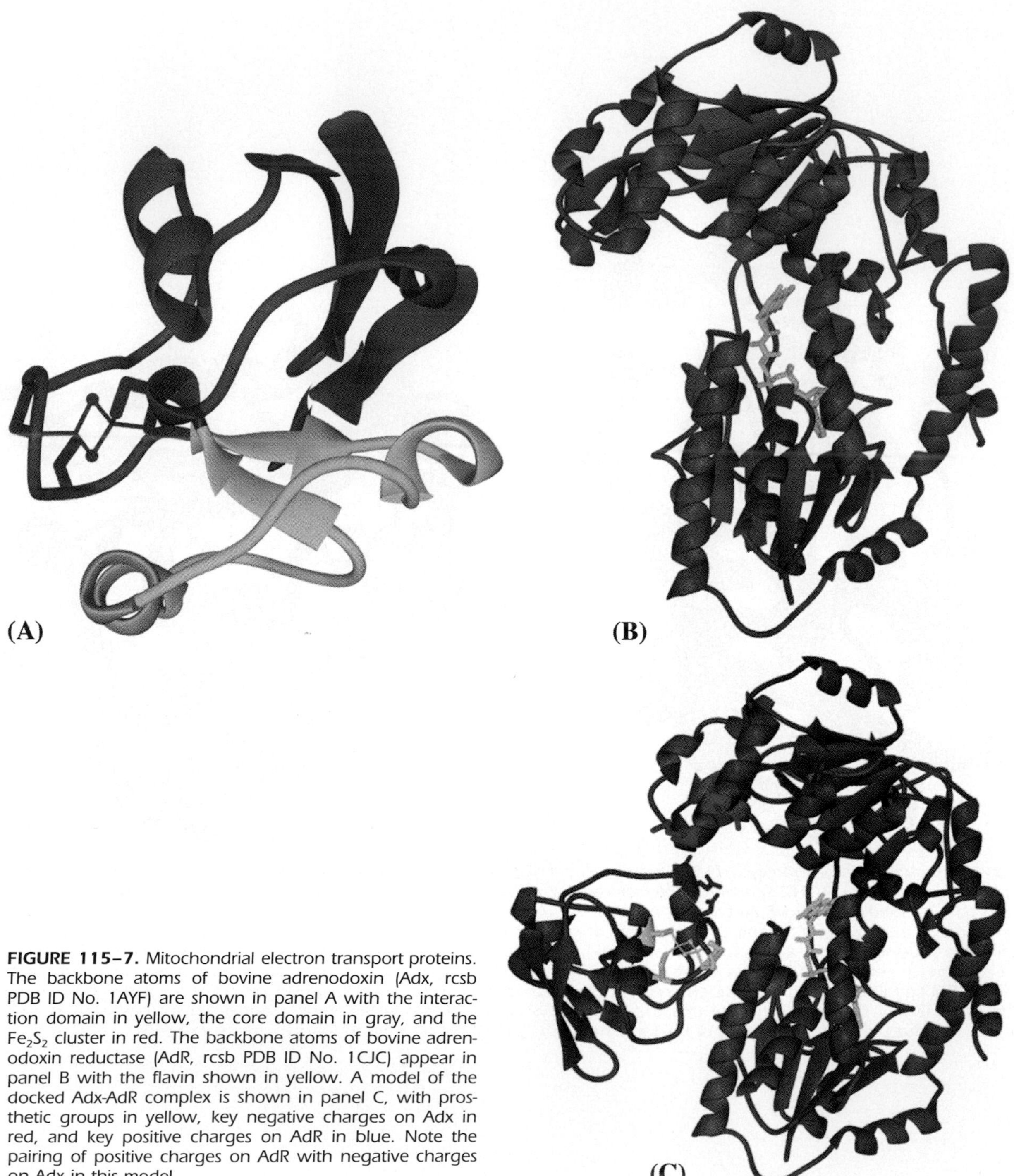

FIGURE 115–7. Mitochondrial electron transport proteins. The backbone atoms of bovine adrenodoxin (Adx, rcsb PDB ID No. 1AYF) are shown in panel A with the interaction domain in yellow, the core domain in gray, and the Fe_2S_2 cluster in red. The backbone atoms of bovine adrenodoxin reductase (AdR, rcsb PDB ID No. 1CJC) appear in panel B with the flavin shown in yellow. A model of the docked Adx-AdR complex is shown in panel C, with prosthetic groups in yellow, key negative charges on Adx in red, and key positive charges on AdR in blue. Note the pairing of positive charges on AdR with negative charges on Adx in this model.

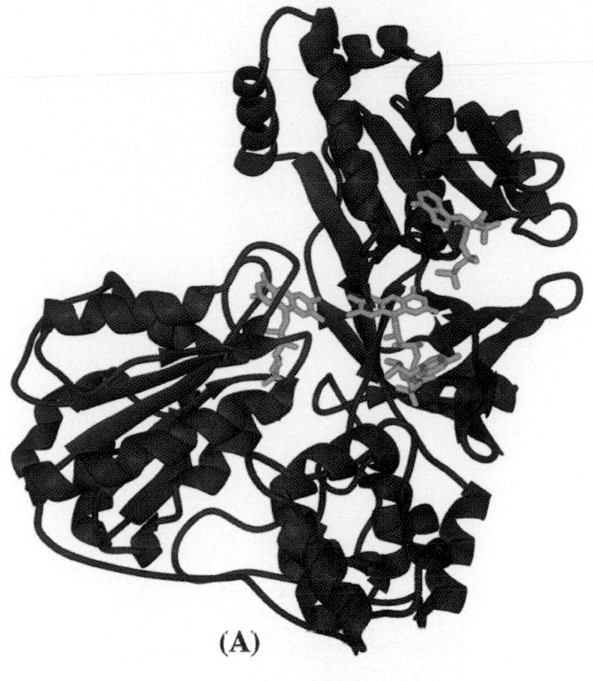

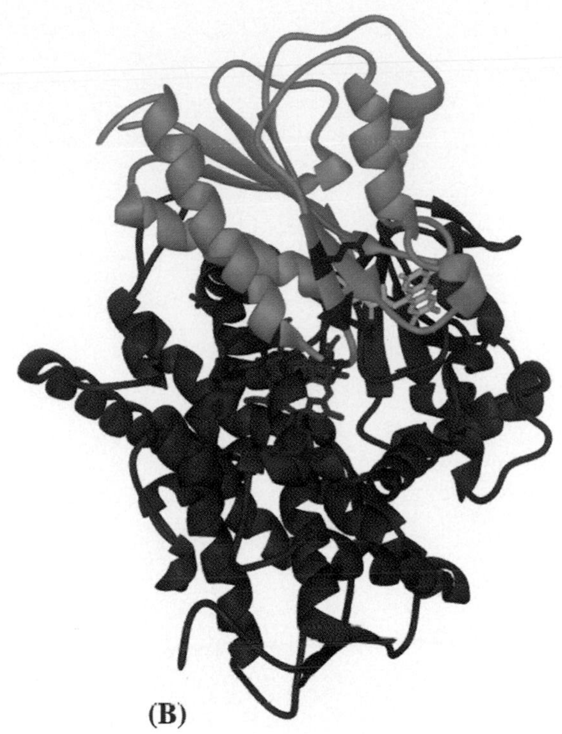

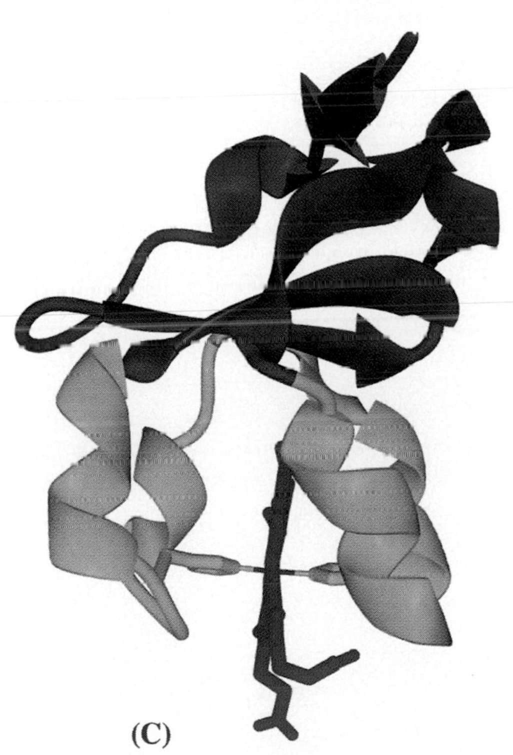

FIGURE 115–8. Flavoproteins and hemoproteins that interact with type II P450 enzymes. Panel A shows a ribbon diagram of rat liver P450-OR structure (rcsb PDB ID No. 1AMO), with (clockwise from lower right) bound nicotinamide adenine dinucleotide phosphate, reduced form (NADPH), flavin adenine dinucleotide (FAD), and flavin mononucleotide (FMN) cofactors in yellow. Panel B shows the structure of the complex between the FMN domain (green) and P450 domain (gray) of $P450_{BM3}$ (rcsb PDB ID No. 1BVY). The flavin is shown in yellow; the heme is shown in magenta; and positive and negative charges in the interaction surface are highlighted with blue and red, respectively. The hemoprotein cytochrome b_5 is shown in panel C, with the heme-binding core 1 domain in yellow and the core 2 domain in gray; the heme is shown in red.

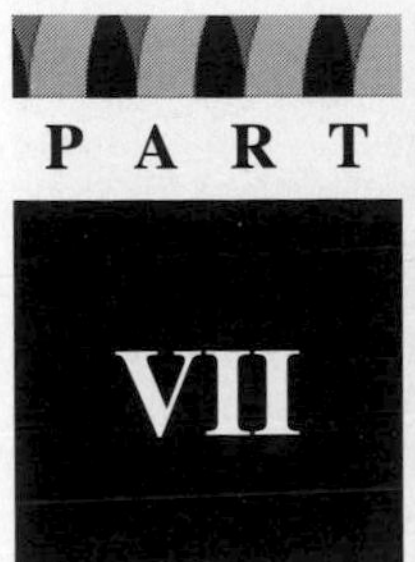

PART VII

Parathyroid Gland, Calciotropic Hormones, and Bone Metabolism

John T. Potts, Jr.

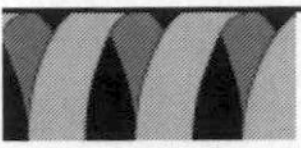

BASIC PHYSIOLOGY

Chapter 70

Parathyroid Hormone and Parathyroid Hormone–Related Peptide in the Regulation of Calcium Homeostasis and Bone Development

Harald W. Jüppner ▪ Thomas J. Gardella ▪ Edward M. Brown
Henry M. Kronenberg ▪ John T. Potts, Jr.

Parathyroid hormone (PTH) and PTH-related peptide (PTHrP), along with other calciotropic hormones, play critical roles in calcium homeostasis and bone biology. First discovered as a calcium-regulating hormone in the 1920s,[1–3] PTH is secreted by the parathyroid glands and is one of the most important regulators of blood calcium concentration in all terrestrial vertebrate species from amphibians to mammals. PTHrP, a slightly larger molecule than PTH, was discovered more recently through efforts to identify the factor that causes, when produced in excess by certain tumors, the humoral hypercalcemia of malignancy syndrome. In contrast to PTH, which is produced by discrete endocrine glands, PTHrP is produced as a paracrine/autocrine factor in many different adult and fetal tissues and has, unlike PTH, multiple functions.[4–6]

PTH and PTHrP most likely evolved from a common ancestral precursor. Despite this common evolutionary origin, both peptides share only limited overall amino acid sequence identity, yet at least their N-terminal regions are sufficiently homologous to enable them to bind to and activate a common G protein–coupled receptor, the PTH/PTHrP receptor (also referred to as PTH1R).[7–9] This receptor mediates the most important biologic actions of both peptides: PTH-dependent

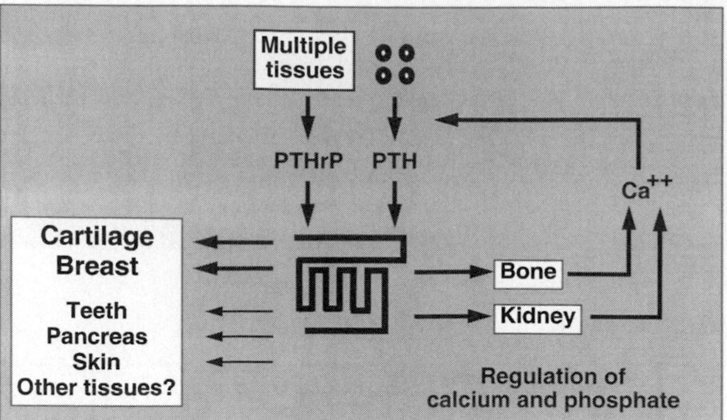

FIGURE 70–1. The parathyroid hormone (PTH)/PTH-related peptide (PTHrP) receptor interacts with indistinguishable efficiency and efficacy with PTH and PTHrP, and it activates at least two distinct second messenger systems, cyclic adenosine monophosphate and Ca^{2+}/inositol 1,4,5-triphosphate. The receptor is abundantly expressed in bone and kidney, where it mediates the endocrine actions of PTH, and in the metaphyseal growth plate and numerous other tissues, where it mediates the autocrine/paracrine actions of PTHrP.

regulation of calcium homeostasis and PTHrP-dependent regulation of endochondral bone formation[10–14] (Fig. 70–1).

This chapter reviews (1) the comparative chemistry of PTH and PTHrP, their genes, and their interactions with PTH1R; (2) the current molecular models of productive interactions between the two ligands and their common receptor; and (3) the different biologic roles of both peptides on target tissues, such as the role of PTH in calcium homeostasis and bone turnover and the role of PTHrP in bone and cartilage development. However, the chapter does not review the potentially numerous and still incompletely characterized biologic roles of PTHrP outside the field of calcium and bone biology. The evolutionary history of the principal PTH/PTHrP receptor is reviewed, as well as the functional characteristics of two novel, closely related receptors and the pharmacologic and physicochemical evidence for several additional, still incompletely characterized receptors for PTH and PTHrP.

REGULATION OF MINERAL ION HOMEOSTASIS—GENERAL CONSIDERATIONS

To ensure a multitude of essential cellular functions, the extracellular concentration of calcium is maintained within narrow limits.[15, 16] In terrestrial vertebrates, calcium is necessary for adequate mineralization of the skeleton, which provides mechanical support and protection for internal organs and acts as levers for the various muscle groups involved in locomotion. Because of its high calcium content, 99% of the body's supply, the skeleton also serves as the most important reservoir from which calcium can be rapidly mobilized. Because food intake and thus the nutritional supply of calcium are usually discontinuous, intestinal calcium absorption occurs only intermittently. Maintenance of a constant blood calcium concentration thus constitutes a major homeostatic challenge, which during evolution led to the development of highly efficient mechanisms to increase intestinal calcium absorption, reduce urinary calcium losses, and facilitate, if necessary, rapid mobilization of calcium from the skeletal reservoir (see work by Neer[16] and Chapter 74).

In contrast to these environmental challenges of most terrestrial vertebrates, marine animals, which are usually exposed to a high environmental calcium concentration, had to adopt mechanisms by which extracellular calcium could be reduced.[17, 18] Unlike the diet of terrestrial animals, seawater provides only a very limited supply of phosphate, and this environmental deficiency resulted in the development of mechanisms to conserve phosphate. It thus appears plausible that the efficient intestinal absorption of phosphate and the impressive capacity of the mammalian kidney to retain phosphate[15, 19] are remnants of earlier evolutionary adaptations to life in the low phosphate environment of the oceans. To reduce blood calcium concentrations fish use stanniocalcin (STC1), which is produced by the corpuscles of Stannius, as well as several other hormonal factors.[17, 18, 20] Recent data indicate that the mammalian homologue of STC1 has similar properties when tested in rodents, but it remains uncertain whether this peptide hormone has a significant physiologic role in mammalian mineral ion homeostasis.[21] A widely expressed mammalian peptide, STC2, that was recently discovered because of its structural homology with STC1[22, 23] appears to inhibit phosphate uptake in renal epithelial cells,[24] but it is unlikely that this peptide is the long-sought phosphaturic hormone. Calcitonin, made by the ultimobranchial bodies in fish, has a calcium-lowering function in this vertebrate species, but its biologic role(s) in mammals remains uncertain (for review see Martin et al.[25]).

PARATHYROID HORMONE

PTH and the active form of vitamin D, 1,25-dihydroxyvitamin D_3 [$1,25(OH)_2D_3$], are the principal physiologic regulators of calcium homeostasis in humans and all terrestrial vertebrates.[11, 26, 27] Synthesis and secretion of PTH are stimulated by any decrease in blood calcium, and conversely, secretion of the hormone is inhibited by an increase in blood calcium.[28–30] This rapid negative feedback regulation of PTH production, along with the biologic actions of the hormone on different target tissues, represents the most important homeostatic mechanism for minute-to-minute control of calcium concentration in the extracellular fluid (ECF).[31–33] In contrast to the rapid actions of PTH, $1,25(OH)_2D_3$ is of critical importance for long-term, day-to-day, and week-to-week calcium balance (see Chapter 72). The actions of both hormones are coordinated, and each influences the synthesis and secretion of the other. Calcitonin, the third of the calciotropic hormones known to be important in the regulation of vertebrate mineral ion homeostasis (see Chapter 71), may be vestigial in humans with respect to calcium homeostasis and will not be discussed in this brief review of physiology.

At least three distinct, but coordinated actions of PTH increase the flow of calcium into the ECF and thus increase the concentration of blood calcium[28–30] (Fig. 70–2). Through its rapid actions on the kidney and bone, which are all mediated through the PTH/PTHrP receptor

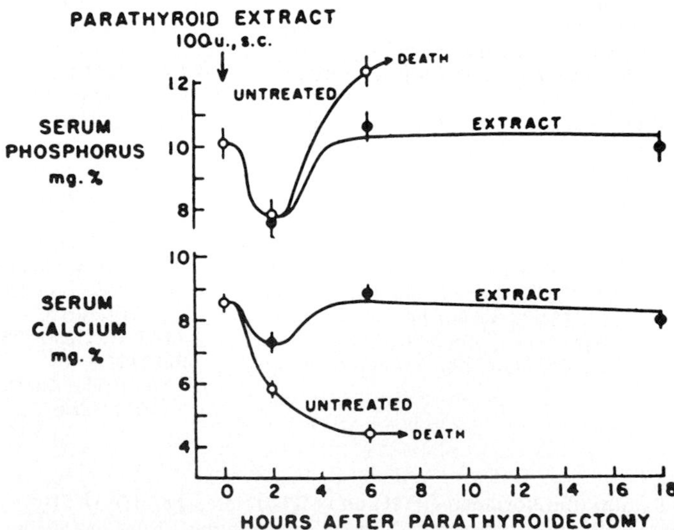

FIGURE 70–2. Rate of change in blood phosphorus and calcium levels in rats with stressed calcium homeostasis (low calcium diet) after parathyroidectomy without treatment or with 100 U of parathyroid hormone extract given in addition at the time of parathyroidectomy. Rapid and usually fatal hypocalcemia and hyperphosphatemia result within hours unless hormone is given. (From Munson PL: Studies on the role of the parathyroids in calcium and phosphorus metabolism. Ann N Y Acad Sci 60:776–796, 1955.)

and subsequent secondary messages in specific and highly specialized cells, PTH increases the release of calcium from bone, reduces the renal clearance of calcium, and stimulates the production of $1,25(OH)_2D_3$ by activating the gene encoding 25-hydroxyvitamin D-1α-hydroxylase (1α-hydroxylase) in the kidney. The relative importance of the first two actions of PTH on the rapid, minute-to-minute regulation of calcium is not definitively resolved, but most physiologists have stressed the importance of the effects of PTH on bone in maintaining hour-to-hour calcium homeostasis in the ECF. Several lines of evidence, such as that provided by calcium kinetic analysis, indicate a transfer between ECF and bone of as much as 500 mg calcium daily, which is equivalent to one-fourth to one-half the total ECF calcium content.[15] Besides regulating this transfer of calcium from bone through direct breakdown of bone tissue (mineral and matrix), PTH influences the rates of exchange of calcium adsorbed to the surface of bone; this exchangeable calcium pool can be stimulated to provide a rapid and substantial rate of entry of calcium into blood. In addition to these PTH-dependent actions on bone, Nordin and colleagues were the first to emphasize that the actions of PTH on the kidney may also be extremely important in the precise hourly regulation of ECF calcium.[34] The third action of PTH on calcium homeostasis—namely, enhancement of intestinal calcium absorption—is indirect and involves the synthesis of $1,25(OH)_2D_3$ from the biologically inactive precursor 25-OHD_3. However, it is difficult to quantitatively analyze or to proportionately contrast the relative physiologic importance of the direct and indirect actions of PTH on the three principal target tissues, kidney, bone, and intestine.

The complexity of bone as a tissue and the many detectable rates of exchange of calcium between the skeleton and the ECF have made the action of PTH on the skeleton difficult to analyze. The state of calcium in blood is complex; much of the calcium is present as chelates or is bound to plasma proteins (for detailed review see Chapter 73). Because actual filtered loads depend on the ratio of free and bound forms of calcium, it is difficult to calculate renal calcium clearance accurately. The different PTH-dependent actions to promote calcium entry into the ECF are most clearly defined in conditions of deficiency or excess of PTH, such as during experiments in animals or during controlled observations in patients with disorders of parathyroid gland function. The experimental data in these extremes abundantly affirm the crucial calcium homeostatic role of PTH. However, because of continuous and rapid adjustments in mineral ion concentration, it can be difficult to observe the consequences of hormone action under normal physiologic conditions. For example, the rate of PTH secretion changes continually and rapidly so that the controlled variable, calcium, remains constant, and it may therefore be difficult to experimentally detect small corrective changes.

Teleologically, the action of PTH on the regulation of blood phosphate concentration in terrestrial species is best understood as a secondary rather than homeostatic action. Phosphate is abundant in the food chain in terrestrial existence. Phosphate deficiency, unlike calcium deficiency, in the absence of specific organ dysfunction is therefore an unlikely environmental challenge (see Chapter 73 for detailed review of the regulation of phosphate homeostasis). To correct a deficiency in calcium, calcium phosphate stores in bone can be rapidly dissolved; such activity results, however, in the simultaneous liberation of ionic calcium and phosphate. Because a high blood phosphate level tends to lower the calcium concentration through multiple mechanisms, the rise in blood calcium that occurs after bone dissolution (desirable homeostatically) is therefore beneficial only if the concomitant increase in blood phosphate concentration (undesirable) can be rapidly corrected. To maximize the control of calcium homeostasis, PTH thus has divergent actions on renal tubular handling of the two mineral ions: it increases the retention of calcium and, at the same time, promotes the excretion of phosphate. Through these mechanisms, namely, increased renal phosphate clearance to prevent hyperphosphatemia and increased tubular calcium reabsorption, PTH guarantees that an elevation in blood calcium results from the increased release of calcium from bone. The renal action of PTH on phosphate homeostasis is biologically predominant over the increased phosphate flux from bone. Consequently, parathyroidectomy (experimentally, in animals) or renal resistance to PTH, as in patients with pseudohypoparathyroidism or renal failure, leads not only to hypocalcemia but also to an increase in blood phosphate and a marked reduction in urinary phosphate excretion (see Fig. 70–1). This finding demonstrates the importance of the PTH-dependent action on phosphate homeostasis in the kidney, which becomes particularly important in disease states when high bone turnover is the result of dietary calcium deficiency or lack of biologically active vitamin D.

Evolution

To maintain extracellular calcium and phosphate concentrations within narrow limits, the sophisticated regulatory system outlined above, in which PTH plays the most important role, developed in terrestrial animals. In mammals, PTH is produced almost exclusively by the parathyroid glands (only small amounts of its mRNA have been detected elsewhere[35, 36]). During evolution these glands first appear as discrete organs in amphibians, that is, with the migration of vertebrates from an aquatic to a terrestrial existence, and their appearance most likely represents an evolutionary adaptation to an environment that is, by comparison to seawater, low in calcium.[17, 18, 37] Although parathyroid glands could not be identified in fish or invertebrate species, there is immunologic evidence for a PTH like protein in the pituitary of different fish species,[17, 18, 38] and a partial nucleotide sequence with significant homology to the mammalian PTH gene has been identified in trout genomic DNA.[39] In addition to a PTH-like substance, several investigations provided immunologic evidence for a PTHrP-like molecule in nonmammalian vertebrate species,[40–43] and a peptide with considerable amino acid sequence homology to mammalian PTH and PTHrP was recently discovered as part of the Fugu Genome Project. The N-terminal portion of this teleost peptide contains eight amino acid residues that are common to all PTH and PTHrP species sequenced thus far. It also contains amino acid residues characteristic of mammalian PTH, as well as residues characteristic of mammalian PTHrP; these residues are never found together in mammalian PTH or PTHrP. This pattern suggests that the fugu protein may be phylogenetically closer to a common PTH/PTHrP precursor (see below).

Chemistry

The first extracts from bovine parathyroid glands were described in 1925, and the content of biologically active PTH was assessed by their hypercalcemic and phosphaturic properties.[2, 44] However, it was not until 1959, when Aurbach[45] and Rasmussen and Craig[46] developed improved extraction procedures, that it became possible to isolate and purify sufficient quantities to determine the primary structure of bovine, porcine, and human PTH through sequential Edman degradation and analysis of the released amino acid.[47–52] Based on these amino acid sequences, the PTH(1–34) fragments of the different species were synthesized, and their biologic activities were compared in vitro and in vivo with those of highly purified intact PTH from the same species (Table 70–1). Nucleotide sequence analysis of genomic and complementary DNA later confirmed the amino acid sequences obtained through peptide sequence analysis; the only exception was residue 76 in human PTH, which was determined to be glutamine instead of glutamic acid.[53–55] Molecular cloning techniques also led to deduction of the amino acid sequences of rat and chicken and, more recently, dog PTH.[56–59] Shown in Figure 70–3 are the sequences for bovine, porcine, and human hormones reported by only one group[48, 49, 51, 52] and not the points of difference between these structural findings and those by a different laboratory[47, 50] (see an earlier review for more details[10]). The synthetic peptides used in parathyroid research today are based on the hormone sequences shown in Figure 70–3 and were confirmed independently by nucleotide sequence analysis of the genes and/or the cDNAs (see below).

Extensive sequence homology is present in the known mammalian PTH species (see Fig. 70–3, left panel); all these molecules consist of a single-chain polypeptide with 84 amino acids and a molecular weight of approximately 9400 Da (that of human PTH[1–84] is 9425 Da). The middle portions of the different molecules are relatively hydropho-

TABLE 70–1. Comparison of the Biologic Activity of Parathyroid Peptides from Different Species

Peptide	Potency (MRC U/mg)*	
	In Vitro Rat Renal Adenyl Cyclase Assay	*In Vivo Chick Hypercalcemia Assay*
Native hormones		
Bovine 1–84	3000 (2500–4000)	2500 (2100–4000)
Porcine 1–84	1000 (850–1250)	4800 (3300–7000)
Human 1–84	350 (275–425)	10,000 (9060–13,400)
Synthetic fragments		
Bovine 1–34	5400 (3900–8000)	7700 (5200–11,100)
Human 1–34	1700 (1400–2150)	7400 (5200–9700)
[Ala¹]–human 1–34	4300 (3400–5400)	—

*Values expressed as mean potency with 95% confidence intervals and are based on Medical Research Council research standard A for parathyroid hormone. From Rosenblatt M, Kronenberg HM, Potts JT Jr: Parathyroid hormone. *In* DeGroot L (ed): Endocrinology, ed 2. Philadelphia, WB Saunders, 1989, p 853.

bic and exhibit the greatest structural differences among species, which could suggest that this portion of PTH is only of limited functional importance. The only nonmammalian homologue isolated thus far is from the chicken, and it shows significant differences in comparison to mammalian homologues. For example, chicken PTH contains two deletions in the hydrophobic middle portion of the sequence and an additional 22 amino acids near the C terminus, which replaces the stretch of 9 amino acids (residues 62–70) in the mammalian hormones. The N-terminal region of PTH, which is necessary and sufficient for the regulation of mineral ion homeostasis, shows high sequence conservation among all vertebrate species; only few amino acid changes are noted in the 13–22 region. In comparison to the known PTHrP species, however, the degree of sequence preservation in PTH is considerably less, particularly in the middle region and toward the C terminus (see Fig. 70–3, right panel).

The three-dimensional structures of intact PTH(1–84) and the N-terminal, biologically active fragments of both PTH and PTHrP have been analyzed by various solution-based methods, including nuclear magnetic resonance (NMR) imaging. However, interpretation of these results is uncertain because the ligand does interact with the membrane-embedded receptor and the hydrophobicity of this environment, as well as the receptor-induced conformational changes, is unknown. Furthermore, the results of different studies have been in disagreement, even under apparently similar solvent conditions. Of particular interest has been the question whether some common structural features might be discerned for both ligands that would explain the equivalent binding of PTH and PTHrP to the common PTH/PTHrP receptor, but no consistent similarities in structure were observed in earlier and more recent studies. For example, a two-dimensional NMR study of the 1–34 fragment of PTHrP reported that residues 3 to 9 are α helical when in an aqueous solution (pH 4.5), residues 10 to 13 and 16 to 19 each form type I β turns, and residues 20 to 34 form a nonhelical but ordered conformation.[60] Earlier NMR studies of PTH(1–34) failed to detect an ordered structure under similar solvent conditions,[61] but subsequent studies with PTH being dissolved in the helix-promoting solvent trifluoroethanol found an ordered structure.[62]

More recent NMR studies using human PTH(1–37) or human PTH(1–34) with a C-terminal carboxamide revealed evidence of helical regions in the N and C termini of both peptides and furthermore provided evidence of a tertiary "U-shaped" structure. This conformation of the peptide was thought to be due to long-range interactions that brought the N-terminal and the C-terminal regions into closer proximity, at least in saline solution.[63, 64] A third group, however, failed to find significant evidence of such long-range interactions under similar conditions[65] but confirmed the previously obtained evidence of N-terminal and C-terminal helixes.

Therefore, consistent with their rather limited homology in primary structure (see Fig. 70–3), convincing evidence has not yet been provided for the conclusion that the N-terminal fragments of PTH and PTHrP display a similar secondary structure in solution. Because of their equivalent potency at the PTH/PTHrP receptor, it appears likely, however, that both ligands adopt a very similar and highly specific conformation when part of an active hormone-receptor complex. Ideally, either hormone should be cocrystallized with the PTH/PTHrP receptor (or one of the other cloned receptors that interact with these peptides [see below]) to permit analysis by x-ray diffraction of those intermolecular interactions that are characteristic of the biologically active hormone-receptor complex. Such analysis has been done with growth hormone and nerve growth factor and their respective receptors.[66, 67] However, G protein–coupled receptors, such as the PTH/PTHrP receptor (or the closely related receptors), have multiple membrane-embedded domains and are likely to have a significantly more complex three-dimensional structure. Interaction with either PTH or PTHrP appears to involve several distinct receptor domains (see be-

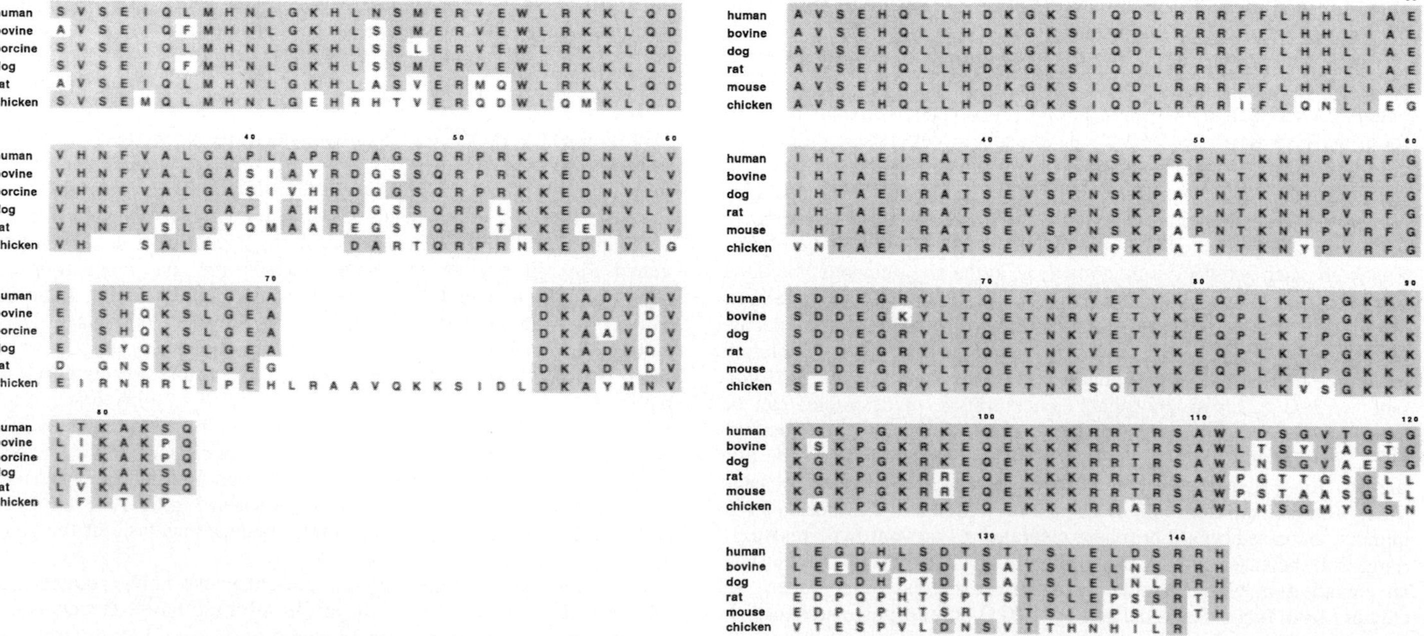

FIGURE 70–3. Alignment of the amino acid sequences of all known parathyroid hormone (PTH) *(left panel)* and PTH-related peptide species *(right panel)*. Conserved residues are *shaded;* numbers indicate the positions of amino acids in the mammalian peptide sequences.

low) that may undergo significant conformational changes after ligand binding has occurred, which makes it even more challenging to conduct x-ray or multidimensional NMR analyses. The only structure of such a complex lipid-embedded, multidomain protein obtained to date is the crystal structure of bacteriorhodopsin.[68]

The PTH Gene and Its mRNA

The human PTH gene consists of three exons located on chromosome 11p15.[69–72] The first exon is 85 nucleotides in length and is noncoding (Fig. 70–4). Exon 2 (90 bp) encodes most amino acids of the prepropeptide sequence, whereas the third exon (612 bp) encodes the remainder of the propeptide sequence and all amino acids of the mature peptide, and it constitutes the 3′ noncoding region.[73] Several frequent intragenic polymorphisms (*Taq*I and *Pst*I,[74] *Bst*BI,[75] *Dra*III,[76] *Xmn*I[77]) and a tetranucleotide repeat ([AAAT]n[78]) have been identified in the human PTH gene, and some were shown to be informative in genetic linkage studies.[79–81] Two mRNAs that are 822 and 793 bp in length are derived in the human gene from two transcriptional start sites that follow two different functional TATA boxes separated by 29 base pairs.[73] Two closely spaced TATA boxes giving rise to two distinct transcripts are also present in the bovine PTH gene, whereas rat and chicken PTH genes give rise to only one transcript; as a consequence of a long 3′ noncoding region, the transcript from the chicken PTH gene is unusually long and comprises 2.3 kb.[26, 82]

PTH Biosynthesis and Intraglandular Processing

During synthesis of the prepro-PTH molecule, the signal sequence, which comprises the 25 amino acids contained in the "pre" sequence, is cleaved off after entry of the nascent peptide chain into the intracisternal space bounded by the endoplasmic reticulum. A heterozygous mutation in this leader sequence that changes a cysteine to an arginine at position 8 and thus impairs processing of prepro-PTH to pro-PTH has been identified as the most plausible molecular cause of an autosomal dominant familial form of hypoparathyroidism.[83, 84] Although it remains uncertain how this missense mutation can cause a dominant disorder, it illustrates the importance of the signal peptide in normal processing of the hormonal precursor.

Subsequent to removal of the prepeptide sequence, the propeptide is transported to the trans-Golgi network, where the propeptide sequence (amino acid residues −6 through −1) is removed.[85] This latter process may involve furin (paired basic amino acid–cleaving enzyme) and/or proprotein convertase-7, which are both expressed in parathyroid tissue; their levels of expression do not appear to be regulated by either calcium or 1,25(OH)$_2$D$_3$.[86, 87] After removal of the basic propeptide sequence, the mature polypeptide, PTH(1–84), is packaged into secretory granules. Two proteases, cathepsins B and H, are subsequently

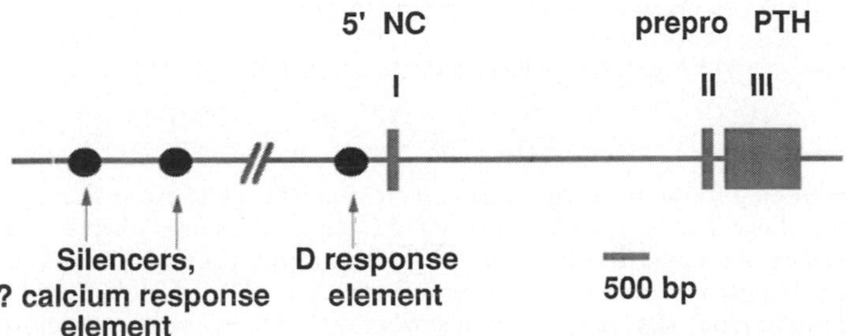

FIGURE 70–4. Schematic of the parathyroid hormone (PTH) gene along several thousand base pairs (approximate length shown by the scale marker for 500 bp). The three exons in the mRNA are represented as numbered *rectangles*. Control elements are identified in the 5′ noncoding region (5′ NC). A region responsive to vitamin D is within a few hundred base pairs of exon 1; far upstream are silencers involved in calcium regulation.

involved in intraglandular generation of C-terminal PTH fragments from the intact hormone; no N-terminal PTH fragments appear to be released from the gland.[88–90] Because C-terminal fragments of PTH are unlikely to be involved in the regulation of calcium homeostasis, intraglandular degradation of intact PTH is thought to represent an inactivating pathway, at least with regard to the regulation of mineral ion homeostasis. Consistent with this conclusion, hypercalcemia results in a substantial decrease in PTH secretion and, furthermore, favors the secretion of C-terminal PTH fragments, including a previously undetected large-molecular-weight species (see the section below on N-terminally truncated PTH).[90–93]

The pool of stored, intracellular PTH is small, so the parathyroid cell must have mechanisms to increase hormone synthesis and release in response to sustained hypocalcemia. One such adaptive mechanism is to reduce intracellular degradation of the hormone, thereby increasing the net amount of intact, biologically active PTH that is available for secretion. During hypocalcemia the bulk of the hormone that is released from the parathyroid cell is intact PTH(1–84).[88–90, 92, 93] As the level of extracellular calcium ion (Ca^{2+}_o) increases, a greater fraction of intracellular PTH is degraded, and with overt hypercalcemia, most of the secreted immunoreactive PTH consists of C-terminal fragments (for review, see elsewhere[10, 26, 27]).

Regulation of PTH Gene Expression

Another adaptive mechanism of the parathyroid cell to sustained reductions in Ca^{2+}_o is to increase cellular levels of PTH mRNA, a response that takes several hours. A reduction in Ca^{2+}_o increases whereas an elevation in Ca^{2+}_o reduces the cellular levels of PTH mRNA by affecting both its stability and the transcriptional rate of its gene.[11, 27, 94, 95] Available data suggest that phosphate ions also regulate, directly or indirectly, PTH gene expression. Hypophosphatemia and hyperphosphatemia in the rat respectively lower and raise the levels of mRNA for PTH through a mechanism that is independent of changes in Ca^{2+}_o or 1,25(OH)$_2$D$_3$.[11, 95–99] An elevated extracellular phosphate concentration could thus contribute importantly to the secondary hyperparathyroidism frequently encountered in patients with end-stage renal failure, who often have chronically elevated serum phosphate concentrations.

Metabolites of vitamin D, principally 1,25(OH)$_2$D$_3$, also play an important role in the long-term regulation of parathyroid function and may act at several levels: by affecting the secretion of PTH and regulation of its gene, by regulating transcriptional activity of the genes encoding the calcium-sensing receptor (CaR) and the vitamin D receptor (VDR), as well as by regulating parathyroid cellular proliferation.[11, 27, 94, 100] 1,25(OH)$_2$D$_3$ is by far the most important vitamin D metabolite that modulates parathyroid function. It acts through a nuclear receptor, the VDR, often in concert with other such receptors (i.e., those for retinoic acid or glucocorticoids), on DNA sequences upstream from the PTH gene[101, 102] (see Chapter 72). 1,25(OH)$_2$D$_3$-induced upregulation of VDR expression in the parathyroid could potentiate its inhibitory action(s) on PTH synthesis and secretion.[11, 27, 94] Recently developed noncalcemic or less calcemic analogues of 1,25(OH)$_2$D$_3$ (e.g., 22-oxacalcitriol and calcipotriol) inhibit PTH secretion while producing relatively little stimulation of intestinal calcium absorption and bone resorption[103–105] and may thus be attractive candidates for treating the hyperparathyroidism of chronic renal insufficiency.

Regulation of Parathyroid Cellular Proliferation

Adjustment of the rate of parathyroid cellular proliferation is the third adaptive mechanism contributing to changes in the overall secretory activity of the parathyroid gland. Under normal conditions, parathyroid cells have little or no proliferative activity. The parathyroid glands, however, can enlarge greatly during states of chronic hypocalcemia, particularly in the setting of renal failure, probably because of a combination of hypocalcemia, hyperphosphatemia, and low levels of $1{,}25(OH)_2D_3$ in the latter condition (for review, see Diaz et al.[27]).

Regulation of PTH Secretion

A large number of factors modulate PTH secretion in vitro, as reviewed in detail elsewhere,[11, 27, 106] but most of these factors are not thought to control hormonal secretion in vivo in a biologically relevant manner. Therefore we focus in this section principally on factors that are the most physiologically meaningful regulators of PTH secretion, namely, the extracellular ionized calcium concentration itself (Ca^{2+}_o), $1{,}25(OH)_2D_3$, and the level of extracellular phosphate ions. Of these three, Ca^{2+}_o is most important in the minute-to-minute control of PTH secretion. Indeed, the actions of $1{,}25(OH)_2D_3$ and phosphate ions on the secretion of PTH probably result, at least in part, from their effects on hormonal biosynthesis rather than secretion.[11, 27, 106] Ca^{2+}_o also modulates several other aspects of parathyroid function that indirectly affect PTH secretion, including PTH gene expression, the hormone's intracellular degradation, and parathyroid cellular proliferation, as described in more detail in earlier sections.

Physiologic Control of PTH Secretion by Ca^{2+}_o

As illustrated in Figure 70–5A, the relationship between PTH and Ca^{2+}_o is represented by a steep inverse sigmoidal curve that can be quantitatively described by four parameters.[107–109] These parameters are the maximal rate of PTH secretion at low Ca^{2+}_o (parameter A), the slope of the curve at its midpoint (parameter B), the value of Ca^{2+}_o at the midpoint (e.g., the "set-point" or the level of Ca^{2+}_o half-maximally suppressing PTH release) (parameter C), and the minimal secretory rate at high Ca^{2+}_o (parameter D) (Fig. 70–5B). Parameter A in vivo is the sum of the maximal rates of PTH release from all individual parathyroid chief cells, as reflected by the resultant, maximally stimulated level of circulating PTH. Because of the large value of parameter B in the Ca^{2+}_o-PTH relationship (i.e., the curve is very steep), small alterations in Ca^{2+}_o evoke large changes in PTH release, thereby contributing importantly to the near constancy of Ca^{2+}_o in vivo. Indeed, parathyroid cells can readily detect reductions in Ca^{2+}_o of a few percentage points,[108] and the percent coefficient of variation in Ca^{2+}_o in humans is less than 2%.[110] The set-point of the parathyroid gland is the key determinant of the level at which Ca^{2+}_o is "set" in vivo, although the parathyroid set-point is usually slightly lower than the ambient blood Ca^{2+}_o.[111] Thus the parathyroid cell is normally more than half-maximally suppressed at normal levels of Ca^{2+}_o and has a large secretory reserve for responding to hypocalcemic stress. Nevertheless, PTH levels in vivo also fall dramatically (e.g., by 80%) when Ca^{2+}_o rises to frankly hypercalcemic levels,[107, 108] which contributes importantly to the mineral ion homeostatic system's defense against hypercalcemia.[111] Furthermore, elevating Ca^{2+}_o also decreases the proportion of secreted hormone that is the intact, biologically active form of PTH because of increased intraglandular degradation to inactive fragments (see the earlier section PTH Biosynthesis and Intraglandular Processing and the later section Metabolism of PTH).[91, 112] Even with severe hypercalcemia, however, some residual release of intact PTH(1–84) still occurs in vivo and persists at a level approximately 5% of that observed with a maximal hypocalcemic stimulus[30, 93, 113] (see Fig. 70–5A). This nonsuppressible basal component of PTH release may contribute to the hypercalcemia caused by hyperparathyroidism when the mass of abnormal parathyroid tissue is very great.[109, 114, 115]

The parathyroid cell has a temporal hierarchy of responses to low Ca^{2+}_o that permits it to secrete progressively larger amounts of hormone during prolonged hypocalcemia.[11, 27, 106] To meet acute hypocalcemic challenges, PTH is released within seconds from preformed secretory vesicles by exocytosis as dictated by the sigmoidal curve (see Fig. 70–5A). Sufficient PTH is stored in the parathyroid chief cell to sustain maximal, low Ca^{2+}_o-stimulated PTH release for about 60 to 90 minutes.[111] Another rapid response of the parathyroid cell to hypocalcemia that enhances its net synthetic rate of PTH is reduced intracellular hormonal degradation—the opposite of what occurs at high levels of Ca^{2+}_o—which occurs within minutes to an hour.[91, 112] Hypocalcemia

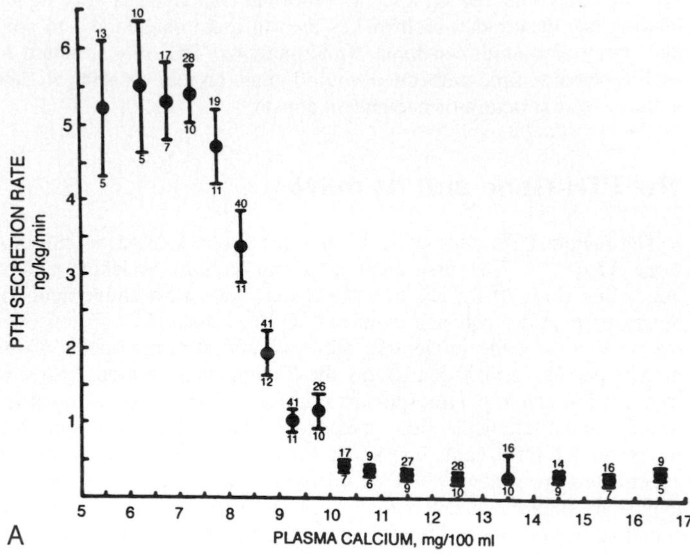

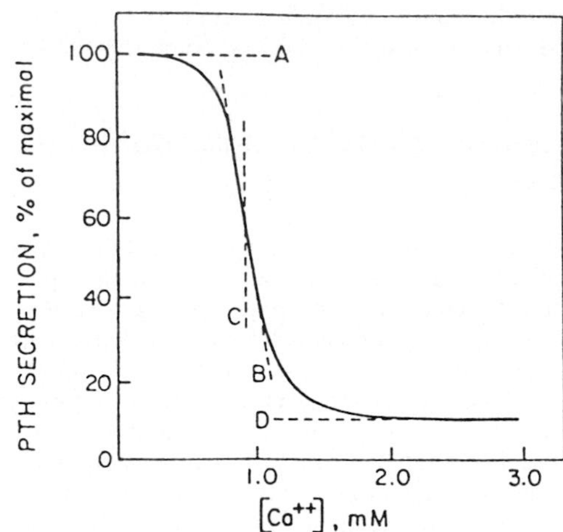

FIGURE 70–5. Inverse sigmoidal relationship between Ca^{2+}_o and parathyroid hormone (PTH) release and the four-parameter model describing these curves. *A*, Secretory response of bovine parathyroid glands to induced alterations in plasma calcium concentration. Calves were infused with calcium or ethylenediaminetetraacetic acid, and PTH secretion was assessed by measuring PTH levels in the parathyroid venous effluent. The *symbols* and *vertical bars* indicate the secretory rate (mean ±SE) in calcium concentration ranges of 1.0 or 0.5 mg/100 mL. The number of calves and samples are indicated, respectively, by numbers below and above. *B*, Sigmoidal curve generated by the equation $Y = [(A - D)/(1 + (X/C^B)] + D$; the significance of A, B, C, and D are described in the text. (*A* from Hurst JG: Sigmoidal relationship between parathyroid hormone secretion rate and plasma calcium concentration in calves. Endocrinology 10:10, 1978; *B* from Brown EM: PTH secretion in vivo and in vitro. Miner Electrolyte Metab 8:130–150, 1982.)

persisting for hours to days elicits increased PTH gene expression (see the above section Regulation of PTH Gene Expression), whereas that lasting for days to weeks or longer stimulates parathyroid cellular proliferation (see the earlier section Regulation of Parathyroid Cellular Proliferation) (for review, see elsewhere[11, 27, 106]). A greater secretory capacity for PTH on a per-cell basis (e.g., as a result of enhanced PTH gene expression) increases maximal hormonal secretion (e.g., parameter A), as does an increase in cell number as a result of parathyroid cellular proliferation (see Fig. 70–5). In severe secondary hyperparathyroidism, very large increases in parathyroid cellular mass can elevate circulating PTH levels by 100-fold or more.

In addition to responding to changes in Ca^{2+}_o per se, the parathyroid cell also appears to sense the rate of change in $Ca^{2+}{}_o$ such that rapid decrements in calcium promote more vigorous secretory responses than do changes of a similar magnitude occurring more slowly.[116] Furthermore, during dynamic testing of parathyroid function in vivo by induced increases or decreases in $Ca^{2+}{}_o$, PTH in blood is higher at a given serum calcium concentration when $Ca^{2+}{}_o$ is falling than when it is rising (e.g., hysteresis is occurring in this relationship).[117, 118] The latter results in an apparent direction dependence of the secretory response, which when combined with the rate dependence just described, may allow for a physiologically appropriate, more vigorous secretory response to large rapid decrements in $Ca^{2+}{}_o$. Also present are circadian[119] (for review, see Diaz et al.[27]) and more rapid (i.e., occurring at rates of one to six pulses per hour) phasic changes in circulating PTH levels,[27, 120] but the physiologic significance of these changes is not known.

Molecular Mechanism of $Ca^{2+}{}_o$ Sensing by Parathyroid Cells and Other Cells Involved in Mineral Ion Homeostasis

The molecular mechanism underlying $Ca^{2+}{}_o$-regulated PTH secretion involves activation of a G protein–coupled, cell surface $Ca^{2+}{}_o$-sensing receptor (abbreviated as CaR or sometimes as CaSR). The CaR was first isolated from bovine parathyroid glands[121] and subsequently from human parathyroid and several other tissues (for review, see Brown et al.[122, 123]). The receptor exhibits the characteristic "serpentine" motif (seven membrane-spanning domains) of the superfamily of G protein–coupled receptors (Fig. 70–6). Its long, N-terminal extracellular domain contains the major determinants of $Ca^{2+}{}_o$ binding.[124, 125] Changes in $Ca^{2+}{}_o$ modulate a number of second messenger systems via coupling of CaR through its intracellular domains to the relevant G proteins regulating these signaling pathways.[122, 123] These functions include activation of phospholipases C, A_2, and D,[126] stimulation of mitogen-activated protein kinase,[127] and inhibition of adenylate cyclase.[128] Despite numerous studies conducted over the past 25 years, a full understanding of the major second messenger pathway(s) through which changes in $Ca^{2+}{}_o$, acting via the CaR, regulate various aspects of the function of parathyroid and other CaR-expressing cells remains elusive (see below).

In the parathyroid the CaR mediates the inhibitory actions of $Ca^{2+}{}_o$ on PTH secretion and parathyroid cellular proliferation and probably also on PTH gene expression.[122, 123] The CaR is likewise expressed in several additional tissues involved in systemic mineral ion homeostasis, including the calcitonin-secreting cells of the thyroid,[129] diverse cells within the kidney,[130] bone cells and/or their precursors,[94] and intestinal epithelial cells.[131] In the C cell the CaR mediates the stimulatory action of high $Ca^{2+}{}_o$ on calcitonin secretion, thereby increasing the circulating level of this $Ca^{2+}{}_o$-lowering hormone. In the kidney, the CaR is present in the cortical thick ascending limb of the nephron. Here it is thought to mediate direct, high $Ca^{2+}{}_o$-induced inhibition of the tubular reabsorption of Ca^{2+} and Mg^{2+}.[130, 132] Therefore, raising $Ca^{2+}{}_o$ both directly inhibits renal tubular reabsorption of Ca^{2+} via actions on the CaR expressed in portions of the nephron involved in hormonal regulation of Ca^{2+} reabsorption (e.g., by PTH) and indirectly inhibits its reabsorption by reducing PTH secretion (see the later section Renal Calcium Reabsorption). The CaR probably also mediates the long-recognized, but poorly understood inhibitory effect of hypercalcemia on renal water conservation, probably exerting this action by inhibiting vasopressin-stimulated water flow in the distal collecting duct. A possible physiologic relevance of this action is to prevent the development of excessively high concentrations of calcium in the distal collecting system, thereby perhaps mitigating the risk of renal stone formation.[132] Elevating $Ca^{2+}{}_o$ is known to stimulate osteoblastic bone formation and inhibit osteoclastic bone resorption.[94, 133] Although the CaR is expressed in osteoblasts and osteoclasts and/or their precursors,[94] its role in mediating the actions of $Ca^{2+}{}_o$ on bone turnover remain to be established. Similarly, it is not currently known whether the CaR that is expressed in intestinal epithelial cells plays any role in regulating $1,25(OH)_2D_3$-mediated absorption of calcium.

The identification of hypercalcemic (e.g., familial hypocalciuric hypercalcemia and neonatal severe hyperparathyroidism[134]) and hypocalcemic (i.e., autosomal dominant hypocalcemia[135]) disorders caused by inactivating and activating mutations of the CaR, respectively, has provided incontrovertible proof of the receptor's central, nonredundant role in setting the serum calcium concentration (for review, see Brown

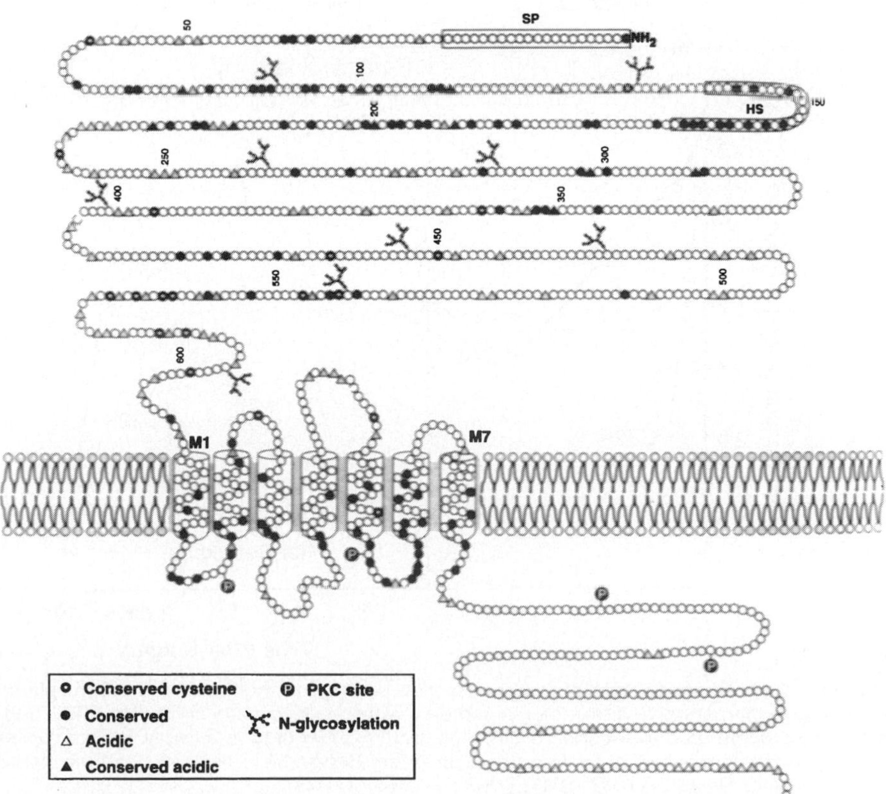

FIGURE 70–6. Schematic representation of the predicted topology of the calcium-sensing receptor cloned from human parathyroid gland. HS, hydrophobic segment; PKC, protein kinase C; SP, signal peptide. (From Brown EM, Gamba G, Riccardi D, et al: Cloning and characterization of an extracellular Ca^{2+}-sensing receptor from bovine parathyroid. Nature 366:575–580, 1993.)

et al.[122, 123]). Patients with these disorders have characteristic abnormalities in parathyroid and renal $Ca^{2+}{}_o$ sensing/handling that have clarified the receptor's normal role in these tissues that was outlined above. Targeted disruption of the CaR gene has also enabled the generation of mouse models of familial hypocalciuric hypercalcemia and neonatal severe hyperparathyroidism via inactivation of one or both alleles of the CaR,[136] further supporting its importance in $Ca^{2+}{}_o$ homeostasis.

1,25(OH)$_2$D$_3$, Phosphate, and Other Factors Regulating PTH Secretion

In addition to directly inhibiting PTH gene expression, 1,25(OH)$_2$D$_3$ also reduces PTH secretion[137, 138] (for review, see elsewhere[11, 27, 106]). It is not known whether this latter action is solely secondary to the effect of 1,25(OH)$_2$D$_3$ on biosynthesis of the hormone and/or represents a direct action on the secretory process per se. Recent studies have provided evidence that increasing the ambient level of phosphate in vitro, independent of concomitant changes in $Ca^{2+}{}_o$, enhances parathyroid cellular proliferation, PTH gene expression, and hormonal secretion.[96–98] Phosphate-induced changes in PTH secretion, however, take several hours and may result secondarily from changes in hormonal biosynthesis rather than secretion per se.[98] Finally, $Mg^{2+}{}_o$ clearly functions as a CaR agonist in vitro when tested in cells containing an endogenous CaR[139] (e.g., parathyroid cells) or expressing the cloned CaR,[121] although it is twofold to threefold less potent than $Ca^{2+}{}_o$ on a molar basis. Because levels of serum ionized $Mg^{2+}{}_o$ are, if anything, lower than those of $Ca^{2+}{}_o$, it is at present unclear whether $Mg^{2+}{}_o$ acts as a physiologically relevant CaR agonist at the parathyroid gland in vivo under normal circumstances. Patients with inactivating or activating CaR mutations, however, can exhibit mild hypermagnesemia or hypomagnesemia,[122, 123] respectively, thus suggesting that the CaR does contribute to setting $Mg^{2+}{}_o$ in vivo, as previously suggested.[140] It may do so, at least in part, in the kidney, where $Mg^{2+}{}_o$ in the tubular fluid of the thick ascending limb exceeds that in blood and may be sufficient to activate the CaR that regulates tubular reabsorption of $Ca^{2+}{}_o$ and $Mg^{2+}{}_o$ in this nephron segment.[122, 123, 132] In addition to the inhibitory effect of elevated $Mg^{2+}{}_o$ on PTH secretion, low concentrations of $Mg^{2+}{}_o$—as in patients with overt magnesium deficiency—also reduce PTH secretion.[141] The mechanism(s) underlying this effect of hypomagnesemia remains uncertain, although it is not thought to involve the CaR.[27]

Metabolism of PTH

Studies performed over more than three decades by several laboratories have focused on the heterogeneity of circulating forms of PTH, which was first identified by Berson and Yalow in 1968[142] (Fig. 70–7). From these investigations it is now apparent that in addition to the full-length polypeptide PTH(1–84), which is the biologically active hormone, much of the circulating hormone lacks an intact N terminus and these fragments are thus devoid of biologic activity, at least with regard to the PTH1R-mediated regulation of mineral ion homeostasis (for a detailed review see Potts et al.[26]). C-terminal PTH fragments are produced in and released from the parathyroid gland, but they are also derived from circulating intact hormone by efficient, high-capacity degradative systems in the liver and kidney and most likely at other peripheral sites (Fig. 70–8).

Until recently, most evidence had indicated that the circulating PTH fragments, which can be detected by immunologic techniques, consist of only the middle and C-terminal regions of the molecule. Biologically active, N-terminal fragments are essentially undetectable, even when highly sensitive techniques are used.[143, 144] Furthermore, intact PTH does not require prior cleavage to be biologically active, and the peripheral metabolism of PTH and the intraglandular generation of hormone fragments, which are then secreted, therefore appeared to be largely a catabolic process. Accordingly, intensive study of the enzymes involved in hormonal cleavage and the cellular mechanisms of uptake and release slowed down more than a decade ago. However, recent studies, summarized later in this chapter, indicate that full-length PTH interacts through its middle and C-terminal regions with other receptors that have been identified and partially character-

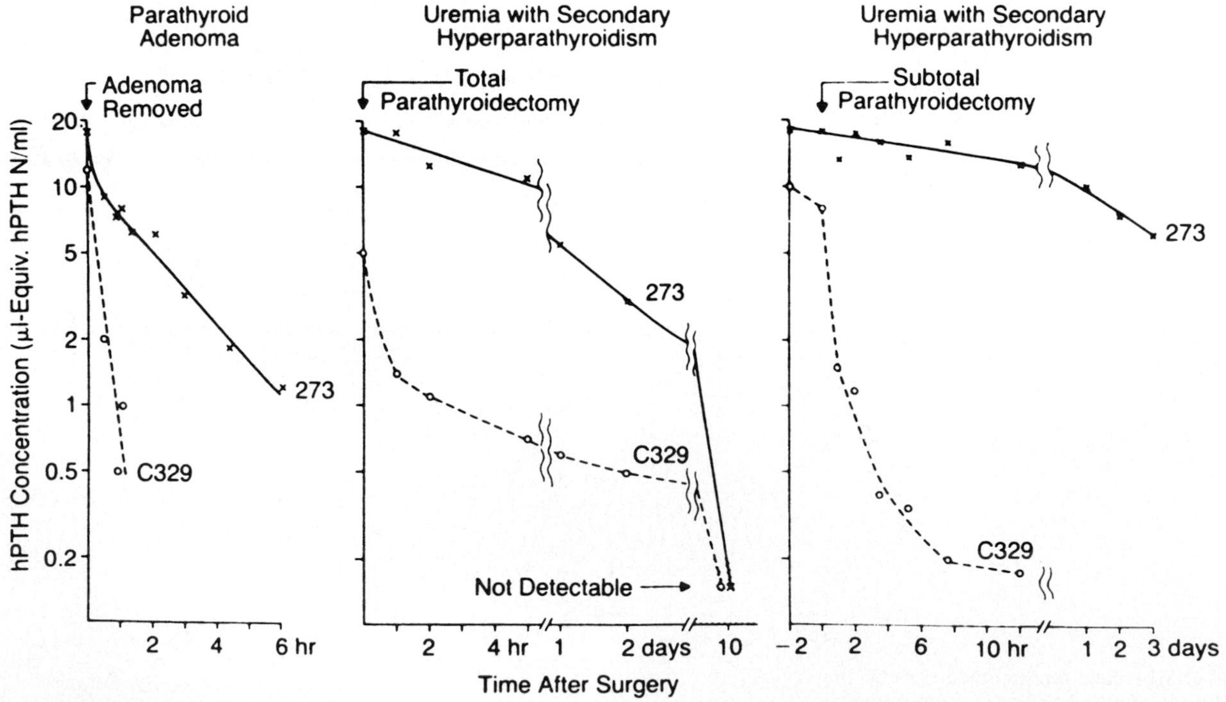

FIGURE 70–7. Disappearance of immunoreactive parathyroid hormone (PTH) from plasma after parathyroidectomy in patients with primary or secondary hyperparathyroidism. Plasma samples were assayed with antiserum C329 and antiserum 273, with an extract of a normal human parathyroid gland used as a standard (hPTH N) and ^{125}I-bPTH used as a tracer. Plasma concentrations of hormone are given as microliter equivalents of the plasma standard of hPTH (see the text). (From Berson SA, Yallow RS: Immunochemical heterogenicity of parathyroid hormone in plasma. J Clin Endocrinol Metab 28:1037–1047, 1968.)

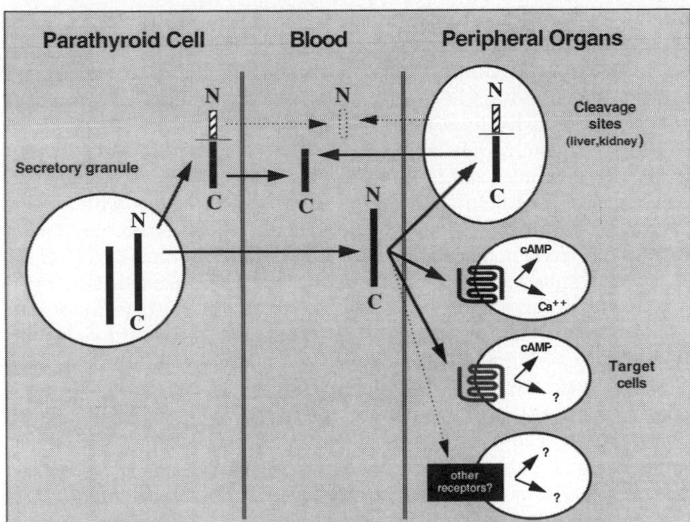

FIGURE 70–8. Scheme of peripheral parathyroid hormone (PTH) cleavage and the interaction of PTH with the PTH/PTH-related peptide receptor and with other putative receptors on target cells; cleavage of the intact hormone into N-terminal (N) *(diagonal stripes)* and C-terminal fragments (C) *(solid bar)* by the parathyroid gland and by peripheral organs. cAMP, cyclic adenosine monophosphate.

ized.[145–148] By activating these (yet uncloned) receptors, C-terminal fragments of PTH appear to have several different effects; for example, they may affect the maturation of preosteoclasts, as well as the biologic activity of chondrocytes, osteoblasts, and possibly other bone cells.[147–151]

Because of the lack of evidence of circulating forms of biologically active, N-terminal fragments, it was feasible to introduce immunometric assays that use two different antibodies, an immobilized capturing antibody directed against the C-terminal portion of PTH(1–84) and a radiolabeled or enzyme-labeled detection antibody that is directed against an epitope within the N-terminal portion of the intact molecule.[152, 153] In addition to other advantages (for example, higher sensitivity and specificity), such assays detect predominantly full-length PTH, thereby reducing or eliminating the detection of smaller, mainly C-terminal fragments that accumulate in certain clinical conditions, particularly in patients with renal failure. Recently, however, large-molecular-weight forms of PTH have been described that are N-terminally truncated and show an elution profile on high-performance liquid chromatography (HPLC) that is largely indistinguishable from that of synthetic PTH(7–84).[93, 113, 154] These large PTH fragments are readily detectable by several different two-site antibody assays that were previously believed to detect only the intact hormone. In individuals with normal renal function, only small amounts of these fragments are detectable, but the same PTH fragments can contribute significantly, depending on the level of blood calcium, to the concentration of immunoreactive "intact" PTH in patients with renal failure.[93, 113, 154] The biologic activity, if any, of these N-terminally truncated PTH molecules has not yet been established. However, because of the recognition of such N-terminally modified PTH molecules, interest has been restimulated in the metabolism of PTH, as outlined below.

PTH Fragments Derived from the Parathyroid Glands

Two seemingly contradictory lines of evidence developed regarding the origin of circulating fragments of hormones. After the original observation of Berson and Yalow,[142] another group showed that most of the PTH found in the venous effluent of parathyroid glands in cows or in humans with parathyroid tumors contained hormone that was indistinguishable in size and immunologic properties from that extracted from the parathyroid glands.[155] In contrast, some immunoreactive hormone found in the circulation was smaller and lacked immunologic determinants corresponding to the N-terminal portion of PTH. These results were interpreted as evidence that PTH heterogeneity is a postsecretory event. Shortly thereafter, however, Silverman and Yalow[156] and DiBella et al.[157] reported that multiple immunoreactive forms of PTH, similar to those found in the peripheral blood, can be found in crude extracts of human parathyroid glands (see Fig. 70–7). These studies suggested that most, if not all circulating immunoreactive forms of the hormone originate from secretion by the parathyroid glands, although subsequent work (see below) showed that PTH fragments also arise from peripheral sites, especially the liver and kidney. Direct measurement of arterial and venous differences in parathyroid effluent blood (with vigorous conditions to prevent any ex vivo cleavage of hormone after sample collection) performed in cattle confirmed that C-terminal fragments and intact hormone, but not N-terminal fragments, are secreted into the circulation. The relative concentration of C-terminal fragments released from the gland increases under conditions of systemic hypercalcemia, when overall secretion rates of intact hormone are lower[90, 158]; these C-terminal PTH fragments are similar to those generated by peripheral metabolism (see below) but were not chemically characterized.

Hepatic and Renal Origin of Circulating PTH Fragments

The peripheral metabolism of PTH has been analyzed by injecting intact hormone into the circulation of test animals. Such experiments have not been performed in human subjects, but it is assumed that the similar metabolism of PTH in rats, dogs, and cows is reflective of its metabolism in humans.[159] Clearance of intact PTH from plasma was found to be very rapid (half-life, 2–4 minutes),[143, 144] the major sites of clearance being the liver and kidney. Clearance by the liver predominates over clearance by the kidney; the two organs together account for virtually all clearance of intact hormone. Hepatic clearance of intact hormone has been estimated to be 40% to 75% and renal clearance, 20% to 30% (for detailed review see Potts et al.[26]).

The two major circulating C terminal fragments found resulted from peripheral cleavage of the hormone between residues 33 and 34 and between residues 36 and 37, respectively[160, 161]; Kupffer cells, but not hepatocytes were found to be responsible.[162] Liver- and kidney-specific cleavage of intact PTH also involves cathepsins, which generate both N- and C-terminal PTH fragments; however, only C-terminal PTH fragments reappear in the circulation.[88, 89, 162, 163] Clearance of C-terminal fragments occurs principally by glomerular filtration (half-life, 20–40 minutes), hence the central role of renal failure in elevating the concentration of C-terminal fragments.[147] PTH metabolism was evaluated in rats with biologically active intact hormone labeled biosynthetically at known sites. The rapid disappearance of intact hormone from the circulation was followed by the appearance of C-terminal fragments, but without evidence of re-entry of N-terminal fragments, even if the animals had undergone partial or total nephrectomy.[143, 144]

In summary, current evidence indicates that intact PTH and multiple C-terminal fragments, which are derived from glandular and peripheral cleavage and may not be identical, are the principal circulating hormonal forms. However, recent data suggest the presence of a previously unrecognized, large, N-terminally truncated form of the hormone (see below). Biologically active, N-terminal fragments of PTH, if found in the circulation at all, are likely to circulate only at extremely low concentrations (less than 10^{-13} to 10^{-14} mol/L), thus causing considerable doubt regarding their physiologic significance. It is for this reason that immunoassays for clinical use are now frequently designed to detect the intact hormone predominantly or exclusively and to largely ignore other circulating fragments (see Fig. 70–8).[152, 153]

Most earlier in vivo evidence regarding the renal clearance and metabolism of intact PTH (as distinct from C-terminal fragments) indicates a peritubular uptake process rather than glomerular filtration followed by uptake from the tubular lumen and subsequent cleavage.[164] Recent studies indicate that megalin, a multifunctional endocytic receptor expressed in the proximal renal tubules, can mediate the reuptake and subsequent degradation of the portion of PTH that is subject to glomerular filtration.[165] Megalin-mediated uptake depends on an intact N terminus of PTH; C-terminal fragments that are eliminated by glomerular filtration are not recognized by megalin. Although homozygous ablation of megalin has been accomplished, the resulting animals are not yet sufficiently robust or uniform for in vivo studies of PTH clearance and metabolism. The potential significance, quantitatively and biologically, of glomerular filtration and megalin-mediated uptake of intact PTH therefore remains uncertain. However, megalin-ablated mice excrete fourfold more N-terminal PTH in the urine than do wild-type animals.[165]

N-Terminally Truncated Fragments of PTH

Recent studies have demonstrated the presence of circulating PTH fragments that are different in character and composition from any of the hormone fragments discussed above.[93, 113, 154] The studies that led to the detection of these PTH species were at least partly stimulated by the clinical observations that two-site immunometric assays to measure intact PTH frequently seemed to give surprisingly high levels of nonsuppressible PTH in patients with end-stage renal disease and histologic changes consistent with adynamic bone disease[93, 166–169] (see Chapter 86).

HPLC analysis of blood samples from such uremic patients and from patients with other forms of hyperparathyroidism revealed two distinct immunoreactive peaks in column effluent that were detectable (although with differing sensitivity) by different commercial assays. One peak corresponded to intact PTH(1–84), whereas the other peak migrated close to the position occupied chromatographically by synthetic PTH(7–84).[93, 113] This finding suggested that the epitope of the detection antibody in these assays did not require the presence of the first six or more amino acids of PTH(1–84).[113, 154] The results were interpreted as being consistent with the view that the molecular entity or entities detected besides PTH(1–84) are N-terminally truncated forms of the intact molecule that are similar, but not necessarily identical to synthetic PTH(7–84).[113] More detailed chromatographic studies performed with one of these "intact" PTH assays showed significant variation in the ratio of the N-terminally truncated PTH to PTH(1–84). Individuals with normal renal function showed a lower ratio than did patients with uremia; furthermore, the percentage of immunoreactivity representing N-terminally truncated forms of PTH rose in both groups when hypercalcemia was present.[93]

Recently, a novel immunoradiometric assay that uses a radiolabeled detection antibody raised against the amino acid sequence 1–6 of human PTH was used to analyze samples from patients with end-stage renal disease in the basal state and during dynamic testing to lower and raise blood calcium acutely. The results were compared with those achieved with an established commercial assay.[113, 152] Characterization of both assays with synthetic PTH fragments showed that the novel assay did not detect PTH(7–84) and furthermore required the presence of position 1 in the PTH sequence. The other widely used assay detected PTH(7–84) and was not sensitive to the presence of the first N-terminal amino acid. The newer immunoradiometric assay showed significantly lower PTH concentrations during stimulation and suppression of glandular activity with alterations in calcium, a result consistent with the conclusion that only PTH(1–84) is detected by this assay system.[154]

Even at this stage, the findings outlined above may have considerable significance for the management of patients with parathyroid dysfunction, especially in the presence of renal failure. Treatment of patients with end-stage renal disease with large amounts of vitamin D and/or calcium is frequently associated with adynamic bone disease, which can be deleterious, particularly in growing children.[170–172] Particularly during hypercalcemia, N-terminally truncated forms of PTH become a significant, if not the dominant PTH species. Measurement of "intact" PTH by earlier assays[152] may therefore overestimate the concentrations of biologically active PTH and could result in the overtreatment of uremic patients with vitamin D analogues and/or calcium. The resulting suppression of the parathyroid gland (even without evoking an inhibitory effect of a PTH[7–84]-like fragment), combined with resistance toward PTH, possibly due to reduced expression of the PTH/PTHrP receptor[173, 174] and other yet unknown mechanisms,[175, 176] could be acting together to excessively reduce PTH-dependent bone turnover.

The origin (glandular vs. peripheral), biologic properties (weak agonist or inhibitor), and precise structure, distribution, and clearance of the N-terminally truncated PTH (sometimes referred to as "non-PTH[1–84]") are as yet unknown. To the extent that in vitro studies with defined cellular and receptor characteristics predict biologic properties in vivo (see below) and that earlier animal studies with biosynthetically labeled PTH reflect the peripheral clearance and cleavage of PTH(1–84), certain speculations about N-terminally truncated PTH are possible. Similar to PTH(7–34), the N-terminally truncated PTH(7–84) is unlikely to have agonist activity at the PTH/PTHrP receptor, and would be predicted to have only weak antagonist activity in vivo.[177, 178]

The concentration of C-terminal fragments (called C-terminal fragments because the entire N-terminal PTH region of 30 to 40 amino acids is missing) in the parathyroid effluent in cows was reported to be higher than that of intact PTH under conditions of induced hypercalcemia, consistent with a continuing process of cleavage and release of preformed hormone during hypercalcemia while the release of intact hormone is sharply suppressed.[90, 158] Such information is more consistent with a glandular origin of the N-terminally truncated PTH and could explain its increased fractional concentration relative to PTH(1–84) in hypercalcemic conditions (as noted above). However, no studies have as yet been reported in which samples of effluent blood from the parathyroids had been analyzed by HPLC or with selective immunoassays, which would be critical to support any such conclusion. Determining the chemical nature and biologic roles of this N-terminally truncated PTH fragment(s) may contribute to understanding its biologic significance and will support a more precise interpretation of PTH assay results, especially in uremic patients.

PTH-DEPENDENT REGULATION OF MINERAL ION HOMEOSTASIS MEDIATED THROUGH THE PTH/PTHrP RECEPTOR (TYPE 1 RECEPTOR)

PTH is, as outlined above, the most important peptide regulator of mineral ion homeostasis in mammals. Through its actions on the kidney and bone, PTH maintains blood calcium concentration within narrow limits. In bone it stimulates the release of calcium and in the kidney it enhances renal tubular reabsorption of calcium and stimulates the urinary excretion of phosphate. Furthermore, in the kidney it increases the synthesis of renal 1α-hydroxylase, which stimulates $1,25(OH)_2D_3$ production and thus increases, albeit indirectly, intestinal absorption of calcium (and phosphate). These direct and indirect endocrine actions of PTH are mediated through the PTH/PTHrP receptor (PTH1R), a G protein–coupled receptor that is abundantly expressed in both major target tissues of PTH action. In addition to regulating renal calcium and phosphate transport, PTH modifies the tubular handling of magnesium, sodium, potassium, bicarbonate, and water and moreover stimulates renal gluconeogenesis.

Specific regions of the nephron that are involved in each of the PTH-dependent actions have been defined through in vivo micropuncture analyses and through in vitro studies with nephron segments that have been dissected from the remainder of the kidney. Furthermore, cell lines from specific regions of the kidney have also been used. However, interpretation of these results has to take into account the complexity of the organization of the kidney as an organ (for example, the complex anatomic relationship involving different renal tubular segments spanning both the cortex and medulla and the effects of countercurrent distribution that modify solute and water transport), particularly since certain in vivo features of renal tubules are not readily imitated in vitro through the use of isolated tubules or cells (see Chapter 73 for details regarding transport functions in different tubular regions).

Renal Calcium Reabsorption

Most of the calcium in the glomerular filtrate is reabsorbed. The bulk of this reabsorption (65%) occurs via passive, paracellular mechanisms, both in the proximal tubules and, to a lesser extent, in the thick ascending limb of Henle's loop and the distal convoluted tubule.[179–183] As noted by Diaz et al.,[27] the calcium sensor plays an important, PTH-independent role in the adjustment of renal calcium reabsorption in the cortical thick ascending limb. The physiologically important stimulation of renal calcium reabsorption by PTH occurs almost entirely in the distal nephron.[184–187] In the cortical thick ascending limb, PTH increases the magnitude of the lumen positive potential that drives the passive, paracellular reabsorption of calcium and magnesium. In the distal convoluted tubule, in contrast, PTH promotes increased transcellular calcium reabsorption. PTH enhances passive uptake of calcium into the tubular cells via the apical (luminal) plasma membrane, as well as its active extrusion against a steep electrochemical gradient at the basolateral membrane. This latter process of extrusion involves two types of transporters. One is the plasma membrane calcium pump (Ca^{2+}, Mg^{2+}-ATPase) and the second is a Na^+/Ca^{2+} exchanger that, in turn, is indirectly regulated by Na^+, K^+-ATPase(s), which maintains the transcellular Na^+ gradient. Studies performed with membrane vesicles from the distal region of the kidney show increased activity of the Na^+/Ca^{2+} exchanger in response to PTH.[188] PTH also stimulates the translocation of preformed calcium channels sequestered within the interior of certain distal tubular cells to the apical surface[189] (Fig. 70–9). These calcium channels translocate to the apical (i.e., luminal) surface of the renal tubular epithelial cell and mediate increased cellular calcium uptake. Because PTH simultaneously enhances the activity of Na^+/Ca^{2+} exchangers in the basolateral (antiluminal) membrane, the overall process promotes an increase in transcellular calcium uptake from the lumen to blood, that is, from the apical surface to the basolateral membrane.

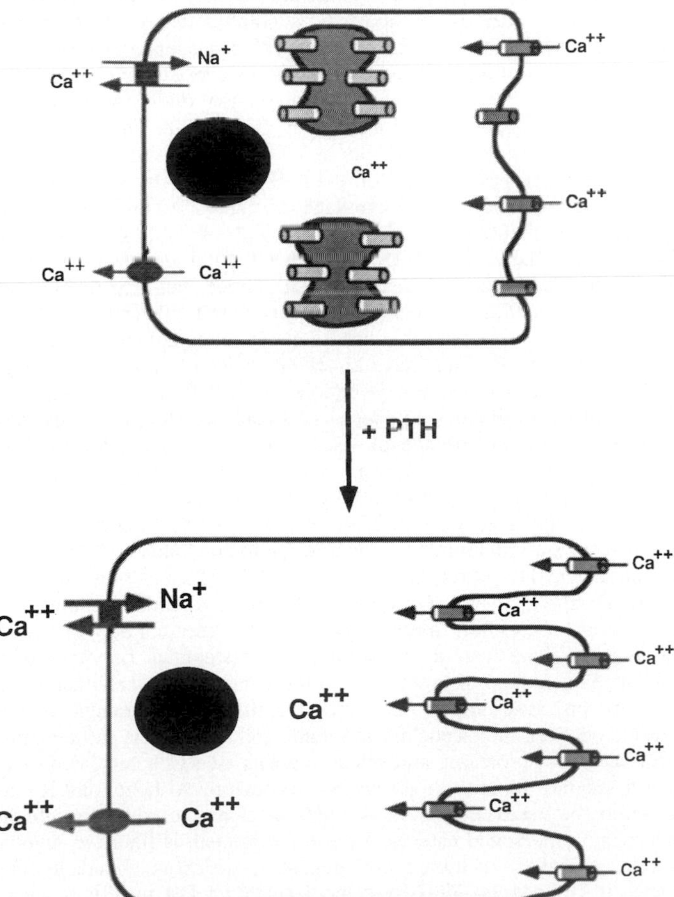

FIGURE 70–9. Parathyroid hormone (PTH) triggers the translocation of preformed voltage-dependent calcium channels from sites of intracellular sequestration to the apical membrane, which also undergoes rapid morphologic changes that greatly increase its surface area. Intracellular free calcium levels rise significantly, and increased net transepithelial calcium transport occurs, mainly via enhanced Na^+/Ca^{2+} exchange at the basolateral membrane, supported in turn by Na^+,K^+-ATPase. Analogous events underlie PTH regulation of proximal tubular phosphate transport.

Regulation of 1α- and 24-Hydroxylase Activity

PTH is a major inducer of the activity of proximal tubular 1α-hydroxylase,[190, 191] a microsomal cytochrome P450 enzyme that synthesizes biologically active $1,25(OH)_2D_3$ from the substrate 25-hydroxyvitamin D_3.[192–194] This effect of PTH on synthesis of the renal enzyme shows longer lag times than its effect on renal Ca^{2+} transport and is mediated, at least in part, by the protein kinase A (PKA) signaling pathway of the PTH/PTHrP receptor.[195, 196] Although 1α-hydroxylase activity has been detected in several nonrenal tissues, its mRNA was found in abundant concentrations only in the kidney, thus confirming that this organ is the most important site for the generation of $1,25(OH)_2D_3$.[196] PTH-dependent synthesis of new 1α-hydroxylase protein requires several hours and is blocked by $1,25(OH)_2D_3$ and actinomycin D, a blocker of protein synthesis.[196–200] Hypophosphatemia is, similar to PTH, a major inducer of 1α-hydroxylase, whereas hypercalcemia, as would be generated by sustained increases in circulating levels of PTH or PTHrP, suppresses synthesis of the enzyme, thus limiting overall $1,25(OH)_2D_3$ synthesis in a homeostatic manner. $25(OH)D_3$ and $1,25(OH)_2D_3$ can also be hydroxylated by the 24-hydroxylase, but the resulting metabolites, $24,25(OH)_2D_3$ and $1,24,25(OH)_3D_3$, appear to have no major role in the regulation of mineral ion homeostasis (see Chapter 72). However, PTH has an inhibitory effect on the 24-hydroxylase, thus reducing the inactivation of $1,25(OH)_2D_3$; in contrast, $1,25(OH)_2D_3$ stimulates the synthesis of 24-hydroxylase, thereby inducing its own metabolism.[201, 202]

Renal Phosphate Transport

PTH is of major importance for maintaining normal blood calcium levels, but it is not the principal regulator of the serum phosphate concentration, which appears to depend to a significant extent on the actions of a poorly characterized phosphaturic factor.[19, 203] However, when PTH causes an increase in bone resorption (as might occur with prolonged dietary calcium deprivation), calcium and phosphate increase simultaneously in the blood circulation. Although calcium is needed, phosphate is best excreted, which is mainly accomplished by a PTH-stimulated increase in renal phosphate clearance.

The potent, PTH-dependent reduction in renal phosphate reabsorption occurs in both the proximal and distal tubules,[185] although the proximal effects of the hormone are quantitatively more important.[204–207] Details of the mechanism(s) whereby PTH modifies phosphate transport remain incompletely defined but involve the sodium-dependent phosphate cotransporter NPT-2 (previously named NaPi-2); the cDNA encoding this protein has been cloned,[208–210] and homozygous ablation of the murine homologue has been accomplished [211] (see Chapter 73). PTH decreases the amount of NPT-2 transporter protein at the apical (luminal) surface of the cell, probably by blocking its synthesis and by increasing its intracellular translocation via endocytosis and subsequent degradation. This action inhibits the capacity of the cell to transport phosphate from the renal tubular lumen to the basolateral cell surface and leads to increased urinary phosphate excretion. Thus current explanations of the bidirectional renal actions of PTH, namely, the increase in tubular reabsorption of calcium and stimulation of renal phosphate excretion, may be explained partly by a hormone-directed increase or reduction, respectively, in critical apical membrane transport channels. Similar mechanisms may apply to other known renal effects of PTH, such as inhibition of the reabsorption of other minerals, water, and bicarbonate.[26, 212]

Actions of PTH on Bone

PTH affects a wide variety of the highly specialized bone cells, including osteoblasts, osteoclasts, and stromal cells. Some of these effects reflect direct actions of PTH; others are indirect and mediated in an autocrine/paracrine manner through factors released by cells expressing PTH/PTHrP receptors that regulate the activity of yet other cells that lack these receptors.[213–215]

It is still unclear which specific cellular actions explain the physiologic actions known to follow PTH administration to animals in vivo. Earlier studies had shown that the administration of PTH leads within minutes to a transient lowering of blood calcium caused by uptake of the mineral by bone cells, [216] which is rapidly followed by increased mobilization of calcium from the mineral phase into the blood stream.[217] Although there continue to be uncertainties regarding the cellular/anatomic basis of these rapid responses of PTH, considerable progress has been made in elucidating the mechanisms through which bone cells respond to PTH and to other autocrine/paracrine factors, such as cytokines (see Chapter 74). The major pathway for calcium release from bone involves osteoclasts, the only cells capable of resorbing bone; osteoclasts undergo multiple cellular changes involving the activation of cellular transporters and pumps, as well as the secretion of enzymes such as cathepsin K and collagenases.

Effects on Osteoblasts

Osteoblasts express the PTH/PTHrP receptor most abundantly and show the most vigorous response to the hormone. Earlier in vitro studies had indicated that PTH stimulates the generation of cyclic adenosine monophosphate (cAMP), inositol triphosphate (IP_3), and diacylglycerol and furthermore induces a change in membrane potential and intracellular pH[214, 218–221]; the PTH-induced increases in cAMP and IP_3 were confirmed in cells expressing the cloned PTH/PTHrP receptor.[5, 9, 222] A remarkable number of cellular activities of osteoblasts are influenced by PTH, including cellular metabolic activity, ion transport, cell shape, gene transcriptional activity, and secretion of multiple proteases (Table 70–2). Osteoblasts are known to have much heterogeneity, and the developmental cascade of cellular proliferation/differentiation events that result in mature osteoblasts is likely to be affected by PTH.[223–227] The cellular effects on osteoblasts caused by PTH depend on the cell line studied in vitro and the pattern of exposure to hormone, that is, continuous vs. intermittent.[224–226, 228] Continuous PTH administration in vivo results in decreased bone mass, whereas intermittent administration of PTH leads to an increase.[26, 229, 230] The cellular mechanisms whereby intermittent PTH administration selectively enhances bone formation remain unknown at present, as is the correlation between in vivo and in vitro responses. Further exploration of these mechanisms is clearly of great interest for understanding the hormone's therapeutic potential as a bone anabolic agent.

TABLE 70–2. Osteoblast Functions Regulated by Parathyroid Hormone

Proliferation
Cellular metabolism
  Glucose and amino acid transport
  Citrate, ornithine decarboxylation
  Creatine kinase activity
  Glycogen synthesis, glucose oxidation
  Synthesis of RNA, protein, lipids
Ion transport
  Calcium, phosphate, hydrogen ions
  Na^+, K^+-ATPase
Cytoskeletal and membrane structure
  Actin, vimentin, tubulin, and actinin synthesis
  Phosphatidylethanolamine synthesis
Hormonal responsiveness
  PTH/PTHrP receptor expression
  EGF receptor expression
  1,25-Dihydroxyvitamin D receptor expression
Matrix protein synthesis and secretion
  Collagen
  Osteonectin
  Osteopontin
Enzyme synthesis and secretion
  Alkaline phosphatase
  Collagenase
  Plasminogen activator/inhibitor
  Metalloproteinase inhibitor
Release of paracrine growth factors, cytokines, and other factors
  IGF-1, IGF-2, IGF-binding proteins
  TGF-β
  M-CSF
  Prostaglandin E_2, others
  Interleukin-6
  Osteoclast differentiation factor
  Osteoprotegerin

EGF, epidermal growth factor; IGF, insulin-like growth factor; M-CSF, macrophage colony-stimulating factor; PTH, parathyroid hormone; TGF, transforming growth factor.

Effects on Osteoclasts

Some reports had provided evidence for PTH receptors, at least on early differentiating precursors of osteoclasts.[231–234] Most investigators believe, however, that mature osteoclasts do not have PTH/PTHrP receptors and that these cells do not respond to PTH.[218, 223, 235] It was therefore suggested that PTH signals to osteoclasts indirectly through osteoblasts, which clearly have abundant PTH/PTHrP receptors on their surface and respond to the hormone with a dramatic change in cellular activity[214, 219–221, 236–239] (see Chapter 74). Consistent with the previously suggested indirect effects of PTH and other hormones,[213–215] several molecules were recently identified that are involved in the paracrine signaling cascade from osteoblasts and/or osteoblast precursors to recruit/activate osteoclasts.

These molecules include osteoclast-differentiating factor (ODF; also termed TRANCE or RANKL),[240, 241] a membrane-associated protein with homology to the family of tumor necrosis factors (TNFs) that induces—upon cell-to-cell contact and in the presence of macrophage colony-stimulating factor—the differentiation of osteoclast precursors into mature bone-resorbing osteoclasts.[242–244] These effects of ODF are likely to be mediated through RANK, a member of the TNF receptor family that is expressed on osteoclast precursors.[241, 242] However, ODF also interacts with osteoprotegerin, a soluble decoy receptor with homology to the TNF receptor family.[245] Transgenic expression of osteoprotegerin in mice leads to impaired osteoclastogenesis and thus to osteopetrosis,[246, 247] whereas ablation of the osteoprotegerin gene through homologous recombination in mice results in osteoporosis associated with arterial calcifications.[248] ODF gene ablation results in severe osteopetrosis because of the lack of osteoclasts, a defect in tooth eruption, and a complete lack of lymph nodes, but without obvious abnormalities in mineral ion homeostasis.[249] In contrast, ablation of the ODF receptor (RANK), leads to osteopetrotic changes similar to those observed in ODF-ablated mice, but also to hypocalcemia and secondary hyperparathyroidism and to renal phosphate wasting.[250] It appears plausible that challenging the homeostatic control mechanisms of either of these knockout mice, in particular, through dietary calcium and vitamin D deficiency, will further aggravate the degree of hypocalcemia and urinary phosphate excretion. However, despite the present absence of such experimental data, the outlined findings further illustrate the importance of osteoclastic bone resorption for maintaining blood calcium concentrations.

Some of the factors previously noted to have an important role in the paracrine stimulation of osteoclast formation, such as interleukin-6, interleukin-11, prostaglandin E_2, $1,25(OH)_2D_3$, and other peptides including PTH,[251–253] were recently shown to directly stimulate the production of ODF by osteoblasts.[242, 245, 254] Other cellular responses involved in bone resorption include the development of vitronectin-mediated anchorage of osteoclasts to the bone surface, acidification of the circumscribed and sealed-off extracellular environment that is created between the osteoclast and bone, and in addition, the secretion of a variety of proteases and other enzymes (see Chapter 74). Osteoclasts may not be able to get access to mineralized bone, and it may therefore be necessary for osteoblasts to clear the way through the overlying mineralized osteoid. Such a mechanism is likely to involve several enzymes, including collagenase-3, which is abundantly secreted in response to PTH by osteoblasts.[255, 256] The resulting "clearing" of the mineralized surface appears to be coordinated with the previously described PTH-induced retraction of osteoblasts from the bone surface.[218]

PARATHYROID HORMONE–RELATED PEPTIDE

Analysis of the physiologic actions of PTH and the molecular basis of its biologic activity requires consideration of the functions of

PTHrP. This peptide, discovered and characterized more than a decade ago, most probably shares an evolutionary origin with PTH. PTHrP has, at least in mammals, both chemical and functional overlaps with PTH, but its biologic roles are most likely quite different. When secreted in large concentrations, for example, by certain tumors, PTHrP has PTH-like properties. Typically, however, it functions as an autocrine/paracrine rather than an endocrine factor. PTHrP is a larger, more complex protein than PTH and is synthesized at multiple sites in different organs and tissues. The still evolving story of this protein and its proteolytic fragments is beyond the scope of this chapter (for comprehensive review see elsewhere[4–6, 257]). However, novel features and selective functions in the regulation of mineral ion homeostasis and bone development are reviewed below.

A substance with biologic properties similar to those of PTH was first proposed in the early 1940s, when Albright discussed a patient with malignancy-associated humoral hypercalcemia.[258] The clinical and biochemical characterization of similarly affected patients subsequently established the syndrome of humoral hypercalcemia of malignancy[259] and eventually led to the amino acid sequence analysis and molecular cloning of PTHrP from several different tumors.[260–263] It is now generally accepted that PTHrP is the most frequent humoral cause of hypercalcemia in malignancies.[4, 257, 264] PTHrP interacts with the same receptor used by PTH, and when large amounts of the peptide are released from certain tumors, it mimics some or all of the effects of excess PTH. However, PTHrP is also expressed in a remarkable variety of normal fetal and adult tissues,[4, 257, 263, 265–269] which suggested, already shortly after its discovery, that it has additional biologic role(s) that are unrelated to calcium and phosphorus homeostasis and that these role(s) are distinct from those mediated by PTH. One of its most prominent functions is the regulation of chondrocyte proliferation and differentiation and, consequently, bone elongation and growth.[12, 13, 270, 271]

The PTHrP Gene in Comparison to the PTH Gene

The human PTHrP gene is located on chromosome 12p12.1-11.2,[263] which has a region analogous to that containing the human PTH gene on chromosome 11p15.[69–71] Both the PTH and the PTHrP genes have a similar organization, including equivalent positions of the boundaries between some of the coding exons and the adjacent introns[11, 73, 263, 272] (Fig. 70–10).

Like the PTH gene, the PTHrP gene contains a single exon that encodes most amino acid residues of the prepropeptide sequence, and both genes have an exon that encodes the remainder of the propeptide sequence, that is, two basic residues (Lys and Arg) that are required for endoproteolytic cleavage of the mature peptide, and either all or most of the amino acids of the secreted peptides. The similarities in their protein sequence and in the structure of their genes, as well as the overlap in some of their functional properties, confirmed that both peptides are derived from a common ancestor.[4, 6, 257] By now, both mammalian genes have diverged considerably; for example, in contrast to the less complex PTH gene, which gives rise to a single gene product, the PTHrP gene uses at least three different promoters and alternative splice patterns that lead to the synthesis of several different mRNA species encoding peptides with different C-terminal ends.[6, 257, 263, 272] A polymorphic dinucleotide repeat sequence that has been used for genetic linkage studies is located downstream of exon 4 (which is exon 6 according to a different nomenclature) of the human PTHrP gene[273] (see Fig. 70–10); thus far, no human disorder has been discovered that is caused by mutations in the PTHrP gene.

Chemistry and Metabolism

The primary structures of several mammalian and chicken PTHrP species are known[6, 59, 274] (see Fig. 70–3, right panel). Furthermore, antibodies against human PTHrP have been used to detect PTHrP-like immunoreactivity in fish and frogs, which indicates that at least some portions of PTHrP remained homologous throughout evolution.[40–43] In fact, a peptide with considerable homology to the N-terminal portion of mammalian PTHrP was recently identified as part of the Fugu Genome Project (FUGU Landmark Mapping Project Database; http://www.fugu.hgmp.mrc.ac.uk). This puffer fish peptide contains eight residues common to all PTH and PTHrP molecules. Five amino acid residues are found only in the known PTH species, whereas nine residues are found only in PTHrP, thus suggesting that this teleost peptide could represent a common precursor of both mammalian peptides (see below). However, a synthetic peptide based on this fugu sequence was recently shown to have functional properties similar to those of mammalian PTHrP, not PTH, which suggests that this peptide represents the teleost homologue of PTHrP and not PTH[275, 276] and that the predicted evolutionary divergence of both peptides occurred yet earlier in evolution.

When compared with each other, chicken PTHrP and the known mammalian species of PTHrP show strong amino acid sequence homology within the first 111 residues; the degree of amino acid sequence conservation of PTHrP is considerably higher than that of the known PTH species. The amino acid sequence homology between

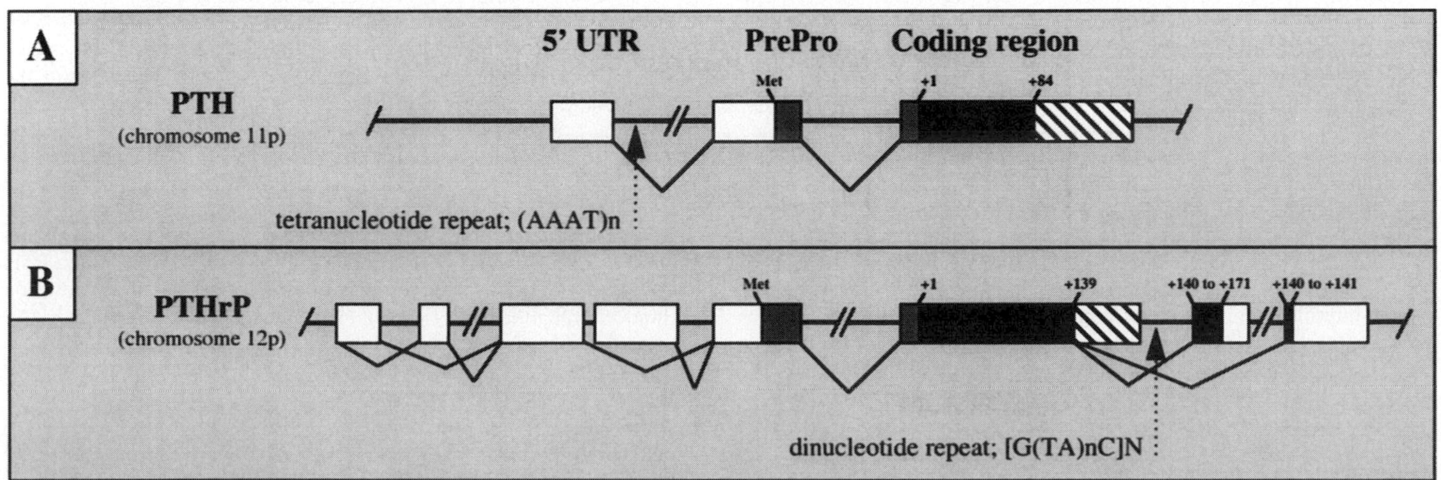

FIGURE 70–10. Schematic representation of the intron/exon organization of the genes encoding parathyroid hormone (PTH) *(A)* and PTH-related peptide (PTHrP) *(B)*. The introns are represented by a *solid line*, and the coding and noncoding exons are shown *(boxes)*; Met indicates the initiator methionine of the prepropeptide sequences *(shaded boxes)*, and numbers indicate the first and the last amino acid residues of the secreted peptides that are encoded by the different exons *(filled boxes)*. The approximate locations of frequent microsatellite polymorphisms in either the *PTH*[78] or the *PTHrP*[273] gene are indicated.

both peptide families is restricted to the N-terminal portion, where 6 of the first 12 amino acid residues are conserved in all PTH and PTHrP species (see Fig. 70–3); the middle and C-terminal regions of both peptides share no recognizable similarity.

Despite the limited structural homology between PTH and PTHrP, N-terminal fragments of both peptides containing residues 1 to 34 have largely indistinguishable biologic properties in vivo, at least with respect to their roles in regulating extracellular concentrations of calcium and phosphorus.[277–280] Furthermore, N-terminal fragments of both peptides interact, albeit with different efficiencies, with at least three different receptors (see below).

Interestingly, analogues of PTH(1–34) and PTHrP(1–34) that are truncated at the N terminus (containing only residues 15–34 of either peptide) and thus share only minimal amino acid sequence homology interact equivalently with PTH1R,[281, 282] and PTHrP(7–34) interacts with the human PTH1R and PTH2R.[283, 284] Such receptor interaction is presumably due to the capacity of both peptides to adopt similar conformations when binding to either receptor. This structural and/or functional similarity between both peptides allowed the construction of hybrids between PTH and PTHrP, some of which had, when tested with cells expressing the PTH1R, similar or even higher biologic potencies than the native ligands.[285] These overall findings indicate that biologically active, N-terminal fragments of both peptides display, despite a very limited number of conserved amino acid residues, a similar secondary structure that is not restricted to the conserved first 12 residues.

PTHrP is likely to undergo extensive posttranslational processing resulting in peptide fragments, some of which may have biologic properties distinct from those involved in the regulation of extracellular calcium. Best studied is the N-terminal PTHrP fragment, functionally homologous to PTH, that is derived through cleavage at amino acid residue Arg37.[286, 287] The resulting PTHrP(1–36) interacts efficiently with the PTH1R,[7–9, 288] and it has an in vivo efficacy similar to that of PTH(1–34).[277, 278, 280] Longer, glycosylated fragments of N-terminal PTHrP were also described; however, these forms appear to be generated predominantly by skin-derived cells, and their biologic role(s), if different from that of PTHrP(1–34) or PTHrP(1–36), remains to be established.[289]

In addition to the biologically active N-terminal PTHrP fragment, different C-terminal fragments are generated and accumulate in patients with end-stage renal disease.[290] A PTHrP fragment consisting of amino acids 107 to 139 and a shorter peptide, PTHrP(107–111), may be relevant to the control of bone metabolism because both fragments were shown to inhibit osteoclastic bone resorption[291, 292] and to stimulate osteoblast activity and proliferation.[293] Although some investigators, using modified experimental conditions, were unable to confirm the in vitro findings with osteoclasts,[294] more recent data indicate that PTHrP(107–139) reduces the number of osteoclasts and inhibits bone resorption in vivo.[295] Taken together, these findings suggest that C-terminal PTHrP fragments may have a role in regulating bone resorption and/or formation (Table 70–3).

Cleavage at amino acid residue Arg37 also generates PTHrP(38–94)amide, a PTHrP fragment that could be of considerable importance in maintaining fetal calcium homeostasis.[286, 309] This peptide is found in the circulation[310] and appears to interact with a distinct receptor that signals through changes in intracellular free calcium and is likely to be an important regulator of transplacental calcium transfer.[286, 302, 303, 309, 311] Studies with PTHrP(38–94)amide and PTHrP(67–86)amide have shown that these fragments increase the blood calcium concentrations of parathyroidectomized fetal lambs and PTHrP-ablated murine fetuses, respectively[286, 302, 311] (see below). These results confirmed earlier data that had provided the first evidence for an important role of PTHrP in the regulation of fetal calcium homeostasis.[312]

Functions of PTHrP

The first actions of PTHrP to be defined were the PTH-like actions associated with the humoral hypercalcemia of malignancy.[4–6, 257] In this pathologic circumstance, PTHrP acts like a hormone, that is, it is secreted from the tumor into the blood stream and then acts on bone and kidney to raise calcium levels (see Chapter 77). Whether PTHrP circulates at high enough levels in normal adults to contribute at all as a hormone to normal calcium homeostasis is an unanswered question; the levels are certainly low, and patients with congenital or acquired hypoparathyroidism are hypocalcemic despite the presence of PTHrP. Although incomplete and somewhat conflicting, growing evidence suggests, however, that PTHrP may act as a hormone in two special circumstances—during fetal life and during lactation as outlined below.

Role of PTHrP in Placental Calcium Transport

During intrauterine life, fetal blood calcium is higher than maternal blood calcium, at least partly because of active transport of calcium across the placenta. In fetal life, in contrast to adulthood, PTHrP is made in easily detectable amounts in the parathyroid gland. Parathyroidectomy lowers the blood level of calcium in fetal sheep and abolishes active calcium transport across the experimentally perfused placenta. PTHrP from human tumors and synthetic PTHrP(1–84), PTHrP(1–108), PTHrP(1–141), and PTHrP(67–86)amide acutely restored placental transport of calcium in a perfused placenta preparation.[313, 314] PTHrP with an intact N terminus, PTHrP extracts, or synthetic peptides such as PTHrP(1–34) or PTHrP(1–36), as well as intact PTH and PTH(1–34), had no effect on placental calcium transport. These results suggest that PTHrP secreted from the fetal parathyroids acts on the placenta to induce calcium transfer from the mother to the fetus.

The role of PTHrP in placental calcium transport is also supported by studies in mice missing both alleles of the PTHrP gene. The blood calcium of fetal PTHrP-ablated mice is identical to maternal blood calcium, i.e., the transport of calcium from the mother into the fetus is diminished.[302] The defect in placental calcium transport can be corrected acutely by injecting PTHrP(1–86) or PTHrP(67–86) into the fetal blood circulation, but not by injecting PTHrP(1–34) or PTH(1–84) (Fig. 70–11). These studies in mice and sheep suggest that a receptor distinct from the cloned PTH/PTHrP receptor mediates the action of PTHrP on placental calcium transport. Consistent with this hypothesis, placental calcium transport is actually increased in mice missing the PTH/PTHrP receptor.[302] The possible role of the fetal parathyroid gland as the crucial source of the PTHrP is suggested by the above-mentioned experiments in sheep,[312, 313] but no measurements of PTHrP in fetal sheep blood have been made.

Role of PTHrP in Lactation

The second possible setting for humoral actions of PTHrP is during pregnancy and lactation. During lactation, transfer of calcium from bone into milk results in a measurable decline in bone mineral content.[311] In experimental animals, PTH and $1,25(OH)_2D_3$ have been eliminated as possible agents responsible for directing this transfer.[315, 316] Furthermore, the lactating breast secretes PTHrP into the circulation,[317] and urinary cAMP rises in response to suckling.[318] Postpartum lactating women have elevated levels of PTHrP in the blood stream,[319–322] and hypoparathyroid patients who are maintained normocalcemic by treatment with $1,25(OH)_2D_3$ can become hypercalcemic during lactation. Thus PTHrP in the blood stream may act on bone to release calcium and on the kidney to increase reabsorption of calcium from the urine, thus retaining the calcium for transport into milk. PTH alone cannot effectively serve these roles because the slight elevation in ionized calcium during lactation suppresses PTH levels.[319–323] An exaggeration of this lactational elevation of PTHrP may explain the rare occurrence of hypercalcemia and high PTHrP levels in pregnant and lactating women.[324, 325]

However, PTHrP is likely to have additional roles in the breast. For example, PTHrP is synthesized by breast tissue and is excreted in enormous amounts into breast milk; the role of PTHrP in milk is unknown, but newborn calves showed increased immunoreactive PTHrP in the circulation after feeding.[326] Furthermore, in fetal life, PTHrP, acting through the PTH/PTHrP receptor, is required for the normal development of breast tissue.[327] Thus PTHrP in the breast may have both paracrine and endocrine roles. These roles may be subverted

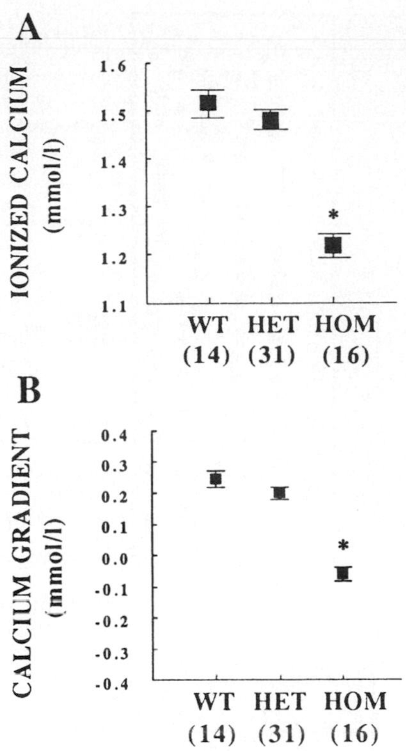

FIGURE 70–11. Ionized blood calcium and placental calcium gradient of wild-type mice (WT) and mice lacking either one (HET) or both alleles (HOM) of the gene encoding parathyroid hormone–related peptide. **P* << .001 vs. WT or HET; the number of observations is indicated in parenthesis. (From Kovacs CS, Lanske B, Hunzelman JL, et al: Parathyroid hormone–related peptide (PTHrP) regulates fetal placental calcium transport through a receptor distinct from the PTH/PTHrP receptor. Proc Natl Acad Sci U S A 93:15233–15238, 1996. Copyright 1996 National Academy of Sciences.)

in breast cancer, a setting in which PTHrP may facilitate the growth of metastases in bone[328] and also cause humoral hypercalcemia.

PTHrP in Bone and Tooth Development

PTHrP has an essential role in bone development. This role is best illustrated by the phenotype of mice missing both copies of the PTHrP gene.[270, 329, 330] These mice die at birth and have diffuse abnormalities in all bones that form by the replacement of a cartilage mold with true bone (endochondral bone formation). The original cartilage molds form normally, but the chondrocytes within the molds stop dividing prematurely and differentiate into hypertrophic chondrocytes at an accelerated pace. Consequently, the growth plates of these bones show dramatically truncated columns of proliferating chondrocytes. The resultant bones are short and mineralize sooner than normal. Growth plates of mice missing the PTH/PTHrP receptor look similar to those of the PTHrP knockout mouse,[12] which suggests that the PTH/PTHrP receptor mediates the actions of PTHrP on chondrocytes. PTHrP is made by perichondrial cells, particularly those at the ends of bones near the joint surfaces and, to a lesser extent, by chondrocytes, again particularly those at the ends of bones. The PTH/PTHrP receptor is expressed at low levels in adjacent chondrocytes in the proliferating columns and is dramatically expressed in chondrocytes just leaving the proliferative pool and becoming hypertrophic. The PTHrP made by the perichondrial cells and some chondrocytes thus acts on proliferating chondrocytes to keep cells in the proliferative pool, to slow differentiation into hypertrophic chondrocytes, and to also slow the subsequent death of hypertrophic chondrocytes by apoptosis. This hypothesis is further supported by the phenotypes of transgenic mice that express the PTHrP gene at high levels in chondrocytes.[271] In these mice, chondrocyte differentiation is dramatically slowed. An analogous phenotype is demonstrated by transgenic mice in which chondrocytes express a constitutively active PTH/PTHrP receptor.[331] Both these transgenes can at least temporarily reverse the growth plate abnormalities in PTHrP knockout mice and allow the mice to live for several months postnatally.[331, 332]

Mice with abnormal PTHrP genes and abnormal PTH/PTHrP receptors have helped clarify the pathogenesis of two human diseases, Blomstrand's lethal chondrodystrophy, in which homozygous or compound heterozygous mutations of the PTH/PTHrP receptor gene are found,[333–336] and Jansen's osteochondrodystrophy, in which heterozygous, constitutively active PTH/PTHrP receptors lead to hypercalcemia and short stature.[337–340] Both these diseases are discussed in detail in Chapter 75.

The potent effects of locally produced PTHrP on bone development and the abnormalities associated with too little or too much PTHrP action suggest a need for careful local regulation of PTHrP production (Fig. 70–12). One major determinant of PTHrP production in the growth plate is Indian hedgehog (Ihh). Ihh belongs to the hedgehog family of secreted proteins that are important for embryonic patterning[341] and acts through Patched, a receptor with 12 membrane-spanning helixes that associates physically with Smoothened and thereby suppresses its constitutive activity.[342, 343] In growth plates, expression of Ihh is restricted to the transition zone within the growth plate, where proliferating chondrocytes differentiate into hypertrophic cells.[13] Ihh, directly or indirectly, stimulates the production of PTHrP by perichondrial cells and chondrocytes near the ends of long bones. This PTHrP then slows the differentiation of chondrocytes and slows the differentiation of cells capable of synthesizing Ihh. Thus a negative feedback loop controlled by Ihh and PTHrP ensures proper pacing of the proliferation and differentiation of chondrocytes. Ihh also has actions on chondrocytes independent of the effects of PTHrP; Ihh is a powerful stimulator of chondrocyte proliferation.

The feedback loop model in Figure 70–12 is supported by a variety of data. Overexpression of Ihh in fetal chicken limbs or the addition of a hedgehog fragment to fetal murine bone explants increases PTHrP expression and slows chondrocyte differentiation.[13] Ihh has no such action on chondrocyte differentiation when added to limbs from either PTHrP or PTH/PTHrP receptor knockout mice. Furthermore, Ihh knockout mice have no detectable PTHrP gene expression in their growth plates and have an accelerated transition from the proliferative pool to the hypertrophic pool of cells.[344] Studies of mice with chimeric growth plates containing both normal cells and cells missing the PTH/PTHrP receptor further confirm the hypothesis.[345] These experiments support a model in which physiologic changes in the secretion of PTHrP and Ihh regulate chondrocyte differentiation and proliferation in a way that ensures optimal bone growth.

PTHrP is made by normal cells of the osteoblast lineage[346] and is likely to have a number of functions in normal osteoblast development and function. These functions have not yet been fully characterized, however. One function of PTHrP in the bones adjacent to developing teeth has been clarified. The mice described earlier, in which transgenic production of PTHrP or a constitutively activated PTH/PTHrP receptor by chondrocytes reverses the growth plate abnormalities of PTHrP-ablated mice and allows postnatal survival, have failure of normal tooth eruption.[331, 332] Normally, the developing tooth elicits PTHrP production in the bone in which the tooth is embedded. This PTHrP then stimulates cells of the osteoblast lineage, which in turn stimulate the development and activity of osteoclasts, the bone-resorbing cells. This stimulation of bone resorption allows the tooth to erupt normally. PTH, a circulating endocrine factor, is unable to compensate for the lack of high local concentrations of PTHrP and thus cannot adequately stimulate the local bone resorption needed for tooth eruption.

It is likely that the local actions of PTHrP in the growth plate and bone are representative of the local actions of PTHrP to control cellular differentiation and proliferation in a number of organs. Still not fully characterized is the amount of crosstalk between the distinct ligands PTH and PTHrP, which can both activate the PTH/PTHrP receptor. Just as such crosstalk certainly explains PTHrP-mediated hypercalcemia of malignancy, it is likely that normally PTH and PTHrP both activate the PTH/PTHrP receptor in a number of tissues in a way that allows integration of the signals from locally produced PTHrP and systemically provided PTH.

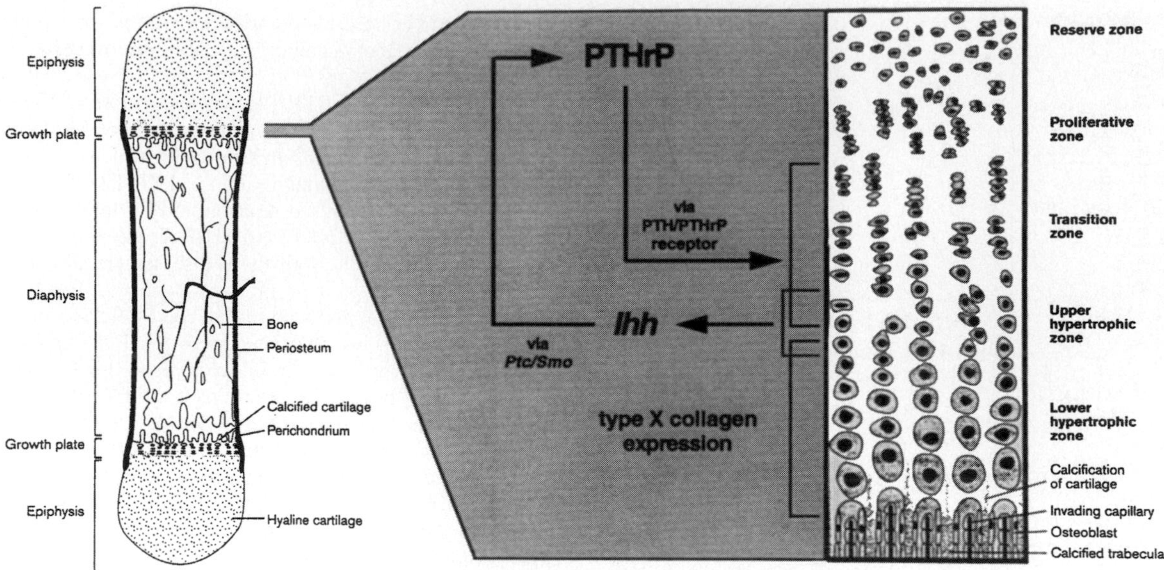

FIGURE 70–12. Schematic regulation of chondrocyte differentiation within the metaphyseal growth plate by parathyroid hormone (PTH)-related peptide (PTHrP) and *Indian Hedgehog (Ihh)*. Ptc, patched; Smo, smoothened.

Other Paracrine Actions of PTHrP

Most of the actions of PTHrP are not thought to be hormonal, but rather to be paracrine or autocrine.[347] PTHrP is synthesized at one time or another during fetal life in virtually every tissue. This widespread expression of PTHrP in fetal life probably explains the extensive expression of PTHrP in a great variety of malignancies. Malignant tissues often revert to a fetal pattern of gene expression; synthesis of PTHrP may be part of this pattern. PTHrP is also synthesized by many adult tissues.[4, 257, 347] In tissues such as skin and hair, it is likely that PTHrP regulates cell proliferation and differentiation.[348] PTHrP is also synthesized widely in the smooth muscle of blood vessels and in the gastrointestinal tract, uterus, and bladder, and transgenic expression of PTHrP in smooth muscle cells leads to severe defects in cardiac development.[349, 350] In these tissues, PTHrP is synthesized in response to stretch and acts on smooth muscle in an autocrine fashion to relax the muscle.[351] PTHrP is also widely expressed in neurons of the central nervous system; its function in the brain is unknown. In mice missing the PTHrP gene, widespread degeneration of neurons occurs postnatally; as explained above, these mice survive postnatally through expression of PTHrP only in cartilage cells.[332] This result and subsequent data suggest that PTHrP might normally be neuroprotective.[352]

RECEPTORS FOR PTH AND PTHrP

Because of the diverse actions of PTH, which were shown to be either direct or indirect and to involve multiple signal transduction mechanisms, it was initially thought that several different receptors mediate the pleiotropic actions of this peptide hormone. Although some of these actions were subsequently shown to be PTHrP rather than PTH dependent, it was somewhat surprising that the initial cloning approaches led to the isolation of cDNAs encoding only a single G protein–coupled receptor, the common PTH/PTHrP receptor (see Fig. 70–1). The recombinant PTH/PTHrP receptor is now known to interact equivalently with PTH and PTHrP and to activate at least two distinct second messenger pathways, namely, adenylate cyclase/PKA and phospholipase C (PLC)/protein kinase C (PKC).[7–9] These findings with recombinant receptors confirmed earlier studies using different clonal cell lines or renal membrane preparations that had shown that PTH and PTHrP bind to and activate a common G protein–coupled receptor with similar efficiency and efficacy.[288, 353–355] Based on these and subsequent findings, such as the similar phenotypes observed in mice that are null for either PTHrP or the PTH/PTHrP receptor,[12, 13] it is very likely that most of the endocrine actions of PTH and most of the paracrine/autocrine actions of PTHrP are mediated through the PTH/PTHrP receptor. However, recent studies have led to the isolation of two novel, closely related G protein–coupled receptors. One of these receptors, the PTH2 receptor (PTH2R), mediates the actions of TIP39 (tubular infundibular peptide of 39 amino acids), a recently discovered hypothalamic peptide[356]; human PTH2R, but not the rat receptor homologue, is also efficiently activated by PTH.[283, 284, 357, 358] The second novel receptor, the PTH3 receptor (PTH3R), has thus far only been cloned from zebrafish, and it responds to human PTHrP more efficiently than to human PTH.[276] Furthermore, functional and physicochemical evidence of additional receptors that interact with different fragments of either PTH or PTHrP is growing (see Table 70–3). However, cDNAs encoding these novel receptors have not yet been isolated.

The PTH/PTHrP Receptor

The PTH/PTHrP receptor (PTH1R) belongs to a distinct family of G protein–coupled receptors, and it interacts equivalently with PTH and PTHrP. The first cDNAs encoding mammalian PTH/PTHrP receptor species were isolated through expression cloning techniques from opossum kidney cells and rat osteoblast-like osteosarcoma cells.[7, 8] Subsequently, cDNAs encoding human,[9, 359, 360] mouse,[361] rat,[362] chicken,[13] porcine,[363] dog,[364] frog,[365] and fish PTH/PTHrP receptors[276] were isolated through hybridization techniques from very different tissue sources: kidney, osteoblast-like cells, brain, embryonic stem cells, and/or whole embryos. Northern blot and in situ studies[237, 269, 366] and data provided through available public EST (expressed sequence tag) databases confirmed that the PTH/PTHrP receptor is expressed in a wide variety of fetal and adult tissues. Except for the tetraploid African clawed frog *Xenopus laevis*, which expresses two nonallelic isoforms of the PTH/PTHrP receptor,[365] all investigated species have only one copy of this receptor per haploid genome.

The existence of PTH/PTHrP receptors with distinct, organ-specific characteristics had been suggested by distinct ligand-binding properties[367–369] and by the activation of distinct second messenger pathways by different clonal cell lines.[370–372] However, the molecular cloning of identical full-length PTH/PTHrP receptor cDNAs from human kidney, brain, and bone-derived cells[9, 359, 360] suggested that the previously observed pharmacologic differences are due to species-specific variations in primary sequence rather than the tissue-specific expression of distinct receptors.

The gene encoding the human PTH/PTHrP receptor is located on chromosome 3p (within the region 3p21.1-3p24.2). Its intron/exon structure has been analyzed in detail,[373–375] and it was shown to have an organization similar to that of the genes encoding the rat and mouse homologues[376, 377] (Fig. 70–13). Each of these three mammalian genes spans at least 20 kb of genomic DNA and consists of 14 coding exons and at least 3 noncoding exons. The size of the coding exons in the human PTH/PTHrP receptor gene ranges from 42 bp (exon M7) to more than 400 bp (exon T); the size of the introns varies from 81 bp (intron between exons M6/7 and M7) to more than 10,000 bp (intron between exons S and E1). Two promoters for the PTH/PTHrP receptor, P1 and P2, have been described in rodents.[376–379] P1 (also referred as U3) activity is mainly restricted to the adult kidney, whereas P2 (also referred to as U1) activity is detected in several fetal and adult tissues, including cartilage and bone. In humans, a third promoter (P3, also referred to as S) appears to control PTH/PTHrP receptor expression in some tissues, including kidney and bone.[375, 380, 381] Several frequent polymorphisms were identified within the human PTH/PTHrP receptor gene, these include an intronic *Bsm*I polymorphism located between the 5′ noncoding exon U1 and the coding exon S[382] and a silent *BsrD*I polymorphism in exon M7 (nucleotide 1417 of human PTH/PTHrP receptor cDNA).[383]

All mammalian PTH/PTHrP receptors have a relatively long N-terminal extracellular domain that is encoded by five exons (S, E1, E2, E3, and G) (see Fig. 70–13). The genes encoding other members of this family of G protein–coupled receptors for which the genomic structure has been explored have a similar organization except that the equivalent of exon E2 is lacking.[384, 385] Interestingly, this exon is also missing in PTH/PTHrP receptors from the frog *X. laevis* and from zebrafish,[275, 365] and earlier in vitro studies had shown that the region corresponding to exon E2 can be modified or deleted without a measurable impact on receptor expression and function.[386, 387] Taken together, these findings supported the conclusion that the addition of a nonessential exon, as observed in all mammalian PTH/PTHrP receptors, represents a relatively recent evolutionary modification.[276]

Molecular cloning of the PTH/PTHrP receptor,[7, 8] along with the receptors for secretin[388] and calcitonin,[389] established a distinct family of G protein–coupled receptors called class B receptors[390] (G protein–coupled receptor database: http://www.gcrdb.uthacsa.edu). Except for a similar overall structure consisting of seven membrane-spanning helixes, members of this family share virtually no amino acid sequence homology with most other G protein–coupled receptors. All members of this secretin/calcitonin/PTH receptor family, including insect and other invertebrate receptors,[391–393] share about 45 strictly conserved amino acid residues. Furthermore, all receptors of this family have a relatively long N-terminal extracellular domain, and most use at least two different signal transduction pathways, adenylate cyclase and PLC.[384, 385] All these related receptors contain up to four sites for potential asparagine-linked glycosylation, 8 conserved extracellular cysteine residues that appear to affect ligand-receptor interaction and/or proper receptor processing,[386, 394] and several other "signature" residues. An overall topologic similarity is predicted between this class B family of heptahelical receptors and other G protein–coupled receptor families, such as those represented by the β-adrenergic receptors (class A receptors) or those represented by the metabotropic glutamate receptor and the CaR (termed class C receptors) (reviewed in Chapter 80).

Recently, a distinctive subgroup of class B receptors has been identified. In addition to the usual hallmarks of the peptide hormone–binding class B receptors, these receptors have very large (>600 amino acid) extensions of the N-terminal extracellular domain in which are found a variety of sequence motifs typically involved in cell adhesion and seen in other single membrane-spanning proteins (e.g., epidermal growth factor modules, cadherin, laminin, thrombospondin, lectin, and mucin).[395–398] The biologic roles of these novel receptors in mammals, the identity of their cognate ligands, and their evolutionary relationship to the other class B receptors remain to be established.

Mapping Sites of Ligand Interaction in the PTH/PTHrP Receptor

Initial clues regarding how PTH interacts with its receptor came soon after PTH(1–34) was synthesized and shown to be fully active,[399] as scores of synthetic peptide fragments and analogues were subsequently prepared to explore the structure-activity relationships in the hormone.[177, 400–403] Quantification of ligand-binding affinity through radioreceptor studies showed that receptor affinity progressively decreased as PTH(1–34) was truncated, particularly from the C termi-

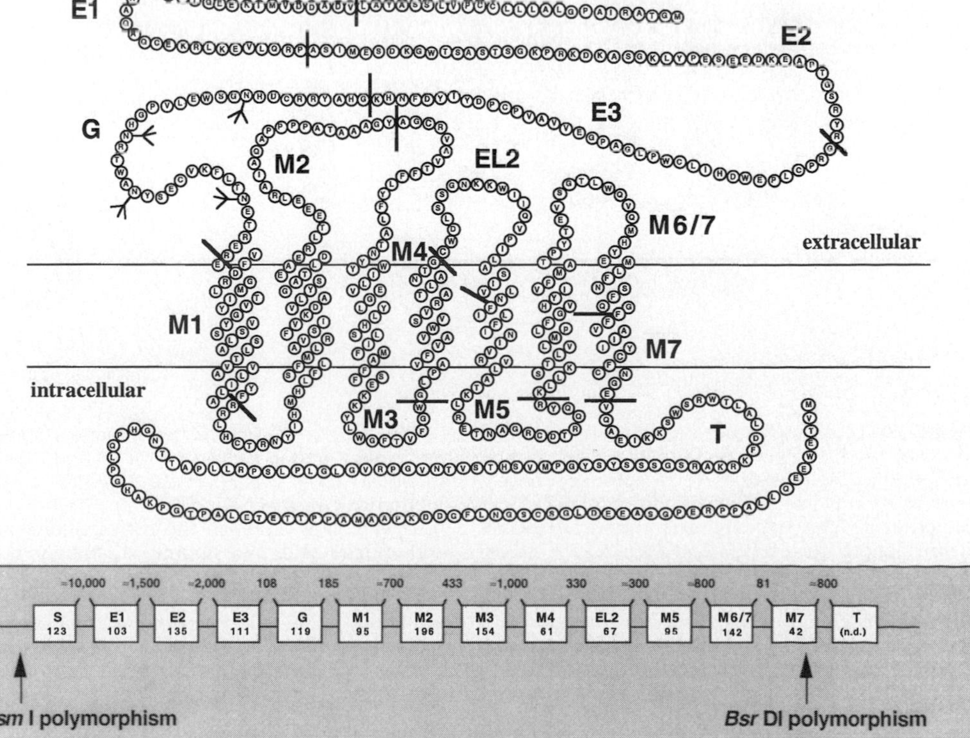

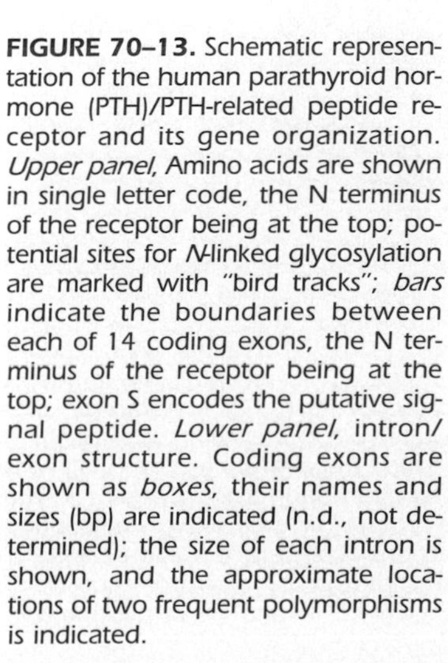

FIGURE 70–13. Schematic representation of the human parathyroid hormone (PTH)/PTH-related peptide receptor and its gene organization. *Upper panel,* Amino acids are shown in single letter code, the N terminus of the receptor being at the top; potential sites for *N*-linked glycosylation are marked with "bird tracks"; *bars* indicate the boundaries between each of 14 coding exons, the N terminus of the receptor being at the top; exon S encodes the putative signal peptide. *Lower panel,* intron/exon structure. Coding exons are shown as *boxes,* their names and sizes (bp) are indicated (n.d., not determined); the size of each intron is shown, and the approximate locations of two frequent polymorphisms is indicated.

nus.[177, 401, 404] Furthermore, fragments such as PTH(7–34), which show little or no agonist activity, proved to inhibit the actions of PTH(1–34), at least when present in high molar excess.[178, 402, 405] These early studies, which broadly defined the structural requirements for biologically active PTH, suggested that the receptor-binding and receptor-activating functions resided in separable domains, and provided the groundwork for the subsequent evaluation of cloned PTH/PTHrP receptors and closely related members of this receptor family.

The initial isolation of cDNAs corresponding to PTH/PTHrP receptors from three different species (opossum, rat, and human) and the subsequent finding that these receptor variants often exhibited altered responses to different PTH ligand analogues enabled a general strategy for mapping interactions that was based largely on the use of receptor chimeras. For the construction of such chimeras, unique restriction sites were introduced at various positions through oligonucleotide-directed, site-specific mutagenesis.[406] This technique allowed the generation of several chimeras between the human and rat PTH/PTHrP receptors to experimentally determine which portions of these two receptors confer the divergent binding affinities for PTH(7–34). These functional studies provided the first clues that the N-terminal extracellular domain of the receptor interacted with the C-terminal region of PTH(1–34).[387] Similarly, experiments on opossum/rat PTH/PTHrP receptor chimeras and the analogue [Arg2]hPTH(1–34), which exhibits impaired activation of the rat receptor in comparison to the opossum receptor,[407] provided evidence that the ligand's N terminus interacts with the membrane-embedded/extracellular loop portion of the receptor; residues Ser370, Val371, and Thr427 were particularly important for this selectivity[408] (Fig. 70–14). Extensions of these experiments using PTH/PTHrP receptors that had small segments systematically deleted or replaced with corresponding sequences from other receptors, combined with point mutation analyses of the receptor, identified Trp437 and Gln440 in the third extracellular loop as being important for interaction with residues 1 and 2 of PTH(1–34).[416] Since then, several other key residues have been identified in the PTH/PTHrP receptor that contribute to ligand interaction[414, 422–424] (see Fig. 70–14).

A general scheme of interaction between ligand and receptor, which may apply to the entire class B family of G protein–coupled receptors, was established when a hybrid ligand, calcitonin(1–11)/PTH(15–34), was shown to activate a chimeric calcitonin-PTH/PTHrP receptor. The chimeric receptor contained the N-terminal extracellular domain of the PTH/PTHrP receptor fused to the portion of the calcitonin receptor containing the seven membrane-embedded helixes, the connecting loops, and the tail region of the calcitonin receptor; the wild-type PTH/PTHrP receptor or a reciprocal receptor chimera was not activated.[425] Likewise, a reciprocal peptide, PTH(1–13)/calcitonin(12–32), selectively activated a chimeric receptor that had the N-terminal extracellular domain of the calcitonin receptor joined to the region of the PTH/PTHrP receptor containing the seven transmembrane domains,

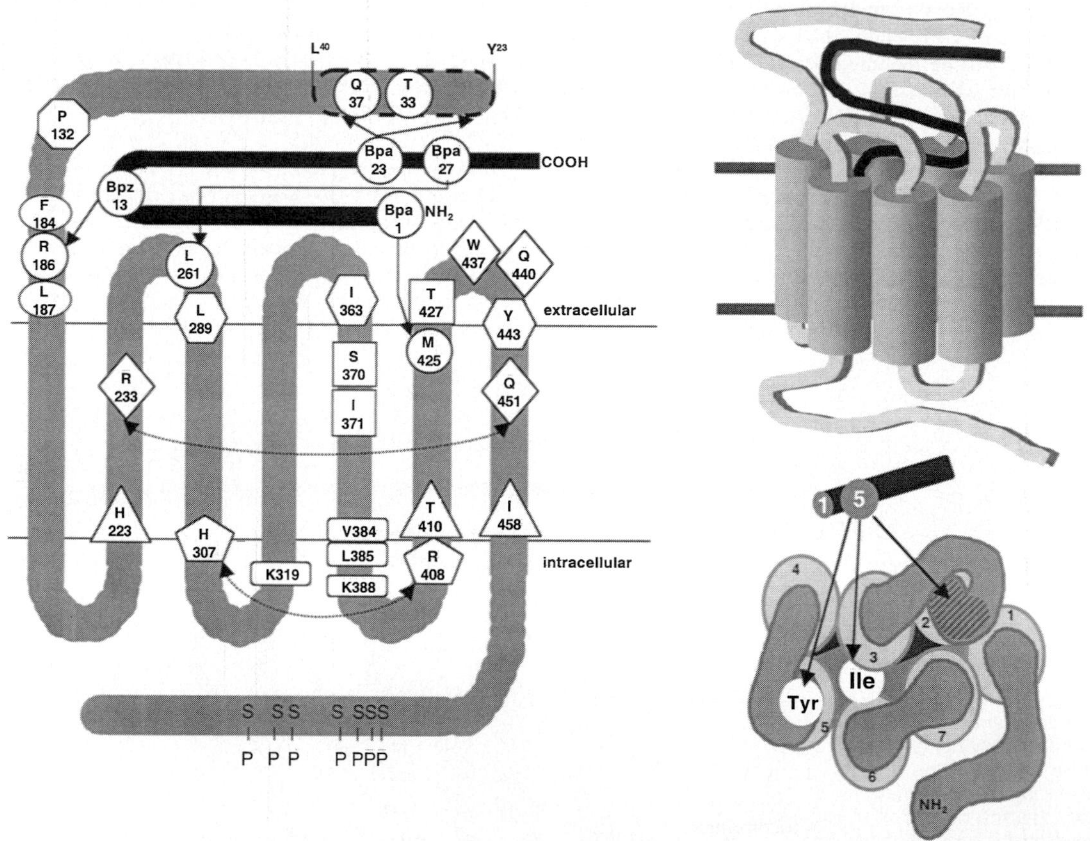

FIGURE 70–14. Complex between parathyroid hormone (PTH) and its PTH/PTH-related peptide (PTHrP) receptor (PTH1R). The schematic on the *left* shows key residues involved in the interaction between the receptor and its two ligands, PTH and PTHrP (amino acid residues and position numbers correspond to the human PTH1 receptor sequence and to either PTH or PTHrP): *circles,* residues identified in cross-linking studies[409–412]; *octagon,* a site involved in Blomstrand's chondrodysplasia[334]; *ovals,* hydrophobic residues important for PTH(1–34) and PTH(1–14) binding[413]; *triangles,* residues mutated in patients with Jansen's chondrodysplasia[340]; *hexagons,* sites at which the corresponding residues in the PTH-2 receptor play a role in discriminating between PTH and PTHrP[414, 415]; *squares,* residues that determine agonist vs. antagonist action of Arg2-PTH(1–34)[408]; *diamonds,* sites at which mutations impair PTH(1–34) binding but not PTH(3–34) binding[416]; *rectangles,* residues that when mutated alter G protein coupling[417, 418]; residues connected by *dashed curves with arrows,* sites involved in interdomain interactions, as determined by paired mutations affecting PTH(1–34) interaction (R233 and Q451)[416] or zinc chelation (H307 and R408)[419]; S-P, agonist serine residues phosphorylated upon agonist exposure.[420, 421] The panel on the *upper right* shows an idealized three-dimensional view of the ligand docking to the receptor; the receptor, in side view, is embedded in the cell membrane; the *barrels* represent the membrane-spanning helical domains; the *lightly shaded* sections represent the extracellular or intracellular domains, and the *dark wavy line* represents the ligand. The panel on the *lower right* depicts the receptor in top view from outside of the cell; the *white circles* represent two residues in the PTH-2 receptor (Ile244 and Tyr318) that modulate selectivity for Ile and His at position 5 in the ligand, as found in PTH and PTHrP, respectively.[414]

connecting loops, and cytoplasmic tail. These data confirmed that for both PTH and calcitonin, the N terminus of the ligand interacts with the membrane-embedded receptor region, whereas the C terminus of the ligand interacts with the receptor's N terminus (see Fig. 70–14). The overall interaction is certain to be more complex; nevertheless, these observations demonstrated that the domains for ligand-receptor interaction can function with some degree of autonomy.

The above conclusion is underscored by the finding that a mutant PTH/PTHrP receptor lacking the N terminus nearly up to the beginning of the first membrane-spanning helix can respond to high concentrations of either PTH(1–34) or PTH(1–14) with a maximal increase in intracellular cAMP accumulation similar to that observed with the wild-type receptor.[426] Because of the low-affinity interaction between the N-terminal residues of PTH and this membrane-embedded portion of the PTH/PTHrP receptor, conventional radioreceptor assays have not demonstrated competitive displacement of radiolabeled PTH analogues by small peptides such as PTH(1–14) and truncated receptors. These data led to the conclusion that the intrinsic signaling efficacy of the PTH(1–14) fragment is very high, such that even a brief encounter with the receptor triggers signal transduction. These considerations also suggested that the PTH(1–14) fragment could be modified to improve interaction with the receptor and enhance potency. Indeed, among over 100 different monosubstituted PTH(1–14) analogues that were prepared and assayed, several activity-enhancing substitutions were found and, when combined, improved overall activity as much as 200-fold relative to that of native PTH(1–14). These substitutions conferred activity to even shorter peptides previously found to be inactive, such as PTH(1–11)[427] (Fig. 70–15). Further design of such short N-terminal peptide fragments of PTH could help probe essential features of the ligand-receptor interaction and could be useful in efforts to design low-molecular-weight agonists (see below).

The above studies demonstrate an important role for the N-terminal residues of PTH (and PTHrP) in activating the PTH receptor, and the strong evolutionary conservation of the N-terminal residues of PTH and PTHrP is consistent with this notion. However, earlier studies using N-terminal peptides that were shorter in length than PTH(1–27) failed to detect a second messenger response. These in vitro bioassays were probably much less sensitive than current assays, which use transfected cells with high numbers of receptors.[426] An important contribution of C-terminal amino acid residues to the overall biologic activity of the PTH(1–34) peptide has been demonstrated by multiple studies.[277, 281, 282, 428] Clearly, removal of the critical C-terminal of PTH(1–34) eliminates high-affinity ligand-receptor interaction, thus preventing a detectable response in the earlier assays with such truncated peptides.[177, 401] The C-terminal 15–34 portion of PTH(1–34) presumably provides docking interactions that stabilize the association of hormone and receptor and thereby position the ligand's N-terminal signaling domain within proximity of the receptor's activation core located within the body of the receptor formed by the seven transmembrane domains and the connecting loops[425, 429] (see Fig. 70–14). Direct evidence for this role of the C-terminal domain of PTH(1–34) is shown by studies in which the PTH(1–9) segment was linked by a short glycine spacer to the PTH(15–31) sequence, resulting in a peptide analogue that was considerably more active than PTH(1–9) (Gardella and Potts, unpublished observations).[427]

Further insight into the ligand-receptor interaction mechanism was provided by experiments using photoaffinity cross-linking and peptide-mapping techniques. The first of these studies used a radioiodinated PTH(1–34) analogue containing the photoreactive benzophenone moiety attached to the side chain of lysine 13. Digestion of the complex formed between this ligand and the PTH/PTHrP receptor with cyanogen bromide and/or other proteolytic reagents led to the conclusion that the modified lysine 13 side chain interacts with a region in the receptor's N-terminal extracellular domain that is close to the first membrane-spanning helix.[409, 430] Functional, mutation-based studies of this receptor region confirmed and extended these findings by showing that several hydrophobic residues in this receptor region (particularly Phe184 and Leu187) contribute to PTH(1–34) and PTH(1–14) binding

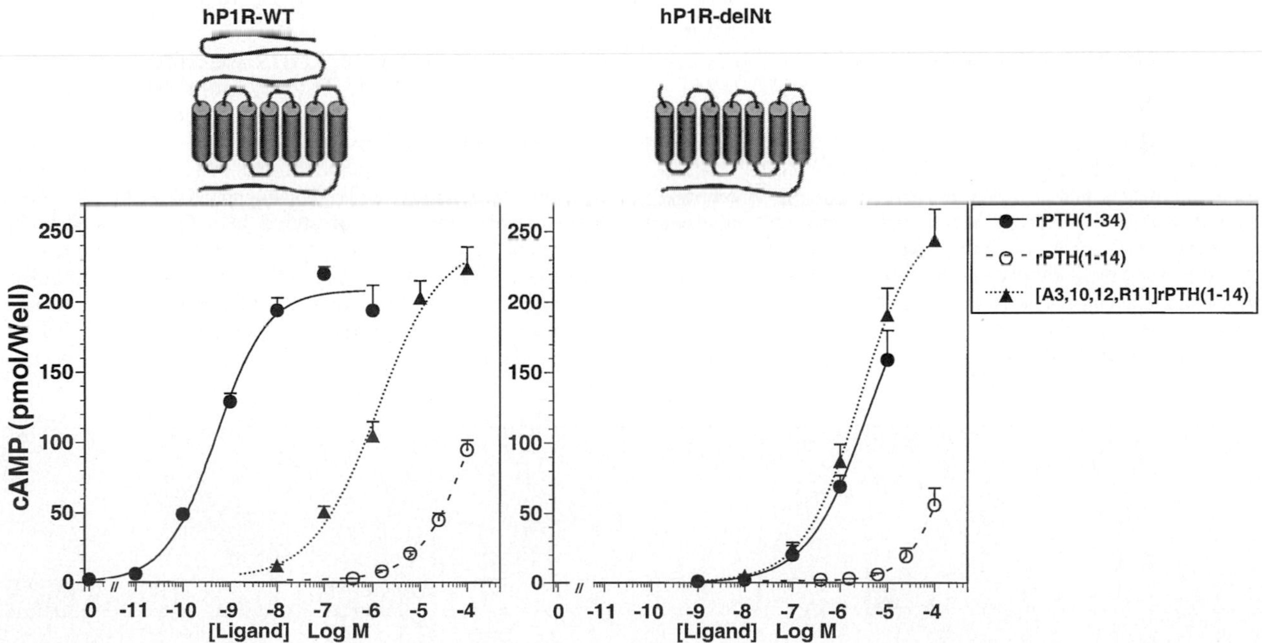

FIGURE 70–15. Interaction of the N-terminal (1–14) domain of parathyroid hormone (PTH) with the membrane-spanning and loop region of the PTH/PTH-related peptide receptor (PTH1R) is sufficient for activating a cyclic adenosine monophosphate (cAMP) response. The findings shown used a mutant human PTH1R in which most of the N-terminal extracellular domain (hP1R-delNt) had been deleted through oligonucleotide-directed, site-specific mutagenesis *(right panel)* and, for comparison, the wild-type human PTH1R (hP1R-WT) *(left panel)*. Receptors were expressed in COS-7 cells and then tested for the ability to respond to varying doses of intact PTH(1–34) or two PTH(1–14) analogues in cAMP formation assays. The peptides used, rPTH(1–34)NH_2, rPTH(1–14)NH_2, or a modified PTH(1–14) analogue, (Ala3, Ala10, Ala12, Arg11) rPTH(1–14)NH_2, which contain several activity-enhancing substitutions, are indicated in the figure key. In comparison to the responses seen with the wild-type receptor, the potency of PTH(1–34) is severely diminished with the truncated receptor whereas the potency of PTH(1–14) is largely unaffected. Thus the PTH(1–14) analogues, in contrast to PTH(1–34), do not require the receptor's N-terminal domain for activity. (Modified from Shimizu M, Potts JT Jr, Gardella TJ: Minimization of parathyroid hormone: Novel amino-terminal parathyroid hormone fragments with enhanced potency, in activating the type-1 parathyroid hormone receptor. Biol Chem, in press.)

and signaling.[413] An independent study suggested that this receptor domain may define an amphipathic α helix that is partially embedded in the lipid membrane bilayer[429] (see Fig. 70–14).

Another study showed that benzoylphenylalanine (Bpa), when introduced at position 1 of PTH(1–34), cross-linked to the extracellular end of the sixth membrane-spanning helix of the PTH/PTHrP receptor and that residue M425 in this region was required for reactivity.[410] This finding is again consistent with results from functional studies with mutant PTH/PTHrP receptors and PTH analogues that identified key residues in the receptor involved in an interaction between the N-terminal residues of PTH and this receptor region.[408, 416] A third study using a PTHrP(1–36) analogue containing Bpa instead of tryptophan at position 23 mapped the site of cross-linking to the region near the extreme end of receptor's N terminus (residues 23–40).[411] Complementary mutational analysis of the receptor region consisting of residues 31 through 39 identified Thr33 and Gln37 as the receptor residues that are most likely involved in ligand-receptor interaction[411] (see Fig. 70–14). In another study, a Bpa27 analogue of PTH was recently predicted to interact with Leu261 in the first extracellular loop of the PTH/PTHrP receptor, which suggests that the C-terminal portion of PTH(1–34), as well as possibly PTHrP(1–34), contacts both the interhelical extracellular loops and the extreme N terminus.[411, 412]

Cross-linking data[409–411, 412, 430] do not necessarily identify the precise contacts used by the native hormone but rather establish the proximity of certain receptor and ligand residues. Similarly, mutational data demonstrating altered ligand-receptor interactions[408, 411, 413, 416] need not reflect direct roles for specific residues but could involve regional conformation effects, such as on the receptor. Thus the general concurrence of the results obtained with these two independent methodologies increases confidence in the emerging model of ligand-receptor interactions summarized in Figure 70–14. Definition of additional points of contact will most likely be provided by a combination of further cross-linking and functional studies with mutant receptors. Advances in techniques of crystallographic analysis of heptahelical receptors may eventually permit high-resolution analysis of the PTH/PTHrP receptor.[68]

The PTH2 Receptor: A Receptor for TIP39

Although the PTH/PTHrP receptor is almost certainly the most important receptor in mediating the actions of PTH and PTHrP, considerable evidence indicates that several other receptors could potentially respond to either PTH or PTHrP or to both. However, only two cDNAs encoding novel PTH receptors have been isolated thus far. The biologic functions mediated by these two receptors remain uncertain but are presumably unrelated to the control of calcium and phosphorus (see also below).

Best characterized is PTH2R, which shares 51% amino acid identity with the PTH/PTHrP receptor[357] and was therefore thought to represent a novel receptor for PTH and/or PTHrP. Support for this conclusion was derived from the initial characterization studies showing that PTH, but not PTHrP, activated human PTH2R with an efficacy similar to that which it displays for the PTH/PTHrP receptor.[283, 284, 357] However, rat PTH2R showed only poor activation by PTH. It was later shown that both the rat and the human receptor were activated with high efficacy by a partially purified peptide from the bovine hypothalamus. These findings indicated that PTH was not necessarily the principal ligand for PTH2R.[358, 432] In fact, the recently isolated hypothalamic peptide TIP39 activates human and rat PTH2R with higher efficiency and efficacy than does PTH and is therefore likely to be the natural ligand for this receptor.[356] Despite very limited overall sequence homology with PTH and PTHrP and an extension by two residues at the N terminus, TIP39 contains several amino acid residues that correspond to functionally important residues in PTH and PTHrP. In particular, Glu19, Trp23, and Leu24 in PTH are found in TIP39 at positions 21, 25, and 26, respectively; Arg21 in PTHrP and Arg20 in PTH and PTHrP are found in TIP39 at positions 23 and 22, respectively (Fig. 70–16). Furthermore, Lys11 in mammalian PTHrP and Lys13 in mammalian PTH and PTHrP are Arg13 and Arg15 in TIP39. These structural similarities made it plausible that TIP39 could cross-react, possibly with reduced affinity, with the PTH/PTHrP receptor; in fact, some activation by TIP39 is observed with the human, but not the rat PTH/PTHrP receptor.[356] It remains unclear whether PTH, which efficiently activates human PTH2R in vitro,[283, 284, 357] stimulates this receptor in vivo.

Expression of PTH2R is restricted to relatively few tissues, such as the placenta, pancreas, blood vessels, testis, and brain, and its mRNA is typically much less abundant than that encoding the PTH/PTHrP receptor.[357, 433] The biologic functions mediated by PTH2R in these and possibly other tissues are currently unknown, but based on localization studies of PTH2R mRNA and protein, the receptor may be involved in pain perception.[356] On the other hand, previous studies in parathyroidectomized dogs had shown that PTH increases the pancreatic secretion of bicarbonate without affecting amylase production.[434] It thus appears possible that PTH2R mediates these exocrine pancreatic functions.

Interestingly, portions of PTH2R were first identified in a catfish genomic DNA clone.[275, 435] The two exons that were available at the time showed considerably higher amino acid sequence homology with the mammalian PTH/PTHrP receptors than with other members of this family of G protein–coupled receptors. Subsequent comparison with the full-length human PTH2R sequence led to the conclusion that a novel receptor had been identified in a teleost species; that is, the amino acid sequence encoded by three exons of the catfish PTH2R gene (M3, M4, and EL2) shared 83% homology with human PTH2R, but only 72% with the human PTH/PTHrP receptor.[275] The available genomic sequence furthermore indicated that the catfish PTH2R gene has exactly the same intron/exon borders and the same exon length

			1				5					10					15					20					25					30				
Human PTH			S	V	S	E	I	Q	L	M	H	N	L	G	K	H	L	N	S	M	E	R	V	E	W	L	R	K	K	L	Q	D	V	H	N	F
Bovine			A	-	-	-	-	-	F	-	-	-	-	-	-	-	-	S	-	-	-	-	-	-	-	-	-	-	-	-	-	-	-	-	-	-
Porcine			-	-	-	-	-	-	-	-	-	-	-	-	-	-	-	S	-	L	-	-	-	-	-	-	-	-	-	-	-	-	-	-	-	-
Dog			-	-	-	-	-	-	F	-	-	-	-	-	-	-	-	S	-	-	-	-	-	-	-	-	-	-	-	-	-	-	-	-	-	-
Rat			A	-	-	-	-	-	-	-	-	-	-	-	-	-	-	A	-	V	-	-	M	Q	-	-	-	-	-	-	-	-	-	-	-	-
Chicken			-	-	-	-	M	-	-	-	-	-	-	-	E	-	R	H	T	V	-	-	Q	D	-	-	Q	M	-	-	-	-	-	-	S	A
fugu PTHrP			S	V	S	H	A	Q	L	M	H	D	K	G	R	S	L	Q	E	F	R	R	R	M	W	L	H	K	L	L	?	?	V	H	T	?
bovine TIP39	S	L	A	L	A	D	D	A	A	F	R	E	R	A	R	L	L	L	L	A	A	L	E	R	R	H	W	L	N	S	Y	M	H	K	L	L	V	L
Human PTHrP			A	V	S	E	H	Q	L	L	H	D	K	G	K	S	I	Q	D	L	R	R	R	F	F	L	H	H	L	I	A	E	I	H	T	A
Bovine			-	-	-	-	-	-	-	-	-	-	-	-	-	-	-	-	-	-	-	-	-	-	-	-	-	-	-	-	-	-	-	-	-	-
Rat			-	-	-	-	-	-	-	-	-	-	-	-	-	-	-	-	-	-	-	-	-	-	-	-	-	-	-	-	-	-	-	-	-	-
Mouse			-	-	-	-	-	-	-	-	-	-	-	-	-	-	-	-	-	-	-	-	-	-	-	-	-	-	-	-	-	-	-	-	-	-
Dog			-	-	-	-	-	-	-	-	-	-	-	-	-	-	-	-	-	-	-	-	-	-	-	-	-	-	-	-	-	-	-	-	-	-
Chicken			-	-	-	-	-	-	-	-	-	-	-	-	-	-	-	-	-	-	-	-	I	-	-	-	Q	N	-	-	E	G	V	N	-	-

FIGURE 70–16. Alignment of the (1–34) amino acid sequences of all known vertebrate parathyroid hormone (PTH) and PTH-related peptide (PTHrP) species, as well as fugu PTHrP and bovine TIP39. Amino acid residues that are conserved in all PTH and PTHrP species are shown in *white boxes.* Amino acid residues found in either fugu PTHrP or bovine Tip39 that are also found in all known PTH species are shown in *black boxes with white letters,* and residues found either in fugu PTHrP or in bovine Tip39 that are also found in all PTHrP species are *boxed;* numbers indicate amino acid positions in mammalian PTH or PTHrP.

as genes encoding the previously isolated mammalian PTH/PTHrP receptors.[373, 376, 377] It therefore appears that organization of the genes encoding the PTH/PTHrP receptor and PTH2R, and most likely the genes encoding other members of this receptor family, has remained largely unchanged during evolution.

Subsequent to the isolation of partial genomic catfish DNA clones, cDNAs encoding full-length zebrafish PTH2Rs were isolated and functionally characterized.[275] As for the amino acid sequence encoded by the available exons of the catfish PTH2R gene, the amino acid sequence encoded by the zebrafish cDNA showed overall highest identity with the human and rat PTH2R (63% and 60%, respectively) and significantly less homology with the frog and human PTH/PTHrP receptor (52% and 47%, respectively). Similar to the human PTH2R, the zebrafish receptor homologue was activated by PTH (albeit with very low efficacy) and not by human or fugu PTHrP (see Fig. 70–18). It thus appears likely that a teleost homologue of TIP39 is the physiologic ligand for this receptor.

The initial observation with human PTH2R regarding PTH and PTHrP selectivity enabled a strategy to be devised for mapping the residues in PTH and PTHrP involved in receptor selectivity. The resulting studies with analogues of both peptides revealed that positions 5 and 23 in either peptide represent key residues for determining PTH2R binding and activation selectivity. All known PTH molecules contain isoleucine at position 5 (with the exception of chicken PTH) and tryptophan at position 23, whereas all PTHrP molecules (with the exception of fugu PTHrP) contain at these positions histidine and phenylalanine, respectively (see Figs. 70–3 and 70–16). Introduction of PTHrP-specific residues at these sites into PTH dramatically reduced the binding affinity and cAMP-signaling potency of the resulting ligand at the human PTH2R. Conversely, introduction of the corresponding PTH-specific residues into PTHrP dramatically improved binding affinity and signaling interactions with PTH2R.[283, 284] Nature thus "designed" PTHrP to allow interaction with the PTH/PTHrP receptor, but not with the PTH2R. To identify receptor regions and subsequently amino acid residues that prevent PTH2R activation by PTHrP, chimeras between the human PTH/PTHrP receptor and human PTH2R were evaluated, and these studies led to the identification of two amino acid residues (Ile244 and Tyr318) in PTH2R that are largely responsible for the PTH-PTHrP selectivity of this receptor; their replacement by the residues found in the corresponding position in the PTH/PTHrP receptor, leucine and isoleucine, respectively, conferred activation by PTHrP[414, 415] (see Fig. 70–14).

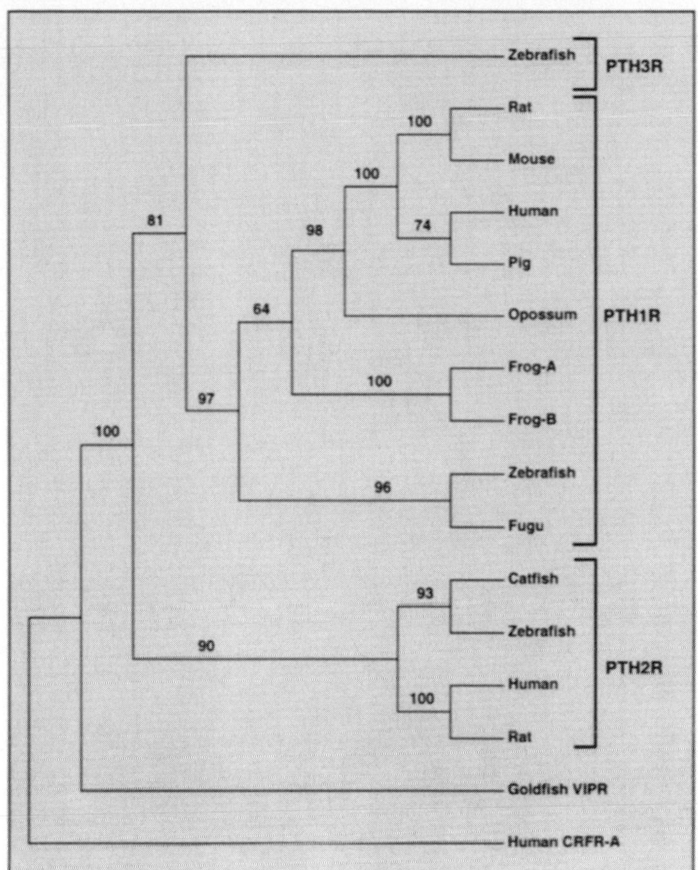

FIGURE 70–17. Phylogenetic tree of all known receptors for parathyroid hormone (PTH) and PTH-related peptide (PTHrP). A strict consensus cladogram for aligning the known PTH/PTHrP receptors (PPR) and PTH2 receptors, the zebrafish PTH3R, the human corticotropin-releasing hormone receptor, and the mouse calcitonin receptor was used. (From Rubin DA, Jüppner H: Zebrafish express the common parathyroid hormone/parathyroid hormone–related peptide (PTH1R) and a novel receptor (PTH3R) that is preferentially activated by mammalian and fugufish parathyroid hormone–related peptide. J Biol Chem 84:28185–28190, 1999.)

Additional Receptors for PTH and/or PTHrP

Evidence is accumulating for the presence of additional receptors and/or binding proteins that interact with different portions of either PTH or PTHrP, but thus far only one cDNA encoding a novel PTH/PTHrP receptor (type 3 receptor, PTH3R) has been isolated—from zebrafish.[276] To isolate portions of the zebrafish homologue of the type 1 PTH/PTHrP receptor (PTH1R), genomic DNA was amplified by polymerase chain reaction (PCR) with the use of degenerate primers located in two highly conserved exons, M6/7 and M7, that are separated in all investigated mammalian PTH/PTHrP receptor genes by a short intron of about 80 nucleotides. However, despite relatively stringent conditions, two PCR products were amplified and subsequently led to the isolation of two distinct, full-length cDNAs. One of these teleost receptors was, at the amino acid level, 76% identical to the human PTH/PTHrP receptor whereas the other receptor showed only 67% homology. These findings indicated that the first cDNA encodes the zebrafish homologue of the mammalian PTH/PTHrP receptor, or zPTH1R (Fig. 70–17). This assignment was confirmed through functional studies that revealed that this teleost receptor interacts equivalently with human PTH and PTHrP (Fig. 70–18). In contrast, the second teleost cDNA encoding zPTH3R bound human and fugu PTHrP with higher affinity than it did human PTH, and it was more efficiently activated by PTHrP than by PTH. Furthermore, in contrast to zPTH1R, which showed PTH- and PTHrP-activated accumulation of IP_3, zPTH3R failed to activate this second messenger pathway.[276]

Interestingly, zPTH3R contains the amino acids DKNC in the second intracellular loop of the receptor, whereas zPTH1R contains the amino acids DRKY. Previous studies with the rat PTH/PTHrP receptor had indicated that replacement of the sequence EKKY by DSEL in the equivalent receptor region abolishes agonist-induced accumulation of IP_3 but has no effect on cell surface expression, ligand binding, and agonist-induced cAMP accumulation.[417] These data indicated that this receptor region, particularly the equivalent of residue Lys319 (the second lysine in the EKKY sequence of the rat PTH1R, which is preserved in zPTH2R; see Fig. 70–14), is important for efficient coupling to the PLC/PKC second messenger pathway. It thus appears plausible that the sequence variation present at this site in zPTH3R is associated with its lack of PLC/PKC activation. It remains uncertain whether the equivalent of the teleost type 3 PTH/PTHrP receptor exists in the mammalian genome, but recent studies in rats have indicated that the release of vasopressin from the supraoptic nucleus is stimulated in vitro and in vivo by PTHrP but not by PTH and that this effect is dependent on the cAMP/PKA signaling pathway.[305, 306] These latter findings support the conclusion that a PTHrP-selective receptor exists; this putative receptor may be homologous to the teleost PTH3R, but no such receptor has as yet been reported in humans or other mammals.

Receptors with Specificity for Non–N-Terminal PTH and PTHrP

Considerable information has accumulated that indicates that regions of PTH(1–84) other than the N-terminal residues may be responsible

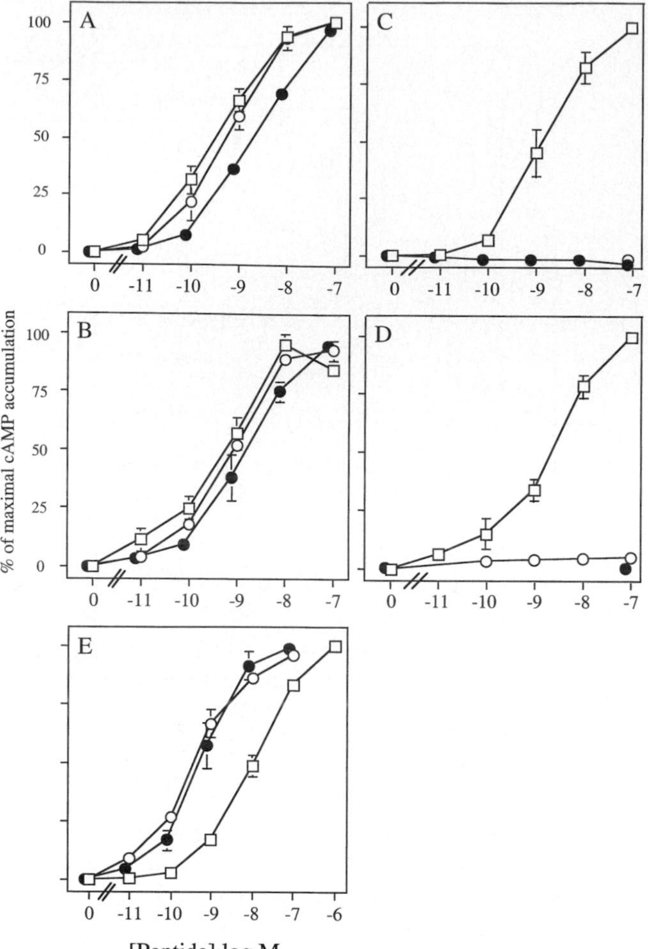

FIGURE 70–18. Agonist-induced cyclic adenosine monophosphate (cAMP) accumulation. COS-7 cells transiently expressing hPTH1R *(A)*, zPTH1R *(B)*, hPTH2R *(C)*, zPTH2R *(D)*, or zPTH3R *(E)* were evaluated for agonist-stimulated cAMP production. *Squares,* human parathyroid hormone (PTH); *open circles,* human PTH-related peptide (PTHrP); *filled circles,* fugu PTHrP. Data are expressed as percentages of maximal. (Data from Rubin et al.[275] and Rubin and Jüppner.[276])

for novel biologic actions (Table 70–3). However, analysis of these effects is still largely limited to in vitro studies. For example, a series of synthetic peptides forming the central region of PTH were reported to delineate a core domain, PTH(30–34), that stimulates the proliferation of chondrocytes but does not appear to involve the cAMP/PKA pathway.[150, 298–301] Early competition binding assays with renal plasma membranes and rat osteosarcoma cells have demonstrated binding sites for C-terminal PTH(53–84) that are discrete from those that bind PTH(1–34).[436–439] The observation that N- and C-terminal fragments of PTH elicited contrasting effects on alkaline phosphatase activity[440–442] further supports the existence of a receptor with specificity for the C-terminal portion of PTH.

In addition, considerable evidence suggests that the C-terminal portion of intact PTH has distinct biologic properties. For example, C-terminal PTH fragments such as PTH(39–84) and PTH(53–84) stimulate the formation of bone-resorbing osteoclasts from precursor cells,[149] and the same PTH fragments were previously shown to enhance the influx of ^{45}Ca into SaOS-2 cells.[443] Several different clonal cell lines, including bone- and cartilage-derived cells, in which the common PTH/PTHrP receptor had been deleted through homologous recombination were shown to increase their proliferative activity in response to intact PTH and C-terminal fragments.[147, 148] Furthermore, PTH(1–84) was shown to be more potent than PTH(1–34) in increasing the concentration of fibronectin in vivo,[444] and finally C-terminal PTH fragments increased type I procollagen expression.[151]

In direct support of a biologic role for C-terminal PTH fragments, ROS 17/2.8 cells and rat PT-r3 cells were shown to specifically interact with the C-terminal portion of PTH. With the use of radiolabeled [Tyr34]hPTH(19–84), which does not bind to cells that express high concentrations of the PTH/PTHrP receptor, these cells were shown to bind PTH(1–84) and PTH(19–84) with equivalent high affinity, whereas fragments of PTH(19–84) that were truncated at the N-terminal end showed a progressive loss of binding affinity.[145] However, even PTH(53–84) showed some displacement of the radiolabeled [Tyr34]hPTH(19–84), whereas the midregional fragment PTH(44–68) failed to do so. Other studies using ROS 17/2.8 cells, but with [^{35}S-Met]hPTH(1–84) instead of ^{125}I-labeled [Tyr34]hPTH(19–84), showed similar binding characteristics of C-terminal PTH fragments, and these studies indicated that residue 84 contributes to the overall ligand-binding affinity.[146] Photoaffinity cross-linking experiments led to the identification of approximately 80- and 30-kDa proteins that show high-affinity interaction with the C-terminal portion of PTH, but not with the N-terminal PTH(1–34).[145] These findings clearly indicate that the C-terminal portion of PTH interacts specifically with a novel receptor/binding protein that is distinct from the known, cloned receptors for PTH and PTHrP. Complementary DNA clones encoding this novel receptor/binding protein have not yet been isolated, and little or nothing is known about the signal transduction systems that mediate the actions of these midregional/C-terminal PTH fragments with yet unknown biologic importance.

Additional, as yet uncloned receptors most likely mediate the actions of midregional PTHrP, which is important for placental calcium transport[286, 302] (see above) and may have biologic functions in skin.[303] Likewise, actions of the C-terminal PTHrP portion on osteoclasts and osteoblasts[291–293, 295] and on the central nervous system[304] appear to be mediated through a specific receptor(s), and other receptors have been characterized that interact equivalently with the N-terminal portions of PTH and PTHrP but signal only through changes in intracellular free calcium.[308, 309, 445]

SUMMARY

The actions of N-terminal fragments of PTH and PTHrP are mediated through at least three different receptors that all belong to a distinct family of G protein–coupled receptors (Fig. 70–19). The PTH/PTHrP receptor mediates the actions of N-terminal PTH and PTHrP fragments equivalently, and it signals through two second messenger

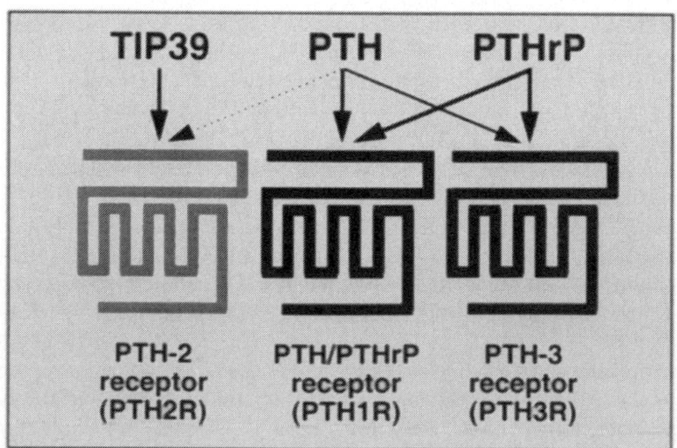

FIGURE 70–19. Parathyroid hormone (PTH), PTH-related peptide (PTHrP), and TIP39 mediate their actions through at least three distinct G protein–coupled receptors, the PTH/PTHrP receptor (PTH1R) *(black)*, the PTH2 receptor (PTH2R) *(shaded)*, and a novel receptor that was recently isolated from zebrafish (PTH3R). All three receptors are closely related and belong to a distinct family of G protein–coupled receptors. In contrast to the PTH/PTHrP receptor, which is expressed in mammals in a large variety of fetal and adult tissues, the PTH2 receptor is expressed in only few organs and its biologic functions are not yet established; the pattern of expression and the biologic role of PTH3R in fish (and in other vertebrate species) remains unknown.

TABLE 70–3. Selective Characteristics of Other Receptors for PTH and/or PTHrP Distinct from the PTH/PTHrP Receptor and the PTH2 Receptor

Receptor	Target Tissue	Ligand Specificity	Function	Signaling Properties	Reference
PTH-specific receptors	Bone, cartilage, parathyroid gland–derived fibroblasts	C-terminal fragments of PTH, i.e., 19–84 and 39–84	Unknown	Unknown	145–151
	Bone, cartilage	Midregional fragments of PTH	Cell proliferation	PLC	296, 298–301
PTHrP-specific receptors	Placenta	Midregional fragments of PTHrP, i.e., (38–94)NH_2 or (67–86)NH_2	Transplacental calcium transfer	Unknown	286, 302
	Keratinocytes, squamous cell carcinoma	Midregional fragments of PTHrP, i.e., (38–94)NH_2 or (67–86)NH_2	Unknown	Ca^{2+}, IP_3	303
	Bone cells	PTHrP(107–139)NH_2 PTHrP(107–111)NH_2, and other peptides	Inhibition of osteoclasts Stimulation of osteoblasts	Unknown	291–293, 294, 297
	Hippocampus	PTHrP(107–139)NH_2	Unknown	Ca^{2+}	304
	Supraoptic nucleus	N-terminal fragments of PTHrP; PTH is considerably less active	Vasopressin release	cAMP	305, 306
Other receptors that interact with PTH and PTHrP	Pancreatic cells, keratinocytes, squamous cell carcinoma	N-terminal fragments of PTH or PTHrP	Unknown	Ca^{2+}	307, 308
	Unknown (isolated thus far only from zebrafish)	Human PTHrP(1–36) and fugu PTHrP(1–36); human PTH(1–34) is considerably less active	Unknown	cAMP	276

cAMP, cyclic adenosine monophosphate; IP_3, inositol 1,4,5-triphosphate; PLC, phospholipase C; PTH, parathyroid hormone; PTHrP, PTH-related peptide.

pathways, cAMP and IP_3. The mRNA encoding the PTH/PTHrP receptor is found in a large variety of fetal and adult tissues, but its expression is most abundant in three tissues; in the first two, kidney and bone, the receptor mediates the endocrine actions of PTH in mineral ion homeostasis. At the third site, the metaphyseal growth plate, it mediates the autocrine/paracrine actions of locally synthesized PTHrP. Although "knockout" studies have clearly demonstrated the critical role played by PTHrP in the embryonic and postnatal development of cartilage and bone,[12, 13, 270, 271] the biologic role of this paracrine PTHrP-PTH/PTHrP receptor interaction system in the adult, if any, remains incompletely understood. Further studies are needed, such as conditional gene "knockout" or gene transplacement approaches. In contrast to the equivalent activation of the PTH/PTHrP receptor by PTH and PTHrP, the closely related PTH2R is activated predominantly by the recently isolated TIP39.[356] Only the human PTH2R,[283, 284, 357] not the rat receptor homologue,[358] is activated by PTH. Expression of PTH2R is restricted to relatively few tissues, its mRNA levels are typically much less abundant than those encoding the PTH/PTHrP receptor, and its biologic role remains to be determined. A third PTH/PTHrP receptor has thus far only been isolated from zebrafish. It interacts preferentially with PTHrP and appears to signal predominantly through the cAMP/PKA pathway.[276] At least three closely related G protein–coupled receptors thus mediate the actions of at least three different polypeptide ligands, PTH, PTHrP, and TIP39. Whereas the roles of the PTH/PTHrP receptor in the regulation of mineral ion homeostasis and growth plate development are well documented, the biologic roles of PTH2R and PTH3R remain to be defined.

REFERENCES

1. Hansen AM: The hydrochloric X sicca: A parathyroid preparation for intramuscular injection. Mil Surg 54:218–219, 1924.
2. Collip JB: Extraction of a parathyroid hormone which will prevent or control parathyroid tetany and which regulates the level of blood calcium. J Biol Chem 63:395–438, 1925.
3. Albright F, Ellsworth R: Studies on the physiology of the parathyroid glands. I. Calcium and phosphorus studies on a case of idiopathic hypoparathyroidism. J Clin Invest 7:183–201, 1929.
4. Broadus AE, Stewart AF: Parathyroid hormone–related protein: Structure, processing, and physiological actions. *In* Bilezikian JP, Levine MA, Marcus R (eds): The Parathyroids. Basic and Clinical Concepts. New York, Raven, 1994, pp 259–294.
5. Moseley JM, Martin TJ: Parathyroid hormone–related protein: Physiological actions. *In* Bilezikian JP, Raisz LG, Rodan RA (eds): The Parathyroids. Basic and Clinical Concepts. New York, Raven, 1996, pp 363–376.
6. Yang KH, Stewart AF: Parathyroid hormone–related protein: The gene, its mRNA species, and protein products. *In* Bilezikian JP, Raisz LG, Rodan RA: Principles of Bone Biology. New York, Academic, 1996, pp 347–362.
7. Jüppner H, Abou-Samra AB, Freeman MW, et al: A G protein–linked receptor for parathyroid hormone and parathyroid hormone–related peptide. Science 254:1024–1026, 1991.
8. Abou-Samra AB, Jüppner H, Force T, et al: Expression cloning of a common receptor for parathyroid hormone and parathyroid hormone–related peptide from rat osteoblast-like cells: A single receptor stimulates intracellular accumulation of both cAMP and inositol triphosphates and increases intracellular free calcium. Proc Natl Acad Sci U S A 89:2732–2736, 1992.
9. Schipani E, Karga H, Karaplis AC, et al: Identical complementary deoxyribonucleic acids encode a human renal and bone parathyroid hormone (PTH)/PTH-related peptide receptor. Endocrinology 132:2157–2165, 1993.
10. Potts JT Jr, Jüppner H: Parathyroid hormone and parathyroid hormone–related peptide in calcium homeostasis, bone metabolism, and bone development: The proteins, their genes, and receptors. *In* Avioli LV, Krane SM (eds): Metabolic Bone Disease, ed 3. New York, Academic, 1997, pp 51–94.
11. Silver J, Kronenberg HM: Parathyroid hormone—molecular biology and regulation. *In* Bilezikian JP Raisz LG, Rodan GA (eds): Principles of Bone Biology. New York, Academic, 1996, pp 325–346.
12. Lanske B, Karaplis AC, Luz A, et al: PTH/PTHrP receptor in early development and Indian hedgehog–regulated bone growth. Science 273:663–666, 1996.
13. Vortkamp A, Lee K, Lanske B, et al: Regulation of rate of cartilage differentiation by Indian hedgehog and PTH-related protein. Science 273:613–622, 1996.
14. Kronenberg HM, Lanske B, Kovacs CS, et al: Functional analysis of the PTH/PTHrP network of ligands and receptors. Recent Prog Horm Res 53:283–301, 1998.
15. Bringhurst FR: Calcium and phosphate distribution, turnover, and metabolic actions. *In* DeGroot LJ (ed): Endocrinology, ed 2. Philadelphia, WB Saunders, 1989, pp 805–843.
16. Neer RM: Calcium and inorganic phosphate homeostasis. *In* DeGroot LJ (ed): Endocrinology, ed 2. Philadelphia, WB Saunders, 1989, pp 927–953.
17. Wendelaar-Bonga SE, Pang PK: Control of calcium regulating hormones in the vertebrates: Parathyroid hormone, calcitonin, prolactin, and stanniocalcin. Int Rev Cytol 128:139–213, 1991.
18. Pang PTK, Pang RK: Hormones and calcium regulation in vertebrates: An evolutionary and overall consideration. *In* Pang PKT, Schreibman MP (eds): Regulation of Calcium and Phosphate. San Diego, Academic, 1989, pp 343–352.
19. Drezner MK: Phosphorus homeostasis and related disorders. *In* Bilezikian JP Raisz LG, Rodan GA (eds): Principles of Bone Biology. New York, Academic, 1996, pp 263–276.
20. Wagner G, Dimattia G, Davie J, et al: Molecular cloning and cDNA sequence analysis of coho salmon stanniocalcin. Mol Cell Endocrinol 90:7–15, 1992.
21. Olsen H, Cepeda M, Zhang Q, et al: Human stanniocalcin: A possible hormonal regulator of mineral metabolism. Proc Natl Acad Sci U S A 93:1792–1796, 1996.
22. Chang A, Reddel R: Identification of a second stanniocalcin cDNA in mouse and human: Stanniocalcin 2. Mol Cell Endocrinol 141:95–99, 1998.
23. DiMattia G, Varghese R, Wagner G: Molecular cloning and characterization of stanniocalcin-related protein. Mol Cell Endocrinol 146:137–140, 1998.

24. Ishibashi K, Miyamoto K, Taketani Y, et al: Molecular cloning of a second human stanniocalcin homologue (STC2). Biochem Biophys Res Commun 250:252–258, 1998.
25. Martin JT, Findley DM, Moseley JM, et al: Calcitonin. *In* Avioli LV, Krane SM (eds): Metabolic Bone Disease, ed 3. New York, Academic, 1998, pp 95–121.
26. Potts JT Jr, Bringhurst FR, Gardella TJ, et al: Parathyroid hormone: Physiology, chemistry, biosynthesis, secretion, metabolism, and mode of action. *In* DeGroot LJ (ed): Endocrinology, ed 3. Philadelphia, WB Saunders, 1996, pp 920–965.
27. Diaz R, El-Hajj GF, Brown E: Parathyroid hormone and polyhormones: Production and export. *In* Fray JCS (ed): Handbook of Physiology: Endocrine Regulation of Water and Electrolyte Balance. New York, Oxford University Press, 2000, pp 607–662.
28. Nordin BEC, Peacock M: Role of kidney in regulation of plasma calcium. Lancet 2:1280–1283, 1969.
29. Peacock M, Robertson W, Nordin B: Relation between serum and urinary calcium with particular reference to parathyroid activity. Lancet 1:384–386, 1969.
30. Mayer G, Habener J, Potts JT Jr: Parathyroid hormone secretion in vivo. Demonstration of a calcium-independent nonsuppressible component of secretion. J Clin Invest 57:678–683, 1976.
31. Parsons JA, Potts JT Jr: Physiology and chemistry of parathyroid hormone. *In* MacIntyre I (ed): Calcium Metabolism and Bone Disease. Philadelphia, WB Saunders, 1972, pp 33–78.
32. Potts JT Jr, Deftos LJ: Parathyroid hormone, calcitonin, vitamin D, bone and bone mineral metabolism. *In* Bondy PK, Rosenberg LE (eds): Duncan's Disease of Metabolism, ed 3. Philadelphia, WB Saunders, 1974, pp 1225–1430.
33. Rasmussen H, Bordier P: The Physiological and Cellular Basis of Metabolic Bone Disease. Baltimore, Williams & Wilkins, 1974.
34. Nordin BEC, Marshall DH, Peacock M, et al: Plasma calcium homeostasis. *In* Talmage RB, Owen M, Parsons JA (eds): Calcium-Regulating Hormones. Amsterdam, Excerpta Medica, 1975, pp 239–253.
35. Fraser RA, Kronenberg HM, Pang PK, et al: Parathyroid hormone messenger ribonucleic acid in the rat hypothalamus. Endocrinology 127:2517–2522, 1990.
36. Nutley MT, Parimi SA, Harvey S: Sequence analysis of hypothalamic parathyroid hormone messenger ribonucleic acid. Endocrinology 136:5600–5607, 1995.
37. Roth SI, Schiller AL: Comparative anatomy of the parathyroid glands. *In* Greep RO, Ashwood EB (eds): Handbook of Physiology. Washington, DC, American Physiological Society; 1981, pp 281–311.
38. Fraser RA, Kaneko T, Pang PKT, et al: Hypo- and hypercalcemic peptides in fish pituitary glands. Am J Physiol 260:R622–R626, 1991.
39. Rosenberg J, Kronenberg HM: Parathyroid hormone without parathyroid glands: A sequence resembling PTH in a teleost fish. J Bone Miner Res 6(suppl 1):379, 1991.
40. Danks JA, Devlin AJ, Ho PMW, et al: Parathyroid hormone–related protein is a factor in normal fish pituitary. Gen Comp Endocrinol 92:201–212, 1993.
41. Devlin AJ, Danks JA, Faulkner MK, et al: Immunochemical detection of parathyroid hormone–related protein in the saccus vasculosus of a teleost fish. Gen Comp Endocrinol 101:83–90, 1996.
42. Danks JA, McHale JC, Martin JT, et al: Parathyroid hormone–related protein in tissues of the emerging frog (*Rana temporaria*): Immunohistochemistry and in situ hybridization. J Anat 190:229–238, 1997.
43. Trivett M, Officer R, Clement J, et al: Parathyroid hormone–related protein (PTHrP) in cartilaginous and bony fish tissues. J Exp Zool 284:541–548, 1999.
44. Albright F, Bauer W, Ropes M, et al: Studies of calcium and phosphorus metabolism. IV. The effect of the parathyroid hormone. J Clin Invest 7:139–181, 1929.
45. Aurbach GD: Isolation of parathyroid hormone after extraction with phenol. J Biol Chem 234:3179, 1959.
46. Rasmussen H, Craig LC: Purification of parathyroid hormone by use of countercurrent distribution. J Am Chem Soc 81:5003, 1959.
47. Brewer HB Jr, Ronan R: Bovine parathyroid hormone: Amino acid sequence. Proc Natl Acad Sci U S A 67:1862, 1970.
48. Niall HD, Keutmann HT, Sauer RT, et al: The amino-acid sequence of bovine parathyroid hormone I. Hoppe-Seyler's Z Physiol Chem 351:1586–1588, 1970.
49. Sauer RT, Niall HD, Hogan ML, et al: The amino acid sequence of porcine parathyroid hormone. Biochemistry 13:1994, 1974.
50. Brewer HB Jr, Fairwell T, Ronan R, et al: Human parathyroid hormone: Amino acid sequence of the amino-terminal residues 1–34. Proc Natl Acad Sci U S A 69:3585, 1972.
51. Niall HD, Sauer RT, Jacobs JW, et al: The amino acid sequence of the amino-terminal 37 residues of human parathyroid hormone. Proc Natl Acad Sci U S A 71:384, 1974.
52. Keutmann HT, Sauer MM, Hendy GN, et al: The complete amino acid sequence of human parathyroid hormone. Biochemistry 17:552, 1978.
53. Kronenberg HM, McDevitt BE, Majzoub JA, et al: Cloning and nucleotide sequence of DNA coding for bovine preproparathyroid hormone. Proc Natl Acad Sci U S A 76:4981–4985, 1979.
54. Hendy GN, Kronenberg HM, Potts JT Jr, et al: Nucleotide sequence of cloned cDNAs encoding human preproparathyroid hormone. Proc Natl Acad Sci U S A 78:7365–7369, 1981.
55. Vasicek T, McDevitt BE, Freeman MW, et al: Nucleotide sequence of genomic DNA encoding human parathyroid hormone. Proc Natl Acad Sci U S A 80:2127–2131, 1983.
56. Heinrich G, Kronenberg HM, Potts JT Jr, et al: Gene encoding parathyroid hormone: Nucleotide sequence of the rat gene and deduced amino acid sequence of rat preproparathyroid hormone. J Biol Chem 259:3320–3329, 1984.
57. Khosla S, Demay M, Pines M, et al: Nucleotide sequence of cloned cDNAs encoding chicken preproparathyroid hormone. J Bone Miner Res 3:689–698, 1988.
58. Russell J, Sherwood LM: Nucleotide sequence of the DNA complementary to avian (chicken) preproparathyroid hormone mRNA and the deduced sequence of the hormone precursor. Mol Endocrinol 3:325–331, 1989.
59. Rosol TJ, Steinmeyer CL, McCauley LK, et al: Sequences of the cDNAs encoding canine parathyroid hormone–related protein and parathyroid hormone. Gene 160:241–243, 1995.
60. Barden JA, Kemp BE: NMR study of a 34-residue N-terminal fragment of the parathyroid-hormone–related protein secreted during humoral hypercalcemia of malignancy. Eur J Biochem 184:379–394, 1989.
61. Lee SC, Russell AF: Two-dimensional ^{1}H-NMR study of the 1–34 fragment of human parathyroid hormone. Biopolymers 28:1115–1127, 1989.
62. Klaus W, Dieckmann T, Wray V, et al: Investigation of the solution structure of the human parathyroid hormone fragment (1–34) by ^{1}H NMR spectroscopy, distance geometry, and molecular dynamics calculations. Biochemistry 30:6936–6942, 1991.
63. Barden JA, Kemp BE: NMR solution structure of human parathyroid hormone(1–34). Biochemistry 32:7126–7132, 1993.
64. Marx UC, Austermann S, Bayer P, et al: Structure of human parathyroid hormone 1–37 in solution. J Biol Chem 270:15194–15202, 1995.
65. Pellegrini M, Royo M, Rosenblatt M, et al: Addressing the tertiary structure of human parathyroid hormone-(1–34). J Biol Chem 273:10420–10427, 1998.
66. DeVos DM, Ultsch M, Kossiakoff AA: Human growth hormone and extracellular domain of its receptor: Crystal structure of the complex. Science 255:306–312, 1992.
67. Wiesmann C, Ultsch MH, Bass SH, et al: Crystal structure of nerve growth factor in complex with the ligand-binding domain of the TrkA receptor. Nature 401:184–188, 1999.
68. Pebay-Peyroula E, Rummel G, Rosenbusch J, et al: X-ray structure of bacteriorhodopsin at 2.5 angstroms from microcrystals grown in lipidic cubic phases. Science 277:1676–1681, 1997.
69. Antonarakis SE, Phillips JA, Mallonee RL, et al: β-Globin locus is linked to the parathyroid hormone (PTH) locus and lies between insulin and PTH loci in man. Proc Natl Acad Sci U S A 80:6615–6619, 1983.
70. Naylor SL, Sakaguchi AU, Szoka P, et al: Human parathyroid hormone gene (PTH) is on short arm of chromosome 11. Somat Cell Gene 9:609–616, 1983.
71. Mayer H, Breyel E, Bostock C, et al: Assignment of the human parathyroid hormone gene to chromosome 11. Hum Genet 64:283–285, 1983.
72. Zabel BU, Kronenberg HM, Bell GI, et al: Chromosome mapping of genes on the short arm of human chromosome 11: Parathyroid hormone gene is at 11p15 together with the genes for insulin, c-Harvey-ras 1, and β-hemoglobin. Cytogenet Cell Genet 39:200–205, 1985.
73. Kronenberg HK, Igarashi T, Freeman MW, et al: Structure and expression of the human parathyroid hormone gene. Recent Prog Horm Res 42:641–663, 1986.
74. Schmidtke J, Pape B, Krengel U, et al: Restriction fragment length polymorphism at the human parathyroid hormone gene locus. Hum Genet 67:428–431, 1984.
75. Gong G, Johnson M, Barger-Lux M, et al: Association of bone dimensions with a parathyroid hormone gene polymorphism in women. Osteoporos Int 9:307–311, 1999.
76. Kanzawa M, Sugimoto T, Kobayashi T, et al: Parathyroid hormone gene polymorphisms in primary hyperparathyroidism. Clin Endocrinol (Oxf) 50:583–588, 1999.
77. Mullersman J, Shields J, Saha B: Characterization of two novel polymorphisms at the human parathyroid hormone gene locus. Hum Genet 88:589–592, 1992.
78. Parkinson D, Shaw N, Himsworth R, et al: Parathyroid hormone gene analysis in autosomal hypoparathyroidism using an intragenic tetranucleotide (AAAT)n polymorphism. Hum Genet 91:281–284, 1993.
79. Ahn TG, Antonarakis SE, Kronenberg HM, et al: Familial isolated hypoparathyroidism: A molecular genetic analysis of 8 families with 23 affected persons. Medicine (Baltimore) 65:73–81, 1986.
80. Miric A, Levine MA: Analysis of the preproPTH gene by denaturing gradient gel electrophoresis in familial isolated hypoparathyroidism. J Clin Endocrinol Metab 74:509–516, 1992.
81. Bilous R, Murty G, Parkinson D, et al: Brief report: Autosomal dominant familial hypoparathyroidism, sensorineural deafness, and renal dysplasia. N Engl J Med 327:1069–1074, 1992.
82. Kronenberg HM, Bringhurst FR, Nussbaum S, et al: Parathyroid hormone: Biosynthesis, secretion, chemistry, and action. *In* Mundy GR, Martin TJ (eds): Handbook of Experimental Pharmacology: Physiology and Pharmacology of Bone. Heidelberg, Germany, Springer-Verlag, 1993, pp 185–201.
83. Arnold A, Horst SA, Gardella TJ, et al: Mutation of the signal peptide–encoding region of the preproparathyroid hormone gene in familial isolated hypoparathyroidism. J Clin Invest 86:1084–1087, 1990.
84. Karaplis AC, Lim SK, Baba H, et al: Inefficient membrane targeting, translocation, and proteolytic processing by signal peptidase of a mutant preproparathyroid hormone protein. J Biol Chem 270:1629–1635, 1995.
85. Habener JF, Rosenblatt M, Potts JT Jr: Parathyroid hormone: Biochemical aspects of biosynthesis, secretion, and metabolism. Physiol Rev 64:985–1053, 1984.
86. Hendy GN, Bennett HP, Gibbs BF, et al: Proparathyroid hormone is preferentially cleaved to parathyroid hormone by the prohormone convertase furin. A mass spectrometric study. J Biol Chem 270:9517–9525, 1995.
87. Canaff L, Bennett HP, Hou Y, et al: Proparathyroid hormone processing by the proprotein convertase-7: Comparison with furin and assessment of modulation of parathyroid convertase messenger ribonucleic acid levels by calcium and 1,25-dihydroxyvitamin D_3. Endocrinology 140:3633–3642, 1999.
88. MacGregor RR, Hamilton JW, Kent GN: The degradation of proparathormone and parathormone by parathyroid and liver cathepsin B. J Biol Chem 254:4428–4433, 1979.
89. MacGregor RR, Hamilton JW, Shofstall RE, et al: Isolation and characterization of porcine parathyroid cathepsin B. J Biol Chem 254:4423–4427, 1979.
90. Mayer GP, Keaton JA, Hurst JG, et al: Effects of plasma calcium concentration on the relative proportion of hormone and carboxyl fragments in parathyroid venous blood. Endocrinology 104:1778–1784, 1979.
91. Habener JF, Kemper B, Potts JT Jr: Calcium-dependent intracellular degradation of parathyroid hormone: A possible mechanism for the regulation of hormone stores. Endocrinology 97:431–441, 1975.

92. D'Amour P, Palardy J, Bahsali G, et al: The modulation of circulating parathyroid hormone immunoheterogeneity in man by ionized calcium concentration. J Clin Endocrinol Metab 74:525–532, 1992.
93. Brossard JH, Clouthier M, Roy L, et al: Accumulation of a non-(1–84) molecular form of parathyroid hormone (PTH) detected by intact PTH assay in renal failure: Importance in the interpretation of PTH values. J Clin Endocrinol Metab 81:3923–3929, 1996.
94. Yamaguchi T, Chattopadhyay N, Brown EM: G protein–coupled extracellular Ca^{2+} ($Ca^{2+}{}_o$)-sensing receptor (CaR): Roles in cell signaling and control of diverse cellular functions. Adv Pharmacol 47:209–253, 2000.
95. Moallem E, Kilav R, Silver J, et al: RNA-protein binding and post-transcriptional regulation of parathyroid hormone gene expression by calcium and phosphate. J Biol Chem 273:5253–5259, 1998.
96. Naveh-Many T, Rahaminov R, Livini N, et al: Parathyroid cell proliferation in normal and chronic renal failure in rats. The effects of calcium, phosphate, and vitamin D. J Clin Invest 96:1786–1793, 1995.
97. Almaden Y, Canalejo A, Hernandez A, et al: Direct effect of phosphorus on PTH secretion from whole rat parathyroid glands in vitro. J Bone Miner Res 11:970–976, 1996.
98. Slatopolsky E, Finch J, Denda M, et al: Phosphorus restriction prevents parathyroid gland growth. High phosphorus directly stimulates PTH secretion in vitro. J Clin Invest 97:2534–2540, 1996.
99. Estepa J, Aguilera-Tejero E, Lopez I, et al: Effect of phosphate on parathyroid hormone secretion in vivo. J Bone Miner Res 14:1848–1854, 1999.
100. Brown A, Zhong M, Finch J, et al: Rat calcium-sensing receptor is regulated by vitamin D but not by calcium. Am J Physiol 270:F454–F460, 1996.
101. Russell J, Sherwood L: The effects of 1,25-dihydroxyvitamin D_3 and high calcium on transcription of the pre-proparathyroid hormone gene are direct. Trans Assoc Am Physicians 100:256 262, 1987.
102. Okazaki T, Igarashi T, Kronenberg HM: 5′-Flanking region of the parathyroid hormone gene mediates negative regulation by $1,25(OH)_2$ vitamin D_3. J Biol Chem 263:2203–2208, 1989.
103. Slatopolsky E, Finch J, Ritter C, et al: A new analog of calcitriol, 19-nor-1,25-$(OH)_2D_2$, suppresses parathyroid hormone secretion in uremic rats in the absence of hypercalcemia. Am J Kidney Dis 26:852–860, 1995.
104. Slatopolsky E: The role of calcium, phosphorus and vitamin D metabolism in the development of secondary hyperparathyroidism. Nephrol Dial Transplant 13(suppl 3):3–8, 1998.
105. Llach F, Keshav G, Goldblat M, et al: Suppression of parathyroid hormone secretion in hemodialysis patients by a novel vitamin D analogue: 19-nor-1,25-dihydroxyvitamin D_2. Am J Kidney Dis 32(suppl 2):48–54, 1998.
106. Silver J, Moallem E, Epstein E, et al: New aspects in the control of parathyroid hormone secretion. Curr Opin Nephrol Hypertens 3:379–385, 1994.
107. Mayer GP, Hurst JG: Sigmoidal relationship between parathyroid hormone secretion rate and plasma calcium concentration in calves. Endocrinology 102:1036–1042, 1978.
108. Brent GA, LeBoff MS, Seely EW, et al: Relationship between the concentration and rate of change of calcium and serum intact parathyroid hormone levels in normal humans. J Clin Endocrinol Metab 67:944 950, 1988.
109. Brown EM: Four-parameter model of the sigmoidal relationship between the parathyroid hormone release and extracellular calcium concentration in normal and abnormal parathyroid tissue. J Clin Endocrinol Metab 56:572–581, 1983.
110. Parfitt AM: Bone and plasma calcium homeostasis. Bone 8(suppl 1):1–8, 1987.
111. Brown EM: Extracellular Ca^{2+} sensing, regulation of parathyroid cell function, and role of Ca^{2+} and other ions as extracellular (first) messengers. Physiol Rev 71:371–411, 1991.
112. Hanley D, Takatsuki K, Sultan J, et al: Direct release of parathyroid hormone fragments from functioning bovine parathyroid glands in vitro. J Clin Invest 62:1247–1254, 1978.
113. Lepage R, Roy L, Brossard JH, et al: A non-(1–84) circulating parathyroid hormone (PTH) fragment interferes significantly with intact PTH commercial assay measurements in uremic samples. Clin Chem 44:805–809, 1998.
114. Parfitt AM: Hypercalcemic hyperparathyroidism following renal transplantation: Differential diagnosis, management, and implications for cell population control in the parathyroid gland. Miner Electrolyte Metab 8:92–112, 1982.
115. Gittes RF, Radde IC: Experimental model for hyperparathyroidism: Effect of excessive numbers of transplanted isologous parathyroid glands. J Urol 95:595–603, 1966.
116. Grant FD, Conlin PR, Brown EM: Rate and concentration dependence of parathyroid hormone dynamics during stepwise changes in serum ionized calcium in normal humans. J Clin Endocrinol Metab 71:370–378, 1990.
117. Conlin PR, Fajtova VT, Mortensen RM, et al: Hysteresis in the relationship between serum ionized calcium and intact parathyroid hormone during recovery from induced hyper- and hypocalcemia in normal humans. J Clin Endocrinol Metab 69:593–599, 1989.
118. Cunningham J, Altmann P, Gleed J, et al: Effect of direction and rate of change of calcium on parathyroid hormone secretion in uremia. Nephrol Dial Transplant 4:339–344, 1989.
119. El-Hajj Fuleihan G, Klerman E, Brown E, et al: The parathyroid hormone circadian rhythm is truly endogenous—a general clinical research center study. J Clin Endocrinol Metab 82:281–286, 1997.
120. Harms HM, Kaptaina U, Kulpmann WR, et al: Pulse amplitude and frequency modulation of parathyroid hormone in plasma. J Clin Endocrinol Metab 69:843–851, 1989.
121. Brown EM, Gamba G, Riccardi D, et al: Cloning and characterization of an extracellular Ca^{2+}-sensing receptor from bovine parathyroid. Nature 366:575–580, 1993.
122. Brown EM, Vassilev PM, Quinn S, et al: G-protein–coupled, extracellular Ca^{2+}-sensing receptor: A versatile regulator of diverse cellular functions. Vitam Horm 55:1–71, 1999.
123. Brown EM: Physiology and pathophysiology of the extracellular calcium-sensing receptor. Am J Med 106:238–253, 1999.
124. Nemeth EF: Calcium receptors as novel drug targets. *In* Bilezikian JP, Raisz LG, Rodan GA (eds): Principles of Bone Biology. San Diego, CA, Academic, 1996, pp 1019–1035.
125. Brauner-Osborne H, Jensen AA, Sheppard PO, et al: The agonist-binding domain of the calcium-sensing receptor is located at the amino-terminal domain. J Biol Chem 274:18382–18386, 1999.
126. Kifor O, Diaz R, Butters R, et al: The Ca^{2+}-sensing receptor (CaR) activates phospholipases C, A_2, and D in bovine parathyroid and CaR-transfected, human embryonic kidney (HEK293) cells. J Bone Miner Res 12:715–725, 1997.
127. McNeil SE, Hobson SA, Nipper V, et al: Functional calcium-sensing receptors in rat fibroblasts are required for activation of SRC kinase and mitogen-activated protein kinase in response to extracellular calcium. J Biol Chem 273:1114–1120, 1998.
128. Chen CJ, Barnett JV, Congo DA, et al: Divalent cations suppress 3′,5′-adenosine monophosphate accumulation by stimulating a pertussis toxin–sensitive guanine nucleotide–binding protein in cultured bovine parathyroid cells. Endocrinology 124:233–240, 1989.
129. Garrett JE, Tamir H, Kifor O, et al: Calcitonin-secreting cells of the thyroid express an extracellular calcium receptor gene. Endocrinology 136:5202–5211, 1995.
130. Riccardi D, Hall AE, Chattopadhyay N, et al: Localization of the extracellular Ca^{2+}/polyvalent cation–sensing protein in rat kidney. Am J Physiol 274:F611–F622, 1998.
131. Chattopadhyay N, Cheng I, Rogers K, et al: Identification and localization of extracellular Ca^{2+}-sensing receptor in rat intestine. Am J Physiol 274:G122–G130, 1998.
132. Hebert SC, Brown EM, Harris HW: Role of the Ca^{2+}-sensing receptor in divalent mineral ion homeostasis. J Exp Biol 200:295–302, 1997.
133. Quarles LD: Cation-sensing receptors in bone: A novel paradigm for regulating bone remodeling? J Bone Miner Res 12:1971–1974, 1997.
134. Pollak MR, Brown EM, Chou YH, et al: Mutations in the human Ca^{2+}-sensing receptor gene cause familial hypocalciuric hypercalcemia and neonatal severe hyperparathyroidism. Cell 75:1297–1303, 1993.
135. Pollak MR, Brown EM, Estep HL, et al: Autosomal dominant hypocalcaemia caused by a Ca^{2+}-sensing receptor gene mutation. Nat Genet 8:303–307, 1994.
136. Ho C, Conner DA, Pollak M, et al: A mouse model for familial hypocalciuric hypercalcemia and neonatal severe hyperparathyroidism. Nat Genet 11:389–394, 1995.
137. Cantley LK, Russell J, Lettieri D, et al: 1,25-Dihydroxyvitamin D_3 suppresses parathyroid hormone secretion from bovine parathyroid cells in tissue culture. Endocrinology 117:2114–2119, 1985.
138. Chan YL, McKay C, Dye E, et al: The effect of 1,25 dihydroxycholecalciferol on parathyroid hormone secretion by monolayer cultures of bovine parathyroid cells. Calcif Tissue Int 38:27–32, 1986.
139. Habener JF, Potts JT Jr: Relative effectiveness of magnesium and calcium on the secretion and biosynthesis of parathyroid in vitro. Endocrinology 98:197–202, 1976.
140. Suewler GJ: Familial benign hypocalciuric hypercalcemia—from the clinic to the calcium sensor (editorial). West J Med 160:579 580, 1994.
141. Anast CS, Winnacker JL, Forte LF, et al: Impaired release of parathyroid hormone in magnesium deficiency. J Clin Endocrinol Metab 42:707–717, 1976.
142. Berson SA, Yalow RS: Immunochemical heterogeneity of parathyroid hormone in plasma. J Clin Endocrinol Metab 28:1037–1947, 1968.
143. Bringhurst FR, Stern AM, Yotts M: Peripheral metabolism of PTH: Fate of the biologically active amino-terminus in vivo. Am J Physiol 255:E886–E893, 1988.
144. Bringhurst FR, Stern AM, Yotts M: Peripheral metabolism of [^{35}S]PTH in vivo: Influence of alterations in calcium availability and parathyroid status. Endocrinology 122:237–245, 1989.
145. Inomata N, Akiyama M, Kubota N, et al: Characterization of a novel PTH-receptor with specificity for the carboxyl-terminal region of PTH(1–84). Endocrinology 136:4732–4740, 1995.
146. Takasu H, Baba H, Inomata N, et al: The 69–84 amino acid region of the parathyroid hormone molecule is essential for the interaction of the hormone with the binding sites with carboxyl-terminal specificity. Endocrinology 137:5537–5543, 1996.
147. Guo J, Lanske B, Liu B, et al: Ablation of PTH/PTHrP receptors in conditionally immortalized, PTH-responsive chondrocyte cell lines. J Bone Miner Res 10(suppl 1):172, 1995.
148. Guo J, Lanske B, Liu B, et al: A functional carboxyl-terminal PTH receptor regulates growth of conditionally immortalized hypertrophic chondrocytes. J Bone Miner Res 11(suppl 1):305, 1996.
149. Kaji H, Sugimoto T, Kanatani M, et al: Carboxyl-terminal PTH fragments stimulate osteoclast-like cell formation and osteoclastic activity. Endocrinology 134:1897–1904, 1994.
150. Erdmann S, Muller W, Bahrami S, et al: Differential effects of parathyroid hormone fragments on collagen gene expression in chondrocytes. J Cell Biol 135:1179–1191, 1996.
151. Nasu M, Sugimoto T, Kaji H, et al: Carboxyl-terminal parathyroid hormone fragments stimulate type-1 procollagen and insulin-like growth factor–binding protein-5 mRNA expression in osteoblastic UMR-106 cells. Endocr J 45:229–234, 1998.
152. Nussbaum SR, Zahradnik RJ, Lavigne JR, et al: Highly sensitive two-site immunoradiometric assay of parathyrin, and its clinical utility in evaluating patients with hypercalcemia. Clin Chem 33:1364–1367, 1987.
153. Blind E, Schmidt-Gayk H, Scharla S, et al: Two-site assay of intact parathyroid hormone in the investigation of primary hyperparathyroidism and other disorders of calcium metabolism compared with a midregion assay. J Clin Endocrinol Metab 67:353–360, 1988.
154. John M, Goodman W, Gao P, et al: A novel immunoradiometric assay detects full-length human PTH but not amino-terminally truncated fragments: Implications for PTH measurements in renal failure. J Clin Endocrinol Metab 84:4287–4290, 1999.
155. Habener JF, Powell D, Murray TM, et al: Parathyroid hormone secretion and metabolism in vivo. Proc Natl Acad Sci U S A 68:2986–2991, 1971.

156. Silverman R, Yalow RS: Heterogeneity of parathyroid hormone: Clinical and physiologic implications. J Clin Invest 52:1958–1971, 1973.
157. DiBella FP, Gilkinson JB, Flueck J, et al: Carboxy-terminal fragments of human parathyroid tumors: Unique new source of immunogens for the production of antisera potentially useful in the radioimmunoassay of parathyroid hormone in human serum. J Clin Endocrinol Metab 46:604–612, 1978.
158. Flueck JA, Dibella FB, Edis AJ, et al: Immunoheterogeneity of parathyroid hormone in venous effluent serum from hyperfunctioning parathyroid glands. J Clin Invest 60:1367–1375, 1977.
159. Brasier A, Wang C, Nussbaum S: Recovery of parathyroid hormone secretion after parathyroid adenomectomy. J Clin Endocrinol Metab 66:495–500, 1988.
160. Segre GV, Niall HD, Habener JR: Metabolism of parathyroid hormone: Physiological and clinical significance. Am J Med 56:774, 1974.
161. Segre GV, Niall HD, Sauer RT: Edman degradation of radioiodinated parathyroid hormone: Application to sequence analysis and hormone metabolism in vivo. Biochemistry 16:2417, 1977.
162. Segre GV, Perkins AS, Witters LA, et al: Metabolism of parathyroid hormone by isolated rat Kupffer cells and hepatocytes. J Clin Invest 67:449–457, 1981.
163. Zull JE, Chuang J: Characterization of parathyroid hormone fragments produced by cathepsin D. J Biol Chem 260:1608, 1985.
164. Martin KJ, Hruska KA, Freitag JJ, et al: The peripheral metabolism of parathyroid hormone. N Engl J Med 301:1092–1098, 1979.
165. Hilpert J, Nykjaer A, Jacobsen C, et al: Megalin antagonizes activation of the parathyroid hormone receptor. J Biol Chem 274:5620–5625, 1999.
166. Hercz G, Pei Y, Greenwood C, et al: Aplastic osteodystrophy without aluminum: The role of "suppressed" parathyroid function. Kidney Int 44:860–866, 1993.
167. Goodman WG, Ramirez JA, Belin TR, et al: Development of adynamic bone in patients with secondary hyperparathyroidism after intermittent calcitriol therapy. Kidney Int 46:1160–1166, 1994.
168. Wang M, Hercz G, Sherrard D, et al: Relationship between intact 1–84 parathyroid hormone and bone histomorphometric parameters in dialysis patients without aluminum toxicity. Am J Kidney Dis 26:836–844, 1995.
169. Goodman W, Veldhuis J, Belin T, et al: Suppressive effect of calcium on parathyroid hormone release in adynamic renal osteodystrophy and secondary hyperparathyroidism. Kidney Int 51:1590–1595, 1997.
170. Kuizon BD, Salusky IB: Intermittent calcitriol therapy and growth in children with chronic renal failure. Miner Electrolyte Metab 24:290–295, 1998.
171. Kuizon BD, Goodman WG, Jüppner H, et al: Diminished linear growth during intermittent calcitriol therapy in children undergoing CCPD. Kidney Int 53:205–211, 1998.
172. Sanchez CP, Salusky IB, Kuizon BD, et al: Growth of long bones in renal failure: Roles of hyperparathyroidism, growth hormone and calcitriol. Kidney Int 54:1879–1887, 1998.
173. Urena P, Kubrusly M, Mannstadt M, et al: The renal PTH/PTHrP receptor is down-regulated in rats with chronic renal failure. Kidney Int 45:605–611, 1994.
174. Urena P, Ferreira A, Morieux C, et al: PTH/PTHrP receptor mRNA is down-regulated in epiphyseal cartilage growth plate of uraemic rats. Nephrol Dial Transplant 11:2008–2016, 1996.
175. Massry S, Coburn J, Lee D, et al: Skeletal resistance to parathyroid hormone in renal failure. Studies in 105 human subjects. Ann Intern Med 78:357–364, 1973.
176. Llach F, Massry S, Singer F, et al: Skeletal resistance to endogenous parathyroid hormone in patients with early renal failure. A possible cause for secondary hyperparathyroidism. J Clin Endocrinol Metab 41:339–345, 1975.
177. Rosenblatt M, Segre GV, Tyler GA, et al: Identification of a receptor-binding region in parathyroid hormone. Endocrinology 107:545–550, 1980.
178. Doppelt SH, Neer RM, Nussbaum SR, et al: Inhibition of the in vivo parathyroid hormone–mediated calcemic response in rats by a synthetic hormone antagonist. Proc Natl Acad Sci U S A 83:7557–7560, 1986.
179. Friedman PA, Gesek FA: Calcium transport in renal epithelial cells. Am J Physiol 264:F181–F198, 1993.
180. Bourdeau J: Mechanisms and regulation of calcium transport in the nephron. Semin Nephrol 13:191–201, 1993.
181. Suki WN: Calcium transport in the nephron. Am J Physiol 237:F1–F6, 1979.
182. Torikai S, Wang M-S, Klein KL, et al: Adenylate cyclase and cell cyclic AMP of rat cortical thick ascending limb of Henle. Kidney Int 20:649–654, 1981.
183. Morel F, Imbert-Teboul M, Chabardes D: Distribution of hormone-dependent adenylate cyclase in the nephron and its physiological significance. Annu Rev Physiol 43:569–581, 1981.
184. Greger R, Lang F, Oberleithner H: Distal site of calcium reabsorption in the rat nephron. Pfluegers Arch Eur J Physiol 374:153–157, 1978.
185. Agus ZS, Gardner LB, Beck LH, et al: Effects of parathyroid hormone on renal tubular reabsorption of calcium, sodium and phosphate. Am J Physiol 224:1143–1148, 1973.
186. Imai M: Effects of parathyroid hormone and N6,O2-dibutyryl cyclic AMP on Ca^{2+} transport across the rabbit distal nephron segments perfused in vitro. Pfluegers Arch Eur J Physiol 390:145–151, 1981.
187. Shareghi GR, Stoner LC: Calcium transport across segments of the rabbit distal nephron in vitro. Am J Physiol 235:F367–F375, 1978.
188. Bouhtiauy I, LaJeunesse D, Brunette MG: The mechanism of parathyroid hormone action on calcium reabsorption by the distal tubule. Endocrinology 128:251–258, 1991.
189. Bacskai BJ, Friedman PA: Activation of latent Ca^{2+} channels in renal epithelial cells by parathyroid hormone. Nature 347:388–391, 1990.
190. Fraser DR, Kodicek E: Regulation of 25-hydroxycholecalciferol-1-hydroxylase activity in kidney by parathyroid hormone. Nature 241:163–166, 1973.
191. Garabedian M, Holick MF, Deluca HF, et al: Control of 25-hydrocholecalciferol metabolism by parathyroid glands. Proc Natl Acad Sci U S A 69:1673–1676, 1972.
192. Takeyama K, Kitanaka S, Sato T, et al: 25-Hydroxyvitamin D_3 1α-hydroxylase and vitamin D synthesis. Science 277:1827–1830, 1997.
193. St Arnaud R, Messerlian S, Moir JM, et al: The 25-hydroxyvitamin D 1-alpha-hydroxylase gene maps to the pseudovitamin D–deficiency rickets (PDDR) disease locus. J Bone Miner Res 12:1552–1559, 1997.
194. Fu GK, Lin D, Zhang MY, et al: Cloning of human 25-hydroxyvitamin D-1 alpha-hydroxylase and mutations causing vitamin D–dependent rickets type 1. Mol Endocrinol 11:1961–1970, 1997.
195. Henry H: Parathyroid hormone modulation of 25-hydroxyvitamin D_3 metabolism by cultured chick kidney cells is mimicked and enhanced by forskolin. Endocrinology 116:503–510, 1985.
196. Murayama A, Takeyama K, Kitanaka S, et al: Positive and negative regulations of the renal 25-hydroxyvitamin D_3 1alpha-hydroxylase gene by parathyroid hormone, calcitonin, and $1\alpha,25(OH)_2D_3$ in intact animals. Endocrinology 140:2224–2231, 1999.
197. Fox J, Mathew MB: Heterogeneous response to PTH in aging rats: Evidence for skeletal PTH resistance. Am J Physiol 260:E933–E937, 1991.
198. Norman AW, Roth J, Orci L: The vitamin D endocrine system: Steroid metabolisms, hormone receptors and biological response. Endocr Rev 3:331–366, 1982.
199. Brenza HL, Kimmel-Jehan C, Jehan F, et al: Parathyroid hormone activation of the 25-hydroxyvitamin D_3-1α-hydroxylase gene promoter. Proc Natl Acad Sci U S A 95:1387–1391, 1998.
200. Kong XF, Zhu XH, Pei YL, et al: Molecular cloning, characterization, and promoter analysis of the human 25-hydroxyvitamin D_3-1α-hydroxylase gene. Proc Natl Acad Sci U S A 96:6988–6993, 1999.
201. Tanaka Y, Lorenc RS, Deluca HF: The role of 1,25-dihydroxyvitamin D_3 and parathyroid hormone in the regulation of chick renal 25-hydroxy-vitamin D_3-24-hydroxylase. Arch Biochem Biophys 171:521–526, 1975.
202. Shigematsu T, Horiuchi N, Ogura Y: Human parathyroid hormone inhibits renal 24-hydroxylase activity of 25-hydroxyvitamin D_3 by a mechanism involving adenosine 3′,5′-monophosphate in rats. Endocrinology 118:1583–1589, 1986.
203. Econs M, Drezner M: Tumor-induced osteomalacia—unveiling a new hormone. N Engl J Med 330:1679–1681, 1994.
204. Wen SF: Micropuncture studies of phosphate transport in the proximal tubule of the dog: The relationship to sodium reabsorption. J Clin Invest 53:143–153, 1974.
205. Amiel C, Kuntziger H, Richet G: Micropuncture study of handling of phosphate by proximal and distal nephron in normal and parathyroidectomized rat: Evidence for distal reabsorption. Pflugers Arch 317:93–109, 1970.
206. Bengele HH, Lechene CP, Alexander EA: Phosphate transport along the inner medullary collecting duct of the rat. Am J Physiol 237:F48–F54, 1979.
207. Pastoriza-Munoz E, Colindres RE, Lassiter WE, et al: Effect of parathyroid hormone on phosphate reabsorption in rat distal convolution. Am J Physiol 235:F321–F330, 1978.
208. Gmaj P, Murer H: Cellular mechanisms of inorganic phosphate transport in kidney. Physiol Rev 66:36–70, 1986.
209. Malmström K, Murer H: Parathyroid hormone inhibits phosphate transport in OK cells but not in LLC-PK1 and JTC-12.P3 cells. Am J Physiol 251:C23–C31, 1986.
210. Caverzasio J, Rizzoli R, Bonjour JV: Sodium-dependent phosphate transport inhibited by parathyroid hormone and cyclic AMP stimulation in an opossum kidney cell line. J Biol Chem 261:3233–3237, 1986.
211. Beck L, Karaplis AC, Amizuka N, et al: Targeted inactivation of *Ntp2* in mice leads to severe renal phosphate wasting, hypercalciuria, and skeletal abnormalities. Proc Natl Acad Sci U S A 95:5372–5377, 1998.
212. Jaeger P, Jones W, Kashgarian M, et al: Parathyroid hormone directly inhibits tubular reabsorption of bicarbonate in normocalcemic rats with chronic hyperparathyroidism. Eur J Clin Invest 17:415–420, 1987.
213. Chambers TJ, Athanasou NA, Fuller K: Effect of parathyroid hormone and calcitonin on the cytoplasmic spreading of isolated osteoclasts. J Endocrinol 102:281–286, 1984.
214. Wong GL: Paracrine interactions in bone-secreted products of osteoblasts permit osteoclasts to respond to parathyroid hormone. J Biol Chem 259:4019–4022, 1984.
215. Perry HM III, Skogen W, Chappel J, et al: Partial characterization of a parathyroid hormone–stimulated resorption factor(s) from osteoblast-like cells. Endocrinology 125:2075–2082, 1989.
216. Parsons JA, Robinson CJ: Calcium shift into bone causing transient hypocalcaemia after injection of parathyroid hormone. Nature 230:581–582, 1971.
217. Talmage RV, Doppelt SH, Fondren FB: An interpretation of acute changes in plasma ^{45}Ca following parathyroid hormone administration to thyroparathyroidectomized rats. Calcif Tissue Res 22:117–128, 1976.
218. Rodan GA, Martin TJ: Role of osteoblasts in hormonal control of bone resorption—a hypothesis. Calcif Tissue Int 33:349–351, 1981.
219. Howard GA, Bottemiller BL, Turner RT, et al: Parathyroid hormone stimulates bone formation and resorption in organ culture: Evidence for a coupling mechanism. Proc Natl Acad Sci U S A 78:3208, 1981.
220. Bingham PJ, Brazell IA, Owen M: The effect of parathyroid extract on cellular activity and plasma calcium levels in vivo. J Endocrinol 45:387–400, 1969.
221. Feldman RS, Krieger NS, Tashjian AH Jr: Effects of parathyroid hormone and calcitonin on osteoclast formation in vitro. Endocrinology 107:1137–1143, 1980.
222. Iida-Klein A, Guo J, Xie LY, et al: Truncation of the carboxyl-terminal region of the parathyroid hormone (PTH)/PTH-related peptide receptor enhances PTH stimulation of adenylate cyclase but not phospholipase C. J Biol Chem 270:8458–8465, 1995.
223. Rouleau MF, Mitchell L, Goltzman D: In vivo distribution of parathyroid hormone receptors in bone: Evidence that a predominant osseous target cell is not the mature osteoblast. Endocrinology 123:187–191, 1988.
224. Guenther HL, Hofstetter W, Stutzer A, et al: Evidence for heterogeneity of the osteoblastic phenotype determined with clonal rat bone cells established from transforming growth factor-β–induced cell colonies grown anchorage independently in semisolid medium. Endocrinology 125:2092–2102, 1989.
225. Rodan GA, Heath JK, Yoon K, et al: Diversity of the osteoblastic phenotype. *In* Cell and Molecular Biology of Vertebrate Hard Tissues. Ciba Foundation Symposium 136. New York, Wiley & Sons, 1988, p 78.

226. Civitelli R, Hruska KA, Jeffrey JJ, et al: Second messenger signaling in the regulation of collagenase production by osteogenic osteosarcoma cells. Endocrinology 124:2928–2934, 1989.
227. Bellows CG, Ishida H, Aubin JE, et al: Parathyroid hormone reversibly suppresses the differentiation of osteoprogenitor cells into functional osteoblasts. Endocrinology 127:3111–3116, 1990.
228. Yoon K, Buenaga R, Rodan GA: Tissue specificity and developmental expression of rat osteopontin. Biochem Biophys Res Commun 148:1129–1136, 1987.
229. Habener JF, Potts JT Jr: Parathyroid physiology and primary hyperparathyroidism. *In* Avioli LV, Krane SM (eds): Metabolic Bone Disease. New York, Academic, 1978, pp 1–147.
230. Finkelstein JS: Pharmacological mechanisms of therapeutics: Parathyroid hormone. *In* Bilezikian JP, Raisz LG, Rodan GA (eds): Principles of Bone Biology. New York, Academic, 1996, pp 993–1005.
231. Mears DC: Effects of parathyroid hormone and thyrocalcitonin on the membrane potential of osteoclasts. Endocrinology 88:1021–1028, 1971.
232. Ferrier J, Ward A, Kanehisa J, et al: Electrophysiological responses of osteoclasts to hormones. J Cell Physiol 128:23–26, 1986.
233. Teti A, Rizzoli R, Zallone AZ: Parathyroid hormone binding to cultured avian osteoclasts. Biochem Biophys Res Commun 174:1217–1222, 1991.
234. Hakeda Y, Hiura K, Sato T, et al: Existence of parathyroid hormone binding sites on murine hemopoietic blast cells. Biochem Biophys Res Commun 163:1481–1486, 1989.
235. Silve CM, Hradek GT, Jones AL, et al: Parathyroid hormone receptor in intact embryonic chicken bone: Characterization and cellular localization. J Cell Biol 94:379–386, 1982.
236. Lomri A, Marie PJ: Distinct effects of calcium- and cyclic AMP–enhancing factors on cytoskeletal synthesis and assembly in mouse osteoblastic cells. Biochim Biophys Acta 1052:179–186, 1990.
237. Urena P, Kong XF, Abou-Samra AB, et al: Parathyroid hormone (PTH)/PTH-related peptide (PTHrP) receptor mRNA are widely distributed in rat tissues. Endocrinology 133:617–623, 1993.
238. Urena P, Iida-Klein A, Kong XF, et al: Regulation of parathyroid hormone (PTH)/PTH-related peptide receptor messenger ribonucleic acid by glucocorticoids and PTH in ROS 17/2.8 and OK cells. Endocrinology 134:451–456, 1994.
239. Lee K, Deeds JD, Chiba S, et al: Parathyroid hormone induces sequential *c-fos* expression in bone cells in vivo: In situ localization of its receptor and *c-fos* messenger ribonucleic acids. Endocrinology 134:441–450, 1994.
240. Wong BR, Rho J, Aaron J, et al: TRANCE is a a novel ligand of the tumor necrosis factor receptor family that activates c-Jun N-terminal kinase in T cells. J Biol Chem 272:25190–25194, 1997.
241. Anderson DA, Maraskovsky E, Billingsley WL, et al: A homologue of the TNF receptor and its ligand enhance T-cell growth and dendritic-cell function. Nature 390:175–179, 1997.
242. Yasuda H, Shima N, Nakagawa N, et al: Osteoclast differentiation factor is a ligand for osteoprotegerin/osteoclastogenesis-inhibitory factor and is identical to TRANCE/RANKL. Proc Natl Acad Sci U S A 95:3597–3602, 1998.
243. Quinn JM, Elliott J, Gillespie MT, et al: A combination of osteoclast differentiation factor and macrophage-colony stimulating factor is sufficient for both human and mouse osteoclast formation in vitro. Endocrinology 139:4424–4427, 1998.
244. Fuller K, Wong B, Fox S, et al: OC activation by TRANCE is necessary and sufficient for osteoblast-mediated activation of bone resorption in osteoclasts. J Exp Med 188:997–1001, 1998.
245. Lacey DL, Timms E, Tan HL, et al: Osteoprotegerin ligand is a cytokine that regulates osteoclast differentiation and activation. Cell 93:165–176, 1998.
246. Simonet SW, Lacey DL, Dunstan CR, et al: Osteoprotegerin: A novel secreted protein involved in the regulation of bone density. Cell 89:309–319, 1997.
247. Suda ET, Goto M, Mochizuki S, et al: Isolation of a novel cytokine from human fibroblasts that specifically inhibits osteoclastogenesis. Biochem Biophys Res Commun 234:137–142, 1997.
248. Bucay N, Sarosi I, Dunstan DR, et al: Osteoprotegerin-deficient mice develop early onset osteoporosis and arterial calcification. Genes Dev 12:1260–1268, 1998.
249. Kong Y, Yoshida H, Sarosi I, et al: OPGL is a key regulator of osteoclastogenesis, lymphocyte development and lymph-node organogenesis. Nature 397:315–323, 1999.
250. Li J, Sarosi I, Yan XQ, et al: RANK is the intrinsic hematopoietic cell surface receptor that controls osteoclastogenesis and regulation of bone mass and calcium metabolism. Proc Natl Acad Sci U S A 15:1566–1571, 2000.
251. Löwik CWGM, van der Pluijm G, Bloys H, et al: Parathyroid hormone (PTH) and PTH-like protein (PLP) stimulate interleukin-6 production by osteogenic cells: A possible role of interleukin-6 in osteoclastogenesis. Biochem Biophys Res Commun 162:1546–1552, 1989.
252. Paliwal I, Insogna K: Partial purification and characterization of the 9,000-dalton bone-resorbing activity from parathyroid hormone–related protein-treated SaOS2 cells (abstract 245). J Bone Miner Res 6(suppl 1):144, 1991.
253. Felix R, Fleisch H, Elford PR: Bone-resorbing cytokines enhance release of macrophage colony-stimulating activity by the osteoblastic cell MC3T3-E1. Calcif Tissue Int 44:356–360, 1989.
254. Lee S, Lorenzo J: Parathyroid hormone stimulates TRANCE and inhibits osteoprotegerin messenger ribonucleic acid expression in murine bone marrow cultures: Correlation with osteoclast-like cell formation. Endocrinology 140:3552–3561, 1999.
255. Partridge N, Walling H, Bloch S, et al: The regulation and regulatory role of collagenase in bone. Crit Rev Eukaryot Gene Expr 6:15–27, 1996.
256. Zhao W, Byrne M, Boyce B, et al: Bone resorption induced by parathyroid hormone is strikingly diminished in collagenase-resistant mutant mice. J Clin Invest 103:517–524, 1999.
257. Martin JT, Moseley JM, Gillespie MT: Parathyroid hormone–related protein: Biochemistry and molecular biology. Crit Rev Biochem Mol Biol 26:377–395, 1991.
258. Albright F: Case records of the Massachusetts General Hospital; case 27461. N Engl J Med 255:789–791, 1941.
259. Stewart AF, Horst R, Deftos LJ, et al: Biochemical evaluation of patients with cancer-associated hypercalcemia. Evidence for humoral and non-humoral groups. N Engl J Med 303:1377–1381, 1980.
260. Moseley JM, Kubota M, Diefenbach-Jagger H, et al: Parathyroid hormone–related protein purified from a human lung cancer cell line. Proc Natl Acad Sci U S A 84:5048–5052, 1987.
261. Suva LJ, Winslow GA, Wettenhall RE, et al: A parathyroid hormone–related protein implicated in malignant hypercalcemia: Cloning and expression. Science 237:893–896, 1987.
262. Strewler GJ, Stern PH, Jacobs JW, et al: Parathyroid hormone–like protein from human renal carcinoma cells. Structural and functional homology with parathyroid hormone. J Clin Invest 80:1803–1807, 1987.
263. Mangin M, Webb AC, Dreyer BE, et al: Identification of a cDNA encoding a parathyroid hormone–like peptide from a human tumor associated with humoral hypercalcemia of malignancy. Proc Natl Acad Sci U S A 85:597–601, 1988.
264. Burtis WJ, Brady TG, Orloff JJ, et al: Immunochemical characterization of circulating parathyroid hormone related protein in patients with humoral hypercalcemia of cancer. N Engl J Med 322:1106–1112, 1990.
265. Ikeda K, Weir EC, Mangin M, et al: Expression of messenger ribonucleic acids encoding a parathyroid hormone–like peptide in normal human and animal tissues with abnormal expression in human parathyroid adenomas and rat keratinocytes. Mol Endocrinol 2:1230–1236, 1988.
266. Thiede MA, Rodan GA: Expression of a calcium-mobilizing parathyroid hormone–like peptide in lactating mammary tissue. Science 242:278–280, 1988.
267. Burton PBJ, Moniz C, Quirke P, et al: Parathyroid hormone–related peptide in the human fetal urogenital tract. Mol Cell Endocrinol 69:R13–R17, 1990.
268. Ferguson JE, Gorman JV, Bruns DE, et al: Abundant expression of parathyroid hormone–related protein in human amnion and its association with labor. Physiology 89:8384–8388, 1992.
269. van de Stolpe A, Karperien M, Löwik CWGM, et al: Parathyroid hormone–related peptide as an endogenous inducer of parietal endoderm differentiation. J Cell Biol 120:235–243, 1993.
270. Karaplis AC, Luz A, Glowacki J, et al: Lethal skeletal dysplasia from targeted disruption of the parathyroid hormone–related peptide gene. Genes Dev 8:277–289, 1994.
271. Weir EC, Philbrick WM, Amling M, et al: Targeted overexpression of parathyroid hormone–related peptide in chondrocytes causes skeletal dysplasia and delayed endochondral bone formation. Proc Natl Acad Sci U S A 93:10240–10245, 1996.
272. Mangin M, Ikeda K, Dreyer BE, et al: Isolation and characterization of the human parathyroid hormone–like peptide gene. Proc Natl Acad Sci U S A 86:2408–2412, 1989.
273. Pausova Z, Morgan K, Fujiwara TM, et al: Molecular characterization of an intragenic minisatellite (VNTR) polymorphism in the human parathyroid hormone–related peptide gene in chromosome 12p12.1-11.2. Genomics 17:243–244, 1993.
274. Wojcik SF, Schanbacher FL, McCauley LK, et al: Cloning of bovine parathyroid hormone–related peptide (PTHrP) cDNA and expression of PTHrP mRNA in the bovine mammary gland. J Mol Endocrinol 20:271–280, 1998.
275. Rubin DA, Hellman P, Zon LI, et al: A G protein–coupled receptor from zebrafish is activated by human parathyroid hormone and not by human or teleost parathyroid hormone–related peptide: Implications for the evolutionary conservation of calcium-regulating peptide hormones. J Biol Chem 274:23035–23042, 1999.
276. Rubin DA, Jüppner H: Zebrafish express the common parathyroid hormone/parathyroid hormone–related peptide (PTH1R) and a novel receptor (PTH3R) that is preferentially activated by mammalian and fugufish parathyroid hormone–related peptide. J Biol Chem 84:28185–28190, 1999.
277. Kemp BE, Moseley JM, Rodda CP, et al: Parathyroid hormone–related protein of malignancy: Active synthetic fragments. Science 238:1568–1570, 1987.
278. Horiuchi N, Caulfield MP, Fisher JE, et al: Similarity of synthetic peptide from human tumor to parathyroid hormone in vivo and in vitro. Science 238:1566–1568, 1987.
279. Fraher LJ, Hodsman AB, Jonas K, et al: A comparison of the in vivo biochemical responses to exogenous parathyroid hormone-(1–34) [PTH-(1–34)] and PTH-related peptide-(1–34) in man. J Clin Endocrinol Metab 75:417–423, 1992.
280. Everhart-Caye M, Inzucchi SE, Guinness-Henry J, et al: Parathyroid hormone (PTH)-related protein(1–36) is equipotent to PTH(1–34) in humans. J Clin Endocrinol Metab 81:199–208, 1996.
281. Abou-Samra A-B, Uneno S, Jüppner H, et al: Non-homologous sequences of parathyroid hormone and the parathyroid hormone related peptide bind to a common receptor on ROS 17/2.8 cells. Endocrinology 125:2215–2217, 1989.
282. Caulfield MP, Rosenblatt M: Parathyroid hormone-receptor interactions. Trends Endocrinol Metab 2:164–168, 1990.
283. Gardella TJ, Luck MD, Jensen GS, et al: Converting parathyroid hormone–related peptide (PTHrP) into a potent PTH-2 receptor agonist. J Biol Chem 271:19888–19893, 1996.
284. Behar V, Nakamoto C, Greenberg Z, et al: Histidine at position 5 is the specificity "switch" between two parathyroid hormone receptor subtypes. Endocrinology 137:4217–4224, 1996.
285. Gardella TJ, Luck MD, Wilson AK, et al: Parathyroid hormone (PTH)/PTH-related peptide hybrid peptides reveal functional interactions between the 1–14 and 15–34 domains of the ligand. J Biol Chem 270:6584–6588, 1995.
286. Wu TL, Vasavada RC, Yang K, et al: Structural and physiological characterization of the mid-region secretory species of parathyroid hormone–related protein. J Biol Chem 271:24371–24381, 1996.
287. Yang KH, dePapp AE, Soifer NE, et al: Parathyroid hormone–related protein: Evidence for isoform- and tissue-specific posttranslational processing. Biochemistry 33:7460–7469, 1994.
288. Jüppner H, Abou-Samra AB, Uneno S, et al: The parathyroid hormone–like peptide associated with humoral hypercalcemia of malignancy and parathyroid hormone bind

to the same receptor on the plasma membrane of ROS 17/2.8 cells. J Biol Chem 263:8557–8560, 1988.
289. Wu TL, Soifer NE, Burtis WJ, et al: Glycosylation of parathyroid hormone–related peptide secreted by human epidermal keratinocytes. J Clin Endocrinol Metab 73:1002–1007, 1991.
290. Orloff JJ, Soifer NE, Fodero JP, et al: Accumulation of carboxy-terminal fragments of parathyroid hormone–related protein in renal failure. Kidney Int 43:1371–1376, 1993.
291. Fenton AJ, Kemp BE, Hammonds RG Jr, et al: A potent inhibitor of osteoclastic bone resorption within a highly conserved pentapeptide region of parathyroid hormone–related protein PTHrP(107–111). Endocrinology 129:3424–3426, 1991.
292. Fenton AJ, Kemp BE, Kent GN, et al: A carboxyl-terminal peptide from the parathyroid hormone–related protein inhibits bone resorption by osteoclasts. Endocrinology 129:1762–1768, 1991.
293. Cornish J, Callon K, Lin C, et al: Stimulation of osteoblast proliferation by C-terminal fragments of parathyroid hormone–related protein. J Bone Miner Res 14:915–922, 1999.
294. Sone T, Kohno H, Kikuchi H, et al: Human parathyroid hormone–related peptide-(107–111) does not inhibit bone resorption in neonatal mouse calvariae. Endocrinology 131:2742–2746, 1992.
295. Cornish J, Callon KE, Nicholson GC, et al: Parathyroid hormone–related protein-(107–139) inhibits bone resorption in vivo. Endocrinology 138:1299–1304, 1997.
296. Somjen D, Binderman I, Schlüter K, et al: Stimulation by defined parathyroid hormone fragments of cell proliferation in skeletal-derived cell cultures. Biochem J 272:781–785, 1990.
297. Kaji H, Sugimoto T, Kanatani M, et al: Carboxyl-terminal peptides from parathyroid hormone–related protein stimulate osteoclast-like cell formation. Endocrinology 136:842–848, 1995.
298. Schlüter K-D, Hellstern H, Wingender E, et al: The central part of parathyroid hormone stimulates thymidine incorporation of chondrocytes. J Biol Chem 264:11087–11092, 1989.
299. Jouishomme H, Whitfield JF, Chakravarthy B, et al: The protein kinase-C activation domain of the parathyroid hormone. Endocrinology 130:53–59, 1992.
300. Neugebauer W, Surewicz WK, Gordon HL, et al: Structural elements of human parathyroid hormone and their possible relation to biological activities. Biochemistry 31:2056–2063, 1992.
301. Rixon RH, Whitfield JF, Gagnon L, et al: Parathyroid hormone fragments may stimulate bone growth in ovariectomized rats by activating adenylyl cyclase. J Bone Miner Res 9:1179–1189, 1994.
302. Kovacs CS, Lanske B, Hunzelman JL, et al: Parathyroid hormone–related peptide (PTHrP) regulates fetal placental calcium transport through a receptor distinct from the PTH/PTHrP receptor. Proc Natl Acad Sci U S A 93:15233–15238, 1996.
303. Orloff JJ, Ganz MB, Nathanson H, et al: A midregion parathyroid hormone–related peptide mobilizes cytosolic calcium and stimulates formation of inositol trisphosphate in a squamous carcinoma cell line. Endocrinology 137:5376–5385, 1996.
304. Fukayama S, Tashjian AH, Davis JN: Signaling by N- and C-terminal sequences of parathyroid hormone–related protein in hippocampal neurons. Proc Natl Acad Sci U S A 92:10182–10186, 1995.
305. Yamamoto S, Morimoto I, Yanagihara N, et al: Parathyroid hormone–related peptide-(1–34) [PTHrP-(1–34)] induces vasopressin release from the rat supraoptic nucleus in vitro through a novel receptor distinct from a type I or type II PTH/PTHrP receptor. Endocrinology 138:2066–2072, 1997.
306. Yamamoto S, Morimoto I, Zeki K, et al: Centrally administered parathyroid hormone (PTH)-related protein (1–34) but not PTH(1–34) stimulates arginine-vasopressin secretion and its messenger ribonucleic acid expression in supraoptic nucleus of the conscious rats. Endocrinology 139:383–388, 1998.
307. Orloff JJ, Ganz MB, Ribaudo AE, et al: Analysis of PTHrP binding and signal transduction mechanisms in benign and malignant squamous cells. Am J Physiol 262:E599–E607, 1992.
308. Gaich G, Orloff JJ, Atillasoy EJ, et al: Amino-terminal parathyroid hormone–related protein: Specific binding and cytosolic calcium responses in rat insulinoma cells. Endocrinology 132:1402–1409, 1993.
309. Soifer NE, Dee K, Insogna KL, et al: Parathyroid hormone–related protein. Evidence for secretion of a novel mid-region fragment by three different cell types. J Biol Chem 267:18236–18243, 1992.
310. Burtis WJ, Dann P, Gaich GA, et al: A high abundance midregion species of parathyroid hormone–related protein: Immunological and chromatographic characterization in plasma. J Clin Endocrinol Metab 78:317–322, 1994.
311. Kovacs CS, Kronenberg HM: Maternal-fetal calcium and bone metabolism during pregnancy, puerperium, and lactation. Endocr Rev 18:832–872, 1997.
312. Rodda CP, Kubota M, Heath JA, et al: Evidence for a novel parathyroid hormone–related protein in fetal lamb parathyroid glands and sheep placenta: Comparison with a similar protein implicated in humoral hypercalcemia of malignancy. J Endocrinol 117:261–271, 1988.
313. Care A, Caple I, Abbas S, et al: The effect of fetal thyroparathyroidectomy on the transport of calcium across the ovine placenta to the fetus. Placenta 4:271–277, 1986.
314. Abbas SK, Pickard DW, Rodda CP, et al: Stimulation of ovine placental calcium transport by purified natural and recombinant parathyroid hormone–related protein (PTHrP) preparations. Q J Exp Physiol 74:549–552, 1989.
315. Garner S, Boass A, Toverud SU: Parathyroid hormone is not required for normal milk composition or secretion or lactation-associated bone loss in normocalcemic rats. J Bone Miner Res 5:69–75, 1990.
316. Halloran B, DeLuca HF: Calcium transport in small intestine during pregnancy and lactation. Am J Physiol 239:E64–E68, 1980.
317. Ratcliffe WA, Thompson GE, Care AD, et al: Production of parathyroid hormone–related protein by the mammary gland of the goat. J Endocrinol 133:87–93, 1980.
318. Yamamoto M, Duong LT, Fisher JE, et al: Suckling-mediated increases in urinary phosphate and 3′, 5′-cyclic adenosine monophosphate excretion in lactating rats: Possible systemic effect of parathyroid hormone–related protein. Endocrinology 129:2614–2622, 1991.
319. Grill V, Hillary J, Ho PMW, et al: Parathyroid hormone–related protein: A possible endocrine function in lactation. Clin Endocrinol 37:405–410, 1992.
320. Dobnig H, Kainer F, Stepan V, et al: Elevated parathyroid hormone–related peptide levels after human gestation: Relationship to changes in bone and mineral metabolism. J Clin Endocrinol Metab 80:3699–3707, 1995.
321. Kovacs C, Chik C: Hyperprolactinemia caused by lactation and pituitary adenomas is associated with altered serum calcium, phosphate, parathyroid hormone (PTH), and PTH-related peptide levels. J Clin Endocrinol Metab 80:3036–3042, 1995.
322. Sowers M, Hollis B, Shapiro B, et al: Elevated parathyroid hormone–related peptide associated with lactation and bone density loss. JAMA 276:549–554, 1996.
323. Cross N, Hillman L, Allen S, et al: Calcium homeostasis and bone metabolism during pregnancy, lactation, and postweaning: A longitudinal study. Am J Clin Nutr 61:514-523, 1995.
324. Reid I, Wattie D, Evans M, et al: Post-pregnancy osteoporosis associated with hypercalcaemia. Clin Endocrinol (Oxf) 37:298–303, 1992.
325. Khosla S, van Heerden JA, Gharib H, et al: Parathyroid hormone–related protein and hypercalcemia secondary to massive mammary hyperplasia. N Engl J Med 322:1157, 1990.
326. Goff J, Reinhardt T, Lee S, et al: Parathyroid hormone–related peptide content of bovine milk and calf blood assessed by radioimmunoassay and bioassay. Endocrinology 129:2815–2819, 1991.
327. Wysolmerski J, Philbrick W, Dunbar M, et al: Rescue of the parathyroid hormone–related protein knockout mouse demonstrates that parathyroid hormone–related protein is essential for mammary gland development. Development 125:1285–1294, 1998.
328. Guise TA, Yin JJ, Taylor SD, et al: Evidence for a causal role of parathyroid hormone–related protein in the pathogenesis of human breast cancer–mediated osteolysis. J Clin Invest 98:1544–1549, 1996.
329. Amizuka N, Warshawsky H, Henderson JE, et al: Parathyroid hormone–related peptide–depleted mice show abnormal epiphyseal cartilage development and altered endochondral bone formation. J Cell Biol 126:1611–1623, 1994.
330. Lee K, Lanske B, Karaplis AC, et al: Parathyroid hormone–related peptide delays terminal differentiation of chondrocytes during endochondral bone development. Endocrinology 137:5109–5118, 1996.
331. Schipani E, Lanske B, Hunzelman J, et al: Targeted expression of constitutively active PTH/PTHrP receptors delays endochondral bone formation and rescues PTHrP-less mice. Proc Natl Acad Sci U S A 94:13689–13694, 1997.
332. Philbrick WM, Dreyer BE, Nakchbandi IA, et al: Parathyroid hormone–related protein is required for tooth eruption. Proc Natl Acad Sci U S A 95:11846–11851, 1998.
333. Jobert AS, Zhang P, Couvineau A, et al: Absence of functional receptors for parathyroid hormone and parathyroid hormone–related peptide in Blomstrand chondrodysplasia. J Clin Invest 102:34–40, 1998.
334. Zhang P, Jobert AS, Couvineau A, et al: A homozygous inactivating mutation in the parathyroid hormone/parathyroid hormone–related peptide receptor causing Blomstrand chondrodysplasia. J Clin Endocrinol Metab 83:3365–3368, 1998.
335. Karaplis AC, Bin He MT, Nguyen A, et al: Inactivating mutation in the human parathyroid hormone receptor type 1 gene in Blomstrand chondrodysplasia. Endocrinology 139:5255–5258, 1998.
336. Karperien MC, van der Harten HJ, van Schooten R, et al: A frame-shift mutation in the type I parathyroid hormone/parathyroid hormone–related peptide receptor causing Blomstrand lethal osteochondrodysplasia. J Clin Endocrinol Metab 84:3713–3720, 1999.
337. Schipani E, Kruse K, Jüppner H: A constitutively active mutant PTH-PTHrP receptor in Jansen-type metaphyseal chondrodysplasia. Science 268:98–100, 1995.
338. Schipani E, Langman CB, Parfitt AM, et al: Constitutively activated receptors for parathyroid hormone and parathyroid hormone–related peptide in Jansen's metaphyseal chondrodysplasia. N Engl J Med 335:708–714, 1996.
339. Minagawa M, Arakawa K, Minamitani K, et al: Jansen-type metaphyseal chondrodysplasia: Analysis of PTH/PTH-related protein receptor messenger RNA by the reverse transcription–polymerase chain reaction method. Endocr J 44:493–499, 1997.
340. Schipani E, Langman CB, Hunzelman J, et al: A novel PTH/PTHrP receptor mutation in Jansen's metaphyseal chondrodysplasia. J Clin Endocrinol Metab 84:3052–3057, 1999.
341. Bitgood MJ, McMahon AP: *Hedgehog* and *Bmp* genes are coexpressed at many diverse sites of cell-cell interaction in the mouse embryo. Dev Biol 172:126–138, 1995.
342. Stone DM, Hynes M, Armanini M, et al: The tumour-suppressor gene *patched* encodes a candidate receptor for Sonic hedgehog. Nature 384:129–134, 1996.
343. Marigo V, Davey RA, Zuo Y, et al: Biochemical evidence that Patched is the Hedgehog receptor. Nature 384:176–179, 1996.
344. St-Jacques B, Hammerschmidt M, McMahon A: Indian hedgehog signaling regulates proliferation and differentiation of chondrocytes and is essential for bone formation. Genes Dev 13:2072–2086, 1999.
345. Chung UI, Lanske B, Lee K, et al: The parathyroid hormone/parathyroid hormone–related peptide receptor coordinates endochondral bone development by directly controlling chondrocyte differentiation. Proc Natl Acad Sci U S A 95:13030–13035, 1998.
346. Suda N, Gillespie MT, Traianedes K, et al: Expression of parathyroid hormone–related protein in cells of osteoblast lineage. J Cell Physiol 166:94–104, 1996.
347. Philbrick WM, Wysolmerski JJ, Galbraith S, et al: Defining the roles of parathyroid hormone–related protein in normal physiology. Physiol Rev 76:127–173, 1996.
348. Wysolmerski JJ, Broadus AE, Zhou J, et al: Overexpression of parathyroid hormone–related protein in the skin of transgenic mice interferes with hair follicle development. Proc Natl Acad Sci U S A 91:1133–1137, 1994.
349. Qian J, Lorenz J, Maeda S, et al: Reduced blood pressure and increased sensitivity of the vasculature to parathyroid hormone–related protein (PTHrP) in transgenic mice overexpressing the PTH/PTHrP receptor in vascular smooth muscle. Endocrinology 140:1826–1833, 1999.

350. Maeda S, Sutliff R, Qian J, et al: Targeted overexpression of parathyroid hormone–related protein (PTHrP) to vascular smooth muscle in transgenic mice lowers blood pressure and alters vascular contractility. Endocrinology 140:1815–1825, 1999.
351. Thiede MA, Daifotis AG, Weir EC, et al: Intrauterine occupancy controls expression of the parathyroid hormone–related peptide gene in preterm rat myometrium. Proc Natl Acad Sci U S A 87:6969–6973, 1990.
352. Brines ML, Broadus AE: Parathyroid hormone–related protein markedly potentiates depolarization-induced catecholamine release in PC12 cells via L-type voltage-sensitive Ca^{2+} channels. Endocrinology 140:646–651, 1999.
353. Shigeno C, Yamamoto I, Kitamura N, et al: Interaction of human parathyroid hormone–related peptide with parathyroid hormone receptors in clonal rat osteosarcoma cells. J Biol Chem 34:18369–18377, 1988.
354. Nissenson RA, Diep D, Strewler GJ: Synthetic peptides comprising the amino-terminal sequence of a parathyroid hormone–like protein from human malignancies: Binding to parathyroid hormone receptors and activation of adenylate cyclase in bone cells and kidney. J Biol Chem 263:12866–12871, 1988.
355. Orloff JJ, Wu TL, Heath HW, et al: Characterization of canine renal receptors for the parathyroid hormone–like protein associated with humoral hypercalcemia of malignancy. J Biol Chem 264:6097–6103, 1989.
356. Usdin TB: Tip39: A new neuropeptide and PTH2-receptor agonist from hypothalamus. Nat Neurosci 2:941–943, 1999.
357. Usdin TB, Gruber C, Bonner TI: Identification and functional expression of a receptor selectively recognizing parathyroid hormone, the PTH2 receptor. J Biol Chem 270:15455–15458, 1995.
358. Hoare SR, Bonner TI, Usdin TB: Comparison of rat and human parathyroid hormone 2 (PTH2) receptor activation: PTH is a low potency partial agonist at the rat PTH2 receptor. Endocrinology 140:4419–4425, 1999.
359. Schneider H, Feyen JHM, Seuwen K, et al: Cloning and functional expression of a human parathyroid hormone (parathormone)/parathormone-related peptide receptor. Eur J Pharmacol 246:149–155, 1993.
360. Eggenberger M, Flühmann B, Muff R, et al: Structure of a parathyroid hormone/parathyroid hormone–related peptide receptor of the human cerebellum and functional expression in human neuroblastoma SK-N-MC cells. Brain Res Mol Brain Res 36:127–136, 1997.
361. Karperien M, van Dijk TB, Hoeijmakers T, et al: Expression pattern of parathyroid hormone/parathyroid hormone related peptide receptor mRNA in mouse postimplantation embryos indicates involvement in multiple developmental processes. Mech Dev 47:29–42, 1994.
362. Pausova Z, Bourdon J, Clayton D, et al: Cloning of a parathyroid hormone/parathyroid hormone–related peptide receptor (PTHR) cDNA from a rat osteosarcoma (UMR106) cell line: Chromosomal assignment of the gene in the human, mouse, and rat genomes. Genomics 20:20–26, 1994.
363. Smith DP, Zang XY, Frolik CA, et al: Structure and functional expression of a complementary DNA for porcine parathyroid hormone/parathyroid hormone–related peptide receptor. Biochim Biophys Acta 1307:339–347, 1996.
364. Smock S, Vogt G, Castleberry T, et al: Molecular cloning and functional characterization of the canine parathyroid hormone receptor 1 (PTH1). J Bone Miner Res 14(suppl 1):288, 1999.
365. Bergwitz C, Klein P, Kohno H, et al: Identification, functional characterization, and developmental expression of two nonallelic parathyroid hormone (PTH)/PTH related peptide (PTHrP) receptor isoforms in *Xenopus laevis* (Daudin). Endocrinology 139:723–732, 1998.
366. Tian J, Smorgorzewski M, Kedes L, et al: Parathyroid hormone–parathyroid hormone related protein receptor messenger RNA is present in many tissues besides the kidney. Am J Nephrol 13:210–213, 1993.
367. McKee RL, Goldman MF, Caulfield MP, et al. The 7–34 fragment of human hypercalcemia factor is a partial agonist/antagonist for parathyroid hormone–stimulated cAMP production. Endocrinology 122:3008–3010, 1988.
368. Chorev M, Goodman ME, McKee RL, et al. Modifications of position 12 in parathyroid hormone and parathyroid hormone related protein: Toward the design of highly potent antagonists. Biochemistry 29:1580–1586, 1990.
369. Chorev M, Roubini E, Goodman ME, et al: Effects of hydrophobic substitutions at position 18 on the potency of parathyroid hormone antagonists. Int J Pept Protein Res 36:465–470, 1990.
370. Yamaguchi DT, Hahn TJ, Iida-Klein A, et al: Parathyroid hormone–activated calcium channels in an osteoblast-like clonal osteosarcoma cell line. cAMP-dependent and cAMP-independent calcium channels. J Biol Chem 262:7711–7718, 1987.
371. Yamaguchi DT, Kleeman CR, Muallem S: Protein kinase C–activated calcium channel in the osteoblast-like clonal osteosarcoma cell line UMR-106. J Biol Chem 262:14967–14973, 1987.
372. Cole JA, Eber SL, Poelling RE, et al: A dual mechanism for regulation of kidney phosphate transport by parathyroid hormone. Am J Physiol 253:E221–E227, 1987.
373. Schipani E, Weinstein LS, Bergwitz C, et al: Pseudohypoparathyroidism type Ib is not caused by mutations in the coding exons of the human parathyroid hormone (PTH)/PTH-related peptide receptor gene. J Clin Endocrinol Metab 80:1611–1621, 1995.
374. Bettoun JD, Minagawa M, Kwan MY, et al: Cloning and characterization of the promoter regions of the human parathyroid hormone (PTH)/PTH-related peptide receptor gene. Analysis of deoxyribonucleic acid from normal subjects and patients with pseudohypoparathyroidism type Ib. J Clin Endocrinol Metab 82:1031–1040, 1997.
375. Manen D, Palmer G, Bonjour J, et al: Sequence and activity of parathyroid hormone/parathyroid hormone–related protein receptor promoter region in human osteoblast-like cells. Gene 218:49–56, 1998.
376. McCuaig KA, Clarke JC, White JH: Molecular cloning of the gene encoding the mouse parathyroid hormone/parathyroid hormone–related peptide receptor. Proc Natl Acad Sci U S A 91:5051–5055, 1994.
377. Kong XF, Schipani E, Lanske B, et al: The rat, mouse and human genes encoding the receptor for parathyroid hormone and parathyroid hormone–related peptide are highly homologous. Biochem Biophys Res Commun 200:1290–1299, 1994.
378. McCuaig KA, Lee H, Clarke JC, et al: Parathyoid hormone/parathyroid hormone related peptide receptor gene transcripts are expressed from tissue-specific and ubiquitous promotors. Nucleic Acids Res 23:1948–1955, 1995.
379. Joun H, Lanske B, Karperien M, et al: Tissue-specific transcription start sites and alternative splicing of the parathyroid hormone (PTH)/PTH-related peptide (PTHrP) receptor gene: A new PTH/PTHrP receptor splice variant that lacks the signal peptide. Endocrinology 138:1742–1749, 1997.
380. Bettoun JD, Minagawa M, Hendy GN, et al: Developmental upregulation of the human parathyroid hormone (PTH)/PTH-related peptide receptor gene expression from conserved and human-specific promoters. J Clin Invest 102:958–967, 1998.
381. Giannoukos G, Williams L, Chilco P, et al: Characterization of an element within the rat parathyroid hormone/parathyroid hormone–related peptide receptor gene promoter that enhances expression in osteoblastic osteosarcoma 17/2.8 cells. Biochem Biophys Res Commun 258:336–340, 1999.
382. Hustmyer FG, Schipani E, Peacock M: BsmI polymorphism at the parathyroid hormone receptor locus (PTHR) in three populations. Hum Mol Genet 2:1330, 1993.
383. Schipani E, Hustmyer FG, Bergwitz C, et al: Polymorphism in exon M7 of the PTHR gene. Hum Mol Genet 3:1210, 1994.
384. Jüppner H: Molecular cloning and characterization of a parathyroid hormone (PTH)/PTH-related peptide (PTHrP) receptor: A member of an ancient family of G protein–coupled receptors. Curr Opin Nephrol Hypertens 3:371–378, 1994.
385. Jüppner H, Schipani E: Receptors for parathyroid hormone and parathyroid hormone–related peptide: From molecular cloning to definition of diseases. Curr Opin Nephrol Hypertens 5:300–306, 1996.
386. Lee C, Gardella TJ, Abou-Samra AB, et al: Role of the extracellular regions of the parathyroid hormone (PTH)/PTH-related peptide receptor in hormone binding. Endocrinology 135:1488–1495, 1994.
387. Jüppner H, Schipani E, Bringhurst FR, et al: The extracellular, amino-terminal region of the parathyroid hormone (PTH)/PTH-related peptide (PTHrP) receptor determines the binding affinity for carboxyl-terminal fragments of PTH(1–34). Endocrinology 134:879–884, 1994.
388. Ishihara T, Nakamura S, Kaziro Y, et al: Molecular cloning and expression of a cDNA encoding the secretin receptor. EMBO J 10:1635–1641, 1991.
389. Lin HY, Harris TL, Flannery MS, et al: Expression cloning of an adenylate cyclase–coupled calcitonin receptor. Science 254:1022–1024, 1991.
390. Kolakowski LFJ: GCRDb: A G-protein–coupled receptor database. Receptors Channels 2:1–7, 1994.
391. Sulston J, Du Z, Thomas K, et al: The *C. elegans* genome sequencing project: A beginning. Nature 356:37–41, 1992.
392. Reagan JD: Expression cloning of an insect diuretic hormone receptor. A member of the calcitonin/secretin receptor family. J Biol Chem 269:9–12, 1994.
393. Reagan JD: Molecular cloning and function expression of a diuretic hormone receptor from the house cricket, *Acheta domesticus*. Insect Biochem Mol Biol 26:1–6, 1996.
394. Qi LJ, Leung A, Xiong Y, et al: Extracellular cysteines of the corticotropin-releasing factor receptor are critical for ligand interaction. Biochemistry 36:12442–12448, 1997.
395. Baud V, Chissoe SL, Viegas-Pequignot E, et al: EMR1, an unusual member in the family of hormone receptors with seven transmembrane segments. Genomics 26:334–344, 1995.
396. Hamann J, Eichler W, Hamann D, et al: Expression cloning and chromosomal mapping of the leukocyte activation antigen CD97, a new seven-span transmembrane molecule of the secretin receptor superfamily with an unusual extracellular domain. J Immunol 155:1942–1950, 1995.
397. Abe J, Suzuki H, Notoya M, et al: Ig-hepta, a novel member of the G protein–coupled hepta-helical receptor (GPCR) family that has immunoglobulin-like repeats in a long N-terminal extracellular domain and defines a new subfamily of GPCRs. J Biol Chem 274:19957–19964, 1999.
398. Usui T, Shima Y, Shimada Y, et al: Flamingo, a seven-pass transmembrane cadherin, regulates planar cell polarity under the control of Frizzled. Cell 98:585–595, 1999.
399. Potts JT Jr, Tregear GW, Keutmann HT, et al: Synthesis of a biologically active N-terminal tetratriacontapeptide of parathyroid hormone. Proc Natl Acad Sci U S A 68:63–67, 1971.
400. Tregear GW, Van Rietschoten J, Greene E, et al: Bovine parathyroid hormone: Minimum chain length of synthetic peptide required for biological activity. Endocrinology 93:1349–1353, 1973.
401. Nussbaum SR, Rosenblatt M, Potts JT Jr: Parathyroid hormone/renal receptor interactions: Demonstration of two receptor-binding domains. J Biol Chem 255:10183–10187, 1980.
402. Goltzman D, Peytremann A, Callahan E, et al: Analysis of the requirements for parathyroid hormone action in renal membranes with the use of inhibiting analogues. J Biol Chem 250:3199–3203, 1975.
403. Rosenblatt M, Callahan EN, Mahaffey JE, et al: Parathyroid hormone inhibitors: Design, synthesis, and biologic evaluation of hormone analogues. J Biol Chem 252:5847–5851, 1977.
404. Segre GV, Rosenblatt M, Reiner BL, et al: Characterization of parathyroid hormone receptors in canine renal cortical plasma membranes using a radioiodinated sulfur-free hormone analogue: Correlation of binding with adenylate cyclase activity. J Biol Chem 254:6980–6986, 1979.
405. Horiuchi N, Holick MF, Potts JT Jr, et al: A parathyroid hormone inhibitor in vivo: Design and biologic evaluation of a hormone analog. Science 220:1053–1055, 1983.
406. Kunkel TA: Rapid and efficient site-specific mutagenesis without phenotypic selection. Proc Natl Acad Sci U S A 82:488–492, 1985.
407. Gardella TJ, Axelrod D, Rubin D, et al: Mutational analysis of the receptor-activating region of human parathyroid hormone. J Biol Chem 266:13141–13146, 1991.
408. Gardella TJ, Jüppner H, Wilson AK, et al: Determinants of [Arg²]PTH-(1–34) binding and signaling in the transmembrane region of the parathyroid hormone receptor. Endocrinology 135:1186–1194, 1994.

409. Adams A, Bisello A, Chorev M, et al: Arginine 186 in the extracellular N-terminal region of the human parathyroid hormone 1 receptor is essential for contact with position 13 of the hormone. Mol Endocrinol 12:1673–1683, 1998.
410. Bisello A, Adams AE, Mierke DF, et al: Parathyroid hormone-receptor interactions identified directly by photocross-linking and molecular modeling studies. J Biol Chem 273:22498–22505, 1998.
411. Mannstadt M, Luck M, Gardella TJ, et al: Evidence for a ligand interaction site at the amino-terminus of the PTH/PTHrP receptor from crosslinking and mutational studies. J Biol Chem 273:16890–16896, 1998.
412. Greenberg Z, Bisello A, Rosenblatt M, et al: Identification of a novel contact domain between a residue in the principal binding domain of parathyroid hormone (PTH) and the first extracellular loop of the PTH-1 receptor. J Bone Miner Res 14(suppl):F393, 1999.
413. Carter P, Shimizu M, Luck M, et al: The hydrophobic residues phenylalanine 184 and leucine 187 in the type-1 parathyroid hormone (PTH) receptor functionally interact with the amino-terminal portion of PTH-(1–34). J Biol Chem 274:31955–31960, 1999.
414. Bergwitz C, Jusseaume SA, Luck MD, et al: Residues in the membrane-spanning and extracellular regions of the parathyroid hormone (PTH)-2 receptor determine signaling selectivity for PTH and PTH-related peptide. J Biol Chem 272:28861–28868, 1997.
415. Turner PR, Mefford S, Bambino T, et al: Transmembrane residues together with the amino-terminus limit the response of the parathyroid hormone (PTH) 2 receptor to PTH-related peptide. J Biol Chem 273:3830–3837, 1998.
416. Lee C, Luck MD, Jüppner H, et al: Homolog-scanning mutagenesis of the parathyroid hormone (PTH) receptor reveals PTH-(1–34) binding determinants in the third extracellular loop. Mol Endocrinol 9:1269–1278, 1995.
417. Iida-Klein A, Guo J, Takamura M, et al: Mutations in the second cytoplasmic loop of the rat parathyroid hormone (PTH)/PTH-related protein receptor result in selective loss of PTH-stimulated phospholipase C activity. J Biol Chem 272:6882–6889, 1997.
418. Huang Z, Chen Y, Pratt S, et al: The N-terminal region of the third intracellular loop of the parathyroid hormone (PTH)/PTH-related peptide receptor is critical for coupling to cAMP and inositol phosphate/Ca^{2+} signal transduction pathways. J Biol Chem 271:33382–33389, 1996.
419. Sheikh SP, Vilardarga JP, Baranski TJ, et al: Similar structures and shared switch mechanisms of the beta2-adrenoceptor and the parathyroid hormone receptor. Zn(II) bridges between helices III and VI block activation. J Biol Chem 274:17033–17041, 1999.
420. Malecz N, Bambino T, Bencsik M, et al: Identification of phosphorylation sites in the G protein–coupled receptor for parathyroid hormone. Receptor phosphorylation is not required for agonist-induced internalization. Mol Endocrinol 12:1846–1856, 1998.
421. Qian F, Leung A, Abou-Samra A: Agonist-dependent phosphorylation of the parathyroid hormone/parathyroid hormone–related peptide receptor. Biochemistry 37:6240–6246, 1998.
422. Gardella TJ, Luck MD, Fan M-H, et al: Transmembrane residues of the parathyroid hormone (PTH)/PTH-related peptide receptor that specifically affect binding and signaling by agonist ligands. J Biol Chem 271:12820–12825, 1996.
423. Turner PR, Bambino T, Nissenson RA: A putative selectivity filter in the G-protein–coupled receptors for parathyroid hormone and secretin. J Biol Chem 271:9205–9208, 1996.
424. Turner PR, Bambino T, Nissenson RA: Mutations of neighboring polar residues on the second transmembrane helix disrupt signaling by the parathyroid hormone receptor. Mol Endocrinol 10:132–139, 1996.
425. Bergwitz C, Gardella TJ, Flannery MR, et al: Full activation of chimeric receptors by hybrids between parathyroid hormone and calcitonin. J Biol Chem 271:26469–26472, 1996.
426. Luck M, Carter P, Gardella T: The (1–14) fragment of parathyroid hormone (PTH) activates intact and amino-terminally truncated PTH-1 receptors. Mol Endocrinol 13:670–680, 1999.
427. Shimizu M, Potts JT Jr, Gardella TJ: Minimization of parathyroid hormone: Novel amino-terminal parathyroid hormone fragments with enhanced potency in activating the type-1 parathyroid hormone receptor. J Biol Chem (in press).
428. Rosenblatt M: Parathyroid hormone: Chemistry and structure-activity relations. *In* Ioachim HL (ed): Pathobiology Annual. New York, Raven, 1981, pp 53–84.
429. Rölz C, Pellegrini M, Mierke DF: Molecular characterization of the receptor-ligand complex for parathyroid hormone. Biochemistry 38:6397–6405, 1999.
430. Zhou AT, Bessalle R, Bisello A, et al: Direct mapping of an agonist-binding domain within the parathyroid hormone/parathyroid hormone–related protein receptor by photoaffinity crosslinking. Proc Natl Acad Sci U S A 94:3644–3649, 1997.
431. Ferrari S, Behar V, Chorev M, et al: Endocytosis of ligand-human parathyroid hormone receptor 1 complexes is protein kinase C–dependent and involves arrestin2. J Biol Chem 274:29968–29975, 1999.
432. Usdin TB: Evidence for a parathyroid hormone-2 receptor selective ligand in the hypothalamus. Endocrinology 138:831–834, 1997.
433. Usdin TB, Bonner TI, Harta G, et al: Distribution of PTH-2 receptor messenger RNA in rat. Endocrinology 137:4285–4297, 1996.
434. Kuroda T, Shiohara E, Haba Y, et al: Effects of parathyroid hormone on pancreatic exocrine secretion. Pancreas 8:732–737, 1993.
435. Hellman P, Jüppner H: Molecular Cloning of the PTH/PTHrP Receptor in Fish. Uppsala, Sweden, Departments of Surgery and Medical Cell Biology. University of Uppsala, 1993.
436. Rao LG, Murray TM, Heersche JNM: Immunohistochemical demonstration of parathyroid hormone binding to specific cell types in fixed rat bone tissue. Endocrinology 113:805–810, 1983.
437. Demay M, Mitchell J, Goltzman D: Comparison of renal and osseous binding of parathyroid hormone and hormonal fragments. Am J Physiol 249:E437–E446, 1985.
438. Rao LG, Murray TM: Binding of intact parathyroid hormone to rat osteosarcoma cells: Major contribution of binding sites for the carboxyl-terminal region of the hormone. Endocrinology 117:1632–1638, 1985.
439. Murray TM, Rao LG, Rizzoli RE: Interaction of parathyroid hormone, parathyroid hormone–related peptide, and their fragments with conventional and nonconventional receptor sites. *In* Bilzikian JP, Levine MA, Marcus R (eds): The parathyroids. Basic and Clinical Concepts. New York, Raven, 1994, pp 185–211.
440. Murray TM, Rao LG, Muzaffar SA, et al: Human parathyroid hormone carboxyterminal peptide (53–84) stimulates alkaline phosphatase activity in dexamethasone-treated rat osteosarcoma cells in vitro. Endocrinology 124:1097–1099, 1989.
441. Murray TM, Rao LG, Muzaffar SA: Dexamethasone-treated ROS 17/2.8 rat osteosarcoma cells are responsive to human carboxylterminal parathyroid hormone peptide hPTH(53–84): Stimulation of alkaline phosphatase. Calcif Tissue Int 49:120–123, 1991.
442. Nakamoto C, Baba H, Fukase M, et al: Individual and combined effects of intact PTH, amino-terminal, and a series of truncated carboxyl-terminal PTH fragments on alkaline phosphatase activity in dexamethasone-treated rat osteoblastic osteosarcoma cells, ROS 17/2.8. Acta Endocrinol 128:367–372, 1993.
443. Fukayama S, Schipani E, Jüppner H, et al: Role of protein kinase-A in homologous down-regulation of parathyroid hormone (PTH)/PTH-related peptide receptor messenger ribonucleic acid in human osteoblast-like SaOS-2 cells. Endocrinology 134:1851–1858, 1994.
444. Sun BH, Mitnick M, Eielson C, et al: Parathyroid hormone increases circulating levels of fibronectin in vivo: Modulating effect of ovariectomy. Endocrinology 138:3918–3924, 1997.
445. Orloff JJ, Kats Y, Urena P, et al: Further evidence for a novel receptor for amino-terminal parathyroid hormone–related protein on keratinocytes and squamous carcinoma cell lines. Endocrinology 136:3016–3023, 1995.

Chapter 71

Calcitonin

T. John Martin ▪ Jane M. Moseley ▪ Patrick M. Sexton

BACKGROUND

In the course of experiments seeking to find some factor in addition to parathyroid hormone that might contribute to the tight control of serum calcium in mammals, Copp and colleagues[1] discovered calcitonin. In perfusing the thyroparathyroid axis in dogs and sheep they obtained evidence for the secretion, in response to a high calcium stimulus, of a factor which rapidly lowered blood calcium; they called it calcitonin and suggested that it was produced by the parathyroid gland. This exciting discovery was quickly confirmed, but calcitonin was found to be a thyroid hormone in mammals.

When they performed parathyroidectomy on rats by cautery, Hirsch et al.[2] had noted that these animals underwent a more rapid and profound fall in calcium level than did animals whose parathyroids were surgically removed. When they showed that acid extracts of rat thyroid caused a lowering of calcium when injected into young rats, they concluded that the cautery was releasing a hypocalcemic factor, which they called "thyrocalcitonin." The work of MacIntyre's group, using thyroparathyroid perfusions in dogs and goats, established the thyroid origin of the hypocalcemic agent.[3] It was by then apparent that calcitonin and thyrocalcitonin were identical. The accepted usage became calcitonin, describing a new hormone of thyroid gland origin, and probably important in calcium homeostasis.

CHEMISTRY

The calcitonin sequence has been determined for many species, the common features being that it is a 32–amino acid peptide with a C-terminal proline amide and a disulfide bridge between cysteine residues at positions 1 and 7. Based on their amino acid sequence homologies, the different species (Fig. 71–1) are classified into three groups:

1. Artiodactyl, which includes swine, cattle, and sheep, differing by four amino acids
2. Primate and rodent, which includes human and rat, differing by two amino acids
3. Teleost and avian, which includes salmon, eel, goldfish, and chicken, differing by four amino acids

The common structural features are essential to biologic activity, with the standard assay used since the discovery of calcitonin measuring the hypocalcemic response in the young rat. Subsequently, receptor-based assays have been used also, and structure-function relationships are preserved in these various assays. The order of biologic potency of the calcitonins is teleost>artiodactyl>human, although absolute biologic activities vary considerably among calcitonin receptors of different species and receptor isoforms within species. Studies of substituted, deleted, and otherwise modified calcitonins have provided considerable information regarding structure-activity relationships of the calcitonin molecule, showing, for example, that the ring structure serves to stabilize the molecule. The disulfide bridge of the ring can be substituted by an N—N bond, as in aminosuberic eel calcitonin, which is extremely stable and fully potent.[4]

The sequence differences among species are concentrated in the middle portion of the molecule, and these differences contribute to the wide variations in biologic potencies. However, the outcomes of studies of structural requirements for biologic activity have varied with the different biologic assays used and it has become clear that the type of receptor used can profoundly influence the results. For example, residues in the C-terminal half of salmon calcitonin are more important for binding competition with the two rat receptor isoforms and the human receptor, whereas residues in the N-terminus are more important with the porcine receptor.[5]

SYNTHESIS, SECRETION, AND CELLS OF ORIGIN

Calcitonin arises from the C cells of mammalian thyroid, with its secretion dependent upon the prevailing serum calcium level.[6] Al-

hCT	C	G	N	L	S	T	C	M	L	G	T	Y	T	Q	D	F	N	K	F	H	T	F	P	Q	T	A	I	G	V	G	A	P
bCT	C	S	N	L	S	T	C	V	L	S	A	Y	W	K	D	L	N	N	Y	H	R	F	S	G	M	G	F	G	P	E	T	P
pCT	C	S	N	L	S	T	C	V	L	S	A	Y	W	R	N	L	N	N	F	H	R	F	S	G	M	G	F	G	P	E	T	P
rCT	C	G	N	L	S	T	C	M	L	G	T	Y	T	Q	D	L	N	K	F	H	T	F	P	Q	T	S	I	G	V	G	A	P
cCT	C	A	S	L	S	T	C	V	L	G	K	L	S	Q	E	L	H	K	L	Q	T	Y	P	R	T	D	V	G	A	G	T	P
sCT	C	S	N	L	S	T	C	V	L	G	K	L	S	Q	E	L	H	K	L	Q	T	Y	P	R	T	N	T	G	S	G	T	P
eCT	C	S	N	L	S	T	C	V	L	G	K	L	S	Q	E	L	H	K	L	Q	T	Y	P	R	T	D	V	G	A	G	T	P

FIGURE 71–1. Amino acid sequences of calcitonins of several species: human (hCT), bovine (bCT), porcine (pCT), rat (rCT), chicken (cCT), salmon (sCT), and eel (eCT). Boxes indicate residues different from those of hCT.

though the dominant site of production of calcitonin in mammals is the thyroid C cell, the distribution of these cells throughout the thyroid gland varies considerably among mammalian species, and there is evidence that in some animals calcitonin-producing cells might be found in other parts of the neck, including the thymus. In fish and in most birds calcitonin is produced by the ultimobranchial glands. Whereas in mammalian development the ultimobranchial bodies fuse with the posterior lobes of the developing thyroid to become the C cells, in submammalian vertebrates these bodies remain separate, and the ultimobranchial glands constitute a separate endocrine system. The calcitonins of ultimobranchial origin are highly potent in their actions upon mammalian targets, even though the physiologic significance of calcitonin in fish and birds remains uncertain.

Although there is little doubt that calcium is an important secretagogue for calcitonin in normal or tumor C cells, the exact mechanisms by which calcium provokes exocytosis of calcitonin have not been fully elucidated. It has recently been shown, however, that the same extracellular calcium-sensing receptor, which leads to decreased parathyroid hormone secretion from parathyroid cells, is also found in C cells.[7] This calcium receptor is likely to represent the primary molecular entity through which C cells detect changes in extracellular calcium and control calcitonin release, showing that activation of the same receptor can either stimulate or inhibit hormone secretion in different cell types.

Agents that elevate C cell cyclic adenosine monophosphate (cAMP) may stimulate calcitonin secretion, since cAMP analogues have been shown to have this effect in vivo and in vitro. Probably the most important calcitonin secretagogues apart from calcium, however, are the gastrointestinal hormones. In the pig, gastrin appears to be an effective physiologic secretagogue, contributing to a view of calcitonin's physiologic role as a hormone important postprandially, capable of counteracting the effect of a calcium meal by preventing the efflux of calcium from bone into blood.[8] Although there is some evidence in favor of this role in the pig and rat, it is difficult to envisage it as being important in adult humans. However, this awaits further study. Other gastrointestinal hormones, including glucagon, cholecystokinin, and secretin, are also capable of promoting calcitonin secretion. The gastrin analogue pentagastrin has been used clinically as a provocative test for calcitonin secretion in patients with medullary carcinoma of the thyroid. Other hormones that influence calcium homeostasis may also directly or indirectly influence calcitonin secretion. 1,25-Dihydroxyvitamin D_3 ($1,25(OH)_2D_3$) administration has been reported to increase plasma calcitonin levels; this was suggested to occur via specific thyroid C cell receptors for $1,25(OH)_2D_3$, which modify secretion of calcitonin.[9] Both calcitonin and $1,25(OH)_2D_3$ levels are raised in pregnancy and lactation, and it has been suggested that calcitonin may act to protect the skeleton in the face of increased calcium demand by the fetus.

The serum and thyroid concentrations of calcitonin increase markedly with age in the rat, and this is associated with substantial increases in thyroid content of calcitonin messenger RNA (mRNA).[10] In normal rats subjected to acute calcium stimulation in vivo, thyroid calcitonin mRNA was increased. On current evidence it seems that calcium can stimulate both synthesis and secretion of calcitonin by thyroid C cells.

Although calcitonin secretion has been studied extensively in patients with medullary carcinoma of the thyroid, who have clearly assayable hormone levels (see below), it has been difficult to establish the circulating hormone level in normal human subjects. With the most sensitive and specific assays available, the level of calcitonin in normal human blood appears to be less than 10 pg/mL (3 pM).

CALCITONIN GENE

As with other hormonal peptides, calcitonin is synthesized as a precursor which is processed by cleavage and amidation before secretion (Fig. 71–2). Calcitonin is synthesized as a high-molecular-weight precursor (136 amino acids), with a leader sequence at the N-terminus, which is cleaved during transport of the molecule into the endoplasmic reticulum. A potentially important posttranslational modification of calcitonin is that of glycosylation. It had been noted that the tripeptide sequence, Asn-Leu-Ser, found within the N-terminal ring structure of calcitonin, is invariate among the calcitonins of different species. This sequence is an acceptor site for N-linked glycosylation. This, together with evidence for glycosylation of tumor calcitonin, led to detailed studies showing that the calcitonin precursor is indeed a glycoprotein and that the only N-linked glycosylation site in the entire precursor was within the calcitonin portion itself.[11] The biologic significance of calcitonin glycosylation has yet to be determined.

The complete sequences of the complementary DNA (cDNA) for human, rat, chicken, and sheep calcitonins and the DNA sequence of the full human calcitonin gene, have been determined.[12–14] These show that the hormone is flanked in the precursor by N- and C-terminal peptides, but the biologic significance of these peptides is unknown. The human calcitonin gene has been located in the p14-qter region of chromosome 11.[15]

Calcitonin Gene–Related Peptide

The calcitonin gene transcript actually encodes a second distinct peptide known as calcitonin gene–related peptide (CGRP), which is produced by tissue-specific alternative splicing of the gene (see Fig. 71–2). The mature CGRP and calcitonin mRNAs predict proteins which share sequence identity in the N-terminal regions, but in the C-terminal regions the nucleotide sequences are almost entirely different. The mature, secreted 32– and 37–amino acid calcitonin and CGRP peptides, respectively, result from cleavage of both N- and C-terminal flanking sequences, at cleavage sites depicted in Figure 71–2.[16]

Calcitonin mRNA is found almost exclusively in the thyroid and CGRP mRNA is found primarily in the nervous system.[17] However, aberrant expression of CGRP may be seen in medullary thyroid carcinoma.[18] Two different calcitonin-CGRP genes, CALC 1 and CALC 2, have been identified in man and rat. CALC 1 produces either calcitonin or CGRP and CALC 2 gives rise to CGRP II, which in humans differs from CGRP I in three amino acids.

Processing of the pre-mRNA to the calcitonin mRNA transcript involves usage of exon 4 as a 3′-terminal exon with concomitant polyadenylation at the end of exon 4. Processing to produce the CGRP mRNA involves the exclusion of exon 4 and direct ligation of exon 3 to exon 5, with polyadenylation at the end of exon 6. Much work has been done on the mechanisms of differential splicing. The human calcitonin–CGRP exon 4 has been characterized as having weak processing signals, like many differentially incorporated exons. Weak differential exons are frequently associated with special enhancer sequences that facilitate exon recognition in the presence of accessory factors that bind to the enhancer. Indeed, such an enhancer, located in the intron downstream of exon 4, has been described for the calcitonin-CGRP gene. In addition, sequences within exon 4 are necessary for the inclusion of exon.[19]

PHYSIOLOGY

Our concept of the physiologic role of calcitonin is that it is an inhibitor of bone resorption, whose function is to prevent bone loss at times of stress on calcium conservation. This includes pregnancy, lactation, and growth. When calcitonin was discovered, it seemed to provide the necessary further explanation for the tight control of serum calcium, but events proved otherwise. Concepts of the role of bone in maintaining extracellular fluid calcium had relied upon observations made in the young, growing rat, in which it was clear that if accretion continued at the same rate and resorption was inhibited, the result would be a lowering of plasma calcium. The younger the animal, the more rapid the bone resorption rate. It would therefore be expected that the calcium-lowering effect of calcitonin should be greater in younger than in older animals. This was indeed the case in the rat, in which it was noted that in the biologic assay of calcitonin, which depends on the calcium-lowering effect of the hormone, the response became less marked with increasing age of the animal.[20] It should be noted, however, that the ability of calcitonin to counteract the effects of a calcium load was not impaired in older animals, at least in the

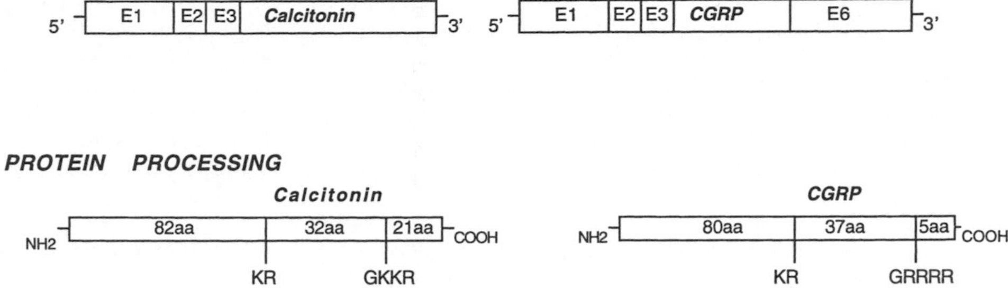

FIGURE 71–2. Cartoon depicting the alternate splicing of the calcitonin gene and the subsequent processing of the messenger RNA and protein, which give rise to mature sequences of calcitonin or calcitonin gene–related peptide (CGRP). Exon sequences are represented by the boxes numbered E1 to E6 and the protein precursors are shown with the basic sequences which are cleaved to generate biologically active peptides of calcitonin or CGRP.

rat,[21] an observation that has not been explained and that has not been extended to other species.

In normal adult human subjects even quite large doses of calcitonin have little effect on serum calcium levels. In those subjects in whom bone turnover is increased (e.g., in thyrotoxicosis or Paget's disease), calcitonin treatment acutely inhibits bone resorption and lowers the serum calcium.[22] Given that the acute effect of calcitonin on serum calcium is related to the prevailing rate of bone resorption, it is not surprising that calcitonin has little or no effect on calcium in the mature animal or human subject, since the process of bone resorption is a slow one in maturity. It may be that the role of calcitonin in its effect on bone throughout life is that of a regulator of the bone resorptive process, whatever the overall rate of the latter. In the young, or in pathologic states of increased bone resorption in maturity (e.g., Paget's disease, thyrotoxicosis), calcitonin inhibition of bone resorption can lower the serum calcium level, and there may even be a calcium homeostatic role for endogenous calcitonin in those circumstances. In a normal adult animal, however, when bone turnover is slow, no effect on serum calcium is obtained with calcitonin. The physiologic function of calcitonin in maturity may nevertheless be to regulate the bone resorptive process, in either a continuous or intermittent manner. It follows that calcitonin should not necessarily be regarded as a "calcium-regulating hormone" in maturity, but may yet be shown to be such in stages of rapid growth (e.g., in the young or in states of increased bone turnover). It is nevertheless important that bone resorption be regulated, and calcitonin is the only hormone known to be capable of carrying out this function by a direct action on bone. Such a role might become more important in circumstances in which skeletal loss particularly needs to be prevented (e.g., in pregnancy and lactation). Evidence in support of such an important physiologic role for endogenous calcitonin in protecting against bone loss is provided by experiments showing that cancellous bone loss in thyroparathyroidectomized rats treated with parathyroid hormone was greater than that in similarly treated sham-operated controls.[23] Further evidence for a role for calcitonin in conservation of bone comes from a recent preliminary report that mice homozygous null for the calcitonin gene were found to have a significant reduction in bone mass at ages 12 months and more.[24]

Bone

The first evidence of the mechanism of action of calcitonin was obtained by organ culture of bone in vitro which showed that calcitonin inhibited bone resorption.[25] The inhibition of resorption appeared to be explained by a direct action on osteoclasts. Calcitonin treatment of resorbing bone in vitro resulted in rapid loss of osteoclast ruffled borders and decreased release of lysosomal enzymes. In vivo evidence was also consistent with an inhibitory action upon bone resorption. Thus, calcitonin infused into rats led to an immediate reduction in the rate of excretion of hydroxyproline, consistent with inhibition of breakdown of bone collagen.[26] Furthermore, kinetic studies in rats led to similar conclusions, with no evidence to suggest any increase in the active uptake of calcium by bone.[27]

Studies of the actions of hormones on isolated bone cell populations established that calcitonin acts directly on osteoclasts, with receptor autoradiography establishing osteoclasts as the only discernible bone cell targets.[28] Consistent with this are observations of its actions in organ culture, especially the demonstration that calcitonin-treated osteoclasts in cultured mouse calvaria rapidly lose their ruffled borders. A similar in vivo observation of loss of ruffled border in osteoclasts has been made in patients with Paget's disease, in whom bone biopsies were taken before and 30 minutes after an injection of calcitonin.[29] In the same clinical study, calcitonin was noted to reduce the number of osteoclasts in addition to altering their ultrastructure.

Studies using isolated osteoclast preparations point to a direct effect of calcitonin upon the osteoclast, in which the hormone rapidly inhibits the activity of osteoclasts. In further experiments it was also noted that, while isolated osteoclasts remained quiescent in calcitonin as long as the hormone was present, they regained activity when osteoblasts were added to the culture.[30] This escape of osteoclasts from inhibition by calcitonin took place at a rate proportional to the number of osteoblasts with which they were in contact. Calcitonin reduced the cytoplasmic spreading of isolated osteoclasts in a dose-dependent manner. Parathyroid hormone had no effect unless osteoblasts were cocultivated with the osteoclasts, in which case addition of parathyroid hormone resulted in a marked increase in cytoplasmic spreading of osteoclasts. It cannot be assumed that these phenomena reflect the responses of cells in bone in vivo, but this work provided for the first time some useful direct observations of actions of hormones on isolated bone cell preparations containing osteoclasts.

The molecular mechanisms by which calcitonin decreases osteoclast function have yet to be fully defined. The rapid effects of the hormone may be brought about through actions on a cytoskeletal function of osteoclasts, after initial events involving generation of several intracellular second messengers. Early events in calcitonin signal transduction have been studied in a variety of cell types and are described later. With the development of improved methods of studying isolated osteoclasts, it has been possible to establish clearly that mammalian osteoclasts possess abundant, specific, high-affinity receptors for calcitonin and that calcitonin stimulates cAMP formation in a sensitive and dose-dependent manner, as well as increasing intracellular Ca^{2+} levels.[28, 30]

The other means by which calcitonin could inhibit resorption is through inhibition of osteoclast formation. In vivo data and results from calcitonin inhibition of resorption in organ culture are consistent with this. The development of methods of studying osteoclast formation in vitro from hemopoietic precursor cells has allowed this question to be addressed directly. There were several reports of calcitonin inhibiting osteoclast-like cell formation in bone marrow cultures of human, baboon, and mouse origin.[31, 32] However, these experiments were all conducted at relatively high calcitonin concentrations and the effects were not convincing. In recent studies using lower concentrations of calcitonin, which nevertheless reduced calcitonin receptor mRNA expression in developing mouse osteoclasts, there was no reduction in osteoclast formation.[33–35] The multinucleated osteoclasts formed under calcitonin treatment, however, had fewer nuclei, and, notably in this and in other studies, evidence was obtained for the generation of osteoclasts deficient in calcitonin receptor mRNA and protein, but nevertheless capable of resorbing bone. This observation may be relevant to the mechanism of "escape" from calcitonin action. There are still some reports appearing of calcitonin inhibition of osteoclast formation in bone marrow and co-culture systems, but technical reasons might explain these apparent discrepancies, for example, the misleading definition of osteoclasts as "TRAP positive cells with three or more nuclei."[36, 37]

The mechanism of calcitonin-induced receptor mRNA loss appeared to be due principally to destabilization of receptor mRNA.[35] The 3′-untranslated region of the mouse and rat calcitonin receptor mRNA contains four AUUUA motifs, as well as other A/U-rich domains and a large number of poly-U regions. Such motifs, commonly found in cytokines and oncogenes, function as signals for rapid mRNA inactivation. We have noted that the calcitonin receptor behaves in a manner similar to the β_2-adrenergic receptor. In the latter case, A/U-rich elements in the 3′-untranslated region have been shown to bind to a number of cytosolic proteins, some of which have been characterized, and which probably accelerate mRNA degradation.

An additional interesting aspect of the work on calcitonin-induced receptor regulation is that glucocorticoid treatment substantially prevented the calcitonin receptor loss.[35] In that work glucocorticoid treatment was shown by nuclear run-on analysis to increase transcription of the calcitonin receptor gene. It is worth noting the clinical evidence suggesting that glucocorticoids, given together with calcitonin, might prevent, to some extent, the calcitonin-induced resistance to its own action.

It should be stressed that the failure of calcitonin to inhibit osteoclast formation in osteoclast-generating cell culture systems, except perhaps at very high calcitonin concentrations, does not exclude the possibility that inhibition of osteoclastogenesis contributes to calcitonin action in vivo. The emergence in vitro of osteoclasts deficient in calcitonin receptors complicates such experiments. It is interesting to consider that development of receptor-deficient osteoclasts might take place also in vivo, and even contribute to calcitonin resistance.

Renal Actions

When infused into rats that have undergone thyroparathyroidectomy, calcitonin caused a dose-dependent phosphaturia, but the effect on phosphate excretion was only a minor one in comparison with the phosphaturic effect of parathyroid hormone.[38] Although it was demonstrated in human subjects also, in several species calcitonin failed to have any effect on phosphate excretion. Thus, it seems unlikely that the phosphaturic effect is of any major physiologic significance.

A number of other renal effects of calcitonin have been noted, including a transient increase in calcium excretion, due probably to inhibition of renal tubular calcium reabsorption.[39] Although this has not usually been regarded as an important effect of calcitonin, recent observations link it to the calcium-lowering effect of calcitonin in hypercalcemic patients with metastatic bone disease. The use of calcitonin in the treatment of hypercalcemia due to cancer has been based exclusively on the inhibition of osteolysis by calcitonin. Some evidence has been produced that failure of the kidneys to excrete the calcium load derived from bone breakdown is a major contributor to the hypercalcemia. This prompted careful studies of the relative contributions to the hypocalcemic effect of calcitonin of its renal and skeletal components. It was concluded that inhibition of renal tubular reabsorption by calcitonin can induce a rapid fall in serum calcium, and that the magnitude of this effect depends upon the correction of volume depletion, which inevitably accompanies hypercalcemia.[40] Thus, the calciuretic action of calcitonin may assume greater importance than hitherto suspected.

Calcitonin receptors have been demonstrated clearly in rat kidney,[41] and a further action on the kidney is to enhance 1-hydroxylation of 25-hydroxyvitamin D in the proximal straight tubule of the kidney.[42] Since autoradiographic studies and polymerase chain reaction (PCR) analysis of calcitonin receptor mRNA expression have failed to localize calcitonin receptors in the proximal tubules (Fig. 71–3), it seems unlikely that these actions are mediated by direct actions on calcitonin receptors. The action of calcitonin upon adenylate cyclase activity has been localized in the human nephron predominantly to the medullary and cortical portions of the thick ascending limb and to the early portion of the distal convoluted tubule. The co-localization of the calcitonin receptor mRNA expression and cell surface receptors with G protein–sensitive adenylate cyclase is consistent with cAMP being an important mediator of calcitonin action in this organ.

PEPTIDES RELATED TO CALCITONIN

The calcitonin peptides are homologous with the related peptides CGRP, amylin, and adrenomedullin. Highest identity is observed between the teleost calcitonins and amylin (~33%) with approximately 22% identity with the CGRPs and 16% with adrenomedullin. Less

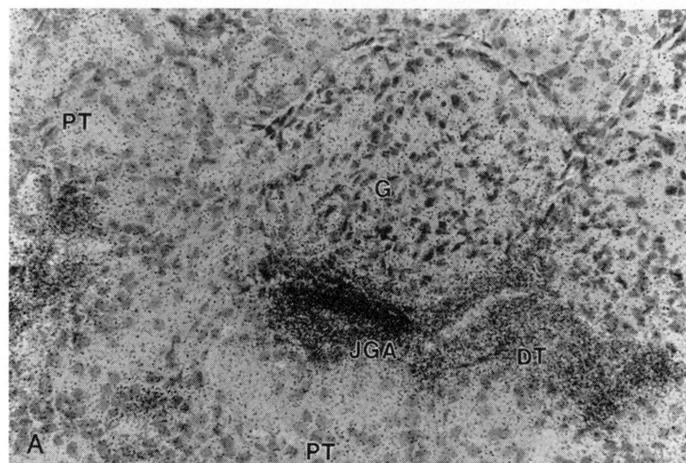

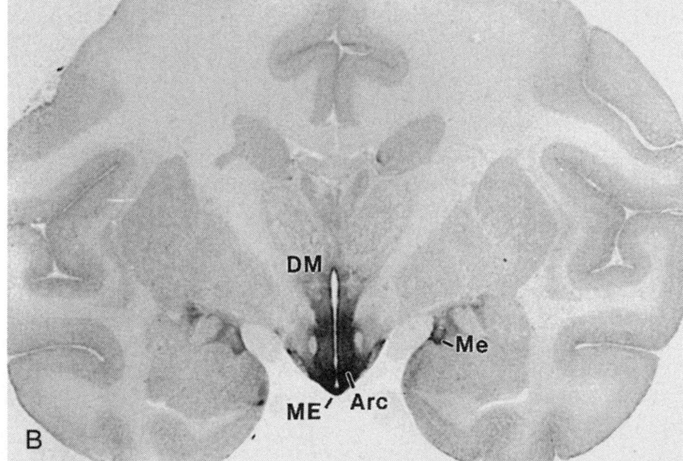

FIGURE 71–3. In vitro autoradiographic localization of calcitonin receptors in rhesus monkey kidney cortex *(upper panel)* and brain stem *(lower panel)*. Receptor binding sites are identified using ^{125}I–salmon calcitonin as the radioligand. Binding to renal cortex is localized principally to the distal tubule, with little binding in glomeruli or the proximal tubule. In the brain section high-density binding is associated with parts of the hypothalamus and amygdala. *Upper panel*: DT, distal tubule; G, glomerulus; JGA, juxtaglomerular apparatus; PT, proximal tubule. *Lower panel*: Arc, arcuate nucleus; DM, dorsomedial hypothalamic nucleus; Me, medial amygdaloid nucleus; ME, median eminence.

homology is observed between the mammalian calcitonins and the other peptides. Consistent with the homology between peptides there is a limited degree of overlap in specificity between the binding sites for the peptide receptors, with calcitonin-like actions seen with high concentrations of amylin and CGRP.

Amylin is a 37–amino acid peptide that is co-secreted with insulin from pancreatic β cells following nutrient ingestion. Amylin acts to inhibit insulin secretion from the pancreas, but its most studied actions are in skeletal muscle where amylin acts to promote glycogen breakdown and decrease insulin-stimulated incorporation of glucose into glycogen. Thus, amylin is thought to act as a partner to insulin in metabolic regulation.[43] Evidence is also emerging for a role for amylin in other tissues, including the intestinal tract, where it potently inhibits gastric emptying, and kidney, where it has a diverse range of actions, including modulation of Ca^{2+} excretion and thiazide receptor levels, proliferative effects on tubule epithelium, and increasing renin activity.[44] Furthermore, a possible role in bone turnover has been highlighted by the work of Cornish et al.[45] who have described effects on bone resorption in vivo.

Amylin receptors are also widely expressed in brain, where administered peptide induces many potent effects. These include decreased appetite and gastric acid secretion, hyperthermia, adipsia, and reduction in growth hormone–releasing hormone release of growth hormone. Central amylin injection may also modulate memory and the extrapyramidal motor system. The receptors mediating these actions of amylin, termed C3, have a unique specificity, displaying high affinity for amylin, but also high affinity for the teleost calcitonins and moderate affinity for CGRP.[46] The interaction with CGRP appears to vary among tissues and this may reflect the presence of subtypes of amylin receptors. Only very weak interaction is seen with human or rat calcitonin. The molecular identity of the receptor for amylin is unclear, but a number of lines of evidence link amylin receptors and calcitonin receptors (CTRs) and it appears likely that generation of the amylin receptor phenotype(s) derives from association of CTRs and the novel receptor activity modifying proteins (see below).

CGRP is a pleiotropic neuropeptide with a diverse range of actions, including potent dilation of vascular beds, as well as relaxation of other smooth muscle, inotropy and chronotropy in the heart, paracrine regulation of pituitary hormone release, and many central effects, such as suppression of appetite and gastric acid secretion, modulation of body temperature, and modulation of sympathetic outflow. CGRP also acts to modulate nicotinic acetylcholine receptor levels at neuromuscular junctions. CGRP weakly modulates calcium homeostasis, although this is likely to reflect mainly its low-affinity interaction with CTRs. The actions of CGRP have been extensively reviewed elsewhere.[46, 47] Specific CGRP receptors have been characterized in many tissues, including bone, and it is likely that more than one subtype of receptor exists.[47, 48]

Adrenomedullin was originally isolated from human pheochromocytoma and is abundant in the normal adrenal medulla, hence its name. The full-length peptide is approximately 50 amino acids in length and it shares approximately 25% homology with CGRP across its N-terminal 37 amino acids.[48] Adrenomedullin is a potent dilator of many vascular beds, although its actions outside the cardiovascular system are not well characterized.

CALCITONIN IN THE CENTRAL NERVOUS SYSTEM

Both immunoreactive calcitonin-like peptide and CTRs have been demonstrated in the brain and nervous system of rats, humans, and other species.[49] Immunoreactive calcitonin related antigenically to human calcitonin (hCT) has also been demonstrated in the nervous systems of protochordates, lizards, and pigeons, and low levels have been found in human and rat brain extracts. Furthermore, radioimmunoassay analyses point to the presence of salmon calcitonin (sCT)–like peptide material in human and rat brain (reviewed in Sexton[50]).

Low levels of immunoreactive hCT (hCTI) occur in extracts of postmortem human brain. However, in addition to hCTI, low levels of material chromatographically and immunologically similar to sCT (sCTI) also occurred, with concentrations in the brain approximately 10 times greater than those in serum and cerebrospinal fluid. Similarly, extracts of rat brain diencephalon contain an sCT-like peptide. Although hCTI has been detected in rat brain, there is only limited evidence for the presence of rat calcitonin (rCT) mRNA. Immunoreactive calcitonin-like material also occurs in the pituitary of both mammals and lower vertebrates, although the identity of the pituitary calcitonin remains to be established. The physiologic significance of calcitonin-like immunoreactivity in the pituitary remains uncertain; however, CTRs are present in the intermediate pituitary and therefore the calcitonin-like material may act as a paracrine regulator of these receptors.

Central Calcitonin Receptors

In addition to the well-characterized CTRs of kidney and bone, CTRs are also abundant in the central nervous system (CNS), where administration of calcitonin generates potent effects that include analgesia and inhibition of appetite and gastric acid secretion, as well as modulation of hormone secretion and the extrapyramidal motor system (reviewed in Sexton[50]). The centrally mediated actions of calcitonin correlate well with the location of calcitonin binding sites. Autoradiographic mapping revealed high binding densities associated with parts of the ventral striatum and amygdala and the hypothalamic and preoptic areas, as well as most of the circumventricular organs (see Fig. 71–3). High-density binding also occurs in parts of the periaqueductal gray, the reticular formation, most of the midline raphe nuclei, parabrachial nuclei, locus caeruleus, and solitary tract nucleus.

Cloning studies have revealed that CTRs in rat brain exist as two distinct isoforms. Calcitonin-specific binding sites in brain have been termed Cl sites and the two receptor isoforms are termed Cla and Clb receptor.[50] The two receptors are identical, except that the Clb sequence encodes a 37–amino acid insert in the second extracellular domain, which confers altered ligand recognition. Both receptors demonstrate high affinity for sCT, but differ greatly in their affinity for hCT. Cla receptors have moderate affinity for hCT, whereas Clb receptors have negligible affinity for hCT. The distribution of CTR mRNA confirmed that message for both receptor isoforms is present in rat brain.

CALCITONIN RECEPTORS

Distribution

Direct evidence for binding of calcitonin to osteoclasts was obtained from the work of Nicholson et al.[38] who demonstrated, by in vitro autoradiography, binding specifically to osteoclasts and precursor cells but not to other cell types. Radioligand binding studies in tissue sections, membranes, or cultured cells have revealed an extensive extraskeletal distribution of CTRs. These sites include kidney, brain, pituitary, placenta, testis and spermatozoa, lung, and lymphocytes, as well as cancer-derived cells from lung, breast, pituitary, bone (giant cell tumor), and embryonal carcinoma.

Following the cloning of the CTR, presence of mRNA for the receptor has been confirmed in many of these sites, including kidney, brain, lung, placenta, and osteoclasts, along with many of the cancer cell lines. However, CTR mRNA studies have also provided evidence for previously uncharacterized sites of CTR expression, including prostate, normal and cancerous breast, thyroid and thyroid carcinoma, skeletal muscle, stomach, ovary, and early rat embyo.

As alluded to elsewhere, it is probable that both calcitonin and amylin receptors derive from the CTR gene product, and consequently care needs to be taken in extrapolating the potential significance of CTR mRNA expression for calcitonin biology. The same is also true for receptor localization studies where ^{125}I-sCT is used as the radioligand.

Receptor Cloning

Our knowledge of the molecular basis of calcitonin action, both in terms of ligand binding and postbinding events, has been greatly augmented by the recent cloning of cDNAs encoding the receptor(s). The first cloned receptor was the porcine CTR, which was isolated by expression cloning from a cDNA library derived from the renal epithelial cell line LLC-PK1.[51] Subsequently, CTR cDNAs from man, rat, mouse, rabbit, and guinea pig have been isolated.

Analysis of the predicted protein translation product(s) revealed that these receptors comprise approximately 500 amino acids and belong to the class II (family B) subclass of G protein–coupled receptors, which include the receptors for other peptide hormones such as secretin, parathyroid hormone, glucagon, glucagon-like peptide 1, vasoactive intestinal polypeptide, pituitary adenylate cyclase–activating peptide, and gastric inhibitory peptide.

Receptor Isoforms

Receptor cloning also provided direct evidence for receptor heterogeneity and the existence of multiple receptor isoforms that arise from alternative splicing of the CTR gene (Fig. 71–4). The human receptor is the most extensively studied and at least five splice variants have been described. The most common splice variant occurs in intracellular domain 1 generating a 16–amino acid insert in this domain (I_{1+}).[51, 53] Additional splice variants have been identified in other species. In rodents alternate splicing leads to two receptor isoforms (termed Cla and Clb) which differ by the presence (Clb; E_{2+}) or absence (Cla) of an additional 37 amino acids in the second extracellular domain. However, it is unlikely that expression of the rodent Clb isoform occurs in humans. In rabbits, an additional splice variant has been isolated in which the exon encoding transmembrane domain 7 is spliced out (ΔTM7).

Functional characterization of the significance of the splice variants reveals that occurrence of inserts or deletions in the basic receptor structure leads into alterations in either ligand binding (E_{2+}, Δamino47), signal transduction (I_{1+}), or both (ΔTM7). For the E_{2+} variants, there is a loss of affinity for peptides exhibiting weak α-helical secondary structure, such as calcitonin, while peptides with strong helical secondary structure, such as sCT, maintain high affinity at this receptor.[50] In contrast, the I_{1+} receptor isoform displays similar affinity for peptides to the I_{1-} variant but has markedly altered G protein–coupling efficiency. Presence of the 16–amino acid insert leads to complete loss of intracellular calcium mobilization. Signaling via Gs is maintained but with decreased efficiency leading to 10- to 100-fold reduction in potency of peptides for stimulation of cAMP production.[53]

Calcitonin Receptor Gene

The gene for the CTR in the pig has been mapped. The CTR gene, like the genes for other class II G protein–coupled receptors, is complex, comprising at least 14 exons with introns ranging in size from 78 nucleotides to more than 20,000 nucleotides. The total receptor gene is estimated to exceed 70 kb in length.[54] The human CTR gene has recently been completely sequenced as part of the human genome project (AC003078). The organization and size of the human gene is similar to the pig CTR gene, although some interspecies difference in organization does occur. For instance, in the pig the I1 insert is generated by selective use of alternate splice sites located on exon 8. However, in humans, the I1 insert occurs on a separate exon, with at least one additional exon proximal to exon 7 in the pig.[53] It is also likely that the pig CTR gene was not completely characterized, as additional exons in the 5′ region of the gene have now been identified in the mouse. Control of gene transcription and mRNA splicing is also likely to be complicated, with preliminary evidence in the mouse for at least three promoters that engender specific exon splicing.

The human CTR gene is located on chromosome 7 at 7q21.3 (AC003078). In the mouse it is in the proximal region of chromosome 6 and in chromosomal band 9q11-12 in the pig, which are homologous to 7q in humans.

Polymorphisms and Osteoporosis

Restriction fragment length polymorphism (RFLP) studies from a Japanese population sample, using the Alu I restriction enzyme, identified a polymorphism arising from a single nucleotide substitution, which leads to either a proline (CC genotype) or a leucine (TT genotype) at amino acid 447. Heterozygotes were designated TC. In this population, the proline heterozygote was the most prevalent (~70%), with the leucine homozygote accounting for approximately 10% of the population and the heterozygote for approximately 20%.[55]

A number of studies have analyzed this polymorphism in postmenopausal women of Italian or French descent. Unlike the Japanese population, the dominant phenotypes were the heterozygote and the leucine homozygote. The proline homozygote accounted for only 7% to 20% of these white populations.[56, 57] In these studies patients who were homozygous for leucine 447 had lower lumbar spine bone mineral density (BMD) in comparison to either heterozygotes or proline homozygotes. Division of patients into osteoporotic and normal or those with fractures vs. those without indicated that heterozygotes had lower fracture risk than the leucine homozygotes,[57] and that the leucine homozygotes may be more represented in the osteoporotic population.[56] However, the finding of increased frequency of the leucine genotype in osteoporotic patients needs to be treated with caution as an earlier study from the same laboratory, which sampled a larger population, found no change in frequency of leucine homozygotes between normal and osteoporotic patients. Nonetheless, the finding of lower lumbar BMD in the leucine homozygotes is a consistent finding in each of the studies, and polymorphism in the CTR gene may contribute to the change in BMD which accompanies polygenic disorders such as osteoporosis.

Amylin and Calcitonin Gene–Related Peptide Receptors

Recent work revealed that the CTR-like receptor, which has highest homology with the cloned CTR, is a CGRP receptor. Expression of

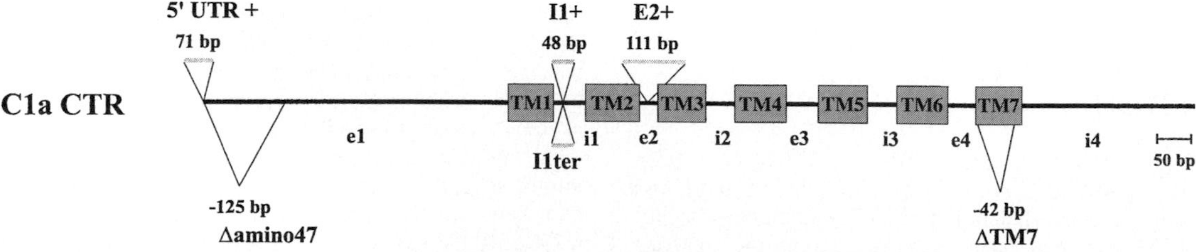

FIGURE 71–4. Linear schematic representation of the coding region of the calcitonin receptor (CTR) gene, indicating identified sites of alternate receptor splicing. The template receptor is the most common form of the CTR in rats and humans and is denoted C1a. Alternate splicing has been identified in multiple species, although differences in splicing patterns between species do occur. At least six different sites of variance occur: (1) an insert in the 5′ untranslated region of the receptor which delivers an upstream, in frame, potential translation initiation AUG (5′ UTR+); (2) a deletion of 125 bp in the 5′ region of the coding sequence leading to a loss of the first 47 amino acids in the first extracellular domain (amino47); (3) an insert in the first intracellular domain of the receptor leading to an addition of 16 amino acids (I1+); (4) an insert in the first intracellular domain leading to termination of the receptor at this position (I1ter); (5) an insert in the second extracellular domain (E2+); and (6) deletion of part of the transmembrane domain (TM7). e, extracellular domain; I, intracellular domain; bp, base pair; TM, transmembrane domain.

this phenotype, however, requires the co-expression of a novel protein, termed receptor activity modifying protein 1 (RAMP 1). RAMP 1 is a member of a family of three single transmembrane spanning proteins and acts to modify the glycosylation of CTR-like receptor (CRLR), enhance the trafficking of the receptor protein to the cell surface, and potentially contribute directly to the cell surface phenotype of the receptor. RAMP 2 and RAMP 3 also enhance the trafficking of CRLR to the cell surface, but do not alter the pattern of glycosylation of the receptor. The RAMP 2– and RAMP 3–induced receptor phenotypes are adrenomedullin-like receptor.[58]

There are a number of lines of evidence that link amylin receptors and CTRs suggesting that the receptors for amylin and calcitonin are related and that expression of appropriate phenotype may be dependent upon a cell specific factor(s). The logical candidate for this was a RAMP and indeed preliminary experiments cotransfecting RAMP with CTRs demonstrate that RAMPs can induce amylin receptor phenotype.[44, 59] The degree to which RAMPs may dynamically regulate receptor phenotype remains to be elucidated. Nonetheless, RAMPs present a novel mechanism for alteration or generation of receptor phenotype, and regulation of RAMPs may be important in the regulation of the physiologic response to the calcitonin family of peptides.

Signaling

The predominance of the cAMP pathway in mediating the action of calcitonin on osteoclasts has been discussed. Calcitonin also stimulates adenylate cyclase activity in kidney, with the pattern of calcitonin responsiveness paralleling the distribution of CTRs in this tissue. Calcitonin induction of cAMP has now been documented in a large number of cultured CTR-bearing cells that include LLC-PK1 pig kidney cells, and cancers of lung, breast, and bone. Receptor cloning and expression studies have confirmed that cAMP production is a principal component of CTR-mediated signaling.[51–53]

It is now apparent that many G protein–coupled receptors interact with and signal through multiple G proteins. In the case of the CTR there is evidence that signaling through both cAMP or intracellular calcium may be important in calcitonin action on the osteoclast. Although controversial and potentially species-specific, the osteoclast retraction component of calcitonin action may be regulated by alternate signaling pathways. In mice, this response appears to be mediated by the protein kinase A pathway.[60] On the other hand, inhibition of osteoclast-mediated bone resorption by calcitonin can be mimicked by both dibutyryl cAMP and phorbol esters or blocked by protein kinase inhibitor.[61] These results suggest that alternative coupling of receptor to different G proteins can activate either adenylate cyclase or phospholipase C, in the latter case leading to increased intracellular triphosphate levels and thence increased cytosolic calcium, which, concurrently with co-liberated diacylglycerol, activate protein kinase C. Direct evidence for the interaction of CTRs with the Gq family of G proteins leading to activation of phospholipase C has recently been described.[62] Expression of cloned receptors in a variety of cell types has now conclusively shown that CTRs of human, rat, and porcine origin are capable of signaling through both cAMP- and calcium-activated second messenger systems. It is important to note that comparison of the calcium response in cell lines expressing different CTR levels has suggested that the magnitude of the response is proportional to the receptor density and it is therefore possible that relative receptor density in target tissues may influence the signaling pathway(s) activated.

Calcitonin can potently modulate the growth of some CTR-bearing cells. It stimulates the growth of human prostate cancer cells, in which calcitonin increases both intracellular calcium and cAMP levels.[63] On the other hand, calcitonin treatment represses growth of T47D human breast cancer cells, an action believed to be mediated by the specific activation of the type II isoenzyme of the cAMP-dependent protein kinase.[64]

Regulation

Regulation of the level or affinity of cell surface receptors is a key component in the physiologic and pathophysiologic responses to both endogenous and pharmacologically administered agents. The CTR is subject to both homologous (calcitonin-induced) and heterologous regulation. Calcitonin-induced CTR downregulation was initially demonstrated in various transformed cell lines and subsequently in primary kidney cell cultures. Downregulation was mediated by specific loss of cell surface receptors, which occurred via an energy-dependent internalization of the ligand-receptor complex, in which the principal internalization pathway involves processing of the receptor-ligand complex into lysosomes and subsequent degradation of the receptor.[65] Receptor regulatory responses to calcitonin are likely to be cell- or tissue-dependent. For example, in mouse or rat osteoclasts, there is a potent downregulation of CTR mRNA, which appears to be mediated by a cAMP-dependent mechanism, in addition to downregulation of the receptor by internalization.[66] This contrasts to CTRs in UMR106-06 cells and T47D cells where no alteration or a small rise in the level of CTR mRNA is observed. Preliminary studies have indicated that the CTR gene in the mouse has at least three promoters and that one of these appears specific for osteoclasts. This may provide at least one mechanism for differences in tissue-specific regulatory responses, although as discussed earlier mRNA stability may also play a key role in regulation of protein levels. It is also worth noting that the degree of internalization of human CTRs appears to be isoform-specific, with the I_{1+} variant being resistant to internalization.[53] Thus, the regulation of receptors and consequently peptide responses may also vary according to the level of specific receptor isoforms present in each tissue.

There are only limited data on regulation of CTR by other agents. In mouse osteoclast cultures the glucocorticoid dexamethasone increases the level of cell surface CTR, following upregulation of receptor mRNA levels, an effect mediated at the level of transcription.[35] Similarly, the calcitonin-mediated decrease in cell surface receptor and mRNA is attenuated by dexamethasone. Increased production of CTR in response to glucocorticoid stimulation also occurs in the human T47D cell line where cortisol is required for the expression of CTRs, suggesting that this may be a common regulatory mechanism for induction of CTR expression.

CALCITONIN AND ITS RECEPTOR IN CANCER

Medullary Carcinoma of the Thyroid

The classic syndrome of calcitonin excess is medullary carcinoma of the thyroid (MCT). This tumor clearly differs in origin from all other thyroid cancers, and it was the intuition of Williams[67] that raised suspicions that MCT might be a tumor of the C cells, derived from the ultimobranchial bodies.[68]

The MCT may occur as either a sporadic or a genetic (familial) tumor.[69–71] The latter can be part of a dominantly inherited syndrome characterized by bilateral, often multifocal, thyroid tumors and diffuse C cell hyperplasia throughout the thyroid gland, and accompanied to a varying degree by hyperplasia or tumor formation in the adrenal medulla and parathyroid glands. The fullest expression of this syndrome (Sipple's syndrome)[72] may include also a characteristic phenotype, with other evidence of neuroectodermal dysplasia, including multiple mucosal neuromas and structural and functional abnormalities of the autonomic nervous system. The prevalence of medullary carcinoma is low, constituting approximately 5% to 12% of all thyroid malignancies.

The genetic variety of MCT tends toward two distinct clinical forms[69, 73–75]: one has a readily recognizable phenotype in the form of a marfanoid appearance, with mucosal neuromas, the syndrome of multiple endocrine neoplasia type-2B (MEN-2B). The other variant, the syndrome of MEN-2A, includes the polyendocrine involvement, but lacks the marfanoid habitus or neuromatosis. MEN-2A, MEN-2B, and familial MCT are all associated with germline mutations in the *RET* proto-oncogene.[76] The classification of the MEN-1 and MEN-2 syndromes is based on the fact that they have in common an autosomal dominant inheritance, with hyperplasia preceding tumor formation. The MEN-3 syndromes exhibit an inherited predisposition to tumor

74. Chong GC, Beahrs OH, Sizemore GW, et al: Medullary carcinoma of the thyroid gland. Cancer 35:695–704, 1975.
75. Tsai MS, Ledger GA, Khosla S, et al: Identification of multiple endocrine neoplasia type 2 gene carriers using linkage analysis and analysis of the rRET proto-oncogene. J Clin Endocrinol Metab 78:1261–1264, 1994.
76. Melvin KEW, Tashjian AH Jr: The syndrome of excessive thyrocalcitonin produced by medullary carcinoma of the thyroid. Proc Natl Acad Sci U S A 59:1216–1222, 1968.
77. Lippman SM, Mendelsohn G, Trump DL, et al: The prognostic and biological significance of cellular heterogeneity in medullary thyroid carcinoma: A study of calcitonin, 1-dopa decarboxylase and histaminase. J Clin Endocrinol Metab 54:233–240, 1982.
78. Tasjian AH Jr, Howland BG, Melvin KEW, et al: Immunoassay of human calcitonin: Clinical measurement, relation to serum calcium and studies in patients with medullary carcinoma. N Engl J Med 283:890–895, 1970.
79. Melvin KEW, Tashjian AH Jr: Studies in familial (medullary) thyroid carcinoma. Rec Prog Horm Res 28:399–470, 1972.
80. Rude RK, Singer F: Comparison of serum calcitonin levels after a 1-minute calcium injection and after pentagastrin injection in the diagnosis of medullary thyroid carcinoma. J Clin Endocrinol Metab 44:980–983, 1977.
81. Jackson CE, Talpos GB, Kambouris A, et al: The clinical course after definitive operation for medullary thyroid carcinoma. Surgery 94:995–1001, 1983.
82. Saad MF, Ordonex NA, Guido JJ, et al: The prognostic value of calcitonin immunostaining in medullary carcinoma of the thyroid. J Clin Endocrinol Metab 59:850–856, 1984.
83. Deftos JL: Radioimmunoassay for calcitonin in medullary thyroid carcinoma. JAMA 227:403–406, 1974.
84. Sizemore GW, Carney JA, Heath H III: Epidemiology of medullary carcinoma of the thyroid gland: A 5 year experience (1971–1976). Surg Clin North Am 57:633–645, 1977.
85. Di Batholomeo M, Bajetta E, Bochicchio AM, et al: A phase II trial of decarbazine, fluorouracil and epirubicin in patients with neuroendocrine tumours. A study by the Italian Trials on Medical Oncology (ITMO) group. Ann Oncol 6:77–79, 1995.
86. Samaan NA, Schultz PN, Hickey RC: Medullary thyroid carcinoma: Prognosis of familial versus sporadic disease and the role of radiotherapy. J Clin Endocrinol Metab 67:801–804, 1988.
87. Marx SJ, Aurbach GD, Gavin JR, et al: Calcitonin receptors on cultured human lymphocytes. J Biol Chem 249:6812–6816, 1974.
88. Findlay DM, DeLuise M, Michelangeli VP, et al: Properties of a calcitonin receptor and adenylate cyclase in BEN cells, a human lung cancer cell line. Cancer Res 40:1311–1318, 1980.
89. Wu G, Burzon DT, di Sant'Agnese PA, et al: Calcitonin receptor mRNA expression in the human prostate. Urology 47:376–381, 1966.
90. Findlay DM, Michelangeli VP, Eisman JA, et al: Calcitonin and 1,25-dihydroxyvitamin D receptors in human breast cancer cell lines. Cancer Res 40:4764–4767, 1980.
91. Gillespie MT, Thomas RJ, Pu ZY, et al: Calcitonin receptors, bone sialoprotein and osteopontin are expressed in primary breast cancers. Int J Cancer 73:812–815, 1977.
92. Iwasaki Y, Iwasaki J, Freake HC: Growth inhibition of human breast cancer cells induced by calcitonin. Biochem Biophys Res Commun 110:235–242, 1983.
93. Lacroix M, Siwek B, Body JJ: Breast cancer cell responses to calcitonin: Modulation by growth-regulating agents. Eur J Pharmacol 5:279–286, 1998.
94. Cho Chung YS, Clair T, Zubialde JP: Increase of cyclic AMP–dependent protein kinase type II as an early event in hormone-dependent mammary tumor regression. Biochem Biophys Res Commun 85:1150–1155, 1978.
95. Cho Chung YS, Clair T, Bodwin JS, et al: Growth arrest and morphological change of human breast cancer cells by dibutyryl cyclic AMP and L-arginine, Science 214:77–79, 1981.
96. Tiegs RD, Body J-J, Rolfe J, Heath D: Do calcitonin levels decrease with age? Reassessment with new techniques. Calcif Tiss Int 36:479–483, 1984.
97. Overgaard K, Hansen MA, Jensen SB, et al: Effect of calcitonin given intranasally on bone mass and fracture rates in established osteoporosis. A dose response study. BMJ 305:556–561, 1992.
98. Kraenzlin ME, Siebel MJ, Trechsel U, et al: Inhibition of bone turnover by salmon calcitonin in postmenopausal women: Maximum effect in eight weeks of treatment (abstract). Eur J Clin Invest 24:A11, 1994.
99. Azaria M, Copp DH, Zanelli JM: 25 years of salmon calcitonin: From synthesis to therapeutic use. Calcif Tiss Int 57:405–408, 1995.
100. Fornasier RL, Stapleton K, Williams CC: Histologic changes in Paget's disease treated with calcitonin. Hum Pathol 9:455–461, 1978.
101. Doyle FH, Pennock J, Greenberg PB, et al: Radiological evidence of a dose-related response to long term treatment of Paget's disease with human calcitonin. Br J Radiol 47:1–8, 1974.
102. Binstock ML, Mundy GR: Effects of calcitonin and glucorticoids in combination in hypercalcemia of malignancy. Ann Intern Med 93:209–272, 1980.
103. Ralston SH, Alzaid AA, Gardner MD, et al: Treatment of cancer associated hypercalcemia with combined aminohydroxypropylidene diphosphonate and calcitonin. BMJ 292:1549–1550, 1986.

Chapter 72

Vitamin D: From Photosynthesis, Metabolism, and Action to Clinical Applications

Roger Bouillon

HISTORY

Rickets as a bone disease of young children was clearly described by Whistler in 1645[1] and by Glisson in 1650.[2] The relation of this disease to lack of exposure to rural life or sunlight was already recognized in the 19th century since in the United Kingdom, as in Poland, a higher incidence of rickets was observed in children living in large industrialized towns than in children living in more rural districts.[3, 4] Early in the 20th century Huldschinsky,[5] Chick and Hume,[6] and Hess and Weinstock[7] demonstrated radiologic improvement of rachitic children after exposure to sunlight. Following an independent line of research in search of essential nutritional factors, Mellanby and Cantag[8] in the United Kingdom raised dogs on a diet of oatmeal (the basic food in the parts of the United Kingdom where rickets was endemic) and observed that they developed rickets curable by cod liver oil, then recently discovered to contain vitamin A.[9] McCollum et al.,[9] however, demonstrated that vitamin A–deficient (by aeration and heating) cod liver oil was still able to cure rickets and thus contained a new essential nutrient called vitamin D.[10] The two discoveries of vitamin D were unified by Goldblatt and Soames[11] who demonstrated that irradiation of 7-dehydrocholesterol in the skin of animals could produce the antirachitic vitamin D. Similar observations were made by Hess and Weinstock.[7] Windaus, a German chemist, then identified the structure of vitamins D_2 and D_3 after irradiation of plant sterols (ergosterol) or 7-dehydrocholesterol.[12] For his contribution Windaus would receive, in 1928, the Nobel Prize for chemistry.

The elucidation of the mode of action of vitamin D can be separated in two phases: the discovery of (1) the endogenous activation of vitamin D by sequential hydroxylation at C-25 and C-1 and (2) the molecular mechanisms following the binding of 1, 25-hydroxyvitamin D_3 ($1,25(OH)_2D_3$) to a specific and quite ubiquitous receptor. This receptor is now known to be a nuclear transcription factor, which regulates the expression of a very large number of genes involved in either calcium homeostasis or related to cell proliferation or differentiation.

ORIGIN OF VITAMIN D: NUTRITION AND PHOTOSYNTHESIS

Vitamin D can be obtained from dietary sources of vegetal (vitamin D_2 or ergocalciferol) or animal origin (vitamin D_3 or cholecalciferol). About 50% of dietary vitamin D is absorbed by the enterocytes and transported to the blood circulation via chylomicrons. Part of this vitamin D is taken up by a variety of tissues (fat and muscle) before the chylomicron remnants and its vitamin D finally reach the hepatocytes.

The best food sources are fatty fish or its liver oils but it is also found in small amounts in butter, cream, and egg yolk. Both human and cow's milk are poor sources of vitamin D, providing only 15 to 40 IU/L. Milk or colostrum has indeed a low vitamin D (315 and 197 ng/L) concentration and the 25OHD concentration is even lower (188 ng/mL), with negligible $1,25(OH)_2D$ concentration.[13] A higher vitamin D intake only slightly increased the vitamin D concentration of milk. A fairly good correlation is found between vitamin D intake and serum 25OHD concentrations, at least when subjects with widely variable intake are studied, whereas when subjects with intakes between 2 and 20 μg/day are selected only a poor correlation is observed.[14] It is very difficult to obtain adequate vitamin D from a natural diet; however, in North America 98% of fluid and dried milk (400 IU/L), as well as some margarines, butter, and certain cereals, are fortified with vitamin D_2 (irradiated ergosterol) or D_3. However, the real vitamin D content was frequently quite different from the labeling standard. Especially skimmed milk had frequently no detectable vitamin D.[15] Moreover, even proprietary infant formulas frequently did not contain the required 10 μg/L.[16] Vitamin D is remarkably stable and does not deteriorate when food is heated or stored for long periods. The National Health and Nutritional Examination Survey (NHANES) II reported a median intake of about 3 μg/day in adults (range, 0 to 49 μg!),[17] whereas a slightly lower median intake (2.3 μg) was recorded in older women.[18] In view of the low vitamin D content of a vegetarian diet (natural vitamin D intake is indeed related to intake of animal fat), vitamin D deficiency and rickets are a possible risk for strict vegetarian children with insufficient sun exposure or vitamin D supplementation.[19]

The normal adult will obtain sufficient vitamin D from solar exposure and from the ingestion of small amounts with food. However, during pregnancy and lactation and for newborns and young children (especially in industrialized cities where exposure to sunlight is limited and in dark-skinned children living in northern countries), extra supplementation is required. The recommended dietary allowances by the U.S. Food and Nutrition Board of the National Research Council and the 1998 updated recommendations are given in Table 72–1.

TABLE 72–1. Adequate Intake (AI), Previous Recommended Dietary Allowance (RDA), Reasonable Daily Allowance, and Tolerable Upper Limit (UL) for Vitamin D

	Age (yr)	RDA (μg/day [IU])	AI (μg/day [IU])	Reasonable Daily Allowance (IU)	UL (μg/day [IU])
Infants	0.0–1.0	7.5 (300)	5 (200)	200–400	25 (1000)
Children	1–10	10 (400)	5 (200)	200–400	50 (2000)
Adults	11–24	10 (400)	5 (200)	200–400	50 (2000)
	25–50	5 (200)	5 (200)	200–400	50 (2000)
	51–70	5 (200)	10 (400)	400–600	50 (2000)
	70+	5 (200)	15 (600)	600–800	50 (2000)
Pregnant or lactating women		10 (400)	5 (200)	200–400	50 (2000)

From the Food and Nutrition Board, National Research Council, National Academy of Sciences: Recommended Dietary Allowances, ed 10. Washington, DC, National Academy Press, 1989; and Dietary Reference Intakes for Calcium, Phosphorus, Magnesium, Vitamin D and Fluoride, Washington, DC, National Academy Press, 1997.

Hypervitaminosis can occur when pharmaceutical vitamin D is taken in excess, with a wide variety of symptoms and signs related to hypercalciuria, hypercalcemia, and metastatic calcifications (Table 72–2). The toxic dosage has not been established for all ages, but infants and children are more susceptible. Toxicity should always be monitored when daily doses of 50 μg or more of vitamin D are given for a longer period.

Most vertebrates accomplish their needs for vitamin D by photochemical synthesis in the skin.[20] Therefore vitamin D is not a true vitamin. It is formed from 7-dehydrocholesterol (7-DHC or provitamin D_3), which is present in large amounts in cell membranes of keratinocytes of the basal or spinous epidermal layers. By the action of ultraviolet B (UVB) light (290 to 315 mm) the B ring of 7-DHC can be broken to form previtamin D_3. Previtamin D_3 is unstable and in the lipid bilayer of membranes it is rapidly isomerized to vitamin D_3 by thermal energy. The conformational change due to this isomerization can deliver vitamin D to the circulation, where it is caught by the vitamin D binding protein and then transported to the liver for further metabolization.[20]

The production of previtamin D_3 is a nonenzymatic photochemical reaction, which is not subject to regulation other than substrate (7-DHC) availability and intensity of UVB irradiation. 7-DHC is the last precursor in the de novo biosynthesis of cholesterol. The enzyme 7-DHC-Δ7-reductase (or sterol-Δ7-reductase) catalyzes the production of cholesterol from 7-DHC. Inactivating mutations of the recently cloned 7-DHC-Δ7-reductase gene[21] are the hallmark of the autosomal recessive Smith-Lemli-Opitz syndrome, characterized by high tissue and serum 7-DHC levels and multiple anomalies including craniofacial dysmorphism and mental retardation, due to lack of cholesterol synthesis.[22] These patients exhibit increased vitamin D and 25OHD concentrations in their serum.[23] Likewise, animals pretreated with a specific sterol-Δ7-reductase inhibitor also exhibit an augmented vitamin D synthesis following UVB irradiation.[24] To maintain high provitamin D levels, skin in vivo exhibits low sterol-Δ7-reductase activity, probably by the presence of an endogenous inhibitor of the enzyme.[25] With increasing age, however, the cutaneous stores of provitamin D decrease together with decreased photoproduction of vitamin D.[20] In cats, the high cutaneous sterol-Δ7-reductase activity hampers photoproduction of vitamin D, making it a true vitamin.[26] Apart from substrate (7-DHC) availability, the photochemical synthesis of vitamin D_3 in the skin largely depends on the amount of UVB photons that strike the basal epidermal layers. Glass, sunscreens, clothes, and skin pigment absorb UVB and blunt vitamin D synthesis. Latitude, time of day, and season are factors that influence the intensity of solar radiation and the cutaneous production of vitamin D. Therefore there is a risk of shortage of vitamin D supply during winter and springtime.[20, 27, 28] In both the Northern and Southern Hemispheres above 40° latitude, the vitamin D_3 synthesis of the skin decreases or disappears during the winter months due to the lower inclination of the sun and the atmospheric filtration of the shortest (but effective for vitamin D synthesis) UV waves of sunlight. The importance of skin synthesis of vitamin D for maintenance of a normal vitamin D status is best reflected by the vitamin D deficiency observed in personnel of submarines during prolonged absence of sun exposure[20] and also by the extremely high prevalence of vitamin D deficiency in countries where exposure to sunlight is extremely low for cultural and religious reasons, as in several Arabian countries with strict adherence to Islamic rules.[29] An "efficient" sun exposure of 2 hours per week of the face and hands is probably sufficient for maintaining normal 25OHD concentrations in children[30] and adults.

Nature has built in several feedback mechanisms to minimize the risk that prolonged sun exposure would cause vitamin D intoxication. Cutaneous vitamin D and especially previtamin D are photosensitive and are photodegraded to inactive sterols (lumisterol, tachysterol), when they are not translocated to the circulation (Fig. 72–1). Therefore only a maximum of 10% to 15% of the provitamin D will be converted to vitamin D. Sunlight-induced melanin synthesis, acting as a natural sunscreen, provides an additional negative feedback.[20]

TABLE 72–2. Symptoms of Vitamin D Toxicity

Symptoms
Hypercalciuria
Kidney stones
Hypercalcemia
Hyperphosphatemia
Polyuria
Polydipsia
Decalcification of bone
Metastatic calcification of soft tissues (kidney and lung)
Nausea and vomiting
Anorexia
Constipation
Headache
Hypertension

METABOLISM

Vitamin D_3 is biologically inert and requires two successive hydroxylations in the liver (on C-25) and kidney (on the α position of C-1) to form its hormonally active metabolite, $1,25(OH)_2D_3$ (see Fig. 72–1). Liver vitamin D-25-hydroxylase and kidney 25OHD-1α-hydroxylase belong to the large family of cytochrome P450 enzymes.[31, 32]

25-Hydroxylation

25OHD was the first metabolite identified after the availability of radiolabeled vitamin D.[33, 34] Although the liver is probably the main tissue responsible for 25-hydroxylation of vitamin D, extrahepatic 25-hydroxylation has been observed in vitro in a large number of tissues. In vivo observations after hepatectomy in rats also revealed that the conversion rate of [$^{-3}$H]-vitamin D was still about 10% when compared with intact rats.[34] The hepatic 25-hydroxylation step is probably performed by more than one enzyme, localized either in the inner mitochondrial membrane (CYP27A1 or sterol-27-hydroxylase) or in

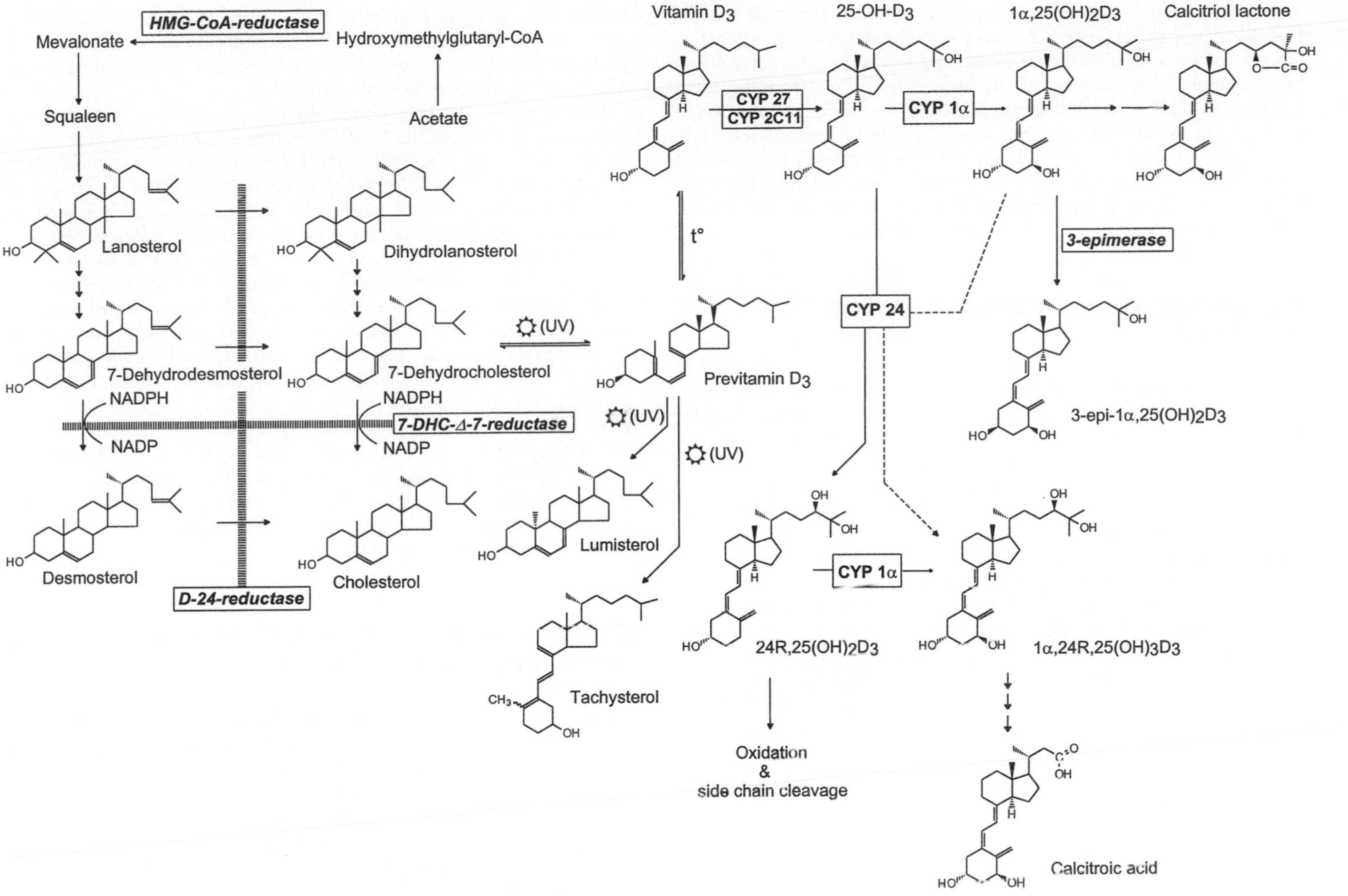

FIGURE 72–1. Origin of vitamin D: photosynthesis and metabolism of vitamin D.

the microsomes (CYP2C11, and probably other enzymes related to the CYP2D family).[31, 35] CYP27A1 is a multifunctional enzyme with broad substrate specificity and is mainly involved in the 26- or 27-hydroxylation of cholesterol and bile acid precursors.[31] CYP27A1 is present in the liver and several other tissues (e.g., fibroblasts, kidney, duodenum, bone cells) of all mammalian species tested. Its capacity for 25-hydroxylation of vitamin D is lower than that of 1α-OHD but still much lower than its high capacity for hydroxylation of bile acid intermediates or cholesterol. Moreover CYP27A1 can easily hydroxylate side-chain analogues of 1,25$(OH)_2D_3$.[36] CYP27A1 gene (human chromosome 2q33) expression is regulated by insulin (negatively), corticosteroids, and growth hormone (positively), but the influence of vitamin D is unclear. Genetic deficiency of CYP27A1 results in a lipid (cholestanol) storage disease, cerebrotendinous xanthomatosis, characterized by prominent neurologic symptoms, accelerated atherosclerosis, cataract, and tendon xanthomas. In some, but not all, cases slightly reduced 25OHD levels and premature osteoporosis[37] have been observed. The rather mild (if any) disturbance of vitamin D metabolism in this disease, as well as the lack of defects in the vitamin D metabolism of CYP27A1 knockout mice,[38] indicates that the 25-hydroxylation of vitamin D does not rely exclusively on the activity of CYP27A1. It is therefore likely that a microsomal enzyme is the more physiologic enzyme as initially suspected on the basis of hepatic enzyme activity being much higher and with lower K_m in the microsomal fraction when compared with mitochondrial 25-hydroxylase activity.[39] The microsomal enzyme activity is upregulated by vitamin D deficiency or by prior exposure to phenobarbital. A purified male-specific CYP2C11 is able to 25-hydroxylate vitamin D[40, 41] but is again unlikely to be the sole or even main hydroxylase responsible for this reaction.

1α-Hydroxylation

25$(OH)D_3$ is biologically inactive and requires further hydroxylation in the kidney[43, 45, 65] to the active hormone, 1,25$(OH)_2D_3$, by 25-hydroxyvitamin D-1α-hydroxylase (CYP27B1). The production of 1,25$(OH)_2D_3$ is regulated primarily at this final step by several factors (see below). The rat, mouse, and CYP27B1 have recently been cloned by several groups[60–64] and the human $P450_{1\alpha}$ is mapped on the human chromosome 12q13.3 in close vicinity to the vitamin D receptor (VDR) gene. The proximal renal tubule is the principle site of 1α-hydroxylation, but high levels of 1α-hydroxylase messenger RNA (mRNA) have also been found in human keratinocytes,[61] and its gene expression is also observed in mouse macrophages.[314] 1α-Hydroxylase activity is under tight control by 1,25$(OH)_2D_3$ (negative but probably indirect feedback), parathyroid hormone (PTH), calcitonin and insulin-like growth factor I (positive feedback), and phosphate and calcium (negative regulation, but may be indirect through suppression of PTH secretion).[32, 66] The promoter of the mouse and human 1α-hydroxylase gene has very recently been characterized with a profound responsiveness to PTH and a weak regulation by 1,25$(OH)_2D_3$[67, 68] despite suppression of its renal activity by 1,25$(OH)_2D_3$ in vivo[62, 63] and high levels of expression in VDR knockout mice.[63] Furthermore, the strong suppression of 1α-hydroxylase activity by calcitriol in cultured keratinocytes is not accompanied by changes in its transcript levels (Bikle, unpublished and our own unpublished results). These findings indicate that the robust feedback of 1,25$(OH)_2D_3$ on 1α-hydroxylase gene expression and function occurs through multiple mechanisms (direct gene suppression through an as yet unidentified vitamin D response element [VDRE] or indirectly via inhibition of enhancer binding transcription factor or through changes in calcium and PTH levels).

Pseudovitamin D–deficiency rickets (PDDR), also known as vitamin D–dependency rickets type I, is an autosomal recessive disease characterized by failure to thrive, muscle weakness, skeletal deformities, hypocalcemia, secondary hyperparathyroidism, normal to high serum levels of $25(OH)D_3$ and low serum $1,25(OH)_2D_3$ concentrations caused by impaired activity of the renal 1α-hydroxylase[69] (see Chapter 84). These patients recover with supplementation of physiologic doses of $1,25(OH)_2D_3$. The human CYP27B1 maps to the previously identified PDDR locus and mutations found in this gene in patients with PDDR provide the molecular genetic basis for this disease.[61, 70]

24-Hydroxylation: Catabolism or Specific Function?

An alternative hydroxylation of $25(OH)D_3$ occurs on C-24 by the multifunctional enzyme, 24-hydroxylase mapped on human chromosome 20q13.[71] This enzyme not only initiates the catabolic cascade of $25(OH)D_3$ and $1,25(OH)_2D_3$[72, 73] by 24-hydroxylation but catalyzes also the dehydrogenation of the 24-OH group and performs 23-hydroxylation resulting in 24-oxo-$1,23,25(OH)_2D_3$.[74] This C-24 oxidation pathway finally leads to calcitroic acid, which is the major end-product of $1,25(OH)_2D_3$ (Fig. 72–2). In vivo evidence for this catabolic role of 24-hydroxylase was provided by treating mice deficient in the 24-hydroxylase gene with $1,25(OH)_2D_3$, which resulted in kidney changes consistent with hypervitaminosis D.[75] The expression of the 24-hydroxylase gene has been detected in kidney, intestine, bone, placenta, skin, and macrophages,[76] tissues that also contain the VDR. The induction of the CYP24 belongs to the most sensitive biomarkers for $1,25(OH)_2D_3$ responsiveness and is explained by the presence of at least two collaborative vitamin D–responsive elements in its promoter.[76] As a consequence CYP24 mRNA levels appear to fall under the detection limits in VDR knockout mice.[63] From this it is clear that the fate of 25OHD to $1,25(OH)_2D_3$ or to $24,25(OH)_2D_3$ largely depends on the presence of $1,25(OH)_2D_3$ and its action through VDR. Regarding potential specific, noncatabolic function for $24,25(OH)_2D_3$ there is evidence from knockout of the 24-hydroxylase gene,[75] that intramembranous bone formation is deficient in certain regions.[77]

Other Metabolic Pathways

Apart from the multifunctional 24-hydroxylation pathway, C-23 and C-26 hydroxylation of $1,25(OH)_2D_3$ is also possible in the absence of prior 24-hydroxylation. The 23-hydroxylation becomes probably only important in case of vitamin D excess. Its major locus is the kidney. In contrast, 26-hydroxylation is mainly performed outside the kidney. Both activities are necessary for the formation of 25OHD- or $1,25(OH)_2D$-23,26-lactones (see Fig. 72–2). The A-ring metabolism involves the oxidation of C-19 and the recently discovered 3-epimerization. The latter, irreversible reaction occurs only in a limited number of cells (e.g., keratinocytes, bone, and parathyroid cells) and is performed by an enzyme resembling hydroxysteroid dehydrogenases.[78] The enzymes involved in the metabolic degradation of $1,25(OH)_2D$ do not recognize all vitamin D analogues in the same way. Indeed, analogues with either 20-epi or 20-methyl configuration or 16-ene structure show an impaired 23-hydroxylation. These or other analogues are then preferentially hydroxylated on C-26 or on new terminal carbons of the side chain. Such alternative metabolism can certainly explain part of the specific selectivity profile of a number of analogues (see below). Vitamin D is mainly excreted in the bile after esterification in the liver but some of its more polar metabolites (e.g., calcitroic acid) are excreted via the urine. The enterohepatic recirculation of vitamin D esters is probably devoid of biologic relevance.

VITAMIN D TRANSPORT

Nutritional vitamin D is absorbed by the gut and then transported via the lymphatic system by chylomicrons[79] and stored in several tissues (e.g., fat), but especially in the liver where it is hydroxylated and thereafter released as 25OHD. Skin-produced vitamin D binds probably directly to a α-globulin known as vitamin D–binding protein (DBP) and is then transported to the liver.

Human DBP[52] detected immunologically in 1959 as group-specific component or Gc-globulin[80] belongs to the serum α_2-globulins synthesized by the liver. This 458–amino acid glycoprotein has a calculated molecular weight of 51300 Da.[81] Long before DBP's functions had been characterized, its polymorphicity was already used in population genetics, parentage testing, and forensic medicine.[82] Worldwide, over 120 Gc alleles have been detected,[83] making the DBP locus one of the most polymorphic known. Gc1F, Gc1S, and Gc2 are the three most common alleles. Since in the many thousands of sera tested none had been found with DBP deficiency, such a mutation was for a long time considered to be lethal, but this was contradicted by the generation of viable and fertile homozygous, DBP-deficient mice (DBP null animals).[84]

The existence of similarity among the genes and protein structure of DBP, albumin, and α-fetoprotein has been well recognized.[52] A fourth member of this family was discovered rather recently and named afamin, or α-albumin. In all these proteins there is a nearly identical positioning of the cysteine residues predicting that the overall folding should be very homologous.[85]

Role of Vitamin D–Binding Protein in Vitamin D Homeostasis

DBP, the major plasma carrier of vitamin D_3, of all its metabolites, and the vitamin D_3 analogues, has one vitamin D sterol-specific binding site.[86, 87] There is only a single binding site for all vitamin D metabolites.[52] The relative binding affinity is $25OHD_3$-23,26-lactone>25OHD = $24,25(OH)_2D$ = $25,26(OH)_2D$ ($K_a = 5.10^8 M^{-1}$ at 4°C for human DBP)>>$1,25(OH)_2D(4.10^7M^{-1})$>>vitamin D>>previtamin D.[88] The affinity for D_2 metabolites is slightly lower than for D_3 metabolites in mammals, but especially in birds. Since probably only non–DBP-bound vitamin D metabolites can readily cross the plasma membrane and since the VDR has a much higher affinity for $1,25(OH)_2D$ than for 25OHD (100-fold difference), whereas the opposite is true for DBP, it is clear that $1,25(OH)_2D$ has substantially higher cellular uptake than 25OHD. This is also confirmed by the distribution space of (radiolabeled) metabolites: 25OHD has a distribution space similar to that of DBP and the plasma volume, whereas the distribution space of $1,25(OH)_2D$ is closer to that of intracellular water. The half-life of 25OHD and $1,25(OH)_2D$ in the human circulation is about 2 to 3 weeks and 4 to 6 hours respectively.[89, 90] This can probably largely be explained by their relative affinity for DBP. Affinity labeling methods and chemical or proteolytic digestions have demonstrated that the sterol-binding domain is located in the N-terminal region and more specifically from amino acid 35 to 49.[91, 92] Moreover, tryptophan 145 is essential for the binding of $25(OH)D_3$.[54]

DBPs function in the vitamin D endocrine system is assumed to reflect the "free hormone hypothesis," which states that the unbound (free) rather than the protein-bound fraction of the active vitamin D hormone is responsible for the biologic activity. On the other hand, vitamin D compounds trapped by DBP in the extracellular compartment provide a readily available reservoir of these molecules. The plasma concentration of DBP is relatively large (~5 μM) compared with other hormone carrier plasma proteins. The plasma concentration of DBP is increased by estrogens in most mammalian species and birds, but in rodents (mice and rats) androgens increase the DBP concentration. In women the DBP concentration therefore doubles at the end of pregnancy.[53] Recent studies with megalin knockout mice indicate that megalin, a lipoprotein-like receptor present at the surface of the proximal tubular cells in the kidney, is responsible for the reabsorption of DBP and of DBP complexed with vitamin D sterols from the urine. This megalin reabsorption mechanism may control the availability of the $25(OH)D_3$-DBP complex for the $25(OH)D_3$-1α-hydroxylation enzyme and explain the severe bone disease of megalin-deficient mice.

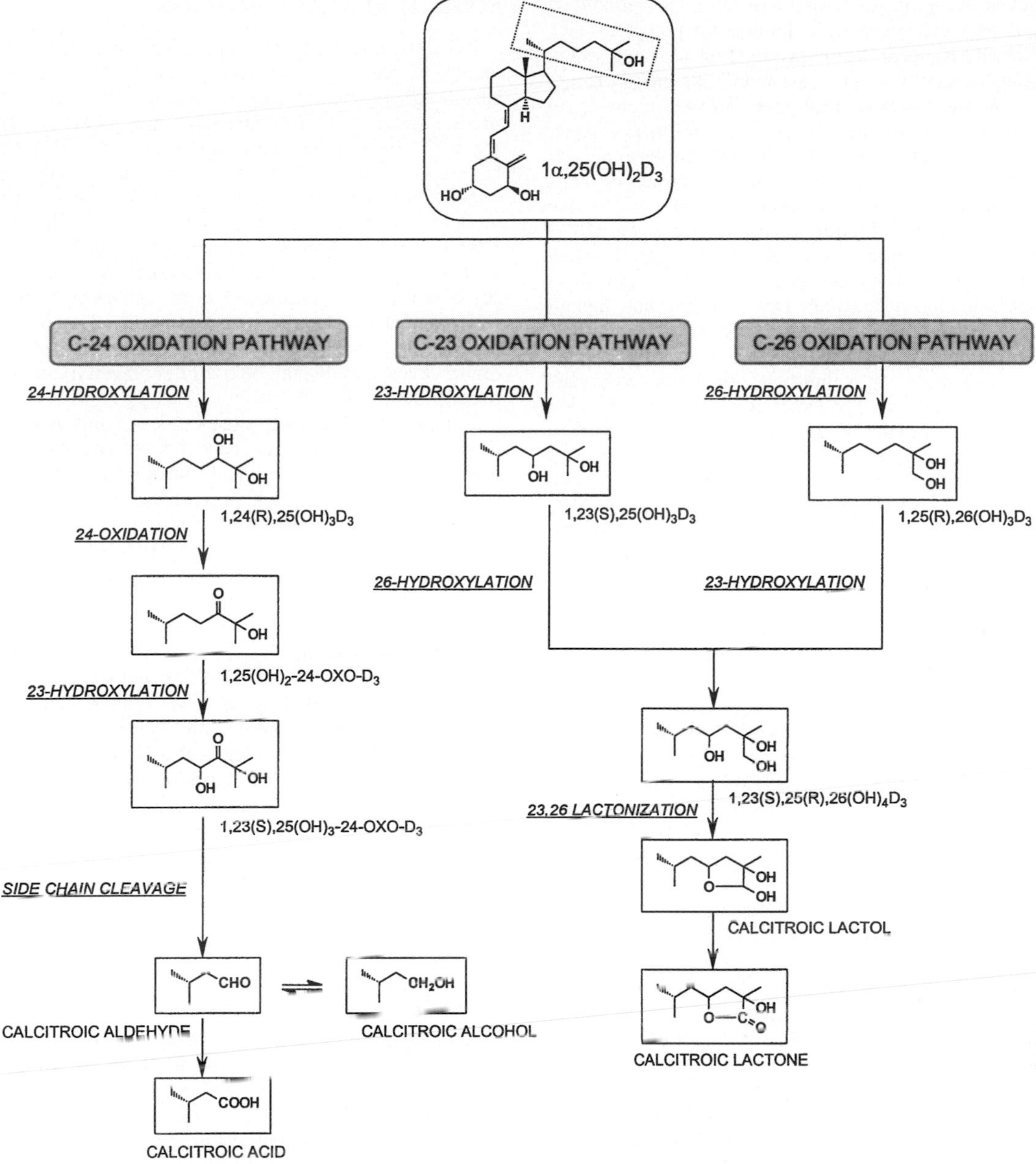

FIGURE 72–2. Catabolism of 1,25-dihydroxyvitamin D_3.

Other Functions of Vitamin D–Binding Protein

DBP, and more specifically its C-terminal part, binds globular actin with a high affinity ($K_a = 2 \times 10^9\ M^{-1}$).[55, 93] This actin-DBP interaction is independent of the presence of vitamin D metabolites. Actin is the most abundant intracellular protein. The cell motility, shape, and size depend on the ability of globular actin to polymerize into filaments (F-actin). Upon cell injury or cell necrosis, actin is released into extracellular space. However, when actin is released from cells, its strong tendency to polymerize is no longer an advantage because the presence of these filaments in blood vessels could be detrimental to the microcirculation. Although multiple intracellular proteins bind actin, only two plasma proteins, DBP and gelsolin, bind actin avidly, thereby acting as an "actin-scavenger system." Whereas gelsolin severs the actin filaments, the generated globular actin is sequestered by DBP, thereby preventing the spontaneous filament formation.[57, 94]

DBP was found to be a precursor of a macrophage-activating factor (MAF)[95] and also enhances the neutrophil chemotactic activity of C5a, a member of the complement family.[96] DBP may also play a role in osteoclastogenesis[97] and osteoclastic bone resorption.[59]

DBP-deficient (knockout) mice, however, develop normally. They are nevertheless more sensitive to vitamin D deficiency and less sensitive to vitamin D excess, probably due to an enhanced urinary loss of vitamin D metabolites.[84] Human DBP has been recently crystallized and its binding and docking sites will soon be available.[98] The DBP and megalin knockout mice, however, suggest that indeed the main function of DBP is to transport all vitamin D metabolites and preserve them from rapid clearance or urinary loss.

ACTION AND MODE OF ACTION

General Characteristics of the Vitamin D Receptor

Protein

$1,25(OH)_2D_3$, the hormonally active form of vitamin D, exerts its effects mainly by activating the nuclear VDR. Human VDR is a 55-kDa (427 amino acids) member of the nuclear receptor superfamily of ligand-activated transcription factors. More specifically, VDR belongs to the class II nuclear receptors that dimerize with the retinoid X receptor (RXR) and also comprise thyroid hormone receptor (TR), retinoic acid receptor (RAR), peroxisome proliferator activated receptor (PPAR), farnesoid X receptor (FXR), and numerous orphan receptors. Based on structure and function similarities between members of this family, plus evidence from disease-causing mutation (see Chapter 84), different functional domains can be distinguished in these nuclear receptor proteins. The short A/B domain at the N-terminus of VDR lacks the usual ligand-independent activation function (AF1). Two highly conserved zinc finger DNA binding motifs constitute the DNA-binding C domain, which also harbors the nuclear localization signal (see Fig. 84–7 in Chapter 84). The D domain or hinge region may regulate the receptor's flexibility between DNA-binding and ligand-binding domains and may be crucial to allow the heterodimer complex of the ligand-binding domains to interact with two differently oriented response elements (direct repeat or palindrome orientation with variable number of spacer nucleotides). The large multifunctional E region contains the ligand-binding domain, as well as a dimerization surface and a ligand-dependent activation function (AF2) at the extreme C-terminus, represented by helix 12.[99] VDR usually acts as a heterodimer with RXR, for which the natural ligand is 9-*cis*-retinoic acid. RXR can also form heterodimers with other class II nuclear receptors (RAR, TR, PPAR) or homodimerize in response to 9cRA.[100] Competition for RXR therefore represents an important mechanism for crosstalk between nuclear receptors.[101]

Gene

The human VDR gene, consisting of 14 exons, spans more than 60 kb on chromosome 12.[102, 103] The main promoter of the gene lacks a TATA box and contains several binding sites for transcription factor Sp1 and other factors such as AP1, AP2, C/EBP, or NFκB.[102] The major VDR transcript is a 4.8-kb mRNA species, but multiple promoters and alternative splicing give rise to a multitude of less abundant transcripts that mostly vary in their 5′ untranslated region, but encode the same 427-amino acid protein.[103] However, two of these mRNAs are translated into VDR proteins that contain an additional 23 or 50 amino acids at the N-terminus.[103] The occurrence of multiple, functionally distinct isoforms is a conserved feature of most nuclear receptors, which is thought to contribute to the tissue- or developmental stage–specific effects of steroid hormones.[104] Among the tissues investigated, the most distal VDR promoter (5′ region of exon 1f) exhibited exclusive activity in calciotropic vitamin D target cells (kidney, gut, and parathyroid gland).[103] Although 1f transcripts encode for the regular VDR protein,[103] differential stability or translation from these mRNAs may underlie a concept for distinct action of vitamin D in calcemic target cells.

Genomic Actions

General Mechanism

The binding of $1,25(OH)_2D_3$ to VDR triggers a sequence of events, eventually leading to changes in the transcription of $1,25(OH)_2D_3$-regulated genes. The mechanism of this transcriptional regulation is very complex and only beginning to be unraveled by site-directed mutagenesis and by extrapolation of crystallographic studies performed on other nuclear receptors.[105] Upon ligation with $1,25(OH)_2D_3$, VDR undergoes conformational changes, heterodimerizes with non–ligand-bound RXR, interacts with VDREs in the promoter region of vitamin D target genes, releases corepressors, and recruits coactivators and general transcription factors for the assembly of an active transcriptional complex[106] (Fig. 72–3). A putative crucial event in this respect is the mousetrap–like intramolecular folding of helix 12, closing off the ligand-binding pocket and exposing the AF2 domain to interaction with coactivators.[107] Concomitantly, the RXR mousetrap will also "spring" and expose its AF2 to coactivators while preventing 9-*cis*-retinoic acid binding.[108] Coactivators serve as bridging factors between RXR-VDR (bound to a VDRE) and the basal transcriptional machinery, but direct interaction between VDR and general transcription factors (e.g., TFIIB) also takes place.

Coactivators and Corepressors

Recently, a vast amount of putative coactivators for VDR have been identified, which are ligand-dependent or ligand-independent, VDR-specific or common to other nuclear receptors. Among these, members of the steroid receptor coactivator group (SRC1, SRC2, and SRC3) are well characterized and appear to regulate the function of most nuclear receptors. Coactivators characteristically possess or recruit histone acetyltransferase activity, which is required for chromatin remodeling (disruption of nucleosomes by dissociation of histones from DNA) in the proximity of vitamin D target genes to augment their accessibility to the basal transcriptional machinery.[109] The large number of coactivators implicated in the action of VDR and other nuclear receptors indicates overlapping and redundant roles for the different coactivators. In this regard, SRC1 knockout animals express SRC2 at higher levels and display only a mild phenotype with partial resistance to steroid hormones.[110]

Corepressors bind and silence non–ligand-bound steroid receptors by recruitment of histone deacetylases maintaining chromatin in a transcriptional repressive state.[111] SMRT (silencing mediator of retinoic acid and TR) was shown to interact with VDR-RXR,[112] whereas NCoR (nuclear receptor corepressor) was not.[113] Of special interest also is the negative impact of SUG1 on VDR transcriptional activity; this subunit of the 26S proteasome competes with coactivators in its ligand-dependent interaction with the VDR AF2 domain and additionally directs VDR to proteasome-mediated degradation.[114] This could provide an important mechanism for the termination of signaling by ligand-bound VDR, in which $1,25(OH)_2D_3$ is trapped in the ligand-binding pocket covered by helix 12. Finally, calreticulin, a multifunctional calcium-binding protein, and the translational regulator L7 were reported to interact with VDR and inhibit its DNA binding.[115, 116]

Distinct regulation of transcriptional coregulators may provide species-, tissue- or developmental stage–specific regulation of nuclear receptor function.[117] Furthermore, the expression or the recruitment of these regulatory proteins are regulated by several intracellular signaling pathways[118] and by steroids themselves,[119] with receptor agonists or antagonists inducing preferential recruitment of coactivators or corepressors respectively.[118]

Vitamin D Response Element

A hexanucleotide direct repeat spaced by three nucleotides (DR3) is the cognate VDRE to which RXR and VDR bind the 5′ and 3′ half-sites respectively. It is possible that a reversal of the orientation of RXR and VDR mediates suppression of gene expression by $1,25(OH)_2D_3$).[106] Although VDR-RXR complexes that interact with DR3 VDRE predominate the transcriptional response to $1,25(OH)_2D_3$, alternative routes appear to be possible both with respect to dimer formation (VDR-VDR, VDR-RAR) and target gene VDRE structure (DR4, DR6; IP9).[119]

The pleiotropic effects of vitamin D cannot entirely be explained by ligand-bound VDR that interacts with VDREs to modulate the transcription of target genes. Indeed, over the last years it has become increasingly clear that transcriptional regulation by $1,25(OH)_2D_3$ also involves indirect mechanisms that are jointly designated as transcriptional crosstalk. In this context, it was presumed that gene activation by vitamin D depends greatly on synergism with other transcription factors.[120] Furthermore, competition for RXR (the promiscuous partner for several nuclear receptors) will give rise to crosstalk between VDR and other class II nuclear receptors.[101] Functional interference between VDR and nuclear receptors, as well as non–receptor transcription factors such as NFAT (nuclear factor of activated T cells), AP-1 (activating protein 1), and NF-κB (nuclear factor κB), may also take place, by inhibiting transcriptional complex formation and DNA binding[121] or by competing for overlapping DNA binding sites[122] for common coactivators, as shown for nuclear receptor–AP1 antagonism,[123] for interaction with the basal transcriptional machinery.[124] To list a few specific examples, VDR regulates interleukin(IL)-2 gene transcription by inhibiting the formation and DNA binding of an NFATp-AP-1 complex[121]; competition between AP-1 and VDR for an overlapping binding site occurs in the promoter of the osteocalcin gene[122]; YY1 is

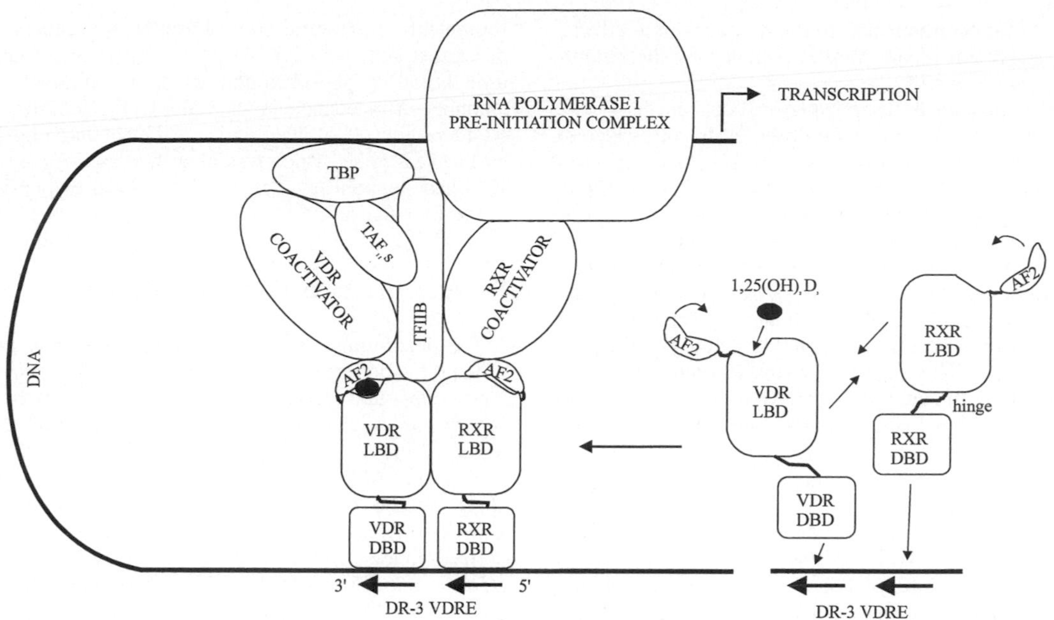

FIGURE 72–3. Mechanism of transcriptional regulation by the vitamin D receptor (VDR). Upon binding its ligand, 1,25-dihydroxyvitamin D_3, VDR undergoes conformational changes, heterodimerizes with non–ligand-bound retinoid X receptor (RXR), interacts with VDR response elements in the promoter region of vitamin D target genes, releases corepressor complexes (not shown), and recruits coactivators and general transcription factors for the assembly of an active transcriptional complex. Interaction with most coactivators is only possible after the crucial intramolecular folding of helix 12 in both VDR and RXR, closing off the ligand-binding pocket and exposing the AF2 domain. Coactivators not only stabilize the preinitiation complex as bridging factors but also exert or recruit histone acetyltransferase activity (not shown), ensuring site-directed chromatin remodeling and access to the core promoter for the general transcriptional apparatus.

a transcription factor that can interfere with the interactions of VDR with both the VDRE and TFIIB[124]; and finally, VDR is able to decrease the levels of NF-κB components[125] and to repress NF-κB binding to DNA and NF-κB–driven transcription of the IL-8[126] and IL-12 gene.[127] It needs to be emphasized that transcriptional crosstalk is predominantly based on protein-protein interactions, which do not require DNA binding or direct transcriptional modulation. Meanwhile, increasing evidence indicates that the desired anti-inflammatory actions of corticosteroids and the antitumoral and growth-inhibitory effects of retinoids are highly related to antagonism to AP-1 or NF-κB, or both.[128] Likewise, it is also appealing to invoke inhibition of NFAT, NF-κB, and AP-1 in the anti-inflammatory and antiproliferative capacities of active vitamin D compounds.

Other critical parameters in the control of the vitamin D response in vitamin D target tissues include, of course, the local $1,25(OH)_2D_3$ concentration (as regulated by the activity of 1α-hydroxylase) and the VDR abundance, which is also highly regulated by a diversity of signals[129]: heterologous regulation mostly occurs by transcriptional mechanisms while autologous upregulation by calcitriol emerges from ligand-dependent stabilization of the receptor protein.[130] Phosphorylation of the VDR finally constitutes an additional mechanism for crosstalk with extracellular signals that originate at membrane receptors: the VDR protein contains two phosphorylation sites implicated in fine-tuning its function via casein kinase (positive regulation), protein kinase C (negative), or protein kinase A (negative).[99] These phosphorylation events may also be involved in ligand-independent activation of VDR,[131] which is also supported by the occurrence of symptoms (alopecia) in VDR knockout mice that do not occur in vitamin-dependent rickets type I or in severe nutritional rickets.

Vitamin D–dependent rickets type II (vitamin D–resistant rickets)[132] is an autosomal recessive disease caused by end-organ unresponsiveness to $1,25(OH)_2D_3$ due to inactivation of the VDR. Such patients present with severe early-onset, postnatal rickets (with hypocalcemia, high circulating levels of $1,25(OH)_2D_3$, and secondary hyperparathyroidism) frequently accompanied by alopecia (see Chapter 84). At present, 18 different natural mutations in the VDR gene have been described, most of which lead to amino acid substitutions in the zinc finger region of the DNA-binding domain or in the ligand-binding domain. Interestingly, some patients with all the clinical and biochemical hallmarks of vitamin D resistance exhibit a normal VDR cDNA. Presumably, this subtype is caused by mutations that either impair VDR expression or target VDR cofactors necessary for its function (VDR promoter, coactivators, RXR).

Several polymorphic allelic variants of the VDR gene have been described, some of which are linked to metabolic bone disease (osteoporosis or osteoarthritis), hyperparathyroidism, prostate or breast cancer, diabetes mellitus, or psoriasis (reviewed in Haussler et al.[106]). This issue remains highly controversial and unresolved, especially with respect to polymorphism at the 3′ end of the gene (BsmI, ApaI, TaqI RFLP and mRNA polyA microsatellite polymorphism, which are often present as a cluster). The unrelated FokI RFLP at the 5′ translation initiation site in exon 2 only recently developed in evolution and exists exclusively in humans. The somewhat more frequent F allele (absence of FokI restriction site) directs initiation of translation only at the fourth codon, giving rise to the M4 VDR isoform containing 424 amino acid residues instead of 427. Recent studies indicate that M4 VDR is transcriptionally more active and that its presence is associated with an increased bone mineral density (BMD).[133] However, further investigation is warranted as a more recent study could not confirm a simple association between BMD and FokI VDR gene polymorphism.[134]

Nongenomic Actions

Besides the VDR transcriptional or genomic effects, several research groups have described rapid effects by $1,25(OH)_2D_3$ that are independent of transcription and would be mediated by a membrane receptor for $1,25(OH)_2D_3$[135] or by the localization of the nuclear VDR near the membrane.[136] These so-called nongenomic effects include the opening of calcium or chloride channels and the activation of second messenger signaling pathways (phosphoinositide turnover, activation of protein kinase C, and the Ras-Raf-ERK MAPK pathway).[137] Recently, $1,25(OH)_2D_3$ was also shown to antagonize the JNK signaling pathway contributing to AP-1 antagonism, most likely by a transcription-independent mechanism.[138] Sometimes there is a close interplay between genomic and nongenomic signals; for example, some phospholipase C genes are transcriptionally regulated by $1,25(OH)_2D_3$.[139] Furthermore, the nuclear VDR itself can be implicated in rapid nongenomic effects, for example, in the activation of the MAPK pathway by the recruitment of the adapter protein Shc.[140]

A wide variety of rapid and transient modifications in the second messenger signaling system have also been observed for other steroid hormones.[141] Since genomic and nongenomic activation or antagonism can be generated by different analogues of $1,25(OH)_2D$ it is highly likely that a different receptor molecule is involved. Annexin 2 was recently identified, based on photoaffinity studies, as a candidate membrane receptor,[142] but others have identified proteins with other characteristics. At the tissue or cellular level, however, nongenomic activity of vitamin D and its analogues or metabolites have only been described for intestinal calcium absorption (transcaltachia) or cellular differentiation of leukemia cells.[143–145] This pathway seems to prefer 6-*s-cis* to the 6-*s-trans*-configuration of vitamin D.[143] Moreover the agonist/antagonist specificity differs for that of the genomic pathway.[146]

Classic Target Tissues

The classic function of $1,25(OH)_2D_3$ in maintaining serum calcium and phosphate levels and as the safeguard of skeletal integrity is the result of its effects on intestine (calcium and phosphate absorption), kidney (phosphate and calcium reabsorption), parathyroid glands (suppression of PTH secretion), and bone (osteoclastogenesis and the incompletely understood effects on osteoblasts and mineralization of bone matrix). In this respect, target genes with a prominent VDRE in their promoter are the calcium-binding proteins calbindin D_{9K} (intestine), calbindin D_{28K} (kidney and other tissues), the noncollagenous bone-specific matrix protein osteocalcin, matrix GLA protein, osteopontin (extracellular matrix protein in bone and other tissues) to which osteoclasts adhere through $\alpha_v\beta_3$ integrin (the promoter for the β_3 gene contains VDRE), and carbonic anhydrase, which generates protons required for osteoclast bone resorption.[106]

Recently, *osf2*/*cbfa*1 transcription factor was identified as the cleidocranial dysostosis gene, which is a master regulator for the differentiation of mesenchymal cells into osteoblasts. Levels of *cbfa*1 mRNA are strongly suppressed by $1,25(OH)_2D_3$, which reveals possible new mechanisms for regulation of gene expression in bone by $1,25(OH)_2D_3$.[147] Exciting new developments in the field of osteoclastogenesis also identified three novel vitamin D–regulated genes in bone osteoblasts and stromal cells. Osteoclast differentiation factor–osteoprotegerin ligand is a $1,25(OH)_2D_3$-induced, membrane-associated member of the tumor necrosis factor (TNF) family enhancing osteoclast formation by mediating direct interactions between osteoblasts and stromal cells and osteoclast progenitor cells.[148, 149] Conversely, osteoclastogenesis inhibitory factor and osteoprotegerin, secreted proteins of the TNF receptor family which block osteoclastogenesis by antagonizing osteoprotegerin ligand function, are downregulated by $1,25(OH)_2D_3$.[149] Moreover the receptor for osteoclast differentiation factor on osteoclast (precursors), RANK, is also upregulated by vitamin D.[150] The broad tissue distribution (e.g., thymus) of the paracrine osteoprotegerin–osteoprotegerin ligand system may indicate that it might also participate in nonclassic vitamin D effects in the immune system or the skin. *Id1* is another critical gene that was shown to be suppressed by $1,25(OH)_2D_3$ in bone cells by the assembly of a silencing complex binding to a specific sequence in the Id1 promoter.[151] Id proteins are important negative regulators of differentiation by their ability to interfere with the action of helix-loop-helix transcription factors.

The classic action of $1,25(OH)_2D_3$ on bone, intestine, kidney, and parathyroid glands and its role in mineral metabolism are the result of a complex interplay between $1,25(OH)_2D_3$, PTH, calcium, and phosphate. PTH induces calcium mobilization from bone and stimulates $1,25(OH)_2D_3$ production, but its secretion is inhibited by the action of $1,25(OH)_2D_3$ on the parathyroid glands (negative feedback). In a second negative feedback loop $1,25(OH)_2D_3$ limits its own availability by inhibition of 1α-hydroxylase and stimulation of 24-hydroxylase, inducing $1,25(OH)_2D$ catabolism. In the last few years, considerable progress has been made in the understanding of phosphate homeostasis. The *NPT2* gene encodes a renal sodium–phosphate cotransporter responsible for resorption of phosphate and represents a newly identified target gene for $1,25(OH)_2D_3$.[152] The poorly characterized phosphaturic hormone phosphatonin, which is putatively produced in large amounts in osteomalacia of malignancy, inhibits the activity of the NPT2 protein. Phosphatonin can be inactivated by a protease encoded by the *PEX* gene, which was identified as the gene that is defective in X-linked hypophosphatemic rickets. *PEX* expression is probably induced by calcitriol.[153]

Effects on Intestine and Kidney

The absorption capacity of calcium along the gastrointestinal tract of the rat is dependent on the segment and follows the following order: ileum>jejunum>duodenum. The efficiency of the small intestine to absorb dietary calcium is increased by $1,25(OH)_2D_3$[154] and the abundance of the VDR is highest in the duodenum followed by jejunum and ileum. Although the exact mechanism by which $1,25(OH)_2D_3$ alters the flux of calcium across the intestinal absorptive cell is not known, $1,25(OH)_2D_3$ increases the production and activity of several proteins in the small intestine, including calbindin-D9K, alkaline phosphatase, and low-affinity calcium-adenosinetriphosphatase (Ca^{2+}-ATPase) (PMCA). The entry of Ca^{2+} from the intestinal lumen across the brush border membrane into the enterocyte is a diffusional process and $1,25(OH)_2D_3$ is suggested to increase the rate of entry by a nongenomic process. The intracellular calcium transfer is considered to be dependent mainly on calbindin-D9K.[155] The regulation of calbindin-D9K by $1,25(OH)_2D_3$ involves both transcriptional and post-transcriptional mechanism.[156] In vivo evidence for the transcriptional regulation was provided by the dramatically reduced levels of calbindin-D9K mRNA in the intestine of VDR-ablated mice and the absence of induction after $1,25(OH)_2D_3$ injection.[157] A classic VDRE was identified in the rat calbindin-D9K.[158] The intestinal calbindin-D9K expression in VDR null mice could, however, be restored by a high lactose, high calcium, high phosphorus diet, suggesting that multiple factors interact to regulate its expression. The transfer of Ca^{2+} from the cytoplasm to the extracellular space requires energy input because of an uphill concentration gradient and an unfavorable electrochemical gradient. Both the plasma membrane calcium pump and a sodium-calcium exchanger play important roles in this process. The stimulatory effect of $1,25(OH)_2D_3$ on the adenosine triphosphate(ATP)–dependent uptake of Ca^{2+} at the basolateral membrane involves an increase in *PMCA* gene expression.[159]

The kidney is important for the metabolism of $1,25(OH)_2D_3$ as well as for the reabsorption of calcium, a process regulated by $1,25(OH)_2D_3$. The kidney, more specifically the proximal tubule, is the central tissue for 1α-hydroxylation of 25OHD[160] and the renal 1α-hydroxylase gene has recently been cloned by several groups.[60–64] Renal disorders such as acquired chronic renal failure result in reduced 1α-hydroxylase activity with renal rickets and hyperphosphatemia as symptoms. In addition, the kidney is the major, although not exclusive, site of 24-hydroxylase activity. Several in vivo and in vitro studies suggest that $1,25(OH)_2D_3$ has an effect on the distal tubular reabsorption of calcium.[161, 162] The exact underlying mechanism is, however, not yet defined. Elements of the calcium transport system, including calbindin-D9K, calbindin-D28K, and the plasma membrane Ca^{2+}-ATPase are present in the distal tubule, where VDRs are also found. The expression of both calbindins is regulated by $1,25(OH)_2D_3$ in the kidney while its effect on Ca^{2+}-ATPase is not known. Whereas in the intestine active calcium absorption in the duodenum takes place before the less regulated diffusion process in the ileum, reabsorption of filtered calcium follows a more logical sequence of massive calcium-sodium reabsorption in the proximal convoluted tubules followed by specific, actively regulated calcium reabsorption in the distal parts of the nephron.

Effects on Bone and Bone-Derived Cells

The effect of $1,25(OH)_2D_3$ on bone homeostasis is less clear. The general concept is that $1,25(OH)_2D_3$ has a biphasic effect on osteoblasts: it abrogates or stimulates the normal developmental pathway or gene expression profiles depending upon whether it is given, respectively, during the proliferation[163] or differentiation stage.[164] $1,25(OH)_2D_3$ given during the proliferative period of rat calvaria osteoblast cultures inhibits proliferation and downregulates collagen synthesis and alkaline phosphatase activity; osteocalcin expression is not stimulated[165] and nodule formation is blocked,[163] suggesting a stop in osteoblast differentiation. In contrast, $1,25(OH)_2D_3$ treatment of mature osteoblasts, results in upregulation of osteoblast-associated genes, such as osteopontin and osteocalcin, and in stimulation of calcium accumulation.[164] At this stage of differentiation $1,25(OH)_2D_3$ may "push" the osteoblast toward an even more mature state. A comparable result was found in a conditionally transformed adult human osteoblast cell line.[166] The in vivo consequence of these in vitro observations is problematic at present, mainly because of the paucity of detailed information. Local factors involved in bone remodeling are also modulated by $1,25(OH)_2D_3$, but again different responses have been observed depending on the system used and on the stage of cell differentiation: as an example, the effect on insulin-like growth factor 1 (IGF-1) production is either stimulatory or inhibitory, whereas the effect on transforming growth factor-β (TGF-β) is mainly stimulatory,[167] and on vascular endothelial growth factor it is always stimulatory.

Osteoclast-like cell formation in co-culture systems, existing of bone marrow, spleen, or peripheral blood and osteoblastic stromal cells, is dependent on osteotrophic factors like $1,25(OH)_2D_3$, and osteoblastic stromal cells are critical in this process. The proposed mechanism is that $1,25(OH)_2D_3$ acts directly on osteoblasts and stromal cells to induce the expression of osteoclast differentiation factor–osteoprotegerin ligand (Fig. 72–4). Interestingly, the action of $1,25(OH)_2D_3$ is not essential to osteoclast formation in vivo since VDR-deficient mice have a normal number of osteoclasts.[168] This can now be explained by the stimulatory effects of either cytokines (e.g., IL-1, IL-6, IL-11) or PTH or PTH-related protein (PTHrP) on osteoclast differention factor and osteoprotegerin expression via their respective receptor and second signaling pathway.

The overall effects of vitamin D metabolites on bone are thus extremely complex. An attractive hypothesis[169] could be that $1,25(OH)_2D$ is mainly responsible for mineralization of bone at the time of endochondral bone formation and during later bone remodeling, whereas $24R,25(OH)_2D$ might have unique properties for mineralization of bone matrix generated by the intramembraneous pathway.[77] Such a mechanism might hypothetically also explain some important effects of $24R,25(OH)_2D$ on fracture healing.

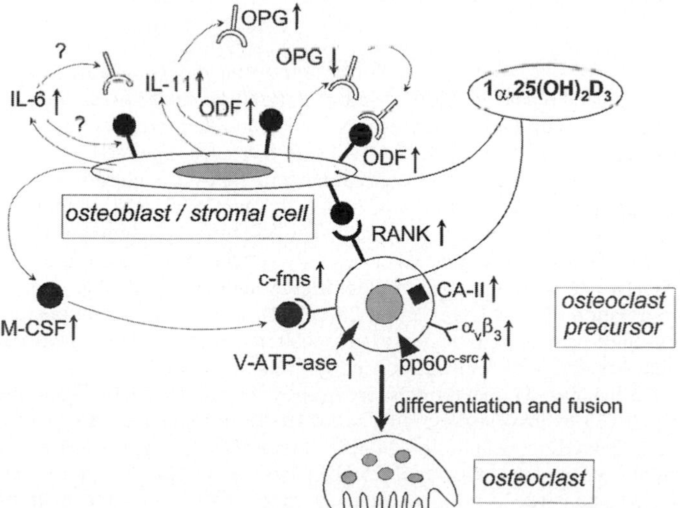

FIGURE 72–4. Effect of 1,25-dihydroxyvitamin D_3 on bone cells and osteoclastogenesis. In osteoblast and stromal cells $1,25(OH)_2D_3$ induces osteoclast differentiation factor (ODF) expression, downregulates osteoprotegerin (OPG), and stimulates macrophage colony-stimulating factor (M-CSF) production. It also stimulates production of interleukins (IL) IL-6 and IL-11, which represent distinct signals in osteoclastogenesis. On osteoclast precursors, $1,25(OH)_2D_3$ induces the expression of RANK (or ODF receptor) and of several osteoclast differentiation markers such as the vitronectin receptor $\alpha_v\beta_3$ and carbonic anhydrase-II. c-fms, M-CSF receptor; CA-II, carbonic anhydrase-II; V-ATP-ase, vacuolar ATPase.

From in vivo observation in man and animals it is clear that vitamin D deficiency or resistance impairs bone matrix mineralization, whereas osteoblast activity and matrix synthesis are stimulated. From in vitro studies $1,25(OH)_2D$ clearly enhances osteoclastogenesis and bone resorption, whereas positive effects on bone matrix formation and mineralization are difficult to observe unless fully mature osteoblasts are used. Osteoclastogenesis and osteoblastogenesis as well as their function can obviously take place in the absence of vitamin D. Bone mineralization can largely be induced by a sufficient supply of minerals via active or passive intestinal calcium absorption. Therefore it would seem that direct effects of vitamin D metabolites on chondrocytes and bone cells are redundant. The present data, however, cannot exclude that some of the vitamin D–regulated genes allow a better fine-tuning of bone mineral homeostasis. Moreover, pharmacologic use of vitamin D metabolites or analogues might positively influence bone balance, as shown by human and animal experiments[170, 171] and transgenic mice overexpressing osteoblast VDR.[172]

Vitamin D Receptor Knockout Mice

Recently, two different groups[168, 173] have created VDR knockout mice. Although the VDR is widely expressed early during embryonic development, no major developmental abnormalities are observed in the VDR-/- mice. Homozygous mice are phenotypically normal at birth and show normal growth until weaning. Demay, however, describes an expanded zone of hypertrophic chondrocytes in the growth plate already at day 15.[62] By day 21, the mice become hypocalcemic and PTH levels begin to rise. Rickets develops progressively and surviving mice have 10-fold elevated levels of $1,25(OH)_2D_3$ together with very low $24,25(OH)_2D_3$ levels. These mice show marked growth retardation and decreased survival rates. The development of alopecia, although not to the same extent, is observed in the two groups, but uterine hypoplasia is only present in Kato's animals.[168] When VDR null mice were fed a diet containing high calcium, high phosphorus, and high lactose, growth and serum Ca^{2+} levels were normalized.[174] In addition, such a diet prevented the development of rickets in VDR-ablated mice, while alopecia was still observed. These data suggest that in the absence of genomic actions of $1,25(OH)_2D_3$, normalization of mineral absorption and extracellular mineral homeostasis can prevent the development of hyperparathyroidism and rickets as has also been observed in vitamin D–resistant patients treated with high doses of intravenous (IV) or oral calcium.[175]

DIAGNOSTIC AND THERAPEUTIC ASPECTS OF VITAMIN D

Assays for Vitamin D and Metabolites: Methodology and Applications

Vitamin D and about 30 of its metabolites are found in plasma. Measurements of their concentrations may be essential to clinical or research purposes.[46, 176] All techniques require a lipid extraction to free these compounds from their binding proteins (especially DBP). In view of the high molar extinction of vitamin D, UV absorptiometry can be used for measurement of vitamin D_2, vitamin D_3, or 25OHD after high-performance liquid chromatography (HPLC). However, competitive binding assays or radioimmunoassay (RIA) is preferred for measurements of 25OHD, $1,25(OH)_2D_3$, or $24,25(OH)_2D$.[47] These assays remain difficult as demonstrated by remarkably poor intra- and especially interlaboratory quality-control studies. Nonchromatographic assays using DBP overestimate the true 25OHD concentration by 10% to 20%, but nonspecific interferences (DBP, lipids?) in some assays can result in up to 100% higher values. The measurement of serum concentrations of vitamin D_2 or D_3 is of little clinical value. Indeed, because of their short half-life in plasma, it reflects only recent exposure to UV light or nutritional intake. Serum 25OHD concentration is, however, an excellent reflection of the vitamin D status because of the rapid conversion of vitamin D into 25OHD and its long plasma half-life.[47, 176] Its plasma concentration varies widely in normal subjects because of large variations in the endogenous and exogenous supply of vitamin D (Table 72–3).

Plasma 25OHD concentration thus behaves as a true vitamin whose concentration depends on "nutritional" (endo- and exogenous) supply. Combined deficiency of exposure to UV light and low vitamin D intake is quite common in infants and elderly subjects if food sources are not supplemented with vitamin D. Plasma 25OHD concentrations are indeed low at birth (about half the maternal concentration because of the 2:1 ratio of maternal to fetal DBP concentration) and the natural vitamin D content of milk is low. Sun exposure was therefore evolution's solution to prevent rickets. However, in view of the relation between exposure to UVB light (especially in young children) and the subsequent risk for skin malignancies, it is probably wise to advocate systematic vitamin D supplementation for all infants and young children. Whereas widespread vitamin D deficiency in infants was recognized and prevented at the beginning of the 20th century, a similar endemic deficiency in the elderly has only recently been recognized and is starting to be tackled at the beginning of the 21st century (see below). Intestinal malabsorption of fat-soluble vitamins interrupts the absorption of the exogenous but probably also the endogenous hepatobiliary excretion of vitamin D and therefore requires either substitution with large amounts of vitamin D or more physiologic doses (10 to 20 μg/day) of the more soluble 25OHD. A low calcium intake can markedly (two fold) increase the catabolism of 25OHD and will therefore facilitate substrate deficiency if the "nutritional" supply is marginal.[48]

TABLE 72–3. Plasma Concentration of 25-Hydroxyvitamin D

Normal fluctuation according to
- Dietary intake (+)*
- Sun (UV light) exposure (+) influenced by seasonal life-style and cultural habits
- Age (−)
- Skin pigmentation (−)
- Latitude (−)
- Sunscreen use (−)

Increased 25OHD concentration
- Exposure to pharmaceutic vitamin D†
- Excess exposure to nutritional vitamin D
- Excess exposure to UV light

Decreased 25OHD concentration‡
- Combined deficiency of access or exposure to nutritional vitamin D and UV light
- Major risk groups include
  - Infants, especially those born in late winter
  - Women and children of immigrants with pigmented skin living in temperate climates
  - Elderly population with limited mobility
  - Subset of population with low exposure to sunshine because of socioeconomic, religious, or cultural reasons
- Decreased intestinal absorption of vitamin D associated with fat malabsorption, e.g., associated with
  - Biliary cirrhosis
  - Short-bowel syndrome
  - Exocrine pancreas insufficiency
  - Gluten enteropathy
- Increased loss or catabolism of vitamin D
  - Nephrotic syndrome
  - Chronic liver P450 activation by drugs (e.g., barbiturates or antiepileptic drugs)
- Low calcium intake or absorption

*Positive or negative effects are indicated by + or −, respectively.

†Vitamin D toxicity with hypercalciuria, hypercalcemia, nephrocalcinosis, kidney stones, metastatic calcification, etc. are only observed if 25OHD concentrations exceed 100 ng/mL. Without access to pharmaceutic vitamin D clinical vitamin D toxicity is unlikely.

‡For definition of vitamin D insufficiency or deficiency, see chapter recommended daily intake and Table 72–1.

TABLE 72–4. Plasma Concentration of 1,25-Dihydroxyvitamin D_3

Decreased Concentrations	Increased Concentrations
*Substrate Deficiency**	*Substrate Excess†*
E.g., nutritional rickets, intestinal malabsorption	
25OHD-1α-Hydroxylase Enzyme Deficiency	*25OHD-1α-Hydroxylase Enzyme Excess*
Inborn	Functional
Vitamin D–dependent rickets	Primary or tertiary hyperparathyroidism
Organic	Hypothyroidism
Renal insufficiency or anephric patients	Glucocorticoid excess
Functional	Acromegaly
Hypoparathyroidism	Granulomatous diseases‡
Pseudohypoparathyroidism	Idiopathic hypercalciuria
Hypomagnesemia	Hypophosphatemic rickets type II (+ hypercalciuria)
Tumoral osteomalacia	Pregnancy
Hypercalcemia of malignancy	Nutritional calcium deficiency
Hyperthyroidism	William's syndrome
Addison's disease (acute)	
Severe insulin deficiency	
X-linked hypophosphatemia	
Rhabdomyolysis	
Tumoral calcinosis	
Vitamin D–Binding Protein (DBP) Deficiency	*DBP Excess*
Fetus	Pregnancy
Nephrotic syndrome	Oral estrogen use
Liver cirrhosis	
Unknown or Disputed Origin	*End-Organ Resistance*
Primary osteoporosis	True vitamin D resistance (so-called vitamin D–dependent rickets type II)

*In many cases of rickets or osteomalacia, $1,25(OH)_2D_3$ concentrations are still measurable or even nearly normal. This may be due to recent and insufficient access to vitamin D after long-term vitamin D deficiency. Nevertheless, such concentration is too low in comparison with the degree of secondary hyperparathyroidism. In any case 25OHD is a better marker for vitamin D deficiency than $1,25(OH)_2D_3$. A similar situation is observed in hypothyroidism when the precursor hormone thyroxine is a better marker for clinical hypothyroidism than the real hormone, triiodothyronine.

†Vitamin D excess only increases serum $1,25(OH)_2D_3$ when renal function remains normal and/or parathyroid hormone secretion is elevated. Frequently, $1,25(OH)_2D_3$ levels are low or normal in vitamin D toxicity.

‡Monocyte activation can result in extrarenal synthesis of $1,25(OH)_2D_3$ as in sarcoidosis, tuberculosis, foreign body inflammation, lymphoma, and some fungal infections.

The metabolism of 25OHD into $1,25(OH)_2D_3$ and $24R,25(OH)_2D_3$ is tightly controlled by hormones, ions, and humoral factors. The plasma concentration of $1,25(OH)_2D_3$ is therefore regulated as a true hormone (Table 72–4) and measurements of its concentration can be useful for clinical exploration of (unusual) cases of rickets, osteopenia, and hypo- or hypercalcemia. The serum concentration of $24,25(OH)_2D_3$ and $25,26(OH)_2D$ usually reflects the concentration of 25OHD and therefore does not contribute additional valuable clinical information. The 25OHD and $1,25(OH)_2D$-lactone concentrations are only increased in case of important substrate excess but their measurement has not (yet) been introduced in clinical practice.

All vitamin D metabolites are tightly bound to DBP. Since the hepatic 25-hydroxylase activity is not feedback-regulated, the free (or total) 25OHD concentration largely fluctuates according to substrate supply. In contrast, the renal 25OHD-1α-hydroxylase is tightly controlled and since access to VDR in target tissues is dependent on the circulating free concentrations, free and not total $1,25(OH)_2D_3$ concentration is important.[53, 177] The circulating DBP concentration is, however, fairly stable except when stimulated by estrogens (or pregnancy) or decreased by reduced synthesis (liver cirrhosis) or increased urinary loss (nephrotic syndrome). The major arguments for the importance of free rather than total $1,25(OH)_2D_3$ are (1) in vitro experiments (biologic activity of $1,25(OH)_2D_3$ on cultured cells[178, 179]) and (2) in vivo observations such as increased steady-state concentration of $1\alpha,25(OH)_2D_3$ without signs of increased action during chronic estrogen use or in animals immunized against the $1,25(OH)_2D$-hapten-protein complex.[180]

Pharmacology of Vitamin D and Metabolites

Recommended Daily Intake

Whereas earlier recommendations by various official nutritional boards around the world have been variable for adults, a daily intake of 10 μg of vitamin D has been recommended for infants and children. In 1997 the Standing Committee on the Scientific Evaluation of Dietary Reference of the Food and Nutrition Board[181] intakes carefully reevaluated vitamin D requirements and recommendations (see Table 72–1). Since vitamin D is in fact not a true vitamin for people regularly exposed to efficient sunlight, guidelines are intended as a recommendation for those who are, willingly or unwillingly, not sufficiently exposed to sunlight. Moreover the expert committee distinguished adequate intake from reasonable daily allowance and also tried to define a tolerable upper limit (see Table 72–1). In view of the lower efficacy of UV light for synthesis of vitamin D in the skin of elderly subjects and the worldwide observation of high prevalence of vitamin D deficiency in elderly people, a higher recommended dietary allowance (600 IU or 15 μg/day) has been recommended for people above 71 years of age. The average intake represents the mean intake that is considered to maintain adequate serum 25OHD in a group of sex- and age-specified subjects with limited sun exposure. While this average intake is an overestimation of the true minimal need, it may nevertheless not be adequate for some (e.g., those with exceptionally low calcium intake). The introduction of upper limits of daily intake is quite appropriate because an intake higher than 50 μg (2000 IU) is not associated with improved health but increases the risk of vitamin D toxicity due to its extremely long retention time as a fat-soluble vitamin. Individuals, therefore, who have a high intake of vitamin D–rich or vitamin D–fortified food should not combine this with (multi)vitamin D preparations.

Clinical Use

Vitamin D_3 and vitamin D_2 are probably the most commonly used drugs because of their widespread addition to foods and their generalized use in newborns and children. The indication is simple: to prevent or cure vitamin D deficiency. Defining mild deficiency of a vitamin is somewhat arbitrary, as is well known for iodine or iron deficiency. The threshold concentration of 25OHD used to define vitamin D deficiency is therefore controversial. Overt clinical rickets or osteomalacia is usually only found when 25OHD levels fall below 5 ng/mL (12.5 nmol/L). Milder degrees of vitamin D deficiency cause secondary hyperparathyroidism with increased bone turnover. Cross-sectional studies comparing serum PTH and 25OHD levels indicated secondary hyperparathyroidism starting from 25OHD levels below 15 ng/mL (37 nmol/L).[47, 182–184] In a French epidemiologic study, however, PTH started (very slowly) to rise when 25OHD levels fell below 78 nmol/L, but the increase was minimal until values fell below 40 to 60 nmol/L.[185] This difference might also be due to differences in calcium intake. On a high calcium intake (800 to 1000 mg/day) PTH only increased when 25OHD concentrations fell below 12 to 15 ng/mL,[186] whereas on a low calcium intake, higher 25OHD levels were needed to prevent secondary hyperparathyroidism.[185] Intervention studies indicated that serum $1,25(OH)_2D_3$ increased and PTH decreased when 25OHD or vitamin D was given to subjects with 25OHD levels below 30 nmol/L.[27, 47, 182] Moreover, in a large cross-sectional study BMD of the femoral neck only decreased when 25OHD levels fell below 30 nmol/L.[186]

Short-term intervention studies revealed that vitamin D supplementation during winter months to maintain high summer levels of 25OHD (90 nmol/L) could prevent a (unusually high) seasonal BMD decrease.[187, 188] Pending further studies it is probably wise to recommend serum 25OHD concentrations (using assays with validated accuracy and lack of nonspecific interferences) above 15 ng/mL throughout the year. Using this definition a very large number of elderly people, especially when institutionalized or homebound, are mildly to even severely vitamin D–deficient; this is the case also in North America[189] and Europe.[27, 185, 186, 190] Vitamin D status is certainly better in a healthy independent, and mobile elderly population, but low levels are still not exceptional.[191]

Vitamin D substitution can easily be obtained by daily administration of 400 to 800 IU or the equivalent dose given once per week or month. Monitoring therapy is usually not recommended except in special cases (e.g., fat malabsorption) but this can be easily performed by measuring serum 25OHD concentration. Somewhat higher doses are used in case of rickets or osteomalacia or in patients on chronic P450 enzyme–inducing drugs (e.g., for epilepsy). A loading dose equivalent to the mass of 25OHD present in the extracellular pool (200 to 300 μg of 25OHD) could also be used. 25OHD rather than vitamin D can be used in case of fat malabsorption. The efficacy of vitamin D substitution (800 IU/day) for the prevention of osteoporotic fractures (29% decrease after 36 months) has been well demonstrated when given in combination with calcium (1200 mg/day) to vitamin D–and calcium-deficient elderly women.[192, 193] In a large Dutch study, however, vitamin D 400 IU/day was able to increase hip BMD but not to reduce the incidence of hip fracture in an elderly vitamin D–deficient population already on a high calcium diet (1000 mg/day).[186] In a much smaller group of elderly (>65 years old) non–vitamin D-deficient (25OHD = 30 ng/mL) American women, calcium and vitamin D (500 mg + 700 IU/day) reduced the incidence of nonvertebral fractures. However, the number of subjects was small, and the effects of calcium and vitamin D cannot be distinguished.[188] Vitamin D metabolites [$1,25(OH)_2D$] or analogues (1α-OHD) with an already present 1α-hydroxyl group are not used for the prevention or treatment of simple vitamin D deficiency. They are, however, the treatment of choice in case of structural, genetic, or functional deficiency of renal 1α-hydroxylase activity. Therefore 1α-OHD or $1,25(OH)_2D_3$ is widely used to prevent or correct secondary hyperparathyroidism of chronic renal failure. The drugs can be used either orally or by IV administration during hemodialysis. Control of phosphate retention and monitoring serum calcium are mandatory.[194, 195] Hypoparathyroidism or pseudohypoparathyroidism (PTH resistance) are also effectively treated by 1α-hydroxylated vitamin D compounds to replace the lack of endogenous production of $1,25(OH)_2D$ in the absence of PTH. In the absence of PTH's beneficial effect on renal calcium reabsorption, serum calcium has to be maintained at slightly lower than normal concentration to avoid hypercalciuria, and frequent monitoring of calcium homeostasis is needed to avoid nephrocalcinosis or hypercalcemia. In contrast, however, such vitamin D treatment in the absence of PTH is usually beneficial for bone. Dihydrotachysterol had for a long time been used before 1α-hydroxylated compounds became available because the rotated 3-hydroxyl group of this vitamin D analogues mimics a 1α-OH group. However, much higher doses are needed (0.1 mg/day) when compared to $1,25(OH)_2D_3$ (1 μg/day).

1α-Hydroxylated vitamin D compounds are also beneficial for the treatment of primary or secondary (glucocorticoid-induced) osteoporosis.[196–198] The incidence of vertebral fracture could indeed be markedly reduced by the administration of $1,25(OH)_2D_3$ (0.5 μg/day) in postmenopausal osteoporotic women.[170] Extensive Japanese and European experience with 1α-OHD (usually 1 μg/day) also demonstrated a beneficial effect on BMD or osteoporotic fractures.[199–201] The magnitude of the effect on the incidence of both BMD and fracture, however, seems to be lower than that of newer bisphosphonates, although no direct comparative studies are available. 1α-Hydroxylated vitamin D compounds are also needed when high oral phosphate therapy is used in patients with hypoposphatemic rickets or osteomalacia to prevent secondary hyperparathyroidism.[202] The choice between $1,25(OH)_2D$ and 1α-OHD is not based on comparative studies. There are differences in pharmacokinetics, as 1α-OHD has no first-pass effect on intestinal calcium absorption since it needs prior 25-hydroxylation in the liver. The therapeutic dose of 1α-OHD needed is usually twice that of 1,25(OH)D for the same indication.

THERAPEUTIC POTENTIAL OF 1,25-DIHYDROXYVITAMIN D_3 ANALOGUES

The combined presence of 25OHD-1α-hydroxylase[61] as well as VDR in several tissues (e.g., keratinocytes, monocytes, bone, placenta, glial cells) introduced the concept of a paracrine role for $1,25(OH)_2D_3$.[203] Moreover, $1,25(OH)_2D_3$ was found to be capable of regulating cell differentiation and proliferation of both normal[204] and malignant cells.[205] These newly discovered functions of $1,25(OH)_2D_3$ create possible new therapeutic applications for immune modulation (e.g., for the treatment of autoimmune diseases or prevention of graft rejection), inhibition of cell proliferation (e.g., psoriasis), and induction of cell differentiation (cancer). To achieve growth inhibition or cell differentiation, supraphysiologic doses of $1,25(OH)_2D$ are needed, causing calcemic side effects. Therefore new analogues of $1,25(OH)_2D$ have been developed to dissociate the antiproliferative and prodifferentiating effects from the calcemic and bone metabolism effects.[206]

The secosteroid $1,25(OH)_2D$ with its open B-ring and side chain of eight carbon atoms is a very flexible molecule. Different modifications have already been introduced in the A-, B-, C-, and D-rings and in the side chain by addition or transposition of hydroxyl groups, introducing unsaturation, replacing a carbon atom with a hetero atom, inverting the stereochemistry, and/or shortening or lengthening the side chain.[206] During the last decade some three hundred analogues were synthesized and their biologic potency reported in the nonpatent literature.[206] Moreover, several thousand analogues have been synthesized by pharmaceutic and academic research groups and reported briefly in the patent literature. Some of these analogues demonstrate a clear dissociation between antiproliferative and calcemic effects. In the meantime, nonsteroidal analogues were synthesized with a totally new structure lacking the full CD-region of $1,25(OH)_2D_3$.[207]

No single or simple mechanism can explain the exact mechanism of superagonistic and selective activity profile (calcemic vs. noncalcemic effects) of the new vitamin D analogues. Most of the biologic effects of $1,25(OH)_2D$ are believed to be mediated via binding to the VDR, but surprisingly the binding affinity of the analogues to the VDR does not always correlate with their potency. Some analogues extend the VDR half-life and induce different conformational changes to the VDR-ligand complex as assessed by limited proteolytic digestion and site-directed mutagenesis.[130, 208, 209] Wurtz et al.[105] described a three-dimensional model of the ligand-binding domain of the VDR using the hRARγ receptor as template. The binding capacity of different analogues of $1,25(OH)_2D$ was investigated and suggested that the VDR-ligand pocket can accommodate the steric requirements of the ligand, which in turn induce subtle deformations of the ligand-binding pocket altering their ligand affinity, their capacity to heterodimerize with RXR, and to bind DNA. The biologic potency of superanalogues or analogues with a molar potency 10- to 100-fold higher than that of $1,25(OH)_2D$ can best be explained by a combination of decreased intracellular catabolism, enhanced VDR stability, and especially enhanced transcriptional activity. The selective action of analogues, however, requires different mechanisms such as different metabolism in different target cells, cell- or gene-specific regulation depending on the VDR: homo- or heterodimer configuration induced by specific analogues, the presence or selective interaction with coactivator or corepressor proteins, and so forth.[206, 210, 211] Some analogues are selective agonist or antagonists for nongenomic rapid actions while being devoid of significant genomic activity.[142] Since for other steroid hormones (e.g., estrogens, androgens, glucocorticoids) it is now well established that analogue-specific gene regulation can be generated by chemical modification of the parent ligand molecule, it is likely that among the many powerful selective vitamin D analogues at least some will be found to be clinically useful for noncalcemic indications.

Bone Disorders

The role of vitamin D or its metabolites in the treatment of bone disorders characterized by defective mineralization, such as rickets and renal osteodystrophy, is well established. The exact mechanism of action of vitamin D and its metabolites on bone is, however, not exactly known. If, as VDR-deficient mice experiments suggest, intestinal calcium and phosphorus absorption are the sole essential role of vitamin D on bone and growth plate homeostasis, then analogues with a good intestinal profile are to be selected. However, it is more likely that an analogue with selective agonist activity on intestinal calcium and phosphate absorption and inhibitory effects on PTH synthesis and osteoclastogenesis might be superior to $1,25(OH)_2D_3$. Presently only a few analogues are being evaluated in preclinical or human phase II trials for the prevention or cure of osteoporosis. The vitamin D analogue 2β-(3-hydroxypropoxy)-$1,25(OH)_2D_3$ (ED-71) is characterized by high calcemic activity and strong binding to DBP (twice that of $1,25(OH)_2D_3$.[169] The effect of ED-71 on growth plate thickness in rachitic rats was 15- to 20-fold greater than that of $1,25(OH)_2D_3$; the BMD of the femur was increased and the serum calcium elevation was less than with $1,25(OH)_2D_3$ administration.[212] In studies employing either normal or ovariectomized rats, ED-71 stimulates bone mass and bone formation rates.[213] Based on the in vitro and in vivo data, ED-71 is being tested in clinical osteoporosis trials. Several other vitamin D analogues such as 1α-OHD_2 and 19-nor-$1,25(OH)_2D_3$ analogues are being evaluated for the same purpose in preclinical or early clinical settings.[214]

Renal Osteodystrophy

Bone disease in patients with chronic renal failure is due to a complex set of mechanisms such as impaired $1,25(OH)_2D$ synthesis, vitamin D resistance, secondary hyperparathyroidism, and abnormal mineral handling (hyperphosphatemia, aluminum or fluoride excess, acidosis). Whereas 1α-OHD_3 and $1,25(OH)_2D_3$ are widely used for the prevention and cure of renal osteodystrophy, several analogues have been evaluated for this indication with the aim of better PTH suppression with less risk of inducing hypercalcemia or hyperphosphatemia. 22-Oxacalcitriol (OCT) has similar effects to $1,25(OH)_2D_3$ on cell proliferation and inhibition of PTH secretion in vitro and in vivo[215] in experimental animals and patients with chronic renal failure.[216] Similarly, the vitamin D_2 analogue 19-nor-$1,25(OH)_2D_3$ has been evaluated for suppressing secondary hyperparathyroidism and is now being marketed in the United States for this indication.[217] However, none of the available analogues have been shown to be marked superantagonists on PTH gene expression and detailed long-term comparison between either 1α-OHD_3 or $1,25(OH)_2D_3$ vs. the new analogues on parathyroid and bone homeostasis are still largely missing.

Cancer

A large number of $1,25(OH)_2D_3$ analogues have been developed with potent antiproliferative and prodifferentiating effects on cancer cells in vitro[205] and reduced effects on calcium and bone metabolism.[206] Several potent analogues have already been tested in animal models for the treatment of different cancers (Table 72–5). A low vitamin D status has been found to be associated in some but not all studies with an increased risk of breast or colon cancer.[218, 219] Besides growth inhibition, $1,25(OH)_2D_3$ and its analogues may exert their antitumor effects via inhibition of angiogenesis[220] and by reducing the invasiveness of cancer cells.[221] An additional anticancer effect of $1,25(OH)_2D_3$ analogues could be the inhibition of PTHrP. Ogata[222] demonstrated that the $1,25(OH)_2D_3$ analogue OCT not only suppresses PTHrP production but also the action of PTHrP in bone, and that treatment with OCT reduced the incidence of bone metastases in a squamous cell lung cancer model in nude mice.[222] Based on the promising results obtained in animal models of cancer, a few clinical cancer trials have been performed with $1,25(OH)_2D_3$ analogues. The analogue calcipotriol (MC 903) has been evaluated for topical treatment of advanced breast cancer.[223] A phase I clinical trial of oral seocalcitol (EB 1089) in patients with advanced breast ($n = 25$) and colorectal cancer ($n = 11$) has been completed in the United Kingdom.[224] Patients received the analogue EB 1089 twice daily for 5 days with a 3-week postdosing follow-up. Unfortunately no clear antitumor effects were seen, whereas

TABLE 72–5. Antitumoral Effects of 1,25-Dihydroxyvitamin D_3 Analogues and Derivates in Animal Models (From 1996–1998)

Tumor Model	Analogue	Results	Reference
Pancreatic cancer			
BXPC-3 cell line	OCT	Decreased tumor growth (−62%)	274
GER cell line	EB 1089	Inhibition of tumor growth	275
Colon cancer			
LoVo cell line	EB 1089	Decreased tumor growth (−50%)	276
Human HT-29 tumor xenograft	Ro 25-6760	Tumor disappearance in 30% of mice	277
Stomach cancer			
Induced by MNNG and NaCl	$24R,25(OH)_2D_3$	Reduced incidence	278
Breast cancer			
MCF-7 cell line	ZXY 1106		
	SDB 112	Decreased tumor growth (−50%)	279
NMU-induced	CB 1093	Decreased tumor growth (−50%)	280
NMU-induced	EB 1089	Regression of tumors at high doses	281
MCF-7 cell line	EB 1089	Decreased tumor growth (−75%)	282
MCF-7 cell line	CB 1093	Decreased tumor growth	283
Prostate cancer			
Dunning MLL and AT-2 cell lines	$1,25(OH)_2D_3$	Inhibition of tumor volume	284
	Ro 25-6760	Reduction in number and size of lung metastases	284
Skin cancer			
Murine SCCVII/SF cells (SCCV II ISF cells)	$1,25(OH)_2D_3$	Decreased tumor growth (−70%)	285
	Ro 23-7553	Reduction in tumor volume and tumor regrowth delay	226
Renal cancer			
	$1,25(OH)_2D_3$	Inhibition of tumor growth	286
	$1(OH)D_3$	Prolongation of life span	286
Retinoblastoma			
	Ro 23-7553	Smaller cross-sectional area of tumor (−21%)	287
	Ro 23-7553	Decreased tumor growth (−45%)	288

MNNG, *N*-methyl-*N*′-nitra-*N*-nitrosoguanidine; OCT, 27-oxacalcitrial.

the maximum tolerable dose was 10 to 20 μg/day vs. 1 to 2 μg/day for $1,25(OH)_2D_3$ Phase I/II trials of EB 1089 are currently underway in patients with advanced pancreatic and hepatocellular carcinoma, as well as breast cancer and myelodysplasia.

The data obtained so far on $1,25(OH)_2D_3$ analogues as potent inhibitors of cancer cell growth, angiogenesis, metastasis, and PTHrP synthesis with reduced calcemic activity are promising for the use of analogues in cancer treatment. Moreover, the synergistic effects of $1,25(OH)_2D_3$ analogues with retinoids,[225] antiestrogens, and conventional chemotherapeutic agents[226] may result in better response rates and reduce the concentration used for conventional anticancer drugs, thereby reducing the risk of side effects.

Skin

Epidermal keratinocytes are not only endowed with the capacity to produce vitamin D_3, they also possess VDRs.[204] Furthermore, they express 25OHD-1α-hydroxylase and also CYP27[227] and 25-hydroxylase activity.[228] The combined presence of vitamin D production, 25-hydroxylase, 1α-hydroxylase, and VDR in the epidermis suggests the existence of a unique vitamin D intracrine system in which UVB-irradiated keratinocytes may supply their own needs for $1,25(OH)_2D_3$. A role for vitamin D in epidermal homeostasis can also be expected from the prominent effects of vitamin D compounds on keratinocyte growth and differentiation.[204] Finally, in view of the close interplay between UVB and the generation of vitamin D (and calcitriol), active vitamin D compounds may serve as an endogenous defense mechanism against harmful events caused by UVB. Indeed, a strong photoprotective effect of calcitriol against UVB-mediated events in cultured keratinocytes was recently identified that may be related to its capability to induce metallothionein, a protein with antioxidant properties.[229, 230]

The epidermal keratinocyte represents the major cell type in the epidermis and most likely the major cutaneous target cell for vitamin D. Calcitriol at pharmacologic concentrations potently induces growth arrest and differentiation of the epidermal keratinocyte.[204] Calcitriol-treated keratinocytes fail to progress from the G_1 to the S phase of the cell cycle (Fig. 72–5), leaving retinoblastoma protein in its dephosphorylated growth-suppressive state.[231] E1A-binding proteins such as retinoblastoma family members (and/or the transcriptional cointegrator p300/CBP) are probably also required for the vitamin D action.[232] The suppression of phosphorylation of the retinoblastoma protein by vitamin D is preceded by induction of the cyclin dependent kinase inhibitors $p21^{WAF1}$ and $p27^{KIP1}$,[231] which prevent the activity of G_1 cyclin-dependent kinases on retinoblastoma. The effects of calcitriol on p21 accumulation and on cell cycle kinetics take 24 hours to several days[231]

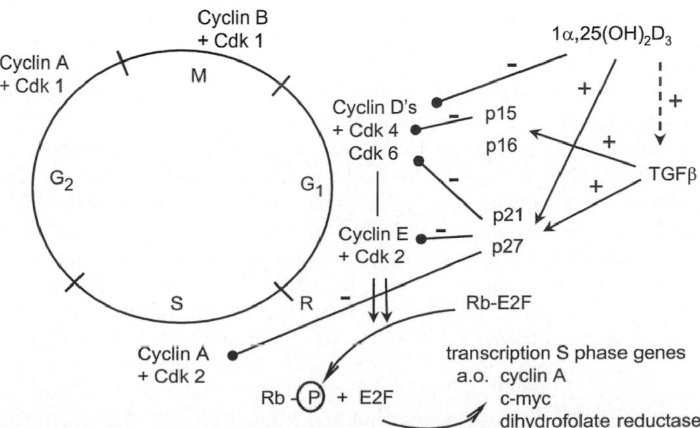

FIGURE 72–5. Effect of 1,25-dihydroxyvitamin D_3 on cell cycle regulatory genes. $1,25(OH)_2D_3$ has a cell cycle phase-specific effect leading to accumulation of cells in G_1. (—●), downregulation; (→), upregulation; p21, p27, p15, p16, cyclin-dependent kinase inhibitors; Cdk, cyclin-dependent kinase; TGFβ, transforming growth factor-β; Rb, retinoblastoma tumor suppressor gene.

and are preceded by changed expression of immediate early genes such as *c-myc* and *c-fos*[233, 234] and by upregulation of phospholipase C with increased phosphoinositide turnover.[139] Indirect effects through autocrine or paracrine growth factors such as TGF-β1 and -β2,[231, 235] TNF-α,[236] and PTHrP[237] are also likely to contribute to the antimitotic vitamin D effect. Increased differentiation is illustrated by induction of type I transglutaminase and cornified envelope precursors such as involucrin.[204] A stimulatory effect on stratification by the translocation of E-cadherin to assembling adherens junction[238] will enhance the prodifferentiative actions of calcitriol, which are also dependent on a functional protein kinase C.[238, 239] The increased secretion of extracellular matrix molecules such as fibronectin and osteopontin in vitamin D–treated keratinocytes[235, 240] may prove beneficial for wound healing but also enhances anchorage-independent growth and possibly invasiveness of transformed keratinocyte.[240]

Most of the studies concerning growth and differentiation were carried out with rather high pharmacologic concentrations of 1,25$(OH)_2$D. Increased proliferation was, however, observed following application of vitamin D compounds to normal mouse skin.[241] In contrast, hyperproliferative epidermis (in psoriasis or induced by application of hyperplasiogens) responds to vitamin D derivatives with growth arrest.[242, 243] These observations indicate that the activation state of the keratinocyte (noncycling vs. actively cycling) appears to determine the vitamin D effects with respect to proliferation and differentiation.

The expression of the VDR in the skin is not confined to keratinocytes but extends to almost every cell type residing in the skin, including hair follicle cells, melanocytes, fibroblasts, endothelial cells, sebocytes, sweat gland cells, smooth muscle cells (vascular walls and arrector pili muscles), Langerhans cells, and activated lymphocytes or monocytes, that takes part in inflammatory skin reaction.[242, 244]

The relation between vitamin D and hair growth has been a focus of primary interest. The hair follicle contains abundant VDR in keratinocytes of the outer root sheath and of the proximal hair matrix, as well as in fibroblasts of the dermal papilla.[245] Furthermore, hair follicle growth in organ culture is stimulated by calcitriol in the nanomolar range, while higher concentrations are growth inhibitory.[246] But the most compelling evidence for the vitamin D system as a guardian of the integrity of the hair follicle is provided by the total alopecia in VDR knockout mice[167, 172] and in patients with vitamin D–dependent rickets type II.[131] The hair loss, which develops only a few weeks after birth, is accompanied by dilation of the piliary canals, progressing to the formation of large dermal cysts and profound wrinkling.[172] Alopecia is most remarkably absent in vitamin D–dependent rickets type I (defective 1α-hydroxylase) or in severe nutritional rickets, indicating a ligand-independent role for VDR in the hair follicle. Interest in the issue was further raised by the observation that topical vitamin D compounds alleviate[247] or even induce resistance against chemotherapy-dependent alopecia.[248] At present, the mechanisms for the vitamin D actions on hair growth remain essentially unknown; suppression of PTHrP expression might be involved, because PTHrP antagonists markedly enhance hair growth.[249]

The profound effects of calcitriol on keratinocyte proliferation and differentiation have led to the application of vitamin D analogues for skin diseases with disturbed keratinocyte proliferation and differentiation, primarily psoriasis.[242] Topical vitamin D analogues that display decreased calcemic activity (calcipotriol and tacalcitol) are now widely used for mild to moderate forms of psoriasis. Monotherapy with these vitamin D compounds achieves an equal effectiveness to topical medium-potency glucocorticoids, without risk of skin atrophy, tachyphylaxis, or rebound phenomena. When the use of vitamin D does not surpass the recommended amount (100 g ointment per week), there is no repercussion on calcium homeostasis. Mild irritation is the only frequently observed side effect.[242] During treatment with vitamin D analogues, the dysregulated epidermal homeostasis is fully restored: keratinocyte proliferation is inhibited; the perturbed psoriatic differentiation profile is normalized with a decrease in the premature expression of involucrin and type I transglutaminase and enhancement of filaggrin expression[250]; and the aberrant expression of cell adhesion molecules (integrins, ICAM1) also returns back to normal.[251] The concomitant decrease in the inflammatory infiltrate is, however, incomplete, leaving a certain amount of (mostly dermal) immune cells and some dilated blood vessels,[250, 251] which may account for the residual redness of the lesions after completion of therapy.

The putative involvement of calcitriol in the hair cycle offers promising prospectives for using vitamin D analogues in the treatment of alopecia. Topical calcitriol prevents hair loss or enhances hair regrowth after chemotherapy-induced alopecia,[247, 248] but no data are yet available from human patients.

Immunology

The detection of VDR in almost all cells of the immune system, especially antigen-presenting cells (macrophages and dendritic cells) and activated T lymphocytes, led to the investigation of the potential for 1,25$(OH)_2D_3$ as an immunomodulator.[252] Application of the molecule in vitro and in vivo has led to interesting observations confirming a role for 1,25$(OH)_2D_3$ and its analogues in the immune system. Not only is VDR present in all cells of the immune system but activated macrophages are able to synthesize and secrete 1,25$(OH)_2D_3$. These cells express the enzyme 1α-hydroxylase, as recently demonstrated on the molecular level by reverse transcriptase–polymerase chain reaction (RT-PCR) in activated macrophages.[314] Although cloning and sequencing of the mRNA clearly demonstrated this enzyme to be identical to the known renal form, its regulation seems to be under completely different control. Indeed the macrophage enzyme mainly runs through immune signals, with interferon-γ (IFN-γ) being a powerful stimulator. In macrophages no clear downregulation of the enzyme by 1,25$(OH)_2D_3$ could be observed, which explains the hypercalcemia occurring in situations of macrophage overactivation such as tuberculosis C or sarcoidosis. The secretion of classic macrophage products such as cytokines (IL-1, TNF-α, and IL-12) precedes the transcription of the enzyme and as a consequence the secretion of 1,25$(OH)_2D_3$.[314] Therefore, its timing is compatible with that of a suppressive signal, allowing first an activation and further recruitment of the other members of the immune system, followed by downtapering signals, such as prostaglandin E_2 (PGE_2), to limit the extend of the reaction (Fig. 72–6).

A true immunomodulator not only interacts with T cells but also targets the central cell in the immune cascade, the antigen-presenting cell. Here 1,25$(OH)_2D_3$ stimulates differentiation of monocytes and dendritic cells toward good phagocytosis and killing of bacteria, but suppresses the antigen-presenting capacity of these cells.[253] Essential

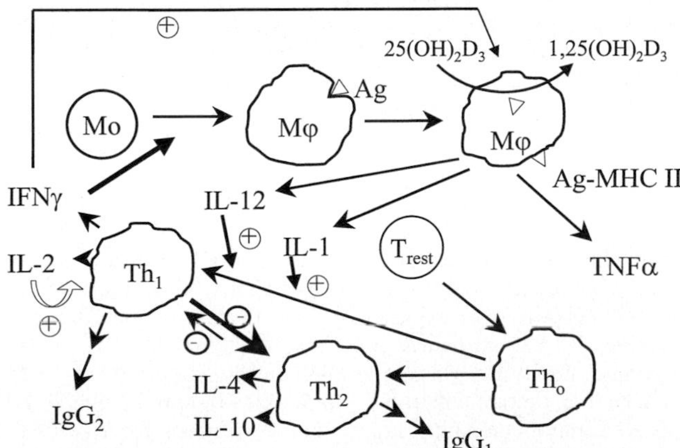

FIGURE 72–6. Action of 1,25-dihydroxyvitamin D_3 in the immune system—a possible scenario for the physiologic role of 1,25$(OH)_2D_3$ as a messenger molecule. Activated macrophages recruit and stimulate the rest of the immune cells through antigen presentation and the secretion of second messenger molecules, especially interleukin-12. In a second stage the immune reaction is tapered down by signals coming from the antigen-presenting cells and from T lymphocytes. We suggest that 1,25$(OH)_2D_3$, produced by activated macrophages, is such a negative signal, downregulating antigen presentation, macrophage cytokine production, T cell proliferation, and Th_1 cytokine production. Immunoglobulin production by B lymphocytes is inhibited in part directly and in part by inhibition of T cell helped by 1,25$(OH)_2D_3$.

here is the suppression of expression of HLA class II molecules and of classic adhesion molecules necessary for full T cell stimulation, such as B7.2.[254] Also, the crucial signals secreted by antigen-presenting cells for recruitment and activation of T cells are directly influenced by $1,25(OH)_2D_3$. A key cytokine in the immune system, IL-12, is clearly inhibited by $1,25(OH)_2D_3$ and analogues.[127, 255, 256] This monocyte-produced substance is the major determinant of the direction in which the immune system will be activated. IL-12 stimulates the development of CD4 T_H1 cells and inhibits the development of CD4 T_H2 lymphocytes.[257] T_H1 lymphocytes mainly secrete IL-2 and IFN-γ and are considered to be the most important cells in graft rejection and autoimmunity. T_H2 cells secrete IL-4, IL-5, and IL-10 and are considered to be regulator cells. The observation of clear inhibition of IL-12 by $1,25(OH)_2D_3$ and its analogues (in vitro by enzyme-linked immunosorbent assay and by intracellular fluorescence-activated cell sorting (FACS) analysis; in vivo by RT-PCR) is essential to understanding the observed effects of these substances in vitro on T cell proliferation and cytokine production and in vivo on graft survival and autoimmunity prevention[252, 258–262] (Table 72–6). By inhibiting IL-12 secretion $1,25(OH)_2D_3$ directly interferes with the heart of the immune cascade and shifts the reaction toward a T_H2 profile. Also, $1,25(OH)_2D_3$ influences the secretion of other cytokines secreted by monocytes: the suppressive PGE_2 is stimulated while the monocyte recruiter granulocyte-macrophage colony-stimulations factor is suppressed.[263, 264] Several T cell cytokines, especially the T_H1 type, are also direct targets for $1,25(OH)_2D_3$ and its analogues. $1,25(OH)_2D_3$-mediated inhibition of IL-2 secretion is through impairment of NFAT complex formation, since the receptor complex itself binds to the distal NFAT binding site in the human IL-2 promoter.[121, 265, 266] Another key T cell cytokine, IFN-γ, which by itself further stimulates antigen presentation, is directly (via a VDRE) downregulated by $1,25(OH)_2D_3$. Moreover, progressive deletion analysis of the IFN-γ promotor revealed that negative regulation by $1,25(OH)_2D_3$ is also present at the level of an upstream region containing an enhancer element.[267]

In conclusion, these data suggest a physiologic role for $1,25(OH)_2D_3$ in the immune system as a downtapering signal secreted by activated macrophages and received by activated T cells, thus limiting the immune reaction (see Fig. 72–6). Although these immune effects are typically mediated through the VDR, VDR knockout mice have no apparent immune abnormalities, probably suggesting a redundancy of $1,25(OH)_2D_3$ as a signal in the immune system.[314] The fact that $1,25(OH)_2D_3$ and its analogues influence the immune system, not by pure immunosuppression but by immunomodulation through induction of immune shifts and regulator cells, makes these products very appealing for clinical use, especially in the treatment and prevention of autoimmune diseases (see Table 72–6). In autoimmune diabetes in the NOD (non-obese diabetic) mouse, upregulation of regulator cells and a shift from T_H1 toward T_H2 locally in the pancreases and islet grafts of treated mice could be observed, but other effects on the immune system have also been described, the most important being a restoration of defective apoptosis sensitivity in lymphocytes, leading to better elimination of potentially dangerous autoimmune effector cells.[268] This increase in immunocyte apoptosis in NOD mice by $1,25(OH)_2D_3$ and its analogues has been described after different apoptosis-inducing signals and could explain why an early short-term treatment with these products, before the onset of autoimmunity, can lead to long-term protection and a restoration of tolerance.[269]

Finally, clear additive and even synergistic effects were observed between $1,25(OH)_2D_3$ or its analogues and other more classic immunomodulators, such as cyclosporine A and sirolimus.[270, 271] These effects were observed in vitro and could be confirmed in vivo in models of autoimmunity (diabetes and experimental allergic encephalitis) and in graft destruction[270, 272, 273] (see Table 72–6).

TABLE 72–6. Effects of 1,25-Dihydroxyvitamin D_3 and Its Analogues in Animal Models of Autoimmunity and Transplantation

Autoimmunity	References
Autoimmune diabetes mellitus	272, 289–291
Chemically induced diabetes mellitus	292
Experimental autoimmune thyroiditis	293
Experimental allergic encephalitis	254, 270, 298
Arthritis	298, 299
Lupus nephritis	253, 300, 301
Heymann's nephritis	302
Nephrotoxic serum nephritis	303
$HgCl_2$-induced glomerulonephritis	304
Transplantation	
Islet, in diabetes mellitus	259, 270, 306, 307
Heart	307–309
Vascular	310
Skin	311, 312
Renal	313
Small bowel	261

SUMMARY

Vitamin D is a flexible secosteroid, which starts as an essential nutritional factor if its endogenous synthesis from 7-dehydrocholesterol in the skin is insufficient because of the absence of short-wave UVB sunlight. Two consecutive hydroxylations by two different P450 enzymes result in the production of $1,25(OH)_2D$. This steroid hormone acts via a ligand-activated nuclear transcription factor present in almost all cells and regulates a large number of genes involved in calcium and bone homeostasis. However, numerous other genes involved in cell cycle control, cell differentiation, or implicated in humoral cell-cell interaction (e.g., in the immune system) are also under the direct or indirect control of $1,25(OH)_2D$. Moreover, $1,25(OH)_2D$ also regulates several rapid and transient nongenomic biochemical reactions typically involved in second messenger signaling in a variety of cells.

A number of other P450 or yet-to-be-identified enzymes convert vitamin D or its hormone into more than 30 other metabolites, some of which may have specific activity [e.g., $24,25(OH)_2D_3$]. Two essential vitamin D target tissues have been identified based on VDR knockout mouse experiments: (1) the intestine for calcium and phosphorus absorption and secondarily for parathyroid function and bone mineralization, and (2) the skin and especially the hair follicle for postnatal hair growth. The function of the vitamin D endocrine system in other tissues is at first sight apparently redundant. However, chemical modifications of the parent $1,25(OH)_2D$ molecule resulted in several thousands of analogues, some of which have a superagonist and/or selective activity profile. They are actually already in use for the treatment of hyperproliferative skin disorders or are being explored for their potential use in a variety of other applications (cancer, immunology, inflammatory or bone diseases).

Vitamin D was discovered at the beginning of the 20th century and allowed the eradication of the then widespread endemic disease rickets. At the beginning of the 21st century it is now increasingly realized that another endemic disease, vitamin D deficiency in the osteoporotic elderly, can and should be similarly eradicated by a similar widespread supplementation program.

Acknowledgments

The efficient help of my collaborators G. Carmeliet, C. Mathieu, S. Segaert, C. Verboven, L. Verlinden, and A. Verstuyf and the financial support from the K.U. Leuven and Fonds Wetenschappelijk Onderzoek Vlaanderen are highly appreciated as is the secretarial assistance of A. Laeremans and B. Minten.

REFERENCES

1. Whistler D: *De morbo puerili anglorum, quem patrio idiomate indigenae vocant* the Rickets. Leiden, 1645, pp 1–13.
2. Glisson F: *De rachitide sive morbo puerili, qui vulgo* the Rickets *dicitur, tractatus, opera primo ac potissimum Francisci Glissinii/././adscitis in operis societatem Georgio Bate et Ahasevo Regemortero*. London, 1650, pp 1–416.
3. Mozolowski W: Jedrzej Sniadecki (1768–1883) on the cure of rickets. Nature 143:121, 1939.

4. Palm TA: The geographic distribution and etiology of rickets. Practitioner 45:321–342, 1890.
5. Huldschinsky K: Heilung von Rachitis durch künstliche Höhensonne. Dtsch Med Wochenschr 45:712–713, 1919.
6. Chick HPEJ, Hume EM: Studies of rickets in Vienna 1919–1922. Med Res Counc Special Rep 77, 1923.
7. Hess AF, Weinstock M: Antirachitic properties imparted to lettuce and to growing wheat by ultraviolet irradiation. Proc Soc Exp Biol Med 22:5–6, 1924.
8. Mellanby E, Cantag MD: Experimental investigation on rickets. Lancet 196:407–412, 1919.
9. McCollum EV, Simmonds N, Pitz W: The relation of unidentified dietary factors, the fat-soluble A and water-soluble B of the diet to the growth promoting properties of milk. J Biol Chem 27:33–38, 1916.
10. McCollum EV, Simmonds N, Becker JE, et al: Studies on experimental rickets. XXI. An experimental demonstration of the existence of a vitamin which promotes calcium deposition. J Biol Chem 53:293–312, 1922.
11. Goldblatt H, Soames KN: A study of rats on a normal diet irradiated daily by the mercury vapor quartz lamp or kept in darkness. Biochem J 17:294–297, 1923.
12. Windaus A, Linsert O: Vitamin D_1. Ann Chem 465:148, 1928.
13. Specker BL, Tsang RC, Hollis BW: Effect of race and diet on human-milk vitamin-D and 25-hydroxyvitamin D. Am J Dis Child 139:1134–1137, 1985.
14. Holick MF: Vitamin D and the kidney. Kidney Int 32:912–929, 1987.
15. Chen TC, Shao Q, Heath H, et al: An update on the vitamin-D content of fortified milk from the United States and Canada. N Engl J Med 329:1507, 1993.
16. Holick MF, Shao Q, Liu WW, et al: The vitamin D content of fortified milk and infant formula. N Engl J Med 326:1178–1181, 1992.
17. Murphy SP, Calloway DH: Nutrient intakes of women in NHANES II, emphasizing trace minerals, fiber, and phytate. J Am Diet Assoc 86:1366–1372, 1986.
18. Krall EA, Sahyoun N, Tannenbaum S, et al Effect of vitamin D intake on seasonal variations in parathyroid hormone secretion in postmenopausal women. N Engl J Med 321:1777–1783, 1989.
19. Lamberg-Allardt C, Karkkainen M, Seppanen R, et al: Low serum 25-hydroxyvitamin D concentrations and secondary hyperparathyroidism in middle-aged white strict vegetarians. Am J Clin Nutr 58:684–689, 1993.
20. Holick MF: Vitamin D. *In* Shils ME, Olson JA, Shike M (eds): Modern Nutrition in Health and Disease. Philadelphia, Lea & Febiger, 1994, pp 308–325.
21. Kelley RI: RXH/Smith-Lemli-Opitz syndrome: Mutations and metabolic morphogenesis. Am J Hum Genet 63:322–326, 1998.
22. Cunniff C, Kratz LE, Moser A, et al: Clinical and biochemical spectrum of patients with RSH/Smith-Lemli-Opitz syndrome and abnormal cholesterol metabolism. Am J Med Genet 68:263–269, 1997.
23. Chen TC, Lu Z, Shao Q, et al: Vitamin D metabolism in patients with Smith-Lemli-Opitz syndrome (abstract). Photodermatol Photoimmunol Photomed 11:63, 1995.
24. Bonjour JP, Trechsel U, Granzer E, et al: The increase in skin 7-dehydrocholesterol induced by an hypocholesterolemic agent is associated with elevated 25-hydroxyvitamin D_3 plasma level. Pflugers Arch 410:165–168, 1987.
25. Pillai S, Bikle DD, Elias PM: Vitamin D and epidermal differentiation: Evidence for a role of endogeously produced vitamin D metabolites in keratinocyte differentiation. Skin Pharmacol 1:149–160, 1988.
26. Morris JG: Ineffective synthesis of vitamin D in kittens exposed to sun or UV light is reversed by an inhibitor of 7-dehydrocholesterol-Δ7-reductase. *In* Norman AW, Bouillon R, Thomasset M (eds): Vitamin D, Chemistry, Biology and Clinical Applications of the Steroid Hormone. Riverside, University of California, 1997, pp 721–722.
27. Bouillon R, Auwerx J, Lissens W, et al: Vitamin D status in the elderly: Seasonal substrate deficiency causes 1,25-dihydroxycholecalciferol deficiency. Am J Clin Nutr 45:755–763, 1987.
28. McKenna MJ, Freaney R, Byrne P, et al: Safety and efficacy of increasing wintertime vitamin D and calcium intake by milk fortification. Q J Med 88:895–898, 1995.
29. Ben Mekhbi H, Zeghoud F, Guillozo H, et al: Prevalence, possible causes, and prevention of infantile rickets in Constantine, Algeria. *In* Norman AW, Bouillon R, Thomasset M (eds): Vitamin D, Chemistry, Biology and Clinical Applications of the Steroid Hormone. Riverside, University of California, 1997, pp 921–924.
30. Specker BL, Valanis B, Hertzberg V, et al: Sunshine exposure and serum 25-hydroxyvitamin D concentrations in exclusively breast-fed infants. J Pediatr 107:372–376, 1985.
31. Gascon-Barré M: The vitamin D 25-hydroxylase. *In* Feldman D, Glorieux FH, Pike JW (eds): Vitamin D. San Diego, Academic Press, 1997, pp 41–55.
32. Henry HL: The 25-hydroxyvitamin D 1α-hydroxylase. *In* Feldman D, Glorieux FH, Pike JW (eds): Vitamin D. San Diego, Academic Press, 1997, pp 57–68.
33. Blunt JW, DeLuca HF, Schnoes HK: 25-Hydroxycholecalciferol. A biologically active metabolite of vitamin D_3. Biochemistry 7:3317–3322, 1968.
34. Ponchon G, Kennan AL, DeLuca HF: "Activation" of vitamin D by the liver. J Clin Invest 48:2032–2037, 1969.
35. Postlind H, Axen E, Bergman T, et al: Cloning, structure, and expression of a cDNA encoding vitamin D_3 25-hydroxylase. Biochem Biophys Res Commun 241:491–497, 1997.
36. Dilworth FJ, Scott I, Green A, et al: Different mechanisms of hydroxylation site selection by liver and kidney cytochrome P450 species (CYP27 and CYP24) involved in vitamin D metabolism. J Biol Chem 14:16766–16774, 1995.
37. Leitersdorf E, Meiner V: Cerebrotendinous xanthomatosis. Curr Opin Lipidol 5:138–142, 1994.
38. Maeda N, Reshef A, Lippoldt A, et al: Markedly reduced bile acid synthesis but maintained levels of cholesterol and vitamin D metabolites in mice with disrupted sterol 27-hydroxylase gene. J Biol Chem 273:14805–14812, 1998.
39. Bhattacharyya MH, DeLuca HF: The regulation of calciferol-25-hydroxylase in the chick. Biochem Biophys Res Commun 59:734–741, 1974.
40. Hayashi SI, Noshiro M, Okuda K: Isolation of a cytochrome P-450 that catalyzed the 25-hydroxylation of vitamin D_3 from rat liver microsomes. J Biochem (Tokyo) 99:1753–1763, 1986.
41. Andersson S, Holmberg I, Wikvall K: 25-Hydroxylation of C_2 steroids and vitamin D_3 by a constitutive cytochrome P-450 from rat liver microsomes. J Biol Chem 258:6777–6781, 1983.
42. Hess A: Influence of light on the prevention of rickets. Lancet 2:1222, 1922.
43. Fraser DR, Kodicek E: Unique biosynthesis by kidney of a biologically active vitamin D metabolite. Nature 228:764–766, 1970.
44. Nicolaysen R: XV. Studies upon the mode of action of vitamin D. III. The influence of vitamin D on the absorption of calcium and phosphorus in the rat. Biochem J 31:122–129, 1937.
45. Nicolaysen R, Eeglarsen N, Malm J: Physiology of calcium metabolism. Physiol Rev 33:424–444, 1953.
46. Porteous CE, Coldwell RD, Trafford DJH, et al: Recent developments in the measurement of vitamin D and its metabolites in human body fluids. J Steroid Biochem 28:785–801, 1987.
47. Schmidt-Gayk H, Bouillon R, Roth HJ: Measurement of vitamin D and its metabolites (calcidiol and calcitriol) and their clinical significance. Scand J Clin Lab Invest 57:35–45, 1997.
48. Clements MR, Johnson L, Fraser DR: A new mechanism for induced vitamin-D deficiency in calcium deprivation. Nature 325:62–65, 1987.
49. Schoentgen F, Metz-Boutigue M, Jolles J, et al: Homology between the human vitamin D–binding protein (group specific component), alpha-fetoprotein and serum albumin. FEBS Lett 185:47–50, 1985.
50. Yang F, Brune JL, Bowman BH, et al: Human group-specific component (Gc) is a member of the albumin family. Proc Natl Acad Sci U S A 82:7994–7998, 1985.
51. Witke FW, Gibbs PEM, Zielinski R, et al: Complete structure of the human Gc gene: Differences and similarities between the members of the albumin gene family. Genomics 16:751–754, 1993.
52. Cooke NE, Haddad JG: Vitamin D binding protein. *In* Feldman D, Glorieux FH, Pike JW (eds): Vitamin D. San Diego, Academic Press, 1997, pp 87–101.
53. Bouillon R, Van Assche FA, Van Baelen H, et al: Influence of the vitamin D–binding protein on the serum concentration of 1,25-dihydroxyvitamin D_3. J Clin Invest 67:589–596, 1981.
54. Swamy N, Brisson M, Ray R: Trp-145 is essential for the binding of 25-hydroxyvitamin D_3 to human serum vitamin D–binding protein. J Biol Chem 270:2636–3639, 1995.
55. McLeod JF, Kowalski MA, Haddad JG: Interactions among serum vitamin D binding protein, monomeric actin, profilin, and profilactin. J Biol Chem 264:1260–1267, 1989.
56. Kew RR, Fisher JA, Webster RO: Co-chemotactic effect of Gc globulin (vitamin D binding protein) for C5a: Transient conversion into an active co-chemotaxin by neutrophils. J Immunol 155:5369–5374, 1995.
57. Lee WM, Galbraith RM: The extracellular actin-scavenger system and actin toxicity. N Engl J Med 326:1335–1341, 1992.
58. Yamamoto N, Lindsay DD, Naraparaju VR, et al: A defect in the inflammation-primed macrophage-activation cascade in osteopetrotic rats. J Immunol 152:5100–5107, 1994.
59. Adebanjo OA, Moonga BS, Haddad JG, et al: A possible new role for the vitamin D–binding protein in osteoclast control: Inhibition of extracellular Ca^{2+} sensing at low physiological concentrations. Biochem Biophys Res Commun 249:668–671, 1998.
60. Monkawa T, Yoshida T, Wakino S, et al: Molecular cloning of cDNA and genomic DNA for human 25-hydroxyvitamin D_3 1α-hydroxylase. Biochem Biophys Res Commun 239:527–533, 1997.
61. Fu GK, Lin D, Zhang MYH, et al: Cloning of human 25-hydroxyvitamin D-1α-hydroxylase and mutations causing vitamin D–dependent rickets type 1. Mol Endocrinol 11:1961–1970, 1997.
62. St-Arnaud R, Messerlian S, Moir JM, et al: The 25-hydroxyvitamin D 1α-hydroxylase gene maps to the pseudovitamin D–deficiency rickets (PDDR) disease locus. J Bone Miner Res 12:1552–1559, 1997.
63. Takeyama K, Kitanaka S, Sato T, et al: 25-Hydroxyvitamin D_3 1α-hydroxylase and vitamin D synthesis. Science 277:1827–1830, 1997.
64. Shinki T, Shimada H, Wakino S, et al: Cloning and expression of rat 25-hydroxyvitamin D_3-1α-hydroxylase cDNA. Proc Natl Acad Sci U S A 94:12920–12925, 1997.
65. Parfitt AM: Vitamin D "resistance" and bioavailability of calciferol tablets. BMJ 1:1470–1471, 1977.
66. Bell NH: 25-Hydroxyvitamin D-1α-hydroxylases and their clinical significance. J Bone Miner Res. 13:350–353, 1998.
67. Brenza HL, Kimmel-Jehan C, Jehan F, et al: Parathyroid hormone activation of the 25-hydroxylation D_3-1α-hydroxylase gene promoter. Proc Natl Acad Sci U S A 95:1387–1391, 1998.
68. Murayama A, Takeyama K, Kitanaka S, et al: The promoter of the human 25-hydroxyvitamin D_3 1α-hydroxylase gene confers positive and negative responsiveness to PTH, calcitonin, and 1α,25$(OH)_2D_3$. Biochem Biophys Res Commun 249:11–16, 1998.
69. Fraser D, Kooh SW, Kind HP, et al: Pathogenesis of hereditary vitamin-D–dependent rickets. An inborn error of vitamin D metabolism involving defective conversion of 25-hydroxyvitamin D to 1α,25-dihydroxyvitamin D. N Engl J Med 289:817–822, 1973.
70. Kitanaka S, Takeyama K, Murayama A, et al: Inactivating mutations in the 25-hydroxyvitamin D_3 1α-hydroxylase gene in patients with pseudovitamin D–deficient rickets. N Engl J Med 338:653–661, 1998.
71. Ohyama Y, Noshiro M, Eggertsen G, et al: Structural characterization of the gene encoding rat 25-hydroxyvitamin-D(3) 24-hydroxylase. Biochemistry 32:76–82, 1993.
72. Lohnes D, Jones G: Side chain metabolism of vitamin D_3 in osteosarcoma cell line UMR-106. J Biol Chem 262:14394–14401, 1987.
73. Reddy GS, Tserng KY: Calcitroic acid, end product of renal metabolism of 1,25-dihydroxyvitamin D_3 through C-24 oxidation pathway. Biochemistry 28:1763–1769, 1989.

74. Akiyoshi-Shibata M, Sakaki T, Ohyama Y, et al: Further oxidation of hydroxycalcidiol by calcidiol 24-hydroxylase. A study with the mature enzyme expressed in *Escherichia coli*. Eur J Biochem 224:335–343, 1994.
75. Barletta F, Arrigo C, Parker GA, et al: Administration of 1,25-dihydroxyvitamin D_3 to mice deficient in the 24-hydroxylase gene results in kidney pathology consistent with hypervitaminosis D and altered responsiveness of vitamin D dependent genes (abstract). Bone 23:S185, 1998.
76. Omdahl J, May B: The 25-hydroxyvitamin D 24-hydroxylase. *In* Feldman D, Glorieux FH, Pike JW (eds): Vitamin D. San Diego, Academic Press, 1997, pp 69–85.
77. St Arnaud R: 24,25-Dihydroxyvitamin D—Active metabolite or inactive catabolite? Endocrinology (editorial). 139:3371–3374, 1998.
78. Reddy GS, Siucaldera ML, Schuster, et al: Target tissue specific metabolism of $1{,}25(OH)_2D_3$ through A-ring modification. *In* Norman AW, Bouillon R, Thomasset M (eds): Vitamin D: Chemistry, Biology and Clinical Applications of the Steroid Hormone. Riverside, University of California, 1997, pp 139–146.
79. Dueland S, Pedersen JI, Helgerud P, et al: Absorption, distribution, and transport of vitamin-D_3 and 25-hydroxyvitamin-D_3 in the rat. Am J Physiol 245:E463–E467, 1983.
80. Hirschfeld J: Immune-electrophoretic demonstration of qualitative differences in human sera and their relation to the haptoglobins. Acta Pathol Microbiol 47:160–168, 1959.
81. Cooke NE, Murgia A, McLeod JF: Vitamin D binding-protein. Structure and pattern of expression. Ann N Y Acad Sci 538:49–59, 1988.
82. Westwood WAWDJ: Group-specific component:A review of the isoelectric focusing methods and auxiliary methods available for the separation of its phenotypes. Forensic Sci Int 32:135–150, 1986.
83. Cleve H, Constants J: The mutants of the vitamin-D–binding protein: More than 120 variants of the GC/DBP system. Vox Sang 54:215–225, 1988.
84. Cooke NE, Safadi FF, Magiera HM, et al: Biological consequences of vitamin D binding protein deficiency in a mouse model. *In* Norman AW, Bouillon R, Thomasset M (eds): Vitamin D: Chemistry, Biology and Clinical Applications of the Steroid Hormone. Riverside, University of California, 1997, pp 105–111.
85. Dugaiczyk A, Law SW, Dennison OE: Nucleotide sequence and the encoded amino acids of human serum albumin mRNA. Proc Natl Acad Sci U S A 79:71–75, 1982.
86. Daiger SP, Schanfield MS, Cavalli-Sforza LL: Group-specific component (Gc) proteins bind vitamin D and 25-hydroxyvitamin D. Proc Natl Acad Sci U S A 72:2076–2080, 1975.
87. Bouillon R, Van Baelen H, Rombauts W, et al: The purification and characterisation of the human-serum binding protein for the 25-hydroxycholecalciferol (transcalciferin): Identity with group-specific component. Eur J Biochem 66:285–291, 1976.
88. Bouillon R, Van Baelen H: The transport of vitamin D: Significance of free and total concentrations of vitamin D metabolites. *In* Norman AW, Schaefer K, v Herrath D, et al (eds): Vitamin D. Chemical, Biochemical and Clinical Endocrinology of Calcium Metabolism. Berlin, Walter de Gruyter, 1982, pp 1181–1186.
89. Vicchio D, Yergey A, Obrien K, et al: Quantification and kinetics of 25-hydroxyvitamin-D_3 by isotope dilution liquid chromatography/thermospray mass spectrometry. Biol Mass Spectrom 22:53–58, 1993.
90. Kumar R: The metabolism and mechanism of action of 1,25-dihydroxyvitamin-D_3. Kidney Int 30:793–803, 1986.
91. Ray R, Bouillon R, Van Baelen H, et al: Photoaffinity labeling of human serum vitamin-D binding protein and chemical cleavages of the labeled protein—identification of an 11.5-kDa peptide containing the putative 25-hydroxyvitamin-D_3 binding site. Biochemistry 30:7638–7642, 1991.
92. Haddad JG, Hu YZ, Kowalski MA, et al: Identification of the sterol and actin-binding domains of plasma vitamin D binding protein (Gc-globulin). Biochemistry 31:7174–7181, 1992.
93. Van Baelen H, Bouillon R, De Moor P: Vitamin D-binding protein (Gc-globulin) binds actin. J Biol Chem 255:2270–2272, 1980.
94. Goldschmidt-Clermont PJ, Van Baelen H, Bouillon R, et al: Role of group-specific component (vitamin D binding protein) in clearance of actin from the circulation in the rabbit. J Clin Invest 81:1519–1527, 1988.
95. Yamamoto N, Homma S: Vitamin D_3 binding protein (group-specific component) is a precursor for the macrophage-activating signal factor from lysophosphatidylcholine-treated lymphocytes. Proc Natl Acad Sci U S A 88:8539–8543, 1991.
96. Kew RR, Webster RO: Gc-Globulin (vitamin D–binding protein) enhances the neutrophil chemotactic activity of C5a and C5a des Arg. J Clin Invest 82:364–369, 1988.
97. Schneider GB, Benis KA, Flay NW, et al: Effects of vitamin D binding protein-macrophage activating factor (DBP-MAF) infusion on bone resorption in two osteopetrotic mutations. Bone 6:657–662, 1995.
98. Verboven C: Three-Dimensional Crystal Structure Determination of the Human Vitamin D Binding Protein, thesis, Katholieke Universiteit Leuven, Belgium, 1998.
99. Haussler MR, Jurutka PW, Hsieh J-C, et al: Nuclear vitamin D receptor: Structure-function, phosphorylation, and control of gene transcription. *In* Feldman D, Glorieux FH, Pike JW (eds): Vitamin D. San Diego, Academic Press, 1997, pp 149–177.
100. Mangelsdorf DJ, Evans RM: The RXR heterodimers and orphan receptors. Cell 83:841–850, 1995.
101. Schräder M, Nayeri S, Kahlen J-P, et al: Natural vitamin D_3 response elements formed by inverted palindromes: Polarity-directed ligand sensitivity of vitamin D_3 receptor–retinoid X receptor heterodimer-mediated transactivation. Mol Cell Biol 15:1154–1161, 1995.
102. Miyamoto K, Kesterson RA, Yamamoto H, et al: Structural organization of the human vitamin D receptor chromosomal gene and its promoter. Mol Endocrinol 11:1165–1179, 1997.
103. Crofts LA, Hancock MS, Morrison NA, et al: Multiple promoters direct the tissue-specific expression of novel N-terminal variant human vitamin D receptor gene transcripts. Proc Natl Acad Sci U S A 95:10529–10534, 1998.
104. Keightley M-C: Steroid receptor isoforms: exception or rule? Mol Cell Endocrinol 137:1–5, 1998.
105. Wurtz J-M, Guillot B, Moras D: 3D model of the ligand binding domain of the vitamin D nuclear receptor based on the crystal structure of holo RAR-gamma. *In* Norman AW, Bouillon R, Thomasset M (eds): Vitamin D. Chemistry, Biology and Clinical Applications of the Steroid Hormone. California, University of Riverside, 1997, pp 165–172.
106. Haussler MR, Whitfield GK, Haussler CA, et al: The nuclear vitamin D receptor: Biological and molecular regulatory properties revealed. J Bone Miner Res 13:325–349, 1998.
107. Masuyama H, Jefcoat SC Jr, MacDonald PN: The N-terminal domain of transcription factor IIB is required for direct interaction with the vitamin D receptor and participates in vitamin D–mediated transcription. Mol Endocrinol 11:218–228, 1997.
108. Thompson PD, Jurutka PW, Haussler CA, et al: Heterodimeric DNA binding by the vitamin D receptor and retinoid X receptors is enhanced by 1,25-dihydroxyvitamin D_3 and inhibited by 9-*cis*-retinoic acid. Evidence for allosteric receptor interactions. J Biol Chem 274:8483–8491, 1998.
109. Chen H, Lin RJ, Schiltz RL, et al: Nuclear receptor coactivator ACTR is a novel histone acetyltransferase and forms a multimeric activation complex with P/CAF and CBP/p300. Cell 90:567–580, 1997.
110. Xu J, Qiu Y, DeMayo FJ, et al: Partial hormone resistance in mice with disruption of the steroid receptor coactivator-1 (SRC-1) gene. Science 279:1922–1925, 1998.
111. Nagy L, Kao J-YCD, Lin RJ, et al: Nuclear receptor repression mediated by a complex containing SMRT, mSin3A, and histone deacetylase. Cell 89:373–380, 1997.
112. Schulman IG, Juguilon H, Evans RM: Activation and repression by nuclear hormone receptors: Hormone modulates an equilibrium between active and repressive states. Mol Cell Biol 16:3807–3813, 1996.
113. Hörlein AJ, Näär AM, Heinzel T, et al: Ligand-independent repression by the thyroid hormone receptor mediated by a nuclear receptor co-repressor. Nature 377:397–404, 1995.
114. Masuyama H, MacDonald PN: Proteasome-mediated degradation of the vitamin D receptor (VDR) and a putative role for SUG1 interaction with the AF-2 domain of VDR. J Cell Biochem 71:429–440, 1998.
115. St-Arnaud R, Candeliere GA, Dedhar S: New mechanisms of regulation of the genomic actions of vitamin D in bone cells: Interaction of the vitamin D receptor with non-classical response elements and with the multifunctional protein calreticulin. Front Biosci 1:177–188, 1996.
116. Berghöfer-Hochheimer Y, Zureck C, Wölfl S, et al: L7 protein is a coregulator of vitamin D receptor–retinoid X receptor-mediated transactivation. J Cell Biochem 69:1–12, 1998.
117. Li H, Chen JD: The receptor-associated coactivator 3 activates transcription through CREB-binding protein recruitment and autoregulation. J Biol Chem 273:5948–5954, 1998.
118. Lavinsky RM, Jepsen K, Heinzel T, et al: Diverse signaling pathways modulate nuclear receptor recruitment of N-CoR and SMRT complexes. Proc Natl Acad Sci U S A 95:2920–2925, 1998.
119. Carlberg C: The concept of multiple vitamin D signaling pathways. J Invest Dermatol Symp Proc 1:10–14, 1996.
120. Liu M, Freedman LP: Transcriptional synergism between the vitamin D_3 receptor and other nonreceptor transcription factors. Mol Endocrinol 8:1593–1604, 1994.
121. Alroy I, Towers TL, Freedman LP: Transcriptional repression of the interleukin-2 gene by vitamin D_3: Direct inhibition of NF-ATp/AP-1 complex formation by a nuclear hormone receptor. Mol Cell Biol 15:5789–5799, 1995.
122. Schule R, Umesono K, Mangelsdorf DJ, et al: *Jun-Fos* and receptors for vitamins A and D recognize a common response element in the human osteocalcin gene. Cell 61:497–504, 1990.
123. Kamei Y, Xu L, Heinzel T, et al: A CBP integrator complex mediates transcriptional activation and AP-1 inhibition by nuclear receptors. Cell 85:403–414, 1996.
124. Guo B, Aslam F, Van Wijnen AJ, et al: YY1 regulates vitamin D receptor/retinoid X receptor mediated transactivation of the vitamin D responsive osteocalcin gene. Proc Natl Acad Sci U S A 94:121–126, 1997.
125. Yu X, Bellita T, Manolagas SC: Down-regulation of NF-κB protein levels in activated human lymphocytes by 1,25-dihydroxyvitamin D_3. Proc Natl Acad Sci U S A 92:10990–10994, 1995.
126. Harant H, Andrew PJ, Reddy GS, et al: 1α,25-Dihydroxyvitamin D_3-induced and a variety of its natural metabolites transcriptionally repress nuclear-factor-κB-mediated interleukin-8 gene expression. Eur J Biochem 250:63–71, 1997.
127. D'Ambrosio D, Cippitelli M, Cocciolo MG, et al: Inhibition of IL-12 production by 1,25-dihydroxyvitamin D_3. Involvement of NF-κB downregulation in transcriptional repression of the p40 gene. J Clin Invest 101:252–262, 1998.
128. Huang C, Ma W-YDMI, Rincon M, et al: Blocking activator protein-1 activity, but not activating retinoic acid response element, is required for the antitumor promotion effect of retinoic acid. Proc Natl Acad Sci U S A 94:5826–5830, 1997.
129. Krishnan AV, Feldman D: Regulation of vitamin D receptor abundance. *In* Feldman D, Glorieux FH, Pike JW (eds): Vitamin D. San Diego, Academic Press, 1997, pp 179–200.
130. van den Bemd GJCM, Pols HAP, Birkenhager JC, et al: Conformational change and enhanced stabilization of the vitamin D receptor by the 1,25-dihydroxyvitamin D_3 analog KH1060. Proc Natl Acad Sci U S A 93:10685–10690, 1996.
131. Matkovits T, Christakos S: Ligand occupancy is not required for vitamin D receptor and retinoid receptor–mediated transcriptional activation. Mol Endocrinol 9:232–242, 1990.
132. Malloy PJ, Pike JW, Feldman D: Hereditary 1,25-dihydroxyvitamin D resistant rickets. *In* Feldman D, Glorieux FH, Pike JW (eds): Vitamin D. San Diego, Academic Press, 1997, pp 765–787.
133. Arai H, Miyamoto K-I, Taketani Y, et al: A vitamin D receptor gene polymorphism in the translation initiation codon: Effect on protein activity and relation to bone mineral density in Japanese women. J Bone Miner Res 12:915–921, 1997.
134. Ferrari S, Rizzoli R, Manen D, et al: Vitamin D receptor gene start condon polymorphisms *(FokI)* and bone mineral density: Interaction with age, dietary calcium, and 3′-end region polymorphisms. J Bone Miner Res 13:925–930, 1998.

135. Nemere I, Schwartz Z, Pedrozo H, et al: Identification of a membrane receptor for 1,25-dihydroxyvitamin D_3 which mediates rapid activation of protein kinase C. J Bone Miner Res 13:1353–1359, 1998.
136. Barsony J, Renyi I, McKoy W: Subcellular distribution of normal and mutant vitamin D receptors in living cells. J Biol Chem 272:5774–5782, 1997.
137. Norman AW: Receptors for 1α,25(OH)$_2$D$_3$: Past, present, and future. J Bone Miner Res 13:1360–1369, 1998.
138. Caelles C, Gonzalez-Sancho JM, Munoz A: Nuclear hormone receptor antagonism with AP1 by inhibition of the JNK pathway. Genes Dev 11:3351–3364, 1997.
139. Xie Z, Bikle DD: Cloning of the human phospholipase C-γ1 promoter and identification of a DR6-type vitamin D–responsive element. J Biol Chem 272:6573–6577, 1997.
140. Gniadecki R: Activation of Raf-mitogen–activated protein kinase signaling pathway by 1,25-dihydroxyvitamin D_3 in normal human keratinocytes. J Invest Dermatol 106:1212–1217, 1996.
141. Revelli A, Massobrio M, Tesarik J: Nongenomic effects of 1α,25-dihydroxyvitamin D_3. Trends Endocrinol Metab 9:419–422, 1998.
142. Baran D, Quail J, Ray R, et al: Identification of the membrane protein that binds 1α,25-dihydroxyvitamin D_3 and is involved in the rapid actions of the hormone (abstract). Bone 25:S176, 1998.
143. Norman AW, Zanello LP, De Song X, et al: Effectiveness of 1α,25(OH)$_2$-vitamin D_3–mediated signal transduction for genomic and rapid biological responses is dependent upon the conformation of the signaling ligand. *In* Norman AW, Bouillon R, Thomasset M (eds): Vitamin D. Chemistry, Biology and Clinical Applications of the Steroid Hormone. Riverside, University of California, 1997, pp 331–333.
144. Norman AW, Bouillon R, Farach-Carson MC, et al: Demonstration that 1β,25-dihydroxyvitamin D_3 is an antagonist of the nongenomic but not genomic biological responses and biological profile of the three A-ring diastereomers of 1α,25-dihydroxyvitamin D_3. J Biol Chem 268:20022–20030, 1993.
145. Song X, Bishop JE, Okamura WH, et al: Stimulation of phosphorylation of mitogen-activated protein kinase by 1α,25-dihydroxyvitamin D_3 in promyelocytic NB4 leukemia cells: A structure-function study. Endocrinology 139:457–468, 1998.
146. Norman AW, Okamura WH, Farach-Carson MC, et al: Structure-function studies of 1,25-dihydroxyvitamin D_3 and the vitamin-D endocrine system. 1,25-Dihydroxy-pentadeuterio-previtamin D_3 (as a 6-s-*cis* analog) stimulates nongenomic but not genomic biological responses. J Biol Chem 268:13811–13819, 1993.
147. Ducy P, Zhang R, Geoffroy V, et al: Osf2/Cbfa1: A transcriptional activator of osteoblast differentiation. Cell 89:747–754, 1997.
148. Yasuda H, Shima N, Nakagawa N, et al: Osteoclast differentiation factor is a ligand for osteoprotegerin/osteoclastogenesis-inhibitory factor and is identical to TRANCE/RANKL. Proc Natl Acad Sci U S A 95:3597–3602, 1998.
149. Yasuda H, Shima N, Nakagawa N, et al: Identity of osteoclastogenesis inhibitory factor (OCIF) and osteoprotegerin (OPG): A mechanism by which OPG/OCIF inhibits osteoclastogenesis *in vitro*. Endocrinology 139:1329–1337, 1998.
150. Horwood NJ, Elliott J, Martin TJ, et al: Osteotropic agents regulate the expression of osteoclast differentiation factor and osteoprotegerin in osteoblastic stromal cells. Endocrinology 139:4743–4746, 1998.
151. Ezura Y, Tournay O, Nifuji A, et al: Identification of a novel suppressive vitamin D response sequence in the 5′-flanking region of the murine *Id1* gene. J Biol Chem 272:29865–29872, 1997.
152. Taketani T, Miyamoto K-I, Tanaka K, et al: Gene structure and functional analysis of the human Na^+/phosphate co-transporter. Biochem J 324:927–937, 1997.
153. Rowe PSN, Goulding JN, Francis F, et al: The gene for X-linked hypophosphataemic rickets maps to a 200–300 kb region in Xp22.1, and is located on a single YAC containing a putative vitamin D response element (VDRE). Hum Genet 97:345–352, 1996.
154. Wasserman RH: Vitamin D and the intestinal absorption of calcium and phosphorus. *In* Feldman D, Glorieux FH, Pike JW (eds): Vitamin D. San Diego, Academic Press, 1997, pp 259–273.
155. Feher JJ: Facilitated calcium diffusion by intestinal calcium-binding protein. Cell Physiol 13:C303–C307, 1983.
156. Dupret J-M, Brun P, Perret C, et al: Transcriptional and post-transcriptional regulational regulation of vitamin D–dependent calcium-binding protein gene expression in the rat duodenum by 1,25-dihydroxycholecalciferol. J Biol Chem 262:16553–16557, 1987.
157. Li YC, Pirro AE, Demay MB: Analysis of vitamin D–dependent calcium-binding protein messenger ribonucleic acid expression in mice lacking the vitamin D receptor. Endocrinology 139:847–851, 1998.
158. Darwish IIM, DeLuca IIF: Identification of a 1,25-dihydroxyvitamin D_3–response element in the 5′-flanking region of the rat calbindin D_{9K} gene. Proc Natl Acad Sci U S A 89:603–607, 1992.
159. Pannabecker TL, Chandler JS, Wasserman RH: Vitamin D–dependent transcriptional regulation of the intestinal plasma membrane calcium pump. Biochem Biophys Res Commun 213:499–505, 1995.
160. Brunette MG, Chan M, Ferriere C, et al: Site of 1,25(OH)$_2$ vitamin D_3 synthesis in the kidney. Nature 276:287–289, 1978.
161. Yamamoto M, Kawanobe Y, Takahashi H, et al: Vitamin-D deficiency and renal calcium-transport in the rat. J Clin Invest 74:507–513, 1984.
162. Mivaver J, Sylk DB, Robertson JS, et al: Micropuncture study of the acute renal tubular transport effects of 25-hydroxyvitamin D_3 in the dog. Miner Electrolyte Metab 4:178–188, 1980.
163. Owen TA, Aronow MS, Barone LM, et al: Pleiotropic effects of vitamin D on osteoblast gene expression are related to the proliferative and differentiated state of the bone cell phenotype: Dependency upon basal levels of gene expression, duration of exposure, and bone matrix competency in normal rat osteoblast cultures. Endocrinology 128:1496–1504, 1991.
164. Matsumoto T, Igarashi C, Taksuchi Y, et al: Stimulation by 1,25-dihydroxyvitamin D_3 of in vitro mineralization induced by osteoblast-like MC3T3-E1 cells. Bone 12:27–32, 1991.
165. Ishida H, Bellows CG, Aubin JE, et al: Characterization of the 1,25-(OH)$_2$D$_3$-induced inhibition of bone nodule formation in long-term cultures of fetal rat calvaria cells. Endocrinology 132:61–66, 1993.
166. Bodine P, Henderson R, Green J, et al: 1,25(OH)$_2$D$_3$ promotes osteoblast differentiation and matrix mineralization of a conditionally transformed adult human osteoblast cell line. *In* Norman AW, Bouillon R, Thomasset M (eds): Vitamin D: Chemistry, Biology and Clinical Applications of the Steroid Hormone. Riverside, University of California, 1997, pp 665–666.
167. Stern PH: 1,25-Dihydroxyvitamin D_3 interactions with local factors in bone remodeling. *In* Feldman D, Glorieux FH, Pike JW (eds): Vitamin D. San Diego, Academic Press, 1997, pp 341–352.
168. Yoshizawa T, Handa Y, Uematsu Y, et al: Mice lacking the vitamin D receptor exhibit impaired bone formation, uterine hypoplasia and growth retardation after weaning. Nat Genet 16:391–396, 1997.
169. Bouillon R: The many faces of rickets. N Engl J Med 338:681–682, 1998.
170. Okano T, Tsugawa N, Masuda S, et al: Regulatory activities of 2β-(3-hydroxypropoxy)-1α,25-dihydroxy-vitamin D_3, a novel synthetic vitamin D_3 derivative, on calcium metabolism. Biochem Biophys Res Commun 163:1444–1449, 1989.
171. Tilyard MW, Spears GFS, Thomson J, et al: Treatment of postmenopausal osteoporosis with calcitriol or calcium. N Engl J Med 326:357–362, 1992.
172. Gardiner EM, Sims NA, Thomas GP, et al: Elevated osteoblastic vitamin D receptor in transgenic mice yields stronger bones (abstract). Bone 23:S176, 1998.
173. Li YC, Pirro AE, Amling M, et al: Targeted ablation of the vitamin D receptor:An animal model of vitamin D dependent rickets type II with alopecia. Proc Natl Acad Sci U S A 94:9831–9835, 1997.
174. Li YC, Amling M, Pirro AE, et al: Normalization of mineral ion homeostasis by dietary means prevents hyperparathyroidism, rickets, and osteomalacia, but not alopecia in vitamin D receptor–ablated mice. Endocrinology 139:4391–4396, 1998.
175. Balsan S, Garabedian M, Larchet M, et al: Long-term nocturnal calcium infusions can cure rickets and promote normal mineralization in hereditary resistance to 1,25-dihydroxyvitamin D. J Clin Invest 77:1661–1667, 1999.
176. Bouillon R: Radiochemical assays for vitamin D metabolites: Technical possibilities and clinical applications. J Steroid Biochem 19:921–927, 1983.
177. Bouillon R, Van Baelen H: Transport of vitamin D: significance of free and total concentrations of the vitamin D metabolites. Calcif Tissue Int 33:451–453, 1981.
178. Bikle DD, Gee E: Free, and not total, 1,25-dihydroxyvitamin D regulates 25-hydroxyvitamin D metabolism by keratinocytes. Endocrinology 124:649–654, 1989.
179. Vanham G, Van Baelen H, Tan BK, et al: The effect of vitamin D analogs and of vitamin D–binding protein on lymphocyte proliferation. J Steroid Biochem 29:381–386, 1988.
180. Bouillon R, Van Baelen H: The transport of vitamin D. *In* Norman AW, Schaefer K, v Herrath D, et al (eds): Vitamin D: Basic Research and Its Clinical Application. Berlin, Walter de Gruyter, 1979, pp 137–143.
181. Food and Nutrition Board, National Research Council, National Academy of Sciences: Dietary Reference Intakes for Calcium, Phosphorous, Magnesium, Vitamin D and Fluoride. Washington, DC, National Academy Press, pp 1–30.
182. Bouillon R, Carmeliet G, Boonen S: Ageing and calcium metabolism. *In* Vermeulen A (ed): Endocrinology of Ageing, 1983, pp 341–365.
183. Gloth FM: Vitamin D deficiency in homebound elderly persons. JAMA 274:1683–1686, 1995.
184. Gloth FM: Vitamin D deficiency in older people. J Am Geriatr Soc 43:822–828, 1999.
185. Chapuy MC, Preziosi P, Maamer M, et al: Prevalence of vitamin D insufficiency in an adult normal population. Osteoporos Int 7:439–443, 1997.
186. Lips P, Graafmans WC, Ooms ME, et al: Vitamin D supplementation and fracture incidence in elderly persons. A randomized, placebo-controlled clinical trial. Ann Intern Med 124:400–406, 1996.
187. Dawson-Hughes B, Dallal GE, Krall EA, et al: Effect of vitamin D supplementation on wintertime and overall bone loss in healthy postmenopausal women. Ann Intern Med 115:505–512, 1991.
188. Dawson-Hughes B, Harris S, Krall E, et al: Effect of calcium and vitamin D supplementation on bone density in men and women 65 years of age or older. N Engl J Med 337:670–676, 1997.
189. Thomas MK, Lloyd-Jones DM, Thadhani RI, et al: Hypovitaminosis D in medical inpatients. N Engl J Med 338:777–783, 1998.
190. McKenna MJ: Differences in vitamin D status between countries in young adults and the elderly. Am J Med 93:69–77, 1992.
191. Looker AC, Gunter EW: Hypovitaminosis D in medical inpatients. N Engl J Med 339:344, 1998.
192. Chapuy MC, Arlot ME, Duboeuf F, et al: Vitamin D_3 and calcium to prevent hip fractures in elderly women. N Engl J Med 327:1637–1642, 1992.
193. Chapuy MC, Arlot ME, Delmas PD, et al: Effect of calcium and cholecalciferol treatment for three years on hip fractures in elderly women. BMJ 308:1081–1082, 1994.
194. Slatopolsky ES, Brown AJ: Vitamin D and renal failure. *In* Feldman D, Glorieux FH, Pike JW (eds): Vitamin D. San Diego, Academic Press, 1997, pp 849–865.
195. Kanis JA, McCloskey EV, Beneton MN: Vitamin D and analogues in renal bone disease and implications for osteoporosis. Osteoporos Int 7 (suppl 3):S179–S183, 1997.
196. Ringe JD: Active vitamin D metabolites in glucocorticoid-induced osteoporosis. Calcif Tissue Int 60:124–127, 1997.
197. Eastell R, Reid DM, Compston J, et al: A UK consensus group on management of glucocorticoid-induced osteoporosis: An update. J Intern Med 244:271–292, 1998.
198. Reid IR: Glucocorticoid effects on bone (editorial). J Clin Endocrinol Metab 83:1860–1862, 1998.
199. Fujita T: Vitamin D in the treatment of osteoporosis. Proc Soc Exp Biol Med 199:394–399, 1992.
200. Lips P: Vitamin D deficiency and osteoporosis: The role of vitamin D deficiency and

treatment with vitamin D and analogues in the prevention of osteoporosis-related fractures. Eur J Clin Invest 26:436–442, 1996.

201. Nakamura T: Vitamin D for the treatment of osteoporosis. Osteoporos Int 7:S155–S158, 1997.
202. Glorieux FH, Marie PJ, Pettifor JM, et al: Bone response to phosphate salts, ergocalciferol, and calcitriol in hypophosphatemic vitamin D–resistant rickets. N Engl J Med 303:1023–1031, 1980.
203. Bouillon R, Garmyn M, Verstuyf A, et al: Paracrine role for calcitriol in the immune system and skin creates new therapeutic possibilities for vitamin D analogs. Eur J Endocrinol 133:7–16, 1995.
204. Bikle DD, Pillai S: Vitamin D, calcium, and epidermal differentiation. Endocr Rev 14:3–19, 1993.
205. Abe E, Miyaura C, Sakagami H, et al: Differentiation of mouse myeloid leukemia cells induced by 1α,25-dihydroxyvitamin D_3. Proc Natl Acad Sci U S A 78:4990–4994, 1981.
206. Bouillon R, Okamura WH, Norman AW: Structure-function relationships in the vitamin D endocrine system. Endocr Rev 16:200–257, 1995.
207. Verstuyf A, Verlinden L, Van Baelen H, et al: The biological activity of nonsteroidal vitamin D hormone analogs lacking both the C- and D-rings. J Bone Miner Res 13:549–558, 1998.
208. Liu Y-Y, Collins ED, Norman AW, et al: Differential interaction of 1α,25-dihydroxyvitamin D_3 analogues and their 20-epi homologues with the vitamin D receptor. J Biol Chem 272:3336–3345, 1997.
209. Peleg S, Nguyen C, Woodard BT, et al: Differential use of transcription activation function 2 domain of the vitamin D receptor by 1,25-dihydroxyvitamin D_3 and its A ring–modified analogs. Mol Endocrinol 12:525–535, 1998.
210. Bouillon R, Allewaert K, Xiang DZ, et al: Vitamin D analogs with low affinity for the vitamin D binding protein: Enhanced in vitro and decreased in vivo activity. J Bone Miner Res 6:1051–1057, 1991.
211. Dusso AS, Negrea L, Gunawardhana S, et al: On the mechanisms for the selective action of vitamin D analogs. Endocrinology 128:1687–1692, 1991.
212. Kubodera N, Sato K, Nishii Y: Characteristics of 22-oxacalcitriol (OCT) and 2β-(3-hydroxypropoxy)-calcitriol (ED-71). *In* Feldman D, Glorieux FH, Pike JW (eds): Vitamin D. San Diego, Academic Press, 1997, pp 1071–1086.
213. Tsurukami H, Nakamura T, Suzuki K, et al: A novel synthetic vitamin D analogue, 2β-(3-hydroxypropoxy)1α,25-dihydroxyvitamin D_3 (ED-71), increases bone mass by stimulating the bone formation in normal and ovariectomized rats. Calcif Tissue Int 54:142–149, 1994.
214. Bain S, Smith C, Humphal-Winter J, et al: Two novel vitamin D analogues reverse established osteopenia in the ovariectomized rat (abstract). Bone 23:S571, 1998.
215. Brown AJ, Ritter CR, Finch JL, et al: The noncalcemic analogue of vitamin D, 22-oxacalcitriol, suppresses parathyroid hormone synthesis and secretion. J Clin Invest 84:728–732, 1989.
216. Kurokawa K, Akizawa T, Suzuki M, et al: Effect of 22-oxacalcitriol on hyperparathyroidism of dialysis patients: Results of a preliminary study. Nephrol Dial Transplant 11:121–124, 1996.
217. Llach F, Keshav G, Goldblat MV, et al: Suppression of parathyroid hormone secretion in hemodialysis patients by a novel vitamin D analogue: 19-nor-1,25-dihydroxyvitamin D_2. Am J Kidney Dis 32:340–354, 1998.
218. Garland FC, Garland CF, Gorham ED, et al: Geographic variation in breast cancer mortality in the United States. A hypothesis involving exposure to solar radiation. Prev Med 19:614–622, 1990.
219. Garland C, Barrett-Connor E, Rossof AH, et al: Dietary vitamin-D and calcium and risk of colorectal-cancer—A 19-year prospective-study in men. Lancet 9:307–309, 1985.
220. Mantell DJ, Mawer EB, Bundred NJ, et al: The effects of 1,25-dihydroxyvitamin D_3 on angiogenesis in vitro. *In* Norman AW, Bouillon R, Thomasset M (eds): Vitamin D. Chemistry, Biology and Clinical Applications of the Steroid Hormone. Riverside, University of California, 1997, pp 471–472.
221. Schwartz GG, Lokeshwar BL, Selzer MG, et al: 1α,25-$(OH)_2$ vitamin D and EB1089 inhibit prostate cancer metastasis in vivo. *In* Norman AW, Bouillon R, Thomasset M (eds): Vitamin D. Chemistry, Biology and Clinical Applications of the Steroid Hormone. Riverside, University of California, 1997, pp 489–490.
222. Ogata E: The potential use of vitamin D analogs in the treatment of cancer. Calcif Tissue Int 60:130–133, 1997.
223. Bower M, Colston KW, Stein RC, et al: Topical calcipotriol treatment in advanced breast cancer. Lancet 337:701–702, 1991.
224. Gulliford T, English J, Colston KW, et al: A phase I study of the vitamin D analogue EB 1089 in patients with advanced breast and colorectal cancer. Br J Cancer 78:6–13, 1998.
225. Elstner E, Linker-Israeli M, Le J, et al: Synergistic decrease of clonal proliferation, induction of differentiation, and apoptosis of acute promyelocytic leukemia cells after combined treatment with novel 20-epi vitamin D_3 analogs and 9-*cis* retinoic acid. J Clin Invest 99:349–360, 1997.
226. Light BW, Yu W-D, McElwain MC, et al: Potentiation of cisplatin antitumor activity using a vitamin D analogue in a murine squamous cell carcinoma model system. Cancer Res 57:3759–3764, 1997.
227. Ichikawa F, Sato K, Nanjo M, et al: Mouse primary osteoblasts express vitamin D_3 25-hydroxylase mRNA and convert 1α-hydroxyvitamin D_3 into 1α,25-dihydroxyvitamin D_3. Bone 16:129–135, 1995.
228. Rudolph T, Lehmann B, Pietzsch J, et al: Normal human keratinocytes in organotypic culture metabolize vitamin D_3 to 1α,25-dihydroxyvitamin D_3. *In* Norman AW, Bouillon R, Thomasset M (eds): Vitamin D. Chemistry, Biology and Clinical Applications of the Steroid Hormone. Riverside, University of California, 1997, pp 581–582.
229. Hanada K, Sawamura D, Nakano H, et al: Possible role of 1,25-dihydroxyvitamin D_3–induced metallothionein in photoprotection against UVB injury in mouse skin and cultured keratinocytes. J Dermatol Sci 9:203–208, 1995.
230. Lee J-H, Youn JI: The photoprotective effect of 1,25-dihydroxyvitamin D_3 on ultraviolet light B–induced damage in keratinocyte and mechanism of action. J Dermatol Sci 18:11–18, 1998.
231. Segaert S, Garmyn M, Degreef H, et al: Retinoic acid modulates the antiproliferative effect of 1,25-dihydroxyvitamin D_3 in cultured human epidermal keratinocytes. J Invest Dermatol 109:46–54, 1997.
232. Park K, Bae H, Heydemann A, et al: The E1A oncogene induces resistance to the effects of 1,25-dihydroxyvitamin D_3 on inhibition of growth of mouse keratinocytes. Cancer Res 54:6087–6089, 1994.
233. Matsumoto K, Hashimoto K, Nishida Y, et al: Growth-inhibitory effects of 1,25-dihydroxyvitamin D_3 on normal human keratinocytes cultured in serum-free medium. Biochem Biophys Res Commun 166:916–923, 1990.
234. Sebag M, Gulliver W, Kremer R: Effects of 1,25 dihydroxyvitamin D_3 and calcium on growth and differentiation and on *c-fos* and *p53* gene expression in normal human keratinocytes. J Invest Dermatol 103:323–329, 1994.
235. Kim H-J, Abdelkader N, Katz M, et al: 1,25-Dihydroxy-vitamin D_3 enhances antiproliferative effect and transcription of TGF-β1 on human keratinocytes in culture. J Cell Physiol 151:579–587, 1992.
236. Geilen CC, Bektas M, Wieder T, et al: 1,25-Dihydroxyvitamin D_3 induces sphingomyelin hydrolyis in HaCaT cells via tumor necrosis factor α. J Biol Chem 272:8997–9001, 1997.
237. Kremer R, Karaplis AC, Henderson J, et al: Regulation of parathyroid hormone–like peptide in cultured normal human keratinocytes. J Clin Invest 87:884–893, 1991.
238. Gniadecki R, Gajkawska B, Hansen M: 1,25-Dihydroxyvitamin D_3 stimulates the assembly of adherens junctions in keratinocytes: Involvement of protein kinase C. Endocrinology 138:2241–2248, 1997.
239. Ohba M, Ishino K, Kashiwagi M, et al: Induction of differentiation in normal human keratinocytes by adenovirus-mediated introduction of the η and δ isoforms of protein kinase C. Mol Cell Biol 18:5199–5207, 1998.
240. Chang PL, Prince CW: 1α,25-Dihydroxyvitamin-D(3) enhances 12-*O*-tetradecanoylphorbol-13-acetate–induced tumorigenic transformation and osteopontin expression in mouse JB6 epidermal cells. Cancer Res 53:2217–2220, 1993.
241. Gniadecki R, Serup J: Stimulation of epidermal proliferation in mice with 1α,25-dihydroxyvitamin D_3 and receptor-active analogues of 1α,25-dihydroxyvitamin D_3. Biochem Pharmacol 49:621–624, 1995.
242. Fogh K, Kragballe K: Vitamin D_3 analogues. Clin Dermatol 15:705–713, 1997.
243. Sato H, Sugimoto I, Matsunaga T, et al: Tacalcitol (1,25$(OH)_2D_3$, TV-02) inhibits phorbol ester–induced epidermal proliferation and cutaneous inflammation and induces epidermal differentiation in mice. Arch Dermatol Res 288:656–663, 1996.
244. Milde P, Hauser U, Simon T, et al: Expression of 1,25-dihydroxyvitamin D_3 receptors in normal and psoriatic skin. J Invest Dermatol. 97:230–239, 1991.
245. Reichrath J, Schilli M, Kerber A, et al: Hair follicle expression of 1,25-dihydroxyvitamin D_3 receptors during the murine hair cycle. Br J Dermatol 131:477–482, 1994.
246. Harmon CS, Nevins TD: Biphasic effect of 1,25-dihydroxyvitamin D_3 on human hair follicle growth and hair fiber production in whole-organ cultures. J Invest Dermatol 103:318–322, 1994.
247. Paus R, Schilli MB, Handjiski B, et al: Topical calcitriol enhances normal hair regrowth but does not prevent chemotherapy-induced alopecia in mice. Cancer Res 56:4438–4443, 1996.
248. Jimenez JJ, Yunis AA: Protection from chemotherapy-induced alopecia by 1,25-dihydroxyvitamin D_3. Cancer Res 52:5123–5125, 1992.
249. Holick MF, Ray S, Chen TC, et al: A parathyroid hormone antagonist stimulates epidermal proliferation and hair growth in mice. Proc Natl Acad Sci U S A 91:8014–8016, 1994.
250. Van de Kerkhof PCM: Reduction of epidermal abnormalities and inflammatory changes in psoriatic plaques during treatment with vitamin D_3 analogs. J Invest Dermatol Symp Proc 1:78–81, 1996.
251. Lu I, Gilleaudeau P, McLane JA, et al: Modulation of epidermal differentiation, tissue inflammation, and T-lymphocyte infiltration in psoriatic plaques by topical calcitriol. J Cutan Pathol 23:419–430, 1996.
252. Casteels K, Bouillon R, Waer M, et al: Immunomodulatory effects of 1,25-dihydroxyvitamin D_3. Curr Opin Nephrol Hypertens 4:313–318, 1995.
253. Lemire JM: Immunomodulatory role of 1,25-dihydroxyvitamin D_3. J Cell Biochem 49:26–31, 1992.
254. Clavreul A, D'Hellencourt CLM-MC, Potron G, et al: Vitamin D differentially regulates B7.1 and B7.2 expression on human peripheral blood monocytes. Immunology 95:272–277, 1998.
255. Lemire JM, Beck L, Faherty D, et al: 1,25-Dihydroxyvitamin D_3 inhibits the production of IL-12 by human monocytes and B cells. *In* Norman AW, Bouillon R, Thomasset M (eds): Vitamin D, a Pluripotent Steroid Hormone: Structural Studies, Molecular Endocrinology and Clinical Applications. Berlin, Walter de Gruyter, 1994, pp 531–539.
256. Panina-Bordignon P, D'Ambrosio D, Di Lucia P, et al: 1α,25$(OH)_2D_3$ inhibits the development of T helper 1 cells by selective inhibition of interleukin-12(IL-12) production. *In* Norman AW, Bouillon R, Thomasset M (eds): Vitamin D. Chemistry, Biology and Clinical Applications of the Steroid Hormone. Riverside, University of California, 1997, pp 525–526.
257. Trembleau S, Germann T, Gately MK, et al: The role of IL-12 in the induction of organ-specific autoimmune diseases. Immunol Today 16:383–386, 1995.
258. Mathieu C, Waer M, Laureys J, et al: Activated form of vitamin D [1,25-$(OH)_2D_3$] and its analogs are dose-reducing agents for cyclosporine in vitro and in vivo. Transplant Proc 26:3048–3049, 1994.
259. Thien R, Willheim M, Bajna E, et al: Regulatory effects of 1α,25-dihydroxyvitamin D_3 on the cytokine production of human peripheral blood lymphocytes. *In* Norman AW, Bouillon R, Thomasset M (eds): Vitamin D. Chemistry, Biology and Clinical Applications of the Steroid Hormone. Riverside, University of California, 1997, pp 523–524.
260. Mathieu C, Casteels K, Branisteanu D, et al: Immunomodulatory effects of 1,25$(OH)_2D_3$ and its analogues: Mechanisms of action and possible clinical applica-

tion. *In* Norman AW, Bouillon R, Thomasset M (eds): Vitamin D. Chemistry, Biology and Clinical Applications of the Steroid Hormone. Riverside, University of California, 1997, pp 507–512.

261. Johnsson C, Binderup L, Tufveson G: Immunosuppression with the vitamin D analogue MC 1288 in experimental transplantation. Transplant Proc 28:888–891, 1996.
262. Larsson P, Klareskog L, Johnsson C: MC1288—a vitamin D analogue with immunosuppressive effects which suppresses collagen arthritis. *In* Norman AW, Bouillon R, Thomasset M (eds): Vitamin D. Chemistry, Biology and Clinical Applications of the Steroid Hormone. Riverside, University of California, 1997, pp 537–538.
263. Koren R, Ravid A, Rotem C, et al: 1,25-Dihydroxyvitamin D_3 enhances prostaglandin E_2 production by monocytes. A mechanism which partially accounts for the antiproliferative effect of 1,25$(OH)_2D_3$ on lymphocytes. FEBS Lett 205:113–116, 1986.
264. Towers TL, Freedman LP: Granulocyte-macrophage colony-stimulating factor gene transcription is directly repressed by the vitamin D_3 receptor. J Biol Chem 273:10338–10348, 1998.
265. Park J, Takeuchi A, Sharma S: Characterization of a new isoform of the NFAT (nuclear factor of activated T cells) gene family member NFATc. J Biol Chem 271:20914–20921, 1996.
266. Takeuchi A, Reddy GS, Kobayashi T, et al: Nuclear factor of activated T cells (NFAT) as a molecular target for 1α,25-dihydroxyvitamin D_3–mediated effects. J Immunol 160:209–218, 1998.
267. Cippitelli M, Santoni A: Vitamin D_3: A transcriptional modulator of the interferon-γ gene. Eur J Immunol 28:3017–3030, 1995.
268. Casteels K, Waer M, Bouillon R, et al: 1,25-Dihydroxyvitamin D_3 restores sensitivity to cyclophosphamide-induced apoptosis in NOD mice and protects against diabetes. Clin Exp Immunol 112:181–187, 1998.
269. Casteels K, Waer M, Laureys J, et al: Prevention of autoimmune destruction of syngeneic islet grafts in spontaneously diabetic nonobese diabetic mice by a combination of a vitamin D_3 analog and cyclosporine. Transplantation 65:1225–1232, 1998.
270. Branisteanu D, Mathieu C, Bouillon R: Synergism between sirolimus and 1,25-dihydroxyvitamin D_3 in vitro and in vivo. J Neuroimmunol 79:138–147, 1997.
271. Branisteanu D, Mathieu C, Casteels K, et al: Combination of vitamin D analogues and immunosuppressants. Potential clinical use. Clin Immunother 6:465–478, 1996.
272. Casteels K, Bouillon R, Waer M, et al: Prevention of type I diabetes by late intervention with non-hypercalcemic analogues of vitamin D_3 in combination with cyclosporin A. Endocrinology 139:95–102, 1998.
273. Raisanen-Sokolowski AK, Pakkala IS, Samila SP, et al: A vitamin D analog, MC1288, inhibits adventitial inflammation and suppresses intimal lesions in rat aortic allografts. Transplantation 63:936–941, 1997.
274. Kawa S, Yoshizawa K, Tokoo M, et al: Inhibitory effect of 22-oxa-1,25-dihydroxyvitamin D_3 on the proliferation of pancreatic cancer cell lines. Gastroenterology 110:1605–1613, 1996.
275. Colston KW, James SY, Ofori-Kuragu EA, et al: Vitamin D receptors and antiproliferative effects of vitamin D derivatives in human pancreatic carcinoma cells in vivo and in vitro. Br J Cancer 76:1017–1020, 1997.
276. Akhter J, Chen X, Bowrey P, et al: Vitamin D_3 analog, EB1089, inhibits growth of subcutaneous xenografts of the human colon cancer cell line, LoVo, in a nude mouse model. Dis Colon Rectum 40:317–321, 1997.
277. Evans SR, Schwartz AM, Shchepotin EI, et al: Growth inhibitory effects of 1,25-dihydroxyvitamin D_3 and its synthetic analogue, 1α,25-dihydroxy-16-ene-23-yne-26,27-hexafluoro-19-nor-cholecalciferol (Ro 25-6760), on a human colon cancer xenograft. Clin Cancer Res 4:2869–2876, 1998.
278. Ikezaki S, Nishikawa A, Furukawa F, et al: Chemopreventive effects of 24R,25-dihydroxyvitamin D_3, a vitamin D_3 derivative, on glandular stomach carcinogenesis induced in rats by *N*-methyl-*N*′-nitro-N-nitrosoguanidine and sodium chloride. Cancer Res 56:2767–2770, 1996.
279. Verstuyf A, Verlinden L, Marcelis S, et al: In vitro and in vivo effects of two new 14-epi analogs on human breast adenocarcinoma. *In* Norman AW, Bouillon R, Thomasset M (eds): Vitamin D. Chemistry, Biology and Clinical Applications of the Steroid Hormone. Riverside, University of California, 1997, pp 467–468.
280. Danielsson C, Mathiasen IS, James SY, et al: Sensitive induction of apoptosis in breast cancer cells by a novel 1,25-dihydroxyvitamin D_3 analogue shows relation to promoter selectivity. J Cell Biochem 66:552–562, 1997.
281. James SY, Mercer E, Brady M, et al: EB1089, a synthetic analogue of vitamin D, induces apoptosis in breast cancer cells in vivo and in vitro. Br J Pharmacol 125:953–962, 1998.
282. VanWeelden K, Flanagan L, Binderup L, et al: Apoptotic regression of MCF-7 xenografts in nude mice treated with the vitamin D_3 analog, EB1089. Endocrinology 139:2102–2110, 1998.
283. Koshizuka K, Koike M, Kubota T, et al: Novel vitamin D_3 analog (CB1093) when combined with paclitaxel and cisplatin inhibit growth of MCF-7 human breast cancer cells in vivo. Int J Oncol 13:421–428, 1998.
284. Getzenberg RH, Light BW, Lapco PE, et al: Vitamin D inhibition of prostate adenocarcinoma growth and metastasis in the Dunning rat prostate model system. Urology 50:999–1006, 1997.
285. Yu WD, McElwain MC, Modzelewski RA, et al: Enhancement of 1,25-dihydroxyvitamin D_3–mediated antitumor activity with dexamethasone. J Natl Cancer Inst 90:134–141, 1998.
286. Fujioka T, Hasegawa M, Ishikura K, et al: Inhibition of tumor growth and angiogenesis by vitamin D_3 agents in murine renal cell carcinoma. J Urol 160:247–251, 1998.
287. Shternfeld IS, Lasudry JG, Chappell RJ, et al: Antineoplastic effect of 1,25-dihydroxy-16-ene-23-yne-vitamin D_3 analogue in transgenic mice with retinoblastoma. Arch Ophthalmol 114:1396–1401, 1996.
288. Wilkerson CL, Darjatmoko SRLMJ, Albert DM: Toxicity and dose-response studies of 1,25-$(OH)_2$-16-ene-23-yne vitamin D_3 in transgenic mice. Clin Cancer Res 4:2253–2256, 1998.
289. Mathieu C, Laureys J, Sobis H, et al: 1,25-Dihydroxyvitamin D_3 prevents insulitis in NOD mice. Diabetes 41:1491–1495, 1992.
290. Mathieu C, Waer M, Laureys J, et al: Prevention of autoimmune diabetes in NOD mice by 1,25 dihydroxyvitamin D_3. Diabetologia 37:552–558, 1994.
291. Mathieu C, Waer M, Casteels K, et al: Prevention of type I diabetes in NOD mice by non-hypercalcemic doses of a new structural analogue of 1,25-$(OH)_2D_3$, KH1060. Endocrinology 136:866–872, 1995.
292. Inaba M, Nishizawa Y, Song K, et al: Partial protection of 1α-hydroxyvitamin D_3 against the development of diabetes induced by multiple low-dose streptozotocin injection in CD-1 mice. Metabolism 41:631–635, 1992.
293. Fournier C, Gepner P, Sadouk M, et al: *In vivo* beneficial effects of cyclosporin A and 1,25-dihydroxyvitamin D_3 on the induction of experimental autoimmune thyroiditis. Clin Immunol Immunopathol 54:53–63, 1990.
294. Lemire JM, Archer DC: 1,25-Dihydroxyvitamin D_3 prevents the *in vivo* induction of murine experimental autoimmune encephalomyelitis. J Clin Invest 87:1103–1107, 1991.
295. Branisteanu D, Waer M, Sobis H, et al: Prevention of murine experimental allergic encephalomyelitis: Cooperative effects of cyclosporine and 1α,25-$(OH)_2D_3$. J Neuroimmunol 61:151–160, 1995.
296. Lemire JM, Archer DC, Reddy GS: 1,25-Dihydroxy-24-oxo-16ene-vitamin D_3, a renal metabolite of the vitamin D analog 1,25-dihydroxy-16ene-vitamin D_3, exerts immunosuppressive activity equal to its parent without causing hypercalcemia *in vivo*. Endocrinology 135:2818–2821, 1994.
297. Garcion E, Sindji L, Montero-Menei C, et al: Expression of inducible nitric oxide synthase during rat brain inflammation: Regulation by 1,25-dihydroxyvitamin D_3. Glia 22:282–294, 1998.
298. Ylikomi T, Bocquel MT, Berry M, et al: Cooperation of proto-signals for nuclear accumulation of estrogen and progesterone receptors. EMBO J 11:3681–3694, 1992.
299. Larsson P, Mattsson LKL, Johnsson C: A vitamin D analogue (MC1288) has immunomodulatory properties and suppresses collagen-induced arthritis (CIA) without causing hypercalcemia. Clin Exp Immunol 114:277–284, 1998.
300. Koizumi T, Nakao Y, Matsui T, et al: Effects of corticosteroid and 1,24R-dihydroxyvitamin D_3 administration on lymphoproliferation and autoimmune disease in MRL/MP lpr/lpr mice. Int Arch Allergy Appl Immunol 77:396–404, 1985.
301. Abe J, Takita Y, Nakano T, et al: 22-Oxa-1α-25-dihydroxyvitamin D_3: A new synthetic analogue of vitamin D having a potent immunoregulating activity without inducing hypercalemia in mice. *In* Cohn DV, Glorieux FH, Martin TJ (eds): Calcium Regulation and Bone Metabolism. Amsterdam, Elsevier, 1990, pp 146–151.
302. Branisteanu DD, Leenaerts P, van Damme B, et al: Partial prevention of active Heymann nephritis by 1α,25 dihydroxyvitamin D_3. Clin Exp Immunol 94:412–417, 1993.
303. Hattori M: Effect of 1α,25$(OH)_2D_3$ on experimental rat nephrotoxic serum nephritis. Nippon Jinzo Gakkai, Shi 32:147–159, 1990.
304. Lillevang ST, Rosenkvist J, Andersen CB, et al: Single and combined effects of the vitamin D analogue KH1060 and cyclosporin A on mercuric-chloride–induced autoimmune disease in the BN rat. Clin Exp Immunol 88:301–306, 1992.
305. Mathieu C, Laureys J, Waer M, et al: Prevention of autoimmune destruction of transplanted islets in spontaneously diabetic NOD mice by KH 1060, a 20-epi analog of vitamin D: Synergy with cyclosporin. Transplant Proc 26:3128–3129, 1994.
306. Mathieu C, Casteels K, Waer M, et al: Prevention of diabetes recurrence after islet transplantation in NOD mice by analogues of 1,25$(OH)_2D_3$ in combination with CyA. Transplant Proc 28:3095, 1997.
307. Lemire JM, Archer DC, Khulkarni A, et al: Prolongation of the survival of murine cardiac allografts by the vitamin D_3 analogue 1,25-dihydroxy-delta^{16}-cholecalciferol. Transplantation 54:762–763, 1992.
308. Jordan SC, Nigata M, Mullen Y: 1,25-Dihydroxyvitamin D_3 prolongs rat cardiac allograft survival. *In* Norman AW, Schaefer K, Grigoleit HG, et al (eds): Vitamin D. Molecular, Cellular and Clinical Endocrinology. Berlin, Walter de Gruyter, 1988, pp 334–335.
309. Hullett DACMT, Redaelli C, Humphal-Winter J, et al: Prolongation of allograft survival by 1,25-dihydroxyvitamin D_3. Transplantation 66:824–828, 1998.
310. Räisanen-Sokolowski AK, Pakkala IS, Samila SP, et al: A vitamin D analog, MC1288, inhibits adventitial inflammation and suppresses intimal lesions in rat aortic allografts. Transplantation 63:936–941, 1997.
311. Jordan SC, Shibuka R, Mullen Y: 1,25-Dihydroxyvitamin D_3 prolongs skin graft survival in mice. *In* Norman AW, Schaefer K, Grigoleit H-G, et al (eds): Vitamin D. Molecular, Cellular and Clinical Endocrinology. Berlin, Walter de Gruyter, 1988, pp 346–347.
312. Veyron P, Pamphile R, Binderup L, et al: Two novel vitamin D analogues, KH 1060 and CB 966, prolong skin allograft survival in mice. Transpl Immunol 1:72–76, 1993.
313. Lewin E, Olgaard K: The in vivo effect of a new, in vitro, extremely potent vitamin D_3 analog Kh1060 on the suppression of renal allograft rejection in the rat. Calcif Tissue Int 54:150–154, 1994.
314. Overbergh L, Decallone B, Valckx D, et al: Identification and immune regulation of 25-hydroxyvitamin $D_{1\alpha}$-hydroxylase in murine macrophages. Clin Exp Immunol, in press.

Chapter 73

Regulation of Calcium and Phosphate Homeostasis

F. Richard Bringhurst

Nearly all of the calcium and phosphate ions in the body reside in insoluble form within the mineral phase of bone, where they determine the mechanical properties of the skeleton and serve also as a source of additional extracellular mineral ions. Normal mineralization of bone and cartilage, both during development and in the adult, requires adequate concentrations of extracellular calcium and phosphate. Soluble calcium and phosphate present within the extracellular and intracellular fluids constitute less than 1% of the total body content of each ion but are crucial for a broad range of physiologic processes. Thus, acute depletion or excess of extracellular calcium, phosphate, or both leads to profound clinical consequences due to disruption of critical metabolic and regulatory pathways, whereas chronic depletion of either or both of these ions produces significant skeletal disease, including osteomalacia, osteoporosis, fracture, and rickets. Accordingly, a network of tightly integrated hormonal systems has evolved to closely regulate the blood concentrations of calcium and phosphate. The key elements of this network include parathyroid hormone (PTH), active forms of vitamin D, and a still-unidentified phosphaturic hormone (phosphatonin).

Details of the distribution, absorption, excretion, and metabolic actions of calcium and phosphate, including the adverse clinical consequences of excessive or deficient concentrations in extracellular fluid, are reviewed in this chapter. PTH and vitamin D biochemistry, physiology, and action are reviewed in Chapters 70 and 72, respectively, whereas discussions of specific clinical disorders of bone and mineral metabolism can be found in Chapters 75 through 89.

CALCIUM

Distribution and Metabolic Actions of Calcium

The total body content of calcium in a normal adult is approximately 1000 g, of which nearly all exists within the crystal structure of bone mineral and less than 1% is soluble in extracellular and intracellular fluid[1, 2] (Fig. 73–1) (Table 73–1). On average, bone mineral closely approximates the composition of hydroxyapatite [$Ca_{10}(PO_4)_6(OH)_2$], which means that 6 mmol of phosphate are released with every 10 mmol of calcium mobilized during bone resorption (or about 1:2 on a milligram-per-milligram basis).[1, 3]

In blood, calcium is partly bound to proteins (Table 73–2). Albumin accounts for about 70% of the protein-bound fraction.[4] Another portion (about 6%) is associated with diffusable ion complexes.[1] Thus, only half of total plasma calcium normally is freely ionized, but it is this fraction that is most important physiologically and thus subject to stringent endocrine regulation. The normal ranges of total and ionized serum calcium in the adult are 8.5 to 10.5 mg/dL and 1.17 to 1.33 mM, respectively.[5] The usual 2:1 ratio of total to ionized calcium may be disturbed by disorders such as metabolic acidosis (calcium binding to proteins is reduced at acid pH) or by changes in serum protein concentrations, as in starvation, cirrhosis, dehydration, or multiple

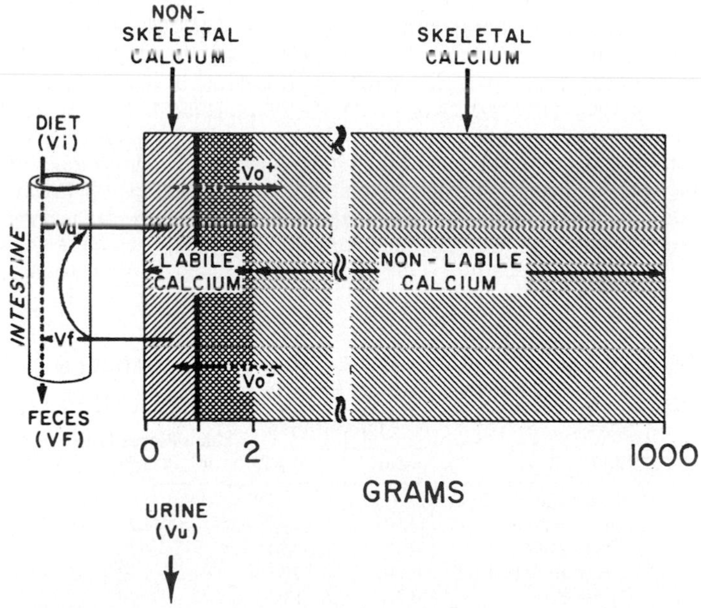

FIGURE 73–1. Schematic representation of the distribution of calcium in the body and its exchange among the different compartments that have been inferred through calcium kinetic studies. The double cross-hatched area shown in the skeletal calcium compartment just to the right of the heavy vertical line is the small skeletal component of labile calcium, the surface, freely diffusible component. Not represented in this diagram is the nonlabile, nonskeletal pool of calcium that is found in sites such as renal stones. Vi, dietary calcium intake; VF, fecal calcium; Va, calcium absorption; Vf, endogenous fecal calcium; Vo^+, bone calcium accretion; Vo^-, bone calcium release; Vu, urinary calcium excretion. (Modified from Potts JT Jr, Deftos LJ: Parathyroid hormone, thyrocalcitonin, vitamin D, bone and mineral metabolism. *In* Bondy PK, Rosenberg LE (eds): Duncan's Diseases of Metabolism, ed 7. Philadelphia, WB Saunders, 1974, pp 1225–1430.)

TABLE 73–1. Distribution of Calcium and Phosphate in Body Tissues

	Calcium	Phosphorus
Total body content (g/kg of fat-free tissue)	20–25	11–14
Relative Distribution		
Skeleton	99%	85%
Muscle	0.3%	6%
Other tissue	0.7%	9%

myeloma. Thus, when precise knowledge of the ionized calcium concentration is clinically important, direct measurement with calcium-selective electrodes should be performed.

Serum calcium is higher during childhood and adolescence than in the adult[6] but does not change at puberty or, in women, during the menstrual cycle. During pregnancy, total serum calcium and albumin decline progressively, but ionized calcium is minimally affected.[7, 8] Fetal calcium content rises dramatically during the third trimester (to about 30 g at term),[9] and fetal serum total and ionized calcium concentrations both are higher than maternal levels, consistent with active placental transport of calcium.[10] Despite daily losses of 200 to 300 mg/day of calcium in breast milk, lactating women maintain normal levels of ionized calcium in blood by increasing intestinal calcium absorption in response to augmented production of 1,25-dihydroxyvitamin D [1,25$(OH)_2$D].[11, 12]

Calcium entry into cells is strongly favored by a steep electrochemical gradient. Thus, the cell interior is electronegative, and cytosolic free calcium is in the range of 10^{-7} M, which is 10,000-fold lower than extracellular calcium concentrations. Calcium traverses the plasma membrane through various channels, including voltage-, receptor- and store-operated forms, the regulation of which is complex and tissue-specific.[13, 14] Intracellularly, nearly all (99%) calcium is sequestered in pools within mitochondria, endoplasmic reticula, or sarcoplasmic reticula or is tightly bound to the inner surface of the plasma membrane.[15] Sequestered calcium, especially that within the endoplasmic reticulum, may be released rapidly into the cytosol following activation of cell-surface receptors. In this way, it plays a critical role in signal transduction and in controlling calcium entry via store-operated channels. The extremely low cytosolic free calcium concentration is maintained by active calcium transport into intracellular pools or by extrusion out of the cell via high-affinity, low-capacity Ca^{2+}, H^+-adenosinetriphosphatases (ATPases) and low-affinity, high-capacity Na^+-Ca^{2+} exchangers driven by the transmembrane sodium gradient.[16]

With the discovery of a G protein–coupled calcium-sensing receptor expressed in parathyroid, renal epithelial, and other cells, it has become clear that calcium can act as an extracellular ligand to directly control cellular function.[17] The principal actions of the calcium sensor include suppression of PTH secretion and, in the thick ascending loop of the renal tubule, inhibition of calcium, magnesium, and sodium chloride (NaCl) reabsorption. Extracellular calcium also is utilized directly for normal matrix mineralization in bone and cartilage and is required for activation of important circulating or extracellular enzymes and proteases. Intracellular calcium exerts a broad range of effects via interaction with key enzymes and effector molecules, including kinases, phosphatases, calmodulins, transcription factors, ion channels (including calcium channels), and troponins and other proteins involved in contraction, microtubule and microfilament assembly, and motility. The steep gradients between intracellular calcium and both extracellular and intracellular sequestered calcium are crucial for normal neuromuscular activity and provide the potential required for rapid transients and waves of cytosolic free calcium that serve key second messenger functions in both excitable and nonexcitable cells.[14, 18] Disturbances in extracellular calcium concentration therefore may cause a variety of symptoms, the most common of which reflect abnormal neuromuscular activity. Thus, hypercalcemia may lead to muscle weakness and areflexia, anorexia, constipation, vomiting, drowsiness, depression, confusion, other cognitive dysfunction, and coma. Renal effects of hypercalcemia are especially common and include impaired urinary concentration (via calcium sensor activation,[17] nocturia and, when severe, medullary calcification, nephrocalcinosis, and renal failure. Hypocalcemia, conversely, may cause anxiety, seizures, muscle twitching, Chvostek's and Trousseau's signs, carpal or pedal spasm, stridor, bronchospasm, or intestinal cramps.

TABLE 73–2. Distribution of Calcium and Phosphate in Normal Human Plasma

State	Concentration *mmol*	*mg/dL*	Percentage of Total
Phosphorus			
Free HPO_4^{2-}	0.50	1.55	44
Free $H_2PO_4^-$	0.11	0.34	10
Protein-bound	0.14	0.43	12
$NaHPO_4^-$	0.33	1.02	28
$CaHPO_4$	0.04	0.12	3
$MgHPO_4$	0.03	0.10	3
Total	1.15	3.56	
Calcium			
Free Ca^{2+}	1.18	4.72	48
Protein-bound	1.14	4.56	46
Complexed	0.08	0.32	3
Unidentified	0.08	0.32	3
Total	2.48	9.92	

Adapted from Walser M: Ion association. VI. Interaction between calcium, magnesium, inorganic phosphate, citrate and protein in normal human plasma. J Clin Invest 40:732, 1961.

Calcium Absorption

Daily calcium intake in the United States ranges rather broadly between 300 and 1500 mg and tends to decline with age. Women generally consume less calcium than men,[19] although awareness of the importance of adequate dietary calcium intake has led to widespread use of calcium supplements to achieve or exceed the recommended daily allowance (RDA) of 1000 mg/day.[19] Intestinal calcium absorption has been measured by a variety of techniques, including use of everted gut sacs, isolated bowel loops, and isolated intestinal cells or subcellular organelles in animals[20–23] and, in humans, via classic balance studies, single- or double-isotope radiocalcium kinetic techniques, or multiple-lumen intestinal tubes.[24] Such studies have shown that intestinal calcium absorptive efficiency in humans ranges broadly between 20% and 70%, declines steadily with age, and is strongly influenced by previous calcium intake, the presence of other nutrients, pregnancy, lactation, overall calcium balance, and the availability of vitamin D.[19, 24–27] Fecal calcium includes the residual fraction of dietary calcium that is not absorbed, as well as a contribution from secreted calcium present in bile and other digestive juices (endogenous fecal calcium). Endogenous fecal calcium in humans normally amounts to 100 to 200 mg/day and is relatively unaffected by changes in dietary or serum calcium.[28, 29]

Intestinal calcium absorption is adjusted physiologically in response to variations in calcium intake, as shown by radiocalcium kinetic and balance studies in normal subjects[30, 31] (Table 73–3). Obligate renal and intestinal excretion of calcium is such that calcium balance cannot be maintained if dietary calcium consistently falls below 200 to 400 mg/day, even though the percentage of calcium absorbed may be very high (i.e., 70%) (Fig. 73–2). As calcium intake increases, overall calcium absorption (in milligrams per day) rises, but the fractional absorption of ingested calcium declines progressively such that, within the physiologic range of calcium intake, total net calcium absorption tends to plateau at approximately 400 mg/day. Consequently, urinary calcium excretion tends also to plateau at higher intakes (Fig. 73–3). Additional buffering of changes in dietary calcium results from control of renal tubular calcium reabsorption and skeletal calcium release (see Table 73–3), but regulation of intestinal absorptive efficiency accounts for 75% to 90% of the homeostatic response.[30] The mechanisms of

TABLE 73–3. Normal Adult Response to Varying Dietary Calcium Intake

Dietary Ca (mg/day)	220 (low)	850 (normal)	2100 (high)
Absorbed Ca (mg/day)*	150	340	490
Efficiency (%)†	68%	40%	23%
Renal Ca excretion (mg/day)	150	210	260
Efficiency (arbitrary units)‡	.75	1.0	1.1
Total Ca balance (mg/day)	−110	0	+70
Skeletal Ca uptake (mg/day)§	420	420	420
Efficiency (arbitrary units)‡	1.9	1.9	1.9
Skeletal Ca release (mg/day)§	530	420	350

*Diet minus fecal calcium corrected for endogenous fecal calcium.
†Absorbed calcium/dietary calcium.
‡Rate constant for ^{47}Ca removal from plasma into urine or nonexchanging bone.
§Values given were calculated with a compartmental model.[30, 31]

this inverse regulation of intestinal absorptive efficiency by changes in calcium availability are considered further below.

Mechanisms and Sites of Calcium Absorption

Calcium is absorbed throughout the intestine. In terms of rates of transport per unit length of mucosa, absorption is most efficient in the duodenum and proximal jejunum, which exhibit the highest levels of vitamin D–dependent calcium-binding proteins and in which lower luminal pH (5 to 6) promotes dissociation of calcium from complexes with food constituents and other ions.[23, 32] On the other hand, longer residence times in the more distal small bowel segments may allow absorption of a larger proportion of total calcium intake in the distal jejunum and ileum.[33, 34] The ileum, for example, may become an important site of net calcium absorption during dietary restriction of calcium or when the residence time of luminal contents in more proximal bowel segments is reduced.[33, 35]

The overall kinetics of duodenal calcium absorption can be approximated by the sum of a saturable and a nonsaturable component[23, 26, 36]:

$$J_{ms} = \frac{J_{max}\,[Ca]}{K_t + [Ca]} + D\,[Ca]$$

where J_{ms} = mucosal-to-serosal absorptive flux, J_{max} = the maximum transport rate of the saturable mechanism, [Ca] = luminal calcium concentration, K_t = [Ca] at which the active transport rate is half-maximal, and D = the diffusion constant for the nonsaturable mechanism. This relation is depicted schematically in Figure 73–4. Actual measurements of duodenal or jejunual K_t in humans and animals are in the range of 2 to 3 mmol,[22, 23, 26] and similar values probably apply to other intestinal segments involved in the active transport of calcium.[22] The essential feature illustrated by Figure 73–4 is that the active transport process, the J_{max} of which is regulated mainly by vitamin D (see below), accounts for most of the calcium transport when luminal (dietary) calcium is low (i.e., well below 3 mM), whereas the passive diffusional component predominates when calcium intakes are high (when the active mechanism is saturated). Luminal calcium concentration in the proximal small bowel of humans following a low calcium meal is in the range of 0.3 to 2.0 mM but, for example, may rise to 3 to 9 mM after drinking a glass of milk.[32]

The molecular correlates of these kinetically defined entities are not yet completely understood. The saturable component likely reflects transcellular calcium transport, whereas the nonsaturable component, common to most or all segments of the intestine, likely results from net voltage-dependent paracellular diffusion down an electrochemical gradient across the tight junctions between enterocytes.[23] Transcellular transport of large amounts of calcium by the intestinal epithelium poses a unique challenge, in that cytosolic free calcium must be maintained at the normal submicromolar level to avoid cytotoxicity. Thus, the transported calcium, which can enter the apical side of the cell from the intestinal lumen down a highly favorable gradient, must be effectively sequestered from the cytosolic compartment as it traverses the cell to be extruded into the extracellular fluid by high-affinity, energy-requiring Ca^{2+}, Mg^{+}-ATPases.[37]

Two mechanisms for preventing transported calcium from flooding the cytosol of the enterocyte have been proposed. Some evidence supports a vesicular flow mechanism, whereby calcium at the apical membrane is endocytosed into vesicles that later fuse with lysozymes, traverse the cytosol, and then release the transported calcium via exocytosis across the basolateral membrane.[38] Other work supports a buffered diffusional model, in which calcium entering the cell via apical membrane channels becomes tightly associated with the cytosolic vitamin D–dependent calcium-binding protein (calbindin-D9k). The calbindin-calcium complex then diffuses across the cytosol to the basolateral membrane, where free calcium dissociates into the low cytosolic calcium environment maintained immediately subjacent to the basolateral membrane by high-affinity membrane Ca^{2+}-ATPases located there that actively extrude calcium out of the cell.[23] The known cellular concentrations and kinetic properties of the calbindin-D9k molecule would support observed rates of duodenal calcium transport at submicromolar concentrations of cytosolic free calcium.[39]

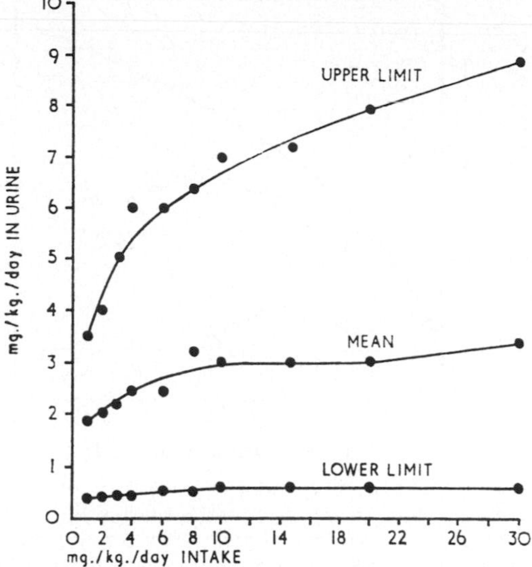

FIGURE 73–3. Urinary calcium excretion as a function of dietary calcium intake in healthy subjects. Note the asymmetry of the normal range about its mean. (From Peacock M, Hodgkinson A, Nordin BEC: Importance of dietary calcium in the definition of hypercalciuria. BMJ 3:469–471, 1967.)

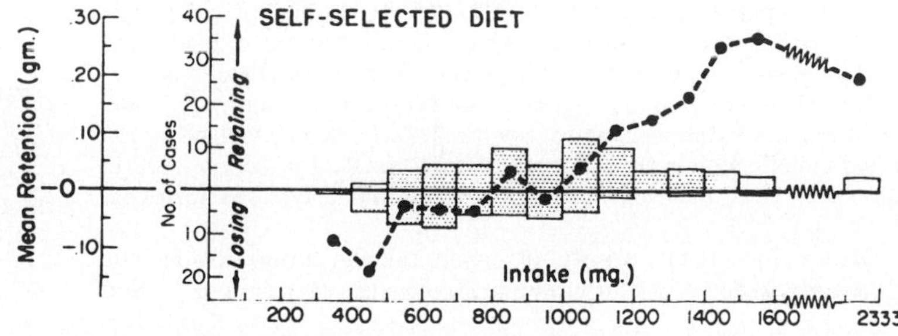

FIGURE 73–2. Mean calcium retention or loss *(interrupted line)* as a function of dietary calcium intake in healthy young adult women studied on a metabolic ward and consuming their customary diets. The shaded bars above and below the zero line show the number of subjects with net calcium retention or loss, respectively, at each calcium intake. Note losses at intakes of less than 500 mg/day, retentions at intakes greater than 1100 mg/day, and apparent homeostatic adaptation between these limits. (From Ohlson MA, Stearns G: Calcium intake of children and adults. Fed Proc 18:1077–1085, 1959.)

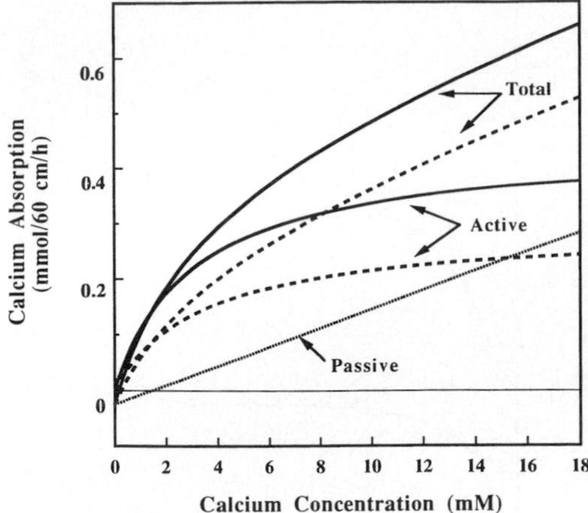

FIGURE 73–4. The kinetics of intestinal calcium absorption in humans. Total net proximal jejunal mucosal-to-serosal calcium flux, measured by an intubation-perfusion technique in normal human subjects, is resolved into its active and passive (diffusional) components for individuals on a low (300 mg/day; *solid curves*) or high (2000 mg/day; *dashed curves*) calcium intake. Passive calcium flux is shown as a linear function of intraluminal calcium concentration that is assumed to be identical during consumption of high and low calcium diets.[34] Passive flux is assumed to be zero in the absence of a transmucosal chemical gradient ([Ca] = 1.5 mM) and actually becomes slightly negative (net secretion) when intraluminal calcium is zero. Active transport is calculated by subtracting passive from total flux. For low and high calcium intakes, kinetic parameters employed were: K_t = 3.1 and 3.5 mM; V_{max} = 0.44 and 0.29 mmol/60 cm/hour, respectively.[37]

The buffered diffusional model predicts that enterocyte calbindin-D9k content would be the main determinant of the rate of calcium transport via this saturable, transcellular route. In fact, intestinal content of calbindin-D9k correlates extremely well with the rate of duodenal calcium absorption.[23] The buffered diffusion model also assumes that the mechanism (channel) for apical calcium entry has a finite conductance and is inhibited by high local cytosolic calcium concentrations. A candidate apical calcium transporter with a K_m for calcium of 0.4 mM recently was isolated from a rat duodenal complementary DNA (cDNA) library.[40] At the basolateral aspect of the cell, Na^+-Ca^{2+} exchange, driven by the Na^+,K^+-ATPase, may supplement the action of the high-affinity Ca^{2+}-ATPases, especially at high rates of calcium transport.[23, 41]

Factors That Affect Calcium Absorption

BIOAVAILABILITY. Calcium is transported across the intestinal epithelium as the free ion and therefore must be released from existing complexes with other dietary constituents prior to absorption.[42] Gastric acid may be important in promoting dissociation of such calcium complexes in food,[43] although the slightly acidic (pH 4 to 6) intestinal environment that follows a typical meal, even in achlorhydric individuals, may be all that is required.[32, 44] In fact, the extremely insoluble but commonly prescribed calcium carbonate salt is not well absorbed in achlorhydric subjects unless it is taken with meals.[44] Calcium citrate, in contrast, is much more readily soluble, even in the absence of gastric acid.[45] Available H_2-receptor blockers, however, appear not to interfere significantly with the absorption of calcium from food or calcium carbonate preparations.[46] The lower solubility of calcium at neutral or alkaline pH may contribute to the reduced efficiency of calcium absorption by intestinal segments distal to the duodenum.[47, 48]

Bile salts increase dietary calcium solubility and absorption,[49, 50] and compromise of this mechanism contributes to calcium malabsorption in individuals with gastrointestinal disease[51] or ileal resection[35] and in those who consume high fiber diets (which impair bile salt reabsorption).[52]

Dietary constituents known to impair calcium absorption include plant-derived fibers rich in uronic acid, phytates, or cellulose[53–56] and oxalate (present in leafy green vegetables, rhubarb, and tea) the calcium salt of which is nonabsorbable.[57] Binding of calcium by long-chain saturated free fatty acids released during lipid digestion normally does not impair calcium absorption but may do so in individuals with steatorrheic disorders.[51, 58] Lactose in milk and infant formulas augments calcium absorption via enhanced paracellular diffusion in the distal small bowel.[59] Dietary protein and phosphate do not directly alter intestinal calcium absorption, although both have important effects on bone remodeling and urinary calcium excretion.[60–63]

VITAMIN D. 1,25 $(OH)_2D$ is the prime physiologic regulator of intestinal epithelial calcium transport.[64, 65] It is the efferent arm of the homeostatic loop that links adaptive changes in intestinal absorptive efficiency to alterations in dietary calcium availability via the control of PTH secretion and subsequent regulation, by PTH, of the renal 1α-hydroxylase. The duodenum is most responsive to $1,25(OH)_2D$, although the hormone regulates calcium absorption in most intestinal segments.[22] In the duodenum, $1,25(OH)_2D$ increases the J_{max} of the saturable, transcellular component of calcium absorption[66] by increasing calcium flux across the apical brush border membrane[67] (see Fig. 73–4), calbindin-D9k messenger RNA (mRNA) and protein levels,[68–70] and basolateral Ca^{2+}-ATPase activity.[71, 72] Some of these effects involve regulation of gene transcription by the $1,25(OH)_2D$–vitamin D receptor complex, whereas others occur very rapidly and likely involve nongenomic mechanisms, including actions upon membrane phospholipid metabolism, cytosolic free calcium, or the biomechanical properties of the membrane.[73, 74] Quantitatively, the increase in calbindin-D9k may be the most important of these actions of $1,25(OH)_2D$, as the cytosolic calbindin-D9k concentration correlates closely with intestinal calcium absorptive efficiency (Fig. 73–5) and may be rate-limiting for active transport of calcium by the enterocyte.[23]

In jejunum and ileum, as well as in duodenum, however, $1,25(OH)_2D$ also may increase the paracellular, passive, voltage-dependent component of calcium flux, which predominates at high intraluminal calcium concentrations.[75] This action of $1,25(OH)_2D$ to facilitate passive, paracellular transport would have particular clinical importance in humans because the level of dietary calcium, especially when supplemented (as in most clinical situations), usually is sufficient to saturate the active, transcellular component of intestinal calcium absorption.[76] The mechanism whereby $1,25(OH)_2D$ augments paracellular calcium flux is unknown but could involve changes in membrane fluidity.[73]

Finally, an extremely rapid (minutes) action of $1,25(OH)_2D$ to increase duodenal calcium absorption, termed "transcaltachia," has been

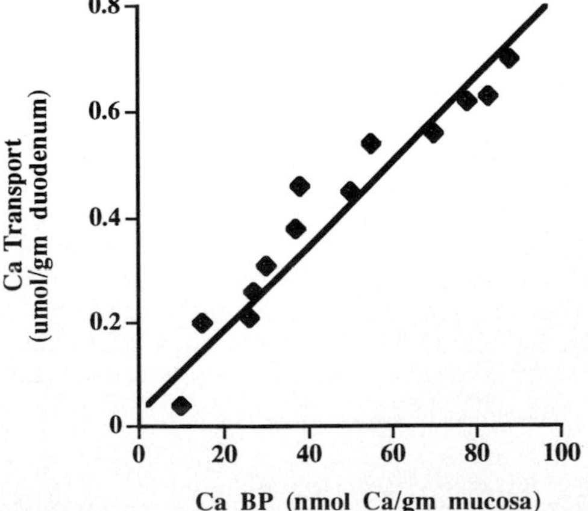

FIGURE 73–5. Relation between intestinal calcium transport and mucosal calbindin content. The absorption of radiocalcium in vitro by everted duodenal gut sacs is shown as a function of the duodenal content of calbindin (Ca BP) for intestines obtained from young male rats equilibrated on a high calcium diet with or without added vitamin D. (Data are replotted from Bronner F, Pansu D, Stein WD: An analysis of intestinal calcium transport across the rat intestine. Am J Physiol 250:G561–G569, 1986.)

demonstrated in perfused chick duodenum.[77] This mechanism is initiated by delivery of 1,25$(OH)_2$D to the basolateral (vascular) but not the mucosal surface of the chick duodenum. It is inhibited at very high concentrations of basolateral extracellular calcium and is mimicked by analogues of 1,25$(OH)_2$D that bind poorly to the classic vitamin D receptor but that do activate calcium channels in other systems.[78, 79] These rapid effects of 1,25$(OH)_2$D, although not fully understood, may be complementary to the slower genomic effects of the hormone, such as increased synthesis of calbindin.[80]

OTHER FACTORS. Intestinal calcium absorption declines strikingly with age.[25, 81] Aging also impairs the adaptive upregulation of intestinal calcium absorption that normally follows dietary calcium restriction, predisposing to negative calcium balance and loss of bone mass.[26, 82, 83] This failure of adaptation to calcium restriction involves diminished capacity for renal synthesis of 1,25$(OH)_2$D in response to PTH,[84, 85] although defective action of 1,25$(OH)_2$D at the level of the intestinal mucosa also may play a role.[86, 87]

In postmenopausal women, estrogens increase calcium absorption, principally via a PTH-mediated increase in synthesis of 1,25$(OH)_2$D, although a direct effect of estrogen on the gut also has been proposed.[88, 89] Estrogens may be partly responsible for the early increase in serum 1,25$(OH)_2$D and calcium absorption characteristic of pregnancy and lactation,[90, 91] although elevated PTH, prolactin, placental factors, and placental synthesis of 1,25$(OH)_2$D have been implicated as well.[92, 93] Intestinal calcium absorption may be augmented independently of vitamin D during pregnancy and lactation,[94, 96] although this effect cannot fully compensate for the complete absence of 1,25$(OH)_2$D.[94, 96] This vitamin D–independent response is accompanied by hypertrophy of intestinal villi and is specific for calcium and phosphorus (magnesium absorption is unaffected, for example).[94] Active placental calcium transport also is vitamin D–independent[97] and, in the developing neonate, normal intestinal calcium absorption and avid whole-body calcium retention can occur independently of vitamin D.[98, 99]

Pharmacologic doses of glucocorticoids depress calcium absorption without impairing the production or intestinal localization of 1,25$(OH)_2$D.[100–102] In rats, glucocorticoids were found to reduce resistance to paracellular calcium diffusion, creating increased serosal-to-mucosal backflux of calcium at low luminal calcium concentrations but actually increasing passive absorption at high calcium intakes.[103]

Impaired calcium absorption in thyrotoxicosis[104] and metabolic acidosis[105] is attributable to diminished renal 1,25$(OH)_2$D synthesis, although direct intestinal effects of acidosis also may play a role.[106] Increased 1,25$(OH)_2$D may occur in hypothyroidism.[101] Ethanol reduces calcium absorption, possibly by a direct toxic effect on enterocytes,[107, 108] but the clinical significance of this effect remains to be determined. The same is true of phenytoin[109] and verapamil.[110]

Calcium Excretion

Regulation of renal calcium excretion is the major mechanism for homeostatic control of blood ionized calcium in the face of fluctuations in filtered load, as derived from intestinal calcium absorption and net bone resorption. When urinary calcium is viewed as a function of the amount of calcium actually absorbed by the gut (i.e., after regulation of intestinal absorptive efficiency has been factored out), the precision with which the kidney adjusts tubular calcium reabsorption to residual changes in filtered load becomes obvious (Fig. 73–6). Ordinarily, the daily load of calcium filtered at the glomerulus (the product of the glomerular filtration rate [GFR] and ultrafilterable calcium[111]) is approximately 10,000 mg/day in adult humans, which means that the extracellular calcium pool is completely filtered several times a day. As urinary calcium excretion (and net intestinal calcium absorption) is approximately 200 mg/day, only 2% of filtered calcium is excreted normally. This high ratio of filtered to excreted calcium affords ample opportunity for finely tuned hormonal control of calcium excretion, even though it may be difficult to measure the small changes involved.

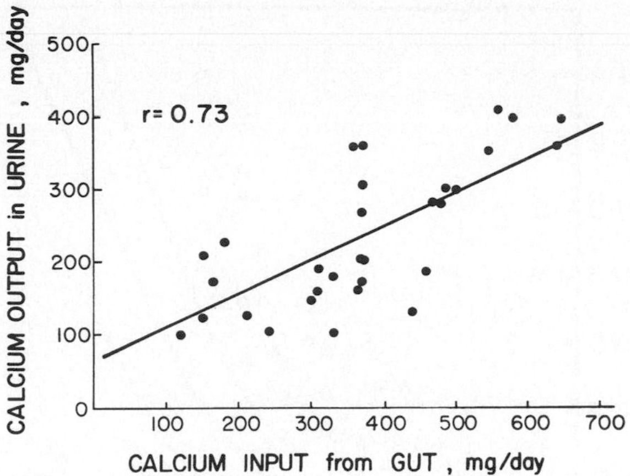

FIGURE 73–6. Urinary calcium excretion as a function of calcium input from the intestine in normal adults studied on various dietary calcium intakes. (Plotted from data in Neer et al.[2] and Pheng et al.[30])

Sites and Mechanisms of Renal Calcium Reabsorption

Calcium is reabsorbed at multiple sites and by different mechanisms along the nephron. As in the intestine, the challenge of transporting calcium across the renal epithelium requires that adequate rates of transport be achieved without substantially increasing the concentration of calcium within the cytosol of the epithelial cell. This is accomplished mainly by use of paracellular diffusional mechanisms that are supplemented, in some nephron segments, by active transcellular transport, especially in response to hormonal stimulation.

Approximately 60% of tubular calcium reabsorption, like that of sodium, occurs in the proximal tubule.[111] The fractional reabsorption rates for sodium and calcium, although highly correlated, are dissociable.[112] Proximal tubular calcium reabsorption occurs mainly via passive diffusion along paracellular pathways, down the ambient (lumen-positive) electrochemical gradient, and thus does not display a saturable maximum, or T_m.[112, 113]

Another 25% of the filtered calcium load is reabsorbed in Henle's loop.[111] This occurs mainly by diffusional transport in the thick ascending limb, particularly in the cortical portion,[114–116] although active, transcellular transport also may play a role.[117] Calcium (and magnesium) reabsorption in this segment is inhibited directly by extracellular calcium and magnesium, which activate calcium-sensing receptors expressed on the basolateral aspect of the tubular cells and thereby reduce the transepithelial voltage gradient via inhibition of Na-K-Cl_2 reabsorption.[17]

Only about 8% of filtered calcium is reabsorbed in more distal segments of the tubule, but calcium transport here clearly involves active, saturable mechanisms that are major sites for hormonal regulation[118–120] (see below). Consonant with these observations, the distribution of several putative components of the active transport mechanism(s), including basolateral membrane Na^+-Ca^{2+} exchangers and the 1,25$(OH)_2$D-dependent calcium-binding protein calbindin-D28k, is limited to the distal tubules.[121, 122] Further heterogeneity exists within this segment, however, as actions of various hormones and diuretics on tubular calcium reabsorption indicate that cells of the distal tubule express functionally distinct mechanisms of calcium transport.[119, 120, 123, 124]

Regulation of Renal Calcium Reabsorption

Calcium excretion is affected by a variety of hormones, nutrients, and drugs.[125, 126] Among these, PTH is the principal physiologic regulator of renal tubular calcium transport, acting mainly to enhance tubular calcium reabsorption at multiple locations beyond the proximal tubule.[115, 116, 119, 127, 128] The critical importance of PTH in the control of renal calcium handling is emphasized by the abnormal overall relation of serum to urinary calcium in hyper- and hypoparathyroidism[125, 129, 130] (Fig. 73–7). The homeostatic role of PTH in calcium excretion is

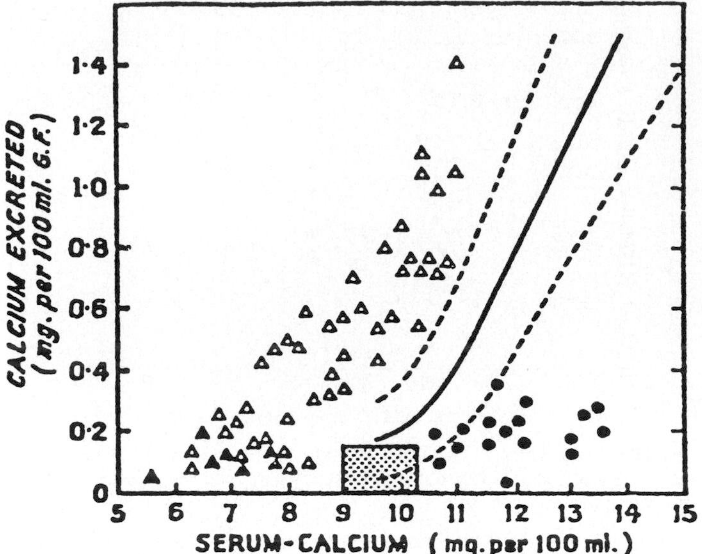

FIGURE 73–7. Relation between urinary calcium excretion and serum calcium during calcium loading in normal subjects and in patients with hypoparathyroidism *(open triangles)* and hyperparathyroidism *(closed circles)*. The solid and broken lines show the mean values (±2 SD) obtained in normal subjects, and the shaded area represents the normal basal range. (From Nordin BEC, Peacock M: Role of kidney in regulation of plasma-calcium. Lancet 2:1280–1283, 1969.)

reviewed in more detail in Chapter 70. The cellular mechanisms whereby PTH regulates calcium reabsorption have been analyzed extensively, especially in cells of the distal tubule and connecting tubule. Here, PTH increases basolateral Na^+-Ca^{2+} exchange,[112, 131, 132] increases the affinity for calcium of the basolateral Ca^{2+}-ATPase,[133] causes insertion into the apical membrane of new dihydropyridine-sensitive membrane calcium channels,[134] and increases cytosolic free calcium.[135] These actions all are consistent with an increased rate of active transcellular transport of calcium, although PTH also may increase paracellular, diffusional calcium transport by augmenting the transepithelial electrical gradient, at least in some segments and species.[136] The action of PTH in the distal tubule thus may involve enhanced apical calcium influx via exocytotic insertion of previously sequestered membrane calcium channels, with stimulated basolateral extrusion of calcium via activated Ca^{2+}-ATPase. In connecting tubules, a major role for stimulated basolateral Na^+-Ca^{2+} exchange in PTH action has been demonstrated.[137] Studies in patients with inactivating vitamin D receptor mutations have demonstrated that vitamin D action is required for the calcium-reabsorptive response to PTH.[138]

Calcitonin, in large doses, acutely reduces proximal tubular calcium reabsorption by a mechanism independent of PTH,[139] but an important role for calcitonin in the physiologic regulation of calcium reabsorption is thought to be unlikely. Vitamin D intoxication causes hypercalciuria,[140, 141] but this is due to an increased filtered load from stimulated intestinal absorption and net bone resorption. Decreased tubular calcium reabsorption may occur because of parathyroid suppression, however, and direct renal tubular effects of vitamin D metabolites have not been excluded. Similarly, hypercalciuria observed in states of excess growth hormone or cortisol seem likely to be secondary to an increased filtered load of calcium rather than to direct tubular actions of these hormones.[101, 142–146] Estrogen treatment of normal postmenopausal women lowers urinary calcium excretion by increasing tubular calcium reabsorption.[147, 148] This occurs partly via an increase in PTH, although PTH-independent effects of estrogen on tubular calcium handling are suggested by additive actions of estrogen and endogenous or administered PTH.[148, 149] Reported effects on tubular calcium reabsorption of insulin,[150] glucagon,[136] and antidiuretic hormone[136] are of uncertain physiologic or clinical significance.

High sodium intake and extracellular fluid volume expansion are calciuric, whereas dehydration exerts the opposite effect.[151, 152] Sodium loading inhibits sodium and calcium reabsorption by the proximal tubule,[153] but filtered load also is increased via secondary parathyroid activation and increased $1,25(OH)_2D$ and intestinal calcium absorption.[154] High intakes of phosphate (or phosphate infusion) lower urinary calcium by several mechanisms, including parathyroid stimulation, reduction in $1,25(OH)_2D$, and a direct renal tubular effect.[155–157] Conversely, dietary phosphate restriction increases calcium excretion,[158] although here the effect is mainly due to an increased filtered load (see below). Alterations in dietary calcium induce corresponding changes in urinary calcium excretion, but, as noted above, the magnitude of the urinary changes is strongly damped by efficient intestinal adaptation to changes in dietary calcium intake.

Hypercalciuria and even hypocalcemia may result from hypermagnesemia, which inhibits calcium reabsorption by activating the calcium-sensing receptor in the thick ascending loop[17] and by suppressing endogenous PTH secretion and, thereby, PTH-mediated tubular calcium reabsorption.[159, 160] Metabolic acidosis directly impairs tubular calcium reabsorption and also increases filtered load by causing mobilization of bone mineral.[161, 162] Chronic respiratory acidosis also reduces renal calcium reabsorption, although the effect is not as great as in metabolic acidosis.[125, 163] Respiratory alkalosis causes hypocalciuria,[164] whereas reported effects of metabolic alkalosis have been inconsistent.[125, 129]

Calcium excretion is predictably enhanced during osmotic diuresis in proportion to the accompanying natriuresis.[165] Furosemide and ethacrynic acid, inhibitors of chloride reabsorption in the loop of Henle, also reduce calcium transport, an effect that has been employed clinically in the urgent therapy of severe hypercalcemia.[166–169] In striking contrast, thiazide diuretics and amiloride both enhance calcium reabsorption in the distal tubule.[170–172] Thiazides directly inhibit apical chloride entry, which hyperpolarizes the distal tubular cell and stimulates calcium influx via opening of apical voltage-dependent calcium channels such as those induced by PTH.[134, 173] Because they reduce calcium excretion, these agents may be useful in therapy for hypercalciuric stone disease and hypoparathyroidism.[174, 175]

Several other drugs may modify renal calcium reabsorption. Cyclosporine and tacrolimus reduce calcium reabsorption, possibly by lowering renal calbindin-D28k levels.[176] Though not clinically significant, digitalis glycosides do impair distal tubular calcium reabsorption, presumably by inhibiting basolateral Na^+,K^+-ATPase, increasing intracellular Na^+ and thereby inhibiting basolateral Na^+-Ca^{2+} exchange.[177, 178] Intravenous aminoglycosides induce a prompt and striking calciuria that is independent of PTH and may reflect competitive displacement of calcium from apical channels or inhibition of basolateral ion pumps.[179] Inhibitors of prostaglandin synthesis have been found to reduce renal calcium clearance and have been advocated in the treatment of hypercalciuria.[180, 181] The action of these drugs is independent of PTH and appears to involve interference with a poorly understood prostaglandin-dependent mechanism of tubular calcium (and magnesium) excretion in the thick ascending limb of Henle.[181]

PHOSPHATE

Distribution and Metabolic Actions of Phosphate

In contrast to calcium, phosphate is widely distributed in nonosseous tissues, both in inorganic form and as a component of numerous organic molecules, ranging from nucleic acids and membrane phospholipids to small phosphoproteins and intermediates of carbohydrate metabolism. These soft tissue phosphates nevertheless make up only about 15% of the total body content (see Table 73–1), the remainder of which is deposited as inorganic phosphate in the mineral phase of bone.

In serum (see Table 73–2), phosphate exists almost exclusively as the free ion or in association with cations. Unlike calcium, only a small fraction (12%) of phosphate is protein-bound,[182] and, further, serum phosphate concentrations may vary by as much as 50% through the day. As discussed below, carbohydrate ingestion may strikingly lower serum phosphate by provoking internal redistribution of phosphate from the extracellular to the intracellular space. Moreover, serum phosphate undergoes a diurnal variation of as much as 1.5 mg/dL (Fig. 73–8), with the nadir between 8 AM and 11 AM.[183] Nocturnal feeding reverses this rhythm,[184] although the timing of meals seems not to be entirely responsible as it is not abolished by evenly spaced feedings.[185]

Interference with the measurement of phosphate in serum may occur during hypertriglyceridemia,[186] hypergammaglobulinemia,[187] or mannitol therapy,[188] depending upon the method of analysis.

Fasting serum phosphate remains stable throughout the menstrual cycle and during pregnancy.[7, 189–192] The placenta actively transports phosphate into the fetus, as reflected in the higher phosphate concentrations of newborn cord arterial and venous blood compared with maternal blood levels.[190] Animal studies indicate that transplacental phosphate transport is upregulated by elevated fetal blood calcium and by $1,25(OH)_2D_3$.[193] Lactating women, who may lose 100 to 500 mg of phosphorus daily in milk, nevertheless maintain normal levels of serum phosphate.[11, 12] Serum phosphate concentrations are relatively high in the newborn (5 to 7 mg/dL),[10, 190] fall gradually thereafter, and then rise again briefly at puberty before reaching adult levels by the age of 18 to 20. Serum phosphate typically increases in women after menopause but decreases in the elderly.[194, 195]

Phosphate is a ubiquitous constituent of a vast array of biomolecules, including phospholipids, phosphoproteins, nucleic acids, enzyme cofactors, and glycolytic intermediates, that are critical for cellular structure, energy metabolism and storage, signal transduction, growth, information transfer, and specialized functions such as ion transport, muscle contraction, and the transmission of nerve impulses. Indeed, the evolution of aerobic prokaryotes and eukaryotes is said to have awaited the availability of adequate soluble environmental phosphate.[196] Of particular importance is the fundamental role of inorganic phosphate as a substrate for intracellular enzymes involved in glycolysis and respiration that synthesize high-energy phosphate bonds for storage of chemical energy in organophosphate compounds such as adenosine triphosphate (ATP), creatine phosphate, diphosphoglycerate, phosphoenolpyruvate, and others. Phosphate also is a component of such important enzyme cofactors as NAD, NADP, and pyridoxal phosphate and of such regulatory molecules as cyclic nucleotides, phosphoinositides, kinases, transcription factors, and other phosphoproteins critical for normal development and cellular metabolism. In addition, intracellular orthophosphate per se exerts major direct effects on cellular energy metabolism. Glucose uptake, lactate production, and levels of ATP and diphosphoglycerate vary directly with the concentration of intracellular phosphate,[197–199] and phosphate inhibits the activity of adenosine monophosphate deaminase, thereby controlling the degradation of adenine nucleotides to inosine and uric acid.[200] Accordingly, free intracellular inorganic phosphate must be maintained at concentrations (1 to 2 mM) adequate to support these many roles, and depletion of intracellular phosphate has profound and wide-ranging clinical consequences. For example, as shown in erythrocytes (Fig. 73–9A), phosphate entering the cell is incorporated into 1,3-diphosphoglycerate by membrane-bound glyceraldehyde 3-phosphate dehydrogenase and therefore is critical for the progress of glycolysis.[201] Severe phosphate depletion leads to a concentration-dependent inhibition of glycolysis, accumulation of "triose phosphates" immediately proximal to glyceraldehyde 3-phosphate dehydrogenase, and consequent arrest of ATP synthesis (Fig. 73–9B).

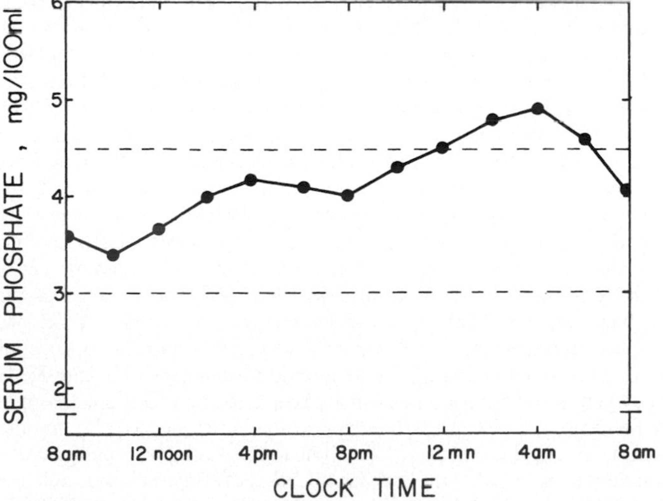

FIGURE 73–8. The diurnal variation in serum phosphate concentration. The curve shows the average values at 2-hour intervals for 10 nonfasting normal humans with nocturnal sleep patterns and self-selected diets. The dashed lines indicate the normal limits of fasting serum phosphate concentration. (Adapted from data of Jubiz W, Canterbury JM, Reiss E, Tyler FH: Circadian rhythm in serum parathyroid hormone concentration in human subjects: Correlation with serum calcium, phosphate, albumin and growth hormone levels. J Clin Invest 51:2040, 1972.)

Adequate extracellular phosphate is required for normal mineralization of bone and cartilage,[202, 203] and chronic hypophosphatemia of any cause therefore may lead to osteomalacia or, in children, rickets (see Chapter 87). Although no direct evidence yet exists for a plasma membrane "phosphate sensor," extracellular phosphate regulates PTH secretion in a manner independent of calcium or vitamin D,[204] controls renal 1α-hydroxylation of 25(OH)D (see Chapter 72), and directly affects bone resorption.[205–208] Further, as reviewed later (see Phosphate Excretion), dietary phosphate availability powerfully modulates renal phosphate excretion via an unknown mechanism that seems to be independent of the serum concentration of phosphate per se.

Phosphate Absorption

The average dietary intake of phosphate, derived largely from dairy products, cereals, and meats, is 800 to 900 mg/day,[1] roughly twice the estimated minimum requirement of 400 mg/day.[209] Absorptive efficiency is high, averaging about 70%, and may increase further (up to 90%) if the intake of dietary phosphate falls below 2 mg/kg/day[1, 210] (Fig. 73–10).

Mechanisms and Sites of Phosphate Absorption

Phosphate is avidly absorbed throughout the small intestine, but especially in the jejunum, in animals and humans.[211–213] As shown in young rabbits, the capacity of the intestine for phosphate absorption declines markedly over the first few weeks post partum as expression of active phosphate transport, initially located throughout the small intestine, becomes more restricted to the duodenum and proximal jejunum.[214] As is true for calcium, phosphate absorption by the intestine of neonatal animals occurs independently of vitamin D.[215, 216]

Intracellular and typical intraluminal free phosphate concentrations in the proximal small intestine are not strikingly different (1 vs. 2 to 5 mM, respectively). Thus, the chemical gradient per se would favor passive cellular uptake.[217] The marked electronegativity of the cytosolic compartment of the enterocyte, however, dictates that phosphate uptake across the apical membrane of the cell must occur by active transport. This is especially true in segments distal to the duodenum, where the alkaline intraluminal pH shifts the valence of phosphate to the more electronegative dibasic form (HPO_4^{2-}). On the other hand, diffusional paracellular transport is highly favored thermodynamically throughout the intestine, given that the intestinal lumen is slightly electronegative with respect to the serosa and that intraluminal phosphate concentrations generally exceed those in extracellular fluid. Unlike that of calcium and other small cations, however, the phosphate permeability of the intercellular junctions is extremely low.[218] Consequently, paracellular absorption of phosphate contributes only slightly to overall phosphate absorption.[217]

In the jejunum, overall phosphate uptake consists of two components: a saturable, sodium-dependent process that is responsive to vitamin D (see below) and a nonsaturable, sodium-independent mechanism thought to represent paracellular diffusional transport.[211, 219] The kinetic analysis is similar to that previously discussed for calcium absorption (see Fig. 73–3). The saturable mechanism reflects active transport via the transcellular route, the energy for which is derived

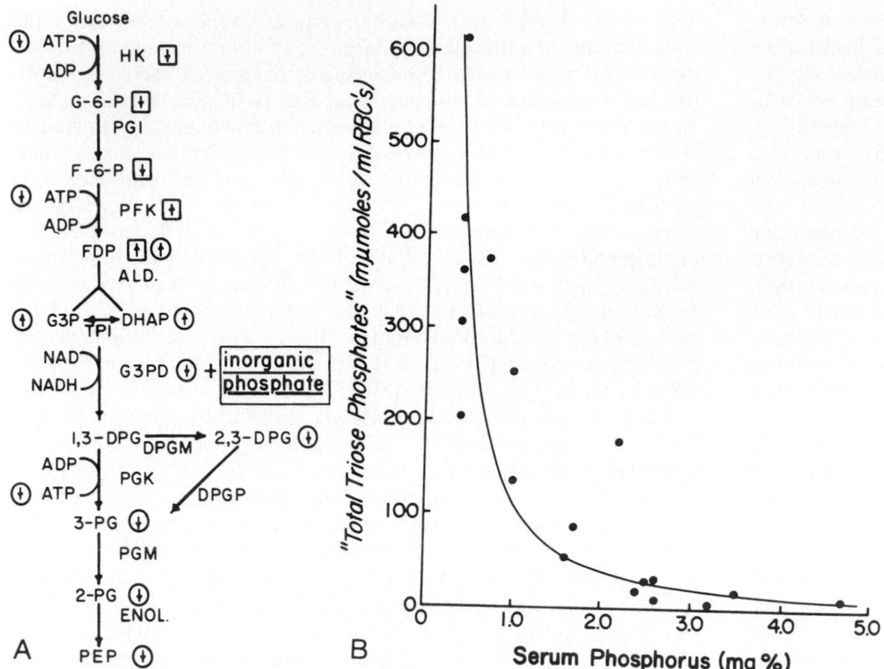

FIGURE 73–9. The importance of inorganic phosphate in intracellular carbohydrate and energy metabolism. *A,* Inorganic phosphate enters the glycolytic pathway as a substrate for glyceraldehyde 3-phosphate dehydrogenase. This phosphorylation yields the precursor (1,3-diphosphoglycerate (DPG) for the key high-energy compounds adenosine triphosphate (ATP) and 2,3-DPG (see text). The arrows within circles indicate changes postulated to result directly from hypophosphatemia, whereas those in squares depict alterations secondary to lowered ATP concentrations. Abbreviations are as defined in the original publication. *B,* Severe hypophosphatemia induced by hyperalimentation in humans blocks the formation of erythrocyte 1,3-DPG, ATP, and 2,3-DPG (data not shown) and leads to an accumulation of precursor triose phosphates. As shown, this blockade becomes significant at serum phosphate levels below 1.0 mg/dL. (From Travis SF, Sugarman HJ: Alterations of red-cell glycolytic intermediates and oxygen transport as a consequence of hypophosphatemia in patients receiving intravenous hyperalimentation. N Engl J Med 285:763–768, 1971.)

from the transmembrane sodium gradient. In animal tissues and in human jejunal biopsies, the sodium phosphate cotransporter exhibits a K_m of approximately 0.05 mM, half-maximal stimulation by 30 to 50 mM of sodium and a ratio of two sodium molecules per molecule of phosphate transported.[211, 220, 221] The sodium phosphate cotransporter(s) present in intestine apparently is different from the predominant form expressed in the renal proximal tubule, however, as mice lacking the renal cotransporter manifest striking hyperphosphaturia due to continued intestinal phosphate absorption, and mRNA encoding that molecule cannot be detected in intestine.[222] Recently, a unique functional sodium phosphate cotransporter cloned from human intestine was found to be the product of a gene different from, but closely related to, that encoding the renal transporter.[223] This sodium phosphate cotransporter may mediate active transport across the apical brush border membrane of the enterocyte and would be fully saturated at intraluminal phosphate concentrations of 1 to 2 mM, which are easily achieved following most typical meals. Subsequent transport across the basolateral membrane into the extracellular fluid does not require active transport and is thought to proceed via facilitated diffusion, although the transporter or channel involved has not been characterized.[224]

Phosphate may be secreted via paracellular pathways in some intestinal segments,[225, 226] but the quantitative physiologic significance of this process remains to be clarified. Efficient absorption of phosphate may require the presence of intraluminal glucose,[225] potassium,[225] and calcium.[227] The requirement for intraluminal calcium once had led to speculation that calcium and phosphate transport might be linked,[225, 228] but much evidence suggests otherwise[211–213] and it seems likely that the apparent coordinate stimulation of calcium and phosphate absorption simply reflects the action of common hormonal influences such as vitamin D (see below).

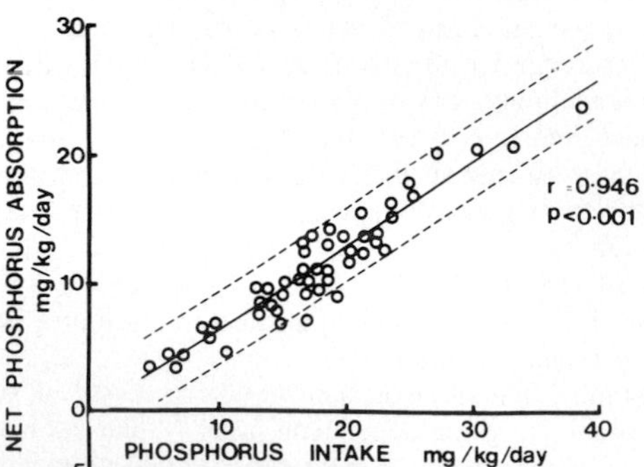

FIGURE 73–10. Intestinal phosphorus absorption vs. dietary intake in normal adults. Note the linearity observed. (From Wilkinson R: Absorption of calcium, phosphorus and magnesium. *In* Nordin BEC (ed): Calcium, Phosphate, and Magnesium Metabolism. New York, Churchill-Livingstone, 1976.)

Regulation of Phosphate Absorption

The central role of vitamin D in the regulation of intestinal phosphate transport was recognized years ago,[225] and it now is clear that the absorption of phosphate, like that of calcium, is strikingly augmented by $1,25(OH)_2D$.[41, 211, 212, 228–230] Basal fractional phosphate absorption in the absence of $1,25(OH)_2D$ is much higher than that of calcium, however. More than 60% of dietary inorganic phosphate is absorbed in anephric ($1,25(OH)_2D$-deficient) humans, for example, and it has been difficult to demonstrate a relation between measured plasma $1,25(OH)_2D$ levels and intestinal absorption of phosphate.[210] The action of $1,25(OH)_2D$ on phosphate transport has been studied in vitro using intact intestinal segments, isolated enterocytes, and brush border membrane vesicles.[219, 226, 231–234] In each case, stimulation by $1,25(OH)_2D$ was shown to result from activation of the sodium-dependent active transport mechanism and not the passive diffusional component. Specifically, $1,25(OH)_2D$ increases the maximal velocity of the sodium-dependent phosphate cotransporter, presumably via a genomic action of the vitamin D metabolite, although it is not known whether this involves transcriptional or post-transcriptional regulation of the presumptive cotransporter.[218, 224] Other studies have pointed to an additional, very rapid (minutes), nongenomic mechanism of $1,25(OH)_2D$-dependent stimulation of intestinal phosphate transport, analogous to its nongenomic effect on duodenal calcium transport.[77, 235] Another component of vitamin D–induced phosphate transport could involve stimulation of basolateral membrane Na^+,K^+-ATPase, an action that would lower intracellular sodium concentration and increase the transmembrane sodium potential that drives phosphate transport.[233]

Restriction of dietary phosphate leads to enhanced intestinal phosphate absorption, due in part to augmented renal synthesis of $1,25(OH)_2D$.[224] Phosphate restriction does increase the V_{max} of the saturable sodium-dependent cotransporter, which is analogous to the action of $1,25(OH)_2D$.[236–238] On the other hand, dietary phosphate (or calcium) deprivation can increase phosphate absorption in some circumstances without increasing $1,25(OH)_2D$ and can do so in vitamin

D–deficient animals.[81, 215, 239] Thus, other mechanisms, independent of vitamin D and not currently understood, must also be available for these adaptations.

Many studies of the effects of PTH[227, 240, 241] or calcitonin[242, 243] have failed to provide convincing evidence for an important direct role of either hormone in the physiologic control of intestinal phosphate absorption. On the other hand, recent work with perfused chick duodenal loops implicates a rapid effect of intravascular PTH on phosphate transport.[244] Animal work indicates that small intestinal phosphate absorption, like that of calcium, declines with age because of a reduction in the capacity of the saturable, active transport mechanism.[81] The effects of pharmacologic doses of glucocorticoids on intestinal phosphate absorption are complex: both increased and decreased absorption have been reported.[245–248] These disparities reflect the fact that glucocorticoids exert two independent actions, the net result of which depends upon the concentration of intraluminal phosphate (i.e., dietary phosphate). Thus, glucocorticoids decrease the maximal rate of saturable transcellular phosphate absorption, as demonstrated in apical brush border membrane vesicles,[221] but they also increase the passive permeability of the intestine to phosphate, which can lead to increased phosphate absorption at high levels of dietary phosphate.[248] Phosphate absorption is impaired progressively by increasing dietary calcium, a maneuver commonly employed to control phosphate absorption in patients with renal failure, but this becomes significant in humans only at calcium intakes exceeding 2 g/day.[249, 250] Aluminum and magnesium hydroxide antacids also bind phosphate in the intestinal lumen, and doses as low as 90 mL/day may induce negative phosphate balance in humans.[251]

Phosphate Excretion

Inorganic phosphate is excreted mainly by the kidney, although small amounts (up to 200 to 300 mg/day in humans) may be lost in sweat, saliva, and stool. Renal tubular reabsorption is the overriding determinant of serum phosphate concentration and is subject to elaborate regulation by a wide variety of hormonal and metabolic factors. The efficiency of intestinal phosphate absorption is not closely regulated. Consequently, unlike calcium, urinary phosphate excretion is tightly correlated with phosphate intake (Fig. 73–11).

The ultrafilterability of total plasma phosphate at the glomerulus is determined by the extent of binding to plasma proteins, complexation with plasma cations, Donnan's membrane equilibrium effects, and the fraction of total plasma volume occupied by solids.[252] Direct micropuncture of surface glomeruli in rats has demonstrated that the concentration of phosphate in ultrafiltrate normally is about 94% of that in plasma water (or 87% of total plasma phosphate),[253] which agrees well with results obtained by ultrafiltration of normal plasma

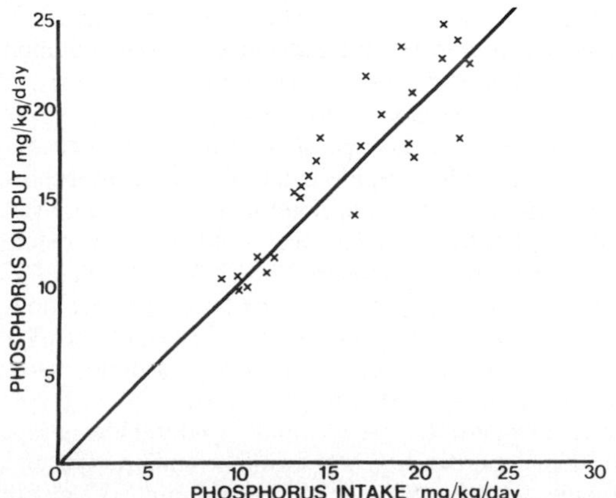

FIGURE 73–11. Phosphate retention as a function of dietary phosphate intake in healthy adults similarly studied. Note homeostatic adaptation at all intakes. (From Wilkinson R: Absorption of calcium, phosphorus and magnesium. *In* Nordin BEC (ed): Calcium, Phosphate, and Magnesium Metabolism. New York, Churchill-Livingstone, 1976.)

through artificial semipermeable membranes.[252, 253] During hypercalcemia, however, ultrafilterable phosphate may be reduced by up to 20%, possibly through increased formation of calcium phosphate complexes, and in vitro membrane ultrafiltration of hypercalcemic plasma may lead to gross underestimation of ultrafilterable phosphate.[254]

Mechanisms and Sites of Renal Phosphate Transport

About 80% of filtered phosphate is reabsorbed by the proximal tubule, and the capacity for phosphate transport appears to diminish between the early convoluted and the straight (pars recta) portions of the proximal tubule.[255–257] Additional phosphate is reabsorbed in the distal tubule or cortical collecting tubule, or both,[258–263] but not in Henle's loop.[264] Participation of the medullary and papillary collecting ducts in phosphate reabsorption remains controversial.[265–267] In addition to this axial or intranephron heterogeneity, internephron differences also exist. Thus, phosphate reabsorption by "deep" or juxtamedullary nephrons may be more responsive to hormonal and other stimuli than that in the more superficial nephrons accessible to micropuncture.[259, 267–269]

The concentration of phosphate in the intraluminal fluid of the proximal tubule of the rat normally equals 1 to 2 mM but may be reduced to 0.2 mM in the absence of PTH or during dietary phosphate restriction.[270–273] Tissue ^{32}P–nuclear magnetic resonance (NMR) studies[274] indicate that free cytosolic concentrations of inorganic phosphate are approximately 30% of the total renal cellular content of about 5 mM,[275, 276] that is, comparable to, or higher than, luminal phosphate levels. This, together with the strongly negative membrane potential of the cell, means that cytosolic free phosphate exceeds by at least 10-fold the intracellular concentration predicted to be at equilibrium with intraluminal (extracellular) phosphate.[277] Accordingly, as in the intestine, phosphate must be actively transported across the luminal brush border membrane against a steep electrochemical gradient. Consistent with this, renal phosphate transport requires luminal sodium ions and is blocked by inhibitors of Na^+,K^+-ATPase.[257, 278–281]

Sodium-dependent cotransport of phosphate can be demonstrated in isolated brush border membrane vesicles (BBMV) prepared from several mammalian species, including humans, and shown to correlate well with changes in tubular phosphate reabsorption induced in vivo by various dietary, hormonal, and metabolic manipulations.[282–286] At physiologic pH, sodium-coupled phosphate transport into BBMVs is electroneutral,[284, 287–289] which is consistent with a carrier stoichiometry of two sodium ions per molecule of dibasic phosphate (HPO_4^{2-}). This is supported by observations that BBMV phosphate transport becomes electrogenic at more acid pH (i.e., 2 Na^+ + $H_2PO_4^-$ = 1 positive charge transported).[283] Moreover, dibasic phosphate is preferentially transported by the rat proximal tubule.[282–284] Studies with isolated perfused tubules have shown that increased intraluminal pH and decreased intracellular pH accelerate phosphate reabsorption by the intact cell.[290]

The molecular mechanism of sodium phosphate cotransport has been elucidated recently with the cloning from several species of cDNAs encoding functional sodium-dependent phosphate cotransporters (NaPis). These currently comprise three families of genes, the products of which are multiple membrane-spanning molecules that have been termed types I, II, and III NaPis. The type I and II NaPi molecules were isolated from renal cDNA libraries by expression cloning in *Xenopus* oocytes, whereas the type III molecules originally were identified as cell-surface virus receptors (gibbon ape leukemia viruses; i.e., Glvr-1 and Ram-1) and only subsequently were found to be phosphate carriers.[291–293] These various NaPis all are expressed in kidney, but they manifest different kinetic properties. Importantly, only the type II molecules exhibit the regulation by PTH and dietary phosphate previously ascribed to the major physiologically important cotransporters in the apical brush border of the proximal tubular cells.[293]

Phosphate transported across the brush border membrane of proximal tubular cells appears not to be sequestered or compartmentalized (as in vesicles) but intermixes freely with cytosolic phosphate. Thus, removal of phosphate from the luminal fluid of isolated perfused tubules leads to an arrest of tubular cell oxidative phosphorylation, a phenomenon that is dependent on the presence of glucose in the tubular fluid. The occurrence of this "Crabtree effect"[294] indicates that phosphate entering across the luminal membrane is critical for the maintenance of normal levels of cytosolic phosphate required for glycolysis and respiration in the tubular cells.

The final step in the renal epithelial transport of phosphate involves passive transfer across the basolateral membrane of the tubular cell down an electrochemical gradient. It is presumed that this transport is facilitated by specific high-capacity membrane carriers, and some evidence exists for both an anion exchange carrier and an electrogenic transporter in the basolateral membrane.[281, 283, 295–298]

Regulation of Renal Phosphate Transport

For clinical purposes, measures of overall renal excretion of phosphate in relation to filtered load, such as tubular reabsorption of phosphate (TRP) or fractional excretion of phosphate (FE_p), commonly are employed to characterize alterations in renal tubular function due to effects of hormones, drugs, and other factors. In light of the complexity of tubular phosphate reabsorption, discussed above, it is clear that such measures constitute a gross oversimplification and cannot distinguish important differences in site(s) or mechanisms of regulatory influences. Nevertheless, such expressions continue to provide useful approximations of overall renal phosphate handling.

When phosphate infusions are employed experimentally to raise the filtered load, overall renal phosphate reabsorption in humans exhibits an apparent transport maximum (Tm_p, in milligrams per minute). It is useful to express this tubular saturation in terms of a theoretical phosphate threshold concentration [$(P_i)_{Th}$, in milligrams per deciliter], which would correspond to the level of plasma phosphate above which any additional filtered phosphate would be quantitatively excreted by an idealized kidney that reabsorbed all filtered phosphate (milligrams per minute) up to the Tm_p. At this point of saturation,

$$TM_p = (Pi)_{Th} \times GFR \quad \text{or} \quad (P_i)_{Th} = Tm_p/GFR$$

Because changes in GFR may alter Tm_p (in the same direction), $(P_i)_{Th}$ is a more reliable measure of phosphate reabsorption than is Tm_p alone.[299] In most clinical situations involving hypophosphatemia and grossly impaired tubular phosphate reabsorption (i.e., TRP $< 80\%$), the $(P_i)_{Th}$ is simply the product of serum phosphate and the measured TRP (Fig. 73–12B):

$$(P_i)_{Th} = P_i \times TRP = P_i(1\text{-}FE_p)$$

More subtle alterations in renal phosphate clearance require correction for the curvature, or "splay," that characterizes actual overall renal phosphate excretion (Fig. 73–12A). The normal range of $(P_i)_{Th}$ has been found to be 2.5 to 4.2 mg/dL. Changes in $(P_i)_{Th}$ account for nearly 80% of the variation in fasting serum phosphate among patients with disorders of blood phosphate and normal subjects, the remainder being attributable to differences in GFR or the filtered load of phosphate.[300–302] Thus, regulation of serum phosphate normally proceeds via the integrated actions of various hormonal, ionic, and metabolic factors that influence the number or activity of the NaPi transporters in the apical membranes of renal tubular cells. The biochemical details of these controlling influences are beginning to yield to intensive investigation, although most available information is limited to studies of proximal tubular cell function. The relative importance of the various regulating factors is only partially defined, but a variety of clinical and experimental observations have clearly demonstrated the dominant roles of PTH and dietary phosphate availability in the control of phosphate excretion. Further details of the regulation of renal phosphate reabsorption are available in several excellent reviews.[277, 303–305]

Regulation of Renal Phosphate Reabsorption

PARATHYROID HORMONE. The central role of PTH in the regulation of serum phosphate was recognized clinically in the 1920s, when early studies with parathyroid extracts indicated that PTH was acutely phosphaturic in normal humans and in patients with hypoparathyroidism.[306–308] The dramatic reduction in renal tubular phosphate transport induced by PTH has been amply demonstrated since in several species and experimental models, both in vivo and in vitro.[309–318] The overall phosphaturic effect of PTH results from actions at multiple sites along the nephron. Proximal tubular phosphate reabsorption is strongly inhibited by PTH,[309, 311] and particular attention has been focused on the role of PTH in regulating phosphate reabsorption in the late proximal tubule.[258, 260, 315, 319, 320] Phosphate reabsorption in the distal nephron seems also to be depressed by PTH,[258, 266, 309, 321] although this has not been demonstrated in all studies.[322] In general, however, the sites at which PTH inhibits phosphate transport correspond to the known distribution of PTH and PTH-related protein (PTHrP) receptors and PTH-responsive adenylate cyclase along the nephron (i.e., early and late proximal tubule, distal convoluted tubule, and the distal regions of the collecting tubules).[323–325] In the proximal tubule, PTH rapidly (15 to 60 minutes) reduces the number of type II NaPi cotransporters on the apical surface of the cell via a microtubule-dependent internalization into endocytic vesicles and subsequent destruction of the transporters.[326] This acute downregulation of NaPi transporters seems not to involve reduction in NaPi gene transcription.[327] Following parathyroidectomy, rats manifest a two- to three-increase in both protein and mRNA levels of type II NaPi, which correlates with a striking increase in phosphate reabsorption.[327] Details of the intracellular mechanisms involved in PTH-PTHrP receptor signaling that lead to regulation of renal phosphate reabsorption are discussed in Chapter 70.

PHOSPHATE. Renal phosphate excretion is extremely sensitive to changes in dietary phosphate availability. Thus, dietary phosphate deprivation[309, 310, 328–333] or supplementation[310, 329, 334] rapidly evokes a compensatory increase or decrease, respectively, in renal phosphate reabsorption [$(P_i)_{Th}$]. Of course, low and high phosphate intakes induce secondary alterations in parathyroid activity—suppression[335, 336] and stimulation[155, 337] respectively—that potentially could account for the observed changes in $(P_i)_{Th}$. Compelling clinical and experimental evidence, however, has established that these adaptations to dietary phosphate occur quite independently of PTH.[285, 309, 310, 327–329, 338] Acute phosphate infusion also lowers $(P_i)_{Th}$ independently of PTH,[339] a response that may be mediated in part by transient phosphate-induced depression of serum calcium.[340]

Withdrawal of phosphate from the diet is rapidly followed by an increased rate of phosphate reabsorption in all segments of the nephron ordinarily involved in phosphate transport.[267, 269, 321, 341, 342] The magnitude of this effect may differ between superficial and deep nephrons[267, 342] and it occurs most quickly in the distal convoluted tubule.[321] This adaptation to phosphate deprivation does not depend upon secondary changes in PTH, calcitonin,[310] vitamin D metabolites,[343, 344] or renal content of inorganic phosphate or adenine nucleotides.[345] It can be observed in isolated renal tubules, BBMVs, and cultured renal epithelial cells.[344, 346, 348] Increased sodium-dependent phosphate transport by isolated BBMVs occurs within a few hours of phosphate deprivation[333, 349] and reflects increased maximal velocity (rather than affinity) of the phosphate carrier,[349, 351] consistent with an increased number of membrane transporters. This has been corroborated by direct immunohistologic demonstration that institution of a low phosphate diet causes rapid (within 2 hours) insertion of type II NaPi cotransporters into the apical plasma membrane of rat proximal tubular cells, especially in midcortical and superficial nephrons, by a microtubule-dependent mechanism.[352, 353] Upregulation of NaPi gene transcription occurs subsequently during more chronic phosphate restriction (i.e., several days).[338] Similarly, high dietary phosphate rapidly reduces apical membrane NaPi protein levels, with no change in NaPi transcription for at least several hours.[338]

The likely mediator of these rapid renal tubular adaptations to dietary phosphate availability is a new hormone, as yet unidentified, that commonly is referred to as "phosphatonin." Compelling functional evidence of phosphatonin has been obtained from studies of the human disorder oncogenous osteomalacia and the murine *Hyp* model of human X-linked hypophosphatemic rickets (see Chapter 87), both of which can be adequately explained only by the existence of a circulating humoral factor capable of potently inhibiting proximal

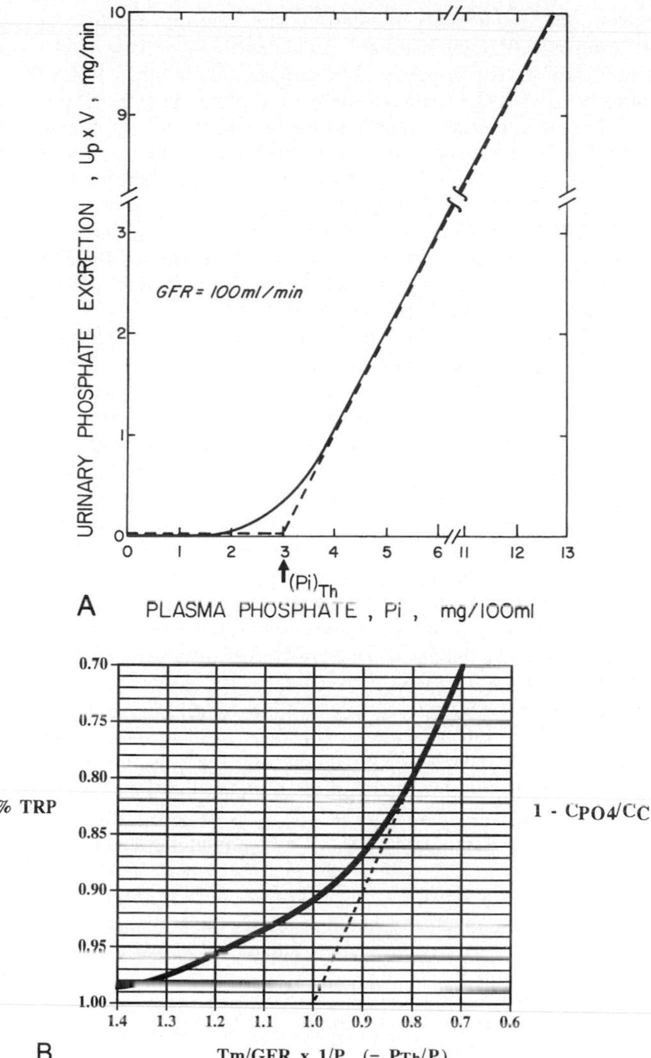

FIGURE 73–12. Quantitative aspects of renal phosphate excretion. *A,* The relation between plasma concentration and urinary excretion of phosphate for a real *(solid line)* and idealized *(broken line)* kidney with a glomerular filtration rate (GFR) of 10 mg/min. Because total plasma and ultrafilterable phosphate are nearly equal, the filtered load equals $P_i \times$ GFR, and the slope of the excretion curve equals the GFR at high (saturating) filtered loads. The Tm_p is equivalent to the filtered load (mg/min) at which phosphate begins to appear in the urine of the idealized kidney (that is, $Tm_i = (P_i)_{Th} \times GFR$). In reality, the excretion curve is curvilinear, and phosphate actually appears in urine at concentrations of plasma phosphate well below $(P_i)_{Th}$. This may reflect internephron heterogeneity as well as the intrinsic saturation kinetics of the phosphate transporter(s). *B,* Nomogram of Bijvoet for estimation of renal $(P_i)_{Th}$. Phosphate excretion curves were determined during graded phosphate infusions in normal subjects and patients with disorders of phosphate clearance. The shape of the splay region *(solid curve)* vs. idealized kidney *(broken line)* was found to be constant when the data were expressed parametrically as tubular reabsorption of phosphorus (TRP) vs. $(Tm_p/GFR \times 1/P_i)$. [Note that $(P_i)_{Th} = Tm_p/GFR$]. Above saturation (TRP<0.8), phosphate excretion is linearly related to plasma phosphate; that is, $U_p \times V = GFR \times (P_i - (P_i)_{Th} = P_i - (U_p \times V)/GFR$. In this case, measurement of phosphate and creatinine in simultaneous serum (P_i Cr) and "spot" urine (U_p, U_{Cs}) samples permits calculation of fractional excretion of phosphate (FE_p) (or TRP): $FE_p = C_p/C_{Cs} = U_p/P_i \times C_r/U$; $_{Cs}$; TRP = 1 − FE_p, and, then, $(P_i)_{Th} = P_i(1 - FE_p) = P_i \times$ TRP. When TRP is greater than 0.8 ($FE_p < 0.2$), however, $(P_i)_{Th}$ is obtained by multiplying serum phosphate by the factor $[Tm_p/GFR \times (1/P_i)]$, as defined by the TRP and the curve for splay *(solid line)*. This nomogram obviates the need to perform phosphate infusions routinely for determination of $(P_i)_{Th}$. The validity of the single curve has been established only in normal subjects and in patients with a limited variety of disorders affecting phosphate clearance, however, and it may not apply to all situations of abnormal phosphate excretion. (Adapted from Bijvoet OLM, Morgan DB: *In* Hioco DJ (ed): Phosphate et Métabolisme Phosphocalcique. Paris, L'Expansion Scientifique Francaise, 1971.)

tubular type II NaPi expression. This concept remains unproven at present, however, as the demonstration of a direct link between altered dietary phosphate and changes in phosphatonin levels awaits the capacity, as yet unrealized, to measure this hormone and to identify its site of secretion and the mechanisms whereby it responds to phosphate intake.

Other Factors

CALCIUM. Infusion of calcium acutely reduces phosphate excretion in normal individuals but increases it in hypoparathyroid subjects.[354–358] This suggests that that antiphosphaturic effect of calcium in normal subjects results from parathyroid suppression. This concept is supported by the fact that the antiphosphaturic effect of calcium is especially pronounced in secondary hyperparathyroidism induced by low dietary calcium or vitamin D deficiency[355, 359] and that it can be prevented by exogenous PTH administration.[356] In micropuncture studies, however, calcium directly impairs tubular phosphate reabsorption, particularly at distal tubular sites, which is consistent with the phosphaturic effect of calcium infusion observed in hypoparathyroidism.[309, 360, 362] Such a direct tubular effect of hypercalcemia could contribute to hypophosphatemia in primary hyperparathyroidism or malignancy, augmenting the direct phosphaturic tubular action(s) of PTH and tumor-derived PTHrP, respectively (see Chapters 76 and 77).[363] The possible involvement of the renal tubular calcium-sensing receptor in mediating this effect has not been directly studied. On the other hand, patients with constitutively active calcium-sensing receptors exhibit mild hyperphosphatemia rather than hypophosphatemia, which points to relative hypoparathyroidism rather than any direct actions of the calcium sensor on the renal tubule.[364]

VITAMIN D. Vitamin D therapy corrects the hypophosphatemia and lowered $(P_i)_{Th}$ in vitamin D deficiency[365, 366] by restoring normal intestinal calcium absorption and reversing secondary hyperparathyroidism. Evidence for more direct effects of active vitamin D metabolites on renal tubular phosphate reabsorption is conflicting, probably because of the difficulties of controlling the many secondary effects of vitamin D administration in vivo.[367–369] In vitamin D–deficient rats, administered $1,25(OH)_2D$ increases phosphate uptake by isolated renal BBMVs, even if the blood calcium is held constant by dietary manipulations,[369] and induces increased mRNA expression of the type II NaPi gene, the promoter for which includes a stimulatory vitamin D receptor DNA binding element.[370] Other work involving direct addition of vitamin D metabolites to rat renal BBMVs supports the notion that a rapid, nongenomic action, perhaps an alteration of membrane fluidity, may partly underlie the stimulation of renal phosphate reabsorption by $1,25(OH)_2D$.[371] Also, in parathyroidectomized animals subjected to volume expansion (to reduce ambient phosphate reabsorption), $1,25(OH)_2D$ increases phosphate reabsorption.[372]

ACID-BASE STATUS. Metabolic acidosis causes phosphaturia and impairs proximal tubular phosphate reabsorption.[373–376] It has been suggested that this is an adaptive mechanism to increase the renal excretion of titratable acid.[377] Recent studies in rats indicate that the type II NaPi protein is rapidly downregulated within several hours of ammonium chloride loading and that more chronic acidosis leads to reduced NaPi mRNA expression by a mechanism that does not involve PTH and that can be overridden by a low phosphate diet.[378] Respiratory acidosis also reduces phosphate reabsorption by mechanisms independent of filtered phosphate, PTH, or plasma bicarbonate.[379, 380]

In general, metabolic and respiratory alkaloses increase phosphate reabsorption, presumably by mechanisms opposite to those invoked by acidosis, although here the dependence on dietary intake (total urinary phosphate) is particularly striking. Bicarbonate infusion, for example, may induce directionally opposite changes in phosphate excretion in subjects whose phosphate intakes are at opposite extremes.[381–383] In the case of acute respiratory alkalosis, accelerated tubular phosphate reabsorption has been shown to involve β-adrenergic receptor activation, as it is blocked by propranolol.[384]

OTHER HORMONES. Calcitonin given in large doses is acutely phosphaturic, an action that may partly reflect increased PTH secretion but that also occurs in hypoparathyroid subjects and in patients with malignancy-associated hypercalcemia.[139, 385–387]

Chronic growth hormone administration and acromegaly both increase renal phosphate reabsorption and the V_{max} of the sodium-dependent phosphate transporter in isolated proximal tubule BBMVs.[312, 388, 389] Growth hormone increases intestinal calcium absorption, but its effect on renal phosphate handling appears not to be secondary to PTH suppression.[142, 390, 391] Phosphate excretion does not change during acute (2 hours) infusion of growth hormone but does decrease after 10 to 12 hours of administration, in association with increases in insulin and insulin-like growth factor-1 (IGF-1).[143, 392] It therefore is likely that the antiphosphaturic effect of growth hormone is mediated indirectly by one or both of these latter factors, both of which promote phosphate reabsorption.[393] Adults with growth hormone deficiency do not manifest impaired renal phosphate reabsorption, however.[394]

Glucocorticoids depress renal phosphate reabsorption by a mechanism that overrides the opposing effect of a low intake of phosphate.[396–400] This action of glucocorticoids in vivo is evident as a reduction in the V_{max} of sodium-dependent phosphate transport in isolated proximal tubular BBMVs and is associated with suppression of type II NaPi expression.[399–401] A role for an intracellular alkaline shift induced by glucocorticoid stimulation of both Na^+-H^+ exchange and gluconeogenesis also has been postulated.[399, 402] Relief of cortisol-dependent inhibition of phosphate reabsorption probably accounts for the rise in $(P_i)_{Th}$ that accompanies successful therapy of Cushing's syndrome,[146] although concomitant decreases in serum PTH, plasma $1,25(OH)_2D$, and filtered phosphate also may be important.

Serum phosphate rises significantly after oophorectomy or at menopause and is lowered by estrogen therapy.[149, 194, 403, 404] This action of estrogen may be due partly to secondary stimulation of PTH secretion via estrogen-induced inhibition of bone turnover.[88, 405, 406] On the other hand, the effects of estrogen on phosphate and PTH in postmenopausal women may be temporally dissociated,[405] and estrogen-mediated lowering of serum phosphate in normal or hyperparathyroid women may occur without changes in PTH or urinary cyclic adenosine monophosphate (cAMP) excretion.[149] Estrogens also oppose the relative hyperphosphatemia in acromegaly without altering levels of growth hormone.[407] These observations suggest a direct effect of estrogen on the renal tubule, but this possibility has not been adequately addressed in appropriate in vitro systems.

A variety of other hormones have been found to affect renal tubular phosphate reabsorption, although the relative importance of these effects in the normal regulation of serum phosphate concentration has not been established. Thyroxine directly increases type II NaPi expression in proximal tubules, and its antiphosphaturic effect in vivo occurs in the absence of the parathyroid glands.[408, 409] Correspondingly, hyperthyroidism is accompanied, in both animals and humans, by increases in $(P_i)_{Th}$ and serum phosphate which are reversed with reestablishment of euthyroidism.[410–412] Insulin also increases $(P_i)_{Th}$[413] and BBMV phosphate transport,[414] despite which serum phosphate typically declines because of insulin-induced increased cellular uptake of extracellular phosphate. Acute administration of glucagon,[415, 416] vasopressin,[417] atriopeptin,[418] angiotensin,[419] mineralocorticoids,[309, 420] norepinephrine,[421] dopamine,[422] acetylcholine,[423] or prostaglandin[423] results in phosphaturia, although the mechanisms and physiologic significance of these effects are unknown.

MISCELLANEOUS FACTORS. Acute extracellular fluid volume expansion with intravenous saline provokes decreased proximal tubular phosphate transport and a striking phosphaturia.[313, 420, 423–426] Intact parathyroid function is necessary for full expression of this phenomenon, and it is thought that parathyroid secretion is stimulated indirectly by dilutional lowering of total and ionized serum calcium.[159, 271, 315, 420, 424–426] Experimental evidence also exists for an additional, PTH-independent inhibitory effect of volume expansion on proximal tubular phosphate reabsorption, however.[427] Thus, in parathyroidectomized animals, volume expansion also inhibits proximal phosphate transport, but this is not reflected by phosphaturia in the final urine, presumably because of avid distal phosphate reabsorption by a mechanism ordinarily inhibited by PTH.[313, 315, 365, 420]

Experimental magnesium depletion leads to phosphaturia, and a reduction in Tm_p occurs in magnesium-deprived rats.[428, 429] Overt hypophosphatemia is unusual in this setting, however, possibly because of the opposing effect of magnesium deficiency to impair parathyroid function.[430–434] Magnesium infusions transiently raise $(P_i)_{Th}$ in dogs, but this effect is not observed in parathyroidectomized animals and is thus presumably mediated via parathyroid suppression.[159, 160, 435, 436] Severe hypokalemia also may induce renal phosphate wasting,[437, 438] possibly through a nonspecific tubular dysfunction that also blocks the phosphaturic responses to PTH and dibutyryl cAMP.[439]

A number of drugs and chemical agents are known to alter renal phosphate handling. Among the diuretics, acetazolamide is a potent phosphaturic agent that acts in a manner similar,[313, 440] but not identical,[441] to PTH, mainly on the proximal tubule. Reports of effects of mercurial, thiazide, and loop diuretics on phosphate reabsorption, which may have variable effects on renal calcium excretion, often have not controlled for possible secondary changes in extracellular fluid volume or parathyroid status.[165–167, 442] Osmotic diuresis with mannitol is accompanied by phosphaturia that is mediated by secondary parathyroid stimulation due to lowered serum ionized calcium.[443] Probenecid transiently lowers serum phosphate over several days in patients with hypoparathyroidism and certain other hyperphosphatemic disorders,[444] although this has not been reported in normal subjects. The bisphosphonate etidronate may raise $(P_i)_{Th}$ in humans without altering the phosphaturic response to PTH.[445, 446] Chronic heparin therapy has been associated with hyperphosphatemia and a raised $(P_i)_{Th}$.[447]

DISORDERS OF PHOSPHATE METABOLISM

Hyperphosphatemia

Most commonly, hyperphosphatemia results from renal insufficiency, wherein a greatly reduced GFR requires that phosphate accumulate in blood until the obligate daily phosphate load, derived from the diet and from bone, can be excreted.[448] Thus, renal failure is the major exception to the general rule that fasting serum phosphate is controlled primarily by the rate of tubular reabsorption [i.e., $(P_i)_{Th}$].[449–452] Another circumstance in which an abnormal filtered load of phosphate preempts tubular mechanisms is that in which massive amounts of phosphate are delivered into the extracellular fluid. This can result from intravenous, oral, or rectal administration of large amounts of phosphate salts (cathartics, enemas, or overvigorous attempts to replete phosphate in hypophosphatemic patients); from extensive cellular injury, lysis, or necrosis (as in trauma, burns, rhabdomyolysis, chemotherapy, hemolysis, or fulminant hepatitis); or from the egress of phosphate from cells in response to metabolic or respiratory alkalosis[453–462] (see Table 73–4). In these situations, hyperphosphatemia is especially likely when renal function also is impaired.[455, 456, 458, 459, 461] Azotemia also may contribute to the development of severe hyperphosphatemia in situations where modestly increased filtered phosphate otherwise might be well tolerated, such as intravenous phosphate infusion, vitamin D therapy, or sarcoidosis.[463–466] Phosphate "poisoning" may produce a significant metabolic acidosis.[467]

Hyperphosphatemia is characteristic of all forms of hypoparathyroidism and reflects loss of the tonic inhibitory effect of PTH on $(P_i)_{Th}$. Reduction of serum phosphate during therapy of hypoparathyroidism with active vitamin D metabolites is attributed to the phosphaturic effect of the raised serum calcium rather than to a direct tubular effect of vitamin D.[354, 355, 468–470] As discussed above, an increase in $(P_i)_{Th}$ probably also underlies the hyperphosphatemia observed in acromegaly[312, 388, 471] and during chronic therapy with etidronate[446, 472] or with heparin.[447] Rarely, "pseudohyperphosphatemia" may result from the presence of a phosphate-binding immunoglobulin in some patients with multiple myeloma.[473, 474]

Among the most interesting and unusual of causes of hyperphosphatemia is the spectrum of disorders that includes tumoral calcinosis, isolated hyperostosis, or both, in association with normocalcemia and normal renal and parathyroid function. In tumoral calcinosis, ectopic (often extensive) calcification of periarticular soft tissue occurs together with elevated plasma $1,25(OH)_2D$ and increased intestinal calcium absorption (despite normal or low serum PTH) and, often, striking hyperphosphatemia.[475–479] Hyperphosphatemia does not occur in all cases of tumoral calcinosis, however, and some patients with hyperphosphatemia and hyperostosis lack evidence of soft tissue lesions.[478, 480, 481] This disorder appears to result from a recessively inherited defect in regulation of both the renal 25(OH)D 1α-hydroxylase and renal tubular phosphate reabsorption.[478] Interestingly, renal responsiveness to both endogenous and exogenous PTH is preserved,[475–479] as is the stimulatory effect of phosphate depletion on $1,25(OH)_2D$ levels.[479] Therapy is problematic, although some success has been reported with combined use of acetazolamide and oral phosphate binders.[482]

The major clinical consequences of acute severe hyperphosphatemia are those of the associated hypocalcemia—that is, paresthesias, muscle cramps, tetany, Q–T interval prolongation, and others—induced directly by severe hyperphosphatemia.[483, 484] Suppression of serum $1,25(OH)_2D$ may contribute to the hypocalcemia as well.[485] In the tumor lysis syndrome, it may be difficult to separate the consequences of hyperphosphatemia per se from those of the associated hyperkalemia and hyperuricemia or of the chemotherapeutic agents involved.[454, 457, 486, 487] Soft tissue deposition of calcium phosphate complexes is particularly likely in patients with preexisting hypercalcemia[488] and may lead to renal failure independent of hyperuricemia.[459, 489] Chronic hyperphosphatemia, especially with associated hypercalcemia, may lead to diffuse visceral deposition of calcium phosphates demonstrable on bone scans.[466] In infants, high phosphate formula may cause hypocalcemia and tetany followed by the development of secondary hyperparathyroidism.[490]

TABLE 73–4. Causes of Hyperphosphatemia

Impaired Renal Phosphate Excretion
- Renal insufficiency
- Tumoral calcinosis
- Hypoparathyroidism, pseudohypoparathyroidism
- Acromegaly
- Etidronate
- Heparin

Increased Extracellular Phosphate
- Rapid administration of phosphate (IV, oral, rectal)
- Rapid cellular catabolism or lysis
  - Catabolic states
  - Tissue injury
    - Hyperthermia
    - Crush injuries
    - Fulminant hepatitis
  - Cellular lysis
    - Hemolytic anemia
    - Rhabdomyolysis
    - Cytotoxic therapy
- Transcellular shifts of phosphate
  - Metabolic acidosis
  - Respiratory acidosis

Hypophosphatemia

Chronic

Phosphate is so abundant in available foods and intestinal phosphate absorption is so efficient, even in the absence of vitamin D, that hypophosphatemia can virtually never be ascribed to inadequate phosphate intake. The only exception to this general rule occurs in the setting of protracted and excessive use of oral phosphate binders, such as nonabsorbable aluminum or magnesium hydroxide antacids, which may lead to significant selective phosphate depletion by binding of phosphate in the intestinal lumen and preventing its absorption.[491–494] With the advent of H_2-receptor and proton pump inhibitors, drugs that directly inhibit gastric acid secretion, this situation now rarely occurs clinically. Fasting or starvation alone does not induce hypophosphatemia, presumably because the release of endogenous osseous and intracellular phosphate during soft tissue and bone catabolism provides more than adequate compensation for obligate phosphate losses.[311, 495] Thus, chronic hypophosphatemia in ambulatory patients not consuming oral phosphate binders or experiencing accelerated net bone formation (see below) invariably results from ongoing renal tubular phosphate wasting.

Most often, the cause of chronic hypophosphatemia (Table 73–5) can be traced to a high circulating concentration of either PTH, as in primary or secondary hyperparathyroidism (see Chapters 76, 82, and 87), or PTHrP, in hypercalcemia of malignancy (see Chapter 77). Hypercalcemia, when present, may exert an additional, PTH-independent tubular effect to lower $(P_i)_{Th}$. In vitamin D deficiency, loss of a modest direct positive renal effect of vitamin D metabolites on $(P_i)_{Th}$ also might contribute (see Phosphate Excretion).

In the absence of elevated blood PTH or PTHrP, chronic hypophosphatemia is attributable either to increased bioactive phosphatonin[196, 500] or to an intrinsic renal tubular defect in phosphate reabsorption. Phosphatonin is believed to mediate the hypophosphatemia associated with X-linked hypophosphatemic rickets, a disorder which, like its murine homologues *Hyp* and *Gy*, results from mutation of the *phex* gene (see Chapter 87). *Phex* encodes a putative cell-surface endopeptidase that has been postulated to play a role in inactivating circulating phosphatonin, although this has not been directly demonstrated and the pathophysiology of these disorders thus remains speculative. High circulating levels of phosphatonin also are believed to be responsible for the tubular phosphate wasting that is the hallmark of the rare disorder oncogenous osteomalacia, in which $1,25(OH)_2D$ levels are inappropriately normal or even low despite the prevailing hypophosphatemia, serum calcium typically is low-normal, PTH may be normal or slightly elevated, and there may be evidence of other proximal tubular dysfunction, including glycosuria and aminoaciduria.[496–500] All of these alterations are presumed to be direct or indirect consequences of the renal actions of phosphatonin.

Intrinsic renal tubular defects in phosphate reabsorption may occur in the Fanconi syndromes or as a consequence of genetic or acquired tubular injury or dysfunction induced by underlying systemic disorders (Wilson's disease, cystinosis, Dent's disease,[501] Lowe's syndrome,[502] hereditary hypophosphatemic rickets with hypercalciuria,[503] hypophosphatemic bone disease,[504] autosomal dominant hypophosphatemic rickets or osteomalacia,[505] multiple myeloma,[506] amyloidosis, neurofibromatosis,[507] etc.); associated with various metabolic, hormonal, or electrolyte disturbances (poorly controlled diabetes,[508] hypokalemia,[437, 438, 509, 510] hypomagnesemia,[428, 511–513]) hyperthermia or heat stroke,[514–517] excessive estrogen[518] or glucocorticoids; or induced by exposure to certain drugs or toxins (e.g., ethanol,[519–522] toluene,[523] heavy metals, cisplatin, foscarnet[524]) (see Table 73–4). The cause of the mild hypophosphatemia often observed in patients with nephrolithiasis due to idiopathic hypercalciuria is unclear.[525]

Chronic hypophosphatemia, together with hypocalcemia, may occasionally accompany extensive osteoblastic metastases due to prostate, breast, lung, or other malignancies.[526–529] Rapid bone formation also may lead to hypophosphatemia following successful surgery for primary hyperparathyroidism or during treatment of severe vitamin D deficiency. In these patients, urinary phosphate excretion is low, and accelerated deposition of calcium and phosphate into new bone mineral by activated osteoblasts is believed to be responsible for the ongoing drain of phosphate from the extracellular fluid.

Acute

Hypophosphatemia is common among hospitalized patients,[530–533] although the frequency of severe hypophosphatemia (<1 mg/dL) is less than 0.1%.[522] Acute, severe hypophosphatemia in this setting usually results from translocation of phosphate into cells and formation of various organophosphate intermediates upon stimulation of glycolysis by respiratory alkalosis, intravenous glucose administration, gram-negative sepsis, or insulin therapy of diabetic ketoacidosis. Antecedent phosphate depletion, due to oral antacids or ongoing renal losses, predisposes to the development of severe acute hypophosphatemia.

Hypophosphatemia may develop rapidly during acute respiratory alkalosis. Serum phosphate may decline by 2 to 3 mg/dL during hyperventilation to a P_{CO_2} of less than 20 mm Hg, and the simultaneous reduction in urinary phosphate excretion confirms that cellular uptake of phosphate is the responsible mechanism.[534–536] The same phenomenon may occur in metabolic alkalosis, although here the hypophosphatemia is less dramatic and may result, in part, from increased phosphate excretion.[535] In both types of acute alkalosis, however, stimulation of glycolysis reduces available inorganic phosphate via accelerated phosphate incorporation into organic intermediates.[537, 538] Exchange of extracellular phosphate salts for intracellular organic acids required to buffer the extracellular alkalosis also may contribute to hypophosphatemia in this setting.[535] Respiratory alkalosis probably contributes to hypophosphatemia associated with salicylate intoxication, gram-negative sepsis, toxic shock syndrome, and heat stroke,[515, 539–541] although other factors also may be involved, as discussed below.

Severe acute hypophosphatemia has been documented within 6 to 12 hours of intubation and mechanical ventilation for severe respiratory acidosis.[542] This may reflect accelerated glycolysis that follows rapid correction of acidosis in the setting of phosphate depletion. Acidosis can lead to phosphate depletion by inhibiting glycolysis, promoting phosphate exit from cells and increasing renal tubular excretion (see Phosphate Excretion).

Perhaps the most common cause of acute hypophosphatemia is the intravenous administration of carbohydrate (usually glucose) as a sole energy source[531] (Table 73–5). This presumably is an exaggeration of the otherwise moderate (<1.5 mg/dL) hypophosphatemic response seen in the first 1 to 2 hours after the administration of oral glucose,[543–545] which is attributed to insulin-dependent stimulation of glycolysis.[546–548] Thus, the glucose-induced fall in serum phosphate is blunted in diabetic patients,[549] whereas that caused by fructose, the cellular uptake of which is not insulin-dependent, provokes striking hypophosphatemia in diabetic patients.[550] The major site of phosphate uptake after glucose loads appears to be peripheral tissues (especially muscle) rather than the liver.[547, 548, 551–553] Hyperalimentation with highly concentrated glucose solutions formerly was an important cause of acute hypophosphatemia in hospitalized patients, especially in those with underlying malnutrition. This now is prevented by routine supplementation of hyperalimentation fluids with phosphate, which averts progressive hypophosphatemia and also improves the utilization of administered nitrogen.[554–556] This mechanism likely also underlies the moderate hypophosphatemia commonly observed in postsurgical patients receiving intravenous glucose solutions,[557–559] although other evidence suggests that trauma per se may induce a humorally mediated cellular uptake of phosphate, independent of glucose, that may be mediated by catecholamines.[560–562] Other factors that may contribute to hypophosphatemia in the postoperative state include respiratory alkalosis, fever, volume expansion, sepsis, and hypokalemia. Catecholamine-mediated cellular phosphate uptake also might explain the hypophosphatemia that can accompany serious nonsurgical illnesses, such as myocardial infarction.[563]

Significant hypophosphatemia commonly develops within hours of initiating therapy of hyperglycemic diabetic coma syndromes.[564–566] In these patients, accelerated glucose- and insulin-dependent cellular phosphate uptake and utilization are engrafted upon underlying phosphate depletion caused by tissue catabolism and renal losses (osmotic diuresis, insulin lack, metabolic acidosis, and competition of acetoacetate with phosphate for tubular reabsorption).[538, 567–571] The magnitude of the phosphate deficit in severe diabetic ketoacidosis may approach several grams of elemental phosphorus.[565, 567, 570] The hypophosphatemic effect of insulin therapy, which is dose- and time-dependent, may be minimized by phosphate supplementation, although this must be undertaken cautiously, as there is no proven mortality benefit and

TABLE 73–5. Causes of Hypophosphatemia

Inadequate Intestinal Phosphate Absorption
- Aluminum-containing antacids
- Sucralfate

Impaired Renal Tubular Phosphate Reabsorption
- Hyperparathyroidism
  - Primary hyperparathyroidism
  - PTHrP-dependent hypercalcemia of malignancy
  - Secondary hyperparathyroidism
    - Vitamin D deficiency/resistance
    - Calcium starvation/malabsorption
    - Aminobisphosphonate therapy (Paget's disease)
- Phosphatonin-mediated phosphaturia
  - X-linked hypophosphatemic rickets
  - Oncogenous osteomalacia
  - Linear sebaceous nevus syndrome
- Renal tubular disorders
  - Fanconi syndromes
  - Dent's disease/X-linked recessive nephrolithiasis
  - Autosomal dominant hypophosphatemic rickets/osteomalacia
  - Hypophosphatemic bone disease
  - Hereditary hypophosphatemic rickets with hypercalciuria
  - Idiopathic hypercalciuria (some forms)
  - Lowe's syndrome
  - Wilson's disease
  - Cystinosis
  - Other
    - Amyloidosis
    - Multiple myeloma
    - Heat stroke/hyperthermia
    - Post renal transplantation
    - Post hemolytic uremic syndrome
    - Rewarming from hypothermia
- Metabolic, hormonal, and electrolyte disorders
  - Poorly controlled diabetes
  - Hypomagnesemia
  - Hypokalemia, Bartter's syndrome, hyperaldosteronism
  - High-dose estrogen
- Drugs and toxins
  - Ethanol
  - Acetazolamide, other diuretics
  - Theophylline
  - Calcitonin
  - Toluene
  - Heavy metals (lead, cadmium)
  - Cisplatin
  - Ifosfamide
  - Suramin
  - Foscarnet
  - *N*-methyl formamide

Shifts of Extracellular Phosphate into Cells or Bone
- Rapid translocation into cells
  - Acute respiratory alkalosis
  - Recovery from respiratory acidosis
  - Intravenous glucose
  - Insulin therapy for hyperglycemia, diabetic ketoacidosis
  - Catecholamines
  - Rapid cellular proliferation
- Accelerated net bone formation
  - Post parathyroidectomy
  - Treatment of vitamin D deficiency
  - Osteoblastic metastases

PTHrP, parathyroid hormone–related protein.

intravenous phosphate therapy is potentially hazardous in the setting of abnormal renal function.[565, 572–574] Phosphate depletion also is thought to cause the lowered levels of intracellular organophosphates (especially 2,3-diphosphoglycerate, 2,3-DPG) in diabetic ketoacidosis, although the acidosis per se, which directly inhibits phosphofructokinase, may be more important.[573, 575, 576] Improvement in glycemic control during chronic insulin therapy actually may raise serum phosphate in diabetic patients by reducing ongoing urinary calcium losses and eliminating secondary hyperparathyroidism.[508, 577]

Hypophosphatemia occurs very frequently in hospitalized alcoholic patients[521, 578, 579] and typically is most obvious 1 or more days after admission. Several factors may contribute to the phosphate depletion and hypophosphatemia in these patients, including malnutrition, use of aluminum-containing antacids, secondary hyperparathyroidism due to malabsorption or vitamin D deficiency, magnesium depletion,[428, 429, 513, 519, 580, 581] respiratory alkalosis, and abnormal shunting of glucose uptake from the liver to peripheral tissues, caused by fasting or undernourishment.[548, 553, 582, 583] Alcoholic patients with hypophosphatemia may develop rhabdomyolysis without experiencing generalized neuromuscular or other symptoms of profound hypophosphatemia (see below), perhaps because the phosphate released by necrotic muscle rapidly corrects the hypophosphatemia.[584]

Rapid cell proliferation, especially in otherwise ill patients with antecedent nutritional deprivation or catabolism, may produce severe hypophosphatemia. Examples include rapidly progressive or relapsing leukemia or lymphoma[585–587] and the use of hemopoietic granulocyte-macrophage colony-stimulating factor (GM-CSF) or erythropoietin in severely ill subjects.[588, 589]

Occasionally, parenteral administration of magnesium for treatment of hypomagnesemia alone in the setting of associated parathyroid secretory dysfunction and hypocalcemia may suddenly evoke a surge of PTH secretion, dramatic phosphaturia, and severe hypophosphatemia, especially in the setting of phosphate depletion. Concurrent treatment of both hypocalcemia and hypomagnesemia is necessary to prevent hypophosphatemia in this circumstance.[512, 590]

Clinical Consequences of Hypophosphatemia

The clinical manifestations of severe hypophosphatemia result from a generalized impairment of cellular energy metabolism and associated tissue or organ dysfunction. When phosphate becomes limiting for the formation of ATP and glucose is introduced (as commonly occurs clinically), overall ATP generation declines and energy metabolism shifts away from oxidative phosphorylation and toward glycolysis, whereby fewer moles of phosphate are required for metabolism of each mole of glucose (even though ATP production from glucose is less efficient than via oxidative phosphorylation).[198, 199, 591] The obligation of phosphate for expansion of the intracellular pool of organophosphates (i.e., glucose-6-phosphate, fructose-1,6-diphosphate, 1,3-DPG) contributes to the depletion of free intracellular inorganic phosphate and further slows ATP generation. The net result is a global decline in cellular function.

As already discussed, these sequelae of *acute* hypophosphatemia occur mainly or exclusively in hospitalized patients with underlying serious medical or surgical illness and preexisting phosphate depletion due to unusual urinary losses, severe malabsorption, malnutrition, or antacid abuse. The obvious clinical consequences of *chronic* hypophosphatemia are largely limited to disordered mineral and bone metabolism (as discussed below), although the possibility of ongoing subtle dysfunction of other organ systems in this setting probably has not been adequately addressed.

Neuromuscular signs and symptoms are among the most commonly recognized abnormalities that accompany the hypophosphatemic syndrome. Muscle weakness responsive to phosphate therapy is a common complaint among patients with both acute and chronic hypophosphatemia, and acute rhabdomyolysis may develop during rapidly progressive hypophosphatemia, notably in hospitalized alcoholic patients.[491, 493, 540, 592–594] In one study, 36% of 129 patients (none were alcoholic) with serum phosphate of 2 mg/dL or less developed asymptomatic elevations of serum creatine kinase (CPK, MM fraction) that were maximal 2 days, on average, after the nadir of the serum phosphate, by which time serum phosphate often had returned to normal.[595] Such findings emphasize the frequency with which unrecognized hypophosphatemia may complicate serious medical illness. Acute, severe hypophosphatemia may lead to a wide array of generalized and focal neurologic findings, including lethargy, confusion, disorientation, hallucinations, dysarthria, dysphagia, oculomotor palsies, anisocoria, nystagmus, ataxia, cerebellar tremor, ballismus, hyporeflexia, impaired sphincter control, distal sensory deficits, paresthesia, hyperesthesia, generalized or Guillain Barré–like ascending paralysis, seizures, coma, and death.[596–607] Confusion, flaccid paralysis, areflexia, seizures, and other major sequelae generally are observed only when serum phosphate falls below 0.8 mg/dL, although abnormalities in muscle electrolyte content and membrane potential are demonstrable in dogs with experimental phosphate depletion and much less severe hypophosphatemia (1.5 to 2.0 mg/dL).[596] Reversible respiratory failure also may occur in severely hypophosphatemic patients because of respiratory muscle weakness,[603] and treatment of hypophosphatemia (serum phosphate <2.5 mg/dL) in patients with acute respiratory failure (serum phosphate <2 mg/dL) or in general inpatients (serum phosphate <2.5 mg/dL) significantly improves respiratory muscle strength.[608, 603]

Reversible left ventricular dysfunction may occur with both acute and chronic severe hypophosphatemia[604] but often is not significant in patients with serum phosphate greater than 1.5 mg/dL.[610, 611] In patients with septic shock and severe hypophosphatemia (<2 mg/dL, average of 1.0 mg/dL), correction of hypophosphatemia acutely improved left ventricular stroke work index and systolic blood pressure.[612]

Various abnormalities in renal tubular function have been detected in phosphate-depleted animals, including tubular acidosis[328, 613–615] and impaired reabsorption of glucose,[616, 617] sodium,[328] and calcium.[158, 328, 618, 619] Defective calcium reabsorption may be partially corrected by phosphate infusion,[158, 328, 619] but also may reflect renal resistance to the action of PTH. The latter has been ascribed to uncoupling of the PTH receptor–guanine nucleotide regulatory subunit–adenylate cyclase complex.[620] Analogous clinical abnormalities in renal function in severely phosphate-depleted hypophosphatemic patients have not been widely described and might be difficult to detect in the typical critically ill patient.

Erythrocyte concentrations of ATP and 2,3-DPG are directly linked to that of extracellular inorganic phosphate, and severe hypophosphatemia may lead to increased erythrocyte fragility, abnormal membrane composition, and excessive oxyhemoglobin affinity. Thus, hemolysis, with membrane rigidity and microspherocytosis, may occur when serum phosphate is below 0.5 mg/dL,[621–623] whereas oxyhemoglobin dissociation may be sufficiently impaired when serum phosphate is less than 1.0 mg/dL to provoke a substantial increase in the cardiac output required for maintenance of adequate oxygen delivery to peripheral tissues.[209, 622, 624, 625] Studies in animals have disclosed significant impairment of critical leukocyte functions (chemotaxis, phagocytosis, bacterial killing), platelet and hemostatic dysfunction, and spontaneous gastrointestinal bleeding during severe hypophosphatemia (<1 mg/dL). The appearance of these abnormalities correlates with reductions in leukocyte and platelet ATP content.[626, 627]

Bone pain was a prominent complaint of the phosphate-depleted patients reported by Lotz et al.[491] Classic osteomalacia, with waddling gait, bone tenderness, and pseudofractures, may occur in patients with chronic hypophosphatemia due to renal phosphate wasting or antacid abuse.[206, 492, 628–630] The abnormal bone mineralization may be due to specific defects in osteoblastic function in addition to a lower chemical potential for calcium-phosphate crystallization.[631] As noted earlier, animal studies have demonstrated that excessive bone resorption also occurs during phosphate depletion, and this has been confirmed by radiokinetic and balance studies in humans.[206, 336] This osteolysis, and associated hypercalciuria, is not mediated by PTH, as underscored by Lotz et al.,[491] who documented substantial increments in serum calcium during phosphate depletion in hypoparathyroid subjects. Indeed, except in primary hyperparathyroidism, chronic phosphate depletion typically leads to parathyroid suppression, as reviewed earlier. The finding of parathyroid suppression also argues that accelerated bone resorption, and not defective renal tubular calcium reabsorption (which also occurs in phosphate depletion), is the cause of the negative calcium balance. It is possible also that increased production of $1,25(OH)_2D$,[618, 630, 632, 633] or lower levels of other vitamin D metabolites,[630] may contribute to the osteolysis induced by phosphate depletion.

The accumulated evidence suggests that severe hypophosphatemia (<2 mg/dL), particularly when it occurs in the setting of underlying phosphate depletion, constitutes a dangerous electrolyte abnormality that should be corrected promptly. In diabetic ketoacidosis, adjunctive intravenous phosphate therapy leads to more rapid repletion of erythrocyte 2,3-DPG concentrations,[573] even though significant clinical benefit (duration of acidosis, glucose disposal rates, morbidity, or mortality) has not been consistently documented.[565, 574] Nevertheless, the frequent association of severe phosphate depletion and hypophosphatemia with global depression of neuromuscular, cardiac, respiratory, and hematologic functions, together with evidence of positive effects of phosphate repletion upon cardiopulmonary function,[608, 609, 612] would seem to provide adequate justification for aggressive treatment of severe hypophosphatemia, particularly when it coexists with neurologic deterioration, heart failure, respiratory failure, severe infection, or hemorrhage. The cumulative deficit in body phosphate in such patients cannot be accurately predicted from knowledge of the serum phosphate, however,[634] and intravenous phosphate therapy thus is necessarily empirical. Available data in humans, derived mainly from studies of diabetic ketoacidosis, indicate that phosphate may be safely administered intravenously at initial doses of 0.2 to 0.8 mmol/kg of elemental phosphorus over 6 hours (i.e., 10 to 50 mmol over 6 hours), with doses greater than 4 mmol/hour reserved for those with serum phosphate less than 1.5 mg/dL and normal renal function.[558, 573, 574, 608, 609, 612, 635–640] Higher doses (1.5 to 3.0 mmol/kg/12 hours) can cause significant hyperphosphatemia, particularly when renal function is diminished, are not necessary for prevention of severe hypophosphatemia, and should be avoided.[641, 642] The threshold for intravenous phosphate therapy and the dose administered should reflect consideration of renal function, the likely severity and duration of the underlying phosphate depletion, and the presence and severity of symptoms consistent with those of hypophosphatemia. Serum phosphate and calcium must be monitored closely throughout the treatment. Less severe hypophosphatemia (1.5 to 2.5 mg/dL) usually can be treated with oral phosphate in divided doses of 750 and 2000 mg/day, although more information is needed to guide the need for and extent of such therapy in specific clinical situations.

REFERENCES

1. Krane SM: Calcium, phosphate and magnesium. *In* Rasmussen H (ed): The International Encyclopedia of Pharmacology and Therapeutics. London, Pergamon Press, 1970, p 19.
2. Neer R, Berman M, Fisher L, Rosenberg LE: Multicompartmental analysis of calcium kinetics in normal adult males. J Clin Invest 46:1364–1379, 1967.
3. Glimcher MK, Krane SM: Organization and structure of bone and the mechanism of calcification. *In* Gould BS, Ramachandran GN (eds): Treatise on Collagen: B. New York, Academic Press; 1968, pp 68–241.
4. Carr CW: Electrochemistry in Biology and Medicine. New York, John Wiley & Sons, 1955.
5. Bowers GN, Brassard C, Sena SF: Measurement of ionized calcium in serum with ion-selective electrodes: A mature technology that can meet the daily service needs. Clin Chem 32:1437–1447, 1986.
6. Krabbe S, Transbol I, Christiansen C: Bone mineral homeostasis, bone growth, and mineralization during years of pubertal growth: A unifying concept. Arch Dis Child 57:359–363, 1982.
7. Pitkin RM, Reynolds WA, Williams GA, Hargis CK: Calcium metabolism in normal pregnancy: A longitudinal study. Am J Obstet 133:781–790, 1979.
8. Gertner JM, Coustan OR, Kliger AS, et al: Pregnancy as a state of physiologic absorptive hypercalcemia. Am J Med 81:451–456, 1986.
9. Forbes GB: Calcium accumulation by the human fetus. Pediatrics 57:976–977, 1976.
10. Pitkin RM, Cruikshank DP, Schauberger CW, et al: Fetal calciotropic hormones and neonatal calcium homeostasis. Pediatrics 66:77–82, 1980.
11. Hillman L, Sateesha S, Haussler M, et al: Control of mineral homeostasis during lactation: Interrelationships of 25-hydroxyvitamin D, 24,25-dihydroxyvitamin D, 1,25-dihydroxyvitamin, parathyroid hormone, calcitonin, prolactin, and estradiol. Am J Obstet Gynecol 139:471–476, 1981.
12. Greer FR, Tasang RC, Searcy JE, et al: Mineral homeostasis during lactation—relationship to serum 1,25-dihydroxyvitamin D, 25-hydroxyvitamin D, parathyroid hormone, and calcitonin. Am J Clin Nutr 36:431–437, 1982.
13. Barritt GJ: Receptor-activated Ca^{2+} inflow in animal cells: A variety of pathways tailored to meet different intracellular Ca^{2+} signalling requirements. Biochem J 337(pt 2):153–169, 1999.
14. Berridge MJ: Elementary and global aspects of calcium signaling. J Physiol 499:291–306, 1997.
15. Carafoli E: Intracellular calcium homeostasis. Annu Rev Biochem 56:395–433, 1987.
16. Rasmussen H, Barrett PQ: Calcium messenger system: An integrated view. Physiol Rev 64:938–984, 1984.
17. Brown E, Pollack A, Hebert S: The extracellular calcium-sensing receptor: Its role in health and disease. Annu Rev Med 49:15–29, 1998.
18. Rasmussen H: The calcium messenger system. N Engl J Med 314:1094–1101, 1986.
19. Heaney RP, Gallagher JC, Johnston CC, et al: Calcium nutrition and bone health in the elderly. Am J Clin Nutr 36:986–1013, 1982.
20. Rasmussen H, Fontaine O, Max EE, Goodman DP: The effect of 1α-hydroxy-vitamin D_2 administration on calcium transport in chick intestine branch border membrane vesicles. J Biol Chem 254:2993–2999, 1979.
21. Bikle DD, Askey EW, Zolock PT, et al: Calcium accumulation by chick intestinal mitochondria. Regulation by vitamin D_3 and 1,25-dihydroxy vitamin D_3. Biochim Biophys Acta 598:561–574, 1980.
22. Favus MJ: Factors that influence absorption and secretion of calcium in the small intestine and colon. Am J Physiol 248:G147–G157, 1985.
23. Bronner F, Pansu D, Stein WD: An analysis of intestinal calcium transport across the rat intestine. Am J Physiol 250:G561–G569, 1986.
24. Allen LH: Calcium bioavailability and absorption: A review. Am J Clin Nutr 35:783–808, 1982.
25. Avioli LV, McDonald FE, Lee SW: The influence of age on the intestinal absorption of ^{47}Ca absorption in postmenopausal osteoporosis. J Clin Invest 44:1960–1967, 1965.
26. Ireland P, Fordtran JS: Effect of dietary calcium and age on jejunal calcium absorption in humans studied by intestinal perfusion. J Clin Invest 52:2672–2681, 1973.
27. Gallagher JC, Riggs BL, Eisman J, et al: Intestinal calcium absorption and serum vitamin D metabolites in normal subjects and osteoporotic patients: Effect of age and dietary calcium. J Clin Invest 64:729–736, 1979.
28. Heaney RP, Skillman TG: Secretion and excretion of calcium by the human gastrointestinal tract. J Lab Clin Med 64:29–41, 1964.
29. Rose GA, Reed GW, Smith AH: Isotopic method for measurement of calcium absorption from the gastrointestinal tract. BMJ 1:690–692, 1965.
30. Phang J, Berman M, Finerman G: Dietary perturbation of calcium metabolism in normal man: Compartmental analysis. J Clin Invest 48:67–77, 1969.
31. Jung A, Bartholdi P, Mermillod B: Critical analysis of methods of analyzing human calcium kinetics. J Theor Biol 73:131–157, 1978.
32. Fordtran JS, Locklear TW: Ionic constituents and osmolality of gastric and small-intestinal fluids after eating. Am J Dig Dis 11:503–521, 1966.
33. Marcus CS, Lengemann FW: Absorption of Ca^{45} and Sr^{85} from solid and liquid food at various levels of the alimentary tract of the rat. J Nutr 77:155–160, 1962.
34. Birge J, Peck WA, Berman M, Whedon DG: Study of calcium absorption in man: A kinetic analysis and physiologic model. J Clin Invest 48:1705–1713, 1969.
35. Dano P, Christiansen C: Calcium absorption and bone mineral content following intestinal shunt operations for obesity: A comparison of three types of procedures. Scand J Gastroenterol 9:775–779, 1974.
36. Pansu D, Bellaton C, Bronner F: Effect of Ca intake on saturable and nonsaturable components of duodenal Ca transport. Am J Physiol 240:G32–G37, 1981.
37. Ghijsen WEJM, DeJong MD, Vanos CH: ATP-dependent calcium transport and its correlation with Ca-ATPase activity in basolateral plasma membranes of rat duodenum. Biochim Biophys Acta 689:327–336, 1982.
38. Nemere I, Leathers V, Norman AW: 1,25-Dihydroxyvitamin D3–mediated intestinal calcium transport. Biochemical identification of lysosomes containing calcium and calcium-binding protein (calbindin-D28K). J Biol Chem 261:16106–16114, 1986.
39. Feher JJ, Fullmer CS, Wasserman RH: Role of facilitated diffusion of calcium by calbindin in intestinal calcium absorption. Am J Physiol 262:C517–C526, 1992.
40. Peng JB, Chen XZ, Berger UV, et al: Molecular cloning and characterization of a channel-like transporter mediating intestinal calcium absorption. J Biol Chem 274:22739–22746, 1999.
41. Murer H, Hildmann B: Transcellular transport of calcium and inorganic phosphate in the small intestinal epithelium. Am J Physiol 240:G409–G416, 1981.
42. Schacter D, Dowdle E, Schenker H: Active transport of calcium by the small intestine of the rat. Am J Physiol 198:263–268, 1960.
43. Mahoney AW, Holbrook RS, Hendricks DG: Effects of calcium solubility on absorption by rats with induced achlorhydria. Nutr Metab 18:310–317, 1975.
44. Recker RR: Calcium absorption and achlorhydria. N Engl J Med 313:70–73, 1985.
45. Nicar MJ, Pak CYC: Calcium bioavailability from calcium carbonate and calcium citrate. J Clin Endocrinol Metab 61:391–393, 1985.
46. Bo-Lin GW, Davis GR, Buddrus DJ, et al: An evaluation of the importance of gastric acid secretion in the absorption of dietary calcium. J Clin Invest 73:640–647, 1984.
47. Wensel RH, Rich C, Brown AC, Volwiler W: Absorption of calcium measured by intubation and perfusion of the intact human small intestine. J Clin Invest 48:1768–1775, 1969.
48. Ammann P, Rizzoli R, Fleisch H: Calcium absorption in rat large intestine in vivo: Availability of dietary calcium. Am J Physiol 251:G14–G18, 1986.
49. Webling D, Holdsworth ES: Bile salts and calcium absorption. Biochem J 100:652–660, 1966.
50. Wills MR: Intestinal absorption of calcium. Lancet 1:820–823, 1973.
51. Agnew JE, Holdsworth CD: The effect of fat on calcium absorption from a mixed meal in normal subjects, patients with malabsorptive disease, and patients with partial gastrectomy. Gut 12:973–977, 1971.
52. Cummings JH, Hill MJ, Jivrat T, et al: The effect of meat protein and dietary fiber on colonic function and metabolism. I. Changes in bowel habit, bile acid excretion and calcium absorption. Am J Clin Nutr 32:2086–2093, 1979.
53. McCance RA, Widdowson EM: Mineral metabolism of healthy adults on white and brown bread dietaries. J Physiol 101:44–85, 1942.
54. Reinhold JG, Faradji B, Abadi P, Ismail-Beigi F: Decreased absorption of calcium, magnesium, zinc and phosphorus by humans due to increased fiber and phosphorus consumption as wheat bread. J Nutr 106:493–503, 1976.
55. James WPT, Branch WJ, Southgate DAT: Calcium binding by dietary fiber. Lancet 1:638–639, 1978.
56. Slavin JL, Marlett JA: Influence of refined cellulose on human small bowel function and calcium and magnesium balance. Am J Clin Nutr 33:1932–1939, 1980.
57. Johnston FA, McMillan TJ, Falconer CD: Calcium retained by young women before and after adding spinach to the diet. J Am Diet Assoc 28:933–938, 1952.
58. Patton JS, Carey MC: Watching fat digestion. Science 204:145–148, 1979.
59. Pansu D, Chapuy MC, Milani M, Bellaton C: Transepithelial calcium transport enhanced by xylose and glucose in the rat jejunal ligated loop. Calcif Tissue Res 45:52, 1976.

60. Spencer H, Kramer L, Osis D, Norris C: Effect of phosphorus on the absorption of calcium and on the calcium balance in man. J Nutr 108:447–457, 1978.
61. Allen LH, Oddoye EA, Margen S: Protein-induced hypercalciuria: A long term study. Am J Clin Nutr 32:741–749, 1979.
62. Johnson NE, Allantra EN, Linkswiler H: Effect of level of protein intake on urinary and fecal calcium and calcium retention of young adult males. J Nutr 100:1425–1430, 1979.
63. Heaney RP, Recker RR: Effects of nitrogen, phosphorus and caffeine on calcium balance in women. J Lab Clin Med 99:46–55, 1982.
64. Omdahl JL, DeLuca HF: Regulation of vitamin D metabolism and function. Physiol Rev 53:327–372, 1973.
65. Norman AW, Henry H: 1,25-Dihydroxycholecalciferol—a hormonally active form of vitamin D. Recent Prog Horm Res 80:431–480, 1974.
66. Pansu D, Bellaton C, Roche C, Bronner F: Duodenal and ileal calcium absorption in the rat and effects of vitamin D. Am J Physiol 244:G695–G700, 1983.
67. Miller A, Bronner F: Calcium uptake in isolated brush-border vesicles from rat small intestine. Biochem J 196:391–401, 1981.
68. Wasserman RH, Corradino RA, Taylor AN: Vitamin D-dependent calcium-binding protein: Purification and some properties. J Biol Chem 243:3978–3986, 1968.
69. Bronner F, Freund T: Intestinal CaBP: A new quantitative index of vitamin D deficiency in the rat. Am J Physiol 229:689–694, 1975.
70. Meyer J, Fullmer CS, Wasserman RH, et al: Dietary restriction of calcium, phosphorus and vitamin D elicits differential regulation of the mRNAs for avian intestinal calbindin-D28k and the 1,25-dihydroxyvitamin D3 receptor. J Bone Miner Res 7:441–448, 1992.
71. Ghijsen WEJM, VanOs CH: 1,25-Dihydroxyvitamin D_3 regulates ATP-dependent calcium transport in basolateral plasma membranes of rat enterocytes. Biochim Biophys Acta 689:170–172, 1982.
72. Wasserman RH, Smith CA, Brindak ME, et al: Vitamin D and mineral deficiencies increase the plasma membrane calcium pump of chicken intestine. Gastroenterology 102:886–894, 1992.
73. Norman AW, Roth J, Orci L: The vitamin D endocrine system: Steroid metabolism, hormone receptors and biological response (calcium binding proteins). Endocr Rev 3:331–366, 1982.
74. Wali RK, Baum CL, Sitrin MD, Brasitus TA: 1,25-(OH)2vitamin D3 stimulates membrane phosphoinositide turnover, activates protein kinase C and increases cytosolic calcium in rat colonic epithelium. J Clin Invest 85:1296–1303, 1990.
75. Karbach U: Paracellular calcium transport across the small intestine. J Nutr 122:672–677, 1992.
76. Sheikh MS, Ramirez A, Emmett M, et al: Role of vitamin D–dependent and vitamin D–independent mechanisms in absorption of food calcium. J Clin Invest 81:126–132, 1988.
77. Nemere I, Yoshimoto Y, Norman AW: Studies on the mode of action of calciferol. LIV. Calcium transport in perfused duodena from normal chicks: Enhancement within 14 minutes of exposure to 1,25-dihydroxyvitamin D3. Endocrinology 115:1476–1483, 1984.
78. Farach-Carson MC, Sergeev I, Norman AW: Non-genomic actions of 1,25(OH)2D3 in rat osteosarcoma cells: Structure-function studies using ligand agonist analogs. Endocrinology 129:1876–1884, 1991.
79. Zhou L, Nemere I, Norman AW: 1,25-Dihydroxyvitamin D3 analog structure-function assessment of the rapid stimulation of intestinal calcium absorption (transcaltachia). J Bone Miner Res 7:457–463, 1992.
80. Yoshimoto Y, Nemere I, Norman AW: Hypercalcemia inhibits the rapid stimulatory effect on calcium transport in perfused duodena from normal chicks mediated in vitro by 1,25-dihydroxyvitamin D_3. Endocrinology 118:2300–2304, 1986.
81. Armbrecht HJ: Age-related changes in calcium and phosphorus uptake by rat small intestine. Biochim Biophys Acta 882:281–286, 1986.
82. Armbrecht HJ, Zenser TV, Bruns MEH, Davis BB: Effect of age on intestinal calcium absorption and adaptation to dietary calcium. Am J Physiol 239:E322–E327, 1979.
83. Horst RL, DeLuca HF, Jorgenson NA: The effect of age on calcium absorption and accumulation of 1,25-dihydroxyvitamin D in intestinal mucosa of rats. Metab Bone Dis Rel Res 1:29–33, 1978.
84. Gallagher JC, Riggs BL, Eisman J, et al: Intestinal calcium absorption and serum vitamin D metabolites in normal subjects and osteoporotic patients. J Clin Invest 64:729–736, 1979.
85. Armbrecht HJ, Forte LR, Halloran BP: Effect of age and dietary calcium on renal 25(OH)D metabolism, serum 1,25(OH)2D and serum PTH. Am J Physiol 246:E266–E270, 1984.
86. Eastell R, Yergey A, Vieira NE, et al: Interrelationship among vitamin D metabolism, true calcium absorption, parathyroid function, and age in women: Evidence of an age-related intestinal resistance to 1,25-dihydroxyvitamin D action. J Bone Miner Res 6:125–132, 1991.
87. Wood RJ, Fleet JC, Cashman K, et al: Intestinal calcium absorption in the aged rat: Evidence of intestinal resistance to 1,25(OH)2 vitamin D. Endocrinology 139:3843–3848, 1998.
88. Gallagher JC, Riggs BL, DeLuca HF: Effect of estrogen on calcium absorption and serum vitamin D metabolites in postmenopausal osteoporosis. J Clin Endocrinol Metab 51:1359–1364, 1980.
89. Liel Y, Shany S, Smirnoff P, Schwartz B: Estrogen increases 1,25-dihydroxyvitamin D receptors expression and bioresponse in the rat duodenal mucosa. Endocrinology 140:280–285, 1999.
90. Heaney RP, Skillman TG: Calcium metabolism in normal human pregnancy. J Clin Endocrinol Metab 33:661–669, 1971.
91. Lund B, Selnes A: Plasma 1,25-dihydroxy vitamin D levels in pregnancy and lactation. Acta Endocrinol 92:330–335, 1979.
92. Spanos E, Brown DJ, Stevenson JC, MacIntyre I: Stimulation of 1,25-dihydroxycholecalciferol production by prolactin and related peptides in intact cell preparations in vitro. Biochim Biophys Acta 672:7–15, 1981.
93. Kohlmeier L, Marcus R: Calcium disorders of pregnancy. Endocrinol Metab Clin North Am 24:15–39, 1995.
94. Brommage R, Baxter DC, Gierke LW: Vitamin D–independent intestinal calcium and phosphorus absorption during reproduction. Am J Physiol 259:G631–G638, 1990.
95. Bruns M, Boass A, Toverud SU: Regulation by dietary calcium of vitamin D–dependent calcium-binding protein and active calcium transport in the small intestine of lactating rats. Endocrinology 121:278–283, 1987.
96. Halloran BP, DeLuca HF: Calcium transport in small intestine during pregnancy and lactation. Am J Physiol 239:E64–E68, 1980.
97. Brommage R, DeLuca HF: Placental transport of calcium and phosphorus is not regulated by vitamin D. Am J Physiol 246:F526–F529, 1984.
98. Dostal LA, Toverud SU: Effect of vitamin D3 on duodenal calcium absorption in vivo during early development. Am J Physiol 246:G528–G534, 1984.
99. Halloran BP, DeLuca HF: Calcium transport in small intestine during early development: Role of vitamin D. Am J Physiol 239:G473–G479, 1980.
100. Adams JS, Wahl TO, Lukert BP: Effect of hydrochlorothiazide and dietary sodium restriction on calcium metabolism in corticosteroid treated patients. Metabolism 30:217, 1981.
101. Hahn TJ, Halstead LR, Baran DT: Effects of short-term glucocorticoid administration on intestinal calcium absorption and circulating vitamin D metabolite concentrations in man. J Clin Endocrinol Metab 52:111–114, 1981.
102. Favus MJ, Kimberg DV, Millar GN, Gershon E: Effects of cortisone administration on the metabolism and localization of 25-hydroxycholecalciferol in the rat. J Clin Invest 52:1328–1335, 1973.
103. Yeh JK, Aloia JF, Semla HM: Interrelation of cortisone and 1,25-dihydroxycholecalciferol on intestinal calcium and phosphate absorption. Calcif Tissue Int 36:608–614, 1984.
104. Bouillon R, Muls E, DeMoor P: Influence of thyroid function on the serum concentration of 1,25-dihydroxyvitamin D_3. J Clin Endocrinol 51:793–797, 1980.
105. Bushinsky DA, Favus MJ, Schneider AB, et al: Effects of metabolic acidosis on PTH and 1,25(OH)2D3 response to low calcium diet. Am J Physiol 243:F570–F575, 1982.
106. Favus MJ, Bushinsky DA, Coe FL: Effects of medium pH on duodenal and ilieal calcium active transport in the rat. Am J Physiol 251:G695–G700, 1986.
107. Krawitt EL: Effect of ethanol ingestion on duodenal calcium transport. J Lab Clin Med 85:665–671, 1975.
108. Krawitt EL, Sampson HW, Katagiri CA: Effect of 1,25-dihydroxycholecalciferol on ethanol-mediated suppression of calcium absorption. Calcif Tissue Res 18:119–124, 1975.
109. Corradino RA: Diphenylhydantoin: Direct inhibition of the vitamin D_3–mediated calcium absorptive mechanism in organ-cultured duodenum. Biochem Pharmacol 25:863, 1976.
110. Fox J, Green DT: Direct effects of calcium channel blockers on duodenal calcium transport in vivo. Eur J Pharmacol 129:159–164, 1986.
111. Lassiter WE, Gottschalk CW, Mylle M: Micropuncture study of renal tubular reabsorption on calcium in normal rodents. Am J Physiol 204:771–775, 1963.
112. Bomsztyk K, George JP, Wright FS: Effects of luminal fluid anions on calcium transport by proximal tubule. Am J Physiol 246:F600–F608, 1984.
113. Ng RCK, Rouse D, Suki WN: Calcium transport in the rabbit superficial proximal convulated tubule. J Clin Invest 74:834, 1984.
114. Bourdeau JE, Burg MB: Effects of PTH on calcium transport across the cortical thick ascending limb of Henle's loop. Am J Physiol 238:F350, 1979.
115. Suki WN, Rouse D, Ng RC, Kokko JP: Calcium transport in the thick ascending limb of Henle: Heterogeneity of function in the medullary and cortical segments. J Clin Invest 66:1004–1009, 1980.
116. Shareghi GR, Agus ZS: Magnesium transport in the cortical thick ascending limb of Henle's loop of the rabbit. J Clin Invest 69:759, 1982.
117. Friedman PA: Basal and hormone-activated calcium absorption in mouse renal thick ascending limbs. Am J Physiol 254:F62–F70, 1988.
118. Agus ZS, Chiu PJS, Goldberg M: Regulation of urinary calcium excretion in the rat. Am J Physiol 232:F545, 1977.
119. Costanzo LS, Windhager EE: Effects of PTH, ADH and cyclic AMP on distal tubular Ca and Na reabsorption. Am J Physiol 239:F478, 1980.
120. Costanzo LS: Comparison of calcium and sodium transport in early and late rat distal tubules: Effect of amiloride. Am J Physiol 246:F937–F945, 1984.
121. Borke JL, Caride A, Verma AK, et al: Plasma membrane calcium pump and 28-kDa calcium binding protein in cells of rat kidney distal tubules. Am J Physiol 257:F842–F849, 1989.
122. Ramachandran C, Brunette MG: The renal Na^+/Ca^{++} exchange system is located exclusively in the distal tubule. Biochem J 257:259–264, 1989.
123. Shimizu T, Yoshitomi K, Nakamura M, Imai M: Effect of parathyroid hormone on the connecting tubule from the rabbit kidney: Biphasic response of transmural voltage. Pfluegers Arch 416:254–261, 1990.
124. Barry EL, Gesek FA, Yu ASL, et al: Distinct calcium channel isoforms mediate parathyroid hormone and chlorothiazide-stimulated calcium entry in transporting epithelial cells. J Membr Biol 161:55–64, 1998.
125. Epstein FH: Calcium and the kidney. Am J Med 45:700–715, 1968.
126. Torikai S, Wang MS, Klein KL, Kurokawa K: Adenylate cyclase and cell cyclic AMP of rat cortical thick ascending limb of Henle. Kidney Int 20:649–654, 1981.
127. Shareghi GR, Stoner LC: Calcium transport across segments of the rabbit distal nephron in vitro. Am J Physiol 235:F367–F375, 1978.
128. Suki WN, Rouse D: Hormonal regulation of calcium transport in thick ascending limb renal tubules. Am J Physiol 241:F171, 1981.
129. Bijvoet OLM: Kidney function in calcium and phosphate metabolism. *In* Avioli LV, Krane SM (eds): Metabolic Bone Disease, vol 1. New York, Academic Press, 1977, pp 49–140.
130. Peacock M, Robertson WG, Nordin BEC: Relation between serum and urinary calcium with particular reference to parathyroid activity. Lancet 1:384–386, 1969.
131. Scoble JE, Mills S, Hruska KA: Calcium transport in canine renal basolateral

membrane vesicles. Effect of parathyroid hormones. J Clin Invest 75:1096–1105, 1985.
132. Bouhtiauy I, LaJeunesse D, Brunette MG: The mechanism of parathyroid hormone action on calcium reabsorption by the distal tubule. Endocrinology 128:251–258, 1991.
133. Tsukamoto Y, Saka S, Saitoh M: Parathyroid hormone stimulates ATP-dependent calcium pump activity by a different mode in proximal and distal tubules of the rat. Biochim Biophys Acta 1103:163–171, 1992.
134. Bacskai BJ, Friedman PA: Activation of latent Ca^{2+} channels in renal epithelial cells by parathyroid hormone. Nature 347:388–391, 1990.
135. Bourdeau JE, Lau K: Effects of parathyroid hormone on cytosolic free calcium concentration in individual rabbit connecting tubules. J Clin Invest 83:373–379, 1989.
136. de Rouffignac C, DiStefano A, Wittner M, et al: Consequences of differential effects of ADH and other peptide hormones on thick ascending limb of mammalian kidney. Am J Physiol 260:R1023–R1035, 1991.
137. Shimizu T, Nakamura M, Yoshitomi K, Imai M: Interaction of trichlormethiazide or amiloride with PTH in stimulating Ca^{2+} absorption in rabbit CNT. Am J Physiol 261:F36–F43, 1991.
138. Even L, Weisman Y, Goldray D, Hochberg Z: Selective modulation by vitamin D of renal response to parathyroid hormone: A study in calcitriol-resistant rickets. J Clin Endocrinol Metab 81:2836–2840, 1996.
139. Singer FR, Woodhouse NJ, Parkinson DK, Joplin GF: Some acute effects of administered porcine calcitonin in man. Clin Sci 37:181–190, 1969.
140. Litvak J: Hypocalcemic hypercalciuria during vitamin D and dihydrotachysterol therapy of hypoparathyroidism. J Clin Endocrinol Metab 18:246–252, 1958.
141. Edwards NA, Hodgkinson A: Metabolic studies in patients with idiopathic hypercalciuria. Clin Sci (Colch) 29:143–154, 1965.
142. Chipman JJ, Zerwekh J, Nicar M, et al: Effect of growth hormone administration: Reciprocal changes in serum 1α,25-dihydroxyvitamin D and intestinal calcium absorption. J Clin Endocrinol Metab 51:321–324, 1980.
143. Gertner JM, Tamborlane WV, Hintz RL, et al: The effects on mineral metabolism of overnight growth hormone infusion in growth hormone deficiency. J Clin Endocrinol Metab 53:818–822, 1981.
144. Wright NM, Papadea N, Wentz B, et al: Increased serum 1,25-dihydroxyvitamin D after growth hormone administration is not parathyroid hormone–mediated. Calcif Tissue Int 61:101–103, 1997.
145. Lemann J Jr, Piering WF, Lennon EJ: Studies of the acute effects of aldosterone and cortisol on the interrelationship between renal sodium, calcium and magnesium excretion in normal man. Nephron 7:117–130, 1970.
146. Findley JW, Adams ND, Lemann J Jr, et al: Vitamin D metabolites and parathyroid hormone in Cushing's syndrome: Relationship to calcium and phosphorus homeostasis. J Clin Endocrinol Metab 54:1039–1044, 1982.
147. Gallagher JC, Nordin BEC: Treatment with oestrogens of primary hyperparathyroidism in post-menopausal women. Lancet 1:503–507, 1972.
148. McKane W, Khosla S, Burritt M, et al: Mechanism of renal calcium conservation with estrogen replacement therapy in women in early menopause—a clinical research center study. J Clin Endocrinol Metab 80:3458–3464, 1995.
149. Marcus R, Madvig P, Crim M, et al: Conjugated estrogens in the treatment of postmenopausal women with hyperparathyroidism. Ann Intern Med 100:633–640, 1984.
150. DeFronzo RA, Cooke CR, Andres R, et al: The effect of insulin on renal handling of sodium, potassium, calcium and phosphate in man. J Clin Invest 55:845–853, 1975.
151. Blythe WB, Gittleman HJ, Welt LG: Effect of expansion of the extracellular space on the rate of urinary excretion of calcium. Am J Physiol 214:52–57, 1968.
152. McCarron DA, Rankin LI, Bennett WM, et al: Urinary calcium excretion at extremes of sodium intake in normal man. Am J Nephrol 1:84–90, 1981.
153. Duarte CG, Watson JF: Calcium reabsorption in proximal tubule of the dog nephron. Am J Physiol 212:1355–1360, 1967.
154. Breslau NA, McGuire JL, Zerwekh JE, Pak CYC: The role of dietary sodium on renal excretion and intestinal absorption of calcium and on vitamin D metabolism. J Clin Endocrinol Metab 55:369–373, 1982.
155. Jowsey J, Balasubramaniam P: Effect of phosphate supplements on soft-tissue calcification and bone turnover. Clin Sci 42:289, 1972.
156. Lau K, Agus ZS, Goldberg M, Goldfarb S: Renal tubular sites of altered Ca transport in phosphate depleted rats. J Clin Invest 64:1681–1687, 1979.
157. Van Den Berg CJ, Kumar R, Wilson DM, et al: Orthophosphate therapy decreases urinary calcium excretion and serum 1,25-dihydroxy vitamin D concentrations in idiopathic hypercalciuria. J Clin Endocrinol Metab 51:998–1001, 1980.
158. Coburn JW, Massry SG: Changes in serum and urinary calcium during phosphate depletion: Studies on mechanisms. J Clin Invest 1619–1629, 1970.
159. Massry SG, Coburn JW, Kleeman CR: Evidence for suppression of parathyroid gland activity by hypermagnesemia. J Clin Invest 49:1619–1629, 1970.
160. Cholst IN, Steinberg SF, Tropper PJ: The influence of hypermagnesemia on serum calcium and parathyroid hormone levels in human subjects. N Engl J Med 310:1221–1225, 1984.
161. Lemann J Jr, Litzow JR, Lennon EJ: The effects of chronic acid loads in normal man: Further evidence for the participation of bone mineral in the defense against chronic metabolic acidosis. J Clin Invest 45:1608, 1966.
162. Sutton RAL, Wong NLM, Dirks JH: Effects of metabolic acidosis and alkalosis on sodium and calcium transport in the dog kidney. Kidney Int 15:520, 1979.
163. Canzanello VJ, Bodvarsson M, Kraut JA, et al: Effect of chronic respiratory acidosis on urinary calcium excretion in the dog. Kidney Int 38:409–416, 1990.
164. Siggard-Anderson O: Acute experimental acid-base disturbances in dogs. Scand J Clin Lab Invest 41:1–20, 1962.
165. Wesson LG Jr: Magnesium, calcium and phosphate excretion during osmotic diuresis in the dog. J Lab Clin Med 60:422–433, 1962.
166. Duarte CG: Effects of ethacrynic acid and furosemide on urinary calcium, phosphate and magnesium. Metabolism 17:867–876, 1968.
167. Eknoyan G, Suki WN, Martinez-Madonado M: Effect of diuretics on urinary excretion of phosphate, calcium and magnesium in thyroparathyroidectomized dogs. J Lab Clin Med 76:257–266, 1970.
168. Bourdeau JE, Buss SL, Vurek GG: Inhibition of calcium absorption in the cortical thick ascending limb of Henle's loop by furosemide. J Pharmacol Exp Ther 221:815–819, 1982.
169. Suki WN, Yium JJ, VonMinden M, et al: Acute treatment of hypercalcemia with furosemide. N Engl J Med 283:836–840, 1970.
170. Lamberg BA, Kuhlback B: Effect of chlorothiazide and hydrochlorothiazide on the excretion of calcium in urine. Scand J Clin Lab Invest 11:351–357, 1959.
171. Costanzo LS, Weiner IM: On the hypercalciuric action of chlorothiazide. J Clin Invest 54:628–637, 1974.
172. Costanzo LS, Weiner IM: Relationship between clearances of Ca and Na: Effect of distal diuretics and PTH. Am J Physiol 230:67–73, 1976.
173. Gesek FA, Friedman PA: Mechanism of calcium transport stimulated by chlorothiazide in mouse distal convoluted tubule cells. J Clin Invest 90:429–438, 1992.
174. Yendt ER, Cohanim M: Prevention of calcium stones with thiazides. Kidney Int 13:397–409, 1978.
175. Maschio G, Tessitore N, D'Angelo A, et al: Prevention of calcium nephrolithiasis with low-dose thiazide, amiloride and allopurinol. Am J Med 71:623–626, 1981.
176. Aicher L, Meier G, Norcross AJ, et al: Decrease in kidney calbindin-D 28kDa as a possible mechanism mediating cyclosporine A- and FK-506-induced calciuria and tubular mineralization. Biochem Pharmacol 53:723–731, 1997.
177. Kupfer S, Kosovsky JD: Effects of cardiac glycosides on renal tubular transport of calcium, magnesium, inorganic phosphate and glucose in the dog. J Clin Invest 44:1132–1143, 1965.
178. Shimizu T, Yoshitomi K, Nakamura N, Imai M: Effects of PTH, calcitonin, and cAMP on calcium transport in rabbit distal nephron segments. Am J Physiol 259:F408–F414, 1990.
179. Elliott WC, Patchin DS: Aminoglycoside-mediated calciuresis. J Pharmacol Exp Ther 262:151–156, 1992.
180. Buck AC, Lote CJ, Sampson WF: The influence of renal prostaglandin on urinary calcium excretion in idiopathic urolithiasis. J Urol 129:421–426, 1983.
181. Friedlander G, Amiel C: Decreased calcium and magnesium urinary excretion during prostaglandin synthesis inhibition in the rat. Prostaglandins 29:123–132, 1985.
182. Walser M: Ion association. VI. Interaction between calcium, magnesium, inorganic phosphate, citrate and protein in normal human plasma. J Clin Invest 40:723, 1961.
183. Somell A, Alveryd A: Diurnal variation in the urinary excretion of calcium and phosphate in hyperparathyroidism. Acta Chir Scand 142:357, 1976.
184. Dossetor JB, Gorman HM, Beck JC: The diurnal rhythm of urinary electrolyte excretion. I. Observations in normal subjects. Metabolism 12:1083, 1963.
185. Birkenhager WH, Hellendoorn HBA, Gerbrandy J: Enkle aspecten van de calciumen fosfaatstofwisseling, in het bijzonder na intraveneuze injectie van calcium-levulinaat. Ned Tijdschr Geneeskd 101:1294, 1957.
186. Adam A, Boulanger J, Azzouzi M, Ers P: Colorimetric vs enzymatic determination of serum phosphorus. Clin Chem 30:1724–1725, 1984.
187. Landowne RA: Immunoglobulin interference with phosphorus and chloride determinations with the Coulter chemistry. Clin Chem 25:1189–1190, 1979.
188. Donhowe JM, Freier EF, Wong ET, Steffes MW: Factitious hypophosphatemia related to mannitol therapy. Clin Chem 27:1765–1769, 1981.
189. MacDonald RG, MacDonald HN: Erythrocyte 2,3-diphosphoglycerate and associated haematological parameters during the menstrual cycle and pregnancy. Br J Obstet Gynaecol 84:427, 1977.
190. Reitz RE, Daane TA, Woods JR, Weinstein RL: Calcium, magnesium, phosphorus, and parathyroid hormone interrelationships in pregnancy and newborn infants. Obstet Gynecol 50:701–705, 1977.
191. Cruikshank DP, Pitkin RM, Reynolds WA, et al: Altered maternal calcium homeostasis in diabetic pregnancy. J Clin Endocrinol Metab 50:264–267, 1980.
192. Baran DT, Whyte MP, Haussler MR, et al: Effect of the menstrual cycle on calcium-regulating hormones in the normal young woman. J Clin Endocrinol Metab 50:377–379, 1980.
193. Stulc J: Placental transfer of inorganic ions and water [review]. Physiol Rev 77:805–836, 1997.
194. Aitken JM, Gallagher MJ, Hart DM, et al: Plasma growth hormone and serum phosphorus concentration in relation to the menopause and to oestrogen therapy. J Endocrinol 59:593, 1973.
195. Halloran BP, Lonergan ET, Portale AA: Aging and renal responsiveness to parathyroid hormone in healthy men. J Clin Endocrinol Metab 81:2192–2197, 1996.
196. Griffith EJ, Ponnamperuma C, Gobel N: Phosphorus, a key to life on the primitive earth. Orig Life 8:71–85, 1977.
197. Lichtman MA, Miller DR, Freeman RB: Erythrocyte adenosine triphosphate depletion during hypophosphatemia in a uremic subject. N Engl J Med 280:240–244, 1969.
198. Erecinska M, Stubbs M, Miyata Y, et al: Regulation of cellular metabolism by intracellular phosphate. Biochem Biophys Acta 462:20–35, 1977.
199. Morris RC, Nigon K, Reed EB: Evidence that the severity of depletion of inorganic phosphate determines the severity of the disturbance of adenine nucleotide metabolism in the liver and renal cortex of the fructose-loaded rat. J Clin Invest 61:209–220, 1978.
200. Chapman AG, Atkinson DE: Stabilization of adenylate energy charge by the adenylate deaminase reaction. J Biol Chem 248:8309–8312, 1973.
201. Niehaus WG, Hammerstedt RN: Mode of orthophosphate uptake and ATP labeling by mammalian cells. Biochem Biophys Acta 443:515–524, 1976.
202. Boskey AL, Posner AS: The role of synthetic and bone extracted Ca-phospholipid-PO_4 complexes in hydroxyapatite formation. Calcif Tissue Res 23:251–258, 1977.
203. Lian JB, Cohen-Solal L, Kossiva K, Glimcher MJ: Changes in phosphoproteins of chicken bone matrix in vitamin D–deficient rickets. FEBS Lett 149:123–125, 1982.
204. Moallem E, Kilav R, Silver J, Naveh-Many T: RNA-protein binding and post-transcriptional regulation of parathyroid hormone gene expression by calcium and phosphate. J Biol Chem 273:5253–5259, 1998.

205. Hughes MR, Brumbaugh PF, Haussler MR, et al: Regulation of serum 1 α,25-dihydroxyvitamin D_3 by calcium and phosphate in the rat. Science 190:578, 1975.
206. Lotz M, Ney R, Bartter FC: Osteomalacia and debility resulting from phosphorus depletion. Trans Assoc Am Physiol 77:281–295, 1964.
207. Baylink D, Wergedal JE, Stauffer M: Formation, mineralization and resorption of bone in hypophosphatemic rats. J Clin Invest 50:2519–2530, 1971.
208. Raisz LG, Niemann I: Effect of phosphate, calcium and magnesium on bone resorption and hormonal responses in tissue culture. Endocrinology 85:446–452, 1969.
209. Marshall DH, Nordin BEC, Speed R: Calcium, phosphorus and magnesium requirements. Proc Nutr Soc 35:163–173, 1976.
210. Wilz DR, Gray RW, Dominguez JH, Lemann J Jr: Plasma 1,25-$(OH)_2$-vitamin D concentrations and net intestinal calcium, phosphate, and magnesium absorption in humans. Am J Clin Nutr 32:2052–2060, 1979.
211. Wasserman RH, Taylor AN: Intestinal absorption of phosphate in the chick: Effect of vitamin D and other parameters. J Nutr 103:586–599, 1973.
212. Kowarski S, Schacter D: Effects of vitamin D on phosphate transport and incorporation into mucosal constituents of rat intestinal mucosa. J Biol Chem 244:211–217, 1969.
213. Hurwitz S, Bar A: Absorption of calcium and phosphorus along the gastrointestinal tract of the laying fowl as influenced by dietary calcium and egg shell formation. J Nutr 86:433, 1965.
214. Borowitz SM, Granrud GS: Ontogeny of intestinal phosphate absorption in rabbits. Am J Physiol 262:G847–G853, 1992.
215. Lee DBN, Walling MW, Brautbar N: Intestinal phosphate absorption: Influence of vitamin D and non–vitamin D factors. Am J Physiol 250:G369–G373, 1986.
216. Schroder B, Hattenhauer O, Breves G: Phosphate transport in pig proximal small intestines during postnatal development: Lack of modulation by calcitriol. Endocrinology 139:1500–1507, 1998.
217. Cross HS, Debiec H, Peterlik M: Mechanism and regulation of intestinal phosphate absorption. Miner Electrolyte Metab 16:115–124, 1990.
218. Fuchs R, Peterlik M: Vitamin D–induced transepithelial phosphate and calcium transport by chick jejunum. Effect on microfilamentous and microtubular inhibitors. FEBS Lett 100:357–359, 1979.
219. Lee DBN, Walling DW, Corry DB, Coburn JW: 1,25-dihydroxyvitamin D_3 stimulates calcium and phosphate absorption by different mechanisms: Contrasting requirement for sodium. Adv Exp Med Biol 178:189–193, 1984.
220. Danisi G, Murer H, Straub RW: Effects of pH and sodium on phosphate transport across brush border membrane vesicles of small intestine. Adv Exp Med Biol 178:173–180, 1984.
221. Borowitz SM, Ghishan FK: Phosphate transport in human jejunal brush-border membrane vesicles. Gastroenterology 96:4–10, 1989.
222. Beck L, Karaplis AC, Amizuka N, et al: Targeted inactivation of Npt2 in mice leads to severe renal phosphate wasting, hypercalciuria, and skeletal abnormalities. Proc Natl Acad Sci USA 95:5372–5377, 1998.
223. Feild JA, Zhang L, Brun KA, et al: Cloning and functional characterization of a sodium-dependent phosphate transporter expressed in human lung and small intestine. Biochem Biophys Res Commun 258:578–582, 1999.
224. Peterlik M, Wasserman RH: Effect of vitamin D on transepithelial phosphate transport in chick intestine. Am J Physiol 234:E379–388, 1978.
225. Harrison HE, Harrison HC: Intestinal transport of phosphate: Action of vitamin D, calcium and potassium. Am J Physiol 201:1007–1012, 1961.
226. Walling MW: Intestinal Ca and phosphate transport: Differential responses to vitamin D_3 metabolites. Am J Physiol 233:E488–E494, 1977.
227. Fox J, Swaminathan R, Murray TM, Care AD: The role of parathyroid hormone in the adaptation of phosphate absorption from the jejunum of conscious pigs. Adv Exp Med Biol 81:133–136, 1976.
228. Chen TC, Castillo L, Korycka-Dahl M: DeLuca HF: Role of vitamin D metabolites in phosphate transport of rat intestine. J Nutr 104:1056–1060, 1974.
229. Corradino RA: Embryonic chick intestine in organ culture: A unique system for the study of the intestinal calcium absorptive mechanism. J Cell Biol 58:64, 1973.
230. Brickman AS, Hartenbower DL, Norman AW, Coburn JW: Actions of 1 α-hydroxyvitamin D_3 and 1,25 dihydroxyvitamin D_3 on mineral metabolism in men. I. Effects on net absorption of phosphorus. Am J Clin Nutr 30:1064, 1977.
231. Birge JJ, Miller R: The role of phosphate in the action of vitamin D in the intestine. J Clin Invest 60:980–988, 1977.
232. Danisi G, Straub RW: Unidirectional influx of phosphate across the mucosal membrane of rabbit small intestine. Pflugers Arch 385:117–122, 1980.
233. Cross HS, Peterlik M: Vitamin D activates (Na^+-K^+)ATPase: A possible regulation of phosphate and calcium uptake by cultured embryonic chick small intestine. Adv Exp Med Biol 178:163–171, 1984.
234. Karsenty G, Lacour B, Ulmann A, et al: Early effects of vitamin metabolites on phosphate fluxes in isolated rat enterocytes. Am J Physiol 248:G40–G45, 1985.
235. Nemere I: Apparent nonnuclear regulation of intestinal phosphate transport: Effects of 1,25-dihydroxyvitamin D_3, 24,25-dihydroxyvitamin D_3, and 25-hydroxyvitamin D_3. Endocrinology 137:2254–2261, 1996.
236. Quamme GA: Phosphate transport in intestinal brush-border membrane vesicles: Effect of pH and dietary phosphate. Am J Physiol 249:G168–G175, 1985.
237. Caverzasio J, Danisi G, Straub RW, et al: Adaptation of phosphate transport to low phosphate diet in renal and intestinal brush border membrane vesicles: influence of sodium and pH. Pflugers Arch 409:333–336, 1987.
238. Danisi G, Caverzasio J, Trechsel U, et al: Phosphate transport adaptation in rat jejunum and plasma levels of 1,25-dihydroxyvitamin D3. Scand J Gastroenterol 25:210–215, 1990.
239. Cramer C, McMillan J: Phosphorus adaptation in rats in the absence of vitamin D or parathyroid glands. Am J Physiol 239:G261–G265, 1980.
240. Borle AB, Keutmann HT, Neumann WF: Role of parathyroid hormone in phosphate transport across rat duodenum. Am J Physiol 204:705, 1963.
241. Clark I, Rivera-Cordero F: Effect of parathyroid function on absorption and excretion of calcium, magnesium and phosphate by rats. Endocrinology 88:302–308, 1971.
242. Tanzer FS, Navia JM: Calcitonin inhibition of intestinal phosphate absorption. Nature 242:221, 1973.
243. Juan D, Liptak P: Absorption of inorganic phosphate in the human jejunum. J Clin Endocrinol Metab 43:517–522, 1976.
244. Nemere I: Parathyroid hormone rapidly stimulates phosphate transport in perfused duodenal loops of chicks: Lack of modulation by vitamin D metabolites. Endocrinology 137:3750–3755, 1996.
245. Ferraro C, Ladizesky M, Cabrejas M, et al: Intestinal absorption of phosphate: Action of protein synthesis inhibitors and glucocorticoids in the rat. J Nutr 106:1752–1756, 1976.
246. Corradino RA: Hydrocortisone and vitamin D3 stimulation of 32Pi-phosphate accumulation by organ-cultured chick embryo duodenum. Horm Metab Res 11:519–523, 1979.
247. Fox J, Bunnett NW, Farrar AR, Care AD: Stimulation by low phosphorus and low calcium diets of duodenal absorption of phosphate in betamethasone treated chicks. J Endocrinol 88:147–153, 1981.
248. Yeh JK, Aloia JF: Effect of glucocorticoids on the passive transport of phosphate in different segments of the intestine in the rat. Bone Miner 2:11–19, 1987.
249. Clark I, Rivera-Cordero F: Effects on endogenous parathyroid hormone on calcium, magnesium and phosphate metabolism in rats. Endocrinology 92:62–71, 1973.
250. Spencer H, Kramer L, Osis D: Effect of calcium on phosphorus metabolism in man. Am J Clin Nutr 40:219–225, 1984.
251. Spencer H, Kramer L, Norris C, Osis D: Effect of small doses of aluminum-containing antacids on calcium and phosphorus metabolism. Am J Clin Nutr 36:32–40, 1982.
252. Walser M: Protein-binding of inorganic phosphate in plasma of normal subjects and patients with renal disease. J Clin Invest 39:501–506, 1960.
253. Harris CA, Baer PG, Chirito E, Dirks JH: Composition of mammalian glomerular filtrate. Am J Physiol 227:972–976, 1974.
254. Harris CA, Sutton RAL, Dirks JH: Effects of hypercalcemia on calcium and phosphate ultrafilterability and tubular reabsorption in the rat. Am J Physiol 233:F201–F206, 1977.
255. Knox FG, Osswald H, Marchand GR, et al: Phosphate transport along the nephron. Am J Physiol 233:F261–F268, 1977.
256. Dennis VW, Stead WW, Myers JL: Renal handling of phosphate and calcium. Annu Rev Physiol 41:257–271, 1979.
257. Dennis VW, Brazy PC: Divalent anion transport in isolated renal tubules. Kidney Int 22:498–506, 1982.
258. Amiel C, Kuntziger H, Richet G: Micropuncture study of handling of phosphate by proximal and distal nephron in normal and parathyroidectomized rat. Evidence for distal reabsorption. Pflugers Arch 317:93–109, 1970.
259. Haas JA, Berndt T, Knox FG: Nephron heterogeneity of phosphate reabsorption. Am J Physiol 234:F287–F290, 1978.
260. LeGrimellec C, Roinel N, Morel F: Simultaneous Mg, Ca, P, K, Na, and Cl analysis in rat tubular fluid IV. During acute phosphate plasma loading. Pflugers Arch 346:189–204, 1974.
261. Pastoriza-Munoz E, Colindres RE, Lassiter WE, Lechene C: Effect of parathyroid hormone on phosphate reabsorption in rat distal convolution. Am J Physiol 235:F321–F330, 1978.
262. Peraino RA, Suki WN: Phosphate transport by isolated rabbit cortical collecting tubule. Am J Physiol 238:F358–F362, 1980.
263. Shareghi GR, Agus ZS: Phosphate transport in the light segment of the rabbit cortical collecting tubule. Am J Physiol 242:F379–F384, 1982.
264. Rocha AS, Magaldi JB, Kokko JP: Calcium and phosphate transport in isolated segments of rabbit Henle's loop. J Clin Invest 59:975, 1977.
265. Haas JA, Berndt T, Knox FG: Nephron heterogeneity of phosphate reabsorption. Am J Physiol 234:F287–F290, 1978.
266. Bengele HH, Lechene CP, Alexander EA: Phosphate transport along the inner medullary collecting duct of the rat. Am J Physiol 237:F48–F54, 1979.
267. Haramati A, Haas JA, Knox FG: Adaptation of deep and superficial nephrons to changes in dietary phosphate intake. Am J Physiol 244:F265–F269, 1983.
268. Knox FG, Haas JA, Berndt T, et al: Phosphate transport in superficial and deep nephrons in phosphate-loaded rats. Am J Physiol 233:F150–F153, 1977.
269. Muhlbauer RC, Bonjour JP, Fleisch H: Tubular localization of adaptation to dietary phosphate in rats. Am J Physiol 233:F342–F348, 1977.
270. Baumann K, DeRouffignac C, Roinel N, et al: Renal phosphate transport: Inhomogeneity of local proximal transport rates and sodium dependence. Pflugers Arch 356:287–298, 1985.
271. Beck LH, Goldberg M: Mechanism of the blunted phosphaturia in saline-loaded thyroparathyroidectomized dogs. Kidney Int 6:18–23, 1974.
272. Haas JA, Berndt TJ, Haramati A, Knox FG: Nephron sites of action of nicotinamide on phosphate reabsorption. Am J Physiol 246:F27–F31, 1984.
273. Ullrich KJ, Rumrich G, Kloess S: Phosphate transport in the proximal convolution of the rat kidney. I. Tubular heterogeneity, effect of parathyroid hormone in acute and chronic parathyroidectomized animals and effect of phosphate diet. Pflugers Arch 372:269–274, 1977.
274. Freeman D, Bartlett S, Radda G, Ross B: Energetics of sodium transport in the kidney. Saturation transfer ^{31}P-NMR. Biochim Biophys Acta 762:325–336, 1983.
275. Hems DA, Gaja G. Carbohydrate metabolism in the isolated perfused rat kidney. Biochem J 128:412–426, 1972.
276. Hoppe A, Metler M, Berndt TJ, et al: Effect of respiratory alkalosis on renal phosphate excretion. Am J Physiol 243:F471–F475, 1982.
277. Gmaj P, Murer H: Cellular mechanisms of inorganic phosphate transport in kidney. Physiol Rev 66:36–70, 1986.
278. Schneider EG, McLane LA: Evidence for a peritubular-to-luminal flux of phosphate in the dog kidney. Am J Physiol 232:F159–F166, 1977.
279. Ullrich KJ: Mechanisms of cellular phosphate transport in the renal proximal tubule. Adv Exp Med Biol 103:21–35, 1978.

280. Ullrich KJ, Capasso G, Rumrich G, et al: Coupling between proximal tubular transport processes: Studies with ouabain, SITS and HCO_3-free solutions. Pflugers Arch 368:245–252, 1977.
281. Ullrich KJ, Murer H: Sulfate and phosphate transport in the renal proximal tubule. Philos Trans R Soc Lond B Biol Sci 229:549–488, 1982.
282. Hoffman N, Thies M, Kinne R: Phosphate transport by isolated renal brush border vesicles. Pflugers Arch 362:147–156, 1976.
283. Burckhardt G, Stern H, Murer H: The influence of pH on phosphate transport into rat renal brush border membrane vesicles. Pflugers Arch 390:191–197, 1981.
284. Cheng L, Sacktor B: Sodium gradient–dependent phosphate transport in renal brush border membrane vesicles. J Biol Chem 256:1556–1564, 1981.
285. Hruska KA, Klahr S, Hammerman MR: Decreased luminal membrane transport of phosphate in chronic renal failure. Am J Physiol 242:F17–F22, 1982.
286. Beliveau R, Brunette MG: The renal brush border membrane in man. Protein pattern, inorganic phosphate binding and transport: Comparison with other species. Renal Physiol 7:65–71, 1984.
287. Murayama Y, Morel F, LeGrimellec C: Phosphate, calcium and magnesium transfers in proximal tubules and loops of Henle, as measured by single nephron microperfusion experiments in the rat. Pflugers Arch 333:1–16, 1972.
288. Amstutz M, Mohrmann M, Gmaj P, Murer H: The effect of pH on phosphate transport in rat renal brush border membrane vesicles. Am J Physiol 248:F705–F710, 1985.
289. Cheng L, Liang CT, Sacktor B: Phosphate uptake by renal membrane vesicles of rabbits adapted to high and low phosphorus diets. Am J Physiol 245:F175–F180, 1983.
290. Ullrich KJ, Rumrich G, Kloss S: Phosphate transport in the proximal convolution of the rat kidney. III. Effect of extracellular and intracellular pH. Pflugers Arch 377:33–42, 1978.
291. Kavanaugh MP, Miller DG, Zhang W, et al: Cell-surface receptors for gibbon ape leukemia virus and amphotropic murine retrovirus are inducible sodium-dependent phosphate symporters. Proc Natl Acad Sci U S A 91:7071–7075, 1994.
292. Olah Z, Lehel C, Anderson WB, et al: The cellular receptor for gibbon ape leukemia virus is a novel high affinity sodium-dependent phosphate transporter. J Biol Chem 269:25426–25431, 1994.
293. Murer H, Biber J: A molecular view of proximal tubular inorganic phosphate (Pi) reabsorption and of its regulation [review]. Pflugers Arch 433:379–389, 1997.
294. Koobs DH: Phosphate mediation of the Crabtree and Pasteur effects. Science 178:127–133, 1972.
295. Grinstein S, Turner RJ, Silverman M, Rothstein A: Inorganic anion transport in kidney and intestinal brush border and basolateral membranes. Am J Physiol 238:F452–F460, 1980.
296. Schwab SJ, Klahr S, Hammerman MR: Na^+ gradient–dependent Pi uptake in basolateral membrane vesicles from dog kidney. Am J Physiol 246:F663–F669, 1984.
297. Ullrich KJ, Rumrich G, Kloess S: Contraluminal sulfate transport in the proximal tubule of the rat kidney. I. Kinetic effect of K^+, Na^+, Ca^{2+}, H^+ and anions. Pflugers Arch 402:264–271, 1984.
298. Murer H, Burckhardt G: Membrane transport of anions across epithelia of mammalian small intestine and kidney proximal tubule. Rev Physiol Biochem Pharmacol 96:1–51, 1983.
299. Anderson J, Parsons V: The tubular maximal resorptive rate for inorganic phosphate in normal subjects. Clin Sci (Colch) 25:431, 1963.
300. Bijvoet OLM: Relation of plasma phosphate concentration to renal tubular reabsorption of phosphate. Clin Sci (Colch) 37:23, 1969.
301. Bijvoet OLM, Morgan DB, Fourman P, et al: The assessment of phosphate reabsorption. Clin Chim Acta 26:15, 1969.
302. Stamp TC, Stacey TE: Measurement of the theoretical renal phosphorus threshold in the investigation and treatment of osteomalacia. Clin Sci (Colch) 38:34P, 1970.
303. Mizgala CL, Quamme GQ: Renal handling of phosphate. Physiol Rev 65:431–466, 1985.
304. Quamme GA, Shapiro RJ: Membrane controls of epithelial phosphate transport. Can J Physiol Pharmacol 65:275–286, 1987.
305. Murer H, Werner A, Reshkin S, et al: Cellular mechanisms in proximal tubular reabsorption of inorganic phosphate. Am J Physiol 260:C885–C899, 1991.
306. Collip JB: The excretion of a parathyroid hormone which will prevent or control parathyroid tetany and which regulates the level of blood calcium. J Biol Chem 63:395, 1925.
307. Albright F, Bauer W, Ropes M, et al: Studies of calcium and phosphorus metabolism IV. The effect of the parathyroid hormone. J Clin Invest 7:139, 1929.
308. Ellsworth R, Howard JE: Studies on the physiology of parathyroid glands. VII. Some responses of normal human kidneys and blood to intravenous parathyroid extract. Bull Johns Hopkins Hosp 55:296, 1934.
309. Wen SF: Micropuncture studies of phosphate transport in the proximal tubule of the dog: The relationship to sodium reabsorption. J Clin Invest 53:143, 1974.
310. Trohler U, Bonjour JP, Fleisch H: Inorganic phosphate homeostasis: Renal adaptation to the dietary intake in intact and thyroparathyroidectomized rats. J Clin Invest 57:264–273, 1976.
311. Agus ZS, Gardner LB, Beck LH, Goldberg M: Effects of parathyroid hormone on renal tubular reabsorption of calcium, sodium, and phosphate. Am J Physiol 224:1143–1148, 1973.
312. Hammerman MR, Karl IE, Hruska KA: Regulation of canine renal vesicle Pi transport by growth hormone and parathyroid hormone. Biochim Biophys Acta 603:322–335, 1980.
313. Agus ZS, Puschett JB, Senesky D, Goldberg M: Mode of action of parathyroid hormone and cyclic adenosine-5-monophosphate on renal tubular phosphate reabsorption in the dog. J Clin Invest 50:617–626, 1971.
314. Brunette MG, Taleb L, Carriere S: Effect of parathyroid hormone on phosphate reabsorption along the nephron at the rat. Am J Physiol 225:1076–1081, 1973.
315. Knox FG, Lecheme C: Distal site of action of parathyroid hormone on phosphate reabsorption. Am J Physiol 229:1556–1560, 1975.
316. Pullman T, Lavender AR, Aho I, Rasmussen H: Direct renal action of a purified parathyroid extract. Endocrinology 67:570–582, 1960.
317. Hiatt HH, Thompson DD: The effects of parathyroid extract on renal function in man. J Clin Invest 36:557–565, 1956.
318. Evers J, Murer H, Kinne R: Effect of parathyrin on the transport properties of isolated renal brush-border vesicles. Biochem J 172:49–56, 1978.
319. Lang RP, Yanagawa N, Nord EP, et al: Nucleotide inhibition of phosphate transport in the renal proximal tubule. Am J Physiol 245:F263–F271, 1983.
320. Strickler JC, Thompson DD, Klose RM, Giebisch G: Micropuncture study of inorganic phosphate excretion in the rat. J Clin Invest 43:1596–1606, 1964.
321. Pastoriza-Munoz E, Mishler DR, Lechene C: Effect of phosphate deprivation on phosphate reabsorption in rat nephron: Role of PTH. Am J Physiol 244:F140–F149, 1983.
322. Greger R, Lang F, Marchand G, Knox FG: Site of renal phosphate reabsorption. Micropuncture and microinfusion study. Pflugers Arch 369:111–118, 1977.
323. Chabardes D, Gagnon Brunette M, et al: Adenylate cyclase responsiveness to hormones in various portions of the human nephron. J Clin Invest 65:439–448, 1980.
324. Morel F: Sites of hormone action in the mammalian nephron. Am J Physiol 240:F159–F164, 1981.
325. Yang T, Hassan S, Huang YG, et al: Expression of PTHrP, PTH/PTHrP receptor, and Ca(2+)-sensing receptor mRNAs along the rat nephron. Am J Physiol 272(6 pt 2):F751–F758, 1997.
326. Lotscher M, Scarpetta Y, Levi M, et al: Rapid downregulation of rat renal Na/P(i) cotransporter in response to parathyroid hormone involves microtubule rearrangement. J Clin Invest 104:483–494, 1999.
327. Takahashi F, Morita K, Katai K, et al: Effects of dietary Pi on the renal Na^+-dependent Pi transporter NaPi-2 in thyroparathyroidectomized rats. Biochem J 333(pt 1):175–181, 1998.
328. Goldfarb S, Westby GR, Goldberg M, Agus ZS: Renal tubular effects of chronic phosphate depletion. J Clin Invest 59:770, 1977.
329. Steele TH, DeLuca HF: Influence of dietary phosphorus on renal phosphate reabsorption in the parathyroidectomized rat. J Clin Invest 57:867–874, 1976.
330. Crawford JD, Osborne MMJ, Talbot NG, et al: The parathyroid glands and phosphorus homeostasis. J Clin Invest 29:1448, 1950.
331. Chambers EL Jr, Gordan GS, Goldman L, Reifenstein EC Jr: Tests for hyperparathyroidism: Tubular reabsorption of phosphate, phosphate deprivation and calcium infusion. J Clin Endocrinol Metab 16:1507, 1956.
332. McCrory WW, Forman C, McNamara H, et al: Renal excretion of inorganic phosphate in newborn infants. J Clin Invest 31:357, 1952.
333. Caverzasio J, Bonjour JP: Mechanism of rapid phosphate (Pi) transport adaptation to a single low Pi meal in rat renal brush border membranes. Pflugers Arch 404:227–231, 1985.
334. Thompson DD, Hiatt HH: Effect of phosphate loading and depletion on the renal excretion and reabsorption of inorganic phosphate. J Clin Invest 36:566–572, 1957.
335. Cuisinier-Gleizes P, Thomasset M, Sainteny F, Mathieu H: Phosphorus deficiency, parathyroid hormone and bone resorption in the growing rat. Calcif Tissue Res 20:235–249, 1976.
336. Dominguez JH, Gray RW, Lemann J: Dietary phosphate deprivation in women and men: Effects on mineral and acid balances, parathyroid hormone and the metabolism of 25-OH-vitamin D. J Clin Endocrinol Metab 43:1056–1068, 1976.
337. Drake TG, Albright F, Castleman B: Parathyroid hyperplasia in rabbits produced by parenteral phosphate administration. J Clin Invest 16:203, 1937.
338. Lotscher M, Wilson P, Ngyuen S, et al: New aspects of adaptation of rat renal Na-Pi cotransporter to alterations in dietary phosphate. Kidney Int 49:1012–1018, 1996.
339. Frick A, Durasin I: Maximal reabsorptive capacity for inorganic phosphate (Tm_{pi}) in the absence of parathyroid hormone in the rat: Decrease of the Tm_{pi} during prolonged administration of phosphate and the role of calcium. Pflugers Arch 377:9–14, 1978.
340. Oberleithner H, Greger R, Lang F: Role of calcium in the decline of phosphate reabsorption during phosphate loading in acutely thyroparathyroidectomized rats. Pflugers Arch 374:249–254, 1978.
341. Wong NLM, Quamme GA, O'Callaghan TJ, et al: Renal tubular transport in phosphate depletion, a micropuncture study. Can J Physiol Pharmacol 58:1063–1071, 1980.
342. Knox FG, Haas JA, Haramati A: Nephron sites of adaptation to changes in dietary phosphate. Adv Exp Med Biol 151:13–19, 1982.
343. Brautbar N, Walling MW, Coburn JW: Interaction between vitamin D deficiency and phosphorus depletion in the rat. J Clin Invest 63:335, 1979.
344. Brazy PC, McKeown JW, Harris RH, Dennis VW: Comparative effects of dietary phosphate, unilateral nephrectomy, and parathyroid hormone on phosphate transport by the rabbit proximal tubule. Kidney Int 17:778–880, 1980.
345. Kreusser WJ, Kurokawa K, Aznar E, Massry SG: Phosphate depletion. Miner Electrolyte Metab 5:30, 1978.
346. Stoll R, Kinne R, Murer H, et al: Phosphate transport by rat renal brush border membrane vesicles: Influence of dietary phosphate, thyroparathyroidectomy and 1,25-dihydroxyvitamin D_3. Pflugers Arch 380:47–52, 1979.
347. Kempson SA, Curthoys NP: NAD_+-dependent ADP-ribosyltransferase in renal brush-border membranes. Am J Physiol 245:C449–C456, 1983.
348. Quamme GA, Biber J, Murer H: Sodium-phosphate cotransport in OK cells: Inhibition by PTH and adaptation to low phosphate. Am J Physiol 257:F957–F973, 1989.
349. Levine BS, Ho K, Hodsman A, et al: Early renal brush border membrane adaptation to dietary phosporus. Miner Electrolyte Metab 10:222–227, 1984.
350. Brunette MG, Chan M, Muag U, Beliveau R: Phosphate uptake by superficial and deep nephron brush-border membranes. Effect of dietary phosphate and parathyroid hormone. Pfluegers Arch 400:356–362, 1984.
351. Murer H, Stern H, Burckhardt G, et al: Sodium dependent transport of inorganic phosphate across the renal brush border membrane. Adv Exp Med Biol 128:11–23, 1980.
352. Lotscher M, Kaissling B, Biber J, et al: Role of microtubules in the rapid regulation

of renal phosphate transport in response to acute alterations in dietary phosphate content. J Clin Invest 99:1302–1312, 1997.
353. Ritthaler T, Traebert M, Lotscher M, et al: Effects of phosphate intake on distribution of type II Na/Pi cotransporter mRNA in rat kidney. Kidney Int 55:976–983, 1999.
354. Howard JE, Hopkins T, Connor T, et al: On certain physiologic responses to intravenous injection of calcium salts into normal, hyperparathyroid and hypoparathyroid persons. J Clin Endocrinol Metab 13:1, 1953.
355. Nordin BEC, Fraser R: The effect of intravenous calcium on phosphate excretion. Clin Sci (Colch) 13:477, 1954.
356. Hiatt HH, Thompson DD: Some effects of intravenously administered calcium on inorganic phosphate metabolism. J Clin Invest 36:573, 1957.
357. Eisenberg E: Effects of serum calcium level and parathyroid extracts on phosphate and calcium excretion in hypoparathyroid patients. J Clin Invest 44:942, 1965.
358. Pak CYC: Parathyroid hormone and thyrocalcitonin: Their mode of action and regulation. Ann N Y Acad Sci 179:450, 1971.
359. Bernstein D, Kleeman C, Rockney R, et al: Studies of the renal clearance of phosphate and the role of parathyroid glands in its regulation. J Clin Endocrinol Metab 22:641, 1962.
360. Amiel C, Kuntziger H, Couette S, et al: Evidence for a parathyroid hormone–independent calcium modulation of phosphate transport along the nephron. J Clin Invest 57:256–263, 1976.
361. Edwards BR, Sutton RAL, Dirks JH: Effect of calcium infusion on renal tubular reabsorption in the dog. Am J Physiol 227:13, 1974.
362. Goldfarb S, Bosanac P, Goldberg M, Agus ZS: Effects of calcium on renal tubular phosphate reabsorption. Am J Physiol 234:22, 1978.
363. Schussler GC, Verso MA, Nemoto T: Phosphaturia in hypercalcemic breast cancer patients. J Clin Endocrinol Metab 35:497–504, 1972.
364. Pearce SH, Williamson C, Kifor O, et al: A familial syndrome of hypocalcemia with hypercalciuria due to mutations in the calcium-sensing receptor [see comments]. N Engl J Med 335:1115–1122, 1996.
365. Gerkle C, Stroder J, Rostock D: The effect of vitamin D on renal inorganic phosphate reabsorption of normal rats, parathyroidectomized rats, and rats with rickets. Pediatr Res 5:40–52, 1971.
366. Morgan DB, Paterson CR, Woods CG, et al: Osteomalacia after gastrectomy: A response to very small doses of vitamin D. Lancet 2:1089, 1965.
367. Muhlbauer RC, Bonjour JP, Fleisch H: Tubular handling of Pi, localization of effects of $1,25(OH)_2D_3$ and dietary Pi in TPTX rats. Am J Physiol 241:F123–F128, 1981.
368. Liang CT, Barnes J, Balakir R, et al: *In vitro* stimulation of phosphate uptake in isolated chick renal cells by 1,25-dihydroxycholecalciferol. Proc Natl Acad Sci U S A 79:3532, 1982.
369. Kurnik BRC, Hruska KA: Effects of 1,25-dihydroxycholecalciferal on phosphate transport in vitamin D–dependent rats. Am J Physiol 247:F177–F182, 1984.
370. Taketani Y, Segawa H, Chikamori M, et al: Regulation of type II renal Na^+-dependent inorganic phosphate transporters by 1,25-dihydroxyvitamin D3. Identification of a vitamin D–responsive element in the human NAPi-3 gene. J Biol Chem 273:14575–14581, 1998.
371. Suzuki M, Kawaguchi Y, Momose M, et al: 1,25 Dihydroxyvitamin D stimulates sodium-dependent phosphate transport by renal outer cortical brush-border membrane vesicles by directly affecting membrane fluidity. Biochem Biophys Res Commun 150:1193–1198, 1988.
372. Puschett JB, Beck WS, Jelonek A, Fernandez PC: Study of the renal tubular interaction of thyrocalcitonin, cyclic adenosine 3′,5′-monophosphate, 25-hydroxycholecalciferol and calcium ion. J Clin Invest 53:756, 1974.
373. Lemann J, Litzow JR, Lennon EJ: Studies of the mechanism by which chronic metabolic acidosis augments urinary calcium excretion in man. J Clin Invest 46:1318–1328, 1967.
374. Kempson SA: Effect of metabolic acidosis on renal brush border membrane adaptation to low phosphorus diet. Kidney Int 22:225–233, 1982.
375. Levine BS, Ho K, Kraut JA, et al: Effect of metabolic acidosis on phosphate transport by the renal brush border membrane. Biochim Biophys Acta 727:7–12, 1983.
376. Quamme GA: Effects of metabolic acidosis, alkalosis and dietary hydrogen ion intake on phosphate transport in the proximal convoluted tubule. Am J Physiol 249:F769–F779, 1985.
377. Hulter HN: Hypophosphaturia impairs the renal defense against metabolic acidosis. Kidney Int 26:302–307, 1984.
378. Ambuhl PM, Zajicek HK, Wang H, et al: Regulation of renal phosphate transport by acute and chronic metabolic acidosis in the rat. Kidney Int 53:1288–1298, 1998.
379. Webb RK, Woodhall PB, Tisher CC, et al: Relationship between phosphaturia and acute hypercapnia in the rat. J Clin Invest 60:829–837, 1977.
380. Quamme GA, Wong NLM: Effect of hypercalcemia and luminal pH on phosphate transport in the proximal tubule of the rat. Kidney Int 17:748, 1980.
381. Quamme GA, Wong NLM: Phosphate transport in the proximal convoluted tubule: Effect of intraluminal pH. Am J Physiol 246:F323–F333, 1984.
382. Quamme GA: Urinary alkalinization may not result in an increase in urinary phosphate excretion. Kidney Int 25:152, 1984.
383. Steele TH: Bicarbonate-induced phosphaturia: Dependence upon the magnitude of phosphate reabsorption. Pflugers Arch 370:291–294, 1977.
384. Tucker RR, Berndt TJ, Thotharthri V, et al: Propranolol blocks the hypophosphaturia of acute respiratory alkalosis in human subjects. J Lab Clin Med 128:423–428, 1996.
385. Sorensen DH, Hindberg I: The acute and prolonged effect of porcine calcitonin on urine electrolyte excretion in intact and parathyroidectomized rats. Acta Endocrinol 70:295, 1972.
386. Bijvoet OLM, Froeling PGAM: Calcitonin, parathyroid hormone and the kidney. *In* Frame B, Parfitt AM, Duncan H (eds): Clinical Aspects of Metabolic Bone Disease. International Conference Series 270. Amsterdam, Excerpta Medica, 1973, 184.
387. Lang R: Renal handling of calcium and phosphate. Klin Wochenschr 58:985–1003, 1980.
388. Schwartz E, Wiedemann E, Simon S, et al: Estrogenic antagonism of metabolic effects of administered growth hormone. J Clin Endocrinol Metab 29:1176, 1969.
389. Corvilain J, Abramow M: Growth and renal control of plasma phosphate. J Clin Endocrinol Metab 34:452, 1972.
390. Corvilain J, Abramow M: Effect of growth hormone on tubular transport of phosphate in normal and parathyroidectomized dogs. J Clin Invest 43:1608, 1964.
391. Gertner JM, Horst RL, Broadus AE, et al: Parathyroid function and vitamin D metabolism during human growth hormone replacement. J Clin Endocrinol Metab 49:185–187, 1979.
392. Westby GR, Goldfarb S, Goldberg M, Agus ZS: Acute effects of bovine growth hormone on renal calcium and phosphate excretion. Metabolism 26:525–530, 1977.
393. Hammerman M: The growth hormone-insulin-like growth factor axis in the kidney. Am J Physiol 257:F503–F514, 1989.
394. de Boer H, Blok GJ, Popp-Snijders C, et al: Intestinal calcium absorption and bone metabolism in young adult men with childhood-onset growth hormone deficiency. J Bone Min Res 13:245–252, 1998.
395. Roberts KE, Randall HT: The effect of adrenal steroids on renal mechanisms of electrolyte excretion. Ann N Y Acad Sci 61:306, 1955.
396. Anderson J, Foster JB: The effect of cortisone on urinary phosphate excretion in man. Clin Sci (Colch) 18:437–439, 1959.
397. Frick A, Durasin I, Neuweg M: Phosphaturic response of hydrocortisone in the presence and the absence of parathyroid hormone. Pflugers Arch 392:99–105, 1981.
398. Durasin I, Frick A, Neuweg M: Glucocorticoid-induced inhibition of the reabsorption of inorganic phosphate in the proximal tubule in the absence of parathyroid hormone. Renal Physiol 7:115–123, 1984.
399. Turner ST, Kiebzak GM, Dousa TP: Mechanism of glucocorticoid effect of renal transport of phosphate. Am J Physiol 243:C227–C236, 1982.
400. Freiberg JM, Kinsella J, Sacktor B: Glucocorticoids increase the Na^+-H^+ exchange and decrease the Na^+-gradient–dependent phosphate uptake system in renal brush border membrane vesicles. Proc Natl Acad Sci U S A 79:4932–4936, 1982.
401. Prabhu S, Levi M, Dwarakanath V, et al: Effect of glucocorticoids on neonatal rabbit renal cortical sodium–inorganic phosphate messenger RNA and protein abundance. Pediatr Res 41:20–24, 1997.
402. Hammerman MR, Hruska KA: Cyclic AMP–dependent protein phosphorylation in canine renal brush border membrane vesicles is associated with decreased phosphate transport. J Biol Chem 257:992–999, 1982.
403. Donaldson IA, Nassim JR: The artificial menopause with particular reference to the occurrence of spinal porosis. BMJ 1:1228, 1954.
404. Stock JL, Coderre JA, Mallette LE: Effects of a short course of estrogen on mineral metabolism in postmenopausal women. J Clin Endocrinol Metab 61:595–600, 1985.
405. Aitken JM, Hart DM, Smith DA: The effect of long-term mestranol administration on calcium and phosphorus homeostasis in oophorectomized women. Clin Sci (Colch) 41:233, 1971.
406. Riggs BL, Jowsey J, Goldsmith RS, et al: Short and long-term effects of estrogen and synthetic anabolic hormones in postmenopausal osteoporosis. J Clin Invest 51:1659, 1972.
407. Schwartz E, Echemendia E, Schiffer M, et al: Mechanism of estrogenic action in acromegaly. J Clin Invest 48:260, 1969.
408. Espinosa RE, Keller MJ, Yusufi ANK, Dousa TP: Effects of thyroxine administration on phosphate transport across renal cortical brush border membrane. Am J Physiol 246:F133–F139, 1984.
409. Alcalde AI, Sarasa M, Raldua D, et al: Role of thyroid hormone in regulation of renal phosphate transport in young and aged rats. Endocrinology 140:1544–1551, 1999.
410. Parsons V, Anderson J: The maximum renal tubular reabsorptive rate for inorganic phophate in thyrotoxicosis. Clin Sci (Colch) 27:313–318, 1964.
411. Adams PH, Jowsey J, Kelly P, et al: Effects of hyperthyroidism on bone and mineral metabolism in man. Q J Med 36:1, 1967.
412. McCaffrey C, Quamme GA: Effects of thyroid status on renal calcium and magnesium handling. Can J Comp Med 48:51–57, 1984.
413. DeFronzo RA, Goldberg M, Agus ZS: The effect of glucose and insulin on renal electrolyte transport. J Clin Invest 58:83–90, 1976.
414. Hammerman MR, Rogers S, Hansen VA, Gavin JR III: Insulin stimulated Pi transport in brush border vesicles from proximal tubular segments. Am J Physiol 247:E616–E624, 1984.
415. Staub A, Springs V, Stoll F, et al: A renal action of glucagon. Proc Soc Exp Biol Med 1957;94:57.
416. Massara F, Tagliabue M, Martina V, Molinatti GM: Glucagon-induced hypophosphatemia is mediated by insulin. Horm Metab Res 14:674–675, 1982.
417. Eisinger AJ, Jones NF, Barraclough MA, et al: Effect of vasopressin on the renal excretion of phosphate in man. Clin Sci (Colch) 39:687, 1970.
418. Hammond TG, Yusufi ANK, Knox FG, Dousa TP: Administration of atrial natriuretic factor inhibits sodium-coupled transport in proximal tubules. J Clin Invest 75:1983–1989, 1985.
419. Brodehl J, Gellissen K: Der Einfluss des Angiotensins II auf die tubuläre Phosphatrückresorption beim Menschen. Ein Beitrag zum Wirkungsmechanismus des Angiotensins. Klin Wochenschr 44:1171, 1966.
420. Maesaka JK, Levitt MF, Abramson RG: Effect of saline infusion on phosphate transport in intact and thyroparathyroidectomized rats. Am J Physiol 225:1421–1429, 1973.
421. Body J, Cryer PE, Offord KP, Heath H III: Epinephrine is a hypophosphatemic hormone in man. J Clin Invest 71:572–578, 1983.
422. Cuche JL, Marchand GR, Greger RF, et al: Phosphaturic effect of dopamine in dogs: Possible role of intrarenally produced dopamine in phosphate regulation. J Clin Invest 58:71–76, 1976.
423. Schneider EG, Strandhoy JW, Willis LR, Knox FG: Relationship between proximal sodium reabsorption and excretion of calcium, magnesium and phosphate. Kidney Int 4:369–376, 1973.
424. Herbert CS, Rouse D, Eknoyan G, et al: Decreased phosphate reabsorption by volume expansion in the dog. Kidney Int 2:247–252, 1972.
425. Schneider EG, Goldsmith RS, Arnaud CD, Knox FG: Role of parathyroid hormone in the phosphaturia of extracellular fluid volume expansion. Kidney Int 7:317–324, 1975.

426. Steel TH: Increased urinary phosphate excretion following volume expansion in normal man. Metabolism 19:129–139, 1970.
427. Knox FG, Schneider EG, Willis LR, et al: Proximal tubular reabsorption after hyperoncotic albumin infusion. J Clin Invest 53:501–508, 1974.
428. Whang R, Welt LG: Observations in experimental magnesium depletion. J Clin Invest 42:305, 1963.
429. Shils ME: Experimental human magnesium depletion. Medicine (Baltimore) 48:61, 1969.
430. Suh SM, Tashjian AH Jr, Matsuo N, et al: Pathogenesis of hypocalcemia and primary hypomagnesemia: Normal end-organ responsiveness to parathyroid hormone, impaired parathyroid gland function. J Clin Invest 52:153, 1973.
431. Anast CS, Winnacker JL, Forte LR, et al: Impaired release of parathyroid hormone in magnesium deficiency. J Clin Endocrinol Metab 42:707, 1976.
432. Rude RK, Oldham SB, Singer FR: Functional hypoparathyroidism and parathyroid hormone end-organ resistance in human magnesium deficiency. Clin Endocrinol 5:209, 1976.
433. Estep H, Shaw WA, Watlington C, et al: Hypocalcemia due to hypomagnesemia and reversible parathyroid hormone unresponsiveness. J Clin Endocrinol 29:842–848, 1969.
434. Chase LR, Slatopolsky E: Secretion and metabolic efficacy of parathyroid hormone in patients with severe hypomagnesemia. J Clin Endocrinol Metab 38:363, 1974.
435. Gitelman HJ, Kukolj S, Welt LG: Inhibition of parathyroid gland activity by hypermagnesemia. Am J Physiol 215:483–485, 1968.
436. Donovan EF, Tsang RC, Steichen JJ, et al: Neonatal hypermagnesemia: Effect on parathyroid hormone and calcium homeostasis. J Pediatr 96:305–310, 1980.
437. Mahler RF, Stanbury SW: Potassium-losing renal disease. Q J Med 25:21, 1956.
438. Anderson DC, Peters TJ, Stewart WK, et al: Association of hypokalemia and hypophosphatemia. BMJ 4:402, 1969.
439. Beck N, Davis BB: Impaired renal response to parathyroid hormone in potassium depletion. Am J Physiol 228:179, 1975.
440. Beck N, et al: Inhibition of carbonic anhydrase by parathyroid hormone and cyclic AMP in rat renal cortex *in vitro*. J Clin Invest 55:149, 1975.
441. Knox FG, et al: Effect of parathyroid hormone on phosphate reabsorption in the presence of acetazolamide. Kidney Int 10:211, 1976.
442. Steele TH: Dual effect of potent diuretics on renal handling of phosphate in man. Metabolism 20:749, 1971.
443. Maesaka JK, et al: Effect of mannitol on phosphate transport in intact and acutely thyroparathyroidectomized rats. J Lab Clin Med 87:680, 1976.
444. Pascale LR, Dubin A, Hoffman WS: Influence of Benemid on urinary excretion of phosphate in hypoparathyroidism. Metabolism 3:462, 1954.
445. Becker RR, et al: The hyperphosphatemic effect of disodium ethane-1-hydroxy-1, 1-diphosphonate (EHDP): Renal handling of phosphorus and the renal response to parathyroid hormone. J Lab Clin Invest 81:258, 1973.
446. Walton RJ, Russell RGG, Smith R: Changes in the renal and extrarenal handling of phosphate induced by disodium etidronate (EHDP) in man. Clin Sci Mol Med 49:45–56, 1975.
447. Bijvoet OLM, et al: The renal phosphate threshold: Its evaluation and application in different clinical conditions. *In* de Graeff J, Leynse B, (eds): Water and Electrolyte Metabolism II. Amsterdam, Elsevier, 1974.
448. Stanbury SW, et al: Elective subtotal parathyroidectomy for renal hyperparathyroidism. Lancet 1:793, 1960.
449. Slatopolsky E, et al: Control of phosphate excretion in uremic man. J Clin Invest 47:1865, 1968.
450. Kleeman CR, et al: Calcium and phosphorus metabolism and bone disease in uremia. Clin Orthop 68:210, 1970.
451. Slatopolsky E, Calgar S, Pennell JP, et al: On the pathogenesis of hyperparathyroidism in chronic experimental renal insufficiency in the dog. J Clin Invest 50:492–506, 1971.
452. Slatopolsky E, Rutherford WE, Rosenbaum R, et al: Hyperphosphatemia. Clin Nephrol 7:138–146, 1977.
453. McConnell TH: Fatal hypocalcemia from phosphate absorption from laxative preparation. JAMA 216:147–148, 1971.
454. Zusman J, Brown DM, Nesbit ME: Hyperphosphatemia, hyperphosphaturia and hypocalcemia in acute lymphoblastic leukemia. N Engl J Med 289:1335, 1973.
455. Chesney RW, Houghton PB: Tetany following phosphate enemas in chronic renal disease. Am J Dis Child 127:584–586, 1974.
456. Oxnard SA, O'Bell J, Grupe WE: Severe tetany in an azotemic child related to a sodium phosphate enema. Pediatrics 53:105–106, 1974.
457. Brereton HD, Anderson T, Johnson RE, et al: Hyperphosphatemia and hypocalcemia in Burkitt's lymphoma. Arch Intern Med 135:307, 1975.
458. O'Connor LR, Klein KL, Bethune JE: Hyperphosphatemia in lactic acidosis. N Engl J Med 297:707–709, 1977.
459. Tsokos GL, Balow JE, Spiegel RJ, Magrath IT: Renal and metabolic complication of undifferentiated and lymphoblastic lymphomas. Medicine (Baltimore) 60:218–229, 1981.
460. Cervantes F, Ribera JM, Granena A, et al: Tumor lysis syndrome with hypocalcemia in accelerated chronic granulocytic leukemia. Acta Haematol 68:157–159, 1982.
461. Nanji AA: Symptomatic hypocalcemia due to hyperphosphatemia associated with alcoholic ketoacidosis. South Med J 77:542, 1984.
462. Biberstein M, Parker BA: Enema induced hyperphosphatemia. Am J Med 79:645–646, 1985.
463. Burnett CH, Commons RR, Albright F, Howard JE: Hypercalcemia without hypercalciuria or hypophosphatemia, calcinosis and renal insufficiency. N Engl J Med 240:787–794, 1947.
464. McMillan DE, Freeman RB: The milk-alkali syndrome: A study of the acute disorder with comment on the development of the chronic condition. Medicine (Baltimore) 44:484–501, 1964.
465. Chernow B, Rainey TG, Georges LP, O'Brian JT: Iatrogenic hyperphosphatemia: A metabolic consideration in critical care medicine. Crit Care Med 9:772–774, 1981.
466. Carroll PR, Clark OH: Milk alkali syndrome. Does it exist and can it be differentiated from primary hyperparathyroidism? Ann Surg 197:427–433, 1983.
467. Kirschbaum B: The acidosis of exogenous phosphate intoxication. Arch Intern Med 158:405–408, 1998.
468. Goldman R, Bassett SH: Effects of intravenous calcium gluconate upon the excretion of calcium and phophorus in patients with idiopathic hypoparathyroidism. J Clin Endocrinol Metab 14:278, 1954.
469. Verbanck M, Toppet N: Study of the regulation of phosphorus metabolism in a hypoparathyroid patient. Effect of calcemia on the urinary excretion of phosphorus and on the variations of serum phosphorus. Rev Fr Etud Clin Biol 6:239–251, 1961.
470. Okano K, Furukawa Y, Hirotoshi M, Fujita T: Comparative efficacy of various vitamin D metabolites in the treatment of various types of hypoparathyroidism. J Clin Endocrinol Metab 55:238–242, 1982.
471. Corvilain J, Abramow M: Some effects of human growth hormone on renal hemodynamics and on tubular phosphate transport in man. J Clin Invest 41:1230–1235, 1962.
472. Bijvoet OLM, Nollen AJ, Slooff TJ, et al: Effect of a diphosphonate on para-articular ossification after total hip replacement. Acta Orthop Scand 45:926, 1974.
473. Mandry J, Posner M, Tucci J, Eil C: Hyperphosphatemia in multiple myeloma due to a phosphate-binding immunoglobulin. Cancer 68:1092–1094, 1991.
474. Larner AJ: Pseudohyperphosphatemia. Clin Biochem 28:391–393, 1995.
475. Lufkin EG, Wilson EM, Smith LH, et al: Phosphorus excretion in tumoral calcinosis: Response to parathyroid hormone and acetazolamide. J Clin Endocrinol Metab 50:648–653, 1980.
476. Mitnick PD, Goldfarb S, Slatopolsky E, et al: Calcium and phosphate metabolism in tumoral calcinosis. Ann Intern Med 92:482–487, 1980.
477. Zerwekh JE, Sanders LA, Townsend J, Pak CYC: Tumoral calcinosis: Evidence for concurrent defects in renal tubular phosphorus transport and in 1 α,25-dihydroxycholecalciferol synthesis. Calcif Tissue Int 32:56, 1980.
478. Prince MG, Schaefer PC, Goldsmith RS, Chausmer AB: Hyperphosphatemic tumoral calcinosis: Association with elevation of serum 1,25-dihydroxycholecalciferol concentration. Ann Intern Med 96:586–591, 1982.
479. Lufkin EG, Kumar R, Heath H III: Hyperphosphatemic tumoral calcinosis: Effects of phosphate depletion on vitamin D metabolism, and of acute hypocalcemia on parathyroid hormone secretion and action. J Clin Endocrinol Metab 56:1319–1322, 1983.
480. Mikati MA, Melhem RE, Najjar SS: The syndrome of hyperostosis and hyperphosphatemia. Pediatrics 99:900–904, 1981.
481. Clarke E, Swischuk LE, Hayden CK Jr: Tumoral calcinosis, diaphysitis and hyperphosphatemia. Radiology 151:643–646, 1984.
482. Yamaguchi T, Sugimoto T, Imai Y, et al: Successful treatment of hyperphosphatemic tumoral calcinosis with long-term acetazolamide. Bone 16(4 suppl):247S–250S, 1995.
483. Hebert LA, Lemann J Jr, Petersen JR, Lennon EJ: Studies of the mechanism by which phosphate infusion lowers serum calcium concentration. J Clin Invest 45:1886–1894, 1966.
484. Cohen L, Balow J, Magrath I, et al: Acute tumor lysis syndrome. A review of 37 patients with Burkitt's lymphoma. Am J Med 68:486–491, 1980.
485. Dunlay R, Camp M, Allon M, et al: Calcitriol in prolonged hypocalcemia due to the tumor lysis syndrome. Ann Intern Med 110:162–164, 1989.
486. Armata J, Depowska T: Hyperphosphatemia and hypocalcemia in neoplastic disorders. N Engl J Med 290:858, 1974.
487. Schilsky RL: Renal and metabolic toxicities of cancer chemotherapy. Semin Oncol 9:75–83, 1982.
488. Libnoch JA, Ajlouni K, Millman WL, et al: Acute myelofibrosis and malignant hypercalcemia. Am J Med 62:432–438, 1977.
489. Kanfer A, Richet G, Roland J, Chatelet F: Extreme hyperphosphatemia causing acute anuric nephrocalcinosis in lymphosarcoma. BMJ 1:1320, 1979.
490. Venkataraman PS, Tsang RC, Greer FR, et al: Late infantile tetany and secondary hyperparathyroidism in infants fed humanized cow milk formula. Am J Dis Child 139:664–668, 1985.
491. Lotz M, Zisman E, Bartter FC: Evidence for a phosphorus depletion syndrome in man. N Engl J Med 278:409–415, 1968.
492. Bloom WL, Flinchum D: Osteomalacia with pseudofractures caused by ingestion of aluminum hydroxide. JAMA 174:1327–1330, 1960.
493. Boelens PA, Norwood W, Kjellstrand C, et al: Hypophosphatemia with muscle weakness due to antacids and hemodialysis. Am J Dis Child 120:350–353, 1970.
494. Sherman RA, Hwang ER, Walker JA, Eisineer RP: Reduction in serum phosphorus due to sucralfate. Am J Gastroenterol 78:210–211, 1983.
495. Spencer H, Lewin I, Samachson J, et al: Changes in metabolism in obese persons during starvation. Am J Med 40:27, 1966.
496. Lyles KW, Berry WR, Haussler M, et al: Hypophosphatemic osteomalacia: Association with prostatic carcinoma. Ann Intern Med 93:275–278, 1980.
497. Ryan EA, Reiss E: Oncogenous osteomalacia: Review of the world literature of 42 cases and report of two new cases. Am J Med 77:501–512, 1984.
498. Miyauchi A, Fukase M, Tsutsumi M, Fujita T: Hemangiopericytoma-induced osteomalacia: Tumor transplantation in nude mice causes hypophosphatemia and tumor extracts inhibit renal 25-hydroxyvitamin D 1-hydroxylase activity. J Clin Endocrinol Metab 67:46–53, 1988.
499. Cai Q, Hodgson S, Kao P, et al: Inhibition of renal phosphate transport by a tumor product in a patient with oncogenic osteomalacia. N Engl J Med 330:1645–1649, 1994.
500. Klein G, Dallas J, Hawkins H, et al: Congenital linear sebaceous nevus syndrome. J Bone Miner Res 13:1056–1057, 1998.
501. Lloyd SE, Gunther W, Pearce SH, et al: Characterisation of renal chloride channel, CLCN5, mutations in hypercalciuric nephrolithiasis (kidney stones) disorders. Hum Mol Genet 6:1233–1239, 1997.
502. Sliman GA, Winters WD, Shaw DW, Avner ED: Hypercalciuria and nephrocalcinosis in the oculocerebrorenal syndrome. J Urol 153:1244–1246, 1995.
503. Tieder M, Modai D, Shaked U, et al: "Idiopathic" hypercalciuria and hereditary hypophosphatemic rickets. N Engl J Med 316:125–129, 1987.
504. Scriver C, MacDonald W, Reade T, et al: Hypophosphatemic nonrachitic bone disease: An entity distinct from X-linked hypophosphatemia in the renal defect, bone involvement, and inheritance. Am J Med Genet 1:101–117, 1977.

505. Econs M, McEnery P: Autosomal dominant hypophosphatemic rickets/osteomalacia: Clinical characterization of a novel renal phosphate-wasting disorder. J Clin Endocrinol Metab 82:674–681, 1997.
506. Dash T, Parker M, Lafayette R: Profound hypophosphatemia and isolated hyperphosphaturia in two cases of multiple myeloma. Am J Kidney Dis 29:445–448, 1997.
507. Konishi K, Nakamura M, Yamakawa H, et al: Case report: hypophosphatemic osteomalacia in von Recklinghausen neurofibromatosis. Am J Med Sci 301:322–328, 1991.
508. Raskin P, Pak CYC: The effect of chronic insulin therapy on phosphate metabolism in diabetes mellitus. Diabetologica 21:50–53, 1981.
509. Black DAK, Milne MD: Experimental potassium depletion in man. Clin Sci (Colch) 11:397, 1952.
510. Dillon MJ, Shah V, Mitchell MD: Bartter's syndrome: 10 cases in childhood. Q J Med 48:429–446, 1979.
511. Nordin BEC, Peacock M: Role of kidney in regulation of plasma calcium. Lancet 2:1280–1283, 1969.
512. Jubiz W, Canterbury JM, Reiss E, et al: Circadian rhythm in serum parathyroid hormone concentration in human subjects: Correlation with serum calcium, phosphate, albumin and growth hormone levels. J Clin Invest 51:2040, 1972.
513. Bijvoet OLM, Morgan DB: *In* Hioco DJ (ed): Phosphate et Métabolisme Phosphocalicique. Paris, L'Expansion Scientifique Francaise, 1971, p 153.
514. Levy L: Severe hypophosphatemia as a complication of the treatment of hypothermia. Arch Intern Med 140:128–129, 1980.
515. Sprung GL, Portocarrero CJ, Fernaine AV, Weinberg PF: The metabolic and respiratory alterations of heat stroke. Arch Intern Med 140:665–669, 1980.
516. Guntupalli KK, Sladen A, Selker RG, et al: Effects of induced total-body hyperthermia on phosphorus metabolism in humans. Am J Med 77:250–254, 1984.
517. Bouchama A, Cafege A, Robertson W, et al: Mechanisms of hypophosphatemia in heat stroke. J Appl Physiol 71:328–332, 1991.
518. Citrin DL, Elson P, Kies MS, Lind R: Decreased serum phosphate levels after high dose estrogens in metastatic prostate cancer. Am J Med 76:787, 1984.
519. Wallach S, Cahill L, Rogan F, et al: Plasma and erythrocyte magnesium in health and disease. J Lab Clin Med 59:195, 1962.
520. Matter BJ, Worona M, Donat P, et al: Effect of ethanol on phosphate excretion in man. Clin Res 12:255, 1965.
521. Stein JN, Smith WO, Ginn HE: Hypophosphatemia in acute alcoholism. Am J Med Sci 252:78, 1966.
522. Larsson L, Rebel K, Sorbo B: Severe hypophosphatemia—a hospital survey. Acta Med Scand 214:221–223, 1983.
523. Weinstein S, Scottolini AG, Bhagavan NV: Low neutrophil alkaline phosphatase in renal tubular acidosis with hypophosphatemia after toluene sniffing. Clin Chem 31:330–331, 1985.
524 Aschan J, Ringden O, Ljungman P, et al: Foscarnet for treatment of cytomegalovirus infections in bone marrow transplant recipients. Scand J Infect Dis 24:143–150, 1992.
525. Williams C, Child D, Hudson P, et al: Inappropriate phosphate excretion in idiopathic hypercalciuria: The key to a common cause and future treatment? J Clin Pathol 49:881–888, 1996.
526. Ludwig GD: Hypocalcemia and hypophosphatemia accompanying osteoblastic metastasis: Studies of calcium and phosphate metabolism and parathyroid function. Ann Intern Med 56:676–677, 1962.
527. Erlich M, Goldstein M, Heinemann HO: Hypocalcemia, hypoparathyroidism and osteoblastic metastasis. Metabolism 12:516–526, 1963.
528. Randall RL Jr, Lierman DS: Hypocalcemia and hypophosphatemia accompanying osteoblastic metastasis. J Clin Endocrinol 24:1331–1333, 1964.
529. Raskin P, McClain CJ, Medsger TA Jr: Hypocalcemia associated with metastatic bone disease. Arch Intern Med 132:539–543, 1973.
530. Gilbert FE, Casey AE, Downey EL, et al: Admission inorganic phosphorus correlated with discharge diagnosis and other metabolic profile components. Ala J Med Sci 7:343–349, 1970.
531. Betro MG, Pain RW: Hypophosphatemia and hyperphosphatemia in a hospital population. BMJ 1:273–276, 1972.
532. Juan D, Elrazak MA: Hypophosphatemia in hospitalized patients. JAMA 242:163–164, 1979.
533. Fisher J, Magid N, Kallman C, et al: Respiratory illness and hypophosphatemia. Chest 83:504–508, 1983.
534. Rapaport S, Stevens C, Endel G, et al: The effect of voluntary overbreathing on the electrolyte equilibrium of arterial blood in man. J Biol Chem 163:411, 1946.
535. Mostellar ME, Tuttle EP Jr: The effects of alkalosis on plasma concentration and urinary excretion of inorganic phosphate in man. J Clin Invest 43:138, 1964.
536. Watchko J, Bifano EM, Bergstrom WH: Effect of hyperventilation on total calcium, ionized calcium, and serum phosphorus in neonates. Crit Care Med 12:1055–1056, 1984.
537. Caniggia A, Gennari C: L'absorption digestive du radiophosphate chez l'homme. *In* Milhaud G (ed): Les Tissus Calcifiés. Paris, Sedes, 1968.
538. Tulin M, Danowski T, Hald P, et al: The distribution and movements of inorganic phosphate between cells and serum of human blood. Am J Physiol 149:678, 1947.
539. Riedler GF, Scheitlin WA: Hypophosphataemia in septicemia: Higher incidence in gram-negative than in gram-positive infections. BMJ 1:753–756, 1969.
540. Knochel JP, Caskey JH: The mechanism of hypophosphatemia in acute heat stroke. JAMA 238:425–426, 1977.
541. Chesney RW, Chesney PJ, Davis JP, Segar WE: Renal manifestations of the staphylococcal toxic shock syndrome. Am J Med 71:583–588, 1981.
542. Storm T: Severe hypophosphatemia during recovery from acute respiratory acidosis. BMJ 289:456–457, 1984.
543. Fiske CH: Inorganic phosphate and acid excretion in the postabsorptive period. J Biol Chem 49:171, 1921.
544. Annino JS, Relman AS: The effect of eating on some of the clinically important chemical constituents of the blood. Am J Clin Pathol 31:155, 1959.
545. Nguyen NU, Dumoulin G, Henriet MT, et al: Calcium phosphorus homeostais during oral glucose load in man. Horm Metab Res 16:264–266, 1984.
546. Bolliger A, Hartman FW: Observations on blood phosphates as related to carbohydrate metabolism. J Biol Chem 64:91, 1925.
547. Pollack H, Millet R, Essex H, et al: Serum phosphate changes induced by injections of glucose into dogs under various conditions. Am J Physiol 110:117, 1934.
548. Danowski TS, Gillespie H, Fergus E, et al: Significance of blood sugar and serum electrolyte changes in cirrhosis following glucose, insulin, glucagon, or epinephrine. Yale J Biol Med 29:361, 1957.
549. Gunderson K, Bradley R, Marble A: Serum phosphorus and potassium levels after intravenous administration of glucose. N Engl J Med 250:547, 1954.
550. Smith LH, Ettinger R, Seligson D: A comparison of the metabolism of fructose and glucose in hepatic disease and diabetes mellitus. J Clin Invest 32:273, 1953.
551. McArdle B: Myopathy due to a defect in muscle glycogen breakdown. Clin Sci (Colch) 10:13, 1951.
552. Groen J, Willebrands A, Kamminga C, et al: Effects of glucose administration of the potassium and inorganic phosphate content of the blood serum and the electrocardiogram in normal individuals and in nondiabetic patients. Acta Med Scand 141:352, 1952.
553. Hill GL, Guinn EJ, Dudrick SJ: Phosphorus distribution in hyperalimentation-induced by hypophosphatemia. J Surg Res 20:527, 1976.
554. Harter HR, Santiago JV, Rutherford WE, et al: The relative roles of calcium, phosphorus, and parathyroid hormone in glucose and tolbutamide-mediated insulin release. J Clin Invest 58:359, 1976.
555. Rudman D, Millikan WJ, Richardson TJ, et al: Elemental balances during intravenous hyperalimentation of underweight adult subjects. J Clin Invest 55:94, 1974.
556. Sheldon GF, Grzyb S: Phosphate depletion and repletion: Relation to parenteral nutrition and oxygen transport. Ann Surg 182:683, 1975.
557. England PC, Duari M, Tweedle DEF, et al: Postoperative hypophosphatemia. Br J Surg 66:340–343, 1979.
558. Hessov I, Jensen NG, Rasmussen A: Prevention of hypophosphatemia during postoperative routine glucose administration. Acta Chir Scand 146:109–114, 1980.
559. Loven L, Gidlof A, Larsson L, et al: Changes in serum phosphate and calcitonin concentrations during elective surgery of the knee. Acta Chir Scand 148:27–31, 1982.
560. Loven L, Larsson L, Sjoberg HE, Lennquist S: Effect of beta-blocking agents on perioperative changes in serum phosphate. Acta Chir Scand 148:339–344, 1982.
561. Loven L, Larsson L, Lennquist S, Liljedahl SO: Hypophosphatemia and muscle phosphate metabolism in severely injured patients. Acta Chir Scand 149:743–749, 1983.
562. Massara F, Camanni F: Propranolol block of adrenaline induced hypophosphatemia in man. Clin Sci (Colch) 38:245, 1970.
563. Yaroslavsky A, Blum M, Peer G, et al: Serum phosphate shift in acute myocardial infarction. Am Heart J 104:884, 1982.
564. Danowski TS, Hald P, Peters J, et al: Sodium, potassium and phosphate in the cell and serum of blood in diabetic acidosis. Am J Physiol 149:667, 1947.
565. Franks M, et al: Metabolic studies in diabetic acidosis. II. The effect of the administration of sodium phosphate. Arch Intern Med 81:42, 1948.
566. Alberti KG, Emerson PM, Darley JH, et al: 2,3-diphosphoglycerate and tissue oxygenation in uncontrolled diabetes mellitus. Lancet 2:391, 1972.
567. Atchley DW, Loeb R, Richards D, et al: On diabetic acidosis: A detailed study of electrolyte balances following the withdrawal and reestablishment of insulin therapy. J Clin Invest 12:297, 1933.
568. Pitts RF, Alexander RS: The renal reabsorptive mechanism for inorganic phosphate in normal and acidotic dogs. Am J Physiol 142:648–662, 1944.
569. Guest GM, Rapoport S: Electrolytes of blood plasma and cells in diabetic acidosis and during recovery. Proc Am Diabetes Assoc 7:95, 1947.
570. Butler AM, Talbott N, Burnett C, et al: Metabolic studies on diabetic coma. Trans Assoc Am Physiol 40:102, 1947.
571. Cohen JJ, Berglund F, Lotspeich W: Renal tubular reabsorption of acetoacetate, inorganic sulfate and inorganic phosphate in the dog as affected by glucose and phlorizin. Am J Physiol 184:91, 1956.
572. Riley MS, Schade DS, Eaton RP: Effects of insulin infusion on plasma phosphate in diabetic patients. Metabolism 28:191–194, 1979.
573. Keller U, Berger W: Prevention of hypophosphatemia by phosphate infusion during treatment of diabetic ketoacidosis and hyperosmolar coma. Diabetes 29:87–95, 1980.
574. Wilson HK, Keuer SP, Lea AS, et al: Phosphate therapy in diabetic ketoacidosis. Arch Intern Med 142:517–520, 1982.
575. Kanter Y, Gerson JR, Bessman AN: 2,3-Diphosphoglycerate, nucleotide phosphate, and organic and inorganic phosphate levels during the early phases of diabetic ketoacidosis. Diabetes 26:429–433, 1977.
576. Kono N, Kuwajima M, Tarui S: Alteration of glycolytic intermediary metabolism in erythrocytes during diabetic ketoacidosis and its recovery phase. Diabetes 30:346–353, 1981.
577. Gertner JM, Tamborlane WV, Horst RL, et al: Mineral metabolism in diabetes mellitus: Changes accompanying treatment with a portable subcutaneous insulin infusion system. J Clin Endocrinol Metab 50:862–866, 1980.
578. Territo MC, Tanaka KK: Hypophosphatemia in chronic alcoholism. Arch Intern Med 134:445, 1974.
579. Knochel TP: Hypophosphatemia in the alcoholic. Arch Intern Med 140:613–614, 1980.
580. Peterson VP: Metabolic studies in clinical magnesium deficiency. Acta Med Scand 173:285, 1963.
581. Lim P, Jocob E: Magnesium status of alcoholic patients. Metabolism 21:1045, 1972.
582. Forsham PH, Thorn GW: Changes in inorganic serum phosphorus during the intravenous glucose tolerance test as an adjunct to the diagnosis of early diabetes mellitus. Proc Am Diabetes Assoc 9:101, 1949.
583. Corredor DG, Sabeh G, Mendelsohn LV, et al: Enhanced post glucose hypophosphatemia during starvation therapy of obesity. Metabolism 18:754, 1969.
584. Knochel J: Hypophosphatemia and rhabdomyolysis (editorial). Am J Med 92:455–457, 1992.
585. Zamkoff KW, Kirshner JJ: Marked hypophosphatemia associated with acute myelomonocytic leukemia. Arch Intern Med 140:1523–1524, 1980.

586. Matzner Y, Procociner M, Polliack A, et al: Hypophosphatemia in a patient with lymphoma in leukemic phase. Arch Intern Med 141:805–806, 1981.
587. Perek J, Mettelman M, Gafter U, Djaldetti M: Hypophosphatemia accompanying blastic crisis in a patient with malignant lymphoma. J Cancer Res Clin Oncol 108:351–353, 1984.
588. Clark R, Lee E: Severe hypophosphatemia during stem cell harvesting in chronic myeloid leukaemia. Br J Haematol 90:450–452, 1995.
589. Kajikawa M, Nonami T, Kurokawa T, et al: Recombinant human erythropoietin and hypophosphatemia in patients with cirrhosis. Lancet 341:503–504, 1993.
590. Giebisch G, Berger L, Pitts RF: The extrarenal response to acute acid base disturbances of respiratory origin. J Clin Invest 34:231, 1955.
591. Dennis V: Phosphate metabolism: Contribution of different cellular compartments. Kidney Int 49:938–942, 1996.
592. Knochel JR, Bilbrey GL, Fuller TJ, et al: The muscle cell in chronic alcoholism: The possible role of phosphate depletion in alcoholic myopathy. Ann N Y Acad Sci 252:274, 1975.
593. Knochel JP: Neuromuscular manifestations of electrolyte disorders. Am J Med 72:521–535, 1982.
594. Gabow PA, Kaehny WD, Kelleher SP: The spectrum of rhabdomyolysis. Medicine (Baltimore) 61:141–152, 1982.
595. Singhal P, Kumar A, Desroches L, et al: Prevalence and predictors of rhabdomyolysis in patients with hypophosphatemia. Am J Med 92:458–464, 1992.
596. Fuller TJ, Carter NW, Barcenas C, Knochel JP: Reversible changes of the muscle cell in experimental phosphorus deficiency. J Clin Invest 57:1019–1024, 1976.
597. Silvis SE, DiBartolomeo AG, Aaker HM: Hypophosphatemia and neurological changes secondary to oral caloric intake. Am J Gastroenterol 73:215–222, 1980.
598. Silvis SE, Paragas PU Jr: Paresthesias, weakness, seizures and hypophosphatemia in patients receiving hyperalimentation. Gastroenterology 62:513, 1972.
599. Prins JG, Schrijver H, Staghouwer JH: Hyperalimentation, hypophosphatemia and coma. Lancet 1:1253, 1973.
600. Weintraub MI, Chakravorty HP: Nutrient deficiencies after intensive parenteral alimentation. N Engl J Med 291:799, 1974.
601. Moser CR, Fessel WJ: Rheumatic manifestations of hypophosphatemia. Arch Intern Med 134:674, 1974.
602. Furlan AJ, Hanson M, Cooperman A, et al: Acute areflexic paralysis. Association with hyperalimentation and hypophosphatemia. Arch Neurol 32:706, 1975.
603. Newman JH, Neff TA, Ziporin P: Acute respiratory failure associated with hypophosphatemia. N Engl J Med 296:1101, 1977.
604. O'Connor LR, Wheeler WS, Bethune JE: Effect of hypophosphatemia on myocardial performance in man. N Engl J Med 297:901, 1977.
605. Scarpa A, Carafoli E: Calcium transport and cell function. Ann N Y Acad Sci 307:1–655, 1980.
606. Aderka D, Shoefeld Y, Santo M, et al: Life-threatening hypophosphatemia in a patient with acute myelogenous leukemia. Acta Haematol 64:117–119, 1980.
607. Vanneste J, Hage J: Acute severe hypophosphatemia mimicking Wernicke's encephalopathy. Lancet 1:44, 1986.
608. Aubier M, Murciano D, Lecocguic Y, et al: Effect of hypophosphatemia on diaphragmatic contractility in patients with acute respiratory failure. N Engl J Med 313:420–424, 1985.
609. Gravelyn T, Brophy N, Siegert C, Peters-Golden M: Hypophosphatemia-associated respiratory muscle weakness in a general inpatient population. Am J Med 84:870–876, 1988.
610. Vered Z, Battler A, Motro M, et al: Left ventricular function in patients with chronic hypophosphatemia. Am Heart J 107:796–798, 1984.
611. Rasmussen A, Buus S, Hessov I: Postoperative myocardial performance during glucose-induced hypophosphatemia. Acta Chir Scand 151:13–15, 1985.
612. Bollaert P-E, Levy B, Nace L, et al: Hemodynamic and metabolic effects of rapid correction of hypophosphatemia in patients with septic shock. Chest 107:1698–1701, 1995.
613. Emmett M, Goldfarb S, Agus ZS, Narins RG: The pathophysiology of acid-base changes in chronically phosphate-depleted rats. J Clin Invest 59:291, 1977.
614. Ginsburg JM: Effect of glucose and free fatty acid on phosphate transport in dog kidney. Am J Physiol 222:1153, 1972.
615. Gold LW, Massry SG, Arieff AI, Coburn JW: Renal bicarbonate wasting during phosphate depletion: A possible cause of altered acid base homeostasis in hyperthyroidism. J Clin Invest 52:2256–2261, 1973.
616. Gold L, Massry SG, Friedler RM: Effect of phosphate depletion on renal glucose reabsorption (abstract). Clin Res 24:400A, 1976.
617. Steele TH, Stromberg BA, Underwood JL, Larmore CA: Renal resistance to parathyroid hormone during phosphorus deprivation. J Clin Invest 58:1461–1464, 1976.
618. Tanaka Y, DeLuca HF: The control of 25-hydroxyvitamin D_3 metabolism by inorganic phosphate. Arch Biochem Biophys 154:566, 1973.
619. Steele TH, Engle JE, Tanaka Y, et al: On the phosphatemic action of 1,25-dihydroxyvitamin D_3. Am J Physiol 229:489–495, 1975.
620. Bellorin-Font E, Tamayo J, Martin KJ: Uncoupling of the parathyroid hormone receptor adenylate cyclase systems of canine kidney during dietary phosphorus deprivation. Endocrinology 115:544–549, 1984.
621. Lichtman MA, Miller DR, Cohen J, Waterhouse C: Reduced red cell glycolysis, 2,3-diphosphoglycerate and adenosine triphosphate concentration and increased hemoglobin oxygen affinity caused by hypophosphatemia. Ann Intern Med 74:562–568, 1971.
622. Klock JC, Williams HE, Mentzer WC: Hemolytic anemia and somatic cell dysfunction in severe hypophosphatemia. Arch Intern Med 134:360–364, 1974.
623. Jacob JS, Amsden P: Acute hemolytic anemia with rigid red cells in hypophosphatemia. N Engl J Med 285:1446, 1971.
624. Garner GB: Dietary phosphorus and salmonellosis in guinea pigs. Fed Proc 26:799, 1967.
625. Rajan KS: Hepatic hypoxia secondary to hypophosphatemia. Clin Res 23:521, 1973.
626. Yawata Y, Hebbel RP, Silvis S, et al: Blood cell abnormalities complicating the hypophosphatemia of hyperalimentation: Erythrocyte and platelet ATP deficiency associated with hemolytic anemia and bleeding in hyperalimented dogs. J Lab Clin Med 84:643–653, 1974.
627. Craddock PR, Yawata Y, VanSanten L, et al: Acquired phagocyte dysfunction. A complication of the hypophosphatemia of parenteral hyperalimentation. N Engl J Med 290:1403–1407, 1974.
628. Dent CE, Winter CS: Osteomalacia due to phosphate depletion from excessive aluminum hydroxide ingestion. BMJ 1:551, 1974.
629. Scriver CR: Rickets and the pathogenesis of impaired tubular transport of phosphate and other solutes. Am J Med 57:43–44, 1974.
630. Godsall JW, Baron R, Insogna KL: Vitamin D metabolism and bone histomorphometry in a patient with antacid-induced osteomalacia. Am J Med 77:747–750, 1984.
631. deVernejoul MC, Marie P, Kuntz D, et al: Nonosteomalacic osteopathy associated with chronic hypophosphatemia. Calcif Tissue Int 34:219–223, 1982.
632. Gray RW, Garthwaite TL: Activation of renal 1,25-dihydroxyvitamin D_3 synthesis by phosphate deprivation: Evidence for a role for growth hormone. Endocrinology 116:189–193, 1985.
633. Castillo L, Tanaka Y, DeLuca HF: The mobilization of bone mineral by 1,25-dihydroxyvitamin D_3 in hypophosphatemic rats. Endocrinology 97:995–999, 1975.
634. Lentz RD, Brown DM, Kjellstrand CM: Treatment of severe hypophosphatemia. Ann Intern Med 89:941–944, 1978.
635. Vanatta JB, Whang R, Papper S: Efficacy of intravenous phosphorus therapy in the severely hypophosphatemic patient. Arch Intern Med 141:885–887, 1981.
636. Vannatta JB, Andress DL, Whang R, Papper S: High-dose intravenous phosphorus therapy for severe complicated hypophosphatemia. South Med J 76:1424–1426, 1983.
637. Becker DJ, Brown DR, Steranka BH, Drash AL: Phosphate replacement during treatment of diabetic ketosis. Am J Dis Child 137:241–246, 1983.
638. Kingston M, Al-Siba'i MB: Treatment of severe hypophosphatemia. Crit Care Med 13:16–18, 1985.
639. Rosen G, Boullata J, O'Rangers E, et al: Intravenous phosphate repletion regimen for critically ill patients with moderate hypophosphatemia. Crit Care Med 23:1204–1210, 1995.
640. Clark C, Sacks G, Dickerson R, et al: Treatment of hypophosphatemia in patients receiving specialized nutrition support using a graduated dosing scheme: Results from a prospective clinical trial. Crit Care Med 23:1504–1511, 1995.
641. Winter RJ, Harris CJ, Phillips LS, Green OC: Diabetic ketoacidosis. Induction of hypocalcemia and hypomagnesemia by phosphate therapy. Am J Med 67:897–900, 1979.
642. Zipp NB, Bacon GE, Spencer ML, et al: Hypocalcemia, hypomagnesemia and transient hypoparathyroidism during therapy with potassium phosphate in diabetic ketoacidosis. Diabetes Care 2:265, 1979.

Chapter 74

Bone Development and Remodeling

Gideon A. Rodan

The skeleton fulfills four major functions in terrestrial animals: (1) Bones provide mechanical support for soft tissues and are levers for muscle action, essential for locomotion and feeding. (2) The skeleton is the site for storage and controlled release of calcium and other ions, essential for the electrolyte homeostasis of the extracellular fluid. (3) Bones house the bone marrow and participate in hematopoiesis through the interaction of stromal cells with hemopoietic precursors. (4) The cranial bones and vertebrae house and protect the central nervous system (brain and spinal cord), its visual, olfactory, and acoustic sensors, and the balance apparatus of the inner ear.

By carrying out these functions the skeleton played a major role in the evolutionary changes that led to the human species. The mineralized skeleton evolved in the marine environment, where calcium is plentiful, probably in order to store phosphate, which is subject to the seasonal variations of plankton in the oceans. Converting the calcium phosphate store into a calcium source was essential for survival on land, where calcium comes from food and feeding is intermittent. The storage of calcium and its release from the skeleton has evolved into a sophisticated endocrine system, covered in other chapters of this book.

The role of the skeleton in providing vertebrates with an extended range of locomotion on land is obvious and offered significant survival advantages. Skeletal evolution is also credited with playing a role in the transition from apes to man. It was suggested that the skeletal changes associated with brachiation, the selective use of upper extremities for climbing trees, development of a thumb which apposes each of the fingers, and bipedalism led to the use of tools and fostered the evolution of the human brain.

In the medical context, normal skeletal function is a mainstay of general well-being, and its failure, often one of the early manifestations of aging, for example, in osteoporosis or osteoarthritis, is associated with and contributes to deteriorating health.

The skeleton seems to be ideally suited for its functions. During embryology it acquires the appropriate structure and relationship to other tissues. Postnatally, the skeleton carries out its functions by continuously turning over. In order to release calcium, or to maintain a structure which provides maximum strength for minimal material, packets of bone are constantly being removed and replaced. This chapter briefly reviews the embryology of bone and the process of bone turnover in the adult, called bone remodeling.

SKELETAL EMBRYOLOGY

Bones develop from two separate embryonic structures. The neural crest–derived branchial arches give rise to all the cranial and facial bones[1] by a process of membranous bone formation (described below). The rest of the skeleton develops by a process in which bone replaces cartilage, called endochondral bone formation (described below). The bony skeleton is preceded by a corresponding complete cartilaginous skeleton. For each bone there is a cartilage anlage, where bone formation starts at a determined time and site.

The axial skeleton (vertebrae and ribs) arises from somite sclerotomes (Fig. 74–1) under the influence of the notochord.[2] The somites contain endoderm-derived mesenchymal cells, which are segmented under the influence of *hox* genes.[3] Experimental mutations in *hox* genes indicate that the shape of each vertebra, and probably of each bone in the body, is coded by separate genes. The appendicular skeleton (limbs) forms from the lateral plate mesoderm, which gives rise to all the structures of each extremity.

The shaping of bones, as different from each other as the semicircular canals of the inner ear and the heel (calcaneus), is the result of several complex processes, which form all organs and are subject to endocrine and paracrine influences. They include cellular proliferation, migration, differentiation, and organ morphogenesis. During differentiation cells express the phenotypic proteins, which determine the tissue-specific cell functions. Morphogenesis (tissue shaping), responsible for the structure of each organ, results from the controlled three-dimensional deployment of differentiated cells. Spontaneous mutations and experimental manipulation of genes, either deletions or overexpression, causing loss or gain of function, have identified many proteins in-

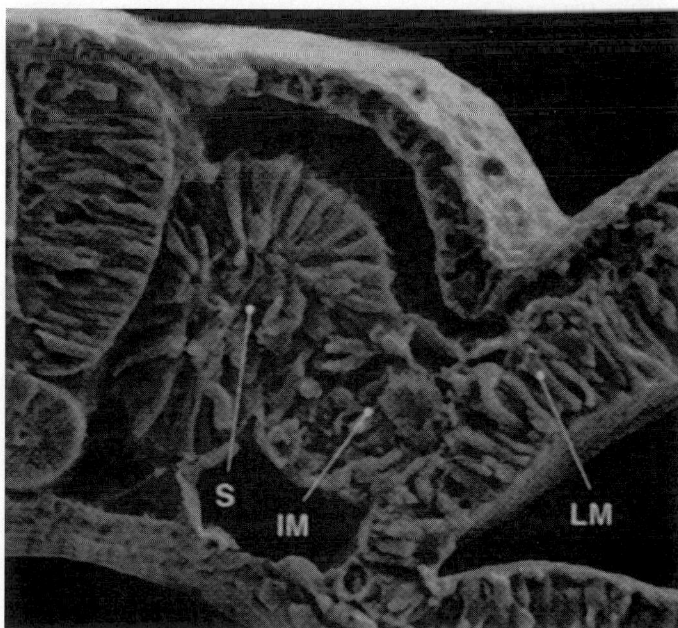

FIGURE 74–1. Cross-section of developing somite (S) in mouse embryo showing the intermediate (IM) and lateral (LM) mesoderm, which will give rise to muscle, dermis, bone, and cartilage, all derived from the same group of embryonic mesenchymal cells. (From Tajbakhsh S, Sporle R: Somite development: Constructing the vertebrate body. Cell 92:9–16, 1998.)

volved in the differentiation of bone-forming cells and in the morphogenesis of individual bones. Examples are presented below.

Limb Development

Limb development from the lateral plate mesoderm is a typical example of morphogenesis. Its investigation, primarily in chicks and mice, has elucidated many aspects of this process and the molecules involved in its regulation. A brief description of the current model[4, 5] follows. Limb development occurs in each of three directions: proximodistal (PD), from shoulders to fingers; dorsoventral (DV), from back of hand to palm; and anteroposterior (AP), from thumb to little finger. PD growth (limb elongation) involves mesenchymal cell proliferation and depends on growth factor(s) produced by a group of epithelial cells in the apical ectodermal ridge (AER). The mitogenic fibroblast growth factors (FGFs) are thought to be responsible for the AER activity for the following reasons: (1) AER cells express FGF-8 and -10, (2) exogenous FGFs can substitute for surgically removed AER, and (3) experimental deletion of the FGF-10 gene in mice results in limbless embryos.[5]

Patterning along the AP axis is controlled by the zone of polarizing activity (ZPA) localized in a group of cells on the posterior aspect of the initial protrusion. ZPA cells produce the growth factor sonic hedgehog (SHH), responsible for this activity.

The DV patterning (back of hand to palm and limb flattening) is, at least in part, controlled by the growth factor WNT7A produced in the dorsal ectoderm. WNT7A acts via the gene *Lmx1* expressed in the underlying mesenchyme.[6, 7]

These are certainly not all the factors involved. For example, there are genes which determine if patterning will form a forelimb (*Tbx5*) or a hindlimb (*Pitx1* and *Tbx4*).[8] There are also several important feedback interactions between these factors. For example, BMP2 (bone morphogenetic protein 2) stimulates the expression of *hox* genes, which induce in ZPA cells the ability to produce SHH. SHH production in ZPA cells is also dependent on FGF, produced in the AER, and on WNT7A, from the dorsal ectoderm. SHH itself stimulates FGF production, establishing a positive feedback loop, most likely interrupted by another factor, yet to be identified.

The result of this patterning is the ordered development of the limb tissues, including cartilage and bone. As mentioned, in the limbs bone replaces cartilage via endochondral bone formation, while in the skull and face bone develops directly from mesenchymal tissue, via intramembranous bone formation.

Intramembranous and Endochondral Bone Formation

In intramembranous bone formation, mesenchymal cells crowd together (condense) at sites destined to become cranial and facial bones and start expressing the proteins characteristic of osteoblasts (see below), the bone-forming cells. The cells deposit the bone extracellular matrix and mineralize it. Through modeling and remodeling (see below) the respective bones will reach their final shape and size.

The other bones in the body are formed by endochondral bone formation. Initially, the embryo has a complete cartilaginous skeleton. Each bone in the axial and appendicular skeleton replaces a cartilage anlage of similar shape. The cartilage anlage also forms by the condensation of mesenchymal cells and their differentiation into matrix-producing cartilage cells. The replacement of cartilage by bone begins at ossification centers in the cartilage anlage, the site and timing of which are genetically determined. The process starts with the hypertrophy of cartilage cells, mineralization of their matrix, followed by vascular invasion, colonization by osteoblast precursors, osteoblastic differentiation on the scaffold of mineralized cartilage, and bone formation.

The Growth Plate

Longitudinal growth of bones also occurs by endochondral bone formation. A segment at each end of the cartilage anlage becomes the epiphysial growth plate (Fig. 74–2). In the proliferative zone of the growth plate cartilage cells divide under the positive and negative control of many growth factors (see below). The daughter cells of proliferating chondrocytes differentiate, deposit the cartilage matrix, hypertrophy, and the matrix mineralizes. As described above, the area is invaded by blood vessels; osteoblasts differentiate on the surface of the mineralized cartilage and start depositing bone, forming the initial cancellous (trabecular) bone, called primary spongiosa. Resorbing cells, chondroclasts, similar to osteoclasts, will gradually remove the remnants of calcified cartilage. The primary spongiosa will be fully replaced by lamellar bone in the secondary spongiosa, which is organized in honeycomb platelike structures in the interior of the bone and is surrounded by bone marrow.

The following growth factors have pronounced effects on the growth plate. IGF-1 (insulin-like growth factor-1), produced in the liver under the control of pituitary growth hormone, promotes chondrocyte proliferation and is responsible for longitudinal growth, thus having a large influence on overall stature.[9] The action of IGF is modulated by IGF binding proteins, which can augment or suppress IGF effects (see Chapter 33).

FGFs (17 genes known so far) are potent mitogens for mesenchymal cells and suppress chondrocyte differentiation, which precedes ossification. Most chondrodystrophies and the associated dwarfism are caused by mutated FGF receptors (FGFRs) which are constitutively active, in the absence of FGF binding. Mutated FGFR1 causes Pfeifer's syndrome; FGFR2, Crouzon's syndrome (craniosynostosis and limb abnormalities); and FGFR3, achondroplasia, thanatophoric dysplasia, and hypochondroplasia.[10]

PTHrP (parathyroid hormone–related protein) under the control of hedgehog (hh) also suppresses chondrocyte differentiation (for review, see Karaplis et al.[11]; see also Chapter 70); its overexpression widens the growth plate and delays ossification. Constitutively active mutated parathyroid hormone (PTH)–PTHrP receptor is the cause of Jansen's metaphyseal chondrodysplasia.[12]

After birth, bones of the axial and appendicular skeleton continue to grow in length, until the age of 18 to 20, when the epiphysial growth plates close. Shaping the bones during growth requires removal of some of the existing bone by the process of bone resorption and, obviously, the formation of additional new bone. The latter can take place either on resorbed surfaces, called remodeling, or de novo, in the absence of resorption, called modeling (see below). In either case, bone resorption is carried out by osteoclasts and bone formation by osteoblasts.

OSTEOCLASTS AND OSTEOBLASTS

Osteoclasts originate from hematopoietic precursors, which can also give rise to the monocyte-macrophage lineage, most likely, cells related to the granulocyte-macrophage colony-forming units (GM-CFU). Genetic mutations, spontaneous or induced, have identified proteins that play rate-limiting roles in osteoclast differentiation. These include the transcription factors c-*fos*,[13] PU-1,[14] and nuclear factor-κB (NF-κB)[15, 16] and the growth factor M-CSF (monocyte-macrophage colony-stimulating factor). The absence of some of these factors also affects monocyte differentiation (e.g., PU-1, M-CSF),[17] indicating that they act upstream of the branching point between the osteoclastic and monocytic lineage (Fig. 74–3). None of these factors have been implicated so far in human osteopetrosis, characterized by excess bone, caused by osteoclast absence or malfunction.

During differentiation, osteoclasts express specific proteins responsible for their unique functions. These include (1) calcitonin[18] and vitronectin receptors[19] (over 10 million each per multinucleated cell), (2) high abundance of lysosomal enzymes, including tartrate-resistant acid phosphatase and cathepsin K,[20, 21] which are preferentially expressed in osteoclasts, and (3) the kinases, c-src[22] and PYK2, which seem to play key roles in osteoclast function.[23] During osteoclast formation in culture these proteins are present in mononucleated osteoclast precursors, which fuse to form the multinucleated bone-resorbing giant cells.

Osteoclast differentiation and function are both under endocrine and

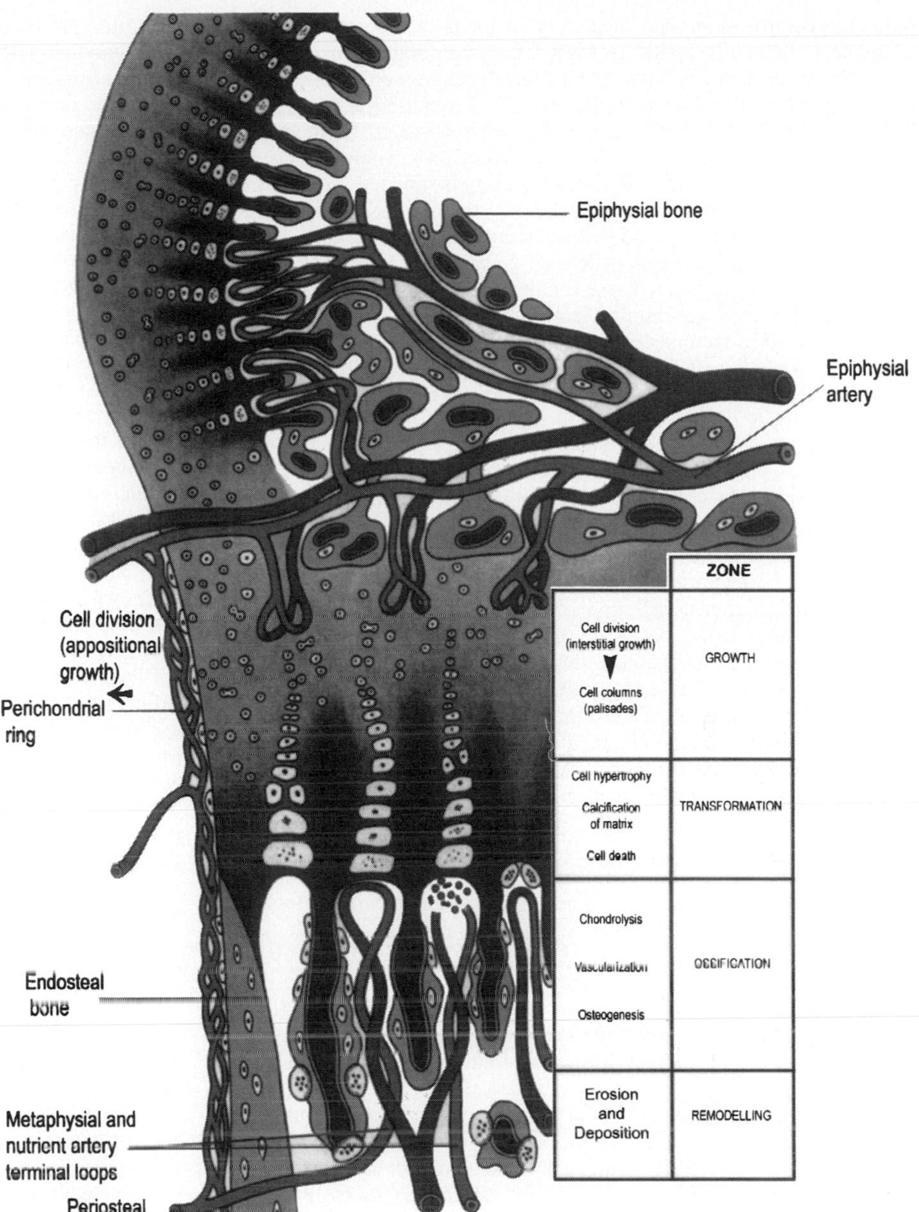

FIGURE 74–2. Diagram of growth plate from a long bone (such as tibia or radius), typical of the growth of all bones in the skeleton through endochondral bone formation, except the craniofacial bones. (From Williams PL, Warwick R (eds): Gray's Anatomy. Philadelphia, WB Saunders, 1989, p 265.)

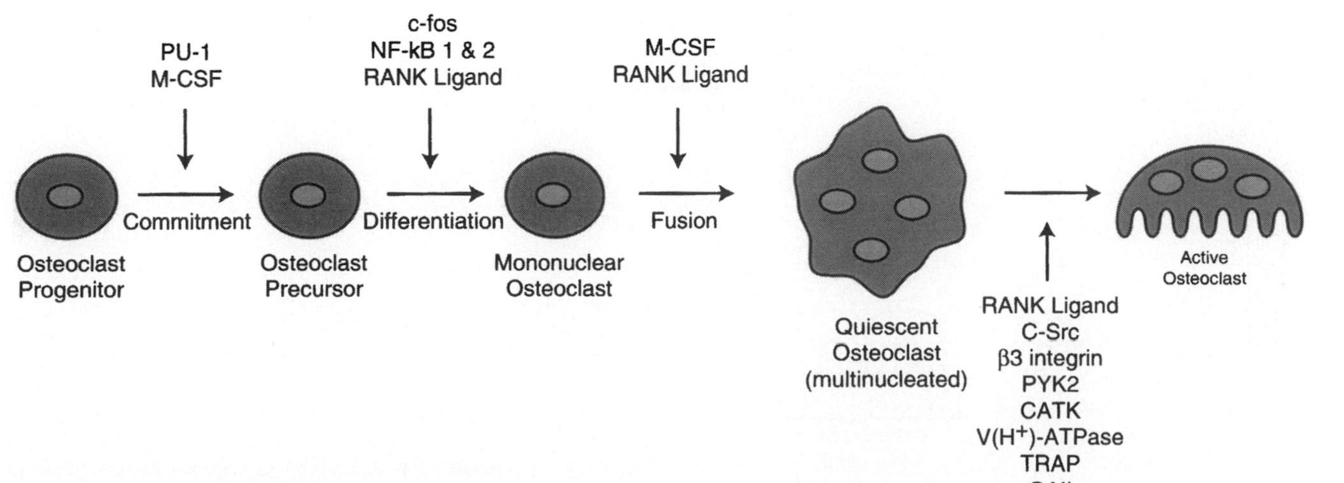

FIGURE 74–3. Schematic differentiation diagram of osteoclasts and some of the factors involved (e.g., monocyte-macrophage colony-stimulating factor and RANK ligand). (Modified from Suda T, Takahashi N, Udagawa N: Modulation of osteoclast differentiation and function by the new members of the tumor necrosis factor receptor and ligand families. Endocr Rev 20:345–367, 1999.)

paracrine control. A crucial regulatory factor is the receptor activator of nuclear factor-κB ligand (RANK-L), a membrane-bound peptide from the tumor necrosis factor (TNF) family, expressed in many cells, including osteoblast lineage cells, which is required for osteoclast differentiation.[24, 25] RANK-L expression was shown to be modulated by factors which influence osteoclast differentiation, such as PTH and 1,25-dihydroxyvitamin D_3.[26] RANK-L activity is blocked by the decoy receptor osteoprotegerin, which was shown to suppress estrogen deficiency bone loss.[27] Osteoprotegerin deletion in mice results in severe osteopenia while the deletion of RANK-L causes osteopetrosis, excessive accumulation of bone. These findings clearly establish, at least in mice, RANK-L as a rate-limiting factor in osteoclastic bone resorption.

Other paracrine factors shown to stimulate osteoclast differentiation include interleukins (ILS) IL-1, IL-6 in the presence of soluble IL-6 receptor, and IL-11, as well as prostaglandin E (PGE), and tumor necrosis factor-α (TNF-α). These factors have all been implicated in estrogen-deficiency bone loss, but their role and relative contribution to postmenopausal osteoporosis remain to be established.[28–30]

Osteoblasts are the bone-forming cells that deposit, in a highly organized fashion, the bone extracellular matrix. Additional cells belonging to the osteoblast lineage include the osteocytes, which are surrounded by mineralized matrix, and the lining cells, which cover the bone surface after completion of the bone formation cycle. Osteocytes and lining cells, based on their location, are best suited to perceive changes in mechanical strain, and were therefore suggested to mediate mechanical effects on bone. Other non–bone-forming cells of the osteoblast lineage are stromal cells, which include osteoblast precursors. These cells are assumed to play a role in osteoclast formation and mediate the effect of various signals on that process.

Embryologically, osteoblasts originate from mesenchymal cells that can also give rise to chondrocytes, adipocytes, myocytes, tendon cells, and various fibroblasts (Fig. 74–4). The decision to follow a given differentiation pathway is determined by the expression of key transcription factors, for example, myo-D and myogenin in muscle cells. Core binding factor A1 (CBFA1), a transcription factor from the acute myeloid leukemia (AML) family, is a key differentiation factor for osteoblasts. Its absence in mice, produced by experimental gene deletion, resulted in the persistence of a nonmineralized cartilaginous skeleton and the total absence of a bony skeleton.[31] CBFA1 expression increases in vitro in cells that differentiate into osteoblasts in response to BMPs.

BMPs can induce bone formation when injected into the muscle or dermis of adult animals and have been implicated as paracrine factors in bone formation.[32] BMPs play a key role in the development of multiple organs, in addition to bone.[33–35] Mutations in BMP family proteins produce skeletal abnormalities in mice, for example, brachypodism (BMP5) and short ear syndrome (growth and development factor 5).[36] BMP-2, -4, and -7, as well as BMP receptors, are expressed during fracture repair.[37–39] BMPs probably play a role in that process and are being developed for the treatment of fracture nonunions. It is still uncertain to what extent BMPs participate in the normal process of bone remodeling (discussed below), and if they could be used therapeutically for systemic bone diseases such as osteoporosis. The situation is similar with the BMP-related transforming growth factor-β (TGF-β) growth factors. These growth factors stimulate bone formation when injected locally in animals, are produced by bone cells and platelets, and were proposed to play a role in bone remodeling (see below).

The pluripotentiality of preosteoblastic mesenchymal cells could be more restricted in vivo in human adults. Bipotent cells in the bone marrow can give rise to adipocytes and to osteogenic cells. Investigation of this phenomenon in vitro showed that adipocyte differentiation is associated with the expression of the transcription factors C/EBPβ, -δ, and -α,[40] and the nuclear receptor PPARγ (peroxisome proliferator–activated receptor-γ),[41] which can be stimulated by specific ligands.[42] It is well documented that with aging there is a relative increase in fatty marrow, but the mechanism for this change is not known, nor is it known if inhibition of adipogenesis in the marrow could increase the pool of osteogenic cells and bone formation. Another group of bipotent cells are the bone-forming periosteal cells, which can form cartilage during fracture repair. The mechanism for inducing cartilage differentiation in these cells is not known.

On differentiation, osteoblast lineage cells express the proteins required for their tissue-specific functions. Bone-forming cells synthesize, secrete, and organize all the molecules of the extracellular matrix. These include predominant expression of type I collagen, which accounts for 90% of the bone matrix proteins, and the noncollagenous proteins, osteocalcin and bone sialoprotein, selectively expressed in bone, as well as osteopontin, biglycan, decorin, osteoadherin, and others. The bone-forming osteoblasts also have very high levels of the ectoenzyme alkaline phosphatase, which plays a key role in matrix mineralization. Mineralization starts about 1 week after matrix deposition and proceeds rapidly to about 70% of maximal mineral content, and more slowly thereafter.

Osteoblast lineage cells, including osteocytes and lining cells, mediate the response of bone to mechanical, endocrine, and paracrine factors and express the appropriate receptors and surface proteins required for these functions. These include receptors for sex steroids, for PTH, for 1,25-dihydroxyvitamin D_3 and for a myriad growth factors, including IGFs, FGFs, BMPs, and TGF-β, mentioned above in the context of bone development. Other factors acting on osteoblasts

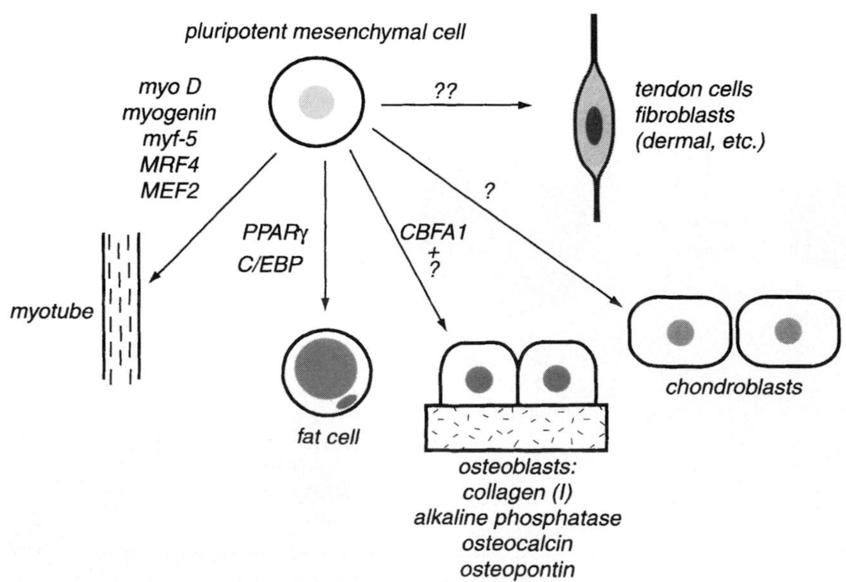

FIGURE 74–4. Scheme of lineages derived from pluripotent mesenchymal precursor cells, pointing to some of the transcription factors involved (e.g., PPRγ NC/EBP for adipocytes; CBFA1, for osteoblasts). (From Rodan GA, Harada S: The missing bone. Cell 89:677–680, 1997.)

include platelet-derived growth factor (PDGF), abundant following fracture; PGE, which can stimulate both resorption and formation and has been implicated in responses to mechanical strain and inflammation; the interleukins, which regulate osteoclast formation; endothelin, nitric oxide, and others.

The effect of these and other factors on the proliferation and differentiation of osteoblastic cells was extensively studied in vitro. As a rule, factors that stimulate proliferation suppress or delay the expression of features associated with differentiation. One should keep in mind that the applicability of in vitro observations to in vivo bone development or remodeling has not always been established. True bone formation and remodeling occur only in vivo. These are three-dimensional phenomena, which probably require vascularization.

The precise contribution of the blood vessels to bone formation has not been fully characterized, but the relationship is well established. In addition to the contribution of cells, such as pericytes, reported to have osteogenic potential, vascular cells produce several paracrine factors, which may play a role in bone formation. FGF-2 can stimulate the proliferation of osteoblast precursors and was shown in vivo to enhance postinjury bone formation in fracture repair.[43, 44] FGF-2 was shown to be produced by bone cells, as well as by vascular endothelial cells, where it would act as part of a positive feedback loop, since it stimulates angiogenesis.

Another factor with autocrine and paracrine action is PGE, a stimulator of bone formation which is produced by and acts on osteoblast lineage cells, most likely via cyclic adenosine monophosphate (cAMP). The mechanism for its osteogenic effects has not been elucidated. Recent information suggests that it may suppress the apoptosis of osteoblast precursors.[45] PGE also stimulates in osteoblastic cells the production of vascular endothelial growth factor, which promotes angiogenesis, providing a further positive feedback link between vascularization and bone formation.[46]

Osteoblast lineage cells interact with other osteoblasts, with other cell types, and with the surrounding matrix via gap junctions, cadherins, and integrins, respectively. Gap junctions produce an osteocyte-osteoblast network, which allows communication mediated by ionic currents and small molecules, such as cAMP.[47] Cadherins play a role in cellular differentiation, connect sheets of osteoblasts, and were reported to connect osteoblast lineage cells to osteoclasts as well.[48, 49] Integrins are heterodimeric transmembrane adhesion receptors,[50, 51] which provide physical continuity between the extracellular matrix and the osteoblast cytoskeleton. These communication features endow the osteoblast lineage cells with the ability to act in concert to deposit a highly organized matrix, consistent with the mechanical needs of each bone, and to coordinate bone remodeling, according to local needs and those of the whole organism.

BONE MODELING AND REMODELING

Structurally (anatomically) one distinguishes between cortical or compact bone, the dense outside envelope of all bones, and cancellous or trabecular bone, the honeycombed interior, exposed to the bone marrow (Fig. 74–5). The human skeleton contains about 80% cortical and 20% cancellous bone. During growth and development there is obviously a substantial amount of bone formation occurring either on the mineralized cartilage under the growth plates, as described above, or in the outside envelope of bones, called periosteum. At the same time there is bone resorption aimed at achieving the genetically prescribed anatomic shape of each bone. This type of bone addition and removal is called modeling and is regulated by the genetic blueprint and by mechanical forces. Furthermore, there is continuous replacement of existing bone, called remodeling, during growth and in the fully formed skeleton.

Remodeling is necessary for the skeletal functions listed at the beginning of this chapter. The removal of calcium from bone, to satisfy homeostatic needs between calcium meals, requires osteoclastic resorption of the calcium-containing bone. Reshaping of the bone for mechanical adaptation requires the replacement of existing bone packets or whole trabeculae with new ones appropriately oriented relative to the prevailing mechanical loads.

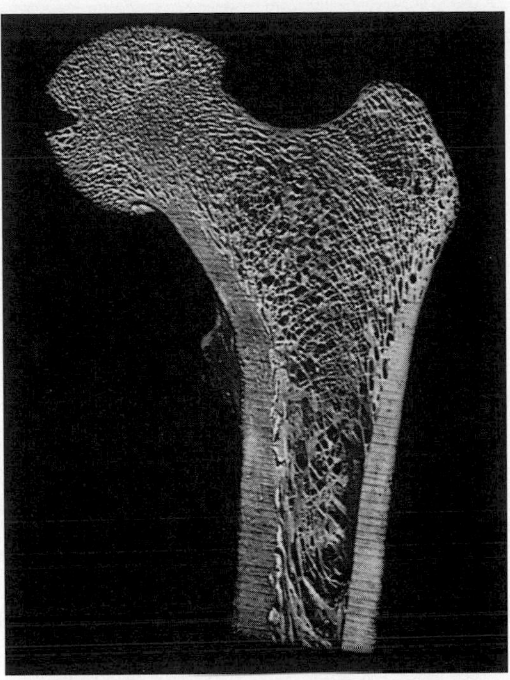

FIGURE 74–5. Cross-section of human femur showing the architecture of bone: a dense envelope of cortical bone and a honeycomb interior of cancellous bone arranged along the lines of mechanical strain. (From Williams PL, Warwick R (eds): Gray's Anatomy. Philadelphia, WB Saunders, 1989, p 232.)

During remodeling osteoblastic bone formation occurs on an exposed bone surface and is preceded by osteoclastic bone resorption on that surface. For cancellous bone, that surface faces the bone marrow and is vastly larger than that of cortical bone, confined to the haversian canals. The haversian canal is at the center of a cylindrical remodeling unit of cortical bone and contains a blood vessel.[52] As a result of these differences in surface area, the remodeling rate for cancellous bone is about 30% per year and for cortical bone is about 3% per year.

During remodeling, packets of bone, called bone remodeling units (BRUs) or bone multicellular units (BMUs), are removed by osteoclastic bone resorption, which lasts 3 to 4 weeks for a packet (Fig. 74–6). The lost bone is replaced by osteoblastic bone formation, which takes 3 to 4 months for one packet. It was estimated that the adult skeleton contains 1.68 million BRUs, 1.4 million in trabecular bone and 0.28 million in cortical bone, occupying a total remodeling space of 12.6 cm^3. The surface area of a single BRU is 0.9 mm^2 in cortical bone and 0.36 mm^2 in cancellous bone.[53] The bone resorption, which starts the remodeling cycle, was proposed to be initiated by osteoblast lineage cells, which perceive and respond to a remodeling signal, such as a change in mechanical strain or an increase in PTH, PGE, or other cytokine. PTH was shown to stimulate collagenase secretion[54] and cause shape changes in osteoblastic cells. If this occurs in lining cells in vivo, a thin protective layer of matrix is removed from the bone surface, exposing the hydroxyapatite.

At the same time, in response to bone resorption stimuli, there could be an increase in the production of RANK-L in osteoblast lineage or other cells, and an increase in osteoclast production. This has not yet been documented in vivo. Assuming that it happens, the newly formed osteoclasts, which are the tissue macrophages of bone, could be activated by the exposed mineral surface, the way macrophages are activated by phagocytic particles. Several osteoclasts are usually seen at the same site, suggesting that, as in inflammation, an active osteoclast could attract additional ones.

In many respects, the bone-remodeling cycle resembles an inflammatory reaction. It probably starts with injury, detected by the fibroblast-related osteoblastic cells, is followed by invasion of the macrophage-related osteoclasts, which, similar to cleaning up debris, resorb the bone, subject to stimulation by the same or similar cytokines

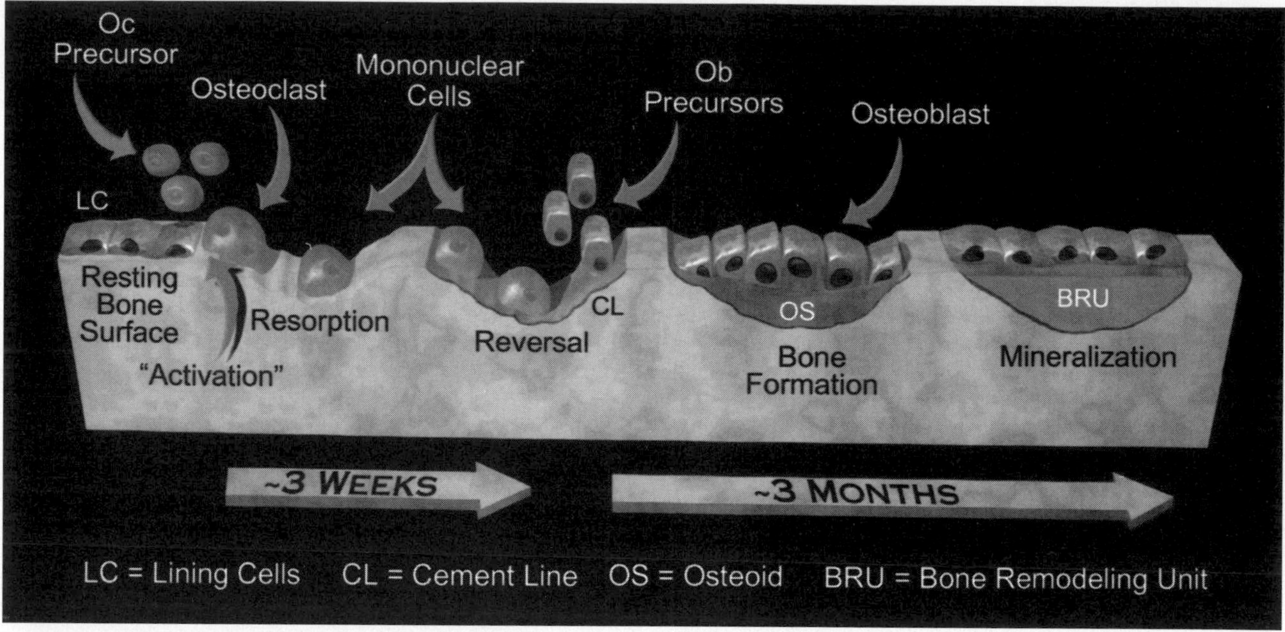

FIGURE 74–6. Diagram of bone-remodeling sequence in a trabecula of cancellous bone and on the surface of a haversian canal in cortical bone.

present in inflammation: e.g., interleukins, prostaglandins, and TNFs. When resorption is completed, the osteoblastic cells deposit bone matrix on the resorbed surface, a process analogous to scar formation or encapsulation of an inflammatory lesion.

The signal responsible for the completion of resorption in a remodeling cycle has not been determined in vivo. The following factors reduce osteoclast formation or activity and could play a role in stopping bone resorption: (1) calcitonin, secreted from the thyroid clear cells in response to elevated calcium concentrations (see Chapter 71), (2) high calcium concentrations in the vicinity of the osteoclast,[55] (3) osteoprotogerin, a decoy receptor of RANK-L,[24] and (4) occupancy of the osteoclast integrin $\alpha_v\beta_3$ by soluble ligands.[56] These factors are not mutually exclusive.

During remodeling, by definition, cessation of resorption is followed by bone formation. However, this is not always the case, which explains the disappearance of trabeculae and the bone loss occurring with age, estrogen deficiency, and other conditions (see below). Histologically, there seems to be a time lag between the end of resorption and the beginning of formation, the reversal phase, during which small cells are seen on the resorbed surface. The plane of reversal can be recognized histologically by the change in direction of the collagen fibers, and was shown to contain osteopontin and bone sialoprotein. Osteopontin is produced both by osteoblasts and osteoclasts and is one of the ligands of the osteoclastic $\alpha_v\beta_3$ integrins, but it is not known if it plays a role in the transition of bone resorption to formation.

At this stage of the remodeling cycle, the plump cuboidal osteoblastic cells appear on the bone surface and deposit the organized matrix. The activity of the osteoclastic layer is clearly coordinated, since the dimension of collagen fibrils exceeds the size of single osteoblasts. The rate of bone formation per osteoblast is usually constant, the overall rate of bone formation being determined by the osteoblast number. Osteoblast recruitment or survival is therefore believed to be the rate-limiting factor in bone formation.

Mineralization starts approximately 7 days after matrix elaboration and continues rapidly to about 70% of maximum mineral content and slowly thereafter, through replacement of water by hydroxyapatite. Bone with a low turnover rate will therefore reach a higher level of mineralization.

The bone formation period is completed after approximately 4 months, when the respective packet of bone, either on the surface of a trabecula or in the haversian canal, enters a quiescent period until the next remodeling cycle. The signal for termination of the bone formation period and the remodeling cycle is not known. The adaptation of bone structure to mechanical loads suggests that mechanical strain must contribute to the control of bone formation.[58]

The sequential occurrence of bone formation following resorption is called coupling. Coupling was proposed to be mediated by local humoral factors released during resorption, such as IGF[59] or TGF-β,[60] or to be due to molecules deposited by osteoclasts at the end of the resorption period.[61] These possibilities are not mutually exclusive and require further in vivo documentation. Mechanical effects on bone could also contribute to the "coupling" phenomenon (see below).

MECHANICAL EFFECTS ON BONE REMODELING

The adaptation of bone structure to mechanical forces has been recognized for a long time and was described in the medical literature about 100 years ago. The adaptation to prevailing mechanical loads is accomplished through bone remodeling. The only way to explain the close, dynamic relationship between bone structure and the lines of "force" in bone is the removal of bone exposed to low strain (force per unit area) and the addition of bone where strain is high. Histologically, it was indeed observed that during cancellous bone remodeling, there is extensive resorption of trabeculae, which are not exposed to mechanical loads, and active bone formation in loaded trabeculae.[62] Bone resorption increases and formation decreases during immobilization, contributing to the bone loss associated with frailty and prolonged bedrest. This regulation of bone resorption and formation by a mechanical strain threshold[63] would in effect produce a coupling effect between the two processes.[64] A reduction in trabecular thickness or increased cortical porosity, caused by bone resorption, would increase the strain in that bone and stimulate or extend the bone formation phase of the remodeling cycle.

The signals for initiation and termination of the bone-remodeling cycle are not known. A change in mechanical load, in either direction, or a microfracture[65] could be the initiating event for specifying the site of a remodeling cycle, and its cessation could be signaled by the dissipation of mechanical strain.[64]

The mechanism for transducing a mechanical stimulus into a biochemical signal in osteoblastic and osteocytic cells has not been clearly identified. The following have been implicated: shearing forces produced by fluid movement,[66, 67] stretch-sensitive ion channels,[68, 69] and integrins.[70, 71] These are not mutually exclusive and can act in tandem; for example, shearing forces on the lining cells can stretch the integrin-mediated attachment of the cells to the matrix and initiate integrin-mediated signaling.

BONE REMODELING AND BONE DISEASES

Postmenopausal Osteoporosis

Bone loss, the most common pathologic bone condition, is always the result of an imbalance between bone resorption and bone formation, due most often to increased bone resorption. This is the case in postmenopausal osteoporosis, where estrogen deficiency increases the number of osteoclasts. Estrogen deficiency increases both the number of sites at which remodeling is initiated, and the extent of resorption at a given site. This process of accelerated bone resorption and increased remodeling is most pronounced during the first few years of estrogen deficiency,[72] but continues thereafter. Biochemical markers, which measure total bone destruction by following bone collagen degradation products in the urine or blood (e.g., N-telopeptides, C-telopeptides, or deoxypyridinoline) are elevated in osteoporotic women, regardless of age or years after menopause.[73, 74]

The accelerated bone loss can be caused by natural menopause, surgical menopause, or cessation of estrogen replacement therapy (ERT). In younger subjects it can be due to amenorrhea caused by vigorous exercise, anorexia, or other causes. Increased bone resorption is accompanied by increased bone formation, presumably as a result of coupling. In the context of bone remodeling this increase is reflected in a larger fraction of the bone surface being involved in bone formation (normally 5% to 10%). The increase in bone formation is not sufficient to maintain bone balance and prevent bone loss. The reason for this "skeletal insufficiency" is not known; it could be due to lack of estrogen or other hormones, such as androgens, required for fully effective bone formation. It could also be due to a kinetic imbalance. It takes about 4 months to form the bone resorbed in 3 weeks. This could explain the faster loss during the first 2 years of estrogen deficiency until a new steady state is reached. Frost et al.[63] suggested that it is due to a different estrogen-dependent strain threshold for mechanical effects on bone remodeling.

In cancellous bone the loss caused by the sustained imbalance results in thinner trabeculae, which become rod-shaped rather than plates, and in trabecular discontinuity which deprive them of mechanical function. In cortical bone, endosteal bone resorption causes thinning of the cortex and sometimes "trabecularization" of the endosteal surface. Enhanced resorption increases the size of haversian canals and the porosity of the bone. The result of these changes is significant weakening of the respective bones and increased fracture risk. It should be mentioned that virtually all the histopathologic information is derived from iliac crest biopsies, the only site practically accessible in patients, and it is assumed that the observed changes are representative of those occurring in other bones.

Glucocorticoid-Induced Osteoporosis

Cushing's disease, and more commonly glucocorticoid treatment, causes significant bone loss due to effects on several systems.[75] Direct action on osteoblast lineage cells suppresses bone formation. Glucocorticoids suppress gonadal function, causing a relative deficiency in estrogens or androgens, or both. Glucocorticoids reduce calcium absorption in the gut and calcium reabsorption in the kidney, which can lead to secondary hyperparathyroidism. The relative sex steroid and calcium deficiencies stimulate bone resorption and bone turnover. These effects are more pronounced in postmenopausal women, who also have a higher incidence of certain autoimmune diseases that often necessitate steroid treatment, such as systemic lupus erythematosus.

The net result of glucocorticoid treatment, usually greater than 7.5 mg prednisolone per day or equivalent for over 6 months, is increased bone resorption with bone formation in the low-normal range. The reduction in bone formation has recently been attributed to osteoblast apoptosis.[76] This imbalance is the cause of bone loss.

Histologically, based on iliac crest biopsies, glucocorticoid-induced osteoporosis is characterized by thinner trabeculae in cancellous bone, rather than a reduction in trabecular number.[77] In postmenopausal osteoporosis, both trabecular thickness and number are reduced, possibly because of higher turnover, longer duration, and multiple remodeling cycles. It has been reported that the return to normal bone mass is more likely in glucocorticoid-induced osteoporosis, after cessation of treatment, than in postmenopausal osteoporosis. This could be due to the fact that usually bone formation only takes place on existing bone surfaces.

Localized Bone Loss

Several pathologic conditions are characterized by localized bone loss. The major ones are periodontal disease, tumor metastases in bone, rheumatoid arthritis, and Paget's disease. In all cases the local bone loss is due to increased osteoclast activity. The mechanism of local osteoclast activation can differ.

In periodontal disease there is a loss of the alveolar bone in the mandible and maxilla, which is the major cause of tooth loss. The increased osteoclast activity was proposed to be due to inflammatory cytokines, such as PGE and IL-1. Attempts to prevent bone loss by locally inhibiting PGE production have not yet been successful.[78] This is also true for the periarticular bone loss in rheumatoid arthritis,[79] attributed to inflammatory cytokines produced in the joint.

Bone metastases are most common in breast and prostate cancer.[80] The reason for the preferential seeding of these tumors in bone is not known; however, local bone destruction is required for the local growth of these tumors. A relatively high percentage of breast cancer bone metastases were shown to produce PTHrP,[81, 82] which stimulates osteoclastic bone resorption via the same mechanism as PTH (see Chapters 70, 75, 76, and 81). The production of cytokines, such as TNF-α, which can stimulate osteoclast formation, either by the tumor cells or macrophages in their vicinity, has also been implicated in tumor osteolysis.

Prostate cancer metastases can produce lytic lesions, as well as sclerotic lesions, the latter via stimulation of bone formation. The molecular mechanisms for osteoclast and osteoblast stimulation have not been elucidated. Another tumor which produces extensive bone destruction is multiple myeloma, wherein IL-6 is elevated and could play a role in osteoclast stimulation.

Paget's disease produces characteristic osteoclastic lesions and is discussed in detail in Chapter 89. In the context of bone remodeling, the pathologic bone resorption is accompanied by localized rapid woven (nonlamellar) bone formation. Following control of the pagetic lesions with bisphosphonate treatment, the woven bone is remodeled and replaced by lamellar bone.

CONCLUSIONS

The skeleton is a vital organ system essential to survival and well-being. Its major functions, mechanical support and ion homeostasis, are achieved by continuous remodeling, destruction, and rebuilding, at the rate of close to 10% per year. Most bone disorders are due to bone loss, either systemic, for example, osteoporosis, or local, for example, rheumatoid arthritis, resulting from an imbalance in the remodeling cycle, bone resorption exceeding bone formation.

Acknowledgments

I thank Dianne E. McDonald for preparation of this manuscript, Raffaella Balena for sketching and Jeff Campbell for drawing the bone remodeling sequence, and Le Duong for input on osteoclast differentiation.

REFERENCES

1. Hall BK: Location of the skeleton within the embryo. *In* Developmental and Cellular Skeletal Biology. London, Academic Press, 1978, pp 37–85.

2. Richardson MK, Allen SP, Wright GM, et al: Somite number and vertebrate evolution. Development 125:151–160, 1998.
3. Christ B, Schmidt C, Huang RJ et al: Segmentation of the vertebrate body. Anat Embryol 1971:1–8, 1998.
4. Hogan BLM: Morphogenesis. Cell 96:225–233, 1999.
5. Martin GR: The roles of FGFs in the early development of vertebrate limbs. Genes Dev 12:1571–1586, 1998.
6. Kengaku M, Capdevila J, Rodrigues Esteban C, et al: Distinct WNT pathways regulating AER formation and dorsoventral polarity in the chick limb bud. Science 280:1274–1277, 1998.
7. Yang YZ, Niswander L: Interaction between the signaling molecules WNT7a and SHH during vertebrate limb development: Dorsal signals regulate anteroposterior patterning. Cell 80:939–947, 1995.
8. Logan M, Tabin CJ: Role of Pitx1 upstream of Tbx4 in specification of hindlimb identity. Science 283:1736–1739, 1999.
9. Daughaday WH: Evolving concepts of GH and IGF-I regulation of skeletal growth. Endocrine 2:767–769, 1994.
10. Burke D, Wilkes D, Blundell TL, Malcolm S: Fibroblast growth factor receptors: Lessons from the genes. Trends Biochem Sci 23:59–62, 1998.
11. Karaplis AC, Deckelbaum RA: Role of PTHrP and PTH-1 receptor in endochondral bone development. Front Biosci 3:d795–803, 1998.
12. Schipani E, Kruse K, Juppner H: A constitutively active mutant PTH-PTHrP receptor in Jansen-type metaphyseal chondrodysplasia. Science 268:98–100, 1995.
13. Grigoriadis AE, Wang ZQ, Cecchini MG, et al: C-fos—A key regulator of osteoclast-macrophage lineage determination and bone remodeling. Science 266:443–448, 1994.
14. Tondravi MM, McKercher SR, Anderson K, et al: Osteopetrosis in mice lacking haematopoietic transcription factor PU.1. Nature 386:81–84, 1997.
15. Franzoso G, Carlson L, Xing LP, et al: Requirement for NF-kappa B in osteoclst and B-cell development. Genes Dev 11:3482–3496, 1997.
16. Iotsova V, Caamano J, Loy J, et al: Osteopetrosis in mice lacking NF-kappa B1 and NF-kappa B2. Nat Med 3:1285–1289, 1997.
17. Wiktorjedrzejczak W, Urbanowska E, Szperl M: Granulocyte-macrophage colony-stimulating factor corrects macrophage deficiencies, but not osteopetrosis, in the colony-stimulating factor-1–deficient op/op mouse. Endocrinology 134:1932–1935, 1994.
18. Ikegame M, Rakopoulos M, Zhou H, et al: Calcitonin receptor isoforms in mouse and rat osteoclasts. J Bone Miner Res 10:59–65, 1995.
19. Horton MA: The alpha v beta 3 integrin "vitronectin receptor." Int J Biochem Cell Biol 29:721–725, 1997.
20. Saftig P, Hunziker E, Wehmeyer O, et al: Impaired osteoclastic bone resorption leads to osteopetrosis in cathepsin-K–deficient mice. Proc Natl Acad Sci U S A 95:13453–13458, 1998.
21. Drake FH, Dodds RA, James IE, et al: Cathepsin K, but not cathepsins B, L, or S, is abundantly expressed in human osteoclasts. J Biol Chem 271:12511–12516, 1996.
22. Soriano P, Montgomery C, Geske R, et al: Targeted disruption of the c-src proto-oncogene leads to osteopetrosis in mice. Cell 64:693–702, 1991.
23. Duong LT, Lakkakorpi PT, Nakamura I, et al: PYK2 in osteoclasts is an adhesion kinase, localized in the sealing zone, activated by ligation of $\alpha v\beta 3$ integrin, and phosphorylated by src kinase. J Clin Invest 102:881–892, 1998.
24. Kong YY, Yoshida H, Sarosi I, et al: OPGL is a key regulator of osteoclastogenesis, lymphocyte development and lymph-node organogenesis. Nature 397:315–323, 1999.
25. Lacey DL, Timms E, Tan HL, et al: Osteoprotegerin ligand is a cytokine that regulates osteoclast differentiation and activation. Cell 93:165–176, 1998.
26. Horwood NJ, Elliott J, Martin TJ, et al: Osteotropic agents regulate the expression of osteoclast differentiation factor and osteoprotegerin in osteoblastic stromal cells. Endocrinology 139:4743–4746, 1998.
27. Simonet WS, Lacey DL, Dunstan CR, et al: Osteoprotegerin: A novel secreted protein involved in the regulation of bone density. Cell 89:309–319, 1997.
28. Martin TJ, Romas E, Gillespie MT: Interleukins in the control of osteoclast differentiation. Crit Rev Eukaryot Gene Expr 8:107–123, 1998.
29. Horowitz MC: Cytokines and estrogen in bone: anti-osteoporotic effects. Science 260:626–627, 1993.
30. Rifas L: Bone and cytokines: beyond IL-1, IL-6 and TNF-alpha. Calcif Tissue Int 64:1–7, 1999.
31. Ducy P, Karsenty G: Genetic control of cell differentiation in the skeleton. Curr Opin Cell Biol 10:614–619, 1998.
32. Wozney JM, Rosen V: Bone morphogenetic protein and bone morphogenetic protein gene family in bone formation and repair. Clin Orthop 346:26–37, 1998.
33. Furuta Y, Hogan BLM: BMP4 is essential for lens induction in the mouse embryo. Genes Dev 2:3764–3775, 1998.
34. Furuta Y, Piston DW, Hogan BL: Bone morphogenetic proteins (BMPs) as regulators of dorsal forebrain development. Development 124:2203–2212, 1997.
35. Luo G, Hofmann C, Bronckers AL, et al: BMP-7 is an inducer of nephrogenesis, and is also required for eye development and skeletal patterning. Genes Dev 9:2808–2820, 1995.
36. Storm EE, Kingsley DM: Joint patterning defects caused by single and double mutations in members of the bone morphogenetic protein (BMP) family. Development 122:3969–3979, 1996.
37. Sakou T: Bone morphogenetic proteins: From basic studies to clinical approaches. Bone 22:591–603, 1998.
38. Onishi T, Ishidou Y, Nagamine T, et al: Distinct and overlapping patterns of localization of bone morphogenetic protein (BMP) family members and a BMP type II receptor during fracture healing in rats. Bone 22:605–612, 1998.
39. Nakase T, Nomura S, Yoshikawa H, et al: Transient and localized expression of bone morphogenetic protein 4 messenger RNA during fracture healing. J Bone Miner Res 9:651–659, 1994.
40. Jiang MS, Tang QQ, McLenithan J, et al: Derepression of the C/EBPalpha gene during adipogenesis: Identification of AP-2alpha as a repressor. Proc Natl Acad Sci U S A 95:3467–3471, 1998.
41. Spiegelman BM: Peroxisome proliferator-activated receptor gamma: A key regulator of adipogenesis and systemic insulin sensitivity. Eur J Med Res 2:457–464, 1997.
42. Shao D, Rangwala SM, Bailey ST, et al: 1998 Interdomain communication regulating ligand binding by PPAR-gamma. Nature 396:377–380, 1997.
43. Bolander ME: Regulation of fracture repair by growth factors. Proc Soc Exp Biol Med 200:165–170, 1992.
44. Nakamura T, Hara Y, Tagawa M, et al: Recombinant human basic fibroblast growth factor accelerates fracture healing by enhancing callus remodeling in experimental dog tibial fracture. J Bone Miner Res 13:942–949, 1998.
45. Machwate M, Rodan SB, Rodan GA, et al: Sphingosine kinase mediates cyclic AMP suppression of apoptosis in rat periosteal cells. Mol Pharmacol 54:70–77, 1998.
46. Harada S, Nagy JA, Sullivan KA, et al: Induction of vascular endothelial growth factor expression by prostaglandin E2 and E1 in osteoblasts. J Clin Invest 93:2490–2496, 1994.
47. Lecanda F, Towler DA, Ziambaras K, et al: Gap junctional communication modulates gene expression in osteoblastic cells. Mol Biol Cell 9:2249–2258, 1998.
48. Mbalaviele G, Nishimura R, Myoi A, et al: Cadherin-6 mediates the heterotypic interactions between the hemopoietic osteoclast cell lineage and stromal cells in a murine model of osteoclast differentiation. J Cell Biol 141:1467–1476, 1998.
49. Cheng SL, Lecanda F, Davidson MK, et al: Human osteoblasts express a repertoire of cadherins, which are critical for BMP-2-induced osteogenic differentiation. J Bone Miner Res 13:633–644, 1998.
50. Hughes PE, Pfaff M: Integrin affinity modulation. Trends Cell Biol 8:359–364, 1998.
51. Hynes RO: Targeted mutations in cell adhesion genes: What have we learned from them? Dev Biol 180:402–412, 1996.
52. Parfitt M: Osteonal and hemi-osteonal remodeling: The spatial and temporal framework for signal traffic in adult human bone. J Cell Biochem 55:273–286, 1994.
53. Parfitt M: Stereologic basis of bone histomorphometry: Theory of quantitative microscopy and reconstruction of the third dimension. *In* Recker RR (ed): Bone Histomorphometry: Techniques and Interpretation, Boca Raton, FL, CRC Press, 1983, pp 53–87.
54. Partridge NC, Walling HW, Bloch SR, et al: The regulation and regulatory role of collagenase in bone. Crit Rev Eukaryot Gene Expr 6:15–27, 1996.
55. Zaidi M, Shankar VS, Tunwell R, et al: A ryanodine receptor-like molecule expressed in the osteoclast plasma membrane functions in extracellular Ca^{2+} sensing. J Clin Invest 96:1582–1590, 1995.
56. Fisher JE, Caulfield MP, Sato M, et al: Inhibition of osteoclastic bone resorption in vivo by echistatin, an "arginyl-glycyl-aspartyl" (RGD)-containing protein. Endocrinology 132:1411–1413, 1993.
57. Frost HM: On our age-related bone loss: Insights from a new paradigm. J Bone Miner Res 12:1539–1546, 1997.
58. Rodan GA: Bone homeostasis. Proc Natl Acad Sci U S A 95:13361–13362, 1998.
59. Mohan S, Farley JR, Baylink DJ: Age-related changes in IGFBP-4 and IGFBP-5 levels in human serum and bone: Implications for bone loss with aging. Prog Growth Factor Res 6:465–473, 1995.
60. Bonewald LF, Mundy GR: Role of transforming growth factor-beta in bone remodeling. Clin Orthop 250:261–276, 1990.
61. Baron R, Vignery A, Horowitz M: Lymphocytes, macrophages and the regulation of bone remodeling. *In* Peck W (ed): Bone and Mineral Research, vol 2. New York, Elsevier, 1984, pp 175–243.
62. Mosekilde L: Consequences of the remodelling process for vertebral trabecular bone structure: A scanning electron microscopy study (uncoupling of unloaded structures). Bone Miner 10:13–35, 1990.
63. Frost HM, Ferretti JL, Jee WS: Perspectives: Some roles of mechanical usage, muscle strength, and the mechanostat in skeletal physiology, disease, and research (editorial). Calcif Tissue Int 62:1–7, 1998.
64. Rodan GA: Mechanical loading, estrogen deficiency, and the coupling of bone formation to bone resorption. J Bone Miner Res 6:527–530, 1991.
65. Mori S, Burr DB: Increased intracortical remodeling following fatigue damage. Bone 14:103–109, 1993.
66. Li YS, Shyy JY, Li S, et al: The ras-JNK pathway is involved in shear-induced gene expression. Mol Cell Biol 16:5947–5954, 1993.
67. Gudi S, Nolan JP, Frangos JA: Modulation of TGPase activity of G proteins by fluid shear stress and phospholipid composition. Proc Natl Acad Sci U S A 95:2515–2519, 1998.
68. Ypey DL, Weidema AF, Hold KM, et al: Voltage, calcium, and stretch activated ionic channels and intracellular calcium in bone cells. J Bone Miner Res 7(suppl 2) S377–387, 1992.
69. Rawlinson SC, Pitsillides AA, Lanyon LE: Involvement of different ion channels in osteoblasts' and osteocytes' early responses to mechanical strain. Bone 19:609–614, 1996.
70. Schmidt C, Pommerenke H, Durr F, et al: Mechanical stressing of integrin receptors induces enhanced tyrosine phosphorylation of cytoskeletally anchored proteins. J Biol Chem 273:5081–5085, 1998.
71. Huang S, Chen CS, Ingber DE: Control of cyclin D1, p27(Kip1), and cell cycle progression in human capillary endothelial cells by cell shape and cytoskeletal tension. Mol Biol Cell 9:3179–3193, 1998.
72. Guthrie JR, Ebeling PR, Hopper JL, et al: A prospective study of bone loss in menopausal Australian-born women. Osteoporos Int 8:282–290, 1998.
73. Arlot ME, Sornay-Rendu E, Garnero P, et al: Apparent pre- and postmenopausal bone loss evaluated by DXA at different skeletal sites in women: the OFELY cohort. J Bone Miner Res 12:683–690, 1997.
74. Garnero P, Hausherr E, Chapuy MC, et al: Markers of bone resorption predict hip fracture in elderly women: The EPIDOS prospective study. J Bone Miner Res 11:1531–1538, 1996.

75. Canalis E: Mechanisms of glucocorticoid action in bone: Implications to glucocorticoid-induced osteoporosis. J Clin Endocrinol Metab 81:3441–3447, 1996.
76. Weinstein RS, Jilka RL, Parfitt AM, et al: Inhibition of osteoblastogenesis and promotion of apoptosis of osteoblasts and osteocytes by glucocorticoids. Potential mechanisms of their deleterious effects on bone. J Clin Invest 102:274–282, 1998.
77. Dempster DW: Bone histomorphometry in glucocorticoid-induced osteoporosis. J Bone Miner Res 4:137–141, 1989.
78. Cavanaugh PF Jr, Meredith MP, Buchanan W, et al: Coordinate production of PGE2 and IL-1 beta in the gingival crevicular fluid of adults with periodontitis: Its relationship to alveolar bone loss and disruption by twice daily treatment with ketorolac tromethamine oral rinse. J Periodontal Res 33:75–82, 1998.
79. Deodhar AA, Woolf AD: Bone mass measurement and bone metabolism in rheumatoid arthritis: A review. Br J Rheumatol 35:309–322, 1996.
80. Bloomfield DJ: Should bisphosphonates be part of the standard therapy of patients with multiple myeloma or bone metastases from other cancers? An evidence-based review. J Clin Oncol 16:1218–1225, 1996.
81. Guise TA, Yin JJ, Taylor SD, et al: Evidence for a causal role of parathyroid hormone–related protein in the pathogenesis of human breast cancer-mediated osteolysis. J Clin Invest 98:1544–1549, 1996.
82. Vargas SJ, Gillespie MT, Powell GJ, et al: Localization of parathyroid hormone–related protein mRNA expression in breast cancer and metastatic lesions by in situ hybridization. J Bone Miner Res 7:971–979, 1992.

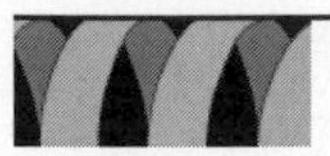

CLINICAL DISORDERS

Chapter 75

Genetic Disorders of Calcium Homeostasis Caused by Abnormal Regulation of Parathyroid Hormone Secretion or Responsiveness

Rajesh V. Thakker ▪ Harald Jüppner

Extracellular calcium ion concentration is tightly regulated through the actions of parathyroid hormone (PTH) on kidney and bone. The intact peptide is secreted by the parathyroid glands at a rate that is appropriate to and dependent upon the prevailing extracellular calcium ion concentration. Hypercalcemia or hypocalcemic disorders can be classified according to whether they arise from an excess or a deficiency of PTH, a defect in the PTH receptor (i.e., the PTH/PTH-related peptide [PTHrP] receptor), or an insensitivity to PTH caused by defects downstream of the PTH/PTHrP receptor (Table 75–1). Recent advances in understanding the biologic importance of key proteins involved in the regulation of PTH secretion and the responsiveness to PTH in target tissues has led to the identification of molecular defects in a variety of disorders and have therefore enabled the characterization of some of the mechanisms involved in the regulation of parathyroid gland development, parathyroid cell proliferation, PTH secretion, and PTH-mediated actions in target tissues. Thus, mutations in the calcium-sensing receptor gene (CaSR) have been reported in patients with familial benign (hypocalciuric) hypercalcemia (FBH or FHH), neonatal severe hyperparathyroidism, and autosomal dominant hypocalcemia. Furthermore, the roles of the oncogene PRAD1, which encodes a novel cyclin, and of the multiple endocrine neoplasia type 1 (MEN1) gene in the pathogenesis of some parathyroid tumors have been revealed (Fig. 75–1). In addition, mutations in the PTH gene and the mitochondrial genome have been demonstrated to be associated with some forms of hypoparathyroidism; mutations in the PTH/PTHrP receptor gene have been identified in patients with two rare genetic disorders, Jansen's and Blomstrand's chondrodysplasia, and mutations in the stimulatory G protein ($G_{S\alpha}$) have been found in individuals with McCune-Albright syndrome, pseudohypoparathyroidism type Ia, and pseudo-pseudohypoparathyroidism. Furthermore, candidate genes have been identified for the DiGeorge syndrome and pseudohypoparathyroidism type Ib, and the chromosomal locations for the susceptibility genes that are responsible for the hereditary hyperparathyroidism and jaw tumors (HPT-JT) syndrome, and for other less frequent variants of FBH, and DiGeorge and Williams syndrome, have been established. Molecular genetic studies thus have provided unique opportunities to elucidate the pathogenesis of rare disorders of calcium homeostasis. These advances, together with the exploration of structure and function of the PTH gene, the genes encoding the PTH/PTHrP and the calcium-sensing receptors, and the effector molecules downstream of these G protein–coupled receptors, are reviewed in this chapter.

PTH GENE STRUCTURE AND FUNCTION

The PTH gene is located on chromosome 11p15 and consists of three exons that are separated by two introns.[1] Exon 1 of the PTH gene is 85 base pairs (bp) in length and is untranslated (Fig. 75–2), whereas exons 2 and 3 encode the 115–amino acid preproPTH peptide. Exon 2 is 90 bp in length and encodes the initiation (ATG) codon, the prehormone sequence, and part of the prohormone sequence. Exon 3 is 612 bp in size and encodes the remainder of the prohormone sequence, the mature PTH peptide, and the 3′ untranslated region.[2] The 5′ regulatory sequence of the human PTH gene contains a vitamin D response element 125 bp upstream of the transcription start site that downregulates PTH messenger ribonucleic acid (mRNA) transcription in response to vitamin D receptor binding.[3, 4] PTH gene transcription (as well as PTH peptide secretion) is also dependent on the extracellular calcium and phosphate[5–8] concentrations, although the presence of specific upstream calcium or phosphate response element(s) has not yet been demonstrated.[9, 10] The secretion of mature PTH, an 84–amino acid peptide, from the parathyroid chief cell is regulated through a G protein–coupled calcium-sensing receptor, which is also expressed in renal tubules and in several other tissues, albeit in less abundance. PTH mRNA is first translated into a preproPTH peptide. The "pre" sequence consists of a 25–amino acid signal peptide (leader sequence), which is responsible for directing the nascent peptide into the endoplasmic reticulum to be packaged for secretion from the cell.[11] The "pro" sequence is 6 amino acids in length and, although its function

TABLE 75–1. Diseases of Calcium Homeostasis and Their Chromosomal Locations

Metabolic Abnormality	Disease	Inheritance	Gene Product	Chromosomal Location
Hypercalcemia	MEN1	Autosomal dominant	Menin	11q13
	MEN2	Autosomal dominant	RET	10q11.2
	Hereditary hyperparathyroidism and jaw tumors (HPT-JT)	Autosomal dominant	Unknown	1q21-31
	Sporadic hyperparathyroidism	Sporadic	PRAD1/CCND1	11q13
			Retinoblastoma	13q14
			Unknown	1p32-pter
	Familial benign hypercalcemia			
	FBH3q	Autosomal dominant	CaSR	3q13-21
	FBH19p	Autosomal dominant	Unknown	19p13
	FBHOk	Autosomal dominant	Unknown	19q13
	Neonatal severe hyperparathyroidism (NSHPT)	Autosomal recessive	CaSR	3q13-21
	Jansen's disease	Autosomal dominant	PTH/PTHrPR	3p21.1-p24.2
	Williams syndrome	Autosomal dominant	Elastin, LIMK (and other genes)	7q11.23
	McCune-Albright syndrome	Mutations during early embryonic development?	Gsα	20q13.2-13.3
Hypocalcemia	Isolated hypoparathyroidism	Autosomal dominant	PTH	11p15*
		Autosomal recessive	PTH	11p15*
		X-linked recessive	Unknown	Xq26-27
	Hypocalcemic hypercalciuria	Autosomal dominant	CaSR	3q13-21
	Hypoparathyroidism associated with polyglandular autoimmune syndrome (APECED)	Autosomal recessive	AIRE	21q22.3
	Hypoparathyroidism associated with Kearns-Sayre and MELAS	Maternal	Mitochondrial genome	
	Hypoparathyroidism associated with complex congenital syndromes			
	DiGeorge syndrome	Autosomal dominant	*rnex40*‡	22q11/10p
			nex2.2-nex3‡	
			UDF1L‡	
	Blomstrand's lethal chondrodysplasia	Autosomal recessive	PTH/PTHrPR	3p21.1-p24.2
	Kenny-Caffey syndrome	Autosomal dominant†	Unknown	?
	Barakat's syndrome	Autosomal recessive†	Unknown	?
	Lymphedema	Autosomal recessive	Unknown	?
	Nephropathy, nerve deafness	Autosomal dominant†	Unknown	?
	Nerve deafness without renal dysplasia	Autosomal dominant	Unknown	?
	Dysmorphology, growth failure	Autosomal recessive	Unknown	1q42-43
	Pseudohypoparathyroidism (type Ia)	Autosomal dominant, paternally imprinted	Gsα	20q13.2-13.3
	Pseudohypoparathyroidism (type Ib)	Autosomal dominant, paternally imprinted	Unknown	20q13.3

*Mutations of PTH gene identified only in some families.
†Most likely inheritance shown.
‡Most likely candidate genes.
MELAS, mitochondrial encephalopathy, strokelike episodes and lactic acidosis; ?, location not known.

is less well defined than that of the "pre" sequence, it is also essential for correct PTH processing and secretion.[11] After the 84–amino acid mature PTH peptide is secreted from the parathyroid cell, it is cleared from the circulation (with a short half-life of about 2 minutes), via nonsaturable hepatic uptake and renal excretion. PTH mediates its actions through a receptor that it shares with PTHrP (also known as PTHrH or PTH-related hormone).[12, 13] This PTH/PTHrP receptor (see Fig. 75–1) is a member of a subgroup of G protein–coupled receptors, and its gene is located on chromosome 3p21-p24.[14, 15] The PTH/PTHrP receptor is highly expressed in kidney and bone, where it mediates the endocrine actions of PTH. However, the most abundant expression of the PTH/PTHrH receptor occurs in chondrocytes of the metaphyseal growth plate, where it predominantly mediates the autocrine and/or paracrine actions of PTHrP.[16, 17] Mutations involving the genes that encode PTH, the calcium-sensing receptor, the PTH/PTHrP receptor, and $G_{s\alpha}$ protein all affect the regulation of calcium homeostasis (see Fig. 75–1) and can thus be associated with genetic disorders characterized by hypercalcemia or hypocalcemia (see Table 75–1).

HYPERCALCEMIC DISEASES

Similar to the findings in other tumor syndromes, the abnormal expression of an oncogene or the loss of a tumor suppressor gene can result in abnormal proliferative activity of parathyroid cells, and the molecular exploration of these genes has provided important new insights into the pathogenesis of different forms of hyperparathyroidism. Oncogenes are genes whose abnormal expression may transform a normal cell into a tumor cell. The normal form of the gene is referred to as a *proto-oncogene,* and a single mutant allele may affect the phenotype of the cell; these genes may also be referred to as *dominant oncogenes* (Fig. 75–3A). The mutant versions (i.e., the oncogene), which are usually excessively or inappropriately active, may arise because of point mutations, gene amplifications, or chromosomal translocations. Tumor suppressor genes, also referred to as *recessive oncogenes* or *anti-oncogenes,* normally inhibit cell proliferation, whereas their mutant versions in cancer cells have lost their normal function. To transform a normal cell to a tumor cell, both

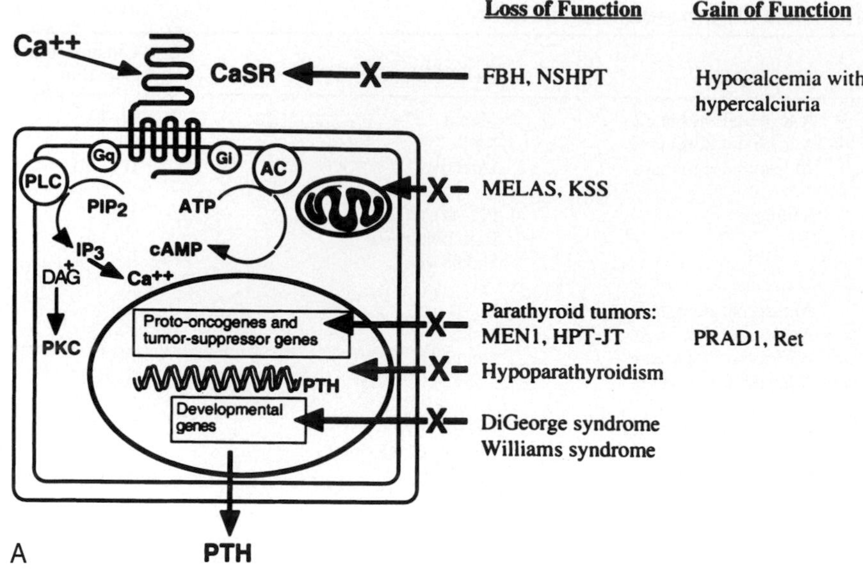

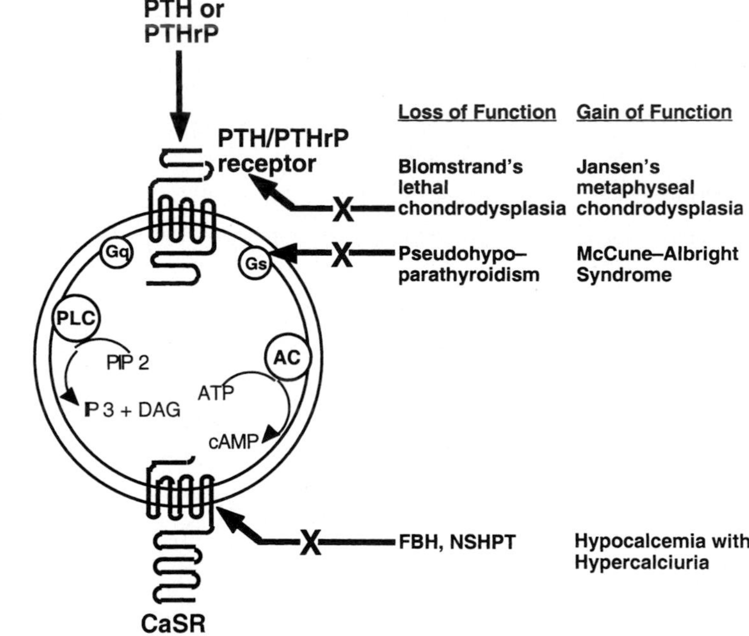

FIGURE 75–1. Schematic representation of some of the components involved in calcium homeostasis in parathyroid cells (A) and target (e.g., renal tubular) cells (B). Alterations in extracellular calcium are detected by the calcium-sensing receptor (CaSR), which is a 1078–amino acid G protein–coupled receptor. The PTH/PTHrP receptor, which mediates the actions of PTH and PTHrP, is also a G protein–coupled receptor. Thus, Ca^{2+}, PTH, and PTHrP involve G protein–coupled signaling pathways, and interaction with their specific receptors can lead to activation of G_s, G_i, and G_q, respectively. G_s stimulates adenylyl cyclase (AC), which catalyzes the formation of cAMP from ATP. G_i inhibits AC activity. cAMP stimulates PKA, which phosphorylates cell-specific substrates. Activation of G_q stimulates PLC, which catalyzes the hydrolysis of the phosphoinositide (PIP_2) to inositol triphosphate (IP_3) (which increases intracellular calcium) and diacylglycerol (DAG) (which activates PKC). These proximal signals modulate downstream pathways, which result in specific physiologic effects. Abnormalities in several genes, which lead to mutations in proteins in these pathways, have been identified in specific disorders of calcium homeostasis (see Table 75–1). (Adapted from Thakker RV: Parathyroid disorders: Molecular genetics and physiology. *In* Morris PJ, Wood WC [eds]: Oxford Textbook of Surgery. New York, Oxford University Press [in press]).

alleles of the tumor suppressor gene must be inactivated. Inactivation arises by point mutations or, alternatively, by small intragenic or larger deletions that can involve substantial genomic portions or a whole chromosome. Larger deletions may be detected by cytogenetic methods, by Southern blot analysis, or by polymerase chain reaction (PCR)-based analysis of polymorphic markers. Typically, genomic DNA from the patient's tumor cells lack certain chromosomal regions, in comparison to genomic DNA from other normal cells (e.g., lymphocytes), and this finding is therefore referred to as *loss of heterozygosity* (LOH) (see Fig. 75–3B). The transformation of a normal cell to a tumor cell requires inactivation of both alleles of the tumor suppressor gene; therefore, the finding of LOH suggests a point mutation in the other allele.

Parathyroid Tumors

Parathyroid tumors may occur as an isolated and sporadic endocrinopathy, or as part of an inherited tumor syndrome[18] (e.g., MEN or HPT-JT),[19] or in response to chronic overstimulation (e.g., uremic hyperparathyroidism).[20] Genetic analyses of kindreds with MEN1 and MEN2A and of tumor tissue from patients with single parathyroid adenomas have shown that some of the known molecular mechanisms known to be involved in tumorigenesis can also be responsible for the development of hyperparathyroidism.

Our current understanding indicates that sporadic parathyroid tumors are caused by single somatic mutations that lead to the activation or overexpression of proto-oncogenes such as PRAD1 (*para*thyroid *a*denoma *1*) or RET (see Fig. 75–3A). Furthermore, different tumor suppressor genes affecting the parathyroid glands are predicted to be located on several different chromosomes, and in a significant number of patients, LOH has been documented for one of these loci. For all these somatic mutations, a single point mutation or a deletion provides a growth advantage of a single parathyroid cell and its progeny, leading to their clonal expansion.

In hereditary forms of the disease, two distinct, sequentially occurring molecular defects are observed. The first "hit" (point mutation or deletion) is an inherited genetic defect that affects only one allele

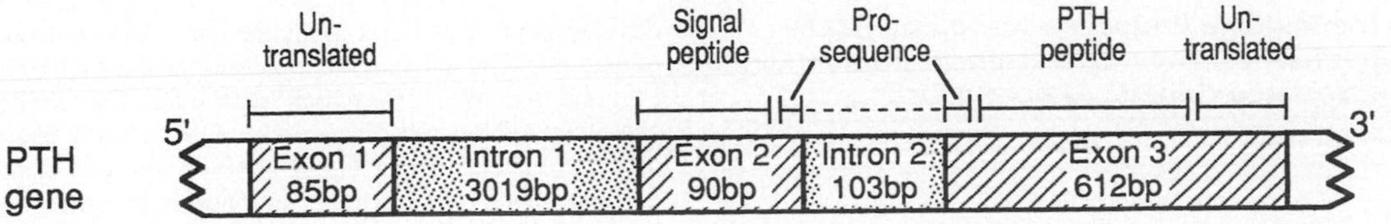

FIGURE 75–2. Schematic representation of the PTH gene. The PTH gene consists of three exons and two introns; the peptide is encoded by exons 2 and 3. The PTH peptide is synthesized as a precursor that contains a "pre" and a "pro" sequence. The mature PTH peptide, which contains 84 amino acids, and larger C-terminal PTH fragments are secreted from the parathyroid cell. (Adapted from Parkinson DB, Thakker RV: A donor splice mutation in the parathyroid hormone gene is associated with autosomal recessive hypoparathyroidism. Nat Genet 1:149–153, 1992).

that comprises a gene encoding an anti-oncogene (see Fig. 75–3B). Subsequently, a somatic mutation or deletion affecting the second allele occurs in a single parathyroid cell, and because of the resulting growth advantage, this mutation leads to its monoclonal expansion and thus the development of parathyroid tumors. Examples of the latter molecular mechanism in the development of hyperparathyroidism are the inactivation of tumor suppressor genes (e.g., MEN1 and retinoblastoma [Rb] genes) or an as-yet-unknown gene located on chromosome 1p.

PRAD1 Gene

Investigations of the PTH gene in sporadic parathyroid adenomas detected abnormally sized restriction fragment length polymorphisms (RFLPs) with a DNA probe for the 5′ part of the PTH gene in some adenomas,[21] indicating disruption of the gene. Further studies of the tumor DNA demonstrated that the first exon of the PTH gene (Fig. 75–2) was separated from the fragments containing the second and third exons, and that a rearrangement had occurred to juxtapose the 5′ PTH regulatory elements with "new" non-PTH DNA.[22] This rearrangement was not found in the DNA from the peripheral leukocytes of the patients, thereby indicating that it represented a somatic event and not an inherited germline mutation. Investigation of this rearranged DNA sequence localized it to chromosome 11q13, and detailed analysis revealed that it was highly conserved in different species and expressed in normal parathyroids and in parathyroid adenomas. The protein expressed as a result of this rearrangement, which was designated PRAD1, was demonstrated to encode a 295–amino acid member of the cyclin D family of cell-cycle regulatory proteins. Cyclins were initially characterized in the dividing cells of budding yeast, where they controlled the G_1 to S transition of the cell cycle, and in marine mollusks, where they regulated the mitotic phase (M phase) of the cell cycle.[23] Cyclins have also been identified in man and have an important role in regulating many stages of cell-cycle progression. Thus, PRAD1, which encoded a novel cyclin, referred to as *cyclin D1* (CCND1), is an important cell-cycle regulator, and overexpression of PRAD1 may be an important event in the development of at least 15% of sporadic parathyroid adenomas.[24] Interestingly, more than 66% of the transgenic mice overexpressing PRAD1 under the control of a mammary tissue–specific promoter were found to develop breast carcinoma in adult life,[25] and expression of this proto-oncogene under the control of the 5′ regulatory region of the PTH gene resulted in mild-to-moderate chronic hyperparathyroidism.[26] Taken together, these findings in transgenic animals provide further evidence for the conclusion that PRAD1 can be involved in the development of a significant number of parathyroid adenomas.

The MEN1 Gene

Multiple endocrine neoplasia type 1 (MEN1) is characterized by the combined occurrence of tumors of the parathyroids, pancreatic islet cells, and anterior pituitary (Table 75–2).[27, 28] Parathyroid tumors occur in 95% of MEN1 patients, and the resulting hypercalcemia is the first manifestation of MEN1 in about 90% of patients. Pancreatic islet cell tumors occur in 40% of MEN1 patients, and gastrinomas, leading to the Zollinger-Ellison syndrome, are the most common type of tumor and also the most important cause of morbidity and mortality in MEN1 patients. Anterior pituitary tumors, most commonly prolactinomas, occur in 30% of MEN1 patients. Associated tumors, which may also occur in MEN1, include adrenal cortical tumors, carcinoid tumors, lipomas, angiofibromas, and collagenomas.[28, 29] The gene causing MEN1 was localized to a less than 300 kb region on chromosome

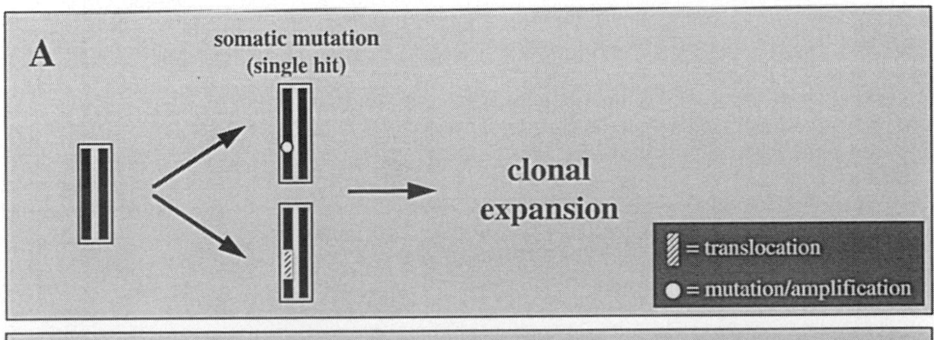

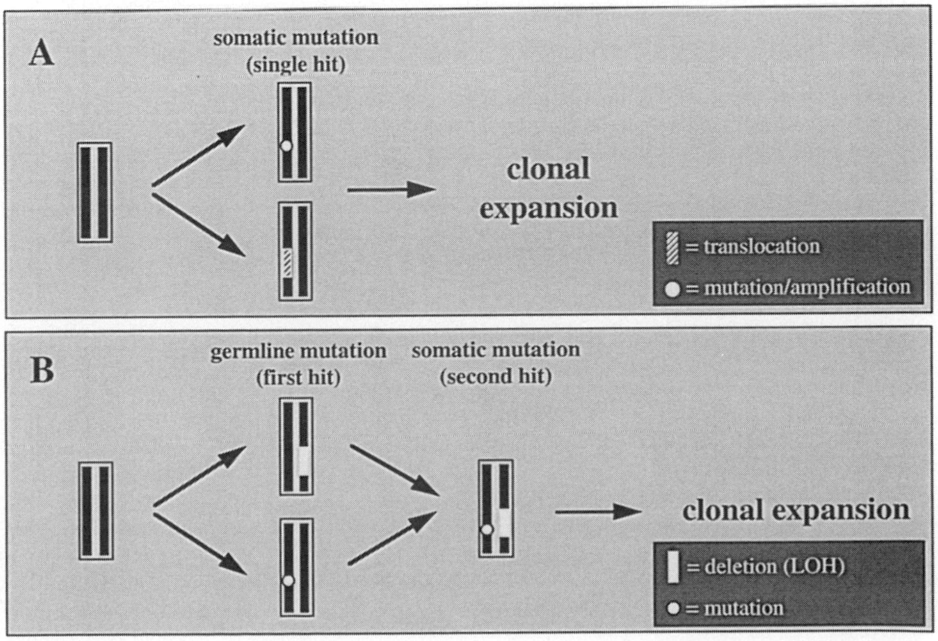

FIGURE 75–3. Schematic illustration of the molecular defects that can lead to the development of parathyroid tumors. *A*, A somatic mutation (point mutation or translocation) affecting a proto-oncogene (for example, PRAD1 or *RET*) results in a growth advantage of single parathyroid cell and thus its clonal expansion. *B*, An inherited single point mutation or deletion affecting a tumor suppressor gene (first hit) makes the parathyroid cell susceptible to a second, somatic "hit" (point mutation or deletion) (i.e., LOH), which then leads to the clonal expansion of a single cell.

TABLE 75–2. The Multiple Endocrine Neoplasia (MEN) Syndromes, Their Characteristic Tumors, and Associated Genetic Abnormalities*

Type (Chromosomal Location)	Tumors
MEN1 (11q13)	Parathyroids
	Pancreatic islets
	Gastrinoma
	Insulinoma
	Glucagonoma
	VIPoma
	PPoma
	Pituitary (anterior)
	Prolactinoma
	Somatotrophinoma
	Corticotrophinoma
	Nonfunctioning
	Associated tumors
	Adrenal cortical
	Carcinoid
	Lipoma
	Angiofibromas
	Collagenomas
MEN2 (10 cen-10q11.2)	
MEN2A	Medullary thyroid carcinoma
	Pheochromocytoma
	Parathyroid
MTC-only	Medullary thyroid carcinoma
MEN2B	Pheochromocytoma
	Medullary thyroid carcinoma
	Associated abnormalities
	Mucosal neuromas
	Marfanoid habitus
	Medullated corneal nerve fibers
	Megacolon

*Autosomal dominant inheritance of the MEN syndromes has been established.

11q13 both by genetic mapping studies that investigated MEN1-associated tumors for LOH and by segregation studies in MEN1 families.[30] The results of these studies, which were consistent with Knudson's model for tumor development, indicated that the MEN1 gene represented a putative tumor suppressor gene (see Fig. 75–3B). Characterization of genes from this region led to the identification of the MEN1 gene,[31, 32] which consists of 10 exons that encode a novel 610–amino acid protein, referred to as MENIN. The majority (>80%) of the germline MEN1 mutations in the families are inactivating and are consistent with its role as a tumor suppressor gene. These mutations are diverse in their types and approximately 25% are nonsense, approximately 45% are deletions, approximately 15% are insertions, less than 5% are donor splice mutations, and approximately 10% are missense mutations.[30] In addition, the MEN1 mutations are scattered throughout the 1830 bp coding region of the gene with no evidence for clustering. Correlations between the MEN1 germline mutations and the clinical manifestations of the disorder appear to be absent.[33] Tumors from MEN1 patients and non-MEN1 patients have been observed to harbor the germline mutation together with a somatic LOH involving chromosome 11q13, as expected from both Knudson's model and the proposed role of the MEN1 gene as a tumor suppressor.[34–43] MENIN has been shown to be located in the nucleus,[44] where it directly interacts with the N terminus of the AP-1 transcriptional factor Jun-D.[45] MENIN suppresses Jun-D–activated transcription and, thus, acts via the transcriptional regulation pathway to control cell proliferation.[45]

The MEN2 Gene (c-*RET*)

MEN2 describes the association of medullary thyroid carcinoma (MTC), pheochromocytomas, and parathyroid tumors.[27, 30] Three clinical variants of MEN2 are recognized: MEN2A, MEN2B, and MTC-only (see Table 75–2). MEN2A is the most common variant, and the development of MTC is associated with pheochromocytomas (in 50% of patients), which may be bilateral, and parathyroid tumors (in 20% of patients). MEN2B, which represents 5% of all MEN2 cases, is characterized by the occurrence of MTC and pheochromocytoma in association with a marfanoid habitus, mucosal neuromas, medullated corneal fibers, and intestinal autonomic ganglion dysfunction leading to multiple diverticula and megacolon. Parathyroid tumors do not usually occur in MEN2B. MTC-only is a variant in which medullary thyroid carcinoma is the sole manifestation of the syndrome. The gene causing all three MEN2 variants was mapped to chromosome 10cen-10q11.2, a region containing the c-*RET* proto-oncogene which encodes a tyrosine kinase receptor with cadherin-like and cysteine-rich extracellular domains and a tyrosine kinase intracellular domain.[46, 47] Specific mutations of c-*RET* have been identified for each of the three MEN2 variants. Thus, in 95% of patients, MEN2A is associated with mutations of the cysteine-rich extracellular domain, and mutations in codon 634 (Cys→Arg) account for 85% of MEN2A mutations. However, a search for c-*RET* mutations in sporadic non-MEN2A parathyroid adenomas revealed no codon 634 mutations.[48, 49] MTC-only is also associated with missense mutations in the cysteine-rich extracellular domain, and most mutations are in codon 618. However, MEN2B is associated with mutations in codon 918 (Met→Thr) of the intracellular tyrosine kinase domain in 95% of patients. Interestingly, the c-*RET* proto-oncogene is also involved in the etiology of papillary thyroid carcinomas and in Hirschsprung's disease. Mutational analysis of c-*RET* to detect mutations in codons 609, 611, 618, 634, 768, and 804 in MEN2A and MTC-only and codon 918 in MEN2B has been used in the diagnosis and management of patients and families with these disorders.[47, 50]

Rb Gene

The Rb gene, which is a tumor suppressor gene[51] located on chromosome 13q14, is involved in the pathogenesis of retinoblastomas and a variety of common sporadic human malignancies, including ductal breast, small cell lung, and bladder carcinomas. Allelic deletion of the Rb gene has been demonstrated in all parathyroid carcinomas and in 10% of parathyroid adenomas[52, 53] and was accompanied by abnormal staining patterns for the RB protein in 50% of the parathyroid carcinomas but in none of the parathyroid adenomas.[52] These results demonstrate an important role for the Rb gene in the development of parathyroid carcinomas and may be of help in the histologic distinction of parathyroid adenoma from carcinoma.[52] However, the findings of extensive deletions of the long arm of chromosome 13 (including the Rb locus) in some parathyroid adenomas and carcinomas,[53] and similar findings in pituitary carcinomas[54] suggest that other tumor suppressor genes on chromosome 13q may also have a role in the development of such tumors.

Gene on Chromosome 1p

LOH studies have revealed allelic loss of chromosome 1p32-pter in 40% of sporadic parathyroid adenomas.[55] This region is estimated to be about 110 centiMorgans (cM), equivalent to about 110 million base pairs (Mbp) of DNA, but recent studies have narrowed the interval containing this putative tumor suppressor gene to an approximate 4 cM (i.e., about 4 Mbp) region.[56]

Autosomal Dominant Hyperparathyroidism Syndromes

HPT-JT syndrome is an autosomal dominant disorder characterized by the occurrence of parathyroid adenomas and carcinomas in association with fibro-osseous mandibular or maxillary jaw tumors and occasional Wilms' tumors or adult nephroblastomas.[19] Genetic linkage studies of five HPT-JT families have mapped the gene causing this disorder to chromosome 1q21-q31.[19] An analysis of parathyroid tumors from affected HPT-JT family members did not detect LOH of the chromosome 1q21-q31 region, thereby suggesting that this gene (designated HRPT2) may be a proto-oncogene rather than a tumor suppressor. Familial isolated primary hyperparathyroidism (FIPH) has been reported in several kindreds, and studies have been pursued to identify the genes causing this disorder. Some FIPH families have been shown to harbor mutations involving the MEN1 gene,[34, 57] whereas in other families, linkage to polymorphic loci from chromosome 1q21-q31 has been established.[58, 59] In addition, an analysis of parathyroid tumors from FIPH patients has revealed LOH involving chromosome 1q21-q31 loci. FIHP, located on chromosome 1q21-q31, has a high incidence of early-onset parathyroid carcinomas.[59] Thus, two genes on chromosome 1q may be involved in the etiology of parathyroid tumors, or FIHP and HPT-JT may be allelic variants. The identification of the FIHP gene and the HPT-JT gene will help to elucidate these possibilities.

Hyperparathyroidism in Chronic Renal Failure

Chronic renal failure is often associated with a form of secondary hyperparathyroidism that may subsequently result in the hypercalcemic state of "tertiary" hyperparathyroidism. The parathyroid proliferative response in this condition led to the proposal that the autonomous parathyroid tissue might have undergone hyperplastic change, and might therefore be polyclonal in origin. However, studies of X-chromosome inactivation in parathyroids from patients undergoing hemodialysis with refractory hyperparathyroidism have revealed at least one monoclonal parathyroid tumor in more than 60% of patients.[20] In addition, LOH involving several loci on chromosome Xp11 was detected in one of these parathyroid tumors, thereby suggesting the involvement of a tumor suppressor gene from this region in the pathogenesis of such tumors.[20] Interestingly, none of the parathyroid tumors from these patients with chronic renal failure had LOH involving loci from chromosome 11q13. This unexpected finding of monoclonal parathyroid tumors in the majority of patients with "tertiary" hyperparathyroidism suggests that an increased turnover of parathyroid cells in secondary hyperparathyroidism may render the parathyroid glands more susceptible to mitotic non-disjunction or to other mechanisms of somatic deletions, which may involve loci other than those located on chromosome 11q13 (MEN1 and PRAD1).

Disorders of the Calcium-Sensing Receptor (CaSR)

Two hypercalcemic disorders due to mutations of the calcium-sensing receptor (CaSR) have been reported[60–65]: familial benign hypercalcemia (FBH), which is also referred to as familial hypocalciuric hypercalcemia (FHH), and neonatal severe hyperparathyroidism (NSHPT). Mutational analyses of the human CaSR, which is a G–protein coupled receptor located on chromosome 3q13-q21,[66] have revealed different mutations that result in a loss of function of the CaSR in patients with FBH and NSHPT (see Fig. 75–1).[60–65] Many of these mutations cluster around the aspartate- and glutamate-rich regions (codons 39 to 300) within the extracellular domain of the receptor, and this has been proposed to contain low affinity calcium-binding sites, based on similarities to that of calsequestrin, in which the ligand-binding pockets also contain negatively charged amino acid residues.[67] Approximately two-thirds of the FBH kindreds investigated have been found to have unique heterozygous mutations of the CaSR, and expression studies of these mutations have demonstrated a loss of CaSR function, whereby an increase occurs in the calcium ion–dependent set-point for PTH release from the parathyroid cell.[60, 65, 68, 69] NSHPT occurring in the offspring of consanguineous FBH families has been shown to be due to homozygous CaSR mutations.[60, 61, 63, 70, 71] However, sporadic neonatal hyperparathyroidism in some patients has been reported to be associated with de novo heterozygous CaSR mutations,[62] thereby suggesting that factors other than mutant gene dosage[70] (e.g., the degree of set-point abnormality, the bony sensitivity to PTH, and the maternal extracellular calcium concentration), may also play a role in the phenotypic expression of a CaSR mutation in the neonate. The remaining one-third of FBH families in whom a mutation within the coding region of the CaSR has not been demonstrated may either have an abnormality in the promoter of the gene or a mutation at one of the two other FBH loci that have been revealed by family linkage studies. One of these FBH loci is located on chromosome 19p and is referred to as *FBH19p*.[72] Studies of another FBH kindred from Oklahoma whose members also suffered from progressive elevations in PTH, hypophosphatemia, and osteomalacia[73, 74] demonstrated that this variant, designated FBHOk, was linked to chromosome 19q13.[75] These three FBH loci located on chromosomes 3q, 19p, and 19q have also been referred to as FBH (or FHH) types 1, 2 and 3, respectively.[75]

Jansen's Disease

Jansen's disease (Figs. 75–4 and 75–5) is an autosomal dominant disease that is characterized by short-limbed dwarfism resulting from an abnormal regulation of chondrocyte proliferation and differentiation in the metaphyseal growth plate and associated severe hypercalcemia and hypophosphatemia, despite normal or undetectable serum levels of PTH or PTHrP.[76–79] These abnormalities are caused by mutations in the PTH/PTHrP receptor that lead to constitutive PTH- and PTHrP-independent receptor activation. Three different mutations of the PTH/PTHrP receptor have been identified, and these involve codon 223 (His→Arg), codon 410 (Thr→Pro), and codon 458 (Ile→Arg)[76–79] (Fig. 75–6). Expression of the mutant receptors in COS-7 cells resulted in constitutive, ligand-independent accumulation of cAMP, while the basal accumulation of inositol phosphates was not increased.[76–78] Because the PTH/PTHrP receptor is most abundantly expressed in kidney, bone, and the metaphyseal growth plate, these findings provide a likely explanation for the abnormalities observed in mineral homeostasis and growth plate development in this disorder. This conclusion is supported further by observations in mice that express the human PTH/PTHrP receptor with the H223R mutation under the control of the rat α_1(II) promoter.[80] This promoter targeted expression of the mutant receptor to the layer of proliferative chondrocytes and delayed their differentiation into hypertrophic cells, which led, at least in animals with multiple copies of the transgene, to a mild impairment in growth of long bones. These observations are consistent with the conclusion that expression of a constitutively active human PTH/PTHrP receptor in growth plate chondrocytes causes the characteristic metaphyseal changes in patients with Jansen's disease.

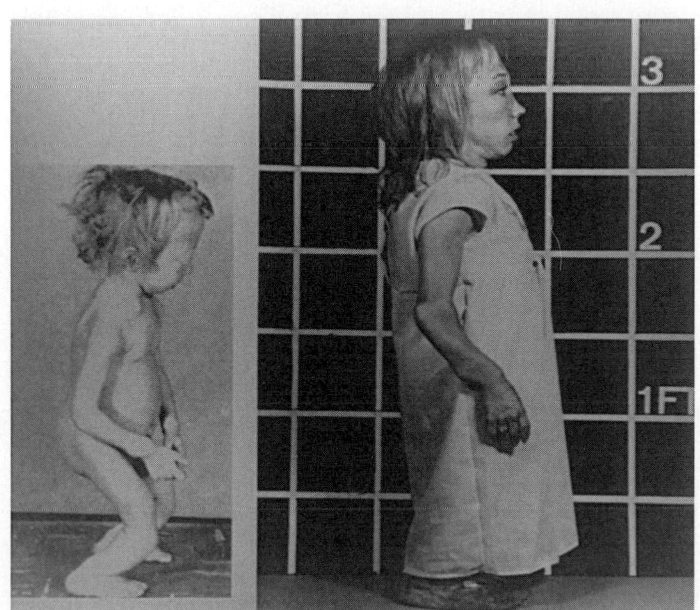

FIGURE 75–4. Patient with Jansen's metaphyseal chondrodysplasia at ages 5 *(left)* and 22 *(right)* years. (From Frame B, Poznanski AK: Conditions that may be confused with rickets. *In* DeLuca HF, Anast CS [eds]: Pediatric Diseases Related to Calcium. New York, Elsevier, 1980, pp 269–289.)

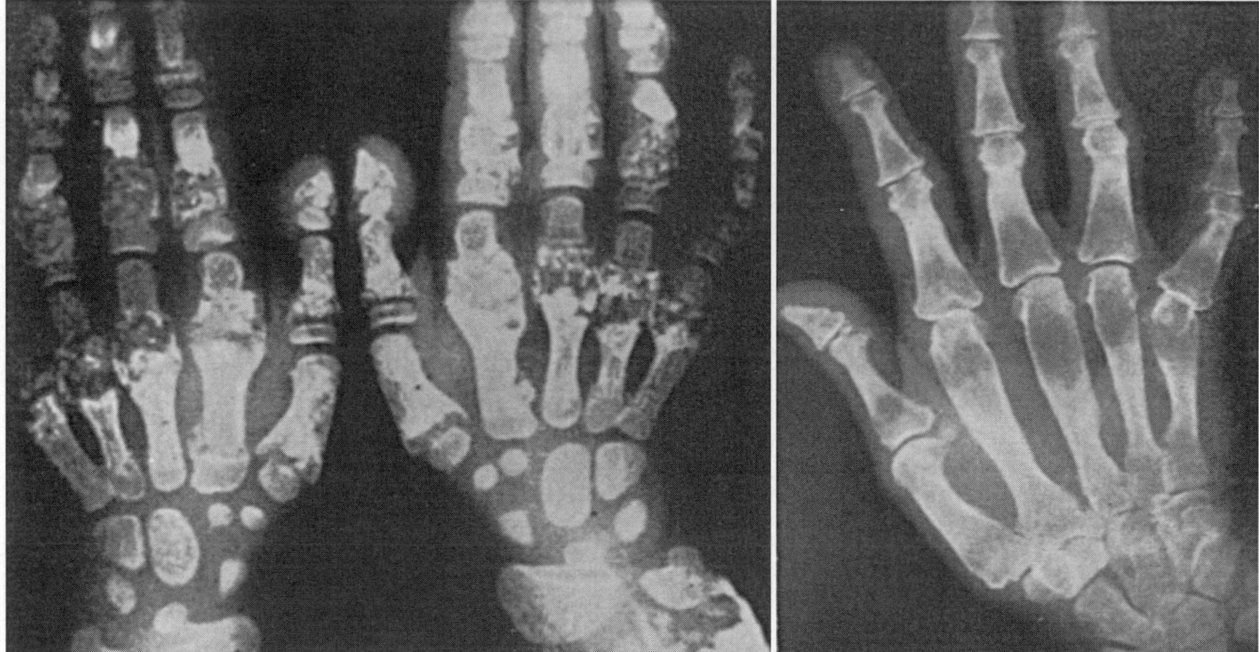

FIGURE 75–5. Hand radiographs of the patient first described by Jansen, at age 10 *(left)* and 44 *(right)* years. (From De Haas WHD, De Boer W, Griffioen F: Metaphysial dysostosis: A late follow-up of the first reported case. J Bone Joint Surg Br 51:290–299, 1969.)

Williams Syndrome

Williams syndrome is an autosomal dominant disorder characterized by supravalvular aortic stenosis, elflike facies, psychomotor retardation, and infantile hypercalcemia. The underlying abnormality of calcium metabolism remains unknown, but abnormal 1,25-dihydroxyvitamin D_3 metabolism or decreased calcitonin production have been implicated, although none has been consistently demonstrated. Studies have demonstrated hemizygosity at the elastin locus on chromosome 7q11.23 in more than 90% of patients with the classical Williams phenotype,[81–83] and only one patient had a cytogenetically identifiable deletion, thereby indicating that the syndrome is usually due to a microdeletion of 7q11.23.[83] Interestingly, ablation of the elastin gene in mice results in vascular abnormalities similar to those observed in patients with Williams syndrome.[84] However, the microdeletions that have been reported involve also another gene, designated *LIM-kinase,* that is expressed in the central nervous system.[85] The calcitonin receptor gene, which is located on chromosome 7q21, is not involved in the deletions found in Williams syndrome and is therefore unlikely to be implicated in the hypercalcemia of such children.[86] Although the involvement of the elastin and LIM-kinase genes in the deletions seen in Williams syndrome patients can explain the respective cardiovascular and neurologic features of this disorder, it seems likely that another, as-yet-uncharacterized gene that is within this contiguously deleted region is likely to explain the abnormalities of calcium metabolism.

HYPOCALCEMIC DISORDERS

Hypoparathyroidism

Hypoparathyroidism may occur as part of a pluriglandular autoimmune disorder or as a complex congenital defect, as, for example, in the DiGeorge syndrome. In addition, hypoparathyroidism may develop as a solitary endocrinopathy, and this has been called *isolated* or *idiopathic hypoparathyroidism.* Familial occurrences of isolated hypoparathyroidism with autosomal dominant, autosomal recessive, and X-linked recessive inheritances have been established (see Table 75–1).

Parathyroid Hormone Gene Abnormalities

DNA sequence analysis of the PTH gene (see Fig. 75–2) from one patient with autosomal dominant isolated hypoparathyroidism has revealed a single base substitution (T→C) in exon 2,[87] which resulted in the substitution of arginine (*C*GT) for cysteine (*T*GT) in the signal peptide. The presence of this charged amino acid in the midst of the hydrophobic core of the signal peptide impeded the processing of the mutant preproPTH, as demonstrated by in vitro studies. These revealed that the mutation impaired the interaction with the nascent protein and the translocation machinery, and that cleavage of the mutant signal sequence by solubilized signal peptidase was ineffective.[87, 88] Another abnormality of the PTH gene, involving a donor splice site at the exon

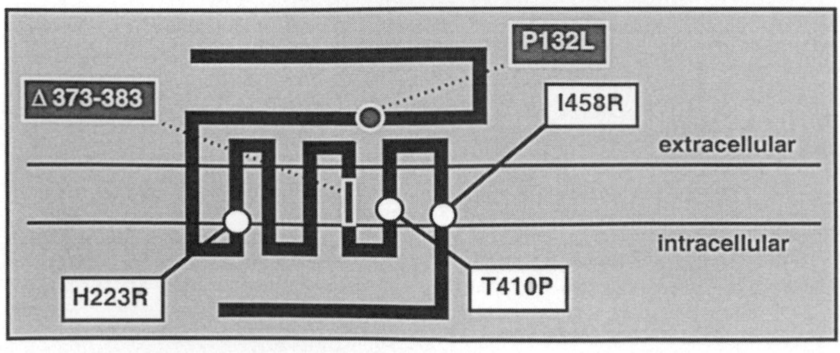

FIGURE 75–6. Schematic representation of the human PTH/PTHrP receptor. The approximate locations of heterozygous missense mutations that lead to constitutive receptor activation in patients with Jansen's disease are indicated by *open circles.* A homozygous loss of function mutation that was identified in a patient with Blomstrand's disease is indicated by a *stippled circle.* In a second patient with this disorder, a nucleotide exchange in exon M5 of the maternal PTH/PTHrP receptor allele introduces a novel splice acceptor site that leads to the synthesis of an abnormal receptor protein, which lacks portions of the fifth membrane-spanning domain *(stippled box).* For as-yet-unknown reasons, the paternal allele is not expressed in this patient (see text for details). H, histidine; R, arginine; T, threonine; P, proline; I, isoleucine.

2–intron 2 boundary, has been identified in one family with autosomal recessive isolated hypoparathyroidism.[89] This mutation involved a single base transition (g→c) at position 1 of intron 2, and an assessment of the effects of this alteration in the invariant gt dinucleotide of the 5′ donor splice site consensus on mRNA processing revealed that the mutation resulted in exon skipping, in which exon 2 of the PTH gene was lost and exon 1 was spliced to exon 3. The lack of exon 2 would lead to a loss of the initiation codon (ATG) and the signal peptide sequence (see Fig. 75–2), which are required, respectively, for the commencement of PTH mRNA translation and for the translocation of the PTH peptide.

X-Linked Recessive Hypoparathyroidism

X-linked recessive hypoparathyroidism has been reported in two multigenerational kindreds from Missouri.[90, 91] In this disorder, only males are affected, and they suffer from infantile onset of epilepsy and hypocalcemia, which is due to an isolated defect in parathyroid gland development.[92] Relatedness of the two kindreds has been established by demonstrating an identical mitochondrial DNA sequence, inherited via the maternal lineage, in affected males from the two families.[93] Studies utilizing X-linked polymorphic markers in these families localized the mutant gene to chromosome Xq26-q27,[94] and a 1.5 Mbp region that contains this gene, which is likely to have a role in parathyroid gland development, has been defined.

Pluriglandular Autoimmune Hypoparathyroidism

Hypoparathyroidism may occur in association with candidiasis and autoimmune Addison's disease, and the disorder has been referred to as either the *autoimmune polyendocrinopathy-candidiasis-ectodermal dystrophy* (APECED) *syndrome* or the *polyglandular autoimmune type 1 syndrome.*[95] This disorder has a high incidence in Finland, and a genetic analysis of Finnish families indicated autosomal recessive inheritance of the disorder.[96] In addition, the disorder has been reported to have a high incidence among Iranian Jews, although the occurrence of candidiasis was less common in this population.[97] Linkage studies of Finnish families mapped the APECED gene to chromosome 21q22.3.[98] Further positional cloning studies led to the isolation of a novel gene from chromosome 21q22.3. This gene, referred to as AIRE (*a*uto*i*mmune *re*gulator), encodes a 545–amino acid protein that contains motifs suggestive of a transcriptional factor and includes two zinc-finger motifs, a proline-rich region, and three LXXLL motifs.[99, 100] Six AIRE mutations have been reported in the APECED families, and a codon 257 (Arg→Stop) mutation was the predominant abnormality in 82% of the Finnish families.[99, 100] The identification of the genetic defect causing APECED will not only facilitate genetic diagnosis but will also enhance the elucidation of the mechanisms causing autoimmune disease.

Mitochondrial Disorders Associated with Hypoparathyroidism

Hypoparathyroidism has been reported to occur in two disorders associated with mitochondrial dysfunction: the Kearns-Sayre syndrome (KSS) and the MELAS syndrome. KSS is characterized by progressive external ophthalmoplegia and pigmentary retinopathy before the age of 20 years, and is often associated with heart block or cardiomyopathy. The MELAS syndrome consists of a childhood onset of *m*itochondrial *e*ncephalopathy, *l*actic *a*cidosis, and *s*trokelike episodes. In addition, varying degrees of proximal myopathy can be seen in both conditions. Both the KSS and MELAS syndromes have been reported to occur with insulin-dependent diabetes mellitus and hypoparathyroidism.[101, 102] A point mutation in the mitochondrial gene tRNA leucine (UUR) has been reported in one patient with the MELAS syndrome who also suffered from hypoparathyroidism and diabetes mellitus.[103] A large deletion, consisting of 6903 base pairs and involving 39% of the mitochondrial genome, has been reported in another patient who suffered from KSS, hypoparathyroidism, and sensorineural deafness.[102] The role of these mitochondrial mutations in the etiology of hypoparathyroidism remains to be further elucidated.

DiGeorge Syndrome

Patients with the DiGeorge syndrome (DGS) typically suffer from hypoparathyroidism, immunodeficiency, congenital heart defects, and deformities of the ear, nose, and mouth. The disorder arises from a congenital failure in the development of the derivatives of the third and fourth pharyngeal pouches with resulting absence or hypoplasia of the parathyroids and thymus. Most cases of DGS are sporadic, but an autosomal dominant inheritance of DGS has been observed, and an association between the syndrome and an unbalanced translocation and deletions involving 22q11.2 have also been reported.[104] In some patients, deletions of another locus on chromosome 10p have been observed in association with DGS.[105] Mapping studies of the DGS-deleted region on chromosome 22q11.2 have defined a 250 kb minimal critical region,[106] and cloning of the translocation breakpoint on 22q11.21 from a DGS patient[107] has revealed that there are probably two genes (*rnex40* and *nex2.2-nex3*), transcribed in opposite directions, that are disrupted by this breakpoint.[108] The coding region of one of these genes, designated *rnex40,* has homology to the mouse and rat androgen receptors and contains a leucine-zipper motif, suggesting that the DGS candidate gene may be a DNA-binding protein. Eleven nucleotides of the rnex40 gene are deleted at the translocation junction, making it likely that loss of function of this gene is responsible for at least part of the DGS phenotype.[108] Another partial transcript, referred to as *nex2.2-nex3,* was also identified from this breakpoint. Both *rnex40* and *nex2.2-nex3* are deleted in all DGS patients with 22q11 deletions, and studies aimed at assessing the presence of hemizygosity and mutations in these two genes in DGS patients who do not have detectable 22q11 deletions are required to demonstrate the role of these genes in the etiology of DGS. Such studies have been performed for a human homologue of a yeast gene that encodes a protein involved in the degradation of ubiquinated proteins, referred to as *UDF1L.*[109] UDF1L is located on 22q11, and has been found to be deleted in all of 182 patients with the 22q11 deletion syndrome,[109] which includes patients with DGS, velocardiofacial syndrome, and conotruncal-anomaly face syndrome.[104, 106] However, a smaller deletion of approximately 20 kb that removed exons 1 to 3 of *UDF1L* was detected in one patient.[109] This patient, who had a de novo deletion resulting in haploinsufficiency of *UDF1L,* suffered from neonatal-onset cleft palate, small mouth, low-set ears, broad nasal bridge, interrupted aortic arch, persistent truncus arteriosus, hypocalcemia, T lymphocyte deficiency, and syndactyly of the toes.[109] These results indicate that abnormalities of the *UDF1L* gene are likely to contribute to the etiology of DGS.

Patients with late-onset DGS have recently been described.[110, 111] These patients, who present later in childhood or during adolescence with symptomatic hypocalcemia but only subtle phenotypic abnormalities, were shown to have similar microdeletions in the 22q11 region, and the molecular definition of these variants of DGS may well provide additional insights into the regulation of PTH secretion and/or parathyroid gland development.

Additional Familial Syndromes

Several familial syndromes have been reported in which hypoparathyroidism forms a component of a complex multisystem developmental disorder that is unique to that kindred (see Table 75–1). For example, hypoparathyroidism may occur as an autosomal dominant disorder in association with sensorineural deafness and renal dysplasia[112, 113] or with sensorineural deafness alone and without renal dysplasia[114]; alternatively, hypoparathyroidism may occur as an autosomal recessive disorder in association with growth retardation, developmental delay, and dysmorphic features.[115] The latter syndrome, which was identified in families of Bedouin origin,[115] has been mapped to chromosome 1q42–43[115] by homozygosity and linkage-disequilibrium mapping studies. In some other families, the inheritance of the disorder has been established and abnormalities of the PTH gene excluded,[112]

REFERENCES

1. Naylor SL, Sakaguchi AY, Szoka P, et al: Human parathyroid hormone gene (PTH) is on the short arm of chromosome 11. Somat Cell Genet 9:609–616, 1983.
2. Vasicek TJ, McDevitt BE, Freeman MW, et al: Nucleotide sequence of the human parathyroid hormone gene. Proc Natl Acad Sci U S A 80:2127–2131, 1983.
3. Okazaki T, Igarahi T, Kronenberg HM: 5′-Flanking region of the parathyroid hormone gene mediates negative regulation by 1,25 $(OH)_2$ vitamin D_3. J Biol Chem 263:2203–2208, 1988.
4. Demay MB, Kiernan MS, DeLuca HF, et al: Sequences in the human parathyroid hormone gene that bind the 1,25 dihydroxyvitamin D_3 receptor and mediate transcriptional repression in response to 1,25 dihydroxyvitamin D_3. Proc Natl Acad Sci U S A 89:8097–8101, 1992.
5. Neveh-Many T, Rahaminov R, Livini N, et al: Parathyroid cell proliferation in normal and chronic renal failure in rats: The effects of calcium, phosphate, and vitamin D. J Clin Invest 96:1786–1793, 1995.
6. Silver J, Kronenberg HM: Parathyroid hormone: Molecular biology and regulation. *In* Bilezikian JP, Raisz LG, Rodan GA (eds): Principles of Bone Biology. New York, Academic Press, 1996, pp 324–346.
7. Slatopolsky E, Finch J, Denda M, et al: Phosporus restriction prevents parathyroid gland growth: High phosphorus directly stimulates PTh secretion in vitro. J Clin Invest 97:2534–2540, 1996.
8. Almaden Y, Canalejo A, Hernandez A, et al: Direct effect of phosphorus on PTH secretion from whole rat parathyroid glands in vitro. J Bone Miner Res 11:970–976, 1996.
9. Russell J, Lettieri D, Sherwood LM: Direct regulation of calcium of cytoplasmic messenger ribonucleic acid coding for pre-proparathyroid hormone in isolated bovine parathyroid cells. J Clin Invest 72:1851–1855, 1983.
10. Naveh-Many T, Friedlander MM, Mayer H, et al: Calcium regulates parathyroid hormone messenger ribonucleic acid (mRNA) but not calcitonin mRNA in vivo in the rat: Dominant role of 1,25-dihydroxyvitamin D. Endocrinology 125:275–280, 1989.
11. Kemper B, Habener JF, Mulligan RC, et al: Preproparathyroid hormone: A direct translation product of parathyroid messenger RNA. Proc Natl Acad Sci U S A 71:3731–3735, 1974.
12. Jüppner H, Abou-Samra AB, Freeman M, et al: A G protein-linked receptor for parathyroid hormone and parathyroid hormone-related peptide. Science 254:1024–1026, 1991.
13. Gelbert L, Schipani E, Jüppner H, et al: Chromosomal localisation of the parathyroid hormone/parathyroid hormone related protein receptor gene to human chromosome 3p21.1-p24.2. J Clin Endocrinol Metab 79:1046–1048, 1994.
14. Abou-Samra AB, Jüppner H, Force T, et al: Expression cloning of a common receptor for parathyroid hormone and parathyroid hormone related peptide from rat osteoblast-like cells. Proc Natl Acad Sci U S A 89:2732–2736, 1992.
15. Pausova Z, Bourdon J, Clayton D, et al: Cloning of a parathyroid hormone/parathyroid hormone-related peptide receptor (PTHR) cDNA from a rat osteosarcoma (UMR106) cell line: Chromosomal assignment of the gene in the human, mouse and rat genomes. Genomics 20:20–26, 1994.
16. Segre GV: Receptors for parathyroid hormone and parathyroid hormone-related protein. *In* Bilezikian JP, Raisz LG, Rodan GA (eds): Principles in Bone Biology. New York, Academic Press, 1996, pp 377–403.
17. Potts JT Jr, Jüppner H: Parathyroid hormone and parathyroid hormone-related peptide in calcium homeostasis, bone metabolism, and bone development: The proteins, their genes, and receptors. *In* Avioli LV, Krane SM (eds): Metabolic Bone Disease. New York, Academic Press, 1997, pp 51–94.
18. Thakker RV: Molecular genetics of parathyroid disease. Curr Opin Endocrinol Diabetes 3:521–528, 1996.
19. Szabo J, Heath B, Hill VM, et al: Hereditary hyperparathyroidism: Jaw tumor syndrome: The endocrine tumor gene HRPT2 maps to chromosome 1q21-q31. Am J Hum Genet 56:944–950, 1995.
20. Arnold A, Brown MF, Urena P, et al: Monoclonality of parathyroid tumors in chronic renal failure and in primary parathyroid hyperplasia. J Clin Invest 95:2047–2053, 1995.
21. Arnold A, Kim HG, Gaz RD, et al: Molecular cloning and chromosomal mapping of DNA rearranged with the parathyroid hormone gene in a parathyroid adenoma. J Clin Invest 83:2034–2040, 1989.
22. Motokura T, Bloom T, Kim HG, et al: A novel cyclin encoded by a bc11-linked candidate oncogene. Nature 350:512–515, 1991.
23. Nurse P: Universal control mechanism regulating the onset of M-phase. Nature 344:503–507, 1990.
24. Hsi ED, Zukerberg LR, Yang WI, et al: Cyclin D1/PRAD1 expression in parathyroid adenomas: An immunohistochemical study. J Clin Endocrinol Metab 81:1736–1739, 1996.
25. Wang TC, Cardiff RD, Zukerberg L, et al: Mammary hyperplasia and carcinoma in MMTV-cyclin D1 transgenic mice. Nature 369:669–671, 1994.
26. Hosokawa Y, Yoshimoto K, Bronson R, et al: Chronic hyperparathyroidism in transgenic mice with parathyroid-targeted overexpression of cyclinD1/PRAD1. J Bone Miner Res 12(suppl 1):S110, 1997.
27. Thakker RV: The molecular genetics of the multiple endocrine neoplasia syndromes. Clin Endocrinol 38:1–14, 1993.
28. Trump D, Farren B, Wooding C, et al: Clinical studies of multiple endocrine neoplasia type 1 (MEN1) in 220 patients. Q J Med 89:653–669, 1996.
29. Marx SJ: Multiple endocrine neoplasia type 1. *In* Vogelstein B, Kinzler KW (eds): The Genetic Basis of Human Cancer. New York, McGraw Hill. 1998, pp 489–506.
30. Thakker RV: Multiple endocrine neoplasia: Syndromes of the 20th century. J Clin Endocrinol Metab 83:2617–2620, 1998.
31. Chandrasekharappa SC, Guru SC, Manickam P, et al: Positional cloning of the gene for multiple endocrine neoplasia–type 1. Science 276:404–407, 1997.
32. The European Consortium on MEN1: Identification of the multiple endocrine neoplasia type 1 (MEN1) gene. Hum Mol Genet 6:1177–1183, 1997.
33. Bassett JHD, Forbes SA, Pannett AAJ, et al: Characterization of mutations in patients with multiple endocrine neoplasia type 1 (MEN1). Am J Hum Genet 62:232–244, 1998.
34. Teh BT, Farnebo F, Phelan C, et al: Mutation analysis of the MEN1 gene in multiple endocrine neoplasia type 1, familial acromegaly and familial isolated hyperparathyroidism. J Clin Endocrinol Metab 83:2621–2626, 1998.
35. Heppner C, Kester MB, Agarwal SK, et al: Somatic mutation of the MEN1 gene in parathyroid tumours. Nature Genet 16:375–378, 1997.
36. Zhuang Z, Vortmeyer AO, Pack S, et al: Somatic mutations of the MEN1 tumor suppressor gene in sporadic gastrinomas and insulinomas. Cancer Res 57:4682–4686, 1997.
37. Zhuang Z, Ezzat SZ, Vortmeyer AO, et al: Mutations of the MEN1 tumor suppressor gene in pituitary tumors. Cancer Res 57:5446–5451, 1997.
38. Prezant TR, Levine J, Melmed S: Molecular characterization of the MEN1 tumor suppressor gene in sporadic pituitary tumors. J Clin Endocrinol Metab 83:1388–1391, 1998.
39. Debelenko LV, Brambilla E, Agarwal SK, et al: Identification of MEN1 gene mutations in sporadic carcinoid tumors of the lung. Hum Mol Genet 6:2285–2290, 1997.
40. Vortmeyer AO, Boni R, Pak E, et al: Multiple endocrine neoplasia 1 alterations in MEN1-associated and sporadic lipomas. J Natl Cancer Inst 90:398–399, 1998.
41. Farnebo F, Teh BT, Kytola S, et al: Alterations of the MEN1 gene in sporadic parathyroid tumors. J Clin Endocrinol Metab 83:2627–2630, 1998.
42. Carling T, Correea P, Hessman O, et al: Parathyroid MEN1 gene mutations in relation to clinical characteristics of non-familial primary hyperparathyroidism. J Clin Endocrinol Metab 83:2951–2954, 1998.
43. Tanaka C, Kimura T, Yang P, et al: Analysis of loss of heterozygosity on chromosome 11 and infrequent inactivation of MEN1 gene in sporadic pituitary adenomas. J Clin Endocrinol Metab 83:2631–2634, 1998.
44. Guru SC, Goldsmith PK, Burns AL, et al: Menin, the product of the MEN1 gene, is a nuclear protein. Proc Natl Acad Sci U S A 95:1630–1634, 1998.
45. Agarwal SK, Guru SC, Heppner C, et al: Menin interacts with AP1 transcriptional factor JunD and represses JunD-activated transcription. Cell 96:143–152, 1999.
46. Mulligan LM, Kwok JBJ, Healey CS, et al: Germline mutations of the RET proto-oncogene in multiple endocrine neoplasia type 2a (MEN2a). Nature 363:458–460, 1993.
47. Mulligan LM, Ponder BAJ: Multiple endocrine neoplasia type 2. J Clin Endocrinol Metab 80:1989–1995, 1995.
48. Pausova Z, Janicic N, Konrad E, et al: Analysis of the RET proto-oncogene in sporadic parathyroid tumours. J Bone Miner Res 9:S151, 1994.
49. Padberg BC, Schroder S, Jochum W, et al: Absence of RET proto-oncogene point mutations in sporadic hyperplastic and neoplastic lesions of the parathyroid gland. Am J Pathol 147:1539–1544, 1995.
50. Heshmati HM, Gharib H, Khosla S, et al: Genetic testing in medullary thyroid carcinoma syndromes: Mutation types and clinical significance. Mayo Clin Proc 72:430, 1997.
51. Weinberg RA: Tumor suppressor genes. Science 254:1138–1145, 1991.
52. Cryns VL, Thor A, Xu HJ, et al: Loss of the retinoblastoma tumor-suppressor gene in parathyroid carcinoma. N Engl J Med 330:757–761, 1994.
53. Pearce SHS, Trump D, Wooding C, et al: Loss of heterozygosity studies at the retinoblastoma gene and hereditary breast cancer susceptibility (BRCA2) locus in pituitary, parathyroid, pancreatic and carcinoid tumors. Clin Endocrinol 45:195–200, 1996.
54. Pei L, Melmed S, Scheithauer B, et al: Frequent loss of heterozygosity at the retinoblastoma susceptibility gene (RB) locus in aggressive pituitary tumors: Evidence for a chromosome 13 tumor suppressor gene other than RB. Cancer Res 55:1613–1616, 1995.
55. Cryns VL, Yi SM, Tahara H, et al: Frequent loss of chromosome arm 1p DNA in para-thyroid adenomas. Genes Chromosomes Cancer 13:9–17, 1995.
56. Williamson C, Pannett AAJ, Pang JT, et al: Localisation of a gene causing endocrine neoplasia to a 4 cM region on chromosome 1p35–36. J Med Genet 34:617–619, 1997.
57. Teh BT, Esapa CT, Houlston R, et al: A family with isolated hyperparathyroidism segregating a missense MEN1 mutation and showing loss of the wild-type alleles in the parathyroid tumors. Am J Hum Genet 63:1544–1549, 1998.
58. Wassif WS, Moniz CF, Friedman E, et al: Familial isolated hyperparathyroidism: A distinct genetic entity with an increased risk of parathyroid cancer. J Clin Endocrinol Metab 77:1485–1489, 1993.
59. Williamson C, Cavaco BM, Jauch A, et al: Mapping the gene causing hereditary primary hyperparathyroidism in a Portuguese kindred to chromosome 1q22-q31. J Bone Miner Res 14:230–239, 1998.
60. Pollak MR, Brown EM, Chou YWH, et al: Mutations in the human Ca^{2+}-sensing receptor gene cause familial hypocalciuric hypercalcemia and neonatal severe hyperparathyroidism. Cell 75:1297–1303, 1993.
61. Chou YWH, Pollak MR, Brandi ML, et al: Mutations in the human Ca^{2+}-sensing receptor gene that cause familial hypocalciuric hypercalcaemia. Am J Hum Genet 56:1075–1079, 1995.
62. Pearce SHS, Trump D, Wooding C, et al: Calcium-sensing receptor mutations in familial benign hypocalcaemia and neonatal hyperparathyroidism. J Clin Invest 96:2683–2692, 1995.
63. Janicic N, Pausova Z, Cole DEC, et al: Insertion of an Alu sequence in the Ca^{2+}-sensing receptor gene in familial hypocalciuric hypercalcaemia and neonatal severe hyperparathyroidism. Am J Hum Genet 56:880–886, 1995.
64. Aida K, Koishi S, Inoue M, et al: Familial hypocalciuric hypercalcemia associated with mutation in the human Ca^{2+}-sensing receptor gene. J Clin Endocrinol Metab 80:2594–2598, 1995.
65. Heath H III, Odelberg S, Jackson CE, et al: Clustered inactivating mutations and

benign polymorphisms of the calcium receptor gene in familial benign hypocalciuric hypercalcaemia suggest receptor functional domains. J Clin Endocrinol Metab 81:1312–1317, 1996.

66. Janicic N, Soliman E, Pausova Z, et al: Mapping of the calcium-sensing receptor gene (CASR) to human chromosome 3q13.3–21 by fluorescent in situ hybridization, and localization to rat chromosome 11 and mouse chromosome 16. Mamm Genome 6:798–801, 1995.
67. Brown EM, Gamba G, Riccardi D, et al: Cloning and characterization of an extracellular Ca^{2+}-sensing receptor from bovine parathyroid. Nature 366:575–580, 1993.
68. Pearce SHS, Bai M, Quinn SJ, et al: Functional characterisation of calcium-sensing receptor mutations expressed in human embryonic kidney cells. J Clin Invest 98:1860–1866, 1996.
69. Bai MS, Quinn S, Trivedi O, et al: Expression and characterisation of inactivating and activating mutations of the human Ca_o^{2+} sensing receptor. J Biol Chem 271:19537–19545, 1996.
70. Pollak MR, Chou YHW, Marx SJ, et al: Familial hypocalciuric hypercalcaemia and neonatal severe hyperparathyroidism: Effects of mutant gene dosage on phenotype. J Clin Invest 93:1108–1112, 1994.
71. Bai M, Pearce SHS, Kifor O, et al: In vivo and in vitro characterisation of neonatal hyperparathyroidism resulting from a de novo, heterozygous mutation in the Ca^{2+} sensing receptor gene: Normal material calcium homeostasis as a cause of secondary hyperparathyroidism in familial benign hypocalciuric hypercalcaemia. J Clin Invest 99:88–96, 1997.
72. Heath H, Jackson CE, Otterud B, et al: Genetic linkage analysis of familial benign (hypocalciuric) hypercalcemia: Evidence for locus heterogeneity. Am J Hum Genet 53:193–200, 1993.
73. McMurtry CT, Schranck FW, Walkenhorst DA, et al: Significant developmental elevation in serum parathyroid hormone levels in a large kindred with familial benign (hypocalciuric) hypercalcemia. Am J Med 93:247–258, 1992.
74. Trump D, Whyte MP, Wooding C, et al: Linkage studies in a kindred from Oklahoma, with familial benign (hypocalciuric) hypercalcaemia (FBH) and developmental elevations in serum parathyroid hormone levels, indicate a third locus for FBH. Hum Genet 96:183–187, 1995.
75. Lloyd SE, Pannett AAJ, Dixon PH, et al: Localisation of the Oklahoma variant of familial benign hypercalcaemia (FBH_{Ok}) to chromosome 19q13. Am J Hum Genet 64:189–195, 1999.
76. Schipani E, Kruse K, Jüppner H: A constitutively active mutant PTH-PTHrP receptor in Jansen type metaphyseal chondrodysplasia. Science 268:98–100, 1995.
77. Schipani E, Langman CB, Parfitt AM, et al: Constitutively activated receptors for parathyroid hormone and parathyroid hormone-related peptide in Jansen's metaphyseal chondrodysplasia. N Engl J Med 335:708–714, 1996.
78. Jüppner H: Jansen's metaphyseal chondrodysplasia: A disorder due to a PTH/PTHrP receptor gene mutation. Trends Endocrinol Metab 7:157–162, 1996.
79. Schipani E, Langman CB, Hunzelman J, et al: A novel parathyroid hormone (PTH)/ PTH-related peptide receptor mutation in Jansen's metaphyseal chondrodysplasia. J Clin Endocrinol Metab 84:3052–3057, 1999.
80. Schipani E, Lanske B, Hunzelman J, et al: Targeted expression of constitutively active PTH/PTHrp receptors delays endochondral bone formation and rescues PTHrP-less mice. Proc Natl Acad Sci U S A 94:13689–13694, 1997.
81. Ewart AK, Morris CA, Atkinson D, et al: Hemizygosity at the elastin locus in a developmental disorder, Williams syndrome. Nature Genet 5:11–17, 1993.
82. Nickerson E, Greenberg F, Keating MT, et al: Deletions of the elastin gene at 7q11.23 occur in 90% of patients with Williams syndrome. Am J Hum Genet 56:1156–1161, 1995.
83. Lowery MC, Morris CA, Ewart A, et al: Strong correlation of elastin deletions, detected by FISH, with Williams syndrome: Evaluation of 235 patients. Am J Hum Genet 57:49–53, 1995.
84. Li D, Brooke B, Davis E, et al: Elastin is an essential determinant of arterial morphogenesis. Nature 393:276–280, 1998.
85. Tassabehji M, Metcalfe K, Fergusson WD, et al: LIM-kinase deleted in Williams syndrome. Nat Genet 5:272–273, 1996.
86. Perez Jurado LA, Li X, Francke U: The human calcitonin receptor gene (CALCR) at 7q21.3 is outside the deletion associated with Williams syndrome. Cytogenet Cell Genet 70:246–249, 1995.
87. Arnold A, Horst SA, Gardella TJ, et al: Mutations of the signal peptide encoding region of preproparathyroid hormone gene in isolated hypoparathyroidism. J Clin Invest 86:1084–1087, 1990.
88. Karaplis AC, Lim SC, Baba H, et al: Inefficient membrane targeting, translocation, and proteolytic processing by signal peptidase of a mutant preproparathyroid hormone protein. J Biol Chem 27:1629–1635, 1995.
89. Parkinson DB, Thakker RV: A donor splice site mutation in the parathyroid hormone gene is associated with autosomal recessive hypoparathyroidism. Nat Genet 1:149–153, 1992.
90. Peden VH: True idiopathic hypoparathyroidism as a sex-linked recessive trait. Am J Hum Genet 12:323–337, 1960.
91. Whyte MP, Weldon VV: Idiopathic hypoparathyroidism presenting with seizures during infancy: X-linked recessive inheritance in a large Missouri kindred. J Pediatr 99:608–611, 1981.
92. Whyte MP, Kim GS, Kosanovich M: Absence of parathyroid tissue in sex-linked recessive hypoparathyroidism. J Paediatr 109:915, 1986.
93. Mumm S, Whyte MP, Thakker RV, et al: mtDNA analysis shows common ancestry in two kindreds with X-linked recessive hypoparathyroidism and reveals a heteroplasmic silent mutation. Am J Hum Genet 60:153–159, 1997.
94. Thakker RV, Davies KE, Whyte MP, et al: Mapping the gene causing X-linked recessive idiopathic hypoparathyroidism to Xq26-Xq27 by linkage studies. J Clin Invest 86:40–45, 1990.
95. Ahonen P, Myllarniemi S, Sipila I, et al: Clinical variation of autoimmune polyendocrinopathy-candidiasis ectodermal dystrophy (APECED) in a series of 68 patients. N Engl J Med 322:1829–1836, 1990.
96. Ahonen P: Autoimmune polyendocrinopathy candidiasis ectodermal dystrophy (APECED): Autosomal recessive inheritance. Clin Genet 27:535–542, 1985.
97. Zlotogora J, Shapiro MS: Polyglandular autoimmune syndrome type 1 among Iranian Jews. J Med Genet 29:824–826, 1992.
98. Aaltonen J, Bjorses P, Sandkuijl L, et al: An autosomal locus causing autoimmune disease: Autoimmune polyglandular disease type 1 assigned to chromosome 21. Nat Genet 8:83–87, 1994.
99. Nagamine K, Peterson P, Scott HS, et al: Positional cloning of the APECED gene. Nat Genet 17:393–398, 1997.
100. The Finnish-German APECED Consortium: An autoimmune disease, APECED, caused by mutations in a novel gene featuring two PHD-type zinc finger domains. Nat Genet 17:399–403, 1997.
101. Moraes CT, DiMauro S, Zeviani M, et al: Mitochondrial deletions in progressive external ophthalmoplegia and Kearns-Sayre syndrome. N Engl J Med 320:1293–1299, 1989.
102. Zupanc ML, Moraes CT, Shanske S, et al: Deletions of mitochondrial DNA in patients with combined features of Kearns-Sayre and MELAS syndromes. Ann Neurol 29:680–683, 1991.
103. Morten KJ, Cooper JM, Brown GK, et al: A new point mutation associated with mitochondrial encephalomyopathy. Hum Mol Genet 2:2081–2087, 1993.
104. Scambler PJ, Carey AH, Wyse RKH, et al: Microdeletions within 22q11 associated with sporadic and familial DiGeorge syndrome. Genomics 10:201–206, 1991.
105. Monaco G, Pignata C, Rossi E, et al: DiGeorge anomaly associated with 10p deletion. Am J Med Genet 39:215–216, 1991.
106. Gong W, Emanuel BS, Collins J, et al: A transcription map of the DiGeorge and velocardiofacial syndrome minimal critical region on 22q11. Hum Mol Genet 5:789–800, 1996.
107. Augusseau S, Jouk S, Jalbert P, et al: DiGeorge syndrome and 22q11 rearrangements. Hum Genet 74:206, 1986.
108. Budarf ML, Collins J, Gong W, et al: Cloning a balanced translocation associated with DiGeorge syndrome and identification of a disrupted candidate gene. Nat Genet 10:269–278, 1995.
109. Yamagishi H, Garg V, Matsuoka R, et al: A molecular pathway revealing a genetic basis for human cardiac and craniofacial defects. Science 283:1158–1161, 1999.
110. Scire G, Dallapiccola B, Iannetti P, et al: Hypoparathyroidism as the major manifestation in two patients with 22q11 deletions. Am J Med Genet 52:478–482, 1994.
111. Sykes K, Bachrach L, Siegel-Bartelt J, et al: Velocardiofacial syndrome presenting as hypocalcemia in early adolescence. Arch Pediatr Adolesc Med 151:745–747, 1997.
112. Bassett JHD, Thakker RV: Molecular genetics of disorders of calcium homeostasis. *In* Thakker RV (ed): Ballière's Clinical Endocrinology and Metabolism. London, Ballière Tindall, 1995, pp 581–608.
113. Bilous RW, Muty G, Parkinson DB, et al: Autosomal dominant familial hypoparathyroidism, sensorineural deafness and renal dysplasia. N Engl J Med 327:1069–1074, 1992.
114. Watanabe T, Mochizuki H, Kohda N, et al: Autosomal dominant familial hypoparathyroidism and sensorineural deafness without renal dysplasia. Eur J Endocrinol 139:101–106, 1999.
115. Parvari R, Hershkovitz E, Kanis A, et al: Homozygosity and linkage-disequilibrium mapping of the syndrome of congenital hypoparathyroidism, growth and mental retardation, and dysmorphism to a 1cM interval on chromosome 1q42–43. Am J Hum Genet 63:163–169, 1998.
116. Pollak MR, Brown EM, Estep HL, et al: Autosomal dominant hypocalcaemia caused by a calcium-sensing receptor gene mutation. Nat Genet 8:303–307, 1994.
117. Finegold DN, Armitage MM, Galiani M, et al: Preliminary localisation of a gene for autosomal dominant hypo-parathyroidism to chromosome 3q13. Pediatr Res 36:414–417, 1994.
118. Perry YM, Finegold DN, Armitage MM, et al: A missense mutation in the Ca-sensing receptor causes familial autosomal dominant hypoparathyroidism. Am J Hum Genet 55:A17, 1994.
119. Pearce SHS, Williamson C, Kifor O, et al: A familial syndrome of hypocalcaemia with hypocalciuria due to mutations in the calcium-sensing receptor gene. N Engl J Med 335:1115–1122, 1996.
120. Baron J, Winer KK, Yanovski JA, et al: Mutations in the Ca^{2+}-sensing receptor gene cause autosomal dominant and sporadic hypoparathyroidism. Hum Mol Genet 5:601–606, 1996.
121. Okazaki R, Chikatsu N, Nakatsu M, et al: A novel activating mutation in calcium-sensing receptor gene associated with a family of autosomal dominant hypocalcemia. J Clin Endocrinol Metab 84:363–366, 1999.
122. Albright F, Burnett CH, Smith PH, et al: Pseudohypoparathyroidism: An example of "Seabright-Bantam syndrome." Endocrinology 30:922–932, 1942.
123. van Dop C: Pseudohypoparathyroidism: Clinical and molecular aspects. Semin Nephrol 9:168–178, 1989.
124. Levine MA: Pseudohypoparathyroidism. *In* Bilezikian JP, Raisz LD, Rodan GA (eds): Principles of Bone Biology. New York, Academic Press, 1996, pp 853–876.
125. Weinstein LS: Albright hereditary osteodystrophy, pseudohypoparathyroidism, and Gs deficiency. *In* Spiegel AM (ed): G Proteins, Receptors, and Disease. Totowa, NJ, Humana Press, 1998, pp 23–56.
126. Schuster V, Eschenhagen T, Kruse K, et al: Endocrine and molecular biological studies in a German family with Albright hereditary osteodystrophy. Eur J Pediatr 152:185–189, 1993.
127. Miric A, Bechio JD, Levine MA: Heterogeneous mutations in the gene encoding the α-subunit of the stimulatory G protein of adenylyl cyclase in Albright hereditary osteodystrophy. J Clin Endocrinol Metab 76:1560–1568, 1993.
128. Weinstein LS, Gejman PV, Friedman E, et al: Mutations of the Gs α-subunit gene in Albright hereditary osteodystrophy detected by denaturing gradient gel electrophoresis. Proc Natl Acad Sci U S A 87:8287–8290, 1990.
129. Davies AJ, Hughes HE: Imprinting in Albright's hereditary osteodystrophy. J Med Genet 30:101–103, 1993.

TABLE 76–1. Changing Profile of Primary Hyperparathyroidism

	Study			
Symptomatology	*Cope[2] (1930–1965)*	*Heath et al.[8] (1965–1974)*	*Mallette et al.[11] (1965–1972)*	*Silverberg et al. (1984–1999)*
Nephrolithiasis (%)	57	51	37	17
Skeletal disease (%)	23	10	14	1.4
Hypercalciuria (%)	NR	36	40	39
Asymptomatic (%)	0.6	18	22	80

NR, not reported.

bone involvement is readily detected by bone mass measurement. This chapter describes the clinical picture of primary hyperparathyroidism as it presents today, how it can be differentiated from other causes of hypercalcemia, our current understanding of the etiology of this disease, and its clinical course. Issues in management, many of which are still unresolved, are also addressed.

ETIOLOGY

Clonal expansion of individual cells which have undergone a shift in their sensitivity to calcium appears to be a regular cellular feature of the disease.[12–18] The work of Arnold et al.[15, 16] suggests, however, that the molecular abnormalities leading to clonal emergence are heterogeneous. Among the alterations identified are genetic rearrangement of the PRAD1 (parathyroid adenomatosis 1) oncogene, also known as cyclin D1, which places it in proximity to the 5′ regulatory region of the gene for PTH[15–17] (Fig. 76–2). The expression of the resulting oncogene is then increased or otherwise poorly regulated. The realignment of DNA now associates a growth promoter (PRAD1) with a regulatory element that normally controls only PTH synthesis. Only a small percentage of parathyroid adenomas have been demonstrated to harbor this genetic rearrangement.

Alterations in tumor suppressor genes have been more commonly identified as molecular mechanisms to account for tumorigenesis. Both alleles of the tumor suppressor gene must be inactivated to render its gene product completely deficient. The initially recognized tumor suppressor gene in the etiology of primary hyperparathyroidism is that associated with the multiple endocrine neoplasia, type 1 (MEN-1) syndrome.[19–21] Abnormalities have been detected in as many as 20% of patients with primary hyperparathyroidism.[22, 23] Even more commonly found is evidence of loss of function of another putative tumor suppressor gene on chromosome 1p[24, 25] (see Chapter 75). Such patients should be predisposed to the same multiplicity of glandular involvement as in the MEN-1 syndrome and acquire the disease at an earlier age. Information is lacking on these different views. Nevertheless, it is evident that tumor suppressor genes are the focus of great attention in sporadic parathyroid adenomas. Probable abnormalities in other tumor suppressor genes have been identifed in parathyroid adenomas, including those at chromosomal sites 1q, 6q, 9p, and 15q[24, 25] (see Chapter 75).

Mutations in the calcium-sensing receptor seemed a potential molecular mechanism for altered calcium-sensing in primary hyperparathyroidism.[26] Point mutations, reducing the activity of this gene, have provided a clear understanding of the underlying basis for familial hypocalciuric hypercalcemia (FHH) and neonatal severe hyperparathyroidism.[26–27] Conversely, activating point mutations in this gene have helped to elucidate the cause of hypoparathyroidism in some patients. However, in primary hyperparathyroidism, mutation or allelic loss in the calcium-sensing receptor gene has not been seen.[28–30] Although structural aspects of the calcium-sensing gene appear to be normal in primary hyperparathyroidism, it is still possible that a promoter region of the calcium receptor gene is defective, as suggested by a recent report by Chikatsu et al.[31] Another hypothesis relating the calcium-sensing receptor to the cellular pathogenesis of primary hyperparathyroidism is a postgenomic reduction in the RNA transcript or the protein itself in the abnormal parathyroid cell clone.[32] This observation needs to be explored further because it is possible that the reduction in calcium-sensing receptor RNA or protein is a secondary cause of the hypercalcemia and not etiologic.

Several recent reports have implicated an abnormality in the parathyroid cell's vitamin D receptor in the pathogenesis of primary hyperparathyroidism.[33–35] The data are conflicting, however, with different allelic polymorphisms being inconsistently described. Post-transcript reductions in vitamin D gene products, which have also been described, are subject to interpretations that place them secondary to, but not primary consequences of, the hyperparathyroid process.

PATHOLOGY

Parathyroid Adenomas

By far the most common lesion found in patients with primary hyperparathyroidism is the solitary parathyroid adenoma, occurring in 80% of patients.[7] Several risk factors have been identified in the development of primary hyperparathyroidism. These include a history of neck irradiation,[36] and prolonged use of lithium therapy for affective disorders.[37–40] While in most cases, a single adenoma is found, multiple parathyroid adenomas have been reported in 2% to 4% of cases.[41–43] These may be familial or sporadic. Parathyroid adenomas can be discovered in many unexpected anatomic locations (see Chapter 79). Embryonal migration patterns of parathyroid tissue account for a plethora of possible sites of ectopic parathyroid adenomas. The most common sites are within the thyroid gland, the superior mediastinum, and within the thymus.[44, 45] Occasionally, the adenoma may ultimately be identified in the retroesophageal space, the pharynx, the lateral neck, and even the alimentary submucosa of the esophagus.[46–48] On histologic examination, most parathyroid adenomas are encapsulated, and composed of parathyroid chief cells. Adenomas containing mainly

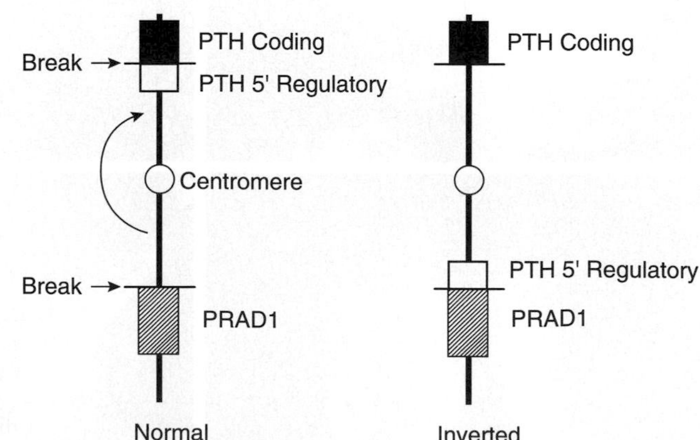

FIGURE 76–2. A genetic rearrangement of the parathyroid hormone (PTH) gene in primary hyperparathyroidism. Normal and inverted chromosome showing relative loci of *PRAD1* and PTH genes. This molecular rearrangement has been described in a small subset of parathyroid adenomas (From Arnold A: Molecular genetics of parathyroid gland neoplasia. J Clin Endocrinol Metab 77:1108–1112, 1993.)

oxyphilic or oncocytic cells are rare, but can give rise to clinical primary hyperparathyroidism.

Multiglandular Parathyroid Disease

In approximately 15% of patients with primary hyperparathyroidism, all four parathyroid glands are involved. There are no clinical features which differentiate single vs. multiglandular disease. The etiology of four-gland parathyroid hyperplasia is multifactorial. In nearly one-half of cases, it is associated with a familial hereditary syndrome, such as MEN-1 or MEN-2a. These syndromes are discussed in detail in Chapters 188 and 189, respectively.

CLINICAL PRESENTATION

Incidence

The incidence of primary hyperparathyroidism has changed dramatically over the past three decades.[8, 9, 49] Prior to the advent of the multichannel autoanalyzer in the early 1970s, Heath et al.[8] reported an incidence of 7.8 cases per 100,000 persons in Rochester, Minnesota. With the introduction of routine calcium measurements in the mid-1970s, this rate rose precipitously to 51.1 cases per 100,000 in the same community. Once prevalent cases were diagnosed (the "sweeping" effect), the incidence declined to approximately 27 per 100,000 persons per year. A recent report from Rochester, Minnesota suggests that newly diagnosed cases of primary hyperparathyroidism have been declining continuously since the mid-1970s.[50] The decline in incidence is not explained by a change in the use of multichannel chemical screening because in the United States, it is only in the very late 1990s that use of this technique became limited. Moreover, such declines in incidence are not being appreciated in other medical centers. It is possible that the special demographics of Rochester, Minnesota combined with the rather complete discovery of primary hyperparathyroidism in a population that receives virtually all of its care in one system (ideal epidemiologic surveillence) would naturally be associated with declining numbers for years thereafter. The analogy here might be to overfishing a small pond. For reasons not related to the Rochester, Minnesota experience, but rather because multichannel screening is now becoming limited, the United States may be about to experience a general decline in new cases of primary hyperparathyroidism; however, other forces are also likely to influence the incidence of primary hyperparathyroidism in the future, so one can only speculate about future changes in incidence figures (see later discussion).

Clinical Features

Primary hyperparathyroidism mainly affects people in their middle years, with a peak incidence between ages 50 and 60 years. However, the disease can be seen from infancy throughout all ages of life. Women are affected more frequently than men, in a ratio of approximately 3:1. Typically, they are discovered with elevated serum calcium concentration in the context of a routine health screen or in connection with an evaluation for an unrelated medical problem. At the time of diagnosis, most patients with primary hyperparathyroidism do not have classic symptoms or signs associated with disease. Kidney stones are uncommon and fractures are rare.[7] Diseases associated epidemiologically with primary hyperparathyroidism, such as hypertension,[8, 51–53] peptic ulcer disease, gout, or pseudogout,[54, 55] are seen commonly. It is not established, however, that any of these associated disorders are etiologically linked to the disease unless one is dealing with the MEN syndromes. In MEN-1, peptic ulcer disease is seen; in MEN-2, hypertension might be an indication of pheochromocytoma. Constitutional complaints such as weakness, easy fatigability, depression, and intellectual weariness are seen with some regularity (see below for further discussion).[56–61]

Physical examination is generally unremarkable. Band keratopathy, a hallmark of classic primary hyperparathyroidism due to deposition of calcium phosphate crystals in the cornea, is virtually never seen grossly. Even by slit-lamp examination it is rare. The neck shows no masses. The neuromuscular system is normal.

Differential Diagnosis

The diagnosis of primary hyperparathyroidism is made when hypercalcemia and elevated PTH levels are present. The other major cause of hypercalcemia, malignancy, is readily distinguished from primary hyperparathyroidism. Patients with hypercalcemia of malignancy typically have advanced disease which has already been diagnosed. An exception is multiple myeloma in which hypercalcemia can be the initial manifestation. Biochemically, PTH levels are suppressed. Improved testing for PTH, especially the immunoradiometric (IRMA) and immunochemiluminometric (ICMA) assays, have facilitated the distinction between hyperparathyroidism and hypercalcemia of malignancy. These assays measure predominantly the intact 84-amino acid molecule and do not detect, in general, inactive fragments of PTH, although the specificity of these tests, especially in renal failure, has recently become an issue (see Chapter 70). They give a more accurate profile of biologically active hormone in hyperparathyroidism than the older displacement-type assays.[62]

However, even using the IRMA, PTH is frankly elevated in only 85% to 90% of patients with primary hyperparathyroidism.[7] In the small percentage of patients whose PTH is "normal," it tends to be in the upper range of normal. With a normal range of 10 to 65 pg/mL for most IRMA and ICMA assays, the PTH concentration tends to be greater than 45 pg/mL. In primary hyperparathyroidism, such values, although "normal," are clearly abnormal in a hypercalcemic setting. This is even more evident in those under the age of 45 years when the normal range is more accurately considered to be up to 45 pg/mL, not up to 65 pg/mL. Because PTH levels normally rise with age, the broader normal range is inclusive of the entire population.

Ninety percent of patients with hypercalcemia will be shown either to have primary hyperparathyroidism or malignancy. Although there are many other causes of hypercalcemia (Table 76–2), they constitute only approximately 10% of the hypercalcemic population. Here also, the PTH assay is useful. With the exception of lithium, thiazide use, and FHH, virtually all other causes of hypercalcemia are associated with suppressed levels of PTH. If the patient can be safely withdrawn from lithium or thiazide, this should be attempted. Serum calcium and PTH levels are reassessed 3 months later. If the serum calcium and PTH levels continue to be elevated, the diagnosis of primary hyperparathyroidism is made. While patients can generally be readily withdrawn from a thiazide diuretic, a safe alternative to lithium therapy is not always feasible. FHH is differentiated from primary hyperparathy-

TABLE 76–2. Differential Diagnosis of Hypercalcemia

- Primary hyperparathyroidism
  - Benign
  - Parathyroid carcinoma
- Hypercalcemia of malignancy
- Nonparathyroid endocrine causes
  - Thyrotoxicosis
  - Pheochromocytoma
  - Addison's disease
  - Islet cell tumors
- Drug-related hypercalcemia
  - Vitamin D
  - Vitamin A
  - Thiazide diuretics
  - Lithium
  - Estrogen and antiestrogens
- Familial hypocalciuric hypercalcemia
- Miscellaneous
  - Immobilization
  - Milk-alkali syndrome
  - Parenteral nutrition

roidism by (1) family history, (2) markedly lowered urinary calcium excretion, and (3) the specific gene abnormality (see Chapter 80).

Rarely, a patient with malignancy will be shown to have elevated PTH levels due to ectopic secretion of native PTH from the tumor itself.[63] Much more commonly, the malignancy is associated with the secretion of parathyroid hormone–related protein (PTHrP), a molecule that does not cross-react in the IRMA and ICMA assay.[62] Finally, it is possible that a malignancy is present in association with primary hyperparathyroidism. When the PTH level is elevated in someone with a malignancy, this is more likely to be the case than a true ectopic PTH syndrome.

Occasionally, a patient with primary hyperparathyroidism has normal calcium levels. This can be a vexing problem. Besides considering a secondary hyperparathyroid state, the diagnosis of primary hyperparathyroidism is aided by finding an elevated ionized calcium concentration. When these patients are followed, elevations in the total serum calcium concentration typically emerge.[7]

Frankly low or low-normal serum calcium concentrations suggest an adaptive response to hypocalcemia with high PTH levels. Secondary hyperparathyroidism can be seen in patients with renal insufficiency, malabsorption, or any of the other vitamin D deficiency states. Rarely, patients with primary hyperparathyroidism and coexisting vitamin D deficiency will present with low calcium concentration. PTH levels are high. In such patients, correction of the vitamin D deficiency is associated with a rise in serum calcium concentration into the hypercalcemic range.[64]

Other Biochemical Features

In primary hyperparathyroidism, the serum phosphorus tends to be in the lower range of normal but frank hypophosphatemia is present in less than one-fourth of patients. Average total urinary calcium excretion is at the upper end of the normal range, with less than half of all patients having hypercalciuria. Serum 25-hydroxyvitamin D levels tend to be in the lower end of the normal range. While mean values of 1,25-dihydroxyvitamin D_3 are in the high-normal range, approximately one-third of patients have frankly elevated levels of 1,25-dihydroxyvitamin D_3.[65] A mild hyperchloremia is seen occasionally, due to the effect of PTH on renal acid-base balance. A typical biochemical profile is shown in Table 76–3.

TABLE 76–3. Biochemical Profile in Primary Hyperparathyroidism (N = 137)

	Patients (mean ± SEM)	Normal Range
Serum calcium	10.7 ± 0.1 mg/dL	8.2–10.2 mg/dL
Serum phosphorus	2.8 ± 0.1 mg/dL	2.5–4.5 mg/dL
Total alkaline phosphatase	114 ± 5 IU/L	<100 IU/L
Serum magnesium	2.0 ± 0.1 mg/dL	1.8–2.4 mg/dL
PTH (IRMA)	119 ± 7 pg/mL	10–65 pg/mL
25(OH) vitamin D	19 ± 1 ng/mL	9–52 ng/mL
1,25(OH)$_2$ vitamin D	54 ± 2 pg/mL	15–60 pg/mL
Urinary calcium	240 ± 11 mg/g creatinine	
Urine DPD	17.6 ± 1.3 nmol/mmol creatinine	<14.6 nmol/mmol creatinine
Urine PYD	46.8 ± 2.7 nmol/mmol creatinine	<51.8 nmol/mmol creatinine

PTH (IRMA), parathyroid hormone (immunoradiometric assay); DPD, deoxypyridinoline; PYD, pyridinoline.

THE SKELETON

The classic radiologic bone disease of primary hyperparathyroidism, osteitis fibrosa cystica, is rarely seen today in the United States. Most series place the incidence of osteitis fibrosa cystica at less than 2% of patients with primary hyperparathyroidism. The absence of classic radiographic features (salt-and-pepper skull, tapering of the distal third of the clavicle, brown tumors) does not mean that the skeleton is not involved in the metabolic processes associated with hyperparathyroid bone disease. With more sensitive techniques, it has become clear that skeletal involvement in the hyperparathyroid process is actually quite common. This section reviews the profile of the skeleton in primary hyperparathyroidism as it is reflected in assays for bone markers, bone densitometry, and bone histomorphometry.

Bone Markers

Both bone resorption and bone formation are increased by PTH. Markers of bone turnover, which reflect those dynamics, provide clues to the extent of skeletal involvement in primary hyperparathyroidism. The study of bone markers in primary hyperparathyroidism has been of considerable interest for several reasons. First, this inquiry sheds light on which markers accurately reflect skeletal activity in the patient with primary hyperparathyroidism. Second, the evaluation of markers of bone turnover in primary hyperparathyroidism has provided insight into the hyperparathyroid process in bone. Finally, clues to the extent of postoperative improvements in bone mineral density might be provided by markers of bone turnover.

Bone Formation Markers

Bone formation is reflected by osteoblast products, including bone-specific alkaline phosphatase activity, osteocalcin, and type 1 procollagen peptide.[66] Despite the availability of these sensitive measurements of bone formation, the total alkaline phosphatase activity is still widely assessed in primary hyperparathyroidism.[67] In primary hyperparathyroidism, levels can be mildly elevated, but in many patients, total alkaline phosphatase values are within normal limits.[68–70] The bone-specific isoenzyme of alkaline phosphatase is far more sensitive, and is clearly elevated in many patients with mild primary hyperparathyroidism.[71, 72] In a small study from our group, bone-specific alkaline phosphatase correlated with PTH levels and bone mineral density (BMD) at the lumbar spine and femoral neck.[71] Osteocalcin is also generally increased in patients with primary hyperparathyroidism.[72–75] Osteocalcin correlates with other indices of bone formation. Assays for procollagen extension peptides reflect osteoblast activation and bone formation, but have not been shown to have significant predictive or clinical utility in primary hyperparathyroidism.[76] In a small study of patients with primary hyperparathyroidism, C-terminal propeptide of human type 1 procollagen (PICP) levels were higher than in control subjects, but distinct elevations were much less impressive than those seen for alkaline phosphatase, osteocalcin, or even hydroxyproline (see below).

Bone Resorption Markers

Markers of bone resorption include the osteoclast product, tartrate-resistant acid phosphatase (TRAP), and collagen breakdown products such as hydroxyproline, hydroxypyridinium cross-links of collagen, and N- and C-telopeptides of type 1 collagen.[66] Urinary hydroxyproline, once the only available marker of bone resorption,[77–79] no longer offers sufficient sensitivity or specificity to make it a useful tool in the assessment of patients with primary hyperparathyroidism. Although urinary hydroxyproline was frankly elevated in patients with osteitis fibrosa cystica, in mild, asymptomatic primary hyperparathyroidism it is now typically entirely normal. Hydroxypyridinium cross-links of collagen, pyridinoline (PYD) and deoxypyridinoline (DPD), on the other hand, are often elevated in primary hyperparathyroidism. They return to normal after parathyroidectomy.[80] DPD and PYD both correlate positively with PTH concentrations. The fact that urinary concentrations of PYD and DPD seem to correlate closely with disease activity, coupled with their usefulness in longitudinal follow-up (see below), make the hydroxypyridinium cross-links of collagen an attractive choice as bone resorptive markers in primary hyperparathyroidism.

Studies of TRAP are limited, although levels have been shown to be elevated.[66] Assays for the N-telopeptide of type I collagen (NTX) have yet to be systematically explored in this disease. In the case of the PYD cross-linked telopeptide domain of type I collagen (ICTP), pooled data from patients with high turnover diseases (i.e., primary hyperparathyroidism as well as hyperthyroidism) suggest that this marker may reflect calcium kinetics and histomorphometric indices.[66] Data specifically relevant to primary hyperparathyroidism alone are not yet available.

Recently, bone sialoprotein, a phosphorylated glycoprotein which makes up approximately 5% to 10% of the noncollagenous bone protein, has been the focus of interest. Bone sialoprotein is thought to reflect bone resorption, although it may also be regarded as an integrated function of bone turnover. In primary hyperparathyroidism, bone sialoprotein levels are elevated and correlate with urinary PYD and DPD.[81] Thus, sensitive assays reflecting bone formation and bone resorption show both to be increased in mild primary hyperparathyroidism.

Longitudinal Bone Marker Studies

Studies of bone markers in the longitudinal follow-up of patients with primary hyperparathyroidism are limited, but indicate a reduction in these markers of bone turnover following parathyroidectomy. Information from our group,[80] Guo et al.,[82] and Tanaka et al.[83] all report declining levels of bone markers following surgery, although the choice of markers in the individual studies differed. Data are also emerging concerning the kinetics of change in bone resorption vs. bone formation following parathyroidectomy. We have found that markers of bone resorption decline rapidly following cure of primary hyperparathyroidism, while indices of bone formation follow a more gradual decrease.[80] Urinary PYD and DPD decreased significantly as early as 2 weeks following parathyroidectomy, preceding reductions in alkaline phosphatase (Fig. 76–3). Similar data were reported from Tanaka et al.,[83] who demonstrated a discrepancy between changes in NTX (reflecting bone resorption) and osteocalcin (reflecting bone formation) following parathyroidectomy, and Minisola et al.,[77] who reported a drop in bone resorptive markers and no significant change in alkaline phosphatase or osteocalcin. Short-term studies reported a brief increase in PICP immediately following parathyroidectomy, while bone resorptive markers fell promptly. The persistence of elevated bone formation markers coupled with rapid declines in bone resorption markers indicates a shift in the coupling between bone formation and bone resorption toward an anabolic build-up of bone mineral postoperatively. Increases in bone density postoperatively provide support for this idea.

Cytokines

Although studies of bone markers shed light on the skeletal manifestations of primary hyperparathyroidism, other molecules have been studied to elucidate the mechanism underlying the effects of PTH excess on bone. These factors, or cytokines, released in response to PTH, lead to important direct and indirect effects on bone cells. Some, such as interleukins (ILs) IL-1, IL-6, and IL-11, transforming growth factor-α (TGF-α), epidermal growth factor (EGF), and tumor necrosis factor (TNF), stimulate bone resorption. Others, including IL-4, insulin-like growth factor-1 (IGF-1), TGF-β, and interferons, may be anabolic for bone. Alterations in the levels of some or all of these cytokines may account for the mechanism of accelerated bone turnover and selective bone loss in primary hyperparathyroidism.

IL-6 and TNF-α have been studied as possible mediators of bone resorption in primary hyperparathyroidism. In vitro and in vivo data support an effect of PTH in stimulating production of IL-6, which in turn leads to increased osteoclastogenesis.[84–86] Furthermore, antibodies to IL-6 prevent PTH-mediated bone resorption. Reports from Grey et al.[87] have shown circulating IL-6 and TNF-α levels to be elevated in primary hyperparathyroidism. These cytokines correlate with PTH levels preoperatively and fall following parathyroidectomy. Although cytokine levels did not correlate significantly with bone density measurements in this report, it should be noted that bone density was not assessed at the site containing mostly cortical bone (the radius) where the catabolic effects of excess PTH would be expected to be seen most clearly. More information is needed to confirm these observations, especially with appropriate control subjects, and to test for potential involvement of other bone resorptive cytokines in primary hyperparathyroidism.

The involvement of other factors in the anabolic effect of primary hyperparathyroidism on bone is also being studied. Levels of IGF-1, which is well documented to be a direct mediator of PTH action in bone, and insulin-like growth factor binding protein 3 (IGFBP3, the major binding protein for IGF-1) change following parathyroidectomy in primary hyperparathyroidism.[88] The alteration in the ratio of IGF-1 to IGFBP3 supports enhanced delivery of IGF-1 to tissues following surgery, an increase inversely proportional to the observed rise in lumbar spine and femoral neck bone density. It is not known whether the anabolic properties of PTH at cancellous sites (e.g., lumbar spine) can be explained by IGF-1 prior to surgery.

Bone Densitometry

The advent of bone mineral densitometry as a major diagnostic tool for osteoporosis occurred at a time when the clinical profile of primary

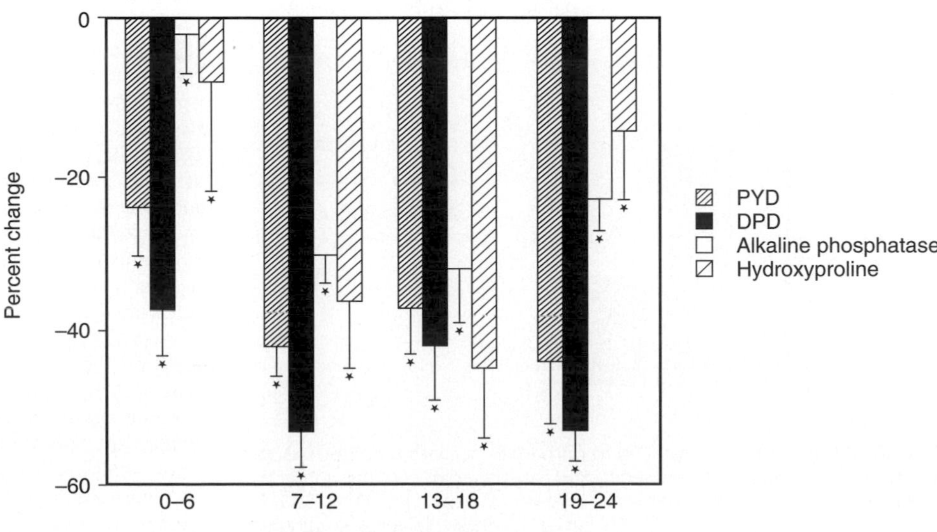

FIGURE 76–3. Bone turnover markers following parathyroidectomy. Data are presented as percentage change from preoperative baseline measurement. *Asterisk* denotes change significant at $P < .05$. (From Seibel MJ, Gartenberg F, Silverberg SJ, et al: Urinary hydroxypyridinium cross-links of collagen in primary hyperparathyroidism. J Clin Endocrinol Metab 74:481–486, 1992.)

hyperparathyroidism was changing from a symptomatic to an asymptomatic disease. This fortuitous timing allowed questions about skeletal involvement in primary hyperparathyroidism to be addressed when specific radiologic features of primary hyperparathyroidism had all but disappeared. Bone mass measurements could provide information about the actual state of bone mineral with great accuracy and precision. The known physiologic proclivity of PTH to be catabolic at sites of cortical bone make a cortical site essential to any complete densitometric study of primary hyperparathyroidism. By convention, the distal third of the radius is the site used. The early densitometric studies in primary hyperparathyroidism also took advantage of another physiologic property of PTH, namely, to be anabolic at cancellous sites. The lumbar spine, enriched in cancellous bone, became an important site, not only because of its composition and the design of central densitometric equipment (dual energy x-ray absorptiometry, computed tomography [CT] scanning) but also because the lumbar spine is a site of early bone loss in the early postmenopausal years.

In primary hyperparathyroidism, bone density at the distal third of the radius is diminished.[89, 90] Bone density at the lumbar spine is only minimally reduced. The hip region, containing a relatively equal mixture of cortical and cancellous elements, shows bone density intermediate between the cortical and cancellous sites (Fig. 76–4). The results support not only the notion that PTH is catabolic in cortical bone but also the view that PTH is anabolic in cancellous bone.[91–93] In postmenopausal women, the same pattern was observed.[89] Postmenopausal women with primary hyperparathyroidism, therefore, show a reversal of the pattern typically associated with postmenopausal bone loss, namely preferential loss of cancellous bone. The reduced bone density at the distal radius (cortical bone), and preserved density at the lumbar spine (cancellous bone) suggest that primary hyperparathyroidism helps to protect postmenopausal women from bone loss due to estrogen deficiency.

Observations of skeletal health in primary hyperparathyroidism made by bone mineral densitometry have established the importance of this technology in the evaluation of all patients with primary hyperparathyroidism. Without this information, the data set on which recommendations are made regarding surgery is incomplete. The Consensus Development Conference on Asymptomatic Primary Hyperparathyroidism implicity acknowledged this point when bone mineral densitometry was included as a separate criterion for clinical decision making.[94]

The bone density profile in which there is relative preservation of skeletal mass at the vertebrae and diminution at the more cortical distal radius is not always seen in primary hyperparathyroidsm. While this pattern is evident in the vast majority of patients, a small group of patients have evidence of vertebral osteopenia at the time of presentation. In our natural history study, approximately 15% of patients had a lumbar spine Z score of less than −1.5 at the time of diagnosis.[95] Although the majority of these patients were postmenopausal women, not all vetebral bone loss could be attributed entirely to estrogen deficiency. These patients are of interest with regard to changes in bone density following parathyroidectomy, and are discussed in further detail later. The extent of vertebral bone involvement will vary as a function of disease severity. In the typical mild form of the disease, the pattern described above is seen. When primary hyperparathyroidism is more advanced, there will be more generalized involvement, and the lumbar spine will not appear to be protected. When primary hyperparathyroidism is severe or more symptomatic, all bones can be extensively involved.

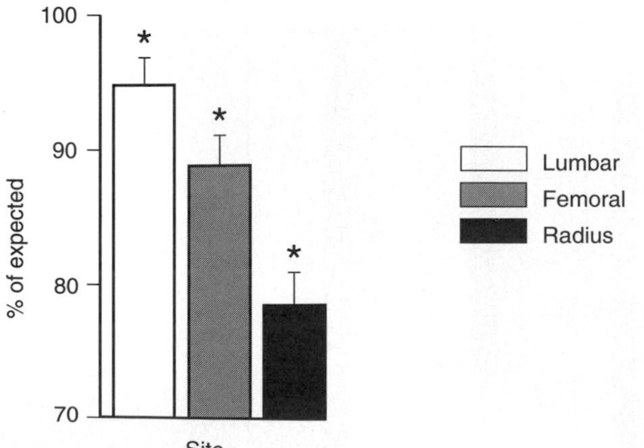

FIGURE 76–4. Bone densitometry in primary hyperparathyroidism. Data are shown in comparison to age- and sex-matched normal subjects. Divergence from expected values is different at each site (P = .0001). (From Silverberg SJ, Shane E, DeLaCruz L, et al: Skeletal disease in primary hyperparathyroidism. J Bone Miner Res 4:283–291, 1989.)

Bone Histomorphometry

Analyses of percutaneous bone biopsies from patients with primary hyperparathyroidism have provided confirmatory information obtained by bone densitometry and by bone markers. Both static and dynamic parameters give a picture of cortical thinning, maintenance of cancellous bone volume (Fig. 76–5), and a very dynamic process associated with high turnover and accelerated bone remodeling.

Cortical thinning, inferred by bone mineral densitometry, is clearly documented in a quantitative manner by iliac crest bone biopsy.[96–98] Van Doorn et al.[99] demonstrated a positive correlation between PTH levels and cortical porosity. These findings are consistent with the known effect of PTH to be catabolic at endocortical surfaces of bone. Osteoclasts are thought to erode more deeply along the corticomedullary junction under the influence of PTH.

Histomorphometric studies have contributed most by elucidating the nature of cancellous bone preservation in primary hyperparathyroidism. Again, as suggested by bone densitometry, cancellous bone volume is clearly well preserved in primary hyperparathyroidism. This is seen as well among the postmenopausal women with primary hyperparathyroidism. Several studies have shown that cancellous bone is actually increased in primary hyperparathyroidism as compared to normal subjects.[96, 100, 101] When cancellous bone volume is compared among age- and sex-matched subjects with primary hyperparathyroidism or postmenopausal osteoporosis, a dramatic difference is evident (Fig. 76–6). Whereas postmenopausal women with osteoporosis have reduced cancellous bone volume, women with primary hyperparathyroidism have higher cancellous bone volume.[100] It is this kind of observation that suggests that while primary hyperparathyroidism is said to be a risk factor for postmenopausal osteoporosis, it is a syndrome of bone loss. The region(s) of bone loss in primary hyperparathyroidism is directed toward the cortical bone compartment, with good maintenance of cancellous bone volume unless the primary hyperparathyroidism is unusually active.

Preservation of cancellous bone volume even extends to comparisons with the expected losses associated with the effects of aging on cancellous bone physiology. In a study of 27 patients with primary hyperparathyroidism (10 men and 17 women), static parameters of bone turnover (osteoid surface, osteoid volume, and eroded surface) were increased, as expected, in patients relative to control subjects.[96] However, in control subjects, trabecular number varied inversely with age, while trabecular separation increased with advancing age. Both of these observations are expected concomitants of aging. In marked contrast, in the patients with primary hyperparathyroidism, no such age dependency was seen. There was no relationship between trabecular number or separation and age in primary hyperparathyroidism, suggesting that the actual plates and their connections were being maintained over time more effectively than one would have expected through the aging process. Thus, primary hyperparathyroidism seems to retard the normal age-related processes associated with trabecular loss.

Further insights into the nature of the effect of PTH on trabecular architecture was obtained by the histomorphometric technique called "strut analysis."[102] This approach assesses the extent to which trabecular plates are connected to each other by measuring two-dimensional indices of cancellous structure, including trabecular nodes (sites at which two trabecular plates come together) and trabecular termini

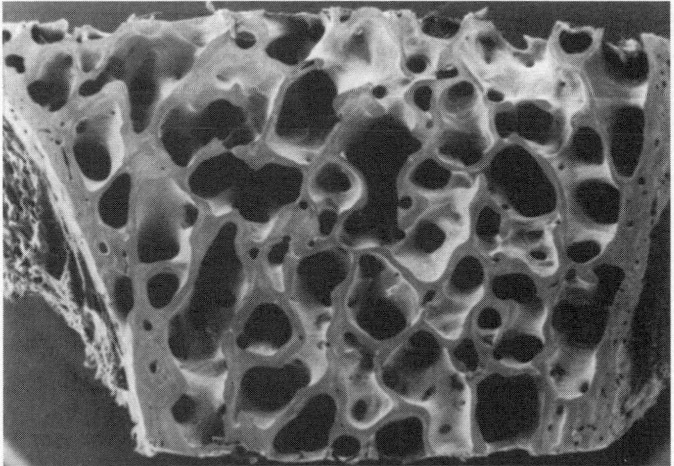

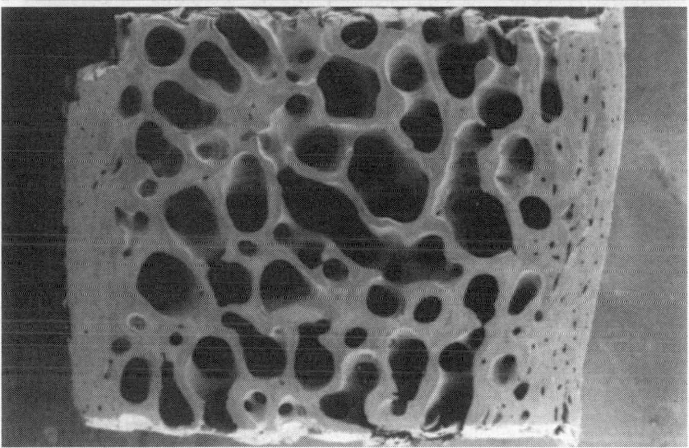

FIGURE 76–5. Scanning electron micrograph of bone biopsy specimens in a normal subject *(top panel)* and age- and sex-matched patient with primary hyperparathyroidism *(bottom panel)*. The cortices of the hyperparathyroid sample are markedly thinned, but cancellous bone and trabecular connectivity appear to be well preserved. (Magnification X31.25.) (From Parisien MV, Silverberg SJ, Shane E, et al: Bone disease in primary hyperparathyroidism. Endocrinol Metab Clin North Am 19:19–34, 1990.)

(sites at which a trabecular plate comes to an end, and is not connected to another plate). Node number, and node-to-node strut length are primary indices of bone connectivity. Terminus number and terminus-to-terminus strut length are primary indices of trabecular disconnectivity. In primary hyperparathyroidism, indices of trabecular connectivity are greater than expected, while indices of disconnectivity are decreased. When three matched groups of postmenopausal women were assessed (a normal group, a group with postmenopausal osteoporosis, and a group with primary hyperparathyroidism), women with primary hyperparathyroidism were shown to have trabeculae with less evidence of disconnectivity compared with normals, despite increased levels of bone turnover.[100, 102] Thus cancellous bone is preserved in primary hyperparathyroidism through the maintenance of well-connected trabecular plates.

In order to determine the mechanism for cancellous bone preservation in primary hyperparathyroidism, static and dynamic histomorphometric indices were compared between normal and hyperparathyroid postmenopausal women. In normal postmenopausal women, there is an imbalance in bone formation and resorption which favors excess bone resorption. In postmenopausal women with primary hyperparathyroidism, on the other hand, the adjusted apposition rate is increased. Bone formation, thus favored, may explain the efficacy of PTH at cancellous sites in patients with osteoporosis.[91, 93, 103–105] Assessment of bone remodeling variables in patients with primary hyperparathyroidism shows increases in active bone formation period.[101] (Table 76–4). The increased bone formation rate and total formation period may explain the preservation of cancellous bone seen in this disease.

Fractures

While fractures were an integral element of classic primary hyperparathyroidism, their importance in modern-day disease is unclear. In a case-control study published in 1975, Dauphine et al.[106] suggested that back pain and vertebral crush fractures might be part of the presenting clinical profile of primary hyperparathyroidism. Since that time, reports on fracture incidence have been conflicting. A retrospective review of lateral chest radiographs of patients who underwent parathyroidectomy showed an increased incidence of vertebral fractures in one study,[107] while Wilson et al.[108] found no increase in such fractures in a cohort of 174 consecutive patients who had mild asymptomatic primary hyperparathyroidism.

In the only study that considered hip fracture, a population-based prospective analysis (mean of 17 years' duration; 23,341 person-years) showed women with primary hyperparathyroidism in Sweden not to be at increased risk.[109] In a much smaller study (46 patients, 44 controls), fractures at any site were increased in hyperparathyroidism.[110] This study is flawed not only by its small sample size but also by the unusually high fracture incidence in both patients (48%) and control subjects (28%), and by the use of thyroid medication in a significantly greater number of patients (28%) relative to control subjects.

Most recently, the Mayo Clinic experience with primary hyperparathyroidism and risk of fracture was published. Khosla et al.[111] reviewed 407 cases of primary hyperparathyroidism recognized during the 28-year period 1965 to 1992. Fracture risk was assessed by comparing fractures at a number of sites with numbers of fractures expected on the basis of sex and age from the general population. The clinical features of these patients with primary hyperparathyroidism was typical of the mild form of the disease, with the serum calcium being only modestly elevated at 10.9 ± 0.6 mg/dL. The data from this retrospective epidemiologic study indicate that overall fracture risk was significantly increased at many sites such as the vertebral spine, the distal forearm, the ribs, and the pelvis. There was no increase in hip fractures. After multivariate analysis, age and female sex remained significant independent predictors of fracture risk. These data, however, are subject to potential ascertainment bias. Patients with primary hyperparathyroidism are typically followed more conscientiously and thus fractures at some of these sites may have been recognized by greater surveillance. This may certainly be true of the vertebral spine

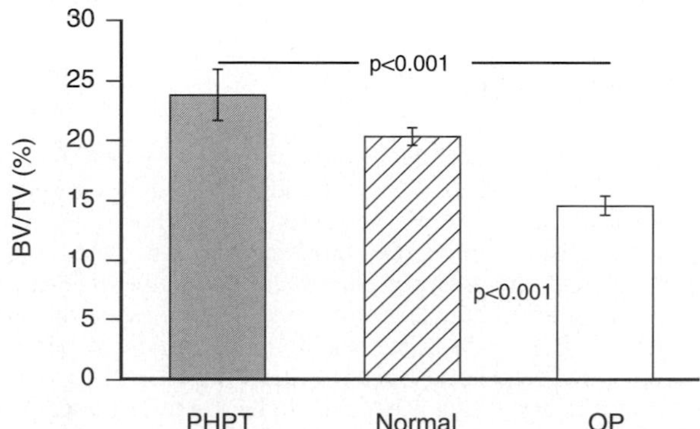

FIGURE 76–6. Cancellous bone volume in primary hyperparathyroidism. Cancellous bone volume was analyzed from bone biopsy specimens of the iliac crest. Comparisons are between 16 women with primary hyperparathyroidism, 17 women with postmenopausal osteoporosis, and 31 women with no known disorder of bone metabolism. Subjects were matched for age and other indices. (From Parisien M, Cosman F, Mellish RWE, et al: Bone structure in postmenopausal hyperparathyroid, osteoporotic and normal women. J Bone Miner Res 10:1393–1399, 1995.)

TABLE 76–4. Wall Width and Remodeling Variables in Primary Hyperparathyroidism (PHPT) and Control Groups (Mean ± SEM)

Variable	PHPT (n = 19)	Control (n = 34)	P
Wall width (μm)	40.26 ± 0.36	34.58 ± 0.45	<.0001
Eroded perimeter (%)	9.00 ± 0.86	4.76 ± 0.39	<.0001
Osteoid perimeter (%)	26.84 ± 2.79	15.04 ± 1.09	<.0001
Osteoid width (μm)	13.39 ± 0.54	9.92 ± 0.36	<.0001
Single-labeled perimeter (%)	11.56 ± 1.63	4.47 ± 0.48	<.0001
Double-labeled perimeter (%)	10.41 ± 1.28	4.45 ± 0.65	<.0001
Mineralizing perimeter (%)*	16.19 ± 1.75	6.68 ± 0.83	<.0001
Mineralizing perimeter/osteoid perimeter (%)	63.0 ± 5.0	44.0 ± 4.0	<.01
Mineral apposition rate (μm/day)	0.63 ± 0.03	0.63 ± 0.02	NS
Bone formation rate (μm²/μm · day)	0.10 ± 0.01	0.042 ± 0.006	<.0001
Adjusted apposition rate (μm/day)	0.40 ± 0.04	0.29 ± 0.03	<.015
Activation frequency/yr	0.95 ± 0.12	0.45 ± 0.06	<.0002
Mineralization lag time (days)	44.0 ± 6.5	57.0 ± 8.9	NS
Osteoid maturation time (days)	22.5 ± 1.8	16.6 ± 0.9	<.003
Total formation period (days)	129.2 ± 21.0	208.8 ± 32.5	NS
Active formation period (days)	67.8 ± 5.1	57.3 ± 2.3	<.05
Resorption period (days)	48.4 ± 7.3	84.8 ± 25.0	NS
Remodeling period (days)	172.5 ± 25.2	299.9 ± 55.1	NS

*Mineralizing perimeter = double-labeled perimeter ÷ ½ (single-labeled perimeter).
NS, not significant.
Modified from Dempster DW, Parisien M, Silverberg SJ, et al: On the mechanism of cancellous bone preservation in postmenopausal women with mild primary hyperparathyroidism. J Clin Endocrinol Metab 84:1562–1566, 1999.

and the ribs but unlikely in the case of fractures of the forearm. One might expect in fact to see an increased incidence of distal forearm fractures since the hyperparathyroid process tends to lead to reduction of cortical bone (distal forearm) in preference to cancellous bone (vertebral spine). Unfortunately, there were no densitometric data provided in this study so one could not relate bone density to fracture incidence. Thus, it is difficult to know whether in fact this study confirms an expectation of preferential distal forearm fractures in primary hyperparathyroidism or whether some other process is at work confirming universally greater fracture risk in these patients.

The conflicting data on fractures in hyperparathyroidism comes, in part, from the heterogeneous groups of patients described by the various studies, as well as from the specific control groups chosen by some of the studies. Important questions remain regarding the implications of the bone densitometry and histomorphometry findings discussed above for fractures in this disease. Ultimately, will there be shown any increase in fractures associated with mild asymptomatic disease? Will there be an increase in fractures at more cortical sites, with possibly a decrease in vertebral fractures in affected postmenopausal women? To obtain the answers to some of these questions, a multicenter trial with sufficient statistical power will be necessary.

NEPHROLITHIASIS

In the past, classic clinical descriptions of primary hyperparathyroidism emphasized skeletal involvement and kidney stones as principal complications of the disease.[112] The cause of nephrolithiasis in primary hyperparathyroidism is probably multifactorial. An increase in the amount of calcium filtered at the glomerulus due to the hypercalcemia of hyperparathyroidism may lead to hypercalciuria despite the physiologic actions of PTH to facilitate calcium reabsorption. A component of absorptive hypercalciuria exists in this disorder. The enhanced intestinal calcium absorption is believed to be due to increased production of 1,25-dihydroxyvitamin D, a consequence of another physiologic action of PTH.[113, 114] Urinary calcium excretion is correlated with 1,25-dihydroxyvitamin D levels.[114, 115] In addition, increased intestinal calcium absorption seen in nephrolithiasis of other causes[116] may also occur in primary hyperparathyroidism. The skeleton provides yet another possible source for the increased levels of calcium in the glomerular filtrate. Hyperparathyroid bone resorption might contribute to hypercalciuria, and subsequently to nephrolithiasis. Previously, however, there has been no convincing evidence to support this hypothesis.[115, 117, 118] Finally, alteration in local urinary factors, such as a reduction in inhibitor activity or an increase in stone-promoting factors, may predispose some patients with primary hyperparathyroidism to nephrolithiasis.[118, 119] It remains unclear whether the urine of patients with hyperparathyroid stone disease is different in this regard from that of other stone formers.

Studies in the 1970s and 1980s documented a higher incidence of renal stone disease (30%,[11] 57%,[117] and 44%[115]) than do reports of more recent experience. With the decreased incidence of osteitis fibrosa cystica, studies in the modern era have tended to focus on patients with kidney stones. Conflicting results have emerged, with one group providing evidence that 1,25-dihydroxyvitamin D_3 plays an etiologic role in the development of nephrolithiasis in primary hyperparathyroidism,[115] and other groups unable to document differences in 1,25-dihydroxyvitamin D_3 levels between those with and without renal stone disease.[112, 118]

Although the incidence of nephrolithiasis is reduced from that seen in classic primary hyperparathyroidism, kidney stones remain the most common manifestation of symptomatic primary hyperparathyroidism (see Table 76–1). Estimates in recent studies place the incidence of kidney stones at 15% to 20% of all patients.[120] Other renal manifestations of primary hyperparathyroidism include hypercalciuria, which is seen in approximately 40% of patients, and nephrocalcinosis, the frequency of which is unknown.

In the 1930s, it was generally accepted that bone and stone disease did not coexist in the same patient[1, 6] with classic primary hyperparathyroidism. Albright and Reifenstein[1] postulated that low dietary calcium intake would lead to bone disease, while adequate or high dietary calcium levels would be associated with stone disease. Dent et al.[121] who provided convincing evidence against this construct, proposed the existence of two forms of cirulating PTH, one causing renal stones and the other causing bone disease. A host of mechanisms, including differences in dietary calcium, calcium absorption, forms of circulating PTH, and levels of 1,25-dihydroxyvitamin D_3, were proposed to account for the clinical distinction between bone and stone disease in primary hyperparathyroidism.[1, 6, 115, 117, 121] Today, there is no clear evidence for two distinct subtypes of primary hyperparathyroidism. In our patients with primary hyperparathyroidism, we could not identify a distinctive set of biochemical data for patients with stone disease.[112] Furthermore, although our population did not include patients with classic hyperparathyroid bone disease, we found no evidence to support the notion that the processes affecting the skeleton and kidneys in hyperparathyroidism occur in different subsets of patients. Urinary calcium excretion per gram of creatinine, levels of 1,25-dihydroxyvitamin D, and BMD at all sites (Fig. 76–7) were indistinguishable among patients with and without nephrolithiasis. Cortical bone demineralization is as common and as extensive in those with and without nephrolithiasis.[112, 118]

OTHER ORGAN INVOLVEMENT

Over the years, primary hyperparathyroidism has been associated with complaints referable to many different organ systems. Perhaps the most common complaints have been those of weakness and easy fatigability. Classic primary hyperparathyroidism used to be associated with a distinct neuromuscular syndrome, characterized by type II muscle cell atrophy.[122, 123] Originally described by Vicale in 1949,[124] the syndrome consisted of easy fatigability, symmetrical proximal muscle weakness, and muscle atrophy. Both the clinical and electromyographic features of this disorder were reversible after parathyroid surgery.[125–127] In the milder, less symptomatic form of the disease that is common today, this disorder is rarely seen.[128] In a group of 42 patients with mild disease, none had complaints consistent with the neuromuscular dysfunction described above. However, over half of all patients had nonspecific complaints of paresthesias and muscle cramps. Electromyographic studies in 9 patients did not show the myopathy or motor unit denervation typical of past observations. Instead, carpal tunnel syndrome was demonstrated in 3 of the 9 subjects, a percentage higher than expected in the general population, but of dubious significance.

The neuropsychiatric abnormalities of primary hyperparathyroidism have yet to be thoroughly characterized, although it remains an area of active interest.[129–134] Many patients, families, and physicians note features of depression, cognitive difficulties, and anxiety in those with the disease. Furthermore, many of these complaints have been described as being reversible after parathyroidectomy. Attempts to characterize these abnormalities using various psychopathologic rating scales, both in the disease state and after cure, have been fraught with difficulties. The study of Solomon et al.[135] is perhaps the best attempt at studying this problem in a prospective manner. Using the SL-149 rating scale, the authors observed a constellation of neuropsychologic abnormalities, most of which improved after successful surgery. A group of euparathyroid subjects, who underwent neck surgery for removal of a thyroid nodule, had similar postoperative improvement. Thus, this study could not easily attribute the improvement in neuropsychologic symptomatology to hyperparathyroidism or to the effects of the surgical procedure per se. Thus, neuropsychologic functioning in primary hyperparathyroidism remains an important but unresolved issue.

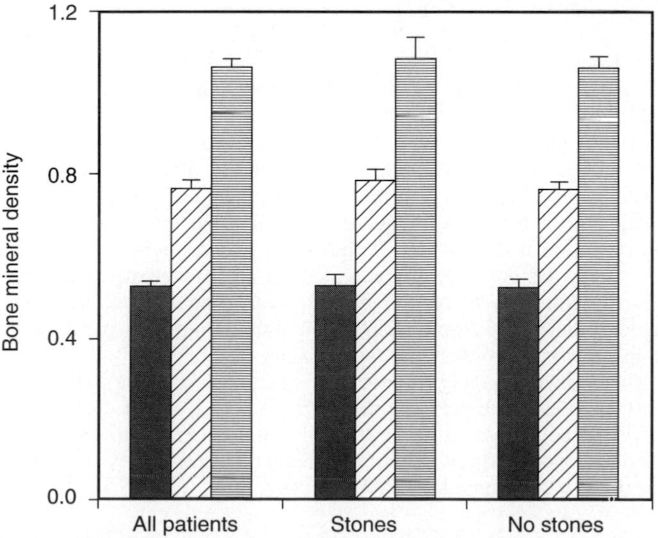

FIGURE 76–7. Bone density in patients with primary hyperparathyroidism with and without stone disease. Bone mineral density is shown at the forearm *(solid bars)*, femoral neck *(diagonally hatched bars)*, and lumbar spine *(horizontally hatched bars)*. Values are shown as mean (±SEM) for the entire cohort and the subgroups with and without nephrolithiasis. (From Silverberg SJ, Shane E, Jacobs TP, et al: Nephrolithiasis and bone involvement in primary hyperparathyroidism, 1985–1990. Am J Med 89:327–334, 1990.)

Interest in the effect of primary hyperparathyroidism on cardiovascular function has its root in pathophysiologic observations of the hypercalcemic state. Hypercalcemia has been associated with increases in blood pressure, left ventricular hypertrophy, heart muscle hypercontractility, and arrhythmias.[136–139] Furthermore, evidence of calcium deposition has been documented in the form of calcifications in the myocardium, heart valves, and coronary arteries. The effect of primary hyperparathyroidism on these parameters is less clear. Stefanelli et al.[140] prospectively studied 64 patients and found that myocardial calcifications were markedly increased (69% of patients vs. 17% of controls). Valvular calcifications were also seen in a significantly higher percentage of patients than controls (63% at the aortic, and 49% at the mitral valve). Regression in left ventricular hypertrophy was seen in nonhypertensive patients 1 year after successful parathyroid surgery. The results of this study, however, may have limited applicability to patients with the mild form of primary hyperparathyroidism observed most commonly in the United States today because the population of Stefanelli et al. was more severely affected. Forty percent had kidney stones. Serum calcium levels (mean, 12 mg/dL) and PTH (10 times normal) were both substantially higher than the values we see today. Potential cardiovascular effects of asymptomatic primary hyperparathyroidism must await studies focused on a population with much milder disease.

Many other pathologic features have been described in patients with primary hyperparathyroidism. First among these disorders is hypertension, which has been noted to be present in a higher percentage of hyperparathyroid patients than expected.[8, 54–56] However, hypertension does not remit with cure of the underlying hyperparathyroid process, and the hypertension is not generally easier to control. A similar association has been made between primary hyperparathyroidism and peptic ulcer disease. Today, it is felt that a significant relationship exists only in patients with primary hyperparathyroidism and MEN-1. Finally, gout and pseudogout have been described in primary hyperparathyroidism, both in the setting of untreated disease, as well as at the time of surgical cure.[57, 58] Again, verifiable etiologic relationships between primary hyperparathyroidism and uric acid or pyrophosphate arthropathy remain to be established.

MORTALITY

Early data supporting the idea of higher mortality rates in primary hyperparathyroidism came from a retrospective study of limited size in Scandinavia and in the United States.[141, 142] More recent data from the United States did not show any increase in mortality in affected patients.[143] The study in question assessed survival in a population-based study of hyperparathyroidism in Rochester, Minnesota over a 28-year period. There was no increase in mortality in the 435 patients with surgically confirmed hyperparathyroidism, hypercalcemia with inappropriately elevated PTH levels, or unexplained hypercalcemia of more than 1 year's duration. It is possible that the change in clinical profile to a largely asymptomatic disease is responsible for this apparent reduction in mortality rates. Consistent with this notion, in the aforementioned survival study, a higher maximal serum calcium level was found to be an independent predictor of mortality. Thus the very mild elevations in serum calcium found today could account for the improved survival rates.

Much of this chapter has focused on asymptomatic primary hyperparathyroidism as the predominating clinical profile in the modern era. Certainly in countries where biochemical screening tests are routinely employed, this description is accurate. However, reports from other countries have revisited the older, more classic descriptions of primary hyperparathyroidism as a disease of "stones, bones, and groans."[144–146] The lack of routine screening tests does not explain completely this older form of the disease in the 1990s in these other countries. Rather, patients who have been described from China, Brazil, India, and Saudi Arabia have a common underlying deficiency in vitamin D. Years ago, primary hyperparathyroidism and vitamin D deficiency were described as a potent negative combination by Lumb and Stanbury.[147] Even in mild, asymptomatic primary hyperparathyroidism, we have shown that indices of disease activity are generally higher among those whose 25-hydroxyvitamin D levels are low.[64] Mechanisms to explain this clinical observation are speculative, but it is intriguing to consider vitamin D–PTH gene interactions. An endogenous regulator of PTH gene function is 1,25-dihydroxyvitamin D.[148, 149] When vitamin D deficiency is present in primary hyperparathyroidism, it is possible that the abnormal PTH cells are stimulated further to produce PTH. With the emergence of vitamin D deficiency as a growing problem in developed countries, it is conceivable that primary hyperparathyroidism will become once again a more symptomatic disease throughout the world.

EVALUATION

The diagnosis of primary hyperparathyroidism is confirmed by demonstrating an elevated PTH level in the face of hypercalcemia. Further biochemical assessment should include serum phosphorus, alkaline phosphatase, vitamin D metabolites, albumin, and creatinine. A morning 2-hour or 24-hour urine collection should be obtained for calcium and creatinine. A urinary bone resorption marker such as DPD or N-telopeptide can be helpful. Radiographs of the skeleton are not routinely obtained in view of the rarity of radiologically evident bone disease. Bone densitometry, on the other hand, is performed in all patients. It is preferable to obtain densitometry at three sites: the lumbar spine, hip, and distal third of the radius. Because of the differing amounts of cortical and cancellous bone at the three sites and the different effects of PTH on cortical and cancellous bone, measurement at all three sites allows a picture of the total effect of the hyperparathyroid process on the skeleton. Bone biopsy is not part of the routine evaluation of primary hyperparathyroidism. While kidney stones are present in only 20% of patients by history, it is not unreasonable to obtain a radiographic view or ultrasound of the abdomen to determine the presence of occult nephrolithiasis.

THERAPY

Parathyroidectomy remains the only currently available option for cure of primary hyperparathyroidism. As the disease profile has changed, questions have been raised concerning the advisability of surgery in asymptomatic patients. If asymptomatic patients have a benign natural history, the surgical alternative is not an attractive one. On the other hand, asymptomatic patients may display levels of hypercalcemia or hypercalciuria that cause concern for the future. Similarly, bone mass measurements can be frankly low at cortical or, less commonly, at cancellous sites. In an effort to address such issues, in 1990 the National Institutes of Health (NIH) held a consensus development conference on the management of asymptomatic primary hyperparathyroidism. The guidelines which emerged from that conference have been helpful to the clinician faced with the hyperparathyroid patient.[94] Surgery is advised in patients meeting the following criteria: (1) serum calcium greater than 12 mg/dL; (2) marked hypercalciuria (>400 mg/day); (3) any overt manifestation of primary hyperparathyroidism (nephrolithiasis, osteitis fibrosa cystica, classic neuromuscular disease); (4) markedly reduced cortical bone density (Z score <-2); (5) reduced creatinine clearance in the absence of other cause; (6) age less than 50 years.

Although these guidelines were not based on long-term prospective data, they nevertheless are reasonable. The only modification by clinicians over the years has been to restate the critical calcium value in relation to the normal assay range for the serum calcium. Since the upper limit of normal for serum calcium has fallen to approximately 10 to 10.2 mg/dL in most diagnostic chemistry laboratories, the serum calcium concentration above which many practitioners will recommend surgery is 1.0 to 1.5 mg/dL above that reference limit.

Surgery

Approximately 50% of patients presenting with primary hyperparathyroidism today will meet one or more of the surgical guidelines listed earlier (Fig. 76–8). A large percentage of these surgical candidates are asymptomatic. Some asymptomatic patients who meet surgical guidelines elect not to have surgery. Among the reasons why surgery is not sought are (1) personal choice; (2) intercurrent medical conditions; (3) previous unsuccessful parathyroid surgery. Conversely, there are patients who meet none of the NIH guidelines for parathyroidectomy, but opt for surgery nevertheless. Physician and patient input remain very important factors in the decision regarding parathyroid surgery.

Preoperative Localization of Hyperfunctioning Parathyroid Tissue

A number of imaging tests have been developed and applied singly or in combination to the challenge of preoperative localization.[150–159] The rationale for locating abnormal parathyroid tissue prior to surgery is that the glands can be notoriously unpredictable in their location. Although the majority of parathyroid adenomas are identified in regions proximate to their embryologically intended position (the four poles of the thyroid gland), many are not. In such situations, previous surgical experience and skill are needed to locate the ectopic parathyroid gland. In such hands, 95% of abnormal parathyroid glands will be discovered and removed at the time of initial parathyroid surgery. However, in the patient with previous neck surgery, such high success rates are not generally achieved, even by expert parathyroid surgeons. Preoperative localization of the abnormal parathyroid tissue can be extremely helpful under these circumstances.

Noninvasive parathyroid imaging studies include technetium Tc-99m sestamibi, ultrasound, CT scanning, and magnetic resonance imaging (MRI). Tc-99m sestamibi is generally regarded to be the most sensitive and specific imaging modality, especially when it is combined with single photon emission computed tomography (SPECT). For the single parathyroid adenoma, sensitivity has ranged from 80% to 100% with a 5% to 10% false-positive rate. On the other hand, sestamibi scintigraphy and the other localization tests have a relatively poor record in the context of multiglandular disease.

The availability of an imaging agent like sestamibi has tempted some to limit the extent of parathyroid surgery to the side or site of uptake. Intraoperative imaging with sestamibi administered 2 to 3 hours prior to surgery has been achieved in some cases with a hand-held gamma counter probe. A small incision is made over the site of the putative adenoma, as defined by the radioactive emissions. If radioactivity subsequently equilibrates in all quadrants of the neck, the surgery is ended. Another intraoperative approach is to measure PTH with a "quick" ICMA after removal of the abnormal parathyroid tissue. If the PTH level returns to normal, the single gland removed is considered to be the sole source of abnormal parathyroid tissue and the operation is terminated. It should be underscored that these new approaches are not generally accepted yet and most expert parathyroid surgeons continue to recommend the conventional total parathyroid exploration, with identification of all four parathyroid glands in the course of parathyroidectomy (see Chapter 79).

These newer imaging technologies clearly are valuable in the patient who has undergone previous neck surgery, but it is not clear whether they will be shown to be beneficial in the patient who has not had previous neck surgery. Claims of higher success rates and shorter operating time remain to be substantiated.

Immediate Postoperative Course

After surgery, biochemical indices return rapidly to normal.[160] Serum calcium and PTH levels normalize and urinary calcium excretion falls by as much as 50%. The serum calcium no longer tends to become abnormally low, a situation characteristic of an earlier time when primary hyperparathyroidism was a symptomatic disease with overt skeletal involvement. The acute reversal of hyperparathyroidism was

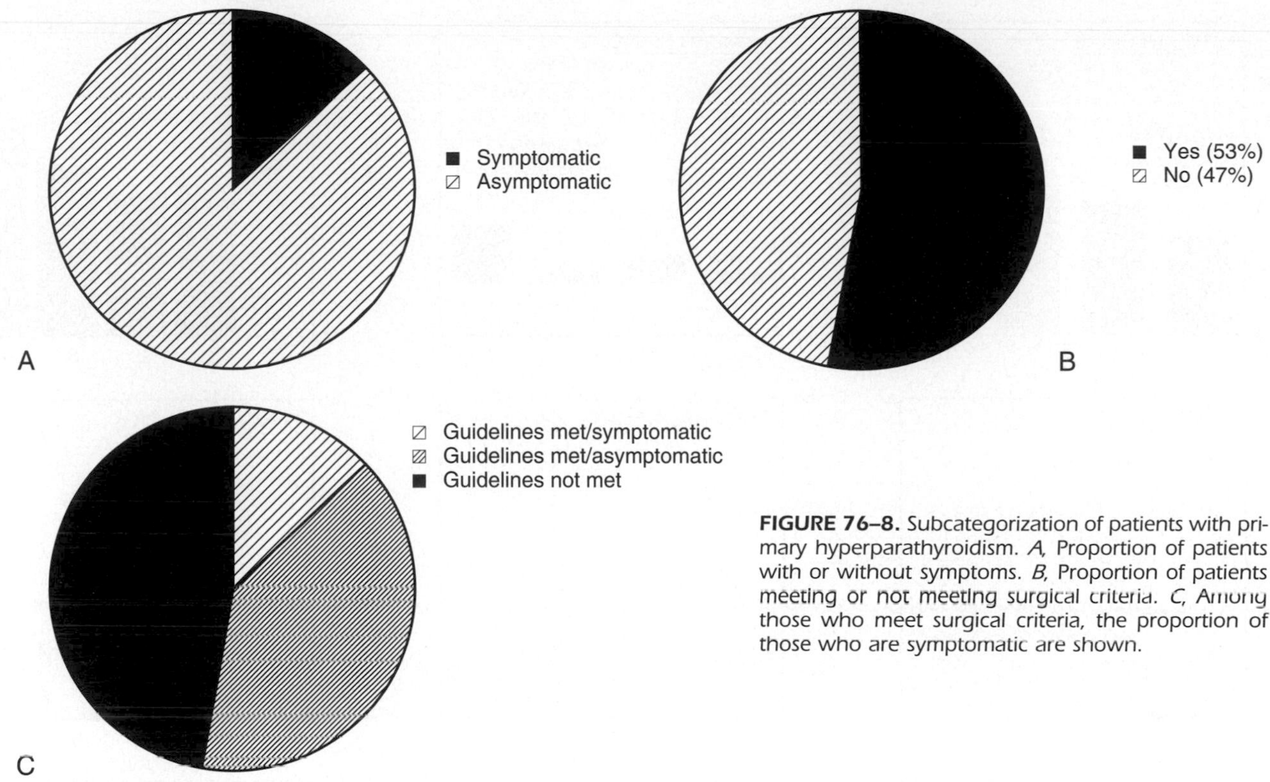

FIGURE 76–8. Subcategorization of patients with primary hyperparathyroidism. *A*, Proportion of patients with or without symptoms. *B*, Proportion of patients meeting or not meeting surgical criteria. *C*, Among those who meet surgical criteria, the proportion of those who are symptomatic are shown.

associated with a robust deposition of calcium into the skeleton at a pace that could not be compensated for by supplemental calcium. Thus, postoperative hypocalcemia was routine and sometimes a serious short term complication ("hungry bone syndrome"). Occasionally, postoperative hypocalcemia still occurs especially if preoperative bone turnover markers are elevated. More typically, however, the early postoperative course is not complicated by symptomatic hypocalcemia.

Long-Term Results

Vague or constitutional symptoms may or may not improve after surgery, while hypertension and peptic ulcer disease, if present, are unlikely to remit. Surgery is of clear benefit in reducing the incidence of recurrent nephrolithiasis.[120, 161] Over 90% of patients with stone disease and hyperparathyroidism do not form additional stones after parathyroid surgery. The 5% to 10% of patients who continue to form kidney stones after parathyroidectomy are thought to have a different cause for their stone disease, which persists despite cure of their hyperparathyroidism.[162, 163]

Surgery also leads to an improvement in BMD in patients with primary hyperparathyroidism.[160] Data are now available from our group spanning a decade of postoperative follow-up.[164] Parathyroidectomy leads to a 10% to 12% rise in bone density at the lumbar spine and femoral neck (Fig. 76–9). This increase occurs mainly within the first few years of surgery and is sustained over a decade after surgery. Postmenopausal women show a similar pattern of increased cancellous bone density. Thus, removing the "protection" afforded these postmenopausal women at the cancellous spine by virtue of PTH excess was not associated with bone loss postoperatively. On the contrary, they gained more cancellous bone mass. A satisfying explanation for why a site protected by PTH excess should gain even more skeletal mineral content when PTH is no longer present in excess is not clear. Histomorphometrically, osteoid width is increased, as is the osteoid surface, a feature of accelerated bone turnover. When bone turnover is returned to normal postoperatively, the "space" occupied by unmineralized osteoid is reduced. Remineralization of this remodeling transient can lead to marked increases in bone mass such as those seen after successful parathyroid surgery. Other potential explanations for the postoperative anabolic course include speculations about restoration of normal pulsatility and amplitude of the secretory patterns of PTH. Smaller gains in bone density are seen at cortical sites, a paradoxical observation considering the fact that cortical bone is diminished most by the hyperparathyroid state.

In patients with primary hyperparathyroidism who have vertebral osteopenia or osteoporosis at the time of diagnosis, the postoperative increase in vertebral bone density is even greater.[95] In our longitudinal study of primary hyperparathyroidism, we observed a substantial number of patients (15%) whose lumbar spine bone density was different from the majority in that they had more markedly reduced bone density (Z score < -1.5) than the group as a whole. Osteopenia of the lumbar spine is not to be expected because of the proclivity of PTH to be anabolic at cancellous sites. This subgroup of patients was representative of patients with primary hyperparathyroidism in that postmenopausal women, as well as premenopausal women and men, were included. There were no demographic or biochemical characteristics which set them apart from other patients other than their low vertebral bone density. Postmenopausal women with osteopenia of the lumbar spine could perhaps be explained by the action of postmenopausal bone loss due to estrogen deficiency, a syndrome associated initially with cancellous bone loss. If one speculates that primary hyperparathyroidism subsequently developed, it would be occurring at a time when lumbar spine osteopenia had already become established. Thus, it is conceivable that osteopenia of the lumbar spine is not directly a function of PTH excess in these patients. Certainly, if primary hyperparathyroidism is severe enough, it would affect all bones, including the cancellous skeleton, but these patients do not present in a way that would suggest that they are more severely involved than the group as a whole. In any event, these patients in fact experience a greater increase in bone mass of the lumbar spine, 21% $\pm$4% 4 years following parathyroidectomy (see Fig. 76–9C), than the group as a whole. The more impressive increase in this subgroup of patients with hyperparathyroidism argues for this being another guideline for surgery in this condition. The marked improvement seen in patients with low vertebral bone density argues for surgery in those who present with cancellous as well as cortical bone loss (see Table 76–5).

The capacity of the skeleton to restore itself is seen dramatically in young patients with severe primary hyperparathyroidism. Kulak et

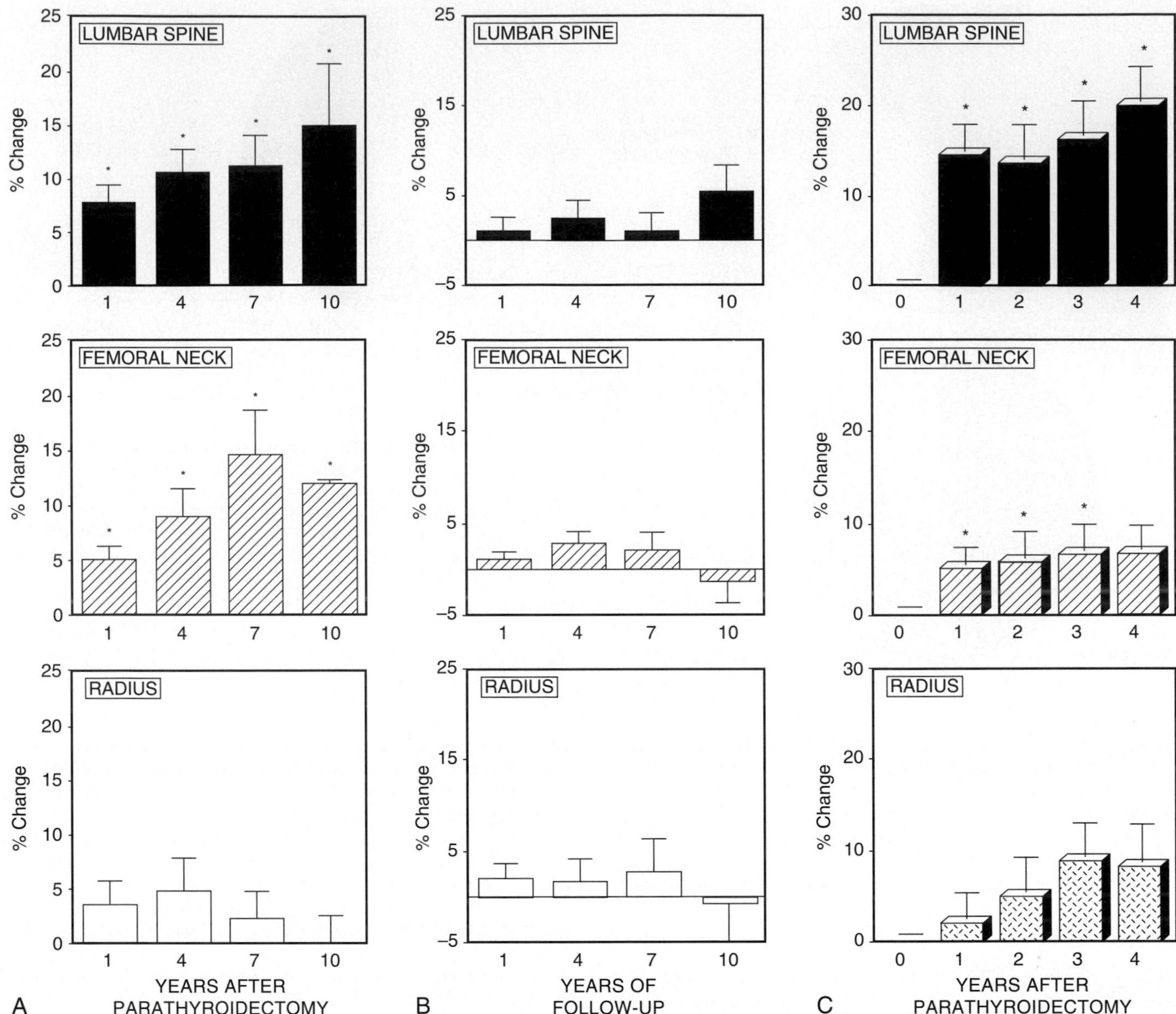

FIGURE 76–9. Longitudinal course of bone density in primary hyperparathyroidism. Data are presented as percentage change from preoperative baseline bone density measurement by site following parathyroidectomy *(A)* or in patients followed with no intervention *(B)*. *Asterisk* denotes significant differences between the two groups at $P < .05$. (*A* and *B* modified with permission from Silverberg SJ, Shane E, Jacobs TP, et al: Primary hyperparathyroidism: 10-year course with or without parathyroid surgery. N Engl J Med 341:1249–1255,1999. Copyright © 1999 Massachusetts Medical Society. All rights reserved.) *C*, Bone mineral density following parathyroidectomy in 14 primary hyperparathyroid patients with vertebral osteopenia. (*C* from Silverberg SJ, Locke FG, Bilezikian JP: Vertebral osteopenia: A new indication for surgery in primary hyperparathyroidism. J Clin Endocrinol Metab 81:4007–4012, 1996.) The cumulative percentage change from preoperative baseline (year 0) is shown for each site. *Asterisk* denotes change from baseline at $P < .05$.

al.[165] reported two patients with osteitis fibrosa cystica who experienced increases in bone density that ranged from 260% to 430% 3 to 4 years following surgery. More recently, similar observations have been made by Tritos and Hartzband[166] and by DiGregorio.[167]

Medical Management

Surgery is generally not recommended in patients who do not meet any surgical guidelines. Among typical cohorts in the United States, about 50% of patients with primary hyperparathyroidism will fit into this category. According to the consensus development conference, it was considered reasonable to pursue a nonsurgical course of management. Data are now available for comment on the longitudinal follow-up of such patients with mild primary hyperparathyroidism.[68, 164, 168, 169] We have found that in up to a decade of follow-up without intervention, there was no change in serum calcium, phosphorus, PTH, vitamin D, or alkaline phosphatase; or in urinary calcium, hydroxyproline, or hydroxypyridinium cross-link excretion. In sharp contrast to the change in BMD seen in patients after parathyroidectomy, lumbar spine, femoral neck, and radius BMD also showed stability in this group (see Fig. 76–9B). No change in biochemical indices or bone density at any of the three sites was seen in the subset of postmenopausal women. This finding is particularly striking in view of the expectation of menopause- and age-related declines in BMD in female patients as they progress through their middle years.

There are preliminary data suggesting a less benign course in a minority of patients who are followed without intervention. First, those patients with coexisting primary hyperparathyroidism and vitamin D insufficiency seem to have evidence of a more active hyperparathyroid process.[64] Certainly, it is difficult to replete vitamin D in a patient who is already hypercalcemic. This raises the question as to the advisability of surgery in these patients (Table 76–5). Second, women with primary hyperparathyroidism who go through menopause tend to lose bone

TABLE 76–5. Guidelines for Parathyroidectomy

*NIH Consensus Conference Guidelines**

- Serum calcium > 12 mg/dL
- Marked hypercalciuria (>400 mg/day)
- Any overt manifestation of primary hyperparathyroidism (nephrolithiasis, osteitis fibrosa cystica, classic neuromuscular disease)
- Markedly reduced cortical bone density (Z score < −2)
- Reduced creatinine clearance in the absence of other cause
- Age < 50 yr

Other Suggested Guidelines

- Vertebral osteopenia
- Perimenopause
- Vitamin D deficiency

*Data from National Institutes of Health: Consensus development conference statement on primary hyperparathyroidism. J Bone Miner Res 6:s9–s13, 1991.

just as their normocalcemic healthy counterparts do. The hyperparathyroid state does not protect the cancellous skeleton of these women, as it does in postmenopausal women years after menopause.[164] Therefore, surgery might be an appropriate alternative in this group (see Table 76–5). It is not known whether hormone replacement therapy (see below) can prevent the bone loss in this group.

General Measures

In patients followed without surgery, serum calcium should be obtained every 6 months, while urinary calcium excretion and bone densitometry should be repeated annually. Patients should be instructed to remain well hydrated and to avoid thiazide diuretics. Prolonged immobilization, which can increase hypercalcemia and hypercalciuria, should also be avoided.

Diet

Dietary management of primary hyperparathyroidism has long been an area of controversy. Many patients are advised to limit their dietary calcium intake because of the hypercalcemia. However, it is well-known that low dietary calcium can lead to increased PTH levels in normal individuals.[170–172] In patients with primary hyperparathyroidism, even though the abnormal PTH tissue is not as sensitive to slight perturbations in the circulating calcium concentration,[173] it is still possible that PTH levels will rise when dietary calcium is tightly restricted. Conversely, diets enriched in calcium could suppress PTH levels in primary hyperparathyroidism, as shown by Insogna et al.[174] Dietary calcium could also be variably influenced by ambient levels of 1,25-dihydroxyvitamin D. In patients with normal levels of 1,25-dihydroxyvitamin D_3, Locker et al.[175] noted no difference in urinary calcium excretion between those on high (1000 mg/day) and low (500 mg/day) calcium intake diets. On the other hand, in those with elevated levels of 1,25-dihydroxyvitamin D_3, high calcium diets were associated with worsening hypercalciuria (Fig. 76–10). This observation suggests that dietary calcium intake in patients can be liberalized to 1000 mg/day if 1,25-dihydroxyvitamin D_3 levels are not increased, but should be more tightly controlled if 1,25-dihydroxyvitamin D levels are elevated.

Pharmaceuticals

PHOSPHATE. Oral phosphate can lower the serum calcium by up to 1 mg/dL.[176–178] A complex interplay of mechanisms leads to this moderating effect of oral phosphate. First, calcium absorption falls in the presence of intestinal phosphorus. Second, concomitant increases in serum phosphorus will tend to reduce circulating 1,25-dihydroxyvitamin D_3 levels. Third, phosphate can be an antiresorptive agent. Finally, increased serum phosphorus reciprocally lowers serum calcium. Problems with oral phosphate include limited gastrointestinal tolerance, possible further increase in PTH levels, and the possibility of soft tissue calcifications after long-term use.[179] Such concerns have limited the chronic use of oral parathyroid in primary hyperparathyroidism.

BISPHOSPHONATES. Bisphosphonates are conceptually attractive in primary hyperparathyroidism because they are antiresorptive agents with an overall effect to reduce bone turnover. Although they do not affect PTH secretion directly, bisphosphonates could reduce serum and urinary calcium levels. Early studies with the first-generation bisphosphonates were disappointing. Etidronate has no effect.[180] Clodronate use was associated in several studies with a reduction in serum and urinary calcium,[181] but the effect was transient.[182] The second-generation bisphosphonates, characterized by alendronate, have not yet been studied systematically. Hassani et al.[183] reported on an open-label pilot study of seven men with primary hyperparathyroidism. After 6 months, lumbar spine bone density—but not hip or radius density—increased by Z score from -0.84 ± 1.9 to -0.3 ± 1.8 ($P < .05$). However, ionized calcium concentration actually increased while the alkaline phosphatase activity declined. In an open-label, unmatched, nonrandomized trial of 32 patients, Parker et al.[184] observed a significant 4.5% increase in lumbar spine bone density after 12 months. Mean serum calcium concentration fell only transiently, returning to baseline by 3 months.[184] Risedronate, a third-generation bisphosphonate, has been used in a very short 7-day study of 19 patients with primary hyperparathyroidism. In this acute experience, risedronate lowered serum and urinary calcium, as well as hydroxyproline excretion, significantly, while the PTH concentration rose.[185] The remarkably limited data on the effects of bisphosphonates in primary hyperparathyroidism need to be pursued by adequate clinical trials to ascertain the potential therapeutic benefit of potent bisphosphonates in primary hyperparathyroidism.

ESTROGENS. The earliest studies on the use of estrogen replacement therapy in primary hyperparathyroidism date back to the early 1970s. A 0.5 to 1.0 mg/dL reduction in total serum calcium levels in postmenopausal women with primary hyperparathyroidism who receive estrogen replacement therapy is generally seen. Gallagher and Nordin[186] first reported a calcium-lowering effect in 10 postmenopausal women given ethinyl estradiol. A prompt lowering of both serum and urinary calcium excretion was noted after 1 week of therapy, with continued reductions at 4 weeks (mean serum calcium [normal range, 8.9 to 10.2 mg/dL]: 12.0 to 11.6 to 11.3 mg/dL; $P < .0025$; and mean urinary calcium, 402 to 291 to 283 mg/g creatinine; $P < .0005$). Subsequent studies have reported similar declines in serum and urinary calcium in response to both ethinyl estradiol, and conjugated equine

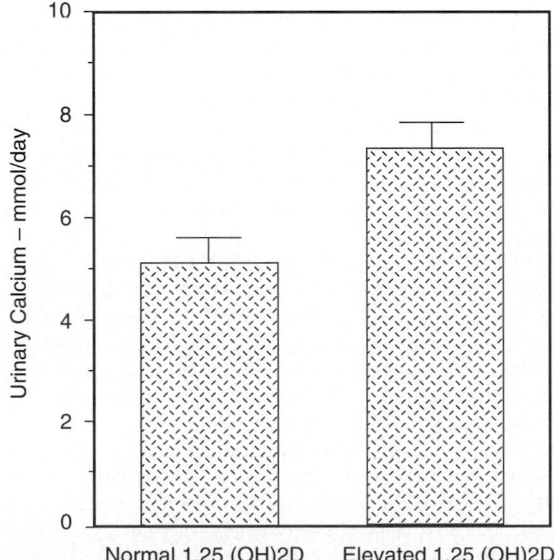

FIGURE 76–10. Urinary calcium excretion (mmol/day) in patients with normal and increased levels of 1,25-dihydroxyvitamin D. Groups differ at $P < .05$. (From Locker FG, Silverberg SJ, Bilezikian P: Optimal dietary calcium intake in primary hyperparathyroidism. Am J Med 102:543–550, 1997.)

estrogens.[187] Although levels of PTH were not measured in the earlier studies, Marcus et al.[187] and Selby and Peacock[188] reported no change in PTH as measured by a C-terminal radioimmunoassay. More recently, Grey et al.[189] also found no changes in intact PTH levels.

Only one study of estrogen replacement therapy in primary hyperparathyroidism has measured changes in other calciotropic hormones. Selby and Peacock found that 1,25-dihydroxyvitamin D concentration did rise after treatment with estrogen replacement therapy, but the increase could be accounted for entirely by the estrogen-induced increase in vitamin D–binding protein.[188]

Various approaches to skeletal dynamics have been used in studies of metabolic and skeletal responses to estrogen replacement therapy in women with primary hyperparathyroidism. Gallagher and Wilkinson[190] demonstrated normalization of calcium balance, with a decrease in output relative to intake. Early isotopic bone turnover studies using calcium[47] showed decreases in both bone resorption and mineralization rates. Markers of bone turnover, including alkaline phosphatase activity, urinary hydroxyproline, and urinary N-telopeptide, have been uniformly documented to decline. Finally, studies of BMD in estrogen-treated patients with primary hyperparathyroidism have documented a salutary effect of treatment on BMD at the femoral neck and lumbar spine.[189]

Estrogen has become a well-accepted means of treating postmenopausal women with mild primary hyperparathyroidism. The ability of estrogen to lower serum calcium levels raises the possibility that the newer selective estrogen receptor modulators (SERMs) might have similar effects. No data are yet available in this regard. However, given that raloxifene has been shown to be an estrogen agonist in bone, similar effects in the hyperparathyroid patient might be expected. The protection that agents in the SERM class seem to confer against breast cancer would make these agents a particularly attractive addition to the therapeutic arsenal in this disease.

The role of cytokines in the skeletal response to estrogen therapy in primary hyperparathyroidism is unknown. While the local anabolic actions of PTH may be mediated in part by IGF-1, estrogens play an important independent role in regulating the synthesis of this cytokine. Moreover, postmenopausal women have lower levels of IGF-1 than their premenopausal counterparts. A further decrease is found in osteoporotic postmenopausal women, arguing against a simple age-related effect. The precise role of IGF-1 in mediating the response to estrogen replacement in primary hyperparathyroidism remains unclear, with decreased (oral administration of ethinyl estradiol, conjugated equine estrogen, or estradiol valerate) or slightly increased (transdermal estrogen) levels reported.

Finally, the effects of estrogen in postmenopausal women with primary hyperparathyroidism could have a counterpart in the mechanisms postulated to account for accelerated bone loss in the early postmenopausal years. The local release of bone-resorbing cytokines is controlled by estrogens, an effect believed to account for their antiresorptive actions. Similarly, in primary hyperparathyroidism, estrogens in postmenopausal women with primary hyperparathyroidism could regulate the local production of cytokines, some of which have been shown to be elevated in primary hyperparathyroidism (see earlier discussion).

INHIBITION OF PARATHYROID HORMONE. The most specific pharmacologic approach to primary hyperparathyroidism is to inhibit the synthesis and secretion of PTH from the parathyroid glands. There was early interest in the organic thiophosphate agent WR-2721, which inhibits PTH release in vitro and has been used for malignancy-associated hypercalcemia.[191–193] Unfortunately, unacceptable side effects have terminated studies with this agent.

Interest has now turned to compounds that act on the parathyroid cell calcium-sensing receptor. This G protein–coupled receptor recognizes calcium as its cognate ligand.[194–196] When activated by increased extracellular calcium, the calcium-sensing receptor signals the cell via a G protein–transducing pathway to raise the intracellular calcium concentration, which inhibits PTH secretion. Molecules that mimic the effect of extracellular calcium could also activate this receptor, and inhibit parathyroid cell function.[197, 198] The phenylalkylamine (*R*)-*N*-(3-methoxy-α-phenylethyl)-3-(2-chlorophenyl)-1-propylamine (R-568) is one such calcimimetic compound. R-568 was found to increase cytoplasmic calcium and reduce PTH secretion in vitro.[199] Furthermore, inhibition of PTH secretion and decreases in serum calcium concentrations were documented in rats and in normal postmenopausal women.[200, 201] In vitro this drug also was shown to inhibit PTH secretion from adenomatous and hyperplastic parathyroid cells.[198] Recently, we reported on an investigation of the ability of single, ascending oral doses of this compound to inhibit PTH secretion and lower serum calcium concentrations in postmenopausal women with primary hyperparathyroidism.[202] The results of this study demonstrated that this calcimimetic drug inhibits secretion of PTH in postmenopausal women with mild primary hyperparathyroidism, and, at higher doses, also leads to a hypocalcemic response (Fig. 76–11). These data suggest that a drug of this type may become a useful alternative to parathyroidectomy in patients with primary hyperparathyroidism.

UNUSUAL PRESENTATIONS

Neonatal Primary Hyperparathyroidism

Neonatal primary hyperparathyroidism is a rare form of primary hyperparathyroidism caused by homozygous inactivation of the calcium-sensing receptor.[203, 204] When present in a heterozygous form, it is a benign hypercalcemic state, known as FHH. However, in the homozygous, neonatal form, hypercalcemia is severe and the outcome is fatal unless it is recognized early. The treatment of choice is early subtotal parathyroidectomy to remove the majority of hyperplastic parathyroid tissue.

Primary Hyperparathyroidism in Pregnancy

Primary hyperparathyroidism in pregnancy is primarily of concern for its potential effect on the fetus and neonate.[205–209] Complications of primary hyperparathyroidism in pregnancy include spontaneous

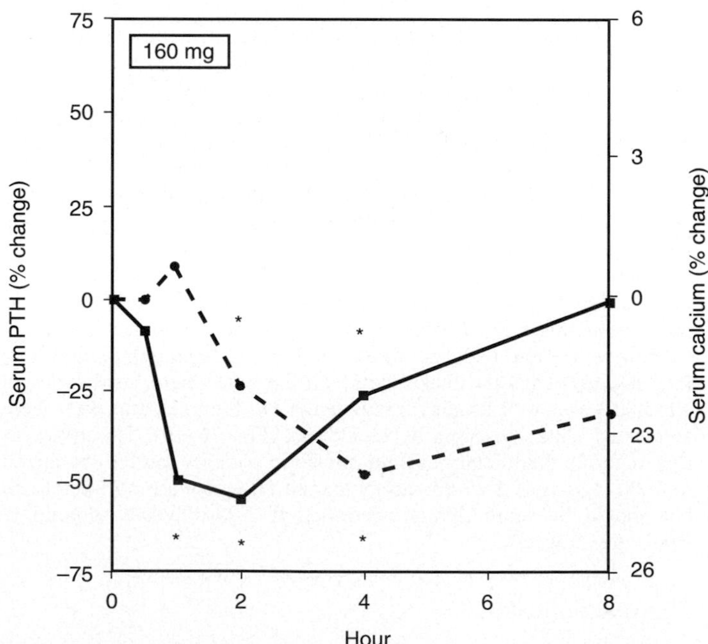

FIGURE 76–11. Percentage changes in serum parathyroid hormone *(broken line)* and serum ionized calcium *(solid line)* concentrations before and after administration of 160 mg of the calcimimetic drug R-568 in postmenopausal women with primary hyperparathyroidism. *Asterisk* denotes $P < .05$ for comparison with the response to placebo. (Modified with permission from Silverberg SJ, Marriott TB, Bone HG III, et al: Short term inhibition of parathyroid hormone secretion by a calcium receptor agonist in primary hyperparathyroidism. N Engl J Med 307:1506–1510, 1997. Copyright © 1997 Massachusetts Medical Society. All rights reserved.)

abortion, low birth weight, supravalvular aortic stenosis, and neonatal tetany. The last condition is a result of fetal parathyroid gland suppression by high levels of maternal calcium, which readily crosses the placenta during pregnancy. These infants, used to hypercalcemia in utero, have functional hypoparathyroidism after birth, and can develop hypocalcemia and tetany in the first few days of life. Today, with most patients (pregnant or not) presenting with a mild form of primary hyperparathyroidism, an individualized approach to the management of the pregnant patient with primary hyperparathyroidism is advised. Many of those with very mild disease can be followed safely, with successful neonatal outcomes without surgery. However, parathyroidectomy during the second trimester remains the traditional recommendation for this condition.

Acute Primary Hyperparathyroidism

Acute primary hyperparathyroidism is known variously as parathyroid crisis, parathyroid poisoning, parathyroid intoxication, and parathyroid storm. Acute primary hyperparathyroidism describes an episode of life-threatening hypercalcemia of sudden onset in a patient with primary hyperparathyroidism.[210–213] Clinical manifestations of acute primary hyperparathyroidism are mainly those associated with severe hypercalcemia. Nephrocalcinosis or nephrolithiasis is frequently seen. Radiologic evidence of subperiosteal bone resorption is also commonly present. Laboratory evaluation is remarkable not only for very high serum calcium levels but for extreme elevations in PTH to approximately 20 times normal.[214] In this way, acute primary hyperparathyroidism resembles parathyroid carcinoma. A history of persistent mild hypercalcemia has been reported in 25% of patients. However, given the rarity of this condition, the risk of developing acute primary hyperparathyroidism in a patient with mild asymptomatic primary hyperparathyroidism is very low. Intercurrent medical illness with immobilization may precipitate acute primary hyperparathyroidism. Early diagnosis, with aggressive medical management followed by surgical cure, is essential for a successful outcome.

Parathyroid Cancer

An indolent, yet potentially fatal disease, parathyroid carcinoma accounts for less than 0.5% of cases of primary hyperparathyroidism. The cause of the disease is unknown, and no clear risk factors have been identified. There is no evidence to support the malignant degeneration of previously benign parathyroid adenomas. Manifestations of hypercalcemia are the primary effects of parathyroid cancer. The disease does not tend to have a bulk tumor effect, spreading slowly in the neck. Metastatic disease is a late finding, with lung (40%), liver (10%), and lymph node (30%) involvement seen most commonly.

The clinical profile of parathyroid cancer differs from that of benign primary hyperparathyroidism in several important ways.[215–222] First, no female predominance is seen among patients with carcinoma. Second, elevations in serum calcium and PTH are far greater. As a consequence, the hyperparathyroid disease tends to be much more severe, with the classic targets of PTH excess involved in most cases. Nephrolithiasis or nephrocalcinosis is seen in up to 60% of patients, while overt radiologic evidence of skeletal involvement is seen in 35% to 90% of patients. A palpable neck mass, distinctly unusual in benign primary hyperparathyroidism, has been reported in 30% to 76% of patients with parathyroid cancer.[223]

Grossly, malignant glands are large, often exceeding 12 g. They tend to be adherent to adjacent structures. Microscopically, the trabecular arrangement of the tumor cells is divided by thick, fibrous bands. Capsular and blood vessel invasion is common by these cells which often contain mitotic figures.[224]

Loss of the retinoblastoma tumor suppressor gene used to be considered a marker for parathyroid cancer[225] but more recent studies do not unequivocally support this impression.[226, 227]

Surgery is the only effective therapy currently available for this disease. The greatest chance for cure occurs with the first operation. Once the disease recurs, cure is unlikely, although the disease may smolder for many years thereafter. The tumor is not radiosensitive, although there are isolated reports of tumor regression with localized radiation therapy.[223, 228] Traditional chemotherapeutic agents have not been useful. When metastasis occurs, isolated removal is an option, especially if only one or two nodules are found in the lung. Such isolated metastatectomies are never curative but they can lead to prolonged remissions, sometimes lasting for several years. Similarly, local debulking of tumor tissue in the neck can be palliative although malignant tissue is invariably left behind. Recently, our group[228] reported on a single patient treated with the calcimimetic R-568. In this patient, who had widely metastatic disease, serum calcium levels were maintained in a range that allowed him to return to normal functioning for nearly 2 years. Finally, Bradwell and Harvey[229] have attempted an immunotherapeutic approach by injecting a patient who had severe hypercalcemia due to parathyroid cancer with immunogenic PTH. Coincident with a rise in antibody titer to PTH, previous refractory hypercalcemia fell impressively.[229]

SUMMARY

This chapter has presented a comprehensive summary of the modern-day presentation of primary hyperparathyroidism. As an asymptomatic disorder in economically more developed countries, its presentation has raised issues regarding the extent to which patients who are asymptomatic may, nevertheless, show involvement in target organs; who should be recommended for parathyroid surgery; who can be safely followed without surgical intervention; as well as newer pharmacologic approaches to management. Questions about the natural history and pathophysiology of the disorder continue to be of great interest. As this disorder appears to be evolving in several different ways, it is clear that additional careful studies are required to continue to gain new insights into this disease.

REFERENCES

1. Albright F, Reifenstein EC: The Parathyroid Glands and Metabolic Bone Disease. Baltimore, Williams & Wilkins, 1948.
2. Cope O: The story of hyperparathyroidism at the Massachusetts General Hospital. N Engl J Med 21.1174–1182, 1966.
3. Bauer W: Hyperparathyroidism: Distinct disease entity. J Bone Joint Surg 15:135–141, 1933.
4. Bauer W, Federman DD: Hyperparathyroidism epitomized: Case of Captain Charles E. Martell. Metabolism 11:21–22, 1962.
5. Mandl F: Therapeutische Versuch bei Ostitis fibrosa generalisata mittels Extirpation eines Epithelkörperchentumors. Wien Klin Wochenschr 50:1343–1344, 1925.
6. Albright F, Aub JC, Bauer W: Hyperparathyroidism: A common and polymorphic condition as illustrated by seventeen proven cases from one clinic. JAMA 102:1276–1287, 1934.
7. Bilezikian JP, Silverberg SJ, Gartenberg F, et al: Clinical presentation of primary hyperparathyroidism. *In* Bilezikian JP, Marcus R, Levine MA (eds): The Parathyroids. New York, Raven Press, 1994, pp 457–470.
8. Heath H, Hodgson SF, Kennedy MA: Primary hyperparathyroidism: Incidence, morbidity, and economic impact in a community. N Engl J Med 302:189–193, 1980.
9. Mundy GR, Cove DH, Fisken R: Primary hyperparathyroidism: Changes in the pattern of clinical presentation. Lancet 1:1317–1320, 1980.
10. Scholz DA, Purnell DC: Asymptomatic primary hyperparathyroidism. Mayo Clin Proc 56:473–478, 1981.
11. Mallette LE, Bilezikian JP, Heath DA, Aurbach GD: Hyperparathyroidism: A review of 52 cases. Medicine (Baltimore) 53:127–147, 1974.
12. Brown EM, Gardner DG, Brennan MF, et al: Calcium-regulated parathyroid hormone release in primary hyperparathyroidism. Studies in vitro with dispersed parathyroid cells. Am J Med 66:923–931, 1979.
13. Lloyd HM, Parfitt AM, Jacobi JM, et al: The parathyroid glands in chronic renal failure: A study of their growth and other properties made on the basis of findings in patients with hypercalcemia. J Lab Clin Med 114:358–367, 1989.
14. Parfitt AM, Willgoss D, Jacob J, Lloyd HM: Cell kinetics in parathyroid adenomas: Evidence for decline in rates of cell birth and tumor growth, assuming clonal origin. Clin Endocrinol 35:151–157, 1991.
15. Arnold A, Staunton CE, Kim HG, et al: Monoclonality and abnormal parathyroid hormone genes in parathyroid adenomas. N Engl J Med 318:658–662, 1988.
16. Arnold A, Kim HG, Gaz RD, et al: Molecular cloning and chromosomal mapping of DNA rearranged with the parathyroid hormone gene in a parathyroid adenoma. J Clin Invest 83:2034–2040, 1989.
17. Friedman E, Bale AE, Marx SJ, et al: Genetic abnormalities in sporadic parathyroid adenoma. J Clin Endocrinol Metab 71:293–297, 1990.
18. Arnold A, Kim HG: Clonal loss of one chromosome 11 in a parathyroid adenoma. J Clin Endocrinol Metab 69:496–499, 1989.
19. Chandrasekharappa SC, Guru SC, Manickam P, et al: Positional cloning of the gene for multiple endocrine neoplasia type 1. Science 276:404–407, 1997.

20. European consortium on MEN1 gene. Hum Mol Genet 6:1177–1183, 1997.
21. Tahara H, Smith AP, Gax RD, et al: Genomic localization of novel candidate tumor suppressor gene loci in human parathyroid adenomas. Cancer Res 56:599–605, 1996.
22. Carling T, Correa P, Hessman O, et al: Parathyroid MEN1 gene mutations in relation to clinical characteristics of nonfamilial primary hyperparathyroidism. J Clin Endocrinol Metab 83:2960–2963, 1998.
23. Farnebo F, The BT, Kytola S, et al: Alterations of the MEN1 gene in sporadic parathyroid tumors. J Clin Endocrinol Metab 83:2627–2630, 1998.
24. Arnold A, Kim HG: Clonal loss of one chromosome 11 in a parathyroid adenoma. J Clin Endocrinol Metab 69:496–499, 1989.
25. Cryns VL, Yi SM, Tahara H, et al: Frequent loss of chromosome arm 1p in parathyroid adenomas. Genes Chromosomes Cancer (in press).
26. Parfitt AM: Parathyroid growth, normal and abnormal. *In* Bilezikian JP, Marcus R, Levine MA (eds): The Parathyroids. New York, Raven Press, 1994, pp 373–405.
27. Pollak MR, Brown EM, Chou Y-HW, et al: Mutations in the human Ca^{2+}-sensing receptor gene cause familial hypocalciuric hypercalcemia and neonatal severe hyperparathyroidism. Cell 75:1297–1303, 1993.
28. Hosokawa Y, Pollak MR, Brown EM, Arnold A: The extracellular calcium-sensing receptor gene in human parathyroid tumors. J Clin Endocrinol Metab 80:3107–3110, 1995.
29. Thompson DB, Samowitz WS, Odelberg S, et al: Genetic abnormalities in sporadic parathyroid adenomas: Loss of heterozygosity for chromosome 3q markers flanking the calcium receptor locus. J Clin Endocrinol Metab 80:3377–3380, 1995.
30. Cetani F, Pinchera A, Pardi E, et al: No evidence for mutations in the calcium-sensing receptor gene in sporadic parathyroid adenomas. J Bone Miner Res 14:878–882, 1999.
31. Chikatsu N, Fukumoto S, Suzawa M, et al: Cloning and characterization of two promoters for human calcium-sensing receptor (CaSR) and changes of CaSR expression in parathyroid adenomas (abstract). Bone 23 (suppl):S249, 1998.
32. Kifor O, Moore FD, Wang P, et al: Reduced immunostaining for the extraceullalar calcium sensing receptor in primary and uremic secondary hyperparathyroidism. J Clin Endocrinol Metab 81:1598–1606, 1996.
33. Carling T, Ridefelt P, Hellman P, et al: Vitamin D receptor polymorphisms correlate to parathyroid cell function in primary hyperparathyroidism. J Clin Endocrinol Metab 82:1772–1775, 1997.
34. Gennari L, Mansani R, Becherini L, Brandi ML: Gene polymorphisms in parathyroid diseases. *In* Brandi ML (ed): Parathyroid Diseases: From the Gene to the Cure. Florence, Italy, SEE Editrice-Firenze, 1997, pp 191–201.
35. Rao DD, Philips Z-H, Han E, et al: Loss of calcitriol receptor expression in parathyroid adenomas: Implications for pathogenesis. J Bone Miner Res 12:S522, 1997.
36. Rao SD, Frame B, Miller MJ, et al: Hyperparathyroidism following head and neck irradiation. Arch Intern Med 140:205–207, 1980.
37. Seely EW, Moore TJ, LeBoff MS, Brown EM: A single dose of lithium carbonate acutely elevates intact parathyroid hormone levels in humans. Acta Endocrinol 121:174–176, 1989.
38. Nordenstrom J, Strigard K, Perbeck L, et al: Hyperparathyroidism associated with treatment of manic-depressive disorders by lithium. Eur J Surg 158:207–211, 1992.
39. McHenry CR, Rosen IB, Rotstein LE, et al: Lithiumogenic disorders of the thyroid and parathyroid glands as surgical disease. Surgery 108:1001–1005, 1992.
40. Krivitzky A, Bentata-Pessayre M, Sarfati E, et al: Multiple hypersecreting lesions of the parathyroid glands during treatment with lithium. Ann Med Interne (Paris) 137:118–122, 1986.
41. Verdonk CA, Edis AJ: "Double adenomas": Fact or fiction? Surgery 90:523–526, 1981.
42. Harness JK, Ramsburg SR, Nishiyama RH, Thompson NW: Multiple adenomas of the parathyroids: Do they exist? Arch Surg 114:468–474, 1979.
43. Attie JN, Bock G, Auguste L: Multiple parathyroid adenomas: Report of 33 cases. Surgery 108:1014–1019, 1990.
44. Nudelman IL, Deutsch AA, Reiss R: Primary hyperparathyroidism due to mediastinal parathyroid adenoma. Int Surg 72:104–108, 1987.
45. Attie JN, Bock G, Auguste L: Multiple parathyroid adenoomas: Report of 33 cases. Surgery 108:1014–1019, 1990.
46. Sloane JA: Parathyroid adenoma in submucosa of esophagus. Arch Pathol Lab Med 102:242–243, 1978.
47. Joseph MP, Nadol JB, Pilch BZ, Goodman ML: Ectopic parathyroid tissue in the hypopharyngeal mucosa (pyriform sinus). Head Neck Surg 5:70–74, 1982.
48. Gilmour JR: Some developmental abnormalities of the thymus and parathyroids. J Pathol Bacteriol 52:213–218, 1941.
49. Christensson T, Hellstrom K, Wengle B, et al: Prevalence of hypercalcaemia in a health screening in Stockholm. Acta Med Scand 200:131–137, 1976.
50. Wermers RA, Khosla S, Atkinson EJ, et al: The rise and fall of primary hyperparathyroidism. Ann Intern Med 126:433–440, 1997.
51. Ringe JD: Reversible hypertension in primary hyperparathyroidism: Pre- and postoperative blood pressure in 75 cases. Klin Wochenschr 62:465–469, 1984.
52. Broulik PD, Horky K, Pacovsky V: Blood pressure in patients with primary hyperparathyroidism before and after parathyroidectomy. Exp Clin Endocrinol 86:346–352, 1985.
53. Rapado A: Arterial hypertension and primary hyperparathyroidism. Am J Nephrol 6(suppl 1):49–50, 1986.
54. Bilezikian JP, Aurbach GD, Connor TB, et al: Pseudogout following parathyroidectomy. Lancet 1:445–447, 1973.
55. Geelhoed GW, Kelly TR: Pseudogout as a clue and complication in primary hyperparathyroidism. Surgery 106:1036–1041, 1989.
56. Joborn C, Hetta J, Johansson H, et al: Psychiatric morbidity in primary hyperparathyroidism. World J Surg 12:476–481, 1988.
57. Joborn C, Hetta J, Frisk P, et al: Primary hyperparathyroidism in patients with organic brain syndrome. Acta Med Scand 219:91–98, 1986.
58. Alarcon RD, Franceschini JA: Hyperparathyroidism and paranoid psychosis: Case report and review of the literature. Br J Psychiatry 145:477–486, 1986.
59. Ljunghall S, Jakobsson S, Joborn C, et al: Longitudinal studies of mild primary hyperparathyroidism. J Bone Miner Res 6(suppl 2):S111–S116, 1991.
60. Brown GG, Preisman RC, Kleerekoper MD: Neurobehavioral symptoms in mild primary hyperparathyroidism: Related to hypercalcemia but not improved by parathyroidectomy. Henry Ford Hosp Med J 35:211–215, 1987.
61. Kleerekoper M: Clinical course of primary hyperparathyroidism. *In* Bilezikian JP (ed): The Parathyroids: Basic and Clinical Concepts. New York, Raven Press 1994, pp 471–484.
62. Nussbaum S, Potts JT Jr: Advance in immunoassays for PTH. *In* Bilezikian JP (ed): The Parathyroids: Basic and Clinical Concepts. New York, Raven Press, 1999, pp 157–170.
63. Burtis WJ, Kai HY, Stewart AF: Nonparathyroid hypercalcemia. *In* Becker KL (ed): Principles and Practice of Endocrinology and Metabolism, ed 2. Philadelphia, JB Lippincott, 1995, pp 520–531.
64. Silverberg SJ, Shane E, Dempster DW, Bilezikian JP: Vitamin D deficiency in primary hyperparathyroidism. Am J Med 107:561–567, 1999.
65. Vieth R, Bayley TA, Walfish PG, et al: Relevance of vitamin D metabolite concentrations in supporting the diagnosis of primary hyperparathyroidism. Surgery 110:1043–1046, 1991.
66. Silverberg SJ, Bilezikian JP: Primary hyperparathyroidism. *In* Seibel MJ, Robins SP, Bilezikian JP (eds): Dynamics of Bone and Cartilage Metabolism. San Diego, Academic Press, 1999, pp 571–580.
67. Parfitt AM, Rao DS, Kleerekoper M: Asymptomatic primary hyperparathyroidism discovered by multichannel biochemical screening: Clinical course and considerations bearing on the need for surgical intervention. J Bone Miner Res 6(suppl 2):s97–s101, 1991.
68. Silverberg SJ, Gartenberg F, Jacobs TP, et al: Longitudinal measurements of bone density and biochemical indices in untreated primary hyperparathyroidism. J Clin Endocrinol Metab 80:723–728, 1995.
69. Deftos LJ: Markers of bone turnover in primary hyperparathyroidism. *In* Bilezikian JP (ed): The Parathyroids: Basic and Clinical Concepts. New York, Raven Press, 1994, pp 485–492.
70. Moss DW: Perspectives in alkaline phosphatase research. Clin Chem 38:2486–2492, 1992.
71. Silverberg SJ, Deftos LJ, Kim T, Hill CS: Bone alkaline phosphatase in primary hyperparathyroidism (abstract). J Bone Miner Res 6:A624, 1991.
72. Duda RJ, O'Brien JF, Katzman JA, et al: Concurrent assays of circulating bone Gla-protein and bone alkaline phosphatase: Effects of sex, age, and metabolic bone disease. J Clin Endocrinol Metab 5:1–7, 1988.
73. Price PA, Parthemore JG, Deftos LJ: New biochemical marker for bone metabolism. Measurement by radioimmunoassay of bone Gla-protein in the plasma of normal subjects and patients with bone disease. J Clin Invest 66:878–883, 1980.
74. Deftos LJ, Parthemore JG, Price PA: Changes in plasma bone Gla-protein during treatment of bone disease. Calcif Tissue Int 34:121–124, 1982.
75. Eastell R, Delmas PD, Hodgson S, et al: Bone formation rate in older normal women: Concurrent assessment with bone histomorphometry, calcium kinetics, and biochemical markers. J Clin Endocrinol Metab 67:741–748, 1994.
76. Ebeling PR, Peterson JM, Riggs BL: Utility of type 1 procollagen propeptide assays for assessing abnormalities in metabolic bone diseases. J Bone Miner Res 7:1243–1250, 1992.
77. Minisola S, Romagnoli E, Scarnecchia L, et al: Serum CITP in patients with primary hyperparathyroidism: Studies in basal conditions and after parathyroid surgery. Eur J Endocrinol 130:587–591, 1994.
78. Deftos LJ: Bone protein and peptide assays in the diagnosis and management of skeletal disease. Clin Chem 37:1143–1148, 1991.
79. Delmas PH: Biochemical markers of bone turnover: Methodology and clinical use in osteoporosis. Am J Med 1:169–174, 1991.
80. Seibel MJ, Gartenberg F, Silverberg SJ, et al: Urinary hydroxypyridinium cross-links of collagen in primary hyperparathyroidism. J Clin Endocrinol Metab 74:481–486, 1992.
81. Seibel MJ, Woitge HW, Pecherstorfer M, et al: Serum immunoreactive bone sialoprotein as a new marker of bone turnover in metabolic and malignant bone disease. J Clin Endocrinol Metab 81:3289–3294, 1996.
82. Guo CY, Thomas WER, Al-Dehaimi AW, et al: Longitudinal changes in bone mineral density and bone turnover in women with primary hyperparathyroidism. J Clin Endocrinol Metab 81:3487–3491, 1996.
83. Tanaka Y, Funahashi H, Imai T, et al: Parathyroid function and bone metabolic markers in primary and secondary hyperparathyroidism. Semin Surg Oncol 13:125–133, 1997.
84. Roodman GD: Interleukin-6: An osteotropic factor? J Bone Miner Res 7:475–478, 1992.
85. Greenfield EM, Shaw SM, Gornik SA, Banks MA: Adenyl cyclase and interleukin 6 are downstream effectors of PTH resulting in stimulation of bone resorption. J Clin Invest 96:1238–1244, 1995.
86. Pollock JH, Blaha MJ, Lavish SA, et al: In vivo demonstration that PTH and PTHrP stimulate expression by osteoblasts of IL-6 and LIF. J Bone Miner Res 11:754–759, 1996.
87. Grey A, Mitnick M, Shapses S, et al: Circulating levels of IL-6 and TNF-alpha are elevated in primary hyperparathyroidism and correlate with markers of bone resorption. J Clin Endocrinol Metab 81:3450–3454, 1996.
88. Rosen CJ, Bing-you R, Silverberg SJ, Bilezikian JP: Enhancement of cancellous bone mass after parathyroidectomy is associated with changes in circulating insulin-like growth factor binding proteins. J Bone Miner Res 9 (suppl I):C424, 1994.
89. Silverberg SJ, Shane E, DeLaCruz L, et al: Skeletal disease in primary hyperparathyroidism. J Bone Miner Res 4:283–291, 1989.
90. Bilezikian JP, Silverberg SJ, Shane E, et al: Characterization and evaluation of asymptomatic primary hyperparathyroidism. J Bone Miner Res 6(suppl I): 585–589, 1991.

91. Dempster DW, Cosman F, Parisien M, et al: Anabolic actions of parathyroid hormone on bone. Endocr Rev 14:690–709, 1993.
92. Canalis E, Hock JM, Raisz LG: Anabolic and catabolic effects of PTH on bone and interactions with growth factors. *In* Bilezikian JP (ed): The Parathyroids: Basic and Clinical Concepts. New York, Raven Press, 1994, pp 65–82.
93. Slovik DM, Rosenthal DI, Doppelt SH, et al: Restoration of spinal bone in osteoporotic men by treatment with human PTH (1–34) and vitamin D. J Bone Miner Res 1:377–381, 1989.
94. National Institutes of Health: Consensus development conference statement on primary hyperparathyroidism. J Bone Miner Res 6:s9–s13, 1991.
95. Silverberg SJ, Locker FG, Bilezikian JP: Vertebral osteopenia: A new indication for surgery in primary hyperparathyroidism. J Clin Endocrinol Metab 81:4007–4012, 1996.
96. Parisien M, Silverberg SJ, Shane E, et al: The histormorphometry of bone in primary hyperparathyroidism: Preservation of cancellous bone structure. J Clin Endocrinol Metab 70:930–938, 1990.
97. Parfitt AM: Accelerated cortical bone loss: Primary and secondary hyperparathyroidism. *In* Uhthoff H, Stahl E (eds): Current Concepts of Bone Fragility. Berlin, Springer-Verlag, 1986, pp 279–285.
98. Parfitt AM: Surface specific bone remodeling in health and disease. *In* Kleerekoper M (ed): Clinical Disorders of Bone and Mineral Metabolism. New York, Mary Ann Liebert, 1989, pp 7–14.
99. Van Doorn L, Lips P, Netelenbos JC, Hackengt WHL: Bone histomorphometry and serum intact PTH (I-84) in hyperparathyroid patients. Calcif Tissue Int 44S:N36, 1989.
100. Parisien M, Cosman F, Mellish RWE, et al: Bone structure in postmenopausal hyperparathyroid, osteoporotic and normal women. J Bone Miner Res 10:1393–1399, 1995.
101. Dempster DW, Parisien M, Silverberg SJ, et al: On the mechanism of cancellous bone preservation in postmenopausal women with mild primary hyperparathyroidism. J Clin Endocrinol Metab 84:1562–1566, 1999.
102. Parisien M, Mellish RWE, Silverberg SJ, et al: Maintenance of cancellous bone connectivity in primary hyperparathyroidism: Trabecular and strut analysis. J Bone Miner Res 7:913–920, 1992.
103. Lindsay R, Nieves, J, Formica C, et al: Randomised controlled study of effect of parathyroid hormone on vertebral-bone mass and fracture incidence among postmenopausal women on oestrogen with osteoporosis. Lancet 350:550–555, 1997.
104. Kurland ES, Cosman F, McMahon DJ, et al: Parathyroid hormone (PTH1–34) increases cancellous bone mass markedly in men with idiopathic osteoporosis (abstract). Bone 23(suppl 5):1039A, 1998.
105. Roe EB, Sanchez SD, del Puerto GA, et al: Treatment of postmenopausal osteoporosis with human parathyroid hormone 1–34 and estrogen. Presented at the Endocrine Society, 81st Annual Meeting, San Diego, CA, 1999, S63-1.
106. Dauphine RT, Riggs BL, Scholz DA: Back pain and vertebral crush fractures: An unemphasized mode of presentation for primary hyperparathyroidism. Ann Intern Med 83:365–367, 1975.
107. Kochesberger G, Buckley NJ, Leight GS, et al: What is the clinical significance of bone loss in primary hyperparathyroidism. Arch Intern Med 147:1951–1953, 1987.
108. Wilson RJ, Rao S, Ellis B, et al: Mild asymptomatic primary hyperparathyroidism is not a risk factor for vertebral fractures. Ann Intern Med 109:959–962, 1988.
109. Larsson K, Ljunghall S, Krusemo UB, et al: The risk of hip fractures in patients with primary hyperparathyroidism: A population-based cohort study with a follow-up of 19 years. J Intern Med 234:585–593, 1993.
110. Kenny AM, MacGillivray DC, Pilbeam CC, et al: Fracture incidence in postmenopausal women with primary hyperparathyroidism. Surgery 118:109–114, 1995.
111. Khosla S, Melton LJ, Wermers RA, et al: Primary hyperparathyroidism and the risk of fracture: A population-based study. J Bone Miner Res 14:1700–1707, 1999.
112. Silverberg SJ, Shane E, Jacobs TP, et al: Nephrolithiasis and bone involvement in primary hyperparathyroidism, 1985–1990. Am J Med 89:327–334, 1990.
113. Pak CYC, Ohata M, Lawrence EC, Snyder W: The hypercalciurias: Causes, parathyroid functions and diagnostic criteria. J Clin Invest 54:387–391, 1974.
114. Kaplan RA, Haussler MR, Deftos LJ, et al: The role of 1,25(OH)2D in the mediation of intestinal hyperabsorption of calcium in primary hyperparathyroidism and absorptive hypercalciuria. J Clin Invest 59:756–760, 1977.
115. Broadus AE, Horst RL, Lang R, et al: The importance of circulating 1,25(OH)2D in the pathogenesis of hypercalciuria and renal stone formation in primary hyperparathyroidism. N Engl J Med 302:421–426, 1980.
116. Pak CYC, Holt K: Nucleation and growth of brushite and calcium oxalate in urine of stone formers. Metabolism 25:665–673, 1976.
117. Peacock M: Renal stone disease and bone disease in primary hyperparathyroidism and their relationship to the action of PTH on calcium absorption. *In* Talmadge R (ed): Calcium Regulating Hormones. Amsterdam, Excerpta Medica, 1975, pp 78–81.
118. Pak CYC, Nicar MJ, Peterson R, et al: Lack of unique pathophysiologic background for nephrolithiaisis in primary hyperparathyroidism. J Clin Endocrinol Metab 53:536–542, 1981.
119. Pak CYC: Effect of parathyroidectomy on crystallization of calcium salts in urine of patients with primary hyperparathyroidism. Invest Urol 17:146–151, 1979.
120. Klugman VA, Favus M, Pak CYC: Nephrolithiasis in primary hyperparathyroidism. *In* Bilezikian JP (ed): The Parathyroids: Basic and Clinical Concepts. New York, Raven Press 1994, pp 505–518.
121. Dent CE, Hartland BV, Hicks J, Sykes ED: Calcium intake in patients with primary hyperparathyroidism. Lancet 2:336–342, 1961.
122. Aurbach GD, Mallette LE, Patten BM, et al: Hyperparathyroidism: Recent studies. Ann Intern Med 79:566–581, 1973.
123. Patten BM, Bilezikian JP, Mallette LE, et al: The neuromuscular disease of hyperparathyroidism. Ann Intern Med 80:182–194, 1974.
124. Vicale CT: Diagnostic features of muscular syndrome resulting from hyperparathyroidism, osteomalacia owing to renal tubular acidosis and perhaps to related disorders of calcium metabolism. Trans Am Neurol Assoc 74:143–147, 1949.
125. Cholod EJ, Haust MD, Husdon AJ, Lewis FN: Myopathy in primary familial hyperparathyroidism: Clnical and morphologic studies. Am J Med 48:700–707, 1970.
126. Frame B, Heinze EG, Block MA, Manson AGA: Myopathy in primary hyperparathyroidism: Observations in three patients. Ann Intern Med 68:1022–1027, 1968.
127. Rollinson RD, Gilligan BS: Primary hyperparathyroidism presenting as a proximal myopathy. Aust N Z J Med 7:420–421, 1977.
128. Turken SA, Cafferty M, Silverberg SJ, et al: Neuromuscular involvement in mild, asymptomatic primary hyperparathyroidism. Am J Med 87:553–557, 1989.
129. Joborn C, Hetta J, Johansson H, et al: Psychiatric morbidity in primary hyperparathyroidism. World J Surg 12:476–481, 1988.
130. Joborn C, Hetta J, Frisk P, et al: Primary hyperparathyroidism in patients with organic brain syndrome. Acta Med Scand 219:91–98, 1986.
131. Alarcon RD, Franceschini JA: Hyperparathyroidism and paranoid psychosis case report and review of the literature. Br J Psychiatry 145:477–486, 1984.
132. Ljunghall S, Jakobsson S, Joborn C, et al: Longitudinal studies of mild primary hyperparathyroidism. J Bone Miner Res 6(suppl 2):S111–S116, 1991.
133. Brown GG, Preisman RC, Kleerekoper MD: Neurobehavioral symptoms in mild primary hyperparathyroidism: Related to hypercalcemia but not improved by parathyroidectomy. Henry Ford Hosp Med J 35:211–215, 1987.
134. Kleerekoper M: Clinical course of primary hyperparathyroidism. *In* Bilezikian JP (ed): The Parathyroids: Basic and Clinical Concepts. New York, Raven Press, 1994, pp 471–484.
135. Solomon BL, Schaaf M, Smallridge RC: Psychologic symptoms before and after parathyroid surgery. Am J Med 96:101–106, 1994.
136. Lafferty FW: Primary hyperparathyroidism: Changing clinical spectrum, prevalence of hypertension, and discriminant analysis of laboratory tests. Arch Intern Med 141:1761–1766, 1981.
137. Rapado A: Arterial hypertension and primary hyperparathyroidism: Incidence and follow-up after parathyroidectomy. Am J Nephrol 6(suppl I).49–50, 1986.
138. Symons C, Fortune F, Greenbaum RA, Dandona P: Cardiac hypertrophy, hypertrophic cardiomyopathy and hyperparathyroidism—an association. Br Heart J 54:539–542, 1985.
139. Diamond TH, Kawalski DL, van der Merwe TL, Myburgh DP: Hypercalcemia due to parathyroid adenoma and hypertrophic cardiomyopathy. S Afr Med J 71:448–449, 1987.
140. Stefenelli T, Mayr H, Bergler Klein J, et al: Primary hyperparathyroidism: Incidence of cardiac abnormalities and partial reversibility after successful parathyroidectomy. Am J Med 95:197–202, 1993.
141. Palmer M, Adami HO, Bergstrom R, et al: Mortality after surgery for primary hyperparathyroidism: A follow up of 441 patients operated on from 1956 to 1979. Surgery 102:1–7, 1987.
142. Palmer M, Adami HO, Bergstrom G, et al: Survival and renal function in untreated hypercalcemia. Lancet I (8524):59–62, 1987.
143. Wermers RA, Khosla S, Atkinson EJ, et al: Survival after the diagnosis of hyperparathyroidism. Am J Med 104:115–122, 1998.
144. Harinarayan DV, Gupta N, Kochupillai N: Vitamin D status in primary hyperparathyroidism in India. Clin Endocrinol 43:351–358, 1995.
145. Meng XW, Xing XP, Liu SQ, Shan ZW: The diagnosis of primary hyperparathyroidism—analysis of 134 cases. Acta Acad Med Sin 16:116–122, 1994.
146. Luong KVQ, Nguyen LTH: Coexisting hyperthyroidism and hyperparathyroidism with vitamin D deficient osteomalacia in a Vietnamese immigrant. Endocr Pract 2:250–254, 1996.
147. Lumb GA, Stanbury SW: Parathyroid function in vitamin D deficiency in primary hyperparathyroidism. Am J Med 54:833–839, 1974.
148. Beckerman P, Silver J: Vitamin D and the parathyroid. Am J Med Sci 317:363–369, 1999.
149. Feldman D: Vitamin D, parathyroid hormone and calcium: A complex regulatory network. Am J Med 107:637–639, 1999.
150. Casas AT, Burke GJ, Sathyanarayana, et al: Prospective comparison of technetium-99m-sestamibi/iodine 123 radionuclide scan versus high resolution ultrasonography for the preoperative localization of abnormal parathyroid glands in patients with previously unoperated primary hyperparathyroidism. Am J Surg 166:369–373, 1993.
151. Doppman JL: Preoperative localization of parathyroid tissue in primary hyperparathyroidism. *In* Bilezikian JP (ed): The Parathyroids: Basic and Clinical Concepts. New York, Raven Press, 1994, pp 553–566.
152. Halvorson DJ, Burke GJ, Mansberger AR: Use of technetium Tc 99m sestamibi and iodine 123 radionuclide scan for preoperative localization of abnormal parathyroid glands in primary hyperparathyroidism. South Med J 87:336–339, 1994.
153. Wei JP, Burke GJ, Mansberger AR: Preoperative imaging of abnormal parathyroid glands in patients with hyperparathyroid disease using combination Tc-99m-pertechnate and Tc-99m-sestamibi radionuclide scans. Ann Surg 219:568–573, 1994.
154. Johnston LM, Carroll MJ, Britton KE, et al: The accuracy of parathyroid gland localization in primary hyperparathyroidism using sestamibi radionuclide imaging. J Clin Endocrinol Metab 81:346–352, 1996.
155. Thule P, Thakore K, Vansant J, et al: Preoperative localization of parathyroid tissue with technetium-99m sestamibi 123 I subtraction scanning. J Clin Endocrinol Metab 78:77–82, 1994.
156. Johnston LB, Carroll MJ, Brittan KE, et al: The accuracy of parathyroid gland localization in primary hyperparathyroidism using sestamibi radionuclide imagery. J Clin Endocrinol Metab 81:346–352, 1996.
157. Calcutt VG, Franco-Saenz R, Morrow LB, Mulrow PJ: Localization of abnormal parathyroid tissue with the use of techetium-99m-sestamibi. Endocr Pract 4:184–189, 1998.
158. McIntyre RC, Ridgway EC: Sestamibi: Operning a new era of parathyroid surgical procedures. Endocr Pract 4:241–244, 1998.
159. Javaid A, Arfaj AA: Technetium-99m-sestamibi scintigraphy and bone densitometry in primary hyperparathyroidism. Endocr Pract 5:169–173, 1999.

160. Silverberg SJ, Gartenberg F, Jacobs TP, et al: Increased bone mineral density following parathyroidectomy in primary hyperparathyroidism. J Clin Metab 80:729–734, 1995.
161. Deaconson TF, Wilson SD, Lemann J: The effect of parathyroidectomy on the recurrence of nephrolithiasis. Surgery 215:241–251, 1987.
162. Kaplan RA, Snyder WH, Stewart A, et al: Metabolic effects of parathyroidectomy in asymptomatic primary hyperparathyroidism. J Clin Endocrinol Metab 42:415–426, 1976.
163. Siminovich JMP, James RE, Esselsytne CBJ, et al: The effect of parathyroidectomy in patients with normocalcemic calcium stones. J Urol 23:335–337, 1980.
164. Silverberg SJ, Shane E, Jacobs TP, et al: Primary hyperparathyroidism: 10-year course with or without parathyroid surgery. N Engl J Med 341:1249–1255, 1999.
165. Kulak CAM, Bandeira C, Voss D, et al: Marked improvement in bone mass after parathyroidectomy in osteititis fibrosa cystica. J Clin Endocrinol Metab 83:732–735, 1998.
166. Tritos NA, Hartzband P: Rapid improvement of osteoporosis following parathyroidectomy in a premenopausal woman with acute primary hyperparathyroidism. Arch Intern Med 139:1498, 1999.
167. DiGregorio S: Hiperparatiroidismo primario: Dramatico incremento de la masa ostea post paratiroidectomia. Diagn Osteol 1:11–15, 1999.
168. Rao DS, Wilson RJ, Kleerekoper M, Parfitt AM: Lack of biochemical progression or continuation of accelerated bone loss in mild asymptomatic primary hyperparathyroidism. J Clin Endocrinol Metab 67:1294–1298, 1988.
169. Parfitt AM, Rao DS, Kleerekoper M: Asymptomatic primary hyperparathyroidism discovered by multichannel biochemical screening: Clinical course and considerations bearing on the need for surgical intervention. J Bone Miner Res 6(suppl 2):S97–S101, 1991.
170. Dawson-Hughes B, Stern DT, Shipp CC, Rasmussen HM: Effect of lowering dietary calcium intake on fractional whole body calcium retention. J Clin Endocrinol Metab 67:62–68, 1998.
171. Barger-Lux MJ, Heaney RP: Effects of calcium restriction on metabolic characteristics of premenopausal women. J Clin Endocrinol Metab 76:103–107, 1993.
172. Calvo MS, Kumar R, Heath H: Persistently elevated parathyroid hormone secretion and action in young women after four weeks of ingesting high phosphorus, low calcium diets. J Clin Endocrinol Metab 70:1334–1340, 1990.
173. Brown EM: Homeostatic mechanisms regulating extracellular and intracellular calcium metabolism. *In* Bilezikian JP (ed): The Parathyroids: Basic and Clinical Concepts. New York, Raven Press, 1994, pp 15–54.
174. Insogna KL, Mitnick ME, Stewart AF, et al: Sensitivity of the parathyroid hormone-1, 25-dihydroxyvitamin D axis to variations in calcium intake in patients with primary hyperparathyroidism. N Engl J Med 313:1126–1130, 1985.
175. Locker FG, Silverberg SJ, Bilezikian JP: Optimal dietary calcium intake in primary hyperparathyroidism. Am J Med 102:543–550, 1997.
176. Stock JL, Marcus R: Medical management of primary hyperparathyroidism. *In* Bilezikian JP (ed): The Parathyroids: Basic and Clinical Concepts. New York, Raven Press 1994, pp 519–530.
177. Purnell DC, Scholz DA, Smith LM, et al: Treatment of primary hyperparathyroidism. Am J Med 56:800–809, 1984.
178. Broadus AE, Magee JS, Mallette LE, et al: A detailed evaluation of oral phosphate therapy in selected patients with primary hyperparathyroidism. J Clin Endocrinol Metab 56:953–961, 1983.
179. Vernava AM III, O'Neal LW, Palermo V: Lethal hyperparathyroid crisis: Hazards of phosphate administration. Surgery 102:941–948, 1987.
180. Kaplan RA, Geho WB, Poindexter C, et al: Metabolic effects of diphosphonate in primary hyperparathyroidism. J Clin Pharmacol 17:410–419, 1977.
181. Shane E, Baquiran DC, Bilezikian JP: Effects of dichloromethylene diphosphonate on serum and urinary calcium in primary hyperparathyroidism. Ann Intern Med 95:23–27, 1981.
182. Adami S, Mian M, Bertoldo F, et al: Regulation of calcium-parathyroid hormone feedback in primary hyperparathyroidism: Effects of bisphosphonate treatment. Clin Endocrinol 33:391–397, 1990.
183. Hassani S, Brickman AS, Hershman JM: Alendronate therapy of primary hyperparathyroidism. Presented at the Endocrine Society, 80th Annual Meeting, New Orleans, LA, 1998, P3-537.
184. Parker CR, Blackwell PJ, Hosking DJ: Alendronate in the treatment of primary hyperparathyroid-related osteoporosis. Bone 23(suppl):F286, 1998.
185. Reasner CA, Stone MD, Hosking DJ, et al: Acute changes in calcium homeostasis during treatment of primary hyperparathyroidism with risedronate. J Clin Endocrinol Metab 77:1067–1071, 1993.
186. Gallagher JC, Nordin BEC: Treatment with oestrogens of primary hyperparathyroidism in post-menopausal women. Lancet 1:503–507, 1972.
187. Marcus R, Madvig P, Crim M, et al: Conjugated estrogens in the treatment of postmenopausal women with hyperparathyroidism. Ann Intern Med 100:633–640, 1984.
188. Selby PL, Peacock M: Ethinyl estradiol and norethinedrone in the treatment of primary hyperparathyroidism in postmenopausal women. N Engl J Med 314:1481–1485, 1986.
189. Grey AB, Stapleton JP, Evans MC, et al: Effect of hormone replacement therapy on BMD in post-menopausal women with primary hyperparathyroidism. Ann Intern Med 125:360–368, 1996.
190. Gallagher JC, Wilkinson R: The effect of ethinyl estradiol on calcium and phosphorus metabolism of post-menopausal women with primary hyperparathyroidism. Clin Sci Mol Med 45:785–802, 1973.
191. Glover D, Riley L, Carmichael K, et al: Hypocalcemia and inhibition of parathyroid hormone secretion after administration of WR-2721 (a radioprotective and chemoprotective agent). N Engl J Med 309:1137–1141, 1983.
192. Glover DJ, Shaw L, Glick JH, et al: Treatment of hypercalcemia or parathyroid cancer with WR-2721, S-2-(3-aminopropylamino) ethylphosphorothioic acid. Ann Intern Med 103:55–57, 1985.
193. Hirschel-Scholz S, Jung A, Fischer A, et al: Suppression of parathyroid secretion after administration of WR-2721 in a patient with parathyroid carcinoma. Clin Endocrinol 23:313–318, 1985.
194. Nemeth EF, Scarpa A: Rapid mobilization fo cellular calcium in bovine parathyroid cells evoked by extracellular divalent cations. Evidence for a cell surface calcium receptor. J Biol Chem 262:5188–5196, 1987.
195. Brown EM, Gamba G, Riccardi D, et al: Cloning and characterization of an extracellular Ca^{2+} sensing receptor from bovine parathyroid. Nature 366:575–580, 1993.
196. Brown EM, Pollak M, Seidman CE: Calcium ion sensing cell surface receptors. N Engl J Med 333:234–240, 1995.
197. Brown EM, Katz C, Butters R, Kifor O: Polyarginine, polylysine, and protamine mimic the effects of high extracellular calcium concentration on dispersed bovine parathyroid cells. J Bone Miner Res 6:1217–1225, 1991.
198. Nemeth EM: Calcium receptors as novel drug targets. *In* Bilezikian JP, Raisz LG, Rodan GA (eds): Principles of Bone Biology. New York, Academic Press, 1996, pp 1019–1036.
199. Steffey ME, Fox J, Van Wagenen BC, et al: Calcimimetics: Structurally and mechanistically novel compounds that inhibit hormone secretion from parathyroid cells. J Bone Miner Res 8:S175, 1993.
200. Fox J, Hadfield S, Petty BA, Nemeth EF: A first generation calcimimetic compound (NPS R-568) that acts on the parathyroid cell calcium receptor: A novel therapeutic approach for hyperparathyroidism. J Bone Miner Res 8:S181, 1993.
201. Heath H III, Sanguinetti EL, Oglseby S, Marriott TB: Inhibition of human parathyroid hormone secretion in vivo by NPS R-568, a calcimimetic drug that targets the parathyroid cell surface calcium receptor. Bone 16:85S, 1995.
202. Silverberg SJ, Marriott TB, Bone HG III, et al: Short term inhibition of parathyroid hormone secretion by a calcium receptor agonist in primary hyperparathyroidism. N Engl J Med 307:1506–1510, 1997.
203. Marx SJ: Etiologies of parathyroid gland dysfunction in primary hyperparathyroidism. J Bone Miner Res 6(suppl 2):S19–S24, 1991.
204. Marx SJ, Fraser D, Rapoport A: Familial hypocalciuric hypercalcemia: Mild expression of the gene in heterozygotes and severe expression in homozygotes. Am J Med 78:15–22, 1985.
205. Kristoffersson A, Dahlgren S, Lithner F, Jarhult J: Primary hyperparathyroidism in pregnancy. Surgery 97:326–330, 1985.
206. Delmonicco FL, Neer RM, Cosmi AB, et al: Hyperparathyroidism during pregnancy. Am J Surg 131:328–332, 1976.
207. Gaeke RK, Kaplan EL, Lindheimer MD, et al: Maternal primary hyperparathyroidism of pregnancy. JAMA 238:508–511, 1977.
208. Lowe DK, Orwoll ES, McClung MR, et al: Hyperparathyroidism and pregnancy. Am J Surg 145:611–619, 1983.
209. Ficinski ML, Mestman JH: Primary hyperparathyroidism during pregnancy. Endocr Pract 2:362–367, 1996.
210. Fitzpatrick LA, Bilezikian JP: Acute primary hyperparathyroidism. Am J Med 82:275–282, 1987.
211. Bayat-Mokhtari F, Palmieri GMA, Moinuddin M, et al: Parathyroid storm. Arch Intern Med 140:1092–1095, 1980.
212. Wang CA, Guyton SW: Hyperparathyroid crisis: Clinical and pathologic study of 14 patients. Ann Surg 190:782–790, 1979.
213. Maselly MJ, Lawrence AM, Brooks M, et al: Hyperparathyroid crisis: Successful treatment of ten comatose patients. Surgery 90:741–746, 1981.
214. Fitzpatrick LA: Acute primary hyperparathyroidism. *In* Bilezikian JP (ed): The Parathyroids: Basic and Clinical Concepts. New York, Raven Press, 1994, pp 583–590.
215. Holmes EC, Morton DL, Ketcham AS: Parathyroid carcinoma: A collective review. Ann Surg 169:631–640, 1969.
216. Schantz A, Castleman B: Parathyroid carcinoma: A study of 70 cases. Cancer 31:600–605, 1973.
217. Shane E, Bilezikian JP: Parathyroid carcinoma: A review of 62 patients. Endocr Rev 3:218–226, 1982.
218. Cohn K, Silverman M, Corrado J, Sedgewick C: Parathyroid carcinoma: The Lahey Clinic experience. Surgery 98:1095–1110, 1985.
219. Wang C, Gaz R: Natural history of parathyroid carcinoma: Diagnosis, treatment, and results. Am J Surg 149:522–527, 1985.
220. Shane E, Bilezikian JP: Parathyroid carcinoma. *In* Williams CJ, Krikorian JC, Green MR, Raghaven D (eds): Textbook of Uncommon Cancer. New York, John Wiley & Sons, 1987, pp 763–771.
221. Obara T, Fujimoto Y: Diagnosis and treatment of patients with parathyroid carcinoma: An update and review. World J Surg 15:738–744, 1991.
222. Wynne AG, van Heerden J, Carney JA, Fitzpatrick LA: Parathyroid carcinoma: Clinical and pathological features in 43 patients. Medicine (Baltimore) 71:197–205, 224, 1992.
223. Levin KE, Galante M, Clark OH: Parathyroid carcinoma versus parathyroid adenoma in patients with profound hypercalcemia. Surgery 101:647–660, 1987.
224. LiVolsi V: Morphology of the parathyroid glands. *In* Becker KL (ed): Principles and Practice of Endocrinology and Metabolism, ed 3. Philadelphia, Lippincott Williams & Wilkins, 2000.
225. Cryns VL, Thor A, Xu H, et al: Loss of the retinoblastoma tumor-suppressor gene in parathyroid carcinoma. N Engl J Med 330:757–761, 1994.
226. Favia G, Lumachi F, Polistina F, D'Amico DF: Parathyroid Carcinoma: Sixteen new cases and suggestions for correct management. World J Surg 22:1225–1230, 1998.
227. Dotzenrath C, Teh BT, Farnebo F, et al: Allelic loss of the retinoblastoma tumor suppressor gene: A marker for aggressive parathyroid tumors? J Clin Endocrinol Metab 81:3194, 1996.
228. Collins MT, Skarulis MC, Bilezikian JP, et al: Treatment of hypercalcemia secondary to parathyroid carcinoma with a novel calcimimetic agent. J Clin Endocrinol Metab 83:1083–1088, 1998.
229. Bradwell AR, Harvey TC: Control of hypercalcemia of parathyroid carcinoma by immunisation. Lancet 353:370–373, 1999.

Chapter 77

Malignancy-Associated Hypercalcemia

Andrew F. Stewart ▪ Arthur E. Broadus

HISTORY OF MALIGNANCY-ASSOCIATED HYPERCALCEMIA

Malignancy is the second most common cause of hypercalcemia in the general population and by far the most common cause among inpatients. Hypercalcemia was first reported in patients with cancer in the 1920s.[1] The first large series of patients with malignancy-associated hypercalcemia (MAHC) was reported in 1936 by Gutman et al.[2] This group of patients suffered primarily from multiple myeloma and breast cancer, and skeletal invasion by tumor was extensive radiologically. The authors inferred that the cause of the hypercalcemia in these patients was skeletal invasion by the malignancy.

This mechanism was assumed to be operative in all instances of MAHC until 1941, when Albright described a hypercalcemic patient with renal carcinoma and a solitary skeletal metastasis.[3] He reasoned that a single bone metastasis was inadequate to cause hypercalcemia. Furthermore, he noted that the patient was hypophosphatemic, not hyperphosphatemic as would be expected from the combination of rapid dissolution of skeletal phosphate containing hydroxyapatite and parathyroid suppression induced by the hypercalcemia. Albright suggested that the hypercalcemia in this patient was etiologically distinct from the previously described patients with breast cancer and multiple myeloma and proposed that the hypercalcemia resulted from secretion by the renal carcinoma of parathyroid hormone (PTH) or another humoral factor that resembled PTH. Support for Albright's humoral hypothesis was presented in 1956, when two groups reported that surgical or other eradication of tumor reversed hypercalcemia in patients with carcinoma unaccompanied by skeletal involvement.[4, 5] After additional reports supporting the "humoral hypothesis," Lafferty in 1966 reviewed 50 patients with humorally mediated hypercalcemia.[6] By definition, these patients had no detectable skeletal metastases on radiographs and/or manifested disappearance of the hypercalcemia with tumor ablation. Histologically, the patients proved to have predominantly squamous (particularly lung), renal, bladder, and gynecologic malignancies.

Thus by the end of the 1960s, two broad mechanistic categories of MAHC had clearly been demonstrated.[7–9] In one group of patients, hypercalcemia appeared to develop through skeletal invasion and destruction by tumor, a condition we have referred to as "local osteolytic hypercalcemia" (LOH)[2, 7–10] (Table 77–1). In the other group of patients, hypercalcemia develops predominantly through humoral mechanisms, a condition we have referred to as "humoral hypercalcemia of malignancy" (HHM).[11, 12] The observations described above were primarily descriptive. The major areas of interest and investigation in the past two decades have been pathophysiologic or mechanistic. It is implicit in the studies summarized above that the final common pathway leading to hypercalcemia in both LOH and HHM is osteoclastic bone resorption. Studies of bone histology have now amply demonstrated such to be the case[13] (Fig. 77–1).

CLINICAL FEATURES OF MALIGNANCY-ASSOCIATED HYPERCALCEMIA

Hypercalcemia occurring in a patient with cancer indicates that the overall prognosis for the patient in question is very poor. For example, in a study by Ralson and collaborators,[14] the onset of hypercalcemia was associated with a 30-day survival rate of only 50%.

The clinical manifestations of the hypercalcemia that accompanies cancer are no different from those that accompany other hypercalcemic disorders. Polyuria, polydipsia, dehydration, renal compromise, constipation, and varying degrees of neurologic dysfunction ranging from lethargy or confusion to coma are common. The electrocardiogram may show shortening of the QTc interval.[15, 16] The correlation between the degree of hypercalcemia and a given patient's neurologic function is poor. Other factors (such as the rate of development of hypercalcemia, the presence of underlying central nervous system dysfunction, the presence of other metabolic disorders, or the use of a variety of medications) may profoundly influence the effects of a given degree of hypercalcemia. Patients with skeletal metastases may report skeletal

TABLE 77–1. Tumor Histology and Hypercalcemia

Tumors Associated with Local Osteolytic Hypercalcemia	Tumors Associated with $1,25(OH)_2D$ Overproduction	Tumors Associated with Humoral Hypercalcemia of Malignancy	Common Tumors Rarely Associated with Hypercalcemia
Multiple myeloma	Lymphoma*	Squamous carcinoma (lung, head and neck, esophagus, cervix, vulva, skin)	Colon adenocarcinoma
Lymphoma		Renal carcinoma	Stomach adenocarcinoma
Breast cancer		Bladder carcinoma	Prostate adenocarcinoma
		Ovarian carcinoma	Small cell carcinoma
		Breast carcinoma	Thyroid carcinoma
		HTLV-1 lymphoma	CNS malignancies
		Endocrine tumors (pheochromocytoma, adrenocortical carcinoma, islet carcinoma, carcinoids)	

*Has been reported with many different histologic types of lymphoma. CNS, central nervous system, HTLV–1, human T cell lymphoma/leukemia virus-1.

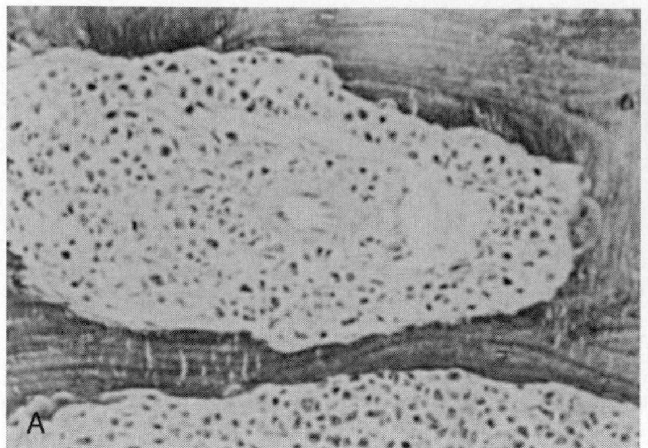

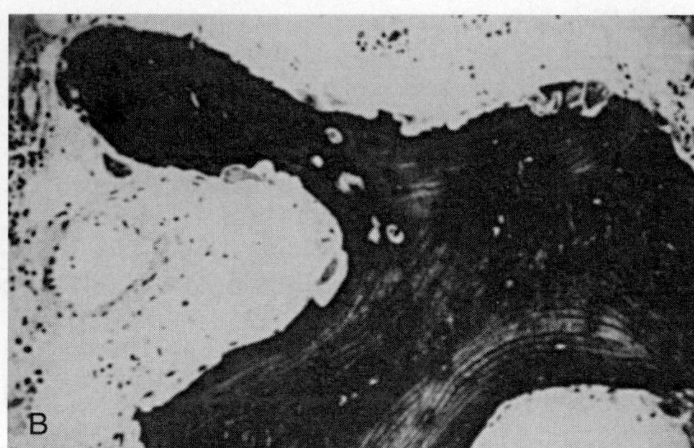

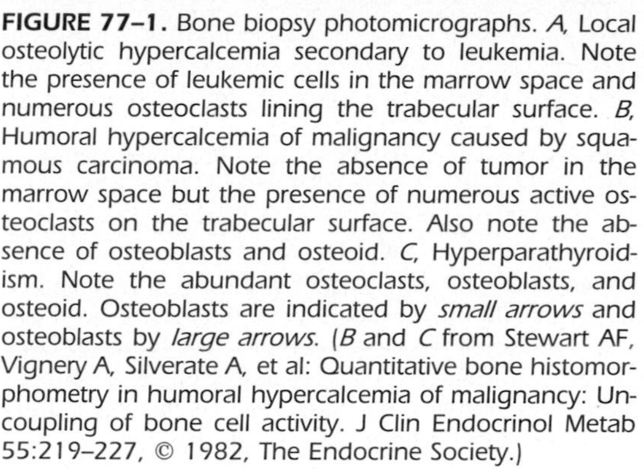

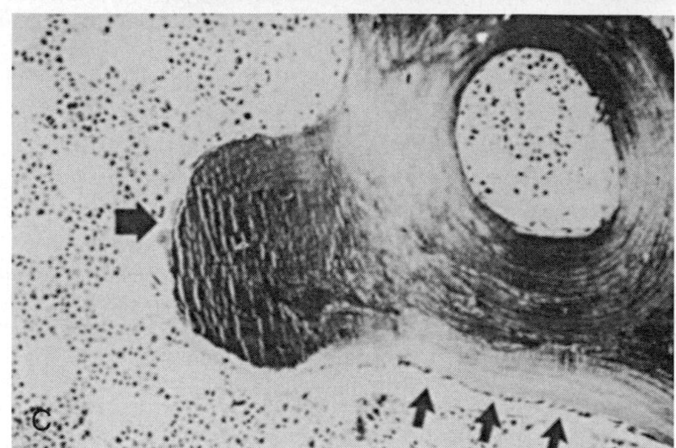

FIGURE 77–1. Bone biopsy photomicrographs. *A*, Local osteolytic hypercalcemia secondary to leukemia. Note the presence of leukemic cells in the marrow space and numerous osteoclasts lining the trabecular surface. *B*, Humoral hypercalcemia of malignancy caused by squamous carcinoma. Note the absence of tumor in the marrow space but the presence of numerous active osteoclasts on the trabecular surface. Also note the absence of osteoblasts and osteoid. *C*, Hyperparathyroidism. Note the abundant osteoclasts, osteoblasts, and osteoid. Osteoblasts are indicated by *small arrows* and osteoblasts by *large arrows*. (*B* and *C* from Stewart AF, Vignery A, Silverate A, et al: Quantitative bone histomorphometry in humoral hypercalcemia of malignancy: Uncoupling of bone cell activity. J Clin Endocrinol Metab 55:219–227, © 1982, The Endocrine Society.)

pain and/or pathologic fractures. Sometimes the onset of hypercalcemia can be ascribed to factors other than tumor progression (e.g., recent immobilization, addition of a thiazide diuretic, prerenal or renal azotemia leading to inadequate renal calcium clearance, hypophosphatemia resulting from inadequate oral intake, gastrointestinal fluid losses, medications, or parenteral calcium administration in the form of "hyperalimentation"). These events should be specifically sought because their correction may reverse a given patient's hypercalcemia.

No studies have precisely defined the relationship of tumor size to the presence or absence of hypercalcemia. Nonetheless, to the extent that tumor size has been studied, it would seem clear that small, occult tumors rarely cause MAHC.[2–12, 17, 18] A corollary of this statement is that when a patient has MAHC, the tumor responsible is usually readily apparent after only a modestly rigorous search; conversely, if a tumor has not been found after 2 or 3 days of evaluation in a hospitalized, hypercalcemic patient, it is unlikely that a malignancy is the cause of the hypercalcemia. Thus a careful history and physical examination with attention to the skin, oropharynx, esophagus, pulmonary system, liver, genitourinary tract, hematopoietic system, and breasts and a limited laboratory and radiologic investigation focused on the hematologic system, esophagus, kidneys, bladder, gynecologic structures, and skeleton will almost invariably lead to rapid definition of the tumor responsible. Occasionally, retroperitoneal tumors (renal carcinomas, lymphomas, pancreatic tumors) may be difficult to demonstrate. Finally, endocrine tumors (e.g., islet carcinomas, pheochromocytomas, ovarian carcinoids) may lead to hypercalcemia and yet may be small and difficult or impossible to localize.

In approaching the evaluation and treatment of a patient with hypercalcemia and cancer, it is important to bear in mind that hypercalcemia may occur in patients with cancer for all the same reasons that it occurs in patients without cancer. For example, in a series of 133 patients with cancer and hypercalcemia encountered between 1978 and 1984, we identified 8 patients in whom hypercalcemia ultimately proved to result from primary hyperparathyroidism.[12] Similarly, we have observed hypercalcemia resulting from tuberculosis, sarcoidosis, immobilization, vitamin D intoxication, hyperthyroidism, thiazide use, Addison's disease, and other causes in patients initially perceived as having MAHC. Thus the entire differential diagnosis of hypercalcemia should be entertained in every patient in whom hypercalcemia is identified, even if it appears at the outset that cancer will prove to be the ultimate cause. This approach is particularly important for the following reasons: (1) in contrast to the ultimate prognosis in MAHC, most causes of hypercalcemia other than cancer are readily treatable; (2) identifying a treatable, nonmalignant cause of hypercalcemia in a patient with cancer may dramatically change the overall perception of a case by the patient's physicians; and (3) treatment will probably be very different.

It is important to say a word about the tumor histologies associated with hypercalcemia (see Table 77–1). Virtually all tumor types have been reported to cause hypercalcemia, but as will be described in the sections on LOH and HHM below, certain tumors types are particularly common causes of hypercalcemia. Conversely, certain tumor types (prostate, colon, oat cell, thyroid, and gastric carcinomas and primary central nervous system malignancies are examples) almost never cause hypercalcemia[2–12, 17, 18] (see Table 77–1). When these tumors are identified in a patient with hypercalcemia, other tumors or other nonmalignant causes of hypercalcemia should be sought.

Major advances have been made over the past two decades in understanding the precise pathophysiologic mechanisms responsible for the various subtypes of MAHC. The sections that follow are divided into four subcategories: LOH, HHM, authentic ectopic hyperparathyroidism, and unusual causes of HHM.

LOCAL OSTEOLYTIC HYPERCALCEMIA

Hypercalcemia can result from direct skeletal involvement by a primary hematologic neoplasm or by skeletal metastases from a nonhematologic neoplasm. Patients with LOH account for approximately 20% of patients in series of patients with MAHC.[2–12, 17–22] The malignancies that most commonly lead to LOH are multiple myeloma, leukemia, lymphoma, and breast cancer[2–12, 17–22] (see Table 77–1). This list is not exclusive, for many other tumor types have been reported to cause hypercalcemia through skeletal metastasis.[2–12, 17–22]

Hypercalcemia occurring in patients with multiple myeloma and breast cancer was initially attributed to the direct physical destruction of bone by malignant cells. This concept is now seen as naive, for it is clear that simply having malignant tumor cells in the bone marrow compartment is insufficient to cause hypercalcemia; certain tumor types typically associated with extensive destructive skeletal metastases (e.g., oat cell and prostate carcinomas)[23, 24] only rarely cause hypercalcemia. Moreover, one large study reported an *inverse* correlation between the number of bone metastases and the serum calcium concentration in a series of hypercalcemic patients with breast cancer.[25] Thus it seems clear that paracrine factors or cytokines that are capable of activating osteoclasts are produced by only certain malignant cells in the bone marrow and it is these factors that lead to LOH.

It has repeatedly been demonstrated by Mundy et al. and others that short-term cultures of bone marrow aspirates from patients with myeloma or lymphoma contain a bone-resorbing factor or family of bone-resorbing factors that have been collectively designated "osteoclast activating factor." [26, 27] Over the past two decades, a number of cytokines have been implicated as being the osteoclast activation factors involved in lymphoma and multiple myeloma. Garrett and collaborators have shown that although human myeloma cells produce a number of bone-resorbing cytokines, the cytotoxicity and bone-resorbing activities in myeloma culture supernatants can be neutralized only by antisera directed against lymphotoxin, also known as tumor necrosis factor-β (TNF-β).[28] These findings strongly suggest a role for lymphotoxin in the hypercalcemia of patients with multiple myeloma. Other bone-resorbing cytokines such as TNF-α (cachectin), interleukin-1 (IL-1), transforming growth factor-α (TGF-α), and IL-6 may play a contributing role as well.[28–30] Similarly, in patients with lymphoma, studies by Dewhirst and others[31] have suggested a role for IL-1.

Progress has also been made in understanding the cellular mechanisms responsible for bone resorption by skeletal metastasis in breast cancer (see Fig. 77–1). Histologic studies of metastatic breast cancer in bone in the Walker 256 rat model of hypercalcemia reveal that breast tumor deposits are surrounded by actively resorbing osteoclasts.[32] Prostaglandin E_2 (PGE_2), a potent bone-resorbing agent, has been suggested as playing a role as the bone-resorbing factor in patients with breast cancer.[33] In addition, direct resorption of devitalized bone by cultured breast cancer cells has been described, a finding that would seem to suggest that at least in some cases, breast cancer cells themselves, in the absence of osteoclastic bone resorption, could lead to hypercalcemia.[34] Finally, increasing evidence suggests a role for PTH-related protein (PTHrP) (see Chapter 70) as a local or intraskeletal mediator of osteoclast activation in women with breast cancer and bone metastases.[35–38] Immunohistochemical analysis by

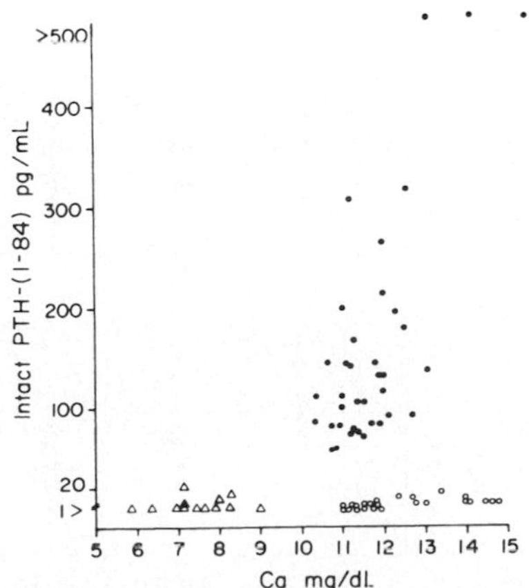

FIGURE 77–2. Immunoreactive parathyroid hormone in the serum of patients with primary hyperparathyroidism *(closed circles)*, hypoparathyroidism *(triangles)*, and hypercalcemia of malignancy *(open circles)* as measured with a two-site immunoradiometric assay for parathyroid hormone (1–84). Note the clear separation of patients with hyperparathyroidism from those with malignancy-associated hypercalcemia. (From Nussbaum SR, Zahradnik RJ, Lavigne JR, et al: Highly sensitive two-site immunoradiometric assay of parathyrin and its clinical utility in evaluating patients with hypercalcemia. Clin Chem 33:1364–1366, 1987.)

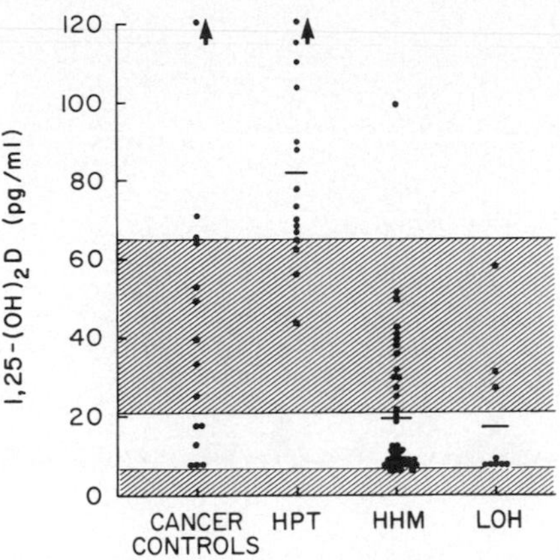

FIGURE 77–3. Plasma 1, 25-dihydroxyvitamin D concentration in the four groups described in Figure 77–6. (Adapted with permission from Stewart AF, Horst R, Deftos LJ, et al: Biochemical evaluation of patients with cancer-associated hypercalcemia: Evidence for humoral and nonhumoral groups. N Engl J Med 303:1377–1383, 1980. Copyright © 1980 Massachusetts Medical Society. All rights reserved.)

Southby et al. demonstrated that 12 of 13 (92%) breast cancer skeletal metastases contained PTHrP whereas only 3 of 18 (17%) nonskeletal breast cancer metastases contained PTHrP.[37] These findings have been confirmed at the in situ hybridization level for PTHrP mRNA in breast cancers metastatic to bone or soft tissue.[38] In addition to suggesting a role for PTHrP as a local bone-resorbing factor, these studies suggest that PTHrP may somehow serve to favor metastasis to the skeleton, as well as tumor growth, in patients with breast cancer. Guise and collaborators have shown this finding to be true[36, 37]: in human breast cancer cell lines bioengineered to express PTHrP at either high or low levels, those producing large quantities of PTHrP were more likely to lead to bone metastasis than those expressing low levels. Moreover, after the development of bone metastases, a local skeletal vicious cycle appeared to develop in which PTHrP induced osteoclastic bone resorption, which in turn led to the local release of TGF-β from resorbed bone. This locally released TGF-β further induced tumor derived PTHrP production and accelerated bone resorption.[35, 36]

Hypercalcemia will develop in approximately one-third of women with breast cancer and bone metastases when treated with either estrogen or antiestrogens such as tamoxifen.[39, 40] The mechanisms responsible for this "estrogen flare" in breast cancer remain undefined. Frequently, hypercalcemia will resolve spontaneously if hypercalcemia can be controlled over the short term and endocrine therapy can be continued. It has been suggested that that the tamoxifen-induced hypercalcemic flare predicts a favorable tumor response. Valentin-Opran and colleagues have suggested, after work with cultured breast cancer cell lines, that estrogen exposure enhances the production of undefined bone-resorbing factors.[41]

From a clinical and biochemical standpoint, LOH is associated with accelerated bone resorption (Fig. 77–1), hypercalcemia, and appropriate suppression of PTH[11] (Fig. 77–2) and 1,25(OH)$_2$ vitamin D (1,25[OH]$_2$D) (Fig. 77–3).[11] PTHrP is not detectable in the circulation[19–22] (Fig. 77–4). In the presence of hypercalcemia and suppressed PTH, fractional calcium excretion is increased[11] (Fig. 77–5). In the presence of bone resorption (delivering a phosphorus load into the extracellular fluid), together with suppression of PTH (limiting phosphorus excretion), one might expect the serum phosphorus concentration to be elevated in patients with LOH. On the other hand, one might expect the serum phosphorus concentration to be low as a reflection of poor dietary intake and the phosphaturic effects of hypercalcemia. In fact, it is usually normal[11] (Fig. 77–6), as is the tubular maximum for phosphorus (TmP/glomerular filtration rate [GFR])[11] (see Fig. 77–6), both of which presumably reflect a balance between these opposing forces. Bone radionuclide scans typically display a diffuse and intense increase in radionuclide uptake in breast cancer associated with LOH. In contrast, bone scans may be entirely negative in patients with multiple myeloma. This difference reflects the uptake of radionuclide in areas of bone formation (e.g., blastic metastases in

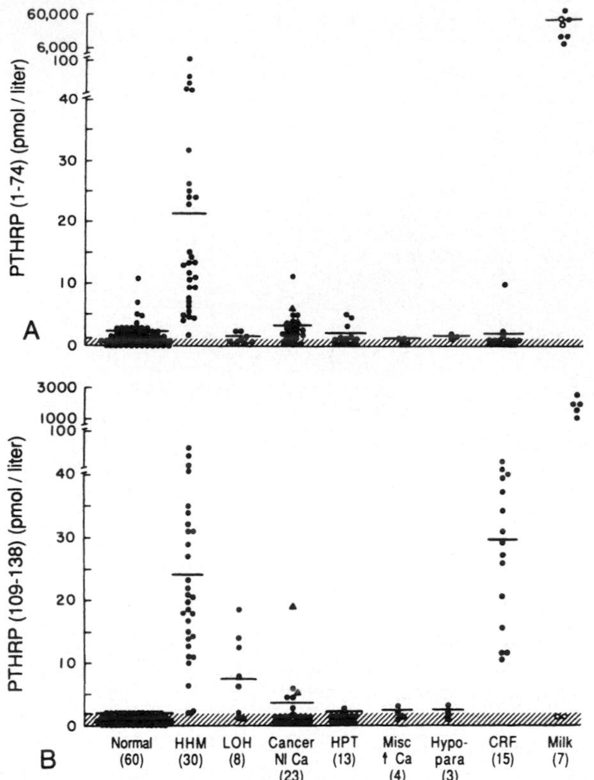

FIGURE 77–4. Immunoreactive parathyroid hormone–related protein (PTHrP) in plasma from patients with the clinical syndromes listed below the x-axis. The *upper panel* shows the results obtained with a two-site PTHrP(1–74) immunoradiometric assay. The *lower panel* shows the results obtained with a carboxyl-terminal PTHrP(109–138) radioimmunoassay. Note that patients with humoral hypercalcemia of malignancy (HHM) have elevated PTHrP values in both the C-terminal and N-terminal assays and that patients with renal failure have elevations in the C-terminal PTHrP. (Reprinted, by permission, from Burtis WJ, Brady TG, Orloff JJ, et al: Immunochemical characterization of circulating parathyroid hormone–related protein in patients with humoral hypercalcemia of malignancy. N Engl J Med 322:1106–1112, 1990. Copyright © 1990 Massachusetts Medical Society. All rights reserved.)

breast cancer) but not areas of osteoclastic activity. Scans may be positive in patients with myeloma in whom fractures and fracture callus formation have developed. As noted above, bone biopsy discloses markedly increased osteoclastic bone resorption in both breast cancer and myeloma associated with LOH (see Fig. 77–1), a finding reflected by increases in biochemical markers of bone resorption such as deoxypyridinoline and N-telopeptide excretion.[42]

HUMORAL HYPERCALCEMIA OF MALIGNANCY

Since the advent of Albright's humoral theory of hypercalcemia of malignancy in the 1940s,[3] several substances have been proposed as candidates for the humoral mediator responsible. In the 1960s, Gordan et al. suggested that elevated circulating levels of four phytosterols (plant-derived vitamin D analogues) were present in patients with breast carcinoma.[43] Subsequent studies showed, however, that these same phytosterols were present in equivalent concentrations in normal and lactating women and that the potency of these analogues was inadequate to cause hypercalcemia.[44] The phytosterol theory thus rapidly lost support.

With the discovery that PGE_2 was a potent stimulator of bone resorption both in tissue culture[45] and in experimental animals in vivo,[46] the possibility arose that the hypercalcemia associated with HHM was due to systemic PGE_2 secretion by tumors. Seyberth et al. and others reported that urinary metabolites of PGE_2 were elevated in patients with MAHC and that therapy with prostaglandin synthesis

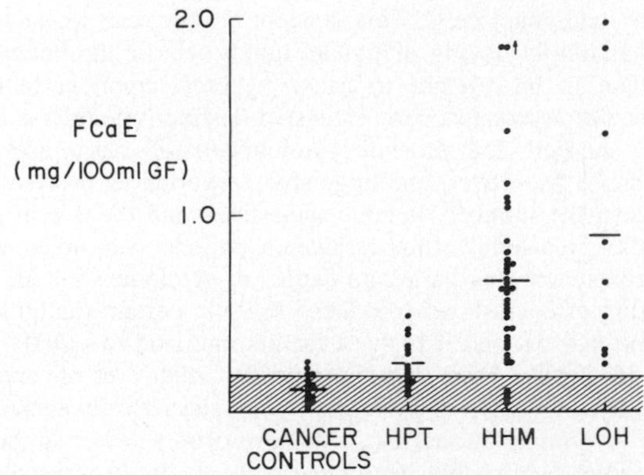

FIGURE 77–5. Fasting calcium excretion in the four groups described in Figure 77–6. Note that on average patients with humoral hypercalcemia of malignancy (HHM) and local osteolytic hypercalcemia (LOH) are far more calciuric than patients with primary hyperparathyroidism (HPT). This result is still true when the groups are matched for serum calcium concentration. (Adapted with permission from Stewart AF, Horst R, Deftos LJ, et al: Biochemical evaluation of patients with cancer-associated hypercalcemia: Evidence for humoral and non-humoral groups. N Engl J Med 303:1377–1383, 1980. Copyright © 1980 Massachusetts Medical Society. All rights reserved.)

inhibitors (aspirin, indomethacin) reversed the hypercalcemia in several patients.[47] However, subsequent, more extensive studies have not shown frequent responses to indomethacin.[48] It is the current view of most investigators that PGE_2 does not act as a systemic mediator of bone resorption in most cases of HHM and that therapy with prostaglandin synthesis inhibitors is usually ineffective. It should be clear, however, that these observations do not exclude a role for PGE_2 or other arachidonate metabolites in HHM at the local level within the skeleton.

As noted above, Albright had initially suggested that PTH was the responsible humoral factor.[3] This concept subsequently gained wide acceptance as evidenced by the entrance into common usage in the 1960s and 1970s of the terms "ectopic hyperparathyroidism" and "pseudohyperparathyroidism."[6] Evidence in support of the "ectopic PTH" thesis included (1) the humoral nature of the syndrome,[4, 5, 10] (2) the hypophosphatemia and renal phosphate wasting characteristic of the syndrome, and (3) the apparent failure of suppression of PTH observed in the early generations of PTH radioimmunoassays.[49, 50] It is now clear, as will be described below, that although bona fide "ectopic hyperparathyroidism" does indeed exist, it is extremely rare and fails to account for most instances of HHM.

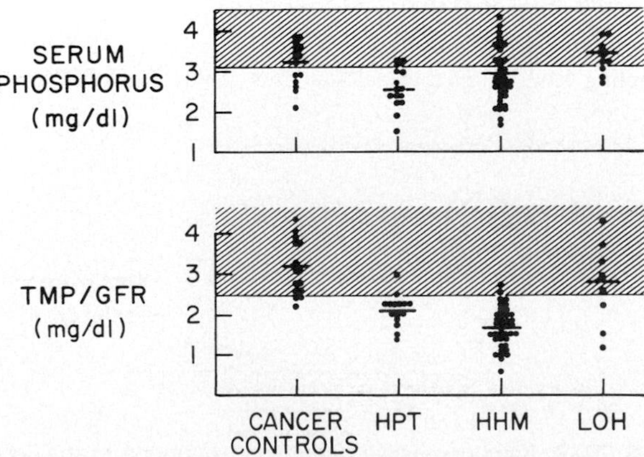

FIGURE 77–6. Serum phosphorus and renal phosphorus threshold in patients with normocalcemia and cancer (cancer controls), primary hyperparathyroidism (HPT), humoral hypercalcemia of malignancy (HHM), and local osteolytic hypercalcemia (LOH). See the text. (Adapted with permission from Stewart AF, Horst R, Deftos LJ, et al: Biochemical evaluation of patients with cancer-associated hypercalcemia: Evidence for humoral and non-humoral groups. N Engl J Med 303:1377–1383, 1980. Copyright © 1980 Massachusetts Medical Society. All rights reserved.)

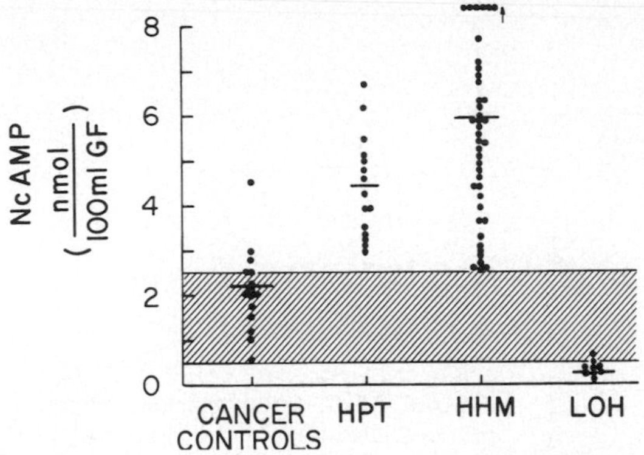

FIGURE 77–7. Nephrogenous cyclic adenosine monophosphate excretion in the four patient groups described in the legend to Figure 77–2. (Adapted with permission from Stewart AF, Horst R, Deftos LJ, et al: Biochemical evaluation of patients with cancer-associated hypercalcemia: Evidence for humoral and non-humoral groups. N Engl J Med 303:1377–1383, 1980. Copyright © 1980 Massachusetts Medical Society. All rights reserved.)

Today, it is widely accepted that the vast majority of cases of HHM are due to the secretion of PTHrP by tumors. Evidence for this theory is as follows: (1) tumors associated with HHM secrete PTHrP, which leads to elevated circulating concentrations of PTHrP[19–22] (see Fig. 77–4); (2) PTHrP infusion into laboratory animals and humans reproduces the key features of the HHM syndrome in vivo[51–53]; and (3) infusion of neutralizing antisera against PTHrP reverses the HHM syndrome in laboratory animals.[54, 55]

HHM accounts for approximately 80% of patients in unselected series of patients with MAHC.[2–12, 17–22] Approximately 50% of patients with HHM have an underlying squamous carcinoma of the lung, cervix, esophagus, larynx, oropharynx, vulva, skin, or other site[2–12, 17–22] (see Table 77–1). Carcinomas of the kidney, ovary, and bladder are also very common.[2–14, 19–22] Interestingly, breast cancer may not only cause MAHC through LOH and skeletal metastases but may also cause hypercalcemia in the absence of skeletal metastases in a classic HHM scenario[56, 57] (see Table 77–1). Human T cell lymphoma/leukemia virus-I lymphomas, 90% of which are associated with hypercalcemia, also operate through this mechanism.[58, 59] Finally, hypercalcemia resulting from endocrine tumors such as pheochromocytomas[60, 61] and islet cell carcinomas[62, 63] may cause hypercalcemia through this mechanism. As is the case with LOH, virtually every tumor type has been reported on occasion to cause HHM.

Patients with HHM display increases in circulating concentrations of PTHrP[19–22] (see Fig. 77–4), and bone biopsies display a marked increase in osteoclastic resorption, accompanied by a decrease in osteoblastic bone formation[13] (see Fig. 77–1). This uncoupling of bone resorption from formation and the quantitatively striking extent of this uncoupling lead to a large calcium flux from the skeleton into the extracellular fluid and account primarily for the degree of hypercalcemia observed in HHM. The cellular basis for this dramatic uncoupling is not known. Circulating PTH concentrations are reduced in patients with HHM[19–22, 64] (see Fig. 77–2), but nephrogenous cyclic adenosine monophosphate (NcAMP) excretion is increased (Fig. 77–7),[11] a reflection of the increases in circulating PTHrP. Although the increase in NcAMP excretion is of little clinical importance today, the elevation in NcAMP and the ability of PTHrP to stimulate adenylyl cyclase in the kidney in vitro led to the identification and purification of PTHrP.[65] HHM is associated with suppression of plasma $1,25(OH)_2D$[11] (see Fig. 77–3), which in turn leads to a reduction in intestinal calcium absorption.[66] The mechanisms responsible for the reduction in $1,25(OH)_2D$ are uncertain because both PTH and PTHrP infusion into humans leads to increases in plasma $1,25(OH)_2D$.[51, 52] Fractional calcium excretion has been reported to be elevated[10, 11] (see Fig. 77–5) or reduced[67, 68] (Fig. 77–8) in patients with HHM. In fact, accurate measurements of the GFR are critical in resolving this issue, but these measurements have not been possible to date in patients with advanced cancer, rapidly declining renal function, markedly reduced skeletal mass (and therefore creatinine release), and aggressive hydration and diuretic therapy. The serum phosphorus concentration is characteristically reduced[13] (see Fig. 77–6) as long as renal function remains normal, a phenomenon reflecting reductions in the TmP/GFR[13] (see Fig. 77–6). This reduction in renal phosphorus reabsorption is a direct effect of PTHrP on the proximal tubule.[51, 52]

Bone radionuclide scans display a complete absence of skeletal metastases or the presence of only a few skeletal metastases,[2–12, 17–22] which is a reflection of the primarily humoral nature of the syndrome. Importantly, the syndrome reverses with successful eradication of the tumor in question, thus underscoring the humoral nature of the syndrome.[2–12, 17, 18] Unfortunately, this outcome is not common.

AUTHENTIC ECTOPIC HYPERPARATHYROIDISM

As noted above, from the 1940s through the 1970s, "ectopic hyperparathyroidism" was believed to be a common cause of paraneoplastic hypercalcemia. By the 1980s the term had fallen into disuse, and the existence of authentic ectopic hyperparathyroidism was in doubt; most authors believed that all cases of what had previously been considered to be "ectopic hyperparathyroidism" were in fact cases of HHM. With the advent of sensitive and specific immunoassays and molecular probes for PTH and PTHrP, the situation has changed. There are now at least seven convincing case reports of patients with cancer (two small cell carcinomas of the lung, one squamous carcinoma of the lung, one thymoma, one undifferentiated neuroendocrine tumor, one clear cell adenocarcinoma of the ovary, and one thyroid papillary carcinoma) who also displayed elevations in immunoreactive PTH in plasma with the use of modern two-site PTH immunoassays and/or expressed PTH mRNA in their tumor.[69–75] In the most thoroughly studied case, reported by Nussbaum et al., immunoreactive PTH values were found to be elevated in plasma by a sensitive and specific two-site PTH immunoradiometric assay.[69] At surgery, a fivefold gradient of PTH was demonstrated across the ovarian tumor. PTH values fell precipitously after tumor resection, and the serum calcium concentra-

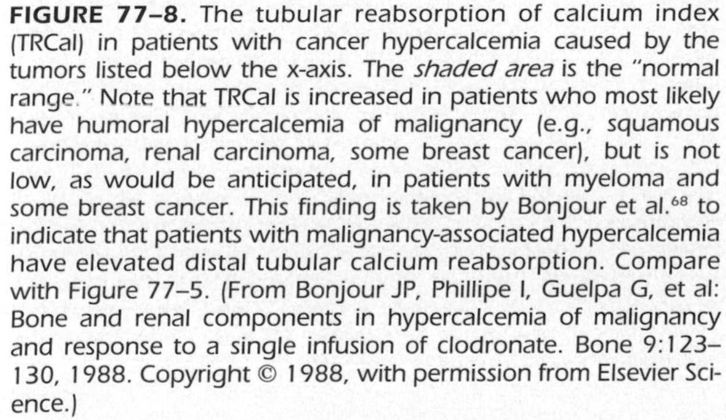
FIGURE 77–8. The tubular reabsorption of calcium index (TRCaI) in patients with cancer hypercalcemia caused by the tumors listed below the x-axis. The *shaded area* is the "normal range." Note that TRCaI is increased in patients who most likely have humoral hypercalcemia of malignancy (e.g., squamous carcinoma, renal carcinoma, some breast cancer), but is not low, as would be anticipated, in patients with myeloma and some breast cancer. This finding is taken by Bonjour et al.[68] to indicate that patients with malignancy-associated hypercalcemia have elevated distal tubular calcium reabsorption. Compare with Figure 77–5. (From Bonjour JP, Phillipe I, Guelpa G, et al: Bone and renal components in hypercalcemia of malignancy and response to a single infusion of clodronate. Bone 9:123–130, 1988. Copyright © 1988, with permission from Elsevier Science.)

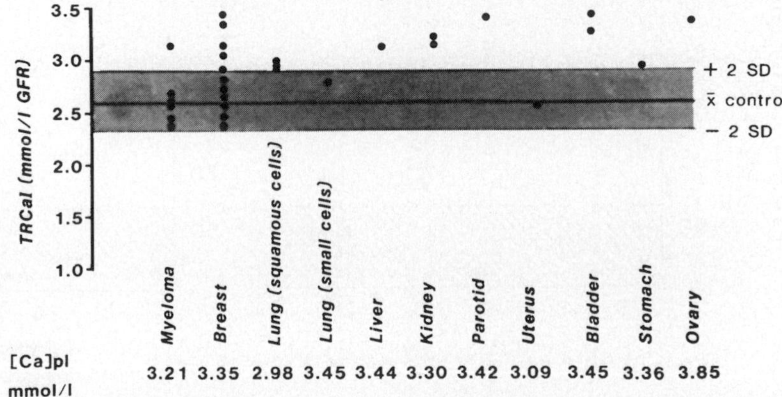

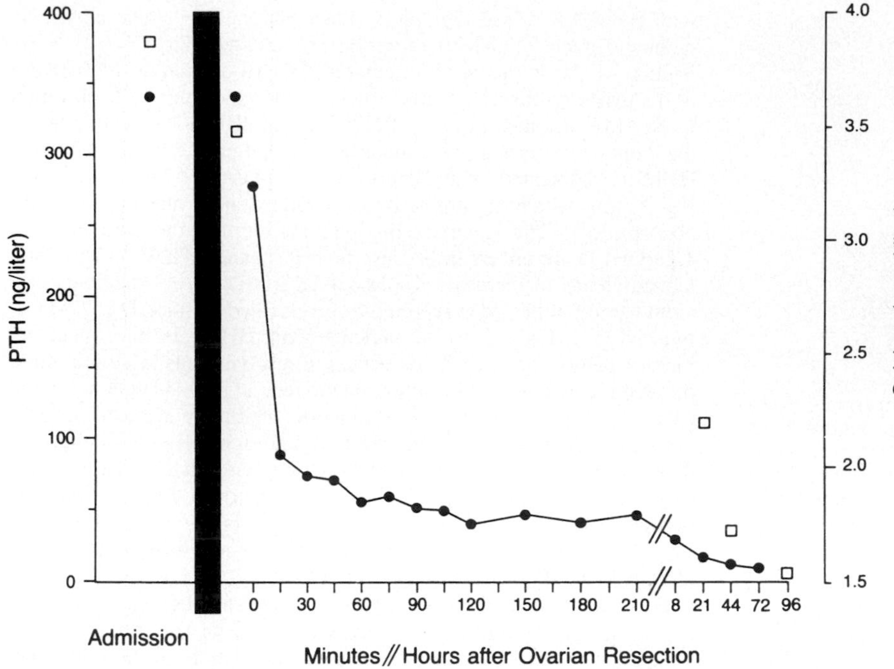

FIGURE 77–9. Serum calcium *(squares)* and immunoreactive parathyroid hormone (PTH) *(circles)* in a patient with an ovarian carcinoma before and after oophrectomy, indicated by the *black bar.* The PTH immunoassay is that shown in Figure 77–2. Prior parathyroidectomy of 3½ glands failed to influence either her hypercalcemia or elevated PTH concentration. (Reprinted, by permission, from Nussbaum SR, Gaz RD, Arnold A: Hypercalcemia and ectopic secretion of PTH by an ovarian carcinoma with rearrangement of the gene for PTH. N Engl J Med 323:1324–1328, 1990. Copyright © 1990 Massachusetts Medical Society. All rights reserved.)

tion normalized (Fig. 77–9). Neck exploration before the ovarian surgery had revealed four normal parathyroid glands, and resection of three and a half parathyroid glands had no effect on the serum calcium concentration. PTH mRNA was present in abundance in the tumor, whereas PTHrP mRNA was undetectable, as was PTHrP in plasma. The basis of PTH gene overexpression in this tumor was found to be twofold. First, a clonal rearrangement in the upstream region of one copy of the PTH gene in the ovarian carcinoma apparently served to either abolish a silencer in this region of the gene or included a promoter region of a normal ovarian gene. Second, the PTH gene was amplified in the tumor. In contrast, in the report by Yoshimoto and coauthors describing ectopic hyperparathyroidism caused by a pulmonary small cell carcinoma, no such gene rearrangement or amplification events were identified, and the cause of the PTH expression was unexplained.[70]

These case reports demonstrate that authentic ectopic hyperparathy-

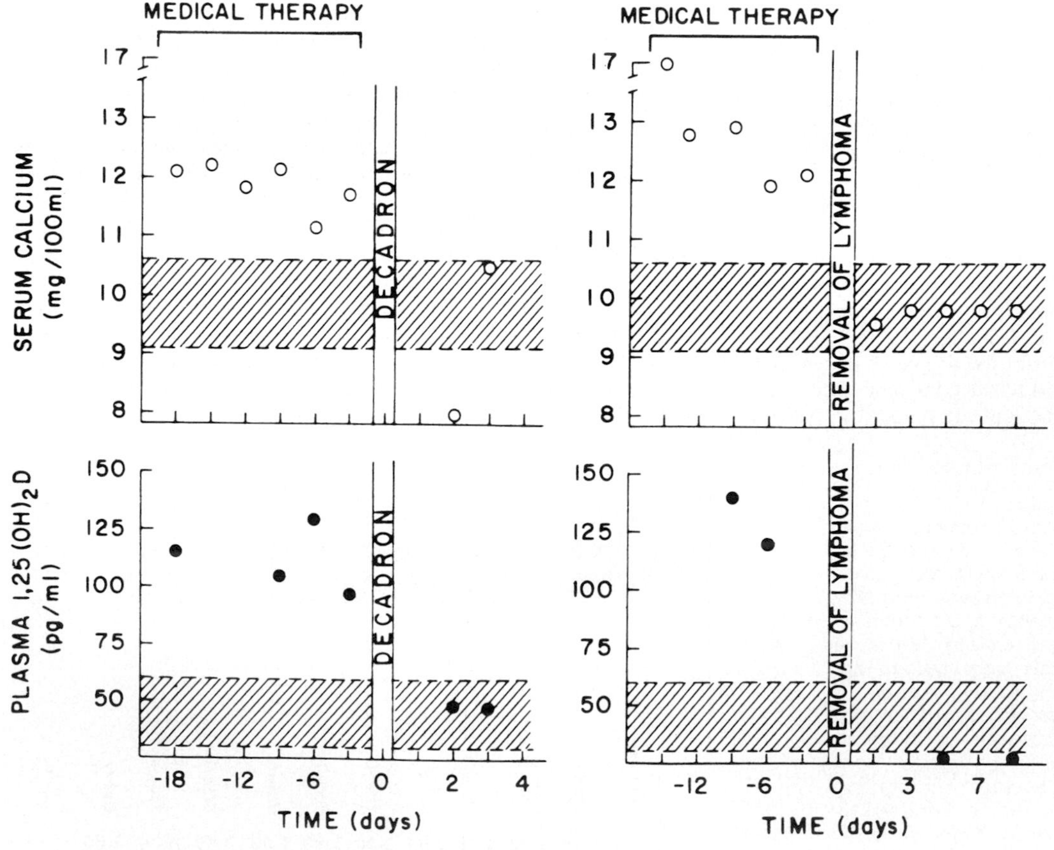

FIGURE 77–10. Serum calcium and plasma 1,25-dihydroxyvitamin ($1,25(OH)_2D$) concentrations in patients with the $1,25(OH)_2D$-induced lymphoma syndrome before and after therapy. The patient shown in the two *left panels* was treated with dexamethasone for systemic lymphoma. The patient in the two *right panels* had a splenectomy for a solitary splenic lymphoma. Note the fall in plasma $1,25(OH)_2D$ concentration after therapy in both patients and the normalization of serum calcium. Also compare the plasma $1,25(OH)_2D$ concentrations in these patients with those in patients with humoral hypercalcemia of malignancy and local osteolytic hypercalcemia shown in Figure 77–3. (From Rosenthal ND, Insogna KL, Godsall JW, et al: Elevations in circulating 1,25 Dihydroxyvitamin D in three patients with lymphoma-associated hypercalcemia. J Clin Endocrinol Metab 60:29–33, © 1985, The Endocrine Society.)

roidism can occur. From a clinical standpoint, because of the elevations in immunoreactive PTH, they are likely to be confused with primary hyperparathyroidism. Unless the offending malignant neoplasm is obvious at the initial evaluation, such confusion may lead to unsuccessful attempts at parathyroidectomy.

UNUSUAL CAUSES OF MALIGNANCY-ASSOCIATED HYPERCALCEMIA

The vast majority of patients with HHM are striking in their homogeneity. As indicated above, the histologic findings (squamous, renal, bladder, and ovarian carcinomas) and biochemical findings (elevated NcAMP, reduced renal phosphorus thresholds, reduced $1,25[OH]_2D$ levels, suppressed immunoreactive PTH levels, elevated immunoreactive PTHrP concentrations) are so uniform that it seems inescapable that most cases of HHM are due to secretion of PTHrP.

It should be clear, however, that other humoral mediators undoubtedly exist in unusual patients. For example, a small number of patients with elevated PGE_2 levels and/or clear responsiveness to prostaglandin synthesis inhibitors have been described,[47, 76] which suggests that in rare instances PGE_2 may act as a humoral, systemic agent. In addition, more than 40 patients with a variety of types of lymphoma have been described in whom hypercalcemia occurred in the absence of bone metastases and with reduced urinary cAMP or NcAMP excretion but elevated circulating levels of $1,25(OH)_2D$[77–79] (Fig. 77–10). These observations suggest that tumor-derived $1,25(OH)_2D$ may have induced intestinal hyperabsorption of calcium and/or led to osteoclastic stimulation. In addition, a patient with an ovarian dysgerminoma, no skeletal involvement, hypercalcemia in the presence of an elevated renal phosphorus threshold, and reduced levels of NcAMP and $1,25(OH)_2D$ has been described.[80] All these abnormalities promptly normalized after eradication of the patient's tumor, which suggests that the tumor produced a humoral agent distinct from that typically associated with HHM. Finally, Bringhurst et al. have described patients with hypercalcemia in the setting of metastatic malignant melanoma and bladder carcinoma.[81, 82] Excision of the tumor reversed the patients' hypercalcemia, thus indicating a humoral mechanism. In culture, the tumors were shown to produce a bone-resorbing protein devoid of adenylate cyclase–stimulating activity or cytochemical PTH-like bioactivity. In the aggregate, these examples indicate that humoral forms of MAHC can occur via the production of factors other than $1,25(OH)_2D$, PTHrP, or PTH; however, these examples appear to be quite rare collectively.

THERAPEUTIC CONSIDERATIONS

This area has received complete attention in several recent reviews[83–85] and in Chapter 78. The mean life expectancy in patients with MAHC is 30 days.[14] Therapy aimed at correcting hypercalcemia is largely palliative and should therefore be aimed at a patient's overall status and not at the serum calcium concentration per se. For example, a patient with a calcium level of 11.5 mg/dL who has been stable and asymptomatic may need no treatment at all, whereas aggressive therapy for a calcium level of 11.0 may be appropriate in a patient with symptoms of hypercalcemia or when a rapid subsequent rise seems likely. Conversely, no antihypercalcemic therapy may be most appropriate in a patient with advanced cancer who has failed all attempts to control the malignancy.

It follows that the most effective long-term therapy for tumor-associated hypercalcemia is successful antitumor therapy. This point should be borne in mind and acted upon early in the management of any given patient. Therapies aimed at treatment of hypercalcemia per se are rarely effective over the long term. Hence long-term control of hypercalcemia depends on tumor eradication or debulking through surgery, chemotherapy, or radiotherapy.

It is useful to conceptualize short-term antihypercalcemic therapy in terms of the three organ systems that regulate calcium homeostasis and whose aggregate homeostatic failure leads to hypercalcemia: the intestine, the kidney, and the skeleton. Therapy should be tailored to a given patient's needs and with the factors in mind that may have precipitated development of the hypercalcemia. For example, the development of hypercalcemia in a patient with MAHC may be traced to recent immobilization or to an episode of dehydration or renal compromise. Therapy aimed at reversing immobilization or increasing the GFR may be all that is necessary to correct such a patient's hypercalcemia. Hemodialysis is effective in selected hypercalcemic patients with treatable tumors and renal failure. Agents that inhibit bone resorption are useful in most patients with MAHC. Dietary calcium restriction is unnecessary in the vast majority of individuals with MAHC because intestinal calcium absorption is reduced. The exception to this generalization would be the rare patient with a lymphoma and $1,25(OH)_2D$-mediated hypercalcemia.[77–79] Most often, combinations of the agents and measures listed in Chapter 78 are used. The brightest stars in the therapeutic armamentarium are the second- and third-generation bisphosphonates. Their general lack of toxicity, their potency, and their ease of use have dramatically improved the management of MAHC in the past 15 years.

Acknowledgment

The authors wish to thank Drs. W.J. Burtis, J.J. Orloff, E.C. Weir, R. Vasavada, K.L. Insogna, N.E. Soifer, and J.J. Wysolmerski for their help in performing the studies and formulating the concepts described herein. We thank the innumerable physicians and patients who have permitted the clinical studies described in this chapter.

REFERENCES

1. Zondek H, Petow H, Siebert W: Die bedeutung der calciumbestimmung im blute fur die diagnose der niereninsuffzientz. Z Klin Med 99:129–138, 1923.
2. Gutman AB, Tyson TL, Gutman EB: Serum calcium, inorganic phosphorus and phosphatase activity in hyperparathyroidism, Paget's disease, multiple myeloma and neoplastic disease of the bones. Arch Intern Med 57:379–413, 1936.
3. Case records of the Massachusetts General Hospital (case 27461). N Engl J Med 225:789–791, 1941.
4. Plimpton CH, Gelhorn A: Hypercalcemia in malignant disease without evidence of bone destruction. Am J Med 21:750–759, 1956.
5. Connors TB, Howard JF: The etiology of hypercalcemia associated with lung carcinoma. J Clin Invest 35:697–698, 1956.
6. Lafferty FW: Pseudohyperparathyroidism. Medicine (Baltimore) 45:247–260, 1966.
7. Rodman JS, Sherwood LM: Disorders of mineral metabolism in malignancy. *In* Avioli LV, Krane SM (eds): Metabolic Bone Disease, vol 2. New York, Academic Press, 1978, pp 555–631.
8. Myers WPL: Hypercalcemia in neoplastic disease. Arch Surg 80:308, 1960.
9. Besarab A, Caro JF: Mechanisms of hypercalcemia in malignancy. Cancer 41:2276–2285, 1978.
10. Powell D, Singer FR, Murray TM, et al: Nonparathyroid humoral hypercalcemia in patients with neoplastic diseases. N Engl J Med 289:176–181, 1973.
11. Stewart AF, Horst R, Deftos LJ, et al: Biochemical evaluation of patients with cancer-associated hypercalcemia: Evidence for humoral and non-humoral groups. N Engl J Med 303:1377–1383, 1980.
12. Godsall JW, Burtis WJ, Insogna KL, et al: Nephrogenous cyclic AMP, adenylate cyclase–stimulating activity, and the humoral hypercalcemia of malignancy. Recent Prog Horm Res 40:705–750, 1986.
13. Stewart AF, Vignery A, Silvergate A, et al: Quantitative bone histomorphometry in humoral hypercalcemia of malignancy: Uncoupling of bone cell activity. J Clin Metab 55:219–227, 1982.
14. Ralson SH, Gallagher SJ, Patel U, et al: Cancer-associated hypercalcemia: Morbidity and mortality. Ann Intern Med 112:499–504, 1990.
15. Nierenberg DW, Ransil BJ: Q-aTc interval as a clinical indicator of hypercalcemia. Am J Cardiol 44:243–248, 1979.
16. Davis TME, Singh B, Choo KE, et al: Dynamic assessment of the electrocardiographic QT intervals during citrate infusion in healthy volunteers. Br Heart J 75:523–526, 1995.
17. Omenn GS, Roth SI, Baker WH: Hyperparathyroidism associated with malignant tumors of non-parathyroid origin. Cancer 24:1004–1012, 1969.
18. Skrabanek P, McPartlin J, Powell DM: Tumor hypercalcemia and ectopic hyperparathyroidism. Medicine (Baltimore) 59:262–282, 1980.
19. Burtis WJ, Brady TG, Orloff JJ, et al: Immunochemical characterization of circulating parathyroid hormone–related protein in patients with humoral hypercalcemia of malignancy. N Engl J Med 322:1106–1112, 1990.
20. Budayr AR, Nissenson RA, Klein RF, et al: Increased serum levels of PTH-like protein in malignancy-associated hypercalcemia. Ann Intern Med 111:807–810, 1989.
21. Blind E, Raue F, Gotzman J, et al: Circulating levels of mid-regional parathyroid hormone–related protein in hypercalcemia of malignancy. Clin Endocrinol 37:290–297, 1992.
22. Pandian MR, Morgan CH, Carlton E, Segre GV: Modified immunoradiometric assay of parathyroid hormone–related protein: Clinical application in the differential diagnosis of hypercalcemia. Clin Chem 38:282–288, 1992.
23. Bender RA, Hansen H: Hypercalcemia in bronchogenic carcinoma. A prospective study of 200 patients. Ann Intern Med 80:205–208, 1974.

24. Mahadevia PS, Pamaswamy A, Greenwald ES, et al: Hypercalcemia in prostatic carcinoma. Arch Intern Med 143:1339–1342, 1983.
25. Ralston S, Fogelman I, Gardner MD, Boyle IT: Hypercalcemia and metastatic bone disease: Is there a link? Lancet 2:903–905, 1982.
26. Mundy GR, Raisz LG, Cooper RA, et al: Evidence for the secretion of an osteoclast stimulating factor in myeloma. N Engl J Med 290:1041–1046, 1974.
27. Mundy GR, Luben RA, Raisz LG, et al: Bone-resorbing activity in supernatants from lymphoid cell lines. N Engl J Med 290:867–871, 1974.
28. Garrett RI, Durie BGM, Nedwin GE, et al: Production of the bone-resorbing cytokine lymphotoxin by cultured human myeloma cells. N Engl J Med 317:526–532, 1987.
29. Mundy GR: Hypercalcemia in hematologic malignancies and in solid tumors associated with extensive localized bone destruction. *In* Favus M (ed): Primer on the Metabolic Bone Disease and Disorders of Mineral Metabolism, ed 3. Philadelphia, Lippincott-Raven, 1996, pp 203–206.
30. Nagai Y, Yamato H, Akaogi K, et al: Role of interleukin-6 in uncoupling of bone in vivo in a human squamous carcinoma coproducing parathyroid hormone–related protein and interleukin-6. J Bone Miner Res 13:664–672, 1998.
31. Dewhirst FE, Stashenko PP, Mole JE, Tsurumachi T: Purification and partial sequence of human osteoclast activating factor: Identity with human interleukin lB. J Immunol 135:2562, 1985.
32. Galasko CSB: Mechanisms of bone destruction in the development of skeletal metastases. Nature 263:507, 1976.
33. Greaves M, Ibbotson KJ, Atkins D, Martin TJ: Prostaglandins as mediators of bone resorption in renal and breast tumors. Clin Sci 58:201–210, 1980.
34. Eilon G, Mundy GR: Direct resorption of bone by human breast cancer cells in vitro. Nature 276:726–728, 1978.
35. Guise TA, Yin JJ, Taylor SD, et al: Evidence for a causal role of parathyroid hormone–related protein in the pathogenesis of human breast cancer–mediated osteolysis. J Clin Invest 98:1544, 1996.
36. Guise TA, Mundy GR: Cancer and bone. Endocr Rev 19:18–54, 1998.
37. Southby J, Kissin MW, Danks JA, et al: Immunohistochemical localization of PTHrP in human breast cancer. Cancer Res 50:7710–7716, 1990.
38. Vargas SJ, Gillespie MT, Powell GJ, et al: Localization of PTHrP mRNA expression in breast cancer and metastatic lesions by in situ hybridization. J Bone Miner Res 7:971–979, 1992.
39. Sztern M, Barkan A, Rakowsky E, et al: Hypercalcemia in carcinoma of the breast without evidence of bone destruction. Cancer 48:2383–2385, 1981.
40. Legha SS, Powell K, Buzdar AU, Blumenschein GR: Tamoxifen-induced hypercalcemia in breast cancer. Cancer 47:2803–2806, 1981.
41. Valentin-Opran A, Eilon G, Saez S, Mundy GR: Estrogens stimulate release of bone-resorbing activity in cultured human breast cancer cells. J Clin Invest 72:726–731, 1985.
42. Nakayama K, Fukumoto S, Takeda S, et al: Differences in bone and vitamin D metabolism between primary hyperparathyroidism and malignancy-associated hypercalcemia. J Clin Endocrinol Metab 81:607–611, 1996.
43. Gordan GS, Fitzpatrick ME, Lubich WP: Identification of osteolytic sterols in human breast cancer. Trans Assoc Am Physicians 80:183–189, 1967.
44. Haddad JG, Couranz SJ, Avioli LV: Circulating phytosterols in normal females, lactating mothers, and breast cancer patients. J Clin Endocrinol Metab 30:174–180, 1970.
45. Klein DC, Raisz LG: Prostaglandins: Stimulation of bone resorption in tissue culture. Endocrinology 86:1436–1440, 1970.
46. Tashjian AH: Role of prostaglandins in the production of hypercalcemia by tumors. Cancer Res 38:4138–4141, 1978.
47. Seyberth WJ, Segre GV, Morgan JL, et al: Prostaglandins as mediators of hypercalcemia associated with certain types of cancer. N Engl J Med 293:1278–1283, 1975.
48. Brenner D, Harvey HA, Lipton A, Demers L: A study of prostaglandin E_2 parahormone, and response to indomethacin in patients with hypercalcemia and malignancy. Cancer 49:556–561, 1982.
49. Benson RC, Riggs BL, Pickard BM, Arnaud CD: Radioimmunoassay of parathyroid hormone in hypercalcemic patients with malignant disease. Am J Med 56:821–826, 1974.
50. Riggs BL, Arnaud CD, Reynolds JC, Smith LH: Immunologic differentiation of primary hyperparathyroidism from hyperparathyroidism due to nonparathyroid cancer. J Clin Invest 50:2079–2083, 197l.
51. Everhart-Caye M, Inzucchi SE, Guinness-Henry J, et al: Parathyroid hormone–related protein[1–36] is equipotent with parathyroid hormone[1–34] in humans. J Clin Endocrinol Metab 81:199, 1996.
52. Henry JG, Mitnick MA, Dann PR, Stewart AF: Parathyroid hormone–related protein[1–36] is biologically active when administered subcutaneously to humans. J Clin Endocrinol Metab 82:900–906, 1997.
53. Stewart A, Mangin M, Wu T, et al: A synthetic human parathyroid hormone–like protein stimulates bone resorption and causes hypercalcemia in rats. J Clin Invest 81:596–600, 1988.
54. Henderson J, Bernier S, D'Amour P, Goltzman D: Effects of passive immunization against PTH-like peptide in hypercalcemic tumor-bearing rats and normocalcemic controls. Endocrinology 127:1310–1316, 1990.
55. Kukreja SC, Shevrin DH, Wimbiscus SA, et al: Antibodies to PTH-related protein lower serum calcium in athymic mouse models of malignancy associated hypercalcemia due to human tumors. J Clin Invest 82:1798–1802, 1988.
56. Grill V, Ho P, Body JJ, et al: PTH-related protein: Elevated levels in both humoral hypercalcemia of malignancy and hypercalcemia complicating metastatic breast cancer. J Clin Endocrinol 73:1309–1315, 1991.
57. Isales C, Carcangiu ML, Stewart AF: Hypercalcemia in breast cancer: A reassessment of the mechanism. Am J Med 82:1143–1147, 1987.
58. Fukumoto S, Matsumoto T, Ikeda T, et al: Clinical evaluation of adult T-cell lymphoma. Arch Intern Med 148:921–925, 1988.
59. Wantabe T, Yamaguchi K, Tatasuki K, et al: Constitutive expression of PTHrP gene in HTLV-1 carriers and adult T-cell leukemia patients that can be trans-activated by HTLV-1 tax gene. J Exp Med 172:759–765, 1990.
60. Mune T, Katakami H, Kato Y, et al: Production and secretion of parathyroid hormone–related protein in pheochromocytoma: Participation of an α-adrenergic mechanism. J Clin Endocrinol Metab 76:757–762, 1993.
61. Stewart AF, Hoecker J, Segre GV, et al: Hypercalcemia in pheochromocytoma: Evidence for a novel mechanism. Ann Intern Med 102:776–779, 1985.
62. Mao C, Carter P, Schaefer P, et al: Malignant islet cell tumor associated with hypercalcemia. Surgery 117:37–40, 1997.
63. Wu T-J, Lin C-L, Taylor RL, et al: Increased parathyroid hormone–related peptide in patients with hypercalcemia associated with islet cell carcinoma. Mayo Clin Proc 72:1111–1115, 1997.
64. Nussbaum SR, Zahradnik RJ, Lavigne JR, et al: Highly sensitive two-site immunoradiometric assay of parathyrin and its clinical utility in evaluating patients with hypercalcemia. Clin Chem 33:1364–1367, 1987.
65. Nissenson RA, Halloran B (eds): Parathyroid Hormone–Related Protein. Boca Raton, FL, CRC Press, 1992.
66. Coombes RC, Ward MK, Greenberg PB, et al: Calcium metabolism in cancer. Studies using calcium isotopes and immunoassay for parathyroid hormone and calcitonin. Cancer 38:2111–2120, 1976.
67. Ralston SH, Fogelman I, Gardner MD, et al: Hypercalcemia of malignancy: Evidence for a non-parathyroid humoral agent with an effect on renal tubular handling of calcium. Clin Sci 66:187–194, 1984.
68. Bonjour J-P, Phillipe J, Guelpa G, et al: Bone and renal components in hypercalcemia of malignancy and response to a single infusion of clodronate. Bone 9:123–130, 1988.
69. Nussbaum SR, Gaz RD, Arnold A: Hypercalcemia and ectopic secretion of PTH by an ovarian carcinoma with rearrangement of the gene for PTH. N Engl J Med 323:1324–1328, 1990.
70. Yoshimoto K, Yamasaki R, Sakai H, et al: Ectopic production of PTH by small cell lung cancer in a patient with hypercalcemia. J Clin Endocrinol Metab 68:976–981, 1989.
71. Strewler GJ, Budayr AA, Clark OH, Nissenson RA: Production of parathyroid hormone by a malignant nonparathyroid tumor in a hypercalcemic patient. J Clin Endocrinol Metab 76:1373–1375, 1993.
72. Iguchi H, Miyagi C, Tomita K, et al: Hypercalcemia caused by ectopic production of parathyroid hormone in a patient with papillary adenocarcinoma of the thyroid gland. J Clin Endocrinol Metab 83:2653–2657, 1998.
73. Nielsen PK, Rasmussen AK, Feldt-Rasmussen U, et al: Ectopic production of intact parathyroid hormone by a squamous cell lung carcinoma in vivo and in vitro. J Clin Endocrinol Metab 81:3793–3796, 1996.
74. Rizzoli R, Pache J-C, Didierjean L, et al: A thymoma as a cause of true ectopic hyperparathyroidism. J Clin Endocrinol Metab 79:912–915, 1994.
75. Schmeltzer HJ, Hesch RD, Mayer H: Parathyroid hormone and PTH mRNA in a human small cell lung cancer. Recent Results Cancer Res 99:88–93, 1985.
76. Metz SA, McRae JR, Robertson RP: Prostaglandins as mediators of paraneoplastic syndromes: Review and update. Metabolism 30:299–316, 1981.
77. Rosenthal N, Insogna KL, Godsall JW, et al: Elevations in circulating 1,25 dihydroxyvitamin D in three patients with lymphoma-associated hypercalcemia. J Clin Endocrinol Metab 60:29–33, 1985.
78. Breslau NA, McGuire JL, Zerwekh JE, et al: Hypercalcemia associated with increased serum 1,25 dihydroxyvitamin D in three patients with lymphoma. Ann Intern Med 100:1, 1984.
79. Seymour JF, Gagel RF, Hagemeister FB, et al: Calcitriol production in hypercalcemia and normocalcemia patients with non-Hodgkin lymphoma. Ann Intern Med 121:633–640, 1994.
80. Stewart AF, Broadus AE, Schwartz PE, et al: Hypercalcemia in gynecologic neoplasms. Cancer 49:2389–2394, 1982.
81. Bringhurst FR, Bierer BE, Godeau F, et al: Humoral hypercalcemia of malignancy. J Clin Invest 77:456–464, 1986.
82. Bringhurst FR, Varner V, Segre GV: Cancer-associated hypercalcemia: Characterization of a new bone-resorbing factor (abstract). Clin Res 30:386, 1982.
83. Yang K, Stewart AF: Therapy of hypercalcemia. *In* Mazzaferri EL, Bar RS, Kreisberg RA (eds): Advances in Endocrinology and Metabolism, vol 4. St Louis, Mosby, 1993, pp 305–334.
84. Shane E: Hypercalcemia: Pathogenesis, clinical manifestations, differential diagnosis, and management. *In* Favus M (ed): Primer on the Metabolic Bone Disease and Disorders of Mineral Metabolism, ed 3. Philadelphia, Lippincott-Raven, 1996, pp 177–181.
85. Bilezikian JP: Management of acute hypercalcemia. N Engl J Med 326:1196–1203, 1992.

Chapter 78

Medical Management of Hypercalcemia

Joel S. Finkelstein

Hypercalcemia is a common clinical disorder that sometimes develops in the setting of an obvious underlying illness or is detected by routine laboratory testing in asymptomatic individuals. Primary hyperparathyroidism is the most common cause of hypercalcemia in the general population. Medical management of patients with primary hyperparathyroidism is discussed in Chapter 76. This chapter will focus on the medical management of patients with hypercalcemia resulting from other disorders.

Understanding the pathogenesis of hypercalcemia in each individual patient is helpful to guide therapy. Hypercalcemia is usually caused by excessive osteoclastic bone resorption. Thus agents that inhibit osteoclastic bone resorption are the mainstays of therapy for hypercalcemia. In some patients, increases in intestinal calcium absorption or alterations in renal calcium excretion may contribute to or even be the sole cause of hypercalcemia. In such patients, restricting dietary calcium intake or increasing renal calcium excretion is beneficial.

Recent advances in the management of skeletal complications in patients with cancer appear to be changing the natural history of hypercalcemia of malignancy. Many patients with skeletal involvement by breast cancer, multiple myeloma, or other malignancies affecting the skeleton receive bisphosphonates on a regular basis to reduce the frequency of skeletal complications. As a consequence, hypercalcemia of malignancy is less common than it was several years ago.

Rapid treatment of hypercalcemia is indicated when the serum calcium level is markedly elevated or if the patient has symptoms attributable to hypercalcemia, particularly alterations in mental status. In patients with mild hypercalcemia who are not symptomatic, treatment may be delayed or may not be necessary at all.

OVERVIEW

Although many agents are available to lower serum calcium levels, the current mainstays of therapy are the bisphosphonates and hydration with or without forced diuresis. In selected patients, calcitonin, glucocorticoids, and/or dialysis may also be useful. Plicamycin, phosphate, gallium nitrate, and indomethacin are rarely used today.

The only methods to lower serum calcium levels rapidly (i.e., within hours) are rehydration, forced diuresis, intravenous infusion of phosphate, administration of calcitonin, or dialysis. Thus when emergency treatment of hypercalcemia is needed, one or more of these therapeutic modalities should be used. Patients with severe hypercalcemia are almost always severely dehydrated. Rapid administration of isotonic saline will lower serum calcium levels in most patients and is generally indicated, except in occasional patients with renal insufficiency or cardiac failure. Because severe hypercalcemia is almost always due to accelerated bone resorption, intravenous bisphosphonate therapy should be administered concurrently with isotonic saline rehydration. The onset of bisphosphonate action is delayed for approximately 24 to 48 hours, however, and the maximal effect is not usually seen for several days. Calcitonin therapy will generally lower serum calcium levels by 1 to 3 mg/dL within a few hours and is helpful in patients with severe hypercalcemia. The effects of calcitonin therapy are generally short-lived, however, because tachyphylaxis develops within a few days. Intravenous phosphate therapy is rarely used today but is very effective and can be used in patients with concomitant hypophosphatemia. Patients with life-threatening hypercalcemia who cannot be managed effectively with saline rehydration and calcitonin administration should undergo dialysis.

In patients with malignancy, hypercalcemia is generally a late event and survival is usually limited to months. Survival is shorter in patients with more severe hypercalcemia[1]; such patients may require vigorous treatment, at least until the overall clinical situation is assessed.[2] Treatment of hypercalcemia in patients with malignancy may improve the quality of life, and if successful in normalizing serum calcium levels, survival may be slightly prolonged.[3] In patients with advanced malignancies that fail to respond to medical or surgical therapy, treatment of hypercalcemia may not be indicated because the effect on longevity is minimal and the sedating effect of hypercalcemia itself may be desirable. The major medical therapies for hypercalcemia are summarized in Table 78–1.

MODES OF THERAPY

Rehydration and Forced Diuresis

Renal calcium reabsorption occurs primarily in the proximal tubule and the ascending limb of the loop of Henle. At these sites, calcium reabsorption is a passive process stimulated by the flow of sodium and water across the intercellular pathway (solvent drag) and by a favorable electrochemical gradient. Therefore, strategies that increase urinary sodium excretion also facilitate urinary calcium excretion. Active calcium reabsorption against a steep electrochemical gradient occurs mainly in the distal tubule and is regulated by parathyroid hormone (PTH). Also playing a significant role in renal calcium transport (see Chapter 80) are the G protein–coupled calcium sensor receptor and perhaps 1,25-$(OH)_2$ vitamin D, among other factors.

Hypercalcemia, especially when severe, is associated with a cycle of decreasing renal concentrating capacity, dehydration, decreased renal blood flow, decreased glomerular filtration rate, and increased calcium reabsorption. If hypercalcemia persists, particularly with elevated serum inorganic phosphate levels, calcium phosphate crystals are deposited in the tubules, which may impair renal tubular function and lead to further losses of sodium and water. Because hypercalcemia is usually due to increased bone resorption, efflux of calcium into the extracellular fluid continues despite increased proximal tubular reabsorption of calcium, and serum calcium levels rise.

Rehydration is generally the first mode of therapy for patients with severe hypercalcemia. Both water and salt need to be replenished. Five to 10 L of isotonic saline is often needed within the initial 24 hours of therapy to restore extracellular volume status. Restoring extracellular volume to normal increases the glomerular filtration rate and the filtered load of calcium in the kidney. Restoring salt and water

TABLE 78–1. Summary of Major Medical Therapies for Hypercalcemia

Treatment	Onset of Action	Duration of Action	Advantages	Disadvantages
Rehydration	Hours	During treatment	Rapid action Rehydration invariably needed	None
Forced saline diuresis (with or without loop diuretics)	Hours	During treatment	Rapid action	Modest calcium-lowering effect Potential for volume overload Electrolyte disturbance Transient efficacy Inconvenient for patients
Etidronate	1–3 days	5–7 days	1st-generation bisphosphonate Well tolerated Normalizes calcium levels in many patients	3-day infusion protocol Less effective than other bisphosphonates
Pamidronate	1–2 days	Weeks to months	2nd-generation bisphosphonate Normalizes calcium levels in most patients Prolonged duration of action Single infusion can be given over 2–4 hr	Fever in 20% of patients Occasional hypocalcemia, hypophosphatemia, and hypomagnesemia
Alendronate	2–3 days	10–14 days	2nd-generation bisphosphonate Normalizes calcium levels in most patients	Fever in 25% of patients Not available for IV use in USA
Zoledronate	1–2 days	Weeks to months	3rd-generation bisphosphonate More potent than 2nd-generation bisphosphonates Normalizes calcium levels in over 90% of patients Can be given in 30 min or less	Fever in 30% of patients Hypophosphatemia in 20% of patients Hypocalcemia in 10% of patients Not currently available in USA
Calcitonin	Hours	3–7 days	Rapid onset of action	Modest calcium-lowering effect Tachyphylaxis develops in a few days Nausea in 10%–15% of patients Occasional flushing or abdominal cramps
Gallium nitrate	5 days	7–10 days	Normalizes calcium levels in most patients	Must be infused continuously over 5 days Occasional nephrotoxicity or hypophosphatemia
Plicamycin	1–2 days	7–10 days	Normalizes calcium levels in most patients	Nephrotoxicity Thrombocytopenia Hepatotoxicity Nausea in 30% of patients
Intravenous phosphate	Hours	During use and for 24–48 hr afterward	Rapid onset of action Highly potent	Ectopic calcifications Hypotension Renal failure Severe hypocalcemia
Oral phosphate	24 hr	During use	Minimal toxicity if serum phosphate is low	Modest calcium-lowering effect Diarrhea
Glucocorticoids	Days	Days to weeks	Oral administration	Only effective in a minority of patients Glucocorticoid side effects
Dialysis	Hours	During use and for 24–48 hr afterward	Rapid onset of action Useful in patients with renal failure and heart failure Useful to treat life-threatening hypercalcemia	Complex procedure Reserved for extreme or special circumstances

balance alone can increase urinary calcium excretion by 100 to 300 mg/day. Serum calcium levels often decrease by 2 to 3 mg/dL. In a series of 16 patients with moderately severe hypercalcemia (mean serum calcium level of 14.6 mg/dL), administration of 4 L of isotonic saline per day lowered serum calcium levels by 2.16 mg/dL.[4] Maintaining adequate hydration is essential to prevent further increases in serum calcium levels.

The clearance of calcium parallels that of sodium. Administering larger amounts of isotonic saline to produce volume expansion inhibits proximal tubular sodium reabsorption and increases the delivery of sodium, calcium, and water to the loop of Henle. A potent loop diuretic such as furosemide or ethacrynic acid can then be administered to block calcium transport at this site and potentiate urinary calcium excretion. The combination of aggressive sodium loading and a potent loop diuretic (e.g., furosemide in doses of 80–120 mg every 3 hours) can increase urinary calcium excretion to 1000 mg/day or more (mean excretion of 1900 mg/day) and decrease serum calcium levels by as much as 4 mg/dL within 24 hours.[5] Careful attention to magnesium and potassium balance is required because significant urinary losses of potassium and magnesium are virtually inevitable. In addition, congestive heart failure can be precipitated, particularly in patients with underlying cardiac disease or severe renal impairment. In such patients, monitoring of central venous pressure or pulmonary capillary wedge pressure may be indicated. Careful monitoring of fluid intake and output, which is facilitated by the use of a bladder catheter, is essential. Loop diuretics should be administered only after intravascular volume has been replenished. Overzealous use of loop diuretics without complete restoration of intravascular volume status will exacerbate hypercalcemia. Before the advent of bisphosphonate therapy, forced diuresis with a loop diuretic was routinely used to treat patients with severe hypercalcemia. With early administration of bisphosphonates and vigorous administration of isotonic saline, forced diuresis with loop diuretics is not routinely required.

Bisphosphonates

The bisphosphonates are analogues of pyrophosphate in which the two phosphate groups are joined by a carbon atom rather than an oxygen atom. Because they are resistant to cleavage by pyrophosphatases, they are stable in the body. The bisphosphonates have two fundamental biologic effects: inhibition of calcification and inhibition of bone resorption. They have a high affinity for the surface of solid-phase calcium phosphate, where they bind to calcium by chemisorption.[6] Bisphosphonates are concentrated in areas of high bone turnover, are taken up by osteoclasts, and are potent inhibitors of bone destruction. Table 78–2 lists the most commonly used bisphosphonates and indicates their relative potency for inhibiting osteoclastic bone resorption.

Bisphosphonates appear to inhibit calcification by a pure physiochemical mechanism whereby they inhibit aggregation of calcium phosphate crystals.[6] Such inhibition requires continuous presence of the bisphosphonate.[6] The more potent bisphosphonates inhibit bone resorption at doses that do not seem to inhibit calcification.[6]

The mechanisms whereby bisphosphonates inhibit osteoclastic bone resorption are complex and not completely understood. At least five mechanisms appear to be involved at the cellular level: (1) inhibition of osteoclast differentiation and recruitment, (2) inhibition of osteoclastic adhesion to the bone surface, (3) a decrease in osteoclast life span, (4) inhibition of osteoclast activity, and (5) a delay in the dissolution of calcium phosphate crystals.[6, 7] All the proposed mechanisms could be due to the direct action of bisphosphonates on osteoclasts or indirect actions on cells that interact with osteoclasts.

The inhibitory effect of bisphosphonates on osteoclast recruitment appears to occur at the terminal step of osteoclastic precursor differentiation and requires the involvement of other cells, probably osteoblasts.[6] When osteoblastic cells are exposed to bisphosphonates, their conditioned medium contains a factor(s) that decreases osteoclastic bone resorption in vitro.[8] The evidence that bisphosphonates decrease adhesion of osteoclasts to the mineralized matrix is ambiguous. A shortening of osteoclast life span could be due to a toxic effect on osteoclasts, which has been demonstrated at very high concentrations of bisphosphonates, or to induction of programmed cell death (apoptosis) of osteoclasts.[9] Finally, bisphosphonates may impair osteoclast activity. Bisphosphonates are selectively taken up by osteoclasts and can induce changes in their morphology.[7] They may inhibit osteoclast activity by altering the osteoclast's proton pump function, which is necessary to dissolve the inorganic component of bone,[10] or by impairing the release of acid hydrolases in the extracellular lysosomes contiguous with mineralized bone.[6]

The molecular events that decrease osteoclast formation, osteoclast life span, and osteoclast activity are currently being investigated. Possibilities include an action of bisphosphonates on a cell surface receptor and/or uptake of bisphosphonates by the cell with subsequent interactions with specific enzymes or other molecules that affect cellular metabolism.[7] No bisphosphonate receptor has been identified, but the observation that effects on osteoblasts occur with short exposure and at low bisphosphonate concentrations is consistent with a receptor-mediated event.[6, 7] Although it is known that bisphosphonates are taken up by osteoclasts, subsequent intracellular events are not well understood. Recent studies indicate that aminobisphosphonates such as pamidronate or alendronate inhibit posttranslational modification of proteins with farnesyl or geranylgeranyl isoprenoid groups, a property that is not shared by bisphosphonates that lack the amino group.[11–13] Moreover, farnesylpyrophosphate or geranylgeranylpyrophosphate prevents aminobisphosphonate-induced apoptosis.[11, 14–16] These findings suggest that aminobisphosphonates cause apoptosis through a mechanism involving prenylation of proteins. Other bisphosphonates appear to work through other mechanisms. For example, tiludronate inhibits the activity of the vacuolar-type proton ATPase in the ruffled border membrane of osteoclasts more effectively than do other bisphosphonates.[17] Clodronate, etidronate, and tiludronate can be metabolized intracellularly to a cytotoxic $\beta\gamma$-methylene analogue of ATP, whereas aminobisphosphonates are not metabolized in this way.[13] Bisphosphonates also inhibit certain protein tyrosine phosphatases that may be involved in c-src activation of osteoclasts.[18]

Disodium dichloromethylene diphosphonate (clodronate) was the first bisphosphonate used to treat hypercalcemia of malignancy in humans. Blood calcium levels decreased in 4 of 5 patients with hypercalcemia secondary to breast or renal cell cancer after treatment for 4 weeks with 3200 mg of oral clodronate.[19] Intravenous clodronate therapy (2.5–5.0 mg/kg for up to 7 days) normalized serum calcium levels in 11 of 12 patients with malignancy-associated hypercalcemia[20] and reduced serum calcium levels markedly in 4 of 5 patients with parathyroid carcinoma.[21] Intravenous clodronate also reduced urinary calcium and hydroxyproline excretion, consistent with its inhibitory effect on bone resorption.[20] Randomized controlled trials subsequently confirmed the efficacy of clodronate for the treatment of hypercalcemia of malignancy.[22] In one study of hypercalcemic patients with breast cancer and bone metastases, serum calcium levels normalized in 17 of 21 patients treated with clodronate as compared with only 4 of 19 controls.[23] Clodronate lowers serum calcium levels more effectively in patients with increased bone resorption and normal tubular reabsorption of calcium than in patients with high tubular reabsorption of calcium.[24] Despite these promising initial results, clodronate was withdrawn from the market in the United States because of preliminary reports that it might be associated with leukemia, although this concern has not been substantiated by subsequent experience in other countries.[25, 26]

Ethane-1-hydroxy-1,1-diphosphonate (etidronate) was the next bisphosphonate to be used for the treatment of hypercalcemia. In noncontrolled studies, serum calcium levels normalized in 73% to 100% of patients with hypercalcemia of malignancy when 7.5 mg/kg/day of etidronate was administered intravenously for up to 7 consecutive days; the mean response time was approximately 3 days.[27, 28] In a small double-blind, placebo-controlled trial, serum calcium levels normalized in 11 of 12 patients with hypercalcemia of malignancy who received intravenous etidronate vs. 2 of 6 controls.[29] In a multicenter, double-blind, placebo-controlled trial involving 202 patients with hypercalcemia of malignancy, serum calcium levels normalized in 63% of etidronate-treated patients and 33% of controls, although the response rates were much lower in both groups when serum calcium levels were adjusted for serum albumin levels.[30] Occasionally, the subsequent administration of oral etidronate may help maintain normocalcemia. Treatment with intravenous etidronate is well tolerated, the only notable side effects being occasional alterations in the sense of taste, nausea, and increases in serum creatinine and phosphate levels.[30] Because it impairs bone mineralization at the doses needed to reduce

TABLE 78–2. Relative Potency of the Major Bisphosphonates for Inhibition of Bone Resorption in the Rat

Compound	Relative Potency
Etidronate	1
Clodronate	10
Tiludronate	10
Pamidronate	100
Neridronate	100
Alendronate	100–1000
EBA-153	100–1000
Incadronate	100–1000
Olpadronate	100–1000
Ibandronate	1000–10,000
Risedronate	1000–10,000
YH 529	>10,000
Zoledronate	>10,000

Reproduced from Rodan GA, Fleisch HA: Bisphosphonates: Mechanisms of action. J Clin Invest 97:2692–2696, 1996 by copyright permission of the American Society for Clinical Investigation.

serum calcium levels and because more potent bisphosphonates are now available, etidronate is rarely used to treat hypercalcemia.

Aminohydroxypropylidene bisphosphonate (pamidronate), one of several aminobisphosphonates, is a much more potent inhibitor of osteoclastic bone resorption than is etidronate and is currently the preferred bisphosphonate for treating hypercalcemia. Pamidronate is usually administered as a single intravenous infusion in a dosage of 30 to 90 mg, depending on the severity of the hypercalcemia. Serum calcium levels normalize in most patients with hypercalcemia of malignancy after the administration of 30 to 90 mg of intravenous pamidronate.[31–38] For example, in 50 patients with cancer and a corrected serum calcium greater than 12 mg/dL, serum calcium levels normalized in all patients treated with 90 mg of pamidronate, 61% of patients treated with 60 mg of pamidronate, and 40% of patients treated with 30 mg of pamidronate[37] (Fig. 78–1). The likelihood that the serum calcium level will normalize is related to both the dose of pamidronate administered and the severity of the initial hypercalcemia.[31–39] In addition, pamidronate is somewhat less effective in patients with increased levels of PTH-related protein (PTHrP) and patients without demonstrable bone metastases.[40–44] The mechanism of relative resistance to bisphosphonates in patients with high PTHrP levels is not known. The major determinant of response duration, however, is the dose of pamidronate.[34, 39] Responsiveness to pamidronate declines with repeated administration.[43, 45, 46]

The most common side effect of intravenous pamidronate therapy is fever, which occurs in approximately 20% of patients and may be related to release of cytokines from osteoclasts, monocytes, and macrophages.[47–49] Fever is generally mild (less than 2°C) and typically occurs only once in a patient's lifetime, even if treatment is discontinued and restarted later.[6] Other side effects of pamidronate include hypocalcemia, hypophosphatemia, hypomagnesemia, and possibly reversible hepatotoxicity.[32, 36–38, 50–52]

Although pamidronate was administered over a 24-hour period in many early studies, subsequent studies have demonstrated that it is equally effective and possibly even more effective when administered over a 2- to 4-hour period.[53–55] In fact, recent studies in patients with breast cancer and Paget's disease suggest that the infusion time for pamidronate can probably be safely reduced to 1 hour,[56–58] although the prevalence of local reactions and fever may be increased.[59]

Several studies have compared the efficacy of different bisphosphonates in patients with hypercalcemia of malignancy. One report indicated that clodronate (500 mg/day intravenously) and etidronate (500 mg/day intravenously) were equally effective in lowering serum calcium levels.[60] In a randomized, double-blind comparison of pamidronate (60 mg intravenously over a 24-hour period) and etidronate (7.5 mg/kg intravenously daily for 3 days), serum calcium levels normalized in 21 of 30 (70%) pamidronate-treated patients vs. only 14 of 34 (41%) etidronate-treated patients.[61] At the doses typically used, pamidronate is also more effective than intravenous clodronate,[51, 62] etidronate,[51] or plicamycin[63–65] in lowering serum calcium levels and maintaining normocalcemia in patients with hypercalcemia of malignancy (Fig. 78–2).

A number of other bisphosphonates have been used to treat patients with cancer-related hypercalcemia. Intravenous alendronate, given as a single dose of 5 to 15 mg over a 2-hour period (or 10 mg over a period of 24 hours), normalizes serum calcium levels in most patients.[52, 66] Intravenous alendronate (7.5 mg) lowers serum calcium levels more effectively than does intravenous clodronate (600 mg).[67] Other bisphosphonates, including ibandronate,[68, 69] neridronate,[70] and cycloheptylaminomethylene bisphosphonate (YM 175),[71] also normalize serum calcium levels in most patients with hypercalcemia of malignancy but do not appear to offer any advantage over pamidronate therapy. In contrast, tiludronate is less effective than other bisphosphonates for the treatment of cancer-related hypercalcemia and may cause nephrotoxicity at the doses required to control serum calcium levels.[72] Zoledronate, a third-generation bisphosphonate claimed to be 100 to

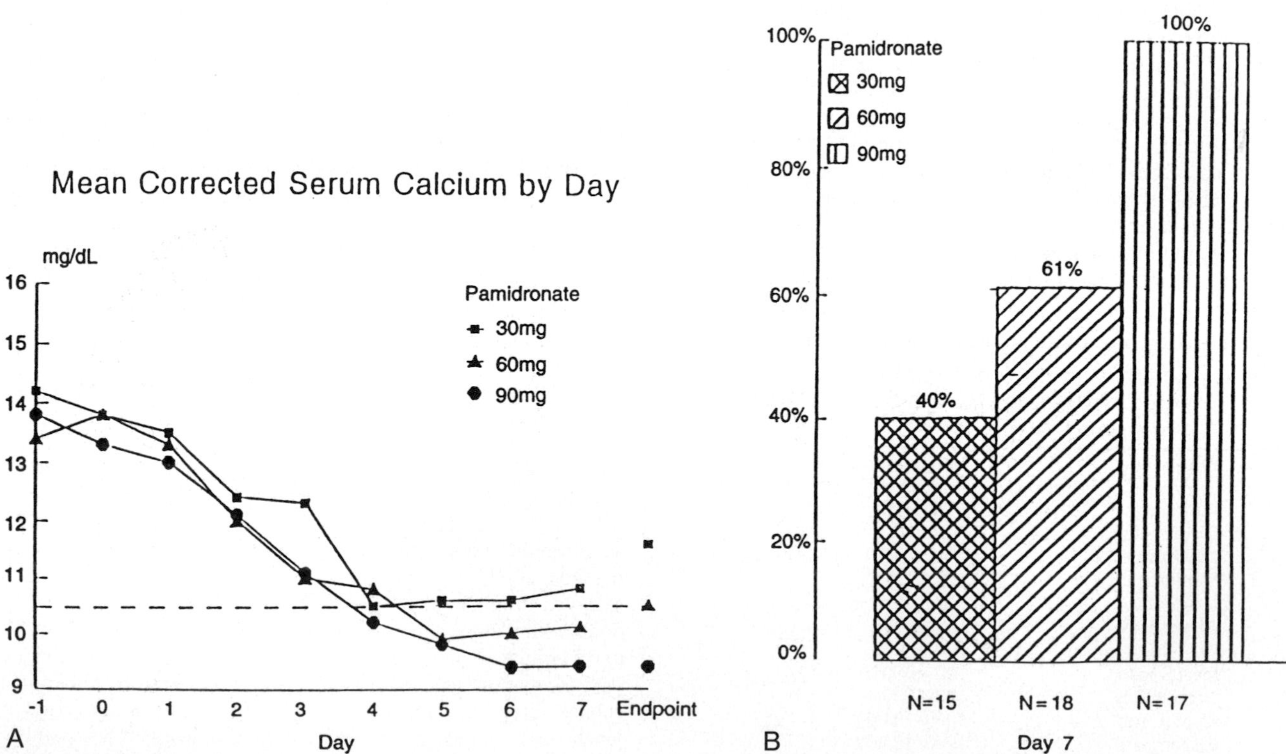

FIGURE 78–1. *A*, Time course of changes in mean corrected serum calcium levels in patients with hypercalcemia of malignancy after treatment with intravenous pamidronate at a dosage of 30 mg *(squares)*, 60 mg *(triangles)*, or 90 mg *(circles)* over a 24-hour period. *B*, Percentage of patients whose serum calcium levels normalized after treatment with 30, 60, or 90 mg of intravenous pamidronate. (From Nussbaum SR, Younger J, Vandepol CJ, et al: Single-dose intravenous therapy with pamidronate for the treatment of hypercalcemia of malignancy: Comparison of 30-, 60-, and 90-mg doses. Am J Med 95:297–304, 1993. Copyright 1993, with permission from Excerpta Medica Inc.)

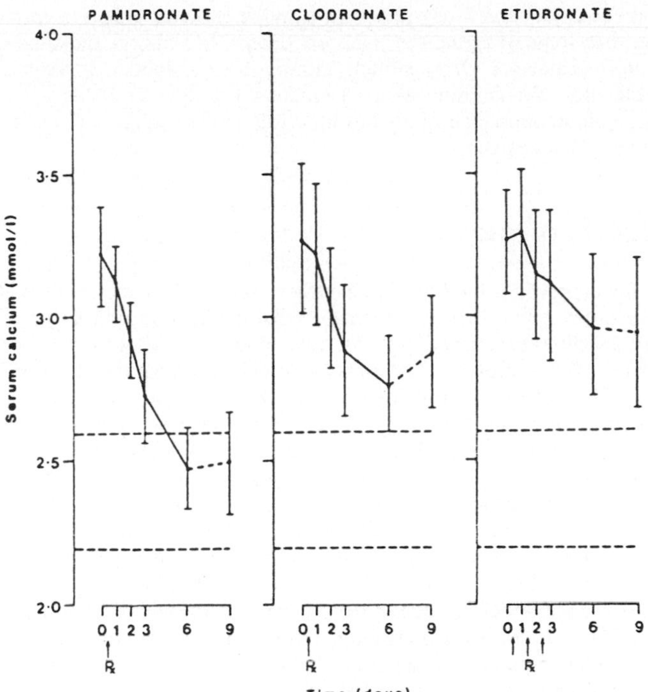

FIGURE 78–2. Time course of changes in serum calcium levels in patients with hypercalcemia of malignancy after treatment with intravenous pamidronate (30 mg over a 4-hour period), clodronate (600 mg over a 6-hour period), or etidronate (7.5 mg/kg over a period of 2 hours for 3 consecutive days). (From Ralston SH, Patel U, Fraser WD, et al: Comparison of three intravenous bisphosphonates in cancer-associated hypercalcaemia. Lancet 2:1180–1182, © by The Lancet Ltd., 1989.)

850 times more potent than pamidronate,[73] may normalize serum calcium levels more rapidly and maintain normocalcemia longer than other agents, however.[74, 75] In an open-label, dose-finding study, serum calcium levels normalized in 19 of 20 patients with cancer-related hypercalcemia after a single infusion of 0.02 or 0.04 mg/kg of zoledronate given over a period of 20 to 50 minutes (median, 30 minutes)[75] (Fig. 78–3). The only detectable side effect was an increase in body temperature in 30% of patients.[75] Zoledronate is currently being tested as a 5- to 10-minute infusion. If zoledronate (or other bisphosphonates) can be administered rapidly with good efficacy and minimal toxicity, it may become the drug of choice for the treatment of cancer-related hypercalcemia in the future.

Bisphosphonates have also been used successfully to treat patients with hypercalcemia that is not associated with malignancy when bone resorption is increased. For example, pamidronate reduces serum calcium levels in patients with vitamin D intoxication[76–79] and is more effective than glucocorticoid therapy.[77] Pamidronate therapy generally normalizes serum calcium levels in patients with hypercalcemia caused by immobilization,[80–83] even after hydration and calcitonin therapy have failed.[81, 82] Pamidronate has also been used to treat hypercalcemia associated with thyrotoxicosis,[84] primary oxalosis,[85] and coccidioidomycosis.[86]

Recently, bisphosphonates have been used to prevent skeletal complications, including hypercalcemia, in patients with malignancies.[87] In patients with stage III multiple myeloma and at least one lytic bone lesion, intravenous pamidronate (90 mg every 4 weeks) reduces the number of skeletal events and improves the quality of life.[88, 89] Similar results have been reported in patients with stage IV breast cancer and at least one lytic bone lesion.[90–92] Oral clodronate therapy (1600 mg daily) also reduces the number of skeletal complications, including hypercalcemia, in patients with recurrent breast cancer.[93, 94] Finally, oral clodronate therapy (1600 mg daily) reduces the number of both osseous and visceral metastases in patients with breast cancer and tumor cells in the bone marrow.[95] As the prophylactic use of bisphosphonates to prevent skeletal complications in patients with malignancies has become more common, the incidence of hypercalcemia of malignancy is declining dramatically.

Plicamycin (Mithramycin)

Plicamycin, which is also known as mithramycin, is a tumoricidal antibiotic derived from an actinomycete of the genus *Streptomyces* and was initially used to treat patients with embryonal cell carcinoma of the testis.[96] Marked hypocalcemia was observed in some patients who received plicamycin therapy. Plicamycin is an inhibitor of RNA synthesis in osteoclasts and may interfere with the differentiation of osteoclast precursors into mature osteoclasts.[26, 96] Plicamycin localizes in areas of active bone resorption and inhibits bone resorption directly. It inhibits the release of $^{45}Ca^{2+}$ from fetal rat bones in response to PTH in vitro,[97] prevents PTH-induced increases in serum calcium in vivo,[98] and may also inhibit renal tubular calcium reabsorption.[96]

Before the clinical availability of potent bisphosphonates, plicamycin was often the preferred agent for the treatment of severe hypercalcemia. When given in doses of 15 to 25 μg/kg intravenously over a period of 4 to 6 hours, the serum calcium level falls within 24 to 48 hours.[26, 65, 99–101] Subsequent studies indicated that it is less effective than pamidronate, however. In a randomized study of patients with cancer-related hypercalcemia, pamidronate normalized serum calcium levels in 88% of patients as compared with only 45% of patients treated with plicamycin. Moreover, the duration of normocalcemia is longer with pamidronate therapy than with plicamycin.[64, 65] Plicamycin is associated with several important side effects, including nephrotoxicity,[102, 103] thrombocytopenia,[102, 104, 105] and hepatic toxicity.[102, 106] Factor II, V, VII, and X levels are often decreased and the prothrombin time is frequently increased.[104] Nausea and vomiting occur in approximately one-third of patients treated with plicamycin[64] but can be minimized by slow intravenous infusion.[26] Toxicity from plicamycin therapy is more common when multiple doses are administered, particularly if given at short intervals.[26] Overall, the advent of more potent agents with less toxicity has led to a marked decline in plicamycin use.

Calcitonin

Calcitonin, a naturally occurring peptide made by the parafollicular cells within the thyroid gland in humans, inhibits bone resorption and

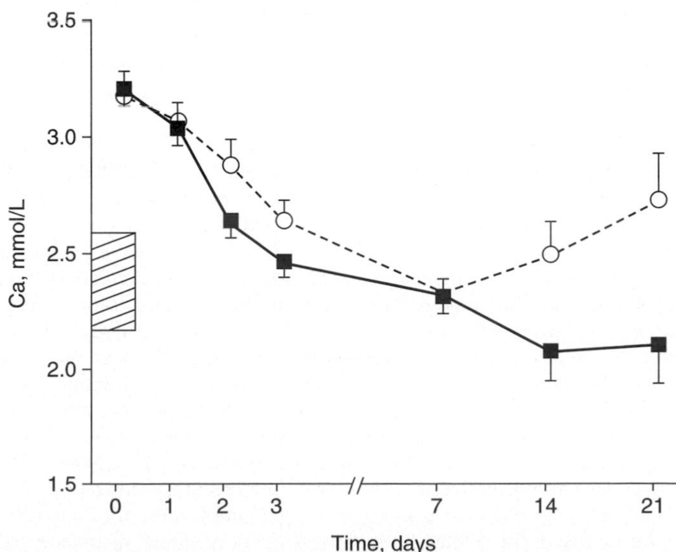

FIGURE 78–3. Time course of changes in serum calcium levels in patients with hypercalcemia of malignancy after treatment with a single intravenous dose of zoledronate, 0.02 mg/kg *(open circles)* or 0.04 mg/kg *(closed squares)*. (From Body JJ, Lortholary A, Romieu G, et al: A dose-finding study of zoledronate in hypercalcemic cancer patients. J Bone Miner Res 14:1557–1561, 1999.)

decreases renal tubular calcium reabsorption.[26, 96, 107, 108] Calcitonin has a rapid onset of action, but its calcium-lowering effect is limited because of rapid tachyphylaxis.[109–111] For example, one early study reported that calcitonin lowered serum calcium levels by an average of 2 mg/dL with a peak effect in 6 hours.[112] In another report, calcitonin lowered serum calcium levels in 75% of subjects within 2 hours, half of whom became normocalcemic in several hours.[113] The calcium-lowering effect of calcitonin is clearly short-lived, however, with an increase in serum calcium levels often occurring within 48 to 96 hours despite continued calcitonin therapy.[26, 113–115] Thus calcitonin is less effective than clodronate[116] or gallium nitrate[114] in patients with hypercalcemia. Coadministration of glucocorticoids has been claimed to enhance or prolong the efficacy of calcitonin,[115, 117] but this combination is still less effective than either pamidronate or plicamycin therapy.[65]

Calcitonin has been used to treat hypercalcemia caused by malignancy,[107, 109, 110, 115, 116, 118–121] hyperparathyroidism,[109, 122, 123] parathyroid carcinoma,[124] thyrotoxicosis,[125] vitamin D intoxication,[123] and immobilization.[126, 127] Calcitonin may be less effective in patients with humoral hypercalcemia of malignancy than in patients with bone metastases[128] and is relatively ineffective in patients with hypercalcemia who are undergoing maintenance hemodialysis.[129]

Because of rapid tachyphylaxis, calcitonin has limited utility as a single agent for the treatment of hypercalcemia. It may be of considerable value, however, when combined with a bisphosphonate in patients with severe hypercalcemia in order to control the hypercalcemia more rapidly.[112, 118, 120, 130] The usual dosage of salmon calcitonin is 4 U/kg every 12 hours, although doses as high as 8 U/kg have been given every 6 hours.[26] Calcitonin also lowers serum calcium levels when administered by rectal suppository,[130, 131] but not when given by intranasal administration.[132] The most common side effects of calcitonin therapy are nausea and vomiting, which occur in approximately 10% to 15% of patients.[113] Other side effects include flushing and abdominal cramps.[26]

Gallium Nitrate

Hypocalcemia develops in many patients who receive anticancer therapy with gallium nitrate. This observation led investigators to examine the potential mechanisms and therapeutic potential of gallium nitrate as a calcium-lowering agent. Gallium nitrate inhibits the release of $^{45}Ca^{2+}$ from fetal rat bones in response to PTH and lymphokines[133] and inhibits the ability of cultured osteoclasts to resorb cortical bone in vitro.[134] It interacts with both hydroxyapatite and the cellular components of bone and accumulates preferentially in areas of active bone formation.[135] Gallium is adsorbed onto hydroxyapatite and appears to decrease hydroxyapatite formation and reduce the solubility of hydroxyapatite crystals.[26, 136]

Several studies have examined the potential efficacy of gallium nitrate in patients with cancer-related hypercalcemia. Continuous infusion of gallium nitrate for 5 to 7 days normalizes serum calcium levels in most patients with cancer-related hypercalcemia, and its effects appear to be dose related.[133, 137–139] Randomized studies have compared the efficacy of gallium nitrate with that of intramuscular salmon calcitonin and intravenous etidronate. In 50 patients with cancer-related hypercalcemia, serum calcium levels normalized in 75% of patients who received a continuous infusion of gallium nitrate (200 mg/m^2 for 5 days) vs. only 31% of patients who received intramuscular calcitonin (8 IU/kg every 6 hours for 5 days).[114] Normal serum calcium levels were maintained for a longer period in patients who received gallium nitrate therapy.[114] In a separate study of 71 patients with cancer-related hypercalcemia, serum calcium levels normalized in 82% of patients who received a continuous infusion of gallium nitrate (200 mg/m^2 infused for 5 days) vs. only 43% of patients who received intravenous etidronate (7.5 mg/kg infused for 5 days).[140] Once again, normal serum calcium levels were maintained for a longer period in patients who received gallium nitrate therapy.[140]

Despite these promising results, gallium nitrate is rarely used to treat hypercalcemia of malignancy. Gallium nitrate may cause nephrotoxicity or hypophosphatemia.[26] Moreover, because it must be infused continuously over a 5-day period, it is much less convenient to administer than some of the newer bisphosphonates. In addition, the duration of normocalcemia after gallium nitrate therapy (about 1 week) is shorter than the duration after treatment with other available agents. Thus gallium nitrate currently has little role in the treatment of patients with hypercalcemia.

Glucocorticoids

Glucocorticoids have multiple effects on calcium metabolism. In large doses, glucocorticoids increase renal calcium clearance and urinary calcium excretion,[141–143] decrease intestinal absorption of calcium,[141, 143] and promote mobilization of calcium from the skeleton.[143] The effects of glucocorticoids on the kidney and the intestine would tend to lower serum calcium levels and may contribute to the beneficial effects of glucocorticoid therapy in selected individuals with hypercalcemia.

Hypercalcemia occurs in approximately 10% of patients with sarcoidosis; hypercalciuria is about three to five times more frequent.[144] Some patients with sarcoidosis who are normocalciuric and normocalcemic have elevated serum 1,25-dihydroxyvitamin D levels.[145, 146] These abnormalities are due to extrarenal conversion of 25-hydroxyvitamin D to 1,25-dihydroxyvitamin D by activated mononuclear cells (predominantly macrophages) in the lungs and lymph nodes.[146–149] Hypercalcemia in association with increased serum 1,25-dihydroxyvitamin D levels is seen in patients with other granulomatous diseases, including tuberculosis,[150, 151] Crohn's disease,[152] and malignant lymphoma.[153–156] Elevated serum 1,25-dihydroxyvitamin D levels appear to be responsible for almost all cases of hypercalcemia in patients with Hodgkin's disease and about one-third of cases of hypercalcemia in patients with non-Hodgkin's lymphoma.[155, 156]

Serum calcium levels do not change when glucocorticoids are administered to normal subjects[141] or subjects with primary hyperparathyroidism, except in some patients with radiographic evidence of osteitis fibrosa cystica.[157–159] Similarly, glucocorticoids have little effect on serum calcium levels in most patients with hypercalcemia of malignancy, except in individuals with multiple myeloma, lymphomas, or other hematologic malignancies.[160–162] Glucocorticoids are highly effective, however, for the treatment of hypercalcemia caused by vitamin D intoxication,[163–165] sarcoidosis,[144, 166–172] tuberculosis,[173] Crohn's disease,[152] Wegener's granulomatosis,[174] and certain hematologic malignancies such as multiple myeloma, Hodgkin's disease, non-Hodgkin's lymphomas, and some leukemias. Low to moderate doses of glucocorticoids (10–40 mg/day of prednisone) reduce serum 1,25-dihydroxyvitamin D levels[168, 169, 175] and are usually sufficient to normalize serum calcium levels in patients with sarcoidosis, although higher doses may be needed in patients with lymphoma[155] or vitamin D intoxication.[163] Serum calcium levels usually begin to fall within the first 2 days of therapy, but the peak response may require 7 to 10 days. In patients with granulomatous diseases, glucocorticoids appear to lower serum calcium levels by inhibiting 1,25-dihydroxyvitamin D synthesis by activated macrophages,[155, 169] although direct inhibition of intestinal calcium absorption may also be important.[143, 176] In patients with hematologic malignancies, glucocorticoids may reduce serum calcium levels by inhibiting the ability of tumor cells to resorb bone[177] or by inhibiting the growth of neoplastic tissue.[178]

Phosphate

Intravenous phosphate is one of the most rapid and dramatically effective therapies for hypercalcemia, but it is potentially dangerous. The ability of phosphate to reduce calcium levels has been known since the 1930s.[179, 180] Calcium kinetic studies demonstrate that calcium disappears from the circulation within minutes after starting a phosphate infusion, thus suggesting that calcium and phosphate are precipitated from the circulation. Phosphate administration lowers serum calcium levels even though urinary calcium excretion is also reduced. The extent to which phosphate administration lowers serum calcium levels is directly proportional to the magnitude by which the hydroxyapatite solubility product is exceeded during the phosphate infusion.[181]

Many studies have demonstrated the efficacy of intravenous phosphate for the treatment of hypercalcemia. Intravenous administration of 100 mmol (3.1 g) of phosphate over a 24-hour period normalized serum calcium levels in 16 of 20 patients with hypercalcemia of malignancy or hyperparathyroidism (average decrease of 5.6 mg/dL) with no adverse effects.[182] Oral or intravenous administration of phosphate normalized serum calcium levels in 7 patients with multiple myeloma,[183] in 7 of 13 patients with solid tumors (mostly breast and squamous cell carcinomas),[184] and in 15 of 18 patients with mixed causes of hypercalcemia.[185] Sodium-potassium phosphate reduces serum calcium levels more effectively than does sodium sulfate or hydrocortisone, and the effects are dose related.[160] The serum calcium level often remains suppressed for several days after a single phosphate infusion, which suggests that precipitation of calcium phosphate is not the only mechanism whereby phosphate therapy lowers serum calcium levels.[160] For example, hypophosphatemia itself can increase bone resorption.

Intravenous phosphate therapy is quite risky, particularly in patients with normal or elevated serum phosphate levels. It may cause precipitation of calcium phosphate in the kidney, heart, lungs, and other soft tissues.[186, 187] Fatal hypotension and acute renal failure have also been reported, particularly when phosphate is infused rapidly.[186, 188] In patients with hypophosphatemia, however, intravenous phosphate therapy is reasonably safe and should be considered in patients with life-threatening hypercalcemia, particularly when concomitant cardiovascular disease or hemodynamic instability might complicate the use of isotonic saline or dialysis.

In contrast to intravenous phosphate therapy, oral phosphate therapy is quite safe but much less effective for the treatment of hypercalcemia. In one study, oral phosphate therapy normalized serum calcium levels in five of six patients with primary hyperparathyroidism but in only one of five patients with hypercalcemia of malignancy.[189] The dose of phosphate should be titrated so that peak serum phosphate levels remain less than 4.0 mg/dL. When given in typical doses of 250 to 500 mg four times daily, troublesome diarrhea develops in many patients. Hyperphosphatemia and azotemia are contraindications to phosphate therapy.

Other Therapies

Prostaglandins, particularly prostaglandin E_2, have been implicated as local mediators of bone resorption in some patients with cancer-related hypercalcemia.[190–193] Circulating prostaglandin E levels or urinary metabolites of prostaglandin E are elevated in some patients with solid tumors, particularly in the setting of hypercalcemia.[194–198] In some patients, prostaglandin inhibitors such as indomethacin or salicylates may help control hypercalcemia. Prostaglandin inhibitors reduce serum calcium levels in occasional patients with renal cell carcinoma,[197, 199–202] multiple myeloma,[200] and other solid tumors,[194, 198, 203] particularly when prostaglandin E levels are elevated.[196, 197] In general, however, prostaglandin inhibitors have little role in the treatment of patients with hypercalcemia of malignancy.

Ketoconazole, an antifungal agent that inhibits steroid hormone synthesis, reduces 1,25-dihydroxyvitamin D levels in normal subjects. Ketoconazole also reduces serum 1,25-dihydroxyvitamin D levels in patients with primary hyperparathyroidism or hypercalcemia of unknown etiology, but the effect on serum calcium levels is small.[204] In patients with sarcoidosis, ketoconazole reduces serum 1,25-dihydroxyvitamin D levels and may lower serum calcium levels,[205, 206] although not all studies have shown this effect.[207] Ketoconazole also reduces serum 1,25-dihydroxyvitamin D and calcium levels in some patients with tuberculosis.[208]

It has been known for many years that the hypercalcemia of sarcoidosis can be treated effectively with chloroquine.[209, 210] Chloroquine reduces serum 1,25-dihydroxyvitamin D levels without altering serum 25-hydroxyvitamin D levels, which suggests that it inhibits 1α-hydroxylase activity.[210, 211] Similar results have been reported with hydroxychloroquine therapy.[212] Chloroquine therapy can also reduce serum calcium and 1,25-dihydroxyvitamin D levels in patients with other granulomatous diseases such as Wegener's granulomatosis.[213] Hydroxychloroquine did not reduce serum calcium or 1,25-dihydroxyvitamin D levels in patients with B cell lymphomas, however.[214] These agents may provide a useful alternative for treating hypercalcemia associated with granulomatous diseases, particularly when glucocorticoid therapy is unsuccessful or contraindicated.

Dialysis

Hemodialysis or peritoneal dialysis against a low calcium bath can lower serum calcium levels rapidly and dramatically. The membranes of artificial kidneys are quite permeable to calcium, and as much as 682 mg of calcium can be cleared per hour with hemodialysis.[215] In a retrospective analysis of 33 patients with severe hypercalcemia of varying etiologies, calcium-free hemodialysis reduced serum calcium levels by an average of 6.9 mg/dL (1.71 mmol/L), but a partial rebound occurred in most patients within the first 24 hours.[216] Transient hypotension was noted in over one-third of patients but resolved with fluid replacement.[216] In another study of six patients with hypercalcemia of malignancy and renal failure, calcium-free hemodialysis reduced serum calcium levels without any adverse effects.[217] Peritoneal dialysis can remove 500 to 2000 mg of calcium and lower the serum calcium level by 3 to 12 mg/dL in 24 to 48 hours if a calcium-free dialysis solution is used.[218–220] In a patient with hypercalcemia and hypophosphatemia caused by primary hyperparathyroidism, hemodialysis using a phosphorus-enriched, conventional calcium solution corrected both the hypercalcemia and the hypophosphatemia.[221] Dialysis should be considered when rapid lowering of serum calcium levels is required, particularly in patients with renal failure or volume overload.

REFERENCES

1. Kristensen B, Ejlertsen B, Mouridsen HT, et al: Survival in breast cancer patients after the first episode of hypercalcaemia. J Intern Med 244:189–198, 1998.
2. Nussbaum SR, Neer RM, Potts JT Jr: Medical management of hyperparathyroidism and hypercalcemia. *In* DeGroot LJ (ed): Endocrinology, ed 3. Philadelphia, WB Saunders, 1995, pp 1094–1105.
3. Ling PJ, A'Hern RP, Hardy JR: Analysis of survival following treatment of tumour-induced hypercalcaemia with intravenous pamidronate (APD). Br J Cancer 72:206–209, 1995.
4. Hosking DJ, Cowley A, Bucknall CA: Rehydration in the treatment of severe hypercalcaemia. Q J Med 50:473–481, 1981.
5. Suki WN, Yium JJ, Von Minden M, et al: Acute treatment of hypercalcemia with furosemide. N Engl J Med 283:836–840, 1970.
6. Fleisch H: Bisphosphonates: Mechanism of action. Endocr Rev 19:80–100, 1998.
7. Rodan GA, Fleisch HA: Bisphosphonates: Mechanisms of action. J Clin Invest 97:2692–2696, 1996.
8. Sahni M, Guenther HL, Fleisch H, et al: Bisphosphonates act on rat bone resorption through the mediation of osteoblasts. J Clin Invest 91:2004–2011, 1993.
9. Hughes DE, Wright KR, Uy HL, et al: Bisphosphonates promote apoptosis in murine osteoblasts in vitro and in vivo. J Bone Miner Res 10:1478–1487, 1995.
10. Zimolo Z, Wesolowski G, Rodan GA: Acid extrusion is induced by osteoclast attachment to bone. Inhibition by alendronate and calcitonin. J Clin Invest 96:2277–2283, 1995.
11. Luckman SP, Hughes DE, Coxon FP, et al: Nitrogen-containing bisphosphonates inhibit the mevalonate pathway and prevent post-translational prenylation of GTP-binding proteins, including Ras. J Bone Miner Res 13:581–589, 1998.
12. van Beek E, Pieterman E, Cohen L, et al: Nitrogen-containing bisphosphonates inhibit isopentenyl pyrophosphate isomerase/farnesyl pyrophosphate synthase activity with relative potencies corresponding to their antiresorptive potencies in vitro and in vivo. Biochem Biophys Res Commun 255:491–494, 1999.
13. Benford HL, Frith JC, Auriola S, et al: Farnesol and geranylgeraniol prevent activation of caspases by aminobisphosphonates: Biochemical evidence for two distinct pharmacological classes of bisphosphonate drugs. Mol Pharmacol 56:131–140, 1999.
14. Rogers MJ, Frith JC, Luckman SP, et al: Molecular mechanisms of action of bisphosphonates. Bone 24(suppl 5):73–79, 1999.
15. Luckman SP, Coxon FP, Ebetino FH, et al: Heterocycle-containing bisphosphonates cause apoptosis and inhibit bone resorption by preventing protein prenylation: Evidence from structure-activity relationships in J774 macrophages. J Bone Miner Res 13:1668–1678, 1998.
16. Ciosek CP Jr, Magnin DR, Harrity TW, et al: Lipophilic 1,1-bisphosphonates are potent squalene synthase inhibitors and orally active cholesterol lowering agents in vivo. J Biol Chem 268:24832–24837, 1993.
17. David P, Nguyen H, Barbier A, et al: The bisphosphonate tiludronate is a potent inhibitor of the osteoclast vacuolar H(+)-ATPase. J Bone Miner Res 11:1498–1507, 1996.
18. Endo N, Rutledge SJ, Opas EE, et al: Human protein tyrosine phosphatase-sigma:

Alternative splicing and inhibition by bisphosphonates. J Bone Miner Res 11:535–543, 1996.

19. Chapuy MC, Meunier PJ, Alexandre CM, et al: Effects of disodium dichloromethylene diphosphonate on hypercalcemia produced by bone metastases. J Clin Invest 65:1243–1247, 1980.
20. Jacobs TP, Siris ES, Bilezikian JP, et al: Hypercalcemia of malignancy: Treatment with intravenous dichloromethylene diphosphonate. Ann Intern Med 94:312–316, 1981.
21. Shane E, Jacobs TP, Siris ES, et al: Therapy of hypercalcemia due to parathyroid carcinoma with intravenous dichloromethylene diphosphonate. Am J Med 72:939–944, 1982.
22. Witte RS, Koeller J, Davis TE, et al: Clodronate. A randomized study in the treatment of cancer-related hypercalcemia. Arch Intern Med 147:937–939, 1987.
23. Rotstein S, Glas U, Eriksson M, et al: Intravenous clodronate for the treatment of hypercalcaemia in breast cancer patients with bone metastases—a prospective randomised placebo-controlled multicentre study. Eur J Cancer 28A:890–893, 1992.
24. Bonjour JP, Philippe J, Guelpa G, et al: Bone and renal components in hypercalcemia of malignancy and responses to a single infusion of clodronate. Bone 9:123–130, 1988.
25. Bonjour JP, Rizzoli R: Clodronate in hypercalcemia of malignancy. Calcif Tissue Int 46(suppl):20–25, 1990.
26. Bilezikian JP: Management of acute hypercalcemia. N Engl J Med 326:1196–1203, 1992.
27. Ryzen E, Martodam RR, Troxell M, et al: Intravenous etidronate in the management of malignant hypercalcemia. Arch Intern Med 145:449–452, 1985.
28. Jacobs TP, Gordon AC, Silverberg SJ, et al: Neoplastic hypercalcemia: Physiologic response to intravenous etidronate disodium. Am J Med 82:42–50, 1987.
29. Hasling C, Charles P, Mosekilde L: Etidronate disodium in the management of malignancy-related hypercalcemia. Am J Med 82:51–54, 1987.
30. Singer FR, Ritch PS, Lad TE, et al: Treatment of hypercalcemia of malignancy with intravenous etidronate. A controlled, multicenter study. The Hypercalcemia Study Group [published erratum appears in Arch Intern Med 1991 Oct;151(10):2008]. Arch Intern Med 151:471–476, 1991.
31. Sleeboom HP, Bijvoet OL, van Oosterom AT, et al: Comparison of intravenous (3-amino-1-hydroxypropylidene)-1,1-bisphosphonate and volume repletion in tumour-induced hypercalcaemia. Lancet 2:239–243, 1983.
32. Body JJ, Borkowski A, Cleeren A, et al: Treatment of malignancy-associated hypercalcemia with intravenous aminohydroxypropylidene diphosphonate. J Clin Oncol 4:1177–1183, 1986.
33. Body JJ, Pot M, Borkowski A, et al: Dose/response study of aminohydroxypropylidene bisphosphonate in tumor-associated hypercalcemia. Am J Med 82:957–963, 1987.
34. Body JJ, Dumon JC: Treatment of tumour-induced hypercalcaemia with the bisphosphonate pamidronate: Dose-response relationship and influence of tumour type. Ann Oncol 5:359–363, 1994.
35. Cantwell BM, Harris AL: Effect of single high dose infusions of aminohydroxypropylidene diphosphonate on hypercalcaemia caused by cancer. BMJ 294:467–469, 1987.
36. Gallacher SJ, Ralston SH, Fraser WD, et al: A comparison of low versus high dose pamidronate in cancer-associated hypercalcaemia. Bone Miner 15:249–256, 1991.
37. Nussbaum SR, Younger J, Vandepol CJ, et al: Single-dose intravenous therapy with pamidronate for the treatment of hypercalcemia of malignancy: Comparison of 30-, 60-, and 90-mg dosages. Am J Med 95:297–304, 1993.
38. Thiebaud D, Jaeger P, Jacquet AF, et al: A single-day treatment of tumor-induced hypercalcemia by intravenous amino-hydroxypropylidene bisphosphonate. J Bone Miner Res 1:555–562, 1986.
39. Thiebaud D, Jaeger P, Jacquet AF, et al: Dose-response in the treatment of hypercalcemia of malignancy by a single infusion of the bisphosphonate AHPrBP. J Clin Oncol 6:762–768, 1988.
40. Body JJ, Dumon JC, Thirion M, et al: Circulating PTHrP concentrations in tumor-induced hypercalcemia: Influence on the response to bisphosphonate and changes after therapy. J Bone Miner Res 8:701–706, 1993.
41. Gurney H, Grill V, Martin TJ: Parathyroid hormone–related protein and response to pamidronate in tumour-induced hypercalcaemia. Lancet 341:1611–1613, 1993.
42. Walls J, Ratcliffe WA, Howell A, et al: Response to intravenous bisphosphonate therapy in hypercalcaemic patients with and without bone metastases: The role of parathyroid hormone–related protein. Br J Cancer 70:169–172, 1994.
43. Thiebaud D, Jaeger P, Burckhardt P: Response to retreatment of malignant hypercalcemia with the bisphosphonate AHPrBP (APD): Respective role of kidney and bone. J Bone Miner Res 5:221–226, 1990.
44. Dodwell DJ, Abbas SK, Morton AR, et al: Parathyroid hormone–related protein(50–69) and response to pamidronate therapy for tumour-induced hypercalcaemia. Eur J Cancer 27:1629-1633, 1991.
45. Yates AJ, Murray RM, Jerums GJ, et al: A comparison of single and multiple intravenous infusions of 3-amino-1-hydroxypropylidene-1,1-bisphosphonate (APD) in the treatment of hypercalcemia of malignancy. Aust N Z J Med 17:387–391, 1987.
46. Ralston SH, Alzaid AA, Gallacher SJ, et al: Clinical experience with aminohydroxypropylidene bisphosphonate (APD) in the management of cancer-associated hypercalcaemia. Q J Med 68:825–834, 1988.
47. Adami S, Bhalla AK, Dorizzi R, et al: The acute-phase response after bisphosphonate administration. Calcif Tissue Int 41:326–331, 1987.
48. Liote F, Boval-Boizard B, Fritz P, et al: Lymphocyte subsets in pamidronate-induced lymphopenia (letter). Br J Rheumatol 34:993–995, 1995.
49. Bijvoet OL, Frijlink WB, Jie K, et al: APD in Paget's disease of bone. Role of the mononuclear phagocyte system? Arthritis Rheum 23:1193–1204, 1980.
50. Cantwell B, Harris AL: Single high dose aminohydroxypropylidene diphosphonate infusions to treat cancer-associated hypercalcaemia (letter). Lancet 1:165–166, 1986.
51. Ralston SH, Patel U, Fraser WD, et al: Comparison of three intravenous bisphosphonates in cancer-associated hypercalcaemia. Lancet 2:1180–1182, 1989.
52. Nussbaum SR, Warrell RP Jr, Rude R, et al: Dose-response study of alendronate sodium for the treatment of cancer-associated hypercalcemia. J Clin Oncol 11:1618–1623, 1993.
53. Body JJ, Magritte A, Seraj F, et al: Aminohydroxypropylidene bisphosphonate (APD) treatment for tumor-associated hypercalcemia: A randomized comparison between a 3-day treatment and single 24-hour infusions. J Bone Miner Res 4:923–928, 1989.
54. Gucalp R, Theriault R, Gill I, et al: Treatment of cancer-associated hypercalcemia. Double-blind comparison of rapid and slow intravenous infusion regimens of pamidronate disodium and saline alone. Arch Intern Med 154:1935–1944, 1994.
55. Dodwell DJ, Howell A, Morton AR, et al: Infusion rate and pharmacokinetics of intravenous pamidronate in the treatment of tumour-induced hypercalcaemia. Postgrad Med J 68:434–439, 1992.
56. Thiebaud D, Portmann L, Burckhardt P: Moderate Paget's disease treated with pamidronate: Comparison of various infusion rates for a 60-mg single dose. Semin Arthritis Rheum 23:279, 1994.
57. Conte PF, Latreille J, Mauriac L, et al: Delay in progression of bone metastases in breast cancer patients treated with intravenous pamidronate: Results from a multinational randomized controlled trial. The Aredia Multinational Cooperative Group. J Clin Oncol 14:2552–2559, 1996.
58. Tyrrell CJ, Collinson M, Madsen EL, et al: Intravenous pamidronate: Infusion rate and safety. Ann Oncol 5(suppl):27–29, 1994.
59. Tyrrell CT, Bruning PF, May-Levin F, et al: Pamidronate infusions as single-agent therapy for bone metastases: A phase II trial in patients with breast cancer. Eur J Cancer 31A:1976–1980, 1995.
60. Jung A: Comparison of two parenteral diphosphonates in hypercalcemia of malignancy. Am J Med 72:221–226, 1982.
61. Gucalp R, Ritch P, Wiernik PH, et al: Comparative study of pamidronate disodium and etidronate disodium in the treatment of cancer-related hypercalcemia. J Clin Oncol 10:134–142, 1992.
62. Purohit OP, Radstone CR, Anthony C, et al: A randomised double-blind comparison of intravenous pamidronate and clodronate in the hypercalcaemia of malignancy. Br J Cancer 72:1289–1293, 1995.
63. Ostenstad B, Andersen OK: Disodium pamidronate versus mithramycin in the management of tumour-associated hypercalcemia. Acta Oncol 31:861–864, 1992.
64. Thurlimann B, Waldburger R, Senn HJ, et al: Plicamycin and pamidronate in symptomatic tumor-related hypercalcemia: A prospective randomized crossover trial. Ann Oncol 3:619–623, 1992.
65. Ralston SH, Gardner MD, Dryburgh FJ, et al: Comparison of aminohydroxypropylidene diphosphonate, mithramycin, and corticosteroids/calcitonin in treatment of cancer-associated hypercalcaemia. Lancet 2:907–910, 1985.
66. Zysset E, Ammann P, Jenzer A, et al: Comparison of a rapid (2-h) versus a slow (24-h) infusion of alendronate in the treatment of hypercalcemia of malignancy. Bone Miner 18:237–249, 1992.
67. Rizzoli R, Buchs B, Bonjour JP: Effect of a single infusion of alendronate in malignant hypercalcaemia: Dose dependency and comparison with clodronate. Int J Cancer 50:706–712, 1992.
68. Ralston SH, Thiebaud D, Herrmann Z, et al: Dose-response study of ibandronate in the treatment of cancer-associated hypercalcaemia. Br J Cancer 75:295–300, 1997.
69. Wuster C, Schoter KH, Thiebaud D, et al: Methylpentylaminopropylidenebisphosphonate (BM 21.0955): A new potent and safe bisphosphonate for the treatment of cancer-associated hypercalcemia. Bone Miner 22:77–85, 1993.
70. O'Rourke NP, McCloskey EV, Rosini S, et al: Treatment of malignant hypercalcaemia with aminohexane bisphosphonate (neridronate). Br J Cancer 69:914–917, 1994.
71. Fukumoto S, Matsumoto T, Takebe K, et al: Treatment of malignancy-associated hypercalcemia with YM175, a new bisphosphonate: Elevated threshold for parathyroid hormone secretion in hypercalcemic patients. J Clin Endocrinol Metab 79:165–170, 1994.
72. Dumon JC, Magritte A, Body JJ: Efficacy and safety of the bisphosphonate tiludronate for the treatment of tumor-associated hypercalcemia. Bone Miner 15:257–266, 1991.
73. Green JR, Muller K, Jaeggi KA: Preclinical pharmacology of CGP 42'446, a new, potent, heterocyclic bisphosphonate compound. J Bone Miner Res 9:745–751, 1994.
74. Body JJ: Clinical research update: Zoledronate. Cancer 80:1699–1701, 1997.
75. Body JJ, Lortholary A, Romieu G, et al: A dose-finding study of zoledronate in hypercalcemic cancer patients. J Bone Miner Res 14:1557–1561, 1999.
76. Tal A, Powers K: Milk-alkali syndrome induced by $1,25(OH)_2D$ in a patient with hypoparathyroidism. J Natl Med Assoc 88:313–314, 1996.
77. Selby PL, Davies M, Marks JS, et al: Vitamin D intoxication causes hypercalcaemia by increased bone resorption which responds to pamidronate. Clin Endocrinol (Oxf) 43:531–536, 1995.
78. Lee DC, Lee GY: The use of pamidronate for hypercalcemia secondary to acute vitamin D intoxication. J Toxicol Clin Toxicol 36:719–721, 1998.
79. Davenport A, Goel S, Mackenzie JC: Treatment of hypercalcaemia with pamidronate in patients with end stage renal failure. Scand J Urol Nephrol 27:447–451, 1993.
80. Varache N, Audran M, Clochon P, et al: Aminohydroxypropylidene bisphosphonate (AHPrBP) treatment of severe immobilization hypercalcaemia in a young patient. Clin Rheumatol 10:328–332, 1991.
81. McIntyre HD, Cameron DP, Urquhart SM, et al: Immobilization hypercalcaemia responding to intravenous pamidronate sodium therapy. Postgrad Med J 65:244–246, 1989.
82. Kedlaya D, Brandstater ME, Lee JK: Immobilization hypercalcemia in incomplete paraplegia: Successful treatment with pamidronate. Arch Phys Med Rehabil 79:222–225, 1998.
83. Gallacher SJ, Ralston SH, Dryburgh FJ, et al: Immobilization-related hypercalcaemia—a possible novel mechanism and response to pamidronate. Postgrad Med J 66:918–922, 1990.
84. Tan TT, Alzaid AA, Sutcliffe N, et al: Treatment of hypercalcaemia in thyrotoxicosis with aminohydroxypropylidene diphosphonate. Postgrad Med J 64:224–227, 1988.

85. Yamaguchi K, Grant J, Noble-Jamieson G, et al: Hypercalcaemia in primary oxalosis: Role of increased bone resorption and effects of treatment with pamidronate. Bone 16:61–67, 1995.
86. Westphal SA: Disseminated coccidioidomycosis associated with hypercalcemia. Mayo Clin Proc 73:893–894, 1998.
87. Body JJ, Bartl R, Burckhardt P, et al: Current use of bisphosphonates in oncology. International Bone and Cancer Study Group. J Clin Oncol 16:3890–3899, 1998.
88. Berenson JR, Lichtenstein A, Porter L, et al: Efficacy of pamidronate in reducing skeletal events in patients with advanced multiple myeloma. Myeloma Aredia Study Group. N Engl J Med 334:488–493, 1996.
89. Berenson JR, Lichtenstein A, Porter L, et al: Long-term pamidronate treatment of advanced multiple myeloma patients reduces skeletal events. Myeloma Aredia Study Group. J Clin Oncol 16:593–602, 1998.
90. Hortobagyi GN, Theriault RL, Porter L, et al: Efficacy of pamidronate in reducing skeletal complications in patients with breast cancer and lytic bone metastases. Protocol 19 Aredia Breast Cancer Study Group. N Engl J Med 335:1785–1791, 1996.
91. Hortobagyi GN, Theriault RL, Lipton A, et al: Long-term prevention of skeletal complications of metastatic breast cancer with pamidronate. Protocol 19 Aredia Breast Cancer Study Group. J Clin Oncol 16:2038–2044, 1998.
92. Theriault RL, Lipton A, Hortobagyi GN, et al: Pamidronate reduces skeletal morbidity in women with advanced breast cancer and lytic bone lesions: A randomized, placebo-controlled trial. Protocol 18 Aredia Breast Cancer Study Group. J Clin Oncol 17:846–854, 1999.
93. Paterson AH, Powles TJ, Kanis JA, et al: Double-blind controlled trial of oral clodronate in patients with bone metastases from breast cancer. J Clin Oncol 11:59–65, 1993.
94. Kanis JA, Powles T, Paterson AH, et al: Clodronate decreases the frequency of skeletal metastases in women with breast cancer. Bone 19:663–667, 1996.
95. Diel IJ, Solomayer EF, Costa SD, et al: Reduction in new metastases in breast cancer with adjuvant clodronate treatment. N Engl J Med 339:357–363, 1998.
96. Nussbaum SR: Pathophysiology and management of severe hypercalcemia. Endocrinol Metab Clin North Am 22:343–362, 1993.
97. Cortes EP, Holland JF, Moskowitz R, et al: Effects of mithramycin on bone resorption in vitro. Cancer Res 32:74–76, 1972.
98. Robins PR, Jowsey J: Effect of mithramycin on normal and abnormal bone turnover. J Lab Clin Med 82:576–586, 1973.
99. Slayton RE, Shnider BI, Elias E, et al: New approach to the treatment of hypercalcemia. The effect of short-term treatment with mithramycin. Clin Pharmacol Ther 12:833–837, 1971.
100. Perlia CP, Gubisch NJ, Wolter J, et al: Mithramycin treatment of hypercalcemia. Cancer 25:389–394, 1970.
101. Ellas EG, Reynoso G, Mittelman A: Control of hypercalcemia with mithramycin. Ann Surg 175:431–435, 1972.
102. Kennedy BJ: Metabolic and toxic effects of mithramycin during tumor therapy. Am J Med 49:494–503, 1970.
103. Benedetti RG, Heilman KJ 3d, Gabow PA: Nephrotoxicity following single dose mithramycin therapy. Am J Nephrol 3:277–278, 1983.
104. Monto RW, Talley RW, Caldwell MJ, et al: Observations on the mechanism of hemorrhagic toxicity in mithramycin (NSC 24559) therapy. Cancer Res 29:697–704, 1969.
105. Yamreudeewong W, Henann NE, Fazio A, et al: Possible severe thrombocytopenia associated with a single dose of plicamycin. Ann Pharmacother 26:1369–1373, 1992.
106. Green L, Donehower RC: Hepatic toxicity of low doses of mithramycin in hypercalcemia. Cancer Treat Rep 68:1379–1381, 1984.
107. Hosking DJ, Gilson D: Comparison of the renal and skeletal actions of calcitonin in the treatment of severe hypercalcaemia of malignancy. Q J Med 53:359–368, 1984.
108. Cochran M, Peacock M, Sachs G, et al: Renal effects of calcitonin. BMJ 1:135–137, 1970.
109. Foster GV, Joplin GF, MacIntyre I, et al: Effect of thyrocalcitonin in man. Lancet 1:107–109, 1966.
110. Milhaud G, Job JC: Thyrocalcitonin: Effect on idiopathic hypercalcemia. Science 154:794–796, 1966.
111. Silva OL, Becker KL: Salmon calcitonin in the treatment of hypercalcemia. Arch Intern Med 132:337–339, 1973.
112. Kammerman S, Canfield RE: Effect of porcine calcitonin on hypercalcemia in man. J Clin Endocrinol Metab 31:70–75, 1970.
113. Wisneski LA, Croom WP, Silva OL, et al: Salmon calcitonin in hypercalcemia. Clin Pharmacol Ther 24:219–222, 1978.
114. Warrell RP Jr, Israel R, Frisone M, et al: Gallium nitrate for acute treatment of cancer-related hypercalcemia. A randomized, double-blind comparison to calcitonin. Ann Intern Med 108:669–674, 1988.
115. Binstock ML, Mundy GR: Effect of calcitonin and glucocorticoids in combination on the hypercalcemia of malignancy. Ann Intern Med 93:269–272, 1980.
116. Ljunghall S, Rastad J, Akerstrom G: Comparative effects of calcitonin and clodronate in hypercalcaemia. Bone 8(suppl):79–83, 1987.
117. Hosking DJ, Stone MD, Foote JW: Potentiation of calcitonin by corticosteroids during the treatment of the hypercalcaemia of malignancy. Eur J Clin Pharmacol 38:37–41, 1990.
118. Ralston SH, Alzaid AA, Gardner MD, et al: Treatment of cancer associated hypercalcaemia with combined aminohydroxypropylidene diphosphonate and calcitonin. BMJ 292:1549–1550, 1986.
119. Wisneski LA: Salmon calcitonin in the acute management of hypercalcemia. Calcif Tissue Int 46(suppl):26–30, 1990.
120. Fatemi S, Singer FR, Rude RK: Effect of salmon calcitonin and etidronate on hypercalcemia of malignancy. Calcif Tissue Int 50:107–109, 1992.
121. Vaughn CB, Vaitkevicius VK: The effects of calcitonin in hypercalcemia in patients with malignancy. Cancer 34:1268–1271, 1974.
122. Bijvoet OL, van der Sluys Veer J, Jansen AP: Effects of calcitonin on patients with Paget's disease, thyrotoxicosis, or hypercalcaemia. Lancet 1:876–881, 1968.
123. West TE, Sinclair L, Joffe M, et al: Treatment of hypercalcaemia with calcitonin. Lancet 1:675–678, 1971.
124. Pak CY, Wills MR, Smith GW 2d, Bartter FC: Treatment with thyrocalcitonin of the hypercalcemia of parathyroid carcinoma. J Clin Endocrinol Metab 28:1657–1660, 1968.
125. Woodhouse NJ, Hoare A, Mohamedally SM, et al: Thyrotoxicosis and hypercalcaemia: Response to antithyroid drugs and salmon calcitonin. Horm Res 7:238–246, 1976.
126. Carey DE, Raisz LG: Calcitonin therapy in prolonged immobilization hypercalcemia. Arch Phys Med Rehabil 66:640–644, 1985.
127. Kaul S, Sockalosky JJ: Human synthetic calcitonin therapy for hypercalcemia of immobilization. J Pediatr 126:825–827, 1995.
128. Nilsson O, Almqvist S, Karlberg BE: Salmon calcitonin in the acute treatment of moderate and severe hypercalcemia in man. Acta Med Scand 204:249–252, 1978.
129. Carney SL, Epstein MT: Effect of calcitonin on hemodialysis patients with hypercalcemia and renal osteodystrophy. Uremia Invest 8:97–101, 1984.
130. Thiebaud D, Jacquet AF, Burckhardt P: Fast and effective treatment of malignant hypercalcemia. Combination of suppositories of calcitonin and a single infusion of 3-amino 1-hydroxypropylidene-1-bisphosphonate. Arch Intern Med 150:2125–2128, 1990.
131. Thiebaud D, Burckhardt P, Jaeger P, et al: Effectiveness of salmon calcitonin administered as suppositories in tumor-induced hypercalcemia. Am J Med 82:745–750, 1987.
132. Dumon JC, Magritte A, Body JJ: Nasal human calcitonin for tumor-induced hypercalcemia. Calcif Tissue Int 51:18–19, 1992.
133. Warrell RP Jr, Bockman RS, Coonley CJ, et al: Gallium nitrate inhibits calcium resorption from bone and is effective treatment for cancer-related hypercalcemia. J Clin Invest 73:1487–1490, 1984.
134. Hall TJ, Chambers TJ: Gallium inhibits bone resorption by a direct effect on osteoclasts. Bone Miner 8:211–216, 1990.
135. Bockman RS, Boskey AL, Blumenthal NC, et al: Gallium increases bone calcium and crystallite perfection of hydroxyapatite. Calcif Tissue Int 39:376–381, 1986.
136. Blumenthal NC, Cosma V, Levine S: Effect of gallium on the in vitro formation, growth, and solubility of hydroxyapatite. Calcif Tissue Int 45:81–87, 1989.
137. Warrell RP Jr, Skelos A, Alcock NW, et al: Gallium nitrate for acute treatment of cancer-related hypercalcemia: Clinicopharmacological and dose response analysis. Cancer Res 46:4208–4212, 1986.
138. Todd PA, Fitton A: Gallium nitrate. A review of its pharmacological properties and therapeutic potential in cancer related hypercalcaemia. Drugs 42:261–273, 1991.
139. Hughes TE, Hansen LA: Gallium nitrate. Ann Pharmacother 26:354–362, 1992.
140. Warrell RP Jr, Murphy WK, Schulman P, et al: A randomized double-blind study of gallium nitrate compared with etidronate for acute control of cancer-related hypercalcemia. J Clin Oncol 9:1467–1475, 1991.
141. Pechet MM, Bowers B, Bartter FC: Metabolic studies with a new series of 1,4-diene steroids. II. Effects in normal subjects of prednisone, prednisolone, and 9-alpha-fluoroprednisolone. J Clin Invest 38:691–701, 1959.
142. Laake H: The action of corticosteroids in the renal reabsorption of calcium. Acta Endocrinol 34:60–64, 1960.
143. Caniggia A, Nuti R, Lore F, et al: Pathophysiology of the adverse effects of glucoactive corticosteroids on calcium metabolism in man. J Steroid Biochem 15:153–161, 1981.
144. Sharma OP: Vitamin D, calcium, and sarcoidosis. Chest 109:535–539, 1996.
145. Basile JN, Liel Y, Shary J, et al: Increased calcium intake does not suppress circulating 1,25-dihydroxyvitamin D in normocalcemic patients with sarcoidosis. J Clin Invest 91:1396–1398, 1993.
146. Insogna KL, Dreyer BE, Mitnick M, et al: Enhanced production rate of 1,25-dihydroxyvitamin D in sarcoidosis. J Clin Endocrinol Metab 66:72–75, 1988.
147. Adams JS, Sharma OP, Gacad MA, et al: Metabolism of 25-hydroxyvitamin D_3 by cultured pulmonary alveolar macrophages in sarcoidosis. J Clin Invest 72:1856–1860, 1983.
148. Adams JS, Singer FR, Gacad MA, et al: Isolation and structural identification of 1,25-dihydroxyvitamin D_3 produced by cultured alveolar macrophages in sarcoidosis. J Clin Endocrinol Metab 60:960–966, 1985.
149. Mason RS, Frankel T, Chan YL, et al: Vitamin D conversion by sarcoid lymph node homogenate. Ann Intern Med 100:59–61, 1984.
150. Gkonos PJ, London R, Hendler ED: Hypercalcemia and elevated 1,25-dihydroxyvitamin D levels in a patient with end-stage renal disease and active tuberculosis. N Engl J Med 311:1683–1685, 1984.
151. Cadranel J, Garabedian M, Milleron B, et al: $1,25(OH)_2D_2$ production by T lymphocytes and alveolar macrophages recovered by lavage from normocalcemic patients with tuberculosis. J Clin Invest 85:1588–1593, 1990.
152. Bosch X: Hypercalcemia due to endogenous overproduction of 1,25-dihydroxyvitamin D in Crohn's disease. Gastroenterology 114:1061–1065, 1998.
153. Breslau NA, McGuire JL, Zerwekh JE, et al: Hypercalcemia associated with increased serum calcitriol levels in three patients with lymphoma. Ann Intern Med 100:1–6, 1984.
154. Rosenthal N, Insogna KL, Godsall JW, et al: Elevations in circulating 1,25-dihydroxyvitamin D in three patients with lymphoma-associated hypercalcemia. J Clin Endocrinol Metab 60:29–33, 1985.
155. Seymour JF, Gagel RF: Calcitriol: The major humoral mediator of hypercalcemia in Hodgkin's disease and non-Hodgkin's lymphomas. Blood 82:1383–1394, 1993.
156. Seymour JF, Gagel RF, Hagemeister FB, et al: Calcitriol production in hypercalcemic and normocalcemic patients with non-Hodgkin lymphoma. Ann Intern Med 121:633–640, 1994.
157. Dent CE: Some problems of hyperparathyroidism. BMJ 2:1419–1425, 1962.
158. Dent CE, Watson L: The hydrocortisone test in primary and tertiary hyperparathyroidism. Lancet 2:662–664, 1968.
159. Watson L, Moxham J, Fraser P: Hydrocortisone suppression test and discriminant analysis in differential diagnosis of hypercalcaemia. Lancet 1:1320–1325, 1980.

160. Fulmer DH, Dimich AB, Rothschild EO, et al: Treatment of hypercalcemia. Comparison of intravenously administered phosphate, sulfate, and hydrocortisone. Arch Intern Med 129:923–930, 1972.
161. Percival RC, Yates AJ, Gray RE, et al: Role of glucocorticoids in management of malignant hypercalcaemia. BMJ 289:287, 1984.
162. Thalassinos NC, Joplin GF: Failure of corticosteroid therapy to correct the hypercalcaemia of malignant disease. Lancet 2:537–538, 1970.
163. Verner JV, Engel FL, McPherson HT: Vitamin D intoxication: Report of two cases treated with cortisone. Ann Intern Med 48:765–773, 1958.
164. Favus MJ: Treatment of vitamin D intoxication. N Engl J Med 283:1468–1469, 1970.
165. Heyburn PJ, Francis RM, Peacock M: Acute effects of saline, calcitonin, and hydrocortisone on plasma calcium in vitamin D intoxication. BMJ 1:232–233, 1979.
166. Dent CE, Flynn FV, Nabarro JDM: Hypercalcemia and impairment of renal function in generalized sarcoidosis. BMJ 2:808, 1953.
167. Anderson J, Harper C, Dent CE, Philpot GR: Effect of cortisone on calcium metabolism in sarcoidosis with hypercalcemia. Possible antagonistic actions of cortisone and vitamin D. Lancet 2:720, 1954.
168. Chesney RW, Hamstra AJ, DeLuca HF, et al: Elevated serum 1,25-dihydroxyvitamin D concentrations in the hypercalcemia of sarcoidosis: Correction by glucocorticoid therapy. J Pediatr 98:919–922, 1981.
169. Sandler LM, Winearls CG, Fraher LJ, et al: Studies of the hypercalcaemia of sarcoidosis: Effect of steroids and exogenous vitamin D_3 on the circulating concentrations of 1,25-dihydroxy vitamin D_3. Q J Med 53:165–180, 1984.
170. Papapoulos SE, Clemens TL, Fraher LJ, et al: 1,25-dihydroxycholecalciferol in the pathogenesis of the hypercalcaemia of sarcoidosis. Lancet 1:627–630, 1979.
171. Bell NH, Stern PH, Pantzer E, et al: Evidence that increased circulating 1 alpha, 25-dihydroxyvitamin D is the probable cause for abnormal calcium metabolism in sarcoidosis. J Clin Invest 64:218–225, 1979.
172. Henneman PH, Dempsey EF, Carroll EL, et al: The cause of hypercalciuria in sarcoid and its treatment with cortisone and sodium phosphate. J Clin Invest 35:1229–1242, 1958.
173. Braman SS, Goldman AL, Schwarz MI: Steroid-responsive hypercalcemia in disseminated bone tuberculosis. Arch Intern Med 132:269–271, 1973.
174. Bosch X, Lopez-Soto A, Morello A, et al: Vitamin D metabolite–mediated hypercalcemia in Wegener's granulomatosis. Mayo Clin Proc 72:440–444, 1997.
175. Zerwekh JE, Pak CY, Kaplan RA, et al: Pathogenetic role of 1 alpha,25-dihydroxyvitamin D in sarcoidosis and absorptive hypercalciuria: Different response to prednisolone therapy. J Clin Endocrinol Metab 51:381–386, 1980.
176. Favus MJ, Walling MW, Kimberg DV: Effects of 1,25-dihydroxycholecalciferol on intestinal calcium transport in cortisone-treated rats. J Clin Invest 52:1680–1685, 1973.
177. Mundy GR, Rick ME, Turcotte R, et al: Pathogenesis of hypercalcemia in lymphosarcoma cell leukemia. Role of an osteoclast activating factor–like substance and a mechanism of action for glucocorticoid therapy. Am J Med 65:600–606, 1978.
178. Goodwin JS, Atluru D, Sierakowski S, et al: Mechanism of action of glucocorticosteroids. Inhibition of T cell proliferation and interleukin 2 production by hydrocortisone is reversed by leukotriene B_4. J Clin Invest 77:1244–1250, 1986.
179. Bulger HA, Dixon HH, Barr DP, et al: Functional pathology of hyperparathyroidism. J Clin Invest 9:143–190, 1930.
180. Albright F, Bauer W, Claflin O, et al: Studies in parathyroid physiology. III. Effect of phosphate ingestion in clinical hyperparathyroidism. J Clin Invest 11:411–435, 1932.
181. Hebert LA, Lemann J Jr, Petersen JR, et al: Studies of the mechanism by which phosphate infusion lowers serum calcium concentration. J Clin Invest 45:1886–1894, 1966.
182. Goldsmith RS, Ingbar SH: Inorganic phosphate treatment of hypercalcemia of diverse etiologies. N Engl J Med 274:1–7, 1966.
183. Goldsmith RS, Bartos H, Hulley SB, et al: Phosphate supplementation as an adjunct in the therapy of multiple myeloma. Arch Intern Med 122:128–133, 1968.
184. Thalassinos N, Joplin GF: Phosphate treatment of hypercalcaemia due to carcinoma. BMJ 3:14–19, 1968.
185. Massry SG, Mueller E, Silverman AG, et al: Inorganic phosphate treatment of hypercalcemia. Arch Intern Med 121:307–312, 1968.
186. Breuer RI, LeBauer J: Caution in the use of phosphates in the treatment of severe hypercalcemia. J Clin Endocrinol Metab 27:695–698, 1967.
187. Carey RW, Schmitt GW, Kopald HH, et al: Massive extraskeletal calcification during phosphate treatment of hypercalcemia. Arch Intern Med 122:150–155, 1968.
188. Shackney S, Hasson J: Precipitous fall in serum calcium, hypotension, and acute renal failure after intravenous phosphate therapy for hypercalcemia. Report of two cases. Ann Intern Med 66:906–916, 1967.
189. Mundy GR, Wilkinson R, Heath DA: Comparative study of available medical therapy for hypercalcemia of malignancy. Am J Med 74:421–432, 1983.
190. Dietrich JW, Goodson JM, Raisz LG: Stimulation of bone resorption by various prostaglandins in organ culture. Prostaglandins 10:231–240, 1975.
191. Klein DC, Raisz LG: Prostaglandins: Stimulation of bone resorption in tissue culture. Endocrinology 86:1436–1440, 1970.
192. Greaves M, Ibbotson KJ, Atkins D, et al: Prostaglandins as mediators of bone resorption in renal and breast tumours. Clin Sci 58:201–210, 1980.
193. Tashjian AH Jr, Voelkel EF, Levine L, et al: Evidence that the bone resorption–stimulating factor produced by mouse fibrosarcoma cells is prostaglandin E_2. A new model for the hypercalcemia of cancer. J Exp Med 136:1329–1343, 1972.
194. Seyberth HW, Segre GV, Morgan JL, et al: Prostaglandins as mediators of hypercalcemia associated with certain types of cancer. N Engl J Med 293:1278–1283, 1975.
195. Robertson RP, Baylink DJ, Marini BJ, et al: Elevated prostaglandins and suppressed parathyroid hormone associated with hypercalcemia and renal cell carcinoma. J Clin Endocrinol Metab 41:164–167, 1975.
196. Robertson RP, Baylink DJ, Metz SA, et al: Plasma prostaglandin E in patients with cancer with and without hypercalcemia. J Clin Endocrinol Metab 43:1330–1335, 1976.
197. Brenner DE, Harvey HA, Lipton A, et al: A study of prostaglandin E_2, parathormone, and response to indomethacin in patients with hypercalcemia of malignancy. Cancer 49:556–561, 1982.
198. Uchida T, Kuwao S, Ishibashi A, et al: Elevated prostaglandin and indomethacin-responsive hypercalcemia in a patient with malignant pheochromocytoma. J Urol 134:712–713, 1985.
199. Brereton HD, Halushka PV, Alexander RW, et al: Indomethacin-responsive hypercalcemia in a patient with renal-cell adenocarcinoma. N Engl J Med 291:83–85, 1974.
200. Dindogru A, Gailani S, Henderson ES, et al: Indomethacin in hypercalcaemia (letter). Lancet 2:365, 1975.
201. Ito H, Sanada T, Katayama T, et al: Indomethacin-responsive hypercalcemia (letter). N Engl J Med 293:558–559, 1975.
202. Chasan SA, Pothel LR, Huben RP: Management and prognostic significance of hypercalcemia in renal cell carcinoma. Urology 33:167–170, 1989.
203. Gibbs J, Dillon MJ, Lang S, et al: Indomethacin responsive hypercalcaemia associated with a renal sarcoma. Arch Dis Child 65:1168–1169, 1990.
204. Glass AR, Eil C: Ketoconazole-induced reduction in serum 1,25-dihydroxyvitamin D and total serum calcium in hypercalcemic patients. J Clin Endocrinol Metab 66:934–938, 1988.
205. Adams JS, Sharma OP, Diz MM, et al: Ketoconazole decreases the serum 1,25-dihydroxyvitamin D and calcium concentration in sarcoidosis-associated hypercalcemia. J Clin Endocrinol Metab 70:1090–1095, 1990.
206. Bia MJ, Insogna K: Treatment of sarcoidosis-associated hypercalcemia with ketoconazole. Am J Kidney Dis 18:702–705, 1991.
207. Glass AR, Cerletty JM, Elliott W, et al: Ketoconazole reduces elevated serum levels of 1,25-dihydroxyvitamin D in hypercalcemic sarcoidosis. J Endocrinol Invest 13:407–413, 1990.
208. Saggese G, Bertelloni S, Baroncelli GI, et al: Ketoconazole decreases the serum ionized calcium and 1,25-dihydroxyvitamin D levels in tuberculosis-associated hypercalcemia. Am J Dis Child 147:270–273, 1993.
209. Hunt BJ, Yendt ER: The response of hypercalcemia in sarcoidosis to chloroquine. Ann Intern Med 59:554–564, 1963.
210. Adams JS, Diz MM, Sharma OP: Effective reduction in the serum 1,25-dihydroxyvitamin D and calcium concentration in sarcoidosis-associated hypercalcemia with short-course chloroquine therapy. Ann Intern Med 111:437–438, 1989.
211. O'Leary TJ, Jones G, Yip A, et al: The effects of chloroquine on serum 1,25-dihydroxyvitamin D and calcium metabolism in sarcoidosis. N Engl J Med 315:727–730, 1986.
212. Barre PE, Gascon-Barre M, Meakins JL, et al: Hydroxychloroquine treatment of hypercalcemia in a patient with sarcoidosis undergoing hemodialysis. Am J Med 82:1259–1262, 1987.
213. Edelson GW, Talpos GB, Bone HG 3d: Hypercalcemia associated with Wegener's granulomatosis and hyperparathyroidism: Etiology and management. Am J Nephrol 13:275–277, 1993.
214. Adams JS, Kantorovich V: Inability of short-term, low-dose hydroxychloroquine to resolve vitamin D–mediated hypercalcemia in patients with B-cell lymphoma. J Clin Endocrinol Metab 84:799–801, 1999.
215. Cardella CJ, Birkin BL, Rapoport A: Role of dialysis in the treatment of severe hypercalcemia: Report of two cases successfully treated with hemodialysis and review of the literature. Clin Nephrol 12:285–290, 1979.
216. Camus C, Charasse C, Jouannic-Montier I, et al: Calcium free hemodialysis: Experience in the treatment of 33 patients with severe hypercalcemia. Intensive Care Med 22:116–121, 1996.
217. Koo WS, Jeon DS, Ahn SJ, et al: Calcium-free hemodialysis for the management of hypercalcemia. Nephron 72:424–428, 1996.
218. Nolph KD, Stoltz M, Maher JF: Calcium free peritoneal dialysis. Treatment of vitamin D intoxication. Arch Intern Med 128:809–814, 1971.
219. Hamilton JW, Lasrich M, Hirszel P: Peritoneal dialysis in the treatment of severe hypercalcemia. J Dial 4:129–138, 1980.
220. Miach PJ, Dawborn JK, Martin TJ, et al: Management of the hypercalcaemia of malignancy by peritoneal dialysis. Med J Aust 1:782–784, 1975.
221. Leehey DJ, Ing TS: Correction of hypercalcemia and hypophosphatemia by hemodialysis using a conventional, calcium-containing dialysis solution enriched with phosphorus. Am J Kidney Dis 29:288–290, 1997.

Chapter 79

Surgical Management of Hyperparathyroidism

Hop N. Le ▪ Jeffrey A. Norton

DIAGNOSIS OF PRIMARY HYPERPARATHYROIDISM

The diagnosis of primary hyperparathyroidism is based on concomitant measurement of elevated serum levels of calcium and intact parathyroid hormone (PTH).

INDICATIONS FOR SURGERY

Primary hyperparathyroidism may have various clinical manifestations: (1) asymptomatic hypercalcemia, (2) nephrolithiasis, (3) osteoporosis, and rarely (4) parathyroid crisis. Surgical intervention is indicated for clear-cut symptoms or signs of the disease complex.[1, 2] Bone disease, evident as bone cysts, elevated serum levels of bony alkaline phosphatase, bone tumors, subperiosteal resorption, and decreased bone density, warrants parathyroidectomy. Nephrolithiasis, nephrocalcinosis, impaired renal function, pancreatitis, peptic ulcer, and parathyroid crisis are clear indications for surgery. A serum calcium level greater than 12 mg/dL and a urinary calcium level greater than 350 mg/24 hours are also indications. Other indications include neuromuscular or musculoskeletal symptoms such as muscle weakness and chondrocalcinosis with pseudogout.

The best treatment for totally asymptomatic patients is still a subject of controversy.[1] This group certainly has no urgent need for surgery, but regular follow-up is indicated to guard against progression. Younger patients with apparently asymptomatic primary hyperparathyroidism require earlier surgery. Symptoms will develop in approximately 20% of these patients with long-term follow-up.[3] Neuromuscular symptoms such as weakness (20%–60%) occur in patients with primary hyperparathyroidism, and successful surgery reverses these symptoms in most patients.[4]

In general, surgical exploration is indicated for all patients with clear biochemical evidence of primary hyperparathyroidism and documented signs or symptoms of the disease. In apparently asymptomatic patients with primary hyperparathyroidism, surgery is indicated for younger patients who have a low operative risk and long temporal exposure to the disease. In apparently asymptomatic, older patients, surgery is reserved for patients in whom evidence of progression and/or symptoms develop. Progression is measured by a decrease in bone density, elevated serum calcium (>12 mg/dL) or bony alkaline phosphatase, or urinary levels of calcium greater than 350 mg/24 hours. (See Chapter 78 for further discussion of this topic.)

PROGNOSTIC INDICATORS OF PARATHYROID PATHOLOGY

Certain symptoms and signs are useful predictors of specific types of parathyroid pathology. Parathyroid adenoma is seldom, if ever palpable, but parathyroid carcinoma is palpable in a high proportion of cases.[5] Exceptionally high concentrations of PTH or calcium in serum also may suggest parathyroid cancer.[5] The diagnosis of familial multiple endocrine neoplasia type 1 (MEN-1) or MEN-2 virtually always predicts parathyroid hyperplasia[6, 7]; however, because of the wide variation in size of the abnormal parathyroid glands in patients with MEN 1, it is important for the surgeon to know whether an individual patient has the syndrome.[8] No physical signs are characteristic of MEN-1 or MEN-2. Recent studies have identified the genetic defect in patients with MEN-2 to be a *MENIN* mutation on chromosome 11q13[9] and in patients with MEN-2, a *RET* proto-oncogene mutation on chromosome 10.[10] MEN-2 must be distinguished from familial MEN-2b because hyperparathyroidism is not part of the latter. Familial hypocalciuric hypercalcemia (FHH) is an autosomal dominant trait usually manifested as asymptomatic hypercalcemia and relative hypocalciuria.[11] Mutations in the calcium-sensing receptor gene on chromosome 3 have been identified in a heterozygous form in benign FHH[12] but not in sporadic adenomas. In patients with FHH, the hypercalcemia is PTH dependent and associated with mild parathyroid hyperplasia; however, subtotal parathyroidectomy is rarely successful in correcting hypercalcemia and is contraindicated. In such cases, measurement of urinary calcium excretion and detection of relative hypocalciuria (<100 mg/24 hours) should lead to postponement of surgery and testing for hypercalcemia in close relatives.[11]

PARATHYROID CRISIS

Parathyroid crisis is an unusual state of progressive, marked hyperparathyroidism producing anorexia, vomiting, dehydration, decrease in renal function, progressive hypercalcemia, deterioration of mental status, confusion, coma, and if untreated, death.[13, 14] Fatigue, muscle weakness, polyuria, and polydipsia are also frequent. Hypercalcemia may have been noted in the past but left untreated or inadequately treated. Often, no apparent reason can be found for the sudden progression of hyperparathyroidism to a state of crisis, but some cases are apparently precipitated by bacterial or viral infection, trauma, or recent surgery. Serum calcium should not be the only defining criteria for a hypercalcemic crisis because asymptomatic patients with serum cal-

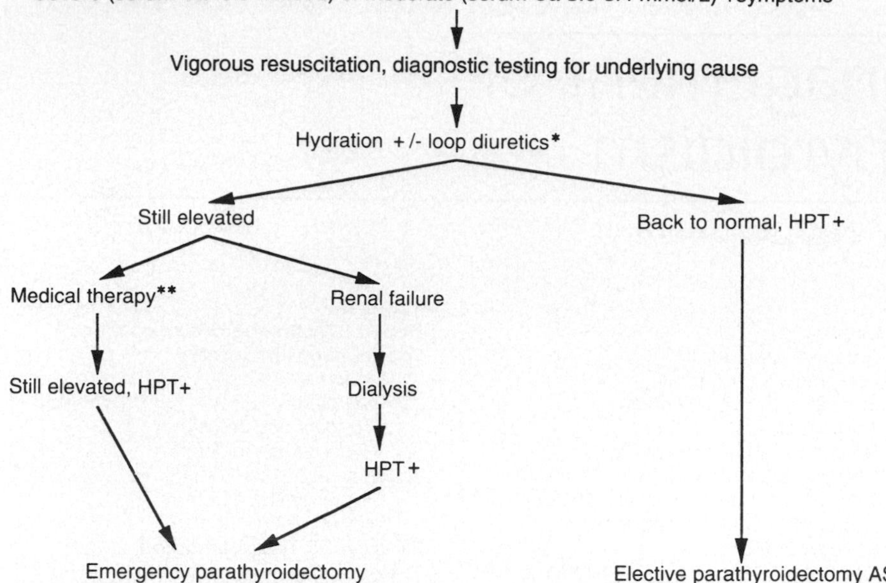

FIGURE 79–1. Flow diagram for management of a hypercalcemic crisis in patients with primary hyperparathyroidism (HPT). *Consider a central venous pressure line/pulmonary artery catheter/urinary catheter for monitoring patients with cardiac/renal failure and/or elderly patients. **That is, calcitonin, diphosphonates, gallium, glucocorticoids, plicamycin as indicated.

cium of 20 mg/dL and patients in hypercalcemic crisis with serum calcium less than 14 mg/dL have been reported.[15] It is almost always attributable to adenoma. Severe hyperparathyroidism may also be a manifestation of parathyroid carcinoma, which should be considered in the differential diagnosis.[5]

Parathyroid crisis is a potentially life-threatening disorder that requires vigorous medical management in preparation for definitive surgery (Fig. 79–1). Attention must first be directed toward hydration, reduction of the hypercalcemia, and stabilization of the clinical state in preparation for surgery. Large amounts of intravenous fluids are administered to ensure rehydration. Intravenous administration of saline followed by furosemide is usually effective in reducing the hypercalcemia. Furosemide should not be given until the patient is clearly rehydrated. In patients with a low serum concentration of phosphate, normal renal function, and moderate hypercalcemia, oral phosphate may also be used. At the same time, the diagnosis of hyperparathyroidism should be definitively established. If hydration and treatment with furosemide intravenously are not effective in reducing the hypercalcemia, treatment with diphosphonates, mithramycin, calcitonin, or gallium should be started as indicated.[14] In most cases, once the clinical condition has been stabilized with rehydration, one can complete the preoperative evaluation, confirm the diagnosis, and proceed with surgery.

PROCEDURES FOR PREOPERATIVE AND INTRAOPERATIVE LOCALIZATION OF ABNORMAL PARATHYROID GLANDS

Parathyroid Localization before Initial Surgery

The introduction of ultrasound (US), computed tomography (CT), magnetic resonance imaging (MRI), and sestamibi scintigraphy for localization of abnormal parathyroid tissue has led to their use before initial surgery. However, most experienced surgeons attempt to identify all four parathyroid glands at the initial procedure and can reliably do so with minimal morbidity. Prospective studies have found preoperative localization to be of minor significance.[16, 17] Because localization studies add expense and do not improve the outcome, they are not indicated before initial operations for hyperparathyroidism.

Parathyroid Localization before Repeat Surgery

In patients with persistent or recurrent hyperparathyroidism, the chance of successful repeat surgery is reduced[18, 19] and the incidence of complications is greater.[20] Therefore, maximum effort at parathyroid gland localization is made, commencing with the noninvasive procedures (US, CT, MRI, sestamibi) and proceeding (if necessary) to the more invasive studies (Fig. 79–2). Currently, noninvasive techniques localize an abnormal gland in about 75% to 80% of patients requiring repeat surgery,[21] whereas invasive studies help in the remainder.[22]

Ultrasound

US is the least expensive and least invasive technique to image abnormal parathyroid glands preoperatively. It is particularly effective for localizing enlarged parathyroid glands in the neck and can be used to identify 30% to 60% of the abnormal glands in patients requiring reoperation.[18, 21, 23] Parathyroid glands appear as hypoechoic masses adjacent to the more echogenic thyroid. The technique is particularly

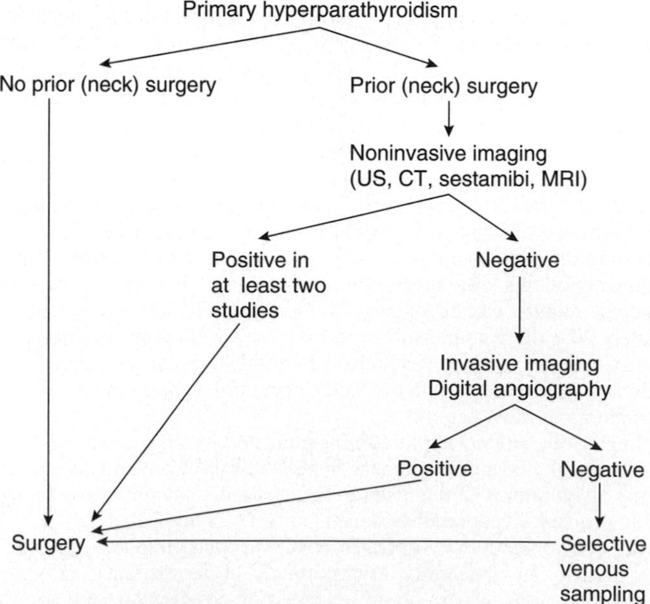

FIGURE 79–2. Flow diagram outlining a suggested radiologic localization strategy for patients with primary hyperparathyroidism undergoing reoperations. CT, computed tomography; MRI, magnetic resonance imaging; US, ultrasound.

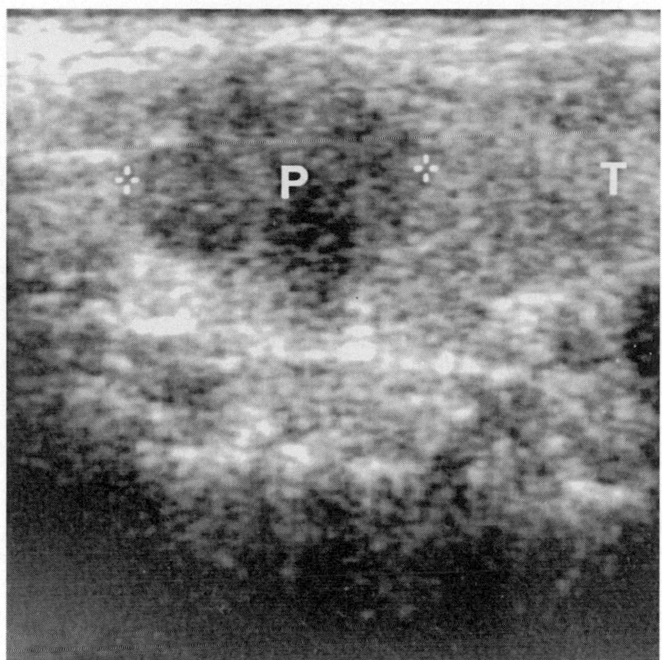

FIGURE 79–3. Ultrasound is best at identifying an intrathyroidal parathyroid adenoma. The hypoechoic mass (P) is an intrathyroidal parathyroid adenoma, and T is the more echogenic right superior thyroid lobe.

effective in identifying either juxtathyroid or intrathyroid parathyroid adenomas (Fig. 79–3).

US does have some disadvantages. It may fail to image ectopic superior glands in the tracheoesophageal groove. Preoperative US cannot image ectopic inferior glands in the anterior mediastinum because the sound waves do not penetrate the sternum. In multiple-gland hyperplasia, it generally demonstrates only the dominant gland. Finally, US is observer dependent and requires an ultrasonographer who is knowledgeable and interested in locating abnormal parathyroid glands.

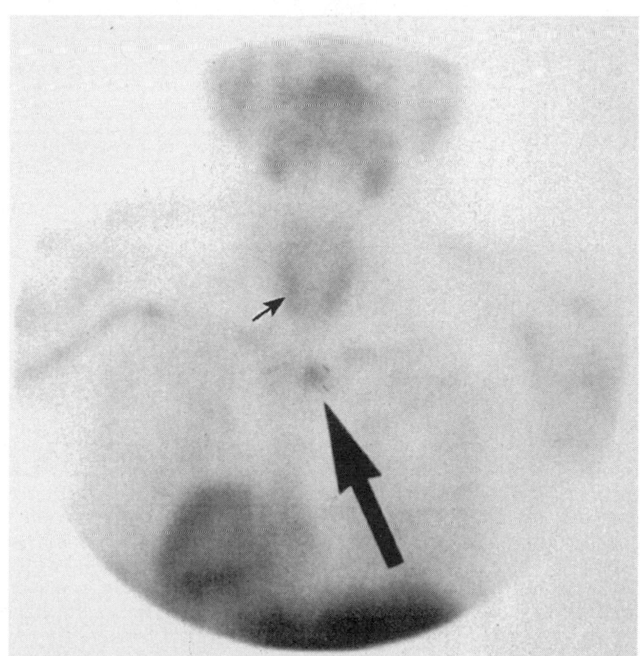

FIGURE 79–4. A positive sestamibi scan demonstrating an intrathymic parathyroid adenoma *(large arrow)* in the mediastinum. The *small arrow* points to the thyroid.

Sestamibi Scintigraphy

Technetium 99m–labeled sestamibi scanning has superior resolution and a sensitivity of 70% to 90% in detecting solitary parathyroid tumors.[24] Both the thyroid and parathyroid will take up sestamibi, but its uptake will be stronger and the signal will persist longer in parathyroid adenomas or hyperplasia (Fig. 79–4). The combination of single-photon emission CT with sestamibi has improved the sensitivity to about 85%, especially for deep cervical and mediastinal parathyroid tumors.[25] Recently, sestamibi has been combined with the gamma probe for hand-held intraoperative localization of abnormal parathyroid glands.[26] Advocates suggest that this approach is less invasive and can be done as an outpatient procedure through a smaller incision. However, early studies have focused primarily on patients who have not had previous surgery, in whom conventional techniques are nearly always efficacious. Furthermore, limited exploration based solely on sestamibi results may miss double adenomas or hyperplasia.

Computed Tomography

CT is particularly effective for identifying ectopic glands in the anterior mediastinum and enlarged glands in the tracheoesophageal groove. Ectopic glands in the anterior mediastinum often lie within the fat-replaced thymus, and even small adenomas are readily visualized (Fig. 79–5A). Ectopic glands in the tracheoesophageal groove are detected as a solid mass adjacent to the esophagus (Fig. 79–5B). Undescended glands near the carotid bifurcation are also identified by CT, provided that the examination is carried up to the level of the hyoid bone. On the other hand, CT is poor at detecting intrathyroid or juxtathyroid tumors and exposes the patient to risks associated with contrast media and radiation.

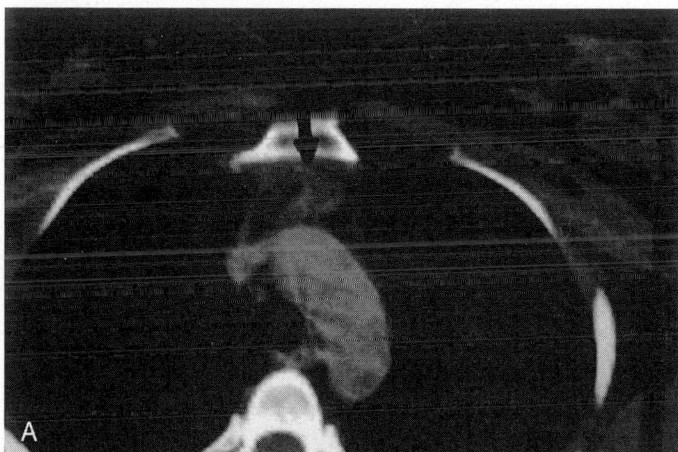

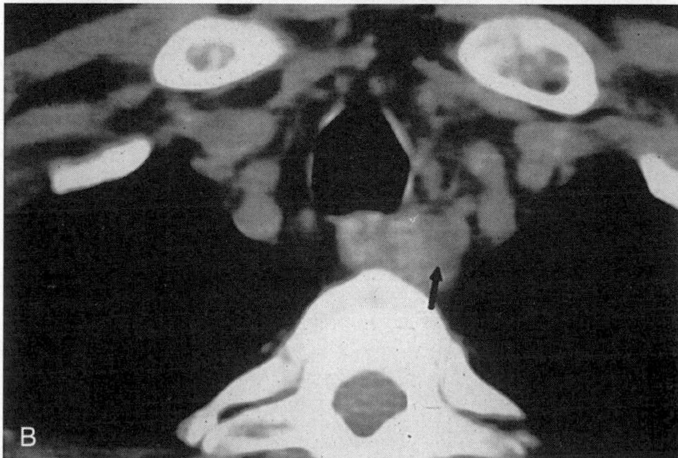

FIGURE 79–5. Computed tomography is the most useful imaging modality for identifying parathyroid adenomas located in the mediastinum *(A)* or in the tracheoesophageal groove *(B)*.

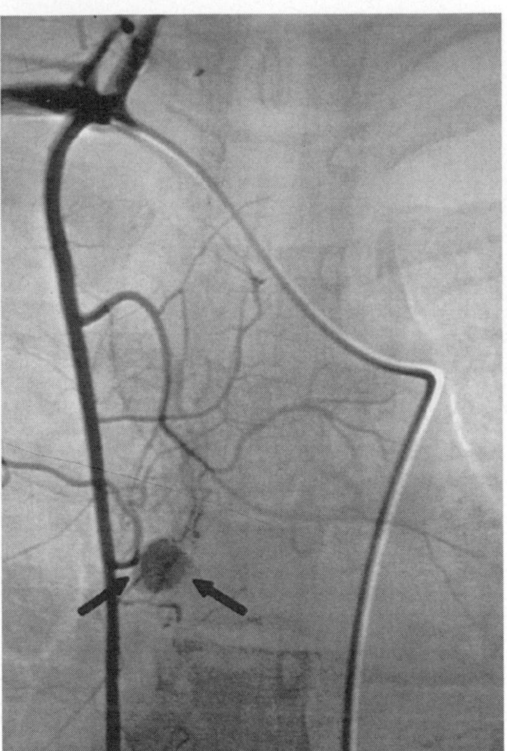

FIGURE 79–6. Angiogram demonstrating a large anterior mediastinal parathyroid adenoma with the right internal mammary artery as its blood supply.

Magnetic Resonance Imaging

Initial experience with MRI of abnormal parathyroid glands has been successful for large parathyroid adenomas, which on T2-weighted or stir-pulse sequences produce a bright signal.[23,26] In the mediastinum this signal may be confused with fat, and a T1-weighted image is required to specifically identify the pathology. With gadolinium-enhanced MRI and T1- and T2-weighted images, MRI can now provide higher sensitivity than CT for identifying ectopic parathyroid tumors. However, MRI is more expensive than CT.

Angiography

The potential for morbidity associated with angiographic procedures to localize parathyroid glands limits its use to patients with symptomatic persistent or recurrent hyperparathyroidism requiring reoperation. Intra-arterial digital techniques have greatly simplified angiographic localization of parathyroid pathology (Fig. 79–6). Because digital examination does not require highly selective catheter positioning, it can be accomplished expeditiously. The improved sensitivity of digital subtraction arteriography makes it possible to significantly reduce the total dose of water-soluble contrast material, thereby decreasing adverse effects on the kidney in a group of patients who may already have compromised renal function.

Selective Venous Sampling for Parathyroid Hormone

Selective venous sampling requires the greatest experience and is the most variably performed of all the localizing procedures in nonreferral centers. Contrast load, radiation exposure, and cost (15 to 20 PTH determinations), in addition to radiography costs, are all significant. Moreover, gradients determined by selective catheterization identify only the region of pathology (e.g., right side of the neck, mediastinum) but do not image the elusive gland. All these reasons have limited the use of selective venous sampling for PTH. It is indicated in only a small proportion of reoperative patients who have significant primary hyperparathyroidism and no apparent localizing information after completing all noninvasive studies and angiography.

Summary of Radiographic Localization

We suggest that parathyroid localization procedures not be used in patients undergoing initial exploration for primary hyperparathyroidism. Preoperative localization studies are expensive and do not improve the outcome. However, in patients undergoing reoperations, preoperative radiologic localization studies are necessary and helpful (see Fig. 79–2). We recommend liberal use of each of the noninvasive imaging studies (US, CT, ^{99m}Tc-sestamibi, and MRI) as an initial imaging cluster. If two studies identify the abnormal parathyroid gland in the same location, we proceed with surgery. If the noninvasive studies are equivocal, we then perform arteriography. If that study is positive, we perform surgery; if negative, we recommend selective venous sampling for PTH.

Intraoperative Determination of Parathyroid Hormone

Intraoperative determination of PTH allows rapid monitoring of parathyroid status during parathyroid surgery.[27]

Generally, after successful removal of a single parathyroid adenoma or adequate resection of hyperplastic glands, serum PTH levels begin to fall immediately and reach normal range within 30 to 90 minutes.[27] Studies demonstrate that serum levels of intact PTH decline rapidly, only 15 minutes after resection of a parathyroid adenoma.[27,28] Furthermore, the rate of decline is less in patients with hyperplasia and may provide an additional intraoperative means of diagnosing hyperplasia[28] (Fig. 79–7).

Intraoperative determination of PTH levels appears to complement surgical skill and histopathologic information and has the potential to provide additional guidance regarding the extent and degree of neck exploration. However, false-negative results or technical difficulties may be encountered, and this information only serves as an adjunct to

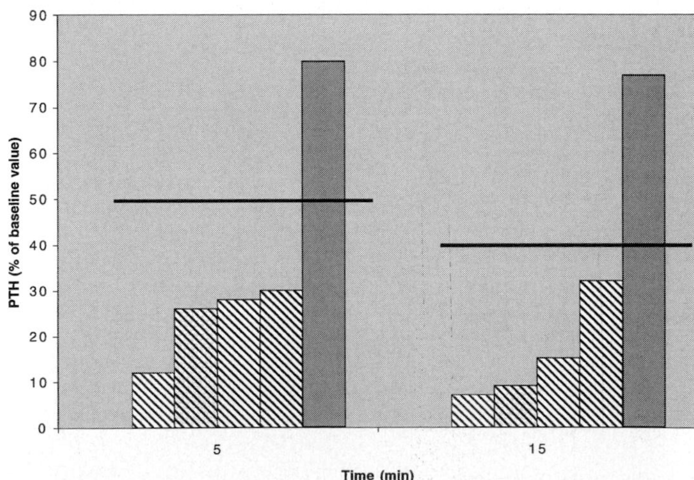

FIGURE 79–7. Intraoperative measurement of intact parathyroid hormone (PTH) in patients who have undergone previous unsuccessful neck exploration: Four patients with persistent primary hyperparathyroidism caused by parathyroid adenoma *(hatched bars)* and one patient with multiglandular disease *(solid bar)*. Measurements were taken 5 and 15 minutes after excision of one enlarged gland. The *bold lines* denote the upper limit for a significant decline in PTH after resection of parathyroid adenoma, which is a decrease of 50% at 5 minutes or at least a 60% decrease at 15 minutes. Note that every patient with an adenoma had a significant decline in PTH after tissue excision, whereas the patient with hyperplasia had only a minimal decrease in PTH, which stayed well above the upper limit for a significant decline. (Data from Bergenfelz A, Isaksson A, Lindblom P, et al: Measurement of parathyroid hormone in patients with primary hyperparathyroidism undergoing first and reoperative surgery. Br J Surg 85:1129–1132, 1998.)

standard judgment. Currently, these determinations are not standard care techniques and should be viewed as potential experimental adjuncts to surgery. Clarification of their exact role, if any, requires additional prospective studies.

SURGICAL MANAGEMENT OF PRIMARY HYPERPARATHYROIDISM

Surgery is the mainstay for treatment of primary hyperparathyroidism. First, the surgeon must identify and determine the exact cause of the hyperparathyroidism. Second, depending on the cause, the surgeon must perform the appropriate operative procedure.

The possible causes of primary hyperparathyroidism are adenoma (83%), hyperplasia (15%), double adenoma (1%–2%), and carcinoma (1%).[29] Some argue that "double adenomas" represent undetected hyperplasia. However, studies have shown that recurrent disease does not develop in patients with resected double adenomas after long follow-up,[30, 31] which suggests that the diagnosis of double adenoma is real and should be included. A family history of parathyroid disease or associated endocrinopathies is associated with hyperplasia. A history of neck irradiation is associated with adenoma.[32]

Before undertaking neck exploration for primary hyperparathyroidism, the surgeon must obtain informed consent, which requires careful discussion of the outcome and complications. A successful outcome is expected in approximately 95% of patients undergoing initial operations[32] and in 78% to 90% of reoperations.[23, 33, 34] Recurrent laryngeal nerve injury occurs in less than 1% of initial operations and more than 5% of repeat operations.[20] Fortunately, the symptoms in many of these nerve injuries are temporary, and full recovery may be seen at the 3- to 6-month follow-up. Hypoparathyroidism rarely occurs after initial explorations but may occur in 2.7% to 16% of reoperations.[23, 33, 34]

Anatomy

Facility in the identification of normal and abnormal parathyroid glands is essential. Parathyroid glands vary in color from light yellow to a reddish brown, and the consistency is usually soft and pliable.[35] A reddish color and dense consistency reflect a high parenchymal cell content (abnormal gland); a yellowish white color is found with a high fat content (normal gland).[35] Typically, four parathyroid glands are present.

Parathyroid glands differ in shape and size. Eighty-three percent are oval or bean shaped, 11% are elongated, 5% are bilobate, and 1% are multilobated.[35] Normal glands tend to be flat and ovoid; with enlargement, they become globular. Normal measurements are 3 × 5 × 7 mm. The combined weight of all parathyroid glands is 90 to 130 mg, and the superior glands are usually smaller than the inferior glands.[32] Most parathyroid glands are suspended by a small vascular pedicle and enveloped by a pad of fatty tissue.[36]

Autopsy series demonstrate that four glands are found in 91% of subjects, five glands in 4%, and three glands in 5%.[37] In studies done by serial sectioning of embryos, at least four parathyroid glands were found in every specimen.[37] Approximately 5% of humans have supernumerary (more than four) parathyroid glands.[38] Supernumerary glands and fragments of parathyroid glands are most commonly found within the thymus.

Although gland distribution may deviate widely, the location of parathyroid glands is predictable from knowledge of embryology.[36] Originating from the fourth pharyngeal pouch,[39] the superior parathyroid glands are commonly found along the posterior surface of the upper two-thirds of the thyroid gland (92%)[35] (Fig. 79–8). Frequently (40%), superior parathyroid gland adenomas migrate posteriorly, behind the inferior thyroid artery, to a position along the esophagus.[29] Division of the superior thyroid artery and mobilization of the superior thyroid pole are usually unnecessary to expose the superior parathyroid glands, but the fascia connecting the lateral portion of the thyroid lobe to the carotid sheath must be incised. The location of the superior glands is relatively constant, and these glands can generally be identified quickly and easily. Superior parathyroid adenomas may have a unique relationship to the recurrent laryngeal nerve such that the nerve is embedded in the anterior medial capsule of the adenoma or the gland can be rounded and tucked into the exact spot where the recurrent nerve enters the larynx.

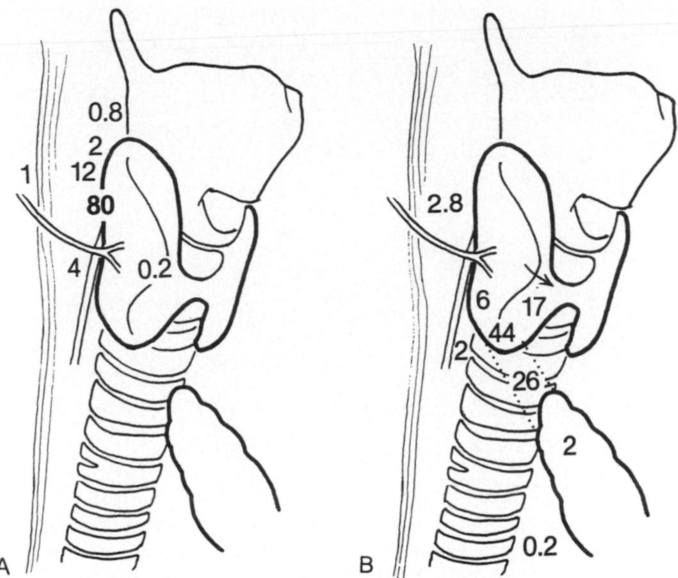

FIGURE 79–8. Diagram of potential locations of superior *(A)* and inferior *(B)* parathyroid glands. Numbers refer to the percentage of glands found at each location. (Data from Akerstrom G, Malmaeus J, Bergstrom R: Surgical anatomy of human parathyroid glands. Surgery 95:14, 1984.)

The inferior parathyroid glands have a more variable distribution than the superior ones (see Fig. 79–8). With the thymus, they originate from the third pharyngeal pouch.[39] As the thymus migrates caudally, the lower glands migrate until they reach the lower pole of the thyroid gland. Seventeen percent of inferior parathyroid glands touch the inferior border of the thyroid, 44% are within 1 cm of the inferior border of the thyroid (also known as the thyrothymic ligament), 26% are within the superior horn of the thymus, and 2% are in the mediastinal thymus.[35, 36] The remainder are either within the thyroid or are undescended in the upper portion of the neck near the carotid bifurcation[40] (see Fig. 79–8). This variable anatomic distribution makes the inferior glands more difficult to locate than the superior ones. An inferior parathyroid adenoma is generally bordered posteriorly and laterally by the recurrent laryngeal nerve and is inferior to the inferior thyroid artery.

General Technique of Exploration

General endotracheal anesthesia is used, although local anesthesia may be effective.[40, 41] The patient is positioned in a manner as for thyroid surgery. A transverse cervical incision is made approximately 2 cm above the sternal notch in a skin crease. The platysma is incised, and flaps are raised cephalad to the thyroid notch and caudad to the sternal notch. A retractor is positioned, and the fascia between the strap muscles is opened in the midline. We recommend identification and biopsy of all four parathyroid glands. Abnormal glands are completely removed. However, others recommend identification of all glands, excision of any abnormal glands, and biopsy of only one normal parathyroid gland. Others recommend a more focused approach based on a hand-held gamma probe to detect labeled sestamibi within an adenoma.[42]

The manner of parathyroid biopsy is very important. Parathyroid glands are usually encircled by an envelope of fat (halo sign). The blood supply is represented by a single small artery and vein that form a discrete pedicle. It is mandatory to gently dissect the fat from the more brown parathyroid gland and to biopsy the side opposite the blood supply. Parathyroid glands must be handled with care because they are delicate structures and the blood supply is easily damaged.

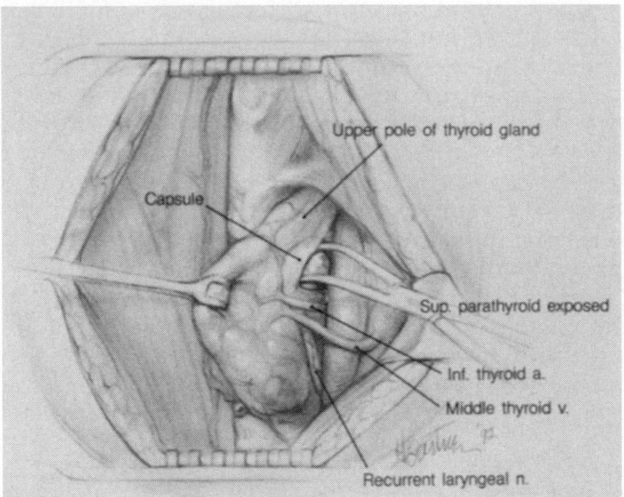

FIGURE 79–9. Identification of a left superior parathyroid adenoma. The thyroid gland is elevated with a Babcock clamp. The investing thyroid fascia is opened posterior to the upper pole of the left lobe. A left upper parathyroid adenoma is identified superior to the inferior thyroid artery and posterolateral to the recurrent laryngeal nerve. The left recurrent laryngeal nerve is shown in its usual location within the tracheoesophageal groove and posterior to the inferior thyroid artery.

After the thyroid gland is exposed, either the right or left thyroid lobe is elevated and rotated medially. The recurrent laryngeal nerve and inferior thyroid artery must be identified. In most patients, the recurrent laryngeal nerve lies in the tracheoesophageal groove, but on the right side it tends to lie more lateral to the trachea and is more susceptible to injury.[43] It may be direct rather than recurrent on the right side.[32] A useful method to identify each recurrent laryngeal nerve is to use its relationship to the inferior cornu of the thyroid cartilage.[43] Dissection of the neck requires meticulous hemostatic technique. Blood-stained tissue alters the color and makes identification of the parathyroid glands more difficult. The upper glands are usually posterior and lateral to the recurrent laryngeal nerve (Fig. 79–9), and the lower glands are generally anteromedial to it (Fig. 79–10). Because the upper glands are most constant in location, they should be identified first. If findings on biopsy of the upper glands are normal but the lower glands cannot be located, the thyrothymic ligament should be carefully explored because 44% of inferior glands are within this ligament. If the ligament does not contain parathyroid tissue, both superior horns of the thymus in the lower part of the neck should be dissected and removed. Seventeen percent of inferior glands are found within the thymus. If the inferior gland is not within the thymus, the thyroid lobe on the side of the missing gland may be removed. Three percent of inferior parathyroid glands are found within the thyroid lobe. Thyroid lobectomy should be performed only as a final step after biopsy identification of three normal parathyroid glands, dissection of the thyrothymic ligament, removal of the superior horn of the thymus, dissection of the usual location inferior to the thyroid along the trachea, and a search high along the carotid sheath near the hyoid bone for a parathymic parathyroid.[40]

Failure of initial exploration, even with diligent search of the areas noted above, calls for stopping the procedure. Re-evaluation of the patient and localization procedures should be performed before initiating a median sternotomy (see Fig. 79–2). Median sternotomy is indicated in only 1% to 2% of patients undergoing initial exploration. In our series of 33 patients who underwent median sternotomy as part of a reoperation for primary hyperparathyroidism, 30% did not have abnormal parathyroid tissue in the mediastinum.[44] Of the abnormal mediastinal glands found, most were discovered in the thymus (64%), and total thymectomy was required. Wells and Cooper[71] have reported the ability to remove the entire thymus (including the mediastinal component) without dividing the sternum by using a special retractor to elevate the sternum. This procedure may be used to explore the anterior mediastinum less invasively.

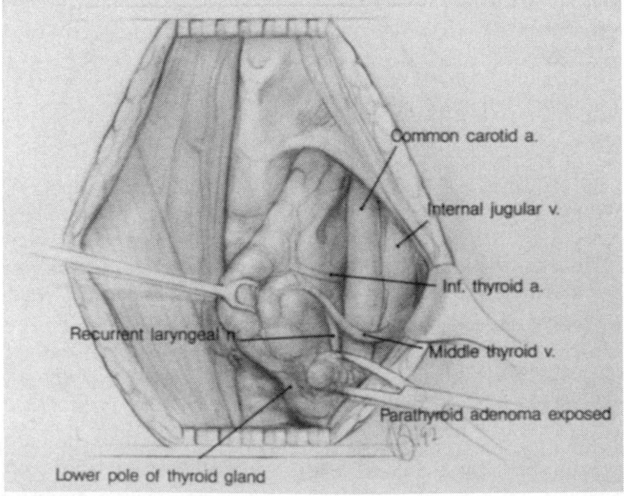

FIGURE 79–10. Identification of a left inferior parathyroid adenoma. The thyroid gland is elevated with a Babcock clamp. A left lower parathyroid adenoma is identified inferior to the inferior thyroid artery and anteromedial to the recurrent laryngeal nerve, which is the most common position for a left inferior parathyroid adenoma, although the inferior parathyroid gland can be located in other positions (see Fig. 79–8).

Special Issues in Surgery

Adenoma

The strategy of parathyroid surgery is controversial. Tibblin and others suggest exploring only one side of the neck. If one abnormal gland is found, it is removed and biopsy is performed on one normal gland.[45] This strategy has the advantage of leaving one side of the neck free and untraumatized. This approach may lead to occasional failure in patients with unrecognized multiple-gland disease. A most recent approach is minimally invasive radioguided parathyroid surgery.[46] Because a high proportion (90%) of parathyroid adenomas are imaged by sestamibi scanning, the technique is used to guide intraoperative localization of the abnormal gland with a hand-held gamma detector. Then, under local anesthesia an incision is made in the area of highest radioactivity and dissection is focused on the abnormal "hot" adenoma. This technique can be combined with immediate parathyroid hormone assay to quickly determine whether all the abnormal parathyroid tissue has been removed. The method relies on radioactive detection and PTH measurement to guide surgery rather than precise operative identification. It may be limited in identification of multiple abnormal glands and glands adjacent to the thyroid, which may also be hot. Paloyan et al. advocate 3.5-gland parathyroidectomy in all patients.[47] Long-term follow-up of patients treated with this more radical approach is comparable to that in other series, but a higher (3%) incidence of permanent hypoparathyroidism is reported.[47] In approximately 80% to 90% of patients, a single adenoma is the cause of hyperparathyroidism, and for these patients a 3.5-gland parathyroidectomy is clearly too much surgery and may result in an inordinately high incidence of hypoparathyroidism. Another strategy is to identify all four parathyroid glands visually, biopsy one normal gland, and remove one abnormal gland.[48, 49] If, however, persistent or recurrent disease develops later and requires repeat surgery, it is more difficult to plan the repeat surgical approach based merely on earlier visualization of glands without biopsy.[19, 23, 34, 50] We recommend exploration of the neck bilaterally and biopsy of four glands. Any enlarged or abnormal glands are removed.[32] The most important indicator of normal or abnormal parathyroid tissue is the appearance of the gland. Pathologists may find it difficult to differentiate normal from hypercellular parathyroid tissue or hyperplasia from adenoma, but they can reliably confirm that whatever tissue was biopsied is parathyroid.[32] If two glands are enlarged (double adenoma), both are removed. Long-term results with this method of management have been highly satisfactory.[30–32]

Hyperplasia

In generalized four-gland enlargement or hyperplasia, surgical management is more difficult and the results less satisfactory. Two possible surgical procedures designed for this diagnosis are subtotal (3.5-gland) parathyroidectomy and four-gland parathyroidectomy with immediate autografting. The results of subtotal parathyroidectomy have been variable, with a 13% incidence of persistent disease, a 15% incidence of recurrent disease, and a similar incidence of hypoparathyroidism. Moreover, in patients with MEN-1, subtotal parathyroidectomy led to a recurrence rate of 50% by 12 years after surgery.[6, 51] These data led others[52] to suggest total parathyroidectomy with autotransplantation rather than subtotal parathyroidectomy for patients with hyperplasia. Wells and colleagues reported results on 21 patients with hyperplasia who underwent this procedure.[53] Hypocalcemia developed in 20 of the 21 patients immediately postoperatively and necessitated vitamin D and calcium replacement. Within 2 months, 20 had a detectable PTH gradient between the grafted and nongrafted arm, indicative of normal autograft function, and were able to discontinue vitamin D and calcium supplementation. However, recurrent disease developed in 2 of 10 patients with nonfamilial hyperplasia and 7 of 11 with familial hyperplasia. Four patients with recurrent disease underwent partial graft resection, and all 4 were again rendered normocalcemic.

Our approach to nonfamilial parathyroid hyperplasia is subtotal (3.5-gland) parathyroidectomy, with approximately 30 to 50 mg of the most normal-appearing parathyroid tissue left and marked with a surgical clip in the neck. The incidence of either persistent disease or hypoparathyroidism has been low, and we expect the rate of recurrent disease to be between 10% and 20%. For familial hyperplasia we use total parathyroidectomy and immediate placement of a parathyroid autograft in the forearm because the incidence of recurrent disease is high (38%–64%).[51, 53] If recurrent hypercalcemia develops, a portion of the transplanted tissue can be removed under local anesthesia. In patients with recurrent disease after subtotal parathyroidectomy, total parathyroidectomy with cryopreservation of resected tissue is required.[48] It is important to prove that all hyperplastic tissue has been removed before reimplantation.[54] Unfortunately, cryopreserved parathyroid autotransplantation appears to have a high incidence of failure inasmuch as only 70% of human cryopreserved autografts function normally.[55]

Secondary and Tertiary Hyperparathyroidism

Almost all patients with advanced renal failure who are maintained by chronic dialysis have evidence of bone disease secondary to hyperparathyroidism and elevated serum levels of PTH. Secondary hyperparathyroidism should be suppressed in these individuals by measures that normalize serum levels of calcium and phosphorus. These measures include the use of a dialysate calcium concentration of 3.5 mEq/L, oral calcium supplementation, dietary restriction of phosphorus (<600 mg/day), phosphate-binding antacids, and vitamin D analogues to promote intestinal absorption of calcium.[56] Failure of these strategies occurs in a minority of individuals, and tertiary hyperparathyroidism is diagnosed when serum levels of ionized calcium and intact PTH are elevated. Subtotal parathyroidectomy is then used to decrease the mass of hyperplastic parathyroid tissue.

Potential indications for parathyroidectomy in these patients include (1) hypercalcemia in prospective renal transplant patients; (2) pathologic fractures secondary to renal osteodystrophy; (3) symptoms such as pruritus, bone pain, and extensive soft tissue calcification and calciphylaxis; (4) hypercalcemia in patients with well-functioning renal transplants; and (5) a calcium times phosphate product greater than 70.[57, 58] Improvements in medical management have reduced the need for surgery.

Controversy exists about whether to perform subtotal parathyroidectomy,[56] total parathyroidectomy without an autograft, or total parathyroidectomy with an immediate autograft.[53] We recommend total (four-gland) parathyroidectomy with an immediate parathyroid autograft in the treatment of secondary hyperparathyroidism.[59] In one study of 30 patients with secondary hyperparathyroidism treated by total parathyroidectomy and an immediate autograft, 80% showed symptomatic relief, and immediate postoperative hypoparathyroidism develop in all. The autograft functioned in 87% of patients at the 20-month follow-up, as determined by PTH concentrations in the venous blood of the arm bearing the graft, and patients were withdrawn from supplemental calcium or vitamin D by the 9-month follow-up. Biopsy of the autografts in 10 patients showed hyperplasia.[59] It is particularly important to avoid permanent hypoparathyroidism in these patients because of the increased likelihood of aluminum-related bone disease.[57]

Reoperations for Primary Hyperparathyroidism

Reoperations for primary hyperparathyroidism should be classified as operations for either persistent disease or recurrent disease. Persistent disease means that hypercalcemia never resolved after the initial neck exploration. Recurrent disease means that hypercalcemia recurs after an initial period of hypocalcemia or normalization of serum calcium. The complexity of repeat neck surgery for primary hyperparathyroidism makes it imperative to confirm the diagnosis and presence of symptoms and to order preoperative localization studies.[19, 23] The prior operative record and pathology reports are reviewed.

The first operative report, pathology results, and localization studies are used to plan the re-exploration. For example, if two abnormal parathyroid glands were removed and the family history is positive for parathyroid disease, the working diagnosis is hyperplasia. A biopsy-proven normal gland found at the initial procedure and radiologic localization studies suggesting a mediastinal adenoma prompt a direct mediastinal approach. Designing the operation—right side, left side, median sternotomy, all or any—can be done only by putting all the data together. We use an alternative route in the neck along the medial border of the sternocleidomastoid muscle instead of between the strap muscles.[19, 23, 50] This technique requires a separate approach on each side of the neck. It is especially important to look for intrathyroid, intrathymic, and paraesophageal parathyroid adenomas because ectopic locations are more common in reoperations.

A new strategy for reoperations is minimally invasive radioguided parathyroidectomy. Norman and Denham recently reported their experience in 21 patients with primary hyperparathyroidism who had undergone previous neck exploration for parathyroid or thyroid disease.[46] The neck re-exploration is guided by a hand-held gamma probe. Possible advantages of this technique include smaller incisions, less operative time, decrease risk of nerve injury and complications, outpatient surgery, and no frozen section analysis. However, the results are preliminary and the reported series is small.

Finally, it should be remembered that even during reoperations for primary hyperparathyroidism, most abnormal glands can be removed through a cervical incision[26] (Fig. 79–11). Abnormal parathyroid glands may be retroesophageal or posterior along the tracheoesophageal groove, which is the most common missed position.[19, 23, 29] They may be intrathyroidal,[60] or they may be located in an undescended parathymic remnant high in the carotid sheath.[61, 62] If these abnormal glands are not in the neck, they may be in the thymus.[36, 44] Slow, meticulous exploration in a bloodless field is generally necessary to find these "ectopic" glands (see Fig. 79–11).

Cryopreservation of removed parathyroid tissue during reoperations is indicated. One cannot predict from prior records whether normal parathyroid tissue remains in the neck. In our experience with reoperations on 175 patients, 35% left the hospital taking vitamin D medication and 43% taking supplemental calcium.[23, 61] Twenty-two patients (12%) were ultimately found to be permanently hypoparathyroid and required cryopreserved autologous parathyroid grafts. This outcome fits well with other published reports in which the rate of hypoparathyroidism after reoperative parathyroid surgery is between 2.7% and 16%. Cryopreservation with delayed autografting is a standard approach, although the overall success rate with cryopreserved grafts is only approximately 50% to 60%; this rate appears to be less than for fresh grafts, which have a 75% to 100% success rate.[55]

Reoperative parathyroid disease remains a major challenge. It is

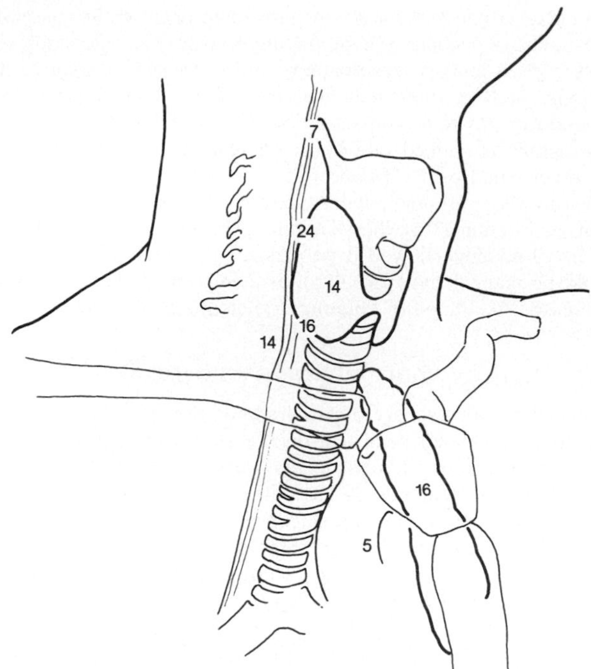

FIGURE 79–11. Location of abnormal parathyroid glands found during reoperations for primary hyperparathyroidism. Numbers refer to the percentage of glands found at each location.

clear that operative risk increases with each succeeding re-exploration. With careful attention, however, to confirmation of the diagnosis, prior operative records, judicious use of preoperative localization, and postoperative autografting, a successful outcome may be achieved in approximately 80% to 90% of reoperations.[23, 61]

Parathyroid Carcinoma

Parathyroid carcinoma should be considered in the working diagnosis of patients with primary hyperparathyroidism when the serum level of calcium is very high (>13 mg/dL), in patients with evidence of local recurrence of the abnormal gland, or when a palpable neck mass is present.[5, 63]

It is difficult to accurately assess the spectrum of clinical manifestations, degree of malignancy, and prognosis of parathyroid carcinoma. The incidence is very low, and the malignancy appears to be diagnosed at an earlier stage as a result of earlier detection of hypercalcemia. A major problem is failure to properly identify the correct pathologic diagnosis during the operation and, therefore, failure to perform adequate resection of the carcinomatous parathyroid tissue along with the ipsilateral lobe of the thyroid.[64] Unequivocal pathologic features of parathyroid carcinoma include the identification of mitoses in several high-power microscopic fields, fibrous bands or desmoplasia, and evidence of distant metastases or direct local invasion of the capsule, adjacent structures, and blood vessels.[65] However, not all patients with parathyroid carcinoma have all these features, so the diagnosis must be ascertained from clinical as well as pathologic evidence.[5] Furthermore, the natural history of patients with parathyroid cancer appears to be variable. Some tumors disseminate rapidly and have a poor prognosis,[66] whereas others tend to recur locally and have a long disease-free interval.[5]

Literature reports involving single cases tend to emphasize more serious tumors, either intrinsically malignant or long-standing, with clear evidence of extraglandular spread at the initial operation. The cancer is usually invading along the tracheoesophageal groove, and the patient may have hoarseness secondary to a recurrent laryngeal nerve injury. At neck exploration, the carcinomatous tissue appears gray with a thick, hard capsule. We recommend, based on suspicion (e.g., mass, local recurrence, high serum level of calcium), wide excision, including thyroid lobectomy in continuity with the tumor.[5, 64, 65] If one has doubt about the diagnosis, biopsy of tumor extrinsic from the main tumor mass either within lymph nodes or invading local strap muscle provides clear evidence of cancer. Recurrent laryngeal nerve injury, either from the tumor itself or from the surgeon attempting to completely resect the tumor mass with the ipsilateral thyroid lobe, is probable and occurs in 75% of patients.[5] Locally recurrent benign parathyroid adenomas may occur and be confused with parathyroid carcinomas. Recurrent adenomas generally have a longer disease-free interval, a lower serum level of calcium, and a history of either incomplete resection or spillage of tumor at the time of initial surgery.[5] Nevertheless, both locally recurrent parathyroid adenoma and cancer appear to respond favorably to aggressive local re-resection, and most patients can be rendered either hypocalcemic or normocalcemic for a reasonable period.[5] Once disease has spread to distant sites, surgery appears to have less of a role in treatment. Resection of pulmonary metastatic disease has been tried,[66] but with minimal gain. In patients with distant metastases, chemotherapy has been used with some benefit.[65] Therapy for these patients has been primarily directed at controlling the severe hypercalcemia.

Parathyroid Transplantation

Halsted performed the first experimental parathyroid transplant in 1909. Since then, many successful transplants in laboratory animals and in humans have been reported.[52, 53] Parathyroid glands have been successfully cryopreserved, stored for long periods, and then transplanted back into humans.[67] Finally, parathyroid tissue has been successfully allografted into immunosuppressed human hosts.[68]

The clinical indications for autotransplantation at the time of surgery or delayed cryopreserved transplantation are primary or secondary parathyroid hyperplasia, re-exploration for persistent or recurrent hyperparathyroidism, and total thyroidectomy for thyroid carcinoma.

The function of immediate (stored in the operating room in iced saline) parathyroid autografts is between 75% and 100%.[55, 69] The function of delayed cryopreserved autografts varies from 54%[69] to 83%.[53] Immediate autografts of either adenoma or hyperplastic glands may lead to recurrent hypercalcemia and may require partial re-excision. Cryopreserved abnormal parathyroid tissue has not appeared to result in recurrent disease but has a higher likelihood of reduced function. In vitro studies demonstrating reasonable function of cryopreserved parathyroid tissue do not appear to correlate with the outcome of human grafts.

The procedure for parathyroid transplantation and cryopreservation is as follows: maintain the tissue on the operating table chilled in sterile saline, and slice the tissue into slivers 1 × 1 × 3 mm in size (Fig. 79–12). For immediate autografting, 20 pieces are implanted into the sternocleidomastoid muscle of the neck (only normal parathyroid tissue during thyroidectomy) or the brachioradialis muscle of the forearm (abnormal hyperplastic parathyroid tissue during total parathyroidectomy) (see Fig. 79–12). Care is taken to not induce bleeding, and each implantation site is closed with 6-0 silk suture. Should graft-dependent hyperparathyroidism subsequently develop, a portion of the graft can be removed under local anesthesia. For cryopreservation, the parathyroid slivers are put into 3-mL glass vials, 10 pieces each, with 1.5 mL of solution containing 10% dimethyl sulfoxide, 10% autologous serum, and 80% tissue culture medium. The vials are immediately placed in an automated freezing chamber and the temperature programmed to decrease 1°C/min to −80°C. The vials are then stored in a liquid nitrogen freezer at −190°C.

Postoperative Hypocalcemia

Most patients who have undergone successful surgery for primary hyperparathyroidism have some (albeit mild) symptoms of hypocalcemia, and a positive Chvostek sign may develop. These symptoms should initiate measurement of the serum level of calcium and phosphorus. Treatment is guided primarily by the serum level of calcium, which should be maintained above 8.0 mg/dL. Initially, dietary calcium is used. However, dietary calcium, primarily milk products, is associ-

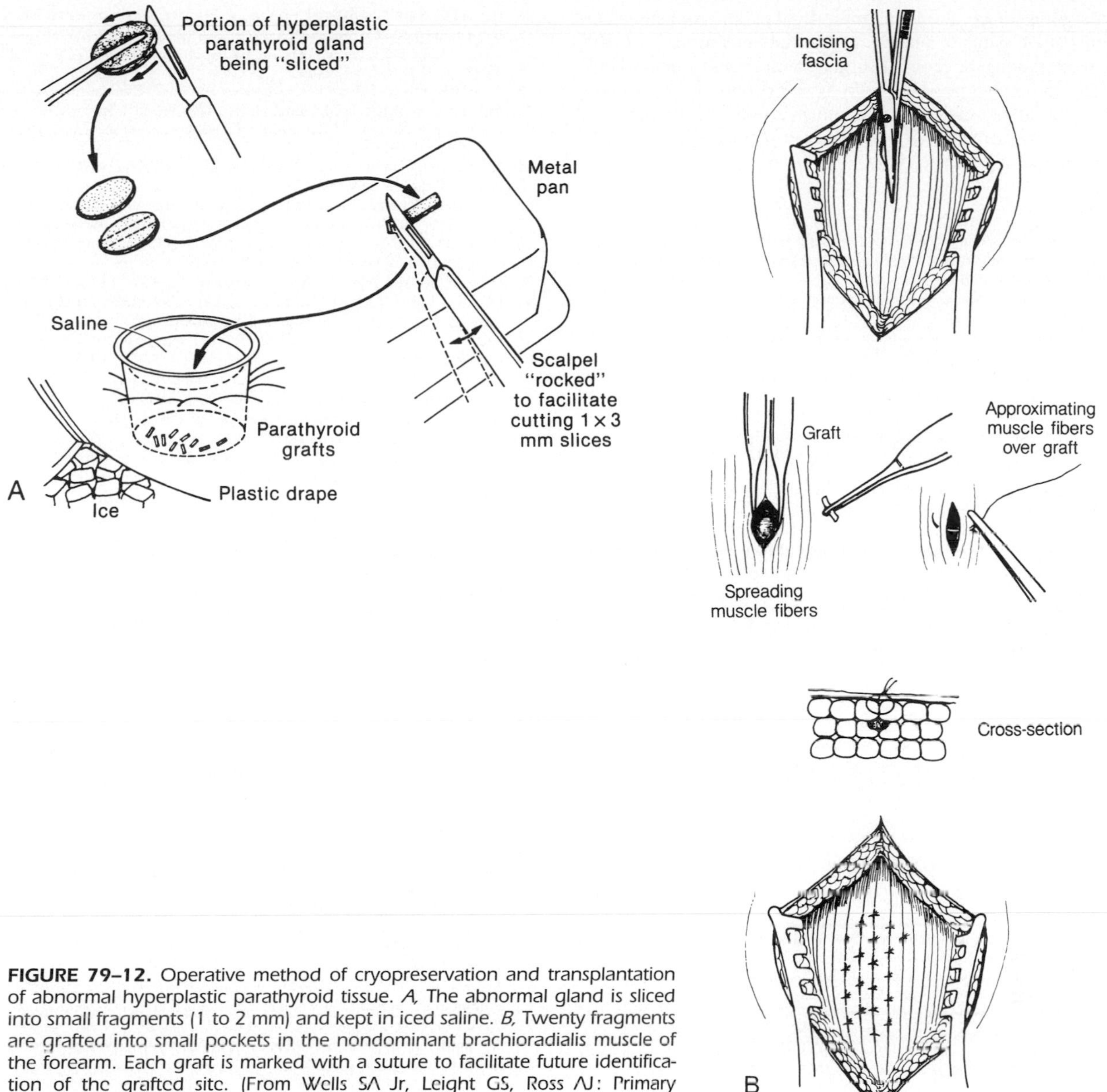

FIGURE 79–12. Operative method of cryopreservation and transplantation of abnormal hyperplastic parathyroid tissue. *A,* The abnormal gland is sliced into small fragments (1 to 2 mm) and kept in iced saline. *B,* Twenty fragments are grafted into small pockets in the nondominant brachioradialis muscle of the forearm. Each graft is marked with a suture to facilitate future identification of the grafted site. (From Wells SA Jr, Leight GS, Ross AJ: Primary hyperparathyroidism. Curr Probl Surg 17:398–463, 1980.)

ated with a large phosphate load and may result in hyperphosphatemia. If this complication occurs, elemental calcium may be given in the usual oral doses of 1 to 2 g/day. Recently, patients have not been hospitalized after parathyroidectomy. Instead, they have been given prescriptions for oral calcium and calcitriol to minimize hypocalcemia and the symptoms from it. This practice has resulted in shorter hospitalizations and fewer symptoms of tetany.

If the symptoms of hypocalcemia are severe and the patient appears to be on the verge of tetany (occurring most frequently in patients with "hungry bone syndrome"), the clinician may need to treat with intravenous calcium. These symptoms can usually be rapidly corrected by the infusion of 2 mg/kg of elemental calcium over a 15-minute period. Symptoms return unless a longer infusion is used. Approximately 15 mg/kg of elemental calcium is then infused over a 24-hour period, with half the total amount administered in the initial 6 hours. Serum levels of calcium should be monitored closely during the infusion, and infusion rates and amounts may be adjusted accordingly. Only approximately 13% of patients have severe symptoms of hypoparathyroidism after surgery; these patients appear to be older; have higher preoperative serum levels of calcium, PTH, alkaline phosphatase, and urea nitrogen; and have large adenomas removed at surgery.[15] They typically require intravenous calcium. Most patients do not need this type of calcium replacement.

When hypocalcemia persists despite maximal oral replacement doses and hyperphosphatemia develops, we recommend the use of a rapidly acting form of vitamin D.[70] We use $1,25(OH)_2D_3$ (calcitriol), which is the major biologically active metabolite of vitamin D_3. We recommend this drug with the expectation that we need rapid onset of action and short duration of use. The usual initial dose of calcitriol is 0.25 to 1.0 μg/day given on a twice-daily schedule. The dose can be increased to a maximum of 2.0 μg/day, depending on the response in terms of serum levels of calcium and phosphorus. In general, the lowest possible dose that produces low normal serum levels and no hypocalcemic symptoms should be used. Serum levels of calcium should be monitored weekly after discharge to further adjust oral calcium and calcitriol doses.

RESULTS OF SURGERY FOR PRIMARY HYPERPARATHYROIDISM

Despite the complexity and decision making required, the results of surgery for primary hyperparathyroidism are excellent. The success rate is between 85% and 100%, with a greater probability of success during initial procedures. Recurrent laryngeal nerve injuries have been reported in approximately 1% of patients undergoing initial operations and 5% undergoing reoperations. Chronic hypoparathyroidism occurs in less than 1% of patients undergoing initial operations and 10% undergoing reoperations. Successful surgery with reasonable morbidity appears to require experience inasmuch as the results of larger series are better than those of smaller ones. Evidence indicates that the vast majority of patients with primary hyperparathyroidism are cured by surgery and few suffer complications.

REFERENCES

1. Consensus Development Conference Panel: Diagnosis and management of asymptomatic primary hyperparathyroidism: Consensus Development Conference statement. Ann Intern Med 114:593–597, 1991.
2. Norton JA: Controversies and advances in primary hyperparathyroidism. Ann Surg 215:1–3, 1992.
3. Scholz DA, Purnell DC: Asymptomatic primary hyperparathyroidism: 10 year prospective study. Mayo Clin Proc 56:473–478, 1981.
4. Delbridge LW, Marshman D, Reeve TS, et al: Neuromuscular symptoms in elderly patients with hyperparathyroidism: Improvement with parathyroid surgery. Med J Aust 149:74–76, 1988.
5. Fraker DL, Travis WD, Merendino JJ Jr, et al: Locally recurrent parathyroid neoplasms as a cause for recurrent and persistent primary hyperparathyroidism. Ann Surg 213:58–65, 1991.
6. Rizzoli R, Green J III, Marx SJ: Primary hyperparathyroidism in familial multiple endocrine neoplasia type I: Long-term follow-up of serum calcium levels after parathyroidectomy. Am J Med 78:467–474, 1985.
7. Keiser HR, Beaven MA, Doppman J, et al: Sipple's syndrome: Medullary thyroid carcinoma, pheochromocytoma and parathyroid disease. Ann Intern Med 78:561–579, 1973.
8. Marx SJ, Menczel J, Campbell G, et al: Heterogeneous size of the parathyroid glands in familial multiple endocrine neoplasia type 1. Clin Endocrinol 35:521–526, 1991.
9. The European Consortium on MEN 1: Identification of the multiple endocrine neoplasia type 1 (MEN1) gene. Hum Mol Genet 6:7, 1997.
10. Lairmore TC, Howe JR, Korte JA, et al: Familial medullary thyroid carcinoma and multiple endocrine neoplasia type 2B map to the same region of chromosome 10 as multiple endocrine neoplasia type 2A. Genomics 9:181–192, 1991.
11. Marx SJ, Spiegel AM, Levine MA, et al: Primary hyperparathyroidism in familial multiple endocrine neoplasia type I: Long-term follow-up of serum calcium after parathyroidectomy. Am J Med 307:416–426, 1982.
12. Hosokawa Y, Pollak MR, Brown EM, et al: Mutational analysis of the extracellular Ca^{++} sensing receptor gene in human parathyroid tumors. J Clin Endocrinol Metab 80:11, 1995.
13. Fitzpatrick LA, Bilezikian JP: Acute primary hyperparathyroidism: A review of 48 patients. Am J Med 82:272–282, 1987.
14. Bilezikian JP: Management of acute hypercalcemia. N Engl J Med 326:1196–1203, 1992.
15. Brasier AR, Nussbaum SR: Hungry bone syndrome: Clinical and biochemical predictors of its occurrence after parathyroid surgery. Am J Med 84:654–660, 1988.
16. van Heerden JA, James EM, Caselle PR, et al: Small part ultrasonography in primary hyperparathyroidism. Ann Surg 195:774–780, 1982.
17. Serpell JW, Campbell PR, Young AE: Preoperative localization of parathyroid tumours does not reduce operating time. Br J Surg 78:589–590, 1991.
18. Carty SE, Norton JA: Management of patients with persistent or recurrent primary hyperparathyroidism. World J Surg 15:716–723, 1991.
19. Shen W, Duren M, Morita E, et al: Reoperation for persistent or recurrent primary hyperparathyroidism. Arch Surg 131:861–869, 1996.
20. Patow CA, Norton JA, Brennan MF: Vocal cord paralysis and reoperative parathyroidectomy. Ann Surg 203:282–285, 1986.
21. Miller DL, Doppman JL, Shawker TH, et al: Localization of parathyroid adenomas in patients who have undergone surgery: Part I. Noninvasive imaging methods. Radiology 162:133–137, 1987.
22. Miller DL: Preoperative localization and interventional treatment of parathyroid tumors: When and how? World J Surg 15:706–715, 1991.
23. Lange JR, Norton JA: Surgery for persistent or recurrent primary hyperparathyroidism. Curr Pract Surg 4:56–62, 1992.
24. Wei JP, Burke GJ, Mansberger AR: Preoperative imaging of abnormal parathyroid glands in patients with hyperparathyroid disease using combination Tc-99m-pertechnetate and Tc-99m-sestamibi radionuclide scans. Ann Surg 219:5, 1994.
25. McBiles M, Lambert AT, Cote MG, Kim SY: Sestamibi parathyroid imaging. Semin Nucl Med 25:221–234, 1995.
26. Norman J, Chheda H, Farrell C: Minimally invasive parathyroidectomy for primary hyperparathyroidism: Decreasing operative time and potential complications while improving cosmetic results. Am Surg 64:391–396, 1998.
27. Patel PC, Pellitteri PK, Patel NM, Fleetwood MK: Use of rapid intraoperative parathyroid hormone assay in the surgical management of parathyroid disease. Arch Otolaryngol Head Neck Surg 123:559–562, 1998.
28. Bergenfelz A, Isaksson A, Lindblom P, et al: Measurement of parathyroid hormone in patients with primary hyperparathyroidism undergoing first and reoperative surgery. Br J Surg 85:1129–1132, 1998.
29. Thompson NW, Eckhauser F, Harness J: Anatomy of primary hyperparathyroidism. Surgery 92:814, 1982.
30. Attie JN, Bock G, Auguste L-J: Multiple parathyroid adenomas: Report of thirty-three cases. Surgery 108:1014–1020, 1990.
31. Roses DF, Karp NS, Sudarsky LA, et al: Primary hyperparathyroidism associated with two enlarged parathyroid glands. Arch Surg 124:1261–1265, 1989.
32. Wells SA, Leight GF, Ross A: Primary hyperparathyroidism. Curr Probl Surg 17:398, 1980.
33. Grant CS, van Heerden JA, Charboneau JW, et al: Clinical management of persistent and/or recurrent primary hyperparathyroidism. World J Surg 10:555–565, 1986.
34. Brennan MF, Norton JA: Reoperation for persistent and recurrent hyperparathyroidism. Ann Surg 201:40–44, 1985.
35. Akerstrom G, Malmaeus J, Bergstrom R: Surgical anatomy of human parathyroid glands. Surgery 95:14, 1984.
36. Wang CA: The anatomic basis of parathyroid surgery. Ann Surg 183:271, 1975.
37. Alveryd A: Parathyroid glands in thyroid surgery. Acta Chir Scand 389:1, 1968.
38. Wang CA, Mahaffey JE, Axelrod L, et al: Hyperfunctioning supernumerary parathyroid glands. Surg Gynecol Obstet 148:711, 1979.
39. Gilmour JR: The gross anatomy of parathyroid glands. J Pathol 46:133, 1938.
40. Edis AJ, Purnell DC, van Heerden JA: The undescended parathymus: An occasional cause of failed neck exploration of hyperparathyroidism. Ann Surg 190:64–68, 1979.
41. Saxe A, Brown E, Hamburger SW: Thyroid and parathyroid surgery performed with patient under regional anesthesia. Surgery 103:415–420, 1988.
42. Norman J, Chheda H: Minimally invasive parathyroidectomy facilitated by intraoperative nuclear mapping. Surgery 122:998–1004, 1997.
43. Wang CA: The use of the interior cornu of the thyroid cartilage in identifying the recurrent laryngeal nerve. Surg Gynecol Obstet 140:91, 1975.
44. Norton JA, Schneider PD, Brennan MF: Median sternotomy in reoperations for primary hyperparathyroidism. World J Surg 9:807–813, 1985.
45. Tibblin S, Bondeson A, Ljungberg O: Unilateral parathyroidectomy due to single adenoma. Ann Surg 195:245, 1982.
46. Norman J, Denham D: Minimally invasive radioguided parathyroidectomy in the reoperative neck. Surgery 124:1088–1093, 1998.
47. Paloyan E, Lawrence AM, Baker WH, et al: Near-total parathyroidectomy. Surg Clin North Am 49:43, 1969.
48. McGarity WC, Bostwick J: Technique of parathyroidectomy. Ann Surg 42:657, 1976.
49. Satava RM Jr, Beahrs OH, Scholz DA: Success rate of cervical exploration for hyperparathyroidism. Arch Surg 110:625–628, 1975.
50. Saxe AW, Brennan MF: Strategy and technique of reoperative parathyroid surgery. Surgery 89:417, 1981.
51. Lamers CBHW, Froeling PGAM: Clinical significance of hyperparathyroidism in familial multiple endocrine adenomatosis type I (MEA I). Am J Med 66:422, 1979.
52. Wells SA, Ellis GJ, Gunnells JC, et al: Parathyroid autotransplantation in primary parathyroid hyperplasia. N Engl J Med 295:57, 1976.
53. Wells SA Jr, Farndon JR, Dale JK, et al: Long-term evaluation of patients with primary parathyroid hyperplasia managed by total parathyroidectomy and heterotopic autotransplantation. Ann Surg 192:451, 1980.
54. Saxe AW, Brennan MF: Reoperative parathyroid surgery for primary hyperparathyroidism caused by multiple-gland disease: Total parathyroidectomy and autotransplantation with cryopreserved tissue. Surgery 91:616–621, 1982.
55. Senapati A, Young AE: Parathyroid autotransplantation. Br J Surg 77:1171–1174, 1990.
56. Johnson WJ, McCarthy JT, van Heerden JA, et al: Results of subtotal parathyroidectomy in hemodialysis patients. Am J Med 84:23–32, 1988.
57. Andress DL, Ott SM, Maloney NA, et al: Effect of parathyroidectomy on bone aluminum accumulation in chronic renal failure. N Engl J Med 312:468–473, 1985.
58. Clark OH: Secondary hyperparathyroidism. *In* Clark OH (ed): Endocrine Surgery of the Thyroid and Parathyroid Glands. St Louis, Mosby, 1985, p 241.
59. Romanus ME, Farndon JR, Wells SA Jr: Transplantation of the parathyroid glands. *In* Johnston IDA, Thompson NW (eds): Endocrine Surgery. Stoneham, MA, Butterworth, 1983, pp 25–40.
60. Wang C, Gaz RD, Moncure AC: Mediastinal parathyroid exploration: A clinical and pathologic study of 47 cases. World J Surg 10:687–695, 1986.
61. Jaskowiak N, Norton JA, Alexander HR, et al: A prospective trial evaluating a standard approach to reoperation for missed parathyroid adenoma. Ann Surg 224:308–322, 1996.
62. Fraker DL, Doppman JL, Shawker TH, et al: Undescended parathyroid adenoma: An important etiology for failed operations for primary hyperparathyroidism. World J Surg 14:342–348, 1990.
63. Wang C, Gaz RD: Natural history of parathyroid carcinoma: Diagnosis, treatment, and results. Am J Surg 149:522–527, 1985.
64. Cohn K, Silverman M, Corrado J, et al: Parathyroid carcinoma: The Lahey Clinic experience. Surgery 98:1095, 1985.
65. Calandra DB, Chejfec G, Foy BK, et al: Parathyroid carcinoma: Biochemical and pathologic response to DTIC. Surgery 96:1132, 1984.
66. Flye MW, Brennan MF: Surgical resection of metastatic parathyroid carcinoma. Ann Surg 193:425, 1981.
67. Leight GS, Parker GA, Sears HF, et al: Experimental cryopreservation and autotransplantation of parathyroid glands: Technique and demonstration of function. Ann Surg 188:16, 1978.
68. Wells SA, Burdick JF, Hattler BG, et al: The allografted parathyroid gland: Evaluation of function in the immunosuppressed host. Ann Surg 180:805, 1974.
69. Niederle B, Roka R, Brennan MF: The transplantation of parathyroid tissue in man: Development, indications, techniques, and results. Endocr Rev 3:345, 1982.
70. Reichel H, Koeffler HP, Norman AW: The role of the vitamin D endocrine system in health and disease. N Engl J Med 320:980–991, 1989.
71. Wells SA Jr, Cooper JD: Closed mediastinal exploration in patients with persistent hyperparathyroidism. Ann Surg 214:555–561, 1991.

Chapter 80

Familial Hypocalciuric Hypercalcemia and Other Disorders Due to Calcium-Sensing Receptor Mutations

Ruben Diaz ▪ Edward M. Brown

One of the features that distinguishes the hormonal regulation of serum calcium from other endocrine regulatory systems is the capacity of tissues involved in calcium homeostasis to respond to or "sense" changes in extracellular calcium ion concentration (Ca^{2+}_o). Although this ability to sense changes in Ca^{2+}_o was long observed to be crucial for the maintenance of mineral ion homeostasis, the mechanism(s) underlying Ca^{2+}_o-sensing was not understood until recently. The cloning of the parathyroid Ca^{2+}_o sensing receptor (CaR), a guanine nucleotide (G) protein–coupled receptor (GPCR) that has Ca^{2+}_o as its principal physiologic ligand, has helped explain the mechanism of Ca^{2+}_o-sensing and the role of Ca^{2+}_o as a first messenger, much like a peptide hormone. Several previously described inherited disorders of Ca^{2+}_o homeostasis have been linked to activating or inactivating mutations of this recently recognized receptor. Inactivating mutations of the CaR produce hypercalcemic syndromes, while activating mutations produce a form of hypocalcemia resembling hypoparathyroidism. Furthermore, the identification of inherited diseases due to changes in receptor function has afforded "experiments in nature" that have clarified substantially the role of Ca^{2+}_o-sensing in the normal regulation of the function of parathyroid and other organs (e.g., kidney) involved in calcium homeostasis. This chapter briefly describes the physiologic role of the CaR in mineral ion homeostasis and delineates in more detail the principal clinical and biochemical features of inherited disorders caused by changes in CaR function.

CALCIUM-SENSING AND MINERAL ION HOMEOSTASIS

Calcium ions modulate or are essential for a vast array of intra- and extracellular processes.[1, 2] Calcium ions represent a key intracellular second messenger and serve as cofactors for various proteins and enzymes, thereby participating in functions as diverse as neurotransmission, cellular motility, hormonal secretion, muscular contraction, and cell division. Ca^{2+}_o also serves as a cofactor for adhesion molecules, clotting factors, and other serum proteins. Neuronal and muscular excitability are affected by Ca^{2+}_o. Calcium is also an essential component of the mineral phase of bone. The skeleton is a large reservoir of mineral ions that can be mobilized in times of need. The blood level of Ca^{2+}_o of most terrestrial animals remains almost invariant under normal circumstances, fluctuating from its mean value of approximately 1 mmol/L by only a few percent, despite only intermittent access to calcium in the diet. A complex homeostatic mechanism that functions to ensure near constancy of Ca^{2+}_o is present in most higher organisms.[1–3] This system adjusts the fluxes of calcium ions between the extracellular fluid and the outside environment, in kidney and intestine, as well as with the mineral phase of bone so as to maintain Ca^{2+}_o within a few percent of its average, normal level. Specific cells of the mineral ion homeostatic system detect (i.e., "sense") and respond in homeostatically appropriate ways to changes in the plasma calcium ion concentration. Classic examples of Ca^{2+}_o-sensing cells are the parathyroid hormone (PTH)–secreting chief cells of the parathyroid glands and the calcitonin (CT)-secreting C cells of the thyroid gland, which secrete less and more of these calciotropic hormones, respectively, when Ca^{2+}_o rises.[3] There is a steep inverse sigmoidal curve relating circulating PTH levels to induced changes in Ca^{2+}_o in normal humans, allowing for a very narrow range within which Ca^{2+}_o is maintained in vivo. Even very small perturbations in Ca^{2+}_o, on the order of a few percent, elicit large alterations in PTH secretion to restore Ca^{2+}_o to its set-point.

Extracellular calcium ions also have direct actions on other important components of the calcium homeostatic system. For instance, the activation of 25-hydroxyvitamin D 25(OH)D by 1-hydroxylation in the proximal tubular cells of the kidney is directly regulated by Ca^{2+}_o.[4] Raising the peritubular but not the luminal level of Ca^{2+}_o to which tubules of the renal thick ascending limb of Henle's loop are exposed diminishes tubular reabsorption of calcium and magnesium ions,[5] enhancing calcium excretion—a homeostatically appropriate response. High Ca^{2+}_o also inhibits the resorption of bone in organ culture[6] and by isolated osteoclasts, the cells that break down bone mineral and matrix.[7, 8] Since Ca^{2+}_o beneath a resorbing osteoclast can be as high as 8 to 40 mmol/L,[9] this resorbed calcium, upon release into the extracellular fluid of the bone microenvironment, could limit further bone breakdown by a direct feedback regulation of osteoclasts. Raising Ca^{2+}_o also stimulates several functions of the bone-forming osteoblasts, including cellular proliferation,[10–12] chemotaxis,[13] release of insulin-like growth factor-2,[14] and bone formation in organ culture.[6] These data strongly suggest that Ca^{2+}_o, like the more classic hormones, PTH, CT, and 1,25-dihydroxy vitamin D [$1,25(OH)_2D$] can act, in effect, as a local or systemic calciotropic "hormone" that plays a central role in maintaining extracellular calcium homeostasis.

CALCIUM-SENSING RECEPTOR

Cloning and Characterization of a G Protein–Coupled CaR

Ca^{2+}_o-sensing by parathyroid cells has been the focus of extensive research for several decades, but the description of a mechanism underlying this capacity has been elusive until very recently. Several lines of evidence suggested that a cell-surface receptor mediated Ca^{2+}_o-sensing by parathyroid cells. Exposure to lectins that bind protein-bound carbohydrate chains blocked the parathyroid cell's ability to sense Ca^{2+}_o,[2] pointing to a cell-surface protein as a putative sensor. Parathyroid cells respond to elevations of Ca^{2+}_o with activation of a number of signaling pathways often mediated by G proteins, intracellular proteins involved in receptor-mediated signal transduction. Elevations of Ca^{2+}_o are linked to increases in inositol phosphates[15, 16] with concomitant rises in intracellular calcium,[17] and inhibition of cyclic adenosine monophosphate (cAMP) production that is sensitive to pertussis toxin, an inactivator of the inhibitory G protein G_i,[18] suggesting that the sensor was a GPCR linked to stimulation and inhibition of phospholipase C and adenylate cyclase, respectively. Furthermore, expression of messenger RNAs (mRNAs) extracted from parathyroid glands in *Xenopus laevis* oocytes rendered them responsive to Ca^{2+}_o,[19, 20] as assessed by the activation of similar G protein–coupled signaling pathways. Brown and colleagues[21] made use of an expression cloning strategy in *X. laevis* oocytes, to isolate a complementary DNA (cDNA) clone coding for a protein with functional properties of a Ca^{2+}_o-sensor. Subsequently, other highly homologous CaRs have been characterized from human[22] and chicken parathyroid.[23] Expression of the CaR is not limited to the parathyroid or even tissues involved in calcium homeostasis. Functionally active CaRs have been isolated from human,[24] rat,[25] and rabbit kidney,[26] rat C cell,[27] and rat brain.[28] In addition to calcium ions, these CaRs are activated by magnesium ions, as well as by a variety of inorganic (e.g., the trivalent cation gadolinium) and organic polycations (i.e., spermine and neomycin). Of these various polycations, both magnesium[29] and spermine[30] are present in vivo at levels that might permit them to act as physiologic agonists of the CaR.

The predicted topology from the amino acid sequences of the bovine parathyroid CaR and its various species homologues reveal very similar overall structures (Fig. 80–1). A large (~600 amino acids) amino (N)-terminal extracellular domain (ECD) is followed by a central core of some 250 amino acids with seven predicted transmembrane domains (TMDs), characteristic of the GPCR superfamily, and a carboxyl (C)-terminal intracellular domain (ICD) of approximately 200 amino acids.[21] The CaR shares many features that are present in other GPCRs. The ECD has at its N-terminus a hydrophobic signal peptide sequence for membrane translocation during synthesis and several predicted sites for N-linked glycosylation that are necessary for its efficient expression on the cell surface. A number of putative protein kinase C and protein kinase A phosphorylation sites are present in both the intracellular loops between the TMDs and within the ICD, rendering the receptor potentially susceptible to regulation by cellular kinases. No high-affinity calcium-binding sites, such as EF hands, are present within the receptor's ECD or extracellular loops between the TMDs; however, this is not surprising, since the affinity of the receptor for Ca^{2+}_o is only in the millimolar range. Instead, the receptor's ECD and extracellular loops contain clusters of negatively charged amino acids (i.e., aspartate and glutamate) that might conceivably represent sites contributing to the sensing of calcium and other polycationic agonists. Similar clusters of acidic residues are thought to bind calcium in other low-affinity calcium-binding proteins.[31] These clusters of negatively charged amino acids could also contribute to the highly cooperative nature of the control of PTH secretion by Ca^{2+}_o,[32] since very small increases in Ca^{2+}_o can fully activate the receptor. Such positive cooperativity could result from the presence of multiple binding sites in a single receptor or by the interaction between receptor monomers. Recent findings have demonstrated that the CaR is present as dimers on the cell surface, with receptor monomers likely held together by disulfide bonds.[33] Dimerization may be important for functional activity of the CaR since co-expression and heterodimerization of two functionally inactive forms of the CaR bearing two different mutations has been shown to restore Ca^{2+}_o-dependent activation of CaR-dependent signaling pathways.[34]

Activation of the CaR is thought to recruit the binding of heterotrimeric G proteins to its intracellular loops and ICD, linking it to modulation of various intracellular effector systems (most likely $G_{q/11}$ for activation of phospholipase C and G_i for inhibition of adenylate cyclase[18, 35]). The CaR also activates phospholipase A_2 and phospholipase D, most likely indirectly through a protein kinase C–mediated mechanism.[36, 37] The receptor has also recently been shown to activate the mitogen-activated protein kinase pathway in rat-1 fibroblasts, probably via tyrosine phosphorylation of a member of the c-SRC tyrosine kinase family.[38] Only a single isoform of the CaR has been described to date that is apparently capable of activating all of these diverse signal transduction pathways.

The CaR shows striking topological similarities to the metabotropic glutamate receptors (mGluRs), despite sharing a modest 20% to 30% sequence homology. Additional members of a growing family of the GPCRs to which the CaR and the mGluRs belong, the so-called family C (or family 3) GPCRs, are the recently cloned G-protein–coupled γ-aminobutyric acid B ($GABA_B$) receptors[39] and a subfamily of putative pheromone receptors cloned from the rat vomeronasal organ.[40, 41] All of the family C GPCRs have large ECDs that likely evolved from the bacterial periplasmic binding proteins.[42] The latter bind a variety of extracellular ligands involved in chemotaxis or destined for cellular uptake by associated bacterial transport systems.

Tissue Distribution and Physiologic Roles of the CaR

The CaR is present in a wide variety of tissues, some of which play no obvious roles in mineral ion metabolism.[43] These tissues and cell types include the parathyroid glands; C cells; kidney, stomach, and intestinal epithelia; lung; both neurons and glial cells in the brain, as well as lens epithelial cells; fibroblasts; and diverse cells within the bone marrow. In addition to playing a central role in the regulation of calcium homeostasis, the CaR has been shown to modulate a variety of cellular functions such as cell proliferation and ion transport.

In parathyroid cells, the CaR appears to mediate the inhibitory effects of high Ca^{2+}_o on PTH secretion; however, the intracellular signals that regulate this inverse relationship remain unexplained. Several observations support the role of the CaR in the regulation of PTH secretion. In addition to Ca^{2+}_o, other ligands for the receptor also affect PTH secretion in a similar fashion. In instances when CaR expression is diminished or absent in parathyroid cells (e.g., in vitro culture, adenomatous and hyperplastic parathyroid glands), PTH secretion is poorly inhibited by elevations in Ca^{2+}_o.[44, 45] The more compelling evidence for the role of CaR in regulating PTH secretion comes from the marked impairment of high Ca^{2+}_o-induced inhibition of PTH secretion in patients that harbor inactivating mutations of the receptor discussed later in this chapter. In addition, the use of "calcimimetic" CaR agonists has shown that the CaR is probably also responsible for the high Ca^{2+}_o-mediated reduction in preproPTH mRNA levels.[46] Interestingly, in the C cell the CaR couples to stimulation, rather than inhibition, of CT secretion,[47] as it does in the adrenocorticotropic hormone (ACTH)–secreting AtT-20 cell line.[48] Thus, depending upon the cellular context in which it is expressed, the CaR can either stimulate or inhibit hormonal secretion. Finally, the pronounced chief cell hyperplasia seen in humans who are homozygous for inactivating mutations of the receptor[49] and mice with homozygous "knockout" of the CaR gene[50] provide indirect evidence for an important role of this receptor in tonically suppressing parathyroid cellular proliferation.

The CaR is present along much of the nephron, although there are some discrepancies as to which segments along the tubule express the receptor. In the cortical thick ascending limb (CTAL), where CaR is present at the highest levels, the receptor is located mainly on the basolateral plasma membrane where it can sense systemic (e.g., blood) levels of Ca^{2+}_o. The CaR in the CTAL and perhaps also in the distal convoluted tubule (DCT) regulates the tubular handling of calcium and magnesium, enhancing their reabsorption if Ca^{2+}_o is low and reducing it when Ca^{2+}_o is high.[51] The CaR and PTH receptors are both expressed in CTAL and DCT, which may permit mutually antagonistic

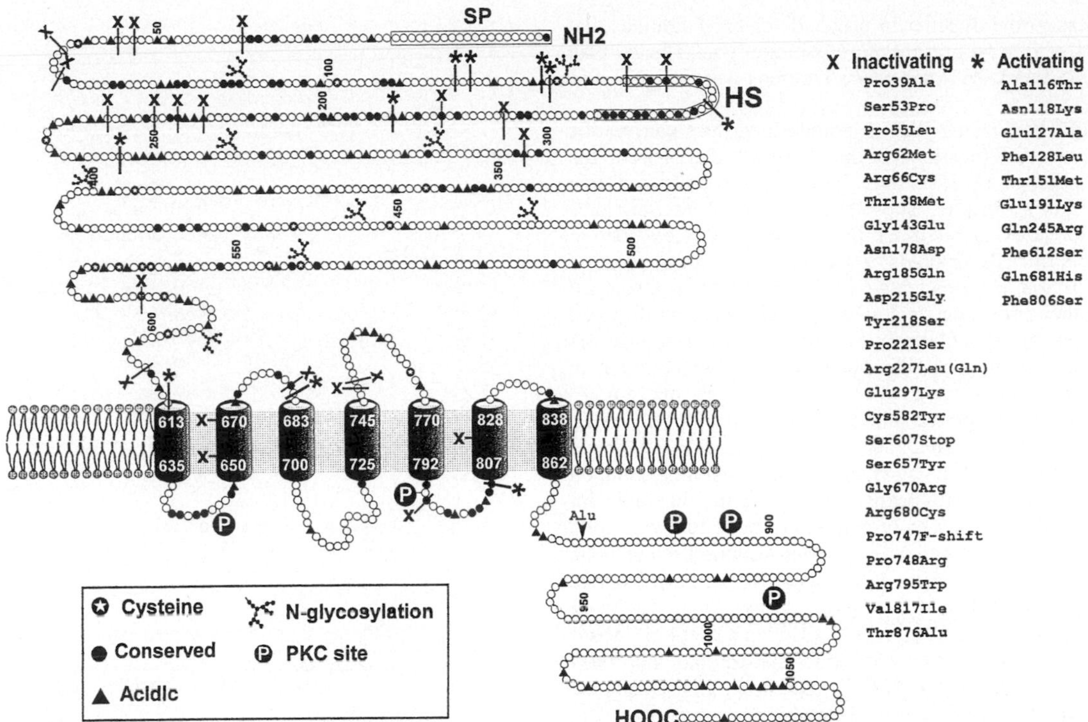

FIGURE 80–1. Schematic representation of the proposed topological structure of the extracellular Ca^{2+}_o-sensing receptor cloned from human parathyroid gland. SP, signal peptide; HS, hydrophobic segment. Also shown are missense and nonsense mutations causing either familial hypocalciuric hypercalcemia (FHH) or autosomal dominant hypocalcemia (ADH), which are indicated using the three-letter amino acid code, with the normal amino acid indicated before and the mutated amino acid causing FHH or ADH shown after the number of the relevant codon. (Modified from Brown EM, Harris HW Jr, Vassilev PM, et al: The biology of the extracellular Ca^{2+}_o-sensing receptor. *In* Raisz LG, Rodan G, Bilezikian JP (eds): Principles of Bone Biology. New York, Academic Press, 1996, p 243.)

interactions between the actions of these two receptors on the reabsorption of calcium in the distal nephron.[52] In the inner medullary collecting duct (IMCD), the CaR is situated largely on the apical (e.g., luminal) cell surface, thereby permitting monitoring of the level of Ca^{2+}_o within the final urine.[53] This apical CaR likely mediates the reduction in vasopressin-stimulated reabsorption of water that is observed when isolated tubules from the rat IMCD are perfused with high Ca^{2+}_o, an action that could potentially diminish the risk of renal stone formation when renal calcium excretion is increased. Moreover, through inhibition of NaCl reabsorption in the medullary thick ascending limb,[3] the CaR may further diminish maximal urinary concentrating capacity by decreasing the medullary hypertonicity that drives vasopressin-mediated, transepithelial water flow in the renal collecting duct.

DISORDERS OF CALCIUM RESISTANCE

Familial Hypocalciuric Hypercalcemia

In 1966, Jackson and Boonstra[54] described a patient with hypercalcemia that was not corrected despite the removal of three-and-one-half hyperplastic parathyroid glands. Multiple members in three generations of the patient's family were found to have hypercalcemia without having any symptoms or complications of hyperparathyroidism. The pattern of inheritance was suggestive of an autosomal dominant disorder. In 1972, Foley et al.[55] described a similar family with an unusually benign form of familial hypercalcemia. The proband was a 5-year-old boy who underwent resection of three normal parathyroid glands without correction of hypercalcemia. The proband had persistent hypocalciuria and the PTH levels of affected family members were within normal limits. The authors termed the condition *familial benign hypercalcemia* (FBH). This report was the first to outline clearly the characteristic clinical features of this syndrome. Later studies confirmed and extended the initial description of FBH. Marx and coworkers[56] called this syndrome of mild and largely asymptomatic hypercalcemia, *familial hypocalciuric hypercalcemia (FHH)*, because of the characteristic alteration in renal handling of calcium exhibited by affected family members. Both FHH and FBH are still used to describe this syndrome, but the former term is used in this chapter.

FHH is an uncommon genetic syndrome, occurring with a frequency that is probably about 1% of that of primary hyperparathyroidism.[56–58] It is inherited in an autosomal dominant fashion, being characterized by lifelong, usually asymptomatic hypercalcemia that is mild to moderate in its severity (usually <12 mg/dL). There is some variability in the degree of severity from family to family that appears to result from the particular functional properties of a given family's defective gene. A few families exhibit serum calcium concentrations that are minimally elevated or even consistently within the upper part of the normal range,[59] and occasional kindreds have serum calcium concentrations averaging greater than 12 or even 13 mg/dL.[49, 60, 61] FHH is often diagnosed serendipitously in the setting of a general laboratory screen or as a result of the diagnosis of hypercalcemia in other members of the family since it seldom causes any clinical symptoms.

Clinical Features of FHH

Despite the diagnosis of hypercalcemia, the symptoms and complications characteristic of other hypercalcemic disorders (i.e., gastrointestinal abnormalities, especially anorexia, nausea and constipation; mental disturbances; renal complications such as nephrolithiasis or nephrocalcinosis; impaired renal function; and defective urinary concentrating ability) are not commonly reported in affected individuals.[1, 62, 63] Even in FHH families with higher-than-average concentrations of serum calcium, affected members are generally remarkably asymptomatic. Nonspecific manifestations present in other forms of hypercalcemia, that is, fatigue, weakness, and arthralgia, were reported in some early clinical descriptions of FHH,[56] but more thorough evaluation of large families has failed to show any symptoms that are more common in affected family members.[58, 63] It is possible that ascertainment bias attributed symptoms to the disorder in probands of FHH families that were not, in fact, found to be present more commonly in affected than in unaffected family members when those kindreds were subjected to closer scrutiny.

Affected individuals in some FHH kindreds have had pancreatitis or chondrocalcinosis (calcification of the cartilage that covers the joint surfaces),[57] perhaps because these conditions represented true complications of this syndrome. Subsequent studies, however, have revealed that pancreatitis is no more prevalent in affected than in unaffected members of FHH kindreds or, for that matter, in the general population.[63] In addition, most patients with FHH who have developed pancreatitis had other coexistent factors that might have predisposed to this condition, such as alcoholism or gallstone.[63] Further studies have also not confirmed that chondrocalcinosis is more common in FHH than in the population as a whole.[58, 63] Although one study[58] described an apparently increased incidence of gallstones in FHH, most large series of FHH kindreds have not reported this to be a complication of the disorder. The incidence of hypertension, a common complication seen in patients with primary hyperparathyroidism, is not increased in FHH.[64] Mild elevations in markers of bone turnover, such as urinary hydroxyproline excretion, have been reported,[65] but bone mineral density is normal and there is no apparent increase in bone fracture rate or other complications of bone disease.[58, 65, 66] Several members of a recently reported FHH kindred from Oklahoma manifested osteomalacia, but this form of bone disease has not been encountered in other FHH kindreds.[67] In addition, this Oklahoma kindred has a form of FHH that is a genetically distinct from that present in the majority of families with this condition (see below). Life expectancy is normal in family members affected with FHH.

Biochemical Features

SERUM CALCIUM. The degree of elevation in the serum calcium concentration in FHH is similar to that encountered in patients with primary hyperparathyroidism of mild to moderate severity. There are equivalent increases in both the serum total and ionized calcium concentrations in the two conditions,[57, 58] suggesting that FHH is not caused by changes in serum calcium binding proteins. Hypercalcemia is typically present since birth and is persistent throughout life, a feature differentiating FHH from familial forms of primary hyperparathyroidism, in which affected family members do not develop hypercalcemia during their first decade.

SERUM PHOSPHATE AND MAGNESIUM. Persons with FHH often have some degree of reduction in serum phosphate concentration, although the latter value generally remains within the lower half of the normal range, and the degree of reduction in serum phosphate concentration is less than that found in primary hyperparathyroidism.[56, 58, 68, 69] Serum magnesium concentrations in FHH can be in the upper half of the normal range or in some cases frankly, albeit mildly, elevated. Unlike primary hyperparathyroidism, there is a positive correlation between the serum calcium and magnesium concentrations in FHH, so that hypermagnesemia may be more common in kindreds with more severe hypercalcemia[56] (Fig. 80–2).

SERUM ELECTROLYTES. In general, serum sodium, potassium, chloride, and bicarbonate levels are within the normal range in FHH patients.[56, 68] In some instances, older patients have been noted to have mildly elevated serum chloride, consistent with mild hyperchloremic acidosis, which can also be seen in primary hyperparathyroidism. Foley et al.[55] also noted a tendency toward increased citrate concentrations in adult FHH patients when compared with unaffected family members.

SERUM PTH. A very characteristic biochemical finding in FHH is an inappropriately "normal" intact PTH level in the face of concomitant hypercalcemia.[63, 70] Occasionally, PTH levels are in the lower part of the normal range or are frankly elevated.[71] Patients with FHH who exhibit overtly elevated PTH levels are difficult to differentiate from patients with mild primary hyperparathyroidism on the basis of their PTH levels alone. This is especially true in the 5% to 10% of patients with primary hyperparathyroidism whose intact PTH levels are in the upper part of the normal range. In addition, PTH levels have been noted to increase with age in FHH patients, further complicating the discrimination of FHH from primary hyperparathyroidism. Studies

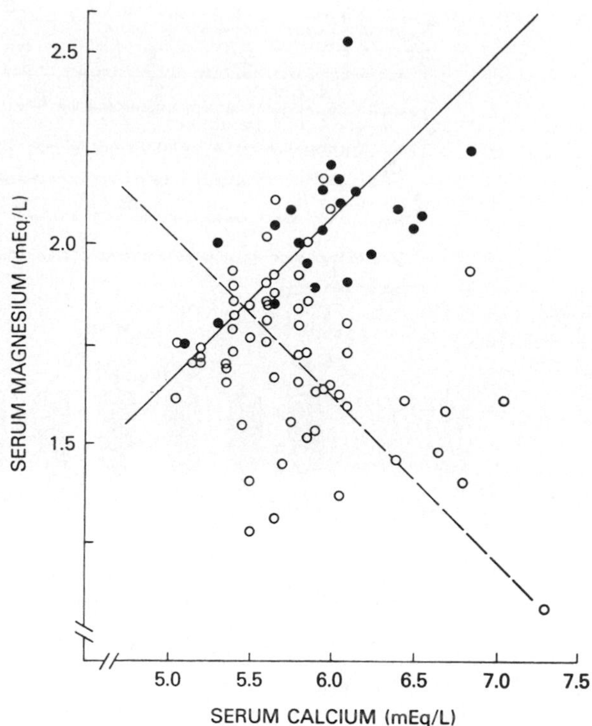

FIGURE 80–2. Relationship of serum calcium and magnesium concentrations in familial hypocalciuric hypercalcemia (FHH) *(closed symbols)* and primary hyperparathyroidism *(open symbols)*. Each point represents data from one patient. Note that among patients with primary hyperparathyroidism there is an inverse relationship between serum calcium and magnesium concentrations, whereas a positive relationship is present in FHH patients. (From Marx S, Spiegel A, Brown EM, et al: Divalent cation metabolism. Familial hypocalciuric hypercalcemia versus typical primary hyperparathyroidism. Am J Med 65:235, 1978. Copyright 1978, with permission from Excerpta Medica Inc.)

utilizing induced changes in serum calcium concentration have confirmed that patients with FHH exhibit dysregulation of Ca^{2+}_o-regulated PTH secretion, showing an increase in the level of Ca^{2+}_o half-maximally suppressing circulating PTH levels, that is, the set-point.[72, 73] Therefore, there is mild to moderate resistance of the parathyroid glands to the inhibitory effects of Ca^{2+}_o on PTH secretion in FHH. Although a similar, but somewhat more severe increase in set-point is exhibited by most patients with primary hyperparathyroidism,[32] these pathologic parathyroid glands have additional defects in PTH secretion, including increases in the maximal and minimal secretory rates observed at low and high Ca^{2+}_o, respectively.

Patients with FHH who have undergone partial or total parathyroidectomy because they were thought to have primary hyperparathyroidism often show normal histology of the parathyroid glands or only mild chief cell hyperplasia.[74, 75] Such patients have exhibited a distinctly atypical course following surgical intervention, providing additional indirect evidence that this disorder differs in some fundamental way from primary hyperparathyroidism. In 27 patients with FHH, each of whom had undergone from one to four neck explorations, recurrence of hypercalcemia took place within a few days or weeks in the majority of them (21 patients); only 2 of these patients remained permanently normocalcemic without any additional therapy.[57] More commonly, long-term remission of hypercalcemia in FHH patients required total removal of parathyroid tissue and treatment with vitamin D (5 of the 27 patients). Recurrent hypercalcemia following resection of a parathyroid adenoma, in contrast, occurs in less than 10% of cases, and, although recurrence of hypercalcemia occurs more commonly in the various forms of primary parathyroid hyperplasia, it generally occurs only after several years.

VITAMIN D. Serum 25(OH)D and $1,25(OH)_2D$ levels in patients with FHH are most commonly within the normal range[76–78] and their intestinal absorption of calcium is normal or modestly reduced. Some patients with FHH exhibit a blunted homeostatic response to a decrease in dietary intake of calcium, showing smaller-than-expected increases in their gastrointestinal absorption of calcium and $1,25(OH)_2D$ levels.[78] Patients with primary hyperparathyroidism, in contrast, frequently show elevated levels of the latter two parameters.

RENAL FUNCTION. Another characteristic biochemical feature of patients with FHH is their excessively avid renal tubular reabsorption of calcium and magnesium despite the concomitant hypercalcemia.[56] The marker of renal calcium handling that is employed most commonly to demonstrate this abnormality is the ratio of the renal clearance of calcium to that of creatinine[57] (Fig. 80–3A). The calcium-to-creatinine clearance ratio is less than 0.01 in about 80% of patients with FHH, while it is higher than this value in the great majority of patients with primary hyperparathyroidism. This ratio is generally even markedly greater in hypercalcemic conditions without parathyroid gland abnormality since the accompanying inhibition of PTH secretion further reduces renal tubular calcium reabsorption. In some instances, relative hypocalciuria can be observed in patients with what otherwise appears to be typical primary hyperparathyroidism. Causes of relative hypocalciuria in the setting of hypercalcemia that can be a source of diagnostic confusion include concomitant vitamin D deficiency, very low intake of calcium, use of thiazides or lithium, and hypothyroidism. Alternatively, occasional kindreds with FHH have been encountered in which there is hypercalciuria and even overt renal stone disease in some family members.[79] These families may have a variant of FHH or two separate disease genes—one conferring the FHH trait and the other promoting increased urinary calcium excretion, thereby outweighing the hypocalciuric effect of the FHH gene(s). This avid renal tubular calcium reabsorption in patients with FHH persists even after total parathyroidectomy[76, 80] (Fig. 80–3B), suggesting that the characteristic abnormality in renal calcium handling in this disorder is not dependent upon PTH but is an independent derangement in renal sensing or handling of Ca^{2+}_o. Thus, the combination of a low urinary calcium-to-creatinine clearance ratio and a normal PTH level in the setting of an autosomal dominant pattern of inheritance of mild, asymptomatic hypercalcemia usually makes the diagnosis of FHH straightforward.

Several additional parameters of renal function in patients with FHH also suggest altered responsiveness of the kidney to Ca^{2+}_o. Renal blood flow and glomerular filtration rate are both normal in FHH, even though these parameters are reduced in a sizable proportion of patients with other causes of chronic hypercalcemia.[57] Moreover, renal concentrating ability in patients with FHH is normal,[81] despite the fact that hypercalcemia of other causes not infrequently diminishes urinary concentrating ability and can sometimes cause overt nephrogenic diabetes insipidus.[82]

Treatment of FHH

Both the clinical and biochemical features of patients with FHH provide compelling evidence that this disorder represents an inherited abnormality in the sensing or handling of Ca^{2+}_o by parathyroid, kidney, and perhaps other tissues. Afflicted individuals are relatively spared the other gastrointestinal or mental symptoms encountered in the more usual forms of hypercalcemia, as though a similar loss of sensitivity were displayed by these organs. Because of the benign clinical course of patients with FHH and because it is so difficult to achieve a biochemical "cure," which would be of dubious value in an otherwise asymptomatic patient, a consensus has evolved that surgical intervention should be avoided in FHH. However, it is imperative that FHH be differentiated from primary hyperparathyroidism to avoid unnecessary and inadvisable exploration of the neck in patients with the former condition.

Neonatal severe hyperparathyroidism appears to be a very rare complication in FHH that in some instances represents the homozygous form of FHH (see below). In instances where both parents have FHH, their offspring have a higher risk (≈25%) of presenting with symptomatic hypercalcemia in the neonatal period. Alternatively, late-presenting hypocalcemia, possibly due to transient hypoparathyroidism, has been reported in at least one infant born to a mother with FHH.[83] Therefore, offspring of afflicted mothers with FHH should probably be carefully observed for symptoms of hyper- or hypocalcemia during the neonatal period.

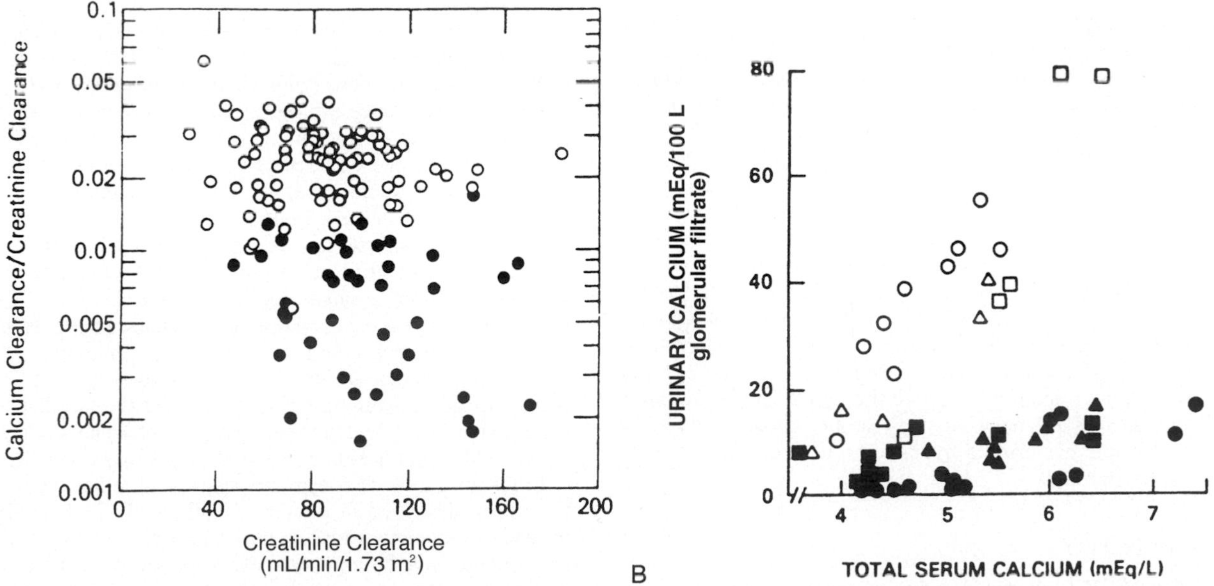

FIGURE 80–3. Altered renal handling of calcium in patients with familial hypocalciuric hypercalcemia (FHH) compared to other conditions. *A*, The urinary calcium-to-creatinine clearance ratio in patients with FHH expressed as a function of creatinine clearance relative to the values for patients with typical primary hyperparathyroidism. Approximately 80% of patients with FHH show a clearance ratio of less than 0.01, while only one patient with primary hyperparathyroidism had a value this low. (From Marx SJ, Attie MF, Levine MA, et al: The hypocalciuric or benign variant of familial hypercalcemia: Clinical and biochemical features in fifteen kindreds. Medicine (Baltimore) 60:397, 1981.) *B*, The relationship between serum calcium concentration and urinary calcium excretion in patients with FHH rendered surgically aparathyroid *(closed symbols)* compared with those with hypoparathyroidism alone *(open symbols)*. Note that there is persistent hypocalciuria in FHH patients. (From Attie MF, Gill J Jr, Stock JL, et al: Urinary calcium excretion in familial hypocalciuric hypercalcemia. Persistence of relative hypocalciuria after induction of hypoparathyroidism. J Clin Invest 72:667, 1983.)

Neonatal Severe Primary Hyperparathyroidism

Even before the description of FHH, a form of primary hyperparathyroidism had been described in a number of infants presenting with severe, symptomatic hypercalcemia that was associated with hyperparathyroid bone disease before the age of 6 months—the clinical syndrome of neonatal severe hyperparathyroidism (NSHPT).[84] A recent review of 49 cases of NSHPT showed that most infants present clinically at birth or shortly thereafter, often during the first week of life.[63] Common presenting symptoms include anorexia, constipation, failure to thrive, hypotonia, and respiratory distress. Additional clinical features that may be encountered include chest wall deformity and, occasionally, dysmorphic facies, craniotabes, and anovaginal or rectovaginal fistula.[49, 85–88] Thoracic deformity from multiple rib fractures can sometimes result in flail chest syndrome, a cause of substantial morbidity.[84, 85] Skeletal radiographs in afflicted infants often show profound reductions in bony mineralization, accompanied by fractures of the long bones and ribs, widening of the metaphyses, subperiosteal erosion, and, occasionally, rickets.[85, 89] Skeletal histology usually reveals the typical osteitis fibrosa cystica that is seen in severe primary hyperparathyroidism.[87] At the time of parathyroidectomy, all four parathyroid glands are usually enlarged, and their combined mass may be many times that of the parathyroid glands of normal children of this age, exhibiting chief cell or water-clear cell hyperplasia. In instances when the parathyroid enlargement is less marked, the low content of fat that is normally present in the parathyroid glands of children can complicate interpretation of the parathyroid histology.[63, 87, 90] Parathyroid adenomas have never been described in cases of NSHPT.

Biochemical Features of NSHPT

In contrast to FHH, serum PTH levels have been markedly elevated in most cases of NSHPT, often being 5- to 10-fold elevated, although the degree of the increase can be more modest on occasion.[91, 92] The hypercalcemia in NSHPT is most commonly severe, greater than 14 mg/dL, and levels as high as 30.8 mg/dL have been recorded.[86] In spite of this marked hypercalcemia, some cases have exhibited relative hypocalciuria, even in the absence of a family history of FHH.[93] Serum magnesium concentrations, when available, have sometimes been elevated well above the normal range.[59] In some cases, the hypercalcemia encountered in neonatal hyperparathyroidism is less severe, in the range of 11 to 12 mg/dL; and occasional cases have run a self-limited course, reverting to a milder form of hypercalcemia at the age of 6 to 7 months following only conservative medical therapy.[85] Recently, cases have been reported that were not diagnosed until adulthood. A 32-year-old woman, diagnosed serendipitously, was the offspring of a consanguineous union between two individuals with unrecognized FHH. Both of the parents' serum calcium concentrations were in the upper range of normal.[59] This homozygous patient did not initially present as having NSHPT and was only diagnosed as an adult. Despite serum calcium concentrations between 15 and 17 mg/dL, the patient was thought to be asymptomatic, although she was characterized as mildly retarded. Her serum magnesium concentration was also elevated to a substantial degree (about 50% above the upper limit of normal), and her serum intact PTH level was just at the upper limit of the normal range. Despite her marked hypercalcemia, renal function was apparently entirely normal.

Treatment of NSHPT

Before 1982, NSHPT often had a fatal outcome unless there was prompt and aggressive combined medical and surgical treatment. This has been less true in the more recent clinical experience, however, and wider recognition of the broadening clinical spectrum of the disease, combined with improvements in the medical treatment of severe hypercalcemia, has resulted in successful medical management in a number of cases during the past 15 years.[63] In symptomatic cases, initial management includes vigorous hydration, the use of inhibitors of bone resorption, and respiratory support. If the infant's condition is very severe or deteriorates during medical therapy, total parathyroidectomy with autotransplantation of part of one of the glands is generally recommended within the first month of life.[63, 92, 94] Since persistent hypercalcemia is often observed when parathyroid tissue is left behind following partial parathyroidectomy or autotransplantation, some authors recommend total parathyroidectomy followed by lifelong management of the resultant hypoparathyroidism with oral calcium and vitamin D therapy [generally with $1,25(OH)_2D$] as needed to prevent symptomatic hypocalcemia.[87, 91] There is usually rapid and dramatic clinical improvement after parathyroidectomy, with rapid healing of the skeletal lesions. Similar clinical improvement has been observed more recently in infants with NSHPT managed medically,[63] indicating that biochemical improvement in the degree of hyperparathyroidism can be part of the natural history of NSHPT.

Genetics of Calcium Resistance

Genetics of FHH

FHH is an autosomal dominant inherited trait with a penetrance approaching 100%.[57, 58, 63] Linkage analysis mapped the disease gene in four large FHH kindreds to chromosome 3 (band q21–24).[95] Furthermore, formal genetic analysis proved that persons with FHH are heterozygous for the FHH gene.[96] Subsequent studies revealed that 90% or more of kindreds sufficiently large for genetic analysis exhibited a similar linkage of the FHH gene to the locus on chromosome 3.[97, 98] One family, however, has linkage of a disorder phenotypically indistinguishable from FHH to the short arm of chromosome 19 (band 19p13.3),[97] suggesting that this condition can be genetically heterogeneous. Furthermore, an Oklahoma kindred that exhibits some atypical clinical features not commonly seen in most afflicted families (e.g., osteomalacia in a few affected family members and a tendency toward progressive elevation in serum PTH with increasing age) initially showed linkage to neither the chromosome 3 nor the chromosome 19 loci.[67, 99] More recently, linkage has been established to another locus on chromosome 19 in this family.[100]

Since the features described for FHH are consistent with a defect in Ca^{2+}_o-sensing by kidney, parathyroid, and probably other tissues, the CaR was clearly a good candidate for the disease gene in this condition. Furthermore, the localization of the human CaR gene on the long arm of chromosome 3,[101] the site linked to FHH, pointed to defects in the CaR gene as a plausible cause of FHH. This suspicion was confirmed with the description of three different missense mutations in the coding sequence of CaR (i.e., an alteration in a single nucleotide base substituting a new amino acid for the one normally encoded) when the CaR gene of three unrelated families with a form of FHH linked to chromosome 3 was examined. Furthermore, these mutations were not present in the genomic DNA of 50 normocalcemic control subjects. Additional studies have subsequently identified between two and three dozen additional mutations in the CaR of families with the form of FHH that is linked to chromosome 3.[59, 98, 102–105] Each family most commonly has its own unique mutation, and only occasional, apparently unrelated families share the same mutation. Most are missense mutations that are present within several distinct portions of the predicted CaR protein (see Fig. 80–1)—(a) the first half of the ECD, (b) a region of the ECD that immediately precedes the first TMD, and (c) the TMDs, intracellular or extracellular loops or ICD.

In addition to missense mutations, several other types of mutations have been described in affected members of FHH families. In some instances, mutations result in truncated forms of the receptor that are not likely to have biologic activity. A nonsense mutation (i.e., substitution of a stop codon for the serine that is normally encoded by this codon) and a frameshift mutation (i.e., a deletion of a single nucleotide and transversion of an adjacent nucleotide) have been described.[98] In both instances truncated forms of the receptor would be expected that terminate either before the first TMD or within the fifth TMD, respectively. Alternatively, a family living in Nova Scotia harbors the insertion at codon 876 of a 383-bp Alu repetitive sequence.[104] The Alu element is present in an orientation opposite to that of the CaR gene and contains a very long polyadenosine sequence. Stop signals within all three reading frames of the Alu sequence would generate a truncated CaR protein that contains a long stretch of repeated phenylalanines within its C-terminus (resulting from the AAA codons encoded by the polyadenylate tract). Interestingly, the length of the Alu repetitive element has approximately doubled in size in a subsequent generation of this family.[106] Although the vast majority of FHH kindreds have their disease gene linked to the locus on chromosome 3, only about two-thirds of these families have identifiable mutations in the CaR's coding sequence. In the remainder, it is probable that mutations reside within the receptor's noncoding sequence or its upstream or downstream regulatory elements and interfere with the normal level of expression of the CaR gene. Of note, benign polymorphisms of the CaR have been described in individuals that have no alterations in Ca^{2+}_o-sensing[103]; some of these benign polymorphisms slightly modify Ca^{2+}_o in the normal range and may be linked to a higher genetic predisposition to bone and mineral disorders.[107]

The functional evaluation of these mutations, an important step in confirming a change in receptor activity as opposed to benign polymorphism of the CaR, has been made possible by the expression of normal and mutant CaRs in human embryonic kidney (HEK293).[60, 61, 108, 109] HEK293 cells expressing the normal CaR respond to elevations of Ca^{2+}_o by showing transient elevations of intracellular calcium, resembling the response observed in parathyroid cells. Figure 80–4 illustrates the impact of several point mutations on high Ca^{2+}_o-evoked increases in intracellular calcium when expressed in HEK293 cells. Some of the mutations, including Arg185Gln and Arg795Trp (see Fig. 80–1 for localization within the protein receptor sequence), substantially diminish the apparent affinity or maximal activity of the mutated CaRs. Others (e.g., Thr138Met or Arg62Met) only modestly reduce apparent affinity and produce no obvious changes in the receptor's maximal response.[60] In many cases, the mutant CaRs showing the most marked decreases in biologic activity exhibit substantial reductions in the cell-surface expression of the putatively mature, glycosylated form of the receptor. Paradoxically, those mutations which markedly reduce the biologic activity of the CaR despite having a normal expression pattern tend to be those producing the greatest degree of elevation in serum calcium concentration. The Arg795Trp or Arg185Gln mutations,[60, 61] for example, produce serum calcium concentrations in affected family members that are about 2 mg/dL and 3 mg/dL higher, respectively, than the levels in unaffected members. These mutant receptors appear to exert a so-called dominant negative effect on the wild-type (i.e., normal) receptor when the two CaRs are expressed together, a condition that mimics the heterozygous state that is present in vivo in FHH patients. This dominant negative action of the latter two mutant receptors probably results from some interference by the mutant receptor with the wild-type CaR's expression or action. Such interference could take place in several possible ways, singly or in combination: (1) a reduction in the quantity of the normal CaR that reaches the cell surface, (2) a decrease in the effective concentration of the G protein(s) that is available to the wild-type CaR as a result of the formation of an inactive complex of G protein(s) with the mutant receptor, or (3) the presence of inactive, presumably heterodimeric complexes of the normal and mutant CaRs on the cell surface. Since many FHH families have serum calcium levels that are higher than in FHH kindreds harboring what are effectively null mutations (e.g., there is essentially no receptor protein produced from the abnormal allele, as in the Ser607stop mutation), it is quite possible that some degree of dominant negative interaction of mutant and wild-type receptors is the rule rather than the exception in FHH.

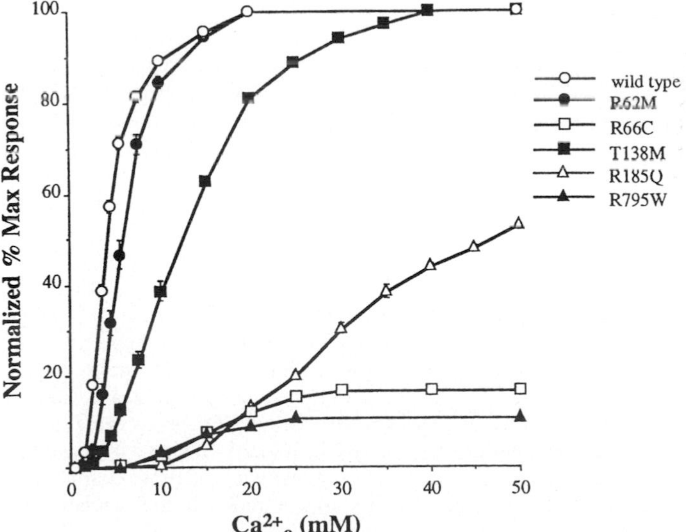

FIGURE 80–4. Expression of Ca^{2+}_o-sensing receptors (CaRs) bearing familial hypocalciuric hypercalcemia (FHH) mutations in human embryonic kidney (HEK293) cells. Each curve shows the effects of varying levels of Ca^{2+}_o on the intracellular calcium level in HEK293 cells transiently expressing the wild-type CaR or mutant CaRs bearing the indicated FHH mutation. Note that CaRs containing the FHH mutations show varying degrees of increase in EC_{50} (the level of Ca^{2+}_o required to produce a half-maximal increase in intracellular calcium) or reduction of the maximal intracellular calcium response, thereby showing resistance to Ca^{2+}_o. (From Bai M, Quinn S, Trivedi S, et al: Expression and characterization of inactivating and activating mutations in the human Ca^{2+}_o-sensing receptor. J Biol Chem 271:19537, 1996.)

Several general conclusions can be drawn about the role of CaR mutations in causing autosomal dominant FHH. This disorder is genetically heterogeneous; however, about 90% of families having FHH are linked to chromosome 3. Two-thirds of these families, in turn, have inactivating mutations in the CaR's coding region. Each family usually has its own unique mutation. Most mutations reside within the CaR's ECD and probably reduce the affinity of the receptor for calcium, interfere with its biosynthesis or cell surface expression, or lead to the formation of heterodimers with the wild-type CaR that have reduced biologic activity. Some mutations present within the CaR's TMDs, intracellular loops, or ICDs may impair the processes required for productive signal transduction. The remaining persons with the form of FHH that is linked to chromosome 3 who do not have detectable mutations in the receptor's coding region may have mutations in promoter or enhancer sequences of the CaR gene that normally regulate its expression. In all instances when FHH is caused by CaR mutations, tissues involved in calcium homeostasis are rendered mildly to moderately "resistant" to the normal actions of Ca^{2+}_o that are mediated by the CaR. PTH secretion is less sensitive to the inhibitory effects of high Ca^{2+}_o in the parathyroid cell. The normal role of Ca^{2+}_o in the PTH-independent regulation of renal calcium, magnesium, and water handling is affected in the kidney. There is an excessive renal tubular reabsorption of these two divalent cations despite hypercalcemia and an absence of the normally inhibitory action of high Ca^{2+}_o on urinary concentration. Finally, in occasional families with conditions phenotypically nearly indistinguishable from FHH, the disease gene maps to two other, as yet undefined genetic loci on chromosome 19. Identifying these genes may enable isolation of additional Ca^{2+}_o-sensing receptors or other molecular elements required for the CaR's normal biologic activities.

Since a significant fraction of patients with FHH do not have mutations that can be identified within the CaR's coding region, and given that mutations can occur in most of the CaR's coding sequence, genetic analysis may not be practical to diagnose FHH in all patients with mild hypercalcemia. The diagnosis of FHH will likely continue to require documenting the presence of mild, PTH-dependent hypercalcemia in combination with relative hypocalciuria that exhibits an autosomal dominant pattern of inheritance. Direct mutational analysis may be of utility in specific clinical settings, as in the differentiation of FHH from primary hyperparathyroidism in persons who do not have relatives available for biochemical and genetic screening or in patients with apparently de novo CaR mutations (see next section). Finally, because persons with FHH usually have a benign clinical course, parathyroidectomy should only be carried out in very unusual clinical circumstances, that is, in cases where patients are suffering adverse consequences of their hypercalcemia.

Genetics of NSHPT

Early descriptions of NSHPT showed that affected infants could occur in FHH kindreds.[57, 87, 110, 111] In 15 kindreds with FHH, Marx et al.[57, 87] identified three patients with NSHPT in two of the families, providing strong indirect evidence that NSHPT can, in some cases, be the homozygous form of FHH. In another family with two children exhibiting NSHPT, the parents, who were related, showed mild increases in their levels of serum ionized calcium and relative hypocalciuria,[110] again suggesting that NSHPT could represent homozygous FHH. Pollak and coworkers[112] subsequently showed that, among 11 FHH families in whom the disease gene mapped to chromosome 3, consanguineous unions of affected individuals in four families produced NSHPT in some offspring. The inheritance of specific genetic markers, closely linked to the FHH gene, provided very strong evidence that NSHPT in these families was the homozygous form of FHH. In separate studies, FHH documented to arise from CaR mutations confirmed that inheritance of two abnormal copies of the mutant gene can cause NSHPT.[101, 102, 104] Because such infants have no normal CaR genes, they exhibit much more severe clinical and biochemical manifestations than observed in the heterozygous state (FHH), typical of the classic description of NSHPT, principally as a result of having a greater degree of resistance of the parathyroid glands to Ca^{2+}_o.

Because a large number of CaR mutations are associated with FHH, inheritance of two different mutations of the CaR (i.e., a compound heterozygote) can occur in the absence of consanguinity. Kobayashi et al.[105] recently described an infant with the clinical picture of NSHPT, each of whose parents had a separate mutation in the coding region of the CaR gene—Arg185stop in the father and Gly670Glu in the mother. The maternal serum calcium concentration averaged 10.4 mg/dL (with an upper limit of 10.5 mg/dL), suggesting the presence of a very mild FHH phenotype, while the father had mild hypercalcemia (averaging 10.6 mg/dL). Co-expression in the infant of the mother's mutant CaR and the father's CaR nonsense mutation caused the NSHPT phenotype, with a serum calcium concentration as high as 26.5 mg/dL. At the time of parathyroidectomy, four hyperplastic parathyroid glands were identified.

In most instances, NSHPT occurs sporadically or in FHH kindreds in which there is only one affected parent,[49, 113, 114] suggesting that a single abnormal CaR allele in the affected neonate(s) can result in a phenotype of severe hyperparathyroidism, although this has been formally proved in only a minority of cases. Such children could also potentially have been compound heterozygotes, harboring two distinct different mutant CaR alleles—as in the case of Kobayashi et al.[105]—the first producing clear-cut hypercalcemia in one parent, but the second being so mild as to be biochemically silent in the other parent. Alternatively, there could conceivably be a mutation in one CaR allele combined with a separate mutation in one allele of another gene causing an FHH-like clinical picture (e.g., those on chromosome 19). No such cases, however, have been documented to date.

Another scenario that can contribute to the development of NSHPT is the exposure of a fetus with a single mutant CaR allele arising from a father with FHH to normal maternal calcium homeostasis. The fetal serum calcium concentration is maintained by the flux of calcium from maternal blood across the placenta.[115] A normal mother would expose the fetal parathyroid glands to a level of Ca^{2+}_o that would be sensed as relatively hypocalcemic owing to the presence of the FHH mutation in one allele of the CaR expressed in those glands. The latter would lead to "overstimulation" of the fetal parathyroids, causing an additional degree of "secondary" fetal or neonatal hyperparathyroidism that would be superimposed on the abnormal Ca^{2+}_o-sensing already present in those parathyroid glands as a result of the inherited FHH mutation. Support for this explanation has been provided by the occurrence of cases of NSHPT with an autosomal dominant pattern of inheritance in cases where the father had FHH and the mother was thought to be normal.[63, 87] In the postnatal period, the "secondary" hyperparathyroidism would gradually resolve over a period of several months, eventually returning to the clinical and biochemical characteristics of FHH. It seems clear, however, that most children with FHH born to normal mothers do not have any greater severity of their hypercalcemia. Some families may be more susceptible to the development of NSHPT in heterozygous infants because their CaR mutations exert a dominant negative action on the normal CaR, thereby causing a more severe defect in Ca^{2+}_o-sensing and hypercalcemia.

Finally, neonatal hyperparathyroidism can occur in the setting of heterozygous de novo CaR mutations[98] (i.e., with a spontaneous, apparently germline CaR mutation occurring de novo in the child of normal parents). Two such infants have been described who exhibited hyperparathyroid bone disease but had less severe hypercalcemia than is generally observed in NSHPT resulting from homozygous FHH. Another case of de novo heterozygous NSHPT has been described in a child who harbored the same Arg185Gln mutation that has previously been associated with a greater degree of elevation in serum calcium concentration than seen in most FHH kindreds.[61, 87, 112]

Therefore, there is genetic hetereogeneity in infants with clinical and biochemical features of NSHPT, which in homozygous or compound heterozygous cases can be equivalent to knockout of the human CaR gene. The central role of CaR function in this disorder points to the importance of this receptor in fetal and neonatal calcium metabolism. In addition, beyond its role in Ca^{2+}_o-regulated PTH release, which is markedly deranged in NSHPT, particularly that resulting from homozygous FHH, the CaR likely serves to inhibit parathyroid cellular proliferation tonically, because there is often florid parathyroid hyperplasia in NSHPT.

Mouse Models of FHH and NSHPT

In 1995, Ho et al.[50] utilized targeted disruption of the CaR gene to create mice that are either heterozygous or homozygous for inactivation of the CaR gene. These mice provide animal models of FHH and NSHPT, respectively. Phenotypically, the heterozygous mice appeared normal, were fertile, and had a normal life span. The level of their serum calcium concentration was 10.4 mg/dL, a value about 10% higher than that of their normal littermates. The heterozygous mice also had mild, but significant, approximately 10% elevations in their serum magnesium concentrations. Serum PTH levels were about 50% higher in the heterozygous mice than in normal mice of the same age; despite the hypercalcemia, the calcium concentration in bladder urine was slightly lower than that in the normal mice. Skeletal radiographs in the wild-type and heterozygous mice were essentially indistinguishable. The heterozygous mouse, probably similar to its human counterpart, showed no significant upregulation of CaR protein expression in parathyroid and kidney by the remaining normal CaR allele, since the levels of expression of the CaR protein in these two tissues were approximately one-half of those in the wild-type animals. This approximately 50% reduction in the level of expression of the CaR protein in the parathyroid led to a mild (~10%) elevation in the apparent set-point of Ca^{2+}_o-regulated PTH release. Therefore, mice that are heterozygous for knockout of the CaR gene appear to share many of the phenotypic and biochemical features of individuals with FHH.

Mice homozygous for inactivation of the CaR, in contrast, while nearly normal in size at birth, subsequently grew much more slowly than their normal or heterozygous littermates. This poor growth may have resulted, in part, from their inability to compete successfully with their more vigorous normal and heterozygous littermates for their mother's milk. The homozygous mice exhibited severe hypercalcemia, with serum calcium levels averaging 14.8 mg/dL. Their serum magnesium levels, in contrast, were only slightly, and not significantly, higher than those in the heterozygous mice. Serum PTH levels were almost 10-fold greater than those observed in normal mice, an increase that was comparable to what is seen in infants with NSHPT. Despite their severe hypercalcemia, the calcium concentration in the bladder urine of the homozygous mice was lower than that in normal mice. Skeletal radiographs showed striking abnormalities, with appreciable reductions in mineral density, bowing of the long bones, and kyphoscoliosis. The majority of the homozygous mice died within the first 2 postnatal weeks, and only occasional homozygotes survived for up to 3 or 4 weeks. Therefore, the biochemical and clinical characteristics of mice homozygous for knockout of the CaR gene exhibited numerous similarities to those of the human disorder, NSHPT. This animal model should prove useful in the investigation of alterations in Ca^{2+}_o-sensing in a variety of tissues that express the CaR, both those involved in, and those not thought to play any role in, systemic calcium homeostasis, such as the brain.

AUTOSOMAL DOMINANT HYPOCALCEMIA

Heritable disorders of calcium metabolism that are distinguished by hypocalcemia are rare. In the pediatric population, sporadic cases of hypoparathyroidism are often seen in the setting of parathyroid gland dysgenesis or agenesis (e.g., DiGeorge's syndrome). Other causes include parathyroid tissue degeneration as part of autoimmune (e.g., polyglandular syndromes) or systemic disease processes. Familial isolated hypoparathyroidism is an uncommon disorder that occurs in several forms—autosomal recessive, autosomal dominant, and X-linked.[116] The molecular pathogenesis of the autosomal recessive and X-linked forms is unknown. In a study of eight families with autosomal dominant hypoparathyroidism, there was linkage of the disorder to the PTH gene in two of them.[117] One of these two families was subsequently shown to harbor a mutation within the region of the preproPTH gene encoding the signal peptide.[118] Another family has since been described with a mutation in a splice junction of the preproPTH gene.[119] The identification of inactivating mutations in the CaR gene as the cause of FHH, combined with the discovery of activating mutations in other G protein–coupled receptors, suggested the possibility that activating mutations of the CaR might also exist. Such mutations would be expected to produce hypocalcemia due to increased sensitivity of the parathyroid cell to Ca$^{2+}_o$. In fact, a form of familial hypocalcemia, autosomal dominant hypocalcemia (ADH), has been shown to be caused by activating mutations of the CaR (Fig. 80–5). ADH, prior to its recognition as the clinical expression of activating mutations in the CaR, had been lumped together with other forms of familial isolated hypoparathyroidism. Nevertheless, families subsequently shown to harbor CaR mutations exhibit certain clinical features that might have been predicted to be the result of "resetting" downward of the set-points of both parathyroid and kidney for Ca$^{2+}_o$.[108, 120–125] In effect, this disorder represents the clinical expression of mild to moderate increases in the responsiveness of CaR-expressing tissues to Ca$^{2+}_o$ as opposed to the resistance to Ca$^{2+}_o$ that is present in FHH.

Clinical Features of ADH

The most prominent clinical feature of ADH is the presence of mild to moderate hypocalcemia (~6 to 8 mg/dL),[120, 124–126] although occasional patients have more severe hypocalcemia (4 to 6 mg/dL).[120] Some individuals with this disorder experience relatively little symptomatology despite their hypocalcemia,[125] while others share many of the signs and symptoms exhibited by patients with hypocalcemia due to other causes, including seizures, paresthesias, muscle cramps, and laryngospasm.[120, 124] The seizures appear to be more common within the first few weeks or months of life. In several cases seizures occurred during febrile episodes and in the majority of patients were not difficult to control. As opposed to hypoparathyroidism caused by defects in parathyroid gland development or PTH production, intact PTH levels are measurable but inappropriately remain in the lower part of the normal range.[125] In one case of ADH, reducing serum calcium further caused a brisk rise in serum PTH, consistent with the presence of a leftward shift in the set-point for Ca$^{2+}_o$-regulated PTH release without frank parathyroid failure.[127] Patients with ADH, similar to those with classic hypoparathyroidism, exhibit hyperphosphatemia, although in some kindreds the serum phosphate levels of affected individuals can be normal,[125] especially in those families that tend to have mild hypocalcemia and normal PTH levels. Serum magnesium levels are often in the lower half of the normal range and may be overtly low in the untreated state.[120, 122, 124, 125] 1,25(OH)$_2$D levels have been measured in relatively few cases and were usually normal.[124] In two studies, the urinary excretion of calcium in the untreated state was approximately twice as high in patients with ADH as in those with other causes of hypoparathyroidism, despite the fact that PTH levels are often higher in the former than in the latter.[120, 124, 126] The increased excretion of calcium is thought to reflect direct inhibition of renal tubular calcium (and magnesium) reabsorption by mutant CaRs activated at inappropriately low levels of Ca$^{2+}_o$, the opposite of the effect of inactivating FHH mutations on renal handling of calcium by the same nephron segments.

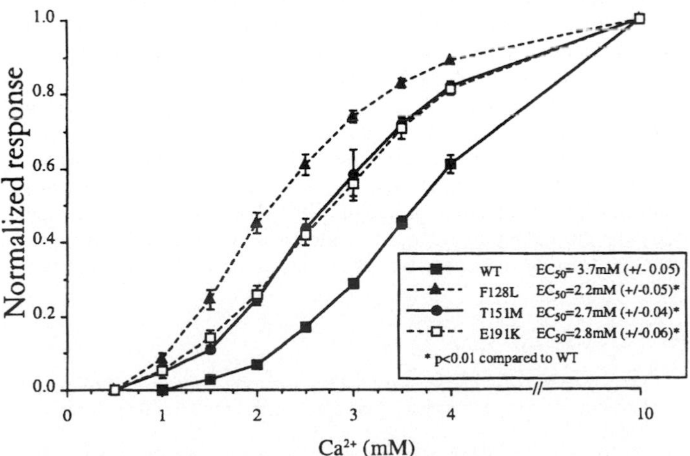

FIGURE 80–5. Expression of CaRs bearing autosomal dominant hypocalcemia (ADH) mutations in HEK293 cells. Each curve shows the effects of varying levels of Ca$^{2+}_o$ on the intracellular calcium level in HEK293 cells transiently expressing the wild-type CaR or mutant CaRs bearing the indicated ADH mutation. CaRs containing ADH mutations show varying degrees of decrease in EC$_{50}$, (see legend to Fig. 80–4), thereby showing increased sensitivity to Ca$^{2+}_o$. (From Pearce SHS, Bai M, Quinn SJ, et al: Functional characterization of calcium-sensing receptor mutations expressed in human embryonic kidney cells. J Clin Invest 98:1860, 1996.)

Genetics of ADH

Finegold and colleagues[128] first identified a family with a form of ADH that was linked to a locus on chromosome 3 close to that of the CaR gene. Shortly afterward, Pollak et al.[123] identified a heterozygous missense mutation in another family with ADH that had previously been postulated to have an inherited reduction in the set-point of the parathyroid glands for Ca$^{2+}_o$.[127] Subsequent studies have identified a total of approximately a dozen heterozygous missense, activating mutations in the CaR gene, which cause either ADH or de novo sporadic cases of hypocalcemia[108, 120, 122, 123, 125, 129] (see Fig. 80–1). The majority are present within the CaR's ECD, providing further indirect evidence for the importance of this region of the receptor in the mechanisms underlying its activation by Ca$^{2+}_o$, while several families harbor mutations residing within the receptor's TMDs.[120, 125] To date, no cases of homozygous activating CaR mutations have been identified in sporadic cases of hypocalcemia or in kindreds with ADH. In several instances, individuals have been described with apparently sporadic hypoparathyroidism due to activating mutations of the CaR, suggesting the presence of de novo mutations in these cases.

Analysis of the functional properties of several of the known mutations in the CaR causing ADH showed a clear increase in the apparent affinity of the CaR for activation by Ca$^{2+}_o$,[60, 108, 121, 123] confirming the effect of these mutations on receptor function. Activating mutations present in other GPCRs, such as the thyroid-stimulating hormone (TSH) or luteinizing hormone (LH) receptors, are most commonly found in the TMDs, where they presumably facilitate the activation of signal transduction or mimic the receptor's active state if there is ligand-independent activation of the receptor. Those mutations present in the TMDs of the CaR may act in a similar manner. Mutations within the CaR's ECD, in contrast, may increase its affinity for Ca$^{2+}_o$, or favor the active conformation of the receptor, thereby promoting subsequent events in signal transduction at levels of Ca$^{2+}_o$ too low to produce similar effects on the wild-type CaR.

Further studies are also needed to determine the true prevalence of hypocalcemia due to activating CaR mutations among the hypocalcemic population previously thought to have hypoparathyroidism. It may well be that a larger number of families with ADH or individual cases arising from de novo activating mutations in the CaR will be uncovered that were previously identified as familial isolated or sporadic hypoparathyroidism. To date, only about one-third as many activating as inactivating CaR mutations have been identified, but there has been a more systematic family screening in hypercalcemic patients after the cloning of the CaR and recognition of it as the disease gene in FHH. Perhaps more vigorous family screening of hypocalcemic probands will identify a larger reservoir of both sporadic hypocalcemia and autosomal dominant forms of hypocalcemia resulting from activating CaR mutations.

Clinical Diagnosis and Treatment of ADH

Hypocalcemia as a consequence of the presence of activating CaR mutations is an entity that is distinct from typical hypoparathyroidism in both its clinical and biochemical manifestations. The inappropriately low levels of PTH are due to the excessive sensitivity of the parathyroid to Ca^{2+}_o, even though further reductions in Ca^{2+}_o can elicit substantial increases in PTH that are probably larger than those that would be encountered in most hypoparathyroid subjects. There are also differences in renal handling of calcium that can help differentiate hypocalcemia due to activating mutations of the CaR from hypoparathyroidism. The presence of "overresponsive" CaRs in the kidney, particularly in the distal tubule, elevates urinary calcium excretion substantially above that generally present in hypoparathyroidism, at least in the untreated state. Further increases in serum calcium elevate urinary calcium excretion even further, producing a substantial risk of nephrolithiasis and nephrocalcinosis. Activating mutations of the CaR, in effect, reset the Ca^{2+}_o homeostatic system, maintaining a level of Ca^{2+}_o that is probably defended just as vigorously as that maintained by the Ca^{2+}_o-resistant homeostatic mechanism that has been reset upward in FHH. Thus ADH should probably be thought of as a form of "hypocalcemia" instead of "hypoparathyroidism".

This distinction of hypocalcemia due to activating CaR mutations from that due to classic isolated hypoparathyroidism is clinically important because of the reversible or even irreversible renal damage that can occur in the former following aggressive correction of hypocalcemia.[124] Identifying individuals with activating CaR mutations requires a prepared mind and careful clinical, biochemical, and genetic evaluation. The most helpful diagnostic clues are the presence of hypocalcemia in other family members with a pattern of inheritance consistent with an autosomal dominant trait. Hypocalcemia is accompanied by hypomagnesemia in some cases, intact PTH levels in the lower half of the normal range, and urinary calcium excretion, which, on average, is greater than that observed in classic hypoparathyroidism. Nevertheless, differentiation from the usual case of hypoparathyroidism may not be straightforward, and in some cases the diagnosis has only been entertained subsequent to the development of severe hypercalciuria or renal impairment following correction of hypocalcemia. The use of mutational analysis to distinguish activating mutations of the CaR may prove useful in this setting.

Treatment should be tailored to eliminate symptoms associated with hypocalcemia. The therapeutic choices are similar to those used in the treatment of primary hypoparathyroidism and include calcium and vitamin D supplementation. Patients with ADH appear to respond to vitamin D supplementation in a manner that differs in a characteristic way from that observed in patients with true hypoparathyroidism. The former are unusually susceptible to the development of marked hypercalciuria and other renal complications of overtreatment with vitamin D, even in the absence of frank hypercalcemia.[124] These deleterious effects of vitamin D therapy include renal stones, nephrocalcinosis, and reversible (and, in some cases, irreversible) reductions in renal function. Polydipsia, enuresis, and polyuria, probably as a result of poor urinary concentrating ability, can develop in these patients during treatment. They often occur more commonly and at lower levels of Ca^{2+}_o than in patients being treated for classic hypoparathyroidism. Thus Ca^{2+}_o should be raised only sufficiently to eradicate symptoms of hypocalcemia or be maintained in the low-normal range to diminish the risk of hypercalciuria with its adverse effects on renal function.

SUMMARY

The description of the CaR, coupled with the identification of naturally occurring syndromes of Ca^{2+}_o resistance and oversensitivity, has provided direct evidence that a variety of cell types can sense small changes in Ca^{2+}_o via a receptor-mediated mechanism. Thus Ca^{2+}_o can function in a hormone-like role as an extracellular first messenger. Several important components of the mineral ion homeostatic system, such as parathyroid and C cells, have now been shown to sense Ca^{2+}_o by this mechanism. The CaR appears to mediate the effects of Ca^{2+}_o on PTH and CT secretion. Furthermore, the presence of CaR in several types of renal cells strongly supports the notion that several of the long-recognized but poorly understood effects of Ca^{2+}_o on the function of the kidney may likewise be CaR-mediated. These effects include the enhanced excretion of calcium and magnesium that occurs with hypercalcemia and the diminished urinary concentrating capacity exhibited by some hypercalcemic individuals.

The inherited human syndromes of Ca^{2+}_o "resistance" or "overresponsiveness" represented by FHH and ADH, respectively, offer interesting "experiments in nature". They are, in effect, syndromes in which the body's "calciostat" has been reset upward or downward, respectively, producing predictable alterations in the regulation of parathyroid and kidney by Ca^{2+}_o. The lack of obvious symptoms of hypercalcemia in most patients with FHH suggests that the CaR, in addition to playing a central role in the regulation of parathyroid and renal function by Ca^{2+}_o, may also mediate other symptoms of hypercalcemia. Conversely, it is clear that individuals with activating mutations can exhibit classic symptoms of hypocalcemia; therefore, neuromuscular manifestations, such as seizures and tetany, are presumably, at least in part, CaR-independent. Much more remains to be learned, however, about the role of CaR in the brain and in other parts of the body, where in many cases it likely responds to local rather than systemic changes in Ca^{2+}_o.

Finally, novel therapeutic approaches to managing disorders of calcium homeostasis may develop based on our current understanding of Ca^{2+}_o-sensing. The development of therapeutic agents that stimulate or inhibit the CaR has substantial potential clinical utility for treating conditions in which the receptor is under- or overactive, respectively. For example, clinical trials are currently in progress on the efficacy of calcimimetic positive modulators of CaR activation for the medical therapy of primary and secondary hyperparathyroidism.[130–132] Based on clinical clues provided by inherited disorders of Ca^{2+}_o-sensing, there are several settings where CaR antagonists, so-called calcilytics, would be of clinical utility. If such agents increased the set-point of the parathyroid and kidney in a manner reciprocal to the decrease in set-point produced by the calcimimetics, calcilytics would represent an effective means of resetting the parathyroid and kidney in individuals with activating mutations. Thus it should be possible by this means to raise the level of Ca^{2+}_o in those individuals who experience complications of hypocalcemia (i.e., seizures) without, presumably, incurring undue hypercalciuria. Similarly, in view of the markedly enhanced renal tubular reabsorption of calcium in FHH, a calcilytic with specificity for the kidney as opposed to the parathyroid could represent an effective form of treatment for renal stones caused by hypercalciuria.

REFERENCES

1. Stewart AF, Broadus AE: Mineral Metabolism. *In* Felig P, Baxter JD, Broadus AE, Frohman LA (eds): Endocrinology and Metabolism, ed 2. New York, McGraw-Hill, 1987, p 1317.
2. Brown EM: Extracellular Ca^{2+} sensing, regulation of parathyroid cell function, and role of Ca^{2+} and other ions as extracellular (first) messengers. Physiol Rev 71:371, 1991.
3. Hebert SC, Brown EM, Harris HW: Role of the Ca^{2+}-sensing receptor in divalent mineral ion homeostasis. J Exp Biol 200:295, 1997.
4. Weisinger JR, Favus MJ, Langman CB, et al: Regulation of 1,25-dihydroxyvitamin D3 by calcium in the parathyroidectomized, parathyroid hormone–replete rat. J Bone Miner Res 4:929, 1989.
5. Quamme GA: Effect of hypercalcemia on renal tubular handling of calcium and magnesium. Can J Physiol Pharmacol 60:1275, 1982.
6. Raisz LG, Niemann I: Effect of phosphate, calcium, and magnesium on bone resorption and bone formation in tissue culture. Endocrinology 85:446, 1969.
7. Zaidi M, Datta HK, Patchell A, et al: "Calcium-activated" intracellular calcium

elevation: A novel mechanism of osteoclast regulation. Biochem Biophys Res Commun 183:1461, 1989.

8. Malgaroli A, Meldolesi J, Zambone-Zallone A, et al: Control of cytosolic free calcium in rat and chicken osteoclasts. The role of extracellular calcium and calcitonin. J Biol Chem 264:14342, 1989.
9. Silver IA, Murrils RJ, Etherington DJ: Microelectrode studies on the acid microenvironment beneath adherent macrophages and osteoclasts. Exp Cell Res 175:266, 1988.
10. Quarles LD, Hartle JE II, Siddhanti SR, et al: A distinct cation-sensing mechanism in MC3T3-E1 osteoblasts functionally related to the calcium receptor. J Bone Miner Res 12:393, 1997.
11. Sugimoto T, Kanatani M, Kano J, et al: Effects of high calcium concentration on the functions and interactions of osteoblastic cells and monocytes and on the formation of osteoclast-like cells. J Bone Miner Res 8:1445, 1993.
12. Kanatani M, Sugimoto T, Fukase M, et al: Effect of extracellular calcium on the proliferation of osteoblastic MC3T3-E1 cells: Its direct and indirect effects via monocytes. Biochem Biophys Res Commun 181:1425, 1991.
13. Godwin SL, Soltoff SP: Extracellular calcium and platelet-derived growth factor promote receptor-mediated chemotaxis in osteoblasts through different signaling pathways. J Biol Chem 272:11307, 1997.
14. Honda Y, Fitzsimmons RJ, Baylink DJ, et al: Effects of extracellular calcium on insulin-like growth factor II in human bone cells. J Bone Miner Res 10:1660, 1995.
15. Kifor O, Kifor I, Brown EM: Effects of high extracellular calcium concentrations on phosphoinositide turnover and inositol phosphate metabolism in dispersed bovine parathyroid cells. J Bone Miner Res 7:1327, 1992.
16. Shoback D, Membreno LA, McGhee J: High calcium and other divalent cations in increased inositol trisphosphate in bovine parathyroid cells. Endocrinology 123:382, 1988.
17. Nemeth E, Wallace J, Scarpa A: Stimulus-secretion coupling in bovine parathyroid cells. Dissociation between secretion and net changes in cytosolic Ca^{++}. J Biol Chem 261:2668, 1986.
18. Chen C, Barnett J, Congo D, et al: Divalent cations suppress 3′,5′-adenosine monophosphate accumulation by stimulating a pertussis toxin–sensitive guanine nucleotide–binding protein in cultured bovine parathyroid cells. Endocrinology 124:233, 1989.
19. Chen T, Pratt S, Shoback D: Injection of bovine parathyroid poly(A)+ RNA into *Xenopus* oocytes confers sensitivity to high extracellular calcium. J Bone Miner Res 9:293, 1994.
20. Racke F, Hammerland L, Dubyak G, et al: Functional expression of the parathyroid cell calcium receptor in *Xenopus* oocytes. FEBS Lett 333:132, 1993.
21. Brown EM, Gamba G, Riccardi D, et al: Cloning and characterization of an extracellular Ca^{2+}-sensing receptor from bovine parathyroid. Nature 366:575, 1993.
22. Garrett JE, Capuano IV, Hammerland LG, et al: Molecular cloning and functional expression of human parathyroid calcium receptor cDNAs. J Biol Chem 270:12919, 1995.
23. Diaz R, Hurwitz S, Chattopadhyay N, et al: Cloning, expression, and tissue localization of the calcium-sensing receptor in chicken (*Gallus domesticus*). Am J Physiol 273:R1008, 1997.
24. Aida K, Koishi S, Tawata M, et al: Molecular cloning of a putative Ca^{2+}-sensing receptor cDNA from human kidney. Biochem Biophys Res Commun 214:524, 1995.
25. Riccardi D, Park J, Lee WS, et al: Cloning and functional expression of a rat kidney extracellular calcium/polyvalent cation–sensing receptor. Proc Natl Acad Sci USA 92:131, 1995.
26. Butters RR, Jr., Chattopadhyay N, Nielsen P, et al: Cloning and characterization of a calcium-sensing receptor from the hypercalcemic New Zealand white rabbit reveals unaltered responsiveness to extracellular calcium. J Bone Miner Res 12:568, 1997.
27. Garrett JE, Tamir H, Kifor O, et al: Calcitonin-secreting cells of the thyroid express an extracellular calcium receptor gene. Endocrinology 136:5202, 1995.
28. Ruat M, Molliver ME, Snowman AM, et al: Calcium sensing receptor: Molecular cloning in rat and localization to nerve terminals. Proc Natl Acad Sci USA 92:3161, 1995.
29. Strewler GJ. Familial hypocalciuric hypercalcemia—from the clinic to the calcium sensor. West J Med 160:579, 1994.
30. Quinn SJ, Ye CP, Diaz R, et al: The calcium-sensing receptor: A target for polyamines. Am J Physiol 273:C1315, 1997.
31. Fliegel L, Ohnishi M, Carpenter MR, et al: Amino acid sequence of rabbit fast-twitch skeletal muscle calsequestrin from its cDNA and peptide sequencing. Proc Natl Acad Sci USA 84:1167, 1987.
32. Brown EM: Four parameter model of the sigmoidal relationship between parathyroid hormone release and extracellular calcium concentration in normal and abnormal parathyroid tissue. J Clin Endocrinol Metab 56:572, 1983.
33. Fan GF, Ray K, Zhao XM, et al: Mutational analysis of the cysteines in the extracellular domain of the human Ca^{2+} receptor: Effects on cell surface expression, dimerization and signal transduction. FEBS Lett 436:353, 1998.
34. Bai M, Trivedi S, Kifor O, et al: Functional reconstitution of two inactive mutant Ca^{2+}_o-sensing receptors via heterodimerization. Proc Natl Acad Sci USA 96:2834, 1999.
35. Varrault A, Pena MS, Goldsmith PK, et al: Expression of G protein alpha-subunits in bovine parathyroid. Endocrinology 136:4390, 1995.
36. Kifor O, Diaz R, Butters R, et al: The Ca^{2+}-sensing receptor (CaR) activates phospholipases C, A2, and D in bovine parathyroid and CaR-transfected, human embryonic kidney (HEK293) cells. J Bone Miner Res 12:715, 1997.
37. Ruat M, Snowman AM, Hester LD, et al: Cloned and expressed rat Ca^{2+}-sensing receptor. J Biol Chem 271:5972, 1996.
38. McNeil L, Hobson S, Nipper V, et al: Functional calcium-sensing receptor expression in ovarian surface epithelial cells. Am J Obstet Gynecol 178:305, 1998.
39. Kaupmann K, Huggel K, Heid J, et al: Expression cloning of GABAB receptors uncovers similarity to metabotropic glutamate receptor. Nature 386:239, 1997.
40. Ryba NJP, Trindell R: A new multigene family of putative pheromone receptors. Neuron 19:371, 1997.
41. Matsunami H, Buck LB: A multigene family encoding a diverse array of putative pheromone receptors in mammals. Cell 90:775, 1997.
42. O'Hara P, Sheppard P, Thogersen H, et al: The ligand binding domain in metabotropic glutamate receptors is related to bacterial periplasmic binding proteins. Neuron 11:41, 1993.
43. Chattopadhyay N, Vassilev PM, Brown EM: Calcium-sensing receptor: Roles in and beyond systemic calcium homeostasis. Biol Chem 378:759, 1997.
44. Kifor O, Moore FD Jr, Wang P, et al: Reduced immunostaining for the extracellular Ca^{2+}-sensing receptor in primary and uremic secondary hyperparathyroidism [see comments]. J Clin Endocrinol Metab 81:1598, 1996.
45. Mithal A, Kifor O, Kifor I, et al: The reduced responsiveness of cultured bovine parathyroid cells to extracellular Ca^{2+} is associated with marked reduction in the expression of extracellular Ca^{2+}-sensing receptor messenger ribonucleic acid and protein. Endocrinology 136:3087, 1995.
46. Garrett J, Steffey M, Nemeth E: The calcium receptor agonist R-568 suppresses PTH mRNA levels in cultured bovine parathyroid cells (abstract). J Bone Miner Res 10 (suppl. 1):S387, 1995.
47. McGehee DS, Aldersberg M, Liu KP, et al: Mechanism of extracellular Ca^{2+} receptor–stimulated hormone release from sheep thyroid parafollicular cells. J Physiol (Lond) 502:31, 1997.
48. Emanuel RL, Adler GK, Kifor O, et al: Calcium-sensing receptor expression and regulation by extracellular calcium in the AtT-20 pituitary cell line. Mol Endocrinol 10:555, 1996.
49. Spiegel AM, Harrison HE, Marx SJ, et al: Neonatal primary hyperparathyroidism with autosomal dominant inheritance. J Pediatr 90:269, 1977.
50. Ho C, Conner DA, Pollak MR, et al: A mouse model of human familial hypocalciuric hypercalcemia and neonatal severe hyperparathyroidism [see comments]. Nat Genet 11:389, 1995.
51. Brown EM, Hebert SC: A cloned Ca^{2+}-sensing receptor: A mediator of direct effects of extracellular Ca^{2+} on renal function? J Am Soc Nephrol 6:1530, 1995.
52. Champigneulle A, Siga E, Vassent G, et al: Relationship between extra- and intracellular calcium in distal segments of the renal tubule. Role of the Ca^{2+} receptor RaKCaR. J Membr Biol 156:117, 1997.
53. Sands JM, Naruse M, Baum M, et al: Apical extracellular calcium/polyvalent cation–sensing receptor regulates vasopressin-elicited water permeability in rat kidney inner medullary collecting duct. J Clin Invest 99:1399, 1997.
54. Jackson CE, Boonstra CE: Hereditary hypercalcemia and parathyroid hyperplasia without definite hyperparathyroidism. J Lab Clin Med 68:883, 1966.
55. Foley T Jr, Harrison H, Arnaud C, et al: Familial benign hypercalcemia. J Pediatr 81:1060, 1972.
56. Marx S, Spiegel A, Brown EM, et al: Divalent cation metabolism. Familial hypocalciuric hypercalcemia versus typical primary hyperparathyroidism. Am J Med 65:235, 1978.
57. Marx SJ, Attie MF, Levine MA, et al: The hypocalciuric or benign variant of familial hypercalcemia: Clinical and biochemical features in fifteen kindreds. Medicine (Baltimore) 60:397, 1981.
58. Law WM Jr, Heath H III: Familial benign hypercalcemia (hypocalciuric hypercalcemia). Clinical and pathogenetic studies in 21 families. Ann Intern Med 105:511, 1985.
59. Aida K, Koishi S, Inoue M, et al: Familial hypocalciuric hypercalcemia associated with mutation in the human Ca^{2+}-sensing receptor gene. J Clin Endocrinol Metab 80:2594, 1995.
60. Bai M, Quinn S, Trivedi S, et al: Expression and characterization of inactivating and activating mutations in the human Ca^{2+}_o-sensing receptor. J Biol Chem 271:19537, 1996.
61. Bai M, Pearce SH, Kifor O, et al: In vivo and in vitro characterization of neonatal hyperparathyroidism resulting from a de novo, heterozygous mutation in the Ca^{2+}-sensing receptor gene: Normal maternal calcium homeostasis as a cause of secondary hyperparathyroidism in familial benign hypocalciuric hypercalcemia. J Clin Invest 99:88, 1997.
62. Aurbach GD, Marx SJ, Spiegel AM: Parathyroid hormone, calcitonin, and the calciferols. *In* Wilson JD, Foster DW (eds): Textbook of Endocrinology, ed 7. Philadelphia, WB Saunders, 1985, p 1137.
63. Heath DA: Familial hypocalciuric hypercalcemia. *In* Bilezikian JP, Marcus R, Levine MA (eds): The Parathyroids: Basic and Clinical Concepts. New York, Raven Press, 1994, p 699.
64. Toss G, Arnqvist H, Larsson L, et al: Familial hypocalciuric hypercalcemia: A study of four kindreds. J Intern Med 225:201, 1989.
65. Kristiansen JH, Rodbro P, Christiansen C, et al: Familial hypocalciuric hypercalcemia. III: Bone mineral metabolism. Clin Endocrinol (Oxf) 26:713, 1987.
66. Abugassa S, Nordenstrom J, Jarhult J: Bone mineral density in patients with familial hypocalciuric hypercalcaemia (FHH). Eur J Surg 158:397, 1992.
67. McMurtry C, Schranck F, Walkenhorst D, et al: Significant developmental elevation in serum parathyroid hormone levels in a large kindred with familial benign (hypocalciuric) hypercalcemia. Am J Med 93:247, 1992.
68. Menko FH, Bijouvet OLM, Fronen JLHH, et al: Familial benign hypercalcemia: Study of a large family. Q J Med 206:120, 1983.
69. Lyons TJ, Crookes PF, Postlethwaite W, et al: Familial hypocalciuric hypercalcemia as a differential diagnosis of hyperparathyroidism: Studies in a large kindred and a review of surgical experience in the condition. Br J Surg 73:188, 1986.
70. Gunn IR, Wallace JR: Urine calcium and serum ionized calcium, total calcium and parathyroid hormone concentrations in the diagnosis of primary hyperparathyroidism and familial benign hypercalcaemia [see comments]. Ann Clin Biochem 29:52, 1992.
71. Heath D: Familial benign hypercalcemia. Trends Endocrinol Metab 1:6, 1989.
72. Auwerx J, Demedts M, Bouillon R: Altered parathyroid set point to calcium in familial hypocalciuric hypercalcaemia. Acta Endocrinol (Copenh) 106:215, 1984.
73. Khosla S, Ebeling PR, Firek AF, et al: Calcium infusion suggests a "set-point" abnormality of parathyroid gland function in familial benign hypercalcemia and more complex disturbances in primary hyperparathyroidism. J Clin Endocrinol Metab 76:715, 1993.

74. Law WM Jr, Carney JA, Heath H III: Parathyroid glands in familial benign hypercalcemia (familial hypocalciuric hypercalcemia). Am J Med 76:1021, 1984.
75. Thogeirsson U, Costa J, Marx SJ: The parathyroid glands in familial hypocalciuric hypercalcemia. Hum Pathol 12:229, 1981.
76. Davies M, Adams PH, Lumb GA, et al: Familial hypocalciuric hypercalcemia: Evidence for continued enhanced renal tubular reabsorption of calcium following total parathyroidectomy. Acta Endocrinol (Copenh) 106:499, 1984.
77. Kristiansen JH, Rodbro P, Christiansen C, et al: Familial hypocalciuric hypercalcemia. II: Intestinal calcium absorption and vitamin D metabolism. Clin Endocrinol 23:511, 1985.
78. Law WM Jr, Bollman S, Kumar R, et al: Vitamin D metabolism in familial benign hypercalcemia (hypocalciuric hypercalcemia) differs from that in primary hyperparathyroidism. J Clin Endocrinol Metab 58:744, 1984.
79. Pasieka JL, Andersen MA, Hanley DA: Familial benign hypercalcemia: Hypercalciuria and hypocalciuria in affected members of a small kindred. Clin Endocrinol 33:429, 1990.
80. Attie MF, Gill J Jr, Stock JL, et al: Urinary calcium excretion in familial hypocalciuric hypercalcemia. Persistence of relative hypocalciuria after induction of hypoparathyroidism. J Clin Invest 72:667, 1983.
81. Marx SJ, Attie MF, Stock JL, et al: Maximal urine-concentrating ability: Familial hypocalciuric hypercalcemia versus typical primary hyperparathyroidism. J Clin Endocrinol Metab 52:736, 1981.
82. Suki WM, Eknoyan G, Rector FC Jr, et al: The renal diluting and concentrating mechanism in hypercalcemia. Nephron 6:50, 1969.
83. Powell BR, Buist NR: Late presenting, prolonged hypocalcemia in an infant of a woman with hypocalciuric hypercalcemia. Clin Pediatr (Phila) 29:241, 1990.
84. Landon JF: Parathyroidectomy in generalized osteitis fibrosa cystica. J Pediatr 1:544, 1932.
85. Eftekhari F, Yousefzadeh D: Primary infantile hyperparathyroidism: Clinical, laboratory, and radiographic features in 21 cases. Skeletal Radiol 8:201, 1982.
86. Gaudelus J, Dandine M, Nathanson M, et al: Rib cage deformity in neonatal hyperparathyroidism (letter). Am J Dis Child 137:408, 1983.
87. Marx S, Attie M, Spiegel A, et al: An association between neonatal severe primary hyperparathyroidism and familial hypocalciuric hypercalcemia in three kindreds. N Engl J Med 306:257, 1982.
88. Steinmann B, Gnehm HE, Rao VH, et al: Neonatal severe primary hyperparathyroidism and alkaptonuria in a boy born to related parents with familial hypocalciuric hypercalcemia. Helv Paediatr Acta 39:171, 1984.
89. Grantmyre E: Roentgenographic features of "primary" hyperparathyroidism in infancy. J Can Assoc Radiol 24:257, 1973.
90. Fujita T, Watanabe N, Fukase M, et al: Familial hypocalciuric hypercalcemia involving four members of a kindred including a girl with severe neonatal primary hyperparathyroidism. Miner Electrolyte Metab 9:51, 1983.
91. Marx S, Lasker R, Brown E, et al: Secretory dysfunction in parathyroid cells from a neonate with severe primary hyperparathyroidism. J Clin Endocrinol Metab 62:445, 1986.
92. Fujimoto Y, Hazama H, Oku K: Severe primary hyperparathyroidism in a neonate having a parent with hypercalcemia: treatment by total parathyroidectomy and simultaneous heterotopic autotransplantation. Surgery 108:933, 1990.
93. Mallette LA: The functional and pathologic spectrum of parathyroid abnormalities in hyperparathyroidism. *In* Bilezikian JP, Marcus R, Levine MA (eds): The Parathyroids: Basic and Clinical Concepts. New York, Raven Press, 1994, p 423.
94. Cooper L, Wertheimer J, Levey R, et al: Severe primary hyperparathyroidism in a neonate with two hypercalcemic parents: Management with parathyroidectomy and heterotopic autotransplantation. Pediatrics 78:263, 1986.
95. Chou YH, Brown EM, Levi T, et al: The gene responsible for familial hypocalciuric hypercalcemia maps to chromosome 3q in four unrelated families. Nat Genet 1:295, 1992.
96. Pollak MR, Chou YH, Marx SJ, et al: Familial hypocalciuric hypercalcemia and neonatal severe hyperparathyroidism. Effects of mutant gene dosage on phenotype. J Clin Invest 93:1108, 1994.
97. Heath H, Jackson C, Otterud B, et al: Genetic linkage analysis of familial benign (hypocalciuric) hypercalcemia: Evidence for locus heterogeneity. Am J Hum Genet 53:193, 1993.
98. Pearce S, Trump D, Wooding C, et al: Calcium-sensing receptor mutations in familial benign hypercalcaemia and neonatal hyperparathyroidism. J Clin Invest 96:2683, 1995.
99. Trump D, Whyte MP, Wooding C, et al: Linkage studies in a kindred from Oklahoma, with familial benign (hypocalciuric) hypercalcaemia (FBH) and developmental elevations in serum parathyroid hormone levels, indicate a third locus for FBH. Hum Genet 96:183, 1995.
100. Lloyd SE, Pannett AA, Dixon PH, et al: Localization of familial benign hypercalcemia, Oklahoma variant (FBHOk), to chromosome 19q13. Am J Hum Genet 64:189, 1999.
101. Pollak MR, Brown EM, Chou YH, et al: Mutations in the human Ca^{2+}-sensing receptor gene cause familial hypocalciuric hypercalcemia and neonatal severe hyperparathyroidism [see comments]. Cell 75:1297, 1993.
102. Chou YH, Pollak MR, Brandi ML, et al: Mutations in the human Ca^{2+}-sensing-receptor gene that cause familial hypocalciuric hypercalcemia. Am J Hum Genet 56:1075, 1995.
103. Heath HI, Odelberg S, Jackson CE, et al: Clustered inactivating mutations and benign polymorphisms of the calcium receptor gene in familial benign hypocalciuric hypercalcemia suggest receptor functional domains. J Clin Endocrinol Metab 81:1312, 1996.
104. Janicic N, Pausova Z, Cole DEC, et al: Insertion of an Alu sequence in the Ca^{2+}-sensing receptor gene in familial hypocalciuric hypercalcemia and neonatal severe hyperparathyroidism. Am J Hum Genet 56:880, 1995.
105. Kobayashi M, Tanaka H, Tsuzuki K, et al: Two novel missense mutations in calcium-sensing receptor gene associated with neonatal severe hyperparathyroidism. J Clin Endocrinol Metab 82:2716, 1997.
106. Janicic N, Pausova Z, Cole DEC, et al: De novo expansion of an Alu insertion mutation of the Ca^{2+}-sensing receptor gene in familial hypocalciuric hypercalcemia and neonatal severe hyperparathyroidism. J Bone Miner Res 10 (suppl. 1):S191, 1995.
107. Cole DEC, Peltekova VD, Rubin LA, et al: Genetic determinants of serum calcium concentration: Potential roles for the A986S and R990G polymorphisms of the calcium-sensing receptor (CASR) gene (abstract). J Bone Miner Res 12:S257, 1997.
108. Pearce SH, Bai M, Quinn SJ, et al: Functional characterization of calcium-sensing receptor mutations expressed in human embryonic kidney cells. J Clin Invest 98:1860, 1996.
109. Bai M, Janicic N, Trivedi S, et al: Markedly reduced activity of mutant calcium-sensing receptor with an inserted Alu element from a kindred with familial hypocalciuric hypercalcemia and neonatal severe hyperparathyroidism. J Clin Invest 99:1917, 1997.
110. Marx SJ, Fraser D, Rapoport A: Familial hypocalciuric hypercalcemia. Mild expression of the gene in heterozygotes and severe expression in homozygotes. Am J Med 78:15, 1985.
111. Matsuo M, Okita K, Takemine H, et al: Neonatal primary hyperparathyroidism in familial hypocalciuric hypercalcemia. Am J Dis Child 136:728, 1982.
112. Pollak M, Chou YH, Marx SJ, et al: Familial hypocalciuric hypercalcemia and neonatal severe hyperparathyroidism. Effects of mutant gene dosage on phenotype. J Clin Invest 93:1108, 1994.
113. Page L, Haddow J: Self-limited neonatal hyperparathyroidism in familial hypocalciuric hypercalcemia. J Pediatr 111:261, 1987.
114. Harris SS, D'Ercole AJ: Neonatal hyperparathyroidism: The natural course in the absence of surgical intervention. Pediatrics 83:53, 1989.
115. Kovacs CS, Ho-Pao CL, Hunzelman JL, et al: Regulation of murine fetal-placental calcium metabolism by the calcium-sensing receptor. J Clin Invest 101:2812, 1998.
116. Eastell R, Heath H III: The hypocalcemic states: Their differential diagnosis and management. *In* Coe F, Favus M (eds): Disorders of Bone Metabolism. New York, Raven Press, 1992, p 571.
117. Ahn TJ, Antonarakis SE, Kronenberg HM, et al: Familial isolated hypoparathyroidism: A molecular genetic analysis of 8 families with 23 affected persons. Medicine (Baltimore) 65:573, 1986.
118. Arnold A, Horst SA, Gardella TJ, et al: Mutation of the signal peptide-encoding region of the preproparathyroid hormone gene in familial isolated hypoparathyroidism. J Clin Invest 86:1084, 1990.
119. Parkinson DB, Thakker RV: A donor splice site mutation in the parathyroid hormone gene is associated with autosomal recessive hypoparathyroidism. Nat Genet 1:149, 1992.
120. Baron J, Winer KK, Yanovski JA, et al: Mutations in the Ca^{2+}-sensing receptor gene cause autosomal dominant and sporadic hypoparathyroidism. Hum Mol Genet 5:601, 1996.
121. De Luca F, Ray K, Mancilla EE, et al: Sporadic hypoparathyroidism caused by *de novo* gain-of-function mutations in the Ca^{2+}-sensing receptor. J Clin Endocrinol Metab 82:2710, 1997.
122. Lovlie R, Eiken HG, Sorheim H: The Ca^{2+}-sensing receptor gene (PCAR1) mutation T151M in isolated autosomal dominant hypoparathyroidism. Hum Genet 98:129, 1996.
123. Mancilla EE, De Luca F, Ray K, et al: A Ca^{2+}-sensing receptor mutation causes hypoparathyroidism by increasing receptor sensitivity to Ca^{2+} and maximal signal transduction. Pediatr Res 42:443, 1997.
124. Pearce SH, Williamson C, Kifor O, et al: A familial syndrome of hypocalcemia with hypercalciuria due to mutations in the calcium-sensing receptor [see comments]. N Engl J Med 335:1115, 1996.
125. Pollak MR, Brown EM, Estep HL, et al: Autosomal dominant hypocalcaemia caused by a Ca^{2+}-sensing receptor gene mutation. Nat Genet 8:303, 1994.
126. Davies M, Mughal Z, Selby P, et al: Familial benign hypocalcemia. J Bone Miner Res 10 (suppl 1):S507, 1995.
127. Estep H, Mistry Z, Burke P: Familial idiopathic hypocalcemia. *In* Proceedings and Abstracts of the 63rd Annual Meeting of the Endocrine Society, Cincinnati. Endocrine Society, 1981, p 275.
128. Finegold DN, Armitage MM, Galiani M, et al: Preliminary localization of a gene for autosomal dominant hypoparathyroidism to chromosome 3q13. Pediatr Res 36:414, 1994.
129. Perry YM, Finegold DM, Armitage MM, et al: A missense mutation in the Ca-sensing receptor causes familial autosomal dominant hypoparathyroidism (abstract). Am J Hum Genet 55 (suppl):A17, 1994.
130. Nemeth EF, Steffey ME, Hammerland LG, et al: Calcimimetics with potent and selective activity on the parathyroid calcium receptor. Proc Natl Acad Sci USA 95:4040, 1998.
131. Nemeth EF: Ca^{2+} receptor-dependent regulation of cellular functions. News Physiol Sci 10:1, 1995.
132. Silverberg SJ, Bone HG III, Marriott TB, et al: Short-term inhibition of parathyroid hormone secretion by a calcium-receptor agonist in patients with primary hyperparathyroidism. N Engl J Med 337:1506, 1997.

Chapter 81

Hypoparathyroidism and Pseudohypoparathyroidism

Michael A. Levine

The term *functional hypoparathyroidism* refers to a group of metabolic disorders in which hypocalcemia and hyperphosphatemia occur either from a failure of the parathyroid glands to secrete adequate amounts of biologically active parathyroid hormone (PTH) or, less commonly, from an inability of PTH to elicit appropriate biologic responses in its target tissues. Plasma concentrations of PTH are low or absent in patients with true hypoparathyroidism. By contrast, plasma concentrations of PTH are typically elevated in patients with pseudohypoparathyroidism (PHP), and reflect the failure of target tissues to respond appropriately to the biologic actions of PTH. Thus true hypoparathyroidism differs fundamentally and biochemically from PHP.

Hypocalcemia is the biochemical hallmark of functional hypoparathyroidism. The concentration of calcium in the extracellular fluid is critical for many physiologic processes, and therefore the concentration is normally maintained within narrow limits despite wide variations in dietary intake, the demands of the skeleton during growth, and losses during pregnancy and lactation (see Chapter 73 for details of calcium and phosphorus metabolism). Approximately 99% of total body calcium is in the skeleton in the form of hydroxyapatite, leaving only 1% of the total body calcium within extracellular fluids and soft tissues. Calcium is distributed among three interconvertible fractions in the circulation. Approximately 45% to 50% of total serum calcium is in the ionized form at normal serum protein concentrations, and represents the biologically active component of the total serum calcium concentration. Another 8% to 10% is complexed to organic and inorganic acids (e.g., citrate, sulfate, and phosphate); together, the ionized and complexed calcium fractions represent the diffusible portion of circulating calcium. Approximately 40% of serum calcium is protein-bound, primarily to albumin (80%) but also to globulins (20%).[1] The protein-bound calcium is not biologically active but provides a reserve of available calcium should a need for increased ionized calcium arise acutely. Although conventional measurement of serum calcium implies determination of the total serum calcium concentration, more physiologically relevant information is obtained by measurement of the ionized calcium concentration. From a practical point of view, measurement of total serum calcium concentration provides a reasonable estimate of the ionized calcium concentration, but several caveats are worth noting. For example, decreased concentration of serum albumin, the major calcium-binding protein in the circulation, accounts for most cases of low serum calcium in hospitalized patients.

This work has been supported in part by grants from the National Institutes of Health (DK-34281, DK-56178, and GCRC M01-RR00052).

Sudden changes in the distribution of calcium between ionized and bound fractions may cause symptoms of hypocalcemia, even in patients with functioning hormonal mechanisms for the regulation of the ionized calcium concentration. Increases in the extracellular fluid concentration of anions, such as phosphate, citrate, bicarbonate, or edetic acid, will increase the proportion of bound calcium and decrease ionized calcium. Extracellular fluid pH also affects the distribution of calcium between ionized and bound fractions. Alkalosis increases the affinity of albumin for calcium, and thereby decreases the concentration of ionized calcium. By contrast, acidosis increases the ionized calcium concentration by decreasing the binding of calcium to albumin. Therefore, measurement of ionized calcium is preferred when evaluating symptoms of hypocalcemia in patients who have abnormal circulating proteins or acid-base and electrolyte disorders.[2] Plasma levels of ionized calcium can be measured in most clinical chemistry laboratories using now-standardized techniques.[3–5] However, when it is not possible, or practical, to determine the ionized calcium concentration directly, a "corrected" total calcium concentration can be derived using one of several proposed algorithms that are based on albumin or total protein concentrations.[2, 6] None of these correction factors is absolutely accurate, but they often provide useful estimates of the true concentration of calcium in serum.[7] One widely used algorithm estimates that total serum calcium declines by approximately 0.8 mg/dL for each 1 g/dL decrease in albumin concentration, without a change in ionized calcium.

PATHOPHYSIOLOGY OF HYPOCALCEMIA

The concentration of extracellular ionized calcium is tightly regulated by PTH and 1,25-dihydroxyvitamin D ([$1,25(OH)_2D$], calcitriol). PTH is synthesized in the four parathyroid glands as a preprohormone (115 amino acids), converted to a prohormone (90 amino acids) as it is transported across the rough endoplasmic reticulum, and stored in secretory granules as the mature 84–amino acid hormone. PTH is secreted at a rate inversely proportional to the ambient serum ionized calcium concentration. Hormone secretion is tightly regulated through the interaction of extracellular calcium (and to a lesser extent other divalent cations) with specific calcium-sensing receptors[8–10] that are present on the surface of the parathyroid cell. Extracellular calcium stimulates a receptor-dependent signaling pathway that leads to the rapid but transient increase in intracellular calcium; the increase in cytosolic calcium inhibits release of PTH from the parathyroid cell. By contrast, PTH synthesis and secretion are increased when the extracellular calcium concentration is low. Over time, protracted hypocalcemia leads not only to increased PTH secretion but also to increased parathyroid gland mass.

Fluctuations in the serum calcium concentration provoke rapid changes in PTH secretion that within minutes affect distal tubular calcium reabsorption and osteoclastic bone resorption. In contrast to this short-loop feedback system, adjustments in the rate of gastrointestinal absorption of calcium via PTH-stimulated synthesis of $1,25(OH)_2D$ require 24 to 48 hours to become maximal and constitute a long-loop feedback system. The integrated actions of PTH on these target tissues provide a precise system of control and maintain the serum ionized calcium concentration within a narrow range.

PTH has direct effects on bone to regulate calcium exchange at osteocytic sites and to enhance osteoclast-mediated bone resorption. In the kidney, PTH directly enhances distal tubular reabsorption of calcium, decreases the proximal tubular reabsorption of phosphate, and stimulates the metabolic conversion of 25-hydroxyvitamin D [25(OH)D] to $1,25(OH)_2D$, the active vitamin D metabolite. $1,25(OH)_2D$ acts on bone to enhance bone resorption and on the gastrointestinal mucosa to increase absorption of dietary calcium.

PTH regulates mineral metabolism and skeletal homeostasis by modulating the activity of specialized target cells that are present in bone and kidney. PTH action first requires binding of the hormone to specific receptors that are expressed on the plasma membrane of target cells. The classic PTH receptor (PTHR) is an approximately 75-kDa glycoprotein that is often referred to as the PTH–PTH-related protein (PTHrP), or type 1 PTHR. Molecular cloning of complementary DNAs (cDNAs) encoding PTHRs from several species[11–14] has indicated that the type 1 receptor expressed on bone and kidney cells is identical. The type 1 PTHR binds both PTH and PTHrP, a factor made by diverse tumors that cause humorally mediated hypercalcemia, with equivalent affinity, which accounts for the similar activities of both hormones. By contrast, a second PTHR, termed the type 2 receptor protein, is not expressed in conventional PTH target tissues (i.e., bone and kidney), and interacts with PTH but not PTHrP.[15, 16] (See Chapter 70.) Both PTHRs are members of a large family of receptors that can bind hormones, neurotransmitters, cytokines, light photons, and taste and odor molecules. These receptors consist of a single polypeptide chain that is predicted by hydrophobicity plots to span the plasma membrane seven times (i.e., heptahelical), forming three extracellular and three or four intracellular loops and a cytoplasmic C-terminal tail. The heptahelical receptors are coupled by heterotrimeric ($\alpha\beta\gamma$) G proteins[17] to signal effector molecules localized to the inner surface of the plasma membrane (Fig. 81–1). The heterotrimeric G proteins share a common structure consisting of an α subunit and a tightly coupled $\beta\gamma$ dimer. The α subunit interacts with detector and effector molecules, binds guanosine triphosphate (GTP), and possesses intrinsic GTPase activity.[18] Mammals have over 20 different G protein α chains encoded by 16 genes; additional protein diversity results from the generation of alternatively spliced messenger RNAs (mRNAs). The various G protein α chains can be grouped into four major classes (G_s, G_i, G_q, G_{12}) according to structural and functional homologies. The ligand-bound GTP α chain is the primary regulator of membrane-bound ion channels and enzymes that generate intracellular second messengers. The α subunits associate with a smaller group of β (at least 5) and γ (>12) subunits.[19] The β and γ subunits combine tightly with one another[20, 21] and the resultant $\beta\gamma$ dimers demonstrate specific associations with different α subunits.[22, 23] Combinatorial specificity in the associations between various G protein subunits provides the potential for enormous diversity, and may allow distinct heterotrimers to interact selectively with only a limited number of the more than one thousand G protein–coupled receptors.[24, 25] At present, it is unknown whether specific G protein subunit associations occur randomly or if there are regulated mechanisms that determine the subunit composition of heterotrimers.

The binding and hydrolysis of GTP regulate the activity of G proteins (Fig. 81–2). In the basal (nonstimulated) state, G proteins exist in the heterotrimeric form with guanosine diphosphate (GDP) tightly bound to the α chain. Upon receptor activation, a conformational change occurs in the α chain that facilitates the exchange of bound GDP for GTP, with subsequent dissociation of the α-GTP chain from the $\beta\gamma$ dimer and the receptor. The free α-GTP chain is able to interact with effector enzymes and ion channels to regulate their activity. In addition, free $\beta\gamma$ dimers can also participate in downstream signaling events[26, 27]; for example, $\beta\gamma$ dimers can influence activity of certain forms of adenylate cyclase and phospholipase C, open potassium channels,[28] participate in receptor desensitization,[29, 30] mediate mitogen-activated protein (MAP) kinase phosphorylation,[31, 32] and modulate leukocyte chemotaxis.[33] The interaction of α-GTP with the effector molecule is terminated by the hydrolysis of GTP to GDP by an endogenous GTPase. With hydrolysis of GTP to GDP, the α-GDP chain reassociates with the $\beta\gamma$ dimer and the heterotrimeric G protein is ready for another cycle of receptor activation.

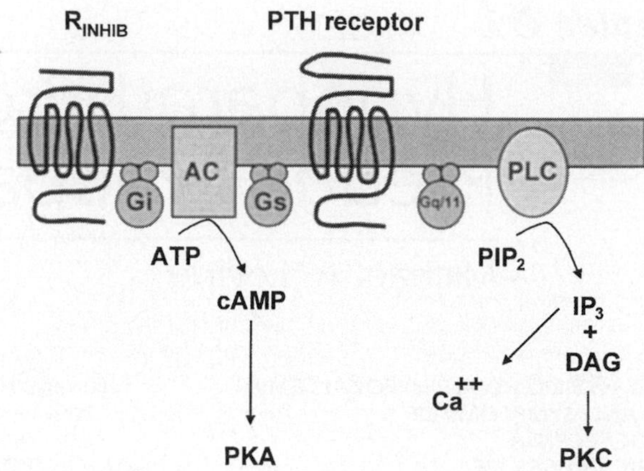

FIGURE 81–1. Cell-surface receptors for parathyroid hormone (PTH) are coupled to two classes of G proteins. G_s mediates stimulation of adenylate cyclase (AC) and the production of cyclic adenosine monophosphate (cAMP), which in turn activates protein kinase A (PKA). G_q stimulates phospholipase C (PLC) to form the second messengers inositol-(1,4,5)-trisphosphate (IP_3) and diacylglycerol (DAG) from membrane- bound phosphatidylinositol-(4,5)-bisphosphate. IP_3 increases intracellular calcium (Ca^{2+}) and DAG stimulates protein kinase C (PKC) activity. Each G protein consists of a unique α chain and a $\beta\gamma$ dimer.

Interaction of PTH with its receptor activates intracellular signal effector systems that generate the second messengers cyclic adenosine monophosphate (cAMP),[34, 35] inositol 1,4,5-trisphosphate and diacylglycerol,[36, 37] and cytosolic calcium[38–41] (see Fig. 81–1). The best-characterized mediator of PTH action is cAMP, which rapidly activates protein kinase A.[42] The relevant target proteins that are phosphorylated by protein kinase A and the precise mode(s) of action of these proteins remain uncharacterized, though proteins that activate genes responsive to cAMP and ion channel proteins are strong candidates. In contrast to the well-recognized biologic effects of cAMP in PTH target tissues, the physiologic importance of metabolites of phosphotidylinositol hydrolysis and intracellular calcium as PTH-induced second messengers has not yet been established. Studies of the expressed type 1 PTHR have revealed that ligand activation of these diverse second messengers derives from the ability of the receptor to interact with several different G proteins. The agonist-bound type 1 PTHR can activate members of the Gq/11 family, and thereby stimulate phospholipase C, and can activate G_s to stimulate adenylate cyclase.[43, 44] These studies have revealed that the number of PTHRs expressed, as well as the concentration of G protein and PTH, cooperate to determine the precise signal response.

Clinical disorders that cause hypocalcemia reflect defects either in the production of biologically active PTH or $1,225(OH)_2D$ or in the ability of specific target tissues to respond appropriately to these hormones, either because of a specific biochemical defect or because of generalized target organ damage (Table 81–1).

In states of functional hypoparathyroidism, in which PTH secretion or action is deficient, the normal effects of PTH on bone and kidney are absent. Bone resorption and release of calcium from skeletal stores are diminished. Renal tubular reabsorption of calcium is decreased,

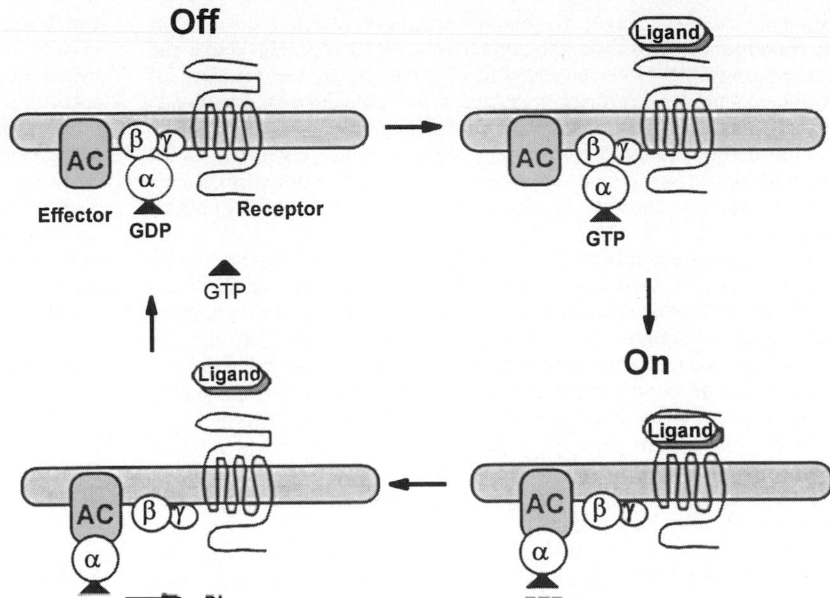

FIGURE 81–2. The G protein GTPase regulatory cycle. In the nonstimulated, basal (Off) state, guanosine diphosphate (GDP) is tightly bound to the α chain of the heterotrimeric G protein. Binding of an agonist (ligand) to its receptor (depicted with seven transmembrane spanning domains) induces a conformational change in the receptor, and enables it to activate the G protein. The G protein now releases GDP and binds guanosine triphosphate (GTP) present in the cytosol. The binding of GTP to the α chain leads to dissociation of the α-GTP from the βγ dimer, and each of these molecules is now free to regulate downstream effector proteins. The hydrolysis of GTP to GDP by the intrinsic GTPase of the α chain promotes reassociation of α-GDP with βγ and the inactive state is restored. The heterotrimeric G protein is ready for another cycle of hormone-induced activation.

but because of hypocalcemia and low filtered load, urinary calcium excretion is low. In the absence of PTH action, urinary clearance of phosphate is decreased, and hyperphosphatemia occurs. The deficiency of PTH action and the hyperphosphatemia together impair renal synthesis of 1,25$(OH)_2$D, and absorption of calcium from the intestine is markedly impaired. 1,25$(OH)_2$D is also a potent stimulator of bone resorption, and its absence also decreases the availability of calcium from bone. Because the parathyroid glands are intact in states of vitamin D deficiency, hypocalcemia induces secondary hyperparathyroidism, and renal phosphate clearance is enhanced. Thus, hypocalcemia in vitamin D deficiency results from decreased intestinal absorption of calcium and a limited availability of calcium from bone despite secondary hyperparathyroidism; characteristically, it is accompanied by hypophosphatemia.

TABLE 81–1. *Causes of Functional Hypoparathyroidism*

A. Surgery
B. Toxic agents
 1. High dose radiation (rarely)
 2. Asparaginase
 3. Amifostine
C. Infiltrative processes
 1. Iron deposition
 2. Copper deposition
 3. Tumor or granuloma
D. Defective secretion of parathyroid hormone (PTH)
 1. Magnesium deficiency
 2. Magnesium excess
 3. Activating mutation of calcium-sensing receptor gene (MIM 145980)
 4. Alcohol
 5. Maternal hypercalcemia
 6. Neonatal hypocalcemia
E. Autoimmune destruction of the parathyroid glands
 1. Autoimmune hypoparathyroidism
 2. Autoimmune polyglandular syndrome, type 1 (APECED, MIM 240300)
F. Idiopathic hypoparathyroidism
 1. Autosomal recessive (MIM 241400)
 2. X-linked (MIM 307700)
G. Embryologic defects in parathyroid gland development
 1. DiGeorge syndrome (del 22q), DGS1 (MIM 188400)
 2. DiGeorge syndrome (del 10p), DGS2 (MIM 601362)
 3. Velocardiofacial syndrome (del 22q) (MIM 192430)
H. Defective synthesis of PTH (MIM 168450)
 1. Autosomal dominant mutation in preproPTH gene
 2. Autosomal recessive mutation in preproPTH gene
I. Metabolic defects and mitochondrial neuromyopathies
 1. Kearn-Sayre syndrome
 2. Pearson's syndrome
 3. t-RNA leu mutations
J. Resistance to PTH
 1. Pseudohypoparathyroidism type 1a (MIM 103580)
 2. Pseudohypoparathyroidism type 1b
 3. Pseudohypoparathyroidism type 1c
 4. Pseudohypoparathyroidism type 2

APECD, autoimmune polyendocrinopathy-condidiasis-ectodermal dystrophy; MIM, Mendelian inheritance in man.

SIGNS AND SYMPTOMS OF HYPOCALCEMIA

The clinical presentation of hypocalcemia can vary from an asymptomatic biochemical finding to a life-threatening condition. The manifestations of hypocalcemia are due primarily to enhanced neuromuscular excitability (tetany), and in general reflect the level of ionized calcium, rather than total calcium, as well as the rate of decline. In addition, the signs and symptoms of hypocalcemic tetany can be potentiated by other electrolyte abnormalities, particularly hypomagnesemia.[45]

There is substantial variation among patients in the severity of symptoms, and there does not appear to be an absolute level of serum calcium at which symptoms can be expected. Patients with chronic hypocalcemia sometimes have few, if any, symptoms of neuromuscular irritability despite markedly depressed serum calcium concentrations. By contrast, patients with acute hypocalcemia frequently manifest many symptoms of tetany. Most patients with hypocalcemia will have some mild features of tetany, including circumoral numbness, paresthesias of the distal extremities, or muscle cramps. Symptoms of fatigue, hyperirritability, anxiety, and depression are also common. Clinical manifestations of marked hypocalcemia consist of carpopedal spasm, muscle cramps, and rarely laryngospasm. Syncope and seizures of all types may occur, including focal and sometimes life-threatening generalized seizures (which must be distinguished from the generalized tonic muscle contractions that occur in severe tetany).

Clinical signs of the neuromuscular irritability associated with latent tetany include *Chvostek's sign* and *Trousseau's sign*. Chvostek's sign is elicited by tapping the facial nerve just anterior to the ear to produce ipsilateral contraction of the facial muscles. Slightly positive reactions occur in 10% to 30% of adults with normal serum calcium levels[46]; thus, a mildly positive sign may not be diagnostic of hypocalcemia unless it is known that the sign was absent when the serum calcium was normal. Trousseau's sign is present if carpal spasm occurs after compression of the nerves in the upper arm. A typical protocol consists of inflation of a cuff on the upper arm to 20 mm Hg above the patient's systolic blood pressure for 3 minutes. In the presence of hypocalcemia, the neuroischemia caused by application of pressure to the upper arm induces sufficient irritability to yield a positive response: flexion of the wrist and metacarpophalangeal joints, extension of the interphalangeal joints, and adduction of the digits. Both Chvostek's and Trousseau's signs can be absent in patients with definite hypocalcemia.

Hypocalcemia is also associated with nonspecific electroencephalographic changes, increases in intracranial pressure, and papilledema. A markedly depressed serum calcium concentration can have profound affects on the heart. The corrected Q–T (Q–Tc) interval may be prolonged on the electrocardiogram (Fig. 81–3), and may be associated with arrhythmias or cardiac dysfunction that is generally reversible with treatment of the hypocalcemia.[47–49] Cardiac dysfunction can range from a mild abnormality that is noted only with exercise,[50] to life-threatening heart failure.[51] The somatosensory evoked potential recovery period may provide a useful tool for assessing the effects and recovery from hypocalcemia.[52]

Additional signs may be associated with long-standing hypocalcemia. Ectodermal findings such as dry skin, coarse hair, and brittle nails are common, but they are frequently overlooked. Dental and enamel hypoplasia and delayed or absent eruption of adult teeth indicate that hypocalcemia has been present since childhood.[53–55] The pattern of dental abnormality can be used to determine the age at which the patient first developed hypocalcemia. Visual impairment may occur in patients with long-standing untreated hypocalcemia and hyperphosphatemia due to the development of posterior subcapsular cataracts. Treatment of hypoparathyroidism may reverse or decrease progression of cataracts. Calcification of the basal ganglia, and to a lesser extent the cerebral cortex, occurs in all forms of hypoparathyroidism and can be detected by computed tomographic (CT) scanning, even when routine skull radiographs do not demonstrate intracerebral calcification.[56, 57] Cerebral calcifications may be associated with significant neuropsychiatric or cognitive deficits.[58] Rarely, calcification of the basal ganglia leads to development of neurologic signs or symptoms that resemble Parkinson's disease or chorea.[59] An unusual neurologic manifestation of hypocalcemia is an increased susceptibility to dystonic reactions induced by phenothiazines.[60] Rickets and osteomalacia, although not characteristic, do occur occasionally in patients with long-standing hypoparathyroidism and marked hypocalcemia.[61, 62] Patients with chronic hypoparathyroidism have been reported to have significantly increased bone mineral density[63] whether they are treated[64] or not.[65]

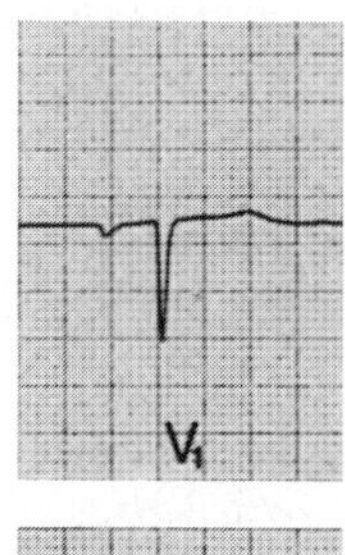

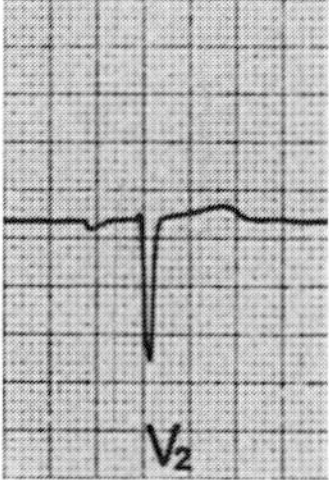

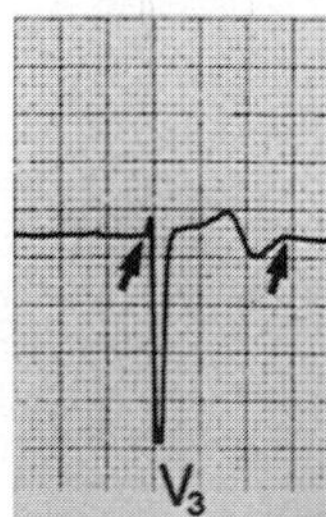

FIGURE 81–3. Electrocardiogram of a patient with severe hypocalcemia. This ECG demonstrates the characteristic prolongation of the (corrected) Q–T interval, measured from the beginning of the QRS complex to the end of the T wave (*arrows* in bottom panel). The Q–T interval corresponds to the duration of ventricular depolarization and repolarization. The interval increases with decreasing heart rate and may be corrected (Q–Tc) by measuring the R–R interval and employing the following formula: $Q\text{–}Tc = Q\text{–}T/\sqrt{(R\text{–}R)}$. The second or plateau phase (ST segment) of the action potential is influenced by the serum calcium, and is of greater duration in hypocalcemic subjects. As the exact end of the T wave may be difficult to determine, some clinicians utilize the $Q_a\text{–}T_c$ interval, which comprises the onset of the QRS complex to the apex of the T wave. (Reprinted by permission from Becker KL, Bilezikian LC [eds]: Principles and Practice of Endocrinology and Metabolism, ed 2. Philadelphia, JB Lippincott, 1992, p 534.)

SPECIFIC CAUSES OF HYPOPARATHYROIDISM

The term *hypoparathyroidism* refers to a group of disorders in which the relative or absolute deficiency of PTH leads to hypocalcemia and hyperphosphatemia. There are many different causes of hypoparathyroidism, as discussed below and listed in Table 81–1.

Surgery and Toxic Agents

Surgery is the most common cause of acquired hypoparathyroidism. Hypoparathyroidism may occur after parathyroid or thyroid surgery or after radical surgery for laryngeal or esophageal carcinoma.[66] The resulting hypoparathyroidism can be transient or permanent, and sometimes may not develop for many years.[67] The degree of hypoparathyroidism may be more profound after treatment of laryngeal cancer with surgery plus radiotherapy than with surgery alone.[68] A chronic state of "decreased parathyroid reserve"[67] may exist in some patients who manifest hypocalcemia only when mineral homeostasis is stressed further by other factors such as pregnancy, lactation, or illness. Surgical removal or biophysical ablation of a hyperfunctioning parathyroid adenoma can precipitate symptomatic hypocalcemia within hours. Hypocalcemia occurs because the remaining normal parathyroid tissue remains "suppressed" by previous hypercalcemia and is unable to secrete PTH appropriately. Hypoparathyroidism is usually transient because the normal parathyroid glands recover function quickly (generally within 1 week), even after long-term suppression. Transient postoperative hypocalcemia may be exaggerated or prolonged in those patients who have significant preexisting hyperparathyroid bone disease. In these patients the acute reduction of previously elevated serum levels of PTH results in an increased movement of serum calcium (and phosphorus) into remineralizing "hungry bones."[69] Treatment with calcium and a short-acting vitamin D metabolite may be required until the bones heal.

Permanent hypoparathyroidism is unusual after an initial neck exploration for primary hyperparathyroidism and develops in less than 1% to 2% of patients. The incidence is greatly increased with repeated neck surgery for recurrent or persistent hyperparathyroidism, after subtotal parathyroidectomy for parathyroid hyperplasia, or when an inexperienced operator performs surgery.

The incidence of permanent hypoparathyroidism after thyroid surgery varies widely, and reflects the underlying thyroid lesion, the extent of surgery, and the experience of the surgeon. Hypoparathyroidism may occur as a result of direct injury or inadvertent removal or devascularization of the parathyroid glands. Permanent hypoparathyroidism is unlikely to occur after a hemithyroidectomy and should be relatively uncommon even after total thyroidectomy.[70, 71] By contrast, transient hypoparathyroidism may occur in up to 33% of patients who undergo a total thyroidectomy for thyroid cancer[72] or thyrotoxicosis. The fall in plasma calcium level generally occurs within 24 to 48 hours after surgery and often is sufficient to provoke symptoms of tetany. The basis for this acute hypocalcemia is not well understood. One mechanism that has been proposed for patients with thyrotoxicosis is similar to the "hungry bones" phenomenon that occurs after parathyroid surgery in patients with marked primary hyperparathyroidism.[73] Patients with severe hyperthyroidism often have increased bone resorption, elevated plasma ionized calcium levels, and suppressed parathyroid function. Although it has been proposed that hypocalcemia occurs as calcium moves rapidly into remineralizing bones after surgical correction of thyrotoxicosis,[74] the early development of hypocalcemia after surgery often precedes significant reduction of serum levels of thyroid hormones. A more likely explanation is that unappreciated damage has occurred to the parathyroid glands during surgery. Whatever the initiating cause, the development of hypocalcemia must indicate that the secretory response of the parathyroid glands is inadequate to maintain a normal serum calcium concentration.[75, 76]

Radiation and Drugs

In contrast to many other endocrine tissues, the parathyroid glands are particularly resistant to damage by a great many toxic agents. The administration of radioactive iodine for the treatment of benign or malignant thyroid disease or for the deliberate induction of hypothyroidism has only rarely caused permanent, symptomatic hypoparathyroidism. Similarly, external beam radiation appears to have little or no effect on parathyroid gland function. Parathyroid tissue is remarkably resistant to most chemotherapeutic or cytotoxic agents, with the notable exceptions of asparaginase, which causes parathyroid necrosis, and amifostine (ethiofos), a radio- and chemoprotector that causes reversible inhibition of PTH secretion.[77, 78] Along with its effects on the parathyroid gland, amifostine also inhibits osteoclast activity. Thus, a significant component of the calcium-reducing effect of this agent derives from its ability to inhibit osteoclast-directed bone resorption and calcium release from skeletal stores. The most common toxic agent to affect parathyroid function is alcohol.[79] Transient hypoparathyroidism has been associated with ingestion of large quantities of alcohol and may be related to either direct effects of alcohol on the parathyroids or through induction of hypomagnesemia.[78, 80, 81]

Infiltrative Disease of the Parathyroids

Infiltrative processes that affect the parathyroid gland can diminish the ability of the gland to secrete PTH. Idiopathic hemochromatosis and chronic transfusion therapy are often associated with significant deposition of iron in the parathyroid glands.[82] Patients occasionally develop clinical hypoparathyroidism, but more commonly manifest decreased "parathyroid reserve" as a consequence of iron infiltration.[83] A similar pathophysiologic process has been described in one patient with Wilson's disease and increased copper storage who developed symptomatic hypoparathyroidism.[84] Pathologic involvement of the parathyroid glands can also occur in metastatic neoplasia, miliary tuberculosis, amyloidosis, and sarcoid, but clinical hypoparathyroidism rarely occurs in these conditions.

Magnesium Deficiency and Excess

Although calcium is the principal physiologic regulator of PTH secretion, magnesium, as a divalent cation, can also modulate secretion of PTH from the parathyroid glands. Recent studies show that at equimolar concentrations, magnesium has approximately 30% to 50% of the effect of calcium on either stimulating or suppressing PTH secretion.[85] Hypermagnesemia can cause reversible hypocalcemia. This situation is most commonly encountered in obstetric practice when high-dose magnesium infusions are used for the treatment of toxemia or premature labor, and likely reflects the ability of elevated serum levels of magnesium to stimulate calcium-sensing receptors expressed by parathyroid cells and thereby inhibit PTH secretion.[86–88] Because the hypocalcemia is accompanied by significant hypermagnesemia, neuromuscular irritability should be less than that expected when similar calcium concentrations occur with normal magnesium; clinical tetany usually does not occur.[45] While elevations in extracellular magnesium can suppress PTH secretion and reduce serum calcium levels, hypocalcemia is more often a manifestation of magnesium depletion.[89] Symptomatic hypocalcemia frequently occurs in patients with magnesium depletion due to chronic alcoholism[78] or burn injury,[90] and is also a feature of Gitelman syndrome,[91, 92] as well as other forms of hereditary renal or intestinal hypomagnesemia.[93] As the serum magnesium level falls, the parathyroid gland responds by increasing secretion of PTH. However, as intracellular magnesium depletion develops, the ability of the parathyroid gland to secrete PTH is impaired, and hypocalcemia may ensue.[94] Magnesium depletion must be severe before hypocalcemia occurs, but hypomagnesemia in the absence of hypocalcemia has been reported to cause neuromuscular hyperexcitability and tetany. The majority of patients with magnesium depletion have low levels of PTH, or "normal" levels of PTH that are in fact inappropriate for the degree of hypocalcemia. Therefore, a state of relative or functional hypoparathyroidism exists in these patients. By contrast, serum levels of PTH are elevated in some hypocalcemic patients with more severe magnesium depletion.[85, 95] These patients show diminished renal and skeletal responses to exogenous PTH, suggesting that refractoriness to PTH may develop with increasing degrees of magnesium depletion. Hypocalcemia can be readily reversed by magnesium therapy alone, but is not corrected by administration of calcium or vitamin D.

Idiopathic Hypoparathyroidism

The term *idiopathic hypoparathyroidism* describes a heterogeneous group of rare disorders that share in common deficient secretion of PTH. The use of the word "idiopathic" to describe this group of disorders has greater historical than scientific relevance at present, as recent molecular and biochemical studies have revealed the cause of hypoparathyroidism in many of these disorders. Accordingly, "idiopathic" is a misnomer for many of these conditions. Although most cases are sporadic, the familial occurrence of idiopathic hypoparathyroidism has been reported. Within these families, hypoparathyroidism may occur as part of a complex autoimmune disorder associated with multiple endocrine deficiencies (i.e., type 1 polyglandular syndrome) or in association with diverse developmental abnormalities (e.g., nephropathy, lymphedema, nerve deafness, or branchial pouch dysembryogenesis). The pleiotropic nature of many of these various syndromes has suggested that the genetic basis of PTH deficiency is not related to defects in the PTH gene or in genes that are specific to parathyroid gland development.

Autoimmune Hypoparathyroidism

Autoimmune hypoparathyroidism may occur alone or in association with additional features, including mucocutaneous candidiasis and adrenal insufficiency, as a component of the autoimmune polyglandular syndrome (APS) type 1 (APS-1).[96] APS-1 may be sporadic or familial with an autosomal recessive inheritance pattern.[97] By contrast, APS-2 is characterized by adult-onset adrenal insufficiency associated with insulin-dependent diabetes mellitus and thyroid disease, and is believed to be polygenic with apparent autosomal dominant inheritance. The APS-1 syndrome is typically considered as a clinical triad of hypoparathyroidism, adrenal insufficiency, and mucocutaneous candidiasis (HAM), but many affected patients have additional autoimmune features (below). The syndrome is generally first recognized in early childhood, although a few individuals have developed the condition after the first decade of life. The clinical onset of the three principal components of the syndrome typically follows a predictable pattern, in which mucocutaneous candidiasis first appears at a mean age of 5 years, followed by hypoparathyroidism at a mean age of 9 years, and adrenal insufficiency at a mean age of 14 years.[96] Patients may not manifest all three components of the clinical triad. On the other hand, some patients will develop additional features, such as alopecia, keratoconjunctivitis, malabsorption and steatorrhea, gonadal failure, pernicious anemia, chronic active hepatitis, thyroid disease, and insulin-requiring diabetes mellitus. Enamel hypoplasia of teeth is also common, and appears to be unrelated to hypoparathyroidism.[98] The presence of these additional defects in patients with APS-1 has led to the suggestion that a more inclusive term be used to describe the syndrome: autoimmune polyendocrinopathy-candidiasis-ectodermal dystrophy (APECED).[97, 99] Antibodies directed against the parathyroid, thyroid, and adrenal glands are present in many patients[100] and a T cell abnormality has been described.[101] The presence of organ-specific autoantibodies may not correlate well with the clinical findings. In those cases that have been examined pathologically, complete parathyroid atrophy or destruction has been demonstrated. In some patients, treatment of hypoparathyroidism has been complicated by apparent vitamin D "resistance," possibly related to coexistent hepatic disease or steatorrhea, or both. The molecular defect in patients with APS-1 has been identified, thus facilitating genetic diagnosis of the syndrome. Based on linkage analyses, the APS-1 candidate gene was first assigned to 21q22.3.[102] Subsequent studies used positional cloning to identify the APS-1 gene, termed *AIRE* for *a*uto*i*mmune *r*egulator, and sequence analysis of genomic DNA from affected subjects has disclosed common *AIRE* mutations in different geoethnic patient groups.[103–107] The *AIRE* gene encodes a predicted 57.7-kDa protein that is expressed in thymus, lymph nodes, and fetal liver, and which contains motifs, including two PHD zinc fingers, that are suggestive of a role as a transcriptional regulator. Mutations in the *AIRE* gene are predicted to lead to truncated forms of the protein that lack at least one of the PHD zinc fingers, and which fail to localize to the cell nucleus or to demonstrate gene activation.[108]

Isolated Hypoparathyroidism

Isolated hypoparathyroidism, in which PTH deficiency is not associated with other endocrine disorders or developmental defects, is usually sporadic, but it may occur on a familial basis. The age of onset is generally within the first decade, although hypocalcemia may not be first discovered until later in adult life.

There is a high incidence of parathyroid antibodies in patients with isolated idiopathic hypoparathyroidism, and some cases may be examples of autoimmune hypoparathyroidism or represent incomplete expression of the APS-1 syndrome (see above). Some patients may possess antibodies that inhibit the secretion of PTH[109] rather than cause parathyroid gland destruction.[110] In other cases that have been examined pathologically, fatty replacement[111] or atrophy with fatty infiltration and fibrosis[112] has been described.

Isolated hypoparathyroidism may be sporadic or familial, with inheritance of PTH deficiency by autosomal dominant, autosomal recessive, or X-linked modes of transmission.[113] The age at onset covers a broad range (1 month to 30 years), but the condition is most commonly diagnosed during childhood. Moreover, it is not unusual in familial cases to discover affected adult relatives who have few if any symptoms of hypocalcemia. Parathyroid antibodies are absent. As the preproPTH gene is located at 11p15, molecular genetic studies of familial isolated hypoparathyroidism have focused on kindreds in which inheritance of hypoparathyroidism is consistent with an autosomal mode of transmission. Defects in the preproPTH gene are an uncommon cause of isolated hypoparathyroidism. Genetic analysis of eight pedigrees in which hypoparathyroidism was inherited in an autosomal manner showed linkage of hypoparathyroidism to the preproPTH gene locus in only one family.[114] Subsequent DNA sequence analysis of the preproPTH gene in this kindred revealed that affected members had a heterozygous mutation consisting of a single base substitution (T→ C) in exon 2.[115] This mutation results in the substitution of arginine (CGT) for cysteine (TGT) in the leader sequence of preproPTH. The substitution of a charged amino acid in the midst of the hydrophobic core of the leader sequence inhibits processing of the mutant preproPTH molecule to proPTH by signal peptidase[115] and is presumed to impair translocation of not only the mutant hormone but also the wild-type protein across the plasma membrane of the endoplasmic reticulum. Thus, this heterozygous mutation results in a dominant inhibitor phenotype that prevents processing of the wild-type preproPTH molecule. Expression of this defect was variable within affected members of this kindred, and resulted in inappropriately low or undetectable levels of circulating PTH in hypocalcemic patients.

Other novel mutations in the preproPTH gene have been found to be the cause of autosomal recessive hypoparathyroidism in two unrelated families. In one family affected children were found to be homozygous for a novel mutation in exon 2 that is predicted to disrupt normal processing of the preproPTH molecule. The mutant allele carries a T→C transition in the first base of codon 23 that results in the replacement of serine (TCG) by proline (CCG) at the–3 position of the signal peptide of preproPTH. This change is hypothesized to inhibit cleavage by signal peptidase at the normal position, and thereby lead to rapid degradation of the preproPTH protein in the rough endoplasmic reticulum.[116] Affected patients who are homozygous for this allele present with symptomatic hypocalcemia within the first few weeks of life. In a second family,[117] hypoparathyroidism occurred in members who were homozygous for a single base transversion (G→C) at the exon 2–intron 2 boundary. This mutation alters the invariant gt dinucleotide of the 5′ donor splice site that presumably affects annealing of the U1-snRNP (small nuclear ribonucleoprotein) recognition component of the nuclear RNA splicing enzyme. The use of a highly sensitive modification of reverse transcriptase–polymerase chain reaction (RT-PCR) allowed detection of very small amounts of preproPTH mRNA in cultured lymphoblasts from these patients, and revealed a PTH cDNA in affected subjects that was 90 bp shorter than the corresponding wild-type form.[117] Nucleotide sequence analysis of the shortened cDNA revealed that exon 1 had been spliced to exon 3 in the mutant PTH mRNA, a process that resulted in the deletion of exon 2 from the mature transcript (i.e., exon skipping).[117] The loss of exon 2 eliminates both the initiation codon and the signal peptide sequence from the aberrant preproPTH mRNA, and explains the molecular basis for autosomal recessive hypoparathyroidism in this family.

Although the molecular pathophysiology of hypoparathyroidism has been defined in these families, both linkage analysis and gene sequencing have failed to disclose defects in the preproPTH gene in affected members of other autosomal kindreds.[114, 118, 119] New insights into the molecular pathology of hypoparathyroidism have come from the recent cloning and characterization of the cDNA[9] and gene[120] encoding the calcium-sensing receptor, the cell surface protein that determines the calcium set-point of the parathyroid cell and thereby controls calcium-sensitive secretion of PTH. Heterozygous mutations that result in the *loss of function* of the calcium-sensing receptor are present in most patients with familial (benign) hypocalciuric hypercalcemia (FHH), an autosomal dominant disorder associated with decreased ability of calcium to suppress PTH secretion.[120–123] In several families some affected members have homozygous mutations that cause severe neonatal hyperparathyroidism,[124] a life-threatening hypercalcemic disorder in which parathyroid hyperplasia occurs. Remarkably, contrasting mutations in the calcium-sensing receptor gene that lead to *gain of function* have been identified in many kindreds with autosomal dominant hypocalcemia, a syndrome associated with low serum levels of PTH.[125, 126] In other cases, linkage of hypocalcemia to the chromosomal locus for the calcium-sensing receptor (3q21-24) has provided indirect evidence for the involvement of this gene with familial hypoparathyroidism.[127] Subsequent studies have identified similar activating mutations of the calcium-sensing receptor gene in many patients with sporadic hypoparathyroidism. In both familial and sporadic cases, each affected propositus has demonstrated a unique mutation, suggesting that new mutations must sustain this disorder in the population. These results suggest that mutation of the calcium-sensing receptor gene may be the most common cause of genetic hypoparathyroidism.

The calcium-sensing receptor is expressed not only in the parathyroid gland but also in the kidney, where it appears to play an important role in regulating calcium reabsorption.[10, 128, 129] Thus, loss-of-function mutations of the calcium-sensing receptor in patients with FHH is associated with decreased calcium clearance and hypocalciuria. By contrast, gain-of-function mutations in the calcium-sensing receptor are likely to account for the increased calcium clearance and relative hypercalciuria noted in patients with autosomal dominant hypocalcemia. These patients are therefore at increased risk of nephrocalcinosis or nephrolithiasis especially when treated with calcium and vitamin D to increase serum calcium (see Chapters 75 and 80).

Familial hypoparathyroidism can also be inherited as an X-linked disorder that is of course unrelated to specific defects in the preproPTH gene on chromosome 11.[130] Using an ordered series of polymorphic markers on the X chromosome, linkage studies of two large multigenerational families with X-linked hypoparathyroidism that share a common ancestry have localized a candidate gene to within a 1.5-Mb interval in the region of Xq26-27.[131, 132] These results imply that the defective gene or genes in this syndrome may be important for parathyroid cell development or function. The early onset of hypocalcemia in affected individuals and the apparent inability to identify parathyroid tissue in a single patient with this disorder at autopsy[113] are consistent with a role for this genetic locus in the embryologic development of the parathyroid glands (see below).

Developmental Disorders of the Parathyroid Gland

Hypoparathyroidism may result from agenesis or dysgenesis of the parathyroid glands. The best-described examples of parathyroid gland dysembryogenesis are the DiGeorge and velocardiofacial syndromes, in which maldevelopment of the third and fourth branchial pouches is frequently associated with congenital absence of not only the parathyroids but also the thymus. Because of thymic aplasia, T cell–mediated immunity is impaired, and affected infants have an increased susceptibility to recurrent viral and fungal infections. Despite the emphasis on thymus dysgenesis in these syndromes, clinically significant immune defects occur in very few patients. The basic embryologic defect is inadequate development of the facial neural crest tissues that results in maldevelopment of branchial pouch derivatives, producing characteristic facial (Fig. 81–4) and aortocardiac anomalies, including hypertelorism, antimongoloid slant of the eyes, low-set and notched ears, short philtrum of the lip, and micrognathia (first branchial pouch), or aortic arch abnormalities, such as right-sided arch, truncus arteriosus, or tetralogy of Fallot. Most cases of DiGeorge syndrome are sporadic, but familial occurrence with apparent autosomal dominant inheritance has been described.[133, 134] Although many affected children with DiGeorge syndrome die of infections or cardiac failure by the age of 6, survival into adolescence or adulthood is possible, particularly when the syndrome is only partially expressed.[135]

Molecular mapping studies have demonstrated an association between the syndrome and deletions involving 22q11.2 (DGS1)[136–140] in the great majority of patients with DiGeorge syndrome, but deletions at a second locus at 10p13, termed DGS2, have been found in some patients.[141–143] Microdeletions in 22q11 can be readily identified by fluorescent in situ hybridization (FISH), but similar molecular testing for the 10p13 microdeletion is not widely available. The loss of genetic material at 22q11 on one chromosome results in haploinsufficiency for genes located in this region, and is associated with contiguous gene deletion syndromes that include not only the DiGeorge syndrome but also the overlapping conotruncal anomaly and velocardiofacial syndromes.[144] The associated embryologic defects that characterize these overlapping syndromes caused by loss of genes in the 22q11 region have been compiled to create the acronym CATCH22, which refers to *c*ardiac anomalies, *a*bnormal facies, *t*hymic aplasia, *c*left palate, and *h*ypocalcemia with deletion at 22q. More than 20 candiate genes from the 22q11 region have been identified and none have been shown to cause DiGeorge syndrome. Recently, evidence from both the *hand2* knockout mouse that resembles DiGeorge syndrome and a patient with a small deletion in the region of the *UFD1L* (ubiquitin fusion degradation 1) gene has implicated haploinsufficiency of this gene as the basis for the DGS1 phenotype.[145–151] *UFD1L* regulates the accumulation of protein substrates via control of degradative pathways, and accumulation of excess protein(s) may lead to aberrant cell signaling, abnormal cellular proliferation, or apoptosis of the pharyngeal arches where *UFD1L* is expressed. Further investigation demonstrating mutations in the *UFD1L* gene alone in patients with DiGeorge syndrome will be needed to validate *UFD1L* as a gene responsible for the DiGeorge syndrome phenotype.

Hypoparathyroidism occurs in more than 50% of patients who have the Kenney-Caffey syndrome, an unusual syndrome characterized by short stature, osteosclerosis, basal ganglion calcifications, and ophthalmic defects.[113, 152] Recent studies indicate that the Kenney-Caffey syndrome is related to the Sanjad-Sakati syndrome, in which congenital hypoparathyroidism is associated with growth and mental retardation. Both of these autosomal recessive disorders are linked to the same 2.6 cM region on chromosome 1q42-q43, and are therefore likely to be allelic.[153] Hypoparathyroidism is a variable component of several other developmental syndromes. Barakat syndrome, also termed the HDR syndrome because of the association of *h*ypoparathyroidism with *d*eafness and *r*enal dysplasia,[154] has been assigned in some patients to a chromosomal region on 10p14 that is very near the DGS2 locus.[150, 151] Hypoparathyroidism also has been described in patients with rare familial syndromes that are associated with collateral developmental defects such as lymphedema, prolapsing mitral valve, brachytelephalangy, and nephropathy,[133] or microcephaly, beaked nose, and micrognathia.[156] Congenital hypoparathyroidism also occurs as a feature of several generalized metabolic defects and in several mitochondrial neuromyopathies (see Table 81–1).

Neonatal Hypocalcemia

Shortly after birth there is a physiologic fall in the serum calcium concentration, and during the first 3 days of life many normal infants will have serum calcium levels that are less than 8 mg/dL. Hypocal-

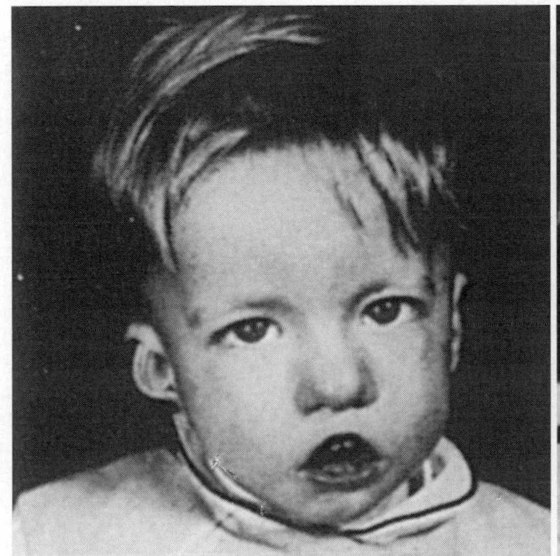
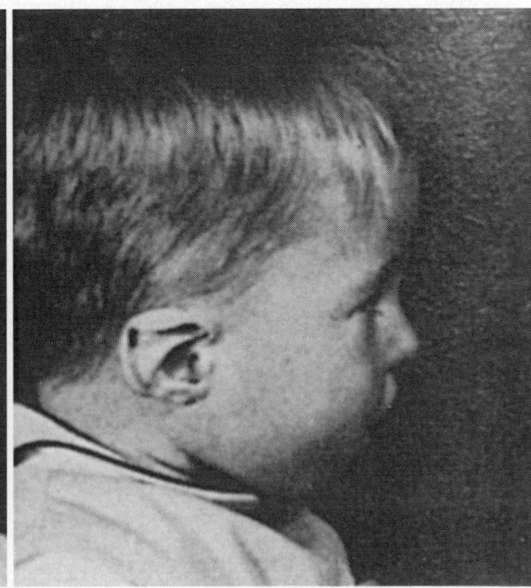

FIGURE 81–4. Photograph of an 18-month-old boy with DiGeorge syndrome. This photograph illustrates the characteristic features, including mild hypertelorism; increased antimongoloid slant of the eyes; low-set, asymmetrical, malformed ears; and a short philtrum. Other features depicted are a broad nose, Cupid's bow mouth, and mandibular hypoplasia. Chest radiograph revealed a right-sided aortic arch and an absent thymic shadow. (From Kretschmer R, Say B, Brown D, Rosen F: Congenital aplasia of the thymus gland (DiGeorge's syndrome). N Engl J Med 279:1295, 1968. Copyright © 1968 Massachusetts Medical Society. All rights reserved.)

cemia in the neonate can be divided into early hypocalcemia, starting within the first 24 to 72 hours of life before feedings have been given, and late hypocalcemia, usually appearing after several days to weeks of feeding.[157, 158]

Early Neonatal Hypocalcemia

Early neonatal hypocalcemia represents an exaggeration of the normal fall in serum calcium concentration and theoretically is due to deficient release of PTH by immature parathyroid glands.[159] Prematurity, low birth weight, hypoglycemia, maternal diabetes, difficult delivery, and respiratory distress syndrome are frequently associated findings. Hypocalcemia may be asymptomatic, but can manifest as irritability, muscular twitching, or convulsive seizures. Although the course is self-limited, symptomatic infants should be treated with oral or intravenous calcium. A more severe form of transient neonatal hypoparathyroidism and tetany can occur in children born to mothers with primary hyperparathyroidism or other causes of hypercalcemia. In these infants, exposure in utero to maternal hypercalcemia suppresses parathyroid activity and apparently leads to impaired responsiveness of the parathyroid glands to hypocalcemia after birth.[160, 161]

Late Neonatal Hypocalcemia

Transient hypocalcemia that occurs 4 to 6 days (or later) after birth is considered to be a manifestation of relative immaturity of renal phosphorus handling or of the renal adenylate cyclase system. Hypocalcemia may be precipitated by a high phosphate diet and appears to occur particularly in those infants who are fed with artificial foods such as cow's milk–based formulas that are often high in phosphorus.[162] In these infants, the renal response to PTH is inadequate and hypocalcemia ensues. The reduction of serum calcium ion concentration is probably secondary to elevated serum phosphate levels and should result in increased parathyroid gland activity. This form of hypocalcemia is the most common cause of seizures in the newborn period. Spontaneous recovery of normal mineral homeostasis typically occurs after a few weeks, but the serum calcium levels of symptomatic infants can be increased within 1 to 2 days by supplementing artificial formulas with sufficient calcium to achieve a high (3:1 to 4:1) calcium-to-phosphorus ratio.

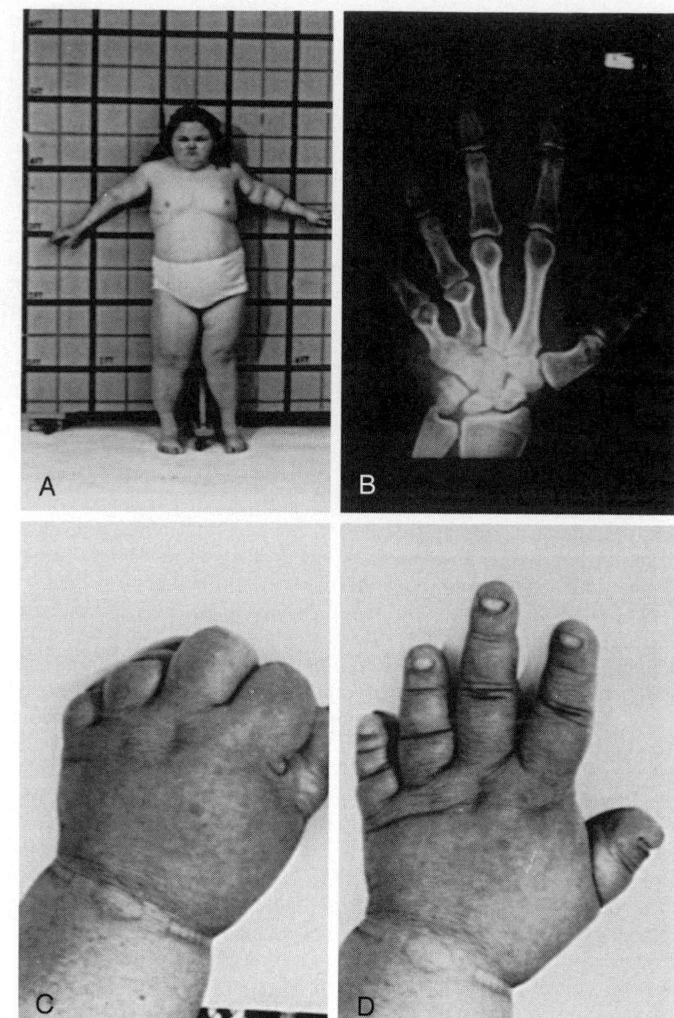

FIGURE 81–5. Typical features of Albright's hereditary osteodystrophy (AHO). *A,* A young woman with characteristic features of AHO; note the short stature, disproportionate shortening of the limbs, obesity, and round face. *B,* Radiograph showing marked shortening of the fourth and fifth metacarpals. *C,* Archibald's sign, the replacement of "knuckles" with "dimples" due to the marked shortening of the metacarpal bones. *D,* Brachydactyly of the hand; note thumb sign ("murderer's thumb" or "potter's thumb") and shortening of the fourth and fifth digits.

PSEUDOHYPOPARATHYROIDISM

The term *pseudohypoparathyroidism* describes a collection of disorders that share in common biochemical hypoparathyroidism (i.e., hypocalcemia and hyperphosphatemia), increased secretion of PTH, and target tissue unresponsiveness to the biologic actions of PTH. Thus the pathophysiology of PHP differs fundamentally from true hypoparathyroidism, in which PTH secretion rather than PTH responsiveness is defective.[163]

In addition to functional hypoparathyroidism, many patients with PHP exhibit a distinctive constellation of developmental and skeletal defects. These characteristics are collectively termed *Albright's hereditary osteodystrophy* (AHO),[164] and include a round face; short, stocky physique; brachydactyly; heterotopic ossification; and mental retardation (Fig. 81–5). There does not appear to be a relationship between the biochemical abnormalities (hypocalcemia and hyperphosphatemia) of PHP and the somatic features of AHO. Indeed, in certain families some affected members manifest both AHO and PTH resistance (i.e., PHP), whereas other family members have AHO without evidence of any endocrine dysfunction, a disorder termed *pseudopseudohypoparathyroidism* (pseudoPHP).[165]

Various variants and subcategories of PHP have been described, and have led to the development of a diagnostic classification that is based on clinical, biochemical, and genetic characteristics (Table 81–2).

Pathophysiology

The first insights into the molecular basis for PHP emerged from the parallel observations that cAMP mediates many of the actions of PTH on kidney and bone, and that administration of PTH to normal subjects markedly increases the urinary excretion of nephrogenous cAMP as well as phosphate.[166] This modification of the original PTH infusion test remains the most reliable test available for the diagnosis of PHP, and enables distinction between several variants of the syndrome (Fig. 81–6). Patients with PHP type 1 fail to show an appropriate increase in urinary excretion of both nephrogenous cAMP and phosphate,[166] suggesting that an abnormality in the renal PTH receptor–adenylate cyclase complex that produces cAMP is the basis for impaired PTH responsiveness. This hypothesis was subsequently confirmed by the finding that administration of dibutyryl cAMP to patients with PHP type 1 produced a phosphaturic response, which clearly demonstrated that the renal response mechanism to cAMP was intact.[167] These studies have led to the conclusion that proximal renal tubule cells are unresponsive to PTH. By contrast, cells in other regions of the kidney appear to respond normally to PTH. For example, the observation that urinary calcium excretion is less in subjects with PHP type 1 than in patients with hormonopenic hypoparathyroidism[168, 169] has been interpreted as evidence that distal renal tubular cells can respond to PTH, Other studies have shown that renal handling of calcium (and sodium) in response to exogenous PTH is normal in patients with PHP type 1.[170] These results suggest that calcium reab-

TABLE 81–2. Classification of the Various Forms of Pseudohypoparathyroidism (PHP) Based on Clinical, Biochemical, and Genetic Features

	PHP Type 1a	PseudoPHP	PHP Type 1b	PHP Type 1c	PHP Type 2
Physical appearance	Albright's hereditary osteodystrophy typical, but may be subtle or (rarely) absent		Normal	Albright's hereditary osteodystrophy	Normal
Response to PTH					
Urine cAMP	Defective	Normal	Defective	Defective	Normal
Urine phosphorus	Defective	Normal	Defective	Defective	Defective
Serum calcium level	Low or (rarely) normal	Normal	Low	Low	Low
Hormone resistance	Generalized	Absent	Limited to PTH target tissues	Generalized	Limited to PTH target tissues
$G_{s\alpha}$ activity	Reduced	Reduced	Normal	Normal	Normal
Inheritance	Autosomal dominant		Autosomal dominant (most cases)	Unknown	Unknown
Molecular defect	Heterozygous mutations in the *GNAS1* gene		Unknown (see text)	Unknown	Unknown

PTH, parathyroid hormone; cAMP, cyclic adenosine monophasphates.

sorption in the distal renal tubule is responsive to circulating PTH in subjects with PHP type 1, and imply that adequate amounts of cAMP are produced in these cells or that other second messengers (e.g., cytosolic calcium or diacylglycerol, see above and Fig. 81–1) may be responsible for these PTH responses.

Administration of PTH to subjects with the less common form of the disorder, PHP type 2, produces a normal increase in urinary cAMP but fails to elicit an appropriate phosphaturic response.[171] These observations have suggested that PTH resistance in PHP type 2 results from a biochemical defect that is either unrelated or distal to the PTH-stimulated generation of cAMP.

It has been generally assumed that bone cells in patients with PHP type 1 are innately resistant to PTH, but this remains unproved. In fact, cultured bone cells from a patient with PHP type 1 have been shown to increase intracellular cAMP normally in response to PTH treatment in vitro.[172] Evidence that bone cells are unresponsive to PTH is largely inferred from the observation that patients with PHP type 1 are hypocalcemic and that administration of PTH does not increase the plasma calcium level. However, clinical, radiographic, or histologic evidence of increased bone turnover and demineralization (Fig. 81–7) occurs in some patients with PHP type 1. Some subjects have apparently normal-appearing bone while others have radiologic or histologic evidence of significant bone resorption (see below).[173] It is generally

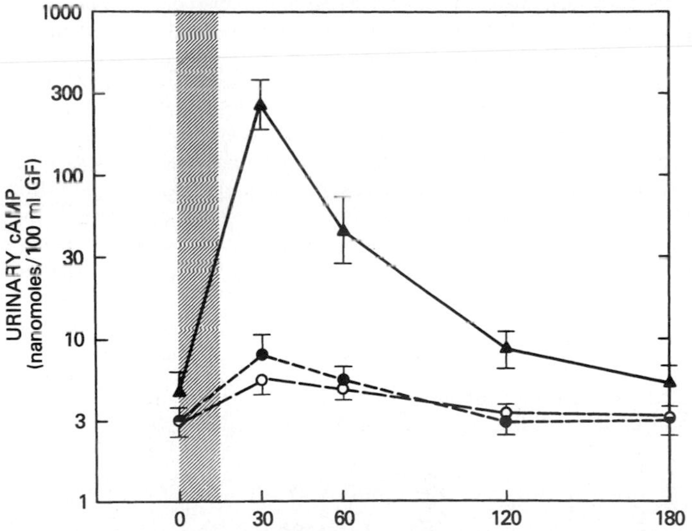

Figure 81–6. Urinary cyclic adenosine monophosphate (cAMP) excretion in response to an infusion of bovine parathyroid extract (300 USP U). The peak response in normal subjects *(solid triangles)* as well as those with pseudopseudohypoparathyroidism (pseudoPHP) (not shown) is 50- to 100-fold times basal. Subjects with PHP type Ia *(open circles)* or PHP type Ib *(solid circles)* show only a two- to fivefold increase. Urinary cAMP is expressed as nanomoles per 100 mL glomerular filtrate (GF), U_{cAMP} (nmol/100 mL, GF) = U_{cAMP} (nmols/dL) X S_{Cre} (mg/dL) / U_{Cre} (mg/dL). (From Levine MA, Jap TS, Mauseth RS, et al: Activity of the stimulatory guanine nucleotide–binding protein is reduced in guanine erythrocytes from patients with pseudohypoparathyroidism and pseudopseudohypoparathyroidism: Biochemical, endocrine, and genetic analysis of Albright's hereditary osteodystrophy in six kindreds. J Clin Endocrinol Metab 62:497–502, 1986.)

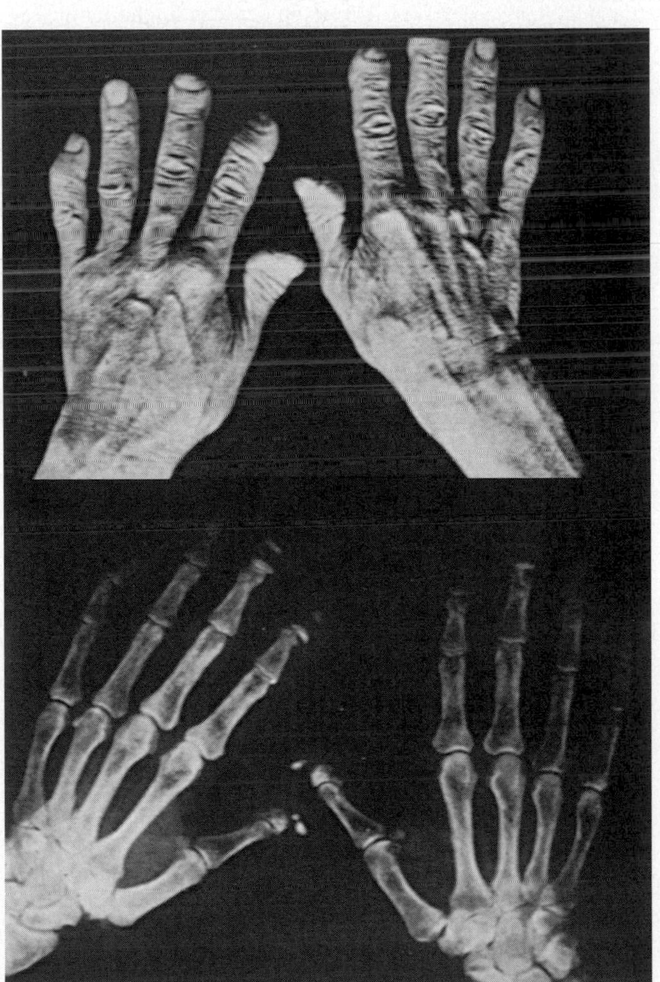

FIGURE 81–7. Photograph (*inset*) and radiograph of hands of a patient with marked hyperparathyroid bone disease. Marked periosteal bone erosion in terminal phalanges has resulted in "pseudoclubbing." (From Levine MA, Parfrey NA, Feinstein RS: Pseudohypoparathyroidism. Johns Hopkins Med J 151:137–146, 1982.)

believed that increased bone resorption is seen more often in the subset of patients with PHP type 1b (see below) who have distinctive features, including absence of the AHO features.

Patients with PHP may develop additional abnormalities in bone metabolism, including osteomalacia,[173] rickets,[174] renal osteodystrophy,[175] and osteopenia.[176] These skeletal abnormalities result from excessive PTH or deficient $1,25(OH)_2D_3$.

One theory offered for the variable bone responsiveness to PTH is the existence of two distinct cellular systems in bone upon which PTH exerts action: the remodeling system and the mineral mobilization or homeostatic system. The bone remodeling system is argued be more responsive to PTH in patients with PHP type 1 than the homeostatic system. This variability may reflect the lesser dependence of the remodeling system upon normal plasma levels of $1,25(OH)_2D$. Plasma levels of $1,25(OH)_2D$ are reduced in hypocalcemic patients with PHP type 1,[62] and could explain the concurrence of hypocalcemia and increased skeletal remodeling in some of these patients. Hypocalcemia leads to a compensatory overproduction of PTH, which could eventually overcome the $1,25(OH)_2D$ dependency for remodeling but not for PTH-stimulated calcium mobilization.

A role for $1,25(OH)_2D$ in modulating the responsiveness of the calcium homeostatic system to PTH is suggested by several observations. First, the calcemic response to PTH is deficient not only in some patients with PHP type 1 but also in patients with other hypocalcemic disorders in which plasma levels of $1,25(OH)_2D$ are low. Moreover, normalization of the plasma calcium level in patients with PHP type 1 by administration of physiologic amounts of $1,25(OH)_2D$ or pharmacologic amounts of vitamin D restores calcemic responsiveness.[177] Second, patients with PHP type 1 who have normal serum levels of calcium and $1,25(OH)_2D_3$ without vitamin D treatment (so-called normocalcemic PHP) show a normal calcemic response to administered PTH.[177] These findings suggest that $1,25(OH)_2D$ deficiency is the basis for the lack of a calcemic response to PTH in some hypocalcemic patients with PHP type 1, and challenge the premise that bone cells are intrinsically resistant to the actions of PTH.

Subjects with PHP type 1 have increased serum levels of phosphate owing to an inability of PTH to decrease phosphate reabsorption in the kidney. Hypocalcemia per se may also contribute to the development of hyperphosphatemia, as renal phosphate clearance is impaired by very low levels of intracellular calcium. Accordingly, restoration of plasma calcium levels to normal by chronic treatment with calcium and vitamin D can reduce elevated levels of serum phosphorus. Similar therapy has been shown to reverse the defective phosphaturic response to administered PTH in certain patients with PHP type 1, although the urinary cAMP response remains markedly deficient.[178] Therefore, persistence of a blunted urinary cAMP response to PTH in PHP type 1 patients in whom chronic vitamin D therapy has led to normalization of plasma calcium levels and restoration of a phosphaturic response need not imply, as has been at least suggested,[178] that there is no relationship between cAMP production and phosphate clearance.

The overall evidence suggests that the disturbances in calcium, phosphorus, and vitamin D metabolism in most patients with PHP type 1 result directly or indirectly from reduced responsiveness of both bone and kidney to PTH. Hypocalcemia results from impaired mobilization of calcium from bone, reduced intestinal absorption of calcium [via deficient generation of $1,25(OH)_2D$], and urinary calcium loss. Of these defects, the diminished movement of calcium out of bone stores into the extracellular fluid probably has the greatest role in producing hypocalcemia. Intensive treatment with $1,25(OH)_2D$ or other vitamin D analogues improves intestinal calcium absorption and bone calcium mobilization, restores plasma calcium to normal, and reduces circulating PTH levels. Thus, although PTH resistance appears to be the proximate biochemical defect, the major abnormalities in mineral metabolism found in patients with PHP type 1 can be largely explained on the basis of deficiency of circulating $1,25(OH)_2D$.

Pseudohypoparathyroidism Type 1a

PHP type 1 can be subclassified into two apparently distinct disorders based on several important clinical and biochemical characteristics: (1) the absence or presence of AHO; (2) hormone resistance that is limited to PTH alone or which is more generalized; and (3) tissue expression of $G_{s\alpha}$ protein. Subjects with the type 1a variant have an approximately 50% reduction in expression or activity of $G_{s\alpha}$ protein in membranes from a wide variety of cells and tissues[179] (Fig. 81–8). The generalized deficiency of $G_{s\alpha}$ may impair the ability of PTH, as well as many other hormones and neurotransmitters, to activate adenylate cyclase and thereby may account for the multihormone resistance that typically occurs in these patients. In addition to hormone resistance, patients with PHP type 1a also manifest the peculiar constellation of developmental and somatic defects that are collectively termed AHO[163] (see Fig. 81–5). By contrast, patients with PHP type 1b lack features of AHO, have hormone resistance that is limited to PTH, and have normal levels of $G_{s\alpha}$ protein in cell membranes.

Early studies of PHP type 1a led to the identification of families in which some individuals had signs of AHO but lacked apparent hormone resistance (i.e., pseudoPHP). The observation that PHP type 1a and pseudoPHP can occur in the same family first suggested that these two disorders might reflect variability in expression of a single genetic lesion. Further support for this view derives from recent studies indicating that within a given kindred, subjects with either pseudoPHP or PHP type 1a have equivalent functional $G_{s\alpha}$ deficiency[179, 180] (see Fig. 81–8), and that a transition from hormone responsiveness to hormone resistance may occur.[181] It therefore seems appropriate to apply the term AHO to both of these variants in acknowledgment of the clinical and biochemical characteristics that patients with PHP type 1a and pseudoPHP share.[164]

Molecular Defect in AHO (PHP Type 1a and PseudoPHP)

The discovery that $G_{s\alpha}$ deficiency results from inactivating mutations in the *GNAS1* gene, located at 20q13.2→13.3,[182] provided confirmation of autosomal dominant transmission of the molecular defect in AHO and resolved long-standing controversies regarding the inheritance of this disorder.[164, 183–185] *GNAS1* is a complex gene[186] comprised of at least 15 exons, including three alternative first exons.[187, 188] Alternative splicing of nascent transcripts derived from exons 1 to 13 generates four mRNAs that encode $G_{s\alpha}$. Deletion of exon 3 results in the loss of 15 codons from the mRNA, while use of an alternative splice site in exon 4 results in the insertion of a single additional codon into the mRNA. This produces two $G_{s\alpha}$ proteins with apparent molecular weights of 45 kDa and two isoforms of apparent molecular weights of 52 kDa[186] that exhibit specific patterns of tissue expression.[189] Both long and short forms of $G_{s\alpha}$ can stimulate adenylate cyclase and open calcium channels,[190] but biochemical characterization of these isoforms has revealed subtle differences in the binding constant for GDP, the

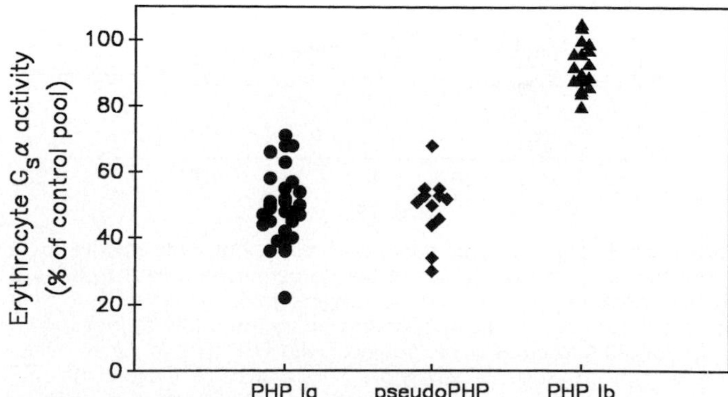

FIGURE 81–8. $G_{s\alpha}$ activity of erythrocyte membranes. $G_{s\alpha}$ is quantified in complementation assays with S49 cyc⁻ membranes, which genetically lack $G_{s\alpha}$ but retain all other components necessary for hormone-response adenylate cyclase activity. Activity is reduced approximately 50% in patients with Albright's hereditary osteodystrophy including subjects with either pseudohypoparathyroidism (PHP) type 1a or pseudoPHP, but is normal in patients with PHP type 1b.

rate at which the forms are activated by agonist binding, efficiency of adenylate cyclase stimulation, and the rate of GTP hydrolysis. The significance of these differences remains unknown,[190–192] but these distinctions imply the existence of as yet unknown roles for these G proteins.[193]

Additional complexity in the processing of the *GNAS1* gene derives from the use of alternative first exons that generate novel transcripts. Because these proteins lack amino acid sequences encoded by exon 1, which are required for interaction of $G_{s\alpha}$ with $G_{\beta\gamma}$ and attachment to the plasma membrane, it is unlikely that these proteins can function as transmembrane signal transducers. In one case, a $G_{s\alpha}$ transcript is produced with an alternative first exon that lacks an initiator ATG; thus, a truncated, nonfunctional $G_{s\alpha}$ protein is translated from an inframe ATG in exon 2.[194] The role of this $G_{s\alpha}$ chain is unknown. In two other instances unique transcripts are generated using additional coding exons that are present upstream of the exon 1 used to generate functional $G_{s\alpha}$ protein. The more 5′ of these exons encodes the neuroendocrine secretory protein NESP55, a chromogranin-like protein, and is generated from a transcript that contains sequences derived from exon 2 of *GNAS1* in the 3′ nontranslated region.[195, 196] Accordingly, NESP55 shares no protein homology with $G_{s\alpha}$. The more downstream alternative exon encodes a 51-kDa protein, and when spliced inframe to exons 2 to 13 results in a transcript that generates a larger $G_{s\alpha}$ isoform that is termed $XL_{\alpha s}$.[197] Both NESP55 and $XL_{\alpha s}$ have been implicated in regulated secretion in neuroendocrine tissues.

Molecular studies of DNA from subjects with AHO have disclosed inactivating mutations in the *GNAS1* gene[198–211] that account for a 50% reduction in expression or function of $G_{s\alpha}$ protein (Fig. 81–9). All patients are heterozygous, and have one normal *GNAS1* allele and one defective allele. A large variety of mutations in the *GNAS1* gene have been identified, including missense mutations,[201, 203–205, 210] point mutations that disrupt efficient splicing[202] or terminate translation prematurely,[208] and small deletions.[202, 203, 206, 212, 213] Although novel mutations have been found in nearly all of the kindreds studied, a four-base deletion in exon 7 has been detected in multiple families[211, 212, 214] and an unusual missense mutation in exon 13 (A366S; see below) has been identified in two unrelated young boys,[199] suggesting that these two regions may be genetic "hot spots."

Most gene mutations lead to reduced expression of $G_{s\alpha}$ mRNA,[180, 215] but in some subjects the mutant allele produces normal levels of $G_{s\alpha}$ mRNA[180, 215, 216] that encode dysfunctional $G_{s\alpha}$ proteins.[199, 204, 205, 210] The replacement of arginine by histidine at codon 385 in the C-terminal tail of $G_{s\alpha}$ selectively "uncouples" G_s from receptors and prevents receptor activation.[204] Substitution of histidine by arginine at position 231 also prevents receptor activation of G_s, but by an entirely different mechanism.[210] The replacement of histidine 231 hinders binding of GTP to the α chain, and thereby inhibits receptor-induced dissociation of $G_{s\alpha}$ from $G_{\beta\gamma}$.

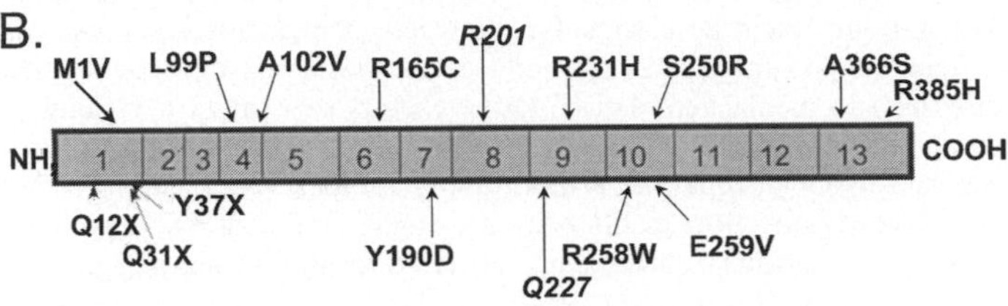

FIGURE 81–9. Mutations in the *GNAS1* gene. The upper panel (*A*) depicts the human *GNAS1* gene, which spans over 20-kb and contains at least 13 exons and 12 introns. Unique mutations that result in *loss of* $G_{s\alpha}$ *function* are depicted; missense mutations are denoted by the *asterisk*. The lower panel (*B*) indicates the position of missense mutations above the protein structure. Two polymorphisms are denoted by the symbol +, and the position of the unchanged amino acid is denoted beneath the predicted $G_{s\alpha}$ protein (*B*). The site of two missense mutations that result in *gain of function* (replacement of either Arg201 or Gln227) in patients with McCune-Albright syndrome[266, 267, 328–330] or in sporadic tumors[331, 332] are depicted in italics. The mutation in exon 1 eliminates the initiator methionine codon and prevents synthesis of a normal $G_{s\alpha}$ protein.[201] The four base-pair deletions in exon 7[212, 214] and exon 8,[203] and the one base-pair deletion and insertion in exon 10 all shift the normal reading frame and prevent normal messenger RNA (mRNA) or protein synthesis. Mutations in intron 3 and at the donor splice junction between exon 10 and intron 10 cause splicing abnormalities that prevent normal mRNA synthesis.[202] The mutations indicated with an *asterisk* represent missense mutations[199, 203, 204]; the resultant amino acid substitutions are indicated in the schematic diagram of the $G_{s\alpha}$ protein at the bottom of the figure. Some of these mutations may prevent normal protein synthesis by altering protein secondary structure; the R231H substitution in exon 9 prevents normal interaction of the α chain with the βγ dimer[205]; the R385H substitution in exon 13 appears to encode an altered protein that cannot couple normally to receptors,[204] and the A366S mutation encodes an activated $G_{s\alpha}$ protein that is unstable at 37 °C.[199]

Multiple Hormone Resistance in PHP Type 1a

Although biochemical hypoparathyroidism is the most commonly recognized endocrine deficiency in PHP type 1a, early clinical studies described additional hormonal abnormalities, such as hypothyroidism[217, 218] and hypogonadism.[219] Because available evidence suggests that $G_{s\alpha}$ is present in all tissues, generalized deficiency of this protein could be the basis for not only PTH resistance, the hallmark of PHP type 1a, but could also explain the decreased responsiveness of diverse tissues (e.g., kidney, thyroid gland, gonads, and liver) to hormones that act via activation of adenylate cyclase (e.g., PTH, thyroid-stimulating hormone [TSH], gonadotropins, and glucagon).[169, 220, 221] Primary hypothyroidism occurs in most patients with PHP type 1a.[220] Typically, patients lack a goiter or antithyroid antibodies and have an elevated serum TSH with an exaggerated response to thyrotropin-releasing hormone (TRH). Serum levels of thyroxine (T_4) may be low or low normal. Hypothyroidism may occur early in life prior to the development of hypocalcemia, and elevated serum levels of TSH are not uncommonly detected during neonatal screening.[222–224] Unfortunately, early institution of thyroid hormone replacement does not seem to prevent the development of mental retardation.[223]

Reproductive dysfunction occurs commonly in subjects with PHP type 1a. Women may have delayed puberty, oligomenorrhea, and infertility.[220] Plasma gonadotropins may be elevated, but are more commonly normal. Some patients show an exaggerated serum gonadotropin response to gonadotropin-releasing hormone (GnRH).[219, 225] Features of hypogonadism may be less obvious in men. Serum testosterone may be normal or reduced. Testes may show evidence of a maturation arrest or may fail to descend normally. Fertility appears to be decreased in men with PHP type 1a. Deficiency of prolactin secretion (basal and in response to secretagogues such as TRH) had been reported in some patients with PHP type 1,[226] but later studies have not confirmed these early findings.[220]

Obesity is common in subjects with PHP type 1a and pseudoPHP, and may reflect a defective lipolytic response to hormonal stimulation due to $G_{s\alpha}$ deficiency.[227, 228] By contrast, abnormal hormone responsiveness may occur in some tissues without obvious clinical sequelae. For example, the hepatic glucose response to glucagon is normal, although plasma cAMP concentrations fail to increase normally.[220, 229] In other tissues significant hormone resistance does not occur despite the apparent reduction in $G_{s\alpha}$. Diabetes insipidus is not a feature of AHO, and urine is concentrated normally in response to vasopressin in patients with PHP type 1a.[230] Although there is a report of adrenal insufficiency in a single individual with PHP type 1a,[231] hypoadrenalism is not a typical feature of PHP type 1a and adrenocortical responsiveness to adrenocorticotropic hormone (ACTH) is normal.[220]

Neurosensory Defects in PHP Type 1a

Patients with PHP type 1a frequently manifest distinctive olfactory,[232] gustatory,[233] and auditory[234] abnormalities that are apparently unrelated to endocrine dysfunction. The molecular basis of these neurosensory deficits is unknown. Unique G proteins have been identified that regulate signal transduction pathways related to vision,[235, 236] olfaction,[237] and taste.[238]

Mild to moderate mental retardation is common in patients with PHP type 1a. Farfel and Friedman[239] assessed intelligence in 25 patients with PHP type 1 whose $G_{s\alpha}$ activity had been determined. The authors found an association between mental deficiency and $G_{s\alpha}$ deficiency, and speculated that reduced cAMP levels in cortical tissue may lead to mental retardation. Other factors that might contribute to mental retardation in patients with PHP type 1a include hypothyroidism and hypocalcemia, but efforts to control these have not prevented cognitive dysfunction in all patients, suggesting that $G_{s\alpha}$ deficiency may cause a primary abnormality of neurotransmitter signaling.

The Somatic Phenotype of AHO

Subjects with PHP type 1a or pseudoPHP typically manifest a characteristic constellation of developmental defects, termed *Albright's hereditary osteodystrophy,* that includes short stature, obesity, a round face, shortening of the digits (brachydactyly), subcutaneous ossification, and dental hypoplasia[163, 165] (see Fig. 81–5). Considerable variability occurs in the clinical expression of these features, even among affected members of a single family, and all of these features may not be present in every case.[240] On rare occasions, it may be impossible to detect any features of AHO in an individual with $G_{s\alpha}$ deficiency.[202, 203]

Although patients with AHO may be of normal height and weight, approximately 66% of children and 80% of adults are below the 10th percentile for height. This reflects a disproportionate shortening of the limbs, as arm span is less than height in the majority of patients. Obesity is a common feature of AHO and about one-third of all patients with AHO are above the 90th percentile of weight for their age, despite their short stature[241] (see Fig. 81–5). Patients with AHO typically have a round face, a short neck, and a flattened bridge of the nose. Numerous other abnormalities of the head and neck have also been noted. Ocular findings include hypertelorism, strabismus, nystagmus, unequal pupils, diplopia, microphthalmia, and a variety of abnormal findings on funduscopic examination that range from irregular pigmentation to optic atrophy and macular degeneration. Head circumference is above the 90th percentile in a significant minority of children.[241] Dental abnormalities are common in subjects with PHP type 1a and include dentin and enamel hypoplasia, short and blunted roots, and delayed or absent tooth eruption.[242]

Brachydactyly is the most reliable sign in the diagnosis of AHO, and may be symmetrical or asymmetrical and involve one or both hands or feet (see Fig. 81–5). Shortening of the distal phalanx of the thumb is the most common abnormality; this is apparent on physical examination as a thumb in which the ratio of the width of the nail to its length is increased (so-called murderer's thumb or potter's thumb; see Fig. 81–5D). Shortening of the metacarpals causes shortening of the digits, particularly the fourth and fifth digits. Shortening of the metacarpals may also be recognized on physical examination as dimpling over the knuckles of a clenched fist (Archibald's sign; see Fig. 81–5C). Often a definitive diagnosis requires careful examination of radiographs of the hands and feet (see Fig. 81–5B). A specific pattern of shortening of the bones in the hand has been identified, in which the distal phalanx of the thumb and third through fifth metacarpals are the most severely shortened.[243, 244] This may be useful in distinguishing AHO from other unrelated syndromes in which brachydactyly occurs, such as familial brachydactyly, Turner's syndrome, and Klinefelter's syndrome.[243]

In addition to brachydactyly, several other skeletal abnormalities are present in AHO. Numerous deformities of the long bones have been reported, including a short ulna, bowed radius, deformed elbow or cubitus valgus, coxa vara, coxa valga, genu varum, and genu valgus deformities.[241] The most common abnormalities of the skull are hyperostosis frontalis interna and a thickened calvarium. It has been reported that the skeletal abnormalities of AHO may not be apparent until a child is 5 years old.[245] Bone age is advanced 2 to 3 years in the majority of patients.[241] Spinal cord compression has been reported in several patients with AHO.[246]

Patients with AHO develop heterotopic ossifications of the soft tissues or skin (osteoma cutis) that are unrelated to abnormalities in serum calcium or phosphorus levels. Osteoma cutis is present in 25% to 50% of cases of AHO, and is usually first noted in infancy or early childhood. Ossification of the skin and subcutaneous tissues may be the presenting feature of AHO in infancy or childhood and may occur in the absence of hypocalcemia or other features of AHO.[247, 248] Blue-tinged, stony-hard papular or nodular lesions that range in size from pinpoint up to 5 cm in diameter often occur at sites of minor trauma and may appear to be migratory on repeated examinations.[247] Biopsy of these lesions reveals heterotopic ossification with spicules of mineralizing osteoid and calcified cartilage. More extensive and progressive ossification that affects the deep connective tissues occurs in subjects with progressive osseous heteroplasia, an unusual genetic disorder with apparent autosomal dominant inheritance.[249]

One or more of the developmental and skeletal abnormalities of AHO can occur in subjects who do not have AHO or a defect in the *GNAS1* gene, and thus need not imply that the subject has PHP or pseudoPHP. Features of AHO, particularly shortened metacarpals or metatarsals, may be present in normal subjects, and have been described in patients with hormone-deficient hypoparathyroidism,[250–253] renal hypercalciuria,[254] and primary hyperparathyroidism.[255] Furthermore, obesity, round face, brachydactyly, and mental retardation, are also present in several other genetic disorders (e.g., Prader-Willi syndrome, acrodysostosis, Ullrich-Turner syndrome, Gardner's syndrome), many of which are associated with unique chromosomal defects. In some instances overlapping clinical features between AHO and other syndromes may lead to confusion. For example, an AHO-like syndrome has been described in a mother and her daughter who have a proximal 15q chromosomal deletion that resembles that found in Prader-Willi syndrome.[256] A growing number of reports have described small terminal deletions of chromosome 2q in patients with variable AHO-like phenotypes. Terminal deletion of 2q37 [del(2)(q37.3)] is the first consistent karyotypic abnormality that has been documented in patients with an AHO-like syndrome.[257, 258] These patients have normal endocrine function and normal $G_{s\alpha}$ activity, however.[258] Thus, high-resolution chromosome analysis, biochemical and molecular analysis, and careful physical and radiologic examination are essential in discriminating between these phenocopies and AHO.

Phenotypic Variability in AHO: The Paradox of PHP Type 1a and PseudoPHP

Molecular studies have provided a basis for $G_{s\alpha}$ deficiency, but they do not explain the striking variability in biochemical and clinical phenotype. Why do some $G_{s\alpha}$-coupled pathways show reduced hormone responsiveness (e.g., PTH, TSH, gonadotropins), whereas other pathways are clinically unaffected (ACTH in the adrenal gland and vasopressin in the renal medulla)? Perhaps even more intriguing is the paradox that $G_{s\alpha}$ deficiency can be associated with hormone resistance and AHO (PHP type 1a), AHO only (pseudoPHP), or no apparent consequences at all.[203] These observations, when considered in the context of studies showing that the number of G_s molecules in cell membranes greatly exceeds the number of either receptor or adenylate cyclase molecules,[259] raise issue with the hypothesis that a 50% deficiency of $G_{s\alpha}$ can impair hormone responsiveness. Indeed, in vitro studies of tissues and cells from subjects with PHP type 1a have often demonstrated normal hormonal responsiveness despite a 50% reduction in $G_{s\alpha}$ expression.[260]

Although the basis for the variable expression of $G_{s\alpha}$ deficiency remains unknown, several observations provide important insights. First, clinical genetic studies have documented that PHP type 1a and pseudoPHP frequently occur in the same family, but are not present in the same generation. Second, analysis of published pedigrees has indicated that in most cases maternal transmission of $G_{s\alpha}$ deficiency leads to PHP type 1a, whereas paternal transmission of the defect leads to pseudoPHP.[179, 209, 261, 262] These findings are inconsistent with models in which chance determines phenotype or in which a second gene is interactive with the defective *GNAS1* gene, as both PHP type 1a and pseudoPHP would be expected to occur with equal frequency and in the same sibship. A more conforming hypothesis suggests that genomic imprinting of the *GNAS1* gene can explain the variable phenotypic expression of a single genetic defect.[262] Recent studies have indeed confirmed that the *GNAS1* gene is imprinted, but in a far more complex manner than had been anticipated (see Chapter 75). Two upstream promoters, each associated with a large coding exon, lie 35 kb upstream of *GNAS1* exon 1. These promoters are only 11 kb apart, yet show opposite patterns of allele-specific methylation and monoallelic transcription. The more 5′ of these exons encodes NESP55, which is expressed exclusively from the maternal allele. By contrast, the $XL_{\alpha s}$ exon is paternally expressed.[187, 188] Despite the simultaneous imprinting in both the paternal and maternal directions of the *GNAS1* gene, expression of $G_{s\alpha}$ appears to be biallelic in all human tissues that have been examined thus far.[187, 188, 263] Moreover, the lack of access to relevant tissues from subjects with PHP type 1a has prevented direct analysis of $G_{s\alpha}$ expression in patients with this disorder.

To overcome these difficulties, murine models of PHP type 1a have been developed through disruption of a single *Gnas* gene in embryonic stem cells.[264, 265] Although these mice have reduced levels of $G_{s\alpha}$ protein, they lack many of the features of the human disorder. Biochemical analyses of these heterozygous *Gnas* knockout mice suggest that $G_{s\alpha}$ expression may derive from only the maternal allele in some tissues (e.g., renal cortex) and from both alleles in other tissues (e.g., renal medulla). Accordingly, mice that inherit the defective *Gnas* gene maternally express only that allele in imprinted tissues, such as the PTH-sensitive renal proximal tubule, in which there is no functional $G_{s\alpha}$ protein. By contrast, the 50% reduction in $G_{s\alpha}$ expression that occurs in nonimprinted tissues, which express both *Gnas* alleles, may account for more variable and moderate hormone resistance in these sites (e.g., the thyroid). Thus, variable hormonal responsiveness implies that haploinsufficiency of $G_{s\alpha}$ is tissue-specific; that is, in some tissues a 50% reduction in $G_{s\alpha}$ is still sufficient to facilitate normal signal transduction. Confirmation of this proposed mechanism in patients with AHO will require demonstration that the human $G_{s\alpha}$ transcript is paternally imprinted in the renal cortex.

In AHO, inherited *GNAS1* gene mutations reduce expression or function of $G_{s\alpha}$ protein. By contrast, in the McCune-Albright syndrome, postzygotic somatic mutations in the *GNAS1* gene (see Fig. 81–9) enhance activity of the protein.[266, 267] These mutations lead to constitutive activation of adenylate cyclase, and result in proliferation and autonomous hyperfunction of hormonally responsive cells. The clinical significance of $G_{s\alpha}$ activity as a determinant of hormone action is emphasized by the description by Iiri et al.[199] of two boys with both precocious puberty and PHP type 1a. These two unrelated boys had identical *GNAS1* gene mutations in exon 13 (A366S; see Fig. 81–9) that resulted in a temperature-sensitive form of $G_{s\alpha}$. This $G_{s\alpha}$ is constitutively active in the cooler environment of the testis, while being rapidly degraded in other tissues at normal body temperature. Thus, different tissues in these two individuals could show hormone resistance (to PTH and TSH), hormone responsiveness (to ACTH), or hormone-independent activation (to luteinizing hormone).

Pseudohypoparathyroidism Type 1b

Subjects with PHP type 1 who lack features of AHO typically manifest hormone resistance that is limited to PTH target organs (see Fig. 81–6) and have normal $G_{s\alpha}$ activity[220] (see Fig. 81–8). This variant is termed PHP type 1b.[268] Although patients with PHP type 1b fail to show a nephrogenous cAMP response to PTH, they often manifest osteopenia or skeletal lesions similar to those that occur in patients with hyperparathyroidism, including osteitis fibrosa cystica[269] (see Fig. 81–7). By contrast, patients with PHP type 1a typically have little or no evidence of diffuse skeletal involvement. Cultured bone cells from one patient with PHP type 1b and osteitis fibrosa cystica were shown to have normal adenylate cyclase responsiveness to PTH in vitro.[172] These observations have suggested that at least one intracellular signaling pathway coupled to the PTHR may be intact in patients with PHP type 1b.

Specific resistance of target tissues to PTH, and normal activity of $G_{s\alpha}$, had implicated decreased expression or function of the PTH-PTHrP receptor as the cause of hormone resistance. In addition, cultured fibroblasts from some, but not all, PHP type 1b patients were shown to accumulate reduced levels of cAMP in response to PTH[270] and contain decreased levels of mRNA encoding the PTH-PTHrP receptor.[271] Several lines of evidence suggest that the primary defect in PHP type 1b is not in the gene encoding the PTH-PTHrP receptor, however. First, pretreatment of cultured fibroblasts from subjects with PHP type 1b with dexamethasone was found to normalize the PTH-induced cAMP response and to increase expression of PTH-PTHrP receptor mRNA.[271] Second, molecular studies have failed to disclose mutations in the coding exons[272] and promoter regions[273] of the PTH-PTHrP receptor gene or its mRNA.[274] Third, mice[275] and humans[276] that are heterozygous for inactivation of the gene encoding the PTH-PTHrP receptor do not manifest PTH resistance or hypocalcemia. And finally, inheritance of two defective type PTH-PTHrP receptor genes results in Blomstrand chondrodysplasia, a lethal genetic disorder characterized by advanced endochondral bone maturation.[276] Thus, it is likely that the molecular defect in PHP type 1b resides in other gene(s) that regulate expression or activity of the PTH-PTHrP receptor.

Although most cases of PHP type 1b appear to be sporadic, familial cases have been described in which transmission of the defect is most consistent with an autosomal dominant pattern.[277, 278] Recent studies have used gene mapping to identify the molecular defect in PHP type 1b.[279] In one study the unknown gene was mapped to a small region of chromosome 20q13.3 near the *GNAS1* gene, thus raising the possibility that some patients with PHP type 1b have inherited a defective promoter or enhancer that regulates expression of $G_{s\alpha}$ in the kidney.[279]

Pseudohypoparathyroidism Type 1c

Resistance to multiple hormones has been described in several patients with AHO who do not have a demonstrable defect in G_s or G_i.[220, 248, 280] This disorder is termed PHP type 1c. The nature of the lesion in such patients is unclear, but it could be related to some other general component of the receptor–adenylate cyclase system, such as the catalytic unit.[281] Alternatively, these patients could have functional defects of G_s (or G_i) that do not become apparent in the assays presently available.

Pseudohypoparathyroidism Type 2

PHP type 2 is the least common form of PHP. This variant of PHP is typically a sporadic disorder, although one case of familial PHP type 2 has been reported.[282] Patients do not have features of AHO. Renal resistance to PTH in PHP type 2 patients is manifested by a reduced phosphaturic response to administration of PTH, despite a normal increase in urinary cAMP excretion.[171] These observations suggest that the PTHR–adenylate cyclase complex functions normally to increase cAMP in response to PTH, and is consistent with a model in which PTH resistance arises from an inability of intracellular cAMP to initiate the chain of metabolic events that result in the ultimate expression of PTH action.

Although supportive data are not yet available, a defect in cAMP-dependent protein kinase A has been proposed as the basis for this disorder.[171] Alternatively, the defect in PHP type 2 may not reside in an inability to generate a physiologic response to intracellular cAMP: a defect in another PTH-sensitive signal transduction pathway may explain the lack of a phosphaturic response. One candidate is the PTH-sensitive phospholipase C pathway that leads to increased concentrations of the intracellular second messengers inositol 1,4,5-trisphosphate and diacylglycerol[36, 37] and cytosolic calcium[38–41] (see Fig. 81–1).

In some patients with PHP type 2 the phosphaturic response to PTH has been restored to normal after serum levels of calcium have been normalized by treatment with calcium infusion or vitamin D.[283] These results point to the importance of Ca^{2+} as an intracellular second messenger. Finally, a similar dissociation between the effects of PTH on generation of cAMP and tubular reabsorption of phosphate has been observed in patients with profound hypocalcemia due to vitamin D deficiency,[284] suggesting that some cases of PHP type 2 may in fact represent vitamin D deficiency.

Circulating Inhibitors of PTH Action as a Possible Cause of Pseudohypoparathyroidism

A circulating inhibitor of PTH action has been proposed as a cause of PTH resistance on the basis of studies showing an apparent dissociation between plasma levels of endogenous immunoreactive and bioactive PTH in subjects with PHP type 1. Despite high circulating levels of immunoreactive PTH, the levels of bioactive PTH in many patients with PHP type 1 have been found to be within the normal range when measured with highly sensitive renal[285] and metatarsal[286] cytochemical bioassay systems. Furthermore, plasma from many of these patients has been shown to diminish the biologic activity of exogenous PTH in these in vitro bioassays.[287] Currently, the nature of this putative inhibitor or antagonist remains unknown. The observation that prolonged hypercalcemia can remove or reduce significantly the level of inhibitory activity in the plasma of patients with PHP has suggested that the parathyroid gland may be the source of the inhibitor. In addition, analysis of circulating PTH immunoactivity after fractionation of patient plasma by reversed phase high-performance liquid chromatography has disclosed the presence of aberrant forms of immunoreactive PTH in many of these patients.[288] Although it is conceivable that a PTH inhibitor may cause PTH resistance in some patients with PHP, it is more likely that circulating antagonists of PTH action arise as a consequence of the sustained secondary hyperparathyroidism that results from the primary biochemical defect. The recent identification of circulating fragments of PTH that may act as competitive antagonists of intact PTH in uremic patients with secondary hyperparathyroidism now provides at least a theoretical basis for this hypothesis.[289]

In contrast to these studies, molecular analyses have confirmed that defects in the PTH-PTHrP receptor–G protein–coupled signaling pathway are responsible for PTH resistance in many patients with PHP type 1.

NATURAL HISTORY OF PSEUDOHYPOPARATHYROIDISM

The natural history of PHP is quite variable. Although PHP is congenital, hypocalcemia is not present from birth, and the biochemical defects arise gradually during childhood. The initial manifestations of tetany typically occur between 3 and 8 years of age, but the significance of these findings may not be appreciated and the diagnosis of hypocalcemia may be delayed for months or even years. A progressive decline in serum calcium, preceded by increasing levels of serum phosphate, PTH, and $1,25(OH)_2D_3$, has been documented in one child as he advanced from 3 to 3½ years of age.[290] In a second report serial PTH infusions were used to evaluate hormone responsiveness. This child was shown to have a normal cAMP response at age 3 months when serum levels of calcium, phosphorus, and PTH were normal, but was found to have an abnormal cAMP response when retested at age 2.6 years after he had developed tetany and was found to be hypocalcemic.[181] At the time of his second PTH infusion, the child had markedly elevated serum concentrations of phosphorus and PTH and was receiving T_4 for recently diagnosed hypothyroidism.[181] Some affected children show few symptoms of tetany and the diagnosis of PHP is recognized only later in life after hypocalcemia is inadvertently discovered or when features of AHO become obvious. Hypocalcemia may not always provide a clue to the clinical diagnosis of PHP, however, as some PHP patients are able to maintain a normal serum calcium level without treatment (i.e., normocalcemic PHP).[177]

DIAGNOSIS

The diagnosis of hypoparathyroidism should be considered in any patient who has hypocalcemia and hyperphosphatemia. A low serum calcium level may be found during an evaluation of unexplained paresthesias or seizures, or may be discovered after multichannel analysis of a blood specimen obtained as part of a routine examination. PHP should be strongly suspected if the serum concentration of PTH is elevated, although occasionally serum levels of PTH are "inappropriately" normal in subjects with PHP owing to confounding hypomagnesemia[277] or other factors.[291] Hypocalcemia may be precipitated or worsened during times of "stress" on calcium homeostasis, such as during early pregnancy, lactation, or during an episode of acute pancreatitis. Although hypocalcemia is present in most patients with hypoparathyroidism by the end of the first decade of life, this biochemical finding may go undetected for many years.

Cataracts and intracranial calcification, particularly of the basal ganglion, are common in patients with all forms of chronic hypoparathyroidism. Thus the presence of these ectopic or metastatic calcifications does not help to discriminate among the various causes of hypocalcemia and hyperphosphatemia.[292] Intracranial calcifications are readily detected when CT scanning is employed,[293, 294] and may occasionally be associated with symptoms such as those seen in Parkinson's disease.[295] Unusual presenting manifestations of PHP include neonatal hypothyroidism,[222, 223] unexplained cardiac failure,[296] Parkinson's disease,[295] and spinal cord compression.[297]

A diagnosis of hypoparathyroidism can be made with reasonable certainty when hypocalcemia is accompanied by normal serum levels of phosphorus and magnesium and the plasma PTH concentration is low or inappropriately normal. By contrast, an elevated level of PTH should suggest the diagnosis of PHP, particularly when clinical features of AHO are present. Further corroboration of the diagnosis of PHP requires demonstration of normal renal function and normal serum levels of magnesium and 25(OH) D. The presence of AHO or manifestations of multihormone resistance, such as hypothyroidism or hypogonadism, favors a diagnosis of PHP type 1a.[220] When most or all of these features are present, more sophisticated tests may not be necessary to confirm the clinical diagnosis. Serum calcium levels can fluctuate in patients with PHP, and may spontaneously change from low to normal and vice versa, thus contributing to the confusion regarding the distinction between PHP and pseudoPHP.[177, 298] However, the abnormal cAMP response to administered PTH (below) does not become normal in PHP patients who become normocalcemic with or without treatment. Thus, the PTH infusion remains the most reliable test to distinguish between these two variants (see Fig. 81–6).

Specialized Tests

The biochemical hallmark of PHP is the failure of the target organs, bone and kidney, to respond normally to PTH. Additional tests have been developed to identify subjects with PHP type 1a; these research tests, which are based on analysis of $G_{s\alpha}$ protein or the *GNAS1* gene, are only rarely indicated under typical clinical circumstances. The classic tests of Ellsworth and Howard, and of Chase, Melson, and Aurbach involved the intravenous infusion of 200 to 300 USP units of bovine parathyroid extract (parathyroid injection, USP; Lilly) and subsequent measurement of urinary excretion of nephrogenous (or total) cAMP (see Fig. 81–6) and phosphate. This relatively crude PTH preparation is no longer available, and has been replaced by synthetic peptides corresponding to the N-terminal region of human PTH (e.g., hPTH(1–34)).[299–301] A standard protocol involves the infusion of synthetic hPTH(1–34) peptide, 200 U in an adult and 3 U/kg body weight (200 U maximum) in children over the age of 3 years, intravenously over 10 minutes.[299, 302] Test subjects should be in a fasting state and active urine output should be initiated and maintained by the ingestion of 200 mL of water per hour, 2 hours prior to the infusion of PTH and continuing through the study. A baseline urine collection should be made in a 60-minute period preceding the PTH infusion. Starting at time 0 urine should be collected in separate collections at the 0- to 30-minute, 30- to 60-minute, and 60- to 120-minute time periods.

Blood samples should be obtained at time 0 and at 2 hours after the start of PTH infusion for measurement of serum creatinine and phosphorus concentrations. Urine samples should be analyzed for cAMP, phosphorus, and creatinine concentrations.

The preferred unit for expression of urinary cAMP is nanomoles per 100 mL (or L) of glomerular filtrate (nanomoles per 100 mL glomerular filtrate [GF]). The cAMP response during the first 30 minutes after the start of PTH infusion best differentiates patients with PHP type 1 from those with hypoparathyroidism and from normal subjects compared with other parameters of cAMP metabolism.[302] Normal subjects and patients with hormonopenic hypoparathyroidism usually display a 10- to 20-fold increase in urinary cAMP excretion, whereas patients with PHP type 1 (type 1a and type 1b) show a markedly blunted response regardless of their serum calcium concentration. The urinary cAMP response to infusion of synthetic hPTH fragments in patients with PHP type 1 is unrelated to serum calcium levels, but may be related to endogenous serum PTH levels. The maximal urinary cAMP response to PTH increases after suppression of endogenous PTH in patients with PHP type 1, but nevertheless does not reach that of the normal range.[170] Thus, this test can distinguish patients with so-called normocalcemic PHP (i.e., patients with PTH resistance who are able to maintain normal serum calcium levels without treatment) from subjects with pseudoPHP (who will have a normal urinary cAMP response to PTH[166, 179] (see Fig. 81–6). Subjects with PHP type 2 typically manifest a normal urinary cAMP response to infused PTH but fail to demonstrate an appropriate phosphaturic response. Several metabolic abnormalities such as hypo- and hypermagnesemia and metabolic acidosis may interfere with the renal generation and excretion of cAMP in response to PTH.[303–306] These abnormalities should be corrected if possible, but probably do not interfere with the interpretation of the test.

Calculation of the phosphaturic response to PTH as the percent decrease in tubular maximum for phosphate reabsorption (percent fall in TMP/GFR) during the first hour after PTH infusion yields the best separation between normal subjects and patients with PHP or hypoparathyroidism.[302] However, distinction between groups is also possible when the results are expressed as the fall in percent tubular reabsorption of phosphorus (decrease in percent TRP). A nomogram has been developed that facilitates calculation of TMP/GFR.[307] TMP/GFR is elevated in patients with PHP and hypoparathyroidism. Patients with hormone-deficient hypoparathyroidism have a steep fall in TMP/GFR during the first hour after beginning the infusion of PTH. This fall does not occur in patients with PHP (for further details see Mallette et al.[299, 302]). Although a normal phosphate response may occur in PHP type 1 patients with serum calcium or PTH levels in the normal range,[170] in patients with PHP type 2 the phosphaturic response to PTH is not changed despite at least a 10-fold increase in cAMP excretion. Unfortunately, interpretation of the phosphaturic response to PTH is often complicated by random variations in phosphate clearance, and it is sometimes not possible to classify a phosphaturic response as normal or subnormal regardless of the criteria employed. More perplexing yet is the observation that biochemical findings that resemble PHP type 2 have been found in patients with various forms of vitamin D deficiency.[284] In these patients, marked hypocalcemia is accompanied by hyperphosphatemia due presumably to an acquired dissociation between the amount of cAMP generated in the renal tubule and its effect on phosphate clearance.

The plasma cAMP response to PTH can also be used to differentiate patients with PHP type 1 from normal subjects and from patients with hypoparathyroidism.[301, 308, 309] Patients with PHP type 2 can be expected to have normal responsiveness, however. This test offers few advantages over protocols that assess the urinary excretion of cAMP, as changes in plasma cAMP in normal subjects and patients with hypoparathyroidism are much less dramatic than changes in urinary cAMP, and urine must still be collected if one wishes to assess the phosphaturic response to PTH. One reasonable indication for measuring the plasma cAMP response to PTH is the evaluation of patients in whom proper collection of urine is not possible, such as young children.[309]

The plasma $1,25(OH)_2D_3$ response to PTH has been used to differentiate between hormone-deficient and hormone-resistant hypoparathyroidism.[300, 310] In contrast to normal subjects and patients with hypoparathyroidism, patients with PHP had no significant increase in circulating levels of $1,25(OH)_2D_3$. This proposed test readily demonstrates the difference in the pathophysiology between hypoparathyroidism and PHP. Its clinical relevance is probably limited to distinguishing type 1 from type 2 PHP where the expected increase in the latter form of PHP might be a more reliable parameter than the phosphaturic response to PTH.

TREATMENT

Urgent treatment of acute or severe symptomatic hypocalcemia in patients with hypoparathyroidism is best accomplished by the intravenous infusion of calcium. Vitamin D is not required. The goal is alleviation of symptoms and prevention of laryngeal spasm and seizures. Hyperphosphatemia, alkalosis, and hypomagnesemia should be corrected. The serum calcium should be increased to the mid-normal range. The desired serum calcium levels can usually be obtained by injecting 1 to 3 g of calcium gluconate (93 to 279 mg of elemental calcium, 10 to 30 mL of 10% calcium gluconate) over a 10-minute period followed by continuous infusion of calcium (up to 100 mg/hour) using a solution of 5% dextrose in water containing 100 mL of 10% calcium gluconate (930 mg of elemental calcium) per liter. A 10% solution of calcium chloride is available for intravenous use but it is very irritating to the veins. The serum calcium level should be measured at frequent intervals, and the amount of intravenous calcium should be adjusted accordingly. Electrocardiographic monitoring is advisable when patients are receiving digitalis-like drugs because increasing serum calcium levels can predispose to digitalis toxicity. Oral calcium and vitamin D therapy should be started as soon as possible and gradually adjusted to replace the need for intravenous calcium.[311]

The long-term treatment of hypocalcemia in patients with hypoparathyroidism involves the administration of oral calcium and vitamin D or analogues. Patients with PHP may require less intensive therapy than patients with PTH deficiency.

The goals of therapy are to maintain serum ionized calcium levels in the normal range, to avoid hypercalciuria, and, in patients with PHP, to suppress PTH levels. Patients with hypoparathyroidism have increased urinary calcium excretion in relation to serum calcium and are therefore prone to hypercalciuria.[312] By contrast, patients with PHP have significantly lower urinary calcium in relation to serum calcium[312, 313] and can tolerate serum calcium levels that are within the normal range without developing hypercalciuria.[168]

Once normocalcemia has been attained attention should be directed toward suppression of PTH levels to normal. This is important because elevated PTH levels in patients with PHP are frequently associated with increased bone remodeling. Hyperparathyroid bone disease, including osteitis fibrosa cystica[245, 269, 314] and cortical osteopenia[176] (see Fig. 81–7), can occur in patients with PHP type 1b. These subjects may have elevated serum levels of alkaline phosphatase[314] and urine hydroxyproline.[176] In this regard calcitriol has an advantage over other vitamin D preparations since it may inhibit PTH release directly[315] in addition to the indirect inhibition caused by elevating the serum calcium.

Oral calcium is usually administered in amounts of from 1 to 3 g of elemental calcium per day in divided doses. To assure optimal absorption, oral calcium supplements should be taken with water or other fluids, and with food in the stomach.[316] Many considerations are involved in the selection of a calcium supplement, and none are unique to the treatment of hypoparathyroidism. Calcium carbonate is an inexpensive form of calcium that is very convenient owing to its high content of elemental calcium (40%). When taken with food, absorption of calcium from calcium carbonate is adequate even in achlorhydric patients. Due to the low content of elemental calcium in calcium lactate (13%) and calcium gluconate (9%), patients must take many tablets to obtain adequate amounts of calcium. Thus, these salts are inconvenient and are often not acceptable to the patients. Calcium citrate is 21% calcium and is well absorbed even in the absence of gastric acid.[317] Although more expensive than many other forms of calcium, calcium citrate has the advantage of causing fewer gastrointestinal side effects. For those who prefer a liquid calcium supplement, calcium glubionate is very palatable and contains 252 mg calcium per 10 mL. Ten to 30 mL of a 10% calcium chloride solution (360 to 1080 mg calcium) every 8 hours may be very effective in patients with achlorhydria.[318] Hyperchloremic acidosis may occur which can be prevented by giving half of the calcium as chloride and half as carbonate simultaneously.[318] Calcium phosphate salts should be avoided.

All patients with hypoparathyroidism who are hypocalcemic will require vitamin D or analogues in addition to calcium. Calcitriol, the active form of vitamin D, is the most physiologic treatment choice. Patients with PHP require about 75% as much calcitriol to maintain normocalcemia as do patients with hypoparathyroidism.[319] Almost all patients with hypoparathyroidism or PHP can be effectively treated with calcitriol in the amount of 0.25 μg twice a day to 0.5 μg four times a day. Because of the expense of calcitriol and the need to administer the drug several times per day, other vitamin D preparations may be preferred. Patients with all forms of hypoparathyroidism and PHP will respond to pharmacologic doses of ergocalciferol (vitamin D_2) and calcifediol. Ergocalciferol is the least expensive choice for vitamin D therapy, and provides a long duration of action (with corresponding prolonged potential toxicity). Patients with PHP require lower doses of vitamin D than patients with hypoparathyroidism,[319] an observation that reflects the response of bone and renal distal tubular cells to endogenous PTH.[320] Treatment with calcium and vitamin D usually decreases the elevated serum phosphate to a high-normal level because of a favorable balance between increased urinary phosphate excretion and decreased intestinal phosphate absorption. In general, phosphate-binding gels such as aluminum hydroxide are not necessary.

Attention should be directed to a number of special situations. Because thiazide diuretics can increase renal calcium reabsorption in patients with hypoparathyroidism,[321–323] the inadvertent institution or discontinuation of these drugs may respectively increase or decrease plasma calcium levels.[324] By contrast, furosemide and other loop diuretics can increase renal clearance of calcium and depress serum calcium levels. The administration of glucocorticoids antagonizes the action of vitamin D (and analogues) and may also precipitate hypocalcemia. The development of hypomagnesemia may also interfere with the effectiveness of treatment with calcium and vitamin D.[325]

Experimental treatments for hypoparathyroidism include transplantation of cultured human parathyroid cells[326] and daily injection of synthetic human PTH(1–34).[327] PTH(1–34) has been shown to effectively normalize serum concentrations of calcium and phosphorus while causing less hypercalciuria than treatment with comparable doses of calcitriol.[327] Unfortunately, uncertainties regarding the future availability of human PTH(1–34), and the need to administer the drug by injection, lessen overall enthusiasm for this form of treatment.

Patients with AHO may require specific treatment for unusual problems related to their developmental and skeletal abnormalities. Patients with PHP type 1a should be treated for their associated hypogonadism and hypothyroidism. Ectopic calcification occurs in about 30% of patients with AHO,[241] but rarely causes a problem. However, at times large extraskeletal osteomas may occur.[247] These may require surgical removal to relieve pressure symptoms.

CONCLUSION

The evolving characterization of the signal transduction pathways that regulate PTH secretion and action has led to a new understanding of the molecular basis of some forms of hypoparathyroidism and PHP. Hand in hand with this experimental approach have come unexpected insights gained through careful study of patients with disorders of mineral metabolism. These unusual patients continue to provide us with an opportunity to discover new genetic mechanisms that control embryologic development of the parathyroid glands and that regulate PTH signaling pathways in classic target tissues, such as bone and kidney, as well as in nonclassic targets.

As the disease genes for these metabolic disorders are identified, and genetic tests are developed that can diagnose these disorders at a molecular level, it is likely that the clinical spectrum of disease will rapidly expand. This prediction has already been fulfilled through our understanding of defects in genes encoding $G_{s\alpha}$ and the calcium-sensing receptor. Future work will be directed toward identification of the molecular basis of other forms of hypoparathyroidism and PTH resistance so that all disorders of PTH action can be described on the basis of their pathophysiology.

REFERENCES

1. Marshall RW: Plasma fractions. *In* Nordin BCE (ed): Calcium, Phosphate and Magnesium Metabolism. London, Churchill Livingstone, 1976, p 162.
2. Berry EM, Gupta MM, Turner SJ, Burns RR: Variations in plasma calcium with induced changes in plasma specific gravity, total protein, and albumin. BMJ 4:640, 1973.
3. Bowers GN, Brassard C, Sena S: Measurement of ionized calcium in serum with ion-selective electrodes: A mature technology that can meet the daily service needs. Clin Chem 32:1437–1447, 1986.
4. Boink ABTJ, Buckley BM, Christiansen TF, et al: IFC recommendation: Recommendation on sampling, transport and storage for the determination of the concentration of ionized calcium in whole blood, plasma and serum. Clin Chim Acta 202:S13–S22, 1991.
5. Moore EW: Ionized calcium in normal serum, ultrafiltrates, and whole blood determined by ion-exchange electrodes. J Clin Invest 49:318, 1970.
6. Nordin BE, Need AG, Hartley TF, et al: Improved method for calculating calcium fractions in plasma: Reference values and effect of menopause [erratum appears in Clin Chem 35:670, 1989]. Clin Chem 35:14–17, 1989.
7. Ladenson JH, Lewis JW, Boyd JC: Failure of total calcium corrected for protein, albrumin, and pH to correctly assess free calcium status. J Clin Endocrinol Metab 46:986, 1978.
8. Hebert SC, Brown EM: The extracellular calcium receptor [review]. Curr Opin Cell Biol 7:484–492, 1995.
9. Brown EM, Gamba G, Riccardi D, et al: Cloning and characterization of an extracellular Ca^{2+}-sensing receptor from bovine parathyroid. Nature 366:575–580, 1993.
10. Chattopadhyay N, Mithal A, Brown EM: The calcium-sensing receptor: A window into the physiology and pathophysiology of mineral ion metabolism [review]. Endocr Rev 17:289–307, 1996.
11. Schipani E, Karga H, Karaplis AC, et al: Identical complementary deoxyribonucleic acids encode a human renal and bone parathyroid hormone (PTH)/PTH-related peptide receptor. Endocrinology 132:2157–2165, 1993.
12. Abou Samra AB, Juppner H, Force T, et al: Expression cloning of a common receptor for parathyroid hormone and parathyroid hormone–related peptide from rat osteoblast-like cells: A single receptor stimulates intracellular accumulation of both cAMP and inositol trisphosphates and increases intracellular free calcium. Proc Natl Acad Sci USA 89:2732–2736, 1992.
13. Juppner H, Abou Samra AB, Freeman M, et al: A G protein–linked receptor for parathyroid hormone and parathyroid hormone–related peptide. Science 254:1024–1026, 1991.
14. Adams AE, Pines M, Nakamoto C, et al: Probing the bimolecular interaction of parathyroid hormone (PTH) and the human PTH/PTHrP receptor. II. Cloning, characterization of, and photoaffinity crosslinking to the recombinant human PTH/PTHrP receptor. Biochemistry 34:10553–10559, 1995.
15. Behar V, Pines M, Nakamoto C, et al: The human PTH2 receptor: Binding and signal transduction properties of the stably expressed recombinant receptor. Endocrinology 137:2748–2757, 1996.
16. Usdin TB, Gruber C, Bonner TI: Identification and functional expression of a receptor selectively recognizing parathyroid hormone, the PTH2. J Biol Chem 270:15455–15458, 1995.
17. Neer EJ: Heterotrimeric G proteins: Organizers of transmembrane signals. Cell 80:249–257, 1995.
18. Bohm A, Gaudet R, Sigler PB: Structural aspects of heterotrimeric G-protein signaling. Curr Opin Biotechnol 8:480–487, 1997.
19. Clapham DE, Neer EJ: G protein beta gamma subunits. Annu Rev Pharmacol Toxicol 37:167–203, 1997.
20. Schmidt CJ, Neer EJ: In vitro synthesis of G protein beta gamma dimers. J Biol Chem 266:4538–4544, 1991.
21. Schmidt CJ, Thomas TC, Levine MA, Neer EJ: Specificity of G protein beta and gamma subunit interactions. J Biol Chem 267:13807–13810, 1992.
22. Rahmatullah M, Robishaw JD: Direct Interaction of the α and γ subunits of the G proteins. J Biol Chem 269:3574–3580, 1994.
23. Rahmatullah M, Ginnan R, Robishaw JD: Specificity of G protein alpha-gamma subunit interactions. N-terminal 15 amino acids of gamma subunit specifies interaction with alpha subunit. J Biol Chem 270:2946–2951, 1995.
24. Taussig R, Zimmermann G: Type-specific regulation of mammalian adenylyl cyclases by G protein pathways. Adv Second Messenger Phosphoprotein Res 32:81–98, 1998.
25. Wess J: Molecular basis of receptor/G-protein–coupling selectivity. Pharmacol Ther 80:231–264, 1998.
26. Gautam N, Downes GB, Yan K, Kisselev O: The G-protein betagamma complex. Cell Signal 10:447–455, 1998.
27. Clapham DE, Neer EJ: New roles for G-protein beta gamma–dimers in transmembrane signalling [review]. Nature 365:403–406, 1993.
28. Wickman KD, Iniguez-Lluhl JA, Davenport PA, et al: Recombinant G-protein beta gamma–subunits activate the muscarinic-gated atrial potassium channel. Nature 368:255–257, 1994.
29. Pitcher J, Lohse MJ, Codina J, et al: Desensitization of the isolated beta 2-adrenergic receptor by beta-adrenergic receptor kinase, cAMP-dependent protein kinase, and protein kinase C occurs via distinct molecular mechanisms. Biochemistry 31:3193–3197, 1992.

30. Pitcher J, Inglese J, Higgins CF, et al: Role of βγ subunits of G proteins in targeting the beta-adrenergic receptor kinase to membrane bound receptors. Science 257:1264–1267, 1992.
31. Faure M, Voyno-Yasenetskaya TA, Bourne HR: cAMP and beta gamma subunits of heterotrimeric G proteins stimulate the mitogen-activated protein kinase pathway in COS-7 cells. J Biol Chem 269:7851–7854, 1994.
32. Ford CE, Skiba NP, Bae H, et al: Molecular basis for interactions of G protein betagamma subunits with effectors. Science 280:1271–1274, 1998.
33. Neptune ER, Bourne HR: Receptors induce chemotaxis by releasing the betagamma subunit of Gi, not by activating Gq or Gs. Proc Natl Acad Sci USA 94:14489–14494, 1997.
34. Melson GL, Chase LR, Aurbach GD: Parathyroid hormone–sensitive adenyl cyclase in isolated renal tubules. Endocrinology 86:511–518, 1970.
35. Chase LR, Fedak SA, Aurbach GD: Activation of skeletal adenyl cyclase by parathyroid hormone in vitro. Endocrinology 84:761–768, 1969.
36. Civitelli R, Reid IR, Westbrook S, et al: PTH elevates inositol polyphosphates and diacylglycerol in a rat osteoblast-like cell line. Am J Physiol 255:E660–E667, 1988.
37. Dunlay R, Hruska K: PTH receptor coupling to phospholipase C is an alternate pathway of signal transduction in bone and kidney. Am J Physiol 258:F223–F231, 1990.
38. Gupta A, Martin KJ, Miyauchi A, Hruska KA: Regulation of cytosolic calcium by parathyroid hormone and oscillations of cytosolic calcium in fibroblasts from normal and pseudohypoparathyroid patients. Endocrinology 128:2825–2836, 1991.
39. Civitelli R, Martin TJ, Fausto A, et al: Parathyroid hormone–related peptide transiently increases cytosolic calcium in osteoblast-like cells: Comparison with parathyroid hormone. Endocrinology 125:1204–1210, 1989.
40. Reid IR, Civitelli R, Halstead LR, et al: Parathyroid hormone acutely elevates intracellular calcium in osteoblastlike cells. Am J Physiol 253:E45–E51, 1987.
41. Yamaguchi DT, Hahn TJ, Iida-Klein A, et al: Parathyroid hormone–activated calcium channels in an osteoblast-like clonal osteosarcoma cell line. J Biol Chem 262:7711–7718, 1987.
42. Bringhurst FR, Zajac JD, Daggett AS, et al: Inhibition of parathyroid hormone responsiveness in clonal osteoblastic cells expressing a mutant form of 3′,5′-cyclic adenosine monophosphate–dependent protein kinase. Mol Endocrinol 3:60–67, 1989.
43. Schwindinger WF, Fredericks J, Watkins L, et al: Coupling of the PTH/PTHrP receptor to multiple G-proteins. Direct demonstration of receptor activation of Gs, Gq/11, and Gi(1) by [alpha-32P]GTP-gamma-azidoanilide photoaffinity labeling. Endocrine 8:201–209, 1998.
44. Offermanns S, Iida-Klein A, Segre GV, Simon MI: G alpha q family members couple parathyroid hormone (PTH)/PTH-related peptide and calcitonin receptors to phospholipase C in COS-7 cells. Mol Endocrinol 10:566–574, 1996.
45. Abbott LG, Rude RK: Clinical manifestations of magnesium deficiency [review]. Miner Electrolyte Metab 19:314–322, 1993.
46. Hoffman E: The Chvostek sign: A clinical study. Am J Surg 96:33, 1958.
47. Rimailho A, Bouchard P, Schaison G, et al: Improvement of hypocalcemic cardiomyopathy by correction of serum calcium level. Am Heart J 109:611, 1985.
48. Giles TD, Iteld BJ, Rives KL: The cardiomyopathy of hypoparathyroidism. Another reversible form of heart muscle disease. Chest 79:225–229, 1981.
49. Suzuki T, Ikeda U, Fujikawa H, et al: Hypocalcemic heart failure: A reversible form of heart muscle disease [see comments]. Clin Cardiol 21:227–228, 1998.
50. Wong CK, Lau CP, Cheng CH, et al: Hypocalcemic myocardial dysfunction: Short and long-term improvement with calcium replacement. Am Heart J 120:381, 1990.
51. Levine SN, Rheams CN: Hypocalcemic heart failure. Am J Med 78:1022, 1975.
52. Kanda F, Jinnai J, Fujita T: Somatosensory evoked potentials in patients with hypocalcemia after parathyroidectomy. J Neurol 235:136, 1988.
53. Nikiforuk G, Fraser D: Chemical determinants of enamel hypoplasia in children with disorders of calcium and phosphate homeostasis. J Dent Res 58(B):1014, 1979.
54. Brown MD, Aaron G: Pseudohypoparathyroidism: Case report. Pediatr Dent 13:106–109, 1991.
55. Ranggard L: Dental enamel in relation to ionized calcium and parathyroid hormone. Studies of human primary teeth and rat maxillary incisors. Swed Dent J Suppl 101:1–50, 1994.
56. Nekula J, Urbanek K, Buresova J: Radiological findings in pseudohypoparathyroidism (in German). Rofo Fortschr Geb Rontgenstr Neuen Bildgeb Verfahr 157:34–36, 1992.
57. Illum F, Dupont E: Prevalences of CT-detected calcification in the basal ganglia in idiopathic hypoparathyroidism and pseudohypoparathyroidism. Neuroradiology 27:32–37, 1985.
58. Kowdley KV, Coull BM, Orwoll ES: Cognitive impairment and intracranial calcification in chronic hypoparathyroidism. Am J Med Sci 317:273–277, 1999.
59. Simpson JA: The neurologic manifestations of idiopathic hypoparathyroidism. Brain 75:76, 1952.
60. Schaaf M, Payne C: Dystonic reactions to prochlorperazine in hypoparathyroidism. N Engl J Med 275:991, 1966.
61. Schutt-Aine JC, Young MA, Pescovitz DH, et al: Hypoparathyroidism: A possible cause of rickets. J Pediatr 106:255, 1985.
62. Drezner MK, Neelon FA, Haussler M, et al: 1,25-Dihydroxycholecalciferol deficiency: The probable cause of hypocalcemia and metabolic bone disease in pseudohypoparathyroidism. J Clin Endocrinol Metab 42:621–628, 1976.
63. Abugassa S, Nordenstrom J, Eriksson S, Sjoden G: Bone mineral density in patients with chronic hypoparathyroidism. J Clin Endocrinol Metab 76:1617, 1993.
64. Shukla S, Gillespy TI, Thomas WC Jr: The effect of hypoparathyroidism on the aging skeleton. J Am Geriatr Soc 38:884, 1990.
65. Orr-Walker B, Harris R, Holdaway IM, et al: High peripheral and axial bone densities in a postmenopausal woman with untreated hypoparathyroidism. Postgrad Med J 66:1061, 1990.
66. Isaacson SR: Hypocalcemia in surgery for carcinoma of the pharynx and larynx. Otolaryngol Clin North Am 13:181–191, 1980.
67. Wade J, Fourman P, Deane L: Recovery of parathyroid function in patients with "transient" hypoparathyroidism after thyroidectomy. Br J Surg 52:493, 1965.
68. Thorp MA, Levitt NS, Mortimore S, Isaacs S: Parathyroid and thyroid function five years after treatment of laryngeal and hypopharyngeal carcinoma. Clin Otolaryngol 24:104–108, 1989.
69. Dent CE: Some problems of hyperparathyroidism. BMJ 2:1419, 1962.
70. Edis AJ: Prevention and management of complications associated with thyroid and parathyroid surgery. Surg Clin North Am 59:83–92, 1979.
71. Loré JM Jr: Complications in management of thyroid cancer. Semin Surg Oncol 7:120, 1991.
72. Gann DS, Paone JF: Delayed hypocalcemia after thyroidectomy for Graves disease is prevented by parathyroid autotranplantation. Ann Surg 190:508, 1979.
73. Dembinski TC, Yatscoff RW, Blandford DE: Thyrotoxicosis and hungry bone syndrome—a cause of posttreatment hypocalcemia. Clin Biochem 27:69–74, 1994.
74. Michie W, Stowers JM, Duncan T, et al: Mechanism of hypocalcemia after thyroidectomy for thyrotoxicosis. Lancet 1:508, 1971.
75. Watson CG, Steed DL, Robinson AG, Deftos LJ: The role of calcitonin and parathyroid hormone in the pathogenesis of post-thyroidectomy hypocalcemia. Metabolism 30:588, 1981.
76. Percival RC, Haregreaves AW, Kanis JA: The mechanism of hypocalcemia following thyroidectomy. Acta Endocrinol 109:220, 1985.
77. Attie MF, Fallon MD, Spar B, et al: Bone and parathyroid inhibitory effects of S-2(3-aminopropylamino)ethylphosphorothioic acid. J Clin Invest 75:1191, 1985.
78. Hermans C, Lefebvre C, Devogelaer JP, Lambert M: Hypocalcaemia and chronic alcohol intoxication: Transient hypoparathyroidism secondary to magnesium deficiency. Clin Rheumatol 15:193–196, 1996.
79. Manfredini R, Bariani L, Bagni B, et al: Hypoparathyroidism in chronic alcohol intoxication: A preliminary report. Riv Eur Sci Med Farmacol 14:293–296, 1992.
80. Laitinen K, Tahtela R, Valimaki M: The dose-dependency of alcohol-induced hypoparathyroidism, hypercalciuria, and hypermagnesuria. Bone Miner 19:75–83, 1992.
81. Laitinen K, Lamberg-Allardt C, Tunninen R, et al: Transient hypoparathyroidism during acute alcohol intoxication. N Engl J Med 324:721–727, 1991.
82. Italian Working Group on Endocrine Complications in Non-endocrine Diseases: Multicentre study on prevalence of endocrine complications in thalassaemia major. Clin Endocrinol (Oxf) 42:581–586, 1995.
83. Gertner JM, Broadus AE, Anast CS, et al: Impaired parathyroid response to induced hypocalcemia in thalassemia major. J Pediatr 95:210–213, 1979.
84. Carpenter, TO, Carnes DL, Jr, Anast CS: Hypoparathyroidism in Wilson's disease. N Engl J Med 309:873–877, 1983.
85. Rude RK: Mg deficiency in parathyroid function. *In* Bilezikian JP, Marcus R, Levine MA (eds): The Parathyroids: Basic and Clinical Concepts. New York, Raven Press, 1994, pp 829–842.
86. Cruikshank DP, Chan GM, Doerrfeld D: Alterations in vitamin D and calcium metabolism with magnesium sulfate treatment of preeclampsia. Am J Obstet Gynecol 168:1170–1176, 1993.
87. Cholst IN, Steinberg SF, Tropper PJ, et al: The influence of hypermagnesemia on serum calcium and parathyroid hormone levels in human subjects. N Engl J Med 310:1221–1225, 1984.
88. Mayan H, Hourvitz A, Schiff E, Farfel Z: Symptomatic hypocalcaemia in hypermagnesaemia-induced hypoparathyroidism, during magnesium tocolytic therapy—possible involvement of the calcium-sensing receptor. Nephrol Dial Transplant 14:1764–1766, 1999.
89. Fatemi S, Ryzen E, Flores J, et al: Effect of experimental human magnesium depletion on parathyroid hormone secretion and 1,25-dihydroxyvitamin D metabolism. J Clin Endocrinol Metab 73:1067–1072, 1991.
90. Klein GL, Herndon DN: Magnesium deficit in major burns: Role in hypoparathyroidism and end-organ parathyroid hormone resistance. Magnes Res 11:103–109, 1998.
91. Bianchetti MG, Bettinelli A, Casez JP, et al: Evidence for disturbed regulation of calciotropic hormone metabolism in Gitelman syndrome. J Clin Endocrinol Metab 80:224–228, 1995.
92. Bettinelli A, Basilico E, Metta MG, et al: Magnesium supplementation in Gitelman syndrome. Pediatr Nephrol 13:311–314, 1999.
93. Meij IC, Saar K, van den Heuvel LP, et al: Hereditary isolated renal magnesium loss maps to chromosome 11q23. Am J Hum Genet 64:180–188, 1999.
94. Matsumoto T: Magnesium deficiency and parathyroid function (editorial; comment). Intern Med 34:603–604, 1995.
95. Rude RK, Oldham SB, Sharp Jr CF, Singer FR: Parathyroid hormone secretion in magnesium deficiency. J Clin Endocrinol Metab 47:800–806, 1978.
96. Neufield RB, Maclaren N, Blizzard R: Two types of autoimmune Addison's disease associated with different polyglandular autoimmune syndromes. Medicine (Baltimore) 60:355, 1981.
97. Ahonen P: Autoimmune polyendocrinopathy–candidosis–ectodermal dystrophy (APECED): Autosomal recessive inheritance. Clin Genet 27:535–542, 1985.
98. Perniola R, Tamborrino G, Marsigliante S, De Rinaldis C: Assessment of enamel hypoplasia in autoimmune polyendocrinopathy–candidiasis–ectodermal dystrophy (APECED). J Oral Pathol Med 27:278–282, 1998.
99. Ahonen P, Myllarniemi S, Sipila I, Perheentupa J: Clinical variation of autoimmune polyendocrinopathy–candidiasis–ectodermal dystrophy (APECED) in a series of 68 patients. N Engl J Med 322:1829–1836, 1990.
100. Blizzard RM, Chee D, Davis W: The incidence of parathyroid and other antibodies in the sera of patients with idiopathic hypoparathyroidism. Clin Exp Immunol 1:119–128, 1966.
101. Verghese MW, Ward FE, Eisenbarth GS: Lymphocyte suppressor activity in patients with polyglandular failure. Hum Immunol 3:173–179, 1981.
102. Chen QY, Lan MS, She JX, Maclaren NK: The gene responsible for autoimmune polyglandular syndrome type 1 maps to chromosome 21q22.3 in US patients. J Autoimmun 11:177–183, 1998.

103. Scott HS, Heino M, Peterson P, et al: Common mutations in autoimmune polyendocrinopathy–candidiasis–ectodermal dystrophy patients of different origins. Mol Endocrinol 12:1112–1119, 1998.
104. Obermayer-Straub P, Manns MP: Autoimmune polyglandular syndromes. Baillieres Clin Gastroenterol 12:293–315, 1998.
105. Ward L, Paquette J, Seidman E, et al: Severe autoimmune polyendocrinopathy–candidiasis–ectodermal dystrophy in an adolescent girl with a novel AIRE mutation: Response to immunosuppressive therapy. J Clin Endocrinol Metab 84:844–852, 1999.
106. Pearce SH, Cheetham T, Imrie H, et al: A common and recurrent 13-bp deletion in the autoimmune regulator gene in British kindreds with autoimmune polyendocrinopathy type 1. Am J Hum Genet 63:1675–1684, 1998.
107. Rosatelli MC, Meloni A, Devoto M, et al: A common mutation in Sardinian autoimmune polyendocrinopathy–candidiasis–ectodermal dystrophy patients. Hum Genet 103:428–434, 1998.
108. Rinderle C, Christensen HM, Schweiger S, et al: AIRE encodes a nuclear protein co-localizing with cytoskeletal filaments: Altered sub-cellular distribution of mutants lacking the PHD zinc fingers. Hum Mol Genet 8:277–290, 1999.
109. Posillico JT, Wortsman J Srikanta S, et al: Parathyroid cell surface autoantibodies that inhibit parathyroid hormone secretion from dispersed human parathyroid cells. J Bone Miner Res 1:475–483, 1986.
110. Brandi ML, Aurbach GD, Fattorossi A, et al: Antibodies cytotoxic to bovine parathyroid cells in autoimmune hypoparathyroidism. Proc Natl Acad Sci USA 83:8366–8369, 1986.
111. Drake TG, Albright F, Bauer W: Chronic idiopathic hypoparathyroidism: Report of 6 cases with autopsy findings in one. Ann Intern Med 12:1751, 1934.
112. Treusch JV: Idiopathic hypoparathyroidism: Follow-up study including autopsy findings of a case previously reported. Ann Intern Med 56:484, 1962.
113. Thakker RV: Molecular basis of PTH underexpression. *In* Bilezikian JP, Raisz LG, Rodan GA, (eds): Principles of Bone Biology. San Diego, Academic Press, 1996, pp 837–851.
114. Ahn TG, Antonarakis SE, Kronenberg HM, et al: Familial isolated hypoparathyroidism: A molecular genetic analysis of 8 families with 23 affected persons. Medicine (Baltimore) 65:73–81, 1986.
115. Arnold A, Horst SA, Gardella TJ, et al: Mutation of the signal peptide–encoding region of the preproparathyroid hormone gene in familial isolated hypoparathyroidism. J Clin Invest 86:1084–1087, 1990.
116. Sunthornthepvarakul T, Churesigaew S, Ngowngarmratana S: A novel mutation of the signal peptide of the preproparathyroid hormone gene associated with autosomal recessive familial isolated hypoparathyroidism. J Clin Endocrinol Metab 84:3792–3796, 1999.
117. Parkinson DB, Thakker RV: A donor splice site mutation in the parathyroid hormone gene is associated with autosomal recessive hypoparathyroidism. Nat Genet 1:149–152, 1992.
118. Parkinson DB, Shaw NJ, Himsworth RL, Thakker RV: Parathyroid hormone gene analysis in autosomal hypoparathyroidism using an intragenic tetranucleotide (AAAT)n polymorphism. Hum Genet 91:281–284, 1993.
119. Miric A, Levine MA: Analysis of the preproPTH gene by denaturing gradient gel electrophoresis in familial isolated hypoparathyroidism. J Clin Endocrinol Metab 74:509–516, 1992.
120. Pollak MR, Brown EM, Chou YW, et al: Mutations in the human Ca^{2+}-sensing receptor gene cause familial hypocalciuric hypercalcemia and neonatal severe hyperparathyroidism. Cell 75:1297–1303, 1993.
121. Pollak MR, Chou YH, Marx SJ, et al: Familial hypocalciuric hypercalcemia and neonatal severe hyperparathyroidism. Effects of mutant gene dosage on phenotype. J Clin Invest 93:1108–1112, 1994.
122. Chou YH, Pollak MR, Brandi ML, et al: Mutations in the human Ca(2+)-sensing-receptor genes that cause familial hypocalciuric hypercalcemia. Am J Hum Genet 56:1075–1079, 1995.
123. Pearce SH, Bai M, Quinn SJ, et al: Functional characterization of calcium-sensing receptor mutations expressed in human embryonic kidney cells. J Clin Invest 98:1860–1866, 1996.
124. Pollak MR, Seidman CE, Brown EM: Three inherited disorders of calcium sensing [review]. Medicine (Baltimore) 75:115–123, 1996.
125. Pearce SH, Williamson C, Kifor O, et al: A familial syndrome of hypocalcemia with hypercalciuria due to mutations in the calcium-sensing receptor [see comments]. N Engl J Med 335:1115–1122, 1996.
126. Bai M, Quinn S, Trivedi S, et al: Expression and characterization of inactivating and activating mutations in the human $Ca^{2+}{}_o$-sensing receptor. J Biol Chem 271:19537–19545, 1996.
127. Finegold DN, Armitage MM, Galiani M, et al: Preliminary localization of a gene for autosomal dominant hypoparathyroidism to chromosome 3q13. Pediatr Res 36:414–417, 1994.
128. Brown EM, Hebert SC: A cloned Ca(2+)-sensing receptor: A mediator of direct effects of extracellular Ca^{2+} on renal function? [review]. J Am Soc Nephrol 6:1530–1540, 1995.
129. Riccardi D, Lee WS, Lee K, et al: Localization of the extracellular Ca(2+)-sensing receptor and PTH/PTHrP receptor in rat kidney. Am J Physiol 271 (pt 2):F951–956, 1996.
130. Mumm S, Whyte MP, Thakker RV, et al: mtDNA analysis shows common ancestry in two kindreds with X-linked recessive hypoparathyroidism and reveals a heteroplasmic silent mutation. Am J Hum Genet 60:153–159, 1997.
131. Thakker RV, Davies KE, Whyte MP, et al: Mapping the gene causing X-linked recessive idiopathic hypoparathyroidism to Xq26-Xq27 by linkage studies. J Clin Invest 86:40–45, 1990.
132. Trump D, Dixon PH, Mumm S, et al: Localisation of X linked recessive idiopathic hypoparathyroidism to a 1.5 Mb region on Xq26-q27. J Med Genet 35:905–909, 1998.
133. Rohn RD, Leffell MS, Leadem P, et al: Familial third-fourth pharyngeal pouch syndrome with apparent autosomal dominant transmission. J Pediatr 105:47, 1984.
134. Raatikka M, Ropola J, Tuteri L, et al: Familial third and fourth pharyngeal pouch syndrome with truncus arteriosus: DiGeorge syndrome. Pediatrics 67:173, 1981.
135. Cuneo BF, Driscoll DA, Gidding SS, Langman CB: Evolution of latent hypoparathyroidism in familial 22q11 deletion syndrome. Am J Med Genet 69:50–55, 1997.
136. de la Chapelle A, Herra R, Kiovisto M, Aula P: A deletion in chromosome 22 can cause DiGeorge syndrome. Hum Genet 57:253, 1981.
137. Kelley RI Zackai FH, Emanuel BS: The association of the DiGeorge anomalad with partial monosomy of chromosome 22. J Pediatr 101:197, 1982.
138. Driscoll DA, Budarf ML, Emanuel BS: A genetic etiology for DiGeorge syndrome: Consistent deletions and microdeletions of 22q11. Am J Hum Genet 50:924, 1991.
139. Greig F, Paul E, DiMartino-Nardi J, Saenger P: Transient congenital hypoparathyroidism: Resolution and recurrence in chromosome 22q11 deletion. J Pediatr 128:563–567, 1996.
140. Hur H, Kim YJ, Noh CI, et al: Molecular genetic analysis of the DiGeorge syndrome among Korean patients with congenital heart disease. Mol Cells 9:72–77, 1999.
141. Monaco G, Pignata C, Rossi E, et al:. DiGeorge anomaly associated with 10p deletion. Am J Med Genet 19:215, 1991.
142. Lai MMR, Scriven PN, Ball C, Berry AC: Simultaneous partial monosomy 10p and trisomy 5q in a case of hypoparathyroidism. J Med Genet 29:586, 1992.
143. Daw SC, Taylor C, Kraman M, et al: A common region of 10p deleted in DiGeorge and velocardiofacial syndromes. Nat Genet 13:458–460, 1996.
144. Stevens CA, Carey JC, Shigeoka AO: DiGeorge anomaly and velocardiofacial syndrome. Pediatrics 85:526–530, 1990.
145. Pizzuti A, Novelli G, Ratti A, et al: UFD1L, a developmentally expressed ubiquitination gene, is deleted in CATCH 22 syndrome. Hum Mol Gene 6:259–265, 1997.
146. Pizzuti A, Novelli G, Ratti A, et al: Isolation and characterization of a novel transcript embedded within HIRA, a gene deleted in DiGeorge syndrome. Mol Genet Metab 67:227–235, 1999.
147. Yamagishi H, Garg V, Matsuoka R, et al: A molecular pathway revealing a genetic basis for human cardiac and craniofacial defects [see comments]. Science 283:1158–1161, 1999.
148. Baldini A: Is the genetic basis of DiGeorge syndrome in HAND? (news). Nat Genet 21:246–247, 1999.
149. Lindsay EA, Botta A, Jurecic V, et al: Congenital heart disease in mice deficient for the DiGeorge syndrome region. Nature 401:379–383, 1999.
150. Van Esch H, Groenen P, Daw S, et al: Partial DiGeorge syndrome in two patients with a 10p rearrangement. Clin Genet 55:269–276, 1999.
151. Fujimoto S, Yokochi K, Morikawa H, et al: Recurrent cerebral infarctions and del(10)(p14p15.1) de novo in HDR (hypoparathyroidism, sensorineural deafness, renal dysplasia) syndrome. Am J Med Genet 86:427–429, 1999.
152. Franceschini P, Testa A, Bogetti G, et al: Kenny-Caffey syndrome in two sibs born to consanguineous parents: Evidence for an autosomal recessive variant. Am J Med Genet 42:112–116, 1992.
153. Diaz GA, Gelb BD, Ali F, et al: Sanjad-Sakati and autosomal recessive Kenny-Caffey syndromes are allelic: Evidence for an ancestral founder mutation and locus refinement. Am J Med Genet 85:48–52, 1999.
154. Barakat AY, D'Albora JB, Martin MM, Jose PA: Familial nephrosis, nerve deafness, and hypoparathyroidism. J Pediatr 91:61, 1977.
155. Dahlberg PJ, Borer WZ, Newcomer KL, Yutac WR: Autosomal or X-linked recessive syndrome of congenital lymphedema, hypoparathyroidism, nephropathy, prolapsing mitral valve, and brachytelephalangy. Am J Med Genet 16:99, 1983.
156. Sanjad SA, Sakati NA, Abu-Osba YK, et al: A new syndrome of congenital hypoparathyroidism, severe growth failure, and dysmorphic features [see comments]. Arch Dis Child 66:193–196, 1991.
157. Salle BL, Delvin E, Glorieux F, David L: Human neonatal hypocalcemia [review]. Biol Neonate 58(suppl 1):22–31, 1990.
158. Noe DA: Neonatal hypocalcemia and related conditions [review]. Clin Lab Med 1:227–238, 1981.
159. Venkataraman PS, Tsang RC, Chen IW, Sperling MA: Pathogenesis of early neonatal hypocalcemia: Studies of serum calcitonin, gastrin, and plasma glucagon. J Pediatr 110:599–603, 1987.
160. Kaplan EL, Burrington JD: Klementschitsch P, et al: Primary hyperparathyroidism, pregnancy, and neonatal hypocalcemia. Surgery 96:717–722, 1984.
161. Thomas BR, Bennett JD. Symptomatic hypocalcemia and hypoparathyroidism in two infants of mothers with hyperparathyroidism and familial benign hypercalcemia. J Perinatol 15:23–26, 1995.
162. Specker BL, Tsang RC, Ho ML, et al: Low serum calcium and high parathyroid hormone levels in neonates fed "humanized" cow's milk–based formula. Am J Dis Child 145:941–945, 1991.
163. Albright F, Burnett CH, Smith PH: Pseudohypoparathyroidism: An example of "Seabright-Bantam syndrome." Endocrinology 30:922–932, 1942.
164. Mann JB, Alterman S, Hills AG: Albright's hereditary osteodystrophy comprising pseudohypoparathyroidism and pseudopseudohypoparathyroidism with a report of two cases representing the complete syndrome occurring in successive generations. Ann Intern Med 56:315–342, 1962.
165. Albright F, Forbes AP, Henneman PH: Pseudopseudohypoparathyroidism. Trans Assoc Am Physicians 65:337–350, 1952.
166. Chase LR, Melson GL, Aurbach GD: Pseudohypoparathyroidism: Defective excretion of 3′,5′-AMP in response to parathyroid hormone. J Clin Invest 48:1832–1844, 1969.
167. Bell NH, Avery S, Sinha T, et al: Effects of dibutyryl cyclic adenosine 3′,5′-monophosphate and parathyroid extract on calcium and phosphorous metabolism in hypoparathyroidisma and pseudohypoparathyroidism. J Clin Invest 51:816–816, 1972.
168. Mizunashi K, Furukawa Y, Sohn HE, et al: Heterogeneity of pseudohypoparathyroidism type I from the aspect of urinary excretion of calcium and serum levels of parathyroid hormone. Calcif Tissue Int 46:227–232, 1990.
169. Shima M, Nose O, Shimizu K, et al: Multiple associated endocrine abnormalities in a patient with pseudohypoparathyroidism type 1a. Eur J Pediatr 147:536–538, 1988.

170. Stone MD, Hosking DJ, Garcia-Himmelstine, C, et al: The renal response to exogenous parathyroid hormone in treated pseudohypoparathyroidism. Bone 14:727–735, 1993.
171. Drezner MK, Neelon FA, Lebovitz HE: Pseudohypoparathyroidism type II: A possible defect in the reception of the cyclic AMP signal. N Engl J Med 280:1056–1060, 1973.
172. Murray TM, Rao LG, Wong MM, et al: Pseudohypoparathyroidism with osteitis fibrosa cystica: Direct demonstration of skeletal responsiveness to parathyroid hormone in cells cultured from bone. J Bone Miner Res 8:83–91, 1993.
173. Burnstein MI, Kottamasu SR, Pettifor JM, et al: Metabolic bone disease in pseudohypoparathyroidism: Radiologic features. Radiology 155:351–356, 1985.
174. Dabbaugh S, Chesney RW, Langer LO, et al: Renal–non-responsive, bone-responsive pseudohypoparathyroidism. A case with normal vitamin D metabolite levels and clinical features of rickets. Am J Dis Child 138:1030–1033, 1984.
175. Hall FM, Segall-Blank M, Genant HK, et al: Pseudohypoparathyroidism presenting as renal osteodystrophy. Skeletal Radiol 6:43–46, 1981.
176. Breslau NA, Moses AM, Pak CYC: Evidence for bone remodeling but lack of calcium mobilization response to parathyroid hormone in pseudohypoparathyroidism. J Clin Endocrinol Metab 57:638–644, 1983.
177. Drezner MK, Haussler MR: Normocalcemic pseudohypoparathyroidism. Am J Med 66:503–508, 1979.
178. Stogmann W, Fischer JA: Pseudohypoparathyroidism. Disappearance of the resistance to parathyroid extract during treatment with vitamin D. Am J Med 59:140–144, 1975.
179. Levine MA, Jap TS, Mauseth RS, et al: Activity of the stimulatory guanine nucleotide–binding protein is reduced in erythrocytes from patients with pseudohypoparathyroidism and pseudopseudohypoparathyroidism: Biochemical, endocrine, and genetic analysis of Albright's hereditary osteodystrophy in six kindreds. J Clin Endocrinol Metab 62:497–502, 1986.
180. Levine MA, Ahn TG, Klupt SF, et al: Genetic deficiency of the alpha subunit of the guanine nucleotide–binding protein Gs as the molecular basis for Albright hereditary osteodystrophy. Proc Natl Acad Sci USA 85:617–621, 1988.
181. Barr DG, Stirling HF, Darling JA: Evolution of pseudohypoparathyroidism: An informative family study. Arch Dis Child 70:337–338, 1994.
182. Levine MA, Modi WS, O Brien SJ: Mapping of the gene encoding the alpha subunit of the stimulatory G protein of adenylyl cyclase (GNAS1) to 20q13.2→ q13.3 in human by in situ hybridization. Genomics 11:478–479, 1991.
183. Weinberg AG, Stone RT: Autosomal dominant inheritence in Albright's hereditary osteodystrophy. J Pediatr 79:996–999, 1971.
184. Cedarbaum SD, Lippe BM: Probable autosomal recessive inheritance in a family with Albright's hereditary osteodystrophy and an evaluation of the genetics of the disorder. Am J Hum Genet 25:638–645, 1973.
185. Van Dop C, Bourne HR, Neer RM: Father to son transmission of decreased Ns activity in pseudohypoparathyroidism type Ia. J Clin Endocrinol Metab 59:825–828, 1984.
186. Kozasa T, Itoh H, Tsukamoto T, Kaziro Y: Isolation and characterization of the human Gs alpha gene. Proc Natl Acad Sci USA 85:2081–2085, 1988.
187. Hayward BE, Moran V, Strain L, Bonthron DT: Bidirectional imprinting of a single gene: GNAS1 encodes maternally, paternally, and biallelically derived proteins. Proc Natl Acad Sci USA 95:15475–15480, 1998.
188. Hayward BE, Kamiya M, Strain L, et al: The human GNAS1 gene is imprinted and encodes distinct paternally and biallelically expressed G proteins. Proc Natl Acad Sci USA 95:10038–10043, 1998.
189. Bhatt B, Burns J, Flanner D, McGee J: Direct visualization of single copy genes on banded metaphase chromosomes by nonisotopic in situ hybridization. Nucleic Acids Res 16:3951–3961, 1988.
190. Mattera R, Graziano MP, Yatani A, et al: Splice variants of the alpha subunit of the G protein Gs activate both adenylyl cyclase and calcium channels. Science 243:804–807, 1989.
191. Jones DT, Masters SB, Bourne HR, Reed RR: Biochemical characterization of three stimulatory GTP-binding proteins. J Biol Chem 265:2671–2676, 1990.
192. Graziano MP, Freissmuth M, Gilman AG: Expression of Gs alpha in *Escherichia coli*. Purification and properties of two forms of the protein. J Biol Chem 264:409–418, 1989.
193. Novotny J, Svoboda P: The long (Gs(alpha)-L) and short (Gs(alpha)-S) variants of the stimulatory guanine nucleotide–binding protein. Do they behave in an identical way? J Mol Endocrinol 20:163–173, 1998.
194. Ishikawa Y, Bianchi C, Nadal-Ginard B, Homcy CJ: Alternative promoter and 5′ exon generate a novel G_s alpha mRNA. J Biol Chem 265:8458–8462, 1990.
195. Leitner B, Lovisetti-Scamihorn P, Heilmann J, et al: Subcellular localization of chromogranins, calcium channels, amine carriers, and proteins of the exocytotic machinery in bovine splenic nerve. J Neurochem 72:1110–1116, 1999.
196. Ischia R, Lovisetti-Scamihorn P, Hogue-Angeletti R, et al: Molecular cloning and characterization of NESP55, a novel chromogranin-like precursor of a peptide with 5-HT1B receptor antagonist activity. J Biol Chem 272:11657–11662, 1997.
197. Kehlenbach RH, Matthey J, Huttner WB: XLαs is a new type of G protein. Nature 372:804–808, 1994.
198. Lin CK, Hakakha MJ, Nakamoto JM, et al: Prevalence of three mutations in the Gs alpha gene among 24 families with pseudohypoparathyroidism type Ia. Biochem Biophys Res Commun 189:343, 1992.
199. Iiri T, Herzmark P, Nakamoto JM, et al: Rapid GDP release from Gsα in patients with gain and loss of function. Nature 371:164–168, 1994.
200. Luttikhuis ME, Wilson LC, Leonard JV, Trembath RC: Characterization of a de novo 43-bp deletion of the Gs alpha gene (GNAS1) in Albright hereditary osteodystrophy. Genomics 21:455–457, 1994.
201. Patten JL, Johns DR, Valle D, et al: Mutation in the gene encoding the stimulatory G protein of adenylate cyclase in Albright's hereditary osteodystrophy. N Engl J Med 322:1412–1419, 1990.
202. Weinstein LS, Gejman PV, Friedman E, et al: Mutations of the Gs alpha-subunit gene in Albright hereditary osteodystrophy detected by denaturing gradient gel electrophoresis. Proc Natl Acad Sci USA 87:8287–8290, 1990.
203. Miric A, Vechio JD, Levine MA: Heterogeneous mutations in the gene encoding the alpha subunit of the stimulatory G protein of adenylyl cyclase in Albright hereditary osteodystrophy. J Clin Endocrinol Metab 76: 1560–1568, 1993.
204. Schwindinger WF, Miric A, Zimmerman D, Levine MA: A novel Gsα mutant in a patient with Albright hereditary osteodystrophy uncouples cell surface receptors from adenylyl cyclase. J Biol Chem 269:25387–25391, 1994.
205. Farfel Z, Iiri T, Shapira H, et al: Pseudohypoparathyroidism, a novel mutation in the betagamma-contact region of Gs alpha impairs receptor stimulation. J Biol Chem 271:19653–19655, 1996.
206. Shapira H, Mouallem M, Shapiro MS, et al: Pseudohypoparathyroidism type Ia: Two new heterozygous frameshift mutations in exons 5 and 10 of the Gs alpha gene. Hum Genet 97:73–75, 1996.
207. Fischer JA, Egert F, Werder E, Born W: An inherited mutation associated with functional deficiency of the alpha-subunit of the guanine nucleotide–binding protein Gs in pseudo- and pseudopseudohypoparathyroidism. J Clin Endocrinol Metab 83:935–938, 1998.
208. Jan de Beur SM, Deng Z, Ding CL, Levine MA: Amplification of the GC-rich exon 1 of GNAS1 and identification of three novel nonsense mutations in Albright's hereditary osteodystrophy. Endocrine Society, June 24–27, 1998, New Orleans, LA.
209. Nakamoto JM, Sandstrom AT, Brickman AS, et al: Pseudohypoparathyroidism type Ia from maternal but not paternal transmission of a Gs alpha gene mutation. Am J Med Genet 77:261–267, 1998.
210. Warner DR, Weng G, Yu S, et al: A novel mutation in the switch 3 region of Gs alpha in a patient with Albright hereditary osteodystrophy impairs GDP binding and receptor activation. J Biol Chem 273:23976–23983, 1998.
211. Ahmed SF, Dixon PH, Bonthron DT, et al: GNAS1 mutational analysis in pseudohypoparathyroidism. Clin Endocrinol (Oxf) 49:525–531, 1998.
212. Weinstein LS, Gejman PV, de Mazancourt P, et al: A heterozygous 4-bp deletion mutation in the $G_s\alpha$ gene (GNAS1) in a patient with Albright hereditary osteodystrophy. Genomics 13:1319–1321, 1992.
213. Yu D, Yu S, Schuster V, et al: Identification of two novel deletion mutations within the Gs alpha gene (GNAS1) in Albright hereditary osteodystrophy. J Clin Endocrinol Metab 84:3254–3259, 1999.
214. Yu S, Yu D, Hainline BE, et al: A deletion hot-spot in exon 7 of the Gs alpha gene (GNAS1) in patients with Albright hereditary osteodystrophy. Hum Mol Genet 4:2001–2002, 1995.
215. Carter A, Bardin C, Collins R, et al: Reduced expression of multiple forms of the alpha subunit of the stimulatory GTP-binding protein in pseudohypoparathyroidism type Ia. Proc Natl Acad Sci USA 84:7266–7269, 1987.
216. Mallet E, Carayon P, Amr S, et al: Coupling defect of thyrotropin receptor and adenylate cyclase in a pseudohypoparathyroid patient. J Clin Endocrinol Metab 54:1028–1032, 1982.
217. Marx SJ, Hershman JM, Aurbach GD: Thyroid dysfunction in pseudohypoparathyroidism. J Clin Endocrinol Metab 33:822–828, 1971.
218. Werder EA, Illig R, Bernasconi S, et al: Excessive thyrotropin-releasing hormone in pseudohypoparathyroidism. Pediatr Res 9:12–16, 1975.
219. Wolfsdorf JI, Rosenfield RL, Fang VS, et al: Partial gonadotrophin-resistance in pseudohypoparathyroidism. Acta Endocrinol 88:321–328, 1978.
220. Levine MA, Downs RW Jr, Moses AM, et al: Resistance to multiple hormones in patients with pseudohypoparathyroidism. Association with deficient activity of guanine nucleotide regulatory protein. Am J Med 74:545–556, 1983.
221. Tsai KS, Chang CC, Wu DJ, et al: Deficient erythrocyte membrane Gs alpha activity and resistance to trophic hormones of multiple endocrine organs in two cases of pseudohypoparathyroidism. Taiwan I Hsueh Hui Tsa Chih 88:450–455, 1989.
222. Levine MA, Jap TS, Hung W. Infantile hypothyroidism in two sibs: An unusual presentation of pseudohypoparathyroidism type Ia. J Pediatr 107:919–922, 1985.
223. Weisman Y, Golander A, Spirer Z, Farfel Z: Pseudohypoparathyroidism type Ia presenting as congenital hypothyroidism. J Pediatr 107:413–415, 1985.
224. Yokoro S, Matsuo M, Ohtsuka T, Ohzeki T: Hyperthyrotropinemia in a neonate with normal thyroid hormone levels: The earliest diagnostic clue for pseudohypoparathyroidism. Biol Neonate 58:69–72, 1990.
225. Downs RW Jr, Levine MA, Drezner MK, et al: Deficient adenylate cyclase regulatory protein in renal membranes from a patient with pseudohypoparathyroidism. J Clin Invest 71:231–235, 1983.
226. Carlson HE, Brickman AS, Bottazzo CF: Prolactin deficiency in pseudohypoparathyroidism. N Engl J Med 296:140–144, 1977.
227. Carel JC, Le Stunff C, Condamine L, et al: Resistance to the lipolytic action of epinephrine: A new feature of protein Gs deficiency. J Clin Endocrinol Metab 84:4127–4131, 1999.
228. Kaartinen JM, Kaar ML, Ohisalo JJ: Defective stimulation of adipocyte adenylate cyclase, blunted lipolysis, and obesity in pseudohypoparathyroidism 1a. Pediatr Res 35:594–597, 1994.
229. Brickman AS, Carlson HE, Levin SR: Responses to glucagon infusion in pseudohypoparathyroidism. J Clin Endocrinol Metab 63:1354–1360, 1986.
230. Moses AM, Weinstock RS, Levine MA, Breslau NA: Evidence for normal antidiuretic responses to endogenous and exogenous arginine vasopressin in patients with guanine nucleotide–binding stimulatory protein-deficient pseudohypoparathyroidism. J Clin Endocrinol Metab 62:221–224, 1986.
231. Ridderskamp P, Schlaghecke R: Pseudohypoparathyroidism and adrenal cortex insufficiency: A case of multiple endocrinopathy due to peripheral hormone resistance. Klin Wochenschr 68:927–931, 1990.
232. Weinstock RS, Wright HN, Spiegel AM, et al: Olfactory dysfunction in humans with deficient guanine nucleotide–binding protein. Nature 322:635–636, 1986.
233. Henkin RI: Impairment of olfaction and of the tastes of sour and bitter in pseudohypoparathyroidism. J Clin Endocrinol Metab 28:624–624, 1968.
234. Koch T, Lehnhardt E, Bottinger H, et al: Sensorineural hearing loss owing to deficient G proteins in patients with pseudohypoparathyroidism: Results of a multicentre study. Eur J Clin Invest 20:416–421, 1990.

235. Lerea CL, Somers DE, Hurley JB, et al: Identification of specific transducin alpha subunits in retinal rod and cone photoreceptors. Science 234:77–80, 1986.
236. Lochrie MA, Hurley JB, Simon MI: Sequence of the alpha subunit of photoreceptor G protein: Homologies between transducin, ras, and elongation factors. Science 228:96–99, 1985.
237. Jones DT, Reed RR: Golf: An olfactory neuron–specific G protein involved in odorant signal transduction. Science 244:790–795, 1989.
238. McLaughlin SK, McKinnon PJ, Margolskee RF: Gustducin is a taste-cell specific G protein closely related to the transducins. Nature 357:563–568, 1992.
239. Farfel Z, Friedman E: Mental deficiency in pseudohypoparathyroidism type I is associated with Ns-protein deficiency. Ann Intern Med 105:197–199, 1986.
240. Faull CM, Welbury RR, Paul B, Kendall Taylor P: Pseudohypoparathyroidism: Its phenotypic variability and associated disorders in a large family. Q J Med 78:251–264, 1991.
241. Fitch N: Albright's hereditary osteodystrophy: A review. Am J Med Genet 11:11–29, 1982.
242. Croft LK, Witkop CJ, Glas JE: Pseudohypoparathyroidism. Oral Surg Oral Med Oral Pathol 20:758–770, 1965.
243. Poznanski AK, Werder EA, Giedion A: The pattern of shortening of the bones of the hand in PHP and PPHP—A comparison with brachydactyly E, Turner syndrome, and acrodysostosis. Radiology 123:707–718, 1977.
244. Graudal N, Galloe A, Christensen H, Olesen K: The pattern of shortened hand and foot bones in D- and E-brachydactyly and pseudohypoparathyroidism/pseudopseudohypoparathyroidism. Rofo Fortschr Geb. Rontgenstr Neven Bildgeb Verfahr 148:460–462, 1988.
245. Steinbach HL, Rudhe U, Jonsson M, et al: Evolution of skeletal lesions in pseudohypoparathyroidism. Radiology 85:670–676, 1965.
246. Alam SM, Kelly W: Spinal cord compression associated with pseudohypoparathyroidism. J R Soc Med 83:50–51, 1990.
247. Prendiville JS, Lucky AW, Mallory SB, et al: Osteoma cutis as a presenting sign of pseudohypoparathyroidism. Pediatr Dermatol 9:11–18, 1992.
248. Izraeli S, Metzker A, Horev G, et al: Albright hereditary osteodystrophy with hypothyroidism, normocalcemia, and normal Gs protein activity. Am J Med 43:764–767, 1992.
249. Kaplan FS, Craver R, MacEwen GD, et al: Progressive osseous heteroplasia: A distinct developmental disorder of heterotopic ossification. Two new case reports and follow-up of three previously reported cases. J Bone Joint Surg [Am] 76:425–436, 1994.
250. Moses AM, Rao KJ, Coulson R, Miller R: Parathyroid hormone deficiency with Albright's hereditary osteodystrophy. J Clin Endocrinol Metab 39:496–500, 1974.
251. Isozaki O, Sato K, Tsushima T, et al: A patient of short stature with idiopathic hypoparathyroidism, round face and metacarpal signs. Endocr J 31:363–367, 1984.
252. Shapira H, Friedman E, Mouallem M, Farfel Z: Familial Albright's hereditary osteodystrophy with hypoparathyroidism: Normal structural Gs alpha gene. J Clin Endocrinol Metab 81:1660–1662, 1996.
253. Le Roith D, Burshell AC, Ilia R, Glick SM: Short metacarpal in a patient with idiopathic hypoparathyroidism. Isr J Med Sci 15:460–461, 1979.
254. Moses AM, Notman DD: Albright's osteodystrophy in a patient with renal hypercalciuria. J Clin Endocrinol Metab 49:794–797, 1979.
255. Sasaki H, Tsutsu N, Asano T, et al: Co-existing primary hyperparathyroidism and Albright's hereditary osteodystrophy—an unusual association. Postgrad Med J 61:153–155, 1985.
256. Hedeland H, Berntorp K, Arheden K, Kristoffersson U: Pseudohypoparathyroidism type I and Albright's hereditary osteodystrophy with a proximal 15q chromosomal deletion in mother and daughter. Clin Genet 42:129–134, 1992.
257. Wilson LC, Leverton K, Oude Luttikhuis ME, et al: Brachydactyly and mental retardation: An Albright hereditary osteodystrophy–like syndrome localized to 2q37. Am J Hum Genet 56:400–407, 1995.
258. Phelan MC, Rogers RC, Clarkson KB, et al: Albright hereditary osteodystrophy and del(2)(q37.3) in four unrelated individuals. Am J Med Genet 58:1–7, 1995.
259. Levis MJ, Bourne HR: Activation of the alpha subunit of Gs in intact cells alters its abundance, rate of degradation, and membrane avidity. J Cell Biol 119:1297–1307, 1992.
260. Levine MA: Pseudohypoparathyroidism. *In* Bilezikian JP, Raisz LG, Rodan GA (eds): Principles of Bone Biology. San Diego, Academic Press, 1996, pp 853–876.
261. Wilson LC, Oude Luttikhuis ME, Clayton PT, et al: Parental origin of Gs alpha gene mutations in Albright's hereditary osteodystrophy. J Med Genet 31:835–839, 1994.
262. Davies SJ, Hughes HE: Imprinting in Albright's hereditary osteodystrophy. J Med Genet 30:101–103, 1993.
263. Campbell R, Gosden CM, Bonthron DT: Parental origin of transcription from the human GNAS1 gene. J Med Genet 31:607–614, 1994.
264. Yu S, Yu D, Lee E, et al: Variable and tissue-specific hormone resistance in heterotrimeric Gs protein alpha-subunit (Gs alpha) knockout mice is due to tissue-specific imprinting of the Gs alpha gene. Proc Natl Acad Sci USA 95:8715–8720, 1998.
265. Schwindinger WF, Lawler AM, Gearhart JD, Levine MA: A murine model of Albright hereditary osteodystrophy. Endocrine Society, June 24–27, 1998, New Orleans, LA.
266. Schwindinger WF, Francomano CA, Levine MA: Identification of a mutation in the gene encoding the alpha subunit of the stimulatory G protein of adenylyl cyclase in McCune-Albright syndrome. Proc Natl Acad Sci USA 89:5152–5156, 1992.
267. Weinstein LS, Shenker A, Gejman PV, et al: Activating mutations of the stimulatory G protein in the McCune-Albright syndrome. N Engl J Med 325:1688–1695, 1991.
268. Silve C, Santora A, Breslau N, et al: Selective resistance to parathyroid hormone in cultured skin fibroblasts from pateints with pseudohypoparathyroidism type 1b. J Clin Endocrinol Metab 62:640–644, 1986.
269. Kidd GS, Schaaf M, Adler RA, et al: Skeletal responsiveness in pseudohypoparathyroidism: A spectrum of clinical disease. Am J Med 68:772–781, 1980.
270. Silve C, Suarez F, el Hessni A, et al: The resistance to parathyroid hormone of fibroblasts from some patients with type 1b pseudohypoparathyroidism is reversible with dexamethasone. J Clin Endocrinol Metab 71:631–638, 1990.
271. Suarez F, Lebrun JJ, Lecossier D, et al: Expression and modulation of the parathyroid hormone (PTH)/PTH–related peptide receptor messenger ribonucleic acid in skin fibroblasts from patients with type Ib pseudohypoparathyroidism. J Clin Endocrinol Metab 80:965–970, 1995.
272. Schipani E, Weinstein LS, Bergwitz C, et al: Pseudohypoparathyroidism type Ib is not caused by mutations in the coding exons of the human parathyroid hormone (PTH)/PTH–related peptide receptor gene. J Clin Endocrinol Metab 80:1611–1621, 1995.
273. Bettoun JD, Minagawa M, Kwan MY, et al: Cloning and characterization of the promoter regions of the human parathyroid hormone (PTH)/PTH–related peptide receptor gene: Analysis of deoxyribonucleic acid from normal subjects and patients with pseudohypoparathyroidism type 1b. J Clin Endocrinol Metab 82:1031–1040, 1997.
274. Fukumoto S, Suzawa M, Takeuchi Y, et al: Absence of mutations in parathyroid hormone (PTH)/PTH–related protein receptor complementary deoxyribonucleic acid in patients with pseudohypoparathyroidism type Ib. J Clin Endocrinol Metab 81:2554–2558, 1996.
275. Lanske B, Karaplis AC, Lee K, et al: PTH/PTHrP receptor in early development and Indian hedgehog–regulated bone growth. Science 273:663–666, 1996.
276. Jobert AS, Zhang P, Couvineau A, et al: Absence of functional receptors for parathyroid hormone and parathyroid hormone–related peptide in Blomstrand chondrodysplasia. J Clin Invest 102:34–40, 1998.
277. Allen DB, Friedman AL, Greer FR, Chesney RW: Hypomagnesemia masking the appearance of elevated parathyroid hormone concentrations in familial pseudohypoparathyroidism. Am J Med Genet 31:153–158, 1988.
278. Winter JSD, Hughes IA: Familial pseudohypoparathyroidism without somatic anomalies. Can Med Assoc J 123:26–31, 1980.
279. Juppner H, Schipani E, Bastepe M, et al: The gene responsible for pseudohypoparathyroidism type Ib is paternally imprinted and maps in four unrelated kindreds to chromosome 20q13.3. Proc Natl Acad Sci USA 95:11798–11803, 1998.
280. Farfel Z, Brothers VM, Brickman AS, et al: Pseudohypoparathyroidism: Inheritance of deficient receptor-cyclase coupling activity. Proc Natl Acad Sci USA 78:3098–3102, 1981.
281. Barrett D, Breslau NA, Wax MB: et al: New form of pseudohypoparathyroidism with abnormal catalytic adenylate cyclase. Am J Physiol 257:E277–E283, 1989.
282. Van Dop C: Pseudohypoparathyroidism: Clinical and molecular aspects. Semin Nephrol 9:168–178, 1989.
283. Kruse K, Kracht U, Wohlfart K, et al: Biochemical markers of bone turnover, intact serum parathyroid hormone and renal calcium excretion in patients with pseudohypoparathyroidism and hypoparathyroidism before and during vitamin D treatment. Eur J Pediatr 148:535–539, 1989.
284. Rao DS, Parfitt AM, Kleerekoper M, et al: Dissociation between the effects of endogenous parathyroid hormone on adenosine 3′, 5′-monophosphate generation and phosphate reabsorption in hypocalcemia due to vitamin D depletion: An acquired disorder resembling pseudohypoparathyroidism type II. J Clin Endocrinol Metab 61:285–290, 1985.
285. de Deuxchaisnes CN, Fischer JA, Dambacher MA, et al: Dissociation of parathyroid hormone bioactivity and immunoreactivity in pseudohypoparathyroidism type I. J Clin Endocrinol Metab 53:1105–1109, 1981.
286. Bradbeer JN, Dunham J, Fischer JA, et al: The metatarsal cytochemical bioassay of parathyroid hormone: Validation, specificity, and application to the study of pseudohypoparathyroidism type I. J Clin Endocrinol Metab 67:1237–1243, 1988.
287. Loveridge N, Fischer JA, Nagant de Deuxchaisnes C, et al: Inhibition of cytochemical bioactivity of parathyroid hormone by plasma in pseudohypoparathyroidism type I. J Clin Endocrinol Metab 54:1274–1275, 1982.
288. Mitchell J, Goltzman D: Examination of circulating parathyroid hormone in pseudohypoparathyroidism. J Clin Endocrinol Metab 61:328–334, 1985.
289. John MR, Goodman WG, Gao P, et al: A novel immunoradiometric assay detects full-length human PTH but not amino-terminally truncated fragments: Implications for PTH measurements in renal failure. J Clin Endocrinol Metab 84:4287–4290, 1999.
290. Tsang RC, Venkataraman P, Ho M, et al: The development of pseudohypoparathyroidism. Am J Dis Child 138:654–658, 1984.
291. Attanasio R, Curcio T, Giusti M, et al: Pseudohypoparathyroidism. A case report with low immunoreactive parathyroid hormone and multiple endocrine dysfunctions. Minerva Endocrinol 11:267–273, 1986.
292. Litvin Y, Rosler A, Bloom RA: Extensive cerebral calcification in hypoparathyroidism. Neuroradiology 21:271, 1981.
293. Sachs C, Sjoberg HE, Ericson K: Basal ganglia calcifications on CT: Relation to hypoparathyroidism. Neurology 32:779–782, 1982.
294. Korn-Lubetzki I, Rubinger D, Siew F: Visualization of basal ganglion calcification by cranial computed tomography in a patient with pseudohypoparathyroidism. Isr J Med Sci 16:40–41, 1980.
295. Pearson DWM, Durward WF, Fogelman I, et al: Pseudohypoparathyroidism presenting as severe Parkinsonism. Postgrad Med J 57:445–447, 1981.
296. Miano A, Casadel G, Biasini G: Cardiac failure in pseudohypoparathyroidism. Helv Paediatr Acta 36:191–192, 1981.
297. Cavallo A, Meyer WJ III, Bodensteiner JB, Chesson AL: Spinal cord compression: An unusual manifestation of pseudohypoparathyroidism. Am J Dis Child 134:706–707, 1980.
298. Breslau NA, Notman D, Canterbury JM, Moses AM: Studies on the attainment of normocalcemia in patients with pseudohypoparathyroidism. Am J Med 68:856–860, 1980.
299. Mallette LE: Synthetic human parathyroid hormone 1–34 fragment for diagnostic testing. Ann Intern Med 109:800–804, 1988.
300. McElduff A, Lissner D, Wilkinson M, et al: A 6-hour human parathyroid hormone (1–34) infusion protocol: Studies in normal and hypoparathyroid subjects. Calcif Tissue Int 41:267–273, 1987.

301. Furlong TJ, Seshadri MS, Wilkinson MR, et al: Clinical experiences with human parathyroid hormone 1–34. Aust N Z J Med 16:794–798, 1986.
302. Mallette LE, Kirkland JL, Gagel RF, et al: Synthetic human parathyroid hormone-(1–34) for the study of pseudohypoparathyroidism. J Clin Endocrinol Metab 67:964–972, 1988.
303. Rude RK, Oldham SB, Singer FR: Functional hypoparathyroidism and parathyroid hormone end-organ resistance in human magnesium deficiency. Clin Endocrinol 5:209–224, 1976.
304. Slatopolsky E, Mercado A, Morrison A, et al: Inhibitory effects of hypomagnesemia on the renal action of parathyroid hormone. J Clin Invest 58:1273–1279, 1976.
305. Beck N, Davis BB: Impaired renal response to parathyroid hormone in potassium depletion. Am J Physiol 228:179–183, 1975.
306. Beck N, Kim HP, Kim KS: Effect of metabolic acidosis on renal action of parathyroid hormone. Am J Physiol 228:1483–1488, 1975.
307. Walton RJ, Bijvoet OLM: Nomogram for derivation of renal threshold phosphate concentration. Lancet 309:310; 1975.
308. Sohn HE, Furukawa Y, Yumita S, et al: Effect of synthetic 1–34 fragment of human parathyroid hormone on plasma adenosine 3′,5′-monophosphate (cAMP) concentrations and the diagnostic criteria based on the plasma cAMP response in Ellsworth-Howard test. Endocr J 31:33–40, 1984.
309. Stirling HF, Darling JA, Barr DG: Plasma cyclic AMP response to intravenous parathyroid hormone in pseudohypoparathyroidism. Acta Paediatr Scand 80:333–338, 1991.
310. Miura R, Yumita S, Yoshinaga K, Furukawa Y: Response of plasma 1,25-dihydroxyvitamin D in the human PTH(1–34) infusion test: An improved index for the diagnosis of idiopathic hypoparathyroidism and pseudohypoparathyroidism. Calcif Tissue Int 46:309–313, 1990.
311. Lebowitz MR, Moses AM: Hypocalcemia. Semin Nephrol 12:146–158, 1992.
312. Litvak J, Moldawer MP, Forbes AP, Henneman PH: Hypocalcemic hypercalciuria during vitamin D and dihydrotachysterol therapy of hypoparathyroidism. J Clin Endocrinol Metab 18:246–252, 1958.
313. Yamamoto M, Takuwa Y, Masuko S, Ogata E: Effects of endogenous and exogenous parathyroid hormone on tubular reabsorption of calcium in pseudohypoparathyroidism. J Clin Endocrinol Metab 66:618–625, 1988.
314. Kolb FO, Steinbach HL: Pseudohypoparathyroidism with secondary hyperparathyroidism and osteitis fibrosa. J Clin Endocrinol Metab 22:59–64, 1962.
315. Slatopolsky E, Weerts C, Thielan J, et al: Marked suppression of secondary hyperparathyroidism by intravenous administration of 1,25-dihydroxycholecalciferol in uremia patients. J Clin Invest 74:2136–2143, 1984.
316. Shangraw RF: Factors to consider in the selection of a calcium supplement. Public Health Rep (suppl) 104:46–50, 1989.
317. Harvey JA, Zobitz MM, Pak CYC: Dose dependency of calcium absorption: A comparison of calcium carbonate and calcium citrate. J Bone Miner Res 3:253–258, 1988.
318. Komindr S, Schmidt LW, Palmieri GMA: Case report: Oral calcium chloride in hypoparathyroidism refractory to massive doses of calcium carbonate and vitamin D. Am J Med Sci 296:182–184, 1989.
319. Okano K, Furukawa Y, Morii H, Fujita T: Comparative efficacy of various vitamin D metabolites in the treatment of various types of hypoparathyroidism. J Clin Endocrinol Metab 55:238–243, 1982.
320. Breslau NA: Pseudohypoparathyroidism: Current concepts. Am J Med Sci 298:130–140, 1989.
321. Breslau N, Moses AM: Renal calcium reabsorption caused by bicarbonate and by chlorothiazide in patients with hormone resistant (pseudo) hypoparathyroidism. J Clin Endocrinol Metab 46:389–395, 1978.
322. Porter RH, Cox BG, Heaney D, et al: Treatment of hypoparathyroid patients with chlorthalidone. N Engl J Med 298:577–581, 1978.
323. Parfitt AM: The interactions of thiazide diuretics with parathyroid hormone and vitamin D. Studies in patients with hypoparathyroidism. J Clin Invest 51:1879–1888, 1972.
324. Parfitt AM: Thiazide-induced hypercalcemia in vitamin D–treated hypoparathyroidism. Ann Intern Med 77:557–563, 1972.
325. Rosler A, Rabinowitz D: Magnesium-induced reversal of vitamin D resistance in hypoparathyrodisim. Lancet 1:803–805, 1973.
326. Tolloczko T, Woniewics B, Sawicki A, et al: Clinical results of human cultured parathyroid cell allotransplantation in the treatment of surgical hypoparathyroidism. Transplant Proc 28:3545–3546, 1996.
327. Winer KK, Yanovski JA, Cutler Jr GB. Synthetic human parathyroid hormone 1–34 vs calcitriol and calcium in the treatment of hypoparathyroidism. JAMA 276:631–636, 1996.
328. Shenker A, Weinstein LS, Sweet DE, Spiegel AM: An activating Gsα mutation is present in fibrous dysplasia of bone in McCune-Albright syndrome. J Clin Endocrinol Metab 79:750–755, 1994.
329. Shenker A, Weinstein LS, Moran A, et al: Severe endocrine and nonendocrine manifestations of the McCune-Albright syndrome associated with activating mutations of stimulatory G protein GS. J Pediatr 123:509–518, 1993.
330. Levine MA, Schwindinger WF, Downs RW Jr, Moses AM: Pseudohypoparathyroidism: Clinical, biochemical, and molecular features. *In* Bilezikian JP, Marcus R, Levine MA (eds): The Parathyroids: Basic and Clinical Concepts. New York, Raven Press, 1994, pp 781–800.
331. Landis CA, Masters SB, Spada A, et al: GTPase inhibiting mutations activate the alpha chain of Gs and stimulate adenylyl cyclase in human pituitary tumours. Nature 340:692–696, 1989.
332. Lyons J, Landis CA, Griffith H, et al: Two G protein oncogenes in human endocrine tumors. Science 249:655–659, 1990.

Chapter 82

Hereditary Defects in Vitamin D Metabolism and Action

René St-Arnaud ▪ Francis H. Glorieux

Vitamin D is a key regulator of mineral homeostasis and bone development, and perturbation of the vitamin D endocrine system leads to rickets and/or osteomalacia. To gain a complete perspective of the clinical manifestations of genetic anomalies involving vitamin D endocrine function, this chapter will review the mechanisms of bone formation during development and present a short overview of the salient aspects of the vitamin D metabolic pathways. The reader is referred to Chapters 72, 73, and 74 for an in-depth discussion of these topics. The brief notions presented here will lay the groundwork for discussion of the clinical, pathophysiologic, and molecular aspects of hereditary rickets involving the vitamin D endocrine system.

OVERVIEW OF BONE DEVELOPMENT

The coordinated action of three cell types is required for proper development of the skeleton: chondrocytes, which form cartilage; osteoblasts, which form bone; and osteoclasts, which resorb bone. Chondrocytes and osteoblasts share a common mesenchymal origin.[1] Osteoclasts, on the other hand, derive from the hematopoietic lineage.[2]

Bone forms via two mechanisms during embryogenesis: intramembranous bone formation and endochondral bone formation.[3] Intramembranous formation allows growth of the surface of flat bones, as well as thickening of cortical bone, whereas endochondral formation provides for the lengthening of long bones. The major difference between the two is the presence or absence of an intermediate cartilaginous phase. Intramembranous bone formation occurs when mesenchymal precursor cells proliferate and differentiate directly into osteoblasts that produce a mucoprotein matrix, called osteoid, in which collagen fibrils are enmeshed. The osteoblasts then begin to mineralize the osteoid by depositing inorganic crystals of calcium phosphate on, between, and within the collagen fibers, whereupon a primary immature bone tissue called woven bone is formed. This woven bone is characterized by a loosely textured matrix with irregular bundles of small, randomly oriented collagen fibers. The mineral is deposited in roughly spherical clusters of varying size termed calcospherulites. These mineral clusters are associated with small membrane-bound particles termed matrix vesicles.[4] It has been proposed that these matrix vesicles might play an active role in promoting mineralization.[4] Subsequent to its removal by osteoclasts, the woven bone is progressively replaced by mature, lamellar bone. In lamellar bone, the matrix is compact and contains virtually no vesicles. The collagen fibers are long and highly ordered. The crystals of mineral are aligned with their long axis parallel to the collagen fibrils and are initially deposited within holes in the matrix by heterogeneous nucleation.[5] Longer and wider crystals are subsequently formed on and between the fibrils.[5] Lamellar bone is always formed by apposition to an existing surface.

Endochondral bone formation entails the conversion of a cartilaginous template, the "anlage," into bone. Mesenchymal cells condense and differentiate into chondroblasts that secrete the cartilaginous matrix. The chondroblasts embed themselves within the matrix they produce and become chondrocytes. Because of the malleable nature of the cartilaginous matrix, chondrocytes can continue to proliferate in their lacunae. The embryonic anlage, a template of the future bone piece, is avascular. During its early development, a ring of woven bone (the bony collar) is formed by intramembranous ossification in the future midshaft area. This calcified woven bone is then invaded by vascular tissue, and this process of angiogenesis brings to the bone rudiment the precursors of the osteoclastic lineage. The osteoclasts excavate the hematopoietic bone marrow cavity while new osteoblasts are recruited to replace the cartilage scaffold with bone matrix.

At the extremities of long bones (epiphyses), longitudinal growth occurs by a similar process of endochondral bone formation at the growth plates (Fig. 82–1). Four anatomic zones can be distinguished at the epiphysis: the zone of resting cartilage cells, which firmly adheres to the overlying bone; the proliferative zone, where chondroblasts are actively dividing; the hypertrophic zone, composed of larger, vacuolated chondrocytes; and the zone of provisional calcification. Starting within the proliferative zone, growth plate chondrocytes form regular columns known as isogenous groups. The cartilaginous matrix becomes mineralized just below the hypertrophic zone of the growth plate and the chondrocytes then undergo apoptosis.[6] Once calcified, the cartilage matrix is partially resorbed by osteoclasts. After resorption, osteoblasts differentiate to form a layer of woven bone on top of the mineralized cartilage remnants of the longitudinal septa. This phase is the first activation-resorption-formation sequence of remodeling the cartilage into woven bone. The trabeculae that will be formed through this process are known as the primary spongiosa. Further down in the growth plate, this immature bone will undergo subsequent remodeling to replace the woven bone and calcified cartilage remnants with lamellar bone. The mature state of trabecular bone is known as the secondary spongiosa. Essentially, whereas the growth plate is expanded by interstitial growth in the proliferative zone, it becomes replaced by bone on the metaphyseal side. This process results in elongation of the shaft.[3]

RICKETS AND OSTEOMALACIA

The term "rickets" is often used to describe all the skeletal abnormalities associated with defective mineralization in the growing skeleton, but it is more precise to restrict the term to changes in the growth plate and adjacent metaphysis. When mineralization is impaired, the accumulation of unmineralized osteoid at sites other than the growing

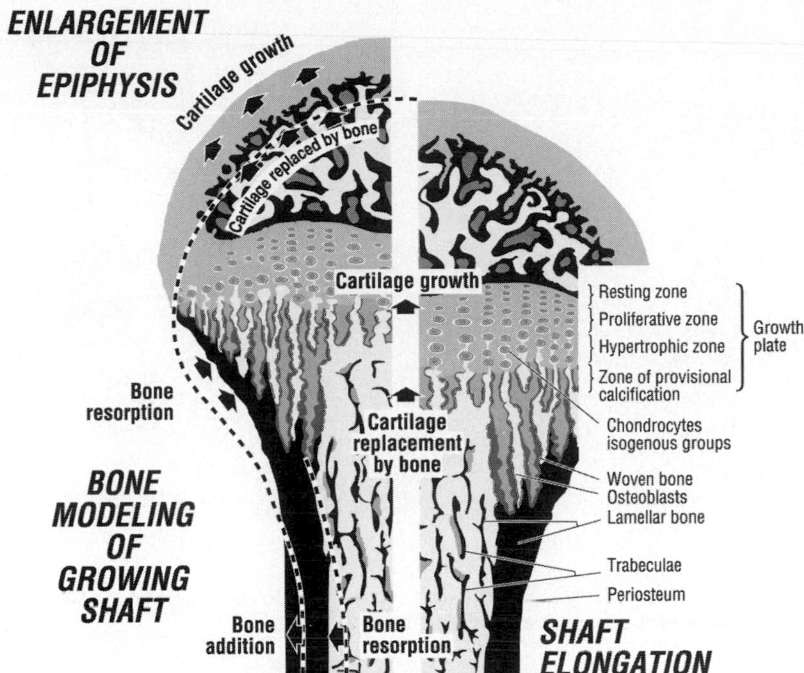

FIGURE 82–1. Endochondral ossification in long bones. Longitudinal bone growth occurs at the epiphyseal growth plate, where chondrocytes appear in regular columns that initially proliferate and progressively hypertrophy. The four anatomic zones of the epiphysis are identified. The mineralized cartilaginous matrix is resorbed by osteoclasts, and osteoblasts differentiate to deposit woven bone on top of the calcified cartilage remnants.

metaphysis should be referred to as osteomalacia, not as rickets. Thus defective mineralization can lead to both rickets and osteomalacia in a growing skeleton, but only to osteomalacia in a mature skeleton.

Rickets is characterized by inadequate calcification of the growth plate and adjacent metaphysis. The impaired mineralization of the growth plate cartilage in the zone of provisional calcification prevents this zone from being resorbed. As cartilage continues to be formed but not resorbed, the growth plate begins to widen. Simultaneously, the trabecular bone directly underneath the cartilage fails to mineralize properly, and vascularization of this tissue becomes aberrant. These defects are accompanied by similar abnormalities in cortical bone leading to the full spectrum of skeletal symptoms associated with the pathology (see below).

OVERVIEW OF VITAMIN D METABOLISM

In humans, 80% of vitamin D requirements can be produced endogenously in the skin upon exposure to ultraviolet light (sunlight). The rest must be acquired through dietary sources such as fish, plants, and grains.[7] After exposure to sunlight, both plants and animals are able to synthesize vitamin D. Vitamin D_2 is generated in yeast and plants; vitamin D_3 is produced in fish and mammals. The slight differences in the chemical structure of the two compounds do not affect function or metabolism. The generic term vitamin D (without subscript) will be used hereafter.

Ultraviolet B photons penetrate the epidermis and induce photolysis of 7-dehydrocholesterol into previtamin D, which rapidly becomes a more thermodynamically stable molecule, vitamin D. Vitamin D then exits the keratinocyte cells and enters the dermal capillary bed, where it becomes bound to the vitamin D–binding protein DBP. Once associated with DBP in the circulation, vitamin D is transported to the liver where the enzyme vitamin D–25-hydroxylase (*CYP27*) adds a hydroxyl group on carbon 25 to produce 25-hydroxyvitamin D, or 25(OH)D. The 25(OH)D metabolite also circulates in the blood stream bound to DBP. It is an abundant, but *relatively* inactive vitamin D metabolite. Its circulating concentration provides the most readily available evaluation of the vitamin D status in a given individual. 25(OH)D must be further hydroxylated at a different site in the convoluted and straight portions of the proximal kidney tubule to gain hormonal bioactivity. Hydroxylation at position 1α by the mitochondrial cytochrome P-450 enzyme 25-hydroxyvitamin D–1α-hydroxylase (*CYP27B1* or P-450c1α) converts 25(OH)D to 1α,25-dihydroxyvitamin D, or $1,25(OH)_2D$, the active, hormonal form of vitamin D that plays an essential role in mineral homeostasis, bone growth, and cellular differentiation.[7]

Upon reaching a target tissue, $1,25(OH)_2D$ binds a specific receptor (vitamin D receptor [VDR]) that is a member of the nuclear hormone receptor superfamily.[8] The VDR is considered a class II nuclear hormone receptor because it needs to form a heterodimer with the retinoid X receptor (RXR) to bind specific DNA sequence elements with high affinity.[9] These target sequences are termed vitamin D response elements, and the best characterized of these binding sites consist of two tandemly repeated hexanucleotide sequences separated by 3 bp.[8] Transcriptional coactivators[10, 11] and components of the basal transcriptional machinery[12, 13] interact with the liganded, DNA-bound, VDR-RXR heterodimer to activate transcription of the vitamin D target genes responsible for carrying out the physiologic actions of $1,25(OH)_2D$.

It should be noted that $1,25(OH)_2D$ can also induce rapid membrane responses in certain target cells.[7] These responses, which involve ionic transport across membranes or the stimulation of particular signal transduction pathways, have been termed "nongenomic" effects of vitamin D. It is unclear whether the nuclear VDR or a distinct, specific receptor is involved in these types of responses. Their physiologic significance remains uncertain.

VITAMIN D DEFICIENCY RICKETS

It is evident from the brief overview presented above that vitamin D metabolism can be affected at several levels: inadequate exposure to sunlight, inadequate dietary intake, malabsorption of dietary vitamin D, impaired hepatic 25-hydroxylation, defects in renal 1α-hydroxylation, or defects in receptor function (Fig. 82–2). Of these, only the last two types of defects have been associated with specific mutations in genes involved in regulating vitamin D metabolism and action and will be discussed in this chapter. Detailed recent reviews on nonhereditary disorders of the vitamin D endocrine system have been published recently[7] (see also Chapters 86 and 87).

The prime metabolic consequence of vitamin D deficiency is reduced net intestinal absorption of calcium.[7] Calcium malabsorption leads to a fall in plasma calcium, secondary hyperparathyroidism, reduced renal tubular reabsorption of phosphate, hypophosphatemia, and thus a reduction in the calcium × phosphate product. Eventually, deposition of mineral in osteoid is impaired because the supply of

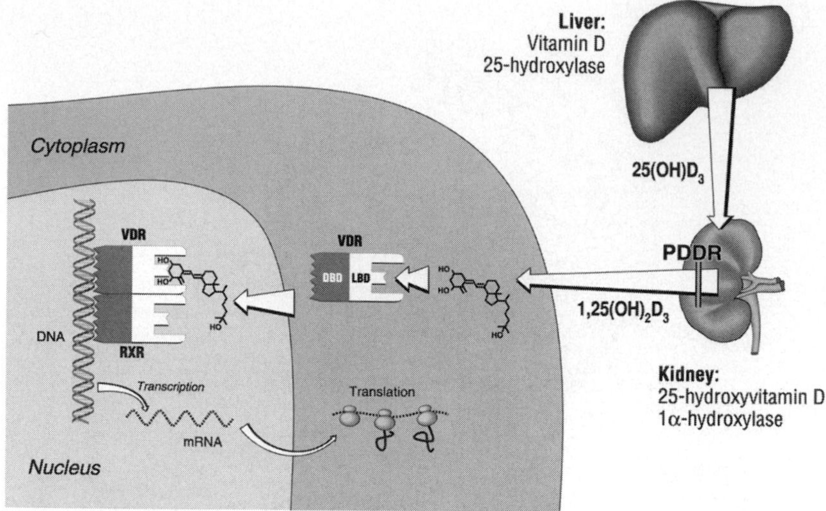

FIGURE 82–2. Schematic representation of the main steps of the vitamin D biosynthetic pathway, where genetic aberrations may lead to rickets and osteomalacia. The renal defect in pseudo–vitamin D deficiency rickets (PDDR) is indicated by the break in the 1,25-dihydroxyvitamin D_3 *(arrow)* arising in the kidney. The mutation leads to insufficient synthesis of 1,25-dihydroxyvitamin D. The *left* part of the figure represents a target cell where schematic coupling of the ligand to its receptor (vitamin D receptor [VDR]) takes place in the cytosol or, more likely, in the nucleus. The VDR then heterodimerizes with the retinoid X receptor (RXR). For ease of representation, the RXR ligand (9-*cis*-retinoic acid) is not depicted. The complex then binds to DNA. Various mutations affecting either of the two VDR domains (DBD, DNA-binding domain; LBD, ligand-binding domain) cause hereditary vitamin D–resistant rickets.

the relevant ions is reduced. The impaired mineralization triggers development of the rachitic and/or osteomalacic phenotype.

Nomenclature

After the description by Albright and colleagues of the first case of "rickets resistant to vitamin D,"[14] which turned out to be the hypophosphatemic type, further clinical observations established that other cases of vitamin D–resistant rickets differed significantly from hypophosphatemic rickets in their clinical and biologic symptoms and response to therapy. Studies of Prader et al. clearly identified this disease as a new hereditary form, which they termed "pseudo-deficiency rickets."[15] Over the years, the nomenclature and terminology was modified to "vitamin D–dependent rickets type I "(VDD I) and then to "pseudovitamin D–deficiency rickets." Recent characterization of the molecular defects responsible for the disease (see below) has started a new onslaught on the vocabulary, and the term "1α-hydroxylase deficiency" has been proposed.[16] Although attractive, this newly introduced nomenclature may prove confusing if the full name of the enzyme, 25-hydroxyvitamin D–1α-hydroxylase, is not specified (steroid hydroxylases abound and naming only the modified carbon without identifying the substrate is imprecise). For this reason, we believe it more appropriate to return to the original terminology of Prader and use the term pseudo–vitamin D deficiency rickets (PDDR) to describe this form of rickets.

In 1978, Brooks et al. described a patient with rickets who exhibited hypocalcemia despite markedly increased serum levels of $1,25(OH)_2D$.[17] The authors suggested that the rickets was due to impaired responsiveness of target organs to $1,25(OH)_2D$ and named this disease vitamin D–dependent rickets type II (VDD II) to distinguish it from the pathology described by Prader,[15] which was then termed VDD I (see above). Since the original report, many cases of patients with end-organ resistance to $1,25(OH)_2D$ have been described in the literature, and the molecular etiology of the disease is now well understood (see below). A number of different terms have been used through the years to describe this syndrome: vitamin D–dependent rickets type II (VDD II or VDDR-II), calcitriol-resistant rickets, vitamin D–resistant rickets, and hereditary hypocalcemic vitamin D–resistant rickets. We agree with the authors of recent reviews on the subject[18] and prefer the term hereditary vitamin D–resistant rickets (HVDRR) to describe this syndrome caused by genetic resistance to vitamin D.

Clinical Features of Pseudo–Vitamin D Deficiency Rickets

The clinical symptoms of PDDR are similar to those of common vitamin D deficiency rickets, including failure to thrive, hypotonia, and growth retardation. Affected babies lay supine because of severe muscle weakness and bone pain. At this age, gross skeletal deformities are rare; however, if diagnosis and treatment are delayed, severe deformities of the spine and long bones occur, together with generalized muscle weakness simulating myopathy. Motor problems translate into regression in head control and the ability to stand. In some patients the initial event is generalized convulsions, tremulations, Bravais-jacksonian fits, or tetany. Pathologic fractures may occur (Fig. 82–3). The onset in most cases takes place early during the third trimester of life; the patients look healthy at birth.

Physical examination reveals a small, hypotonic child with a wide anterior fontanelle, frontal bossing, and frequent craniotabes (easy depression of the softened parieto-occipital region). Tooth eruption is delayed, and erupted teeth show evidence of enamel hypoplasia. A rachitic rosary is either visible or palpable. In limbs, widening of the metaphyseal areas is evidenced by enlargement of the wrists and ankles, and long bone diaphyses show a variable degree of deformity (bowing). Deformities of the thorax may interfere with ventilation and predispose to pulmonary infection; infant death by pulmonary infection was not infrequent in the past when the diagnosis was either missed (confused with a neurologic or respiratory condition) or made too late. The Chvostek sign (twitching of the upper lip upon light finger tapping of the facial nerve) reflects nerve irritability, a consequence of a rapid fall in serum calcium.

The x-ray features include diffuse osteopenia (mild to severe hypomineralization of the skeleton) and classic rachitic metaphyseal changes: fraying, cupping, widening, and fuzziness of the zone of provisional calcification immediately under the growth plate (see Fig. 82–3). These changes are seen better and detected earlier in the most active growth plates, namely, the distal ends of the ulna and femur and the proximal and distal ends of the tibia. Changes in the diaphyses may not be evident when metaphyseal changes are first detected. However, they will appear a few weeks later as rarefaction, coarse trabeculation, cortical thinning, and subperiosteal erosion. Looser-Milkman pseudofractures and curvature of the shafts of long bones may be observed, especially in children older than 1 to 2 years.

Hypocalcemia is the main biochemical feature in PDDR. A rapid decrease in serum calcium concentration may give rise to tetany and convulsions, which may occur before any radiologic evidence of rickets. Prolonged hypocalcemia triggers secondary hyperparathyroidism and hyperaminoaciduria.[19] Urinary calcium excretion is very low, whereas fecal calcium is high as a consequence of impaired intestinal calcium absorption. Elevated urinary cyclic adenosine monophosphate is not a consistent finding, and normal values have been measured in patients with PDDR despite high circulating parathyroid hormone levels.[20]

Serum phosphate concentrations may be normal or low. When reduced, the hypophosphatemia is usually of a lesser degree than that measured in X-linked hypophosphatemic rickets.[7] It results from the

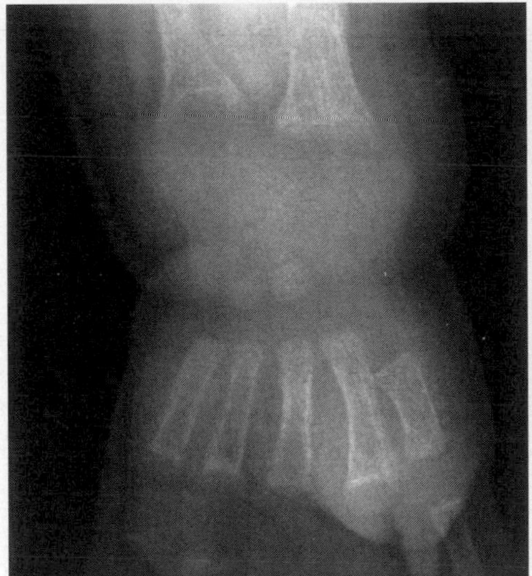
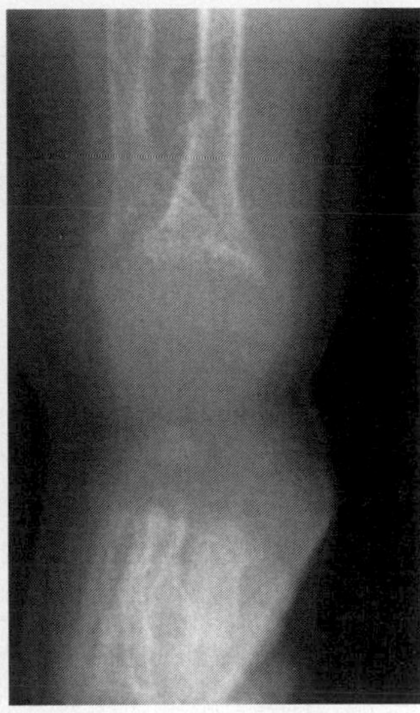

FIGURE 82–3. Radiographs of the wrist of a 19-month-old boy with pseudo–vitamin D deficiency rickets at diagnosis. Severe rickets and demineralization are evident. Pronounced hypocalcemia and secondary hyperparathyroidism were documented, the latter causing a metaphyseal pseudofracture clearly seen on the lateral view, *right.*

combination of impaired intestinal absorption and increased urinary loss induced by the secondary hyperparathyroidism. Serum alkaline phosphatase activity is consistently elevated, and its increase precedes the appearance of clinical symptoms.

Patients with PDDR have normal serum levels of 25(OH)D after exposure to sunlight or oral intake of small doses of vitamin D; concentrations increase if higher doses are given.[20] Circulating levels of 24,25-dihydroxyvitamin D, or 24,25(OH)$_2$D (see Chapter 72), are normal and correlate with those of 25(OH)D.[21] Serum levels of 1,25(OH)$_2$D are low in untreated patients.[20, 22] This condition is evident immediately after birth, months before any clinical evidence of rickets appears. Even when patients are treated with high enough doses of vitamin D to cause major increases in circulating levels of 25(OH)D, the blood concentration of 1,25(OH)$_2$D does not reach the normal range. These characteristic features of serum vitamin D metabolites have provided key insight into the pathogenesis of PDDR (discussed below).

Clinical Features of Hereditary Vitamin D–Resistant Rickets

Many of the clinical findings in patients with HVDRR are identical to those described for patients with PDDR, including bone pain, muscle weakness, hypotonia, and occasional convulsions.[18] Children are often growth retarded, and hypoplasia of the teeth is observed. The radiologic features of rickets are present. A major difference is that many children with HVDRR have sparse body hair and some have total scalp and body alopecia (Fig. 82–4), sometimes even including the eyebrows and eyelashes. Hair loss may be evident at birth or occur during the first months of life. Patients with alopecia generally have more severe resistance to vitamin D. In families with a prior history of the disease, the absence of scalp hair in newborns can provide initial diagnostic clues to HVDRR. The lack of 1,25(OH)$_2$D action at a critical stage of hair follicle development is the hypothesized cause of alopecia, but the precise mechanism remains unknown.

Serum biochemistry reveals low concentrations of calcium and phosphate and elevated alkaline phosphatase activity. Secondary hyperparathyroidism with elevated circulating parathyroid hormone is measurable. The key difference concerns circulating levels of vitamin D metabolites. 25(OH)D values are normal, and in cases in which it has been measured, 24,25(OH)$_2$D levels have been low. Importantly, serum levels of 1,25(OH)$_2$D are elevated. This clinical feature clearly distinguishes HVDRR from PDDR, where circulating concentrations of 1,25(OH)$_2$D are depressed. Additionally, patients with HVDRR are resistant to supraphysiologic doses of all forms of vitamin D therapy. Table 82–1 outlines the similarities and differences between the two forms of hereditary rickets involving the vitamin D endocrine system.

PSEUDO–VITAMIN D DEFICIENCY RICKETS

Molecular Etiology

As previously mentioned, serum levels of 25(OH)D are normal in untreated patients with PDDR and elevated in patients receiving large daily amounts of vitamin D.[20] These results indicate that intestinal absorption of vitamin D and its hydroxylation in the liver are not impaired in patients with PDDR. Circulating levels of 24,25(OH)$_2$D are also normal and highly correlated with those of 25(OH)D, thus indicating a fully functional 25-hydroxyvitamin D–24-hydroxylase enzyme.[21] However, serum concentrations of 1,25(OH)$_2$D are low in untreated patients and remain low even when they are treated with high doses of vitamin D.[20, 22, 23] This finding clearly identifies defective activity of the 25-hydroxyvitamin D–1α-hydroxylase enzyme (*CYP27B1* or P-450c1α; hereafter referred to as 1α-hydroxylase) as the basic abnormality in PDDR and differentiates it from HVDRR.

PDDR is inherited as a simple autosomal recessive trait.[24] No phenotypic abnormalities are observed in heterozygotes.[19] By taking advantage of the unusual frequency of PDDR in the French-Canadian population and the availability of sample material from relatively large

TABLE 82–1. Comparison of PDDR and HVDRR

Feature	PDDR	HVDRR
Mutations	25-Hydroxyvitamin D–1α-hydroxylase	Vitamin D receptor
Genetic inheritance	Autosomal recessive	Autosomal recessive
Age of onset	Early	Early
Rickets	Yes	Yes
Hypocalcemia	Yes	Yes
Serum alkaline phosphatase	Elevated	Elevated
Secondary hyperparathyroidism	Yes	Yes
Alopecia	No	Yes
Serum 25(OH)D	Normal	Normal
Serum 1,25(OH)$_2$D	Low	Elevated
Response to 1,25(OH)$_2$D therapy	Yes	No

Reference range, serum biochemistry (child): calcemia (total calcium), 2.2 to 2.7 mmol/L; alkaline phosphatase, 20 to 150 U/L; 25(OH)D, 35 to 200 nmol/L; 1,25(OH)$_2$D, 12 to 46 μmol/L.

HVDRR, hereditary vitamin D–resistant rickets; PDDR, pseudo–vitamin D deficiency rickets.

From Favus MJ: Primer on the Metabolic Bone Diseases and Disorders of Mineral Metabolism, ed. 3. Philadelphia, Lippincott-Raven, 1996, pp 451–452.

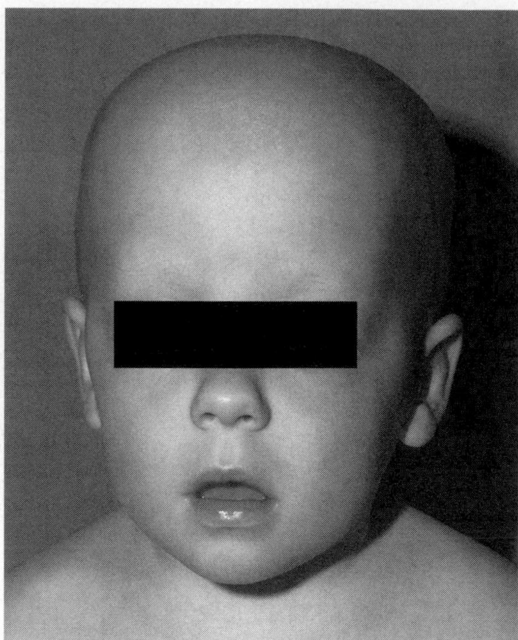

FIGURE 82–4. Alopecia in a patient with hereditary vitamin D–resistant rickets.

kindreds, the PDDR locus was mapped to the region of band 14 on the long arm of chromosome 12 (12q13-14).[25] The mapping was first performed by restriction fragment length polymorphism analysis[25] and subsequently by multipoint linkage analysis and studies of haplotypes.[26] Haplotypes are groups of tightly linked markers segregating together over the generations. These methods allowed the PDDR locus to be placed between the gene coding for the α1 chain of type II collagen (*COL2A1*) and a cluster of microsatellite markers (*D12S90*, *D12S305*, and *D12S104*), which segregate as a three-marker haplotype.[26] Linkage disequilibrium, or the occurrence of combinations of closely linked genes at higher frequency than expected with random distribution, has been observed between the PDDR locus and the three-marker haplotype in the French-Canadian kindreds that were studied from the Charlevoix-Saguenay-Lac Saint Jean area of the province of Quebec.[26]

Tremendous progress has been achieved in studying the molecular etiology of PDDR through recent cloning of the cDNA encoding for the 1α-hydroxylase enzyme. 1α-Hydroxylase cDNA was cloned from rat kidney,[27, 28] mouse kidney,[29] and human keratinocytes and kidney.[30] The human gene has also been cloned, sequenced, and located on chromosome 12 with the use of somatic cell hybrids[31] and then mapped to 12q13.1-13.3 by fluorescence in situ hybridization,[27, 32, 33] consistent with the earlier mapping of the disease to this locus by linkage analysis.

The ultimate proof that mutations in the 1α-hydroxylase gene were responsible for the PDDR phenotype required the identification of such mutations in patients with PDDR and in carriers of the disease. The first mutation identified was reported by Fu et al.[30] in 1997; several additional mutations in various ethnic groups have since been published.[32–35] These findings unequivocally establish the molecular genetic basis of PDDR as inactivating mutation(s) in the 1α-hydroxylase gene. The mutations and their effect on the activity of the 1α-hydroxylase enzyme will be discussed in detail below.

25-Hydroxyvitamin D–1α-Hydroxylase

Characteristics

The 25-hydroxyvitamin D–1α-hydroxylase (1α-hydroxylase) enzyme catalyzes the addition of a hydroxyl group at position 1α of the secosteroid backbone of 25(OH)D (Fig. 82–5A). The enzyme belongs to the mixed-function oxidase class because it reduces molecular oxygen to water and to the hydroxyl group to be incorporated into the steroid (see Fig. 82–5B). 1α-Hydroxylase is a mitochondrial cytochrome P-450 enzyme that requires electrons from reduced nicotinamide-adenine dinucleotide phosphate (NADPH) to promote catalysis (see Fig. 82–5B). These electrons are delivered to the P-450 moiety by the flavoprotein NADPH–ferredoxin reductase[36] and by the nonheme iron protein ferredoxin.[37] Expression of these cofactors is ubiquitous, and their genes were mapped to chromosomes 17 and 11,[36, 37] respectively, which rapidly excluded them in the search for PDDR mutations because the PDDR locus was previously mapped to chromosome 12.[25]

The main site for the 1α-hydroxylation of 25(OH)D is the proximal tubule of the renal cortex.[38] Expression of the enzyme has also been reported in bone cells,[39] keratinocytes,[30] and cells of the lymphohematopoietic system.[40] Identification of these extrarenal sites of expression of 1α-hydroxylase has led investigators to hypothesize that local production of $1,25(OH)_2D$ could play an important autocrine or paracrine role in the differentiation or function of these cells. In the kidney, expression of the 1α-hydroxylase gene is subject to complex regulation by parathyroid hormone, calcium, phosphorus, and $1,25(OH)_2D$ itself.[7]

Cloning of 1α-hydroxylase has been made difficult by the low levels of gene expression. Several ingenious strategies coalesced to enable the cloning of cDNA for 1α-hydroxylase from several species. Reduced-stringency hybridization cloning using a probe derived from the heme-binding domain of the rat 25-hydroxyvitamin D–24-hydroxylase (24-hydroxylase) cDNA[41] first allowed identification and characterization of full-length 1α-hydroxylase cDNA from the kidney of vitamin D–deficient rats.[27] Similar strategies that used polymerase chain reaction (PCR) with degenerate oligonucleotide primers led to cloning of rat kidney cDNA by a different laboratory and also to cloning of human cDNA from keratinocytes.[28, 30] The PCR primers used were derived from the amino acid sequence of conserved regions of the 25-hydroxylase and 24-hydroxylase enzymes. For their part, Takeyama et al. took advantage of the unique animal model (discussed below) that they had engineered by inactivating the VDR gene through homologous recombination.[29] Mice lacking the VDR show abnormally high serum concentrations of $1,25(OH)_2D$ because the negative feedback loop through which $1,25(OH)_2D$ downregulates 1α-hydroxylase expression is impaired in these animals.[29] The authors reasoned that the elevated $1,25(OH)_2D$ levels reflected excessive 1α-hydroxylase expression and thus that the cDNA coding for 1α-hydroxylase would be represented at an increased frequency in cDNA libraries prepared from kidneys of VDR-deficient mice. The screening method used a chimeric transcription factor that contained the ligand-binding domain (LBD) of the VDR. This chimeric factor activates the transcription of a reporter gene only in the presence of $1,25(OH)_2D$. Cells were transfected with the reporter, the chimeric factor, and clones from the kidney cDNA library and treated with 25(OH)D. Cells expressing 1α-hydroxylase activity converted the 25(OH)D precursor to $1,25(OH)_2D$, activated the chimeric protein, and turned on the reporter gene.[29] This elegant strategy led to cloning of mouse 1α-hydroxylase cDNA.

cDNA from all species examined to date shows high sequence similarity. For example, the sequence of the coding region of human cDNA is 82% identical to that of mouse 1α-hydroxylase at both the nucleotide and the amino acid levels. Human 1α-hydroxylase cDNA is 2469 bp in length and codes for a deduced protein of 508 amino acids containing a ferredoxin-binding domain and a heme-binding domain. The deduced amino acid sequence has substantial homology with members of the mitochondrial P-450 family,[42] particularly human vitamin D–25-hydroxylase[43] (*CYP27*, 40%); 25-hydroxyvitamin D–24-hydroxylase[41] (*CYP24*, 32%); P-450scc, the cholesterol side chain cleavage enzyme[44] (*CYP11A*, 33%); and P-450c11β, the steroid 11β-hydroxylase[45] (*CYP11B1*, 30%).

All laboratories that isolated 1α-hydroxylase cDNA rapidly obtained the sequence of the 1α-hydroxylase gene in various species. The gene exists in a single copy in the human genome and contains nine exons spanning 5 kb of sequence. The ferredoxin-binding domain is encoded by sequences contained in exons 6 and 7, whereas the heme-binding domain is contained in exon 8. The 1α-hydroxylase 5′ flanking sequence containing the promoter and its regulatory elements has also been cloned and should soon allow deciphering of the molecular control of expression of the 1α-hydroxylase gene in various cells.[46]

FIGURE 82–5. The vitamin D biosynthetic pathway. *A,* Activation of the vitamin D molecule. *B,* Mechanism of hydroxylation of 25-hydroxyvitamin D at C-1 by the renal 25-hydroxyvitamin D–1α-hydroxylase. FDX, ferredoxin; FR, ferredoxin reductase; NADP, nicotinamide-adenine dinucleotide phosphate; NADPH, dihydronicotinamide-adenine dinucleotide phosphate; ox, oxidized; red, reduced.

Mutations

To date, 20 different 1α-hydroxylase mutations have been described in patients with PDDR and their parents (Table 82–2). All patients have mutations on both alleles, but a high frequency of compound heterozygosity (a different mutation on each allele) has been observed (12 of 32 cases reported). Nucleotide deletions and duplications, as well as several missense and one nonsense mutation, have been reported (see Table 82–2). The mutations are dispersed throughout the 1α-hydroxylase sequence and affect all exons except exon 5. The functional consequence of the mutations will be discussed below.

The mutation that was detected at the highest frequency, in various ethnic groups, is located at codons 438 to 442 in exon 8. These codons are composed of the duplicated 7-bp sequence 5′-CCCACCC CCCACCC-3′. In eight families described to date,[33–35] three rather than two copies of the 7-bp sequence are present, which alters the downstream reading frame (Fig. 82–6). Careful analysis of the correlation between ethnic origin, microsatellite haplotyping, and presence of the 7-bp duplication mutation suggested that the mutation had arisen

TABLE 82–2. 1α-Hydroxylase Gene Mutations in Patients with Pseudo–Vitamin D Deficiency Rickets

Mutation*	Ethnic Group	Reference
212ΔG (codon 46)	Hispanic	34
Q65H	Chinese	34
958ΔG (codon 88)	White American, French-Canadian	33, 34
R107H	Japanese	32
G125E	Japanese	32
E189L	Polish	34
1921ΔG (codon 211)	White American	30, 34
1984ΔC (codon 231)	White American	30, 34
W241X	Polish	34
S323Y	British	35
R335P	Japanese	32
P382S	Japanese	32
R389H	White American, French-Canadian	34
T409I	Filipino	34
R429P	Black American	34
7-bp duplication (codons 438–442)	Filipino, Polish, Chinese, British, White American, Black American, Hispanic, French-Canadian, Acadian	33–35, herein
2-bp duplication (codon 442)	White American	34
R453C	Haitian	34
V478G	British	35
P497R	Polish	34

*The one-letter amino acid code is used.
Δ, deletion; X, premature stop codon.

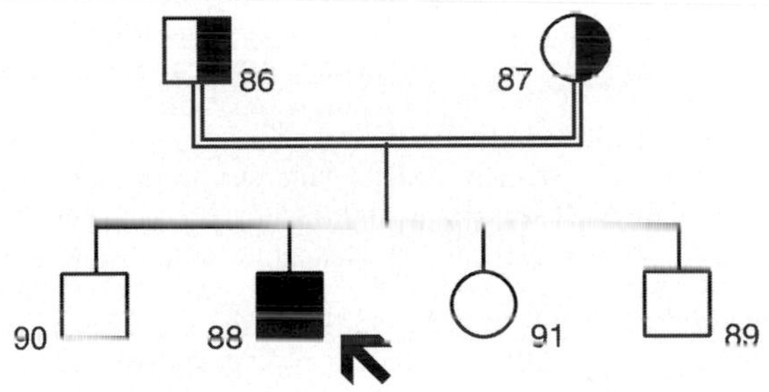

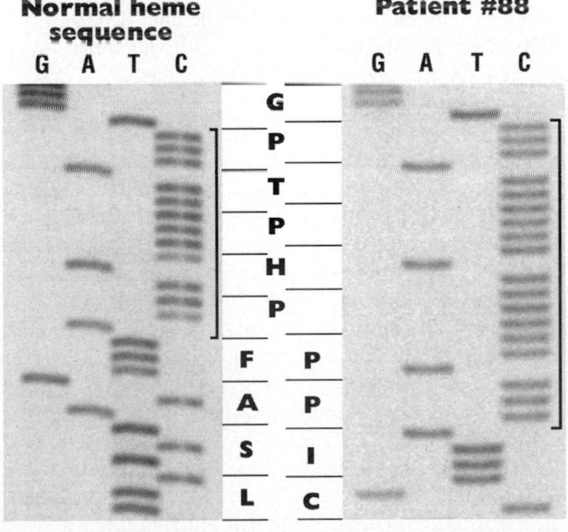

FIGURE 82–6. Identification of the molecular defect in a pseudo–vitamin D deficiency rickets pedigree. *Upper panel,* the heterozygote parents are identified by half-filled boxes (male parent, *square symbol,* no. 86; female parent, *round symbol,* no. 87). The affected patient (male, no. 88) is identified by a *filled square with an arrow. Lower panel,* DNA sequence analysis of the mutation within the heme-binding domain of the 25-hydroxyvitamin D–1α-hydroxylase gene. The 7-bp duplication is *bracketed.* The amino acid sequence (one-letter code) is highlighted in the center of the figure. Note the change in reading frame leading to an aberrant protein sequence and premature termination in the affected patient.

by several independent de novo events[33] and points to this region of the 1α-hydroxylase gene as a mutational hot spot.

As previously mentioned, PDDR is unusually frequent in a subset of the French-Canadian population located in the Charlevoix-Saguenay-Lac Saint Jean region of Quebec.[47] The prevalence of PDDR in that population was estimated at 1 in 2358 live births, with a carrier rate of 1 in 26.[47] This high prevalence was attributed to a founder effect that would have taken place in the second half of the 17th century. Microsatellite haplotyping supported the notion of such a founder effect.[26] Combined analysis of 1α-hydroxylase mutations and haplotypes confirmed that the Charlevoix haplotype is strongly associated with this ethnic group and confirms the founder effect.[33, 34]

Structure/Function Relationships

An important aspect of the identification of mutations in the 1α-hydroxylase gene is to attempt to correlate the genotype of the patients with their phenotype, that is, the severity of the disease with the circulating levels of 1,25(OH)$_2$D. In several cases, although 1,25(OH)$_2$D serum levels were low, they were not undetectable,[20, 22, 48] thus suggesting some degree of residual 1α-hydroxylase activity. Presumably, some 1α-hydroxylase mutations affect the structural integrity of the enzyme and result in a modification of its kinetics. This reasoning cannot apply to the frameshift (deletions and duplications) and nonsense mutations described to date. All such mutations eliminate the heme-binding site of the protein and thus completely abolish 1α-hydroxylase enzymatic activity. The apparent residual 1α-hydroxylase activity observed in some patients could be attributable to the several missense mutations that have been characterized. So far, these missense mutations have been tested only by using expression vectors in transient transfection assays.[32, 34] The mutant proteins were entirely devoid of enzymatic activity in the assays used and thus prevented a clear understanding of the mechanisms responsible for the apparent low residual 1α-hydroxylase activity in certain patients. It is expected that future avenues of research will include purification of the mutant enzyme in recombinant form and careful analysis of enzyme kinetics.

Wang et al. have explained the lack of activity of the missense mutants by comparing the sequence of the 1α-hydroxylase protein (a mitochondrial class I cytochrome P-450) with the sequence of bacterial class I cytochrome P-450s for which x-ray crystallographic data are available.[34] The tertiary structures of these enzymes show remarkable conservation despite low amino acid sequence identity.[42] The comparison revealed that mutations Q65H, T409I, and R389H all lie in the clustered β sheet domain that interacts with the inner mitochondrial membrane and defines the substrate entry channel. These mutations are likely to disrupt the ability of the enzyme to bind substrate. Mutation E189L should cause significant disruption of the P-450 structure because it breaks a domain called the four-helix bundle. Similarly, mutation R429P inserts a proline residue, which disrupts α helical structures, at the junction of two critical domains and should change the direction of the carbon backbone in those domains. The mutant R453C is hypothesized to disrupt a salt bridge involving the heme propionate. Finally, the P497R mutation affects a β sheet that defines the top of the substrate-binding pocket and probably affects substrate binding. Thus many of the missense mutations identified to date are predicted to severely affect 1α-hydroxylase structure and function. The relatively insensitive assays used so far to test the function of mutant enzymes revealed an apparent complete lack of activity.[34] It is probable, however, that substrate-binding pocket mutants such as Q65H, T409I, R389H, and P497R will exhibit residual activity in more refined enzyme kinetics biochemical assays involving a wide range of substrate concentrations.

Treatment

Vitamin D$_2$, at high doses, was initially used to treat PDDR. With such treatment, circulating levels of 25(OH)D increase sharply, and it is likely that massive concentrations of 25(OH)D can bind to the VDR and induce the response of the target organs to normalize calcium homeostasis. The risk of overdose is high because vitamin D progressively accumulates in fat and muscle, and therapeutic doses are close to toxic doses, which ultimately places the patient at risk for nephrocalcinosis and impaired renal function. The use of 25(OH)D$_3$ as a therapeutic agent in PDDR has been reported.[49] The mechanism of action is likely to be similar to the one described for vitamin D above. The low availability and high cost of the metabolite have not encouraged its widespread use as long-term therapy for PDDR.

The treatment of choice is long-term (lifelong) replacement therapy with 1,25(OH)$_2$D$_3$.[20, 50] Such treatment results in rapid and complete correction of the abnormal phenotype by eliminating hypocalcemia, secondary hyperparathyroidism, and radiographic evidence of rickets. Strikingly, the myopathy disappears within days after the initiation of therapy. Restoration of bone mineral content is equally rapid, and histologic evidence of healing of the bone structure has been reported.[20] Correction of tooth enamel hypoplasia is only partial. An important aspect of treatment is to ensure adequate calcium intake during the bone-healing phase. Needs can be monitored by frequent assessment of urinary calcium excretion. It should be noted that hypercalciuria is common during treatment with 1,25(OH)$_2$D$_3$, particularly during the first year of administration. Close monitoring for hypercalciuria is required to adjust the dose of 1,25(OH)$_2$D$_3$. The initial dose will be 1 to 2 μg/day, whereas the maintenance dose will vary between 0.5 and 1 μg/day. High levels of calcium excretion may amplify the pattern of calcium deposition in the kidney; thus frequent renal imaging and assessment of renal function are essential during the course of treatment.

Before 1,25(OH)$_2$D$_3$ became available from commercial sources, several investigators used the monohydroxylated analogue 1α(OH)D$_3$,[51] which requires only liver hydroxylation at position 25 to be activated to the hormonally active metabolite. It should be remembered that the 25-hydroxylation step is not affected by the PDDR mutation. Response to treatment with 1α(OH)D$_3$ is rapid, with healing of rickets in 7 to 9 weeks, and this compound is still used in several countries. On a weight basis, 1α(OH)D$_3$ is about half as potent as 1,25(OH)$_2$D$_3$, which nullifies any possible economic advantage in favor of the monohydroxylated compound.

HEREDITARY VITAMIN D–RESISTANT RICKETS

Molecular Etiology

Patients with HVDRR have normal 25(OH)D and low, but measurable 24,25(OH)$_2$D serum values. Circulating levels of 1,25(OH)$_2$D are elevated three to five times the normal values. These biochemical findings demonstrate that all the vitamin D metabolic enzymes (25-hydroxylase, 24-hydroxylase, and 1α-hydroxylase) are active in patients with HVDRR. Most patients with the disease are resistant to all forms of vitamin D therapy. This lack of response to vitamin D treatment led Albright et al. to introduce the concept of hormonal resistance.[14] The molecular basis of vitamin D end-organ resistance became clearer as the mechanism of action of the hormonal form of vitamin D was elucidated.

Ligand-binding studies first established that the 1,25(OH)$_2$D hormone, like other sex steroid hormones studied at the time, binds to a high-affinity receptor located in the nucleus.[52] It was later discovered that this receptor could bind to DNA.[53] This property was used to purify sufficient quantities of the VDR to raise antibodies.[54, 55]

The observation that binding sites for 1,25(OH)$_2$D could be detected in many tissues in addition to the classic vitamin D target tissues helped define the etiology of HVDRR. Investigators began to study the VDR from cultured fibroblasts of patients and relatives by using ligand-binding assays, radioimmunoassays, and DNA-cellulose chromatography. Other fibroblast responses measured included induction of 24-hydroxylase enzyme activity and vitamin D–mediated growth arrest. These methodologies led to several milestone observations. In the first studies reported, ^{3}H-1,25(OH)$_2$D$_3$ binding was undetectable in fibroblasts from patients with HVDRR, and high doses of 1,25(OH)$_2$D failed to induce the 24-hydroxylase biomarker.[56] The diminished hormone binding provided a clear rationale for the end-organ resistance reported in patients. Subsequent reports continued to describe a lack of response of the patient's cells to $1,25(OH)_2D$, but some patients' fibroblasts exhibited normal ^3H-$1,25(OH)_2D_3$ binding.[57] From these early reports it was concluded that at least two classes of patients with HVDRR could be recognized: "receptor-negative" patients and "receptor-positive" patients. The development of a sensitive radioimmunoassay for the VDR protein[58] demonstrated that these semantic differences were incorrect. With this assay it was shown that fibroblasts from "receptor-negative" patients expressed normal levels of receptor protein. Pike et al. hypothesized that the VDR defect in the patients' cells was due to a structural abnormality in the ligand-binding domain (LBD) that prevented ^3H-$1,25(OH)_2D_3$ from binding to the receptor and not due to defective synthesis of the VDR protein.[59] The two classes of HVDRR were more adequately described by the terminology "ligand binding positive" and "ligand binding negative."

A second type of VDR structural abnormality was identified in cultured cells from patients displaying the "ligand binding–positive" HVDRR phenotype. The VDR from these cells showed reduced affinity for heterologous DNA as measured by DNA-cellulose chromatography.[60] It was suspected that the defect in those patients would likely be a point mutation in the DNA-binding domain (DBD) of the VDR. Interestingly, measurements of DNA-binding affinities of the VDR from parents of "ligand binding–positive" patients clearly identified two forms of the VDR molecule, one with normal, wild-type affinity for DNA and the second with reduced, defective DNA binding.[60] This finding was the first clear evidence establishing the heterozygous state of parents with HVDRR. Binding and antibody-based assays had failed to reconcile the genotype and phenotype of carriers in the past.

Eventually, the purified receptor was used to obtain monoclonal antibodies that led to the cloning of VDR cDNA from various species.[61–63] In turn, the VDR genomic structure was analyzed. Interestingly, the VDR gene maps close to the PDDR locus at 12q13-14.[64] Eight exons spanning approximately 50 kb of genomic DNA constitute the entire coding region.[65] The translation start site is contained within exon 2. At least three short exons designated 1a, 1b, and 1c lie upstream of exon 2.[66] These noncoding exons are differentially spliced to produce various VDR mRNA transcripts, all containing the full-length protein coding sequence. Type I transcripts contain exons 1a and 1c, type II transcripts contain exons 1a, 1b, and 1c, and type III transcripts contain only exon 1a fused to exon 2.[66] The guanosine/cytosine-rich promoter of the VDR gene lies immediately upstream of exon 1a.[66, 67]

Analysis of the VDR cDNA sequence soon established that the VDR is a member of the nuclear hormone receptor superfamily, and its mechanism of action was subsequently unraveled.[8] The ligand-bound receptor forms a heterodimer with the RXR, and the dimer contacts specific sites within the regulatory domains of responsive genes. This interaction results in positive or negative modulation of the transcription of target genes. The VDR is essential to transduce the biologic effects of $1,25(OH)_2D$, such as promoting calcium and phosphate transport across the small intestine and maintaining calcium homeostasis. The underlying molecular basis of the hormone resistance described in patients with HVDRR is mutations in the VDR that render the receptor nonfunctional or less functional than the wild-type VDR.

HVDRR follows an autosomal recessive pattern of inheritance. Parents of patients who are heterozygous for the mutation show no symptoms and have normal bone development. In many cases, parental consanguinity is associated with the disease. Families often have several affected children, and males and females are affected equally.

Vitamin D Receptor

Characteristics

Structure/function analysis, sequence comparison alignments, and recent crystallographic studies have contributed to our understanding of the domain structure of the members of the nuclear hormone receptor superfamily, to whom the VDR belongs. A discussion of the structural and functional aspects of each domain is in order to allow a full understanding of the consequences of the natural VDR mutations responsible for HVDRR that have been identified and characterized to date.

The different domains of nuclear receptors have been labeled A to E/F (Fig. 82–7). Some of these domains exhibit high sequence similarity between individual family members, whereas others vary considerably or are altogether absent. This diversity is manifested most strongly in domains A/B, D, and F. Domain A/B includes all residues that are N-terminal to the receptor's DBD. The size of this domain is highly variable and ranges from hundreds of residues in the progesterone receptor, for example, to only 24 amino acids in the VDR. The function of the A/B domain remains somewhat uncertain, but recent results suggest that polymorphisms in the VDR A/B segment could modulate its transcriptional activity.[68] Domain C contains the highly conserved zinc finger DBD, the hallmark feature of nuclear receptor family members, and will be discussed in detail below. Region D serves as a flexible hinge domain between the DBD and domain E and is the least conserved among nuclear receptors. Interestingly, the D segment of the VDR is 50 amino acids longer than that of classic steroid receptors because an additional exon has been spliced in.[66] Residues within the D domain of the VDR are subject to posttranslational modification in the form of reversible serine phosphorylation.[69, 70] This regulation provides an additional degree of control of VDR activity.[8] The E region encodes the LBD of ligand-activated receptors and exhibits several additional functional activities that will be detailed below. The small F domain is not highly conserved between nuclear receptor family members and is in fact absent in the VDR.

Structure/Function Relationships

The VDR DNA-Binding Domain

The DBD of the VDR consists of two zinc finger motifs located between residues 24 to 90. The zinc fingers are of the C2C2 type,

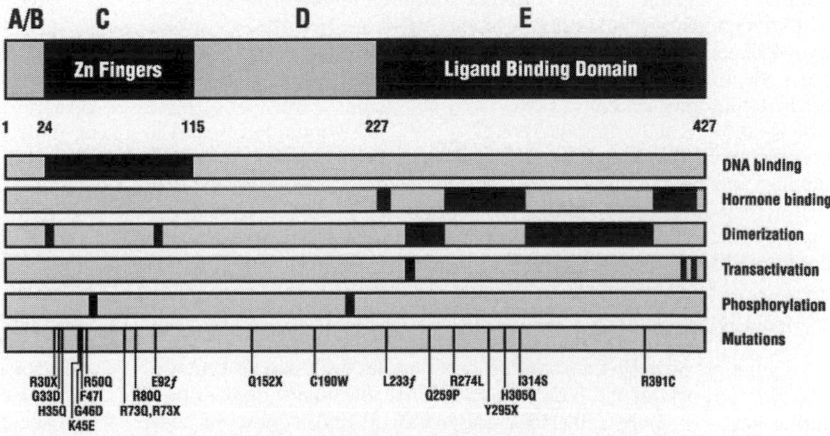

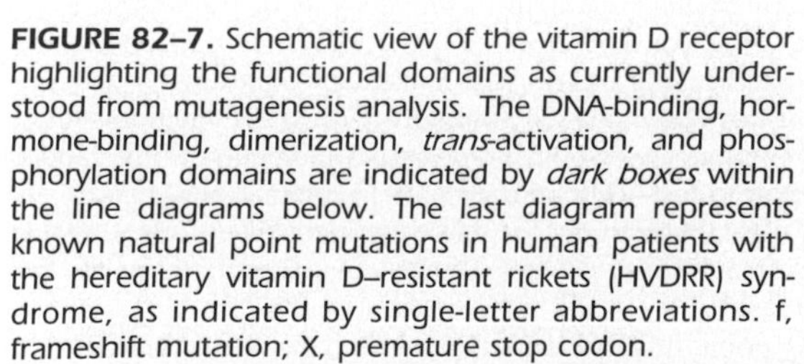

FIGURE 82–7. Schematic view of the vitamin D receptor highlighting the functional domains as currently understood from mutagenesis analysis. The DNA-binding, hormone-binding, dimerization, *trans*-activation, and phosphorylation domains are indicated by *dark boxes* within the line diagrams below. The last diagram represents known natural point mutations in human patients with the hereditary vitamin D–resistant rickets (HVDRR) syndrome, as indicated by single-letter abbreviations. f, frameshift mutation; X, premature stop codon.

with two zinc atoms tetrahedrally coordinated through four cysteine residues, each of which serves to stabilize the finger structure itself. Based on structural homology with the thyroid hormone receptor (TR), for which x-ray crystallographic data are available,[71] it is hypothesized that the α helical motifs residing on the C-terminal side of each zinc finger would constitute the DNA recognition and phosphate backbone–binding helices, respectively.[8] The region immediately C-terminal to the second zinc finger, which includes residues 91 to 115, also forms an α helical structure that could contribute to DNA contact. The functional importance of these helical domains is confirmed by analysis of the HVDRR mutations described below.

The VDR exhibits a unique characteristic when compared with other nuclear receptors: a cluster of five basic amino acids is located at residues 49 to 55, in the intervening sequence between the two zinc fingers. This domain is predicted to make DNA contact[71] and regulate nuclear localization of the receptor.[72] Interestingly, this cluster contains residue serine 51, a site of posttranslational modification through phosphorylation by protein kinase C.[73, 74]

Besides their well-characterized role in binding of the DNA response element, residues within the zinc finger motifs of the VDR also contribute to association with the partner receptor, RXR, to form the functional heterodimer[75, 76] (see Figs. 82–2 and 82–7). The α helical domain immediately C-terminal to the second zinc finger also provides interactions with partner proteins.[76] These specific contact sites in the DBD of the VDR facilitate weak heterodimerization between the VDR and the RXR, whereas stronger, ligand-dependent heterodimerization interactions are provided by residues located within the LBD.

The VDR Ligand-Binding Domain

The E region of the VDR (see Fig. 82–7) represents a complex multifunctional domain involved in binding of the $1,25(OH)_2D$ ligand, heterodimerization with the RXR, and *trans*-activation. The structure of the LBD of the retinoic acid receptor (RAR), TR, and RXR has been modeled after x-ray crystallographic analysis.[77–79] It consists of 12 α helices and several short β strands organized as a "sandwich" around a lipophilic hormone-binding pocket. By analogy, the LBD of the VDR would contain three regions that would be in closest contact with the $1,25(OH)_2D$ ligand: residues 227 to 240 (helix 3), 268 to 316 (helices 4–7), and 396 to 422 (helices 10–12). Several of the mutations characterized in HVDRR coincide with hormone contact sites in the RAR and/or TR (discussed below). The conclusion from the analysis of several natural and artificial VDR mutations that compromise ligand binding is that the structure of the VDR LBD closely resembles that of its nuclear receptor family cousins RAR and TR. One exception is the relatively unconserved stretch encoded by exon 5, between residues 155 and 194.[66]

It is hypothesized that ligand binding leads to conformational changes that expose, enhance, or produce novel dimerization and/or *trans*-activation interfaces. Proteolytic digestion assays have provided indirect evidence that binding of $1,25(OH)_2D$ induces changes in conformation of the VDR.[80, 81] It is unlikely that ligand-induced conformational changes are restricted to the E domain. Interestingly, different vitamin D analogues induce different conformational changes.[82]

Two regions within the LBD of the VDR are involved in strong, ligand-dependent heterodimerization with the RXR. These areas have been identified by mutagenesis experiments and by analogy to the RXR homodimer crystal.[79] These two subdomains consist of residues 244 to 263[83–85] and amino acids 317 to 395,[85, 86] which correspond to portions of helices 3 and 4 and 7 to 10, respectively. Thus the ligand-binding and heterodimerization functions of the VDR are interrelated within the context of the tertiary structure of the molecule, presumably through allosteric effects that ultimately generate an active receptor conformation.

Trans-activation

Regulation of gene transcription requires three classes of proteins. The first consists of the basal transcriptional machinery used to transcribe genes in every cell. RNA polymerase II and a series of basal factors serve to ensure transcription of protein-coding genes. Precise control of the transcription of particular genes is ensured by sequence-specific DNA-binding transcription factors. The VDR is such a factor, and its activity is further regulated through ligand binding. Finally, recent progress in our understanding of the molecular control of gene expression has unveiled a third class of proteins, generally known as transcriptional coactivators, that provide protein-protein contact between the basal factors and the sequence-specific DNA-binding factors. The players involved in this tightly orchestrated choreography are just beginning to be identified for VDR-mediated transcription.

As previously mentioned, ligand binding probably serves to induce conformational changes that allow the VDR to contact pertinent partners. Mutagenesis experiments have identified some of the key residues involved in these contacts. Two regions of the receptor are required exclusively for transcriptional activation. One of these regions is located between residues 244 and 263, a domain also involved in heterodimerization with the RXR.[83–85] However, residue lysine 246 is not involved in contact with the RXR partner, and its alteration severely compromises *trans*-activation.[84] This residue, highly conserved among nuclear receptors, must form part of the binding interface with transcriptional coactivators.[84, 87]

The second region is known as activator function-2 (AF-2) and corresponds to helix 12 (residues 416–422).[88–90] Alteration of residues leucine 417 and glutamic acid 420 does not affect hormone binding or heterodimeric DNA binding but completely abrogates *trans*-activation.[89, 90] These residues also function to stimulate transcription by a mechanism involving coactivators. Some of the proteins interacting with the VDR to allow ligand-activated transcription have recently been identified. Within the basal transcriptional machinery, the VDR interacts with transcription factor TFIIB.[12, 13] This contact involves the AF-2 domain of the VDR, but also requires the wild-type residue arginine 391, located N-terminal to the AF-2 region within helix 10/11.[90]

A series of novel transcriptional coactivators interacting with the VDR have been identified, such as the DRIPs (D receptor–interacting proteins)[11] or NCoA-62 (nuclear receptor coactivator of 62 kDa).[10] The role of these accessory proteins in vitamin D–regulated transcription will require additional experimental work. Based on their interaction with different members of the nuclear receptor family, it has also been shown that the VDR interacts with coactivators that have been cloned, including SRC-1 (steroid receptor coactivator-1) and TIF1 (transcriptional mediator/intermediary factor-1).[90–93] It is also hypothesized that the unliganded VDR in the nucleus is bound by a repressor molecule related to SMRT (silencing mediator for retinoid and thyroid hormone receptors).[8, 94] Such interactions would maintain chromatin in a repressed transcriptional state. The availability of cell-free systems in which VDR-RXR dimers can activate transcription in a ligand-dependent fashion should facilitate analysis of the molecular mechanisms of VDR-mediated transcription. In particular, the relevance of the interactions between the VDR and coactivators, basal factors, and repressors can be tested. The availability of natural VDR mutations isolated from HVDRR patient material, combined with engineered mutations, also provides a powerful tool to identify the pertinent molecular interactions.

Mutations

Our understanding of the structural and functional consequences of HVDRR-causing mutations in the VDR has followed the introduction of molecular biologic techniques as routine detection methods. For example, amplification of mRNA by reverse transcription-coupled PCR has been of tremendous help in the analysis of mutations. Similarly, the functional consequences of particular mutations, first analyzed with ligand-binding assays and nonspecific binding to calf thymus DNA, can now be analyzed routinely with transient transfection assays on real vitamin D–responsive promoter elements. Some laboratories have begun to test VDR protein-protein interactions. Finally, the availability of crystal structures for related nuclear receptors allows an understanding of the consequences of particular mutations at the tertiary structure level.

Close to 20 point mutations in the VDR have been described in

TABLE 82–3. VDR Mutations in Patients with Hereditary Vitamin D–Resistant Rickets

Mutation*	Exon	VDR Domain	Ligand Binding	Reference
R30X	2	DBD	−	95, 96, herein
G33D	2	DBD	+	65
H35Q	2	DBD	+	97
K45E	2	DBD	+	98
G46D	2	DBD	+	99
F47I	2	DBD	+	98
R50Q	3	DBD	+	100
R73Q	3	DBD	+	65
R73X	3	DBD	−	101, 102
R80Q	3	DBD	+	103, 104
E92fs	Intron	Hinge	−	105
Q152X	4	Hinge	−	106
L233fs	6	LBD	−	101
Q259P	7	LBD	+	101
R274L	7	LBD	+	106
Y295X	7	LBD	−	102, 107–109
H305Q	8	LBD	+	110
I314S	8	LBD, dimer	+	111
R391C	9	LBD, dimer	+	111

*The one-letter amino acid code is used.
DBD, DNA-binding domain; dimer, domains involved in heterodimerization; fs, frameshift; LBD, ligand binding domain; VDR, vitamin D receptor; X, premature stop codon

patients with HVDRR (see Fig. 82–7 and Table 82–3; reviewed in depth by Malloy et al.[18]). Six of these genetic alterations are nonsense (X) or frameshift (fs) mutations that introduce premature stop codons in the receptor: R30X (Fig. 82–8), R73X, E92fs, Q152X, L233fs, and Y295X. The premature translation termination codons lead to truncated VDRs that lack the DBD (R30X and R73X) or the LBD (E92fs, Q152X, L233fs, and Y295X); in most cases, the mRNAs for these truncated receptors are unstable.[107] Mutations involving amino acid substitutions (missense mutations) have been more revealing in terms of structure/function relationships.

DNA-Binding Domain Mutations

The first VDR mutation ever reported was described by Hughes et al. and affected the DBD of the receptor.[65] The mutation substitutes a polar uncharged glutamine for a positively charged arginine at position 73 (R73Q) within the second zinc finger of the DBD. The VDR mutation identified by Hughes et al. was the first natural disease-causing mutation reported for the entire steroid-thyroid-retinoid receptor gene superfamily.[65]

Several additional missense mutations affecting the DBD have since been reported (G33D through R80Q; Table 82–3). Based on the crystal structure of the related glucocorticoid receptor (GR), RXR, and TR molecules,[77–79] the H35Q, K45E, R50Q, R73Q, and R80Q mutations are thought to affect residues that contact DNA.[8, 18, 98] The conversion of residue glycine 46 to aspartic acid (G46D) introduces a bulky, charged amino acid that would create unfavorable electrostatic interactions with the negatively charged phosphate backbone of the DNA helix.[101] The G33D mutation would be expected to have the same effect.[98] The F47I mutation is a relatively conserved substitution, but loss of the phenylalanine ring structure may disrupt the hydrophobic core of the DBD and affect the proposed α helical structure at the base of the first zinc finger.[98]

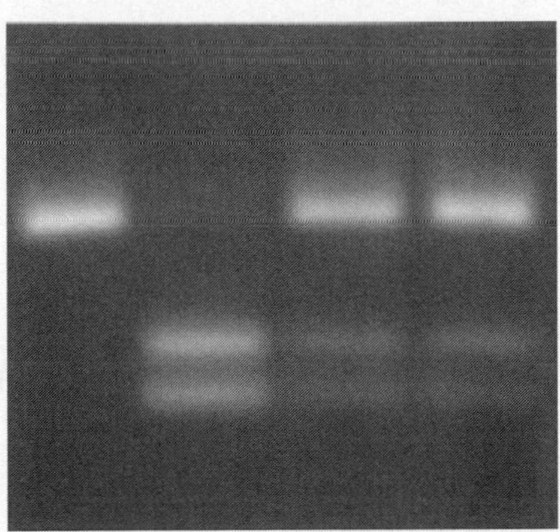

FIGURE 82–8. Prenatal diagnosis in a family where a first child had hereditary vitamin D–resistant rickets caused by a R30X mutation. This mutation in the vitamin D receptor (VDR) gene (C-to-T substitution in exon 2) has introduced a recognition site for the restriction endonuclease DdeI. By using primers internal to the affected exon, an 89-bp DNA fragment was amplified by polymerase chain reaction with 100 ng of genomic DNA prepared from amniotic cells (A) or from whole blood of an unrelated control (C), the mother (M), or the father (F). An aliquot of each amplimer was incubated with the restriction endonuclease DdeI. The digested fragments were visualized on 2.5% agarose gel. The data show unambiguous homozygosity for the R30X mutation in the fetus, with both parents carriers for the mutation.

Ligand-Binding Domain Mutations

The first mutation identified that affected the LBD was the Y295X mutation reported by Ritchie et al.[108] This mutation truncates 132 amino acids from the C terminus of the VDR, which results in the deletion of a major portion of the LBD. This mutation has been described in seven families forming a large kindred in which consanguineous marriages occurred.[107] The mutation was also identified in three additional families unrelated to the extended kindred.[102, 109] As previously mentioned, the mutant mRNA is unstable and the truncated VDR is undetectable with immunology-based assays.[107]

The crystallographic data on the related RXR, RAR, and TR LBDs[77–79] can again be used to understand the structural consequences of missense mutations in the VDR LBD described in patients with HVDRR. The canonic structure of the LBD of nuclear receptors is composed of a hydrophobic core formed by helix 3 (H3), H4, H5, H8, and H9 and the loops between H3 and H4 (loop 3–4) and H8 and H9 (loop 8–9).[112] The lipophilic pocket accommodating the ligand is formed by residues in H1, H3, H5, the β turn, loop 6–7, H11, loop 11–12, and H12. Once the ligand enters the pocket, a "lid" formed by H11 and H12 closes over the pocket (the so-called mouse trap model).[77]

The Q259P mutation occurs in H4 and is involved in stabilizing the hydrophobic core by interacting with residues in loop 8–9.[77] The R274L mutation in the core of H5 affects a residue involved in hydrogen bonding with the ligand.[77] The H305Q mutation occurs in loop 6–7 and causes a decrease in affinity for the ligand, presumably by increasing the flexibility of the ligand-binding pocket.

The I314S mutation occurs in H7 and affects both hormone binding and receptor heterodimerization.[111] The mutation lies between a ligand-binding contact observed in the TR[78] and a dimerization interface detected in the RXR.[79] Similarly, the R391C mutation is positioned within the H10 dimerization surface, but close to C-terminal ligand-binding contacts. Consistently, the R391C mutant receptor has a primary heterodimerization defect and a milder, secondary ligand-binding deficiency.[111]

Additional Mutations

The Q152X mutation, located within the hinge domain (see Fig. 82–7), deletes 306 residues from the VDR and results in a mutant receptor unresponsive to ligand in gene transcription assays.[102, 106] Two splice-site mutations have been described in patients of unrelated origin. In one case (E92fs), the nucleotide change eliminated the donor splice site from the 5′ end of the intron between exons 3 and 4. Loss of the 5′ donor splice site causes exon 4 to be skipped in processing of the VDR transcript and thereby results in a frameshift and premature stop codon within exon 5.[105] In the second case (L233fs), a cryptic 5′ donor splice site in exon 6 caused a 56-bp deletion in exon 6 that led to a frameshift within exon 7.[101] A partial VDR gene deletion affecting exons 7, 8, and 9 has been reported in conference proceedings but has not been published elsewhere.

Conceptually, because the signal transduction pathway of $1,25(OH)_2D$ involves accessory molecules such as the RXR, coactivators, and components of the basic transcriptional machinery, it is possible that target organ resistance to $1,25(OH)_2D$ may be due to mutations in other proteins involved in the *trans*-activation process. When the proteins interact with numerous partners, such as RXR, the phenotype associated with mutations would be expected to be broader than the clinical symptoms of HVDRR. The recent identification of transcriptional coactivators with specificity toward the VDR[10] widens the range of putative targets for mutations that could cause HVDRR. It is interesting to note that Hewison et al. described a case of HVDRR in an English patient in which a mutation could not be found in the VDR.[113] The patient exhibited all the clinical features of HVDRR, including alopecia. The patient's fibroblasts expressed wild-type VDR mRNA, and the receptor bound ligand with normal affinity. Ligand-dependent transcriptional activation by the VDR was deficient in the patient's cells but normal when the patient's VDR was expressed in heterologous cells. These results clearly demonstrate that the patient's VDR was normal and suggest that the vitamin D resistance is the result of a mutation affecting an accessory protein specific for $1,25(OH)_2D$-dependent transcriptional activation.

Animal Models of Disease

Two laboratories have independently engineered an animal model of HVDRR by inactivating the VDR gene through homologous recombination in embryonic stem cells.[114, 115] In one case, exon 2, which encodes the first zinc finger, was deleted,[114] whereas the other group targeted the second zinc finger, encoded by exon 3.[115] Both strategies, of course, lead to complete loss of function of the VDR, and the reported phenotypes are close to identical, with the main difference being the longevity of the mutant mice, a factor that could be influenced by genetic background, diet, or environmental conditions. Mice with targeted deletion of exon 2 die within 15 weeks,[114] whereas the mice lacking exon 3 can survive longer provided that the rachitic phenotype is rescued (see below).

Animals that are heterozygous for the engineered mutation are phenotypically normal. Homozygous VDR mutant mice display a phenotype very similar to HVDRR, including the progressive development of alopecia. Postweaning, VDR-null mice exhibit low bone mass, hypocalcemia, hypophosphatemia, secondary hyperparathyroidism, and elevated circulating $1,25(OH)_2D$.[114, 115] Serum levels of $24,25(OH)_2D$ are extremely low.

Feeding the mutant mice a "rescue" diet containing high levels of calcium, phosphate, and lactose can normalize mineral ion homeostasis and prevent rickets, osteomalacia, and secondary hyperparathyroidism in VDR-ablated mice.[116] The diet also normalized growth of the mutant animals. Rescue of the bone phenotype of VDR-deficient mice by dietary intervention[116, 117] aimed at normalizing circulating mineral concentrations parallels the results obtained in patients with HVDRR, in whom bone defects are resolved by therapy with intravenous calcium infusions (see below). The VDR-mutant mice thus represent a valid and potentially very useful animal model of the disease.

Study of the VDR-ablated mice has led to several key findings concerning the vitamin D endocrine system. Indeed, despite a lack of VDR throughout embryogenesis, VDR-null mice are born phenotypically normal.[114, 115] It is only after weaning that the symptoms of rickets and secondary hyperparathyroidism begin to develop. This observation suggests that vitamin D affects bone development principally by maintaining mineral ion homeostasis.

The genomic effects of $1,25(OH)_2D$ appear essential, however, for hair and skin development, independent of bone mineral homeostasis.[116] Dietary normalization of circulating mineral ion concentrations fails to correct alopecia in VDR-ablated mice, and the skin of these mice appears abnormal.[116] The VDR is expressed in the outer root sheath and the bulb of hair follicles, as well as in sebaceous glands,[118] but the role of vitamin D or the VDR in hair growth is not understood. Studies of the molecular basis for the effects of the VDR on keratinocytes in cells from normal and VDR-mutant mice will further our understanding of the physiologic actions of $1,25(OH)_2D$ and its nuclear receptor.

Treatment

Therapies consisting of pharmacologic doses of vitamin D metabolites, including vitamin D itself, 25(OH)D, 1α(OH)D, and $1,25(OH)_2D$, have been used in attempts to overcome the target organ resistance to vitamin D associated with HVDRR. Patients with HVDRR but without alopecia are generally more responsive to treatment with high doses of vitamin D preparations than are patients with alopecia.[119] Doses reported to be effective range from 5000 to 40,000 IU/day for vitamin D, 20 to 200 μg/day for 25(OH)D, and 17 to 20 μg/day for $1,25(OH)_2D$.[120–122] The efficacy of treatment with high doses of vitamin D metabolites can be reconciled with the molecular cause of HVDRR. When the resistance to vitamin D is caused by mutations in the VDR that moderately decrease the affinity of the receptor for its ligand, such as the H305Q or I314S mutations,[110, 111] high doses of the hormone can apparently overcome the low-affinity binding defect and achieve adequate VDR occupancy to mediate normal $1,25(OH)_2D$ responses.

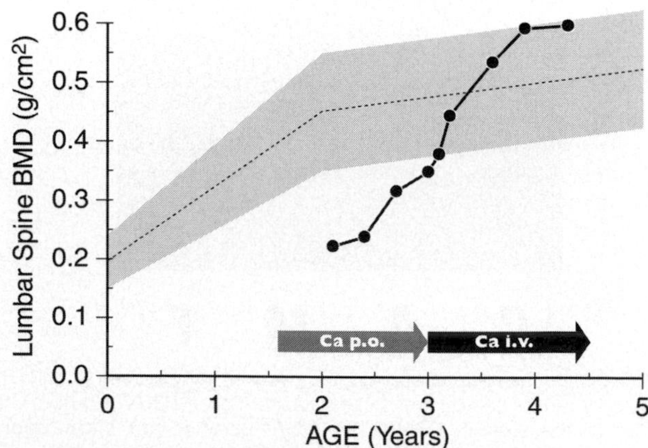

FIGURE 82–9. Bone mineral density (BMD) response in a patient with hereditary vitamin D–resistant rickets treated with oral and intravenous calcium. BMD of the lumbar spine was measured by dual-energy x-ray absorptiometry. The patient received oral calcium (Ca p.o., 2 g/day) for 17 months before treatment with intravenous calcium (Ca i.v.). The *shaded area* represents the reference values for the corresponding ages. Note the rapid correction of BMD upon initiation of intravenous calcium therapy.

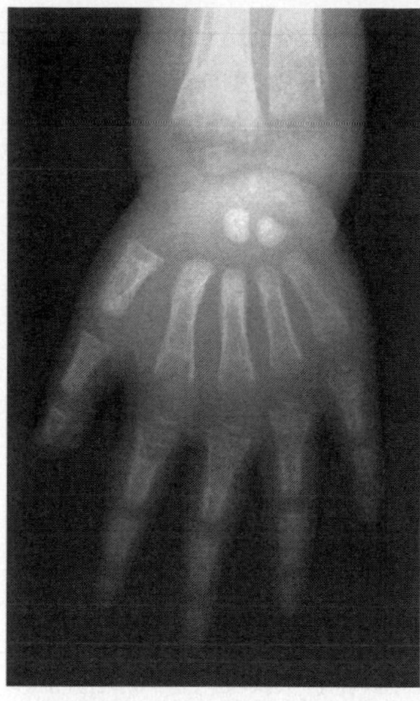 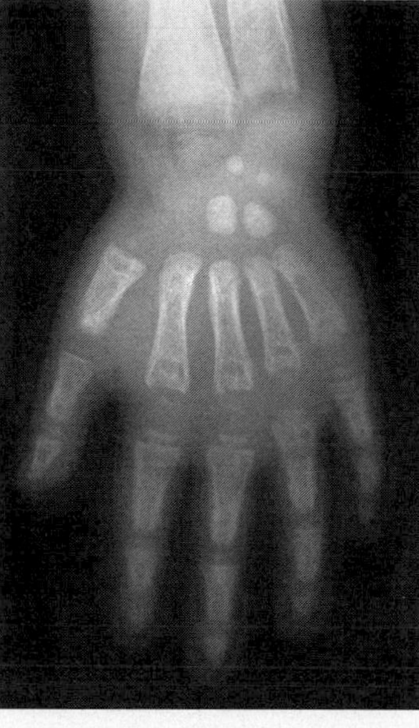 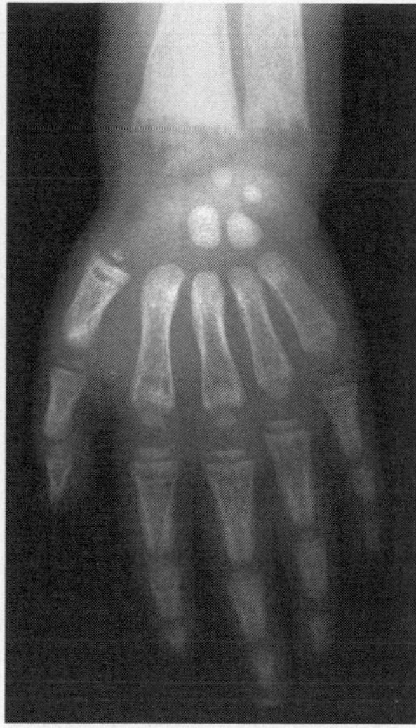 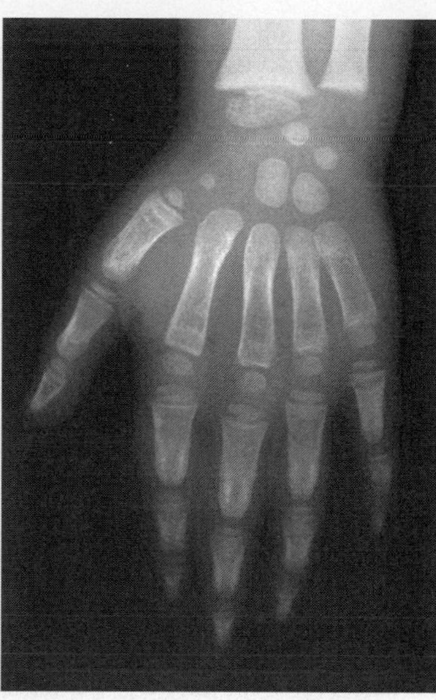

FIGURE 82–10. Radiographic analysis of response to calcium therapy in a patient with hereditary vitamin D–resistant rickets. From left to right, *first panel,* at referral, the patient had been treated for 3 months with $1,25(OH)_2D_3$ (15 μg/day). Rickets is still active, and the bone is demineralized. *Second panel,* after 6 months of $1,25(OH)_2D_3$ (30 μg/day) and oral calcium (2 g/day), no significant improvement was seen. *Third panel,* after 2 months of continuous intravenous calcium (without $1,25[OH]_2D_3$), mineralization is improved. *Last panel,* after 11 months of continuous infusion, mineralization is adequate but the growth plate remains irregular. Clinical status is satisfactory and maintained with oral calcium (2 g/day).

A few patients with HVDRR and alopecia have also been treated successfully with vitamin D metabolites.[57, 65, 123–127]

When vitamin D therapy proves ineffective, intensive calcium therapy is the alternative treatment of choice. Some success has been achieved with high-dose oral calcium[128] (Fig. 82–9). To bypass the calcium absorption defect in the intestine caused by the mutant VDR, long-term intravenous calcium infusions should be considered (see Fig. 82–9). High doses of calcium are infused intravenously during the night over a several-month period. Rapid disappearance of bone pain has been documented, as well as gradual improvement in calcemia and parathyroid function, followed by improvement of the rickets (Fig. 82–10) and weight and height gain.[129–132] The syndrome can recur when the intravenous infusions are discontinued.[129] After the serum calcium level normalizes and radiologic control of the rickets has been achieved with intravenous calcium infusions, high-dose oral calcium therapy is effective in maintaining normocalcemia.[131] For patients with HVDRR who do not respond to high-dose vitamin D therapy, the two-step calcium protocol (intravenous infusions followed by high oral doses) appears to be the preferred therapeutic approach.

One report has described a successful response to oral phosphorus in a patient in whom $1,25(OH)_2D$ therapy was ineffective.[133] It is also interesting to note that in several reports, spontaneous improvement was seen in the disease of patients with HVDRR.[57, 134, 135] This spontaneous healing of rickets usually happens between 7 and 15 years of age and has not been consistently associated with the onset of puberty. Spontaneous recovery does not appear to be related to treatment because therapy was often ineffective and improvement occurred after the treatment was discontinued. These patients appear to remain normocalcemic without therapy and show no evidence of rickets or osteomalacia. Spontaneous improvement has been reported for both ligand binding–positive and ligand binding–negative patients with HVDRR.[57, 134, 135] The alopecia persists despite healing of the rickets.[57, 134, 135] It is not uncommon for children to "outgrow" genetic diseases, and the organism appears able to compensate for the loss of VDR function after skeletal growth has been completed. This apparent functional redundancy does not apply to the hair follicle, however, a situation analogous to what has been described in the VDR-ablated animal model of the disease.[116]

PERSPECTIVES: ROLE OF VITAMIN D IN BONE DEVELOPMENT

The skeleton of VDR-deficient mice develops normally,[114, 115] and the bone abnormalities appearing after weaning can be cured by normalization of circulating mineral ion concentrations via dietary manipulation.[116, 117] These observations dramatically support the concept that the major physiologic effect of $1,25(OH)_2D$ concerns intestinal absorption of calcium and phosphate and that the effects of vitamin D on bone development are indirect. On the contrary, the well-documented effects of $1,25(OH)_2D$ on bone cells in vitro[7] suggest that $1,25(OH)_2D$ plays an important role in the regulation of osteoblast and osteoclast activity, as well as in the control of bone matrix protein synthesis. Because the metabolic enzymes responsible for the synthesis and degradation of $1,25(OH)_2D$ are expressed in the osteoblast,[39, 136, 137] it is possible that vitamin D metabolites can influence bone formation via paracrine or autocrine effects. The recent engineering of transgenic mice overexpressing the VDR specifically in bone tissue support this hypothesis.[138] Osteoblastic expression of a VDR transgene caused elevated periosteal bone formation and therefore wider and stronger bones, consistent with an autocrine anabolic effect of $1,25(OH)_2D$ on bone formation in vivo.

Evidence gathered in vivo also support a physiologic role for another vitamin D metabolite, $24,25(OH)_2D$, during embryogenesis and in processes regulating bone growth, development, and repair (reviewed elsewhere[139]). The power of molecular genetic approaches, including the engineering of loss-of-function and gain-of-function mutations for the VDR and the vitamin D metabolic enzymes 1α-hydroxylase and 24-hydroxylase, should unravel novel molecular mechanisms implicated in the regulation of bone development by vitamin D metabolites and generate useful animal models of hereditary defects in vitamin D metabolism and action.

REFERENCES

1. Bruder SP, Fink DJ, Caplan AI: Mesenchymal stem cells in bone development, bone repair, and skeletal regeneration therapy. J Cell Biochem 56:283–294, 1994.
2. Suda T, Udagawa N, Nakamura I, et al: Modulation of osteoclast differentiation by local factors. Bone 17(suppl):87–91, 1995.
3. Bilezikian JP, Raisz LG, Rodan GA: Principles of Bone Biology. San Diego, CA, Academic Press, 1996, 1398 pp.
4. Anderson HC, Morris DC: Mineralization. *In* Mundy GR, Martin TJ (eds): Handbook of Experimental Pharmacology, vol 107, Physiology and Pharmacology of Bone. Heidelberg, Springer-Verlag, 1993, pp 267–298.
5. Christoffersen J, Landis WJ: A contribution with review to the description of mineralization of bone and other calcified tissues in vivo. Anat Rec 230:435–450, 1991.
6. Roach HI, Erenpreisa J, Aigner T: Osteogenic differentiation of hypertrophic chondrocytes involves asymmetric cell divisions and apoptosis. J Cell Biol 131:483–494, 1995.
7. Feldman D, Glorieux FH, Pike JW: Vitamin D. San Diego, CA, Academic Press, 1997, 1285 pp.

8. Haussler MR, Whitfield GK, Haussler CA, et al: The nuclear vitamin D receptor: Biological and molecular regulatory properties revealed. J Bone Miner Res 13:325–349, 1998.
9. Mangelsdorf DJ, Thummel C, Beato M, et al: The nuclear receptor superfamily: The second decade. Cell 83:835–839, 1995.
10. Baudino TA, Kraichely DM, Jefcoat SC, et al: Isolation of a novel coactivator, NCoA-62, involved in vitamin D–mediated transcription. J Biol Chem 273:16434–16441, 1998.
11. Rachez C, Suldan Z, Ward J, et al: A novel protein complex that interacts with the vitamin D_3 receptor in a ligand-dependent manner and enhances VDR transactivation in a cell-free system. Genes Dev 12:1787–1800, 1998.
12. Blanco J, Wang I, Tsai S, et al: Transcription factor TFIIB and the vitamin D receptor cooperatively activate ligand-dependent transcription. Proc Natl Acad Sci U S A 92:1535–1539, 1995.
13. MacDonald PN, Sherman DR, Dowd DR, et al: The vitamin D receptor interacts with general transcription factor IIB. J Biol Chem 270:4748–4752, 1995.
14. Albright F, Butler AM, Bloomberg E: Rickets resistant to vitamin D therapy. Am J Dis Child 54:529–547, 1937.
15. Prader A, Illig R, Heierli E: Eine besondere form des primäre vitamin D–resistenten rachitis mit hypocalcämie und autosomal-dominanten Erbgang: Die hereditäre PseudoMangelrachitis. Helv Paediatr Acta 16:452–468, 1961.
16. Portale AA, Miller WL: Hereditary rickets revealed (editorial). Kidney Int 54:1762–1764, 1998.
17. Brooks MH, Bell NH, Love L, et al: Vitamin-D–dependent rickets type II. Resistance of target organs to 1,25-dihydroxyvitamin D. N Engl J Med 298:996–999, 1978.
18. Malloy PJ, Pike JW, Feldman D: The vitamin D receptor and the syndrome of hereditary 1,25-dihydroxyvitamin D resistant rickets. Endocr Rev 20:156–188, 1999.
19. Arnaud C, Maijer R, Reade TM, et al: Vitamin D dependency: An inherited postnatal syndrome with secondary hyperparathyroidism. Pediatrics 46:871–880, 1970.
20. Delvin EE, Glorieux FH, Marie PJ, et al: Vitamin D–dependency: Replacement therapy with calcitriol. J Pediatr 99:26–34, 1981.
21. Mandla S, Jones G, Tenenhouse HS: Normal 24-hydroxylation of vitamin D metabolites in patients with vitamin D–dependency rickets type I. Structural implications for vitamin D hydroxylases. J Clin Endocrinol Metab 74:814–820, 1992.
22. Scriver CR, Reade TM, Hamstra AJ, et al: Serum 1,25-dihydroxyvitamin D levels in normal subjects and in patients with hereditary rickets or bone disease. N Engl J Med 299:976–979, 1978.
23. Glorieux FH, St-Arnaud R: Vitamin D pseudodeficiency. *In* Feldman D, Glorieux FH, Pike JW (eds): Vitamin D. San Diego, CA, Academic Press, 1997, pp 755–764.
24. Scriver CR: Vitamin D dependency. Pediatrics 45:361–363, 1970.
25. Labuda M, Morgan K, Glorieux FH: Mapping autosomal recessive vitamin D dependency type I to chromosome 12q14 by linkage analysis. Am J Hum Genet 47:28–36, 1990.
26. Labuda M, Labuda D, Korab-Laskowska M, et al: Linkage disequilibrium analysis in young populations: Pseudovitamin D deficiency rickets (PDDR) and the founder effect in French Canadians. Am J Hum Genet 59:633–643, 1996.
27. St-Arnaud R, Messerlian S, Moir JM, et al: The 25-hydroxyvitamin D 1-alpha-hydroxylase gene maps to the pseudovitamin D–deficiency rickets (PDDR) disease locus. J Bone Miner Res 12:1552–1559, 1997.
28. Shinki T, Shimada H, Wakino S, et al: Cloning and expression of rat 25-hydroxyvitamin D_3–1α-hydroxylase cDNA. Proc Natl Acad Sci U S A 94:12920–12925, 1997.
29. Takeyama K-I, Kitanaka S, Sato T, et al: 25-hydroxyvitamin D_3–1α-hydroxylase and vitamin D synthesis. Science 277:1827–1830, 1997.
30. Fu GK, Lin D, Zhang MYH, et al: Cloning of human 25-hydroxyvitamin D-1α–hydroxylase and mutations causing vitamin D–dependent rickets type I. Mol Endocrinol 11:1961–1970, 1997.
31. Fu GK, Portale AA, Miller WL: Complete structure of the human gene for the vitamin D 1alpha-hydroxylase, P450c1alpha. DNA Cell Biol 16:1499–1507, 1997.
32. Kitanaka S, Takeyama K-I, Murayama A, et al: Inactivating mutations in the 25-hydroxyvitamin D_3 1α-hydroxylase gene in patients with pseudovitamin D–deficiency rickets. N Engl J Med 338:653–661, 1998.
33. Yoshida T, Monkawa T, Tenenhouse HS, et al: Two novel 1α-hydroxylase mutations in French-Canadians with vitamin D dependency rickets type I. Kidney Int 54:1437–1443, 1998.
34. Wang JT, Lin C-J, Burridge SM, et al: Genetics of vitamin D 1α-hydroxylase deficiency in 17 families. Am J Hum Genet 63:1694–1702, 1998.
35. Smith SJ, Rucka AK, Berry JL, et al: Novel mutations in the 1α-hydroxylase (P450c1) gene in three families with pseudovitamin D–deficiency rickets resulting in loss of functional enzyme activity in blood-derived macrophages. J Bone Miner Res 14:730–739, 1999.
36. Solish SB, Picado-Leonard J, Morel Y, et al: Human adrenodoxin reductase: Two mRNAs encoded by a single gene on chromosome 17cen-q25 are expressed in steroidogenic tissues. Proc Natl Acad Sci U S A 85:7104–7108, 1988.
37. Chang C, Wu D-A, Mohandas TK, et al: Structure, sequence, chromosomal location and evolution of the human ferredoxin gene. DNA Cell Biol 9:205–212, 1990.
38. Brunette MG, Chan M, Ferriere C, et al: Site of $1,25(OH)_2$ vitamin D_3 synthesis in the kidney. Nature 276:287–289, 1978.
39. Puzas JE, Turner RT, Howard GA, et al: Synthesis of 1,25-dihydroxycholecalciferol and 24,25-dihydroxycholecalciferol by calvarial cells: Characterization of the enzyme systems. Biochem J 245:333–338, 1987.
40. Reichel H, Bishop JE, Koeffler HP, et al: Evidence for 1,25-dihydroxyvitamin D_3 production by cultured porcine alveolar macrophages. Mol Cell Endocrinol 75:163–167, 1991.
41. Ohyama Y, Noshiro M, Okuda K: Cloning and expression of cDNA encoding 25-hydroxyvitamin D_3 24-hydroxylase. FEBS Lett 278:195–198, 1991.
42. Hasemann CA, Kurumbail RG, Boddupalli SS, et al: Structure and function of cytochromes P450: A comparative analysis of three crystal structures. Structure 3:41–62, 1995.
43. Su P, Rennert H, Shayiq RM, et al: A cDNA encoding a rat mitochondrial cytochrome P450 catalyzing both the 26-hydroxylations of cholesterol and 25-hydroxylation of vitamin D_3: Gonadotropic regulation of the cognate mRNA in ovaries. DNA Cell Biol 9:657–665, 1990.
44. Chung B, Matteson KJ, Voutilainen R, et al: Human cholesterol side-chain cleavage enzyme, P450cc: cDNA cloning, assignment of the gene to chromosome 15, and expression in the placenta. Proc Natl Acad Sci U S A 83:8962–8966, 1986.
45. Mornet E, Dupont J, Vitek A, et al: Characterization of two genes encoding human steroid 11β-hydroxylase (P45011β). J Biol Chem 264:20961–20967, 1989.
46. Brenza HL, Kimmel-Jehan C, Jehan F, et al: Parathyroid hormone activation of the 25-hydroxyvitamin D_3–1α-hydroxylase promoter. Proc Natl Acad Sci U S A 95:1387–1391, 1998.
47. De Braekeleer M: Hereditary disorders in Saguenay-Lac-St-Jean (Quebec, Canada). Hum Hered 41:141–146, 1991.
48. Rosen JF, Finberg L: Vitamin D–dependent rickets: Actions of parathyroid hormone and 25-hydroxycholecalciferol. Pediatr Res 6:552–562, 1972.
49. Balsan S, Garabedian M, Lieberherr M, et al: Serum 1,25-dihydroxyvitamin D concentrations in two different types of pseudo-deficiency rickets. *In* Norman AW, Schaefer K, Herrath DV, et al (eds): Vitamin D: Basic Research and Its Clinical Application. New York, Walter de Gruyter, 1979, pp 1143–1149.
50. Glorieux FH: Calcitriol treatment in vitamin D–dependent and vitamin D–resistant rickets. Metabolism 39(suppl):10–12, 1990.
51. Reade TM, Scriver CR, Glorieux FH, et al: Response to crystalline 1α-hydroxyvitamin D_3 in vitamin D dependency. Pediatr Res 9:593–599, 1975.
52. Haussler MR, Norman AW: Chromosomal receptor for a vitamin D metabolite. Proc Natl Acad Sci U S A 62:155–162, 1969.
53. Pike JW, Haussler MR: Purification of chicken intestinal receptor for 1,25-dihydroxyvitamin D. Proc Natl Acad Sci U S A 76:5485–5489, 1979.
54. Pike JW, Marion SL, Donaldson CA, et al: Serum and monoclonal antibodies against the chick intestinal receptor for 1,25-dihydroxyvitamin D_3. Generation by a preparation enriched in a 64,000-dalton protein. J Biol Chem 258:1289–1296, 1983.
55. Dame MC, Pierce EA, Prahl JM, et al: Monoclonal antibodies to the porcine intestinal receptor for 1,25-dihydroxyvitamin D_3: Interaction with distinct receptor domains. Biochemistry 25:4523–4534, 1986.
56. Feldman D, Chen T, Cone C, et al: Vitamin D resistant rickets with alopecia: Cultured skin fibroblasts exhibit defective cytoplasmic receptors and unresponsiveness to $1,25(OH)_2D_3$. J Clin Endocrinol Metab 55:1020–1022, 1982.
57. Hirst MA, Hochman HI, Feldman D: Vitamin D resistance and alopecia: A kindred with normal 1,25-dihydroxyvitamin D binding, but decreased receptor affinity for deoxyribonucleic acid. J Clin Endocrinol Metab 60:490–495, 1985.
58. Dokoh S, Haussler MR, Pike JW: Development of a radioligand immunoassay for 1,25-dihydroxycholecalciferol receptors utilizing monoclonal antibody. Biochem J 221:129–136, 1984.
59. Pike JW, Dokoh S, Haussler MR, et al: Vitamin D_3–resistant fibroblasts have immunoassayable 1,25-dihydroxyvitamin D_3 receptors. Science 224:879–881, 1984.
60. Malloy PJ, Hochberg Z, Pike JW, et al: Abnormal binding of vitamin D receptors to deoxyribonucleic acid in a kindred with vitamin D–dependent rickets, type II. J Clin Endocrinol Metab 68:263–269, 1989.
61. McDonnell DP, Mangelsdorf DJ, Pike JW, et al: Molecular cloning of complementary DNA encoding the avian receptor for vitamin D. Science 235:1214–1217, 1987.
62. Baker AR, McDonnell DP, Hughes M, et al: Cloning and expression of full-length cDNA encoding human vitamin D receptor. Proc Natl Acad Sci U S A 85:3294–3298, 1988.
63. Burmester JK, Maeda N, DeLuca HF: Isolation and expression of rat 1,25-dihydroxyvitamin D_3 receptor cDNA. Proc Natl Acad Sci U S A 85:1005–1009, 1988.
64. Labuda M, Fujiwara TM, Ross MV, et al: Two hereditary defects related to vitamin D metabolism map to the same region of human chromosome 12q13-14. J Bone Miner Res 7:1447–1453, 1992.
65. Hughes MR, Malloy PJ, Kieback DG, et al: Point mutations in the human vitamin D receptor gene associated with hypocalcemic rickets. Science 242:1702–1705, 1988.
66. Miyamoto K, Kesterson RA, Yamamoto H, et al: Structural organization of the human vitamin D receptor chromosomal gene and its promoter. Mol Endocrinol 11:1165–1179, 1997.
67. Jehan F, DeLuca HF: Cloning and characterization of the mouse vitamin D receptor promoter. Proc Natl Acad Sci U S A 94:10138–10143, 1997.
68. Arai H, Miyamoto K-I, Taketani Y, et al: A vitamin D receptor gene polymorphism in the translation initiation codon: Effect on protein activity and relation to bone mineral density in Japanese women. J Bone Miner Res 12:915–921, 1997.
69. Jurutka PW, Hsieh JC, MacDonald PN, et al: Phosphorylation of serine 208 in the human vitamin D receptor. The predominant amino acid phosphorylated by casein kinase II, in vitro, and identification as a significant phosphorylation site in intact cells. J Biol Chem 268:6791–6799, 1993.
70. Hilliard GM, Cook RG, Weigel NL, et al: 1,25-dihydroxyvitamin D_3 modulates phosphorylation of serine 205 in the human vitamin D receptor: Site-directed mutagenesis of this residue promotes alternative phosphorylation. Biochemistry 33:4300–4311, 1994.
71. Rastinejad F, Perlamann T, Evans RM, et al: Structural determinants of nuclear receptor assembly on DNA direct repeats. Nature 375:203–211, 1995.
72. Hsieh J-C, Shimizu Y, Minoshima S, et al: Novel nuclear localization signal between the two DNA-binding zinc fingers in the human vitamin D receptor. J Cell Biochem 70:94–109, 1998.
73. Hsieh J-C, Jurutka PW, Galligan MA, et al: Human vitamin D receptor is selectively phosphorylated by protein kinase C on serine 51, a residue crucial to its *trans*-activation function. Proc Natl Acad Sci U S A 88:9315–9319, 1991.
74. Hsieh J-C, Jurutka PW, Nakajima S, et al: Phosphorylation of the human vitamin D receptor by protein kinase C: Biochemical and functional evaluation of the serine 51 recognition site. J Biol Chem 268:15118–15126, 1993.
75. Nishikawa J, Kitaura M, Imagawa M, et al: Vitamin D receptor contains multiple

dimerization interfaces that are functionally different. Nucleic Acids Res 23:606–611, 1995.
76. Hsieh J-C, Jurutka PW, Selznick SH, et al: The T-box near the zinc fingers of the human vitamin D receptor is required for heterodimeric DNA binding and transactivation. Biochem Biophys Res Commun 215:1–7, 1995.
77. Renaud J-P, Rochel N, Ruff M, et al: Crystal structure of the RAR-γ ligand-binding domain bound to all-*trans* retinoic acid. Nature 378:681–689, 1995.
78. Wagner RL, Apriletti JW, McGrath ME, et al: A structural role for hormone in the thyroid hormone receptor. Nature 378:690–697, 1995.
79. Bourguet W, Ruff M, Chambon P, et al: Crystal structure of the ligand-binding domain of the human nuclear receptor RXR-α. Nature 375:377–382, 1995.
80. Allegretto EA, Pike JW: Trypsin cleavage of chick 1,25-dihydroxyvitamin D_3 receptors. Generation of discrete polypeptides which retain hormone but are unreactive to DNA and monoclonal antibody. J Biol Chem 260:10139–10145, 1985.
81. Allegretto EA, Pike JW, Haussler MR: Immunochemical detection of unique proteolytic fragments of the chick 1,25-dihydroxyvitamin D_3 receptor. Distinct 20-kDa DNA-binding and 45-kDa hormone-binding species. J Biol Chem 262:1312–1319, 1987.
82. Peleg S, Sastry M, Collins ED, et al: Distinct conformational changes induced by 20-epi analogues of 1 alpha,25-dihydroxyvitamin D_3 are associated with enhanced activation of the vitamin D receptor. J Biol Chem 270:10551–10558, 1995.
83. Rosen ED, Beninghof EG, Koenig RJ: Dimerization interfaces of thyroid hormone, retinoic acid, vitamin D, and retinoid X receptors. J Biol Chem 268:11534–11541, 1993.
84. Whitfield GK, Hsieh J-C, Nakajima S, et al: A highly conserved region in the hormone binding domain of the human vitamin D receptor contains residues vital for heterodimerization with retinoid X receptor and for transcriptional activation. Mol Endocrinol 9:1166–1179, 1995.
85. Jin CH, Kerner SA, Hong MH, et al: Transcriptional activation and dimerization functions in the human vitamin D receptor. Mol Endocrinol 10:945–957, 1996.
86. Nakajima S, Hsieh J-C, MacDonald PN, et al: The C-terminal region of the vitamin D receptor is essential to form a complex with a receptor auxiliary factor required for high affinity binding to the vitamin D responsive element. Mol Endocrinol 8:159–172, 1994.
87. Henttu PM, Kalkhoven E, Parker MG: AF-2 activity and recruitment of steroid receptor coactivator 1 to the estrogen receptor depend on a lysine residue conserved in nuclear receptors. Mol Cell Biol 17:1832–1839, 1997.
88. Danielian PS, White R, Lees JA, et al: Identification of a conserved region required for hormone dependent transcriptional activation by steroid hormone receptors. EMBO J 11:1025–1033, 1992.
89. Jurutka PW, Hsieh J-C, Remus LS, et al: Mutations in the 1,25-dihydroxyvitamin D_3 receptor identifying C-terminal amino acids required for transcriptional activation that are functionally dissociated from hormone binding, heterodimeric DNA binding and interaction with basal transcription factor IIB, in vitro. J Biol Chem 272:14592–14599, 1997.
90. Masuyama H, Brownfield CM, St-Arnaud R, et al: Evidence for ligand-dependent intramolecular folding of the AF-2 domain in vitamin D receptor–activated transcription and coactivator interaction. Mol Endocrinol 11:1507–1517, 1997.
91. Hong H, Kohli K, Garabedian MJ, et al: GRIP 1, a transcriptional coactivator for the AF-2 transactivation domain of steroid, thyroid, retinoid, and vitamin D receptors. Mol Cell Biol 17:2735–2744, 1997.
92. Chen H, Lin RJ, Schiltz RL, et al: Nuclear receptor coactivator ACTR is a novel histone acetyltransferase and forms a multimeric activation complex with P/CAF and CBP/p300. Cell 90:569–580, 1997.
93. Le Douarin B, Zechel C, Garnier J-M, et al: The N-terminal part of TIF1, a putative mediator of the ligand-dependent activation function (AF-2) of nuclear receptors, is fused to B-raf in the oncogenic protein T18. EMBO J 14:2020–2033, 1995.
94. Schulman IG, Juguilon H, Evans RM: Activation and repression by nuclear hormone receptors: Hormone modulates an equilibrium between active and repressive states. Mol Cell Biol 16:3807–3813, 1996.
95. Zhu WJ, Malloy PJ, Delvin E, et al: Hereditary 1,25-dihydroxyvitamin D–resistant rickets due to an opal mutation causing premature termination of the vitamin D receptor. J Bone Miner Res 13:259–264, 1998.
96. Mechica JB, Leite MO, Mendonca BB, et al: A novel nonsense mutation in the first zinc finger of the vitamin D receptor causing hereditary 1,25-dihydroxyvitamin D_3–resistant rickets. J Clin Endocrinol Metab 82:3892–3894, 1997.
97. Yagi, H, Ozono K, Miyake H, et al: A new point mutation in the deoxyribonucleic acid–binding domain of the vitamin D receptor in a kindred with hereditary 1,25-dihydroxyvitamin D–resistant rickets. J Clin Endocrinol Metab 76:509–512, 1993.
98. Rut AR, Hewison M, Kristjansson K, et al: Two mutations causing vitamin D resistant rickets: Modeling on the basis of steroid hormone receptor DNA-binding domain crystal structures. Clin Endocrinol 41:581–590, 1994.
99. Lin NU-T, Malloy PJ, Sakati N, et al: A novel mutation in the deoxyribonucleic acid–binding domain of the vitamin D receptor gene causes hereditary 1,25-dihydroxyvitamin D resistant rickets. J Clin Endocrinol Metab 81:2564–2569, 1996.
100. Saijo T, Ito M, Takeda E, et al: A unique mutation in the vitamin D receptor gene in three Japanese patients with vitamin D–dependent rickets type II: Utility of single-strand conformation polymorphism analysis for heterozygous carrier detection. Am J Hum Genet 49:668–673, 1991.
101. Cockerill FJ, Hawa NS, Yousaf N, et al: Mutations in the vitamin D receptor gene in three kindreds associated with hereditary vitamin D resistant rickets. J Clin Endocrinol Metab 82:3156–3160, 1997.
102. Wiese RJ, Goto H, Prahl JM, et al: Vitamin D–dependency rickets type II: Truncated vitamin D receptor in three kindreds. Mol Cell Endocrinol 90:197–201, 1993.
103. Sone T, Marx SJ, Liverman UA, et al: A unique point mutation in the human vitamin D receptor chromosomal gene confers hereditary resistance to 1,25-dihydroxyvitamin D_3. Mol Endocrinol 4:623–631, 1990.
104. Malloy PJ, Weisman Y Feldman D, et al: Hereditary 1 alpha, 25-dihydroxyvitamin D–resistant rickets resulting from a mutation in the vitamin D receptor deoxyribonucleic acid–binding domain. J Clin Endocrinol Metab 78:313–316, 1994.
105. Hawa, NS, Cockerill FJ, Vadher S, et al: Identification of a novel mutation in hereditary vitamin D resistant rickets causing exon skipping. Clin Endocrinol 45:85–92, 1996.
106. Kristjansson K, Rut AR, Hewison M, et al: Two mutations in the hormone binding domain of the vitamin D receptor cause tissue resistance to 1,25 dihydroxyvitamin D_3. J Clin Invest 92:12–16, 1993.
107. Malloy PJ, Hochberg Z, Tiosano D, et al: The molecular basis of hereditary 1,25-dihydroxyvitamin D_3 resistant rickets in seven related families. J Clin Invest 86:2071–2079, 1990.
108. Ritchie HH, Hughes MR, Thompson ET, et al: An ochre mutation in the vitamin D receptor gene causes hereditary 1,25-dihydroxyvitamin D_3–resistant rickets in three families. Proc Natl Acad Sci U S A 86:9783–9787, 1989.
109. Malloy PJ, Hughes MR, Pike JW, et al: Vitamin D receptor mutations and hereditary 1,25-dihydroxyvitamin D resistant rickets. *In* Norman AW, Bouillon R, Thomasset M (eds): Vitamin D: Gene Regulation, Structure-Function Analysis, and Clinical Application. Eighth Workshop on Vitamin D. New York, Walter de Gruyter, 1991, pp 116–124.
110. Malloy PJ, Eccleshall TR, Gross C, et al: Hereditary vitamin D resistant rickets caused by a novel mutation in the vitamin D receptor that results in decreased affinity for hormone and cellular hyporesponsiveness. J Clin Invest 99:297–304, 1997.
111. Whitfield GK, Selznick SH, Haussler CA, et al: Vitamin D receptors from patients with resistance to 1,25-dihydroxyvitamin D_3: Point mutations confer reduced transactivation in response to ligand and impaired interaction with the retinoid X receptor heterodimeric partner. Mol Endocrinol 10:1617–1631, 1996.
112. Wurtz JM, Bourguet W, Renaud JP, et al: A canonical structure for the ligand-binding domain of nuclear receptors. Nat Struct Biol 3:87–94, 1996.
113. Hewison M, Rut AR, Kristjansson K, Walker RE, et al: Tissue resistance to 1,25-dihydroxyvitamin D receptor gene. Clin Endocrinol 39:663–670, 1993.
114. Yoshizawa T, Handa Y, Uematsu Y, et al: Mice lacking the vitamin D receptor exhibit impaired bone formation, uterine hypoplasia and growth retardation after weaning. Nat Genet 16:391–396, 1997.
115. Li YC, Pirro AE, Amling M, et al: Targeted ablation of the vitamin D receptor: An animal model of vitamin D–dependent rickets type II with alopecia. Proc Natl Acad Sci U S A 94:9831–9835, 1997.
116. Li YC, Amling M, Pirro AE, et al: Normalization of mineral ion homeostasis by dietary means prevents hyperparathyroidism, rickets, and osteomalacia, but not alopecia in vitamin D receptor ablated mice. Endocrinology 139:4391–4396, 1998.
117. Priemel M, Amling M, Holzmann T, et al: Rescue of the skeletal phenotype of vitamin D receptor–ablated mice in the setting of normal mineral ion homeostasis: Formal histomorphometric and biomechanical analyses. Endocrinology 140:4982–4987, 1999.
118. Reichrath J, Schilli M, Kerber A, et al: Hair follicle expression of 1,25-dihydroxyvitamin D_3 receptor during the murine hair cycle. Br J Dermatol 131:477–482, 1994.
119. Marx SJ, Bliziotes MM, Nanes M, et al: Analysis of the relation between alopecia and resistance to 1,25-dihydroxyvitamin D. Clin Endocrinol 25:373–381, 1986.
120. Brooks MH, Bell NH, Love L, et al: Vitamin-D–dependent rickets type II. Resistance of target organs to 1,25-dihydroxyvitamin D. N Engl J Med 298:996–999, 1978.
121. Marx SJ, Spiegel AM, Brown EM, et al: A familial syndrome of decrease in sensitivity to 1,25-dihydroxyvitamin D. J Clin Endocrinol Metab 47:1303–1310, 1978.
122. Zerwekh JE, Glass K, Jowsey J, et al: An unique form of osteomalacia associated with end organ refractoriness to 1,25-dihydroxyvitamin D and apparent defective synthesis of 25-hydroxyvitamin D. J Clin Endocrinol Metab 49:171–175, 1979.
123. Kudoh T, Kumagai T, Uetsuji N, et al: Vitamin D dependent rickets: Decreased sensitivity to 1,25-dihydroxyvitamin D. Eur J Pediatr 137:307–311, 1981.
124. Balsan S, Garabedian M, Liberman UA, et al: Rickets and alopecia with resistance to 1,25-dihydroxyvitamin D: Two different clinical courses with two different cellular defects. J Clin Endocrinol Metab 57:803–811, 1983.
125. Tsuchiya Y, Matsuo N, Cho H, et al: An usual form of vitamin D–dependent rickets in a child: Alopecia and marked end-organ hyposensitivity to biologically active vitamin D. J Clin Endocrinol Metab 51:685–690, 1980.
126. Castells S, Greig F, Fusi MA, et al: Severely deficient binding of 1,25-dihydroxyvitamin D to its receptors in a patient responsive to high doses of this hormone. J Clin Endocrinol Metab 63:252–256, 1986.
127. Takeda E, Kuroda Y, Saijo T, et al: 1 alpha-hydroxyvitamin D_3 treatment of three patients with 1,25-dihydroxyvitamin D-receptor–defect rickets and alopecia. Pediatrics 80:97–101, 1987.
128. Sakati N, Woodhouse NJY, Niles N, et al: Hereditary resistance to 1,25-dihydroxyvitamin D: Clinical and radiological improvement during high-dose oral calcium therapy. Horm Res 24:280–287, 1986.
129. Balsan S, Garabedian M, Larchet M, et al: Long-term nocturnal calcium infusions can cure rickets and promote normal mineralization in hereditary resistance to 1,25-dihydroxyvitamin D. J Clin Invest 77:1661–1667, 1986.
130. Weisman Y, Bab I, Gazit D, et al: Long-term intracaval calcium infusion therapy in end-organ resistance to 1,25-dihydroxyvitamin D. Am J Med 83:984–990, 1987.
131. Hochberg Z, Tiosano D, Even L: Calcium therapy for calcitriol-resistant rickets. J Pediatr 121:803–808, 1992.
132. Bliziotes M, Yergey AL, Nanes MS, et al: Absent intestinal response to calciferols in hereditary resistance to 1,25-dihydroxyvitamin D: Documentation and effective therapy with high dose intravenous calcium infusions. J Clin Endocrinol Metab 66:294–300, 1988.
133. Rosen JF, Fleischman AR, Finberg L, et al: Rickets with alopecia: An inborn error of vitamin D metabolism. J Pediatr 94:729–735, 1979.
134. Hochberg Z, Benderli A, Levy J, et al: 1,25-Dihydroxyvitamin D resistance, rickets, and alopecia. Am J Med 77:805–811, 1984.
135. Chen TL, Hirst MA, Cone CM, et al: 1,25-dihydroxyvitamin D resistance, rickets,

and alopecia: Analysis of receptors and bioresponse in cultured fibroblasts from patients and parents. J Clin Endocrinol Metab 59:383–388, 1984.

136. Turner RT, Puzas JE, Forte MD, et al: In vitro synthesis of 1α,25-dihydroxycholecalciferol and 24,25-dihydroxycholecalciferol by isolated calvarial cells. Proc Natl Acad Sci U S A 77:5720–5724, 1980.

137. Bolt MA, Armbrecht HJ, Hodam TL, et al: Induction of the vitamin D 24-hydroxylase (CYP24) by 1,25-dihydroxyvitamin D_3 is regulated by parathyroid hormone in UMR 106 osteoblastic cells. Endocrinology 134:3375–3381, 1998.

138. Gardiner EM, Sims NA, Thomas GP, et al: Elevated osteoblastic vitamin D receptor in transgenic mice yields stronger bones. Bone 23(suppl):176, 1998.

139. St-Arnaud R: 24, 25-Dihydroxyvitamin D–active metabolite or inactive catabolite (editorial)? Endocrinology 139:3371–3374, 1998.

Chapter 83

Nephrolithiasis

Jill S. Lindberg ▪ Stuart M. Sprague

Kidney stone disease is a common, painful, and costly condition. The upper renal tract is the primary location of stones in industrialized, developed countries, opposed to the bladder, which is the primary site of stones in less developed countries.[1–3] Lower tract stones are composed predominantly of ammonium acid urate and calcium oxalate, whereas upper tract stones are predominantly calcium oxalate and calcium phosphate (Table 83–1). The incidence of upper tract stones has not been well defined, but it is estimated that 12% of men and 5% of woman will have at least one symptomatic stone by the age of 70 years.[4] Unfortunately, the natural history of stone disease is that once a patient passes their first calcium stone, the likelihood of forming a second stone is approximately 15% at 1 year, 35% at 5 years, 50% at 10 years, and 75% at 20 to 30 years.[4–6] For most stone types there is a clear male predominance, the exception being the triple phosphate stone where the higher incidence in females may reflect the role of urinary tract infections in its etiology.

Recent years have seen tremendous advances in techniques for stone removal and fragmentation, notably extracorporeal shock wave lithotripsy (ESWL). However, the enthusiasm surrounding such advances has resulted in many clinicians losing sight of the need to search for metabolic causes of stone formation. The impact of patient morbidity and the costs due to acute nephrolithiasis, coupled with the success of medical management, reinforce the premise that stone formers should be evaluated and appropriately treated.

EPIDEMIOLOGY

The incidence and prevalence of kidney stones may be affected by genetic,[7–23] environmental,[24–27] and nutritional[28–33] factors (Table 83–2). A positive family history has been reported in 16% to 37% of patients who have formed a kidney stone. Curhan et al. (34) evaluated 37,999 males in the health professional follow-up study and found that the relative risk for stone formation in men with a positive family history of nephrolithiasis vs. those without was 2.57 (95% CI, 2.19 to 3.02).

TABLE 83–1. Relative Frequency of Different Stone Types in Industrialized Countries

Stone Type	Frequency of Occurrence (%)
Calcium oxalate	67
Triple phosphate	12
Calcium phosphate	8
Uric acid	8
Cystine	1–2
Complex mixed	2–3
Other	1

It is important to note that that not all patients with familial hypercalciuria, a major risk for nephrolithiasis, form stones. Thus, environmental and dietary factors contribute heavily to stone formation. Nutritional factors (see Table 83–2) have also been shown to be important in predisposing to new stone formation and may explain, in large part, the rising incidence of nephrolithiasis in Western countries and Japan.[24, 29] Environmental factors, such as climate, occupation, and medication, also contribute to the risk of stone formation (see Table 83–2). Further analysis of the health professional follow-up data revealed that dietary calcium restriction may further increase the risk of stone formation, even among individuals with a family history of stones.[28, 29, 34]

The patient who forms their first stone is young. The incidence of nephrolithiasis begins to rise in early teenage years with the average age for the onset of nephrolithiasis between 30 and 60 years and a mean age for a first calcium stone being 35 years for males and 33 years for females. The incidence of new stone formers declines later in life.[4, 35] Except for triple phosphate stones, the incidence of nephrolithiasis is two to three times more likely in men than in women.[35]

PATHOGENESIS

Kidney stones consist of approximately 98% crystalline material. Based upon the crystalline composition, some 50 types of stones, most of them extreme rarities, have been recognized. However, calcium salts (calcium oxalate and calcium phosphate) are most often found as the crystalline components of stones, followed by uric acid, struvite, and cystine. A number of theories have been proposed to explain the pathogenesis of stone formation. The formation of kidney stones is a result of a complex biologic process that involves the physicochemical process of crystallization. Crystalluria is very common in both normal individuals and stone formers and will not distinguish kidney stone formers from nonformers,[36–38] as crystalluria is often absent in stone formers.[38]

Most stones do not contain one single crystal type but rather a mixture of several different types with one or two that are predominant. Furthermore, kidney stones do not consist of crystals alone, as biomineralization requires an organic material whereupon the mineral is deposited.[39] In fact, loosely clustered crystals would never become a dense stone if they were not tightly glued together by some organic material.[40] This matrix accounts for approximately 2% of the weight of a stone and is found in concentric layers throughout the stone.[41] The chemical analysis of the matrix has proved to be unrewarding as the dissolution of the stone for analysis requires aggressive procedures such as acid hydrolysis. Thus, most of the knowledge of matrix composition emerges from the substances that are found soluble in urine. The matrix is believed to be composed predominantly of protein, with small amounts of nonamino sugars, glucosamine, water, and organic ash.[42]

TABLE 83–2. Genetic, Nutritional, and Environmental Factors in the Incidence and Prevalence of Kidney Stones

I. Genetic
  A. Hypercalciuria[7, 8]
    1. Absorptive hypercalciuria[9]
      a. Mechanism controversial
      b. Increase in vitamin D receptors in activated lymphcytes[9]
      c. Genetic hypercalciuric rats via enhanced intestinal absorption in enhanced bone demineralization[10]
    2. Defect in renal chloride transporter gene[9, 11, 12]
      a. *CLCN5*
      b. Dent's disease: X-linked recessive disease characterized by hypercalciuric nephrolithiasis, rickets, nephrocalcinosis, hypophosphatemia
    3. Defective oxalate transport in red blood cells[13]
    4. Distal renal tubular acidosis[14]
  B. Uric acid nephrolithiasis
    1. Primary gout—an inherited disorder[15]
    2. Inborn errors of metabolism[16]
      a. Hypoxanthine-guanine phosphoribosyl-transferase deficiency
      b. Phosphoribosylpyrophosphate synthetase overactivity
      c. Glucose-6-phosphatase deficiency
  C. Oxalate[17–19]
    1. Primary hyperoxaluria
    2. Defect in *AGXT* gene in coding liver-specific peroxisomal enzyme
    3. Abnormal activation of pyridoxine to pyridoxal 5′-phosphate
  D. Cystine[9, 20, 21]
    Mutations in *SLC3AL* gene causing types I, II, III cystinuria
  E. Abnormal inhibitors[22, 23]
    1. Abnormal inhibitory macromolecules
      a. Nephrocalcin lacking λ-carboxyglutamic acid radicals
      b. Reduced carbohydrate Tamm-Horsfall protein content
II. Environmental[24–27]
  A. Regional—most common in southeastern states
  B. Hypertension
  C. Occupational
  D. Climate
  E. Medication
  F. Stress
III. Dietary[28–33]
  A. Calcium intake high vs. low
  B. Protein
  C. Salt
  D. Beverage intake

As mentioned above, kidney stones predominantly consist of calcium oxalate or calcium phosphate, or both, and the majority of studies on the process of stone formation have focused on the crystallization of calcium oxalate. Thus, the following discussion of the principles of stone formation will primarily focus on the calcium oxalate crystallization process. The formation of crystalline particles in tubular fluid and urine comprises two major physicochemical aspects: a thermodynamic one, supersaturation, which results in the nucleation of microcrystals; and a kinetic one, comprising rates of crystal growth and aggregation, which also depends, in part, on solution supersaturation.[43]

Crystal Formation

The formation of crystals in the urine is largely a function of supersaturation. A solution that contains any material at a concentration above that material's solubility is said to be supersaturated with respect to that material.[44] Supersaturation is often expressed as the ratio of a dissolved material to its solubility concentration; thus a solution that contains a dissolved material at exactly its solubility concentration has a supersaturation of 1. In tubular fluid and urine, the supersaturation may rise to between 2 and 8 without new solid phase formation (Fig. 83–1). Such a solution is called metastably supersaturated and if a solid phase is placed into metastable solution, crystalline growth of the particle will occur. At supersaturation values above the metastable upper limit, crystals will form spontaneously, a process called nucleation. Once nucleation occurs, the kinetic phase, which is comprised of growth and aggregation, will proceed. If such a supersaturated solution is in the tubular fluid or urine, the spectrum of crystalluria, gravel, stones, and nephrocalcinosis will result. With respect to supersaturation, each substance acts as if it is alone; thus a solution may be simultaneously supersaturated with respect to multiple substances.[45]

Calcium oxalate is the most prevalent solid phase in stones, with both calcium phosphate and uric acid occurring as minor constituents.[45, 46] Some patients may produce pure crystalline stones, but most stones contain several crystalline forms with a single predominant crystal.

Factors That Affect Supersaturation

Urinary pH strongly controls the crystallization of uric acid and calcium phosphate, but seems to have little effect on calcium oxalate. Thus most patients who form uric acid and calcium phosphate stones appear to be unsupersaturated with respect to uric acid and calcium phosphate.[35] The causes of low urine pH which promote uric acid crystallization include extrarenal losses of alkali (usually gastrointestinal) and renal disorders that limit the availability of ammonium ions for excretion of acids. The low urinary pH can usually be easily corrected. High urinary pH, which increases the supersaturation of calcium phosphate, may result from infection, or some form of incomplete renal tubular acidosis, but exact mechanisms have not been fully explored in stone formers. Other than treating infection, therapy for elevated pH is difficult. Calcium oxalate supersaturation is very dependent on urinary volume and increasing the volume to greater than 2 L/day is of practical benefit in reducing the supersaturation and incidence of stones. However, volume has only a modest effect on uric acid and calcium phosphate supersaturation, as pH is such a powerful factor.

Several other disorders, which directly affect supersaturation, could be found in a large number of stone formers.[45, 47] Hypercalciuria arises from intestinal hyperabsorption and increased bone resorption. This is further discussed below. Primary hyperparathyroidism may be found in 5% of stone formers.[47, 48] Hyperparathyroidism raises urine calcium and phosphorus by increasing bone resorption and indirectly increasing their intestinal absorption via increased production of calcitriol (1,25-dihydroxyvitamin D_3).[48] Hyperparathyroidism also causes bicarbonaturia and the increased urinary pH results in increasing the supersaturation for calcium phosphate as well as calcium oxalate. Hypocitraturia is very common among stone formers.[49] A low urine citrate raises the theoretical risk of stones by decreasing the concentration of soluble calcium citrate[50] and because citrate may also act as an inhibitor of crystallization. Hyperoxaluria will proportionately increase the supersaturation of calcium oxalate.[44] This may result from dietary excess, low calcium diet, enteric diseases with small bowel malabsorption, or primary overproduction. Hyperuricosuria is also common among stone formers and is usually the result of a high purine diet.[51] Surprisingly, high urine urate appears to contribute to calcium oxalate stones and reduction of urine uric acid is quite effective in reducing calcium oxalate stone formation.[52] There are numerous theories as to how high uric acid levels could influence calcium oxalate formation. Coe et al.[53] and Pak and Arnold[54] have proposed that uric acid causes the heterogeneous nucleation of calcium oxalate.

Other Factors

Recent studies have demonstrated that factors that modulate crystal–renal cell interaction may be critical determinants in the formation of renal calculi. Cultured Madin-Darby canine kidney (MDCK) cells adsorb and internalize uric acid crystals,[55] whereas both MDCK and BSC-1 renal cells internalize calcium oxalate monohydrate crystals.[56] The attachment of crystals to cells appears to involve the extrusion of microvilli from the cell surface up and over the crystal. Calcium oxalate crystals competitively inhibit the binding of urate crystals, suggesting competition for some fixed array of binding sites. The crystals localize inside vacuoles and cause the release of lysosomal

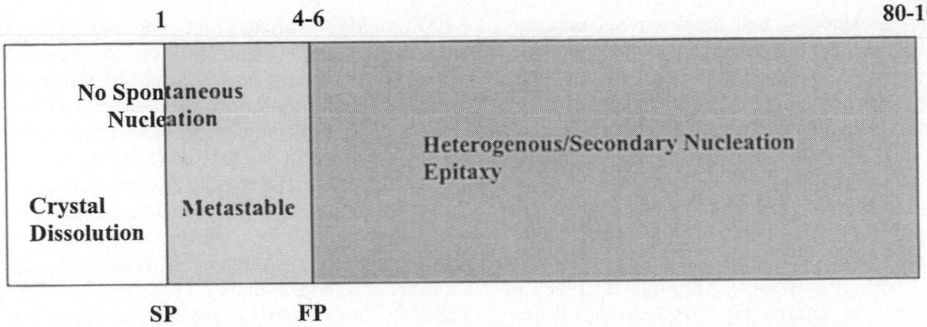

FIGURE 83–1. Relative supersaturation (RS) and crystal nucleation. Illustrated is the scenario of calcium oxalate supersaturation in human urine. The solubility product (SP) is the RS of substances in a solution below which there is complete crystal dissolution. Above the SP, the solution becomes metastable, a condition in which crystals could be induced but spontaneous nucleation does not occur. Once the RS exceeds a threshold value, formation product (FP), nucleation, and growth of crystals will ensue. Heterogeneous nucleation is the process by which crystals nucleate on foreign substances. Secondary nucleation is the nucleation of new crystals on preexisting surfaces of the same species and epitaxy is the phenomenon by which one crystal type is precipitated upon the surface of another crystal. (Adapted from Hess B, Kok BJ: Nucleation, growth, and aggregation of stone-forming crystals. *In* Coe FL, Favus MJ, Pak CYC, et al (eds): Kidney Stones. Medical and Surgical Management. Philadelphia, Lippincott-Raven, 1996, p 6.)

enzymes. The crystals also induce cell proliferation and the expression of early-response genes that seem to regulate extracellular matrix formation. This cell adhesion could be blocked by many of the identified crystal inhibitors that are described below.[56] Tubular fluid normally passes quickly through the tubule, but the adherence of crystals to epithelial cells may set up sites that permit crystal growth over months or years to form stones.

Another recent and interesting finding is that of the potential of nanobacteria to act as a crystallization nidus for the formation of apatite crystals.[57] Nanobacteria are the smallest cell-walled bacteria that produce biogenic apatite on their cell envelope. This mineralized envelope is then shed. In in vitro cultures nanobacteria have been shown to produce stonelike growths of apatite, even in unsupersaturated solutions. Live nanobacteria are detectable in human urine and nanobacteria antigens have been identified in 30 of 30 human kidney stones.[57]

Inhibition of Crystallization

Normal urine is generally supersaturated in regard to multiple substances. If it were not for the remarkable ability of the urine to inhibit crystallization it would be expected that the majority of the population, rather than the minority, would continuously form stones. This inhibition is generally kinetic, a delaying rather than a permanent stoppage of crystal formation, growth, and aggregation. Since the transit time through the nephron is measured in minutes, these delaying mechanisms permit the excretion of supersaturated urine. The molecules that stabilize and prevent crystallization within the tubules and urinary tract are a poorly defined collection. Which ones predominate, how they function, and how they are regulated is not well understood. Whether defects in these inhibitors cause stone disease is presently under intense investigation. The effects of these inhibitors are broad and include reductions in nucleation, growth, and aggregation. Although not complete, Table 83–3 lists the inhibitors considered as potentially important modifiers of crystallization.

TABLE 83–3. Inhibitors of Urinary Crystallization

	Nucleation	Growth	Aggregation
Citrate	No	Yes	Yes
Glycosaminoglycans	Yes	Yes	Yes
Tamm-Horsfall protein	No	No	Yes
Uropontin	Yes	Yes	Yes
Nephrocalcin	Yes	Yes	Yes
Calgranulin	?	Yes	Yes
Uronic acid–rich protein	Yes	Yes	?

The primary effect of citrate is to complex with calcium to form a soluble complex, thereby reducing supersaturation. Although citrate is not an inhibitor of nucleation, at physiologic concentrations it inhibits crystal growth and aggregation.[58, 59] The glycosaminoglycans, chondroitin sulfate and heparan sulfate, have a mild inhibitory effect on nucleation, as well as inhibitory actions on growth and aggregation at concentrations present in urine.[59, 60] Tamm-Horsfall protein is produced and secreted by the ascending limb of the loop of Henle and inhibits the aggregation of calcium oxalate crystals.[23, 61] It has no effect on nucleation or growth.[62] Uropontin is nearly identical to bone osteopontin and inhibits the formation of hydroxyapatite,[63, 64] as well as the nucleation, growth, and aggregation of calcium oxalate crystals.[65, 66] Because it is active against both kinds of crystals at concentrations typically found in urine, it is likely to contribute to the overall defense against supersaturation. Whether defects of uropontin contribute to stone formation is unknown. Nephrocalcin is an acidic glycoprotein that has been purified but not yet sequenced or cloned.[67] It inhibits nucleation, growth, and aggregation of calcium oxalate crystals.[62] Nephrocalcin exists in multiple isoforms and normally contains γ-carboxyglutamic acid, but this unusual amino acid substitution is absent in stone formers.[22, 68, 69] Calgranulin, an S100 calcium-binding protein, has recently been isolated from human kidney and urine and found to be a potent inhibitor of calcium oxalate crystal growth and aggregation.[70] Uronic acid rich protein is a portion of the interalpha-trypsin inhibitor, which has been isolated from urine.[71] It appears to inhibit nucleation and growth at relatively low concentrations, but normal levels in urine are not known. Although this molecule is a candidate as an inhibitor, its in vivo activity cannot be estimated.

EVALUATION OF STONE FORMERS

Evaluation of the stone former is usually divided into the single stone former, or "inactive stone former," vs. the active stone former.[72, 73] Traditionally, active stone formers have been described as patients with greater than two to three stones formed over a 2-year period. Although a person who presents with their first stone may not be an active stone former, there is a high incidence of subsequent stone formation.[4–6] It has also been demonstrated that single stone formers have the same incidence of metabolic abnormalities as patients who form multiple stones.[74] In addition, some urologists have recommended that in view of the technological achievements in stone removal, it is better to treat the stones as they appear than to spend money on expensive investigations and lifelong management.[73] However, this reasoning is not tenable. Spontaneous passage of stones is a common feature among recurrent stone formers and although such stones by definition are delivered without surgical procedures they definitely do not pass without pain and, in most cases, require some kind of medical assistance.[73, 75] Furthermore, small stones can obstruct the ureter, thereby resulting in infection and altered renal function. Repeated ESWL, which is the standard procedure for stone removal, is thought to be a gentle procedure. However, it is expensive and may cause some damage to the renal parenchyma.[76] Long-term medical treatment will, in most cases, prevent stones and be less expensive than commonly used procedures for stone removal. Every attempt should also be made to avoid development of a complicated stone, such as a very large, obstructive, or infected stone, which may require considerable efforts to remove. Finally, the recurrent stone former always suffers from the threat of a new painful stone episode that might jeopardize his or her normal activities. Although all types of recurrent nephrolithiasis cannot be completely arrested, the disease can often be converted to a less serious form.

When evaluating patients, it may be useful to divide stone formers into either the single (first time) stone former or the recurrent stone former. There may be a reason for further subgrouping of single stone formers into those who experience uncomplicated and complicated passage of the stone. Obviously, the first group represents patients in whom the stone passes spontaneously, whereas the second group represents patients in whom the stone becomes lodged in the ureter, which may lead to complications of residual stone in the kidney or infection.

Regardless, a thorough history must be obtained from both single and multiple stone formers that includes family history, medication history, and stone formation history. In addition, the history should address other conditions such as malabsorption, chronic diarrhea, hyperparathyroidism, history of neoplasm, and history of recurrent urinary tract infections. Physical examination should include blood pressure, along with evaluation of evidence of loss of height and kyphosis of the thoracolumbar spine. One must also evaluate the patient for evidence of subcutaneous calcification. The laboratory approach to the patient with a single uncomplicated stone should include urinalysis and culture, serum calcium, phosphorus, uric acid, electrolytes, and creatinine. Parathyroid hormone (PTH) should be evaluated if calcium and phosphorus levels are abnormal. In addition, one may consider a spot urine test for cystine. The laboratory approach to those with multiple or complex stones should include the same laboratory workup described for the single stone former. In addition, it is recommended that duplicate 24-hour urine collections be obtained for volume, calcium, phosphate, sodium, uric acid, oxalate, citrate, creatinine, and pH. The necessity of a 24-hour urine quantitation of cystine and magnesium depends on the patient's clinical situation. A single 24-hour urine collection and serum chemistries should be repeated in 3 to 4 months after initiation of preventive therapy. Once the stone burden is stable, the patient can be followed with periodic imaging studies and the 24-hour urine test may be repeated every 1 to 2 years. If there is a change in the stone burden, more frequent evaluations should be performed.

Radiologic analysis varies depending on whether the physician has information on the type of stone the patient forms. Uric acid stones are not visible on plain KUB (kidneys, ureter, bladder) films. However, plain KUB films with tomograms with or without intravenous (IV) urography are the most common radiologic methods utilized to evaluate stones both in the acute situation and for follow-up of stone burden after therapy. If the patient has uric acid stones or is pregnant, certainly renal ultrasound has been an excellent method by which to evaluate both uric acid and calcium oxalate stones.

Recently, spiral computed tomography (CT) and helical CT have become available for evaluation of kidney stones. The CT examination has many advantages over the other methods mentioned above, as it is more accurate. It evaluates both uric acid and calcium oxalate stones without the use of IV contrast. It is also an excellent means to utilize in follow-up of kidney stones after initiation of preventive therapy.

CALCAREOUS STONES

Hypercalciuric Nephrolithiasis

Hypercalciuria is defined as urinary calcium excretion greater than 300 mg/day in men, 250 mg/day in women,[77] or 4 mg/kg/day on a 1000 mg/day[33] calcium diet. The majority of patients with stones have primary idiopathic calcium stone disease. Less than 10% of the calcium stone formers have a predisposing disease such as hyperparathyroidism, renal tubular acidosis, or primary hyperoxaluria.[1, 47, 75] Current understanding of the pathogenesis emphasizes the multifactorial nature of nephrolithiasis. Various investigators[47, 74] have proposed the diagnostic categorization of stones. Pak and colleagues[74] conducted an ambulatory evaluation of 241 patients and classified their nephrolithiases into 10 metabolic etiologic groups. Since that classification the understanding of the pathophysiology of renal stone disease has progressed and a more recent ambulatory evaluation of 1270 patients was reported in 1995.[72] An extensive ambulatory evaluation was performed, as well as a fasting and calcium load test for assessment of renal calcium leak and intestinal hyperabsorption. The resulting classification of nephrolithiasis is shown in Table 83–4. Hypercalciuria was the most common disorder, but, it should be noted that hypocitraturia was encountered in 41% of patients. Some of these patients suffered from renal tubular acidosis or chronic diarrheal syndrome, but the majority of hypocitraturia was idiopathic.

As described above, idiopathic hypercalciuria can be classified into specific diagnostic groups (see Table 83–4). However, many general concepts have emerged from studies of patients with excessive calcium excretion, which allows for patients to be divided into more general categories. For the purposes of this discussion we use the classification proposed by Bushinksy[75]: idiopathic hypercalciuria, hormonal hypercalciuria, and renal hypercalciuria.

IDIOPATHIC HYPERCALCIURIA

Though the cause of idiopathic hypercalciuria is not known, it results from disordered regulation of calcium handling at sites where large fluxes of calcium must be tightly regulated.[75, 78] This disordered regulation may occur in the intestine, the kidney, or the bone, resulting in an increase in urinary calcium. Increased intestinal calcium absorption may occur either by a direct mechanism or mediated by excess $125(OH)_2D_3$-induced intestinal calcium absorption. This increase in calcium absorption results in a slight increase in serum calcium, suppressed PTH secretion, and an increase in the calcium filtered by the glomerulus and delivered to the renal tubule. In this process, the suppressed PTH causes decreased tubular calcium reabsorption, further contributing to the hypercalciuria. Most investigators agree that patients with idiopathic hypercalciuria have an increase in net intestinal calcium absorption, increased $1,25(OH)_2D_3$ levels, and increased number of intestinal vitamin D receptors.[35, 75, 78, 79] Some investigators prefer to differentiate patients into those with dietary (absorptive) hypercalciuria; those who have hypercalciuria following exposure to increased oral calcium but have normal urinary calcium when on a low calcium diet; those with resorptive hypercalciuria; and those with hypercalciuria on a calcium-restricted diet. In addition, most of these patients also have low bone mineral density[79, 80] and may be at increased risk for fracture.[81] These abnormalities appear to point to a systemic dysregulation of the effect of $1,25(OH)_2D_3$ acting on the intestine, bone, and possibly the kidney.[75] In those patients with resorptive hypercalciuria, increased production of bone-resorbing cytokines may be responsible for the increased filtered load of calcium.[80–82]

Therapy for Idiopathic Hypercalciuria

For all patients with nephrolithiasis, there are several dietary adjustments that should be made (Table 83–5). Medical therapy may be initiated with either a long-acting thiazide diuretic such as chlorthalidone or twice-daily dosing of hydrochlorthiazide to lower calcium excretion.[35, 75, 84] Sodium restriction (<100 mEq/day) is necessary for thiazides to be effective. Triamterene, an alternative potassium-sparing diuretic, should be avoided in patients with a history of stones, as it or its metabolites can precipitate in urine and contribute to stone formation.[85] This occurs in approximately 0.5% of all stones submitted for analysis. Potassium citrate or bicarbonate (20 mEq, two to three

TABLE 83–4. Classification of Nephrolithiases

	Occuring Alone (%)	Occurring with Multiple Stone Diagnosis (%)	Percent Incidence in Single Stone and Multiple Stone Diagnosis	
Absorptive hypercalciuria				*n*
Type I	2.2	9.9	12.1	(154)
Type II	3.9	13.2	17.2	(218)
Renal hypercalciuria	0.3	1.3	1.7	(21)
Primary hyperparathyroidism	0.8	1.3	2.1	(27)
Unclassified hypercalciuria				
Renal phosphate leak	2.1	7.6	9.7	(123)
Fasting hypercalciuria	4.3	13.9	18.1	(230)
Hyperuricosuric Ca nephrolithiasis	8.3	27.6	35.8	(455)
Gouty diathesis	3.1	6.9	10.0	(127)
Hyperoxaluric Ca nephrolithiasis				
Enteric hyperoxaluria	0.2	1.4	1.6	(20)
Primary hyperoxaluria	0.0	0.4	0.4	(5)
Dietary hyperoxaluria	0.4	5.7	6.1	(78)
Hypocitraturic Ca nephrolithiasis				
Distal renal tubular acidosis				
Complete	0.08	0.16	0.24	(3)
Incomplete	0.0	1.1	1.1	(14)
Chronic diarrheal syndrome	0.2	1.8	2.0	(26)
Idiopathic	3.5	24.4	28.0	(355)
Hypomagnesiuric Ca nephrolithiasis	0.3	6.5	6.8	(86)
Infection stones	1.6	4.3	5.9	(75)
Cystinuria	0.7	0.2	0.9	(11)
Low urine volume	1.7	13.5	15.3	(194)
No metabolic abnormality	4.0	0.0	4.0	(51)
Difficult to classify	3.5	0.0	3.5	(45)
Total	41.3	141.3	182.5	(1270)

Adapted from Levy FL, Adams-Huet B, Pak CYC: Ambulatory evaluation of nephrolithiasis: An update for a 1980 protocol. Am J Med 98:50–59, 1995.

times daily) may be given with a thiazide to prevent hypokalemia and improve citrate excretion.[86]

The importance of monitoring urinary calcium is unclear. Thiazide diuretics do not reduce intestinal calcium hyperabsorption in patients with absorptive hypercalciuria and urinary calcium tends to increase during the first year of therapy.[87] However, therapy with thiazides also increases the mineral content of bone.[88] Outcome studies of thiazide intervention have been both positive and negative. In two double-blinded trials, lasting 1 and 1½ years, thiazide therapy failed to decrease hypercalciuria.[87, 89] However, other studies have shown a clear benefit of thiazides over placebo in decreasing stones in patients with recurrent nephrolithiasis.[90] In a prospective study of patients receiving thiazides for reasons other than stone formation, a 44% decrease in likelihood to form a stone was observed.[91]

The use of orthophosphate[92, 93] in patients with absorptive idiopathic hypercalciuria is controversial. Only the neutral potassium salt should be used, as both sodium and acid have a calciuric effect. The phosphate causes a reduction in urinary calcium by decreasing the production of $1,25(OH)_2D_3$. However, this therapy should be reserved as a last resort and is probably indicated only for patients who have a documented phosphate-losing state and subsequent stimulation of $1,25(OH)_2D_3$, in other words those with type III absorptive hypercalciuria.

Cellulose phosphate[93] is a calcium-binding resin that decreases intestinal calcium hyperabsorption resulting in lower urine calcium excretion and higher urine oxalate. It is the only therapy that actually corrects the basic abnormality of absorptive hypercalciuria. Two potential complications of sodium cellulose phosphate are magnesium depletion by binding dietary magnesium,[92, 93] and secondary hyperoxaluria by binding divalent cations in the intestinal tract, thus reducing divalent cation oxalate complexation and making more oxalate available for absorption.[93] These complications may be overcome by oral magnesium supplementation. This drug therapy is contraindicated in other forms of hypercalciuria such as a renal leak or resorptive hypercalciuria because decreased absorption of calcium at the gut may cause stimulation of the parathyroid gland.[94]

TABLE 83–5. Dietary Modifications and Conservative Therapy for Nephrolithiasis

Fluid intake
- Two to 3 L of fluid per day or enough to produce more than 2 L of urine each day
- Possibly higher coffee or alcohol intake is associated with decreased risk of stone formation

Obtain RDA requirement of calcium of 1000–1200 mg/day
- Reduce calcium intake only if >2–3 g/day

Reduce sodium to 100 mEq or 2–3 g/day of sodium

Reduce animal proteins to a maximum of 1.5 g/kg/day

Reduce oxalate (ice tea, nuts, roughage, chocolate)

RDA, recommended dietary allowance.

HORMONAL HYPERCALCIURIA

There are several conditions that may lead to hormonally mediated hypercalciuria (Table 83–6). Patients with primary hyperparathyroidism develop hypercalcemia and hypercalciuria due to overproduction of PTH, which stimulates osteoclast turnover and results in net bone resorption.[48, 95] In addition, there is usually a decreased serum phosphorus secondary to decreased phosphorus reabsorption by the renal tubule. The increased PTH and decreased serum phosphorus also cause an increase in synthesis of $1,25(OH)_2D_3$. These factors contribute to the development of resorptive hypercalciuria. This occurs despite the increase in renal tubular calcium reabsorption. This disorder is most

TABLE 83–6. Hormonally Mediated Hypercalciuria

Primary hyperparathyroidism

Granulomatous tissue conversion of $25(OH)_2D_3$ to $1,25(OH)_2D_3$
- Sarcoidosis
- Tuberculosis

Excessive vitamin D supplementation

Lithium therapy

Malignancy with parathyroid hormone–related peptide increase in resorptive hypercalciuria

TABLE 83–7. Stone Disease in Renal Tubular Acidosis (RTA)

Type of RTA	Stone Composition	Bone Lesion	Urine Composition
Type I classic distal RTA	Calcium phosphate		Increased urine calcium ± decreased urine citrate
Proximal renal tubular acidosis type II	Rare stone formation	Osteomalacia or rickets	
Distal RTA type IV	Calcium oxalate, calcium phosphate	High turnover of bone lesion due to increased bone resorption	Increased urine calcium and phosphorus; high urine pH; decreased urine citrate excretion

common in elderly women who at surgery are generally found to have a single parathyroid adenoma.[96]

There is no established medical treatment for the nephrolithiasis of primary hyperparathyroidism. Parathyroidectomy should be undertaken to correct this abnormality. In the future, agents such as the calcimimetics may have a role in the medical management of nephrolithiasis associated with hyperparathyroidism.[97] Postmenopausal women with primary hyperparathyroidism who cannot undergo surgery may respond to oral estrogen therapy, which should decrease the osteoclastic bone resorption.

RENAL HYPERCALCIURIA

Renal hypercalciuria is characterized by "primary" impairment of the renal tubular reabsorption of calcium, secondary hyperparathyroidism, and compensatory intestinal hyperabsorption of calcium from the PTH-dependent stimulation of $1,25(OH)_2D_3$ synthesis. This is a rare disorder, with an incidence of approximately 0.3%.[98] These patients also tend to have decreased bone density due to PTH stimulation of osteoclast resorption.[78]

Thiazide diuretics are the agents of choice for the treatment of renal hypercalciuria.[93] This diuretic corrects the renal calcium leak by increasing calcium reabsorption in the distal tubule, causing extracellular volume depletion resulting in proximal tubular reabsorption of sodium and calcium. Correction of the renal calcium leak results in decreasing PTH secretion, thus normalizing serum $1,25(OH)_2D_3$ levels and intestinal calcium absorption. Thiazide therapy should be administered as mentioned previously. Potassium citrate should also be administered to avoid hypokalemia and hypocitraturia.

Renal tubular acidosis is also a cause of hypercalciuria. The stone composition and bone lesion is described in Table 83–7. Treatment of patients with renal tubular acidosis consists of administration of potassium alkali salt to replace citrate deficiency and administration of thiazide diuretic if hypercalciuria persists.

HYPOCITRATURIA

As noted above (see Table 83–4), hypocitraturia is fairly common in calcium stone formation, affecting between 20% and 60% of patients.[86] It is known that urinary citrate has inhibitory activity with respect to calcium oxalate and calcium phosphate growth and aggregation (see Table 83–3) and low levels of citrate predispose to calcareous stone formation.[86] The mechanisms of citrate action are important in promoting the formation of a soluble calcium citrate salt rather than the insoluble calcium oxalate and calcium phosphate crystals. In addition, citrate inhibits sodium urate–induced calcium oxalate crystallization.[99] Oral citrate supplementation also provides an alkali load that leads to an increase in renal calcium reabsorption, therefore reducing urinary calcium.

There are multiple causes of hypocitraturia (Table 83–8). The hypocitraturia seen with distal renal tubular acidosis (usually an incomplete form), metabolic acidosis of chronic diarrhea (from intestinal alkali loss), hypokalemia (from intracellular acidosis), and physical exercise (from lactic acidosis) is rare. In industrialized nations, however, the most common cause of hypocitraturia is from the consumption of a diet rich in meat (increased acid-ash diet).[1] Urinary tract infection can also cause degradation of citrate by bacterial enzymes. Whether defective intestinal citrate absorption occurs has not been confirmed.[100] In addition, the use of the carbonic anhydrase inhibitor, acetazolamide, has also been shown to lower urinary citrate.

Several studies have clearly shown that there is an effect of citrate in preventing new stone formation.[1, 86, 101] However, this has not been a universal finding.[100, 102] Recent studies have demonstrated that the administration of citrate decreases aggregation of crystals and thus the incidence of stone formation.[103–106] Barcelow and colleagues[101] randomized hypocitraturic stone formers to potassium citrate 30 to 60 mEq/day or placebo for 3 years. Of the 38 patients who completed 3 years of study, 13 (72%) of the 18 patients in the treatment group had no further stone formation compared with 20% in the placebo group.[101] Similarly, Pak[86] showed remission rates after potassium citrate therapy of 67% in patients with chronic diarrheal syndromes and 92% in those with idiopathic hypocitraturia.

Hypocitraturia should be treated with potassium citrate at a starting dose of 40 to 60 mEq/day, in divided doses, in an attempt to normalize or increase urinary citrate. This therapy also causes a slight decrease in urinary calcium, further improving the saturation profile of calcium oxalate.[107]

HYPEROXALURIA

Dietary Hyperoxaluria

Oxalate is produced by the oxidation of ascorbic acid and glycolate (Fig. 83–2). Normal excretion of oxalate is 20 to 40 mg/day (222 to 444 μmol/day).[98] In otherwise normal persons, urinary oxalate could be increased by dietary excess of oxalate from foods such as spinach, rhubarb, Swiss chard, cocoa, beets, peppers, wheat germ, pecans, peanuts, okra, chocolate, and lime peel. A diet low in calcium may also increase urinary oxalate excretion.[28, 29] Whether the ingestion of supplemental dietary ascorbic acid increases urinary oxalate in some individuals has been controversial.[95, 99] However, a recent large-scale clinical trial has refuted this concept.[108] A not uncommon cause of acute calcium oxalate crystal deposition in the form of nephrolithiasis or nephrocalcinosis is the ingestion, either accidental or intentional, of the antifreeze ethylene glycol, which is metabolized to oxalate.

Treatment of dietary hyperoxaluria consists in altering the diet to avoid an excess of oxalate or administering calcium carbonate or citrate with meals. Patients should undergo follow-up measurements of urinary oxalate and stone burden. No trials have proved the efficacy of this therapy.

Enteric Hyperoxaluria

Malabsorption by the small bowel from any cause, including resection, intrinsic disease (Crohn's disease, celiac sprue, ulcerative colitis), and jejunoileal bypass, exposes the colonic mucosa to detergents in

TABLE 83–8. Causes of Hypocitraturia

1. Chronic diarrheal state
2. Renal tubular acidosis
3. Hypokalemia
4. Physical exercise
5. High acid-ash diet
6. Thiazide diuretic or acetazolamide administration

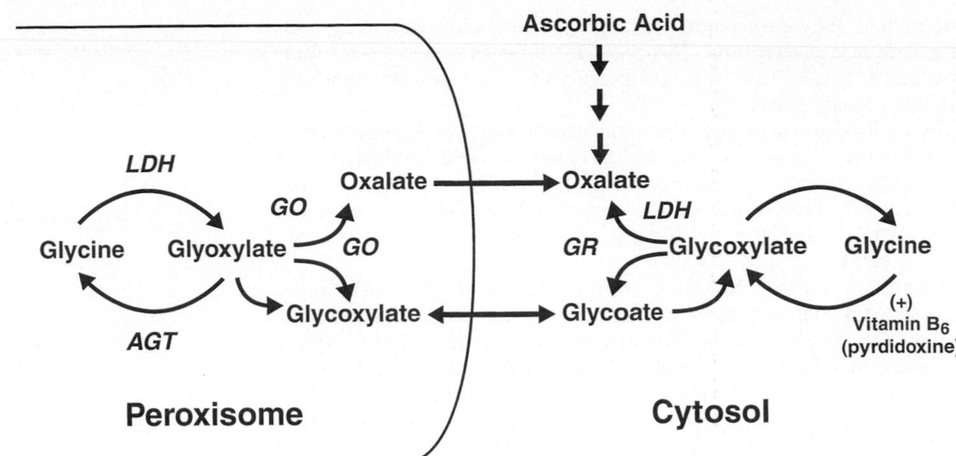

FIGURE 83–2. Metabolic pathways leading to the formation of oxalate. (Adapted from Ruml LA, Pearle MS, Pak CYC: Medical therapy for calcium oxalate nephrolithiasis. Urol Clin North Am 24:117–133, 1997.)

the form of biosalts and fatty acids. These increase the mucosal permeability to charged and uncharged molecules which include sugars, amino acids, and especially oxalate.[109] There is also a decrease in the amount of *Oxalobacter formigenes*, an oxalate-degrading intestinal bacterium.[110] The hyperoxaluria from small bowel malabsorption often exceeds 100 mg/day and provokes frequent stone formation and even tubulointerstitial renal disease from intrarenal calcification.

Treatment includes reducing dietary oxalate in fat and administering agents that bind oxalate in the intestinal lumen, thus preventing absorption. This includes the administration of oral calcium supplements (1 to 4 g of calcium as the carbonate or citrate salt given with meals), or cholestyramine.[95, 98] The calcium supplement of choice is calcium citrate because of the additional benefit of citrate supplementation, which increases citrate inhibition with respect to calcium oxalate crystallization.[111] Careful monitoring of urinary calcium and oxalate should be performed if calcium supplementation is given in significant amounts to these patients. Magnesium supplements may also be used as they act via an identical mechanism, binding and preventing the absorption of free oxalate.[112] Care should be taken that magnesium supplementation does not worsen or cause diarrhea in patients with intestinal disease; diarrhea can attenuate any beneficial effect of magnesium by contributing to a lower urinary pH, reducing citrate, and diminishing urinary volume.[99] In patients with diarrheal syndromes (inflammatory bowel disease, pancreatic insufficiency) and an associated low urinary pH and hypocitraturia, supplementation with potassium citrate 40 to 60 mEq/day in divided doses should be given.[99] Often patients with short-bowel syndrome require potassium citrate in a powder or liquid preparation as opposed to tablet because of difficulty in tolerating the tablets.

Primary Hyperoxaluria

Type I primary hyperoxaluria, an autosomal recessive trait, results from molecular abnormalities that reduce the activity of the hepatic peroxisomal alanine-glyoxylate aminotransferase; this results in increased availability of glyoxalase which is irreversibly converted to oxylalic acid[17–19] (see Fig. 83–2). Type II is a rare form resulting from a deficiency of d-glycerate dehydrogenase or glyoxylate reductase.[95] Both forms cause a high level of oxalate production causing urinary oxalate excretion to increase to 135 to 270 mg/day (1.3 to 3 mmol/day.) Stone formation often begins in childhood with the development of tubular interstitial nephropathy that ultimately progresses to chronic renal failure. Pyridoxine (vitamin B_6) supplementation reduces the production of oxalate by enhancing the conversion of glyoxylate to glycine (see Fig. 83–2), thereby reducing the substrate available for metabolism to oxalate.[113] Another approach that has been studied is magnesium supplementation. Both magnesium oxide and magnesium hydroxide have been effective in lowering urinary oxalate.[114] The mechanism of action involves complexation of magnesium with oxalate in the urine, thereby reducing free ion activity and decreasing calcium oxalate supersaturation. Orthophosphate and pyridoxine have also been used in combination in patients with primary hyperoxaluria with some success. In addition, increasing urinary volume to 3 L/day, supplemental oral citrate, and thiazide diuretics for those with hypercalciuria have also been utilized in treating this severe disease with some success. In patients who develop end-stage renal disease, a combined liver-kidney transplant is necessary for definitive treatment. A normal liver is required for normal glyoxylate metabolism to prevent recurrent nephrocalcinosis in the transplanted kidney.[115]

HYPERURICOSURIA

Hyperuricosuria is the excretion of more than 800 mg (4.8 mmol) of uric acid per day in men and more than 750 mg (4.5 mmol) in women and may be a major predisposing factor to the formation of calcium oxalate stones.[109] The pathogenesis of hyperuricosuria associated with calcium oxalate nephrolithiasis depends on the presence of hyperuricosuria and a urinary pH greater than 5.5.[99, 116, 117] The crystallization of monosodium urate can directly induce the heterogeneous nucleation of calcium oxalate[118] or directly promote calcium oxalate crystallization by complexing urinary inhibitors.[116] In general, excess urine uric acid excretion is a result of increased dietary purine intake derived from meat, poultry, and fish.

Therapy for hyperuricosuric calcium oxalate nephrolithiasis is directed at reducing urinary uric acid. For mild hyperuricosuria, dietary purine restriction may suffice; reduction in the intake of red meat, fish, and poultry limits the substrate available for uric acid synthesis, thereby reducing the urinary saturation of monosodium urate.[117] However, dietary restriction is frequently not adhered to. Therefore, potassium citrate (30 to 60 mEq/day in divided doses) may be used to treat mild hyperuricosuria, particularly in patients unable to tolerate allopurinol or in those with associated hypocitraturia.[119] Allopurinol, if tolerated, is the preferred therapy when dietary restriction fails. It has been shown that allopurinol reduces monosodium urate and urinary supersaturation in treating patients with hyperuricosuric calcium oxalate nephrolithiasis.[99, 117] Doses range from 100 to 300 mg/day and routine monitoring of 24-hour urine uric acid, along with radiologic evaluation of stone burden, should be performed. Side effects are few and include a rash, reversible elevation of liver enzymes, and leukopenia. In the event of the rash, the therapy should be discontinued immediately due to concerns over development of Stevens-Johnson syndrome.[99]

URIC ACID STONES

Urine pH is a major determinant of uric acid supersaturation and subsequent stone formation.[99, 116, 117] Uric acid is a weak acid; the solubility of fully protonated uric acid in urine at a temperature of 37°C, is 96 mg/L. The pK_a approximates at 5.35. At this pH, half the uric acid is fully protonated, making supersaturation inevitable even at a normal excretion rate. Mean pH for urine in patients who form uric acid stones is 5.5[16, 117] as compared with 6.0 in patients who form calcium oxalate stones.[16, 117]

In addition to urine pH, the main determinants of supersaturation with respect to uric acid are endogenous uric acid production and subsequent decrease in urine volume. In healthy persons, uric acid production is directly related to consumption of dietary purine from meat, poultry, and fish. Increasing purine intake will increase uric acid excretion.

There are varying levels of overproduction of uric acid. Some patients with gout may have mild overproduction of uric acid, whereas others with genetic defects of purine reutilization, as in Lesch-Nyhan syndrome (see Table 83–2), will suffer from substantial overproduction of uric acid.[14, 120] Patients with myeloproliferative disorders often overproduce uric acid and may have massive release of preformed uric acid during effective treatment, the so-called tumor lysis syndrome.[16] Renal excretion is responsible for more than 50% of daily uric acid elimination while the remainder is degraded in the intestine.[16, 117] There are some patients who have a relative decrease in renal tubule uric acid reabsorption, resulting in increased uric acid excretion. Approximately 25% of patients with clinical gout have uric acid nephrolithiasis.[15, 16, 117] These patients tend to have excess uric acid excretion even while consuming a low purine diet and have a very acidic urine pH. Patients with chronic diarrhea are particularly at risk for uric acid stones because they are often dehydrated and the alkaline diarrheal fluid causes chronic metabolic acidosis and an acidic urine.[16] Both probenecid and large doses of salicylates promote uric acid excretion and predispose to stone formation.

Treatment should be focused on first decreasing dietary uric acid (purine intake) and increasing fluid intake. If unsuccessful, alkalization with bicarbonate or a bicarbonate precursor (citrate) should be introduced. The goal is to maintain urinary pH greater than 6 but less than 7 throughout the day and night. During the day, multiple doses of bicarbonate, to match the endogenous acid production of approximately 1 mEq/kg/24 hours, should be used.[117] However, one must avoid a urine pH greater than 7 to avoid increasing the risk of calcium oxalate nephrolithiasis.[117] As mentioned above, allopurinol 100 to 300 mg/day should be added for patients in whom these measures fail and whose uric acid excretion remains at 800 to 1200 mg/24 hours and whose urine pH will not increase to greater than 6.5 with bicarbonate or citrate alone.

STRUVITE STONES

Struvite stones, or what are commonly referred to as infection stones, form when the urinary tract is infected with urea-splitting bacteria such as *Proteus mirabilis, Klebsiella pneumoniae,* or *Providencia* species.[121] Bacteria produce urease, which hydrolyzes urea, resulting in the production of struvite ($MgNH_4PO_4$-H_2O) (Fig. 83–3). This cascade of events is totally dependent upon the presence of urease.[121] *Escherichia coli* does not cause struvite stones because it does not product urease. Struvite stones may occur secondary to previous stone disease, which causes obstruction and subsequent infection. In the presence of bacteria, local supersaturation occurs and crystals form around the bacteria. The infection is difficult to control because normal urine flow, which can wash away bacteria, is disrupted. Struvite stones may rapidly increase in size and can fill the renal collecting system, resulting in staghorn calculi.[121] Patients often present with hematuria, obstruction, and infection. Contralateral spread is common.

Struvite stones require removal for definitive therapy. ESWL and percutaneous nephrolithotomy (PCNL) can be used to reduce the damage incurred by the growth and spread of these stones. The American Urological Association Nephrolithiasis Clinical Guidelines Panel[122] recommends a combination of PCNL and ESWL for the management of struvite debris and calculi in most situations. Open surgery and ESWL monotherapy should not be a first-line choice. An infected struvite stone is similar to a foreign body. Thus, prolonged use of antibiotics may slow the progression of the disease but is rarely

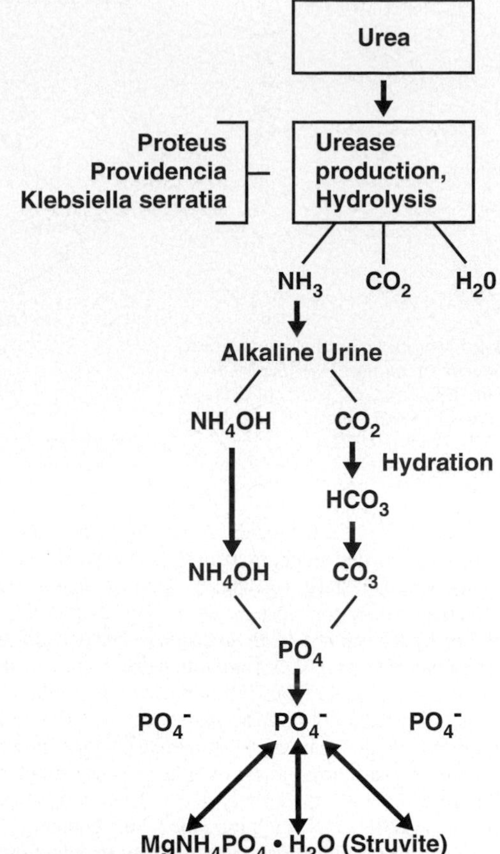

FIGURE 83–3. Formation of struvite stones. (Adapted from Cohen TD, Preminger GM: Struvite calculi. Semin Nephrol 16:424–434, 1996.)

curative. Bacterial urease can be inhibited by acetohydroxamic acid (AHA).[95, 98, 122] AHA has been shown to be effective in reducing the rate of stone growth, but this compound has numerous side effects.

CYSTINE STONES

Cystine stones account for 1% to 2% of kidney stones. They result from an uncommon autosomal recessive inborn error of metabolism wherein renal tubular reabsorption of dibasic amino acids is abnormal. These amino acids include cystine, ornithine, arginine, and lysine.[123] Only the excretion of cystine is clinically significant. Normal cystine excretion is less than 18 mg/day, heterozygotes may excrete up to 100 mg/day, and homozygotes may excrete more than 1 g/day. Cystine solubility is about 250 mg/L, thus heterozygotes do not necessarily form cystine stones; however, cystine excretion in heterozygotes may be sufficient to promote calcium stone formation. Nephrolithiasis in these patients usually presents by the fourth decade, although a later presentation has been reported.[95] Due to the sulfur content of the cystine molecule the stones are visible on plain radiographs and will often present as staghorn calculi or multiple bilateral stones. Cystinuria, in which cystine accumulates only in the lumen of the renal tubules, is distinct from cystinosis, in which there is widespread intracellular cystine accumulation.[95]

Genetic studies show that there are at least three distinct types of cystinuria that can be classified by intestinal transport studies.[9] In addition, genomic organization of the human cystine transporter gene (*SLC3AL*) and de novo mutations have been identified[20] (see Table 83–2).

Treatment of cystinuria must be directed at decreasing the urinary cystine concentration below the limits of solubility.[123] The metabolic precursor of cystine is methionine, an essential amino acid; thus it is impractical to reduce its intake. Increasing urinary volume so that cystine remains below the limits of solubility is the first approach to treatment and is generally practical.[95, 123] However, sometimes it requires 4 L of urine per day. Increasing the urine pH above 7.5 will increase cystine solubility. However, this pH is often difficult to maintain in the long term. Tiopronin or D-penicillamine will both bind cystine and reduce urine supersaturation; however, side effects[95, 123] limit their use.

MANAGEMENT OF STONE DISEASE

Historical features which differentiate acute abdominal and flank pain secondary to urolithiasis and urinary tract obstruction from other causes include (1) family history of nephrolithiasis; (2) prior history of stone disease; (3) dehydration; (4) frequent urinary tract infections; (5) persistent abdominal and flank pain; (6) nausea and vomiting; and (7) unresolved bacteriuria or hematuria.[124] Physical examination is characterized by (1) occasional flank tenderness; (2) usually no rebound tenderness; (3) normal active bowel sounds or minimally decreased bowel sounds; (4) occasional testicular tenderness; and (5) fever (rarely).

Diagnostic Testing: Laboratory and Radiology

Laboratory testing should include urinalysis and a complete blood count (CBC). Hematuria is usually present but may be absent if the ureter is completely obstructed.[124] There is some controversy over the choice of radiologic test to diagnose nephrolithiasis and obstruction. This issue must be approached from the standpoint of the most appropriate test in the acute setting, and must take into consideration the expertise of the radiology department and the test's safety and efficacy in patients with impaired renal function. The objective should be to determine whether an obstruction exists, the level of obstruction, and whether the obstruction is due to stones or other causes.

Noncontrast helical CT probably is the most rapid and cost-effective method of quickly diagnosing nephrolithiasis and obstruction in the acute setting.[125–127] Since contrast is not required it is safe in patients with decreased renal function. A disadvantage, however, is that it is not readily available in some institutions. In addition, it is performed in the early stages of evaluation for following stone burden after urologic intervention or preventive intervention (i.e., for comparison of stone burden after appropriate medical management).[125] Although the noncontrast helical CT scan is replacing the intravenous pyelogram (IVP) the latter remains the most common approach to the acute diagnosis of nephrolithiasis and ureteral obstruction. It is important to note that some studies have shown that ultrasound in combination with plain KUB film is also an excellent choice, especially in the patient with renal impairment or radiocontrast sensitivity.

Management of Acute Nephrolithiasis

There are two components to the acute management of stone disease and renal colic. The first involves the appropriate and safe choice of analgesia and the second is appropriate referral to the urologist or decision to hospitalize. Parenteral pain control is essential for these patients in that their pain is severe, and associated nausea and vomiting prevent the utilization of oral analgesia in the acute setting.[124, 128, 129] Parenteral narcotics have been the gold standard for pain management. However, the downside to utilizing parenteral narcotics is the side effects such as nausea and lethargy. There is also controversy regarding sedation and the need for prolonged emergency room stay, hospitalization, and assistance in transporting the patient back to his or her home. Because of these concerns, the newer parenteral nonsteroidal anti-inflammatory drugs (NSAIDs, e.g., ketorolac) have been used for analgesia management of acute stone passage. Unfortunately, some case reports have demonstrated an increased risk of renal dysfunction with ketorolac administration, both in patients receiving this medication for renal colic and in those receiving it for non–renal-related analgesia. Acute tubular necrosis or acute interstitial nephritis has occurred in young normal subjects and in patients who are renally impaired.[130, 131] The risk of parenteral NSAIDs may be increased in states of dehydration, decreased renal function, or associated with radiocontrast administration in the acute setting.[131]

The current literature suggests that meperidine and morphine sulfate are the gold standard for pain control for renal colic. In the patient who has known addiction to narcotics, or in the patient who has the need to immediately return to a setting where he or she cannot be under the influence of narcotics, ketorolac or other parenteral NSAIDs may be appropriate.

Early referral to the urologist should be made if the patient has (1) infection, (2) persistent pain, (3) inability to pass the stone, (4) urinary extravasation detected on IVP study, (5) high-grade obstruction with a large stone, (6) a solitary kidney, or (7) failure of medical management (analgesia and hydration) to induce passage of a stone.[124]

In summary, new methods for the diagnosis of ureteral obstruction are important in the acute management of stone disease. However, expertise and availability must be considered in the utilization of noncontrast helical CT scan of the kidneys. It is important that patient issues such as renal impairment and sensitivity to radiocontrast be considered when choosing radiologic methods that utilize contrast, such as IVP. Appropriate hydration and choice of analgesia must be made in light of the renal impairment and volume status of each individual patient in the emergent setting.

Surgical Management

Advances in surgical techniques have dramatically altered the management of patients with urolithiasis requiring intervention. ESWL, PCNL, and ureteroscopy allow virtually any stone to be removed from the upper urinary tract without resorting to open surgery.[132, 133] ESWL is the preferred initial treatment for 80% to 85% of calculi, particularly if the stone is less than 2 cm. PCNL should be considered as initial therapy for stones greater than 2 cm or smooth dense calculi located in the lower calix. Residual fragments less than 4 mm were once considered insignificant; not surprisingly, their presence increased the risk of symptomatic recurrence. Ureteroscopy is generally more effective and less costly for distal ureteral calculi or a large ureteral stone burden. Staghorn calculi are best managed initially with PCNL followed by ESWL. Although there is still not a consensus as to the extent of renal injury following ESWL, growth measures of renal function and morphology have not been able to detect long-term effects.[124]

There has been some concern that residual stone debris after ESWL serves as a nidus for further stone formation. Carr et al.[133] reported an increase in the stone recurrence rate after ESWL as compared to PCNL. However, ESWL still remains excellent therapy for the resolution of large intraparenchymal and intraureteral kidney stones.[76, 132, 133]

SPECIAL CONSIDERATIONS

Kidney Graft Lithiasis

The occurrence of lithiasis in renal grafts is an infrequent complication, appearing in only 0.1% of cases.[134] There has been concern that supplementation with calcium and vitamin D to prevent osteopenia post renal transplant may contribute to nephrolithiasis secondary to increased urinary calcium oxalate supersaturation in long-term kidney transplant recipients. The risk of calcium stone formation associated with calcium supplementation is not increased in renal transplant recipients compared to healthy subjects receiving calcium supplementation for prevention of osteopenia.[135] Twenty-four-hour urine calcium excretion was lower in transplant recipients than in healthy subjects despite calcium supplementation. Because of the hypocitraturia that is common in the transplant population, it is recommended that replacement of calcium be with calcium citrate as there is less propensity for crystallization with calcium citrate compared to other calcium preparations.[136]

Surgical treatment for renal graft lithiasis has been studied by Benoit and colleagues.[134] In 12 cases of lithiasis from a series of 1500 kidney transplant patients, they showed that renal graft calculi must be treated surgically in the same way as calculi in native kidneys. The presence of small calculi in renal grafts discovered before transplantation does not contraindicate for transplantation. The treatment of the calculus depends on the type of urinary anastomosis. In the case of ureteroureteral anastomosis, ureteroscopy can be performed, while ESWL is preferable in cases of ureterovesical anastomosis. The routine use of ureterovesical anastomosis with absorbable sutures and the early treatment of hyperparathyroidism by many transplant teams has reduced the overall rate of kidney graft stones and facilitated their treatment with ESWL.[134] In addition, it is important to note that patients may have asymptomatic urinary obstruction due to denervation of the kidney. This requires close observation after ESWL is carried out.

Pregnancy

The development of a symptomatic stone during pregnancy is a rare event, occurring in 0.03% to 0.24% of pregnancies, similar to the percentage in nonpregnant women of the same age.[137–139] Affected patients usually present in the second or third trimester with acute flank pain and microscopic or gross hematuria. Although urinary calculi are uncommon in pregnancy, renal colic is one of the most common causes of nonobstetric abdominal pain requiring hospitalization.[140] Most (approximately 85%) stones pass spontaneously due, in part, to the normally dilated urinary tract in pregnant patients.[132]

Several physiologic changes may affect stone formation in gravid females. An increase in renal plasma flow and glomerular filtration rate occurs, reaching a peak at 9 to 11 weeks of gestation.[138] This increased filtration rate causes an increase in the filtered load of sodium, calcium, and uric acid, resulting in hypercalciuria and hyperuricosuria. Thus, calcium excretion can increase by twofold during pregnancy.[137] There is also an increase in urinary citrate, magnesium, glycosaminoglycans, and acidic glycoproteins that inhibit calcium oxalate stone formation.[137] In addition, the alkaline urine, which results from the respiratory alkalosis of pregnancy, helps to prevent the formation of uric acid stones.[137] Although there is an increased incidence of hypercalciuria and hyperuricosuria in pregnancy, there is not an overall increase in the incidence of symptomatic stones because of other physiologic changes that occur in the composition of the urine (alkalization, increased magnesiuria, citraturia, and increased nephrocalcin).

There are special considerations that pertain to the diagnosis of stones in the pregnant patient to ensure minimal radiation exposure. Ultrasonography is the preferred diagnostic procedure[132, 137] but may not be satisfactory for immediate diagnosis in the case of a pregnant patient who is suffering from decreased renal function, obstruction, and severe pyelonephritis. Should this be the case, then a tailored IVP is appropriate and presents only 0.4- to 1.0-rad exposure. After the second trimester of a pregnancy, radiation is of minimal risk to the patient.

Early urologic referral is very important in pregnancy.[137] Lithotripsy is contraindicated in the pregnant woman, due to the risk of high-energy sound waves to the fetus.[137] The most appropriate approach to the removal of a stone in a pregnant patient is cystoscopy followed by urethral passage of a stent to relieve obstruction. Percutaneous nephrostomy or open surgery is utilized as the last resort. It is recommended that pregnant women who are at risk for forming stones, or are known active stone formers, increase their fluid intake and receive adequate citrate replacement for prevention of stones. Potassium citrate is safe therapy during pregnancy.

REFERENCES

1. Pak CYC: Kidney stones. Lancet 351:1797–1801, 1998.
2. Anderson DA: Historical and geographical differences in the pattern of incidence of urinary stones considered in relation to possible aetiological factors. *In* Hodgkinson A, Nordin BEC (eds): Renal Stone Research Symposium. London, J&A Churchill, 1969, p 7.
3. Scott R: Prevalence of calcified upper urinary tract stone disease in a random population survey. Br J Urol 59:111–117, 1987.
4. Johnson CM, Wilson DM, O'Fallon WM, et al: Renal stone epidemiology: A 25-year study in Rochester, Minnesota. Kidney Int 16:624–631, 1979.
5. Uribarri J, Oh MS, Carroll HJ: The first kidney stone. Ann Intern Med 111:1006–1011, 1989.
6. Sutherland JW, Parks JH, Coe FL: Recurrence after a single renal stone in a community practice. Miner Electrolyte Metab 11:267–269, 1985.
7. Trinchieri A, Mandresi A, Luongo P, et al: Familial aggregation of renal calcium stone disease. J Urol 139:478–481, 1998.
8. Resnick M, Pridgen DB, Goodman HO: Genetic predisposition to formation of calcium oxalate renal calculi. N Engl J Med 278:1313–1318, 1968.
9. Lloyd SE, Pearce SH, Fisher SE, et al: A common molecular basis for three inherited kidney stone diseases. Nature 379:445–449, 1996.
10. Bushinsky DA, Grynpas MD, Nilsson EL, et al: Stone formation in genetic hypercalciuric rats. Kidney Int 48:1705–1713, 1995.
11. Schurman SJ, Norden AG, Scheinman SJ: X-linked recessive nephrolithiasis: Presentation and diagnosis in children. J Pediatr 132:859–862, 1998.
12. Scheinman SJ: X-linked hypercalciuric nephrolithiasis: Clinical syndromes and chloride channel mutations. Kidney Int 53:3–17, 1998.
13. Baggio B, Gambero G, Marchini F, et al: An inheritable anomaly of red cell oxalate transport in "primary" calcium nephrolithiasis correctable with diuretics. N Engl J Med 314:599–604, 1986.
14. Coe FL, Parks JH: Stone disease in hereditary distal renal tubular acidosis. Ann Intern Med 93:60–61, 1980.
15. Stoller ML: Gout and stones or stones and gout. J Urol 154:1670, 1995.
16. Lo RK, Stoller ML: Uric acid-related nephrolithiasis. Urol Clin North Am 24:135–148, 1997.
17. von Schnakenburg C, Rumsby G: Primary hyperoxaluria type I: A cluster of new mutations in exon 7 of the AGXT gene. J Med Genet 34:489–492, 1997.
18. Danpure CJ: Advances in enzymology and molecular genetics of primary hyperoxaluria type I. Prospects for gene therapy. Nephal Dial Transplant 10(suppl 8):24–29, 1995.
19. Hoppe B, Danpure CJ, Rumsby G: A vertigo (pseudo) dominant pattern of inheritance in primary hyperoxaluria type I. Am J Kidney Dis 29:36–44, 1997.
20. Endsley JK, Phillips JA, Hruska KA, et al: Genomic organization of a human cystine transporter gene (SLC3AL) and identification of novel mutations causing cystinuria. Kidney Int 51:1893–1899, 1997.
21. Bisceglia L, Calonge MJ, Totaro A, et al: Localization, by linkage analysis, of the cystinuria type III gene to chromosome 19q13.1. Am J Hum Genet 60:1611–1616, 1997.
22. Nakagawa Y, Abram V, Parks JH, et al: Urine glycoprotein crystal growth inhibitors: Evidence for molecular abnormality in calcium oxalate nephrolithiasis. J Clin Invest 76:1455–1462, 1985.
23. Hess B, Hasler-Strub U, Ackermann D, et al: Metabolic evaluation of patients with recurrent idiopathic calcium nephrolithiasis. Nephrol Dial Transplant 12:1362–1368, 1997.
24. Jaeger P: Genetic versus environmental factors in renal stone disease. Curr Opin Nephrol Hypertens 5:342–346, 1996.
25. Soucie JM, Thun MJ, Coats RJ, et al: Demographic and geographic variability of kidney stones in the United States. Kidney Int 46:893–899, 1994.
26. Strazzulo P, Cappucio FP: Hypertension and kidney stones: Hypothesis and implications. Semin Nephrol 15:519–525, 1995.
27. Najem GR, Seebode JJ, Samady AJ, et al: Stressful life events and risk of symptomatic kidney stones. Int J Epidemiol 26:1017–1023, 1997.
28. Curhan GC: Dietary calcium, dietary protein in kidney stone formation. Miner Electrolyte Metab 23:261–264, 1997.
29. Curhan GC, Willett T, Speizer FE, et al: Comparison of dietary calcium with supplemental calcium and other nutrients as factors affecting the risk for kidney stones in women. Ann Intern Med 126:497–504, 1997.
30. Hess B: Bad dietary habits and recurrent calcium oxalate nephrolithiasis. Nephrol Dial Transplant 13:1033–1038, 1998.
31. Cirillo M, Laurenzi M, Panarelli W, et al: Urinary sodium to potassium ratio in urinary stone disease. Kidney Int 46:1133–1139, 1994.
32. Curhan GC, Willett WC, Speizer F, et al: Beverage use and risk for kidney stones in women. Ann Intern Med 128:534–540, 1998.
33. Peacock M, Hodgkinson A, Nordan BEC: Importance of dietary calcium in the definition of hypercalciuria. BMJ 3:469–471, 1967.
34. Cuhran GC, Willett WC, Rimm EB, et al: Family history and risk of kidney stones. J Am Soc Nephrol 8:1568–1573, 1997.
35. Coe FL, Parks JH: New insights into the pathophysiology and treatment of nephrolithiasis: New research venues. J Bone Miner Res 12:522–533, 1997.
36. Elliot JS, Rabinowitz IN: Calcium oxalate–crystalluria: Crystal size in urine. J Urol 123:324–327, 1980.
37. Werness PG, Bergert JH, Smith LH: Crystalluria. J Crystal Growth 53:166–181, 1981.
38. Hermann U, Schwille PO, Kuch P: Crystalluria determined by polarization microscopy: Technique and results in healthy control subjects and patients with idiopathic recurrent calcium urolithiasis classified in accordance with calciuria. Urol Res 19:151–158, 1991.
39. Boskey AL: Current concepts of the physiology and biochemistry of calcification. Clin Orthop 157:225–257, 1981.
40. Morse RM, Resnick MI: Urinary stone matrix. J Urol 139:602–605, 1988.
41. Malek RS, Boyce WH: Observations on the ultrastructure and genesis of urinary calculi. J Urol 117:336–341, 1977.

42. Boyce WH: Organic matrix of human urinary concentrations. Am J Med 45:673–683, 1968.
43. Kok DJ, Papapoulos SJ, Blomen LJMJ, et al: Modulation of calcium oxalate monohydrate crystallization kinetics in vitro. Kidney Int 34:346–350, 1988.
44. Tiselius H: Solution chemistry of supersaturation. *In* Coe FL, Favus MJ, Pak CYC, et al (eds): Kidney Stones: Medical and Surgical Management. Philadelphia, Lippincott-Raven, 1996, p 33.
45. Parks JH, Coward M, Coe FL: Correspondence between stone composition and urine supersaturation in nephrolithiasis. Kidney Int 51:894–900, 1997.
46. Herring LC: Observations on the analysis of ten thousand urinary calculus. J Urol 88:545–555, 1962.
47. Coe FL, Parks JH, Asplin JR: The pathogenesis and treatment of kidney stones. N Engl J Med 327:1141–1152, 1992.
48. D'Angelo A, Calo L, Cantaro S, et al: Calciotropic hormones and nephrolithiasis. Miner Electrolyte Metab 23:269–272, 1997.
49. Parks JH, Coe FL: A urinary calcium-citrate index for the evaluation of nephrolithiasis. Kidney Int 30:85–90, 1986.
50. Meyer JL, Smith LH: Growth of calcium oxalate crystals. II. Inhibition by natural urinary crystal growth inhibitors. Invest Urol 13:36–39, 1975.
51. Coe LF, Moran E, Kavalich AG: The contribution of dietary purine over-consumption to hyperuricosuria in calcium oxalate stone formers. J Chronic Dis 29:793–800, 1976.
52. Coe FL, Raisen L: Allopurinol treatment of uric-acid disorders in calcium-stone formers. Lancet 1:129–131, 1993.
53. Coe FL, Lawton RL, Goldstein RB, et al: Sodium urate accelerates precipitation of calcium oxalate in vitro. Proc Soc Exp Biol Med 149:926–929, 1975.
54. Pak CYC, Arnold LH: Heterogeneous nucleation of calcium oxalate by seeds of monosodium urate. Proc Soc Exp Biol Med 149:930–932, 1975.
55. Emmerson BT, Cross M, Osborne JM, et al: Reaction of MDCK cells to crystals of monosodium urate monohydrate and uric acid. Kidney Int 37:36–43, 1990.
56. Lieske JC, Hammes MS, Toback FG: Role of calcium oxalate monohydrate crystal interactions with renal epithelial cells in the pathogenesis of nephrolithiasis: A review. Scannins Microsc 10:519–534, 1996.
57. Kajander EO, Ciftcioglu N: Nanobacteria: An alternative mechanism for the pathogenic intra- and extracellular calcification and stone formation. Proc Natl Acad Sci U S A 95:8274–8279, 1998.
58. Kok DJ, Papapoulos SE, Blomen LJ, et al: Modulation of calcium oxalate monohydrate crystallization kinetics in vitro. Kidney Int 34:346–350, 1988.
59. Worcester E: Urinary calcium oxalate crystal growth inhibitors. J Am Soc Nephrol 5:46–53, 1994.
60. Lieske JC, Leonard R, Swift H, et al: Adhesion of calcium oxalate monohydrate crystals to anionic sites on the surface of renal epithelial cells. Am J Physiol 39:F192–199, 1996.
61. Hess B, Nakagawa Y, Coe FL: Inhibition of calcium oxalate monohydrate crystal aggregation by urine proteins. Am J Physiol 257:F99–106, 1989.
62. Asplin J, Deganello S, Nakagawa YN, et al: Evidence that nephrocalcin and urine inhibit nucleation of calcium oxalate monohydrate crystals. Am J Physiol 261:F824–830, 1991.
63. Worcester EM, Blumenthal SS, Beshensky AM, et al: The calcium oxalate crystal growth inhibitor protein produced by mouse kidney cortical cells in culture is osteopontin. J Bone Miner Res 7:1029–1036, 1992.
64. Goldberg HA, Hunter GK: The inhibitory activity of osteopontin on hydroxyapatite formation in vitro. Ann N Y Acad Sci 760:305–308, 1995.
65. Worcester EM, Beshensky AM: Osteopontin inhibits nucleation of calcium oxalate crystals. Ann N Y Acad Sci 760:375–377, 1995.
66. Asplin JR, Arsenault D, Parks JH, et al: Contribution of human uropontin to inhibition of calcium oxalate crystallization. Kidney Int 53:194–199, 1998.
67. Nakagawa Y, Margolis HC, Yokoyama S, et al: Purification and characterization of a calcium oxalate monohydrate crystal inhibitor from human kidney tissue culture medium. J Biol Chem 256:3936–3944, 1981.
68. Nakagawa Y, Ahmed M, Hall SL, et al: Isolation from human calcium oxalate renal stones of nephrocalcin, a glycoprotein inhibitor of calcium oxalate crystal growth: Evidence that nephrocalcin from patients with calcium oxalate nephrolithiasis is deficient in gamma-carboxy-glutamic acid. J Clin Invest 79:1782–1787, 1987.
69. Nakagawa Y: Properties and function of nephrocalcin: Mechanism of kidney stone inhibition or promotion. Keio J Med 46:1–9, 1997.
70. Pillay SN, Asplin JR, Coe FL: Evidence that calgranulin is produced by kidney cells and is an inhibitor of calcium oxalate crystallization. Am J Physiol 275:F255–F261, 1998.
71. Atmani F, Khan SR: Characterization of uronic-acid-rich inhibitor of calcium oxalate crystallization isolated from rat urine. Urol Res 23:95–101, 1995.
72. Levy FL, Adams-Huet B, Pak CYC: Ambulatory evaluation of nephrolithiasis: An update of a 1980 protocol. Am J Med 98:50–59, 1995.
73. Tiselius HG: Investigation of single and recurrent stone formers. Miner Electrolyte Metab 20:321–327, 1994.
74. Pak CYC, Britton F, Peterson R, et al: Ambulatory evaluation of nephrolithiasis: Classification, clinical presentation and diagnostic criteria. Am J Med 69:19–30, 1980.
75. Bushinsky DA: Nephrolithiasis. J Am Soc Nephrol 9:917–924, 1998.
76. Wilson WT, Preminger GM: Extracorporeal shock wave lithotripsy, an update. Urol Clin North Am 17:231–242, 1990.
77. Hodgkinson A, Pyra LN: The urinary excretion of calcium and organic phosphate in 334 patients with calcium stone of renal origin. Br J Surg 48:10–18, 1958.
78. Coe FL, Bushinsky DA: Pathophysiology of hypercalciuria. Am J Physiol 247:F1–13, 1984.
79. Bataille P, Achard JM, Fournenier A: Diet, vitamin D and vertebral bone mineral density in hypercalciuric stone formers. Kidney Int 39:1193–2005, 1991.
80. Ghazali A, Fuentes V, Desaint C, et al: Low bone mineral density and peripheral blood monocyte activation profile in calcium stone formers with idiopathic hypercalciuria. J Clin Endocrinol Metab 82:32–38, 1997.
81. Weisinger JR, Alonzo E, Bellorinfont E, et al: Possible role of cytokines on the bone mineral loss in idiopathic hypercalciuria. Kidney Int 49:244–250, 1996.
82. Pacifici R: Idiopathic hypercalciuria and osteoprorsis—Distinct clinical manifestations of increased cytokine-induced bone resorption? (editorial). J Clin Endocrinol Metab 82:29–31, 1997.
83. Melton LJ, Crowson CS, Khosla S, et al: Fracture risk among patients with urolithiasis: A population-based cohort study. Kidney Int 53:459–464, 1998.
84. Costanza LS, Weiner IM: On the hypocalciuric action of chlorothiazide. J Clin Invest 34:628–637, 1979.
85. Ettinger B, Oldroyd NO, Sorgel F: Triamterene nephrolithiasis. JAMA 244:2443–2445, 1980.
86. Pak CYC: Citrate and renal calculi: An update. Miner Electrolyte Metab 20:371–377, 1994.
87. Preminger GM, Pak CYC: Eventual attenuation of hypocalciuric response to hydrochlorothiazide and absorptive hypercalciuria. J Urol 137:1104–1109, 1987.
88. Wasnich RD, Benfante RJ, Yano K: Thiazide effect on the mineral content of bone. N Engl J Med 309:344–347, 1983.
89. Scholz D, Schwille PO, Sigel A: Double-blind study with thiazide and recurrent calcium lithiasis. J Urol 128:903–907, 1982.
90. Brocks P, Dahl C, Wolf H: Do thiazides prevent recurrent idiopathic renal calcium stones? Lancet 2:124–125, 1983.
91. Ettinger B, Citton JT, Livermore B: Chlorthalidone reduces calcium oxalate calculus recurrence but magnesium hydroxide does not. J Urol 139:679–684, 1988.
92. Pak CYC: Etiology and treatment of urolithiasis. Am J Kidney Dis 18:624–637, 1991.
93. Pak CYC: Nephrolithiasis: Current therapeutic. Endocrinol Metab 6:572–576, 1997.
94. Mallette LE, Dagel RF: Parathyroid hormone and calcitonin. *In* Favis MJ (ed): Primer on the Metabolic Bone Diseases and Disorders of Mineral Metabolism. Philadelphia, Lippincott-Raven, 1996, pp 96–105.
95. Asplin J, Chandhoke PS: The stone forming patient. *In* Coe FL, Favus MJ, Pak CYC (eds): Kidney Stones: Medical and Surgical Management. Philadelphia, Lippincott-Raven, 1996, pp 773–786.
96. Bilezikan JP: Primary hyperparathyroidism. *In* Favis MJ (ed): Primer on the Metabolic Bone Diseases and Disorders of Mineral Metabolism. Philadelphia, Lippincott-Raven, 1996, pp 181–186.
97. Silverberg SJ, Bone HG, Marriott TB, et al: Short-term inhibition of parathyroid hormone secretion by a calcium-receptor agonist in patients with primary hyperparathyroidism. N Engl J Med 337.1506–1510, 1997.
98. Pak CYC: Pathogenesis, prevention, and treatment. *In* Pak CYC (ed): Renal Stone Disease. Boston, Martinus Nijhoff, 1987, pp 52–58.
99. Ruml LA, Pearle MS, Pak CYC: Medical therapy for calcium oxalate nephrolithiasis. Urol Clin North Am 24:117–133, 1997.
100. Bedeir J, Lindberg J, Cole F, et al: Low gastrointestinal absorption of alkali as a cause of idiopathic hypocitraturia (abstract). J Am Soc Nephrol 8:101A, 1997.
101. Barcelow P, Wuhl O, Servitage, et al: Randomized double-blind study of potassium citrate in idiopathic hypocitraturic calcium nephrolithiasis. J Urol 150:1761–1764, 1993.
102. Abdulhadi MD, Hall PM, Streem SB: Can citrate therapy prevent nephrolithiasis? Urology 41:221–224, 1993.
103. Kok DJ, Papoulos SE, Bijovoet OL: Crystal agglomeration is a major element in calcium oxalate urinary stone formation. Kidney Int 37:51–56, 1990.
104. Erwin DT, Kok DJ, Alam J, et al: Calcium oxalate stone agglomeration reflects stone-forming activity: Citrate inhibition depends on macromolecules >30kD. Am J Kidney Dis 24:893–900, 1996.
105. Fuselier HA, Allen JM, Marcucci PA, et al: Urinary Tamm-Horsfall protein increased after potassium citrate therapy of calcium oxalate stone formers. Urology 45:942–946, 1995.
106. Fuselier HA, Moore K, Lindberg J, et al: Agglomeration inhibition reflected stone forming activity during long-term potassium citrate therapy in hypocitraturic calcium stone formers. Adult Urol 52:988–994, 1998.
107. Nicar R, Hsu MC: Urinary response to oral potassium citrate therapy for urolithiasis in a private practice setting. Clin Ther 8:219–225, 1986.
108. Gerster H: No contribution of ascorbic acid to renal calcium oxalate stones. Ann Nutr Metab 41:269–282, 1997.
109. Asplin JR, Favis MJ, Coe FL: Nephrolithiasis. *In* Brenner BM (ed): The Kidney. Philadelphia, WB Saunders, 1996, pp 1893–1935.
110. Sutton RAL, Walker VR: Enteric and mild hyperoxaluria. Miner Electrolyte Metab 20:352–360, 1994.
111. Harvey JA, Zobitz MM, Pak CYC: Calcium citrate: Reduced propensity for the crystallization of calcium oxalate in urine resulting from induced hypercalciuria of calcium supplementation. J Clin Endocrinol Metab 61:1223–1225, 1985.
112. Khan FR, Shevock PN, Hackett RL: Magnesium oxide administration and prevention of calcium oxalate nephrolithiasis. J Urol 149:412–416, 1993.
113. Watts RWE, Chalmers RA, Gibbs DA, et al: Studies on some possible biochemical treatments of primary hyperoxaluria. Q J Med 48:259–272, 1979.
114. Silver L, Brendler H: Use of magnesium oxide in management of familial hyperoxaluria. J Urol 106:274–279, 1971.
115. McDonald JC, Landreneau MD, Rohr MS, et al: Reversal by liver transplantation of the complications of primary hyperoxaluria as well as the metabolic defect. N Engl J Med 321:1100–1103, 1989.
116. Pak CYC, Holt K, Britton F, et al: Assessment of pathogenic genetic roles of uric acid, mono-potassium urate, mono-ammonium urate and monosodium urate in hyperuricosuric calcium oxalate nephrolithiasis. Miner Electrolyte Metab 4:130–136, 1980.
117. Asplin JR: Uric acid stones. Semin Nephrol 16:412–424, 1996.
118. Zerwekh JE, Holt K, Pak CYC: Attenuation by monosodium urate of the inhibitory effective glucosaminoglycans on calcium oxalate nucleation. Invest Urol 17:138–140, 1979.
119. Pak CYC, Peterson R: Successful treatment of hyperuricosuria calcium oxalate nephrolithiasis with potassium citrate. Arch Intern Med 146:863–867, 1986.

120. Lesch M, Nyhan WL: A familial disorder of uric acid, and metabolism in central nervous system function. Am J Med 36:561–568, 1964.
121. Cohen TD, Preminger GM: Struvite calculi. Semin Nephrol 16:424–434, 1996.
122. Wang LP, Wong HY, Griffith D: Treatment options in struvite stones. Urol Clin North Am 24:149–162, 1997.
123. Sakhaee K: Pathogenesis and medical management of cystinuria. Semin Nephrol 16:435–447, 1996.
124. Stewart C, Summers JL: Acute urolithiasis: Current strategies for diagnosis and therapy. Emerg Med Clin North Am 12:97–104, 1996.
125. Zagoria RJ: Helical CT of urolithiasis: Leaving no stone unturned. Appl Radiat Isot 5:8–13, 1998.
126. Smith RC, Verga M, Dalrymple N, et al: Acute ureteral obstruction: Value of secondary signs on helical unenhanced CT. AJR 167:1109–1113, 1996.
127. Smith RC, Rosenfield, Arthur T, et al: Acute flank pain: Comparison of noncontrast enhanced CT and intravenous urography. Radiology 194:789–794, 1995.
128. Begun FP, Foley WD, Peterson A, et al: Patient evaluation laboratory and imaging studies. Urol Clin North Am 24:97–116, 1997.
129. Cordell WH, Wright SW, Wolfson AB, et al: Comparison of intravenous ketorolac, meperidine and both (balanced analgesia) for renal colic. Ann Emerg Med 28:151–158, 1996.
130. Buck ML, Norwood V: Ketorolac induced renal failure in a previous healthy adolescent. Pediatrics 98:294–296, 1996.
131. Heyman SN, Fuchs S, Jaffe R, et al: Renal microcirculation and tissue damage during acute ureteral obstruction in the rat: Effect of saline infusion, indomethacin and radiocontrast. Kidney Int 51:653–663, 1997.
132. Carr LK, Honey JDA, Jewett MAS, et al: New stone formation: A comparison of extracorporeal shock wave lithotripsy and percutaneous nephrolithotomy. J Urol 155:1565–1567, 1996.
133. Psihramis KE, Jewett MAS, Bombardier C, et al: Lithostar extracorporeal shock wave lithotripsy: The first 1,000 patients. J Urol 147:1006–1009, 1992.
134. Benoit G, Dergham R, Blanchet P, et al: Treatment of kidney graft lithiasis. Transplant Proc 27:1743, 1995.
135. Dumoulin G, Hory B, Nguyen NU, et al: Lack of increased urinary calcium oxalate supersaturation in long term kidney transplant recipients. Kidney Int 51:804–810, 1997.
136. Harvey JA, Zobitz MA, Pak CYC: Calcium citrate: Reduced propensity for crystallization of calcium oxalate in urine resulting from induced hypercalciuria of calcium supplementation. J Clin Endocrinol Metab 61:1223–1225, 1985.
137. Maikranz P, Lindheimer M, Coe F: Nephrolithiasis in pregnancy. Ballicres Clin Obstet Gynaecol 8:375–386, 1994.
138. Gorton E, Whitfield HN: Renal calculi in pregnancy. Br J Urol 80:4–9, 1997.
139. Rodriguez PN, Klein S: Management of urolithiasis during pregnancy. Surg Gynecol Obstet 166:103–106, 1988.
140. Dafnis E, Sabatini S: The effect of pregnancy on renal function: Physiology and pathophysiology. Am J Med Sci 303:184–205, 1992.

Chapter 84

Clinical Approach to Metabolic Bone Disease

Murray J. Favus

Metabolic bone disease refers to a group of seemingly unrelated inherited and acquired disorders that primarily affect the skeleton and the levels of circulating minerals and calciotropic hormones. The metabolic bone diseases are defined by their diffuse bone involvement, but the presenting signs and symptoms may be diffuse or localized to one or more sites. The skeletal symptoms may appear alone, or be accompanied by manifestations resulting from altered mineral or calciotropic hormone levels. Because of their similar symptoms, localized bone diseases such as Paget's disease and fibrous dysplasia are included in the differential diagnosis of metabolic bone disorders. Some metabolic bone diseases and mineral disorders are of genetic origin and may become manifest early in life. As some acquired disorders may appear at certain ages, the diagnosis of metabolic bone disease must be considered in infants, children, adolescents, and adults of all ages.

CLINICAL PRESENTATIONS

The presenting manifestations of metabolic bone diseases and mineral disorders are important clues to the underlying pathologic process and dictate the physician's initial approach to diagnosis. This chapter describes the more common presenting signs, symptoms, and laboratory tests and offers a differential diagnosis for each of the major presentations. The approaches to reach a specific diagnosis are discussed and, where appropriate, the reader is directed to the other chapters in this book that contain detailed descriptions of the diagnostic approach to the major disorders of bone and mineral diseases.

Metabolic bone diseases may present with physical signs and symptoms of bone involvement such as fracture, skeletal pain, tenderness, or progressive deformity. These initial symptoms are not specific to metabolic bone disease and may be indistinguishable from those of bone disorders due to tumor, infection, vasculopathy, or secondary to adjacent joint disease. Elevations or decreases in one or more of the blood minerals (calcium, phosphorus, magnesium) may accompany the skeletal symptoms or alone may be responsible for the presenting symptoms.

Metabolic bone and mineral disorders present to the physician in a limited number of ways (Table 84–1). At least six syndromes can be recognized by their cluster of well-recognized signs and symptoms that suggest a specific metabolic bone disorder. The syndromes of osteoporosis, osteomalacia, rickets, uremic osteodystrophy, nephrolithiasis, and soft tissue calcification each has several causes that may or may not be distinguished by the initial clinical information alone. Metabolic bone and mineral diseases may also present as individual signs or symptoms (skeletal deformity, fracture, tenderness, muscle weakness), while others are revealed initially by abnormal laboratory tests (abnormal mineral levels, radiographs, bone densitometry). In this chapter, all of the potential symptoms and physical findings are described, but in practice, patients rarely exhibit all of the features of the syndrome.

Osteoporosis

There are many causes of osteoporosis in both women and men, of which postmenopausal osteoporosis is by far the most common. Postmenopausal osteoporosis is recognized by the presence in a postmenopausal woman of fracture with minimal or no trauma, thoracic kyphosis, and shifting of the thorax anteriorly and downward with the lower ribs at or below the iliac crest. Chronic back pain may result from multiple vertebral compression fractures, but vertebral fractures may also occur without back pain and in the absence of a clinical fracture event. Chronic thoracic or lumbar back pain in the absence of acute or chronic vertebral fracture is not due to osteoporosis, and other causes of back pain should be considered. Pain, deformity, or limitation of motion of the cervical spine is almost never due to cervical vertebral osteoporosis. However, extensive thoracic kyphosis that pitches the head forward may cause chronic neck and upper back pain. Positioning the head forward in the absence of thoracic kyphosis is more likely the result of weakness of the upper back, shoulder, and neck muscles due to lack of exercise or intrinsic neuromuscular disease.

The history of a fracture with minimal or no trauma suggests osteoporosis, and demonstration of low bone mass confirms the diagnosis. The diagnosis of osteoporosis is more difficult when the fracture occurred in the presence of some trauma. A fall from the standing position should not result in a fracture. Therefore, a fracture that occurs while standing or walking should raise suspicion of osteoporosis. The contribution to fracture is less clear when a person sustains a fracture upon being propelled either by tripping, or falling either downstairs or from some height. Under these conditions, low bone mass by bone densitometry can be diagnostic of osteoporosis.

Secondary causes of osteoporosis represent a diverse group of disorders, and their detection requires a careful history and thorough examination. Signs and symptoms that suggest secondary osteoporosis are listed in Table 84–2. Other metabolic bone diseases may present with fracture and low bone mass, such as primary hyperparathyroidism, rickets, and osteomalacia. The course of a malignancy with skeletal metastases may present with vertebral compression fracture and raise the question of osteoporosis until the underlying disease is recognized.

TABLE 84–1. Presentations of Metabolic Bone Diseases

Osteoporosis
Rickets
Osteomalacia
Uremic osteodystrophy
Nephrolithiasis
Soft tissue calcification
Fracture
Skeletal deformity
Radiographic abnormalities
Abnormal blood test
Low bone density

TABLE 84–2. Signs and Symptoms Suggestive of Secondary Osteoporosis

History

Medical conditions, including malabsorption syndromes, rheumatoid arthritis, long-term immobilization, chronic renal failure, calcium oxalate nephrolithiasis, thyrotoxicosis, Cushing's syndrome, chronic liver disease, prostate cancer treated with orchiectomy or antiandrogens

Gynecologic history of oligomenorrhea or amenorrhea, galactorrhea, pituitary tumor, gonadotropin-releasing hormone (GnRH) agonist use

Surgical history of terminal ileal resection, partial gastrectomy, small bowel bypass for obesity

Diet and nutrition, including eating disorders, malnutrition, frequent dieting, alcoholism

Medications: glucocorticoids, anticonvulsants, heparin, GnRH agonists, vitamin A, cytotoxic agents, antiandrogens

Physical examination

Skin: eruption of mastocytosis; bruising and thin skin of Cushing's syndrome; bronze coloration of hemochromatosis

Head: blue sclerae of osteogenesis imperfecta, displaced lens of Marfan's syndrome, Sturge-Weber changes accompanying chronic seizure disorder

Neck: enlarged thyroid gland of thyrotoxicosis; adenopathy of malignancy

Abdominal: surgical scar of partial gastrectomy, ileal resection, small bowel bypass surgery, enlarged liver of chronic liver disease

Extremities: fracture deformities of osteogenesis imperfecta

Genitalia: absent secondary sex characteristics of hypogonadism, absent testes following orchiectomy, small firm testes of Klinefelter's syndrome

Musculoskeletal: thoracic kyphosis, lumbar lordosis or scoliosis, proximal muscle weakness, muscle wasting of myopathies, immobilization

Of special consideration is myeloma, whose presenting constellation of back pain, vertebral compression fracture, and low bone mass may masquerade as osteoporosis. Chapters 85 and 88 discuss the differential diagnosis of low bone mass and osteoporosis.

The osteoporosis syndrome occurs in men, but at a lower frequency than in women. Men with the osteoporosis syndrome should be examined for evidence of hypogonadism. Small testes suggest primary gonadal failure, due either to a genetic disorder such as Klinefelter's syndrome,[1] or to an acquired condition such as orchiectomy as treatment of prostate cancer.[2] The examination should include a search for evidence of secondary hypogonadism due to pituitary or hypothalamic hypofunction. The presence of hypothyroidism or adrenal insufficiency should raise the possibility of hypopituitarism and possible hypogonadism. An anamnesis including the mileposts in pubertal development should be obtained, as a history of delayed puberty increases the risk for osteoporosis in men.[3]

Idiopathic hypercalciuria (IH) is frequent (5% to 7%) in the general population, with men and women equally affected.[4, 5] IH increases the risk for calcium oxalate nephrolithiasis and is associated with low bone mass and fracture.[6–8] Thus, IH should be considered in a man or woman with the osteoporosis syndrome and a history of calcium stone formation.

Rickets

The syndrome of rickets appears in infants and children as a collection of signs and symptoms that depend upon the stage of demineralization of the growth plates, the extent of hypocalcemia, and the age at onset. The classic skeletal changes of rickets are listed in Table 84–3. Fraser et al.[9] offer a classification of vitamin D deficiency rickets based upon the clinical manifestations. In stage I, the signs and symptoms of hypocalcemia dominate the clinical picture. Stage II is due primarily to the defective mineralization of the growth plates. The presence of both hypocalcemia and rickets characterizes stage III. Infants under age 6 months often present as stage I with the consequences of hypocalcemia such as tetany and convulsions and no sign of skeletal rickets. As the disease progresses, rachitic changes become manifest as irritability, hypotonia, and progressive deformity of the long bones, skull, and chest. Softening of the skull bones (craniotabes) is accompanied by delay in closure of the fontanelles and frontal bossing (prominence of the frontal bone and lengthening of the anteroposterior axis).

Compared to infants, older children present in stage II, as they are less likely to become symptomatic with hypocalcemia before the skeletal manifestations appear. Signs suggestive of the rickets syndrome are short stature, delayed growth, skeletal tenderness, bowing of the long bones, and muscle weakness with waddling gait. The rachitic changes depend upon the state of ambulation of the child. In younger children, skeletal changes tend to be prominence of the wrists, bowing of the upper extremities, and bowing of the femur and tibia (genu varum or bowleg deformity). In the older child, genu valgum deformity (knock-knees) or valgum deformity in one leg and varum deformity in the other are more common.

Both infants and older children may demonstrate a protuberant abdomen due to muscle weakness. Weakness of the pelvic girdle muscles and proximal weakness of the lower extremities contribute to the waddling gait. Several deformities of the chest may be found in the child with rickets. Enlargement of the cartilaginous costochondral junctions (rachitic rosary) may be palpable and tender. Infants and young children with severe rickets may develop Harrison's groove or sulcus, which is a flaring of the lower ribs as the diaphragmatic muscle attachments at the lower ribs pull inward. Severe respiratory compromise may result from muscle weakness, hyperflexibility of the ribs, or narrowing of the lateral aspect of the chest cavity.

Dentition may be abnormal in rachitic children. Hypoplasia of the enamel may be present if rickets develops before the deposition of enamel is completed. Delayed tooth eruption and decreased bone density of the alveolar ridge are often present as well.

Vitamin D therapy improves or reverses the rachitic changes, but some deformities, such as bowlegs and frontal bossing, persist as stigmata of childhood rickets. The many diseases that cause rickets and the tests to reach specific diagnoses are discussed in Chapters 82 and 87.

Osteomalacia

Complications of a variety of diseases, including disorders of the gastrointestinal tract, may result in the osteomalacia syndrome. At some time during the course of the primary disease, patients may develop the osteomalacic syndrome of bone pain and tenderness, generalized weakness, waddling gait, and symptoms of hypocalcemia. The diagnosis is often delayed because the presenting symptoms are nonspecific, vague, and may be attributed to the underlying disease, arthritis, or hypochondriasis. Skeletal tenderness may be elicited by pressing on the thorax, pelvis, or pretibial region. Tenderness may be so severe as to limit motion and cause a limp. Limping may also be due to tarsal or metatarsal fractures. In addition to a gait disturbance, muscle weakness of the pelvic girdle may result in pain, difficulty in arising from a chair, climbing stairs, or reaching to a high shelf. In other patients, multiple vertebral compression fractures cause thoracic kyphosis, loss of lumbar lordosis, or scoliosis suggestive of osteoporosis. Most of the skeletal changes of childhood rickets do not occur in osteomalacia, as the bones become less soft and pliable in adults.

TABLE 84–3. Physical Findings in Clinical Rickets

General: listlessness, irritability, crying, Chvostek's and Trousseau's signs of hypocalcemia, carpopedal spasm

Skin: alopecia and absence of eyelashes in VDRR type II

Head: frontal bossing, parietal flattening, soft skull bones (craniotabes), delayed tooth eruption

Chest: horizontal indentation along the lower border of the chest wall (Harrison's groove); palpable cartilage accumulation at the costochondral junction (rachitic rosary); indentation of the sternum (pigeon breast)

Abdomen: protuberance, umbilical hernia

Extremities: tenderness to palpation; thickness, swelling, and tenderness at wrists, ankles, knees; bowing deformity of the long bones; reduced muscle strength, lax ligaments, waddling gait

VDRR, vitamin D–resistant rickets.

Occasionally, symptoms of hypocalcemia may be the presenting features of osteomalacia. The many causes, differential diagnosis, and clinical evaluation of osteomalacia are discussed in Chapter 87.

Renal Osteodystrophy

Renal osteodystrophy refers to the signs and symptoms of bone changes that accompany chronic renal failure. Bone pain, tenderness, and fractures with minimal trauma may result from a variety of bone pathologic processes, including osteitis fibrosa, childhood rickets, osteomalacia, adynamic bone disease, or sclerosing bone disease. In children with renal insufficiency, skeletal changes may be indistinguishable from those of classic rickets, including growth retardation, bowing of the lower extremities, enlargement of the epiphyses of the long bones, and rachitic rosary. In older children, genu valgum or genu varum of the lower extremities may occur with long-standing renal insufficiency. In extreme cases, widening of the proximal femoral epiphyses may result in slipped epiphysial plates, avascular necrosis of the femoral head, and hip pain.

In adults, bone pain and tenderness and muscle weakness are common, whereas deformities of the long bones are more common in affected children. Multiple vertebral fractures result in kyphoscoliosis and chronic back pain. After several years of hemodialysis, complications of an amyloid syndrome of periarticular β_2-microglobulin accumulation may appear as pain and pathologic fracture through the protein-laden cystic lesions.[10] Oral aluminum administration is highly effective in binding intestinal luminal phosphate and minimizing hyperphosphatemia. However, because aluminum ingestion in renal failure may induce a syndrome of aluminum toxicity, including encephalopathy, proximal muscle weakness, symptoms of osteomalacia, and anemia,[11] its use has been all but eliminated in recent years.

Chapter 86 discusses causes of renal osteodystrophy, how each can be diagnosed, and the indications for bone biopsy; Chapter 83 discusses bone disease seen in nephrolithiasis.

Extraskeletal Calcification

Calcification of the soft tissue may be located at sites of earlier injury, or in a periarticular distribution. Vascular calcification that may complicate uremic osteodystrophy may be palpable over the radial or ulnar arteries. Calcified masses may be large and bulky, or small and scattered at multiple sites. There may be painless skin breakdown and spontaneous extrusion of calcific masses. Three distinct syndromes represent separate processes that may result in soft tissue calcification or mineralization[12–17] (Table 84–4).

Metastatic calcification may complicate any hypercalcemic or hyperphosphatemic state. Precipitation of amorphous calcium phosphate may occur when the solubility product of calcium phosphate calculated as the product of blood or tissue calcium and phosphate levels is exceeded. There are a number of exceptions that remain unexplained,

TABLE 84–4. Causes of Extraskeletal Calcification*

Metastatic calcification[12]
- Hypercalcemic states
- Tumoral calcinosis[13]
- Other hyperphosphatemias

Dystrophic calcification
- Sites of injection[14]
- Calcinosis universalis or circumscripta[14]
- Dermatomyositis[15]
- Scleroderma
- Systemic lupus erythematosus

Ectopic calcification
- Post-traumatic myositis ossificans
- Fibrodysplasia ossificans progressiva[16]

*For an overview of this topic, see Whyte.[17]

such as hyperphosphatemia in the presence of hypocalcemia in hypoparathyroid states in which the calcium phosphate product in blood is not exceeded. Certain tissues are more prone to calcification, including skin, kidney, lung, gastric mucosa, conjunctiva, periarticular tissue, endocardium, and the vasculature. Tumoral calcinosis is a specific entity that is often familial and is characterized by hyperphosphatemia and normal serum calcium (see Table 84–4).

Dystrophic calcification occurs at the site of injured tissue in the presence of normal serum calcium and phosphate. Microscopic examination of the deposited crystals reveals either amorphous calcium phosphate or, if the process is more prolonged, crystals of hydroxyapatite. Microscopic examination of a tissue biopsy or a concretion also distinguishes a gouty mass (tophus) from calcium-rich soft tissue deposition.

Ectopic calcification refers to painful epidermal or dermal calcification deposits that occur in the course of other diseases (see Table 84–4). Distribution may be circumscribed, around the joints or at the fingertips, or more generalized, in the skin and deeper into the soft tissues around joints and in areas of prior trauma. Ectopic calcification or the development of histologically proven bone (see Table 84–4) may occur following injury (burns, surgery, neurologic trauma, general trauma) or as an inherited condition of unknown cause (fibrodysplasia myositis ossificans progressiva).

Fracture

Fracture is a common presenting event in osteoporosis and osteogenesis imperfecta, while rickets, osteomalacia, primary hyperparathyroidism, states of secondary hyperparathyroidism, and uremic osteodystrophy present less frequently with fracture. Those fractures due to a metabolic bone disease may occur with minimal or no trauma and may involve either the appendicular or axial skeleton, or both. Fractures due to motor vehicle accidents and other events in which there is major trauma do not raise the suspicion of an underlying bone disorder. Some patterns of fracture suggest the underlying disease. For example, osteoporotic fractures commonly involve the trabecular-rich, weight bearing regions of the skeleton such as the thoracic and lumbar spine, proximal femur, tibia, fibula, and pelvis, and non–weight-bearing areas, including the humerus, distal radius, ulna, and ribs. Green stick fractures and subtrochanteric fractures of the proximal femur occur, especially in osteomalacia.[18] Fractures of the tarsal and metatarsal bones are also common in osteomalacia. In the early part of the 20th century when primary hyperparathyroidism was first characterized, fractures were a common presenting feature, but the pattern is changing[19, 20] (see Chapter 76).

Glucocorticoid excess either from endogenous Cushings' syndrome or from glucocorticoid administration as treatment of a variety of diseases accelerates loss of trabecular bone in excess of that of cortical bone.[21, 22] Therefore, presenting clinical fractures often involve the thoracic and lumbar vertebral bodies, ribs, and proximal femur. Among the cortical fractures, those of the small bones of the feet (tarsals and metatarsals) may occur early in the course of glucocorticoid therapy.

The initial evaluation of a low-impact or nontraumatic fracture should include a careful history and physical examination to search for evidence of metabolic bone disease. Fractures at the site of metastatic lesions, or "pathologic fractures," occur most commonly in patients with known malignancy, and may be the first manifestation of skeletal metastases.

In children, multiple fractures suggest osteogenesis imperfecta, childhood osteoporosis, rickets, uremic osteodystrophy, or a variety of less common heritable skeletal lesions.

Skeletal Deformity

Asymmetrical skull enlargement may occur from acromegaly, or during active Paget's disease. Flattening of the base of the skull (craniotabes) or frontal bossing in adults suggests inadequately treated rickets during early childhood. Premature closure of the cranial sutures and the resulting deformity often accompanies X-linked hypophosphatemic rickets. Maxillary and mandibular deformity or asymmetrical growth of the orbital bones may be caused by fibrous dysplasia of bone[23] or Paget's disease.

Axial or appendicular deformities may be due either to fracture or gradual curvature or bending. Vertebral compression fracture with loss of height results in thoracic kyphosis and shifting of the rib cage anteriorly and downward. Extensive kyphosis may displace the lower ribs over the epigastrum and cause a protrusion of the lower abdomen. The patient may complain of a rubbing pain of the lower ribs on or below the iliac crest. Thoracic deformity may also occur following multiple rib fractures as due to osteogenesis imperfecta, or bowing of the ribs at the costochondral junction in rickets.

Bowing and other deformities commonly affect the lower extremities due to the effects of weight-bearing on long bones softened by rickets, osteomalacia, osteogenesis imperfecta, Paget's disease, or chronic hyperparathyroidism. Hip pain and limp may result from changes in the hip joint such as protrusio acetabuli (softened acetabulum with indentation into the pelvis) or change in the angle of the femoral neck that may occur secondary to bowing of the mid- and distal femur. Slipped capital femoral epiphysis may result from hypothyroidism, glucocorticoid excess, and renal osteodystrophy.[24–26] Distal femur and proximal tibia softening and bending may present as genu valgum, or knockknee deformity. Childhood rickets, and especially vitamin D–resistant (X-linked hypophosphatemic, XLH) rickets results in bowing of the femur or tibia and fibula and shortening of the lower extremities.[27] Rickets appearing during the rapid growth phase of adolescence may result in bilateral knockknee deformity. If not completely treated during early childhood, the deformities persist and may eventually cause sclerosis and degenerative arthritis of the hip and knee joints. The waddling gait of rickets is the result of bowing of the lower extremities and proximal muscle weakness. In children with rickets, the absence of proximal muscle weakness suggests XLH as the specific cause.

In adults, osteomalacia may be manifest as skeletal tenderness, proximal muscle weakness, and waddling gait, but there is less curvature of the long bones than occurs in rickets of infancy or childhood. Also, epiphysial widening, and chest wall and skull deformities that are characteristic of childhood rickets do not occur in adult osteomalacia.

Radiographic Abnormalities

The first suggestion of the presence of metabolic bone disease may come from radiographs obtained either to investigate a painful or tender region of the skeleton, a skeletal deformity, a fracture, or to evaluate symptoms unrelated to bone disease. Several radiographic patterns suggest metabolic bone disease and include compression fracture of the vertebral bodies, curvature or other deformity of the long bones, vertebral or cortical osteopenia, pagetoid pattern involving cortical or trabecular bone, or sclerotic or cystic lesions (Table 84–5). Inspection of the immediate bony structure around the site of a fracture may suggest its cause by the presence of cystic lesions, extreme deformity, metastatic lesion, pagetoid patterns, or osteopenia.

The osteoporosis syndrome is suggested by the presence of vertebral compression fracture, thoracic kyphosis, proximal femur fracture, or osteopenia with or without fracture. Careful inspection of cortical bone of the phalanges may reveal cortical thinning or porosity, both of which strongly suggest excessive bone loss. Estimates of bone mass on standard radiographs are at best qualitative, and bone mass must be reduced by 30% to 40% before it can be detected by standard radiographs. Therefore, quantification of bone mass by bone densitometry is required to make the diagnosis of osteoporosis.

Osteomalacia may cause one or more radiographic changes that are highly suggestive of a mineralization defect, including protrusio acetabuli, bowing of the lower extremities, and Looser's zones or pseudofractures (areas of cortical lucency surrounded by sclerosis that does not go completely through the cortex) involving the pelvic rami, ribs, proximal femur, or proximal or distal long bones.

Abnormal Blood Test

An abnormal serum calcium, phosphate, magnesium, or alkaline phosphatase level may be the first suggestion of a metabolic bone disorder. As these measurements are often performed as part of screening biochemical tests, many patients found to have an abnormal blood mineral level have no apparent symptoms of a bone or mineral disorder.[29, 30] A careful history and examination, including a review of signs and symptoms, should be undertaken; additional diagnostic approaches must be considered (Table 84–6). (See also Chapters 73, 76, 77, and 87 for discussion of disorders of calcium and phosphate.)

TABLE 84–5. Common Radiographic Changes in Metabolic Bone Disease

Finding	Site	Disorders
Osteopenia	Ax, Ap	OP, OM, HPT, OI
Vertebral fracture in children	Ax	OP, OM, OI, HPT ME/T
Vertebral fracture in adults	Ax	OP, OM, HPT ME/T
Vertebral sclerosis	Ax	HPT (uremia)
Cortical thinning	Ap, Ax	OP, OI
Subperiosteal resorption	Ap	HPT
Endosteal scalloping	Ap	OP
Expansile mass	Ap > Ax	FD
Intracortical resorption	Ap	HPT, OM
Brown tumor	Ax, Ap	HPT, OM
Bowing and cortical fracture	Ap	Rickets, OI, OM, FD
Metaphyseal Ap widening		Rickets, HPT
Looser's zones	Ap	OM, FD, Paget's disease
Sclerosis	Ap, Ax	Uremia, OPET, Dys*
CNS calcification	Brain	CAIID, PHP, IHP

Ax, axial; Ap, appendicular; OP, osteoporosis, both 1° and 2°; OM, osteomalacia; ME/T, marrow expansion/tumor; HPT, hyperparathyroidism; OI, osteogenesis imperfecta; FD, fibrous dysplasia; OPET, osteopetrosis; Dys, bone dysplasias; CAIID, carbonic anhydrase II deficiency; PHP, pseudohypoparathyroidism; IHP, idiopathic hypoparathyroidism.

*There are many causes of bone dysplasias; see Whyte and Murphy.[28]

Low Bone Density

The growing number of postmenopausal women undergoing bone density measurements to assess the risk of osteoporosis fracture is becoming the most frequent way in which metabolic bone disease is being discovered. Although most perimenopausal women have low bone mass due to estrogen deficiency, it is well to remember that bone mass measurements cannot establish bone structure or histology and, therefore, diagnosis. Other metabolic bone diseases such as osteomalacia, osteitis fibrosa cystica, uremic osteodystrophy, and osteogenesis imperfecta also have low bone mass. Further, low bone mass may result from one of several causes of secondary osteoporosis, as listed in Table 84–2. Thus, the physician must be prepared to search for other causes of low bone mass if information from the history, physical examination, or initial blood tests suggests a diagnosis other than postmenopausal osteoporosis. A detailed discussion of current methods used to detect low bone mass and to diagnose osteoporosis are contained in Chapters 85 and 88.

Other Signs and Symptoms Suggestive of Specific Disorders

Several physical findings accompanied by symptoms or specific history along with abnormal routine laboratory test results may lead to a specific diagnosis. The lack of one or more clinical findings may obscure the identification of the diseases; therefore they were not included as one of the well-recognized clinical syndromes. Paget's disease of bone (see Chapter 89) may be recognized by the presence of an enlarged skull, prominent temporal arteries, hearing loss, bowing of one or both legs, and focal extremity warmth and pain. An elevated

TABLE 84–6. Diagnosis of Metabolic Bone Disease Based upon Presenting Signs and Symptoms

Presenting Syndrome/Sign	Suggested Evaluation
Osteoporosis	BMD; exclude secondary causes; serum Ca, creatinine; see Chapters 85, 88
Rickets	Serum 25(OH)D, phos, alk phos, wrist radiographs; see Chapters 82, 86, 87
Osteomalacia	Serum 25(OH)D, phos, alk phos, creatinine, wrist radiographs, bone biopsy; see Chapters 82, 86, 87
Uremic osteodystrophy	Serum PTH, Ca, phos, creatinine, 25(OH)D; consider tetracycline bone biopsy; see Chapters 79, 86
Nephrolithiasis	Serum Ca, phos, PTH, 1,25(OH)D; 24-hr urine Ca, oxalate, uric acid, pH, citrate, phos, cystine, stone analysis; see Chapter 83
Soft tissue calcification	Serum Ca, phos, creatinine, skin biopsy
Fracture	Tc 99m bone scan, radiograph fracture site; consider biopsy of fracture site; serum Ca, phos, creatinine, 25(OH)D, BMD, skin biopsy; see Chapters 77, 82, 85, 87–89
Skeletal deformity	Radiographs of affected areas; serum Ca, phos, alk phos, creatinine, BMD, bone or skin biopsy; see Chapters 76, 82, 86–89
Radiographic abnormality	Tc 99m bone scan, radiograph fracture site; consider biopsy of fracture site; serum Ca, phos, creatinine, 25(OH)D, BMD; see Chapters 75, 79, 82, 85–89
Hypercalcemia	Serum PTH, phos, alk phos, creatinine, $1,25(OH_2)D$, PTHrP, thyroid, SPIE, CXR; see Chapters 75–80
Hypocalcemia	Serum PTH, phos, alk phos, creatinine, albumin; see Chapters 75, 81, 82, 86, 87, 92
Hyperphosphatemia	Serum PTH, CPK, Ca, alk phos; creatinine, 24-hr urine Ca, phos; see Chapters 81, 86
Hypophosphatemia	Serum and 24-hr urine Ca, creatinine, phos, Mg, 25(OH)D, PTH, urine pH, $1,25(OH_2)D$; see Chapters 76, 82, 83, 87
Hypermagnesemia	Serum and 24-hr urine Ca, Mg, phos, creatinine, serum PTH; see Chapters 75, 76, 80, 81, 86
Hypomagnesemia	Serum Ca, phos, PTH, $1,25(OH_2)D$, creatinine, 24-hr urine Mg, phos; see Chapters 76, 80, 87
Elevated alkaline phosphatase	Serum Ca, PTH, phos, creatinine, Tc 99m bone scan, radiograph symptomatic and scan abnormal sites; see Chapters 76, 77, 82, 86, 87, 89

BMD, bone mineral density; PTH, parathyroid hormone; $1,25(OH_2)D$, 1,25-dihydroxyvitamin D; 25(OH)D, 25-hydroxyvitamin D; phos, phosphate; alk phos, alkaline phosphatase; SPIE, serum protein immunoelectrophoresis; CXR, chest x-ray film; CPK, creatine phosphokinase; PTHrP, parathyroid hormone–related protein.

serum alkaline phosphatase may also be obtained and support the diagnosis.

The combination of blue or gray sclerae and deformity of the long bones and spine in an infant or child with a history of multiple fractures is virtually diagnostic of osteogenesis imperfecta (see Chapter 92). However, OI may present with a range of clinical symptoms in age groups from the newborn to postmenopausal women and with varying degrees of severity.

The presence of café au lait spots with highly irregular borders (coast of Maine), precocious development of secondary sex characteristics, fracture, and appendicular deformity strongly suggest McCune-Albright syndrome.[31] Skeletal lesions may be widespread, involving the appendicular and axial skeleton. There may be other endocrinopathies, including hyperparathyroidism and low serum phosphate with renal phosphate wasting. Café au lait spots with smooth borders (coast of California) suggest neurofibromatosis.

DIAGNOSTIC EVALUATION

The initial findings from history, physical examination, radiographs, or routine laboratory analysis suggestive of metabolic bone disease should lead to tests that will provide a specific diagnosis. The cause of the bone disease may be a primary disorder of bone or of one of the calciotropic hormones. However, the disorder may also be a complication of a disease primarily involving another organ system such as celiac sprue causing vitamin D malabsorption and osteomalacia. Table 84–6 suggests diagnostic tests and refers to other chapters for detailed discussions of the differential diagnosis based upon the presenting clinical findings and the tests needed to arrive at a specific diagnosis.

1. Bone biopsy. The histomorphometric analysis of a transiliac bone biopsy following tetracycline labeling remains the gold standard for diagnosis of metabolic bone diseases. However, because of the availability of improved diagnostic biochemical tests, few indications for bone biopsy remain. Currently, bone biopsy may be indicated in separating the various forms of vitamin D–resistant rickets (see Chapter 82) and in identifying the several entities that compose uremic osteodystrophy (see Chapter 86). The extensive differential diagnosis of osteomalacia may require bone biopsy to make a specific diagnosis (see Chapter 87). Anticonvulsant osteomalacia may be caused by vitamin D depletion or be a direct effect of the agents on bone, and a specific diagnosis permits a more rational therapeutic approach.

2. Bone mineral density. Measurement of bone mineral density of the lumbar spine and proximal femur is indicated in patients who sustain a fracture occurring with little or no trauma; to assess the extent of bone loss in patients treated with pharmacologic doses of glucocorticoids (see Chapter 88); in patients with primary hyperparathyroidism (see Chapter 76); and in patients with vertebral compression fracture or other deformity that may be due to osteoporosis.

3. Serum 25-hydroxyvitamin D [25(OH)D]. When the clinical presentation suggests osteomalacia in adults or rickets in children or infants, serum 25(OH)D is the best estimate of vitamin D body stores. Because of the seasonal variation in 25(OH)D, the normative range must take into account the lower average values at the end of winter compared to the values at the end of summer (see Chapter 87). 25(OH)D may also be low in states of vitamin D malabsorption such as celiac sprue, following distal ileal resection, chronic pancreatitis, and chronic obstructive liver disease (Table 84–7). Nephrotic syndrome is associated with low serum 25(OH)D due to renal losses of the vitamin D binding protein. In some cases, the urinary losses are sufficiently severe to cause vitamin D depletion and osteomalacia.[32, 33] Accelerated metabolism of vitamin D to inactive vitamin D metabolites or metabolism of 25(OH)D to inactive metabolites, as during chronic anticonvulsant therapy,[34] may reduce vitamin D body stores sufficiently to cause rickets or osteomalacia.

4. Serum 1,25-dihydroxyvitamin D [$1,25(OH)_2D$]. The normal range of serum $1,25(OH)_2D$ may vary by fourfold which is due in part to variation in age, sex, estrogen status in women, and dietary calcium intake (see Chapter 72). Further, values cover a broad range even when physiologic factors that cause variation in $1,25(OH)_2D$ are taken into consideration. Very low serum $1,25(OH)_2D$ levels are anticipated in vitamin D deficiency, but serum levels in patients are often within the so-called normal range (see Chapters 72 and 87). Thus, the mea-

TABLE 84–7. Disorders Characterized by Low Serum 25-Hydroxyvitamin D

Nutritional vitamin D deficiency
Celiac sprue
Pancreatic insufficiency
Inflammatory bowel disease
Distal ileal resection or bypass
Chronic obstructive liver disease
Accelerated metabolism of vitamin D via alternative pathways
Nephrotic syndrome

surement of serum 1,25$(OH)_2$D levels has limited the application to the diagnosis of vitamin D deficiency states and 25(OH)D levels are consistently more reliable.

Elevated serum 1,25$(OH)_2$D levels can be useful in the differential diagnosis of hypercalcemic states (see Chapter 78). Elevated 1,25$(OH)_2$D may be seen in sarcoidosis, or other granulomatous diseases, or B cell lymphoma (see Chapters 76 and 77).

5. Serum parathyroid hormone (PTH). A PTH assay that measures intact PTH in the physiologic range may provide elevated serum PTH levels in over 90% of patients with primary hyperparathyroidism (see Chapter 76).

6. Serum parathyroid hormone–related protein (PTHrP). The value of measuring serum PTHrP in patients with hypercalcemia is discussed in Chapter 77.

7. The diagnostic utility of technetium Tc 99m bone scanning and other imaging procedures in the diagnosis of metabolic bone diseases is discussed in Chapter 85.

REFERENCES

1. Delmas P, Meunier PJ: Osteoporosis in Klinefelter's syndrome. Quantitative bone histologic data in 5 cases and relationship with hormonal deficiency. Nouv Presse Med 10:687–690, 1981.
2. Manni A, Santen RJ: Endocrine aspects of prostate cancer. *In* Becker KL (ed): Principles and Practice of Endocrinology and Metabolism, ed 2. Philadelphia, JB Lippincott, 1995, pp 1875–1884.
3. Finkelstein JS, Neer RM, Biller BMK, et al: Osteopenia in men with a history of delayed puberty. N Engl J Med 326:763–773, 1992.
4. Bulusu L, Hodgkinson A, Nordin BEC, et al: Urinary excretion of calcium and creatinine in relation to age and body weight in normal subjects and patients with renal calculus. Clin Sci (Colch) 38:601–612, 1970.
5. Coe FL, Parks JH, Asplin JR: Medical progress: The pathogenesis and treatment of kidney stones. N Engl J Med 327:1141–1152, 1992.
6. Pietschmann F, Breslau NA, Pak CYC: Reduced vertebral bone density in hypercalciuric nephrolithiasis. J Bone Miner Res 7:1383–1388, 1992.
7. Jaeger P, Lippuner K, Casez JP, et al: Low bone mass in idiopathic renal stone formers: Magnitude and significance. J Bone Miner Res 9:1525–1532, 1994.
8. Ghazali A, Fuentes V, Desaint C, et al: Low bone mineral density and peripheral blood monocyte activation profile in calcium stone formers with idiopathic hypercalciuria. J Clin Endocrinol Metab 82:32–38, 1997.
9. Fraser D, Kooh SW, Scriver CR: Hyperparathyroidism as the cause of hyperaminoaciduria and phosphaturia in human vitamin D deficiency. Pediatr Res 1:425–435, 1976.
10. Koch KM: Dialysis-related amyloidosis. Kidney Int 41:1416–1429, 1992.
11. Goodman WG, Coburn JW, Slatopolsky E, et al: Renal osteodystrophy in adults and children. *In* Favus MJ (ed): Primer on Metabolic Bone Disease and Disorders of Mineral Metabolism, ed 4. Philadelphia, Lippincott-Raven, 1999, pp 347–363.
12. Block GA, Hulbert-Shearon TE, Levin NW, et al: Association of serum phosphorus and calcium x phosphorus product with mortality risk in chronic hemodialysis patients: A national study. Am J Kidney Dis 31:607–617, 1998.
13. Paksas NM, Kalengayi RM: Tumoral calcinosis: A clinicopathological study of 111 cases with emphasis on the earliest changes. Histopathology 31:18–24, 1997.
14. Kanda A, Uchimiya H, Ohtake N, et al: Two cases of gigantic dystrophic calcinosis cutis caused by subcutaneous and/or intramuscular injections. J Dermatol 26:371–374, 1999.
15. Pachman LM: Juvenile dermatomyositis: Pathophysiology and disease expression. Pediatr Clin North Am 42:1071–1098, 1995.
16. Smith R: Fibrodysplasia (myositis) ossificans progressiva: Clinical lessons from a rare disease. Clin Orthop 346:7–14, 1998.
17. Whyte MP: Extraskeletal (ectopic) calcification and ossification. *In* Favus MJ (ed): Primer on Metabolic Bone Disease and Disorders of Mineral Metabolism, ed 4, Philadelphia, Lippincott-Raven, 1999, pp 427–429.
18. Steinbach HL, Noetzli M: Roentgen appearance of the skeleton in osteomalacia and rickets. AJR 91:955–966, 1964.
19. Steinbach HL, Gordan GS, Eisenberg E, et al: Primary hyperparathyroidism: A correlation of roentgen, clinical and pathologic features. AJR 86:239–243, 1961.
20. Dauphine RT, Riggs BL, Scholz DA: Back pain and vertebral crush fractures: An unemphasized mode of presentation for primary hyperparathyroidism. Ann Intern Med 83:365–367, 1975.
21. Curtiss PH, Clark WS, Herndon CH: Vertebral fractures resulting from prolonged cortisone and corticotrophin therapy. JAMA 156:467–469, 1954.
22. Laan RF, Buijs WC, van Erning LJ: Differential effects of glucocorticoids on cortical appendicular and cortical vertebral bone mineral content. Calcif Tiss Int 52:5–9, 1993.
23. Waldron CA: Fibro-osseous lesions of the jaws. J Oral Maxillofac Surg 51:828–835, 1993.
24. Chew FS: Radiologic manifestations in the musculoskeletal system of miscellaneous endocrine disorders. Radiol Clin North Am 29:135–147, 1991.
25. Heiman WG, Freiberger RH: Avascular necrosis of the femoral and humeral heads after high-dose corticosteroid therapy. N Engl J Med 263:672–674, 1969.
26. Loder RT, Hensinger RN: Slipped capital femoral epiphysis associated with renal failure osteodystrophy. J Pediatr Orthop 17:205–211, 1997.
27. Econs MJ, Drezner MK: Bone disease resulting from inherited disorders of renal tubule transport and vitamin D metabolism. *In* Coe FL, Favus MJ (eds): Disorders of Bone and Mineral Metabolism. Philadelphia, Raven Press, 1992, pp 935–950.
28. Whyte MP, Murphy WA: Osteopetrosis and other sclerosing bone disorders. *In* Avioli LV, Krane SM (eds): Metabolic Bone Disease, ed 2. Philadelphia, WB Saunders, 1990, pp 616–658.
29. Bilezikian JP, Singer FR: Acute management of hypercalcemia due to parathyroid hormone and parathyroid hormone–related protein. *In* Bilezikian JP, Levine MA, Marcus R (eds): The Parathyroids: Basic and Clinical Concepts. New York, Raven Press, 1994, pp 359–372.
30. Eastell R, Heath H III: The hypocalcemic states: Their differential diagnosis and management. *In* Coe FL, Favus MJ (eds): Disorders of Bone and Mineral Metabolism. New York, Raven Press, 1992, pp 571–585.
31. Yu D, Yu S, Schuster V, et al: Identification of two novel deletion mutations within the Gs alpha gene (GNAS1) in Albright hereditary osteodystrophy. J Clin Endocrinol Metab 84:3254–3259, 1999.
32. Malluche HH, Goldstein DA, Massry SG: Osteomalacia and hyperparathyroid bone disease in patients with nephrotic syndrome. J Clin Invest 63:494–500, 1979.
33. Mittal SK, Dash SC, Tiwari SC, et al: Bone histology in patients with nephrotic syndrome and normal renal function. Kidney Int 55:1912–199, 1999.
34. Valimaki MJ, Tiihonen M, Laitinen K, et al: Bone mineral density measured by dual-energy x-ray absorptiometry and novel markers of bone formation and resorption in patients on antiepileptic drugs. J Bone Miner Res 9:631–637, 1994.

Chapter 85

Bone Density and Imaging of Osteoporosis

Christopher F. Njeh ▪ Michael Jergas ▪ Harry K. Genant

Metabolic diseases, particularly osteoporosis, are a growing public health problem. The term *osteoporosis* is widely used clinically to mean generalized loss of bone, or osteopenia. Because of uncertainties of specific radiologic interpretation, the term *osteopenia* ("poverty of bone") has been used as a generic designation for radiographic signs of decreased bone density. The currently accepted conceptual definition of osteoporosis is that it is a systemic skeletal disease characterized by low bone mass and microarchitectural deterioration of bone tissue with a consequent increase in bone fragility and susceptibility to low-trauma or atraumatic fractures.[1] Fractures, especially those of the spine, hip, and wrist, are the clinical complications of osteoporosis. Initially, spine fractures tend to be asymptomatic, but they are associated with significant morbidity as the severity and number of fractures increase. The most serious fractures are those of the hip, which contribute substantially to morbidity, mortality, and healthcare cost. Within a year of a hip fracture the mortality rate is as high as 20%, with reduced functional capacity in 50% of patients.[2] Osteoporosis is a major and growing health problem worldwide that causes approximately 2.3 million fractures annually at a cost of more than $23 billion dollars per annum in the United States and Europe alone.[3] One in three postmenopausal women and most elderly women are affected, as well as a substantial number of men.[3] Furthermore, the progressive aging of the population has led to the prediction of increasing fracture rates and associated cost.[4, 5]

Osteoporosis is often called the silent epidemic because early osteoporosis is asymptomatic and significant bone loss may become evident only after a hip or vertebral fracture has occurred. Even the presence of clinical risk factors (see Chapter 88) such as life-style, diet, and a family history of osteoporosis are relatively insensitive in predicting the presence of osteopenia.[6] The pathophysiology of osteoporosis is multifactorial and complex. The clinical manifestations of osteoporosis (i.e., fractures) depend on a variety of factors, including the propensity to fall, visual acuity, response to falling, and bone mass[7, 8] (see Chapter 88). However, studies have shown that bone mass is the most important determinant of bone strength and accounts for up to 80% of its variance.[9] Reduced bone mass is therefore a useful predictor of increased fracture risk.[10] Many prospective studies have shown that a decrease in bone density at the spine or hip of 1 SD increases the risk by a factor of 2 to 3.[11] Methods of measuring bone mineral density (BMD) are therefore pertinent to the detection of osteopenia, identification of individuals at risk for atraumatic fracture, and assessment of the efficacy of either prevention or treatment of osteoporosis.

Radiographic findings suggestive of osteopenia and osteoporosis are frequently encountered in daily medical practice and can result from a wide spectrum of diseases ranging from highly prevalent causes such as postmenopausal and involutional osteoporosis to very rare endocrinologic and hereditary or acquired disorders (see Chapter 88). Histologically, the result in each of these disorders is a deficient amount of osseous tissue, although different pathogenic mechanisms may be involved. Conventional radiography is readily available, and alone or in conjunction with other modern quantitative imaging techniques it is widely used for the detection of complications of osteopenia, for the differential diagnosis of osteopenia, or for follow-up examinations in specific clinical settings. Radionuclide imaging, computed tomography (CT), and magnetic resonance imaging (MRI) are additional diagnostic methods that are applied almost routinely to aid in the differential diagnosis of bone diseases and their sequelae.

TECHNICAL PRINCIPLES OF BONE MEASUREMENT MODALITIES

Conventional radiographs are readily available and fairly inexpensive. However, estimation of spinal BMD from appearances on conventional radiographs is insensitive and inaccurate if vertebral fractures are not present because the subjective assessment is influenced by radiographic exposure factors, patient size, and film processing techniques.[12] BMD must decline by as much as 35% before it can be detected on radiographs. These factors have supported the need for objective, noninvasive methods of bone density measurements. Such methods should be accurate, precise (reproducible), sensitive, and inexpensive and involve minimal exposure to ionizing radiation.

In the last 25 years, considerable effort has been expended on the development of noninvasive methods for assessing bone status in the axial and peripheral skeleton. Current techniques include radiographic absorptiometry (RA), single x-ray absorptiometry (SXA), dual x-ray absorptiometry (DXA), quantitative CT (QCT), and quantitative ultrasound (QUS)[13–17] (Table 85–1). These techniques vary in precision,

TABLE 85–1. Comparison of Available Modalities for Bone Status Assessment

Technique	Precision Error (%)	Accuracy Error (%)	Effective Dose (μSv)*	Advantages	Disadvantages
RA				Low cost per test/equipment	Limited to the phalanges
Phalanx/metacarpal	1–2	5	~5	Equipment mobile	
SXA/pDXA				Low cost per test/equipment	Limited to wrist or heel area density
Radius/calcaneus	1–2	4–6	<1	Equipment mobile	Limited correlation to spine/hip
				Low radiation dose	
DXA				Multiple-site capability	Limited mobility
PA spine	1–1.5	4–10	~1	Low radiation exposure	Areal density
Lateral spine	2–3	5–15	~3		Moderate cost of equipment
Proximal femur	1.5–3	6	~1		
Forearm	~1	5	<1		
Whole body	~1	3	~3		
QCT				Volumetric density	High radiation exposure
Spine, trabecular	2–4	5–15	~50		Recalibration between tests
Spine, integral	2–4	4–8	~50		Difficulty measuring the hip
pQCT				Volumetric density	Limited to wrist
Radius, trabecular	1–2	?	~1	Equipment mobile	Limited correlation with spine/hip
Radius, total	1–2	2–8	~1	Low radiation dose	
QUS				Radiation-free	Limited to peripheral sites
SOS, calcaneus/tibia	0.3–1.2	?	0	Low cost per test/equipment	Limited correlation to the spine/hip
BUA, calcaneus	1.3–3.8	?	0	Equipment mobile	

*Dose for annual background, ~2000 μSv; for abdominal radiograph, ~500 μSv; and for abdominal CT, ~4000 μSv.[14]

BUA, broadband ultrasound attenuation; DXA, dual x-ray absorptiometry; PA, posteroanterior; pDXA, peripheral DXA; pQCT, peripheral QCT; QCT, quantitative computed tomography; QUS, quantitative ultrasonography; RA, radiographic absorptiometry; SOS, speed of sound; SXA, single x-ray absorptiometry.

Adapted from Genant HK, Engelke K, Fuerst T, et al: Noninvasive assessment of bone mineral and structure: State of the art. J Bone Miner Res 11:707–730, 1996 and Scheiber LB, Torregrosa L: Evaluation and treatment of postmenopausal osteoporosis. Semin Arthritis Rheum 27:245–261, 1998.

accuracy, and discrimination and differ substantially in fundamental methodology, in clinical and research utility, and in general availability.

Radiographic Absorptiometry

This method, the first quantitative technique to assess integral bone, has recently attracted interest as a simpler, readily available screening tool (see Table 85–1). In RA, standardized hand radiographs are taken with an aluminum step-wedge placed on the film and the image analyzed with an optical densitometer. BMD is determined by comparison with the defined density of the aluminum step-wedge. The results are expressed in aluminum equivalent values or arbitrary units. RA is a low-cost and potentially widely available technique but is restricted to the appendicular bones such as the metacarpals and phalanges, which are surrounded by a relatively small amount of soft tissue. Improvements in obtaining radiographs under standard conditions and recently developed computer-assisted methods have reduced operator errors and improved precision.[19] RA appears to be suitable for measuring the BMD of phalanges and metacarpals.[13, 20]

Single X-Ray Absorptiometry

SXA with its high photon flux superseded single photon absorptiometry (SPA), first introduced in the 1960s. Replacement of the photon source ^{125}I with an x-ray tube has imparted better precision, improved the spatial resolution of these systems, and reduced examination time. The method overcame the problems of RA caused by nonuniformity of film sensitivity and development artifacts. To correct for overlying soft tissue, the anatomic site at which BMD is being measured has to be surrounded by either water, water bags, or water-equivalent moldable material.[16] SXA makes possible quantitative assessment of bone mineral content (BMC) only at peripheral sites of the skeleton. At the radius BMD measurements are carried out at the ultradistal, distal (midradius), and shaft (one-third radius) regions. The precision of 1% to 2% depends on the site, with better precision at the shaft region. The calcaneus is also a site of interest because it is weight bearing and has a high cancellous bone content. SXA has proved to be a valuable method in the diagnosis of osteoporosis because of its reasonable precision and low radiation exposure.

Dual X-Ray Absorptiometry

Sites with variable soft tissue thickness and composition such as the axial skeleton, hip, or whole body cannot be measured accurately with SXA. Dual photon absorptiometry (DPA), which uses a radionuclide source, typically ^{153}Gd, was introduced to overcome this restriction of constant overall thickness of the measurement site. DXA (Fig. 85–1) was first available commercially in 1987 as the direct successor to DPA. The fundamental physical principle behind DXA is the simultaneous measurement of x-rays with two different energies through the body. The dual x-ray spectrum can be generated by using either K-edge filters or kVp switching.[21] The main advantages of an x-ray system over a DPA radionuclide system are a shortened examination time, greater accuracy and precision, and the elimination of errors caused by source decay corrections.

The preferred anatomic sites for DXA measurement of bone mineral include the lumbar spine (L1-4), the proximal end of the femur (neck, trochanter, Ward's triangle, and total hip), and the whole body, but peripheral sites can also be scanned (Figs. 85–2 to 85–4). DXA does not measure true density but rather areal density, which is an integral of both cortical and cancellous BMC normalized to the size of the projected bone area.

A more recent development in DXA technology has been the introduction of a new generation of fan-beam scanners such as the Hologic QDR 4500 (Hologic Inc., Waltham, MA) and the Lunar Expert-XL (Lunar Corp., Madison, WI) (Fig. 85–1B). Fan-beam scanners perform a single sweep across the patient instead of the two-dimensional raster scan required by pencil-beam geometry. As a result, scan times have been shortened from about 10 to 5 minutes for the pencil-beam scanners to about 10 to 30 seconds for the fan-beam system, with a consequently higher patient throughput. Another advantage of the fan-beam system is its higher image resolution, which allows easier identification of vertebral structures and artifacts caused by degenerative disease.

DXA is also used for measurements of the appendicular skeleton. Most standard DXA densitometers allow for highly precise measurement of the radius or calcaneus by using regions of interest such as those derived from SXA measurements, as well as user-defined subregions.[22, 23] Recently, peripheral DXA (pDXA) (Fig. 85–1C) densitometers specially designed for forearm or calcaneal measurements have been introduced and may provide these measurements at a lower cost and with greater portability. Low radiation dose, availability, and

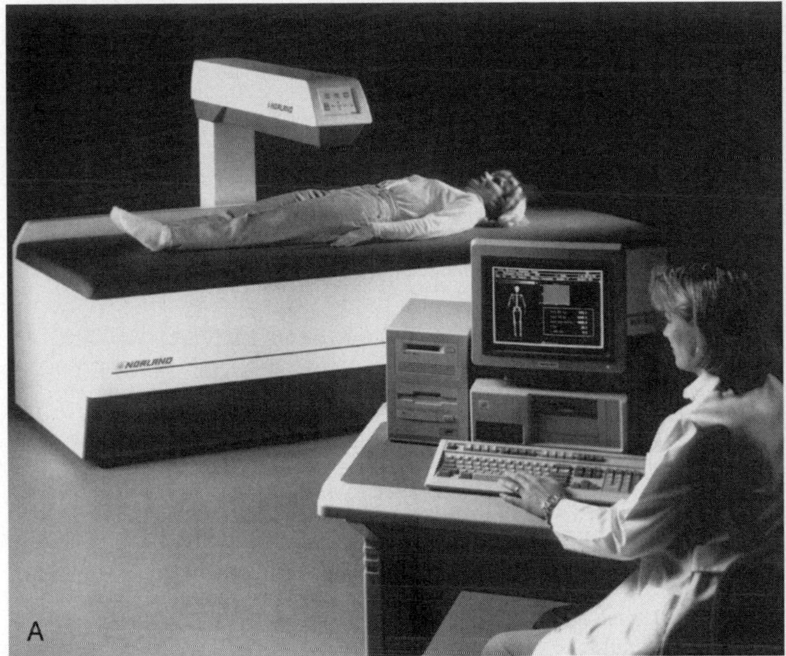

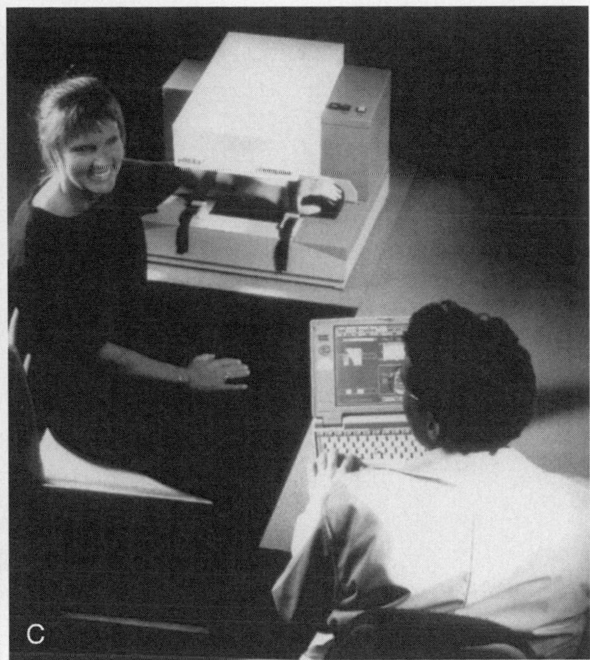

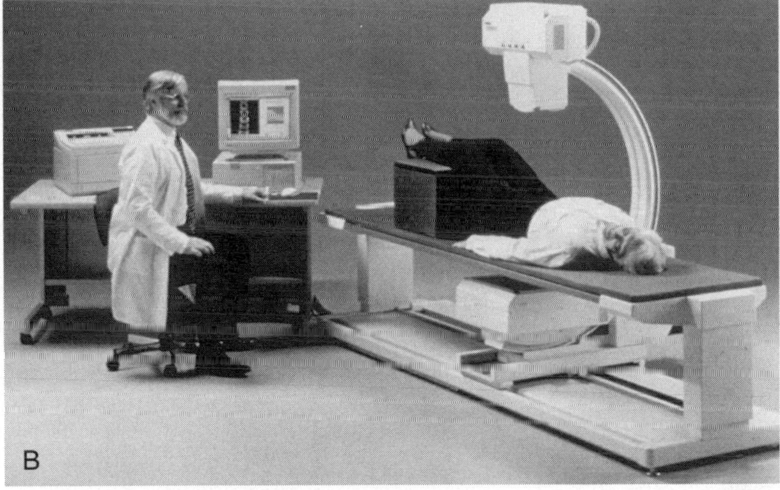

FIGURE 85–1. *A,* A pencil-beam dual x-ray absorptiometry (DXA) scanner (Norland XR 36; courtesy of Norland) demonstrating patient positioning for total body measurement. *B,* A fan-beam DXA scanner (Lunar Expert-XL; courtesy of Lunar Corp.) demonstrating patient positioning for anteroposterior spine measurement. *C,* Peripheral DXA scanner (pDEXA; courtesy of Norland Corp.) demonstrating patient positioning for forearm measurement.

ease of use have made DXA the most widely used technique for measurement of bone density in clinical trials and epidemiologic studies, with a worldwide distribution of over 10,000 systems.[13]

Quantitative Computed Tomography

Spinal QCT

QCT can be performed on clinical CT scanners to determine in three dimensions the true volumetric density (milligrams per cubic centimeter) of cancellous or cortical bone. However, because of the high responsiveness of vertebral cancellous bone and its importance for vertebral strength, QCT has been principally used to determine cancellous bone density in the vertebral body.[24] A spinal QCT examination requires that an external bone mineral reference phantom be scanned along with the patient to calibrate the CT number measurements to bone-equivalent values. In carrying out the QCT examination, a sagittal scout view encompassing the lumbar spine is first obtained. Then the sagittal location of the midplane of the vertebral bodies (typically L1-3) is marked and axial midvertebral slices are acquired.

QCT's ability to selectively assess the metabolically active and structurally important trabecular bone in the vertebral body results in an excellent ability to discriminate vertebral fracture and measure bone loss, generally with better sensitivity than projectional methods such as DXA.[24, 25] It has been found that the cross-sectional bone loss rate in females is typically 1.2% per year when measured with QCT and a little over half that value when measured with DXA. QCT for measurement of vertebral cancellous bone is widely accepted and is used at over 4000 centers worldwide. Consequently, QCT has been used for the assessment of vertebral fracture risk[26] and for measurement and follow-up of osteoporosis and other metabolic bone diseases. However, QCT scanners are much more expensive than DXA devices, the precision of BMD measurement is poorer, and the radiation dose to the patient, although acceptable, is much higher (See Table 85–1).

Peripheral QCT

To some extent the high cost and limited access to conventional all-purpose CT scanners has prompted the development of dedicated peripheral QCT (pQCT) instrumentation specifically for the measurement of purely trabecular and cortical BMC and BMD in the radius. pQCT has the advantage of delivering a lower dose of radiation to the patient than standard spinal QCT does because only the appendicular skeleton is irradiated. Unlike SPA or SXA, pQCT uses a transaxial image to allow separate measurement of the true volumetric density (milligrams per cubic centimeter) and cross-sectional area of trabecular and cortical bone without superimposition of other tissues and provides exact three-dimensional localization of the target volume. The ability to measure the metabolically more active trabecular bone and determine geometric parameters related to the cortical shell, such as the

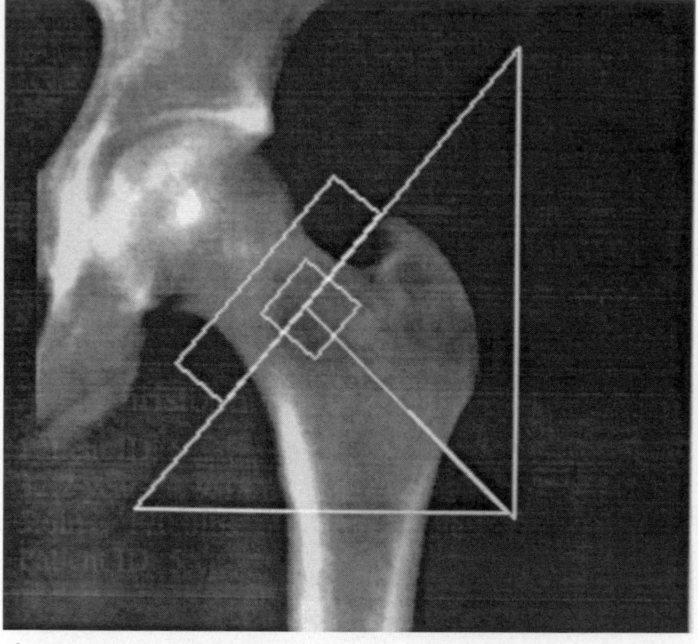

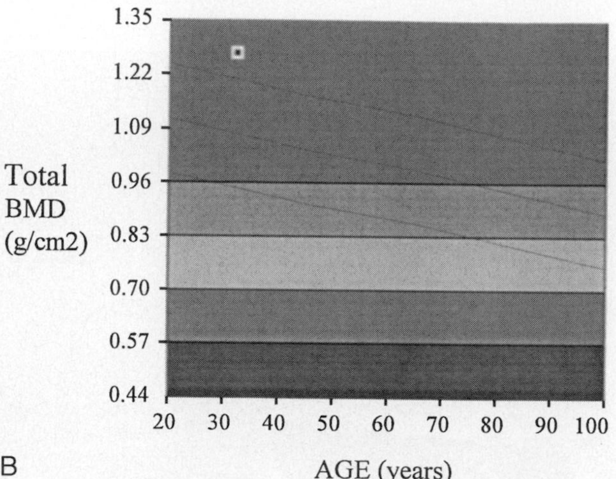

Region	BMD[1] (g/cm2)	Young-Adult[2] (%)	(T)	Age-Matched[3] (%)	(Z)
Neck	1.259	118	+1.5	119	+1.5
Ward's	1.045	109	+0.7	110	+0.7
Troch	1.037	111	+1.0	112	+1.0
Shaft	1.499	-	-	-	-
Total	1.275	117	+1.4	118	+1.5

C

FIGURE 85–2. Dual x-ray absorptiometry of the proximal end of the femur of a 32-year-old man. *A,* The region of interest analyzed consisted of the femoral neck *(oblong box),* Ward's area *(box),* trochanter, shaft, and total. *B,* Bone mineral density (BMD) plotted on a normal distribution curve. *C,* BMD values expressed as percentages of young normal individuals' values (T-scores) or age-matched values (Z-score).

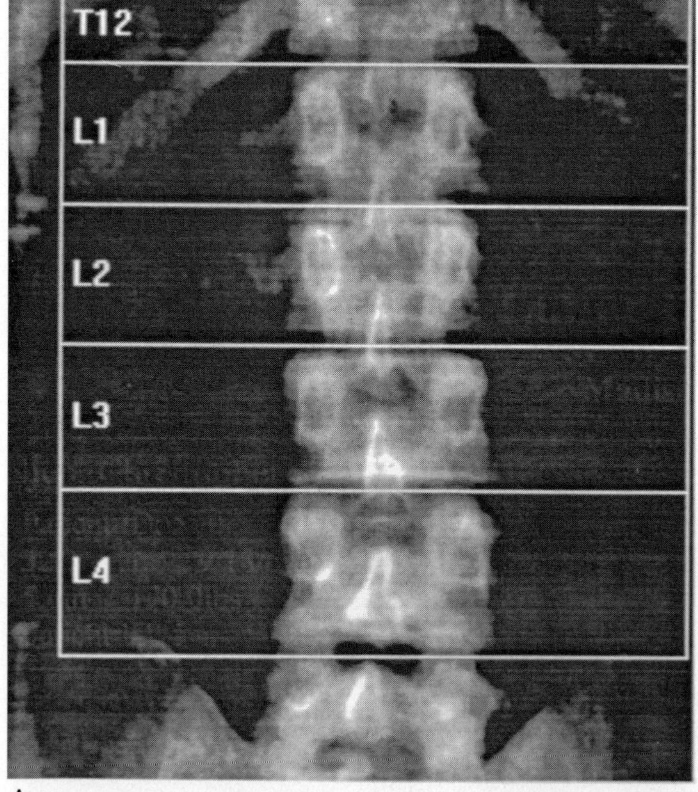

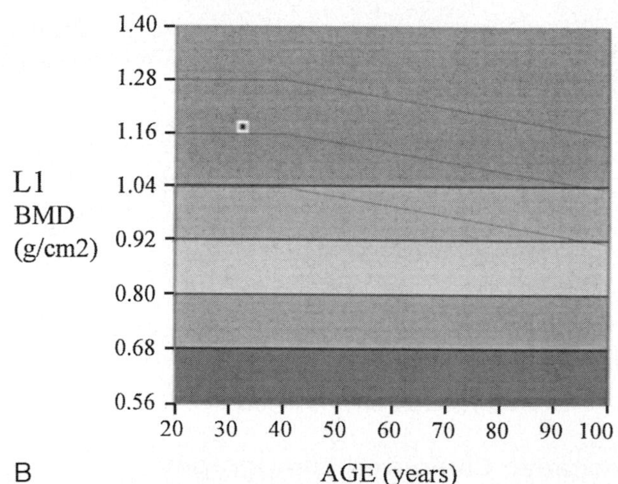

Region	BMD[1] (g/cm^2)	Young-Adult[2] (%)	(T)	Age-Matched[3] (%)	(Z)
L1	1.178	102	+0.1	102	+0.1
L2	1.463	118	+1.9	118	+1.9
L3	1.332	107	+0.8	107	+0.8
L4	1.399	113	+1.3	113	+1.3
L2-L4	1.395	113	+1.3	113	+1.3

C

FIGURE 85–3. A typical anteroposterior spine dual x-ray absorptiometry printout. *A,* The region of interest analyzed (L1-4). *B,* Bone mineral density (BMD) plotted on a normal distribution curve. *C,* BMD values expressed as percentages of young normal individuals' values (T-scores) or age-matched values (Z-score).

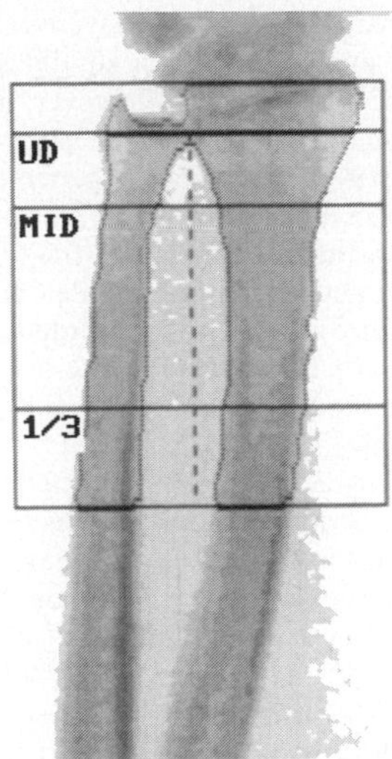

RADIUS + ULNA	Area (cm2)	BMC (grams)	BMD (gms/cm2)
UD	5.29	1.84	0.348
MID	9.48	4.61	0.486
1/3	4.95	2.81	0.568
TOTAL	19.72	9.26	0.470

FIGURE 85–4. Left forearm dual/single x-ray absorptiometry scan of a 76-year-old woman showing the region of interest analyzed. MID, mid-shaft; 1/3, shaft; UD, ultradistal.

moment of inertia and mean thickness, and its ease of use make pQCT an interesting alternative to SPA or SXA.[13]

Quantitative Ultrasound

QUS has experienced renewed interest in its application to skeletal status assessment since the work of Langton et al.[27] Interest in QUS comes from the fact that the equipment is inexpensive, small, and portable and does not involve the use of ionizing radiation. Also, indirect and/or in vitro studies have suggested that ultrasound may give information about architecture and elasticity as well as about bone density.[13, 28, 29] These benefits, combined with clinical results showing good diagnostic sensitivity for fracture discrimination, have encouraged further basic investigation and commercial development.

Bone tissue may be characterized in terms of speed of sound (SOS) and broadband ultrasound attenuation (BUA). It is currently accepted that QUS parameters are influenced by bone structure in addition to bone density.[15] However, the exact mechanisms of ultrasound interaction with bone and which physical properties are measured remain unclear. A number of manufacturers have developed several different QUS systems since the late 1980s (Fig. 85–5). Although all QUS devices measure either BUA and/or SOS, they exhibit differences in the sites measured, coupling, calibration methods, analysis software, scanner design, and algorithms for BUA and SOS calculations. Because of these variations, different instruments will give different readings, even from the same site on the same patient.[15, 30] Most of the commercial QUS systems measure the calcaneus submerged in a water bath or with ultrasonic gel as couplant and use a fixed single-point transmission transducer system. Recent developments include calcaneal transmission imaging and phalangeal, tibial, and multisite measuring devices.

QUS parameters are significantly positively correlated with BMD in vivo. Site-matched comparisons of BMD and QUS measurements have produced correlations of about 0.7 to 0.90.[15] Both cross-sectional and prospective studies have demonstrated that QUS can be used to discriminate normal from osteoporotic subject groups as effectively as traditional bone densitometry approaches do.[29, 31, 32] The ability of QUS to discriminate between normal and osteoporotic patients is independent of BMD in some cases.[32]

Contraindications and Problems in BMD Measurement

Contraindications for spinal BMD include pregnancy (abdominal thickness, radiation dose), recent administration of oral contrast media or radioisotopes, spinal deformity, and orthopedic hardware. BMD results could be affected by metal objects such as belts, buttons, and brassieres, as well as by recent ingestion of calcium-containing tablets. The presence of osteomalacia and osteoarthritis will cause underestimation and overestimation of BMD, respectively. Previous fracture, severe scoliosis, small stature, and obesity will also affect BMD measurements.

Radiation Dose

Studies of the radiation dose to patients from DXA confirm that the patient dose is small (0.08–4.6 μSv) when compared with that from many other investigations involving ionizing radiation. Fan-beam technology with increased resolution has resulted in increased patient radiation dose (6.7–31 μSv), but this dose is still relatively small. Measuring vertebral morphometry by DXA also incurs less radiation dose (<60 μSv) than standard lateral radiographs do. QCT has a radiation dose (<60 μSv) comparable to that of a simple radiologic

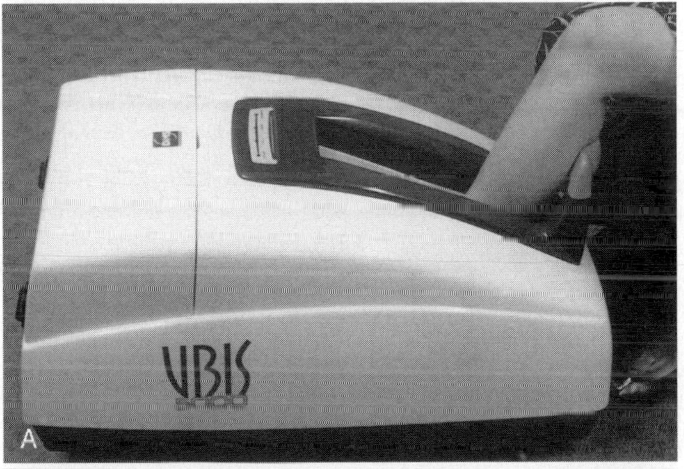

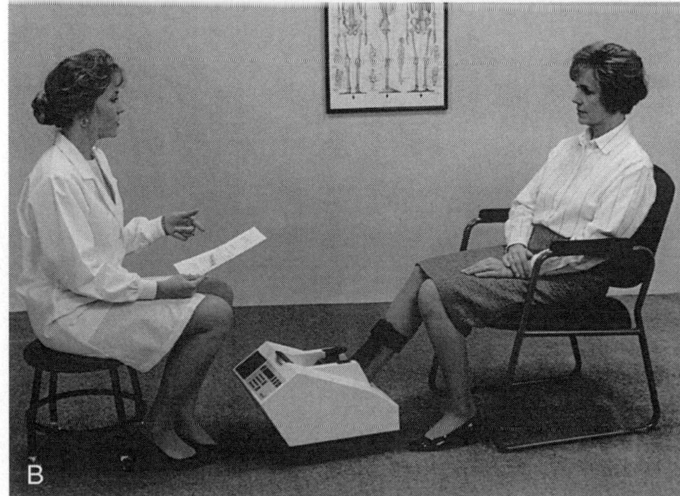

FIGURE 85–5. *A,* Imaging and water-coupled quantitative ultrasound (QUS) system (UBIS-5000; courtesy of DMS). *B,* A gel-coupled contact QUS system (SAHARA; courtesy of Hologic) illustrating patient positioning for calcaneus measurement.

examination, such as a chest radiograph, but lower than standard CT imaging. Radiation doses from other techniques such as RA and SXA are of the same order of magnitude as pencil-beam DXA. For pencil-beam DXA and SXA systems the time-average dose to staff from scatter is very low, even with the operator sitting as close as 1 m from the patient during measurement. However, the scatter dose from fan-beam DXA systems is considerably higher and approaches the limits set by regulatory bodies for occupational exposure.[33]

CLINICAL UTILITY OF DENSITOMETRY

Interpretation of BMD Results

No consensus has been reached on how BMD measurements should be presented. To be clinically useful, BMD results for individual patients must be related to similar values obtained from a healthy reference population. The reference population is usually described in terms of the mean BMD and the population standard matched for age, sex, and race as T- and Z-scores. The T-score as used by the World Health Organization (WHO) osteoporosis definition (Table 85–2) represents the number of standard deviations that a BMD measurement is above or below the mean peak bone mass of a young normal population matched for sex and race. Z-scores express the number of standard deviations that a subject differs from the mean value for an age-, sex-, and race-matched reference population. Z-scores should not be used to define osteoporosis because their use would result in the apparent prevalence of the disease not increasing with age.

With the WHO criteria, osteoporosis can be diagnosed in women if the value for BMD or BMC is 2.5 SD or more below the mean value of a young reference population[34] (T-score of -2.5 SD) (see Table 85–2). These figures are general guidelines for diagnosis and are not intended to require or restrict therapy for individual patients. Rather, the physician and the patient should use the BMD information in conjunction with knowledge of the patient's specific medical and personal history to determine the best course of action for each individual. This cutoff approach is certainly easy to apply. However, such a simplistic approach is associated with inherent problems. It is heavily dependent on estimates of young adult reference means and standard deviations, different patterns of bone loss at specific sites are not taken into consideration,[35] and it ignores the continuous increase in risk with decreasing BMD. Today, the diagnosis of osteoporosis relies mainly on bone mass measurements, and in a clinical setting the essential role of bone densitometry (and QUS) is to identify patients at risk for osteoporotic fractures.

Which Site to Measure

Different skeletal sites contain different proportions of trabecular and cortical bone, which differ in their rate of bone loss. However, osteoporosis is a systemic disease, and loss of bone occurs at all sites albeit at different rates. So one could assume that for diagnostic purposes bone density could be measured at any site. Low bone density at different anatomic sites is significantly associated with the risk of osteoporotic fracture.[11, 36] However, BMD assessed in areas remote from the fracture site generally has weaker predictive power, except for the lumbar spine, where degenerative disease may falsely elevate DXA BMD in elderly women.[11, 37] In a meta-analysis, Marshal et al. showed that to predict the risk of fracture occurring at any site, risk ratios for different measurement sites are similar.[38] So for predicting overall fracture risk in any individual, any bone density measurement can be used. However, for site-specific fracture prediction, the site of interest should be measured (i.e., measure the hip when predicting hip fracture).[39]

The question of whether more information would be gained by making multiple measurements has also been addressed. Several studies have documented the discordance of diagnosis from measurements at different sites and the possibility of frequent misdiagnosis of women if BMD is measured at a single site.[13, 40–42] Other reports suggest that for hip fractures, BMD at the hip is the superior measurement and that the addition of measurements at the spine, calcaneus, or radius adds little new information.[13, 41] In contrast, Davis and colleagues found that combining BMC measurements from multiple sites improved the prediction of incident vertebral fracture.[40] Further investigation will be required to clarify the role of multiple measurements, with particular attention paid to the type of fracture, the characteristics of the population studied, and the statistical techniques used. Until these points are resolved, it is advisable to scan several sites, if practical, when screening for osteoporosis.

The clinician should be aware of the limitations of BMD, such as the effect of disease or medication on the type of bone. For example, changes in BMD that occur in the immediate postmenopausal period or as a result of treatment are often more marked in the spine and can be detected earlier than at the hip or wrist. In the elderly, where degenerative disease may be prevalent, BMD assessed by spinal QCT or at a remote site such as the femur may be more effective for risk assessment. Alternatively, lateral scanning of the lumbar spine reduces the influence of degenerative changes and may be a more suitable measurement in an osteoarthritic individual.[26]

TABLE 85–2. WHO Definitions of Osteoporosis Based on BMD or BMC Values

Normal	A BMD/BMC value greater than 1 SD below the average value of a young adult ($T > -1$)
Low bone mass (osteopenia)	A BMD/BMC value more than 1 SD below the young adult average but not more than 2.5 SD below ($-2.5 < T < -1$)
Osteoporosis	A BMD/BMC value more than 2.5 SD below the young adult average value ($T < -2.5$)
Severe (established) osteoporosis	A BMD/BMC value more than 2.5 SD below the young adult average with one or more osteoporotic fractures

Adapted from World Health Organization: Assessment of Fracture Risk and Its Application to Screening for Postmenopausal Osteoporosis, WHO Technical Report Series 843. Geneva, WHO, 1994.

BMC, bone mineral content; BMD, bone mineral density.

Which Technique to Use

As previously discussed, a number of techniques are available for the assessment of bone status. Some prospective studies have shown that these techniques are comparable in their ability to identify patients at risk for fracture.[13, 29, 38] Even though these techniques can classify different groups of patients according to their bone status, none of these techniques can provide absolute discrimination between fracture and nonfracture patients.[42, 43] Once a measurement site has been chosen, the best technique to measure that site will depend on the precision, accuracy, availability, and cost of the technique, as well as many other parameters.[39] It is important to recognize that bone density or ultrasound measurement provides only an estimate of the patient's fracture risk. The clinician should interpret the scan findings along with other clinical risk factors (see Chapter 88) to determine the best treatment for the individual patient.

When to Measure BMD

Given the current awareness of osteoporosis, bone densitometry is becoming widely used in routine medical practice. A consensus is forming regarding when a bone density scan is appropriate, and four indications have emerged.[13]

- Evaluation of perimenopausal women for initiation of estrogen therapy
- Detection of osteoporosis and assessment of its severity
- Evaluation of patients with metabolic diseases that affect the skeleton
- Monitoring of treatment and evaluation of disease course

BMD for Monitoring

Serial measurements are very useful for monitoring the natural history of the condition and assessing response to therapy. The choice of site for longitudinal testing depends on two variables: first, the rate of change in bone mass within the skeleton itself and, second, the precision of bone density testing at particular sites. In general, the measured change in bone density should be 2.8 times the long-term precision error for the measured variable.[44, 45] The precision of serial DXA scans is approximately 1% to 2% when performed by an experienced technologist. Thus a change in bone mass of at least 3% to 6% in the spine and 6% to 8% at the femoral neck is required to be considered significant. The rate of bone loss in early menopause is on average 2% per year but may range from less than 1% to more than 5% per year.[34] So measurements at 1- to 2-year intervals may be sufficient at this stage to document the natural history of bone change.[46] Testing too infrequently may mean that patients who are rapidly losing bone in the range of 5% per year may be missed and go untreated. For a patient with borderline bone mass measurements, repeated measurements may help clarify decisions on intervention. In patients with secondary conditions producing osteoporosis, such as corticosteroid therapy, a rapid rate of bone loss can sometimes be expected, and more frequent measurements such as every 6 months may be useful.[47]

Repeated measurements are also useful for assessing response to therapy. Most patients respond to the most widely prescribed therapies, hormone replacement therapy (HRT) and bisphosphonates. Measurement of the spine at 1- to 2-year intervals will detect significant improvement in most patients commencing HRT or bisphosphonate therapy because the spine is the optimal site for monitoring therapy. On the whole, follow-up measurements should be used to establish that the therapeutic intervention is effective, as well as to provide incentive for the patient to maintain treatment. It is difficult for individuals to continue long-term treatment programs, especially when the disease is asymptomatic and it has no direct impact on their sense of well-being.

How to Use BMD

It should be recognized that the best use of each bone densitometry technique depends on the nature of the clinical problem and the age of the patient, as well as technical factors.[39] The primary purpose of measuring bone status should be to assess fracture risk in individual patients in order to make clinical decisions about intervention to minimize that risk. In fact, a recent meta-analysis demonstrated that BMD is a better predictor of the risk of fracture than cholesterol is for the risk of coronary disease.[38] Bone densitometry is appropriate in the evaluation of perimenopausal women if the result will influence subsequent clinical decisions. As an example, it would be appropriate to treat a patient who has severe symptoms of estrogen deficiency with estrogen regardless of bone density. However, if the density value will affect a decision to undertake HRT (or an alternative such as alendronate or raloxifene), testing is clearly defensible. An international panel has recently formulated guidelines on the clinical use and interpretation of BMD.[36] The main consensus statements are listed below.

- Bone mass measurements predict a patient's future risk of fracture.
- Osteoporosis can be diagnosed on the basis of bone mass measurements even in the absence of prevalent fractures.
- Bone mass measurements provide information that can affect the management of patients.
- Choice of the appropriate skeletal measurement site(s) may vary depending on the specific circumstances of the patient.
- The technique chosen for bone mass measurement should be based on an understanding of the strength and limitations of the different techniques.
- Bone mass data should be accompanied by a clinical interpretation.

VERTEBRAL FRACTURE ASSESSMENT

Vertebral fractures are one of the most common consequences of osteoporosis. Patients have loss of height, possibly with acute pain and disability, but in many cases they are completely asymptomatic.[48] Although hip fractures may be identified unambiguously on radiographs, criteria for identifying osteoporotic fractures in the spine are less well defined. The conventional practice is for radiologists to diagnose vertebral fractures by reading lateral radiographs of the lumbar and thoracic spine. Alteration in the normally rectangular shape of the vertebral body is identified as a fracture. Vertebral fractures are commonly grouped by fracture type (wedge, biconcavity, or compression) and by the degree of deformity.

To accurately assess the presence, type, and severity of a vertebral fracture, measurements of the anterior, middle, and posterior heights of the vertebral bodies from T4 to L4 on lateral spine radiographs are classically performed in clinical trials. This measurement technique is called vertebral morphometry. It requires digitizing conventional radiographs obtained under carefully standardized conditions.[49] Over the years a number of proposals have been published for interpreting vertebral morphometry measurements,[50] including the Minne method,[51] Eastell method,[52] Black method,[53] and McCloskey method.[54] These methods usually have satisfactory sensitivity at the expense of poorer specificity, which leads to a high number of false positives. These morphometric approaches are of comparable validity; no standard has been adopted, however, but guidelines have been established.[55]

None of the quantitative morphometry methods outlined can discriminate between vertebral fractures and other causes of vertebral deformity. The radiologist viewing the radiographs has a long list of potential differential diagnoses for vertebral deformities to contend with, and only visual inspection and expert interpretation of the radiograph can ensure the correct classification. This viewpoint is the basis of the semiquantitative technique of Genant et al.[56] In the Genant method, each vertebra from T4 to L4 is assessed visually without any direct vertebral measurement and graded as either normal or mildly, moderately, or severely fractured (Fig. 85–6). After visual assessment, a spinal fracture index can be calculated as the sum of all grades divided by the number of vertebrae that can be evaluated. The advantage of the method is that it makes a trained human observer the basis of interpretation while also providing a quantitative index that allows for meaningful interpretation of changes on follow-up films.

Morphometric X-Ray Absorptiometry

In the past 5 years, technical advances (fan beam) in DXA scanners have improved image quality to the extent that it is now possible to use DXA images for vertebral morphometry.[57] The rotating C-arm enables the acquisition of both posteroanterior and lateral images of the thoracic and lumbar spine (T4-L4) with the patient lying in the supine position. Morphometric x-ray absorptiometry is relatively new but has several potential advantages over conventional radiography, including a low radiation dose, reduced beam distortion, and ease of storage.[58] However, resolution is lower and noise is higher.

BONE TURNOVER BIOCHEMICAL MARKERS

Bone mass depends on the balance between resorption and formation within a remodeling unit. The rate of bone activity can be assessed either by measuring the enzymatic activity of osteoblastic or osteoclastic cells or by measuring components of the bone matrix released into the circulation during formation or resorption (see Chapter 88). These tests are particularly useful in research studies or clinical drug trials to better understand bone metabolism or the response of bone to the clinical agent. They may also be useful to specialists in complex cases to determine whether a patient is losing bone rapidly, responding to therapy, or continuing with therapy. Some studies performed in postmenopausal women suggest that increased bone turn-

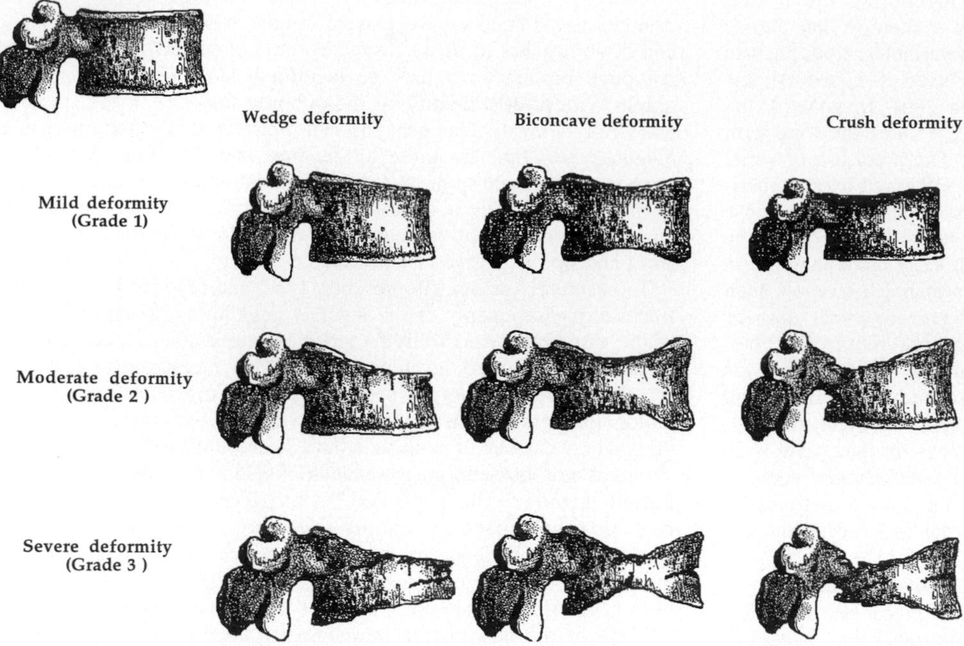

FIGURE 85–6. Schematic representations of wedge, biconcave, and crush vertebral deformities. The figure illustrates the semiquantitative visual grading system of Genant.[55] (Drawn by C. Y. Wu.)

over is associated with increased bone loss and lower bone mass in the elderly and, eventually, more osteoporotic fractures.[58] At the present time the optimal and cost-effective use of biochemical markers in individual primary care is less clear.

RADIOLOGIC ASSESSMENT OF OSTEOPOROSIS: PRINCIPAL RADIOGRAPHIC FINDINGS

The absorption of x-rays by a tissue depends on the quality of the x-ray beam, the character of the atoms composing the tissue, the physical density of the tissue, and the thickness of the penetrated structure. The amount of x-ray absorption defines the density of x-ray shadow that a tissue casts on the film. Because absorption increases with the third power of the atomic number and because calcium has a high atomic number, it is primarily the amount of calcium that affects the x-ray absorption of bone. The amount of calcium per unit mineralized bone volume in osteoporosis remains constant at about 35%.[60, 61] Therefore, a decrease in mineralized bone volume results in a decrease in total bone calcium and, consequently, decreased absorption of the x-ray beam. On the x-ray film this phenomenon is referred to as increased radiolucency.

At the same time as bone mass is lost, changes in bone structure occur and can be observed radiographically. Bone is composed of two compartments: cortical bone and trabecular bone. The structural changes seen in cortical bone represent bone resorption at different sites (e.g., the inner and outer surfaces of the cortex or within the cortex in the haversian and Volkmann canals). These three sites (endosteal, intracortical, and periosteal) may react differently to distinct metabolic stimuli, and careful investigation of the cortices may be of value in the differential diagnosis of metabolic disease affecting the skeleton.

Cortical bone remodeling typically occurs in the endosteal "envelope," and interpretation of subtle changes in this layer may be difficult at times. With increasing age comes widening of the marrow canal because of an imbalance in endosteal bone formation and resorption that leads to "trabeculization" of the inner surface of the cortex. Endosteal scalloping caused by resorption of the inner bone surface can be seen in high bone turnover states such as reflex sympathetic dystrophy (Fig. 85–7).

Intracortical bone resorption may cause longitudinal striation or tunneling, predominantly in the subendosteal zone. These changes are seen in various high-turnover metabolic diseases affecting the bone such as hyperparathyroidism, osteomalacia, renal osteodystrophy, and acute osteoporosis from disuse or the reflex sympathetic dystrophy syndrome, as well as in postmenopausal osteoporosis. Intracortical

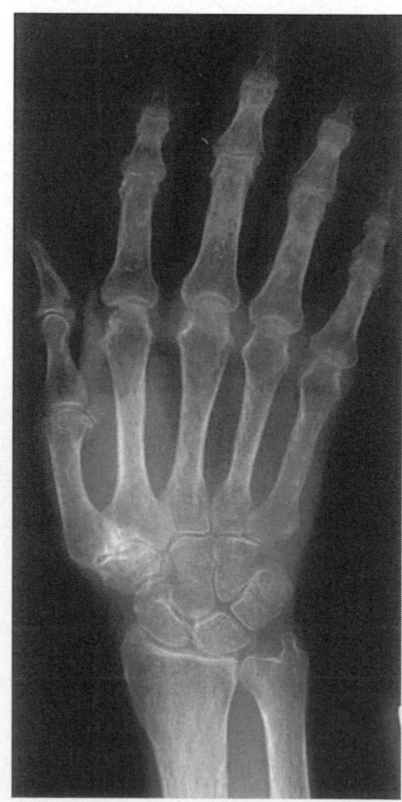

FIGURE 85–7. Cortical thinning in senile osteoporosis, as shown in this hand radiograph of a 77-year-old woman, is primarily the result of endosteal bone resorption.

tunneling is a hallmark of rapid bone turnover. It is not usually apparent in disease states with relatively low bone turnover such as senile osteoporosis. Accelerated endosteal and intracortical resorption with intracortical tunneling and an indistinct border of the inner cortical surface is best depicted with high-resolution radiographic techniques. Intracortical tunneling must be distinguished from nutritional foramina, which are isolated and occur with an oblique orientation. Intracortical resorption is also a sign of bone viability and is not seen in necrotic or allograft bone.

Subperiosteal bone resorption is associated with an irregular definition of the outer bone surface. This finding is pronounced in diseases with high bone turnover, principally primary and secondary hyperparathyroidism. However, it may also rarely be present in other diseases. Cortical thinning with expansion of the medullary cavity occurs as endosteal bone resorption exceeds periosteal bone apposition in most adults. In the late stages of osteoporosis, the cortices appear paper thin, with the endosteal surface usually being smooth.

Trabecular bone responds faster to metabolic changes than cortical bone does.[62] Trabecular bone changes are most prominent in the axial skeleton and in the ends of the long and tubular bones of the appendicular skeleton (juxta-articular), such as the proximal end of the femur and distal third of the radius. These sites have a relatively great proportion of trabecular bone. Loss of trabecular bone (in cases of low rates of loss) occurs in a predictable pattern. Non–weight-bearing trabeculae are resorbed first, which leads to a relative prominence of the weight-bearing trabeculae. The remaining trabeculae may even become thicker and result in a distinct radiographic trabecular pattern. For example, early changes of osteopenia in the lumbar spine typically include rarefaction of the horizontal trabeculae accompanied by relative accentuation of the vertical trabeculae. These changes may lead to an appearance of vertical striation of the bone (Fig. 85–8). With decreasing density of trabecular bone the cortical rim of the vertebrae is more accentuated, and the vertebrae may have a "picture-frame" appearance (Fig. 85–9). In addition to the changes in trabecular bone, thinning of cortical bone occurs. Changes in bone structure at distinct skeletal sites are assessed for the differential diagnosis of various skeletal conditions. For the evaluation of very subtle changes, such as different forms of bone resorption, high-resolution radiographic techniques with optical or geometric magnification may be required.[63–65]

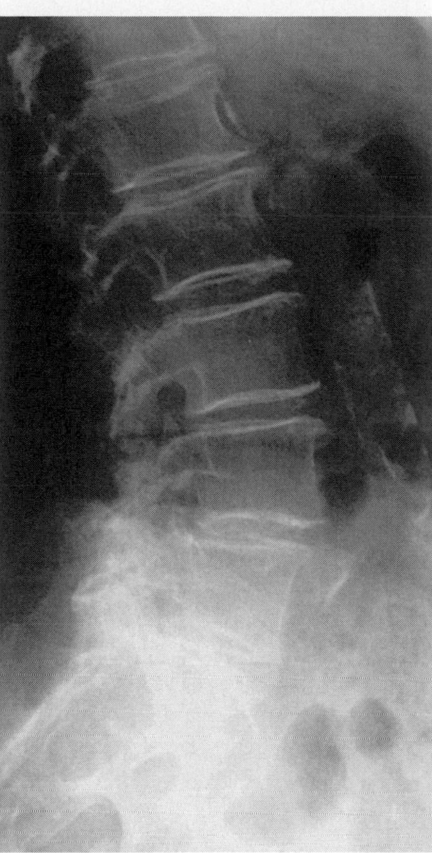

FIGURE 85–9. Loss of trabecular bone and relative accentuation of the cortices result in the appearance of "picture framing" of the vertebrae in postmenopausal osteoporosis.

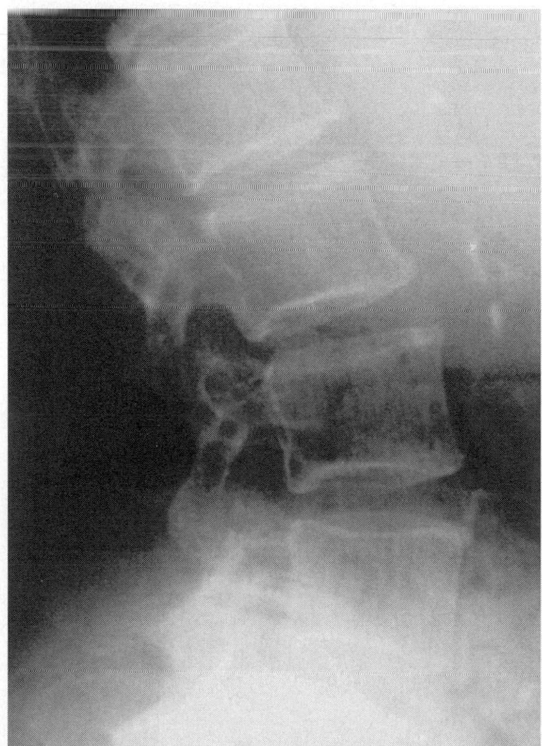

FIGURE 85–8. Reinforcement of the vertical primary trabeculae and loss of the horizontal trabeculae in postmenopausal osteoporosis lead to vertical striations on a radiograph of the spine, combined with an overall loss of bone density.

The anatomic distribution of the osteopenia or osteoporosis depends on the underlying cause. Osteopenia can be generalized and affect the whole skeleton or it can be regional and affect only part of the skeleton, usually in the appendicular skeleton. Typical examples of generalized osteopenia are involutional and postmenopausal osteoporosis and osteoporosis caused by endocrine disorders such as hyperparathyroidism, hyperthyroidism, osteomalacia, and hypogonadism. Regional forms of osteoporosis result from factors affecting only parts of the appendicular skeleton, such as disuse, reflex sympathetic syndrome, and transient osteoporosis of large joints. The distribution of osteopenia may vary considerably between different diseases and may be suggestive of a specific diagnosis. Focal osteopenia primarily reflects the underlying cause, such as inflammation, fracture, or tumor, and is not the subject of this chapter.

Thus it seems that a number of characteristic features by conventional radiography make the diagnosis of osteopenia or osteoporosis possible. However, detection of osteopenia by conventional radiography is inaccurate because it is influenced by many technical factors such as radiographic exposure, film development, soft tissue thickness of the patient, and other factors[66] (Table 85–3). It has been estimated that as much as 20% to 40% of bone mass must be lost before a decrease in bone density can be seen on lateral radiographs of the thoracic and lumbar spine.[67] Finally, the diagnosis of osteopenia from conventional radiographs is also dependent on the experience of the reader and the reader's subjective interpretation.[68]

In summary, a radiograph may reflect the amount of bone mass, histology, and gross morphology of the skeletal part examined. The principal findings of osteopenia are increased radiolucency, changes in bone microstructure such as rarefaction of trabeculae, and thinning of the cortices, all of which eventually result in changes in gross bone morphology, namely, changes in shape of the bone and fractures.

TABLE 85–3. Factors Influencing the Radiographic Appearance of Objects

Radiation source	Exposure time
	Film-focus distance
	Anode characteristics
	Voltage
	Beam filtration
Object	Thickness of bone
	Bone mineral content
	Soft tissue composition
	Scattering
Film and screen	Film granularity
	Emulsion of film
	Film speed
	Screen properties
Film processing	Developing time
	Temperature of developer
	Type of developer
	Type of fixer
	Type of processing (automated vs. manual)

Adapted from Heuck F, Schmidt E: Die quantitative Bestimmung des Mineralgehaltes des Knochens aus dem Röntgenbild. Fortschr Rontgenstr 93:523–554, 1960.

Further characteristics of osteopenic and osteoporotic disease conditions and specific techniques for their radiologic assessment are described in greater detail below.

DISEASES CHARACTERIZED BY GENERALIZED OSTEOPENIA: INVOLUTIONAL OSTEOPOROSIS

Involutional osteoporosis is the most common generalized skeletal disease. It has been classified as type I, or postmenopausal osteoporosis, and type II, or senile osteoporosis.[61, 69] Gallagher added a third type, secondary osteoporosis.[70] Even though the importance of estrogen deficiency in postmenopausal osteoporosis has been established, the distinction between the first two types of osteoporosis is not generally accepted. Distinctions between postmenopausal and senile osteoporosis may sometimes be arbitrary, and the assignment of fracture sites to the different types of osteoporosis is uncertain. Postmenopausal osteoporosis is believed to represent that process occurring in a subset of postmenopausal women typically between the ages of 50 and 65 years. Trabecular bone resorption related to estrogen deficiency is accelerated, and the fracture pattern in this group of women primarily involves the spine and the wrist. Senile osteoporosis is associated with a proportionate loss of cortical and trabecular bone. The characteristic fractures of senile osteoporosis include fractures of the hip, the proximal end of the humerus, the tibia, and the pelvis in elderly women and men, usually 75 years or older (Fig. 85–10). Major factors in the etiology of senile osteoporosis include an age-related decrease in bone formation, diminished adrenal function, reduced intestinal calcium absorption, and secondary hyperparathyroidism.

The radiographic appearance of the skeleton in involutional osteoporosis may include all of the aforementioned characteristics of generalized osteoporosis. The high prevalence of involutional osteoporosis with its typical radiographic manifestations has led to numerous attempts to base diagnosis and quantification of osteoporosis on its radiographic characteristics.

OSTEOPENIA AND OSTEOPOROSIS OF THE AXIAL SKELETON

The radiographic manifestation of osteopenia of the axial skeleton includes increased radiolucency of the vertebrae (Fig. 85–11), which may assume the radiographic density of the intervertebral disk space. Further findings include vertical striation of the vertebrae as a result of reinforcement of vertical trabeculae in the osteopenic vertebra, framed appearance of the vertebrae (picture framing or empty box) caused by accentuation of the cortical outline, and increased biconcavity of the vertebral end plates (see Figs. 85–8 and 85–9). Biconcavity of the vertebrae results from protrusion of the intervertebral disk into the weakened vertebral body. A classification of these characteristics can be found with the Saville index.[71] This index, however, has never gained widespread acceptance because it is prone to great subjectivity and experience of the reader. Doyle and colleagues found that none of the aforementioned signs of osteopenia reflects the bone mineral status of an individual reliably and cannot be used for the follow-up of osteopenic patients.[72] Thus bone density measurements using dedicated densitometric methods have widely replaced subjective analysis of bone density from conventional radiographs. Densitometric results may suggest osteopenia even if the bone loss is not detectable on a spine radiograph. Nevertheless, the aforementioned radiographic signs of osteoporosis have been found to be significantly related to measured bone density, and normal bone densitometry measurements may sometimes have to be considered false if the radiograph displays clear characteristic changes of osteopenia.[73, 74]

Vertebral Fractures and Their Diagnosis

Vertebral fractures are the hallmarks of osteoporosis, and even though one may argue that osteopenia per se may not be diagnosed reliably from spinal radiographs, spinal radiography continues to be a substantial aid in diagnosing and monitoring vertebral fractures.[56] Changes in the gross morphology of the vertebral body have a wide range of appearances from increased concavity of the end plates to complete destruction of the vertebral anatomy in vertebral crush fractures (see Figs. 85–6 and 85–11). In clinical practice, conventional radiographs of the thorax and lumbar region in the lateral projection are analyzed qualitatively by radiologists or experienced clinicians to identify vertebral deformities or fractures. For an experienced radiologist, this assessment is generally uncomplicated, and it can be aided by additional radiographic projections such as anteroposterior and oblique views or by complementary examinations such as bone scintig-

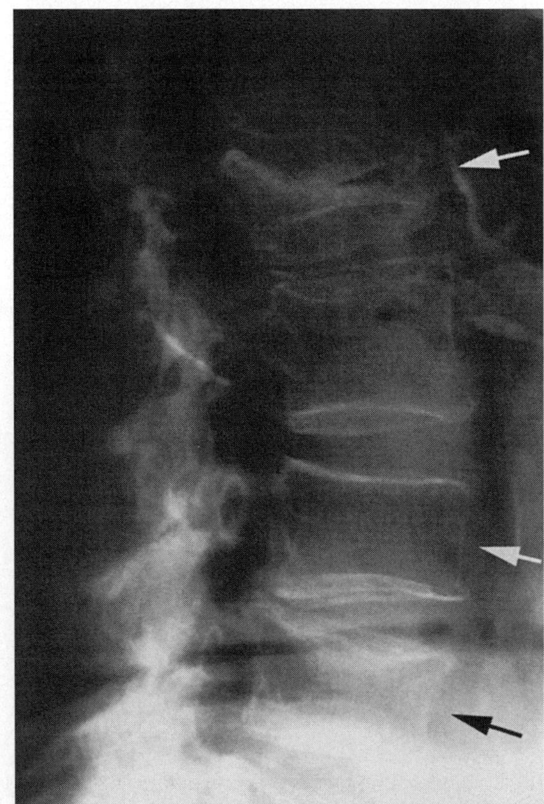

FIGURE 85–10. Advanced involutional osteoporosis with osteopenia and multiple fractures in the lumbar spine *(white and black arrows)*.

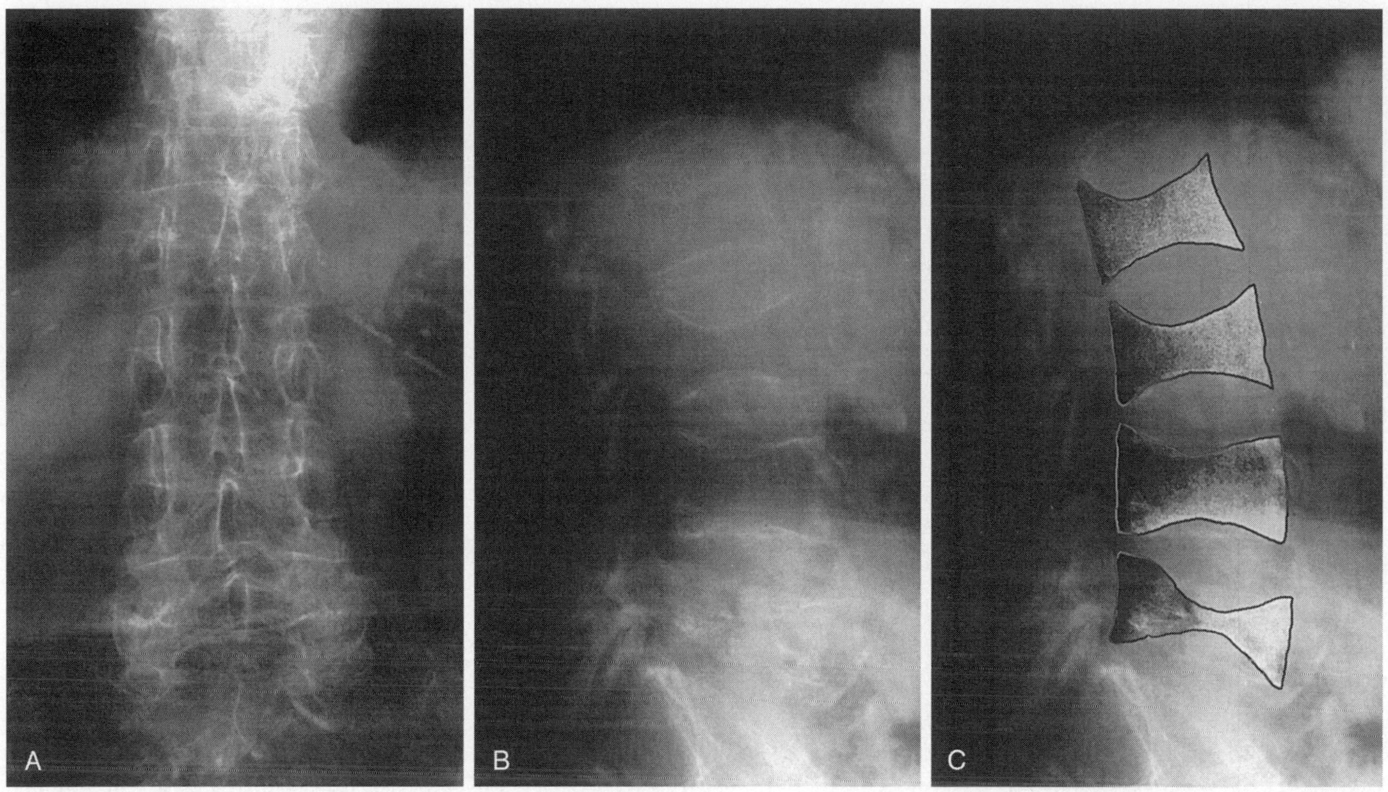

FIGURE 85–11. Conventional radiography of the lumbar spine in a patient with severe osteoporosis. The anteroposterior *(A)* and lateral *(B)* projections clearly display increased radiolucency of the vertebrae and multiple biconcave fractures of the spine. *C,* Outlines and areas of the lumbar vertebrae in the lateral projection.

raphy, CT, and even MRI[75–77] (Figs. 85–12 and 85–13). Because vertebral fractures are the most frequent fractures in early postmenopausal women, they have become the most important endpoints in epidemiologic studies and clinical drug trials. In these settings, conventional radiography is usually the only method applied to assess vertebral fractures. Several quantitative morphometric methods that rely entirely on measurements of vertebral height for vertebral fracture diagnosis have been proposed to reduce the subjectivity that is inherent

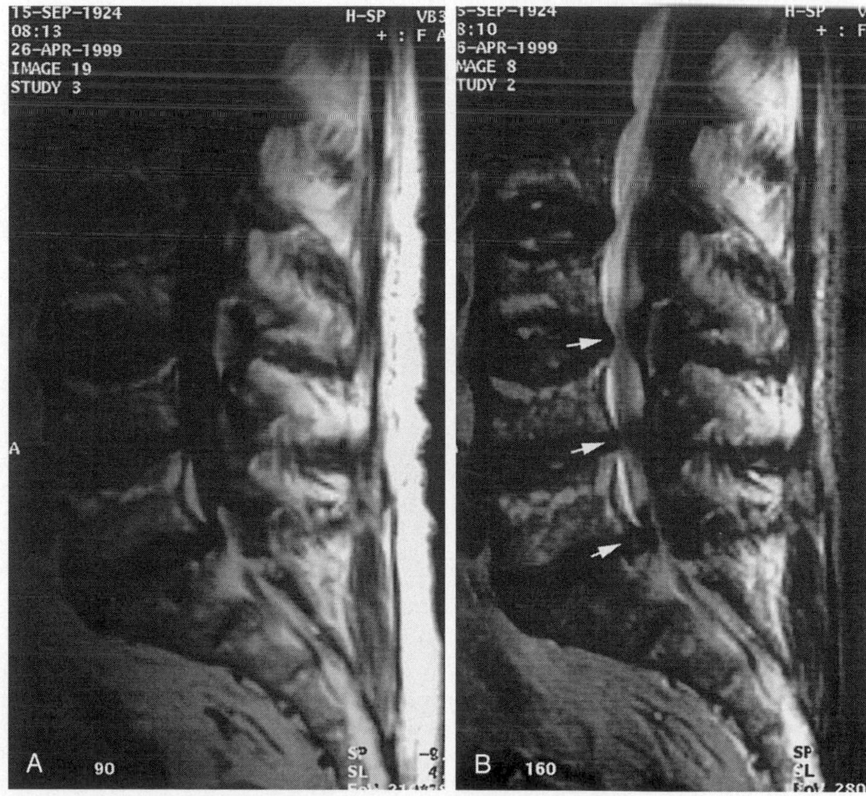

FIGURE 85–12. Magnetic resonance appearance of an osteoporotic spine in a 75-year-old man. Multiple biconcave vertebrae are seen in T1-*(A)*, and T2-weighted *(B)* images. Disk extrusions (*arrows* in *B*) led to spinal stenosis in this patient.

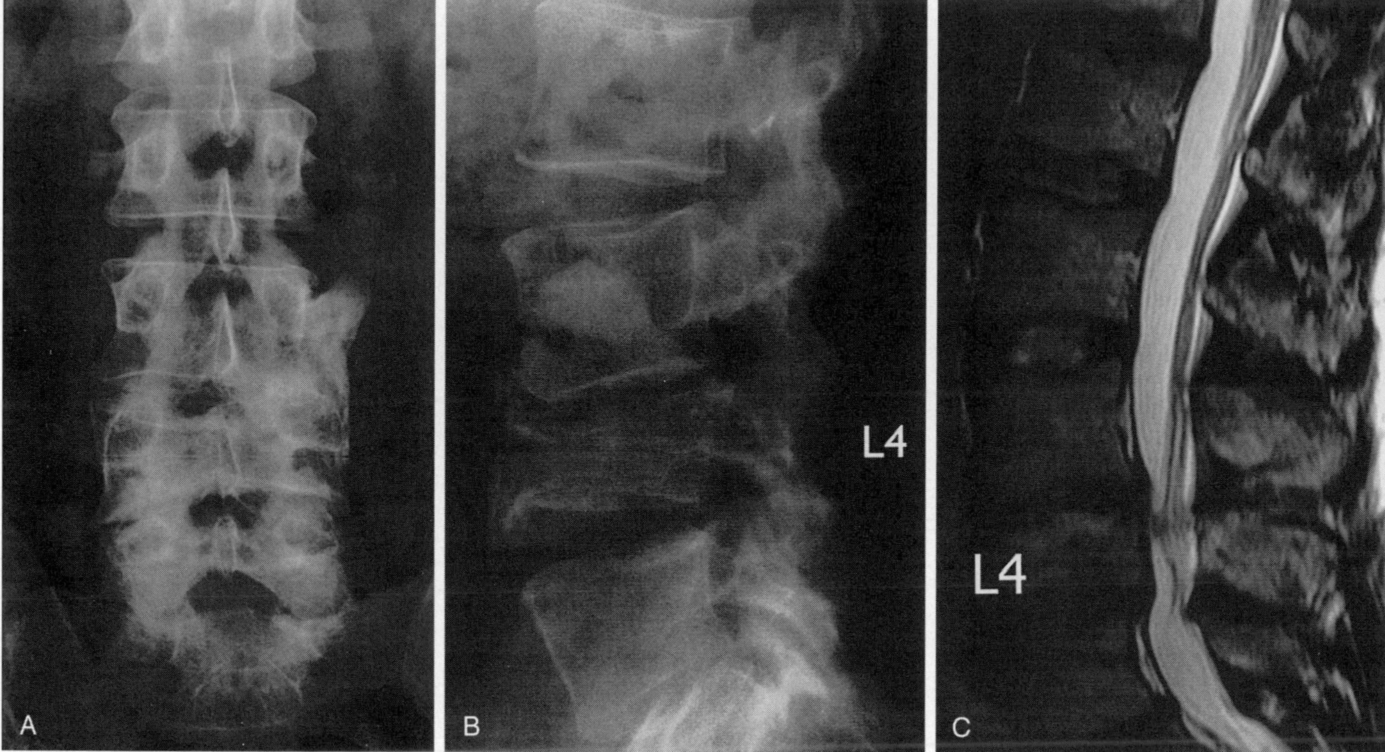

FIGURE 85–13. Conventional radiographs of the lumbar spine in the anteroposterior *(A)* and lateral *(B)* view reveal an old traumatic fracture of the fourth lumbar vertebra resulting in instability of the lumbar spine and spinal stenosis as shown on the corresponding magnetic resonance image *(C)*.

in a radiologist's reading.[51, 54, 78] Especially with respect to its specificity, the usefulness of a purely morphometric analysis of vertebral deformities has been somewhat controversial.[79, 80] Drawing on the strength of each of the approaches, a quantitative approach as well as a standardized visual approach may be applied in combination to reliably diagnose vertebral fractures in clinical drug trials.[13, 81]

Osteopenia and Osteoporosis at Other Skeletal Sites

The axial skeleton is not the only site where characteristic changes of osteopenia and osteoporosis can be depicted radiographically. Changes in trabecular and cortical bone can also be seen in the appendicular skeleton. It is first apparent at the ends of long and tubular bones because of the predominance of cancellous bone in these regions. Endosteal resorption has a prominent role, particularly in senile osteoporosis. The net result of this chronic process is widening of the medullary canal and thinning of the cortices. In the late stages of senile osteoporosis, the cortices are paper thin and the endosteal surfaces are smooth. In rapidly evolving postmenopausal osteoporosis, accelerated endosteal and intracortical bone resorption may be seen and can be directly assessed by high-resolution radiographic techniques. Methods to quantify changes in the peripheral skeleton have been proposed and also clinically applied (e.g., Singh index, radiogrammetry). Conventional radiography is the basis for a number of recent studies exploring new aspects of assessing bone structure by using sophisticated image analysis procedures such as fractal analysis or fast Fourier transforms.[82–85] These techniques have also been applied to the study of bone structure with high-resolution images acquired with MRI or CT.[86–88] This scientific field is relatively young, and application of these techniques in a clinical setting awaits validation.

DIFFERENTIAL DIAGNOSIS OF RADIOGRAPHIC OSTEOPOROSIS

Aside from senile and postmenopausal states, various other conditions may be accompanied by generalized osteoporosis. Although most of the previously mentioned radiographic characteristics are shared by a variety of conditions, some apparent differences may be seen in the appearance of osteoporosis vs. involutional osteoporosis.

Endocrine Disorders Associated with Osteoporosis

Increased serum concentrations of parathyroid hormone in hyperparathyroidism may result from autonomous hypersecretion by a parathyroid adenoma or diffuse hyperplasia of the parathyroid glands (primary hyperparathyroidism). A long, sustained hypocalcemic stimulus may result in hyperplasia of all parathyroid glands and secondary hyperparathyroidism. The cause of hypocalcemia is usually chronic renal failure or rarely malabsorption states. Autonomous function and hypercalcemia (tertiary hyperparathyroidism) may develop in patients with long-standing hyperparathyroidism. Although it is the increase in serum parathyroid hormone and calcium that establishes the diagnosis, radiographs document the severity and the course of the disease. Hyperparathyroidism leads to both increased bone resorption and bone formation. Changes induced by hyperparathyroidism may affect all bone surfaces and result in subperiosteal, intracortical, endosteal, subchondral, subepiphyseal, subligamentous and subtendinous, and trabecular bone resorption.[89–91]

Subperiosteal bone resorption is the most characteristic radiographic feature of hyperparathyroidism.[92] It is especially prominent in the hand, wrist, and foot but may also be seen in other sites. Radiographically, the outer margin of the bone becomes indistinct. Scalloping and spiculations of the cortex may occur in later stages. Undermineralization of the tela ossea leads to the distinctive radiographic appearance of acro-osteolysis.[93, 94] Intracortical resorption results in longitudinally oriented linear striations within the cortex, and endosteal bone resorption leads to scalloping of the inner cortex, cortical thinning, and widening of the medullary canal[95] (Fig. 85–14).

Subchondral bone resorption also frequently affects the joints of the axial skeleton and causes undermineralization of the tela ossea. For example, it may mimic widening of the sacroiliac joint space and lead to "pseudo-widening" of the joint.[96] The osseous surface may collapse

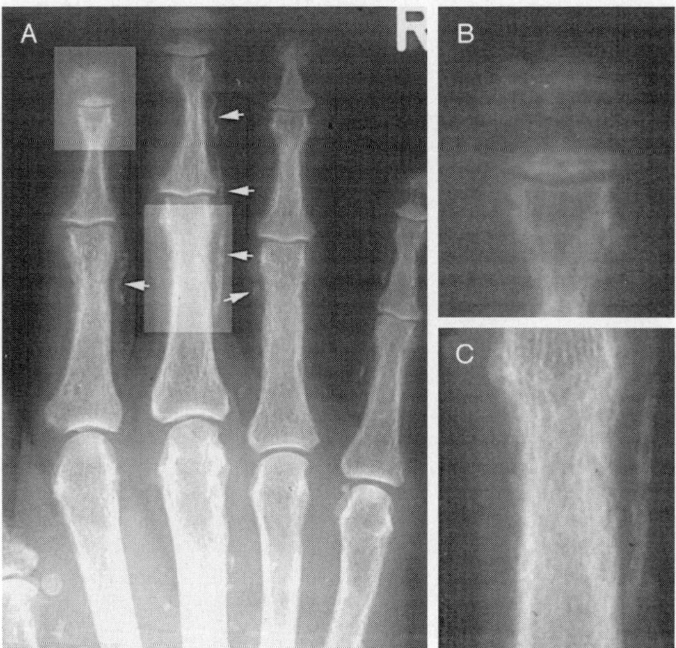

FIGURE 85–14. Hand radiograph of a patient with hyperparathyroidism *(A)* showing characteristic findings, including scalloping and spiculations of the cortex *(B)*, as well as undermineralization of the tela ossea resulting in the radiographic appearance of acro-osteolysis *(C)*. Calcified blood vessels are outlined by *small arrows* in *A*. *B* and *C* represent magnifications of the highlighted areas in *A*.

and may thus simulate subchondral lesions of inflammatory disease. Osteopenia occurs frequently in hyperparathyroidism and may be observed throughout the skeleton. Other radiographic signs of hyperparathyroidism include focal bone lesions ("brown tumors"), cartilage calcification, and also bone sclerosis.[97] Increased amounts of trabecular bone leading to bone sclerosis may occur, especially in patients with renal osteodystrophy and secondary hyperparathyroidism.[98, 99] Increased bone density may occur preferentially in the axial skeleton and sometimes leads to the deposition of bone in subchondral areas of the vertebral body, with the subsequent appearance of radiodense bands across the superior and inferior border and normal or decreased density in the center[100] (rugger-jersey spine) (Fig. 85–15).

Whereas osteoporosis is defined by a reduction in regularly mineralized osteoid, findings in osteomalacia include an abnormally high amount of nonmineralized osteoid and a reduction in mineralized bone volume. Thus radiographic abnormalities in osteomalacia include osteopenia (reduction of mineralized bone), coarsened indistinct trabeculae and unsharp delineation of cortical bone (excessive apposition of nonmineralized osteoid), deformities, insufficiency fractures, and true fractures (bone softening and weakening). The deformations include bowing and bending of the long bones and biconcave deformities of the vertebrae.[101] Pseudofractures, or Looser's zones (focal accumulations of osteoid in compact bone at right angles to the long axis), are diagnostic of osteomalacia and are often bilateral and symmetrical. Of the more than 50 different diseases and conditions that may cause osteomalacia, chronic renal insufficiency, hemodialysis, and renal transplantation are the most common.[102, 103] A decrease in vitamin D and reduced responsiveness in chronic renal insufficiency result in osteomalacia and rickets. The additional secondary hyperparathyroidism leads to a superimposition of radiographic changes from both osteomalacia and secondary hyperparathyroidism.[104] This radiographic appearance is termed *renal osteodystrophy*. A common finding in secondary hyperparathyroidism associated with renal osteodystrophy is osteosclerosis resulting in a typical appearance of the vertebral bodies as seen in the rugger-jersey spine[102] (see Fig. 85–15). Several other radiographic abnormalities may be frequently seen in renal osteodystrophy, including amyloid deposits, destructive spondyloarthropathy, inflammatory changes, avascular necrosis, soft tissue calcification, and arteriosclerosis.[105, 106]

Hyperthyroidism is a high-turnover disease that is associated with an increase in both bone resorption and bone formation.[107] Because bone resorption exceeds bone formation, rapid bone loss may occur and result in generalized osteoporosis.[108, 109] This effect is especially pronounced in patients with thyrotoxicosis or with a history of thyrotoxicosis.[109, 110] Thyroid-stimulating hormone–suppressive doses of thyroid hormone have been reported to decrease or have no effect on bone density.[111] Radiologic findings of hyperthyroidism-induced osteoporosis are those commonly seen in involutional or senile osteoporosis and include generalized osteopenia and cortical thinning and tunneling. Fractures associated with this condition affect the spine, the hip, and the distal end of the radius.[112, 113]

Medication-Induced Osteoporosis

Hypercortisolism is probably the most common cause of medication-induced generalized osteoporosis, whereas the endogenous form of hypercortisolism, Cushing's disease, is relatively rare,[114–117] which is why hypercortisolism is listed in this section on medication-induced osteoporosis. Decreased bone formation and increased bone resorption have been observed in hypercortisolism. These findings have been attributed to inhibition of osteoblast formation, either direct stimulation of osteoclast activity or increased secretion of parathyroid hormone. The typical radiographic appearance of steroid-induced osteoporosis consists of generalized osteoporosis at predominantly trabecular sites, with decreased bone density and fractures of the axial but also the appendicular skeleton. A characteristic finding in steroid-induced osteoporosis is marginal condensation of the vertebral bodies resulting from exuberant callus formation. Osteonecrosis, another complication of hypercortisolism, most frequently involves the femoral head and to a lesser extent the humeral head and the femoral condyles.[118, 119]

Generalized osteoporosis has been observed in patients receiving high-dose heparin therapy.[120, 121] The radiologic features of heparin-induced osteoporosis include generalized osteopenia and vertebral compression fractures.[122] The pathomechanism of heparin-induced os-

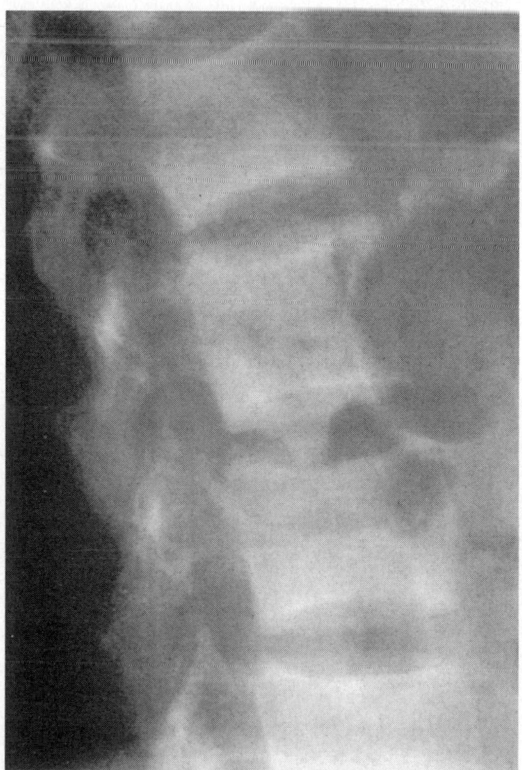

FIGURE 85–15. Renal dystrophy is usually a combination of osteomalacia and secondary hyperparathyroidism, and it may result in a "rugger-jersey" appearance of the spine with sclerosis of the end plates.

teoporosis is not completely clear, and the changes may be reversible with cessation of therapy.[123]

Other Causes of Generalized Osteoporosis

Other causes of generalized osteoporosis include malnutrition,[124] chronic alcoholism (if associated with malnutrition),[124, 125] smoking[126] and caffeine intake, Marfan syndrome,[127] and rather uncommonly, pregnancy.[128] Marrow abnormalities associated with osteoporosis are anemias (sickle cell anemia, thalassemia), plasma cell myeloma, leukemia, Gaucher's disease, and glycogen storage disease.[129, 130] This list is certainly far from being complete, but it represents some of the major causes of osteoporosis. Additional imaging techniques such as CT, magnetic resonance tomography, and bone scintigraphy, as well as clinical information, may be helpful in the differential diagnosis of the various conditions associated with osteoporosis[131–135] (Figs. 85–16 and 85–17).

Some conditions of the juvenile skeleton result in generalized osteoporosis. Rickets is characterized by inadequate mineralization of the bone matrix, and some of its radiographic appearance may resemble that of osteomalacia.[136] Widening of the growth plates, cupping of the metaphysis, and decreased density and irregularities of the metaphyseal margins may be present.[137] Epiphyseal ossification centers may show delayed ossification and unsharp borders.[138] Overgrowth of hyaline cartilage may lead to prominence of the costochondral junctions of the ribs (rachitic rosary). The child's age at the onset of the disease determines the pattern of bone deformity, with bowing of the long bones being more pronounced in infancy and early childhood and vertebral deformities and scoliosis more prominent in older children.[139] Further deformities that may be observed in rickets include pseudofractures, basilar invagination, and a triradiate configuration of the pelvis.

Idiopathic juvenile osteoporosis is a self-limited disease of childhood, with recovery occurring as puberty progresses.[140] A typical feature of this condition is increased vulnerability of the metaphyses, often resulting in metaphyseal injuries in the knees and ankles. Idiopathic juvenile osteoporosis must be distinguished from osteogenesis imperfecta, another disease often seen with radiographic signs of generalized osteoporosis.[141] The pathogenesis of osteogenesis imperfecta is quantitative or qualitative abnormalities in type I collagen. Osteogenesis imperfecta is divided into four major types, and the degree of osteoporosis in osteogenesis imperfecta depends strongly on the type of disease.[142] The clinical features of each type usually correspond to the type of mutation. The abnormal maturation of collagen seen in this disorder results in a primary defect in bone matrix. This defect in bone matrix, combined with defective mineralization, results in overall loss of bone density involving both the axial and peripheral skeleton. Patients with type III disease have significantly decreased bone density manifested as generalized osteopenia, thinned cortices, fractures of the long bones and ribs, exuberant callus formation, and bone deformation.[143] The degree of osteopenia is highly variable, however, and at the mildest end of the spectrum some patients do not have any radiographic signs of osteopenia.[144]

Regional Osteoporosis

Osteoporosis may also be confined to only a segment of the body. This type of osteoporosis is called regional osteoporosis, and it is commonly caused by some disorder of the appendicular skeleton.

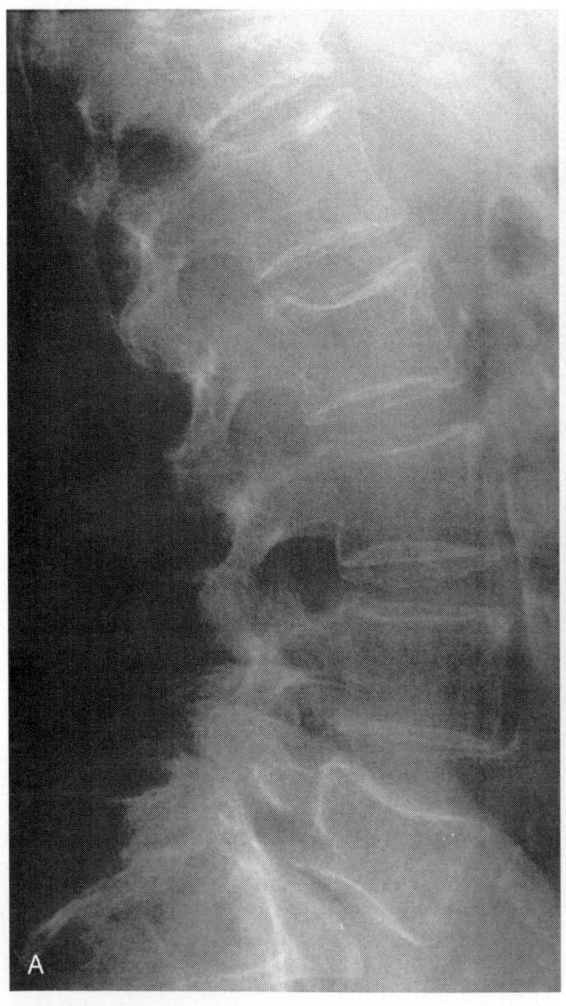

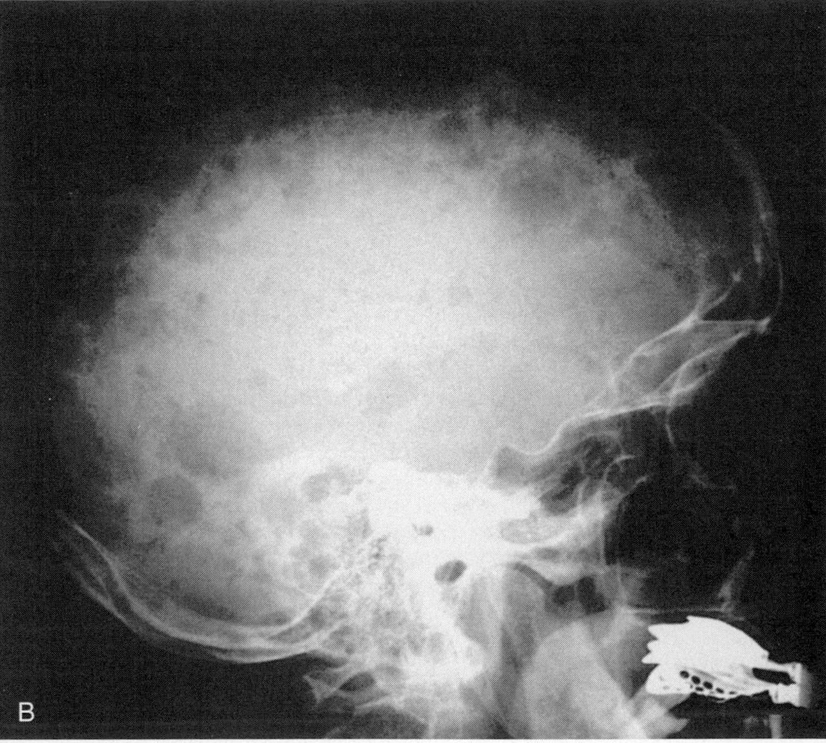

FIGURE 85–16. Changes in the spine in multiple myeloma *(A)*, here seen with increased radiolucency and vertebral deformities, may easily be confused with osteoporotic changes. However, additional typical lesions at other sites (besides clinical features and relatively typical laboratory values) may reveal the nature of the underlying disease. In this example, multiple osteolytic lesions in the skull *(B)* support the diagnosis of multiple myeloma.

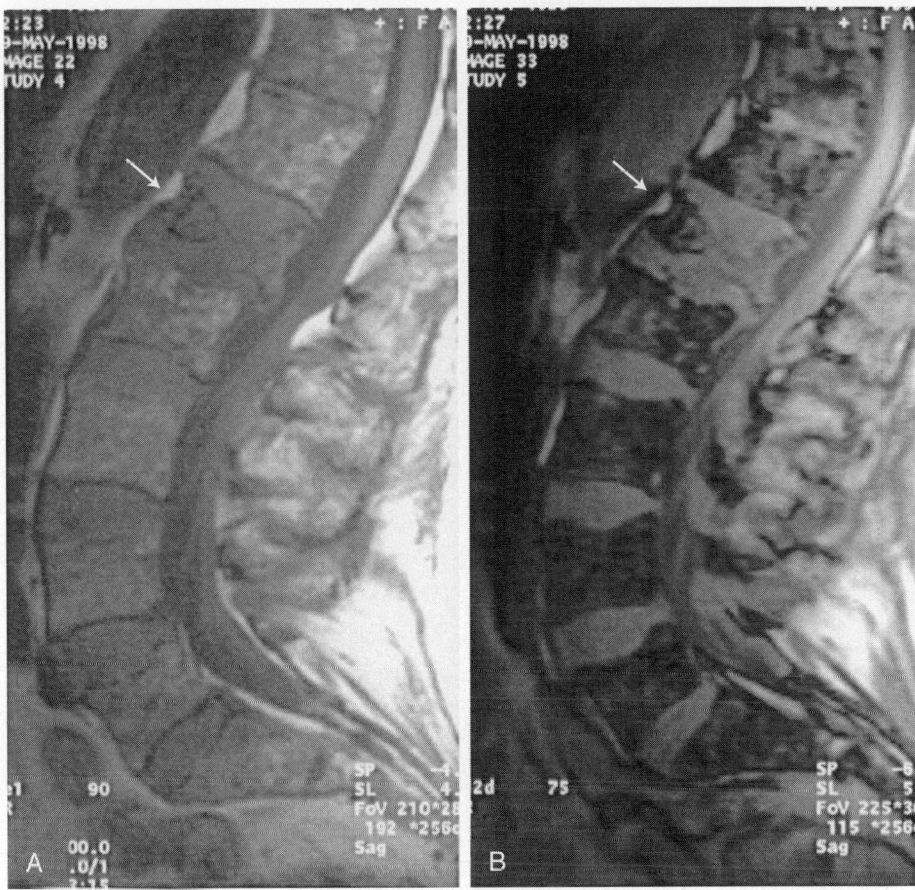

FIGURE 85–17. Magnetic resonance imaging of the spine in patients with multiple myeloma may give information on the infiltration of spinal bone marrow. In this patient a diffuse infiltration pattern may be seen on T1-weighted spin echo *(A)* and gradient echo *(B)* images. In addition, the patient has a fracture of the first lumbar vertebra *(arrow)*.

Osteoporosis resulting from immobilization or disuse characteristically occurs in the immobilized regions of patients with fractures, motor paralysis secondary to central nervous system disease or trauma, and bone and joint inflammation[145] (Fig. 85–18). Chronic and acute disease may vary in their radiographic appearance somewhat and show diffuse osteopenia, linear radiolucent bands, speckled radiolucent areas, and cortical bone resorption.

Reflex sympathetic dystrophy, sometimes also termed Sudeck's atrophy or algodystrophy, has the radiographic appearance of a high-turnover process. It most often occurs in patients with trauma, such as Colles' fracture, but also in patients with any neurally related musculoskeletal, neurologic, or vascular condition such as hemiplegia or myocardial infarction.[146–149] This condition is probably related to overactivity of the sympathetic nervous system with increased blood flow and increased intravenous oxygen saturation in the affected extremity.[150, 151] Its radiographic appearance includes soft tissue swelling, as well as regional effects consisting of bandlike, patchy, or periarticular osteoporosis. Additional radiographic features include subperiosteal bone resorption, intracortical tunneling, endosteal bone resorption with initial excavation and scalloping of the endosteal surface, and subsequent remodeling and widening of the medullary canal, as well as subchondral and juxta-articular erosion.[152] Especially in the early stages of reflex sympathetic dystrophy, bone scintigraphy may be helpful in establishing the diagnosis.[153–155]

Transient regional osteoporosis includes conditions that have in common the development of self-limited pain and radiographic osteopenia affecting one or several joints, most commonly the hip. Transient osteoporosis typically occurs in middle-aged men and in women in the third trimester of pregnancy.[156, 157] At the onset of clinical symptoms the radiographic findings may be normal, and within several weeks variable osteopenia of the hip develops, sometimes involving the acetabulum. Some patients later have similar changes in the opposite hip or in other joints, in which case the term *regional migratory osteoporosis* may be used.[158] No specific therapy is required because all patients recover. The cause of transient regional osteoporosis is not known, and it appears that it may be related to reflex sympathetic dystrophy. In some patients with clinically similar or identical manifestations, MRI shows transient regional bone marrow edema.[159, 160] Because regional osteoporosis does not develop in all patients with identical clinical symptoms, its sensitivity regarding the detection of regional osteoporosis has to be questioned, as well as the interrelationship between transient regional osteoporosis and transient bone marrow edema. Transient bone marrow edema also seems to be related to ischemic necrosis of bone, and criteria must be established to allow differentiation of transient bone marrow edema and the edema pattern associated with osteonecrosis.[161–163]

BONE SCINTIGRAPHY IN METABOLIC BONE DISEASES

Of the different modes of radionuclide imaging, planar scintigraphy and single-photon emission computed tomography (SPECT) have found clinical application in metabolic bone diseases. Technetium 99m–labeled diphosphonate bone imaging provides a means of visualizing physiology and pathophysiology within the skeleton and may be of value in detecting metabolic bone diseases and monitoring the response to therapy. Metabolic bone diseases are mostly associated with increased bone turnover and increased uptake of radiolabeled diphosphonate. The increased uptake produces heightened contrast between bone and soft tissues.[164] The uniform nature of the pathologic process of metabolic bone disease results in scans that may be extremely difficult to differentiate from normal.[165] More severe cases may have characteristic patterns of abnormality, including some of the following identified by Fogelman et al.[166]:

1. Symmetrically increased tracer uptake in axial and long bones
2. Faint or almost absent kidney images
3. Increased uptake in periarticular areas
4. Increased tracer uptake in the vault of the skull and mandible

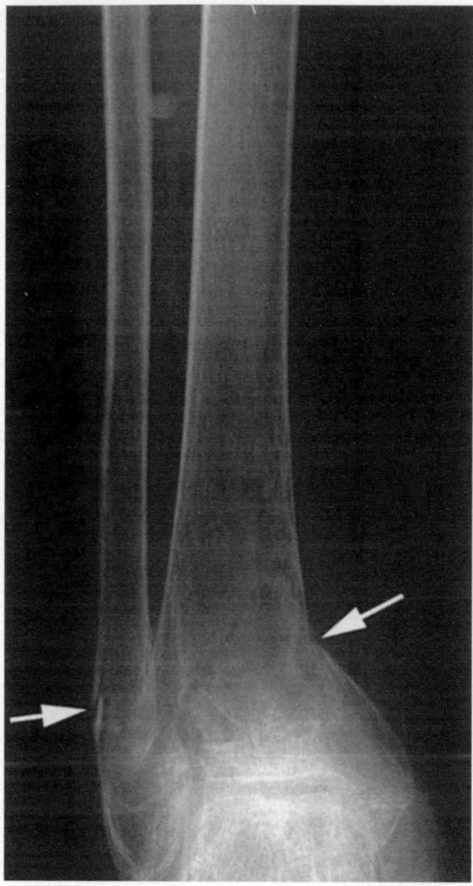

FIGURE 85–18. Fracture of the ankle in an osteoporotic patient. *Arrows* highlight the outer borders of the fracture. Osteoporosis resulted from disuse of the lower extremities in this female wheelchair driver.

5. Prominent uptake at costochondral junctions
6. Reduced soft tissue uptake
7. "Tie" sign in the sternum

Although these scan features are classic in patients with severe metabolic diseases, they are rarely all present and in mild forms of the disease may be extremely difficult to identify. Hence interpretations are highly subjective and therefore the bone scan is rarely used for the detection of metabolic bone diseases. However, although the sensitivity of the bone scan for generalized metabolic bone disease may be poor, its sensitivity for focal metabolic diseases such as Paget's disease or for focal complications such as fracture or pseudofracture is good. These applications are the major uses of bone radionuclide imaging in clinical practice.[164]

Bone Radionuclide Imaging in Osteoporosis

Uptake of ^{99m}Tc-diphosphonate usually fails to show any abnormality in the absence of fractures.[167] A few patients may show a generalized increase in skeletal uptake qualitatively. However, such uptake is often difficult to interpret because of marked normal variation, especially in older individuals.[168] Bone scans are therefore not used for the detection of reduced bone mass (osteopenia), for which bone densitometry, as previously discussed, is the modality of choice. Vertebral collapse is associated with a characteristic intense linear pattern of tracer uptake corresponding to the site of the fracture. This activity then fades over a period of 6 to 8 months, which allows the intensity to be of help in assessing the age of the fracture.[169] In the evaluation of a patient with known osteoporosis and back pain, the bone scan can be of particular value in clarifying whether further fracture has occurred or whether some other explanation should be sought. For example, a normal scan excludes a recent fracture, and in this situation another cause should be determined. Microfractures may cause bone pain without visible radiographic changes, and a bone scan may show localized increased uptake in this instance.[170] Total body images are also useful in assessing all fracture locations throughout the body (Fig. 85–19). It has also been found that back pain in osteoporosis may often be due to coexistent degenerative disease that can be unrelated to the site of fracture.[171] In the osteoporosis of postmenopausal women with rheumatoid arthritis, elevation of serum phosphorus and alkaline phosphatase is usually seen, as well as increased urinary excretion of hydroxyproline and mucupolysaccharides.[172] Although generalized osteoporosis is not generally evident by imaging, the increased periarticular activity of the involved joints is obvious in the presence of active disease.

On occasion the bone scan will identify coexistent disease such as a rib fracture or metastases that may be the cause of or contribute to the symptoms. It should always be remembered that even when scan appearances are typical of a vertebral fracture, the findings are not specific to osteoporosis and coexistent lesions cannot be excluded. However, when multiple vertebral fractures are present, osteoporosis is the probable diagnosis. Occasionally a disease that causes generalized demineralization, such as myeloma, can mimic this situation.

The bone scan is of value in confirming suspected fractures when initial radiographs are negative at sites such as the forearms or hips. Bone scans may also provide diagnostic information in other less common situations such as osteoporosis of pregnancy, transient osteoporosis,[173] and the detection of microfractures in patients receiving fluoride therapy.[174]

SPECT

The addition of SPECT has improved the diagnostic value of the bone scan, particularly in the lumbar spine.[164] Images are acquired at multiple positions around the patient with a rotating gamma camera.

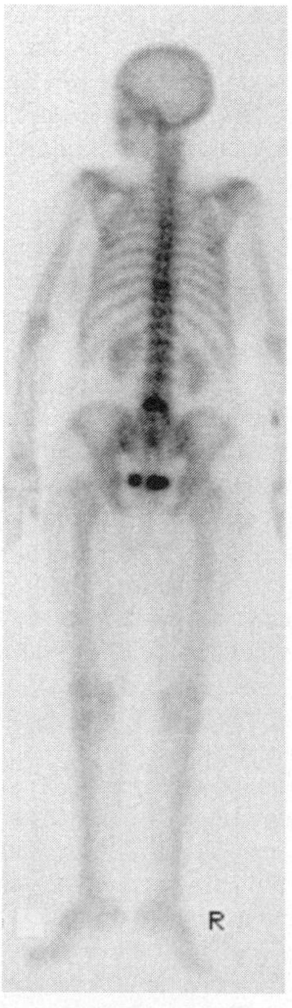

FIGURE 85–19. The radionuclide bone scan in osteoporosis is nonspecific. However, it may reveal recent fractures by showing increased radionuclide uptake. This bone scan shows a recent vertebral fracture in the lower lumbar spine of a 76-year-old woman.

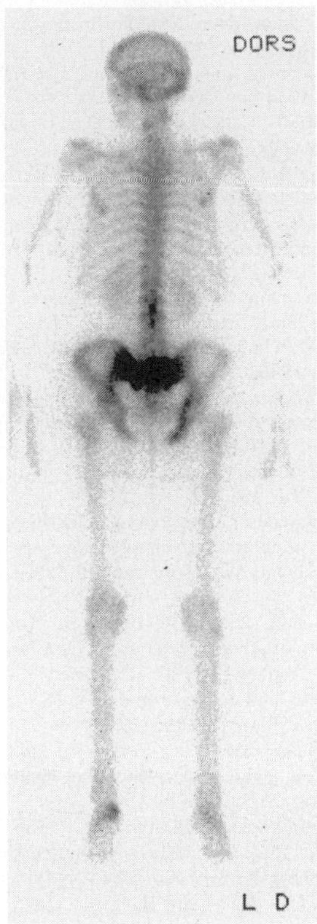

FIGURE 85–20. This radionuclide bone scan of a 57-year-old woman with Paget's disease shows increased radionuclide accumulation in the pelvis, as well as some lumbar vertebrae and the base of the skull.

This technique leads to greatly improved image contrast and the ability to separate activity above and below the areas of interest, which in the spine means that uptake can be separately identified in the vertebral body, pedicle, facet joint, pars interarticularis, lamina, and spinous process.[164] SPECT is particular useful in the diagnosis of chronic back pain caused by benign disorders.[175, 176] In particular, activity in a pars defect enables pain to be attributed to spondylolysis,[177] and activity in a facet joint identifies this structure as the likely source of pain that may be used to target therapy.[178] A further use has been to identify nonunion or facet joint disease in patients after spinal fusion.[179]

In summary, bone scan is of value in confirming suspected fractures when initial radiographs are negative at sites such as the arms or hips.

Radionuclide Imaging in Paget's Disease

Bone scan appearances in Paget's disease are well known, and the exquisite sensitivity of bone scanning and clear visualization of the whole skeleton make this technique the imaging modality of choice.[164, 180] However, radiographs are necessary in patients with unexplained bone pain or other suspicion of fracture or sarcomatous change. The bone scan appearance in Paget's disease is usually characteristic, with the predominant feature being strikingly increased uptake distributed throughout most or all of the affected bone (Fig. 85–20).

SUMMARY

Awareness of osteoporosis and its economic and social costs has increased. The value of bone status assessment for prediction of fracture risk is as good as the ability of blood pressure to predict stroke. Currently, DXA is the most widely used technique for bone densitometry. The momentum to establish the role of peripheral techniques such as QUS and pDXA has increased because of their low cost and potentially wide availability. This impetus is also driven by the availability of effective and acceptable therapies for osteoporosis. Clinical questions, availability, and cost should govern the choice of site, the number of sites, and the technique. BMD or ultrasound should not be used in isolation in the management of osteoporosis. These measurements should be considered along with other risk factors, the patient's medical history, a physical examination, and other laboratory tests.[181, 182]

Conventional radiographs are principally useful for diagnosing fractures and deformities. The sensitivity of diagnosing osteoporosis from conventional radiographs is low. Nevertheless, conventional radiography is widely available, and it remains useful for the detection of specific alterations in certain instances. Alone and in conjunction with modern imaging techniques such as bone scintigraphy and MRI, conventional radiography is still widely used for the detection of complications of osteopenia such as fracture, for the differential diagnosis of osteopenia, and for follow-up examinations in specific clinical settings.

The bone scan has well-recognized appearances in metabolic bone diseases, with its main clinical value found in focal conditions or the focal complications of disease. Radionuclide bone scans have no role in the initial diagnosis of osteoporosis, but they could be used to detect/confirm osteoporotic fractures and pseudofractures in osteomalacia and to evaluate Paget's disease.

REFERENCES

1. Consensus Development Conference: Diagnosis, prophylaxis and treatment of osteoporosis. Am J Med 94:646–650, 1993.
2. Cooper C, Atkinson EJ, Jacobsen SJ, et al: Population-based study of survival after osteoporotic fractures. Am J Epidemiol 137:1001–1005, 1993.
3. Consensus Development Statement: Who are candidates for prevention and treatment for osteoporosis? Osteoporos Int 7:1–6, 1997.
4. Ray NF, Chan JK, Thamer M, Melton LJ 3rd: Medical expenditures for the treatment of osteoporotic fractures in the United States in 1995: Report from the National Osteoporosis Foundation. J Bone Miner Res 12:24–35, 1997.
5. Cummings SR, Rubin MPH, Black D: The future of hip fractures in the United States. Clin Orthop 252:163–166, 1990.
6. Cooper C, Shah S, Hand DJ, et al: Screening for vertebral osteoporosis using individual risk factors. The Multicentre Vertebral Fracture Study Group. Osteoporos Int 2:48–53, 1991.
7. Prudham D, Evans JG: Factors associated with falls in the elderly: A community study. Age Ageing 10:141–146, 1981.
8. Kelsey JL, Hoffman S: Risk factors for hip fracture (editorial). N Engl J Med 316:404–406, 1987.
9. Hodgskinson R, Njeh CF, Currey JD, Langton CM: The ability of ultrasound velocity to predict the stiffness of cancellous bone in vitro. Bone 21:183–190, 1997.
10. Ross PD, Davis JW, Vogel JM, Wasnich RD: A critical review of bone mass and the risk of fractures in osteoporosis. Calcif Tissue Int 46:149–161, 1990.
11. Cummings SR, Black DM, Nevitt MC, et al: Bone density at various sites for prediction of hip fractures. The Study of Osteoporotic Fractures Research Group. Lancet 341:72–75, 1993.
12. Masud T, Mootoosamy I, McCloskey EV, et al: Assessment of osteopenia from spine radiographs using two different methods: The Chingford Study. Br J Radiol 69:451–456, 1996.
13. Genant HK, Engelke K, Fuerst T, et al: Noninvasive assessment of bone mineral and structure: State of the art. J Bone Miner Res 11:707–730, 1996.
14. Blake GM, Fogelman I: Technical principles of dual energy x-ray absorptiometry. Semin Nucl Med 27:210–328, 1997.
15. Njeh CF, Boivin CM, Langton CM: The role of ultrasound in the assessment of osteoporosis: A review. Osteoporos Int 7:7–22, 1997.
16. Adams JE: Single and dual energy X-ray absorptiometry. Eur Radiol 7(suppl 2):20–31, 1997.
17. Levis S, Altman R: Bone densitometry: Clinical considerations. Arthritis Rheum 41:577–587, 1998.
18. Scheiber LB 2nd, Torregrosa L: Evaluation and treatment of postmenopausal osteoporosis. Semin Arthritis Rheum 27:245–261, 1998.
19. Matsumoto C, Kushida K, Yamazaki K, et al: Metacarpal bone mass in normal and osteoporotic Japanese women using computed x-ray densitometry. Calcif Tissue Int 54:324–329, 1994.
20. Yates AJ, Ross PD, Lydick E, Epstein RS: Radiographic absorptiometry in the diagnosis of osteoporosis. Am J Med 98(suppl 2A):41–47, 1995.
21. Wahner HW, Fogelman I: The Evaluation of Osteoporosis: Dual Energy X-ray Absorptiometry in Clinical Practice. London, Martin Dunitz, 1994.
22. Yamada M, Ito M, Hayashi K, et al: Dual energy x-ray absorptiometry of the calcaneus: Comparison with other techniques to assess bone density and value in predicting risk of spine fracture. AJR 163:1435–1440, 1994.
23. Faulkner KG, McClung MR, Schmeer MS, et al: Densitometry of the radius using single and dual energy absorptiometry. Calcif Tissue Int 54:208–211, 1994.
24. Genant HK, Cann CE, Ettinger B, Gordan GS: Quantitative computed tomography of vertebral spongiosa: A sensitive method for detecting early bone loss after oophorectomy. Ann Intern Med 97:699–705, 1982.
25. Guglielmi G, Grimston SK, Fischer KC, Pacifici R: Osteoporosis: Diagnosis with lateral and posteroanterior dual x-ray absorptiometry compared with quantitative CT. Radiology 192:845–850, 1994.

26. Yu W, Glüer CC, Grampp S, et al: Spinal bone mineral assessment in postmenopausal women: A comparison between dual x-ray absorptiometry and quantitative computed tomography. J Bone Miner Res 9(suppl 1):406, 1994.
27. Langton CM, Palmer SB, Porter RW: The measurement of broadband ultrasonic attenuation in cancellous bone. Eng Med 13:89–91, 1984.
28. Hans D, Schott AM, Meunier PJ: Ultrasonic assessment of bone: A review. Eur J Med 2:157–163, 1993.
29. Gregg EW, Kriska AM, Salamone LM, et al: The epidemiology of quantitative ultrasound: A review of the relationships with bone mass, osteoporosis and fracture risk. Osteoporos Int 7:89–99, 1997.
30. Gluer CC, Consensus G: Quantitative ultrasound techniques for the assessment of osteoporosis: Expert agreement on current status. J Bone Miner Res 12:1280–1288, 1997.
31. Bauer DC, Gluer CC, Cauley JA, et al: Broadband ultrasound attenuation predicts fractures strongly and independently of densitometry in older women. A prospective study. Study of Osteoporotic Fractures Research Group. Arch Intern Med 157:629–634, 1997.
32. Hans D, Dargent-Molina P, Schott AM, et al: Ultrasonographic heel measurements to predict hip fracture in elderly women: The EPIDOS prospective study. Lancet 348:511–514, 1996.
33. Njeh CF, Fuerst T, Hans D, et al: Radiation exposure in bone mineral density assessment. Appl Radiat Isot 50:215–236, 1999.
34. World Health Organization: Assessment of Fracture Risk and Its Application to Screening for Postmenopausal Osteoporosis, WHO Technical Report Series 843. Geneva, WHO, 1994.
35. Slosman DO, Rizzoli R, Pichard C, et al: Longitudinal measurement of regional and whole body bone mass in young healthy adults. Osteoporos Int 4:185–190, 1994.
36. Miller PD, Bonnick SL, Rosen CJ, et al: Clinical utility of bone mass measurements in adults: Consensus of an international panel. The Society for Clinical Densitometry. Semin Arthritis Rheum 25:361–372, 1996.
37. Melton LJI, Atkinson EJ, O'Fallon WM, et al: Long-term fracture prediction by bone mineral assessed at different skeletal sites. J Bone Miner Res 8:1227–1233, 1993.
38. Marshall D, Johnell O, Wedel H: Meta-analysis of how well measures of bone mineral density predict occurrence of osteoporotic fractures. BMJ 312:1254–1259, 1996.
39. Baran DT, Faulkner KG, Genant HK, et al: Diagnosis and management of osteoporosis: Guidelines for the utilization of bone densitometry. Calcif Tissue Int 61:433–440, 1997.
40. Davis JW, Ross PD, Wasnich RD: Evidence for both generalized and regional low bone mass among elderly women. J Bone Miner Res 9:305–309, 1994.
41. Black D, Bauer D, Lu Y, et al: Should BMD be measured at multiple sites to predict fracture risk in elderly women? J Bone Mineral Res 10(suppl):7, 1995.
42. Grampp S, Genant HK, Mathur A, et al: Comparisons of noninvasive bone mineral measurements in assessing age-related loss, fracture discrimination, and diagnostic classification. J Bone Miner Res 12:697–711, 1997.
43. Kleerekoper M, Nelson DA: Which bone density measurement? (editorial). J Bone Miner Res 12:712–714, 1997.
44. Blake GM, Jagathesan T, Herd RJ, Fogelman I: Dual x-ray absorptiometry of the lumbar spine: The precision of paired anteroposterior/lateral studies. Br J Radiol 67:624–630, 1994.
45. Hassager C, Jensen SB, Gotfredsen A, Christiansen C: The impact of measurement errors on the diagnostic value of bone mass measurements: Theoretical considerations. Osteoporos Int 1:250–256, 1991.
46. He YF, Ross PD, Davis JW, et al: When should bone density measurements be repeated? Calcif Tissue Int 55:243–248, 1994.
47. Eastell R: Management of corticosteroid-induced osteoporosis. UK Consensus Group Meeting on Osteoporosis. J Intern Med 237:439–447, 1995.
48. Ross PD, Davis JW, Epstein RS, Wasnich RD: Pain and disability associated with new vertebral fractures and other spinal conditions. J Clin Epidemiol 47:231–239, 1994.
49. Banks LM, Van Kuijk C, Genant HK: Radiographic technique for assessing osteoporotic vertebral deformity. *In* Genant HK, Jergas M, Van Kuijk C (eds): Vertebral Fracture in Osteoporosis. San Francisco, Radiology Research and Education Foundation, 1995, pp 131–147.
50. Ziegler R, Scheidt-Nave C, Leidig-Bruckner G: What is a vertebral fracture? Bone 18(suppl):169–177, 1996.
51. Minne HW, Leidig G, Wüster C, et al: A newly developed spine deformity index (SDI) to quantitate vertebral crush fractures in patients with osteoporosis. Bone Miner 3:335–349, 1988.
52. Eastell R, Cedel SL, Wahner HW, et al: Classification of vertebral fractures. J Bone Miner Res 6:207–215, 1991.
53. Black DM, Cummings SR, Stone K, et al: A new approach to defining normal vertebral dimensions. J Bone Miner Res 6:883–892, 1991.
54. McCloskey EV, Spector TD, Eyres KS, et al: The assessment of vertebral deformity: A method for use in population studies and clinical trials. Osteoporos Int 3:138–147, 1993.
55. Kiel D: Assessing vertebral fractures. National Osteoporosis Foundation Working Group on Vertebral Fractures. J Bone Miner Res 10:518–523, 1995.
56. Genant HK, Wu CY, van Kuijk C, Nevitt MC: Vertebral fracture assessment using a semiquantitative technique. J Bone Miner Res 8:1137–1148, 1993.
57. Steiger P, Cummings SR, Genant HK, Weiss H: Morphometric x-ray absorptiometry of the spine: Correlation in vivo with morphometric radiography. Study of Osteoporotic Fractures Research Group. Osteoporos Int 4:238–244, 1994.
58. Blake GM, Rea JA, Fogelman I: Vertebral morphometry studies using dual-energy x-ray absorptiometry. Semin Nucl Med 27:276–290, 1997.
59. Garnero P, Delmas PD: Bone markers. Baillieres Clin Rheumatol 11:517–537, 1997.
60. LeGeros RZ: Biological and synthetic apatites. *In* Brown PW, Constantz B (eds): Hydroxyapatite and Related Materials. Boca Raton, FL, CRC, 1994, pp 3–28.
61. Albright F, Smith PH, Richardson AM: Postmenopausal osteoporosis. Its clinical features. JAMA 116:2465–2474, 1941.
62. Frost HM: Dynamics of bone remodelling. *In* Frost HM (ed): Bone Biodynamics. Boston, Little, Brown, 1964, pp 315–334.
63. Genant HK, Doi K, Mall JC, Sickles EA: Direct radiographic magnification for skeletal radiology. Radiology 123:47–55, 1977.
64. Genant HK, Doi K, Mall JC: Comparison of non-screen techniques (medical vs. industrial film) for fine-detail skeletal radiography. Invest Radiol 11:486–500, 1976.
65. Link TM, Rummeny EJ, Lenzen H, et al: Artificial bone erosions: Detection with magnification radiography versus conventional high resolution radiography. Radiology 192:861–864, 1994.
66. Heuck F, Schmidt E: Die quantitative Bestimmung des Mineralgehaltes des Knochens aus dem Röntgenbild. Fortschr Rontgenstr 93:523–554, 1960.
67. Lachmann E, Whelan M: The roentgen diagnosis of osteoporosis and its limitations. Radiology 26:165–177, 1936.
68. Jergas M, Uffmann M, Escher H, et al: Visuelle Beurteilung konventioneller Röntgenaufnahmen und duale Röntgenabsorptiometrie in der Diagnostik der Osteoporose. Z Orthop Ihre Grenzgeb 132:91–98, 1994.
69. Riggs BL, Melton LJ: Evidence for two distinct syndromes of involutional osteoporosis. Am J Med 75:899–901, 1983.
70. Gallagher JC: The pathogenesis of osteoporosis. Bone Miner 9:215–227, 1990.
71. Saville PD: A quantitative approach to simple radiographic diagnosis of osteoporosis: Its application to the osteoporosis of rheumatoid arthritis. Arthritis Rheum 10:416–422, 1967.
72. Doyle FH, Gutteridge DH, Joplin GF, Fraser R: An assessment of radiological criteria used in the study of spinal osteoporosis. Br J Radiol 40:241–250, 1967.
73. Jergas M, Uffmann M, Escher H, et al: Interobserver variation in the detection of osteopenia by radiography and comparison with dual x-ray absorptiometry (DXA) of the lumbar spine. Skeletal Radiol 23:195–199, 1994.
74. Ahmed AIH, Ilic D, Blake GM, et al: Review of 3530 referrals for bone density measurements of spine and femur: Evidence that radiographic osteopenia predicts low bone mass. Radiology 207:619–624, 1998.
75. McAfee PC, Yuan HA, Fredrickson BE, Lubicky JP: The value of computed tomography in thoracolumbar fractures. An analysis of one hundred consecutive cases and a new classification. J Bone Joint Surg Am 65:461–473, 1983.
76. Campbell SE, Phillips CD, Dubovsky E, et al: The value of CT in determining potential instability of simple wedge-compression fractures of the lumbar spine. AJNR Am J Neuroradiol 16:1385–1392, 1995.
77. Ballock RT, Mackersie R, Abitbol JJ, et al: Can burst fractures be predicted from plain radiographs? J Bone Joint Surg Br 74:147–150, 1992.
78. Jergas M, Fuerst T, Grampp S, et al: Assessment of spinal osteoporosis with dual x-ray absorptiometry of the spine and femur. Radiology 197(suppl):362, 1995.
79. Black D, Palermo L, Nevitt MC, et al: Comparison of methods for defining prevalent vertebral deformities: The study of osteoporotic fractures. J Bone Miner Res 10:890–902, 1995.
80. Wu CY, Li J, Jergas M, Genant HK: Comparison of semiquantitative and quantitative techniques for the assessment of prevalent and incident vertebral fractures. Osteoporos Int 5:354–370, 1995.
81. Cummings SR, Melton LJ III, Felsenberg D, National Osteoporosis Foundation Working Group on Vertebral Fracture: Report: Assessing vertebral fractures. J Bone Miner Res 10:518–523, 1995.
82. Ruttimann UE, Webber RL, Hazelrig JB: Fractal dimension from radiographs of peridental alveolar bone. A possible diagnostic indicator of osteoporosis. Oral Surg Oral Med Oral Pathol 74:98–110, 1992.
83. Geraets WGM, Van der Stelt PF, Elders PJM: The radiographic trabecular bone pattern during menopause. Bone 14:859–864, 1993.
84. Geraets W, Van der Stelt P, Lips P, Van Ginkel F: The radiographic trabecular pattern of hips in patients with hip fractures and in elderly control subjects. Bone 22:165–173, 1998.
85. Lespessailles E, Roux JP, Benhamou CL, et al: Fractal analysis of bone texture on os calcis radiographs compared with trabecular microarchitecture analyzed by histomorphometry. Calcif Tissue Int 63:121–125, 1998.
86. Majumdar S, Kothari M, Augat P, et al: High-resolution magnetic resonance imaging: Three-dimensional trabecular bone architecture and biomechanical properties. Bone 22:445–454, 1998.
87. Link TM, Majumdar S, Augat P, et al: Proximal femur: Assessment for osteoporosis with T2* decay characteristics at MR imaging. Radiology 209:531–536, 1998.
88. Millard J, Augat P, Link TM, et al: Power spectral analysis of vertebral trabecular bone structure from radiographs: Orientation dependence and correlation with bone mineral density and mechanical properties. Calcif Tissue Int 63:482–489, 1998.
89. Genant HK, Heck LL, Lanzl LH, et al: Primary hyperparathyroidism. A comprehensive study of clinical, biochemical and radiographic manifestations. Radiology 109:513–519, 1973.
90. Genant HK, Vander Horst J, Lanzl LH, et al: Skeletal demineralization in primary hyperparathyroidism. *In* Mazess RB (ed): Proceedings of International Conference on Bone Mineral Measurement. Washington, DC, National Institute of Arthritis, Metabolism and Digestive Diseases, 1974, pp 177.
91. Richardson ML, Pozzi-Mucelli RS, Kanter AS, et al: Bone mineral changes in primary hyperparathyroidism. Skeletal Radiol 15:85–95, 1986.
92. Camp JD, Ochsner HC: The osseous changes in hyperparathyroidism associated with parathyroid tumor: A roentgenologic study. Radiology 17:63, 1931.
93. Resnick D, Niwayama G: Parathyroid disorders and renal osteodystrophy. *In* Resnick D (ed): Diagnosis of Bone and Joint Disorders, ed 3. Philadelphia, WB Saunders, 1995, pp 2012–2075.
94. Heuck FHW: Endokrine, metabolische und medikamentös induzierte Knochen- und Gelenkerkrankungen. *In* Heuck A (ed): Radiologie der Knochen- und Gelenkerkrankungen. Stuttgart, Germany, Georg Thieme Verlag, 1998, pp 51–150.
95. Meema HE, Meema S: Microradioscopic and morphometric findings in the hand

bones with densitometric findings in the proximal radius in thyrotoxicosis and in renal osteodystrophy. Invest Radiol 7:88, 1972.
96. Hayes CW, Conway WF: Hyperparathyroidism. Radiol Clin North Am 29:85–96, 1991.
97. Steinbach HL, Gordan GS, Eisenberg E, et al: Primary hyperparathyroidism: A correlation of roentgen, clinical, and pathologic features. AJR 86:239–243, 1961.
98. Crawford T, Dent CE, Lucas P: Osteosclerosis associated with chronic renal failure. Lancet 2:981, 1954.
99. Davis JG: Osseous radiographic findings of chronic renal insufficiency. Radiology 60:406, 1953.
100. Resnick D: The "rugger jersey" vertebral body. Arthritis Rheum 24:1191–1194, 1981.
101. Kienböck R: Osteomalazie, Osteoporose, Osteopsathyrose, porotische Kyphose. Fortschr Rontgenstr 61:159, 1940.
102. Pitt MJ: Rickets and osteomalacia are still around. Radiol Clin North Am 29:97–118, 1991.
103. Kainberger F, Traindl O, Baldt M, et al: Renale Osteodytrophie: Spektrum der Röntgensymptomatik bei modernen Formen der Nierentransplantation und Dauerdialysetherapie. Fortschr Rontgenstr 157:501–505, 1992.
104. Sundaram M: Renal osteodystrophy. Skeletal Radiol 18:415–426, 1989.
105. Kriegshauser JS, Swee RG, McCarthy JT, Hauser MF: Aluminum toxicity in patients undergoing dialysis: Radiographic findings and prediction of bone biopsy results. Radiology 164:399–403, 1987.
106. Murphey MD, Sartoris DJ, Quale JL, et al: Musculoskeletal manifestations of chronic renal insufficiency. Radiographics 13:357–379, 1993.
107. Mosekilde L, Eriksen EF, Charles P: Effects of thyroid hormones on bone and mineral metabolism. Endocrinol Metab Clin North Am 19:35–63, 1990.
108. Eriksen EF: Normal and pathological remodeling of human trabecular bone: Three dimensional reconstruction of the remodeling sequence in normals and in metabolic bone disease. Endocr Rev 7:379–408, 1986.
109. Toh SH, Claunch BC, Brown PH: Effect of hyperthyroidism and its treatment on bone mineral content. Arch Intern Med 145:883–886, 1985.
110. Linde J, Friis T: Osteoporosis in hyperthyroidism estimated by photon absorptiometry. Acta Endocrinol 91:437–448, 1979.
111. Krølner B, Jørgensen JV, Nielsen SP: Spinal bone mineral content in myxoedema and thyrotoxicosis. Effects of thyroid hormone(s) and antithyroid treatment. Clin Endocrinol 18:439–446, 1983.
112. Chew FS: Radiologic manifestations in the musculoskeletal system of miscellaneous endocrine disorders. Radiol Clin North Am 29:135–147, 1991.
113. Solomon BL, Wartofsky L, Burman KD: Prevalence of fractures in postmenopausal women with thyroid disease. Thyroid 3:17–23, 1993.
114. Laan RF, Buijs WC, van Erning LJ, et al: Differential effects of glucocorticoids on cortical appendicular and cortical vertebral bone mineral content. Calcif Tissue Int 52:5–9, 1993.
115. Brandli DW, Golde G, Greenwald M, Silverman SL: Glucocorticoid-induced osteoporosis: A cross-sectional study. Steroids 56:518–523, 1991.
116. Saito JK, Davis JW, Wasnich RD, Ross PD: Users of low-dose glucocorticoids have increased bone loss rates: A longitudinal study. Calcif Tissue Int 57:115–119, 1995.
117. Adachi JD, Bensen WG, Hodsman AB: Corticosteroid-induced osteoporosis. Semin Arthritis Rheum 22:375–384, 1993.
118. Heimann WG, Freiberger RH: Avascular necrosis of the femoral and humeral heads after high-dosage corticosteroid therapy. N Engl J Med 263:672–674, 1969.
119. Hurel SJ, Kendall-Taylor P: Avascular necrosis secondary to postoperative steroid therapy. Br J Neurosurg 11:356–358, 1997.
120. Griffith GC, Nichols G, Ashey JD, Flannagan B: Heparin osteoporosis. JAMA 193:85–88, 1965.
121. Rupp WM, McCarthy HB, Rohde TD, et al: Risk of osteoporosis in patients treated with long-term intravenous heparin therapy. Curr Surg 39:419–422, 1982.
122. Sackler JP, Liu L: Heparin-induced osteoporosis. Br J Radiol 46:548–550, 1973.
123. Walenga JM, Bick RL: Heparin-induced thrombocytopenia, paradoxical thromboembolism, and other side-effects of heparin therapy. Med Clin North Am 82:635–658, 1998.
124. Seeman E, Szmukler GI, Formica C, et al: Osteoporosis in anorexia nervosa: The influence of peak bone density, bone loss, oral contraceptive use, and exercise. J Bone Miner Res 7:1467–1474, 1992.
125. Diez A, Puig J, Serrano S, et al: Alcohol-induced bone disease in the absence of severe chronic liver damage. J Bone Miner Res 9:825–831, 1994.
126. Hopper JL, Seeman E: The bone density of twins discordant for tobacco use. N Engl J Med 330:387–392, 1994.
127. Kohlmeyer L, Gasner C, Marcus R: Bone mineral status of women with Marfan syndrome. Am J Med 95:568–572, 1993.
128. Smith R, Stevenson JC, Winearls CG, et al: Osteoporosis of pregnancy. Lancet 1:1178–1180, 1985.
129. Resnick D: Hemoglobinopathies and other anemias. *In* Resnick D (ed): Diagnosis of Bone and Joint Disorders, ed 3. Philadelphia, WB Saunders, 1995, pp 2107–2146.
130. Resnick D: Plasma cell dyscrasias and dysgammaglobulinemias. *In* Resnick D (ed): Diagnosis of Bone and Joint Disorders, ed 3. Philadelphia, WB Saunders, 1995, pp 2147–2189.
131. Stäbler A, Baur A, Bartl R, et al: Contrast enhancement and quantitative signal analysis in MR imaging of multiple myeloma: Assessment of focal and diffuse growth patterns in marrow correlated with biopsies and survival rates. AJR 167:1029–1036, 1996.
132. Baur A, Stabler A, Steinborn M, et al: Magnetresonanztomographie beim Plasmozytom: Wertigkeit verschiedener Sequenzen bei diffuser und lokaler Infiltrationsform. Rofo Fortschr Geb Rontgenstr Neuen Bildgeb Verfahr 168:323–329, 1998.
133. Moulopoulos LA, Dimopoulos MA: Magnetic resonance imaging of the bone marrow in hematologic malignancies. Blood 90:2127–2147, 1997.
134. Lecouvet F, Malghem J, Michaux L, et al: Vertebral compression fractures in multiple myeloma. Part II: Assessment of fracture risk with MR imaging of spinal bone marrow. Radiology 204:201–205, 1997.
135. Lecouvet F, Van de Berg B, Maldague B, et al: Vertebral compression fractures in multiple myeloma. Part I: Distribution and appearance at MR imaging. Radiology 204:195–199, 1997.
136. Molpus WM, Pritchard RS, Walker CW, Fitzrandolph RL: The radiographic spectrum of renal osteodystrophy. Am Fam Physician 43:151–158, 1991.
137. Pitt MJ: Rickets and osteomalacia. *In* Resnick D (ed): Diagnosis of Bone and Joint Disorders, ed 3. Philadelphia, WB Saunders, 1995, pp 1885–1922.
138. Steinbach HL, Kolb FO, Gilfillan R: A mechanism of the production of pseudofractures in osteomalacia (milkman's syndrome). Radiology 62:388, 1954.
139. Rosenberg AE: The pathology of metabolic bone disease. Radiol Clin North Am 29:19–35, 1991.
140. Smith R: Idiopathic juvenile osteoporosis: Experience of twenty-one patients. Br J Rheumatol 34:68–77, 1995.
141. Norman ME: Juvenile osteoporosis. *In* Favus MJ (ed): Primer on the Metabolic Diseases and Disorders of Mineral Metabolism, ed 3. Philadelphia, Lippincott-Raven, 1996, pp 275–278.
142. Minch CM, Kruse RW: Osteogenesis imperfecta: A review of basic science and diagnosis. Orthopedics 21:558–567, 1998.
143. Hanscom DA, Winter RB, Lutter L, et al: Osteogenesis imperfecta. Radiographic classification, natural history, and treatment of spinal deformities. J Bone Joint Surg Am 74:598–616, 1992.
144. Zionts LE, Nash JP, Rude R, et al: Bone mineral density in children with mild osteogenesis imperfecta. J Bone Joint Surg Br 77:143–147, 1995.
145. Kiratli BJ: Immobilization osteopenia. *In* Marcus R, Feldman D, Kelsey J (eds): Osteoporosis. San Diego, CA, Academic, 1996, pp 833–853.
146. Sudeck P: Über die akute (reflectorische) Knochenatrophie nach entzündungen und Verletzungen an den Extremitäten und ihre klinischen Erscheinungen. Rofo Fortschr Geb Rontgenstr Neuen Bildgeb Verfahr 5:277, 1901.
147. Miller DS, DeTakats G: Post-traumatic dystrophy of the extremities: Sudeck's atrophy. Surg Gynecol Obstet 75:558, 1942.
148. Oyen WJ, Arntz IE, Claessens RM, et al: Reflex sympathetic dystrophy of the hand: An excessive inflammatory response? Pain 55:151–157, 1993.
149. Sarangi PP, Ward AJ, Smith EJ, et al: Algodystrophy and osteoporosis after tibial fractures. J Bone Joint Surg Br 75:450–452, 1993.
150. Gellman H, Keenan MA, Stone L, et al: Reflex sympathetic dystrophy in brain-injured patients. Pain 51:307–311, 1992.
151. Schwartzman RJ, McLellan TL: Reflex sympathetic dystrophy: A review. Arch Neurol 44:555–561, 1987.
152. Resnick D, Niwayama G: Osteoporosis. *In* Resnick D (ed): Diagnosis of Bone and Joint Disorders, ed 3. Philadelphia, WB Saunders, 1995, pp 1783–1853.
153. Todorovic Tirnanic M, Obradovic V, Han R, et al: Diagnostic approach to reflex sympathetic dystrophy after fracture: Radiography or bone scintigraphy? Eur J Nucl Med 22:1187–1193, 1995.
154. Steinert H, Hahn K: Wertigkeit der Drei Phasen Skelettszintigraphie zur Fruhdiagnostik des Morbus Sudeck. Rofo Fortschr Geb Rontgenstr Neuen Bildgeb Verfahr 164:318–323, 1996.
155. Leitha T, Staudenherz A, Korpan M, Fialka V: Pattern recognition in five-phase bone scintigraphy: Diagnostic patterns of reflex sympathetic dystrophy in adults. Eur J Nucl Med 23:256–262, 1996.
156. Rosen RA: Transitory demineralization of the femoral head. Radiology 94:509–512, 1970.
157. Hunder GG, Kelly PJ: Roentgenologic transient osteoporosis of the hip. Ann Intern Med 68:539–552, 1968.
158. Gupta RC, Popovtzer MM, Huffer WE, Smyth CJ: Regional migratory osteoporosis. Arthritis Rheum 21:363–368, 1973.
159. Hayes CW, Conway WF, Daniel WW: MR imaging of bone marrow edema pattern: Transient osteoporosis, transient bone marrow edema syndrome, or osteonecrosis. Radiographics 13:1001–1011, 1993.
160. Boos S, Sigmund G, Huhle P, Nurbakhsch I: Magnetresonanztomographie der sogenannten transitorischen Osteoporose. Primärdiagnostik und Verlaufskontrolle nach Therapie. Rofo Fortschr Geb Rontgenstr Neuen Bildgeb Verfahr 158:201–206, 1993.
161. Trepman E, King TV: Transient osteoporosis of the hip misdiagnosed as osteonecrosis on magnetic resonance imaging. Orthop Rev 21:1089–1091, 1094–1098, 1992.
162. Froberg PK, Braunstein EM, Buckwalter KA: Osteonecrosis, transient osteoporosis, and transient bone marrow edema: Current concepts. Radiol Clin North Am 34:273–291, 1996.
163. Guerra JJ, Steinberg ME: Distinguishing transient osteoporosis from avascular necrosis of the hip. J Bone Joint Surg Am 77:616–624, 1995.
164. Ryan PJ, Fogelman I: Bone scintigraphy in metabolic bone disease. Semin Nucl Med 27:291–305, 1997.
165. Clarke SE, Fogelman I: Bone scanning in metabolic and endocrine bone disease. Endocrinol Metab Clin North Am 18:977–993, 1989.
166. Fogelman I, Citrin DL, Turner JG, et al: Semi-quantitative interpretation of the bone scan in metabolic bone disease: Definition and validation of the metabolic index. Eur J Nucl Med 4:287–289, 1979.
167. Schneider R: Radiologic methods of evaluating generalized osteopenia. Orthop Clin North Am 15:631–651, 1984.
168. McAfee JG: Radionuclide imaging in metabolic and systemic skeletal diseases. Semin Nucl Med 17:334–349, 1987.
169. Fogelman I, Carr D: A comparison of bone scanning and radiology in the evaluation of patients with metabolic bone disease. Clin Radiol 31:321–326, 1980.
170. Lane JM, Vigorita VJ: Osteoporosis. Orthop Clin North Am 15:711–728, 1984.
171. Ryan PJ, Evans P, Gibson T, Fogelman I: Osteoporosis and chronic back pain: A study with single-photon emission computed tomography bone scintigraphy. J Bone Miner Res 7:1455–1460, 1992.

172. Verstraeten A, Dequeker J: Mineral metabolism in postmenopausal women with active rheumatoid arthritis. J Rheumatol 13:43–46, 1986.
173. Kim SM, Desai AG, Krakovitz M, et al: Scintigraphic evaluation of regional migratory osteoporosis. Clin Nucl Med 14:36–39, 1989.
174. Schulz EE, Libanati CR, Farley SM, et al: Skeletal scintigraphic changes in osteoporosis treated with sodium fluoride: Concise communication. J Nucl Med 25:651–655, 1984.
175. Ryan PJ, Evans PA, Gibson T, Fogelman I: Chronic low back pain: Comparison of bone SPECT with radiography and CT: Radiology 182:849–854, 1992.
176. Ryan RJ, Gibson T, Fogelman I: The identification of spinal pathology in chronic low back pain using single photon emission computed tomography. Nucl Med Commun 13:497–502, 1992.
177. Collier BD, Johnson RP, Carrera GF, et al: Painful spondylolysis or spondylolisthesis studied by radiography and single-photon emission computed tomography. Radiology 154:207–211, 1985.
178. Dolan AL, Ryan PJ, Arden NK, et al: The value of SPECT scans in identifying back pain likely to benefit from facet joint injection. Br J Rheumatol 35:1269–1273, 1996.
179. Lusins JO, Danielski EF, Goldsmith SJ: Bone SPECT in patients with persistent back pain after lumbar spine surgery. J Nucl Med 30:490–496, 1989.
180. Fogelman I, Collier BD, Brown ML: Bone scintigraphy: Part 3. Bone scanning in metabolic bone disease. J Nucl Med 34:2247–2252, 1993.
181. Kanis JA, Delmas P, Burckhardt P, et al: Guidelines for diagnosis and management of osteoporosis. Osteoporos Int 7:390–406, 1997.
182. Pande I, Close JCT, Woolf AD: How to investigate a patient with osteoporosis. Osteoporos Rev 5:1–4, 1997.

Chapter 86

The Renal Osteodystrophies

Isidro B. Salusky ▪ William G. Goodman ▪ Jack W. Coburn

The kidneys play a central role in mineral homeostasis: they (1) maintain the external balance of calcium, phosphorus, and magnesium; (2) synthesize 1,25-dihydroxyvitamin D_3 (1,25$(OH)_2D_3$) and 24,25$(OH)_2D_3$; and (3) serve as a target organ for the action and degradation of parathyroid hormone (PTH) and the clearance of PTH from the circulation. In addition, the kidneys provide the major, if not the only route for the elimination of certain substances (e.g., aluminum and α_2-microglobulin) that can adversely affect mineral homeostasis and bone when retained in high concentration.[1] Therefore, it is not surprising that a progressive reduction in nephron mass is associated with altered mineral homeostasis. The term *renal osteodystrophies* is used in a global sense to include all the skeletal syndromes and alterations in mineral metabolism that appear as renal function declines.

The renal bone diseases represent a spectrum of skeletal disorders ranging from high-turnover lesions arising predominantly from excess PTH secretion to low-turnover lesions of diverse etiology that are most often associated with normal or reduced serum PTH levels[2] (Fig. 86–1). The transition from one histologic subtype to another is determined by one or more dominant pathogenic factors, and such changes can be documented in individual patients by periodically obtaining bone biopsy samples for quantitative histology. Because the serum level of PTH represents the major regulator of bone formation and turnover in patients with chronic renal disease, alterations in parathyroid gland function associated with renal failure play a pivotal role in the pathogenesis and evolution of renal osteodystrophy.[3, 4]

In this chapter the pathogenesis, histologic features, clinical symptoms, radiologic characteristics, and prevention and treatment of renal osteodystrophy are reviewed.

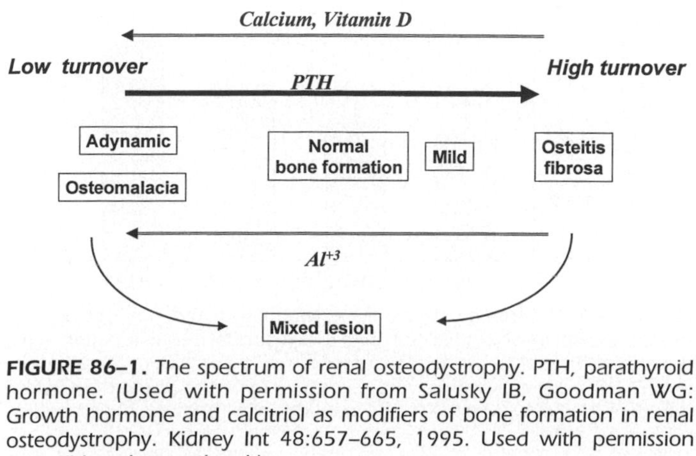

FIGURE 86–1. The spectrum of renal osteodystrophy. PTH, parathyroid hormone. (Used with permission from Salusky IB, Goodman WG: Growth hormone and calcitriol as modifiers of bone formation in renal osteodystrophy. Kidney Int 48:657–665, 1995. Used with permission from Kidney International.)

PATHOGENESIS OF HIGH BONE TURNOVER (SECONDARY HYPERPARATHYROIDISM)

Several factors contribute to sustained increases in PTH secretion and, ultimately, to the development of high-turnover lesions of bone in patients with chronic renal failure. Among these factors are hypocalcemia, impaired renal calcitriol production, skeletal resistance to the calcemic actions of PTH, alterations in the regulation of prepro-PTH gene transcription, reductions in calcium-sensing receptor (CaSR) expression in the parathyroids, and hyperphosphatemia resulting from diminished renal phosphorus excretion[5] (Fig. 86–2).

The kidney is responsible for the production of 1,25$(OH)_2D_3$, the most active metabolite of vitamin D[6–8] (see Chapter 72). Generation of 1,25$(OH)_2D_3$ from 25$(OH)D_3$ is normally stimulated by PTH, by hypocalcemia per se, and by a reduction in dietary phosphate intake. With renal disease, the decreased ability of the kidney to generate 1,25$(OH)_2D_3$ is an important factor leading to the development of secondary hyperparathyroidism.[9–11] Low serum levels of 1,25$(OH)_2D_3$ can both impair intestinal absorption of calcium, thereby causing hypocalcemia, and cause increased PTH synthesis via stimulation of mRNA for prepro-PTH.[12] Although 1,25$(OH)_2D_3$ has been recognized for many years to be a key negative regulator of PTH transcription, more recent evidence indicates that the serum levels of both calcium and phosphorus influence posttranscriptional events that also affect PTH synthesis.[13, 14] Thus hypocalcemia increases, whereas hypophosphatemia decreases, the half-life of PTH mRNA.[14] Administration of small, physiologic amounts of 1,25$(OH)_2D_3$ increases the intestinal absorption of calcium in patients with advanced renal failure.[15] Patients with advanced renal failure have reduced or even undetectable plasma levels of 1,25$(OH)_2D_3$, and deficiency of this sterol plays a key role in the development of secondary hyperparathyroidism and bone disease in these patients by directly affecting PTH gene transcription and indirectly modifying message translation.[9–11, 16]

In patients with creatinine clearances above 50 mL/min, however, intestinal absorption of calcium is subnormal in only a small fraction of patients.[17] Plasma levels of 1,25$(OH)_2D_3$ have been reported to be either slightly reduced or normal in adults with mild to moderate renal insufficiency.[9, 10] Portale et al. found that mean plasma 1,25$(OH)_2D_3$ levels were lower in children with moderate renal failure than in age-matched controls.[16] Also, dietary phosphate restriction increased levels of 1,25$(OH)_2D_3$ and reduced serum PTH concentrations in children with moderate renal failure.[18] Similar findings were noted by Llach

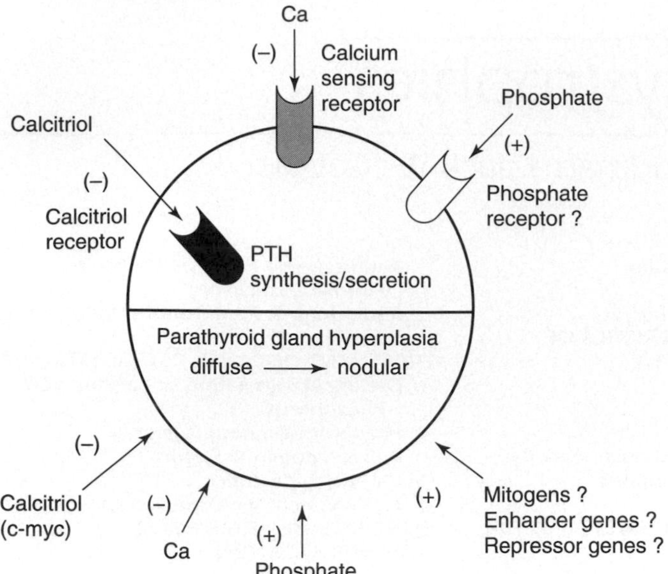

FIGURE 86–2. Pathogenesis of secondary hyperparathyroidism. PTH, parathyroid hormone. (Courtesy of Tilman B. Drüeke, M.D.)

and Massry[19] in adults with mild renal insufficiency. These findings provide evidence for a link between dietary phosphate intake and altered vitamin D metabolism in patients with early to moderate renal failure. Other observations indicate that dogs with experimentally induced advanced renal failure had low serum levels of $1,25(OH)_2D_3$ despite being fed a diet low in phosphate[20]; however, a slight increase was noted in the ionized calcium level, as well as significant suppression of serum PTH levels. Lucas et al. noted a fall in serum PTH and a rise in $1,25(OH)_2D_3$ levels when patients with advanced renal failure were fed a low protein, low PO_4 diet.[21] On the other hand, Schaefer et al. demonstrated decreased levels of plasma phosphorus and PTH after 8 weeks of therapy with a low phosphate ketoacid diet in patients with advanced renal failure without any changes in serum levels of calcium or $1,25(OH)_2D_3$.[22] These data suggest that the factors that contribute to secondary hyperparathyroidism may differ with the degree of renal impairment. Studies by Lopez-Hilker et al. in dogs with advanced renal failure demonstrated that a reduction in dietary phosphorus can improve secondary hyperparathyroidism by a mechanism independent of the levels of both calcitriol and serum ionized calcium.[20]

The kidney is the major organ responsible for the production of $24,25(OH)_2D_3$, although this sterol may be produced in the intestine and bone as well.[23] The physiologic role of this vitamin D metabolite is uncertain, and it has not been consistently effective in suppression of secondary hyperparathyroidism caused by renal failure[24] (see Chapter 72).

The development and progression of parathyroid gland hyperplasia are particularly important aspects of renal secondary hyperparathyroidism.[25] Once established, parathyroid enlargement is difficult to reverse because the rate of apoptosis in parathyroid glands is quite low, and the half-life of parathyroid cells has been estimated to be approximately 30 years.[26] Clinical assessment of parathyroid gland function suggests that differences in functional parathyroid size contribute substantially to the wide variation in serum PTH levels in patients with chronic renal failure.[27] Excess PTH secretion may become uncontrollable clinically if the parathyroid glands become greatly enlarged because the nonsuppressible component of PTH release from a very large number of parathyroid cells can be sufficient to produce hypercalcemia and progressive bone disease in patients with end-stage renal disease.

Because 1,25-dihydroxyvitamin D is a potent inhibitor of cell proliferation, disturbances in renal calcitriol production and/or changes in vitamin D receptor (VDR) expression may be particularly important determinants of the degree of parathyroid hyperplasia and the extent of parathyroid gland enlargement in chronic renal failure.[28] VDR expression is markedly reduced in parathyroid tissues that exhibit a nodular pattern of tissue hyperplasia, whereas lesser reductions in VDR expression are seen in glands with a diffuse pattern of hyperplasia.[29] Interestingly, the extent of glandular enlargement is generally greater in nodular parathyroid hyperplasia.[30] Clonal expansion of subpopulations of parathyroid cells and selected chromosomal deletions represent additional mechanisms that may influence the extent of parathyroid gland enlargement in end-stage renal disease.[31]

Expression of the CaSR is reduced by 30% to 70% as judged by immunohistochemical methods in hyperplastic parathyroid tissue obtained from human subjects with renal failure.[32] As such, the primary mechanism by which parathyroid cells detect and respond to changes in blood ionized calcium is abnormal in advanced renal secondary hyperparathyroidism, possibly rendering parathyroid tissue less sensitive to the inhibitory effect of calcium on PTH release. In addition, decreased expression of the putative calcium-sensing CAS (gp330/megalin) protein has been demonstrated in parathyroid adenomas.[33] These findings have to be confirmed on parathyroid glands obtained from uremic patients. In this regard, CaSR mRNA levels in the parathyroid gland have been reported to increase in vitamin D–deficient rats given exogenous 1,25-dihydroxyvitamin D, which suggests that alterations in vitamin D metabolism in renal failure could account for changes in calcium sensing by the parathyroids.[34] Reductions in CaSR expression have not been a consistent finding, however, in animals with renal failure,[35] and further work is needed to clarify the role of 1,25-dihydroxyvitamin D as a modifier of CaSR expression in parathyroid tissue.

The temporal relationship between the duration and/or the severity of renal failure and the decrease in parathyroid CaSR expression has yet to be determined. In vivo studies of parathyroid gland function in patients with end-stage renal disease indicate that calcium sensing by the parathyroid glands is altered in advanced, but not in mild to moderate secondary hyperparathyroidism[36, 37] (Fig. 86–3). Such findings are consistent with in vitro assessments demonstrating that calcium-regulated PTH release is altered in dispersed parathyroid cells obtained from hyperplastic tissue removed from patients undergoing parathyroidectomy for severe secondary hyperparathyroidism.[38] In contrast, evidence of alterations in CaSR expression is not found in patients with moderate renal insufficiency who do not require dialysis, as judged by in vivo studies of parathyroid gland function.[39] These in vivo findings in mild to moderate secondary hyperparathyroidism have yet to be confirmed by in vitro assessment of either calcium-regulated PTH release or CaSR expression because parathyroid tissue from such individuals is not available for study. It remains uncertain, therefore, whether alterations in CaSR expression fully account for disturbances in PTH secretion in mild to moderate chronic renal failure.

Skeletal resistance to the calcemic action of PTH contributes to the

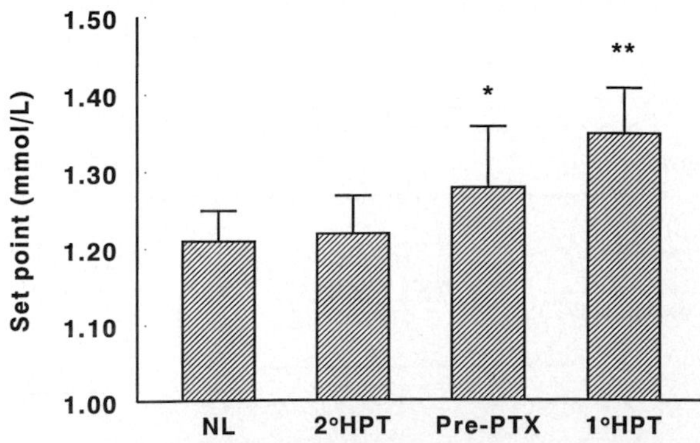

FIGURE 86–3. Set-point values for calcium-regulated parathyroid hormone release in volunteer subjects with normal renal function (NL), patients with mild to moderate degrees of secondary hyperparathyroidism (2° HPT), patients with severe secondary hyperparathyroidism before parathyroidectomy (Pre-PTX), and patients with primary hyperparathyroidism (1° HPT).

hypocalcemia and secondary hyperparathyroidism in renal failure. The calcemic response to a standardized infusion of parathyroid extract is subnormal in patients with moderate and advanced renal failure and in those undergoing maintenance dialysis.[40] Recovery from induced hypocalcemia in patients with mild renal insufficiency is delayed in comparison to that in normal individuals[40]; this phenomenon occurs despite a marked increment in serum PTH concentrations in these patients. These observations indicate that skeletal resistance to the action of PTH appears early in the course of renal failure; indeed, higher serum PTH levels are required to elicit equivalent biologic responses in patients with chronic renal failure.[41, 42] Abnormalities in vitamin D metabolism have been reported to account for these changes, but alterations in VDR expression could also contribute. In addition, expression of the receptor for PTH/PTH-related protein (PTHrP) is reduced in renal failure; this abnormality is probably attributable to renal failure per se rather than PTH-mediated downregulation of its own receptor because receptor expression is low in uremic animals regardless of the prevailing serum level of PTH.[43] Decreases in PTH/PTHrP receptor expression may therefore contribute to tissue resistance to the actions of PTH in renal failure.

Phosphorus retention and hyperphosphatemia have been recognized for many years as important factors in the pathogenesis of secondary hyperparathyroidism. The development of secondary hyperparathyroidism is prevented in experimental animals with chronic renal failure when dietary phosphorus intake is lowered in proportion to the glomerular filtration rate (GFR),[44] and dietary phosphate restriction can reduce previously elevated serum PTH levels in patients with moderate renal failure.[18, 19] Phosphorus retention and hyperphosphatemia indirectly promote the secretion of PTH in several ways. First, hyperphosphatemia lowers blood ionized calcium levels and stimulates PTH release as free calcium ions form complexes with excess amounts of inorganic phosphate. Second, phosphorus impairs renal 1α-hydroxylase activity, which diminishes the conversion of 25-dihydroxyvitamin D to 1,25-dihydroxyvitamin D; high rates of transepithelial phosphate transport in the proximal tubule when the GFR is reduced may account for this change and thereby contribute to reductions in renal calcitriol production.[18] In addition, recent evidence suggests that phosphorus can directly enhance PTH synthesis by the parathyroid cell. The amount of PTH released from parathyroid glands maintained in tissue culture increases at high medium phosphorus concentrations; this response appears to be mediated by a posttranscriptional mechanism because the rate of prepro-PTH gene transcription is not affected by the level of phosphorus in the culture medium.[45]

PATHOGENESIS OF LOW BONE TURNOVER (ADYNAMIC BONE AND OSTEOMALACIA)

In the 1970s and 1980s, aluminum intoxication was largely responsible for the development of adynamic bone and osteomalacia in patients with chronic renal failure. Two distinct patterns of aluminum intoxication have been identified: (1) from the aluminum content of water used to prepare dialysate solution[46–48] and (2) intestinal aluminum absorption after the ingestion of large doses of aluminum hydroxide.[49–55] The neurologic syndrome of "dialysis encephalopathy" and a bone disease manifested by fractures, pain, persistent hypercalcemia, and osteomalacia were the main clinical features.

In addition, factors that may substantially augment the absorption of aluminum and increase the risk of aluminum toxicity should be taken into consideration.[56] The most important factor known to augment aluminum absorption is citrate, either as citric acid or as one of its salts; citrate forms a complex with aluminum that enhances its absorption from the gut, but it may also hasten its movement into intracellular sites, particularly in the central nervous system. The absorption of aluminum is augmented 5- to 20-fold, as indicated by increments in urinary aluminum after citrate ingestion by normal subjects. Such increased absorption can occur with any salt of citrate (e.g., sodium, calcium). Treatment with a combination of oral aluminum gels to control serum phosphorus and with Shohl solution or Bicitra to treat metabolic acidosis can lead to severe aluminum toxicity in patients with advanced renal failure not yet needing dialysis.[57] Vitamin D may have a small effect of enhancing aluminum absorption,[56] and the presence of iron deficiency also results in enhanced aluminum absorption. Other factors such as previous parathyroidectomy, an earlier renal transplantation that has failed, bilateral nephrectomy, and the presence of diabetes mellitus[58] are more prevalent with aluminum-related bone disease than with other types of bone disease.

The prevalence of adynamic renal osteodystrophy not associated with aluminum intoxication has increased substantially in recent years in adult patients receiving regular dialysis.[59] The widespread use of large doses of oral calcium carbonate to control hyperphosphatemia and treatment with active vitamin D sterols to lower serum PTH levels have probably contributed to the increased prevalence of adynamic bone in patients with end-stage renal disease[60] (Fig. 86–4). High concentrations of calcium in dialysis solutions may also play a role. Approximately 40% of those treated with hemodialysis and more than half of adult patients undergoing peritoneal dialysis have serum PTH levels that are only minimally elevated or fall within the normal range; such values are typically associated with normal or reduced rates of bone formation and turnover.[61]

Because PTH is the major determinant of bone formation and skeletal remodeling in renal failure, oversuppression of PTH secretion can result in adynamic renal osteodystrophy. Calcitriol may also directly suppress osteoblastic activity when given intermittently in large doses to patients receiving regular dialysis.[62]

The long-term consequences of adynamic renal osteodystrophy not attributable to aluminum toxicity remain to be determined, but concerns have been raised about increases in the risk of skeletal fracture and delayed fracture healing because of low rates of bone remodeling.[62] The development of soft tissue and vascular calcifications may be facilitated by frequent episodes of hypercalcemia. Recent work suggests that calcification of the coronary arteries and cardiac valves is common in patients undergoing long-term dialysis, but the relationship between these changes and the presence of adynamic renal osteodystrophy is uncertain.[63] In children, adynamic renal osteodystrophy has been associated with a reduction in linear growth in prepubertal patients.[64]

Additional factors have been identified in patients with osteomalacia. In England, the most important predictive factor for the development of osteomalacia in patients with advanced renal failure or those undergoing dialysis is low serum levels of 25(OH)D_2 in patients with advanced uremia or low serum phosphorus levels in those undergoing dialysis.[65] On the other hand, studies in the United States have not generally noted a relationship between serum levels of 25(OH)D_2 and

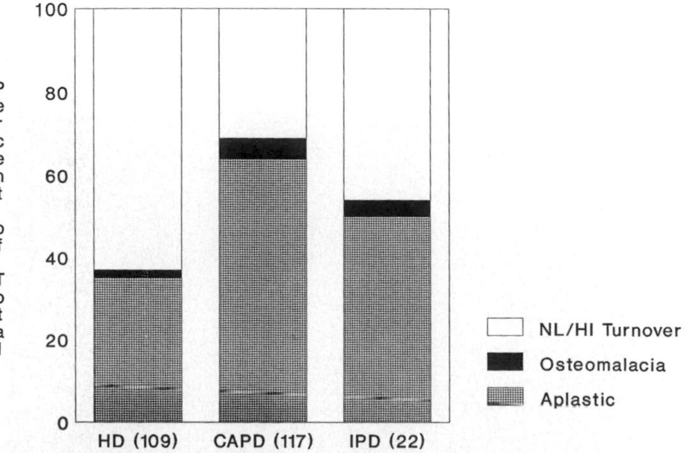

FIGURE 86–4. Distribution of bone lesions in patients treated with hemodialysis (HD), continuous ambulatory peritoneal dialysis (CAPD), and intermittent peritoneal dialysis (IPD). NL/HI, normal-to-high bone formation rates. (Modified from Sherrard DJ, Hercz G, Pei Y, et al: The spectrum of bone disease in end-stage renal failure—an evolving disorder. Kidney Int 43:436–442, 1993. Used with permission from Kidney International.)

the appearance of osteomalacia, probably because of the greater sunlight exposure and supplementation of more foods with vitamin D_2 or D_3 in the United States. With the appropriate management of patients with advanced renal failure and those undergoing hemodialysis, plasma levels of calcium and phosphorus are not usually low, and growing evidence indicates that the osteomalacia of vitamin D deficiency can be healed when serum calcium and phosphorus levels are raised to normal.[66, 67] Thus alterations in vitamin D metabolism and a reduction in sunlight exposure and/or reduced intake of vitamin D can predispose to osteomalacia in patients with advanced renal failure.

Treatment with phenytoin may contribute to the development of osteomalacia in patients with renal failure. Long-term ingestion of phenytoin and/or phenobarbital is associated with a high incidence of osteomalacia in nonuremic patients.[68] Jubiz et al. found low serum levels of $25(OH)D_3$ but normal levels of $1,25(OH)_2D_3$ in patients with normal renal function who were receiving anticonvulsant therapy and had clinical evidence of osteomalacia.[69] Furthermore, Pierides et al. reported a higher incidence of symptomatic bone disease in dialysis patients who were being treated with barbiturates and phenytoin than in dialysis patients not receiving such treatment.[70]

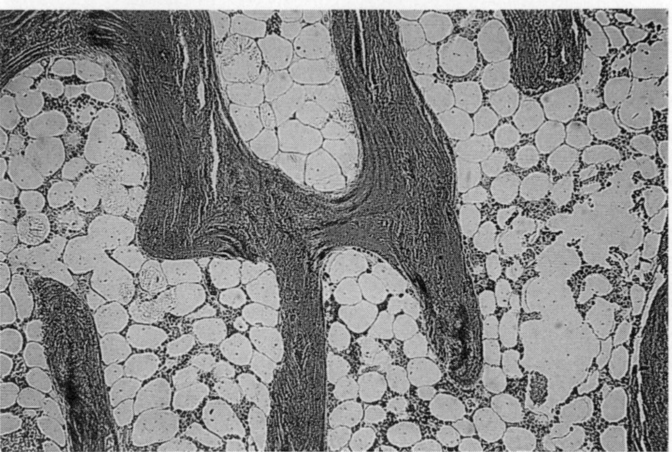

FIGURE 86–6. Histologic lesion of adynamic bone characterized by a diminished amount of osteoid formation, osteoblasts, and osteoclasts.

HISTOLOGIC CHARACTERISTICS OF RENAL OSTEODYSTROPHY

Evaluation of skeletal histology provides both a method for understanding the pathophysiology of renal bone disease and a guide to its proper management. Currently, bone biopsy procedures are done on an outpatient basis, and morbidity is minimal in both adult and pediatric patients.[59, 71, 72] Double tetracycline labeling in conjunction with quantitative histomorphometric techniques provides the best method to identify defective mineralization.[73] Tetracycline is given on two occasions separated by a specific time interval, usually 10 to 17 days. The tetracycline is identified in bone sections by its fluorescent characteristics; separation of the two bands of tetracycline and the length of bone surface showing the double label allow a determination of the bone formation rate, thereby providing a dynamic approach to the evaluation of bone disease.

Several forms of skeletal pathology occur in patients with advanced renal failure. One of the most common types of pathology in adult uremic patients is osteitis fibrosa cystica arising from an excess of PTH.[74] The bone in osteitis fibrosa cystica exhibits a marked increase in turnover with increased numbers of osteoblasts and osteoclasts and variable degrees of peritrabecular fibrosis (Fig. 86–5). Activation of osteoclasts is mediated through PTH[75–78]; the result is increased resorption of both mineral and matrix along the trabecular surface and within the haversian canals of cortical bone.[79] Such increased cellular activity can occur secondary to a nonspecific reaction to local factors, such as insulin-like growth factor-1 (IGF-1), cytokines, or fracture, or from systemic stimuli such as increased thyroxine or PTH.[80] One characteristic of bone showing fibro-osteoclasia is increased quantities of woven osteoid, which exhibits a haphazard arrangement of collagen fibers in contrast to the usual lamellar pattern of osteoid in normal bone. Woven osteoid can become mineralized in patients with advanced renal failure in the absence of vitamin D[81]; however, the calcium may be deposited as amorphous calcium phosphate rather than hydroxyapatite.[82]

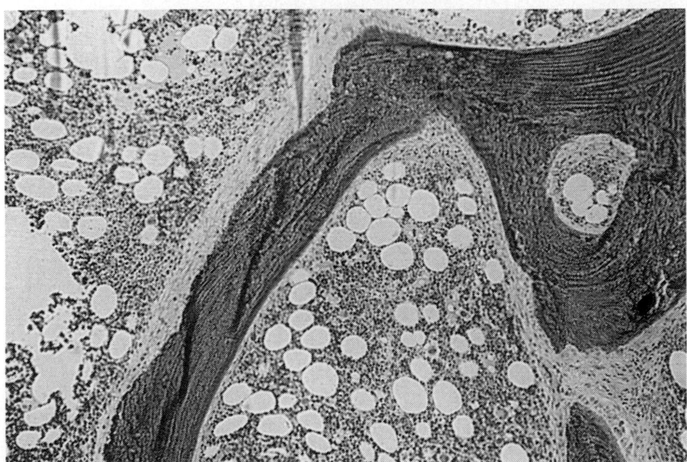

FIGURE 86–5. Histologic lesion of osteitis fibrosa characterized by increased resorptive surface on mineralized bone by osteoclasts and fibrosis.

Another group of patients with asymptomatic bone disease may show normal osteoid volume, absence of fibrosis, and a reduced bone formation rate, as indicated by a reduced or absent double tetracycline label (Fig. 86–6). This group has been classified as having "aplastic" or "adynamic" bone lesions.[61] If substantial staining with aluminum is seen along the bone surfaces, as well as a paucity of osteoblasts and osteoclasts, patients exhibit all the clinical features of aluminum-related bone disease.[73] Pei et al. suggest that the aplastic or adynamic lesion of renal osteodystrophy not related to aluminum is a predominant skeletal lesion in adult patients undergoing long-term peritoneal dialysis[61] (see Fig. 86–4). These initial findings have been confirmed by other group of investigators.[83, 84] In addition, the adynamic bone lesion was predominant after intermittent calcitriol therapy in a substantial proportion of pediatric patients treated with maintenance peritoneal dialysis.[85] The histologic features of adynamic renal osteodystrophy, in the absence of aluminum deposition in bone, cannot be distinguished from the histologic features of corticosteroid-induced osteoporosis or either age-related or postmenopausal osteoporosis. As such, it is not possible to determine whether osteoporosis accounts for decreases in osteoblastic activity and bone formation in patients with adynamic renal osteodystrophy unless the amount of trabecular bone is reduced. Decreases in bone mass and histologic evidence of trabecular bone loss are not, however, integral features of the adynamic lesion of renal osteodystrophy when other causes of osteoporosis can be excluded.

Osteomalacia is another feature of uremic bone; the characteristics of osteomalacia include the presence of wide osteoid seams, an increased number of osteoid lamellae, an increase in the trabecular surface covered with osteoid, and a diminished rate of mineralization or bone formation, as assessed by double tetracycline labeling. Fibrosis is often absent.[73] When osteomalacia is refractory to therapy with vitamin D in a patient who has had long-term treatment with dialysis, it most often arises as a result of aluminum intoxication.[86]

Osteitis fibrosa cystica, a finding of secondary hyperparathyroidism, can coexist with osteomalacia in some patients; this pattern is called a "mixed" lesion.[73] When mixed lesions are associated with hypocalcemia and elevated serum PTH levels, the condition generally responds to therapy with calcitriol or another active vitamin sterol. Such lesions can also occur as a transition from osteitis fibrosa cystica to aluminum-related bone disease.

CLINICAL MANIFESTATIONS

The symptoms and signs of renal osteodystrophy are usually nonspecific, and laboratory and radiographic abnormalities generally predate clinical manifestations. Some specific symptoms and syndromes do occur, however.

Bone Pain

Bone pain is a common manifestation of severe bone disease in patients with advanced renal failure. It is usually insidious in appearance and is often aggravated by weight bearing or a change in posture. Physical findings are often absent. The pain is most common in the lower part of the back, hips, and legs, but it may occur in the peripheral skeleton. Occasionally, sudden appearance of pain around the knee, ankle, or heel can suggest acute arthritis; such pain is not usually relieved by massage or local heat. Bone pain is more common and often more marked in patients with aluminum-related bone disease than in those with osteitis fibrosa cystica, but marked variability is seen from one patient to another.[1]

In long-term dialysis patients, carpal tunnel syndrome and chronic arthralgias often occur in association with the deposition of β_2-microglobulin amyloid in articular and periarticular structures (see below).[87] The arthralgias are usually bilateral and most commonly affect the shoulders, knees, wrists, and small joints of the hand; symptoms are typically worse with inactivity and at night.[88, 89]

Muscle Weakness

Proximal myopathy can be marked in patients with advanced renal failure. Symptoms appear slowly. Patients may note difficulty climbing stairs or rising from a low chair, or they may have difficulty raising their arms to comb their hair. This proximal muscle weakness resembles that of nutritional vitamin D deficiency and is also reported in primary hyperparathyroidism. Plasma levels of muscle enzymes are usually normal, and electromyographic changes are nonspecific.

The pathogenesis of this myopathy is not clear, and several different mechanisms have been implicated, including secondary hyperparathyroidism, phosphate depletion,[90] abnormal vitamin D metabolism, and aluminum intoxication.[91] Improvement in gait posture has been reported in children with moderate renal failure after treatment with $1,25(OH)_2D_3$, and muscle weakness improves rapidly in affected adult patients with end-stage renal disease. Expression of VDRs in muscle may account for these findings.[92] Improvement in muscular strength has also been observed after treatment with $25(OH)D_3$, after subtotal parathyroidectomy, after successful renal transplantation, and after chelation therapy with deferoxamine for aluminum intoxication. Nonetheless, the favorable response of certain patients to $25(OH)D_3$ or $1,25(OH)_2D_3$ suggests that a therapeutic trial with an active vitamin D sterol is warranted in uremic patients with myopathy. Aluminum intoxication and severe secondary hyperparathyroidism must also be excluded.

Skeletal Deformities

Bone deformities are common in uremic children because their bones undergo growth, modeling, and remodeling; in adult patients, skeletal deformities also arise from abnormal remodeling or recurrent fractures.[93] In children, bone deformities of the femur and wrists arise from slipped epiphyses.[94] This problem is most common during the preadolescent period and is most frequent in patients with long-standing congenital renal disease. In adults with renal failure, particularly those with aluminum-related bone disease, skeletal deformities may be characterized by lumbar scoliosis, kyphosis, and deformities of the thoracic cage.[93]

Growth Retardation

Growth retardation is common in children with chronic renal failure. Factors that have been thought to contribute to growth failure include protein and calorie malnutrition, metabolic acidosis, end-organ growth hormone resistance, anemia, and the renal bone diseases.[95] In addition, linear growth is influenced by the age of onset of chronic renal failure and primary renal disease. Children in whom renal failure develops in infancy are more growth impaired than those in whom renal disease develops later in childhood.[96] Correction of certain of these abnormalities has been associated with improvement in growth velocity, but such improvement does not occur in all cases. Improved or even catch-up growth has been observed in a few children after treatment with calcitriol,[97] but the number of patients studied was small and subsequent reports have not confirmed the original findings.[98] Moreover, diminished linear growth has been demonstrated after intermittent calcitriol therapy in children with bone biopsy–proven secondary hyperparathyroidism. The greatest reductions in height were observed in patients in whom adynamic bone developed after intermittent use of calcitriol.[64] Overall, such findings suggest that the therapeutic administration of calcitriol can directly affect epiphyseal growth plate chondrocytes.

Extraskeletal Calcification

An association between extraskeletal calcification and uremia has been recognized for many years, but this problem increased significantly after the initiation of long-term dialysis treatment.[99] The three different varieties of calcification are (1) visceral, (2) tumoral or periarticular, and (3) vascular. Pain, joint stiffness, and soft tissue swelling may occur with calcific periarthritis, which is described below. The chemical and crystallographic composition of visceral calcifications is consistent with amorphous or microcrystalline material; pyrophosphate is a major constituent.

Calcific periarthritis, a clinical syndrome arising from periarticular calcifications, is characterized by attacks of acute arthritis with periarticular warmth and redness. Small-joint effusions are often present, and radiographs usually show periarticular calcifications. The characteristics of these patients include increased serum phosphorus levels, an increase in the Ca × P product in serum, and serum PTH levels higher than those seen in other dialysis patients. On the other hand, because patients with adynamic bone have a tendency for hypercalcemia, it may be consider an additional factor in the pathogenesis of vascular calcifications.

Visceral calcifications most commonly involve the lungs, heart, kidneys, skeletal muscle, and stomach. Pulmonary calcifications can cause restrictive lung disease[99] (Fig. 86–7). Visceral calcifications have shown little relationship to hyperphosphatemia, the product of Ca × P in serum, or circulating levels of PTH.[99] On the other hand, Milliner et al. demonstrated a relationship between the development of soft tissue calcifications and the Ca × P product in serum in autopsy studies performed in pediatric patients with end-stage renal disease.[100]

The most characteristic form of vascular calcification in patients with renal failure is medial calcification.[101] Most patients are asymptomatic; however, because of rigidity of the vessel wall the pulse and blood pressure may be difficult to feel or hear, or the blood pressure measurement may be falsely elevated. Vascular calcifications are best detected by lateral radiographs of the ankle or an anteroposterior view of the feet or hands.[102] Uremic patients with diabetes mellitus are particularly prone to such calcifications. The calcifications occasionally regress very slowly after parathyroidectomy; more commonly, no change is seen in the vascular calcification after either parathyroidectomy or successful kidney transplantation.[102, 103] The importance of a high calcium-phosphorus ion product in the development of vascular calcifications has been emphasized,[104] and a major effort should be made to avoid values above 60 to 70.[105] Newer radiographic imaging techniques such as electron beam computed tomography can detect calcifications in coronary arteries and cardiac valves, and these methods may prove useful in the future assessment of vascular calcification in subjects with renal failure.[63]

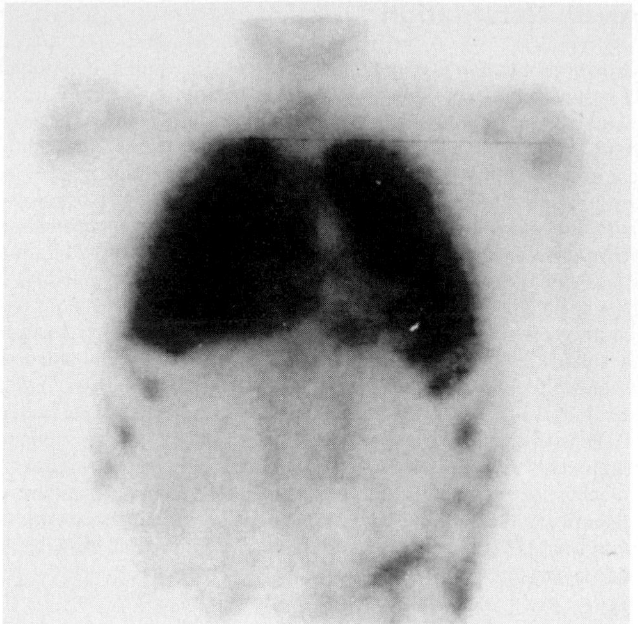

FIGURE 86–7. Diffuse bilateral lung calcifications diagnosed by bone scan in a patient with severe secondary hyperparathyroidism.

Calciphylaxis

This unique syndrome, which is characterized by ischemic necrosis of the skin, subcutaneous fat, and muscles, can develop in patients with advanced renal failure not yet treated by dialysis, in those treated with regular dialysis, and in patients with well-functioning kidney transplants.[106] The pathogenesis of this syndrome is uncertain. Extensive medial calcifications of medium-sized arteries are noted; such calcifications commonly exist in patients with renal disease without causing gangrene or ulcerations, and it is not clear that vascular calcifications per se are the cause of the ischemic necrosis. Two rather distinct types of the syndrome are recognized: *proximal calciphylaxis*, with the thighs, abdomen, and chest wall affected, and the *acral* variety, which involves sites distal to the knees and elbows, such as the toes, fingers, and ankles.[107] The former has a terrible prognosis, with death occurring in more than 80% to 90% of affected patients. This syndrome may be limited to white patients, and morbid obesity is common; also, hypoalbuminemia is observed. With acral or distal calciphylaxis, many patients have severe secondary hyperparathyroidism, and the great majority have a history of severe and uncontrolled hyperphosphatemia.[107, 108] Some patients may have a thrombotic diathesis or defective regulation of coagulation.[109] A significant number of patients have improved after parathyroidectomy; a few have healed after substantial reductions in serum phosphorus levels. The appearance of this syndrome in renal transplant recipients receiving glucocorticoids suggests that these steroids may play a role. Patients with calciphylaxis frequently die of secondary infection. Because of the poor prognosis, urgent parathyroidectomy is indicated in the face of evidence of severe secondary hyperparathyroidism. Ischemic lesions and medial vascular calcifications are common in uremic patients with diabetes; such lesions rarely improve after parathyroidectomy; thus parathyroid surgery should be reserved for those with clear evidence of severe secondary hyperparathyroidism.

Dialysis-Related Amyloidosis

Several clinical syndromes that arise as a consequence of dialysis-related amyloidosis can mimic the clinical features of renal osteodystrophy, or this type of amyloidosis can occur concurrently with uremic bone disease. Dialysis-related amyloidosis arises from the deposition in bone and periarticular structures of a specific type of amyloid composed of β_2-microglobulin.[110] In addition to β_2-microglobulin, the amyloid deposits contain advanced glycosylation end products,[111] which may account for their uptake by certain collagen-rich structures.[112, 113] The frequency of its clinical manifestation rises markedly in patients treated with regular dialysis for more than 5 to 10 years, and it is much more common in patients who start dialysis when older than 50 years.[114] Blood levels of β_2-microglobulin are strikingly elevated in all patients with end-stage renal disease because of failure of normal renal clearance and catabolism of this normal plasma protein. Clinical manifestations include (1) carpal tunnel syndrome; (2) destructive or erosive arthropathy involving the large and medium-sized joints, with shoulder, knee, hip, or back pain being the common manifestations; (3) spondyloarthropathy, most commonly affecting the cervical spine; and (4) subchondral, thin-walled cysts of bone, most commonly affecting the carpal bones, the humoral and femoral heads, the distal end of the radius, the acetabulum, and the tibial plateau. These subchondral cysts are at times confused with brown tumors of secondary hyperparathyroidism, although their location and occurrence in multiple sites make them quite different from brown tumors. Nonetheless, in a patient who has undergone long-term dialysis, this syndrome may be a potential cause of neuromuscular and periarticular symptoms usually considered to be due to secondary hyperparathyroidism or aluminum accumulation. A pitfall to avoid is the recommendation of parathyroid surgery for a dialysis patient whose severe musculoskeletal symptoms have not improved after variable lowering of PTH levels with calcitriol therapy; the symptoms of such patients are actually due to dialysis-related amyloidosis. Specific diagnosis of the latter is made from the biopsy demonstration of amyloid composed of β_2-microglobulin; however, the diagnosis can be strongly suspected from the clinical features, the presence of multiple thin-walled cysts, or the demonstration in periarticular sites of presumed amyloid tissue on ultrasonography.[115] Its management is difficult and largely unsatisfactory, but successful renal transplantation leads to rapid disappearance of symptoms and no further progression on radiographs of the bone lesions.[116]

BIOCHEMICAL CHARACTERISTICS OF RENAL OSTEODYSTROPHY

Serum Phosphorus

Hyperphosphatemia is frequent when the GFR decreases below 30% of normal; however, in patients with early renal failure, serum phosphorus levels may be normal or even below normal.[117–119] With advanced renal insufficiency, dietary intake of phosphorus contributes significantly to the degree of hyperphosphatemia. Moreover, hyperphosphatemia has been found to be an independent risk factor for mortality in patients treated with maintenance dialysis.[104] Therefore, dietary phosphate restriction and the use of phosphate-binding agents are required to control serum phosphorus levels.[120] Hemodialysis and continuous ambulatory peritoneal dialysis (CAPD) remove substantial amounts of phosphate, but dietary phosphate restriction and the use of phosphate-binding agents are required by 90% to 95% of patients undergoing treatment with dialysis. Serum phosphorus levels should be maintained within age-adjusted normal range.

Serum Calcium

Serum calcium levels are often decreased in patients with advanced renal failure, but wide variation exists among individual patients. After initiation of regular therapy with hemodialysis, serum calcium levels increase into the normal range in most patients. The degree of elevation of serum calcium immediately after hemodialysis is related to the calcium concentration in the dialysate solution. In patients treated with CAPD who are not receiving vitamin D supplements, serum calcium levels are generally normal to slightly above normal.[121] Because of reduced serum albumin levels, measurement of ionized calcium levels discloses hypercalcemia more commonly in patients treated with peritoneal dialysis.[122]

The development of hypercalcemia in patients undergoing regular dialysis warrants prompt and thorough investigation. Conditions associated with hypercalcemia include marked hyperplasia of the parathyroid glands as a result of severe secondary hyperparathyroidism, aluminum-related bone disease, adynamic renal osteodystrophy, therapy with calcitriol or other vitamin D sterols, administration of large doses of calcium carbonate or other calcium-containing compounds, immobilization, malignancy, and granulomatous disorders such as sarcoidosis or tuberculosis, in which extrarenal production of 1,25-dihydroxyvitamin D occurs.[5] Basal serum calcium levels are higher in patients with adynamic bone than in subjects with other lesions of renal osteodystrophy, and episodes of hypercalcemia are common.[123] Because skeletal calcium uptake is limited in adynamic lesions, calcium entering the extracellular fluid from dialysate or after intestinal absorption cannot adequately be buffered in bone, and serum calcium levels rise.[124] Lowering the dose of calcium-containing, phosphate-binding agents and decreasing dialysate calcium concentrations usually correct the hypercalcemia.

Serum Magnesium

The net intestinal absorption of magnesium is generally normal or only very slightly reduced in patients with renal failure,[120] and serum magnesium levels often increase with advanced renal failure. During hemodialysis, serum magnesium levels are generally increased if the dialysate is 1.75 mEq/L; however, magnesium levels remain within the upper range of normal with dialysate magnesium concentrations of 0.5 mEq/L. The use of magnesium-containing laxatives or antacids can abruptly raise serum magnesium levels in patients with renal failure,[125] so these medications should be avoided. Serum magnesium levels should be measured frequently and regularly if magnesium-containing medications are used. Rarely, hypomagnesemia can develop in uremic patients with severe malabsorption or diarrhea.[120]

Plasma Alkaline Phosphatase Activity

Serum alkaline phosphatase values are fair markers of the severity of secondary hyperparathyroidism in patients with renal failure. Osteoblasts normally express large amounts of the bone isoenzyme of alkaline phosphatase, and serum levels are usually elevated when osteoblastic activity and bone formation rates are increased. High levels generally reflect the extent of histologic change in patients with high turnover lesions of renal osteodystrophy, and values frequently correlate with serum PTH levels.[126] Serum total alkaline phosphatase measurements are also useful for monitoring the skeletal response to treatment with vitamin D sterols in patients with osteitis fibrosa; values that decrease over several months usually indicate histologic improvement. Serum alkaline phosphatase levels may increase early in the course of treating aluminum-related bone disease with the chelating agent deferoxamine. Also, serum alkaline phosphatase levels increased during therapy with recombinant human growth hormone in pediatric patients with renal failure.[127]

Newer assays for bone-specific alkaline phosphatase and measurements of serum osteocalcin levels provide additional information about the level of osteoblastic activity in patients with chronic renal failure.[128] Osteocalcin levels are generally elevated in renal failure, but values may help distinguish between patients with high-turnover or low-turnover skeletal lesions.[128, 129] If these assays are not available, measurement of the heat-stabile and heat-labile fractions of alkaline phosphatase helps separate skeletal from hepatic causes of elevated total alkaline phosphatase levels.

Serum Parathyroid Hormone

Serum PTH levels are substantially increased in most patients with advanced renal failure, and serum PTH may be elevated during the early course of renal insufficiency.[1, 22, 130] Double-antibody immunoradiometric serum PTH assays are generally better than other methods for separating patients with secondary hyperparathyroidism from those with adynamic lesions of bone.[41, 123, 131] In untreated patients and in those receiving small daily oral doses of calcitriol, bone biopsy evidence of secondary hyperparathyroidism is found when serum intact PTH levels are above 250 to 300 pg/mL (25 to 30 pmol/L). In contrast, values in patients with adynamic lesions are usually below 150 pg/mL (15 pmol/L), and levels frequently fall below 100 pg/mL (10 pmol/L). Both in children and in adults with chronic renal failure, intact serum PTH levels that are two to three times the upper limit of normal generally correspond to normal rates of bone formation as documented by bone biopsy.[41, 131]

Despite their superiority over the older radioimmunoassays, some evidence indicates that several immunoradiometric assays for PTH detect peptide fragments that are not the full-length 84–amino acid hormone[132–134] (see Chapter 70). The N-terminally truncated PTH molecules may be as much as 50% of what is measured as PTH by several immunoradiometric assays, especially under conditions of induced hypercalcemia.[135] Because the large fragment is not believed to be biologically active, its detection as intact PTH could be misleading and lead to excessive suppression of PTH in renal failure patients.[135]

Plasma Aluminum

Several investigators have shown that plasma aluminum levels are elevated both in patients with chronic renal failure and in those receiving treatment with maintenance dialysis.[53, 54, 136–138] Substantial differences exist in the normal values reported from different laboratories.[139] Electrothermic atomic absorption spectroscopy provides the most accurate method of measurement of aluminum levels in both plasma and tissues, and normal values are always below 10 μg/L, whereas dialysis patients without any exposure to aluminum usually have serum aluminum levels of 15 to 30 μg/L.[140] Plasma aluminum levels probably reflect a recent load of aluminum, either from dialysate contaminated with aluminum or from the ingestion of aluminum-containing phosphate-binding agents.[53, 54, 136] Plasma aluminum concentrations do not provide a close prediction of tissue stores of aluminum,[141] but infusion of deferoxamine results in a substantial elevation in plasma aluminum levels in patients with aluminum-related bone disease.[142] The deferoxamine infusion test is performed as follows: patients receive a standardized intravenous dose of deferoxamine (40 mg/kg dissolved in 100 mL of 5% dextrose solution) infused for 2 hours immediately after a hemodialysis procedure. Plasma aluminum levels are measured before and 24 to 48 hours after the infusion.[142] Increments in plasma aluminum levels after the administration of deferoxamine more closely predict the total bone aluminum content than does the basal plasma concentration of aluminum.[142] Malluche et al. found that the results of the deferoxamine infusion test were not specific in all cases,[143] and Hodsman et al. noted that dialysis patients with secondary hyperparathyroidism exhibited a substantial increment in plasma aluminum after the infusion of deferoxamine.[144] Moreover, Pei et al. conducted an extensive survey of the value of the deferoxamine infusion test in the diagnosis of aluminum-related bone disease.[61] Bone biopsies, the deferoxamine infusion test, and measurements of intact PTH were carried out in 259 patients, 142 undergoing peritoneal dialysis and 117 undergoing hemodialysis, selected from 445 patients at three large dialysis centers in Toronto. An increment in serum aluminum of 100 μg/L or more had a positive predictive value of 75% for aluminum bone disease in peritoneal dialysis patients and 88% in hemodialysis patients, but the sensitivity was only 10% and 37%, respectively. The best results were found when they combined the deferoxamine test, using an increment of 150 μg/L or more, with an intact PTH concentration of 200 pg/mL or less. When both markers were used, a 95% to 100% positive predictive value for aluminum bone disease was achieved in the groups of hemodialysis and peritoneal dialysis patients; the sensitivity was 53% and 39%, respectively. However, when patients had been withdrawn from therapy with aluminum gels for more than 6 months, the sensitivity and specificity of the test decreased substantially. In such patients, a bone biopsy may be needed to identify the presence of aluminum-related bone disease.[73]

RADIOLOGIC CHARACTERISTICS OF RENAL OSTEODYSTROPHY

Radiographic Features of Osteitis Fibrosa Cystica

The most consistent radiographic feature of secondary hyperparathyroidism is the presence of subperiosteal erosions.[93, 126, 145] The degree of subperiosteal erosion can correlate with serum PTH and alkaline phosphatase levels, but radiographs can be normal in patients with moderate to severe histologic features of osteitis fibrosa cystica on bone biopsy.[146]

In pediatric patients, metaphyseal changes (i.e., growth zone lesions that are termed "rickets-like lesions") are common.[93] These findings are best detected by hand radiographs. Several techniques are used to enhance the sensitivity of hand radiographs. Meema et al. use fine-grain films and then magnify them sixfold to sevenfold with a hand lens.[147] Direct-magnification radiographs are also used.[147]

Subperiosteal erosions also occur in the distal ends of clavicles, on the surface of the ischium and pubis, at the sacroiliac joints, and at the junction of the metaphysis and diaphysis of long bones.[145, 146] Subperiosteal erosions can also be found in patients with aluminum-related bone disease.[148] This finding represents the residual of earlier hyperparathyroidism with osteitis fibrosa cystica; however, because of aluminum toxicity, remineralization and normalization of the skeletal radiograph could not occur when the secondary hyperparathyroidism was reversed by treatment with either vitamin D sterols or parathyroidectomy.[148]

Radiographic abnormalities of the skull in secondary hyperparathyroidism can include (1) a diffuse "ground-glass" appearance, (2) a generalized mottled or granular appearance, (3) focal radiolucencies, and (4) focal sclerosis.

In children with renal failure, abnormalities of the growth zone are common.[93] The radiographic changes arising from secondary hyperparathyroidism are difficult to differentiate from true rachitic abnormalities; however, Mehls et al. demonstrated that the histologic features of slipped epiphyses in uremic children are those of osteitis fibrosa cystica and that the radiographic features differ from those of rickets resulting from vitamin D deficiency.[94]

Radiographic Features of Osteomalacia

The radiographic features of osteomalacia are both less specific and less common than those of secondary hyperparathyroidism. Typical rachitic lesions, with widening of the epiphyseal growth plate and other deformities, can occur in children with open epiphyses.[93] Looser's zones or pseudofractures, the only pathognomonic radiographic features of osteomalacia in adult patients, are rare in renal patients with osteomalacia; they occur as straight, wide bands of radiolucency that are perpendicular to the long axis of the bone.[149] Fractures, particularly of the ribs, vertebral bodies, and hips, are more common in patients with osteomalacia than in patients with osteitis fibrosa cystica or mixed osteodystrophy.[150] Another common radiographic feature present in patients with advanced renal failure is a decrease in bone density, which may arise from secondary hyperparathyroidism, osteomalacia, or osteoporosis.[151] Paradoxically, localized osteosclerosis is quite common in patients with renal failure and more frequent in patients with osteitis fibrosa cystica.

Bone Scan

Scintiscan of bone using technetium 99–labeled diphosphonate can be used to detect and judge the severity of skeletal disease in patients with advanced renal failure.[152] Also, the response to a specific treatment can be monitored by bone scan.[153] In one study, scintiscans were abnormal in 13 of 14 dialysis patients, with symmetrically increased activity over the skull, mandible, sternum, shoulders, vertebrae, and distal aspects of the femur and tibia. Osteitis fibrosa cystica is usually manifested by symmetrical increases in the uptake of diphosphonate by the axial skeleton and around the epiphyseal areas of the long bones, an appearance resulting in the so-called super scan. A diffuse decrease in uptake is common in patients with osteomalacia.[153] However, Hodson et al. compared bone scans and bone histology and concluded that bone scans did not provide useful information on the severity and type of renal osteodystrophy.[154] On the other hand, Karsenty et al. demonstrated differentiation in uptake by bone scan between patients with osteitis fibrosa cystica and those with osteomalacia secondary to aluminum intoxication.[155] No differentiation in uptake was seen in patients with mixed lesions. The scintiscan can also be used to detect nondisplaced fractures (pseudofractures) in the ribs and elsewhere in patients with osteomalacia.[93] At the present time, the bone scan can be used as a noninvasive diagnostic method to establish the severity or precise type of bone disease in certain, but not all patients and to detect ectopic calcifications. Bone biopsies are still needed, however, to delineate the histologic type of renal osteodystrophy in many cases.

TREATMENT OF RENAL OSTEODYSTROPHY

The specific aims of the management of renal osteodystrophy are (1) to maintain blood levels of serum calcium and phosphorus near normal limits, (2) to prevent hyperplasia of the parathyroid glands and to maintain serum PTH at levels corresponding to the appropriate indices of bone remodeling, (3) to avoid the development of extraskeletal calcifications, and (4) to prevent or reverse the accumulation of toxic substances such as aluminum and β_2-microglobulin.

Dietary Manipulation of Calcium and Phosphorus

In patients with advanced renal failure, a substantial increase in calcium intake, usually by adding calcium salts, is useful for two reasons. First, calcium salts, either calcium carbonate or calcium acetate, are effective and safe when used as phosphate-binding agents in patients with end-stage renal disease,[156] and second, calcium supplements are often indicated because of impaired calcium absorption and suboptimal calcium intake by most patients with end-stage renal disease.[17] As a result of their reduced ingestion of dairy products, dietary calcium intake can be as low as 400 to 700 mg/day in patients with renal failure.[17] Furthermore, studies of net intestinal calcium absorption indicate that a neutral or positive calcium balance can be achieved when dietary calcium is increased to above 1.5 μg/day with calcium carbonate, calcium citrate, or calcium lactate.[156]

Long-term treatment with large doses of calcium supplements has been shown to reduce the incidence of erosive lesions of bone, fractures, and episodes of extraskeletal calcification.[157] On the other hand, treatment with oral calcium did not restore a normal "calcification front" to bone biopsies when compared with the effect of vitamin D.[158] Calcium supplements should be used with caution when serum phosphorus levels are above 7.5 to 8.0 mg/dL. This admonition is particularly appropriate when serum calcium levels are in the normal range inasmuch as one wants to avoid hypercalcemia with an increment in the Ca × P product and thereby predispose to extraskeletal calcification. In addition, Block et al. demonstrated that an elevated Ca × P product is associated with an increased risk of mortality in patients undergoing maintenance dialysis.[104] Mild hypercalcemia (10.5–11.0 mg/dL) is usually associated with no symptoms,[138] but attention should be paid to the presence of severe pruritus.[159] In addition, nausea, anorexia, vomiting, mental confusion, and lethargy can occur when serum calcium levels are high.

Control of hyperphosphatemia is important for the prevention of soft tissue calcifications and secondary hyperparathyroidism, as well as mortality.[104] Dietary phosphorus is derived primarily from meat and dairy products, and phosphorus intake commonly ranges from 1.0 to 1.8 μg/day in normal adults in the United States and Western Europe.

To prevent hyperphosphatemia, dietary intake of phosphorus should be reduced below 1000 mg/day in patients with mild to moderate renal failure by limiting the intake of dairy products. The ingestion of a highly restricted phosphate diet (e.g., <600 mg/day) would be useful, but such a diet is unpalatable, particularly to patients who are accustomed to the typical high protein diet consumed in the United States. For these reasons, phosphate-binding agents must be given to most patients with advanced renal failure and those treated with maintenance dialysis.

Phosphate-Binding Agents

In the past, the aluminum-containing phosphate-binding agents aluminum hydroxide and aluminum carbonate have been the primary drugs used to control hyperphosphatemia in patients with advanced renal failure and those treated with dialysis.[1] It is now recognized, however, that the intake of aluminum-containing gels is a major risk factor for the development of aluminum intoxication, particularly that causing osteomalacia and other low-turnover states.[49, 51–54] Therefore, at present several calcium-containing compounds, calcium carbonate, calcium acetate, and calcium citrate, have been used to reduce intestinal phosphorus absorption.

Calcium carbonate is one of the most commonly used compounds and is given to approximately 70% to 80% of adult and pediatric dialysis patients. Calcium carbonate should be ingested together with a meal, both to maximize phosphate-binding efficiency and to minimize absorption of calcium. The required dosage of calcium carbonate varies from patient to patient, but the initial dose ranges from 4 to 7 g/day and can be adjusted by age according to subsequent serum levels of phosphorus.[138, 160, 161] The other forms of calcium salts, calcium acetate and calcium citrate, have also been shown to be effective phosphate-binding agents. When the efficacy and side effects of calcium acetate were compared with those of calcium carbonate in patients treated with maintenance hemodialysis, however, Schaefer et al. did not find major advantages for either compound.[162]

Hypercalcemia is the major side effect associated with the long-term use of calcium salts with or without vitamin D therapy. The use of dialysate solutions with the level of calcium reduced has proved to be of value in patients treated by hemodialysis[163] and in patients undergoing peritoneal dialysis.[164]

Recently, sevelamar (RenaGel), a hydrogel of cross-linked polyallylamine that is an effective phosphate-binding agent containing neither calcium nor aluminum, has been introduced.[165, 166] Its efficacy has been shown in studies carried out only in patients undergoing hemodialysis. This new compound has been found to be an effective phosphate-binding agent that results in a reduction in serum PTH levels without causing changes in serum calcium levels. In addition, serum cholesterol and low-density lipoprotein cholesterol levels decreased during therapy.[167] Thus the diminished calcium load and changes in the lipid pattern may have potential important implications in the prevention of vascular and soft tissue calcification in patients treated with long-term hemodialysis.

Discontinuation of the use of aluminum-containing phosphate-binding agents has been recommended, but such agents are still required in a small proportion (10%–20%) of patients. Although guidelines for the safe use of aluminum hydroxide have been proposed,[54, 168] when the recommended doses for pediatric patients were prospectively evaluated, they were associated with progressive increases in the body burden of aluminum.[169] Thus aluminum-containing drugs should be avoided in the vast majority of patients with renal failure. If these agents are to be used, great caution should be taken with the combined use of aluminum-containing gels and agents that enhance aluminum absorption, among which the most important is citrate, as either citric acid or various citrate salts.[170] Other sources of citrate should be avoided in advanced renal failure as well. Thus although calcium citrate may be an effective phosphate-binding agent,[142] it should be avoided because of the potential risk of aluminum intoxication if aluminum gels are coincidentally ingested. Other drugs commonly ingested by patients with gastric discomfort contain citric acid, such as Alka-Seltzer, and increase the risk for aluminum intoxication.

Active Vitamin D Sterols

Despite dietary phosphate restriction, the intake of phosphate-binding agents, the use of an appropriate level of calcium in dialysate solution, and an adequate intake of calcium, severe and progressive osteitis fibrosa cystica develops in a significant number of uremic patients. Adequate treatment with an active vitamin D sterol can control progression of the bone disease in patients with overt secondary hyperparathyroidism. Serum PTH levels have been used as surrogates for diagnosis of the different subtypes of renal osteodystrophy and to monitor response to vitamin D therapy. Although many patients with renal insufficiency will require vitamin D therapy, target PTH levels are different for patients with stable renal failure than for those treated with maintenance dialysis. Indeed, serum PTH levels between 150 and 200 pg/mL are associated with skeletal lesions of secondary hyperparathyroidism in adult and pediatric patients with stable chronic renal failure.[171] By contrast, such values correspond to low-turnover bone lesions in patients undergoing maintenance dialysis.[41, 123, 172] Moreover, the schedule of vitamin D administration, daily vs. intermittent, should be taken into consideration in patients receiving dialysis.[85] As listed above and reviewed in Chapter 70, the heterogeneity of PTH even with immunoradiometric assays may contribute to low bone turnover by inadvertent excessive supression.[135]

Although calcifediol, or 25-hydroxyvitamin D, 1α-hydroxyvitamin D_3, and dihydrotachysterol have all proved to be effective in the management of secondary hyperparathyroidism, calcitriol is by far the most widely used agent in the United States.

The efficacy of daily oral doses of calcitriol for the treatment of patients with symptomatic renal osteodystrophy has been documented in several clinical trials.[173, 174] Bone pain diminishes, muscle strength and gait-posture improve, and osteitis fibrosa frequently resolves either partially or completely.[86] When measured by reliable assays, serum PTH levels decrease in patients who respond favorably to treatment. Growth velocity has been reported to increase during calcitriol therapy in some children with severe bone disease,[97] but other investigators have failed to find improvement in growth velocity.[98]

Similar findings have been reported in patients treated with daily doses of oral 1α-hydroxyvitamin D_3 (alfacalcidol), which undergoes 25-hydroxylation in the liver to form calcitriol[175, 176], this agent is widely used in Europe, Japan, and Canada. Calcitriol and 1α-hydroxyvitamin D_3 are similarly effective for the treatment of secondary hyperparathyroidism in patients with chronic renal failure. Doses of oral calcitriol in most clinical trials have ranged from 0.25 to 1.5 μg/day. Hypercalcemia is the most common side effect, but most adult patients tolerate daily doses of 0.25 to 0.50 μg/day without marked increases in serum calcium levels; children may require somewhat larger daily oral doses of calcitriol.

Treatment is started with small doses, which are periodically adjusted to maintain serum calcium levels between 10.0 and 10.5 mg/dL; such an approach lowers serum PTH levels in many patients.[177] Because the biologic half-life of calcitriol is relatively short, episodes of hypercalcemia resolve within several days after treatment is withheld.

The development of hypercalcemia during calcitriol therapy may predict the underlying type of skeletal lesion. When hypercalcemia occurs after several months of treatment and previously elevated serum PTH and alkaline phosphatase levels have returned toward normal, it is likely that osteitis fibrosa has substantially resolved. In contrast, hypercalcemia that occurs within the first several weeks of treatment suggests the presence of either low-turnover bone disease, which in some cases is due to bone aluminum deposition, or severe secondary hyperparathyroidism.[86] Bone biopsy and measurements of bone aluminum content are needed to exclude aluminum-related bone disease. If evidence of autonomous hyperparathyroidism is found, parathyroidectomy may be required.

In adult hemodialysis patients, intravenous administration of calcitriol three times weekly effectively lowers serum PTH levels.[178] A portion of this response appears to be independent of changes in serum ionized calcium, thus suggesting that calcitriol directly reduces PTH synthesis and/or release.[178] Intravenous calcitriol is now the most widely used approach for the treatment of secondary hyperparathyroidism in patients undergoing regular hemodialysis. Advantages of intravenous calcitriol include ensured patient compliance, convenience of therapy because doses are given during regularly scheduled hemodialysis treatments, and the ability to achieve high serum levels of 1,25-dihydroxyvitamin D after bolus intravenous injections.[179] Despite these theoretic considerations, when the intravenous route of calcitriol was compared with the oral route given intermittently, similar reductions in serum PTH levels were observed.[180] As with intermittent oral calcitriol therapy, the rise in serum calcium levels during treatment with three-times-weekly doses of intravenous calcitriol appears to be less than with daily oral doses of calcitriol; thus larger amounts of 1,25-$(OH)_2D_3$ can be given each week, which may enhance delivery of calcitriol to the parathyroid glands and promote the suppressive effect of 1,25-dihydroxyvitamin D on PTH secretion.[179]

Use of the intravenous form of calcitriol is impractical for patients receiving maintenance peritoneal dialysis; therefore, large intermittent doses of oral calcitriol have also been used to treat secondary hyperparathyroidism in those patients.[181, 182] When given two or three times per week, the cumulative weekly dose of calcitriol is greater, and higher peak serum levels of 1,25-dihydroxyvitamin D are achieved after each dose. As such, large intermittent oral doses of calcitriol may be more effective than smaller daily oral doses for reducing PTH gene transcription and lowering serum PTH levels in patients with secondary hyperparathyroidism. Dosage regimens have ranged from 0.5 to 1.0 μg to 3.5 to 4.0 μg three times weekly or 2.0 to 5.0 μg twice weekly; low doses should be used initially, and dosage adjustments must be based on frequent measurements of serum calcium and phosphorus levels.

Most clinical trials have used reductions in serum PTH levels as an index of efficacy during treatment with active vitamin D sterols in patients with secondary hyperparathyroidism. Although serum PTH levels generally correspond to the severity of osseous changes associated with secondary hyperparathyroidism in untreated patients and in those receiving small daily oral doses of calcitriol, similar relationships may not apply during treatment with larger intermittent doses of vitamin D sterols given twice or three times weekly.[62] Bone formation and turnover may fall dramatically during intermittent calcitriol therapy, and adynamic renal osteodystrophy develops in a substantial proportion of patients.[62, 85] In some patients, adynamic lesions are seen with marked reductions in basal serum PTH levels, but PTH values remain substantially elevated in others in the face of subnormal rates of bone formation.[62] Such findings suggest that large intermittent doses of calcitriol diminish osteoblastic activity directly and lower bone formation and turnover by PTH-independent mechanisms. Accordingly, serum PTH levels should be monitored regularly during intermittent calcitriol therapy, and the dose of calcitriol should be lowered when serum PTH levels fall to values four to five times the upper limit of normal to reduce the risk of adynamic bone. Immunoradiometric assays that detect only intact PTH and not the N-terminally truncated variant may help in this monitoring.[135]

Increases in serum calcium and phosphorus levels often limit the dose of calcitriol that can be given to patients with end-stage renal disease. Several newer vitamin D analogues, however, have been shown to effectively lower serum PTH levels with only minor increases in serum calcium concentration in patients with renal secondary hyperparathyroidism.[183] As such, 1α-hydroxyvitamin D_2 and 19-*nor*-1α,25-dihydroxyvitamin D_2 may provide wider margins of safety than calcitriol does when treating patients with overt renal secondary hyperparathyroidism. Whether these compounds diminish osteoblastic activity and lower bone formation in a manner similar to that observed during intermittent calcitriol therapy remains to be determined. Moreover, combined use of these new vitamin D analogues and the calcium-aluminum–free phosphate-binding agent (RenaGel) may have important implications in the long-term management of secondary hyperparathyroidism in patients treated with maintenance dialysis.

Novel therapeutic agents called "calcimimetics" are also being developed[184]; these compounds activate the CaSR, with subsequent prompt reductions in PTH release from the parathyroid glands. Serum PTH levels fall within 1 to 2 hours after drug administration.[185, 186] In contrast to the response to vitamin D sterols, serum calcium concentrations decline rather than increase as PTH-mediated calcium release from bone diminishes. Although not yet available for clinical use, calcimimetic agents may in the future permit clinicians to diminish PTH secretion more reliably and to more precisely regulate serum PTH levels in patients with secondary hyperparathyroidism caused by chronic renal failure.

Parathyroidectomy

Certain features of secondary hyperparathyroidism indicate a need for parathyroid surgery. The presence of hyperplasia and/or hypertrophy of the parathyroid glands should be documented by the presence of biochemical and radiographic features and, if necessary, the findings of osteitis fibrosa cystica on bone biopsy. Recent data reviewed in Chapter 79 suggest that in many cases when parathyroid surgery is needed and undertaken, the tumor has become monoclonal, that is, growth autonomous, which explains the intractability to medical therapy. Indications for parathyroid surgery include elevated serum PTH levels within the context of at least one or more of the following criteria: (1) persistent hypercalcemia (serum calcium levels between 11.5 and 12.0 mg/dL), particularly when symptomatic; (2) intractable pruritus that does not respond to dialysis or other medical treatment; (3) progressive extraskeletal calcifications when the Ca × P product in serum exceeds 75 to 80 mg/dL despite appropriate phosphate restriction; (4) severe skeletal pain or fractures; and (5) the appearance of calciphylaxis. Algorithms that provide guidelines for deciding whether to pursue parathyroid surgery are given in Figure 86–8. Persistent hypercalcemia in patients receiving low doses of calcitriol can occur in patients with aluminum-related bone disease[187]; therefore, the presence of aluminum toxicity must be excluded before parathyroid surgery. Other causes of hypercalcemia such as sarcoidosis, malignancy-related hypercalcemia, intake of calcium supplements, and the presence of adynamic/aplastic bone lesions not related to aluminum should also be considered.[79]

When a decision to perform parathyroid surgery has been made, it is essential to avoid a marked postoperative fall in serum calcium levels caused by the "hungry bone" syndrome. Because of the severity of the bone disease, this fall can be much more marked and more prolonged than that after parathyroidectomy for primary hyperparathyroidism. Renal patients should receive oral calcitriol, 0.5 to 1.0 μg, or intravenous calcitriol, 1.5 to 2.0 μg, per hemodialysis treatment for 2 to 6 days before parathyroid surgery to stimulate intestinal calcium absorption during the postoperative period and maximize the effectiveness of oral calcium salts. After surgery, serum calcium and potassium levels should be monitored every 8 to 12 hours and serum phosphorus and magnesium measured daily. By 24 to 36 hours after surgery, marked hypocalcemia with serum calcium levels below 7 to 8 mg/dL can develop; this condition can be associated with serious symptoms, including major seizures with fractures and tendon avulsion. For reasons that are not certain, these seizures most often occur during the last 1 to 2 hours of a hemodialysis procedure or immediately thereafter. To reduce the risk of this serious problem, an infusion containing calcium gluconate should be given when the serum calcium concentration falls below 7.5 to 8.0 mg/dL. The initial calcium gluconate should be given to provide 100 mg of calcium ion per hour and the infusion continued for at least 48 to 74 hours according to the magnitude of the hypocalcemia. Serum calcium should be measured every 4 to 6 hours; the calcium gluconate infusion should be increased if the serum calcium level continues to fall, and the infusion rate could be 200 mg/hr or higher. Recommended doses of infused calcium have also been based on the degree of preoperative elevation in serum alkaline phosphatase [188] or the size of the parathyroid glands found at surgery.[73] Oral calcium carbonate in doses as high as 1.0 g Ca given four to six times daily is often needed, and oral calcitriol in doses of 1.0 to 2.0 μg/day or even higher should be added in patients with marked hypocalcemia. Simultaneous administration of intravenous calcitriol may be beneficial in diminishing the degree of hypocalcemia and the need for calcium salt infusions. The length of time that intravenous calcium is required varies greatly: most patients require it for only 2 to 3 days, but severe hypocalcemia can persist for several weeks or months, and a "permanent" central catheter may be needed for daily

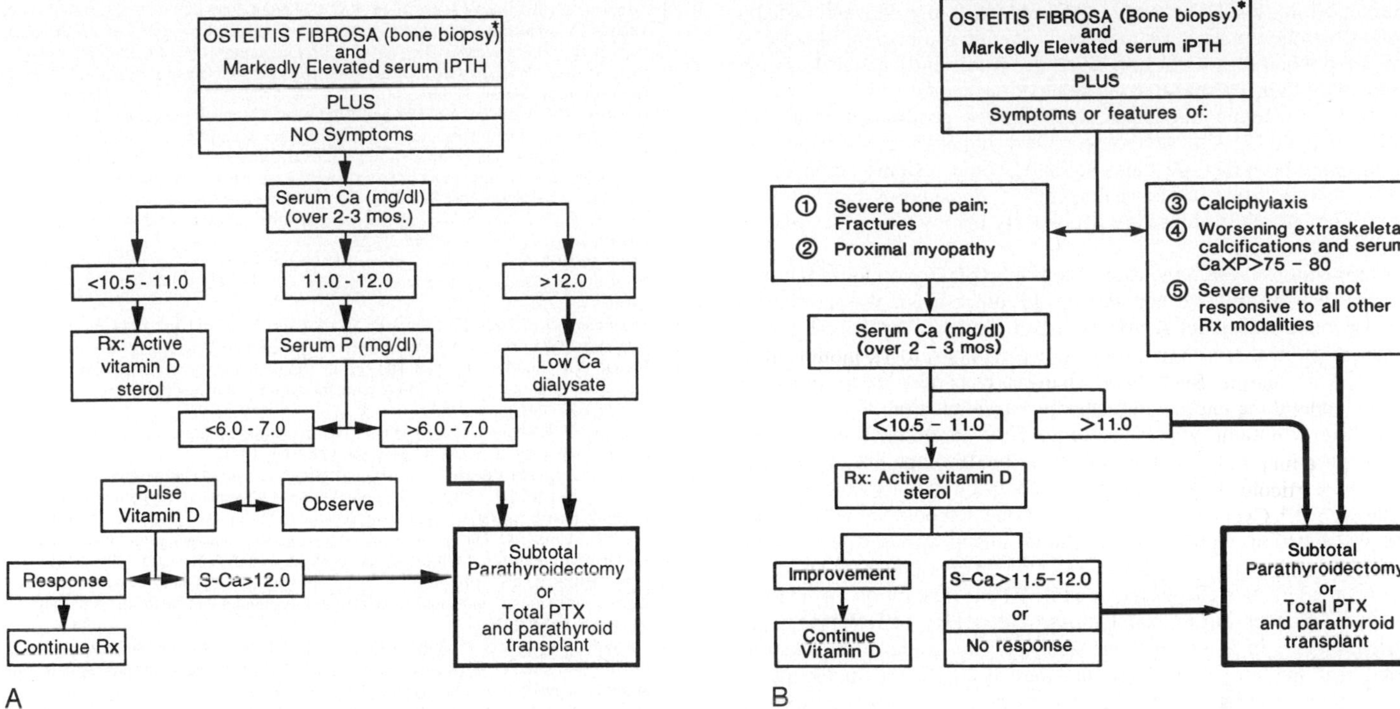

FIGURE 86–8. Algorithm showing an approach to a decision for parathyroidectomy in patients with end-stage renal disease. *A*, Patients with various symptoms of hyperparathyroidism; *B*, Patients without symptoms. *Aluminum-related bone disease must be excluded. iPTH, immunoreactive parathyroid hormone; PTX, parathyroidectomy.

home infusions of 800 to 1000 mg of calcium ion. When the serum calcium concentration begins to rise toward normal, intravenous calcium can be discontinued, the calcitriol treatment can be reduced or stopped, and the dosage of oral calcium can be adjusted to prevent hyperphosphatemia.

Serum phosphorus levels can fall to subnormal levels postoperatively; phosphate treatment will markedly aggravate the hypocalcemia, and patients should not be treated with phosphate unless serum phosphorus falls below 2.0 mg/dL. Therefore, serum phosphorus should be maintained between 3.5 and 4.0 mg/dL because of the risk of aggravating hypocalcemia. Calcium carbonate or calcium acetate should be the phosphate-binding agent of choice, and $Al(OH)_3$ should be avoided.[189, 190]

Management of Aluminum Intoxication

After the report of using deferoxamine for aluminum removal in dialysis patients,[191] several reports documented significant improvement in both symptoms and bone histology after long-term treatment in patients undergoing maintenance dialysis.[192–194] A substantial increase in the removal of aluminum is produced by both hemodialysis and CAPD after the administration of deferoxamine[195, 196]; this finding contrasts with the relatively small amount of aluminum removed during a standard dialysis procedure without deferoxamine.[195]

After 4 to 6 months of therapy with deferoxamine, substantial clinical improvement was observed in a large proportion of affected patients. The use of analgesics decreased, and patients who had been confined to bed or a wheelchair were able to walk without assistance.[192] The biochemical changes after treatment with deferoxamine included a decrease in serum calcium levels and a rise in serum alkaline phosphatase levels, observations that suggest increased mineralization of bone. Repeat bone biopsies have shown improvement in the bone formation rate and a significant reduction in surface staining for aluminum in most patients[194]; indeed, osteitis fibrosa cystica has developed in some patients. Responses to deferoxamine can be much less marked in patients who have undergone earlier parathyroidectomy.[192]

Although deferoxamine is well tolerated in most patients, a number of adverse reactions have been documented. Hypotension, skin rash and/or urticaria, headache, fever, abdominal pain, or diarrhea may occur within the first several hours after deferoxamine infusion. Changes in visual or auditory acuity can occur with both short-term and long-term therapy; these disturbances are often, but not always reversible on withdrawal of deferoxamine therapy.[197–199]

The most serious risk of therapy with deferoxamine in dialysis patients with aluminum or iron overload is the development of severe and fatal infections, particularly disseminated cerebral mucormycosis.[200] *Rhizopus* species have been well documented in patients receiving deferoxamine for the treatment of aluminum or iron overload.[201] The chelation of iron by deferoxamine enhances iron delivery to certain organisms, thereby increasing their pathogenic potential.[202–204] Therefore, therapy with deferoxamine should be recommended only to patients with severe, life-threatening manifestations of aluminum toxicity.

If deferoxamine is absolutely required, the dose should be limited to 0.250 to 1.0 g every 7 to 10 days, and plasma aluminum levels should be measured regularly. In asymptomatic patients with aluminum deposition in bone, bone histology and bone formation can improve solely by withdrawing therapy with aluminum-containing medications and using calcium carbonate to control serum phosphorus levels.[205]

BONE DISEASE AFTER RENAL TRANSPLANTATION

Successful kidney transplantation corrects many of the abnormalities associated with renal osteodystrophy, but disorders of bone and mineral metabolism remain a major problem in such patients. Several factors have been implicated in the development of bone disease after organ transplantation, including persistent secondary hyperparathyroidism, prolonged immobilization, graft function, and most importantly, use of the different immunosuppressive agents.

Hypercalcemia is not uncommon after renal transplantation. During the first several months it can be quite severe, and patients with severe secondary hyperparathyroidism before renal transplantation are at greatest risk. More often, hypercalcemia may be less severe, with serum calcium levels between 10.5 and 12.0 mg/dL, and usually resolves within the first 12 months.[206] Parathyroidectomy should be considered when serum calcium levels are persistently above 12.5 mg/dL for more than 1 year after transplantation.[207]

Hypophosphatemia may occur early in the posttransplant period, mainly in patients with severe secondary hyperparathyroidism. The clinical manifestations are quite variable; some patients complain of malaise, fatigue, and muscle weakness.[208–210] Phosphorus supplementation is required when values are persistently below 2.0 mg/dL, mainly in pediatric patients.

Osteopenia is common after renal transplantation in adult patients[208–210]; bone mineral content, on the other hand, was normal in pediatric renal transplant recipients when corrected by height age.[211] Decreases in bone mass have been shown within 6 to 18 months after renal transplantation. Such bone changes have also been found in patients undergoing cardiac and hepatic transplantation.[212]

The use of immunosuppressive drugs after transplantation has been considered a major contributing factor to the development of osteopenia. Glucocorticoid directly inhibits osteoblastic activity and collagen synthesis.[213, 214] Cyclosporine increases bone remodeling with reductions in cancellous bone volume without changes in serum calcium, magnesium, calcitriol, or PTH in rats.[214] Furthermore, Stewart et al. demonstrated that cyclosporine inhibited bone resorption in a dose-dependent manner during incubations with PTH, $1,25(OH)_2D_3$, and interleukin-1.[215] In a retrospective analysis, Landmenn et al. demonstrated that the use of cyclosporine may decrease the incidence of osteonecrosis in renal transplant recipients because of the use of lower doses of prednisone with the present immunosuppressive regimens.[216]

Osteonecrosis, or avascular necrosis, is by far the most debilitating skeletal complication associated with organ transplantation. In approximately 15% of patients osteonecrosis will develop within 3 years of renal transplantation.[217, 218] The occurrence of osteonecrosis in inpatients after cardiac, hepatic, and bone marrow transplantation suggests that glucocorticoids play a critical role in the pathogenesis of this disorder.[219, 220]

The effect of the combined use of prednisone and cyclosporine on bone mass has been evaluated after liver-related kidney transplants in 18 adult patients.[221] Such data demonstrated a loss of bone mass during the first 6 months after transplantation, and bone density values remained low during the 18 months of follow-up. Growth retardation persists in the vast majority of pediatric kidney recipients with normal graft function; although the prednisone dosage has been implicated, the previous subtype of renal osteodystrophy and the growth hormone/IGF-1 system may also have a role.

Therapeutic agents that prevent bone loss after renal transplantation have yet to be carefully evaluated. Synthetic compound derivatives of prednisolone, such as deflazacort, appear to have fewer adverse effects on bone and mineral metabolism.[222, 223] Bisphosphonates such as pamidronate and alendronate diminish bone resorption by lowering osteoclastic activity in bone, but their efficacy in preserving bone mass after renal transplantation awaits further clinical trial.

REFERENCES

1. Coburn JW, Slatopolsky E: Vitamin D, parathyroid hormone, and renal osteodystrophy. *In* Brenner B, Rector F (eds): The Kidney. Philadelphia, WB Saunders, 1986, pp 1657–1729.
2. Sherrard DJ, Ott SM, Maloney NA, et al: Uremic osteodystrophy: Classification, cause and treatment. *In* Frame B, Potts J (eds): Clinical Disorders of Bone and Mineral Metabolism. Amsterdam, Excerpta Medica, 1983, pp 254–259.
3. Salusky IB, Goodman WG: Growth hormone and calcitriol as modifiers of bone formation in renal osteodystrophy. Kidney Int 48:657–665, 1995.
4. Goodman WG, Belin TR, Salusky IB: In vivo assessments of calcium-regulated parathyroid hormone release in secondary hyperparathyroidism. Kidney Int 50:1834–1844, 1996.
5. Coburn JW, Slatopolsky E: Vitamin D, parathyroid hormone, and the renal osteodystrophies. *In* Brenner B, Rector F (eds): The Kidney. Philadelphia, WB Saunders, 1990, p 2076.
6. Fraser DR, Kodicek E: Unique biosynthesis by kidney of a biologically active vitamin D metabolite. Nature 228:764–776, 1970.
7. Gray R, Boyle I, DeLuca HF: Vitamin D metabolism: The role of kidney tissue. Science 172:1232–1234, 1971.
8. Norman AW, Midgett RJ, Myrtle JF, et al: Studies on calciferol metabolism. I. Production of vitamin D metabolite 4B from 25-OH-cholecalciferol by kidney homogenates. Biochem Biophys Res Commun 19:1082–1087, 1971.
9. Juttmann JR, Buurman CJ, De Kam E, et al: Serum concentrations of metabolites of vitamin D in patients with chronic renal failure (CRF). Consequences for the treatment with 1-alpha-hydroxy derivatives. Clin Endocrinol (Oxf) 14:225–236, 1981.
10. Cheung AK, Manolagas SC, Catherwood BD: Determinants of serum $1,25(OH)_2D$ levels in renal disease. Kidney Int 24:104–109, 1983.
11. Chesney RW, Hamstra AJ, Mazess RB, et al: Circulating vitamin D metabolite concentrations in childhood renal diseases. Kidney Int 21:65–69, 1982.
12. Silver J, Russell J, Sherwood LM: Regulation by vitamin D metabolites of messenger ribonucleic acid for preproparathyroid hormone in isolated bovine parathyroid cells. Proc Natl Acad Sci U S A 82:4270–4273, 1985.
13. Kilav R, Silver J, Naveh-Many T: Parathyroid hormone gene expression in hypophosphatemic rats. J Clin Invest 96:327–333, 1995.
14. Moallem E, Kilav R, Silver J, et al: RNA-protein binding and post-transcriptional regulation of parathyroid hormone gene expression by calcium and phosphate. J Biol Chem 273:5253–5259, 1998.
15. Brickman AS, Coburn JW, Massry SG, et al: 1,25-dihydroxyvitamin D_3 in normal man and patients with renal failure. Ann Intern Med 80:161–168, 1974.
16. Portale AA, Boothe BE, Tsai HC, et al: Reduced plasma concentration of 1,25-dihydroxy-vitamin D in children with moderate renal insufficiency. Kidney Int 21:627–632, 1982.
17. Coburn JW, Hartenbower DL, Massry SG: Intestinal absorption of calcium and the effect of renal insufficiency. Kidney Int 4:96–103, 1973.
18. Portale AA, Booth BE, Halloran BP, et al: Effect of dietary phosphorus on circulating concentrations of 1,25-dihydroxyvitamin D and immunoreactive parathyroid hormone in children with moderate renal insufficiency. J Clin Invest 73:1580–1589, 1984.
19. Llach F, Massry SG: On the mechanism of secondary hyperparathyroidism in moderate renal insufficiency. J Clin Endocrinol Metab 61:601–606, 1985.
20. Lopez-Hilker S, Dusso A, Rapp N, et al: Phosphorus restriction reverses hyperparathyroidism in uremia independent of changes in calcium and calcitriol. Am J Physiol 259:F432–F437, 1990.
21. Lucas PA, Brown RC, Woodhead JS, et al: 1,25-Dihydroxycholecalciferol and parathyroid hormone in advanced renal failure: Effect of simultaneous protein and phosphorus restriction. Clin Nephrol 25:7–10, 1986.
22. Schaefer K, Erley CM, von Herrath D, et al: Calcium salts of ketoacids as a new treatment strategy for uremic hyperphosphatemia. Kidney Int Suppl 27:136–139, 1989.
23. Horst RL, Littledike ET, Gray RW, et al: Impaired 24,25-dihydroxyvitamin D production in anephric man and pig. J Clin Invest 67:274–280, 1981.
24. Olgaard K, Finco D, Schwartz J, et al: Effect of $24,25(OH)_2D_3$ on PTH levels and bone histology in dogs with chronic uremia. Kidney Int 26:791–797, 1984.
25. Parfitt AM: The hyperparathyroidism of chronic renal failure: A disorder of growth. Kidney Int 52:3–9, 1997.
26. Lloyd HM, Parfitt AM, Jacobi JM, et al: The parathyroid glands in chronic renal failure: A study of their growth and other properties made on the basis of findings in patients with hypercalcemia. J Lab Clin Med 114:358–367, 1989.
27. Sanchez CP, Goodman WG, Ramirez JA, et al: Calcium-regulated parathyroid hormone secretion in adynamic renal osteodystrophy. Kidney Int 48:838–843, 1995.
28. Szabo A, Merke J, Beier E, et al: $1,25(OH)_2$ vitamin D_3 inhibits parathyroid cell proliferation in experimental uremia. Kidney Int 35:1049–1056, 1989.
29. Fukuda N, Tanaka H, Tominaga Y, et al: Decreased 1,25-dihydroxyvitamin D_3 receptor density is associated with a more severe form of parathyroid hyperplasia in chronic uremic patients. J Clin Invest 92:1436–1443, 1993.
30. DeFrancisco AM, Ellis HA, Owen JP, et al: Parathyroidectomy in chronic renal failure. Q J Med 55:289–315, 1985.
31. Arnold A, Brown MF, Urĕna P, et al: Monoclonality of parathyroid tumors in chronic renal failure and in primary parathyroid hyperplasia. J Clin Invest 95:2047–2053, 1995.
32. Kifor O, Moore FD Jr, Wang P, et al: Reduced immunostaining for the extracellular Ca^{2+}-sensing receptor in primary and uremic secondary hyperparathyroidism. J Clin Endocrinol Metab 81:1598–1606, 1996.
33. Farnebo F, Hoog A, Sandelin K, et al: Decreased expression of calcium-sensing receptor messenger ribonucleic acids in parathyroid adenomas. Surgery 124:1094–1098, 1998.
34. Brown AJ, Zhong M, Finch J, et al: Rat calcium-sensing receptor is regulated by vitamin D but not by calcium. Am J Physiol 270:F454–F460, 1996.
35. Rogers KV, Dunn CK, Conklin RL, et al: Calcium receptor messenger ribonucleic acid levels in the parathyroid glands and kidney of vitamin D–deficient rats are not regulated by plasma calcium or 1,25-dihydroxyvitamin D_3. Endocrinology 136:499–504, 1995.
36. Goodman WG, Veldhuis JD, Belin TR, et al: Calcium-sensing by parathyroid glands in secondary hyperparathyroidism. J Clin Endocrinol Metab 83:2765–2772, 1998.
37. Ramirez JA, Goodman WG, Gornbein J, et al: Direct in vivo comparison of calcium-regulated parathyroid hormone secretion in normal volunteers and patients with secondary hyperparathyroidism. J Clin Endocrinol Metab 76:1489–1494, 1993.
38. Brown EM, Wilson RE, Eastmen RC, et al: Abnormal regulation of parathyroid hormone release by calcium in secondary hyperparathyroidism due to chronic renal failure. J Clin Endocrinol Metab 54:172–179, 1982.
39. Messa P, Vallone C, Mioni G, et al: Direct in vivo assessment of parathyroid hormone–calcium relationship curve in renal patients. Kidney Int 46:1713–1720, 1994.
40. Massry SG, Coburn JW, Lee DBN, et al: Skeletal resistance to parathyroid hormone in renal failure. Ann Intern Med 78:357–364, 1973.
41. Quarles LD, Lobaugh B, Murphy G: Intact parathyroid hormone overestimates the presence and severity of parathyroid-mediated osseous abnormalities in uremia. J Clin Endocrinol Metab 75:145–150, 1992.
42. Cohen-Solal ME, Sebert JL, Boudailliez B, et al: Comparison of intact, midregion, and carboxy-terminal assays of parathyroid hormone for the diagnosis of bone disease in hemodialyzed patients. J Clin Endocrinol Metab 73:516–524, 1991.

43. Linkhart TA, Mohan S: Parathyroid hormone stimulated release of insulin-like growth factor I (IGF-I) and IGF-II from neonatal mouse calvaria in organ culture. Endocrinology 125:1484–1491, 1989.
44. Slatopolsky E, Caglar S, Pennell JP, et al: On the pathogenesis of hyperparathyroidism in chronic experimental renal insufficiency in the dog. J Clin Invest 50:492–499, 1971.
45. Denda M, Finch J, Slatopolsky E: Phosphorus accelerates the development of parathyroid hyperplasia and secondary hyperparathyroidism in rats with renal failure. Am J Kidney Dis 28:596–602, 1996.
46. Ward MK, Feest TG, Ellis HA, et al: Osteomalacic dialysis osteodystrophy: Evidence for a water-borne etiological agent, probably aluminum. Lancet 1:841–845, 1978.
47. Parkinson IS, Feest TG, Ward MK, et al: Fracturing dialysis osteodystrophy and dialysis encephalopathy: An epidemiological survey. Lancet 1:406–409, 1979.
48. Pierides AM, Edwards WG Jr, Cullu US Jr, et al: Hemodialysis encephalopathy with osteomalacic fractures and muscle weakness. Kidney Int 18:115–124, 1980.
49. Nathan E, Pederson SE: Dialysis encephalopathy in a non-dialysed uremic boy treated with aluminum hydroxide orally. Acta Paediatr Scand 69:793–796, 1980.
50. Felsenfeld AJ, Gutman RA, Llach F, et al: Osteomalacia in chronic renal failure: A syndrome previously reported only with maintenance dialysis. Am J Nephrol 2:147–154, 1982.
51. Griswold WR, Reznik V, Mendoza SA, et al: Accumulation of aluminum in a nondialyzed uremic child receiving aluminum hydroxide. Pediatrics 71:56–58, 1983.
52. Kaye M: Oral aluminum toxicity in a non-dialyzed patient with renal failure. Clin Nephrol 20:208–211, 1983.
53. Andreoli SP, Bergstein JM, Sherrard DJ: Aluminum intoxication from aluminum-containing phosphate binders in children with azotemia not undergoing dialysis. N Engl J Med 310:1079–1084, 1984.
54. Sedman AB, Miller NL, Warady BA, et al: Aluminum loading in children with chronic renal failure. Kidney Int 26:201–204, 1984.
55. Kaehny WD, Hegg P, Alfrey AC: Gastrointestinal absorption of aluminum from aluminum-containing antacids. N Engl J Med 296:1389–1390, 1977.
56. Ittel TH, Buddington B, Miller NL, et al: Enhanced gastrointestinal absorption of aluminum in uremic rats. Kidney Int 32:821–826, 1987.
57. Bakir AA, Hryhorczuk DO, Berman E, et al: Acute fatal hyperaluminemic encephalopathy in undialyzed and recently dialyzed uremic patients. Trans Am Soc Artif Intern Organs 32:171–176, 1986.
58. Norris KC, Crooks PW, Nebeker HG, et al: Clinical and laboratory features of aluminum-related bone disease: Differences between sporadic and "epidemic" forms of the syndrome. Am J Kidney Dis 6:342–347, 1985.
59. Salusky IB, Coburn JW, Brill J, et al: Bone disease in pediatric patients undergoing dialysis with CAPD or CCPD. Kidney Int 33:975–982, 1988.
60. Pei Y, Hercz G, Greenwood C, et al: Non-invasive prediction of aluminum bone disease in hemo- and peritoneal dialysis patients. Kidney Int 41:1374–1382, 1992.
61. Goodman WG, Ramirez JA, Belin TR, et al: Development of adynamic bone in patients with secondary hyperparathyroidism after intermittent calcitriol therapy. Kidney Int 46:1160–1166, 1994.
62. Atsumi K, Kushida K, Yamazaki K, et al: Risk factors for vertebral fractures in renal osteodystrophy. Am J Kidney Dis 33:287–293, 1999.
63. Braun J, Oldendorf M, Moshage W, et al: Electron beam computed tomography in the evaluation of cardiac calcifications in chronic dialysis patients. Am J Kidney Dis 27:394–401, 1996.
64. Kuizon BD, Goodman WG, Jüppner H, et al: Diminished linear growth during treatment with intermittent calcitriol and dialysis in children with chronic renal failure. Kidney Int 53:205–211, 1998.
65. Eastwood JB, Harris E, Stamp TCB, et al: Vitamin D deficiency in the osteomalacia of chronic renal failure. Lancet 2:1209–1211, 1976.
66. Howard GA, Baylink DJ: Matrix formation and osteoid maturation in vitamin D–deficient rats made normocalcemic by dietary means. Miner Electrolyte Metab 3:44–50, 1980.
67. Weinstein RS, Underwood JL, Hutson MS, et al: Bone histomorphometry in vitamin D–deficient rats infused with calcium and phosphorus. Am J Physiol 246:E499–E505, 1984.
68. Genuth SM, Klein L, Rabinovich S, et al: Osteomalacia accompanying chronic anticonvulsant therapy. J Clin Endocrinol Metab 35:378–378, 1972.
69. Jubiz W, Haussler MR, McCaw TA, et al: Plasma 1,25-dihydroxyvitamin D levels in patients receiving anticonvulsant drugs. J Clin Endocrinol Metab 44:617–617, 1977.
70. Pierides AM, Ellis HA, Ward M, et al: Barbiturate and anticonvulsant treatment in relation to osteomalacia with haemodialysis and renal transplantation. BMJ 1:190–193, 1976.
71. Hodgson SF: Skeletal remodeling and renal osteodystrophy. Semin Nephrol 6:42–55, 1986.
72. Norris KC, Goodman WG, Howard N, et al: The iliac crest bone biopsy for the diagnosis of aluminum toxicity and a guide to the use of deferoxamine. Semin Nephrol 6(suppl 1):27–34, 1986.
73. Sherrard DJ: Renal osteodystrophy. Semin Nephrol 6:56–67, 1986.
74. Sherrard DJ, Baylink DJ, Wergedal JE, et al: Quantitative histological studies on the pathogenesis of uremic bone disease. J Clin Endocrinol Metab 39:119–135, 1974.
75. Parfitt AM: The actions of parathyroid hormone on bone: Relation to bone remodeling and turnover, calcium homeostasis, and metabolic bone disease. IV. The state of the bones in uremic hyperparathyroidism—the mechanisms of skeletal resistance to PTH in renal failure and pseudohypoparathyroidism and the role of PTH in osteoporosis, osteopetrosis, and osteofluorosis. Metabolism 25:1157–1188, 1976.
76. Parfitt AM: The actions of parathyroid hormone on bone: Relation to bone remodeling and turnover, calcium homeostasis, and metabolic bone disease. I. Mechanisms of calcium transfer between blood and bone and their cellular basis: Morphologic and kinetic approaches to bone turnover. Metabolism 25:809–844, 1976.
77. Parfitt AM: The actions of parathyroid hormone on bone: Relation to bone remodeling and turnover, calcium homeostasis, and metabolic bone disease. II. PTH and bone cells: Bone turnover and plasma calcium regulation. Metabolism 25:909–955, 1976.
78. Parfitt AM: The actions of parathyroid hormone on bone: Relation to bone remodeling and turnover, calcium homeostasis, and metabolic bone disease. III. PTH and osteoblasts, the relationship between bone turnover and bone loss, and the state of the bones in primary hyperparathyroidism. Metabolism 25:1033–1068, 1976.
79. Malluche H, Faugere MC: Renal bone disease 1990: An unmet challenge for the nephrologist. Kidney Int 38:193–211, 1990.
80. Hruska KA, Teitelbaum SL: Renal osteodystrophy. N Engl J Med 333:166–174, 1995.
81. Ball JH, Garner A: Mineralization of woven bone in osteomalacia. J Pathol Bacteriol 91:563–567, 1966.
82. Bordier P, Rasmussen H, Marie P, et al: Vitamin D metabolites and bone mineralization in man. J Clin Endocrinol Metab 46:284–294, 1976.
83. Torres A, Lorenzo V, Hernandez D, et al: Bone disease in predialysis, hemodialysis, and CAPD patients: Evidence of a better bone response to PTH. Kidney Int 47:1434–1442, 1995.
84. Hernandez D, Concepcion MT, Lorenzo V, et al: Adynamic bone disease with negative aluminum staining in predialysis patients: Prevalence and evolution after maintenance dialysis. Nephrol Dial Transplant 9:517–523, 1994.
85. Salusky IB, Kuizon BD, Belin T, et al: Intermittent calcitriol therapy in secondary hyperparathyroidism: A comparison between oral and intraperitoneal administration. Kidney Int 54:907–914, 1998.
86. Ott SM, Maloney NA, Coburn JW, et al: The prevalence of bone aluminum deposition in renal osteodystrophy and its relation to the response to calcitriol therapy. N Engl J Med 307:709–713, 1982.
87. Noel LH, Zingraff J, Bardin T, et al: Tissue distribution of dialysis amyloidosis. Clin Nephrol 27:175–178, 1987.
88. Kleinman KS, Coburn JW: Amyloid syndromes associated with hemodialysis. Kidney Int 35:567–575, 1989.
89. Hampl H, Lobeck H, Bartel-Schwarze S, et al: Clinical, morphologic, biochemical, and immunohistochemical aspects of dialysis-associated amyloidosis. Trans Am Soc Artif Intern Organs 33:250–259, 1987.
90. Baker LR, Ackrill P, Cattell WR: Iatrogenic osteomalacia and myopathy due to phosphate depletion. BMJ 3:150–150, 1974.
91. Coburn JW, Nebeker HG, Hercz G, et al: Role of aluminum accumulation in the pathogenesis of renal osteodystrophy. *In* Robinson RR (ed): Nephrology, vol 2. New York, Springer-Verlag, 1984, pp 1383–1395.
92. Zanello SB, Collins ED, Marinissen MJ, et al: Vitamin D receptor expression in chicken muscle tissue and cultured myoblasts. Horm Metab Res 29:231–236, 1997.
93. Wright RS, Mehls O, Ritz E, et al: Musculoskeletal manifestation of chronic renal failure, dialysis and transplantation. *In* Bacon P, Hadler N (eds): Renal Manifestations in Rheumatic Disease. London, Butterworth, 1982, pp 352–352.
94. Mehls O, Ritz E, Krempien B, et al: Slipped epiphyses in renal osteodystrophy. Arch Dis Child 50:545, 1975.
95. Tonshoff B, Schaefer F, Mehls O: Disturbance of growth hormone insulin like growth factor axis in uremia. Pediatr Nephrol 4:654–662, 1990.
96. Betts PR, Magrath G: Growth pattern and dietary intake of children with chronic renal insufficiency. BMJ 2:189, 1974.
97. Chesney RW, Moorthy AV, Eisman JA, et al: Increased growth after long-term oral 1,25-vitamin D_3 in childhood renal osteodystrophy. N Engl J Med 298:238–242, 1978.
98. Bulla M, Delling G, Offermann G: Renal bone disorders in children: Therapy with vitamin D_3 or 1,25 dihydroxycholecalciferol. *In* Norman AW, Shaefer K, Herrath DV (eds): Basic Research and Its Clinical Application. Berlin, Walter de Gruyter, 1979, pp 853–853.
99. Conger JD, Hammond WS, Alfrey AC, et al: Pulmonary calcification in chronic dialysis patients. Clinical and pathologic studies. Ann Intern Med 83:330–336, 1975.
100. Milliner DS, Zinsmeister AR, Lieberman E, et al: Soft tissue calcification in pediatric patients with end-stage renal disease. Kidney Int 38:931–936, 1990.
101. Kuzela DC, Huffer WE, Conger JD, et al: Soft tissue calcification in chronic dialysis patients. Am J Clin Pathol 86:403–424, 1977.
102. Meema HE, Oreopoulos DG, DeVeber GA: Arterial calcification in severe chronic renal disease and their relationship to dialysis treatment, renal transplant and parathyroidectomy. Radiology 121:315–321, 1976.
103. Katz AI, Hampers CH, Merrill JP: Secondary hyperparathyroidism and renal osteodystrophy in chronic renal failure. Analysis of 195 patients with observations on the effects of chronic dialysis, kidney transplantation and subtotal parathyroidectomy. Medicine (Baltimore) 48:333–337, 1969.
104. Block GA, Hulbert-Shearon TE, Levin NW, et al: Association of serum phosphorus and calcium × phosphorus product with mortality risk in chronic hemodialysis patients: A national study. Am J Kidney Dis 31:607–617, 1998.
105. Ibels LS, Alfrey AC, Huffer WE, et al: Arterial calcification and pathology in uremic patients undergoing dialysis. Am J Med 66:790–796, 1979.
106. Gipstein RM, Coburn JW, Adams JA, et al: Calciphylaxis in man: A syndrome of tissue necrosis and vascular calcification in 11 patients with chronic renal failure. Arch Intern Med 136:1273–1280, 1976.
107. Bleyer AJ, Choi M, Igwemezie B, et al: A case control study of proximal calciphylaxis. Am J Kidney Dis 32:376–383, 1998.
108. Hafner J, Keusch G, Wahl C, et al: Uremic small-artery disease with medial calcification and intimal hyperplasia (so-called calciphylaxis): A complication of chronic renal failure and benefit from parathyroidectomy. J Am Acad Dermatol 33:954–962, 1999.
109. Goldsmith DJA: Calciphylaxis, thrombotic diathesis and defects in coagulation regulation. Nephrol Dial Transplant 12:1082–1083, 1997.
110. Bardin T, Kuntz D, Zingraff J, et al: Synovial amyloidosis in patients undergoing long-term hemodialysis. Arthritis Rheum 28:1052–1058, 1985.
111. Hou FF, Boyce J, Chertow GM, et al: Aminoguanidine inhibits advanced glycation end products formation on beta2 microglobulin. J Am Soc Nephrol 9:277–283, 1998.
112. Hou FF, Chertow GM, Kay J, et al: Interaction between beta 2-microglobulin and advanced glycation end products in the development of dialysis-related amyloidosis. Kidney Int 51:1514–1519, 1997.

113. Miyata T, Inagi R, Iida Y, et al: Involvement of β_2-microglobulin modified with advanced glycation end products in the pathogenesis of hemodialysis-associated amyloidosis. Induction of human monocyte chemotaxis and macrophage secretion of tumor necrosis factor-α and interleukin-1. J Clin Invest 93:521–528, 1994.
114. van Ypersele de Strihou CA, Jadoul M, Malghem J, et al: Effect of dialysis membrane and patient's age on signs of dialysis-related amyloidosis. Kidney Int 41:1012–1019, 1991.
115. McMahon LP, Radford J, Dawborn JK: Shoulder ultrasound in dialysis-related amyloidosis. Clin Nephrol 35:227–232, 1991.
116. Bindi P, Chanard J: Destructive spondyloarthropathy in dialysis patients: An overview. Nephron 55:104–109, 1990.
117. Goldman R, Bassett SH: Phosphorus excretion in renal failure. J Clin Invest 33:1623–1628, 1954.
118. Coburn JW, Popovtzer M, Massry SG, et al: The physiochemical state and renal handling of divalent ions in chronic renal failure. Arch Intern Med 124:302–311, 1969.
119. Fournier AE, Arnaud CD, Johnson WJ: Etiology of hyperparathyroidism and bone disease during chronic hemodialysis. II. Factors affecting serum immuno-reactive parathyroid hormone. J Clin Invest 50:599–599, 1971.
120. Alfrey AC, Miller NL, Butkus D: Evaluations of body magnesium stores. J Lab Clin Med 84:153–162, 1974.
121. Buccianti G, Bianchi ML, Valenti G: Progress of renal osteodystrophy during continuous ambulatory peritoneal dialysis. Clin Nephrol 22:279–283, 1984.
122. Nilsson P, Danielson BG, Grefberg N, et al: Secondary hyperparathyroidism in diabetic and nondiabetic patients on long-term continuous ambulatory peritoneal dialysis (CAPD). Scand J Urol Nephrol 19:59–65, 1985.
123. Salusky IB, Ramirez JA, Oppenheim WL, et al: Biochemical markers of renal osteodystrophy in pediatric patients undergoing CAPD/CCPD. Kidney Int 45:253–258, 1994.
124. Kurz P, Monier-Faugere MC, Bognar B, et al: Evidence for abnormal calcium homeostasis in patients with adynamic bone disease. Kidney Int 46:855–861, 1994.
125. Guillot AP, Hood VL, Runge CF, et al: The use of magnesium-containing phosphate binders in patients with end-stage renal disease on maintenance hemodialysis. Nephron 30:114–117, 1982.
126. Hruska KA, Teitelbaum SL, Kopelman R, et al: The predictability of the histological features of uremic bone disease by non-invasive techniques. Metab Bone Dis Relat Res 1:39–44, 1978.
127. van Renen MJ, Hogg RJ, Sweeney AL, et al: Accelerated growth in short children with chronic renal failure treated with both strict dietary therapy and recombinant growth hormone. Pediatr Nephrol 6:451–458, 1992.
128. Charhon SA, Delmas PD, Malaval L, et al: Serum bone Gla-protein in renal osteodystrophy: Comparison with bone histomorphometry. J Clin Endocrinol Metab 63:892–897, 1986.
129. Epstein S, Traberg H, Raja R, et al: Serum and dialysate osteocalcin levels in hemodialysis and peritoneal dialysis patients and after renal transplantation. J Clin Endocrinol Metab 60:1253–1256, 1985.
130. Hercz G, Coburn JW: Prevention of phosphate retention and hyperphosphatemia in uremia. Kidney Int Suppl 22:215–220, 1987.
131. Broman GE, Trotter M, Peterson RR: The density of selected bones of the human skeleton. Am J Phys Anthropol 16:197–211, 1958.
132. Brossard JH, Cloutier M, Roy L, et al: Accumulation of a non-(1–84) molecular form of parathyroid hormone (PTH) detected by intact PTH assay in renal failure: Importance in the interpretation of PTH values. J Clin Endocrinol Metab 81:3923–3929, 1996.
133. Lepage R, Roy L, Brossard JH, et al: A non-(1–84) circulating parathyroid hormone (PTH) fragment interferes significantly with intact PTH commercial assay measurements in uremic samples. Clin Chem 44:805–809, 1998.
134. D'Amour P, Rousseau L, Rocheleau B, et al: Influence of Ca^{2+} concentration on the clearance and circulating levels of intact and carboxy-terminal iPTH in pentobarbital-anesthetized dogs. J Bone Miner Res 11:1075–1085, 1996.
135. John M, Goodman WG, Gao P, et al: A novel immunoradiometric assay detects full-length human PTH but not amino-terminally truncated fragments: Implications for PTH measurements in renal failure. J Clin Endocrinol Metab 84:4287–4290, 1999.
136. Salusky IB, Coburn JW, Paunier L, et al: Role of aluminum hydroxide in raising serum aluminum levels in children undergoing continuous ambulatory peritoneal dialysis. J Pediatr 105:717–720, 1984.
137. Moriniere PH, Roussel A, Tahiri Y, et al: Substitution of aluminum hydroxide by high doses of calcium carbonate in patients on chronic hemodialysis: Disappearance of hyperaluminemia and equal control of hyperparathyroidism. Proc Eur Dial Transplant Assoc 19:784–787, 1982.
138. Salusky IB, Coburn JW, Foley J, et al: Effects of oral calcium carbonate on control of serum phosphorus and changes in plasma aluminum levels after discontinuation of aluminum-containing gels in children receiving dialysis. J Pediatr 108:767–770, 1986.
139. Versiek J, Cornelis R: Measuring aluminum levels. N Engl J Med 302:468–469, 1980.
140. Alfrey AC: Aluminum. Adv Clin Chem 23:69–91, 1983.
141. Coburn JW, Mischel MG, Goodman WG, et al: Calcium citrate markedly enhances aluminum absorption from aluminum hydroxide. Am J Kidney Dis 17:708–711, 1991.
142. Cushner HM, Copley JB, Lindberg JS, et al: Calcium citrate, a nonaluminum-containing phosphate-binding agent for treatment of CRF. Kidney Int 33:95–99, 1988.
143. Malluche HH, Smith AJ, Abreo K, et al: The use of deferoxamine in the management of aluminum accumulation in bone in patients with renal failure. N Engl J Med 311:140–144, 1984.
144. Hodsman AB, Hood SA, Brown P, et al: Do serum aluminum levels reflect underlying skeletal aluminum accumulation and bone histology before or after chelation by deferoxamine? J Lab Clin Med 106:674–681, 1985.
145. Dent CE, Hodson CJ: Radiological changes associated with certain metabolic bone diseases. Br J Radiol 27:605–608, 1954.
146. Parfitt AM, Kleerekoper M, Cruz C: Reduced phosphate reabsorption unrelated to parathyroid hormone after renal transplantation: Implications for the pathogenesis of hyperparathyroidism in chronic renal failure. Miner Electrolyte Metab 12:356, 1986.
147. Meema HE, Rabinovich S, Meema S, et al: Improved radiological diagnosis of azotemic osteodystrophy. Radiology 102:1–10, 1972.
148. Shimada H, Nakamura M, Marumo F: Influence of aluminum on the effect of 1-alpha-$(OH)D_3$ on renal osteodystrophy. Nephron 35:163–170, 1983.
149. Parfitt AM: Clinical and radiographic manifestations of renal osteodystrophy. *In* David DS (ed): Calcium Metabolism in Renal Failure and Nephrolithiasis. New York, John Wiley & Sons, 1977, pp 150–190.
150. Simpson W, Ellis HA, Kerr DNS, et al: Bone disease in long-term hemodialysis: The association of radiological with histologic abnormalities. Br J Radiol 49:105–110, 1976.
151. Parfitt AM, Massry SG, Winfield AC: Osteopenia and fractures occurring during maintenance hemodialysis: A "new" form of renal osteodystrophy. Clin Orthop 87:287–302, 1972.
152. Vanherweghem JL, Schoutens A, Bergman P, et al: Usefulness of ^{99m}Tc-pyrophosphate bone scintigraphy in aluminum bone disease. Trace Elements Med 1:80–83, 1984.
153. Botella J, Gallego JL, Fernandez-Fernandez J, et al: The bone scan in patients with aluminum-associated bone disease. Proc Eur Dial Transplant Assoc Eur Ren Assoc 21:403–409, 1985.
154. Hodson EM, Howman-Gilles RB, Evans RB, et al: The diagnosis of renal osteodystrophy: A comparison of technetium99 pyrophosphate bone scintigraphy with other techniques. Clin Nephrol 16:24–28, 1981.
155. Karsenty G, Vigneron N, Jorgetti V, et al: Value of the 99m-Tc-methylene diphosphonate bone scan in renal osteodystrophy. Kidney Int 29:1058–1065, 1986.
156. Clarkson EM, McDonald SJ, de Wardener HE: The effect of a high intake of calcium carbonate in normal subjects and patients with chronic renal failure. Clin Sci 30:425–438, 1966.
157. Meyrier A, Marsac J, Richet G: The influence of a high calcium carbonate intake on bone disease in patients undergoing hemodialysis. Kidney Int 4:146–153, 1973.
158. Bordier PJ, Marie PJ, Arnaud CD: Evolution of renal osteodystrophy: Correlation of bone histomorphometry and serum mineral and immunoreactive parathyroid hormone values before and after treatment with calcium carbonate or 25-hydroxycholecalciferol. Kidney Int Suppl 7:102, 1975.
159. Massry SG, Popovtzer MM, Coburn JW, et al: Intractable pruritus as a manifestation of secondary hyperparathyroidism in uremia. Disappearance of itching following subtotal parathyroidectomy. N Engl J Med 279:697–700, 1968.
160. Slatopolsky E, Weerts C, Lopez-Hilker S, et al: Calcium carbonate is an effective phosphate binder in patients with chronic renal failure undergoing dialysis. N Engl J Med 315:157–161, 1986.
161. Fournier A, Moriniere PH, Sebert JL, et al: Calcium carbonate, an aluminum-free agent for control of hyperphosphatemia, hypocalcemia and hyperparathyroidism in uremia. Kidney Int Suppl 18:115–119, 1986.
162. Schaefer K, Scheer J, Asmus G, et al: The treatment of uraemic hyperphosphataemia with calcium acetate and calcium carbonate: A comparative study. Nephrol Dial Transplant 6:171–175, 1991.
163. Slatopolsky E, Weerts C, Norwood K, et al: Long-term effects of calcium carbonate and 2.5 mEq/liter calcium dialysate on mineral metabolism. Kidney Int 36:897–903, 1989.
164. Hercz G, Pei Y, Greenwood C, et al: Aplastic osteodystrophy without aluminum: The role of "suppressed" parathyroid function. Kidney Int 44:860–866, 1993.
165. Burke TJ, Slatopolsky EA, Goldberg DI: RenaGel, a novel calcium- and aluminum-free phosphate binder, inhibits phosphate absorption in normal volunteers. Nephrol Dial Transplant 12:1640–1644, 1997.
166. Chertow GM, Dillon M, Burke SK, et al: A randomized trial of sevelamer hydrochloride (RenaGel) with and without supplemental calcium. Strategies for the control of hyperphosphatemia and hyperparathyroidism in hemodialysis patients. Clin Nephrol 51:18–26, 1999.
167. Slatopolsky EA, Burke SK, Dillon MA: RenaGel, a nonabsorbed calcium- and aluminum-free phosphate binder, lowers serum phosphorus and parathyroid hormone. The RenaGel Study Group. Kidney Int 55:299–307, 1999.
168. Winney RJ, Cowie JF, Robson JS: The role of plasma aluminum in the detection and prevention of aluminum toxicity. Kidney Int Suppl 18:91–95, 1986.
169. Salusky IB, Foley J, Nelson P, et al: Aluminum accumulation during treatment with aluminum hydroxide and dialysis in children and young adults with chronic renal disease. N Engl J Med 324:527–531, 1991.
170. Ott SM, Recker RR, Coburn JW, et al: Vitamin D therapy in aluminum-related osteomalacia. Kidney Int 32:107–107, 1983.
171. Hofbauer LC, Heufelder AE: Antibodies targeting the calcium sensing receptor: Acquired hypoparathyroidism—an autoimmune disease at last? Eur J Endocrinol 135:172–173, 1996.
172. Sherrard DJ, Hercz G, Pei Y, et al: The spectrum of bone disease in end-stage renal failure—an evolving disorder. Kidney Int 43:436–442, 1993.
173. Baker LR, Muir JW, Sharman VL, et al: Controlled trial of calcitriol in hemodialysis patients. Clin Nephrol 26:185–191, 1986.
174. Berl T, Berns AS, Huffer WE, et al: 1,25-dihydroxycholecalciferol effects in chronic dialysis. A double-blind controlled study. Ann Intern Med 88:774–780, 1978.
175. Pierides AM, Simpson W, Ward MK, et al: Variable response to long-term 1α-hydroxycholecalciferol in hemodialysis osteodystrophy. Lancet 1:1092–1095, 1976.
176. Kanis JA, Henderson RG, Heynen G, et al: Renal osteodystrophy in nondialysed adolescents: Long-term treatment with 1α-hydroxycholecalciferol. Arch Dis Child 52:473–481, 1977.
177. Salusky IB, Fine RN, Kangarloo H, et al: "High-dose" calcitriol for control of renal osteodystrophy in children on CAPD. Kidney Int 32:89–95, 1987.
178. Slatopolsky E, Weerts C, Thielan J, et al: Marked suppression of secondary hyperparathyroidism by intravenous administration of 1,25-dihydroxycholecalciferol in uremic patients. J Clin Invest 74:2136–2143, 1984.

179. Salusky IB, Goodman WG, Horst R, et al: Pharmakokinetics of calcitriol in CAPD/CCPD patients. Am J Kidney Dis 16:126–132, 1990.
180. Quarles LD, Yohay DA, Carroll BA, et al: Prospective trial of pulse oral versus intravenous calcitriol treatment of hyperparathyroidism in ESRD. Kidney Int 45:1710–1721, 1994.
181. Fukagawa M, Kitaoka M, Kaname S, et al: Suppression of parathyroid gland hyperplasia by $1,25(OH)_2D_3$ pulse therapy. N Engl J Med 315:421–422, 1990.
182. Martin KJ, Bullal HS, Domoto DT, et al: Pulse oral calcitriol for the treatment of hyperparathyroidism in patients on continuous ambulatory peritoneal dialysis: Preliminary observations. Am J Kidney Dis 19:540–545, 1992.
183. Tan AU Jr, Levine BS, Mazess RB, et al: Effective suppression of parathyroid hormone by 1 alpha-hydroxy-vitamin D_2 in hemodialysis patients with moderate to severe secondary hyperparathyroidism. Kidney Int 51:317–323, 1997.
184. Nemeth EF: Calcium receptors as novel drug targets. *In* Bilezikian JP, Raisz LG, Rodan GA (eds): Principles in Bone Biology. New York, Academic Press, 1996, pp 1019–1035.
185. Silverberg SJ, Bone HG III, Marriott TB, et al: Short-term inhibition of parathyroid hormone secretion by a calcium-receptor agonist in patients with primary hyperparathyroidism. N Engl J Med 337:1506–1510, 1997.
186. Antonsen JE, Sherrard DJ, Andress DL: A calcimimetic agent acutely suppresses parathyroid hormone levels in patients with chronic renal failure. Rapid communication. Kidney Int 53:223–227, 1998.
187. Froment DPH, Molitoris BA, Buddington B, et al: Site and mechanism of enhanced gastrointestinal absorption of aluminum by citrate. Kidney Int 36:978–984, 1989.
188. Dawborn JK, Brown DJ, Douglas MC, et al: Parathyroidectomy in chronic renal failure. Nephron 33:100–105, 1983.
189. Andress DL, Ott SM, Maloney NA, et al: Effect of parathyroidectomy on bone aluminum accumulation in chronic renal failure. N Engl J Med 312.468–473, 1985.
190. de Vernejoul MC, Marchais S, London G, et al: Increased bone aluminum deposition after subtotal parathyroidectomy in dialyzed patients. Kidney Int 27:785–791, 1985.
191. Ackrill P, Ralston AJ, Day JP, et al: Successful removal of aluminum from a patient with dialysis encephalopathy. Lancet 2:692–693, 1980.
192. Ott SM, Andress DL, Nebeker HG, et al: Changes in bone histology after treatment with desferrioxamine. Kidney Int Suppl 18:108–113, 1986.
193. Ackrill P, Day JP, Garstang FM, et al: Treatment of fracturing renal osteodystrophy by desferrioxamine. Proc Eur Dial Transplant Assoc 19:203–207, 1983.
194. Andress DL, Nebeker HG, Ott SM, et al: Bone histologic response to deferoxamine in aluminum-related bone disease. Kidney Int 31:1344–1350, 1987.
195. Milliner DS, Hercz G, Miller JH, et al: Clearance of aluminum by hemodialysis: Effect of deferoxamine. Kidney Int Suppl 18:100–103, 1986.
196. Hercz G, Salusky IB, Norris KC, et al: Aluminum removal by peritoneal dialysis: Intravenous vs. intraperitoneal deferoxamine. Kidney Int 30:944–948, 1986.
197. Simon P, Ang KS, Meyrier A, et al: Desferrioxamine, ocular toxicity and trace metals. Lancet 2:512–513, 1983.
198. Olivieri NF, Buncic J, Chew E, et al: Visual and auditory neurotoxicity in patients receiving subcutaneous deferoxamine infusions. N Engl J Med 314:869–873, 1986.
198. Guerin A, London G, Marchais S, et al: Acute deafness and desferrioxamine. Lancet 2:39–40, 1985.
200. Veis JH, Contiguglia R, Klein M, et al: Mucormycosis in deferoxamine treated patients on dialysis. Ann Intern Med 107:258–258, 1987.
201. Windus DW, Stokes TJ, Julian BA, et al: Fatal *Rhizopus* infections in hemodialysis patients receiving deferoxamine. Ann Intern Med 107:678–680, 1987.
202. Abe F, Inaba H, Katoh T, et al: Effects of iron and desferrioxamine of *Rhizopus* infection. Mycopathologica 110:81–91, 1990.
203. Van Cutsem J, Boelaert JR: Effects of deferoxamine, feroxamine and iron on experimental mucormycosis (zygomycosis). Kidney Int 36:1061–1068, 1989.
204. Robins-Browne RM, Prpic JK, Stuart SJ: Yersiniae and iron. A study in host-parasite relationships. Contrib Microbiol Immunol 9:254–258, 1987.
205. Hercz G, Andress DL, Nebeker HG, et al: Reversal of aluminum-related bone disease after substituting calcium carbonate for aluminum hydroxide. Am J Kidney Dis 11:70–75, 1988.
206. Diethelm AG, Edwards RP, Whelchel JD: The natural history and surgical treatment of hypercalcemia before and after renal transplantation. Surg Gynecol Obstet 154:481–490, 1982.
207. D'Alessandro AM, Melzer JS, Pirsch JD, et al: Tertiary hyperparathyroidism after renal transplantation: Operative indications. Surgery 106:1049–1056, 1989.
208. Kober M, Schneider H, Reinold HM, et al: Development of renal osteodystrophy after kidney transplantation. Kidney Int 28:378, 1985.
209. Bonomini V, Felelli C, DiFelice A, et al: Bone remodelling after renal transplantation. Adv Exp Med Biol 178:207–216, 1984.
210. Nielsen HE, Melsen F, Christensen MS: Aseptic necrosis of bone following renal transplantation. Acta Med Scand 202:27, 1977.
211. Sanchez CP, Salusky IB, Kuizon BD, et al: Bone disease in children and adolescents undergoing successful renal transplantation. Kidney Int 53:1358–1364, 1998.
212. McDonald JA, Dunstan CR, Dilworth P, et al: Bone loss after liver transplantation. Hepatology 14:613–619, 1991.
213. Lukert BP, Raisz LG: Glucocorticoid-induced osteoporosis: Pathogenesis and management. Ann Intern Med 112:352–364, 1990.
214. Pocock NA, Eisman JA, Dunstan CR, et al: Recovery from steroid-induced osteoporosis. Ann Intern Med 107:319–323, 1987.
215. Stewart PJ, Green OC, Stern PH: Cyclosporine A inhibits calcemic hormone-induced bone resorption in vitro. J Bone Miner Res 1:285–291, 1986.
216. Landmenn J, Renner N, Gacher A, et al: Cyclosporin A and osteonecrosis of the femoral head. J Bone Joint Surg Am 69:1226–1228, 1987.
217. Slatopolsky E, Martin K: Glucocorticoids and renal transplant osteonecrosis. Adv Exp Med Biol 171:353–359, 1984.
218. Parfrey PS, Farge D, Parfrey NA, et al: The decreased incidence of aseptic necrosis in renal transplant recipients: A case control study. Transplantation 41:182–187, 1986.
219. Isono SS, Woolson ST, Schurman DJ: Total joint arthroplasty for steroid-induced osteonecrosis in cardiac patients. Clin Orthop 217:201–208, 1987.
220. Enright H, Haake R, Weisort D: Avascular necrosis of bone: A common serious complication of allogeneic bone marrow transplantation. Am J Med 89:733–738, 1990.
221. Julian BA, Laskow DA, Dubovsky J, et al: Rapid loss of vertebral mineral density after renal transplantation. N Engl J Med 325:544–550, 1991.
222. Gray RE, Doherty SM, Galloway J, et al: A double-blind study of deflazacort and prednisone in patients with chronic inflammatory disorders. Arthritis Rheum 34:287–295, 1991.
223. Montecucco C, Baldi F, Fortina A, et al: Serum osteocalcin (bone Gla-protein) following corticosteroid therapy in post-menopausal women with rheumatoid arthritis. Comparison of the effect of prednisone and deflazacort. Clin Rheumatol 7:366–371, 1988.

Chapter 87

Disorders of Calcification: Osteomalacia and Rickets

Steven R. Goldring ▪ Stephen M. Krane ▪ Louis V. Avioli

Osteomalacia and rickets are disorders of calcification. Osteomalacia is a failure to mineralize the newly formed organic matrix (osteoid) of bone in a normal manner. In rickets, a disease of children, the growth plate at the epiphysis is also involved in a process characterized by defective calcification of cartilage, delayed maturation of the cellular sequence in the growth plate, and disorganization of the arrangement of the cartilage cells, resulting in thickening of the growth plate. A number of different disorders are associated with osteomalacia in adults and rickets in children.[1–5] The pathogenesis of the mineralization defect, the biochemical alterations, the clinical manifestations, and the therapeutic approaches differ in these conditions, and a systematic approach to osteomalacia is therefore essential.

MINERALIZATION DEFECT

Mineralization of bone is a complex process in which the calcium-phosphate inorganic mineral phase is deposited in relation to the organic matrix in a highly ordered fashion. Optimal mineralization can take place at bone-forming surfaces only if (1) cellular activity of bone-forming cells is adequate, (2) matrix is normal in composition and is synthesized at a normal rate, (3) the supply of mineral ions (calcium and inorganic phosphate) from the extracellular fluid is sufficient, (4) the pH at sites of mineralization is appropriate (approximately 7.6), and (5) the concentration of inhibitors of calcification is controlled. These regulatory mechanisms have already been considered in Chapter 74 and have been reviewed by Glimcher[6] and Slavkin and Price.[7] It is possible that clinical disorders of mineralization can be attributed to defects at several of these control steps, examples of which are shown in Table 87–1.

Because the mechanism of defective mineralization is not the same in all of the above disorders, biochemical indices such as serum levels of calcium and phosphate also differ. Moreover, the relative imbalance in matrix synthesis and its mineralization vary, depending upon the underlying disease mechanism. Thus although it is clinically useful to consider changes in a "calcium-phosphate product" in certain forms of rickets and osteomalacia, it should be emphasized that there are other conditions in which defective mineralization occurs in the face of normal or even elevated "calcium-phosphate products." Even when a low "product" is raised, for example, by increasing the serum phosphate concentration in phosphate-depleted animals, the rise in the product itself may not be the only biologic event to explain the change in mineralization because profound alterations in metabolic behavior and modifications of the matrix accompany phosphate depletion and repletion.[8]

Rickets and osteomalacia are disorders of skeletal turnover. The defects can all be ascribed to insufficient mineralization of newly forming matrix (cartilage and bone), not to the removal of mineral from mature bone. In the rachitic growth plate, the characteristic changes occur in the maturation zone, whereas the resting and proliferative zones show normal histologic features (Fig. 87–1). In the maturation zone, the height of the cell columns is increased, and the cells

TABLE 87–1. Examples of Disorders with Different Mechanisms for Mineralization Control

Disorder	Possible Mechanism
1. Postoperative hyperparathyroidism	1. Rate of matrix synthesis exceeds rate of mineralization
2. Fibrogenesis imperfecta ossium	2. Defective collagenous matrix
3. Adult phosphate diabetes	3. Phosphate concentration deficient at mineralization sites
4. Nutritional (vitamin D–deficient) osteomalacia	4. Calcium and phosphate concentrations deficient (? role of deficient vitamin D itself)
5. Systemic acidosis	5. pH inadequate for mineralization
6. Hypophosphatasia	6. Concentration of inhibitor (? inorganic pyrophosphate) excessive

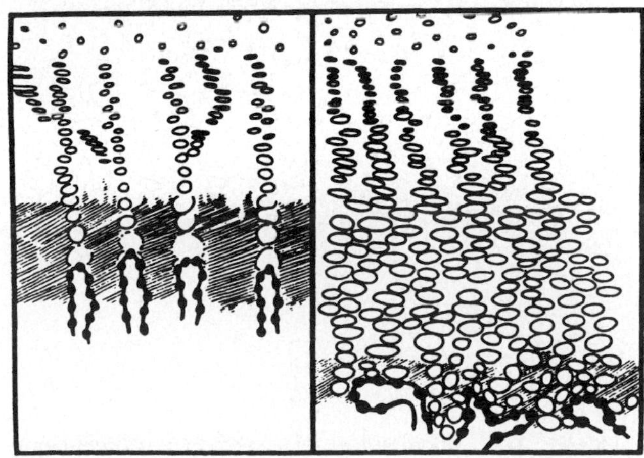

FIGURE 87–1. Diagram of postulated mechanism involved in causing increased length of cartilage columns in the growth plate in rickets. In the normal plate *(left)*, the calcified zone *(shaded area)* provides tunnels for the ingrowth of vascular buds, which are presumably involved in destruction of the cells of the hypertrophic zone most distal from the growth plate, thereby limiting growth in the length of the column. In the rachitic plate *(right)*, the calcium-deficient zone does not provide tunnels, and the normal vascular mechanism limiting the growth in length of the columns is lost. (From Mankin HJ: Rickets, osteomalacia and renal osteodystrophy. J Bone Joint Surg [AM] 56:101–129, 352–386, 1974.)

are closely packed and irregularly aligned. The hypertrophic cells are sparse in number and irregularly distributed. The increase in thickness of the plate is also accompanied by an increase in the transverse diameter, which may extend beyond the ends of the bone, resulting in characteristic cupping or flaring. In experimental rickets, the water content of the plate is increased,[9] and a number of metabolic abnormalities have been observed, including decreased glycogen content and an altered pattern of glycolysis.[8]

Estimates from tetracycline labeling indicate that the appositional growth rate in normal bone is about 1 μm/day.[10] It has also been suggested that complete mineralization of the osteoid in normal bone requires approximately 10 to 21 days.[11] Thus, the thickness of the osteoid seam normally does not exceed 15 to 20 μm and is usually no greater than 13 μm. The surface of bone covered by osteoid is normally less than 20%, and the active surface covered by osteoid is considerably less.[12–14] The major histologic criteria for establishment of osteomalacia are the increased osteoid surface and the increased thickness of the osteoid seam[12–17] (Fig. 87–2). The "calcification front" at the junction of mineralized bone and osteoid is also abnormal in osteomalacia, and some consider this alteration critical to diagnosis.[13]

In applying kinetic criteria to the diagnosis of osteomalacia, it has been suggested that a mean osteoid seam width greater than 15 μm and a mineralization lag time of greater than 100 days are appropriate diagnostic criteria.[15] Boyce et al.[16] and Frame and Parfitt[17] have suggested that more stringent criteria be applied to establish the diagnosis of osteomalacia. They presented evidence that reduced mineral apposition rate, reduced fractional extent of the mineralization front (determined by tetracycline fluorescence or toluidine blue staining), and prolongation of the mineralization lag time are indices reflecting impaired matrix synthesis by osteoblasts rather than specific features of osteomalacia. They stressed that the diagnosis of osteomalacia must include evidence of an absolute increase in the total osteoid volume and an increased number of osteoid lamellae.[16, 17] The architecture of the bone cells and matrix in osteomalacic bone is usually normal. The collagen of the osteoid is largely lamellar, although foci of woven bone are occasionally seen (Fig. 87–3).[14] Although some cellular abnormalities have been described, such as osteocyte perilacunar defects,[18, 19] these defects are probably nonspecific.[20] Hypomineralized periosteocytic lesions have been observed in individuals with hypophosphatemic vitamin D–resistant rickets (VDRR). The persistence of this defect in patients in whom the abnormality in bone mineralization has been corrected with therapy supports the hypothesis that osteocyte function may be abnormal in VDRR. This periosteocytic defect is probably not a feature of other forms of osteomalacia, however.[21]

When bone is examined histologically, it is essential that undemineralized sections be used. In usual practice, however, with classic clinical, radiologic, and biochemical findings, bone biopsy is not necessary to arrive at the diagnosis of osteomalacia. Techniques for biopsy have been standardized in several laboratories and have been facilitated by the design of special trocars for this purpose. The most commonly biopsied site is the iliac crest; sample size ranges from 5 to 10 mm in diameter and should include both inner and outer cortices. Growth plates from long bones in children are usually not biopsied, although an open-wedge biopsy of growth cartilage of the iliac apophysis may occasionally be obtained without the possible hazard of altering subsequent skeletal proportions. Mineralized specimens of bone are most satisfactorily embedded in plastic media, which provide preservation of tissue architecture not usually attained with paraffin-embedding techniques, because the tinctorial distinction between mineralized and unmineralized bone is markedly decreased by decalcification of the specimen. Undecalcified sections should therefore be obtained to adequately differentiate osteoid from mineralized bone, although in severely affected patients, undecalcified paraffin sections may show the osteoid satisfactorily if the samples can be properly cut. Plastic-embedded specimens can be prepared using grinding procedures or sectioning with a heavy-duty sledge microtome. A number of different staining techniques can then be used to demonstrate the osteoid and apply quantitative morphometric analysis (Fig. 87–4).[16, 17, 22]

In normal bone, a "calcification front" is seen at the junction of the osteoid seam and newly mineralized bone.[12, 13, 16, 17] This region can be

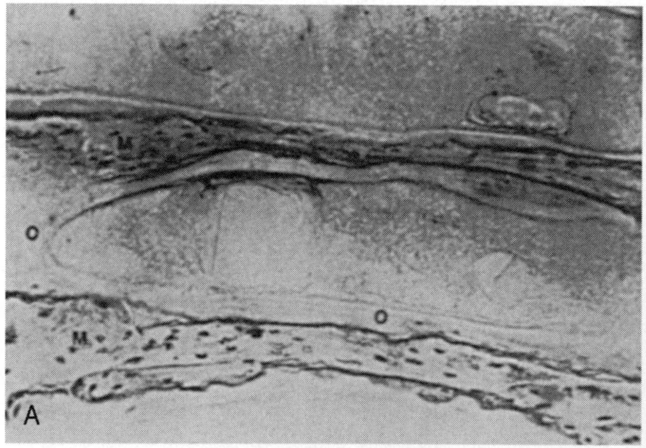

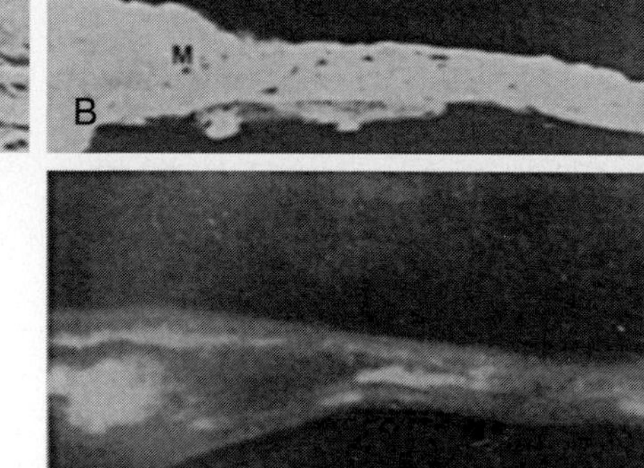

FIGURE 87–2. Undecalcified thick sections of a bone biopsy from a patient with adult-onset hypophosphatemic osteomalacia (renal tubular phosphate leak) (case 1 in Barnes et al.[26]). Sections were examined under different conditions. *A*, Unstained. *B*, Microradiograph. *C*, Ultraviolet photomicrograph demonstrating fluorescence (F) of tetracycline administered 14 days prior to biopsy. Note mineralized bone (M) and osteoid (O).

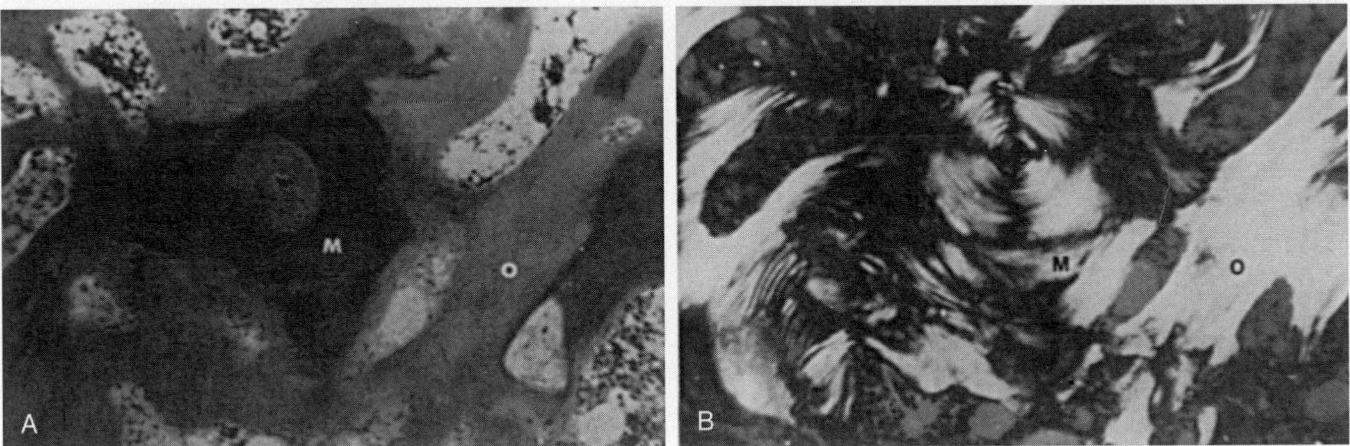

FIGURE 87–3. Biopsy of bone from a patient with nutritional osteomalacia (partially decalcified sections stained with hematoxylin-eosin). *A,* Viewed with transmitted nonpolarized light. *B,* Viewed under polarized light with analyzer. Note that most of bone is lamellar whether mineralized (M) or osteoid (O).

demonstrated by an intense fluorescence of tetracycline, which is deposited in this zone if the antibiotic is administered prior to obtaining the biopsy (Fig. 87–5). In normal persons, the osteoid seam–bone junctions fluoresce intensely, whereas in osteomalacia the fluorescence is less well defined (more diffuse) or even absent (see Fig. 87–2C). The calcification front may also be demonstrated by staining the sections with toluidine blue or the dye Solochrome-cyanine R. There is not universal agreement, however, concerning the requirement of abnormality in the calcification front in the diagnosis of osteomalacia.[3]

It is apparent that if a wide osteoid seam is demonstrated in osteomalacia, the rate at which matrix is formed must be greater than that at which it is mineralized. In most forms of human osteomalacia, matrix biosynthesis is probably not occurring at a normal rate, even though the total osteoid surface is increased. In rats, in which the process can be adequately quantitated, the osteomalacia of vitamin D deficiency is associated with a decreased rate of matrix formation. Similar observations have been made in humans.[16, 17] Despite these observations,[23] the level of serum alkaline phosphatase is elevated in many but not all forms of human rickets and osteomalacia. Although the level of alkaline phosphatase in serum probably reflects osteoblastic "activity" in bone, the rate of matrix biosynthesis cannot be adequately estimated from the levels of this enzyme alone. Because the lag time in mineralization is also prolonged, and the rate of mineralization slowed, the net results is an increase in the thickness of the osteoid seam. Not only is the rate of matrix synthesis altered in such situations, but the matrix itself may be modified. Indeed, the hydroxylation of certain lysyl residues of bone collagen is increased

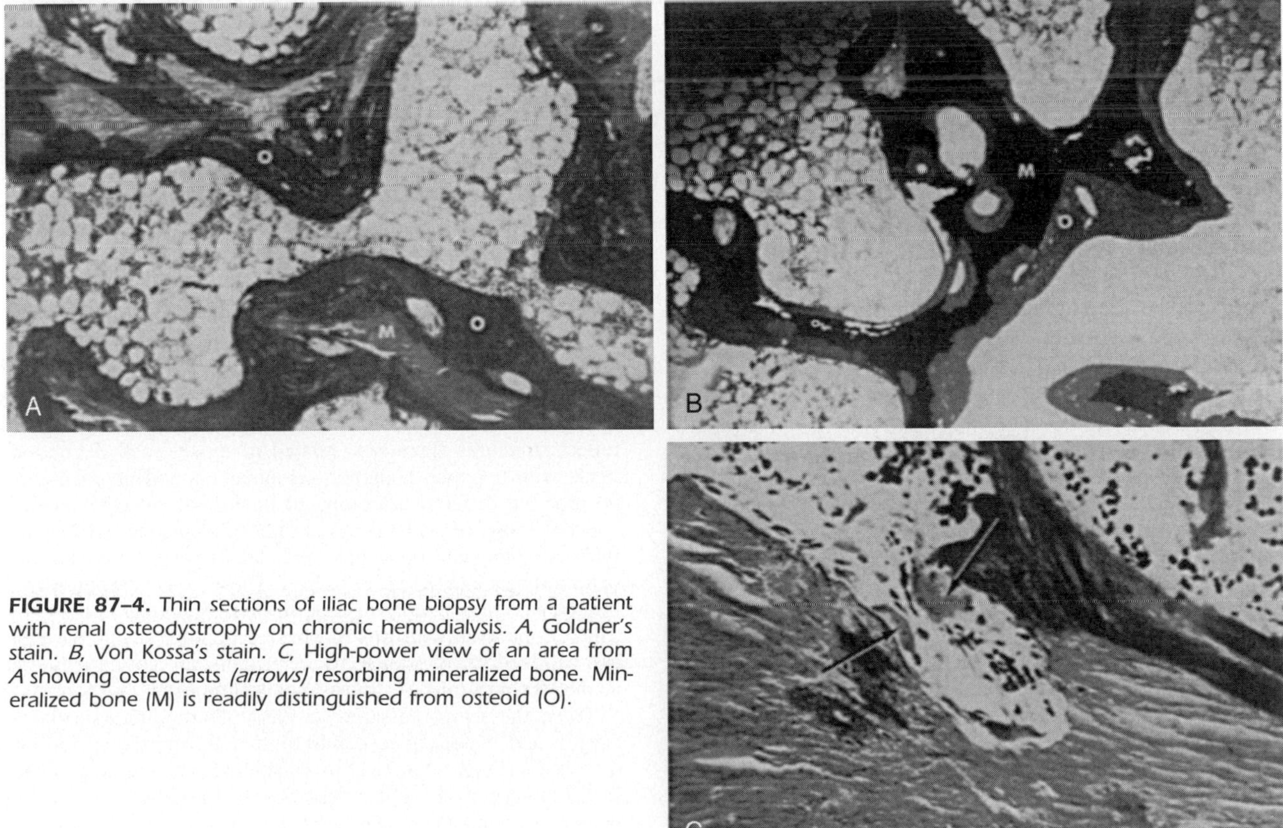

FIGURE 87–4. Thin sections of iliac bone biopsy from a patient with renal osteodystrophy on chronic hemodialysis. *A,* Goldner's stain. *B,* Von Kossa's stain. *C,* High-power view of an area from *A* showing osteoclasts *(arrows)* resorbing mineralized bone. Mineralized bone (M) is readily distinguished from osteoid (O).

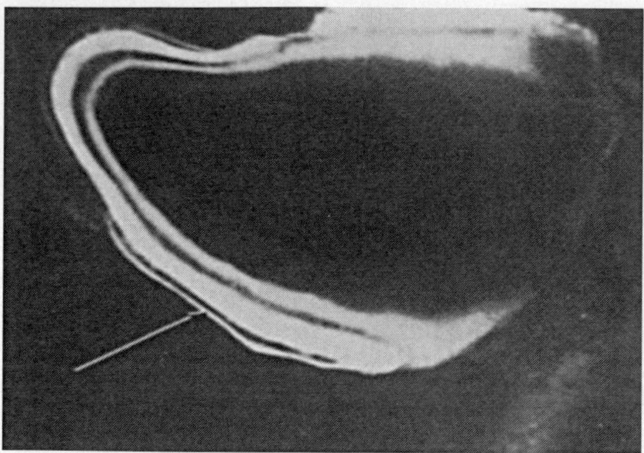

FIGURE 87–5. Thick section of undermineralized bone from a man with mild phosphate diabetes (case 4, in Jaworski et al.[22]). This patient received tetracycline on several occasions months before the biopsy was taken. The fluorescence of the region corresponding to the earliest dose of tetracycline *(arrow)* is sharp and characteristic of a normal calcification front. Compare with Figure 87–2C, in which the tetracycline deposition is irregular and diffuse.

in vitamin D deficiency, as well as in other experimental hypocalcemic states.[24–26]

CLINICAL FEATURES OF RICKETS AND OSTEOMALACIA

The clinical manifestations of rickets, although they vary to some extent depending upon the underlying disorder, are mainly related to skeletal pain and deformity, fracture of the abnormal bones, slippage of epiphyses, and disturbances in growth.[1–3] Hypocalcemia when it occurs may be symptomatic. In some children, especially those with vitamin D deficiency, muscular weakness and hypotonia may be prominent. Dent and Stamp[2] have indicated nine factors that underlie the clinical manifestations of rickets, and they are modified here as follows:

1. Failure of the calcification mechanism affects predominantly those parts of the skeleton whose growth is most rapid.
2. Rickets affects endochondral bone more than intramembranous bone, possibly because of the more rapid growth of the former. Furthermore, only when rickets is severe is bone such as that in the midshaft involved clinically.
3. Proximal and distal ends of bones do not grow at the same rate, and rickets affects the most rapidly growing area.
4. Different bones grow at different rates at different stages of development. At the time when rickets is active, these factors determine the clinical expression. For example, the skull is growing rapidly at birth, and craniotabes is therefore a manifestation of congenital rickets. During the first year the upper limbs and rib cage grow rapidly, and therefore abnormalities at these sites are prominent, for example, rachitic rosary. Signs of rickets at the wrist are usually seen at the ulnar side, because the growth rate of the distal ulnar epiphysis is relatively greater than that of the distal radial epiphysis.
5. Deformities in mild chronic rickets are most often due to disordered growth at the epiphysial plate rather than to bending at the shafts.
6. In some forms of rickets the radiologic changes include those of secondary hyperparathyroidism (subperiosteal resorption, most commonly at the metaphyses).
7. Deformities that occur before the age of 4 years correct themselves if the rickets is cured, whereas if rickets persists to a later age, the deformities are permanent (dwarfism, bowleg, and knock-knee).
8. "Late" rickets, which occurs at the time of the pubescent growth spurt, produces dramatic disturbances and results in knock-knee.
9. Adult manifestations of osteomalacia, such as Looser's zones and increased bioconcavity of vertebral bodies, are seen in young children only when the rickets is very severe.

In infants and young children, especially in severe, classic rickets, listlessness and irritability are common. In infants, myopathy is characteristic and is manifested by floppiness and hypotonia. In older children, the weakness may present as a proximal myopathy similar to that observed in the adult. Other findings in infants include parietal flattening or frontal bossing, softening of the calvarium (craniotabes), and widening of the sutures. The thickened growth plates may be evident clinically as the rachitic rosary at the rib ends and may even simulate juvenile rheumatoid arthritis when areas such as the wrists are involved. Indentation of the lower ribs at the site of attachment of the diaphragm is known as Harrison's groove or sulcus. Pelvic deformities also occur, and the skeleton is more prone to fractures. Pain may not be prominent and, when present, is greater at the knees and other weight-bearing joints. Dental eruption may be delayed, and enamel defects are common.

In contrast, osteomalacia in adults may be difficult to detect on clinical grounds alone. Diffuse skeletal pain and muscular weakness may be present in the absence of a specific pattern. Pain is often prominent about the hips and may produce a waddling or antalgic gait. Fractures may occur about the rib cage and vertebral bodies, as well as in long bones, and lead to progressive deformities. Affected individuals have localized pain and swelling in joints, some only in a single joint. Synovial fluid is noninflammatory and crystals are not seen. Other patients may have symmetrical polyarthralgias resembling those of rheumatoid arthritis or polymyalgia rheumatica.[27] Muscular weakness is particularly prominent[28]; in one series of 45 patients with osteomalacia, it was present in almost half.[29] The weakness is primarily proximal in distribution (which contributes to the waddling gait) and is often associated with wasting, discomfort on movement, and hypotonia with preservation of brisk reflexes.[30] The same myopathy is seen in patients with all types of osteomalacia, with the exception of those with X-linked hypophosphatemic osteomalacia. In adults with acquired renal tubular phosphate leak, in contrast to children with the X-linked form, proximal muscle weakness may also be profound and is correctable by phosphate repletion.[31] Although electro-myograms occasionally show myopathic changes and muscle biopsies rarely show denervation,[27, 29] in one series of six patients with osteomalacia of different causes, muscle biopsies revealed nonspecific changes, including neurogenic atrophy or type II fiber atrophy of uncertain cause.[32] These patients had electromyographic changes of neurogenic muscle disease consistent with the histologic changes. None of these patients had severe hypophosphatemia (lowest recorded phosphatemia was 2.7 mg/dL).

Similar changes in muscle fiber morphology have been described in patients with renal failure on chronic hemodialysis, and the relationship to the bone disorder is difficult to evaluate.[33] The presence of so-called lobulated fibers has also been described in the muscle biopsies from patients with osteomalacia.[34] These fibers are characterized by small subsarcolemmal triangular aggregates. These changes are not unique to patients with osteomalacia and are detected in several different neuromuscular disorders, including some forms of muscular dystrophy and glucocorticoid-associated myopathy. These changes may reflect structural alterations related to muscle cell disruption. In patients with hypophosphatemic osteomalacia and myopathy, there was no reported difference (compared to normal subjects) in the relative concentrations of skeletal muscle phosphocreatine, adenosine triphosphate, or inorganic phosphate estimated by phosphorus nuclear magnetic resonance (MR) spectroscopy. These levels change with exercise, but the pattern of changes is not different from that in normal subjects. Thus, in patients with low plasma phosphorus levels the myocellular and extracellular phosphate concentrations are not directly related and cannot account for the clinical manifestations.[35]

Thus, the neuromuscular disease of osteomalacia has multiple causes, and it usually responds to specific therapy of the underlying disorder, such as vitamin D in nutritional osteomalacia, alkalinization in acidosis, and phosphate repletion in the adult form of hypophosphatemic osteomalacia. There may be a role for the secondary hyperparathyroidism (when it occurs) in the production of the neuromuscu-

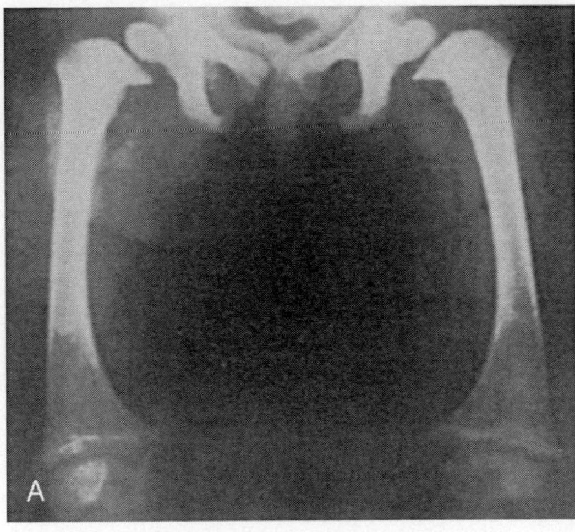

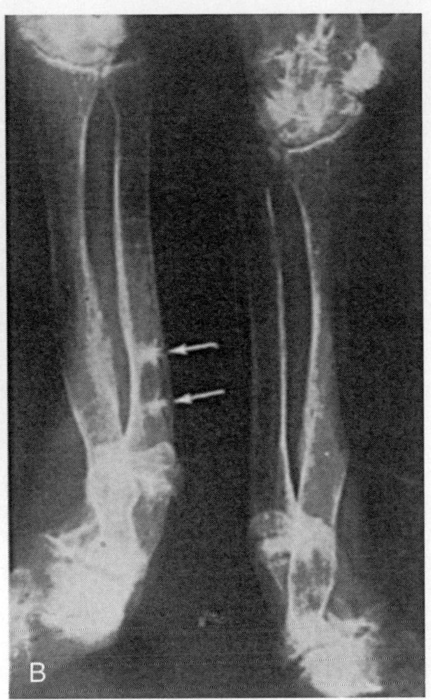

FIGURE 87–6. *A,* Rickets in a child with Fanconi's syndrome showing typical cupping of distal femoral epiphyses. *B,* Osteomalacia in an 80-year-old woman who had a history compatible with hypophosphatemic rickets dating to early childhood. Note multiple pseudofractures *(arrows).*

lar disease because changes similar to those described in osteomalacia have also been found in primary hyperparathyroidism.[36] The role of hypophosphatemia per se in muscular weakness is discussed in Chapter 73.

RADIOLOGIC FEATURES

Radiologic changes in the skeleton in rickets and osteomalacia reflect the histopathologic changes.[1, 8] In rickets, the alterations are most evident at the epiphyseal growth plate, which is increased in thickness, is cupped, and reveals a haziness at the diaphyseal border due to decreased calcification of the hypertrophic zone and inadequate mineralization of the primary spongiosa (Fig. 87–6). Variation in the pattern of the rachitic changes is influenced by differences in rates of growth of bones or portions of bones, as discussed earlier. The trabecular pattern of the metaphyses is abnormal, the cortices of the diaphyses may be thinned, and bowing of the shafts may be present.

Osteomalacia usually demonstrates some decrease in bone density associated with loss of trabeculae, blurring of trabecular margins, and variable degrees of thinning of the cortices.[1, 2, 8] In some patients, the radiologic changes are indistinguishable from those seen in osteoporosis. The finding that suggests osteomalacia more specifically is the presence of radiolucent bands ranging from a few millimeters to several centimeters in length, usually oriented perpendicularly to the surface of the bone (Fig. 87–7). They tend to occur symmetrically and are particularly common at the inner aspects of the femur, especially near the femoral neck; in the pelvis; in the outer edge of the scapula; in the upper fibula; and in the metatarsals. These translucent bands are referred to as *pseudofractures*, *Looser's zones*, or *umbauzonen*. They are often multiple, occasionally occurring at 10 to 15 sites in a single individual.[31, 37] Such multiple symmetrical pseudofractures occurring in individuals with osteomalacia of a variety of causes have been referred to as *Milkman's syndrome*.[38, 39] The abnormalities in Milkman's original case[40, 41] were also considered by Albright and Reifenstein[39] to be manifestations of osteomalacia. The pseudofractures most often occur at sites where major arteries cross the bones and have been thought to be secondary to the mechanical stress of the pulsating vessel. Arteriography in some cases,[31, 42, 43] but not all,[44] has indicated that the origins of the pseudofractures correspond to the location of major arteries (Fig. 87–8). Trauma of some sort, whether related to arterial pulsation or other factors, such as weight-bearing stress, must be responsible for the symmetry of the lesions and their predilection for the described sites. The histopathology of Looser's zones, according to Ball and Garner,[45] is that of premalacic lamellar bone, some of which is surrounded by lamellar osteoid at the edge of the defect. In addition, there are foci of woven bone, some of which is mineralized and some not. This accounts for the lower radiologic mineral density of the pseudofracture compared with the surrounding bone. Subperiosteal erosions along the diaphyseal cortices extending to the metaphyses may be seen when secondary hyperparathyroidism is present. Widening (or pseudowidening) of the sacroiliac joints with hazy margins has also been observed, sometimes suggesting ankylosing spondylitis (which osteomalacia may mimic clinically).[31]

In some patients with osteomalacia, increased rather than decreased radiologic density of bones may be observed.[37] This is seen particularly in patients with renal tubular phosphate leaks, as opposed to vitamin D deficiency (Fig. 87–9). In such patients there may be a striking degree of thickening of the cortices and trabeculae of the spongy bone, at time associated with exostotic spurs. This hyperostosis has been noted in untreated patients. It is not usually observed in patients with generalized defects in proximal renal tubular reabsorption. Despite the increase in mass of bone per unit volume, microscopically the trabeculae are covered with abnormally thickened osteoid seams typical of

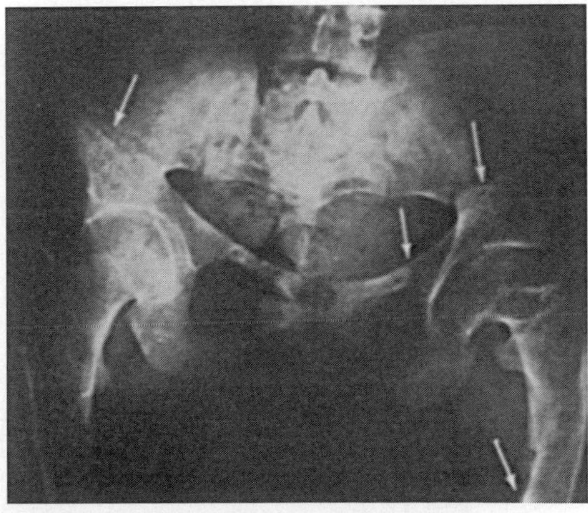

FIGURE 87–7. Radiograph of the pelvis and proximal femora in a patient with adult phosphate diabetes (case 2 in Jaworski et al.[22]). Note pseudofractures or Looser's zones *(arrows).*

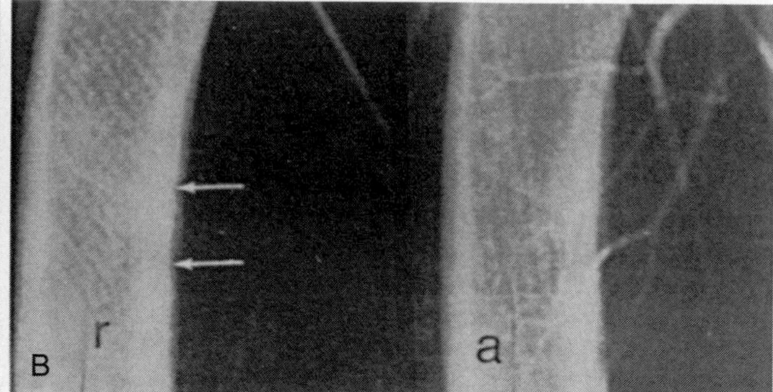

FIGURE 87–8. Radiograph (r) and corresponding arteriograms (a) in a patient with adult-onset phosphate diabetes (case 2 in Jaworski et al.[22]; see Fig. 87–1). *A*, Pelvis. *B*, Femur. Note that origin of Looser's zones *(arrows)* corresponds with crossing of major vessels.

osteomalacia. Similar findings may be noted in patients with chronic renal failure. The reason for the hyperostosis is unknown; the bone is still architecturally abnormal and subject to fracture with relatively minimal trauma.

In patients with X-linked hypophosphatemic osteomalacia (or rickets), an additional finding has been the presence of a generalized involvement of the entheses with exuberant calcification (more likely ossification) of tendon and ligament insertions.[46, 47] The absence of inflammatory cells, as well as other clinical features, differentiate this disorder from degenerative joint disease and the seronegative spondyloarthropathies.

A comprehensive classification of rickets and osteomalacia is shown in Table 87–2. A detailed discussion of all these conditions is not included here because selected areas are covered in other chapters.

NUTRITIONAL OSTEOMALACIA

Writings of the 17th century in Scotland and England vividly documented the association between poverty, undernutrition, and the occurrence of infantile rickets. Reports from Glasgow in the late 1800s and early 1900s drew further attention to the widespread prevalence of infantile rickets in the industrialized regions of Britain. In 1923, the work of the Vienna Council finally established the link between rickets, dietary deficiency of vitamin D, and correction of vitamin D deficiency by irradiation with sunlight. Following the discovery that rickets was a vitamin-deficiency disease, fortification of certain foods with vitamin D reduced the incidence of nutritional rickets in Europe and the United States to negligible levels, and by the 1940s, deficiency of vitamin D was no longer regarded as an important cause of osteomalacia and rickets.[39] Vitamin D metabolism and the role of specific metabolites in bone development, mineralization, and remodeling are discussed elsewhere (see Chapters 72–74, 82). Nevertheless, the role of vitamin D in the development of osteomalacia and rickets is pertinent to the discussion in this chapter.

The studies of Dunnigan et al.[48] and of Arneil and Crosbie[49] in Glasgow and Benson et al.[50] in London have documented the reappearance of nutritional osteomalacia and rickets as a public health problem in Britain.[51] The new population at risk exists primarily among the large number of immigrants to Britain since the 1950s from India, Pakistan, and other Commonwealth countries. Unique dietary and social customs have played a significant role in the emergence of osteomalacia and rickets in this population.[48–54] Another large group of people in whom nutritional osteomalacia is being recognized with increasing frequency include housebound and other elderly subjects.[55–59] Cases are also being recognized among food faddists, especially those on certain inadequate vegetarian or fat-free diets.[55, 56] Ralston et al.[60] have also noted an unexpectedly high prevalence of osteomalacia in patients with rheumatoid arthritis. All of the affected patients in their series were elderly women who were housebound and had poor nutritional status. They noted that biochemical screening was of limited value in establishing the diagnosis of osteomalacia, which was confirmed by transiliac bone biopsy. Prior gastrectomy and occult celiac disease were additional risk factors in two of the cases.

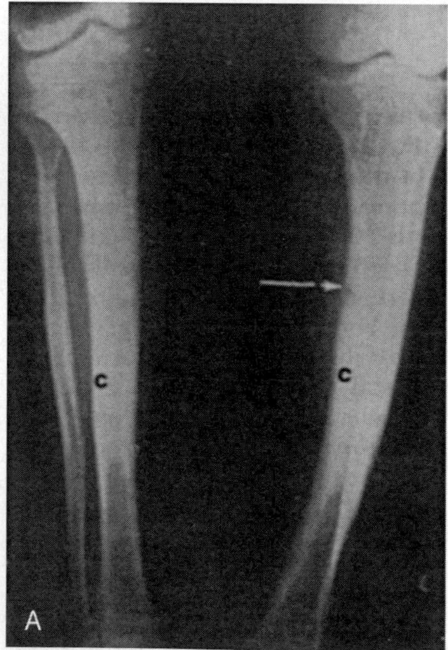

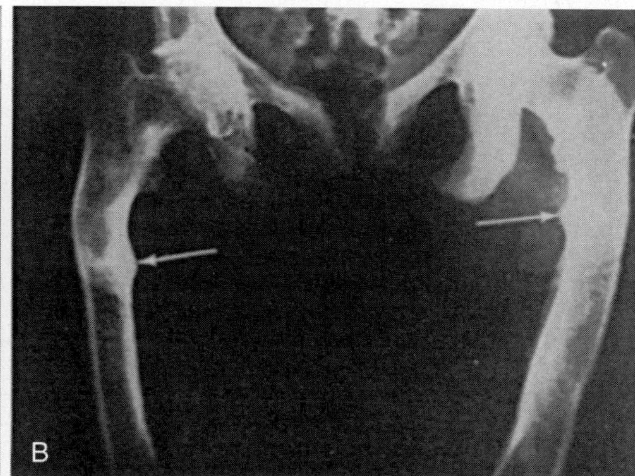

FIGURE 87–9. Increased bone mass in patients with osteomalacia. *A*, Radiographs of femora of a 15-year-old boy with X-linked hypophosphatemia. Note thick tibial cortex (c) and Looser's zone *(arrow)*. *B*, Radiograph of pelvis and femora of a 38-year-old woman with hypophosphatemia present since childhood. No hypophosphatemia was detected in members of a large family. Note Looser's zones *(arrows)*.

An additional population risk for the development of osteomalacia on the basis of nutritional deficiency are individuals who have undergone intestinal bypass surgery for treatment of severe obesity.[61–63] In one series, iliac bone biopsies revealed the presence of osteomalacia in nearly one-third of the 21 patients studied.[62] In another study, it was shown that with treatment with vitamin D_2 (36,000 IU/day), as well as supplemental calcium (27 mmol/day), a more positive calcium balance could be achieved.[63] An increased frequency of osteomalacia has also been observed in patients after gastrectomy.[64, 65] Bisballe et al.[64] examined a population of 68 patients following gastrectomy, using histomorphometric evaluation of transiliac bone biopsy specimens. Overall, 18% of the patients fulfilled the histologic criteria for the diagnosis of osteomalacia. The authors noted that the severity of the mineralization defect was positively correlated with the 25-hydroxyvitamin D [25(OH)D] level, but not the levels of 1,25-dihydroxyvitamin D [1,25$(OH)_2$D], and that the serum level of 25(OH)D, the age of the patient, and the duration of the postoperative follow-up were the most significant determinants of the mineralization defect in a given patient. They emphasized the limited value of serum markers in the diagnosis of osteomalacia, because six of eight patients with established bone disease had normal serum levels of calcium and alkaline phosphatase. Although the 25(OH)D levels were positively correlated with the presence of a mineralization defect in five of eight patients with documented osteomalacia, these levels were within the range of normal. The authors stressed the need for vitamin D and calcium supplementation after gastric resection.

Osteomalacia is also detected with increased frequency among low-birth-weight infants. The incidence has been reported to be between 13% and 32%. Insufficient intake of calcium, phosphorus, and vitamin D probably plays a role. It is important that this condition be detected early and that prompt adjustment in nutritional supplement in the infants be effected.[66] Infants of Asian mothers are at greatest risk for neonatal osteomalacia.[67] Vitamin D deficiency in the mothers appears to be the critical factor in the development of this disorder. In one study, supplements of 1000 IU of vitamin D daily during pregnancy significantly increased plasma 25(OH)D concentrations at delivery and averted development of osteomalacia in the neonates.

In normal persons, vitamin D is provided from two sources: (1) dietary supplementation with ergocalciferol (D_2), which is an irradiation product obtained from plants, and (2) the natural vitamin, cholecalciferol (D_3), produced in human skin by the action of ultraviolet light on the physiologic precursor, 7-dehydrocholesterol. Because most foods (with the exception of fatty fish) contain only small amounts of vitamin D_3, individuals must rely upon either adequate sunlight exposure or dietary supplements of ergocalciferol for maintenance of an adequate vitamin D supply.

With the availability of a reliable assay for 25(OH)D, it has become possible to study vitamin D status in persons who have no evidence of clinical disease. There is marked seasonal variation in the levels of plasma 25(OH)D independent of age and sex.[52–54, 68–73] These variations parallel changes in sun exposure, with higher levels occurring in late summer months and fall.

More recent detailed studies have confirmed and extended earlier observations. For example, although men and women have similar levels of 25(OH)D during winter months, overall the levels in men are higher than in women.[74] Plasma levels of 25(OH)D are almost twice as high in American white women compared to black women during winter months and the increment during summer months is significantly lower in black women compared to white women.[75] The plasma levels of 25(OH)D and those of parathyroid hormone (PTH) are inversely correlated, implying that the changes in 25(OH)D are metabolically significant.[74] Measurements of plasma levels of 25(OH)D in patients hospitalized in a general medical ward showed, surprisingly, that over half of the subjects had levels consistent with vitamin D deficiency.[76] These observations point out the crucial role played by irradiation from sunlight in maintaining adequate vitamin D homeostasis in those on marginal intake of vitamin D. Estimates by the World Health Organization suggest that the daily vitamin D requirement in a nonlactating woman is 70 to 100 IU ($\sim$2.5 μg).[77] In the elderly populations described above, estimated vitamin D intakes often fall below 100 IU/day.[56, 69,78, 79] These findings of low dietary vitamin D intake are of particular relevance because several investigators have suggested that daily vitamin D requirements may be greater in the elderly than in young adults, in part related to the frequency of previous gastric surgery, occult malabsorption, and possible alterations in vitamin D metabolism.[55, 57, 64, 71, 73, 80] In an attempt to determine the optimal plasma levels of 25(OH)D and how much vitamin D must be produced or ingested to achieve such levels, Vieth[81] conducted an exhaustive review of published data. He concluded, as is also summarized in an accompanying editorial by Heaney,[82] that total daily intake and production of vitamin D of 2.5 to 5.0 μg (100 to 200 IU) and plasma 25(OH)D levels of greater than 20 to 25 nmol/L (1 nmol/L = 1 ng/mL $\times$2.5) are sufficient to prevent clinical rickets or osteomalacia. Higher levels of vitamin D intake or production would be necessary, however, to prevent secondary hyperparathyroidism, bone loss, and subclinical osteomalacia. Therefore, it may be necessary to maintain 25(OH)D levels of 100 nmol/L or greater to avoid bone loss and subclinical osteomalacia. How much vitamin D is necessary to attain these levels would vary widely in different populations in different parts of the world.

In the Asian immigrant populations of Britain, rickets and osteomalacia secondary to vitamin D deficiency are seen most commonly in neonates, infants, and adolescents during pubertal growth and less frequently among adults.[48–51, 55, 66, 67, 83–86] Multiple factors have been implicated in the development of bone disease, including insufficient intake of vitamin D[51, 66, 67, 82]; racial pigmentation,[87] which presumably interferes with ultraviolet transmission through the epidermis; genetic factors[88, 89]; and social customs such as avoidance of sun exposure and consumption of chapatis, a dietary staple of this population, high in phytate content, which may bind calcium in the gut and thus interfere with calcium absorption.[90] Clements et al.[91] have speculated that diets high in cereal content might adversely affect vitamin D utilization, thus contributing to the mineralization defect. They showed in rats that the rate of inactivation of vitamin D in the liver was increased by calcium deprivation. These alterations are probably mediated by the 1,25$(OH)_2$D produced in response to secondary hyperparathyroidism, and they suggested that this vitamin D metabolite might promote hepatic conversion of vitamin D to polar inactivation products.

Sly et al.[92] compared the effects of diets containing high cereal content on the development of vitamin D deficient rickets and osteomalacia in young baboons. They found that, although all animals fed vitamin D–deficient diets developed rickets and osteomalacia, the rapidity and severity of the bone disease was much greater in the animals receiving maize. The mechanism of this effect of maize is not defined, but these results offer further evidence that diets of predominantly cereal (which contain a high content of phytates) may exacerbate the effects of vitamin D deficiency. As noted in two more recent studies,[52, 53] the presence of osteomalacia is strongly correlated with a vegetarian diet, and the wheat cereal content is a risk factor for the development of mineralization defect only in the pediatric age group. It was also noted that individuals on a vegetarian diet had an impaired seasonal rise in 25(OH)D levels.

Studies by Dent et al.[93] strongly suggest that insufficient sunlight exposure plays a pivotal role in the development of nutritional rickets and osteomalacia in addition to the rickets and osteomalacia observed in patients on long-term anticonvulsant therapy.[94] In two carefully studied individuals, Dent et al. were able to demonstrate healing of rickets and positive calcium balance following therapy with ultraviolet light, despite a vitamin D–deficient, high phytate diet. Substitution of a low phytate diet did not affect the plasma biochemical abnormalities or the calcium balance.[93] Similar observations by Stanbury et al.[84] confirmed the important role of adequate exposure to sunlight in prevention of bone disease in this population.

Vitamin D is crucial to homeostatic control of calcium and phosphorus metabolism through regulatory mechanisms involving the small intestine, skeleton, and kidney. Vitamin D indirectly affects bone mineralization by increasing the availability of calcium and phosphorus through actions on these organ systems. Data also suggest a direct effect of vitamin D on the mineralization process per se, independent of indirect effects on mineral ion concentrations. In vitamin D–deficient states, formation of the calcification front is defective, as manifested by deficient tetracycline uptake. Treatment with phosphate alone results in patchy mineralization without producing a normal calcification front. Addition of vitamin D results in the rapid appearance of normal mineralization and calcification front.[95, 96]

The role of the individual metabolites of vitamin D in regulating the process of mineralization has not been firmly elucidated. For example, $1,25(OH)_2D$ levels have been reported to be in the normal range in some individuals with established vitamin D–deficient osteomalacia.[97, 98] and in a single patient with antacid-induced osteomalacia. In a series of patients with postgastrectomy osteomalacia,[64] levels of this metabolite were markedly elevated.[99] These findings suggest that $1,25(OH)_2D$ is not the only metabolite of vitamin D responsible for the maintenance of normal mineralization. There may also be a role in the mineralization process for other metabolites of vitamin D such as 25(OH)D or $24,25(OH)_2D$.[99–103]

Scriver[104] divides the evolution of vitamin D deficiency in infancy into three stages. In stage 1, serum calcium tends to be low, serum phosphorus normal, and aminoaciduria absent. If the disorder is untreated, it progresses to stage 2, in which tubular reabsorption of phosphorus and amino acids is impaired and aminoaciduria and hypophosphatemia appear. In this stage, serum calcium levels tend to return to normal associated with an increase in serum alkaline phosphatase activity, presumably related to the stimulation of PTH release and resultant increase in bone turnover. Stage 3 is characterized by the return of hypocalcemia. The effect of lowered concentrations of serum phosphorus in stage 2 and lowered concentrations of phosphorus and calcium in stage 3 are presumably responsible for the production of the mineralization defect.

Rao et al.[15] have reviewed the findings in a series of 65 patients with vitamin D depletion diagnosed on the basis of plasma levels of 25(OH)D less than 10 ng/mL. They found that in early vitamin D depletion the effects on bone are manifested principally by the occurrence of secondary hyperparathyroidism. With increasing severity or duration of the vitamin D deficiency, the mineralization process becomes progressively impaired, bone formation rates decline, and osteoid surface and thickness increase.

Immunoreactive PTH levels measured during stage 1 are usually within normal limits.[105] In stage 2, levels of PTH are usually elevated, and the tubular dysfunction (aminoaciduria, phosphaturia) has, at least in part, been attributed to elevated circulating levels of this hormone.[105, 106] The abnormal phosphate excretion and hyperaminoaciduria can be suppressed by transient increases in serum calcium. Although the improvement in tubular dysfunction may be related primarily to inhibition of PTH release by the increased levels of serum calcium, the calcium ion itself may act directly on tubular epithelial cells to restore proper function.[104]

Other studies by Rao et al.[107] have shown that in patients with severe hypocalcemia and osteomalacia due to vitamin D depletion, basal excretion of nephrogenous cyclic adenosine monophosphate (cAMP) is increased, but the steady-state phosphaturic response to endogenous PTH is impaired. Correction of hypocalcemia by administration of vitamin D and calcium restores the normal phosphaturic response to endogenous PTH.

The level of $1,25(OH)_2D$ may not be a reliable indicator of the metabolism of vitamin D because, as previously mentioned, individuals with vitamin D deficiency may have normal levels of this metabolite.[97, 98] The occurrence of a mineralization defect in the presence of apparently normal levels of $1,25(OH)_2D$ is paradoxical. One explanation for this paradox is that the activity of the renal 1α-hydroxylase may be increased in the presence of the secondary hyperparathyroidism. Indeed, serum levels of $1,25(OH)_2D$ higher than normal result from ultraviolet irradiation in these subjects.[98]

Administration of vitamin D to patients with vitamin D–deficient rickets of osteomalacia invariably results in healing of the bone disease, although the patterns of response, particularly with regard to changes in levels of serum calcium, phosphorus, alkaline phosphatase, and immunoreactive PTH, show marked variation. In general, with treatment, serum phosphorus levels rapidly rise. There may be delayed normalization of serum calcium levels, presumably secondary to the deposition of calcium in the healing bone. The fall in alkaline phosphatase and immunoreactive PTH levels is often delayed, as is improvement in the radiographic abnormalities. Therefore, failure of alkaline phosphatase or radiographic findings to return to normal during the first several months of therapy should not be misinterpreted as a lack of response to treatment.

Several protocols are recommended for treatment of vitamin D–deficient bone disease. In general, a trial with small daily doses of vitamin D 50 μg (2000 IU), orally, for 3 to 4 weeks is suggested because a clear biochemical response occurs in classic rickets and osteomalacia secondary to simple vitamin D deficiency. This dose is not sufficient to produce an effect in any of the metabolic forms of rickets associated with renal insufficiency, malabsorption, and various hereditary and acquired forms of vitamin D resistance or dependency. Patients on chronic anticonvulsant therapy may also require higher doses.[108] Moreover, unlike adults, in whom the effects of anticonvulsant drugs in producing osteomalacia may be self-limited, children may require persistent therapy because long-term anticonvulsant therapy has a greater effect on growing children than on adults.[109] Although twice-yearly supplementation with 2.5 mg of vitamin D_2 orally has been suggested as prophylaxis against vitamin D deficiency in institutionalized elderly people,[110] as little as 500 IU (12.5 μg) of vitamin D per day can reduce bone loss in adults,[111] especially in elderly subjects who are predisposed to subclinical vitamin D deficiency syndrome.[112] Osteomalacia can also be corrected with relatively low doses of $1\alpha(OH)D_3$ (0.5 μg/day) or vitamin D_2 (25 μg/day) for 3 months.[113] Gallagher[73] has recommended that more potent analogues of vitamin D be reserved for patients with more pronounced forms of calcium malabsorption. Chronic maintenance therapy in patients subjected to long-term anticonvulsant therapy in doses of 800 to 1000 U of vitamin D or 10 μg of 25(OH)D per day can reduce bone loss in epileptic populations.[114–116]

Whittle and associates[117] and others[113] have suggested the use of intravenous vitamin D for the detection of early stages of osteomalacia in the elderly. They claim that a favorable response to 40,000 IU (1 mg) of vitamin D, as measured by a greater than 15% increase in serum phosphorus within 6 days after the dose, strongly supports the diagnosis of vitamin D–deficient osteomalacia and helps distinguish this disorder from other forms of osteomalacia discussed here. Occasionally, oral calcium supplement and higher doses of vitamin D are required during the early treatment phase, especially in children with severe vitamin D–deficient rickets, in order to avoid the development of tetany.

Other investigators[113, 118, 119] have reported successful treatment of nutritional rickets and osteomalacia with either 1,25 (OH)D or 1α(OH)D. Similar beneficial effects have not been achieved with dihydrotachysterols,[120] which are no longer of clinical use. Because the role of other metabolites of vitamin D in regulating the process of mineralization has not been established, treatment with vitamin D alone is probably preferable. Phosphate supplements are not indicated in deficiency rickets or osteomalacia because of the potential hazard of severe hypocalcemia and tetany.

In summary, rickets and osteomalacia are being recognized with increasing frequency in selected populations. The availability of assays of serum 25(OH)D has also permitted detection of these disorders prior to the development of overt clinical disease.[78, 79, 113]

ACIDOSIS AND OSTEOMALACIA

Acidosis resulting from a number of different causes has been associated with osteomalacia. The mechanisms of bone loss and the mineralization defects are complex, and the problem is by no means settled. Albright and Reifenstein[39] originally suggested that acidosis produces slow dissolution of the mineral phase of bone in an attempt to buffer retained hydrogen ion. This process is associated with hypercalciuria. Support for this suggestion has been obtained by studies of patients with renal tubular acidosis in whom retention of hydrogen ion is greater than that theoretically required to produce the observed decrease in plasma bicarbonate concentrations.[121] On the basis of measurements in normal subjects in whom metabolic acidosis is induced, it has been proposed that the excess of retained hydrogen ion is balanced by the increase in urinary calcium excretion.[122, 123] This has been ascribed to increased bone dissolution. The effects of acidosis on increasing bone resorption may also be cellularly mediated.[124, 125] For example, in vitro comparable small decrements in pH produce greater calcium release from living than from dead bones. The hypercalciuria and increased bone resorption that accompany most acidotic states do not directly result in osteomalacia; therefore, other mechanisms must be invoked to explain the occurrence of clinically significant skeletal mineralization defects.

Maintenance of pH within a critical range is essential for mineralization to proceed normally. In rats, in which it is possible to obtain micropuncture samples at calcification sites in the growth plate, the pH is approximately 7.6.[126, 127] An independent decrease in systemic pH alone could thus inhibit mineralization by lowering pH at calcification sites. It has been demonstrated that chronic extracellular acidosis activates vacuolar hydrogen ion pumps in isolated osteoclasts. These data are consistent with the concept that acidosis induces the vacuolar-type adenosinetriphosphatase (ATPase) and stimulates osteoclastic bone resorption.[128] Furthermore PTH and acidosis have independent yet additive effects on bone resorption.[129] Acidosis can also affect phosphate metabolism[130] by altering renal tubular handling of the anion and changing the species of phosphate in solution (see Chapter 73). In patients with chronic acidosis (e.g., with ureterosigmoidostomy, an operation that is no longer performed), treatment with alkali alone can restore a low serum phosphate level to normal when the acidosis is alleviated. Currently, the use of ileal bladder substitutes is not associated with hyperchloremia, acidosis, or vitamin D deficiency.[131] This is accomplished by increased renal tubular phosphate reabsorption, accompanied by an increased phosphate maximal tubular excretory capacity. Secondary hyperparathyroidism may be an important factor in the altered phosphate handling in systemic acidosis.[130] Harrison and Harrison[132] have emphasized that acidosis may also alter the response to exogenous vitamin D. They showed that doses of vitamin D that were ineffective in producing rises in intestinal calcium absorption and serum calcium levels in the presence of acidosis were effective when the acidosis was corrected. In rats made acidotic with ammonium chloride feeding, conversion of cholecalciferol to 1,25$(OH)_2$ cholecalciferol measured in the intestine is diminished[133] despite the presence of hypocalcemia and hypophosphatemia, both of which usually stimulate formation of this metabolite.

Rickets and osteomalacia secondary to acidosis are most often a complication of distal renal tubular acidosis.[1, 2, 134–136] In most of the reported cases,[2, 137] healing of the bone disease can result from correction of the acidosis with sodium bicarbonate alone (5 to 10 g/day). Healing is slow, and the response may be hastened by the addition of vitamin D or 1,25$(OH)_2$D. Occasionally, vitamin D toxicity may develop unexpectedly, and these patients must therefore be carefully monitored. Although treatment with vitamin D is usually not necessary once the osteomalacia is cured, continued use of vitamin D may be required to complete healing in those individuals in whom the glomerular filtration rate is low.[137, 138]

In several of the syndromes associated with more widespread renal tubular reabsorptive defects, systemic acidosis may contribute to the pathogenesis of osteomalacia. Some of these are inherited, such as various forms of Fanconi's syndrome, with and without cystinosis, and Lowe's syndrome (oculocerebrorenal syndrome). Some patients with renal tubular phosphate leaks may also have mild acidosis, especially those associated with excessive urinary excretion of glycine.[139–142] The clinical picture is variable in these cases, and the specificity of the hyperglycinuria has not been established. Detailed considerations of the general features of these syndromes have been published,[1, 134–136, 143] and other aspects are considered elsewhere in this chapter.

As mentioned, osteomalacia may also be a complication of the acidosis produced by ureterosigmoidostomy, a procedure formerly used in the treatment of patients with carcinoma of the bladder.[130] Reabsorption of chloride and hydrogen ions from urine in the colon is responsible for the acidosis. An example of Looser's zones seen in such individuals is shown in Figure 87–10. Keeping the rectosigmoid empty by frequent drainage may prevent or correct the acidosis and thus prevent the development of osteomalacia. Although it is rarely used at present as a diuretic, we have encountered typical osteomalacia (Fig. 87–11) in a patient with acidosis presumably resulting from chronic acetazolamide therapy. This patient was receiving phenobarbital and phenytoin as well for a severe seizure disorder, but when the acetazolamide alone was discontinued and the plasma bicarbonate increased, the osteomalacia showed evidence of healing both radiologically and clinically. Acetazolamide has direct inhibitory effects on bone resorption in animals independent of pH,[144] and carbonic anhydrase inhibitors do prevent bone loss in humans.[195] Therefore an exact interpretation of the course in this patient is not possible at this time. More recent evidence for the role of carbonic anhydrase in bone resorption will be considered in the discussion on osteopetrosis.

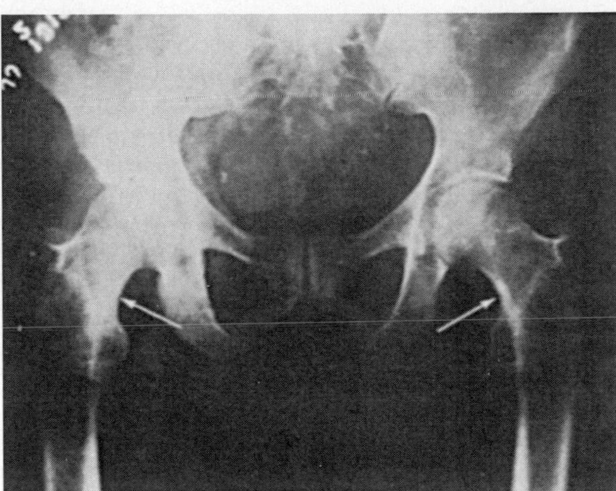

FIGURE 87–10. Radiograph of pelvis and femora of a 60-year-old man with ureterosigmoidostomy. Note Looser's zones *(arrows)*.

DIETARY PHOSPHATE DEPLETION

In humans, phosphate depletion and resultant hypophosphatemia may lead to the development of rickets or osteomalacia by mechanisms discussed earlier. A state of phosphate depletion can be produced either by inadequate dietary supply of this element or by excessive losses through urine or stool (see Chapter 73). It is difficult to produce selective deficiency of phosphorus by dietary means alone because most foods contain this element in concentrations sufficient to prevent hypophosphatemia and bone disease (see Chapter 73). Several authors[99, 146 153] have reported the occurrence of severe phosphate depletion and hypophosphatemia associated with osteomalacia in patients ingesting large quantities of nonabsorbable antacids, usually as a form of self-medication for dyspepsia. Studies in these patients, as well as in normal volunteers, have revealed that ingestion of nonabsorbable

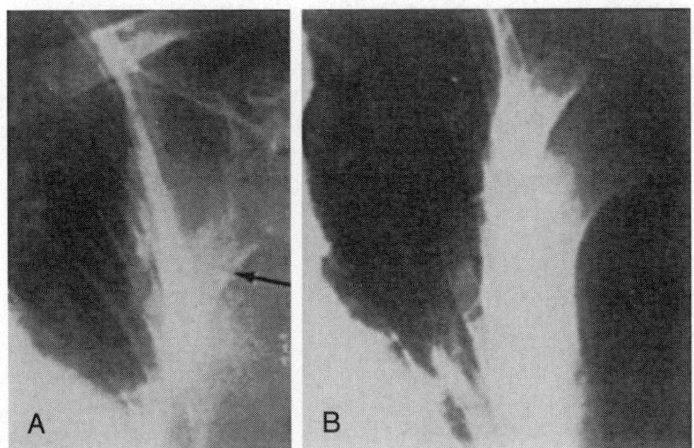

FIGURE 87–11. Radiograph of left scapula from a 42-year-old woman with acidosis due in part to chronic acetazolamide therapy. *A,* Before and *B,* six months after discontinuing acetazolamide. Note Looser's zone *(arrow)* in pretreatment radiograph.

antacids in large doses is associated with a rapid decline in urinary phosphorus to undetectable levels.[147, 148] This is accompanied by a marked increase in fecal phosphorus content, presumably related to binding of dietary phosphate by the antacid, resulting in a complex that is poorly absorbed from the gastrointestinal tract. With continued ingestion of the antacid, serum phosphorus levels gradually decrease, eventually leading to symptomatic hypophosphatemia. The early decline in urinary phosphorus excretion cannot be accounted for entirely by a decrease in filtered load because decreases in glomerular filtration rates are not observed initially. In addition to the changes in phosphorus handling, these individuals also develop hypercalciuria. Because serum calcium levels also do not change despite marked hypophosphatemia, the hypercalciuria cannot be attributed to changes in filtered load of calcium. The levels of urinary calcium excretion occasionally exceed that of dietary calcium intake; therefore, a portion of the urinary calcium excreted must be of skeletal origin. Most of the affected individuals show no evidence of increased bone resorption, however, although a small increase in osteoclastic surface and number of osteoclasts has been reported in one patient studied.[99] It is more likely that the rise in urinary calcium excretion is related primarily to impaired bone mineralization, a concept that is supported by the association of this syndrome with osteomalacia. Godsall et al.[99] also measured the serum levels of 1,25- and 24,25$(OH)_2D$ in this patient with antacid-induced osteomalacia. Although levels of 1,25$(OH)_2D$ were elevated, the levels of the 24,25$(OH)_2D$ metabolite were reduced. It is therefore possible that altered vitamin D metabolism could have a role in the pathogenesis of this disorder. Several other authors[151–153] have documented elevated or high-normal levels of 1,25$(OH)_2D$ in patients with antacid-induced osteomalacia. In general, however, clinically significant bone disease is quite rare, despite the wide use of nonabsorbable antacids for treatment of peptic ulcer disease. This suggests that despite interference with intestinal phosphate absorption, an ample supply of dietary phosphorus in milk and dairy products compensates for the absorptive defect. A similar syndrome of phosphate depletion has been described in patients with renal failure receiving large quantities of aluminum hydroxide gel (see following section), but osteomalacia in these patients may be related to aluminum intoxication.

Hypophosphatemia has also been observed in both chronic and acute alcoholism[154, 155] (see Chapter 73). Bone densitometric studies and tetracycline-labeled bone biopsies obtained from chronic alcoholic patients have revealed an increased frequency of bone disease compared to sex- and race-matched controls.[156] The bone abnormalities include changes consistent with mixtures of osteoporosis, osteomalacia, and osteitis fibrosa.

The bone disease in alcoholism may be part of the generalized skeletal disorder associated with chronic liver disease of diverse origin, which has been termed "hepatic osteodystrophy."[157–159] The syndrome comprises osteomalacia, osteitis fibrosa, osteoporosis, and periosteal new bone formation in the presence of chronic liver disease.[157, 160] Osteomalacia is most common in patients with cholestasis (particularly primary biliary cirrhosis), but is also observed in patients with alcoholic liver disease and other forms of cirrhosis. In most patients, the serum levels of 25(OH)D are low, ascribable to impaired intestinal absorption of vitamin D, but reduced exposure to ultraviolet light and reduced dietary intake also contribute. Healing of hepatic osteomalacia can be induced using various metabolities of vitamin D_2 or D_3, such as 25$(OH)D_3$, 1$\alpha(OH)D_3$, and 1,25$(OH)_2D_3$.

IMPAIRED RENAL TUBULAR PHOSPHATE REABSORPTION

In 1937, Albright and co-workers[161] reported their studies of a 16-year-old boy with long-standing rickets in whom standard doses of vitamin D failed to produce clinical improvement. Healing of the bone disease eventually occurred, but only after administration of extremely high doses of vitamin D. The results of their studies led to the introduction of the concept of "vitamin D resistance" in certain types of rickets. Since this initial report, so-called vitamin D–resistant rickets has been classified into several clinical and biochemical subtypes, the most common of which is the X-linked, dominantly inherited form discussed in detail in Chapter 82. Affected individuals usually present with clinical and radiographic evidence of rickets within the second or third year of life. Another X-linked form has been identified in which the bone disease first becomes manifest in the fourth or fifth decade without evidence of earlier rachitic abnormalities.[162] In still other patients, the disease occurs sporadically in the absence of an associated family history of bone disease or hypophosphatemia. As in the X-linked form of the disease, the cardinal biochemical disturbance is the abnormally low serum phosphorus level, which can be accounted for by a primary renal tubular phosphorus leak. Plasma calcium levels are normal, but serum alkaline phosphatase activity is usually increased, although in some individuals the elevations are minimal.[163, 164] The calcium balance in untreated patients tends to be slightly negative or zero and the urinary excretion of hydroxyproline peptides is usually normal.[30, 164, 165] The diagnosis depends upon the demonstration of impaired renal tubular phosphorus absorption and the presence of osteomalacia (i.e., widened osteoid seams and increased osteoid surface on bone biopsy). As in the X-linked disease other causes of osteomalacia, such as those listed in Table 87–2, must be excluded, particularly primary vitamin D deficiency, malabsorption, renal insufficiency, generalized renal tubular disorders, neurofibromatosis, and the presence of certain mesenchymal tumors. Evaluation of patients with possible adult-onset hypophosphatemic osteomalacia should thus include general tests of renal function (creatinine clearance, acidification, and concentrating ability, and analysis of urinary amino acid excretion), tests of intestinal absorptive capacity (fecal fat, D-xylose absorption), and careful search for the presence of occult tumors.

The mode of presentation of patients with adult hypophosphatemic osteomalacia or phosphate diabetes, as it has occasionally been termed, is characteristic. In contrast to individuals with the X-linked form, patients with the sporadic disease often develop prominent myopathy similar to that seen in other forms of rickets or osteomalacia. Deformities of the limbs are usually absent (possibly indicating normophosphatemia during the growth period), but these patients may experience severe bone pain related to vertebral body collapse or femoral neck fractures. As in other forms of osteomalacia, radiographs often reveal extensive pseudofractures. Some subjects may also have isolated renal hyperglycinuria and occasionally renal glycosuria in addition to the hypophosphatemia. Generalized aminoaciduria or acidification defects are not usually seen in these individuals.

With regard to the pathogenesis of the hypophosphatemia in individuals with the X-linked disorder, early studies had suggested that there was a primary defect in the renal tubular membrane transport of inorganic phosphate[161, 166, 167] and an associated defect in intestinal membrane transport.[168–170] A model for the human disease is the *Hyp* mouse in which there is a demonstrable impairment of the high-affinity, low-capacity, Na^+-dependent phosphate co-transport system.[171–173] Later it was found that there was a reduction of approximately 50% in levels of the messenger RNA (mRNA) and protein encoded by the sodium-phosphate co-transporter, *Npt2*. Later, the human *NPT2* gene was mapped to chromosome 5q35, thereby excluding it as a candidate for X-linked hypophosphatemia. Later, targeted inactivation of the *Npt2* gene was accomplished.[174] This resulted in hypercalcemia, hypercalciuria, and decreased serum PTH levels and increased serum alkaline phosphatase levels, findings also not found in the X-linked disease but typical of patients with a syndrome termed *hereditary hypophosphatemia rickets with hypercalciuria* (HHRH), a mendelian disorder of renal tubular phosphate reabsorption.[175]

The positional cloning approach was then utilized by a consortium of investigators to identify the gene for X-linked hypophosphatemia and map the gene to Xp22.1.[176, 177] The gene was structurally similar to a group of membrane-bound metalloendopeptidases and was termed *PEX*. Later, the name was changed to *PHEX* to avoid confusion with other genes. Many mutations have now been shown in the *PHEX* genes in patients with X-linked hypophosphatemia as well as in the murine *Phex* gene in the *Hyp* mouse.[178–180] It is still not clear how the mutations in the *PHEX* genes account for the excessive renal tubular phosphate losses, but this issue should be resolved in the next few years. One of the putative phosphaturia factors has been termed *phos-*

phatonin[181] and will be considered further in the discussion of oncogenic osteomalacia.

Another disorder with isolated renal tubular phosphate wasting and inappropriately normal plasma 1,25$(OH)_2$D levels has been termed *autosomal dominant hypophosphatemic rickets* (ADHR). In contrast to X-linked hypophosphatemia, ADHR displays variable and incomplete penetrance, as well as other clinical manifestations.[179, 182] The locus for ADHR is on chromosome 12p13, firmly establishing the distinction from the X-linked disorder, although so far the gene responsible has not been identified. Patients with so-called adult-onset X-linked hypophosphatemia also have been shown to have mutations in the *PHEX* gene and therefore do not represent a distinct entity.[183] Although a missense mutation in the gene for voltage-gated chloride channel, *CLCN5* had been previously reported in X-linked recessive hypophosphatemic rickets, in an additional kindred with an inherited syndrome of hypercalciuria, nephrocalcinosis, low-molecular-weight proteinuria, renal tubular acidosis and renal failure, but *without* hypophosphatemia or rickets, the same mutation in *CLCN5* was found in affected members.[184]

It has been suggested that alterations in 1α-hydroxylase activity secondary to impaired phosphate handling by the proximal renal tubules are responsible for the apparent abnormalities in vitamin D metabolism in this condition.[185] The possible role of PTH and altered vitamin D metabolism in the pathogenesis of the X-linked form of hypophosphatemia is considered in Chapter 82. In these patients, serum levels of 25(OH)D are normal, whereas the levels of 1,25$(OH)_2$D are in the low-normal range. The latter may be inappropriately low for the level of serum phosphorus, however. Based on these observations, Harrell et al.[186] have evaluated the therapeutic effects of high doses of 1,25$(OH)_2$D in patients with X-linked hypophosphatemic rickets. Affected patients were treated with 1,25$(OH)_2D_3$ (more than 1 μg/day) plus oral phosphate (1 to 2 g/day phosphorus equivalent), and all demonstrated complete healing, by radiographic as well as by histologic criteria. Hypercalcemia and hypercalciuria developed in four of five patients, necessitating reduction in the dose of 1,25$(OH)_2D_3$. Subsequently, normal mineralization could be maintained with lower doses of the vitamin D metabolites plus phosphorus supplements. Verge and coworkers,[187] who treated 24 children with 1,25$(OH)_2D_3$ and phosphate for at least 2 years, noted a 79% incidence of nephrocalcinosis detected by renal ultrasonography; of note is that heterozygous girls appear to respond better than hemizygous boys to 1,25$(OH)_2D_3$ and phosphate therapy.[188]

Although abnormal metabolism of vitamin D or altered renal and intestinal response to this vitamin may exist in patients with adult sporadic hypophosphatemia, nearly complete healing of the bone disease (as shown by biopsy) can be effected with oral phosphate supplements alone in some individuals[31] (Fig. 87–12). The first changes associated with the institution of oral phosphate therapy are a rise in serum phosphorus level, often accompanied by a fall in serum calcium level and a decrease in urinary calcium excretion. Initially, fecal calcium excretion remains high, but with prolonged phosphate supplements, fecal calcium excretion decreases and positive calcium balance develops.

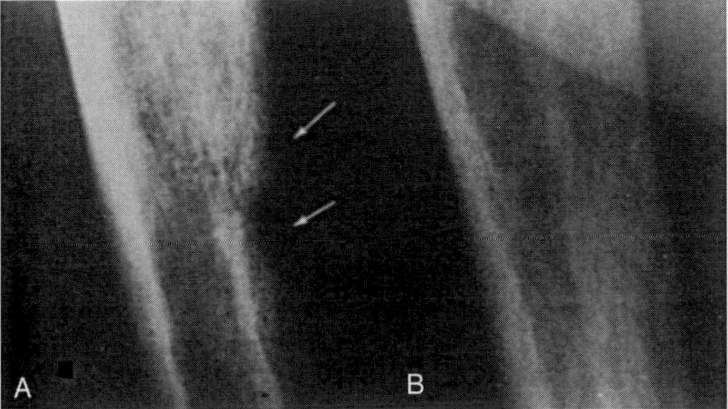

FIGURE 87–12. Radiograph of right femur of a patient with phosphate diabetes (case 2 in Jaworshi et al.[22]). *A,* Before therapy. *B,* Eleven weeks after starting phosphate therapy. *Arrows* indicate Looser's zones.

Although usually normal prior to treatment, serum immunoreactive PTH levels are elevated during the initial stage of therapy with phosphate, suggesting that phosphate supplementation results in stimulation, to some degree, of increased secretion of PTH by inducing hypocalcemia. The mechanism of the hypocalcemia may be related to a phosphate-induced increased rate of mineralization and increased net movement of calcium into bone. An increase in urinary hydroxyproline excretion also accompanies initiation of therapy, presumably reflecting increased bone (matrix) resorption related either to a primary effect of phosphate supplementation or to a secondary effect of increased PTH secretion. Cessation of phosphate supplementation results in a rapid fall in urinary hydroxyproline excretion and return of the immunoreactive PTH levels to normal. These findings suggest that PTH plays a secondary rather than a primary role in the genesis of the renal tubular phosphate leak.

A variety of neutral phosphate salts are available for oral supplementation, including sodium and potassium salts or mixtures of the two. We have compared the relative efficacy of the neutral sodium and potassium phosphate salts and have observed consistently greater elevations in serum phosphorus levels in individuals receiving the potassium salt.[189] The less favorable results with the sodium salt are most likely related to the effects of the sodium ion on increasing renal phosphate clearance. The rise in serum phosphorus level after a single oral dose of phosphate is transient,[31, 167, 189, 190] and therefore phosphate supplements must be administered at frequent intervals. The precise amount of phosphate must be individualized in each patient; in individuals with severe leaks, as much as 1000 mg of elemental phosphorus is required every 4 to 6 hours to effect sustained elevations of serum phosphorus levels.

The efficacy of therapy cannot be assessed with a single fasting determination of phosphatemia; multiple measurements of serum levels at various times after each dose are required. Emptying the capsules and dissolving the salt in water or other liquid may improve intestinal absorption and enhance serum phosphorus levels. Most patients experience some degree of gastrointestinal distress, such as cramps and diarrhea, when therapy is initiated. Therefore initial doses should be low and increments gradually introduced as tolerated. Glorieux et al.[191] have shown that simultaneous use of phosphate and vitamin D has resulted in accelerated healing in children with the X-linked form of hypophosphatemic osteomalacia. Vitamin D itself or various analogues have a "phosphate-sparing" effect, allowing the use of lower doses of oral phosphate supplements. Whether the improved serum phosphorus levels seen with vitamin D or 1,25$(OH)_2$D are accounted for by increased intestinal absorption of phosphate or decreased renal loss (due to decreased secondary hyperparthyroidism) has not been established. Sullivan et al.[192] and Glorieux et al.[191] have reviewed the outcome of treatment of symptomatic adults with X-linked hypophosphatemia. Prior studies[193] documented the efficacy of combined therapy with oral phosphate and 1,25$(OH)_2$D in children, but comparable data were not available in adults. It was noted that, although most patients tolerated this therapy, 1 patient of the original 16 developed parathyroid hyperplasia and hypercalcemia during treatment and renal insufficiency that progressed despite cessation of therapy. We have also noted the development of this type of secondary hyperparathyroidism with hypercalcemia in patients with this condition, treated for extended periods with phosphate supplementation.

Although over the past decade most patients have been treated with 1,25$(OH)_2$D, we have also observed improved phosphate tolerance in our patients on oral phosphate with vitamin D, 1α(OH)D, and dihydrotachysterol.[189] The doses have been adjusted to produce maximal serum phosphorus levels without raising urinary calcium excretion. In our hands, calcium supplements, as suggested by others,[164] are not required during early phases of treatment. With healing of the osteomalacia, serum phosphorus levels can be maintained with lower doses of supplemental phosphorus, at least in some patients. Decreased phosphate requirements have not been related to decreased glomerular filtration rate, because renal function has usually been well maintained.

TUMOR-ASSOCIATED RICKETS AND OSTEOMALACIA

In 1959, Prader et al.[194] described the case of an 11-year-old girl who, over the course of a year, developed severe symptomatic rickets accompanied by hypophosphatemia, increased renal phosphate clearance, and mild hypocalcemia. The child was found to have a large tumor in the left chest that on biopsy was interpreted as a reparative giant cell granuloma of a rib. Following excision of the tumor, the rickets healed without any specific therapy. It was postulated that the giant cell reparative granuloma may have produced a "rachitogenic substance." A case reported earlier by McCance[195] was subsequently considered to be an example of this situation,[196] as was the patient reported by Hauge.[197]

Since that time numerous patients have been described in whom osteomalacia has been associated with the presence of various types of tumor.[198–212] One review included 69 reported cases and 3 additional cases of the authors.[213] Of the 72 tumors, 40 were localized to bone and 31 to soft tissues; two-thirds of the tumors occurred in the extremities. More than one-third of the tumors were classified as vascular tumors, and half of these were hemangiopericytomas. Other common pathologic diagnoses were nonossifiying fibromas and "mesenchymal" and giant cell tumors. All of the tumors exhibited prominent vascularity and the presence of multinucleated giant cells and primitive stromal cells. Ten of the tumors were classified as malignant.

Although most neoplasms associated with this syndrome have been exclusively of mesenchymal origin, Lyles et al.[214] have reported two cases of hypophosphatemic osteomalacia associated with prostatic carcinoma. As in other forms of tumor-associated osteomalacia, $1,25(OH)_2D$ levels were low. They speculated that the high frequency of hypophosphatemia in patients with prostate carcinoma could be related to the effects of tumor products that influence renal phosphate handling. Stone et al.[215] reported the occurrence of osteomalacia in a patient with a spinal tumor that exhibited histologic features of a neuroendocrine tumor. In most of the reported cases, the removal of the tumor results in clinical cure of the osteomalacia or rickets, although, in some, early recurrence of the tumor or inadequate removal of the malignancy presumably prevents a good clinical response.[3] In the patient reported from our service[199] (Fig. 87–13), the tumor was a malignant giant cell sarcoma that was first detected clinically after the osteomalacia was successfully treated with phosphate supplements and vitamin D. When the tumor, which involved the upper femur, was resected by hindquarter amputation, the hypophosphatemia improved, despite cessation of phosphate and vitamin D therapy. Four years later, hypophosphatemia recurred, associated with the reappearance of pulmonary metastases. The patient died 2 years thereafter of a massive pulmonary embolus, at which time the lungs were filled with metastatic tumor.

All of these patients had hypophosphatemia, high phosphate clearance, and normal or nearly normal serum calcium levels. In a few, renal glycosuria was also present. When measured, serum immunoreactive PTH levels have usually been normal,[200, 203, 205] although high values have also been reported in some cases.[202] The size of the tumors has ranged from very large, in the original case of Prader et al.,[194] to one as small as 1×1 cm. In several instances the tumor was not detected until years after development of clinical osteomalacia.[3, 205] On the other hand, clinical response to resection of the tumor is observed by an average of 16 weeks (range 24 hours to 17 months).[3, 205]

Measurements in most patients with tumor-associated osteomalacia usually reveal low or undetectable levels of serum $1,25(OH)_2D$.[206, 216–218] Oral administration of $1,25(OH)_2D$ in amounts sufficient to raise serum levels of this metabolite decreases the renal phosphorus clearance and increases serum phosphorus concentrations, although not into the normal range.[206] It has been suggested that these tumors release products that impair renal function, including 1α-hydroxylation of 25(OH)D and phosphate transport. Evidence to support this hypothesis is provided by studies by Miyauchi et al.,[219] who transplanted into nude mice tumor tissue excised from a patient with classic clinical and laboratory features of oncogenic osteomalacia. Nodules formed in all animals, and the nodules demonstrated histologic features of the original tumor (a hemangiopericytoma.) The tumor-bearing animals demonstrated hypophosphatemia and increased urinary phosphate excretion consistent with the development of the tumor-associated syndrome. Addition of extracts of the tumor to renal tubular cells resulted in inhibition of 25(OH)D 1α-hydroxylase activity. Nitzan et al.[220] reported the development of a similar sequence of events in nude mice in whom tumor tissue (fibrosarcoma) from a patient with oncogenic osteomalacia had been transferred, although they did not investigate the effects of the murine tumors on vitamin D metabolism. That the tumor is the source of the factor(s) is suggested by the increase in circulating levels of $1,25(OH)_2D$ and restoration of serum phosphorus concentrations following removal of the tumor. Others have also provided evidence for the secretion of a phosphaturic factor by the tumors in tumor-induced osteomalacia.[221, 222] Although this factor, which Econs and Drezner[179, 181] termed *phosphatonin*, has not yet been identified, it could also be responsible for the renal phosphate leak in the *Hyp* mouse. Econs[179] pointed out that since *PHEX* mutations that result in the X-linked hypophosphatemia phenotype are loss-of-function mutations, then *PHEX* could not be "phosphatonin." Nevertheless, he raised the possibility that the *PHEX* gene product could have a role in regulating the production of "phosphatonin." Kumar et al.[223] postulated that a gene product called HEM-1 might be a factor responsible for the hypophosphatemia of tumor-induced osteomalacia. Nelson et al.,[224] however, were subsequently unable to detect the expression of HEM-1 in two tumors excised from patients with tumor-associated osteomalacia.

Hypophosphatemic osteomalacia may also occur in association with neurofibromatosis, although the nature of the association is unclear.[225–230] Dent and Gertner[231] also described three patients with fibrous dysplasia who had concomitant hypophosphatemic osteomalacia or rickets. Two of the patients were adults with polyostotic fibrous dysplasia, and the third was an 8-year-old child with fibrous dysplasia of the facial bones and rickets. In the child, resection of most of the dysplastic bone was accompanied by improvement in the metabolic bone disease. The authors were aware of five previously reported cases in which fibrous dysplasia in children was associated with hypophosphatemia and rickets. The immunoreactive PTH levels in the cases of Dent and Gertner[231] were not elevated. These authors suggested that the occurrence of hypophosphatemia and bone disease in patients with fibrous dysplasia is analogous to other forms of oncogenic osteomalacia.

GENERAL RENAL TUBULAR DISORDERS

In addition to the individuals previously described with so-called vitamin D–resistant rickets and osteomalacia attributable solely to a primary renal phosphate leak, a further subset of patients with rickets or osteomalacia of renal origin can be identified. The disorder in these individuals is characterized by a generalized dysfunction of the proximal renal tubules leading to excessive loss of amino acids, glucose, phosphate, uric acid, and bicarbonate in the absence of a primary disturbance in glomerular function. The metabolic consequences of these disturbances are systemic acidosis, hypophosphatemia, and dehydration, which in turn lead to growth disturbance and development of rickets or osteomalacia. These disorders have been classified under the general heading of de Toni-Debre-Fanconi syndrome or renal Fanconi's syndrome. They may be further classified into primary renal types, in which the underlying defect is located within the tubular cells, and prerenal types, in which toxic metabolic substances outside the kidney lead to derangements in tubular function (see Table 87–2). These disorders occur in adults as well as in children.

Dent and Harris[232] were the first to describe a patient with presumed adult-onset idiopathic Fanconi's syndrome with an autosomal recessive pattern of inheritance. These patients usually present at age 40 with signs and symptoms of hypokalemia and osteomalacia. They do not have cystinosis, and no other systemic disease has been identified. Healing of the bone disease has occurred with the use of vitamin D, alkali, and potassium. Brodehl[233] described another patient with presumed idiopathic Fanconi's syndrome of the sporadic type who presented at age 7 with muscle weakness and bone pain attributable to

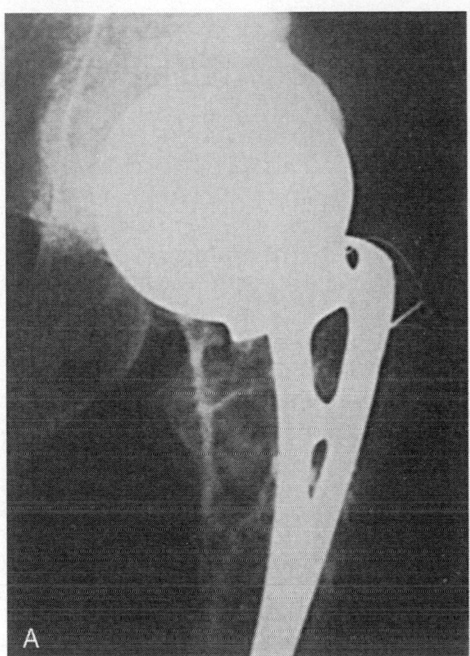

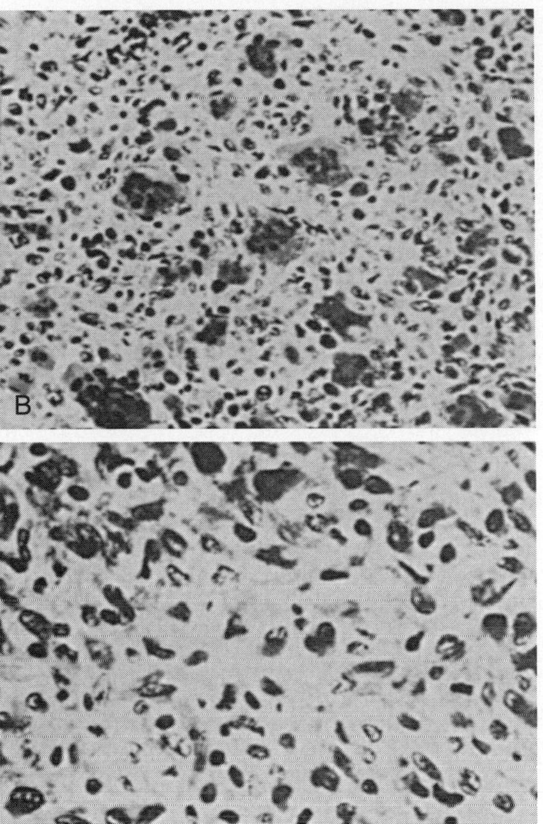

FIGURE 87–13. Radiograph of the left femur of a 56-year-old woman showing irregularity of cortex at site of giant cell sarcoma.[155] *B,* Sections of the tumor showing giant cells surrounded by atypical stromal cells. The latter are seen at higher power in *C.*

osteomalacia. Renal biopsy showed no crystalline material, and electron microscopic studies revealed the presence of abnormal giant mitochondria. This grouping of patients with idiopathic renal Fanconi's syndrome is somewhat artificial, and in time the specific biochemical derangements responsible for the tubular dysfunction may be identified.

In cystinosis (Lignac-de Toni-Fanconi syndrome),[143] glycogenosis,[233] and Lowe's syndrome,[234] the renal disease is associated with a more generalized systemic metabolic disorder. The precise metabolic defect in each of these diseases is unknown. In cystinosis, there is an accumulation of cystine in many tissues, including the kidneys, resulting in tubular dysfunction and later in renal glomerular failure. Recent experience with renal transplantation in patients with cystinosis has shown reaccumulation of cystine in the transplanted kidney without the reappearance of Fanconi's syndrome, suggesting that a primary renal tubular cell defect may exist in these patients.[235] Whether a similar pathogenic mechanism occurs in glycogenosis and in Lowe's syndrome is not known because the underlying metabolic defect in those syndromes remains obscure.

In Wilson's disease, tyrosinemia,[236] and the other inborn errors of metabolism outlined in Table 87–2, Fanconi's syndrome may be an accompaniment of the generalized systemic disease and lead to the development of bone disease. In Wilson's disease, the clinical and pathologic manifestations are presumably related to the toxic effects of excessive accumulation of copper in liver, kidney, brain, and cornea. Most patients present with signs and symptoms secondary to liver disease, hemolytic anemia, or neurologic disease. Occasionally, however, renal dysfunction and associated osteomalacia may predominate. Morgan et al.[237] were the first to describe a patient with Wilson's disease in whom Fanconi's syndrome and rickets were the initial presenting features. Although the bone disease responded promptly to oral vitamin D supplementation, the tubular dysfunction persisted. Renal biopsy from this patient did not reveal evidence of swan-neck deformity. The renal tubular abnormalities in these patients include aminoaciduria, glucosuria, uricosuria, hypercalciuria, and renal tubular acidosis. Studies by Wilson and Goldstein[238] have suggested that the defect in acidification is presumably related to a distal rather than a proximal tubular defect. The presence of hypercalciuria and the frequent occurrence of renal lithiasis are consistent with a distal tubular abnormality. Several investigators[238, 239] have shown that treatment of Wilson's disease with D-penicillamine significantly improves the renal tubular acidification defect. As mentioned earlier, in patients with coexistent rickets or osteomalacia, healing of the bone disease can be accomplished with oral vitamin D supplements alone.

The development of Fanconi's syndrome in plasma cell myeloma has been attributed to the toxic effects of Bence Jones protein on the proximal renal tubules.[240] Although extremely rare, osteomalacia may develop as a consequence of the renal phosphate wasting and resultant hypophosphatemia. Osteomalacia associated with renal tubular acidosis has also been reported in a patient with Sjögren's syndrome[241] with documented increased urinary excretion of β_2-microglobulin and retinol-binding protein. The patient showed clinical improvement after treatment with oral potassium citrate, calcium supplements, and glucocorticoids.

Fanconi's syndrome and osteomalacia have been observed in patients with heavy metal poisoning, particularly cadmium.[242, 243] The bone disease is presumably secondary to hypophosphatemia and systemic acidosis produced by impaired tubular function. A similar syndrome has been described in lead intoxication[244] and in patients exposed to outdated tetracycline.[245]

In the various types of so-called prerenal Fanconi's syndrome, the specific treatment of the underlying disorder often results in disappearance or improvement in the renal tubular dysfunction, thus allowing healing of the associated bone disease. In several of the above disorders, improvement in the bone disease can also be achieved by correcting the acidosis and hypophosphatemia (i.e., supplementation with alkali, oral phosphate, and vitamin D).

HYPOPHOSPHATASIA

Hypophosphatasia is a heritable disorder characterized by deficiency in alkaline phosphatase, increased urinary excretion of phosphoryl-

TABLE 87–2. Classification of Rickets and Osteomalacia

I. Vitamin D lack
  A. Dietary deficiency
    1. "Classic" nutritional
    2. Fat-phobic
  B. Deficient endogenous synthesis
    1. Inadequate solar irradiation
    2. Other factors, e.g., genetic, aging
II. Gastrointestinal
  A. Intestinal
    1. Small intestine diseases with malabsorption, e.g., celiac disease (gluten-sensitive enteropathy)
    2. Partial or total gastrectomy
    3. Intestinal bypass
  B. Hepatobiliary
    1. Cirrhosis
    2. Biliary fistula
    3. Biliary atresia
  C. Pancreatic
    1. Chronic pancreatic insufficiency
III. Disorders of vitamin D metabolism
  A. Hereditary
    1. "Pseudovitamin D deficiency" (vitamin D dependency)—recessive inheritance
  B. Acquired
    1. Anticonvulsants
    2. Renal insufficiency (see below)
IV. Acidosis
  A. Distal renal tubular acidosis (classic or type I)
    1. Primary (specific cause not determined)
      a. Sporadic
      b. Familial
    2. Secondary
      a. Galactosemia (after galactose ingestion)
      b. Hereditary fructose intolerance with nephrocalcinosis (after chronic fructose ingestion)
      c. Fabry's disease
    3. Hypergammaglobulinemic states
    4. Medullary sponge kidney
    5. Following renal transplantation
  B. Acquired
    1. Ureterosigmoidostomy
    2. Drug-induced
      a. Chronic acetazolamide administration
      b. Chronic ammonium chloride administration
V. Chronic renal failure
VI. Phosphate depletion
  A. Dietary
    1. Low phosphate intake
    2. Aluminum hydroxide ingestion (or other nonabsorbable hydroxides)
  B. Impaired renal tubular phosphate reabsorption (? intestinal)
    1. Hereditary
      a. X-linked hypophosphatemic rickets (vitamin D–resistant rickets)—dominant inheritance
      b. Adult-onset vitamin D–resistant hypophosphatemic osteomalacia—dominant inheritance
    2. Acquired
      a. Sporadic hypophosphatemic osteomalacia (phosphate diabetes)
      b. Tumor-associated rickets and osteomalacia (? includes neurofibromatosis and fibrous dysplasia)
VII. General renal tubular disorders (Fanconi's syndrome)
  A. Primary renal
    1. Idiopathic
      a. Sporadic
      b. Familial
    2. Associated with systemic metabolic process
      a. Cystinosis
      b. Glycogenosis
      c. Lowe's syndrome
  B. Systemic disorder with associated renal disease (prerenal)
    1. Hereditary
      a. Inborn errors
        i. Wilson's disease
        ii. Tyrosinemia
      b. Neurofibromatosis
    2. Acquired
      a. Multiple myeloma
      b. Nephrotic syndrome
      c. Transplanted kidney
    3. Intoxications
      a. Cadmium
      b. Lead
      c. Outdated tetracycline
VIII. Primary mineralization defects
  A. Hereditary
    1. Hypophosphatasia
  B. Acquired
    1. Diphosphonate administration
    2. Fluoride treatment
IX. States of rapid bone formation with or without a relative defect in bone resorption
  A. Postoperative hyperparathyroidism with osteitis fibrosa cystica
  B. Osteopetrosis
X. Defective matrix synthesis
  A. Fibrogenesis imperfecta ossium
XI. Miscellaneous
  A. Magnesium-dependent
  B. Steroid-sensitive
  C. Axial osteomalacia
  D. Aluminum intoxication
    1. Chronic renal failure
    2. Total parenteral nutrition

ethanolamine, and skeletal disease that includes osteomalacia and rickets.[246–250] The disease may present in infancy, when it is associated with hypercalcemia, renal failure, and increased intracranial pressure. These infants may show enlarged sutures of the skull, craniostenosis, delayed dentition, enlarged epiphyses, and prominent costochondral junctions. Genu valgum or varum may develop subsequently. The histologic picture is indistinguishable from other forms of rickets. In older children, it is manifested in a less severe form and may present as rickets alone. In this group, serum calcium and phosphorus levels are usually normal. In the infantile forms, the disorder is inherited as an autosomal recessive trait. The disorder in the adult, however, is probably distinct from the infantile and childhood forms and is inherited as an autosomal dominant trait with variable penetrance. In adults, even though osteopenia may be seen, the disorder tends to be mild, and osteomalacia may not be the primary pathologic process.[248, 251, 252]

Activity of the tissue-nonspecific (bone, kidney, or liver) alkaline phosphatase isoenzyme in blood and tissues is reduced. Phosphorylethanolamine and phosphorylcholine are excreted in excessive amounts in the urine, and the circulating levels of pyridoxal-5′-phosphate are markedly elevated.[252–256] Serum phosphorus levels are normal, and it is not clear how these biochemical findings are related to the inadequate skeletal mineralization. Alkaline phosphatase from bone cartilage and other tissues is a pyrophosphatase at neutral pH,[257, 258] and patients with hypophosphatasia demonstrate deficient pyrophosphatase activity.[259, 260] It is possible that the concentrations of inorganic pyrophosphate (which is the substrate for this enzyme and is a potent inhibitor of mineralization)[261] are too high to allow normal mineralization at sites of bone formation.[262]

Since the alkaline phosphatase cDNA was cloned, it has been possible to study the defects in the gene in patients with hypophosphatasia. Characterization of the patterns of clinical expression with the specific gene or mutation in humans has provided insights into the molecular basis for the high degree of phenotypic heterogeneity in this disorder. Observations in human subjects have been correlated with results of transfection studies using missense mutations as well as computer-assisted modeling to localize the crucial functions of domains of the enzyme. The results indicate that the extreme heterogeneity in phenotype among patients with hypophosphatasia are due to residual enzyme activity encoded by certain of the missense mutations.[263, 264] In several individuals with the lethal form, different missense mutations were identified.[265, 266]

Therapy is a problem. Vitamin D has been ineffective, and phosphate supplements are probably not indicated. Glucocorticoids are probably also ineffective.[199] When osteotomies are performed, healing has been slow.[125]

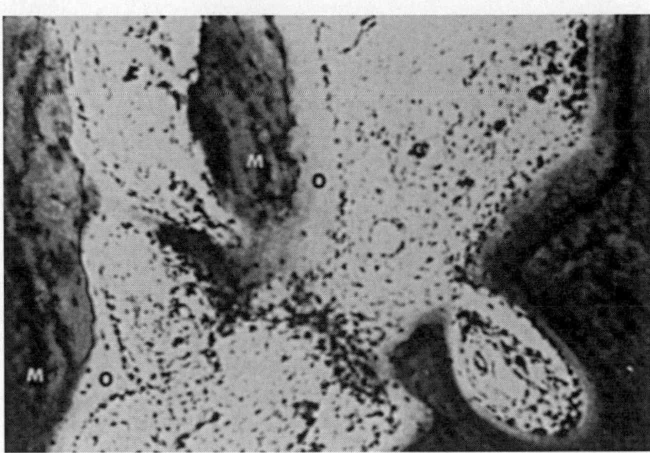

FIGURE 87–15. Section of bone from a patient with hyperparathyroidism and osteitis fibrosa cystica taken 8 days following removal of a parathyroid adenoma.[32] Even in this demineralized section stained with hematoxylin-eosin, mineralized bone (M) can be distinguished from the thickened osteoid seam (O).

CALCIFICATION INHIBITORS

The skeletal abnormalities that result from ingestion of excessive amounts of fluoride ion include increases in total osteoid surface.[267] These occur despite adequate vitamin D intake. When fluoride ion in doses of 13 to 41 mg/day is administered to patients with osteoporosis, the new bone formed is poorly mineralized and has other histologic features of osteomalacia.[268] These findings are reproduced in normal individuals consuming excessive amounts of fluoride. Evidence suggests that the mineralization defect can be overcome by increasing dietary intake of calcium and vitamin D (50,000 U twice weekly).

The diphosphonate etidronate disodium (EHDP) has been used in the treatment of a large number of patients with Paget's disease of bone.[269–275] In patients who have received 10 to 20 mg/kg/day for several months or longer, bone biopsies in a number of individuals have revealed increased osteoid surface as well as increased thickness of the osteoid seams.[271–274] Individuals who received the drug for periods of 3 to 17 months, especially at the higher dose range, have had an increased incidence of fractures associated with spotty increased radiolucency of involved bones.[274] An example of changes in bone histology produced after 18 months of therapy with EHDP at 10 to 20 mg/kg/day is shown in Figure 87–14. Here the mineralized pagetic bone is encased by lamellar osteoid, which in some instances exceeds 150 μm. The thick osteoid is located almost entirely around the pagetic bone, not around normal bone.[273] In patients with osteoporosis who have been treated with EHDP, broad osteoid seams have also been observed surrounding osteoporotic bone within 3 months of starting the drug.[276] Others have noted decreased tetracycline uptake at the calcification fronts.[273] The data suggested that EHDP acts primarily by inhibiting osteoclastic resorption, although at first bone formation continues at a high rate.[272, 274] The new bone is poorly mineralized as a result of an additional direct effect of EHDP on mineralization or an imbalance of bone resorption and formation, or both. At some time in the course of therapy, osteoblastic activity decreases, the rate of matrix synthesis slows, and the osteoid seams decrease. The gross radiologic abnormalities are reversed within months after EHDP is discontinued.[274] It is also possible that the mineralization defect is due in part to altered metabolism of vitamin D and inadequate formation of 1,25$(OH)_2$ cholecalciferol, as has been shown in animals receiving large doses of EHDP.[3, 277]

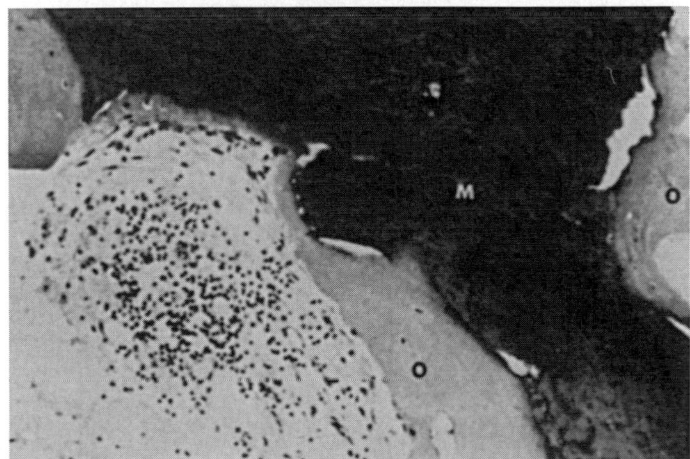

FIGURE 87–14. Undemineralized section stained with hematoxylin-eosin of femoral head from a patient with Paget's disease of bone who had been treated with the diphosphonate, etidronate disodium, initially for 12 months with 1 mg/kg/day followed by an additional 12 months with 10 mg/kg/day. He had no therapy for 3 months prior to total hip replacement when this specimen was obtained. Note mineralized pagetic bone (M) surrounded by lamellar nonpagetic osteoid (O).

HYPERPARATHYROIDISM AND HYPOPARATHYROIDISM

In individuals with hyperparathyroidism who have excessive bone resorption and high rates of bone formation, thick osteoid seams may be seen. The mineralization defects are especially prominent in the early period following operative therapy of the hyperparathyroidism when chemical osteomalacia (low levels of serum calcium and phosphorus) is associated with histologic changes in bone, as discussed by Albright and Reifenstein.[39] An example of this finding is shown in Figure 87–15. In some patients, however, frank osteomalacia has coexisted with untreated hyperparathyroidism.[3] Radiologic findings have included typical Looser's zones and vertebral hyperostosis. Some of the cases have been associated with intestinal malabsorption or "privational" vitamin D deficiency. Serum calcium levels have tended to be relatively or absolutely low. Standbury,[3] who reviewed the problem in detail, proposed that the syndrome is the bony expression of primary hyperparathyroidism modified by vitamin D deficiency.

It should also be noted that hypercalcemia and autonomous hyperparathyroidism may be associated with hypophosphatemic rickets and osteomalacia.[142, 278] It has been suggested that primary hyperparathyroidism is a chance occurrence in these individuals rather than a manifestation of the hypophosphatemic rickets or a complication of therapy.[279]

Hypoparathyroidism has also been associated with osteomalacia on rare occasions.[280] The mechanism may be related to a decrease in formation of $1,25(OH)_2D$ owing to lack of PTH per se as well as hyperphosphatemia.[281]

OSTEOPETROSIS

The association of radiologically dense bones and increased bone mass with rickets and osteomalacia has been discussed previously. Rickets also may occur in the severe (recessive) form of osteopetrosis.[282] Affected children may have low levels of serum phosphorus and calcium and increased activity of alkaline phosphatase.[283, 284] Dent[284] described an osteopetrotic child with gross aminoaciduria and increased urinary hydroxyproline excretion whose rickets failed to respond to a high dosage of vitamin D (15 μg/day).

The morphologic changes in cartilage and bone include, in addition to rickets, decreased osteoclastic and chondroclastic resorption and abnormal-appearing osteoclasts.[285] Considerable evidence indicates that this disorder is heterogeneous and that several different cellular or biochemical defects may account for the clinical manifestations. It is not clear why abnormal matrix mineralization should occur in these patients. One possible explanation is a decreased local supply of mineral ions secondary to decreased resorption in the face of relatively high rates of bone formation. Sly et al.[286] have characterized the biochemical defect in a series of 18 patients with the autosomal recessive syndrome of osteopetrosis with renal tubular acidosis and cerebral calcification. They found a virtual absence of the isoenzyme II of carbonic anhydrase. Reduced levels of isoenzyme II were also detected in obligate heterozygotes. Because these patients all had a mixed form of renal tubular acidosis, the contribution of the systemic acidosis to the mineralization defect remains uncertain.

FIBROGENESIS IMPERFECTA OSSIUM

Fibrogenesis imperfecta ossium[287–291] is a rare disorder characterized by progressively disabling skeletal pain and tenderness, forced immobilization, muscular weakness and atrophy, and contractures. It has been described in men over age 50. Levels of calcium and phosphorus in the serum are normal, but alkaline phosphatase activity is increased. The radiographic abnormalities are generalized and consist of thickened and amorphous-appearing trabeculae with spotty increase in density, reduced cortical thicknesses, and occasional pseudofractures. The abnormal "fishnet" trabecular pattern seen on conventional radiographs combined with MR imaging of low signal–intensity bone marrow on T1-weighted as well as T2-weighted images are helpful in diagnosis.[292] Histologically, there is an increase in thickness of "osteoid" which occurs diffusely on bone surfaces. Its appearance is distinctive and it is best seen using polarized light microscopy. The "osteoid" lacks the lamellar structure and typical birefringence that is characteristic of the other osteomalacic states. Electron microscopic studies[291] of the "osteoid" region have shown small-diameter collagen fibers that are immature and arranged in loops and dense areas that have been termed *whorls.* A single study of bone from a patient with fibrogenesis imperfecta ossium has revealed that the collagen was more soluble in neutral salt and dilute acetic acid. This was interpreted as indicative of defective cross-linking.[293] However, direct evidence for defective cross-linking or the chemical nature of the putative defect has not been obtained.

Of interest are observations that among the 17 cases of fibrogenesis imperfecta ossium reported by 1996, five had associated monoclonal gammopathy.[294] In the most recent reported case,[294] melphalan and calcitriol were ineffective in therapy. In an earlier report,[295] the use of glucocorticoids and intermittent melphalan appeared to be efficacious.

AXIAL OSTEOMALACIA

Axial osteomalacia is a term introduced by Frame et al.[296] in 1961 to describe a disorder occurring in three patients, all males. The characteristic radiographic findings included a coarsened and spongelike trabecular pattern in the bones of the cervical spine and, to a lesser degree, in the ribs, lumbar spine, and pelvis. The skull and appendicular skeleton were uninvolved. Bone biopsies revealed wide osteoid seams compatible with osteomalacia. The authors interpreted the serum chemical findings as inconsistent with other forms of osteomalacia. It should be emphasized, however, that the serum phosphorus level in one of the original cases was 2.6 mg/dL and in the other two, 3.1 mg/dL. Two cases have since been reported by Whyte et al.[297] and the literature reviewed. They described the findings in a family study of a black mother and son with axial osteomalacia associated with polycystic liver and kidney disease. Although they speculated that an abnormality of vitamin D action may be involved in the pathogenesis of the disorder, the actual levels of vitamin metabolites were normal.[18, 297, 298] It has been suggested[289] that axial osteomalacia and fibrogenesis imperfecta ossium are the same conditions, although others[290] have disputed this idea. The presence of definite or borderline hypophosphatemia in the reported cases raises questions as to whether axial osteomalacia is a distinct entity or belongs in one of the several categories of hypophosphatemic osteomalacia discussed earlier.

ALUMINUM INTOXICATION

Several distinct patterns of renal osteodystrophy have been identified on the basis of characteristic clinical, biochemical, and bone histologic features. Although some patients develop only secondary hyperparathyroidism and osteitis fibrosa, osteomalacia is present in the majority, most often accompanied by some component of hyperparathyroid bone disease.[298–302] In untreated children with chronic renal disease, skeletal features of advanced nutritional rickets such as "rosary ribs," Harrison's groove, and knoblike enlargements of the wrists and ankles are among the clinical manifestations of the bone disease.[302] Among adult patients with osteomalacia, two patterns have been identified.[300, 303] In one group, identified as osteomalacia type I, there are markedly increased osteoid seams, and plasma calcium and phosphorus levels tend to be relatively low. In the second group, termed osteomalacia type II, the osteoid seams are thin and there is often a dramatic reduction in the double-tetracycline–labeled surfaces, reflecting a low mineralization rate. Bone formation rates are decreased at both the tissue and basic multicellular unit level.[303–305] In contrast to patients with type I osteomalacia, patients with type II osteomalacia tend to have normal or slightly elevated serum concentrations of calcium and phosphorus and clinically manifest a high frequency of skeletal pain, fractures, and vertebral collapse. An additional feature associated with the type II pattern of osteomalacia has been the accumulation of aluminum at the osteoid-bone interfaces. The source of the aluminum may be the water used in the hemodialysis or the consumption of aluminum-containing antacids.[295, 296, 303–309] Although osteomalacia due to antacid-induced phosphate depletion has been well characterized, osteomalacia with stainable aluminum in bone biopsies in an individual with normal renal function who ingested approximately 8 kg of aluminum over several years has only recently been reported.[310] Very little orally administered aluminum is absorbed and most of the latter is rapidly excreted in the urine.

Although aluminum is an apparent pathogenic factor in the development of dialysis osteomalacia, the mechanism by which aluminum impairs mineralization has not been elucidated.[300, 301, 303–307] The deposition of aluminum at the calcification front suggests that it may interfere with the mineralization process in addition to its ability to impair osteoblastic function.[311] This view is supported by the frequent occurrence of hypercalcemia with only moderate doses of vitamin D and calcium given to treat the osteomalacia.[303] Alternatively, deposition at this site could reflect deposition of aluminum in preexistent osteomalacic bone without direct effects on the mineralization process. For example, it has been shown[312] that in vitamin D–deficient dogs fed aluminum chloride, aluminum is localized at the osteoid-bone interface of the osteomalacic bone. The induction of bone healing by repletion with vitamin D was not, however, prevented by the continued administration of aluminum. In fact, aluminum could be demonstrated in the cement lines of the healed bone. Felsenfeld et al.[313] and Rodriquez et al.[314] have suggested a role for relative PTH deficiency in the pathogenesis of aluminum-associated osteomalacia. They demonstrated that, in rats with experimentally induced renal insufficiency, for equivalent aluminum exposure, treatment with PTH markedly reduced the severity of the low-turnover aluminum bone disease.

Identification of patients with aluminum-related bone disease cannot be predicted by plasma aluminum levels, and bone biopsy is necessary for definitive diagnosis.[315, 316] Some authors have suggested the use of a desferrioxamine infusion test to diagnose aluminum intoxication.[317–318] The extent to which plasma aluminum levels increase following infusion of a standard dose of desferrioxamine is measured. The magnitude of the increase correlates with the extent of accumulation of the bone aluminum. Desferrioxamine has also been used to treat patients with aluminum-related bone disease; the mobilization of aluminum from bone has been reported to improve the bone disease.

Other metals in addition to aluminum accumulate in tissues of dialyzed patients, and some of these may also play a role in the pathogenesis of the bone disease. For example, zirconium[320] has been detected in the skeletal tissues of patients with dialysis osteomalacia type II. It has also been suggested that aluminum may be responsible for a similar syndrome of osteomalacia in burn patients[321] and others on total parenteral nutrition,[322] but this association has not been fully established.[323, 324]

REFERENCES

1. Mankin HJ: Rickets, osteomalacia and renal osteodystrophy. J Bone Joint Surg [Am] 56:101–128, 352–386, 1974.
2. Dent CE, Stamp TCB: Vitamin D, rickets and osteomalacia. *In* Avioli LV, Krane SM (eds): Metabolic Bone Disease. New York, Academic Press, 1977.
3. Stanbury SW: Osteomalacia. Clin Endocrinol Metab 1:239–266, 1972.
4. Parfitt AM: Osteomalacia and related disorders. *In* Avioli LV, Krane SM (eds): Metabolic Bone Disease. San Diego, Academic Press, 1998, pp 328–386.
5. Hutchinson FN, Bell NH: Osteomalacia and rickets. Semin Nephrol 12:127–145, 1992.
6. Glimcher MJ: The nature of the mineral phase in bone: Biological and clinical implications. *In* Avioli LV, Krane SM (eds): Metabolic Bone Disease. San Diego, Academic Press, 1988, pp 23–50.
7. Slavkin H, Price P: Chemistry and Biology of Mineralized Tissues. Amsterdam, Excerpta Medica, 1992.
8. Krane SM, Parsons V, Kunin AS: Studies of the metabolism of epiphyseal cartilage. *In* Basset CAL (ed): Cartilage Degradation and Repair. Washington, DC, National Research Council, 1967, p 43.
9. Howell DS: Histologic observations and biochemical composition of rachitic cartilage with special reference to mucopolysaccharides. Arthritis Rheum 8:337–354, 1965.
10. Lee WR: Bone formation in Paget's disease: A quantitative microscopic study using tetracycline markers. J Bone Joint Surg [Br] 49:146–153, 1967.
11. Frost HM: Tetracycline-based histological analysis of bone remodeling. Calcif Tissue Res 3:211–237, 1969.
12. Rasmussen H, Bordier P: The Physiological and Cellular Basis of Metabolic Bone Disease. Baltimore, Williams & Wilkins, 1974.
13. Bordier PJ, Tun Chot S: Quantitative histology of metabolic bone disease. Clin Endocrinol Metab 1:197–215, 1972.
14. Byers PD: The diagnostic value of bone biopsies. *In* Avioli LV, Krane SM (eds): Metabolic Bone Disease. New York, Academic Press, 1977, p 184.
15. Rao DS, Villanueva A, Mathews M: Histological evolution of vitamin D-depletion in patients with intestinal malabsorption or dietary deficiency. *In* Frame B, Potts JT Jr (eds): Clinical Disorders of Bone and Mineral Metabolism. Amsterdam, Excerpta Medica, 1983, pp 224–226.
16. Boyce BF, Smith L, Fogelman I: Focal osteomalacia due to low-dose diphosphonate therapy in Paget's disease. Lancet 1:821–824, 1984.
17. Frame B, Parfitt AM: Osteomalacia: Current concepts. Ann Intern Med 89:966–982, 1978.
18. Arnstein AR, Frame B, Frost H: Recent progress in osteomalacia and rickets. Ann Intern Med 67:1296–1330, 1967.
19. Engfeldt B, Zetterstrom R, Winberg J: Primary vitamin-D resistant rickets: III. Biophysical studies of skeletal tissues. J Bone Joint Surg [Am] 38:1323–1334, 1956.
20. Bohr HH: Microradiographic studies in osteomalacia. *In* Hioco DJ (ed): L'Ostéomalacie. Paris, Masson, 1967, p 117.
21. Marie PJ, Glorieux FH: Relation between hypomineralization periosteocytic lesions and bone mineralization in vitamin D–resistant rickets. Calcif Tissue Int 35:443–448, 1983.
22. Jaworski ZFG, Kloswvych S, Cameron E: Proceedings of the First Workshop on Bone Morphometry. Ottawa, University of Ottawa Press, 1973.
23. Baylink D, Stauffer M, Wergedal J, Rich C: Formation mineralization and resorption of bone in vitamin-D deficient rats. J Clin Invest 49:1122–1134, 1970.
24. Toole BP, Kang AH, Trelstad RL, Gross J: Collagen heterogeneity within different growth regions of long bones of rachitic and nonrachitic chicks. Biochem J 127:715–720, 1972.
25. Barnes MJ, Constable BJ, Morton LF, Kodicek E: Bone collagen metabolism in vitamin-D deficiency. Biochem J 132:113–115, 1973.
26. Barnes MJ, Constable BJ, Morton LF, Kodicek E: The influence of dietary calcium deficiency and parathyroidectomy on bone structure. Biochim Biophys Acta 328:373–382, 1973.
27. Reginato AJ, Falasca GF, Pappu R, et al: Musculoskeletal manifestations of osteomalacia: Report of 26 cases and literature review. Semin Arthritis Rheum 28:287–304, 1999.
28. Prineas W, Stuart Mason A, Henson RA: Myopathy in metabolic bone disease. BMJ 1:1034–1036, 1965.
29. Smith R, Stern G: Myopathy osteomalacia and hyperparathyroidism. Brain 90:593–602, 1967.
30. Schott GD, Wills MR: Muscle weakness in osteomalacia. Lancet 1:626–629, 1976.
31. Nagant de Deuxchaisnes C, Krane SM: The treatment of adult phosphate diabetes and Fanconi syndrome with neutral sodium phosphate. Am J Med 43:508–543, 1967.
32. Mallett LE, Pattern BM, King Engel W: Neuromuscular disease in secondary hyperparathyroidism. Ann Intern Med 82:474–483, 1975.
33. Bautista J, Gil-Necija E, Castilla J: Dialysis myopathy. Acta Neuropathol 61:71–75, 1983.
34. Guerard MJ, Sewry CA, Dubowitz V: Lobulated fibers in neuromuscular disease. J Neurol Sci 69:345–356, 1985.
35. Smith R, Newman RJ, Radda GK: Hypophosphataemic osteomalacia and myopathy: Studies with nuclear magnetic resonance spectroscopy. Clin Sci 67:505–509, 1984.
36. Aurbach GD, Mallette LE, Patten BM: Hyperparathyroidism: Recent studies. Ann Intern Med 79:566–581, 1973.
37. Steinbach HL, Noetzli M: Roentgen appearance of the skeleton in osteomalacia and rickets. AJR 91:955–972, 1964.
38. de Seze S, Lichtwitz A, Ryckewaert A: Le syndrome de Looser-Milkman: Etude de 60 cas. Sem Hop 34:2005–2025, 1962.
39. Albright F, Reifenstein EC Jr: The Parathyroid Gland and Metabolic Bone Disease. Baltimore, Williams & Wilkins, 1948.
40. Milkman LA: Pseudofractures (hunger osteopathy, late rickets, osteomalacia): Report of a case. AJR 24:29–37, 1930.
41. Milkman LA: Multiple spontaneous idiopathic symmetrical fractures. AJR 32:622–634, 1934.
42. Steinbach HL, Kolb FO, Gilfillan R: A mechanism of the production of pseudofractures in osteomalacia (Milkman's syndrome). Radiology 62:388–394, 1954.
43. LeMay M, Blunt JWJ: Factor determining the location of pseudofractures in osteomalacia. J Clin Invest 28:521–525, 1949.
44. Jackson WPU, Dowdle E, Linder GC: Vitamin-D resistant osteomalacia. BMJ 1:1269–1274, 1958.
45. Ball J, Garner A: Mineralization of woven bone in osteomalacia. J Pathol Bacteriol 91:562–568, 1966.
46. Polisson RP, Martinez S, Khoury M: Calcification of entheses associated with X-linked hypophosphatemic osteomalacia. N Engl J Med 313:1–6, 1985.
47. Burnstein MI, Lawson JP, Kottamasu SR, et al: The enthesopathic changes of hypophosphatemic osteomalacia in adults: Radiologic findings. AJR 153:785–790, 1989.
48. Dunnigan MG, Paton JOJ, Haase S: Late rickets and osteomalacia in the Pakistani community in Glasgow. Scott Med J 7:159–167, 1962.
49. Arneil GC, Crosbie JC: Infantile rickets returns to Glasgow. Lancet 2:423–425, 1963.
50. Benson PF, Stroud CE, Mitchell NJ, Nicolaides A: Rickets in immigrant children in London. BMJ 5337:1054–1056, 1963.
51. Shaunak S, Colston K, Ang L: Vitamin D deficiency in adult British Hindu Asians: A family disorder. BMJ 291:1166–1168, 1985.
52. Henderson JB, Dunnigan MG, McIntosh WB, et al: Asian osteomalacia is determined by dietary factors when exposure to ultraviolet radiation is restricted: A risk factor model. Q J Med 76:923–933, 1990.
53. Finch PJ, Ang L, Colston KW, et al: Blunted seasonal variation in serum 25-hydroxy vitamin D and increased risk of osteomalacia in vegetarian London Asians. Eur J Clin Nutr 46:509–515, 1992.
54. Nisbet JA, Eastwood JB, Colston KW, et al: Detection of osteomalacia in British Asians: A comparison of clinical score with biochemical measurements. Clin Sci 78:383–389, 1990.
55. Chanarin I, Malkowska V, Ohea AM: Megaloblastic anaemia in a vegetarian Hindu community. Lancet 2:1168–1172, 1985.
56. Dent CE, Smith R: Nutritional osteomalacia. Q J Med 38:195–209, 1969.
57. Chalmers J, Conacher WDH, Gardner DL, Scott PJ: Osteomalacia—a common disease in elderly women. J Bone Joint Surg [Br] 49:403–423, 1967.
58. Gough KR, Lloyd OC, Wills MR: Nutritional osteomalacia. Lancet 2:1261–1264, 1964.
59. Haddad JG, Chyu KJ: Competitive protein-binding radioassay for 25-hydroxycholecalciferol. J Clin Endocrinol Metab 33:992–996, 1971.
60. Ralston SH, Willocks L, Pitkeathly DA, et al: High prevalence of unrecognized osteomalacia in hospital patients with rheumatoid arthritis. Br J Rheumatol 27:202–205, 1988.
61. Crowley LV, Seay J, Mullin G: Late effects of gastric bypass for obesity. Am J Gastroenterol 79:850–860, 1984.
62. Parfitt AM, Pdenphant J, Villanueva AR, Frame B: Metabolic bone disease with and without osteomalacia after intestinal bypass surgery: A bone histomorphometric study. Bone 6:211–220, 1985.
63. Charles P, Mosekilde L, Sondergard K, Jensen FT: Treatment with high-dose oral vitamin D_2 in patients with jejunoileal bypass for morbid obesity: Effects on calcium and magnesium metabolism, vitamin D metabolites, and faecal lag time. Scand J Gastroenterol 19:1031–1038, 1984.
64. Bisballe S, Ericksen EF, Melsen F, et al: Osteopenia and osteomalacia after gastrectomy: Interrelations between biochemical markers of bone remodelling, vitamin D metabolites, and bone histomorphometry. Gut 32:1303–1307, 1991.
65. Tovey FL, Godfrey JE, Lewin MR: A gastrectomy population: 25–30 years on. Postgrad Med J 66:450–456, 1990.
66. Roberts WA, Badger VM: Osteomalacia of very-low-birth-weight infants. J Pediatr Orthop 4:593–598, 1984.
67. Heckmatt JZ, Peacock M, Davies AEJ: Plasma 25-hydroxyvitamin D in pregnant Asian women and their babies. Lancet 2:546–549, 1979.

68. Corless D, Boucher BJ, Beer M: Vitamin D status in long-stay geriatric patients. Lancet 1:1404–1406, 1975.
69. Hodkinson HM, Round P, Stanton BR, Morgan C: Sunlight, vitamin D and osteomalacia in the elderly. Lancet 1:910–912, 1973.
70. Stamp TCB, Round JM: Seasonal changes in human plasma levels of 25-hydroxyvitamin D. Nature 247:563–565, 1974.
71. Lester E, Skinner RK, Wills MR: Seasonal variation in serum 25-hydroxyvitamin D in the elderly in Britain. Lancet 1:979–988, 1977.
72. Haddad JG, Stamp TCB: Circulating 25-hydroxyvitamin D in man. Am J Med 57:57–62, 1974.
73. Gallagher JC: Vitamin D metabolism and therapy in elderly subjects. South Med J 85:2S43–2S47, 1992.
74. Dawson-Hughes B, Harris SS, Dallal GE: Plasma calcidiol, season, and serum parathyroid hormone concentrations in healthy elderly men and women. Am J Clin Nutr 65:67–71, 1997.
75. Harris SS, Dawson-Hughes B: Seasonal changes in plasma 25-hydroxyvitamin D concentrations of young American black and white women. Am J Clin Nutr 67:1232–1236, 1998.
76. Thomas MK, Lloyd-Jones DM, Thadhani RI, et al: Hypovitaminosis D in medical inpatients. N Engl J Med 338:777–783, 1998.
77. WHO Tech Rep Ser 452:34, 1970.
78. Exton-Smith AN, Hodkinson HM, Stanton BR: Nutrition and metabolic bone disease in old age. Lancet 2:999–1001, 1966.
79. McLennan WJ, Caird FI, MacLeod CC: Diet and bone rarefaction in old age. Age Ageing 1:131–140, 1972.
80. Harris SS, Dawson-Hughes B, Perrone GA: Plasma 25-hydroxyvitamin D responses of younger and older men to three weeks of supplementation with 1800 IU/day of vitamin D. J Am Coll Nutr 18:470–474, 1999.
81. Vieth R: Vitamin D supplementation, 25-hydroxyvitamin D concentrations, and safety. Am J Clin Nutr 69:842–856, 1999.
82. Heaney RP: Lessons for nutritional science from vitamin D (editorial). Am J Clin Nutr 69:825–826, 1999.
83. Arneil GC: Symposium on osteomalacia and rickets: Nutritional rickets in children in Glasgow. Proc Nutr Soc 34:101–109, 1975.
84. Stanbury SW, Torkington P, Lumb GA: Asian rickets and osteomalacia: Patterns of parathyroid response in vitamin D deficiency. Proc Nutr Soc 34:111–117, 1975.
85. Goel KM, Logan RW, Arneil GC: Florid and subclinical rickets among immigrant children in Glasgow. Lancet 1:1141–1145, 1976.
86. Lawson M, Thomas M: Vitamin D concentrations in Asian children aged 2 years living in England: Population survey. BMJ 318:28, 1999.
87. Loomis WF: Skin-pigment regulation of vitamin D biosynthesis in man. Science 157:501–506, 1967.
88. Ford JA, Calhoun EM, McIntosh WB, Dunnigan MG: Rickets and osteomalacia in the Glasgow Pakistani community: 1961–1971. BMJ 2:677–680, 1967.
89. Doxiadia S, Angelis C, Karatzaz P: Genetic aspects of nutritional rickets. Arch Dis Child 51:83–90, 1976.
90. Wills MR, Day RC, Phillips JB, Bateman EC: Phytic acid and nutritional rickets in immigrants. Lancet 1:771–773, 1972.
91. Clements MR, Johnson L, Fraser DR: A new mechanism for induced vitamin D deficiency in calcium deprivation. Nature 325:62–65, 1987.
92. Sly MR, van der Walt WH, du Bruyn DB: Exacerbation of rickets and osteomalacia by maize: A study of bone histomorphology and composition in young baboons. Calcif Tissue Int 36:370–379, 1984.
93. Dent CE, Rowe DJF, Round JM, Stamp TCB: Effect of chapattis and ultraviolet irradiation on nutritional rickets in an Indian immigrant. Lancet 1:1282–1284, 1973.
94. Dent CE, Richens A, Rowe DJF, Stamp TCB: Osteomalacia with long term anticonvulsant therapy in epilepsy. BMJ 4:69–72, 1970.
95. Bordier PL, Hioco D, Hepner GW, Thompson GR: Effect of intravenous vitamin D on bone and phosphate metabolism in osteomalacia. Calcif Tissue Res 4:78–83, 1969.
96. Teitelbaum SL, Rosenberg EM, Bates M, Avioli LV: The effects of phosphate and vitamin D therapy in osteopenic, hypophosphatemic osteomalacia of childhood. Clin Orthop 116:38–47, 1976.
97. Eastwood JB, de Wardener HE, Gray RW, Lemann JLJ: Normal plasma-1, 25-$(OH)_2$-vitamin-D concentrations in nutritional osteomalacia. Lancet 1:1377–1378, 1979.
98. Adams JS, Clemens TL, Parrish JA, Holick MF: Vitamin-D synthesis and metabolism after ultraviolet irradiation of normal and vitamin-D–deficient subjects. N Engl J Med 306:722–725, 1982.
99. Godsall JW, Baron R, Insogna KL: Vitamin D metabolism and bone histomorphometry in a patient with antacid-induced osteomalacia. Am J Med 77:747–750, 1984.
100. Rasmussen H, Baron R, Broadus A: 1,25$(OH)_2D_3$ is not the only D metabolite involved in the pathogenesis of osteomalacia. Am J Med 69:360–368, 1980.
101. Rasmussen H, Baron R, Broadus A: 1,25$(OH)_2D_3$ in the pathogenesis of osteomalacia. *In* Frame B, Potts JT Jr (eds): Clinical Disorders of Bone and Mineral Metabolism. Amsterdam, Excerpta Medica, 1983, pp 82–89.
102. Bordier P, Rasmussen R, Marie P: Vitamin D metabolites and bone mineralization in man. J Clin Endocrinol Metab 46:284–294, 1978.
103. Hodsman AB, Wong EGC, Sherrard DJ: Preliminary trials with 24, 25-dihydroxyvitamin D_3 in dialysis osteomalacia. Am J Med 74:407–414, 1983.
104. Scriver CR: Rickets and the pathogenesis of impaired tubular transport of phosphate and other solutes. Am J Med 57:43–49, 1974.
105. Arnaud CD, Glorieux F, Scriver CR: Serum parathyroid hormone levels in acquired vitamin D deficiency of infancy. Pediatrics 49:837–840, 1972.
106. Muldowney FP, Freaney R, McGeeney D: Renal tubular acidosis and aminoaciduria in osteomalacia of dietary or intestinal origin. Q J Med 148:517–548, 1968.
107. Rao DS, Parfitt AM, Kleerekoper M: Dissociation between the effects of endogenous parathyroid hormone on adenosine 3′,5′-monophosphate generation and phosphate reabsorption in hypocalcemia due to vitamin D depletion: An acquired disorder resembling pseudohypoparathyroidism type II. J Clin Endocrinol Metab 6:285–290, 1985.
108. Collins N, Maher J, Cole M, et al: A prospective study to evaluate the dose of vitamin D required to correct low 25-hydroxyvitamin D levels, calcium, and alkaline phosphatase in patients at risk of developing antiepileptic drug–induced osteomalacia. Q J Med 78:113–122, 1991.
109. Bareen HS, Mazess RB, Chesney RW, et al: Bone status of children receiving anticonvulsant therapy. Metab Bone Dis Rel Res 4:43–47, 1982.
110. Davies M, Mawer EB, Hahn JT: Vitamin D prophylaxis in the elderly: A simple effective method suitable for large populations. Age Ageing 14:349–354, 1985.
111. Dawson-Hughes B, Dallal GE, Krall EA, Harris S: Effects of vitamin D supplementation on winter time and overall bone loss in healthy postmenopausal women. Ann Intern Med 115:505–512, 1991.
112. Villareal DT, Civitelli R, Chines A, Avioli LV: Subclinical vitamin D deficiency in postmenopausal women with low vertebral bone mass. J Clin Endocrinol Metab 72:628–634, 1991.
113. Hosking DJ, Campbell GA, Kemm JR: Safety of treatment for subclinical osteomalacia in the elderly. BMJ 289:785–787, 1984.
114. Barden HS, Mazees RB, Ross PG, McAweeney W: Bone mineral status measured by direct photon absorptiometry in institutionalized adults receiving long term anticonvulsant therapy and multivitamin supplementation. Calcif Tissue Int 31:117–121, 1980.
115. Christiansen C, Rodbro P, Lund P: Incidence of anticonvulsant osteomalacia and effect of vitamin D: Controlled therapeutic trial. BMJ 4:695–701, 1973.
116. Hahn TJ, Hendin BA, Sharp CR, Haddad J: Effects of chronic anticonvulsant therapy on serum 25$(OH)D_3$ levels in adults. N Engl J Med 287:900–906, 1972.
117. Whittle H, Neale G, McLaughlin M: Intravenous vitamin D in the detection of vitamin D deficiency. Lancet 1:747–750, 1969.
118. Balsan S, Garabedian M, Sorgniard R: 1,25-Dihydroxyvitamin D_3 and 1α-hydroxyvitamin D_3 in children: Biologic and therapeutic effects in nutritional rickets and different types of vitamin D resistance. Pediatr Res 9:586–593, 1975.
119. Bordier PH, Pechet MM, Hesse R: Response of adult patients with osteomalacia to treatment with crystalline 1α-hydroxyvitamin D_3. N Engl J Med 291:866–871, 1974.
120. Stamp TCB: Factors in human vitamin D nutrition and in the production and cure of classical rickets. Proc Nutr Soc 34:119–130, 1975.
121. Goodman AD, Lemann JJ, Lennon EJ, Relman AS: Production, excretion and net balance of fixed acid in patients with renal acidosis. J Clin Invest 44:495–506, 1965.
122. Lemann JJ, Lennon EJ, Goodman AD: The net balance of acid in subjects given large loads of acid or alkali. J Clin Invest 44:507–517, 1965.
123. Lemann JJ, Litzow JR, Lennon EJ: The effects of chronic acid loads in normal man: Further evidence for the participation of bone minerals in the defense against chronic metabolism acidosis. J Clin Invest 45:1608–1614, 1966.
124. Raisz LG: Physiologic and pharmacologic regulation of bone resorption. N Engl J Med 282:909–916, 1970.
125. Raisz LG: Mechanisms of bone resorption. *In* Aurbach GD (ed): Handbook of Physiology: Endocrinology, Parathyroid Gland. Washington, DC, American Physiological Society, 1976, p 117.
126. Howell DS, Pita JC, Marquez JF, Madruga JE: Partition of calcium, phosphate, and protein in the fluid phase aspirated at calcifying sites in epiphyseal cartilage. J Clin Invest 47:1121–1132, 1968.
127. Howell DS: Review article: Current concepts of calcification. J Bone Joint Surg [Am] 53:250–258, 1971.
128. Nordstrom T, Shrode LD, Rotstein OD, et al: Chronic extracellular acidosis induces plasmalemmal vacuolar type H^+ ATPase activity in osteoclasts. J Biol Chem 272:6354–6360, 1997.
129. Bushinsky DA, Nilsson EL: Additive effects of acidosis and parathyroid hormone on mouse osteoblastic and osteoclastic function. Am J Physiol 269:C1364–C1370, 1995.
130. Donohoe JF, Freaney R, Muldowney FP: Osteomalacia in ureterosigmoidostomy. Ir J Med Sci 2:523–530, 1969.
131. Tschopp AB, Lippuner K, Jaeger P, et al: No evidence of osteopenia 5 to 8 years after ileal orthotopic bladder substitution. J Urol 155:71–75, 1996.
132. Harrison HE, Harrison HC: Physiology of vitamin D. *In* Rodahl K, Nicholson JT, Brown EMJ (eds): Bone as a Tissue. New York, McGraw-Hill, 1960, p 300.
133. Lee SW, Russell J, Avioli LV: 25-Hydroxycholecalciferol to 1,25-dihydroxycholecalciferol: Conversion impaired by systemic metabolic acidosis. Science 195:994–996, 1977.
134. Morris RCJ: Renal tubular acidosis: Mechanisms, classification and implications. N Engl J Med 281:1405–1413, 1969.
135. Morris RCJ, Sebastian A, McSherry E: Renal acidosis. Kidney Int 1:322–340, 1972.
136. Seldin DW, Wilson JD: Renal tubular acidosis. *In* Stanbury JB, Wyngaarden JB, Frederickson DS (eds): The Metabolic Basis of Inherited Disease. New York, McGraw-Hill, 1972, p 1548.
137. Richards P, Chamberlain MJ, Wrong OM: Treatment of osteomalacia of renal tubular acidosis by sodium bicarbonate alone. Lancet 2:994–997, 1972.
138. York SE, Yendt ER: Osteomalacia associated with renal bicarbonate loss. Can Med Assoc J 94:1329–1342, 1966.
139. Dent CE, Harris H: Hereditary forms of rickets and osteomalacia. J Bone Joint Surg [Br] 38:204–226, 1956.
140. Kallmeyer J, Dunea G, Schwartz FD: Hypophosphatemic osteomalacia with hyperglycosuria. Ann Intern Med 66:136–141, 1967.
141. Scriver CR, Goldbloom RB, Roy CC: Hypophosphatemic rickets with renal hyperglycosuria, renal glycosuria and glycyl-prolinuria: A syndrome with evidence for renal tubular secretion of phosphorus. Pediatrics 34:357–371, 1964.
142. Henneman PH, Dempsey EF, Carroll EL, Henneman DH: Acquired vitamin D–resistant osteomalacia: A new variety characterized by hypercalcemia, low sodium bicarbonate and hyperglycinuria. Metabolism 11:103–116, 1962.
143. Schneider JA, Seegmiller JE: Cystinosis and the Fanconi syndrome. *In* Stanbury JB, Wyngaarden JB, Frederickson D (eds): The Metabolic Basis of Inherited Disease. New York, McGraw-Hill, 1972, p 1581.
144. Waite LC, Volkert WA, Kenny AD: Inhibition of bone resorption by acetazolamide in the rat. Endocrinology 87:1129–1139, 1970.

145. Pierce WM, Nardin GF, Fuqua MF, et al: Effect of chronic carbonic anhydrase inhibitor therapy on bone mineral density in white women. J Bone Miner Res 6:347–394, 1991.
146. Bloom WL, Flinchum D: Osteomalacia with pseudofractures caused by ingestion of aluminum hydroxide. JAMA 174:1327–1330, 1960.
147. Lotz M, Zisman E, Bartter FC: Evidence for a phosphorus-depletion syndrome in man. N Engl J Med 278:409–415, 1968.
148. Lotz M, Ney R, Bartter FC: Osteomalacia and debility resulting from phosphorus depletion. Trans Assoc Am Physicians 77:281–295, 1964.
149. Dent CE, Winter CE: Osteomalacia due to phosphate depletion from excessive aluminium hydroxide. BMJ 1:551–552, 1974.
150. Baker LRI, Ackrill P, Cattell WR: Iatrogenic osteomalacia and myopathy due to phosphate depletion. BMJ 3:150–152, 1974.
151. Chines A, Pacifici R: Antacid and sucralfate-induced hypophosphatemic osteomalacia: A case report and review of the literature. Calcif Tissue Int 47:291–295, 1990.
152. Kassem M, Eriksen EF, Melsen F, Mosekilde L: Antacid-induced osteomalacia: A case report with a histomorphometric analysis. J Intern Med 229:275–279, 1991.
153. Levy Y, Bansal M, Zackson DA, et al: Phosphate depletion syndrome: Case report and muscle histology findings and review of the literature. JPEN 12:313–317, 1988.
154. Territo MC, Tanaka KR: Hypophosphatemia in chronic alcoholism. Arch Intern Med 134:445–447, 1974.
155. Stein JH, Smith WO, Ginn HE: Hypophosphatemia in acute alcoholism. Am J Med Sci 252:78–83, 1966.
156. de Vernejoul MC, Bielakoff J, Herve M: Evidence for defective osteoblast function: A role for alcohol and tobacco consumption in osteoporosis in middle age men. Clin Orthop 179:286–291, 1983.
157. Kumar R: Hepatic and intestinal osteodystrophy and the hepatobiliary metabolism of vitamin D. Ann Intern Med 98:662–663, 1983.
158. Bonkovsky HL, Hawkins M, Steinberg K, et al: Prevalence and prediction of osteopenia in chronic liver disease. Hepatology 12:273–280, 1990.
159. Diamond TH: Metabolic bone disease in primary biliary cirrhosis. J Gastroenterol Hepatol 5:66–81, 1990.
160. Hepatic osteomalacia and vitamin D (editorial). Lancet 1:943–944, 1982.
161. Albright F, Butler AM, Bloomberg E: Rickets resistant to vitamin D therapy. J Clin Dis Child 54:529–547, 1937.
162. Robertson BR, Harris RC, McCune DJ: Refractory rickets: Mechanism of therapeutic action of calciferol. Am J Dis Child 64:948–952, 1942.
163. Frymoyer JW, Hodgkin W: Adult-onset vitamin-D–resistant hypophosphatemic osteomalacia. J Bone Joint Surg [Am] 59:101–106, 1977.
164. Dent CE, Stamp TCB: Hypophosphatemic osteomalacia presenting in adults. Q J Med 158:303–329, 1971.
165. Ray RD, Mueller KH, SanKaran B: Metabolic diseases of bone: Kinetic studies. Med Clin North Am 49:241–258, 1965.
166. Glorieux F, Scriver CR: Loss of a parathyroid-sensitive component of phosphate transport in X-linked hypophosphatemia. Science 175:997–1000, 1972.
167. Dent CE: Rickets and osteomalacia from renal tubular defects. J Bone Joint Surg [Br] 34:266–274, 1952.
168. Condon JR, Nassim JR, Rutter A: Pathogenesis of rickets and osteomalacia in familial hypophosphatemia. Arch Dis Child 46:269–272, 1971.
169. Short EM, Binder HJ, Rosenberg LE: Familial hypophosphatemic rickets: Defective transport of inorganic phosphate by intestinal mucosa. Science 179:700–702, 1973.
170. Glorieux FH, Morin CL, Travere R: Intestinal phosphate transport in familial hypophosphatemic rickets. Pediatr Res 10:691, 1976.
171. to 173. References omitted.
174. Beck L, Karaplis AC, Amizuka N, et al: Targeted inactivation of *Npt2* in mice leads to severe renal phosphate wasting, hypercalciuria, and skeletal abnormalities. Proc Natl Acad Sci U S A 95:5372–5377, 1998.
175. and 176. References omitted.
177. The Hyp Consortium: A gene *(PEX)* with homologies to endopeptidases is mutated in patients with X-linked hypophosphatemic rickets. Nat Genet 11:130–136, 1995.
178. Dixon PH, Christie PT, Wooding C, et al: Mutational analysis of PHEX gene in X-linked hypophosphatemia. J Clin Endocrinol Metab 83:3615–3623, 1998.
179. Econs MJ: New insights into the pathogenesis of inherited phosphate wasting disorders. Bone 25:131–135, 1999.
180. Glorieux FH, Karsenty G, Thakker RV: Metabolic Bone Disease in Children. *In*: Avioli LV, Krane SM (eds): Metabolic Bone Disease and Clinically Related Disorders. San Diego, Academic Press 1998, pp 759–783.
181. Econs MJ, Drezner MK: Tumor-induced osteomalacia—unveiling a new hormone. N Engl J Med 330:1679–1681, 1994.
182. Econs MJ, McEnery PT: Autosomal dominant hypophosphatemic rickets/osteomalacia: Clinical characterization of a novel renal tubular wasting disorder. J Clin Endocrinol Metab 82:1674–1681, 1997.
183. Econs MJ, Friedman NE, Rowe PS, et al: A PHEX gene mutation is responsible for adult-onset vitamin D–resistant hypophosphatemic osteomalacia: Evidence that the disorder is not a distinct entity from X-linked hypophosphatemic rickets. J Clin Endocrinol Metab 83:3459–3462, 1998.
184. Kelleher CL, Buckalew VM, Frederickson ED, et al: CLCN5 mutation Ser244Leu is associated with X-linked renal failure without X-linked recessive hypophosphatemic rickets. Kidney Int 53:31–37, 1998.
185. Pettifor JM: Recent advances in pediatric metabolic bone disease: The consequences of altered phosphate homeostasis in renal insufficiency and hypophosphatemic vitamin D–resistant rickets. Bone Miner 9:199–214, 1990.
186. Harrell RM, Lyles KW, Harrelson JM: Healing of bone disease X-linked hypophosphatemic rickets/osteomalacia: Induction and maintenance with phosphorus and calcitriol. J Clin Invest 75:1858–1868, 1985.
187. Verge CF, Albert L, Simpson JM: Effects of therapy in X-linked hypophosphatemic rickets. N Engl J Med 325:1843–1848, 1991.
188. Peterson DJ, Boneface AM, Schranck FW, et al: X-linked hypophosphatemic rickets: A study (with literature review) of linear growth response to calcitrol and phosphate therapy. J Bone Miner Res 7:583–596, 1992.
189. Goldring SR, Krane SM: Cation effects on phosphate homeostasis in hypophosphatemic subjects. *In* Massry SG, Ritz E, Jahn H (eds): Phosphate and Minerals in Health and Disease. New York, Plenum Press, 1980, pp 361–368.
190. Frame F, Manson G: Refractory rickets and osteomalacia. Henry Ford Hosp Med Bull 8:293–298, 1960.
191. Glorieux FM, Scriver CR, Reade TM: Use of phosphate and vitamin D to prevent dwarfism and rickets in X-linked hypophosphatemia. N Engl J Med 87:481–487, 1972.
192. Sullivan W, Carpenter T, Glorieux F, et al: A prospective trial of phosphate and 1,25-dihydroxyvitamin D_3 therapy in symptomatic adults with X-linked hypophosphatemic rickets. J Clin Endocrinol Metab 75:879–885, 1992.
193. Glorieux FH: Calcitriol treatment in vitamin D–dependent and vitamin D–resistant rickets. Metabolism 39:10–12, 1990.
194. Prader A, Illig R, Uehlinger E, Stalder G: Rachitis infolge Knochen-tumors. Helv Paediatr Acta 14:554–565, 1959.
195. McCance RA: Osteomalacia with Looser's nodes (Milkman's syndrome) due to raised resistance to vitamin-D acquired about the age of 15 years. Q J Med 16:33–50, 1947.
196. Dent CE, Friedman M: Hypophosphatemic osteomalacia with complete recovery. BMJ 1:1676–1679, 1964.
197. Hauge BN: Vitamin-D resistant osteomalacia. Acta Med Scand 153:271–282, 1956.
198. Yoshkiawa S, Kawabata M, Hatsuyama Y: Atypical vitamin-D resistant osteomalacia: Report of a case. J Bone Joint Surg [Am] 46:998–1007, 1964.
199. Case Records of the Massachusetts General Hospital (Case 38-1965): N Engl J Med 273:494–504, 1965.
200. Salassa RM, Jowsey J, Arnaud CD: Hypophosphatemic osteomalacia associated with "nonendocrine" tumors. N Engl J Med 283:65–70, 1970.
201. Evans SJ, Azzopardi JG: Distinctive tumors of bone and soft tissue causing acquired vitamin-D osteomalacia. Lancet 1:353–354, 1972.
202. Olefsky J, Kempson R, Jones H, Reavan G: "Tertiary" hyperparathyroidism and apparent "cure" of vitamin-D resistant rickets after removal of an ossifying mesenchymal tumor of the pharynx. N Engl J Med 286:740–745, 1972.
203. Pollack JA, Schiller AL, Crawford JD: Rickets and myopathy cured by removal of a nonossifying fibroma of bone. Paediatrics 52:364–371, 1973.
204. Moser CR, Fessel WJ: Rheumatic manifestations of hypophosphatemia. Arch Intern Med 134:674–678, 1974.
205. Linovitz RJ, Resnick D, Keissling P: Tumor-induced osteomalacia and rickets: A surgically curable syndrome. J Bone Joint Surg [Am] 58:419–423, 1976.
206. Ryan EA, Reiss E: Oncogenous osteomalacia. Am J Med 77:501–512, 1984.
207. Weidner N: Review and update: Oncogenic osteomalacia-rickets. Ultrastruct Pathol 15:317–333, 1991.
208. Taylor HC, Santa-Cruz D, Teitelbaum SL, et al: Assessment of calcitriol and inorganic phosphate therapy before cure of oncogenous osteomalacia by resection of a mixed mesenchymal tumor. Bone 9:37–43, 1988.
209. Leicht E, Biro G, Langer HJ: Tumor-induced osteomalacia: Pre- and postoperative biochemical findings. Horm Metab Res 22:640–643, 1990.
210. Schapira D, Ben Izhak O, Nachtigal A, et al: Tumor-induced osteomalacia. Semin Arthritis Rheum 25:35–46, 1995.
211. Ohashi K, Ohnishi T, Ishikawa T, et al: Oncogenic osteomalacia presenting as bilateral stress fractures of the tibia. Skeletal Radiol 28:46–48, 1999.
212. Zura RD, Minasi JS, Kahler DM: Tumor-induced osteomalacia and symptomatic Looser zones secondary to mesenchymal chondrosarcoma. J Surg Oncol 71:58–62, 1999.
213. Nuovo MA, Dorfman HD, Sun CC, Chalew SA: Tumor-induced osteomalacia and rickets. Am J Surg Pathol 13:588–599, 1989.
214. Lyles KW, Berry WR, Haussler M: Hypophosphatemic osteomalacia: Association with prostatic carcinoma. Ann Intern Med 93:275–278, 1980.
215. Stone MD, Quincey C, Hosking DJ: A neuroendocrine cause of oncogenic osteomalacia. J Pathol 167:181–185, 1992.
216. Sweet RA, Males JL, Hamstra AJ, DeLuca HF: Vitamin D metabolite levels in oncogenic osteomalacia. Ann Intern Med 93:279–280, 1980.
217. Drezner MK, Feinglos MN: Osteomalacia due to 1α, 25-dihydroxycholecalciferol deficiency. J Clin Invest 60:1046–1053, 1977.
218. Fukumoto Y, Tarui S, Tsukiyama K: Tumor-induced vitamin D–resistant hypophosphatemic osteomalacia associated with proximal renal tubular dysfunction and 1,25-dihydroxyvitamin D deficiency. J Clin Endocrinol Metab 49:873–878, 1979.
219. Miyauchi A, Fukase M, Tsutsumi M, Fujita T: Hematopericytoma-induced osteomalacia: Tumor extracts inhibit renal 25-hydroxyvitamin D 1-hydroxylase activity. J Clin Endocrinol Metab 67:46–53, 1988.
220. Nitzan DW, Horowitz AT, Darmon D, et al: Oncogenous osteomalacia: A case study. Bone Miner 6:191–197, 1989.
221. Nelson AE, Namkung HJ, Patava J, et al: Characteristics of tumor cell bioactivity in oncogenic osteomalacia. Mol Cell Endocrinol 124:17–23, 1996.
222. Nelson AE, Robinson BG, Mason RS: Oncogenic osteomalacia: Is there a new phosphate regulating hormone? Clin Endocrinol 47:635–642, 1997.
223. Kumar R, Haugen JD, Wieben E, et al: Inhibitors of renal epithelial phosphate transport in tumor-induced osteomalacia and uremia. Proc Assoc Am Physicians 107:296–305, 1995.
224. Nelson AE, Mason RS, Hogan JJ, et al: Tumor expression studies indicate that HEM-1 is unlikely to be the active factor in oncogenic osteomalacia. Bone 23:549–553, 1998.
225. Hernberg CA, Edgren W: Looser-Milkman's syndrome with neurofibromatosis Recklinghausen and general decalcification of the skeleton. Acta Med Scand 136:26–33, 1949.
226. Swann GF: Pathogenesis of bone lesions in neurofibromatosis. Br J Radiol 27:623–629, 1954.

227. Saville PD, Nassim JR, Stevenson FH: Osteomalacia in von Recklinghausen's neurofibromatosis: Metabolic study of a case. BMJ 1:1311–1313, 1955.
228. Lambert J, Lips P: Adult hypophosphataemic osteomalacia with Fanconi syndrome presenting in a patient with neurofibromatosis. Neth J Med 35:309–316, 1989.
229. Weinstein RS, Harris RL: Hypercalcemic hyperparathyroidism and hypophosphatemic osteomalacia complicating neurofibromatosis. Calcif Tissue Int 46:361–366, 1990.
230. Konishi K, Nakamura M, Yamakawa H, et al: Hypophosphatemic osteomalacia in von Recklinghausen neurofibromatosis. Am J Med Sci 301:322–328, 1991.
231. Dent CE, Gertner JM: Hypophosphatemic osteomalacia in fibrous dysplasia. Q J Med 45:411–420, 1976.
232. Dent CE, Harris M: Hereditary forms of rickets and osteomalacia. J Bone Joint Surg [Br] 38:204–226, 1956.
233. Brodehl J: Tubular Fanconi syndromes with bone involvement. *In* Bickel H, Stern J (eds): Inborn Errors of Calcium and Bone Metabolism. Baltimore, University Park Press, 1976, pp 191–213.
234. Lowe CU, Ferrey M, MacLachlin EA: Organic aciduria, decreased renal ammonia production, hydrophthalmos and mental retardation. Am J Dis Child 83:164, 1952.
235. Briggs WA, Kominami N, Merrill JP, Wilson RE: Kidney transplantation in Fanconi syndrome. N Engl J Med 286:25, 1972.
236. Rosenberg LE, Scriver CR: Disorders of amino acid metabolism. *In* Bondy PK (ed): Duncan's Diseases of Metabolism. Philadelphia, WB Saunders, 1969, pp 366–515.
237. Morgan HG, Stewart WK, Lowe KG: Wilson's disease and the Fanconi syndrome. Q J Med 31:361–383, 1962.
238. Wilson DM, Goldstein NP: Bicarbonate excretion in Wilson's disease (hepatolenticular degeneration). Mayo Clin Proc 49:394–400, 1974.
239. Walshe JM: Effect of penicillamine on failure of renal acidification in Wilson's disease. Lancet 1:775–778, 1968.
240. Snapper I, Kahn A: Determination of Bence Jones protein in urine and serum. *In* Myelomatosis, Fundamentals and Clinical Features. Baltimore, University Park Press, 1971, pp 203–204.
241. Monte Neto JT, Sesso R, Kirsztajn GM, et al: Osteomalacia secondary to renal tubular acidosis in a patient with primary Sjögren's syndrome. Clin Exp Rheumatol 9:625–627, 1991.
242. Adams RG, Harrison JF, Scott P: The development of cadmium-induced proteinuria, impaired renal function, and osteomalacia in alkaline-battery workers. Q J Med 38:425–443, 1969.
243. Emerson BT: "Ouch-Ouch" disease: The osteomalacia of cadmium nephropathy. Ann Intern Med 73:854–855, 1970.
244. Chisolm JJJ, Leahy NB: Aminoaciduria as a manifestation of renal tubular lead injury in lead intoxication and a comparison with patterns of aminoaciduria seen in other diseases. J Pediatr 160:1–17, 1962.
245. Gross JM: Fanconi syndrome (adult type) developing secondary to the ingestion of outdated tetracycline. Ann Intern Med 48:523–528, 1963.
246. Rathbun JR: Hypophosphatasia. Am J Dis Child 75:822–831, 1948.
247. Sobel EH, Clark LC, Fox RP, Robinow M: Rickets, deficiency of "alkaline" phosphatase activity and premature loss of teeth in childhood. Pediatrics 11:309–321, 1953.
248. Fraser D: Hypophosphatasia. Am J Med 22:730–746, 1957.
249. Bartter FC: Hypophosphatasia. *In* Stanbury JB, Wyngaarden JB, Frederickson DS (eds): The Metabolic Basis of Inherited Disease. New York, McGraw-Hill, 1972, p 1295.
250. Whyte MP: Hypophosphatasia. *In* Scriver CR, Beaudent AL, Sly WS, Valle D (eds): The Metabolic Basis of Inherited Disease. New York, McGraw-Hill, 1989, pp 2843–2856.
251. Bethune JE, Dent CE: Hypophosphatasia in the adult. Am J Med 28:615–622, 1960.
252. Birtwell VMJ, Riggs BL, Peterson LFA, Jones JD: Hypophosphatasia in an adult. Arch Intern Med 120:90–93, 1967.
253. Whyte MP, Mahuren JD, Vrabel LA, Coburn SP: Markedly increased circulating pyridoxal-5′-phosphate levels in hypophosphatasia. J Clin Invest 76:752–756, 1985.
254. Fraser D, Yendt ER, Christie FHE: Metabolic abnormalities in hypophosphatasia. Lancet 1:286, 1955.
255. McCance RA: The excretion of phosphorylethanolamine and hypophosphatasia. Lancet 1:131, 1955.
256. McCance RA, Fairweather DVI, Barrett AM, Morrison AB: Genetic, clinical, biochemical and pathological features of hypophosphatasia. Q J Med 25:523–538, 1956.
257. Fernley HN, Walker PG: Studies on alkaline phosphatase: Inhibition by phosphate derivatives and the substrate specificity. Biochem J 104:1011–1018, 1967.
258. Moss DW, Eaton RH, Smith JK, Whitby LG: Association of inorganic pyrophosphatase activity with human alkaline phosphatase preparation. Biochem J 102:53–57, 1967.
259. Russell RGG, Bisaz S, Donath A: Inorganic pyrophosphate in plasma in normal persons and in patients with hypophosphatasia, osteogenesis imperfecta and other disorders of bone. J Clin Invest 50:961–969, 1971.
260. Russell RGG: Excretion of inorganic pyrophosphate in hypophosphatasia. Lancet 2:899–902, 1970.
261. Fleisch H, Neuman WF: Mechanisms of calcification: Role of collagen, polyphosphates and phosphatase. Am J Physiol 200:1291–1300, 1961.
262. Russell RGG: Metabolism of inorganic pyrophosphate (PPi). Arthritis Rheum 19:465–478, 1976.
263. Zurutuza L, Muller F, Gibrat JF, et al: Correlations of genotype and phenotype in hypophosphatasia. Hum Mol Genet 8:1039–1046, 1999.
264. Girschick HJ, Schneider P, Kruse K, Huppertz HI: Bone metabolism and bone mineral density in childhood hypophosphatasia. Bone 25:361–367, 1999.
265. Weiss MJ, Cole DEC, Ray K, et al: A missense mutation in the human liver/bone/kidney alkaline phosphatase gene causing a form of lethal hypophosphatasia. Proc Natl Acad Sci U S A 85:7666–7669, 1988.
266. Henthorn PS, Raducha M, Fedde KN, et al: Different missense mutations at the tissue-nonspecific alkaline phosphatase gene locus in autosomal recessively inherited forms of mild and severe hypophosphatasia. Proc Natl Acad Sci U S A 89:9924–9928, 1992.
267. Teotia SPS, Teotia M: Endemic skeletal fluorosis in children: Evidence of secondary hyperparathyroidism. *In* Frame B, Parfitt AM, Duncan H (eds): Clinical Aspects of Metabolic Bone Disease. Amsterdam, Excerpta Medica, 1973, p 232.
268. Riggs BL, Jowsey J: Treatment of osteoporosis with fluoride. Semin Drug Treat 2:27–33, 1972.
269. Smith R, Russell RGG, Bishop M: Diphosphonates and Paget's disease of bone. Lancet 1:945–947, 1971.
270. Smith R, Russell RGG, Bishop MC: Paget's disease of bone: Experience with a diphosphonate (disodium etidronate) in treatment. Q J Med 42:235–256, 1973.
271. Khairi MRA, Johnston CCJ, Altman RD: Treatment of Paget's disease of bone (osteitis deformans). JAMA 230:562–567, 1974.
272. deVries HR, Bijvoet OLM: Results of prolonged treatment of Paget's disease of bone with disodium ethane-1-hydroxy-1, 1-diphosphonate (EHDP). Neth J Med 171:281–298, 1974.
273. Guncaga J, Lauffenburger T, Lentnen C: Diphosphonate treatment of Paget's disease of bone: A correlated metabolic, calcium kinetic and morphometric study. Horm Metab Res 6:62–69, 1974.
274. Kantrowitz FG, Byrne MH, Schiller AL, Krane SM: Clinical and biochemical effects of diphosphonate in Paget's disease of bone. Arthritis Rheum 18:407, 1975.
275. Canfield R, Rosner W, Skinner J: Diphosphonate therapy of Paget's disease. J Clin Endocrinol Metab 44:96–106, 1977.
276. Jowsey J, Riggs BL, Kelly PJ: Treatment of osteoporosis with disodium ethane-1-hydroxy-1, 1-diphosphonate. J Lab Clin Med 78:514–584, 1971.
277. Hill LF, Lumb GA, Mawer EB, Stanbury SW: Indirect inhibition of the biosynthesis of 1,25-dihydroxycholecalciferol in rats treated with a diphosphonate. Clin Sci 44:335–347, 1973.
278. Thomas WC, Fry RM: Parathyroid adenomas in chronic rickets. Am J Med 49:404–407, 1970.
279. Kleerekoper M, Coffey R, Greco T: Hypercalcemic hyperparathyroidism in hypophosphatemic rickets. J Clin Endocrinol Metab 45:86–94, 1977.
280. Albright F: Hypoparathyroidism as a cause of osteomalacia. J Clin Endocrinol Metab 16:419–425, 1956.
281. Drezner MK, Neelon FA, Jowsey J, Lebovitz HE: Hypoparathyroidism: A possible cause of osteomalacia. J Clin Endocrinol Metab 45:114–122, 1977.
282. Whyte MP, Murphy WA: Osteopetrosis and other sclerosing bone disorders. *In* Avioli LV, Krane SM (eds): Metabolic Bone Disease. Philadelphia, WB Saunders, 1990, pp 616–658.
283. Pincus JB, Gittleman IF, Kramer B: Juvenile osteopetrosis: Metabolic studies in two cases and further observations on the composition of bones in this disease. Am J Dis Child 73:458–472, 1947.
284. Dent CE: Problems in metabolic bone disease. *In* Frame B, Parfitt AM, Duncan H (eds): Clinical Aspects of Metabolic Bone Disease. Amsterdam, Excerpta Medica, 1973, p 1.
285. Bonucci E, Sartori E, Spina M: Osteopetrosis fetalis: Report on a case with special references to ultrastructure. Virchows Arch 368:109–121, 1975.
286. Sly WS, Whyte MD, Sundaram V: Carbonic anhydrase II deficiency in 12 families with the autosomal recessive syndrome of osteopetrosis with renal tubular acidosis and cerebral calcification. N Engl J Med 313:139–145, 1985.
287. Baker SL, Turnbull HM: Two cases of a hitherto undescribed disease characterized by a gross defect with collagen of the bone matrix. J Pathol Bacteriol 62:132–134, 1950.
288. Baker SL, Dent CE, Friedman M, Watson L: Fibrogenesis imperfecta ossium. J Bone Joint Surg [Br] 48:804–825, 1966.
289. Thomas WCJ, Moore TH: Fibrogenesis imperfecta ossium. Trans Am Clin Climatol Assoc 80:54–62, 1968.
290. Frame B, Frost HM, Pak CYC: Fibrogenesis imperfecta ossium: A collagen defect causing osteomalacia. N Engl J Med 285:769–772, 1971.
291. Swan CHJ, Cooke WT: Fibrogenesis imperfect ossium. *In* Frame B, Parfitt AM, Duncan H (eds): Clinical Aspects of Metabolic Bone Disease. Amsterdam, Excerpta Medica, 1973, p 465.
292. Reference omitted.
293. Henneman DH, Pak CYC, Bartter FC: Collagen composition, solubility and biosynthesis in fibrogenesis imperfecta ossium. *In* Frame B, Parfitt AM, Duncan H (eds): Clinical Aspects of Metabolic Bone Disease. Amsterdam, Excerpta Medica, 1973, p 469.
294. and 295. References omitted.
296. Frame B, Frost HM, Ormord RS, Hunter RB: Atypical osteomalacia involving the axial skeleton. Ann Intern Med 55:632–639, 1961.
297. Whyte MP, Fallon MD, Murphy WA, Teitelbaum SL: Axial osteomalacia. Am J Med 71:1041–1049, 1981.
298. Goodman WC: Bone disease and aluminum: Pathogenic considerations. Am J Kidney Dis 6:330–335, 1985.
299. Chan YL, Furlong TJ, Cornish CJ, Posen S: Dialysis osteodystrophy: A study involving 94 patients. Medicine (Baltimore) 64:296–309, 1985.
300. Dunstan CR, Hills E, Norman AW: The pathogenesis of renal osteodystrophy: Role of vitamin D, aluminum, parathyroid hormone, calcium and phosphorus. Q J Med 55:127–144, 1985.
301. Charhon SA, Berland YF, Olmer MJ: Effects of parathyroidectomy on bone formation and mineralization in hemodialyzed patients. Kidney Int 27:426–435, 1985.
302. Chesney RW, Avioli LV: Childhood renal osteocystrophy. *In* Edelmann CMJ, Bernstein J, Meadow SR, et al (eds): Pediatric Kidney Disease, vol I. Boston, Little, Brown, 1992, pp 647–684.
303. Hodsman AB, Sherrard DJ, Alfrey AC: Bone aluminum and histomorphometric features of renal osteodystrophy. J Clin Endocrinol Metab 54:539–546, 1982.
304. de Vernejoul MC, Belenguer R, Halkidou H: Histomorphometric evidence of deleterious effect of aluminum on osteoblasts. Bone 6:15–20, 1985.

305. Charhon SA, Chavassieux PM, Chapuy MC: Low rate of bone formation with or without histologic appearance of osteomalacia in patients with aluminum intoxication. J Lab Clin Med 106:123–131, 1985.
306. Vick KE, Johnson CA: Aluminum-related osteomalacia in renal-failure patients. Clin Pharmacol Ther 4:434–439, 1985.
307. Alfrey AC: The case against aluminum affecting parathyroid function. Am J Kidney Dis 6:309–312, 1985.
308. Chan MK, Varghese Z, Li MK, et al: Newcastle bone disease in Hong Kong: A study of aluminum associated osteomalacia. Int J Artif Organs 13:162–168, 1990.
309. Turner MW, Ardila M, Hutchinson T, et al: Sporadic aluminum osteomalacia: Identification of patients at risk. Am J Kidney Dis 11:51–56, 1988.
310. Woodson GC: An interesting case of osteomalacia due to antacid use associated with stainable bone aluminum in a patient with normal renal function. Bone 22:695–698, 1998.
311. Parisien M, Charhon SA, Maninetti E, et al: Evidence for a toxic effect of aluminum on osteoblasts. J Bone Miner Res 3:259–267, 1988.
312. Quarles LD, Dennis VW, Gitelman HJ: Aluminum deposition at the osteoid-bone interface: An epiphenomenon of the osteomalacic state in vitamin D–deficient dogs. J Clin Invest 75:1441–1447, 1985.
313. Felsenfeld AJ, Machado L, Rodriguez M: The effect of high parathyroid hormone levels on the development of aluminum-induced osteomalacia in the rat. J Am Soc Nephrol 1:970–979, 1991.
314. Rodriquez M, Lorenzo V, Felsenfeld AJ, Llach F: Effect of parathyroidectomy of aluminum toxicity and azotemic bone disease in the rate. J Bone Miner Res 5:379–386, 1990.
315. Charhon SA, Chavassieux PM, Meunier PJ, Accominotti M: Serum aluminium concentration and aluminium deposits in bone in patients receiving haemodialysis. BMJ 290:1613–1614, 1985.
316. Heaf JG, Nielsen LP: Serum aluminium in haemodialysis patients: Relation to osteodystrophy, encephalopathy and aluminium hydroxide consumption. Miner Electrolyte Metab 10:345–350, 1984.
317. Fournier A, Fohrer P, Leflon P: The desferrioxamine test predicts bone aluminium burden induced by $A1(OH)_3$ in uraemic patients but not mild histological osteomalacia. Proc Eur Dial Transplant Assoc Eur Renal Assoc 21:371–376, 1985.
318. Milliner DS, Nebeker HG, Ott SM: Use of the desferrioxamine infusion test in the diagnosis of aluminum-related osteodystrophy. Ann Intern Med 101:775–780, 1984.
319. de Vernejoul MC, Marchais S, London G, et al: Deferoxamine test and bone disease in dialysis patients with mild aluminum accumulation. Am J Kidney Dis 14:124–130, 1989.
320. Ham KN, Brown DJ, Dawborn JK: Dialysis osteomalacia: A possible role for zirconium as well as aluminum. Pathology 17:458–463, 1985.
321. Klein GL, Herndon DN, Rutman TL: Bone disease in burn patients. J Bone Miner Dis 8:337–345, 1993.
322. Lipkin EW, Ott SM, Klein GL: Heterogeneity of bone histology in parenteral nutrition patients. Am J Clin Nutr 46:673–680, 1987.
323. Klein GL, Coburn JW: Metabolic bone disease associated with total parenteral nutrition. Adv Nutr Res 6:67–92, 1984.
324. de Vernejoul MC, Messing B, Modrowski D: Multifactorial low remodeling bone disease during cyclic total parenteral nutrition. J Clin Endocrinol Metab 60:109–113, 1985.

Chapter 88

Osteoporosis

Pierre D. Delmas ▪ Roland D. Chapurlat

DEFINITION

Osteoporosis is defined as a "systemic skeletal disease characterized by low bone mass and microarchitectural deterioration of bone tissue, leading to enhanced bone fragility and a consequent increase in fracture risk."[1] The etymology is descriptive of the alteration in bone tissue: osteoporosis is derived from the Greek *osteon*, or bone, and *poros*, or small hole. The term *osteoporosis* was first used in France and Germany in the 19th century to describe bone of the elderly, thus emphasizing its visible porosity. Bone fragility increases the risk of fractures resulting from moderate trauma, defined as a fall from standing height or less, which has led to the concept of "fragility fracture."

The concept of osteoporosis has progressively evolved from criteria based on histology, to the occurrence of fractures, and finally to the assessment of bone mass. Indeed, a fracture-based diagnosis unacceptably delays intervention in a condition for which prevention of fracture is essential. Changes encountered in osteoporosis can be assessed by noninvasive techniques measuring bone mineral density (BMD), such as bone densitometry. BMD accounts for 75% to 85% of the variance in ultimate strength of bone tissue[2] and is well correlated with the load-bearing capacity of the skeleton in vitro.[3] Prospective studies demonstrate that the risk of fragility fractures increases as BMD declines, with a 1.5- to 3-fold increased risk of fracture for each standard deviation (SD) fall in BMD.[4] The main advantage of a density-based diagnosis is the possibility of an early intervention, before fractures.

This approach has been carried out by the World Health Organization (WHO) in its definition of osteoporosis in 1994.[5] In women, osteoporosis can be diagnosed if the BMD or the bone mineral content is 2.5 SD or more below the mean value of a reference population of young healthy premenopausal women, with the following categories:

1. Normal: BMD higher than 1 SD below the young adult mean
2. Osteopenia, or low bone mass: BMD between 1 and 2.5 SD below the young adult mean
3. Osteoporosis: BMD lower than 2.5 SD below the young adult mean
4. Established (or severe) osteoporosis: BMD lower than 2.5 SD below the young adult mean and the presence of one or more fragility fractures

Thus osteoporosis is defined in practice by a surrogate marker (i.e., BMD), not a health outcome (fracture), even if other factors can influence the likelihood of fractures. Therefore, the relationship between BMD and fractures is very similar to that between hypertension and stroke and stronger than that between serum cholesterol and coronary heart disease (Fig. 88–1). The gradient of the risk of fracture with decreasing BMD is as steep as that between diastolic blood pressure and stroke.

It is estimated that with this 2.5-SD threshold, 30% of white women older than 30 years have osteoporosis,[6] a fraction that is similar to the lifetime risk of fracture at the hip, spine, and forearm for a 50-year-old woman.[7] By this definition about 0.6% of young adult women have osteoporosis and 16% have low bone mass. The prevalence of osteoporosis increases with age because of the decline in bone mass. Not all women who have osteoporosis by the WHO criteria will sustain fractures, and, conversely, some women who do not have osteoporosis by this definition might deserve treatment because of other risk factors that will increase their risk of fracture. Thus the

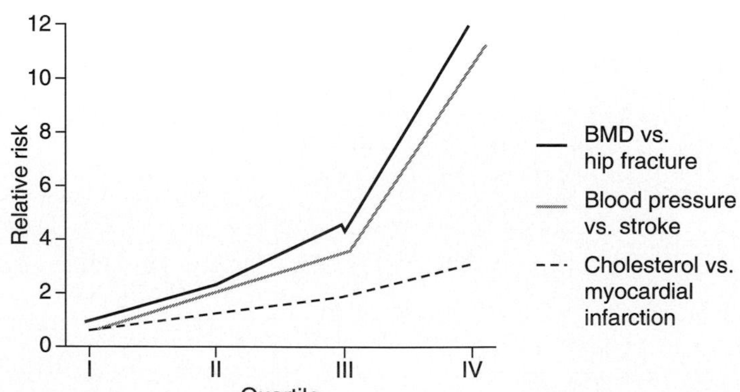

FIGURE 88–1. Comparison of the relationship between low bone mineral density (BMD) and the risk of hip fracture, between blood pressure and stroke, and between serum cholesterol and myocardial infarction. Quartiles I to IV represent increasing values for blood pressure and cholesterol and decreasing values for BMD. Relative risks of hip fracture, stroke, and myocardial infarction are expressed in fold increase over the risk in quartile I. The gradient of risk for hip fracture is similar to the one for stroke and steeper than the one for myocardial infarction. (Adapted from Cooper C, Aihie A: Osteoporosis: Recent advances in pathogenesis and treatment. Q J Med 87:203–209, 1994.)

current WHO definition of osteoporosis provides the concept of osteoporosis as a risk factor for fractures, which is important for assessing the number of affected individuals.

EPIDEMIOLOGY

Magnitude of the Problem

According to the WHO criteria, osteoporosis is rare in women before menopause. With aging, more and more women are affected by osteoporosis: by the age of 80 years 27% have low bone mass and 70% have osteoporosis at the hip, spine, or forearm.[7] Sixty percent of osteoporotic women will experience one or more fragility fractures. In the United States it is estimated that 16.8 million (54%) of postmenopausal white women have low bone mass and 9.4 million (30%) have osteoporosis.[7] These rates of prevalence are lower in nonwhite women and in men. NHANES III (Third National Health and Nutritional Examination Survey) data indicate that 10,103,000 Americans (8,021,000 women and 2,082,000 men) have osteoporosis and that 18,557,000 (15,434,000 women and 3,123,000 men) have low bone mass and thus an increased risk of osteoporosis in comparison to those who do not have low bone mass.[8] The prevalence of vertebral fractures can vary according to the definition of fracture used. Thus 10% to 25% of women older than 50 years are estimated to have vertebral fractures.[9, 10] In 1990, 1.66 million hip fractures were estimated worldwide in those older than 35 years.[11]

Osteoporosis results in high rates of morbidity. In 1986 in the United States, osteoporosis was responsible for an estimated 321,909 hospitalizations in white women 45 years and older, 167,421 for hip fractures, 35,106 for fragility vertebral fractures, 120,636 for wrist fractures, and 20,369 for humerus fractures.[12] Osteoporosis-related fractures also significantly contribute to the economic burden of health care. In 1995, direct costs for osteoporosis fractures were estimated to be $13.8 billion,[13] whereas it was 5 to 6 billion annually 10 years ago.[12] Being elderly, patients with hip fractures often have other medical conditions, thus increasing their risk of complications such as pressure sores or infections. Hip fractures often result in admission to nursing homes.[14] The number of hip fractures and their associated costs are expected to sharply increase and could triple by the year 2040. Indeed, the number of elderly people increases quickly, and fracture incidence rates increase with age.[15] This phenomenon is observed in developed countries, but the projected rapid expansion of the elderly populations of Latin America and Asia could lead to an increase in hip fractures from 1.66 million worldwide in 1990 to 6.26 million in 2050, with only 25% occurring in North America and Europe.[11]

The lifetime risk of fractures can be estimated, given the probability of fracture and the odds of reaching a given age. Most data have been generated in white populations of western countries. The lifetime risk of sustaining an osteoporotic fracture has been estimated in the United States to be close to 40% for women and 13% for men. For vertebral fractures, the estimated risk is 15.6% for women and 5% for men. The risk of hip fracture is 17.5% for women and 6% for men, and it is 16% for women and 2.5% for men for wrist fracture.[7]

Site-Specific Fractures

Hip Fracture

Hip fracture is the most serious complication of osteoporosis. It results in high morbidity and sometimes mortality. The most striking characteristic of hip fractures is that they are associated with a 12% to 20% reduction in expected survival.[16] Many of the deaths after hip fractures are related to other diseases,[17] and few deaths are actually due to or hastened by the fracture, but the risk of dying of another disease is sometimes increased by the hip fracture. About 5% of women sustaining a hip fracture die during the following year as a consequence of fracture. In women living in nursing homes, 36% of those having a hip fracture will die within a year. Thirty percent to 50% of these patients are unable to regain the level of function that they had before the hip fracture. The patient's physical condition before the fracture may be the best predictor of postfracture functional outcome.

The incidence of hip fracture increases exponentially with age in both genders. In women younger than 35 years, the incidence is 2 per 100,000 person-years, whereas it is 3032 per 100,000 person-years in women older than 85 years.[18] In men the rates are 4 and 1909 per 100,000 person-years, respectively. Most hip fractures occur in elderly people: 52% after age 80 years (and 90% after age 50 years).[18] The decline in BMD and the increase in frequency of falls in elderly people are responsible for this high incidence of hip fracture. Only 1% of falls lead to a hip fracture, but 90% of hip fractures are related to a fall from standing height or less.[19] Hip fractures tend to be the consequence of falls on hard surfaces, the fall not being stopped by protective reflexes of upper limbs.[20] Fifty percent of the falls leading to hip fractures result from slipping or tripping, 20% from loss of consciousness, and 20% to 30% of loss of balance and other factors.

The incidence of hip fracture varies among different countries and populations. Rates are higher in Scandinavia than in Western Europe and Oceania.[21] A north-south gradient in age-standardized risk is found in Europe and the United States,[22] with a higher rate in the north. The age-adjusted increase in incidence that has been observed in several countries over the past 50 years appears to have leveled off in some of these countries. The incidence increases with socioeconomic difficulties, decreased winter sunlight, and water fluoridation. Fractures are more frequent in winter months. This seasonal trend could be due to altered neuromuscular coordination and vitamin D deficiency in winter months, because most fractures occur indoors and thus cannot be explained only by slippery winter conditions.[22] The incidence of hip fracture is markedly lower in black and Asian people. About 80% of hip fractures occur in women, because the age-adjusted incidence in men is two times lower than in women, and more elderly women are alive than are elderly men.

The estimate of cost for care during the first year after a hip fracture is $20,000 per person (in U.S. dollars) and is much higher in women older than 80 years. If the cost of the subsequent nursing home is attributed to the hip fracture, the cost of care for those who stay in nursing homes after 1 year is $93,378 per person.

Vertebral Fracture

The epidemiology of vertebral fractures is less well characterized than that for hip fractures because of the absence of symptoms after a vertebral fracture in up to 70% of cases and a lack of standardized diagnostic criteria for vertebral fractures on radiographs. Less than a third of patients with vertebral deformities seek medical assistance, and only 2% to 8% need hospital admission.[23] In women, 90% of vertebral deformities are a consequence of mild to moderate trauma, whereas this proportion is only 50% in men.[24]

The incidence of clinical vertebral fractures increases gradually with age in both genders. The age-adjusted prevalence is thought to be between 8% and 25% in women older than 50 years. The difference in prevalence figures is due to the definition used.[24] Early definitions of vertebral fracture were based on the type of deformity and thus had poor precision. New techniques using vertebral morphometry give more reliable results.[25] Vertebral deformities are mostly noted in women, with a ratio of 2:1, but this ratio becomes narrower in elderly people older than 80 years. It has been suggested in a large epidemiologic study involving 15,570 European men and women that the incidence of vertebral deformities might be equal in both genders.[26] Changes in the gross appearance of the vertebral body encompass a wide range of morphologic characteristics, from increased concavity of the end plates to complete destruction of the vertebral anatomy in vertebral crush fractures. Several approaches have been developed to standardize visual qualitative readings of radiographs. Smith et al. proposed a three-grade description of vertebral fractures.[27] Meunier and colleagues have described an approach in which vertebrae are graded according to their shape or deformity.[28] Kleerekoper et al. modified this index by introducing a deformity score.[29] Hedlund and Gallagher used percent reduction in vertebral height, wedge angles, and areas.[30] It must be kept in mind that vertebral deformity is not synonymous with vertebral fracture; for example, Scheuermann's disease is frequently discussed as a differential diagnosis.[31]

New vertebral fractures, even those not recognized clinically, are associated with substantial increases in back pain and functional limitation because of back pain, at least in elderly women.[32] Ten percent to 20% of elderly women with worsening of their functional status because of back pain have had a vertebral fracture. Common complications of vertebral deformities are chronic back pain, back disability, height loss, limitations in activity, emotional difficulties stemming from physical appearance, and more medical consumption. Kyphosis from vertebral fractures adds to the overall back pain. For instance, after adjustment for age, a 15% increase in kyphosis increases the odds ratio of severe upper back pain 2.1-fold. However, no association has been found between the number of fractures and impairment in quality of life. Vertebral fractures are associated with increased mortality at 5 years, as for hip fracture. The increase in mortality is progressive over this period, however, as opposed to hip fracture.

Wrist Fracture

Wrist fractures, also called distal forearm fractures or Colles' fractures, are very common. The incidence of wrist fracture is hard to calculate because only a minority of patients are hospitalized. A Norwegian study showed that it was the most common fracture responsible for admission to a local university hospital.[33] The incidence varies among different ethnic groups. Wrist fracture risk is lower in black people than white people.[34] An increasing incidence has been observed between 1950 and 1982,[35] but this trend seemed to have leveled off during the second part of the 1980s.

The pattern of incidence of wrist fracture is different from that in hip or vertebral fractures. The age-adjusted female-to-male ratio is 4:1, with a linear increase in incidence in women from ages 40 to 60 years, followed by a plateau.[36] In men, the incidence is almost constant between the ages of 20 and 80 years, for unknown reasons. Wrist fractures are not associated with an increase in mortality and are usually thought to be free of long-term poor outcome.[37] However, other data suggest that half of the patients do not report good functional status at 6 months because of complications such as algodystrophy, neuropathies, and posttraumatic osteoarthritis.[38]

Wrist fractures must be considered an important predictor of subsequent vertebral and hip fractures. Indeed, it has been shown that men and women with distal forearm fractures have on average a twofold increase in the risk of sustaining a hip fracture.[35] Previous wrist fractures are also significant predictors of overall osteoporotic fractures, with a relative risk of 1.54 (1.11–2.09) for people between 50 and 59 years of age and 1.75 (1.2–2.56) after 70 years of age.[39] In younger women, the predictive value of a previous wrist fracture for subsequent osteoporotic fractures seems even more important, with a relative risk of 2.67 (1.02–6.94) for women aged 40 to 49 years. This predictive value is of the same magnitude as that provided by a 1-SD decrease in BMD measured by bone densitometry.[40] Thus the occurrence of a wrist fracture in an early postmenopausal woman is suggestive of osteoporosis and should trigger appropriate investigation, such as BMD measurement.

Other Fractures

Other fractures include proximal humerus, pelvis, proximal tibia, and rib fractures. An excess of these fractures is noted in postmenopausal women, their rates increase with aging, and they are often a consequence of minimal trauma. These fractures are related to low bone mass, similar to hip and vertebral fracture,[41] and they should also motivate BMD measurement because any of them could be the first symptom of osteoporosis.

PATHOPHYSIOLOGY OF POSTMENOPAUSAL OSTEOPOROSIS

Osteoporosis is a multifactorial disease. Most, but not all risk factors influence the level of bone mass, but some may have an impact on bone structure (the so-called quality of bone) and some increase the risk of fragility fracture through extraskeletal mechanisms.

Clinical Risk Factors

Clinical risk factors can shed light on the pathophysiology of fragility fractures. Numerous studies have evaluated risk factors for fractures apart from bone density.[16, 42–50] The use of such factors (Table 88–1) to identify high-risk subjects is frequently advocated. Different types of fractures have different risk factor profiles.[43]

Estrogen Deficiency

Estrogen deficiency has been associated with osteoporosis since first suggested by Fuller Albright in the 1940s. It is the main cause of bone loss in women after menopause. Premature menopause—natural or surgically induced—extends the period during which a woman is exposed to a hypogonadal state, thus increasing the total duration of bone loss occurring after menopause.[51] Similarly, late menarche and primary or secondary amenorrhea also increase the risk for osteoporosis.[52] Luteal deficiency in premenopausal women has been suggested to be associated with bone loss,[53] but the evidence is still controversial.

Other Factors

Among the long list of risk factors for osteoporosis, four have been suggested to be the most important to search for in postmenopausal women because of their high prevalence and strong independent association with a risk of hip fracture.[54] These four factors are history of a prior fracture after age 40 years; history of a fracture of the hip, wrist, or vertebra in a first-degree relative ("family history"); thinness (being in the lowest quartile in weight, i.e., below 57 kg); and current cigarette smoking. Of these four clinical risk factors, personal history of fracture is the clinically most significant. Combinations of risk factors account for only 20% to 40% of the variability in bone mass, but they also influence the risk of fracture independently of low BMD.

TABLE 88–1. Risk Factors for Hip Fracture with and without Adjustment for Calcaneal Bone Density and History of Prior Fracture

	Relative Risk (95%) Confidence Interval	
Factor	*Base Model*	*Adjustment for Fracture and BMD*
Age (per 5 y)	1.5 (1.3–1.7)	1.4 (1.2–1.6)
History of maternal hip fracture	2.0 (1.4–2.9)	1.8 (1.2–2.7)
Increase in weight since age 25	0.6 (0.5–0.7)	0.8 (0.6–0.9)
Height at age 25 yr	1.2 (1.1–1.4)	1.3 (1.1–1.5)
Self-rated health	1.7 (1.3–2.2)	1.6 (1.2–2.1)
Previous hyperthyroidism	1.8 (1.2–2.6)	1.7 (1.2–2.5)
Current use of long-acting benzodiazepines	1.6 (1.1–2.4)	1.6 (1.1–2.4)
Current use of anticonvulsant drugs	2.8 (1.2–6.3)	2.0 (0.8–4.9)
Current caffeine intake	1.3 (1.0–1.5)	2.0 (0.8–4.9)
Walking for exercise	0.7 (0.5–0.9)	1.2 (1.0–1.5)
On feet <4 hr/day	1.7 (1.2–2.4)	0.7 (0.5–1.0)
Inability to rise from chair	2.1 (1.3–3.2)	1.7 (1.2–2.4)
Lowest quartile for distant depth perception	1.5 (1.1–2.0)	1.4 (2.0–1.9)
Low-frequency contrast sensibility	1.2 (1.0–1.5)	1.2 (1.0–1.5)
Resting pulse rate >80 beats/min	1.8 (1.3–2.5)	1.7 (1.2–2.4)
Any fracture since age 50 yr		1.5 (1.1–2.0)
Calcaneal bone density (per 1-SD decrease)		1.6 (1.3–1.9)

BMD, bone mineral density.
Data from Study of Osteoporotic Fractures.

Many other factors increase the risk of fracture. For instance, the Study of Osteoporotic Fractures[48] identified 16 independent risk factors for hip fracture in addition to low BMD (see Table 88–1). Numerous studies have described risk factors such as female gender, white or Asian race, age, previous fractures, thinness, cigarette smoking, family history of hip fracture, use of sedative hypnotics, and impairment in visual and neuromuscular function. Lack of physical activity may also be an important cause of bone loss,[55, 56] and it has been hypothesized that some of the age-related bone loss and the burden of skeletal fragility resulted from a decline in physical activity, in particular, in Western societies. Black people have less osteoporosis and fewer fractures than white and Asian people do. Excessive alcohol consumption increases the risk of fractures, whereas moderate intake may exert a protective effect. Undernutrition in the elderly may contribute to bone loss, the risk of falling, or the response to injury.[57] It is widely believed that inadequate calcium intake throughout life is a significant risk factor.[58]

In a cohort of 7575 French women aged 75 years or older, the risk of subsequent hip fracture was significantly increased, even after adjustment for femoral hip BMD, in women with a slow gait speed, in women who have difficulty performing a tandem (heel-to-toe) walk (i.e., neuromuscular impairment), and in women with visual acuity less than 2/10.[50] The incidence of hip fracture among women classified as being at high risk because of both a high fall risk status and a low BMD was found to be 29 per 1000 women-years; it was 11 per 1000 in women at risk because of either a high fall risk status or low BMD, and the risk was 5.4 per 1000 women-years in those at low risk according to both criteria.[50] Even with this combined approach, about a third of women with a hip fracture had not been identified as being at high risk, thus indicating that other factors are important in the pathogenesis of hip fracture. Although these clinical risk factors can be easily assessed with a rapid questionnaire and physical examination, they are probably of limited value in younger women. A personal history of hip fracture is still predictive, but its prevalence is much lower in women younger than 65 years. Fall-related factors have not been tested but are likely to be poor discriminants in younger and healthier women.

Peak Bone Mass

Peak bone mass is the amount of bone acquired at the end of skeletal growth, and it is followed by bone loss throughout the rest of life (Fig. 88–2). Bone mass at a given age is a function of the peak bone mass achieved and the amount of bone lost as a consequence of menopause and aging. Peak bone mass, which is reached in early adult life, primarily depends on genetic factors. It is also influenced by dietary calcium intake during adolescence and by physical activity.

Blacks achieve higher peak bone mass than whites do, who have greater peak bone mass than Asians, particularly Japanese. Twin studies have shown a strong correspondence of peak bone mass in monozygotic twins, who have closer concordance in BMD than dizygotic twins do.[59] Which genes are the most important is still unknown. It has been reported by Morrison et al. that polymorphism of a noncoding sequence of the vitamin D receptor gene was associated with peak bone mass variance in monozygotic twins and that these polymorphisms accounted for most of the genetic effect.[60] This association has not been confirmed by most subsequent studies[61–63] but has initiated searches for other candidate genes, including the estrogen receptor, interleukin-6 (IL-6), transforming growth factor-β (TGF-β), and type I collagen. For example, the collagen Iα1 Sp1 polymorphism appears to be associated with bone mass but accounts for only a small part of the variability in BMD.[64, 65]

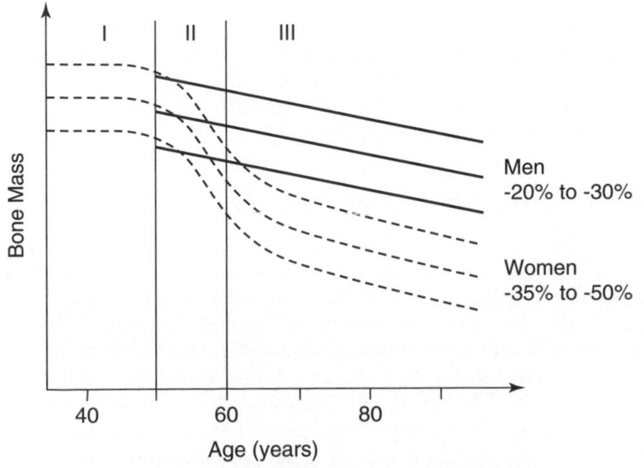

FIGURE 88–2. Bone loss during adult life.

Dietary calcium intake may be important for attaining optimal peak bone mass. Three placebo-controlled trials in children or in adolescents, including one performed in twins, have shown a modest, but significant increase in BMD in those receiving calcium supplementation.[66–68] Children with very low calcium intake are more likely to benefit from an increase in calcium intake, preferably a dietary source.

Other ill-defined factors may be important, such as those influencing the progression of puberty. Exercise during growth may contribute to the level of peak bone mass. It has been shown that intensive exercise before puberty may enhance bone acquisition, which might persist in adulthood,[69] but the role of exercise in the normal physiologic range is unknown.

Bone Loss with Aging

Changes in bone mass as a function of age are presented in Figure 88–2. Throughout life, women lose 35% to 50% of their bone mass, depending on the skeletal site. Although osteoporosis is a systemic disease affecting the whole skeleton (with the exception of the bones of the skull and face), the pattern of bone loss differs slightly and depends on the type of bone. Minimal or no bone loss is seen before menopause, with the exception of some sites of predominantly cancellous bone such as the vertebral bodies and Ward's triangle at the hip. Menopause induces accelerated bone loss within 5 to 8 years, followed by a linear rate of bone loss that may accelerate after the age of 75 years.[70] Because of a much slower rate of bone remodeling, cortical bone loss may start later, but the total amount of cortical bone mass that is lost in women in their 80s is probably similar to the amount of cancellous bone lost. The proportion of overall bone loss related to menopause and to the estrogen-independent aging process is debated, but clearly bone loss in the elderly is still under the influence of estrogen deficiency and can be prevented by hormone replacement therapy (HRT).[71]

Two major mechanisms underlie bone loss in women. First, an age-related decrease in osteoblast activity occurs and leads to an imbalance between the amount of bone resorbed and the amount of bone formed within a remodeling unit. Second, menopause induces a marked increase in the number of remodeling units activated within the cancellous and cortical bone envelopes per unit of time, which will amplify the small deficits observed at each remodeling unit. This overall increase in bone turnover peaks within the first 2 to 3 years after menopause but persists throughout life, even in women in their 80s, as shown by the sustained increase in bone markers of resorption and formation in elderly postmenopausal women. The mechanism by which estrogen deficiency results in increased bone resorption and bone loss is not yet completely understood, but evidence indicates that estrogens could act indirectly through cytokines and growth factors such as IL-1α, IL-1 receptor antagonist, tumor necrosis factor (TNF), IL-6, and TGF-β. It is not yet clear whether human osteoclasts have functional estrogen receptors.[72, 73] IL-1 production by peripheral blood monocytes is enhanced after menopause and decreases with estrogen replacement therapy.[74] In the rat, treatment with IL-1 receptor antagonist prevents bone loss induced by estrogen withdrawal.[75] Estrogen also inhibits IL-6 production by bone cells and stromal cells, and neutralizing antibodies to IL-6 counteract the effects of estrogen deficiency.[76] Estrogen may also regulate TGF-β production by bone cells and osteoclasts.[77] Thus estrogen deficiency induces upregulation and downregulation of the secretion of several cytokines in the marrow microenvironment that may be responsible for the increased bone remodeling and the imbalance between resorption and formation.[78]

Serum intact parathyroid hormone (PTH) levels increase with advanced age in both genders. This hyperparathyroidism is secondary to the calcium and/or vitamin D deficiency commonly found in the elderly, especially in those institutionalized, and may contribute to bone loss in both women and men. A classification of osteoporotic fractures based on clinical features and underlying mechanisms was proposed by Riggs and Melton.[42] Type I osteoporosis includes mainly wrist and vertebral fractures, occurring mostly in women younger than 70 years, and is predominantly due to loss of cancellous bone because of estrogen deficiency. Type II osteoporosis includes mainly hip fractures that occur in both elderly men and women as a result of cancellous and cortical bone loss driven primarily by secondary hyperparathyroidism. It has been proposed that this model should be unitary, with bone loss caused by estrogen deficiency in both phases and in both genders.[79] In this model, the accelerated phase of bone loss after menopause involves a disproportionate loss of cancellous bone and is mainly due to estrogen deficiency. The subsequent phase of slow bone loss involves proportionate losses of cancellous and cortical bone and is associated with secondary hyperparathyroidism. In aging men, low testosterone and estrogen levels may contribute to bone loss.

Mechanism of Fracture

Fractures occur because of low bone mass, architectural abnormalities of the skeleton, and trauma. Thus factors that influence the frequency of falls (such as the propensity to fall) and those associated with trauma (such as protective factors, including neuromuscular function and soft tissues) will influence the occurrence of fractures.

Bone loss occurring with menopause and aging is associated with disturbances in bone microarchitecture.[80] Osteoclastic resorption leads to focal perforations in cancellous bone plates, which results in loss of connection of the horizontal plates, along with detachment of vertical bars throughout the bone marrow cavity. Thus the probability of crush fracture is increased in bones rich in cancellous bone, such as vertebrae. The thickness of cancellous bone plates is about 100 to 150 μm, and osteoclasts dig resorption defects of 50 to 100 μm during normal remodeling. Perforations in cancellous plates could be a consequence of increased osteoclast activity and could lead to impairment in bone mechanical properties and therefore to an increased risk of fracture.

The geometry of the hip (hip axis length) influences the risk of hip fractures. Femoral neck length is a predictor of future fracture, and individuals with particularly long femoral necks are more likely to have hip fractures. This feature has been noted in white women from the United States[81] and France.[82] The increase in height over the second part of the 20th century could partly explain the increase in the incidence of hip fracture during this period.[83]

Skeletal determinants of bone strength do not reflect all the factors related to fracture risk. For any given bone density, the risk of fracture is greater in the elderly. The increased frequency of falling, the type of fall that occurs among the elderly, and the loss of protective soft tissue may all explain the larger contribution of age and the less important role of bone mass in the elderly. Among postmenopausal women in the United States, the frequency of at least one annual fall rises from about one in five at 60 to 64 years of age to one in three at 80 to 84 years of age.[83] Propensity for falling has been assessed in several studies[48, 50] with parameters such as gait speed, inability to rise from a chair without using one's arms, and of course, visual impairment. These parameters are associated with a risk of falling. The increase in falling is nevertheless not sufficient to account for the increasing incidence of fractures because only 5% to 6% of falls result in a fracture (1% of hip fractures and 4%–5% for other fractures). Fracture risk is also related to the seriousness of the trauma on the femur and the direction of the fall. Indeed, the risk of hip fracture is 13 times higher when the impact is delivered directly over the hip.[84] A great amount of force can be dissipated by the thickness of soft tissue over the femur, and patients with low fat mass may be at higher risk of hip fracture.

CLINICAL SYNDROMES

Postmenopausal Osteoporosis

The most common clinical form of osteoporosis is postmenopausal. Typically, women sustain a wrist fracture about 10 years after menopause, a vertebral fracture 15 to 20 years after menopause, and eventually, after 70 years of age, a hip fracture.

Wrist fractures, or distal forearm fractures, are mainly of two types: a Colles fracture is a consequence of dorsal angulation, and the less frequent type, a Smith fracture, results from volar angulation. These fractures usually have a favorable outcome, but some patients suffer from algodystrophy, osteoarthritis, or neuropathies.[33]

Two types of hip fracture are cervical and trochanteric. The femoral trochanter is composed of more cancellous bone than the femoral neck is. It seems that the predictive value of BMD and ultrasonic parameters may be higher for trochanteric fracture than for cervical fracture.[85] Hip fractures are associated with more morbidity and mortality, and the prefracture functional state is restored in less than half of the patients (see above in Epidemiology).

Vertebral fracture requires separate consideration. Vertebral fracture results in back pain, which often appears after some strain on the back, such as lifting a suitcase or working in the garden. The pain is generally very severe and often confines the patient to bed. This pain is commonly localized to the back and rarely radiates to the legs; cord compression is exceptional, and one must consider other diagnoses such as metastases or myeloma. Pain from the fracture usually eases over a period of 6 to 8 weeks and disappears. Nevertheless, it has been estimated that about half of vertebral fractures are asymptomatic.[23] Loss of height is another main feature of vertebral fracture, but often patients do not report it spontaneously, so it needs to be sought by asking about the individual's height in early adulthood. Therefore, it is worthwhile to record the patient's height at each clinical visit. Height loss of 1 cm or more should alert the physician to the possibility of a new vertebral fracture. Detection of asymptomatic vertebral fractures is clinically relevant because they are associated with a threefold to fivefold increased risk of new vertebral fractures, independent of the level of BMD. Kyphosis is generally a consequence of vertebral crush fractures in the thoracic spine and sometimes results in decreased lung capacity. Vertebral fractures in the lumbar spine result in decreased abdominal volume, which causes protrusion of the abdomen, and in impingement of the costal margin on the iliac crest. This iliocostal contact provokes pain and a grating sensation.[86]

Diseases and Treatments Contributing to Osteoporosis

A variety of disorders are associated with an increased risk of osteoporosis (Table 88–2). In most of these cases, osteoporosis appears to be multifactorial and cannot be attributed to only a specific disease ("secondary osteoporosis"). We will discuss only the most common disorders associated with osteoporosis.

Glucocorticoid-Induced Osteoporosis

Consistent evidence indicates that glucocorticoids impair bone formation[87] by directly inhibiting osteoblastic activity. Osteoblast synthesis of type I collagen, osteocalcin, and alkaline phosphatase is decreased; the production of insulin-like growth factor-1 (IGF-1) and IGF-2 is also inhibited by glucocorticoids. Measurement of serum osteocalcin provides a good index of this osteoblast inhibition by glucocorticoids. The effect of corticosteroids on bone resorption is less clear. High doses have been associated in some, but not all, studies with an increased rate of bone resorption, which may be a consequence of secondary hyperparathyroidism resulting from de-

TABLE 88–2. Diseases and Treatments Contributing to Osteoporosis

Endocrine disorders	Bone marrow disorders
Hyperthyroidism	Multiple myeloma
Hyperparathyroidism	Mastocytosis
Type 1 diabetes mellitus	Leukemia
Conditions associated with hypogonadism	Disorders of connective tissues
Hemochromatosis	Osteogenesis imperfecta
Turner's syndrome	Marfan's syndrome
Klinefelter's syndrome	Homocystinuria
Postchemotherapy	Drugs
Hypopituitarism	Corticosteroids
Anorexia nervosa	Medroxyprogesterone acetate
Inflammatory disorders	Anticonvulsants
Rheumatoid arthritis	Methotrexate
Ankylosing spondyloarthritis	Heparin
Lupus erythematosus	Cyclosporine
Disorders associated with malabsorption	Miscellaneous
Celiac disease	Pregnancy/lactation
Gastrectomy	Hypercalciuria
Chronic liver diseases	Alcohol
Total parenteral nutrition	Caffeine
Inflammatory bowel disease	
Conditions associated with immobilization	
Parkinson's disease	
Poliomyelitis	
Cerebral palsy	
Paraplegia	

creased calcium intestinal absorption. Urine calcium excretion is usually increased. Glucocorticoids contribute to adrenal and gonadal deficiency because of inhibition of pituitary hormone secretion, with a dose-dependent reduction in free testosterone in men. Consequently, exposure to supraphysiologic doses of glucocorticoids leads to substantial and rapid bone loss in most individuals, especially in the first year of therapy and with doses above 7.5 mg of prednisone. Thus fractures are very common, especially vertebral fractures, which occur in 30% to 50% of corticosteroid-treated patients.[88] The risk of hip fracture is increased 2.7-fold.[89] Patients undergoing organ transplantation may have a higher fracture risk than other steroid-treated patients, perhaps because of the preexisting condition and the osteopenic effect of other immunosuppressive drugs such as cyclosporine. One of the main problems with corticosteroid treatment is the minimal effective dose to avoid side effects. Some evidence suggests that corticosteroid-induced inhibition of bone formation occurs even with low doses of inhaled corticosteroids, with a marked decrease in serum osteocalcin.[90] Data from cross-sectional studies suggest that the bone mass of asthmatic patients treated with low oral doses of corticosteroids or with inhaled corticosteroids is lower than that of controls. However, prospective studies are lacking.

Endocrine Diseases

Sex hormone deficiency in both genders results in bone loss. All diseases and drugs that reduce sex hormone levels are associated with bone loss, and the list includes athletic amenorrhea, anorexia nervosa, hemochromatosis, Turner's syndrome, Klinefelter's syndrome, numerous chemotherapeutic regimens, hypopituitarism, or treatment with luteinizing hormone–releasing hormone analogues for endometriosis. In type 1 diabetes mellitus, small and variable decreases in bone density have been reported. In type 2 diabetes, BMD seems to be increased, perhaps because of increased body weight and hyperinsulinemia. Cushing's syndrome leads to bone loss that is reversible after treatment of the disease. Thyroid hormones are major activators of bone remodeling.

Patients with hyperthyroidism are subject to high-turnover osteoporosis with or without mild hypercalcemia, and they have an increased risk of fracture.[48, 91] The decrease in BMD in thyrotoxic patients is reversible after treatment of the hyperthyroidism. The deleterious effects of supraphysiologic doses of thyroid hormone on bone may also occur, but to a lesser extent, in patients who receive suppressive doses of thyroxin for the treatment of thyroid carcinomas and nontoxic goiter. Conversely, hypothyroidism does not seem to significantly affect BMD. The potential role of calcitonin deficiency in bone loss after thyroidectomy is unclear.

Studies by dual x-ray absorptiometry (DXA) in mild primary hyperparathyroidism have shown that bone density is reduced in regions of cortical bone but is normal in areas of cancellous bone. This decrease in BMD is likely to increase the risk of fracture. Skeletal recovery after surgical treatment of parathyroid adenoma is very significant, with an increased BMD of about 10% to 12% at most sites.[92] These patients were the more severely affected patients whose surgery was dictated by the guidelines of the National Institutes of Health.[92] Nonetheless, the result raises the question of whether asymptomatic hyperparathyroidism is a risk factor for osteoporosis (see Chapter 76).

Gastrointestinal Diseases

All diseases associated with impairment in calcium and/or vitamin D absorption may induce bone loss and include disorders such as celiac disease, inflammatory bowel syndromes, jejuno-ileal bypasses, pancreatic insufficiency, gastrectomy, chronic liver diseases, or prolonged total parenteral nutrition. The decrease in bone density is sometimes due to osteomalacia rather than osteoporosis per se. The origin of gastrointestinal-induced osteoporosis can be multifactorial and could include, for example, the role of corticosteroid therapy in the case of inflammatory bowel diseases.

Bone Marrow Diseases

Multiple myeloma is generally characterized by osteolytic lesions but often induces generalized bone loss. Vertebral crush fractures are also very common. Histomorphometric studies of bone have shown a marked uncoupling between increased resorption and decreased formation that may be due to the secretion of IL-1, IL-6, and TNF-β by plasma cells and other cells of the marrow environment. Corticosteroid therapy and immobilization can also contribute to this bone loss. Acute leukemia in children and adolescents, rather than lymphomas, is sometimes associated with generalized osteoporosis with or without osteolytic lesions. Systemic mastocytosis is a rare disease caused by the proliferation of mast cells infiltrating the skin, bone marrow, spleen, liver, and lymph nodes. Skeletal involvement may be focal or generalized, and about 70% of patients have radiographic abnormalities, including osteosclerotic lesions but also generalized osteopenia and vertebral fractures. In the absence of typical skin lesions, bone biopsy is often the only way to diagnose mastocytosis.

Other Conditions

Rheumatologic conditions such as rheumatoid arthritis and ankylosing spondylitis are associated with osteoporosis and with an increased rate of fracture. Pregnancy is very uncommonly associated with bone loss in the last trimester. At intakes higher than 40 g of ethanol per day, alcoholism increases the risk of osteoporotic fractures, particularly in men. In addition to the direct effect of alcohol on osteoblasts, the role of hypogonadism and liver disease may be of importance. Caffeine consumption has also been associated with reduced bone mass and hip fracture risk in some studies.[48, 55] Medroxyprogesterone acetate is a progestational agent that suppresses gonadotropin, thus causing anovulation and hypoestrogenemia. Its prolonged use is associated with decreased spinal bone density in about 10%. Other drugs, such as some anticonvulsants, methotrexate, heparin, and cyclosporine, may increase the risk of osteoporosis.

Osteoporosis in Young Adults

A few young adults have osteoporotic fractures corresponding to either mild osteogenesis imperfecta or idiopathic osteoporosis. Osteogenesis imperfecta is an inherited syndrome characterized by fragile bones and recurrent fractures that can lead to skeletal deformities.[89]

Inheritance and phenotypic expression are very heterogeneous.[89] Clinical features of osteogenesis imperfecta also include short stature, blue sclerae, dentinogenesis imperfecta, hearing loss, scoliosis, and joint laxity. Osteogenesis imperfecta generally results from mutations of type I collagen.

Idiopathic juvenile osteoporosis is a very rare condition[93] of children and adolescents before puberty. This disease does not seem to be familial. Vertebral fractures usually occur over a 2- to 4-year period. In severe cases, patients may have deformities of the extremities and kyphoscoliosis.

Idiopathic adult osteoporosis is more often recognized because bone densitometry is more widely available. Although the condition may resemble mild osteogenesis imperfecta, these patients do not have dentinogenesis imperfecta, blue sclerae, or hearing loss. They do, however, have joint laxity and mild scoliosis, and a familial history is sometimes found.[94]

Osteoporosis in Men

Fractures are more prevalent in men than in women from childhood to middle life, probably because of a higher incidence of trauma. After 40 years of age, fractures are less common in men than in women, but the incidence of fracture as a result of mild trauma increases with aging. The incidence of hip fracture in men rises exponentially with age, as in women. The sex ratio (female to male) is about 2:1 in northern Europe, but it may vary in other areas and reflects the lower life expectancy of men. Mortality related to hip fracture is significantly higher in men than in women. Although vertebral deformities are common in men, many of them are unrelated to osteoporosis. Vertebral fractures in men are associated with height loss, kyphosis, and increased disability, as in women. The incidence of osteoporotic vertebral fractures seems to be half that in women.[23] Vertebral fracture in men is associated with lower BMD than in controls.[95] The incidence of limb fracture begins to rise at a later age in men than in women.

As in women, osteoporosis in men can result from an inadequate peak bone mass and/or accelerated bone loss. As discussed below, gonadal status may be critical for the achievement of peak bone mass in the male. Age-related bone loss is less pronounced in men than in women, around 15% to 20% from 30 to 80 years of age. The mechanisms underlying bone loss with aging in men are unknown, but some evidence indicates decreased osteoblastic activity in males with idiopathic osteoporosis.[96] In elderly men, secondary hyperparathyroidism may contribute to bone loss.

The same risk factors for fragility fractures have been described in men and women and include smoking and excessive alcohol intake, and these factors are often combined in a man with osteoporosis. About 50% of men with osteoporosis are considered to have secondary osteoporosis. The most common causes are chronic glucocorticoid therapy, hypogonadism, alcoholism, gastrectomy, and other gastrointestinal disorders. Male hypogonadism has a major influence on the occurrence of osteoporosis. Peak bone mass may be impaired by disorders of puberty, and men with abnormal or delayed puberty have reduced bone mass.[97] Estrogen status is believed to be critical for the acquisition of peak bone mass in men since the observation that aromatase deficiency in a man, resulting in estrogen deficiency, led to the absence of epiphyseal closure and to osteopenia, abnormalities that can be successfully treated with estrogen.[98] Androgens are also essential for the maintenance of bone mass in adult men inasmuch as hypogonadism in men is associated with low bone mass. Osteoporosis is encountered in many forms of hypogonadism, such as hyperprolactinemia, castration, anorexia, hemochromatosis, and Klinefelter's syndrome. Prolonged abuse of alcohol has detrimental effects on the skeleton, with reduced bone mass resulting mainly from impaired osteoblast activity, nutritional deficiencies, and hypogonadism. Gastrointestinal disorders, particularly gastrectomy, are also associated with osteoporosis in men. Some, but not all, studies have linked nephrolithiasis or hypercalciuria with reduced bone mass, but their impact on the mechanisms of bone loss remains unclear.

The diagnosis of osteoporosis in men is somewhat different from that in women.[99] Indeed, the WHO criteria proposed for women cannot be used in men. Peak bone mass is higher in men than in women, so T-score thresholds may not be the same. No international consensus has been reached on the definition of osteoporosis in men, but the increase in fracture risk starts to rise at the same volumic density as in women.

DIAGNOSIS

Investigation of patients with osteoporosis is intended to fulfill the following purposes:

- To establish the diagnosis and eliminate the possibility of conditions mimicking osteoporosis
- To identify factors contributing to osteoporosis
- To determine the prognosis of the disease, with quantification of bone mass, identification of previous fractures, identification of factors that influence the risk of fractures independently of bone mass, and assessment of the rate of bone loss with biochemical markers
- To select the most appropriate treatment
- To obtain baseline measurements that can be useful for monitoring treatment efficacy

Differential Diagnosis and Causes of Osteoporosis

Evaluation of a patient suspected of having osteoporosis includes an adequate history and physical examination, and it must assess the potential causes of secondary osteoporosis and diseases mimicking osteoporosis. A minimum biochemical profile is necessary in patients with vertebral fractures, including assays of serum calcium, phosphate, creatinine, and alkaline phosphatase; serum protein electrophoresis; test for proteinuria; and, in some cases, urine protein immunoelectrophoresis and blood cell count. Thyroid-stimulating hormone measurement and, in men, free testosterone and prolactin assays may be useful in some cases. In the elderly, 25-hydroxycholecalciferol (25-OHD) and PTH assays are appropriate when vitamin D deficiency is suspected. Assessment is guided by the clinical findings because some patients with apparent primary osteoporosis turn out to have mild hyperparathyroidism, systemic mastocytosis, late appearance of atypical osteogenesis imperfecta, or osteomalacia.

A complete examination of the spine is often necessary in patients with osteoporosis and includes height measurement and assessment of pain, paraspinal muscle contraction, thoracic kyphosis and lumbar lordosis, scoliosis, and the gap between the costal margin and the iliac crest, as well as the abdomen protrusion that can result from multiple vertebral fractures. Blue sclerae, joint hyperelasticity, and signs in favor of hyperthyroidism or hyperadrenocorticism should be looked for. A general examination is also important to rule out a neoplasm (e.g., lymph node and breast palpation) or other conditions.

Radiographs are important tools to confirm fractures and their potential etiology. Plain radiographs with anteroposterior and lateral views are required for both the thoracic and lumbar spine. Vertebral fractures include wedge deformities, end-plate ("biconcave") deformities, and compression (or crush) fractures (see Chapter 85). Some vertebral deformities unrelated to osteoporosis include Scheuermann's disease, malignancies, and osteomalacia. The diagnosis of mild vertebral fracture can be difficult because of overlap with the normal range of vertebral body shape. Algorithms to define vertebral fractures that were developed for epidemiologic studies and clinical trials have led to a consensus proposal for the radiologic diagnosis of vertebral fractures.[100]

Bone Mass Measurements

Measurement of bone mass is a critical step in the investigation of an osteoporotic patient to (1) confirm the reduction in bone mass and (2) assess the magnitude of bone loss and therefore the risk of further fracture (see extensive discussion in Chapter 85).

Dual X-ray Absorptiometry

Since its development over a decade ago, DXA has emerged as the technique of choice for measuring BMD because it is rapid, precise, and relatively accurate, involves exposure to a low radiation dose, and allows measurement of sites that commonly fracture, such as the lumbar spine, hip, and radius. DXA can be applied to the entire skeleton, and measurement of attenuation of the x-ray photons of two distinct energies also allows accurate assessment of body fat content.[101] Smaller DXA devices measuring peripheral sites only (forearm and/or calcaneum) have been developed and may play an important role in screening. DXA measures BMD as grams of hydroxyapatite content per square centimeter, that is, the local density of bone.

As mentioned above, several prospective studies have shown that BMD measured by DXA at various skeletal sites (spine, hip, forearm, calcaneus, total body) predicts the risk of fragility fractures, with a relative risk of 1.5 to 3.0 for each 1-SD decrease in BMD.[4] The prediction of fracture is higher when BMD is measured at the site of fracture, for example, measuring hip BMD for hip fracture. Although BMD is commonly measured at the spine and hip, measuring multiple sites has little advantage.

The most convenient way to describe BMD is by T-scores and Z-scores. The T-score is the number of standard deviations above or below the mean for young adults. The WHO definition of osteoporosis is based on the T-score (see above). The T-score declines with aging. The Z-score is the number of standard deviations above or below the mean for people of the same age. The Z-score permits a comparison of patients with a reference population of the same age and therefore permits detection of bone loss that is excessive for age. The high prevalence of osteoporosis in the elderly, however, as well as the difficulty in selecting a population adequate to establish a reference range of values in the elderly, limits use of the Z-score. From a practical perspective, the diagnostic thresholds proposed by the WHO can be applied effectively to spine and hip DXA measurement. Therapeutic thresholds should include not only the BMD T-score but also age and risk factors that predict the risk of fracture independently of BMD.[102]

DXA has some limitations (see Chapter 85). First, measurement of the spine is often more difficult to interpret in persons older than 65 years because of the high prevalence of degenerative osteoarthritic lesions, which will increase the apparent BMD reading without accurately measuring trabecular bone. Second, the accuracy of the technique is reduced in obese subjects. Third, repeated measurements may have limited value in assessing the rate of change in BMD because the expected percent change in BMD is the same magnitude as the precision error of the technique. A 3- to 5-year interval between two measurements may be necessary in untreated postmenopausal women to detect fast BMD losers. In patients treated with antiresorptive therapy, a 2-year interval is usually necessary to detect a significant increase in BMD.

Other Techniques

Quantitative computed tomography measures the volumetric BMD of the lumbar spine vertebral bodies and allows differentiation between cortical and trabecular BMD; however, it has several drawbacks, including relatively high radiation exposure, a high precision error, and an inability to measure the hip.

Quantitative ultrasonography may be a surrogate technique for DXA and may provide additional information on the material properties of bone. Ultrasound velocity (speed of sound) and ultrasound attenuation through bone (broadband attenuation) are recorded at various peripheral bones such as the os calcis, patella, phalanges, and tibia.[103] In general, ultrasound devices have a low precision error, but their accuracy is unknown. Both speed of sound and broadband attenuation decrease with age, with a magnitude that varies considerably from device to device. Two prospective studies have shown that ultrasound measurement of the os calcis is a valid predictor of hip fracture risk in elderly women.[85, 104] Quantitative ultrasonography is a promising technique for the broad diagnosis of osteoporosis, with the availability of cheap and portable devices. Until each device is adequately validated and until precise diagnostic and therapeutic thresholds are defined, quantitative ultrasound should be still considered a research tool.

Biochemical Markers

Different Types of Markers

Bone markers are usually classified as markers of bone formation and markers of bone resorption (Table 88–3).

Markers of bone formation are serum total and bone measurements of alkaline phosphatase, osteocalcin, and procollagen I extension peptides. Serum alkaline phosphatase is the most commonly used marker of bone formation but lacks sensitivity and specificity. New assays have been developed to improve specificity in order to separate bone and the liver isoenzymes, in particular, immunoassays using monoclonal antibodies with a cross-reactivity of only 15% to 20%.[105] Thus bone alkaline phosphatase is a sensitive marker of increased turnover in postmenopausal women. Serum osteocalcin, also called bone Gla protein, is a small noncollagenous protein that is specific for bone tissue and dentin and only produced by osteoblasts and odontoblasts. Serum osteocalcin levels correlate with skeletal growth during puberty, as well as with increases in conditions characterized by increased bone turnover, such as primary and secondary hyperparathyroidism, hyperthyroidism, or acromegaly. Conversely, osteocalcin is decreased in hypothyroidism, hypoparathyroidism, and glucocorticoid-treated patients, conditions associated with a decreased rate of bone formation. When resorption and formation are coupled, serum osteocalcin is a good marker of bone turnover. The most robust and sensitive assays measure both the intact molecule and the N-midfragment (which is the largest product of degradation of osteocalcin).[106] N-terminal and C-terminal extension peptides of type I collagen are cleaved during the extracellular processing of collagen. They also reflect bone formation because type I collagen is the most abundant organic component of bone matrix. These assays have variable sensitivity.

Markers of bone resorption are fasting urinary calcium and hydroxyproline, plasma tartrate-resistant acid phosphatase (TRAP), and collagen pyridinium cross-links. Fasting urinary calcium, corrected by creatinine excretion, is the cheapest marker of bone resorption but lacks sensitivity in osteoporosis. Hydroxyproline is derived from the degradation of collagen and has long been used as a routine marker of resorption, but it also lacks sensitivity and specificity. Technical drawbacks and the lack of specificity limit the use of plasma TRAP to reflect osteoclast activity; the development of new immunoassays could improve the ability of serum TRAP to assess bone resorption. Pyridinoline (Pyr) and deoxypyridinoline (D-Pyr) are nonreducible pyridinium cross-links in the mature form of collagen (Fig. 88–3). This posttranslational covalent cross-linking creates interchain bonds stabilizing the molecule of collagen. Concentration of Pyr and D-Pyr in biologic fluids is derived predominantly from bone. Pyr and D-Pyr are released from bone matrix during osteoclastic bone resorption. They are excreted in urine in a free form (around 40%) and in a

TABLE 88–3. Biochemical Markers of Bone Turnover

Formation	Resorption
Serum	Plasma
Osteocalcin (bone Gla protein)	Tartrate-resistant acid phosphatase
Total and bone-specific alkaline phosphatase	Free pyridinoline and deoxypyridinoline
Procollagen I C- and N-terminal extension peptides (PICP and PINP)	Type I collagen N- and C- telopeptide breakdown products (NTX and CTX)
Urine	
Free pyridinoline and deoxypyridinoline	
Type I collagen N- and C-telopeptide breakdown products (NTX and CTX)	
Fasting urinary calcium and hydroxyproline	
Urinary hydroxylysine products	

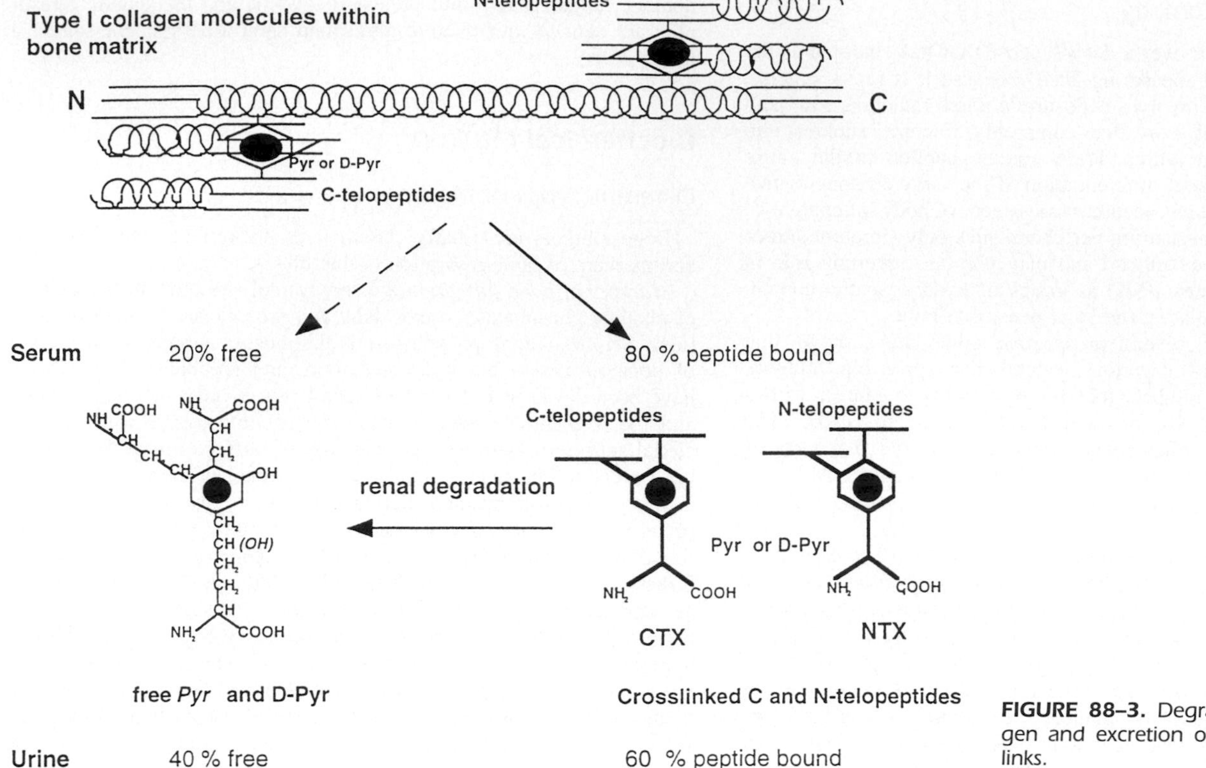

FIGURE 88–3. Degradation of type I collagen and excretion of type I collagen cross-links.

peptide-bound form (60%). Urinary enzyme-linked immunosorbent assays have been developed against the N-telopeptide to helix (NTX) and against breakdown products of type I collagen C-telopeptide (CTX). These cross-links are markedly increased at the time of menopause and return to premenopausal levels with estrogen and bisphosphonate therapy.[107]

Clinical Use of Bone Markers

BONE MARKERS FOR ASSESSMENT OF BONE LOSS. A sharp increase in bone markers occurs after menopause. This increase is sustained long after the start of menopause, even in elderly women, and markers are negatively correlated with bone mass assessed by DXA,[108] which suggests that a high bone turnover rate is associated with increased bone loss. A long-term study suggested that the rate of bone loss measured over 12 years by densitometry is increased in women classified as rapid losers at baseline and significantly higher than that of slow losers.[109] Thus a combination of markers and BMD measurement could be useful in assessment of the risk of osteoporosis.[110]

BONE MARKERS FOR THE ASSESSMENT OF FRACTURE RISK. It has been reported that women classified as fast losers have a vertebral and wrist fracture risk double that of those classified as normal or slow losers.[111] In elderly healthy women, those with higher baseline measurements of urinary CTX and free D-Pyr excretion had an increased risk of hip fracture, even after adjustment for mobility status and BMD.[112] Women with both a low BMD and increased bone resorption had a fourfold to fivefold increase in the risk of hip fracture.

BONE MARKERS FOR MONITORING TREATMENT OF OSTEOPOROSIS. Antiresorptive therapies such as calcitonin, estrogen, and bisphosphonates induce a significant decrease in markers, which return to the premenopausal range within 3 to 6 months for resorption markers and within 6 to 9 months for formation markers. The significant decrease in bone turnover seen after treatment of osteoporotic women with a bisphosphonate significantly correlates with an increase in BMD at the lumbar spine after 2 years, with a low rate of false-positive and false-negative results.[113] Given the precision of bone mass measurement with DXA and the expected change induced by antiresorptive treatment, it is usually necessary to wait 2 years to determine whether the treatment is effective in an individual patient. Determination of markers after a few months of treatment is likely to provide useful information on efficacy and might improve compliance.

Histomorphometry

Bone histomorphometry of the iliac crest allows an assessment of bone structure and turnover and is usually performed on transiliac bone biopsy samples. The specimen is processed without prior decalcification and analyzed with standardized histomorphometric methods. Histomorphometry is the only method to differentiate the cell and tissue level of remodeling. Nowadays, noninvasive techniques such as DXA and bone markers are sufficient for most clinical situations involving osteoporosis, and very few indications for bone biopsy still remain. Histomorphometry should be restricted to patients whose history, examination, radiographs, or biochemical profile suggests the possibility of atypical osteomalacia, mast cell bone disease, nonsecreting myeloma, sarcoidosis, or other rare conditions.[114]

MANAGEMENT

Nonpharmacologic Intervention

Life-Style

Patients who have sustained vertebral fractures need specific guidelines in their daily activities to prevent additional fractures. They should avoid weight lifting and learn how to bend to avoid excessive strain on their spine. All life-style factors that might be deleterious to bone metabolism should be corrected. Thus patients should not smoke, they should consume moderate amounts of alcohol, and conditions predisposing to osteoporosis should be treated. Although no controlled trial has shown that cessation of smoking increases BMD or reduces the risk of osteoporotic fractures, sufficient evidence indicates that smoking is a risk factor for vertebral and hip fractures.[48] Drugs predisposing to osteoporosis should be avoided as much as possible.

Nutrition

No universal consensus has been reached on the daily calcium requirement by age. The 1994 Consensus Development Conference on Optimal Calcium Intake recommended 1200 to 1500 mg/day for adolescents, 1000 mg/day for adults up to 65 years, 1500 mg/day for postmenopausal women not receiving estrogen, and 1500 mg/day after the age of 65 years.[115] Although most studies have shown a beneficial effect of calcium supplementation as discussed below, the long-term effect of a high dietary calcium intake on bone health is unknown. Conversely, there seems to be a threshold of calcium intake—around 400 mg/day—under which increasing calcium intake appears to be beneficial and necessary, both in children and in women older than 60 years.

Several nutritional factors influence the calcium requirement, such as sodium, protein, caffeine, fiber, and vitamin D status. The effect of fiber and caffeine is relatively small, whereas sodium and protein intake may be more relevant because they influence urinary excretion of calcium. The effects of phosphorus and fat intake do not substantially influence bone metabolism. Vitamin D promotes calcium absorption and thereby influences calcium requirements. Vitamin D status commonly deteriorates in older people, with serum levels of 25-hydroxyvitamin D lower than those in young adults because of low vitamin D intake and decreased sunlight exposure. The current recommended daily allowance in the United States is 200 IU for adults, but several studies suggest that this intake should be around 400 to 800 IU/day if sunlight exposure is low.[116–118] The low levels of 25-OHD commonly seen in the elderly, especially those institutionalized, contribute to secondary hyperparathyroidism, which may play a role in bone loss in the elderly.

Exercise

Immobilization induces bone loss, as documented after prolonged bedrest, space flight, paralysis from spinal cord injury, and casting of limbs. The beneficial effect of exercise on bone mass and bone strength in normal and osteoporotic individuals, however, is still unclear.[54] Several controlled trials have looked at the effect of various exercise programs on BMD, including walking, weight training, acrobics, and high-impact and low-impact exercise. Most of them show a small (1%–2%) increase in BMD in comparison to either baseline or the control group at some but not all skeletal sites; the increase is not sustained once the exercise program is stopped. Both clinical trials and observational studies suggest that load-bearing exercise is more effective in preserving or increasing bone mass than other types of exercise are. The dominant arm of tennis players or the limbs of gymnasts usually have higher bone mass than other sites do.[119] Skeletal sites must be directly strained to be affected by exercise. In addition, it is likely that fitness might indirectly preserve individuals from fractures by improving mobility and reducing the risk of falls. No randomized controlled trial has been conducted to assess the effect of exercise on fracture risk. Because of the many nonskeletal benefits of exercise, it seems appropriate to recommend regular and moderate exercise in postmenopausal women, but it cannot replace pharmacologic prevention measures such as estrogen replacement therapy at the time of menopause. After vertebral fracture, a supervised exercise program to maintain strength and flexibility of the thoracic and lumbar spine is recommended in the elderly.

It is critical to develop specific interventions aimed at preventing falls and their consequences in the elderly. So far, few studies have shown that specific strategies prevent falls. However, several intervention strategies are in progress in numerous American sites (FICSIT trials: Frailty and Injuries: Cooperative Studies of Intervention Techniques).[120] Results published to date show that these targeted interventions can be effective in reducing falls,[120] but no controlled study has shown that they reduce the risk of fracture, and their cost-effectiveness has not been evaluated. Given the multifactorial etiology of falls, interventions have to be multidimensional.

An adequate exercise program may decrease the risk of falling in the elderly, who should be encouraged to walk at least half an hour per day. Indeed, a sedentary life-style leads to low muscle mass, postural alterations, and deconditioning of lower limbs and increases the incidence of falls. Visual impairment is a risk factor for falls and fractures because it results in tripping or slipping accidents and decreases postural stability. Therefore, glasses should be checked regularly and cataracts detected early. Whenever possible, the use of drugs that increase the risk of falling should be reduced; such drugs include benzodiazepines, hypnotics, antidepressant agents, and medications that can induce hypotension. Patients should be instructed to avoid slippery floors and to have adequate lights and handrails in bathrooms and on stairs at home. Experimental studies have shown that the soft tissues covering the hip could have an impact on energy absorption of the fall. One controlled study performed in institutionalized elderly has shown that the risk of hip fracture could be reduced as much as 50% with the use of energy-absorbing external hip protectors.[121] Long-term compliance with these devices is unknown.

Pharmacologic Intervention

Evaluation of Drug Efficacy

The goal of therapy is to prevent fragility fractures, and drugs for osteoporosis should demonstrate their ability to significantly decrease the incidence of fractures in adequately powered, prospective randomized placebo-controlled studies. The diagnosis of nonvertebral fractures is easy, whereas the diagnosis of existing and new vertebral fractures requires adequate morphometric evaluation of spinal radiographs to exclude vertebral deformities unrelated to osteoporosis. Changes in BMD are commonly monitored and are usually seen as a surrogate marker of treatment efficacy. Actually, most drugs that inhibit bone turnover induce a small increase in BMD (i.e., 2% 10% according to the skeletal site of measurement) that does not account for their marked reduction in fracture rate (i.e., 30%–50% for vertebral fractures). In addition, some drugs—such as fluoride—may induce a marked increase in BMD without decreasing the fracture rate. Bone turnover markers are another surrogate for treatment efficacy of antiresorptive drugs. High bone turnover is associated with an increased risk of fractures that is independent of the level of BMD,[112] and antiresorptive therapy such as HRT and bisphosphonates induces a dose-dependent decrease in bone markers that is sustained throughout treatment. The antifracture efficacy of the most commonly used treatments of postmenopausal osteoporosis is indicated in Table 88–4.

Calcium

Calcium partially decreases the rate of bone loss, especially in women in late postmenopause. It is generally prescribed as an adjunct to other drugs such as bisphosphonates, and in most clinical trials both the active and placebo groups receive calcium supplements.

Calcium is likely to be partially effective in preventing bone loss, particularly in older women and those with low calcium intake.[122] Two

TABLE 88–4. Antifracture Efficacy of Treatments of Postmenopausal Osteoporosis in Addition to the Effects of Calcium and/or Vitamin D Supplementation, as Derived from Randomized Controlled Trials

Agents	Vertebral Fractures	Hip Fracture
HRT*	+	+
Etidronate	+	0
Alendronate	+ +	+
Raloxifene	+ +	0
Calcitonin	+	0
Fluoride	±	−
Vitamin D derivatives	±	0

*Evidence derived mainly from observational studies.

+ +, strong evidence; +, some evidence; ±, variable effects reported; 0, no effect or not studied; −, negative effect.

HRT, hormone replacement therapy.

studies have shown a slight reduction in the incidence of fractures in patients receiving calcium supplements.[123, 124] In one study, women older than 60 years were supplemented with 1200 mg/day when their calcium intake was below 1000 mg/day, and this regimen resulted in prevention of bone loss from the forearm over a 4-year period and decreased the rate of vertebral fractures by 59% in women who had vertebral fractures at baseline but not in those without existing vertebral fractures.[125] Calcium supplementation on the order of 500 to 1500 mg/day is safe. Mild gastrointestinal disturbances such as constipation are commonly reported. The risk of kidney stone disease related to hypercalciuria appears to be minimally increased if any. Bioavailability is greater during meals and varies with different calcium salts, but this factor is probably of little clinical significance.

Vitamin D

In a French study of 3270 institutionalized women with a mean age of 84 years who were treated with calcium (1200 mg/day) and vitamin D (800 IU/day) for 1.5 years, the risk of hip fracture and other nonvertebral fractures was decreased 43% and 32%, respectively, when compared with the placebo group.[117] Treatment increased serum 25-OHD, decreased serum PTH, and increased femoral neck BMD. However, in a Dutch study of 2578 women of similar age treated with 400 IU of vitamin D or placebo for 3.5 years but without supplemental calcium because of higher dietary calcium intake, the rate of hip fracture was the same in the two groups.[126] These women were healthier and more ambulatory, and the hip fracture rate was much lower than in the French study. In a recent smaller study, 389 men and women older than 63 years were treated with vitamin D (700 IU/day) and calcium (500 mg/day); the study noted a trend toward a decrease in nonvertebral fractures.[127] Another study showed a decrease in nonvertebral fractures when vitamin D was given annually by intramuscular injection.[128] These studies show the utility of adequate calcium (500–1500 mg/day) and vitamin D (700 IU or equivalent) in calcium– and vitamin D–deficient elderly women and probably men.

Vitamin D should be used routinely in institutionalized patients because they have low vitamin D intake, low sunshine exposure, and impaired vitamin D synthesis in the skin. When compliance is reduced, oral or intramuscular dosing of 150,000 to 300,000 U can be administered once or twice a year. Vitamin D is safe and does not require monitoring. The utility of calcium and vitamin D supplementation in healthy elderly persons with adequate dairy product intake and normal BMD has not been established.

Estrogen

The benefits and risks of HRT have to be explained to patients (Table 88–5). Menopausal symptoms are a common reason to prescribe HRT, and the duration of HRT to control these symptoms is far shorter (1–2 years) than the duration of treatment required to reduce the risk of fragility fractures (5–10 years or even longer). Women who have undergone hysterectomy can be given estrogen alone. Those with an intact uterus should be given both estrogen and a progestin either in a combined cyclic regimen (in women close to menopause) or in a combined continuous regimen (especially in those menopausal for more than 5 years) to prevent the risk of endometrial carcinoma. Several observational studies have shown a small increase in the risk of breast cancer after 10 years of use. Several observational studies suggest a significant reduction of the risk of coronary heart disease in women taking HRT, which was not confirmed in a randomized secondary prevention trial.[129]

Several controlled trials have shown that estrogen stops bone loss in early and late postmenopausal women by inhibiting bone resorption and that it results in a small increment in BMD (5%–10% over a period of 1–3 years). Results from observational studies[130] and one randomized placebo-controlled trial[131] show that estrogen decreases the risk of hip fracture by about 30% and the risk of spine fracture by about 50%. The reduction in fracture risk exceeds that expected by BMD alone. Estrogen reduces bone turnover and increases bone density in postmenopausal women of all ages, as well as improving calcium homeostasis. Calcium supplements enhance the effect of estrogen on BMD.[127, 132] When HRT is stopped, bone loss resumes at the same rate as after menopause. In the Study of Osteoporotic Fractures, the relative risk for nonspinal fracture was 0.66 in postmenopausal women currently taking HRT as compared with those not taking HRT,[133] but it was not decreased in previous users regardless of the duration of treatment. This positive effect was not affected by age and was more significant for women who started HRT soon after menopause (within 5 years).

TABLE 88–5. Benefits and Risks of Long-Term Hormone Replacement Therapy in Postmenopausal Women

Benefits	Risks
Relief of climacteric symptoms	Vaginal bleeding
Prevention of bone loss and fractures	Breast tenderness
	Migraine
Prevention of ischemic heart disease?	Deep venous thrombosis and pulmonary embolism
Prevention of Alzheimer's disease?	Moderate risk of breast cancer
	Moderate risk of endometrial cancer

Each patient should be explained the advantages and risks of hormone replacement therapy before prescription.

Bisphosphonates

Bisphosphonates are stable analogues of pyrophosphate characterized by two P-C-P bonds. By substituting for hydrogens on the carbon atom, a variety of bisphosphonates have been synthesized, the potency of which depends on the length and structure of the side chain. Bisphosphonates have a strong affinity for bone apatite, both in vitro and in vivo, which is the basis for their clinical use. Bisphosphonates are potent inhibitors of bone resorption and produce their effect by reducing the recruitment and activity of osteoclasts and increasing their apoptosis. This activity varies greatly from compound to compound and ranges from 1 to 10,000. The mechanism of action on osteoclasts includes inhibition of the proton vacuolar ATPase of some phosphatases and alteration of the cytoskeleton and the ruffled border. Aminobisphosphonates also inhibit several steps of the mevalonate pathway, thereby modifying the isoprenylation of guanosine triphosphatate–binding proteins.[134]

Oral bioavailability is low, between 1% and 3% of the dose ingested, and is impaired by food, calcium, iron, coffee, tea, and orange juice. Bisphosphonates are quickly cleared from plasma, about 50% being deposited in bone and the remainder excreted in urine. Their half-life in bone is very prolonged. Aminobisphosphonates can induce a 24- to 48-hour period of fever when administered intravenously and, rarely, esophagitis when given orally.

- Etidronate, given in an intermittent regimen, has led to an increase of about 3.5% in spine BMD after 2 years, with a reduction in the vertebral fracture rate[135]; this reduction in vertebral fracture rate was no longer significant after 3 years of treatment.[136] Etidronate does not appear to be effective in preventing bone loss at the hip and in reducing nonvertebral fractures. Inhibition of mineralization can occur when etidronate is given in high dose.
- Alendronate at 5 mg/day is effective in preventing bone loss in postmenopausal women to nearly the same extent as HRT.[137] In women with vertebral fractures, alendronate given for 3 years resulted in an 8.8% increase in BMD at the lumbar spine and at the hip[138] (Fig. 88–4). This treatment reduced the incidence of new vertebral, wrist, and hip fractures by half and prevented height loss. Alendronate also reduces fracture risk in postmenopausal women at the highest risk of fracture (i.e., those older than 75 years or those with very low BMD).[139] In women without preexisting vertebral fracture but with a hip T-score lower than 2.5, alendronate is able to decrease clinical fractures of all types.[140] Alendronate is approved in most countries for the treatment of osteoporosis at the 10-mg/day dose and for the prevention of osteoporosis at the 5-mg/day dose in

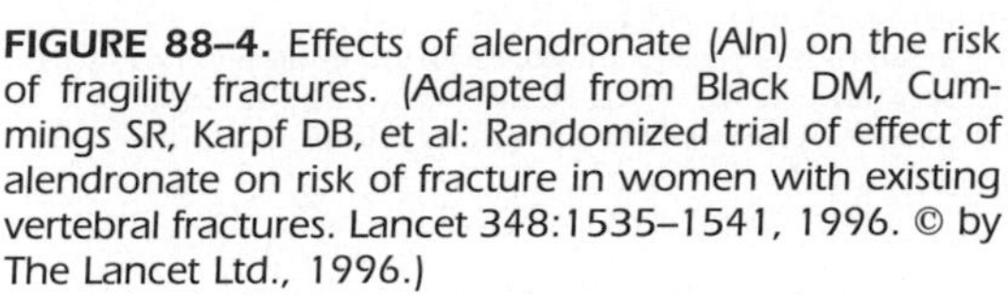

FIGURE 88–4. Effects of alendronate (Aln) on the risk of fragility fractures. (Adapted from Black DM, Cummings SR, Karpf DB, et al: Randomized trial of effect of alendronate on risk of fracture in women with existing vertebral fractures. Lancet 348:1535–1541, 1996. © by The Lancet Ltd., 1996.)

the United States. Alendronate is safe but can induce mild upper gastrointestinal tract disturbances and heartburn; on rare occasion these side effects are related to the esophagitis sometimes caused by inappropriate administration of the drug.

- Other bisphosphonates have been studied in the treatment of osteoporosis. Clodronate and pamidronate can increase BMD, but no adequate data on their antifracture efficacy have been presented. Risedronate and ibandronate are currently under phase III evaluation in osteoporosis. They have been reported to increase BMD and reduce bone turnover. Fracture data should be available soon.

Bisphosphonates can also be used in secondary osteoporosis, such as corticosteroid-induced osteoporosis. Etidronate prevents bone loss at the spine in men and women receiving corticosteroids, but not entirely at the femoral neck.[141] At a dose of 5 to 10 mg/day, alendronate is an effective therapy for the prevention and the treatment of glucocorticoid-induced osteoporosis. It prevents bone loss at all skeletal sites in men and women and reduces the rate of new vertebral fractures in postmenopausal women.[118]

Selective Estrogen Receptor Modulators

These compounds, also called estrogen analogues, act as estrogen agonists or antagonists, depending on the target tissue. Tamoxifen, which has long been used for the adjuvant treatment of breast cancer, is an estrogen antagonist in breast tissue but a partial agonist of bone, cholesterol metabolism, and endometrium. Tamoxifen does not entirely prevent bone loss in postmenopausal women and increases the risk of endometrial cancer, which precludes its use in healthy postmenopausal women. Raloxifene is a benzothiophene that competitively inhibits the action of estrogen in the breast and the endometrium and also acts as an estrogen agonist of bone and lipid metabolism. In a large 2-year randomized controlled study of raloxifene in postmenopausal women,[143] raloxifene increased lumbar spine (2.4%), total hip (2.4%), and total body (2.0%) BMD and significantly reduced markers of bone turnover. Serum cholesterol concentrations and its low-density lipoprotein (LDL) fraction were reduced without stimulation of the endometrium.[143] The ongoing RUTH study will determine whether the decrease in LDL cholesterol and fibrinogen can result in a reduction in coronary heart disease in an at-risk population of postmenopausal women. Raloxifene is now approved for the prevention of postmenopausal osteoporosis in the United States and Europe. Results of the MORE study (Multiple Outcomes of Raloxifene Evaluation) performed in 7705 osteoporotic women show that the incidence of breast cancer is reduced by half in postmenopausal women.[144] In this study, raloxifene also lowered the incidence of vertebral fractures in osteoporotic women with or without existing fracture but had no significant effect on nonvertebral fractures.[145] Other selective estrogen receptor modulators are currently under investigation.[146]

Calcitonin

Calcitonin, a peptide produced by thyroid C cells, reduces bone resorption by inhibiting osteoclast activity. It is traditionally given by subcutaneous or intramuscular injection, with poor tolerance (nausea, facial flushes, diarrhea). The development of intranasal salmon calcitonin may make this therapy more acceptable with fewer side effects. The minimum intranasal dose to have an effect on BMD is 200 IU/day. Calcitonin is less effective in preventing cortical bone loss than cancellous bone loss in postmenopausal women.[147] A small controlled study in osteoporotic women suggested a reduction in new vertebral fractures.[148] In the PROOF (Prevent Recurrence of Osteoporotic Fractures) study, which is a 5-year double blind, randomized, placebo-controlled study of 1255 postmenopausal women with osteoporosis, 200 IU/day of intranasal salmon calcitonin significantly reduced the rate of vertebral, but not peripheral, fractures by about 30% in comparison to placebo, but doses of 100 and 400 IU had no effect, and no consistent effect on BMD and bone turnover markers was seen.[149] Thus the role of nasal calcitonin in the management of postmenopausal osteoporosis is not yet clearly documented.

Others

VITAMIN D ANALOGUES. The effect of vitamin D analogues on BMD appears to be small and limited to the spine. Alfacalcidol and calcitriol are used in some countries for the treatment of osteoporosis. Data on reduction of fracture risk are scarce and conflicting. In one randomized, non–placebo-controlled study,[150] the rate of vertebral fractures was reduced in osteoporotic patients receiving calcitriol in comparison to those receiving calcium alone because of an increased fracture rate in the calcium group with time. No study has compared the effect of vitamin D derivatives vs. calcium plus vitamin D. Vitamin D derivatives expose patients to the risk of hypercalcemia and hypercalciuria. Calcium supplementation should be avoided and serum and urine calcium levels should be monitored.

FLUORIDE SALTS. Fluoride stimulates osteoblast recruitment and activity, thus increasing bone formation. In several studies sodium fluoride has resulted in a large increase in spine BMD that is linear, with little effect on femoral neck BMD. Fluoride effects on fractures are conflicting. In one randomized, nonblinded study of postmenopausal osteoporotic women treated with 50 mg/day of sodium fluoride over a 2-year period, the vertebral fracture rate was significantly reduced by 44%, but numerous patients were lost to follow-up.[151] Another study using intermittent slow-release sodium fluoride has also shown a small reduction in vertebral fracture incidence.[152] Larger placebo-controlled randomized trials using low or high doses of fluoride given as sodium salt or monofluorophosphate[153, 154] have shown that fluoride does not decrease the vertebral fracture rate and may have a negative effect on hip fracture. Current evidence does not support the use of fluoride in the treatment of postmenopausal osteoporosis.

OTHER TREATMENTS. Ipriflavone is a synthetic compound that belongs to the family of isoflavones. It inhibits bone resorption and prevents bone loss at a daily oral dose of 600 mg. No fracture data are available yet. Tibolone is a synthetic analogue of anabolic steroids with estrogen-like, androgen-like, and progestin-like properties. It prevents postmenopausal bone loss and has positive effects on hot flashes, but data on fractures are lacking.

PTH stimulates bone formation. It can be administered as the intact hormone or as the 1–34 fragment. Treatment with PTH results in an increase in cancellous BMD, with no clear positive effect on cortical BMD. Its activity on fracture rates is not yet conclusive. The combination of PTH with HRT might be appropriate, as shown by a small randomized study over a 3-year period in which the vertebral fracture rate was decreased in the PTH + HRT group.[155] Growth hormone has been used for its alleged bone and muscle anabolic properties. However, growth hormone has produced conflicting results in the prevention of bone loss in postmenopausal osteoporosis.[156, 157] Thiazide diuretics reduce tubular reabsorption of calcium and may decrease bone turnover and bone loss. Although they could be useful in patients with hypercalciuria, the role of thiazides in the management of osteoporosis has not been established.

Which Treatment for which Woman?

The following recommendations apply only to postmenopausal women. No treatment has been validated for male osteoporosis. The decision-making process should be based on an analysis of the patient's risk of fracture and the efficacy and tolerance of the drugs likely to be prescribed. This decision should rely on age, the existence of clinical risk factors, the magnitude of bone loss as assessed by the level of BMD, and the presence or not of previous fragility fractures.[54]

Patients with Previous Fragility Fractures

The existence of a previous fragility fracture requires, as an initial diagnostic step, investigation of the differential diagnosis and measurement of BMD. The first-line treatment, based on the current evidence for antifracture efficacy, should be alendronate (10 mg/day). HRT is a valid alternative, especially in younger women. An alternative, in case of contraindication or intolerance, is cyclic etidronate. Calcitonin is another option, although evidence of efficacy is limited. Based on results of the MORE study, raloxifene is likely to soon be approved for the treatment of osteoporosis. General measures including fall prevention and adequate nutrition should be implemented. The potential benefits of osteoporosis therapy may be limited if life expectancy is short, and the decision may be to not treat in very elderly women. Whatever the treatment option, adequate calcium and vitamin D supplementation is warranted.

Patients without Fractures

- Women with a T-score lower than −2.5 at the spine and hip have osteoporosis and should be treated as indicated above, unless their life expectancy is short and therefore their lifetime risk of fracture is low. For example, women older than 80 years with no additional risk factor for fractures may be treated with calcium and vitamin D alone.
- Women with a T-score above −1 have normal BMD and should not be treated, which does not preclude the use of HRT for other reasons such as treatment of hot flashes.
- Management of women with a low bone mass, that is, with a T-score ranging between −1 and −2.5, is more complex. The decision to treat or not is based on the individual's fracture risk, which depends on the magnitude of the deficit in BMD (the fracture risk at a T-score of −2 is double the risk of fracture at a T-score of −1) and on additive risk factors such as age, maternal history of hip fracture, low body weight, and increased bone resorption as assessed by a biochemical marker. Although treating elderly women with low bone mass might be more cost-effective than treating younger ones, treating women in their late fifties and sixties who have a high lifetime risk of fracture is recommended. If HRT is contraindicated or not accepted, raloxifene, 60 mg/day, or alendronate, 5 mg/day, is an excellent alternative.

REFERENCES

1. Consensus Development Conference: Prophylaxis and treatment of osteoporosis. Am J Med 90:107–110, 1991.
2. Hayes WC: Biomechanics of fractures. *In* Riggs BL, Melton LJ III (eds): Osteoporosis Diagnosis and Management, ed 2. Philadelphia, Lippincott-Raven, 1995, pp 93–114.
3. Mosekilde L, Bentzen SM, Ortoft G, et al: The predictive value of quantitative computed tomography for vertebral body compressive strength and ash density. Bone 10:465–470, 1989.
4. Cummings SR, Black DM, Nevitt MC, et al: Bone density at various sites for prediction of hip fractures. Lancet 341:72–75, 1993.
5. World Health Organization: Assessment of fracture risk and its application to screening for postmenopausal osteoporosis. World Health Organ Tech Rep Ser 1994.
6. Kanis JA, Melton LJ III, Christiansen C, et al: The diagnosis of osteoporosis. J Bone Miner Res 9:1137–1141, 1994.
7. Melton LJ III: How many women have osteoporosis now? J Bone Miner Res 10:175–177, 1995.
8. National Osteoporosis Foundation: 1996 and 2015: Osteoporosis Prevalence Figures: State-by-State Report. Washington, DC, National Osteoporosis Foundation, 1997.
9. O'Neill TW, Felsenberg D, Varlow J, et al: The prevalence of vertebral deformity in European men and women: The European vertebral osteoporosis study. J Bone Miner Res 11:1010–1018, 1996.
10. Spector TD, McCloskey EV, Doyle DV, Kanis JA: Prevalence of vertebral fractures in women and the relationship with bone density and symptoms: The Chingford study. J Bone Miner Res 7:817–822, 1993.
11. Cooper C, Campion G, Melton LJ III: Hip fractures in the elderly: A worldwide projection. Osteoporos Int 2:285–289, 1992.
12. Phillips S, Fox N, Jacobs J, Wright WE: The direct medical costs for osteoporosis for American women aged 45 and older, 1986. Bone 9:271–279, 1988.
13. Ray NF, Chan JK, Thaemer M, Melton LJ III: Medical expenditures for the treatment of osteoporotic fractures in the United States in 1994. J Bone Miner Res 12:24–35, 1997.
14. Jensen JS, Bagger J: Long-term social prognosis after hip fractures. Acta Orthop Scand 53:97–101, 1982.
15. Schneider EL, Guralnik JM: The aging of America: Impact on health care costs. JAMA 263:2335–2350, 1990.
16. Cummings SR, Kelsey JL, Nevitt MC, O'Dowd KJ: Epidemiology of osteoporosis and osteoporotic fractures. Epidemiol Rev 7:178–208, 1985.
17. Browner WS, Pressman AR, Nevitt MC, et al: Mortality following fractures in older women: The Study of Osteoporotic Fractures. Arch Intern Med 156:1521–1525, 1996.
18. Cooper C, Melton LJ III: Epidemiology of osteoporosis. Trends Endocrinol Metab 314:224–229, 1992.
19. Gallagher JC, Melton LJ, Riggs BL, Bergstralh E: Epidemiology of fractures of the proximal femur in Rochester, Minnesota. Clin Orthop 150:163–171, 1980.
20. Nevitt MC, Cummings SR, Study of Osteoporotic Fractures Research Group: Type of fall and risk of hip and wrist fractures: The study of osteoporotic fractures. Am J Geriatr Soc 41:1226–1234, 1993.
21. Melton LJ III: Differing patterns of osteoporosis across the world. *In* Chesnut CH III (ed): New Dimensions in Osteoporosis in the 1990s. Asia Pacific Conference Series No 125. Hong Kong, Excerpta Medica, 1991, pp 13–18.
22. Melton LJ III: Epidemiology of age-related fractures. *In* Avioli LV (ed): The Osteoporotic Syndrome: Detection, Prevention and Treatment. New York, Wiley-Liss, 1993, pp 17–18.
23. Cooper C, Atkinson EJ, O'Fallon WM, Melton LJ III: The incidence of clinically diagnosed vertebral fractures: A population-based study in Rochester, Minnesota, 1985–1989. J Bone Miner Res 7:221–227, 1992.
24. Melton LJ III, Lane AW, Cooper C, et al: Prevalence and incidence of vertebral deformities. Osteoporos Int 3:113–119, 1993.
25. McCloskey EV, Spector TD, Eyres KS, et al: The assessment of vertebral deformity. A method for use in population studies and clinical trials. Osteoporos Int 3:138–147, 1993.
26. O'Neill TW, Felsenberg D, Varlow J et al: The prevalence of vertebral deformity in European men and women: The European vertebral osteoporosis study. J Bone Miner Res 11:1010–1018, 1996.
27. Smith RW, Eyler WR, Mellinger RC: On the incidence of senile osteoporosis. Ann Intern Med 52:773–781, 1960.
28. Meunier PJ, Bressot C, Vignon E: Radiological and histological evolution of post-menopausal osteoporosis treated with sodium fluoride–vitamin D–calcium. Preliminary results. *In* Courvoisier B, Donath A, Baud CA (eds): Fluoride and Bone. Bern, Switzerland, Hans Huber, 1978, pp 263–276.
29. Kleerekoper M, Parfitt AM, Ellis BI: Measurement of vertebral fracture rates in osteoporosis. *In* International Symposium on Osteoporosis, vol 1. Copenhagen, June 3–8, 1984, pp 103–108.
30. Hedlund LR, Gallagher JC: Vertebral morphometry in diagnosis of spinal fractures. Bone Miner 5:59–67, 1988.
31. Kleerekoper M, Nelson DA: Vertebral fracture or vertebral deformity? Calcif Tissue 50:5–6, 1992.
32. Nevitt MC, Ettinger B, Black DM, et al: The association of radiographically detected vertebral fractures with back pain and function: A prospective study. Ann Intern Med 128:793–800, 1998.
33. Sahlin Y: Occurrence of fractures in a defined population: A 1-year study. Injury 21:158–160, 1990.
34. Baron JA, Barrett J, Malenka D, et al: Racial differences in fracture risk. Epidemiology 5:42–47, 1994.
35. Bengnér U, Johnell O: Increasing incidence of forearm fractures. Acta Orthop Scand 56:158–160, 1985.

36. Owen RA, Melton LJ III, Johnson KA, et al: Incidence of Colle's fracture in a North American Community. Am J Public Health 72:605–607, 1982.
37. Cooper C, Atkinson EJ, Jacobsen SJ, et al: Population-based study of survival following osteoporotic fractures. Am J Epidemiol 137:1001–1005, 1993.
38. Kaukonen JP, Karaharju EO, Porras M, et al: Functional recovery after fractures of the distal forearm. Ann Chir Gynaecol 77:27–31, 1988.
39. Gärdsell P, Johnell O, Nilsson BE, Nilsson JA: The predictive value of fracture, disease, and falling tendency for fragility fractures in women. Calcif Tissue Int 45:327–330, 1989.
40. Cummings SR, Black DM, Nevitt MC, et al: Bone densitometry at various sites for prediction of hip fractures. Lancet 341:72–75, 1993.
41. Seeley DG, Browner WS, Nevitt MC, et al: Which fractures are associated with low appendicular bone mass in elderly women ? Ann Intern Med 115:837–842, 1991.
42. Riggs BL, Melton LJ III: Medical progress: Involutional osteoporosis. N Engl J Med 314:1676–1686, 1986.
43. Kelsey JL, Browner WS, Seeley DG, et al: Risk factors for fractures of the distal forearm and proximal humerus. Am J Epidemiol 135:477–489, 1992.
44. Cooper C, Barker DJP, Wickham C: Physical activity, muscle strength, and calcium intake in fracture of the proximal femur in Britain. BMJ 297:1443–1446, 1988.
45. Farmer ME, Harris T, Madans JH, et al: Anthropometric indicators and hip fracture: The NHANES I epidemiologic follow-up study. J Am Geriatr Soc 37:9–16, 1989.
46. Paganini-Hill A, Chao A, Ross RK, Henderson BE: Exercise and other factors in the prevention of hip fracture: The Leisure World study. Epidemiology 2:16–25, 1991.
47. Grisso JA, Kelsey JL, Strom BL, et al: Risk factors for falls as a cause for hip fractures in women. N Engl J Med 324:1326–1331, 1991.
48. Cummings SR, Nevitt MC, Browner WS, et al: Risk factors for hip fracture in white women. N Engl J Med 332:767–773, 1995.
49. Johnell O, Gullberg B, Kanis JA, et al: Risk factors for hip fracture in European women—the MEDOS study. J Bone Miner Res 10:1802–1815, 1995.
50. Dargent-Molina P, Favier F, Grandjean H et al: Fall-related factors and risk for hip fracture: The EPIDOS prospective study. Lancet 348:145–149, 1996.
51. Ohta H, et al: Which is more osteoporosis-inducing, menopause or oophorectomy? Bone Miner 19:273–285, 1992.
52. Davies MC, Hall ML, Jacobs HS: Bone mineral loss in young women with amenorrhea. BMJ 301:790–793, 1990.
53. Prior JC, Vigna YM, Schechter MT, Burgess AE: Spinal bone loss and ovulatory disturbances. N Engl J Med 323:1211–1227, 1990.
54. Eddy DH, Johnston CC, Cummings SR, et al: Osteoporosis: Review of the evidence for prevention, diagnosis and cost-effectiveness analysis. Osteoporos Int 8S4:1–88, 1998.
55. Bauer DC, Browner WS, Cauley JA, et al: Factors associated with appendicular bone mass in older women. Ann Intern Med 118:657–665, 1993.
56. Mosekilde L: Osteoporosis and exercise. Bone 17:193–195, 1995.
57. Tinetti ME, Speechley M, Ginter SF: Risk factors for falls among persons living in the community. N Engl J Med 319:1701–1707, 1988.
58. Nordin BEC, Heaney RP: Calcium supplementation of the diet: Justified by the present evidence. BMJ 300:1056–1060, 1990.
59. Smith DM, Nance WE, Kang KW, et al: Genetic factors in determining bone mass. J Clin Invest 52:2800–2808, 1973.
60. Morrison NA, Qi JC, Tokita A, et al: Prediction of bone density from vitamin D receptor alleles. Nature 367:284–287, 1994.
61. Morrison NA, Qi JC, Tokita A, et al: Prediction of bone density from vitamin D alleles. Nature 387:106, 1997.
62. Peacock M: Vitamin D receptor gene alleles and osteoporosis: A contrasting view. J Bone Miner Res 10:1294–1297, 1995.
63. Garnero P, Borel O, Sornay-Rendu E, et al: Vitamin D receptor gene polymorphisms are not related to bone turnover, rate of bone loss, and bone mass in post-menopausal women: The OFELY study. J Bone Miner Res 11:827–834, 1996.
64. Uitterlinden AG, Burger H, Huang Q, et al: Relation of alleles of the collagen type $I\alpha 1$ gene to bone density and the risk of osteoporotic fractures in post-menopausal women. N Engl J Med 338:1016–1021, 1998.
65. Garnero P, Borel O, Grant SFA, et al: Collagen $I\alpha 1$ Sp1 polymorphism, bone mass, and bone turnover in healthy French premenopausal women: The OFELY study. J Bone Miner Res 13:813–817, 1998.
66. Bonjour J-P, Carrie A-L, Ferrari S, et al: Calcium-enriched foods and bone mass growth in prepubertal girls: A randomized, double-blind, placebo-controlled trial. J Clin Invest 99:1287–1294, 1997.
67. Cadogan J, Eastell R, Jones N, Barker ME: Milk intake and bone mineral acquisition in adolescent girls: Randomised, controlled intervention trial. BMJ 315:1255–1260, 1997.
68. Johnston CC, Miller JZ, Slemenda CW, et al: Calcium supplementation and increases in bone mineral density in children. N Engl J Med 327:82–87, 1992.
69. Bass S, Pearce G, Bradney M, et al: Exercise before puberty may confer residual benefits in bone density in adulthood: Studies in active prepubertal and retired female gymnasts. J Bone Miner Res 13:500–507, 1998.
70. Riggs BL, Wahner HW, Dunn WL, et al: Differential changes in bone mineral density of the appendicular and axial skeleton with ageing: Relationship to spinal osteoporosis. J Clin Invest 67:328–335, 1981.
71. Lindsay R, Hart DM, Forrest C, et al: Prevention of spinal osteoporosis in oophorectomised women. Lancet 2:1151–1153, 1980.
72. Oursler MJ, Osdoby P, Pyfferoen J, et al: Avian osteoclasts as estrogen target cells. Proc Natl Acad Sci U S A 88:6613–6617, 1991.
73. Collier FM, Huang WH, Holloway WR, et al: Osteoclasts from human giant cell tumors of bone lack estrogen receptors. Endocrinology 139:1258–1267, 1998.
74. Pacifici R, Rifas L, McCraken R, et al: Ovarian steroid treatment blocks a postmenopausal increase in blood monocyte interleukin-1 release. Proc Natl Acad Sci U S A 86:2398–2402, 1989.
75. Pacifici R, Vannice JL, Rifas L, et al: Monocytic secretion of interleukin-1 receptor antagonist in normal and osteoporotic women—effects of menopause and estrogen-progesterone therapy. J Clin Endocrinol Metab 77:1135–1141, 1993.
76. Manolagas SC, Jilka RL: Mechanisms of disease: Bone marrow, cytokines, and bone remodeling—emerging insights into the pathophysiology of osteoporosis. N Engl J Med 332:305–311, 1995.
77. Oursler MJ: Osteoclast synthesis and secretion and activation of latent transforming growth factor β. J Bone Miner Res 9:443–452, 1994.
78. Jilka RL, Takahashi K, Munshi M, et al: Loss of estrogen upregulates osteoblastogenesis in the murine bone marrow. J Clin Invest 101:1942–1950, 1998.
79. Riggs BL, Khosla S, Melton LJ III: A unitary model for involutional osteoporosis: Estrogen deficiency causes both type I and type II osteoporosis in postmenopausal women and contributes to bone loss in aging men. J Bone Miner Res 13:763–773, 1998.
80. Parfitt AM, Matthews CHE, Villanueva AR, et al: Relationship between surface, volume and thickness of iliac trabecular bone on aging and in osteoporosis: Implications for the micro-anatomic and cellular mechanism of bone loss. J Clin Invest 72:1396–1409, 1983.
81. Faulkner KG, Cummings SR, Black D, et al: Simple measurement of femoral geometry predicts hip fracture: The Study of Osteoporotic Fractures. J Bone Miner Res 8:1211–1217, 1993.
82. Reid IR, Chin K, Evans MC, et al: Relation between increase in length of hip axis in older women between 1950s and 1990s and increase in age specific rates of hip fracture. BMJ 309:508–509, 1994.
83. Cummings SR, Nevitt MC: Epidemiology of hip fractures and falls. *In* Kleerekoper M, Krane SM (eds): Clinical disorders of bone and mineral metabolism. New York, Mary Ann Liebert, 1989, pp 231–236.
84. Hayes WC, Piazza SJ, Zysset PK, et al: Biomechanics of fracture risk prediction of the hip and spine by quantitative computed tomography. Radiol Clin North Am 29:1–18, 1991.
85. Hans D, Dargent-Molina P, Schott AM, et al: Ultrasonographic heel measurements to predict hip fracture in elderly women: The EPIDOS prospective study. Lancet 348:511–514, 1996.
86. Hirschberg GG, Williams KA, Byrd JG: Medical management of iliocostal pain. Geriatrics 47:62–67, 1992.
87. Dempster DW: Bone histomorphometry in glucocorticoid-induced osteoporosis. J Bone Miner Res 4:137–141, 1989.
88. Adinoff AD, Hollister JR: Steroid-induced fractures and bone loss in patients with asthma. N Engl J Med 309:265–268, 1983.
89. Cooper C, Coupland C, Mitchell M: Rheumatoid arthritis, corticosteroid therapy and hip fracture. Ann Rheum Dis 54:49–52, 1995.
90. Teelucksingh S, Padfield PL, Tibi L, et al: Inhaled corticosteroids, bone formation, and osteocalcin. Lancet 338:60–61, 1991.
91. Toh SH, Claunch BC, Brown PH: Effect of hyperthyroidism and its treatment on bone mineral content. Arch Intern Med 145:883–886, 1985.
92. Silverberg SJ, Gartenberg F, Jacobs TP, et al: Increased bone mineral density after parathyroidectomy in primary hyperparathyroidism. J Clin Endocrinol Metab 80:729–734, 1995.
93. Norman ME. Juvenile osteoporosis. *In* Primer on the Metabolic Bone Diseases and Disorders of Mineral Metabolism, ed 3. Philadelphia, Lippincott-Raven, 1998, pp 275–278.
94. Shapiro JR: Osteogenesis imperfecta and other defects of bone development as occasional causes of adult osteoporosis. *In* Marcus R, Feldman D, Kelsey J (eds): Osteoporosis. San Diego, CA, Academic, 1996, pp 899–921.
95. Mann T, Oviatt SK, Wilson D, et al: Vertebral deformity in men. J Bone Miner Res 7:1259–1265, 1992.
96. Marie PJ, De Vernejoul MC, Connes C, et al: Decreased DNA synthesis by cultures of osteoblastic cells in eugonadal osteoporotic men with defective bone formation. J Clin Invest 88:1167–1172, 1991.
97. Finkelstein JS, Klibanski A, Neer RM, et al: Osteoporosis in men with idiopathic hypogonadotrophic hypogonadism. Ann Intern Med 106:354–361, 1987.
98. Bilezikian JP, Morishima A, Bell J, Grumbach MM: Increased bone mass as a result of estrogen therapy in a man with aromatase deficiency. N Engl J Med 339:599–603, 1998.
99. Seeman E: Advances in the study of osteoporosis in men. *In* Meunier PJ (ed): Osteoporosis, Diagnosis and Management. London, Martin Dunitz, 1998, pp 211–232.
100. National Osteoporosis Foundation Working Group on Vertebral Fractures: Assessing vertebral fractures. J Bone Miner Res 10:518–523, 1995.
101. Wahner HW: Use of densitometry in management of osteoporosis. *In* Marcus R, Feldman D, Kelsey J (eds): Osteoporosis. San Diego, CA, Academic, 1996, pp 1055–1074.
102. Kanis JA, Delmas PD, Burkhardt P, et al: Guidelines for diagnosis and management of osteoporosis. Osteoporos Int 7:390–406, 1997.
103. Hans D, Gluer CC, Njeh CF: Ultrasonic evaluation of osteoporosis. *In* Meunier PJ (ed): Osteoporosis, Diagnosis and Management. London, Martin Dunitz, 1998, pp 59–78.
104. Bauer DC, Glüer CC, Cauley JA, et al: Bone ultrasound predicts fractures strongly and independently of densitometry in older women: A prospective study. Arch Intern Med 157:629–634, 1997.
105. Garnero P, Delmas PD: Assessment of the serum levels of bone alkaline phosphatase with a new immunometric assay in patients with metabolic bone disease. J Clin Endocrinol Metab 77:1046–1053, 1993.
106. Garnero P, Grimaux M, Demiaux B, et al: Measurement of serum osteocalcin with a human-specific two-site immunoradiometric assay. J Bone Miner Res 7:1389–1398, 1992.
107. Uebelhart D, Schlemmer A, Johansen J, et al: Effect of menopause and hormone replacement therapy on the urinary excretion of pyridinium crosslinks. J Clin Endocrinol Metab 72:367–373, 1991.

108. Garnero P, Sornay-Rendu E, Chapuy MC, Delmas PD: Increased bone turnover in late post-menopausal women is a major determinant of osteoporosis. J Bone Miner Res 11:337–349, 1996.
109. Hansen MA, Kirsten O, Riis BJ, Christiansen C: Role of peak bone mass and bone loss in postmenopausal osteoporosis: 12 years study. BMJ 303:961–964, 1991.
110. Garnero P, Dargent-Molina P, Hans D, et al: Do markers of bone resorption add to bone mineral density and ultrasonographic heel measurement for the prediction of hip fracture in elderly women? The EPIDOS prospective study. Osteoporos Int 8:563–569, 1998.
111. Riis SBL, Hansen AM, Jensen K, et al: Low bone mass and fast rate of bone loss at menopause—equal risk factors for future fracture. A 15 year follow-up study. Bone 19:9–12, 1996.
112. Garnero P, Hausher E, Chapuy MC, et al: Markers of bone resorption predict fractures in elderly women: The EPIDOS prospective study. J Bone Miner Res 11:1531–1538, 1996.
113. Garnero P, Shih WJ, Gineyts E, et al: Comparison of new biochemical markers of bone turnover in late postmenopausal osteoporotic women in response to alendronate treatment. J Clin Endocrinol Metab 79:1693–1700, 1994.
114. Chavassieux P, Arlot M, Meunier PJ: Clinical use of bone biopsy. *In* Marcus R, Feldman D, Kelsey J (eds): Osteoporosis. San Diego, CA, Academic Press, 1996, pp 899–921.
115. NIH Consensus Conference: Optimal calcium intake. JAMA 272:1942–1948, 1994.
116. Ooms ME, Roos JC, Bezemer PD, et al: Prevention of bone loss by vitamin D supplementation in elderly women: A randomized double-blind trial. J Clin Endocrinol Metab 80:1052–1058, 1995.
117. Chapuy MC, Arlot ME, Duboeuf, et al: Vitamin D_3 and calcium to prevent hip fractures in elderly women. N Engl J Med 237:1637–1642, 1992.
118. Dawson-Hugues B, Dallal GE, Krall EA, et al: Effects of vitamin D supplementation on overall bone loss in healthy postmenopausal women. Ann Intern Med 115:505–512, 1991.
119. Kannus P, Haapasalo H, Sankelo M, et al: Effect of starting age of physical activity on bone mass in the dominant arm of tennis and squash players. Ann Intern Med 123:27–31, 1995.
120. Miller PD: Diagnostic prediction of increased risk of hip fracture: A clinician perspective. *In* Ringe JD, Meunier PJ (eds): Osteoporotic Fractures in the Elderly: Clinical Management and Prevention. Stuttgart, Germany, Georg Thième, 1996, pp 17–24.
121. Lauritzen JB, Pettersen MM, Lund B: Effect of external hip protectors on hip fracture. Lancet 341:11–13, 1993.
122. Tinetti ME, Baker DI, McAvay G, et al: A multifactorial intervention to reduce the risk of falling among elderly people living with community. N Engl J Med 331:821–827, 1994.
123. Dawson-Hugues B, Dallal GE, Krall EA, et al: A controlled trial of the effect of calcium supplementation on bone density in postmenopausal women. N Engl J Med 323:878–883, 1990.
124. Reid IR, Ames RW, Evans MC, et al: Long-term effects of calcium supplementation on bone loss and fractures in postmenopausal women: A randomized controlled trial. Am J Med 98:331–335, 1995.
125. Recker RR, Hinders S, Davies KM, et al: Correcting calcium nutritional deficiency prevents spine fractures in elderly women. J Bone Miner Res 11:1961–1966, 1996.
126. Lips P, Graafmans WC, Ooms ME, et al: Vitamin D supplementation and fracture incidence in elderly persons: A randomized, placebo-controlled clinical trial. Ann Intern Med 124:400–406, 1996.
127. Dawson-Hugues B, Harris SS, Krall EA, et al: Effect of calcium and vitamin D supplementation on bone density in men and women 65 years of age or older. N Engl J Med 337:670–676, 1997.
128. Heikinheimo RJ, Inkovaraa JA, Harju EJ, et al: Annual injection of vitamin D and fractures of aged bones. Calcif Tissue Int 51:105–110, 1992.
129. Hulley S, Grady D, Bush T, et al: Randomized trial of estrogen plus progestin for secondary prevention of coronary heart disease in postmenopausal women. JAMA 280:605–613, 1998.
130. Grady D, Rubin SM, Pettiti DB, et al: Hormone therapy to prevent disease and prolong life in postmenopausal women. Ann Intern Med 117:1016–1037, 1992.
131. Lufkin EG, Wahner HW, O'Fallon WM, et al: Treatment of postmenopausal osteoporosis with transdermal estrogen. Ann Intern Med 117:1–9, 1992.
132. Nieves JW, Komar L, Cosman F, Lindsay R: Calcium potentiates the effect of estrogen and calcitonin on bone mass: Review and analysis. Am J Clin Nutr 67:18–24, 1998.
133. Cauley JA, Seeley DJ, Ensrud K, et al: Estrogen replacement therapy and fractures in older women: Study of Osteoporotic Fractures Research Group. Ann Intern Med 122:9–16, 1995.
134. Luckman SP, Hugues DE, Coxon FP, et al: Nitrogen-containing bisphosphonates inhibit the mevalonate pathway and prevent post-translational prenylation of GTP-binding proteins, including Ras. J Bone Miner Res 13:581–589, 1998.
135. Watts NB, Harris ST, Genant HK, et al: Intermittent cyclical etidronate treatment of postmenopausal osteoporosis. N Engl J Med 323:73–79, 1990.
136. Harris ST, Watts NB, Jackson RD, et al: Four years of intermittent cyclical etidronate treatment of postmenopausal osteoporosis: Three years of blinded therapy followed by one year of open therapy. Am J Med 95:557–567, 1993.
137. Hosking D, Chilvers CED, Christiansen C, et al: Prevention of bone loss with alendronate in postmenopausal women under 60 years of age. N Engl J Med 338:485–492, 1998.
138. Black DM, Cummings SR, Karpf DB, et al: Randomised trial of effect of alendronate on risk of fracture in women with existing vertebral fractures. Lancet 348:1535–1541, 1996.
139. Ensrud KE, Black DM, Palermo L, et al: Treatment with alendronate prevents fractures in women at highest risk. Arch Intern Med 157:2617–2624, 1997.
140. Cummings SR, Black DM, Thompson DE, et al: Effect of alendronate on risk of fracture in women with low bone density but without vertebral fractures. JAMA 280:2077–2082, 1998.
141. Adachi JD, Bensen WG, Brown J, et al: Intermittent etidronate therapy to prevent corticosteroid-induced osteoporosis. N Engl J Med 337:382–387, 1997.
142. Saag KG, Emkey R, Schnitzer TJ, et al: Alendronate for the prevention and treatment of glucocorticoid-induced osteoporosis. N Engl J Med 339:292–299, 1998.
143. Delmas PD, Bjarnason NH, Mitlak BH, et al: Effects of raloxifene on bone mineral density, serum cholesterol concentrations and uterine endometrium in postmenopausal women. N Engl J Med 337:1641–1647, 1997.
144. Cummings SR, Eckert S, Krueger KA, et al: The effect of raloxifene on risk of breast cancer in postmenopausal women: Results from the MORE randomized trial. Multiple Outcomes on Raloxifene Evaluation. JAMA 281:2189–2197, 1999.
145. Ettinger B, Black DM, Mitlack BH, et al: Reduction of vertebral fracture risk in postmenopausal women with osteoporosis treated with raloxifene. JAMA 282:637–645, 1999.
146. Delmas PD: Clinical use of selective estrogen receptor modulators (SERMs). Bone 1999 (in press).
147. Overgaard K, Riis BJ, Christiansen C, et al: Effect of salcatonin given intranasally on early postmenopausal bone loss. BMJ 299:477–479, 1989.
148. Overgaard K, Hansen MA, Jensen SB, Christiansen C: Effect of salcatonin given intranasally on bone mass and fracture rates in established osteoporosis: A dose-response study. BMJ 305:556–561, 1992.
149. Silverman SL, Chesnut C, Andriano K, et al: Salmon calcitonin nasal spray reduces risk of vertebral fracture in established osteoporosis and has continuous efficacy with prolonged treatment: Accrued 5 year worldwide data of the PROOF study. Bone 23(suppl 5):174, 1998.
150. Tilyard MW, Spears GF, Thomsin J, Dovey S: Treatment of postmenopausal osteoporosis with calcitriol or calcium. N Engl J Med 326:357–362, 1992.
151. Mamelle N, Meunier PJ, Dusan R, et al: Risk-benefit ratio of sodium fluoride treatment in primary vertebral osteoporosis. Lancet 2:361–365, 1988.
152. Pak CY, Sakhaee K, Adams-Huet B, et al: Treatment of postmenopausal osteoporosis with slow release sodium fluoride: Final report of a randomized controlled trial. Ann Intern Med 123:401–408, 1995.
153. Riggs BL, Hodgson SF, O'Fallon WM, et al: Effect of fluoride treatment on the fracture rate in postmenopausal women with osteoporosis. N Engl J Med 322:802–809, 1990.
154. Meunier PJ, Sebert JL, Reginster JY, et al: Fluoride salts are no better at preventing new vertebral fractures than calcium–vitamin D in postmenopausal osteoporosis: The FAVO Study. Osteoporos Int 8:4–12, 1998.
155. Lindsay R, Nieves J, Formica C, et al: Randomized controlled study of effect of parathyroid hormone on vertebral bone mass and fracture incidence among postmenopausal women on estrogen with osteoporosis. Lancet 350:550–555, 1997.
156. Holloway L, Kohlmeier L, Kent K, Marcus R: Skeletal effects of cyclic recombinant human growth hormone and salmon calcitonin on osteopenic postmenopausal women. J Clin Endocrinol Metab 82:1111–1117, 1997.
157. Eastell R: Treatment of postmenopausal osteoporosis. N Engl J Med 338:736–746, 1998.

Chapter 89

Paget's Disease of Bone

Frederick R. Singer

Paget's disease of bone (osteitis deformans) is a common disorder of a focal nature that is an example of physiology gone awry. The primary disturbance appears to be an exaggeration of osteoclastic bone resorption that initially produces localized loss of bone. Usually the disorder is not appreciated until secondary bone formation becomes so pronounced that it results in one or more enlarged and deformed bones. The clinical findings depend on which bones are affected and vary from discovery of an incidental radiologic or biochemical abnormality to devastating musculoskeletal disabilities with a variety of neurologic and systemic complications. Great progress has been made in the ability to treat this disorder, and recently, new information concerning genetic influences has been acquired.

INCIDENCE AND EPIDEMIOLOGY

Studies of the incidence of Paget's disease are inherently imprecise because many affected individuals are asymptomatic.[1] On the basis of autopsy studies[2, 3] and review of radiographs, the prevalence of the disease is believed to be 3% or greater in individuals older than 40 years in countries where the disease is common.[4]

A striking feature of the epidemiology of Paget's disease is the great variability in prevalence estimates in different regions of the world and even within one country. A survey of hospital radiographs in patients older than 55 years in 31 British towns revealed a prevalence of Paget's disease ranging from 2.3% in Aberdeen, Scotland, to 8.3% in Lancaster, England.[5] A similar survey done throughout Europe found that only in France did the prevalence equal the lowest prevalence rates in Britain.[6] Australia, New Zealand, and the United States have a relatively high prevalence, perhaps because of British migration. The disease appears to be rare in Asia. In Japan, since the first description of the disease in 1921, fewer than 200 patients have been reported.[7] In most studies the prevalence of Paget's disease in men slightly exceeds that in women.[2–6]

Much emphasis has been placed on the apparent increase in prevalence of Paget's disease with aging. It has been estimated that the prevalence is nearly 10% by the ninth decade.[2–4] Conversely, the disease has rarely been reported in individuals younger than 20 years. Although Paget's disease is most often recognized after the age of 50, it is probably misleading to conclude that the disease is rare in younger individuals. As will be discussed, the obvious manifestations, such as skeletal deformity, probably evolve over decades. Failure to diagnose the earlier phases of the disease is no doubt due to lack of symptoms and minimal use of the radiologic and biochemical tests that would lead to an early diagnosis in younger individuals.

Since 1883, it has been appreciated that Paget's disease may affect more than one member of a family.[8] In large studies, a positive family history has been obtained in 12.3% of 788 cases[9] (United States), 13.8% of 407 cases[10] (Great Britain), and 22.8% of 658 cases[11] (Australia). In the former two studies, a 7- to 10-fold increase in Paget's disease was noted in relatives of patients in comparison to control groups. In a small study in Spain in which relatives of patients were screened by bone scans, 40% of patients had at least one first-degree relative with Paget's disease.[12] Examination of the overall pattern of apparent transmission suggests an autosomal dominant mode of inheritance.[8]

The search for potential environmental factors in the pathogenesis of Paget's disease has led to a consideration of whether past ownership of dogs might be a risk factor. This possibility was suggested by the finding of greater dog ownership in 50 patients than in 50 control subjects in northwest England.[13] This observation has not generally been confirmed in several subsequent studies. Occupational exposure to lead has been proposed as a possible factor in Paget's disease.[14] In one study, levels of cortical bone lead were higher than those in control subjects, but trabecular bone lead was lower.[15] The relevance of these findings is unknown.

PATHOPHYSIOLOGY

A consideration of the radiologic and pathologic evolution of the lesions of Paget's disease strongly suggests that the primary disturbance is localized acceleration of osteoclastic bone resorption. At the interface of normal bone and an advancing lesion, numerous osteoclasts are found in Howship's lacunae in cortical or trabecular bone.[2] Many of the osteoclasts are larger than normal and may have up to 100 nuclei in cross-section rather than the several found in normal osteoclasts.[16] Examination of the ultrastructure of osteoclasts in specimens of Paget's disease reveals a striking and characteristic feature—the presence of microfilaments in the nucleus and, less frequently, in the cytoplasm.[17, 18] These structures have not been observed in osteoclasts from normal subjects or in the bone of patients with primary or secondary hyperparathyroidism, osteoporosis, or osteomalacia. They have also not been observed in osteoblasts, osteocytes, or bone marrow cells in the lesions of Paget's disease. The inclusions have been found in a small percentage of the multinucleated giant cells (osteoclasts) in giant cell tumors of bone and in the osteoclasts of some patients with osteopetrosis and pyknodysostosis.[19] The structure of the microfilaments most closely resembles the nucleocapsids of viruses of the Paramyxoviridae family, a group of RNA viruses known to cause common childhood infections. Evidence of Paramyxoviridae nucleocapsid proteins[20, 21] and mRNA[22, 23] has been found in pagetic lesions. The relevance of these findings to the cause of Paget's disease is discussed later.

As osteoclastic resorption progresses in the cortex, individual osteons widen and become confluent with adjacent osteons. The resorptive area may thereby extend to the endosteal and periosteal surfaces. In trabecular bone of the medullary cavities, the osteolytic process results in a marked reduction in bone volume. Associated with both early cortical and trabecular lesions is a remarkable proliferation of fibrous tissue that replaces normal fatty or hematopoietic bone marrow. The fibrous stroma is highly vascular, and although arteriovenous shunts were previously thought to be present, this feature has not been confirmed with radiolabeled albumin microspheres.[24]

The earliest recognizable radiologic feature of Paget's disease is a focal osteolytic lesion. The skull was first appreciated to be affected by circumscribed osteolytic lesions, and Schuller applied the term "osteoporosis circumscripta" to this finding.[25] One or more osteolytic foci may be present, most often in the frontal and occipital regions, and may be observed to slowly coalesce over a period of years (Fig. 89–1). Pure osteolytic lesions may also be detected in other regions of the skeleton, but less frequently. They are seldom observed in the vertebral column or pelvis. In the long bones, osteolytic lesions usually develop at either end of the bone, less often in the diaphysis.[26] Occasionally, osteolytic foci can be observed simultaneously at both ends of a bone. The junction of normal bone and the osteolytic lesion shows a characteristic appearance that is nearly diagnostic of Paget's disease. The edge of the lesion usually assumes the shape of a flame or inverted V (Fig. 89–2). Serial radiologic follow-up of untreated lesions has documented an average rate of extension of about 1 cm annually.[26] As the lesion progresses, some individuals have not only cortical thinning but also expansion of the bone in the absence of visible new bone formation. This pattern is more likely to be found in younger individuals with a much more aggressive clinical course. Bone biopsies taken during this earliest phase of Paget's disease not unexpectedly reveal a marked increase in osteoclastic activity and thinning of the trabeculae.[27] Other striking features are a fibrovascular marrow, numerous osteoblasts lining the trabeculae, and prominent woven bone. Thus a discrepancy is found in the results of radiologic and pathologic examination of an osteolytic lesion. Although focal density is decreased on radiographs, histology demonstrates very active bone formation, but not sufficient to overcome the remarkable degree of osteoclastic bone resorption.

A more commonly observed stage of Paget's disease is the mixed phase, in which osteoblastic (or osteosclerotic) features are intermixed with osteolytic features in an individual bone. This phase is best appreciated in long bones, in which one may observe the advancing osteolytic front adjacent to normal bone and, trailing this front, a heterogeneous region of osteosclerosis superimposed on the region that had previously been dominated by the osteolytic process (Fig. 89–3). Biopsies of the mixed phase reveal a characteristic abnormality of lamellar bone in both cortical and trabecular bone. The matrix is transformed into a bizarre "mosaic" pattern of irregularly juxtaposed pieces of lamellar bone separated by cement lines that have a scalloped outline. The irregularity probably reflects areas of previous osteoclastic resorption. The structure of the involved cortex is so disordered that complete osteons are rare, and the outer and inner circumferential lamellae and interstitial lamella may be totally disrupted. The same disordered matrix structure is seen in trabecular bone. Interspersed among the chaotic lamellae are patches of woven bone characterized by a random pattern of deposition of collagen fibers and a larger number of osteocytes per unit area of matrix. It has been suggested

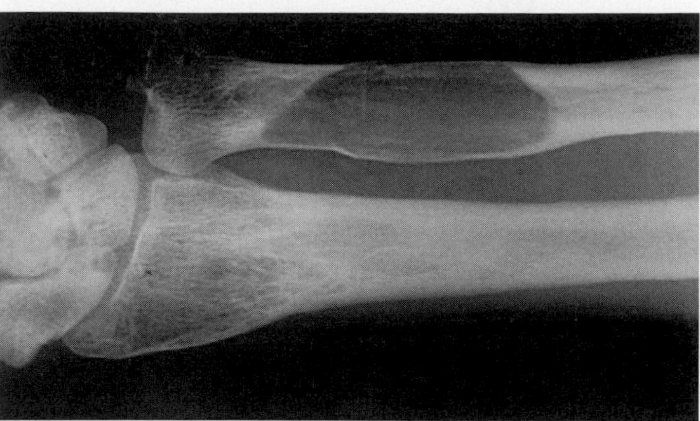

FIGURE 89–2. Radiograph of an osteolytic lesion of Paget's disease that began in the diaphysis of the ulna and exhibits the characteristic flame-shaped or inverted V extension toward the wrist. Note also the expansile nature of the lesion.

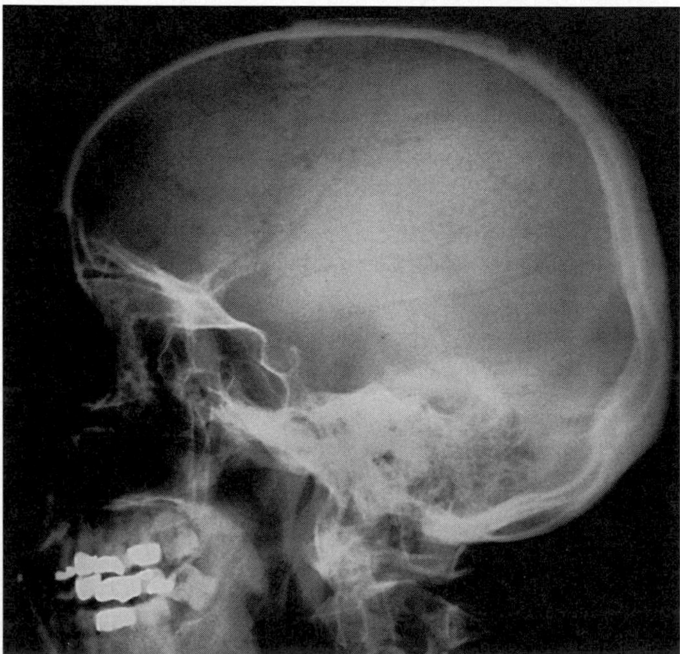

FIGURE 89–1. Radiograph demonstrating osteoporosis circumscripta of the skull affecting the frontal and temporal regions.

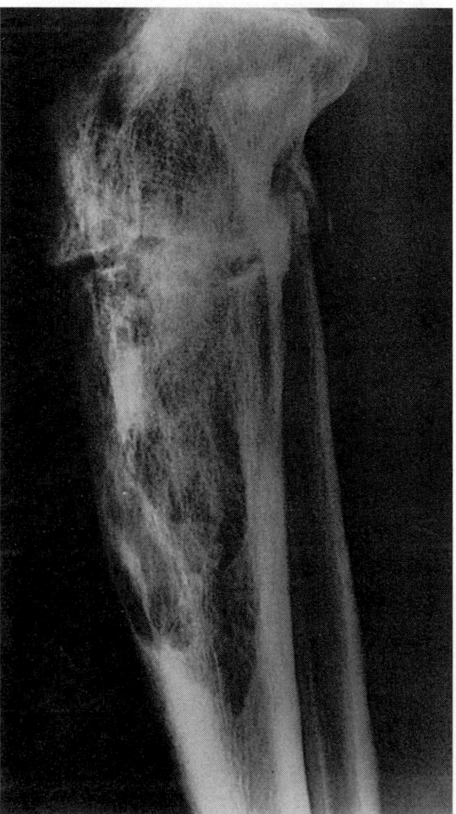

FIGURE 89–3. Radiograph of a tibia exhibiting a distal advancing osteolytic front with proximal sclerotic bone. A partially healed pathologic fracture is present proximally.

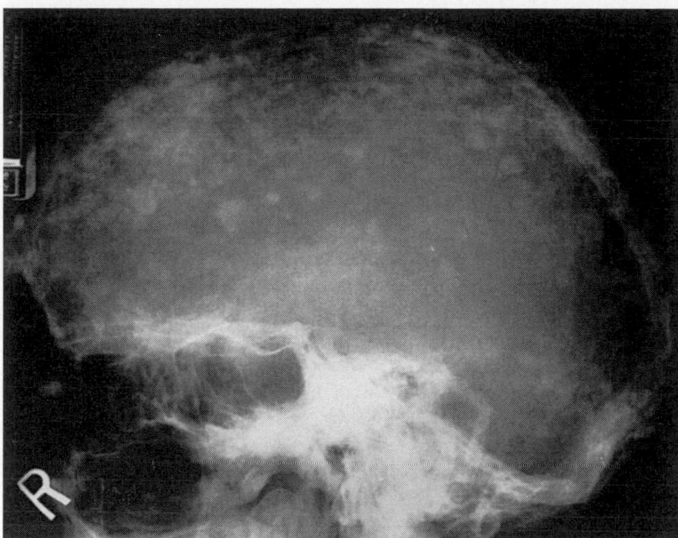

FIGURE 89–4. Radiograph of the sclerotic phase of Paget's disease in the skull exhibiting a "cotton-wool" appearance.

that the lacunae surrounding the osteocytes are larger than normal and that this finding represents osteocytic osteolysis.[28] However, it is more likely that the increased size of the periosteocytic lacunae is simply a characteristic of woven bone and not a second type of bone resorption in Paget's disease. At the surfaces of bone formation, plump osteoblasts are found in great number adjacent to abundant osteoid. This type of bone is seldom found in adults except when associated with rapid remodeling of bone, such as occurs after a fracture or in response to tumor invasion of bone. Studies using quantitative histomorphometry of bone have documented the marked degree of cellular activity underlying the dramatic changes in bone structure in Paget's disease.[29] The total amount of osteoid and the percentage of the bone surface covered by osteoid may be increased 4- to 5-fold. The increase in osteoid is not associated with an increase in osteoid seam width because the rate of calcification is also increased, as established by double labeling of bone-forming surfaces with tetracycline. No dynamic means of defining the rate of bone resorption is available, but the extent of the total bone surface exhibiting evidence of bone resorption averages about 6-fold that of normal individuals, and the number of osteoclasts may be increased as much as 10-fold. In the medullary cavities, the intense resorptive process may produce hemorrhagic cysts with encircling fibrous marrow containing microphages filled with hemosiderin. These cysts are believed to result from rupture of multiple dilated vessels and ensuing microinfarctions.[30]

In the mixed phase of Paget's disease, not only does patchy sclerosis of bone become apparent on radiography, but a bone may also be enlarged. If the osteolytic process extends to the subperiosteal layer, bone formation may be stimulated to such an extent that the thickness and circumference of the bone are increased as a result of periosteal new bone formation. When the skull is affected, this process can produce as much as a fourfold thickening of the calvarium, as was reported by Paget.[31] A patchy form of sclerosis is often of a "cotton-wool" character (Fig. 89–4). The skull may be so severely affected that platybasia, or basilar impression, may be a complication. Long bones may be lengthened, and typically, lateral bowing of the femur and/or anterior bowing of the tibia may develop. Later in the course of the disease, the tibia may also exhibit severe lateral bowing. The pathogenesis of the slowly progressive deformity is not known but must be related to the state of abnormal remodeling of the bone. Frequently, fissure fractures are associated with the bowing deformity. These fractures are linear transverse radiolucencies that are usually present in the cortex of the convex aspect of the deformed bone. They are often multiple and may remain stable in appearance for years. They can be found in either osteopenic or osteosclerotic cortices and may be present even in the absence of deformity. Histologic examination of these lesions suggests that they are incomplete fractures.[2] Only a small percentage of these lesions progress to a complete transverse fracture, which has been more often seen in patients with a sclerotic cortex.

Even after osteosclerotic bone has invaded the previously osteolytic regions of affected bone, evidence of ongoing abnormal bone resorption can be seen in the form of secondary resorption fronts. These secondary fronts are commonly seen as clefts in the cortex of long bones and trail in the path of the primary front.

In the final stage of Paget's disease, termed osteoblastic or sclerotic, the affected bone remains dense and retains the "mosaic" matrix pattern characteristic of Paget's disease. Tubular bones show a loss of differentiation between cortical and trabecular bone, even with enlargement of the bone as a result of periosteal new bone formation, because the new bone is no longer compact bone. Much less cellular activity is present in sclerotic lesions. Osteoclasts are few or absent, but osteoblasts may still be seen to line bone surfaces. The marrow may remain fibrous, but the numbers of blood vessels are greatly reduced. Scattered chronic inflammatory cells may be present. Occasionally, parts of lesions are totally devoid of bone cells, and for this reason, the concept of "burned-out" Paget's disease has arisen. However, it is very unlikely that extensive lesions of Paget's disease ever achieve an entirely burned-out state. On the contrary, the presence of all stages of the disease in a single bone is much more likely.

The evolution of Paget's disease can also be observed by administration of radioactive tracers and scanning of the entire skeleton or selected regions. Bone scans use technetium-labeled bisphosphonates, which after intravenous injection localize to skeletal sites in proportion to the relative blood flow and the rate of bone formation. The scans usually, but not always, demonstrate high uptake of radioactivity in the areas of the skeleton noted to be radiographically abnormal[32] (Fig. 89–5). In a small proportion of patients, increased uptake may be seen when the radiograph is normal, thus illustrating the great sensitivity of bone scans. On the contrary, a small percentage of sclerotic lesions

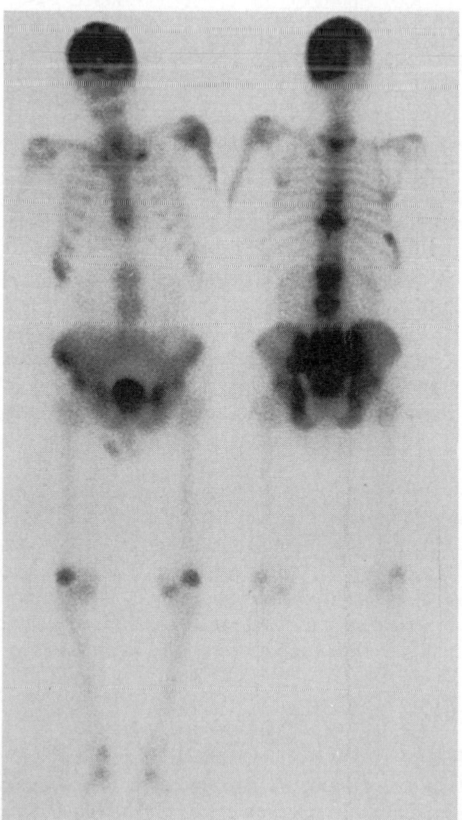

FIGURE 89–5. Anterior and posterior views of a bone scan in a patient with polyostotic Paget's disease. Increased uptake of tracer can be noted in the skull, multiple vertebrae, and the pelvis, areas in which Paget's disease was observed on radiographs. The other abnormal areas probably represent degenerative arthritis and a healed rib fracture.

may not be picked up by a bone scan. These lesions appear to represent areas of inactive disease. Bone scans can be analyzed semiquantitatively or by computer and may thus be used to monitor response to treatment.

Gallium scans, most often used to detect occult infection or tumors, have also been shown to delineate the lesions of Paget's disease.[33] Evidence indicates that tracer gallium is localized to the nuclei of osteoclasts.[34] Therefore, the gallium scan may serve as a direct index of cellular activity in Paget's disease.

CLINICAL FEATURES

A considerable proportion of individuals with Paget's disease have neither symptoms nor signs of the disease. The disease is accidentally discovered in these cases because of radiologic or biochemical abnormalities uncovered during investigation of another disorder.

The most common clinical problems are pain and deformity. The bone pain of Paget's disease, when present, is seldom severe. Usually it is a dull pain, is located deep below the soft tissues, and often persists during the night. In weight-bearing bone, the pain may be slightly worsened by ambulation, but to a lesser extent than pain originating from the joints or from nerve impingement. Deformity of the skeleton is most often noted in the skull and the lower extremity. Over many years, the hat size of an affected individual may be noted to increase. Bowing and enlargement of the femur and tibia may also evolve over a period of years.

Regional Manifestations

The Skull

In the absence of an enlarged cranium, symptoms in the skull are uncommon. Even with an enlarged cranium, symptoms are often absent. Certainly, the most common symptom (30% to 50%) is hearing loss,[35] which is slowly progressive in untreated patients. Vertigo and/or tinnitus is much less common. The mechanism of hearing loss in Paget's disease has recently been attributed to a reduction in bone mineral density of the cochlear capsule.[36]

Much more serious complications of Paget's disease may occur in the advanced stage of the disease in a small number of patients. The weight of the skull may be so great that the ability of the patient to keep the head erect is impaired. Muscle spasm may then produce pain in the neck and tension headaches. Neurologic abnormalities may be found in such patients as a consequence of basilar invagination or platybasia. Although they are unusual complications, even in the presence of radiologic evidence of basilar invagination, compression of structures in the posterior fossa or cerebellar tonsillar herniation may produce ataxia, muscle weakness, and impaired respiration. Hydrocephalus has also been noted to be a rare complication and may be manifested by impaired gait, urinary incontinence, and some degree of dementia.

Finally, severe skull disease may be associated with the vague findings of a withdrawn individual who is somnolent and weak. It has been suggested that this manifestation might be a consequence of shunting of blood from the brain vessels to the external carotid artery system, a possible pagetic steal syndrome.[37] These symptoms could also represent a psychologic response to disability inasmuch as nearly 50% of patients have been reported to have depression in one study.[38]

The Jaws

Paget's disease may affect the facial bones and jaws, but such involvement is uncommon. Leontiasis ossea is the descriptive term applied to a patient with enlargement of all the facial bones, but such deformity is more likely to be found in fibrous dysplasia.

Involvement of the mandible or maxilla may produce progressive root resorption leading to the loss of teeth.[39] In the more advanced stages of Paget's disease, excessive formation of the cementum is associated with absence of the lamina dura and periodontal membranes. Facial disfigurement may occur from enlargement of the maxilla and/or mandible and is associated with spreading of the teeth and malocclusion. Edentulous patients have difficulty acquiring properly fitting dentures. Oral surgery may be complicated by excessive intraoperative bleeding and postoperative osteomyelitis. Tooth extractions may prove difficult because of ankylosis resulting from hyperplasia of the cementum.

The Spine

Neck and back pain are common complaints in an aging population of patients with Paget's disease. Visualization of Paget's disease in one or more vertebrae on radiographic examination often leads clinicians to conclude that they are dealing with bone pain, and treatment is instituted. However, most patients with moderate to severe pain have a complication associated with Paget's disease as the cause of the pain rather than bone pain alone.

Paget's disease affects the lumbar and sacral regions most frequently. One vertebra or many vertebrae may be involved. In the early osteolytic phase, which is not often seen, the vertebral body appears osteoporotic and, in rare cases, may undergo so much resorption that it takes the shape of a thin transverse rod. Much more often, the vertebral bodies become enlarged overall, with thickened margins and coarse vertical striations centrally. Compression of a sclerotic vertebral body may develop because of the abnormal mechanical properties produced by the chaotic microarchitecture.

Severe pain and/or impaired neurologic function may result from compression of the spinal cord or nerve roots.[40] This complication can arise from enlargement of the vertebral bodies, pedicles, or laminae, as well as from compression fractures. It has also been suggested that shunting of blood may occur from the spinal arteries to the highly vascular bone.[41] Neurologic syndromes are more likely to develop with thoracic involvement. Symptoms include back pain, difficult ambulation, numbness, paresthesias of the feet, and progressive paresis of the legs. Later problems can include impaired bladder and bowel function, as well as spastic paraparesis and loss of sensation. Computed tomography (CT) and magnetic resonance imaging (MRI) are particularly helpful in resolving the anatomic abnormalities producing the disturbed function.

A rare complication in the spine is the development of a discrete paraspinal mass consisting of a central narrow cavity surrounded by pagetic bone that extends from the vertebrae.[42] It may appear that the lesion represents a neoplasm, but careful analysis of prior radiologic studies may reveal the chronic nature of the lesion and make it unnecessary to perform a biopsy.

The other major causes of back pain in Paget's disease are intervertebral disk disease and degenerative arthritis. No evidence indicates that disk degeneration is more common in patients with Paget's disease, but it has been reported that the pagetic process can invade the disk and produce bony bridging across the disk space.[43] Back pain in the lumbar region is frequently associated with degenerative arthritis,[44] particularly when distortion of the facet joints is associated with Paget's disease. Large osteophytes may also be found in association with enlarged vertebral bodies or where a compression fracture has occurred. A syndrome mimicking ankylosing spondylitis may occur in the presence of extensive osteophyte formation or with ossification of spinal ligaments,[45] but the HLA-B27 antigen may be absent. However, classic ankylosing spondylitis has been found in association with Paget's disease.[44]

The Pelvis and Extremities

The main symptoms associated with pelvic and lower extremity involvement are pain and impaired ambulation. Pain is seldom a significant symptom in the osteolytic phase of the disease. Hip pain is most common when both the acetabulum and the proximal end of the femur are affected by the sclerotic phase of the disease.[45] Bowing of the femur and protrusio acetabuli are often associated with pain aggravated by weight bearing. Many patients are relatively comfortable when not weight bearing, unlike patients with bone pain, who usually have nocturnal discomfort.

Knee pain and occasionally joint effusions may occur with sclerotic disease affecting the femur and/or tibia. Distortion of the knee joint produced by enlargement of the distal end of the femur or proximal part of the tibia and severe bowing of either bone can induce mechanical strains on the articular cartilage and thereby accelerate the degenerative process. The pagetic process in subchondral bone may also contribute to joint disease. A similar set of circumstances may also account for ankle pain.

Fractures of the lower extremity are more likely to affect the femur than the tibia. In the largest series of reported femoral fractures, the subtrochanteric region was the most common site of fracture (49/182), and the rate of nonunion was noted to be 40%, a figure considerably greater than previously appreciated.[46] Nonunion appears to be less common after tibial fractures.

Involvement of the upper extremity long bones is much less likely to produce symptoms, although deformity may be apparent. At the shoulder, impaired rotator cuff function may be noted when overgrowth of bone leads to anatomic distortion of the glenohumeral joint.

Occasionally, patients who have Paget's disease affecting the foot have pain on weight bearing. Symptoms are seldom encountered in individuals with radiologic evidence of Paget's disease in the hands.

Sarcoma, Giant Cell Tumors, and Nonskeletal Malignancies

The most feared complication in Paget's disease is sarcoma. It has been estimated that 10% of patients with extensive disease may experience this problem,[30] but if all affected individuals are considered, the incidence is probably less than 1%.[47] Sarcomas have rarely been reported to develop in multiple members of families with Paget's disease.

Patients in whom sarcomas develop usually have pain and swelling, always in an area previously affected with Paget's disease. Occasionally, fracture at the tumor site may lead to discovery of the neoplasm. Tumors most often arise in the pelvis, femur, humerus, skull, and facial bones.[48] Multifocal sarcomas are found only in patients with advanced and widespread polyostotic disease and are thought to represent tumors of independent origin rather than metastases.[49]

The histology of sarcomas is quite variable. Fibrosarcomas, chondrosarcomas, osteogenic sarcomas, and anaplastic sarcomas may be found.[30] Variable amounts of multinucleated giant cells (probably osteoclasts) may be scattered throughout the tumor stroma and most likely are not neoplastic in nature. The nuclear inclusions typical of Paget's disease have been observed in giant cells but not in the tumor cells.[50] It is not unusual for several histologic patterns to be present in a single tumor, which suggests that a common stem cell may give rise to a variety of more differentiated mesenchymal cells.

Lymphomas and multiple myelomas have been found in association with Paget's disease[47] but probably represent chance occurrence rather than a complication of the pathologic process.

It is difficult to detect early sarcoma formation by radiologic examination because of the underlying distortion of pagetic bone. Because they appear to arise in medullary bone, an early finding may be a subcortical osteolytic lesion. Only when a radiolucent focus with speckled areas of calcification has broken through the confines of the cortex is it quite apparent that a malignant neoplasm is present. CT or MRI is the best means of determining the extent of the tumor mass.

The rate of change in serum alkaline phosphatase activity has not proved to be a useful marker for the development of sarcomas despite early reports that such might be the case.

The life expectancy for the average patient in whom a sarcoma develops is sadly brief, perhaps because of the difficulty in early detection. In one study, only 7.5% of patients survived 5 years, whereas in elderly patients free of underlying Paget's disease, a 37% 5-year survival rate was noted.[51]

Giant cell tumors of bone, which usually follow a benign course and are most often found at the ends of long bones in otherwise normal individuals, may arise in the lesions of Paget's disease.[52] They appear to be much less common than sarcoma in Paget's disease and have frequently been noted to originate in the skull and facial bones. Rarely, these tumors have been reported in multiple family members who have Paget's disease.

These tumors are characterized by spindle-shaped cells with fusiform nuclei and clumped chromatin or nuclei and by scattered multinucleated giant cells. Mitoses are rarely found in either the mononuclear or giant cells. The giant cells contain the nuclear inclusions of Paget's disease, but the stromal cells do not.[52] The opinion has been expressed that many of the reported cases of giant cell tumor in Paget's disease actually represent giant cell reparative granulomas, which are common lesions arising in the jaw.[53]

Surgery and radiation have been used to treat symptomatic giant cell tumors in Paget's disease, and in a few patients, high doses of dexamethasone have been effective in shrinking the tumors.[54]

Evidence does not indicate a high incidence of cancer in patients with Paget's disease. Metastatic cancer would be expected to be more frequent in the highly vascular lesions of Paget's disease. Although metastasis has been reported, no systematic study of the localization of skeletal metastases has been performed in patients with Paget's disease.

BIOCHEMICAL FEATURES

The intense cellular activity in active lesions of Paget's disease may be reflected in various biochemical markers of bone resorption and bone formation. In most patients who come to clinical attention, biochemical markers do reflect the extent and activity of the disease, although patients with only a small percentage of affected skeleton have no biochemical abnormalities.

Indices of Bone Resorption

The increased bone resorption typical of active Paget's disease might be expected to produce an increase in serum and urinary calcium levels, but in the absence of fractures or immobilization, hypercalcemia and/or hypercalciuria is not a prominent feature of Paget's disease.[55] It is generally believed that this finding is explained by a concomitant increase in bone formation that is demonstrable histologically and by kinetic analysis of plasma disappearance rates and skeletal uptake of radiocalcium[55] or other skeletal tracers. A variety of bone collagen matrix breakdown products have been used as indices of bone resorption. These products include urinary hydroxyproline, total and free pyridinoline and deoxypyridinoline, type I collagen N-telopeptide, and type I collagen C-telopeptide. Recently, serum assays have been developed for some of these collagen components, although few published studies have documented their clinical value as yet. The telopeptide assays appear to be most specific for bone collagen resorption and provide the greatest sensitivity to therapeutic intervention.[56]

Indices of Bone Formation

Since 1929 it has been appreciated that serum alkaline phosphatase activity is usually increased in patients with Paget's disease.[57] It is localized at the plasma membrane in osteoblasts and may participate in the mineralization of bone matrix. In Paget's disease, enzyme activity in the circulation correlates with the extent of the disease on radiographic skeletal surveys,[45] as well as with parameters of bone resorption, including total urinary hydroxyproline[45] and urinary pyridinolines.[58]

During long-term follow-up of untreated patients with Paget's disease, alkaline phosphatase activity usually exhibits a gradual increase or no significant change.[59] In some patients, major fluctuations may represent technical errors rather than changes in disease activity. In the presence of liver disease, hepatic alkaline phosphatase activity may interfere with an accurate assessment of Paget's disease activity. In such patients, measurement of bone-specific alkaline phosphatase levels by immunoassay is preferable.[60]

Serum osteocalcin or bone Gla protein is a nearly specific product of osteoblasts that may be elevated in Paget's disease but not to the same degree as serum alkaline phosphatase activity.[61, 62] Paradoxically, treatment of patients with drugs that reduce turnover may produce a transient increase in osteocalcin levels.[61, 62] No studies have provided any explanation for these surprising observations. It is conceivable that in untreated patients, osteoblast differentiation is such that relatively little osteocalcin is produced.

Serum levels of type I procollagen carboxyl-terminal peptide correlate significantly with other parameters of disease activity and decline with treatment of Paget's disease.[63] However, this parameter of bone formation is not as sensitive as total or bone-specific alkaline phosphatase levels in assessing the response to therapy.[56]

Calciotropic Hormones

It might be suspected that an abnormality in calcitonin secretion in Paget's disease could contribute to increased osteoclast activity. However, circulating calcitonin levels in pagetic patients have been found to not differ from levels in normal subjects.[64]

Parathyroid hormone concentrations are usually found to be within the normal range in most patients. However, in subsets of patients, elevated hormone concentrations may be found.[65, 66] Concomitant renal failure and vitamin D deficiency are two factors that may increase parathyroid secretion. In one study, a positive correlation of serum parathyroid levels with disease activity was found[66]; in another, this relationship was absent.[65] It is possible that at any level of disease activity, if the rate of bone formation exceeds the rate of bone resorption, subtle hypocalcemia could produce secondary hyperparathyroidism.

In patients who ingest adequate amounts of vitamin D or who are exposed to adequate amounts of ultraviolet light, serum 25-hydroxyvitamin D and 1,25-dihydroxyvitamin D levels are normal. However, it has been reported that serum 24,25-dihydroxyvitamin D levels are low in patients with Paget's disease, particularly in those with a high degree of disease activity.[67, 68] The physiologic or pathologic role of 24,25-dihydroxyvitamin D in humans, including patients with Paget's disease, is unknown, as is the pathogenesis of this vitamin D abnormality in Paget's disease.

SYSTEMIC COMPLICATIONS AND ASSOCIATED DISEASES

Hypercalciuria, Hypercalcemia, and Primary Hyperparathyroidism

Urinary calcium excretion is usually normal in patients with Paget's disease, and no compelling evidence has been presented that renal stone formation is increased over that in an age- and sex-matched control group.[55] However, hypercalciuria is readily provoked by immobilization after fractures[69] or neurologic injury. In this setting, bone resorption increases while bone formation falls.

Hypercalcemia is uncommon in patients with Paget's disease but may occur as a consequence of immobilization,[69] nonskeletal malignancy,[70] or primary hyperparathyroidism.[71] Despite some discussion that an increased incidence of primary hyperparathyroidism may occur in Paget's disease, the presence of both diseases in one individual is very likely coincidental.

Hyperuricemia and Gout

Serum uric acid concentrations have been reported to be elevated primarily in men with relatively severe Paget's disease.[45] Nearly half of the hyperuricemic men had clinical episodes of gouty arthritis. Paget's disease was also found to be present in 23% of a group of patients with gout.[72] It is possible that a high turnover of nucleic acids in the lesions of Paget's disease could increase the urate pool sufficiently to account for these observations.[73]

Cardiovascular Abnormalities

Increased cardiac output has been found to be present in patients who have at least 15% of their skeleton affected by Paget's disease.[74] This abnormality is often associated with left ventricular hypertrophy. The excessive vascularity of the soft tissue and adjacent pagetic bone no doubt accounts for these observations. High-output cardiac failure may occur but seems to be unusual.

Calcific aortic stenosis appears to be four to six times more common in patients with Paget's disease than in a control population.[75, 76] It is more likely to be found in patients with severe disease, which suggests that increased cardiac output producing turbulence across the valve may induce calcification. Intracardiac calcification may also occur in the interventricular septum and produce a complete heart block.[76, 77]

DRUG TREATMENT

Indications for Treatment

Indications for drug treatment of Paget's disease are listed in Table 89–1. Perhaps the most common reason for treatment is bone pain. When Paget's disease is adjacent to a joint, it may be difficult to distinguish bone pain from joint pain. In such cases, a therapeutic trial of drug therapy for 1 to 2 months may be particularly useful in clarifying the origin of the pain. Pretreatment of patients who require elective orthopedic surgery may prevent complications such as intraoperative or postoperative hemorrhage and immobilization hypercalcemia. Hypercalciuria and hypercalcemia can be reversed or prevented by drug treatment, but these indications are uncommon.

Some patients with neurologic deficits associated with vertebral disease may have dramatic remissions of their signs and symptoms. Although hearing loss is seldom reversed, preservation of auditory acuity is expected. Reduction of disease activity produces a decrease in cardiac output. It is possible that early treatment could prevent future complications such as skeletal deformity, but no long-term randomized clinical trials have been conducted.

Certainly, many patients do not need to be treated. The decision to treat must take into consideration the present symptoms, the likelihood of future complications, the cost of therapy, and the mode of administration.

Pretreatment Evaluation

Measurement of serum total alkaline phosphatase activity in a reliable laboratory is probably the only biochemical test needed in most patients. Radiographs of known lesions of Paget's disease should be performed to be aware of osteolytic lesions. In patients whose extent of disease is unknown, a bone scan is the best means of defining the regions of the skeleton requiring radiographic evaluation.

Calcitonin

Salmon calcitonin was introduced into clinical use in the United States in 1975. This peptide hormone binds to calcitonin receptors on osteoclasts and rapidly inhibits bone resorption in vivo and in vitro.

TABLE 89–1. Indications for Drug Treatment in Paget's Disease

Bone pain
Preparation for orthopedic surgery
Hypercalciuria
Hypercalcemia
Neurologic deficit from vertebral disease
Prevention of hearing loss
Treatment of high-output congestive heart failure
Prevention of complications in young patients

Salmon calcitonin, 50 to 100 U subcutaneously three to seven times per week, relieves bone pain in a high percentage of patients within 2 to 6 weeks.[78] Cardiac output is reduced,[79] along with increased skin temperature over lower extremity bones. Remarkable improvement of neurologic deficits has been noted,[80] as well as stabilization of hearing deficits.[81] Patients treated preoperatively may have less hemorrhage from orthopedic procedures.[82] An immediate reduction in urinary hydroxyproline excretion reflects inhibition of bone resorption. Serum alkaline phosphatase activity does not begin to decline until 1 month has passed, but within 3 to 6 months both parameters decrease on average by 50%. With cessation of therapy, these biochemical parameters gradually increase toward pretreatment levels over a period of months. In patients with radiologically defined osteolytic lesions, restoration of a more normal bone structure occurs after long-term treatment.[83] However, treatment must be continued indefinitely or the osteolytic focus will recur. Bone scans[84] and gallium scans[32] show reduced activity of the pagetic lesions after chronic treatment. Reduced disease activity is also manifested in bone biopsies by a reduction in the number of bone cells, as well as by a decrease in the extent of woven bone and marrow fibrosis.[85]

As many as 26% of patients administered salmon calcitonin exhibit loss of biochemical responsiveness after an initial period of biochemical improvement.[86] Nearly all these patients have high titers of antibodies specific to salmon calcitonin in the circulation. These patients can be successfully treated with any of the bisphosphonates.

Salmon calcitonin may cause a variety of side effects.[78] The most common are nausea and facial flushing (10% to 20%). Less commonly, vomiting, abdominal pain, diarrhea, and polyuria may occur. Tetany and allergic reactions are very rare. Side effects are less common with a nasal spray mode of administration, but efficacy is also reduced.[87] Presently, the use of salmon calcitonin is much less frequent than in the past because of the availability of potent bisphosphonates.

Bisphosphonates

Bisphosphonates, previously known as diphosphonates, are analogues of inorganic pyrophosphate, a compound thought to participate in the mineralization of bone. By substituting a P-C-P bond for the naturally occurring P-O-P bond, a family of metabolically stable compounds have been produced that bind to hydroxyapatite and inhibit bone resorption and formation in experimental animals and humans. Recent studies suggest that the earliest bisphosphonates, such as clodronate, may inhibit osteoclasts by producing nonhydrolyzable analogues of adenosine triphosphate, whereas the more potent aminobisphosphonates inhibit enzymes in the mevalonate pathway, which results in inhibition of protein prenylation.[88]

Four oral bisphosphonates are now approved for the treatment of Paget's disease in the United States: etidronate[89] (5 mg/kg body weight for 6 months), alendronate[90] (40 mg for 6 months), tiludronate[91] (400 mg for 3 months), and risedronate[92] (30 mg for 2 months). Pamidronate is available in intravenous form and is commonly infused once over a period of several hours at a dose of 60 mg for patients with less than fivefold elevations of serum alkaline phosphatase activity[93] and at a dose of 60 or 90 mg on 2 or more days depending on the level of alkaline phosphatase and the response to each infusion.

The bisphosphonates taken orally must be ingested with water only on an empty stomach because they are poorly absorbed. Generally, side effects are not a major problem and, when present, include abdominal distress, diarrhea, and a temporary increase in bone pain. Patients who receive pamidronate intravenously may experience fever and myalgias for about 24 hours. Allergic reactions are rare and are most often inflammatory eye reactions associated with pamidronate use. Etidronate is the only bisphosphonate reported to produce significant osteomalacia, usually at a dose greater than 5 mg/kg body weight daily. Patients treated with multiple 6-month courses of etidronate may become resistant to therapy, usually between the second and third courses of therapy.[94] Such resistance occurs in about 25% of patients. Preliminary evidence for resistance to pamidronate has recently been presented.

The potent aminobisphosphonates can induce biochemical remissions in the great majority of patients, although patients with very extensive Paget's disease may not exhibit suppression of biochemical parameters to within the normal range. It remains to be seen whether long-term biochemical suppression, an achievable goal in most patients, can reduce the incidence of complications in patients who are most at risk. These individuals include those with skull, vertebral, pelvic, and lower extremity involvement.

Presently, a group of potent bisphosphonates, including olpadronate, ibandronate, and zoledronate, are being studied in a variety of skeletal disorders and may one day be used in patients with Paget's disease.

Miscellaneous Agents

Plicamycin[95] (formerly mithramycin) and gallium nitrate[96] are agents approved for the treatment of hypercalcemia of malignancy and are active in patients with Paget's disease. Given the success of bisphosphonate therapy, there seems to be little need for these agents in treating Paget's disease.

TREATMENT AND POSTTREATMENT EVALUATION

For most patients, measurement of total serum alkaline phosphatase activity is sufficient to determine the success of treatment. In patients with known osteolytic lesions on radiologic examination, an annual evaluation should be adequate.

SURGERY

Certainly, the benefits of surgery for the appropriate indications in patients with Paget's disease outweigh the potential complications of excessive hemorrhage and impaired healing. Probably the most common reason for orthopedic surgery is total hip replacement.[97] The success in relieving intractable hip pain and improving mobility is excellent. Heterotopic ossification may be somewhat more common postoperatively but is seldom a major problem. Total knee replacement is also now achieving good clinical results.[98] Tibial and fibular osteotomies to correct varus deformity of the tibia are quite impressive in relieving knee and ankle pain associated with marked deformity.[82] Because the rate of nonunion is relatively high in femoral fractures, open reduction and fixation of fractures may prove necessary.

Much less commonly required are suboccipital craniectomy and upper cervical vertebral laminectomy in patients with symptomatic basilar impression. Equally uncommon is the need for ventricular shunting in patients with hydrocephalus. An attempted relief of hearing loss in patients with skull loss by stapes mobilization or stapedectomy has been of questionable benefit. Surgery to correct spinal stenosis or nerve root compression has generally been successful.[40]

ETIOLOGY

Genetics

Familial expansile osteolysis (FEO) is a very rare autosomal dominant disorder that bears considerable resemblance to Paget's disease.[99] Genetic linkage analysis has indicated a genetic abnormality on chromosome 18q.[100] Because of this finding, similar studies were done in families with classic Paget's disease, and linkage analysis pointed to a similar abnormality in the same region of chromosome 18 as that for FEO.[101, 102] In other families, no linkage to chromosome 18q was identified.[102] The genetic abnormalities are under study. Recent studies of pagetic osteosarcomas indicate that the same chromosome 18q region may harbor a tumor suppressor gene.[103] Identification of the FEO, Paget's disease, and osteosarcoma susceptibility genes should provide new insight into bone biology.

Slow Virus Infection

The nearly universal finding of nuclear and cytoplasmic nucleocapsid-like microfilaments in pagetic osteoclasts coupled with immunohistologic evidence of measles virus and respiratory syncytial virus antigens and measles virus or canine distemper virus mRNA in pagetic bone cells strongly supports the presence of paramyxoviruses in pagetic bone specimens.[19] Studies continue in an attempt to definitively identify the nature of the nucleocapsid-like microfilaments. If these structures prove to be of viral origin, it must still be determined whether they cause the disease and how the genetic findings relate to them.

REFERENCES

1. Ziegler R, Holz G, Rotzler B, Minne H: Paget's disease of bone in West Germany: Prevalence and distribution. Clin Orthop 194:199–204, 1985.
2. Schmorl G: Über Osteitis deformans Paget. Virchows Arch 283:694–751, 1932.
3. Collins DH: Paget's disease of bone—incidence and subclinical forms. Lancet 2:51–57, 1956.
4. Pygott F: Paget's disease of bone: The radiological incidence. Lancet 1:1170–1171, 1956.
5. Barker DJP, Chamberlain AT, Guyer PB, Gardner MJ: Paget's disease of bone: The Lancashire focus. BMJ 1:1105–1107, 1980.
6. Detheridge FM, Guyer PB, Barker DJP: European distribution of Paget's disease of bone. BMJ 285:1005–1008, 1982.
7. Tohgo O, Ito K, Takeda H, et al: Paget's disease of bone. Orthop Trauma Surg (Jpn) 27:525–530, 1984.
8. McKusick VA: Heritable Disorders of Connective Tissue. St Louis, Mosby, 1972.
9. Siris ES, Ottman R, Flaster E, Kelsey JL: Familial aggregation of Paget's disease of bone. J Bone Miner Res 6:495–500, 1991.
10. Sofoer JA, Holloway SM, Emery AEH: A family study of Paget's disease of bone. J Epidemiol Community Health 37:226–231, 1983.
11. Posen S: Paget's disease: Current concepts. Aust N Z J Surg 62:17–23, 1992.
12. Morales-Piga AA, Rey-Rey JS, Corres-Gonzales J, et al: Frequency and characteristics of familial aggregation of Paget's disease of bone. J Bone Miner Res 10:663–670, 1995.
13. O'Driscoll JB, Anderson DC: Past pets and Paget's disease. Lancet 2:919–921, 1985.
14. Spencer H, O'Sullivan V, Sontag SJ: Does lead play a role in Paget's disease of bone? A hypothesis. J Lab Clin Med 120:798–800, 1992.
15. Adachi JD, Arlen D, Webber CE, et al: Is there any association between the presence of bone disease and cumulative exposure to lead? Calcif Tissue Int 63:429–432, 1998.
16. Rubinstein MA, Smelin A, Freedman AL: Osteoblasts and osteoclasts in bone marrow aspiration. Arch Intern Med 92:684–696, 1953.
17. Rebel A, Malkani K, Basle M: Anomalies nucleaires de la maladie osseuse de Paget. Nouv Presse Med 3:1299–1301, 1974.
18. Mills BG, Singer FR: Nuclear inclusions in Paget's disease of bone. Science 194:201–202, 1976.
19. Singer FR: Paget's disease of bone. Possible viral basis. Trends Endocrinol Metab 7:258–261, 1996.
20. Rebel A, Basle M, Pouplard A, et al: Viral antigens in osteoclasts from Paget's disease of bone. Lancet 2:344–346, 1980.
21. Mills BG, Singer FR, Weiner LP, et al: Evidence for both respiratory syncytial virus and measles virus antigens in the osteoclasts of patients with Paget's disease of bone. Clin Orthop 183:303–311, 1984.
22. Basle MF, Fournier JG, Rozenblatt S, et al: Measles virus RNA detected in Paget's disease bone tissue by in situ hybridization. J Gen Virol 67:907–913, 1986.
23. Gordon MT, Sharpe PT, Anderson DC: Canine distemper virus localised in bone cells of patients with Paget's disease. Bone 12:195–201, 1991.
24. Rhodes BA, Greyson ND, Hamilton CR Jr, et al: Absence of anatomic arteriovenous shunts in Paget's disease of bone. N Engl J Med 287:686–689, 1972.
25. Schuller A: Ueber circumscripte Osteoporose des Schädels. Med Klin 25:631–632, 1929.
26. Maldague B, Malghem J: Dynamic radiologic patterns of Paget's disease of bone. Clin Orthop 217:126–151, 1987.
27. Jacobs P: Osteolytic Paget's disease. Clin Radiol 25:137–144, 1974.
28. Belanger LF, Jarry L, Uhthoff HK: Osteocytic osteolysis in Paget's disease. Rev Can Biol 27:37–44, 1968.
29. Meunier PJ, Coindre JM, Edouard CM, Arlot ME: Bone histomorphometry in Paget's disease: Quantitative and dynamic analysis of pagetic and non-pagetic bone tissue. Arthritis Rheum 23:1095–1103, 1980.
30. Jaffe HL: Metabolic, Degenerative and Inflammatory Diseases of Bones and Joints. Philadelphia, Lea & Febiger, 1972.
31. Paget J: On a form of chronic inflammation of bones (osteitis deformans). Med Chir Trans 60:37–64, 1877.
32. Vellenga CJLR, Bijuoet OLM, Pauwels EKJ: Bone scintigraphy and radiology in Paget's disease of bone: A review. Am J Physiol 3:154–168, 1988.
33. Waxman AD, McKee D, Siemsen JK, Singer FR: Gallium scanning in Paget's disease of bone: Effect of calcitonin. AJR 134:303–306, 1980.
34. Mills BG, Masuoka LS, Graham CC Jr, et al: Gallium-67 citrate localization in osteoclast nuclei of Paget's disease of bone. J Nucl Med 29:1083–1087, 1988.
35. Nager GT: Paget's disease of the temporal bone. Ann Otol Rhinol Laryngol 84(suppl 22):1–32, 1975.
36. Monsell EM, Cody DD, Bone HG, et al: Hearing loss in Paget's disease of bone: The relationship between pure tone thresholds and mineral density of the cochlear capsule. Hearing Res 83:114–120, 1995.
37. Blotman F, Blard J-M, Labauge R, Simon L: Exploration ultrasonique de la circulation encephalique chez le Pagetique. Rev Rhum 42:647–651, 1975.
38. Gold DT, Boisture J, Shipp KM, et al: Paget's disease of bone and quality of life. J Bone Miner Res 11:1897–1904, 1996.
39. Smith NHH: Monostotic Paget's disease of the mandible presenting with progressive resorption of the teeth. Oral Surg Oral Med Oral Pathol 46:246–253, 1978.
40. Hadjipavlou A, Lander P: Paget's disease of the spine. J Bone Joint Surg Am 73:1376–1381, 1991.
41. Douglas DL, Duckworth T, Kanis JA, et al: Spinal cord dysfunction in Paget's disease of bone. J Bone Joint Surg Br 63:495–503, 1981.
42. Samuels MA, Schiller AL: Case records of the Massachusetts General Hospital. N Engl J Med 304:1411–1421, 1981.
43. Lander P, Hadjipavlou A: Intradiscal invasion of Paget's disease of the spine. Spine 16:46–51, 1991.
44. Altman RD, Collins B: Musculoskeletal manifestations of Paget's disease of bone. Arthritis Rheum 23:1121–1127, 1980.
45. Franck WA, Bress NM, Singer FR, Krane SM: Rheumatic manifestations of Paget's disease of bone. Am J Med 56:592–603, 1974.
46. Dove J: Complete fractures of the femur in Paget's disease of bone. J Bone Joint Surg Br 62:12–17, 1980.
47. Hadjipavlou A, Lander P, Srolovitz H, Enker IP: Malignant transformation in Paget disease of bone. Cancer 70:2802–2808, 1992.
48. Haibach H, Farrell C, Dittrich BS: Neoplasms arising in Paget's disease of bone: A study of 82 cases. Am J Clin Pathol 83:594–601, 1985.
49. Choquette D, Haraoui B, Altman RD, Pelletier JP: Simultaneous multifocal sarcomatous degeneration in Paget's disease of bone. Clin Orthop 179:308–311, 1983.
50. Seret P, Basle MF, Rebel A, et al: Sarcomatous degeneration in Paget's bone disease. J Cancer Res Clin Oncol 113:392–399, 1987.
51. Huvos AG: Osteogenic sarcoma of bones and soft tissues in older persons. Cancer 57:1442–1449, 1986.
52. Singer FR, Mills BG: Giant cell tumor in Paget's disease of bone—recurrence after 36 years. Clin Orthop 293:293–301, 1993.
53. Upchurch KS, Simon LS, Schiller AL, et al: Giant cell reparative granuloma of Paget's disease of bone: A unique clinical entity. Ann Intern Med 98:35–40, 1983.
54. Ziambaras K, Totty WA, Teitelbaum SL, et al: Extraskeletal osteoclastomas responsive to dexamethasone treatment in Paget bone disease. J Clin Endocrinol Metab 82:3826–3834, 1997.
55. Nagant de Deuxchaisnes CN, Krane SM: Paget's disease of bone: Clinical and metabolic observations. Medicine (Baltimore) 43:233–266, 1964.
56. Randall AG, Kent GN, Garcia-Webb P, et al: Comparison of biochemical markers of bone turnover in Paget disease treated with pamidronate and a proposed model for the relationships between measurements of the different forms of pyridinoline crosslinks. J Bone Miner Res 11:1176–1184, 1996.
57. Kay HD: Plasma phosphatase in osteitis deformans and in other disease of bone. Br J Exp Pathol 10:253–256, 1929.
58. Alvarez L, Guanabens N, Peris P, et al: Discriminative value of biochemical markers of bone turnover in assessing the activity of Paget's disease. J Bone Miner Res 10:458–465, 1995.
59. Woodard HQ: Long term studies of the blood chemistry in Paget's disease of bone. Cancer 12:1226–1237, 1959.
60. Panigrahi K, Delmas PD, Singer F, et al: Characteristics of a two-site immunoradiometric assay for human skeletal alkaline phosphatase in serum. Clin Chem 40:822–828, 1994.
61. Papapoulos SE, Frolich M, Mudde AH, et al: Serum osteocalcin in Paget's disease of bone: Basal concentrations and response to bisphosphonate treatment. J Clin Endocrinol Metab 65:189–194, 1987.
62. Coulton LA, Preston CJ, Cough M, Kanis JA: An evaluation of serum osteocalcin in Paget's disease of bone and its response to diphosphonate treatment. Arthritis Rheum 31:1142–1147, 1988.
63. Simon LS, Krane SM, Wortman PD, et al: Serum levels of type I and III procollagen fragments in Paget's disease of bone. J Clin Endocrinol Metab 58:110–120, 1984.
64. Kanis JA, Heynen G, Walton RJ: Plasma calcitonin in Paget's disease of bone. Clin Sci 52:329–332, 1977.
65. Chapuy M-C, Zucchelli P, Meunier PJ: Parathyroid function in Paget's disease of bone. Miner Electrolyte Metab 6:112–118, 1981.
66. Siris ES, Clemens TP, McMahon D, et al: Parathyroid function in Paget's disease of bone. J Bone Miner Res 4:75–79, 1989.
67. Guillard-Cumming DF, Beard DJ, Douglas DL, et al: Abnormal vitamin D metabolism in Paget's disease of bone. Clin Endocrinol 22:559–566, 1985.
68. Castro-Errecaborde N, de la Piedra C, Rapado A, et al: Correlation between serum osteocalcin and 24,25-dihydroxyvitamin D levels in Paget's disease of bone. J Clin Endocrinol Metab 72:462–466, 1991.
69. Reifenstein EC Jr, Albright F: Paget's disease: Its pathologic physiology and the importance of this in the complications arising from fracture and immobilization. N Engl J Med 231:343–355, 1944.
70. Rosenkrantz JA, Gluckman EC: Coexistence of Paget's disease of bone and multiple myeloma. AJR 78:30–38, 1957.
71. Posen S, Clifton-Bligh P, Wilkinson M: Paget's disease of bone and hyperparathyroidism: Coincidence or causal relationship. Calcif Tissue Res 26:107–109, 1978.
72. Lluberas-Acosta G, Hansell JR, Schumacher HR Jr: Paget's disease of bone in patients with gout. Arch Intern Med 146:2389–2392, 1986.
73. Fennelly JJ, Hogan A: Pseudouridine excretion—a reflection of high RNA turnover in Paget's disease. Ir J Med Sci 141:103–107, 1972.
74. Arnalich F, Plaza I, Sobrino JA, et al: Cardiac size and function in Paget's disease of bone. Int J Cardiol 5:491–505, 1984.
75. Strickberger SA, Schulman SP, Hutchins GM: Association of Paget's disease of bone with calcific aortic valve disease. Am J Med 82:953–956, 1987.

76. Hultgren HN: Osteitis deformans (Paget's disease) and calcific disease of the heart valves. Am J Cardiol 81:1461–1464, 1998.
77. Harrison CV, Lennox B: Heart block in osteitis deformans. Br Heart J 10:167–176, 1948.
78. Lesh JB, Aldred JP, Bastian JW, Kleszynski RR: Clinical experience with porcine and salmon calcitonin. *In* Taylor S (ed): Endocrinology 1973. Proceedings of the Fourth International Symposium. London, W Heinemann, 1974, pp 409–424.
79. Woodhouse NJY, Crosbie WA, Mohamedally SM: Cardiac output in Paget's disease: Response to long-term salmon calcitonin therapy. BMJ 4:686, 1975.
80. Chen J-R, Rhee RSC, Wallach S, et al: Neurologic disturbances in Paget's disease of bone: Response to calcitonin. Neurology 29:448–457, 1979.
81. El Sammaa M, Linthicum FH Jr, House HP, House JW: Calcitonin as treatment for hearing loss in Paget's disease. Am J Otolaryngol 7:241–243, 1986.
82. Meyers M, Singer F: Osteotomy for tibia vara in Paget's disease under cover of calcitonin. J Bone Joint Surg Am 60:810–814, 1978.
83. Nagant de Deuxchaisnes C, Maldague B, Malghem J, et al: The action of the main therapeutic regimes on Paget's disease of bone with a note on the effect of vitamin D deficiency. Arthritis Rheum 23:1215–1234, 1980.
84. Waxman AD, Ducker S, McKee D, et al: Evaluation of ^{99m}Tc diphosphonate kinetics and bone scans in patients with Paget's disease before and after calcitonin treatment. Radiology 125:761–764, 1977.
85. Fornasier VL, Stapleton K, Williams CC: Histologic changes in Paget's disease treated with calcitonin. Hum Pathol 9:455–461, 1978.
86. Singer FR, Ginger K: Resistance to calcitonin. *In* Singer FR, Wallach S (eds): Paget's Disease of Bone, Clinical Assessment, Present and Future Therapy. New York, Elsevier, 1991, pp 75–85.
87. Nagant de Deuxchaisnes C, Devogelaer JP: Alternative modes of administration of salmon calcitonin in Paget's disease of bone. *In* Singer FR, Wallach S (eds): Paget's Disease of Bone, Clinical Assessment, Present and Future Therapy. New York, Elsevier, 1991, pp 135–165.
88. Rogers MJ, Watts DJ, Russell RGG: Overview of bisphosphonates. Cancer 80(suppl):1652–1660, 1997.
89. Khairi MRA, Altman RD, DeRosa GP, et al: Sodium etidronate in the treatment of Paget's disease of bone: A study of long-term results. Ann Intern Med 87:656–663, 1977.
90. Siris E, Weinstein RS, Altman R, et al: Comparative study of alendronate versus etidronate for the treatment of Paget's disease of bone. J Clin Endocrinol Metab 81:961–967, 1996.
91. Reginster JY, Calson F, Morlock G, et al: Efficacy and safety of oral tiludronate in Paget's disease of bone. A double-blind, multiple-doseage, placebo-controlled study. Arthritis Rheum 35:967–974, 1992.
92. Siris ES, Chines AA, Altman RD, et al: Risedronate in the treatment of Paget's disease of bone: An open label multicenter study. J Bone Miner Res 13:1032–1038, 1998.
93. Thiebaud D, Jaeger P, Gobelet C, et al: A single infusion of the bisphosphonate AHPrBP (APD) as treatment of Paget's disease of bone. Am J Med 85:207–212, 1988.
94. Meunier PJ, Ravault A: Treatment of Paget's disease with etidronate disodium. *In* Singer FR, Wallach S (eds): Paget's Disease of Bone, Clinical Assessment, Present and Future Therapy. New York, Elsevier, 1991, pp 86–99.
95. Ryan WG: Two decades of experience in the treatment of Paget's disease of bone with plicamycin (mithramycin). *In* Singer FR, Wallach S (eds): Paget's Disease of Bone, Clinical Assessment, Present and Future Therapy. New York, Elsevier, 1991, pp 176–190.
96. Warrell RP Jr, Bosco B, Weinerman S, et al: Gallium nitrate for advanced Paget disease of bone: Effectiveness and dose-response analysis. Ann Intern Med 113:847–851, 1990.
97. Ludkowski P, Wilson-MacDonald J: Total arthroplasty in Paget's disease of the hip: A clinical review and review of the literature. Clin Orthop 255:160–167, 1990.
98. Gabel GT, Rand JA, Sim FH: Total knee arthroplasty for osteoarthrosis in patients who have Paget disease of bone at the knee. J Bone Joint Surg Am 73:739–744, 1991.
99. Osterberg PH, Wallace RG, Adams DA, et al: Familial expansile osteolysis—a new dysplasia. J Bone Joint Surg Br 70:255–260, 1988.
100. Hughes AE, Shearman AM, Weber JL, et al: Genetic linkage of familial expansile osteolysis to chromosome 18q. Hum Mol Genet 3:359–361, 1994.
101. Cody JD, Singer FR, Roodman GD, et al: Genetic linkage of Paget's disease of bone to chromosome 18q. Am J Hum Genet 61:1117–1122, 1997.
102. Haslam SI, Van Hul W, Morales-Piga A, et al: Paget's disease of bone: Evidence for a susceptibility locus on chromosome 18q and for genetic heterogeneity. J Bone Miner Res 13:911–917, 1998.
103. Nellisery MJ, Padalecki SS, Branae Z, et al: Evidence for a novel osteosarcoma tumor-suppressor gene in the chromosome 18 region genetically linked with Paget disease of bone. Am J Hum Genet 63:817–824, 1998.

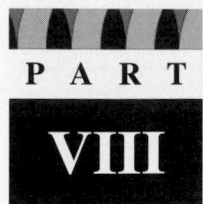

PART VIII Thyroid Gland

Editor: Leslie J. DeGroot

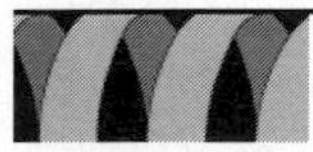

BASIC PHYSIOLOGY

Chapter 90 Anatomy and Development

Roberto Di Lauro ▪ Mario De Felice

ANATOMY OF THE THYROID GLAND

Gross Anatomy

The thyroid gland was first described by Galen (130–210 AD) in his work "De Voce." The name "thyroid," proposed by Thomas Whorton (1614–1673), was given not because of its shape but because of its proximity to the thyroid cartilage.[1] Despite its name (*thyreòs* in Greek means "shield"), the characteristic shape of the thyroid, which consists of two lateral lobes connected by a narrow isthmus, has been proposed to be more reminiscent of a butterfly or a capital H than a shield (Fig. 90–1). The lateral lobes are 3 to 4 cm long and 15 to 20 mm wide and are located between the larynx and the trachea medially and the carotid sheath and the sternomastoid muscles laterally. The upper pole of the lobes reaches the level of the thyroid cartilage, whereas the lower pole reaches the fifth to sixth tracheal ring. The isthmus is 12 to 20 mm long and 20 mm wide and crosses the trachea between the the first and second rings. In a normal adult the entire gland is 6 to 7 cm wide and 3 to 4 cm long and its weight ranges between 15 and 25 g. The thyroid is nearly always asymmetrical: the right lobe may be twice as large as the left, and the upper and lower right poles extend higher up and lower in the neck, respectively, than the left poles. The different size of the lobes could be due to the position of the heart because it has been reported that lobe size was reversed in a patient with dextrocardia.[2] A thin connective capsule encloses the thyroid. Fibrous septa are occasionally detached from this capsule and penetrate the parenchyma to produce incomplete lobulation. This inner capsule is connected to an outer capsule (also called the false capsule of the thyroid) continuous with the pretracheal fascia. Vessels, the parathyroids, and the recurrent laryngeal nerves are located in the space between the two capsules in very close relation to the thyroid: the parathyroids on the posterior surface of the gland and the recurrent laryngeal nerves just medial to the lateral lobes.

Blood Supply

The thyroid is a highly vascularized organ with at least four arteries that provide the gland with an abundant blood supply. Frequent anastomoses among these vessels and an arteriolar network are present on the surface of the gland; from this network small arteries arborize and enter deeply into the tissue. The capillaries are localized in the interfollicular connective tissue and form a basket-like network that surrounds each follicle. The capillary endothelial cells are fenestrated as those of other endocrine glands. Each fenestration is about 50 nm in diameter, and the number and density of fenestration increase during stimulation by thyroid-stimulating hormone (TSH).[3] The veins emerge from the thyroid parenchyma and form a plexus confluent in three groups of veins: the superior, middle, and inferior thyroid veins.

Lymphatics

A rich plexus of lymphatic capillaries surrounds the thyroid follicles and communicates with small lymphatic vessels in the interlobular connective tissue. These deep vessels give rise to a surface network of lymphatics draining to several groups of nodes. The uppermost group of nodes is situated just above the thyroid isthmus and is a constant group of one to five nodes called the Delphian nodes.[2] These nodes are readily palpated if involved by cancer or Hashimoto's thyroiditis. The pretracheal nodes below the isthmus are not as constant as the Delphian nodes. Other node groups are found on the thyroid surface, along the lateral veins or the recurrent laryngeal nerve, or along the carotid sheath.

Innervation

Innervation of the thyroid is provided by sympathetic, parasympathetic, and peptidergic fibers, although few fibers enter the gland.[4, 5] Both sympathetic and parasympathetic fibers extend throughout the tissue among the follicles in close approximation to the follicular cells or around a blood vessel.

Regulator peptides detected in the thyroid are not only produced by neural crest–derived parafollicular cells but are also found in intrathy-

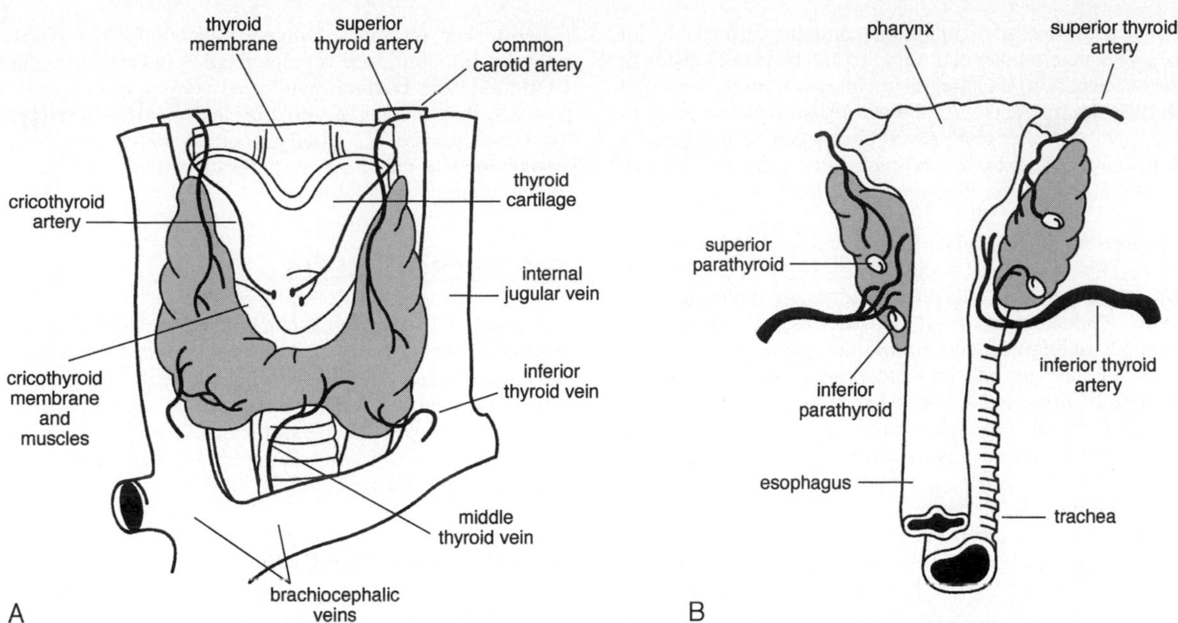

FIGURE 90–1. Gross anatomy of the thyroid. *A,* Anterior view. *B,* Posterior view.

roid peptidergic nerve fibers.[6, 7] Some neuropeptides such as vasoactive intestinal peptide, neuropeptide Y,[8] substance P, or galanin are exclusively produced in nerve fibers distributed throughout the thyroid.[9] These neuropeptides are suspected of regulating follicular cell function via a paracrine pathway. It has been reported that thyroid innervation is very poor in comparison to that of the other endocrine glands.[3]

Anatomic Variants

The variants most frequently discovered in healthy individuals are caused by defects in disappearance of the thyroglossal duct. In this group of anomalies the presence of an accessory lobe (pyramidal lobe) attached to the upper part of the isthmus of the thyroid is a relatively common finding (15% of the population).[2] The pyramidal lobe is a rostrally directed stalk resulting from retention and growth of the caudal end of the thyroglossal duct. Other anomalies can be associated with failure of atrophy of the duct. The entire thyroglossal duct may persist as an epithelial cord connecting the foramen cecum of the tongue to the larynx; in other cases, rests of the duct form isolated or multiple cysts located along the line of descent of the duct. Sometimes, persistent portions of the thyroglossal duct may differentiate into thyroid tissue and form structures called accessory thyroids. This thyroid tissue can be found in different anatomic sites ranging from the posterior of the tongue (lingual thyroid) to the mediastinum (the so-called thyroid retrosternal goiter) or even the trachea (intratracheal thyroid rests).[10] The presence of accessory thyroids in addition to a normally located gland is characteristic of this anomaly. On the contrary, localization of the entire thyroid in an ectopic position is due to a different developmental defect (see the later section Molecular Defects in Thyroid Development).

The other frequent variant (5% of the population) is a thyroid gland that is not developed as a unique mass.[2] The posterior part of the gland is split into two globes of thyroid tissue.

Other anomalies are rare and found in less than 1% of healthy individuals. These variants are absence of the isthmus (the thyroid consists of two separate lateral lobes, a physiologic condition in nonmammalian vertebrates[11]) or absence of a significant portion of a lateral lobe, frequently the lower half of the left lobe.

THE THYROID FOLLICLE

The thyroid gland displays a peculiar, highly organized architecture characterized by the presence of spheroidal structures called follicles that are composed of a single layer of epithelial cells (thyroid follicular cells) surrounding a closed cavity (follicular lumen) filled with colloid, a concentrated solution of thyroglobulin (Tg).[12] The follicle has been defined as the morphofunctional unit of the thyroid.[13] Notably, during intrauterine life the onset of thyroid function coincides with the appearance of differentiated follicles.[14] As seen below, thyroid follicular cells express a specific set of genes whose protein products perform functions essential to thyroid hormone biosynthesis. However, it is the follicular organization together with the polarity of the follicular cells that allows the several biochemical steps required for thyroid hormone biosynthesis (secretion of proteins in the follicular lumen as exocrine cells do, reabsorption and hydrolysis of proteins, release of hormones into blood by endocrine secretion[15]) to occur as a functional chain of events. The follicle cell divides the follicular lumen (where hormone synthesis begins) and the blood stream, from where iodine has to be uploaded and where hormones will be released at the end of the process.

Cell polarity is established by mechanisms that create different specialized regions in the plasma membrane and cytoplasm.[16, 17] The surface of a polarized thyroid follicular cell is divided into two functionally distinct, but physically contiguous regions: an apical and a basolateral domain. Junctional complexes between cells separate these two domains and prevent the mixing of asymmetrically distributed proteins. The apical domain displays a differentiated tissue-specific organization characterized by the presence of apical microvilli and pseudopods and by the localization of thyroperoxidase (TPO)[18] and Na^+ or Cl^- channels.[19, 20] Na^+/I^- symporter (NIS),[21] Na^+/K^+-ATPase,[22] epidermal growth factor,[23] and TSH receptors[24] are located in the basal domain. Thyroid hormone synthesis requires basal-to-apical transport of iodide and Tg.[25] Conversely, hormone secretion is based on apical-to-basal transport of Tg and hormones; in addition, a bidirectional ion transport system controls follicular size. The basal cell plasma membrane is structurally and functionally connected by integrins to the basal lamina surrounding the follicle.[26, 27] The basal lamina consists of laminin, type IV collagen, and fibronectin[28, 29]; a very thin connective space—less than 2 μm wide—separates the basal lamina from the endothelial capillary cells.

To prevent passive backdiffusion and to guarantee efficient transport, particular cell-cell junctions are required.[30] Among the different types of cell junctions, the tight junction (*zonula occludens*), located close to the apical border of the cells, is the structure principally responsible for sealing the intercellular space. Tight junctions not only control the permeability of the paracellular space but are also the boundary between the apical and basolateral domains of the follicular plasma membrane. Tight junctions appear as a complex network of anastomosing fibrils consisting of junctional proteins responsible for cell-cell contact. This macromolecular complex interacts with different cellular structures. Occludin, an integral membrane protein localized in the occluding barrier, interacts with the cytoplasmic plaque proteins ZO-1 and ZO-2.[31] On the other side, microtubules can be functionally linked to tight junctions via cytoskeleton-associated proteins[32] such as cingulin, 7H6 antigen, and actin, also present in the tight junction region.

The adherent junction, another type of cell junction, is located below the tight junction. This junction is necessary for cell-cell association. Cadherins, transmembrane Ca^{2+}-dependent adhesion molecules, are involved in these interactions. In thyroid tissue, as well as in other epithelial tissues,[33] E-cadherin, found around the lateral plasma membrane domain, accumulates in adherent junctions and plays a central role in the induction of these stable adhesions. E-cadherin is linked to the catenins, which participate in signal transduction pathways.[34] This functional bridge could couple physical adhesion to intracellular events.

Desmosomal junctions are the third type of junction present in epithelia. These structures occur on the plasma membrane below the adherent junction. Desmogleins and desmocollins, members of the cadherin superfamily,[35] are present in desmosomal junctions. Desmosomes are linked to the intermediate cytoskeleton filaments, with which they form a network through the tissue that connects different adjacent cells.[36] In addition to these sealing cell junctions, gap junctions are found between follicular cells.[37] At the site of these structures a narrow gap about 2 nm in diameter separates the membranes of adjacent cells. Gap junctions might mediate cell-to-cell communication because small informative molecules can be exchanged through these structures.

Primary culture of porcine thyroid follicular cells provided a helpful in vitro model to understand the mechanisms leading to folliculogenesis and the onset of thyroid cell function.[38, 39] Follicular cells freshly isolated from pig thyroid glands and cultured in the presence of TSH have the capacity to assemble epithelial junctions, polarize, and finally organize themselves into follicle-like structures in which the apical poles of cells delineate a lumen cavity and the basal surface is oriented toward the culture medium. The first and essential step in in vitro folliculogenesis is cell aggregation mediated by E-cadherin. During the first few hours of culture, E-cadherin increases its expression through the lateral cell surface and then accumulates in the subapical regions, where adherent junctions will be assembled.[40] ZO-1 and Na^+/K^+-ATPase initiate their expression, and the earliest stage of cell surface differentiation is marked by the redistribution of these two proteins: ZO-1 is recruited around the future pole of the cell and ATPase is confined to the basal-lateral cell surface. At this stage, apical domain–associated proteins are detected in intracellular vacuoles, which later fuse with the cell surface at the nascent apical pole.

The follicular lumen is generated in two different steps, both consequences of the polarized phenotype of thyroid cells. The first step is triggered by the lack of adhesive properties of the apical cell surface. Analysis of human[41] and chick[42] thyroid morphogenesis has confirmed that in vivo, the primitive follicles also appear after the assembly of focal tight junctions that seal adjacent follicular cells. A second step, which is required for the control of follicular size, is driven by a bidirectional ion transport system that secrets Cl^- in a basal-to-apical direction and absorbs Na^+ in an apical-to-basal direction as well.[13]

In vitro, folliculogenesis is dependent on TSH. In the absence of TSH, thyroid cells will aggregate only transiently.[43] TSH, acting via cyclic adenosine monophosphate (cAMP), seems to modulate different steps to maintain follicle organization.[44] Stimulation of cAMP/protein kinase A inhibits the dissociation of tight and adherent junctions by stabilizing E-cadherin–dependent cell-cell adhesions[45] and inhibiting the production of thrombospodin-1, a matricellular protein that is a negative modulator of cell-cell adhesion.[46] Furthermore, TSH down-regulates the expression of transforming growth factor-β_1 (TGF-β_1),[47] which induces the loss of epithelial polarization.[48] TSH might also control follicular lumen generation because chloride channels localized at the apical pole are regulated by cAMP.[49] However, it would not be correct to extrapolate all the information from in vitro models and refer it to tissue follicles because they display some relevantly different features. For instance, cultured follicles lack a basal lamina surrounding follicles in the thyroid gland,[40] and their structure is unstable. Unless they are cultured with a gel consisting of extracellular matrix proteins, they invert their polarity and manifest a dramatic change in functional properties.[50] Analysis of thyroid development in mutated animal models can help us understand the mechanisms of in vivo folliculogenesis (see below).

THE THYROID CELLS

In addition to the stromal component, the thyroid gland is composed of three epithelial cell populations (the thyroid parenchyma) of different embryologic origin: (1) follicular cells, the largest population, which surround the follicular lumen and are responsible for thyroid hormone synthesis; (2) parafollicular C cells, which are devoted to calcitonin production; and (3) epithelial cell vestiges of the ultimobranchial body (UB).

Thyroid Follicular Cells

Under the light microscope, follicular cells show a neutrophilic cytoplasm, a basal nucleus, and periodic acid–Schiff-positive vacuoles (phagosomes).[51] Follicular cells appear as cuboidal epithelial cells whose height is approximately 15 μm. Cells become flatter (squamous) or higher (columnar) depending on whether they undergo TSH stimulation.

Electron microscopy (Fig. 90–2) reveals the characteristic features of cells actively engaged in protein synthesis,[52] with the rough endoplasmic reticulum and the Golgi apparatus as the dominant organelles in the cell. The apical surface is covered with thin microvilli or pseudopods protruding into the follicular lumen. A distinctive feature of follicular cells is the presence of several vesicles localized in the apical or subapical cytoplasm. Smaller (150–200 nm) vesicles are exocytotic vesicles containing newly synthesized Tg. Fusion of vesicle membranes with the apical plasma membrane leads to the delivery of Tg into the follicle lumen, where TPO- and hydrogen peroxide–producing enzymes are localized[18] and the iodination process can occur. Larger vesicles (500–4000 nm) called colloid droplets filled with dense material are a result of the uptake of iodinated Tg—stored in the follicular lumen—back into the follicular cell. Reabsorption of the colloid involves a macropinocytosis mechanism whose first step is the formation of pseudopods at the apical pole. The pseudopods close and a portion of the colloid is internalized into the cell.[53] TSH induces the uptake of Tg from the follicle lumen, and the number of colloid droplets increases greatly under TSH stimulation.[54]

At a molecular level (Fig. 90–3), a follicular cell can be identified by the presence of a set of proteins—and the corresponding mRNA—necessary for its particular functions.[55] Among such proteins, Tg and TPO are remarkably specific in that they are detectable exclusively in thyroid follicular cells. Other proteins, such as TSH receptor (TSHR), NIS, and pendrin, although usually expressed at the highest level in thyroid follicular cells, are also present in a few other tissues. The exclusive or prevalent expression in thyroid follicular cells of genes necessary for thyroid hormone biosynthesis appears to be due, at least in part, to a combination of transcription factors unique to this cell type.[55] Thyroid transcription factor-1 (TTF-1), TTF-2, and Pax8 have subsequently been found to be relevant in controlling not only differentiation but also morphogenesis of the gland. The relevant features of these transcription factors are summarized below.

Thyroid Transcription Factor-1

TTF-1 is a transcription factor that recognizes and binds to unique DNA sequences in regulatory regions of specific genes and is required for tissue-specific gene expression.[56] It is encoded by the *Titf1* gene in mice and by the *TITF1* gene in humans. This factor belongs to the homeodomain family that contains transcription factors characterized by a 60–amino acid DNA-binding domain (homeodomain) whose sequence is conserved from the fruit fly to humans with very few

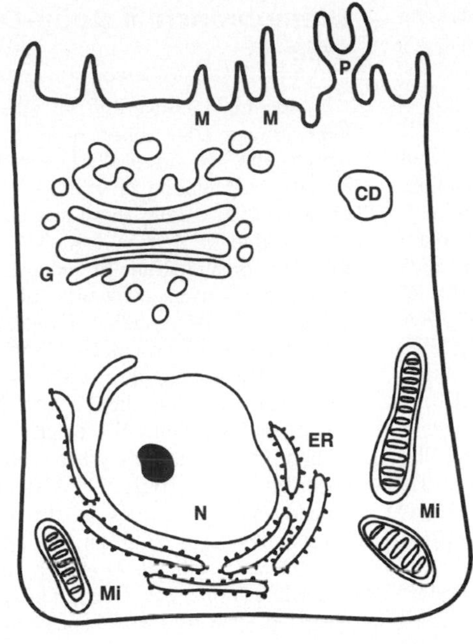

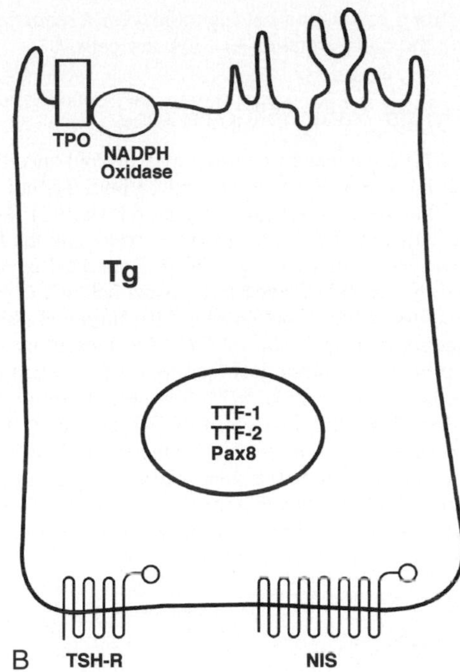

FIGURE 90–2. Electron micrograph of a rat follicular cell. AV, apical vesicles; ER, endoplasmic reticulum; G, Golgi apparatus; L, lumen; Ly, lysosome; M, microvilli; N, nucleus; NADPH, reduced nicotinamide-adenine dinucleotide phosphate; Tg, thyroglobulin; TJ, tight junction; TPO, thyroperoxidase; TTF-1, thyroid transcription factor-1. (Courtesy of Professor L. Nitsch.)

changes. TTF-1 is a member of the NKx2 class of transcription factors because its homeodomain is closely related to that of *Drosophila* NK2 protein.[57] Other proteins of this class have been characterized in mice and humans, all identified by a similar DNA-binding domain.

TTF-1 was initially identified in a rat cell line as a nuclear protein able to bind to specific sequences present in both Tg and TPO gene promoters.[58] This binding is a necessary event for full promoter activity. Functional studies have addressed the question that the homeodomain is responsible only for binding to DNA whereas the transactivating property resides in two apparently redundant domains located at the two ends of the protein.[59] Human *TITF1* is located on chromosome 14q13; it is split into at least three exons that encode for a 371–amino acid protein of 42 kDa.[56] TTF-1 is phosphorylated in serine residues, and a kinase specifically responsible for this activity has been identified.[60] However, the role of this posttranslation modification in thyroid cells is not yet clear.

The presence of TTF-1 in the precursors of follicular cells 5 days before the expression of Tg and TPO[61] led to the hypothesis that this protein could play a crucial role in gland morphogenesis. The agenesis of the thyroid in mutated mice in which both *Titf1* alleles have been disrupted has confirmed this hypothesis.[62] TTF-1 expression is not restricted to the follicular cells; it is also present in embryonic diencephalic neurons and in the lung epithelium,[61] where it is necessary for surfactant protein expression.[63] Recently, TTF-1 mRNA was also identified in parafollicular C cells[64] and the epithelial cell of the UB (De Felice M, Di Lauro R: Unpublished results).

Pax8

Pax8 is a member of the transcription factor family containing a paired domain that can recognize and bind to specific DNA sequences.[65] The paired domain is evolutionarily conserved in the fly, mouse, and human and was identified for the first time in the *Drosophila* segmentation gene *paired*.

The *PAX8* gene maps to human chromosome 2q12-q14[66] and consists of at least 10 exons encoding a protein of 457 amino acids containing the paired domain near the N terminus. Several Pax8 isoforms generated by alternative splicing exist and show different transcriptional activity.[67] Pax8 was identified in the mouse as a protein expressed in the kidney early during development[68] and in the thyroid, where it is maintained throughout adult life. It was later demonstrated that the Pax8 paired domain binds to the Tg and TPO promoter at a site overlapping with a TTF-1 binding site.[60] In transfection assays, Pax8 can activate transcription from the TPO promoter and, to a lesser extent, the Tg promoter.[60] As for TTF-1, gene inactivation experiments in the mouse have revealed that Pax8 is necessary for the formation of follicular cells.[69] Furthermore, Pax8 seems to have a unique role in maintaining the differentiated phenotype of these cells. Studies involving both thyroid neoplasia and experimental models have demonstrated

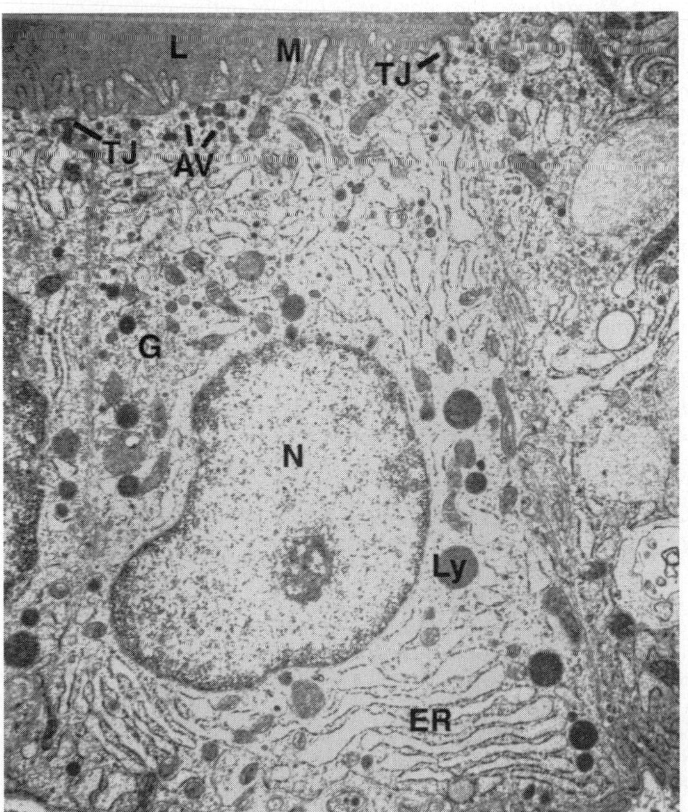

FIGURE 90–3. A thyroid follicular cell. *A,* A schematic structural representation. *B,* A schematic molecular representation. C, colloid droplets; ER, endoplasmic reticulum; G, Golgi apparatus; M, microvilli; MI, mitochondrion; N, nucleus; P, pseudopod.

a strong correlation between a loss (or a reduction) of Pax8 expression and the transformation of follicular cells.[70]

Thyroid Transcription Factor-2

TTF-2 has been identified as a thyroid-specific nuclear protein that can bind to a sequence present on both Tg and TPO promoters under insulin, insulin-like growth factor-1 (IGF-1), and TSH stimulation.[71] Recently, rat TTF-2 cDNA was cloned, and the features of this protein have been characterized.[72] TTF-2, encoded by the *Titf2* gene in mice and by the *TITF2* gene in humans, belongs to the family of forkhead proteins, which contain the 110 amino acids long forkhead DNA binding domain.[73] Human *TITF2* is located on chromosome 9q22[74, 75] and is an intronless gene coding for a 370–amino acid protein with a molecular mass of 42 kDa. In cultured thyroid cell, TTF-2 mRNA is under TSH and insulin or IGF-1 control.[76] TTF-2 is expressed in mouse embryos in the developing thyroid and anterior pituitary[72]; the generation of mutated mice carrying both disrupted *Titf2* alleles has shown that this factor is necessary for thyroid organogenesis.[75] However, the role of TTF-2 in the adult gland has not been fully clarified yet.

C Cells

The other endocrine cells present in the thyroid gland are known as parafollicular or C cells because of their distribution among follicular cells and their ability to secrete calcitonin,[77] a polypeptide hormone involved in calcium metabolism. The ultrastructural features of the cell are peculiar because of the presence of secretion granules 100 to 200 nm in diameter in the cytoplasm.[78] These cells originate from the neural crest[79] and during embryonic life colonize the UB,[80] a transient organ in mammals; finally, they disperse into the thyroid gland.[81] In spite of their name, not all parafollicular cells are located between follicular cells and the basement membrane (a real parafollicular position), but they can also be found among follicles (interfollicular) or in an intrafollicular position. C cells can be found dispersed as individual cells, in small groups, tightly adherent to follicular cells, or even in complex structures consisting of both follicular and C cells. The number of C cells differs among species.[82] In humans, C cells decrease with age: in adults these cells are less than 1% of the follicular cells, whereas in the neonatal thyroid it is possible to observe a value even 10 times greater, usually distributed in the upper two-thirds of the lateral lobe in an intrafollicular and parafollicular position.[83] Synthesis of calcitonin represents the functional marker of parafollicular cells. The calcitonin/calcitonin gene–related peptide gene expresses different mRNA by the tissue-specific process of its primary RNA transcript. Calcitonin mRNA, the main product of C cells, is obtained by splicing of the first three exons to the fourth exon. This mRNA encodes for a protein precursor containing calcitonin and a C-terminal peptide also called katacalcin I. Calcitonin-gene related peptide (CGRP) and katacalcin II are products of the different alternative splicing and are far less abundant than calcitonin in C cells. CGRP is a 37–amino acid, vasoactive peptide with no known effect on calcium metabolism.[84]

Several reports have revealed a more complex role and functional heterogeneity of mammalian parafollicular cells.[7] Production of a large number of regulatory peptides, including somatostatin, gastrin-releasing peptide, thyrotropin-releasing hormone, and helodermin, has been associated with the parafollicular cells, so the term C cells does not seem to be adequate. Whether different subpopulations of parafollicular cells can synthesize different sets of regulatory factors has not been demonstrated yet. In humans, for instance, calcitonin and somatostatin are colocalized only in a few parafollicular cells[85]; however, almost 100% of medullary carcinomas express somatostatin.[86] Because parafollicular cells are distributed among follicular cells and often tightly adherent to them, these biologically active peptides might regulate thyroid function by a paracrine pathway. Somatostatin, calcitonin, CGRP, and katacalcin seem to inhibit thyroid hormone secretion, whereas gastrin-releasing peptide and helodermin act as stimulators in this process.[7]

Ultimobranchial Body–Derived Epithelial Cells

In the mammalian thyroid other epithelial structures are evident. Such structures are absent in the glands of species in which UBs never merge with the thyroid. They probably represent vestiges of a UB endodermal component carried to the thyroid during fetal life.[87] Because of their origin, these structures are known as UB follicles or a second kind of thyroid follicle[88] even if they rarely display a clear follicular organization. In rodents these epithelial cells are organized as squamous cysts consisting of two or more layers of flattened or cuboid cells (also called U cells). This layer surrounds a lumen containing cell debris and amorphous material.[78] In humans, so-called solid cell nests are frequently present in the thyroid gland.[89] These structures are parafollicular or intrafollicular clusters and cords of squamous epithelial cells clearly separated from follicles by a basal lamina. In the gland they are preferentially located in the middle and upper third of the lobes.[90, 91] A significant clustering of C cells is noted around (and sometimes in the wall of) solid cell nests, which is consistent with a common UB origin of both solid cell nests and C cells. Mixed follicles in which follicular cells and epidermoid cells underlie a lumen filled with Tg-containing colloid are also frequently observed. The presence of such mixed follicles[92] and, moreover, the finding of a so-called mixed medullary carcinoma[93] that expresses both Tg and calcitonin have given rise to the hypothesis of a multipotential ultimobranchial endodermal cell able to differentiate toward either a Tg- or calcitonin-producing cell.

DEVELOPMENT OF THE THYROID GLAND

The adult thyroid gland in mammals is assembled from two different embryologic structures: the thyroid bud and UBs. This composite origin reflects the dual endocrine function of the gland. The thyroid bud is derived from the endoderm of the primitive pharynx and will give rise to the Tg-producing follicular cells. The UBs originate from the fourth pharyngeal pouch and contain neural crest–derived cells that will become calcitonin-producing parafollicular cells. These structures migrate from their respective sites of origin, reach their final position in front of the trachea, and fuse to form the definitive thyroid gland. After this early ontogenetic phase, thyroid function begins but remains at a basal level; the later differentiation of hypothalamic nuclei and the organization of the pituitary–portal vascular system guarantee maturation of thyroid system function.[94]

Thyroid development has been extensively studied in animal models, especially mice and rats. In all mammals, formation of the initial primordium, differentiation of follicular cells, and folliculogenesis probably have the same developmental pattern and are mediated by the same mechanisms. On the contrary, pituitary-hypothalamic regulation of thyroid function can be established among the different species at various stages during embryonic or even perinatal life.[94]

Ontogenesis and Differentiation of the Thyroid Follicular Cell

The thyroid primordium of the human embryo is first visible at 20 to 22 embryonic days as a midline endodermal thickening in the floor of the primitive pharynx,[95] caudal to the region of the first branchial arch that forms the tuberculum impar. This thickened bud first forms a small endodermal pit and then an outpouching of the endoderm that is in contact with the endothelium of the developing heart. The epithelium of the thyroid bud is different from that lining the pharynx and does not display a homogeneous structure. In the distal part the cells are arranged more compactly than the cells of the proximal part.[96] These cells rapidly become an endodermal-lined diverticulum that starts from the foramen caecum (in the midline of the dorsum of the tongue) and extends caudally to form the thyroglossal duct. The thyroid anlage develops as a flasklike structure with a narrow neck;

until embryonic day 24 it is still connected with the floor of the pharynx, and at embryonic day 30 it becomes larger and bilobated.[96] At the same time the thyroglossal duct becomes longer and thinner and its lumen narrower, and finally the duct fragments by embryonic day 30 to 40. The gland bifurcates and expands laterally to reach its final destination between embryonic days 45 and 50. At the same stage the UBs have completed their ventrocaudal migration and come in close contact with the primitive thyroid. Around embryonic day 60, the gland exhibits its definitive shape: two lobes connected by a narrow isthmus.[97] The onset of Tg expression in humans is not exactly defined. However, Tg was detected in follicular cells at a stage earlier than 10 weeks, when TSH is first identified,[94] and this finding confirms that Tg synthesis does not require TSH.

Exhaustive analysis of rodent thyroid development has been a useful tool in understanding the mechanism underlying gland morphogenesis. In the mouse (gestational length, 19.5 days), precursors of thyroid follicular cells are identified at embryonic day 8.5 as a thickened region of the endoderm in the ventral wall of the primitive pharynx (thyroid bud) (Fig. 90–4). This median endodermal thickening deepens and at embryonic day 9.5 begins to migrate caudally (thyroid diverticulum). The thyroglossal duct disappears at embryonic day 11.5, and the thyroid primordium, after losing all connection with the floor of the

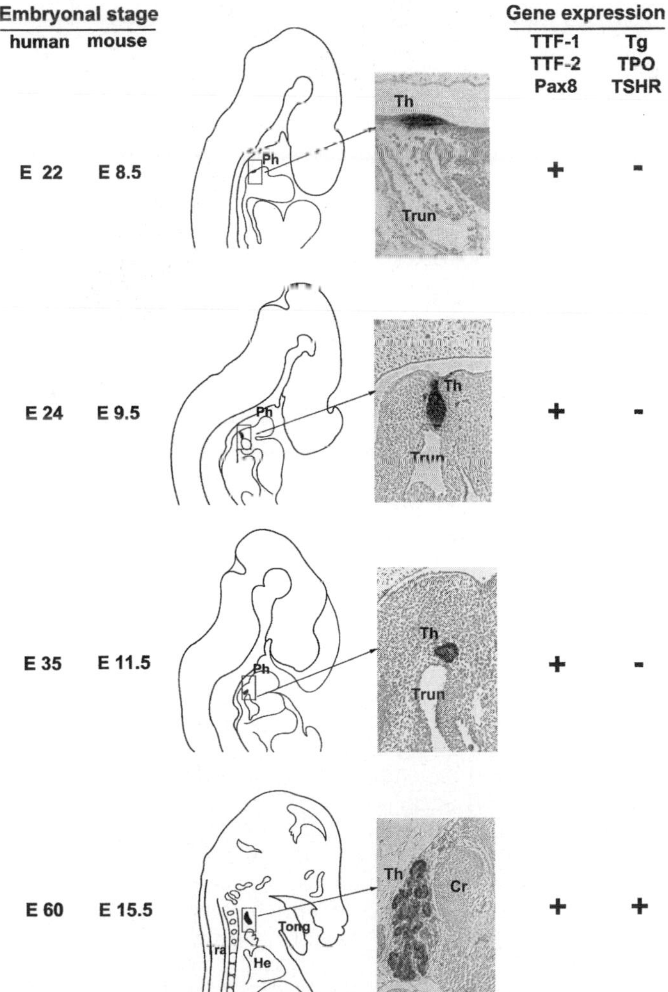

FIGURE 90–4. Thyroid development. In the *middle* is a schematic representation of thyroid organogenesis in mouse embryos and relevant sagittal sections stained with an anti-TTF-1 (thyroid transcription factor-1) antibody, on the *right* is the expression of some thyroid-specific genes for each stage, and on the *left* are the different embryonal stages (E, embryonic day) for the mouse embryo and the correspondent stages in humans. Cr, cricoid cartilage; He, heart; Ph, pharynx; Tg, thyroglobulin; Th, thyroid; Tong, tongue; TPO, thyroperoxidase; Tra, trachea; TSHR, thyroid-stimulating hormone receptor.

pharynx, reaches its destination—in front of the trachea—by embryonic day 13 to 14, where it merges with cells derived from the UBs.[10] At this stage thyroid follicular cells start their final differentiation process and thyroid-specific genes are expressed. Tg is present in follicular cells at embryonic day 14.5, and at the same stage TPO and TSHR genes are expressed[61]; one day later, NIS is detected on the basal pole of these cells.

The discovery that transcription factors relevant for the expression of genes specific to mature thyroid are expressed in the thyroid primordium makes it possible to explore the genetic basis of this developmental process and its defects. At embryonic day 8.5, the epithelial cells fated to form the thyroid are unequivocally identified in the endodermal layer of the primitive pharynx by unique patterns of gene expression which leads to the coexpression of three transcription factors, TTF-1, TTF-2, and Pax8.[61, 72] It is worth noting that these factors are also expressed in other embryonic tissues, but all three are coexpressed only in the presumptive thyroid bud, as soon as endodermal thickening appears on the floor of the primitive pharynx. When the thyroid diverticulum forms and begins its migration, only the thyroid primordium still expresses TTF-1, TTF-2, and Pax8, whereas the thyroglossal duct does not.[61] These three factors will remain for the rest of life as a hallmark of differentiated thyroid follicular cells, and their expression can be downregulated only after transformation of the cells.[98] The hypothesis that these factors are necessary in the early stage of morphogenesis has recently been confirmed. Mice in which homologous recombination in ES cells has disrupted both *Titf1* alleles are born dead; they show impaired lung morphogenesis and lack thyroid tissue.[62] Analyses during development demonstrate that the thyroid bud forms in its correct position but gland organogenesis is arrested and thyroid precursor cells are not detected by embryonic day 12.[99] The thyroid phenotype of *Pax8*$^{-/-}$ mice is similar to that described in *Titf1*$^{-/-}$ animals: the thyroid bud forms and migrates, but mature thyroid follicular cells are absent and the whole thyroid is composed of calcitonin-producing cells.[69] Thus in mice, Pax8 seems to be necessary for the differentiation of endodermal cells into thyroxine-producing cells. No other defects are observed in these mutated mice, which die within a week unless thyroid hormone is supplied to them. *Titf2* null mice died within 48 hours after birth. Examination of these mice revealed severe cleft palate and no thyroid gland in the normal location.[75] The thyroid primordium forms in *Titf2*$^{-/-}$ animals but does not migrate from the pharyngeal cavity; it eventually disappears at embryonic day 11.5, and mutant mice exhibit either a small differentiated sublingual or no thyroid gland at all. Therefore, TTF-1 and Pax8 seem to be relevant in the expansion and/or differentiation of precursors of follicular cells, whereas only TTF-2 plays an essential role in promoting migration of the thyroid follicular cell precursors. The fact that in 50% of *Titf2* null mice the thyroid disappears indicates that this gene, too, is implicated in control of the survival of thyroid cells at a different step from that of TTF-1 and Pax8.[75] At the moment it is not possible to analyze the role of other genes detected in the first stage of thyroid organogenesis, such as Hex,[100] HFN-3β,[101] or Nkx-2.5[102]; indeed, their wide and early expression in embryonic tissue makes it impossible to study the effect of their absence on the developing thyroid. Finally, it has been demonstrated that fibroblast growth factors (FGFs) have a role in thyroid morphogenesis in that functional inactivation of receptor II for FGF results in mice lacking thyroid tissue,[103] but the developmental stage in which thyroid organogenesis is impaired has not been elucidated.

Folliculogenesis

In humans, establishment of the characteristic histologic organization lasts several weeks and can be divided into three phases: the precolloid phase, the beginning colloid phase, and the follicular growth phase, which occur at 7 to 10, at 10 to 11, and after 11 weeks of gestation, respectively.[94] In the precolloid phase, small intracellular canaliculi develop as an accumulation of colloid material. These small canaliculi enlarge and the colloid organizes itself into extracellular spaces. In the last phase, primary follicles are clearly visible and the fetal thyroid is able to concentrate iodide and synthesize thyroid hormone. At midgestation (18–20 weeks in humans) the hypothalamic-pituitary-thyroid axis begins to develop, and hormone production increases. The early stages of folliculogenesis and colloid storage proceed in the absence of TSH. On the contrary, iodide concentration and hormone synthesis appear after pituitary TSH secretion.[94] After morphogenesis, TSH is absolutely necessary for thyroid growth and function.

In the mouse, the first evidence of follicular organization and thyroxine production appears between embryonic days 16 and 17,[104] but unlike humans, thyroid functions are accomplished only in postnatal life.[94] However, the availability of mutated mouse strains affected by congenital hypothyroidism provides a powerful tool for the exploration of some of the steps of in vivo folliculogenesis. Analysis of gland development in two hypothyroid mice, Hyt and Snell, has elucidated the role of TSH in controlling the structure of thyroid follicles. Homozygous *hyt/hyt* mice are characterized by very low serum thyroid hormones, elevated serum TSH, and a hypoplastic thyroid.[105] The genetic lesion inducing this phenotype was recognized as a mutation in the gene coding for TSHR, which causes the expression of a defective receptor whose binding activity for its cognate ligand is almost nonexistent.[106] Snell mice (*dw/dw*) are dwarf mice affected by hypothyroidism secondary to a pituitary defect resulting in impaired expression of prolactin, growth hormone (GH), and TSH because of a mutation in the *PIT-1* gene.[107] Hence, in both these mice thyroid morphogenesis is disturbed by suppression of the TSH-induced cAMP pathway. The *hyt/hyt* thyroid shows both more and much smaller follicles than does the wild-type gland. However, the size of follicles increases during life, and at 6 months follicles are only slightly smaller than normal.[105, 108] More and smaller follicles characterize the Snell mice thyroid phenotype as well.[109] After TSH treatment the number of follicles does not change, but they begin to enlarge; GH treatment has primarily a mitogenic effect and induces the fusion of smaller follicles to form larger ones. After combined GH and TSH treatment, the normal thyroid phenotype is restored. Therefore, TSH and GH (or probably IGF-1) are necessary to guarantee correct morphofunctional organization of the gland,[110] whereas these hormones are not relevant in the first steps of folliculogenesis. Other factors required for assembly and maintenance of follicle structure could be provided by interactions between follicular cells and the surrounding mesenchyme. These interactions have been hypothesized during chick thyroid organogenesis. In fact, follicular cells explanted from a developing chick thyroid can organize a correct histologic pattern in vitro only if cocultured in the presence of fibroblasts obtained from the capsule of a more mature gland.[111] However, in the mouse the ventral thyroid rudiment can give rise to large aggregations of normal thyroid follicles even when grafted in a kidney capsule at an early stage (embryonic day 12).[112] Furthermore, thyroid tissue located in an ectopic position is correctly differentiated even if migration is blocked. An inductive role of surrounding tissues in thyroid differentiation is therefore still a matter of debate.

Molecular Defects in Thyroid Development

Thyroid dysgenesis is responsible for impaired thyroid function in 85% of cases of permanent congenital hypothyroidism detected in newborns. The term "thyroid dysgenesis" indicates an ectopic or hypoplastic thyroid (or both), as well as total thyroid agenesis.[113] These phenotypes are probably due to disturbances during gland organogenesis, and now, at least in some cases, the molecular defects underlying this disease are beginning to be elucidated.[114]

The first examples of genetic lesions responsible for thyroid dysgenesis–associated congenital hypothyroidism were identified as mutations in the *TSHR* gene.[115] A functional TSHR is absent in patients with thyroid hypoplasia caused by the unresponsiveness to TSH. Among the molecular defects causing thyroid dysgenesis identified at present, mutations in the *TSHR* gene represent the most frequent finding.

On the contrary, no mutations in the *TITF1* gene were discovered in patients with thyroid dysgenesis.[116] It is noteworthy that TTF-1 is required for lung morphogenesis as well, and its absence could cause a lethal phenotype in humans. A large chromosomal deletion, including the *TITF* locus, was reported in a patient with congenital hypothyroidism and severe respiratory distress.[117] However, it is hard to conclude that the observed phenotype is a consequence of the absence of TTF-1.

Mutations in the *PAX8* gene have been reported in less than 5% of patients with sporadic and familiar thyroid dysgenesis.[118] These patients have a hypoplastic thyroid and an altered version of Pax8 that is unable to bind DNA. All affected individuals identified thus far are heterozygous for the mutation, in contrast to the animal model, where *Pax8*$^{+/-}$ mice do not display any thyroid phenotype. Thus, in humans both *PAX8* alleles are necessary for correct thyroid morphogenesis. The difference observed between the behavior of heterozygous mutants in mice and humans has not been clarified yet; however, subjects heterozygous for mutations in other *PAX* genes often display abnormal phenotypes.

Two siblings showing thyroid agenesis and cleft palate (Bamforth's syndrome[119]) have been demonstrated to carry a mutation within the *TITF2* gene.[120] The mutant protein has impaired DNA binding and transcriptional activity. Mice in which *Titf2* is disrupted show either an absent or ectopic thyroid gland, which indicates that these two phenotypes represent variable expressivity of the same mutation.[75] However, the association of thyroid dysgenesis and cleft palate is a very rare condition, so it is difficult to confirm the same finding in humans.

All defects described at present account for less than 10% of the thyroid dysgenesis cases reported. Mutations of genes downstream from those already described, somatic mutations, and/or multigenic origins might be implicated in the pathogenesis of other cases of thyroid dysgenesis.

Ontogenesis and Differentiation of the C Cell

In vertebrates, calcitonin-producing cells differentiate in the UB, a structure derived from the fourth pharyngeal pouch. C cells do not originate in the endodermal epithelium but derive from neural crest cells that early in development colonize the ventral part of the fourth pharyngeal pouch and migrate from the most caudal part of the rhombencephalon. The UB is a definitive organ in all vertebrates except in placental mammals, where it is an embryonic transient structure destined to join to the medial thyroid bud. The use of chimeric model systems in birds,[79] experimental transplantation and ablation studies in rodents,[80] and more recently, the generation of mutated animal models[121] have clarified many aspects of the ontogenesis and multistep migration of C cell precursors. The few data available from humans up to now largely appear to match those from these models.

UB primordium is first evident in humans at embryonic day 24 as an outpouching of the ventral component of the fourth pharyngeal pouch. At this stage the primordium of parathyroid IV is visible as a dorsal evagination of the same pouch.[122] Some authors identify a transient fifth pouch as the endodermal origin of the UB.[123] Probably the shape of the UB anlage itself, which appears as an incomplete pouch, has generated these different interpretations. By 5 weeks the ventral extroflexion is a long-necked flask still attached to the pharynx; a few days later the UB primordium loses its connection with the pharyngeal cavity, starts its migration, and at 7 weeks, reaches the posterior surface of the median thyroid. A connective layer separates these two buds, which display different histologic organization: the lateral bud is composed of a compact mass of cells, whereas the median bud is composed of interconnecting sheets of epithelium. Finally, at 8 weeks, UBs are incorporated with the lateral lobes of the thyroid, and the cells from both structures are mixed with each other.[97]

In mice, UB development is similar to that in humans. At embryonic day 9 the fourth pharyngeal pouch consists of a lateral extroflexion of the primitive foregut, at embryonic day 11 the caudal portion of the pouch grows, and at embryonic day 11.5 the fourth pharynx–branchial duct is pinched off to form a UB primordium visible as a vesicle with a lumen lined by columnar epithelium.[124] One day later, the UB is in contact with the median thyroid, and at embryonic day 15, calcitonin-producing cells can be detected between follicular cells. Explant experiments have demonstrated the origin and the complex migration of calcitonin-producing cells in mice. Formal proof of the neural crest origin of these cells was obtained in birds some years ago, and at the present time we have sufficient data to infer that C cell ontogeny follows the same pattern in mammals. In mice, precursors of C cells are first located in the mesenchyme of the fourth branchial pouch around embryonic day 9 to 9.5. Between embryonic days 10.5 and 11, cells that can differentiate into calcitonin-producing cells are present in the endoderm of the pouch. At the same stage, UB primordium initiates its migration and carries the neural crest–derived cells toward the thyroid gland.[80]

Some genes of the Hox family are expressed in rhomboencephalic neural crest cells before their migration and in the pharyngeal regions colonized from them. In particular, Hoxa-3 is detected in mesenchymal, endodermal, and neural crest–derived cells of the third and fourth pharyngeal arches and pouches. Expression of Hoxa-3 might be relevant in the morphogenesis of organs derived from these structures. The generation of a mutated mouse in which the gene had been disrupted has confirmed the role of this gene in development of the UB and its contribution to thyroid organogenesis.[121] In *Hoxa-3*$^{-/-}$ mice, C cells differentiate but their number is severely reduced. In many cases UBs fail to fuse with the thyroid bud and remain as bilateral vesicles composed exclusively of calcitonin-producing cells. These data indicate that the differentiation of C cells and correct migration and fusion are under different genetic control and that Hoxa-3 regulates a step unique only to mammals.[125]

Spontaneous or induced mutations of other genes necessary for the development or migration of neural crest cells, such as *Pax3*[126] or *endothelin I*,[127] can cause defects in the thyroid gland. It is noteworthy that in human diseases such as DiGeorge syndrome[128] or truncus arteriosus syndrome,[129] whose pathogenesis is due to developmental defects in pharyngeal arch– or pouch-derived structures, alterations in the thyroid gland are sometimes described.

Ultimobranchial Body and Follicular Cells

In the past, embryologists considered the UB to be the lateral anlage of a thyroid whose cells were fated to differentiate toward typical follicular cells and become a definitive component of the mature gland. The presence of cystic lateral structures in subjects whose thyroid is absent or ectopically located is not rare. Sometimes these cysts have been described as filled with "a material which appears identical to thyroid colloid."[97] More recently, some authors have confirmed these findings,[130, 131] and moreover, similar structures, such as colloid-containing follicles, have been described in some of the persistent UBs in *Hoxa-3*$^{-/-}$ mice.[125] These data suggest that follicular cells could originate from both median and lateral thyroid anlage. Conclusive demonstration of the presence of Tg in such structures has not been reported. On the contrary, UBs from embryonic day 12 mice, transplanted under kidney capsules, never give rise to the typical thyroid epithelial cells but only to the so-called UB follicles. These data indicate that cells originating from the lateral anlage cannot differentiate into thyroxine-producing cells. However, in *Hoxa-3*$^{-/-}$ mice, in many cases it is possible to also observe several defects in the follicular component of the thyroid. These defects range from a reduction in the number of follicular cells to absence of the isthmus of the entire lateral lobe. Because Hoxa-3 is also expressed in epithelial cells of the UB, these data seem to suggest that the endoderm from the fourth pouch (the lateral thyroid of the past embryologist) is necessary for correct morphogenesis of the thyroid gland. Furthermore, the recent and puzzling discovery that particular follicular cell markers such as TTF-1 and Pax8 are also expressed in the endoderm of the fourth pouch and in the UB (M. De Felice and R. Di Lauro, unpublished results) could support this hypothesis.

PHYLOGENESIS OF THE THYROID GLAND

The morphologic basis of thyroid function is the same in all vertebrates, to the extent that follicular structure remains an invariant particular feature throughout vertebrate evolution. On the contrary, the gross anatomy of the thyroid gland is quite different among the vertebrate classes.[11] In placental mammals and in some reptiles, the thyroid is composed of two lobes connected by an isthmus that crosses the trachea. In nonplacental mammals, birds, and amphibians, the thyroid consists of two isolated lobes. In cartilaginous fish and in some teleosts (mostly marine ones), the thyroid is massed into a compact organ, whereas in many marine and almost all freshwater teleosts and in cyclostomes, the thyroid consists of nonencapsulated follicles scattered in subpharyngeal connective tissue. It is not rare to find heterotopic follicles in nonpharyngeal areas such as the kidneys, heart, esophagus, or spleen. In particular, it has been shown in platyfish that the ability to proliferate in these ectopic areas is genetically controlled and that low iodine intake is a strong inductive stimulus toward this condition.[132]

The ontogeny of the thyroid follows the same pattern in all *Gnathostoma* (higher vertebrates): the thyroid anlage arises from an outpouching of the primitive pharynx, migrates caudally to form a transient thyroglossal duct, and finally reaches its definitive position. In cyclostomes (such as the lamprey), thyroid development does not match this pattern because it derives from the endostyle, an organ present only during larval life. In the larval lamprey at the first stages, the endostyle forms as a ciliated groove in the ventral part of the pharynx. During development the groove becomes a cylinder and then a complex structure connected to the pharyngeal cavity by the ductus hypobranchialis.[133] The epithelium of the endostyle differentiates into many types of cells, a group of which display both peroxidase activity and the ability to bind iodine. These cells are fated to become "typical" follicular cells only after metamorphosis; however, in some species, a 19S iodinated protein can already be identified in the later stages of larval life. Evidence of homology between the cyclostome endostyle and the thyroid gives rise to the possibility of considering the endostyle of protochordates a homologous and a primitive antecedent of the vertebrate thyroid gland as well. In the endostyle of both ascidians and amphioxus, a "protothyroid region" has been identified. In amphioxus this region consists of a group of ciliated microvilli containing cells able to bind iodine. In addition, peroxidase activity is evident on the outer surface of the apical plasma membrane, and autoradiographic studies indicate that iodination is an extracellular process as in the vertebrate thyroid gland.[133] Similarly, in the ascidian endostyle a zone is present in which organification of iodine is accomplished by a membrane peroxidase whose biochemical properties are similar to those of the vertebrate TPO.[134] The presence of iodoproteins or even Tg is not sufficient to guarantee homology between the thyroid gland and the endostyle because the latter does not display any endocrine function. However, recent discovery of the expression of genes homologous to TTF-1[135] and Pax2/5/8[136] in the endostyle of amphioxus and homologous to TTF-1 in the endostyle of the ascidian *Ciona intestinalis*[137] gives strong "molecular" support to a hypothesis of homology suggested more than a century ago solely on morphologic observations.

REFERENCES

1. Werner S: Historical resumè. *In* Ingbar SH, Braverman L (eds): The Thyroid, ed 5. Philadelphia, JB Lippincott, 1986, pp 3–6.
2. Netter F: Anatomy of the thyroid and parathyroid glands. *In* The CIBA Collection of Medical Illustrations, vol 4. West Caldwell, NJ, CIBA, 1965, pp 41–70.
3. Fujita H: Functional morphology of the thyroid. Int Rev Cytol 113:145–185, 1988.
4. Romeo HE, Gonzalez Solveyra C, Vacas MI, et al: Origins of the sympathetic projections to rat thyroid and parathyroid glands. J Auton Nerv Syst 17:63–70, 1986.
5. Cauna N, Naik N: The distribution of cholinesterases in the sensory ganglia of man and some mammals. J Histochem Cytochem 11:129–138, 1963.
6. Sundler F, Grunditz T, Hakanson R, et al: Innervation of the thyroid. A study of the rat using retrograde tracing and immunocytochemistry. Acta Histochem 37(suppl):191–198, 1989.
7. Sawicki B: Evaluation of the role of mammalian thyroid parafollicular cells. Acta Histochem 97:389–399, 1995.
8. Grunditz T, Hakanson R, Rerup C, et al: Neuropeptide Y in the thyroid gland: Neuronal localization and enhancement of stimulated thyroid hormone secretion. Endocrinology 115:1537–1542, 1984.
9. Ahrèn B: Regulatory peptides in the thyroid gland—a review on their localization and function. Acta Endocrinol 124:225–232, 1991.
10. Kaufman MH, Bard J: The thyroid. *In* The Anatomic Basis of Mouse Development. San Diego, CA, Academic Press, 1999, pp 165–166.

11. Gorbman A, Bern H: Thyroid gland. *In* A Texbook of Comparative Endocrinology. New York, John Wiley & Sons, 1962, pp 99–173.
12. Mauchamp J, Mirrione A, Alquier C, et al: Follicle-like structure and polarized monolayer: Role of the extracellular matrix on thyroid cell organization in primary culture. Biol Cell 90:369–380, 1998.
13. Yap AS, Stevenson BR, Armstrong JW, et al: Thyroid epithelial morphogenesis in vitro: A role for butamide-sensitive Cl^- secretion during follicular lumen development. Exp Cell Res 213:319–326, 1994.
14. Shepard T: Onset of function in the human fetal thyroid: Biochemical and radioautographic studies from organ culture. J Clin Endocrinol Metab 27:945–958, 1987.
15. Romagnoli P, Herzog V: Transcytosis in thyroid follicle cells: Regulation and implications for thyroglobulin transport. Exp Cell Res 194:202–209, 1991.
16. Drubin DG, Nelson J: Origins of cell polarity. Cell 84:335–344, 1996.
17. Matter K, Mellman I: Mechanism of cell polarity: Sorting and transport in epithelial cells. Curr Opin Cell Biol 6:545–554, 1994.
18. Ekholm R: Biosynthesis of thyroid hormones. Int Rev Cytol 120:243–288, 1990.
19. Bourke JR, Sand O, Abel KC, et al: Chloride channels in the apical membrane of thyroid epithelial cells are regulated by cyclic AMP. J Endocrinol 147:441–448, 1995.
20. Bourke JR, Abel KC, Huxham GJ, et al: Sodium channel heterogeneity in the apical membrane of porcine thyroid epithelial cells. J Endocrinol 149:101–108, 1996.
21. Paire A, Bernier-Valentin F, Selmi-Ruby S, et al: Characterization of the rat thyroid iodide transporter using anti-peptide antibodies. J Biol Chem 272:18245–18249, 1997.
22. Gerard C, Gabrion J, Verrier B, et al: Localization of the Na^+/K^+-ATPase and of an amiloride sensitive Na^+ uptake on thyroid epithelial cells. Eur J Cell Biol 38:134–141, 1985.
23. Westermack K, Westermack B, Karslsson A, et al: Localization of epidermal growth factor receptors on porcine thyroid follicle cells and receptor regulation by thyrotropin. Endocrinology 118:1040–1046, 1986.
24. Costagliola S, Rodien P, Many MC, et al: Genetic immunization against the human thyrotropin receptor causes thyroiditis and allows production of monoclonal antibodies recognizing the native receptor. J Immunol 160:1458–1465, 1998.
25. Ericson L: Exocytosis and endocytosis in the thyroid follicle cell. Mol Cell Endocrinol 22:1–24, 1981.
26. Lohi J, Leivo I, Franssila K, et al: Changes in the distribution of integrins and their basement membrane ligands during development of human thyroid follicular epithelium. Histochem J 29:337–345, 1997.
27. Vitale M, Casamassima A, Illario M, et al: Cell-to-cell contact modulates the expression of the beta1 integrins in primary cultures of thyroid cells. Exp Cell Res 220:124–129, 1995.
28. Burgi-Saville ME, Gerber H, Peter HJ, et al: Expression patterns of extracellular matrix components in native and cultured normal human thyroid tissue and in human toxic adenoma tissue. Thyroid 7:347–356, 1997.
29. Andre F, Filippi P, Feracci H: Merosin is synthesized by thyroid cells in primary culture irrespective of cellular organization. J Cell Sci 107:183–193, 1994.
30. Gumbiner B: Cell adhesion: The molecular basis of tissue architecture and morphogenesis. Cell 84:345–357, 1996.
31. Denker BM, Nigam S: Molecular structure and assembly of the tight junction. Am J Physiol 274:1–9, 1998.
32. Yap AS, Stevenson BR, Abel KC, et al: Microtubule integrity is necessary for the epithelial barrier function of cultured thyroid cell monolayers. Exp Cell Res 218:540–545, 1995.
33. Boller K, Vestweber D, Kemler R: Cell-adhesion molecule uvomorulin is localized in the intermediate junctions of adult intestinal epithelial cells. Cell Biol 100:327–332, 1985.
34. Kemler K: From cadherins to catenins: Cytoplasmic protein interactions and regulation of cell adhesion. Trends Genet 9:317–321, 1993.
35. Buxton RS, Magee A: Structure and interactions of desmosomal and other cadherins. Semin Cell Biol 3:157–167, 1992.
36. Kowalczyk AP, Bornslaeger EA, Norvell SM, et al: Desmosomes: Intercellular adhesive junctions specialized for attachment of intermediate filaments. Int Rev Cytol 185:237–230, 1999.
37. Munari-Silem Y, Rousset B: Gap junction–mediated cell-to-cell communications in endocrine glands—molecular and functional aspects: A review. Eur J Endocrinol 135:251–264, 1996.
38. Fayet G, Michel-Bechet M, Lissitzky S: Thyrotrophin-induced aggregation and reorganization into follicles of isolated porcine-thyroid cells. II. Ultrastructural studies. Eur J Biochem 24:100–111, 1971.
39. Lissitzky S, Fayet G, Giraud A, et al: Thyrotrophin-induced aggregation and reorganization into follicles of isolated porcine-thyroid cells. I. Mechanisms of action of thyrotrophin and metabolic properties. Eur J Biochem 24:88–99, 1971.
40. Yap AS, Stevenson BR, Keast JR, et al: Cadherin-mediated adhesion and apical membrane assembly define distinct steps during thyroid epithelial polarization and lumen formation. Endocrinology 136:4672–4680, 1995.
41. Chan A: Ultrastructural observations on the formation of follicles in the human fetal thyroid. Cell Tissue Res 233:693–698, 1983.
42. Ishimura K, Fujita H: Development of cell-to-cell relationships in the thyroid gland of the chick embryo. Cell Tissue Res 198:15–25, 1979.
43. Yap AS, Manley S: Contact inhibition of cell spreading: A mechanism for the maintenance of thyroid cell aggregation in vitro. Exp Cell Res 208:121–127, 1993.
44. Yap AS, Abel KC, Bourke JR, et al: Different regulation of thyroid cell-cell and cell-substrate adhesion by thyrotropin. Exp Cell Res 202:366–369, 1992.
45. Nilsson M, Fagman H, Ericson L: Ca^{2+}-dependent and Ca^{2+}-independent regulation of the thyroid epithelial junction complex by protein kinases. Exp Cell Res 225:1–11, 1996.
46. Pellerin S, Croizet K, Rabilloud R, et al: Regulation of the three-dimensional organization of thyroid epithelial cells into follicle structures by the matricellular protein, thrombospondin-1. Endocrinology 140:1094–1103, 1999.
47. Gartner R, Schopohl D, Schaefer S, et al: Regulation of transforming growth factor beta 1 messenger ribonucleic acid expression in porcine thyroid follicles in vitro by growth factors, iodine, or delta iodolactone. Thyroid 7:633–640, 1997.
48. Toda S, Matsumura S, Fujitani N, et al: Transforming growth factor-beta 1 induces a mesenchyma-like cell shape without epithelial polarization in thyrocytes and inhibits thyroid folliculogenesis in collagen gel culture. Endocrinology 138:5561–5575, 1997.
49. Paire A, Bernier-Valentin F, Rabilloud R, et al: Expression of alpha- and beta-subunits and activity of Na^+ K^+ ATPase in pig thyroid cells in primary culture: Modulation by thyrotropin and thyroid hormones. Mol Cell Endocrinol 146:93–101, 1998.
50. Tacchetti C, Zurzolo C, Monticelli C, et al: Functional properties of normal and inverted rat thyroid follicles in suspension culture. J Cell Physiol 126:93–98, 1986.
51. Halmi N: Anatomy and histochemistry. *In* Ingbar SH, Braverman L (eds): The Thyroid. Philadelphia, JB Lippincott, 1986, pp 24–36.
52. Fujita H: Fine structure of the thyroid gland. Int Rev Cytol 40:197–280, 1975.
53. Bernier-Valentine F, Kostrouch Z, Rabilloud R, et al: Analysis of the thyroglobulin internalization process using in vitro reconstituted follicles: Evidence for a coated vesicle-dependent endocytic pathway. Endocrinology 129:2194–2201, 1991.
54. Engstrom G, Ericson L: Effect of graded dose of thyrotropin on exocytosis and early phase of endocytosis in the rat thyroid. Endocrinology 108:399–405, 1981.
55. Damante G, Di Lauro R: Thyroid-specific gene expression. Biochim Biophys Acta 1218:255–266, 1994.
56. Guazzi S, Price M, De Felice M, et al: Thyroid nuclear factor 1 (TTF-1) contains a homeodomain and displays a novel DNA binding specificity. EMBO J 9:3631–3639, 1990.
57. Kim Y, Niremberg M: *Drosophila* NK-homeobox genes. Proc Natl Acad Sci U S A 86:7716–7720, 1989.
58. Civitareale D, Lonigro R, Sinclair AJ, et al: A thyroid-specific nuclear protein essential for tissue-specific expression of the thyroglobulin promoter. EMBO J 8:2537–2542, 1989.
59. De Felice M, Damante G, Zannini MS, et al: Redundant domains contribute to the transcriptional activity of thyroid transcription factor 1 (TTF-1). J Biol Chem 270:26649–26656, 1995.
60. Zannini MS, Francis-Lang H, Plachov D, et al: Pax-8, a paired domain-containing protein, binds to a sequence overlapping the recognition site of a homeodomain and activates transcription from two thyroid-specific promoters. Mol Cell Biol 12:4230–4241, 1992.
61. Lazzaro D, Price M, De Felice M, et al: The transcription factor TTF-1 is expressed at the onset of thyroid and lung morphogenesis and in restricted regions of the foetal brain. Development 113:1093–1104, 1991.
62. Kimura S, Hara Y, Pineau T, et al: The T/ebp null mouse: Thyroid-specific enhancer-binding protein is essential for the organogenesis of the thyroid, lung, ventral forebrain, and pituitary. Genes Dev 10:60–69, 1996.
63. Bohinski RJ, Di Lauro R, Whitsett J: The lung-specific surfactant protein B gene promoter is a target for thyroid transcription factor 1 and hepatocyte nuclear factor 3, indicating common factors for organ-specific gene expression along the foregut axis. Mol Cell Biol 14:5671–5681, 1994.
64. Suzuki K, Kobayashi Y, Katoh R, et al: Identification of thyroid transcription factor-1 in C cells and parathyroid cells. Endocrinology 139:3014–3017, 1998.
65. Frigerio G, Burri M, Bopp D, et al: Structure of the segmentation gene paired and the *Drosophila* PRD gene set a part of a gene network. Cell 47:735–746, 1986.
66. Stapleton P, Weith A, Urbanek P, et al: Chromosomal localization of 7 Pax genes and cloning of a novel family member, Pax-9. Nat Genet 3:292–298, 1993.
67. Kozmik Z, Kurzbauer R, Dörfler P, et al: Alternative splicing of Pax-8 gene transcripts is developmentally regulated and generates isoforms with different transactivation properties. Mol Cell Biol 13:6145–6149, 1993.
68. Plachov D, Chowdhury K, Walther C, et al: Pax8, a murine paired box gene expressed in the developing excretory system and thyroid gland. Development 110:643–651, 1990.
69. Mansouri A, Chowdhury K, Gruss P: Follicular cells of the thyroid gland require Pax8 gene function. Nat Genet 19:87–90, 1998.
70. Fagin J, Tang SH, Zeki K, et al: Reexpression of thyroid peroxidase in a derivative of an undifferentiated thyroid carcinoma cell line by introduction of wild-type p53. Cancer Res 56:765–771, 1996.
71. Santisteban P, Acebron A, Polycarpou-Schwarz M, et al: Insulin and insulin-like growth factor I regulate a thyroid-specific nuclear protein that binds to the thyroglobulin promoter. Mol Endocrinol 6:1310–1317, 1992.
72. Zannini M, Avantaggiato V, Biffali E, et al: TTF-2, a new forkhead protein, shows a temporal expression in the developing thyroid which is consistent with a role in controlling the onset of differentiation. EMBO J 16:3185–3197, 1997.
73. Kaestner KH, Lee KH, Schlondorff J, et al: Six members of the mouse forkhead gene family are developmentally regulated. Proc Natl Acad Sci U S A:7628–7631, 1993.
74. Chadwick BP, Obermayr F, Frischau A: FKHL15, a new human member of the forkhead gene family located on chromosome 9q22. Genomics 41:390–396, 1997.
75. DeFelice M, Ovitt C, Biffali E, et al: A mouse model for hereditary thyroid dysgenesis and cleft palate. Nat Genet 19:395–398, 1998.
76. Ortiz L, Zannini MS, Di Lauro R, et al: Transcriptional control of the forkhead thyroid transcription factor TTF-2 by thyrotropin, insulin and insulin-like growth factor 1. J Biol Chem 272:23334–23339, 1997.
77. Pearse A: The cytochemistry of the thyroid C cells and their relationship to calcitonin. Proc R Soc Biol 164:478–487, 1966.
78. Neve P, Wollman S: Fine structure of ultimobranchial follicles in the thyroid gland of the rat. Anat Rec 171:259–272, 1971.
79. Le Douarin N, Fontaine J, LeLievre C: New studies on the neural crest origin of the avian ultimobranchial glandular cells. Interspecific combinations and cytochemical characterization of C cells based on the uptake of biogenic amine precursors. Histochemie 38:297–305, 1974.
80. Fontaine J: Multistep migration of calcitonin cell precursors during ontogeny of the mouse pharynx. Gen Comp Endocrinol 37:81–92, 1979.

81. Pearse AG, Caralheira A: Cytochemical evidence for an ultimobranchial origin of rodent thyroid C cells. Nature 214:929–930, 1967.
82. Martin-Lacave M, Conde E, Montenero C, et al: Quntitative changes in the frequency and distribution of the C-cell population in the rat thyroid gland with age. Cell Tissue Res 270:73–77, 1992.
83. Wolfe HJ, DeLellis RA, Voelkel EF, et al: Distribution of calcitonin-containing cells in the normal neonatal human thyroid gland: A correlation of morphology with peptide content. J Clin Endocrinol Metab 41:1076–1081, 1975.
84. Minvielle S, Giscard-Dartevelle S, Cohen R, et al: A novel calcitonin carboxyl-terminal peptide produced in medullary thyroid carcinoma by alternative RNA processing of the calcitonin/calcitonin gene–related peptide gene. J Biol Chem 266:24627–24631, 1991.
85. Kameda Y, Oyama H, Endoh M, et al: Somatostatin immunoreactive C cells in thyroid glands from various mammalian species. Anat Rec 204:161–170, 1982.
86. Scopsi L, Ferrari C, Pilotti S, et al: Immunocytochemical localization and identification of prosomatostatin gene products in medullary carcinoma of human thyroid gland. Hum Pathol 21:820–830, 1990.
87. Calvert R: Structure of rat ultimobranchial bodies after birth. Anat Rec 181:561–580, 1974.
88. Wollman SH, Neve P: Postnatal development and properties of ultimobranchial follicles in the rat thyroid. Anat Rec 171:247–258, 1971.
89. Janzer RC, Weber E, Hedinger C: The relation between solid cell nests and C cells of the thyroid gland. Cell tissue Res 197:295–312, 1979.
90. Harach H: Solid cell nests of the thyroid. Acta Anat 122:249–255, 1985.
91. Harach H: Solid cell nests of the thyroid. J Pathol 155:191–200, 1988.
92. Harach H: Thyroid follicles with acid mucins in man: A second kind of follicles. Cell Tissue Res 242:211–215, 1985.
93. Harach H: A study on the relationship between solid cell nests and mucoepidermoid carcinoma of the thyroid. Histopathology 9:195–207, 1985.
94. Fisher DA, JH D, Sach J, et al: Ontogenesis of hypothalamic-pituitary-thyroid function and metabolism in man, sheep and rat. Recent Prog Horm Res 33:59–116, 1977.
95. Ingalls N: A human embryo at the beginning of segmentation, with special reference to the vascular system. Contrib Embryol 11:61–88, 1920.
96. Sgalitzer K: Contribution to the study of the morphogenesis of the thyroid gland. J Anat 75:389–405, 1941.
97. Weller G: Development of the thyroid, parathyroid and thymus glands in man Contrib Embryol 24:93–140, 1933.
98. Francis-Lang H, Zannini MS, DeFelice M, et al: Multiple mechanisms of interference between transformation and differentiation in thyroid cells. Mol Cell Biol 12:5793–5800, 1992.
99. Kimura S, Ward JD, Minoo P: Thyroid-specific enhancer–binding protein/transcription factor 1 is not required for the initial specification of the thyroid and lung primordia. Biochemie 81:321–328, 1999.
100. Thomas PQ, Brown A, Beddington R: Hex: A homeobox gene revealing peri-implantation asymmetry in the mouse embryo and an early transient marker of endothelial cell precursors. Development 125:85–95, 1998.
101. Kaestner KH, Hiemisch H, Luckow B, et al: The HNF-3 gene family of transcription factors in mice: Gene structure, cDNA sequence and mRNA distribution. Genomics 20:377–385, 1994.
102. Lints TJ, Parsons LM, Hartley L, et al: Nkx-2.5: A novel murine homeobox gene expressed in early heart progenitor cells and their myogenic descendants. Development 119:419–431, 1993.
103. Celli G, LaRochelle WJ, Mackem S, et al: Soluble dominant-negative receptor uncovers essential roles for fibroblast growth factors in multi-organ induction and patterning. EMBO J 17:1642–1645, 1998.
104. VanHeyningen H: The initiation of thyroid function in the mouse. Endocrinology 69:720–727, 1961.
105. Stein SA, Shanklin DR, Krulich L, et al: Evaluation and characterization of the hyt/hyt hypothyroid mouse. Nueroendocrinology 49:509–519, 1989.
106. Stuart A, Oates E, Hall C, et al: Identification of a point mutation in the thyrotropin receptor of the hyt/hyt hypothyroid mouse. Mol Endocrinol 8:129–138, 1994.
107. Li S, Crenshaw EBI, Rawson EJ, et al: Dwarf locus mutants lacking three pituitary cell types result from mutations in the POU-domain gene pit-1. Nature 347:528–533, 1990.
108. Beamer WG, Cresswell L: Defective thyroid ontogenesis in fetal hypothyroid (hyt/hyt) mice. Anat Rec 202:387–393, 1982.
109. Cordier AC, Denef JF, Haumont S: Thyroid gland in Dwarf mice. Cell Tissue Res 171:449–475, 1976.
110. Denef JF, Cordier AC, Haumont S, et al: The influence of thyrotropin and growth hormone on the thyroid gland in the hereditary dwarf mouse: A morphometric study. Endocrinology 107:1249–1257, 1980.
111. Hilfer SR, Stern M: Instability of the epithelial-mesenchymal interaction in the eight-day embryonic chick thyroid. J Exp Zool 178:293–305, 1971.
112. Wollman SH, Hilfer S: Embryologic origin of various epithelial cell types in the thyroid gland of the rat. Anat Rec 189:467–478, 1977.
113. Fisher DA, Klein A: Thyroid development and disorders of thyroid function in the newborn. N Engl J Med 304:702–712, 1981.
114. Macchia PE, DeFelice M, DiLauro R: Molecular genetics of congenital hypothyroidism. Curr Opin Genet Dev 9:289–294, 1999.
115. Takeshida J, Nagayama M, Yamashita S, et al: Sequence analysis of the thyrotropin (TSH) receptor gene in congenital primary hypothyroidism associated with TSH unresponsiveness. Thyroid 4:255–259, 1994.
116. Lapi P, Macchia PE, Chiovato L, et al: Mutations in the gene for thyroid transcription factor-1 (TTF-1) are not a frequent cause of congenital hypothyroidism (CH) with thyroid dysgenesis. Thyroid 7:383–387, 1997.
117. Devriendt K, Vanhole C, Matthijs G, et al: Deletion of thyroid transcription factor-1 gene in an infant with neonatal thyroid dysfunction and respiratory failure. N Engl J Med 338:1317–1318, 1998.
118. Macchia PE, Lapi P, Krude H, et al: PAX8 mutations associated with congenital hypothyroidism caused by thyroid dysgenesis. Nat Genet 19:83–86, 1998.
119. Bamforth JS, Hughes IA, Lazarus JH, et al: Congenital hypothyroidism, spiky hair, and cleft palate. J Med Genet 26:49–60, 1989.
120. Clifton-Bligh RJ, Wentworth JM, Heinz P, et al: Mutation of the gene encoding human TTF-2 associated with thyroid agenesis, cleft palate and choanal atresia. Nat Genet 19:399–401, 1998.
121. Manley NR, Capecchi M: The role of Hoxa-3 in mouse thymus and thyroid development. Development 121:1989–2003, 1995.
122. Norris E: The parathyroid glands and the lateral thyroid in man: Their morphogenesis, histogenesis, topographic anatomy and prenatal growth. Contrib Embryol 26:247–294, 1937.
123. Merida-Velasco JA, Garcia-Garcia JD, Espin-Ferra J, et al: Origin of the ultimobranchial body and its colonizing cells in human embryos. Acta Anat 73:325–330, 1989.
124. Cordier AC, Haumont S: Development of thymus, parathyroids, and ultimo-branchial bodies in NMRI and nude mice. Am J Anat 157:227–263, 1980.
125. Manley NR, Capecchi M: Hox group 3 paralogs regulate the development and migration of the thymus, thyroid, and parathyroid glands. Dev Biol 195:1–15, 1998.
126. Conway SJ, Henderson DJ, Copp A: Pax3 is required for cardiac neural crest migration in the mouse: Evidence from the splotch (Sp^{2H}) mutant. Development 124:505–514, 1997.
127. Kurihara Y, Kurihara H, Maemura K, et al: Impaired development of the thyroid and thymus in endothelin-1 knockout mice. J Cardiovasc Pharmacol 26:13–16, 1995.
128. Burke BA, Johnson D, Gilbert EF, et al: Thyrocalcitonin-containing cells in the DiGeorge anomaly. Hum Pathol 4:355–360, 1987.
129. Gamallo C, Garcia M, Palacios J, et al: Decrease in calcitonin containing cells in truncus arteriosus. Am J Med Genet 46:149–153, 1993.
130. Harach H: Thyroglobulin in human thyroid follicles with acid mucins. J Pathol 164:261–263, 1991.
131. Williams ED, Toyn CE, Harach H: The ultimobranchial gland and congenital thyroid abnormalities in man. J Pathol 159:135–141, 1989.
132. Eales J: Thyroid functions in cyclostomes and fishes. *In* Barrington E (ed): Hormones and Evolution, vol 1. New York, Academic Press, 1979, pp 341–436.
133. Ericson LE, Fredriksson G: Phylogeny and ontogeny of the thyroid gland. *In* Greer M (ed): The Thyroid Gland. New York, Raven, 1990, pp 1–35.
134. Dunn A: Properties of an iodinating enzyme in ascidian endostyle. Gen Comp Endocrinol 40:484–493, 1979.
135. Venkatesh TV, Holland ND, Holland LZ, et al: Sequence and developmental expression of amphioxus AmphiNk2–1: Insights into the evolutionary origin of the vertebrate thyroid gland and forebrain. Dev Genes Evol 209:254–259, 1999.
136. Kozmik Z, Holland ND, Kalousova A, et al: Characterization of an amphioxus paired box gene, AmphiPax2/5/8: Developmental expression patterns in optic support cells, nephridium, thyroid-like structures and pharyngeal gill slits, but not in the midbrain-hindbrain boundary region. Development 126:1295–1304, 1999.
137. Ristoratore F, Spagnuolo A, Aniello F, et al: Expression and functional analysis of *Cittf1*, an ascidian *NK-2* class gene, suggest its role in endoderm development. Development 126:5149–5159, 1999.

Chapter 91

Thyrotropin-Releasing Hormone and Thyroid-Stimulating Hormone

Maurice F. Scanlon

Thyrotropin (thyroid-stimulating hormone [TSH]), a glycoprotein hormone, is responsible for normal thyroid function. It is synthesized and secreted by thyrotrophs in the anterior pituitary gland, which are controlled in part by the hypothalamus via thyrotropin-releasing hormone (TRH) and other molecules.

The hypothalamus exerts stimulatory control over thyroid function through the mediation of TSH because hypothyroidism occurs if the hypothalamus is lesioned or diseased or if the pituitary stalk is transected. This stimulatory hypothalamic control is exerted by TRH, a small tripeptide produced by hypothalamic neurons and transported along their axons to specialized nerve terminals in the median eminence of the hypothalamus, where it is released into hypophysial portal blood. It is then carried directly to the anterior pituitary gland. The other major component of the hypothalamic-pituitary-thyroid axis is the powerful inhibitory action of circulating thyroid hormones. This inhibition is exerted primarily on thyrotrophs but also to a lesser extent on TRH-producing neurons of the hypothalamus (Fig. 91–1). In addition, a variety of secondary modulators exert lesser control over TSH secretion, the net result of which is the maintenance of a steady output of TSH and therefore thyroid hormones. Important secondary modulators are somatostatin and dopamine, both of which contribute to inhibition of the function of thyrotrophs, and α-adrenergic pathways, which are, in general, stimulatory. Other modulators of thyroid function include glucocorticoid hormones, the adipocyte-derived peptide leptin, various cytokines, and other inflammatory mediators.

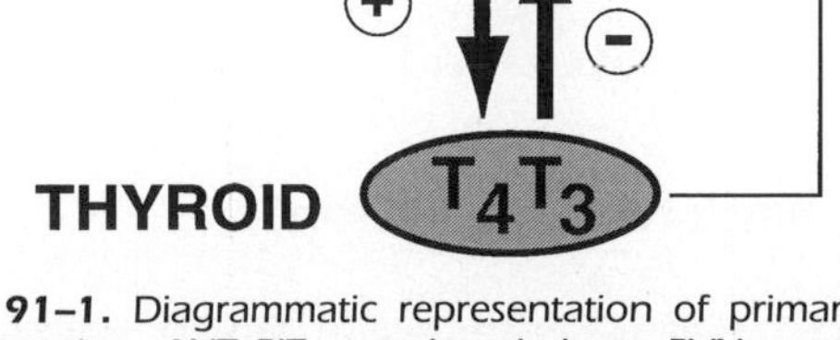

FIGURE 91–1. Diagrammatic representation of primary regulators of thyroid function. ANT PIT, anterior pituitary; PVN, paraventricular nucleus; T_3, triiodothyronine; T_4, thyroxine; TRH, thyrotropin-releasing hormone; TSH, thyroid-stimulating hormone. (From Scanlon MF, Toft AD: Regulation of thyrotropin secretion. *In* Braverman LE, Utiger RD (eds): The Thyroid: A Fundamental and Clinical Text, ed 8. Philadelphia, Lippincott Williams & Wilkins, 1996.)

PHYSIOLOGY OF THYROTROPIN-RELEASING HORMONE

Although the existence of TRH was first suggested about five decades ago,[1] it was not until 15 years later that a porcine hypothalamic extract with TSH-releasing properties was isolated.[2] Elucidation of the structure and subsequent synthesis of porcine[3] and ovine[4] TRH established its nature as the weakly basic tripeptide pyroglutamyl-histidyl prolinamide (Fig. 91–2). The biologic activity of synthetic TRH is identical to that of the natural molecule, which exhibits a lack of phylogenetic specificity common to several other hypothalamic regulatory peptides. The importance of TRH in the maintenance of normal thyroid function and interaction with other neuroregulators of TSH secretion is well established and is also reviewed elsewhere.[5] In addition to its actions on the thyrotroph, TRH may play a physiologic role in the stimulation of prolactin (PRL) release, stimulates growth hormone (GH) release in certain pathophysiologic and experimental conditions (Table 91–1), and can stimulate adrenocorticotropic hormone (ACTH) release in some patients with Cushing's disease. It is also widely distributed throughout the extrahypothalamic brain, spinal cord, pancreatic islets, and other body tissues and probably has important neuromodulatory and paracrine roles in these areas (Table 91–2). This view is supported by evidence from the TRH-deficient knockout mouse, which develops not only hypothyroidism, reversible by TRH, but also hyperglycemia and reduced insulin responses to glucose.[6]

Synthesis and Metabolism

TRH, like other more complex peptides, is derived from posttranslational cleavage of a larger precursor molecule.[7, 8] Investigation of the synthesis of TRH proved difficult for many years, in part because antibodies to this small peptide do not cross-react with precursor molecules. However, antibodies to a peptide sequence present in the pro-TRH molecule, deduced from cloned amphibian skin cDNA,[8] cross-react with neuronal perikarya in the parvocellular division of the medulla oblongata of rats.[7] Similar antibodies have been used to characterize the mammalian (rat) TRH prohormone, and both TRH and pro-TRH have been found in neurons of the paraventricular nucleus, whereas only TRH is present in axon terminals in the median eminence.[7, 9] The cDNA sequence of the rat TRH precursor encodes a protein with a molecular size of 29,247 Da that contains five copies of the sequence Glu-His-Pro-Gly.[10] Rat pro-TRH is processed at paired basic residues to a family of peptides including TRH and flanking and

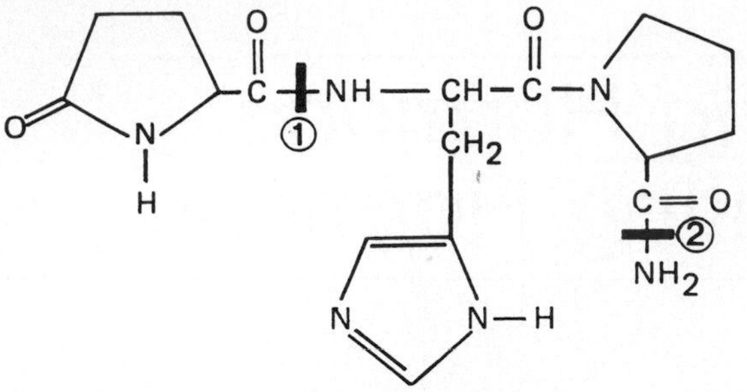

FIGURE 91–2. Structure of thyrotropin-releasing hormone (TRH) and pyroglutamyl-histidyl-prolinamide. Metabolic degradation occurs at site 1 via membrane-bound pyroglutamyl aminopeptidase and at site 2 via TRH deamidase. DA, dopamine; GH, growth hormone; IGF-1, insulin-like growth factor-1; PRL, proline; SS, somatostatin; T_3, triiodothyronine; T_4, thyroxine; TSH, thyroid-stimulating hormone. (From Scanlon MF: Thyroid stimulating hormone. *In* Braverman LE, Utiger RD (eds): The Thyroid: A Fundamental and Clinical Text. Philadelphia, JB Lippincott, 1991, pp 230–256.)

intervening sequences. These peptides may prove to exert important intracellular or extracellular actions,[11, 12] particularly prepro-TRH (160–169), which stimulates TSH gene expression. Indeed, the potentiating effect of this peptide on TRH-induced TSH secretion may be mediated by folliculostellate cells in the anterior pituitary.[13, 14] Pro-TRH may be preferentially processed to produce different peptides in different brain regions.[9]

The gene encoding human prepro-TRH was isolated, cloned, and sequenced from a human lung fibroblast genomic DNA library with the use of a rat prepro-TRH cDNA fragment. Exon 3 contains six copies of the TRH sequence vs. five copies in the rat, and human prepro-TRH contains 242 amino acids whereas the rat molecule contains 255 amino acids. Corresponding homologies with the rat are 73.3% and 59.5% at the nucleic acid and amino acid levels, respectively.[15] Further studies have assigned the gene encoding human prepro-TRH to chromosome 3.[16]

TRH is rapidly degraded to TRH free acid, the stable cyclized metabolite histidyl-proline-diketopiperazine (His-Pro-DKP; cyclo[His-Pro]) and its constituent amino acids.[17, 18] TRH is hydrolyzed at the pyro-Glu-His bond (see Fig. 91–2) by a particulate enzyme, pyroglutamyl aminopeptidase, that is present in synaptosomal and anterior pituitary membrane preparations. This enzyme is similar to the serum-degrading enzyme in that it has great specificity for TRH.[19, 20]

Cyclo(His-Pro) has several pharmacologic actions in rats, including inhibition of dopamine uptake and Na^+,K^+-ATPase activity by brain synaptosomes,[21] and TRH may act as a prohormone for about 50% of this molecule in the rodent hypothalamus and cortex. However, it is generated independently in other brain regions as indicated by studies using the TRH knockout mouse.[22] Also, cyclo(His-Pro) can be absorbed in sufficient quantities from certain foods to achieve biologically significant levels.[23] The relevance of these observations to human physiology is unknown.

TABLE 91–1. Paradoxic Growth Hormone Responses to Thyrotropin-Releasing Hormone

Normal subjects	After GnRH administration, after H_1 agonist drugs, full-term fetus
Endocrine	Acromegaly, primary hypothyroidism (children), diabetes mellitus, carcinoid syndrome, during GnRH infusion
Neuropsychiatric	Anorexia nervosa, depression, schizophrenia
Metabolic	Chronic liver disease, chronic renal failure, protein-calorie malnutrition, thalassemia
Experimental (rats)	Hypothalamic destruction, ectopic pituitary transplantation, hypothyroidism

GnRH, gonadotropin-releasing hormone.

TABLE 91–2. CNS or CNS-Mediated Pharmacologic Actions of Thyrotropin-Releasing Hormone

- Basic neuronal actions
  - Alters firing rate of certain neurons
  - Stimulates rhythmic electrical activity in nucleus tractus solitarius
  - Increases norepinephrine turnover
  - Increases acetylcholine turnover
  - Stimulates dopamine release in nucleus accumbens
  - Acute depolarization of cultured LMNs
  - LMN trophic factor
- Behavioral and vegetative actions
  - Increased locomotor activity (nucleus accumbens)
  - Stimulates respiration (brain stem)
  - Hyperthermia (nucleus accumbens)
  - Suppresses feeding and drinking behavior (ICV)
- Brain-gut actions (vagal cholinergic mechanism)
  - Stimulates gastrointestinal motility (ICV)
  - Increases gastric acid, pepsin, and exocrine pancreatic secretion (ICV)
- Interactions with other drugs and neuropeptides
  - Antagonizes narcosis induced by certain depressant drugs (e.g., pentobarbital and ethanol)
  - Antagonizes the hypothalamic and anti-nociceptive action of neurotensin (ICV and peripheral)
  - Antagonizes the hypothalamic and cataleptic effects of opiates without affecting analgesia (ICV and peripheral)

ICV, intracerebroventricular; LMN, lower motor neuron.

The plasma half-life of TRH is short and ranges from about 2 minutes in thyrotoxic animals to 6 minutes in hypothyroid ones.[24] These differences may be due to the effects of thyroid status on membrane-bound pyroglutamyl aminopeptidase because levels of serum pyroglutamyl aminopeptidase, which also shows high stereospecificity for TRH, are independent of thyroid status.[25] Gene expression and activity of the anterior pituitary TRH-degrading enzyme are rapidly and potently stimulated by thyroid hormones, counterbalanced by an inhibitory effect of estrogen, whereas in the brain, TRH-degrading activity is unaffected.[26–29] This effect is entirely appropriate to the differing roles of TRH within the pituitary and brain. The potency of the thyroid hormone effect on the degradation of TRH by anterior pituitary membranes indicates that this activity is probably an important regulatory mechanism.

Immunoreactive TRH is widely distributed in the hypothalamus, particularly high concentrations being found in the median eminence and in the nuclei of the so-called thyrotropic area or parvocellular division of the paraventricular nucleus, which is a major site of origin of immunoreactive TRH in the median eminence. Lesions of the paraventricular nuclei reduce circulating TSH levels and TSH responses to primary hypothyroidism but increase TRH levels in the nucleus of the tractus solitarius[7, 30–32]; this finding indicates that TRH fibers in this region do not arise in the hypothalamus. TRH and TRH-positive nerve fibers are present in posterior pituitary tissue, and lesions of the thyrotropic area of the hypothalamus reduce TRH levels in both the anterior and posterior pituitary glands.[33, 34] These two observations indicate that the hypothalamus is the source of most immunoreactive TRH in these areas. However, as with several other hypothalamic peptides, the TRH gene is expressed in both normal and adenomatous human anterior pituitary tissue, which can therefore synthesize and secrete very small amounts of immunoreactive TRH.[35, 36] The functional relevance of these observations is unknown, although a paracrine role in the control of pituitary function seems most likely.

Control of Thyrotrope Function

The dominant stimulatory role of the hypothalamus in the control of TSH synthesis and release is mediated by TRH. The direct dose-related action of TRH on TSH release is well known both in vivo and in vitro,[33, 37, 38] and decreased TSH release and hypothyroidism follow hypothalamic-pituitary dissociation by hypothalamic lesions and diseases.[33] This action of TRH occurs at nanomolar concentrations and is mediated by specific high-affinity receptors. TRH is released from nerve terminals in the median eminence into hypophysial portal blood at physiologically relevant concentrations, and sheep in which antibodies to TRH are raised show a decline in thyroid function.[33, 39, 40]

Intravenous administration of 15 to 500 μg of TRH to normal humans causes a dose-related release of TSH from the pituitary. The serum TSH response to TRH given intravenously to normal subjects is detectable within 2 to 5 minutes after TRH administration and is maximal at 20 to 30 minutes, and serum TSH levels return to basal levels by 2 to 3 hours. An elevation in serum thyroid hormone levels follows, with peak serum triiodothyronine (T_3) and thyroxine (T_4) concentrations occurring about 3 and 8 hours, respectively, after TRH administration. In addition to stimulating TSH release, TRH also stimulates TSH synthesis by promoting transcription and translation of the β subunit of the TSH gene.[40–44] The transcriptional protein Pit-1 mediates this stimulatory effect of TRH.[45] Pit-1 is a pituitary-specific transcription factor that also regulates the development and cell-specific expression of the PRL and GH genes and mediates the action of TRH on PRL gene expression in GH_3 cells.[46, 47] Consequently, mutations of the Pit-1 gene are associated with congenital TSH deficiency, as well as deficient function of lactotropes and somatotropes.[48, 49]

TRH plays an important role in the posttranslational processing of the oligosaccharide moieties of TSH and hence exerts an important influence on the biologic activity of the TSH that is secreted.[50, 51] Full glycosylation of TSH is required for complete biologic activity, as assessed by stimulation of adenylate cyclase activity in thyroid membrane preparations or by generation of cyclic adenosine monophosphate (cAMP) in functional rat thyroid (FRTL-5) cells.[52–54] Receptor binding, however, is not impaired by deglycosylation, thus indicating some alternative mechanism for reduced agonist activity.[55] In early studies TRH was found to have differential effects on the glycosylation of TSH and translation of TSH gene products,[56] and subsequent studies showed that TRH can modify the sialic acid, sulfate, and carbohydrate components of TSH.[50] These findings explain the clinical observation that some patients with central hypothyroidism and slightly elevated basal serum TSH levels secrete TSH with reduced biologic activity[57] and that long-term TRH administration increases TSH biologic activity in some of these patients.[58] This situation is analogous to that of the TRH knockout mouse, in which hypothyroidism develops as a result of the production of TSH with reduced biologic activity; the hypothyroidism is reversible by the administration of TRH.[6] Alterations in both hypothalamic TRH secretion and the response of thyrotrophs to TRH contribute to the variable biologic activity of the TSH secreted in different thyroid disorders[59, 60] and in patients with TSH-secreting pituitary adenomas.[61, 62]

Relationship with Thyroid Hormones

Although TRH acts in concert with the inhibitory hypothalamic regulators somatostatin and dopamine to control TSH synthesis and release, thyroid hormones exert the most important negative feedback control via direct pituitary inhibition of the thyrotroph (Fig. 91–3). In this process, local intrapituitary conversion of T_4 to T_3 is particularly important.

In addition to their direct inhibitory actions on TSH subunit gene expression and TSH release, thyroid hormones were shown by early studies to modulate the number of TRH receptors on thyrotrophs. TRH binding to anterior pituitary membranes from hypothyroid animals is increased twofold, and the increase can be reduced by thyroid hormone replacement.[63, 64] This effect is specific because epidermal growth factor and somatostatin receptors are not altered, thus indicating that regulation of TRH receptors by thyroid hormones is not secondary to general changes in membrane structure.[65] T_3 also decreases TRH receptors in TSH-secreting tumors in mice and GH/PRL-secreting GH_3 cells.[65, 66] Conversely, in GH_4C_1 cells, TRH itself causes a dose-related reduction in T_3 receptors and T_3 responsiveness[67] that may represent a further site of feedback interaction between T_3 and TRH at the pituitary level.

In addition to their direct effects on TSH and TRH receptor gene expression, thyroid hormones also exert powerful effects on hypothalamic function. Injection of nanomolar concentrations of T_3 into the hypothalamus of hypothyroid monkeys causes immediate inhibition of TSH release.[68] Whether this acute effect is due to inhibition of TRH secretion or to stimulation of somatostatin or dopamine secretion is unknown, although T_3 can stimulate immediate somatostatin release from hypothalamic tissue in vitro.[69] TRH mRNA levels in the paraventricular nucleus increase in hypothyroidism and are reduced by thyroid hormone treatment.[70, 71] Furthermore, rats with bilateral lesions of the paraventricular nuclei do not show the normal rise in serum TSH and TSH subunit mRNA after induction of primary hypothyroidism,[71] an effect that presumably reflects depletion of TRH. These results indicate that the paraventricular nuclei of the hypothalamus are a target for the action of thyroid hormones and therefore contribute to the neuroregulation of TSH secretion.

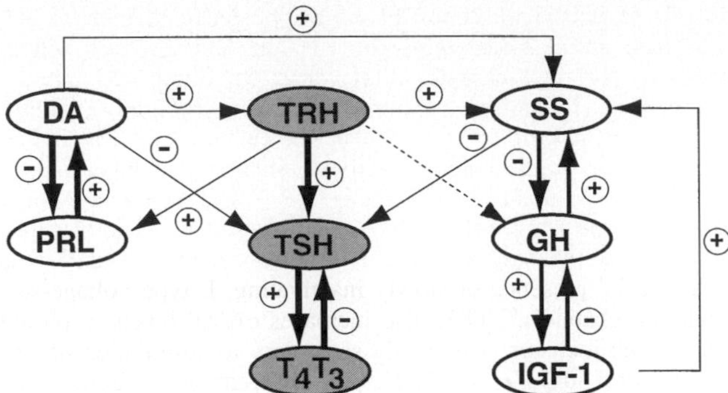

FIGURE 91–3. Schematic representation of the complex interactions that can occur between primary and secondary modulators of thyrotrope function. This figure is a summary of data available from in vivo and in vitro studies in animals and in humans. DA, dopamine; GH, growth hormone; IGF-1, insulin-like growth factor-1; PRL, proline; SS, somatostatin; T_3, triiodothyronine; T_4, thyroxine; TRH, thyrotropin-releasing hormone; TSH, thyroid-stimulating hormone. (From Scanlon MF, Toft AD: Regulation of thyrotropin secretion. *In* Braverman LE, Utiger RD (eds): The Thyroid: A Fundamental and Clinical Text, ed 8. Philadelphia, Lippincott Williams & Wilkins, 1996.)

Mechanism of Action

TRH binds to specific, high-affinity receptors on anterior pituitary membranes, and the TRH receptor is a member of the family of G protein–coupled receptors containing seven membrane-spanning domains and an extracellular N-terminal region with *N*-glycosylation sites.[73–77] The gene encoding the human TRH receptor spans 35 kb and contains three exons and two introns. The 541-bp intron 1 is conserved between the human and mouse.[77] A novel subtype of rat TRH receptor (TRHR2) has recently been cloned and characterized.[78, 79] This gene shares only 50% homology with the pituitary TRH receptor gene and is differentially expressed: whereas the pituitary TRH receptor is expressed in the anterior pituitary, the hypothalamus, and the ventral spinal cord, TRHR2 is expressed only in the dorsal horn of the spinal cord and the spinothalamic tract, where it may subserve the sensory, antinociceptive actions of TRH.[78] A hydrophobic amino acid cluster between transmembrane helixes 5 and 6 holds the TRH receptor in an inactive conformation, and the relative position of these two transmembrane elements is altered after TRH binding to activate the receptor.[80] Studies using fluorescent tagging and confocal microscopy have demonstrated rapid internalization of the TRH–TRH receptor complex via clathrin-coated vesicles after ligand binding.[81–83] The receptor is then recycled to the plasma membrane, the whole process being dependent on the integrity of the intracellular C terminus of the receptor.[83]

Much of the work on the secondary message events involved in TRH action has been performed on GH_3 cells and mouse thyrotroph tumor cells. In these systems TRH stimulates the activity of phospholipase C by coupling to the pertussis toxin–sensitive guanosine triphosphate–binding proteins G_s, G_q, and G_{11}.[84, 85] This action causes rapid hydrolysis of phosphatidylinositol 4,5-bisphosphate to inositol 1,4,5-bisphosphate and 1,2-diacylglycerol.[86, 87] The latter in turn activates intracellular protein kinase C. TRH causes an immediate, rapid increase in intracellular free calcium (which decays rapidly), followed by an extended plateau of intracellular free calcium.[88–92] This biphasic action correlates with secretory activity, electrical changes, and the induction of ^{45}Ca fluxes in GH_3 cells.[89, 93–96] The first phase reflects increased release from intracellular stores caused by inositol triphosphate, whereas the second phase is due to calcium influx[91, 92] and depends on the presence of slowly inactivating, L-type voltage-sensitive calcium channels.[97] TRH also increases cAMP levels in pituitary tissue, but the increase is probably secondary to stimulation of phosphatidylinositol turnover by TRH.[98] In different brain regions, TRH selectively stimulates either cAMP generation or phosphatidylinositol turnover.[99] This diversity indicates that TRH receptors are functionally linked to different intracellular pathways in different sites, which may be relevant to the different subtypes of TRH receptor described above.

Continuous TRH administration both in vivo and in vitro causes marked homologous desensitization of TSH and PRL responses.[100–102] Because this secretory refractoriness occurs in vitro, it cannot be explained by the increase in serum T_4 and T_3 concentrations that accompanies TRH administration in vivo. The biphasic pattern of the TSH response and intracellular free calcium levels to maximal doses of TRH in mouse thyrotropic tumor cells is determined by the number of TRH receptors; downregulation of TRH receptors abolishes the early secretory burst of TSH release and the intracellular free calcium elevation.[103, 104] Also, the inositol triphosphate response to TRH displays homologous desensitization, whereas the intracellular free calcium response displays heterologous desensitization inasmuch as depletion of intracellular calcium stores prevents responses to other stimuli.[105] In anterior pituitary tissue, in TSH-secreting tumors in mice, and in GH_3 cells, TRH can reduce the number of its own receptors after chronic exposure.[65, 104, 106] In GH_3 cells this reduction in receptors is preceded by a decrease in TRH receptor mRNA mediated by protein kinase C.[107, 108] However, neither this mechanism nor rapid internalization of the TRH–TRH receptor complex fully explains the acute desensitization of hormonal responses to TRH, for which other mechanisms have been proposed: uncoupling of the receptor from phospholipase C, which is dependent on the presence of the intracellular C terminus of the receptor.[109] Nevertheless, at least some desensitization is dependent on protein kinase C because staurosporine, a potent inhibitor of protein kinase C, can attenuate the TRH-induced refractoriness of inositol phospholipid hydrolysis in rat anterior pituitary tissue.[110] Therefore, protein kinase C may participate in an intracellular feedback system to limit hydrolysis of inositol phospholipids (Fig. 91–4).

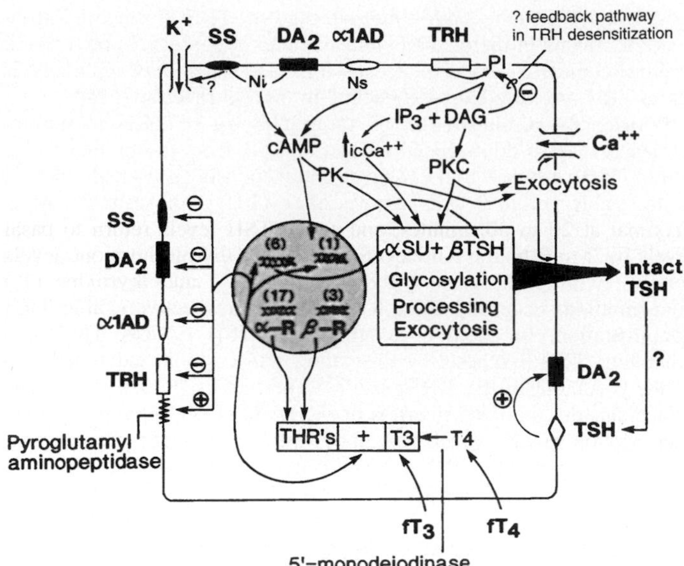

FIGURE 91–4. Thyroid hormones reduce the biologic actions of somatostatin (SS), dopamine (DA), epinephrine, and thyrotropin-releasing hormone (TRH) because of a reduction in number rather than affinity of DA_2, TRH, and α_1-adrenergic (αAD) receptors, and the same may well apply to SS receptors. These actions and the stimulation of pyroglutamyl aminopeptidase by triiodothyronine (T_3) are due to binding of the activated thyroid hormone receptor (TRH) to relevant parts of the genome. Diacylglycerol may participate in feedback inhibition of the functional response to TRH receptor agonism and cause apparent TRH desensitization. TRH and αAD agonism exert additive effects on thyroid-stimulating hormone (TSH) release, thus indicating separate intracellular pathways. The numbers in parentheses indicate the chromosomal origin of the α and β thyroid hormone receptors. T_4, thyroxine. (From Scanlon MF: Thyroid stimulating hormone. *In* Braverman LE, Utiger RD (eds): The Thyroid: A Fundamental and Clinical Text. Philadelphia, JB Lippincott, 1991, pp 230–256.)

OTHER REGULATORS OF THYROID-STIMULATING HORMONE SECRETION

Somatostatin

Somatostatin, which is the major physiologic inhibitor of GH secretion, was initially isolated and characterized from ovine hypothalamus on the basis of its ability to inhibit GH release from anterior pituitary tissue. In addition, somatostatin is an inhibitor of TSH secretion in both animals and humans. Somatostatin-producing hypothalamic neurons are found mainly in the anterior periventricular region. About half the somatostatin in the median eminence arises from the preoptic region, and the remainder arises from the suprachiasmatic and retrochiasmatic regions. A lower density of somatostatin-producing neurons is present in the ventromedial and arcuate nuclei and also in the lateral hypothalamus. The somatostatin gene[111, 112] is widely expressed throughout the extrahypothalamic nervous system and other tissues, where somatostatin exerts a wide array of inhibitory actions. It is secreted in two principal forms: a 14–amino acid peptide (somatostatin-14) and an N-terminal extended peptide (somatostatin-28). Its precursor, preprosomatostatin, is a 116–amino acid peptide[112, 113] that undergoes differential posttranslational processing in different tissues to yield varying amounts of the 14– and 28–amino acid forms of the hormone. Each of these forms is secreted into hypophysial portal blood in physiologically relevant concentrations.[114]

During studies of the effects of somatostatin on other anterior pituitary hormones it was found to inhibit basal and TRH-stimulated TSH release from cultured rat anterior pituitary cells. This finding led to the proposal that TSH release was regulated by the hypothalamus through a dual control system, stimulation by TRH and inhibition by somatostatin, analogous to that demonstrated for GH regulation.[115] The physiologic relevance of this proposal was established in studies using antiserum directed against somatostatin. Incubation of anterior pituitary cells with antisomatostatin serum causes increased secretion of TSH (as well as GH), and administration of antiserum to rats increases basal serum TSH concentrations and serum TSH responses to both cold stress and TRH.[116, 117] In humans, somatostatin administration reduces the elevated serum TSH concentrations in patients with primary hypothyroidism, reduces the serum TSH response to TRH, abolishes the nocturnal elevation in TSH secretion, and prevents TSH release after the administration of dopamine antagonist drugs. Somatostatin-14 and somatostatin-28 exert equipotent effects on TSH release.[118] Furthermore, GH administration in humans decreases basal and TRH-stimulated TSH secretion, probably because of the direct stimulatory effects of GH on hypothalamic somatostatin release. In patients with pituitary disease, TSH secretory status correlates inversely with GH secretory status. Despite these potent acute inhibitory effects of somatostatin on TSH secretion in humans, long-term treatment with somatostatin or the long-acting analogue octreotide does not result in hypothyroidism, presumably because the great sensitivity of thyrotrophs to any decrease in serum thyroid hormone concentration overrides the inhibitory effect of somatostatin in the long term.

Somatostatin binds to at least five distinct types of specific high-affinity receptors that are variably expressed in the anterior pituitary, brain, and other tissues. The receptor subtypes differ in binding specificities, molecular weight, and linkage to adenylyl cyclase through the inhibitory subunit of the guanine nucleotide regulatory protein. However, somatostatin may also act independently of cAMP by inducing hyperpolarization of membranes through modulation of voltage-dependent potassium channels leading to reduced calcium influx and a fall in intracellular calcium levels.[119]

Neurotransmitters

An extensive network of neurotransmitter neurons terminates on the cell bodies of the hypophysiotropic neurons and within the interstitial spaces of the median eminence, where they regulate neuropeptide release into hypophysial portal blood. In addition, dopamine (and possibly other neurotransmitters) is released directly into hypophysial portal blood and exerts direct actions on anterior pituitary cells, particularly as the major physiologic inhibitor of PRL release, but to a lesser extent as a physiologic inhibitor of TSH release.

Studies using central neurotransmitter agonist and antagonist drugs have indicated the existence of stimulatory α-adrenergic and inhibitory dopaminergic pathways in the control of TSH secretion in rats. α-Adrenergic agonists injected systemically or into the third ventricle stimulate TSH release, and α-adrenergic antagonists or catecholamine-depleting drugs block TSH responses to cold.[120] More precisely, it appears that α_2-adrenergic pathways are stimulatory whereas α_1-adrenergic pathways are inhibitory.[121] It has been assumed from such in vivo studies that these neurotransmitter effects are mediated by appropriate modulation of the release of TRH, somatostatin, or both into hypophysial portal blood. A clear example is that the acute TSH release that follows cold stress in rats can be abolished by pretreatment with either anti-TRH antibodies or α-adrenergic antagonists, thus suggesting that adrenergically stimulated TRH release mediates this effect.[33]

However, the results of in vitro studies using rat hypothalamic tissue are not in keeping with this attractive and simple hypothesis. For example, dopamine and dopamine agonist drugs stimulate both TRH and somatostatin release from the rat hypothalamus by acting through the DA_2 class of dopamine receptor.[122, 123] This effect may reflect a general action of DA_2 receptors to mediate enhanced neuropeptide release at the level of the median eminence, in contrast to the usual inhibitory action of DA_2 agonists at the level of the anterior pituitary.

Although little precise knowledge exists about central mechanisms, it is clear that dopamine and epinephrine exert opposing actions on TSH release directly at the anterior pituitary level. Furthermore, both these molecules are present in rat hypophysial portal blood in higher concentrations than in peripheral blood and in concentrations that could exert physiologic actions on thyrotrophs.[124, 125] Dopamine inhibits TSH release from rat[126] and bovine[127] anterior pituitary cells in a dose-related, stereospecific way, and a striking parallelism is seen between the inhibition of TSH and PRL by dopamine and dopamine agonist drugs. As with PRL, this inhibitory action on TSH release is mediated by DA_2 receptors that are negatively coupled to adenylyl cyclase[128] (see Fig. 91–4). TSH release by thyrotroph cells from hypothyroid animals is more sensitive to the inhibitory effects of dopamine, which may reflect increased DA_2 receptor number rather than affinity.[129] In contrast, the sensitivity of PRL to the inhibitory effects of dopamine is reduced in lactotroph cells from hypothyroid animals,[129] a phenomenon that may contribute to the hyperprolactinemia that occurs in some patients with primary hypothyroidism.

Evidence from in vitro studies using rat anterior pituitary cells suggests that TSH may specifically regulate its own release via induction of DA_2 receptors on thyrotroph cells.[130] These data indicate a mechanism for the ultrashort-loop feedback control of TSH secretion that is dependent on functional integrity of the hypothalamic-pituitary axis and consequent catecholamine supply (see Fig. 91–4).

In addition to its acute inhibitory effects on TSH secretion in vitro, dopamine also decreases the levels of α and β subunit TSH mRNA and gene transcription by up to 75% in cultured anterior pituitary cells from hypothyroid rats. These effects occur within a few minutes and can be reversed by the activation of adenylyl cyclase with forskolin.[131] Similar actions of dopamine have been described in relation to PRL gene expression.

In contrast to dopamine, adrenergic activation stimulates TSH release by cultured rat and bovine anterior pituitary cells in a dose-related stereospecific fashion. This effect is mediated by high-affinity, α_1-adrenoreceptors,[132–134] and both α_1-adrenoreceptors and α_1-adrenoreceptor–mediated TSH release are reduced in cells from hypothyroid animals.[135] Quantitatively, the adrenergic release of TSH is almost equivalent to that induced by TRH[132]; together, at maximal dosage these two agents have additive effects on TSH release, which is an indication of activation of separate intracellular pathways. It is likely that dopamine and epinephrine exert their direct actions on thyrotrophs by opposing actions on cAMP generation, with DA_2 receptors being negatively linked to adenylyl cyclase and α_1-adrenoreceptors being positively linked.

In humans, it is well established that dopamine has a physiologic inhibitory role in the control of TSH release, and some data suggest a stimulatory α-adrenergic pathway. In contrast to the situation in animals, evidence for direct effects of dopaminergic and adrenergic manipulation on TSH release by normal human pituitary cells is lacking. Data from the use of dopamine, dopamine agonists, and specific dopamine receptor antagonist drugs such as domperidone, which does not penetrate the blood-brain barrier to any appreciable extent, suggest that dopamine-induced decreases in TSH secretion are a direct pituitary or median eminence action mediated by the DA_2 class of dopamine receptors.[136]

The dopaminergic inhibition of TSH release varies according to sex, thyroid status, time of day, and PRL secretory status. TSH release after endogenous dopamine disinhibition with dopamine receptor–blocking drugs such as metoclopramide and domperidone is greater in women than in men. It is assumed that estrogens determine this effect, but the mechanism of action is unknown. Dopaminergic inhibition of TSH release, like the stimulation of TSH release by TRH, is also greater in patients with mild or subclinical hypothyroidism than in normal subjects or severely hypothyroid patients.[137] The mechanisms that underlie this biphasic relationship between the dopaminergic inhibition of TSH release and thyroid status are not known, but data from in vitro studies of anterior pituitary cells from hypothyroid rats suggest an increase in dopamine receptor capacity rather than affinity.[129] Also, the concentration of dopamine in the hypophysial portal blood of thyroidectomized rats is greater than that of sham-operated rats because of increased activity of tyrosine hydroxylase in the median eminence, an effect that can be reversed by thyroid hormone replacement.[138, 139] In addition to its effects on the release of TSH, dopamine also inhibits the release of TSH α and β subunits, the greatest effect occurring in patients with primary hypothyroidism.[136]

Only limited data are available on the adrenergic control of TSH release in humans. α-Adrenergic blockade with phentolamine, which does not readily cross the blood-brain barrier, or with thymoxamine, which does, inhibits the serum TSH response to TRH[140] and reduces but does not abolish the nocturnal rise in TSH secretion.[141] Overall, these data suggest a small stimulatory role for endogenous adrenergic pathways in TSH control in humans. However, adrenergic activation with epinephrine or α-amphetamine and β-adrenoreceptor blockade with propranolol do not influence the serum TSH response to TRH.[142, 143] The catecholaminergic control of TSH secretion appears to act as a fine-tuning mechanism rather than being of primary importance, which is not to say that the effects of catecholamines are so small as to be without consequence. For example, acute dopaminergic blockade in humans releases enough TSH to elicit the subsequent release of thyroid hormones. As with somatostatin agonist analogues, however, chronic administration of catecholaminergic drugs does not lead to long-term alterations in thyroid status because of the action of compensatory mechanisms to maintain TSH secretion and euthyroidism.

Other Neurotransmitters, Neuropeptides, and Cytokines

The role of the serotoninergic system in the control of TSH release in animals and humans is unclear, both stimulatory and inhibitory actions having been described.[120, 144] Opioid pathways appear to play an important role in the inhibitory control of TSH secretion in rats. Opioid peptides decrease basal TSH secretion, and their action can be blocked by the specific antagonist naloxone,[145] which also blocks the stress-induced fall in TSH secretion.[146] In humans, however, endogenous opioids may have a stimulatory effect on TSH secretion, especially during the nocturnal TSH surge.[147] A variety of other neuropeptides, including neurotensin, vasoactive intestinal polypeptide, bombesin, vasopressin, oxytocin, substance P, and cholecystokinin, can produce small alterations in TSH secretion both in vitro and in vivo in animals, but the lack of suitable specific antagonist drugs has not allowed adequate physiologic studies to be undertaken. These molecules should be added to the list of agents that can affect TSH secretion, but their physiologic relevance is uncertain.

Tumor necrosis factor (TNF, cachectin) is a peptide produced by macrophages that acts as an inflammatory mediator and can cause many of the clinical phenomena that accompany severe systemic illness. Interleukin-1 (IL-1) is a cytokine produced by many cells, including monocytes, that stimulates B and T lymphocytes to produce a range of other cytokines and lymphokines. Both TNF and IL-1β inhibit TSH secretion in rats and mice,[148–150] and IL-1β causes a relative reduction in TRH gene expression in the paraventricular nucleus that is inappropriate in the face of low thyroid hormone concentrations.[151] Similar suppression of the hypothalamic-pituitary-thyroid axis occurs in rats treated with bacterial lipopolysaccharide, an effect that is independent of activation of the hypothalamic-pituitary-adrenal axis.[152]

These molecules each produce a biochemical pattern similar to what occurs in patients with acute nonthyroidal illness,[153, 154] and they also activate the hypothalamic-pituitary-adrenal axis,[155–157] probably via stimulation of the release of hypothalamic corticotropin-releasing hormone.[158] This family of molecules plays a crucial role in mediating and coordinating the thyroidal and adrenal responses to nonthyroidal illness. IL-1β is produced by rat anterior pituitary cells, and its release can be stimulated by bacterial lipopolysaccharide. It colocalizes with TSH in thyrotroph cells.[159] Presumably, IL-1β subserves an important autocrine or paracrine role in anterior pituitary control, as has been suggested for the IL-1–dependent cytokine IL-6, which is also produced by rat anterior pituitary cells,[160] particularly folliculostellate cells.[161]

PHYSIOLOGIC CHANGES IN THYROID-STIMULATING HORMONE RELEASE

Alterations in TSH secretion may be manifested in the pattern and degree of change in basal TSH secretion or in the pattern and degree of serum TSH responses to TRH or dopamine receptor blockade.

Thyroid-Stimulating Hormone Rhythms

A clear circadian variation is evident in serum TSH concentrations. In most humans, serum TSH concentrations begin to rise several hours before the onset of sleep, reach maximal concentrations between 11 PM and 4 AM, and gradually decline thereafter, with the lowest concentrations occurring at about 11 AM. Concentrations during the nocturnal surge are sometimes slightly above the normal range reported by most clinical laboratories. Sleep itself modulates TSH secretion by reducing pulse amplitude rather than frequency,[162] but the underlying mechanisms are not clear. Furthermore, a seasonal variation in TSH secretion has been described in patients with primary hypothyroidism who are receiving T_4 therapy; some of these patients have higher basal serum TSH concentrations in the winter than in the summer.[163] This contrast may be a consequence of temperature effects on the peripheral metabolism of thyroid hormones, but such a difference was not found in euthyroid subjects.[164] Although some evidence indicates that estrogens can enhance and androgens reduce serum TSH responses to TRH,[165, 166] no sex-related difference in the amplitude or frequency of circadian TSH changes has been found.[164]

TSH is secreted in a pulsatile manner, with increases in pulse amplitude and frequency at night.[162, 167–170] Patients with severe primary hypothyroidism have increased pulse amplitude throughout the day but loss of the usual nocturnal increase in pulse amplitude. The pulses of TSH, α subunit, and the gonadotropins are concordant, consistent with the operation of a common hypothalamic pulse generator.[171]

The circadian and pulsatile changes in TSH secretion are not secondary to peripheral factors such as changes in serum T_4 and T_3 concentrations, hemoconcentration, or changes in cortisol secretion,[172] although the latter may modulate TSH rhythms. Furthermore, circadian changes in serum TSH concentrations can be detected in some patients with mild thyrotoxicosis,[173] which suggests that central mechanisms can to some extent override the powerful negative feedback effects of thyroid hormones at the pituitary level.

Basal serum TSH concentrations rise slightly after serum cortisol concentrations are lowered by 11β-hydroxylase inhibition with metyrapone,[174] which suggests that cortisol exerts a small inhibitory influence on TSH secretion. Furthermore, pharmacologic doses of glucocorticoids acutely inhibit basal TSH secretion and abolish the circadian variation in serum TSH concentration.[164] This mechanism may well explain the reduction in basal and TRH-stimulated serum TSH concentrations and in circadian TSH changes that occur in patients with depression,[175, 176] after major surgery,[177] and in nonthyroidal illness. Total abolition of the circadian rhythm of cortisol with metyrapone, however, did not cause disruption of the overall circadian TSH changes, although a small but significant decrease did occur in the acrophase and amplitude of the TSH profile.[178]

The central mechanisms that underlie TSH pulsatility and rhythmicity are unknown. Pulsatile TRH release does not appear to be involved in TSH pulse frequency, although it may influence amplitude.[179] Pulsatility is probably mediated in part by signals from the suprachiasmatic nuclei of the hypothalamus. These nuclei are paired structures situated just above the optic chiasm that initiate intrinsic circadian rhythmicity, the timing of which can be influenced by nonvisual nerve impulses arising in the retina. Although both dopamine and dopamine agonists acutely abolish the circadian change in TSH secretion, endogenous dopaminergic pathways probably do not play a role in determining the circadian changes in TSH secretion. The nocturnal increase in TSH secretion is not due to a decline in dopaminergic inhibition because dopaminergic inhibition of TSH release is greater at night than during the day. Dopamine is, however, a determinant of TSH pulse amplitude (but not frequency).[170] It appears that dopamine acts as a fine-tuning control to dampen TSH pulsatility, presumably to maintain basal TSH concentrations and hence thyroid function in as steady a state as possible. Why the serum TSH response to dopamine blockade is greater at night than during the day is not known. It is unlikely to be due to increased central dopaminergic activity because the serum PRL response to dopamine blockade is the same during the day and night.[172]

Similarly, α-adrenergic pathways do not play a primary role in determining TSH circadian rhythmicity because α-adrenergic blockade with thymoxamine, which penetrates the blood-brain barrier, did not affect the circadian pattern of TSH secretion, although serum TSH concentrations decreased slightly throughout the entire period of study.[141] TSH may regulate its own secretion through an increase in dopamine receptors at the level of the thyrotrophs,[130] a finding that could explain the higher serum TSH and unaltered serum PRL responses to dopamine blockade at the time of greatest TSH secretion.[172] A further possible contributor to the changes in circadian TSH secretion in rats is diurnal variation in the activity of anterior pituitary T_4 5′-deiodinase in this species.[180]

Temperature, Age, and Nutritional Status

Cold exposure in rats causes an acute rise in serum TSH concentration that is accompanied by an increase in hypothalamic TRH gene expression and increased TRH release.[181, 182] A similar phenomenon occurs in human neonates, but it is unusual in adults; when it does occur, the increase is very small. The cold-induced effect in rats can be abolished either by passive immunization with anti-TRH antibodies or by α-adrenergic blockade, thus indicating that adrenergic release of hypothalamic TRH mediates the phenomenon.[33] Cold exposure in rats also increases TRH mRNA levels in the dorsal motor and caudal raphe nuclei, which is evidence of a functional link between the autonomic and neuroendocrine systems involved in thermoregulation.[183] Lesions that affect the temperature-regulating center of the preoptic nucleus of the hypothalamus abolish the serum TSH response to cold stress but do not cause hypothyroidism.[120]

Aging itself causes a slight decrease in TSH secretion because of a resetting of the threshold of TSH inhibition by thyroid hormones as a result of increased pituitary conversion of T_4 to T_3, increased T_4 uptake by thyrotrophs, or decreased T_4 and T_3 clearance.[184] In one study of healthy elderly subjects, 5% had low basal serum TSH concentrations and a reduced serum TSH response to TRH.[185] In addition, TSH pulse amplitude was reduced with preservation of the frequency of pulsatility and the overall pattern of circadian change.[186] These data should introduce caution into the use of TSH assays alone for assessment of thyroid function in the elderly. The underlying mechanism is unclear, but the change in TSH secretion may reflect an adaptive mechanism to the reduced need for thyroid hormones in the elderly.[186]

Caloric restriction causes a small decrease in basal and TRH-stimulated serum TSH concentrations despite a decline in the serum T_3 concentration.[187] In rats this decrease is associated with reduced TSH-β mRNA levels together with reduced nitric oxide synthase and TRH gene expression in the paraventricular nucleus.[188–190] This change may be a consequence of enhanced adrenal secretion of corticosterone.[190] The components of the decrease in TSH secretion in humans are a reduction in the daytime serum TSH concentration and in the nocturnal increase in TSH secretion with an overall decrease in TSH pulse amplitude.[191] In the more extreme clinical setting of anorexia nervosa, the reduced basal and stimulated serum TSH concentrations may be a consequence of increased serum cortisol concentrations. Passive immunization with somatostatin antibodies reduces the starvation-induced decline in TSH secretion in rats,[192] thus indicating a mediating role of hypothalamic somatostatinergic pathways secondary to metabolic feedback signals (Fig. 91-5). Indeed, recent evidence indicates the critical role of leptin, a circulating peptide released by adipocytes, in mediating hypothalamic responses to starvation. The increased sensitivity of paraventricular TRH-producing neurons to negative feedback inhibition by lowered thyroid hormone levels in acutely fasted rats (in which leptin levels are low) is reversed by leptin administration. All these effects are dependent on the integrity of the connections between the arcuate and paraventricular nuclei and indicate an important feedback role for leptin in determining the set-point of

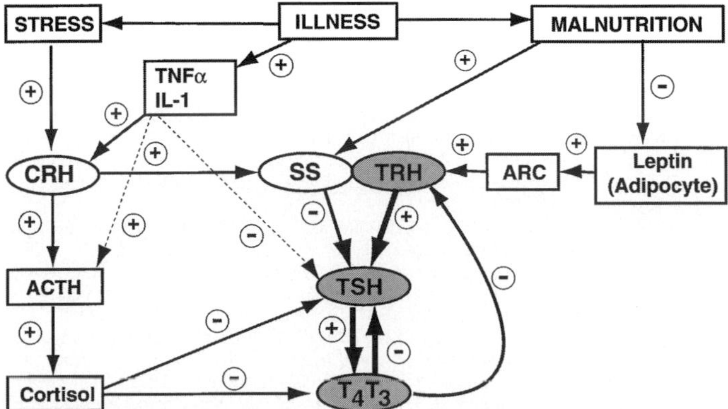

FIGURE 91–5. Schematic representation of probable interacting pathways involved in secondary alterations in hypothalamic-pituitary-thyroid function in response to illness. ACTH, adrenocorticotropic hormone; ARC, arcuate nucleus; CRH, corticotropin-releasing hormone; IL-1, interleukin-1; SS, somatostatin; T_3, triiodothyroxine; T_4, thyroxine; TNFα, tumor necrosis factor-α; TRH, thyrotropin-releasing hormone; TSH, thyroid-stimulating hormone. (From Scanlon MF, Toft AD: Regulation of thyrotropin secretion. *In* Braverman LE, Utiger RD (eds): The Thyroid: A Fundamental and Clinical Text, ed 8. Philadelphia, Lippincott Williams & Wilkins, 1996.)

sensitivity of paraventricular TRH neurons to thyroid hormones.[193, 194] When considered along with suppression of the GH and gonadal axes in acute fasting in rats, which are also reversed by leptin administration, this process can be seen as an important adaptive, energy-conserving mechanism in response to food shortage. The importance of these mechanisms in caloric restriction in humans is unknown, but it seems likely that leptin will also play an important role in mediating some of the adaptive responses to the malnutrition and enhanced catabolism associated with acute and chronic illness.

Stress, Nonthyroidal Illness, and Depression

In rats, stress causes an acute decline in serum TSH concentrations. In humans, surgical stress causes both transient, acute lowering of serum TSH and a longer-term abolition of the nocturnal increase in serum TSH. This decline in TSH occurs despite a fall in serum free T_3 concentrations but no change in serum free T_4 concentrations.[177, 195] In animals, both opioids and dopamine may play a role in this stress phenomenon, whereas in humans, glucocorticoids and dopamine have been implicated.[146, 177, 195] As with the effects of caloric restriction, these stress phenomena bear some resemblance to the altered neuroregulation of TSH that can occur in nonthyroidal illness and in certain neuropsychiatric disorders. Although basal serum TSH concentrations are usually normal in patients with both acute and chronic nonthyroidal illness, they may be either low or slightly raised.[196–198] In addition to the frequent use of pharmacologic agents such as glucocorticoids and dopamine that acutely inhibit TSH secretion, intrinsic central suppression of thyrotroph function is common, as illustrated by abolition of the nocturnal increase in serum TSH concentration in up to 60% of acutely ill patients in the presence of low serum free T_3 concentrations.[198, 199] However, true central hypothyroidism is rare in these patients, who usually but not always have normal serum free T_4 concentrations.[199, 200]

It seems clear that in addition to peripheral alterations in thyroid hormone economy usually manifested as low serum free T_3, high reverse T_3, and normal free T_4 concentrations, central suppression of thyrotroph function occurs in patients with severe nonthyroidal illness, for example, heart failure, infection, diabetes mellitus, and chronic renal failure. Indeed, the fall in free T_3 levels correlates with the severity of disease and predicts mortality, as does the much less commonly encountered fall in free T_4 levels.[201–203] The precise initiating signals and underlying mechanisms are unknown, although alterations in opioidergic, dopaminergic, and somatostatinergic activity may each contribute. In addition, peripheral glucocorticoid-mediated inhibitory feedback plays a role, particularly in acutely ill patients,[204] through activation of the cytokine pathways involving TNF-α and IL-1β, each of which inhibits TSH and stimulates ACTH release in animals,[148, 149] a mechanism that is central to the coordination of thyroidal and adrenal responses to stress and nonthyroidal illness. Finally, changes in leptin concentrations, which modulate adaptive hypothalamic responses to caloric restriction in animals, may well serve as an important metabolic feedback pathway in both acute and chronic nonthyroidal illness (see above and Fig. 91–5).

Alterations in TSH secretion occur in patients with anorexia nervosa and endogenous depression in the form of a reduced serum TSH response to TRH.[205, 206] Even more common is loss of the nocturnal increase in TSH secretion,[175] which together with low serum free thyroid hormones, ferritin, and sex hormone–binding globulin concentrations, may indicate central hypothyroidism. Once again, the mechanisms are unclear. Dopamine is not involved in central TSH suppression in anorexia nervosa, and both serum cortisol and body temperature changes have been implicated in depression.[175, 176]

The debate will probably continue about whether central hypothyroidism exists in patients with stress, severe nonthyroidal illness, depression, or anorexia nervosa. It is therefore of interest that thyroid hormone treatment of patients with nonthyroidal illness is of no benefit or may even be detrimental.[207] In contrast, thyroid hormone administration may enhance the therapeutic benefits of tricyclic antidepressant drug therapy in depression.[208]

REFERENCES

1. Greer MA: Evidence of hypothalamic control of the pituitary release of thyrotrophin. Proc Soc Exp Biol Med 77:603–608, 1951.
2. Schally AV, Bowers CY, Redding TW, Barrett JF: Isolation of thyrotropin releasing factor (TRF) from porcine hypothalamus. Biochem Biophys Res Commun 25:1651–1669, 1966.
3. Folkers K, Enzman F, Boler J, et al: Discovery of modification of the synthetic tripeptide sequence of the thyrotropin releasing hormone having activity. Biochem Biophys Res Commun 37:123–126, 1969.
4. Burgus R, Dunn TF, Desiderio D, et al: Characterisation of the hypothalamic hypophysiotropic TSH-releasing factor (TRF) of ovine origin. Nature 226:321–325, 1970.
5. Scanlon MF, Toft AD: Regulation of thyrotropin secretion. *In* Braverman LC, Utiger RD (eds): The Thyroid: A Fundamental and Clinical Text, ed 8. Philadelphia, Lippincott, Williams & Wilkins.
6. Yamada M, Saga Y, Shibusawa N, et al: Tertiary hypothyroidism and hyperglycaemia in mice with targeted disruption of the thyrotropin-releasing hormone gene. Proc Natl Acad Sci U S A 94:10862, 1997.
7. Jackson IMD, Wu P, Lechan RM: Immunohistochemical localisation in the rat brain of the precursor for thyrotropin-releasing hormone. Science 229:1097–1099, 1985.
8. Richter K, Kawashima E, Egger R, et al: Biosynthesis of thyrotropin releasing hormone in the skin of *Xenopus laevis*: Partial sequence of the precursor deduced from cloned cDNA. EMBO J 3:617–621, 1984.
9. Lechan RM, Wu P, Jackson IMD, et al: Thyrotropin releasing hormone precursor: Characterization in rat brain. Science 231:159–161, 1986.
10. Jackson IMD: Controversies in TRH biosynthesis and strategies toward the identification of a TRH precursor. Ann N Y Acad Sci 553:7–10, 1989.
11. Wu P: Identification and characterization of TRH-precursor peptides. Ann N Y Acad Sci 553:60–63, 1989.
12. Wu P, Jackson IM: Post-translational processing of thyrotropin-releasing hormone precursor in rat brain: Identification of 3 novel peptides derived from pro-TRH. Brain Res 456:22–26, 1988.
13. Carr FE, Reid AH, Wessendorf MW: A cryptic peptide from the preprothyrotropin-releasing hormone precursor stimulates thyrotropin gene expression. Endocrinology 133:809, 1993.
14. Valentyn K, Vandenbulene F, Beauvillain JC, Vaudry H: Distribution, cellular localisation and ontogeny of preprothyrotropin-releasing hormone-(160–169)(PS-4)-binding sites in the rat pituitary. Endocrinology 139:1306, 1998.
15. Yamada M, Radovick S, Wondisford FE, et al: Cloning and structure of human genomic DNA and hypothalamic cDNA encoding human preprothyrotropin-releasing hormone. Mol Endocrinol 4:551–556, 1990.
16. Yamada M, Wondisford FE, Radovick S, et al: Assignment of human preprothyrotropin–releasing hormone (TRH) gene to chromosome 3. Somat Cell Mol Genet 17:97–100, 1991.
17. Jackson IMD, Papapetrou PD, Reichlin S: Metabolic clearance of thyrotropin-releasing hormone in the rat in hypothyroid and hyperthyroid states: Comparison with serum degradation in vitro. Endocrinology 104:1292–1298, 1979.
18. Yanagisawa T, Prasad C, Peterkofsky A: The subcellular and organ distribution and natural form of histidyl-proline-diketopiperazine in rat brain determined by a specific radioimmunoassay. J Biol Chem 255:10290–10298, 1980.
19. Bauer K, Nowak P, Kleinkauf H: Specificity of a serum peptidase hydrolyzing thyroliberin at pyroglutamyl-histidine bond. Eur J Biochem 118:173–177, 1981.
20. O'Connor B, O'Cuinn G: Purification of and kinetic studies on a narrow specificity synaptosomal membrane pyroglutamate aminopeptidase from guinea pig brain. Eur J Biochem 150:47–53, 1985.
21. Battaini F, Peterkofsky A: Inhibition of dopamine (DA) uptake and (Na^+,K^+)-ATPase in rat brain synaptosomes by histidyl-proline diketopiperazine [cyclo(His)-pro], a metabolite of thyrotropin-releasing hormone (TRH). Fed Proc 39:594–598, 1980.
22. Yamada M, Shibusawa N, Hashida T, et al: Abundance of cyclo(His-Pro)-like immunoreactivity in the brain of TRH-deficient mice. Endocrinology 140:538, 1999.
23. Hilton CW, Prasad C, Vo P, Mouton C: Food contains the bioactive peptide, cyclo(His-Pro). J Clin Endocrinol Metab 75:375–378, 1992.
24. Iverson E: Pharmocokinetics of thyrotrophin-releasing hormone in patients in different thyroid states. J Endocrinol 128:153–159, 1991.
25. Yamada M, Mori M: Thyrotropin-releasing hormone–degrading enzyme in human serum is classified as type II of pyroglutamyl aminopeptidase: Influence of thyroid status. Proc Soc Exp Biol Med 194:346–351, 1990.
26. Bauer K: Adenohypophyseal degradation of thyrotropin releasing hormone regulated by thyroid hormones. Nature 330:375–377, 1987.
27. Ponce G, Charli J-L, Pasten JA, et al: Tissue-specific regulation of pyroglutamate aminopeptidase II activity by thyroid hormones. Neuroendocrinology 48:211–213, 1988.
28. Heuer H, Ehrchen J, Bauer K, Schafer MK: Region-specific expression of thyrotropin-releasing hormone–degrading ectoenzyme in the rat central nervous system and pituitary gland. Eur J Neurosci 10:1465–1478, 1998.
29. Schomburg L, Bauer K: Regulation of the adenohyphophyseal thyrotropin-releasing hormone–degrading ectoenzyme by estradiol. Endocrinology 138:3587–3593, 1997.
30. Martin JB, Boshans R, Reichlin S: Feedback regulation of TSH secretion in rats with hypothalamic lesions. Endocrinology 87:1032–1040, 1970.
31. Lechan RM, Jackson IMD: Immunohistochemical localization of thyrotropin-releasing hormone in the rat hypothalamus and pituitary. Endocrinology 111:55–65, 1982.
32. Siaud P, Tapia-Arancibia L, Szafarczyk A, Alonso G: Increase of thyrotropin-releasing hormone immunoreactivity in the nucleus of the solitary tract following bilateral lesions of the hypothalamic paraventricular nuclei. Neurosci Lett 79:47–52, 1987.
33. Jackson IMD: Thyrotropin releasing hormone. N Engl J Med 306:145–155, 1982.
34. Jackson IMD: Thyrotropin-releasing hormone (TRH): Distribution in mammalian species and its functional significance. *In* Griffiths EC, Bennett GW (eds): Thyrotropin-Releasing Hormone. New York, Raven, 1983, pp 3–18.
35. Le Dafniet M, Lefebvre P, Barret A, et al: Normal and adenomatous human pituitaries secrete thyrotropin-releasing hormone in vitro: Modulation by dopamine, haloperidol, and somatostatin. J Clin Endocrinol Metab 71:480–486, 1990.
36. Pagesy P, Croissandeau G, Le Dafniet M, et al: Detection of thyrotropin-releasing hormone (TRH) mRNA by the reverse transcription–polymerase chain reaction in the human normal and tumoral anterior pituitary. J Biochem Biophys Res Commun 182:182 187, 1992.
37. Morley JE: Neuroendocrine control of thyrotropin secretion. Endocr Rev 2:396–436, 1981.
38. Scanlon MF, Lewis M, Weightman DR, et al: The neuroregulation of human thyrotropin secretion. *In* Martini L, Ganong WF (eds): Frontiers in Neuroendocrinology. New York, Raven, 1980, pp 333–380.
39. Sheward WJ, Harmar AJ, Fraser HM, Fink G: TRH in rat pituitary stalk blood and hypothalamus. Studies with high performance liquid chromatography. Endocrinology 113:1865–1869, 1983.
40. Fraser HM, McNeilly AS: Effect of chronic immunoneutralization of thyrotropin-releasing hormone on the hypothalamic-pituitary-thyroid axis, prolactin and reproductive function in the ewe. Endocrinology 111:1964–1974, 1982.
41. Carr FE, Shupnik MA, Burnside J, Chin WW: Thyrotropin-releasing hormone stimulates the activity of the rat thyrotropin β-subunit gene promoter transfected into pituitary cells. Mol Endocrinol 3:717–724, 1989.
42. Franklyn JA, Wilson M, Davis JR, et al: Demonstration of thyrotropin β-subunit messenger RNA in primary culture: Evidence for regulation by thyrotropin-releasing hormone and forskolin. J Endocrinol 111:R1–R4, 1986.
43. Kourides IA, Gurr JA, Wolf O: The regulation and organization of thyroid stimulating hormone genes. Recent Prog Horm Res 40:79–120, 1984.
44. Shupnik MA, Greenspan SL, Ridgway EC: Transcriptional regulation of thyrotropin subunit genes by thyrotropin-releasing hormone and dopamine in pituitary cell culture. J Biol Chem 261:12675–12679, 1986.
45. Steinfelder HJ, Hauser P, Nakayama Y, et al: Thyrotropin-releasing hormone regulation of human TSHβ expression: Role of a pituitary-specific transcription factor (Pit-1/GHF-1) and potential interaction with a thyroid hormone–inhibitory element. Proc Natl Acad Sci U S A 88:3130–3134, 1991.
46. Guo-zai Y, Pan WT, Bancroft C: Thyrotropin-releasing hormone action on the prolactin promoter is mediated by the POU protein Pit-1. Mol Endocrinol 5:535–541, 1991.
47. Guo-zai Y, Bancroft C: Mediation by calcium of thyrotropin-releasing hormone action on the prolactin promoter via transcription factor Pit-1. Mol Endocrinol 5:1488–1497, 1991.
48. Cohen LE, Wondieford FE, Radovick S: Role of Pit-1 in the gene expression of growth hormone, prolactin and thyrotropin. Endocrinol Metab Clin North Am 25:523–540, 1996.
49. Brue T, Vallette S, Pellegrini-Bouiller L, Enjalbert A: Congenital multiple anterior pituitary hormone deficiencies: An approach of pituitary ontogenesis. Ann Endocrinol 58:436–450, 1997.
50. Magner JA: Thyroid-stimulating hormone: Biosynthesis, cell biology and bioactivity. Endocr Rev 11:354–385, 1990.
51. Magner JA, Kane J, Chou ET: Intravenous thyrotropin (TSH)-releasing hormone releases human TSH that is structurally different from basal TSH. J Clin Endocrinol Metab 74:1306–1311, 1992.
52. Amir SM, Kubota K, Tramontano D, et al: The carbohydrate moiety of bovine thyrotropin is essential for full bioactivity but not for receptor recognition. Endocrinology 120:345–352, 1987.
53. Berman MI, Thomas CG, Manjunath P, et al: The role of the carbohydrate moiety in thyrotropin action. Biochem Biophys Res Commun 133:680–687, 1985.
54. Nissim M, Lee KO, Petrick PA, et al: A sensitive thyrotropin (TSH) bioassay based on iodide uptake in rat FRTL-5 thyroid cells: Comparison with the adenosine 3′,5′-monophosphate response to human serum TSH and enzymatically deglycosylated bovine and human TSH. Endocrinology 121:1278–1287, 1987.
55. Amir S, Menezes-Ferreira MM, Shimohigashi Y, et al: Activities of deglycosylated thyrotropin at the thyroid membrane receptor–adenylate cyclase system. J Endocrinol Invest 8:537–541, 1986.
56. Wilber JF: Stimulation of ^{14}C-glucosamine and ^{14}C-alanine incorporation into thyrotropin by synthetic thyrotropin-releasing hormone. Endocrinology 89:873–877, 1971.
57. Faglia G, Bitensky L, Pinchera A, et al: Thyrotropin secretion in patients with central hypothyroidism: Evidence for reduced biological activity of immunoreactive thyrotropin. J Clin Endocrinol Metab 48:989–998, 1979.
58. Beck-Peccoz P, Amir S, Menezes-Ferreira MM, et al: Decreased receptor binding of biologically inactive thyrotropin in central hypothyroidism: Effect of treatment with thyrotropin-releasing hormone. N Engl J Med 312:1085–1090, 1985.
59. DeCherney GS, Gesundheit N, Gyves PW, et al: Alterations in the sialylation and sulfation of secreted mouse thyrotropin in primary hypothyroidism. Biochem Biophys Res Commun 159:755–762, 1989.
60. Miura Y, Perkel VS, Papenberg KA, et al: Concanavalin-A, lentil and ricin affinity binding characteristics of human thyrotropin: Differences in the sialylation of thyrotropin in sera of euthyroid, primary and central hypothyroid patients. J Clin Endocrinol Metab 69:985–995, 1988.
61. Beck-Peccoz P, Piscitelli G, Amir S, et al: Endocrine, biochemical and morphological studies of a pituitary adenoma secreting growth hormone, thyrotropin (TSH), and α-subunit: Evidence for secretion of TSH with increased bioactivity. J Clin Endocrinol Metab 62:704–711, 1986.
62. Gesundheit N, Petrick PA, Nissim M, et al: Thyrotropin-secreting pituitary adenomas: Clinical and biochemical heterogeneity. Ann Intern Med 111:827, 1989.

63. DeLean A, Ferland L, Drouin J, et al: Modulation of pituitary thyrotropin releasing hormone receptor levels by estrogens and thyroid hormones. Endocrinology 100:1496–1504, 1977.
64. Hinkle PM, Perrone MH, Schonbrunn A: Mechanism of thyroid hormone inhibition of thyrotropin-releasing hormone action. Endocrinology 108:199–205, 1981.
65. Hinkle PM, Tashjian AH: Thyrotropin-releasing hormone regulates the number of its own receptors in the GH_3 strain of pituitary cells in culture. Biochemistry 14:3845–3851, 1975.
66. Hinkle PM, Goh KBC: Regulation of thyrotrophin releasing hormone receptors and responses by L-triiodothyronine in dispersed rat pituitary cell cultures. Endocrinology 110:1725–1731, 1982.
67. Kaji H, Hinkle PM: Regulation of thyroid hormone receptors and responses by thyrotropin-releasing hormone in GH_4C_1 cells. Endocrinology 121:1697–1704, 1987.
68. Belchetz PE, Gredley G, Bird D, Himsworth RL: Regulation of thyrotropin secretion by negative feedback of triiodothyronine on the hypothalamus. J Endocrinol 76:439–448, 1977.
69. Berelowitz M, Maeda K, Harris S, Frohman LA: The effect of alterations in the pituitary-thyroid axis on hypothalamic content and in vitro release of somatostatin-like immunoreactivity. Endocrinology 107:24–29, 1980.
70. Koller KJ, Wolff RS, Warden MK, Zoeller RT: Thyroid hormones regulate levels of thyrotropin-releasing hormone mRNA in the paraventricular nucleus. Proc Natl Acad Sci U S A 84:7329–7333, 1987.
71. Segerson TP, Kauer J, Wolfe HC, et al: Thyroid hormone regulates TRH biosynthesis in the paraventricular nucleus of the rat hypothalamus. Science 238:78–80, 1987.
72. Taylor T, Wondisford FE, Blaine T, Weintraub BD: The paraventricular nucleus of the hypothalamus has a major role in thyroid hormone feedback regulation of thyrotropin synthesis and secretion. Endocrinology 126:317–323, 1990.
73. Straub RE, Frech GC, Joho RH, Gershengorn MC: Expression cloning of a cDNA encoding the mouse pituitary thyrotropin releasing hormone receptor. Proc Natl Acad Sci U S A 87:9514–9518, 1990.
74. De La Pena P, Delgado LM, Del Camino D, Barros F: Cloning and expression of the thyrotropin-releasing hormone receptor from GH_3 rat anterior pituitary cells. Biochem J 284:891–899, 1992.
75. De La Pena P, Delgado LM, Del Camino D, Barros F: Two isoforms of the thyrotropin-releasing hormone receptor generated by alternative splicing have indistinguishable functional properties. J Biol Chem 267:25703–25708, 1992.
76. Duthie SM, Taylor PL, Anderson J, et al: Cloning and functional characterisation of the human TRH receptor. Mol Cell Endocrinol 95:11–15, 1993.
77. Matre V, Hovring PI, Orstavik S, et al: Structural and functional organisation of the gene encoding the human thyrotropin-releasing hormone receptor. J Neurochem 72:40–50, 1999.
78. Cao J, O'Donnell D, Vu H, et al: Cloning and characterisation of a cDNA encoding a novel subtype of rat thyrotropin-releasing hormone receptor. J Biol Chem 273:32281–32287, 1998.
79. Itadami H, Nakamura T, Itoh J, et al: Cloning and characterisation of a new subtype of thyrotropin-releasing hormone receptor. Biochem Biophys Res Commun 250:68–71, 1998.
80. Colson AO, Perlman JH, Jinsi-Parimoo A, et al: A hydrophobic cluster between transmembrane helices 5 and 6 constrains the thyrotropin-releasing hormone receptor in an inactive conformation. Mol Pharmacol 54:968–978, 1998.
81. Drmota T, Gould GW, Milligan G: Real time visualisation of agonist-mediated redistribution and internalisation of a green fluorescent protein tagged form of the thyrotropin-releasing hormone receptor. J Biol Chem 273:24000–24008, 1998.
82. Yu R, Ashworth R, Hinkle PM: Receptors for thyrotropin-releasing hormone on lactotropes and thyrotropes. Thyroid 8:887–894, 1998.
83. Ashworth R, Yu R, Nelson EJ, et al: Visualisation of the thyrotropin-releasing hormone receptor and its ligand during endocytosis and recycling. Proc Natl Acad Sci U S A 92:512–516, 1995.
84. Hsieh K-P, Martin TFJ: Thyrotropin-releasing hormone and gonadotropin-releasing hormone receptors activate phospholipase C by coupling to the guanosine triphosphate–binding proteins G_q and G_{11}. Mol Endocrinol 6:1673–1681, 1992.
85. De la Pena P, del Camino D, Pardo LA, et al: Gs couples thyrotropin-releasing hormone receptors expressed in *Xenopus* oocytes to phospholipase C. J Biol Chem 270:3554–3559, 1995.
86. Drummond AH: Inositol lipid metabolism and signal transduction in clonal pituitary cells. J Exp Biol 124:337–342, 1986.
87. Gershengorn MC: Thyrotropin-releasing hormone action: Mechanism of calcium-mediated stimulation of prolactin secretion. Recent Prog Horm Res 41:607–653, 1985.
88. Albert PR, Tashjian AH: Thyrotropin-releasing hormone–induced spike and plateau in cytosolic free Ca^{2+} concentrations in pituitary cells. J Biol Chem 259:5827–5832, 1984.
89. Geras EJ, Gershengorn MC: Evidence that TRH stimulates secretion of TSH by two calcium-mediated mechanisms. Am Physiol 242:109–114, 1981.
90. Akerman SN, Zorec R, Cheeck TR, et al: Fura2 imaging of thyrotropin-releasing hormone and dopamine effects on calcium homeostasis of bovine lactotrophs. Endocrinology 129:475–488, 1991.
91. Tornquist K: Evidence for TRH-induced influx of extracellular Ca^{2+} in pituitary GH4C1 cells. Biochem Biophys Res Commun 180:860–866, 1991.
92. Law GJ, Pachter JA, Thastrup O, et al: Thapsigargin, but not caffeine, blocks the ability of thyrotropin-releasing hormone to release Ca^{2+} from an intracellular store in GH_4C_1 cells. Biochem J 267:359–364, 1990.
93. Gershengorn MC: Thyrotropin releasing hormone stimulation of prolactin release: Evidence for a membrane potential–independent, Ca^{2+}-dependent mechanism of action. J Biol Chem 255:1801–1803, 1980.
94. Tan KN, Tashjian AHJ: Receptor-mediated release of plasma membrane–associated calcium and stimulation of calcium uptake by thyrotropin-releasing hormone in pituitary cells in culture. J Biol Chem 256:8994–9002, 1981.
95. Martin TFJ: Thyrotropin-releasing hormone rapidly activates the phosphodiester hydrolysis of polyphosphoinositides in GH_3 pituitary cells: Evidence for the role of a polyphosphoinositide-specific phospholipase C in hormone action. J Biol Chem 258:14816–14822, 1983.
96. Gershengorn MC, Thaw C: TRH stimulates biphasic elevation of cytoplasmic free calcium in GH_3 cells. Further evidence that TRH mobilizes cellular and extracellular Ca^{2+}. Endocrinology 116:591–596, 1985.
97. Peizhi LI, Thaw CN, Sempowski GD, et al: Characterization of the calcium response to thyrotropin-releasing hormone (TRH) in cells transfected with TRH receptor complementary DNA: Importance of voltage-sensitive calcium channels. Mol Endocrinol 6:1393–1402, 1992.
98. Gershengorn MC, Rebecchi MJ, Geras E, Arevalo CO: Thyrotropin-releasing hormone (TRH) action in mouse thyrotropic tumor cells in culture: Evidence against a role for adenosine 3,5′-monophosphate as a mediator of TRH-stimulated thyrotropin release. Endocrinology 107:665–670, 1980.
99. Iriuchijimia T, Mori M: Regional dissociation of cyclic AMP and inositol phosphate formation in response to thyrotropin-releasing hormone in the rat brain. J Neurochem 52:1944–1949, 1989.
100. Judd AM, Canonico PL, MacLeod RM: Prolactin release from MtTW15 and 731a pituitary tumors is refractory to TRH and VIP stimulation. Mol Cell Endocrinol 36:221–226, 1984.
101. Mongioli A, Aliffi A, Vicari E, et al: Downregulation of prolactin secretion in men during continuous thyrotropin-releasing hormone infusion: Evidence for induction of pituitary desensitization by continuous TRH administration. J Clin Endocrinol Metab 56:904–908, 1983.
102. Sheppard MC, Shennan KJ: Desensitization of rat anterior pituitary gland to thyrotropin releasing hormone. J Endocrinol 101:101–105, 1984.
103. Mori M, Yamada M, Kobayashi S: Role of the hypothalamic TRH in the regulation of its own receptors in rat anterior pituitaries. Neuroendocrinology 48:153–158, 1988.
104. Winikov I, Gershengorn MC: Receptor density determines secretory response patterns mediated by inositol lipid-derived second messengers. Comparison of thyrotropin-releasing hormone and carbamylcholine actions in thyroid-stimulating hormone–secreting mouse pituitary tumor cells. J Biol Chem 264:9438–9442, 1989.
105. Yu R, Hinkle PM: Desensitisation of thyrotropin-releasing hormone receptor–mediated responses involves multiple steps. J Biol Chem 272:28301–28307, 1997.
106. Gershengorn MC: Bihormonal regulation of the thyrotropin-releasing hormone receptor in mouse pituitary thyrotropic tumor cells in culture. J Clin Invest 62:937–943, 1978.
107. Oron Y, Straub RE, Traktman P, Gershengorn MC: Decreased TRH receptor mRNA activity precedes homologous downregulation: Assay in oocytes. Science 238:1406–1408, 1987.
108. Fujimoto J, Straub RE, Gershengorn MC: Thyrotropin releasing hormone (TRH) and phorbol myristate acetate decrease TRH receptor messenger RNA in rat pituitary GH_3 cells: Evidence that protein kinase-C mediates the TRH effect. Mol Endocrinol 5:1527–1532, 1991.
109. Yu R, Hinkle PM: Signal transduction, desensitisation and recovery of responses to thyrotropin-releasing hormone after inhibition of receptor internalisation. Mol Endocrinol 12:737–749, 1998.
110. Iriuchijima T, Mori M: Inhibition by staurosporine of TRH-induced refractoriness of inositol phospholipid hydrolysis by rat anterior pituitaries. J Endocrinol 124:75–79, 1990.
111. Shen L-P, Pictet RL, Rutter WJ: Human somatostatin. I. Sequence of the cDNA. Proc Natl Acad Sci U S A 79:4575–4579, 1982.
112. Montminy MR, Goodman RH, Horovitch SJ, et al: Primary structure of the gene encoding rat pre-prosomatostatin. Proc Natl Acad Sci U S A 81:3337–3340, 1984.
113. Goodman RH, Aron DC, Roos BA: Rat-preprosomatostatin: Structure and processing by microsomal membranes. J Biol Chem 258:5570–5573, 1983.
114. Millar RP, Sheward RJ, Wegener I, Fink G: Somatostatin 28 is a hormonally active peptide secreted into hypophyseal portal vessel blood. Brain Res 260:334–337, 1983.
115. Vale W, Brazeau P, Rivier C, et al: Somatostatin. Recent Prog Horm Res 31:365–397, 1975.
116. Arimura A, Schally AV: Increase in basal and thyrotropin-releasing hormone stimulated secretion of thyrotropin by passive immunization with antiserum to somatostatin. Endocrinology 98:1069–1072, 1976.
117. Ferland L, Labrie F, Jobin M, et al: Physiological role of somatostatin in the control of growth hormone and thyrotropin secretion. Biochem Biophys Res Commun 68:149–156, 1976.
118. Rodriguez-Arnao MD, Gomez-Pan A, Rainbow SJ, et al: Effects of prosomatostatin on growth hormone and prolactin response to arginine in man. Comparison with somatostatin. Lancet 1:353–356, 1981.
119. Hofland LJ, Lamberts SW: Somatostatin receptors and disease: Role of receptor subtypes. Baillieres Clin Endocrinol Metab 10:163–176, 1996.
120. Morley JE: Neuroendocrine control of thyrotropin secretion. Endocr Rev 2:396–436, 1981.
121. Krulich L: Neurotransmitter control of thyrotropin secretion. Neuroendocrinology 35:139–147, 1982.
122. Lewis BM, Dieguez C, Lewis MD, Scanlon MF: Dopamine stimulates release of thyrotropin-releasing hormone from perfused intact rat hypothalamus via hypothalamic D_2 receptors. J Endocrinol 115:419–424, 1987.
123. Lewis BM, Dieguez C, Lewis MD, Scanlon MF: Hypothalamic D2 receptors mediate the preferential release of somatostatin-28 in response to dopaminergic stimulation. Endocrinology 119:1712–1717, 1986.
124. Ben-Jonathan N, Oliver C, Weiner HJ, et al: Dopamine in hypophyseal portal plasma of the rat during the estrous cycle and throughout pregnancy. Endocrinology 100:452–458, 1977.
125. Johnston CA, Gibbs DM, Negro-Vilar A: High concentrations of epinephrine derived from a central source and of 5-hydroxyindole-3-acetic acid in hypophysial portal plasma. Endocrinology 113:819–824, 1983.

126. Foord SM, Peters JR, Scanlon MF, et al: Dopaminergic control of TSH secretion in isolated rat pituitary cells. FEBS Lett 121:257–259, 1980.
127. Cooper DS, Klibanski A, Ridgway EC: Dopaminergic modulation of TSH and its subunits: In vivo and in vitro studies. Clin Endocrinol 18:265–275, 1983.
128. Foord SM, Peters JR, Dieguez C, et al: Dopamine receptors on intact anterior pituitary cells in culture: Functional association with the inhibition of prolactin and thyrotropin. Endocrinology 112:1567–1577, 1983.
129. Foord SM, Peters JR, Dieguez C, et al: Hypothyroid pituitary cells in culture: An analysis of TSH and PRL responses to dopamine and dopamine receptor binding. Endocrinology 115:407–415, 1984.
130. Foord SM, Peters JR, Dieguez C, et al: TSH regulates thyrotroph responsiveness to dopamine in vitro. Endocrinology 118:1319–1326, 1985.
131. Shupnik MA, Greenspan SL, Ridgway EC: Transcriptional regulation of thyrotropin subunit genes by thyrotropin-releasing hormone and dopamine in pituitary cell culture. J Biol Chem 261:12675–12679, 1986.
132. Dieguez C, Foord SM, Peters JR, et al: Interactions among epinephrine, thyrotropin (TSH)-releasing hormone, dopamine and somatostatin in the control of TSH secretion in vitro. Endocrinology 114:957–961, 1984.
133. Klibanski A, Milbury PE, Chin WW, Ridgway EC: Direct adrenergic stimulation of the release of thyrotropin and its subunits from the thyrotrope in vitro. Endocrinology 113:1244–1249, 1983.
134. Peters JR, Foord SM, Dieguez C, et al: α_1-Adrenoreceptors on intact rat anterior pituitary cells: Correlation with adrenergic stimulation of thyrotropin release. Endocrinology 113:133–140, 1983.
135. Dieguez C, Foord SM, Peters JR, et al: α_1-Adrenoreceptors and α_1-adrenoreceptor–mediated thyrotropin release in cultures of euthyroid and hypothyroid rat anterior pituitary cells. Endocrinology 117:1172–1179, 1985.
136. Peters JR, Foord SM, Dieguez C, Scanlon MF: TSH neuroregulation and alterations in disease states. Clin Endocrinol Metab 12:669–694, 1983.
137. Scanlon MF, Lewis M, Weightman DR, et al: The neuroregulation of human thyrotropin secretion. *In* Martini L, Ganong WF (eds): Frontiers in Neuroendocrinology. New York, Raven, 1980, pp 333–357.
138. Reymond MJ, Benotto W, Lemarchand-Beraud T: The secretory activity of the tubero-infundibular dopaminergic neurons is modulated by the thyroid status in the adult rat: Consequence of prolactin secretion. Neuroendocrinology 46:62–68, 1987.
139. Wang PS, Gonzalez HA, Reymond MJ, Porter JC: Mass and in situ molar activity of tyrosine hydroxylase in the median eminence. Neuroendocrinology 49:659–663, 1989.
140. Zgliczynski S, Kaniewski M: Evidence for α-adrenergic receptor mediated TSH release in men. Acta Endocrinol 95:172–176, 1980.
141. Valcavi R, Dieguez C, Azzarito C, et al: Alpha-adrenoreceptor blockade with thymoxamine reduces basal thyrotrophin levels but does not influence circadian thyrotrophin changes in man. J Endocrinol 115:187–191, 1987.
142. Little KY, Garbutt JC, Mayo JP, Mason G: Lack of acute α-amphetamine effects on thyrotropin release. Neuroendocrinology 48:304–307, 1988.
143. Rogol AD, Reeves GD, Varma MM, Blizzard RM: Thyroid stimulating hormone and prolactin response to thyrotropin-releasing hormone during infusion of epinephrine and propranolol in man. Neuroendocrinology 29:413–417, 1979.
144. Smythe GA, Bradshaw JE, Cai WY, Symons RG: Hypothalamic serotoninergic stimulation of thyrotropin secretion and related brain-hormone and drug interactions in the rat. Endocrinology 111:1181–1191, 1982.
145. Scharp B, Morley JE, Carlson HE, et al: The role of opiates and endogenous opioid peptides in the regulation of rat TSH secretion. Brain Res 219:335–344, 1981.
146. Judd AM, Hedge GA: The role of opioid peptides in controlling thyroid stimulating hormone release. Life Sci 31:2529–2536, 1982.
147. Samuels MH, Kramer P, Wilson D, Sexton G: Effects of naloxone infusions on pulsatile thyrotropin secretion. J Clin Endocrinol Metab 78:1249–1252, 1994.
148. Dubuis JM, Dayer JM, Siegrist-Kaiser CA, Burger AG: Human recombinant interleukin-1β decreases plasma thyroid hormone and thyroid stimulating hormone levels in rats. Endocrinology 123:2175–2181, 1988.
149. Ozawa M, Sato K, Han DC, et al: Effects of tumor necrosis factor-α and cachectin on thyroid hormone metabolism in mice. Endocrinology 123:1461–1467, 1988.
150. Pang XP, Hershman JM, Mirell CJ, Pekary AE: Impairment of hypothalamic-pituitary-thyroid function in rats treated with human recombinant tumour necrosis factor-α (cachectin). Endocrinology 125:76–84, 1989.
151. Kakucska I, Romero LI, Clark BD, et al: Suppression of thyrotropin-releasing hormone gene expression by interleukin-1-beta in the rat: Implications for nonthyroidal illness. Neuroendocrinology 59:129–137, 1994.
152. Kondo K, Harbuz MS, Levy A, Lightman SL: Inhibition of the hypothalamic-pituitary-thyroid axis in response to lipopolysaccharide is independent of changes in circulating corticosteroids. Neuroimmunomodulation 4:188–194, 1997.
153. Hermus RM, Sweep CG, van der Meer MJ, et al: Continuous infusion of interleukin-1 beta induces a nonthyroidal illness syndrome in the rat. Endocrinology 131:2139–2146, 1992.
154. Pang XP, Yoshimura M, Hershman JM: Suppression of rat thyrotroph and thyroid cell function by tumor necrosis factor-alpha. Thyroid 3:325–330, 1993.
155. Bernton EW, Beach JE, Holaday JW, et al: Release of multiple hormones by a direct action of interleukin-1 on pituitary cells. Science 238:519–521, 1987.
156. Besedovsky H, Del Rey A, Sorkin E, et al: Immunoregulatory feedback between interleukin-1 and glucocorticoid hormones. Science 233:652–654, 1986.
157. Woloski BM, Smith EM, Meyer WJ III, et al: Corticotropin-releasing activity of monokines. Science 230:1035–1037, 1985.
158. Sapolsky R, Rivier C, Yamamoto G, et al: Interleukin-1 stimulates the secretion of hypothalamic corticotropin-releasing factor. Science 238:522–524, 1987.
159. Koenig JI, Snow K, Clark BD, et al: Intrinsic pituitary interleukin-1 beta is induced by bacterial lipopolysaccharide. Endocrinology 126:3053–3058, 1990.
160. Spangelo BL, MacLeod RM, Isaacson PC: Production of interleukin-6 by anterior pituitary cells in vitro. Endocrinology 126:582–586, 1990.
161. Vankelecom H, Carmeliet P, Van Damme J, et al: Production of interleukin-6 by folliculo-stellate cells of the anterior pituitary gland in a histiotype cell aggregate culture system. Neuroendocrinology 49:102–106, 1989.
162. Brabant G, Frank K, Ranft U, et al: Psychological regulation of circadian and pulsatile thyrotropin secretion in normal man and woman. J Clin Endocrinol Metab 70:403–409, 1990.
163. Konno N, Morikawa K: Seasonal variation of serum thyrotropin concentration and thyrotropin response to thyrotropin-releasing hormone in patients with primary hypothyroidism on constant replacement dosage of thyroxine. J Clin Endocrinol Metab 54:1118–1124, 1982.
164. Brabant G, Ocran K, Ranft U, et al: Psychological regulation of thyrotropin. Biochimie 71:293–301, 1989.
165. LeRoith D, Liel Y, Sack J, et al: The TSH response to TRH is exaggerated in primary testicular failure and normal in the male castrate. Acta Endocrinol 97:103–108, 1981.
166. Spitz IM, Zylber-Haran EA, Trestian S: The thyrotropin (TSH) profile in isolated gonadotropin deficiency: A model to evaluate the effect of sex steroids on TSH secretion. J Clin Endocrinol Metab 57:415–420, 1983.
167. Brabant G, Ranft U, Ocran K, et al: Thyrotropin: An episodically secreted hormone. Acta Endocrinol 112:315–322, 1986.
168. Brabant G, Brabant A, Ranft U, et al: Circadian and pulsatile thyrotropin secretion in euthyroid man under the influence of thyroid hormone and glucocorticoid administration. J Clin Endocrinol Metab 65:83–88, 1987.
169. Greenspan SL, Klibanski A, Schoenfeld D, Ridgway EC: Pulsatile secretion of thyrotropin in man. J Clin Endocrinol Metab 63:661–668, 1986.
170. Rossmanith WG, Mortola JF, Laughlin GA, Yen SS: Dopaminergic control of circadian and pulsatile pituitary thyrotropin release in women. J Clin Endocrinol Metab 67:560–564, 1988.
171. Samuels MH, Veldhuis JD, Henry PO, Ridgway EC: Pathophysiology of pulsatile and copulsatile release of thyroid-stimulating hormone, luteinising hormone, follicle-stimulating hormone and α-subunit. J Clin Endocrinol Metab 71:425–432, 1990.
172. Salvador J, Dieguez C, Scanlon MF: The circadian rhythms of thyrotropin and prolactin secretion. Chronobiol Int 5:85–93, 1988.
173. Evans PJ, Weeks I, Jones MK, et al: The circadian variation of thyrotropin in patients with primary thyroidal disease. Clin Endocrinol 24:343–348, 1986.
174. Re RN, Kourides IA, Ridgway EC, et al: The effect of glucocorticoid administration on human pituitary secretion of thyrotropin and prolactin. J Clin Endocrinol Metab 43:338–346, 1976.
175. Bartalena L, Placidi GF, Martino E, et al: Nocturnal serum thyrotropin (TSH) surge and the TSH response to TSH-releasing hormone: Dissociated behaviour in untreated depressives. J Clin Endocrinol Metab 71:650–655, 1990.
176. Souetre E, Salvati E, Wehr TA, et al: Twenty-four hour profiles of body temperature and plasma TSH in bipolar patients during depression and during remission and in normal control subjects. Am J Psychiatry 145:1133–1137, 1988.
177. Bartalena L, Martino E, Brandi LS, et al: Lack of nocturnal serum thyrotropin surge after surgery. J Clin Endocrinol Metab 70:293–296, 1990.
178. Salvador J, Wilson DW, Harris PE, et al: Relationships between the circadian rhythms of TSH, prolactin and cortisol in surgically treated microprolactinoma patients. Clin Endocrinol 22:265–272, 1985.
179. Samuels MH, Henry P, Luther M, Ridgway EC: Pulsatile TSH secretion during 48-hour continuous TRH infusions. Thyroid 3:201–206, 1993.
180. Murakami M, Tanaka K, Greer MA: There is a nyctohemeral rhythm of type II iodothyronine 5′-deiodinase activity in rat anterior pituitary. Endocrinology 123:1631–1635, 1988.
181. Rage F, Lazaro JB, Benyassi A, et al: Rapid changes in somatostatin and TRH mRNA in whole rat hypothalamus in response to acute cold exposure. J Neuroendocrinol 6:19–23, 1994.
182. Zoeller RT, Kabeer N, Alberts HE: Cold exposure elevates cellular levels of messenger ribonucleic acid encoding thyrotropin-releasing hormone in paraventricular nucleus despite elevated levels of thyroid hormones. Endocrinology 127:2955–2962, 1990.
183. Arancibia S, Rage F, Astier H, Tapia-Arancibia L: Neuroendocrine and autonomous mechanisms underlying thermoregulation in cold environment. Neuroendocrinology 64:257–267, 1996.
184. Lewis GF, Alessi CA, Imperial JG, Refetoff S: Low serum free thyroxine index in ambulating elderly is due to a resetting of the threshold of thyrotropin feedback suppression. J Clin Endocrinol Metab 73:843–849, 1991.
185. Finucane P, Rudra T, Church H, et al: Thyroid function tests in elderly patients with and without an acute illness. Age Ageing 18:398–402, 1989.
186. Van Coevorden A, Laurent E, DeCoster C, et al: Decreased basal and stimulated thyrotropin secretion in healthy elderly men. J Clin Endocrinol Metab 69:177–185, 1989.
187. Borst GC, Osburne RC, O'Brian JT, et al: Fasting decreases thyrotropin responsiveness to thyrotropin-releasing hormone: A potential cause of misinterpretation of thyroid function tests in the critically ill. J Clin Endocrinol Metab 57:380–383, 1983.
188. Shi ZX, Levy A, Lightman SL: The effect of dietary protein on thyrotropin-releasing hormone and thyrotropin gene expression. Brain Res 606:1–4, 1993.
189. Ueta Y, Levy A, Chowdrey HS, Lightman SL: Inhibition of hypokalemic nitric oxide synthase gene expression in the rat paraventricular nucleus by food deprivation is independent of serotonin depletion. J Neuroendocrinol 7:861–865, 1995.
190. van Haasteren GA, Linkels E, Klootwijk W, et al: Starvation-induced changes in the hypothalamic content of prothyrotropin-releasing hormone (proTRH) mRNA and the hypothalamic release of proTRH-derived peptides: Role of the adrenal gland. J Endocrinol 145:143–153, 1995.
191. Romijn JA, Adriaanse R, Brabant G, et al: Pulsatile secretion of thyrotropin during fasting: A decrease of thyrotropin pulse amplitude. J Clin Endocrinol Metab 70:1631–1636, 1990.
192. Hugues JN, Enjalbert A, Moyse E, et al: Differential effects of passive immunization

with somatostatin antiserum on adenohypophysial hormone secretions in starved rats. J Endocrinol 109:169–174, 1986.
193. Legradi G, Emerson CH, Ahima RS, et al: Leptin prevents fasting-induced suppression of prothyrotropin-releasing hormone messenger ribonucleic acid in neurons of the hypothalamic paraventricular nucleus. Endocrinology 138:2569–2576, 1997.
194. Legradi G, Emerson CH, Ahima RS, et al: Arcuate nucleus ablation prevents fasting-induced suppression of ProTRH mRNA in the hypothalamic paraventricular nucleus. Neuroendocrinology 68:89–97, 1998.
195. Zalaga GP, Chernow B, Smallridge RC, et al: A longitudinal evaluation of thyroid function in critically ill surgical patients. Ann Surg 201:456–464, 1985.
196. Wartofsky L, Burman KD: Alterations in thyroid function in patients with systemic illness: The "euthyroid sick syndrome." Endocr Rev 3:164–217, 1982.
197. Hamblin PS, Dyer SA, Mohr VS, et al: Relationship between thyrotropin and thyroxine changes during recovery from severe hypothyroxinemia of critical illness. J Clin Endocrinol Metab 62:717–722, 1986.
198. Wehmann RE, Gregerman RI, Burns WH, et al: Suppression of thyrotropin in the low-thyroxine state of severe non-thyroidal illness. N Engl J Med 312:546–552, 1985.
199. Romijn JA, Wiersinga WM: Decreased nocturnal surge of thyrotropin in nonthyroidal illness. J Clin Endocrinol Metab 70:35–42, 1990.
200. Faber J, Kirkegaard C, Rasmussen B, et al: Pituitary-thyroid axis in critical illness. J Clin Endocrinol Metab 65:315–320, 1987.
201. Maldonado LS, Murata GH, Hershman JM, Braunstein GD: Do thyroid function tests independently predict survival in the critically ill? Thyroid 2:119–123, 1992.
202. Chopra IJ: Clinical review 86: Euthyroid sick syndrome: Is it a misnomer? J Clin Endocrinol Metab 82:329–334, 1997.
203. McIver B, Gorman CA: Euthyroid sick syndrome. An overview. Thyroid 7:125–132, 1997.
204. Delitala G, Tomasi P, Virdis R: Prolactin, growth hormone and thyrotropin-thyroid hormone secretion during stress states in man. Baillieres Clin Endocrinol Metab 1:391–414, 1987.
205. Loosen PT: Thyroid function in affective disorders and alcoholism. Endocrinol Metab Clin North Am 17:55–82, 1988.
206. Jackson IM: The thyroid axis and depression. Thyroid 8:951–956, 1998.
207. Brent GA, Hershman JM: Thyroxine therapy in patients with severe nonthyroidal illness and low serum thyroxine concentration. J Clin Endocrinol Metab 63:1–8, 1986.
208. Joffe RT, Sokolov STH, Singer WT: Thyroid hormone treatment of depression. Thyroid 5:235–239, 1995.

Chapter 92

Biosynthesis and Secretion of Thyroid Hormones

John T. Dunn

The thyroid's major responsibility is to produce the hormones thyroxine (T_4) and triiodothyronine (T_3), which it accomplishes by actively trapping iodine, incorporating iodine into thyroglobulin (Tg), with hormone formed in the process, and then breaking down Tg to release T_4 and T_3 into the circulation.

Figure 92–1 summarizes this process. The Na^+/I^- symporter (NIS) concentrates iodide across the basement membrane from the circulation into the thyroid. Once in the cell, iodide travels to the apical membrane to await incorporation into Tg. Meanwhile, the endoplasmic reticulum (ER) synthesizes the Tg monomer, which matures through folding and the addition of carbohydrates as it also migrates to the apical membrane under the guidance of molecular chaperones. At the apical membrane, thyroperoxidase (TPO) and H_2O_2 oxidize the iodide and, through a complex series of reactions, attach it to selected tyrosyl residues within the structure of Tg to form monoiodotyrosine (MIT) and diiodotyrosine (DIT) (Fig. 92–2). Further action of TPO causes two iodotyrosine residues to couple, both still part of the Tg molecule, to produce the thyroid hormones T_4 and T_3. The iodinated Tg, now a mature glycoprotein containing MIT, DIT, T_4, and T_3, is stored as colloid in the thyroid's follicular lumen. To deliver thyroid hormone to the circulation, endosomal and lysosomal pathways break down Tg and release its T_4 and T_3 across the basal membrane. The DIT and MIT of Tg are deiodinated and their iodide recycled within the cell.

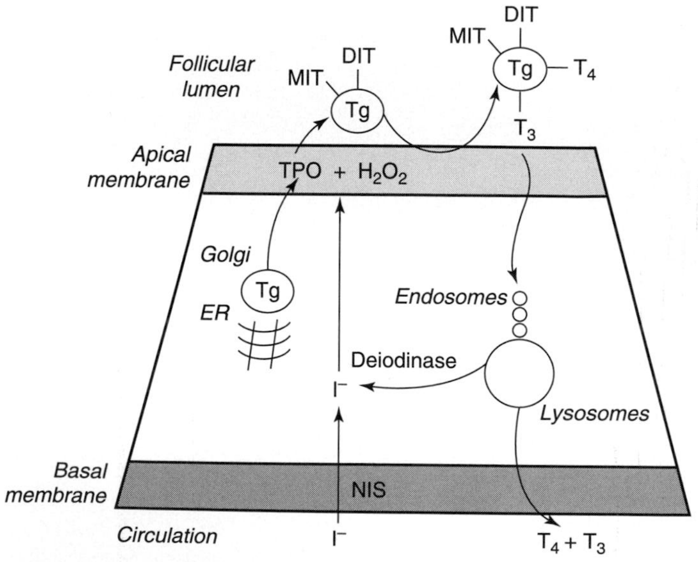

The two major regulators of this overall process are the amount of iodide available, which directly influences the amount of iodide concentrated, and thyroid-stimulating hormone (TSH), which controls most of the steps within the cell. The most important proteins in thyroid hormone formation are Tg, TPO, and NIS. Table 92–1 lists some of their characteristics, and detailed descriptions of each follow in the relevant sections.

This chapter considers thyroid hormone formation under the following headings: (1) iodide concentration, (2) Tg, (3) TPO and H_2O_2 generation, (4) Tg iodination and hormone formation, and (5) Tg proteolysis and hormone release. This division into steps is for convenience of presentation; in fact, hormone synthesis is a dynamic process, and its different components are intimately connected and interdependent. The present summary builds on a comprehensive review by Gentile, DiLauro, and Salvatore[1] in the last edition of this book and explores new developments since 1995.

FIGURE 92–1. Overview of hormone synthesis and release. See the text for details. DIT, 3,5-diiodotyrosine; ER, endoplasmic reticulum; MIT, 3-monoiodotyrosine; NIS, Na/I symporter; T_3, triiodothyronine; T_4, thyroxine; Tg, thyroglobulin; TPO, thyroid peroxidase.

IODIDE CONCENTRATION

The Iodide Pump

An active transport mechanism allows thyroid cells to concentrate I^- some 20- to 40-fold above its levels in the extracellular space against an electrical gradient of approximately −40 mV (for reviews see Wolff[2] and Taurog[3]). The process is inhibited by ouabain, which implies the involvement of Na^+,K^+-ATPase, and it is closely associated with the transport of Na^+ into the thyroid cell. These properties suggest that cotransport of Na^+ and I^- occurs in the thyroid cell and that Na^+,K^+-ATPase serves as the driving force by maintaining the Na^+ ion gradient. The transport process is not specific for I^-, and many other monovalent anions act as competitive inhibitors, for example, ClO_4^-, SCN^-, ReO_4^-.[2] A similar I^- transport system exists in several other tissues such as the salivary gland, mammary gland, and gastric mucosa.[2] Patients with defects in thyroid I^- transport lack the ability to concentrate I^- in these extrathyroidal sites as well, thus pointing to a common genetic determinant.

Studies with porcine thyrocytes cultured in a bicameral system demonstrated that I^- transport was restricted to the basolateral cell membrane.[4] Heat and sonication in the presence of trypsin inactivated transport activity in hybrid vesicles made from porcine thyroid membrane and soybean phospholipids, which suggests that a protein rather than a lipid was involved in the transport system.[5] The task of solubilizing and thus purifying the putative symporter was difficult in these earlier studies, and further characterization of the system awaited the development of genetic cloning and expression techniques.

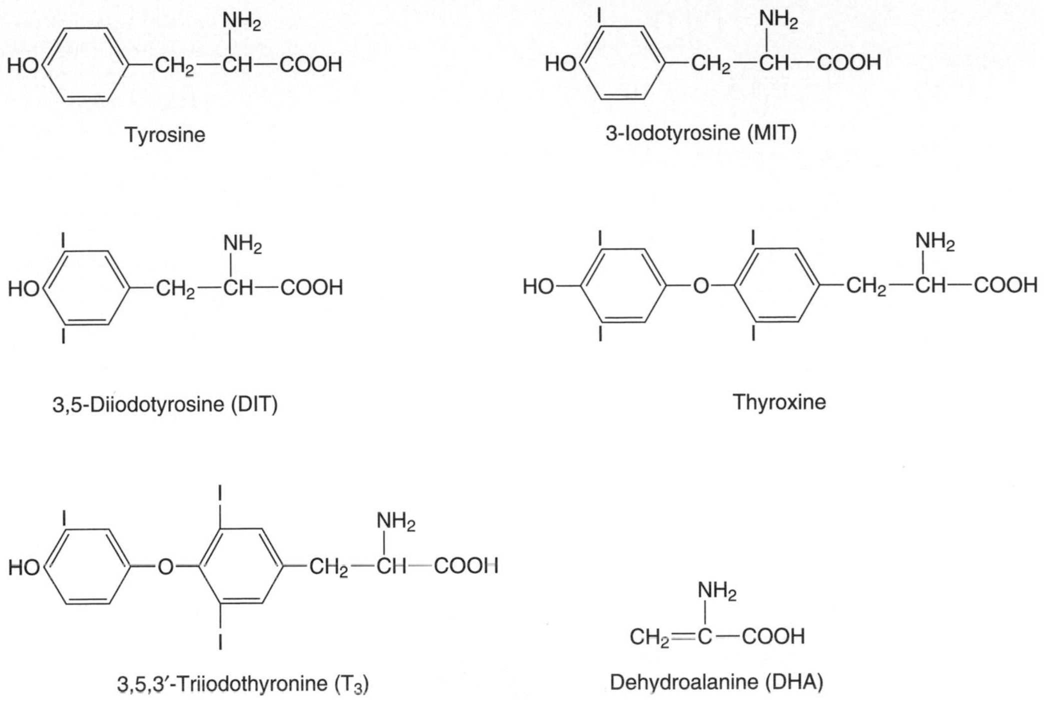

Tyrosine

3-Iodotyrosine (MIT)

3,5-Diiodotyrosine (DIT)

Thyroxine

3,5,3′-Triiodothyronine (T_3)

Dehydroalanine (DHA)

FIGURE 92–2. The thyroid hormones and related compounds.

The *NIS* Gene and Its Expression

In 1989 Vilijn and Carrasco demonstrated I^- transport in *Xenopus laevis* oocytes by transfecting them with RNA from rat FRTL5 cells.[6] Expression cloning with this system eventually led to isolation of the gene coding for the protein responsible for I^- transport in thyroid cells, now known as NIS.[7, 8] In these studies cRNA molecules were synthesized from a cDNA library derived from FRTL5 cells, and testing of successively fewer cDNA clones led to the final isolation. The properties of the expressed protein closely resembled those previously described for the I^- transport process in that they were Na^+ dependent and perchlorate sensitive. Activity after injection of the NIS clone led to greater than a 30-fold increase in the concentration of I^- in oocytes. The apparent K_m for I^- was 36 μmol/L, similar to values reported for FRTL5 cells.[9] The nucleotide sequence of the NIS clone was 2839 bp in length with a predicted open reading frame of 1854 nucleotides coding for a protein of 618 amino acids and an apparent molecular weight of 65.2 kDa.[7] NIS showed 24.6% homology with the human Na^+/glucose transporter. Based on its hydropathic profile and predicted secondary structure, the gene product appeared to be an intrinsic membrane protein originally thought to have 12 membrane-spanning domains with three putative *N*-linked glycosylation consensus sequences.[7] Site-directed mutagenesis of these sites indicated that all were used and led to a modification of the original model to include 13 rather than 12 membrane-spanning domains.[10] The cytosolic location of the C terminus of NIS was demonstrated by indirect immunofluorescence with the use of a site-directed polyclonal antibody against this region of the molecule.[10] The N terminus appeared to be extracellular from experiments using a mutated NIS construct with an N-terminal Flag epitope that was detected by immunofluorescence with an anti-Flag antibody.

Development of the expression system for rat NIS (rNIS) in *X. laevis* oocytes allowed comprehensive investigation of the I^- transport process.[11] rNIS activity depended on Na and was electrogenic. Oocytes expressing NIS in the presence of I^- generated a net inward current of approximately 400 mA. The apparent affinity constants for Na^+ and I^- were 28 ± 3 mmol/L and 33 ± 9 μmol/L, respectively. The stoichiometry of Na^+/I^- was 2:1. Other anions—ClO_3^-, SCN^-, $SeCN^-$, NO_3^-, Br^-, IO_4^-—generated similar steady-state inward currents, but I^- was most active. Surprisingly, ClO_4^- did not generate an inward current, which suggests that it is not transported by NIS despite its potent inhibitory action on I^- transport. The authors proposed a model of Na^+/I^- cotransport based on their kinetic studies[8] (Fig. 92–3). In this model Na^+ binds first to the transporter, at a binding site facing the external milieu. In the absence of I^-, NIS would serve as a uniporter and undergo conformational changes within the plasma membrane to deliver Na^+ into the cell. According to this scheme, in the presence of I^- a complex, CNa_2I, is formed that undergoes conformational changes to deliver I^- and two Na^+ ions to the cell interior. Once empty, NIS undergoes a second conformational change to expose its binding sites again to the cell exterior.[11]

Cloning of the human homologue followed shortly after cloning of the *rNIS* gene.[12] Total RNA from human papillary thyroid carcinoma tissue was reverse-transcribed and used as a template for polymerase

TABLE 92–1. Major Proteins of Hormone Formation—Tg, TPO, NIS

Feature	Tg	TPO	NIS
Function	Matrix for iodination and hormonogenesis	Catalyze oxidation of I^- and coupling	I^- transport into cell
Molecular mass (kDa)	660	103	65
Location	Follicular lumen	Apical membrane	Basal membrane
Transcription factors	TTF-1, TTF-2, Pax-8	TTF-1, TTF-2, Pax-8	Promoter has some homology to TTF-1
Response to TSH	↑ Activity	↑ Activity	↑ Activity
Homology	Acetylcholinesterase (C terminus); nidogens, etc. (N terminus)	Myeloperoxidase	Na^+/glucose transporter
Other features	Protein kinase activity?	I^- release from i-Tg?	Also in breast, other anions also active

i-Tg, insoluble thyroglobulin; NIS, sodium-iodide symporter; TPO, thyroperoxidase; TSH, thyroid-stimulating hormone; TTF-1, thyroid transcription factor-1.

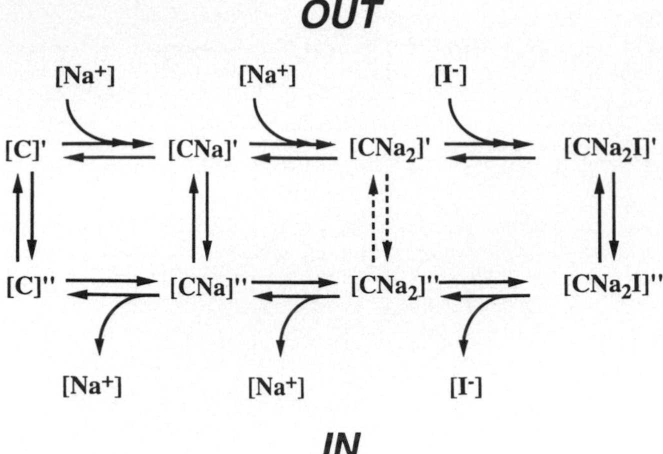

FIGURE 92–3. Model for Na^+/I^- cotransport as proposed by Levy et al. See the text for a description. (From Levy O, de la Vieja A, Carrasco N: The Na^+/I^- symporter: Recent advances. J Bioenerg Biomembr 30:195–206, 1998.)

chain reaction (PCR) amplification with two pairs of primers derived from the then-known nucleotide sequence of the rat gene. The human *NIS* (*hNIS*) gene predicted an open reading frame of 1929 nucleotides encoding for a protein of 643 amino acids with 84% identity with the *rNIS* gene. The coding region of *hNIS* contains 15 exons interrupted by 14 introns. The human gene maps to chromosome 19p.[13] hNIS expression in various thyroid states was studied by reverse transcription PCR[12, 13] and by immunohistochemistry.[14] In normal thyroids hNIS expression was sporadic, being present in relatively few thyrocytes within a given follicle. Immunohistochemical staining localized it to the thyrocyte's basal and lateral membranes.[14] In contrast, most thyrocytes from patients with Graves' disease reacted strongly to the NIS antibody. Thyroid carcinoma tissue had a much lower level of NIS expression relative to normal tissue by Northern blot, thus offering a partial explanation for the reduced I^- uptake seen in thyroid tumor tissue. Expression of hNIS in papillary carcinoma tissue by reverse transcription PCR proved to be quite variable.[13] Saito et al. found hNIS mRNA and protein levels 3.8 and 3.1 times higher, respectively, in thyroid tissue from patients with Graves' disease than in normal thyroid.[15]

TSH stimulation of I^- transport depends at least partly on increased expression of the *NIS* gene. Hypophysectomized rats have decreased levels of NIS protein that are restored by injection of TSH.[16] The addition of TSH (1 mU/mL) to quiescent FRTL5 cells led to an increase in I^- transport after 12 hours, with a maximum effect at 72 hours,[17] accompanied by an increase in NIS mRNA within 3 to 6 hours and a maximum effect at 24 hours, as analyzed by Northern blot with rNIS cDNA as probe. This effect could be mimicked by forskolin and $(Bu)_2$ cyclic adenosine monophosphate (cAMP). The NIS protein, detected by Western blot, increased in parallel with TSH-induced iodide transport. Moderate doses of I^- reduced both NIS and TPO mRNA expression in the TSH-stimulated dog thyroid, whereas expression of mRNA's TSH receptor and Tg were unaffected under the same conditions.[18] Transforming growth factor-β (TGF-β), which is known to inhibit I^- uptake by thyroid cells, suppressed both TSH-stimulated NIS mRNA, by Northern blot, and NIS protein levels, by Western blot.[19] Forskolin or cAMP overcame the inhibitory effect, thus indicating that TGF-β action occurs downstream of cAMP production.

Control of the *NIS* Gene

Control elements include a constitutive promoter within a 0.56-kb segment upstream from the NIS transcription start site and a cell-specific enhancer between nucleotides −2945 and −2264, which responds to cAMP in a cell-type–specific manner and requires protein synthesis.[8] Protein kinase A and CREB (cAMP response element–binding protein) were not essential for transcriptional activity of *rNIS*, thus differing from other thyroid-specific genes (Tg, TPO, and TSH receptor) whose regulatory elements are proximal to the start site and said to be largely independent of cAMP (but see below under Tg). On the other hand, DNA regulatory elements in the 2-kb immediate 5′ flanking region were not sufficient to explain thyroid-selective transcription of the *hNIS* gene,[20] nor were those within 8 kb of the 5′ flanking region of *rNIS*.[21]

Ohmori et al. identified a TSH response element between −420 and −385 bp by transfecting NIS promotor–luciferase chimeric plasmids into FRTL5 cells in the presence or absence of TSH.[22] The addition of TSH to FRTL5 cells caused an increase in one of two groups of protein-DNA complexes in gel mobility shift assays when the −420- to −385-bp fragment was used. The increase was seen within 3 to 6 hours with a maximum of 12 hours in FRTL5 cells. This increase did not occur in the nonfunctioning FRT thyroid or in Buffalo rat liver cell nuclear extracts. The same group reported that thyroid-specific transcription factor-1 (TTF-1) activates the *rNIS* promoter.[23]

Mutations in the Human *NIS* Gene

Defective iodide transport is a rare, but well-documented, cause of congenital goiter.[2] Recent reports have identified mutations in the *hNIS* gene as probable causes for the defect. Fujiwara et al. found a hypothyroid patient with a missense mutation in the *NIS* gene that substituted Pro for Thr at position 354.[24] Transfection of the mutant NIS into a nonthyroid cell line (HEK-293 cells) failed to elicit I^- transport. The authors suggested that the mutation led to a structural change in the putative ninth transmembrane domain. Another patient, euthyroid but with a large goiter, had the same mutation.[25] The mutant NIS cDNA transfected into COS cells showed greatly reduced I^- uptake. On Northern blot analysis, NIS mRNA was increased more than 100-fold over that in normal thyroid, thus suggesting compensatory overexpression in this subject's thyroid. More recently, Levy et al. altered the cDNA to substitute Pro for Thr at residue 354 in the expressed protein by site-directed mutagenesis and transfected it or wild-type NIS cDNA into COS cells.[8] Cells expressing the wild-type, but not the mutant NIS showed perchlorate-sensitive I^- transport. Immunoblot analysis indicated that levels of expression of the wild-type and mutant protein were essentially the same. Substitution of either Ala or Gly for Thr yielded nonfunctioning proteins, which suggests that the absence of Thr itself rather than structural changes in the protein was responsible for the loss of activity. In another patient, substitution of adenine for cytosine at nucleotide 1163 led to a premature stop at codon 272 in *NIS* and a nonfunctional protein.[26] A recent report described compound heterozygosity in a hypothyroid patient with very low I^- uptake.[27] She had a missense mutation in the *NIS* gene, with substitution of Glu for Gln 267 producing a nonfunctional protein, and in addition she had a nonsense mutation causing a downstream cryptic 3′ splice site that led to the loss of 129 C-terminal amino acids. Her isolated mRNA did not increase I^- transport when injected into *X. laevis* oocytes. Her father and brother were heterozygous for the missense mutation, and her mother and sister were heterozygous for the nonsense mutation; all four were euthyroid.

Further Significance of NIS

NIS also occurs outside the thyroid. Reverse transcription PCR shows hNIS expression in several other tissues known to concentrate iodide, including the breast and ovary.[14] The hNIS protein has also been detected in salivary glands, but in ductal rather than acinar cells.[14] NIS occurs in the plasma membrane of mammary gland epithelium, where it differs in molecular mass from thyroid NIS (~75 and ~90 kDa, respectively) and appears to be subjected to different posttranslational processing. NIS expression in the mammary gland is regulated by lactogenic stimuli.[8] This finding correlates with the physiologic need to provide iodine to nursing offspring to avoid iodine deficiency and its consequences in infants. Expression of NIS can increase with increased thyroid activity, such as with Graves' disease or hyperplastic nodules, and decrease with lowered thyroid metabolic activity, as in autoimmune thyroiditis and thyroid cancer. Application of NIS to clinical use appears promising, for example, in improved diagnosis with antibodies and cell targeting.[28]

THYROGLOBULIN

Chemistry

Most of the thyroid's Tg resides in the follicular lumen as a soluble dimer of approximately 660 kDa that sediments as a 19S fragment. It contains two identical polypeptide chains, each of 2750 amino acids (hTg), with slight variations among species. Carbohydrate accounts for about 10% of its weight and iodine for about 0.1% to 1.0%, which represents 5 to 50 atoms of iodine per molecule of 660-kDa Tg (detailed reviews and references up to 1995 can be found elsewhere[1, 29]).

Work from several laboratories deduced the primary structure of the Tg monomer from the cDNA of the human,[30] bovine,[31] rat,[32] and mouse[33] proteins. A recent re-examination of the cDNA for hTg changes 30 nucleotides and 21 amino acid residues, inserts a Gln at residue 966, and substitutes His for Tyr1024.[34] These new data show that hTg has 8307 bp coding for 2750 amino acids, including 66 tyrosyls. Homology among the several mammalian species is 75% or more. The cDNA sequences of nonmammalian species have not been elucidated, but their homology with those of mammals is expected to be fairly high because they share common hormonogenic sites and have similar patterns on gel electrophoresis.[29]

The Tg polypeptide chain has three distinct components, which suggests that the Tg molecule is a fusion of several distinct ancestral genes, at least two and probably three or even more. The N-terminal segment, which consists of the first 1190 residues, contains regions of highly conserved internal homology. The motif CWCVD appears 10 times at intervals of about 50 to 100 residues with slight variation[31] and has also been recently reported at residues 1510 to 1561.[35] This motif, referred to as the Tg type I domain, also occurs in seemingly unrelated proteins, including nidogens, saxiphilin, and testican, and appears to be associated with inhibition of cysteine proteases. Because these proteases are prominent in Tg proteolysis, Molina et al. proposed that this motif has a role in controlling the selective degradation of Tg to release hormone,[36] discussed below under hormone retrieval.

The second part of the polypeptide chain extends from residues 1191 to 2208. This portion does not have known similarity to other proteins but does have some internal homology: a short type 2 motif occurring three times between residues 1436 and 1483, a longer type 3a motif occurring three times between residues 1583 and 2167, and a long type 3c motif occurring twice between residues 1704 and 2109. One of the residues, Tyr1290, is a hormonogenic site[37] (see below). The third portion of the Tg monomer, from about residue 2209 through the terminus at 2750, shares 28% homology with acetylcholinesterases, both vertebrate and invertebrate. Acetylcholinesterase binds to cell membranes, and a similar function has been suggested by analogy for the C-terminal region of Tg. The homology has also invited speculation that Tg's C terminus may have enzymatic activity, perhaps promoting its own degradation.

Tg contains two basic carbohydrate units, similar to those of many other soluble glycoproteins, such as α_2-macroglobulin and IgM.[38] The first, the polymannose or type A unit, has a molecular weight of about 1800 and contains 5 to 11 mannose residues linked by *N*-acetylglucosamine to the polypeptide chain. The second, the complex or type B unit, has a molecular weight of 2100 to 3300 and consists of chains of *N*-acetylglucosamine, galactose, and either fucose or sialic acid attached to a mannose core, also linked through *N*-acetylglucosamine to the polypeptide chain. In hTg, about 75% of the 20 potential glycosylation sites are occupied.[39] Two other types of carbohydrate units have been described: one is type C, which has a molecular weight of 2000 to 3000 and consists chiefly of galactosamine, and the other is a large chondroitin sulfate unit.

Tg is one of the very few proteins that contain iodine in their native state. About 30% of Tg's iodine is in T_4 and T_3, the rest being in the inactive precursors DIT and MIT. A typical distribution for Tg with 0.5% iodine is 5 residues each of MIT and DIT, 2.5 of T_4, and 0.7 of T_3, but these proportions change considerably with different amounts of available iodine and with various thyroid diseases, particularly those with large amounts of Tg stored in colloid. Under physiologic as well as most experimental conditions, the maximum amount of iodine that can be incorporated into Tg is about 1%, or about 60 atoms of iodine per 660-kDa dimer, so less than half of Tg's tyrosyls are capable of iodination.

In addition to the well-characterized soluble 660-kDa molecule, Tg also exists in an insoluble form (i-Tg).[40] After extraction of soluble Tg from the follicular lumen, the i-Tg is found in globules measuring 20 to 120 μm in diameter at an estimated protein concentration of 590 mg/mL. About 30% of the follicular lumen's Tg was in this multimerized form. In comparison with 19S Tg, porcine i-Tg had about 40% more iodine and virtually no T_4 or T_3.[41] The Tg molecules in i-Tg are highly cross-linked, principally by disulfide bonds[42] but also through dityrosine.[41] It has been suggested that multimerization involves protein disulfide isomerase and provides a convenient iodine storage bin. The i-Tg is resistant to the usual proteolytic enzymes that degrade 660-kDa Tg. Baudry et al. exposed i-Tg in vitro to lactoperoxidase and a hydrogen peroxide–generating system designed to simulate the oxidizing conditions present in the thyroid for Tg iodination and found that free iodide was released and that staining on sodium dodecyl sulfate polyacrylamide gel electrophoresis was shifted from the electrophoretic origin to smaller bands, predominantly in 20- and 80-kDa regions, that were identified by immunoblotting as being Tg derived.[41] Those authors suggested that release of iodide from i-Tg by TPO/H_2O_2 may occur naturally in the thyroid and could be an additional function for this enzyme system in addition to its well-established role in Tg iodination and iodotyrosyl coupling (see below).

Tg preparations from rat, bovine, human, and FRTL5 thyroid cells may have protein kinase A activity.[43] A specific and saturable ATP-binding site was found in an N-terminal 64-kDa Tg polypeptide with two glycine-rich sequences (residues 154–160 and 468–475) that may serve as ATP binding sites. Although contaminating protein kinase activity could not be excluded, these investigators concluded that Tg has intrinsic protein kinase activity that can direct autophosphorylation of the Tg molecule. Of Tg's approximately 5 mol phosphate per 660-kDa dimer, about half occurs as mannose 6-phosphate in the high mannose carbohydrate unit, and the remainder is attributed to phosphotyrosine and phosphoserine. Formation of the latter may come from Tg's protein kinase A action. Kohn has suggested that the mannose 6-phosphate may affect lysosomal targeting and that the phosphoserine has a role in intracellular trafficking of Tg or perhaps in ordering Tg proteolysis.[44]

The Thyroglobulin Gene and Its Expression

The *Tg* gene resides on chromosome 8 (human), 15 (mouse), 7 (rat), or 14 (bovine). It consists of more than 200 kb, and its 42 or more exons constitute 10% or less of the gene. Assessment of exon placement thus far in the N-terminal portion of the *Tg* gene suggests its origin from an ancestral unit of 4 exons.[45] The dominant mRNA translates a 2750-residue peptide in hTg, but heterogeneity exists at both the mRNA and protein levels,[46] especially at the 3′ end. Acetylcholinesterase, to which the 3′ end is homologous, has extensive alternative splicing and variability in the translated proteins.[47]

Thyroid-specific transcription factors control the synthesis of Tg, TPO, and the TSH receptor[48, 49] (Fig. 92–4). The promoter is located about 170 bases before the initiation site. The three principal transcription factors identified thus far are TTF-1, TTF-2, and Pax-8. TTF-1 has three binding sites—A, B, and C—to the DNA of the *Tg* gene. Pax-8 has one apparent binding site and increases transcription.[50] Isoforms of Pax-8 mRNA occur in human thyroid from alternative splicing and influence transactivation. TTF-2 recognizes a single site, K, in the *Tg* gene. The binding site for Pax-8 partially overlaps with binding site C of TTF-1. The promoters for Tg and TPO have the same binding sites for TTF-1, TTF-2, and Pax-8. Both also have TTF-1 binding sites in the enhancer regions of the gene.

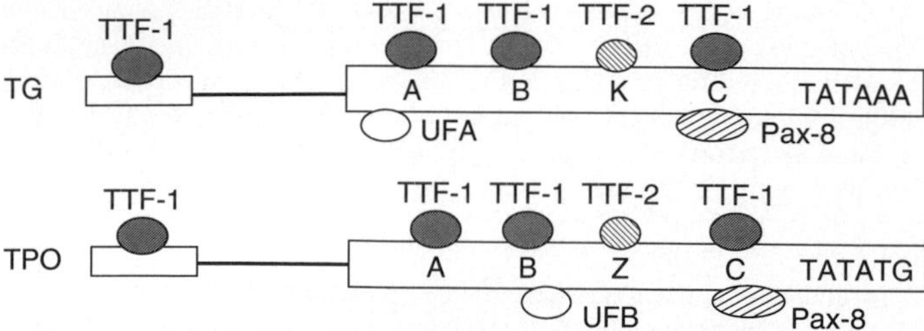

FIGURE 92–4. Thyroid-specific expression of the thyroglobulin (Tg) and thyroperoxidase (TPO) genes showing binding sites. TTF-1, thyroid transcription factor-1. (Adapted from Damante G, Di Lauro R: Thyroid-specific gene expression. Biochim Biophys Acta 1218:255–266, 1994.)

The relative activities of these several factors under varying physiologic conditions are complex.[49] TSH decreases binding of TTF-1 while increasing that of Pax-8, but Tg formation also increases, and TTF-1 appears to be a positive regulator.[51] TTF-1 was more effective in activating the Tg promoter, whereas Pax-8 activated the TPO promoter in one in vitro study. TTF-1 is also necessary for maximal expression of the TSH receptor gene. Additionally, Suzuki et al. suggest that Tg suppresses expression of the TTF-1, TTF-2, and Pax-8 genes and therefore expression of the Tg, TPO, NIS, and TSH receptor genes to create an autoregulatory system that TSH stimulates and Tg suppresses.[51] A role has also been suggested for redox systems in the expression of transcription factors. Reduced Pax-8 and TTF-1 were associated with increased promoter activity in TSH-stimulated FRTL5 cells,[52] which led to the speculation that the thyroid's production of H_2O_2 could affect gene expression in addition to its better known role in Tg iodination (see below).[49]

Work on the transcription factors and their role in thyroid regulation is advancing rapidly. Many results depend on elaborate experiments with rat FRTL5 cells or similar models, and their application to normal mammalian physiology must be established. Still, it is gratifying to glimpse seeming relationships among elements in thyroid physiology that seemed quite disparate a decade ago.

Thyroglobulin Maturation in the Cell

Synthesis of the Tg polypeptide chain occurs on polyribosomes on the surface of the rough ER. The Asn found at the N terminus of secreted Tg is preceded by a 19–amino acid leader that positions the molecule in the rough ER lumen. To become functional, the Tg polypeptide chains must undergo folding and dimerization. Proper ordering of these processes depends on molecular chaperones. Recent careful studies by Kim, Arvan, and others have done much to clarify this process.[53–61] In the ER, newly synthesized Tg appears first in high-molecular-weight aggregates held together by disulfide bonds and is then sequentially transformed into unfolded monomers, folded monomers, and finally stable dimers. Initial glycosylation of the molecule begins in the ER and is completed in the Golgi. Proper folding is directed by specific enzymes, including protein disulfide isomerase and peptidyl-prolyl isomerase. In addition, molecular chaperones are essential both for folding and for sorting the nascent Tg so that only mature and properly folded proteins are allowed to move on from the ER. Key chaperones include BiP, GRP 94, Erp 72, and calnexin. Of these, calnexin associates with Tg early, when it translocates into the ER before forming disulfide bonds.[56] The association with BiP also occurs early, when Tg exists as an unfolded monomer. The chaperone GRP 94 has activity parallel to that of BiP.[57] When glycosylation is inhibited, aggregated and misfolded Tg accumulates in the ER, with increased and prolonged binding of Tg to specific molecular chaperones, including BiP, GRP 94, GRP 72, and GRP 170.[55, 58] Experimentally increased levels of BiP or GRP 94 in Chinese hamster ovary cells impaired the folding and export of Tg, thus showing a direct role for these chaperones in Tg processing.[59, 60] Misfolded Tg that accumulates in the ER is probably abandoned and dumped into the cytoplasm for proteosomal degradation.[61]

The *cog/cog* mouse offers an instructive example of the interaction between Tg and molecular chaperones.[62] Mice homozygous for this defect have goiter, a distended ER, and little follicular glycoprotein.[63] The *Tg* gene appears to be involved, but Tg mRNA is abundant and synthesizes full-length Tg. However, the *cog/cog* Tg showed defective folding and ER export and was associated with increased induction of several molecular chaperones, including BiP, GRP 94, Erp 72, ER 60, and calreticulin. The Tg showed a single base substitution that changed leucine to proline at residue 2263. Site-directed mutagenesis that corrected this mutation restored normal Tg secretion in transfected COS cells. Thus the goiter of the *cog/cog* mouse is due to an abnormal Tg that results in defective folding and export from the ER, which makes this condition one of the so-called ER storage diseases.[53] This mouse model, in which a single amino acid substitution in Tg causes goiter, also emphasizes the enormous importance of Tg's primary structure in ensuring its normal maturation.

Reports of human congenital goiter with hypothyroidism, accumulation of immunoreactive and normally glycosylated Tg in the ER, and increased levels of BiP and GRP 94 suggest a situation similar to that in the *cog/cog* mouse.[64–66] One kindred lacked 138 nucleotides from Tg mRNA, which led to the deletion of residues 1831 to 1876 in the Tg molecule. This defect was distinct from that in the *cog/cog* mice and probably caused an unsatisfactory Tg, which in turn accounted for the increased levels of chaperone and the clinical findings.[66]

After leaving the ER, Tg, properly folded and partly glycosylated, moves to the Golgi for further attachment of carbohydrates. At this point the peripheral monosaccharides of the complex carbohydrate unit and sulfate are added. Phosphorylation probably occurs in either the ER or the Golgi. From the Golgi, glycosylated Tg travels to the apical membrane, where it is iodinated, as described below.

THYROPEROXIDASE AND HYDROGEN PEROXIDE GENERATION

TPO is the enzyme at the apical membrane of the thyroid cell that catalyzes both the iodination of Tg and the subsequent formation of thyroid hormones.[3] Expression of its gene is stimulated by TSH and depends on the same transcription factors—TTF-1, TTF-2, and Pax-8—that regulate the *Tg* gene (see Fig. 92–4). In its native form TPO may exist as dimer.[67] As usually isolated, TPO has a molecular mass of approximately 100 kDa and contains heme. About 10% of its mass is carbohydrate. Its cDNA sequence was first reported for humans[68] and the pig[69] and later for the rat and mouse. Two cDNAs for human TPO were found: TPO_1, which has 3048 nucleotides coding for 933 amino acids that produce a peptide with a molecular weight of 103 kDa, and TPO_2, which differs from TPO_1 only in 1 bp and in the lack of 171 bp representing exon 10. Studies on stable cell lines expressing TPO_1 and TPO_2 showed that only the former reached the cell surface.[70] TPO_2 also did not bind to heme and was rapidly degraded, thus showing that it was enzymatically inactive. The cDNA for pig TPO codes for a protein of 926 residues.[69] TPO is quite similar to myeloperoxidase in both structure and function. The overall homology is 44% but increases to 74% around histidine residue 407 of TPO, the site of the heme group. A highly active form of TPO can be prepared in the laboratory by treatment with trypsin and membrane solubilization to give a peptide of about 90 kDa. Yokoyama and Taurog proposed that the easily solubilized portion of TPO, from residues 1 to 844, is in the thyroid follicular lumen, the portion spanning residues 845 through 870 is in the apical membrane, and the remainder through residue 926 is in the cytoplasm.[71] Although TPO activity occurs at the apical membrane, most of the protein is found within the cell in the ER and perinuclear membrane.[72] Much of the TPO found intracellularly is not folded properly and has only the high mannose–type carbohydrate units, whereas TPO at the cell surface contains complex carbohydrate units. Blocking glycosylation with tunicamycin abolishes 95% of the enzymatic activity.[72]

Hydrogen peroxide is the substrate for TPO and is essential to iodination. H_2O_2 generation occurs at the apical membrane, requires both calcium and reduced nicotinamide-adenine dinucleotide phosphate (NADPH), and is stimulated by TSH. The enzyme responsible for the H_2O_2-generating activity, referred to as thyroid NADPH oxidase, has not been identified, but it appears to be independent of cytochrome *c* reductase activity.[73] TSH stimulates NADPH oxidase activity and H_2O_2 production, but it is uncertain whether this stimulation is through cAMP, as reported in dog thyrocytes,[74] by the phospholipase C/calcium cascade, as described in FRTL5 cells,[75] or by yet another pathway. Different hypotheses also exist for the intermediate steps leading to H_2O_2 generation. In one, O_2 produced by NADPH oxidase is converted to the superoxide ion (O_2^-), which superoxide dismutase converts to H_2O_2 at the membrane surface.[76] A second scheme involves direct electron transfer from NADPH to O_2 on the follicular side of the apical membrane.[77] Experimental approaches for identifying this mechanism are complex and indirect, and a satisfactory scheme is still not available.

IODINATION AND HORMONE FORMATION

Iodide and Tg meet at the apical membrane of the thyrocyte, where iodination of Tg produces thyroid hormone. The process includes the following sequential steps: (1) oxidation of iodide to an iodinating form, (2) transfer of iodine atoms to Tg to produce iodotyrosines, and (3) coupling of two iodotyrosyl molecules within Tg to produce the iodothyronine thyroid hormones.

Oxidation of Iodide

Iodide by itself is unreactive and must be oxidized to attach to proteins and other substrates. Standard in vitro procedures, such as iodinating proteins for radioimmunoassays, add iodine directly to the substrate or, alternatively, combine a peroxidase (e.g., lactoperoxidase), hydrogen peroxide, and iodide to constitute an iodinating system. The overall process is similar in the thyroid: iodide, H_2O_2, and TPO interact to form an iodinating species that attaches iodine to the substrate Tg. Figure 92–5 describes these steps. Although this broad outline is reasonably well established, details are less certain, particularly the chemical form of the iodine intermediate (for detailed reviews, see elsewhere[1, 3]). One proposed mechanism has iodide oxidized to the free radical and then to I_2. Another involves the iodinium ion I^+. A third proposes hypoiodite (OI^-) as an intermediate. Overall, the sequential steps are as follows (Fig. 92–6). TPO reacts with H_2O_2 to produce "compound I," which oxidizes iodide to an activated form that reacts with the tyrosyls in Tg to form iodotyrosines. In the absence of iodide, compound I is converted to compound II, which catalyzes iodotyrosyl coupling to form thyroid hormone. Excess H_2O_2 leads to the inactive compound III, and its formation is inhibited by iodide. Excess iodide prevents conversion of compound I to compound II and iodotyrosyl coupling. Recently, Taurog et al. analyzed the mechanisms of iodination and coupling in detail.[78] From comparisons with two similar peroxidases, cytochrome *c* peroxidase and lignin peroxidase, they suggest that both iodination and coupling catalyzed by TPO could be mediated by the porphyrin π cation radical form of compound I. Coupling was inhibited by excess iodide, which might reflect competition between iodide and iodotyrosines in Tg.

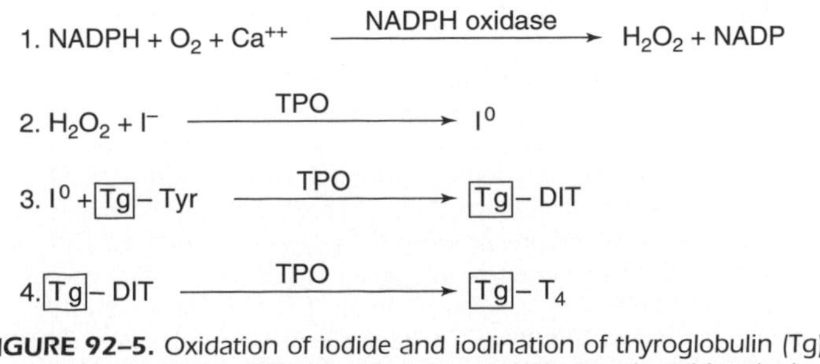

1. $NADPH + O_2 + Ca^{++} \xrightarrow{\text{NADPH oxidase}} H_2O_2 + NADP$

2. $H_2O_2 + I^- \xrightarrow{\text{TPO}} I^0$

3. $I^0 + \boxed{Tg} - Tyr \xrightarrow{\text{TPO}} \boxed{Tg} - DIT$

4. $\boxed{Tg} - DIT \xrightarrow{\text{TPO}} \boxed{Tg} - T_4$

FIGURE 92–5. Oxidation of iodide and iodination of thyroglobulin (Tg) to produce thyroxine. DIT, diiodotyrosine; NADP, nicotinamide-adenine dinucleotide phosphate; NADPH, reduced NADP; TPO, thyroperoxidase.

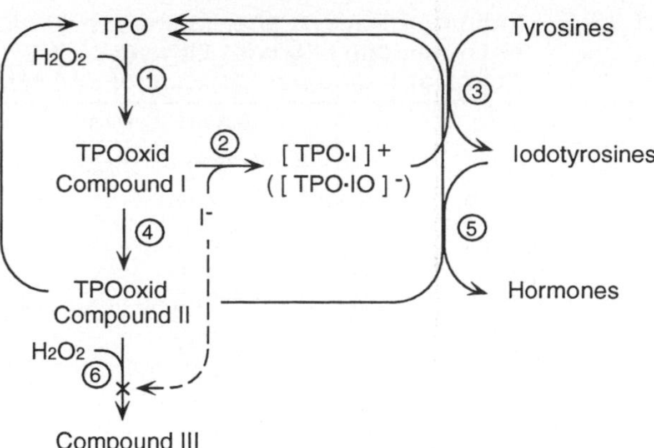

FIGURE 92–6. Compounds of thyroperoxidase (TPO) and H_2O_2 and their reactions. Compound I is formed upon addition of H_2O_2 to TPO (reaction 1) and oxidizes iodide (reaction 2) to an active iodinating form (represented here as either an iodinium ion or a hypoiodite ion bound to TPO) that catalyzes iodination of the tyrosyl residues of thyroglobulin (Tg) (reaction 3). In the absence of iodide, TPO compound I is converted to compound II (reaction 4), which catalyzes the coupling reaction (reaction 5). Excess H_2O_2 causes the conversion of TPO compound II to the inactive compound III (reaction 6). Inactivation is prevented by iodide.

The amount of available iodine is critical for successful Tg iodination. When the iodine supply is low, thyroid hormone synthesis diminishes for want of this indispensable ingredient, and the level of circulating T_4 is low. The pituitary responds by increasing TSH secretion, which stimulates most of the steps of thyroid hormone synthesis, and by producing more T_3 relative to T_4, which requires one less atom of iodine per iodothyronine molecule. Excess iodine acutely interferes with Tg iodination, the so-called Wolff Chaikoff effect. A proposed mechanism is that the excess iodine inhibits H_2O_2 and makes it unavailable for oxidation.[79]

Tyrosine Iodination

Iodotyrosines (MIT and DIT) are the precursors of thyroid hormones. In general, the addition of iodine to proteins iodinates the tyrosyls within the protein and occasionally its histidyls as well. Conditions required for this process are an appropriate substrate, a peroxidase, and a source of H_2O_2. These conditions are readily achieved in vitro, less frequently in vivo. Examples other than the thyroid include inactivation of bacteria by myeloperoxidase and probably the formation of MIT and DIT in kelp and scleral proteins. Thus the thyroid might be predicted to form iodotyrosines on Tg because peroxidase, H_2O_2, and a protein substrate are all present. What is unique about the thyroid is that it carries the process further in that it forms not only iodotyrosines but also thyroid hormones. Iodothyronine formation does not occur naturally anywhere else and only rarely with other proteins, even under favorable in vitro conditions. Thus Tg itself appears to be the critical feature that allows thyroid hormone synthesis in the thyroid.

Several laboratories have investigated the tyrosyls in Tg that are favored for early iodination (for review, see Dunn[29]). The in vitro addition of iodine to an hTG preparation of low iodine content from a goiter showed that several specific tyrosyls were the first to form MIT or DIT.[80] Table 92–2 shows the relative priority of iodination after the addition of two atoms of iodine per 660-kDa molecule to an hTg preparation containing 4.7 atoms per molecule. Figure 92–7 shows the location of these early iodination sites. The most prominent were at residues 2553, 130, 685, 847, 1447, and 5, in that order. The addition of 7.8 atoms of iodine per 660-kDa molecule to the same Tg increased the iodine at these sites, iodinated some new tyrosyl sites,

TABLE 92–2. Iodinated Tyrosyls after Iodination *In Vitro* of Low Iodine hTg with Either 2 or 7.8 Atoms of Iodine per Molecule of 660 kDa

		Residues Formed		
		Iodotyrosines		$T_4 + T_3$
Tyrosyl Residue	Sequence	*2.0 Atoms*	*7.8 Atoms*	*7.8 Atoms*
5	ADYVP	0.17	0.52	0.08
130	EGYVT	0.23	0.45	—
685	ECYCV	0.19	0.67	0.03
847	EPYLF	0.19	0.57	—
1290	ADYAG	0.07	0.25	Trace
1447	GSYSQ	0.19	0.60	—
2553	DDYAS	0.37	0.52	0.06
2567	RDYFI	0.08	0.29	—
2746	KTYSK	0.02	0.22	0.04

hTg, human thyroglobulin; T_3, triiodothyronine; T_4, thyroxine.

and produced thyroid hormone at residues 5, 2553, 2746, and 685, with a trace found at residue 1290.

Under a variety of conditions of both in vitro and in vivo analysis, Tyr5 usually contains from one-third to one-half of Tg's total T_4, and Tyr2553 contains about 20% to 25%. Hormone formation at different sites varies considerably with the experimental conditions. Tyr2746 is of particular interest because it is two residues away from Tg's C terminus and because it is a favorite site for T_3 synthesis in some species. The sequence Ser-Tyr-Ser at Tyr2746, as found in guinea pigs, rabbits, and pigs, may be more susceptible than the Thr-Tyr-Ser of hTg and bovine Tg (bTg). Tyr1290 formed little T_4 in hTg but accounted for 15% to 20% in rabbit and guinea pig Tg, and in these species TSH stimulated T_4 formation more vigorously there than at Tyr5 or Tyr2553.[37] Xiao et al. iodinated low iodine Tg from a human goiter and found iodine at residue Tyr2520, as well as at Tyr5 and Tyr2553.[81] Turtle Tg forms T_4 at residue 532, which has phenylalanine in the human but tyrosine in the rat.[82] These several observations show that the two most important hormonogenic sites are Tyr5 and Tyr2553, but that others exist and are occupied to varying degrees under physiologic and possibly pathologic conditions.

Several amino acid sequences in Tg appear to favor iodination and hormone synthesis.[80] One, Asp/Glu-Tyr, occurs at the two major hormonogenic sites at residues 5 and 2553 and also at residues 1290 and 2567. Another, Ser/Thr-Tyr-Ser, is associated with hormone formation at site 2746, and both of the other two sites where it occurs, around tyrosyls 1447 and 864, are iodinated early. The third consensus sequence, Glu-X-Tyr, occurs seven times in hTg and each was iodinated early. The existence of these consensus sequences points to a strong role of the primary structure of Tg in promoting iodination and hormone formation.

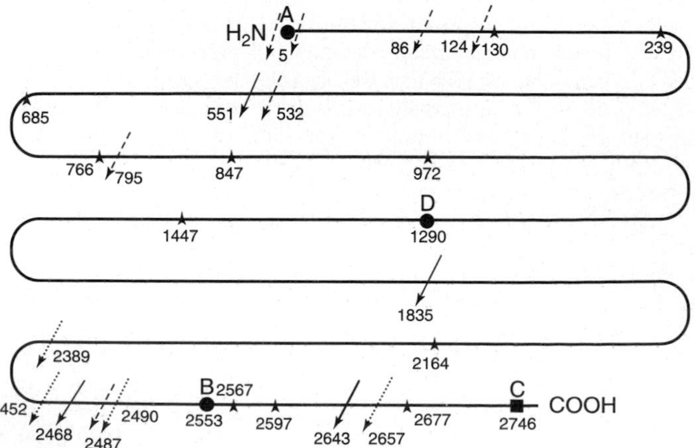

FIGURE 92–7. Diagram of the human thyroglobulin polypeptide chain; residue numbers refer to the human cDNA sequence. *A,* Sites forming thyroxine (sites A, B, D) *(solid circles)* and/or triiodothyronine (site C) *(solid square)*. *B,* Other early iodinated sites *(triangles)*. *C,* Cleavage sites of cathepsins D *(solid arrows)*, B *(dashed broken arrows)*, or L *(dotted broken arrows)*.

FIGURE 92–8. Iodotyrosyl coupling to form thyroxine (T_4). *Above,* The two diiodotyrosines (DITs) within thyroglobulin's peptide chain. *Below,* After coupling. The donor iodophenyl ring (DIT [d]) attaches at the -OH of the acceptor DIT (DIT [a]), with T_4 left at the acceptor site and dehydroalanine at the donor site.

Iodotyrosyl Coupling to Form T_4 and T_3

The next step in hormone formation is the coupling of two DIT residues to form T_4 or one DIT and one MIT to form T_3. This process takes place while both acceptor (providing the inner iodothyronine ring) and donor (providing the outer ring) remain within Tg's polypeptide chain (Fig. 92–8). TPO is involved in this step, as well as in tyrosine iodination. Several schemes have been proposed for the chemical events. In one, TPO and H_2O_2 produce free DIT radicals that interact to form a diphenyl ether across the OH group of the acceptor DIT, with subsequent cleavage from the donor side chain to leave T_4 and dehydroalanine (DHA) at the acceptor and donor sites, respectively.[3] Another scheme proposes formation of the iodine radical I°, which either reacts directly with the phenoxy radical of tyrosine or is first oxidized to I^+ before reacting.[83] Early reports proposed that the "lost side chain" remaining at the donor site is serine, but subsequent work by Gavaret et al. showed it to be DHA.[84] These investigators added 50 atoms of iodine to low iodine human Tg and identified the formation of equimolar amounts of T_4 and DHA, the latter characterized as *S*-benzylcysteine after acid hydrolysis. They also incorporated

^{14}C-tyrosine into hog thyroid slices, isolated the Tg, iodinated it, and recovered one residue of alanine per residue of T_4 formed. Depending on the isolation procedure, DHA could be identified as pyruvic acid, acetic acid, or alanine.

Once the cDNA structure of Tg's polypeptide chain was established and the hormonogenic sites were identified, the location of donor sites received attention. Identifying these sites is a more challenging chemical problem because DHA and its derivatives are less conspicuous than the bulky iodothyronine groups. Several indirect studies suggested possible candidates. Thus treatment of bTg with sodium ^{3}H-borohydride to convert DHA to ^{3}H-alanine led Palumbo to propose Tyr2539 as a donor.[85] Labeling bTg with 4-aminothiophenol suggested DHA at residues 5, 926, 1374, 985, and 1008 (corresponding positions in hTg).[86] However, of these residues, only residues 5 and 986 have Tyr in both hTg and bTg. The data from Table 92–2 show tyrosyls at positions 130, 847, 1447, and 2567 to be among the favored sites for early iodination of hTg in vitro. However, in contrast to tyrosyls 5, 2553, 2746, and 685, these tyrosyls did not seem to be acceptors in thyroid hormone formation and therefore appeared to be attractive possibilities for donors of outer rings. In vitro iodination of a CNBr-derived peptide from low iodine hTg, including residues 1 to 171, produced T_4 and an apparent cleavage in the peptide chain at Tyr130, which led to the suggestion that Tyr130 was a donor to the major hormonogenic site at Tyr5.[87] Other investigators concluded from a similar experiment that Tyr130 was an acceptor rather than donor[88]; these apparently conflicting results suggest that this CNBr peptide may not be a good model for in vivo thyroid hormone formation. Another experimental model expressed the first 198 residues of hTg in a baculovirus system and prepared mutant Tg fragments in which different tyrosyl residues were replaced with phenylalanine.[89] The mutants were iodinated in vitro and examined for T_4 formation. A fragment containing only Tyr5, Tyr107, and Tyr130 had as much T_4 as the intact normal peptide did. However, substitution of phenylalanine for a single tyrosyl at either residue 5 or 130 did not impair hormonogenesis, thus indicating that tyrosyls 5 and 130 were not essential for hormonogenesis in this system. As with the N-terminal CNBr fragments discussed above, this model may not provide the whole picture for in vivo hormone formation.[90]

More direct evidence comes from two recent papers that identify tyrosyls 130 (hTg) and 1375 (bTg) as outer ring donors. For the latter, Gentile et al. isolated a fragment of bTg encompassing residues 1218 to 1591 (bTg numbering) and separated its components by mass spectrometry.[91] Three of the seven tyrosyls in this peptide were iodinated: Tyr1234 containing MIT; Tyr1291 containing MIT, DIT, T_3, and T_4; and Tyr1375 containing MIT, DIT, and DHA. The iodothyronine at Tyr1291 (corresponding to hTg 1290) accounted for 10% of this Tg preparation's T_4 and 8% of its T_3. This hormonogenic site is the same one previously described in rabbits, guinea pigs, and humans.[37] The identification of DHA replacing Tyr1375 was by mass spectrometry, followed by digestion with endoproteinase Lys-C to yield a smaller peptide with DHA substituted for tyrosine. The iodine content at residue 1291 and its distribution among the iodoamino acids allowed a calculation of 0.4 mol of iodothyronine per mole of 660-kDa Tg at this site. After subtracting the amount of iodotyrosine found at residue 1375, the authors concluded that the molar amount of DHA at this site was similar to that of T_4 at position 1291 and therefore that residue 1375 was a plausible donor for the acceptor 1291. Neither human nor mouse Tg has a tyrosyl in a position corresponding to 1375. The primary structures at this portion of Tg in the guinea pig and rabbit, the two species with the most active T_4 formation at the site corresponding to 1390, are not known.

Previous indirect work, summarized above, suggested that Tyr130 may be a donor, probably for Tg's most important hormonogenic site at position 5. Dunn et al. approached this problem by incorporating ^{14}C-Tyr into beef thyroid slices, isolating the Tg, and iodinating it in vitro.[92] Nonlabeled Tg was isolated from the same glands, without in vitro iodination. Production of ^{14}C-T_4 left ^{14}C-DHA at the donor site, identified as its derivative ^{14}C-pyruvate. The N-terminal 22-kDa peptide was obtained by chemical reduction and digested with endoproteinase Glu-C to generate a fragment spanning residues 130 to 146 that contained ^{14}C-labeled pyruvate after pronase digestion. Mass spectrometry of the corresponding unlabeled peptide showed pyruvate replacing tyrosine at residue 130, and tryptic digestion of this peptide gave the expected cleavage and shortened fragment. Tryptic digestion of the 22-kDa fragment showed peptide cleavage between residues 129 and 130. The presence of ^{14}C-pyruvate in a fraction containing residue 130 (and no other tyrosyl) and the demonstration of pyruvate at position 130 in nonlabeled Tg offered convincing evidence that Tyr130 is an outer ring donor. Its most likely acceptor is Tyr5, Tg's principal hormonogenic site. Evidence for this conclusion was that Tyr5 and Tyr130 are the only important early iodination sites in the first 240 residues of hTg, the N terminus appears sufficient by itself to form T_4,[93] and amounts of Tg's ^{14}C-DHA and ^{14}C-pyruvate in the 22-kDa fragment were fairly similar.

Additional Effects of Iodination on Thyroglobulin

The process of Tg iodination is associated with discrete cleavage sites in its peptide chain.[29] Chemical reduction of disulfide bonds in normally iodinated hTg is sufficient to release a 26-kDa N-terminal peptide.[94] This peptide is not evident in poorly iodinated Tg, such as from certain goiters, but appears with progressive iodination in parallel with T_4 formation. Further iodination cleaves the 26-kDa peptide of hTg to an N-terminal 18-kDa peptide, as does TSH stimulation in vivo. These two N-terminal peptide groups—corresponding to human 26- and 18-kDa peptides—have been found in all species examined, including fish, amphibians, reptiles, birds, and a number of mammals.[95] Typically, more than half of their iodine is T_4, all apparently at position 5 in the peptide chain. Reduction of bTg gives discrete peptides, one beginning at residue 81 and another at 233 or 234.[96] These peptides in bTg probably correspond respectively to the 18- and 26-kDa peptides seen in humans, but precise cleavage sites have not been established in other species. The association between iodination and Tg cleavage is found in Tg isolated directly from the thyroid, without in vitro iodination, and is unaffected by proteolytic enzyme inhibitors. Administration of iodide acutely to iodine-deficient rats led to the progressive appearance of both the 20-kDa form (corresponding to 26 kDa in hTg) and T_4, but a low T_4 content in early samples suggested that iodination-associated cleavage may precede hormonogenesis and perhaps even depend on it.[97] The mechanism for this iodine-associated cleavage is not known. Iodination can split model peptides at tryptophanyl residues, and iodine in the presence of myeloperoxidase inactivates bacteria, probably by disruption of protein. A similar process may well exist in the thyroid.

A different type of peptide cleavage at Val129 was described earlier. Marriq et al. also reported a cleavage site between residues 129 and 130 in a CNBr-generated fragment of hTg.[98] As noted above, residue 130 contains DHA, and perhaps the instability of the peptide bond associated with the DHA residue makes it more susceptible to cleavage. Whether this activity occurs naturally after DHA formation or later during subsequent experimental steps is not known. The association of this cleavage may be indirect and result from the formation of DHA rather than a direct attack of iodine on the polypeptide. The details of how the process of iodination cleaves peptide bonds and why particular bonds are susceptible await further investigation.

THYROGLOBULIN PROTEOLYSIS AND HORMONE RELEASE

The thyroid stores its hormone, still part of the peptide structure of Tg, as colloid in the follicular lumen. Observers occasionally speculate on the biologic wisdom of producing a large protein such as Tg merely to iodinate a few tyrosyl residues and form hormone. A partial explanation is that colloid forms a convenient site for storage of both thyroid hormone and iodine, which is not always in constant supply. This storage depot allows the thyroid to dole out thyroid hormone as the body needs it and to rapidly mobilize it when called for. Such mobilization is accomplished by bringing stored Tg back from the follicular lumen into the cell, passing it through endosomal and lysosomal digestive systems, and delivering free hormone to the basal membrane for secretion into the circulation. About 70% of Tg's iodine is in the form of the inactive precursors MIT and DIT, which the thyrocyte deiodinates and then recycles the iodine. The most important enzymes for Tg degradation are the lysosomal proteases.

Proteases

The thyroid contains several proteases that are common to many tissues. The best characterized are the aspartic endopeptidase cathepsin D and the cysteine endopeptidases cathepsin B and L.[99] Additionally, cathepsin H has been described in the thyroid. Dunn et al. used specific enzyme inhibitors to study the activities of cathepsin D, B, and L, in lysosomes purified from human thyroids, against rabbit Tg labeled in vivo with ^{125}I.[100] Inhibition of all three enzymes blocked Tg degradation completely. Studies involving individual inhibitors showed that the cysteine proteases cathepsin L and B were more potent endopeptidases than cathepsin D was in this system. TSH stimulated the activities of cathepsin B and L but had little or no effect on cathepsin D activity. Peptides produced by the individual enzymes purified from human thyroids were isolated and the sites of cleavage identified by analogy to the cDNA sequence of hTg.[101] Figure 92–7 summarizes the major cleavage sites for each enzyme. Cathepsin L attacked near hydrophobic residues, particularly leucine, and its major cleavage sites were within the C-terminal 400 residues of Tg. Cathepsin D preferentially cleaved peptide bonds between hydrophobic residues, particularly aromatic ones, similar to its activity in other tissues. Cathepsin B had its principal cleavage sites in both the N-terminal and C-terminal regions. The presence of major hormonogenic sites at Tg's extreme N and C termini may favor selective release of thyroid hormone during proteolysis. For example, digestion of Tg with lysosomal extracts in vitro showed preferential release of hormone-rich fractions.[102]

The endopeptidases cleave Tg into large peptides that must then be further degraded by exopeptidases. The several exopeptidases identified in the thyroid include dipeptidyl-peptidases I and II, lysosomal dipeptidase I, and the carboxyl exopeptidase *N*-acetyl-L-phenolalanyl-L-tyrosine hydrolase.[99] Also, cathepsin B has exopeptidase activity in addition to its role as an endopeptidase.[101] Extended digestion of labeled rabbit Tg with purified cathepsin B produced the dipeptide T_4-Gln, which corresponds to residues 5 and 6 of the Tg sequence.[103] Incubation of N-terminal Tg with lysosomal dipeptidase I in addition to cathepsin B released free T_4. Thus the combination of cathepsin B and lysosomal dipeptidase I is sufficient to release T_4 from its most important site at residue 5. Dipeptidyl-peptidase II also increased the release of T_4 from Tg, but at a site different from residue 5. Identification of the site(s) and endopeptidase partner(s) awaits further investigation.

Thyroglobulin Degradation

The rat thyroid stimulated by TSH shows prompt and vigorous engulfment of material from the lumen to form colloid droplets, which are then internalized into the thyrocyte and passed through its lysosomal degradative pathway. However, under more usual physiologic conditions, colloid resorption takes place by micropinocytosis, and endocytotic vesicles are formed and pass successively through an endosomal compartment and then into lysosomes.[104–106] The initial event in micropinocytosis appears to involve the entrance of Tg into coated pits, probably without the intervention of receptors, the amount processed depending on the availability of endocytotic vesicles and the amount of Tg in the lumen.[107]

Tg's structure, specifically, the completion of its carbohydrate side chains, is important for its trafficking at the apical membrane. Immature Tg molecules are deficient in both iodine and glycosylation, so they have exposed *N*-acetylglucosamine residues. These residues are recognized by membrane receptors that apparently direct these immature molecules back to the Golgi for glycosylation and subsequent iodination. The Tg domain recognized by this receptor stretches from Ser789 to Met1172.[108] These observations suggest that Tg molecules are sorted in the endosomes, perhaps by iodine content, with immature molecules being recycled and mature ones readied for degradation and hormone release.

Some proteolytic processing may take place in endosomes before Tg enters lysosomes.[105, 106, 108] Lysosomal enzymes are also present in endosomes, where the acidic pH would favor their activity.[109] Some proteolytic processing may occur even before endocytosis. For example, cathepsin B activity has been detected at the cell surface of cultured thyrocytes.[110] In the same experimental model, activation of cysteine proteases permitted T_4 release at extralysosomal sites, as well as in the lysosomes, although T_3 release appeared to be restricted to lysosomes.

This chapter has already described specific cleavages in the peptide chain of Tg associated with its iodination. Such breaks occurred in the presence of protease inhibitors, thus suggesting that proteolytic enzymes were not involved. However, other specific proteolytic cleavages may also occur as early events in Tg degradation. Limited digestion with trypsin has identified several susceptible regions in the Tg molecule, most notably a region after residue 500 and another one around residue 1800.[111] A recent report on mouse Tg describes an initial cleavage after Lys500 that was proteolytic in character and independent of iodination.[112] A further cleavage released a 20-kDa N-terminal fragment containing T_4 and the consensus sequence R-X-K-R, a sequence known to be a substrate for prohormone convertases, which led to the speculation that Tg's iodination may also lead to its autoproteolysis. Also, as described earlier in this chapter, the Tg type 1 motif occurs in certain cysteine proteinase inhibitors.[36] A similar function for this motif in Tg would permit it to influence its own proteolysis.

T_4 emerges from the lysosomal degradative pathway probably as the free hormone or perhaps in small peptides. Most is secreted into the circulation. A specific transport mechanism across the basal membrane has not been identified. While still in the thyroid, some T_4 is converted to T_3 by type I 5′-iodothyronine deiodinase. This enzyme is the same one that in other tissues, such as the liver and kidney, produces T_3, the active form of the hormone, from circulating T_4, as described in Chapter 94.

About 70% of Tg's iodine is in MIT and DIT. Although small amounts of MIT and DIT are secreted into the circulation, most is deiodinated within the thyroid and its iodide returned to the general pool for recycling. This mechanism is important for iodine conservation, as shown by the functional iodine deficiency of patients who have the rare defect that blocks this step.[113] The iodotyrosine deiodinase responsible for this activity is an NADPH-dependent flavoprotein.[114] Its partial purification showed a molecular weight of about 42,000, and it consisted of two possibly identical subunits.

REFERENCES

1. Gentile F, DiLauro R, Salvatore G: Biosynthesis and secretion of thyroid hormones. *In* DeGroot LJ (ed): Endocrinology, ed 3. Philadelphia, WB Saunders, 1995, pp 517–542.
2. Wolff J: Congenital goiter with defective iodide transport. Endocr Rev 4:240–254, 1983.
3. Taurog A: Hormone synthesis. *In* Braverman LE, Utiger RD (eds): The Thyroid, ed 7. Philadelphia, JB Lippincott, 1996, pp 47–81.
4. Chambard M, Verrier B, Gabrion J, et al: Polarization of thyroid cells in culture: Evidence for the basolateral localization of the iodide "pump" and of the thyroid-stimulating hormone receptor–adenyl cyclase complex. J Cell Biol 96:1172–1177, 1983.
5. Saito K, Yamamoto K, Takai T, Yoshida S: Characteristics of the thyroid iodide translocator and of iodide-accumulating phospholipid vesicles. Endocrinology 114:868–872, 1984.
6. Vilijn F, Carrasco N: Expression of the thyroid sodium/iodide symporter in *Xenopus laevis* oocytes. J Biol Chem 264:11901–11903, 1989.
7. Dai G, Levy O, Carrasco N: Cloning and characterization of the thyroid iodide transporter. Nature 379:458–460, 1996.
8. Levy O, de la Vieja A, Carrasco N: The Na^+/I^- symporter (NIS): Recent advances. J Bioenerg Biomembr 30:195–206, 1998.
9. Carrasco N: Iodide transport in the thyroid gland. Biochim Biophys Acta 1154:65–82, 1993.
10. Levy O, de la Vieja A, Ginter CS, et al: *N*-linked glycosylation of the thyroid Na^+/I^- symporter (NIS). J Biol Chem 273:22657–22663, 1998.

11. Eskandari S, Loo DDF, Dai G, et al: Thyroid Na^+/I^- symporter. J Biol Chem 272:27230–27238, 1997.
12. Smanik PA, Liu Q, Furminger TL, et al: Cloning of the human sodium iodide symporter. Biochem Biophys Res Commun 226:339–345, 1996.
13. Smanik PA, Ryu K-Y, Theil KS, et al: Expression, exon-intron organization, and chromosome mapping of the human sodium iodide symporter. Endocrinology 138:3555–3558, 1997.
14. Jhiang SM, Cho J-Y, Ryu KY, et al: An immunohistochemical study of Na^+/I^- symporter in human thyroid tissues and salivary gland tissues. Endocrinology 139:4416–4419, 1998.
15. Saito T, Endo T, Kawaguchi A, et al: Increased expression of the Na^+/I^- symporter in cultured human thyroid cells exposed to thyrotropin and in Graves' thyroid tissue. J Clin Endocrinol Metab 82:3331–3336, 1997.
16. Levy O, Dai G, Riedel C: Characterization of the thyroid Na^+/I^- symporter with an anti-COOH terminus antibody. Proc Natl Acad Sci U S A 94:5568–5573, 1997.
17. Kogai T, Endo T, Saito T, et al: Regulation by thyroid-stimulating hormone of sodium/iodide symporter gene expression and protein levels in FRTL-5 cells. Endocrinology 138:2227–2232, 1997.
18. Uyttersprot N, Pelgrims N, Carrasco N, et al: Moderate doses of iodide in vivo inhibit cell proliferation and the expression of thyroperoxidase and Na^+/I^- symporter mRNAs in dog thyroid. Mol Cell Endocrinol 131:195–203, 1997.
19. Kawaguchi A, Ikeda M, Endo T, et al: Transforming growth factor-beta 1 suppresses thyrotropin-induced Na^+/I^- symporter messenger RNA and protein levels in FRTL-5 rat thyroid cells. Thyroid 7:789–794, 1997.
20. Ryu KY, Tong Q, Jhiang SM: Promoter characterization of the human Na^+/I^- symporter. J Clin Endocrinol Metab 83:3247–3251, 1998.
21. Tong Q, Ryu KY, Jhiang SM: Promoter characterization of the rat Na^+/I^- symporter gene. Biochem Biophys Res Commun 239:34–41, 1997.
22. Ohmori M, Endo T, Harii N, Onaya T: A novel thyroid transcription factor is essential for thyrotropin-induced up-regulation of Na^+/I^- symporter gene expression. Mol Endocrinol 12:727–736, 1998.
23. Endo T, Kaneshige M, Nakazato M, et al: Thyroid transcription factor-1 activates the promoter activity of rat thyroid Na^+/I^- symporter gene. Mol Endocrinol 11:1747–1755, 1997.
24. Fujiwara H, Tatsumi K, Miki K, et al: Congenital hypothyroidism caused by a mutation in the Na^+/I^- symporter (letter). Nat Genet 16:124–125, 1997.
25. Matsuda A, Kosugi S: A homozygous missense mutation of the sodium/iodide symporter gene causing iodide transport defect. J Clin Endocrinol Metab 82:3966–3971, 1997.
26. Pohlenz J, Medeiros-Neto G, Gross JL, et al: Hypothyroidism in a Brazilian kindred due to iodide trapping defect caused by a homozygous mutation in the sodium/iodide symporter gene. Biochem Biophys Res Commun 240:488–491, 1997.
27. Pohlenz J, Rosenthal IM, Weiss RE: Congenital hypothyroidism due to mutations in the sodium/iodide symporter. Identification of a nonsense mutation producing a downstream cryptic 3′ splice site. J Clin Invest 101:1028–1035, 1998.
28. Schmutzler C, Köhrle J: Implications of the molecular characterization of the sodium-iodide symporter (NIS). Exp Clin Endocrinol Diabetes 106(suppl):1–9, 1998.
29. Dunn JT: Thyroglobulin: Chemistry and biosynthesis. *In* Braverman LE, Utiger RD (eds): The Thyroid, ed 7. Philadelphia, JB Lippincott, 1996, pp 85–95.
30. Malthiery Y, Lissitzky S: Primary structure of human thyroglobulin deduced from the sequence of its 8448-base complementary DNA. Eur J Biochem 165:491–498, 1987.
31. Mercken L, Simons M-J, Swillens S, et al: Primary structure of bovine thyroglobulin deduced from the sequence of its 8,431-base complementary DNA. Nature 316:647–651, 1985.
32. DiLauro R, Avvedimento EV, Cerillo R, et al. Structure and function of the rat thyroglobulin gene. *In* Eggo MC, Burrow GN (eds): Thyroglobulin—The Prothyroid Hormone. Progress in Endocrine Research and Therapy, vol 2. New York, Raven, 1985, pp 77–86.
33. Kim PS, Hossain SA, Park Y-N, et al: A single amino acid change in the acetylcholinesterase-like domain of thyroglobulin causes congenital goiter with hypothyroidism in the *cog/cog* mouse: A model of human endoplasmic reticulum storage diseases. Proc Natl Acad Sci U S A 95:9909–9913, 1998.
34. van de Graaf SAR, Pauws E, de Vijlder JJM, Ris-Stalpers C: The revised 8307 base pair coding sequence of human thyroglobulin transiently expressed in eukaryotic cells. Eur J Endocrinol 136:508–515, 1997.
35. Molina F, Bouanani M, Pau B, Granier C: Characterization of the type-1 repeat from thyroglobulin, a cysteine-rich module found in proteins from different families. Eur J Biochem 240:125–133, 1996.
36. Molina F, Pau B, Granier C: The type-1 repeats of thyroglobulin regulate thyroglobulin degradation and T_3, T_4 release in thyrocytes. FEBS Lett 391:229–231, 1996.
37. Fassler CA, Dunn JT, Anderson PC, et al: Thyrotropin alters the utilization of thyroglobulin's hormonogenic sites. J Biol Chem 263:17366–17371, 1988.
38. Spiro MJ, Spiro RG: Synthesis and processing of thyroglobulin carbohydrate units. *In* Eggo MC, Burrow GN (eds): Thyroglobulin—The Prothyroid Hormone. Progress in Endocrine Research and Therapy, vol 2. New York, Raven, 1985, pp 103–113.
39. Yang S-X, Pollock HG, Rawitch AB: Glycosylation in human thyroglobulin: Location of the *N*-linked oligosaccharide units and comparison with bovine thyroglobulin. Arch Biochem Biophys 327:61–70, 1996.
40. Herzog V, Berndorfer U, Saber Y: Isolation of insoluble secretory product from bovine thyroid: Extracellular storage of thyroglobulin in covalently cross-linked form. J Cell Biol 118:1071–1083, 1992.
41. Baudry N, Lejeune PJ, Delom F, et al: Role of multimerized porcine thyroglobulin in iodine storage. Biochem Biophys Res Commun 242:292–296, 1998.
42. Berndorfer U, Wilms H, Herzog V: Multimerization of thyroglobulin (TG) during extracellular storage: Isolation of highly cross-linked TG from human thyroids. J Clin Endocrinol Metab 81:1918–1926, 1996.
43. Alvino CG, Acquaviva AM, Memoli Catanzano AM, Tassi V: Evidence that thyroglobulin has an associated protein kinase activity correlated with the presence of an adenosine triphosphate binding site. Endocrinology 136:3179–3185, 1995.
44. Kohn LD: Thyroglobulin—a new cyclic adenosine monophosphate–dependent protein kinase (editorial)? Endocrinology 136:3177–3178, 1995.
45. Parma J, Christophe D, Pohl V, Vassart G: Structural organization of the 5′ region of the thyroglobulin gene. Evidence for intron loss and "exonization" during evolution. J Mol Biol 196:769–779, 1987.
46. Mason ME, Struyk BP, Dunn JT: mRNA encoding human thyroglobulin's C-terminus is heterogeneous. Thyroid 6:633–637, 1996.
47. Taylor P: The cholinesterases. J Biol Chem 266:4025–4028, 1991.
48. Damante G, Di Lauro R: Thyroid-specific gene expression. Biochim Biophys Acta 1218:255–266, 1994.
49. Kambe F, Seo H: Thyroid-specific transcription factors. Endocr J 44:775–784, 1997.
50. Zannini M, Francis-Lang H, Plachov D, DiLauro R: Pax-8, a paired domain–containing protein, binds to a sequence overlapping the recognition site of a homeodomain and activates transcription from two thyroid-specific promoters. Mol Cell Biol 12:4230–4241, 1992.
51. Suzuki K, Lavaroni S, Mori A, et al: Autoregulation of thyroid-specific gene transcription by thyroglobulin. Proc Natl Acad Sci U S A 95:8251–8256, 1998.
52. Kambe F, Nomura Y, Okamoto T, Seo H: Redox regulation of thyroid-transcription factors, Pax-8 and TTF-1, is involved in their increased DNA-binding activities by thyrotropin in rat thyroid FRTL-5 cells. Mol Endocrinol 10:801–812, 1996.
53. Kim PS, Arvan P: Endocrinopathies in the family of endoplasmic reticulum (ER) storage diseases: Disorders of protein trafficking and the role of ER molecular chaperones. Endocr Rev 19:173–202, 1998.
54. Kim PS, Arvan P: Folding and assembly of newly synthesized thyroglobulin occurs in a pre-Golgi compartment. J Biol Chem 266:12412–12418, 1991.
55. Kim PS, Bole D, Arvan P: Transient aggregation of nascent thyroglobulin in the endoplasmic reticulum: Relationship to the molecular chaperone, BiP. J Cell Biol 118:541–549, 1992.
56. Kim PS, Arvan P: Calnexin and BiP act as sequential molecular chaperones during thyroglobulin folding in the endoplasmic reticulum. J Cell Biol 128:29–38, 1995.
57. Kim PS, Kwon O-Y, Arvan P: An endoplasmic reticulum storage disease causing congenital goiter with hypothyroidism. J Cell Biol 133:517–527, 1996.
58. Kuznetsov G, Chen LB, Nigam SK: Multiple molecular chaperones complex with misfolded large oligomeric glycoproteins in the endoplasmic reticulum. J Biol Chem 272:3057–3063, 1997.
59. Muresan Z, Arvan P: Thyroglobulin transport along the secretory pathway. J Biol Chem 272:26095–26102, 1997.
60. Muresan Z, Arvan P: Enhanced binding to the molecular chaperone BiP slows thyroglobulin export from the endoplasmic reticulum. Mol Endocrinol 12:458–467, 1998.
61. Yoo SE, Hossain SA, Kim YJ, Kim PS: Selective inhibition of proteosomal degradation of misfolded thyroglobulin is associated with induction of heat shock response and P53 mediated apoptosis in cultured thyrocytes (abstract 218). *In* Proceedings of the 71st Annual Meeting of the American Thyroid Association, Portland, Oregon, 1998.
62. Kim PS, Hossain SA, Park YN, et al: A single amino acid change in the acetylcholinesterase like domain of thyroglobulin causes congenital goiter with hypothyroidism in the *cog/cog* mouse: A model of human endoplasmic reticulum storage diseases. Proc Natl Acad Sci U S A 95:9909–9913, 1998.
63. Mayerhofer A, Amador AG, Beamer WG, Bartke A: Ultrastructural aspects of the goiter in *cog/cog* mice. J Hered 79:200–203, 1988.
64. Ohyama Y, Hosoya T, Kameya T, et al: Congenital euthyroid goitre with impaired thyroglobulin transport. Clin Endocrinol 41:129–135, 1994.
65. Targovnik HM, Vono J, Billerbeck AEC, et al: A 138-nucleotide deletion in the thyroglobulin ribonucleic acid messenger in a congenital goiter with defective thyroglobulin synthesis. J Clin Endocrinol Metab 80:3356–3360, 1995.
66. Medeiros-Neto G, Kim PS, Yoo SE, et al: Congenital hypothyroid goiter with deficient thyroglobulin. Identification of an endoplasmic reticulum storage disease with induction of molecular chaperones. J Clin Invest 98:2838–2844, 1996.
67. Baker JR Jr, Arscott P, Johnson J: An analysis of the structure and antigenicity of different forms of human thyroid peroxidase. Thyroid 4:173–178, 1994.
68. Kimura S, Kotani T, McBride OW, et al: Human thyroid peroxidase: Complete cDNA and protein sequence, chromosome mapping, and identification of two alternately spliced mRNAs. Proc Natl Acad Sci U S A 84:5555–5559, 1987.
69. Magnusson RP, Gestautas J, Taurog A, Rapoport B: Molecular cloning of the structural gene for porcine thyroid peroxidase. J Biol Chem 262:13885–13888, 1987.
70. Niccoli P, Fayadat L, Panneels V, et al: Human thyroperoxidase in its alternatively spliced form (TPO2) is enzymatically inactive and exhibits changes in intracellular processing and trafficking. J Biol Chem 272:29487–29492, 1997.
71. Yokoyama N, Taurog A: Porcine thyroid peroxidase: Relationship between the native enzyme and an active, highly purified tryptic fragment. Mol Endocrinol 2:838–844, 1988.
72. Fayadat L, Niccoli-Sire P, Lanet J, Franc JL: Human thyroperoxidase is largely retained and rapidly degraded in the endoplasmic reticulum. Its *N*-glycans are required for folding and intracellular trafficking. Endocrinology 139:4277–4285, 1998.
73. Carvalho DP, Dupuy C, Gorin Y, et al: The Ca^{2+}- and reduced nicotinamide adenine dinucleotide phosphate–dependent hydrogen peroxide generating system is induced by thyrotropin in porcine thyroid cells. Endocrinology 137:1007–1012, 1996.
74. Raspe E, Dumont JE: Tonic modulation of dog thyrocyte H_2O_2 generation and I^- uptake by thyrotropin through the cyclic adenosine 3′,5′-monophosphate cascade. Endocrinology 136:965–973, 1995.
75. Kimura T, Okajima F, Sho K, et al: Thyrotropin-induced hydrogen peroxide production in FRTL-5 thyroid cells is mediated not by adenosine 3′,5′-monophosphate, but by Ca^{2+} signaling followed by phospholipase-A_2 activation and potentiated by an adenosine derivative. Endocrinology 136:116–123, 1995.
76. Nakamura Y, Ohtaki S, Makino R, et al: Superoxide anion is the initial product in the hydrogen peroxide formation catalyzed by NADPH oxidase in porcine thyroid plasma membrane. J Biol Chem 264:4759–4761, 1989.

77. Dupuy C, Virion A, Ohayon R, et al: Mechanism of hydrogen peroxide formation catalyzed by NADPH oxidase in thyroid plasma membrane. J Biol Chem 266:3739–3743, 1991.
78. Taurog A, Dorris ML, Doerge DR: Mechanism of simultaneous iodination and coupling catalyzed by thyroid peroxidase. Arch Biochem Biophys 330:24–32, 1996.
79. Corvilain B, Van Sande J, Dumont JE: Inhibition by iodide of iodide binding to proteins: The "Wolff-Chaikoff" effect is caused by inhibition of H_2O_2 generation. Biochem Biophys Res Commun 154:1287–1292, 1988.
80. Lamas L, Anderson PC, Fox JW, Dunn JT: Consensus sequences for early iodination and hormonogenesis in human thyroglobulin. J Biol Chem 264:13541–13545, 1989.
81. Xiao S, Dorris ML, Rawitch AB, Taurog A: Selectivity in tyrosyl iodination sites in human thyroglobulin. Arch Biochem Biophys 334:284–294, 1996.
82. Roe MT, Anderson PC, Dunn AD, Dunn JT: The hormonogenic sites of turtle thyroglobulin and their homology with those of mammals. Endocrinology 124:1327–1332, 1989.
83. Gavaret J-M, Cahnmann HJ, Nunez J: Thyroid hormone synthesis in thyroglobulin. The mechanism of the coupling reaction. J Biol Chem 256:9167–9173, 1981.
84. Gavaret J-M, Nunez J, Cahnmann HJ: Formation of dehydroalanine residues during thyroid hormone synthesis in thyroglobulin. J Biol Chem 255:5281–5285, 1980.
85. Palumbo G: Thyroid hormonogenesis. Identification of a sequence containing iodophenyl donor site(s) in calf thyroglobulin. J Biol Chem 262:17182–17188, 1987.
86. Ohmiya Y, Hayashi H, Kondo T, Kondo Y: Location of dehydroalanine residues in the amino acid sequence of bovine thyroglobulin. Identification of "donor" tyrosine sites for hormonogenesis in thyroglobulin. J Biol Chem 265:9066–9071, 1990.
87. Marriq C, Lejeune P-J, Venot N, Vinet L: Hormone formation in the isolated fragment 1–171 of human thyroglobulin involves the couple tyrosine 5 and tyrosine 130. Mol Cell Endocrinol 81:155–165, 1991.
88. Xiao S, Pollock G, Taurog A, Rawitch AB: Characterization of hormonogenic sites in an N-terminal, cyanogen bromide fragment of human thyroglobulin. Arch Biochem Biophys 320:96–105, 1995.
89. den Hartog M, Sijmons CC, Bakker O, et al: Importance of the content and localization of tyrosine residues for thyroxine formation within the N-terminal part of human thyroglobulin. Eur J Endocrinol 132:611–617, 1995.
90. Dunn JT: Thyroglobulin, hormone synthesis and thyroid disease. Eur J Endocrinol 132:603–604, 1995.
91. Gentile F, Ferranti P, Mamone G, et al: Identification of hormonogenic tyrosines in fragment 1218–1591 of bovine thyroglobulin by mass spectrometry. J Biol Chem 272:639–646, 1997.
92. Dunn AD, Corsi CM, Myers HE, Dunn JT: Tyrosine 130 is an important outer ring donor for thyroxine formation in thyroglobulin. J Biol Chem 273:25223–25229, 1998.
93. Veenboer GJ, de Vijlder JJ: Molecular basis of the thyroglobulin synthesis defect in Dutch goats. Endocrinology 132:377–381, 1993.
94. Dunn, JT, Kim PS, Dunn AD: Favored sites for thyroid hormone formation on the peptide chains of human thyroglobulin. J Biol Chem 257:88–94, 1982.
95. Kim PS, Dunn JT, Kaiser DL: Similar hormone-rich peptides from thyroglobulins of five vertebrate classes. Endocrinology 114:369–374, 1984.
96. Gregg JD, Dziadik-Turner C, Rouse J, et al: A comparison of 30-kDa and 10-kDa hormone-containing fragments of bovine thyroglobulin. J Biol Chem 263:5190–5196, 1988.
97. Dunn JT, Kim PS, Dunn AD, et al: The role of iodination in the formation of hormone-rich peptides from thyroglobulin. J Biol Chem 258:9093–9099, 1983.
98. Marriq C, Lejeune PJ, Venot N, Vinet L: Hormone synthesis in human thyroglobulin: Possible cleavage of the polypeptide chain at the tyrosine donor site. FEBS Lett 242:414–418, 1989.
99. Dunn AD: Thyroglobulin retrieval and the endocytic pathway. *In* Braverman LE, Utiger RD (eds): The Thyroid, ed 7. Philadelphia, JB Lippincott, 1996, pp 81–84.
100. Dunn AD, Crutchfield HE, Dunn JT: Proteolytic processing of thyroglobulin by extracts of thyroid lysosomes. Endocrinology 128:3073–3080, 1991.
101. Dunn AD, Crutchfield HE, Dunn JT: Thyroglobulin processing by thyroidal proteases. J Biol Chem 266:20198–20204, 1991.
102. Tokuyama T, Yoshinari M, Rawitch AB, Taurog A: Digestion of thyroglobulin with purified thyroid lysosomes: Preferential release of iodoamino acids. Endocrinology 121:714–721, 1987.
103. Dunn AD, Myers HE, Dunn JT: The combined action of two thyroidal proteases releases T_4 from the dominant hormone-forming site of thyroglobulin. Endocrinology 137:3279–3285, 1996.
104. Bernier-Valentin F, Kostrouch Z, Rabilloud R, et al: Coated vesicles from thyroid cells carry iodinated thyroglobulin molecules. J Biol Chem 265:17373–17380, 1990.
105. Bernier-Valentin F, Kostrouch Z, Rabilloud R, Rousset B: Analysis of the thyroglobulin internalization process using in vitro reconstituted thyroid follicles: Evidence for a coated vesicle-dependent endocytic pathway. Endocrinology 129:2194–2201, 1991.
106. Kostrouch Z, Munari-Silem Y, Rajas F: Thyroglobulin internalized by thyrocytes passes through early and late endosomes. Endocrinology 129:2202–2211, 1991.
107. Kostrouch Z, Bernier-Valentin F, Munari-Silem Y, et al: Thyroglobulin molecules internalized by thyrocytes are sorted in early endosomes and partially recycled back to the follicular lumen. Endocrinology 132:2645–2653, 1993.
108. Rousset B, Selmi S, Bornet H, et al: Thyroid hormone residues are released from thyroglobulin with only limited alteration of the thyroglobulin structure. J Biol Chem 264:12620–12626, 1989.
109. Blum JS, Diaz R, Mayorga LS, Stahl PD: Reconstitution of endosomal transport and proteolysis. *In* Bergeron JJM, Harris JR (eds): Subcellular Biochemistry. Endocytic Components: Identification and Characterization, vol 19. New York, Plenum, 1993, pp 69–93.
110. Brix K, Lemansky P, Herzog V: Evidence for extracellularly acting cathepsins mediating thyroid hormone liberation in thyroid epithelial cells. Endocrinology 137:1963–1974, 1996.
111. Gentile F, Salvatore G: Preferential sites of proteolytic cleavage of bovine, human, and rat thyroglobulin. The use of limited proteolysis to detect solvent-exposed regions of the primary structure. Eur J Biochem 218:603–621, 1993.
112. Yoo SE, Hossain SA, Kim PS: Processing of mouse thyroglobulin in the export pathway: Relationship to thyroid hormonogenesis and endocytosis (abstract). *In* Proceedings of the 80th Annual Meeting of the Endocrine Society. 1998, p 88.
113. Medeiros-Neto G, Stanbury JB: The iodotyrosine deiodinase defect. *In* Inherited Disorders of the Thyroid System. Boca Raton, FL, CRC, 1994, pp 139–159.
114. Rosenberg IN, Goswami A: Purification and characterization of a flavoprotein from bovine thyroid with iodotyrosine deiodinase activity. J Biol Chem 254:12318–12325, 1979.

Chapter 93

Thyroid Regulatory Factors

Jacques E. Dumont ▪ Gilbert Vassart

Four major biologic variables are regulated in the thyrocyte as in any other cell type: function, cell size, cell number, and differentiation. The first three variables are quantitative and the latter is qualitative. In this chapter we consider the factors involved in these controls in physiology and in pathology, the main regulatory cascades through which these factors exert their effects, and the regulated processes, which are function, proliferation and cell death, gene expression, and differentiation. Whenever possible, we describe what is known in humans.

THYROID REGULATORY FACTORS

In Physiology

The two main factors that control the physiology of the thyroid are the requirement for thyroid hormones and the supply of its main and specialized substrate iodide (Table 93–1). Thyroid hormone plasma levels and action are monitored by the hypothalamic supraoptic nuclei and by the thyrotrophs of the anterior lobe of the pituitary, where they exert a negative feedback. The corresponding homeostatic control is expressed by thyroid-stimulating hormone (TSH, thyrotropin). Iodide supply is monitored in part through its effects on the plasma level of thyroid hormone, but mainly in the thyroid itself, where it depresses various aspects of thyroid function and the response of the thyrocyte to TSH. These two major physiologic regulators control the function and size of the thyroid—TSH positively, iodide negatively.[1–4] Although the thyroid contains receptors for thyroid hormones and a direct effect of these hormones on thyrocytes would make sense,[5] as yet little evidence has indicated that such control plays a role in physiology. Luteinizing hormone (LH) and human chorionic gonadotropin (hCG) at high levels directly stimulate the thyroid, and this effect accounts for the elevated thyroid activity at the beginning of pregnancy.[6–8]

The thyroid gland is also influenced by various other nonspecific hormones. Hydrocortisone exerts a differentiating action in vitro. Estrogens affect the thyroid by unknown mechanisms, directly or indirectly, as exemplified in the menstrual cycle and in pregnancy. Growth hormone induces thyroid growth, but its effects are thought to be mediated by locally produced somatomedins. Effects of locally secreted neurotransmitters and growth factors on thyrocytes have been demonstrated in vitro and sometimes in vivo, and the presence of some of these agents in the thyroid has been ascertained. However, there is no evidence that such controls have a physiologic role. The set of neurotransmitters acting on the thyrocyte and their effects vary from species to species.[2, 9] In the human, well-defined direct, but short-lived responses to norepinephrine, ATP, adenosine, bradykinin, and thyrotropin-releasing hormone (TRH) have been observed.[2, 10, 11] Similarly, effects of insulin-like growth factor-1 (IGF-1), epidermal growth factor (EGF), hepatocyte growth factor (HGF), tumor growth factor, and fibroblast growth factor (FGF) have been demonstrated on the thyrocytes of human and other species in vitro.[2, 12, 13] The fact that the thyroid is hypertrophied in acromegaly and does not develop into a goiter in endemic goiter areas in pygmies who have a defect of the IGF-1 system suggests that IGF-1 might have a tonic physiologic role in growth of the human thyroid.[2]

HGF does not activate normal human thyrocytes.[14] The physiologic and developmental role of the other growth factors remains to be defined. Thyroid hormone itself may act on the thyroid cell: it induces production of some proteins and its receptor is abundant in these cells.[15]

TABLE 93–1. Thyroid Regulatory Factors

Factor	Function	Differentiation	Proliferation
Specific			
Physiologic			
TSH	↗	↗	↗
LH, hCG (high levels)	↗	↗	↗
I^-	↘	?	↘
T_3, T_4	?	?	?
Pathologic			
TSAb	↗	↗	↗
TBAb	↘	?	↘
Nonspecific			
Physiologic			
Hydrocortisone	0	↗	0
IGF-I	?	↗	↗
EGF	↘/0	↘	↗
FGF	?	↘/0	↗
TGF-β	?	↘/0	↘
Norepinephrine	↗	0	0
PGE	↗	0	0
ATP, bradykinin, TRH	↗/↘	?	?
Pathologic			
IL-1	↘	↘	↘
TNF	↘	↘	↘
IFN-γ	↘	↘	↘

↗, stimulation; ↘, inhibition; 0, no effect; EGF, epidermal growth factor; FGF, fibroblast growth factor; hCG, human chorionic gonadotropin; IFN, interferon; IGF, insulin-like growth factor; IL, interleukin; LH, luteinizing hormone; PGF, prostaglandin F; T_3, triiodothyronine; T_4, thyroxine; TBAb, thyroid-blocking antibody; TGF, transforming growth factor; TRH, thyrotropin-releasing hormone; TSAb, thyroid-stimulating hormone.

In Pathology

Pathologic extracellular signals play an important role in autoimmune thyroid disease. Thyroid-stimulating antibodies (TSAbs), which bind to the TSH receptor and activate it, reproduce the stimulatory effects of TSH on the function and growth of the tissue. Their abnormal generation is responsible for the hyperthyroidism and goiter of Graves' disease. Thyroid-blocking antibodies (TBAbs) also bind to the TSH receptor but do not activate it and hence behave as competitive inhibitors of the hormone. Such antibodies are responsible for some cases of hypothyroidism in thyroiditis. Both stimulating and inhibitory antibodies induce transient hyperthyroidism or hypothyroidism in newborns of mothers with positive sera.[1] The existence of thyroid growth immunoglobulins has been hypothesized to explain the existence of Graves' disease with weak hyperthyroidism and prominent goiter. The thyroid specificity of such immunoglobulins would imply that they recognize thyroid-specific targets. However, despite many reports on the subject, convincing evidence is still lacking.[16–18] Moreover, discrepancies between growth and functional stimulation may instead reflect cell intrinsic factors. Local cytokines have been shown to influence the function, growth, and differentiation of thyrocytes in vitro and thyroid function in vivo. Because they are presumably secreted in loco in autoimmune thyroid diseases, these effects might play a role in the pathology of these diseases, but this notion has not yet been proved.[2, 19]

REGULATORY CASCADES

The great number of extracellular signals acting through specific receptors on cells in fact controls a very limited number of regulatory cascades. We first outline these cascades, along with the signals that control them, and then describe in more detail the specific thyroid cell features: controls by iodide and the TSH receptor.

The Cyclic Adenosine Monophosphate Cascade

The cyclic adenosine monophosphate (cAMP) cascade in the thyroid corresponds, as far as it has been studied, to the canonic model of the β-adrenergic receptor cascade[1] (Fig. 93–1). It is activated in the human thyrocyte by the TSH and the β-adrenergic and prostaglandin E receptors. These receptors are classic seven-transmembrane receptors controlling transducing guanosine triphosphate (GTP)-binding proteins. Activated G proteins belong to the G_s class and activate adenylate cyclase; they are composed of a distinct α_s subunit and nonspecific β and γ monomers. Activation of a G protein corresponds to its release of guanosine diphosphate (GDP) and binding of GTP and to its dissociation into α_{GTP} and βγ dimers. α_{sGTP} directly binds to and activates adenylate cyclase. Inactivation of the G protein follows the spontaneous, more or less rapid hydrolysis of GTP to GDP by α_s GTPase activity and the reassociation of α_{GDP} with βγ. The effect of stimulation of the receptor by agonist binding is to increase the rate of GDP release and GTP binding, thus shifting the equilibrium of the cycle toward the α_{GTP} active form. One receptor can consecutively activate several G proteins (hit-and-run model). A similar system negatively controls adenylate cyclase through G_i. It is stimulated in the human thyroid by norepinephrine through α_2-receptors. Adenosine at high concentrations directly inhibits adenylate cyclase. The cAMP generated by adenylate cyclase binds to the regulatory subunit of protein kinase A (PKA) that is blocking the catalytic subunit and releases this now-active unit. The activated, released catalytic unit of protein kinase phosphorylates serines in the set of proteins containing accessible specific peptides that it recognizes. These phosphorylations, through more or less complicated cascades, lead to the observed effects of the cascade. cAMP-dependent kinases have two isoenzymes (I, II), the first of which is more sensitive to cAMP, but as yet no clear specificity of action of these kinases has been demonstrated.[1] In the case of the thyroid, this cascade is activated through specific receptors by TSH in all species and by norepinephrine receptors and prostaglandin E in humans, with widely different kinetics: prolonged for TSH and short lived (minutes) for norepinephrine and prostaglandins.[2, 20, 21] Other neurotransmitters have been reported to activate the cascade in thyroid tissue, but not necessarily in the thyrocytes of the tissue.[11] Besides PKA, in the thyroid cAMP activates erythromycin propionate-*N*-acetylcysteinate (EPAC) or Rap guanosine nucleotide exchange factor-1 (GEF1) and the less abundant GEF-2, which activate the small G protein Rap.[22] Of the other known effectors of cAMP, cyclic guanosine monophosphate (cGMP)-dependent protein kinases are present in the thyroid but cyclic nucleotide–activated channels have not been looked for.

The Ca^{2+}–Inositol 1,4,5-Triphosphate Cascade

The Ca^{2+}–inositol 1,4,5-triphosphate (IP_3) cascade in the thyroid also corresponds, as far as has been studied, to the canonic model of the muscarinic or α_1-adrenergic receptor–activated cascades. It is activated in the human thyrocyte by TSH, through the same receptors that stimulate adenylate cyclase, and by ATP, bradykinin, and TRH—through specific receptors. In this cascade, as in the cAMP pathway, the activated receptor causes the release of GDP and the binding of GTP by the GTP-binding transducing protein (G_q) and its dissociation into α_q and βγ. α_{GTP} then stimulates phospholipase C. Phospholipase C hydrolyzes membrane phosphatidylinositol 4,5-bis-

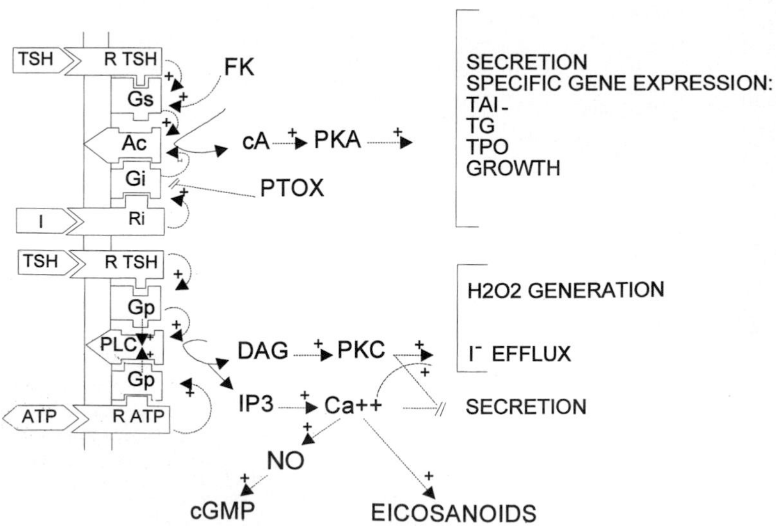

FIGURE 93–1. Regulatory cascades activated by thyroid-stimulating hormone (TSH) in human thyrocytes. In the human thyrocyte, H_2O_2 (H2O2) generation is activated only by the phosphatidylinositol 4,5-bisphosphate (PIP_2) cascade, that is, by the Ca^{2+} (Ca++) and diacylglycerol (DAG) internal signals. In dog thyrocytes, it is activated also by the cyclic adenosine monophosphate (cAMP) cascade. In dog thyrocytes and FRTL-5 cells, TSH does not activate the PIP_2 cascade at concentrations 100 times higher than those required to elicit its other effects. Ac, adenylate cyclase; cA, 3′5′-cAMP; cGMP, 3′5′-cyclic guanosine monophosphate; FK, forskolin; G_i, guanosine triphosphate (GTP)-binding transducing protein inhibiting adenylate cyclase; G_p, GTP-binding transducing protein activating PIP_2 phospholipase C; G_s, GTP-binding transducing protein activating adenylate cyclase; I, extracellular signal inhibiting adenylate cyclase (e.g., adenosine through A_1 receptors); IP_3, myoinositol 1,4,5-triphosphate; PKA, cAMP-dependent protein kinases; PKC, protein kinase C; PLC, phospholipase C; PTOX, pertussis toxin; R ATP, ATP purinergic P_2 receptor; R TSH, TSH receptor; Ri, receptor for I; TAI^-, active transport of iodide; TG, thyroglobulin; TPO, thyroperoxidase.

phosphate (PIP_2) into diacylglycerol and IP_3. IP_3 enhances calcium release from its intracellular stores, followed by an influx from the extracellular medium. The rise in free ionized intracellular Ca^{2+} leads to the activation of several proteins, including calmodulin. The latter protein in turn binds to target proteins and thus stimulates them: cyclic nucleotide phosphodiesterase and, most importantly, calmodulin-dependent protein kinases. These kinases phosphorylate a whole set of proteins exhibiting serines and threonines on their specific peptides and thus modulate them and cause many observable effects of this arm of the cascade.[1] Calmodulin also activates constitutive nitric oxide (NO) synthase in thyrocytes. The generated NO itself enhances soluble guanylate cyclase activity in thyrocytes and perhaps in other thyroid cells and thus increases cGMP accumulation.[21] Nothing is yet known about the role of cGMP in the thyroid cell.

Diacylglycerol released from PIP_2 activates protein kinase C, or rather the family of protein kinases C, which by phosphorylating serines or threonines in specific accessible peptides in target proteins causes the effects of the second arm of the cascade.[23] It inhibits phospholipase C or its G_q, thus creating a negative feedback loop. In the thyroid, the PIP_2 cascade is stimulated through specific receptors by ATP, bradykinin, and TRH and in humans by TSH.[11, 24, 25] The effects of bradykinin and TRH are very short lived. Acetylcholine, which is the main activator of this cascade in the dog thyrocyte, is inactive on the human cell, although it activates nonfollicular (presumably endothelial) cells in this tissue.[11]

Other Phospholipid-Linked Cascades

In dog thyroid cells and in a functional rat thyroid cell line (FRTL5), TSH activates PIP_2 hydrolysis weakly and at concentrations several orders of magnitude higher than those required to enhance cAMP accumulation. Of course, these effects have little biologic significance. However, in dog cells, at lower concentrations TSH increases the incorporation of labeled inositol and phosphate into phosphatidylinositol. Similar effects may exist in human cells, but they would be masked by stimulation of the PIP_2 cascade. They may reflect increased turnover or increased synthesis. Increased turnover would be explained by the reported stimulation by TSH of the hydrolysis of phosphatidylinositol glycan with the release of inositol phosphate glycan as observed in pig cells.[26] No such release is observed in dog or human cells. This explanation therefore does not stand in these systems, and the possible role of inositol phosphate glycan in the mediation of TSH effects remains very doubtful. After elimination of other hypotheses, the only remaining mechanism for the increased incorporation is increased synthesis, which is perhaps coupled to and necessary for cell growth.[1, 27, 28]

Diacylglycerol can be generated by other cascades than the classic Ca^{2+}-IP_3 pathway. Activation of phosphatidylcholine phospholipase D takes place in dog thyroid cells stimulated by carbamylcholine. Because it is reproduced by phorbol esters, that is, by stable analogues of diacylglycerol, it has been ascribed to phosphorylation of the enzyme by protein kinase C, which would represent a positive feedback loop. Although such mechanisms operate in many types of cells, their existence in human thyroid cells has not been demonstrated.[1]

Release of arachidonate from phosphatidylinositol by phospholipase A_2 and the consequent generation of prostaglandins by a substrate-driven process are enhanced in various cell types directly through G protein–coupled receptors, by intracellular calcium, or by phosphorylation by protein kinase C. In dog thyroid cells all agents enhancing intracellular calcium concentration, including acetylcholine, also enhance the release of arachidonate and the generation of prostaglandins. In this species, stimulation of the cAMP cascade by TSH inhibits this pathway. In pig thyrocytes, TSH has been reported to enhance arachidonate release. In human thyroid, TSH, by stimulating PIP_2 hydrolysis and intracellular calcium accumulation, might be expected to enhance arachidonate release and prostaglandin generation, but such effects have not yet been proved.[1, 20]

Regulatory Cascades Controlled by Receptor Tyrosine Kinases

Many growth factors and hormones act on their target cells by receptors that contain one transmembrane segment. They interact with the extracellular domain and activate the intracellular domain, which phosphorylates proteins on their tyrosines. Receptor activation involves in some cases a dimerization and in others a conformational change. The first step in activation is interprotein tyrosine phosphorylation, followed by binding of various protein substrates on the peptides of the receptor, including tyrosine phosphates. Such binding through src homology domains (SH2) leads to phosphorylation of these proteins on their tyrosines. In turn, this phosphorylation causes sequential activation of the *ras* and *raf* proto-oncogenes, mitogen-activated protein (MAP) kinase kinase, MAP kinase, and so on, on the one hand, and phosphatidylinositol-3′-OH kinase (PI-3-kinase), protein kinase B (PKB), and TOR (target of rapamycin) on the other hand. The set of proteins phosphorylated by a receptor defines the pattern of action of this receptor. In thyroids of various species, insulin, IGF-I, EGF, FGF, keratinocyte growth factor, HGF, but not platelet-derived growth factor activate such cascades.[29] In the human thyroid, effects of insulin, IGF-I, EGF, FGF, but not HGF have been demonstrated.[2, 30–32] Transforming growth factor-β, acting through its serine threonine kinase activity and intermediate proteins (Smad), inhibits proliferation and specific gene expression in human thyroid cells.

Cross-Signaling between the Cascades

Calcium, the intracellular signal generated by the PIP_2 cascade, activates calmodulin-dependent cyclic nucleotide phosphodiesterases and thus inhibits cAMP accumulation and its cascade.[33] This activity represents a negative cross-control between the PIP_2 and the cAMP cascades. Activation of protein kinase C enhances the cAMP response to TSH and inhibits the prostaglandin E response, which suggests opposite effects on the TSH and prostaglandin receptors.[34] No important effect of cAMP on the PIP_2 cascade has been detected. On the other hand, stimulation of protein kinase C by phorbol esters inhibits EGF action.

SPECIFIC CONTROL BY IODIDE

Iodide, the main substrate of the specific metabolism of the thyrocyte, is known to control the thyroid. Its main effects in vivo and in vitro are to decrease the response of the thyroid to TSH, acutely inhibit its own oxidation (Wolff-Chaikoff effect), reduce its trapping after a delay (adaptation to the Wolff-Chaikoff effect), and at high concentrations inhibit thyroid hormone secretion (Fig. 93–2). The first effect is very sensitive inasmuch as small changes in iodine intake are sufficient to reset the thyroid system at different serum TSH levels without any other changes (e.g., thyroid hormone levels), which suggests that in physiologic conditions, modulation of the thyroid response to TSH by iodide plays a major role in the negative feedback loop.[3] Iodide in vitro has also been reported to inhibit a number of metabolic steps in thyroid cells.[35, 36] These actions might be direct or indirect as a result of an effect on an initial step of a regulatory cascade. Certainly, iodide inhibits the cAMP cascade at the level of G_s or cyclase and the Ca^{2+}-PIP_2 cascade at the level of G_q or phospholipase C; such effects can account for the inhibition of many metabolic steps controlled by these cascades.[37–39] In one case in which this process has been studied in detail, the control of H_2O_2 generation, that is, the limiting factor of iodide oxidation and thyroid hormone formation, iodide inhibited both the cAMP and the Ca^{2+}-PIP_2 cascades at their first step and the effects of the generated intracellular signals cAMP, Ca^{2+}, and diacylglycerol on H_2O_2 generation.

The mechanism of action of iodide on all the metabolic steps besides secretion fits the "Xi" paradigm of Van Sande. These inhibitions are relieved by agents that block the trapping of iodide (e.g., perchlorate) and its oxidation (e.g., methimazole)—the Van Sande criteria. The

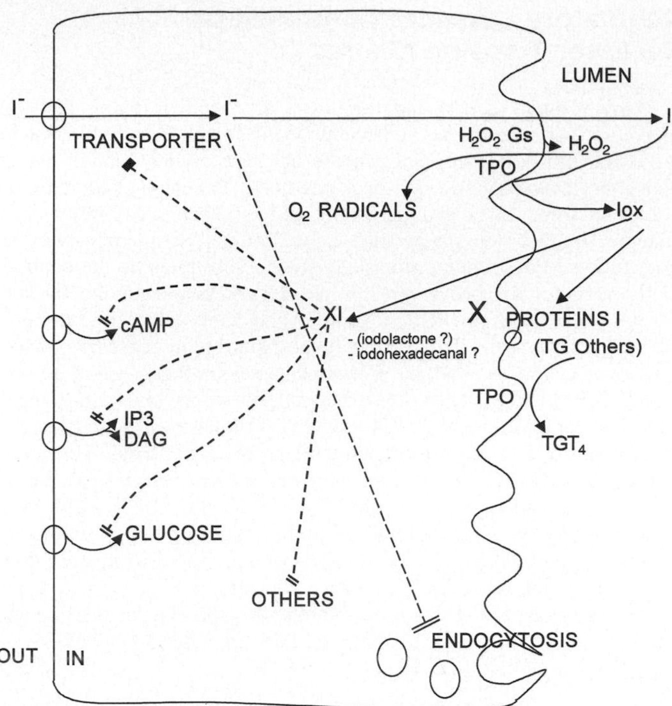

FIGURE 93–2. Effects of iodide on thyroid metabolism. All inhibitory effects of iodide, except in part the inhibition of secretion, are relieved by drugs that inhibit iodide trapping (e.g., perchlorate) or iodide oxidation (e.g., methimazole). Three possible mechanisms corresponding to this paradigm are outlined: generation of O_2 (O2) radicals, synthesis of an Xi compound, and iodination of target proteins. Any of these mechanisms could account for the various steps inhibited by I^- (indicated by *slashes*).

effects are therefore ascribed to one or several postulated intracellular iodinated inhibitors called Xi.[43] The identity of such signals is still unproved. At various times several candidates have been proposed for this role, such as thyroxine, iodinated eicosanoids (iodolactone), and iodohexadecanal.[43] The latter, the predominant iodinated lipid in the thyroid, could certainly account for the inhibition of adenylate cyclase. It should be emphasized that iodination of the various enzymes, as well as a catalytic role of iodide in the generation of O_2 radicals (shown to be involved in the toxic effects of iodide), could account for the Van Sande criteria with no need for the Xi paradigm.[40, 44]

THE THYROID-STIMULATING HORMONE RECEPTOR

As the sensor for the main regulatory agent acting on the thyroid and the target of autoimmune reactions, the TSH receptor had been extensively studied before it was cloned. Studies from affinity-labeling experiments described the receptor quite accurately as an integral membrane protein inserted in the basolateral plasma membrane and consisting of a relatively large extracellular domain responsible for TSH binding that is linked to a membrane-spanning domain.[45] The number of receptors was estimated to be around 1000 per cell. From its coupling to the generation of cAMP, it was classified as a member of the large family of G protein–coupled receptors interacting with G_s (see earlier). It was its belonging to this large receptor family and the expectation that it would display significant sequence similarity with other members of the family (in particular, with the FSH and LH receptors) that allowed cloning of TSH receptor cDNA.[46–51]

Structure of the Protein

The structure of the protein as it can be deduced from the sequence of the cDNA confirms that it belongs to the superfamily of G protein–coupled receptors (Fig. 93–3). Its 346-residue C-terminal half contains seven segments with the potential to constitute transmembrane helices, which is the hallmark of this protein family.[53] However, as predicted before cloning, it contains in addition a large N-terminal extracellular domain, a characteristic that it shares with the other glycoprotein hormone receptors. The cDNA sequence also revealed that contrary to most other G protein–coupled receptors, the TSH receptor (and the LH/chorionic gonadotropin [CG] and follicle-stimulating hormone [FSH] receptors as well) relies on a 20-residue signal peptide for its cotranslational insertion in the membrane of the endoplasmic reticulum. The N-terminal extracellular domain is about 398 residues in length. It consists of the loose repetition of 25–amino acid segments, referred to as *leucine repeats*. This kind of protein motif is found in a variety of intracellular as well as extracellular proteins, in which it is believed to serve in protein-protein or protein-membrane interactions.[54] Six potential acceptor sites for *N*-glycosylation are distributed along the extracellular domain.

The existence of structural variants of the receptor has been postulated from the cloning of several cDNAs with distinctive characteristics. In the dog, a cDNA lacking the potential to encode one leucine repeat is likely to arise from the differential splicing of exon 3.[55] In humans, cDNAs coding for a truncated form of the receptor lacking the transmembrane domains and C-terminal part have been identified.[56, 57] From a comparison of these cDNAs with the structure of the chromosomal gene,[52] it is suggested that they originate from differential splicing and/or polyadenylation of the primary transcript (see later). Similar cDNA variants have been described for the LH/CG receptor.[58] It is presently unclear whether the corresponding truncated proteins do

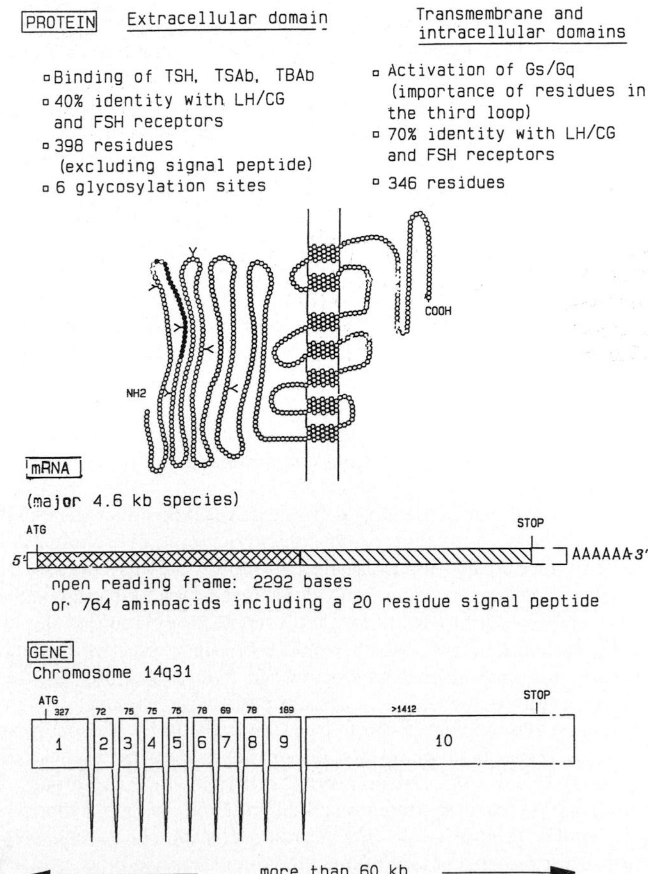

FIGURE 93–3. Schematic representation of the thyroid-stimulating hormone (TSH) receptor and its chromosomal gene. The potential N-glycosylation sites are represented by Y. The black portion of the extracellular domain represents one "leucine motif." The organization of the gene is not represented to scale except for the size of the exons, which are numbered and connected by introns schematized as V. Their sizes are indicated above individual boxes and are taken from Gross et al.[52]

exist or whether these cDNAs represent "noise" of the splicing/maturation pathway of gene expression.

It must be emphasized that the above description is that of a conceptual molecule derived from the mere translation of a reading frame (see Fig. 93–3). Regarding the actual structure of the receptor, as it is inserted in the basolateral membrane of the thyrocyte, the earlier suggestion that the receptor protein consists of two subunits held together by disulfide bonds has been validated in part. This arrangement implies maturation of the molecule by posttranslational cleavage.[58] Whether this cleavage, which affects part of the receptors in transfected cells and in vivo, is necessary for function of the molecule is not known. Sequence comparison of the primary structures of glycoprotein hormone receptors reveals maximal conservation (about 70% identity) within the carboxyl half of the molecules, which contains the transmembrane segments. The N-terminal extracellular domains still display highly significant similarities, in the range of 40% overall identity. A 50-residue insertion specific for the TSH receptor is found at the border between the extracellular domain and the first transmembrane segment. The pattern of these similarities within the glycoprotein hormone receptors immediately suggests that the extracellular domain would be responsible for binding specificity. The C-terminal half of the molecules containing the transmembrane segments would play the role of a transducer leading to G_s protein activation. Structure-function analyses of mutagenized receptors have since confirmed this hypothesis (see below).

Desensitization of some G protein–coupled receptors has been shown to involve phosphorylation of specific residues by G protein receptor kinases (homologous desensitization) or PKA (heterologous desensitization) enzymes.[53] When compared with other G protein–coupled receptors, the TSH receptor contains few phosphorylatable serine or threonine residues in its intracellular loops and C-terminal tail, which probably accounts for the limited desensitization observed after stimulation by TSH.

Structure of the Gene

The gene coding for the human TSH receptor has been localized on the long arm of chromosome 14 (14q31)[59, 60] (see Fig. 93–3). It spreads over more than 60 kb and is organized into 10 exons displaying an interesting correlation with the protein structure.[52] The extracellular domain is encoded by a series of 9 exons, each of which corresponds to one or an integer number of leucine repeats. The C-terminal half of the receptor containing the transmembrane segments is encoded by a single large exon. This finding is reminiscent of the fact that many G protein–coupled receptor genes are intronless. A likely evolutionary scenario derives from this gene organization[52]: the glycoprotein hormone receptor genes would have evolved from the condensation of an intronless classic G protein–coupled receptor with a mosaic gene encoding a protein with leucine repeats. Triplication of this ancestral gene and subsequent divergence led to the receptors for LH/CG, FSH, and TSH.

The gene promoter has been cloned and sequenced in humans and rats.[52, 61] It is too early to draw a precise picture of its structure-function relationships. However, the proximal promoter of the gene has characteristics of "housekeeping" genes in that it is guanine cytosine rich and devoid of TATA boxes; in the rat it was shown to drive transcription from multiple start sites.[61]

Expression of the TSH receptor gene is largely thyroid specific. Constructs made of a chloramphenicol acetyltransferase reporter gene under control of the 5′ flanking region of the rat gene show expression when transfected into FRTL5 cells and FRT cells but not into nonthyroid HeLa or a rat liver cell line (BRL) cells.[61] If one excepts a clear demonstration of TSH receptor mRNA in fat tissue of the guinea pig,[62] reports showing its presence in lymphocytes and extraocular tissue by reverse-transcription polymerase chain reaction are likely to correspond at best to illegitimate transcription because no functional activity has been clearly demonstrated in these cell types. Expression of the receptor in thyroid cells is extremely robust. It is moderately upregulated and downregulated by TSH in vitro and downregulated by iodide in vivo.[63]

Functional Aspects

Activation by Thyroid-Stimulating Hormone

Binding to the receptor of TSH, its natural ligand, results mainly in activation of G_s, which induces the stimulation of adenylyl cyclase. The median effective concentration (EC_{50}) for adenylyl cyclase activation by bovine TSH in human thyrocytes and in Chinese hamster ovary (CHO) cells transfected with the human cDNA is around 0.3 to 0.4 mU/mL.[24, 64] The dissociation constant for TSH binding (bovine TSH) expressed in biologic units is close to the same value (1.5 to 1.8 mU/mL).[65] In the absence of reliable knowledge of the bioactivity of pure intact human TSH,[66] it is difficult to translate this value in molar terms. The consensus is that it must be in the nanomolar range. The bioactivity of TSH is highly dependent on the glycosylation state of the hormone (see Chapter 91). In this respect it is interesting that artificially deglycosylated TSH behaves as a potent antagonist.[67]

In humans but not in the dog, TSH is also able to activate phospholipase C and thereby induce the accumulation of IP_3 and diacylglycerol (see earlier).[24, 25] The EC_{50} for the activation of this pathway is about one order of magnitude higher (about 5 mU/mL) than that for the cAMP cascade. The ability to activate adenylyl cyclase and phospholipase C is an intrinsic property of the receptor inasmuch as the cloned molecule expressed in CHO cells displays both activities.[24] Interestingly, the cloned canine TSH receptor exhibits the same dual potential when expressed in CHO cells, even though it activates only cAMP accumulation in the dog thyrocyte. It is likely that it is the G protein or the RGS (regulators of G protein signaling proteins) complement of cells that determines whether the receptor couples to one cascade, the other, or both.

Activation by Chorionic Gonadotropin

The extensive sequence similarity between glycoprotein hormones and observations of hyperthyroidism in molar pregnancies led to the concept that LH/CG could stimulate the TSH receptor (for references, see Hershman[8]). Although the issue is still controversial, a detailed analysis of TSH and thyroid hormone levels during pregnancy suggests that physiologic levels of CG can activate the thyroid.[6] LH and hCG at high concentrations certainly do it in vitro.

Activation by Autoantibodies

Autoantibodies found in Graves' disease and some types of idiopathic myxedema can stimulate (TSAb) or block (TBAb) TSH receptor, respectively (see Chapter 100). On slices of human thyroid tissue, under the conditions tested TSAbs have been found to stimulate only the cAMP cascade with no effect on phospholipase C activation.[68] However, experiments with the recombinant human TSH receptor expressed in CHO cells have shown that potent TSAb preparations, acting on cells superexpressing the receptor, are capable of activating both cascades, thus demonstrating that binding of TSH or TSAbs results in similar conformational changes within the TSH receptor.[69]

Structure-Function Relationships

It is tempting to exploit our knowledge of the primary structure of the TSH receptor and its belonging to the family of G protein–coupled receptors to try to answer the following questions: what are the domains involved in recognition of the receptor by TSH or TSAbs and what are the mechanisms leading to activation of the receptor and to subsequent activation of G_s? Before doing so, it is appropriate to briefly summarize what has been learned from the study of other G protein–coupled receptors and in particular from the adrenergic receptors.[52] Interaction between the ligand and the receptor takes place within the hydrophobic slit provided in the plasma membrane by the seven transmembrane α helixes. Key hydrophilic residues on some of these helices are implicated in the actual binding; for example, the Asp113 residue of the β-adrenergic receptor (or the homologue in the other receptors for charged amines) interacts with the amino group of norepinephrine. A still undefined change in conformation induced by the binding of agonists triggers activation of $G_{\alpha s}$. Residues of the amino and carboxyl portions of the third intracellular loop are known to play a crucial role in this interaction with G_s.

In view of their common evolutionary origin and extensive sequence similarities, the TSH receptor and the adrenergic receptor are likely to share basic mechanisms implicated in their activation. However, one faces the problem of disproportion of the ligands. The huge dimeric TSH obviously cannot fit within the hydrophobic slit of the TSH receptor. Despite extensive site-directed mutagenesis studies,[70, 71] the problem is still open. Domain-swapping experiments in which the extracellular domains of the LH/CG and TSH receptors were exchanged clearly demonstrated that the extracellular domain is responsible for binding of the hormone. Because the chimeric receptors were competent for adenylyl cyclase stimulation, these experiments also demonstrate that whatever the mechanism of receptor activation, it is compatible with exchange of the extracellular domain–hormone complex. Attempts to identify the hormone-binding domain on a few residues have been unsuccessful, the conclusion being that binding of TSH must involve large portions of tertiary structure. Nevertheless, TSH receptor–LH/CG receptor chimeric constructs led to the identification of short segments of the extracellular domain of the TSH receptor that take part in the interaction. The exact role of carbohydrate chains in the function of the receptor awaits further extension of site-directed mutagenesis experiments to include mutation of each residue in the six potential acceptor sites for *N*-glycosylation.

Identification of the binding sites of TSAbs to the receptor (see Chapter 100) is an example of the difficulties of dealing with discontinuous epitopes. A fair summary is that some epitopes implicated in Graves' disease can be separated from regions involved in the binding of TSH, that TSAbs seem to be heterogeneous in their recognition sites, and that the extreme N-terminal part of the receptor is involved.[72]

Identification of the segments or residues of the receptor responsible for interaction with G_s or with its activation has been difficult because of the great sensitivity of the receptor to mutation of individual residues or segments of its intracellular loops. In agreement with results obtained with the adrenergic receptors, a detailed site-directed mutagenesis study indicated an important role for the C-terminal portion of the third intracellular loop.[71] Recent data suggest that Ala623 in this region would play a role in coupling of the receptor to G_q inasmuch as its mutation to Glu or Lys in the rat receptor destroys its ability to stimulate the Ca^{2+}-IP_3 pathway, thereby leaving stimulation of adenylyl cyclase intact.[73]

CONTROL OF THYROID FUNCTION

Thyroid Hormone Synthesis

Thyroid hormone synthesis requires the uptake of iodide by active transport, thyroglobulin biosynthesis, oxidation and binding of iodide to thyroglobulin, and within the matrix of this protein, oxidative coupling of two iodotyrosines into iodothyronines. All these steps are regulated by the cascades just described.

Iodide Transport

Iodide is actively transported by the iodide Na^+/I^- symporter (NIS) against an electrical gradient at the basal membrane of the thyrocyte and diffuses by a specialized channel (pendrin)[75] from the cell to the lumen at the apical membrane. The opposite fluxes of iodide, from the lumen to the cell and from the cell to the outside, are generally considered to be passive and nonspecific. At least three types of control have been demonstrated[35, 36, 75]:

1. Rapid and transient stimulation of iodide efflux by TSH in vivo, which might reflect a general increase in membrane permeability. The cascade involved is not known.
2. Rapid activation of iodide apical efflux from the cell to the lumen by TSH. This effect, which contributes to the concentration of iodide at the site of its oxidation, is mediated, depending on the species, by Ca^{2+} and/or cAMP.[75] In human cells it is mainly controlled by Ca^{2+} and therefore by the TSH effect on phospholipase C.
3. Delayed increase in the capacity (Vmax) of the active iodide transport NIS in response to TSH. This effect is inhibited by inhibitors of RNA and protein synthesis and is due to activation of iodide transporter gene expression. This effect of TSH is reproduced by cAMP analogues in vitro and is therefore mediated by the cAMP cascade.[4] mRNA expression is enhanced by TSH and cAMP and decreased by iodide.[15, 63] TSH enhancement of thyroid blood flow, more or less delayed depending on the species, also contributes to increase the uptake of iodide.[4] Iodine levels in the thyroid are also inversely related to blood flow.[76]
4. Rapid inhibition by iodide of its own transport in vivo and in vitro. This inhibitory effect requires an intact transport and oxidation function, that is, it fulfills the criteria of an Xi effect. After several hours the capacity of the active transport mechanism is greatly impaired (adaptation to the Wolff-Chaikoff effect).[35] The mechanism of the first effect is unknown but probably initially involves direct inhibition of the transport system itself (akin to the desensitization of a receptor), followed later by inhibition of NIS gene expression and its synthesis (akin to the downregulation of a receptor).[63]

Iodide Binding to Protein and Iodotyrosine Coupling

Iodide oxidation and binding to thyroglobulin and iodotyrosine coupling in iodothyronines are catalyzed by the same enzyme, thyroperoxidase, with H_2O_2 used as a substrate.[77] The same regulations therefore apply to the two steps. H_2O_2 is generated by a still-undefined membrane system. The system is very efficient in the basal state inasmuch as little of the iodide trapped can be chased by perchlorate in vivo. Also, in vitro the amount of iodine bound to proteins mainly depends on the iodide supply. Nevertheless, in human thyroid in vitro, stimulation of the iodination process takes place even at low concentrations of the anion, thus indicating that iodination is a secondary limiting step. Such stimulation is caused in all species by intracellular Ca^{2+} and is therefore a consequence of activation of the Ca^{2+}-PIP_2 cascade. In many species, phorbol esters and diacylglycerol, presumably through protein kinase C, also enhance iodination.[78] It is striking that in a species such as the human, in which TSH activates the PIP_2 cascade, cAMP inhibits iodination, whereas in a species (dog) in which TSH activates only the cAMP cascade, cAMP enhances iodination. Obviously in the latter species a supplementary cAMP control was necessary.[1, 78, 79]

Thyroperoxidase does not contain any obvious phosphorylation site in its intracellular tail. On the other hand, all the agents that activate iodination also activate H_2O_2 generation, and inhibition of H_2O_2 generation decreases iodination, which therefore suggests that iodination is an H_2O_2 substrate–driven process and that it is mainly controlled by H_2O_2 generation.[30, 78] Congruent with the relatively high K_m of thyroperoxidase for H_2O_2, H_2O_2 is generated in disproportionate amounts with regard to the quantity of iodide oxidized. Negative control of iodination by iodide (the Wolff-Chaikoff effect) is accompanied and mostly explained by the inhibition of H_2O_2 generation. This effect of I^- is relieved by perchlorate and methimazole and thus pertains to the Xi paradigm.[21, 40, 78]

Iodotyrosine coupling to iodotyrosines is catalyzed by the same system and is therefore subject to the same regulations as iodination. However, coupling requires that suitable tyrosyl groups in thyroglobulin be iodinated, that is, that the level of iodination of the protein be sufficient. In the case of severe iodine deficiency or when thyroglobulin exceeds the iodine available, insufficient iodination of each thyroglobulin molecule will preclude iodothyronine formation whatever the activity of the H_2O_2 generating system and thyroperoxidase. On the other hand, when the iodotyrosines involved in the coupling are present, coupling is controlled by the H_2O_2 concentration but independent of iodide.[77] In this case, H_2O_2 control has a significance even at very low iodide concentrations.

H_2O_2 generation requires the reduced form of nicotinamide-adenine dinucleotide phosphate (NADPH) as a coenzyme and is thus accompanied by NADPH oxidation. Limitation of the activity of the pentose phosphate pathway by $NADP^+$ leads to stimulation of this pathway by H_2O_2 generation. Also, excess H_2O_2 leaking back into the thyrocyte is reduced by glutathione (GSH) peroxidase, and the oxidized GSH (GSSG) produced is reduced by NADPH-linked GSH reductase. Thus both the generation of H_2O_2 and the disposal of excess H_2O_2 by pulling NADP reduction and the pentose pathway lead to activation of this pathway—historically one of the earliest and unexplained effects of TSH.[4, 78]

In long-term situations in vivo or in vitro, the activity of the whole iodination system obviously also depends on the level of its constitutive enzymes. It is therefore not surprising that activation of thyrocytes by the cAMP cascade increases the corresponding gene expression whereas dedifferentiating treatments with EGF and phorbol esters inhibit this expression and thus reduce the capacity and activity of the system. Apparent discrepancies in the literature about the effects of phorbol esters on iodination are mostly explained by the kinetics of these effects (acute stimulation of the system, delayed inhibition of expression of the involved genes).

Thyroid Hormone Secretion

Secretion of thyroid hormone requires endocytosis of human thyroglobulin, its hydrolysis, and the release of thyroid hormones from the cell. Thyroglobulin can be ingested by the thyrocyte by three mechanisms.[4, 80, 81] In *macropinocytosis*, which is the first, pseudopods engulf clumps of thyroglobulin. In all species this process is triggered by activation of the cAMP cascade and therefore by TSH. Stimulation of macropinocytosis is preceded and accompanied by an enhancement of thyroglobulin exocytosis and thus the membrane surface.[4, 82–85] By *micropinocytosis*, the second process, small amounts of colloid fluid are ingested. This process does not appear to be greatly influenced by acute modulation of the regulatory cascades. It is enhanced in chronically stimulated thyroids. A third (hypothesized) process is *receptor-mediated endocytosis*; its existence is still controversial and its regulation unknown.[86, 87] The protein involved could be megalin.[88]

Contrary to the last named, the first two processes are not specific for the protein. They can be distinguished by the fact that macropinocytosis is inhibited by microfilament and microtubule poisons and by lowering of the temperature (below 23°C). Whatever its mechanism, endocytosis is followed by lysosomal digestion with complete hydrolysis of thyroglobulin. The main iodothyronine in thyroglobulin is thyroxine. However, during its secretion a small fraction is deiodinated by type I 5-deiodinase to triiodothyronine (T_3), thus increasing relative T_3 (the active hormone) secretion.[1, 4]

The free thyroid hormones are released by an unknown mechanism, which may be diffusion or transport. The iodotyrosines are deiodinated by specific deiodinases and their iodide recirculated in the thyroid iodide compartments. Under acute stimulation, a release (spillover) of amino acids and iodide from the thyroid is observed. A mechanism for lysosome uptake of poorly iodinated thyroglobulin on *N*-acetylglucosamine receptors and recirculation to the lumen has been proposed. Under normal physiologic conditions, endocytosis is the limiting step of secretion, but after acute stimulation, hydrolysis might become limiting with the accumulation of colloid droplets. Secretion by macropinocytosis is triggered by activation of the cAMP cascade and inhibited by Ca^{2+} at two levels: cAMP accumulation and cAMP action. It is also inhibited in some thyroids by protein kinase C downstream from cAMP. Thus the PIP_2 cascade negatively controls macropinocytosis.[1, 34]

The thyroid also releases thyroglobulin. Inasmuch as this thyroglobulin was first demonstrated by its iodine, at least part of this thyroglobulin is iodinated; thus it must originate from the colloid lumen. Release is inhibited in vitro by various metabolic inhibitors and therefore corresponds to active secretion.[5, 83] The most plausible mechanism is transcytosis from the lumen to the thyrocyte lateral membranes.[84] As for thyroid hormone, this secretion is enhanced by activation of the cAMP cascade and TSH and inhibited by Ca^{2+} and protein kinase C activation. Because thyroglobulin secretion does not require its iodination, it reflects the activation state of the gland regardless of the efficiency of thyroid hormone synthesis. Thyroglobulin serum levels and their increase after TSH stimulation constitute a very useful index of the functional state of the gland when this synthesis is impaired, as in iodine deficiency, congenital defects in iodine metabolism, treatment with antithyroid drugs, and the like. Regulated thyroglobulin secretion should not be confused with the release of this protein from thyroid tumors, which corresponds in large part to exocytosis of newly synthesized thyroglobulin in the extracellular space rather than in the nonexistent or disrupted follicular lumen. In inflammation or after even mild trauma, opening of the follicles can cause unregulated leakage of lumen thyroglobulin.

CONTROL OF THYROID-SPECIFIC GENE EXPRESSION

Thyroid cell differentiation in the embryo depends on the expression of some well-defined but not specific transcription factors (HNF3, HOXB3, NKX25, MOXa-3) and some almost specific thyroid transcription factors (TTF-1, TTF-2, Pax-8). However, until now there has been little evidence that modulation of these factors is involved in quantitative regulation of thyroid-specific proteins in the normal differentiated thyrocyte.[89] The CREB (cAMP response element–binding protein), CREM (cAMP response element modulator), and transcription factors activated by PKA through phosphorylation modulate the expression of several genes but not those of thyroperoxidase or thyroglobulin.[90, 91]

A positive in vivo effect of TSH on general protein synthesis has been well documented. This effect is mimicked by cAMP agonists and is part of the trophic effect of TSH on the thyrocyte. It involves stimulation of transcription and translation; however, the detailed mechanisms implicated are not known.

Thyroglobulin

Regulation of thyroglobulin gene expression has been studied in depth and reviewed in several publications.[92] Clear evidence has been obtained for regulation by TSH via cAMP at the transcription level, with some evidence for the existence of translational control as well.[92–95] Continuous protein synthesis is required to sustain thyroglobulin gene transcription.[96] Together with the relatively long delay before stimulation by TSH or cAMP (8–16 hours in primary culture of dog thyrocytes, depending on the conditions), this observation suggests that the TSH or cAMP transcriptional effects on the thyroglobulin gene require the synthesis of new proteins. However, provided that the thyroids have first been deprived of TSH, a rapid stimulatory effect on transcription is observed 1 hour after stimulation by TSH or cAMP in incubated tissue slices[96] and in vivo after TSH administration in the rat.[93] Obviously, the proteins necessary for transcription of the gene are present in the normal in vivo situation.

It is likely that TSH or cAMP can exert effects at more than one level, depending on the differentiation state of the cell. In a fully differentiated thyrocyte, as present in vivo or in tissue slices, rapid stimulation may be achieved via a phosphorylation cascade involving preexisting proteins. It is not clear whether de novo protein synthesis is required because in thyroid slices also, the protein synthesis inhibitor cycloheximide abolishes thyroglobulin gene transcription.[96] In primary cultures of thyrocytes, TSH may need to bring the thyroglobulin gene and its complement of transcription factors to a state of differentiation (by mechanisms involving regulation at transcription and/or translation), on which it could exert its stimulatory action.[2] Another possibility is that one level of control is simply lost during the adaptation of thyrocytes to primary culture. Coherent with this view is the observation that expression of the thyroglobulin gene is poorly controlled by TSH or cAMP in the FRTL5 cell line.[97] This immortalized rat thyroid cell line is expected to be one step further down the scale of thyroid differentiation in comparison to primary culture of thyrocytes, which themselves would be less differentiated than thyroid slices or tissue in vivo.

The 250 bp upstream from the transcription start contain DNA sequences implicated in TSH or cAMP stimulation of both thyroglobulin gene transcription and elements responsible for its tissue-specific expression[98–104] (see Chapter 90). Contrary to the case in most of the genes under rapid control by cAMP, thyroglobulin promoter does not contain target sequences for CREB (see Chapter 90). This scenario fits with the relatively slow kinetics of cAMP action and with the dependence of the effect on protein synthesis. An important unanswered question is whether two transcription factors showing some specificity for expression in the thyroid (TTF-1 and Pax-8) and interacting with specific segments of the proximal gene promoter play a role in the control of thyroglobulin gene transcription by cAMP (see Chapter 90). However, there is clear indication that regulation of thyroglobulin gene transcription involves DNA segments situated further upstream. In the bovine species, an enhancer displaying thyroid-specific hypersensitivity to DNAase I has been identified between −1600 and −2000 from the CAP site.[105] Gene constructs containing 2000 bp of 5′ flanking sequences of the thyroglobulin gene have been found very effective in targeting expression of a series of genes for the thyroid in transgenic mice.[106–108] In addition, a similarly positioned enhancer has recently been identified in humans. Whereas the bovine enhancer did not show any sensitivity to stimulation by cAMP, the human one does. This different behavior fits well with the observation that the human proximal promoter seems to be less efficiently controlled by cAMP than is its bovine counterpart, thus suggesting a different spatial organization of the regulatory segments in different species.[109]

It has recently been shown that under stimulation by TSH, a short 0.95-kb thyroglobulin transcript accumulates in the rat thyroid. This transcript results from differential splicing and polyadenylation of the primary transcript, which yields a protein limited to the first five exons.[110] The functional significance of this observation is not completely clear; it could mean that in conditions in which the balance of thyroid metabolism would favor hormone synthesis over iodine storage (e.g., shortage of iodine), the thyrocyte would manufacture a truncated thyroglobulin containing the major hormonogenic site at the C terminus (see Chapter 92) but devoid of the many nonhormonogenic tyrosines.

Thyroperoxidase

TSH has been shown to increase both thyroperoxidase enzymatic activity[111] and steady-state mRNA levels in the thyrocytes of all species studied.[112–114] This effect is mimicked by cAMP analogues and by forskolin. Still no consensus has been reached, however, on whether the thyroperoxidase mRNA accumulation observed after stimulation by TSH or forskolin is entirely due to transcriptional or posttranscriptional mechanisms. According to some data, no transcriptional regulation of thyroperoxidase gene expression is observed in the immortalized rat thyroid FRTL5 cell line.[113] On the contrary, in dog thyrocytes in primary culture, clear transcriptional regulation of the gene has been demonstrated in run-on assays.[115] As already stated, this difference may reflect the less differentiated phenotype of FRTL5 cells more than a true species difference. Contrary to regulation of the thyroglobulin gene, activation of thyroperoxidase gene transcription by cAMP is rapid and does not require ongoing protein synthesis.[95, 116] The thyroperoxidase gene thus behaves as most other genes under rapid control by cAMP. However, its proximal promoter region is conspicuous in that it does not contain any of the cAMP-responsive *cis*-acting sequences known to date (see Chapter 92). Nevertheless, it was shown that the 130-bp 5′ flanking sequence of the gene contains targets for regulation by TSH-cAMP.[115] The TSH- or cAMP-dependent interaction of transcription factors has been localized within this gene segment, which is able to confer regulation by cAMP agonists to reporter genes ligated downstream. Here also, a question remains regarding whether TTF-1 and/or Pax-8, which also bind to the thyroperoxidase gene promoter, have a role in activation of the gene by cAMP or whether their role is limited to establishment and maintenance of the differentiated phenotype of the cell[100, 117] (see Chapter 90). In keeping with this question, an enhancer with binding sites for TTF-1 has been identified 5.5 kb upstream from the CAP site, but its role in cAMP-dependent regulation remains speculative.[118, 119]

Thyrotropin Receptor

It is generally accepted that low concentrations of TSH (<0.2 mU/mL) exert a positive control on TSH receptor number at the surface of thyrocytes whereas high concentrations (>0.2 mU/mL) lead to partial desensitization.[120] Control of TSH receptor gene expression has been studied in the FRTL5 cell line,[121–123] the canine thyrocyte in primary culture,[124] cultured human thyrocytes,[125, 126] and human thyroid cancer.[127, 128] The general conclusion emerging from these studies is the extreme robustness of TSH receptor gene expression as compared with the other markers of thyroid cell differentiation (thyroglobulin and thyroperoxidase). In the dog, levels of TSH receptor mRNA remain virtually unchanged in animals subjected for 28 days to hyperstimulation by TSH secondary to treatment with methimazole or to TSH withdrawal achieved by administration of thyroxine.[124] In the same study, the effect of TSH or forskolin has been investigated in dog thyrocytes in primary culture. This experimental system has the advantage that the differentiation state of the cells can be manipulated at will: cAMP agonists maintain expression of the differentiated phenotype, whereas agents such as EGF, tetradecanoyl phorbol acetate (TPA), and serum lead to "dedifferentiation."[129] The results demonstrate that the dedifferentiating agents strongly reduce accumulation of the receptor mRNA. However, contrary to what is observed with thyroglobulin and thyroperoxidase mRNA, the inhibition is never complete. TSH or forskolin is capable of promoting reaccumulation of the receptor message, a maximum being reached after 20 hours. As with thyroglobulin but at variance with the thyroperoxidase gene, this stimulation requires ongoing protein synthesis.[124] Chronic stimulation of cultured dog thyrocytes by TSH for several days does not lead to any important downregulation in mRNA. Similar data have been obtained with human thyrocytes in primary culture.[124, 126]

Negative regulation of receptor mRNA accumulation has been observed in immortal FRTL5 cells after treatment with TSH or TSAB.[121, 123] The significance of this difference in human and canine cells must probably be interpreted in the general framework of the other known differences in phenotype and regulatory behavior of this cell line as compared with primary cultured thyrocytes (see above). The effect of malignant transformation on the amounts of TSH receptor mRNA has been studied in spontaneous tumors in humans,[127, 128] in a murine transgenic model of thyroid tumor promoted by expression of the simian virus-40 large T oncogene,[107] and in FRTL5 cells transformed with v-*ras*.[122] In the two last models, expression of the TSH receptor gene was suppressed: the tumor or cell growth became TSH independent. In the transgenic animal model, loss of TSH receptor mRNA seemed to take place gradually, with early tumors still displaying some TSH dependence for growth. In the human tumors a spectrum of phenotypes was observed. As expected, anaplastic tumors had completely lost the receptor mRNA, as well as other markers of thyrocyte differentiation (thyroglobulin and thyroperoxidase). In papillary carcinoma, variable amounts of TSH receptor mRNA were invariably found,[127] even in the tumors that had lost the capacity to express the thyroglobulin or thyroperoxidase genes.[127] These data agree well with the observations of thyrocytes in primary culture: expression of the TSH receptor gene is robust and it persists in the presence of agents (or after several steps in tumor progression) that promote extinction of the other markers of thyroid cell differentiation. This evidence leads to the conclusion that the basic marker of the thyroid phenotype is probably the TSH receptor itself, which makes sense: the gene encoding the sensor of TSH—the major regulator of thyroid function, growth, and differentiated phenotype—is virtually constitutive in thyrocytes. From a pragmatic viewpoint, these data provide a rationale for the common therapeutic practice of suppressing TSH secretion in patients with a differentiated thyroid tumor.[130]

CONTROL OF GROWTH AND DIFFERENTIATION

Thyroid Cell Turnover

The thyroid is composed of thyrocytes (70%), endothelial cells (20%), and fibroblasts (10%). In a normal adult the weight and composition of the tissue remain relatively constant. Because a low but significant proliferation is demonstrated in all types of cells, it must be assumed that the generation of new cells is balanced by a corresponding rate of cell death.[2, 4, 131, 132] The resulting turnover is on the order of one per 5 to 10 years for human thyrocytes, that is, six to eight renewals in adult life, as in other species.[132] Cell population can therefore be modulated at the level of proliferation or cell death. In growth situations, that is, either in normal development or after stimulation, the different cell types grow more or less in parallel, which implies coordination between them.[23, 133] Because TSH receptors and iodine metabolism and signaling exist only in the thyrocyte, this cell, sole receiver of the physiologic information, must presumably control the other types of cells by paracrine factors such as FGF, IGF-I, NO, and the like.[2]

The Mitogenic Cascades

In the thyroid at least three families of distinct mitogenic pathways have been well defined (Fig. 93–4): (1) the hormone receptor–adenylate cyclase–cAMP protein kinase system, (2) the hormone receptor–tyrosine protein kinase pathways, and (3) the hormone receptor–phospholipase C cascade.[2, 134] The receptor–tyrosine kinase pathway may be subdivided into two branches; some growth factors, such as EGF, induce proliferation and repress differentiation expression, whereas others, such as FGF or IGF-I and insulin, are either mitogenic or are necessary for the proliferation effect of other factors without being mitogenic by themselves, but they do not inhibit differentiation expression.[135] In human thyroid cells, IGF-I or insulin is required for the mitogenic action of TSH or EGF but does not by itself stimulate proliferation.[136] In FRTL5 and rat cells, IGF-I is weakly stimulatory per se, whereas in pig thyroid cells it produces a strong mitogenic signal.[2, 12]

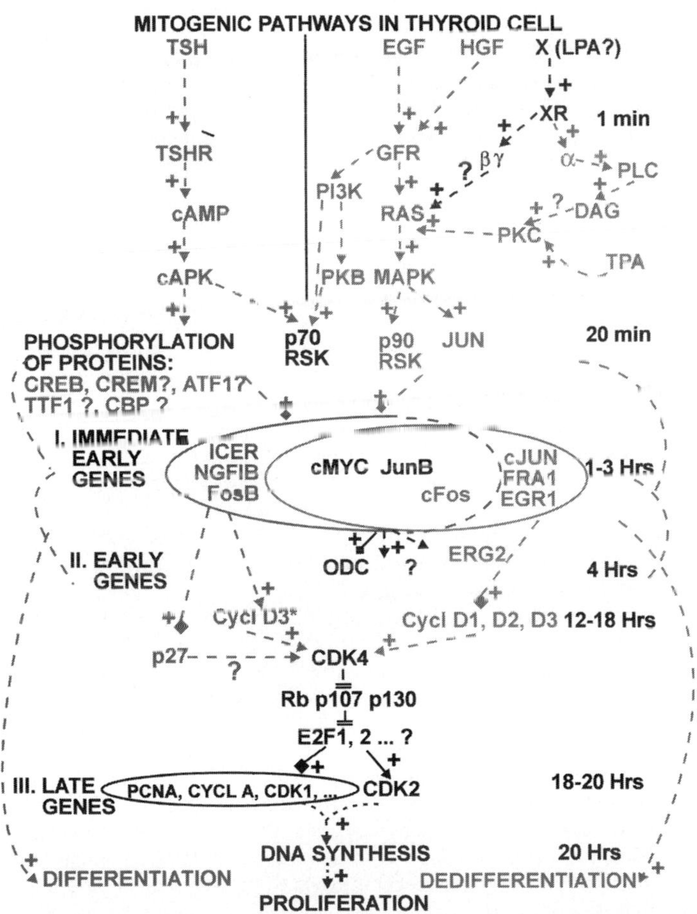

FIGURE 93–4. Mitogenic pathways in the thyroid. Data from the thyroid cell system are integrated into the present general scheme of cell proliferation cascades. In first line, known activators of various cascades in dog and human thyroid cells are shown. Various levels indicate a time sequence and postulated causal relationships from initial interaction of extracellular signal with its receptor to endpoints: proliferation and differentiation expression. Cyclin is now called proliferating cell nuclear antigen (PCNA); cAPK, cyclic adenosine monophosphate–dependent kinase; CDK, cyclin-dependent kinase; DAG, diacylglycerol; =n – – – →+, stimulation; =n – – – ‖, inhibition; =n – – – ◆+, induction; GFR, growth factor receptor; ODC, ornithine decarboxylase; PI3K, phosphatidylinositol 3-kinase; PKB, protein kinase B; PLC, phospholipase C; RSK, ribosomal S6 kinase.

It should be noted that TSH directly stimulates proliferation while maintaining the expression of differentiation. Differentiation expression, as evaluated by NIS or by thyroperoxidase and thyroglobulin mRNA content or nuclear transcription, is induced by TSH, forskolin, cholera toxin, and cAMP analogues.[2] These effects are obtained in all the cells of a culture, as shown by in situ hybridization experiments.[135] They are reversible; they can be obtained either after the arrest of proliferation or during the cell division cycle.[135] Moreover, the expression of differentiation, as measured by iodide transport, is stimulated by concentrations of TSH lower than those required for proliferation.[2]

All the effects of TSH are mimicked by nonspecific modulators of the cAMP cascade, that is, cholera toxin and forskolin (which stimulate adenylate cyclase), cAMP analogues (which activate the cAMP-dependent protein kinases), and even synergistic pairs of cAMP analogues acting on the different sites of these two kinases.[137] They are reproduced in vitro and in vivo by expression of the adenosine A_2 receptor, which is constitutively activated by endogenous adenosine.[108] They are inhibited by antibodies blocking G_s.[138] There is, therefore, no doubt that the mitogenic and differentiating effects of TSH are mainly and probably entirely mediated by cAMP.[2, 136] Inhibition of cAMP-dependent PKA inhibits the proliferation and differentiation effects of cAMP. However, stimulation of this kinase, by microinjection of a constitutively active catalytic subunit of the kinase, is not sufficient to induce thyroglobulin expression or DNA synthesis.[139] Activation of PKA by cAMP is therefore necessary but not sufficient for these effects.

EGF also induces proliferation of thyroid cells from various species.[2, 136] However, the action of EGF is accompanied by a general and reversible loss of differentiation expression assessed as described above. The effects of EGF on differentiation can be dissociated from their proliferative action. Indeed, they are obtained in cells that do not proliferate in the absence of insulin and in human cells, in which the proliferative effects are weaker, or in pig cells at concentrations lower than the mitogenic concentrations.[2]

Finally, the tumor-promoting phorbol esters, the pharmacologic probes of the protein kinase C system, and analogues of diacylglycerol also enhance the proliferation and inhibit the differentiation of thyroid cells (see Table 93–1). These effects are transient because of desensitization of the system by protein kinase C inactivation.[2, 136, 140] Activation of the PIP_2 cascade by physiologic agents such as carbamylcholine and bradykinin in dog thyroid cells does not reproduce all the effects of phorbol esters. In particular, prolonged stimulation of the cascade inhibits rather than stimulates proliferation.[141] Thus we cannot necessarily equate the effects of phorbol esters and prolonged stimulation of the PIP_2 cascade. Similarly, prolonged enhancement of intracellular Ca^{2+} levels might explain the mitogenic effects of IGF-I on FRTL5 cells but does not stimulate growth in dog thyroid cells. The dedifferentiating effects of phorbol esters do not require their mitogenic action either. Thus the effects of TSH, EGF, and phorbol esters on differentiation expression are largely independent of their mitogenic action.[2]

In several thyroid cell models, very high insulin concentrations are necessary for growth even in the presence of EGF. We now know that this prerequisite mainly reflects a requirement for IGF-I receptor.[2, 12, 13, 142] It is interesting that in FRTL5 cells, as in cells from thyroid nodules, this requirement may disappear as the cells secrete their own somatomedins and thus become autonomous with regard to these hormones.[13, 143]

In the action of growth factors on receptor protein tyrosine kinase pathways, the effects on differentiation expression vary with the species and the factor involved: from stimulation (e.g., insulin, as well as

IGF-II in dog and FRTL5 cells) to an absence of effect, to transitory inhibition of differentiation during growth (FGF and HGF in dog cells), to full dedifferentiation effects (EGF in dog and human cells).[2, 136, 142, 143] Ret expression, which is responsible for many papillary cancers constitutively activates a growth factor cascade downstream of the receptor (Src kinase activity[144]).

The kinetics of the induction of thymidine incorporation into nuclear DNA of dog thyroid cells is similar for TSH, forskolin, EGF, and TPA. Whatever the stimulant, a minimal delay of about 16 to 20 hours takes place before the beginning of labeling, that is, the beginning of DNA synthesis. This time is the minimal amount required to prepare the necessary machinery. For the cAMP and EGF pathways, the stimulatory agent has to be present during this whole prereplicative period; any interruption in activation (e.g., by washing out the stimulatory forskolin) greatly delays the start of DNA synthesis. This limitation explains why norepinephrine and prostaglandin E, which also activate the cAMP cascade, do not induce growth and differentiation: the rapid desensitization of their receptors does not allow a sustained rise in cAMP levels.

The three main types of mitogenic cascade, specifically, the growth factor–protein tyrosine kinase, phorbol ester–protein kinase C, and TSH-cAMP cascades, are fully distinct at the level of their primary intracellular signal and/or the first signal-activated protein kinase.[2]

Iodide actually inhibits the cAMP and the Ca^{2+}-phosphatidylinositol cascades and in a more delayed and chronic effect decreases the sensitivity of the thyroid to the TSH growth response. In FRTL5 cells it inhibits TSH, IGF-I, and tumor promoters (TPA, i.e., phorbol myristate ester)-induced cell proliferation; these effects are relieved, according to the general paradigm of Van Sande, by perchlorate and methimazole.[40, 145]

Steps in the Mitogenic Cascades

The phenomenology of EGF, TPA, and TSH proliferative action on dog quiescent cells has been partially elucidated.[2] Three biochemical aspects of the proliferative response occurring at different times of the prereplicative phase have been considered. The pattern of protein phosphorylation induced within minutes by TSH is reproduced by forskolin and cAMP analogues.[146] The serine-threonine phosphorylation of at least 11 proteins is increased or induced. In EGF-stimulated cells, the phosphorylation of five proteins is stimulated, two of them phosphorylated on tyrosines (42 kDa to 44 kDa), the MAP kinases. Phorbol esters induce the phosphorylation of 19 proteins, including the tyrosine-phosphorylated MAP kinases already mentioned. Insulin and IGF-I also activate MAP kinases, but less so than EGF does. No overlap is seen in the patterns of protein phosphorylation induced by TSH and cAMP enhancers on the one hand and by EGF and phorbol esters on the other.[146] In particular, the cAMP cascade does not involve the phosphorylation of MAP kinases. PI-3-kinase and its effector enzyme PKB are activated for several hours only by insulin and IGF-I, the effect of EGF being short lived. This activity is therefore the one specific feature of insulin action and presumably the mechanism of the permissive effect on mitogenicity. Only insulin and IGF-I also markedly enhance general protein synthesis and induce cell hypertrophy.[147]

As in other types of cells, EGF and TPA first enhance c-fos and then c-myc mRNA concentrations. On the other hand, TSH and forskolin strongly, but for a short period enhance the c-myc mRNA concentration and with the same kinetics as enhancement of the c-fos mRNA concentration by EGF/TPA. In fact, cAMP first enhances and then decreases c-myc mRNA accumulation. This second phenomenon is akin to what has been observed in the fibroblast, in which cAMP negatively regulates growth. As in fibroblasts, EGF and TPA enhance c-jun, junB, junD, and egrl expression. However, as in fibroblasts, activators of the cAMP cascade decrease c-jun and egrl expression. c-Jun is therefore not, as has been claimed, a gene whose expression is universally necessary for growth.[2, 148]

The pattern of proteins synthesized in response to the various proliferation stimuli has been studied.[2, 149, 150] Again, two patterns emerge. TSH and forskolin induce the synthesis of at least eight proteins and decrease the synthesis of five proteins. EGF, phorbol ester, and serum induce the synthesis of at least two proteins and decrease the synthesis of two proteins. The only overlap between the two patterns concerns the decrease in synthesis of a protein (18 kDa), which is also reduced by EGF after proliferation has stopped. Only one protein has been shown to be synthesized in response to the three pathways: proliferating cell nuclear antigen (PCNA), the auxiliary protein of DNA polymerase δ. However, the kinetics of this synthesis is very different, with an early synthesis in the cAMP cascade (consistent with a role of signal) and a late S phase synthesis in the other cascades. Thus, obviously two different phenomenologies are involved in the proliferation response to TSH through cAMP on the one hand and EGF and phorbol ester, presumably through protein tyrosine phosphorylation, on the other. Although this conclusion needs to be further substantiated, it certainly suggests that the proliferation of dog thyroid cells is controlled by at least two largely independent pathways. The effects of TSH, EGF, and phorbol esters on specific protein synthesis can be obtained in the absence of insulin in the medium, except for the induction of PCNA synthesis; some are enhanced by insulin. Thus these effects also are not sufficient to induce mitogenesis.[2]

It is now well established that the triggering of DNA synthesis and the cell division program in vertebrate cells involves the generation of cyclin D–dependent kinase (CDK4 and CDK6) complexes and the inactivation of cyclin inhibitors. Phosphorylation of proteins of the Rb family (Rb, p107, p130) releases transcription factors of the E2F family, which together with DP partners will induce the genes coding for the proteins involved in DNA synthesis. These pathways have been well studied in dog thyroid cells. Agents (such as HGF) and combinations of factors (e.g., TSH plus insulin, EGF plus insulin, phorbol esters plus insulin) that trigger DNA synthesis also cause phosphorylation of the three Rb-like pocket proteins, whereas the factors that are not sufficient by themselves (e.g., TSH, EGF, phorbol esters, insulin) do not. Thus phosphorylation of these proteins is a common converging point of the mitogenic cascades. Upstream from these phosphorylations, cyclin D–CDK complex formation is also a common step of the TSH-cAMP, the EGF, and the phorbol ester cascades in the presence of insulin. What is strikingly different between the cascades is the mechanism of complex generation: whereas EGF, as in many growth cascades, induces the synthesis of cyclin D1 and mostly cyclin D3, the TSH-cAMP cascade does not. For the latter pathway an unknown mechanism of activation must be postulated.

Studies of protein phosphorylation, proto-oncogene expression, and protein synthesis in dog thyrocytes allow discrimination between two models of cAMP action on proliferation in this system: a direct effect on the thyrocyte or an indirect effect through the secretion and autocrine action of another growth factor. If the effect of TSH through cAMP involved such an autocrine loop, one would expect to find faster kinetics of action of the growth factor and at least some common parts in the patterns of protein phosphorylation and protein synthesis induced by cAMP and the growth factor. The results do not support such a hypothesis, at least for the growth factors tested[2] (Fig. 93–5).

The validity of these concepts in vivo has been established by using transgenic mice models. Expression in the thyroid of the adenosine A_2 receptor, which behaves as a constitutive activator of adenylate cyclase, induces thyroid growth, goitrogenesis, and hyperthyroidism. The expression of oncogene E7 of HPV-16, which sequestrates Rb protein, leads to thyroid growth and euthyroid goiter. On the other hand, expression of Ret papillary thyroid carcinoma (PTC), which is a constitutive growth factor receptor, leads to growth, cancer, and hypothyroidism.

Proliferation and Differentiation

The incompatibility at the cell level of a proliferation and differentiation program is commonly accepted in biology. In general, cells with a high proliferative capacity are poorly differentiated, and during development such cells lose this capacity as they progressively differentiate. Some cells even lose all potential to divide when reaching their full differentiation, a phenomenon called terminal differentiation. Conversely, in tumor cells, proliferation and differentiation expression are inversely related. It is therefore not surprising that in thyroid cells

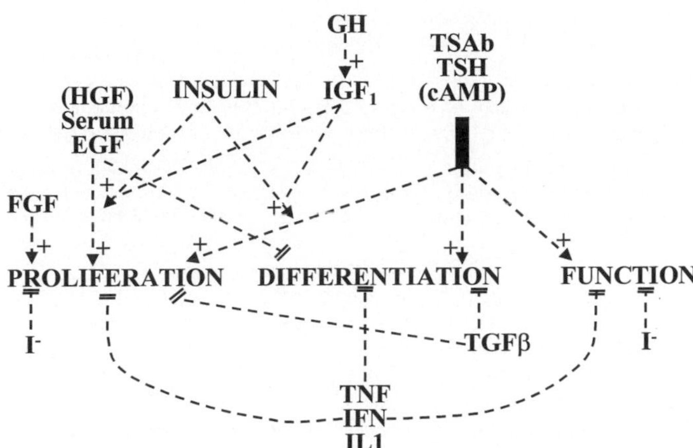

FIGURE 93–5. Main controls of the principal biologic variables of the human thyrocyte. EGF, epidermal growth factor; FGF, fibroblast growth factor; GH, growth hormone; HGF, hepatocyte growth factor; I^-, iodide; IGF-I, insulin-like growth factor-I; IFN, interferon; IL-1, interleukin-1; TGI, thyroid growth immunoglobulins; TGF-β, tumor growth factor-β; TNF, tumor necrosis factor; TSAb, thyroid-stimulating immunoglobulins; +, positive control (stimulation); −, negative control (inhibition).

the general mitogenic agents and pathways, phorbol esters and the protein kinase C pathway, EGF, and in calf and porcine cells, FGF and the protein tyrosine kinase pathway, induce both proliferation and the loss of differentiation expression. The effects of the cAMP cascade are in striking contrast to this general concept. Indeed, TSH and cAMP induce proliferation of dog thyrocytes while maintaining differentiation expression; both proliferation and differentiation programs can be triggered by TSH in the same cells at the same time. This situation is by no means unique because neuroblasts in the cell cycle may simultaneously differentiate. It is tempting to relate this apparent paradox to the role and expression of proto-oncogenes in these cells. C-fos expression is enhanced in a great variety of cell stimulations and leads to either proliferation or differentiation expression. On the other hand, if one generalization could be made about proto-oncogenes, it is the dedifferentiating role of c-myc in all. A rapid and dramatic decrease in c-myc mRNA by antisense myc sequences induces differentiation of a variety of cell types. It is therefore striking that in the case of the thyrocyte, in which activation of the cAMP cascade leads to both proliferation and differentiation, the kinetics of the c-*myc* gene appears to be tightly controlled. After a first phase of 1 hour of higher level of c-myc mRNA, c-myc expression is decreased below control levels. In this second phase, cAMP decreases c-myc mRNA levels, as it does in proliferation-inhibited fibroblasts. It even depresses EGF-induced expression. The first phase could be necessary for proliferation, whereas the second phase could reflect stimulation of differentiation by TSH. This downregulation is suppressed by cycloheximide, which suggests the involvement of a neosynthesized or labile inhibitory protein at the transcriptional level or at the level of mRNA stabilization.[2]

Because the cell renewal rate is very low in the thyroid (once every 8 years in adults), the role of apoptosis is also very low. However, under different circumstances the apoptotic role can greatly increase, such as after the arrest of an important stimulation in vitro[151] and in vivo.[152, 153]

REFERENCES

1. Vassart G, Dumont JE: The thyrotropin receptor and the regulation of thyrocyte function and growth. Endocr Rev 13:596–611, 1992.
2. Dumont JE, Lamy F, Roger PP, et al: Physiological and pathological regulation of thyroid cell proliferation and differentiation by thyrotropin and other factors. Physiol Rev 72:667–697, 1992.
3. Brabant G, Bergmann P, Kirsch CM, et al: Early adaptation of thyrotropin and thyroglobulin secretion to experimentally decreased iodine supply in man. Metabolism 41:1093–1096, 1992.
4. Dumont JE: The action of thyrotropin on thyroid metabolism. Vitam Horm 29:287–412, 1971.
5. Toyoda N, Nishikawa M, Horimoto M: Synergistic effect of thyroid hormone and thyrotropin on iodothyronine 5′-adenosinase in FRTL-5 rat thyroid cells. Endocrinology 127:1199–1205, 1990.
6. Glinoer D, de Nayer P, Bourdoux P, et al: Regulation of maternal thyroid during pregnancy. J Clin Endocrinol Metab 71:276–287, 1990.
7. Hershman JM, Lee HY, Sugawara M, et al: Human chorionic gonadotropin stimulates iodide uptake, adenylate cyclase, and deoxyribonucleic acid synthesis in cultured rat thyroid cells. J Clin Endocrinol Metab 67:74–79, 1988.
8. Hershman JM: Role of human chorionic gonadotropin as a thyroid stimulator (editorial). J Clin Endocrinol Metab 74:258–259, 1992.
9. Ahren B: Regulatory peptides in the thyroid gland—a review on their localization and function. Acta Endocrinol 124:225–232, 1991.
10. Van Sande J, Lamy F, Lecocq R, et al: Pathogenesis of autonomous thyroid nodules: In vitro study of iodine and adenosine 3′,5′-monophosphate metabolism. J Clin Endocrinol Metab 66:570–579, 1988.
11. Raspé E, Andry G, Dumont JE: Adenosine triphosphate, bradykinin, and thyrotropin-releasing hormone regulate the intracellular Ca^{2+} concentration and the $^{45}Ca^{2+}$ efflux of human thyrocytes in primary culture. J Cell Physiol 140:608–614, 1989.
12. Tramontano D, Cushing G, Moses AC, et al: Insulin-like growth factor-I stimulates the growth of rat thyroid cells in culture and synergizes the stimulation of DNA synthesis induced by TSH and Graves' IgG. Endocrinology 119:940–942, 1986.
13. Williams DW, Williams ED, Wynford-Thomas D: Evidence for autocrine production of IGF-1 in human thyroid adenomas. Mol Cell Endocrinol 61:139–147, 1989.
14. Dremier S, Taton M, Coulonval K, et al: Mitogenic, dedifferentiating, and scattering effects of hepatocyte growth factor on dog thyroid cells. Endocrinology 135:135–140, 1994.
15. Paire A, Bernier-Valentin F, Rabilloud R, et al: Expression of alpha- and beta-subunits and activity of Na^+ K^+ ATPase in pig thyroid cells in primary culture: Modulation by thyrotropin and thyroid hormones. Mol Cell Endocrinol 146:93–101, 1998.
16. Dumont JE, Roger PP, Ludgate M: Assays for thyroid growth immunoglobulins and their clinical implications: Methods, concepts and misconceptions. Endocr Rev 8:448–452, 1987.
17. Zakarija M, Jin S, McKenzie JM: Evidence supporting the identity in Graves' disease of thyroid-stimulating antibody and thyroid growth-promoting immunoglobulin G as assayed in FRTL-5 cells. J Clin Invest 81:879–884, 1988.
18. Zakarija M, McKenzie JM: Do thyroid growth-promoting immunoglobulins exist? J Clin Endocrinol Metab 70:308–310, 1990.
19. Zakarija M, McKenzie JM: Influence of cytokines on growth and differentiated function of FRTL-5 cells. Endocrinology 125:1260–1265, 1989.
20. Van Sande J, Mockel J, Boeynaems JM, et al: Regulation of cyclic nucleotide and prostaglandin formation in human thyroid tissues and in autonomous nodules. J Clin Endocrinol Metab 50:776–785, 1980.
21. Esteves R, Van Sande J, Dumont JE: Nitric oxide as a signal in thyroid. Mol Cell Endocrinol 90:R1–R3, 1992.
22. de Rooij J, Zwartkruis FJT, Verheijen MHG, et al: Epac is a Rap1 guanine-nucleotide-exchange factor directly activated by cyclic AMP. Nature 396:474–477, 1998.
23. Munari-Silem Y, Audebet C, Rousset B: Protein kinase C in pig thyroid cells: Activation, translocation and endogenous substrate phosphorylating activity in response to phorbol esters. J Clin Invest 54:81–90, 1987.
24. Van Sande J, Raspe E, Perret J, et al: Thyrotropin activates both the cyclic AMP and the PIP_2 cascades in CHO cells expressing the human cDNA of TSH receptor. J Clin Invest 74:R1–R6, 1990.
25. Laurent E, Mockel J, Van Sande J, et al: Dual activation by thyrotropin of the phospholipase C and cAMP cascades in human thyroid. Mol Cell Endocrinol 52:273–278, 1987.
26. Jacquemin C: Glycosyl phosphatidylinositol in thyroid: Cell signalling or protein anchor? Biochimie 73:37–40, 1991.
27. Lejeune C, Mockel J, Dumont JE: Relative contribution of phosphoinositides and phosphatidylcholine hydrolysis to the actions of carbamylcholine, thyrotropin (TSH), and phorbol esters on dog thyroid slices: Regulation of cytidine monophosphate–phosphatidic acid accumulation and phospholipase-D activity. I. Actions of carbamylcholine, calcium ionophores, and TSH. Endocrinology 135:2488–2496, 1994.
28. Mockel J, Lejeune C, Dumont JE: Relative contribution of phosphoinositides and phosphatidylcholine hydrolysis to the actions of carbamylcholine, thyrotropin, and phorbol esters on dog thyroid slices: Regulation of cytidine monophosphate–phosphatidic acid accumulation and phospholipase-D activity. II. Actions of phorbol esters. Endocrinology 135:2497–2503, 1994.
29. Bidey SP, Hill DJ, Eggo MC: Growth factors and goitrogenesis. J Endocrinol 160:321–332, 1999.
30. Garbi C, Colletta G, Cirafici AM, et al: Transforming growth factor-beta induces cytoskeleton and extracellular matrix modifications in FRTL5 thyroid epithelial cells. Eur J Cell Biol 53:281–289, 1990.
31. Gärtner R, Bechtner G, Stübner D, et al: Growth regulation of porcine thyroid follicles in vitro by growth factors. Horm Metab Res 23:61–67, 1990.
32. Grübeck-Loebenstein B, Buchan G, Sadeghi R: Transforming growth factor beta regulates thyroid growth. J Clin Invest 83:764–770, 1989.
33. Dumont JE, Miot F, Erneux C, et al: Negative regulation of cyclic AMP levels by activation of cyclic nucleotide phosphodiesterases: The example of the dog thyroid. Adv Cyclic Nucl Res 16:325–336, 1984.
34. Mockel J, Van Sande J, Decoster C, et al: Tumor promoters as probes of protein kinase C in dog thyroid cell: Inhibition of the primary effects of carbamylcholine and reproduction of some distal effects. Metabolism 36:137–143, 1987.
35. Wolff J: Iodide goiter and the pharmacologic effects of excess iodide. Am J Med 47:101–124, 1969.
36. Wolff J: Congenital goiter with defective iodide transport. Endocr Rev 4:240, 1983.
37. Bray GA: Increased sensitivity of the thyroid in iodine-depleted rats to the goitrogenic effects of thyrotropin. J Clin Invest 47:1640–1647, 1968.

38. Cochaux P, Van Sande J, Swillens S, et al: Iodide-induced inhibition of adenylate cyclase activity in horse and dog thyroid. Eur J Biochem 170:435–442, 1987.
39. Laurent E, Mockel J, Takazawa K, et al: Stimulation of generation of inositol phosphates by carbamylcholine and its inhibition by phorbol esters and iodide in dog thyroid cells. Biochem J 263:795–801, 1989.
40. Van Sande J, Grenier G, Willems C, et al: Inhibition by iodide of the activation of the thyroid cyclic 3′,5′-AMP system. Endocrinology 96:781–786, 1975.
41. Boeynaems JM, Hubbard WC: Transformation of arachidonic acid into an iodolactone by the rat thyroid. J Biol Chem 255:9001–9004, 1980.
42. Dugrillon A, Bechtner G, Uedelhoven WM, et al: Evidence that an iodolactone mediates the inhibitory effect of iodine on thyroid cell proliferation but not on adenosine 3′,5′-monophosphate formation. Endocrinology 127:337–343, 1990.
43. Pereira A, Braekman JC, Dumont JE, et al: Identification of a major iodolipid from the horse thyroid gland as 2-iodohexadecanal. J Biol Chem 265:17018–17025, 1990.
44. Many MC, Mestdagh C, Van Den Hove MF, et al: In vitro study of acute toxic effects of high iodide doses in human thyroid follicles. Endocrinology 131:621–630, 1992.
45. Rees Smith B, McLachlan SM, Furmaniak J: Autoantibodies to the thyrotropin receptor. Endocr Rev 9:106–121, 1988.
46. Libert F, Lefort A, Gerard C, et al: Cloning, sequencing and expression of the human thyrotropin (TSH) receptor: Evidence for binding of autoantibodies. Biochem Biophys Res Commun 165:1250–1255, 1989.
47. Parmentier M, Libert F, Maenhaut C, et al: Molecular cloning of the thyrotropin (TSH) receptor. Science 296:1620–1622, 1989.
48. Misrahi M, Loosfelt H, Atger M, et al: Cloning, sequencing and expression of human TSH receptor. Biochem Biophys Res Commun 166:394–403, 1990.
49. Nagayama Y, Kaufman KD, Seto P, et al: Molecular cloning, sequence and functional expression of the cDNA for the human thyrotropin receptor. Biochem Biophys Res Commun 165:1184–1190, 1989.
50. Frazier AL, Robbins LS, Stork PJ, et al: Isolation of TSH and LH/CG receptor cDNAs from human thyroid: Regulation by tissue specific splicing. Mol Endocrinol 4:1264–1276, 1990.
51. Rapoport B, Chazenbalk GD, Jaume JC, et al: The thyrotropin (TSH) receptor: Interaction with TSH and autoantibodies. Endocr Rev 19:673–716, 1998.
52. Gross B, Misrahi M, Sar S, et al: Composite structure of the human thyrotropin receptor gene. Biochem Biophys Res Commun 177:679–687, 1991.
53. Raymond JR, Hnatowich M, Lefkowitz RJ, et al: Adrenergic receptors. Models for regulation of signal transduction processes. Hypertension 15:119–131, 1990.
54. McFarland KC, Sprengel R, Phillips HS, et al: Lutropin-choriogonadotropin receptor: An unusual member of the G protein–coupled receptor family. Science 245:494–499, 1989.
55. Libert F, Parmentier M, Maenhaut C, et al: Molecular cloning of a dog thyrotropin (TSH) receptor variant. Mol Cell Endocrinol 68:R15–R17, 1990.
56. Takeshita A, Nagayama Y, Fujiyama K, et al: Molecular cloning and sequencing of an alternatively spliced form of the human TSH receptor transcript. Biochem Biophys Res Commun 188:1214–1219, 1992.
57. Graves PN, Tomer Y, Davies TF: Cloning and sequencing of a 1.3 KB variant of human thyrotropin receptor mRNA lacking the transmembrane domain. Biochem Biophys Res Commun 187:1135–1143, 1992.
58. Loosfelt H, Pichon C, Jolivet A, et al: Two-subunit structure of the human thyrotropin receptor. Proc Natl Acad Sci U S A 89:3765–3769, 1992.
59. Libert F, Passage E, Lefort A, et al: Localization of human thyrotropin receptor gene to chromosome region 14q3 by in situ hybridization. Cytogenet Cell Genet 54:82–83, 1990.
60. Rousseau-Merck MF, Misrahi M, Loosfelt H, et al: Assignment of the human thyroid stimulating hormone receptor (TSHR) gene to chromosome 14q31. Genomics 8:233–236, 1990.
61. Ikuyama S, Niller HH, Shimura H, et al: Characterization of the 5′-flanking region of the rat thyrotropin receptor gene. Mol Endocrinol 6:793–804, 1992.
62. Roselli Rehfuss L, Robbins LS, Cone RD: Thyrotropin receptor messenger ribonucleic acid is expressed in most brown and white adipose tissues in the guinea pig. Endocrinology 130:1857–1861, 1992.
63. Uyttersprot N, Pelgrims N, Carrasco N, et al: Moderate doses of iodide in vivo inhibit cell proliferation and the expression of thyroperoxidase and Na^+/I^- symporter mRNAs in dog thyroid. Mol Cell Endocrinol 131:195–203, 1997.
64. Perret J, Ludgate M, Libert F, et al: Stable expression of the human TSH receptor in CHO cells and characterization of differentially expressing clones. Biochem Biophys Res Commun 171:1044–1050, 1990.
65. Costagliola S, Swillens S, Niccoli P, et al: Binding assay for thyrotropin receptor autoantibodies using the recombinant receptor protein. J Clin Endocrinol Metab 75:1540–1544, 1992.
66. Rapoport B, Seto P: Bovine thyrotropin has a specific bioactivity 5- to 10-fold that of previous estimates for highly purified hormone. Endocrinology 116:1379–1382, 1985.
67. Amr S, Menezez Ferreira M, Shimohigashi Y, et al: Activities of deglycosylated thyrotropin at the thyroid membrane receptor–adenylate cyclase system. J Endocrinol Invest 8:537–541, 1985.
68. Laurent E, Van Sande J, Ludgate M, et al: Unlike thyrotropin, thyroid-stimulating antibodies do not activate phospholipase C in human thyroid slices. J Clin Invest 87:1634–1642, 1991.
69. Van Sande J, Lejeune C, Ludgate M, et al: Thyroid stimulating immunoglobulins, like thyrotropin activate both the cyclic AMP and the PIP_2 cascades in CHO cells expressing the TSH receptor. Mol Cell Endocrinol 88:R1–R5, 1992.
70. Kosugi S, Ban T, Akamizu T, et al: Identification of separate determinants on the thyrotropin receptor reactive with Graves' thyroid-stimulating antibodies and with thyroid-stimulating blocking antibodies in idiopathic myxedema: These determinants have no homologous sequence on gonadotropin receptors. Mol Endocrinol 6:168–180, 1992.
71. Kosugi S, Ban T, Akamizu T, et al: Further characterization of a high affinity thyrotropin binding site on the rat thyrotropin receptor which is an epitope for blocking antibodies from idiopathic myxedema patients but not thyroid stimulating antibodies from Graves' patients. Biochem Biophys Res Commun 180:1118–1124, 1991.
72. Tahara K, Ban T, Minegishi T, et al: Immunoglobulins from Graves' disease patients interact with different sites on TSH receptor/LH-CG receptor chimeras than either TSH or immunoglobulins from idiopathic myxedema patients. Biochem Biophys Res Commun 179:70–77, 1991.
73. Kosugi S, Okajima F, Ban T, et al: Mutation of alanine 623 in the third cytoplasmic loop of the rat TSH receptor results in a loss in the phosphoinositide but not cAMP signal induced by TSH and receptor autoantibodies. J Biol Chem 267:24153–24156, 1992.
74. Scott DA, Wang R, Kreman TM, et al: The Pendred syndrome gene encodes a chloride-iodide transport protein. Nat Genet 21:440–443, 1999.
75. Nilsson M, Björkman U, Ekholm R, et al: Polarized efflux of iodide in porcine thyrocytes occurs via a cAMP-regulated iodide channel in the apical plasma membrane. Acta Endocrinol 126:67–74, 1992.
76. Arntzenius AB, Smit LJ, Schipper J: Inverse relation between iodine intake and thyroid blood flow: Color Doppler flow imaging in euthyroid humans. J Clin Endocrinol Metab 73:1051–1055, 1991.
77. Nunez J, Pommier J: Formation of thyroid hormones. Vitam Horm 39:175–229, 1982.
78. Corvilain B, Van Sande J, Laurent E, et al: The H_2O_2-generating system modulates protein iodination and the activity of the pentose phosphate pathway in dog thyroid. Endocrinology 128:779–785, 1991.
79. Björkman U, Ekholm R: Hydrogen peroxide generation and its regulation in FRTL-5 and porcine thyroid cells. Endocrinology 130:393–399, 1992.
80. Bernier-Valentin F, Kostrouch Z, Rabilloud R, et al: Analysis of the thyroglobulin internalization process using in vitro reconstituted thyroid follicles: Evidence for a coated vesicle-dependent endocytic pathway. Endocrinology 129:2194–2201, 1991.
81. Deshpande V, Venkatesh SG: Thyroglobulin, the prothyroid hormone: Chemistry, synthesis and degradation. Biochim Biophys Acta 1430:157–178, 1999.
82. Björkman U, Ekholm R: Accelerated exocytosis and H_2O_2 generation in isolated thyroid follicles enhance protein iodination. Endocrinology 122:488–494, 1988.
83. Chambard M, Depetris D, Gruffat D, et al: Thyrotropin regulation of apical and basal exocytosis of thyroglobulin by porcine thyroid monolayers. J Mol Endocrinol 4:193–199, 1990.
84. Herzog V: Pathways of endocytosis in thyroid follicle cells. Int Rev Cytol 91:107–139, 1984.
85. Van Den Hove MF, Couvreur M, De Visscher M: A new mechanism for the reabsorption of thyroid iodoproteins: Selective fluid pinocytosis. Eur J Biochem 122:415–422, 1982.
86. Lemansky P, Herzog V: Endocytosis of thyroglobulin is not mediated by mannose-6-phosphate receptors in thyrocytes. Evidence for low-affinity-binding sites operating in the uptake of thyroglobulin. Eur J Biochem 209:111–119, 1992.
87. Consiglio E, Shifrin S, Yavin Z: Thyroglobulin interactions with thyroid membranes. Relationship between receptor recognition of *N*-acetylglucosamine residues and the iodine content of thyroglobulin preparations. J Biol Chem 256:10592–10599, 1981.
88. Marino M, Zheng G, McCluskey RT: Megalin (gp330) is an endocytic receptor for thyroglobulin on cultured Fischer rat thyroid cells. J Biol Chem 274:12898–12904, 1999.
89. Missero C, Cobellis G, De Felice M, et al: Molecular events involved in differentiation of thyroid follicular cells. Mol Cell Endocrinol 140:37–43, 1998.
90. Woloshin PI, Walton KM, Rehfuss RP, et al: 3′,5′-Cyclic adenosine monophosphate–regulated enhancer binding (CREB) activity is required for normal growth and differentiated phenotype in the FRTL5 thyroid follicular cell line. Mol Endocrinol 6:1725–1733, 1992.
91. Uyttersprot N, Costagliola S, Dumont JE, et al: Requirement for cAMP-response element (CRE) binding protein/CRE modulator transcription factors in thyrotropin-induced proliferation of dog thyroid cells in primary culture. Eur J Biochem 259:370–378, 1999.
92. Christophe D, Vassart G: The thyroglobulin gene: Evolutionary and regulatory issues. Trends in Endocrinology and Metabolism 1:10–15, 1990.
93. Van Heuverswyn B, Streydio C, Brocas H, et al: Thyrotropin controls transcription of the thyroglobulin gene. Proc Natl Acad Sci U S A 81:5941–5945, 1984.
94. Van Heuverswyn B, Leriche A, Van Sande J, et al: Transcriptional control of thyroglobulin gene expression by cyclic AMP. FEBS Lett 188:192–196, 1985.
95. Davies E, Dumont JE, Vassart G: Thyrotropin-stimulated recruitment of free monoribosomes on to membrane-bound thyroglobulin-synthesizing polyribosomes. Biochem J 172:227–231, 1978.
96. Gérard CM, Lefort A, Christophe D: Control of thyroperoxidase and thyroglobulin transcription by cAMP: Evidence for distinct regulatory mechanisms. Mol Endocrinol 3:2110–2118, 1989.
97. Avvedimento VE, Tramontano D, Ursini MV: The level of thyroglobulin mRNA is regulated by TSH both in vitro and in vivo. Biochem Biophys Res Commun 122:472–477, 1984.
98. Sinclair AJ, Lonigro R, Civitareale D, et al: The tissue-specific expression of the thyroglobulin gene requires interaction between thyroid-specific and ubiquitous factors. Eur J Biochem 193:311–318, 1990.
99. Civitareale D, Lonigro R, Sinclair AJ, et al: A thyroid specific nuclear protein essential for tissue-specific expression of the thyroglobulin promoter. EMBO J 8:2537–2542, 1989.
100. Zannini M, Francis-Lang H, Plachov D, et al: Pax-8, a paired domain-containing protein, binds to a sequence overlapping the recognition site of a homeodomain and activates transcription from two thyroid-specific promoters. Mol Cell Biol 12:4230–4241, 1992.
101. Lazzaro D, Proce M, De Felice M, et al: The transcription factor TTF-1 is expressed at the onset of thyroid and lung morphogenesis and in restricted regions of the foetal brain. Development 113:1093–1104, 1991.
102. Javaux F, Bertaux F, Donda A, et al: Functional role of TTF-1 binding sites in bovine thyroglobulin promoter. FEBS Lett 3:222–226, 1992.

103. Damante G, Di Lauro R: Several regions of Antennapedia and thyroid transcription factor 1 homeodomains contribute to DNA binding specificity. Proc Natl Acad Sci U S A 88:5388–5392, 1991.
104. Christophe D, Gérard C, Juvenal G, et al: Identification of a cAMP-responsive region in thyroglobulin gene promoter. Mol Cell Endocrinol 64:5–18, 1989.
105. Christophe-Hobertus C, Donda A, Javaux F, et al: Identification of a transcriptional enhancer upstream from the bovine thyroglobulin gene. Mol Cell Endocrinol 88:31–37, 1992.
106. Ledent C, Parmentier M, Vassart G: Tissue-specific expression and methylation of a thyroglobulin-chloramphenicol acetyltransferase fusion gene in transgenic mice. Proc Natl Acad Sci U S A 87:6176–6180, 1990.
107. Ledent C, Dumont JE, Vassart G, et al: Thyroid adenocarcinomas secondary to tissue-specific expression of simian virus-40 large T-antigen in transgenic mice. Endocrinology 129:1391–1401, 1991.
108. Ledent C, Dumont JE, Vassart G, et al: Thyroid expression of an A2 adenosine receptor transgene induces thyroid hyperplasia and hyperthyroidism. EMBO J 11:537–542, 1991.
109. Donda A, Javaux F, Van Renterghem P, et al: Human, bovine, canine and rat thyroglobulin promoter sequences display species-specific differences in an in vitro study. Mol Cell Endocrinol 90:R23–R26, 1993.
110. Graves PN, Davies TF: A second thyroglobulin messenger RNA species (rTg-2) in rat thyrocytes. Mol Endocrinol 4:155–161, 1990.
111. Magnusson RP, Rapoport B: Modulation of differentiated function in cultured thyroid cells: Thyrotropin control of thyroid peroxidase activity. Endocrinology 116:1493–1500, 1985.
112. Chazenbalk G, Magnusson RP, Rapoport B: Thyrotropin stimulation of cultured thyroid cells increases steady state levels of the messenger ribonucleic acid for thyroid peroxidase. Mol Endocrinol 1:913–917, 1987.
113. Damante G, Chazenbalk G, Russo D: Thyrotropin regulation of thyroid peroxidase messenger ribonucleic acid levels in cultured rat thyroid cells: Evidence for the involvement of a nontranscriptional mechanism. Endocrinology 124:2889–2894, 1989.
114. Foti D, Gestaulas J, Rapoport B: Studies on the functional activity of the promoter for the human thyroid peroxidase gene. Biochem Biophys Res Commun 168:281–287, 1990.
115. Abramowicz MJ, Vassart G, Christophe D: Functional study of the human thyroid peroxidase gene promoter. Eur J Biochem 203:467–473, 1992.
116. Gérard C, Lefort A, Libert F: Transcriptional regulation of the thyroperoxidase gene by thyrotropin and forskolin. Mol Cell Endocrinol 60:239–242, 1988.
117. Francis-Lang H, Price M, Polycarpou Schwarz M, et al: Cell-type–specific expression of the rat thyroperoxidase promoter indicates common mechanism for thyroid-specific gene expression. Mol Cell Biol 12:576–588, 1992.
118. Kikkawa F, Gonzalez FJ, Kimura S: Characterization of a thyroid-specific enhancer located 5.5 kilobase pairs upstream of the human thyroid peroxidase gene. Mol Cell Biol 10:6216–6224, 1990.
119. Mizuno K, Gonzalez FJ, Kimura S: Thyroid-specific enhancer-binding protein (T/EBP): cDNA cloning, functional characterization, and structural identity with thyroid transcription factor TTF-1. Mol Cell Biol 11:4927–4933, 1991.
120. Takasu N, Charrier B, Mauchamp J, et al: Modulation of adenylate cyclase/cyclic AMP response by thyrotropin and prostaglandin E_2 in cultured thyroid cells. 2. Positive regulation. Eur J Biochem 90:139–146, 1978.
121. Saji M, Akamizu T, Sanchez M: Regulation of thyrotropin receptor gene expression in rat FRTL-5 thyroid cells. Endocrinology 130:520–533, 1992.
122. Berlingieri MT, Akamizu T, Fusco A: Thyrotropin receptor gene expression in oncogene-transfected rat thyroid cells: Correlation between transformation, loss of thyrotropin dependent growth, and loss of thyrotropin receptor gene expression. Biochem Biophys Res Commun 173:172–178, 1990.
123. Akamizu T, Ikuyama S, Saji M, et al: Cloning, chromosomal assignment, and regulation of the rat thyrotropin receptor: Expression of the gene is regulated by thyrotropin, agents that increase cAMP levels, and thyroid autoantibodies. Proc Natl Acad Sci U S A 87:5677–5681, 1990.
124. Maenhaut C, Brabant G, Vassart G, et al: In vitro and in vivo regulation of thyrotropin receptor mRNA levels in dog and human thyroid cells. J Biol Chem 267:3000–3007, 1992.
125. Kung AW, Collison K, Banga JP, et al: Effect of Graves' IgG on gene transcription in human thyroid cell cultures. Thyroglobulin gene activation. FEBS Lett 232:12–16, 1988.
126. Huber GK, Weinstein SP, Graves PN, et al: The positive regulation of human thyrotropin (TSH) receptor messenger ribonucleic acid by recombinant human TSH is at the intranuclear level. Endocrinology 130:2858–2864, 1992.
127. Brabant G, Maenhaut C, Kohrle J, et al: Human thyrotropin receptor gene: Expression in thyroid tumors and correlation to markers of thyroid differentiation and dedifferentiation. Mol Cell Endocrinol 82:R7–R12, 1991.
128. Ohta K, Endo T, Onaya T: The mRNA levels of thyrotropin receptor, thyroglobulin and thyroid peroxidase in neoplastic human thyroid tissues. Biochem Biophys Res Commun 174:1148–1153, 1991.
129. Roger PP, Van Heuverswyn B, Lambert C, et al: Antagonistic effects of thyrotropin and epidermal growth factor on thyroglobulin mRNA level in cultured thyroid cells. Eur J Biochem 152:239–245, 1985.
130. Mazzaferri EL: Papillary and follicular thyroid cancer: A selective approach to diagnosis and treatment. Annu Rev Med 32:73–91, 1981.
131. Christov K: Cell population kinetics and DNA content during thyroid carcinogenesis. Cell Tissue Kinet 18:119–131, 1985.
132. Coclet J, Foureau F, Ketelbant P, et al: Cell population kinetics in dog and human adult thyroid. Clin Endocrinol 31:655–665, 1989.
133. Smeds S, Wollman SH: ^{3}H-thymidine labeling of endothelial cells in thyroid arteries, veins, and lymphatics during thyroid stimulation. Lab Invest 48:285–291, 1983.
134. Takasu N, Komiya I, Nagasawa Y, et al: Stimulation of porcine thyroid cell alkalinization and growth by EGF, phorbol ester, and diacylglycerol. Am J Physiol 258:E445–E450, 1990.
135. Pohl V, Roger PP, Christophe D, et al: Differentiation expression during proliferative activity induced through different pathways: In situ hybridization study of thyroglobulin gene expression in thyroid epithelial cells. J Cell Biol 111:663–672, 1990.
136. Roger PP, Taton M, Van Sande J, et al: Mitogenic effects of thyrotropin and adenosine 3′,5′-monophosphate in differentiated normal human thyroid cells in vitro. J Clin Endocrinol Metab 66:1158–1165, 1988.
137. Van Sande J, Lefort A, Beebe S, et al: Pairs of cyclic AMP analogs, that are specifically synergistic for type I and type II cAMP-dependent protein kinases, mimic thyrotropin effects on the function, differentiation expression and mitogenesis of dog thyroid cells. Eur J Biochem 183:699–708, 1989.
138. Meinkoth JL, Goldsmith PK, Spiegel AM: Inhibition of thyrotropin-induced DNA synthesis in thyroid follicular cells by microinjection of an antibody to the stimulatory G protein of adenylate cyclase, Gs. J Biol Chem 267:13239–13245, 1992.
139. Dremier S, Pohl V, Poteet-Smith C, et al: Activation of cyclic AMP–dependent kinase is required but may not be sufficient to mimic cyclic AMP–dependent DNA synthesis and thyroglobulin expression in dog thyroid cells. Mol Cell Biol 17:6717–6726. 1997.
140. Bachrach LK, Eggo MC, Mak WW, et al: Phorbol esters stimulate growth and inhibit differentiation in cultured thyroid cells. Endocrinology 116:1603–1609, 1985.
141. Raspe E, Reuse S, Roger PP, et al: Lack of correlation between the activation of the Ca^{2+}-phosphatidylinositol cascade and the regulation of DNA synthesis in the dog thyrocyte. Exp Cell Res 198:17–26, 1992.
142. Ollis CA, Hill DJ, Munro DS: A role for insulin-like growth factor-I in the regulation of human thyroid cell growth by thyrotropin. J Clin Endocrinol 123:495–500, 1989.
143. Maciel RMB, Moses AC, Villone G, et al: Demonstration of the production and physiological role of insulin-like growth factor II in rat thyroid follicular cells in culture. J Clin Invest 82:1546–1553, 1988.
144. Melillo RM, Barone MV, Lupoli G, et al: Ret-mediated mitogenesis requires Src kinase activity. Cancer Res 59:1120–1126, 1999.
145. Becks GP, Eggo MC, Burrow GN: Organic iodide inhibits deoxyribonucleic acid synthesis and growth in FRTL5 cells. Endocrinology 123:545–550, 1988.
146. Contor L, Lamy F, Lecocq R, et al: Differential protein phosphorylation in induction of thyroid cell proliferation by thyrotropin, epidermal growth factor, or phorbol ester. Mol Cell Biol 8:2494–2503, 1988.
147. Deleu S, Pirson I, Coulonval K, et al: IGF-1 or insulin, and the TSH cyclic AMP cascade separately control dog and human thyroid cell growth and DNA synthesis, and complement each other in inducing mitogenesis. Mol Cell Endocrinol 149:41–51, 1999.
148. Tramontano D, Chin WW, Moses AC, et al: Thyrotropin and dibutyryl cyclic AMP increase levels of c-myc and c-fos mRNAs in cultured rat thyroid cells. J Biol Chem 261:3919–3922, 1986.
149. Lamy F, Roger PP, Lecocq R, et al: Differential protein synthesis in the induction of thyroid cell proliferation by thyrotropin, epidermal growth factor or serum. Eur J Biochem 155:265–272, 1986.
150. Lamy F, Roger PP, Lecocq R, et al: Protein synthesis during induction of DNA replication in thyroid epithelial cells: Evidence for late markers of distinct mitogenic pathways. J Cell Physiol 138:568–578, 1989.
151. Dremier S, Golstein J, Mosselmans R, et al: Apoptosis in dog thyroid cells. Biochem Biophys Res Commun 200:52–58, 1994.
152. Riesco JM, Juanes JA, Carretero J, et al: Cell proliferation and apoptosis of thyroid follicular cells are involved in the involution of experimental non-tumoral hyperplastic goiter. Anat Embryol 198:439–450, 1998.
153. Tamura M, Kimura H, Koji T, et al: Role of apoptosis of thyrocytes in a rat model of goiter. A possible involvement of Fas system. Endocrinology 139:3643–3646, 1998.

Chapter 94

Thyroid Hormone Binding and Metabolism

Thyroid Hormone Binding

Jan R. Stockigt

An understanding of thyroid hormone transport and metabolism allows the clinician to better appreciate tissue delivery and interconversion of thyroid hormones, especially when these phenomena change as a result of illness or drug therapy or when treatment is given to alter thyroid status. Knowledge of these fundamentals facilitates the interpretation of (1) atypical thyroid function test results, (2) the effects of critical illness, (3) the influence of medications, and (4) the effects of hereditary and acquired abnormalities of the plasma proteins that bind thyroid hormones. In particular, an insight into thyroid hormone binding is helpful in critically assessing the validity, or otherwise, of abbreviated methods for the estimation of free concentrations of serum triiodothyronine (T_3) and thyroxine (T_4).

THYROID HORMONE TRANSPORT

The evolution of thyroid hormone binding to plasma proteins can be traced from fish, which show only albumin binding, through birds, which show binding to both albumin and transthyretin (TTR, previously known as prealbumin), to most larger mammals, which with the exception of felines have developed a low-capacity, high-affinity protein termed thyroxine-binding globulin (TBG) for the specific carriage of iodothyronines. In humans, only 0.02% to 0.03% (about 1 part in 4000) of T_4 and 0.2% to 0.3% of T_3 are present in the free or unbound state in undiluted normal human serum or plasma at equilibrium and 37°C. Other iodothyronines, both synthetic analogues and metabolites, are also generally highly protein bound.[1]

In normal human serum, about 75% of the total circulating T_4 concentration of 60 to 140 nmol/L or 4 to 11 μg/dL is carried on TBG, with about 10% to 15% attached to TTR and 10% to 15% bound to albumin. It should be noted that the electrophoretic techniques used to make these estimates allow dissociation of labeled hormone during separation and thus tend to underestimate proportional carriage on lower-affinity sites. A minor fraction (<5%) of circulating T_4 and T_3 is associated with lipoprotein.[2]

The assumption that the minute free fraction of the total circulating T_4 and T_3 pool determines hormone action and clearance, as well as feedback on the pituitary secretion of thyroid-stimulating hormone (TSH), is the basis of the free hormone hypothesis (see below). The fact that total hormone concentrations vary widely in response to diverse patterns of protein binding while maintaining relatively constant concentrations of free hormone supports this hypothesis (see Chapter 113).

Concentrations of binding protein can vary for reasons independent of thyroid status. When the concentration of TBG changes, total serum T_4 and T_3 concentrations will be altered to levels that restore the preexisting concentration of free hormone, as determined by the set-point of the feedback relationship with TSH. Hence in theory, free hormone estimates will give a more accurate reflection of thyroid status than will measurement of total hormone. However, an understanding of the dynamic relationship between free and total circulating hormone is useful in maintaining a critical approach to current free hormone techniques in which stored samples are assayed after dilution. Both storage and dilution can create misleading artifacts (see below).

Binding to plasma proteins is noncovalent and rapidly reversible; it is important to emphasize that the much larger bound moiety of hormone has a reservoir function. Dissociation of bound hormone almost instantaneously replenishes the free hormone concentration as this minute fraction is taken up by tissue or irreversibly cleared. Similarly, when serum is progressively diluted in vitro, the free concentration is at first well maintained by progressive dissociation of the large store of bound hormone. A rigid distinction between bound and free hormone moieties may in fact be artificial in light of studies that suggest dissociation and reassociation so rapid that the free and bound moieties interchange several million times per day.[3]

FUNCTION OF BINDING PROTEINS

The large pool of extracellular T_4 that is maintained as a result of plasma protein binding is equivalent to 10 to 15 days of hormone secretion from a normal thyroid. Avid protein binding is the basis for the long plasma half-life of about 7 days and the slow metabolic clearance rate of T_4, properties that favor sustained thyroid hormone action even in the event of gland failure. A high degree of protein binding also serves to protect against the iodine loss that would result from urinary excretion of unbound iodothyronines. It has been suggested that protein binding of T_4 may have a key role in the regulation of T_4 delivery to the fetus in early pregnancy.[4]

Autoradiographic studies suggest that binding proteins facilitate even tissue distribution of iodothyronines.[5] When rat liver lobules were perfused with ^{125}I-labeled T_4 in the absence of binding protein, almost all the T_4 was taken up by periportal cells. When either 4% human serum albumin or human serum was added to the perfusate, the labeled hormone was taken up uniformly by all cells within the lobule. When a competitor was added to displace T_4 from albumin, uptake was again predominantly periportal.[5]

It is notable that the normal free concentration of T_4 is close to its K_d for TBG (see below). When a binding protein is approximately half occupied, the relationship between free and total hormone concentrations will be close and changes in total hormone concentration will have maximum regulatory impact. TBG does not appear to have a role in targeted hormone delivery via specific cellular receptors for this protein, as has been suggested for corticosteroid-binding globulin[6] and for TTR.[7] None of the multiple hereditary human variations in the binding of T_4 and/or T_3 to plasma proteins (see Chapter 113) appear to confer any advantage or disadvantage in terms of nutrition, organ function, or survival.

THE BINDING PROTEINS AND CHARACTERISTICS OF HORMONE BINDING

The characteristics of the three normal major iodothyronine-binding proteins, TBG, TTR, and albumin, are summarized in Table 94–1. Their physical properties and major hereditary variants are described in Chapter 113.

The definition of a number of terms assists the understanding of thyroid hormone binding. *Capacity* expresses the molar concentration of a specific class of ligand-binding site; if one binding site per protein molecule is available, capacity and protein concentration will be identical in molar terms. When about half the binding sites remain empty, the free hormone concentration will increase in direct relationship to the total hormone concentration (i.e., the free fraction will show little change). However, as the total concentration of ligand approaches the binding protein capacity, the free hormone concentration will rise disproportionately, as occurs in thyrotoxicosis, where the total T_4 serum concentration may approach the capacity of TBG.

Proportional carriage, the distribution of total hormone between a number of heterogeneous binding proteins, is influenced by the concentration of binding protein, the affinity of binding, and the free hormone concentration, but it is not directly influenced by the total hormone concentration.[8] In a heterogeneous mixture of binding proteins, as in serum, proportional carriage will change as the free hormone concentration is altered in response to either dilution or hormone loading (see below).

Free fraction describes the percentage of total hormone that is unbound. When serum containing a highly bound ligand is progressively diluted, bound hormone will dissociate; the free hormone concentration is at first well maintained, with an increase in the free fraction proportional to the degree of dilution.

Occupancy, the proportion of a particular class of binding site that is filled with hormone, is a direct function of the free hormone concentration and is fundamental to the definition of affinity, or K_d. TBG is normally about one-third occupied by T_4, TTR is less than 1% occupied by T_4, and albumin shows negligible occupancy (see Table 94–1).

Affinity (K_d, moles per liter) describes the free hormone concentration at which a particular binding site is half occupied. The *association constant* (K_a, liters per mole) is the inverse of K_d. (K_a is a theoretic concept of the number of liters at which 1 mol of ligand would occupy half the sites on 1 mol of binding protein.) By definition, a binding protein is 50% occupied when the free hormone concentration is the inverse of K_a.

The *dissociation rate* ($T_{1/2}$, seconds) or the rate constant (sec^{-1}) defines the rate of unidirectional dissociation or delivery of hormone from a binding site.[3] The unidirectional maximum rate of hormone delivery is relevant under non–steady-state conditions, as for example, when free hormone is rapidly removed from the circulation during tissue transit. The dissociation rate, as well as K_a and K_d, are highly temperature dependent. The free T_4 fraction is higher at 37°C than at room temperature by a factor of up to 2,[9] and dissociation of ligand is much faster.[3]

The reversible interaction between free T_4 (fT_4) and the unoccupied TBG-binding sites (uTBG) can be represented by

$$fT_4 + uTBG \rightleftharpoons TBG \cdot T_4$$

When represented in terms of the association constant k_{TBG}, this relationship becomes

$$k_{TBG} = \frac{[TBG \cdot T_4]}{[fT_4]\,[uTBG]}$$

It follows that

$$[fT_4] = \frac{[TBG \cdot T_4]}{k_{TBG}[uTBG]}$$

At half occupancy of the binding site, [TBG • T_4] will equal [uTBG] and

$$[fT_4] = \frac{1}{K_a} = K_d$$

For the total hormone concentration to have a regulatory influence on tissue function it is appropriate for the K_d of the dominant binding protein and the physiologic concentration of free hormone to be of the same order, as is the case for the relationship between normal serum free T_4 (10 to 25 pmol/L) and the K_d of TBG (~100 pmol/L). If the physiologic free hormone concentration were much lower than the K_d of the dominant binding protein, very large changes in total hormone concentration would be required to achieve regulatory variation. In effect, TBG stabilizes the tissue distribution of T_4 and protects against iodine wastage while allowing normal regulatory variation over an approximately twofold range of total hormone concentration.

THE FREE HORMONE HYPOTHESIS

According to the free hormone hypothesis, it is the free or unbound equilibrium concentration of a hormone that determines its biologic

TABLE 94–1. Properties of the Major Human Thyroid Hormone–Binding Proteins

Property	Thyroxine-Binding Globulin	Transthyretin	Albumin
Molecular weight (kDa)	54	55	66
Structure	Glycoprotein	Peptide tetramer	Single peptide chain
Concentration (mol/L)	3×10^{-7}	2×10^{-6}	6×10^{-4}
Half-life (days)	5	2	15
Degradation rate (mg/day)	15	650	17,000
Proportion of T_4 carried (%)	75	10–15	10–15
Occupancy by T_4 (%)	30	0.5	<0.01
Dissociation constant*			
T_4K_d (mol/L)	10^{-10}	10^{-8}	10^{-6}†
T_3K_d (mol/L)	2×10^{-9}	6×10^{-8}	10^{-5}†
Off rate‡			
$T_4t½$ (sec)	20–40	8	<2
$T_3t½$ (sec)	5–10	<2	<1

*Free hormone concentration at half occupancy of binding sites at equilibrium.
†Highest-affinity site.
‡Unidirectional dissociation rate.
T_3, triiodothyronine; T_4, thyroxine.

activity. The validity of this hypothesis, which is generally well sustained for thyroid hormones, has been analyzed in detail.[10, 11] Earlier liver perfusion experiments that showed the loosely albumin-bound moiety of the total circulating hormone pool to be virtually as readily available as the free hormone[12] have now been refuted.[10] No evidence has indicated that any particular class of binding protein facilitates tissue uptake of thyroid hormones. When isolated rat liver was perfused with T_4 bound to various normal and variant binding proteins,[13] tissue uptake of T_4 was proportional to the spontaneous dissociation of T_4 from each protein.[13]

Under some circumstances, especially when capillary transit is slow or when mixing of layers across the diameter of a vessel is incomplete, tissue uptake of hormone may be limited by dissociation of bound hormone.[10] Under these circumstances, when the local concentration of free hormone at a particular site may be lower than the equilibrium concentration, the albumin-bound moiety that has the fastest rate of unidirectional dissociation (see Table 94–1) will make a large contribution in replenishing the free concentration.[10]

As formulated by Mendel,[10, 11] the unmodified free hormone hypothesis will be valid when tissue uptake of hormone is limited by influx or elimination. When flow or dissociation is the limiting condition, for example, when flow is slow and clearance is rapid in a tissue such as the liver, the free hormone hypothesis still holds, with hormone dissociation as an additional critical variable.

ACQUIRED ALTERATIONS

Numerous drugs can influence the concentrations of TBG and TTR (Table 94–2) by effects that either alter protein synthesis or influence degradation; in most instances the mechanism is not yet clearly defined. The most common acquired change in TBG is an increase in concentration caused by exogenous or endogenous estrogens; this modification results in TBG with a greater proportion of bands having anodal mobility on isoelectric focusing because of an increase in the sialic acid content of the side chains.[14] The reduced TBG degradation rate caused by this oligosaccharide modification appears to be the major mechanism of estrogen-induced TBG excess.[15] Transdermal estrogens do not have this effect.[16]

Serum concentrations of TBG are reduced in thyrotoxicosis and increased in hypothyroidism in humans[17] and in experimental primate studies,[18] whereas serum TBG concentrations are decreased by glucocorticoid excess.[19] Unlike human TBG, rat TBG is strongly repressed during adult life but actively expressed during postnatal development, in senescence, in the face of malnutrition, in hypothyroidism,[20] and also after adrenalectomy.[21]

If the concentration of TBG were to increase acutely, a number of changes would result in re-equilibration of the pituitary-thyroid axis. First, a shift of T_4 from tissues to blood would decrease T_4 clearance, followed by activation of pituitary TSH secretion in response to lower tissue levels of free T_4 and a subsequent increase in T_4 production until the original concentration of serum free T_4 is restored at a higher total T_4. At the new steady state, the intravascular T_4 pool would increase with a decrease in the fractional turnover rate, but the rate of T_4 secretion and degradation would return to baseline. Opposite changes would follow an abrupt decrease in the concentration of TBG, similar to the consequences of occupancy of TBG by an alternative ligand such as a drug competitor (see below).

Acquired changes in TTR concentration are common but have relatively minor effects on the total serum concentrations of T_4 and T_3 because of the low occupancy of this protein. Androgens[22] and glucocorticoids[19] increase whereas estrogens decrease the concentrations of TTR[23]; these agents have the opposite effect on TBG. Hepatic synthesis of TTR decreases abruptly during any major illness. Some islet cell carcinomas can directly synthesize and release sufficient TTR to result in euthyroid hyperthyroxinemia.[24]

TABLE 94–2. Drug Effects on Serum TBG and TTR Concentrations in Humans

Increase TBG	*Decrease TBG*
Estrogens	Thyroid hormones
Tamoxifen	Androgens, anabolic steroids
Heroin	Glucocorticoids
Methadone	L-Asparaginase
5-Fluorouracil	Interleukin-6
Perphenazine	
Clofibrate	
Mitotane	
Increase TTR	*Decrease TTR*
Androgens	Estrogens
Glucocorticoids	

TBG, thyroxine-binding globulin; TTR, transthyretin.

TABLE 94–3. The Principal Drugs that Displace T_4 from TBG Binding in Normal Human Serum

Drug	Mean Percent Increase in Free T_4 Fraction*
Salicylates	
Acetylsalicylic acid (aspirin)	62
Salicylsalicylic acid (salsalate)	>100
Furosemide†	5–30
Fenclofenac	90
Mefenamic acid	31
Flufenamic acid	10
Diclofenac	7
Diflunisal	37
Phenytoin	45
Carbamazepine	30

*Equilibrium dialysis or ultrafiltration of undiluted serum at 37°C in vitro at appropriate therapeutic concentrations of each drug.

†Wide therapeutic range.

T_4, thyroxine; TBG, thyroxine-binding globulin. Data from Munro et al.,[25] Lim et al.,[26, 27] Surks and Defesi,[28] and Wang et al.[29]

COMPETITORS FOR THYROID HORMONE TRANSPORT SITES

In contrast to plasma proteins which bind corticosteroids, vitamin D, and sex hormones and are highly specific for a single family of ligand, the iodothyronine-binding proteins show wide cross-reactivity with unrelated hydrophobic ligands such as nonesterified fatty acids (NEFAs) and numerous drugs (Table 94–3). Each of these substances is itself highly bound to albumin; the unbound rather than the total ligand concentration determines competition.

Competition in Serum

When competition is studied by examining displacement of labeled T_4 or T_3 from an isolated binding protein with the unlabeled hormone used as reference, the affinities of important drug competitors for TBG range from 3 orders of magnitude less (furosemide) to almost 7 orders of magnitude less than T_4 itself in the case of aspirin.[25] However, such direct studies do not reflect in vivo competition because the free serum concentration of a competitor is determined by its binding to sites other than TBG, in particular, albumin. Many highly bound drugs circulate in micromolar concentrations and may occupy 5% to 50% of the albumin-binding sites; the concentration of albumin, or its occupancy by other ligands, then becomes an important determinant of the free drug concentration. Because of differences in albumin binding, the hierarchy of drug competitor potency at relevant therapeutic concentrations in undiluted serum differs markedly from their relative affinity for TBG in isolation.[25, 26] The data shown in Table 94–3 are influenced by the total concentration of each drug and its free fraction, as well as its affinity for T_4-binding proteins.

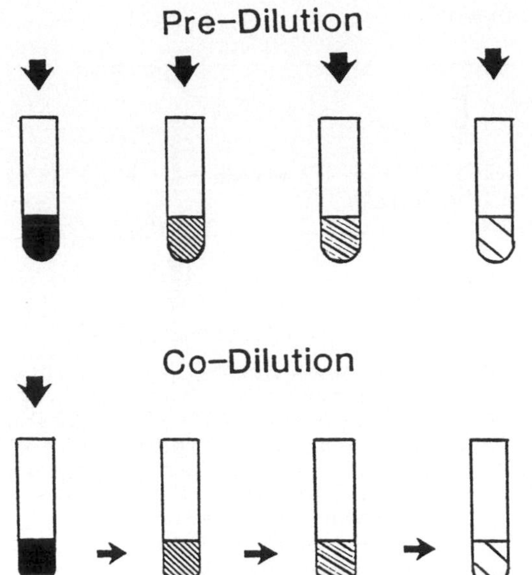

FIGURE 94–1. Predilution: serum is diluted, followed by addition of a particular concentration of competitor. The effect of the competitor will be overestimated as albumin occupancy increases. Codilution: the competitor is added to serum, followed by identical simultaneous dilution of binding proteins, hormone, and competitors. If the competitor is less highly bound than the hormone, its effect will be progressively underestimated. (From Stockigt JR, et al: Thyroid hormone transport. *In* Weetman AP, Grossman A (eds): Pharmacotherapeutics of the Thyroid Gland. Berlin, Springer-Verlag, 1997, pp 119–150.)

Dilution Effects

When working with a highly bound ligand, such as T_4, it is technically easier to study binding in diluted serum. In the absence of competitors, such measurements give useful comparisons between samples with high, normal, and low free hormone concentrations. It is much more difficult to establish a system in which the concentrations of free hormone, competitor(s), and unoccupied binding sites are maintained in the relationships that apply in vivo. The existing literature on competitor effects has become confused because details such as dilution and albumin concentration are often poorly defined. The terms "predilution" and "codilution" are useful in defining potential artifacts.

Predilution occurs when the concentration of binding proteins is progressively decreased before particular concentrations of competitor are added (Fig. 94–1). The lower the concentration of albumin, the higher the occupancy of available binding sites, thus leading to a disproportionate increase in the free competitor concentration which will magnify apparent competitor potency.[30] For example, in the case of a highly albumin-bound competitor, the T_4-displacing effect of 5 mmol/L oleic acid added to undiluted serum could be matched almost exactly by 0.5 mmol/L oleic acid in serum diluted 1:10.[26] In general, predilution of the sample magnifies the apparent competition.

Codilution occurs when a competitor present in whole serum is serially diluted so that *total* concentrations of binding proteins, hormone, and competitors diminish in parallel. Notably, the free concentrations do not maintain this parallelism. The difference becomes clear if a hormone such as T_4 with a free fraction of about 1:4000 is compared with a drug that has a free fraction in serum of 1:50. Progressive dissociation will sustain the free T_4 *concentration* at a 1:100 dilution (although the free *fraction* rises sharply as a result of dissociation). In contrast, the free drug concentration decreases markedly after a dilution of only 1:10. Codilution effects lead to underestimation of the potency of competitors that are less highly protein bound than the hormone itself.

A codilution effect was the initial clue that led to recognition of furosemide as an important inhibitor of T_4 binding in serum.[31] When T_4 binding was studied by serial dilution in critically ill hypothyroxinemic patients, those who had received high-dose furosemide showed a marked increase in the free T_4 fraction that became less obvious with progressive dilution.[31] In comparing the ability of three commercial free T_4 assays to detect the T_4-displacing effect of furosemide, the effect was most obvious in the method with the least sample dilution[32] (Fig. 94–2).

The importance of a codilution effect was demonstrated for therapeutic concentrations of phenytoin and carbamazepine, which increased the free fraction of T_4 by 40% to 50% as determined by ultrafiltration of undiluted serum.[28] During continuing drug therapy, total T_4 was lowered by 25% to 50%, which resulted in calculated free concentrations within the normal range. However, no increase in T_4 free fraction was seen with a commercial single-step free T_4 assay after a 1:5 serum dilution.[28]

Kinetics of the Competitor

The kinetics of the competitor itself will determine how it influences hormone binding in vivo (Fig. 94–3). A competitor with a short half-life such as furosemide or salsalate will show fluctuating effects on hormone binding, so free hormone estimates may vary widely depending on the time between dosage and sampling.[29] In contrast, a competitor with a long half-life will result in a new steady state with a normal free hormone concentration and a lowered total hormone concentration (i.e., an increased free fraction). It is not yet known whether intermittent competitor-induced increases in free hormone concentration can augment hormone action in humans, but it has been shown that a T_3- and T_4-displacing synthetic flavonoid has a transient thyromimetic effect in rats.[34]

Interaction between Competitors

Increasing concentrations of any substance that shares albumin binding sites with a competitor can increase the free concentration of that competitor. Two substances that show potential to exert such a "cascade" effect on T_4 binding in serum are oleic acid[35] and 3-carboxy-4-methyl-5-propyl-2-furanpropanoic acid (CMPF),[27] a naturally occurring furanoid acid that accumulates in renal failure. At concentrations that had only a minimal direct effect on the binding of T_4 in undiluted normal serum, oleic acid and CMPF (Fig. 94–4) augmented the T_4-displacing effect of several drug competitors for T_4 binding in undiluted serum.[27] By such a mechanism, free hormone concentrations can be influenced by substances that have little direct interaction with hormone-binding sites.

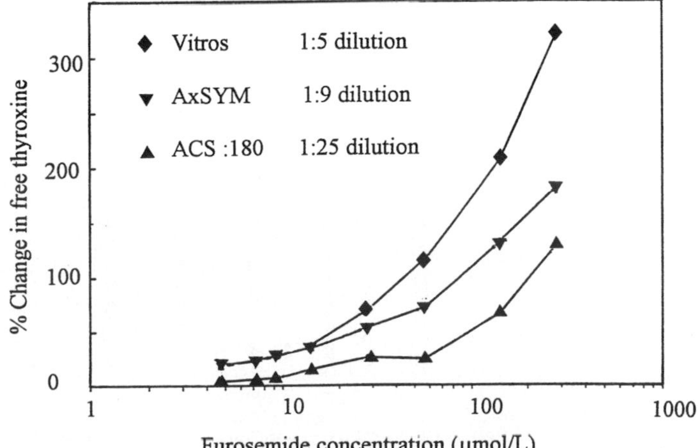

FIGURE 94–2. Effect of addition of furosemide to serum on estimates of free T_4 using three commercial free T_4 methods that involve varying degrees of sample dilution. The effect of the competitor is progressively obscured with increasing sample dilution. (Redrawn from Hawkins RC: Furosemide interference in newer free thyroxine assays. Clin Chem 44:2550–2551, 1998.)

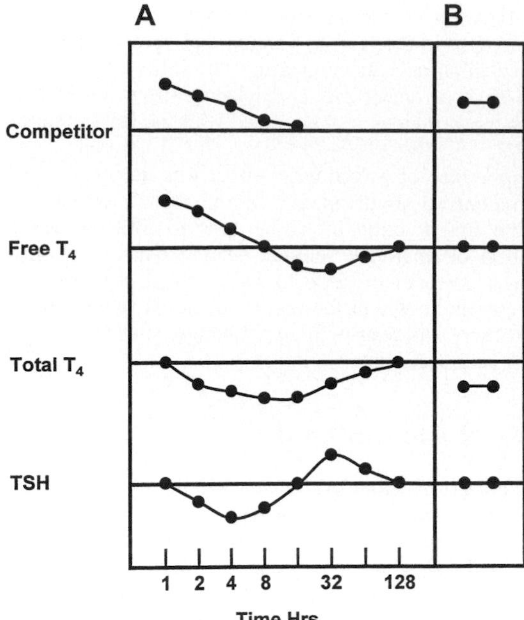

FIGURE 94–3. Representation of the serial changes in serum free T_4, total T_4, and TSH that occur after ingestion of a single dose of a potent competitor for T_4 binding to TBG *(A)*. An initial increase in free T_4 is followed by a decrease in TSH and accelerated T_4 clearance, resulting in a decrease in total and free T_4, followed by a rebound increase in TSH. Note logarithmic time scale. *B* shows the effect of a competitor of long half-life, or frequent dosage of a short half-life competitor: stabilization occurs at a new steady state with normal serum free T_4 and TSH concentrations but a decrease in total T_4. (Data from Wang et al.[29] and Newnham et al.[33])

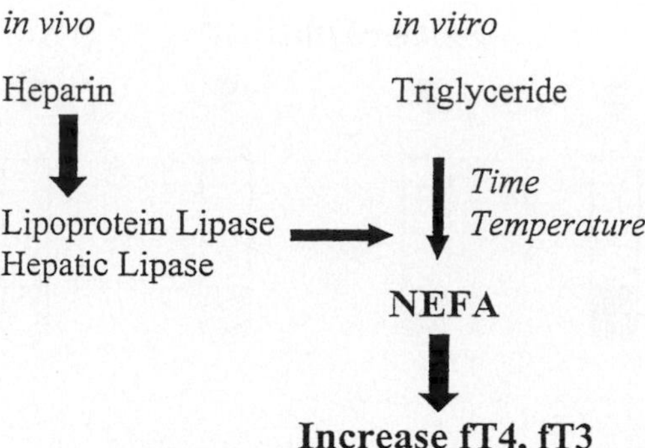

FIGURE 94–5. Summary of the heparin-induced changes that can markedly increase the apparent concentration of serum free T_4. Heparin acts in vivo *(left)* to liberate lipoprotein lipase from vascular endothelium. Lipase acts in vitro *(right)* to increase the concentration of nonesterified fatty acids (NEFA) to levels >3 mmol/L, resulting in displacement of T_4 and T_3 from TBG. In vitro generation of NEFA is increased by sample storage at room temperature, by incubation at 37°C, and by high concentration of serum triglyceride. The T_4-displacing effect of NEFA is accentuated at low albumin concentrations.

Spurious Competition

The effect of heparin to increase the apparent free T_4 concentration in vitro can be misleading because of spurious competition. As summarized in Figure 94–5, increases in free T_4 as a result of heparin treatment appear to cause in vivo release of lipase, followed by in vitro generation of NEFA during assay incubation or storage.[36] As a result of this artifact, serum NEFA concentrations at the time of assay can be much higher than they were in vivo.[37] This effect could account for some reports of apparent increases in free T_4 and free T_3 fractions in critically ill subjects. It remains to be established whether earlier reports of circulating inhibitors of T_4 binding in critical illness can be attributed to the effects of medications, including heparin. When heparin has been given, assays of total T_4 and T_3 are likely to be more informative than assays of free T_4 and T_3, unless special precautions are taken to avoid in vitro generation of NEFA.[37]

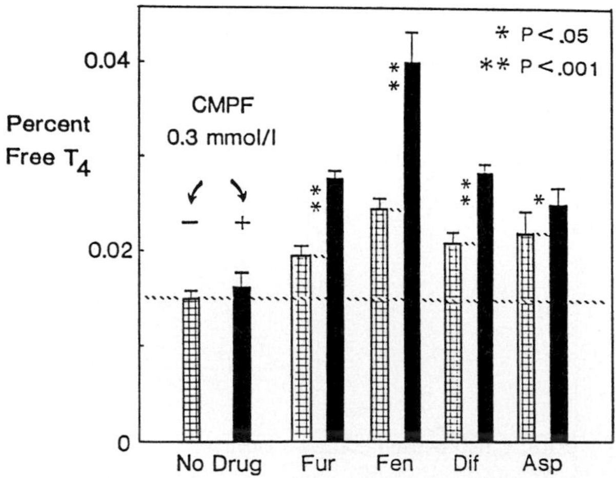

FIGURE 94–4. Influence of 3-carboxy-4-methyl-5-propyl-2 furanpropanoic acid (CMPF) on the T_4-displacing effects of therapeutic concentrations of furosemide (Fur), fenclofenac (Fen), diflunisal (Dif), and aspirin (Asp) in undiluted serum at 37°C (equilibrium dialysis). Percentage of free T_4 is shown in the presence *(solid columns)* and absence *(hatched columns)* of 0.3 mM CMPF. Each drug together with CMPF increased free T_4 more than the sum of drug alone plus CMPF alone (**p <.001). (Data from Lim et al.[27])

STUDIES OF SPECIFIC BINDING SITES

With a knowledge of the capacity and affinity of the heterogeneous thyroid hormone–binding sites in human serum, it is possible to manipulate hormone concentration and sample dilution to effectively characterize a single class of binding site without isolating that protein. Similar approaches may ultimately be applicable to the studies of heterogeneous thyroid hormone–binding sites in the intracellular milieu.

Because the affinity (K_d) of any binding site is defined as the free hormone concentration that achieves half occupancy, it follows that a change in the bound/total or bound/free hormone ratio is analytically optimal when the free hormone concentration is about the same as the K_d and when the concentration of binding sites is approximately double the K_d, that is, when the bound/free hormone ratio is approximately 1 and the bound/total hormone ratio is about 50%.

Because the T_4- binding affinities of TBG and albumin differ by about 4 orders of magnitude, high-affinity binding can be "dissected" from low-affinity sites by high sample dilution. For example, if normal serum with a total T_4 concentration of 100 nmol/L is diluted 5000-fold, the total T_4 concentration will be 20 pmol/L, close to the affinity of TBG. With the use of $[^{125}I]$-T_4 of high specific activity, the effect of drug competitors on specific T_4 binding to TBG can be studied in such a system without a need to isolate the protein. The effects of TTR and albumin are negligible under these conditions.[8] Such a method can be used to measure the minute amounts of TBG produced by cultured cells.[38]

Conversely, low-affinity binding is best examined after hormone loading to achieve a free concentration close to the affinity of that site; at high free hormone concentrations the low-capacity sites are saturated and are not altered by changes in the free hormone concentration. At artificially high hormone concentrations the abnormally avid binding of T_4 to albumin in familial dysalbuminemic hyperthyroxinemia can be readily demonstrated in the presence of a 1000-fold relative excess of unlabeled T_4 (see Chapter 113).

CELL MEMBRANE AND INTRACELLULAR TRANSPORT

Although it is generally assumed that free T_3 and T_4 move passively through cell membranes, many substances, including calcium channel blockers,[8] can be shown to inhibit this process by mechanisms that appear to be competitive.[39] The physiologic significance of these interactions is uncertain and does not necessarily imply specific active transport. The possible identification of a specific cell membrane transport protein[40] needs to be confirmed. It is notable that under pathologic conditions, bilirubin[41] and metabolites that accumulate in renal failure such as indoxyl sulfate and CMPF[42] can inhibit cell entry of T_4 and may, by limiting the amount of available substrate, impair the formation of T_3 during critical illness.

The recent demonstration that some cultured cell lines show a saturable, stereospecific, verapamil-inhibitable mechanism that mediates T_3 efflux in vitro,[43] raises the possibility that variable exit of T_3 from cells could modify thyroid hormone action. A putative transport protein was identified by photoaffinity labeling.[43]

Cytoplasmic T_3 binding can be competitively inhibited by some anti-inflammatory agents and non–bile acid cholephils,[44] but interpretation of these interactions is uncertain because the relevant free concentrations of hormone and competitor at specific cytoplasmic binding sites are unknown.

REFERENCES

1. Robbins J, Cheng S-Y, Gershengorn MC, et al: Thyroxine transport proteins of plasma, molecular properties and biosynthesis. Recent Prog Horm Res 34:477–519, 1978.
2. Benvenga S, Cahnmann HJ, Robbins J: Characterization of thyroid hormone binding to apolipoprotein-E: Localization of the binding site in the exon 3–coded domain. Endocrinology 133:1300–1305, 1993.
3. Hillier AP: Thyroxine dissociation in human plasma: Measurement of its rate by a continuous-flow dialysis method. Acta Endocrinol 78:32–38, 1975.
4. Ekins T: Roles of serum thyroxine-binding proteins and maternal thyroid hormones in foetal development. Lancet 1:1129–1132, 1985.
5. Mendel CM, Weisiger RA, Jones AL, et al: Thyroid hormone–binding proteins in plasma facilitate uniform distribution of thyroxine within tissues: A perfused rat liver study. Endocrinology 120:1742–1749, 1987.
6. Rosner W: The functions of corticosteroid-binding globulin and sex hormone–binding globulin: Recent advances. Endocr Rev 11:80–91, 1990.
7. Divino CM, Schussler GC: Receptor-mediated uptake and internalization of transthyretin. J Biol Chem 265:1425–1429, 1990.
8. Stockigt JR, Lim C-F, Barlow JW, et al: Thyroid hormone transport. *In* Weetman AP, Grossman A (eds): Pharmacotherapeutics of the Thyroid Gland. Berlin, Springer, 1997, pp 119–150.
9. Korcek L, Tabachnick M: Thyroxine-protein interactions. Interaction of thyroxine and triiodothyronine with human TBG. J Biol Chem 251:3558–3562, 1976.
10. Mendel CM: The free hormone hypothesis: A physiologically based mathematical model. Endocr Rev 10:232–274, 1989.
11. Mendel CM: The free hormone hypothesis and free hormone transport hypothesis: Update 1994. *In* Braverman LE Refetoff S (eds): Clinical and Molecular Aspects of Diseases of the Thyroid. Endocrine Reviews Monographs, vol 3. Bethesda, MD, The Endocrine Society, 1994, pp 208–209.
12. Pardridge WM: Transport of protein-bound hormones into tissue in vivo. Endocr Rev 2:103–123, 1981.
13. Mendel CM, Weisiger RA: Thyroxine uptake by perfused rat liver: No evidence for facilitation by five different thyroxine-binding proteins. J Clin Invest 86:1840–1847, 1990.
14. Ain KB, Mori Y, Refetoff S: Reduced clearance rate of thyroxine-binding globulin (TBG) with increased sialylation: A mechanism for estrogen-induced elevation of serum TBG concentration. J Clin Endocrinol Metab 65:689–696, 1987.
15. Ain KB, Refetoff S: Relationship of oligosaccharide modification to the cause of serum thyroxine-binding globulin excess. J Clin Endocrinol Metab 66:1037–1043, 1988.
16. Chetkowski RJ, Meldrum DR, Steingold KA, et al: Biologic effects of transdermal estradiol. N Engl J Med 314:1615–1620, 1986.
17. Konno N, Kakinoki K, Hagiwara K: Serum concentrations of unsaturated thyroxine-binding globulin in hyper- and hypothyroidism. Clin Endocrinol 22:249–255, 1985.
18. Glinoer D, McGuire R, Dubois A, et al: Thyroxine-binding globulin metabolism in Rhesus monkeys: Effects of hyper- and hypothyroidism. Endocrinology 104:175–183, 1979.
19. Oppenheimer J, Werner S: Effect of prednisone on thyroxine-binding proteins. J Clin Endocrinol Metab 26:715–721, 1966.
20. Rouaze-Romet M, Savu L, Vranckx R, et al: Re-expression of thyroxine-binding globulin in post-weaning rats during protein or energy malnutrition. Acta Endocrinol 127:441–448, 1992.
21. Emerson CH, Seiler CM, Alex S, et al: Gene expression and serum thyroxine-binding globulin are regulated by adrenal status and corticosterone in the rat. Endocrinology 133:1192–1196, 1993.
22. Arafah BM: Decreased levothyroxine requirement in women with hypothyroidism during androgen therapy for breast cancer. Ann Intern Med 121:247, 1994.
23. Man EB, Reid WA, Hellegers AE: Thyroid function in human pregnancy. III. Serum thyroxine binding prealbumin (TBPA) and thyroxine-binding globulin (TBG) of pregnant women. Am J Obstet Gynecol 103:338–347, 1969.
24. Maye P, Bisetti A, Burger A, et al: Hyperprealbuminemia, euthyroid hyperthyroxinemia, Zollinger-Ellison–like syndrome and hypercorticism in a pancreatic endocrine tumour. Acta Endocrinol 120:87–91, 1989.
25. Munro SL, Lim C-F, Hall JG, et al: Drug competition for thyroxine binding to transthyretin (prealbumin): Comparison with effects on thyroxine-binding globulin. J Clin Endocrinol Metab 68:1141–1147, 1989.
26. Lim C-F, Bai Y, Topliss DJ, et al: Drug and fatty acid effects on serum thyroid hormone binding. J Clin Endocrinol Metab 67:682–688, 1988.
27. Lim C-F, Stockigt JR, Curtis AJ, et al: Influence of a naturally-occurring furanoid acid on the potency of drug competitors for specific thyroxine binding in serum. Metabolism 42:1468–1474, 1993.
28. Surks MI, Defesi CR: Normal serum free thyroid hormone concentrations in patients treated with phenytoin or carbamazepine: A paradox resolved. JAMA 275:1495–1498, 1996.
29. Wang R, Nelson JC, Wilcox RB: Salsalate administration—a potential pharmacological model of the sick euthyroid syndrome. J Clin Endocrinol Metab 83:3095–3099, 1998.
30. Mendel CM, Frost PH, Cavalieri RR: Effect of free fatty acids on the concentration of free thyroxine in human serum: The role of albumin. J Clin Endocrinol Metab 63:1394–1399, 1986.
31. Stockigt JR, Lim C-F, Barlow JW, et al: High concentrations of furosemide inhibit plasma binding of thyroxine. J Clin Endocrinol Metab 59:62–66, 1984.
32. Hawkins RC: Furosemide interference in newer free thyroxine assays. Clin Chem 44:2550–2551, 1998.
33. Newnham HH, Hamblin PS, Long F, et al: Effect of oral furosemide on diagnostic indices of thyroid function. Clin Endocrinol (Oxf) 26:423–431, 1987.
34. Lueprasitsakul W, Alex S, Fang SL, et al: Flavonoid administration immediately displaces thyroxine (T_4) from serum transthyretin, increases serum free T_4 and decreases serum thyrotropin in the rat. Endocrinology 126:2890–2895, 1990.
35. Lim C-F, Curtis AJ, Barlow JW, et al: Interactions between oleic acid and drug competitors influence specific binding of thyroxine in serum. J Clin Endocrinol Metab 73:1106–1110, 1991.
36. Mendel CM, Frost PH, Kunitake ST, et al: Mechanism of the heparin-induced increase in the concentration of free thyroxine in plasma. J Clin Endocrinol Metab 65:1259–1264, 1987.
37. Zambon A, Hashimoto SI, Brunzell JD: Analysis of techniques to obtain plasma for measurement of levels of free fatty acids. J Lipid Res 34:1021–1028, 1993.
38. Crowe TC, Cowen NL, Loidl NM, et al: Down-regulation of thyroxine-binding globulin messenger ribonucleic acid by 3,5,3′-triiodothyronine in human hepatoblastoma cells. J Clin Endocrinol Metab 80:2233–2237, 1995.
39. Topliss DJ, Kolliniatis E, Barlow JW, et al: Uptake of T_3 cultured rat hepatoma cells is inhibitable by non–bile acid cholephils, diphenylhydantoin and non-steroidal anti-inflammatory drugs. Endocrinology 124:980–986, 1989.
40. Docter R, Friesema CH, Van Stralen PG, et al: Expression of rat liver cell membrane transporters for thyroid hormone in *Xenopus laevis* oocytes. Endocrinology 138:1841–1846, 1997.
41. Lim C-F, Docter E, Visser TJ, et al: Inhibition of thyroxine transport into cultured rat hepatocytes by serum of nonuremic critically ill patients: Effects of bilirubin and nonesterified fatty acids. J Clin Endocrinol Metab 76:1165–1172, 1993.
42. Lim C-F, Bernard BF, de Jong M, et al: A furan fatty acid and indoxyl sulfate are the putative inhibitors of thyroxine hepatocyte transport in uremia. J Clin Endocrinol Metab 76:318–324, 1993.
43. Cavalieri RR, Simeoni LA, Park SW, et al: Thyroid hormone export in rat FRTL-5 thyroid cells and mouse NIH-3T3 cells in carrier-mediated verapamil sensitive, and stereospecific. Endocrinology 140:4948–4954, 1999.
44. Barlow JW, Curtis AJ, Raggatt LE, et al: Drug competition for intracellular triiodothyronine-binding sites. Eur J Endocrinol 130:417–421, 1994.

Thyroid Hormone Metabolism

Donald L. St. Germain

Secretion of thyroxine (T_4) and triiodothyronine (T_3) from the thyroid gland provides an overall "set-point" for the activity of this hormonal axis. However, as in the case of other hormones, in particular, those from the adrenal cortex and gonads, mechanisms governing the cellular uptake and metabolism of thyroid hormones have an important influence on their plasma concentrations. These "prereceptor" processes are also critical determinants of the cellular level of T_3 available for binding to nuclear thyroid hormone receptors. The metabolic fate of thyroid hormones in peripheral tissues thus serves as an important control mechanism of thyroid hormone action.

The principal secretory product of the thyroid gland, T_4, undergoes a complex series of intracellular metabolic alterations in peripheral tissues, as shown in Figure 94–6. Some of these reactions, such as 5′-deiodination of T_4 to form T_3 or decarboxylation and deamination of T_3 to form the acetic acid analogue termed Triac, result in compounds with considerably greater intrinsic biopotency because of their increased affinity for thyroid hormone receptors.[1] Other reactions result in the formation of apparently inactive compounds, such as reverse T_3 (rT_3) formed by 5-deiodination of T_4 or the sulfated and glucuronidated forms of T_4 and T_3 formed by conjugation of the phenolic ring hydroxyl group.[2,3] Progressive deiodination of T_4, T_3, and rT_3 results in the formation of various diiodinated and monoiodinated thyronines and eventually thyronine (T_0) itself.[4] These compounds are generally believed to have little or no biologic activity. An exception to this generalization may be the compounds 3,5-diiodothyronine (3,5-T_2) and 3,3′-T_2, which have been demonstrated to have effects on mitochondrial function.[5,6]

The enzymatic processes shown in Figure 94–6 are not mutually exclusive. Indeed, modification of an iodothyronine molecule at one site may markedly alter its susceptibility to other metabolic reactions. For example, Tetrac and Triac are much better substrates for glucuronidation than are T_4 and T_3.[7] The acetic acid analogues and sulfated conjugates are also markedly better substrates for deiodination in the liver and kidney than are the native compounds.[8,9] In contrast, sulfation of iodothyronines in certain organs may effectively block further metabolism because these conjugates are poorly reactive with the deiodinase isoforms expressed in other tissues.[10,11]

HORMONE KINETICS AND PRODUCTION

Deiodination at either the 5′ or 5 position accounts for approximately 80% of the daily disposal of T_4, with the other processes shown in Figure 94–1 responsible for the remaining metabolism of this compound.[4] Such approximations may underestimate the role of both deiodinative and nondeiodinative pathways, however. Many of the products of these reactions, including T_3 and rT_3, are present primarily in the intracellular compartment and may undergo degradation before they have a chance to exchange with the plasma pool. It is thus difficult in human kinetic studies that use plasma sampling techniques alone to assess the contribution of these processes to overall thyroid hormone metabolism. For example, it has been demonstrated that most of the thyronine (T_0) excreted in the urine is in the form of its

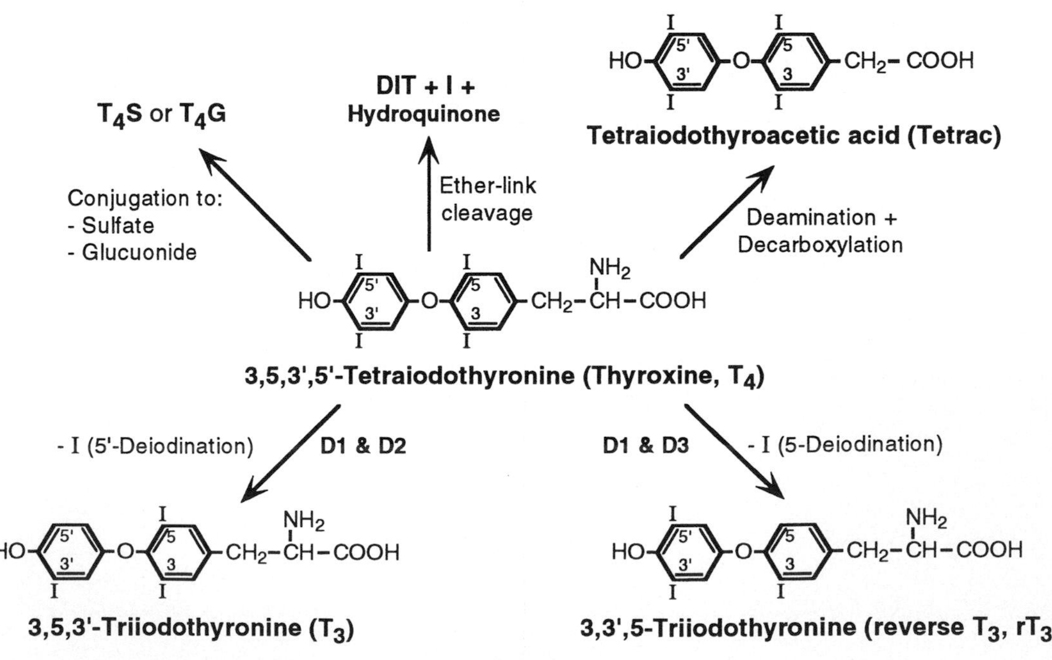

FIGURE 94–6. Graphic representation of the pathways of iodothyronine metabolism. The types 1 and 2 deiodinases (D1, D2) catalyze the removal of the 5′ (or chemically equivalent 3′) iodine from T_4 and other iodothyronine substrates. The types 1 and 3 enzymes catalyze 5 (or chemically equivalent 3) deiodination. A variety of less common reactions occur via alternative enzymatic pathways. The metabolites shown are subject to further deiodination to form diiodothyronines, monoiodothyronines, and tyrosine. (From St. Germain DL, Galton VA: The deiodinase family of selenoproteins. Thyroid 7:655–658, 1997.)

acetic acid analogue,[12] thus suggesting that deamination plays a more prominent role in thyroid hormone metabolism than is apparent from the very low circulating levels of Tetrac and Triac. Such concerns have led to the concept that "hidden pools" of thyroid hormone metabolites may be present in tissues.[13]

Table 94–4 provides estimates of various kinetic parameters of thyroid hormone production and metabolism in humans.[4, 17, 18] The high affinity of T_4 for plasma binding proteins, along with its greater production rate, accounts for its relatively high concentration in serum, as well as its long serum half-life. In contrast, T_3 and rT_3 are present at much lower serum concentrations because of their lower production rates, greater metabolic clearance rates, and lower affinity for TBG. In addition, these two triiodothyronines appear to reside primarily within the intracellular compartment, and thus their volumes of distribution are significantly greater than that of T_4.

The rate of T_4 production remains remarkably constant in healthy adults, with alterations noted only during pregnancy and in the aged. Although not well documented, increased T_4 secretion probably occurs during pregnancy in response to a number of factors, including thyroidal stimulation by human chorionic gonadotropin, an increase in the size of the extrathyroidal T_4 pool resulting from increased TBG levels, and an increase in the rate of T_4 and T_3 degradation because of high levels of 5-deiodinase activity in the placenta.[19] One clinical consequence is the need to increase the replacement dose of T_4 by 25% to 50% in hypothyroid women during pregnancy.[20] Although a slight decrease in T_4 production and clearance is noted after the age of 60 years,[21] the decreased T_4 requirements of elderly hypothyroid patients probably result more from the presence of chronic illness and the use of concurrent medications than from the aging process per se.[22]

DEIODINATION AND THE IODOTHYRONINE DEIODINASES

The potential importance of deiodination to thyroid hormone action was first recognized nearly 50 years ago when Gross and Pitt-Rivers demonstrated that although T_3 was considerably more potent than T_4,[23] it was present in the thyroid in much lower amounts.[24] This observation suggested that T_3 was largely derived from T_4 by metabolism in extrathyroidal tissues. This thesis was later proved by Braverman et al., who demonstrated the presence of T_3 in the serum of athyreotic subjects injected with T_4.[25] Research over the last two decades has confirmed the physiologic importance of the 5′- and 5-deiodination processes, defined the biochemical parameters of these enzymatic reactions, determined important regulatory factors that influence deiodinase activities, and identified key structural determinants of the proteins that catalyze these reactions.

To date, three deiodinase isoforms, termed D1, D2, and D3, have been identified and differ in their catalytic properties, patterns of tissue expression, and mechanisms of regulation.[26] Based on subcellular fractionation studies, the deiodinases appear to be located within the endoplasmic reticulum of the cell, with the exception of the D1 present in the kidney, which colocalizes with markers specific to the plasma membrane.[27] The 5′- and 5-deiodination reactions catalyzed by these enzymes can broadly be considered as activating and inactivating processes, respectively.

TABLE 94–4. Normal Thyroid Hormone Kinetics in Humans

Property	T_4	T_3	rT_3
Total serum concentration (μg/dL)*	8.1	0.11	0.012
Free serum concentration (ng/dL)	1.2	0.29	0.04
Distribution volume (L)	10	35	90
Metabolic clearance rate (L/day/70 kg)	1.2	24	111
Serum half-life (day)	7	1	0.2
Production or disposal rate (μg/day/70 kg)	100	31	39

*Conversion factors: T_4, 1 μg = 1.3 nmol; T_3 and rT_3, 1 μg = 1.5 nmol. rT_3, reverse triiodothyronine; T_4, thyroxine. Data from Chopra[14, 16] and Faber et al.[15]

Biochemical Characteristics

The biochemical properties of the deiodinases are outlined in Table 94–5. They are in essence reductases in that they catalyze the substitution of hydrogen for iodine on the iodothyronine substrate. No other catalytic properties of these enzymes have yet been identified, nor do other known enzymes possess deiodinase activity. The enzymes are remarkable in terms of their substrate specificity and the precise location of the iodine removed.[11] D1 is unique in that it can catalyze either 5′- or 5-deiodination, depending on the reacting substrate. Thus rT_3 is efficiently deiodinated only at the 5′ position. In contrast, T_4 and T_3 are poor substrates for D1 unless they are first sulfated. This reaction markedly enhances their rate of 5-deiodination and further reduces their susceptibility to 5′-deiodination.[32] That D1 is relatively inefficient in converting T_4 to T_3 presents a considerable paradox given that a significant proportion of T_3 production is believed to occur in the liver and other D1-expressing tissues.

D2 catalyzes only 5′-deiodination and very efficiently converts T_4 to T^3.[11] The T_3 thus formed is a poor substrate for 5′-deiodination and is not further metabolized by this enzyme. In contrast, rT_3 is a good substrate for D2 as well as D1 and is frequently used in research assays to quantitate 5′-deiodinase activity. D3 exclusively catalyzes 5-deiodination[11] and thus serves to convert T_4 and T_3 to rT_3 and 3,3′-T_2, respectively, metabolites with little known biologic activity.

The deiodinases all require the availability of reduced thiol cofactors for efficient catalytic cycling.[28] These cofactors presumably function to displace iodine from an enzyme intermediate formed during the reaction and thus to regenerate the active deiodinase.[33] In in vitro assay systems using tissue homogenates or cellular subfractions, dithiothreitol is typically added as cofactor. This small, nonnative four-carbon dithiol efficiently supports deiodination of all three enzymes. Kinetic data derived from broken cell preparations with dithiothreitol used as cofactor has demonstrated Michaelis-Menten constant (K_m) values for D1 of approximately 2.3 μmol/L (for T_4 5′-deiodination), whereas D2 and D3 manifest much lower values in the nanomolar range.[26] Based on this analysis, D1 is sometimes referred to as a "high K_m" enzyme whereas D2 is said to catalyze a "low K_m" process. This distinction is spurious, however, because the kinetic properties of the deiodinases are clearly dependent on the cofactors used in the assay system.[34] Thus when using the native thiol cofactors glutathione or thioredoxin, K_m values for D1 in the nanomolar range are obtained. Unfortunately, the cofactor system(s) supporting deiodination in intact cells remains unknown, and recent evidence suggests that glutathione and thioredoxin may not serve this role.[35] Thus the physiologic significance of the kinetic parameters derived in vitro remains uncertain.

Inhibitors

In addition to differences in their catalytic properties, the deiodinases also show differential susceptibility to certain inhibitors[28] (see Table 94–5). Most notable is the marked sensitivity of D1 to the antithyroid drug propylthiouracil (PTU). This agent forms an inactive complex with D1 by binding covalently to its active site. Notably, D2 and D3 show little or no susceptibility to inhibition by PTU. A related thioureylene drug, methimazole, has very little inhibitory effect on deiodination.[33]

Gold compounds such as aurothioglucose are known to react with the active-site selenocysteine residue in glutathione peroxidase and impair its activity.[36] This compound also inhibits all three deiodinase isoforms, with D1 again showing a significantly greater sensitivity to this effect.[37–39] The structural differences between the deiodinases that govern their differential susceptibility to inhibition by these various compounds remain uncertain.

Other drugs affecting thyroid hormone metabolism include the iodinated radiographic contrast agents iopanoic acid (Telepaque) and sodium ipodate (Oragrafin). These small phenolic compounds act as substrate analogues and inhibit all three deiodinases in a competitive manner. To date, no selective inhibitors of D2 or D3 have been described, a situation that has significantly limited experimental investigations into the physiologic roles of these enzymes.

TABLE 94–5. Characteristics of Iodothyronine Deiodinases

Characteristic	D1	D2	D3
Reaction catalyzed	5′ or 5	5′	5
Substrate preference	5′:$rT_3 > T_3S > T_4$ 5:$T_4S > T_3S$	$T_4 > rT_3$	$T_3 > T_4$
K_m (DTT as cofactor)	rT_3 (5′):0.06 μmol/L T_4 (5′):2.3 μmol/L T_4S (5):0.3 μmol/L	T_4 (5′):1 nmol/L	T_3 (5):6 nmol/L T_4 (5):37 nmol/L
Inhibitors			
PTU	++++	+	+/−
Aurothioglucose	++++	++	++
Iopanoic acid	+++	++++	+++
Location	Liver, kidney, thyroid, pituitary	Pituitary, brain, brown fat, thyroid,* heart,* skeletal muscle*	Brain, skin, uterus, placenta, fetus
Selenocysteine	Present	Present	Present
Molecular mass (kDa)	29	30	32
Chromosome location (human)	1p32-p33	14q24.3	14q32
Activity in hypothyroidism	↓ (Liver, kidney) ↑ (Thyroid)	↑ (All tissues)	↓ (Brain)

*Human only. DTT, dithiothreitol; PTU, propylthiouracil; rT_3, reverse triiodothyronine; T_3S, triiodothyronine sulfate; T_4, thyroxine. Data from St. Germain and Galton,[26] Leonard and Visser,[28] Jakobs et al.,[29] Celi et al.,[30] and Hernández et al.[31]

Tissue Patterns of Expression

An intriguing feature of the deiodinases is their pattern of tissue expression (see Table 94–5). The liver, kidney, thyroid gland, and pituitary gland express high levels of D1, with lesser amounts found in the brain.[11, 40, 41] In contrast, D2 is most abundant in the pituitary gland and brown adipose tissue of rodents, with significant amounts also noted in the central nervous system.[11] Recent studies using in situ hybridization on rat brain sections have demonstrated that D2 expression appears to be confined to certain subpopulations of astroglial cells, which suggests that they serve as the principal site of T_3 production in this tissue.[42, 43] In humans, D2 expression appears more widespread; the mRNA for this enzyme has been noted in the heart, skeletal muscle, and thyroid gland.[39, 44]

In adult mammals, D3 expression occurs primarily in the brain, with significant amounts also present in the skin.[45, 46] The brain is thus the only tissue that expresses all three deiodinases, with their presence suggesting that thyroid hormone metabolism in this tissue is exceedingly complex and perhaps designed to maintain strict control over cellular thyroid hormone levels. Experimental evidence in animal model systems indicates that such is indeed the case.

Finally, as detailed below, a remarkably different pattern of deiodinase expression occurs during development, with high levels of D3 activity being present in the uterus, placenta, and several fetal tissues.[47, 48]

Structural and Genetic Characteristics

Important structural features of the deiodinases have been deduced from the results of molecular cloning experiments.[26] All the enzymes have a molecular mass of approximately 29 to 32 kDa, and all are selenoproteins in that they contain the uncommon amino acid selenocysteine as the reactive residue in the catalytic cleft (Fig. 94–7). The importance of this amino acid to enzymatic activity is demonstrated by experiments in which selenocysteine has been replaced by cysteine. Such a substitution decreases the catalytic efficiency of the mutant protein to less than 1% of that of the native enzyme.[49] This result probably derives from the fact that selenocysteine is ionized at physiologic pH and is thus a much more potent nucleophile than cysteine.[50] Incorporation of selenocysteine into the deiodinases and selenoproteins occurs at the time of translation and is directed by a specific element in the 3′ untranslated region of the mRNA termed a selenocysteine insertion sequence.[50] Each of the deiodinases also contains a hydrophobic transmembrane region near the N terminus[51] (Fig. 94–8). Although overall amino acid identity between the three isoforms is less than 30%, a high degree of homology is noted in the region of the selenocysteine and a conserved histidine residue.

SELENOCYSTEINE: $H_2N—C(H)(CH_2Se^-)—COOH$, pI = 5.5

CYSTEINE: $H_2N—C(H)(CH_2SH)—COOH$, pI = 8.3

FIGURE 94–7. Comparison of the structures of selenocysteine and cysteine. Selenocysteine is ionized at physiologic pH, which may contribute to the catalytic efficiencies of the deiodinases.

The three deiodinase isoforms are coded in mammals by three different genes located on chromosomes 1 (D1) and 14 (D2 and D3).[29–31] Their gene structure is relatively simple in that they contain four, two, and a single exon, respectively. To date, genetic defects resulting in altered deiodinase activity have not been described in humans, although a mouse model of impaired D1 activity has been described.[52, 53] Remarkably, this defect has little effect on overall thyroid hormone homeostasis; although circulating T_4 levels are elevated, T_3 and thyroid-stimulating hormone (TSH) levels are unaltered, which implies that D1 deficiency impairs both T_3 production and degradation.

Regulation

The deiodinases are regulated by multiple hormones, growth factors, and environmental and nutritional factors.[26] Foremost among these

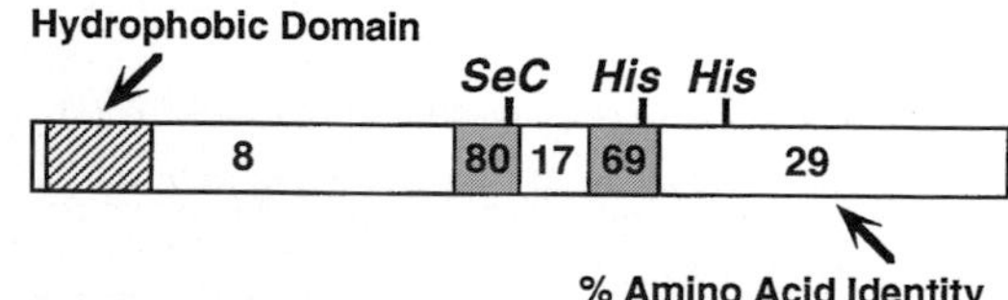

FIGURE 94–8. Structural features of the deiodinase proteins. The proteins are composed of 257 to 278 amino acids with predicted molecular masses of 29 to 32 kDa. The hydrophobic domain near the amino terminus, the selenocysteine residue (SeC), and two histidines (His) essential for catalytic activity are conserved in all three isoforms. The percentage of amino acid identity between the three isoforms in different portions of the molecule is given. A high degree of homology is noted in the regions surrounding the selenocysteine and one of the histidines. (Adapted from St. Germain DL, Galton VA: The deiodinase family of selenoproteins. Thyroid 7:655–658, 1997.)

factors are the thyroid hormones themselves; alterations in thyroid status induce profound changes in enzyme activity (see Table 94–5). Hypothyroidism is associated with a marked decrease in D1 and D3 levels, whereas D2 activity increases severalfold. Opposite changes occur in hyperthyroidism. These changes result from both pretranslational and posttranslational mechanisms.[26] For example, D1 and D3 mRNA levels are increased in the hyperthyroid state,[38, 54] and D2 mRNA is decreased.[39] Hyperthyroidism also results in rapid inactivation of D2 by mechanisms that may involve cellular trafficking or proteolytic degradation.[55, 56]

Other important regulatory effects on deiodinase activity are noted in the thyroid gland, where TSH and thyroid-stimulating immunoglobulins stimulate both D1 and D2 activity[44]; in brown adipose tissue, where cold exposure markedly stimulates D2 activity[57]; and in the liver, where nutritional deprivation and diabetes decrease D1 activity.[54] In addition, D2 activity in the brain and other tissues of experimental animals displays a significant diurnal variation, the physiologic significance of which remains to be determined.[58]

ALTERNATIVE ROUTES OF IODOTHYRONINE METABOLISM

Conjugation of the phenolic ring hydroxyl group to sulfate or glucuronide probably represents the second most prevalent mechanism of thyroid hormone metabolism.[11] Sulfation and glucuronidation are inactivating reactions because the compounds formed are devoid of thyromimetic activity, do not bind to nuclear thyroid hormone receptors, and are rapidly metabolized by D1 or excreted in bile.[3, 11] However, sulfation is a reversible process through the action of tissue sulfatases or bacterial sulfatases in the intestine.[59] Thus T_3 sulfate (T_3S) injected into hypothyroid rats demonstrates approximately 20% of the thyromimetic activity of native T_3 because of liberation of this active hormone.[60]

Sulfotransferases in the cytoplasm of many tissues serve to catalyze the formation of iodothyronine sulfate conjugates. In rat tissue homogenates, 3,3′-T_2 and T_3 appear to be the best substrates for sulfation.[32] Although the exact enzymes mediating iodothyronine sulfation are uncertain, the phenol sulfotransferases found in human liver and kidney have been demonstrated in vitro to possess this activity.[61] Sensitive and specific radioimmunoassays for various iodothyronine sulfates have been developed and used to demonstrate detectable, but very low levels of T_3S, $rT3S$, and T_4S in normal human serum.[32] These low circulating levels probably reflect the rapid metabolism of these compounds by D1 in tissues such as the liver. Evidence for this thesis comes from experiments in animals and humans, where treatment with inhibitors of D1 activity, such as PTU or iopanoic acid, results in marked increases in iodothyronine sulfoconjugate levels in both serum and bile.[62, 63] In other circumstances where D1 activity is low or impaired, such as during fetal life, in hypothyroidism, or in nonthyroidal illness, serum levels of these compounds are also elevated, either in absolute terms or relative to the native, unconjugated iodothyronines.[11] To date, the physiologic role of sulfation in thyroid hormone economy has not been clearly defined, although it appears to represent an important component of the degradative process.

Glucuronidation of iodothyronines followed by their secretion into bile represents another pathway of iodothyronine clearance. Studies in humans, however, suggest that this pathway accounts for less than 1% of the total clearance of T_4 by the liver and only minute amounts of these conjugates are present in plasma.[4, 64]

Two enzymes, L-amino acid oxidase and thyroid hormone aminotransferase, have been implicated in catalyzing the deamination of T_4 and T_3 to their acetic acid analogues Tetrac and Triac, respectively.[65] Current evidence suggests, however, that these reactions occur to only a limited extent in normal humans. Triac has intrinsic biologic activity equivalent to that of T_3 when tested in in vitro assay systems,[65] and it binds with greater avidity than T_3 to the β isoform of the thyroid hormone receptor.[1] Injection of Triac into humans or animals results in significant physiologic effects; however, relatively large doses are required because of its apparent rapid clearance and degradation via deiodination and glucuronidation.[66] Despite its short half-life, Triac has been used successfully in the treatment of thyroid hormone resistance states.[1] As in the case of sulfated conjugates, levels of Triac and its conjugates increase in circumstances in which D1 activity is low or impaired, such as fasting or treatment with PTU or iopanoic acid.[65] The physiologic relevance of these observations is uncertain but could be important given Triac's significant intrinsic activity.

A final mechanism of thyroid hormone metabolism involves oxidative cleavage of the ether link of T_4 and T_3 by phagocytosing leukocytes.[67] Current evidence suggests that this pathway is a minor one for iodothyronine degradation, except in the special circumstances of severe bacterial infection.

AN INTEGRATED VIEW OF THYROID HORMONE METABOLISM

The preceding discussion has served to highlight the extraordinary complexity of thyroid hormone metabolism. Two critical features of this intricate system are apparent. First, the metabolic fate of iodothyronines varies significantly in different organs, thus providing a mechanism whereby thyroid hormone content and action can be individualized from tissue to tissue. Second, these metabolic processes, and in particular the rates of deiodination, are regulated by a number of factors, which suggests that alterations in thyroid hormone metabolism may be important in adapting to internal or external homeostatic challenges.

Altered Thyroid States

Several examples of these principles can be cited, starting first with the response to alterations in thyroid hormone status. Experimental studies, as well as clinical experience, indicate that serum T_3 levels tend to be maintained within the normal range in patients with moderate degrees of hypothyroidism despite the attendant hypothyroxinemia.[68, 69] Several factors appear to be responsible for this finding, including an increase in the relative proportion of T_3 secreted from the thyroid gland and an increase in the proportion of T_4 converted to T_3 in extrathyroidal tissue[70] (Fig. 94–9). Both these effects result from increased rates of 5′-deiodination. Thus in the thyroid gland, D1 and D2 activity is stimulated by the increase in TSH that accompanies

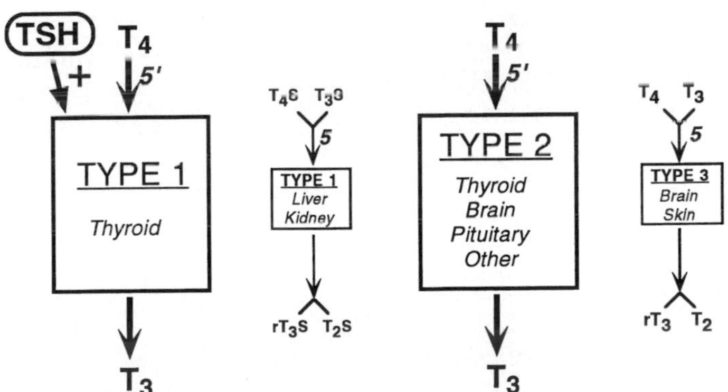

FIGURE 94–9. Autoregulation of thyroid hormone metabolism that accompanies the hypothyroid state, as might occur in iodine deficiency. D1 activity in the thyroid is stimulated by TSH. Although this enzyme is relatively inefficient in converting T_4 to T_3, in the high T_4 environment of the thyroid gland, this may serve to increase the proportion of T_3 formed and secreted by this organ. Concurrently, D1 activity in extrathyroidal tissues is reduced, thereby decreasing the degradation of T_4 and T_3 by the 5-deiodination of their sulfated analogues. D2 activity is increased in all tissues that express this enzyme, which increases the proportion of T_4 to T_3 conversion in both the thyroid and peripheral tissues. Finally, D3 activity is decreased, again serving to diminish T_4 and T_3 degradation by 5-deiodinase processes. The net effect of these changes is to increase the relative rate of T_3 production and decrease T_3 degradation, thereby preserving the circulating and tissue levels of this active hormone in the presence of a diminished supply of T_4.

hypothyroidism.[44] In peripheral tissues, D2 expression is also markedly enhanced.[39] As a result, T_4 is used more efficiently for T_3 production. In addition, the rate of T_3 clearance in extrathyroidal tissues is decreased. This decrease probably results in part from diminished 5-deiodination caused by the decreases in D1 and D3 activity that have been observed in the hypothyroid state. The physiologic importance of these extrathyroidal mechanisms, which in essence act as a form of peripheral autoregulation to help maintain T_3 levels, is easily demonstrated by the administration of varying doses of T_4 to athyreotic individuals. Under such circumstances the circulating T_3/T_4 ratio is highest when low doses of T_4 are given, and the ratio progressively declines as full replacement and then supraphysiologic doses are provided.[68, 69] Alterations in the rates of nondeiodinative pathways may also contribute to this response. The net effect of these metabolic adaptations is to minimize alterations in the circulating T_3 level in the face of either impaired or increased activity of the thyroid gland.

The increases and decreases in D2 activity observed in hypothyroidism and hyperthyroidism, respectively, have an important additional effect. In organs expressing this enzyme, these alterations in activity provide a local mechanism for the maintenance of T_3 concentrations at the cellular level in these tissues. Thus in the hypothyroid rat infused with increasing doses of T_4, normalization of the T_3 content of D2-expressing tissues, such as the cerebral cortex, cerebellum, and brown adipose tissue, is attained at much lower infusion rates than that required by other tissues.[71] This may provide an additional level of autoregulation in tissues where thyroid hormone effects are especially critical.

Development

Thyroid hormones are of unquestioned importance to the developing fetus both in utero and during the immediate neonatal period; hypothyroidism during this period can result in the clinical syndrome of cretinism characterized by severe neurologic impairment.[72] However, throughout most of gestation, circulating levels of T_4 and T_3 in the mammalian fetus are extremely low,[73] perhaps to protect tissues from the premature differentiating effects of these agents. Isolation of the fetus from maternal circulating and tissue thyroid hormones thus appears to be critical for normal development. Such isolation is accomplished by expression in the uterus[74] and the placenta[48] of exceedingly high levels of D3 activity. Certain fetal tissues also express this enzyme early in gestation.[47] During the later stages of gestation and after fetal thyroid function has been initiated, expression of 5′-deiodinases becomes more prevalent and fetal T_3 levels increase. Of potential importance, the high levels of D3 in the placenta do not result in a complete barrier to the transfer of maternal thyroid hormones to the fetus, as evidenced by the finding of significant levels of T_4 and T_3 at term in the serum of athyreotic infants.[75]

An important aspect of thyroid hormone metabolism during development relates to the very high levels of sulfated iodothyronines that circulate in the fetus, most likely as a result of the low D1 levels present during development and the fact that these metabolites are not efficiently degraded by D3.[76] This observation has led to speculation that fetal T_3S could serve as a reservoir of T_3 that becomes available later in pregnancy through the actions of tissue sulfatases.[77]

Fasting and Illness

Profound changes occur in thyroid hormone economy during states of acute illness and fasting, as detailed elsewhere in this volume (Chapter 109). Kinetic studies performed in humans have demonstrated marked decreases in plasma T_3 disposal rates under such circumstances, which has been interpreted to indicate that T_3 production and hence conversion of T_4 to T_3 are also significantly reduced in nonthyroidal illness.[78] Such a suggestion is consistent with in vitro studies in experimental animals, which have shown decreased D1 activity in the liver and kidney of starved rats or those with diabetes.[54] However, a recent report wherein whole body thyroid hormone pool sizes and interconversion rates were determined directly from whole body tissue measurements in fasted rats casts doubt on these concepts.[79] Although in this study the plasma T_3 disposal rate was diminished by fasting, consistent with prior reports, directly measured T_3 production was unchanged and the fraction of T_4 converted to T_3 was approximately doubled. It thus appears, as suggested by the authors, that much of the T_3 produced during fasting remains in the tissues, where it may be metabolized via other pathways, and is not exchanged with the plasma T_3 pool. Such results serve to highlight the methodologic shortcomings inherent in kinetic studies of thyroid hormone metabolism in humans where sampling is limited to the plasma compartment. Caution should also be exercised in inferring in vivo rates of deiodination from deiodinase activities determined in tissue homogenates.

Effects of Selenium

Nutritional selenium deprivation in experimental animals leads to characteristic changes in deiodinase activities and serum thyroid hormone levels.[26] The most profound changes are noted in the liver and kidney, where marked decreases in D1 activity are noted secondary to impaired translation of this and other selenoproteins.[80] In tissues where selenium levels are better preserved, such as the thyroid gland and brain, deiodinase activities are altered to a lesser extent or not at all.[81, 82] Thus the changes in serum thyroid hormone levels in selenium deficiency resemble those observed in other model systems where D1 activity is impaired; namely, T_4 is increased and little change occurs in T_3 or TSH.[83] Similar observations in circulating hormone levels have been noted in human populations susceptible to selenium deficiency.[84, 85] In these circumstances, dietary selenium supplementation results in small, but significant decreases in serum T_4 levels and increases in the T_3/T_4 ratio, thus suggesting restoration of D1 activity. The clinical consequences of these changes have not been determined.

Of note are reported cases of worsening hypothyroidism developing in individuals with combined selenium and iodine deficiency who were given selenium supplements alone.[86] It is postulated that under such circumstances, restoration of D1 activity enhances T_4 metabolism and thereby worsens the iodine-induced hypothyroxinemic state. Thus concurrent iodine and selenium supplementation is required to restore thyroid hormone economy in this situation.

Drug Effects

Numerous drugs are known to affect the metabolism of thyroid hormones either by directly interfering with enzymatic mechanisms or by altering the regulation of these processes. The effect of PTU in inhibiting D1 activity provides it with a theoretic advantage over methimazole and carbimazole for use in the treatment of hyperthyroidism. In this condition, the increased expression of D1, combined with elevations in T_4 levels, probably contributes to the overproduction of T_3 in both the thyroid gland and peripheral tissues. However, this effect of PTU is noted only with relatively high doses of the drug (>1000 mg/day). At the usual doses prescribed for treating hyperthyroidism, methimazole (10 mg three times daily) actually results in more rapid restoration of the euthyroid state than does PTU (100 mg three times daily).[87]

As noted previously, oral radiographic contrast dyes are potent competitive inhibitors of all three deiodinase isoforms. Although they are now rarely used in clinical medicine as diagnostic agents, the rapidity with which they lower circulating T_3 levels makes them extremely useful in the treatment of severe hyperthyroidism. For example, treatment of patients with Graves' disease with sodium ipodate (1 g daily per os) has been noted to lower serum T_3 levels by 58% within 24 hours of initiating therapy, a decrease that is much greater than that noted with PTU (200 mg three times daily)[88] or a saturated solution of potassium iodide (12 drops SSKI daily).[89] Of importance, these decreases in serum T_3 levels are associated with rapid improvement in cardiovascular complications, with beneficial effects on systemic resistance and cardiac output noted within 3 to 6 hours after initiating treatment.[90] However, because of the high iodine content of these dyes, escape from their T_3-lowering effects and exacerbation of hyperthyroidism may occur after several days of therapy.[89] It is thus important that PTU or methimazole be administered concurrently to impair thyroidal secretion and that use of the contrast agent be discontinued when the thyrotoxicosis has been adequately controlled.

Propranolol, in relatively modest doses (80 mg/day), also blocks the conversion of T_4 to T_3 by acting as a competitive inhibitor of 5′-deiodinase activity.[91] This drug therefore results in hyperthyroid patients in a 20% to 30% decrease in serum T_3 levels and a slight elevation in serum T_4. Other commonly used β-blockers do not share this effect.

High doses of glucocorticoids (e.g., 2 mg of dexamethasone four times daily) have also been demonstrated to lower T_3 levels within 24 hours in hyperthyroid patients with Graves' disease,[92] as well as in euthyroid individuals.[18] This activity provides part of the rationale for the use of these agents in severe thyrotoxicosis. Animal studies have demonstrated that this effect is due, at least in part, to diminished total body production of T_3, and indeed, decreased D1 activity in the liver of dexamethasone-treated rats has been observed.[93]

Finally, the antiarrhythmic agent amiodarone is another iodine-rich compound that competitively inhibits the conversion of T_4 to T_3 and thus frequently causes a rise in serum T_4 levels and a modest decrease in serum T_3.[94] Although most patients taking this drug remain euthyroid as judged by normal serum TSH levels, the large quantities of iodine liberated during the course of its metabolism can result in either hypothyroid or hyperthyroid states, with the latter at times being extremely difficult to treat.

SUMMARY

The extrathyroidal systems mediating thyroid hormone metabolism work in concert with the hypothalamic-pituitary-thyroid axis to regulate the availability of thyroid hormones in peripheral tissues. The presence and activity of these metabolic pathways differ significantly between tissues, thus allowing for the T_3 content to vary from organ to organ. These prereceptor processes appear to function in an autoregulatory fashion and thus serve as adaptive mechanisms to help maintain T_3 homeostasis in response to environmental and internal stress. Knowledge of these pathways is important for understanding the changes in thyroid hormone levels that accompany a variety of thyroi dal and nonthyroidal diseases, as well as for optimizing therapy for hypothyroidism and hyperthyroidism. Further studies will probably provide additional insight into the physiologic role and biochemistry of the deiodinase isoforms, as well as a better appreciation of the importance of alternative pathways of thyroid hormone metabolism.

REFERENCES

1. Takeda T, Suzuki S, Liu RT, et al: Triiodothyroacetic acid has unique potential for therapy of resistance to thyroid hormone. J Clin Endocrinol Metab 80:2033–2040, 1995.
2. Pittman HA, Brown RW, Register HBJ: Biological activity of 3,3′,5′-triiodo-DL-thyronine. Endocrinology 70:79–83, 1962.
3. Spaulding SW, Smith TJ, Hinkle PM, et al: Studies on the biological activity of triiodothyronine sulfate. J Clin Endocrinol Metab 74:1062–1067, 1992.
4. Engler D, Burger AG: The deiodination of the iodothyronines and their derivatives in man. Endocr Rev 5:151–184, 1984.
5. Lanni A, Moreno M, Lombardi A, et al: Rapid stimulation in vitro of rat liver cytochrome oxidase activity by 3,5-diiodo-L-thyronine and by 3,3′-diiodo-L-thyronine. Mol Cell Endocrinol 99:89–94, 1994.
6. Lombardi A, Lanni A, Moreno M, et al: Effect of 3,5-di-iodo-L-thyronine on the mitochondrial energy-transduction apparatus. Biochem J 330:521–526, 1998.
7. Moreno M, Kaptein E, Goglia F, et al: Rapid glucuronidation of tri- and tetraiodothyroacetic acid to ester glucuronides in human liver and to ether glucuronides in rat liver. Endocrinology 135:1004–1005, 1994.
8. Sorimachi K, Yasumura Y: High affinity of triiodothyronine (T3) for nonphenolic ring deiodinase and high affinity of tetraiodothyroacetic acid (TETRAC) for phenolic ring deiodinase in cultured monkey hepatocarcinoma cells and in rat liver homogenates. Endocrinol Jpn 28:775–783, 1981.
9. Rutgers M, Heusdens FA, Visser TJ: Metabolism of triiodothyroacetic acid (TA_3) in rat liver. I. Deiodination of TA_3 and TA_3 sulfate by microsomes. Endocrinology 125:424–432, 1989.
10. Santini F, Hurd RE, Chopra IJ: A study of metabolism of deaminated and sulfoconjugated iodothyronines by rat placental iodothyronine 5-monodeiodinase. Endocrinology 131:1689–1694, 1992.
11. Visser TJ: Pathways of thyroid hormone metabolism. Acta Med Aust 23:10–16, 1996.
12. Chopra IJ, Boado RJ, Geffner DL, et al: A radioimmunoassay for measurement of thyronine and its acetic acid analog in urine. J Clin Endocrinol Metab 67:480–487, 1988.
13. LoPresti JS, Anderson KP, Nicoloff JT: Does a hidden pool of reverse triiodothyronine (rT3) production contribute to total thyroxine (T4) disposal in high T4 states in man? J Clin Endocrinol Metab 70:1479–1484, 1990.
14. Chopra IJ: Nature, sources, and relative biologic significance of circulating thyroid hormones. *In* Braverman LE, Utiger RD (eds): The Thyroid. New York, JB Lippincott, 1991, pp 126–143.
15. Faber J, Rogowski P, Kirkegaard C, et al: Serum free T4, T3, rT3, 3,3′-diiodothyronine and 3′,5′-diiodothyronine measured by ultrafiltration. Acta Endocrinol 107:357–365, 1984.
16. Chopra IJ: Simultaneous measurement of free thyroxine and free 3,5,3′-triiodothyronine in undiluted serum by direct equilibrium dialysis/radioimmunoassay: Evidence that free triiodothyronine and free thyroxine are normal in many patients with the low triiodothyronine syndrome. Thyroid 8:249–257, 1998.
17. Nicoloff JT, Low JC, Dussault JH, et al: Simultaneous measurements of thyroxine and triiodothyronine peripheral turnover kinetics in man. J Clin Invest 51:473–483, 1972.
18. LoPresti JS, Eigen A, Kaptein E, et al: Alterations in 3,3′,5′-triiodothyronine metabolism in response to propylthiouracil, dexamethasone, and thyroxine administration in man. J Clin Invest 84:1650–1656, 1989.
19. Glinoer D: The regulation of thyroid function in pregnancy: Pathways of endocrine adaptation from physiology to pathology. Endocr Rev 18:404–433, 1997.
20. Mandel SJ, Larsen PR, Seely EW, et al: Increased need for thyroxine during pregnancy in women with primary hypothyroidism. N Engl J Med 323:91–96, 1990.
21. Gregerman RI, Goffney GW, Schck NW: Thyroxine turnover in euthyroid man with special reference to changes with age. J Clin Invest 41:2065–2074, 1962.
22. Kabadi UM: Variability of L-thyroxine replacement dose in elderly patients with primary hypothyroidism. J Fam Pract 24:473–477, 1987.
23. Gross J, Pitt-Rivers R: 3:5:3′-triiodothyronine. 2. Physiological activity. Biochem J 53:652–656, 1953.
24. Gross J, Pitt-Rivers R: 3:5:3′-triiodothyronine. 1. Isolation from thyroid gland and synthesis. Biochem J 53:645–652, 1953.
25. Braverman LE, Ingbar SH, Sterling K: Conversion of thyroxine to triiodothyronine in athyreotic human subjects. J Clin Invest 49:855–864, 1970.
26. St Germain DL, Galton VA: The deiodinase family of selenoproteins. Thyroid 7:655–668, 1997.
27. Leonard JL, Rosenberg IN: Subcellular distribution of thyroxine 5′-deiodinase in the rat kidney: A plasma membrane location. Endocrinology 103:374–380, 1978.
28. Leonard JL, Visser TJ: Biochemistry of deiodination. *In* Hennemann G (ed): Thyroid Hormone Metabolism. New York, Marcel Dekker, 1986, pp 189–229.
29. Jakobs TC, Koehler MR, Schmutzler C, et al: Structure of the human type I iodothyronine 5′-deiodinase gene and location to chromosome 1p32-p33. Genomics 42:361–363, 1997.
30. Celi FS, Canettieri G, Yarnell DP, et al: Genomic characterization of the coding region of the human type II 5′-deiodinase. Mol Cell Endocrinol 141:49–52, 1998.
31. Hernández A, Park J, Lyon GJ, et al: Localization of the type 3 iodothyronine deiodinase (DIO3) gene to human chromosome 14q32 and mouse chromosome 12F1. Genomics 53:119–121, 1998.
32. Visser TJ: Role of sulfation in thyroid hormone metabolism. Chem Biol Interact 92:293–303, 1994.
33. Visser TJ: Mechanism of inhibition of iodothyronine-5′-deiodinase by thioureylenes and sulfite. Biochim Biophys Acta 611:371–378, 1980.
34. Sharifi J, St Germain DL: The cDNA for the type I iodothyronine 5′-deiodinase encodes an enzyme manifesting both high K_m and low K_m activity. J Biol Chem 267:12539–12544, 1992.
35. Croteau W, Bodwell JE, Richardson JM, et al: Conserved cysteines in the type 1 deiodinase selenoprotein are not essential for catalytic activity. J Biol Chem 273:25230–25236, 1998.
36. Chaudiere J, Tappel AL: Interaction of gold(I) with the active site of selenium-glutathione peroxidase. J Inorg Biochem 20:313–325, 1984.
37. Berry MJ, Kieffer JD, Harney JW, et al: Selenocysteine confers the biochemical properties characteristic of the type I iodothyronine deiodinase. J Biol Chem 266:14155–14158, 1991.
38. Croteau W, Whittemore SL, Schneider MJ, et al: Cloning and expression of a cDNA for a mammalian type III iodothyronine deiodinase. J Biol Chem 270:16569–16575, 1995.
39. Croteau W, Davey JC, Galton VA, et al: Cloning of the mammalian type II iodothyronine deiodinase: A selenoprotein differentially expressed and regulated in the human brain and other tissues. J Clin Invest 98:405–417, 1996.
40. Köhrle J, Schomburg L, Drescher S, et al: Rapid regulation of type I 5′-deiodinase in rat pituitaries by 3,3′,5-triiodo-L-thyronine. Mol Cell Endocrinol 109:17–21, 1995.
41. Visser TJ, Leonard JL, Kaplan MM, et al: Kinetic evidence suggesting two mechanisms for iodothyronine 5′-deiodination in rat cerebral cortex. Proc Natl Acad Sci U S A 79:5080–5084, 1982.
42. Guadaño-Ferraz A, Obregón MJ, St Germain DL, et al: The type 2 iodothyronine deiodinase is expressed primarily in glial cells in the neonatal rat brain. Proc Natl Acad Sci U S A 94:10391–10396, 1997.
43. Tu HM, Kim SW, Salvatore D, et al: Regional distribution of type 2 thyroxine deiodinase messenger ribonucleic acid in rat hypothalamus and pituitary and its regulation by thyroid hormone. Endocrinology 138:3359–3368, 1997.
44. Salvatore D, Tu H, Harney JW, et al: Type 2 iodothyronine deiodinase is highly expressed in human thyroid. J Clin Invest 98:962–968, 1996.
45. Kaplan MM, Yaskoski KA: Phenolic and tyrosyl ring deiodination of iodothyronines in rat brain homogenates. J Clin Invest 66:551–562, 1980.
46. Huang T, Chopra IJ, Beredo A, et al: Skin is an active site of inner ring monodeiodination of thyroxine to 3,3′,5′-triiodothyronine. Endocrinology 117:2106–2113, 1985.
47. Bates JM, St Germain DL, Galton VA: Expression profiles of the three iodothyronine deiodinases, D1, D2 and D3, in the developing rat. Endocrinology 140:844–851, 1999.

48. Roti E, Fang SL, Green K, et al: Human placenta is an active site of thyroxine and 3,3′,5-triiodothyronine tyrosyl ring deiodination. J Clin Endocrinol Metab 53:498–501, 1981.
49. Berry MJ, Maia AL, Kieffer JD, et al: Substitution of cysteine for selenocysteine in type I iodothyronine deiodinase reduces the catalytic efficiency of the protein but enhances its translation. Endocrinology 131:1848–1852, 1992.
50. Stadtman TC: Selenocysteine. Annu Rev Biochem 65:83–100, 1996.
51. Toyoda N, Berry MJ, Harney JW, et al: Topological analysis of the integral membrane protein, type 1 iodothyronine deiodinase (D1). J Biol Chem 270:12310–12318, 1995.
52. Berry MJ, Grieco D, Taylor B, et al: Physiological and genetic analysis of inbred mouse strains with a type I iodothyronine 5′ deiodinase deficiency. J Clin Invest 92:1517–1528, 1993.
53. Schoenmakers CHH, Pigmans IGAJ, Poland A, et al: Impairment of the selenoenzyme type I iodothyronine deiodinase in C3H/He mice. Endocrinology 132:357–361, 1993.
54. O'Mara BA, Dittrich W, Lauterio TJ, et al: Pretranslational regulation of type I 5′-deiodinase by thyroid hormones and in fasted and diabetic rats. Endocrinology 133:1715–1723, 1993.
55. Farwell AP, Safran M, Dubord S, et al: Degradation and recycling of the substrate-binding subunit of type II iodothyronine 5′-deiodinase in astrocytes. J Biol Chem 271:16369–16374, 1996.
56. Steinsapir J, Harney J, Larsen PR: Type 2 iodothyronine deiodinase in rat pituitary tumor cells is inactivated in proteasomes. J Clin Invest 102:1895–1899, 1998.
57. Silva JE, Larsen PR: Adrenergic activation of triiodothyronine production in brown adipose tissue. Nature 305:712–713, 1983.
58. Campos-Barros A, Musa A, Flechner A, et al: Evidence for circadian variations of thyroid hormone concentrations and type II 5′-iodothyronine deiodinase activity in the rat central nervous system. J Neurochem 68:795–803, 1997.
59. Kung MP, Spaulding SW, Roth JA: Desulfation of 3,5,3′-triiodothyronine sulfate by microsomes from human and rat tissues. Endocrinology 122:1195–1200, 1988.
60. Santini F, Hurd RE, Lee B, et al: Thyromimetic effects of 3,5,3′-triiodothyronine sulfate in hypothyroid rats. Endocrinology 133:105–110, 1993.
61. Anderson RJ: Biochemical characterization of triiodothyronine sulfotransferases. *In* Wu S-Y, Visser TJ (eds): Thyroid Hormone Metabolism. Boca Raton, FL, CRC, 1994, pp 155–174.
62. Chopra IJ, Wu SY, Teco GN, et al: A radioimmunoassay for measurement of 3,5,3′-triiodothyronine sulfate: Studies in thyroidal and nonthyroidal diseases, pregnancy, and neonatal life. J Clin Endocrinol Metab 75:189–194, 1992.
63. Eelkman Rooda SJ, Kaptein E, Rutgers M, et al: Increased plasma 3,5,3′-triiodothyronine sulfate in rats with inhibited type I iodothyronine deiodinase activity, as measured by radioimmunoassay. Endocrinology 124:740–745, 1989.
64. Van Middlesworth L: Metabolism and excretion of thyroid hormones. *In* Greer M, Solomon DH (ed): Handbook of Physiology: Endocrinology. Washington, DC, American Physiological Society, 1974, pp 215–231.
65. Siegrist-Kaiser CA, Burger AG: Modification of the side chain of thyroid hormones. *In* Wu S-Y, Visser TJ (eds): Thyroid Hormone Metabolism. Boca Raton, FL, CRC, 1994, pp 175–198.
66. Liang H, Juge-Aubry CE, O'Connell M, et al: Organ-specific effects of 3,5,3′-triiodothyroacetic acid in rats. Eur J Endocrinol 137:537–544, 1997.
67. Green WL: Ether-link cleavage of iodothyronines. *In* Wu S-Y, Visser TJ (eds): Thyroid Hormone Metabolism. Boca Raton, FL, CRC, 1994, pp 199–221.
68. Lum SM, Nicoloff JT, Spencer CA, et al: Peripheral tissue mechanism for maintenance of serum triiodothyronine values in a thyroxine-deficient state in man. J Clin Invest 73:570–575, 1984.
69. Keck FS, Loos U, Duntas L, et al: Evidence for peripheral autoregulation of thyroxine conversion. *In* Medeiros-Neto G, Gaitan E (eds): Frontiers in Thyroidology. New York, Plenum, 1986, pp 525–530.
70. Nicoloff JT, LoPresti JS: Alternate pathways of thyroid hormone metabolism. *In* Wu S-Y (ed): Thyroid Hormone Metabolism. Boston, Blackwell, 1991, pp 55–64.
71. Escobar-Morreale H, Obregn MJ, Escobar del Rey F, et al: Replacement therapy for hypothyroidism with thyroxine alone does not ensure euthyroidism in all tissues, as studied in thyroidectomized rats. J Clin Invest 96:2828–2838, 1995.
72. Porterfield SP, Hendrich CE: The role of thyroid hormones in prenatal and neonatal neurological development—current perspectives. Endocr Rev 14:94–106, 1993.
73. Burrow GN, Fisher DA, Larsen PR: Maternal and fetal thyroid function. N Engl J Med 331:1072–1078, 1994.
74. Galton VA, Martinez E, Hernandez A, et al: Pregnant rat uterus expresses high levels of the type 3 iodothyronine deiodinase. J Clin Invest 103:979–987, 1999.
75. Vulsma T, Gons MH, de Vijlder JJM: Maternal-fetal transfer of thyroxine in congenital hypothyroidism due to a total organification defect or thyroid agenesis. N Engl J Med 321:13–16, 1989.
76. Fisher DA, Polk DH, Wu SY: Fetal thyroid hormone metabolism. Thyroid 4:367–371, 1994.
77. Santini F, Chopra IJ, Wu S-Y, et al: Metabolism of 3,5,3′-triiodothyronine sulfate by tissues of the fetal rat: A consideration of the role of desulfation of 3,5,3′-triiodothyronine sulfate as a source of T3. Pediatr Res 31:541–544, 1992.
78. Kaptein EM, Robinson WJ, Grieb DA, et al: Peripheral serum thyroxine, triiodothyronine and reverse triiodothyronine kinetics in the low thyroxine state of acute nonthyroidal illnesses. A noncompartmental analysis. J Clin Invest 69:526–535, 1982.
79. Yen YM, Distefano J Jr, Yamada H, et al: Direct measurement of whole body thyroid hormone pool sizes and interconversion rates in fasted rats: Hormone regulation implications. Endocrinology 134:1700–1709, 1994.
80. DePalo D, Kinlaw WB, Zhao C, et al: Effect of selenium deficiency on type I 5′-deiodinase. J Biol Chem 269:16223–16228, 1994.
81. Chanoine J, Braverman LE, Farwell AP, et al: The thyroid gland is a major source of circulating T3 in the rat. J Clin Invest 91:2709–2713, 1993.
82. Meinhold H, Campos-Barros A, Walzog B, et al: Effects of selenium and iodine deficiency on type I, type II, and type III iodothyronine deiodinases and circulating thyroid hormones in the rat. Exp Clin Endocrinol 101:87–93, 1993.
83. Chanoine J, Safran M, Farwell AP, et al: Effects of selenium deficiency on thyroid hormone economy in rats. Endocrinology 131:1787–1792, 1992.
84. Olivieri O, Girelli D, Azzini M, et al: Low selenium status in the elderly influences thyroid hormones. Clin Sci 89:637–642, 1995.
85. Kauf E, Dawczynski H, Jahreis G, et al: Sodium selenite therapy and thyroid-hormone status in cystic fibrosis and congenital hypothyroidism. Biol Trace Elem Res 40:247–253, 1994.
86. Contempré B, Duale NL, Dumont JE, et al: Effect of selenium supplementation on thyroid hormone metabolism in an iodine and selenium deficient population. Clin Endocrinol 36:579–583, 1992.
87. Okamura K, Ikenoue H, Shiroozu A, et al: Reevaluation of the effects of methylmercaptoimidazole and propylthiouracil in patients with Graves' hyperthyroidism. J Clin Endocrinol Metab 65:719–723, 1987.
88. Wu S, Shyh T, Chopra IJ, et al: Comparison of sodium ipodate (Oragrafin) and propylthiouracil in early treatment of hyperthyroidism. J Clin Endocrinol Metab 54:630–634, 1982.
89. Roti E, Robuschi G, Manfredi A, et al: Comparative effects of sodium ipodate and iodide on serum thyroid hormone concentrations in patients with Graves' disease. Clin Endocrinol 22:489–496, 1985.
90. Seclen SN, Pretell EA, Tapia FA, et al: Rapid amelioration of severe cardiovascular complications of thyrotoxic patients with sodium ipodate. *In* Medeiros-Neto G, Gaitan E (eds): Frontiers in Thyroidology. New York, Plenum, 1986, pp 1101–1105.
91. Wiersinga WM: Propranolol and thyroid hormone metabolism. Thyroid 1:273–277, 1991.
92. Chopra IJ, Williams DE, Orgiazzi J, et al: Opposite effects of dexamethasone on serum concentrations of 3,3′,5′-triiodothyronine (reverse T3) and 3,3′,5-triiodothyronine (T3). J Clin Endocrinol Metab 41:911–920, 1975.
93. Cavaleri RH, Castle JN, McMahon FA: Effects of dexamethasone on kinetics and distribution of triiodothyronine in the rat. Endocrinology 114:215–221, 1984.
94. Newman CM, Price A, Davies DW, et al: Amiodarone and the thyroid: A practical guide to the management of thyroid dysfunction induced by amiodarone therapy. Heart 79:121–127, 1998.

Chapter 95

Mechanisms of Thyroid Hormone Action

J. Larry Jameson

Thyroid hormones, thyroxine (T_4) and triiodothyronine (T_3), have myriad physiologic effects. They exert actions in all tissues and affect essentially every metabolic pathway. The physiologic actions of thyroid hormones can be largely divided into two broad categories: (1) effects on cellular differentiation and development; and (2) effects on metabolic pathways. Obviously, these two actions of thyroid hormone are interrelated in that alterations in growth and development require concomitant shifts in metabolism. Similarly, changes in cellular differentiation can alter patterns of gene expression, thereby influencing metabolic pathways. Thus, the effects of thyroid hormone represent a complex integration of pathways both at the cellular level and in terms of whole-animal physiology.

Some of the most prominent effects of thyroid hormone occur during fetal development and in early childhood. In animal models, the developmental effects of thyroid hormone have been well documented. For example, in amphibians, the process of metamorphosis from tadpoles to frogs is strictly dependent on thyroid hormone.[1–3] In humans, the requirement for thyroid hormone during development is manifest dramatically in the syndrome of cretinism. Many of these developmental effects are not reversed by later treatment with hormone, indicating that thyroid hormone acts during developmental windows in combination with other differentiation factors that may not be available later in life. Thyroid hormone continues to play a critical role during growth and development in childhood, as illustrated by the characteristic delayed growth curves that occur in hypothyroidism (see Chapter 105). In this case, many of the effects of thyroid hormone may be metabolic rather than developmental, as growth is restored rapidly after the institution of treatment.

In adults, the primary effects of thyroid hormones are manifest by alterations in metabolism, including changes in oxygen consumption, and protein, carbohydrate, lipid, and vitamin metabolism. Thyroid hormones also alter the synthesis and degradation rates of many other hormones and growth factors and they therefore influence other endocrine pathways. The clinical features of hypothyroidism and hyperthyroidism serve as emphatic reminders that thyroid hormones cause pleiotropic effects that reflect their actions on many different pathways and target organs. Alterations in oxygen consumption have long been recognized as one of the hallmarks of thyroid hormone action. Clinically, this aspect of thyroid hormone action forms the basis for measurements of basal metabolic rate (BMR), which is reduced in hypothyroidism and increased in hyperthyroidism. Measurement of oxygen consumption in individual tissues has provided an index of organs that are targets for the metabolic effects of thyroid hormones (Fig. 95–1). Oxygen consumption is stimulated markedly by thyroid hormone in heart, skeletal muscle, liver, kidney, and gastrointestinal organs, whereas brain, spleen, and the gonads are metabolically less responsive.[4, 5] The pituitary gland exhibits a paradoxical response to thyroid hormone with increased metabolic activity in hypothyroidism and decreased activity in hyperthyroidism. This may reflect the unique role of the pituitary in the regulation of the thyroid axis. The reasons for the variable metabolic responses in different organs are not well understood. Each of these tissues depends on aerobic metabolism and contains the enzymes necessary for increasing oxygen consumption. As described below, these variable tissue responses are accounted for in part, but not entirely, by the composition of receptors for thyroid hormone. It is clear, however, that oxygen

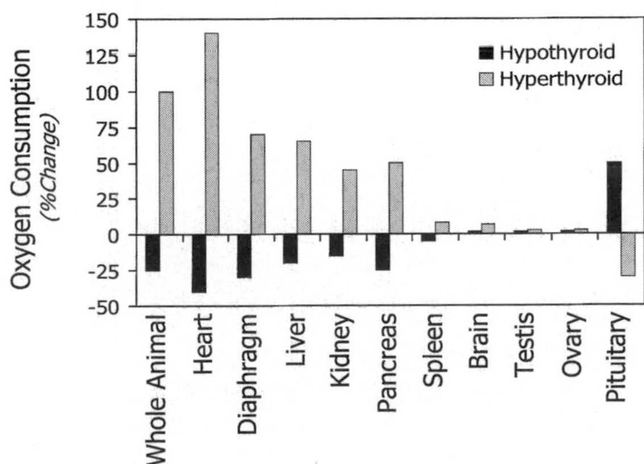

FIGURE 95–1. Oxygen consumption by various rat tissues in hypothyroid and hyperthyroid states. Oxygen consumption was determined in thyroidectomized Sprague-Dawley rats before *(solid bars)* and after *(striped bars)* treatment with thyroxine for 4 to 6 days. (Drawn from data in Barker SB: Physiological activity of thyroid hormones and analogues. *In* Pitt-Rivers R, Trotter WR (eds): The Thyroid Gland. London, Butterworths, 1964, p 200.)

This work was supported by Public Health Service grant DK42144.

consumption is not a comprehensive marker of thyroid hormone effects. This point is particularly apparent in the case of the brain. Although oxygen consumption in brain is altered minimally by thyroid hormone, some of the most prominent clinical effects of thyroid hormone deficiency and excess are manifest as alterations in central nervous system function. More recent studies have identified a number of specific markers of thyroid hormone action in the brain.[6–8]

At a clinical level, it is challenging to identify quantitative markers of thyroid hormone action.[9] At the extreme ends of the clinical spectrum, which extends from hypothyroidism to hyperthyroidism, the clinical diagnosis of a thyroid abnormality is usually apparent, and can be confirmed using laboratory tests for thyroid hormones and thyroid-stimulating hormone (TSH). However, more subtle forms of thyroid dysfunction, often referred to as subclinical hypothyroidism or hyperthyroidism, pose a greater challenge (see Chapter 105). Although the level of circulating TSH provides a sensitive and quantitative indicator of thyroid hormone action at the level of the hypothalamic-pituitary axis, there has been less success in the identification of peripheral markers of thyroid hormone action.[9, 10] The effect of thyroid hormone on basal metabolism has been revisited using measurements of resting energy expenditure (REE). In patients taking varying levels of thyroid hormone replacement, there is a strong inverse correlation between REE and the TSH level.[11] Approximately 20% to 25% of REE is thought to be thyroid hormone–dependent.[11] Thus, it is all the more remarkable that REE represents a relatively sensitive indicator of changes in thyroid hormone levels. Subclinical hypothyroidism has also been associated with lipid abnormalities, decreased cardiac contractility, and neuropsychiatric effects.[12] Subclinical hyperthyroidism increases the risk of atrial fibrillation, particularly in the elderly.[13] TSH remains the most sensitive and useful indicator of thyroid hormone action. As discussed below, evidence for variable metabolism of thyroid hormones and tissue sensitivity to its effects underscore the importance of developing additional markers of thyroid hormone action.

Since the initial description of thyroid hormone effects on metabolic rate by Magnus-Levy in 1895, investigators have searched for a unifying mechanism of hormone action that could explain all of its effects. Not surprisingly, this goal has not been readily achieved, and a number of theories have been put forward over the last century to explain thyroid hormone action. Initially, thyroid hormone was thought to act by uncoupling oxidative phosphorylation. This model has not held up to rigorous quantitative analysis and it has been largely abandoned as a primary action of thyroid hormone. Subsequently, thyroid hormone was proposed to increase energy expenditure by stimulating Na^+, K^+-ATPase (adenosinetriphosphatase) activity. Although thyroid hormone causes alterations in the activity of this and other ATPases,[14–16] these effects are unlikely to account for as much of the energy expenditure as estimated originally. As described below, thyroid hormone may also have direct effects on selected transporters and enzymes in the plasma membrane and mitochondria. However, most of the effects of thyroid hormone are now considered to occur through the actions of nuclear receptors that mediate changes in gene expression. Over the last decade, there has been a remarkable surge of new information subsequent to the cloning of thyroid hormone receptors (TRs)[17, 18] and the identification of regulatory regions in thyroid hormone–responsive genes. The purpose of this chapter is to review how thyroid hormone exerts its action at the cellular level, with particular emphasis on recent developments in our understanding of nuclear receptor action.

CIRCULATING LEVELS AND INTRACELLULAR FORMS OF THYROID HORMONES

Binding Characteristics of Thyroxine and Triiodothyronine

The thyroid gland secretes both T_4 and T_3. T_4 is secreted from the thyroid gland in great excess (at least 20-fold) over T_3 (Table 95–1). Substantial amounts of secreted T_4 are metabolized to T_3 in the peripheral circulation (see Chapter 94).[19–22] However, the plasma T_4/T_3 ratio is about 60:1, reflecting a much greater clearance rate for T_3. Both T_4 and T_3 are bound to plasma proteins and very little hormone circulates in the unbound form. Approximately 99.98% of T_4, and 99.7% of T_3, are bound to plasma proteins, including thyroxine-binding globulin (TBG), thyroxine-binding prealbumin (TBPA), and albumin. The estimated free concentrations of the two forms of thyroid hormone are 2×10^{-11} M for T_4 and 6×10^{-12} M for T_3. T_3 is more active than T_4 when assessed in bioassays of thyromimetic activity.[23] The greater biologic potency of T_3 parallels its affinity for nuclear receptors.[24, 25]

TABLE 95–1. Summary of Metabolic and Kinetic Parameters for Thyroxine (T_4) Triiodothyronine (T_3)

	T_4	T_3
Serum concentrations		
Total hormone (μg/dL)	8	0.14
Fraction of total hormone in the free form (%)	0.02	0.3
Free hormone (pM)	21	6
Distribution volume (L)	12	31
Extrathyroidal pool (μg)	960	43
Fraction, intracellular (%)	~20	~70
Half-life (days)	7	1
Production rate (μg/day)	90	32
Fraction directly from the thyroid	100	5
Relative metabolic potency	0.3	1
Receptor binding in vitro (K_d, M)	10^{-9}	10^{-10}
Receptor binding in vivo (K_d, M)	10^{-10}	10^{-11}

Adapted from DeGroot LJ: Thyroid hormone transport, cellular uptake, metabolism, and molecular action. *In* DeGroot LJ, Larsen PR, Henneman G (eds): The Thyroid and Its Diseases. New York, Churchill Livingstone, 1996, p 73.

T_3 is bound to its receptors with about 10- to 15-fold greater affinity than T_4. The dissociation constants for liver nuclear receptors measured in vitro are 2×10^{-9} M for T_4 and 2×10^{-10} M for T_3. These binding characteristics predict that very little circulating hormone would be bound by receptors. However, nuclear receptors are approximately 75% saturated with thyroid hormone in brain and pituitary and 50% saturated with thyroid hormone in liver and kidney.[26, 27] This apparent discrepancy between circulating concentrations of thyroid hormones and the amounts that are bound to receptors may be accounted for by the challenges of measuring free hormone concentrations or receptor binding constants. Alternatively, there may be mechanisms to facilitate the transport of thyroid hormones into cells. In any event, it is notable that thyroid hormone occupancy of receptors varies in different tissues. The fact that receptors are not fully occupied in most tissues provides a circumstance in which changes in thyroid hormone levels can be expected to alter receptor activity.

Deiodinases Modulate T_4/T_3 Ratios and Hormone Availability to Different Tissues

In many respects, T_4 may be thought of as a precursor of the more potent hormone, T_3. Most of the hormone bound to receptors is in the form of T_3, which is derived either from the peripheral circulation, or from T_4 conversion by 5′-monodeiodinases. As described in Chapter 94, there are three distinct deiodinases, type I, type II, and type III.[20, 22] In view of the relatively greater potency of T_3 vs. T_4, the distribution and regulation of these enzymes can have important effects on thyroid hormone action.

Type I deiodinase is located primarily in thyroid, liver, and kidney and has a low affinity for T_4 (micromolar). It is sensitive to inhibition by propylthiouracil (PTU) and plays an important role in the production of circulating T_3. The type I enzyme is induced by thyroid hormone, which may explain, in part, the relatively high production of T_3 in thyrotoxicosis. Type II deiodinase has a high affinity for T_4 (nanomolar) and is found primarily in the pituitary gland, brain, and

TABLE 95–2. Examples of Extranuclear Sites of Thyroid Hormone Action

Site of Action	Potential Cellular Targets	References
Plasma membrane	Thyroid hormone binding sites	38
	Thyroid hormone transporters	39
	Ca^{2+}-ATPase	14
	Adenylate cyclase	40
	Sugar transport	41
Nuclear membrane	Thyroid hormone transporters	42
Mitochondria		43
Cytosol	Pyruvate kinase	44
	Type II 5′-deiodinase	45
Cytoskeleton	Actin polymerization	46

brown fat, where it may function to convert T_4 to T_3 as a mechanism for modulating the local concentration of T_3. Type II deiodinase is induced by low levels of T_4, thereby increasing the efficiency of T_3 production. These characteristics allow tissues that contain type II deiodinase to respond differently to a given concentration of T_4 than other organs in which exposure to T_3 more closely reflects circulating concentrations of the hormone.[28, 29] Type III deiodinase catalyzes deiodination of the inner ring of T_4 and T_3, leading to inactivation of the hormones. It is located mainly in the skin, placenta, and brain. In the placenta, the type III enzyme is thought to represent an important barrier to the transport of thyroid hormones from the mother to the fetus.[30] Like the type I enzyme, its activity is induced by hyperthyroidism and decreased by hypothyroidism. Therefore, in hypothyroid conditions, the type II and type III enzymes act together to preserve T_3 concentrations in the central nervous system. Induction of type II enhances the conversion of T_4 to T_3, and the reduction of type III deiodinase minimizes the degradation of T_4 and T_3.

EXTRANUCLEAR ACTIONS OF THYROID HORMONES

Although there is general agreement that most of the physiologic effects of thyroid hormones are mediated via high-affinity nuclear receptors,[31–36] there is ongoing consideration of possible extranuclear sites of thyroid hormone action. It should also be noted that nongenomic actions have been described for other nuclear receptor ligands, such as progesterone and estrogen. Some of the proposed nongenomic actions of thyroid hormone are summarized in Table 95–2 and have been reviewed.[37] Because these effects of thyroid hormones are not mediated by its nuclear receptor, the nongenomic actions of thyroid hormone are likely to have different structure-activity relationships of iodothyronines. In addition, one might expect distinct time courses, including more rapid effects, than can occur by alterations in gene transcription followed by protein biosynthesis (see below).

Nongenomic actions of thyroid hormone have been described at the plasma membrane, the cytoskeleton, in mitochondria, and in the cytoplasm. High-affinity thyroid hormone binding sites have been described in the plasma membranes of several different cell types.[38, 47, 48] Thyroid hormones have been shown to induce calcium ATPase activity in red blood cell membranes[14, 48] and in sarcoplasmic reticulum.[49] A 55-kDa membrane protein (p55) has been identified by affinity labeling with analogues of T_3, and the complementary DNA (cDNA) encoding this protein reveals that it is prolyl hydroxylase.[50] Additional immunohistochemical analyses indicate that p55 is localized primarily on the nuclear envelope and endoplasmic reticulum.[51] Thus, this protein is unlikely to participate in thyroid hormone transport across the plasma membrane, but it may serve other T_3-mediated processes. A 58-kDa cytosolic thyroid hormone–binding protein has also been identified.[52] Its cDNA reveals that it is a subunit of pyruvate kinase that binds T_3 when the enzyme is in its monomeric, but not tetrameric, form. The monomer-tetramer interconversion is regulated by glucose via fructose-1,6-bisphosphonate. It has been proposed that pyruvate kinase could regulate the availability of cytosolic T_3 to nuclear receptors.[44] T_4, but not T_3, activates F-actin interactions with proteins involved in the intracellular trafficking of 5′-monodeiodinase.[46] T_4 also regulates the half-life of type II deiodinase. Hypothyroidism induces the enzyme and T_4 (or reverse T_3 [rT_3]) suppresses its activity. Agents that inhibit messenger RNA (mRNA) and protein synthesis do not block these actions of T_4, suggesting that they are post-translational.[45, 53]

There has also been great interest in the possibility that T_4 or T_3 might exert rapid, nongenomic actions on the vascular system[54] or in brain.[55] Several studies have examined whether high doses of T_3 might be useful for preserving cardiac function in conjunction with bypass surgery or transplantation.[55, 56] Although there are few controlled trials in humans, recent studies indicate that raising serum T_3 concentrations in patients undergoing coronary artery bypass surgery increases cardiac output and lowers systemic vascular resistance, but does not alter the outcome or postoperative therapy.[57, 58]

THYROID HORMONE BINDS TO HIGH-AFFINITY NUCLEAR RECEPTORS TO MODULATE GENE EXPRESSION

In 1966, Tata and Widnell[59] proposed a novel nuclear mechanism for thyroid hormone action. In an elegant series of experiments, injected T_3 was shown to first induce gene transcription, followed by incorporation of amino acids into proteins, finally resulting in induction of mitochondrial enzyme activity (Fig. 95–2). These results suggested that alterations in gene expression might be the most proximal step in thyroid hormone action.

In 1972, nuclear binding sites for thyroid hormone were demonstrated and subsequent experiments led to detailed characterization of these receptors.[60] Based on Scatchard analyses, TRs bound hormone as a single class of high-affinity binding sites (K_d approximately 10^{-10} M for T_3) with no evidence of positive or negative cooperativity.[61] The affinity of various thyroid hormones for the receptor parallels their biologic potencies, supporting the view that most biologic effects are mediated via the nuclear receptor.[24, 25, 62] For example, the order of biologic potency and receptor binding is triiodothyroacetic acid (TRIAC) > L-T_3 > L-T_4 > rT_3. The number of TRs per nucleus is relatively low. Tissues such as the anterior pituitary and liver, which are very responsive to thyroid hormone, contain approximately 10,000 receptors per nucleus.[63] In general, there is a correlation between receptor number and tissue responsiveness to T_3, at least as assessed by indices of oxygen consumption (see Fig. 95–1). However, brain is a notable exception in that receptor binding capacity is relatively high,[64] but oxygen consumption in response to thyroid hormone is low, suggesting that other factors modify tissue responses.

Unlike some of the steroid hormone receptors, little TR is found in

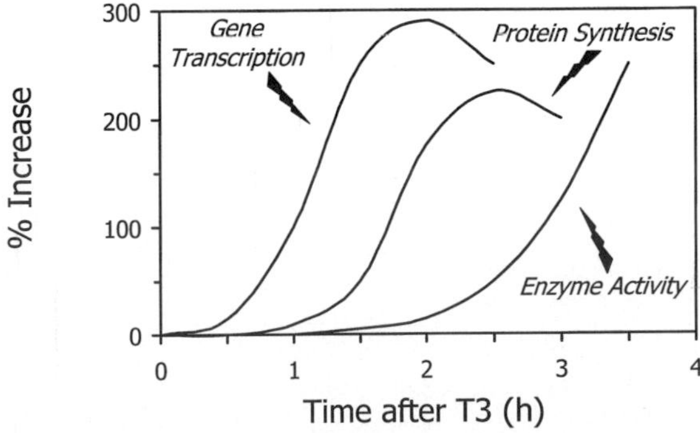

FIGURE 95–2. Kinetics of biosynthetic and enzymatic responses to thyroid hormone. An idealized version of the time course for nuclear RNA polymerase (gene transcription), amino acid incorporation (protein biosynthesis), and cytochrome oxidase activity (enzyme activity) is shown for livers of thyroidectomized rats after a single injection of triiodothyronine. (Modified from Tata J: Thyroid hormone action. *In* Greep RO, Astwood EB (eds): Handbook of Physiology, Section 7: Endocrinology, Vol 3: Thyroid. Washington, DC, American Physiological Society, 1974, p 471.)

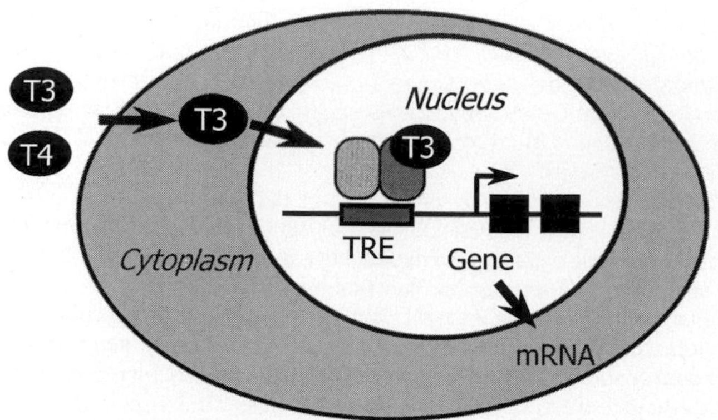

FIGURE 95–3. Mechanism of thyroid hormone action via its nuclear receptor. Thyroid hormone diffuses or is transported across plasma and nuclear membranes to bind to its receptor. The thyroid hormone receptor *(hatched area)* is localized almost exclusively in the nucleus where it is associated with DNA as a homodimer or as a heterodimer with retinoid X receptor (RXR) *(stippled area)*. The hormone-activated receptor binds to thyroid hormone response elements (TREs) to alter rates of gene transcription and, consequently, levels of mRNA.

the cytoplasm, and thyroid hormone binding does not seem to be required for receptor transport into the nucleus.[65] In fact, TRs are tightly associated with chromatin,[66–68] consistent with their proposed role as DNA-binding proteins that act to regulate gene expression. Photoaffinity labeling of receptors reveals two major nuclear binding proteins of approximately 57 and 47 kDa.[69, 70] Physical methods such as sedimentation coefficients confirm this molecular mass and also provide evidence for receptor heterogeneity.[68, 71, 72] As described below, the multiple forms of receptor proteins reflect their production from two distinct genes. Using micrococcal nuclease digestion of chromatin, the receptor is estimated to protect about 35 bp, a surprisingly long segment of DNA sequence given the molecular mass of the receptor.[68] Although these findings may be accounted for by the low degree of resolution of micrococcal nuclease digestion, the results are consistent with a model in which the receptor binds to DNA as a dimer or in association with other cellular proteins. There is growing evidence that chromatin remodeling is an important action of the TR.

The issue of how plasma thyroid hormone enters the cell and subsequently gains access to nuclear receptors has received considerable attention. Because thyroid hormone is lipophilic, it is generally considered to enter cells by diffusion. However, there is also evidence for facilitated transport across the plasma membrane.[39, 73–76] Because these transporters appear to be relatively low-affinity, high-capacity units, they are unlikely to respond to physiologic concentrations of thyroid hormone. In human erythrocytes, T_3 can be concentrated 55-fold inside cells by a mechanism involving facilitated diffusion with intracellular trapping.[39] There is additional evidence for a stereospecific thyroid hormone transporter that pumps hormone from the cytoplasm into the nucleus. Using isotopic dilution techniques, there is 58-fold greater L-T_3 and fourfold greater D-T_3 in the nucleus than in the cytosol.[42] Although these calculations rely on indirect methods, they suggest that the transport of L-T_3 into the nucleus is greatly favored. In different tissues, there are large differences in the thyroid hormone concentration gradient across plasma and nuclear membranes, suggesting that this process may be able to alter thyroid hormone delivery to different target tissues. In cultured cells, the apparent affinity of L-T_3 for its nuclear receptor is increased by about eightfold in whole-cell binding assays compared with measurements in isolated nuclei, suggesting that transport mechanisms may reduce the amount of thyroid hormone required to exert a biologic response.[77] It should also be recalled that the presence of 5′-monodeiodinase in different tissues (e.g., pituitary, brain) is capable of altering the ratio of T_4 to T_3.[29]

TABLE 95–3. Selected Positive Triiodothyronine-Regulated Genes

Positively Regulated Genes*	References
β_1-Adrenergic receptor	83
Fatty acid synthetase	84
Growth hormone	85
Lysozyme silencer	86
Malic enzyme	87
Moloney leukemia virus enhancer	88
mdm2	89
Myelin basic protein	6
Myosin heavy chain α	90
NGFI-A	91
Oxytocin	92
Phospho*enol*pyruvate carboxykinase	93
Prostaglandin D synthase	94
RC3	95
SER Ca^{2+}-ATPase	96
Spot 14 lipogenic enzyme	97
Type I 5′-deiodinase	98
Uncoupling protein	99

*In most cases, thyroid hormone has been shown to induce steady-state mRNA levels, and thyroid hormone response elements have been characterized in the promoter regions of these genes. A large number of other genes (not shown) are also induced by thyroid hormone.

THYROID HORMONE REGULATES PATTERNS AND LEVELS OF GENE EXPRESSION

A simplified model of thyroid hormone action is depicted in Figure 95–3. According to this view, thyroid hormone binds to nuclear receptors, which, in turn, act upon thyroid hormone response elements (TREs) in specific target genes. As described later in the chapter, TRs function in conjunction with a large number of additional proteins that enhance their binding to DNA and modulate their transcriptional activity. After activation by thyroid hormone, the receptor causes alterations in gene expression, either stimulating or repressing the transcriptional activity of a target gene. Changes in gene transcription are reflected by alterations in mRNA levels, and subsequently, changes in protein biosynthesis.

Since the recognition that thyroid hormone acts primarily to modulate gene expression, a variety of different target genes have been studied extensively (for reviews, see references 31, 33, 35, 78, 79). Thyroid hormone has the dual ability to stimulate expression of some genes while causing repression of other genes, even in the same tissue. Thus, mechanisms for TR action must ultimately account for positive and negative regulation by the receptor. Examples of the target genes that are regulated by thyroid hormone are summarized in Tables 95–3 and 95–4. Clearly, many other genes are also regulated by thyroid hormone, and the list continues to expand rapidly.

For the most part, the targets of thyroid hormone action have been analyzed by measuring steady-state mRNA or protein levels. These measurements integrate a number of biosynthetic steps, including gene transcription, mRNA processing and stabilization, and translational

TABLE 95–4. Selected Negative Triiodothyronine-Regulated Genes

Negatively Regulated Genes	References
β-Amyloid	100
Cellular retinoic acid–binding protein-I	101
Epidermal growth factor receptor	102
Myosin heavy chain β	103
Na^+, K^+-ATPase α3 subunit	104
Peroxisomal enoyl-CoA hydratase	105
Prolactin	106
Thyroid-stimulating hormone-α	107
Thyroid-stimulating hormone-β	108
Thyrotropin-releasing hormone	109
Type II 5′-deiodinase	21

efficiency. Thyroid hormone is thought to act at each of these steps. For many genes, such as 3-hydroxy-3-methylglutaryl–coenzyme A (HMG-CoA) reductase[80] and apolipoprotein A-1,[81] thyroid hormone affects both transcription rate and mRNA stability, causing relatively greater increases in steady-state mRNA by affecting both synthesis and degradation. For other genes, the effects of thyroid hormone may be primarily transcriptional or post-transcriptional. Although the net effects of these events are similar in that they increase the amount of newly synthesized protein product, the mechanisms and kinetics are different. Transcriptional events cause rapid changes in mRNA levels, whereas changes in mRNA stability affect the time required to reach a new steady state, as well as the persistence of newly synthesized mRNA.[82] In general, thyroid hormone effects on gene transcription have been studied most extensively, in part because of the availability of methods for analyzing promoter activity in transfected cells. Some of the genes for which thyroid hormone–responsive promoter elements have been defined are listed in Table 95–3.

In the most straightforward model for transcriptional stimulation, the receptor binds directly to specific DNA sequences in the promoter and induces transcription by interactions with other transcription factors on the promoter (Fig. 95–4). Examples of genes that use this type of mechanism include rat growth hormone, malic enzyme, myosin heavy-chain α, and myelin basic protein, among others. These genes share in common the feature that a receptor-binding site is located within several hundred base pairs upstream of the transcriptional start site. Deletion or mutation of the receptor-binding sites in these genes eliminates or greatly reduces thyroid hormone responsiveness. Comparison of these so-called TREs reveals some sequence similarity, allowing derivation of a consensus DNA sequence (see below).[33]

In contrast to positive transcriptional regulation, the mechanism of transcriptional repression by thyroid hormone is less well understood. Thyroid hormone–induced negative regulation should be contrasted with the process of basal repression that occurs for positive TREs that are inhibited in the absence of hormone binding (see below).[88, 110–112] True negative regulation is hormone-dependent. For example, in hypothyroidism, expression of the TSH-α and TSH-β genes is greatly increased.[113] Examples of negatively regulated genes are provided in Table 95–4. Addition of thyroid hormone causes transcriptional repression in a manner that is proportionate to receptor occupancy by hormone.[114] Several lines of evidence suggest that these effects of thyroid hormone are mediated directly, without the induction of intermediate gene products. First, transcriptional repression is very rapid, occurring within 30 minutes after the addition of hormone.[115] Second, protein synthesis inhibitors, such as cycloheximide, do not block transcriptional repression of these genes, suggesting that synthesis of an intermediate gene product is not required.[116] Third, thyroid hormone–responsive regions have been identified in the promoters of the thyrotropin-releasing hormone (TRH) and TSH genes, although these elements appear to differ from traditional positive TREs (see below).[108, 109, 117–121]

Despite these examples of genes that are regulated directly by TRs, the majority of thyroid hormone–responsive genes may be regulated indirectly (see Fig. 95–4). This concept is supported by the fact that, in some cases, the kinetics for changes in gene expression are relatively slow (requiring several hours). Moreover, experiments using cycloheximide to block the induction of intermediate gene products are consistent with an indirect mechanism for stimulation or repression of many thyroid hormone–responsive genes.[82]

Indirect mechanisms for thyroid hormone action provide a powerful means to alter patterns of gene expression. If thyroid hormone first causes induction of a transcription factor or kinase, this protein can, in turn, alter the expression of a cascade of additional genes. Analogously, thyroid hormone can ultimately change patterns of gene expression by participating in the process of cellular differentiation. Of course, indirect mechanisms do not preclude concomitant direct actions of TRs for a given gene. Furthermore, it is possible that some effects of thyroid hormone are direct (e.g., transcription), whereas other effects may be mediated through an indirect pathway (e.g., mRNA stability).

Thyroid hormone also exerts indirect effects at the physiologic level. For example, in the rat, thyroid hormone stimulates hepatic insulin-like growth factor 1 (IGF-1) mRNA. Because thyroid hormone also causes marked stimulation of growth hormone (GH) in this species,[122, 123] the effects of thyroid hormone on IGF-1 are mediated largely by an indirect mechanism involving GH.[124, 125] In hypophysectomized animals, thyroid hormone has little or no effect on IGF-1 mRNA, although it enhances GH stimulation of IGF-1, suggesting that it may also function in concert with GH at the hepatic level.[124] Similarly, thyroid hormone effects on cardiac proteins and enzymes may represent a combination of direct effects on target genes and secondary effects that are the consequences of thyroid hormone–induced alterations in contractility and hemodynamics.[126]

The physiologic setting in which the effects of thyroid hormone are analyzed can have a major impact on its action. For example, thyroid hormone and glucocorticoids stimulate rat GH gene expression in a synergistic manner.[127–129] Many of the effects of thyroid hormone on liver enzymes involve complex interactions with other hormones. Thyroid hormone enhances insulin or IGF-1 stimulation of fatty acid

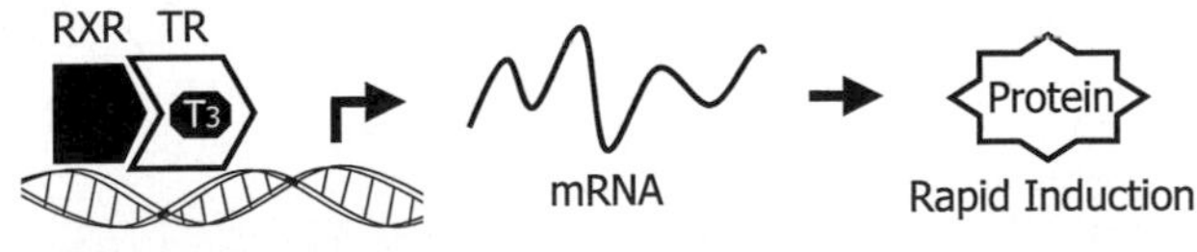

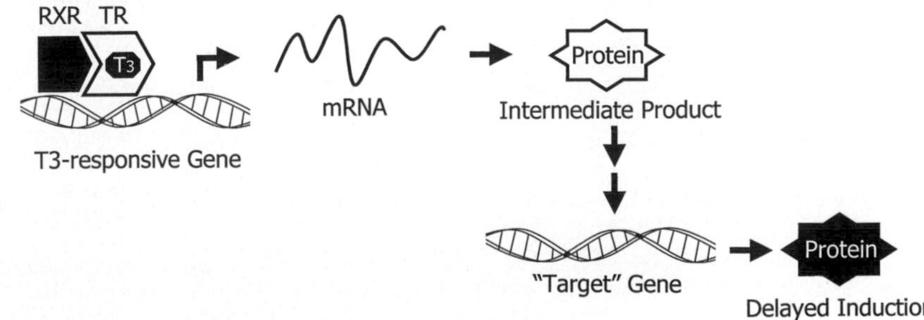

FIGURE 95–4. Direct and indirect mechanisms of thyroid hormone action. The thyroid hormone receptor activates gene expression after binding triiodothyronine. In the model for direct action of thyroid hormone, the receptor acts on the target gene itself to increase transcription. In most cases, genes that are stimulated or repressed directly by thyroid hormone exhibit altered levels of mRNA within 2 to 6 hours after hormone addition. In this case, treatment with protein synthesis inhibitors (e.g., cycloheximide) does not block the effects of thyroid hormone. In the model for indirect action of thyroid hormone, the "target" gene that is being analyzed for thyroid hormone effects is not itself an initial site for thyroid hormone receptor action. Rather, the thyroid hormone receptor stimulates expression of an intermediate gene to make protein, which in turn alters expression of the "target genes," either by changing the concentration of a transcription factor as depicted, or by modifying mRNA stability (not shown). The kinetics of thyroid hormone induction through an indirect mechanism are delayed (>6 hours) and may be inhibited by cycloheximide, assuming that this agent does not also block production of repressors. Not shown are potential effects of thyroid hormone on translation, post-translational modification, or secretion.

synthetase.[130] Activation of protein kinase pathways can block thyroid hormone stimulation of several lipogenic enzymes, including malic enzyme, fatty acid synthetase, and acetyl-CoA carboxylase.[130, 131] Nutritional states also have a profound effect on hepatic enzyme induction by T_3. For example, a high carbohydrate diet amplifies T_3 effects on glucose 6-phosphate dehydrogenase production by 40-fold.[31, 132] Thus, for many, if not most, thyroid hormone–responsive genes, the level of transcriptional activity integrates many signaling pathways in addition to thyroid hormone. Indeed, thyroid hormone often plays the role of a modulator that amplifies the effects of other hormones. At a mechanistic level, this complex hormonal regulation is likely to reflect the large number of signaling pathways and transcription factors that regulate a given gene. Many well-characterized genes have been shown to bind a daunting number of regulatory proteins in their promoter regions in addition to the basal transcription factors that are required by RNA polymerase to initiate transcription. As described later in the chapter, an understanding of how TRs interact with these other proteins is beginning to emerge.

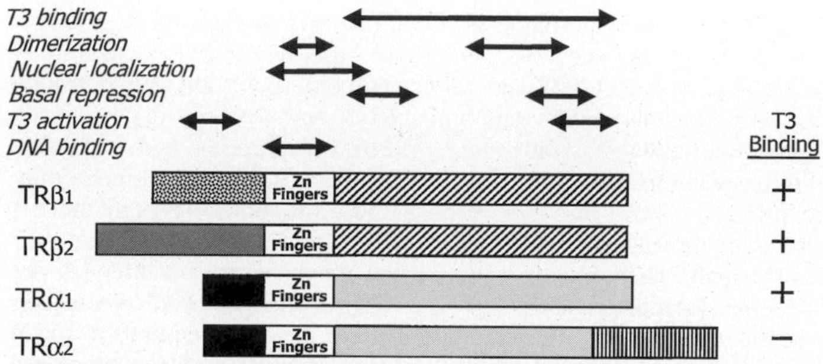

FIGURE 95–5. Functional domains of thyroid hormone receptor isoforms. The thyroid hormone receptor (TR) β and α isoforms are illustrated schematically. The zinc finger DNA-binding regions are indicated. The TRβ2 isoform, which is expressed predominantly in the pituitary and hypothalamus, contains a unique N-terminus. The TRα2 isoform contains unique C-terminal sequences that eliminate hormone binding. *Arrows* at the top of the figure indicate selected functional domains. Other regions of the receptor may be important for these functions in the three-dimensional context of the native receptor.

CLONING, STRUCTURE, AND EXPRESSION OF THYROID HORMONE RECEPTORS

Thyroid Hormone Receptors Are Cellular Homologues of the *v-erbA* Oncogene

The TR cDNAs were cloned in 1986.[17, 18] Although two groups independently isolated receptor clones, neither group had set out explicitly to clone a TR. Rather, in the course of analyzing clones that were related to the *v-erbA* oncogene, TR cDNAs were isolated based upon their high degree of sequence homology with the viral oncogene.

Sap et al.[17] isolated a *v-erbA*-related cDNA from a chicken embryo library. The 46-kDa protein encoded by this cDNA was shown to bind thyroid hormones with high affinity and is referred to as the thyroid hormone receptor α (TRα) isoform. The amino acid sequence of TRα was strikingly similar to the *v-erbA* oncogene, suggesting that the TR is the cellular homologue of the viral oncogene. There are, however, important differences between the *v-erbA* oncogene and the cellular TRα. Comparison of their sequences reveals that the *v-erbA* protein contains 17 amino acid substitutions, including two changes in the DNA-binding domain. In addition, deletion of 9 amino acids at the C-terminus of the *v-erbA* protein eliminates its ability to bind thyroid hormone.[17] These mutations in *v-erbA* likely account for its ability to block cellular differentiation and to function together with the *v-erbB* oncogene to cause erythroleukemia.[133] *V-erbA* exerts constitutive repression of target genes, suggesting that it may act in part by blocking the actions of TRs.[134–136]

In parallel with the isolation of the TRα receptor, Weinberger et al.[18] isolated a β form of the TR from a human placental library. Like TRα, TRβ binds thyroid hormones with high affinity, and with a profile of binding to thyroid hormone analogues that is similar to that of native TRs isolated from tissue sources. The TRα and TRβ isoforms are encoded by separate genes located on chromosomes 17 and 3, respectively.[137, 138]

Structure of the Thyroid Hormone Receptors

In addition to the TRs the *v-erbA*-related superfamily includes receptors for estrogen, progesterone, glucocorticoid, mineralocorticoid, androgen, vitamin D, and retinoic acid, as well as a number of "orphan nuclear receptors" that may or may not bind specific ligands[139, 140] (see also Chapter 10). The members of this receptor family are characterized by a central DNA-binding domain and a C-terminal hormone or ligand-binding domain. Dimerization domains and nuclear localization signals are found in both the DNA- and ligand-binding domains (Fig. 95–5). The N-terminal regions are more variable among different classes of receptors (e.g., glucocorticoid vs. thyroid), as well as within subgroups of receptors (e.g., TRα vs. TRβ). The crystal structure of the ligand-binding domain of the TR has now been solved[141] (Fig. 95–6). This structure reveals a series of α-helical segments surrounding the ligand, which is buried deep in a pocket of the protein. Additional studies suggest that major conformational changes are associated with ligand binding, particularly involving the extreme C-termi-

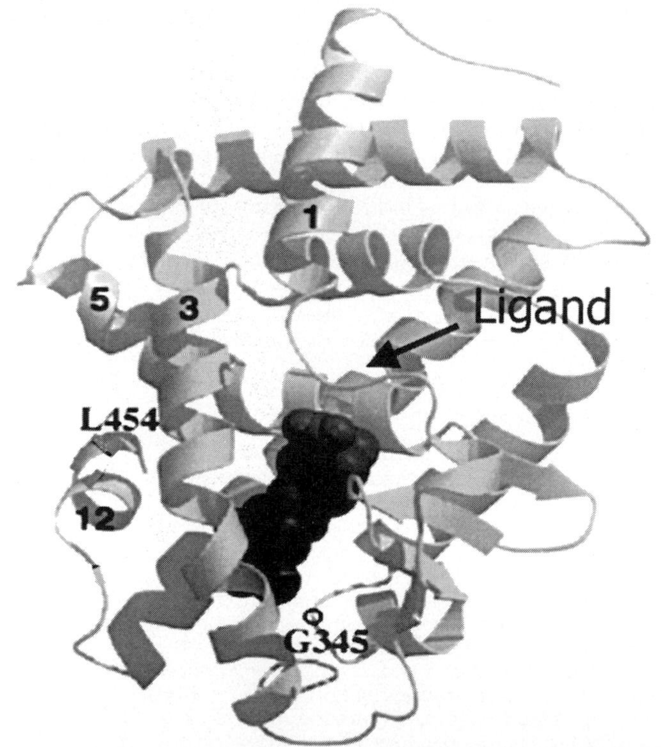

FIGURE 95–6. Three-dimensional structure of the thyroid hormone receptor (TR) ligand–binding domain. A ribbon diagram of the x-ray crystal structure of the TR ligand–binding domain reveals extensive α-helical structure. Helixes 1, 3, 5, and 12 are indicated. The ligand is buried in the central region of the receptor *(solid spheres)*. The location of a mutation, glycine 345 (G345), that eliminates hormone binding and causes resistance to thyroid hormone, is indicated. A second mutation, leucine 454 (L454), is located on the coactivator-binding surface, and disrupts transcriptional activity and causes resistance to thyroid hormone. (Adapted from Tagami T, Gu WX, Peairs PT, West BL, et al: A novel natural mutation in the thyroid hormone receptor defines a dual functional domain that exchanges nuclear receptor corepressors and coactivators. Mol Endocrinol 12:1888, 1998.)

nus of the ligand-binding domain (helix 12).[142] After hormone binding, a hydrophobic surface that includes portions of helixes 3, 5, and 12, is formed and represents a docking site for transcriptional adapter proteins (see below).

The DNA-binding domains of the nuclear receptors are comprised of two distinct zinc fingers in which a single zinc atom is coordinated tetrahedrally with four cysteines. Each of the zinc fingers contains a loop of amino acids, which forms a "finger" that extends from the planar zinc-coordinated complex. The fingers are separated by a 15- to 17-amino acid linker sequence. The crystal structure of the DNA-binding domain of the glucocorticoid receptor–DNA complex was solved in 1991, allowing detailed understanding of the structural features of this domain.[143] More recently, the crystal structure of the DNA-binding domains of the TR and its heterodimeric partner, 9-*cis*-retinoic acid receptor was determined. This study revealed that the two subunits interact with a direct repeat of the TRE in a head-to-tail manner.[144, 145] Thus, as described in greater detail below, the DNA-binding domain of the TR interacts with DNA, and with its heterodimeric partner. This orientation of receptor heterodimers is different from that of the homodimeric steroid receptors such as the glucocorticoid or estrogen receptors (ERs) (see Chapter 10).

In addition to these structural studies, a number of mutational analyses have been very useful in elucidating the functional elements of the DNA-binding domain. Exchanges of sequences between various receptors have been used to define the structural determinants for binding to specific DNA sequences.[146–150] These experiments show that a small stretch of amino acids at the base of the first finger (referred to as the P-box) dictate DNA sequence specificity. Consistent with its role in defining DNA specificity, the P-box sequence is one of the most variable regions in the DNA-binding domain of the nuclear receptors. The P-box sequence is shared by certain receptor subfamilies that bind to similar or identical DNA recognition sites. This finding allows the nuclear receptors to be divided into subfamilies (Table 95–5). In the case of the TRs, the P-box sequence (<u>EG</u>CK<u>G</u>) is also shared with the retinoic acid receptors, the retinoic acid X receptors (RXRs), the rev-erbA protein, the vitamin D receptor (VDR), and NGFI-B. The underlined residues, EGG, which correspond to the sequences that vary among nuclear receptors, are most important for DNA-binding specificity. Detailed mutational analyses of these residues reveal that the glutamic acid residue (E) is particularly important for TR binding to its DNA recognition site.[150]

TABLE 95–5. Subfamilies of Nuclear Receptors Based on Their DNA-Binding Domains and DNA Recognition Sequences*

Receptor	P-Box	Consensus Half-Site
Estrogen-Thyroid Subfamily		AGGTCA
Estrogen	EGCKA	
Thyroid α,β	EGCKG	
Rev-erbA	EGCKG	
Retinoic acid α,β,γ	EGCKG	
Retinoid X α,β,γ	EGCKG	
Vitamin D	EGCKG	
NGFI-B	EGCKG	
v-erbA	EGCKS	
COUP-TF	EGCKS	
ARP-1	EGCKS	
Glucocorticoid Subfamily		AGAACA
Glucocorticoid	GSCKV	
Mineralocorticoid	GSCKV	
Progesterone	GSCKV	
Androgen	GSCKV	

ARP, apolipoprotein A1 regulatory protein; COUP-TF, chicken ovalbumin upstream promoter–transcription factor.

*The P-box refers to a 5–amino acid sequence (in single-letter code) at the base of the first zinc finger in the DNA-binding domain of the nuclear receptors. The half-sites refer to a consensus nucleotide sequence recognized by the DNA-binding domains of the receptor subfamilies. Adapted from Umesono K, Evans RM: Determinants of target gene specificity for steroid/thyroid hormone receptors. Cell 57:1142, 1989.

A second region of the DNA-binding domain (referred to as the D-box) is located between the first two cysteines of the second zinc finger.[147] The D-box is involved in spacing between receptor homodimers or, potentially, heterodimers. Because most DNA recognition sequences for receptors are either palindromic, or direct repeats of the hexameric half-sites, the D-box likely represents one of the receptor determinants that defines the spacing between the half-sites. Thus, for receptor subfamilies that share a common P-box and hexameric half-site, distinct target DNA sequences are defined largely by the spacing between the half-sites rather than by the primary sequence of the receptor binding sites. This hypothesis is supported by data that varying the number of nucleotides in the spacer region between half-sites alters the DNA sequence specificity for members of the thyroid hormone receptor subfamily.[151, 152] Although the length of the spacer sequence clearly has important effects on receptor recognition of binding sites, variations in the composition of the flanking sequences, the core half-site, or the spacer can influence receptor binding.[153, 154] For this reason, one cannot reliably identify TR-binding sites based solely on inspection of the DNA sequence.

Alternate Splicing Results in Multiple Thyroid Hormone Receptor Isoforms

The TRα gene is alternately spliced, resulting in a number of distinct protein products. In mammals, the splicing variants involve only the C-terminal hormone-binding domain (see Fig. 95–5). One variant, referred to as α2, is identical to TRα1 through the first 370 amino acids, but then the sequences diverge completely, reflecting the splicing of alternative exons.[155–158] Another splicing variant, referred to as TRvII or α3, is similar to α2 except that it lacks the first 39 amino acids that are found in the unique region of α2.[157] The functional consequences of substituting the C-terminal sequences of α1 with those of α2 are profound. First, α2 no longer binds thyroid hormone because of substitution of critical amino acids at the extreme C-terminal end of the protein.[159] Consequently, α2 cannot modulate gene transcription in a manner analogous to its TRα1 and TRβ receptor counterparts.[160–162] Second, the sequence substitutions in α2 alter its dimerization properties. Thus, even though the DNA-binding domain is not changed, the affinity of α2 binding to DNA is reduced, presumably because dimerization is important for high-affinity binding to DNA.[154, 163–165] The function of the α2 splicing variant is poorly understood. It is expressed in many tissues, and it is present at particularly high levels in brain, testis, kidney, and brown fat.[166–168] The α2 isoform has been proposed to be an endogenous inhibitor of TR function, and it is notable that the metabolic effects of thyroid hormone are relatively low in some of the tissues in which α2 is highly expressed, such as brain and testis. Consistent with this view, α2 inhibits TRα and TRβ receptor function in transient gene expression assays,[156, 160, 164] but its inhibitory effects are not seen for all target genes.[154, 164, 169] The mechanism by which α2 antagonizes receptor action is controversial. Some studies suggest that α2 acts by competing for active receptor complexes at DNA target sites.[164, 165, 169–171] Other studies indicate that α2 exerts inhibitory activity that is independent of DNA binding.[162, 172, 173] It is likely that the inhibitory effects of α2 involve more than one type of mechanism. Recently, it has been shown that the amino acid substitutions in the C-terminal region of α2 prevent its interactions with transcriptional corepressors.[154] This finding, in conjunction with its variable binding to TREs, provides an explanation for why α2 is not a more potent inhibitor of active TRs. The physiologic significance of the inhibitory effects of α2 remains to be established, although gene knockout experiments may eventually shed light on this topic.

In addition to splicing variants of the TRα gene, a number of isoforms appear to be generated by initiation of translation from internal AUG codons, at least in chicken.[174] Internal translation gives rise to a series of proteins that contain variable amounts of the N-terminal and DNA-binding domains. These receptor fragments are of interest because of their potential to act as receptor antagonists by forming inactive dimers. When coexpressed with full-length receptors, the C-terminal receptor fragments inhibit activation of receptor-dependent gene expression.[175, 176] Dimerization domains are required for the inhibitory activity of the C-terminal fragments. Although C-terminal fragments have not been demonstrated in mammals, or for TRβ, it is important to consider such proteins because they can contribute to thyroid hormone–binding activity and potentially play a role in regulating the activity of the full-length receptor.

Surprisingly, a receptor-like molecule is also encoded on the opposite strand of the TRα genomic locus.[177, 178] This protein, Rev-erbA, is approximately 56 kDa and contains a DNA-binding domain that is homologous to thyroid hormone receptors (see Table 95–5). However, Rev-erbA does not bind thyroid hormone and exhibits relatively low homology to other nuclear receptors in its putative ligand-binding domain. The function of Rev-erbA is unknown and it is currently categorized as an "orphan nuclear receptor." One possibility is that it exerts direct transcriptional control of genes in a manner analogous to other nuclear receptors. Rev-erbA represses some target genes and it interacts with a subset of transcriptional corepressors.[179, 180] Alternatively, because Rev-erbA shares a 269-bp exonic segment of the bidirectionally transcribed TRα gene, it might modulate expression or splicing of TRα1 and TRα2.[181, 182] It is notable that Rev-erbA mRNA cycles rapidly in some tissues with a periodicity of 22.5 hours,[183] although the function of these rapidly changing mRNA levels is unknown.

In contrast to the TRα gene, the splicing variants of the TRβ gene involve the N-terminus of the receptor (see Fig. 95–5). One splicing variant, referred to as TRβ2, is expressed predominantly in the pituitary,[184] hypothalamus,[185, 186] and cochlea.[187] In TRβ2, the N-terminal region of the receptor is distinct, probably reflecting use of a tissue-specific promoter as well as alternate splicing. The function of the N-terminus of the TR is not known. The β1 and β2 isoforms function similarly in most transient gene expression assays.[184, 188] However, differences in the transcriptional activities of the TRβ1 and TRβ2 isoforms have been noted with certain target genes.[189, 190] The significance of the TRβ2 isoform may reflect its expression by a distinct promoter, thereby allowing unique patterns of expression and regulation. As described below, expression of TRβ2 is downregulated by thyroid hormone, whereas expression of TRβ1 is unaffected or increased by thyroid hormone.[168] Thus, expression from the TRβ2 promoter may provide an additional level of thyroid hormone regulation in tissues like the hypothalamus and pituitary that are involved in the control of TSH. It is notable that a large number of N-terminal splicing variants of both TRα and TRβ have been found in *Xenopus*.[191] It is unclear why this degree of TR diversity exists in the frog and not in mammals. However, these findings raise the possibility of unrecognized functions for the N-terminal domain of the receptors. Possibilities include modulation of translational efficiency, interactions with other cellular proteins, promoter-specific expression, and control of receptor turnover.

Regulation of Thyroid Hormone Receptor Expression During Development

The distribution of TRs in adult tissues has been assessed in several species.[82, 168, 192] In general, the α and β receptor isoforms are distributed widely and exhibit overlapping patterns of expression. Spleen and testis are notable for relatively low levels of α1 and β1 receptors, a feature that is consistent with data indicating minimal metabolic responses to thyroid hormone in these tissues. The α2 isoform is highly expressed in many tissues, particularly brain, kidney, and testis. Most studies of receptor isoform expression have involved mRNA analyses and it is possible that expression of the proteins may be different from that predicted by studies of mRNA.[64]

Expression of TRs during development is of great interest in view of the effects of T_3 on cellular differentiation and organogenesis. In particular, the effects of T_3 deficiency on brain maturation have prompted detailed analyses of receptor expression during brain development.[7, 64, 187, 192–194] In the rat, α1 mRNA increases gradually throughout fetal development, peaking in the neonatal period, before declining in the adult. In contrast, β1 mRNA is very low initially, but increases markedly in specific regions of the brain during the neonatal period and there is persistent expression in the adult. Expression of the β receptor correlates temporally with the fetal capacity to make thyroid hormone, but a causal relationship remains to be demonstrated. In addition to its high level of expression in the pituitary gland,[184] β2 mRNA is also expressed in the hypothalamus, hippocampus, and developing striatum.[185, 186, 194]

The patterns of α and β receptor expression in the brain suggest that they may have distinct functions.[7, 194] For example, there is a surge in α1 mRNA expression in cortical neurons that have ceased proliferation, suggesting a possible role in neuronal differentiation. In contrast, β1 mRNA expression is most marked in proliferative zones where a role in neuroblast division has been postulated.[194] The levels of α2 isoform expression are relatively high in brain, but the ratio of α2/α1 is, for the most part, constant during development. Although the patterns of receptor expression are emerging, it remains difficult to propose precise mechanisms for how thyroid hormone deficiency leads to alterations in the central nervous system.[195, 196] As noted above, the expression of other genes that can modify TR action may also play a critical role during development. These include the deiodinases,[22] which can modulate thyroid hormone metabolism, as well as other nuclear receptors, like (COUP-TF) chicken ovalbumin upstream promoter–transcription factor,[197] that could compete for TR interactions with target genes. Models using targeted mutagenesis of the receptors are beginning to shed light on this topic (see below).[198, 199] In particular, there is evidence that the β receptor plays an essential role in development of the auditory system.[198] Identification of T_3-responsive genes in the brain will be an important step for elucidating this process further.[8, 95]

Receptor expression has also been studied extensively during development in *Xenopus laevis*, a species in which thyroid hormone has profound effects on metamorphosis.[1, 2] TRα increases throughout the premetamorphosis stage in the tadpole, reaching maximal levels by prometamorphosis and declining thereafter.[3, 82] In contrast, TRβ expression is very low in premetamorphosis and increases in parallel with endogenous thyroid hormone levels, reaching a peak at metamorphosis. Treatment with exogenous thyroid hormone causes 20-fold induction of TRβ and twofold induction of TRα, suggesting a possible role for autoregulation of TRβ expression by thyroid hormone.[3]

TR expression is also autoregulated by thyroid hormone in mammals, an effect which could have important consequences for biologic responses to T_3.[200] For example, in pituitary GH1 cells, treatment with T_3 decreases receptor number and diminishes T_3-induced GH gene transcription.[201] Thyroid hormone affects expression of the various TR isoforms differentially and in a tissue-specific manner.[168] In most tissues, T_3 causes about a 65% to 70% reduction in TRα1 and TRα2 mRNA levels, whereas expression of TRβ1 is unaffected by T_3. Interestingly, TRα1 and TRα2 levels are not affected by T_3 in brain, a phenomenon that is reminiscent of the diminished metabolic responses in this tissue. Receptor regulation in the pituitary gland is quite different from that in other tissues. In the pituitary, TRβ1 is increased 3.4-fold, TRβ2 is decreased by 43%, and α1 and α2 are decreased by 22% by thyroid hormone. The unique pattern of regulation in the pituitary gland may reflect the presence of TRβ2 and the central role of this tissue in regulating TSH biosynthesis.[190] As in studies of developmental expression, there is little information on T_3-induced changes in the amounts of receptor proteins, but these data should be forthcoming with the availability of isoform-specific antisera.

PHENOTYPIC FEATURES OF MICE DEFICIENT IN TRα OR TRβ

The ability to disrupt genes by targeted mutagenesis provides a powerful strategy for assessing the function of the encoded protein products in vivo (see Chapter 11). In the case of the TRs, this issue is particularly complex because there is more than one gene, there are splicing variants (TRα1, TRα2, TRβ1, TRβ2), and because an additional transcript (Rev-erbA) is derived from the opposite strand of the TRα gene. Moreover, the ability to perform physiologic studies in mice are limited somewhat by their relatively small size. Despite these challenges, remarkable progress has been made toward the creation of these gene knockout models.

Forrest and colleagues[198] disrupted the TRβ locus, creating a mouse deficient in both TRβ1 and TRβ2. These mice reveal functions that specifically require TRβ or are influenced by the total amount of TR in a manner that cannot be compensated by the remaining TRα gene products (Table 95–6). The most striking phenotypic feature in these mice is deafness.[198] Although the cochlea is morphologically normal, additional studies reveal a defect in fast-acting potassium conductance ($I_{K,f}$) in the inner hair cell.[202] An intriguing aspect of these studies is the fact that TRα1 and TRβ exhibit overlapping patterns of expression in the organ of Corti.[194] Thus, the occurrence of deafness in the TRβ-deficient mice, but not in TRα1-deficient mice (see below), suggests that the receptors might elicit specific responses in various target genes. A second major phenotype in these mice is the basal elevation of TSH in conjunction with increased T_4 and T_3.[203, 204] TSH increases when thyroid hormone levels are reduced, indicating that TRβ is not required for this response. On the other hand, thyroid hormone–mediated suppression of TSH is blunted.[204] These features are reminiscent of those seen in patients with resistance to thyroid hormone (RTH) (see below). Indeed, the original report of this disorder, which is most commonly caused by heterozygous, dominant mutations in the TRβ gene, was described in a family with a recessive deletion of the TRβ gene.[205] Members of this family with homozygous deletions of TRβ were deaf and exhibited elevated free thyroid hormone and TSH levels. Thus, the mouse model appears to faithfully replicate some of the features seen in humans who are deficient in TRβ. Other features of the TRβ knockout mice include blunted thyroid hormone induction of alkaline phosphatase, and markedly decreased stimulation of spot 14 and malic enzyme.[206] It is notable that the chronotropic effects of thyroid hormone in the heart, its metabolic effects on energy expenditure, and thyroid hormone–mediated acceleration of myelin basic protein (MBP) and Purkinje cell protein-2 (PCP-2) gene expression are affected minimally by disruption of the TRβ gene.[206, 207]

Targeted disruption of the TRα locus was performed by Wikstrom and colleagues.[199] In this case, the mutation was designed to selectively disrupt expression of TRα1 without altering expression of TRα2, or transcription of Rev-erbA from the opposite strand. TRα1 deficient mice are viable and fertile. In fact, the phenotypic effects of the loss of TRα1 are relatively mild. Unexpectedly, there is no evidence of RTH, as occurs with the TRβ knockout. Rather, thyroid hormone levels are low (32% reduced in males; 16% reduced in females), apparently because of a reduction in expression of the TSH-α gene. In contrast, expression of the TSH-β gene is greater in the TRα1-deficient mice, suggesting potential differences in the mechanism by which TRα1 regulates the TSH subunit genes. As a consequence of these changes in TSH-α and -β gene expression, circulating TSH levels are reduced by about 20% in the TRα1 knockout mice. Disruption of the TRα1 also causes significant changes in cardiac function.[199, 208] These mice have a lower heart rates (19% reduced) and prolonged QRS and Q–T. The cardiac effects are not the consequences of reduced thyroid hormone levels, as they persist after hormone replacement. The molecular basis for these cardiac effects is not known, but the alteration in the Q–T interval is indicative of an effect on ventricular repolarization, a process known to involve multiple ion channels. Thus far, no changes have been found in the levels of known thyroid hormone–responsive genes in the heart (e.g., sarcoplasmic Ca^{2+}, ATPase, Na^+, K^+-ATPase, β-adrenergic receptors).[208] The bradycardic effect of the TRα1 knockout may also reflect alterations in the sympathetic or parasympathetic nervous systems. However, based on pharmacologic studies with adrenergic blockers, it appears to be an intrinsic defect in cardiac myocytes. The TRα1-deficient mice also have a 0.5°C reduction in body temperature that is independent of thyroid hormone levels. The mice have normal amounts of brown adipose tissue and exhibit normal amounts of activity, suggesting that the hypothermia results from alterations in metabolic processes. As summarized in Table 95–6, the phenotypes of the TRα1 and TRβ1 and 2 knockouts are strikingly different, despite their overlapping patterns of expression.

Future studies will examine the effects of selective mutations in the TRα2, TRβ1, or TRβ2 isoforms. It will also be possible, by cross-breeding various knockout lines, to study the consequences of combined deficiencies of TRα and TRβ isoforms. It is notable that severe hypothyroidism causes different, and often more pronounced, physiologic alterations than disruption of the receptor genes. This may reflect the observation in vitro that non–ligand-bound TRs are capable of repressing gene expression.[110, 111] Thus, the absence of hormone may permit receptor-mediated repression, whereas disruption of the receptor is expected to preclude either repression or activation of target genes.

TABLE 95–6. Summary of Phenotypic Traits in Thyroid Hormone Receptor (TR) Knockout Mice

Features	TRα1 Knockout	TRβ1 and TRβ2 Knockout
Thyroid hormone levels	Decreased	Increased
Thyroid-stimulating hormone levels	Mildly decreased	Mildly increased; fail to suppress
Goiter	None	Present
Auditory system	Normal	Deaf
Heart	Bradycardia; prolonged Q–T interval	Normal
Liver enzymes	Unknown	Blunted changes in cholesterol and alkaline phosphatase; markedly reduced responses of malic enzyme and spot 14
Temperature	Decreased	Normal

Data from references 198, 199, 202–204, and 206.

THYROID HORMONE ACTION IS MEDIATED VIA SPECIFIC SEQUENCES IN TARGET GENES

Characterization of Thyroid Hormone Response Elements

In the case of the steroid receptors, high-affinity DNA-binding sites are palindromic,[140] consistent with data showing that the glucocorticoid and estrogen receptors bind to DNA as homodimers.[209, 210] The interactions of the glucocorticoid and estrogen receptors with their respective DNA response elements have been defined by nuclear magnetic resonance (NMR)[211, 212] and x-ray crystallography,[143] confirming that each receptor monomer interacts with one DNA half-site in the palindromic sequence.

Surprisingly, TR interactions with DNA are quite different from those seen with steroid receptors. Although TR can bind to certain TREs as a homodimer, it exhibits preferential binding to most response elements as a heterodimer with other members of the nuclear receptor family, particularly RXRs. This property of TRs has profound implications for the nature of its binding sites, its orientation when bound to DNA, and its ability to exert biologic action in conjunction with heterodimeric partners. Elucidation of TRE-binding sites has been the subject of extensive studies, which have been reviewed.[213]

Initial attempts to define the TREs centered primarily on analyses of the rat growth hormone (rGH) promoter. When the rGH promoter is fused to reporter genes, thyroid hormone stimulates reporter gene activity, indicating that positive TREs (pTREs) are located in this region of the GH gene. The DNA sequences of the GH TRE have been delineated further by extensive mutagenesis studies.[33, 213] This region contains three potential TR-binding half-sites that are related to the hexameric sequence AGGTCA. These three TRE half-sites are arranged as a pair of direct repeats on the left and as a palindromic inverted repeat on the right, with the central element comprising part of each functional element (Fig. 95–7). Mutations in any one of

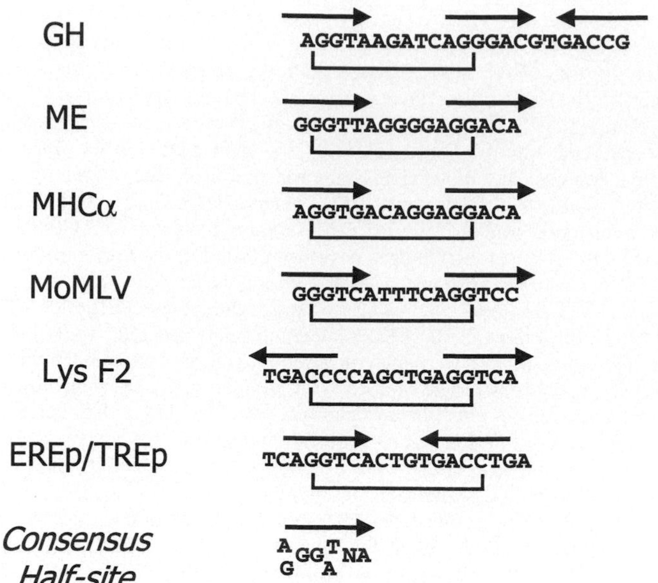

FIGURE 95–7. Sequences of positive thyroid response elements (TREs). Promoter regions involved in thyroid hormone stimulation are shown for several different genes, including rat growth hormone (GH), rat malic enzyme (ME), rat myosin heavy-chain α, Moloney murine leukemia virus (MoMLV), and chicken lysozyme F2 silencer (Lys F2). Although detailed mutagenesis has not been performed for each element, putative TRE half-sites are denoted by *arrows* and a 10-bp interval between pairs of guanines is indicated by *brackets*. A "consensus" TRE half-site sequence is shown at the bottom of the figure. Of note, there is considerable diversity in the sequences of half-sites, orientation of half-sites, and bases that form the spacers between half-sites.

the three half-sites greatly reduces thyroid hormone responsiveness, although mutations in the central element cause the most severe impairment.[85] The functional properties of the TRE mutants correlate well with their binding to TRs.[214]

Subsequent studies of TREs from many other genes reveal a notable lack of sequence conservation among these elements, raising the possibility that native TREs have diverged from the consensus element as a means to modulate the degree of thyroid hormone responsiveness.[85] The sequences of some of these elements are summarized in Figure 95–7. The variations in these sequences affect the affinity of receptor binding, as well as the ability of other nuclear receptors to interact at these sites. Recent studies have used mutagenesis in an attempt to optimize the TR recognition site.[215, 216] Although the TRE half-site has generally been considered to be a hexamer, related to the sequence AGGTCA, binding is optimal with a more extended binding site. Specifically, the sequence TAAGGTCA is optimal for TR binding and T_3 responsiveness. In fact, using artificial reporter genes, a single copy of this optimized element is sufficient for TR function, suggesting that monomeric forms of the receptor may be functional under certain circumstances. Based on the crystal structure of the TR bound to DNA, the 5′-end of the TRE may interact with an α-helical segment at the C-terminal end of the DNA-binding domain.[145]

Surprisingly, the target sequences for several other nuclear receptors are the same or very similar to the TRE. For example, the half-sites for the retinoic acid receptor (RAR), ER, the VDR, and the TR appear to share a similar core consensus hexamer, AGGTCA. A large number of orphan nuclear receptors, such as COUP-TF and steroidogenic factor-1 (SF-1) also bind to sequences similar to this core motif.[139] In contrast, the glucocorticoid receptor (GR), progesterone receptor (PR), and androgen receptor (AR) recognize the half-site AGAACA, which is distinct from the TRE sequence (see Chapter 10).[140] These observations are compatible with the idea that amino acid sequence determinants in the P-box of the DNA-binding domain define interactions with one or the other class of half-sites (see Table 95–5).

Receptor Dimerization and Thyroid Hormone Response Element Half-Site Spacing Are Major Determinants of Receptor Specificity

There is evidence that the TR is capable of binding to half-sites that are arranged in a remarkable array of different configurations. These include palindromic arrangements (head to head), direct repeats (head to tail), as well as inverted repeats (tail to tail). However, most naturally occurring TREs are direct repeats (see Fig. 95–7). The ability of TR dimers to bind to TREs in different orientations raises the possibility of flexible protein structure, or distinct protein surfaces could be involved in the dimeric protein-protein interface. There are naturally occurring examples of each of these TRE configurations. Although the functional consequences of these various response element arrangements are still under investigation, it is notable that some inverted repeats act as TR-mediated silencers in the absence of hormone,[86] whereas most direct repeats function as positive response elements.

Based on inspection of the sequences of naturally occurring response elements for TR, it was proposed that a direct repeat of the TRE half-sites spaced by four nucleotides was optimal. In contrast, the retinoic acid and vitamin D receptors bind to half-sites spaced by 5 or 2 bp, respectively (Fig. 95–8). This concept was dubbed the 3, 4, 5 rule for nuclear receptor specificity to emphasize the importance of the spacing between half-sites as a critical determinant of effective binding by these nuclear receptor heterodimers.[151, 152] Although there are exceptions to this rule, it provides a useful framework for molecular modeling. In addition, the nature of nuclear receptor interaction with the spacer region also confers specificity. Thus, the specificity and affinity for the RXR-TR heterodimer are determined by sequences within the half-site (optimally TAAGGTCA), by the length of the spacer region (optimally 4 bp), and by the sequences within the spacer region.[151–154]

The TR is capable of forming homodimers, analogous to the situation with other members of the steroid receptor family. However, it also interacts with other members of the nuclear receptor family to form heterodimers. An extensive series of studies led to the characterization of the heterodimeric partners for the TR.[217–227] Although TR can interact with a wide variety of other nuclear receptors and transcriptional adapter proteins (see below), the RXR family of proteins are the predominant heterodimeric partner for the TR. There are three different RXR isoforms (α, β, and γ) that are expressed from different genes and have distinct developmental and tissue-specific distributions.[139] Although the RXRs were initially classified as orphan recep-

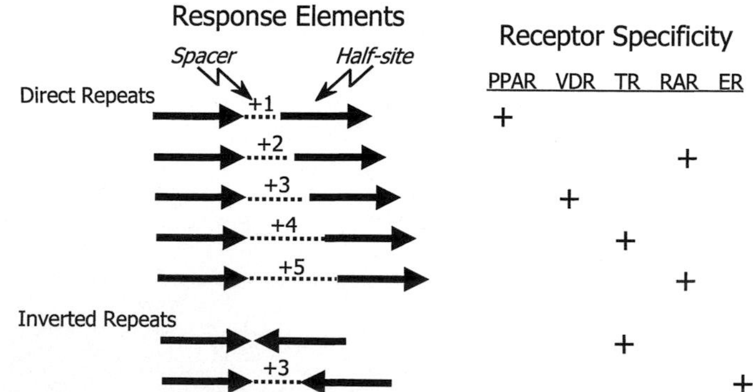

FIGURE 95–8. Nuclear receptor specificity for DNA is defined by the sequences of DNA half-sites and by the spacing between half-sites. Receptor binding to thyroid response elements is dictated by DNA half-sites *(arrows)*, as well as the orientation and spacing between the half-sites. In the idealized example shown, the same half-site (AGGTCA) is arranged as direct repeats or inverted repeats spaced by a variable number of nucleotides. Binding by the peroxisome proliferator–activated receptor (PPAR), vitamin D receptor (VDR), thyroid hormone receptor (TR), retinoic acid receptor (RAR), and estrogen receptor (ER) is depicted by + (see text for details).

tors because they had no apparent ligand, it is now known that these receptors bind the stereoisomer, 9-*cis*-retinoic acid, with high affinity.[228, 229] The RXRs also serve as heterodimeric partners for several other nuclear receptors, including the RARs, the VDR, and the peroxisome-proliferator–activated receptors (PPARs).[139] The role of 9-*cis*-retinoic acid in the transcriptional activity of these heterodimers varies depending on the nuclear receptor partner and the nature of the response element.[230] In the case of the TR, 9-*cis*-retinoic acid potentiates T_3-mediated regulation of some target genes.[231–233] However, the RXR ligand antagonizes the effect of TR, or has little effect on its activity, for other target genes.[234–236] Furthermore, there is little information on the tissue distribution and production of 9-*cis*-retinoic acid in vivo. Additional studies are required to clarify the functional roles of RXRs and their ligands in thyroid hormone action.

Although the functional roles of RXRs are still being defined, there is considerable information on their structural interaction with the TRs. The RXR proteins enhance TR binding to DNA, primarily by reducing the rate of receptor dissociation from DNA.[237] The crystal structure of the DNA-binding domains of the RXR-TR heterodimer bound to a TRE provides considerable insight into the basis for receptor recognition of TREs[145] (Fig. 95–9). Using a direct repeat of the TRE half-site, RXR binds to the 5′-TRE repeat and TR binds to the 3′-TRE repeat.[238, 239] With 4 bp of spacing between the TRE repeats, the centers of the half-sites are 10 bp apart, or nearly one turn of the DNA double helix. Consequently, the DNA-binding domains engage the major grooves of the half-sites on the same face of the DNA. However, the tandem head-to-tail alignment of the half-sites prevents symmetrical protein-protein contacts as are seen for ER-ER or GR-GR homodimers bound to palindromic response elements. In agreement with mutagenesis studies,[239] residues from the second zinc finger of RXR interact with residues of the first zinc finger of the TR. In addition, the C-terminal end of the TR DNA-binding domain forms an α-helical structure that forms extensive interactions with the spacer region in the DNA minor groove between the TRE half-sites. These interactions are important determinants of TR specificity for nucleotides at the 5′-end of the half-site and also for the length of the spacer between the half-sites.

The recognition of the importance of RXR-TR dimers has focused attention on the structural domains that mediate dimerization. Receptor heterodimers form in solution, but are greatly stabilized by binding to DNA.[240] Although the protein-protein contacts described above in the RXR and TR DNA-binding domains are important for aligning the proteins and for mediating DNA interactions, the major forces that govern dimerization reside in the C-terminal ends of the proteins. Mutagenesis studies of this region of the TR initially suggested that a series of conserved hydrophobic sequences might be involved in dimerization.[241] Mutations in some of these residues (e.g., Leu 428 in TRβ) are sufficient to disrupt TR interactions with RXR.[164, 242, 243] However, when the crystal structure of the ligand-binding domain of the TR was solved[141] (see Fig. 95–6), these hydrophobic residues were seen to be buried deep within the protein core, rather than existing on the protein surface where one would expect residues involved in the formation of protein-protein contacts. Consequently, these mutations that disrupt dimerization probably alter protein conformation in a manner that indirectly affects a dimerization interface. Although the dimerization surface of the TR remains to be clearly established, it appears to involve residues that lie along the surfaces of helixes 10 and 11. Whether the same residues that mediate TR-TR homodimerization also mediate RXR-TR heterodimerization is also unknown. T_3 binding appears to facilitate the formation of RXR-TR heterodimers.[244] On the other hand, T_3 dissociates TR-TR homodimers.[245] Assuming that these in vitro observations apply in vivo, these findings suggest that ligand binding might induce disruption of TR homodimers and favor the formation of RXR-TR heterodimers.

The observation that the TR binds to its target sequence as a heterodimer has major implications for physiologic responses to thyroid hormone action. TR action can be influenced potentially by the composition and amounts of RXR proteins, as well as by the presence 9-*cis*-retinoic acid. Moreover, the RXR-TR heterodimer appears to bind preferentially to TREs that are configured as direct repeats, and can therefore influence which target genes are regulated.

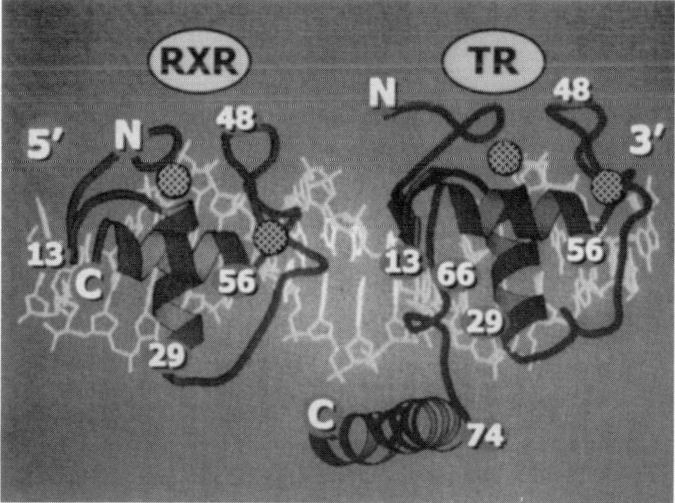

FIGURE 95–9. Structure of the retinoid X receptor (RXR)–thyroid hormone receptor (TR) heterodimer bound to DNA. A ribbon diagram of the x-ray crystal structure of the DNA-binding domains of RXR and TR are shown superimposed on the DNA double helix. The 5′ and 3′ ends of DNA are indicated along with the N-terminal (N) and C-terminal (C) ends of the proteins. Zinc atoms in the zinc fingers are indicated by *hatched circles.* Selected numbered residues are shown in each subunit. (Adapted from Rastinejad F, Perlmann T, Evans RM, Sigler PB: Structural determinants of nuclear receptor assembly on DNA direct repeats. Nature 375:203, 1995.)

ROLE OF TRANSCRIPTIONAL COREPRESSORS AND COACTIVATORS IN THYROID HORMONE RECEPTOR ACTION

The identification of additional proteins that interact with the TR has altered dramatically the concepts of how the TR acts to change gene transcription. These proteins can be classified generally into three groups: (1) corepressors; (2) coactivators; and (3) general transcription factors (GTFs). Many of these factors have been identified based on assays for protein-protein interaction, such as the yeast two-hybrid assay, or by coimmunoprecipitation. There has been remarkably rapid progress in this area, prompting an appropriate degree of caution regarding the interpretation of working models. However, as described below, there is mounting evidence to support the idea that interactions with these cofactors serves, in part, to link TR action to alterations in chromatin structure.[246]

Early studies suggested that in the non–ligand-bound state, the TR repressed basal transcription in proportion to the amount of receptor and the affinity of receptor-binding sites.[110, 111] This property is also referred to as transcriptional silencing.[134] In these experimental systems, the addition of thyroid hormone relieves basal repression and also induces additional transcriptional stimulation relative to that seen in the absence of receptor. These features are illustrated schematically in Figure 95–10.

The mechanism of transcriptional silencing by non–ligand-bound receptor was clarified by the discovery of a family of repressor proteins that bind selectively to the TRs and RARs in the absence of ligand. This corepressor family includes silencing mediator for retinoid and thyroid hormone receptors (SMRT)[247, 248] and nuclear receptor corepressor (NCoR).[249–251] These corepressors, in turn, assemble a repression complex that includes Sin3 and histone deacetylases (HDACs).[252–254] Transcriptional silencing by this receptor-assembled complex is thought to involve chromatin remodeling caused by histone deacetylation (Fig. 95–11). The exact mechanism for this event is not well understood. However, the deacetylation of histones may alter their packing in a manner that forms transcriptionally inactive chromatin. In

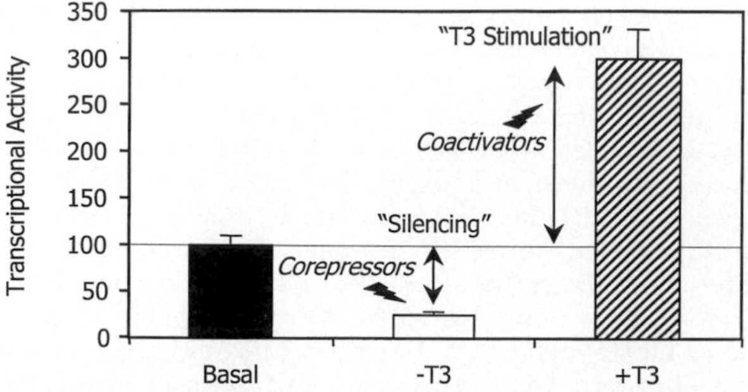

FIGURE 95–10. Thyroid hormone receptor (TR)–mediated silencing and transcriptional activation. In the absence of hormone, the TR silences gene expression in a process that involves interactions with a corepressor complex. Binding of triiodothyronine (T_3) releases corepressors, relieving silencing. T_3 also induces the recruitment of coactivators that mediate transcriptional stimulation.

addition to histones, it is likely that other transcription factors are also targets for acetylation and deacetylation. The repression complex may also function by mechanisms independent of deacetylation.

As noted above, the binding of ligand reverses transcriptional silencing and induces transcriptional activation. When T_3 binds to the receptor, it induces conformational changes that cause dissociation of corepressors. The T_3-bound conformation of the receptor also allows the recruitment of an array of coactivators. Thus, by altering the group of cofactors that bind to the receptor, hormone binding has a dual effect of relieving repression and stimulating transcriptional activation (see Fig. 95–11).

In comparison to the corepressors, many more coactivators have been identified to date. These include steroid receptor coactivator 1 (SRC1),[255] transcriptional intermediary factor 2 (TIF2),[256] glucocorticoid receptor interacting protein 1 (GRIP1),[257] amplified in breast cancer 1 (AIB1),[258] receptor-associated coactivator 3 (RAC3),[259] p300/CBP cointegrator-associated protein (p/CIP),[260] nuclear receptor coactivator (ACTR),[261] thyroid receptor activator molecule 1 (TRAM 1),[262] peroxisome proliferator activated protein–binding protein (PBP),[263] positive cofactors 2 and 4 (PC2, PC4),[264] VDR interacting proteins

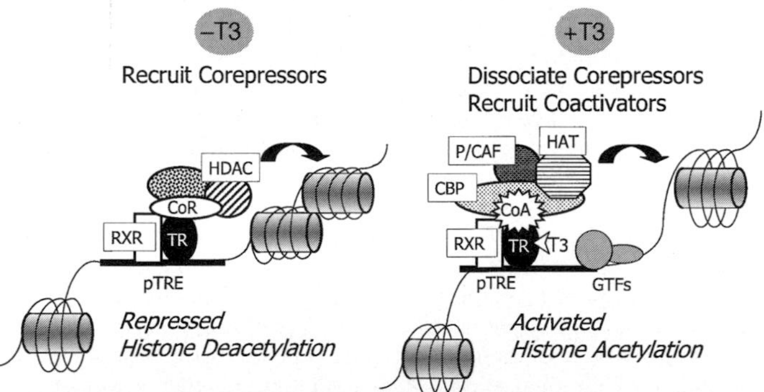

FIGURE 95–11. Role of corepressors and coactivators in the control of triiodothyronine (T_3)-mediated positively regulated genes. A model is presented for how thyroid hormone receptor (TR) interacts with additional proteins to potentially alter chromatin structure, in the context of a positively regulated gene. In the absence of T_3, the retinoid X receptor (RXR)–TR heterodimer recruits corepressors (CoR), which, in turn, assemble additional components of a repressor complex that includes histone deacetylase (HDAC). Deacetylation of histones is postulated to induce transcriptional repression. In the presence of T_3, the corepressor complex dissociates and coactivators (CoA) bind. The coactivator complex can include CREB-binding protein (CBP), p300/CBP-associated factors (P/CAF), and proteins with histone acetyltransferase (HAT) activity. General transcription factors (GTFs) are also indicated. Acetylation of histones is postulated to modify chromatin structure to enhance transcriptional activation.

(DRIPs),[265] p300/CBP-associated factor (p/CAF),[266] cyclic adenosine monophosphate (cAMP) response element–binding protein (CREB), CREB binding protein (CBP),[267] and p300,[268] among others (Table 95–7). The CoAs possess intrinsic histone acetyltransferase (HAT) activity[261, 269–271] and recruit additional HAT enzymes that alter chromatin structure and modulate gene transcription.[272]

The observation that the TR affects the level of gene transcription both in the absence and presence of hormone has important implications for how thyroid hormone exerts its physiologic effects. Rather than acting as a switch that activates a target gene only after thyroid hormone is bound, this model suggests that TR functions more as a modulator of the level of gene expression. For example, at low hormone concentrations as occur in hypothyroidism, the non–ligand-bound receptor is predicted to repress expression in proportion to the amount of expressed receptor and the strength of the TRE sites. On the other hand, at higher concentrations of thyroid hormone, when TRs are more fully occupied by hormone, transcriptional activation would occur. In some respects, the predictions of this model are borne out by the genetic knockout models of TRα and TRβ. The phenotypes of these mice are different, and in many respects less pronounced than the clinical features of hypothyroidism. This may reflect the fact that deletion of the receptor precludes its ability to function as a repressor in the absence of hormone.

UNIQUE ASPECTS OF NEGATIVE REGULATION BY THYROID HORMONE

In contrast to positively regulated genes, the mechanisms that control TR-mediated transcription of negatively regulated genes are not well understood. Because the non–ligand-bound TR also exerts transcriptional repression of positively regulated genes, it is important to further define the concept of a negatively regulated gene. These are genes that are stimulated in the absence of thyroid hormone and repressed in response to the ligand. Examples of negatively regulated genes, such as the TRH or the TSH-α and TSH-β genes, are listed in Table 95–4. Several different mechanisms for T_3-mediated repression have been proposed. And it is possible that different mechanisms apply for various target genes. Proposed mechanisms include competition of nuclear receptors at the binding sites of other transcription factors, receptor binding to so-called negative regulatory elements, direct interactions of nuclear receptors with transcription factors like activating protein 1 (AP-1) or nuclear factor κB (NF-KB), and competition for transcriptional cofactors like CBP.[273]

TABLE 95–7. Transcriptional Coactivators and Corepressors

Cointegrators	*Interacting Proteins*
p300/CBP	Nuclear receptors: (RAR, RXR, ER, TR, PR, GR)
	CREB, c-Fos, c-Jun, JunB, YY1, E1a, SV40 Tag, c-Myb, SRC-1, Sap 1a, STAT2, MyoD, E2F-1, TBP, $TF_{II}B$, p/CAF, $pp90^{RSK}$, Tax, SREBP-2, p53
Coactivators	*Nuclear Receptors*
ARA_{70}	AR
GRIP 95, GRIP 120, GRIP 170	GR
p140 (ERAP 140, RIP 140)	ER, RAR
p160 (ERAP 160, RIP 160)	ER, RAR
SRC-1/Nco-A1	PR, ER, RAR, RXR, TR, GR
Sug 1/Trip 1	TR, RAR, RXR
TIF1	ER, RAR, RXR
TIF2/GRIP1	PR, ER, RAR, RXR
PBP/PC4	TR, PPAR, VDR
Corepressors	*Nuclear Receptors*
NCoR 1	TR, RAR
SMRT	TR, RAR

In the case of the TR, negative regulation of TRH and TSH-α and TSH-β subunit genes have been studied most extensively as models of negatively regulated genes. From a physiologic perspective, negative regulation of these genes represents a critical aspect of feedback control of the thyroid hormone axis. As described above, it is clear that the effect of T_3 on these genes is a direct action of the hormone. The rate of transcription, as measured in nuclear run-on experiments, is decreased within minutes and it is not blocked by treatment with the protein synthesis inhibitor, cycloheximide.[114, 116] The T_3-responsive regions of these negatively regulated genes have been localized to the proximal promoter regions.[108, 109, 119] However, these promoter regions do not contain canonical TRE sequences, and TR binding to potential TREs is relatively weak in comparison to the binding sites in positively regulated genes. These findings have led to the hypothesis that negative regulation might involve receptor interference with the actions of other transcriptions or with the basal transcription apparatus.[274, 275]

The TR has been shown to inhibit the activity of AP-1, a heterodimeric transcription factor composed of Jun and Fos.[231, 276] In this case, there is mutual inhibition such that AP-1 also blocks TR activation of its target genes. T_3-mediated repression of the prolactin promoter has been proposed to occur by preventing AP-1 binding.[106] The TR also interacts with other classes of transcription factors, including NF-1, Oct-1, Sp-1, p53, and Pit-1, a pituitary-specific factor involved in GH and Prl gene expression.[89, 277–280] In the case of the epidermal growth factor (EGF) receptor gene, a negative TRE is located in an upstream region of the promoter and appears to overlap a binding site for the positive transcription factor, Sp-1.[102, 281] Thus, it is possible that the hormone-activated receptor interferes in some manner with the binding or action of Sp-1. By binding to these or other positive transcription factors, the TR may be able to inhibit gene expression in a manner that does not explicitly require receptor binding to DNA. In the case of the alcohol dehydrogenase 3 gene, the TR causes inhibition, probably by blocking access of RARs to their DNA target sites.[282] The COUP-TF, which is a member of the nuclear receptor superfamily, is also able to block TR action by binding to a subset of TREs.[195, 283] Thus, competition for DNA-binding sites among related nuclear receptors may provide an important mechanism for altering gene expression in response to different hormonal signals. Other mechanisms of transcriptional repression may also apply for these and other negatively regulated genes. There is evidence that a negative TRE from the TSH-β gene and the β-amyloid precursor protein resides in an exon downstream of the start site of transcription.[100, 108] These negative TREs bind receptors and may act by occluding the progression of the transcription complex.

It also appears that corepressors and coactivators may be involved in the control of negatively regulated genes. In contrast to the silencing effect of non–ligand-bound TR that is seen with positively regulated genes, corepressors cause basal activation of the TSH and TRH genes in conjunction with non–ligand-bound TRs.[107] In addition, coactivators appear to play a role in T_3-dependent repression of negatively regulated genes.[284] These findings raise the possibility that cofactor-associated changes in histone acetylation, and alterations in chromatin structure, may be involved in negative regulation by TR. A potential model for negative regulation and the role of corepressors and coactivators is depicted in Figure 95–12.

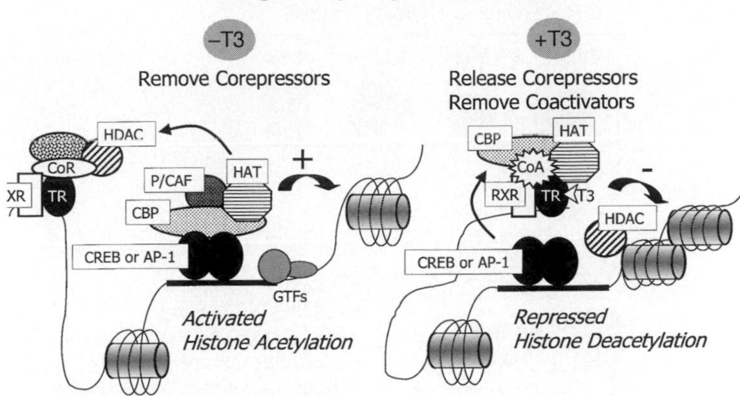

FIGURE 95–12. Role of corepressors and coactivators in the control of triiodothyronine (T_3)-mediated negatively regulated genes. A model is presented for how thyroid hormone receptor (TR) interacts with additional proteins to potentially alter chromatin structure, in the context of a negatively regulated gene. In the absence of T_3, the retinoid X receptor (RXR)–TR heterodimer recruits a corepressor (CoR), including histone deacetylase (HDAC). TR binding of the repressor complex may facilitate acetylation by other transcription factors like cAMP response element–binding protein (CREB) or activating protein 1 (AP-1), which recruit a subset of the coactivator proteins described in Figure 95–11. Acetylation of histones is postulated to modify chromatin structure to enhance transcriptional activation. In the presence of T_3, the corepressor complex dissociates and coactivators (CoA) bind to the TR. This exchange of cofactors may shift the equilibrium to favor chromatin acetylation. Deacetylation of histones is postulated to induce transcriptional repression.

RESISTANCE TO THYROID HORMONE: A DEFECT IN THYROID HORMONE ACTION CAUSED BY MUTATIONS IN TRβ

RTH is characterized by elevated free thyroid hormone levels and inappropriately normal or elevated TSH (assuming that other causes of inappropriate TSH secretion have been excluded). Since the original report, more than 200 cases of RTH have been described.[285–287] An autosomal dominant mode of inheritance is seen in almost all kindreds. Individuals with RTH do not, in general, exhibit signs and symptoms that are typical of hypothyroidism, presumably because the resistant state is compensated by increased levels of thyroid hormone. The clinical features of RTH can include attention-deficit disorder, reduced IQ, delayed skeletal maturation, tachycardia, and altered metabolic responses to thyroid hormone (see Chapter 114).[10, 287, 288]

The availability of the cloned TRs made it possible to demonstrate definitively that RTH is due to a TR abnormality. Mutations in the TRβ gene were initially demonstrated in two different kindreds with amino acid substitutions in the C terminal thyroid hormone binding domain of the receptor.[289, 290] Subsequently, a large number of distinct mutations have been identified in the ligand-binding domain in different kindreds.[286]

Consistent with the autosomal dominant inheritance of RTH, recent studies have shown that mutant β receptors block the activity of normal α and β receptor isoforms when examined in transient gene expression assays.[291, 292] This property is referred to as "dominant negative" activity and represents a novel mechanism for the pathogenesis of an endocrine disease. Several molecular models have been proposed to explain the inhibitory activity of the mutant receptors[292] (Fig. 95–13). Most mutations appear to inactivate the receptor either by reducing thyroid hormone binding or by altering its transactivation properties. As depicted in Figure 95–6, several RTH mutations can be seen to surround the T_3-binding pocket in the x-ray crystal structure of the ligand-binding domain of TR. This figure also shows an example of an RTH mutation of a key residue (Leu 454) involved in transactivation.[284, 293] The dominant negative effects of mutant receptors in RTH were initially thought to result purely from competition between mutant receptors and remaining wild-type α and β receptors. Of note, RTH mutant receptors retain the DNA-binding and receptor dimerization properties, suggesting that their inhibitory effects occur as a result of binding of transcriptionally inactive receptors to target genes.[243, 294] However, more recent studies suggest a previously unappreciated role for corepressors in the inhibitory activity of mutant receptors.[284, 295, 296] The introduction of mutations that disrupt corepressor binding in the background of RTH mutants essentially eliminates the dominant negative effects of these receptors.[295, 297] This finding suggests that the retention of corepressor binding is important, if not necessary, for the dominant negative activity of RTH mutants. As a result of this feature, RTH mutants not only inhibit access of wild-type receptors, but they can also actively silence target genes. These naturally occurring muta-

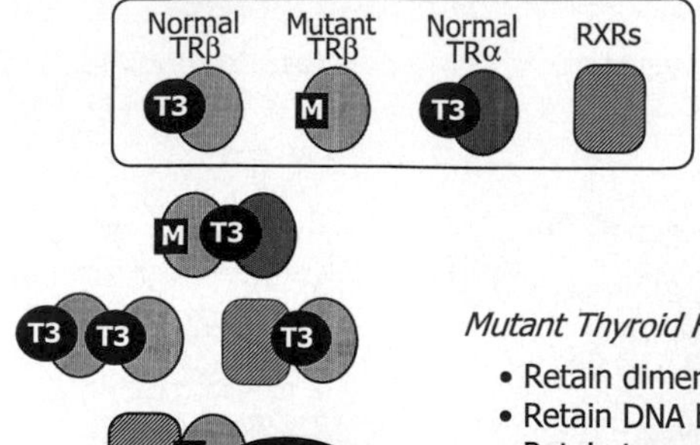

FIGURE 95–13. Mechanism of thyroid hormone resistance (THR) due to mutations in the thyroid hormone receptor (TR). In the autosomal dominant form of resistance to thyroid hormone, mutations occur in the C-terminal ligand-binding domain of TRβ. In this circumstance, the TR genes include one normal and one mutant TRβ allele and two normal TRα alleles. The TRβ mutations disrupt thyroid hormone binding or the transcriptional activity of the receptor to cause inactivation. Because the inactive mutant receptor retains the ability to form dimers and to bind to DNA target sites, it is capable of acting as an antagonist of normal receptors. In addition, the mutant receptors retain binding to corepressor proteins, which causes further inhibition of target genes. This inhibitory property of mutant receptors is referred to as "dominant negative" activity and accounts for expression of THR in the heterozygous state.

tions in the TR have been useful in defining structural domains in the receptor and in confirming their functional importance in vivo.

REFERENCES

1. Gudernatsch JF: Feeding experiments on tadpoles. 1. The influence of specific organs given as food on growth and differentiation. A contribution to the knowledge of organs with internal secretion. Arch Entwickelnde Mech Org 35:457, 1912.
2. Shellabarger CJ, Brown JR: The biosynthesis of thyroxine and 3,5,3′-triiodothyronine in larval and adult toads. J Endocrinol 18:98, 1959.
3. Yaoita Y, Brown DD: A correlation of thyroid hormone receptor gene expression with amphibian metamorphosis. Genes Dev 4:1917–1924, 1990.
4. Barker SB, Klitgaard HM: Metabolism of tissues excised from thyroxine-injected rats. Am J Physiol 170:81–86, 1952.
5. Barker SB, Schwartz HS: Further studies on metabolism of tissues from thyroxine-injected rats. Proc Soc Exp Biol Med 83:500–502, 1953.
6. Farsetti A, Mitsuhashi T, Desvergne B, et al: Molecular basis of thyroid hormone regulation of myelin basic protein gene expression in rodent brain. J Biol Chem 266:23226–23232, 1991.
7. Forrest D, Hallbook F, Persson H, et al: Distinct functions for thyroid hormone receptors alpha and beta in brain development indicated by differential expression of receptor genes. EMBO J 10:269–275, 1991.
8. Munoz A, Rodriguez PA, Perez CA, et al: Effects of neonatal hypothyroidism on rat brain gene expression. Mol Endocrinol 5:273–280, 1991.
9. Zulewski H, Muller B, Exer PM, et al: Estimation of tissue hypothyroidism by a new clinical score: Evaluation of patients with various grades of hypothyroidism and controls. J Clin Endocrinol Metab 82:771–776, 1997.
10. Refetoff S, Weiss RE, Usala SJ: The syndromes of resistance to thyroid hormone. Endocr Rev 14:348–399, 1993.
11. Al-Adsani H, Hoffer LJ, Silva JE: Resting energy expenditure is sensitive to small dose changes in patients on chronic thyroid hormone replacement. J Clin Endocrinol Metab 82:1118–1125, 1997.
12. Ayala AR, Wartofsky L: Minimally symptomatic (subclinical) hypothyroidism. Endocrinologist 7:44–50, 1997.
13. Sawin CT, Geller A, Wolf PA, et al: Low serum thyrotropin concentrations as a risk factor for atrial fibrillation in older persons [see comments]. N Engl J Med 331:1249–1252, 1994.
14. Davis FB, Cody V, Davis PJ, et al: Stimulation by thyroid hormone analogues of red blood cell Ca^{2+}-ATPase activity in vitro. Correlations between hormone structure and biological activity in a human cell system. J Biol Chem 258:12373–12377, 1983.
15. Chaudhury S, Ismail BF, Gick GG, et al: Effect of thyroid hormone on the abundance of Na,K-adenosine triphosphatase alpha-subunit messenger ribonucleic acid. Mol Endocrinol 1:83–89, 1987.
16. Silva JE: Thyroid hormone control of thermogenesis and energy balance. Thyroid 5:481–492, 1995.
17. Sap J, Munoz A, Damm K, et al: The c-erb-A protein is a high-affinity receptor for thyroid hormone. Nature 324:635–640, 1986.
18. Weinberger C, Thompson CC, Ong ES, et al: The *c-erb-A* gene encodes a thyroid hormone receptor. Nature 324:641–646, 1986.
19. Larsen PR, Silva JE, Kaplan MM: Relationships between circulating and intracellular thyroid hormones: Physiological and clinical implications. Endocr Rev 2:87–102, 1981.
20. Berry MJ, Larsen PR: The role of selenium in thyroid hormone action. Endocr Rev 13:207–219, 1992.
21. DeGroot LJ, Larsen PR, Henneman G: The Thyroid and Its Diseases, ed 6. New York, Churchill Livingstone, 1996, p. 793.
22. Kohrle J: Thyroid hormone deiodinases—a selenoenzyme family acting as gate keepers to thyroid hormone action. Acta Med Austriaca 23:17–30, 1996.
23. Selenkow HA, Asper SP: Biological activity of compounds structurally related to thyroxine. Physiol Rev 35:426, 1955.
24. Koerner D, Schwartz HL, Surks MI, et al: Binding of selected iodothyronine analogues to receptor sites of isolated rat hepatic nuclei. High correlation between structural requirements for nuclear binding and biological activity. J Biol Chem 250:6417–6423, 1975.
25. Samuels HH, Stanley F, Casanova J: Relationship of receptor affinity to the modulation of thyroid hormone nuclear receptor levels and growth hormone synthesis by L-triiodothyronine and iodothyronine analogues in cultured GH1 cells. J Clin Invest 63:1229–1240, 1979.
26. Silva JE, Larsen PR: Contributions of plasma triiodothyronine and local thyroxine monodeiodination to triiodothyronine to nuclear triiodothyronine receptor saturation in pituitary, liver, and kidney of hypothyroid rats. Further evidence relating saturation of pituitary nuclear triiodothyronine receptors and the acute inhibition of thyroid-stimulating hormone release. J Clin Invest 61:1247–1259, 1978.
27. Crantz FR, Larsen PR: Rapid thyroxine to 3,5,3′-triiodothyronine conversion and nuclear 3,5,3′-triiodothyronine binding in rat cerebral cortex and cerebellum. J Clin Invest 65:935–938, 1980.
28. Larsen PR, Frumess RD: Comparison of the biological effects of thyroxine and triiodothyronine in the rat. Endocrinology 100:980–988, 1977.
29. Silva JE, Dick TE, Larsen PR: The contribution of local tissue thyroxine monodeiodination to the nuclear 3,5,3′-triiodothyronine in pituitary, liver, and kidney of euthyroid rats. Endocrinology 103:1196–1207, 1978.
30. Burrow GN, Fisher DA, Larsen PR: Maternal and fetal thyroid function. N Engl J Med 331:1072–1078, 1994.
31. Oppenheimer JH, Schwartz HL, Mariash CN, et al: Advances in our understanding of thyroid hormone action at the cellular level. Endocr Rev 8:288–308, 1987.
32. Lazar MA, Chin WW: Nuclear thyroid hormone receptors. J Clin Invest 86:1777–1782, 1990.
33. Brent GA, Moore DD, Larsen PR: Thyroid hormone regulation of gene expression. Annu Rev Physiol 53:17–35, 1991.
34. Lazar M: Thyroid hormone receptors: Multiple forms, multiple possibilities. Endocr Rev 14:184–193, 1993.
35. Brent GA: The molecular basis of thyroid hormone action. N Engl J Med 331:847–853, 1994.
36. Glass CK: Differential recognition of target genes by nuclear receptor monomers, dimers, and heterodimers. Endocr Rev 15:391–407, 1994.
37. Davis PJ, Davis FB: Nongenomic actions of thyroid hormone. Thyroid 6:497–504, 1996.
38. Segal J, Ingbar SH: Specific binding sites for the triiodothyronine in the plasma membrane of rat thymocytes. Correlation with biochemical responses. J Clin Invest 70:919–926, 1982.
39. Osty J, Valensi P, Samson M, et al: Transport of thyroid hormones by human erythrocytes: Kinetic characterization in adults and newborns. J Clin Endocrinol Metab 71:1589–1595, 1990.
40. Segal J, Ingbar SH: 3,5,3′-Triiodothyronine increases cellular adenosine 3′,5′-monophosphate concentration and sugar uptake in rat thymocytes by stimulating adenylate cyclase activity: Studies with the adenylate cyclase inhibitor MDL 12330A. Endocrinology 124:2166–2171, 1989.
41. Segal J, Ingbar SH: In vivo stimulation of sugar uptake in rat thymocytes. An extranuclear action of 3,5,3′-triiodothyronine. J Clin Invest 76:1575–1580, 1985.
42. Oppenheimer JH, Schwartz HL: Stereospecific transport of triiodothyronine from plasma to cytosol and from cytosol to nucleus in rat liver, kidney, brain, and heart. J Clin Invest 75:147–154, 1985.
43. Sterling K: Direct thyroid hormone activation of mitochondria: The role of adenine nucleotide translocase. Endocrinology 119:292–295, 1986.
44. Ashizawa K, Fukuda T, Cheng SY: Transcriptional stimulation by thyroid hormone of a cytosolic thyroid hormone binding protein which is homologous to a subunit of pyruvate kinase M1. Biochemistry 31:2774–2778, 1992.
45. Leonard JL, Silva JE, Kaplan MM, et al: Acute posttranscriptional regulation of cerebrocortical and pituitary iodothyronine 5′-deiodinases by thyroid hormone. Endocrinology 114:998–1004, 1984.
46. Farwell AP, DiBenedetto DJ, Leonard JL: Thyroxine targets different pathways of internalization of type II iodothyronine 5′-deiodinase in astrocytes. J Biol Chem 268:5055–5062, 1993.
47. Horiuchi R, Johnson ML, Willingham MC, et al: Affinity labeling of the plasma membrane 3,3′,5-triiodo-L-thyronine receptor in GH3 cells. Proc Natl Acad Sci U S A 79:5527–5531, 1982.
48. Angel RC, Botta JA, Farias RN: High affinity L-triiodothyronine binding to right-side-out and inside-out vesicles from rat and human erythrocyte membrane. J Biol Chem 264:19143–19146, 1989.
49. Rohrer D, Dillmann WH: Thyroid hormone markedly increases the mRNA coding for sarcoplasmic reticulum Ca^{2+}-ATPase in the rat heart. J Biol Chem 263:6941–6944, 1988.
50. Cheng SY, Gong QH, Parkison C, et al: The nucleotide sequence of a human cellular thyroid hormone binding protein present in endoplasmic reticulum. J Biol Chem 262:11221–11227, 1987.
51. Cheng S-Y, Hasumura S, Willingham MC, et al: Purification and characterization of a membrane-associated 3,3′,5-triiodo-L-thyronine binding protein from a human carcinoma cell line. Proc Natl Acad Sci U S A 83:947–951, 1986.

52. Kato H, Fukuda T, Parkison C, et al: Cytosolic thyroid hormone–binding protein is a monomer of pyruvate kinase. Proc Natl Acad Sci U S A 86:7861–7865, 1989.
53. Leonard JL, Kaplan MM, Visser TJ, et al: Cerebral cortex responds rapidly to thyroid hormones. Science 214:571–573, 1981.
54. Yoneda K, Takasu N, Higa S, et al: Direct effects of thyroid hormones on rat coronary artery: Nongenomic effects of triiodothyronine and thyroxine. Thyroid 8:609–613, 1998.
55. Novitzky D: Novel actions of thyroid hormone: The role of triiodothyronine in cardiac transplantation. Thyroid 6:531–536, 1996.
56. Jeevanandam V: Triiodothyronine: Spectrum of use in heart transplantation. Thyroid 7:139–145, 1997.
57. Klemperer JD, Klein I, Gomez M, et al: Thyroid hormone treatment after coronary-artery bypass surgery. N Engl J Med 333:1522–1527, 1995.
58. Gomberg-Maitland M, Frishman WH: Thyroid hormone and cardiovascular disease. Am Heart J 135:187–196, 1998.
59. Tata JR, Widnell CC: Ribonucleic acid synthesis during the early action of thyroid hormone. Biochem J 98:604–620, 1966.
60. Schadlow AR, Surks MI, Schwartz HL, et al: Specific triiodothyronine binding sites in the anterior pituitary of the rat. Science 176:1252–1254, 1972.
61. Samuels HH, Tsai JS, Casanova J, et al: Thyroid hormone action: In vitro characterization of solubilized nuclear receptors from rat liver and cultured GH1 cells. J Clin Invest 54:853–865, 1974.
62. Schwartz HL, Trence D, Oppenheimer JH, et al: Distribution and metabolism of L- and D-triiodothyronine (T_3) in the rat: Preferential accumulation of L-T_3 by hepatic and cardiac nuclei as a probable explanation of the differential biologic potency of T_3 enantiomers. Endocrinology 113:1236–1243, 1983.
63. Oppenheimer JH, Schwartz HL, Surks MI: Tissue differences in the concentration of triiodothyronine nuclear binding sites in the rat: Liver, kidney, pituitary, heart, brain, spleen, testis. Endocrinology 95:897–903, 1974.
64. Strait KA, Schwartz HL, Perez-Castillo A, et al: Relationship of c-erbA mRNA content to tissue triiodothyronine nuclear binding capacity and function in developing and adult rats. J Biol Chem 265:10514–10521, 1990.
65. Spindler SR, MacLeod KM, Ring J, et al: Thyroid hormone receptors: Binding characteristics and lack of hormonal dependency for nuclear localization. J Biol Chem 250:4113–4119, 1975.
66. MacLeod KM, Baxter JD: Chromatin receptors for thyroid hormones: Interactions of the solubilized proteins with DNA. J Biol Chem 251:7380–7387, 1976.
67. Jump DB, Seelig S, Schwartz HL, et al: Association of thyroid hormone receptor with rat liver chromatin. Biochemistry 20:6781–6789, 1981.
68. Perlman AJ, Stanley F, Samuels HH: Thyroid hormone nuclear receptor: Evidence for multimeric organization in chromatin. J Biol Chem 257:930–938, 1982.
69. Pascual A, Casanova J, Samuels HH: Photoaffinity labeling of thyroid hormone nuclear receptors in intact cells. J Biol Chem 257:9640–9647, 1982.
70. Casanova J, Horowitz ZD, Copp RP, et al: Photoaffinity labeling of thyroid hormone nuclear receptors. Influence of *n*-butyrate and analysis of the half-lives of the 57,000 and 47,000 molecular weight receptor forms. J Biol Chem 259:12084–12091, 1984.
71. Latham KR, Ring JC, Baxter JD: Solubilized nuclear "receptors" for thyroid hormones: Physical characteristics and binding properties, evidence for multiple forms. J Biol Chem 251:7388–7387, 1976.
72. Ichikawa K, DeGroot LJ: Purification and characterization of rat liver nuclear thyroid hormone receptors. Proc Natl Acad Sci U S A 84:3420–3424, 1987.
73. Hennemann G, Krenning EP, Polhuys M, et al: Carrier-mediated transport of thyroid hormone into rat hepatocytes is rate-limiting in total cellular uptake and metabolism. Endocrinology 119:1870–1872, 1986.
74. Blondeau JP, Osty J, Francon J: Characterization of the thyroid hormone transport system of isolated hepatocytes. J Biol Chem 263:2685–2692, 1988.
75. Lakshmanan M, Goncalves E, Lessly G, et al: The transport of thyroxine into mouse neuroblastoma cells, NB41A3: the effect of L-system amino acids. Endocrinology 126:3245–3250, 1990.
76. Zhou Y, Samson M, Osty J, et al: Evidence for a close link between the thyroid hormone transport system and the aromatic amino acid transport system T in erythrocytes. J Biol Chem 265:17000–17004, 1990.
77. Freake HC, Mooradian AD, Schwartz HL, et al: Stereospecific transport of triiodothyronine to cytoplasm and nucleus in GH1 cells. Mol Cell Endocrinol 44:25–35, 1986.
78. Samuels HH, Forman BM, Horowitz ZD, et al: Regulation of gene expression by thyroid hormone. J Clin Invest 81:957–967, 1988.
79. Chin WW: Molecular mechanisms of thyroid hormone action. Thyroid 4:389–393, 1994.
80. Simonet WS, Ness GC: Transcriptional and posttranscriptional regulation of rat hepatic 3-hydroxy-3-methylglutaryl-coenzyme A reductase by thyroid hormones. J Biol Chem 263:12448–12453, 1988.
81. Strobl W, Gorder NL, Lin LY, et al: Role of thyroid hormones in apolipoprotein A-I gene expression in rat liver. J Clin Invest 85:659–667, 1990.
82. Kanamori A, Brown DD: The regulation of thyroid hormone receptor beta genes by thyroid hormone in *Xenopus laevis*. J Biol Chem 267:739–745, 1992.
83. Bahouth SW, Cui X, Beauchamp MJ, et al: Thyroid hormone induces β_1-adrenergic receptor gene transcription through a direct repeat separated by five nucleotides. J Mol Cell Cardiol 29:3223–3237, 1997.
84. Xiong S, Chirala SS, Hsu MH, et al: Identification of thyroid hormone response elements in the human fatty acid synthase promoter. Proc Natl Acad Sci U S A 95:12260–12265, 1998.
85. Brent GA, Harney JW, Chen Y, et al: Mutations of the rat growth hormone promoter which increase and decrease response to thyroid hormone define a consensus thyroid hormone response element. Mol Endocrinol 3:1996–2004, 1989.
86. Baniahmad A, Steiner C, Kohne AC, et al: Modular structure of a chicken lysozyme silencer: Involvement of an unusual thyroid hormone receptor binding site. Cell 61:505–514, 1990.
87. Desvergne B, Petty KJ, Nikodem VM: Functional characterization and receptor binding studies of the malic enzyme thyroid hormone response element. J Biol Chem 266:1008–1013, 1991.
88. Sap J, Munoz A, Schmitt J, et al: Repression of transcription mediated at a thyroid hormone response element by the *v-erb-A* oncogene product. Nature 340:242–244, 1989.
89. Qi JS, Yuan Y, Desai-Yajnik V, et al: Regulation of the *mdm2* oncogene by thyroid hormone receptor. Mol Cell Biol 19:864–872, 1999.
90. Tsika RW, Bahl JJ, Leinwand LA, et al: Thyroid hormone regulates expression of a transfected human alpha-myosin heavy-chain fusion gene in fetal rat heart cells. Proc Natl Acad Sci U S A 87:379–383, 1990.
91. Rodriguez-Manzaneque JC, Perez-Castillo A, Santos A: Control by thyroid hormone of NGFI-A gene expression in lung: Regulation of NGFI-A promoter activity. Mol Cell Endocrinol 141:101–110, 1998.
92. Adan RA, Cox JJ, van Kats JP, et al: Thyroid hormone regulates the oxytocin gene. J Biol Chem 267:3771–3777, 1992.
93. Giralt M, Park EA, Gurney AL, et al: Identification of a thyroid hormone response element in the phosphoenolpyruvate carboxykinase (GTP) gene. Evidence for synergistic interaction between thyroid hormone and cAMP *cis*-regulatory elements. J Biol Chem 266:21991–21996, 1991.
94. Garcia-Fernandez LF, Urade Y, Hayaishi O, et al: Identification of a thyroid hormone response element in the promoter region of the rat lipocalin-type prostaglandin D synthase (beta-trace) gene. Brain Res Mol Brain Res 55:321–330, 1998.
95. Martinez de Arrieta C, Morte B, Coloma A, et al: The human RC3 gene homolog, NRGN contains a thyroid hormone–responsive element located in the first intron. Endocrinology 140:335–343, 1999.
96. Simonides WS, Brent GA, Thelen MH, et al: Characterization of the promoter of the rat sarcoplasmic endoplasmic reticulum Ca^{2+}-ATPase 1 gene and analysis of thyroid hormone responsiveness. J Biol Chem 271:32048–32056, 1996.
97. Zilz ND, Murray MB, Towle HC: Identification of multiple thyroid hormone response elements located far upstream from the rat S14 promoter. J Biol Chem 265:8136–8143, 1990.
98. Jakobs TC, Schmutzler C, Meissner J, et al: The promoter of the human type I 5′-deiodinase gene—mapping of the transcription start site and identification of a DR+4 thyroid-hormone–responsive element. Eur J Biochem 247:288–297, 1997.
99. Rabelo R, Reyes C, Schifman A, et al: Interactions among receptors, thyroid hormone response elements, and ligands in the regulation of the rat uncoupling protein gene expression by thyroid hormone. Endocrinology 137:3478–3487, 1996.
100. Belandia B, Latasa MJ, Villa A, et al: Thyroid hormone negatively regulates the transcriptional activity of the beta-amyloid precursor protein gene. J Biol Chem 273:30366–30371, 1998.
101. Chang L, Wei LN: Characterization of a negative response DNA element in the upstream region of the cellular retinoic acid-binding protein-I gene of the mouse. J Biol Chem 272:10144–10150, 1997.
102. Hudson LG, Santon JB, Glass CK, et al: Ligand-activated thyroid hormone and retinoic acid receptors inhibit growth factor receptor promoter expression. Cell 62:1165–1175, 1990.
103. Ojamaa K, Klemperer JD, MacGilvray SS, et al: Thyroid hormone and hemodynamic regulation of beta-myosin heavy chain promoter in the heart. Endocrinology 137:802–808, 1996.
104. He H, Chin S, Zhuang K, et al: Negative regulation of the rat Na-K-ATPase alpha 3-subunit gene promoter by thyroid hormone. Am J Physiol 271:C1750–1756, 1996.
105. Chu R, Madison LD, Lin Y, et al: Thyroid hormone (T_3) inhibits ciprofibrate-induced transcription of genes encoding beta-oxidation enzymes: Cross talk between peroxisome proliferator and T_3 signaling pathways. Proc Natl Acad Sci U S A 92:11593–11597, 1995.
106. Pernasetti F, Caccavelli L, Van de Weerdt C, et al: Thyroid hormone inhibits the human prolactin gene promoter by interfering with activating protein-1 and estrogen stimulations. Mol Endocrinol 11:986–996, 1997.
107. Tagami T, Madison LD, Nagaya T, et al: Nuclear receptor corepressors activate rather than suppress basal transcription of genes that are negatively regulated by thyroid hormone. Mol Cell Biol 17:2642–2648, 1997.
108. Bodenner DL, Mroczynski MA, Weintraub BD, et al: A detailed functional and structural analysis of a major thyroid hormone inhibitory element in the human thyrotropin beta-subunit gene. J Biol Chem 266:21666–21673, 1991.
109. Hollenberg AN, Monden T, Flynn TR, et al: The human thyrotropin-releasing hormone gene is regulated by thyroid hormone through two distinct classes of negative thyroid hormone response elements. Mol Endocrinol 9:540–550, 1995.
110. Brent GA, Dunn MK, Harney JW, et al: Thyroid hormone aporeceptor represses T3-inducible promoters and blocks activity of the retinoic acid receptor. New Biol 1:329–336, 1989.
111. Damm K, Thompson CC, Evans RM: Protein encoded by *v-erbA* functions as a thyroid-hormone receptor antagonist. Nature 339:593–597, 1989.
112. Shibata H, Spencer TE, Onate SA, et al: Role of co-activators and co-repressors in the mechanism of steroid/thyroid receptor action. Recent Prog Horm Res 52:141–164, 1997.
113. Chin WW, Shupnik MA, Ross DS, et al: Regulation of the alpha and thyrotropin beta-subunit messenger ribonucleic acids by thyroid hormones. Endocrinology 116:873–878, 1985.
114. Shupnik MA, Ardisson LJ, Meskell MJ, et al: Triiodothyronine (T_3) regulation of thyrotropin subunit gene transcription is proportional to T_3 nuclear receptor occupancy. Endocrinology 118:367–371, 1986.
115. Shupnik MA, Chin WW, Habener JF, et al: Transcriptional regulation of the thyrotropin subunit genes by thyroid hormone. J Biol Chem 260:2900–2903, 1985.
116. Shupnik MA, Ridgway EC: Thyroid hormone control of thyrotropin gene expression in rat anterior pituitary cells. Endocrinology 121:619–624, 1987.
117. Burnside J, Darling DS, Carr FE, et al: Thyroid hormone regulation of the rat glycoprotein hormone alpha-subunit gene promoter activity. J Biol Chem 264:6886–6891, 1989.

118. Carr FE, Burnside J, Chin WW: Thyroid hormones regulate rat thyrotropin beta gene promoter activity expressed in GH3 cells. Mol Endocrinol 3:709–716, 1989.
119. Chatterjee VKK, Lee JK, Rentoumis A, et al: Negative regulation of the thyroid-stimulating hormone alpha gene by thyroid hormone: Receptor interaction adjacent to the TATA box. Proc Natl Acad Sci U S A 86:9114–9118, 1989.
120. Wondisford FE, Farr EA, Radovick S, et al: Thyroid hormone inhibition of human thyrotropin beta-subunit gene expression is mediated by a *cis*-acting element located in the first exon. J Biol Chem 264:14601–14604, 1989.
121. Wood WM, Kao MY, Gordon DF, et al: Thyroid hormone regulates the mouse thyrotropin beta-subunit gene promoter in transfected primary thyrotropes. J Biol Chem 264:14840–14847, 1989.
122. Hervas F, Morreale de Escobar G, Escobar Del Ray F: Rapid effects of single small doses of L-thyroxine and triiodo-L-thyronine on growth hormone as studied in the rat by radioimmunoassay. Endocrinology 97:91–101, 1975.
123. Samuels HH, Shapiro LE: Thyroid hormone stimulates *de novo* growth hormone synthesis in cultured GH1 cells: Evidence for the accumulation of a rate limiting RNA species in the induction process. Proc Natl Acad Sci U S A 73:3369–3373, 1976.
124. Wolf M, lngbar SH, Moses AC: Thyroid hormone and growth hormone interact to regulate insulin-like growth factor-I messenger ribonucleic acid and circulating levels in the rat. Endocrinology 125:2905–2914, 1989.
125. Harakawa S, Yamashita S, Tobinaga T, et al: In vivo regulation of hepatic insulin-like growth factor-1 messenger ribonucleic acids with thyroid hormone. Endocrl J 37:205–211, 1990.
126. Balkman C, Ojamaa K, Klein I: Time course of the in vivo effects of thyroid hormone on cardiac gene expression. Endocrinology 130:2001–2006, 1992.
127. Martial JA, Baxter JD, Goodman HM, et al: Regulation of growth hormone messenger RNA by thyroid and glucocorticoid hormones. Proc Natl Acad Sci U S A 74:1816–1820, 1977.
128. Evans RM, Birnberg NC, Rosenfeld MG: Glucocorticoids and thyroid hormones transcriptionally regulate growth hormone gene expression. Proc Natl Acad Sci U S A 79:7659–7663, 1982.
129. Spindler SR, Mellon SH, Baxter JD: Growth hormone gene transcription is regulated by thyroid and glucocorticoid hormones in cultured rat pituitary tumor cells. J Biol Chem 257:11627–11632, 1982.
130. Stapleton SR, Mitchell DA, Salati LM, et al: Triiodothyronine stimulates transcription of the fatty acid synthase gene in chick embryo hepatocytes in culture. Insulin and insulin-like growth factor amplify that effect. J Biol Chem 265:18442–18446, 1990.
131. Swierczynski J, Mitchell DA, Reinhold DS, et al: Triiodothyronine-induced accumulations of malic enzyme, fatty acid synthase, acetyl-coenzyme A carboxylase, and their mRNAs are blocked by protein kinase inhibitors. Transcription is the affected step. J Biol Chem 266:17459–17466, 1991.
132. Mariash CN, Seelig S, Schwartz HL, et al: Rapid synergistic interaction between thyroid hormone and carbohydrate on mRNAS14 induction. J Biol Chem 261:9583–9586, 1986.
133. Zenke M, Munoz A, Sap J, et al: *v-erbA* oncogene activation entails the loss of hormone-dependent regulator activity of c-erbA. Cell 61:1035–1049, 1990.
134. Baniahmad A, Kohne AC, Renkawitz R: A transferable silencing domain is present in the thyroid hormone receptor, in the *v-erbA* oncogene product and in the retinoic acid receptor. EMBO J 11:1015–1023, 1992.
135. Damm K, Evans RM: Identification of a domain required for oncogenic activity and transcriptional suppression by *v-erbA* and thyroid-hormone receptor alpha. Proc Natl Acad Sci U S A 90:10668–10672, 1993.
136. Busch K, Martin B, Baniahmad A, et al: At least three subdomains of *v-erbA* are involved in its silencing function. Mol Endocrinol 11:379–389, 1997.
137. Thompson CC, Weinberger C, Lebo R, et al: Identification of a novel thyroid hormone receptor expressed in the mammalian central nervous system. Science 237:1610–1614, 1987.
138. Drabkin H, Kao FT, Hartz J, et al: Localization of human ERBA2 to the 3p22–3p24.1 region of chromosome 3 and variable deletion in small cell lung cancer. Proc Natl Acad Sci U S A 85:9258–9262, 1988.
139. Mangelsdorf D, Evans R: The RXR heterodimers and orphan receptors. Cell 83:841–850, 1995.
140. Mangelsdorf DJ, Thummel C, Beato M, et al: The nuclear receptor superfamily: The second decade. Cell 83:835–839, 1995.
141. Wagner RL, Apriletti JW, McGrath ME, et al: A structural role for hormone in the thyroid hormone receptor. Nature 378:690–697, 1995.
142. Feng W, Ribeiro RC, Wagner RL, et al: Hormone-dependent coactivator binding to a hydrophobic cleft on nuclear receptors. Science 280:1747–1749, 1998.
143. Luisi BF, Xu WX, Otwinowski Z, et al: Crystallographic analysis of the interaction of the glucocorticoid receptor with DNA. Nature 352:497–505, 1991.
144. Gronemeyer H, Moras D: Nuclear receptors. How to finger DNA. Nature 375:190–191, 1995.
145. Rastinejad F, Perlmann T, Evans RM, et al: Structural determinants of nuclear receptor assembly on DNA direct repeats. Nature 375:203–211, 1995.
146. Mader S, Kumar V, de VH, et al: Three amino acids of the oestrogen receptor are essential to its ability to distinguish an oestrogen from a glucocorticoid-responsive element. Nature 338:271–274, 1989.
147. Umesono K, Evans RM: Determinants of target gene specificity for steroid/thyroid hormone receptors. Cell 57:1139–1146, 1989.
148. Nelson CC, Fans JS, Hendy SC, et al: Functional analysis of the amino acids in the DNA recognition alpha-helix of the human thyroid hormone receptor. Mol Endocrinol 7:1185–1195, 1993.
149. Nelson CC, Hendy SC, Faris JS, et al: The effects of P-box substitutions in thyroid hormone receptor on DNA binding specificity. Mol Endocri 8:829–840, 1994.
150. Nelson CC, Hendy SC, Romaniuk PJ: Relationship between P-box amino acid sequence and DNA binding specificity of the thyroid hormone receptor. The effects of sequences flanking half-sites in thyroid hormone response elements. J Biol Chem 270:16988–16994, 1995.
151. Näär A, Boutin J, Lipkin SM, et al: The orientation and spacing of core DNA-binding motifs dictate selective transcriptional responses to three nuclear receptors. Cell 65:1267–1279, 1991.
152. Umesono K, Murakami KK, Thompson CC, et al: Direct repeats as selective response elements for the thyroid hormone, retinoic acid, and vitamin D receptors. Cell 65:1255–1266, 1991.
153. Katz RW, Subauste JS, Koenig RJ: The interplay of half-site sequence and spacing on the activity of direct repeat thyroid hormone response elements. J Biol Chem 270:5238–5242, 1995.
154. Tagami T, Kopp P, Johnson W, et al: The thyroid hormone receptor variant alpha2 is a weak antagonist because it is deficient in interactions with nuclear receptor corepressors. Endocrinology 139:2535–2544, 1998.
155. Izumo S, Mahdavi V: Thyroid hormone receptor alpha isoforms generated by alternative splicing differentially activate myosin HC gene transcription. Nature 334:539–542, 1988.
156. Lazar MA, Hodin RA, Darling DS, et al: Identification of a rat c-erbAα-related protein which binds deoxyribonucleic acid but does not bind thyroid hormone. Mol Endocrinol 2:893–901, 1988.
157. Mitsuhashi T, Tennyson GE, Nikodem VM: Alternative splicing generates messages encoding rat c-erbA proteins that do not bind thyroid hormone. Proc Natl Acad Sci U S A 85:5804–5808, 1988.
158. Nakai A, Seino S, Sakurai A, et al: Characterization of a thyroid hormone receptor expressed in human kidney and other tissues. Proc Natl Acad Sci U S A 85:2781–2785, 1988.
159. Schueler PA, Schwartz HL, Strait KA, et al: Binding of 3,5,3′-triiodothyronine (T_3) and its analogs to the in vitro translational products of *c-erbA* protooncogenes: Differences in the affinity of the α and β forms for the acetic acid analog and failure of the human testis and kidney products to bind T_3. Mol Endocrinol 4:227–234, 1990.
160. Koenig RJ, Lazar MA, Hodin RA, et al: Inhibition of thyroid hormone action by a non-hormone binding c-erbA protein generated by alternative mRNA splicing. Nature 337:659–661, 1989.
161. Lazar MA, Hodin RA, Chin WW: Human carboxy-terminal variant of α-type c-erbA inhibits trans-activation by thyroid hormone receptors without binding thyroid hormone. Proc Natl Acad Sci U S A 86:7771–7774, 1989.
162. Rentoumis A, Chatterjee VKK, Madison LD, et al: Negative and positive transcriptional regulation by thyroid hormone receptor isoforms. Mol Endocrinol 4:1522–1531, 1990.
163. Katz D, Berrodin TJ, Lazar MA: The unique C-termini of the thyroid hormone receptor variant, c-erbAα2, and thyroid hormone receptor α1 mediate different DNA-binding and heterodimerization properties. Mol Endocrinol 6:805–814, 1992.
164. Nagaya T, Jameson JL: Distinct dimerization domains provide antagonist pathways for thyroid hormone receptor action. J Biol Chem 268:24278–24282, 1993.
165. Yang YZ, Burgos-Trinidad M, Wu Y, et al: Thyroid hormone receptor variant alpha2. Role of the ninth heptad in DNA binding, heterodimerization with retinoid X receptors, and dominant negative activity. J Biol Chem 271:28235–28242, 1996.
166. Santos A, Freake HC, Rosenberg ME, et al: Triiodothyronine nuclear binding capacity in rat tissues correlates with a 6.0 kilobase (kb) and not a 2.6 kb messenger ribonucleic acid hybridization signal generated by a human c-erbA probe. Mol Endocrinol 2:992–998, 1988.
167. Mitsuhashi T, Nikodem VM: Regulation of expression of the alternative mRNAs of the rat alpha-thyroid hormone receptor gene. J Biol Chem 264:8900–8904, 1989.
168. Hodin RA, Lazar MA, Chin WW: Differential and tissue-specific regulation of the multiple rat c-erbA messenger RNA species by thyroid hormone. J Clin Invest 85:101–105, 1990.
169. Farsetti A, Lazar J, Phyillaier M, et al: Active repression by thyroid hormone receptor splicing variant alpha2 requires specific regulatory elements in the context of native triiodothyronine-regulated gene promoters. Endocrinology 138:4705–4712, 1997.
170. Katz D, Lazar MA: Dominant negative activity of an endogenous thyroid hormone receptor variant (alpha 2) is due to competition for binding sites on target genes. J Biol Chem 268:20904–20910, 1993.
171. Reginato MJ, Zhang J, Lazar MA: DNA-independent and DNA-dependent mechanisms regulate the differential heterodimerization of the isoforms of the thyroid hormone receptor with retinoid X receptor. J Biol Chem 271:28199–28205, 1996.
172. Liu RT, Suzuki S, Miyamoto T, et al: The dominant negative effect of thyroid hormone receptor splicing variant alpha 2 does not require binding to a thyroid response element. Mol Endocrinol 9:86–95, 1995.
173. Meier-Heusler SC, Zhu X, Juge-Aubry C, et al: Modulation of thyroid hormone action by mutant thyroid hormone receptors, c-erbA alpha 2 and peroxisome proliferator-activated receptor: Evidence for different mechanisms of inhibition. Mol Cell Endocrinol 107:55–66, 1995.
174. Bigler J, Eisenman RN: *c-erbA* encodes multiple proteins in chicken erythroid cells. Mol Cell Biol 8:4155–4161, 1988.
175. Forman BM, Yang CR, Au M, et al: A domain containing leucine-zipper-like motifs mediate novel in vivo interactions between the thyroid hormone and retinoic acid receptors. Mol Endocrinol 3:1610–1626, 1989.
176. Bigler J, Hokanson W, Eisenman RN: Thyroid hormone receptor transcriptional activity is potentially autoregulated by truncated forms of the receptor. Mol Cell Biol 12:2406–2417, 1992.
177. Lazar MA, Hodin RA, Darling DS, et al: A novel member of the thyroid/steroid hormone receptor family is encoded by the opposite strand of the rat c-erbA alpha transcriptional unit. Mol Cell Biol 9:1128–1136,1989.
178. Miyajima N, Horiuchi R, Shibuya Y, et al: Two erbA homologs encoding proteins with different T_3 binding capacities are transcribed from opposite DNA strands of the same genetic locus. Cell 57:31–39, 1989.
179. Harding HP, Lazar MA: The monomer-binding orphan receptor Rev-Erb represses transcription as a dimer on a novel direct repeat [erratum appears in Mol Cell Biol 15(1):6479, 1995]. Mol Cell Biol 15:4791–4802, 1995.
180. Zamir I, Dawson J, Lavinsky RM, et al: Cloning and characterization of a corepressor

and potential component of the nuclear hormone receptor repression complex. Proc Natl Acad Sci U S A 94:14400–14405, 1997.

181. Lazar MA, Hodin RA, Cardona G, et al: Gene expression from the c-erbA alpha/Rev-ErbA alpha genomic locus. Potential regulation of alternative splicing by opposite strand transcription. J Biol Chem 265:12859–12863, 1990.
182. Munroe SH, Lazar MA: Inhibition of c-erbA mRNA splicing by a naturally occurring antisense RNA. J Biol Chem 266:22083–22086, 1991.
183. Balsalobre A, Damiola F, Schibler U: A serum shock induces circadian gene expression in mammalian tissue culture cells. Cell 93:929–937, 1998.
184. Hodin RA, Lazar MA, Wintman BI, et al: Identification of a thyroid hormone receptor that is pituitary-specific. Science 244:76–79, 1989.
185. Cook CB, Kakucska I, Lechan RM,et al: Expression of thyroid hormone receptor β2 in rat hypothalamus. Endocrinology 130: 1077–1079, 1992.
186. Lechan RM, Qi Y, Berrodin TJ, et al: Immunocytochemical delineation of thyroid hormone receptor beta 2-like immunoreactivity in the rat central nervous system. Endocrinology 132:2461–2469, 1993.
187. Bradley DJ, Towle HC, Young WS III: Alpha and beta thyroid hormone receptor (TR) gene expression during auditory neurogenesis: Evidence for TR isoform-specific transcriptional regulation in vivo. Proc Natl Acad Sci U S A 91:439–443, 1994.
188. Satoh T, Yamada M, Iwasaki T, et al: Negative regulation of the gene for the preprothyrotropin-releasing hormone from the mouse by thyroid hormone requires additional factors in conjunction with thyroid hormone receptors. J Biol Chem 271:27919–27926, 1996.
189. Tomura H, Lazar J, Phyillaier M, et al: The N-terminal region (A/B) of rat thyroid hormone receptors alpha 1, beta 1, but not beta 2 contains a strong thyroid hormone–dependent transactivation function. Proc Natl Acad Sci U S A 92:5600–5604, 1995.
190. Safer JD, Langlois MF, Cohen R, et al: Isoform variable action among thyroid hormone receptor mutants provides insight into pituitary resistance to thyroid hormone. Mol Endocrinol 11:16–26, 1997.
191. Shi YB, Yaoita Y, Brown DD: Genomic organization and alternative promoter usage of the two thyroid hormone receptor beta genes in *Xenopus laevis*. J Biol Chem 267:733–738, 1992.
192. Forrest D, Sjoberg M, Vennstrom B: Contrasting developmental and tissue-specific expression of alpha and beta thyroid hormone receptor genes. EMBO J 9:1519–1528, 1990.
193. Mellstrom B, Naranjo JR, Santos A, et al: Independent expression of the α and β c-erbA genes in developing rat brain. Mol Endocrinol 5:1339–1350, 1991.
194. Bradley DJ, Towle HC, Young WS: Spatial and temporal expression of α- and β-thyroid hormone receptor mRNAs, including the β2-subtype, in the developing mammalian nervous system. J Neurosci 12:2288–2302, 1992.
195. Nicholson JL, Altman J: Synaptogenesis in the rat cerebellum: Effects of early hypo- and hyperthyroidism. Science 176:530–532, 1972.
196. Nunez J: Effects of thyroid hormone during brain differentiation. Mol Cell Endocrinol 37:125–132, 1984.
197. Cooney AJ, Tsai SY, O′Malley BW, et al: Chicken ovalbumin upstream promoter transcription factor (COUP-TF) dimers bind to different GGTCA response elements, allowing COUP-TF to repress hormonal induction of the vitamin D_3, thyroid hormone, and retinoic acid receptors. Mol Cell Biol 12:4153–4163, 1992.
198. Forrest D, Erway LC, Ng L, et al: Thyroid hormone receptor beta is essential for development of auditory function. Nat Genet 13:354–357, 1996.
199. Wikstrom L, Johansson C, Salto C, et al: Abnormal heart rate and body temperature in mice lacking thyroid hormone receptor alpha 1. EMBO J 17:455–461, 1998.
200. Samuels HH, Stanley F, Shapiro LE: Dose-dependent depletion of nuclear receptors by L-triiodothyronine: Evidence for a role in induction of growth hormone synthesis in cultured GH1 cells. Proc Natl Acad Sci U S A 73:3877–3881, 1976.
201. Samuels HH, Stanley F, Shapiro LE: Modulation of thyroid hormone nuclear receptor levels by 3,5,3′-triiodo-L-thyronine in GH1 cells. J Biol Chem 252:6052–6060, 1977.
202. Rusch A, Erway LC, Oliver D, et al: Thyroid hormone receptor beta-dependent expression of a potassium conductance in inner hair cells at the onset of hearing. Proc Natl Acad Sci U S A 95:15758–15762, 1998.
203. Forrest D, Hanebuth E, Smeyne RJ, et al: Recessive resistance to thyroid hormone in mice lacking thyroid hormone receptor beta: Evidence for tissue-specific modulation of receptor function. EMBO J 15:3009–3015, 1996.
204. Weiss RE, Forrest D, Pohlenz J, et al: Thyrotropin regulation by thyroid hormone in thyroid hormone receptor beta–deficient mice. Endocrinology 138:3624–3629, 1997.
205. Refetoff S, DeWind LT, DeGroot LJ: Familial syndrome combining deaf-mutism, stippled epiphyses, goiter and abnormally high PBI: Possible target organ refractoriness to thyroid hormone. J Clin Endocrinol Metab 27:279–294, 1967.
206. Weiss RE, Murata Y, Cua K, et al: Thyroid hormone action on liver, heart, and energy expenditure in thyroid hormone receptor beta–deficient mice. Endocrinology 139:4945–4952, 1998.
207. Sandhofer C, Schwartz HL, Mariash CN, et al: Beta receptor isoforms are not essential for thyroid hormone-dependent acceleration of PCP-2 and myelin basic protein gene expression in the developing brains of neonatal mice. Mol Cell Endocrinol 137:109–115, 1998.
208. Johansson C, Vennstrom B, Thoren P: Evidence that decreased heart rate in thyroid hormone receptor-alpha 1–deficient mice is an intrinsic defect. Am J Physiol 275:R640–646, 1998.
209. Kumar V, Chambon P: The estrogen receptor binds tightly to its responsive element as a ligand-induced homodimer. Cell 55:145–156, 1988.
210. Eriksson P, Wrange O: Protein-protein contacts in the glucocorticoid receptor homodimer influence its DNA binding properties. J Biol Chem 265:3535–3542, 1990.
211. Hard T, Kellenbach E, Boelens R, et al: Solution structure of the glucocorticoid receptor DNA binding domain. Science 249:157–160, 1990.
212. Schwabe JWR, Neuhaus D, Rhodes D: Solution structure of the DNA binding domain of the oestrogen receptor. Nature 348:458–461, 1990.
213. Williams GR, Brent GA: Thyroid hormone response elements. *In* Weintraub BD (ed): Molecular Endocrinology: Basic Concepts and Clinical Correlations. New York, Raven Press, 1994.
214. Williams GR, Harney JW, Forman BM, et al: Oligomeric binding of T3 receptor is required for maximal T3 response. J Biol Chem 266:19636–19644, 1991.
215. Katz RW, Koenig RJ: Nonbiased identification of DNA sequences that bind thyroid hormone receptor alpha 1 with high affinity. J Biol Chem 268:19392–19397, 1993.
216. Katz RW, Koenig RJ: Specificity and mechanism of thyroid hormone induction from an octamer response element. J Biol Chem 269:18915–18920, 1994.
217. Murray MB, Towle HC: Identification of nuclear factors that enhance binding of the thyroid hormone receptor to a thyroid hormone response element. Mol Endocrinol 3:1434–1442, 1989.
218. Burnside J, Darling DS, Chin WW: A nuclear factor that enhances binding of thyroid hormone receptors to thyroid hormone response elements. J Biol Chem 265:2500–2504, 1990.
219. Glass CK, Devary OV, Rosenfeld MG: Multiple cell type-specific proteins differentially regulate target sequence recognition by the α retinoic acid receptor. Cell 63:729–738, 1990.
220. Lazar MA, Berrodin TJ: Thyroid hormone receptors form distinct nuclear protein-dependent and independent complexes with a thyroid hormone response element. Mol Endocrinol 4:1627–1635, 1990.
221. O′Donnell AL, Rosen ED, Darling DS, et al: Thyroid hormone receptor mutations that interfere with transcriptional activation also interfere with receptor interaction with a nuclear protein. Mol Endocrinol 5:94–99, 1991.
222. Yu VC, Delsert C, Andersen B, et al: RXR beta: A coregulator that enhances binding of retinoic acid, thyroid hormone, and vitamin D receptors to their cognate response elements. Cell 67:1251–1266, 1991.
223. Bugge TH, Pohl J, Lonnoy O, et al: RXRa, a promiscuous partner of retinoid acid and thyroid hormone receptors. EMBO J 11:1409–1418, 1992.
224. Kliewer SA, Umesono K, Mangelsdorf DJ, et al: Retinoid X receptor interacts with nuclear receptors in retinoic acid, thyroid hormone and vitamin D3 signalling. Nature 355:446–449, 1992.
225. Leid M, Kastner P, Lyons R, et al: Purification, cloning, and RXR identity of the HeLa cell factor with which RAR or TR heterodimerizes to bind target sequences efficiently. Cell 68:377–395, 1992.
226. Marks MS, Hallenbeck PL, Nagata T, et al: H-2RIIBP (RXR beta) heterodimerization provides a mechanism for combinatorial diversity in the regulation of retinoic acid and thyroid hormone responsive genes. EMBO J 11:1419–1435, 1992.
227. Zhang XK, Hoffmann B, Tran PB, et al: Retinoid X receptor is an auxiliary protein for thyroid hormone and retinoic acid receptors. Nature 355:441–446, 1992.
228. Heyman RA, Mangelsdorf DJ, Dyck JA, et al: 9-*cis* retinoic acid is a high affinity ligand for the retinoid X receptor. Cell 68:397–406, 1992.
229. Levin AA, Sturzenbecker LJ, Kazmer S, et al: 9-*cis* retinoic acid stereoisomer binds and activates the nuclear receptor RXRα. Nature 355:359–361, 1992.
230. Kurokawa R, DiRenzo J, Boehm M, et al: Regulation of retinoid signalling by receptor polarity and allosteric control of ligand binding. Nature 371:528–531, 1994.
231. Claret FX, Antakly T, Karin M, et al: A shift in the ligand responsiveness of thyroid hormone receptor alpha induced by heterodimerization with retinoid X receptor alpha. Mol Cell Biol 16:219–227, 1996.
232. Kakizawa T, Miyamoto T, Kaneko A, et al: Ligand-dependent heterodimerization of thyroid hormone receptor and retinoid X receptor. J Biol Chem 272:23799–23804, 1997.
233. Chin S, Apriletti J, Gick G: Characterization of a negative thyroid hormone response element in the rat sodium, potassium-adenosine triphosphatase alpha3 gene promoter. Endocrinology 139:3423–3431, 1998.
234. Lehmann JM, Zhang XK, Graupner G, et al: Formation of retinoid X receptor homodimers leads to repression of T3 response: Hormonal cross talk by ligand-induced squelching. Mol Cell Biol 13:7698–7707, 1993.
235. Cohen O, Flynn TR, Wondisford FE: Ligand-dependent antagonism by retinoid X receptors of inhibitory thyroid hormone response elements. J Biol Chem 270:13899–13905, 1995.
236. Ulisse S, Iwamura S, Tata JR: Differential responses to ligands of overexpressed thyroid hormone and retinoid X receptors in a *Xenopus* cell line and in vivo. Mol Cell Endocrinol 126:17–24, 1997.
237. Wahlstrom GM, Sjoberg M, Andersson M, et al: Binding characteristics of the thyroid hormone receptor homo- and heterodimers to consensus AGGTCA repeat motifs. Mol Endocrinol 6:1013–1022, 1992.
238. Perlmann T, Rangarajan PN, Umesono K, et al: Determinants for selective RAR and TR recognition of direct repeat HREs. Genes Dev 7:1411–1422, 1993.
239. Zechel C, Shen XQ, Chen JY, et al: The dimerization interfaces formed between the DNA binding domains of RXR, RAR and TR determine the binding specificity and polarity of the full-length receptors to direct repeats. EMBO J 13:1425–1433, 1994.
240. Hermann T, Hoffmann B, Zhang X-K, et al: Heterodimeric receptor complexes determine 3,5,3′-triiodothyronine and retinoid signaling specificities. Mol Endocrinol 6:1153–1162, 1992.
241. Forman BM, Samuels HH: Interactions among a subfamily of nuclear hormone receptors: The regulatory zipper model. Mol Endocrinol 4:1293–1301, 1990.
242. Au-Fliegner M, Helmer E, Casanova J, et al: The conserved ninth C-terminal heptad in thyroid hormone and retinoic acid receptors mediates diverse responses by affecting heterodimer but not homodimer formation. Mol Cell Biol 13:5725–5737, 1993.
243. Nagaya T, Jameson JL: Thyroid hormone receptor dimerization is required for dominant negative inhibition by mutations that cause thyroid hormone resistance. J Biol Chem 268:15766–15771, 1993.
244. Collingwood TN, Butler A, Tone Y, et al: Thyroid hormone–mediated enhancement of heterodimer formation between thyroid hormone receptor beta and retinoid X receptor. J Biol Chem 272:13060–13065, 1997.
245. Yen PM, Darling DS, Carter RL, et al: Triiodothyronine (T_3) decreases binding to DNA by T_3-receptor homodimers but not receptor-auxiliary protein heterodimers. J Biol Chem 267:3565–3568, 1992.
246. Wolffe AP: Transcriptional control. Sinful repression. Nature 387:16–17, 1997.

247. Chen JD, Evans RM: A transcriptional co-repressor that interacts with nuclear hormone receptors. Nature 377:454–457, 1995.
248. Sande S, Privalsky ML: Identification of TRACs (T3 receptor-associating cofactors), a family of cofactors that associate with, and modulate the activity of, nuclear hormone receptors. Mol Endocrinol 10:813–825, 1996.
249. Horlein AJ, Naar AM, Heinzel T, et al: Ligand-independent repression by the thyroid hormone receptor mediated by a nuclear receptor co-repressor [see comments]. Nature 377:397–404, 1995.
250. Kurokawa R, Soderstrom M, Horlein A, et al: Polarity-specific activities of retinoic acid receptors determined by a co-repressor. Nature 377:451–454, 1995.
251. Lee JW, Ryan F, Swaffield JC, et al: Interaction of thyroid-hormone receptor with a conserved transcriptional mediator. Nature 374:91–94, 1995.
252. Alland L, Muhle R, Hou Jr H, et al: Role for N-Cor and histone deacetylase in Sin3-mediated transcriptional repression. Nature 387:49–55, 1997.
253. Heinzel T, Lavinsky RM, Mullen TM, et al: A complex containing N-CoR, mSin3 and histone deacetylase mediates transcriptional repression. Nature 387:43–48, 1997.
254. Nagy L, Kao HY, Chakravarti D, et al: Nuclear receptor repression mediated by a complex containing SMRT, mSin3A, and histone deacetylase. Cell 89:373–380, 1997.
255. Onate SA, Tsai SY, Tsai MJ, et al: Sequence and characterization of a coactivator for the steroid hormone receptor superfamily. Science 270:1354–1357, 1995.
256. Voegel JJ, Heine MJS, Zechel C, et al: TIF2, a 160 kDa transcriptional mediator for the ligand-dependent activation function AF-2 of nuclear receptors. EMBO J 15:3667–3675, 1996.
257. Hong H, Kohli K, Trivedi A, et al: GRIP1, a novel mouse protein that serves as a transcrptional coactivator in yeast for the hormone binding domains of steroid receptors. Proc Natl Acad Sci U S A 93:4948–4952, 1996.
258. Anzick SL, Kononen J, Walker RL, et al: AIB1, a steroid receptor coactivator amplified in breast and ovarian cancer. Science 277:965–968, 1997.
259. Li H, Leo C, Schroen DJ, et al: Characterization of receptor interaction and transcriptional repression by the corepressor SMRT. Mol Endocrinol 11:2025–2037, 1997.
260. Torchia J, Rose DW, Inostrova J, et al: The transcriptional co-activator p/CIP binds CBP and mediates nuclear-receptor function. Nature 387:677–684, 1997.
261. Chen H, Lin RJ, Schiltz RL, et al: Nuclear receptor coactivator ACTR is a novel histone acetyltransferase and forms a multimetric activation complex with P/CAF and CBP/p300. Cell 90:569–580, 1997.
262. Takeshita A, Cardona GR, Koibuchi N, et al: TRAM-1, A novel 160-kDa thyroid hormone receptor activator molecule, exhibits distinct properties from steroid receptor coactivator-1. J Biol Chem 272:27629–27634, 1997.
263. Zhu Y, Qi C, Jain S, et al: Isolation and characterization of PBP, a protein that interacts with peroxisome proliferator-activated receptor. J Biol Chem 272:25500–25506, 1997.
264. Fondell JD, Guermah M, Malik S, et al: Thyroid hormone receptor–associated proteins and general positive cofactors mediate thyroid hormone receptor function in the absence of the TATA box-binding protein-associated factors of TFIID. Proc Natl Acad Sci U S A 96:1959–1964, 1999.
265. Rachez C, Suldan Z, Ward J, et al: A novel protein complex that interacts with the vitamin D3 receptor in a ligand-dependent manner and enhances VDR transactivation in a cell-free system. Genes Dev 12:1787–1800, 1998.
266. Yang X-J, Ogryzko VV, Nishikawa J, et al: A p300/CBP-associated factor that competes with the adenoviral oncoprotein E1A. Nature 382:319–324, 1996.
267. Kwok RP, Lundblad JR, Chrivia JC, et al: Nuclear protein CBP is a coactivator for the transcription factor CREB. Nature 370:223–226, 1994.
268. Eckner R, Ewen ME, Newsome D, et al: Molecular cloning and functional analysis of the adenovirus E1A-associated 300-kD protein (p300) reveals a protein with properties of a transcriptional adaptor. Genes Dev 8:869–884, 1994.
269. Bannister A, Kouzarides T: The CBP co-activator is a histone acetyltransferase. Nature 384:641–643, 1996.
270. Ogryzko VV, Schiltz RL, Russanova V, et al: The transcriptional coactivators p300 and CBP are histone acetyltransferases. Cell 87:953–959, 1996.
271. Spencer TE, Jenster G, Burcin MM, et al: Steroid receptor coactivator-1 is a histone acetyltransferase. Nature 389:194–198, 1997.
272. Struhl K: Histone acetylation and transcriptional regulatory mechanisms. Genes Dev 12:599–606, 1998.
273. Karin M: New twist in gene regulation by glucocorticoid receptor: Is DNA binding dispensable? Cell 93:487–490, 1998.
274. Datta S, Magge SN, Madison LD, et al: Thyroid hormone receptor mediates transcriptional activation and repression of different promoters in vitro. Mol Endocrinol 6:815–825, 1992.
275. Madison LD, Ahlquist JA, Rogers SD, et al: Negative regulation of the glycoprotein hormone alpha gene promoter by thyroid hormone: Mutagenesis of a proximal receptor binding site preserves transcriptional repression. Mol Cell Endocrinol 94:129–136, 1993.
276. Zhang XK, Wills KN, Husmann M, et al: Novel pathway for thyroid hormone receptor action through interaction with *jun* and *fos* oncogene activities. Mol Cell Biol 11:6016–6025, 1991.
277. Schaufele F, West BL, Reudelhuber TL: Overlapping Pit-1 and Sp1 binding sites are both essential to full rat growth hormone gene promoter activity despite mutually exclusive Pit-1 and Sp1 binding. J Biol Chem 265:17189–17196, 1990.
278. Tansey WP, Catanzaro DF: Sp1 and thyroid hormone receptor differentially activate expression of human growth hormone and chorionic somatomammotropin genes. J Biol Chem 266:9805–9813, 1991.
279. Schaufele F, West BL, Baxter JD: Synergistic activation of the rat growth hormone promoter by Pit-1 and the thyroid hormone receptor. Mol Endocrinol 6:656–665, 1992.
280. Barrera-Hernandez G, Zhan Q, Wong R, et al: Thyroid hormone receptor is a negative regulator in p53-mediated signaling pathways. DNA Cell Biol 17:743–750, 1998.
281. Thompson KL, Santon JB, Shephard LB, et al: A nuclear protein is required for thyroid hormone receptor binding to an inhibitory half-site in the epidermal growth factor receptor promoter. Mol Endocrinol 6:627–635, 1992.
282. Harding PP, Duester G: Retinoic acid activation and thyroid hormone repression of the human alcohol dehydrogenase gene ADH3. J Biol Chem 267:14145–14150, 1992.
283. Tran P, Zhang X-K, Salbert G, et al: COUP orphan receptors are negative regulators of retinoic acid response pathways. Mol Cell Biol 12:4666–4676, 1992.
284. Tagami T, Gu WX, Peairs PT, et al: A novel natural mutation in the thyroid hormone receptor defines a dual functional domain that exchanges nuclear receptor corepressors and coactivators. Mol Endocrinol 12:1888–1902, 1998.
285. Weiss RE, Refetoff S: Thyroid hormone resistance. Annu Rev Med 43:363–375, 1992.
286. Kopp P, Kitajima K, Jameson JL: Syndrome of resistance to thyroid hormone: Insights into thyroid hormone action. Proc Soc Exp Biol Med 211:49–61, 1996.
287. Chatterjee VKK, Clifton-Bligh RJ, Gurnell M: Thyroid hormone resistance. *In* Jameson JL (ed): Hormone Resistance Syndromes. Totowa, NJ, Humana Press, 1999, pp 145–163.
288. Brucker-Davis F, Skarulis MC, Grace MB, et al: Genetic and clinical features of 42 kindreds with resistance to thyroid hormone. The National Institutes of Health Prospective Study [see comments]. Ann Intern Med 123:572–583, 1995.
289. Sakurai A, Takeda K, Ain K, et al: Generalized resistance to thyroid hormone associated with a mutation in the ligand-binding domain of the human thyroid hormone receptor beta. Proc Natl Acad Sci U S A 86:8977–8981, 1989.
290. Usala SJ, Tennyson GE, Bale AE, et al: A base mutation of the c-erbA beta thyroid hormone receptor in a kindred with generalized thyroid hormone resistance. Molecular heterogeneity in two other kindreds. J Clin Invest 85:93–100, 1990.
291. Sakurai A, Miyamoto T, Refetoff S, et al: Dominant negative transcriptional regulation by a mutant thyroid hormone receptor-beta in a family with generalized resistance to thyroid hormone. Mol Endocrinol 4:1988–1994, 1990.
292. Chatterjee VK, Nagaya T, Madison LD, et al: Thyroid hormone resistance syndrome. Inhibition of normal receptor function by mutant thyroid hormone receptors. J Clin Invest 87:1977–1984, 1991.
293. Collingwood TN, Rajanayagam O, Adams M, et al: A natural transactivation mutation in the thyroid hormone β receptor: Impaired interaction with putative transcriptional mediators. Proc Natl Acad Sci U S A 94:248–253, 1997.
294. Nagaya T, Madison LM, Jameson JL: Thyroid hormone receptor mutations that cause resistance to thyroid hormone. Evidence for receptor competition for DNA sequences in target genes. J Biol Chem 267:13014–13019, 1992.
295. Yoh SM, Chatterjee VKK, Privalsky ML: Thyroid hormone resistance syndrome manifests as an aberrant interaction between mutant T3 receptors and transcriptional corepressors. Mol Endocrinol 11:470–480, 1997.
296. Clifton-Bligh RJ, de Zegher F, Wagner RL, et al: A novel TR beta mutation (R383H) in resistance to thyroid hormone syndrome predominantly impairs corepressor release and negative transcriptional regulation. Mol Endocrinol 12:609–621, 1998.
297. Tagami T, Jameson JL: Nuclear corepressors enhance the dominant negative activity of mutant receptors that cause resistance to thyroid hormone. Endocrinology 139:640–650, 1998.

Chapter 96

Thyroid-Stimulating Hormone and Regulation of the Thyroid Axis

Bruce D. Weintraub ▪ Rasa Kazlauskaite
Mathis Grossmann ▪ Mariusz W. Szkudlinski

The history of TSH (thyroid-stimulating hormone, thyrotropin) began with the discovery of thyroid-stimulating activity in the pituitary gland. In 1926 Eduard Uhlenhuth[1] from the University of Maryland Medical School was the first to demonstrate that the anterior lobe of the pituitary gland secreted a thyroid stimulator. This was followed in the mid-1960s by the purification, and in the early 1970s by the determination, of the primary amino acid sequence of the TSH subunits. In the 1980s, the cloning of the human α subunit and TSH-β subunit genes, as well as the TSH receptor gene, were important milestones in studies on TSH structure, regulation, and action.

This chapter provides an overview of TSH structure and function. It also summarizes the physiology, as well as the clinical pathophysiology, of TSH synthesis, secretion, and action.

STRUCTURE AND FUNCTION

TSH is a 28- to 30-kDa glycoprotein synthesized and secreted from thyrotrophs (basophil cells) of the anterior pituitary gland. It is a member of the glycoprotein hormone family, which includes follicle-stimulating hormone (FSH), luteinizing hormone (LH), and chorionic gonadotropin (CG). The glycoprotein hormones are heterodimeric cystine knot proteins consisting of a common α subunit and a unique β subunit that confer biologic specificity onto each hormone.

Gene Structure

The common human α and TSH-β subunits are encoded by single genes located on chromosomes 6 and 1, respectively.[2] The organization of the human α subunit and TSH-β subunit genes is shown in Figure 96–1. The α subunit gene contains four exons and three introns, while the TSH-β subunit gene contains three exons and two introns. The α subunit gene is almost two times larger (9.4 kb) than the TSH-β subunit gene (4.9 kb). The first exon is short in both cases, untranslated, and separated from the coding region by a large first intron. Each gene contains a single transcription start site with an upstream TATA box that binds RNA polymerase II. Expression of the TSH-β subunit gene in the anterior pituitary is restricted to thyrotroph cells, which constitute approximately 5% of all adenohypophysial cells.

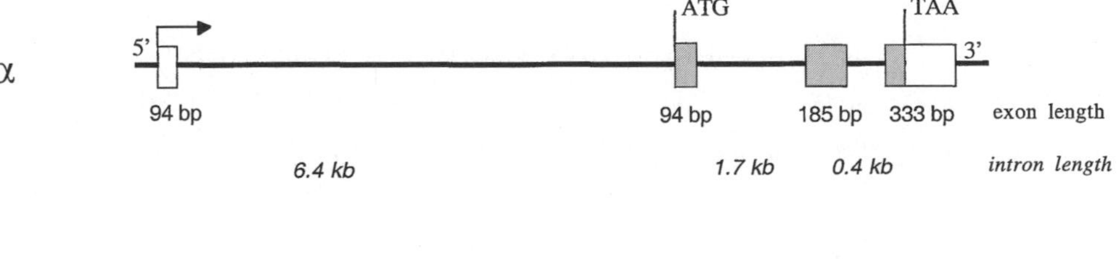

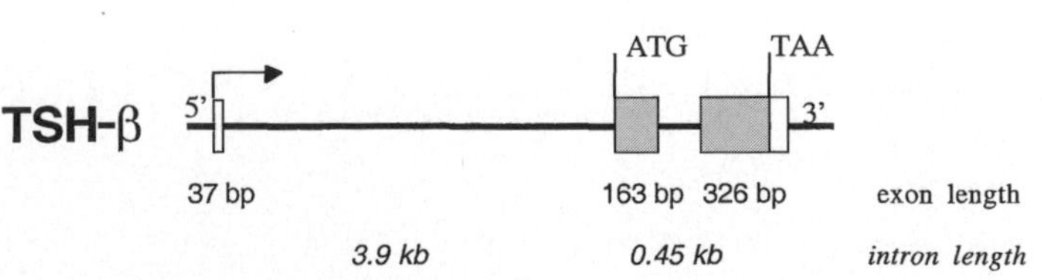

FIGURE 96–1. Structure of the common α and thyroid-stimulating hormone-β subunit genes. Exons are denoted by the *boxes,* and introns or flanking DNA sequences by *lines.* The length of exons is shown in base pairs (bp); the intron length is in italics and depicted in kilobase pairs (kb). Coding regions of exons are shaded; noncoding regions are white. The start of transcription is marked by a *bent arrow.* Location of the sense strand DNA sequence for the initiation codon (AUG) is marked ATG and the sequence for the termination codon (UAA) is marked TAA. This diagram serves to illustrate the general structure of each gene and is drawn to scale.

Protein Structure

Human TSH (hTSH) consists of two noncovalently linked subunits: the α subunit (92 amino acids, in common with other human glycoprotein hormones) and the TSH-β subunit. The coding sequence of the TSH-β subunit gene predicts a 118–amino acid protein. However, β subunit of TSH isolated from cadaver pituitary has 112 amino acids, most likely the result of proteolytic cleavage during purification. In any case, the C-terminal amino acid residues 113–118 are not important in human TSH biologic activity.[3] The primary sequences (see Figure 96–2) of TSH subunits are species-specific. hTSH, for example, differs from bovine TSH by 28 amino acids in the α subunit, and by 12 amino acids in TSH-β subunit.

TSH is a member of the glycoprotein hormone family,[4] structurally classified as a part of the cystine knot growth factor (CKGF) superfamily.[5] The crystal structure of homologous human chorionic gonadotropin (hCG) has revealed that each subunit contains a central cystine knot and three loops: two β hairpin loops (L1 and L3) on one side of a cystine knot and a long loop (L2) on the other (see Figure 96–3). The long loop in the α subunit contains a two-turn α helix. The cystine knot is made up of three central disulfide bridges, where one bond threads through a ring formed by the other two, linked by backbone atoms. This structure has previously been found in several growth factors, including platelet-derived growth factor (PDGF), vascular endothelial growth factor (VEGF), transforming growth factor-β (TGF-β), and nerve growth factor (NGF). In contrast to the other CKGFs, which exist as homo- or heterodimers with interchain disulfide bridges, glycoprotein hormones are noncovalently linked heterodimers stabilized by a unique segment of the β subunit termed "seat belt," because it wraps around the α subunit long loop. This additional stabilization by the seat belt results in doubling of the subunit interface compared to the other CKGFs. This may be necessary because of the extensive glycosylation of glycoprotein hormones, which constitutes up to one third of their molecular weight. In light of the common α subunit, as well as 38% sequence identity between the hCG β and hTSH-β subunits, homology modeling of hTSH was performed and showed expected similarities in the conformation of these two hormones.[6] Accordingly, assignment of disulfide bridges to the bovine TSH-β subunit using a double alkylation strategy revealed bonding analogous to hCG.[7] Thus, in the hTSH-β subunit, three disulfide bridges (2–52, 27–83, and 31–85) form a cystine knot motif that determines the core structure: two disulfide bridges (19–105, 88–95) are involved in seat belt formation and one (17–67) links two β hairpin loops.

hTSH, purified from the cadaver pituitary, has been shown to be heterogeneous at the N-terminus of each subunit. In addition, variable amidation of glutamic and aspartic acid residues contributed to TSH protein heterogeneity. It is now believed that most of these changes are artifactual and result from the delay in collection of human pituitaries, as well as purification procedures.

Structure of Carbohydrate Chains

Like other glycoprotein hormones TSH also contains carbohydrate chains attached to a protein backbone. These oligosaccharides constitute 15% to 22% of the molecular weight of TSH and include three asparagine (N)-linked carbohydrate chains. The human α subunit has two carbohydrate chains linked to asparagine 52 and 78, respectively, and the human TSH-β subunit has one carbohydrate chain attached at asparagine 23 (see Fig. 96–2). Such N-linked oligosaccharides are complex-type structures displaying notable hormone- and species-dependent differences in their terminal carbohydrate residues, as well as antennary structure. It is noteworthy that the heterogeneity of TSH derived from different sources (pituitary or recombinant) depends primarily on the variability in the carbohydrate chains. Terminal sialic acid residues (NeuAc), as well as sulfated *N*-acetylgalactosamine (SO_4-4GalNAc) determine the metabolic clearance rate of TSH and are vitally important to its biologic activity.

Figure 96–4 shows typical biantennary structures of pituitary bovine TSH, which terminate almost exclusively with SO_4-4GalNAc, and recombinant human TSH (rhTSH) expressed in CHO cells containing only NeuAcα2-3Gal terminal sequences. In contrast, pituitary human TSH oligosaccharides contain both SO_4-4GalNAc and NeuAcα2-3/6Gal terminal residues. The presence of sulfated oligosaccharides is a unique feature of pituitary hTSH and LH due to the expression of GalNAc-transferase and sulfotransferase in the anterior pituitary cells.[8, 9]

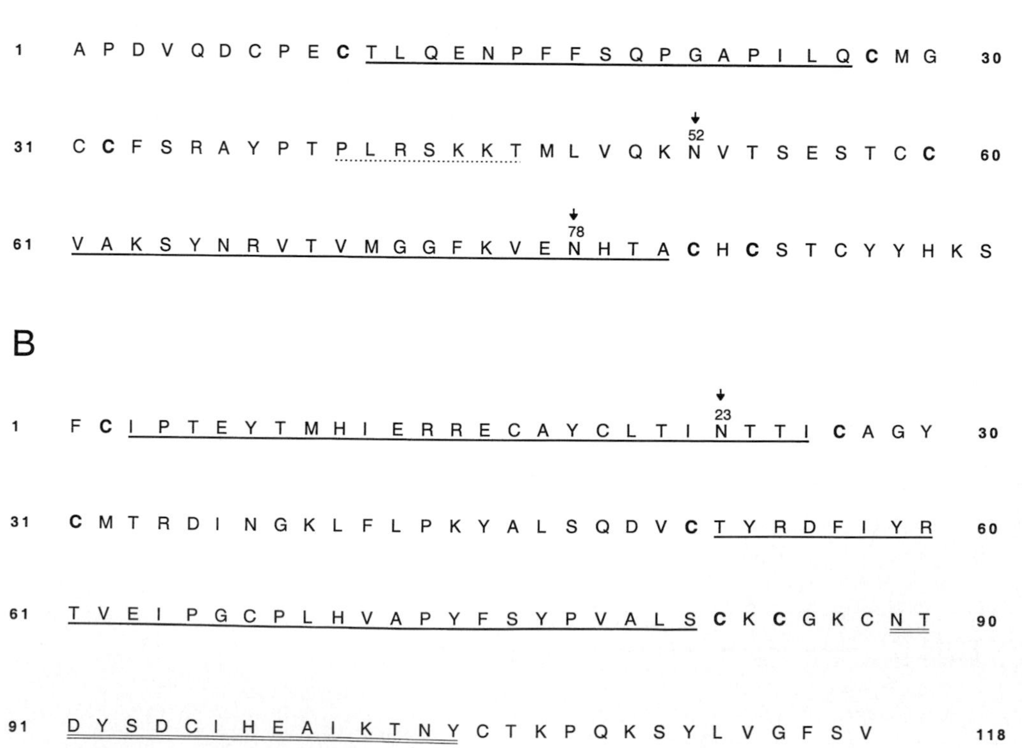

FIGURE 96–2. Primary structure of the human α subunit *(A)* and human thyroid-stimulating hormone-β subunit *(B)*, using the single-letter code for amino acids. Two-turn α helix in the α subunit is underlined with a *dotted line*. The sequences of β hairpin peripheral loops are underlined with a *single solid line*; the seat belt region in the β subunit is underlined with a *double solid line*. Location of asparagine residues linked to oligosaccharide chains are marked with *arrows*. Cysteine residues, involved in the formation of the cystine knot, are boldface.

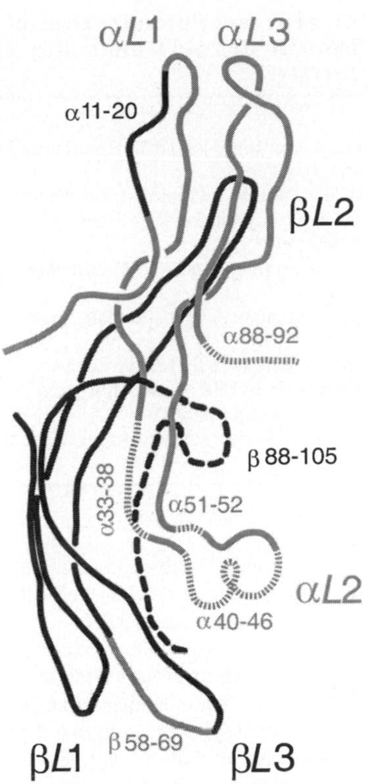

FIGURE 96–3. The schematic drawing of human thyroid-stimulating hormone showing domains important for bioactivity. For clarity the carbohydrate chains are not shown. The α subunit backbone is shown as a gray line; the β subunit chain is shown as a black line. Functionally critical domains are marked directly within the line drawings. The peripheral β hairpin loops are marked: α*L1*, α*L3* in the α subunit and β*L1*, β*L3* in the β subunit. Two long loops are α*L2* with α-helical structure and β*L2*, a loop analogous to the "Keutmann loop" in the human chorionic gonadotropin β subunit.

Functionally Important TSH Protein Domains

TSH expression and biologic activity require a noncovalent association of the α and TSH-β subunits. The free TSH-β subunit, similar to the free LH-β subunit, is degraded intracellularly and less than 10% of it is secreted into the culture medium. Therefore, simultaneous co-expression of the α subunit prevents intracellular degradation of the TSH-β subunit.[10]

Structure-function studies of TSH and gonadotropins involve alteration of coding sequences using molecular biology techniques and various chemical and biochemical modifications, as well as utilization of antibodies or synthetic peptides to disrupt association of subunits or receptor binding.[11] The most important functional domains thus far recognized in TSH are depicted in Figure 96–3. Certain domains are tightly conserved among different species or homologous hormones and even minor modifications of such areas result in decreased expression, receptor binding, or both. Most of these domains are located in close proximity and within the "composite binding domain" as described in hCG.[5] Particularly important domains or residues in receptor activation include the α helix (α40–46), αLys51, αAsn52, the α-C-l terminus (α88–92), α33–38, the "Keutmann loop" (TSH-β 31–52) and the seat belt in the β subunit (TSH-β 88–105).[9, 11] In addition to the stabilizing role of the seat belt, recent studies involving β subunit chimeras have shown that this region is critical in conferring glycoprotein hormone specificity, probably by restricting heterologous ligand-receptor interactions or by influencing the conformation of the composite binding domain.[12] Functionally important residues are also identified in studies of patients with familial hypothyroidism and natural mutations in the TSH-β subunit gene (see Alterations of TSH Bioactivity and Structure).

Several additional regions and residues have been recently recognized to be involved in the modulation of TSH and gonadotropin function. Studies employing the combination of alanine- and proline-scanning mutagenesis have revealed the importance of α-helical conformation (α40–46) in TSH bioactivity. Furthermore, the 11–20 region in the α subunit with a cluster of basic residues (K–K/R--K---K/R), present in all vertebrates except hominoids (apes and humans), has been recognized as an important motif in the evolution of TSH and gonadotropin bioactivity in primates.[6] Of importance, the elimination of basic residues in this region resulted in a decrease in TSH intrinsic activity and coincided with the divergence of apes from Old World monkeys. Identification of such nonconservative amino acid changes during hormone evolution suggested that rapid adaptive mechanisms directed by natural selection were involved. It led to speculation that the attenuation of TSH biologic activity in early apes, due to substitutions in the 11–20 region, may be related to the conservation of iodine for thyroid hormone synthesis during the periods of intermittent feeding. In addition to these evolutionary insights, this study[6] provided the first evidence that selective alteration of the residues in the loop domains to charged residues may permit design of analogs with enhanced bioactivity. Based on that, further analysis suggested that the presence of basic amino acids in the β subunit sequence modulated intrinsic activity of TSH.[13]

Functional Role of Carbohydrate Chains

The carbohydrate chains assume importance in every aspect of the life span of TSH, from early translational events during biosynthesis to its removal from the circulation affecting TSH biologic activity (see also Post-translational Processing and Regulation). Overall, the carbohydrates serve comparable functions among the members of the glycoprotein hormone family.[8] However, more recent work has shown that the oligosaccharides may have structure-, subunit-, and site-dependent roles for hTSH, which are in part different from those for the gonadotropins.[14, 15]

Effect of terminal sialic acid residues in modulation of receptor

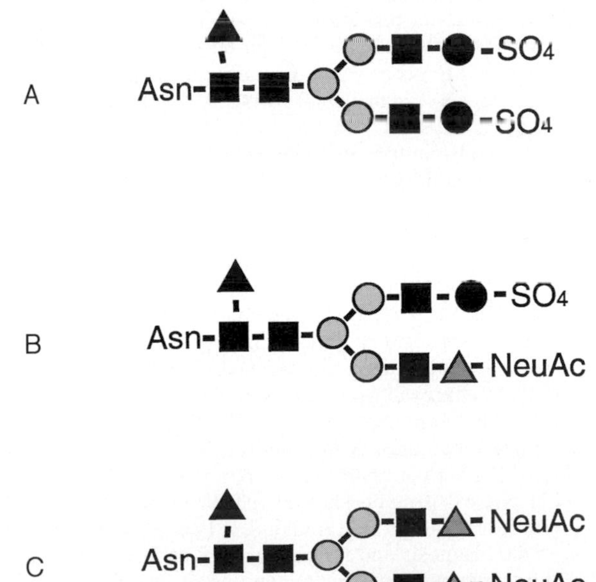

FIGURE 96–4. N-linked oligosaccharides of thyroid-stimulating hormone (TSH). The sulfated biantennary structure *(A)* represents that of bovine TSH. The sulfated and sialylated oligosaccharide *(B)* is more typical of pituitary-derived human TSH (hTSH). The sialylated nonsulfated structure *(C)* represents that of recombinant hTSH expressed in Chinese hamster ovary (CHO) cells. Carbohydrate residues are marked as follows: *gray circle*, mannose; *black square*, *N*-acetylglucosamine; *black circle*, *N*-acetylgalactosamine; *black triangle*, fructose; *gray triangle*, galactose; NeuAc, sialic acid.

activation and signal transduction is different for hTSH as compared to other glycoprotein hormones. In contrast to gonadotropins, receptor binding and signal transduction of desialylated rhTSH occurs undisturbed and even improved.[14, 16] However, the observation that oligosaccharide structures of the α subunit have a more pronounced role than those of the β subunit in signal transduction is still valid for all glycoprotein hormones.[17, 18] Combination of site-directed mutagenesis with expression in glycosylation mutant cell lines has further emphasized the unique roles of individual side chains for hTSH activity, different from the gonadotropins.[15] In particular, the oligosaccharide at Asn52, but not the one at Asn78, and specifically its terminal sialic acid residues, markedly attenuated TSH receptor binding and activation. The carbohydrate chain at Asn52 is positioned close to the putative binding site,[5] explaining why desialylation or removal of this chain affects hormone potency.

Finally, the oligosaccharides play an important role in tissue distribution and clearance mechanisms and thus modulate circulating levels and final biopotency in vivo. In general, effects on clearance are far more important for the final in vivo potency than on intrinsic activity, and even relatively minor changes in clearance can supersede those observed for the in vitro bioactivity. For example, enzymatically desialylated rhTSH has a 5- to 10-fold higher in vitro potency than sialylated rhTSH. However, asialo-rhTSH is cleared significantly faster than rhTSH and exhibits very low in vivo activity.[19] An important lesson from these and similar findings in other glycoprotein hormones is that no correlation exists between the effects of carbohydrates on in vitro and in vivo activities of glycoproteins. Such studies highlight the difficulties of translating results obtained using an in vitro system into whole-organism physiology and illustrate the importance of determining the activity of such hormones in suitable animal models. Moreover, the pulsatile pattern of serum hormone concentrations may affect desensitization and thus may be more important for chronic, as compared to acute, hormone response.[20]

Recombinant Human TSH and Its Analogues

Cloning of the hTSH-β subunit gene permitted expression of bioactive rhTSH in embryonal kidney cells.[21] However, more detailed structural and biologic characterization was possible after larger quantities of rhTSH were produced in Chinese hamster ovary (CHO) cells stably transfected with TSH genes.[19, 22, 23] Commercial preparation of rhTSH (Thyrogen, Genzyme) became available after its production in a large-scale bioreactor.[23]

Since CHO cells, unlike the pituitary thyrotroph cells, have no capacity to add penultimate *N*-acetylgalactosamine or terminal sulfate, rhTSH is predominantly composed of oligosaccharide chains terminating in sialic acid. This is similar to the highly sialylated isoforms of hTSH that circulate in primary hypothyroidism (see below), and rhTSH also has a slower metabolic clearance rate compared with normal pituitary hTSH. rhTSH showed slightly lower potency in vitro, but the maximal stimulatory activity is similar to that of pituitary TSH. Subsequent studies demonstrated that rhTSH exhibits similar or higher biologic activity in vivo due to a slower metabolic clearance rate and higher peak serum concentration.[19, 24] Serum rhTSH concentration after single intramuscular injection in the human peaks within 4 to 6 hours, with a biologic half-life of approximately 24 hours.[25]

An initial phase I/II study showed rhTSH to be safe and demonstrated preliminary efficacy in stimulating ^{131}I uptake and thyroglobulin secretion in the diagnosis and follow-up of 19 patients with differentiated thyroid carcinoma, thus avoiding the side effects of thyroid hormone withdrawal.[25] Subsequent phase III trials[26] with more than 100 patients have shown that rhTSH is virtually equivalent to conventional hormone withdrawal, but leads to considerable improvement in quality of life because it avoids the symptoms of hypothyroidism. These major studies, as well as case reports, including a description of a patient with papillary thyroid carcinoma and hypopituitarism who had metastases detected only after administration of rhTSH, but not thyroid hormone withdrawal, exemplify the diagnostic potential of rhTSH.[27] Thyrogen has been approved by the Food and Drug Administration (FDA) for use in conducting thyroid scanning and thyroglobulin testing in the follow-up of patients with well-differentiated thyroid cancer (Table 96–1) (see also Chapter 109).

TABLE 96–1. Current and Potential Uses of Recombinant Human Thyroid-Stimulating Hormone (rhTSH)

Clinical
Differentiated thyroid cancer follow-up (rhTSH-stimulated thyroglobulin testing and whole-body scanning)
TSH stimulation test (e.g., testing thyroid reserve, identifying "warm" thyroid nodules, detecting thyroid hemiagenesis)
Nonthyroidal illness syndrome[132]
Differentiated thyroid cancer treatment (rhTSH-stimulated radioiodine ablation)
Large euthyroid goiter treatment (rhTSH-stimulated radioiodine ablation)
Laboratory
Standards and ^{125}I–human TSH in TSH immunoassays
TSH-stimulated thyroglobulin mRNA testing in thyroglobulin antibody–positive thyroid cancer patients
TSH binding inhibition (TBI) assay for autoantibodies to the TSH receptor[192]
TSH bioactivity testing

Modification of protein activity using recombinant technologies, often called protein engineering or protein design, started in 1982 after the first results of site-directed mutagenesis had been published. Despite numerous attempts, examples of engineered proteins with desirable or improved properties are quite rare. Szkudlinski et al. constructed the first glycoprotein hormone superagonists (analogs with increased receptor binding and bioactivity).[6, 28] Superagonists of hTSH with major increases in receptor binding affinity as well as in vitro and in vivo bioactivity were constructed based on homology comparisons of various sequences and homology modeling of hTSH. hTSH with quadruple mutations in the α subunit (Q13K + E14K + P16K + Q20K) and an additional replacement in the hTSH-β subunit (L69R) showed 95-fold higher potency and more than a 1.5-fold increase in efficacy compared to the in vitro bioactivity of the wild-type hormone.[6] Moreover, the combination of these four mutations in the α subunit with three mutations in the β subunit (I58R + E63R + L69R) resulted in an analog with greater than a 1000-fold increase in receptor binding and in vitro bioactivity, and a 100-fold increase in in vivo activity.[13] Furthermore, recently found new "gain-of-activity" mutations (four in the αL3 loop and three in βL1 loop) will permit selection of the most optimal combinations of hTSH mutations in all peripheral loops. Such novel hTSH analogs, with combinations of basic residues not present in any natural hormone, are significantly more potent than any natural TSH (bovine or rat) and hold great promise as second-generation therapeutic forms of recombinant TSH, including minimized superagonists as well as superagonists with modified plasma half-life.

PHYSIOLOGIC REGULATION

Hypothalamic-Pituitary-Thyroid Axis

TSH synthesis and secretion is stimulated by thyrotropin-releasing hormone (TRH), and inhibited by thyroid hormone in a classic endocrine negative feedback loop (Fig. 96–5). TSH controls thyroid function upon its interaction with the G protein–coupled TSH receptor. TSH binding to its receptor on thyroid cells leads to the stimulation of second messenger pathways involving predominantly cyclic adenosine 3′,5′-monophosphate (cAMP) and, in high concentrations, inositol 1,4,5-trisphosphate (IP_3) and diacylglycerol (DAG), ultimately resulting in the modulation of thyroidal gene expression.[29]

Physiologic Roles of TSH

- TSH stimulates differentiated thyroid functions, such as iodine uptake and organification, thyroglobulin production, as well as produc-

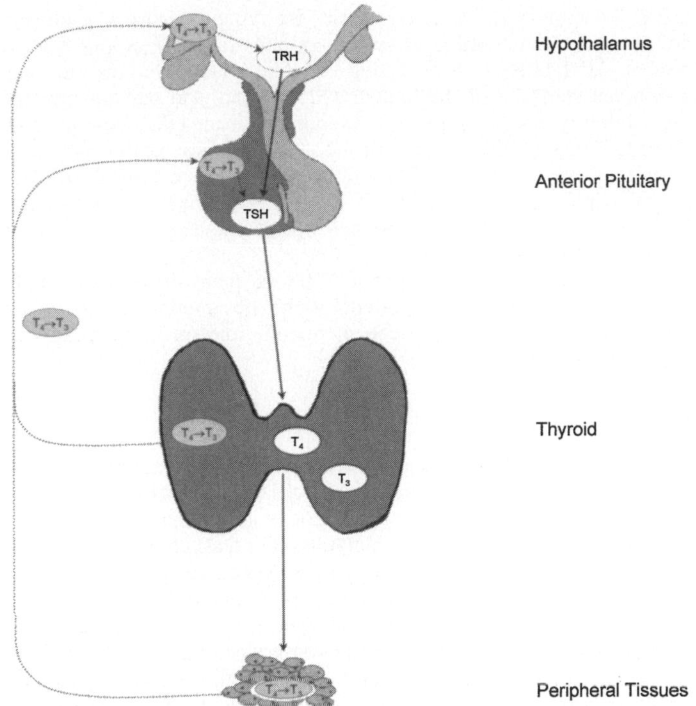

FIGURE 96–5. Hypothalamic-pituitary-thyroid axis. *Solid lines* correspond to stimulatory effect; *dotted lines* depict inhibitory effects. Conversion of thyroxine to triiodothyronine in the pituitary and hypothalamus is mediated via 5′-deiodinase type II. 5′-Deiodinase type II is also important in the rest of the CNS, thyroid, and muscle. 5′-Deiodinase type I (propylthiouracyl sensitive) plays a major role in liver, kidney, and thyroid.

tion and release of iodothyronines from the gland. It also increases activity of thyroid 5′-deiodinase type I (see Chapter 94).

- TSH promotes thyroid growth by inducing hypertrophy and hyperplasia of thyrocytes.
- TSH also acts as a thyrocyte survival factor and protects the cells from apoptosis, perhaps analogously to hCG via regulation of *p53* and the *bcl*-2 gene family.[30]
- TSH plays a critical role in ontogeny. In a mouse model with targeted disruption of the common α subunit gene and thus devoid of circulating glycoprotein hormones, thyroid development was arrested in late gestation.[31]
- Extrathyroidal actions of TSH may be related to the presence of TSH receptors in tissues other than thyroid or extrapituitary TSH subunit production.[32, 33] Thus, the presence of TSH-binding sites in a variety of extrathyroidal tissues, such as lymphocytes, adipocytes, or testicular and adrenal tissue, has long been known.[34] More recently, the expression of hTSH receptor or its splicing variants in nonthyroidal tissues, including adipocytes and lymphocytes, was demonstrated, as well as the extrapituitary expression of the TSH-β subunit gene.[32] Evidence for both hTSH receptor as well as hTSH-β subunit expression in the same tissue, such as lymphocytes, may indicate that such tissues are under paracrine or autocrine TSH regulation. According to one study, proliferative capacity and natural killer cell activity of murine spleen lymphocytes improved upon stimulation with TSH.[35] The presence of TSH receptor in fat may explain the lipolytic effects of TSH, which have been implicated in promoting physiologically occurring lipolysis during the neonatal period.[36] A local TRH-TSH network and expression of TSH receptor was detected in the intestinal mucosa,[37] suggesting that enterocyte-produced TSH may play a role in the regulation of intraepithelial lymphocyte function. This observation is supported by the fact that mice with mutant TSH receptor (*hyt/hyt* mice) have a selective decrease in the number of intraepithelial lymphocytes. Interestingly, thyroid receptor α knockout mice had reduced numbers of epithelial cells or even arrested maturation of small intestine.[38]

Physiologic Conditions Affecting TSH Secretion

The TSH secretion rate varies from 40 to 150 mIU/day and the plasma half-life in euthyroid subjects ranges from 30 to 80 minutes.[39, 40]

AGE AND SEX DIFFERENCES. TSH in the pituitary and serum of the fetus appears at approximately 13 weeks of gestation and can also be detected in amniotic fluid. Mean TSH is higher in cord than in maternal blood. TSH levels during the first 30 minutes of life are severalfold higher than basal TSH concentrations in adults, and decline to the normal adult range by the third day of life. Slight fluctuations in TSH are also observed during puberty. The TSH levels are similar in both sexes, but a clinically insignificant decline may occur with advanced age. In healthy elderly men over age 65 a decrease in pituitary responsiveness to TRH accompanied by a decrease in overall 24-hour TSH secretion has been described,[41] explaining slightly lower TSH levels in older persons.[42] In particular, the TSH response to decreased free thyroid hormone levels is inappropriately low in elderly people, indicative of an apparent resetting of the thyroid hormone feedback regulation threshold of TSH secretion.[43]

EFFECTS OF STRESS AND FASTING. A transient decrease in TSH in serum may occur under stressful conditions such as surgery, trauma, hypoxia, exposure to low temperatures, and fasting. Some of these effects may be related to cortisol secretion, adrenergic stimulation, and TRH decrease.

CIRCADIAN RHYTHM. TSH secretion occurs in a circadian pattern characterized by a nadir in the late afternoon and a peak in late evening, before the onset of sleep.[44] Evidence suggests that the pulsatile nature of TSH secretion is regulated primarily by TRH rather than by dopamine or somatostatin,[45] which may also affect the TSH nocturnal surge. The development of the circadian rhythm begins after the first month of life and persists throughout childhood and adult life.[46] Sleep withdrawal was reported to augment nightly TSH secretion, whereas sleep after a period of sleep withdrawal almost completely suppressed the circadian variation.[47] In addition, TSH appears to be secreted in a pulsatile manner with intervals of 2 to 6 hours between peaks, with a nocturnal increase in the frequency and amplitude of the pulses.[45] Within an individual subject the circadian TSH levels vary within 0.5 and 2.0 times the 24-hour mean value. However, morning TSH levels increase significantly at the age of 9 to 10 years, followed by the onset of puberty and a concomitant increase in triiodothyronine (T_3) and thyroxine (T_4) concentrations.[48]

Transcriptional Regulation of TSH Subunit Genes

Thyroid Hormone

Thyroid hormone, in a classic negative feedback system, is the major negative regulator of TSH subunit gene expression. T_3, bound to its receptor, results in a dramatic decrease in transcription of both the common α and TSH-β subunit genes.[49, 50]

It is important to recognize that the thyrotroph contains a high activity of 5′-deiodinase type II, thereby accounting for 50% to 60% of the nuclear T_3 content.[51] Hence, the inhibitory effects of thyroid hormones on TSH secretion depend not only on T_3 serum levels but also on the serum T_4 concentrations and local deiodinase activity. The negative feedback action of thyroid hormones on TSH synthesis and secretion occurs not only directly at the pituitary level but also by decreasing hypothalamic TRH release.

Cis-acting elements responsible for negative transcriptional regulation by T_3 are located near the transcriptional start site of each gene (Fig. 96–6).[52–57] These elements, referred to as *negative thyroid hormone response elements*, contain two copies of 6-bp consensus DNA sequences [(A/G)GGT(C/A)], which bind the T_3 receptor.[58] The consensus DNA sequence, referred to as a *half-site*, is thought to bind one T_3 receptor molecule. The negative transcriptional regulation of TSH-α and -β genes is mediated through receptor monomers, homodimers, or heterodimers involving retinoid X (RXR) or other nuclear

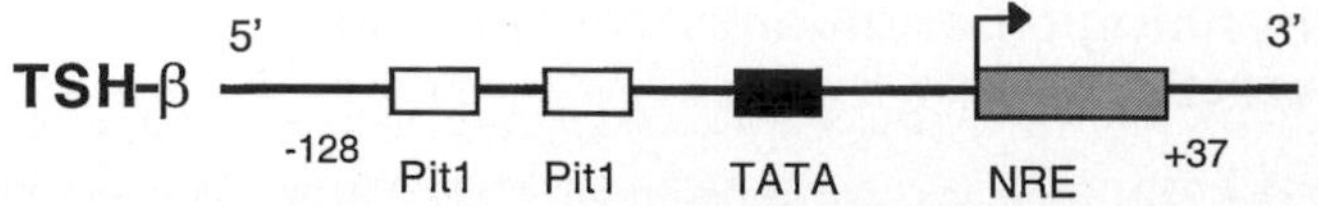

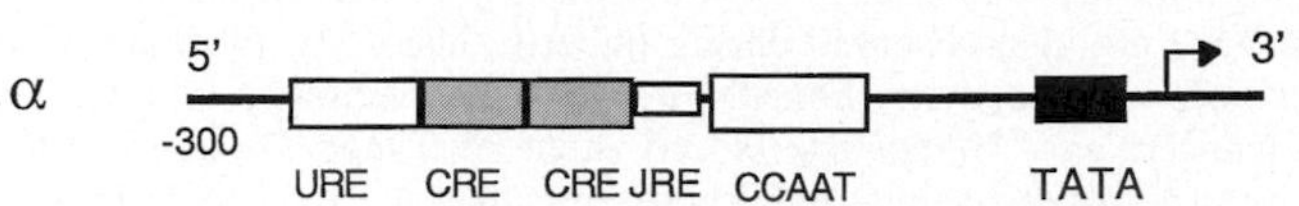

FIGURE 96–6. Schematic representation of human thyroid-stimulating hormone-β (TSH-β) subunit and α subunit gene promoters.

TSH-β subunit promoter: β Subunit gene negative response element (NRE) is marked in gray. Pit-1 on the scheme represents Pit-1 factor binding site. Negative regulation of TSH-β subunit gene by triiodothyronine (T_3) is mediated by thyroid receptor binding to NRE. Transcriptional regulation of the TSH-β subunit gene may also involve recruitment of various corepressors and coactivators, as well as T_3-dependent regulation of histone deacetylase and alterations of chromatin structure.

α Subunit promoter: The α subunit gene cyclic adenosine monophosphate response element (CRE) is marked in gray; the upstream regulatory element (URE), junctional response element (JRE), and CCAAT box element are marked in white. Factors that activate the α subunit promoter exclusively in thyrotrophs have not been described. However, it has been demonstrated[191] that the α subunit promoter contains at least three elements that are functional in human thyrotrophs but not gonadotrophs. The *arrows* represent the transcription initiation sites. (Adapted from Nilson JH, Bokar JA, Clay CM, et al: Different combinations of regulator elements may explain why placenta-specific expression of the glycoprotein hormone alpha-subunit gene occurs only in primates and horses. Biol Reprod 44:231–237, 1991.)

receptors (see Chapter 95). Inhibition of TSH-β subunit expression by RXR-selective ligands was demonstrated in vitro and resulted in decreased TSH secretion in humans.[59] Moreover, the negative regulation of TSH by thyroid hormones may be affected by expression of thyroid hormone receptor isoforms in the thyrotrophs. Transgenic knockout mice experiments suggest that the thyroid receptor β isoform primarily mediates T_3-dependent modulation of TSH levels.[60]

Thyrotropin-Releasing Hormone

The major positive regulator of TSH subunit gene transcription is TRH. At the pituitary, TRH binds to its plasma membrane receptor and increases transcription of the TSH subunit genes three- to fivefold. Most of the cellular effects of TRH on the thyrotrophs are thought to be mediated by activation of the phospholipase C pathway resulting in production of a variety of second messengers that activate protein kinase C and calcium–dependent protein kinases, as well as other possible kinases.

At least two nuclear transcription factors are activated by protein kinase C and, possibly, other kinases to mediate the effect of TRH on transcription of the TSH subunit genes. Pit-1/GHF-1 (hereinafter Pit-1) is a pituitary-specific transcription factor that mediates part of the TRH response in the prolactin and TSH-β subunit genes by binding to 5′ flanking *cis*-acting elements that share homology to the consensus sequences A(A/T) (A/T)TATNCAT.[61–64] Both protein kinase C and protein kinase A pathways phosphorylate Pit-1 at two sites.[65] In the TSH-β subunit gene, phosphorylated Pit-1 binds with greater avidity to these elements than nonphosphorylated Pit-1, providing a mechanism by which transcription can be stimulated by either protein kinase C– or A–dependent pathways.[66]

Activating protein-1 (AP-1) is a heterogeneous group of nuclear transcription factors that is also necessary for TRH stimulation of TSH subunit gene expression.[64, 67] These factors, whose expression is markedly stimulated by activators of the protein kinase C pathway, are primarily composed of c-*jun* homodimers and c-*fos*/c-*jun* heterodimers. AP-1 binds to a *cis*-acting element, which overlaps the transcriptional start site of the human TSH-β gene, and contains part of the inhibitory thyroid hormone response element (Fig. 96–6). AP-1 interacts directly with the thyroid hormone receptor at this site, suggesting crosstalk between TRH and thyroid hormone control of TSH-β gene expression.[68, 69] In addition, thyroid hormone is known to alter TRH receptor number in pituitary cells, providing a second mechanism of integrated control.[70]

The physiologic importance of TRH in maintaining basal TSH secretion in humans is supported by the observation of decreased TSH concentrations and subsequent hypothyroidism in patients with hypothalamic lesions.

Other Factors

Arginine vasopressin is a positive regulator,[71] while dopamine and somatostatin are important negative regulators of TSH secretion in vivo.[72, 73] Receptors for these neuropeptides are thought to be coupled to adenylate cyclase through stimulatory (G_s) and inhibitory (G_i) guanylyl nucleotide–binding proteins, respectively, such that intracellular cAMP levels are altered when these receptors bind their ligand. cAMP-dependent pathways regulate the synthesis of both the common α and TSH-β subunits. Transcription of the human common α subunit gene is stimulated by cAMP-dependent pathways that phosphorylate the cAMP-response DNA-binding protein (CREB) and enhance its binding to a palindromic cAMP-response element (CRE), TGACGTCA, located in the 5′ flanking region.[74, 75] CREB is a ubiquitous transcription factor and is important in cAMP regulation of a number of genes.[76] Unlike that of the common α subunit gene, however, cAMP regulation of the TSH-β gene is mediated by Pit-1, as well as by the ubiquitous factor AP-1 described above. cAMP-dependent pathways phosphorylate Pit-1 as well as AP-1 and enhance binding to their respective *cis*-acting DNA elements, thereby increasing gene transcription.[67, 77] More recent studies suggested that interactions of Pit-1 and GATA-2 factor protein are part of the process restricting the TSH-β gene expression to thyrotroph cells.[78]

Experiments with the transgenic mouse model, exhibiting pituitary-specific resistance to thyroid hormone syndrome,[79] demonstrated that ligand-independent activation of TSH-β expression may be present in vivo.

Post-transcriptional Regulation of TSH Subunit Genes

Thyroid hormone regulates the expression of rat TSH-β subunit messenger RNA (mRNA) by reducing the half-life of the TSH-β subunit mRNA.[80] The mechanism of this alteration in mRNA stability is attributable to the *trans*-acting RNA-binding protein, which may also be involved in regulation of other cytoplasmic mRNAs. The binding activity of this *trans*-acting RNA-binding protein is positively regulated by T_3. It is possible that similar to the effect of gonadotropin-releasing hormone (GnRH) on α subunit mRNA stability in the gonadotroph-derived cell line,[81] TRH may also increase α subunit mRNA stability in thyrotrophs.

Translation of TSH Subunit Genes

α Subunit and TSH-β subunit genes are translated in the thyrotroph from separated mRNAs as precursor molecules with 24– and 20–amino acid N-terminal extensions respectively.[82–87] These N-terminal extensions or leader peptides are necessary for transport of TSH subunit proteins across the membrane of the endoplasmic reticulum (ER). During translation, the leader peptide is cleaved from precursor α and β subunit proteins, and high-mannose oligosaccharide chains are transferred from a dolichol phosphate carrier[88] to asparagine residues on the α and β subunits. Excess α subunit present in the rough endoplasmic reticulum (RER) begins to combine with TSH-β subunit when both subunits contain high mannose oligosaccharide chains. Subunit combination is complete in the RER, and oligosaccharide chains on TSH are processed further in the Golgi apparatus (see below).

Since the production of hTSH-β subunit mRNA is the rate-limiting step in the synthesis of hTSH, the α subunit is synthesized in excess of TSH-β subunit and a small amount of uncombined α subunit is normally secreted from the thyrotroph. Such free α subunit, unlike α subunit found in TSH, contains a third *O*-linked oligosaccharide chain at threonine.[89, 90] Glycosylation at this site appears to prevent combination with the TSH-β subunit; however, the physiologic significance of noncombined forms of the α subunit is unknown.

Post-translational Processing and Regulation

Post-translational processing of TSH is primarily associated with the addition and subsequent modification of carbohydrate chains. Differences in the molecular weight of TSH are primarily due to the heterogeneity of carbohydrate chains. Different degrees in the terminal processing of oligosaccharides give rise to a mixture of circulating glycoforms, which in turn are responsible for the physiologic microheterogeneity of TSH.

High-mannose–type oligosaccharides are attached to asparagine residues in ER.[91] These oligosaccharide chains are processed by glucosidases and mannosidases in the RER.[92] In the proximal Golgi apparatus, specific glycosyltransferases attach galactose, *N*-acetylgalactosamine, or other residues to mannose residues of the "core" oligosaccharide chain, composed of three mannose and two *N*-acetylglucosamine residues. Fucose residues are also added in the RER and proximal Golgi apparatus to the innermost *N*-acetylglucosamine residue attached to asparagine. In the distal Golgi apparatus, terminal sialic acid and sulfate residues are added by specific transferases to acceptor galactose or *N*-acetylgalactosamine sugars, respectively, on the oligosaccharide. The anterior pituitary, unlike the placenta, contains a glycosyltransferase for *N*-acetylgalactosamine and a sulfotransferase and thus is capable of synthesizing oligosaccharide chains capped by sulfate.[93]

Glycoprotein hormones containing "sulfate-capped" oligosaccharide chains (TSH and LH) have a shorter biologic half-life than those capped by sialic acid residues only (CG). This shorter plasma half-life is a result of sulfated *N*-acetylgalactosamine interaction with specific hepatic carbohydrate receptor.[94] By contrast, terminal sialylation enables the glycoprotein hormone to escape such specific receptor-mediated hepatic clearance mechanisms, and the kidney becomes the major organ of hormone clearance.[95] Therefore in vivo bioactivity of TSH isoforms is determined by terminal carbohydrate residues.

The structure of TSH oligosaccharide chains is also known to be regulated during development and by certain hormones. In a rodent model, it was demonstrated that the complexity and number of terminal sialic acid residues on oligosaccharide chains is increased during development.[96] Hypothyroidism has also been shown to increase the number of terminal sialic acid residues while decreasing terminal sulfate residues on both subunits of TSH.[97] These changes have been shown to increase the biologic half-life of TSH, prolong its duration of action, and possibly facilitate adaptation to hypothyroidism.[98] Finally, TRH can affect the glycosylation structure of TSH, but its in vitro effect appears to differ from its in vivo effects. It was also demonstrated that in vitro TRH administration altered the branching of carbohydrate chains on TSH, increasing the number of biantennary forms.[99] However, TRH deficiency in rodents caused by paraventricular nuclear lesions reduced the number of biantennary carbohydrate chains and TRH administration increased the number of multiantennary carbohydrate chains to near-normal levels.[100] The differences between these studies may related to the in vitro (static) vs. in vivo (dynamic) effects of TRH.

CLINICAL PATHOPHYSIOLOGY

Testing TSH Immunoreactivity

The routine measurement of hTSH in clinical practice today is performed by immunometric assays (IMAs) with a lower sensitivity limit of approximately 0.01 mIU/L (third-generation assay) (see also Chapter 97). Radioimmunoassays (RIAs) used in the 1970s, had poor sensitivity (1 mIU/L in the first generation; 0.1 mIU/L in the second generation) and specificity. Second- and first-generation assays did not allow discrimination between euthyroid and thyrotoxic patients and TRH stimulation testing was required to make the distinction.

At present fourth-generation assays, allowing measurements down to the range of 0.005 mIU/L, are also available. However, a properly performed third-generation assay with valid sensitivity is sufficient in the clinical setting. The reference range for TSH measured by IMA is typically 0.5 to 5.0 mIU/L.

The TSH RIAs are used for screening of neonatal hypothyroidism in dry blood spots on filter paper.

Levels of free α subunit in serum are measured by RIA and typically range from 0.5 to 2.0 μg/L. They are higher in postmenopausal women (<5 μg/L). The free α subunit–TSH arbitrary ratio is calculated using free α subunit in micrograms per liter divided by TSH in milliunits per liter and multiplied by 10.[101] Normogonadotropic patients without TSH-secreting tumors have a free α subunit–TSH ratio less than 5.7 μg/L if TSH is within the reference range, and less than 0.7 μg/L if TSH is elevated. Hypergonadotropic patients typically have TSH less than 29.1 μg/L if TSH is within the reference range, and less than 1.0 μg/L if TSH is elevated.[102] The α subunit–TSH molar ratio is usually pathologically increased in TSH-secreting pituitary tumors (see Chapter 24).

Principles of TSH Regulation in Pathologic Conditions

Precise regulation of plasma TSH levels over a wide range of thyroid hormone concentrations is the rationale behind measuring basal serum TSH in the diagnosis of both hypothyroid and hyperthyroid disorders (Table 96–2). Plasma TSH concentration is a function of TSH clearance, as well as thyroid hormone production and clearance rates. Since T_4 has a longer half-life than T_3, TSH levels correlate better with T_4 rather than T_3 concentrations. It has been estimated that a twofold change in plasma T_4 levels prompts a 100-fold change in plasma TSH concentrations.[103] Under physiologic conditions T_4 action in the pituitary is mediated by its more active form T_3, derived from intrapituitary T_4 deiodination by 5′-deiodinase type II.[104] 5′-Deiodinase type II is resistant to inhibition by propylthiouracil, and is regulated by T_4 concentrations[105]; If T_4 production falls, 5′-deiodinase type II activity increases, increasing the T_3/T_4 ratio in thyrotrophs. In the absence of T_4 production, plasma T_3 levels should be doubled to replace half of the pituitary nuclear T_3 that is normally generated from T_4 deiodination.[51]

Similarly, TRH production in the hypothalamus is negatively regulated by the intracellular T_3 pool, generated in part from hypothalamic

TABLE 96–2. Thyroid-Stimulating Hormone and Thyroxine Levels in Hypo- and Hyperthyroid Disorders

Clinical Syndrome	TSH Levels	Free Thyroxine Levels	Clinical Features
Overt hyperthyroidism	Lower than the assay sensitivity	Above the reference range	Hyperthyroidism
Subclinical hyperthyroidism	Higher than the assay sensitivity, but below the reference range	Within the reference range	Mild hyperthyroidism or normal
Euthyroidism	Within the reference range	Within the reference range	Normal
Subclinical hypothyroidism	Above the reference range, but usually <20 mIU/L	Within the reference range	Normal or subtle hypothyroidism
Mild hypothyroidism	Above the reference range, but usually <20 mIU/L	Below the reference range	Minimal hypothyroidism
Overt hypothyroidism	Usually >20 mIU/L	Below the reference range	Hypothyroidism

T_4 deiodination,[106, 107] and is modulated by dopamine, glucocorticoids, and fasting.[108] TRH stimulates thyrotrophs via its action on their membrane receptors, inducing TSH release and synthesis within minutes, while it takes hours for thyroid hormones to inhibit these functions via their nuclear receptors. When thyroid hormone levels are sufficiently high, TRH is unable to overcome the inhibition (see Primary Hyperthyroidism).

Glucocorticoids, somatostatin, and dopamine are of pathophysiologic and pharmacologic importance in regulation of TSH.

CIRCADIAN TSH CHANGES IN DISEASE CONDITIONS. The nocturnal surge in TSH is usually abolished in central hypothyroidism, thyrotoxicosis, levothyroxine suppressive therapy, and fasting.[109–112] Similarly, this nocturnal rise is diminished in states of hypercortisolism (such as Cushing's syndrome), severe nonthyroidal illness, and major depression.[113]

Decreased TSH Secretion

TSH secretion may be decreased via thyrotroph downregulation by excess thyroid hormones or other centrally acting substances, by insufficient TRH production, or by thyrotroph maldevelopment or malfunction (Table 96–3).

Primary Hyperthyroidism

In overt primary hyperthyroidism, serum TSH levels are below the range of detection (by third-generation assay) even after TRH stimulation. The nocturnal TSH surge is also invariably suppressed in the face of elevated thyroid hormone levels. Upregulation of thyroid hormone receptors in the pituitary and hypothalamus by excess thyroid hormones (increased negative feedback) is responsible for the decreased synthesis of TSH, independent of the cause of primary hyperthyroidism.

Mildly elevated T_4 and T_3 concentrations that suppress TSH below the reference range without raising free thyroid hormones above the normal range result in subclinical hyperthyroidism[114] (see Table 96–2). If the basal TSH level is detectable by the third-generation assay, a TSH increment in response to TRH also is measurable; if the basal TSH level is undetectable, a slight increment after TRH stimulation sometimes may be noted.

After treatment of a patient with hyperthyroidism or after discontinuation of suppressive thyroid hormone therapy, the TSH may remain decreased and unresponsive to TRH for several months while the thyroid hormone levels are low or normal.[115] During this period of thyrotroph recovery low free thyroid hormone concentrations are better predictors of impending hypothyroidism.

Central Hypothyroidism

While the causes of central hypothyroidism can be etiologically grouped into TRH deficiency of hypothalamic and TSH deficiency of pituitary origin, the exact site of the abnormality is often difficult to establish in a given patient. Direct TRH measurement in the hypophysial portal circulation is problematic, and peripheral TRH levels reflect predominantly its production from nonhypothalamic sources such as pancreatic islet cells.[116] In most cases, the TRH stimulation test does not help in differentiation of secondary vs. tertiary hypothyroidism. Many patients with pituitary disease have normal responses to TRH.[117–119] In contrast, a delayed TSH response to TRH can be due to TRH deficiency, as well as to impairment in hypophysial portal circulation

TABLE 96–3. Decreased Thyroid-Stimulating Hormone (TSH) Levels in Systemic Circulation

Hormonal Profile	Mechanism	Examples
Primary hyperthyroidism (↓TSH, ↑ free thyroid hormones)	TR upregulation in the pituitary and hypothalamus by the thyroid hormone	Inflammatory or destructive process in the thyroid gland (subacute thyroiditis, radiation thyroiditis, Hashimoto's thyroiditis, etc.) Upregulation of TSH receptor by activating antibodies (Graves' disease) Activating TSH receptor mutations causing thyroid hormone hypersecretion (autonomously hyperfunctioning thyroid adenomas, including toxic multinodular goiter; autosomal dominant toxic thyroid hyperplasia) Exogenous thyroid hormone use Drugs and chemicals inducing excessive thyroid hormone release Ectopic thyroid hormone production (struma ovarii) Activating mutations in $G_s\alpha$ (toxic thyroid adenomas, McCune-Albright syndrome) TSH receptor stimulation by high levels of hCG (e.g., gestational hyperthyroidism, molar pregnancies, etc.) Hypersensitivity to hCG due to TSH receptor mutations (familial gestational hyperthyroidism)
Secondary hypothyroidism (↓TSH, ↓thyroid hormones)	Thyrotroph cell destruction or hypofunction	Neoplastic (adenoma, craniopharyngioma, metastases) Ischemic or hemorrhagic necrosis (post partum, diabetes mellitus, arteritis, sickle-cell anemia, pituitary apoplexy), cavernous sinus thrombosis Infiltrative (hemochromatosis, sarcoidosis) Traumatic (post surgery, radiation necrosis, head injury) Lymphocytic hypophysitis Idiopathic hypopituitarism (panhypopituitarism, isolated TSH deficiency) Drugs and chemicals suppressing thyrotroph function. Combined pituitary hormone deficiency syndrome (*Pit*-1 gene and other transcription factor gene mutations in the pituitary, affecting thyrotroph cells)
	Activating mutations in pituitary TR*	Hypothetical—could present with clinical picture of isolated TSH deficiency if TR activating mutation is selective to the pituitary, or with hormonal profile of secondary hypothyroidism, small thyroid, and clinical hyperthyroidism if TR activation is universal
Tertiary hypothyroidism (↓TSH, ↓thyroid hormones)	Insufficient TRH secretion	Congenital (cysts, midline defects, familial syndromes) Neoplastic (craniopharyngioma, dysgerminoma, meningioma, glioma) Infectious (encephalitis, fungal diseases, tuberculosis) Infiltrative (sarcoidosis, eosinophilic granulomatosis, lipid storage diseases) Vasculitis syndromes Traumatic (closed head injury, radiation necrosis, post surgery) Idiopathic hypothalamic hypothyroidism Nonthyroidal illness syndrome Drugs and chemicals inhibiting TRH secretion

TR, thyroid hormone receptor; hCG, human chorionic gonadotropin; TRH, thyrotropin-releasing hormone.
*Hypothetical—has not been reported.

caused by vascular changes or pituitary stalk compression. This delay could be explained by exogenous TRH reaching the pituitary through the systemic rather than through the hypophysial portal circulation. Of note, thyrotroph responsiveness is not impaired by prolonged TRH deficiency.

In central hypothyroidism, free T_4 levels are low, whereas T_3 concentrations may still be normal. Basal TSH levels are undetectable in 35%, normal in 40%, and slightly elevated up to 10 mIU/L in 25% of these patients.[117] The last may be due to secretion of TSH with a prolonged plasma half-life (see Alterations of TSH Bioactivity and Structure).

On adequate levothyroxine therapy in central hypothyroidism, the patient is clinically euthyroid and TSH levels are undetectable. Therefore, in this situation, free T_4 concentrations are more accurate in evaluation of levothyroxine replacement adequacy.[120]

Isolated TSH deficiency is uncommon, but has been described.[121] Most commonly, however, impaired thyrotroph function is accompanied by growth hormone (GH) and gonadotropin deficiencies, whereas the adrenal axis is less frequently affected.

Most frequently central hypothyroidism is a result of pituitary destruction of various etiology (see Table 96–3). Mutations in the TSH-β subunit gene (see Alterations of TSH Bioactivity and Structure) or Pit-1 and related factors are described in cases of familial central hypothyroidism. Defects in pituitary development due to impaired expression of cell-specific transcription factors such as Pit-1[122–124] and others lead to impaired thyrotroph survival and thyrotropin expression.[125] They are also responsible for decreased GH and prolactin production, resulting in combined pituitary hormone deficiency (CPHD). TSH in these cases may be decreased or inappropriately normal with a blunted TSH response to TRH and clinical hypothyroidism.

Other Disorders

NONTHYROIDAL ILLNESS SYNDROME. About 10% of patients admitted to hospitals have abnormally low or, rarely, suppressed (<0.01 mIU/L) TSH levels.[126, 127] These abnormalities are usually normalized spontaneously within 2 to 5 days.[128] This clinical constellation became known as the nonthyroidal illness syndrome (NTIS), and is discussed in Chapter 106. If elevated TSH concentrations occur in patients with NTIS, they likely represent the rebound in TSH secretion associated with recovery of thyroid function. In critically ill patients the circadian rhythmicity of TSH secretion is altered. Mean 24-hour TSH levels are reduced to 50% of controls, reflecting a decrease in pulse amplitude. Moreover, the nocturnal TSH surge is replaced by peak TSH levels occurring in the later afternoon.[129] It has been hypothesized that the exogenous or endogenous increase in glucocorticoids, dopamine, or adrenergic stimulation may contribute to these alterations in TSH secretion.[130, 131] TSH levels typically remain responsive to TRH stimulation. It is also thought that NTIS may represent a subset of central hypothyroidism.[132]

NEUROPSYCHIATRIC DISORDERS. Patients with acute psychosis may present with subnormal levels of TSH, which is thought to be secondary to increased adrenergic stimulation and stress hormone (cortisol) action. TRH tests were shown to be blunted in one-fourth of patients with primary depression and in one-fourth to one-half of chronic alcoholic patients, compared with only 3% of a healthy control population. However, disease nonspecificity and low sensitivity render this test difficult to interpret in psychiatric patients.[133] In addition, some psychiatric medications (Table 96–4) may have effects on TSH secretion.

TSH AND HIV-RELATED DISEASES. Clinical thyroid disease

TABLE 96–4. Drugs Implicated in Altering Thyroid-Stimulating Hormone (TSH) Concentration

Increase in TSH Concentration		Decrease in TSH Concentration	
Drug	***Class***	***Drug***	***Class***
Aluminum hydroxide	Antacid	Acetylsalicylic acid	NSAID
Aminoglutethimide	Adrenal suppressant	Amiodarone	Antiarrhythmic
Amiodarone	Antiarrhythmic	Bexarotene	Retinoid
Apomorphone	Opioid	Bromocriptine	Dopaminergic
Benserazide	Decarboxylase inhibitor	Carbamazepine	Antiepileptic
Buprenorphine	Opioid	Cimetidine	Histamine-receptor blocker
Calcium carbonate	Calcium supplement	Cyproheptadine	Serotonin antagonist
Carbimazole	Thionamide	Diazepam	Benzodiazepine
Chlorpromazine	Neuroleptic	Dopamine	Dopaminergic
Cholestyramine	Antilipemic	Dobutamine	Adrenergic
Clofibrate	Antilipemic	Fenoclofenac	NSAID
Clomiphene	Antiestrogen	Fluoxetine	SSRI
Colestipol	Antilipemic	Fusaric acid	Dopamine hydroxylase inhibitor
Cyclophosphamide	Cancer chemotherapeutic agent	Growth hormone	Hormone
Domperidone	Dopamine-receptor blocker	Glucocorticoids	Hormone
Ephedrine	Amphetamine	Heparin	Anticoagulant
Ethionamide	Antituberculous	5-Hydroxytryptophan	Serotonin agonist
Haloperidol	Neuroleptic	Interferon	Cytokine
Heroin	Opioid	Interleukins	Cytokine
Iodine, iodide	Radiologic contrast, antiseptic	Iodine, iodide	Radiologic contrast, antiseptic
Iron sulfate	Iron supplement	Levodopa	Dopaminergic
Kelp tablets	Nutritional supplement	Lisuride	Dopaminergic
Ketoconazole	Adrenal suppressant	Lithium	Antipsychotic
Lithium	Antipsychotic	Methylergonovine maleate	Oxytocic
Methimazole	Thionamide	Phentolamine	α-Blocker
Metoclopramine	Dopamine-receptor blocker	Phenytoin	Antiepileptic
Morphine	Opioid	Pirbidil	Dopaminergic
Pentazocine	Opioid	Pyridoxine	Vitamin
Perchlorate	Miscellaneous	Reserpine	Antihypertensive
Propylthiouracil	Thionamide	Sertraline	SSRI
Sulfonamides	Antibiotics	Somatostatin analogues	Hormone
Sulpiride	Dopamine blocker	Spironolactone	Diuretic
Theophylline	Bronchodilator	Thioridazine	Antipsychotic
Thyrotropin-releasing hormone	Hormone	Thyroid hormones and their analogues	Hormone

NSAID, nonsteroidal anti-inflammatory drug; SSRI, selective serotonin reuptake inhibitor.

Data from Surks MI, Sievert R: Drugs and thyroid function. N Engl J Med 333:1688–1694, 1995; and Yeung VTF, Cocram CS: Endocrine disorders. *In* Davis DM (ed): Textbook of Adverse Drug Reactions. New York, Oxford University Press, 1991, p 345.

has been reported in patients with HIV disease: *Pneumocystis*-induced painful thyroiditis, *Mycobacterium avium-intracellulare* and cryptococcus infection, and Kaposi's sarcoma in the thyroid have been described. Secondary hypothyroidism, resulting from pituitary destruction by toxoplasmosis and cytomegalovirus (CMV), has been reported. Medications used in HIV treatment may also interfere with thyroid hormone metabolism and secondarily cause TSH alterations (see Table 96–4).

HCG-INDUCED HYPERTHYROIDISM. Because of the high degree of sequence identity among the glycoprotein hormones in their specific β subunits (30% to 80%), as well as in the extracellular domains of their respective receptors (39% to 46%), glycoprotein hormones can interact with heterologous receptors, albeit with low cross-reactivity (<0.1%). At physiologically occurring hormone levels, this degree of specificity prevents stimulation of heterologous receptors, but cross-activation of heterologous receptors can be observed with high hormone levels.

Increased function of the thyroid gland, goiter, or occasionally frank thyrotoxicosis is observed in patients with high circulating hCG levels, as seen in early pregnancy or trophoblastic tumors.[134] Accordingly, a weak thyrotropic activity of hCG (estimated to be <1% that of TSH on a molar basis) has been demonstrated in a variety of experimental settings, and recent studies using the rhTSH receptor have confirmed direct interaction of hCG with the hTSH receptor.[135]

Familial gestational hyperthyroidism caused by a mutant thyrotropin receptor hypersensitive to hCG has been reported.[136] However, Graves' disease is by far the most common cause of hyperthyroidism in pregnancy.

Endogenous Substances and Drugs Decreasing TSH Production

SOMATOSTATIN. The acute administration of somatostatin or its long-acting analogues, acting through inhibitory G protein, reduces basal TSH, its response to TRH, and the nocturnal peak of TSH secretion.[137] This effect has been exploited in the treatment of patients with TSH-producing pituitary adenomas.[138] In contrast, long-term therapy of acromegalic patients with somatostatin analogues did not alter any of the TSH pulse parameters, indicating that somatostatin is not likely to be primarily responsible for the nocturnal rise in TSH. It has been speculated that compensatory mechanisms are involved in restoring a normal TSH pulse generation during this treatment.[139]

DOPAMINE. Infusion of dopamine into euthyroid subjects lowers the basal TSH and blunts the TSH response to TRH.[140] Studies with various dopamine receptor agonists suggest that the dopaminergic inhibition of basal TSH secretion and TSH pulsatility is predominantly regulated through dopamine D_2 receptors at the pituitary level, and through D_1 receptors at the hypothalamic level,[141] resulting in adenylate cyclase inhibition. However, chronic administration of dopamine agonists for the treatment of prolactinoma does not cause central hypothyroidism.

STEROID HORMONES. Pharmacologic amounts of glucocorticoids reduce basal TSH and blunt the response to TRH. Consequently, patients with Cushing's syndrome often have a suppressed TSH response to TRH, while subjects suffering from Addison's disease have elevated serum TSH levels.[140] Although the decrease in basal and stimulated TSH is inversely related to the serum cortisol levels under these conditions, these effects occur only at supra- or infraphysiologic doses and do not seem to be physiologically significant. It is nevertheless important to recognize the confounding effect of steroids when interpreting thyroid function tests from subjects treated with one of these drugs.

Animal studies suggest that estrogen and testosterone may have some effect on TSH subunit gene expression.[142]

OTHER SUBSTANCES. The T_3 analogue, 3,5,3′-triiodothyroacetic acid (TRIAC) binds in vitro to thyroid β-receptors with 3.5-fold higher affinity than T_3, although its residence time on thyroid receptors is shorter. This selective β_1-receptor binding enables TRIAC to suppress basal TSH levels and TSH response to TRH.[143]

Diphenylhydantoin, carbamazepine, and high doses of salicylates are capable of blunting TSH secretion.[144, 145] Reserpine and phentolamine reduce basal TSH and block the TSH response to cold stimulation. The RXR-selective ligand bexarotene, used for cutaneous T cell lymphoma treatment, decreases TSH production and causes central hypothyroidism.[59]

Interleukin-1β,[146, 147] interleukin-6,[148] and tumor necrosis factor-α[149] inhibit TSH release. Indirectly, via alterations in thyroid hormone levels, TSH secretion is affected by a number of other drugs and chemicals (see Table 96–4).

Increased TSH Secretion

TSH secretion increases are due to lack of inhibition by thyroid hormone activity at the pituitary and hypothalamic levels, or to thyrotroph autonomy (Table 96–5).

Primary Hypothyroidism

The most frequent cause of increased basal TSH levels is primary hypothyroidism. The TSH increase is due to diminished or absent

TABLE 96–5. Increased Thyroid-Stimulating Hormone (TSH) Levels in Systemic Circulation

Hormonal Profile	Mechanism	Examples
Primary hypothyroidism (↑ TSH, ↓ thyroid hormones)	Downregulation of TR in the pituitary/hypothalamus	Post destruction of thyroid gland by surgery; radiation; autoimmune, inflammatory, or infiltrative disease Iodine deficiency and impaired iodine metabolism, causing hypoproduction of thyroid hormone Drugs and chemicals causing thyroid hormone hypoproduction Downregulation of TSH receptor by inactivating antibodies (thyroid blocking antibodies) Resistance to TSH—inactivating TSH receptor mutations (thyroid atresia and hypoplasia), inactivating $G_s\alpha$ mutations (Albright's hereditary osteodystrophy), deficiency of TSH-dependent adenylate cyclase activity of thyroid membranes
Inappropriate TSH secretion (↑ TSH, ↑ thyroid hormones; ↑ TSH, normal thyroid hormones; normal TSH, ↑ thyroid hormones)	Inactivating TR mutations	Central resistance to thyroid hormone Generalized resistance to thyroid hormone
	Autonomous TSH secretion	TSH-secreting pituitary tumors TSH production by ectopic thyrotroph tumors
Tertiary hyperthyroidism (↑ TSH, ↑ thyroid hormones)	TRH hypersecretion*	Hypothetical—most likely to present with normal hormonal profile, if thyroid hormone secretion and TR are intact; potentially could present with thyrotroph hyperplasia if thyroid hormone secretion is markedly impaired secondary to primary thyroid insufficiency

TR, thyroid hormone receptor.
*Hypothetical—has not been reported.

negative feedback by thyroid hormones on thyrotroph cells. The logarithm of the TSH concentration is inversely proportionate to the level of free T_4 and corresponds with the severity of hypothyroidism. The duration of severe clinical hypothyroidism may have dramatic effects on thyrotrophs, leading in rare instances to TSH elevations above 1000 mIU/L and pituitary hyperplasia. However, at TSH levels greater than 50 mIU/L, the severity of hypothyroidism and the degree of TSH elevation do not correlate as well.[130]

In primary hypothyroidism mean 24-hour TSH pulse amplitude is increased, whereas TSH pulse frequency remains unchanged. However, the nocturnal increase in TSH is absent owing to the loss of the nocturnal increase in TSH pulse amplitude and frequency.[150]

In overt primary hypothyroidism, TSH values are invariably greater than 20 mIU/L. In patients who have an intact hypothalamic-pituitary axis, TRH testing does not typically confer any diagnostic advantage over an accurately measured basal TSH value determined by third- or fourth-generation TSH assays.[151]

The diagnosis of subclinical primary hypothyroidism (see Table 96–2) is based on normal free T_4 (and T_3) levels in the face of mildly elevated TSH.[152] The upper limit of the TSH cutoff for patients with this condition is not well defined. Antithyroid antibody testing is useful in prognosis, since, typically, patients with subclinical TSH elevations and positive antibodies develop overt hypothyroidism at a rate of 5% to 10% per year.

Subclinical primary hypothyroidism should be differentiated from central hypothyroidism with slight or modest elevations of immunoreactive TSH. The TRH test may be helpful in differentiating these two conditions. In primary hypothyroidism, the TRH test shows an increased TSH response that peaks at the normal time of 20 to 30 minutes. In central hypothyroidism, the TRH test may be blunted or at least not elevated. Occasionally, patients with central hypothyroidism may have an exaggerated response to TRH, but such patients usually show a delayed peak of 60 minutes or longer.[117, 153]

Serum TSH levels remain a sensitive test for moderate to severe primary hypothyroidism in severely ill hospitalized patients, since TSH levels remain higher than normal, even if partially attenuated.

Following institution of full levothyroxine replacement therapy for overt primary hypothyroidism, TSH levels normalize within 4 to 6 weeks. Adjustments in doses of levothyroxine based on TSH values should not be made at more frequent intervals than this to ensure a true steady-state value.

Resistance to TSH

In rare instances, the thyroid gland is resistant to the action of circulating TSH, as seen in Albright's hereditary osteodystrophy (pseudohypoparathyroidism type I), due to inactivating mutations in $G_s\alpha$, a regulatory subunit of adenylate cyclase, and diseases caused by thyrotropin receptor mutations.[154] A patient with a deficiency in TSH-dependent adenylate cyclase activity of thyroid membranes has been reported.[155]

Clinically, patients with TSH resistance have nongoitrous hypothyroidism, and their serum T_4 does not respond to TRH or TSH stimulation, but increases after the infusion of dibutyryl cAMP.

Inappropriate Secretion of TSH

The most common cause of elevated TSH levels with elevated-to-high-normal free T_4 levels is seen in the noncompliant patient with a non–steady-state TSH who avoids taking levothyroxine therapy at prescribed doses until a few days before hormone values are determined.

Steady-state nonsuppressed TSH in the presence of elevated free thyroid hormone (free T_4, free T_3) concentrations in patients not taking drugs affecting the pituitary-thyroid axis are attributed to a syndrome of inappropriate TSH secretion.[156, 157] This syndrome includes neoplastic (e.g., TSH-secreting adenoma) and non-neoplastic (e.g., resistance to thyroid hormone) diseases.

Syndromes of resistance to thyroid hormones are clinically and biochemically heterogeneous, reflecting differences in the tissue distribution of the refractoriness to thyroid hormones[158–160] (see Chapter 114). In generalized resistance to thyroid hormones, most tissues with thyroid hormone receptors are refractory to T_3 and T_4, and the set-point of the pituitary-thyroid negative feedback axis is increased, that is, the pituitary TSH secretion normalizes only at supraphysiologic circulating thyroid hormone levels ("reset thyrostat"). A subgroup of patients with clinical hyperthyroidism and inappropriately normal or elevated TSH levels in the absence of a TSH-secreting tumor may be characterized as having central resistance to thyroid hormones. In this condition, primarily the pituitary and paraventricular nucleus of the hypothalamus (a site of TRH synthesis) are resistant to thyroid hormone.

The clinical differentiation of resistance to thyroid hormone from neoplastic causes of inappropriate TSH secretion is based on disproportionately high production of glycoprotein hormone common α subunit by the thyrotroph tumor (and an increased α subunit-TSH molar ratio) and exclusion of neoplastic thyrotroph autonomy (diminished or lacking responsiveness to TRH stimulation as well as thyroid hormone suppression).[161] In previously thyroidectomized patients poor responsiveness to short T_3 suppression seems to be most sensitive and specific in documenting the presence of TSH-secreting tumor.[162]

TSH-SECRETING PITUITARY TUMORS. The TSH-secreting pituitary adenoma is the most common cause of secondary hyperthyroidism and accounts for about 1% of all pituitary tumors.[163–165] Co-secretion of prolactin or GH occurs frequently. The presenting clinical symptoms usually follow the pattern of hormone hypersecretion and, dependent on tumor size, consequences of local structure compression. Basal TSH levels are often within the normal range, the pulse frequency is normal, and the pulse amplitude is either increased or normal[166] in the presence of elevated free thyroid hormone levels. This phenomenon is explained by the increased bioactivity of secreted TSH,[167–169] causing clinical hyperthyroidism (sometimes milder than expected given the level of thyroid hormones) and goiter. Although the measurement of TRH in the circulation has limitations, it was found to be undetectable after pituitary surgery in one patient.[170] High levels were detected in another case,[171] suggesting a possible etiologic role of TRH in tumor formation. Thyroid adenomas, multinodular goiter, and differentiated thyroid carcinoma have been documented in several clinical cases, suggesting a potential role of long-standing TSH hypersecretion in thyroid tumorigenesis. Autoimmune thyroid diseases occur with the same incidence as in the general population.

TSH-secreting adenomas have a high density of somatostatin receptors, making them easy to visualize on somatostatin scan. Somatostatin analogue therapy has been used to control TSH secretion and diminish tumor size.[138, 172] Up to 50% of patients cannot be cured by surgery.[162, 167, 173] Despite its unproven benefit, radiotherapy has been used as an adjunct to postoperative medical treatment with somatostatin analogues. Thyroid hormone–lowering therapy should be avoided to prevent conversion of the tumor to a more aggressive form leading to extensive local invasion. Transformation of a TSH-secreting adenoma into a pituitary carcinoma with metastases outside the central nervous system has also been reported in one case.[174] In contrast to paraneoplastic hCG secretion, no paraneoplastic intact TSH production has been reported.

PITUITARY ENLARGEMENT IN PATIENTS WITH THYROID HYPOFUNCTION. Long-standing, severe primary hypothyroidism can lead to a diffuse or nodular sellar mass due to hypertrophy and hyperplasia of TSH-producing cells.[175] Thyrotroph stimulation may be caused in part by augmented TRH secretion in the absence of negative feedback inhibition by thyroid hormones at the level of both the pituitary and hypothalamus. The pituitary enlargement is insidious and typically requires about 10 years to become clinically apparent.

Hyperplasia of thyrotrophs may mimic a neoplastic process in the pituitary, raising a question of thyrotroph autonomy. In cases of dramatic TSH elevations with pituitary enlargement, simple hyperplasia may be differentiated from thyrotroph autonomy by documentation of low free thyroid hormones, proportional α subunit and TSH levels, a short T_3 suppression test, and a TRH stimulation showing an adequate response. Moreover, the significant reduction in pituitary size was documented after 1 week of high-dose thyroid hormone treatment, normalization of the thyroid profile was noted within 4 weeks of therapy, and complete resolution of the pituitary hyperplasia was evident after 3 months of therapy.[176, 177]

Drugs Increasing TSH Levels

Haloperidol, chlorpromazine, and other dopamine receptor blockers can raise basal TSH and enhance the TSH response to TRH.[73] Theophylline increases TSH and T_4, possibly through β-adrenergic stimulation of the hypothalamus. The number of medications induce decrease in thyroid hormone concentrations, which leads to compensatory elevations of TSH.[178]

Alterations of TSH Bioactivity and Structure

Testing the B/I Ratio of TSH

Overall potency of TSH, similar to that of other hormones, has been traditionally quantitated as the B/I ratio (i.e., the ratio of serum TSH bioactivity [B] to immunoreactivity [I]) when samples are simultaneously quantified by in vitro bioassay and sensitive immunoassay (see discussion of bioactivity assays and testing TSH immunoreactivity). When the B/I ratio changes, it is considered to be the result of a change in biologic activity per unit of immunologic activity. A basic assumption in the generation of the B/I ratio is that the immunometric assay does not discriminate between isohormones of TSH. In studies of recombinant TSH isoforms the accuracy of the B/I ratio was validated by mass determination based on amino acid analysis.[19] However, this kind of validation can only be done with purified material.

Decreased biologic activity of TSH may be present in patients with steady-state free thyroid hormone levels disproportionately low relative to the elevation of TSH and a normal thyroid hormone response to TSH stimulation. Analogously, patients with TSH inappropriately normal for markedly elevated levels of thyroid hormones and a normal thyroid hormone response to TSH stimulation may have increased TSH bioactivity, as may be seen in TSH-secreting pituitary tumors or resistance to thyroid hormones. Thus, it seems that an altered steady-state TSH–free T_4 ratio in patients with a normal thyroid hormone response to TSH stimulation may raise a suspicion of changed TSH biologic activity.

Low TSH bioactivity is found in patients lacking TRH. Moreover, variations in TSH bioactivity have been recorded in normal subjects during nocturnal TSH surge, in normal fetuses during the last trimester of pregnancy, in patients with primary hypothyroidism, TSH-secreting pituitary adenoma, and nonthyroidal illness. In conclusion, the secretion of TSH molecules with altered bioactivity plays an important pathogenetic role in various thyroid disorders, while in some particular physiologic conditions the bioactivity of TSH may vary in order to adjust thyroid hormone secretion to temporary needs.[179] Since at present the clinical management of patients with altered TSH bioactivity is the same as that of any patient with hypothyroidism or hyperthyroidism, routine testing of TSH biologic activity in clinical practice is generally not performed.

BIOACTIVITY ASSAYS. Biologic activity of serum TSH can be easily tested using various sensitive in vitro bioassays. In particular, CHO cells stably transfected with human TSH receptor provide a convenient system to measure TSH biologic activity.[180] This assay is based on comparison of differences in cAMP levels after stimulation by TSH in test samples. Differentiated TSH functional activity can be compared in the Fischer rat thyroid line 5 (FRTL-5) cell system[181] by testing stimulation of cell growth, iodine uptake, and deiodinase activity.[19] As a result, the TSH B/I ratio is calculated. The B/I ratio may be altered due to changes in TSH carbohydrate as well as protein structure.

Alterations in TSH Carbohydrate Structure

Variations in the TSH B/I ratio have been associated with alterations in carbohydrate structure in physiologic and pathologic conditions. Synthesis and secretion of TSH isoforms with different carbohydrate structure (glycoforms) are regulated by TRH and the thyroid hormone.[179] It has been shown that TSH has low bioactivity due to an altered glycosylation pattern in some cases of central hypothyroidism. Such patients are thought to suffer from hypothalamic TRH deficiency. TRH administration has been shown to increase TSH bioactivity and subsequently circulating thyroid hormone levels.[153, 182]

TSH is more highly sialylated in patients with primary hypothyroidism,[183] and similarly, TSH glycosylation isoforms with higher bioactivity have been reported in patients with resistance to thyroid hormone.[179] Variable carbohydrate structures of circulating TSH have also been described in TSH-secreting pituitary adenomas, and have also been associated with nonthyroidal illness syndrome, chronic uremia, TRH and somatostatin administration, cranial irradiation, intrauterine stage, and aging.[184] Such regulation of TSH glycosylation may be viewed largely as an adaptive response, thus contributing to the classic negative T_3/T_4–TSH-TRH feedback loop. In primary hypothyroidism, pituitary compensation would not only consist of increased production and release of the hormone, but the secreted TSH would have an altered carbohydrate structure that prolongs its plasma half-life. At the molecular level, this may involve a direct regulation of the transcription of glycosyltransferases by thyroid hormone, as, for example, thyroid hormone status has been shown to modulate α2,3- and α2,6-sialyltransferase messenger RNA levels in mouse thyrotrophs.[185]

CARBOHYDRATE STRUCTURE ANALYSIS. Determination of carbohydrate structure in circulating TSH is based on indirect lectin affinity chromatography, due to limited quantities of the hormone in the serum samples. Despite the limitations of this method it permits partial analysis of oligosaccharide structures in various conditions. Lectin analyses may be complemented by carefully performed TSH metabolic clearance studies in rats. For example, a gradual decrease in the number of sialic acid and an increase in the number of sulfated *N*-acetylgalactosamine residues on TSH correlate with progressive elevation in metabolic clearance rate.[19]

Mutations in the TSH-β Subunit Gene

Familial TSH deficiency has been described in three families with point mutations in the TSH-β subunit gene (Table 96–6). In a Greek kindred described by Dacou-Voutetakis and coworkers,[186] a point mutation converted a glutamic acid codon (GAA, codon 12) to a premature

TABLE 96–6. Mutations in the Thyroid-Stimulating Hormone (TSH)-β Subunit Gene

Gene Alteration	Amino Acid Alteration	Specific Structural Change	hTSH Heterodimer Formation	Bioactivity (B/I)	Clinical Presentation
Point mutation	Gly29Arg	Arginine introduced to the cystine knot region (CA<u>G</u>YC)	Undetected	—	Familial central hypothyroidism[187]
Stop at codon 12	Deletion of residues 12–112	TSH-β subunit 11–amino acid N-terminal peptide produced	Undetected	—	Familial central hypothyroidism[186]
Frameshift mutation	Cys105Val, change in the amino acid sequence	Disulfide bond in the seatbelt region disrupted	Reduced	Reduced	Familial central hypothyroidism[188]
Frameshift mutation and stop at codon 114	Cys105Val, change in the amino acid sequence at positions 106–114	Disulfide bond in the seatbelt region disrupted	Undetected	—	Congenital central hypothyroidism[189]

hTSH, human TSH; B/I, the ratio of TSH bioactivity to immunoreactivity.

stop codon (TAA). No functional TSH-β subunit was produced in patients with two defective alleles, and TSH was not detectable in the serum.

Hayashizaki and associates[187] described several related Japanese families with a point mutation in the CAGY region of the TSH-β subunit gene. The CAGY region is named for the one-letter amino acid codes of a conserved region of pituitary and placental glycoprotein hormone β subunit genes. The CAGY region is thought to be essential for α-β subunit interactions. In this kindred, codon[187] was converted from a GGA (glycine residue) to AGA (arginine residue). This alteration prevents the mutant TSH-β subunit from interacting with the common α subunit, and intact TSH is not secreted from thyrotrophs in patients expressing two defective alleles.

A third kindred with a TSH β point mutation was described by Medeiros-Neto and coworkers.[188] This family had 1-bp frameshift deletion in codon 105 of the TSH-β subunit leading to C105V mutation, which was predicted to enhance intracellular degradation of TSH-β subunit or diminish β subunit ability to interact with the α subunit. In agreement with this prediction TSH was detectable only at trace amounts in the serum. Hypothyroidism in this family might be due to both impaired TSH secretion and secretion of TSH with reduced biologic activity. Identical homozygous base-pair deletion in the TSH-β subunit gene resulting in congenital central hypothyroidism was described by Doecker and coworkers.[189] Analysis of the TSH-β subunit gene in this case demonstrated a frameshift deletion in codon 105 with a premature stop at codon 114, resulting in lack of five terminal amino acids. TSH was undetectable even after administration of TRH; thyroid hormones were below the range of detectability as well.

In contrast, mutations in the common α subunit gene have not been described in humans. They may be lethal in humans, although mice with a targeted disruption of the common α subunit gene were viable and suffered from hypothyroidism and hypogonadism.[31]

REFERENCES

1. Uhlenhuth E: The anterior lobe of the hypophysis as a control mechanism of the function of the thyroid gland. Br J Exp Biol 5:1–5, 1927.
2. Dracopoli NC, Rettig WJ, Whitfield GK, et al: Assignment of the gene for the beta subunit of thyroid-stimulating hormone to the short arm of human chromosome 1. Proc Natl Acad Sci U S A 83:1822–1826, 1986.
3. Takata K, Watanabe S, Hirono M, et al: The role of the carboxyl-terminal 6 amino acid extension of human TSH beta subunit. Biochem Biophys Res Commun 165:1035–1042, 1989.
4. Pierce JG, Parsons TF: Glycoprotein hormones: Structure and function. Annu Rev Biochem 50:465–495, 1981.
5. Lapthorn AJ, Harris DC, Littlejohn A, et al: Crystal structure of human chorionic gonadotropin. Nature 369:455–461, 1994.
6. Szkudlinski MW, Teh NG, Grossmann M, et al: Engineering human glycoprotein hormone superactive analogues. Nat Biotechnol 14:1257–1263, 1996.
7. Fairlie WD, Stanton PG, Hearn MT: The disulphide bond structure of thyroid-stimulating hormone beta-subunit. Biochem J 314:449–455, 1996.
8. Baenziger JU: Glycosylation and glycoprotein hormone function. *In* Lustbader JW, Puett D, Ruddon RW (eds): Glycoprotein hormones: Structure, function and clinical implications. New York, Springer-Verlag, 1994, pp. 167–174.
9. Szkudlinski MW, Grossmann M, Weintraub BD: Structure-function studies of human TSH: New advances in the design of glycoprotein hormone analogs. Trends Endocrinol Metab 7:277–286, 1996.
10. Matzuk MM, Kornmeier CM, Whitfield GK, et al: The glycoprotein alpha-subunit is critical for secretion and stability of the human thyrotropin beta-subunit. Mol Endocrinol 2:95–100, 1988.
11. Grossmann M, Weintraub BD, Szkudlinski MW: Novel insights into the molecular mechanisms of human thyrotropin action: Structural, physiological and therapeutic implications for the glycoprotein hormone family. Endocr Rev 18:476–501, 1997.
12. Grossmann M, Szkudlinski MW, Wong R, et al: Substitution of the seat-belt region of the thyrotropin (TSH)-β subunit with the corresponding regions of choriogonadotropin or follitropin confers luteotropic, but not follitropic activity to chimeric TSH. J Biol Chem 272:15532–15540, 1997.
13. Grossmann M, Leitolf H, Weintraub BD, Szkudlinski MW: A rational design strategy for protein hormone superagonists. Nat Biotechnol 16:871–875, 1998.
14. Szkudlinski MW, Thotakura NR, Weintraub BD: Subunit-specific functions of *N*-linked oligosaccharides in human thyrotropin: Role of terminal residues of alpha and beta-subunit oligosaccharides in metabolic clearance and bioactivity. Proc Natl Acad Sci U S A 92:9062–9066, 1995.
15. Grossmann M, Szkudlinski MW, Tropea JE, et al: Expression of human thyrotropin in cell lines with different glycosylation patterns combined with mutagenesis of specific glycosylation sites. Characterization of a novel role for the oligosaccharides in the in vitro and in vivo bioactivity. J Biol Chem 270:29378–29385, 1995.
16. Thotakura NR, Szkudlinski MW, Weintraub BD: Structure-function studies of oligosaccharides of recombinant human thyrotrophin by sequential deglycosylation and resialylation. Glycobiology 4:525–533, 1994.
17. Thotakura NR, Desai RK, Szkudlinski MW, Weintraub BD: The role of the oligosaccharide chains of thyrotropin alpha- and beta-subunits in hormone action. Endocrinology 131:82–88, 1992.
18. Bielinska M, Boime I: The glycoprotein hormone family: Structure and function of the carbohydrate chains. *In* Montreuil J, Schachter H, Vliegenhart JFG (eds): Glycoproteins. Amsterdam, Elsevier Science 1995, pp 565–587.
19. Szkudlinski MW, Thotakura NR, Bucci I, et al: Purification and characterization of recombinant human thyrotropin (TSH) isoforms produced by Chinese hamster ovary cells: The role of sialylation and sulfation in TSH bioactivity. Endocrinology 133:1490–1503, 1993.
20. Leitolf H, Szkudlinski MW, Hoang-Vu C, et al: Effects of continuous and pulsatile administration of pituitary rat thyrotropin and recombinant human thyrotropin in a chronically cannulated rat. Horm Metab Res 27:173–178, 1995.
21. Wondisford FE, Usala SJ, DeCherney GS, et al: Cloning of the human thyrotropin beta-subunit gene and transient expression of biologically active human thyrotropin after gene transfection. Mol Endocrinol 2:32–39, 1988.
22. Thotakura NR, Desai RK, Bates LG, et al: Biological activity and metabolic clearance of a recombinant human thyrotropin produced in Chinese hamster ovary cells. Endocrinology 128:341–348, 1991.
23. Cole ES, Lee K, Lauziere K, et al: Recombinant human thyroid stimulating hormone: Development of a biotechnology product for detection of metastatic lesions of thyroid carcinoma. Biotechnology 11:1014–1024, 1993.
24. East-Palmer J, Szkudlinski MW, Lee J, et al: A novel, nonradioactive in vivo bioassay of thyrotropin (TSH). Thyroid 5:55–59, 1995.
25. Meier CA, Braverman LE, Ebner SA, et al: Diagnostic use of recombinant human thyrotropin in patients with thyroid carcinoma (phase I/II study). J Clin Endocrinol Metab 78:188–196, 1994.
26. Haugen BR, Pacini F, Reiners C, et al: A comparison of recombinant human thyrotropin and thyroid hormone withdrawal for the detection of thyroid remnant or cancer. J Clin Endocrinol Metab 84:377–385, 1999.
27. Ringel MD, Ladenson PW: Diagnostic accuracy of ^{131}I scanning with recombinant human thyrotropin versus thyroid hormone withdrawal in a patient with metastatic thyroid carcinoma and hypothyroidism. J Clin Endocrinol Metab 81:1724–1725, 1996.
28. Ruddon R: Super hormones. Analysis - research news. Nat Biotechnol 14:1224, 1996.
29. Vassart G, Dumont JE: The thyrotropin receptor and the regulation of thyrocyte function and growth. Endocr Rev 13:596–611, 1992.
30. Kawakami A, Eguchi K, Matsuoka N, et al: Thyroid-stimulating hormone inhibits Fas antigen–mediated apoptosis of human thyrocytes in vitro. Endocrinology 137:3163–3169, 1996.
31. Kendall SK, Samuelson LC, Saunders TL, et al: Targeted disruption of the pituitary glycoprotein hormone alpha-subunit produces hypogonadal and hypothyroid mice. Genes Dev 9:2007–2019, 1995.
32. Davies TF: The thyrotropin receptors spread themselves around (editorial). J Clin Endocrinol Metab 79:1232–1233, 1994.
33. Szkudlinski MW, Grossmann M, Weintraub BD: Progress in understanding structure-function relationships of human thyroid-stimulating hormone. Curr Opin Endocrinol Diabetes 4:354–363, 1997.
34. Pekonen F, Weintraub BD: Thyrotropin binding to cultured lymphocytes and thyroid cells. Endocrinology 103:1668–1677, 1978.
35. Provinciali M, Di Stefano G, Fabris N: Improvement in the proliferative capacity and natural killer cell activity of murine spleen lymphocytes by thyrotropin. Int J Immunopharmacol 14:865–870, 1992.
36. Marcus C, Ehren H, Bolme P, Arner P: Regulation of lipolysis during the neonatal period. Importance of thyrotropin. J Clin Invest 82:1793–1797, 1988.
37. Wang J, Whetsell M, Klein JR: Local hormone networks and intestinal T cell homeostasis. Science 275:1937–1939, 1997.
38. Murata Y: Multiple isoforms of thyroid hormone receptor: An analysis of their relative contribution in mediating thyroid hormone action. Nagoya J Med Sci 61:103–115, 1998.
39. Ridgway EC, Weintraub BD, Maloof F: Metabolic clearance and production rates of human thyrotropin. J Clin Invest 53:895–903, 1974.
40. Kourides IA, Re RN, Weintraub BD, et al: Metabolic clearance and secretion rates of subunits of human thyrotropin. J Clin Invest 59:508–516, 1977.
41. van Coevorden A, Laurent E, Decoster C, et al: Decreased basal and stimulated thyrotropin secretion in healthy elderly men. J Clin Endocrinol Metab 69:177–185, 1989.
42. Sawin CT, Geller A, Kaplan MM, Bacharach P, et al: Low serum thyrotropin (thyroid-stimulating hormone) in older persons without hyperthyroidism. Arch Intern Med 151:165–168, 1991.
43. Lewis GF, Alessi CA, Imperial JG, Refetoff S: Low serum free thyroxine index in ambulating elderly is due to a resetting of the threshold of thyrotropin feedback suppression. J Clin Endocrinol Metab 73:843–849, 1991.
44. Brabant G, Ocran K, Ranft U, et al: Physiological regulation of thyrotropin. Biochimie 71:293–301, 1989.
45. Brabant G, Prank K, Hoang-Vu C, et al: Hypothalamic regulation of pulsatile thyrotropin secretion. J Clin Endocrinol Metab 72:145–150, 1991.
46. Mantagos S, Koulouris A, Makri M, Vagenakis AG: Development of thyrotropin circadian rhythm in infancy. J Clin Endocrinol Metab 74:71–74, 1992.
47. Brabant G, Prank K, Ranft U, et al: Circadian and pulsatile TSH secretion under physiological and pathophysiological conditions. Horm Metab Res Suppl 23:12–17, 1990.
48. Michaud P, Foradori A, Rodriguez-Portales JA, Arteaga E, et al: A prepubertal surge of thyrotropin precedes an increase in thyroxine and 3,5,3′-triiodothyronine in normal children. J Clin Endocrinol Metab 72:976–981, 1991.
49. Gurr JA, Kourides IA: Thyroid hormone regulation of thyrotropin alpha- and beta-subunit gene transcription. DNA 4:301-307, 1985.
50. Shupnik MA, Chin WW, Habener JF, Ridgway EC: Transcriptional regulation of the thyrotropin subunit genes by thyroid hormone. J Biol Chem 260:2900–2903, 1985.

51. Larsen PR, Silva JE, Kaplan MM: Relationships between circulating and intracellular thyroid hormones: Physiological and clinical implications. Endocr Rev 2:87–102, 1981.
52. Chatterjee VK, Lee JK, Rentoumis A, Jameson JL: Negative regulation of the thyroid-stimulating hormone alpha gene by thyroid hormone: Receptor interaction adjacent to the TATA box. Proc Natl Acad Sci U S A 86:9114–9118, 1989.
53. Burnside J, Darling DS, Carr FE, Chin WW: Thyroid hormone regulation of the rat glycoprotein hormone alpha-subunit gene promoter activity. J Biol Chem 264:6886–6891, 1989.
54. Carr FE, Burnside J, Chin WW: Thyroid hormones regulate rat thyrotropin beta gene promoter activity expressed in GH3 cells. Mol Endocrinol 3:709–716, 1989.
55. Wondisford FE, Farr EA, Radovick S, et al: Thyroid hormone inhibition of human thyrotropin beta-subunit gene expression is mediated by a cis-acting element located in the first exon. J Biol Chem 264:14601–14604, 1989.
56. Wood WM, Kao MY, Gordon DF, Ridgway EC: Thyroid hormone regulates the mouse thyrotropin beta-subunit gene promoter in transfected primary thyrotropes. J Biol Chem 264:14840–14847, 1989.
57. Bodenner DL, Mroczynski MA, Weintraub BD, et al: A detailed functional and structural analysis of a major thyroid hormone inhibitory element in the human thyrotropin beta-subunit gene. J Biol Chem 266:21666–21673, 1991.
58. Brent GA, Harney JW, Chen Y, et al: Mutations of the rat growth hormone promoter which increase and decrease response to thyroid hormone define a consensus thyroid hormone response element. Mol Endocrinol 3:1996–2004, 1989.
59. Sherman SI, Gopal J, Haugen BR, et al: Central hypothyroidism associated with retinoid X receptor–selective ligands. N Engl J Med 340:1075–1079, 1999.
60. Abel ED, Kaulbach HC, Campos-Barros A, et al: Novel insight from transgenic mice into thyroid hormone resistance and the regulation of thyrotropin. J Clin Invest 103:271–279, 1999.
61. Nelson C, Albert VR, Elsholtz HP, et al: Activation of cell-specific expression of rat growth hormone and prolactin genes by a common transcription factor. Science 239:1400–1405, 1988.
62. Day RN, Maurer RA: The distal enhancer region of the rat prolactin gene contains elements conferring response to multiple hormones. Mol Endocrinol 3:3–9, 1989.
63. Shupnik MA, Rosenzweig BA, Showers MO: Interactions of thyrotropin-releasing hormone, phorbol ester, and forskolin-sensitive regions of the rat thyrotropin-beta gene. Mol Endocrinol 4:829–836, 1990.
64. Steinfelder HJ, Hauser P, Nakayama Y, et al: Thyrotropin-releasing hormone regulation of human TSHB expression: Role of a pituitary-specific transcription factor (Pit-1/GHF-1) and potential interaction with a thyroid hormone-inhibitory element. Proc Natl Acad Sci U S A 88:3130–3134, 1991.
65. Kapiloff MS, Farkash Y, Wegner M, Rosenfeld MG: Variable effects of phosphorylation of Pit-1 dictated by the DNA response elements. Science 253:786–789, 1991.
66. Steinfelder HJ, Radovick S, Wondisford FE: Hormonal regulation of the thyrotropin beta-subunit gene by phosphorylation of the pituitary-specific transcription factor Pit-1. Proc Natl Acad Sci U S A 89:5942–5945, 1992.
67. Kim MK, McClaskey JH, Bodenner DL, Weintraub BD: An AP-1-like factor and the pituitary-specific factor Pit-1 are both necessary to mediate hormonal induction of human thyrotropin beta gene expression. J Biol Chem 268:23366–23375, 1993.
68. Bodenner DL, McClaskey JH, Kim MK, et al: The proto-oncogenes c-*fos* and c-*jun* modulate thyroid hormone inhibition of human thyrotropin beta subunit gene expression in opposite directions. Biochem Biophys Res Commun 189:1050–1056, 1992.
69. Wondisford FE, Steinfelder HJ, Nations M, Radovick S: AP-1 antagonizes thyroid hormone receptor action on the thyrotropin beta-subunit gene. J Biol Chem 268:2749–2754, 1993.
70. Perrone MH, Hinkle PM: Regulation of pituitary receptors for thyrotropin-releasing hormone by thyroid hormones. J Biol Chem 253:5168–5173, 1978.
71. Lumpkin MD, Samson WK, McCann SM: Arginine vasopressin as a thyrotropin-releasing hormone. Science 235:1070–1073, 1987.
72. Cooper DS, Klibanski A, Ridgway EC: Dopaminergic modulation of TSH and its subunits: In vivo and in vitro studies. Clin Endocrinol (Oxf) 18:265–275, 1983.
73. Scanlon MF, Weightman DR, Shale DJ, et al: Dopamine is a physiological regulator of thyrotrophin (TSH) secretion in normal man. Clin Endocrinol (Oxf) 10:7–15, 1979.
74. Silver BJ, Bokar JA, Virgin JB, et al: Cyclic AMP regulation of the human glycoprotein hormone alpha-subunit gene is mediated by an 18-base-pair element. Proc Natl Acad Sci U S A 84:2198–2202, 1987.
75. Deutsch PJ, Jameson JL, Habener JF: Cyclic AMP responsiveness of human gonadotropin-alpha gene transcription is directed by a repeated 18-base pair enhancer. Alpha-promoter receptivity to the enhancer confers cell-preferential expression. J Biol Chem 262:12169–12174, 1987.
76. Hoeffler JP, Meyer TE, Yun Y, Jameson JL, et al: Cyclic AMP–responsive DNA-binding protein: Structure based on a cloned placental cDNA. Science 242:1430–1433, 1988.
77. Steinfelder HJ, Radovick S, Mroczynski MA, et al: Role of a pituitary-specific transcription factor (pit-1/GHF-1) or a closely related protein in cAMP regulation of human thyrotropin-beta subunit gene expression. J Clin Invest 89:409–419, 1992.
78. Gordon DF, Lewis SR, Haugen BR, et al: Pit-1 and GATA-2 interact and functionally cooperate to activate the thyrotropin beta-subunit promoter. J Biol Chem 272:24339–24347, 1997.
79. Abel ED, Kaulbach HC, Campos-Barros A, et al: Novel insight from transgenic mice into thyroid hormone resistance and the regulation of thyrotropin. J Clin Invest 103:271–279, 1999.
80. Leedman PJ, Stein AR, Chin WW: Regulated specific protein binding to a conserved region of the 3′- untranslated region of thyrotropin beta-subunit mRNA. Mol Endocrinol 9:375–387, 1995.
81. Chedrese PJ, Kay TW, Jameson JL: Gonadotropin-releasing hormone stimulates glycoprotein hormone alpha-subunit messenger ribonucleic acid (mRNA) levels in alpha T_3 cells by increasing transcription and mRNA stability. Endocrinology 134:2475–2481, 1994.
82. Chin WW, Habener JF, Kieffer JD, Maloof F: Cell-free translation of the messenger RNA coding for the alpha subunit of thyroid-stimulating hormone. J Biol Chem 253:7985–7988, 1978.
83. Giudice LC, Waxdal MJ, Weintraub BD: Comparison of bovine and mouse pituitary glycoprotein hormone pre-alpha subunits synthesized in vitro. Proc Natl Acad Sci U S A 76:4798–4802, 1979.
84. Giudice LC, Weintraub BD: Evidence for conformational differences between precursor and processed forms of thyroid-stimulating hormone beta subunit. J Biol Chem 254:12679–12683, 1979.
85. Kourides IA, Weintraub BD: mRNA-directed biosynthesis of alpha subunit of thyrotropin: Translation in cell-free and whole-cell systems. Proc Natl Acad Sci U S A 76:298–302, 1979.
86. Kourides IA, Vamvakopoulos NC, Maniatis GM: mRNA-directed biosynthesis of alpha and beta subunits of thyrotropin. Processing of pre-subunits to glycosylated forms. J Biol Chem 254:11106–11110, 1979.
87. Vamvakopoulos NC, Kourides IA: Identification of separate mRNAs coding for the alpha and beta subunits of thyrotropin. Proc Natl Acad Sci U S A 76:3809–3813, 1979.
88. Behrens NH, Leloir LF: Dolichol monophosphate glucose: An intermediate in glucose transfer in liver. Proc Natl Acad Sci U S A 66:153–159, 1970.
89. Parsons TF, Bloomfield GA, Pierce JG: Purification of an alternate form of the alpha subunit of the glycoprotein hormones from bovine pituitaries and identification of its *O*-linked oligosaccharide. J Biol Chem 258:240–244, 1983.
90. Miura Y, Perkel VS, Magner JA: Rates of processing of the high mannose oligosaccharide units at the three glycosylation sites of mouse thyrotropin and the two sites of free alpha-subunits. Endocrinology 123:1296–1302, 1988.
91. Baenziger JU, Green ED: Pituitary glycoprotein hormone oligosaccharides: Structure, synthesis and function of the asparagine-linked oligosaccharides on lutropin, follitropin and thyrotropin. Biochim Biophys Acta 947:287–306, 1988.
92. Magner JA: Thyroid-stimulating hormone: Biosynthesis, cell biology, and bioactivity. Endocr Rev 11:354–385, 1990.
93. Smith PL, Baenziger JU: A pituitary *N*-acetylgalactosamine transferase that specifically recognizes glycoprotein hormones. Science 242:930–933, 1988.
94. Fiete D, Srivastava V, Hindsgaul O, Baenziger JU: A hepatic reticuloendothelial cell receptor specific for SO4-4GalNAc beta 1, 4GlcNAc beta 1,2Man alpha that mediates rapid clearance of lutropin. Cell 67:1103–1110, 1991.
95. Szkudlinski MW, Thotakura NR, Tropea JE, et al: Asparagine-linked oligosaccharide structures determine clearance and organ distribution of pituitary and recombinant thyrotropin. Endocrinology 136:3325–3330, 1995.
96. Gyves PW, Gesundheit N, Stannard BS, et al: Alterations in the glycosylation of secreted thyrotropin during ontogenesis. Analysis of sialylated and sulfated oligosaccharides. J Biol Chem 264:6104–6110, 1989.
97. Gyves PW, Gesundheit N, Thotakura NR, et al: Changes in the sialylation and sulfation of secreted thyrotropin in congenital hypothyroidism. Proc Natl Acad Sci U S A 87:3792–3796, 1990.
98. Constant RB, Weintraub BD: Differences in the metabolic clearance of pituitary and serum thyrotropin (TSH) derived from euthyroid and hypothyroid rats: Effects of chemical deglycosylation of pituitary TSH. Endocrinology 119:2720–2727, 1986.
99. Gesundheit N, Fink DL, Silverman LA, Weintraub BD: Effect of thyrotropin-releasing hormone on the carbohydrate structure of secreted mouse thyrotropin. Analysis by lectin affinity chromatography. J Biol Chem 262:5197–5203, 1987.
100. Taylor T, Weintraub BD: Altered thyrotropin (TSH) carbohydrate structures in hypothalamic hypothyroidism created by paraventricular nuclear lesions are corrected by in vivo TSH-releasing hormone administration. Endocrinology 125:2198–2203, 1989.
101. Kourides IA, Ridgway EC, Weintraub BD, et al: Thyrotropin-induced hyperthyroidism: Use of alpha and beta subunit levels to identify patients with pituitary tumors. J Clin Endocrinol Metab 45:534–543, 1977.
102. Beck-Peccoz P, Persani L, Faglia G: Glycoprotein hormone alpha-subunit in pituitary adenomas. Trends Endocrinol Metab 2:41–45, 1992.
103. Wehmann RE, Nisula BC: Radioimmunoassay of human thyrotropin: Analytical and clinical developments. Crit Rev Clin Lab Sci 20:243–283, 1984.
104. Silva JE, Larsen PR: Pituitary nuclear 3,5,3′-triiodothyronine and thyrotropin secretion: An explanation for the effect of thyroxine. Science 198:617–620, 1977.
105. Larsen PR, Berry MJ: Nutritional and hormonal regulation of thyroid hormone deiodinases. Annu Rev Nutr 15:323–352, 1995.
106. Dyes SEM, Segerson TP, Liposits Z, et al: Triiodothyronine exerts direct cell-specific regulation of thyrotropin-releasing hormone gene expression in the hypothalamic paraventricular nucleus. Endocrinology 123:2291–2297, 1988.
107. Fliers E, Wiersinga WM, Swaab DF: Physiological and pathophysiological aspects of thyrotropin-releasing hormone gene expression in the human hypothalamus. Thyroid 8:921–928, 1998.
108. Yang H, Yuan P, Wu V, Tache Y: Feedback regulation of thyrotropin-releasing hormone gene expression by thyroid hormone in the caudal raphe nuclei in rats. Endocrinology 140:43–49, 1999.
109. Caron PJ, Nieman LK, Rose SR, Nisula BC: Deficient nocturnal surge of thyrotropin in central hypothyroidism. J Clin Endocrinol Metab 62:960–964, 1986.
110. Bartalena L, Martino E, Falcone M, et al: Evaluation of the nocturnal serum thyrotropin (TSH) surge, as assessed by TSH ultrasensitive assay, in patients receiving long term L-thyroxine suppression therapy and in patients with various thyroid disorders. J Clin Endocrinol Metab 65:1265–1271, 1987.
111. Samuels MH, Lillehei K, Kleinschmidt-Demasters BK, Stears J, et al: Patterns of pulsatile pituitary glycoprotein secretion in central hypothyroidism and hypogonadism. J Clin Endocrinol Metab 70:391–395, 1990.
112. Brabant G: Pulsatile and circadian TSH secretion. Clinical relevance? Internist (Berl) 39:619–622, 1998.
113. Bartalena L, Martino E, Petrini L, et al: The nocturnal serum thyrotropin surge is

abolished in patients with adrenocorticotropin (ACTH)-dependent or ACTH-independent Cushing's syndrome. J. Clin Endocrinol Metab 72:1195–1199, 1991.

114. Caldwell G, Kellett HA, Gow SM, et al: A new strategy for thyroid function testing. Lancet 1:1117–1119, 1985.

115. Davis JR, Black EG, Sheppard MC: Evaluation of a sensitive chemiluminescent assay for TSH in the followup of treated thyrotoxicosis. Clin Endocrinol (Oxf) 27:563–570, 1987.

116. Yamada M, Saga Y, Shibusawa N, et al: Tertiary hypothyroidism and hyperglycemia in mice with targeted disruption of the thyrotropin-releasing hormone gene. Proc Natl Acad Sci U S A 94:10862–10867, 1997.

117. Faglia G, Bitensky L, Pinchera A, et al: Thyrotropin secretion in patients with central hypothyroidism: Evidence for reduced biological activity of immunoreactive thyrotropin. J Clin Endocrinol Metab 48:989–998, 1979.

118. Hall R, Ormston BJ, Besser GM, Cryer RJ: The thyrotrophin-releasing hormone test in diseases of the pituitary and hypothalamus. Lancet 1:759–763, 1972.

119. Snyder PJ, Jacobs LS, Rabello MM, et al: Diagnostic value of thyrotrophin-releasing hormone in pituitary and hypothalamic diseases. Assessment of thyrotrophin and prolactin secretion in 100 patients. Ann Intern Med 81:751–757, 1974.

120. Ferretti E, Persani L, Jaffrain-Rea ML, et al: Evaluation of the adequacy of levothyroxine replacement therapy in patients with central hypothyroidism. J Clin Endocrinol Metab 84:924–929, 1999.

121. Hashimoto K: The etiology of isolated thyroid stimulating hormone deficiency. Intern Med 37:231–232, 1998.

122. Tatsumi K, Miyai K, Notomi T, et al: Cretinism with combined hormone deficiency caused by a mutation in the PIT1 gene. Nat Genet 1:56–58, 1992.

123. Pfaffle RW, DiMattia GE, Parks JS, et al: Mutation of the POU-specific domain of Pit-1 and hypopituitarism without pituitary hypoplasia. Science 257:1118–1121, 1992.

124. Radovick S, Nations M, Du Y, et al: A mutation in the POU-homeodomain of Pit-1 responsible for combined pituitary hormone deficiency. Science 257:1115–1118, 1992.

125. Treier M, Rosenfeld MG: The hypothalamic-pituitary axis: Co-development of two organs. Curr Opin Cell Biol 8:833–843, 1996.

126. Spencer CA: Clinical utility and cost-effectiveness of sensitive thyrotropin assays in ambulatory and hospitalized patients. Mayo Clin Proc 63:1214–1222, 1988.

127. Spencer C, Eigen A, Shen D, et al: Specificity of sensitive assays of thyrotropin (TSH) used to screen for thyroid disease in hospitalized patients. Clin Chem 33:1391–1396, 1987.

128. Nicoloff J, Lopresti J: Nonthyroidal illness. *In* Braverman LE, Utiger RD (eds): The Thyroid. Philadelphia, JB Lippincott, 1991, pp 286–295.

129. Custro N, Scafidi V, Notarbartolo A: Alterations in circadian rhythm of serum thyrotropin in critically ill patients. Acta Endocrinol (Copenh) 127:18–22, 1992.

130. Spencer CA, LoPresti JS, Patel A, et al: Applications of a new chemiluminometric thyrotropin assay to subnormal measurement. J Clin Endocrinol Metab 70:453–460, 1990.

131. Kaptein EM, Spencer CA, Kamiel MB, Nicoloff JT: Prolonged dopamine administration and thyroid hormone economy in normal and critically ill subjects. J Clin Endocrinol Metab 51:387–393, 1980.

132. De Groot LJ: Dangerous dogmas in medicine: The nonthyroidal illness syndrome. J Clin Endocrinol Metab 84:151–164, 1999.

133. Loosen PT: Thyroid function in affective disorders and alcoholism. Neurol Clin 6:55–82, 1988

134. Yoshimura M, Hershman JM: Thyrotropic action of human chorionic gonadotropin. Thyroid 5:425–434, 1995.

135. Tomer Y, Huber GK, Davies TF: Human chorionic gonadotropin (hCG) interacts directly with recombinant human TSH receptors. J Clin Endocrinol Metab 74:1477–1479, 1992.

136. Rodien P, Bremont C, Sanson ML, et al: Familial gestational hyperthyroidism caused by a mutant thyrotropin receptor hypersensitive to human chorionic gonadotropin. N Engl J Med 339:1823–1826, 1998.

137. Morley JE: Neuroendocrine control of thyrotropin secretion. Endocr Rev 2:396–436, 1981.

138. Comi RJ, Gesundheit N, Murray L, et al: Response of thyrotropin-secreting pituitary adenomas to a long-acting somatostatin analogue. N Engl J Med 317:12–17, 1987.

139. Roelfsema F, Frolich M: Pulsatile thyrotropin release and thyroid function in acromegalics before and during subcutaneous octreotide infusion. J Clin Endocrinol Metab 72:77–82, 1991.

140. Hershman J, Pekary A: Regulation of thyrotropin secretion. *In* Imura H (ed): The Pituitary Gland. New York, Raven Press, 1985, pp 149–188.

141. Boesgaard S, Hagen C, Hangaard J, et al: Effect of dopamine and a dopamine D-1 receptor agonist on pulsatile thyrotrophin secretion in normal women. Clin Endocrinol (Oxf) 32:423–431, 1990.

142. Glass CK, Holloway JM, Devary OV, Rosenfeld MG: The thyroid hormone receptor binds with opposite transcriptional effects to a common sequence motif in thyroid hormone and estrogen response elements. Cell 54:313–323, 1988.

143. Takeda T, Suzuki S, Liu RT, DeGroot LJ: Triiodothyroacetic acid has unique potential for therapy of resistance to thyroid hormone. J Clin Endocrinol Metab 80:2033–2040, 1995.

144. Rootwelt K, Ganes T, Johannessen SI: Effect of carbamazepine, phenytoin and phenobarbitone on serum levels of thyroid hormones and thyrotropin in humans. Scand J Clin Lab Invest 38:731–736, 1978.

145. Dussault JH, Turcotte R, Guyda H: The effect of acetylsalicylic acid on TSH and PRL secretion after TRH stimulation in the human. J Clin Endocrinol Metab 43:232–235, 1976.

146. van Haasteren GA, van der Meer MJ, Hermus AR, et al: Different effects of continuous infusion of interleukin-1 and interleukin-6 on the hypothalamic-hypophysial-thyroid axis. Endocrinology 135:1336–1345, 1994.

147. Dubuis JM, Dayer JM, Siegrist-Kaiser CA, Burger AG: Human recombinant interleukin-1 beta decreases plasma thyroid hormone and thyroid stimulating hormone levels in rats. Endocrinology 123:2175–2181, 1988.

148. Stouthard JM, van der Poll T, Endert E, et al: Effects of acute and chronic interleukin-6 administration on thyroid hormone metabolism in humans. J Clin Endocrinol Metab 79:1342–1346, 1994.

149. van der Poll T, Romijn JA, Wiersinga WM, Sauerwein HP: Tumor necrosis factor: A putative mediator of the sick euthyroid syndrome in man. J Clin Endocrinol Metab 71:1567–1572, 1990.

150. Adriaanse R, Brabant G, Prank K, et al: Circadian changes in pulsatile TSH release in primary hypothyroidism. Clin Endocrinol (Oxf) 37:504–510, 1992.

151. Spencer CA, Schwarzbein D, Guttler RB, et al: Thyrotropin (TSH)-releasing hormone stimulation test responses employing third and fourth generation TSH assays. J Clin Endocrinol Metab 76:494–498, 1993.

152. Staub JJ, Althaus BU, Engler H, et al: Spectrum of subclinical and overt hypothyroidism: Effect on thyrotropin, prolactin, and thyroid reserve, and metabolic impact on peripheral target tissues. Am J Med 92:631–642, 1992.

153. Beck-Peccoz P, Amr S, Menezes-Ferreira MM, et al: Decreased receptor binding of biologically inactive thyrotropin in central hypothyroidism. Effect of treatment with thyrotropin-releasing hormone. N Engl J Med 312:1085–1090, 1985.

154. Refetoff S, Sunthornthepvarakul T, Gottschalk ME, Hayashi Y: Resistance to thyrotropin and other abnormalities of the thyrotropin receptor. Recent Prog Horm Res 51:97–120; discussion 120–122, 1996.

155. Codaccioni JL, Carayon P, Michel-Bechet M, et al: Congenital hypothyroidism associated with thyrotropin unresponsiveness and thyroid cell membrane alterations. J Clin Endocrinol Metab 50:932–937, 1980.

156. Gershengorn MC, Weintraub BD: Thyrotropin-induced hyperthyroidism caused by selective pituitary resistance to thyroid hormone. A new syndrome of "inappropriate secretion of TSH." J Clin Invest 56:633–642, 1975.

157. Weintraub BD, Menezes-Ferreira MM, Petrick PA: Inappropriate secretion of TSH. Endocr Res 15:601–617, 1989.

158. Chatterjee VK: Resistance to thyroid hormone. Horm Res 48(suppl 4):43–46, 1997.

159. Beck-Peccoz P, Chatterjee VK, Chin WW, et al: Nomenclature of thyroid hormone receptor beta-gene mutations in resistance to thyroid hormone: Consensus statement from the first workshop on thyroid hormone resistance, July 10–11, 1993, Cambridge, United Kingdom. J Clin Endocrinol Metab 78:990–993, 1994.

160. Refetoff S: Resistance to thyroid hormone. Curr Ther Endocrinol Metab 6:132–134, 1997.

161. Beck-Peccoz P, Brucker-Davis F, Persani L, et al: Thyrotropin-secreting pituitary tumors. Endocr Rev 17:610–638, 1996.

162. Brucker-Davis F, Oldfield EH, Skarulis MC, et al: Thyrotropin-secreting pituitary tumors: Diagnostic criteria, thyroid hormone sensitivity, and treatment outcome in 25 patients followed at the National Institutes of Health. J Clin Endocrinol Metab 84:476–486, 1999.

163. Saeger W, Ludecke DK: Pituitary adenomas with hyperfunction of TSH. Frequency, histological classification, immunocytochemistry and ultrastructure. Virchows Arch 394:255–267, 1982.

164. Wilson CB: A decade of pituitary microsurgery. The Herbert Olivecrona lecture. J Neurosurg 61:814–833, 1984.

165. Samuels MH, Ridgway EC: Glycoprotein-secreting pituitary adenomas. Baillieres Clin Endocrinol Metab 9:337–358, 1995.

166. Samuels MH, Henry P, Kleinschmidt-Demasters BK, et al: Pulsatile glycoprotein hormone secretion in glycoprotein-producing pituitary tumors. J Clin Endocrinol Metab 73:1281–1288, 1991.

167. Gesundheit N, Petrick PA, Nissim M, et al: Thyrotropin-secreting pituitary adenomas: Clinical and biochemical heterogeneity. Case reports and follow-up of nine patients. Ann Intern Med 111:827–835, 1989.

168. Beck-Peccoz P, Piscitelli G, Amr S, et al: Endocrine, biochemical, and morphological studies of a pituitary adenoma secreting growth hormone, thyrotropin (TSH), and alpha-subunit: Evidence for secretion of TSH with increased bioactivity. J Clin Endocrinol Metab 62:704–711, 1986.

169. Nissim M, Lee KO, Petrick PA, et al: A sensitive thyrotropin (TSH) bioassay based on iodide uptake in rat FRTL-5 thyroid cells: Comparison with the adenosine 3′,5′-monophosphate response to human serum TSH and enzymatically deglycosylated bovine and human TSH. Endocrinology 121:1278–1287, 1987.

170. Simard M, Pekary AE, Smith VP, Hershman JM: Thyroid hormones modulate thyrotropin-releasing hormone biosynthesis in tissues outside the hypothalamic-pituitary axis of male rats. Endocrinology 125:524–531, 1989.

171. Kamoi K, Mitsuma T, Sato H, et al: Hyperthyroidism caused by a pituitary thyrotrophin-secreting tumour with excessive secretion of thyrotrophin-releasing hormone and subsequently followed by Graves' disease in a middle-aged woman. Acta Endocrinol (Copenh) 110:373–382, 1985.

172. Chanson P, Weintraub BD, Harris AG: Octreotide therapy for thyroid-stimulating hormone-secreting pituitary adenomas. A follow-up of 52 patients. Ann Intern Med 119:236–240, 1993.

173. McCutcheon IE, Weintraub BD, Oldfield EH: Surgical treatment of thyrotropin-secreting pituitary adenomas. J Neurosurg 73:674–683, 1990.

174. Mixson AJ, Friedman TC, Katz DA, et al: Thyrotropin-secreting pituitary carcinoma. J Clin Endocrinol Metab 76:529–533, 1993.

175. Beck-Peccoz P, Persani L, Asteria C, et al: Thyrotropin-secreting tumors in hyper- and hypothyroidism. Acta Med Austriaca 23:41–46, 1996.

176. Sarlis NJ, Brucker-Davis F, Doppman JL, Skarulis MC: MRI-demonstrable regression of a pituitary mass in a case of primary hypothyroidism after a week of acute thyroid hormone therapy. J Clin Endocrinol Metab 82:808–811, 1997.

177. Levine M, Koppelman MC, Patronas N, Weintraub B: Amenorrhea-galactorrhea due to occult hypothyroidism. South Med J 79:1183–1184, 1986.

178. Surks MI, Sievert R: Drugs and thyroid function. N Engl J Med 333:1688–1694, 1995.

179. Beck-Peccoz P, Persani L: Variable biological activity of thyroid-stimulating hormone. Eur J Endocrinol 131:331–340, 1994.

180. Perret J, Ludgate M, Libert F, et al: Stable expression of the human TSH receptor in

CHO cells and characterization of differentially expressing clones. Biochem Biophys Res Commun 171:1044–1050, 1990.

181. Vitti P, Valente WA, Ambesi-Impiombato FS, et al: Graves' IgG stimulation of continuously cultured rat thyroid cells: A sensitive and potentially useful clinical assay. J Endocrinol Invest 5:179–182, 1982.
182. Magner JA, Kane J, Chou ET: Intravenous thyrotropin (TSH)-releasing hormone releases human TSH that is structurally different from basal TSH. J Clin Endocrinol Metab 74:1306–1311, 1992.
183. Miura Y, Perkel VS, Papenberg KA, et al: Concanavalin-A, lentil, and ricin lectin affinity binding characteristics of human thyrotropin: Differences in the sialylation of thyrotropin in sera of euthyroid, primary, and central hypothyroid patients. J Clin Endocrinol Metab 69:985–995, 1989.
184. Grossmann M, Weintraub BD, Szkudlinski MW: Novel insights into the molecular mechanisms of human thyrotropin action: Structural, physiological, and therapeutic implications for the glycoprotein hormone family. Endocr Rev 18:476–501, 1997.
185. Helton T, Magner J: Sialyltransferase messenger ribonucleic acid increases in thyrotrophs of hypothyroid mice: An in situ hybridization study. Endocrinology 134:2347–2353, 1994.
186. Dacou-Voutetakis C, Feltquate DM, Drakopoulou M, et al: Familial hypothyroidism caused by a nonsense mutation in the thyroid-stimulating hormone beta-subunit gene. Am J Hum Genet 46:988–993, 1990.
187. Hayashizaki Y, Hiraoka Y, Tatsumi K, et al: Deoxyribonucleic acid analyses of five families with familial inherited thyroid stimulating hormone deficiency [see comments]. J Clin Endocrinol Metab 71:792–796, 1990.
188. Medeiros-Neto G, Herodotou DT, Rajan S, et al: A circulating, biologically inactive thyrotropin caused by a mutation in the beta subunit gene. J Clin Invest 97:1250–1256, 1996.
189. Doeker BM, Pfaffle RW, Pohlenz J, Andler W: Congenital central hypothyroidism due to a homozygous mutation in the thyrotropin beta-subunit gene follows an autosomal recessive inheritance. J Clin Endocrinol Metab 83:1762–1765, 1998.
190. Nilson JH, Bokar JA, Clay CM, et al: Different combinations of regulatory elements may explain why placenta-specific expression of the glycoprotein hormone alpha-subunit gene occurs only in primates and horses. Biol Reprod 44:231–237, 1991.
191. Sarapura VD, Strouth HL, Wood WM, et al: Activation of the glycoprotein hormone alpha-subunit gene promoter in thyrotropes. Mol Cell Endocrinol 146:77–86, 1998.
192. Kakinuma A, Chazenbalk GD, Jaume JC, et al: The human thyrotropin (TSH) receptor in a TSH binding inhibition assay for TSH receptor autoantibodies. J Clin Endocrinol Metab 82:2129–2134, 1997.

Chapter 97

Thyroid Function Tests

Neil J.L. Gittoes ▪ Jayne A. Franklyn ▪ David H. Sarne
Samuel Refetoff ▪ Michael C. Sheppard

The possibility of thyroid disease is suggested by signs or symptoms consistent with hyperthyroidism or hypothyroidism or some physical abnormality of the thyroid gland. Evaluation of patients should include a detailed history and physical examination. Because most thyroid diseases require treatment, it is crucial that a firm diagnosis be established. Furthermore, a number of medications, in particular, those used in the treatment of thyroid disease, may alter the results of thyroid function tests in such a way that reinvestigation after therapy has begun may provide ambiguous results.

EVALUATION OF THYROID FUNCTION BY LABORATORY TESTS

During the past three decades, clinical thyroidology has witnessed the introduction of a plethora of diagnostic procedures. These laboratory procedures provide greater sensitivity and specificity that enhance the likelihood of early detection of occult thyroid disease with only minimal clinical findings or obscured by coincidental nonthyroid disease. They also assist in the exclusion of thyroid dysfunction when symptoms and signs closely mimic thyroid pathology. On the other hand, the wide choice of complementary and overlapping tests indicates that each has its limitations and that no single test is always reliable.

Thyroid tests can be classified into broad categories according to the information that they provide at the functional, etiologic, or anatomic levels.

1. Tests that directly assess the level of thyroid gland activity and the integrity of hormone biosynthesis, such as thyroidal radioactive iodide uptake (RAIU) and perchlorate discharge, are carried out in vivo.

2. Tests that measure the concentration of thyroid hormones and their transport in blood are performed in vitro and provide indirect assessment of the level of thyroid hormone–dependent metabolic activity.

3. Tests that attempt to directly measure the impact of thyroid hormone on peripheral tissues are nonspecific because they are often altered by a variety of nonthyroidal processes.

4. Tests that detect substances, such as thyroid autoantibodies, that are generally absent in healthy individuals are useful in establishing the etiology of some thyroid illnesses.

5. Invasive tests for histologic examination or enzymatic studies, such as biopsy, are occasionally required to establish a definite diagnosis. Gross abnormalities of the thyroid gland, detected by palpation, can be assessed by scintiscanning and by ultrasonography.

6. Tests to evaluate the integrity of the hypothalamic-pituitary-thyroid axis at the level of (1) the response of the pituitary gland to thyroid hormone excess or deficiency, (2) the ability of the thyroid gland to respond to thyrotropin (thyroid-stimulating hormone [TSH]), and (3) pituitary responsiveness to thyrotropin-releasing hormone (TRH) are intended to identify the primary organ affected by the disease process that is manifested as thyroid dysfunction—in other words, primary (thyroid), secondary (pituitary), or tertiary (hypothalamic) malfunction.

7. Finally, a number of special tests will be briefly described. Some are valuable in the elucidation of rare inborn errors of hormone biosynthesis, and others are mainly research tools.

Each test has inherent limitations, and no single procedure is diagnostically adequate for the entire spectrum of possible thyroid abnormalities. The choice, execution, application, and interpretation of each test require an understanding of the thyroid physiology and biochemistry dealt with in the preceding chapters. Thyroid tests not only assist in the diagnosis and management of thyroid illnesses but also allow one to better understand the pathophysiology underlying a specific disease.

IN VIVO TESTS OF THYROID GLAND ACTIVITY AND INTEGRITY OF HORMONE SYNTHESIS AND SECRETION

In contrast to all other tests, these procedures provide a means to directly evaluate thyroid gland function. Common to these investigations is the administration of radioisotopes to the patient that cannot be distinguished by the body from the naturally occurring stable iodine isotope (^{127}I). Formerly, these tests were used to diagnose hypothyroidism and thyrotoxicosis, but this application has been supplanted by measurement of serum TSH and thyroid hormone concentrations in blood. Also, alterations in thyroid gland activity and the uptake and metabolism of iodine are not necessarily coupled to the amount of hormone produced and secreted. The tests are time consuming and relatively expensive and expose the patient to radiation. Nevertheless, they still have some specific applications, including the diagnosis of inborn errors of thyroid hormonogenesis. Administration of radioisotopes can also be used to demonstrate ectopic thyroid tissue and to establish the etiology of some forms of thyrotoxicosis. Finally, measurement of tissue uptake of radioiodide is used as a means for estimating the dose of radioiodide to be delivered to the thyroid gland or to metastatic tissue in the treatment of thyrotoxicosis and thyroid carcinoma, respectively.

The physiologic basis for radioisotope thyroid scanning relies on the observations that iodine is an integral part of thyroid hormone molecules, and although several other tissues (salivary glands, mammary glands, lacrimal glands, the choroid plexus, and the parietal cells of the stomach) can extract iodide from blood, only the thyroid gland stores iodine for an appreciable period.[1] Because the kidneys continually filter blood iodide, the final fate of most iodine atoms is either to be trapped by the thyroid gland or to be excreted in urine. When a tracer of iodide is administered to the patient, it rapidly becomes mixed with the stable extrathyroidal iodide pool and is thereafter handled identically as the stable isotope. Thus the thyroidal content of radioiodine gradually increases and that in the extrathyroidal body pool gradually declines until virtually no free iodide is left. This endpoint is normally reached between 24 and 72 hours after administration of the iodide isotope.

A number of important physiologic parameters can be derived from measurement of RAIU by the thyroid gland, measurement of urinary excretion, and/or determination of the stable iodide concentration in plasma and urine: (1) the rate of thyroidal iodine uptake (thyroid iodide clearance), (2) fractional thyroid RAIU, (3) absolute iodide uptake by the thyroid gland, and (4) urinary excretion of radioiodide, or iodide clearance. After complete removal of the administered radioiodide from the circulation, depletion of the radioisotope from the thyroid gland can be monitored by direct counting over the gland. Reappearance of the radioiodine in the circulation in protein-bound form can be measured and used to estimate the intrathyroidal turnover of iodine and the secretory activity of the thyroid gland.

Further useful information can be generated by combining the administration of radioisotopes with agents known to either normally stimulate or inhibit thyroid gland activity, thus providing information on the control of thyroid gland activity. Administration of radioiodide followed by scanning allows examination of the anatomy of functional thyroid tissue. The latter two applications of in vivo tests using radioiodide will be discussed under their respective headings.

A number of radioisotopes are now available for investigative procedures, and the provision of more sophisticated and sensitive detection devices has substantially decreased the dose and radiation exposure required for these studies. The potential hazard of irradiation resulting from the administration of radioisotopes should always be kept in mind, however. Children are particularly vulnerable, and doses of x-rays as small as 20 rad to the thyroid gland are associated with an increased risk of thyroid malignancies.[2] However, no danger from isotopes used for the diagnosis of thyroid diseases has been substantiated.[3] Administration of radioisotopes during pregnancy and breast-feeding is absolutely contraindicated because of placental transport of the isotopes and excretion into breast milk, respectively.

Table 97–1 lists the most commonly used isotopes for in vivo studies of thyroid function.[4–6] Isotopes with slower physical decay, such as ^{125}I and ^{131}I, are particularly suitable for long-term studies. Conversely, isotopes with faster decay, such as ^{123}I and ^{132}I, usually deliver a lower radiation dose and are advantageous in short-term and repeated studies. Because the peak photon energy γ-emission differs among isotopes, simultaneous studies can be performed with two different isotopes.

Thyroidal Radioiodide Uptake

RAIU is the most commonly used thyroid test requiring the administration of a radioisotope. It is usually given orally in a capsule or in liquid form, and the quantity accumulated by the thyroid gland at various intervals is measured with a gamma scintillation counter. It is important to correct for the background activity of isotope circulating in the blood of the neck region (particularly during the early periods after administration). Background correction is achieved by subtracting counts obtained over the region of the thigh. A dose of the same radioisotope, usually 10%, placed in a neck "phantom" is also counted as a "standard." The percentage of RAIU is calculated from the counts accumulated per constant time unit.

The percentage of RAIU 24 hours after the administration of radioiodide is most useful because in most instances the thyroid gland has reached the plateau of isotope accumulation and the best separation between high, normal, and low uptake is obtained at this time. Normal values for 24-hour RAIU in most parts of North America are 5% to 30%. In many other parts of the world, normal values range from 15% to 50%. Lower normal values are due to the increase in dietary iodine intake after the enrichment of foods, particularly mass-produced bread (150 mg of iodine per slice) containing this element.[7] The inverse relationship between the daily dietary intake of iodine and the RAIU test is clearly illustrated in Figure 97–1. The intake of large amounts of iodide (>5 mg/day), mainly from the use of iodine-containing radiologic contrast media, antiseptics, vitamins, and drugs such as

TABLE 97–1. Commonly Used Isotopes for In Vivo Studies and Radiation Dose Delivered

Nuclide	Principal Photon Energy (KeV)	Physical Decay		Estimated Radiation Dose (mrad/μCi) Administered		Average Dose Given for Scanning Purposes (μCi)
		Mode	*Half-Life (Days)*	*Thyroid**	*Total Body*	
$^{131}I^-$	364	β (0.606 MeV)	8.1	1340	0.08	50
$^{125}I^-$	28	Electron capture	60	825	0.06	50
$^{123}I^-$	159	Electron capture	0.55	13	0.03	200
$^{132}I^-$	670	β (2.12 MeV)	0.10	15	0.1	50†
$^{99m}TcO_4^-$	141	Isometric transition	0.25	0.2	0.01	2500

*Calculations take into account the rate of maximal uptake and residence time of the isotope, as well as gland size. For the iodine isotopes, average data for adult euthyroid people used were a t½ uptake of 5 hours, a biologic t½ of 50 days, maximal uptake of 20%, and gland size of 15 g (see also Quimby et al.[4] and MIRD[5,6]).

†Dose used for early thyroid uptake studies.

amiodarone, suppresses RAIU values to a level hardly detectable with the usual equipment and doses of isotope. Depending on the type of iodine preparation and the period of exposure, depression of RAIU can last for weeks, months, or even years. Even external application of iodide may suppress RAIU. It is therefore important to inquire about individual dietary habits and sources of excess iodide intake.

RAIU is a measure of the avidity of the thyroid gland for iodide and its rate of clearance relative to the kidney, but results of this test do not equate with hormone production or release. Disease states resulting in excessive production and release of thyroid hormone are most often associated with increased thyroidal RAIU, and those causing hormone underproduction are generally associated with decreased thyroidal RAIU (Fig. 97–2). Some important exceptions to these rules include the high uptake values seen in certain hypothyroid patients and the low values in some hyperthyroid patients. Increased thyroidal RAIU with hormonal insufficiency can be caused by severe iodide deficiency and by most inborn errors of hormonogenesis (see Chapters 108 and 112). Lack of substrate in the former and a specific enzymatic block of hormone synthesis in the latter cause hypothyroidism poorly compensated by TSH-induced thyroid gland overactivity. Decreased thyroidal RAIU with hormonal excess is typically encountered in the syndrome of transient thyrotoxicosis (both de Quervain's and painless thyroiditis),[8] after the ingestion of exogenous hormone (thyrotoxicosis factitia), with iodide-induced thyrotoxicosis (Jod-Basedow disease),[9] rarely in patients with metastatic functioning thyroid carcinoma or struma ovarii, and also in patients with thyrotoxicosis who have a moderately high intake of iodide. High or low thyroidal RAIU as a result of low or high dietary iodine intake, respectively, may not be associated with significant changes in thyroid hormone secretion.

Various factors, including diseases that affect the value of the 24-hour thyroidal RAIU, are listed in Table 97–2. Several variations of the RAIU test have been devised that have particular value under special circumstances. Some of these variations are briefly described.

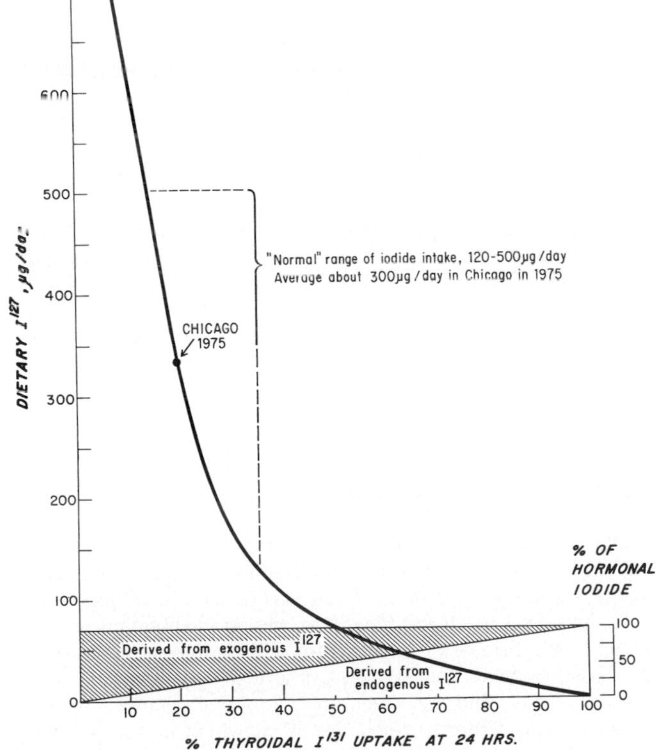

FIGURE 97–1. Relationship of 24-hour thyroidal radioiodide (^{131}I) uptake (RAIU) to dietary content of stable iodine (^{125}I). Uptake increases with decreasing dietary iodine. If iodine intake is below the amount provided from thyroid hormone degradation, the latter contributes a larger proportion of the total iodine taken up by the thyroid. With dietary habits in the United States, the average 24-hour thyroidal RAIU is below 20%. (From DeGroot LJ, Reed Larsen P, Hennemann G, et al: The Thyroid and Its Diseases. New York, John Wiley & Sons, 1984.)

Early Thyroid Radioiodide Uptake and ^{99m}Tc Uptake Measurements

The combination of severe thyrotoxicosis and a low intrathyroidal iodine concentration may result in an accelerated turnover rate of iodine in some patients; the accelerated iodine turnover causes rapid initial uptake of radioiodide, which reaches a plateau before 6 hours, followed by a decline through release of the isotope in hormonal or

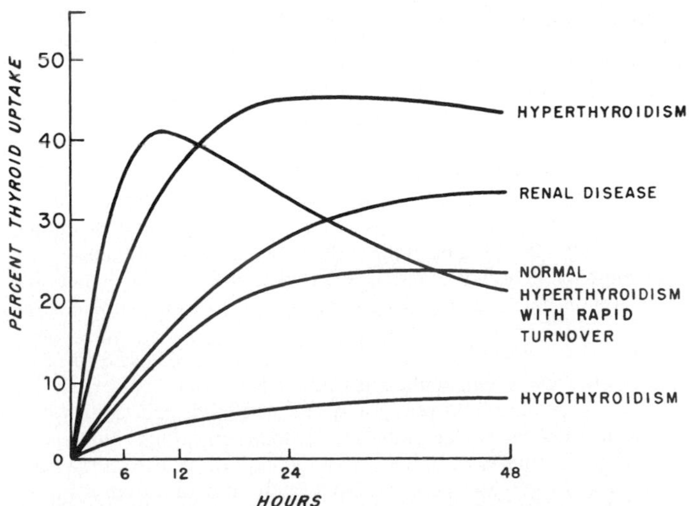

FIGURE 97–2. Examples of thyroidal radioiodide uptake curves under various pathologic conditions. Note the prolonged uptake in renal disease caused by decreased urinary excretion of the isotope and the early decline in thyroidal radioiodide content in some patients with thyrotoxicosis associated with a small, but rapidly turning over intrathyroidal iodine pool. (From DeGroot LJ, Reed Larsen P, Hennemann G, et al: The Thyroid and Its Diseases. New York, John Wiley & Sons, 1984.)

TABLE 97–2. Diseases and Other Factors That Affect 24-Hour Thyroidal RAIU

Increased RAIU
Hyperthyroidism (Graves' disease, Plummer's disease, toxic adenoma, trophoblastic disease, predominantly pituitary resistance to thyroid hormone, TSH-producing pituitary adenoma)
Nontoxic goiter (edemic, inherited biosynthetic defects, generalized resistance to thyroid hormone, Hashimoto's thyroiditis)
Excessive hormonal loss (nephrosis, chronic diarrhea, hypolipidemic resins, diet high in soybean)
Decreased renal clearance of iodine (renal insufficiency, severe heart failure)
Recovery of the suppressed thyroid (withdrawal of thyroid hormone and antithyroid drug administration, subacute thyroiditis, iodine-induced myxedema)
Iodine deficiency (endemic or sporadic dietary deficiency, excessive iodine loss as in pregnancy or in the dehalogenase defect)
TSH administration
Decreased RAIU
Hypothyroidism (primary or secondary)
Defect in iodide concentration (inherited trapping defect, early phase of subacute thyroiditis, transient hyperthyroidism)
Suppressed thyroid gland caused by thyroid hormone (hormone replacement, thyrotoxicosis factitia, struma ovarii)
Iodine excess (dietary, drugs, and other iodine contaminants)
Miscellaneous drugs and chemicals (see Tables 99–10 and 99–12)

RAIU, radioactive iodine uptake; TSH, thyroid-stimulating hormone.

other forms (see Fig. 97–2). Although this phenomenon is rare, some laboratories choose to routinely measure early RAIU, usually at 2, 4, or 6 hours. As mentioned above, early measurements require accurate determination of the background activity contributed by circulating isotope. Radioisotopes with a shorter half-life, such as ^{123}I and ^{132}I, are more suitable in this context.

Because thyroidal uptake in the very early period after administration of radioiodide reflects mainly iodide trapping activity, ^{99m}Tc as the pertechnetate ion ($^{99m}TcO_4^-$) may be used. In euthyroid patients, thyroid trapping is maximal at about 20 minutes and is approximately 1% of the administered dose.[10] This test, when coupled with the administration of triiodothyronine (T_3) has been used to evaluate thyroid gland suppressibility in thyrotoxic patients treated with antithyroid drugs (see below).

Perchlorate Discharge Test

The perchlorate discharge test is used to detect defects in intrathyroidal iodide organification. It is based on the following physiologic principle. Iodide is "trapped" in the thyroid gland by an active transport mechanism mediated by the Na^+-I^- symporter (NIS).[11] Once in the gland, iodine is rapidly bound to thyroglobulin (Tg) and retention no longer requires active transport. Several ions, such as thiocyanate (SCN^-) and perchlorate (ClO_4^-), inhibit NIS-mediated iodide transport and cause release of the intrathyroidal iodide not bound to thyroid protein. Thus intrathyroidal radioiodine loss after the administration of an inhibitor of iodide trapping measures intrathyroidal iodide that is not protein bound and indicates the presence of an iodide-binding defect.

In the standard test, epithyroid counts are obtained every 10 or 15 minutes after the administration of radioiodide. Two hours later, 1 g of $KClO_4$ is administered orally and repeated epithyroid counts continue to be obtained for an additional 2 hours. In normal individuals, radioiodide accumulation in the thyroid gland ceases after administration of the iodide transport inhibitor, and little or no loss of the accumulated thyroidal radioactivity occurs before induction of the "trapping" block. An organification defect is indicated if a loss of 5% or more is noted.[12] The severity of the defect is proportional to the extent of radioiodide discharged from the gland and is complete when virtually all the activity accumulated by the gland is lost. The test is positive in the inborn defect of iodide organification caused by thyroid peroxidase (TPO) defects or by mutations in the chloride/iodide transport protein (pendrin) when associated with sensorineural deafness (Pendred's syndrome).[13, 14] The test may also be positive during the administration of iodide organification–blocking agents or after treatment with radioactive iodide.

MEASUREMENT OF HORMONE CONCENTRATION AND OTHER IODINATED COMPOUNDS AND THEIR TRANSPORT IN BLOOD

The most commonly used tests for evaluating thyroid hormone–dependent metabolic status are measurements of free thyroid hormone concentrations. This approach is used because of the development of simple, sensitive, and specific methods for measuring these iodothyronines and because of the lack of specific tests for direct measurement of the metabolic effect of these hormones in target tissues. Other advantages are the requirement of only a small blood sample and the large number of determinations that can be completed by a laboratory during a regular workday.

The principal source of all hormonal iodine-containing compounds or their precursors is the thyroid gland, whereas peripheral tissues are the source of the products of their degradation. Their chemical structures and normal concentrations in serum are given in Figure 97–3. It is important to note that the concentration of each substance is dependent not only on the amount synthesized and secreted but also on its affinity for carrier serum proteins, distribution in tissues, rate of degradation, and finally, clearance.

Quantitatively, the major secretory product of the thyroid gland is thyroxine (T_4), T_3 being next in relative abundance. They are synthesized and stored in the thyroid gland as part of a larger molecule, Tg, which is degraded to release the two iodothyronines in a ratio favoring T_4 by 10- to 20-fold.[15] Under normal circumstances, only minute amounts of Tg escape into the circulation. On a molar basis, it is the least abundant iodine-containing compound in blood. With the exception of T_4, Tg, and small amounts of diiodotyrosine (DIT) and monoiodotyrosine (MIT), all other iodine-containing compounds found in normal human serum are produced mainly in extrathyroidal tissues by a stepwise process of deiodination of T_4.[16] An alternative pathway of T_4 metabolism that involves deamination and decarboxylation but retention of the iodine residues gives rise to tetraiodothyroacetic acid (TETRAC) and triiodothyroacetic acid (TRIAC).[17, 18] Conjugation to form sulfated iodoproteins also occurs.[19] Circulating iodalbumin is generated by intrathyroidal iodination of serum albumin.[20] Small amounts of iodoproteins may be formed in peripheral tissues[21] or in serum[22, 23] by covalent linkage of T_4 and T_3 to soluble proteins. The physiologic function of circulating iodine compounds other than T_4 and T_3 remains unknown. With the exception of reverse T_3 (rT_3), measurement of changes in their concentration is currently purely of research interest.

Measurement of Total Thyroid Hormone Concentration in Serum

IODOMETRY. Because of the observation that iodine is an integral part of the thyroid hormone molecule, it is not surprising that determination of the iodine content in serum was the first method suggested over six decades ago for the identification and quantitation of thyroid hormone.[24] Measurement of protein-bound iodine was the earliest method used routinely for the estimation of thyroid hormone concentration in serum. This test measured the total quantity of iodine precipitable with serum proteins,[25] 90% of which is T_4. The normal range was 4 to 8 mg of iodine per deciliter of serum.

Efforts to measure serum thyroid hormone levels with greater specificity and with lesser interference from nonhormonal iodinated compounds led to the development of measurement of butanol-extractable iodine and T_4 iodine by column techniques. All such chemical methods for the measurement of thyroid hormone in serum have been replaced by ligand assays, which are devoid of interference by even large quantities of nonhormonal iodine-containing substances.

NAME	Abbreviation	Molecular Weight	FORMULA	NORMAL CONCENTRATION[a] (range) ng / dl	pmol / L
3,5,3',5'-tetraiodothyronine (Thyroxine)	T_4	777	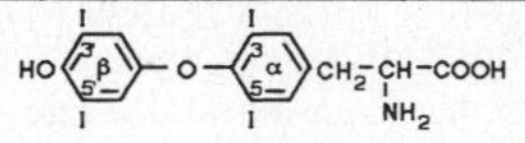	5,000 - 12,000	64,000 - 154,000
3,5,3'-triiodothyronine (Liothyronine)	T_3	651	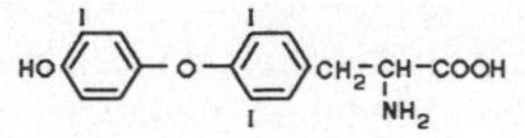	80 - 190[b]	1,200 - 2,900
3,3',5'-triiodothyronine (ReverseT_3)	rT_3	651	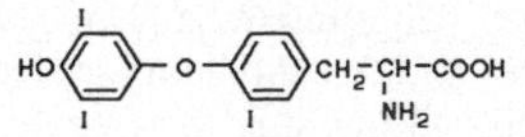	14 - 30	220 - 480
3.5-diiodothyronine	3,5-T_2	525	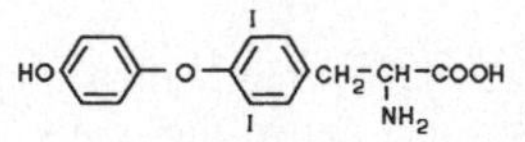	0.2 0- 0.75[b]	3.8 - 14
3,3'-diiodothyronine	3,3'-T_2	525	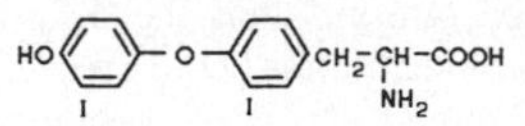	1 - 8[b]	19 - 150
3'5'-diiodothyronine	3'5'-T_2	525	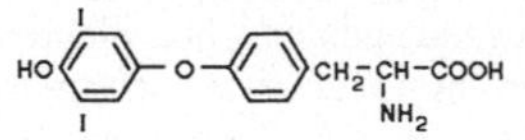	1.5 - 9.0[b]	30 - 170
3'-monoiodothyronine	3'-T_1	399	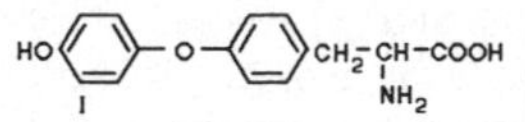	0.6 - 4	15 - 100
3-monoiodothyronine	3-T_1	399	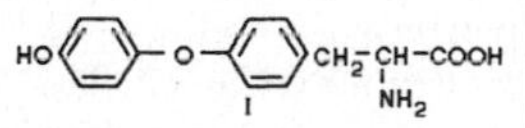	< 0.5 - 7.5	< 13 - 190
3,5,3',5'-tetraiodothyroacetic acid (TETRAC)	T_4A	748	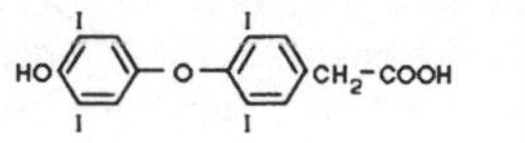	< 8 - 60	< 105 - 800
3,5,3'-triiodothyroacetic acid (TRIAC)	T_3A	622	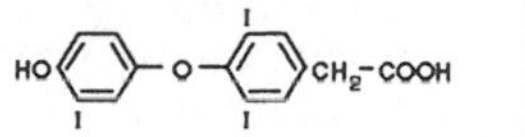	1.6 - 3	26 - 48
3,5-diiodotyrosine	DIT	433	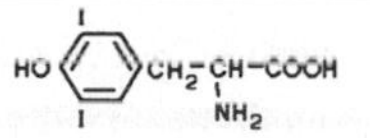	1 - 23	23 - 530
3-monoiodotyrosine	MIT	307	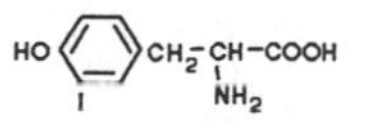	90 - 390[c]	2,900 - 12,700
thyroglobulin	Tg	[illegible]	glycoprotein made of two identical subunits	< 100 - [illegible]	1.5 - [illegible]

FIGURE 97–3. Iodine containing compounds in the serum of healthy adults. [a]Iodothyronine concentrations in the euthyroid population are not normally distributed. Thus calculation of the normal range on the basis of 95% confidence limits for a gaussian distribution is accurate. [b]Significant decline with old age. [c]Probably an overestimation because of cross-reactivity by related substances.

RADIOIMMUNOASSAYS. Concentrations of thyroid hormones in serum can be measured by radioimmunoassays (RIAs). The principle of these assays relies on competition between the hormone being measured with the same isotopically labeled compound for binding to a specific class of IgG molecule present in the antiserum. In assays for thyroid hormones, the hormone needs to be liberated from serum hormone-binding proteins, mainly thyroxine-binding globulin (TBG). Methods to achieve such liberation include extraction, competitive displacement of the hormone being measured, or inactivation of TBG.[26–29] Rarely, circulating antibodies against thyronines develop in some patients and interfere with RIAs carried out on unextracted serum samples. Depending on the method used for the separation of bound from free ligand, values obtained may be either spuriously low or high in the presence of such antibodies.[30, 31]

The wide choice of commercial kits available for most RIA procedures makes these assays accessible to all medical centers. RIAs have been adapted for the measurement of T_4 in small samples of dried blood spots on filter paper and are used in screening for neonatal hypothyroidism.[32]

NONRADIOACTIVE METHODS. More recently, assays have been developed that are based on the principle of the radioligand assay but do not use radioactive material. These assays, which use ligand conjugated to an enzyme, have largely replaced RIAs. The enzyme-linked ligand competes with the ligand being measured for the same binding sites on the antibody. Quantitation is carried out by spectrophotometry of the color reaction developed after addition of the enzyme substrate.[33] Both homogeneous (enzyme-multiplied immunoassay technique) and heterogeneous (enzyme-linked immunosorbent assay) assays for T_4 have been developed.[34–36] In the homogeneous assays, no separation step is required, thus providing easy automation.[34] In one such assay, T_4 is linked to malate dehydrogenase to inhibit enzyme activity. The enzyme is activated when the T_4-enzyme conjugate is bound to T_4-specific antibody. Active T_4 conjugates to other enzymes such as peroxidase[35] and alkaline phosphatase[36] have also been developed. This assay has also been adapted for the measurement of T_4 in dried blood samples used in mass screening programs for neonatal hypothyroidism.[36] Other nonradioisotopic immunoassays use fluorescence excitation for detection of the labeled ligand, a technique that is finding increasing application. Such assay methods use a variety of chemiluminescent molecules such as 1,2-dioxetanes, luminol and derivatives, acridinium esters, oxalate esters, and firefly luciferins, as well as many sensitizers and fluorescent enhancers.[37] One such assay that uses T_4 conjugated to β-galactosidase and fluorescence measurements of the hydrolytic product of 4-methylumbelliferyl-β-D-galactopyranoside has been adapted for use in a microanalytic system requiring only 10 mL of serum.[38]

SERUM TOTAL T_4. The usual concentration of total T_4 (TT_4) in adults ranges from 5 to 12 μg/dL (64–154 nmol/L). When concentrations are below or above this range in the absence of thyroid dysfunction, they are usually the result of an abnormal level of serum TBG. Such abnormalities are commonly seen during the hyperestrogenic state of pregnancy and during the administration of estrogen-containing compounds, which results in a significant elevation of serum TT_4 levels in euthyroid individuals. Far less commonly, TBG excess is inherited.[39] Serum TT_4 is virtually undetectable in the fetus until midgestation. Thereafter, it rapidly increases and reaches high normal adult levels during the last trimester. A further acute, but transient, rise occurs within hours after delivery.[40] Values remain above the adult range until 6 years of age, but subsequent age-related changes are minimal, so in clinical practice the same normal range of TT_4 applies to both sexes and all ages.

Small seasonal variations and changes related to high altitude, cold, and heat have been described. Rhythmic variations in serum TT_4 concentration are of two types: variations related to postural changes in serum protein concentration[41] and true circadian variation.[26] Postural changes in protein concentration do not alter the free T_4 (FT_4) concentration, however.

Although levels of serum TT_4 below the normal range are usually associated with hypothyroidism and above this range are associated with thyrotoxicosis, it must be stressed that the TT_4 level does not always correspond to the FT_4 concentration, which represents the metabolically active fraction (see below). The TT_4 concentration in serum may be altered by independent mechanisms: (1) an increase or decrease in the supply of T_4, as seen in most cases of thyrotoxicosis and hypothyroidism, respectively; (2) changes caused solely by alterations in T_4 binding to serum proteins; and (3) compensatory changes in the serum TT_4 concentration because of high or low serum levels of T_3. Conditions associated with changes in serum TT_4 and their relationship to the metabolic status of the patient are listed in Table 97–3.

Serum TT_4 levels are low in conditions associated with decreased TBG concentrations, in the presence of abnormal TBGs with reduced binding affinity (see Chapter 113), or when the available T_4-binding sites on TBG are partially saturated by competing drugs present in blood in high concentration (Table 97–4). Conversely, TT_4 levels are high when the serum TBG concentration is high. In this situation, the person remains euthyroid provided that feedback regulation of the thyroid gland is intact.

Although changes in transthyretin (TTR) concentration rarely give rise to significant alterations in TT_4 concentration,[67] the presence of a variant serum albumin with high affinity for T_4[68, 69] or antibodies against T_4[26] produce apparent elevations in the measured TT_4 concentration, whereas the metabolic status remains normal. The variant albumin is inherited as an autosomal dominant trait termed familial dysalbuminemic hyperthyroxinemia (FDH; see Chapter 113).

Another possible cause of discrepancy between the observed serum TT_4 concentration and the metabolic status of the patient is divergent changes in the serum total T_3 (TT_3) and TT_4 concentrations with alterations in the serum T_3/T_4 ratio. The most common situation is that of an elevated TT_3 concentration. The source of T_3 may be endogenous, as in T_3 thyrotoxicosis, or exogenous, as during ingestion of T_3. In the former situation, contrary to the common variety of thyrotoxicosis, elevation in the serum TT_3 concentration is not accompanied by an increase in the TT_4 level. In fact, the serum TT_4 level is normal and occasionally low.[70] This finding indicates that the pathogenesis of T_3 thyrotoxicosis is the direct secretion of T_3 from the thyroid rather than peripheral conversion of T_4 to T_3. Ingestion of pharmacologic doses of T_3 results in thyrotoxicosis associated with severe depression of the serum TT_4 concentration. Moderate hypersecretion of T_3 can be associated with euthyroidism and a low serum TT_4 concentration. This situation, occasionally referred to as T_3 euthyroidism, may be more prevalent than T_3 thyrotoxicosis. It is believed to constitute a state of compensatory T_3 secretion as a physiologic adaptation of the failing thyroid gland, such as after treatment of thyrotoxicosis, in some cases of chronic thyroiditis, or during iodine deprivation.[71, 72] The serum TT_4 concentration is also low in normal persons receiving replacement doses of T_3. Conversely, serum TT_4 levels are above the upper limit of normal in 15% to 50% patients treated with exogenous T_4 and having normal serum TSH.[73] Because of the relatively slow rate of metabolism and large extrathyroidal T_4 pool, the serum concentration of the hormone varies little with the time of sampling in relation to ingestion of the daily dose.[74]

SERUM TOTAL T_3. Normal serum TT_3 concentrations in the adult are in the range of 80 to 190 ng/dL (1.2–2.9 nmol/L). Although sex differences are small, those with age are more dramatic. In contrast to

TABLE 97–3. Conditions Associated with Changes in Serum TT_4 Concentration and Relationship to Metabolic Status

	Serum TT_4 Concentration		
Metabolic Status	***High***	***Low***	***Normal***
Thyrotoxic	Hyperthyroidism (all causes, including Graves' disease, Plummer's disease, toxic thyroid adenoma, early phase of subacute thyroiditis) Thyroid hormone leak (early stage of subacute thyroiditis, transient thyrotoxicosis) Excess of exogenous or ectopic T_4 (thyrotoxicosis factitia, struma ovarii) Predominantly pituitary resistance to thyroid hormone	Intake of excess amounts of T_3 (thyrotoxicosis factitia)	Low TBG (congenital or acquired) T_3 thyrotoxicosis (untreated or recurrent posttherapy); more common in iodine-deficient areas Drugs competing with T_4 binding to serum proteins (see also entry under euthyroid with low TT_4 Hypermetabolism of nonthyroidal origin (Luft's syndrome)
Euthyroid	High TBG (congenital or acquired) T_4-binding albumin–like variant Endogenous T_4 antibodies Replacement therapy with T_4 only Treatment with D-T_4 Generalized resistance to thyroid hormone	Low TBG (congenital or acquired) Endogenous T_4 antibodies Mildly elevated or normal T_3 T_3 replacement therapy Iodine deficiency Treated thyrotoxicosis Chronic thyroiditis Congenital goiter Drugs competing with T_4 binding to serum proteins (see Table 97–4)	Normal state
Hypothyroid	Severe generalized resistance to thyroid hormone	Thyroid gland failure Primary (all causes, including gland destruction, severe iodine deficiency, inborn error of hormonogenesis) Secondary (pituitary failure) Tertiary (hypothalamic failure)	High TBG (congenital or acquired) Isolated peripheral tissue resistance to thyroid hormone

T_3, triiodothyronine; T_4, thyroxine; TBG, thyroxine-binding globulin; TT_4, total T_4.

TABLE 97–4. Compounds That Affect Thyroid Hormone Serum Transport Proteins

Substance	Common Use
Increase TBG concentration	
Estrogens[42, 43]	Ovulation suppressants and anticancer
Heroin and methadone[44]	Opiates (in addicts)
Clofibrate[45]	Hypolipidemic
5-Fluorouracil[46]	Anticancer
Perphenazine[47]	Tranquilizer
Decrease TBG concentration	
Androgens and anabolic steroids[48, 49]	Virilizing, anticancer, and anabolic
Glucocorticoids[50]	Anti-inflammatory and immunosuppressive; decrease intracranial pressure
L-Asparaginase[51]	Antileukemic
Nicotinic acid[52]	Hypolipidemic
Interfere with thyroid hormone binding to TBG and/or TTR	
Salicylates and salsalate[53, 54]	Anti-inflammatory, analgesic, and antipyretic
Diphenylhydantoin and analogues[53, 55]	Anticonvulsive and antiarrhythmic
Diazepam[56]	Antianxiety
Furosemide[57]	Diuretic
Sulfonylureas[58]	Hypoglycemic
Dinitrophenol[53]	Uncouples oxidative phosphorylation
Free fatty acids[59]	
o,p′-DDD[60]	Antiadrenal
Phenylbutazone[61]	Anti-inflammatory
Halofenate[62]	Hypolipidemic
Fenclofenac[63]	Antirheumatic
Orphenadrine[64]	Spasmolytic
Monovalent anions (SCN^-, ClO_4^-)[65]	Antithyroid
Thyroid hormone analogues, including dextroisomers[66]	Cholesterol reducing

o,p′-DDD, 2,4′-dichlorodiphenyldichloroethane (mitotane); TBG, thyroxin-binding globulin; TTR, transthyretin.

serum TT_4, the TT_3 concentration at birth is low, about half the normal adult level. It rises rapidly within 24 hours to about double the normal adult value, followed by a decrease over the subsequent 24 hours to a level in the upper adult range, which persists for the first year of life.[40] A decline in the mean TT_3 level has been observed in old age, although not in healthy subjects,[75, 76] which suggests that a fall in TT_3 may reflect the prevalence of nonthyroidal illness rather than an effect of age alone.[77] Although a positive correlation between serum TT_3 level and body weight has been observed, it may be related to overeating.[78] Rapid and profound reductions in serum TT_3 can be produced within 24 to 48 hours of total calorie or carbohydrate-only deprivation.[79–81]

Most conditions causing serum TT_4 levels to increase are associated with high TT_3 concentrations. Thus serum TT_3 levels are usually elevated in thyrotoxicosis and reduced in hypothyroidism. However, in both conditions the TT_3/TT_4 ratio is elevated relative to normal euthyroid persons. This elevation is due to the disproportionate increase in serum TT_3 concentration in thyrotoxicosis and a lesser diminution in hypothyroidism relative to the TT_4 concentration.[82] Accordingly, measurement of the serum TT_3 level is a more sensitive test for the diagnosis of hyperthyroidism, and measurement of TT_4 is more useful in the diagnosis of hypothyroidism.

Under certain conditions, changes in the serum TT_3 and TT_4 concentrations are either disproportionate or in the opposite direction (Table 97–5). Such conditions include the syndrome of thyrotoxicosis with normal TT_4 and FT_4 levels (T_3 thyrotoxicosis). In some patients, treatment of thyrotoxicosis with antithyroid drugs may normalize the serum TT_4 but not the TT_3 level and produce a high TT_3/TT_4 ratio. In areas of limited iodine supply[72] and in patients with limited thyroidal ability to process iodide,[71] euthyroidism can be maintained at low serum TT_4 and FT_4 levels by increased direct thyroidal secretion of T_3. Although these changes have a rational physiologic explanation, the significance of discordant serum TT_4 and TT_3 levels under other circumstances is less well understood.

The most common cause of discordant serum concentrations of TT_3 and TT_4 is a selective decrease in serum TT_3 caused by decreased conversion of T_4 to T_3 in peripheral tissues. This reduction is an integral part of the pathophysiology of a number of nonthyroidal acute and chronic illnesses and calorie deprivation (see Chapter 106). In these conditions the serum TT_3 level is often lower than that commonly found in patients with frank primary hypothyroidism. However, no clear clinical evidence of hypometabolism is found in this situation. In some individuals, decreased T_4-to-T_3 conversion in the pituitary gland[83] or in peripheral tissues[84] is thought to be an inherited condition.

A variety of drugs are responsible for producing changes in the serum TT_3 concentration without apparent metabolic consequences. Drugs that compete with hormone binding to serum proteins decrease serum TT_3 levels, generally without affecting the free T_3 (FT_3) concentration (see Table 97–4). Some drugs such as glucocorticoids[85] depress the serum TT_3 concentration by interfering with the peripheral conversion of T_4 to T_3. Others, such as phenobarbital,[86] depress the serum TT_3 concentration by stimulating the rate of intracellular hormone degradation and clearance. Most have multiple effects. These effects are combinations of those described above, as well as inhibition of the hypothalamic-pituitary axis or thyroidal hormonogenesis.[87]

Changes in serum TBG concentration have an effect on the serum TT_3 concentration similar to that on TT_4 (see Chapter 94). The presence of endogenous antibodies to T_3 may also result in apparent elevation of serum TT_3, but as in the case of high TBG, it does not cause hypermetabolism.[30]

Administration of commonly used replacement doses of T_3, usually on the order of 75 μg/day or 1 μg/kg body weight per day,[88] results in serum TT_3 levels in the thyrotoxic range. Furthermore, because of rapid gastrointestinal absorption and a relatively fast degradation rate, the serum level varies considerably according to the time of sampling in relation to hormone ingestion.[74]

Measurement of Total and Unsaturated Thyroid Hormone–Binding Capacity in Serum

The concentration of thyroid hormone in serum is dependent on its supply, as well as on the abundance of hormone-binding sites on serum proteins; therefore, estimation of the latter has proved useful in the correct interpretation of values obtained from measurement of the total hormone concentration. These results have been used to provide an estimate of the free hormone concentration, which is important in differentiating changes in serum total hormone concentrations caused by alterations in binding proteins in euthyroid patients from those caused by abnormalities in thyroid gland activity giving rise to hypermetabolism or hypometabolism.

IN VITRO UPTAKE TESTS. In vitro uptake tests measure the unoccupied thyroid hormone–binding sites on TBG. They use labeled T_3 or T_4 and some form of synthetic absorbent to measure the proportion of radiolabeled hormone that is not tightly bound to serum proteins. Because ion exchange resins are often used as absorbents, the test became known as the resin T_3 or T_4 uptake test, which describes the technique rather than the entity measured.

The test is usually carried out by incubating a sample of the patient's serum with a trace amount of labeled T_3 or T_4. The labeled hormone, not bound to available binding sites on TBG present in the serum sample, is absorbed onto an anion exchange resin and measured as resin-bound radioactivity. Values correlate inversely with the concentration of unsaturated TBG. Various methods use different absorbing materials to remove the hormone not tightly bound to TBG.[89] Labeled T_3 is generally used because of its less firm, yet preferential, binding to TBG. Depending on the method, typical normal results for T_3 uptake are 25% to 35% or 45% to 55%. Thus it is more valuable to express results of the uptake tests as a ratio of the result obtained in a normal control serum run in the same assay as the test samples.

TABLE 97–5. Conditions That May Be Associated with Discrepancies Between the Concentration of Serum TT_3 and TT_4

Serum			Metabolic Status		
TT_3/TT_4 Ratio	*TT_3*	*TT_4*	*Thyrotoxic*	*Euthyroid*	*Hypothyroid*
↑	↑	N	T_3 thyrotoxicosis (endogenous)	Endemic iodine deficiency (T_3 autoantibodies)*	—
↑	N	↓	—	Treated thyrotoxicosis (T_4 autoantibodies)*	Endemic cretins (severe iodine deficiency)
↑	↑	↓	Pharmacologic doses of T_3 (exogenous T_3 toxicosis) Partially treated thryrotoxicosis	T_3 replacement (especially 1–3 hr after ingestion) Endemic iodine deficiency	T_3 autoantibodies*
↓	↓	N	—	Most conditions associated with reduced conversion of T_4 to T_3 Chronic or severe acute illness† Trauma (surgical, burns) Fasting and malnutrition Drugs‡ (T_3 autoantibodies)	—
↓	N	↑	Severe nonthyroidal illness associated with thyrotoxicosis	Neonates (first three weeks of life) T_4 replacement Familial hyperthyroxinemia resulting from T_4 binding albumin–like variant (T_4 autoantibodies)*	—
↓	↓	↑	—	At birth Acute nonthyroidal illness with transient hyperthyroxinemia	T_4 autoantibodies*

*Artifactual values depend on the method of hormone determination in serum.
†Hepatic and renal failure, diabetic ketoacidosis, myocardial infarction, infectious and febrile illness, cancers.
‡Glucocorticoids, iodinated contrast agents, amiodarone, propranolol, propylthiouracil.
TT_3, total triiodothyronine; TT_4, total thyroxine.

Normal values will then range on either side of 1.0, usually 0.85 to 1.15.

Uptake of tracer by the absorbent is inversely proportional to the amount of unsaturated binding sites (unoccupied by endogenous thyroid hormone) in serum TBG. Thus uptake is increased when the amount of unsaturated TBG is reduced as a result of excess endogenous thyroid hormone or a decrease in the concentration of TBG. In contrast, uptake is decreased when the amount of unsaturated TBG is increased as a result of a low serum thyroid hormone concentration or an increase in the concentration of TBG. Because the test can be affected by either or both independent variables, serum total thyroid hormone and TBG concentrations, the results cannot be interpreted without knowledge of the hormone concentration. As a rule, parallel increases or decreases in both serum TT_4 concentration and the T_3 uptake test indicate hyperthyroidism and hypothyroidism, respectively, whereas discrepant changes in serum TT_4 and T_3 uptake suggest abnormalities in TBG binding. However, abnormalities in hormone and TBG concentrations may coexist in the same patient. For example, a hypothyroid patient with a low TBG level will typically show a low TT_4 level and normal T_3 uptake results (Fig. 97–4). Several nonhormonal compounds, because of structural similarities, compete with thyroid hormone for its binding site on TBG. Some are used as pharmacologic agents and may thus alter the in vitro uptake test, as well as the total thyroid hormone concentration in serum. A list is provided in Table 97–4.

TBG AND TTR MEASUREMENTS. The concentrations of TBG

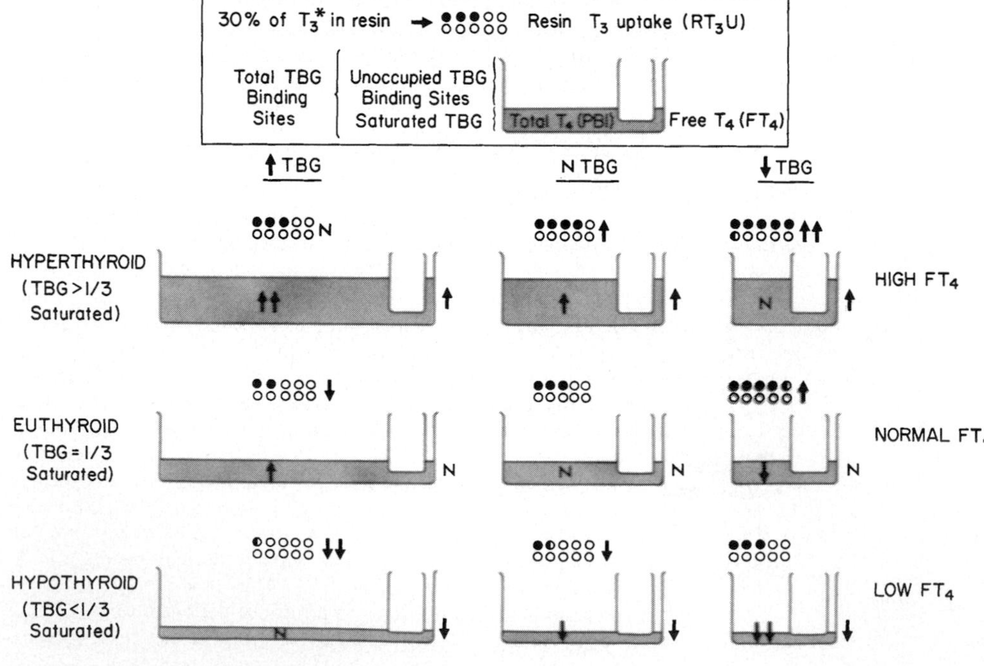

FIGURE 97–4. Graphic representation of the relationship between the serum total thyroxine (T_4) concentration, the reverse triiodothyronine uptake (rT_3U) test, and the free T_4 (FT_4) concentration in various metabolic states and in association with changes in thyroxin-binding globulin (TBG). The principle of communicating vessels is used as an illustration. The height of fluid in the small vessel represents the level of FT_4; the total amount of fluid in the large vessel, the total T_4 concentration; and the total volume of the large vessel, the TBG capacity. *Dots* represent resin beads and *black dots,* those carrying the radioactive T_3 tracer (T_3*). The rT_3U test result *(black dots)* is inversely proportional to the unoccupied TBG-binding sites represented by the unfilled capacity of the large vessel.

and TTR in serum can be either estimated by measurement of their total T_4-binding capacity at saturation or more usually measured directly by immunologic techniques.[90, 91]

The TBG concentration in serum can be determined by RIA,[91] and both TBG and TTR can be measured by Laurell's rocket immunoelectrophoresis,[92, 93] by radial immunodiffusion,[94] or by enzyme immunoassay[90]; commercial methods are available. The true mean value for TBG is 1.6 mg/dL (260 nmol/L), with a range of 1.1 to 2.2 mg/dL (180–350 nmol/L) in serum. In adults, the normal range for TTR is 16 to 30 mg/dL (2.7–5.0 mmol/L). Concentrations of TBG and TTR in serum vary with age, sex, pregnancy status, and posture. Determination of the concentration of these proteins in serum is particularly helpful for evaluation of extreme deviations from normal, as in congenital abnormalities of TBG. In most instances, however, the in vitro uptake test, in conjunction with the serum TT_4 level, gives an approximate estimation of the TBG concentration.

Estimation of Free Thyroid Hormone Concentration

Most thyroid hormones in the blood are bound to serum protein carriers, thus leaving only a minute fraction of free hormone in the circulation that is capable of mediating biologic activities. A reversible equilibrium exists between bound and unbound hormone, and it is the latter that represents the diffusible fraction of the hormone capable of traversing cellular membranes to exert its effects on body tissues.[95] Although changes in serum hormone–binding proteins affect both the total hormone concentration and the corresponding circulating free fraction, in a euthyroid person the absolute concentration of free hormone remains constant and correlates with the tissue hormone level and its biologic effect. Information concerning this value is probably the most important parameter in the evaluation of thyroid function because it relates to the metabolic status of the patient.

With few exceptions, the free hormone concentration is high in thyrotoxicosis, low in hypothyroidism, and normal in euthyroidism, even in the presence of profound changes in TBG concentration,[96] provided that the patient is in a steady state. Notably, the FT_4 concentration may be normal or even low in patients with T_3 thyrotoxicosis and in those ingesting pharmacologic doses of T_3. The concentration of FT_4 may be outside the normal range in the absence of an apparent abnormality in thyroid hormone–dependent metabolic status. This situation is frequently observed in severe nonthyroidal illness, during which both high and low values have been reported.[97–99] As expected, when a euthyroid state is maintained by the administration of T_3 or by predominant thyroidal secretion of T_3, the FT_4 level is also depressed. More consistently, patients with a variety of nonthyroidal illnesses have low FT_3 levels.[100] This decrease is characteristic of all conditions associated with depressed serum TT_3 concentrations caused by diminished conversion of T_4 to T_3 in peripheral tissues by deiodinase enzymes (see Chapter 92). Both FT_4 and FT_3 values may be out of line in patients receiving a variety of drugs (see below). Marked elevations in both FT_4 and FT_3 concentrations in the absence of hypermetabolism are typical of patients with the inherited condition of resistance to thyroid hormone (see Chapter 114). The FT_3 concentration is usually normal or even high in hypothyroid persons living in areas of severe endemic iodine deficiency. Their FT_4 levels are, however, normal or low.[72]

DIRECT MEASUREMENT OF FREE T_4 AND FREE T_3. Direct measurements of the absolute FT_4 and FT_3 concentrations are technically difficult and have until recently been limited to research assays. To minimize perturbations of the relationship between free and bound hormone, these hormones must be separated by ultrafiltration or by dialysis involving minimal dilution and little alteration in pH or the electrolyte composition. The separated free hormone is then measured directly by RIA or chromatography.[96] These assays are probably the most accurate available, but small, weakly bound, dialyzable substances or drugs may be removed from the binding proteins and the free hormone concentration measured in their presence may not fully reflect the free concentration in vivo.

ISOTOPIC EQUILIBRIUM DIALYSIS. This method has been the "gold standard" for the estimation of FT_4 or FT_3 for almost 30 years. It is based on a determination of the proportion of T_4 or T_3 that is unbound, or free, and is thus able to diffuse through a dialysis membrane (i.e., the dialyzable fraction). To carry out the test, a sample of serum is incubated with a trace amount of labeled T_4 or T_3. The labeled tracer rapidly equilibrates with the respective bound and free endogenous hormones. The sample is then dialyzed against buffer at a constant temperature until the concentration of free hormone on either side of the dialysis membrane has reached equilibrium. The dialyzable fraction is calculated from the proportion of labeled hormone in the dialysate. The contribution from radioiodide present as contaminant in the labeled tracer hormone should be eliminated by purification[97] and by various techniques of precipitation of the dialyzed hormone.[101] FT_4 and FT_3 levels can be measured simultaneously by addition to the sample of T_4 and T_3 labeled with two different radioiodine isotopes.[42] Ultrafiltration is a modification of the dialysis technique.[97] Results are expressed as the fraction (dialyzable fraction of T_4 or T_3) or percentage (%FT_4 or %FT_3) of the respective hormones that dialyzed, and the absolute concentrations of FT_4 and FT_3 are calculated from the product of the total concentration of the hormone in serum and its respective dialyzable fraction. Typical normal values for FT_4 in adults range from 1.0 to 3.0 ng/dL (13–39 pmol/L), and those for FT_3 range from 0.25 to 0.65 ng/dL (3.8–10 nmol/L).

Results by these techniques are generally comparable to those determined with direct one-step methods (see below) but are more likely to differ with extremely low or extremely high TBG concentrations or in the presence of circulating inhibitors of protein binding, especially in situations of nonthyroidal illness.[102–104] The measured dialyzable fraction may be altered by the temperature at which the assay is run, the degree of dilution, the time allowed for equilibrium to be reached, and the composition of the diluting fluid.[105] The calculated value is dependent on an accurate measurement of TT_4 or TT_3 and may be incorrect in patients with T_4 or T_3 autoantibodies. Some of these problems, particularly those arising from dilution, may be superseded by commercially available dialysis methods or ultrafiltration methods of free from bound hormone that do not necessitate serum dilution.[106]

INDEX METHODS. Because determination of free hormone by equilibrium dialysis is cumbersome and technically demanding, many clinical laboratories have used a method by which an FT_4 index (FT_4I) or FT_3 index (FT_3I) is derived from the product of the TT_4 or TT_3 (determined by immunoassay) and the value of an in vitro uptake test (see below). Although not always in agreement with the values obtained by dialysis, these techniques are rapid and simple. They are more likely to fail at extremely low or extremely high TBG concentrations, in the presence of abnormal binding proteins, in patients with nonthyroidal illness, or in the presence of circulating inhibitors of protein binding.

The theoretic contention that the FT_4I is an accurate estimate of the absolute FT_4 concentration can be confirmed by the linear correlation between these two parameters. This statement is true provided that results of the in vitro uptake test (T_3 or T_4 uptake) are expressed as the thyroid hormone–binding ratio, which is determined by dividing the tracer counts bound to the solid matrix by counts bound to serum proteins.[107] Values are corrected for assay variations by using appropriate serum standards and are expressed as the ratio of a normal reference pool.[107, 108] The normal range is slightly narrower than the corresponding TT_4 in healthy euthyroid patients with a normal TBG concentration. It is 6.0 to 10.5 mg/dL (77–135 nmol/L) when calculated from TT_4 values measured by RIA. In thyrotoxicosis, the FT_4I is high and in hypothyroidism it is low irrespective of the TBG concentration. Euthyroid patients with TT_4 values outside the normal range as a result of TBG abnormalities have a normal FT_4I.[89] Lack of correlation between the FT_4I and the metabolic status of the patient has been observed in the same circumstances as those described for similar discrepancies when the FT_4 concentration was measured by dialysis.

Methods for estimation of the FT_3I are also available[42] but are rarely used in routine clinical evaluation of thyroid function. Like the FT_4I, it correlates well with the absolute FT_3 concentration. The test corrects for changes in TT_3 concentration resulting from variations in TBG concentration.

ESTIMATION OF FREE T_4 AND FREE T_3 BASED ON TBG MEASUREMENTS. Because most T_4 and T_3 in serum are bound to TBG, their free concentration can be calculated from their binding affinity constants to TBG and molar concentrations of hormones and TBG.[109, 110] A simpler calculation of the T_4/TBG and T_3/TBG ratios yields values that are similar to but less accurate than the FT_4I and FT_3I, respectively.[107]

TWO-STEP IMMUNOASSAYS. In these assays, the free hormone is first immunoextracted by a specific bound antibody (first step), frequently fixed to the tube (coated tube).[111, 112] After washing, labeled tracer is added and allowed to equilibrate between the unoccupied sites on the antibody and those of serum thyroid hormone–binding proteins. The free hormone concentration will be inversely related to the antibody-bound tracer, and values are determined by comparison to a standard curve. Values obtained with this technique are generally comparable to those determined with the direct methods. They are more likely to differ in the presence of circulating inhibitors of protein binding and in sera from patients with nonthyroidal illness.

ANALOGUE (ONE-STEP) IMMUNOASSAYS. In these assays a labeled analogue of T_4 or T_3 directly competes with the endogenous free hormone for binding to antibodies.[113] In theory, these analogues are not bound by the thyroid hormone–binding proteins in serum. However, various studies have found significant protein binding to the variant albumin-like protein,[114] to TTR, and to iodothyronine autoantibodies.[115] Such binding results in discrepant values to other assays in a number of conditions, including nonthyroidal illness, pregnancy, and FDH.[114] A growing number of commercial kits are available, some of which have been modified to minimize these problems.[116, 117] Nonetheless, their accuracy remains controversial, although such commercial methods are being increasingly adopted in the routine clinical chemistry laboratory.[112]

AUTOMATED MEASUREMENT OF FREE T_4 AND FREE T_3. During the 1990s, through the introduction of random-access immunoassay analyzers that operate with chemiluminescent or fluorescent labels, measurements of free thyroid hormones have become automated and therefore allow rapid processing of multiple samples. Although the initial financial burden of such equipment is considerable, they reduce labor costs, demand few handling skills on behalf of the operator, and provide random access so that samples can be tested on demand. Precision studies have shown highly reproducible data with this approach.[118, 119] Comparison of results between different automated analyzers[120] and with manual free thyroid hormone assays, including the gold standard of equilibrium dialysis, has revealed good correlation over a broad range of free thyroid hormone concentrations.[121, 122]

CONSIDERATIONS IN SELECTION OF METHODS FOR THE ESTIMATION OF FREE THYROID HORMONE CONCENTRATION. No single method for the estimation of free hormone concentration in serum is infallible in the evaluation of thyroid hormone–dependent metabolic status. Each test possesses inherent advantages and disadvantages depending on specific physiologic and pathologic circumstances. For example, methods based on measurement of total thyroid hormone and TBG cannot be used in patients with absent TBG secondary to inherited TBG deficiency. Under such circumstances, the concentration of free thyroid hormone is dependent on interaction of the hormone with serum proteins that normally play a negligible role (TTR and albumin). When alterations in thyroid hormone binding do not equally affect T_4 and T_3, discrepant results of FT_4I are obtained when using labeled T_4 or T_3 in the in vitro uptake test. For example, euthyroid patients with the inherited albumin variant (FDH) or having endogenous antibodies with greater affinity for T_4 will have high TT_4 but a normal T_3 uptake test, which will result in an overestimation of the calculated FT_4I. In such instances, calculation of the FT_4I from a T_4 uptake test may provide more accurate results. Conversely, reduced overall binding affinity for T_4, which affects T_3 to a lesser extent, will underestimate the FT_4I derived from a T_3 uptake test. Similarly, use of T_4 and T_3 uptake for estimation of the free hormone concentration is satisfactory in the presence of alterations in TBG concentration but not alterations of the affinity of TBG for the hormone.[123, 124]

Methods based on equilibrium dialysis are most appropriate for estimation of the free thyroid hormone level in patients with all varieties of abnormal binding to serum proteins, provided that the true concentration of total hormone has been accurately determined. All methods for the estimation of FT_4 may give either high or low values in patients with severe nonthyroidal illness who are believed to be euthyroid.[96–99, 125, 126] This finding has been attributed, at least in part, to the presence of inhibitors of thyroid hormone binding to serum proteins, as well as to the various adsorbents used in the test procedures.[127, 128] Some of these inhibitors have been postulated to leak from tissues of the diseased patient.[129, 130] Such discrepancies are even more pronounced during transient states of hyperthyroxinemia or hypothyroxinemia associated with acute illness, after withdrawal of treatment with thyroid hormone, and in patients with acute changes in TBG concentration (see Chapter 94).

The contribution of various drugs that interfere with binding of thyroid hormone to serum proteins or with the in vitro tests should also be taken into account in the choice and interpretation of tests (see Table 97–4). Although the free thyroid hormone concentration in serum would appear to determine the amount of hormone available to body tissues, factors that govern their uptake, transport to the nucleus, and functional interactions with nuclear receptors and cofactors ultimately determine their biologic effects.

Measurements of Iodine-Containing Hormone Precursors and Products of Degradation

The last two decades have witnessed the development of RIAs for the measurement of a number of naturally occurring, iodine-containing substances that possess little, if any thyromimetic activity. Some of these substances are products of T_4 and T_3 degradation in peripheral tissues. Others are predominantly, if not exclusively, of thyroidal origin. Because they are devoid of significant metabolic activity, with the exception of rT_3, measurement of their concentration is of value only in the research setting in detecting abnormalities in the metabolism of thyroid hormone in peripheral tissues, as well as defects of hormone synthesis and secretion.

3,3′,5′-TRIIODOTHYRONINE OR REVERSE T_3. rT_3 is principally a product of T_4 degradation in peripheral tissues (see Chapter 92). It is also secreted by the thyroid gland, but the amounts are practically insignificant.[131] Thus measurement of the rT_3 concentration in serum reflects both tissue supply and metabolism of T_4 and identifies conditions that favor this particular pathway of T_4 degradation.

When total rT_3 (TrT_3) is measured in unextracted serum, a competitor of rT_3 binding to serum proteins must be added.[132] Several chemically related compounds may cross-react with the antibodies. The strongest cross-reactivity is observed with 3,3′-diiodothyronine (3,3′-T_2), but such cross-reactivity does not present a serious methodologic problem because of its relatively low levels in human serum. Although cross-reactivity with T_3 and T_4 is less, these compounds are more often the cause of rT_3 overestimation because of their relative abundance, particularly in thyrotoxicosis.[133] Free fatty acids interfere with the measurement of rT_3 by RIA.[134]

The normal range in adult serum for TrT_3 is 14 to 30 ng/dL (0.22–0.46 nmol/L), although varying values have been reported. It is elevated in subjects with high TBG and in some individuals with FDH.[135] Serum TrT_3 levels are normal in hypothyroid patients treated with T_4, which indicates that peripheral T_4 metabolism is an important source of circulating rT_3.[131, 136] Values are high in thyrotoxicosis and low in untreated hypothyroidism. High values are normally found in cord blood and in newborns.[136, 137]

With only a few exceptions, notably uremia, serum TrT_3 concentrations are elevated in all circumstances that cause low serum T_3 levels in the absence of obvious clinical signs of hypothyroidism. These conditions include, in addition to the newborn period, a variety of acute and chronic nonthyroidal illnesses, calorie deprivation, and the influence of a growing list of clinical agents and drugs (see Table 97–6).

The current clinical application of TrT_3 measurement in serum is in the differential diagnosis of conditions associated with alterations in

TABLE 97–6. Agents That Alter the Extrathyroidal Metabolism of Thyroid Hormone

Substance	Common Use
Inhibit conversion of T_4 to T_3	
PTU[138–140]	Antithyroid
Glucocorticoids (hydrocortisone, prednisone, dexamethasone)[85, 141]	Anti-inflammatory and immunosuppressive; decrease intracranial pressure
Propranolol[142, 143]	Adrenergic blocker (antiarrhythmic, antihypertensive)
Iodinated contrast agents: ipodate (Oragrafin), iopanoic acid (Telepaque)[144, 145]	Radiologic contrast media
Amiodarone[146–148]	Antianginal and antiarrhythmic
Clomipramine[149]	Tricyclic antidepressant
Stimulators of hormone degradation or fecal excretion	
Diphenylhydantoin[150–152]	Anticonvulsive and antiarrhythmic
Carbamazepine[152]	Anticonvulsant
Phenobarbital[86, 152]	Hypnotic, tranquilizing, and anticonvulsive
Cholestyramine,[153] colestipol[154]	Hypolipidemic resins
Soybeans[155, 156]	Diet
Rifampin[157]	Antituberculosis drug

PTU, propylthiouracil; T_3, triiodothyronine; T_4, thyroxine.

serum T_3 and T_4 concentrations when thyroid gland and metabolic abnormalities are not readily apparent.

The dialyzable fraction of rT_3 in normal adult serum is 0.2% to 0.32%, or approximately the same as that of T_3. The corresponding serum free rT_3 (FrT_3) concentration is 50 to 100 pg/dL (0.77–1.5 pmol/L). In the absence of gross TBG abnormalities, variations in serum FrT_3 concentration closely follow those of TrT_3.[100]

3,5-DIIODOTHYRONINE. The normal adult range for total 3,5-diiodothyronine (3,5-T_2) in serum measured by direct RIAs is 0.20 to 0.75 ng/dL (3.8–14 pmol/L).[158] That 3,5-T_2 is derived from T_3 is supported by the observations that conditions associated with high and low serum T_3 levels have elevated and reduced serum concentrations of 3,5-T_2, respectively.[159] Thus high serum 3,5-T_2 levels have been reported in hyperthyroidism and low levels in the serum of hypothyroid patients, in newborns, during fasting, and in patients with liver cirrhosis.

3,3′-DIIODOTHYRONINE. Normal concentrations in adults probably range from 1 to 8 ng/dL (19–150 pmol/L).[160] Levels are clearly elevated in hyperthyroidism and in the newborn. Values have been found to be either normal or depressed in nonthyroidal illnesses,[160] in agreement with the demonstration of reduced monodeiodination of rT_3 to 3,3′-T_2.[161] In vivo turnover kinetic studies and measurement of 3,3′-T_2 in serum after the administration of T_3 and rT_3 have clearly shown that 3,3′-T_2 is the principal metabolic product of these two triiodothyronines.

3′,5′-DIIODOTHYRONINE. Reported concentrations of 3′,5′-diiodothyronine (3′,5′-T_2) in the serum of normal adults have a mean overall range of 1.5 to 9.0 ng/dL (30–170 pmol/L).[162, 163] Values are high in hyperthyroidism and in the newborn.[162, 163] Being the derivative of rT_3 monodeiodination,[162] 3′,5′-T_2 levels are elevated in serum during fasting[164, 165] and in chronic illnesses[136] in which the level of the rT_3 precursor is also high. Administration of dexamethasone also produces an increase in the serum 3′,5′-T_2 level.[162]

3′-MONOIODOTHYRONINE. The concentration of 3′-monoiodothyronine (3′-T_1) in the serum of normal adults, as measured by RIA, has been reported to range from 0.6 to 2.3 ng/dL (15–58 pmol/L)[136] and from less than 0.9 to 6.8 ng/dL (<20–170 pmol/L). Its two immediate precursors, 3,3′-T_2 and 3′,5′-T_2 are the main cross-reactants in the RIA. Serum levels are very high in hyperthyroidism and low in hypothyroidism. The concentration of 3′-T_1 in serum is elevated in all conditions associated with high rT_3 levels, including the newborn period, nonthyroidal illness, and fasting.[137] This finding is not surprising because the immediate precursor of 3′-T_1 is 3′,5′-T_2,[165] a product of rT_3 deiodination, which is also present in serum in high concentration under the same circumstances. The elevated serum levels of 3′-T_1 in renal failure are attributed to decreased clearance inasmuch as the concentrations of its precursors are not increased.

3-MONOIODOTHYRONINE. Experience with the measurement of 3-T_1 in serum is limited. Normal values in the serum of adult humans determined by ^{3}H-labeled 3-T_1 in a specific RIA ranged from less than 0.5 to 7.5 ng/dL (<13–190 pmol/L).[166] The mean concentration of 3-T_1 in the serum of thyrotoxic patients and in cord blood was significantly higher. 3-T_1 appears to be a product of in vivo deiodination of 3,3′-T_2.

TETRAIODOTHYROACETIC ACID AND TRIIODOTHYROACETIC ACID. The iodoamino acids TETRAC (T_4A) and TRIAC (T_3A), products of deamination and oxidative decarboxylation of T_4 and T_3, respectively, have been detected in serum by direct RIA measurements.[18, 84, 167] Reported mean concentrations in the serum of healthy adults have been 8.7 ng/dL[167] and 2.6 ng/dL (range, 1.6–3.0 ng/dL or 26–48 pmol/L)[18] for T_3A and 28 ng/dL (range, <8–60 mg/dL or <105–800 pmol/L)[84] for T_4A. Serum T_4A levels are reduced during fasting and in patients with severe illness,[168] although the percentage of conversion of T_4 to T_4A is increased.[17, 169] The concentration of serum T_3A remains unchanged during the administration of replacement doses of T_4 and T_3.[18] It has been suggested that intracellular rerouting of T_3 to T_3A during fasting is responsible for the maintenance of normal serum TSH levels in the presence of low T_3 concentrations.[170]

3,5,3′-TRIIODOTHYRONINE SULFATE. Sulfation of iodothyronines results in the inactivation of thyroid hormones and enhances their excretion in urine and bile. An RIA procedure to measure 3,5,3′-triiodothyronine sulfate (T_3S) in ethanol extracted serum samples is available.[19, 171] Concentrations in normal adults range from 4 to 10 ng/dL (50–125 pmol/L). Although the principal source of T_3S is T_3 and the former binds to TBG, values are high in the newborn period and low in pregnancy. This observation suggests different rates of T_3S generation or metabolism in the mother and fetus. T_3S values are high in thyrotoxicosis (including patients taking suppressive doses of thyroxine[172]), in patients receiving amiodarone therapy,[173] and in patients with nonthyroidal illness.

DIIODOTYROSINE AND MONOIODOTYROSINE. Although RIA methods for the measurement of DIT and MIT have been developed, because of limited experience their value in clinical practice remains unknown. Early reports gave a normal mean value for DIT in the serum of normal adults of 156 ng/dL (3.6 nmol/L),[174] with a progressive decline caused by refinement of techniques to values as low as 7 ng/dL with a range of 1 to 23 ng/dL (0.02–0.5 nmol/L).[175] Thus the normal range of 90 to 390 ng/dL (2.9–12.7 nmol/L) for MIT[176] is undoubtedly an overestimation. Iodotyrosine that has escaped enzymatic deiodination in the thyroid gland appears to be the principal source of DIT in serum. Iodothyronine degradation in peripheral tissues is probably a minor source of iodotyrosines because the administration of large doses of T_4 to normal subjects produces a decline rather than an increase in the serum DIT level.[175] DIT is metabolized to MIT in peripheral tissues. Serum levels of DIT are low during pregnancy and high in cord blood.

THYROGLOBULIN. RIA methods were the methods first used routinely for measurement of Tg in serum,[177] although other methods using immunoradiometric assay, immunochemiluminescent assay, and enzyme-linked immunosorbent assay technology have been reported[178–181] and are gaining increasing popularity. They are specific and, depending on the sensitivity of the assay, capable of detecting Tg in the serum of approximately 90% of euthyroid healthy adults. When antisera are used in high dilutions, virtually no cross-reactivity with iodothyronines or iodotyrosines occurs. Results obtained from analysis of sera containing Tg autoantibodies may be inaccurate depending on the antiserum used.[182] The presence of TPO antibodies does not interfere with the Tg RIA. Despite the reliability of measurements of serum Tg, it is clear that different assay methods may result in values discrepant by up to 30%, even though reference preparations are available.[183] Typically, ICMA methods underestimate the serum Tg value, whereas RIA methods overestimate it, so it is essential that clinical decisions be based on serial measurements using the same assay.

Tg concentrations in the serum of normal adults range from less than 1 to 25 ng/mL (<1.5–38 pmol/L), with mean levels of 5 to 10 ng/mL.[177, 184–186] On a molar basis, these concentrations of Tg are minute relative to the circulating iodothyronines: 5000-fold lower than the corresponding concentration of T_4 in serum. Values tend to be slightly higher in women than in men.[177] In the neonatal period and during the third trimester of pregnancy, mean values are approximately 4- and 2-fold higher.[185, 187] They gradually decline throughout infancy, childhood, and adolescence.[188] The positive correlation between the levels of serum Tg and TSH indicates that pituitary TSH regulates the secretion of Tg.

Elevated serum Tg levels reflect increased secretory activity by stimulation of the thyroid gland or damage to thyroid tissue, whereas values below or at the level of detectability indicate a paucity of thyroid tissue or suppressed activity. Tg levels in a variety of conditions affecting the thyroid gland have been reviewed[189] and are listed in Table 97–7.

Interpretation of a serum Tg value should take into account the fact that Tg concentrations may be high under normal physiologic conditions or altered by drugs. Administration of iodine and antithyroid drugs increases the serum Tg level, as do states associated with hyperstimulation of the thyroid gland by TSH or other substances with thyroid-stimulating activity. This increased Tg is due to increased thyroidal release of Tg rather than changes in its clearance.[190] Administration of TRH and TSH also transiently increases the serum level of Tg.[191] Trauma to the thyroid gland, such as that occurring during diagnostic and therapeutic procedures, including percutaneous needle biopsy, surgery, or ^{131}I therapy, can produce a striking, although short-lived elevation in the Tg level in serum.[185, 192, 193] Pathologic processes with destructive effect on the thyroid gland also produce transient, although more prolonged increases.[194] Tg is undetectable in serum after total ablation of the thyroid gland, as well as in normal persons receiving suppressive doses of thyroid hormone.[189] It is thus a useful test in the differential diagnosis of thyrotoxicosis factitia,[195] especially when transient thyrotoxicosis with low RAIU or suppression of thyroidal RAIU by iodine is an alternative possibility.

TABLE 97–7. Conditions Associated with Changes in Serum Tg Concentration Listed According to the Presumed Mechanism

- Increased
  - *TSH mediated*
    - Acute and transient (TSH and TRH administration, neonatal period)
    - Chronic stimulation
      - Iodine deficiency, endemic goiter, goitrogens
      - Reduced-thyroidal reserve (lingual thyroid)
      - TSH-producing pituitary adenoma
      - Resistance to thyroid hormone
      - TBG deficiency
  - *Non–TSH mediated*
    - Thyroid stimulators
      - IgG (Graves' disease)
      - hCG (trophoblastic disease)
    - Trauma to the thyroid (needle aspiration and surgery of the thyroid gland, ^{131}I therapy)
    - Destructive thyroid pathology
      - Subacute thyroiditis
      - Painless thyroiditis
      - Postpartum thyroiditis
    - Abnormal release
      - Thyroid nodules (toxic, nontoxic, multinodular goiter)
      - Differentiated nonmedullary thyroid carcinoma
    - Abnormal clearance (renal failure)
- Decreased
  - *TSH suppression*
    - Administration of thyroid hormone
  - *Decreased synthesis*
  - Athyrosis (postoperative, congenital)
  - Tg synthesis defect

hCG, human chorionic gonadotropin; TBG, thyrotropin-binding globulin; Tg, thyroglobulin; TSH, thyroid-stimulating hormone; TRH, thyrotropin-releasing hormone.

The most striking elevations in serum Tg concentrations have been observed in patients with metastatic differentiated nonmedullary thyroid carcinoma, even after total surgical and radioiodide ablation of all normal thyroid tissue.[185, 196] It usually persists despite full thyroid hormone suppressive therapy, thus suggesting excessive autonomous release of Tg by the neoplastic cells. The determination is thus of particular value in the follow-up and management of metastatic thyroid carcinomas, particularly when they fail to concentrate radioiodide.[184, 196] Follow-up of such patients with sequential serum Tg determinations helps in the early detection of tumor recurrence or growth and in assessment of the efficacy of treatment. Measurement of serum Tg is also useful in patients with metastases, particularly to bone, in whom no evidence of a primary site is noted and thyroid malignancy is being considered in the differential diagnosis.[185, 196] On the other hand, serum Tg levels are of no value in the differential diagnosis of primary thyroid cancer because levels may be within the normal range in the presence of differentiated thyroid cancer and high in a variety of benign thyroid diseases.[184, 186, 196] Whether early detection of recurrent thyroid cancer after initial ablative therapy could be achieved by serum Tg measurement without cessation of hormone replacement therapy is debated because Tg secretion by the tumor is modulated by TSH and could be suppressed by the administration of thyroid hormone.[197–199] Although the presence of an elevated Tg level with suppressed TSH is an indicator of probable recurrence, suppressed Tg with suppressed TSH is not a reliable indicator of the absence of recurrence. The introduction of recombinant human TSH allows stimulation of thyroid tissue for the measurement of Tg without cessation of replacement treatment (see Chapter 109).

In the early phase of subacute thyroiditis Tg levels are high.[194] Declining serum Tg levels during the course of antithyroid drug treatment of patients with Graves' disease may indicate the onset of a remission.[193, 200] Tg may be undetectable in the serum of neonates with dyshormonogenetic goiters caused by defects in Tg synthesis,[201] but levels are very high in some hypothyroid infants with thyromegaly or ectopy.[202] Measurement of serum Tg in hypothyroid neonates is useful in the differentiation of infants with complete thyroid agenesis from those with hypothyroidism resulting from other causes and thus in most cases obviates the need for diagnostic administration of radioiodide.[203, 204]

MEASUREMENT OF THYROID HORMONE AND ITS METABOLITES IN OTHER BODY FLUIDS AND IN TISSUES

Clinical experience with measurement of thyroid hormone and its metabolites in body fluids other than serum and in tissues is limited for several reasons. Analyses carried out in urine and saliva do not appear to give information additional to that determined from measurements carried out in serum. Amniotic fluid, cerebrospinal fluid (CSF), and tissues are less readily accessible for sampling. Their likely application in the future will depend on information that they could provide beyond that obtained from similar analyses in serum.

Urine

Because thyroid hormone is filtered in the urine predominantly in free form, measurement of the total amount excreted over 24 hours offers an indirect method for estimation of the free hormone concentration in serum. The 24-hour excretion of T_4 in normal adults ranges from 4 to 13 mg and from 1.8 to 3.7 mg, depending on whether total or only conjugated T_4 is measured. Corresponding normal ranges for T_3 are 2.0 to 4.0 mg and 0.4 to 1.9 mg.[204–206] Striking seasonal variations have been shown for the urinary excretion of both hormones, with a nadir during the hot summer months in the absence of significant changes in serum TT_4 and TT_3. As expected, values are normal in pregnancy and in nonthyroidal illnesses and are high in thyrotoxicosis and low in hypothyroidism.[205–207] The test may not be valid in the presence of gross proteinuria and impairment in renal function.[208]

Amniotic Fluid

All iodothyronines measured in blood have also been detected in amniotic fluid. With the exception of T_3, 3,3′-T_2, and 3′-T_2, the concentration at term is lower than that in cord serum.[162, 163, 165, 209–211] This fact cannot be fully explained by the low TBG concentration in amniotic fluid. Although the source of iodothyronines in amniotic fluid is unknown, the general pattern more closely resembles that found in the fetal than in the maternal circulation.

The TT_4 concentration in amniotic fluid averages 0.5 mg/dL (65 nmol/L) with a range of 0.15 to 1.0 mg/dL and is thus very low when compared with values in maternal and cord serum.[209–211] The FT_4 concentration is, however, twice as high in amniotic fluid relative to serum. The TT_3 concentration is also low relative to maternal serum, being on average 30 ng/dL (0.46 nmol/L) in both amniotic fluid and cord serum.[211] rT_3, on the other hand, is very high in amniotic fluid, on average 330 ng/dL (5.1 nmol/L) during the first half of gestation and declining precipitously at about the 30th week of gestation to an average of 85 ng/dL (1.3 nmol/L), which is also found at term.[210, 211]

Cerebrospinal Fluid

T_4, T_3, and rT_3 concentrations have been measured in human CSF.[212–214] The concentrations of both TT_4 and TT_3 are approximately 50-fold lower than those found in serum. However, the concentrations of these iodothyronines in free form are similar to those in serum. In contrast, the level of TrT_3 in CSF is only 2.5-fold lower than that of serum, whereas that of FrT_3 is 25-fold higher. This difference is probably due to the presence in CSF of a larger proportion of TTR, which has high affinity for rT_3.[213] All the thyroid hormone–binding proteins present in serum are also found in CSF, although in lower concentration.[213] The concentrations of TT_4 and FT_4 are increased in thyrotoxicosis and depressed in hypothyroidism. Severe nonthyroidal illness gives rise to increased TrT_3 and FrT_3 levels.[214]

Milk

The TT_4 concentration in human milk is on the order of 0.03 to 0.5 mg/dL.[215] Analytic artifacts were responsible for the much higher values formerly reported.[215, 216] TT_3 concentrations range from 10 to 200 ng/dL (0.15–3.1 nmol/L).[216, 217] The concentration of TrT_3 ranges from 1 to 30 ng/dL (15–460 pmol/L).[216] Thus it is unlikely that milk would provide a sufficient quantity of thyroid hormone to alleviate hypothyroidism in an infant.

Saliva

It has been suggested that only the free fraction of small nonpeptide hormones that circulate predominantly bound to serum proteins would be transferred to saliva and that their measurement, in this easily accessible body fluid, would provide a simple and direct means to determine their free concentration in blood. This hypothesis was confirmed for steroid hormones not tightly bound to serum proteins.[218] Levels of T_4 in saliva range from 4.2 to 35 ng/dL (54–450 pmol/L) and do not correlate with the concentration of FT_4 in serum.[219] This finding is, in part, due to the transfer of T_4 bound to the small but variable amounts of serum proteins that reach the saliva.

Effusions

TT_4 measured in fluid obtained from serous cavities bears a direct relationship to the protein content and the serum concentration of T_4. Limited experience with Tg measurement in pleural effusions from patients with thyroid cancer metastatic to the lungs suggests that it may be of diagnostic value.[196]

Tissues

Because the response to thyroid hormone is expressed at the cell level via nuclear receptors, it is logical to assume that hormone concentrations in tissues should correlate best with their action. Methods for extraction, recovery, and measurement of iodothyronines from tissues have been developed, but for obvious reasons, data from thyroid hormone measurements in human tissues are limited. Preliminary work has shown that under several circumstances, hormonal levels in tissues such as liver, kidney, and muscle usually correlate with those found in serum.[220]

Measurements of T_3 in cells most accessible for sampling in humans, namely, red blood cells, gave values of 20 to 45 ng/dL (0.31–0.69 nmol/L), or one-fourth those found in serum.[221] They are higher in thyrotoxicosis and lower in hypothyroidism.

The concentrations of all iodothyronines have been measured in thyroid gland hydrolysates.[15, 136, 162] In normal glands, the molar ratios relative to the concentration of T_4 are on average as follows: T_4/T_3 = 10; T_4/rT_3 = 80; T_4/3,5′-T_2 = 1400; T_4/3,3′-T_2 = 350; T_4/3′,5′-T_2 = 1100; and T_4/3′-T_1 = 4400. Information concerning the content of iodothyronines in hydrolysates of abnormal thyroid tissue is limited, and the diagnostic value of such measurements has not been established.

Measurement of Tg in metastatic tissue obtained by needle biopsy may be of value in the differential diagnosis, especially when the primary site is unknown and the histologic diagnosis is not conclusive.

TESTS ASSESSING THE EFFECTS OF THYROID HORMONE ON BODY TISSUES

Because of the ubiquitous expression of thyroid hormone receptors, thyroid hormone regulates a variety of biochemical reactions in virtually all tissues. Thus ideally, the adequacy of hormonal supply should be assessed by tissue responses rather than by parameters of thyroid gland activity or serum hormone concentrations, which are several steps removed from the site of thyroid hormone action. Unfortunately, tissue responses (metabolic indices) are nonspecific because they are altered by a variety of physiologic and pathologic mechanisms unrelated to thyroid hormone deprivation or excess. The following review of biochemical and physiologic changes mediated by thyroid hormone has a dual purpose: (1) to outline some of the changes that may be used as clinical tests in the evaluation of metabolic status and (2) to point out the changes in various determinations commonly used in the diagnosis of a variety of nonthyroidal illnesses that may be affected by the concomitant presence of thyroid hormone deficiency or excess.

Basal Metabolic Rate

The basal metabolic rate (BMR) has a long history in the evaluation of thyroid function. It measures oxygen consumption under basal conditions of overnight fast and rest from mental and physical exertion. Because standard equipment for the measurement of BMR may not be readily available, the BMR can be estimated from the oxygen consumed over a timed interval by analysis of samples of expired air.[222] The test indirectly measures metabolic energy expenditure or heat production.

Results are expressed as the percentage of deviation from normal after appropriate corrections have been made for age, sex, and body surface area. Low values are suggestive of hypothyroidism, and high values reflect thyrotoxicosis. The various nonthyroidal illnesses and other factors affecting the BMR, including sources of errors, have been reviewed.[223] Although this test is no longer a part of the routine diagnostic armamentarium, it is still useful in research.

Deep Tendon Reflex Relaxation Time (Photomotography)

A delay in the relaxation time of the deep tendon reflexes, visible to the experienced eye, occurs in hypothyroidism. Several instruments have been devised to quantitate various phases of the Achilles tendon reflex. Although normal values vary according to the phase of the tendon reflex measured, the apparatus used, and individual laboratory standards, the approximate adult normal range for the half-relaxation time is 230 to 390 msec. Diurnal variation, differences with sex, and changes with age, cold exposure, fever, exercise, obesity, and pregnancy have been reported. However, the main reason for failure of this test as a diagnostic measure of thyroid dysfunction is the large overlap with values obtained in euthyroid patients and alterations caused by nonthyroidal illnesses.[224]

Tests Related to Cardiovascular Function

Thyroid hormone–induced changes in the cardiovascular system can be measured by noninvasive techniques. One such test measures the time interval between the onset of the electrocardiographic QRS complex (Q) and the arrival of the pulse wave at the brachial artery, detected by the Korotkoff sound at the antecubital fossa.[225] Related tests that determine the systolic time interval measure the pre-ejection period (PEP), obtained by subtraction of the left ventricular ejection time (LVET) from the total electromechanical systole.[226] The LVET, which is also affected by thyroid status, can be measured by the M-mode echocardiogram.[227] The PEP/LVET ratio is also useful in the assessment of thyroid hormone action in the cardiovascular system.[228] As with other tests of thyroid hormone action, the principal deficiency of these measurements is their alteration in a variety of nonthyroidal illnesses.

Miscellaneous Biochemical and Physiologic Changes Related to the Action of Thyroid Hormone on Peripheral Tissues

Thyroid hormone affects the function of a variety of peripheral tissues. Thus hormone deficiency or excess may alter a number of determinations used in the diagnosis of illnesses unrelated to thyroid hormone dysfunction. Knowledge of the determinations that may be affected by thyroid hormone is important in the interpretation of laboratory data (Table 97–8).

MEASUREMENT OF SUBSTANCES ABSENT IN NORMAL SERUM

Tests that measure substances present in the circulation only under pathologic circumstances do not provide information on the level of thyroid gland function. They are of value in establishing the cause of the hormonal dysfunction or thyroid gland pathology.

Thyroid Autoantibodies

In clinical practice, the antibodies most commonly measured are directed against Tg or thyroid cell microsomal proteins. The latter is principally represented by TPO.[328–330] More recently, immunoassays have been developed with the use of purified and recombinant TPO.[331–333] Other circulating immunoglobulins, which are less frequently used as diagnostic markers, are those directed against a colloid antigen, T_4, and T_3. Immunoglobulins possessing the property of stimulating the thyroid gland will be discussed in the next section.

A variety of techniques have been developed for the measurement of Tg and microsomal antibodies. These procedures include a competitive binding radioassay, complement fixation reaction,[334] tanned red cell agglutination assay,[335] Coon's immunofluorescent technique,[336] and enzyme-linked immunosorbent assay.[331, 337] Although the competitive binding radioassay[338, 339] is a sensitive test, agglutination methods combine sensitivity and simplicity and have now largely superseded other methods. Current commercial kits use synthetic gelatin beads rather than red cells.[340]

In the assay of Tg and microsomal antibodies by hemagglutination, particulate material is coated with either human Tg or solubilized thyroid microsomal proteins (TPO) and exposed to serial dilutions of the patient's serum. Agglutination of the coated particulate material occurs in the presence of antibodies specific to the antigen attached to their surface. To detect false-positive reactions, it is important to include a blank for each sample consisting of uncoated particles. Because of the common occurrence of a prozone or blocking phenomenon, it is necessary to screen all serum samples through at least six consecutive twofold dilutions.[341] Results are expressed in terms of the highest serum dilution, or titer, showing persistent agglutination. The presence of immune complexes, particularly in patients with high serum Tg levels, may mask the presence of Tg antibodies. Assays for the measurement of such Tg–anti-Tg immune complexes have been developed.[342]

Normally the test response is negative, but results may be positive in up to 10% of the adult population. The frequency of positive test results is higher in women and with advancing age. The presence of thyroid autoantibodies in the apparently healthy population is thought to represent subclinical autoimmune thyroid disease rather than false-positive reactions. Nonetheless, it is difficult to compare results from such studies because some laboratories using agglutination methods report low titers (1/100–1/400) as positive. It is important when reporting values that a method-specific normal range be used and assays calibrated against internationally available reference preparations. The availability of such preparations allows the reporting of results in international units.[340] TPO antibodies are detectable in approximately 95% of patients with Hashimoto's thyroiditis and 85% of those with Graves' disease, irrespective of the functional state of the thyroid gland. Similarly, Tg antibodies are positive in about 60% and 30% of adult patients with Hashimoto's thyroiditis and Graves' disease, respectively.[339–341, 343] Tg antibodies are less frequently detected in children with autoimmune thyroid disease.[344] Although higher titers are more common in Hashimoto's thyroiditis, quantitation of the antibody titer carries little diagnostic implication. The tests are of particular value in the evaluation of patients with atypical or selected manifestations of autoimmune thyroid disease (ophthalmopathy and dermopathy). Positive antibody titers are predictive of postpartum thyroiditis.[345] Low antibody titers occur transiently in some patients after an episode of subacute thyroiditis,[346] presumably caused by antigen exposure. No increased incidence of thyroid autoantibodies is seen in patients with multinodular goiter, thyroid adenomas, or secondary hypothyroidism. In some patients with Hashimoto's thyroiditis and undetectable thyroid autoantibodies in their serum, intrathyroidal lymphocytes have been demonstrated to produce TPO antibodies.

The development of sensitive radioassays and quantitative enzyme-linked immunoassays has allowed measurement of the concentration of antibodies to TPO and Tg in absolute terms.[347–350] Such methods provide sensitive, precise, and antigen-specific means of revealing quantitative fluctuations in autoantibody concentrations.

Other antibodies directed against thyroid components (such as NIS)[351–353] or other tissues have been detected in the serum of some patients with autoimmune thyroid disease, but their diagnostic value has not been fully evaluated. Circulating antibodies capable of binding T_4 and T_3 have also been demonstrated in patients with autoimmune thyroid diseases and may interfere with the measurement of T_4 and T_3 by RIA techniques.[30, 31, 354]

Antibodies reacting with nuclear components, which are not tissue specific, and with cellular components of parietal cells and adrenal, ovarian, and testicular tissue are more commonly encountered in patients with autoimmune thyroid disease.[355] Their presence reflects the frequency of coexistence of several autoimmune disease processes in the same patient (see Chapter 41).

Thyroid-Stimulating Immunoglobulins

A large number of names have been given to tests that measure abnormal γ-globulins present in the serum of some patients with

TABLE 97–8. Biochemical and Physiologic Changes Related to Thyroid Hormone Deficiency and Excess

Entity Measured	During Hypo- thyroidism	During Thyro- toxicosis
Metabolism of various substances and drugs		
Fractional turnover rate (antipyrine,[229] dipyrone,[230] PTU and methimazole,[229] albumin,[231] low-density lipoproteins,[232] cortisol,[233,234] and Fe[235,236])	↓	↑
Serum		
Amino acids		
Tyrosine (fasting level and afterload)[237,238]	↓	↑
Glutamic acid[237]	N	↑
Proteins		
Albumin[239]	↓	↓
Sex hormone–binding globulin[240–242]	↓	↑ ↑
Ferritin[243,244]	↓	↑
Low-density lipoproteins[232]	↓	↑
Fibronectin[245]		↑
Factor VIII–related antigen[245]		↑
Tissue plasminogen activator[245]		↑
TBG[89]	↑	↓
TBPA[106]	N	↓
Hormones		
Insulin		
Response to glucose[246]	↓	↓
Response to glucagon[247]	↑	↓
Estradiol-17β,[248] testosterone,[240,241,248] and gastrin[249]	↓ or N	↑
Parathyroid hormone concentration[250,251]	↑	↓
Response to PTH administration[251]	↓	↑
Calcitonin[252]	↓	↑
Calcitonin response to Ca^{2+} infusion[253]	↓	
Renin activity and aldosterone[254,255]	↓	↑
Catecholamines[256] and noradrenaline[257]	↑	↑
Atrial natriuretic peptide[258,259]	↓	↑
Erythropoietin[236]	N or ↓	↑
LH[248]		N or ↑
Response to GnRH[260]	↑	N
Prolactin and response to stimulation with TRH, arginine, and chlorpromazine[261,262]	↑ or N	↓
Growth hormone		
Response to insulin[263,264]	↓	N or ↓
Response to TRH[265]		No change
Epidermal growth factor[266]	N	↑
Enzymes		
Creatine phosphokinase,[267,268] lactate dehydrogenase,[268] aspartate aminotransferase[268]	↑	↓
Adenylate kinase[269]	N	↑
Dopamine β-hydroxylase[270]	↑	↓
Alkaline phosphatase[251,271]	↓*	↑
Malic dehydrogenase[272]	↑ ↑	↑
Angiotensin-converting enzyme,[245,273] alanine aminotransferase,[274] and glutathione S-transferase[274,275]	N	↑
Coenzyme Q_{10}[276]		↓
Others		
1,25-OH-vitamin D_3[277]	↑	N or ↓
Carotene, vitamin A[278]	↑	↓
cAMP,[279] cGMP,[280] and Fe[235,281]	N or ↓	N or ↑
K[282]		↓
Na[283]	↓	
Mg[284]	↑	↓
Ca[251,285]	↓	↑
P[250,251]		↑
Glucose		
Concentration[247,263]	↓	↑
Fractional turnover during IV tolerance test[246]	↓	
Insulin hypoglycemia[263]	prolonged	
Bilirubin[286,287]	↑†	↑
Creatinine[288]	N or ↑	↓
Creatine[288]	N or ↑	↑
Cholesterol,[278,289] carotene,[278,289] phospholipids and lethicin,[278,289] and triglycerides[289,290]	↑	↓

Entity Measured	During Hypo- thyroidism	During Thyro- toxicosis
Lipoprotein[291]	↑	↓
Apolipoprotein B[291]	↑	↓
Type IV collagen[292]	↓	↑
Type III procollagen[292]	↓	↑
Free fatty acids[293]		↑
Carcinoembryonic antigen[294]	↑	
Osteocalcin[252]	↓	↑
Urine		
cAMP[295]	↓	↑
After epinephrine infusion[296]	No change	↑
cGMP[280]	N or ↓	↑
Mg[284]	↓	↑
Creatinine[288]	N	↓
Creatine[288]	N	↑
Tyrosine[238]	N or ↓	↑
MIT (after administration of ^{131}I-MIT[297]		↑
Glutamic acid[238]	N	↑ ↑
Taurine[298]	↓	
Carnitine[299]	↓	↑
Tyramine, tryptamine, and histamine[300]		↑
17-hydroxycorticoids and ketogenic steroids[301]	↓	↑
Pyridinoline, deoxypyridinoline[302]		↑
Hydroxyproline[303] and hydroxylysyl glycoside[304]		↑
Red blood cells		
Fe[235,281]	↓	↑
Na[305]	N	↑
Zn[306]	N	↓
Hemoglobin[235,281]	↓	↓
Glucose-6-phosphate dehydrogenase activity	N or ↓	↑
Reduced glutathione[308] and carbonic anhydrase[309]	↑	↓
Ca-ATPase activity[310]	↓	↓
White blood cells		
Alkaline phosphatase[311]	? ↑	↓
ATP production in mitochondria[312]	N	↓
Adipose tissue		
cAMP[279]		↑
Lipoprotein lipase[290]	↓	
Skeletal muscle		
cAMP[279]		↑
Sweat glands		
Sweat electrolytes[313]	↑	N
Sebum excretion rate[314]	↓	N
Intestinal system and absorption		
Basic electrical rhythm of the duodenum[315]	↓	↑
Riboflavin absorption[316]	↑*	↓*
Ca absorption[317]		↓*
Intestinal transit and fecal fat[318,319]		↑
Pulmonary function and gas exchange		
Dead space,[320] hypoxic ventilatory drive,[321] and arterial Po_2[320]	↓	
Neurologic system and CSF		
Relaxation time to deep tendon reflexes (photomotography)[322]	↑	↓
CSF proteins[323]	↑	
Cardiovascular and circulatory system		
Timing of the arterial sounds (QKd)[225]	↑	↓
Pre-ejection period, left ventricular ejection time ratio[226]	↑	↓
ECG[324,325]	↓	↑
Heart rate QRS voltage		↓
Q-Tc interval		↑
PR interval	Flat or	Transient
T wave	inverted	abnormalities
Common arrhythmias	Arterio-ventricular block	Atrial fibrillation
Bones		
Osseous maturation (bone age by x-ray film)[326,327]	Delayed (epiphysial dysgenesis)	Advanced

N, normal; ↑, increased; ↓, decreased.

*In children.

†In neonates.

cAMP, cyclic adenosine monophosphate; cGMP, cyclic guanosine monophosphate; CSF, cerebrospinal fluid; ECG, electrocardiogram; GnRH, gonadotropin-releasing hormone; IV, intravenous; LH, luteinizing hormone; MIT, monoiodotyrosine; PTH, parathyroid hormone; PTU, propylthiouracil; TBG, thyrotropin-binding globulin; TBPA, thyroxine-binding prealbumin; TRH, thyrotropin-releasing hormone.

autoimmune thyroid disease, in particular, Graves' disease.[356] The interaction of these unfractionated immunoglobulins with thyroid follicular cells usually results in global stimulation of thyroid gland activity and only rarely causes inhibition. It has been recommended that these assays all be called TSH receptor antibodies with a phrase "measured by . . . assay" to identify the type of method used for their determination.[107] The tests will be described under three general categories: (1) those measuring thyroid-stimulating activity by using in vivo or in vitro bioassays, (2) tests based on competition of the abnormal immunoglobulin with binding of TSH to its receptor, and (3) measurement of the thyroid growth-promoting activity of immunoglobulins. Tests use both human and animal tissue material or cell lines.

THYROID STIMULATION ASSAYS. The earliest assays used various modifications of the McKenzie mouse bioassay.[357, 358] The abnormal γ-globulin with TSH-like biologic properties has relatively longer in vivo activity, hence its name—long-acting thyroid stimulator (LATS). The assay measures the LATS-induced release of thyroid hormone from the mouse thyroid gland prelabeled with radioiodide. The presence of LATS in serum is pathognomonic of Graves' disease. However, depending on assay sensitivity, a variable percentage of untreated patients will show a positive LATS response. LATS activity may be found in the serum of patients with Graves' disease even in the absence of thyrotoxicosis. Although it is more commonly present in patients with ophthalmopathy, especially when accompanied by pretibial myxedema,[359] LATS activity does not appear to correlate with the presence of Graves' disease, its severity, or the course of complications. LATS crosses the placenta and may be found transiently in newborns of mothers possessing the abnormal γ-globulin.[360]

Attempts to improve the ability to detect thyroid-stimulating antibodies (TSAbs) in autoimmune thyroid disease led to the development of several in vitro assays using animal as well as human thyroid tissue. The ability of the patient's serum to stimulate endocytosis in fresh human thyroid tissue is measured by direct count of the intracellular colloid droplets formed. When such a technique is used, human thyroid stimulator activity has been demonstrated in serum samples from patients with Graves' disease that were devoid of LATS activity measured by the standard mouse bioassay.[361] TSAbs can be detected by measuring the accumulation of cyclic adenosine monophosphate (cAMP) or stimulation of adenylate cyclase activity in human thyroid cell cultures and thyroid plasma membranes, respectively.[362] Accumulation of cAMP in the cultured rat thyroid cell line FRTL5 has also been used as an assay for TSAb.[363] Stimulation of release of T_3 from human[364] and porcine[365] thyroid slices is another form of in vitro assay for TSAb. An in vitro bioassay using a cytochemical technique depends on the ability of thyroid-stimulating material to increase lysosomal membrane permeability to a chromogenic substrate, leucyl-β-naphthylamide, which then reacts with the enzyme naphthylamidase. Quantitation is by scanning and integrated microdensitometry.[366]

Cloning of the TSH receptor[367, 368] led to the development of an in vitro assay for TSAb in cell lines that express the recombinant TSH receptor.[369, 370] This assay, based on the generation of cAMP, is specific for the measurement of human TSH receptor antibodies that have thyroid-stimulating activity and thus contrasts with assays based on binding to the TSH receptor (see below), which cannot distinguish between antibodies with thyroid-stimulating and TSH-blocking activity. Accordingly, the recombinant human TSH receptor assay measures antibodies relevant to the pathogenesis of autoimmune thyrotoxicosis and is more sensitive than the formerly used TSAb assays.[371] For example, 94% of serum samples were positive for TSAb vs. 74% when the same samples were assayed by using FRTL5 cells.[372]

One of the major drawbacks with the bioassays mentioned above is that they are unsuitable for use as routine laboratory tools. This problem has largely been circumvented, however, with the advent of a luminescence-linked bioassay for TSAbs.[373] This assay uses Chinese hamster ovary cells stably transfected with the human TSH receptor and a cAMP-dependent luciferase reporter. With the use of an international TSAb standard, the assay responded in a dose-dependent manner, with 10 mIU/mL of standard generating a relative light unit score of greater than 10. The authors also reported that the assay was modified to allow use in a 96-well plate format, thereby permitting automated measurement of relative luminosity in a large number of samples.

THYROTROPIN-BINDING INHIBITION ASSAYS. The principal of binding inhibition assays dates to the discovery of another class of abnormal immunoglobulins in patients with Graves' disease: those that neutralize the bioactivity of LATS tested in the mouse.[374] This material, known as LATS protector, is species specific; it has no biologic effect on the mouse thyroid gland but is capable of stimulating the human thyroid.[375] The original assay was cumbersome, which limited its clinical application.

Techniques used currently, which may be collectively termed radioreceptor assays, are based on competition of the abnormal immunoglobulins and TSH for a common receptor-binding site on thyroid cells. The test is akin in principle to the radioligand assays, in which a natural membrane receptor takes the place of the binding proteins or antibodies. Various sources of TSH receptor are used, including human thyroid cells,[376] their particulate or solubilized membrane,[377, 378] and cell membranes from porcine thyroids[379] or guinea pig fat cells[380] or recombinant human TSH receptor expressed in mammalian cells.[381] The latter have been improved and modified for routine laboratory use.[382, 383] Because the assays do not directly measure thyroid-stimulating activity, the abnormal immunoglobulins determined have been given a variety of names, such as thyroid-binding inhibitory immunoglobulins or antibodies and thyrotropin-displacing immunoglobulins. This type of assay has indicated that not all the antibodies detected stimulate the thyroid, and some are inhibitory. Even with modern techniques,[340] the presence of inhibitory antibody is less sensitive and specific for Graves' disease than is the presence of stimulatory antibody activity.[370] The stimulatory and inhibitory effects can be differentiated only by functional assays, which typically measure the production of cAMP.

THYROID GROWTH-PROMOTING ASSAYS. Assays have also been developed that measure the growth-promoting activity of abnormal immunoglobulins. One such assay is based on the staining of nuclei from guinea pig thyroid cells in S phase by the Feulgen reaction.[384] Another assay measures the incorporation of ^{3}H-thymidine into DNA in FRTL cells.[385] Whether the thyroid growth-stimulating immunoglobulins measured by these assays represent a population of immunoglobulins distinct from those with stimulatory functional activity remains a subject of active debate.

CLINICAL APPLICATIONS. Measurement of abnormal immunoglobulins that interact with thyroid tissue by any of the methods described above is not indicated as a routine diagnostic test for Graves' disease. It is useful, however, in a few selected clinical conditions: (1) in the differential diagnosis of exophthalmos, particularly unilateral exophthalmos, when the origin of this condition is otherwise not apparent; the presence of thyroid-stimulating immunoglobulins would obviate the necessity to undertake more complex diagnostic procedures described elsewhere[386]; (2) in the differential diagnosis of pretibial myxedema or other forms of dermopathy when the etiology is unclear and it is imperative that the cause of the skin lesion be ascertained; (3) in the differentiation of Graves' disease from toxic nodular goiter when both are being considered as the possible cause of thyrotoxicosis, when other tests such as thyroid scanning and thyroid autoantibody tests have been inconclusive, and particularly when such a distinction would play a role in determining the course of therapy; (4) when nonautoimmune thyrotoxicosis is suspected in a patient with hyperthyroidism and diffuse or nodular goiter[387]; (5) in Graves' disease during pregnancy, when high maternal levels of TSAb are a warning for the possible occurrence of neonatal thyrotoxicosis; and (6) in neonatal thyrotoxicosis, where serial TSAb determinations showing a gradual decrease may be helpful in distinguishing between intrinsic Graves' disease in an infant and transient thyrotoxicosis resulting from passive transfer of maternal TSAb.[360, 388] Some investigators have found the persistence of TSAbs to be predictive of relapse of Graves' thyrotoxicosis after a course of antithyroid drug therapy.[389]

Other Substances with Thyroid-Stimulating Activity

Hyperthyroidism develops in some patients with trophoblastic disease as a result of the production and release of a thyroid stimulator that has been termed molar or trophoblastic thyrotropin or big placental TSH.[390] It is likely that the thyroid-stimulating activity in patients with trophoblastic disease is entirely due to the presence of high levels of human chorionic gonadotropin (hCG).[391] Thus an RIA for hCG can be useful in the differential diagnosis of thyroid dysfunction, although the clinical status of the patient is likely to suggest this etiology.

The thyroid-stimulating activity of hCG can be enhanced by mutations in the TSH receptor that increase its affinity for this placental hormone. The consequence is thyrotoxicosis limited to pregnancy and associated with hyperemesis gravidarum in women.[392]

Exophthalmos-Producing Substance

A variety of tests have been developed for measuring exophthalmogenic activity in serum.[493–496] Although great uncertainty still exists regarding the pathogenesis of thyroid-associated eye disease, the role of the immune system appears to be central. Exophthalmogenic activity has also been detected in IgG fractions of some patients with Graves' ophthalmopathy. Autoantibodies directed toward a 64-kDa eye muscle protein have been identified in 73% of patients with active thyroid-associated ophthalmopathy,[497–499] although the role of these antibodies in the diagnosis and management of the ophthalmopathy is at present unclear. The role of assays to detect specific antibodies is discussed further in Chapter 101.

Tests of Cell-Mediated Immunity

Delayed hypersensitivity reactions to thyroid antigens are present in autoimmune thyroid diseases (see Chapter 99). Cell-mediated immunity can be measured in several ways: (1) the migration inhibition test, which measures the inhibition of migration of sensitized leukocytes when exposed to the sensitizing antigen; (2) the lymphotoxic assay, which measures the ability of sensitized lymphocytes to kill target cells when exposed to the antigen; (3) the blastogenesis assay, which scores the formation of blast cells after exposure of lymphocytes to a thyroid antigen, and (4) thymus dependent (T) lymphocyte subset quantitation using monoclonal antibodies. More recently, measurement of T cell proliferation determined by uptake of ^{3}H-thymidine has become the standard test for cell-mediated immunity used in the research setting.[400, 401] The tests require fresh leukocytes from the patient, are variable in their response, and are difficult to perform.

ANATOMIC AND TISSUE DIAGNOSES

The purpose of the procedures described in this section is to evaluate the anatomic features of the thyroid gland, localize and determine the nature of abnormal areas, and eventually provide a pathologic or tissue diagnosis.

Thyroid Scintiscanning

Normal and abnormal thyroid tissue can be externally imaged by three scintiscanning methods: (1) with radionuclides that are concentrated by normal thyroid tissues, such as iodide isotopes and ^{99m}Tc given as the pertechnetate ion; (2) by administration of radiopharmaceutical agents that are preferentially concentrated by abnormal thyroid tissues; and (3) by fluorescent scanning, which uses an external source of ^{241}Am and does not require the administration of radioactive material. Each has specific indications, advantages, and disadvantages.

The physical properties, dosages, and radiation delivered by the most commonly used radioisotopes are listed in Table 97–1. The choice of scanning agent depends on the purpose of the scan, the age of the patient, and the equipment available. Radioiodide scans cannot be performed in patients who have recently ingested iodine-containing compounds. ^{123}I and $^{99m}TcO_4^-$ are the radionuclides of choice because of the low radiation exposure.[402–404] The radioisotope ^{131}I is still used for the detection of functioning metastatic thyroid carcinoma by total body scanning.

RADIOIODIDE AND ^{99m}Tc SCANS. $^{99m}TcO_4^-$ is concentrated, and all iodide isotopes are concentrated and bound by thyroid tissue. Depending on the isotope used, scans are carried out at different times after administration: 20 minutes for $^{99m}TcO_4^-$; 4 or 24 hours for ^{123}I; 24 hours for ^{125}I and ^{131}I; and 48, 72, and 96 hours when ^{131}I is used in the search for metastatic thyroid carcinoma. The appearance of the normal thyroid gland on scan may be best described as a narrow-winged butterfly. Each "wing" represents a thyroid lobe, which in the adult measures 5 ± 1 cm in length and 2.3 ± 0.5 cm in width.[405] Common variants include the absence of a connecting isthmus, a large isthmus, asymmetry between the two lobes, and trailing activity extending to the cricoid cartilage (pyramidal lobe). The latter is more commonly found in conditions associated with diffuse thyroid hyperplasia. Occasionally, collection of saliva in the esophagus during $^{99m}TcO_4^-$ scanning may simulate a pyramidal lobe, but this artifact can be eliminated by drinking water.

Indications for scanning are listed in Table 97–9. In clinical practice, scans are most often requested for evaluation of the functional activity of solitary nodules. Normally, the isotope is homogeneously distributed throughout both lobes of the thyroid gland. This diffuse distribution occurs in the enlarged gland of Graves' disease and may be seen in Hashimoto's thyroiditis. A mottled appearance may be noted in Hashimoto's thyroiditis and can occasionally be seen in Graves' disease, especially after therapy with radioactive iodide. Irregular areas of relatively diminished and occasionally increased uptake are characteristic of large multinodular goiters. The traditional nuclear medicine jargon classifies nodules as "hot," "warm," and "cold," according to their isotope-concentrating ability relative to the surrounding normal parenchyma. Hot, or hyperfunctioning, nodules are typically benign, although the presence of malignancy has been reported.[406, 407] In a large series of patients in whom thyroid scans were undertaken and subsequent surgery was performed irrespective of the scan result, 84% were cold, 11% were warm, and 6% were hot nodules. A histopathologic diagnosis of thyroid cancer was made in 16% of cold, 9% of warm, and 4% of hot nodules.[408, 409] These data demonstrate that cold nodules are most likely to harbor malignancy but most cold nodules are benign and, furthermore, the finding of a hot nodule on thyroid isotope scanning does not exclude the presence of malignancy. Occasionally, a nodule that is functional on a $^{99m}TcO_4^-$ scan will be found to be cold on an iodine scan; this pattern is found with both benign and malignant nodules.

Thyroid isotope scans are of particular value in identifying autonomous thyroid nodules because the remainder of the activity in the gland is suppressed. A search for functioning thyroid metastases is best accomplished by using 2 to 10 mCi of ^{131}I after ablation of normal thyroid tissue and cessation of hormone therapy to allow TSH to increase above the upper limit of normal. Recent studies have addressed the question of whether recombinant human TSH allows scanning without requiring cessation of hormone therapy.[410] Uptake is also found outside the thyroid gland in patients with lingual thyroids and in the rare ovarian dermoid tumor containing functioning thyroid tissue.

The scan can be used as an adjunct during TSH stimulation and T_3 suppression tests to localize suppressed normal thyroid tissue or autonomously functioning areas, respectively (see below). Applications other than those listed in Table 97–9 are of doubtful benefit and

TABLE 97–9. Indications for Radionuclide Scanning

Detection of anatomic variants and search for ectopic thyroid tissue (thyroid hemiagenesis, lingual thyroid, struma ovarii)
Diagnosis of congenital athyrosis
Determination of the nature of abnormal neck or chest (mediastinal) masses
Evaluation of solitary thyroid nodules (functioning or nonfunctioning)
Evaluation of thyroid remnants after surgery
Detection of functioning thyroid metastases
Evaluation of focal functional thyroid abnormalities (suppressed or nonsuppressible tissue)

are rarely justified in view of the radiation exposure, expense, and inconvenience. ^{123}I single photon emission computed tomography may also be useful in the evaluation of thyroid abnormalities.[411]

OTHER ISOTOPE SCANS. Because most test procedures, short of direct microscopic examination of thyroid tissue, fail to detect thyroid malignancy with any degree of certainty, efforts have been made to find other radioactive materials that would possibly be of diagnostic use. Several such agents that are concentrated by metabolically active tissues, irrespective of whether they have iodide-concentrating ability, have been tried. However, despite claims to the contrary, either they have had only limited value or their diagnostic usefulness has not been fully evaluated. These agents include ^{75}Se-methionine, ^{125}Ce, ^{67}Ga-citrate, ^{32}P-pyrophosphate, ^{99m}Tc, and ^{201}Th.[412]

Scanning with ^{131}I-labeled anti-Tg for the detection of occult metastatic thyroid malignancy that fails to concentrate ^{131}I showed early promising results.[413] However, the procedure has not proved clinically useful.

Ultrasonography

Ultrasonography is used to outline the thyroid gland and to characterize lesions differing in density from the surrounding tissue. The technique differentiates interphases of different acoustic densities by using sound frequencies in the megahertz range that are above the audible range. A transducer fitted with a piezoelectric crystal produces and transmits the signal and receives echo reflections. Interfaces of different acoustic densities reflect dense echoes, liquid transmits sound without reflections, and air-filled spaces do not transmit the ultrasound.[414]

One of the most useful applications of the ultrasonogram is in the differentiation of solid from cystic lesions.[414, 415] Purely cystic lesions are entirely sonolucent, whereas solid lesions produce multiple echoes as a result of multiple sonic interphases. Many lesions, however, are mixed (solid and cystic) and are termed complex lesions. Some tumors may have the same acoustic characteristics as the surrounding normal tissue, thus escaping echographic detection. True cystic lesions are usually benign, although most large thyroid nodules contain cystic areas. Carcinomas may also undergo infarction, which causes degenerative cystic change within their substance. In one large series of thyroid nodules, 69% were found to be solid and 21% of these were subsequently shown to be malignant. Similarly, of the 19% of cystic lesions, 7% were malignant and malignancy was also detected in 12% of the mixed lesions.[408, 409] Thus, solid nodules, as determined by ultrasound scanning, were most likely to be malignant, but the majority were benign, and a similar proportion of cystic nodules were also malignant. Ultrasound scanning of thyroid nodules is poorly sensitive and specific as an indicator of the presence of malignancy in a thyroid mass.

Although high-resolution ultrasonography can detect thyroid nodules on the order of a few millimeters,[416] lesions need to be larger than 0.5 cm to allow differentiation between solid and cystic structures. A sonolucent pattern is frequently noted in glands with Hashimoto's thyroiditis, but this pattern has also been described in multinodular glands and in patients with Graves' disease.[414, 417, 418]

Because sonography localizes the position as well as the depth of lesions, the procedure has been used to successfully guide the needle during aspiration biopsy.[419] In complex lesions, sonographic guiding ensures sampling from the solid portion of the nodule. With experience and proper calibration, sonography can be used for estimation of thyroid gland size.[420, 421] Several recent reports have described treatment of toxic nodules by the injection of alcohol under sonographic guidance.[422] Although ultrasonography has found virtually the same applications as scintiscanning, claims that the former may differentiate benign from malignant lesions are unfounded. Also, ultrasonography cannot be used for the assessment of substernal goiters because of interference from overlying bone.

The procedure is simple and painless and, at the frequencies of sound used, does not produce tissue damage. Because it does not require the administration of isotopes, it can be safely used in children and during pregnancy. Also, because the procedure is independent of iodine-concentrating mechanisms, it is valuable in the study of suppressed glands.

X-ray Procedures

A simple X-ray film of the neck and upper part of the mediastinum may provide valuable information regarding the location, size, and effect of a goiter on surrounding structures. Radiographs may show an asymmetrical goiter, an intrathoracic extension of the gland, and displacement or narrowing of the trachea. If any suggestion of posterior extension of the mass is seen, it is useful to take films during the swallow of x-ray contrast material. The soft tissue x-ray technique may disclose calcium deposits. Large deposits in flakes or rings are typical of an old multinodular goiter, whereas foci of finely stippled flecks of calcium are suggestive of papillary adenocarcinoma.

Information not related to anatomic abnormalities of the thyroid gland may be obtained from x-ray studies. In children with a history of hypothyroidism, an x-ray film of the hand to determine bone age could aid in estimating the onset and duration of thyroid dysfunction.[326, 327] Hypothyroidism leads to retardation in bone age and in infants produces a dense calcification of epiphyseal plates most easily seen at the distal end of the radius. Long-standing myxedema produces pituitary hypertrophy, which especially in children but also in adults causes enlargement of the sella turcica demonstrable on imaging of the pituitary region.

COMPUTED TOMOGRAPHY AND MAGNETIC RESONANCE IMAGING. Computed tomography (CT) and magnetic resonance imaging (MRI) provide useful information on the location and architecture of the thyroid gland, as well as its relationship to surrounding tissues.[423] An important application of CT is the assessment and delineation of obscure mediastinal masses and large substernal goiters.[424] The necessity to infuse iodine-containing contrast agents limits the application of CT in patients being considered for radioiodide therapy. CT and MRI have found firm application in another area of thyroid diseases, namely, in the evaluation of ophthalmopathy[386] and mediastinal masses.[424]

Other Procedures

A barium swallow may be useful in evaluating impingement of a goiter on the esophagus, whereas a flow-volume loop[425] may be useful in allowing quantitative documentation of functional impingement on the upper part of the airway.

Biopsy of the Thyroid Gland

Histologic examination of thyroid tissue for diagnostic purposes requires some form of an invasive procedure. The biopsy procedure depends on the intended type of microscopic examination. Core biopsy for histologic examination of tissue with preservation of architecture is obtained by closed needle or open surgical procedures; aspiration biopsy is performed to obtain material for cytologic examination.

CORE BIOPSY. Closed core biopsy is an office procedure carried out under local anesthesia. A large (about 15-gauge) cutting needle of the Vim-Silverman type is most commonly used.[426] The needle is introduced under local anesthesia through a small skin nick, and firm pressure is applied over the puncture site for 5 to 10 minutes after withdrawal of the needle. In experienced hands complications are rare, but they may be serious and include transient damage to the laryngeal nerve, puncture of the trachea, laryngospasm, jugular vein phlebitis, and bleeding.[408] With the improvement in cytology and biopsy techniques, open biopsy carried out under local or general anesthesia has been virtually abandoned.[408]

PERCUTANEOUS FINE-NEEDLE ASPIRATION. The development of more sophisticated staining techniques for cytologic examination, the realization that fear of tumor dissemination along the needle tract was not well founded, and especially the high diagnostic accuracy of the technique are responsible for the increasing popularity of percutaneous fine-needle aspiration (FNA).[406, 408, 427, 428]

The procedure is exceedingly simple and safe. The patient lies supine, with the neck hyperextended by placing a small pillow under the shoulders. Local anesthesia is not usually required. The skin is prepared with an antiseptic solution. The lesion, fixed between two gloved fingers, is penetrated with a fine (22- to 27-gauge) needle attached to a syringe. Suction is then applied while the needle is moved within the nodule. A nonsuction technique using capillary action has also been developed. The small amount of aspirated material, usually contained within the needle or its hub, is applied to glass slides and spread. Some slides are air-dried and others are fixed before staining. Because biopsy of small nodules may be technically more difficult, the use of ultrasound to guide the needle has been suggested.[419, 422] It is important that the slides be properly prepared, stained, and read by a cytologist experienced in the interpretation of material from thyroid gland aspirates. Newer molecular approaches have been used to analyze FNA material to help distinguish benign from malignant pathologies,[429–432] although these techniques are currently in development stages.

The yield of false-positive and false-negative results is variable from one center to another, but both are acceptably low. Various centers have reported that the accuracy of this technique in distinguishing benign from malignant lesions may be as high as 95%.[408, 427] Patients with an initial FNA demonstrating frankly malignant or suspicious cytologic findings (including follicular neoplasms; see below) on first examination are immediately referred for surgery. Some clinicians recommend that repeat FNA be performed 6 to 12 months after the initial biopsy to reduce the risk of false-negative results. In one study the second FNA changed the diagnosis in 7% of patients and an additional four carcinomas were detected.[433]

In one clinic in which the procedure is used routinely, the number of patients operated upon decreased by one-third, whereas the percentage of thyroid carcinomas among the patients who underwent surgery doubled.[434] When the results are suggestive of follicular neoplasia, surgery is required because follicular adenoma cannot be differentiated from follicular cancer by cytologic analysis alone. Because the sample obtained may not always be representative of the lesion, surgical treatment is indicated for lesions highly suspicious of being malignant on clinical grounds. Other uses of aspiration biopsy include presumed lymphoma or invasive anaplastic carcinoma when biopsy may spare the patient an unnecessary neck exploration. Another application of needle aspiration is in the confirmation and treatment of thyroid cysts and autonomous thyroid nodules.[435]

EVALUATION OF THE HYPOTHALAMIC-PITUITARY-THYROID AXIS

The development of an RIA for the routine measurement of TSH in serum and the availability of synthetic TRH[436, 437] have placed increased reliance on tests assessing the hypothalamic-pituitary control of thyroid function. These tests allow the diagnosis of mild and subclinical forms of thyroid dysfunction and provide a means of differentiating between primary, pituitary (secondary), or hypothalamic (tertiary) thyroid gland failure.

Thyrotropin

In recent years dramatic improvements have been made in assays for TSH. The routine measurement of TSH in clinical practice initially used RIA techniques. These first-generation assays had a sensitivity level of 1 mU/L, which did not allow the separation of normal from reduced values. A major problem with early TSH RIAs was cross-reactivity with gonadotropins (luteinizing hormone, follicle-stimulating hormone, and hCG) that share with TSH a common α subunit.[438] Nevertheless, even older RIA methods for measurement of pituitary TSH correlated well with values obtained by bioassay techniques.[439] Another uncommon source of error is the presence in the serum sample of heterophilic antibodies induced by vaccination with materials contaminated with animal serum[440] or the presence of endogenous TSH antibodies.[441] RIA techniques for the measurement of TSH in dry blood spots on filter paper are used for the screening of neonatal hypothyroidism.[28]

Newer techniques have been developed that use multiple antibodies to produce a "sandwich"-type assay in which one antibody (usually directed against the α subunit) serves to anchor the TSH molecule and another (usually monoclonal antibodies directed against the β subunit) is either radioiodinated (immunoradiometric assay) or is conjugated with an enzyme (immunoenzymometric) or a chemiluminescent compound (chemiluminescent assay).[112, 442] In these assays the signal should be directly related to the amount of the ligand present rather than being inversely related as in RIAs measuring the bound tracer.[443] This technique results in decreased background "noise" and greater sensitivity, decreased interference from related compounds, and an expanded useful range.[112, 442, 444] Initial improvements in the TSH assay resulted in assays with a sensitivity limit of 0.1 mU/L, a normal range of approximately 0.5 to 4.5 mU/L, and the ability to distinguish between low and normal TSH values.[112, 442, 444] Recently, commercial assays have been developed with an even higher sensitivity limit of 0.005 to 0.01 mU/L and a similar normal range but an expanded range between the lower limit of normal and the lower limit of sensitivity.[445, 446]

The nomenclature for differentiating these various assays has not been standardized, with manufacturers applying various combinations of "high(ly)," "ultra," and "sensitive." It has been recommended that the sensitivity limit be used in defining the assays, with the early RIAs detecting values of 1 mU/L or greater designated "first-generation assays," those with a lower sensitivity limit of 0.1 mU/L designated as "second-generation assays," and those with a lower sensitivity limit of 0.01 mU/L or less designated as "third-generation assays."[112] Determination of the appropriate sensitivity level has also been controversial. Some base the definition on the level with a coefficient of variation less than 20%, whereas others define it as the lowest level that can be reliably differentiated from the zero TSH standard.[112, 444] At a minimum, for a TSH assay to be considered "sensitive," the overlap of TSH values in sera from clinically hyperthyroid and euthyroid individuals should be less than 5% and preferably less than 1%.[112]

In a number of these "third-generation" assays, TSH detected in clinically toxic patients and elevated values found in euthyroid subjects were not confirmed when the samples were measured in other assays. In some cases these discrepant results have been attributed to the presence of antibodies directed against the animal immunoglobulins used in the assay.[447–449] These immunoglobulins act to bind the anchoring and detecting antibodies and lead to an overestimation of TSH. In some cases this effect may be blocked by the addition of an excess of nonspecific immunoglobulin of the same species.[449]

The availability of random-access immunoassay analyzers has revolutionized TSH measurements. These assays are highly reproducible and provide convenience and rapid throughput of large volumes of serum samples.[118, 119]

TSH appears abruptly in the pituitary and serum of the fetus at midgestation and can also be detected in amniotic fluid.[40, 450, 451] The mean TSH level is higher in cord than in maternal blood. A substantial increase, to levels severalfold above the upper range in adults, is observed during the first half-hour of life.[451] Levels decline to near the normal adult range by the third day of life. Minimal changes reported to occur during adult life and in early adolescence[452] have no significant effect on the overall range of normal. In the absence of pregnancy, no significant sex differences have been observed. Although early studies failed to show diurnal TSH variation,[453] significantly higher values have been recorded during the late evening and early night and are partially inhibited by sleep.[454] This diurnal rhythm of TSH is superimposed on continuous high-frequency, low-amplitude variations. The nocturnal TSH surge persists in patients with mild primary hypothyroidism[455, 456] and is abolished in hypothalamic hypothyroidism[455, 457] and in some patients during fasting[458] and with nonthyroidal illness.[459, 460] It is enhanced by oral contraceptives[461] and is abolished by high levels of glucocorticoids.[462] The presence of seasonal variation has not been a uniform finding, but it is unlikely to affect the clinical interpretation of serum values.[463] Various types of stressful stimuli have no significant effect on the basal serum TSH level, except for a rise during surgical hypothermia in infants but not in adults.[464] Various stimuli that elicit in normal humans a secretory response of some pituitary hormones, such as the administration of insulin, vasopressin, glucagon, bacterial pyrogens, arginine, prostaglandins, and chlorpromazine, have no effect on serum TSH. However, administration of any of a growing list of drugs has been found to alter the basal concentration of serum TSH and/or its response to exogenous TRH (Table 97–10).

TABLE 97–10. Agents That May Affect TSH Secretion

Substance	Common Use
Increase serum TSH concentration and/or its response to TRH	
Iodine (iodide and iodine-containing compounds)[144, 465, 466]	Radiologic contrast media, antiseptic, expectorant, antiarrhythmic, and antianginal
Lithium[467]	Treatment of bipolar psychoses
Dopamine antagonists	
Dopamine receptor blockers (metoclopramide,[468, 469] domperidone[469])	Antiemetic
Dopamine-blocking agent (sulpiride[470])	Tranquilizer
Decarboxylase inhibitor (benserazide[471])	—
Dopamine-depleting agent (monoiodotyrosine[469])	—
L-Dopa inhibitors (chlorpromazine,[472] biperiden,[473] haloperidol[473])	Neuroleptic
Cimetidine (histamine receptor blocker)[474]	Treatment of peptic ulcers
Clomiphene (antiestrogen)[475]	Induction of ovulation
Spironolactone[476]	Antihypertensive
Amphetamines[477]	Anticongestants and antiappetite
Increase serum TSH concentration and/or its response to TRH	
Thyroid hormones (T_4 and T_3)	Replacement therapy, antigoitrogenic, and anticancer
Thyroid hormone analogues (DT_4,[478] 3′,3′,5-TRIAC,[479] etiroxate-HCl,[480] dimethyl-3 isopropyl-L-thyronine[481])	Cholesterol lowering and weight reducing
Dopaminergic agents (agonists)	
Dopamine[468, 482]	Antihypotensive
L-Dopa[261] (dopamine precursor)	Diagnostic agent and antiparkinsonian
Bromocriptine[483]	Antilactation and pituitary tumor suppression
Fusaric acid (inhibitor of dopamine hydroxylase)[484]	—
Pyridoxine (coenzyme of dopamine synthesis)[485]	Vitamin and antineuropathic
Other dopaminergic agents (pirbedil,[486] apomorphine,[486] lisuride[486])	Treatment of cerebrovascular diseases and migraine
Dopamine antagonist (pimozide)[488]	Neuroleptic
α-Noradrenergic blockers (phentolamine,[489] thioridazine[490])	Neuroleptic
Serotonin antagonists (metergoline,[491] cyproheptadine,[492] methysergide[493])	Antimigraine and appetite stimulators
Serotonin agonist (5-hydroxytryptophan)[494]	—
Glucocorticoids[495, 496]	Anti-inflammatory, immunosuppressive, and anticancer; reduction of intracranial pressure
Acetylsalicylic acid[497]	Anti-inflammatory, antipyretic, and analgesic
Growth hormone[498]*	Growth promoting
Somatostatin[499]	—
Opiates (morphine,[500] leu-enkephalin,[501] heroin[502])	Analgesic
Clofibrate[503]	Hypolipidemic
Fenclofenac[63]	Nonsteroidal anti-inflammatory drug

*In hyposomatotrophic dwarfs.

DT_4, dextrothyroxine; T_3, triiodothyronine; T_4, thyroxine; TRH, thyrotropin-releasing hormone; TRIAC, triiodothyroacetic acid; TSH, thyroid-stimulating hormone.

In the presence of a normally functioning hypothalamic-pituitary system, an inverse correlation is found between the serum concentration of FT_4 and TSH. Changes in the serum concentration of TT_4 as a result of TBG abnormalities or drugs competing with T_4 binding to TBG have no effect on the level of serum TSH. The pituitary is exquisitely sensitive to both minimal decreases and increases in thyroid hormone concentration, with a logarithmic change in TSH levels in response to changes in T_4[442, 446, 465, 504] (Fig. 97–5). Thus serum TSH levels should be elevated in patients with primary hypothyroidism and low or undetectable in those with thyrotoxicosis. Indeed, in the absence of hypothalamic pituitary disease, illness, or drugs, TSH is an accurate indicator of thyroid hormone status and the adequacy of thyroid hormone replacement.[442, 505]

In patients with primary hypothyroidism of whatever cause, levels may reach 1000 mU/mL or higher. The magnitude of serum TSH elevation grossly correlates with the severity and in part with the duration of thyroid hormone deficiency.[506, 507] TSH concentrations above the upper limit of normal have been observed in the absence of clinical symptoms and signs of hypothyroidism and in the presence of serum T_4 and T_3 levels well within the normal range.[506, 508] This condition is most commonly encountered in patients with incipient hypothyroidism from Hashimoto's thyroiditis or with limited ability to synthesize thyroid hormone because of prior thyroid surgery, radioiodide treatment, or severe iodine deficiency.[506, 509] No agreement has been reached on whether such patients have subclinical hypothyroidism or a "compensated state" in which euthyroidism is maintained by chronic stimulation of a reduced amount of functioning thyroid tissue through hypersecretion of TSH. Transient hypothyroidism may occur in some infants during the early neonatal period.[510] In two circumstances the usual reverse relationship between the serum level of TSH and T_4 is not maintained in patients with proven primary hypothyroidism. Treatment with replacement doses of T_4 may normalize or even produce serum levels of thyroid hormone above the normal range before the high TSH levels have reached the normal range.[442, 507, 511] This finding is particularly true in patients with severe or long-standing primary hypothyroidism, who may require 3 to 6 months of hormone replacement before TSH levels are fully suppressed. Conversely, serum TSH concentrations may remain low or normal for up to 5 weeks after withdrawal of thyroid hormone replacement when serum levels of T_4 and T_3 have already declined to values well below the lower range of normal.[442, 512] Causes of discrepancies between TSH and FT_4 and FT_3 levels are listed in Table 97–11.

At this time it is uncertain what TSH level is appropriate for suppressive thyroid hormone therapy. The frequency with which patients have subnormal, but detectable, TSH values depends on both

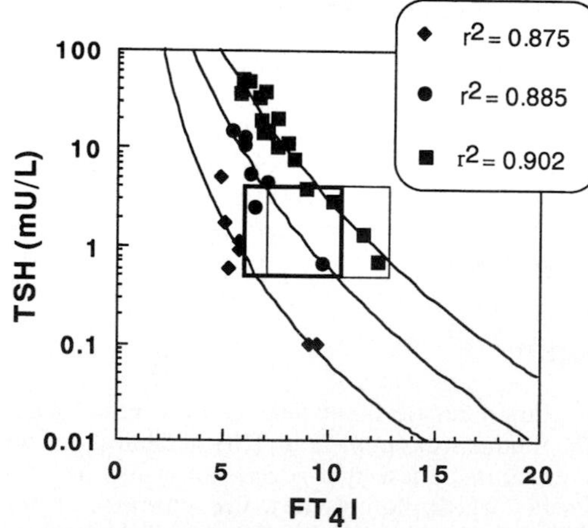

FIGURE 97–5. Correlation of the serum thyroid-stimulating hormone (TSH) concentration and the free thyroxine index (FT_4I) in three persons given increasing doses of levothyroxine. Note the logarithmic correlation between TSH and FT_4I and the variable individual requirement of T_4 to normalize the TSH level. Normal ranges are included in the *heavily lined box* and those for subjects treated by levothyroxine replacement in the *lightly lined box.*

TABLE 97–11. Discrepancies Between TSH and Free Thyroid Hormone Levels

Elevated serum TSH value without low FT_4 or FT_3 values
Subclinical hypothyroidism (inadequate replacement therapy, mild thyroid gland failure)
Recent increase in thyroid hormone dosage
Drugs
Inappropriate TSH secretion syndromes
Laboratory artifact
Subnormal serum TSH value without elevated FT_4 or FT_3 values
Subclinical hyperthyroidism (excessive replacement therapy, mild thyroid gland hyperfunction, autonomous nodule)
Recent decrease in suppressive thyroid hormone dosage
Recent treatment of thyrotoxicosis (Graves' disease, toxic multinodular goiter, toxic nodule)
Resolution of thyrotoxic phase of thyroiditis
Nonthyroidal illness
Drugs
Central hypothyroidism

FT_3, free triiodothyronine; FT_4, free thyroxine; TSH, thyroid-stimulating hormone.

the population studied and the sensitivity of the assay (Fig. 97–6). When an assay is used with a sensitivity limit of 0.1 mU/L, 3% to 4% of hospitalized patients have been noted to have subnormal TSH.[508, 513] When patients with undetectable TSH in such an assay were re-evaluated in an assay with a sensitivity limit of 0.005 mU/L, 3 of 77 (4%) with thyrotoxicosis and 32 of 37 (86%) with nonthyroidal illness or taking drugs were found to have a subnormal, but detectable, TSH level.[445] Thus the more sensitive the assay, the more likely that patients with clinical thyrotoxicosis will have undetectable serum TSH, whereas those with illness will have a subnormal but detectable level. However, with progressively more sensitive assays, the likelihood of a clinically toxic patient to have detectable TSH will increase, and if patients receiving suppressive therapy are treated until the TSH is undetectable, the more likely it is that they will have symptoms of thyrotoxicosis.

Persistent absence of a reverse correlation between the serum thyroid hormone and TSH concentration has a very different connotation. A low serum level of thyroid hormone without clear elevation in the serum TSH concentration is suggestive of trophoprivic hypothyroidism, especially when associated with obvious clinical stigmata of hypothyroidism.[509] An inherited defect in the TSH receptor has been shown to produce marked persistent hyperthyrotropinemia in the presence of normal thyroid hormone levels.[514] In some cases, a mild elevation in the serum TSH level measured by RIA is probably due to the presence of immunoreactive TSH with reduced biologic activity.[515]

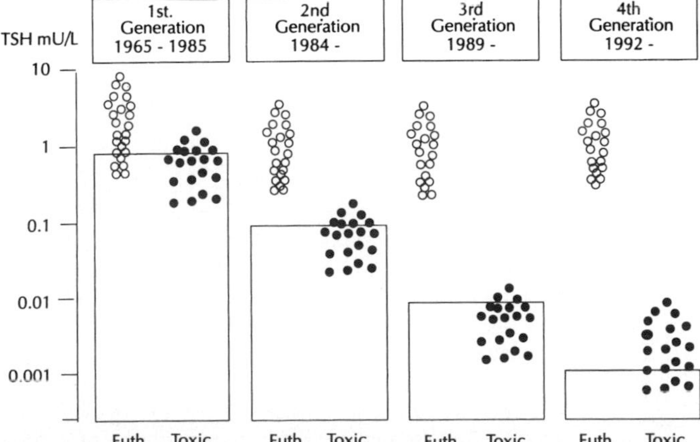

FIGURE 97–6. The effect of serum thyroid-stimulating hormone (TSH) assay sensitivity on the discrimination of euthyroid subjects (Euth) from those with thyrotoxicosis (Toxic). (From Spencer C: Clinical Diagnostics. Rochester, NY, Eastman Kodak, 1992.)

Distinction between pituitary and hypothalamic hypothyroidism can be made on the basis of the TSH response to the administration of TRH (see below).

In another group of pathologic conditions, serum TSH levels may not be suppressed despite a clear elevation of serum free thyroid hormone levels. Because such a finding is incompatible with a normal thyroregulatory control mechanism of the pituitary, which is preserved in the more common forms of thyrotoxicosis, it has been termed inappropriate secretion of TSH.[516] It implicitly suggests defective feedback regulation of TSH. When associated with the clinical and metabolic changes of thyrotoxicosis, it is usually due to one of two rare conditions: TSH-secreting pituitary adenoma or predominantly pituitary resistance to thyroid hormone.[516] The existence of hypothalamic hyperthyroidism can be questioned.[517] Precise diagnosis requires further studies, including radiologic examination of the pituitary gland and a TRH test. In addition, the presence of high circulating levels of the common α subunit of pituitary glycoprotein hormones (α-SU), with a subsequent disproportionately high α-SU/TSH molar ratio in serum, is characteristic, if not pathognomonic of TSH-secreting pituitary tumors.[516, 518] Normal and occasionally high serum TSH levels associated with a clear elevation in serum FT_4 and FT_3 but no clear clinical evidence of hypothyroidism or symptoms and signs suggestive of both thyroid hormone deficiency and excess are typical of resistance to thyroid hormone[519, 520] (see Chapter 114).

Although TSH has been implicated in the pathogenesis of simple, nontoxic goiter, unless hypothyroidism supervenes or iodide deficiency is very severe, TSH levels are characteristically normal. Elevated TSH levels may occur in the presence of normal thyroid hormone levels and apparent euthyroidism in nonthyroidal diseases[513, 521] (see also Chapter 106) and with primary adrenal failure.[522] A more common occurrence in severe acute and chronic illnesses is a normal or low serum TSH concentration despite low levels of T_3 and even low T_4 levels.[445, 505, 523] TSH values may be transiently elevated during the recovery phase.[524] Various hypotheses to explain these anomalous findings have been proposed, but a satisfactory explanation is not at hand.

A specific RIA for the β subunits of human TSH is also available but has not found clinical application.[525]

Thyrotropin-Releasing Hormone

The hypothalamic tripeptide TRH (protirelin) plays a central role in the regulation of pituitary TSH secretion.[437, 457] Several methods have been used for quantitation of TRH,[526–529] but for many reasons, measurement in humans has failed to provide information of diagnostic value. These reasons include high dilution of TRH by the time that it reaches the systemic circulation, rapid enzymatic degradation, and ubiquitous tissue distribution.[526, 528, 529] Mean serum TSH levels of 5 and 6 pg/mL have been reported. It is uncertain whether measurements carried out in urine truly represent TRH.[527]

TRH TEST. The TRH test measures the increase in pituitary TSH in serum in response to the administration of synthetic TRH. The magnitude of the TSH response to TRH is modulated by the thyrotroph response to active thyroid hormone and is thus almost always proportional to the concentration of free thyroid hormone in serum. The response is exquisitely sensitive to minor changes in the level of circulating thyroid hormones, which may not be detected by direct measurement.[465, 504] A direct correlation between basal serum TSH measurements and the maximal response to TRH has been observed even in the absence of thyroid hormone abnormalities, which suggests that the euthyroid state may be associated with a fine modulation of pituitary sensitivity to TRH.[530]

TRH normally stimulates pituitary prolactin secretion and, under certain pathologic conditions, the release of growth hormone and adrenocorticotropic hormone.[437] Accordingly, the test has been used for the assessment of a variety of endocrine functions, some unrelated to the thyroid. In clinical practice, the TRH test is used mainly (1) to assess the functional integrity of pituitary thyrotrophs and thus to aid in differentiating hypothyroidism caused by intrinsic pituitary disease from hypothalamic dysfunction, (2) in the diagnosis of mild thyrotoxicosis when results of other tests are equivocal, and (3) in the differential diagnosis of inappropriate TSH secretion, in particular, when a TSH-secreting adenoma is suspected.

TRH is effective when given intravenously as a bolus or by infusion,[452, 531] intramuscularly,[532] or orally[533] in single or repeated doses. Doses as small as 6 μg can elicit a significant TSH response, and a linear correlation exists between the incremental changes in serum TSH concentration and the logarithm of the TRH dose administered.[452] The standard test uses a single TRH dose of 400 μg/1.73 m^2 body surface area, given by rapid intravenous injection. Serum is collected before and at 15 minutes and then at 30-minute intervals over a period of 120 to 180 minutes, although many clinicians chose to obtain a single postinjection sample at 15, 20, or 30 minutes. Normal persons have a prompt increase in serum TSH, with a peak level at 15 to 40 minutes that is on average 16 mU/mL, or fivefold the basal level. The decline is more gradual, with a return of serum TSH to the preinjection level by 3 to 4 hours.[452, 531] Results can be expressed in terms of the peak level of TSH achieved, the maximal increment above the basal level, the peak TSH value expressed as a percentage of the basal value, or the integrated area of the TSH response curve. Determination of TSH before and 30 minutes after the injection of TRH provides information concerning the presence or absence of TSH responsiveness but cannot detect delayed or prolonged responses.

The stimulatory effect of TRH is specific for pituitary TSH, its free α and β subunits,[525] and prolactin. Under normal circumstances, no significant changes are observed in the serum levels of other pituitary hormones[534] or potential thyroid stimulators.[535] Responsiveness is present at birth,[536] is greater in women than in men, particularly in the follicular phase of the menstrual cycle,[537] and may be blunted in older men,[452, 532, 533] but this finding is not consistent.[538] On the average, the magnitude of the response is greater at 11 PM than at 11 AM,[530] in accordance with the diurnal pattern of the basal TSH level, which correlates with its response to TRH. Repetitive administration of TRH to the same subject at daily intervals causes gradual obtundation of the TSH response,[531] presumably because of the increase in thyroid hormone concentration[539] and also in part because of TSH "exhaustion."[540] However, more than 1 hour must elapse between the increase in thyroid hormone concentration and TRH administration for inhibition of the TSH response to occur. A number of drugs and nonendocrine diseases may affect the magnitude of the response to varying extent.

TRH-induced secretion of TSH is followed by a release of thyroid hormone that can be detected by direct measurement of serum TT_4 and TT_3 concentrations.[191] Peak levels are normally reached approximately 4 hours after the administration of TRH and are accompanied by an increase in serum Tg concentration. The incremental rise in serum TT_3 is relatively greater, and the peak is on average 50% above the basal level. Measurement of changes in serum thyroid hormone concentration after the administration of TRH has been proposed as an adjunctive test and is useful for evaluation of the integrity of the thyroid gland or bioactivity of endogenous TSH.[541] The increase in RAIU is minimal and occurs only with high doses of TRH given orally.[533]

Side effects from the intravenous administration of TRH, in decreasing order of frequency, include nausea, flushing or a sensation of warmth, desire to micturate, peculiar taste, light-headedness or headache, dry mouth, urge to defecate, and chest tightness. They are usually mild, begin within a minute after the injection of TRH, and last for a few seconds to several minutes. A transient rise in blood pressure has been observed on occasion, but no other changes are seen in vital signs, urine analysis, blood count, or routine blood chemistry tests.[534, 542] The occurrence of circulatory collapse is exceedingly rare.[543]

The test provides a means to distinguish between secondary (pituitary) and tertiary (hypothalamic) hypothyroidism (Fig. 97–7). Although the diagnosis of primary hypothyroidism can be easily confirmed by the presence of elevated basal serum TSH levels, secondary and tertiary hypothyroidism are typically associated with TSH levels that are low or normal. On occasion, the serum TSH concentration may be slightly elevated because of the secretion of biologically less potent molecules, but it remains inappropriately low for the degree of thyroid hormone deficiency. Differentiation between secondary and tertiary hypothyroidism cannot be made with certainty without the TRH test. A TSH response is suggestive of a hypothalamic disorder, and failure to respond is compatible with intrinsic pituitary dysfunction.[544] Furthermore, the typical TSH response curve in hypothalamic hypothyroidism shows a delayed peak with a prolonged elevation in serum TSH before return to the basal value (see Fig. 97–7). The finding of a lack of TSH response in association with normal prolactin stimulation may be due to isolated pituitary TSH deficiency.[545] Caution should be exercised in the interpretation of test results after withdrawal of thyroid hormone replacement or after treatment of thyrotoxicosis because despite a low serum thyroid hormone concentration, TSH may remain low and not respond to TRH for several weeks.[442, 509, 512, 546]

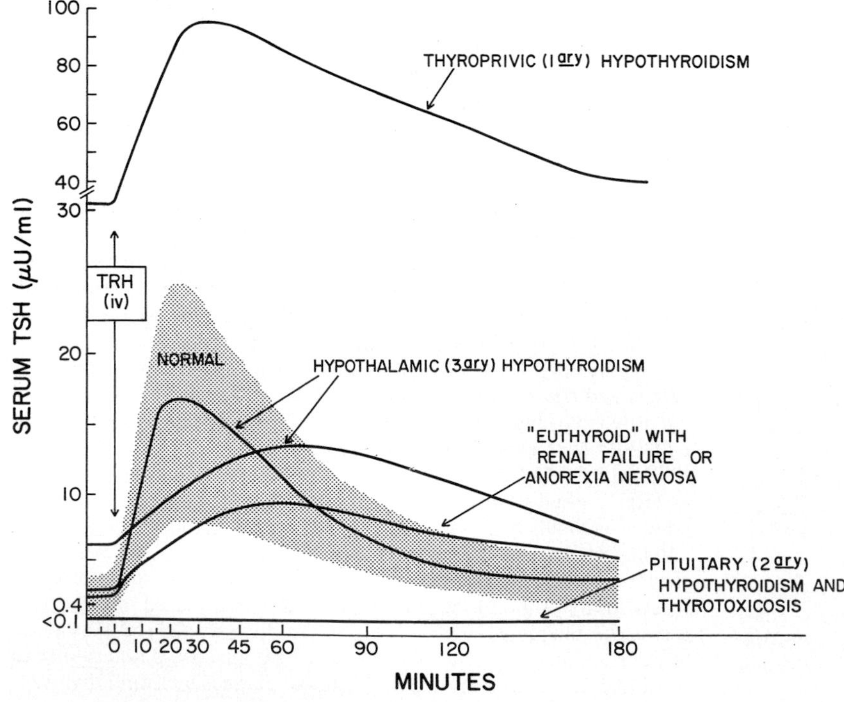

FIGURE 97–7. Typical serum thyroid-stimulating hormone (TSH) responses to the administration of a single intravenous bolus of thyrotropin-releasing hormone at time 0 in various conditions. The normal response is represented by the *shaded area.* Data used for this figure are the average of several studies.

In the most common forms of thyrotoxicosis the mechanism of feedback regulation of TSH secretion is intact but is appropriately suppressed by the excessive amounts of thyroid hormone. Thus both the basal TSH level and its response to TRH are suppressed unless thyrotoxicosis is TSH induced.[442, 445, 455] With the development of more sensitive TSH assays, the TRH test is not generally needed in the evaluation of a thyrotoxic patient with undetectable TSH.[445] The differential diagnosis of conditions leading to inappropriate secretion of TSH may be aided by the TRH test result. Elevated basal TSH values that do not respond to TRH by a further increase are typical of rare TSH-secreting pituitary adenomas.[518] In contrast, patients with inappropriate secretion of TSH resulting from pituitary resistance to thyroid hormone have a normal or exaggerated TSH response to TRH that in most instances is suppressed by supraphysiologic doses of thyroid hormone.[519]

Because of the exquisite sensitivity of the pituitary gland to feedback regulation by thyroid hormone, small changes in the latter profoundly affect the response of TSH to TRH. Thus patients with non–TSH-induced thyrotoxicosis of the mildest degree have a reduced TSH response to TRH, whereas those with primary hypothyroidism exhibit an accentuated response that is prolonged (see Fig. 97–7). These changes may occur in the absence of clinical or other laboratory evidence of thyroid dysfunction.

The TSH response to TRH is subnormal or absent in one-third of apparently euthyroid patients with autoimmune thyroid disease, and even members of their family may not respond to TRH.[547, 548] Most, but not all, patients with a reduced TSH response to TRH will also show thyroid activity that is nonsuppressible by thyroid hormone. A common dissociation between these two tests is typified by a normal TRH response in a nonsuppressible patient. This finding is not surprising because patients with nonsuppressible thyroid glands often have limited capacity to synthesize and secrete thyroid hormone as a result of prior therapy or partial destruction of their glands by the disease process. Clinically, euthyroid patients who do not respond to TRH admittedly have a slight excess of thyroid hormone. It is less easy to reconcile the rare occurrence of TRH unresponsiveness in a patient whose condition is suppressible by exogenous thyroid hormone. It should be remembered, however, that a suppressed pituitary may take a variable amount of time to recover, a phenomenon that may be the basis of such discrepancies.[442, 512, 546] Despite discrepancies between the results of the TRH and T_3 suppression tests,[547, 548] use of the former is much preferred, particularly in elderly patients, in whom administration of T_3 can produce untoward effects.

Other Tests of TSH Reserve

It has been reasoned that by virtue of different mechanisms of action, testing the TSH response by means other than TRH may provide information of diagnostic value not obtainable from stimulation and suppression of the pituitary by TRH and thyroid hormone, respectively.[465] Many trials using various drugs such as metoclopramide, L-dopa, and dexamethasone have been carried out but so far have provided only limited additional information and thus have not found a place in clinical practice. These tests have limited application in the study of patients with inappropriate secretion of TSH, in whom the distinction of autonomous secretion of TSH as compared with selective unresponsiveness to thyroid hormone inhibition is of diagnostic value.[516]

Other tests indirectly measure pituitary TSH reserve during the rebound period after suppression of thyroid hormone synthesis or pituitary TSH secretion. Assessment of thyroid gland activity after withdrawal of antithyroid drugs or T_3 replacement has been proposed.[549, 550]

Thyroid Stimulation Test

The thyroid stimulation test, also known as the TSH stimulation test, measures the ability of thyroid tissue to respond to exogenous TSH by an increase in iodide accumulation and hormone release. Formerly used to differentiate hypothyroidism caused by thyroid gland failure from that caused by TSH deficiency, the test is now almost exclusively done in conjunction with a scintiscan to localize areas of suppressed thyroid tissue. It requires the intramuscular administration of one or three 5- to 10-U doses of bovine TSH. The response is assessed from the change in 24-hour RAIU or the incremental change in serum TT_4 or TT_3 measured before and after the course of TSH treatment.[551, 552] The presence of normal, but nonfunctioning thyroid tissue suppressed by excess hormone from a functioning thyroid nodule, ectopic thyroid tissue, or hormone administration is best demonstrated by scanning after a 3-day course of TSH.

The test may cause discomfort, and some of the reactions to the heterologous TSH may be serious.[552] Repeated administration of bovine TSH can also lead to the production of antibodies that may neutralize its action.[553] Production of neutralizing antibodies is the main reason for not recommending the routine use of exogenous TSH in the search for functioning metastases in patients with thyroid cancer. Whether similar problems will occur with recombinant human TSH remains to be determined.

Thyroid Suppression Test

Maintenance of thyroid gland activity that is independent of TSH can be demonstrated by the thyroid suppression test. Under normal conditions, administration of thyroid hormone in quantities sufficient to satisfy the body requirement suppresses endogenous TSH and results in a reduction in thyroid hormone synthesis and secretion. Because thyrotoxicosis resulting from excessive secretion of hormone by the thyroid gland implies that the feedback control mechanism is not operative or has been perturbed, it is easy to understand why under such circumstances the supply of exogenous hormone would also be ineffective in suppressing thyroid gland activity. The test has very limited applications today, although it may be of value in patients who are euthyroid or only mildly thyrotoxic but suspected of having abnormal thyroid gland stimulation or autonomy, particularly for confirmation of the diagnosis of resistance to thyroid hormone.

Usually the test is carried out with 100 μg of liothyronine given daily in two divided doses over a period of 7 to 10 days. A 24-hour RAIU is determined before and during the last 2 days of T_3 administration.[554] Normal persons show a suppression of RAIU by at least 50% when compared with the pre-liothyronine treatment value. No change or a lesser reduction is typical of not only Graves' disease but also other forms of endogenous thyrotoxicosis, including toxic adenoma, functioning carcinoma, and thyrotoxicosis caused by trophoblastic diseases. The presence of nonsuppressibility indicates thyroid gland activity independent of TSH but not necessarily thyrotoxicosis. Euthyroid patients with autonomous thyroid function have a normal TSH response to TRH before the administration of liothyronine. However, inhibition of TSH secretion by exogenous T_3 does not suppress the autonomous activity of the thyroid gland. This discrepancy is the most commonly encountered difference between the results of the two related tests. When the T_3 suppression test is used in conjunction with a scintiscan, localized areas of autonomous function can be identified. The test can be carried out without the administration of radioisotopes by measuring serum T_4 before and 2 weeks after the ingestion of liothyronine. Although total suppression of T_4 secretion never occurs, even after prolonged treatment with liothyronine, reduction by at least 50% is normal.[555]

Variants of the test have been proposed to reduce the potential risks of liothyronine administration in elderly patients and in those with angina pectoris or congestive heart failure. However, with the availability of sensitive TSH assays, thyroid suppression tests are no longer indicated.

SPECIALIZED THYROID TESTS

A number of specialized tests are available for the evaluation of specific aspects of thyroid hormone biosynthesis, secretion, turnover, distribution, and absorption. Their primary application is investigative. They are only briefly mentioned here for the sake of completeness.

Iodotyrosine Deiodinase Activity

The iodotyrosine deiodinase test involves the intravenous administration of tracer MIT or DIT labeled with radioiodide. Urine collected over a period of 4 hours is analyzed by chromatography or resin column separation. Normally, only 4% to 8% of the radioactivity is excreted as such; the remainder appears in the urine in the form of iodide.[556] Excretion of larger amounts of the parent compound indicates an inability to deiodinate iodotyrosine. The test is useful in the diagnosis of a dehalogenase defect (see Chapter 112).

Test for Defective Hormonogenesis

After the administration of radioiodide, the isotopically labeled compounds synthesized in the thyroid gland and those secreted into the circulation can be analyzed by immunologic, chromatographic, electrophoretic, and density gradient centrifugation techniques.[557] Such tests serve to evaluate the synthesis and release of thyroid hormone, as well as delineate the formation of abnormal iodoproteins.

Iodine Kinetic Studies

The iodine kinetic procedure is used to evaluate overall iodide metabolism and to elucidate the pathophysiology of thyroid diseases. Analysis involves follow-up of the fate of administered radioiodide tracer by measurement of thyroidal accumulation, secretion into blood, and excretion in urine and feces.[558] Double-tracer techniques and programs for computer-assisted analysis of data are available.

Absorption of Thyroid Hormone

Failure to achieve a normal serum thyroid hormone concentration after the administration of replacement doses of thyroid hormone is usually due to poor compliance, occasionally due to the use of inactive preparations, and rarely, if ever, due to malabsorption. The last can be evaluated by simultaneous oral and intravenous administration of the hormone labeled with two different iodine isotope tracers. The ratio of the two isotopes in blood is proportional to the net absorbed fraction of the orally administered hormone.[559, 560] Under normal circumstances, approximately 80% of the T_4 and 95% of the T_3 administered orally are absorbed. Hypothyroidism and a variety of other unrelated conditions have little effect on the intestinal absorption of thyroid hormones. Absorption may be diminished in patients with steatorrhea, in some cases of hepatic failure, during treatment with cholestyramine, and with diets rich in soybeans. Absorption of thyroid hormone can also be evaluated by the administration of a single oral dose of 100 μg of liothyronine or 1 mg of levothyroxine, followed by their measurement in blood sampled at various intervals.[561, 562]

Turnover Kinetics of T_4 and T_3

Turnover kinetic studies require the intravenous administration of isotope-labeled tracer levothyroxine or liothyronine.[563–566] The half-time of disappearance of the hormone is calculated from the rate of decrease in serum trichloroacetic acid–precipitable, ethanol-extractable, or antibody-precipitable isotope counts. Compartmental analysis can be used for calculation of the turnover parameters.[563, 564] The calculated daily degradation or production rate (PR) is the product of the fractional turnover rate (K), the extrathyroidal distribution space (DS), and the average concentration of the hormone in serum. Noncompartmental analysis may be used for the calculation of kinetic parameters.[563] The metabolic clearance rate (MCR) is defined as the dose of the injected labeled tracer divided by the area under its curve of disappearance. The PR is then calculated from the product of the MCR and the average concentration of the respective nonradioactive iodothyronine measured in serum over the period of the study. Simultaneous studies of T_4 and T_3 turnover kinetics can be carried out by injection of both hormones labeled with different iodine isotopes.[563, 565, 566]

Average normal values in adults for T_4 and T_3, respectively, are as follows: $t_{1/2}$ = 7.0 and 0.8 days; K = 10% and 90% per day; DS = 11 and 30 L of serum equivalent; MCR = 1.1 and 25 L/day; and PR = 90 and 25 mg/day.

The hormonal PR is accelerated in thyrotoxicosis and diminished in hypothyroidism. In euthyroid patients with TBG abnormalities, the PR remains normal because changes in serum hormone concentration are accompanied by compensatory changes in the fractional turnover rate and the extrathyroidal hormonal pool.[567] A variety of nonthyroidal illnesses may alter hormone kinetics[566, 568] (see Chapter 106).

Metabolic Kinetics of Thyroid Hormones and Their Metabolites

The kinetics of the production of various metabolites of T_4 and T_3 in peripheral tissues and their further metabolism can be studied. Most methods use radiolabeled iodothyronine tracers injected intravenously.[564–566] Their disappearance is monitored in serum samples obtained at various intervals after injection of the tracers by means of chromatographic and immunologic techniques of separation. Kinetic parameters can be calculated by noncompartmental analysis or by two- or multiple-compartment analysis. Estimates have been made by the differential measurement in urine of the isotopes derived from the precursor and its metabolite. They are in agreement with measurements carried out in serum.[569] Conversion rates of iodothyronines, principally generated in peripheral tissues, can be calculated from the ratio of their PR and that of their respective precursors. Some iodothyronines such as T_3 are secreted by the thyroid gland as well as generated in peripheral tissues. Studies to calculate the conversion rate require the administration of thyroid hormone to block thyroidal secretion.[568]

On average, 35% and 45% of T_4 are converted to T_3 and rT_3, respectively, in peripheral tissues. The conversion of T_4 to T_3 is greatly diminished in a variety of illnesses (see Chapter 106) of nonthyroidal origin and in response to many drugs (see Table 97–6). Degradation and monodeiodination of iodothyronines can be estimated without the administration of isotopes. They are, however, less accurate. The conversion of T_4 to T_3 can be estimated semiquantitatively by the measurement of serum TT_3 after treatment with replacement doses of levothyroxine.[568]

Measurement of the Production Rate and Metabolic Kinetics of Other Compounds

The metabolism and PRs of a variety of compounds related to thyroid physiology can be studied by using their radiolabeled congeners and application of the general principles of turnover kinetics. Studies of TSH have demonstrated changes not only related to thyroid dysfunction but also associated with age and kidney and liver disease.[570, 571] Studies of the turnover kinetics of TBG have shown that the slight increases and decreases in serum TBG associated with hypothyroidism and thyrotoxicosis, respectively, are due to changes in the degradation rate of TBG rather than synthesis.[567]

Transfer of Thyroid Hormone from Blood to Tissues

Transfer of hormone from blood to tissues can be estimated in vivo by two techniques. A direct method monitors accumulation of the administered labeled hormone tracer by surface counting over the organ of interest.[572] An indirect method monitors the early disappearance from plasma of the simultaneously administered hormone and albumin, labeled with different radioisotope tracers.[573] The difference between the rates of disappearance of hormone and albumin represents the fraction of hormone that has left the vascular (albumin) space and presumably has entered tissues.

EFFECTS OF DRUGS ON THYROID FUNCTION

Many drugs can interfere with biochemical tests of thyroid function by interfering with the synthesis, transport, and metabolism of thyroid hormones or by altering the synthesis and secretion of thyrotropin (TSH). Only rarely, however, do these effects cause overt, clinically apparent thyroid disease. This section is not intended to provide exhaustive information on all drugs that can affect tests of thyroid function. Instead, the more commonly encountered agents, those with broad clinical applications, and those helpful in understanding the mechanisms of drug interactions are described.

Mechanisms of Action

All levels of thyroid hormone regulation are affected by drugs, from hormone synthesis and transport to metabolism and excretion. Some drugs and hormones, such as estrogens and androgens, affect thyroid hormone transport in blood by altering the concentration of binding proteins in serum (see Chapter 94). Thyroid hormone transport may also be affected by substances that compete with the binding of thyroid hormone to its carrier proteins (see Table 97–4).

Some of the agents that may alter the extrathyroidal metabolism of thyroid hormone are listed in Table 97–6. Several drugs widely used in clinical practice (e.g., glucocorticoids, amiodarone, and propranolol) inhibit the conversion of T_4 to T_3 in peripheral tissues. As expected, their most profound effect on thyroid function is a decrease in the serum concentration of T_3, usually with a concomitant increase in the rT_3 level.[82, 142, 146, 147] An increase in the serum T_4 concentration has also been observed on occasion.[143, 146, 147] When intrapituitary T_4-to-T_3 conversion is inhibited, the serum TSH concentration may also rise.[146] In the absence of inherent abnormalities in thyroid hormone synthesis or in its secretion, TSH levels should return to normal and hypothyroidism should not ensue from the chronic administration of compounds that only partially interfere with T_4 monodeiodination. Other mechanisms by which some compounds affect the extrathyroidal metabolism of thyroid hormone are acceleration of the overall rates of the deiodinative and nondeiodinative routes of hormone disposal. An example of a drug acting principally through the former mechanism is phenobarbital,[86] and by way of the latter, diphenylhydantoin.[151] In such circumstances, thyroid hormone concentrations should remain unaltered. Furthermore, it has been anticipated, as well as observed, that hypothyroid patients receiving such drugs require higher doses of exogenous hormone to maintain a eumetabolic state. Some drugs have multiple effects.

A large array of drugs act on the hypothalamic-pituitary axis (see Table 97–10), although only a few have a significant effect on thyroid function by way of this central mechanism. Furthermore, people undergoing drug treatment who have no thyroid disease seldom show important changes in the basal serum TSH concentration.

The most potent suppressors of pituitary TSH secretion are thyroid hormone and its analogues. They act on the pituitary by blocking TSH secretion through mechanisms discussed in Chapter 96. Some of the TSH-inhibiting agents listed in Table 97–10—fenclofenac and salicylates—may act by increasing the free thyroid hormone level by interference with its binding to serum proteins. Other agents appear to have a direct inhibitory effect on the pituitary and, possibly, the hypothalamus. The most notable is dopamine and its agonists. They have been shown to suppress basal TSH levels in the euthyroid state[261, 482] and in patients with primary hypothyroidism.[261, 482–485] They also suppress the TSH response to TRH.[261] As expected, dopamine antagonists amplify TSH secretion.[468–473, 574] A notable exception to this rule, which casts some doubt on the assumed mechanism of action of dopamine antagonists, is pimozide. This neuroleptic dopamine blocker has been shown to reduce elevated serum TSH levels in patients with primary hypothyroidism.[488]

Iodide and some iodine-containing organic compounds cause a rapid increase in the basal and TRH-stimulated levels of serum TSH. This effect is undoubtedly caused by a decrease in the serum thyroid hormone concentration either by inhibition of hormone synthesis and secretion by the thyroid gland[465] or by a selective decrease in the intrapituitary concentration of T_3 as with iopanoic acid and amiodarone.[466] Indeed, a predominant block on the intrapituitary conversion of T_4 to T_3 has been demonstrated.[503] It should be noted that iodide and iodine-containing compounds do not stimulate TSH secretion in patients in whom they induce excessive secretion of thyroid hormone.[575, 576] A decrease in the free thyroid hormone concentration in serum, albeit minimal in magnitude, may also be responsible for the increase in TSH levels observed during treatment with clomiphene.[475] An increase in serum TSH concentration during lithium therapy is also believed to be caused by reduced thyroid hormone levels rather than by a direct effect of this ion on the pituitary.[467]

It has been postulated that some agents may act by modifying the effect of TSH on its target tissue. For example, theophylline may potentiate the action of TSH through its inhibitory effect on phosphodiesterase, which may lead to an increase in the intracellular concentration of cAMP.[577] A handful of drugs appear to act by blocking some of the peripheral tissue effects of thyroid hormone. Others appear to mimic one or several manifestations of thyroid hormone effects on tissues. Guanethidine, which releases catecholamines from tissues, has a beneficial effect in thyrotoxicosis by decreasing the BMR, pulse rate, and tremulousness.[578, 579] This agent probably has no direct effect on the thyroid gland but may depress those manifestations of thyrotoxicosis that are mediated by sympathetic pathways. Among the multiple effects of the β-adrenergic blocker propranolol on thyroid hormone economy is a reduction in peripheral tissue responses to thyroid hormone.

Specific Agents

Estrogens

Hyperestrogenism caused by pregnancy, hydatidiform moles, tumors, or treatment with estrogens is the most common cause of increased TBG, the major carrier of thyroid hormone in serum.[107, 109] Estrogens produce a dose-dependent increase in the complexity of oligosaccharide side chains that proportionately increases the number of sialic acids in the TBG molecule, which in turn prolongs its survival in serum.[580] The concentrations of other serum proteins, ceruloplasmin, transferrin, and several that bind hormones (cortisol-binding globulin and testosterone-binding globulin) are also increased.[581] Tamoxifen blocks the estrogen-induced increase in TBG, whereas tamoxifen alone in postmenopausal women increases serum TBG, T_4, and T_3 levels.[582, 583]

The consequences of increased TBG concentration in serum are higher serum levels of both T_4 and T_3 and, to a lesser extent, other metabolites of T_4 deiodination. The fractional turnover rate of T_4 is reduced principally because of an increase in the intravascular T_4 pool. On the other hand, the FT_4 and FT_3 concentrations and the absolute amount of hormone degraded each day remain normal.[567, 585]

Androgens

Androgens decrease the concentration of TBG in serum and thereby reduce levels of T_4 and T_3.[111, 112] As with estrogens, the concentration of free hormone remains unaffected, and the degradation rate of T_4 is normal at the expense of an accelerated turnover rate.[111] TSH levels are normal.[585] Anabolic steroids with weaker androgenic action have the same effect, although similar changes observed during danazol therapy have been attributed to its androgen-like properties.[586]

Salicylates

Salicylate and its noncalorigenic congeners compete for thyroid hormone–binding sites on TTR and TBG in serum and thereby cause a decline in T_4 and T_3 concentrations and an increase in their free fractions.[116, 117] The turnover rate of T_4 is accelerated, but degradation rates remain normal.[587, 588] Furthermore, they suppress thyroidal RAIU but do not retard iodine release from the thyroid gland.[589] Thus the hypermetabolic effect of this drug was attributed to the increase in FT_4 and FT_3 fractions.[497] If this proposed explanation were correct, however, hormonal release from the serum hormone-binding proteins should produce only a temporary suppression of thyroidal RAIU and transient hypermetabolism. In fact, both effects have been observed during chronic administration of salicylates.[587, 588] In addition, this mechanism of action does not explain the lack of calorigenic effect of some salicylate congeners despite their ability to also displace thyroid hormone from its serum hormone-binding proteins. In vitro studies have also demonstrated an inhibitory effect of salicylate on the outer-ring monodeiodination of both T_4 and rT_3,[590] but lack of typical changes in the relative levels of serum iodothyronine suggests that this action is less important in vivo. Similar abnormalities in thyroid function tests have been noted in patients treated with salsalate.[54]

Acetylsalicylic acid mimics the action of thyroid hormone in several ways. For example, it lowers the serum cholesterol level,[591] but it does not provide a therapeutic effect in myxedema or lower TSH levels.[592] Administration of 8 g aspirin daily raises the BMR and accelerates the circulation, which suggests that the changes in blood flow in thyrotoxicosis and myxedema are secondary to heat production rather than to primary effects of the hormone on the circulation.

p-Aminosalicylic acid and *p*-aminobenzoic acid are closely related chemically to salicylate. They inhibit iodide binding in the thyroid gland and are goitrogenic.[593, 594]

Glucocorticoids

Physiologic amounts of glucocorticoids, as well as pharmacologic doses, influence thyroid function. The effects are variable and multiple, depending on the dose and the endocrine status of the person. The type of glucocorticoid and the route of administration may also influence the magnitude of the effect.[595] Known effects include a decrease in the serum concentration of TBG and an increase in that of TTR,[114] inhibition of the outer-ring deiodination of T_4 and probably rT_3,[85, 141] suppression of TSH secretion,[595] a possible decrease in hepatic binding of T_4, and an increase in the renal clearance of iodide.[596]

The decrease in serum concentration of TBG caused by the administration of pharmacologic doses of glucocorticoids results in a decrease in the serum TT_4 concentration and an increase in its free fraction. The absolute concentration of FT_4 and the FT_4I remain normal.

A more profound decrease is noted in the concentration of serum T_3 as opposed to T_4 in association with pharmacologic doses of glucocorticoids, and this difference cannot be ascribed to the reduced serum TBG level. It is caused by decreased conversion of T_4 to T_3 in peripheral tissues. A reduced T_3/T_4 ratio also occurs in hypothyroid patients receiving replacement doses of T_4. It is accompanied by an increase in the serum level of rT_3.[85] This effect of the steroid is rapid and may be seen within 24 hours.[85, 141]

Earlier observations of cortisone-induced depression of uptake and clearance of iodide by the thyroid gland[596] can now be attributed to the effect of this steroid on TSH secretion. Pharmacologic doses of glucocorticoids suppress the basal TSH level in euthyroid subjects and in patients with primary hypothyroidism and decrease their TSH response to TRH.[495, 496] Normal adrenocortical secretion appears to have a suppressive influence on pituitary TSH secretion inasmuch as patients with primary adrenal insufficiency have a significant elevation in serum TSH concentrations.[522] Administration of moderate doses of hydrocortisone reduces the basal release of TSH and the T_3 and TSH response to TRH.[597]

No single change in thyroid function can be ascribed to a specific mode of action of glucocorticoids. For example, diminished thyroidal RAIU may be caused by the combined effects of TSH suppression and increased renal clearance of iodide. Similarly, a low serum TT_4 level is the result of suppressed thyroidal secretion caused by diminished TSH stimulation, as well as the decreased serum level of TBG. One of the common problems in clinical practice is to separate the effect of glucocorticoid action on pituitary function from that of other agents and those caused by acute and chronic illness. This situation arises often because steroids are commonly used in various autoimmune and allergic disorders, as well as in the treatment of septic shock. The diagnosis of coexisting true hypothyroidism is difficult. Because of the suppressive effects of glucocorticoids on the hypothalamic-pituitary axis, the low levels of serum T_4 and T_3 may not be accompanied by an increase in the serum TSH level, which would otherwise be diagnostic of primary hypothyroidism. In such circumstances a depressed rather than an elevated serum rT_3 level may be helpful in the detection of coexistent primary thyroid failure.

Pharmacologic doses of glucocorticoids induce a prompt decline in serum T_4 and T_3 concentrations in thyrotoxic patients with autoimmune thyroid disease.[85] Amelioration of the symptoms and signs in such patients may also be accompanied by a decrease in the elevated thyroidal RAIU and a diminution in TSH receptor antibody titer.[598] This effect of glucocorticoids may be caused in part by its immunosuppressive action because it has been shown that administration of dexamethasone to hypothyroid patients with Hashimoto's thyroiditis causes an increase in the serum concentration of both T_4 and T_3.[599]

Diphenylhydantoin

Diphenylhydantoin competes with thyroid hormone binding to TBG.[117, 120] This effect of diphenylhydantoin and diazepam, a related compound, has been exploited to study the conformational requirements for the interaction of thyroid hormone with its serum carrier protein.[119, 120] Although the affinity of diphenylhydantoin for TBG is far below that of T_4, when used in therapeutic doses the serum concentration achieved is high enough to cause significant occupancy of the hormone-binding sites on TBG. This effect of diphenylhydantoin is only partly responsible for the decrease in TT_4 and TT_3 concentrations in serum.

Diphenylhydantoin reduces the intestinal absorption of T_4 and increases its nondeiodinative metabolism.[151] At the usual therapeutic concentrations this effect of the drug is probably more important than competition with T_4 for binding to TBG and is, by and large, responsible for the reduced concentration of T_4 in serum. Despite these observations, basal and TRH-stimulated TSH levels are within the normal range[600] or only slightly elevated.[151, 152] This finding is partly the result of the increased generation of T_3 from T_4.[150, 151]

Both diphenylhydantoin and diazepam are commonly used in clinical practice, the former as an anticonvulsant and antiarrhythmic agent and the latter as an anxiolytic. Reduced serum levels of thyroid hormone in patients with therapeutic blood levels of diphenylhydantoin should not be viewed as indicative of thyroid dysfunction unless the TSH level is elevated. Treatment with T_4 in such patients does not alter parameters of cardiac function or symptoms that might be caused by hypothyroidism.[601] Diphenylhydantoin may slightly increase the dose required for thyroid hormone replacement in athyrotic subjects.[602]

Lithium

Lithium is a commonly prescribed drug in bipolar affective disorders. It has long been known to cause significant abnormalities in thyroid status[603, 604]; hence thyroid function tests should be performed at 6-month intervals during lithium therapy. Overt hypothyroidism develops in up to 15% of patients,[604–606] and as many as one-third have evidence of subclinical hypothyroidism (elevated serum TSH with a normal free T_4 concentration).

Lithium-induced hypothyroidism that is clinically overt is frequently associated with the presence of autoimmune thyroiditis and high titers of thyroid autoantibodies in 24% of cases.[467] These findings often predate commencement of lithium therapy[607] and occur more frequently in females.[608]

Possible mechanisms of lithium-induced thyroid dysfunction include direct inhibitory actions on thyroid function, including a reduction in iodine-concentrating capacity and inhibition of iodotyrosine and iodothyronine biosynthesis.[609–611] Lithium may also inhibit the secretion of thyroid hormones by stabilizing the follicular cell microtubule system.[612] In vitro studies have suggested that lithium inhibits the peripheral conversion of T_4 to T_3,[613] although this action has not been confirmed in vivo.[614] Despite the predilection of lithium-induced hypothyroidism in females[608] and the high prevalence of thyroid autoantibodies,[467] few data support a primary immunogenic role for lithium. It has been postulated that lithium alters the tertiary structure of macromolecules in thyroid membrane receptors or other membrane proteins, thus making these proteins more immunogenic,[615] although this activity is purely speculative. A central (pituitary or hypothalamic) mechanism of action of lithium has been proposed on the basis of its dopaminergic activity in the central nervous system.[607, 616–618] Although dopamine inhibits TSH secretion,[468] serum prolactin levels are normal in patients treated with lithium,[467] which argues against a central mode of action.

Phenobarbital

Chronic administration of phenobarbital to animals induces increased binding of thyroid hormone to liver microsomes and enhanced deiodinating activity.[619] Phenobarbital administration reduces the biologic effectiveness of the hormone by diverting it to microsomal degradative pathways. In humans, phenobarbital augments fecal T_4 clearance by nearly 100%,[86] but serum T_4 levels and the FT_4I remain near normal because of compensatory increases in T_4 secretion. Barbiturates therefore appear to have no important effect on thyroid-mediated metabolic action in normal humans. The augmented hepatic removal of T_4 induced by phenobarbital increases T_4 clearance and lowers T_4 levels and the FT_4I in patients with Graves' disease but has no effect on the clinical response.[86]

Propranolol

Propranolol, a β-adrenergic blocker, is often used as an adjunct in the treatment of thyrotoxicosis. It is also used, in its own right, in the treatment of cardiac arrhythmias and hypertension. Propranolol does not affect the secretion or overall turnover rate of T_4 or TSH release or its regulatory mechanisms.[86] A small to moderate lowering effect on serum T_4 has been reported in euthyroid subjects, as well as in patients with hyperthyroidism or in those with myxedema receiving liothyronine replacement therapy.[142, 143] Such data, combined with the findings of reciprocal increases in rT_3 and minimal increases in serum T_4 levels, suggest a mild blocking effect of this drug on the 5′-deiodination of iodothyronines in peripheral tissue.[143] This effect does not appear to be related to the β-adrenergic blocking action of propranolol because other β-blocking agents do not share the deiodinase-blocking property.[620, 621]

Clearly, amelioration of the clinical manifestations of thyrotoxicosis is related to the β-adrenergic blocking action of propranolol rather than its effect on thyronine metabolism. Whether it in fact alters the hypermetabolism of thyrotoxicosis is debatable.

Nitrophenols

2,4-Dinitrophenol elevates the BMR, lowers the serum T_4 concentration, accelerates the peripheral metabolism of T_4, and depresses thyroidal RAIU and secretion.[622, 623] Its actions are probably complex. Like T_4, the drug stimulates metabolism by uncoupling oxidative phosphorylation in the mitochondria.[624] Part of the effect of dinitrophenol may be to mimic the action of thyroid hormone on hypothalamic or pituitary receptor control centers; this effect would account for the diminished thyroid activity. Dinitrophenol also displaces thyroid hormone from T_4-binding serum proteins; this action could lower the total hormone concentration in serum but should have no persistent effect on thyroid function. Dinitrophenol increases biliary and fecal excretion of T_4, and this action largely accounts for the rapid removal of hormone from the circulation.[625] Deiodination of T_4 is also increased. 2,4-Dinitrophenol does not share some of the most important properties of T_4. It cannot initiate metamorphosis in tadpoles[626] or provide substitution therapy in myxedema.

Dopaminergic Agents

It is now reasonably well established that endogenous brain dopamine plays a physiologic role in the regulation of TSH secretion through its effect on the hypothalamic-pituitary axis.[468, 627] Dopamine exerts a suppressive effect on TSH secretion and can be regarded as antagonistic to the stimulatory action of TRH at the pituitary level. Much of the information regarding the role of dopamine in the control of TSH secretion in humans has been derived from observations made during the administration of agents with dopamine agonistic and antagonistic activity (see Table 97–10).

Dopamine infusion is commonly used in acutely ill hypotensive patients. It lowers the basal serum TSH level in both euthyroid and hypothyroid patients and blunts its response to the administration of TRH.[468, 482, 628] Levodopa, the precursor of dopamine used in the treatment of Parkinson's disease and as a test agent in the diagnosis of pituitary diseases, also suppresses the basal and TRH-stimulated serum TSH level in euthyroid subjects, as well as in patients with primary hypothyroidism.[261] A similar effect has been observed during the administration of bromocriptine, a dopamine agonist used to treat some pituitary tumors and to suppress lactation during the puerperal period. Although the agent has been shown to diminish high serum TSH levels in patients with primary hypothyroidism,[483] chronic administration does not produce a significant inhibitory effect on TRH-induced TSH secretion.[629] Metoclopramide, a dopamine antagonist used as a diagnostic agent and in the treatment of motility disorders, increases TSH secretion.[630]

Although some authors have cautioned that prolonged infusion of dopamine may induce secondary hypothyroidism and thus worsen the prognosis of severely ill patients,[631] no evidence suggests that chronic treatment with dopaminergic drugs induces hypothyroidism in less critically ill patients. These drugs have been used in the treatment of pituitary-induced thyrotoxicosis.[632] When measurements of basal or stimulated serum TSH levels are used in the differential diagnosis of primary and secondary hypothyroidism, the concomitant use of drugs with dopamine agonistic or antagonistic activity should be taken into account in the interpretation of results.

Iodide and Iodine-Containing Compounds

Iodine has complex effects on the thyroid gland and is recognized as causing both hypothyroidism and hyperthyroidism or inducing goiter formation. The effect of iodine on thyroid function is dependent on a number of variables: the total dose, the rate of administration, previous iodine status, and the presence or absence of underlying thyroid dysfunction.

Uptake and organification of iodine are inhibited in the presence of iodine excess (the Wolff-Chaikoff effect). Under these circumstances the stimulatory effect of TSH, via adenyl cyclase, is also reduced. Excess iodine may also inhibit proteolytic enzymes responsible for cleaving T_3 and T_4 before release.[633] It has been recognized that iodine may also reduce the peripheral conversion of T_4 to T_3 by inhibition of 5′-monodeiodinase.[634] The net effect of excess iodine in some euthyroid individuals is to cause hypothyroidism.

Some of the effects of iodine may have an immune basis. Correction of iodine deficiency in depleted areas results in an increased incidence of autoimmune thyroid disease.[635] One of the proposed mechanisms to explain this phenomenon involves increased iodination of Tg, which results in increased immunogenicity and subsequently leads to autoantibody formation. Indirect evidence for a primary immunogenic role has also been achieved through in vitro studies. Such experiments, which used cultured lymphocytes grown in the presence of iodine, revealed increased quantities of IgG production.[636] Patients with high titers of thyroid autoantibodies are also more likely to acquire hypothyroidism after iodine administration.[637]

Induction of hyperthyroidism by iodine is almost exclusively limited to patients who have underlying thyroid disease,[638] which is often secondary to iodine deficiency in the first place. Administration of iodine to iodine-deficient subjects with nodular goiters can induce the autonomous secretion of excess thyroid hormone.[638] Hyperthyroidism induced via these means is known as the Jod-Basedow phenomenon. Iodine-induced hyperthyroidism may also be seen in the absence of nodular goiter, especially in patients with autoantibodies to thyroid antigens.

Iodine can have profound and variable effects on thyroid function, although rarely in iodine-replete areas do these effects become clinically relevant. Only some drugs containing very large doses of iodine can cause abnormalities in thyroid function in normal, healthy individuals. These drugs are discussed below.

IODINATED CONTRAST AGENTS. Some radiographic contrast media contain large doses of iodine[639, 640]; for example, a 3-g dose of ipodate (used in oral cholecystography) contains 1.8 g of iodine. The principal effect of this agent is to inhibit deiodination of T_4 to T_3 in peripheral tissues[641] and in the pituitary,[642] which results in a profound decrease in the serum T_3 concentration and an increase in rT_3 and T_4 levels[144, 145, 643, 644] in association with a rise in serum TSH.[643] The serum T_4 concentration may reach values well within the thyrotoxic range.[144] These changes are maximal 3 to 4 days after administration[644] and disappear within 14 days.

Iodocontrast agents also decrease the hepatic uptake of T_4[645] and inhibit T_3 binding to its nuclear receptors.[646] The antithyroidal effect of the iodine released from these agents is believed to be responsible for the falling T_4 level and amelioration of the symptoms and signs of thyrotoxicosis when they are administered to patients with Graves' thyrotoxicosis.[145]

AMIODARONE. Amiodarone is a very potent and effective antiarrhythmic agent derived from benzofuran that contains large quantities of iodine (37% by weight). It bears some structural homology with thyroid hormones, and among its array of potential side effects,[647] abnormalities in thyroid function tests are common during its administration.[148] These abnormalities are similar to those seen with iodine-containing contrast agents and include a marked decrease in serum T_3, an increase in rT_3, and a more modest elevation in the T_4 concentration.[145, 147] Basal and TRH-stimulated TSH levels are increased. All these changes can occur as early as 1 week after institution of amiodarone therapy.[648] The principal mechanism of action is believed to be inhibition of T_3 generation from T_4 in peripheral tissues and in the pituitary gland.[649, 650] Amiodarone also directly stimulates TSH secretion from cultured thyrotrophs.[148] Metabolic studies in humans have also shown clearance rates of T_4 and rT_3 to be reduced with a concomitant reduction in the rate of production of T_3.

Despite changes in thyroid function, clinically relevant thyroid dysfunction develops in only a minority of patients taking amiodarone. Hypothyroidism is reported to be more common in iodine-replete areas, whereas hyperthyroidism has a higher prevalence in iodine-deficient areas.[651] The iodine dependence of both these diseases is confirmed by the improvement in both with the use of perchlorate to discharge iodine from the thyroid gland. A second form of thyrotoxicosis that is a destructive thyroiditis does not respond to antithyroid drugs or perchlorate but is responsive to steroid therapy.[652] The development of overt thyroid disease is also more common in subjects with a past history of thyroid disease and in those with goiter or evidence of autoimmune-related thyroid disease. Because most patients taking amiodarone have abnormalities in thyroid function tests, clinical assessment of the patient is extremely important in the diagnosis of overt thyroid disease. Clinical assessment is, however, complicated by the α-adrenergic receptor and β-adrenergic receptor blocking properties of the drug, which mask some of the symptoms and signs of hyperthyroidism.[653] The clinical picture may therefore not be typical, and symptoms of tiredness and weight loss often predominate. Despite a paucity of symptoms, a number of serious and occasionally fatal cases of amiodarone-induced thyrotoxicosis have been reported.[654, 655] Drug-induced thyroiditis may also cause thyrotoxicosis, which is often followed by transient hypothyroidism.[656]

Amiodarone metabolites compete with thyroid hormone for its receptor, but it is uncertain to what extent this action is of physiologic relevance at the concentrations achieved at the level of tissues. The bradycardia that almost invariably occurs when the drug is used in high doses may suggest the presence of hypothyroidism.[147] Measurement of serum TSH, the most useful test in the differential diagnosis of this condition, may also give misleading results, however. If hypothyroidism is suspected, measurement of the serum rT_3 concentration could be helpful. Failure to show high serum levels of this iodothyronine in a patient receiving amiodarone can be considered indicative of hypothyroidism, and a low serum TSH value with a normal serum T_3 concentration may possibly be considered thyrotoxicosis. Overt hyperthyroidism should not be diagnosed on the basis of an elevated T_4 level alone, and similarly, a modestly elevated TSH with a low T_3 concentration is not necessarily indicative of hypothyroidism.

TABLE 97–12. Agents That Inhibit Thyroid Hormone Synthesis and Secretion

Substance	Common Use
Block iodide transport into the thyroid gland	
Monovalent anions (SCN^-, ClO_4^-, NO_3^-)	Not in current use; ClO_4 test agent
Complex anions (monofluorosulfonate, difluorophosphate, fluoroborate)	—
Minerals	In diet
Lithium	Treatment of manic-depressive psychosis
Ethionamide	Antituberculosis drug
Impair Tg iodination and iodotyrosine coupling	
Thionamides and thiourylenes (PTU, methimazole, carbimazole)	Antithyroid drugs
Sulfonamides (acetazolamide, sulfadiazine, sulfisoxazole)	Diuretic, bacteriostatic
Sulfonylureas (carbutamide, tolbutamide, metahexamide, ? chlorpropamide)	Hypoglycemic agents
Salicylamides (aminosalicylic acid)	Antituberculosis drugs
Ethionamide (*p*-aminobenzoic acid)	
Resorcinol	Cutaneous antiseptic
Amphenone and aminoglutethimide	Antiadrenal and anticonvulsive agents
Thiocyanate	No current use; in diet
Antipyrine (phenazone)	Antiasthmatic
Aminotriazole	Cranberry poison
Amphenidone	Tranquilizer
2,3-Dimercaptopropanol (BAL)	Chelating agent
Ketoconazole	Antifungal agent
Inhibitors of thyroid hormone secretion	
Iodide (in large doses)	Antiseptic, expectorant, and others
Lithium	
Mechanism unknown	
p-Bromdylamine maleate	Antihistaminic
Phenylbutazone	Anti-inflammatory agent
Minerals (calcium, rubidium, cobalt)	—
Interleukin-2	Chemotherapeutic agent
γ-Interferon	Antiviral and chemotherapeutic agent

BAL, bronchoalveolar lavage; PTU propylthiouracil; Tg, thyroglobulin.

Interferon and Interleukin

These cytokines have been associated with the development of both hypothyroidism and thyrotoxicosis.[656–662] They are used in the treatment of infectious diseases such as hepatitis, as well as in malignancies, including melanoma and renal cell carcinoma. Acute administration has been used as a model of illness because the effects are similar; interferon-α leads to a decrease in T_3, an increase in rT_3, and a fall in TSH.[662]

Cytokine-induced thyroid disease appears to be immune mediated. The incidence is much greater in females and in patients with positive antiperoxidase and anti-TPO antibodies before the initiation of therapy.[657–659] During therapy, patients who were antibody positive may have a rise in titer, whereas antibody positivity may develop in previously negative patients.[657] In patients treated with interferon, the incidence of thyroid disease is much higher in those with hepatitis C than those with hepatitis B.[657] The thyrotoxicosis often occurs as a manifestation of a destructive thyroiditis.[658, 659] In many patients the thyroid disease resolves within several months after stopping cytokine therapy.[658, 660]

Antithyroid Drugs

Agents that act principally by inhibiting thyroid hormone synthesis are collectively called *goitrogens* or *antithyroid drugs*. A number of these compounds occur naturally in foodstuffs. Others are used in the treatment of thyrotoxicosis. A list of substances that inhibit thyroid hormone synthesis and secretion is provided in Table 97–12.

REFERENCES

1. Brown-Grant K: Extrathyroidal iodide concentrating mechanisms. Physiol Rev 41:189–211, 1961.
2. Modan B, Mart H, Baidatz D: Radiation-induced head and neck tumors. Lancet 1:277–299, 1974.
3. Hall P, Boice JD, Berg G, et al: Leukaemia incidence after iodine-131 exposure. Lancet 340:1–4, 1992.
4. Quimby EH, Feitelberg S, Gross W: Radioactive Nuclides in Medicine and Biology, ed 3. Philadelphia, Lea & Febiger, 1970.
5. MIRD: Dose estimate report no. 5: Summary of current radiation dose estimates to humans from ^{123}I, ^{124}I, ^{126}I, ^{130}I, ^{131}I, and ^{132}I as sodium iodide. J Nucl Med 16:857–860, 1975.
6. MIRD: Dose estimate report no. 8: Summary of current radiation dose estimates to normal humans from ^{99m}Tc as sodium pertechnetate. J Nucl Med 17:74–77, 1976.
7. Pittman JA Jr, Dailey GE III, Beschi RJ: Changing normal values for thyroidal radioiodine uptake. N Engl J Med 280:1431–1434, 1969.
8. Gluck FB, Nusynowitz ML, Plymate S: Chronic lymphocytic thyroiditis, thyrotoxicosis, and low radioactive iodine uptake: Report of four cases. N Engl J Med 293:624–628, 1975.
9. Savoie JC, Massin JP, Thomopoulos P, et al: Iodine-induced thyrotoxicosis in apparently normal thyroid glands. J Clin Endocrinol Metab 41:685–691, 1975.
10. Higgins HP, Ball D, Estham S: 20-min ^{99m}Tc thyroid uptake: A simplified method using the gamma camera. J Nucl Med 14:907–911, 1973.
11. Dai G, Levy O, Carrasco N: Cloning and characterisation of the thyroid iodide transporter. Nature 379:458–460, 1996.
12. Baschieri L, Benedetti G, deLuca F, et al: Evaluation and limitations of the perchlorate test in the study of thyroid function. J Clin Endocrinol Metab 23:786–791, 1963.
13. Bikker H, Vulsma T, Bass F, et al: Identification of 5 novel inactivating mutations in the human thyroid peroxidase gene by denaturing gradient gel electrophoresis. Human Genet 6:9–12, 1995.
14. Scott DA, Wang R, Kreman TM, et al: The Pendred syndrome (PDS) gene encodes a chloride, iodide transport protein. Nat Genet 21:440–443, 1999.
15. Chopra IJ, Fisher DA, Solomon DH, et al: Thyroxine and triiodothyronine in the human thyroid. J Clin Endocrinol Metab 36:311–316, 1973.
16. Engler D, Burger AG: The deiodination of iodothyronines and of their derivatives in man. Endocr Rev 5:151–184, 1984.
17. Pittman CS, Shimizu T, Burger A, et al: The nondeiodinative pathways of thyroxine metabolism: 3,5,3′,5′-tetraiodothyroacetic acid turnover in normal and fasting human subjects. J Clin Endocrinol Metab 50:712–716, 1980.
18. Gavin LA, Livermore BM, Cavalieri RR, et al: Serum concentration, metabolic clearance, and production rates of 3,5,3′-triiodothyroacetic acid in normal and athyreotic man. J Clin Endocrinol Metab 51:529–534, 1980.
19. Chopra IJ, Wu S-Y, Teco GNC, et al: A radioimmunoassay for measurement of 3,5,3′-triiodothyronine sulfate: Studies in thyroidal and nonthyroidal diseases, pregnancy, and neonatal life. J Clin Endocrinol Metab 75:189–194, 1992.
20. deVijlder JJM, Veenboer GJM: Thyroid albumin originates from blood. Endocrinology 131:578–584, 1992.
21. Surks MI, Oppenheimer JH: Formation of iodoprotein during the peripheral metabolism of 3,5,3′-triiodo-L-thyroxine-^{125}I in the euthyroid man and rat. J Clin Invest 48:685–695, 1969.
22. Refetoff S, Matalon R, Bigazzi M: Metabolism of L-thyroxine (T_4) and L-triiodothyronine (T3) by human fibroblasts in tissue culture: Evidence for cellular binding proteins and conversion of T_4 to T_3. Endocrinology 91:934–947, 1972.
23. Koerner D, Surks MI, Oppenheimer JH: In vitro formation of apparent covalent complexes between L-triiodothyronine and plasma protein. J Clin Endocrinol Metab 36:239–245, 1973.
24. Trevorrow V: Studies on the nature of the iodine in blood. J Biol Chem 127:737–750, 1939.
25. Barker SB: Determination of protein-bound iodine. J Biol Chem 173:715–724, 1948.
26. O'Connor JF, Wu GY, Gallagher TF, et al: The 24-hour plasma thyroxin profile in normal man. J Clin Endocrinol Metab 39:765–771, 1974.
27. Fang VS, Refetoff S: Radioimmunoassay for serum triiodothyronine: Evaluation of simple techniques to control interference from binding proteins. Clin Chem 20:1150–1154, 1974.
28. Larsen PR, Dockalova J, Sipula D, et al: Immunoassay of thyroxine in unextracted human serum. J Clin Endocrinol Metab 37:117–182, 1973.
29. Sterling K, Milch PO: Thermal inactivation of thyroxine-binding globulin for direct radioimmunoassay of triiodothyronine in serum. J Clin Endocrinol Metab 38:866–875, 1974.
30. Ikekubo K, Konishi J, Endo K, et al: Anti-thyroxine and anti-triiodothyronine antibodies in three cases of Hashimoto's thyroiditis. Acta Endocrinol 89:557–566, 1978.
31. Sakata S, Nakamura S, Miura K: Autoantibodies against thyroid hormones or iodothyronine. Implications in diagnosis, thyroid function, treatment, and pathogenesis. Ann Intern Med 103:579–589, 1985.
32. Canadian Task Force on the Periodic Health Examination. Periodic health examination, 1990 Update: 1. Early detection of hyperthyroidism and hypothyroidism in adults and screening of newborns for congenital hypothyroidism. J Can Med Assoc 142:955–961, 1990.
33. Schuurs AWM, Van Weemen BK: Enzyme-immunoassay. Clin Chim Acta 81:1–40, 1977.
34. Galen RS, Forman D: Enzyme immunoassay of serum thyroxine with AutoChemist multichannel analyzer. Clin Chem 23:119–121, 1977.
35. Schall RF, Fraser AS, Hausen HW, et al: A sensitive manual enzyme immunoassay for thyroxine. Clin Chem 24:1801–1804, 1978.
36. Miyai K, Ishibashi K, Kawashima M: Enzyme immunoassay of thyroxine in serum and dried blood samples on filter paper. Endocrinol Jpn 27:375–380, 1980.
37. Rongen HA, Hoetelmans RM, Bult A, et al: Chemiluminescence and immunoassays. J Pharm Biomed Anal 12:433–462, 1994.
38. Gonzalez RR, Robaina R, Rodriguez ME, et al: An enzyme immunoassay for determining total thyroxine in human serum using an ultramicroanalytical system. Clin Chim Acta 197:159–170, 1991.
39. Refetoff S: Inherited thyroxine-binding globulin (TBG) abnormalities in man. Endocr Rev 10:275–293, 1989.
40. Abuid J, Klein AH, Foley TP Jr, et al: Total and free triiodothyronine and thyroxine in early infancy. J Clin Endocrinol Metab 39:263–268, 1974.
41. De Costre P, Buhler U, DeGroot LJ, Refetoff S: Diurnal rhythm in total serum thyroxine levels. Metabolism 20:782–791, 1971.
42. Snyder SM, Cavalieri RR, Ingbar SH: Simultaneous measurement of percentage free thyroxine and triiodothyronine: Comparison of equilibrium dialysis and Sephadex chromatography. J Nucl Med 17:660–664, 1976.
43. Oppenheimer JH: Role of plasma proteins in the binding, distribution, and metabolism of the thyroid hormones. N Engl J Med 278:1153–1162, 1968.
44. Azizi F, Vagenakis AG, Portnay GI, et al: Thyroxine transport and metabolism in methadone and heroin addicts. Ann Intern Med 80:194–199, 1974.
45. McKerron CG, Scott RL, Asper SP, et al: Effects of clofibrate (Atromid S) on the thyroxine-binding capacity of thyroxine-binding globulin and free thyroxine. J Clin Endocrinol Metab 29:957–961, 1969.
46. Beex L, Ross A, Smals P, Kloppenborg P: 5-Fluorouracil–induced increase of total thyroxine and triiodothyronine. Cancer Treat Rep 61:1291–1295, 1977.
47. Oltman JE, Friedman S: Protein-bound iodine in patients receiving perphenazine. JAMA 185:726–727, 1963.
48. Braverman LE, Ingbar SH: Effects of norethandrolone on the transport in serum and peripheral turnover of thyroxine. J Clin Endocrinol Metab 27:389–396, 1967.
49. Barbosa J, Seal US, Doe RP: Effects of anabolic steroids on hormone-binding proteins, serum cortisol and serum nonprotein-bound cortisol. J Clin Endocrinol Metab 32:232–240, 1971.
50. Oppenheimer JH, Werner SC: Effect of prednisone on thyroxine-binding proteins. J Clin Endocrinol Metab 26:715–721, 1966.
51. Garnick MB, Larsen PR: Acute deficiency of thyroxine-binding globulin during L-asparaginase therapy. N Engl J Med 301:252–253, 1979.
52. O'Brien T, Silverberg JD, Nguyen TT: Nicotinic acid–induced toxicity associated with cytopenia and decreased levels of thyroxine-binding globulin. Mayo Clin Proc 67:465–468, 1992.
53. Christensen LK: Thyroxine-releasing effect of salicylate and of 2,4-dinitrophenol. Nature 183:1189–1190, 1959.
54. McConnell RJ: Abnormal thyroid function in patients taking salsalate. JAMA 267:1242–1243, 1992.
55. Oppenheimer JH, Tavernetti RR: Displacement of thyroxine from human thyroxine-binding globulin by analogues of hydantoin. Steric aspects of the thyroxine-binding site. J Clin Invest 41:2213–2220, 1962.
56. Schussler GC: Diazepam competes for thyroxine binding. J Pharmacol Exp Ther 178:204–209, 1971.
57. Stockigt JR, Lim CF, Barlow JW, et al: Interaction of furosemide with serum thyroxine-binding sites: In vivo and in vitro studies and comparison with other inhibitors. J Clin Endocrinol Metab 60:1025–1031, 1985.
58. Hershman JM, Craane TJ, Colwell JA: Effect of sulfonylurea drugs on the binding of triiodothyronine and thyroxine to thyroxine-binding globulin. J Clin Endocrinol Metab 28:1605–1610, 1968.
59. Tabachnick M, Hao YL, Korcek L: Effect of oleate, diphenylhydantoin, and heparin on the binding of ^{125}I-thyroxine to purified thyroxine-binding globulin. J Clin Endocrinol Metab 36:392–394, 1973.
60. Marshall JS, Tompkins LS: Effect of *o,p*-DDD and similar compounds on thyroxine-binding globulin. J Clin Endocrinol Metab 28:386–392, 1968.
61. Abiodun MO, Bird R, Havard CW, et al: The effects of phenylbutazone on thyroid function. Acta Endocrinol 72:257–264, 1973.
62. Davis PJ, Hsu TH, Bianchine JR, et al: Effects of a new hypolipidemic agent, MK-185, on serum thyroxine-binding globulin (TBG) and dialyzable fraction thyroxine. J Clin Endocrinol Metab 34:200–208, 1972.
63. Taylor R, Clark F, Griffiths ID, et al: Prospective study of effect of fenclofenac on thyroid function tests. BJM 281:911–912, 1980.
64. Wiersinga WM, Fabius AJ, Touber JL: Orphenadrine, serum thyroxine and thyroid function. Acta Endocrinol 86:522–532, 1977.
65. Michajlovskij N, Langer P: Increase of serum free thyroxine following the administration of thiocyanate and other anions in vivo and in vitro. Acta Endocrinol 75:707–716, 1974.
66. Pages RA, Robbins J, Edelhoch H: Binding of thyroxine and thyroxine analogs to human serum prealbumin. Biochemistry 12:2773–2779, 1973.
67. Bartalena L: Recent achievements in studies on thyroid hormone–binding proteins. Endocr Rev 11:47–64, 1990.
68. Stockigt JR, Topliss DJ, Barlow JW, et al: Familial euthyroid thyroxine excess: An appropriate response to abnormal thyroxine binding associated with albumin. J Clin Endocrinol Metab 53:353–359, 1981.
69. Sunthornthepvarakul T, Angkeow P, Weiss RE, et al: A missense mutation in the albumin gene produces familial disalbuminemic hyperthyroxinemia in 8 unrelated families. Biochem Biophys Res Commun 202:781–787, 1994.
70. Sterling K, Refetoff S, Selenkow HA: T_3 toxicosis: Thyrotoxicosis due to elevated serum triiodothyronine levels. JAMA 213:571–575, 1970.

71. Sterling K, Brenner MA, Newman ES, et al: The significance of triiodothyronine (T_3) in maintenance of euthyroid status after treatment of hyperthyroidism. J Clin Endocrinol Metab 33:729–731, 1971.
72. Delange F, Camus M, Ermans AM: Circulating thyroid hormones in endemic goiter. J Clin Endocrinol Metab 34:891–895, 1972.
73. Parle JV, Franklyn JA, Cross KW, et al: Thyroxine prescription in the community: serum TSH level assays as an indicator of undertreatment or overtreatment. Br J Gen Pract 43:107–109, 1993.
74. Saberi M, Utiger RD: Serum thyroid hormone and thyrotropin concentrations during thyroxine and triiodothyronine therapy. J Clin Endocrinol Metab 39:923–927, 1974.
75. Franklyn JA, Ramsden DB, Sheppard MC: The influence of age and sex on tests of thyroid function. Ann Clin Biochem 22:502–505, 1985.
76. Westgren U, Burger A, Ingemanssons S, et al: Blood levels of 3,5,3′-triiodothyronine and thyroxine: Differences between children, adults, and elderly subjects. Acta Med Scand 200:493–495, 1976.
77. Olsen T, Laurberg P, Weeke J: Low serum triiodothyronine and high serum reverse triiodothyronine in old age: An effect of disease not age. J Clin Endocrinol Metab 47:1111–1115, 1978.
78. Welle S, O'Conell M, Danforth D Jr, Campbell R: Decreased free fraction of serum thyroid hormones during carbohydrate over-feeding. Metabolism 33:837–839, 1984.
79. Portnay GI, O'Brian JT, Bush J, et al: The effect of starvation on the concentration and binding of thyroxine and triiodothyronine in serum and on the response to TRH. J Clin Endocrinol Metab 39:191–194, 1974.
80. Azizi F: Effect of dietary composition on fasting-induced changes in serum thyroid hormones and thyrotropin. Metabolism 27:935–942, 1978.
81. Scriba PC, Bauer M, Emmert D, et al: Effects of obesity, total fasting and re-alimentation of L-thyroxine (T_4), 3,5,3′-L-triiodothyronine (T_3), 3,3′,5′-L-triiodothyronine (rT_3), thyroxine binding globulin (TBG), cortisol, thyrotropin, cortisol binding globulin (CBG), transferrin, α_2-haptoglobin and complement C′3 in serum. Acta Endocrinol 91:629–643, 1979.
82. Larsen PR: Triiodothyronine. Review of recent studies of its physiology and pathophysiology in man. Metabolism 21:1073–1092, 1972.
83. Rösler A, Litvin Y, Hage C, et al: Familial hyperthyroidism due to inappropriate thyrotropin secretion successfully treated with triiodothyronine. J Clin Endocrinol Metab 54:76–82, 1982.
84. Maxon HR, Burman KD, Premachandra BN, et al: Familial elevation of total and free thyroxine in healthy, euthyroid subjects without detectable binding protein abnormalities. Acta Endocrinol 100:224–230, 1982.
85. Chopra IJ, Williams DE, Orgiazzi J, et al: Opposite effects of dexamethasone on serum concentrations of 3,3′,5′-triiodothyronine (reverse T_3) and 3,3′,5-triiodothyronine (T_3). J Clin Endocrinol Metab 41:911–920, 1975.
86. Cavalieri RR, Sung LC, Becker CE: Effects of phenobarbital on thyroxine and triiodothyronine kinetics in Graves' disease. J Clin Endocrinol Metab 37:308–316, 1973.
87. Davies PH, Franklyn JA: Effects of drugs on tests of thyroid function. Eur J Clin Pharmacol 40:439–451, 1991.
88. Busnardo B, Vangelista R, Girelli ME, et al: TSH levels and TSH response to TRH as a guide to the replacement treatment of patients with thyroid carcinoma. J Clin Endocrinol Metab 42:901–906, 1976.
89. Refetoff S, Hagen S, Selenkow HA: Estimation of the T_4 binding capacity of serum TBG and TBPA by a single T_4 load ion exchange resin method. J Nucl Med 13:2–12, 1972.
90. Miyai K, Ito M, Hata N: Enzyme immunoassay of thyroxine-binding globulin. Clin Chem 28:2408–2411, 1982.
91. Refetoff S, Murata Y, Vassart G, et al: Radioimmunoassays specific for the tertiary and primary structures of thyroxine-binding globulin (TBG): Measurement of denatured TBG in serum. J Clin Endocrinol Metab 59:269–277, 1984.
92. Freeman T, Pearson JD: The use of quantitative immunoelectrophoresis to investigate thyroxine-binding human serum proteins. Clin Chim Acta 26:365–368, 1969.
93. Nielsen HG, Buus O, Weeke B: A rapid determination of thyroxine-binding globulin in human serum by means of the Laurell Rocket immunoelectrophoresis. Clin Chim Acta 36:133–138, 1972.
94. Mancini G, Carbonara AO, Heremans JF: Immunochemical quantitation of antigens by single radial immunodiffusion. Immunochemistry 2:235–254, 1965.
95. Ekins R: Measurement of free hormones in blood. Endocr Rev 11:5–6, 1990.
96. Nelson JC, Tomel RT: Direct determination of free thyroxin in undiluted serum by equilibrium dialysis/radioimmunoassay. Clin Chem 34:1737–1744, 1988.
97. Surks MI, Hupart KH, Pan C, et al: Normal free thyroxine in critical nonthyroidal illnesses measured by ultrafiltration of undiluted serum and equilibrium dialysis. J Clin Endocrinol Metab 67:1031–1039, 1988.
98. Melmed S, Geola FL, Reed AW, et al: A comparison of methods for assessing thyroid function in non-thyroidal illness. J Clin Endocrinol Metab 54:300–306, 1982.
99. Wong TK, Pekary E, Hoo GS, et al: Comparison of methods for measuring free thyroxin in nonthyroidal illness. Clin Chem 38:720–724, 1992.
100. Chopra IJ, Chopra U, Smith SR, et al: Reciprocal changes in serum concentration of 3,3′,5′-triiodothyronine (reverse T_3) and 3,3′,5-triiodothyronine (T_3) in systemic illnesses. J Clin Endocrinol Metab 41:1043–1049, 1975.
101. Oppenheimer JH, Squef R, Surks MI, et al: Binding of thyroxine by serum proteins evaluated by equilibrium dialysis and electrophoretic techniques. Alterations in nonthyroidal illness. J Clin Invest 42:1769–1782, 1963.
102. Nelson JC, Bruce WR, Pandian MR: Dependence of free thyroxine estimates obtained with equilibrium tracer dialysis on the concentration of thyroxine-binding globulin. Clin Chem 38:1294–1300, 1992.
103. Nelson JC, Weiss R, Wilcox RB: Underestimates of serum free T_4 concentrations by free T_4 immunoassays. J Clin Endocrinol Metab 79:76–79, 1994.
104. Nelson JC, Nayak SS, Wilcox RB: Variable underestimates of serum free T_4 immunoassays of free T_4 concentrations in simple solutions. J Clin Endocrinol Metab 79:1373–1375, 1994.
105. Van der Sluijs Veer G, Vermes I, Bonte HA, et al: Temperature effects on free-thyroxine measurements: Analytical and clinical consequences. Clin Chem 38:1327–1331, 1992.
106. Faber J, Waetjen I, Siersbaek-Nielsen K: Free T_4 measured in undiluted serum by dialysis and ultrafiltration: Effects of non-thyroidal illness and an acute load of salicylate or heparin. Clin Chim Acta 223:159–167, 1993.
107. Larsen PR, Alexander NM, Chopra IJ, et al: Revised nomenclature for test of thyroid hormones and thyroid-related proteins in serum. Clin Chem 33:2114–2116, 1987.
108. Felicetta JV, Green WL, Mass LB, et al: Thyroid function and lipids in patients with chronic liver disease treated by hemodialysis with comments on the free thyroxine index. Metabolism 28:756–763, 1979.
109. Glinoer D, Fernandez-Deville M, Ermans AM: Use of direct thyroxine-binding globulin measurement in the evaluation of thyroid function. J Endocrinol Invest 1:329–335, 1978.
110. Attwood EC: The T_3/TBG ratio and the biochemical investigation of thyrotoxicosis. Clin Biochem 12:88–92, 1979.
111. Nuutila P, Koskinen P, Irjala K, et al: Two new two-step immunoassays for free thyroxin evaluated: Solid-phase radioimmunoassay and time-resolved fluoroimmunoassay. Clin Chem 36:1355–1360, 1990.
112. Hay ID, Bayer MF, Kaplan MM, et al: American Thyroid Association assessment of current free thyroid hormone and thyrotropin measurements and guidelines for future clinical assays. Clin Chem 37:2002–2008, 1991.
113. Wilkins TA, Midgley JEM, Barron N: Comprehensive study of a thyroxin-analog–based assay for free thyroxin ("Amerlex FT_4"). Clin Chem 31:1644–1653, 1985.
114. Stockigt JR, Stevens V, White E, et al: Unbound analog radioimmunoassays for free thyroxin measure the albumin-bound hormone fraction. Clin Chem 29:1408–1410, 1983.
115. John R: Autoantibodies to thyroxin and interference with free-thyroxin assay. Clin Chem 29:581–582, 1983.
116. Christofides ND, Sheehan CP: Enhanced chemiluminescence labeled-antibody immunoassay (Amerlite-MAB) for free thyroxine: Design, development and technical validation. Clin Chem 41:17–23, 1995.
117. Christofides ND, Sheehan CP: Multicenter evaluation of enhanced chemiluminescence labeled-antibody immunoassay (Amerlite-MAB) for free thyroxine. Clin Chem 41:24–31, 1995.
118. Letellier M, Levesque A, Daigle F, et al: Performance evaluation of automated immunoassays on the Technicon Immuno 1 system. Clin Chem 42:1695–1701, 1996.
119. Costongs G, van Oers R, Leerkes B, et al: Evaluation of the DPC IMMULITE random access immunoassay analyser. Eur J Clin Chem Clin Biochem 33:887–892, 1995.
120. Bock J, Morris D, Cheng D, et al: Evaluation of the Technicon Immuno 1 free thyroxine assay. Am J Clin Pathol 105:583–588, 1996.
121. Vogeser J, Jacob K: Measurements of free triiodothyronine in intensive care patients—comparison of two routine methods. Eur J Clin Chem Clin Biochem 35:873–875, 1997.
122. Liewendahl K, Melamies L, Helenius T, et al: Automated and manual serum free thyroxine assays evaluated with equilibrium dialysis. Scand J Clin Lab Invest 54:347–351, 1994.
123. Sarne DH, Refetoff S, Murata Y, et al: Variant thyroxine-binding globulin in serum of Australian Aborigines. A comparison with familial TBG deficiency in Caucasians and American Blacks. J Endocrinol Invest 8:217–224, 1985.
124. Murata Y, Refetoff S, Sarne DH, et al: Variant thyroxine-binding globulin in serum of Australian Aborigines: Its physical, chemical and biological properties. J Endocrinol Invest 8:225–232, 1985.
125. Kaptein EM, Macintyre SS, Weiner JM, et al: Free thyroxine estimates in nonthyroidal illness: Comparison of eight methods. J Clin Endocrinol Metab 52:1073–1077, 1981.
126. Lehotay DC, Weight CW, Seltman JH, et al: Free thyroxin: A comparison of direct and indirect methods and their diagnostic usefulness in nonthyroidal illness. Clin Chem 28:1826–1829, 1982.
127. Oppenheimer JH, Schwartz HL, Mariash CN, et al: Evidence for a factor in the sera of patients with nonthyroidal illness which inhibits iodothyronine binding by solid matrices, serum proteins, and rat hepatocytes. J Clin Endocrinol Metab 54:757–766, 1982.
128. Woeber KA, Maddux BA: Thyroid hormone binding in nonthyroidal illness. Metabolism 30:412–416, 1981.
129. Chopra IJ, Solomon DH, Teco GNC, et al: An inhibitor of the binding of thyroid hormones to serum proteins is present in extrathyroidal tissues. Science 215:407–409, 1982.
130. Chopra IJ, Chua Teco GN, Mead JF, et al: Relationship between serum free fatty acids and thyroid hormone binding inhibitor in nonthyroidal illnesses. J Clin Endocrinol Metab 60:980–984, 1985.
131. Chopra IJ: An assessment of daily production and significance of thyroidal secretion of 3,3′,5′-triiodothyronine (reverse T_3) in man. J Clin Invest 58:32–40, 1976.
132. Nicod P, Burger A, Staeheli V, et al: A radioimmunoassay for 3,3′,5′-triiodo-L-thyronine in unextracted serum: Method and clinical results. J Clin Endocrinol Metab 42:823–829, 1976.
133. Chopra IJ: A radioimmunoassay for measurement of 3,3′,5′-triiodothyronine (reverse T_3). J Clin Invest 54:583–592, 1974.
134. O'Connell M, Robbins DC, Bogardus C, et al: The interaction of free fatty acids in radioimmunoassays for reverse triiodothyronine. J Clin Endocrinol Metab 55:577–582, 1982.
135. Weiss RE, Angkeow P, Sunthornthepvarakul T, et al: Linkage of familial dysalbuminemic hyperthyroxinemia to the albumin gene in a large Amish family. J Clin Endocrinol Metab 80:116–121, 1995.
136. Chopra IJ: A radioimmunoassay for measurement of 3′-monoiodothyronine. J Clin Endocrinol Metab 51:117–123, 1980.
137. Chopra IJ, Sack J, Fisher DA: Circulating 3,3′,5′-triiodothyronine (reverse T_3) in the human newborn. J Clin Invest 55:1137–1141, 1975.

138. Escobar del Rey F, Morreale de Escobar G: The effect of propylthiouracil, methylthiouracil and thiouracil on the peripheral metabolism of L-thyroxine in thyroidectomized L-thyroxine maintained rats. Endocrinology 69:456–465, 1961.
139. Furth ED, Rives K, Becker DV: Nonthyroidal action of propylthiouracil in euthyroid, hypothyroid, and hyperthyroid man. J Clin Endocrinol Metab 26:239–246, 1966.
140. Oppenheimer JH, Schwartz HL, Surks MI: Propylthiouracil inhibits the conversion of L-thyroxine to L-triiodothyronine. An explanation of the antithyroxine effect of propylthiouracil and evidence supporting the concept that triiodothyronine is the active hormone. J Clin Invest 51:2493–2497, 1972.
141. Duick DS, Warren DW, Nicoloff JT, et al: Effect of a single dose of dexamethasone on the concentration of serum triiodothyronine in man. J Clin Endocrinol Metab 39:1151–1154, 1974.
142. Faber J, Friis T, Kirkegaard C, et al: Serum T_4, T_3 and reverse T_3 during treatment with propranolol in hyperthyroidism, L-T_4 treated myxedema and normal man. Horm Metab Res 11:34–36, 1979.
143. Wiersinga WM, Touber JL: The influence of β-adrenoreceptor blocking agents on plasma thyroxine and triiodothyronine. J Clin Endocrinol Metab 45:293–298, 1977.
144. Bürgi H, Wimpfheimer C, Burger A, et al: Changes of circulating thyroxine, triiodothyronine and reverse triiodothyronine after radiographic contrast agents. J Clin Endocrinol Metab 43:1203–1210, 1976.
145. Wu SY, Chopra IJ, Solomon DH, et al: Changes in circulating iodothyronines in euthyroid and hyperthyroid subjects given ipodate (Oragrafin), an agent for oral cholecystography. J Clin Endocrinol Metab 46:691–697, 1978.
146. Burger A, Dinichert D, Nicod P, et al: Effects of amiodarone on serum triiodothyronine, reverse triiodothyronine, thyroxine and thyrotropin. J Clin Invest 58:255–259, 1976.
147. Nademanee K, Piwonka RW, Singh BN, et al: Amiodarone and thyroid function. Prog Cardiovasc Dis 31:427–437, 1989.
148. Franklyn JA, Davis JR, Gammage M, et al: Amiodarone and thyroid hormone action. Clin Endocrinol 22:257–264, 1985.
149. Schlienger JL, Kapfer MT, Singer L, et al: The action of clomipramine on thyroid function. Horm Metab Res 12:481–482, 1980.
150. Larsen PR, Atkinson AJ, Wellman HN, et al: The effect of diphenylhydantoin on thyroxine metabolism in man. J Clin Invest 49:1266–1279, 1970.
151. Faber J, Lumholtz IB, Kirkegaard C, et al: The effects of phenytoin (diphenylhydantoin) on the extrathyroidal turnover of thyroxine, 3,5,3′-triiodothyronine, 3,3′,5′-triiodothyronine and 3′,5′-diiodothyronine in man. J Clin Endocrinol Metab 61:1093–1099, 1985.
152. Rootwelt K, Ganes T, Johannessen SI: Effect of carbamazepine, phenytoin and phenobarbitone on serum levels of thyroid hormones and thyrotropin in humans. Scand J Clin Lab Invest 38:731–736, 1978.
153. Northcutt RC, Stiel MN, Nollifield JW, et al: The influence of cholestyramine on thyroxine absorption. JAMA 208:1857–1861, 1969.
154. Witztum JL, Jacobs LS, Schonfeld G: Thyroid hormone and thyrotropin levels in patients placed on colestipol hydrochloride. J Clin Endocrinol Metab 46:838–840, 1978.
155. Van Wyk JJ, Arnold MB, Wynn J, et al: The effects of a soybean product on thyroid functions in humans. Pediatrics 24:752–760, 1959.
156. Pinchera A, MacGillivray MH, Crawford JD, et al: Thyroid refractoriness in an athyrotic cretin fed soybean formula. N Engl J Med 273:83–86, 1965.
157. Isley WL: Effect of rifampin therapy on thyroid function tests in a hypothyroid patient on replacement L-thyroxine. Ann Intern Med 107:517–518, 1987.
158. Engler D, Markelbach U, Steiger G, et al: The monodeiodination of triiodothyronine and reverse triiodothyronine in man: A quantitative evaluation of the pathway by the use of turnover rate techniques. J Clin Endocrinol Metab 58:49–61, 1984.
159. Pangaro L, Burman KD, Wartofsky L, et al: Radioimmunoassay for 3,5-diiodothyronine and evidence for dependence on conversion from 3,5,3′-triiodothyronine. J Clin Endocrinol Metab 50:1075–1081, 1980.
160. Faber J, Kirkegaard C, Lumholtz IB, et al: Measurements of serum 3′,5′-diiodothyronine and 3,3′-diiodothyronine concentrations in normal subjects and in patients with thyroid and nonthyroid disease: Studies of 3′,5′-diiodothyronine metabolism. J Clin Endocrinol Metab 48:611–617, 1979.
161. Geola F, Chopra IJ, Geffner DL: Patterns of 3,3′,5′-triiodothyronine monodeiodination in hypothyroidism and nonthyroidal illnesses. J Clin Endocrinol Metab 50:336–340, 1980.
162. Chopra IJ, Geola F, Solomon DH, et al: 3′,5′-Diiodothyroxine in health and disease: Studies by a radioimmunoassay. J Clin Endocrinol Metab 47:1198–1207, 1978.
163. Burman KD, Wright FD, Smallridge RC, et al: A radioimmunoassay for 3′,5′-diiodothyronine. J Clin Endocrinol Metab 47:1059–1064, 1978.
164. Jaedig S, Faber J: The effect of starvation and refeeding with oral versus intravenous glucose on serum 3,5-, 3,3′- and 3′,5′-diiodothyronine and 3′-monoiodothyronine. Acta Endocrinol 100:388–392, 1982.
165. Smallridge RC, Wartofsky L, Green BJ, et al: 3′-L-Monoiodothyronine: Development of a radioimmunoassay and demonstration of in vivo conversion from 3′,5′-diiodothyronine. J Clin Endocrinol Metab 48:32–36, 1979.
166. Corcoran JM, Eastman CJ: Radioimmunoassay of 3-L-monoiodothyronine: Application in normal human physiology and thyroid disease. J Clin Endocrinol Metab 57:66–70, 1983.
167. Nakamura Y, Chopra IJ, Solomon DH: An assessment of the concentration of acetic acid and propionic acid derivatives of 3,5,3′-triiodothyronine in human serum. J Clin Endocrinol Metab 46:91–97, 1978.
168. Burger A, Suter P, Nicod P, et al: Reduced active thyroid hormone levels in acute illness. Lancet 1:163–655, 1976.
169. Pittman CS, Suda AK, Chambers JB Jr, et al: Abnormalities of thyroid hormone turnover in patients with diabetes mellitus before and after insulin therapy. J Clin Endocrinol Metab 48:854–860, 1979.
170. Dlott RS, LoPresti JS, Nicoloff JT: Evidence that triiodoacetate (TRIAC) is the autocrine thyroid hormone in man. Thyroid 2(suppl):94, 1992.
171. Chopra IJ, Tang L: Radioimmunoassay (RIA) for measurement of 3,3′-diiodothyronine sulfate (3,3′-T_2S). Studies in thyroidal and thyroidal illness, pregnancy and fetal/neonatal life. *In* Proceedings of the Annual Meeting of the American Thyroid Association. San Diego, CA, Nov 1997.
172. Huang W, Kuo SW, Chen WL, et al: Increased urinary excretion of sulfated 3,3′,5-triiodothyronine in patients with nodular goiters receiving suppressive thyroxine therapy. Thyroid 6:91–96, 1996.
173. Iervasi G, Clerico A, Manfredi C, et al: Acute effects of intravenous amiodarone on sulphate metabolites of thyroid hormones in arrhythmic patients. Clin Endocrinol 47:699–705, 1997.
174. Nelson JC, Weiss RM, Lewis JE, et al: A multiple ligand-binding radioimmunoassay of diiodothyronine. J Clin Invest 53:416–422, 1974.
175. Nelson JC, Lewis JE: Radioimmunoassay of iodotyrosines. *In* Abraham GE (ed): Handbook of Radioimmunoassay. New York, Marcel Dekker, 1979.
176. Meinhold H, Beckert A, Wenzel W: Circulating diiodotyrosine: Studies of its serum concentration, source, and turnover using radioimmunoassay after immunoextraction. J Clin Endocrinol Metab 53:1171–1178, 1981.
177. Van Herle AJ, Uller RP, Matthews NL, et al: Radioimmunoassay for measurement of thyroglobulin in human serum. J Clin Invest 52:1320–1327, 1973.
178. Spencer CA, Takeuchi M, Kazarosyan M: Current status and performance goals for serum thyroglobulin assays. Clin Chem 42:164–173, 1996.
179. Marquet PY, Daver A, Sapin R et al: Highly sensitive immunoradiometric assay for serum thyroglobulin with minimal interference from autoantibodies. Clin Chem 42:258–262, 1996.
180. Erali M, Bigelow RB, Meikle AW: ELISA for thyroglobulin in serum: Recovery studies to evaluate autoantibody interference and reliability of thyroglobulin values. Clin Chem 42:766–770, 1996.
181. Dai J, Dent W, Atkinson JW, et al: Comparison of three immunoassay kits for serum thyroglobulin in patients with thyroid cancer. Clin Biochem 29:461–465, 1996.
182. Spencer CA, Takeuchi M, Kazarosyan M, et al: Serum thyroglobulin autoantibodies: Prevalence, influence on serum thyroglobulin measurement, and prognostic significance in patients with differentiated thyroid carcinoma. J Clin Endocrinol Metab 83:1121–1127, 1998.
183. Spencer CA, Wang CC: Thyroglobulin measurement: Techniques, clinical benefits and pitfalls. Endocrinol Metab Clin North Am 24:841–863, 1995.
184. Ozata M, Suzuki S, Miyamoto T, et al: Serum thyroglobulin in the follow-up of patients with treated differentiated thyroid cancer. J Clin Endocrinol Metab 79:98–105, 1994.
185. Pacini F, Pinchera A, Giani C, et al: Serum thyroglobulin in thyroid carcinoma and other thyroid disorders. J Endocrinol Invest 3:283–292, 1980.
186. Black EG, Cassoni A, Gimlette TMD, et al: Serum thyroglobulin in thyroid cancer. BMJ 3:443–445, 1981.
187. Pezzino V, Filetti S, Belfiore A, et al: Serum thyroglobulin levels in the newborn. J Clin Endocrinol Metab 52:364–366, 1981.
188. Penny R, Spencer CA, Frasier D, et al: Thyroid-stimulating hormone and thyroglobulin levels decrease with chronological age in children and adolescents. J Clin Endocrinol Metab 56:177–180, 1983.
189. Refetoff S, Lever EG: The value of serum thyroglobulin measurement in clinical practice. JAMA 250:2352–2357, 1983.
190. Izumi M, Kubo I, Taura M, et al: Kinetic study of immunoreactive human thyroglobulin. J Clin Endocrinol Metab 62:400–412, 1986.
191. Uller RP, Van Herle AJ, Chopra IJ: Comparison of alterations in circulating thyroglobulin, triiodothyronine and thyroxine in response to exogenous (bovine) and endogenous (human) thyrotropin. J Clin Endocrinol Metab 37:741–745, 1973.
192. Lever EG, Refetoff S, Scherberg NH, et al: The influence of percutaneous fine needle aspiration on serum thyroglobulin. J Clin Endocrinol Metab 56:26–29, 1983.
193. Uller RP, Van Herle AJ: Effect of therapy on serum thyroglobulin levels in patients with Graves' disease. J Clin Endocrinol Metab 46:747–755, 1978.
194. Smallridge RC, DeKeyser FM, Van Herle AJ, et al: Thyroid iodine content and serum thyroglobulin: Clues to the national history of destruction-induced thyroiditis. J Clin Endocrinol Metab 62:1213–1219, 1986.
195. Mariotti S, Martino E, Cupini C, et al: Low serum thyroglobulin as a clue to the diagnosis of thyrotoxicosis factitia. N Engl J Med 307:410–412, 1982.
196. Van Herle AJ, Uller RP: Elevated serum thyroglobulin: A marker of metastases in differentiated thyroid carcinoma. J Clin Invest 56:272–277, 1975.
197. Schneider AB, Line BR, Goldman JM, et al: Sequential serum thyroglobulin determinations, ^{131}I scans, and ^{131}I uptakes after triiodothyronine withdrawal in patients with thyroid cancer. J Clin Endocrinol Metab 53:1199–1206, 1981.
198. Colacchio TA, LoGerfo P, Colacchio DA, et al: Radioiodine total body scan versus serum thyroglobulin levels in follow-up of patients with thyroid cancer. Surgery 91:42–45, 1982.
199. Black EG, Sheppard MC: Serum thyroglobulin measurements in thyroid cancer: Evaluation of "false" positive results. Clin Endocrinol (Oxf) 35:519–520, 1991.
200. Kawamura S, Kishino B, Tajima K, et al: Serum thyroglobulin changes in patients with Graves' disease treated with long term antithyroid drug therapy. J Clin Endocrinol Metab 56:507–512, 1983.
201. Black EG, Bodden SJ, Hulse JA, et al: Serum thyroglobulin in normal and hypothyroid neonates. Clin Endocrinol 16:267–274, 1982.
202. Heinze HJ, Shulman DI, Diamond FB Jr, et al: Spectrum of serum thyroglobulin elevation in congenital thyroid disorders. Thyroid 3:37–40, 1993.
203. Czernichow P, Schlumberger M, Pomarede R, et al: Plasma thyroglobulin measurements help determine the type of thyroid defect in congenital hypothyroidism. J Clin Endocrinol Metab 56:242, 1983.
204. Burke CW, Shakespear RA, Fraser TR: Measurement of thyroxine and triiodothyronine in human urine. Lancet 2:1177–1179, 1972.
205. Chan V, Landon J: Urinary thyroxine excretion as index of thyroid function. Lancet 1:4–6, 1972.
206. Chan V, Besser GM, Landon J, Ekins RP: Urinary tri-iodothyronine excretion as index of thyroid function. Lancet 2:253–256, 1972.

207. Gaitan JE, Wahner HW, Gorman CA, et al: Measurement of triiodothyronine in unextracted urine. J Lab Clin Med 86:538–546, 1975.
208. Burke CW, Shakespear RA: Triiodothyronine and thyroxine in urine. II. Renal handling, and effect of urinary protein. J Clin Endocrinol Metab 42:504–513, 1976.
209. Sack J, Fisher DA, Hobel CJ, et al: Thyroxine in human amniotic fluid. J Pediatr 87:364–368, 1975.
210. Chopra IJ, Crandall BF: Thyroid hormones and thyrotropin in amniotic fluid. N Engl J Med 293:740–743, 1975.
211. Burman KD, Read J, Dimond RC, et al: Measurement of 3,3′,5′-triiodothyronine (reverse T_3), 3,3′-L-diiodothyronine, T_3, and T_4 in human amniotic fluid and in cord and maternal serum. J Clin Endocrinol Metab 43:1351–1359, 1976.
212. Siersbaek-Nielsen K, Hansen JM: Tyrosine and free thyroxine in cerebrospinal fluid in thyroid disease. Acta Endocrinol 64:126–132, 1970.
213. Hagen GA, Elliott WJ: Transport of thyroid hormones in serum and cerebrospinal fluid. J Clin Endocrinol Metab 37:415–422, 1973.
214. Nishikawa M, Inada M, Naito K, et al: 3,3′,5′-triiodothyronine (reverse T_3) in human cerebrospinal fluid. J Clin Endocrinol Metab 53:1030–1035, 1981.
215. Mallol J, Obregón MJ, Morreale de Escobar G: Analytical artifacts in radioimmunoassay of L-thyroxin in human milk. Clin Chem 28:1277–1282, 1982.
216. Varma SK, Collins M, Row A, et al: Thyroxine, tri-iodothyronine, and reverse tri-iodothyronine concentrations in human milk. J Pediatr 93:803–806, 1978.
217. Jansson L, Ivarsson S, Larsson I, et al: Tri-iodothyronine and thyroxine in human milk. Acta Paediatr Scand 72:703–705, 1983.
218. Riad-Fahmy D, Read GF, Walker RF, et al: Steroids in saliva for assessing endocrine function. Endocr Rev 3:367–395, 1982.
219. Elson MK, Morley JE, Shafer RB: Salivary thyroxine as an estimate of free thyroxine: Concise communication. J Nucl Med 24:700–702, 1983.
220. Reichlin S, Bollinger J, Nejad I, et al: Tissue thyroid hormone concentration of rat and man determined by radioimmunoassay: Biologic significance. Mt Sinai J Med 40:502–510, 1973.
221. Ochi Y, Hachiya T, Yoshimura M, et al: Determination of triiodothyronine in red blood cells by radioimmunoassay. Endocrinol Jpn 23:207–213, 1976.
222. Lim VS, Zavata DC, Flanigan MJ, et al: Basal oxygen uptake: A new technique for an old test. J Clin Endocrinol Metab 62:863–868, 1986.
223. Becker DV: Metabolic indices. *In* Werner SC, Ingbar SH (eds): The Thyroid: A Fundamental and Clinical Text. New York, Harper & Row, 1971, pp 524–533.
224. Waal-Manning HJ: Effect of propranolol on the duration of the Achilles tendon reflex. Clin Pharmacol Ther 10:199–206, 1969.
225. Rodbard D, Fujita T, Rodbard S: Estimation of thyroid function by timing the arterial sounds. JAMA 201:884–887, 1967.
226. Nuutila P, Irjala K, Saraste M, et al: Cardiac systolic time intervals and thyroid hormone levels during treatment of hypothyroidism. Scand J Clin Lab Invest 52:467–477, 1992.
227. Lewis BS, Ehrenfeld EN, Lewis N, et al: Echocardiographic LV function in thyrotoxicosis. Am Heart J 97:460–468, 1979.
228. Tseng KH, Walfish PG, Persand JA, Gilbert BW: Concurrent aortic and mitral valve echocardiography permits measurements of systolic time intervals as an index of peripheral tissue thyroid functional status. J Clin Endocrinol Metab 69:633–638, 1989.
229. Vesell ES, Shapiro JR, Passananti GT, et al: Altered plasma half-lives of antipyrine, propylthiouracil, and methimazole in thyroid dysfunction. Clin Pharmacol Ther 17:48–56, 1975.
230. Brunk SF, Combs SP, Miller JD, et al: Effects of hypothyroidism and hyperthyroidism on dipyrone metabolism in man. J Clin Pharmacol 14:271–279, 1974.
231. Kekki M: Serum protein turnover in experimental hypo- and hyperthyroidism. Acta Endocrinol Suppl 91:1–139, 1964.
232. Walton KW, Scott PJ, Dykes PW, et al: The significance of alterations in serum lipids in thyroid dysfunction. II. Alterations of the metabolism and turnover of ^{131}I-low-density lipoproteins in hypothyroidism and thyrotoxicosis. Clin Sci 29:217–238, 1965.
233. Hellman L, Bradlow HL, Zumoff B, et al: The influence of thyroid hormone on hydrocortisone production and metabolism. J Clin Endocrinol Metab 21:1231–1247, 1961.
234. Gallagher TF, Hellman L, Finkelstein J, et al: Hyperthyroidism and cortisol secretion in man. J Clin Endocrinol Metab 34:919–927, 1972.
235. Kiely JM, Purnell DC, Owen CA Jr: Erythrokinetics in myxedema. Ann Intern Med 67:533–538, 1967.
236. Das KC, Mukherjee M, Sarkar TK, et al: Erythropoiesis and erythropoietin in hypo- and hyperthyroidism. J Clin Endocrinol Metab 40:211–220, 1975.
237. Rivlin RS, Melmon KL, Sjoerdsma A: An oral tyrosine tolerance test in thyrotoxicosis and myxedema. N Engl J Med 272:1143–1148, 1965.
238. Bélanger R, Chandramohan N, Misbin R, et al: Tyrosine and glutamic acid in plasma and urine of patients with altered thyroid function. Metabolism 21:855–865, 1972.
239. Lamberg BA, Gräsbeck R: The serum protein pattern in disorders of thyroid function. Acta Endocrinol 19:91–100, 1955.
240. Ford HC, Cooke RR, Keightley EA, et al: Serum levels of free and bound testosterone in hyperthyroidism. Clin Endocrinol 36:187–192, 1992.
241. Anderson DC: Sex-hormone–binding globulin. Clin Endocrinol 3:69–96, 1974.
242. DeNayer P, Lambot MP, Desmons MC, et al: Sex hormone–binding protein in hypothyroxinemic patients: A discriminator for thyroid status in thyroid hormone resistance and familial dysalbuminemic hyperthyroxinemia. J Clin Endocrinol Metab 62:1309–1312, 1986.
243. Macaron CI, Macaron ZG: Increased serum ferritin levels in hyperthyroidism. Ann Intern Med 96:617–618, 1982.
244. Takamatsu J, Majima M, Miki K, et al: Serum ferritin as a marker of thyroid hormone action on peripheral tissues. J Clin Endocrinol Metab 61:672–676, 1985.
245. Graninger W, Pirich KR, Speiser W, et al: Effect of thyroid hormones on plasma protein concentration in man. J Clin Endocrinol Metab 63:407–411, 1986.
246. Shah JH, Cechio GM: Hypoinsulinemia of hypothyroidism. Arch Intern Med 132:657–661, 1973.
247. Levy LJ, Adesman JJ, Spergel G: Studies on the carbohydrate and lipid metabolism in thyroid disease: Effects of glucagon. J Clin Endocrinol Metab 30:372–379, 1970.
248. Chopra IJ, Tulchinsky D: Status of estrogen-androgen balance in hyperthyroid men with Graves' disease. J Clin Endocrinol Metab 38:269–277, 1974.
249. Seino Y, Matsukura S, Miyamoto Y, et al: Hypergastrinemia in hyperthyroidism. J Clin Endocrinol Metab 43:852–855, 1976.
250. Bouillon R, DeMoor P: Parathyroid function in patients with hyper- or hypothyroidism. J Clin Endocrinol Metab 38:999–1004, 1974.
251. Castro JH, Genuth SM, Klein L: Comparative response to parathyroid hormone in hyperthyroidism and hypothyroidism. Metabolism 24:839–848, 1975.
252. Kojima N, Sakata S, Nakamura S, et al: Serum concentrations of osteocalcin in patients with hyperthyroidism, hypothyroidism and subacute thyroiditis. J Endocrinol Invest 15:491–496, 1992.
253. Body JJ, Demeester-Mirkine N, Borkowski A, et al: Calcitonin deficiency in primary hypothyroidism. J Clin Endocrinol Metab 62:700–703, 1986.
254. Hauger-Klevene JH, Brown H, Zavaleta J: Plasma renin activity in hyper- and hypothyroidism: Effect of adrenergic blocking agents. J Clin Endocrinol Metab 34:625–629, 1972.
255. Ogihara T, Yamamoto T, Miyai K, et al: Plasma renin activity and aldosterone concentration of patients with hyperthyroidism and hypothyroidism. Endocrinol Jpn 20:433–438, 1973.
256. Stoffer SS, Jiang NS, Gorman CA, et al: Plasma catecholamines in hypothyroidism and hyperthyroidism. J Clin Endocrinol Metab 36:587–589, 1973.
257. Christensen NJ: Plasma noradrenaline and adrenaline in patients with thyrotoxicosis and myxoedema. Clin Sci Mol Med 45:163–171, 1973.
258. Zimmerman RS, Gharib H, Zimmerman D, et al: Atrial natriuretic peptide in hypothyroidism. J Clin Endocrinol Metab 64:353–355, 1987.
259. Rolandi E, Santaniello B, Bagnasco M, et al: Thyroid hormones and atrial natriuretic hormone secretion: Study in hyper- and hypothyroid patients. Acta Endocrinol 127:23–26, 1992.
260. Distiller LA, Sagel J, Morley JE: Assessment of pituitary gonadotropin reserve using luteinizing hormone–releasing hormone (LRH) in states of altered thyroid function. J Clin Endocrinol Metab 40:512–515, 1975.
261. Refetoff S, Fang VS, Rapoport B, et al: Interrelationships in the regulation of TSH and prolactin secretion in man: Effects of L-DOPA, TRH and thyroid hormone in various combinations. J Clin Endocrinol Metab 38:450–457, 1974.
262. Honbo KS, Van Herle AJ, Kellett KA: Serum prolactin levels in untreated primary hypothyroidism. Am J Med 64:782–787, 1978.
263. Brauman H, Corvilain J: Growth hormone response to hypoglycemia in myxedema. J Clin Endocrinol Metab 28:301–304, 1968.
264. Rosenfield PS, Wool MS, Danforth E Jr: Growth hormone response to insulin-induced hypoglycemia in thyrotoxicosis. J Clin Endocrinol Metab 29:777–780, 1969.
265. Hamada N, Uoi K, Nishizawa Y, et al: Increase of serum GH concentration following TRH injection in patients with primary hypothyroidism. Endocrinol Jpn 23:5–10, 1976.
266. Kung AEC, Hui WM, Ng ESK: Serum and plasma epidermal growth factor in thyroid disorders. Acta Endocrinol 127:52–57, 1992.
267. Graig FA, Smith JC: Serum creatine phosphokinase activity in altered thyroid states. J Clin Endocrinol Metab 25:723–731, 1965.
268. Fleisher GA, McConahey WM, Pankow M: Serum creatine kinase, lactic dehydrogenase, and glutamic-oxaloacetic transaminase in thyroid diseases and pregnancy. Mayo Clin Proc 40:300–311, 1965.
269. Doran GR, Wilkinson JH: Serum creatine kinase and adenylate kinase in thyroid disease. Clin Chim Acta 35:115–119, 1971.
270. Stolk JM, Hurst JH, Nisula BC: The inverse relationship between serum dopamine-β-hydroxylase activity and thyroid function. J Clin Endocrinol Metab 51:259–264, 1980.
271. Talbot NB, Hoeffel G, Schwachman H, et al: Serum phosphatase as an aid in the diagnosis of cretinism and juvenile hypothyroidism. Am J Dis Child 62:273–278, 1941.
272. Lieberthal AS, Benson SG, Klitgaard HM: Serum malic dehydrogenase in thyroid disease. J Clin Endocrinol Metab 23:211–214, 1963.
273. Yotsumuto H, Imai Y, Kuzuya N, et al: Increased levels of serum angiotensin-converting enzyme activity in hyperthyroidism. Ann Intern Med 96:326–328, 1982.
274. Gow SMG, Caldwell G, Toft AD, et al: Relationship between pituitary and other target organ responsiveness in thyroid patients receiving thyroxine replacement. J Clin Endocrinol Metab 64:364–370, 1987.
275. Beckett GJ, Kellett HA, Gow SM, et al: Elevated plasma glutathione *S*-transferase concentrations in hyperthyroidism and in hypothyroid patients receiving thyroxine replacement: Evidence for hepatic damage. BMJ 2:427–429, 1985.
276. Ogura F, Morii H, Ohmo M, et al: Serum coenzyme Q_{10} levels in thyroid disorders. Horm Metab Res 12:537–540, 1980.
277. Bouillon R, Muls E, DeMoor P: Influence of thyroid function on the serum concentration of 1,25-dihydroxy vitamin D_3. J Clin Endocrinol Metab 51:793–796, 1980.
278. Walton KW, Campbell DA, Tonks EL: The significance of alterations in serum lipids in thyroid function. I. The relation between serum lipoproteins, carotenoids, and vitamin A in hypothyroidism and thyrotoxicosis. Clin Sci 29:199–215, 1965.
279. Karlberg BE, Henriksson KG, Andersson RGG: Cyclic adenosine 3′,5′-monophosphate concentration in plasma, adipose tissue and skeletal muscle in normal subjects and in patients with hyper- and hypothyroidism. J Clin Endocrinol Metab 39:96–101, 1974.
280. Peracchi M, Bamonti-Catena F, Lombardi L, et al: Plasma and urine cyclic nucleotide levels in patients with hyperthyroidism and hypothyroidism. J Endocrinol Invest 6:173–177, 1983.
281. Rivlin RS, Wagner HN Jr: Anemia in hyperthyroidism. Ann Intern Med 70:507–516, 1969.

282. Feldman DL, Goldberg WM: Hyperthyroidism with periodic paralysis. Can Med Assoc J 101:667–671, 1969.
283. Pettinger WA, Talner L, Ferris TF: Inappropriate secretion of antidiuretic hormone due to myxedema. N Engl J Med 272:362–364, 1965.
284. Jones JE, Deser PC, Shane SR, et al: Magnesium metabolism in hyperthyroidism and hypothyroidism. J Clin Invest 45:891–900, 1966.
285. Baxter JD, Bondy PK: Hypercalcemia of thyrotoxicosis. Ann Intern Med 65:429–442, 1966.
286. Weldon AP, Danks DM: Congenital hypothyroidism and neonatal jaundice. Arch Dis Child 47:469–471, 1972.
287. Greenberger NJ, Milligan FD, DeGroot LJ, et al: Jaundice and thyrotoxicosis in the absence of congestive heart failure: A study of four cases. Am J Med 36:840–846, 1964.
288. Kuhlbäch B: Creatine and creatinine metabolism in thyrotoxicosis and hypothyroidism. Acta Med Scand Suppl 331:1–70, 1957.
289. Adlkofer F, Armbrecht U, Schleusener H: Plasma lecithin: Cholesterol acyltransferase activity in hypo- and hyperthyroidism. Horm Metab Res 6:142–146, 1974.
290. Pykälistö O, Goldberg AP, Brunzell JD: Reversal of decreased human adipose tissue lipoprotein lipase and hypertriglyceridemia after treatment of hypothyroidism. J Clin Endocrinol Metab 43:591–600, 1976.
291. De Bruin TWA, Van Barlingen H, Van Linde-Sibenius Trip M, et al: Lipoprotein (a) and apolipoprotein B plasma concentrations in hypothyroid, euthyroid, and hyperthyroid subjects. J Clin Endocrinol Metab 76:121–126, 1993.
292. Inui T, Ochi Y, Chen W, et al: Increased serum concentration of type IV collagen peptide and type III collagen peptide in hyperthyroidism. Clin Chim Acta 205:181–186, 1992.
293. Rich C, Bierman EL, Schwartz IL: Plasma nonesterified fatty acids in hyperthyroid states. J Clin Invest 38:275–278, 1959.
294. Amino N, Kuro R, Yabu Y, et al: Elevated levels of circulating carcinoembryonic antigen in hypothyroidism. J Clin Endocrinol Metab 52:457–462, 1981.
295. Tucci JR, Kopp L: Urinary cyclic nucleotide levels in patients with hyper- and hypothyroidism. J Clin Endocrinol Metab 43:1323–1329, 1976.
296. Guttler RB, Shaw JW, Otis CL, et al: Epinephrine-induced alterations in urinary cyclic AMP in hyper- and hypothyroidism. J Clin Endocrinol Metab 41:707–711, 1975.
297. MacFarlane S, Papadopoulos S, Harden RM, et al: ^{131}I and MIT-^{131}I in human urine, saliva and gastric juice: A comparison between euthyroid and thyrotoxic patients. J Nucl Med 9:181–186, 1968.
298. Hellström K, Schuberth J: The effect of thyroid hormones on the urinary excretion of taurine in man. Acta Med Scand 187:61–65, 1970.
299. Maebashi M, Kawamura N, Sato M, et al: Urinary excretion of carnitine in patients with hyperthyroidism and hypothyroidism: Augmentation by thyroid hormone. Metabolism 26:351–356, 1977.
300. Levine RJ, Oates JA, Vendsalu A, et al: Studies on the metabolism of aromatic amines in relation to altered thyroid function in man. J Clin Endocrinol Metab 22:1242–1250, 1962.
301. Copinschi G, Leclercq R, Bruno OD, et al: Effects of altered thyroid function upon cortisol secretion in man. Horm Metab Res 3:437–442, 1971.
302. Harvey RD, McHardy KC, Reid IW, et al: Measurement of bone collagen degradation in hyperthyroidism and during thyroxine replacement therapy using pyridinium cross-links as specific urinary markers. J Clin Endocrinol Metab 72:1189–1194, 1991.
303. Kivirikko KI, Laitinen O, Lamberg BA: Value of urine and serum hydroxyproline in the diagnosis of thyroid disease. J Clin Endocrinol Metab 23:1347–1352, 1963.
304. Askenasi R, Demeester-Mirkine N: Urinary excretion of hydroxylysyl glycosides and thyroid function. J Clin Endocrinol Metab 40:342–344, 1975.
305. Golden AWG, Bateman D, Torr S: Red cell sodium in hyperthyroidism. BMJ 2:552–554, 1971.
306. Weinstein M, Sartorio G, Stalldecker GB, et al: Red cell zinc in thyroid dysfunction. Acta Endocrinol 20:147–152, 1972.
307. Pearson HA, Druyan R: Erythrocyte glucose-6-phosphate dehydrogenase activity related to thyroid activity. J Lab Clin Med 57:343–349, 1961.
308. Vuopio P, Viherkoski M, Nikkilä E, et al: The content of reduced glutathione (GSH) in the red blood cells in hypo- and hyperthyroidism. Ann Clin Res 2:184–186, 1970.
309. Kiso Y, Yoshida K, Kaise K, et al: Erythrocyte carbonic anhydrase-I concentrations in patients with Graves' disease and subacute thyroiditis reflect integrated thyroid hormone levels over the previous few months. J Clin Endocrinol Metab 72:515–518, 1991.
310. Dube MP, Davis FB, Davis PJ, et al: Effects of hyperthyroidism and hypothyroidism on human red blood cells Ca^{2+}-ATPase activity. J Clin Endocrinol Metab 62:253–257, 1986.
311. Gwinup G, Ogundip O: Preliminary report: Decreased leukocyte alkaline phosphatase in hyperthyroidism. Metabolism 23:659–661, 1974.
312. Jemelin M, Frei J, Scazziga B: Production of ATP in leukocyte mitochondria from hyperthyroid patients before and after treatment with a β-adrenergic blocker and antithyroid drugs. Acta Endocrinol 66:606–610, 1971.
313. Strickland AL: Sweat electrolytes in thyroid disorders. J Pediatr 82:284–286, 1973.
314. Goolamali SK, Evered D, Shuster S: Thyroid disease and sebaceous function. BMJ 1:432–433, 1976.
315. Christensen J, Schedl HP, Clifton JA: The basic electrical rhythm of the duodenum in normal human subjects and in patients with thyroid disease. J Clin Invest 43:1659–1667, 1964.
316. Levy G, MacGillivray MH, Procknal JA: Riboflavin absorption in children with thyroid disorders. Pediatrics 50:896–900, 1972.
317. Singhelakis P, Alevizaki CC, Ikkos DG: Intestinal calcium absorption in hyperthyroidism. Metabolism 23:311–321, 1974.
318. Thomas FB, Caldwell JH, Greenberger NJ: Steatorrhea in thyrotoxicosis: Relation to hypermotility and excessive dietary fat. Ann Intern Med 78:669–675, 1973.
319. Wegener M, Wedmann B, Langhoff T, et al: Effect of hyperthyroidism on the transport of a solid-liquid meal through the stomach, intestine, and the colon in man. J Clin Endocrinol Metab 75:745–749, 1992.
320. Scherrer M, König MP: Pulmonary gas exchange in hypothyroidism. Pneumonologie 151:105–113, 1974.
321. Zwillich CW, Pierson DJ, Hofeldt FD, et al: Ventilatory control in myxedema and hypothyroidism. N Engl J Med 292:662–665, 1975.
322. Lawson JD: The free Achilles reflex in hypothyroidism and hyperthyroidism. N Engl J Med 259:761–764, 1958.
323. Hall R, Owen SG: Thyroid antibodies in cerebrospinal fluid. BMJ 2:710–711, 1960.
324. Hoffman I, Lowrey RD: The electrocardiogram in thyrotoxicosis. Am J Cardiol 6:893–904, 1960.
325. Lee JK, Lewis JA: Myxoedema with complete A-V block and Adams-Stokes disease abolished with thyroid medication. Br Heart J 24:253–265, 1962.
326. Wilkins L: Epiphysial dysgenesis associated with hypothyroidism. Am J Dis Child 61:13–34, 1941.
327. Bonakdarpour A, Kirkpatrick JA, Renzi A, et al: Skeletal changes in neonatal thyrotoxicosis. Radiology 102:149–150, 1972.
328. Mariotti S, Anelli S, Ruf J, et al: Comparison of serum thyroid microsomal and thyroid peroxidase autoantibodies in thyroid diseases. J Clin Endocrinol Metab 65:987–993, 1987.
329. Portmann L, Hamada N, Neinrich G, et al: Antithyroid peroxidase antibody in patients with autoimmune thyroid disease: Possible identity with anti-microsomal antibody. J Clin Endocrinol Metab 61:1001–1003, 1985.
330. Rinke R, Seto P, Rapoport B: Evidence for the highly conformational nature of the epitope(s) on human thyroid peroxidase that are recognized by sera from patients with Hashimoto's thyroiditis. J Clin Endocrinol Metab 71:53, 1990.
331. Kaufman KD, Filetti S, Seto P, et al: Recombinant human thyroid peroxidase generated in eukaryotic cells: A source of specific antigen for the immunological assay of antimicrosomal antibodies in the sera of patients with autoimmune thyroid disease. J Clin Endocrinol Metab 70:724–728, 1990.
332. Chang CC, Huang CN, Chuang LM: Autoantibodies to thyroid peroxidase in patients with type 1 diabetes in Taiwan. Eur J Endocrinol 139:44–48, 1998.
333. Smyth PP, Shering SG, Kilbane MT et al: Serum thyroid peroxidase antibodies, thyroid volume, and outcome in breast carcinoma. J Clin Endocrinol Metab 83:2711–2716, 1998.
334. Trotter WR, Belyavin G, Waddams A: Precipitating and complement fixing antibodies in Hashimoto's disease. Proc R Soc Med 50:961–962, 1957.
335. Boyden SV: The adsorption of proteins on erythrocytes treated with tannic acid and subsequent hemagglutination by antiprotein sera. J Exp Med 93:107–120, 1951.
336. Holborrow EJ, Brown PC, Roitt IM, et al: Cytoplasmic localization of complement-fixing auto-antigen in human thyroid epithelium. Br J Exp Pathol 40:583–588, 1959.
337. Hamada N, Jaeduck N, Portmann L, et al: Antibodies against denatured and reduced thyroid microsomal antigen in autoimmune thyroid disease. J Clin Endocrinol Metab 64:230–238, 1987.
338. Mori T, Kriss JP: Measurements by competitive binding radioassay of serum anti-microsomal and anti-thyroglobulin antibodies in Graves' disease and other thyroid disorders. J Clin Endocrinol Metab 33:688–698, 1971.
339. Mariotti S, Pinchera A, Vitti P, et al: Comparison of radioassay and haemagglutination methods for anti thyroid microsomal antibodies. Clin Exp Immunol 34:118–125, 1978.
340. Miles J, Charles P, Riches P: A review of methods available for the identification of both organ-specific and non organ specific autoantibodies. Ann Clin Biochem 35:19–47, 1998.
341. Amino N, Hagen SR, Yamada N, et al: Measurement of circulating thyroid microsomal antibodies by the tanned red cell haemagglutination technique: Its usefulness in the diagnosis of autoimmune thyroid disease. Clin Endocrinol 5:115, 1976.
342. Ohtaki S, Endo Y, Horinouchi K, et al: Circulating thyroglobulin-antithyroglobulin immune complex in thyroid diseases using enzyme-linked immunoassays. J Clin Endocrinol Metab 52:239–246, 1981.
343. Feldt-Rasmussen U: Analytical and clinical performance goals for testing autoantibodies to thyroperoxidase, thyroglobulin, and thyrotropin receptor. Clin Chem 42:160–163, 1996.
344. Loeb PB, Drash AL, Kenny FM: Prevalence of low-titer and "negative" antithyroglobulin antibodies in biopsy-proved juvenile Hashimoto's thyroiditis. J Pediatr 82:17–21, 1973.
345. Tamaki H, Katsumaru H, Amino N, et al: Usefulness of thyroglobulin antibody detected by ultrasensitive enzyme immunoassay: A good parameter for immune surveillance in healthy subjects and for prediction of post-partum thyroid dysfunction. Clin Endocrinol (Oxf) 37:266–273, 1992.
346. Volpé R, Row VV, Ezrin C: Circulating viral and thyroid antibodies in subacute thyroiditis. J Clin Endocrinol Metab 27:1275–1284, 1967.
347. Kuppers RC, Outschoorn IM, Hamilton RG, et al: Quantitative measurement of human thyroglobulin-specific antibodies by use of a sensitive enzyme-linked immunoassay. Clin Immunol Immunopathol 67:68–77, 1993.
348. Chailurkit LO, Rajatanavin R, Teerarungsikul, K: Evaluation of a new direct radioimmunoassay for serum thyroid peroxidase and thyroglobulin antibodies. J Med Assoc Thailand 77:337–342, 1994.
349. Engler H, Staub JJ, Althaus B, et al: Assessment of antithyroglobulin and antimicrosomal autoantibodies in patients with autoimmune thyroid disease: Comparison of haemagglutination assay, enzyme-linked immunoassay and radioligand assay. Clin Chim Acta 17:9251–9263, 1989.
350. Kousaka T, Higuchi K, Iida Y, et al: Clinical significance of measurements of antithyroid antibodies in the diagnosis of Hashimoto's thyroiditis: Comparison with histological findings. Thyroid 6:445–450, 1996.
351. Ajjan RA, Findlay JC, Metcalfe RA, et al: The modulation of the human sodium iodine symporter activity by Graves' disease sera. J Clin Endocrinol Metab 83:1217–1221, 1998.
352. Raspe E, Costagliola S, Rurf J, et al: Identification of the thyroid Na^+/I^- cotrans-

porter as a potential autoantigen in thyroid autoimmune disease. Eur J Endocrinol 132:399–405, 1995.
353. Morris JC, Bergert ER, Bryant WP.: Binding if immunoglobulin G from patients with autoimmune thyroid disease to rat sodium-iodide symporter peptides: Evidence for the iodide transporter as an autoantigen. Thyroid 7:527–534, 1997.
354. Staeheli V, Vallotton MB, Burger A: Detection of human anti-thyroxine and anti-triiodothyronine antibodies in different thyroid conditions. J Clin Endocrinol Metab 41:669–675, 1975.
355. Bastenie PA, Bonnyns M, Vanhaelst L, et al: Diseases associated with autoimmune thyroiditis. *In* Bastenie PA, Ermans A (eds): Thyroiditis and Thyroid Function. Oxford, Pergamon, 1972.
356. Gupta MK: Thyrotropin receptor antibodies: Advances and importance of detection techniques in thyroid disease. Clin Biochem 25:193–199, 1992.
357. McKenzie JM: The bioassay of thyrotropin in serum. Endocrinology 63:372–381, 1958.
358. Furth ED, Rathbun M, Posillico J: A modified bioassay for the long-acting thyroid stimulator (LATS). Endocrinology 85:592–593, 1969.
359. Kriss JP, Pleshakov V, Rosenblum AL, et al: Studies on the pathogenesis of the ophthalmopathy of Graves' disease. J Clin Endocrinol Metab 27:582–593, 1967.
360. Sunshine P, Kusumoto H, Kriss JP: Survival time of circulating long-acting thyroid stimulator in neonatal thyrotoxicosis: Implications for diagnosis and therapy of the disorder. Pediatrics 36:869–876, 1965.
361. Onaya T, Kotani M, Yamada T, et al: New in vitro tests to detect the thyroid stimulator in sera from hyperthyroid patients by measuring colloid droplet formation and cyclic AMP in human thyroid slices. J Clin Endocrinol Metab 36:859–866, 1973.
362. Hinds WE, Takai N, Rapoport B, et al: Thyroid-stimulating activity and immunoglobulin bioassay using cultured human thyroid cells. J Clin Endocrinol Metab 52:1204–1210, 1981.
363. Leedman PJ, Frauman AG, Colman PG, et al: Measurement of thyroid-stimulating immunoglobulins by incorporation of tritiated-adenine into intact FRTL-5 cells: A viable alternative to radioimmunoassay for the measurement of cAMP. Clin Endocrinol (Oxf) 37:493–499, 1992.
364. Takata I, Suzuki Y, Saida K, et al: Human thyroid-stimulating activity and clinical state in antithyroid treatment of juvenile Graves' disease. Acta Endocrinol (Copenh) 94:46–52, 1980.
365. Kendall-Taylor P, Atkinson S: A biological method for the assay of TSAb in serum. *In* Stockigt JR, Nagataki S (eds): Thyroid Research VIII. Canberra, Australian Academy of Science, 1980.
366. Petersen V, Rees Smith B, Hall R: A study of thyroid-stimulating activity in human serum with the highly sensitive cytochemical bioassay. J Clin Endocrinol Metab 41:199–202, 1975.
367. Libert F, Lefort A, Gerard C, et al: Cloning, sequencing and expression of the human thyrotropin (TSH) receptors: Evidence for binding of autoantibodies. Biochem Biophys Res Commun 165:1250–1255, 1989.
368. Nagayama Y, Kaufman KD, Seto P, et al: Molecular cloning, sequence and functional expression of the cDNA for the human thyrotropin receptor. Biochem Biophys Res Commun 165:1184–1190, 1989.
369. Ludgate M, Perret J, Parmentier M, et al: Use of the recombinant human thyrotropin receptor (TRHr) expressed in mammalian cell lines to assay TSHr autoantibodies. Mol Cell Endocrinol 73:R13–R18, 1990.
370. Filetti S, Foti D, Costante G, et al: Recombinant human thyrotropin (TSH) receptor in a radioreceptor assay for the measurement of TSH receptor antibodies. J Clin Endocrinol Metab 72:1096–1101, 1991.
371. Botero D, Brown RS: Bioassay of TSH receptor antibodies with Chinese hamster ovary cells transfected with recombinant human TSH receptor: Clinical utility in children and adolescents with Graves' disease. J Pediatr 132:612–618, 1998.
372. Vitti P, Elisei R, Tonacchera M, et al: Detection of thyroid-stimulating antibody using Chinese hamster ovary cells transfected with cloned human thyrotropin receptor. J Clin Endocrinol Metab 76:499–503, 1993.
373. Evans C, Morgenthaler NG, Lee S, et al: Development of a luminescent bioassay for thyroid stimulating antibodies. J Clin Endocrinol Metab 84:374–377, 1999.
374. Adams DD, Kennedy TH: Occurrence in thyrotoxicosis of a gamma globulin which protects LATS from neutralization by an extract of thyroid gland. J Clin Endocrinol Metab 27:173–177, 1967.
375. Shishiba Y, Shimizu T, Yoshimura S, et al: Direct evidence for human thyroidal stimulation by LATS-protector. J Clin Endocrinol Metab 36:517–521, 1973.
376. Rapoport B, Greenspan FS, Filetti S, et al: Clinical experience with a human thyroid cell bioassay for thyroid-stimulating immunoglobulins. J Clin Endocrinol Metab 58:332–338, 1984.
377. Smith BR, Hall R: Thyroid-stimulating immunoglobulins in Graves' disease. Lancet 2:427–431, 1974.
378. Zakarija M, McKenzie JM, Munro DS: Evidence of an IgG inhibitor of thyroid-stimulating antibody (TSAb) as a cause of delay in the onset of neonatal Graves' disease. J Clin Invest 72:1352–1356, 1983.
379. Shewring G, Smith BR: An improved radioreceptor assay for TSH receptor antibodies. Clin Endocrinol 17:409–417, 1982.
380. Endo K, Amir SM, Ingbar SH: Development and evaluation of a method for the partial purification of immunoglobulin specific for Graves' disease. J Clin Endocrinol Metab 52:1113–1123, 1981.
381. Kosugi S, Ban T, Akamizu T, et al: Identification of separate determinants on the thyrotropin receptor reactive with Graves' thyroid-stimulating antibodies and with thyroid-stimulating blocking antibodies in idiopathic myxedema: These determinants have no homologous sequence on gonadotropin receptor. Mol Endocrinol 6:166–180, 1992.
382. Michelaangeli VP, Munro DS, Poon CW, et al: Measurement of thyroid stimulating immunoglobulins in a new cell line transfected with a functional human TSH receptor (JPO9), compared with an assay using FRTL-5 cells. Clin Endocrinol 40:645–652, 1994.
383. Costagliola S, Morgenthaler NG, Hoerman R, et al: Second generation assay for thyrotrophin receptor antibodies has superior diagnostic sensitivity for Graves' disease. J Clin Endocrinol Metab 87:90–97, 1999.
384. Drexhage HA, Bottazzo GF, Doniach D: Thyroid growth stimulating and blocking immunoglobulins. In Chayen J, Bitensky L (eds): Cytochemical Bioassays. New York, Marcel Dekker, 1983.
385. Valente WA, Vitti P, Rotella CM, et al: Autoantibodies that promote thyroid growth: A distinct population of thyroid stimulating antibodies. N Engl J Med 309:1028–1034, 1983.
386. Grove AS Jr: Evaluation of exophthalmos. N Engl J Med 292:1005–1013, 1975.
387. Parma J, Duprez L, van Sande J, et al: Diversity and prevalence of somatic mutations in the thyrotropin receptor and Gs alpha genes as a cause of toxic thyroid adenomas. J Clin Endocrinol Metab 82:2695–2701, 1997.
388. McKenzie JM, Zakarija M: Fetal and neonatal hyper- and hypothyroidism due to maternal TSH receptor antibodies. Thyroid 2:155–159, 1992.
389. Cho Y, Shong MH, Yi KH, et al: Evaluation of serum basal thyrotrophin levels and thyrotrophin receptor antibody activities as prognostic markers for discontinuation of antithyroid drug treatment in patients with Graves' disease. Clin Endocrinol (Oxf) 36:585–590, 1992.
390. Hershman JM: Hyperthyroidism induced by trophoblastic thyrotropin. Mayo Clin Proc 47:913–918, 1972.
391. Nisula BC, Ketelslegers JM: Thyroid-stimulating activity and chorionic gonadotropin. J Clin Invest 54:494–499, 1974.
392. Rodien P, Bremont C, Vassant G, et al: Familial gestational hyperthyroidism caused by a mutant thyrotrophin receptor hypersensitive to human chorionic gonadotropin. N Engl J Med 339:1823–1826, 1998.
393. Bahn R, Heufelder AE: Pathogenesis of Graves' ophthalmopathy. N Engl J Med 329:1468–1475, 1993.
394. Miller A, Arthurs B, Boucher A, et al: Significance of antibodies reactive with a 64kDa eye muscle membrane antigen in patients with thyroid autoimmunity. Thyroid 2:197–202, 1992.
395. Winand RJ, Kohn LD: Stimulation of adenylate cyclase activity in retro-orbital tissue membranes by thyrotropin and an exophthalmogenic factor derived from thyrotropin. J Biol Chem 250:6522–6526, 1975.
396. Kodama K, Sikorka H, Bandy-Dafoe P, et al: Demonstration of a circulating antibody against a soluble eye-muscle antigen in Graves' ophthalmopathy. Lancet 2:1353–1356, 1982.
397. Kubota S, Gunji K, Ackrell BA, et al: The 64-kilodalton eye muscle protein is the flavoprotein subunit of mitochondrial succinate dehydrogenase: The corresponding serum antibodies are good markers of an immune-mediated damage to the eye muscle in patients with Graves' hyperthyroidism. J Clin Endocrinol Metab 8:3443–3447, 1998.
398. Wall J, Barsouk A, Stolarski C, et al: Serum antibodies reactive with eye muscle antigens and the TSH receptor in a euthyroid subject who developed ophthalmopathy and Graves' hyperthyroidism. Thyroid 6:353–358, 1996.
399. Kubota S, Gunji K, Stolarski C, et al: Reevaluation of the prevalences of serum autoantibodies reactive with "64-kd eye muscle proteins" in patients with thyroid-associated ophthalmopathy. Thyroid 8:175–179, 1998.
400. Matsuoka N, Eguchi K, Kawakami A, et al: Lack of B7–1/BB1 and B7–2/B70 expression on thyrocytes of patients with Graves' disease. J Clin Endocrinol Metab 81:4137–4143, 1996.
401. Otto EA, Ochs K, Hansen C, et al: Orbital tissue–derived T lymphocytes from patients with Graves' ophthalmopathy recognize autologous orbital antigens. J Clin Endocrinol Metab 81:3045–3050, 1996.
402. Ryo UY, Arnold J, Colman M, et al: Thyroid scintigram: Sensitivity with sodium pertechnetate Tc 99m and gamma camera with pinhole collimator. JAMA 235:1235–1238, 1976.
403. Atkins HL, Klopper JF, Lambrecht RM, et al: A comparison of technetium 99m and iodine 123 for thyroid imaging. AJR 117:195–201, 1973.
404. Nishiyama H, Sodd VJ, Berke RA, et al: Evaluation of clinical value of ^{123}I and ^{131}I in thyroid disease. J Nucl Med 15:261–265, 1974.
405. Tong ECK, Rubenfeld S: Scan measurements of normal and enlarged thyroid glands. AJR 115:706–708, 1972.
406. Mazzaferri EL: Management of a solitary thyroid nodule. N Engl J Med 328:553–559, 1993.
407. Becker FO, Economou PG, Schwartz TB: The occurrence of carcinoma in "hot" thyroid nodules: Report of two cases. Ann Intern Med 58:877–882, 1963.
408. Ashcraft MW, Van Herle AJ: Management of thyroid nodules. II: Scanning techniques, thyroid suppressive therapy, and fine needle aspiration. Head Neck Surg 3:297–322, 1981.
409. Ashcraft MW, Van Herle AJ: Management of thyroid nodules I. History and physical examination, blood tests, x-ray tests and ultrasonography. Head Neck Surg 3:216–230, 1981.
410. Ladenson PW, Braverman LE, Mazzaferri EL, et al: Comparison of administration of recombinant human thyrotropin with withdrawal of thyroid hormone for radioactive iodine scanning in patients with thyroid carcinoma. N Engl J Med 337:888–896, 1997.
411. Chen JJS, LaFrance ND, Allo MD, et al: Single photon emission computed tomography of the thyroid. J Clin Endocrinol Metab 66:1240–1246, 1988.
412. Corstens F, Huysmans D, Kloppenborg P: Thallium-210 scintigraphy of the suppressed thyroid: An alternative for iodine-123 scanning after TSH stimulation. J Nucl Med 29:1360–1363, 1988.
413. Fairweather DS, Bradwell AR, Watson-James SF, et al: Deletion of thyroid tumours using radiolabeled thyroglobulin. Clin Endocrinol 18:563–570, 1983.
414. Barki Y: Ultrasonographic evaluation of neck masses—sonographic pattern in differential diagnosis. Isr J Med Sci 28:212–216, 1992.
415. Watters DAK, Ahuja AT, Evans RM, et al: Role of ultrasound in the management of thyroid nodules. Am J Surg 164:654–657, 1992.

416. Scheible W, Leopold GR, Woo VL, et al: High resolution real-time ultrasonography of thyroid nodules. Radiology 133:413–417, 1979.
417. Sostre S, Reyes MM: Sonographic diagnosis and grading of Hashimoto's thyroiditis. J Endocrinol Invest 14:115–121, 1991.
418. Brander A, Viikinkoski P, Nickels J, et al: Thyroid gland: US screening in a random adult population. Radiology 181:683–687, 1991.
419. Danese D, Sciacchitano S, Farsetti A, et al: Diagnostic accuracy of conventional versus sonography-guided fine-needle aspiration biopsy of thyroid nodules. Thyroid 8:15–21, 1998.
420. Szebeni A, Beleznay EJ: New simple method for thyroid volume determination by ultrasonography. Clin Ultrasound 20:329–337, 1992.
421. Jarlov AE, Hegedus L, Gjorup T, et al: Accuracy of the clinical assessment of thyroid size. Dan Med Bull 38:87–89, 1991.
422. Paracchi A, Ferrari C, Livraghi T, et al: Percutaneous intranodular ethanol injection: A new treatment for autonomous thyroid adenoma. J Endocrinol Invest 15:353–362, 1992.
423. Blum M, Reede DL, Seltzer TF, et al: Computerized axial tomography in the diagnosis of thyroid and parathyroid disorders. Am J Med Sci 287:34–39, 1984.
424. Brown LR, Aughenbaugh GL: Masses of the anterior mediastinum: CT and MR imaging. Am J Radiol 157:1171–1180, 1991.
425. Gittoes NJL, Miller MR, Daykin J, et al: Upper airways obstruction in patients presenting with thyroid enlargement. BMJ 312:484, 1996.
426. Wang C, Vickery AL Jr, Maloof F: Needle biopsy of the thyroid. Surg Gynecol Obstet 143:365–368, 1976.
427. Matos-Godilho L, Kocjan G, Kurtz A: Contribution of fine needle aspiration cytology to diagnosis and management of thyroid disease. J Clin Pathol 45:391–395, 1992.
428. Franklyn JA, Daykin J, Young J, et al: Fine needle aspiration cytology in diffuse or multinodular goitre compared with solitary thyroid nodules. BMJ 307:240–241, 1993.
429. Aogi K, Kitahara K, Buley, et al: Telomerase activity in lesions of the thyroid: Application to diagnosis of clinical samples including fine-needle aspirates. Clin Cancer Res 4:1965–1970, 1998.
430. Saji M, Westra WH, Chen H, et al: Telomerase activity in the differential diagnosis of papillary carcinoma of the thyroid. Surgery 122:1137–1140, 1997.
431. Takiyama Y, Saji M, Clark DP, et al: Polymerase chain reaction–based microsatellite analysis of fine-needle aspirations from Hürthle cell neoplasm. Thyroid 7:853–857, 1997.
432. Lovchik J, Lane MA, Clark DP: Polymerase chain reaction–based detection of B-cell clonality in the fine needle aspiration biopsy of a thyroid mucosa-associated lymphoid tissue (MALT) lymphoma. Hum Pathol 28:989–992, 1997.
433. Dwarakanathan AA, Staren ED, Amore MJ, et al: Importance of repeat fine-needle biopsy in the management of thyroid nodules. Am J Surg 166:350–352, 1993.
434. Hamberger B, Gharib H, Melton LJ 3rd, et al: Fine-needle aspiration biopsy of thyroid nodules: Impact on thyroid practice and cost of care. Am J Med 73:381–384, 1982.
435. Bennedbaek FN, Karstrup S, Hegedus L: Percutaneous ethanol injection therapy in the treatment of thyroid and parathyroid diseases. Eur J Endocrinol 136:240–250, 1997
436. Odell WD, Wilber FJ, Utiger RD: Studies on thyrotropin physiology by means of radioimmunoassay. Recent Prog Horm Res 23:47–83, 1967.
437. Jackson IMD: Thyrotropin releasing hormone. N Engl J Med 306:145–155, 1982.
438. Pierce JG: The subunits of pituitary thyrotropin: Their relation to other glycoprotein hormones. Endocrinology 89:1331–1344, 1971.
439. Miyai K, Fukuchi M, Kumahara Y: Correlation between biological and immunological potencies of human serum and pituitary thyrotropin. J Clin Endocrinol Metab 29:1438–1442, 1969.
440. Gendrel D, Feinstein MC, Grenier J, et al: Falsely elevated serum thyrotropin (TSH) in newborn infants: Transfer from mothers to infants of a factor interfering in the TSH radioimmunoassay. J Clin Endocrinol Metab 52:62–65, 1981.
441. Chaussain JL, Binet E, Job JC: Antibodies to human thyrotrophin in the serum of certain hypopituitary dwarfs. Rev Eur Etud Clin Biol 17:95–99, 1972.
442. Nicoloff JT, Spencer CA: The use and misuse of the sensitive thyrotropin assays. J Clin Endocrinol Metab 71:553–558, 1990.
443. Kricka LJ: Chemiluminescent and bioluminescent techniques. Clin Chem 37:1472–1481, 1991.
444. Spencer CA, Schwarzbein D, Guttler RB, et al: Thyrotropin-releasing hormone stimulation test responses employing third and fourth generation TSH assays. J Clin Endocrinol Metab 76:494–498, 1993.
445. Spencer CA, Takeuchi M, Kazarosyan M et al: Interlaboratory differences in functional sensitivity of immunometric assays of thyrotropin and impact on reliability of measurement of subnormal concentrations of TSH. Clin Chem 41:367–374, 1995.
446. Spencer CA, Takeuchi M, Kazarosyan M: Current status and performance goals for serum TSH assays. Clin Chem 42:140–145, 1996.
447. Brennan MD, Klee GG, Preissner CM, et al: Heterophilic serum antibodies: A cause for falsely elevated serum thyrotropin levels. Mayo Clin Proc 62:894–898, 1987.
448. Wood JM, Gordon DL, Rudinger AN, et al: Artifactual elevation of thyroid-stimulating hormone. Am J Med 90:261–262, 1991.
449. Zweig MH, Csako G, Reynolds JC, et al: Interference by iatrogenically induced anti-mouse IgG antibodies in a two-site immunometric assay for thyrotropin. Arch Pathol Radiol Metab 1165:164–168, 1991.
450. Kourides IA, Heath CV, Ginsberg-Fellner F: Measurement of thyroid-stimulating hormone in human amniotic fluid. J Clin Endocrinol Metab 54:635–637, 1982.
451. Fisher DA, Kleinm AH: Thyroid development and disorders of thyroid function in the newborn. N Engl J Med 304:702–712, 1981.
452. Snyder PJ, Utiger RD: Response to thyrotropin releasing hormone (TRH) in normal man. J Clin Endocrinol Metab 34:380–385, 1972.
453. Hershman JM, Pittman JA Jr: Utility of the radioimmunoassay of serum thyrotrophin in man. Ann Intern Med 74:481–490, 1971.
454. Brabant G, Prank K, Ranft U, et al: Physiological regulation of circadian and pulsatile thyrotropin secretion in normal man and woman. J Clin Endocrinol Metab 70:403–409, 1990.
455. Bartalena L, Martino E, Falcone M, et al: Evaluation of the nocturnal serum thyrotropin (TSH) surge, as assessed by TSH ultrasensitive assay, in patients receiving long term L-thyroxine suppression therapy and in patients with various thyroid disorders. J Clin Endocrinol Metab 65:1265–1271, 1987.
456. Ria AG, Brabant K, Prank E, et al: Circadian changes in pulsatile TSH release in primary hypothyroidism. Clin Endocrinol 37:504–510, 1992.
457. Brabant G, Prank C, Hoang-Vu C, et al: Hypothalamic regulation of pulsatile thyrotropin secretion. J Clin Endocrinol Metab 72:145–150, 1991.
458. Romijn JA, Adriaanse G, Brabant K, et al: Pulsatile secretion of thyrotropin during fasting: A decrease of thyrotropin pulse amplitude. J Clin Endocrinol Metab 70:1631–1636, 1990.
459. Bartalena L, Pacchiarotti A, Palla R, et al: Lack of nocturnal serum thyrotropin (TSH) surge in patients with chronic renal failure undergoing regular maintenance hemofiltration: A case of central hypothyroidism. Clin Nephrol 34:30–34, 1990.
460. Romijn JA, Wiersinga WM: Decreased nocturnal surge of thyrotropin in nonthyroidal illness. J Clin Endocrinol Metab 70:35–42, 1990.
461. Van Cauter E, Golstein J, Vanhaelst L, et al: Effects of oral contraceptive therapy on the circadian patterns of cortisol and thyrotropin (TSH). Eur J Clin Invest 5:115–121, 1975.
462. Brabant G, Brabant A, Ranft U, et al: Circadian and pulsatile thyrotropin secretion in euthyroid man under the influence of thyroid hormone and glucocorticoid administration. J Clin Endocrinol Metab 65:83–88, 1987.
463. Simoni M, Velardo A, Montanini V, et al: Circannual rhythm of plasma thyrotropin in middle-aged and old euthyroid subjects. Horm Res 33:184–189, 1990.
464. Wilber JF, Baum D: Elevation of plasma TSH during surgical hypothermia. J Clin Endocrinol Metab 31:372–375, 1970.
465. Vagenakis AG, Rapoport B, Azizi F, et al: Hyper-response to thyrotropin-releasing hormone accompanying small decreases in serum thyroid hormone concentration. J Clin Invest 54:913–918, 1974.
466. Kleinman RE, Vagenakis AG, Braverman LE: The effect of iopanoic acid on the regulation of thyrotropin secretion in euthyroid subjects. J Clin Endocrinol Metab 51:399–403, 1980.
467. Lazarus JH, Joh R, Bennie EH, et al: Lithium therapy and thyroid function: A long term study. Psychiatr Med 11:85–92, 1981.
468. Scanlon MF, Weightman DR, Shale DJ, et al: Dopamine is a physiological regulator of thyrotropin (TSH) secretion in normal man. Clin Endocrinol 10:7–15, 1979.
469. Scanlon MF, Rodriguez-Arnao MD, Pourmand M, et al: Catecholaminergic interactions in the regulation of thyrotropin (TSH) secretion in man. J Endocrinol Invest 3:125–129, 1980.
470. Massara F, Camanni F, Belforte L, et al: Increased thyrotropin secretion induced by sulpiride in man. Clin Endocrinol 9:419–428, 1978.
471. Delitala G, Devilla L, Lotti G: TSH and prolactin stimulation by the decarboxylase inhibitor benserazide in primary hypothyroidism. Clin Endocrinol 12:313–316, 1980.
472. Kirkegaard C, Bjoerum CN, Cohn D, et al: Studies of the influence of biogenic amines and psychoactive drugs on the prognostic value of the TRH stimulation test in endogenous depression. Psychoneuroendocrinology 2:131–136, 1977.
473. Kirkegaard C, Bjoerum N, Cohn D, et al: TRH stimulation test in manic-depressive illness. Arch Gen Psychiatry 35:1017–1021, 1978
474. Nelis GF, Van DeMeene JG: The effect of oral cimetidine on the basal and stimulated values of prolactin, thyroid stimulating hormone, follicle stimulating hormone and luteinizing hormone. Postgrad Med J 56:26–29, 1980.
475. Feldt-Rasmussen U, Lange AP, Date J, et al: Effect of clomifen on thyroid function in normal men. Acta Endocrinol 90:43–51, 1979.
476. Smals AG, Kloppenborg PW, Hoefnagesl WH, et al: Pituitary-thyroid function in spironolactone treated hypertensive women. Acta Endocrinol (Copenh) 90:577–584, 1979.
477. Morely JE, Shafer RB, Elson MK, et al: Amphetamine-induced hyperthyroxinemia. Ann Intern Med 93:707–709, 1980.
478. Gloebel B, Weinheimer B: TRH-test during D-T_4 application. Nuc-Compact 8:44, 1977.
479. Medeiros-Neto G, Kallas WG, Knobel M, et al: TRIAC (3,5,3-triiodothyroacetic acid) partially inhibits the thyrotropin response to thyrotropin-releasing hormone in normal and thyroidectomized hypothyroid patients. J Clin Endocrinol Metab 50:223–225, 1980.
480. Emrich D: Untersuchungen zum einfluss von Etiroxat-HCL auf den Jodstoffwechsel beim menschen. Arzneim Forsch 27:422–426, 1977.
481. Tamagna EI, Hershman JM, Jorgensen EC: Thyrotropin secretion by 3,5-dimethyl-3-isopropyl-L-thyronine in man. J Clin Endocrinol Metab 48:196–200, 1979.
482. Delitala G: Dopamine and TSH secretion in man. Lancet 2:760–761, 1977.
483. Miyai K, Onishi T, Hosokawa M, et al: Inhibition of thyrotropin and prolactin secretions in primary hypothyroidism by 2-Br-β-ergocryptine. J Clin Endocrinol Metab 39:391–394, 1974.
484. Yoshimura M, Hachiya T, Ochi Y, et al: Suppression of elevated serum TSH levels in hypothyroidism by fusaric acid. J Clin Endocrinol Metab 45:95–98, 1977.
485. Delitala G, Rovasio P, Lotti G: Suppression of thyrotropin (TSH) and prolactin (PRL) release by pyridoxine in chronic primary hypothyroidism. J Clin Endocrinol Metab 45:1019–1022, 1977.
486. Masala A, Delitala G, Devilla L, et al: Effect of apomorphine and piribedil on the secretion of thyrotropin and prolactin in patients with primary hypothyroidism. Metabolism 27:1608–1612, 1978.
487. Delitala G, Wass JAH, Stubbs WA, et al: The effect of lisuride hydrogen maleate, an ergot derivative on anterior pituitary hormone secretion in man. Clin Endocrinol 11:1–9, 1979.
488. Collu R, Jéquier JC, Leboeuf G, et al: Endocrine effects of pimozide, a specific dopaminergic blocker. J Clin Endocrinol Metab 41:981–984, 1975.
489. Nilsson KO, Thorell JI, Hökfelt B: The effect of thyrotrophin releasing hormone on

the release of thyrotrophin and other pituitary hormones in man under basal conditions and following adrenergic blocking agents. Acta Endocrinol 76:24–34, 1974.
490. Lamberg BA, Linnoila M, Fogelholm R, et al: The effect of psychotropic drugs on the SH-response to thyroliberin (TRH). Neuroendocrinology 24:90–97, 1977.
491. Delitala G, Rovasio PP, Masala A, et al: Metergoline inhibition of thyrotropin and prolactin secretion in primary hypothyroidism. Clin Endocrinol 8:69–73, 1978.
492. Ferrari C, Paracchi A, Rondena M, et al: Effect of two serotonin antagonists on prolactin and thyrotropin secretion in man. Clin Endocrinol 5:575–578, 1976.
493. Collu R: The effect of TRH on the release of TSH, PRL and GH in man under basal conditions and following methysergide. J Endocrinol Invest 2:121–124, 1978.
494. Yoshimura M, Ochi Y, Miyazaki T, et al: Effect of intravenous and oral administration of L-DOPA on HGH and TSH release. Endocrinol Jpn 19:543–548, 1972.
495. Re RN, Kourides IA, Ridgway EC, et al: The effect of glucocorticoid administration on human pituitary secretion of thyrotropin and prolactin. J Clin Endocrinol Metab 43:338–346, 1976.
496. Dussault JH: The effect of dexamethasone on TSH and prolactin secretion after TRH stimulation. Can Med Assoc J 111:1195–1197, 1974.
497. Dussault JH, Turcotte R, Guyda H: The effect of acetylsalicylic acid on TSH and PRL secretion after TRH stimulation in the human. J Clin Endocrinol Metab 43:232–235, 1976.
498. Porter BA, Refetoff S, Rosenfield RL, et al: Abnormal thyroxine metabolism in hyposomatotrophic dwarfism and inhibition of responsiveness to TRH during GH therapy. Pediatrics 51:668–674, 1973.
499. Weeke J, Hansen AP, Lundbaek K: Inhibition by somatostatin of basal levels of serum thyrotropin (TSH) in normal men. J Clin Endocrinol Metab 41:168–171, 1975.
500. Thomas JA, Shahid-Salles KS, Donovan MP: Effects of narcotics on the reproduction system. Adv Sex Horm Res 3:169–195, 1977.
501. May P, Mittler J, Manougian A, Erte N: TSH release–inhibiting activity of leucine-enkephalin. Horm Metab Res 11:30–33, 1979.
502. Chan V, Wang C, Yeung RT: Effects of heroin addiction on thyrotropin, thyroid hormones and prolactin secretion in men. Clin Endocrinol 10:557–565, 1979.
503. Kobayashi I, Shimomura Y, Maruta S, et al: Clofibrate and a related compound suppress TSH secretion in primary hypothyroidism. Acta Endocrinol 94:53–57, 1980.
504. Snyder PJ, Utiger RD: Inhibition of thyrotropin response to thyrotropin releasing hormone by small quantities of thyroid hormones. J Clin Invest 51:2077–2084, 1972.
505. Ehrmann DA, Weinberg M, Sarne DH: Limitations to the use of a sensitive assay for serum thyrotropin in the assessment of thyroid status. Arch Intern Med 149:369–372, 1989.
506. Ridgway EC, Cooper DS, Walker H, et al: Peripheral responses of thyroid hormone before and after L-thyroxine therapy in patients with subclinical hypothyroidism. J Clin Endocrinol Metab 53:1238–1242, 1981.
507. Aizawa T, Koizumi Y, Yamada T, et al: Difference in pituitary-thyroid feedback regulation in hypothyroid patients, depending on the severity of hypothyroidism. J Clin Endocrinol Metab 47:560–565, 1978.
508. Spencer CA: Clinical utility and cost-effectiveness of sensitive thyrotropin assays in ambulatory and hospitalized patients. Mayo Clin Proc 63:1214–1222, 1988.
509. Surks MI, Chopra IJ, Mariash CN, et al: American Thyroid Association guidelines for use of laboratory tests in thyroid disorders. JAMA 263:1529–1532, 1990.
510. Delange F, Dodion J, Wolter R, et al: Transient hypothyroidism in the newborn infant. J Pediatr 92:974–976, 1978.
511. Brown ME, Refetoff S: Transient elevation of serum thyroid hormone concentration after initiation of replacement therapy in myxedema. Ann Intern Med 92:491–495, 1980.
512. Sanchez-Franco F, Cacicedo GL, Martin-Zurro A, et al: Transient lack of thyrotropin (TSH) response to thyrotropin-releasing hormone (TRH) in treated hyperthyroid patients with normal or low serum thyroxine (T_4) and triiodothyronine (T_3). J Clin Endocrinol Metab 38:1098–1102, 1974.
513. Spencer CA, Elgen A, Shen D, et al: Specificity of sensitive assays of thyrotropin (TSH) used to screen for thyroid disease in hospitalized patients. Clin Chem 33:1301–1396, 1987.
514. Sunthornthepvarakul T, Gottschalk ME, Hayashi Y, et al: Resistance to thyrotropin caused by mutations in the thyrotropin receptor gene. N Engl J Med 332:115–160, 1995.
515. Beck-Peccoz P, Amr S, Menezes-Ferreira M, et al: Decreased receptor binding of biologically inactive thyrotropin in central hypothyroidism. Effect of treatment with thyrotropin-releasing hormone. J Clin Endocrinol Metab 312:1085–1090, 1985.
516. Refetoff S, Weiss RE, Usala SJ: The syndrome of resistance to thyroid hormone. Endocr Rev 14:378–399, 1993.
517. Mihailovic V, Feller MS, Kourides IA, et al: Hyperthyroidism due to excess thyrotropin secretion: Follow-up studies. J Clin Endocrinol Metab 50:1135–1138, 1980.
518. Kourides IA, Ridgway EC, Weintraub BD, et al: Thyrotropin-induced hyperthyroidism: Use of alpha and beta subunit levels to identify patients with pituitary tumors. J Clin Endocrinol Metab 45:534–543, 1977.
519. Sarne DH, Sobieszczyk S, Ain KB, et al: Serum thyrotropin and prolactin in the syndrome of generalized resistance to thyroid hormone: Responses to thyrotropin-releasing hormone stimulation and short term triiodothyronine suppression. J Clin Endocrinol Metab 70:1305–1311, 1990.
520. Franklyn JA: Syndromes of thyroid hormone resistance. Clin Endocrinol 34:237–245, 1991.
521. Brent GA, Hershman JM, Braunstein GD: Patients with severe nonthyroidal illness and serum thyrotropin concentrations in the hypothyroid range. Am J Med 81:463–466, 1986.
522. Topliss DJ, White EL, Stockigt JR: Significance of thyrotropin excess in untreated primary adrenal insufficiency. J Clin Endocrinol Metab 50:52–56, 1980.
523. Wehmann RE, Gregerman RI, Burns WH, et al: Suppression of thyrotropin in the low-thyroxine state of severe nonthyroidal illness. N Engl J Med 312:546–552, 1985.
524. Bacci V, Schussler GC, Kaplan TB: The relationship between serum triiodothyronine and thyrotropin during systemic illness. J Clin Endocrinol Metab 54:1229–1235, 1982.
525. Kourides IA, Weintraub BD, Ridgway EC, et al: Pituitary secretion of free alpha and beta subunit of human thyrotropin in patients with thyroid disorders. J Clin Endocrinol Metab 40:872–885, 1975.
526. Oliver C, Charvet JP, Codaccioni J-L, et al: Radioimmunoassay of thyrotropin-releasing hormone (TRH) in human plasma and urine. 39:406–410, 1974.
527. Emerson CH, Frohman LA, Szabo M, et al: TRH immunoreactivity in human urine: Evidence for dissociation from TRH. J Clin Endocrinol Metab 45:392–399, 1977.
528. Mitsuma T, Hiraoka Y, Nihei N: Radioimmunoassay of thyrotrophin-releasing hormone in human serum and its application. Acta Endocrinol (Copenh) 83:225–235, 1976.
529. Mallik TK, Wilber JF, Pegues J: Measurements of thyrotropin-releasing hormone–like material in human peripheral blood by affinity chromatography and radioimmunoassay. 54:1194–1198, 1982.
530. Weeke J: The influence of the circadian thyrotropin rhythm on the thyrotropin response to thyrotropin-releasing hormone in normal subjects. Scand J Clin Lab Invest 33:17–20, 1974.
531. Haigler ED Jr, Hershman JM, Pittman JA Jr, et al: Direct evaluation of pituitary thyrotropin reserve utilizing thyrotropin releasing hormone. J Clin Endocrinol Metab 33:573–581, 1971.
532. Azizi F, Vagenakis AG, Portnay GE, et al: Pituitary-thyroid responsiveness to intramuscular thyrotropin-releasing hormone based on analyses of serum thyroxine, triiodothyronine and thyrotropin concentration. N Engl J Med 292:273–277, 1975.
533. Haigler ED Jr, Hershman JM, Pittman JA Jr: Response to orally administered synthetic thyrotropin-releasing hormone in man. J Clin Endocrinol Metab 35:631–635, 1972.
534. Ormston BJ, Kilborn JR, Garry R, et al: Further observations on the effect of synthetic thyrotrophin-releasing hormone in man. BMJ 2:199–202, 1971.
535. Hershman JM, Kojima A, Friesen HG: Effect of thyrotropin-releasing hormone on human pituitary thyrotropin, prolactin, placental lactogen, and chorionic thyrotropin. J Clin Endocrinol Metab 36:497–501, 1973.
536. Jacobsen BB, Andersen H, Dige-Petersen H, et al: Thyrotropin response to thyrotropin-releasing hormone in fullterm, euthyroid and hypothyroid newborns. Acta Paediatr Scand 65:433–438, 1976.
537. Sanchez-Franco F, Garcia MD, Cacicedo L, et al: Influence of sex phase of the menstrual cycle on thyrotropin (TSH) response to thyrotropin-releasing hormone (TRH). J Clin Endocrinol Metab 37:736–740, 1973.
538. Harman SM, Wehmann RE, Blackman MR: Pituitary-thyroid hormone economy in healthy aging men: Basal indices of thyroid function and thyrotropin responses to constant infusions of thyrotropin releasing hormone. J Clin Endocrinol Metab 58:320–326, 1984.
539. Wilber J, Jaffer A, Jacobs L, et al: Inhibition of thyrotropin releasing hormone (TRH) stimulated thyrotropin (TSH) secretion in man by a single oral dose of thyroid hormone. Horm Metab Res 4:508, 1972.
540. Wartofsky L, Dimond RC, Noel GL, et al: Effect of acute increases in serum triiodothyronine on TSH and prolactin responses to TRH, and estimates of pituitary stores of TSH and prolactin in normal subjects and in patients with primary hypothyroidism. J Clin Endocrinol Metab 42:443–458, 1976.
541. Shenkman L, Mitsuma T, Suphavai A, et al: Triiodothyronine and thyroid-stimulating hormone response to thyrotrophin-releasing hormone: A new test of thyroidal and pituitary reserve. Lancet 1:111–113, 1972.
542. Anderson MS, Bowers CY, Kastin AJ, et al: Synthetic thyrotropin-releasing hormone: A potent stimulator of thyrotropin secretion in man. N Engl J Med 285:1279–1283, 1971.
543. McFarland KF, Strickland AL, Metzger WT, et al: Thyrotropin-releasing hormone test: An adverse reaction. Arch Intern Med 142:132–133, 1982.
544. Fleischer N, Lorente M, Kirkland J, et al: Synthetic thyrotropin releasing factor as a test of pituitary thyrotropin reserve. J Clin Endocrinol Metab 34:617–624, 1972.
545. Sachson R, Rosen SW, Cuatrecasas P, et al: Prolactin stimulation by thyrotropin-releasing hormone in a patient with isolated thyrotropin deficiency. N Engl J Med 287:972–973, 1972.
546. Vagenakis AG, Braverman LE, Azizi F, et al: Recovery of pituitary thyrotropic function after withdrawal of prolonged thyroid-suppression therapy. N Engl J Med 293:681–684, 1975.
547. Tamai H, Nakagawa T, Ohsako N, et al: Changes in thyroid function in patients with euthyroid Graves' disease. J Clin Endocrinol Metab 50:108–112, 1980.
548. Tamai H, Suematsu H, Ikemi Y, et al: Responses to TRH and T_3 suppression tests in euthyroid subjects with a family history of Graves' disease. J Clin Endocrinol Metab 47:475–479, 1978.
549. Stein RB, Nicoloff JT: Triiodothyronine withdrawal test—a test of thyroid-pituitary adequacy. J Clin Endocrinol Metab 32:127–129, 1971.
560. Mornex R, Berthezene F: Comments on a proposed new way of measuring thyrotropin (TSH) reserve. J Clin Endocrinol Metab 31:587–590, 1970.
551. Taunton OD, McDaniel HG, Pittman JA Jr: Standardization of TSH testing. J Clin Endocrinol Metab 25:266–277, 1965.
552. Burke G: The thyrotropin stimulation test. Ann Intern Med 69:1127–1139, 1968.
553. Hays MT, Solomon DH, Beall GN: Suppression of human thyroid function by antibodies to bovine thyrotropin. J Clin Endocrinol Metab 27:1540–1549, 1967.
554. Werner SC, Spooner M: A new and simple test for hyperthyroidism employing L-triiodothyronine and the twenty-four hour I-131 uptake method. Bull N Y Acad Med 31:137–145, 1955.
555. Duick DS, Stein RB, Warren DW, et al: The significance of partial suppressibility of serum thyroxine by triiodothyronine administration in euthyroid man. J Clin Endocrinol Metab 41:229–234, 1975.
556. Stanbury JB, Kassenaar AAH, Meijer JWA: The metabolism of iodotyrosines. I. The fate of mono- and di-iodotyrosine in normal subjects and in patients with various diseases. J Clin Endocrinol Metab 16:735–746, 1956.
557. Lissitzky S, Codaccioni JL, Bismuth J, et al: Congenital goiter with hypothyroidism and iodo-serum albumin replacing thyroglobulin. J Clin Endocrinol Metab 27:185–196, 1967.

558. DeGroot LJ: Kinetic analysis of iodine metabolism. J Clin Endocrinol Metab 26:149–173, 1966.
559. Hays MT: Absorption of oral thyroxine in man. J Clin Endocrinol Metab 28:749–756, 1968.
560. Hays MT: Absorption of triiodothyronine in man. J Clin Endocrinol Metab 30:675–677, 1970.
561. Valente WA, Goldiner WH, Hamilton BP, et al: Thyroid hormone levels after acute L-thyroxine loading in hypothyroidism. J Clin Endocrinol Metab 53:527–529, 1981.
562. Ain KB, Refetoff S, Fein HG, et al: Pseudomalabsorption of levothyroxine. JAMA 266:2118–2120, 1991.
563. Oppenheimer JH, Schwartz HL, Surks MI: Determination of common parameters of iodothyronine metabolism and distribution in man by noncompartmental analysis. J Clin Endocrinol Metab 41:319–324, 1172–1173, 1975.
564. Curti GI, Fresco GF: A theoretical five-pool model to evaluate triiodothyronine distribution and metabolism in healthy subjects. Metabolism 41:3–10, 1992.
565. Bianchi R, Mariani G, Molea N, et al: Peripheral metabolism of thyroid hormones in man. I. Direct measurement of the conversion rate of thyroxine to 3,5,3′-triiodothyronine (T_3) and determination of the peripheral and thyroidal production of T_3. J Clin Endocrinol Metab 56:1152–1163, 1983.
566. Faber J, Heaf J, Kirkegaard C, et al: Simultaneous turnover studies of thyroxine, 3,5,3′- and 3,3′,5-triiodothyronine, and 3′-monoiodothyronine in chronic renal failure. J Clin Endocrinol Metab 56:211–217, 1983.
567. Refetoff S, Fang VS, Marshall JS, et al: Metabolism of thyroxine-binding globulin (TBG) in man: Abnormal rate of synthesis in inherited TBG deficiency and excess. J Clin Invest 57:485–495, 1976.
568. Lim VS, Fang VS, Katz AI, et al: Thyroid dysfunction in chronic renal failure: A study of the pituitary-thyroid axis and peripheral turnover kinetics of thyroxine and triiodothyronine. J Clin Invest 60:522–534, 1977.
569. LoPresti JS, Warren DW, Kaptein EM, et al: Urinary immunoprecipitation method for estimation of thyroxine and triiodothyronine conversion in altered thyroid states. J Clin Endocrinol Metab 55:666–670, 1982.
570. Ridgway EC, Weintraub BD, Maloof F: Metabolic clearance and production rates of human thyrotropin. J Clin Invest 53:895–903, 1974.
571. Cuttelod S, Lemarchand-Beraud T, Magnenat P, et al: Effect of age and role of kidneys and liver on thyrotropin turnover in man. Metabolism 23:101–113, 1974.
572. Cavalieri RR, Searle GL: The kinetics of distribution between plasma and liver of ^{131}I-labeled L-thyroxine in man: Observations of subjects with normal and decreased serum thyroxine-binding globulin. J Clin Invest 45:939–949, 1966.
573. Oppenheimer JH, Bernstein G, Hasen J: Estimation of rapidly exchangeable cellular thyroxine from the plasma disappearance curves of simultaneously administered thyroxine-^{131}I and albumin-^{125}I. J Clin Invest 46:762–777, 1967.
574. Delitala G, Devilla L, Lotti G: Domperidone, an extracerebral inhibitor of dopamine receptors, stimulates thyrotropin and prolactin release in man. J Clin Endocrinol Metab 50:1127–1130, 1980.
575. Vagenakis AG, Wang CA, Burger A, et al: Iodide-induced thyrotoxicosis in Boston. N Engl J Med 287:523–527, 1972.
576. Martino E, Safran M, Aghini-Lombardi F, et al: Environmental iodine intake and thyroid dysfunction during chronic amiodarone therapy. Ann Intern Med 101:28–34, 1984.
577. Faglia G, Ambrosi B, Beck-Peccoz P, et al: The effect of theophylline on plasma thyrotropin response (HTSH) to thyrotropin releasing factor (TRF) in man. J Clin Endocrinol Metab 34:906–909, 1972.
578. Gaffney TE, Braunwald E, Kahler RL: Effects of guanethidine on triiodothyronine induced hyperthyroidism in man. N Engl J Med 265:16–20, 1961.
579. Lee WY, Bronsky D, Waldstein SS: Studies of thyroid and sympathetic nervous system interrelationships. II. Effect of guanethidine on manifestations of hyperthyroidism. J Clin Endocrinol Metab 22:879–885, 1962.
580. Ain KB, Mori Y, Refetoff S: Reduced clearance of thyroxine-binding globulin (TBG) with increased sialylation: A mechanism for estrogen induced elevation of serum TBG concentration. J Clin Endocrinol Metab 65:689–696, 1987.
581. Doe RP, Mellinger GT, Swaim WR, et al: Estrogen dosage effects on serum proteins: A longitudinal study. J Clin Endocrinol Metab 27:1081–1086, 1967.
582. Draper MW, Flowers DE, Neild JA, et al: Antiestrogenic properties of raloxifene. Pharmacology 50:209–217, 1995.
583. Anker GB, Lonning PE, Aakvaag A, et al: Thyroid function in postmenopausal breast cancer patients treated with raloxifene. Scand J Lab Clin Invest 58:103–107, 1998.
584. Dowling JT, Frienkel N, Ingbar SH: The effect of estrogens upon the peripheral metabolism of thyroxine. J Clin Invest 39:1119–1130, 1974.
585. Gross HA, Appelman MD, Nicoloff JT: Effect of biologically active steroids on thyroid function in man. J Clin Endocrinol Metab 33:242–248, 1971.
586. Graham RL, Gambrell RD: Changes in thyroid function tests during danazol therapy. Obstet Gynecol 55:395–397, 1980.
587. Austen FK, Rubini ME, Meroney WH, et al: Salicylates and thyroid function. I. Depression of thyroid function. J Clin Invest 37:1131–1143, 1958.
588. Wolff J, Austen FK: Salicylates and thyroid function. II. The effect on the thyroid-pituitary interrelation. J Clin Invest 37:1144–1165, 1958.
589. Woeber KA, Barakat RM, Ingbar SH: Effects of salicylate and its noncalorigenic congeners on the thyroidal release of ^{131}I in patients with thyrotoxicosis. J Clin Endocrinol Metab 224:1163–1168, 1964.
590. Chopra IJ, Solomon DH, Chua Teco GN, Nguyen AH: Inhibition of hepatic outer ring monodeiodination of thyroxine and 3,3′,5′-triiodothyronine by sodium salicylate. Endocrinology 106:1728–1734, 1980.
591. Alexander WD, Johnson KWM: A comparison of the effects of acetylsalicylic acid and DL-triiodothyronine in patients with myxoedema. Clin Sci 15:593–600, 1956.
592. Yamamoto T, Woeber KA, Ingbar SH: The influence of salicylate on serum TSH concentration in patients with primary hypothyroidism. J Clin Endocrinol Metab 34:423–426, 1972.
593. Christensen K: The metabolic effect of *p*-aminosalicylic acid. Acta Endocrinol 31:608–610, 1959.
594. MacGregor AG, Somner AR: The antithyroid action of para-amino salicylic acid. Lancet 2:931–936, 1954.
595. Gemstedt A, Jarnerot A, Kagedal B, et al: Corticosteroids and thyroid function. Acta Med Scand 205:379–383, 1979.
596. Ingbar SH: The effect of cortisone on the thyroidal and renal metabolism of iodine. Endocrinology 53:171–181, 1953.
597. Samuels MH, McDaniel PA: Thyroptrophin levels during hydrocortisone infusions that mimic fasting-induced cortisol elevations: A clinical research study. J Clin Endocrinol Metab 82:3700–3704, 1997.
598. Benoit FL, Greenspan FS: Corticoid therapy for pretibial myxedema. Observations on the long-acting thyroid stimulator. Ann Intern Med 66:711–720, 1967.
599. Yamada T, Ikejiri K, Kotani M, et al: An increase of plasma triiodothyronine and thyroxine after administration of dexamethasone to hypothyroid patients with Hashimoto's thyroiditis. J Clin Endocrinol Metab 46:784–790, 1978.
600. Cavalieri RR, Gavin LA, Wallace A, et al: Serum thyroxine, free T_4, triiodothyronine, and reverse-T_3 in diphenylhydantoin treated patients. Metabolism 28:1161–1165, 1979.
601. Surks MI, DeFesi CR: Normal serum free thyroid hormone concentrations in patients treated with phenytoin or carbamazepine, a paradox resolved. JAMA 275:1495–1498, 1996.
602. Blackshear JL, Schultz AL, Napier JS, et al: Thyroxine replacement requirements in hypothyroid patients receiving phenytoin. Ann Intern Med 99:341–359, 1983.
603. Schou M, Amdisen A, Jensen S, et al: Occurrence of goitre during lithium treatment. BMJ 2:710–713, 1968.
604. Hullin R: The place of lithium in biological psychiatry. *In* Johnson F, Johnson S (eds): Lithium in Medical Practice. Lancaster, MTP, 1978, p 433.
605. Pallisgaard G, Frederiksen P: Thyrotoxicosis in patients treated with lithium carbonate for mental disease. Acta Med Scand 204:141–143, 1978.
606. Barclay M, Brownlie B, Turner J, et al: Lithium associated thyrotoxicosis: A report of 14 cases, with statistical analysis of incidence. Clin Endocrinol 40:759–764, 1994.
607. Schorderet M: Lithium inhibition of cyclic AMP accumulation induced by dopamine in isolated retinae of the rabbit. Biochem Pharmacol 26:167–170, 1977.
608. Joffe R, Kutcher S, MacDonald C: Thyroid function and bipolar affective disorders. Psychiatry Res 25:117–121, 1988.
609. Lazarus JH: The effect of lithium on the iodide concentrating mechanism in the mouse salivary gland. Acta Pharmacol Toxicol 43:55–58, 1978.
610. Leppalnoto J, Mannisto P, Virkkumen P: On the mechanism of goitre formation during lithium treatment in the rat. Acta Endocrinol 74:296–306, 1973.
611. Bagchi N, Brown T, Mack R: Studies on the mechanism of inhibition of thyroid function by lithium. Biochim Biophys Acta 542:163–169, 1978.
612. Bhattacharya B, Wolff J: Stabilisation of microtubules by lithium ion. Biochem Biophys Res Commun 73:383–390, 1976.
613. Voss C, Shober H, Hartmann N: Einfluss von Lithium auf die in vitro Dejodierung von L-thyroxine in der Rattenleber. Acta Biol Med Ger 36:1061–1065, 1977.
614. Blomquist N, Lindstedt G, Lundberg P, et al: No inhibition by lithium of thyroxine monodeiodination to 3,5,3′-triiodothyronine and 3,3′,5′-triiodothyronine (reverse triiodothyronine). Clin Chim Acta 79:457–464, 1977.
615. Singer I, Rotenberg D: Mechanisms of lithium action. N Engl J Med 289:254–260, 1973.
616. Stefanski E, Argiolas A, Gessa G, et al: Effect of lithium on dopamine uptake by brain synaptosomes. J Neurochem 26:443–445, 1976.
617. Geisler A, Klysner R: Influence of lithium and dopamine stimulated adenylate cyclase activity on rat brain. Life Sci 23:635–636, 1978.
618. Hesketh J, Nicolaou N, Arbuthnott G, et al: The effect of chronic lithium administration on dopamine metabolism in rat striatum. Psychopharmacology 56:163–166, 1978.
619. Schwartz HL, Kozyreff V, Surks MI, et al: Increased deiodination of L-thyroxine and L-triiodothyronine by liver microsomes from rats treated with phenobarbital. Nature 221:1262–1263, 1969.
620. Murchison LE, How J, Bewsher PD: Comparison of propranolol and metoprolol in the management of hyperthyroidism. Br J Clin Pharmacol 8:581, 1979.
621. How ASM, Khir AN, Bewsher PD: The effect of atenolol on serum thyroid hormones in hyperthyroid patients. Clin Endocrinol 13:299–302, 1980.
622. Cutting WC, Rytand DA, Tainter ML: Relationship between blood cholesterol and increased metabolism from dinitrophenol and thyroid. J Clin Invest 13:547–552, 1934.
623. Goldberg RC, Wolff J, Greep RO: The mechanism of depression of plasma protein-bound iodine by 2,4-dinitrophenol. Endocrinology 56:560–566, 1955.
624. Lardy HA, Wellman H: Oxidative phosphorylations: Role of inorganic phosphate and acceptor systems in control of metabolic rates. J Biol Chem 195:215–224, 1952.
625. Escobar del Rey F, Morreale de Escobar G: Studies on the peripheral disappearance of thyroid hormone. IV. The effect of 2,4-dinitrophenol on the ^{131}I distribution in thyroidectomized, L-thyroxine maintained rats, 24 hours after the injection of ^{131}I-labeled L-thyroxine. Acta Endocrinol 29:161–175, 1958.
626. Cutting CC, Tainter ML: Comparative effects of dinitrophenol and thyroxine on tadpole metamorphosis. Proc Soc Exp Biol Med 31:97–100, 1933.
627. Morley JE: Neuroendocrine control of thyrotropin secretion. Endocr Rev 2:396–436, 1981.
628. Kaptein EM, Spencer CA, Kamiel MB, et al: Prolonged dopamine administration and thyroid hormone economy in normal and critically ill subjects. J Clin Endocrinol Metab 51:387–393, 1980.
629. Kobberling J, Darrach A, Del Pozo E: Chronic dopamine receptor stimulation using bromocriptine: Failure to modify thyroid function. Clin Endocrinol 11:367–370, 1979.
630. Samuels MH, Kramer P: Effects of metoclopramide on fasting-induced TSH suppression. Thyroid 6:85–89, 1996.
631. Heinen E, Herrmann J, Konigshausen T, et al: Secondary hypothyroidism in severe non-thyroidal illness. Horm Metab Res 13:284–288, 1981.

632. Weintraub BD, Gershengorn MC, Kourides IA, et al: Inappropriate secretion of thyroid stimulating hormone. Ann Intern Med 95:339–351, 1981.
633. Wartofsky L, Ransil B, Ingbar S: Inhibition by iodine of the release of thyroxine from the thyroid glands of patients with thyrotoxicosis. J Clin Invest 49:78–86, 1970.
634. Grubeck-Loebenstein B, Kleiber M: The influence of iodide upon thyroxine metabolism in euthyroid subjects (abstract). Acta Endocrinol 94(suppl 234):21, 1980.
635. McGregor A, Weetman A, Ratanachaiyavov S, et al: Iodine: An influence on the development of autoimmune thyroid disease. *In* Hall R, Kobberling J (eds): Thyroid Disorder Associated with Iodine Deficiency. New York, Raven, 1985, p 209.
636. Sundik R, Hergeden D, Brown T: The incorporation of dietary iodine into thyroglobulin increased its immunogenicity. Endocrinology 120:2078–2080, 1987.
637. Braverman L, Woeber K, Ingbar S: Induction of myxedema by iodine in patients euthyroid after radioiodine or surgical treatment of diffuse toxic goitre. N Engl J Med 281:816–821, 1969.
638. Fradkin J, Walff J: Iodine-induced thyrotoxicosis. Medicine (Baltimore) 62:1–20, 1983.
639. Cavalieri R, Pitt-Rivers R: The effects of drugs on the distribution and metabolism of thyroid hormones. Pharmacol Rev 33:55–79, 1981.
640. Martin FI, Tress BW, Colman PG, et al: Iodine-induced hyperthyroidism due to nonionic contrast radiography in the elderly. Am J Med 95:78–82, 1993.
641. Chopra I: Inhibition of outer ring monodeiodination of T_4 and reverse T_3 (rT_3) by some radiocontrast agents (abstract). Clin Res 26:303, 1978.
642. Obregon M, Pascual A, Mallol J, et al: Marked decrease of the effectiveness of a T_4 dose in iopanoic acid treated rats (abstract). Ann Endocrinol 40:72, 1979.
643. Suzuki H, Kadena N, Takeuchi K, et al: Effects of three day oral cholecystography on serum iodothyronines and TSH concentrations. Acta Endocrinol 92:477–488, 1979.
644. Beng C, Wellby M, Symons R, et al: Effect of ipodate on serum iodothyronine patterns in normal subjects. Acta Endocrinol 93:175–178, 1980.
645. Felicetta JV, Green WL, Nelp WB: Inhibition of hepatic binding of thyroxine by cholecystographic agents. J Clin Invest 65:1032–1040, 1980.
646. DeGroot LJ, Rue PA: Roentgenographic contrast agents inhibit triiodothyronine binding to nuclear receptors in vitro. J Clin Endocrinol Metab 49:538–542, 1979.
647. Vrobel T, Miller P, Mostow N, et al: A general overview of amiodarone toxicity: Its prevention, detection, and management. Prog Cardiovasc Dis 31:393–426, 1989.
648. Melmed S, Nademanee K, Reed A, et al: Hyperthyroxinemia with bradycardia and normal thyrotroph secretion after chronic amiodarone administration. J Clin Endocrinol Metab 53:997–1001, 1981.
649. Sogol P, Hershman J, Reed A, et al: The effects of amiodarone on serum thyroid hormones and hepatic thyroxine 5′-monodeiodination in rats. Endocrinology 113:1464–1469, 1983.
650. Hershman J, Nademanee K, Sugawara M, et al: Thyroxine and triiodothyronine kinetics in cardiac patients taking amiodarone. Acta Endocrinol 3:193–199, 1986.
651. Martino E, Safran M, Aghini-Lombardi F: Environmental iodine intake and thyroid dysfunction during chronic amiodarone therapy. Ann Intern Med 101:28–34, 1984.
652. Bartlena L, Brogoni S, Grasso L, et al: Treatment of amiodarone-induced thyrotoxicosis, a difficult challenge: Result of a prospective study. J Clin Endocrinol Metab 81:2930–2933, 1996.
653. Singh B: Amiodarone: Historical development and pharmacologic profile. Am Heart J 106:788–797, 1983.
654. Georges JL, Normand JP, Lenormand ME, et al: Life-threatening thyrotoxicosis induced by amiodarone in patients with benign heart disease. Eur Heart J 13:129–132, 1992.
655. Hauptman PJ, Fyfe B, Mechanick J, et al: Fatal hyperthyroidism after amiodarone treatment and total lymphoid irradiation in a heart transplant recipient [published erratum appears in J Heart Lung Transplant 1993 Jul-Aug;12:572]. J Heart Lung Transplant 12:513–516, 1993.
656. Roti E, Minelli R, Gardini E, et al: Thyrotoxicosis followed by hypothyroidism in patients treated with amiodarone. Arch Intern Med 153:886–892, 1993.
657. Fernandez-Soto L, Gonzalez A, Escobar-Jimenez F, et al: Increased risk of autoimmune thyroid disease in hepatitis C vs hepatitis B before, during and after discontinuing interferon therapy. Arch Intern Med 158:1445–1448, 1998.
658. Amenomori M, Mori T, Fukuda Y, et al: Incidence and characteristics of thyroid dysfunction following interferon therapy in patients with chronic hepatitis C. Intern Med 37:246–252, 1998.
659. Koh LK, Greenspan FS, Yeo PP: Interferon-alpha induced thyroid dysfunction: Three clinical presentations and a review of the literature. Thyroid 7:891–896, 1997.
660. Schuppert F, Rambusch E, Kirchnwer H, et al: Patients treated with interferon-alpha, interferon-beta, and interleukin-2 have a different autoantibody pattern than patients suffering from endogenous thyroid disease. Thyroid 7:837–842, 1997.
661. Krouse RS, Yoral RE, Heywood G, et al: Thyroid dysfunction in 281 patients with metastatic melanoma or renal carcinoma treated with interleukin-2 alone. J Immunother 18:272–278, 1995.
662. Corssmit EP, Heyligenberg R, Endert E, et al. Acute effects of interferon-alpha on thyroid hormone metabolism in healthy men. J Clin Endcorinol Metab 80:3140–3144, 1995.

Chapter 98

Thyroid Imaging

Ralph R. Cavalieri ▪ Manfred Blum

Several techniques yield clinically useful images of the thyroid gland, including radioisotope scintiscanning, sonography, computed tomography (CT), and magnetic resonance imaging (MRI). Each of these methods provides unique information. The radioisotope scintiscan yields a "function" map. The others provide various kinds of anatomic data. Although each type of imaging modality can answer specific diagnostic questions, any imaging procedure may be unnecessary and may even be misleading when used indiscriminately or inappropriately.

This chapter will discuss how the various thyroid imaging techniques can be integrated into patient management. As a basic principle, thyroid imaging should be used only when needed to arrive at a diagnosis and to assist in planning therapy. Imaging procedures should not be used for the purpose of "screening." Nor should they be done before the clinical history has been taken, a physical examination performed, and a differential diagnosis formulated. They should be used together with other laboratory data to answer specific diagnostic questions. Selection of the proper procedure is predicated on an understanding of the disease under consideration and an awareness of the known capabilities and limitations of the techniques. Imaging tests are not efficient in assessing the presence of cancer in a thyroid nodule. Furthermore, it is essential to precisely correlate the results of palpation with the image. Rarely is more than one imaging modality required to solve a problem. When the information obtained from an imaging examination is inadequate and a different type of imaging is required, the several images should be correlated to optimize their diagnostic value.

RADIOISOTOPE SCINTISCANNING (SCINTIGRAPHY)

Scintigraphy provides information about the *functional* anatomy of an organ. When scintigraphy is applied to the thyroid gland, the resulting image, by showing the pattern of distribution of radioiodine or pertechnetate, reveals the location and volume of functioning thyroid tissue and answers the question of whether a particular nodule is functioning. Thyroid scintiscanning is not to be confused with thyroid radioiodine uptake testing. The latter is a quantitative measure of the function of the entire gland in trapping and retaining iodine.

Common clinical indications for thyroid scintigraphy are listed in Table 98–1. In the assessment of a hyperthyroid patient with a single or multinodular goiter, scintigraphy provides information that no other imaging modality offers, namely, whether a nodule or nodules are the source of the hyperthyroidism.

Radionuclides Used in the Diagnosis of Thyroid Disorders

Several radionuclides can be used for imaging the thyroid (Table 98–2). The choice depends in part on the clinical question to be addressed. Of the isotopes of iodine, ^{123}I is close to an ideal agent both for imaging and for determining thyroid uptake. ^{123}I exposes the gland to relatively low radiation doses.[1,2] The commonly administered activity (orally) of ^{123}I for imaging the thyroid ranges from 200 to 600 μCi (7.4–22 MBq). ^{123}I images of the gland may be obtained any time between 4 hours and 24 hours after administration.

Technetium-99m (^{99m}Tc) in the form of pertechnetate is trapped by the thyroid gland and other sites that concentrate iodide (salivary glands, gastric mucosa), but it is not organified in the thyroid and is therefore not a true tracer of iodine metabolism.[1] The radiation exposure to the thyroid from ^{99m}Tc is even lower than that from ^{123}I. ^{99m}Tc is readily available in all nuclear medicine laboratories and is relatively inexpensive. ^{99m}Tc-pertechnetate is administered intravenously in amounts ranging from 2 to 10 mCi (74–370 MBq), and imaging of the thyroid is usually begun 15 to 30 minutes after injection.[2]

^{123}I and ^{99m}Tc have largely replaced ^{131}I for thyroid scintigraphy. Radiation exposure to the thyroid from ^{131}I per microcurie administered is 100-fold higher than that from ^{123}I, and ^{131}I-labeled images of the gland are generally inferior in quality because of the high γ energy of ^{131}I. The principal diagnostic use of ^{131}I is in whole-body scanning to search for functioning metastases that are potentially treatable with ^{131}I in patients who have had thyroid cancer surgery. The 8-day half-life of ^{131}I permits scanning over a period of several days and allows for dosimetry in preparation for ^{131}I therapy.

TABLE 98–1. Clinical Indications for Thyroid Scintigraphy

Clinical Setting	Purpose of Scintigraphy
1. Hyperthyroid patient with or without a goiter (diffuse or nodular)	To determine function of palpable nodule(s)
	To detect unsuspected cold nodule(s) in a diffusely hyperfunctioning gland
	To distinguish Graves' disease from toxic nodular goiter or other causes of thyrotoxicosis (e.g., destructive thyroiditides)
	To estimate volume of a functional gland before ^{131}I therapy
2. Euthyroid patient with a	
Solitary nodule ("follicular neoplasm" on FNA)	To determine whether the nodule is hyperfunctional
Multinodular goiter	To identify hypofunctional nodule(s) before FNA
	To estimate the volume and location of functional tissue in planning surgery or ^{131}I therapy
3. Patient suspected of having an ectopic thyroid	To identify a mass as functioning thyroid tissue (e.g., substernal goiter, lingual thyroid)
4. Patient who has had thyroid surgery for cancer	To define the amount of thyroid remnant (usually combined with whole-body scintigraphy)

FNA, fine-needle aspiration.
Data from Cavalieri and McDougall[1] and Becker et al.[2]

TABLE 98–2. Radionuclides Used in Thyroid Scintigraphy

Radionuclide/Chemical Form	Physical Half-Life	Type of Emission	Clinical Applications
^{123}I-iodide	13 hr	Gamma	Thyroid scintigraphy (planar or SPECT)
^{131}I-iodide	8 days	Gamma and beta	Whole-body scintigraphy (posttreatment for thyroid cancer) Radioiodine therapy
^{99m}Tc-pertechnetate	6 hr	Gamma	Thyroid scintigraphy
^{99m}Tc-sestamibi*	6 hr	Gamma	Localization of thyroid cancer metastases
^{201}Tl-Cl$^-$	77 hr	Gamma	Localization of thyroid cancer metastases
^{18}F-fluorodeoxyglucose (FDG)	110 min	Positron	Localization of thyroid cancer metastases

*Other radioactive agents that have been used for localizing metastases from thyroid cancer include ^{99m}Tc-tetrofosmin and ^{99m}Tc-labeled dimercaptosuccinic acid (DMSA) (V). Medullary thyroid carcinoma has been imaged with ^{99m}Tc-DMSA (V) and ^{111}In-octreotide (reviewed by Sisson[19]).

SPECT, single-photon emission computed tomography.

Scintiscanning Instrumentation

In most nuclear medicine laboratories the scintillation camera has largely replaced the rectilinear scanner for thyroid imaging. The camera is fitted with a pinhole collimator, which provides a magnified image of the gland and yields higher resolution than that obtained with a parallel-hole collimator or rectilinear scanner[3] (Fig. 98–1). The pinhole technique permits oblique views of the gland, which is an advantage in detecting posterior nodules, but accurate estimation of gland size is not possible. When dealing with thyroid nodules, it is important to correlate the image with the palpable lesion by placing radioactive spot markers on the skin overlying or adjacent to the nodule. Particular care must be taken when placing radioactive markers because parallax errors are possible with the pinhole method and, in the case of small nodules (<1 cm), skin markers may even be misleading.

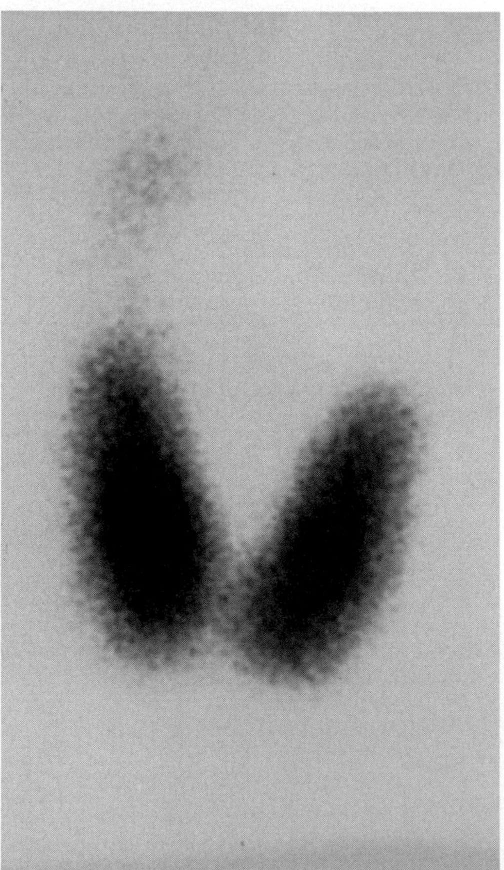

FIGURE 98–1. Scintiscan of the thyroid in a 72-year-old patient with Graves' hyperthyroidism. This image was obtained with a pinhole collimator 6 hours after oral administration of 200 μCi ^{123}I. Thyroid uptake was 24% at 6 hours. Note the diffuse pattern of ^{123}I distribution throughout the gland. The faint activity extending superiorly from the right lobe is a pyramidal lobe.

Rectilinear scanners provide life-size images and allow more accurate placement of markers (over nodules), but the resolution is not as high as that produced by a camera with a pinhole collimator.[3]

Whole-body scintiscans, obtained by using either a scintillation camera or a rectilinear scanner and a special scanning table, are used in surveys for thyroid cancer metastases that involve the administration of ^{131}I or other radiolabeled agents.

Single-photon emission computed tomography (SPECT), which is widely used in nuclear medicine, provides three-dimensional images or tomographic slices through the organ of interest. When used with either ^{99m}Tc or ^{123}I, SPECT of the thyroid has an advantage over other methods of scintigraphy (including the pinhole technique) in defining the function of small nodules that may be obscured by overlying normal thyroid tissue.[4] SPECT is also useful for estimating the volume of functioning thyroid and for identifying thyroid tissue in ectopic sites, such as the substernal area.

Positron emission tomography (PET) requires special tomographic equipment capable of imaging the high-energy γ-rays produced by positron-emitting radionuclides (e.g., ^{18}F and ^{124}I).

Patient Preparation

The patient need not be fasting on the morning of the study. Patients are asked about medications and dietary items that interfere with thyroid radioiodine uptake. When the uptake of radioiodine is low for any reason, the quality of the image is impaired. The most common interfering substances are radiographic contrast dyes and drugs that contain iodine. Thyroid hormone in any form reduces thyroid radioiodine uptake, except when autonomously functioning thyroid tissue is present. Because the administration of radioactive materials is contraindicated during pregnancy and breast-feeding, these aspects of the history should be included in the preliminary interview, when appropriate.

Diagnostic Applications of Thyroid Scintigraphy

THE SOLITARY THYROID NODULE. The terms "cold" and "hot" are commonly used to describe the functional activity of thyroid nodules as revealed by scintigraphy. These descriptors refer to the apparent amount of radionuclide in the lesion relative to that in surrounding normal thyroid tissue. Nearly all malignant tumors in the gland and most benign nodules concentrate less radioiodine or ^{99m}Tc than the normal gland does and therefore appear "cold" (hypofunctional). In general, a cold nodule must be at least 0.5 to 1 cm in diameter to be detected by pinhole imaging. The term "warm" is ambiguous and not helpful because such a lesion may in fact be a cold nodule that is too small to be distinguishable from surrounding normal thyroid.

A "hot" nodule is one that takes up relatively more radionuclide than adjacent tissue; specifically, it is hyperfunctional (Fig. 98–2).

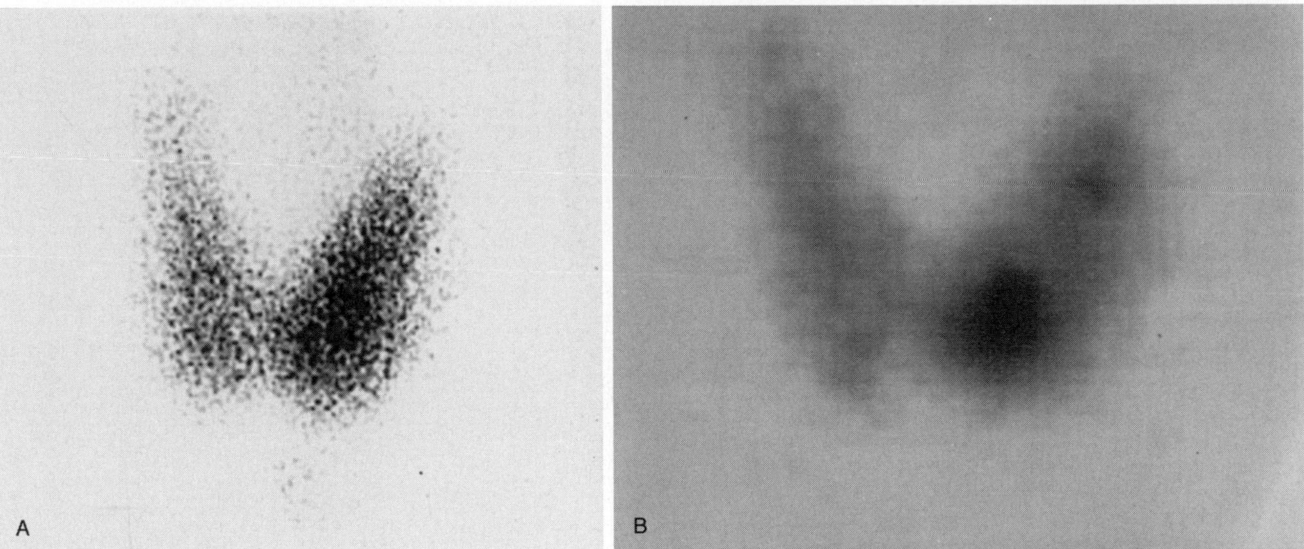

FIGURE 98–2. Thyroid scintiscans in a mildly hyperthyroid patient (suppressed serum thyroid-stimulating hormone, borderline-high free thyroxin and triiodothyronine levels) with a palpable 1.5-cm solitary nodule in the lower portion of the left thyroid lobe. *A*, Pinhole image showing that most of the ^{123}I uptake is in the lower pole of the left lobe, which corresponds to the palpable nodule. *B*, Single-photon emission computed tomographic (SPECT) image showing a more clearly delineated hyperfunctioning nodule in the lower pole and two smaller (nonpalpable) foci of uptake in the upper portion of the left lobe. Both pinhole and SPECT images were obtained 6 hours after administration of ^{123}I (200 μCi). The diagnosis was multiple autonomously functioning nodules.

Nodules that function autonomously (i.e., independent of thyroid-stimulating hormone [TSH]) may over time grow large enough to lead to hyperthyroidism ("toxic" nodule) with suppression of normal paranodular tissue because of low TSH levels.[5] In some cases a hyperfunctioning nodule undergoes degeneration or hemorrhage and becomes hypofunctioning.

Because the great majority of solitary nodules are "cold" on radioisotope scintiscanning and such "cold" nodules may be either benign or malignant, it is not cost effective to obtain a scintiscan as the initial diagnostic test in a euthyroid patient with a solitary nodule. A fine-needle aspiration (FNA) biopsy is usually performed first. However, when the FNA result indicates a "follicular neoplasm," scintigraphy may be helpful if the nodule is "hot."

The chance of malignancy in a "hot" nodule is less than 1%.[1] Some of the reported instances are in fact cases of small coexisting carcinomas in close proximity to a larger, benign hot nodule. Although documented cases have been reported in which the entire hot nodule is malignant, these cases are quite rare. Occasionally, follicular neoplasms (including follicular adenomas and even some carcinomas) may appear hot on a ^{99m}Tc-pertechnetate image but cold on a radioiodine image, presumably because such tumors are able to trap but do not organify iodine. This type of discordance between ^{99m}Tc and radioiodine images occurs infrequently and should not discourage the use of ^{99m}Tc for thyroid scintiscanning.[5–7]

MULTINODULAR GOITER. Scintiscanning has a role in the assessment of multinodular goiter in euthyroid or hyperthyroid patients. When the nodules are discrete and larger than 1 to 2 cm in diameter, the scintiscan reveals the functional activity of a particular nodule relative to that of paranodular tissue (Fig. 98–3). When a nodule is clinically dominant, that is, a nodule that on palpation is different from the others or is growing faster, the finding on scintiscan that this nodule contains all or most of the functional activity helps guide management in that such a nodule is unlikely to be malignant. When a multinodular goiter is large and causing symptoms and signs of compression of the trachea or esophagus, scintiscanning may complement other imaging modalities such as MRI or sonography. Either of the latter two methods depicts the full extent of the goitrous mass, but only scintiscanning can reveal functioning tissue, information that is often helpful in making therapeutic decisions, such as surgery or ^{131}I therapy.

On the other hand, in a hyperthyroid patient with a goiter consisting of many functioning, widely dispersed nodules, none larger than 0.5 cm, scintiscanning is likely to show a diffusely "patchy" or a uniform pattern of uptake not unlike that of Graves' disease. Clearly, in this case, differentiation must be made by other means. When thyroid uptake is low, the scintigraphic image may also show a "patchy" distribution of radioisotope. Scintiscanning by itself does not reveal the etiology of the goiter. In a *hypo*thyroid patient with either a diffuse or nodular goiter, scintigraphy is rarely of any value.

SUBSTERNAL GOITER. A substernal goiter is suspected when chest radiographs or CT reveals an anterior mediastinal mass. A

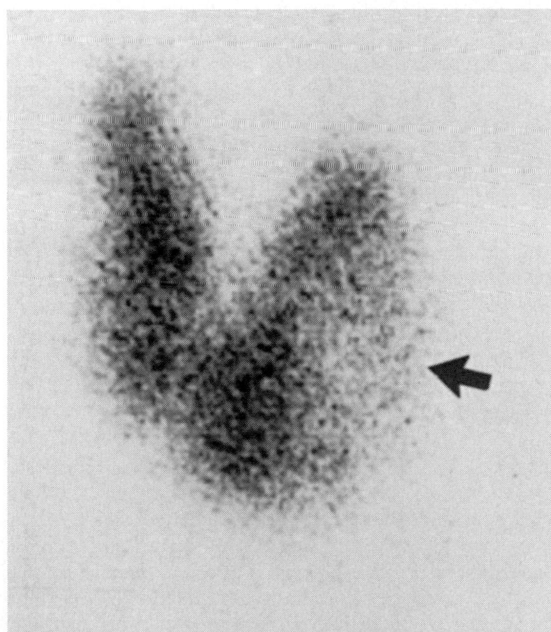

FIGURE 98–3. Anterior pinhole scintiscan of a multinodular goiter in a euthyroid patient. Physical examination revealed many firm nodules with the largest nodule (2×3 cm) in the left lobe. The image, obtained 24 hours after administration of 250 μCi ^{123}I (thyroid uptake, 23%), shows the left lobe nodule to be cold *(arrow)*. A functioning nodule is seen in the isthmus. Surgical excision of the gland showed all nodules to be mixed solid/cystic and benign.

positive radioiodine scintigram definitively identifies such a mass as thyroid tissue. ^{123}I is preferred over ^{99m}Tc in such cases because of interference by circulating ^{99m}Tc in the mediastinal blood vessels. SPECT (using ^{123}I) is of particular value in visualizing substernal thyroid tissue.

SCINTIGRAPHY IN PATIENTS WITH THYROID CARCINOMA. Although in general thyroid carcinoma takes up and retains radioiodine much less efficiently than normal thyroid tissue does, under the stimulation of elevated TSH levels, the uptake in differentiated thyroid carcinoma is often sufficiently high to permit detection by scintigraphy and therapy with ^{131}I. Thus diagnostic imaging with radioiodine is indicated for patients who have recently undergone thyroid surgery for differentiated thyroid carcinoma. The rationale for imaging in such patients is to identify and quantify uptake in the thyroid remnant and to detect any functioning metastases in the neck or in distant sites. This information helps determine the amount of ^{131}I that should be administered to ablate the normal remnant and treat functioning metastases.

To stimulate uptake of radioiodine by malignant thyroid tissue, it is necessary to raise serum TSH levels to 30 mU/L or higher.[7] In routine practice levothyroxine therapy is discontinued for 5 to 6 weeks before administration of the diagnostic dose of radioiodine for imaging. To shorten the period of hypothyroidism, liothyronine (triiodothyronine [T_3]) is often given (50 μg/day in divided doses) for 3 weeks after discontinuation of levothyroxine therapy. T_3 therapy is discontinued 2 weeks before radioiodine administration. Alternatively, patients may be instructed to take one half their usual dosage of thyroid hormone for 6 weeks, until TSH levels reach 30 μU/mL or above.

Recently, recombinant human TSH (rhTSH, Thyrogen, Genzyme Corp., Cambridge, MA) has been developed and in clinical trials has been shown to stimulate uptake of ^{131}I by thyroid remnants and metastases and to raise serum thyroglobulin (Tg) levels in patients who remain euthyroid while taking thyroid hormone therapy.[8, 9] The Food and Drug Administration has recently approved the use of rhTSH for radioiodine imaging and serum Tg testing in such patients.

Patients scheduled to undergo diagnostic whole-body scintigraphy are advised to follow a low iodine diet for 7 to 10 days before administration of the radioiodine. A simple low iodine diet has been described.[10] It is even more important to avoid iodine-containing medications and radiographic contrast agents.

The "Stunning" Effect. Diagnostic administration of ^{131}I may reduce the uptake of subsequent therapeutic ^{131}I by normal thyroid remnants or functioning metastases. This phenomenon, which has been termed "stunning," seems to involve a sublethal, presumably temporary suppression of iodine uptake (reviewed elsewhere[11, 12]). To avoid stunning, many authors recommend limiting the quantity of ^{131}I given for diagnostic imaging to 2 mCi (74 MBq)[11, 13] or even less.[14] An alternative is to use ^{123}I for whole-body imaging,[15] but the present cost of this radionuclide in millicurie amounts is prohibitive for many centers.

Physicians who interpret whole-body radioiodine scintigrams must be familiar with normal sites of uptake, which include the salivary glands, gastric mucosa, and large bowel. Nasal secretions, saliva, sweat, and urine, which contain high concentrations of radioiodine, can cause artifacts. Nonthyroid tumors, inflammatory lesions, and cysts may occasionally concentrate radioiodine and result in false-positive scintigrams.[11, 16]

^{131}I scanning is not 100% sensitive for metastatic thyroid carcinoma. In some series the rate of false-negative radioiodine scans approaches 35%.[17] When diagnostic ^{131}I scans are negative and metastases are suspected on the basis of elevated serum Tg levels, some advocate empiric treatment with ^{131}I. Scans done after ^{131}I therapy are frequently positive in these cases (reviewed by Clark and Hoelting[18]) (Fig. 98–4). The approach that we favor in ^{131}I scan–negative, Tg-positive patients is to search for metastases by performing sonography of the neck and, if negative, performing MRI or CT of the neck and chest. The aim is to find metastases that are either surgically accessible or can be treated by external radiotherapy, if appropriate. When the above imaging techniques do not reveal a source of the elevated Tg, scintiscanning with other radiolabeled agents may succeed in localizing ^{131}I-negative metastases[19] (see Table 101–2).

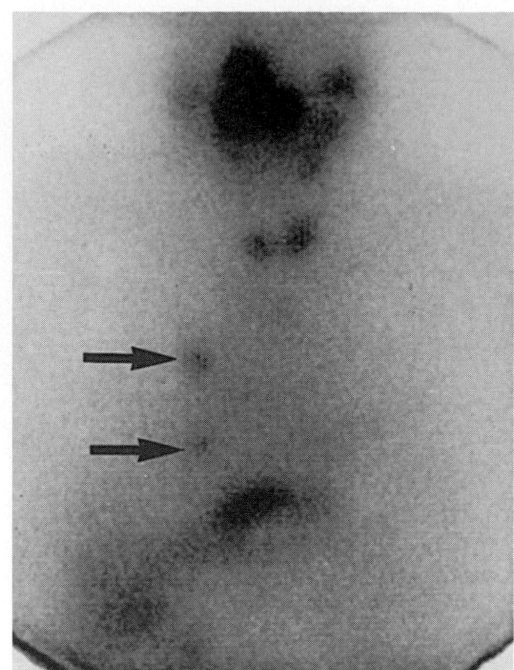

FIGURE 98–4. *Anterior scintiscan of head, neck, chest, and upper part of the abdomen in a male patient who 72 hours previously had received 212 mCi ^{131}I as therapy for follicular thyroid carcinoma metastatic to the lung. The image shows intense activity in the nose, mouth, and salivary glands; small right and left thyroid lobe remnants; two discrete foci of uptake in the right side of the chest (arrows) corresponding to small lung nodules seen on computed tomography; and physiologic radioiodine in the stomach and bowel. The liver is faintly visualized, a common finding in posttherapy scintiscans with no pathologic significance.*

Thallium (^{201}Tl) has been useful in localizing metastases in selected patients (reviewed by Cavalieri[12] and Sisson[19]). However, ^{201}Tl is concentrated by a variety of benign and malignant lesions other than thyroid carcinoma.

^{99m}Tc-sestamibi (MIBI) is a cationic, lipophilic agent that concentrates in normal and neoplastic thyroid tissue and in a variety of other cancers. Experience indicates that like ^{201}Tl, ^{99m}Tc-MIBI may be useful in ^{131}I-negative patients in whom one has reason to suspect persistent or recurrent tumor.[19, 20] ^{99m}Tc-MIBI is the agent of choice for imaging Hürthle cell carcinoma, which typically takes up radioiodine poorly.[21]

Other agents that have been shown to concentrate in some metastatic differentiated thyroid tumors are ^{99m}Tc-tetrofosmin, which like MIBI is a myocardial perfusion imaging agent, and ^{99m}Tc-labeled dimercaptosuccinic acid in the pentavalent form (DMSA [V]) (reviewed by Sisson[19]). Clinical experience with these agents is still limited. Indium-111–labeled octreotide is used to localize metastatic medullary thyroid carcinoma.[22]

^{18}Fluoro-2-Deoxyglucose Positron Emission Scanning. ^{18}F-fluoro-2-deoxyglucose (^{18}FDG), a radiolabeled analogue of glucose, is actively concentrated in a variety of malignant tumors, including thyroid carcinoma.[23] ^{18}FDG uptake tends to be higher in thyroid tumors that are less well differentiated. For this reason, ^{131}I-negative tumors are more often positive with ^{18}FDG, and ^{18}FDG-negative tumors tend to be positive with ^{131}I.[23] ^{18}FDG-PET scans show low background in the chest and liver, which gives this agent a relative advantage over ^{201}Tl and ^{99m}Tc-MIBI.

NONISOTOPIC THYROID IMAGING TESTS

The nonisotopic thyroid imaging tests consist of sonography, CT, and MRI. Sonography reveals how the tissue transmits and/or reflects sound waves, CT is a computerized analysis of the relative density of tissues to x-rays, and MRI depicts the response of hydrogen atoms to a magnetic field. Both CT and MRI provide sectional images that can be electronically assembled in perpendicular planes. None of these techniques are a substitute for histopathology, and none differentiates benign and malignant lesions.

Sonography (Echography)

Sonography is efficiently used to elucidate cryptic findings on physical examination, identify the solid component of a complex nodule for guiding FNA, determine the comparative size of nodules in patients who are under observation, detect small nodules in patients who were exposed to therapeutic irradiation of the head or neck, and evaluate for recurrence of thyroid cancer after surgery, particularly in cervical lymph nodes.

TECHNICAL ASPECTS. Sonography uses high-frequency sound waves (ultrasound) in the megahertz range to produce a photographic image of the internal structure of the thyroid gland and its region.[24, 25] No ionizing radiation is involved, nor is iodinated contrast material given. Sonography is safe; tissue damage has not been reported, and it is less costly than other imaging procedures. Preparation of the patient for the procedure is unnecessary, and it is performed without discontinuing TSH suppressive therapy. To image the thyroid gland and surrounding regions, the patient's neck is examined in the sagittal, transverse, and oblique planes with a probe, called a transducer, that both generates the sound energy and receives the reflected signal. The sound enters the body and is transmitted or reflected by interfaces within the tissues. Air does not transmit ultrasound, and calcified areas block its passage. The images are produced quickly and assembled electronically in "real time." Each frame of the sonogram shows a static image, and sequential pictures depict motion. Swallowing is used to elevate the thyroid to examine the lower pole of an enlarged lobe, and this maneuver may facilitate identification of the esophagus. With the use of a signal having a frequency of 7.5 to 10 MHz, thyroid nodules and lymphadenopathy as small as 2 to 3 mm are identified in shades of gray. Dynamic information such as blood flow is added by using physics principles called the Doppler effect.[26] The signals are translated into colors to differentiate static fluid-filled cystic spaces and blood flowing through the vasculature. Thus the direction and velocity of flow and the degree of vascularity are revealed. Color is assigned to the signal by assuming that venous flow is parallel to but in the opposite direction to arterial flow. Arterial signals are made red and the accompanying venous signals blue. The shade of a color is proportional to the direction of flow as it relates to the transducer and flow velocity.

Routine protocols for ultrasound scanning by a technologist are not satisfactory. Rather, the ultrasound operator must be experienced and aware of the clinical question that has been posed to provide an appropriate answer. Close supervision by a sonographer-physician who is expert in physical examination is needed.

SONOGRAPHY OF THE NORMAL THYROID GLAND AND ENVIRONS. With standard gray-scale technique, the normal thyroid gland has a homogeneous appearance like ground glass (Fig. 98–5). The surrounding muscles are of lower echogenicity. Tissue planes are identified. The air-filled trachea, which does not transmit the ultrasound signal, is poorly imaged and its calcified tracheal ring is represented anteriorly by dense echoes. The carotid artery and other blood vessels are echo-free unless calcified. Lateral and anterior to the carotid arteries is the jugular vein, which is frequently collapsed and can be identified when it is distended during a Valsalva maneuver. Small blood vessels on the surface of the thyroid and the inferior thyroid artery and vein may sometimes be seen. Color Doppler enhances the identification of blood vessels and flow. The esophagus is sometimes detected behind the thyroid and left of center, anteromedial to the longus colli muscle. It can be observed to distend with swallowing. Lymph nodes can be seen normally as less than 1 × 3-mm, elliptical, uniform structures with an echo-dense central hilum. The parathyroid glands are not visualized unless they are enlarged. They are less dense to ultrasound than the thyroid gland because of the absence of iodine.

Generally, imaging procedures are not useful in patients whose thyroid gland is normal to palpation unless the patient has a history of exposure to therapeutic irradiation in youth or if metastatic thyroid cancer has been discovered and a primary lesion in the gland is being sought. However, in selected circumstances, an ultrasound image may be used to supplement or confirm physical examination findings and identify the size and shape of regional structures accurately and relatively inexpensively. This test is useful when thyroid anatomy is in question but clinical perception is confused by obesity, great muscularity, distortion by abnormal adjacent structures, tortuous blood vessels, a prominent thyroid cartilage, metastatic tumor, lymphadenopathy, prior surgery, or examiner inexperience. On the other hand, the sonogram is so sensitive that many small nonpalpable thyroid nodules may be detected. Management of these nodules, which are called incidentalomas, requires mature clinical judgment. Objective diagnostic evaluation of all of them is needless and impractical. Selective attention to those that are found in a patient with a high risk of cancer and those with special characteristics or that grow is prudent. Neglecting all of them is inappropriate and occasionally dangerous.

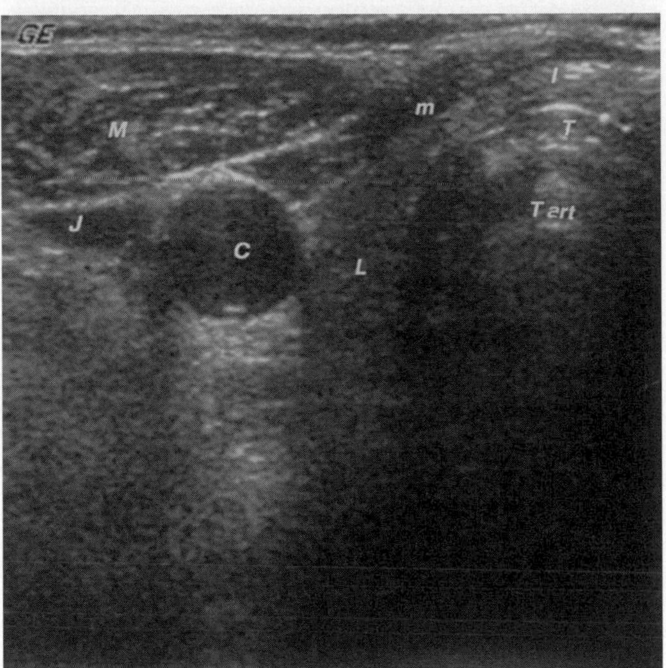

FIGURE 98–5. Sonogram of the neck in the transverse plane showing a normal right thyroid lobe and isthmus. C, carotid artery (note the enhanced echoes deep to the fluid-filled blood vessel); I, isthmus; J, jugular vein; L, thyroid lobe; M, sternocleidomastoid muscle; m, strap muscles; T, anterior portion of the tracheal ring (the dense white arc is calcification); T art, artifact in the trachea.

SONOGRAPHY WITH THYROID ENLARGEMENT (GOITER). Enlargement of the thyroid gland is common. In general terms, enlargement may be diffuse and symmetrical, asymmetrical, smooth and uniform, or nodular. It is not generally necessary to obtain a sonogram to confirm thyroid enlargement unless a specific question has attracted clinical concern. Such questions may involve a dominant nodule, a tender spot, focal hardness, or substernal extension. At times a physician may obtain a sonogram to explain a cryptic finding, such as differentiating goiter from fat or muscle, documenting a controversial observation, estimating the size of the thyroid gland for ^{131}I dosimetry, or assessing volume changes in response to suppressive therapy with thyroid hormone. Sonography has been used in population studies to objectively identify thyroid enlargement as a screen for iodine deprivation.

Sonography can show alterations of the echo pattern of the thyroid gland and its size. Cystic and/or hemorrhagic degeneration, which is depicted by an echo-free zone, is common (Fig. 98–6). These findings are not specific for any particular type of pathology. However, sonography can identify one region in a uniform goiter whose echo pattern is different from the rest of the goiter, which is suggestive of a focal

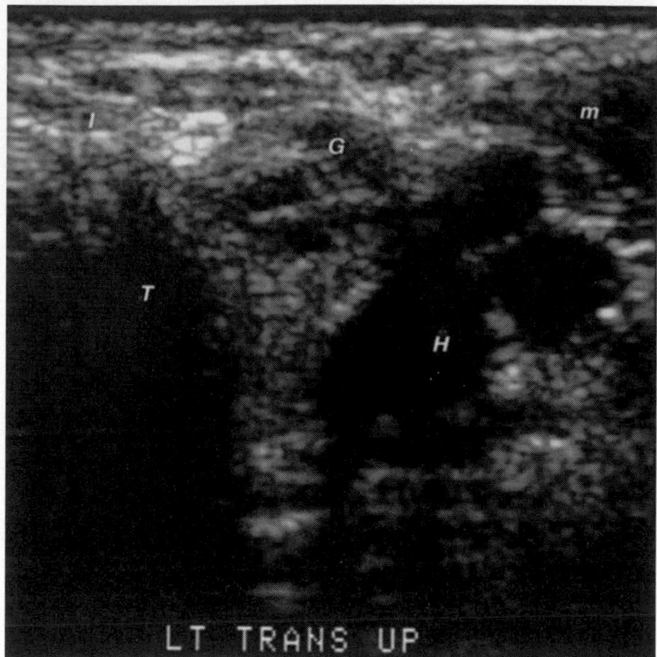

FIGURE 98–6. Sonogram of the left lobe of the thyroid gland in the transverse plane showing a degenerated multinodular goiter. G, heterogeneous goiter; H, hemorrhagic/cystic degenerated area; I, region of lobe adjacent to the enlarged isthmus; m, sternocleidomastoid muscle; T, trachea.

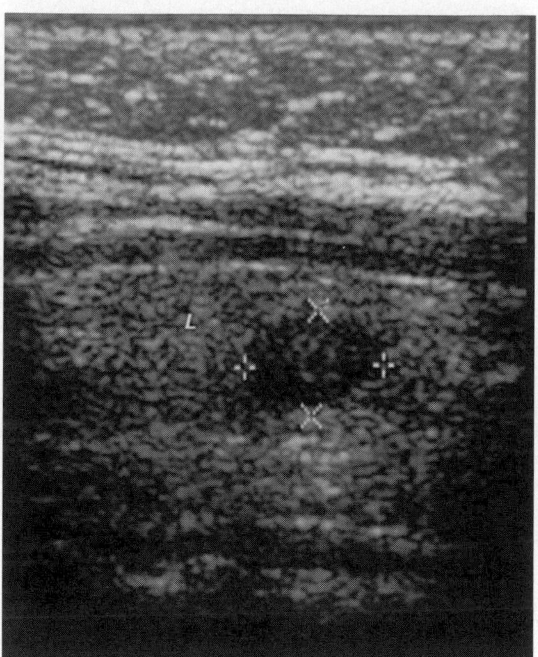

FIGURE 98–7. Sonogram of the right lobe of the thyroid gland in the longitudinal plane from a 33-year-old, 235-lb woman. The serum contained high titers of antithyroid antibodies. The thyroid gland was difficult to palpate, and examiners could not agree on the findings. Therefore, a sonogram was done. It shows a 7.7 × 10.0-mm nodule (× and + symbols) that is less echo dense than the rest of the thyroid lobe. Fine-needle aspiration biopsy demonstrated and surgery confirmed papillary carcinoma. L, thyroid lobe.

lesion, especially if that focus is surrounded by a distinctive rim or halo.

SONOGRAPHY IN PATIENTS WITH THYROIDITIS AND GRAVES' DISEASE. The greatest value of ultrasonography in patients with immune or inflammatory thyroid disease is to identify incidental focal lesions. However, because most focally distinct zones in these glands are not neoplastic, the need for their subsequent management requires judgment. In situations in which localized firm consistency, focal enlargement, or pain call attention to a part of Graves' or Hashimoto's goiter, a sonogram may demonstrate a region that has a distinctive appearance for accurate aspiration biopsy (Fig. 98–7).

Sonography may demonstrate an image of the thyroid gland that highly correlates with subacute thyroiditis, Hashimoto's thyroiditis, and Graves' disease, but such correlation is of limited practical diagnostic importance. Several types of thyroiditis show reduced echogenicity. During the active phase of subacute thyroiditis, the echogram is characterized by a severely reduced echo density of the thyroid gland that returns to a normal pattern with healing.[27] Some patients with Hashimoto's thyroiditis have low echogenicity (see Fig. 98–7). Marcocci et al. reported that only 44 of 238 (18.5%) patients with autoimmune thyroiditis had diffuse hypoechogenicity, especially when they were hypothyroid.[28] Graves' disease goiters and a few goiters without thyroid autoantibodies have a similar appearance. In Graves' disease, color Doppler imaging can detect diffuse hyperemia in the thyroid gland,[29] a condition that has been called a "thyroid inferno."[30] Increased flow velocity in hyperthyroid patients has been demonstrated with duplex Doppler techniques.[31] However, neither the sensitivity nor the specificity of these observations is known.

SONOGRAPHY OF THE THYROID NODULE. Thyroid nodules are identified by sonography because they distort the uniform echo pattern or the shape of the gland. Most nodules have a less dense appearance than normal thyroid tissue does. Most of the remainder are more echogenic, and isoechogenicity is less common. Some nodules have a sonolucent rim called a halo. Nodules may contain regions of calcium (Fig. 98–8) that are extremely echo dense. The echo texture within a small nodule tends to be uniform, but nodules larger than 2.5 cm usually have irregular zones free of echoes. These areas represent cystic and/or hemorrhagic degeneration that may occur in benign or malignant nodules (see Fig. 98–6). Such nodules are called complex. Careful examination of echo-free zones is necessary to discern internal echoes that represent septa or small solid regions that differentiate common, complex "*cystic*" nodules and a true thyroid *cyst*. A cyst is

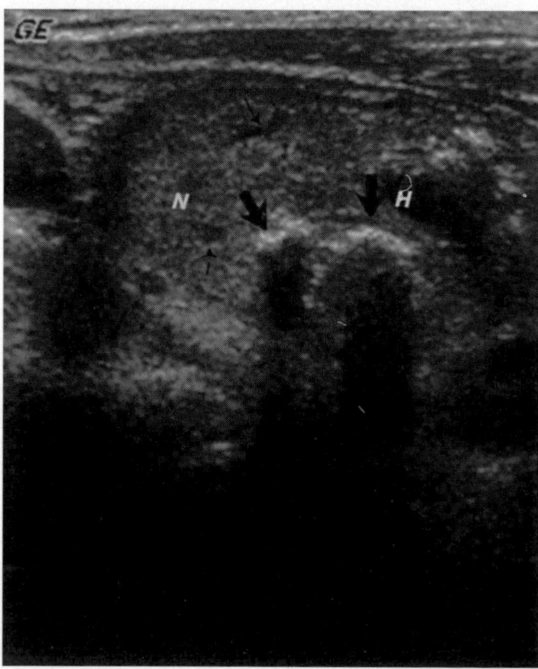

FIGURE 98–8. Sonogram of the neck in the longitudinal plane showing a large nodule. The *small arrows* point to echo-free zones that Doppler examination identified as small blood vessels. The *thick straight arrows* point to calcifications. Note that passage of the ultrasound signal distal to the calcium is blocked in a linear fashion and is creating an artifact. H, hemorrhagic/cystic degenerated area; N, nodule.

encountered once in approximately 500 to 1000 nodules and is globular shaped, smooth walled, and without internal echoes.

The prevalence of palpable thyroid nodules in members of the general population who are screened by palpation is 1.5% to 6.4%.[32] It is 10-fold greater when they have been screened by ultrasonography.[33] The prevalence of sonographically detectable nodules increases with age to around 50% in older adults. The risk of malignancy of palpable nodules is 5% to 15%, and in ultrasonically detected nonpalpable nodules the risk is smaller.[34]

The ultrasonic appearance of a nodule cannot reliably differentiate benign lesions and cancer.[35] Cancers may be minute or large, entirely solid or complex. As a group, malignancies tend to be rather hypoechoic.[36, 37] However, most benign nodules are also of low echo density. Nevertheless, it can be said that hyperdense nodules are probably not cancerous. Deposits of calcium may be seen in benign or malignant nodules. Frequently, large irregular plaques or egg-shell calcifications are found, and because benign nodules are more common than malignant ones, these concretions do not correlate with cancer. In distinction, punctate calcifications or microcalcifications are not common in nodules and reportedly have high specificity for thyroid cancer (95.2%) but low sensitivity (59.3%) and a diagnostic accuracy of 83.8%.[36] They may represent psammoma bodies in papillary cancer. A halo around a nodule is thought to represent a boundary, capsule, or vasculature that may be seen in benign or malignant conditions.[36, 37]

SONOGRAPHY IN PATIENTS WITH A DOMINANT PALPABLE NODULE IN A GOITER. Improved technology has permitted the detection of thyroid nodules as small as 2 mm, which can be the source of problems.[34] Approximately 20% of all adults have nonpalpable micronodules that are of indeterminate significance, usually benign, and of no clinical consequence in most patients (Figs. 98–9 to 98–11). Their discovery, usually by sonography of the neck but sometimes by CT or MRI during an investigation of cervical vascular or neurologic pathology or during thyroid sonography for a palpable thyroid nodule, may occasion needless expense, concern, and therapy. However, rarely, one of these lesions represents occult thyroid cancer and could become a clinically significant malignancy.[38] Therefore, a micronodule, or "incidentaloma," should not be dismissed simply for reasons of cost-effectiveness, as some authorities have suggested. Overreaction and surgery are not suitable either. Rather, yearly reassessment seems appropriate. However, it remains for future investigation to determine the value of periodic sonography in examining for changes in the size or characteristics of a nodule, as well as the benefit, if any, of suppressive therapy with thyroid hormone.

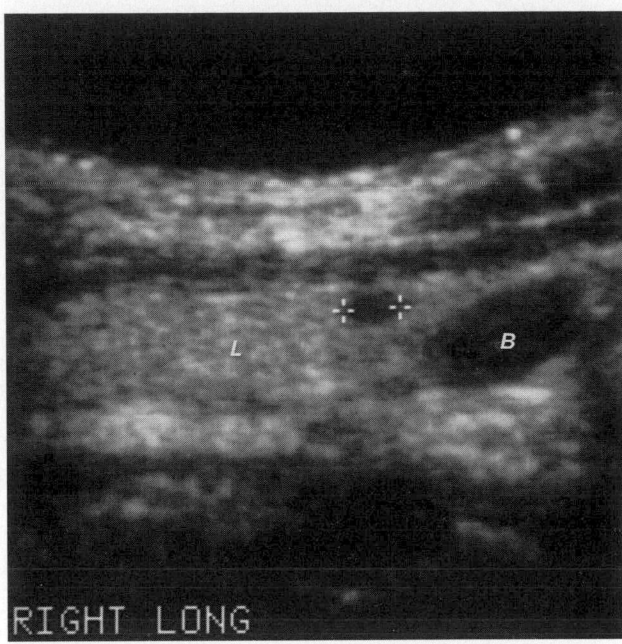

FIGURE 98–10. Sonogram of the right thyroid lobe in the longitudinal plane from a 51-year-old man with a history of radiation therapy in youth. A hypoechoic, 5.2-mm nodule (+ +) is located in the lower pole of the lobe, just above the level of the thoracic inlet. B, blood vessel demonstrated by Doppler examination; L, thyroid lobe.

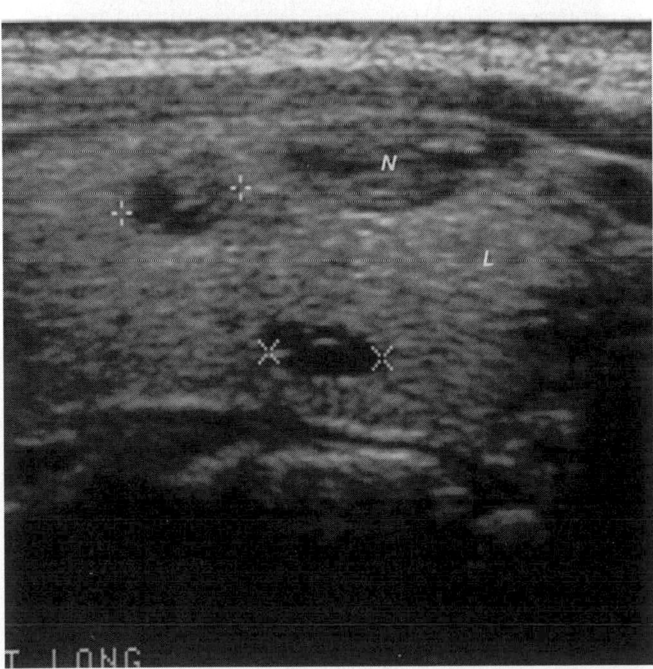

FIGURE 98–9. Sonogram of the right lobe of the thyroid gland in the longitudinal plane from a 44-year-old woman with one palpable nodule in the right thyroid lobe. The sonogram shows two nonpalpable micronodules (+ +, 6.8 mm; x x, 6.5 mm). L, thyroid lobe; N, palpable nodule.

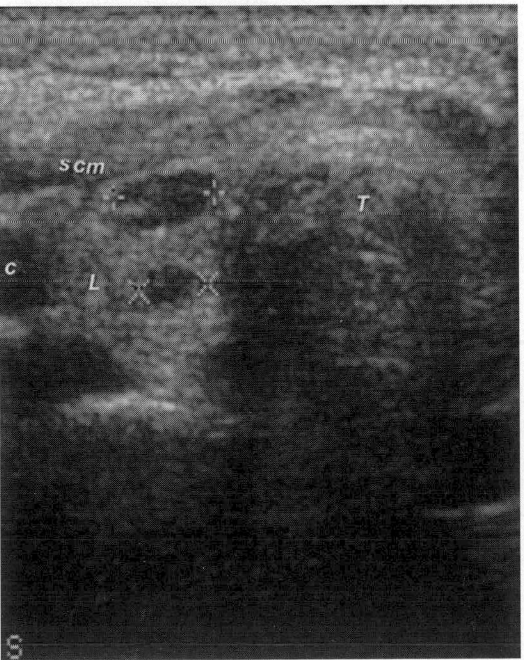

FIGURE 98–11. Sonogram of the left lobe of the thyroid gland in the longitudinal plane showing two hypoechoic micronodules (+ +, 7.1 mm; x x, 4.8 mm) that represent tumor in the contralateral thyroid lobe after partial thyroidectomy for papillary thyroid cancer. C, carotid artery; L, thyroid lobe; scm, sternocleidomastoid muscle, T, artifact in the tracheal region.

It is common when a solitary nodule is palpable for sonography to demonstrate micronodules in the rest of the thyroid (see Fig. 98–9). This occurrence has the same pathologic significance as a dominant nodule in a patient with clinical multinodular goiter. FNA biopsy and cytology of the dominant nodule appear to be the most cost-effective approach.

SONOGRAPHY OF LYMPHADENOPATHY. Ultrasonography may be useful to diagnose and monitor lymphadenopathy in patients, especially if they have thyroid cancer or a history of therapeutic irradiation in youth. However, one must be mindful that even in cancer patients, enlarged benign nodes are more common than malignant ones.

Consensus is growing that the shape of benign lymph nodes tends to be a thin oval whereas malignant ones are "plump" and rounded (Fig. 98–12), but differences in size or homogeneity are not reliable indicators of pathology. Solbiati et al. evaluated 291 lymph nodes in 143 patients before thyroid cancer surgery and reported that the ultrasonic characteristics of lymph nodes correlated with the histologic findings.[39] A ratio of longitudinal diameter to transverse diameter of less than 1.5 was reported in 62% of metastatic nodes and a ratio of greater than 2 in 79% of reactive nodes.[39] The absence of a nodal hilus was observed in 44% of malignant lesions but in only 8% of benign nodes.[40] Thus ultrasound can detect head and neck cancer metastases to cervical nodes with a sensitivity of 92.6%.[41] It is not clear whether additional information about lymphadenopathy may be offered by color and spectral Doppler studies.[42]

SONOGRAPHY IN PATIENTS WITH A HISTORY OF THERAPEUTIC IRRADIATION IN YOUTH. Patients with a history of therapeutic irradiation in youth may have a risk of thyroid cancer that is as high as 30%. Therefore, some clinicians use sonography to screen irradiated people for tiny thyroid nodules before a mass becomes palpable. However, in the process, many more benign nodules are found than malignancies. The inefficiency of the selection process and the indolence of thyroid cancer have resulted in continuing controversy about the clinical relevance of sonographic identification of nodules and subsequent management. The approach to which the authors subscribe is to obtain potentially useful baseline anatomic information but not act on it unless studies at intervals reveal changes or other circumstances arise that heighten suspicion of malignancy.

SONOGRAPHY TO MONITOR CHANGES IN THYROID SIZE. In a patient with thyroid disease, sonography can accurately and objectively assess the size of the thyroid gland or a nodule during the course of therapy or the emergence of a new nodule.[43] Because growth of a nodule may be difficult to perceive clinically, sonography may be useful in this context. Furthermore, inasmuch as most patients change doctors over the years, objective assessment of thyroid size greatly facilitates continuity of care. Comparison of serial records even with different equipment may demonstrate changes in the thyroid gland or in a nodule and lead to a change in treatment earlier than palpation alone would warrant.

SONOGRAPHY IN PATIENTS WITH KNOWN THYROID CANCER. Sonography is useful in the management of a patient with thyroid carcinoma[44] and has became the most frequently used imaging procedure in patients who have had either a partial or a complete thyroidectomy. After a hemithyroidectomy, the procedure will detect even nonpalpable nodules in the contralateral lobe or lymphadenopathy that could represent tumor (see Fig. 98–11). In these patients and also in those who have undergone a total (or near-total) thyroidectomy, sonography done without interrupting thyroid hormone therapy will detect recurrent carcinoma either in the thyroid bed or in lymph nodes before the mass has grown sufficiently large to be palpable[44] (see Fig. 98–12). Sonography is particularly useful in searching for a nonpalpable malignant lesion in a patient who has had a thyroidectomy when periodic assessment has disclosed an elevated Tg concentration. Another circumstance in which sonography is effective is in detecting an occult primary thyroid tumor in a patient with known metastases of thyroid origin and a thyroid gland that is normal by examination.

SONOGRAPHY IN CONJUNCTION WITH NEEDLE BIOPSY. In an attempt to enhance the utility of FNA biopsy, sonographic guidance has been used in selected circumstances to minimize sampling errors[45] (Fig. 98–13). Ultrasound guidance for needle biopsy is generally reserved for (1) unusually deep nodules, particularly in an obese, muscular, or large-framed patient; (2) very small nodules; (3) nonpalpable nodules; (4) ultrasonically detected incidentalomas that are associated with cancer risk factors; (5) complex degenerated nodules if a prior aspiration has not been diagnostic; and (6) nonpalpable adenopathy.[46, 47] A special transducer to guide the needle is available but is cumbersome and not required. It is easier to explore the thyroid area of the neck with a hand-held transducer to locate the nodule and then insert the needle into the lesion under direct vision from another angle. The success rate is low for nodules that are smaller than 8 mm. Generally, correlation of the anatomy with the sonographic film without guided puncture is less costly and adequate for nodules that are palpable unless a prior aspiration has been unsuccessful.

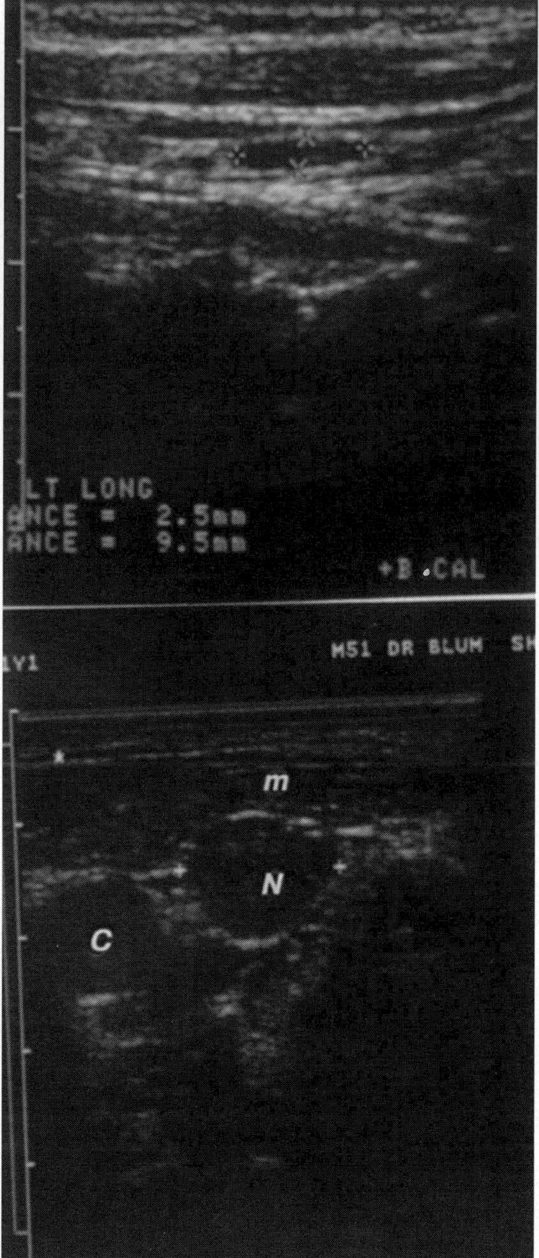

FIGURE 98–12. Sonograms showing lymphadenopathy. *Upper panel,* Sonogram in the longitudinal plane from a patient who had a thyroidectomy. A benign, thin elliptical, 2.5×9.5-mm lymph node (+ + and xx) is present. *Lower panel,* Sonogram of the left side of the neck from a 51-year-old muscular man who had a thyroidectomy because of papillary thyroid carcinoma. The sonogram disclosed a nonpalpable "plump" 13-mm lymph node that was involved with metastatic cancer. The thyroid lobe is absent. C, carotid artery; m, muscle; N, pathologic lymph node.

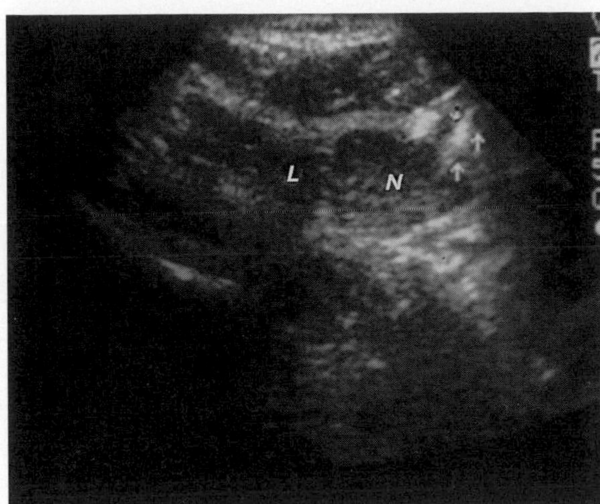

FIGURE 98–13. Sonogram of the right lobe of the thyroid gland in the transverse plane from a patient who is having fine-needle aspiration biopsy of an 8×11-mm nodule. The *arrows* point to the tip of the needle in the nodule. L, thyroid lobe; N, nodule.

Sectional Imaging: Computed Tomography and Magnetic Resonance Imaging

CT and MRI are computer-assisted sectional imaging techniques that may be used to accurately define the regional anatomy of the neck and superior mediastinum, but they are expensive to perform.[48, 49] Although these tests are not usually required in the diagnosis of a patient with a thyroid nodule or goiter, they can be useful in selected cases to answer specific clinical questions that cannot be addressed by sonography.

COMPUTED TOMOGRAPHY. CT images are a reconstruction of a computer-assisted analysis of multiple x-rays of a region. Standard CT represents discontinuous thin slices through an anatomic region, and spiral CT provides a continuous assemblage of pictures.

In CT of the neck, the thyroid gland is distinctive in that it is relatively more radiopaque than the rest of the soft tissues of the neck because of its high iodine content. The thyroid is homogeneous except for regions of enhanced or reduced density that correspond to nodules, cysts, hemorrhage, and calcification. It is clear that sonography is far more sensitive than CT in detecting millimeter-sized nodules. To precisely define the gland for clinical purposes, the regional vasculature must be enhanced by the intravenous administration of iodinated contrast material, which is a major limitation to subsequent management when CT is used for thyroid diagnosis.[50, 51]

MAGNETIC RESONANCE IMAGING. MRI images are generated by computer-produced analysis of the interaction of electromagnetic waves of a specific frequency and the hydrogen atoms in a patient's body. To perform the test, the person must be housed within a magnetic field. Special properties of the hydrogen atoms can be selectively emphasized by varying the magnetic field. The two properties that are conventionally used in MRI are termed T1 and T2. Because the hydrogen atoms of various tissues have specific T1 and T2 properties, differences between "T1-weighted" and "T2-weighted" images can be used to identify the thyroid gland, skeletal muscle, blood vessels, or lymph nodes.[52] The quality and diagnostic value of MRI are enhanced by the intravenous administration of noniodinated contrast agents such as gadolinium-labeled diethylenetriamine pentaacetic acid (DTPA) or by electronically repressing a relatively unique signal derived from fat (short τ inversion recovery [STIR]). As with CT, MRI is not as sensitive as sonography in detecting small nodules.

In general, normal thyroid tissue tends to be slightly more intense than muscle on a T1-weighted image, and thyroid tumor usually appears even more intense, or brighter.[53] Although differences in the MRI characteristics of malignant and benign thyroid tissue have been suggested as a result of investigations in vitro,[53] the distinctions have rarely proved to be of clinical value.

DISTINCTIONS BETWEEN COMPUTED TOMOGRAPHY AND MAGNETIC RESONANCE IMAGING. The relative clinical utility of CT and MRI in thyroid disease has not been examined critically and is controversial. However, one of us (M.B.) is persuaded that when additional imaging is needed to supplement thyroid sonography, MRI is preferred and CT should be used only when specifically needed. The major advantages of MRI are that ionizing radiation and iodinated contrast agents are not required. MRI seems to provide better spatial resolution, and reports have suggested superior differentiation of postoperative scar from recurrent tumor.[54, 55] The use of MRI has been limited by discomfort for a claustrophobic patient, considerable noise, long test time, great demand for the equipment for other types of examinations, relatively high cost, and incompatibility with pacemakers or ferrous prostheses. New "open" MRI systems address some of these problems but provide inferior images. CT is more sensitive in detecting small metastases to lymph nodes[56] and the lungs.[57, 58] The total examination time for CT is shorter than that for MRI, and access to CT scanners outside major centers is superior.

Sectional Imaging in Clinical Management

Sectional imaging is too expensive and insufficiently specific to be useful in the initial diagnosis of the usual thyroid nodule or goiter. MRI or CT becomes necessary only when the results of physical examination and ultrasonography are inadequate to answer a clinical question about anatomy.

When CT is needed, alteration of thyroid function by iodine contrast material is a serious issue. If the patient has not had a thyroidectomy, the excessive iodide may cause hyperthyroidism, including cardiac arrhythmias, or may cause hypothyroidism, depending on the underlying thyroid condition. In patients with thyroid cancer who may need an ^{131}I whole-body scan or therapy, the excess iodine will delay diagnosis or therapy. Therefore, radioiodine studies should precede contrast-enhanced CT. In patients who are taking suppressive therapy and in whom contrast-enhanced CT is required, it is best to continue administration of thyroid hormone for several days after the contrast-enhanced CT to keep TSH suppressed while the dye is excreted. The radiologist and clinician must discuss these aspects before the performance of contrast-enhanced CT and consider a non–contrast-enhanced study, which may be adequate to answer the clinical question. Iodinated dye is not used for MRI examinations, which is a distinct advantage.

A preoperative sectional imaging examination is useful for a thyroid nodule or goiter only for special situations to supplement information from a sonogram. These situations include circumstances in which the clinical examination demonstrates a thyroid or extrathyroid mass that is fixed to surrounding tissues, when an unusually large mass is obstructing the thoracic inlet and impinging on other structures or extending substernally, when tracheal compression or invasion is noted, when evaluating substernal or retrotracheal extension for a possible transthoracic surgical approach, and as a surgical guide for palliation when the sonogram suggests that total excision is precluded.[59]

Although sonography is the primary imaging procedure for assessing patients after thyroid cancer surgery, sectional imaging is useful if recurrence has been demonstrated. The major uses in these patients are to confirm recurrent thyroid cancer when the sonogram is equivocal, detect lymphadenopathy in regions where sonography is technically unsatisfactory such as the mediastinum or near bone, investigate suspected invasion, and evaluate cryptic findings. For instance, after radical surgery, sectional imaging may be required to distinguish whether a palpable deep mass is tumor or part of a vertebra. It has been claimed that after postoperative edema, infection, or bleeding has resolved, recurrent thyroid carcinoma may be differentiated from scarring with MRI.[60]

At times, thyroid lesions are incidentally detected as part of CT or MRI examinations for cervical spine, vascular, or neurologic disease, as is also true of incidentalomas discovered by sonography. They provide no unique diagnostic problem but sometimes engender undue anxiety.

REFERENCES

1. Cavalieri RR, McDougall IR: In vivo isotopic tests and imaging. *In* Braverman LE, Utiger RD (eds): The Thyroid: A Fundamental and Clinical Text, ed 7. Philadelphia, JB Lippincott, 1996, pp 352–376.
2. Becker DV, Charkes ND, Dworkin H, et al: Procedure guideline for thyroid scintigraphy: 1.0. J Nucl Med 37:1264–1266, 1996.
3. Sostre S, Ashare AB, Quinones JD, et al: Thyroid scintigraphy: Pinhole images vs. rectilinear scans. Radiology 129:759–762, 1978.
4. Chen JJS, LaFrance ND, Allo MD, et al: Single photon emission computed tomography of the thyroid. J Clin Endocrinol Metab 66:1240–1246, 1988.
5. Burch HB, Shakir F, Fitzsimmons TR, et al: Diagnosis and management of the autonomously functioning thyroid nodule: The Walter Reed Army Medical Center experience, 1975–1996. Thyroid 8:871–880, 1998.
6. Kusic Z, Becker DV, Saenger EL, et al: Comparison of Tc-99m and iodine-123 imaging of thyroid nodules: Correlation with pathological findings. J Nucl Med 31:393–399, 1990.
7. Singer PA, Cooper DS, Daniels GH, et al: Treatment guidelines for patients with thyroid nodules and well-differentiated thyroid cancer. Arch Intern Med 156:2165–2172, 1996.
8. Meier CA, Braverman LE, Ebner SA, et al: Diagnostic use of recombinant human thyrotropin in patients with thyroid carcinoma (phase I/II study). J Clin Endocrinol Metab 78:188–196, 1994.
9. Ladenson P, Braverman L, Mazzaferri E, et al: Comparison of administration of recombinant human thyrotropin with withdrawal of thyroid hormone for radioactive iodine scanning in patients with thyroid carcinoma. N Engl J Med 337:888–896, 1997.
10. Lakshmanan M, Schaffer A, Robbins J, et al: A simplified low iodine diet in I-131 scanning and therapy of thyroid cancer. Clin Nucl Med 13:866–868, 1988.
11. Maxon HRI, Smith HS: Radioiodine I-131 in the diagnosis and treatment of metastatic well differentiated thyroid cancer. Endocrinol Metab Clin North Am 19:685–719, 1990.
12. Cavalieri RR: Nuclear imaging in the management of thyroid carcinoma. Thyroid 6:485–492, 1996.
13. McDougall IR: 74 MBq radioiodine ^{131}I does not prevent uptake of therapeutic doses of ^{131}I (i.e., does not cause stunning in differentiated thyroid cancer). Nucl Med Commun 18:505–512, 1997.
14. Muratet J-P, Daver A, Minier J-F, et al: Influence of scanning doses of iodine-131 on subsequent first ablative treatment outcome in patients operated on for differentiated thyroid carcinoma. J Nucl Med 39:1546–1550, 1998.
15. Park HM, Park YA, Zhou XH: Detection of thyroid remnants/metastases without stunning: An ongoing dilemma. Thyroid 7:277–280, 1997.
16. McDougall IR: Whole body scintigraphy with radioiodine-131: A comprehensive list of false-positives with some examples. Clin Nucl Med 20:869–875, 1995.
17. Schlumberger M, Parmentier C, de Vathaire F, et al: Iodine-131 and external radiation in the treatment of local and metastatic thyroid cancer. *In* Falk SA (ed): Thyroid Disease, ed 2. Philadelphia, Lippincott-Raven, 1997, pp 601–617.
18. Clark OH, Hoelting T: Management of patients with differentiated thyroid cancer who have positive serum thyroglobulin levels and negative radioiodine scans. Thyroid 4:501–505, 1994.
19. Sisson JC: Selection of the optimal scanning agent for thyroid cancer. Thyroid 7:295–302, 1997.
20. Dadparvar S, Chevres A, Tulchinsky M, et al: Clinical utility of technetium-99m methoxyisobutylisonitrile imaging in differentiated thyroid carcinoma: Comparison with thallium-201 and iodine-131 Na scintigraphy, and serum thyroglobulin quantitation. Eur J Nucl Med 22:1330–1338, 1995.
21. Yen T-C, Lin HD, Lee CH, et al: The role of technetium-99m sestamibi whole-body scans in diagnosis of metastatic Hürtle cell carcinoma of the thyroid gland after total thyroidectomy: A comparison with iodine-131 and thallium-201 whole-body scans. Eur J Nucl Med 21:980–983, 1994.
22. Baudin E, Lubroso J, Schlumberger M, et al: Comparison of octreotide scintigraphy and conventional imaging in medullary thyroid carcinoma. J Nucl Med 36:912–916, 1996.
23. Grunwald F, Schomburg A, Bender H, et al: Fluorine-18 fluorodeoxyglucose positron imaging tomography in the follow-up of differentiated thyroid cancer. Eur J Nucl Med 23:312–319, 1996.
24. Blum M, Goldman AB, Herskovic A, Hernberg J: Clinical applications of thyroid echography. N Engl J Med 287:1164–1169, 1972.
25. Butch RJ, Simeone JF, Mueller PR: Thyroid and parathyroid ultrasonography. Radiol Clin North Am 23:57, 1995.
26. Clarke DK, Cronan J, Scola F: Color Doppler sonography: Anatomic and physiologic assessment of the thyroid. J Clin Ultrasound 23:215–223, 1995.
27. Blum M, Passalaqua AM, Sackler J, Pudiowski R: Thyroid echography of subacute thyroiditis. Radiology 124:795–799, 1977.
28. Marcocci C, Vitti P, Cetani F, et al: Thyroid ultrasonography helps to identify patients with diffuse lymphocytic thyroiditis who are prone to develop hypothyroidism. J Clin Endocrinol Metab 72:209–213, 1991.
29. Fobbe F, Finke R, Reichenstein E, et al: Appearance of thyroid diseases using colour-coded duplex sonography. Eur J Radiol 9:29–31, 1989.
30. Ralls PW, Mayekawa DS, Lee K, et al: Color-flow Doppler sonography in Graves' disease: "Thyroid inferno." AJR 150:781–784, 1988.
31. Hodgson KW, Lazarus JH, Wheeler MH, et al: Duplex scan–derived thyroid blood flow in euthyroid and hyperthyroid patients. World J Surg 12:470–475, 1988.
32. Vander JB, Gaston EA, Dawber TR: The significance of nontoxic thyroid nodules. Final report of a 15-year study of the incidence of thyroid malignancy. Ann Intern Med 69:537–540, 1968.
33. Mazzaferri EL: Management of a solitary thyroid nodule. N Engl J Med 328:553–559, 1993.
34. Ridgway EC: Clinical review 30: Clinician's evaluation of a solitary thyroid nodule. J Clin Endocrinol Metab 74:231–235, 1992.
35. Brander A, Viikinkoski P, Tuuhea LJ, Voutilainen L: Clinical versus ultrasound examination of the thyroid gland in common clinical practice. J Clin Ultrasound 20:37–42, 1992.
36. Solbiati L, Cioffi V, Ballarati E: Ultrasonography of the neck. Radiol Clin North Am 30:941–953, 1992.
37. Simeone JF, Daniels GH, Muller PR, et al: High-resolution real-time sonography of the thyroid. Radiology 145:431–435, 1982.
38. Boehm TM, Rothose L, Wartofsky L: Occult follicular carcinoma of the thyroid with a solitary slowly growing metastasis. JAMA 235:2420, 1976.
39. Solbiati L, Rizzatto G, Bellotti E, et al: High resolution sonography of cervical lymph nodes in head and neck cancer: Criteria for differentiation of reactive versus malignant nodes (abstract). Radiology 169:113, 1988.
40. Vassallo P, Wernecke K, Roos N, Peters PE: Differentiation of benign from malignant superficial lymphadenopathy: The role of high-resolution US. Radiology 183:215–220, 1992.
41. Bruneton JN, Roux P, Caramella E, et al: Ear, nose, and throat cancer: Ultrasound diagnosis of metastasis to cervical lymph nodes. Radiology 152:771–773, 1984.
42. Choi M, Lee JW, Jang KJ: Distinction between benign and malignant causes of cervical, axillary, and inguinal adenopathy: Value of Doppler spectral waveform analysis. AJR 165:981–984, 1995.
43. Blum M: Ultrasonography and computed tomography of the thyroid gland. *In* Ingbar SH, Braverman LE (eds): Werner's the Thyroid, ed 5. New York, JB Lippincott, 1986, pp 576–591.
44. Simeone JF, Daniels GH, Hall DA, et al: Sonography in the follow up of 100 patients with thyroid carcinoma. AJR 148:45–49, 1987.
45. Rizzatto G, Solbiati L, Croce F, Derci LE: Aspiration biopsy of superficial lesions: Ultrasonic guidance with a linear-array probe. AJR 148:623–625, 1987.
46. Takashima S, Yoshida J, Kishimoto H, et al: Nonpalpable lymph nodes of the neck: Assessment with US and US-guided fine-needle aspiration biopsy (abstract). Radiology 197(suppl):270, 1995.
47. Gharib H, Goellner JR, Johnson DA: FNA cytology of the thyroid: A 12 year experience with 11,000 biopsies. Clin Lab Med 13:699–710, 1995.
48. Blum M: Evaluation of thyroid function sonography, computed tomography and magnetic resonance imaging. *In* Becker KL (ed): Principles and Practice of Endocrinology and Metabolism. Philadelphia, JB Lippincott, 1990, pp 289–293.
49. Bahist B, Ellis K, Gold RP: Computed tomography of intrathoracic goiters. AJR 140:455–460, 1983.
50. Blum M, Reede DL, Seltzer TF, et al: Computerized axial tomography in the diagnosis and management of thyroid and parathyroid disorders. Am J Med Sci 287:34, 1984.
51. Blum M, Braverman LE, Holliday RA, et al: The thyroid: Diagnosis. *In* Wagner HN, Szabo Z, Buchanan JW (eds): Principles of Nuclear Medicine, ed 2. Philadelphia, WB Saunders, 1995, pp 595–621.
52. Higgins CB, Auffermann W: MR imaging of thyroid and parathyroid glands: A review of current status. AJR 151:1095–1106, 1988.
53. Tennvall J, Biorklund A, Moller T, et al: Studies of MRI relaxation times in malignant and normal tissues of the human thyroid gland. Prog Nucl Med 8:142–148, 1984.
54. Glazer HS, Niemeyer JH, Balfe DM, et al: Neck neoplasms: MR imaging Part II. Posttreatment evaluation. Radiology 160:349–354, 1986.
55. Freeman M, Toriumi DM, Mafee MF: Diagnostic imaging techniques in thyroid cancer. Am J Surg 155:215–223, 1988.
56. Yousem DM, Som PM, Hackney DB, et al: Central nodal necrosis and extracapsular neoplastic spread in cervical lymph nodes: MR imaging versus CT. Radiology 182:753–759, 1992.
57. Webb WR, Sostman HD: MR imaging of thoracic disease: Clinical uses. Radiology 182:621–630, 1992.
58. Davis SD: CT evaluation of pulmonary metastases in patients with extrathoracic malignancy. Radiology 180:1–12, 1991.
59. Auffernann W, Clark OH, Thurner S, et al: Recurrent thyroid carcinoma: Characteristics on MR images. Radiology 168:753–757, 1988.
60. Takashima S, Morimoto S, Ikezoe J, et al: CT evaluation of anaplastic thyroid carcinoma. Am J Neuroradiol 11:361–367, 1990.

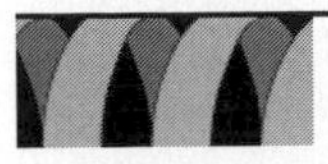

CLINICAL DISORDERS

Chapter 99

Autoimmune Thyroid Disease

Anthony P. Weetman

THE SYNDROMES OF THYROID AUTOIMMUNITY

Thyroid autoimmunity, the original exemplar of an organ-specific autoimmune disorder, arose from the seminal observations of Rose and Witebsky, who showed that thyroid autoantibodies and thyroiditis developed in rabbits immunized with thyroid extract,[1] and from the observations of Doniach and colleagues, who first described thyroglobulin (TG) antibodies in the serum of patients with Hashimoto's thyroiditis.[2] Graves' disease became defined as an autoimmune disorder after the discovery of a long-acting thyroid stimulator in the serum of such patients[3] that was subsequently shown to be a specific IgG directed against the thyroid-stimulating hormone receptor (TSH-R). In the last 40 years a huge volume of work founded on these discoveries has continued to improve our understanding of the etiology and pathogenesis of these disorders. It is now appreciated that autoimmune hypothyroidism and Graves' disease share many features, with some patients progressing from one to the other, and that lesser degrees of thyroid autoimmunity (subclinical hypothyroidism, focal thyroiditis, postpartum thyroiditis) are remarkably common in the general population.

The main types of thyroid autoimmunity are summarized in Table 99-1. The prevalence of subclinical thyroid autoimmunity is difficult to define because the prevalence depends in part on the sensitivity of assays for thyroid autoantibodies, with sensitive assays detecting TG and thyroid peroxidase (TPO) antibodies in up to 20% of women. However, focal thyroiditis, which is closely associated with circulating thyroid autoantibodies, is present in up to 40% of white women and 20% of men at autopsy,[4] thus indicating that these figures do reflect the real prevalence of subclinical thyroid autoimmunity. Careful community studies have shown that such subclinical disease only progresses slowly and infrequently to overt thyroid dysfunction; the weighted prevalence of autoimmune hypothyroidism in the United States is 0.8 per 100, 95% of whom are women.[5]

Subclinical autoimmune thyroiditis may become clinically apparent in the postpartum period as the result of an exacerbation of the autoimmune process for reasons that are not yet clear. Typically, such women have TPO autoantibodies antepartum and experience transient thyroid dysfunction (thyrotoxicosis followed by hypothyroidism, or either phase alone) accompanied by a small painless goiter, with full recovery within a year after delivery.[6] It is now known that postpartum thyroiditis is a risk factor for future permanent hypothyroidism, which ensues in 20% to 30% of cases in the subsequent 5 years. Around 5% of pregnant white women have one or more episodes of postpartum thyroiditis.

Overt hypothyroidism caused by autoimmunity has two main forms: Hashimoto's (or goitrous) thyroiditis and primary myxedema, also known as atrophic thyroiditis. The former is characterized by a variably sized, firm goiter, often with an irregular surface; the goiter is typically painless, although a rare, painful variant occurs that in contrast to subacute thyroiditis, may respond poorly to steroid treatment.[7] Such patients may have a goiter and normal thyroid function or subclinical or overt hypothyroidism, depending on the extent of the autoimmune destructive process. However, in primary myxedema the typical manifestation is clinically evident hypothyroidism, obviously without a goiter. Many attempts have been made to ascribe distinct genetic or pathogenic factors to these two disorders, but in most cases a unique pathogenesis is not evident, and it seems most likely that they are simply at opposite ends of a spectrum of clinical features, with gradual diminution in the size of the goiter as disease progresses.

Similarly, Graves' disease shares many immunologic features with autoimmune hypothyroidism, and even the hallmark of Graves' disease, TSH-R autoantibodies, can be found in some patients with autoimmune hypothyroidism, although their effects are masked by a more vigorous destructive autoimmune process (see below). Graves' disease is the most common autoimmune disorder in the United States, with an estimated weighted prevalence of 1.2 per 100, 88% of whom are women.[5] Many of these individuals progress to hypothyroidism, either spontaneously after successful treatment with antithyroid drugs or iatrogenically after radioiodine therapy or surgery.

TABLE 99–1. Main Types of Thyroid Autoimmunity

Condition	Goiter	Thyroid Function	Features
Focal thyroiditis	No	Normal or subclinical hypothyroidism	May progress to overt hypothyroidism
Hashimoto's thyroiditis	Usually large	Normal or hypothyroid	Usually strongly positive for thyroid autoantibodies
Atrophic thyroiditis	No	Hypothyroid	Probably end-stage disease
Silent thyroiditis; postpartum thyroiditis	Small	Transient thyrotoxicosis and/or hypothyroidism	May progress to permanent hypothyroidism
Graves' disease	Variable size	Hyperthyroid	Associated with ophthalmopathy and thyroid-stimulating antibodies

Further clinical details on these conditions are given in subsequent chapters; this chapter will provide an overview of the basic etiologic and pathologic factors involved in autoimmune thyroid disease.

PATHOLOGY

The typical appearance of Hashimoto's thyroiditis is termed struma lymphomatosa to indicate the extensive infiltration of the thyroid by lymphocytes, plasma cells, and macrophages.[7] As well as a diffuse infiltrate, germinal center formation may be particularly prominent, and giant (Langerhans) cells can occur. The thyroid follicular cells are destroyed to a variable extent, depending on the chronicity of the disease, and during this process the remaining cells become hyperplastic and undergo oxyphil metaplasia, which gives rise to the so-called Askanazy or Hürthle cells. Variable fibrosis and, in rare cases, concurrent changes typical of Graves' disease appear, so-called hashitoxicosis.

Primary myxedema is characterized by extensive fibrosis, loss of normal lobular architecture, and gland atrophy; lymphocytic infiltration varies from minor to moderate. It remains to be established how frequently Hashimoto's thyroiditis progresses to primary myxedema. The extent of fibrosis in autoimmune hypothyroidism is directly correlated with the age of the patient,[8] compatible with the occurrence of such a progression, although little change in the pathologic appearance has been found in sequential biopsies over 10 to 20 years in those with Hashimoto's thyroiditis.[9] The histologic appearances of postpartum thyroiditis and silent thyroiditis resemble Hashimoto's thyroiditis, although oxyphil metaplasia and germinal centers are less frequent, whereas in focal thyroiditis, mild Hashimoto-like changes are seen in localized areas of the thyroid, but most follicles are preserved.

The pathologic features of Graves' disease are usually obscured by prior treatment with antithyroid drugs, whose effects on the autoimmune process are considered later. Hypertrophy and hyperplasia of the thyroid follicles may be noted, the epithelium is columnar, and the colloid shrinks.[7] In addition, a variable degree of lymphocytic infiltration is present, sometimes with germinal center formation. Lymphoid hyperplasia can also be found in the thymus, lymph nodes, and spleen. Follicular involution and reversal of the lymphocytic infiltrate and hyperplasia occur with antithyroid drug treatment.

Thus all forms of thyroid autoimmunity are associated with a lymphocytic infiltrate in the thyroid, and these lymphocytes are largely responsible for generating both T and B cell–mediated autoreactivity, although other sites such as thyroid-draining lymph nodes and bone marrow contain thyroid-autoreactive lymphocytes in autoimmune thyroid disease.[10] Many investigations have used peripheral blood lymphocytes from patients, but although these cells are readily accessible, they will reflect the behavior of only a small proportion of autoreactive lymphocytes migrating in the blood compartment in what is essentially a localized disease.

THE BASIS OF AUTOIMMUNE DISEASE

This section provides only a very attenuated overview of the basic mechanisms underlying autoimmunity; the reader is referred elsewhere for a more comprehensive review.[11] For the purposes of this chapter, however, a brief summary of the normal immune response will be followed by a description of how autoreactivity can arise.

The Normal Immune Response

The essence of the immune response is shown in Figure 99–1. The initial step is presentation of an antigen by an antigen-presenting cell (APC), such as a dendritic cell or macrophage, to a helper T cell, which recognizes the antigen by means of a specific T cell receptor (TCR).[12] Such T cells can be identified phenotypically by expression

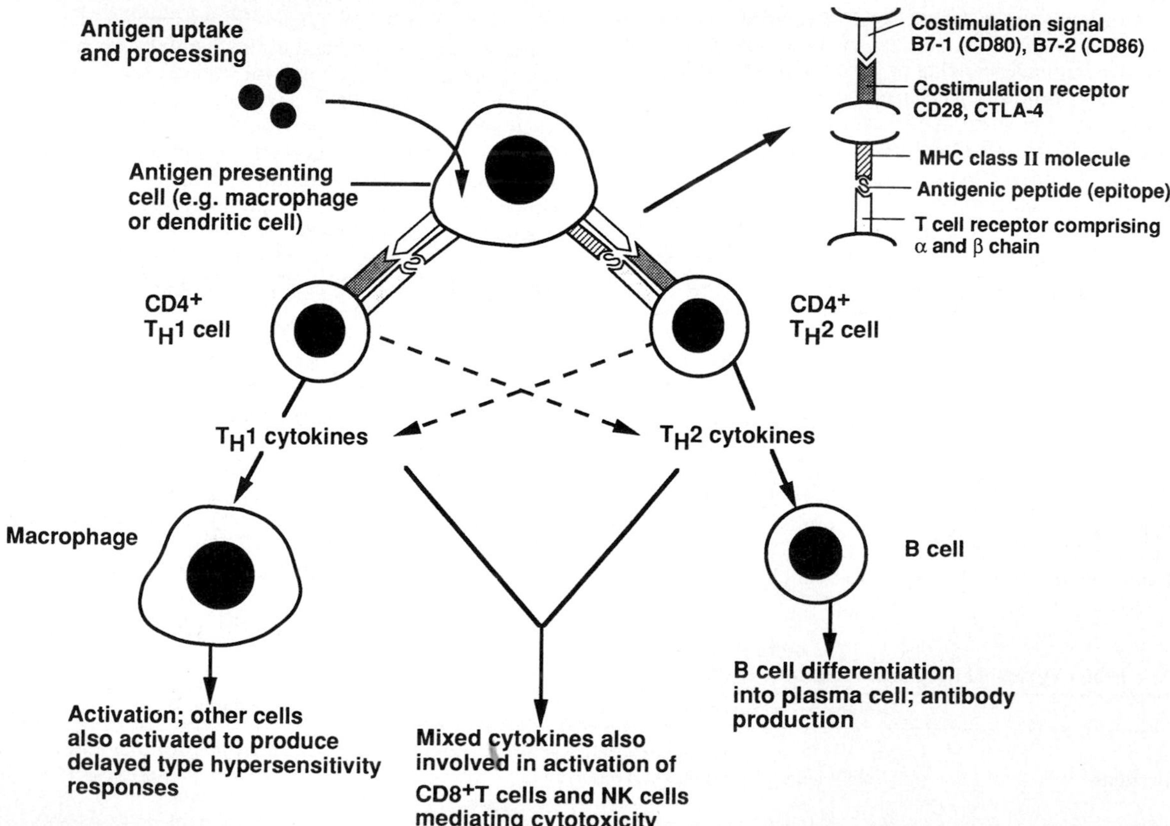

FIGURE 99–1. Simplified diagram of the key elements in a normal immune response, starting with antigen presentation. The type of immune response induced depends on the cytokine profile of the T helper cell that is stimulated. (From Weetman AP: Recent progress in thyroid autoimmunity: An overview for the clinician. Thyroid Today 19(2):1–9, 1996.)

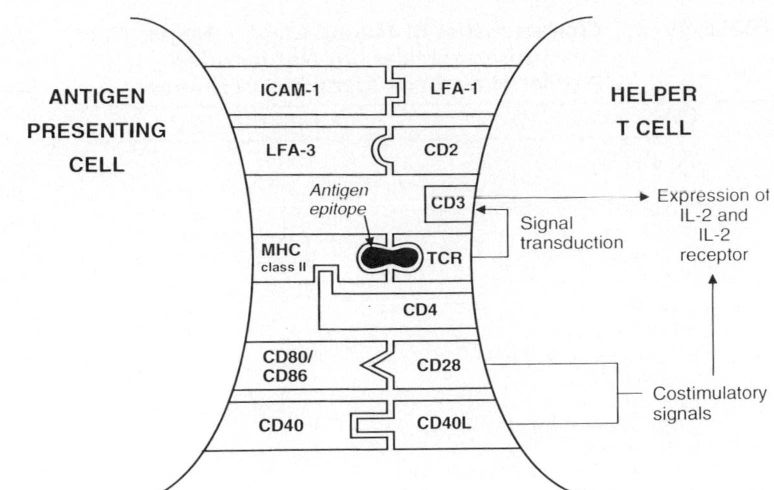

FIGURE 99–2. Diagram of the key molecular interactions in CD4⁺ T cell activation by an antigen-presenting cell (APC).

of the molecule CD4 (CD stands for cluster of differentiation and is used to define an array of surface molecules on lymphocytes and other cells). The antigen is first taken up, either by simple phagocytosis or by involvement of specific surface receptors, and processed by the APC so that fragments of 12 to 18 amino acids are generated. These fragments are the "epitopes" of the antigen, which binds to major histocompatibility complex (MHC) class II molecules expressed constitutively by the APC. The MHC (termed HLA in humans and H-2 in mice) is a huge complex of genes of fundamental immunologic importance because the class I (described below) and class II genes encode polymorphic molecules capable of binding a wide range of antigenic peptides.[13] The ability of an individual to mount an immune response to any given antigen depends in part on the inheritance of class I and II genes, which determine (1) whether appropriate T cells develop in the thymus, because MHC molecules can either positively or negatively select T cells with particular antigenic specificities, as determined by their TCR and stage of development, and (2) whether an antigenic epitope can bind to an appropriate MHC molecule and therefore be presented to a mature T cell in adult life.

Formation of the trimolecular complex between the MHC class II molecule, antigenic epitope, and TCR is followed by activation of the $CD4^+$ T cell, a process that involves expression of interleukin-2 (IL-2) receptor and autocrine stimulation by IL-2 release, and leads to T cell proliferation, secretion of other cytokines, and thus the development of effector function. However, many other molecules are involved in this interaction and act as stabilizers, signal transducers, or providers of so-called costimulatory or second signals (Fig. 99–2). In brief, interaction of a number of adhesion molecule ligands and receptors, such as intercellular adhesion molecule-1 (ICAM-1, CD54)/lymphocyte function-associated antigen-1 (LFA-1, CD11a/CD18) and LFA-3 (CD58)/CD2, allows initial binding of the T cell to an APC. CD4 interacts with a nonpolymorphic region on the MHC molecule to stabilize the trimolecular complex; this activity explains why helper T cells recognize antigen presented by class II rather than class I molecules. CD3 is composed of five peptides expressed uniquely by all T cells and serves to initiate the intercellular events after TCR ligation. Finally, a host of costimulatory signals can determine whether antigen recognition proceeds or is terminated because of either the absence of an essential costimulator or the presence of an inhibitory signal.

The best-defined costimulatory pathway involves the interaction of B7-1 (CD80) and B7-2 (CD86) on the APC with either CD28, which transduces a stimulatory second signal, or cytotoxic T lymphocyte antigen type 4 (CTLA-4), which transduces an inhibitory second signal on the surface of the T cell.[14] Interaction of the TCR on naive T cells with an MHC class II molecule plus epitope, in the absence of CD28 ligation, induces anergy (rather than stimulation) in the T cell; that is, the T cell is paralyzed and unable to respond (Fig. 99–3). Similarly, engagement of CTLA-4 results in T cell anergy. As discussed below, induction of anergy is an important mechanism in preventing autoimmune responses. Other important membrane-bound costimulatory signals exist; for instance, those delivered by the interaction between CD40 and CD40 ligand,[15] and cytokines derived from the APC, such as IL-1, may also act as costimulators for previously activated ("memory") T cells. Thus strikingly different outcomes are possible after antigen presentation, depending on which costimulatory signals are delivered, and the signal delivered in turn depends on the maturity of the T cell and the type of APC involved.

Activated $CD4^+$ T cells can follow two broad pathways of function depending on their pattern of cytokine secretion (Table 99–2). Type 1 helper T (T_H1) cells mediate delayed-type hypersensitivity responses,

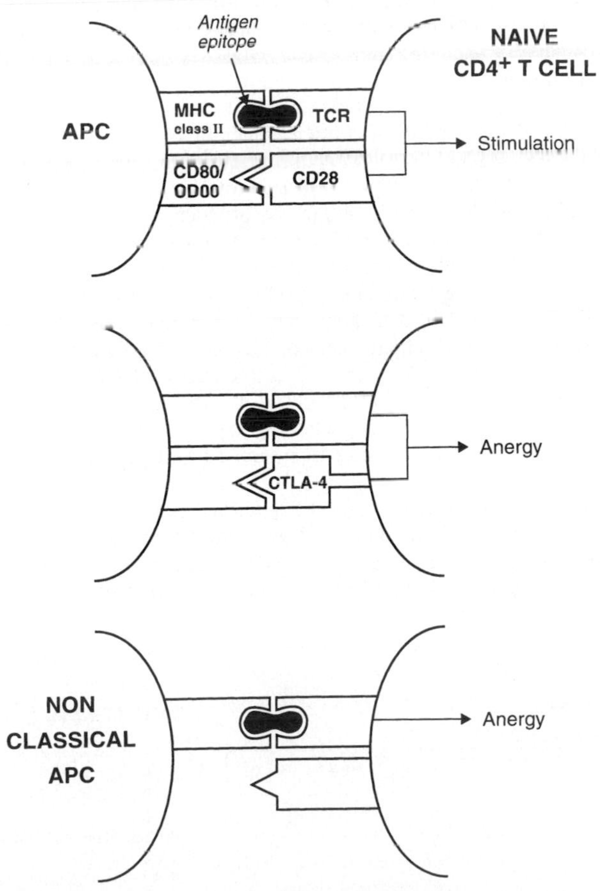

FIGURE 99–3. Mechanisms for anergy induction. The normal pathway for antigen presentation is shown in the *upper panel;* failure to provide an appropriate costimulatory signal *(lower panels)* results in anergy. Classic antigen-presenting cells (APCs) express costimulatory molecules, but class II–positive nonclassic APCs (e.g., thyroid cells) do not.

TABLE 99–2. Characteristics of Murine CD4+ T Helper (T_H) Cell Subsets; Similar but Not Identical Profiles Have Been Identified in Humans

Characteristic	T_H1	T_H2
Cytokine profile		
IL-2	++	−
IL-3	++	++
IL-4	−	++
IL-5	−	++
IL-6	−	++
IL-10	−	++
Interferon-γ	++	−
Tumor necrosis factor	++	+
Lymphotoxin	++	+
Function		
Delayed-type hypersensitivity	++	−
B cell help	+	++
Eosinophil/mast cell production	−	++

IL, interleukin.

essentially the kind of destructive process seen in organ-specific endocrinopathies, whereas T_H2 cells promote antibody production.[16] A number of factors determine which pathway is followed, including TCR affinity and ligand density, the nature of the APC, and the presence of non–T cell–derived IL-4 and IL-12.[17, 18] Although this paradigm is undoubtedly useful, many helper T cells, particularly in humans, cannot be neatly classified into the T_H1/T_H2 dichotomy. For example, a third subset of T_H0 cells produces a mix of T_H1 and T_H2 cytokines and is thought to be a precursor population.[16]

CD8+ T cells have been ascribed both cytotoxic and suppressor functions, but the nature of antigen-specific suppressor T cells remains a clouded issue.[19] T_H1 and T_H2 responses are mutually inhibitory, and therefore many suppressor phenomena may be due to a population of cells capable of secreting appropriate cytokines that can switch off an ongoing immune response (termed immune deviation). CD8+ T cells can also secrete cytokines that have patterns akin to T_H1 and T_H2 cells.[18] More clear is the cytotoxic function of CD8+ T cells that react against antigenic epitopes synthesized within the target cell and presented by MHC class I molecules; the two classic groups of antigens recognized by these cells are the products of viral infection or malignant transformation.[19] Destruction of target cells is mediated by three mechanisms: (1) release of cytokines; (2) release of perforin, a molecule resembling complement proteins in its ability to insert into cell membranes and lead to lysis; and (3) apoptosis, or programmed cell death. In the last, engagement of Fas on the surface of the target cell with Fas ligand (FasL) on the T cell leads to activation of a chain of intracellular events that results in target cell apoptosis[20] (Fig. 99–4). Fas expression is generalized, whereas FasL is restricted to cells of the immune system and to sites of immune privilege, as described in the next section.

Mention should also be made of a further subdivision of T cells. Most T cells have a TCR that is a heterodimer composed of an α and β chain. The genes for these chains are rearranged to ensure adequate diversity for antigen recognition.[21] However, a small proportion of T cells have a TCR composed of a γ and δ chain, and these receptors have a more restricted diversity.[22] The role of γδ T cells is unclear, but they may be important in mucosal immunity and protection against particular microorganisms.

Two other cell types are essential components of the immune response. B cells produce antibodies after differentiation into plasma cells, a process regulated by T_H2 cytokines and CD40/CD40 ligand interaction with a helper T cell. Up to 10^7 different antibody specificities can be generated in humans by recombination and somatic mutation of the immunoglobulin genes.[23] During an immune response, these processes ensure selection of the most appropriate antibodies so that IgG molecules with the highest affinity for antigen are produced. Antibodies generally recognize specific determinants on an antigen that is intact rather than processed or fragmented, and these determinants are termed epitopes; however, unlike T cell epitopes, most B cell epitopes are conformational and formed from discontinuous regions of the molecule.[24] As well as producing antibodies, B cells are important APCs in that they are able to take up antigen via this surface-bound immunoglobulin and enter into cognate recognition of appropriate T cells. This type of antigen presentation may be important in diversifying the T cell response because B cells present multiple epitopes of the antigen to T cells.

Killer and natural killer cells are CD3 negative and spontaneously destroy target cells with altered surface antigens, such as tumor cells.[19] Because killer and natural killer cells express receptors (CD16) for the constant (Fc) region of immunoglobulins, they can also bind to and kill antibody-coated targets, a process called antibody-dependent cell-mediated cytotoxicity (ADCC). This function can also be mediated by macrophages. Thus, although natural killer cells have little antigen specificity, they can be focused on a target via specific antibody (Fig. 99–5).

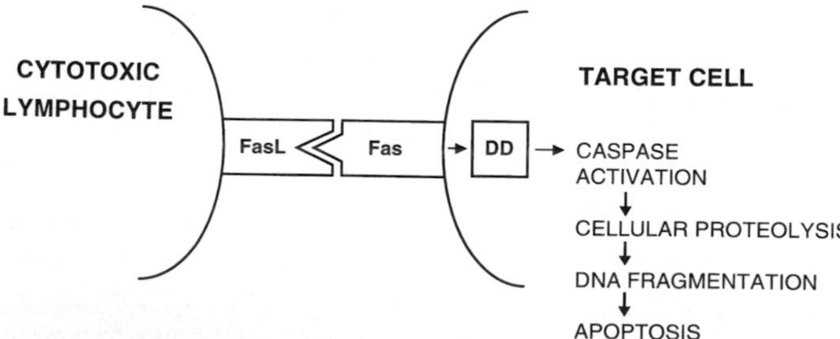

FIGURE 99–4. Interaction between Fas ligand (FasL) on cytotoxic lymphocytes and Fas on a target cell leads to signaling via the death domain (DD) proteins and apoptosis.

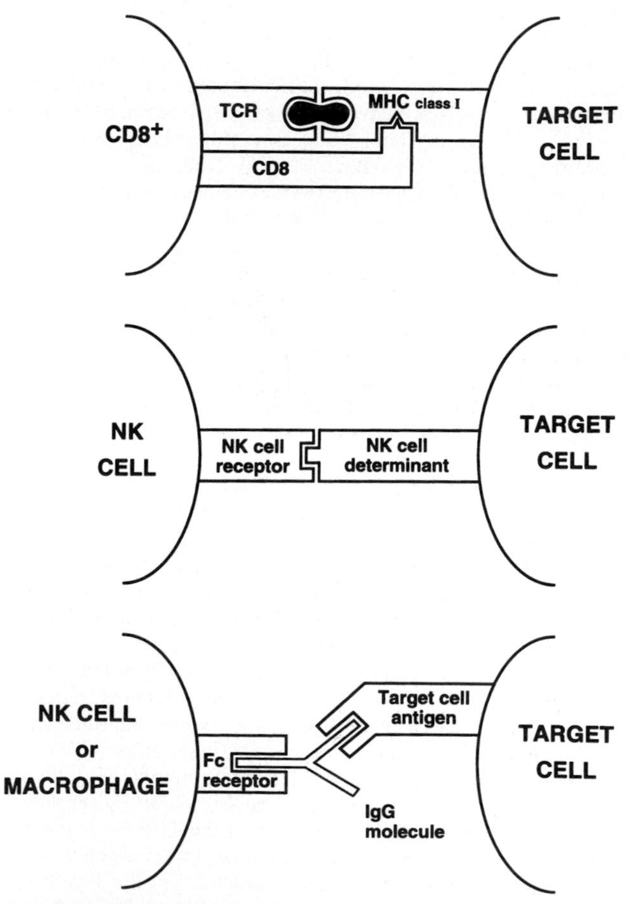

FIGURE 99–5. Recognition mechanisms involved in the interaction between cytotoxic effector cells and target cells in cell-mediated cytotoxicity. Various adhesion molecules are also involved in stabilizing these interactions.

TABLE 99–3. Mechanisms for Maintaining Autoreactive T Cell Nonresponsiveness to Target Tissues

Mechanism	Reversibility
Thymic presentation of self-antigens	
Deletion	No
Anergy	Yes
Peripheral tolerance	
Deletion	No
Anergy	Yes
Clonal ignorance	Yes
Immunologic privilege at a target site	Yes
Active suppression	
Cytokine network	Yes
Idiotype–anti-idiotype networks	Yes
Other suppressor factors	Yes

Self-Tolerance and Autoimmunity

The immune system exists to eliminate foreign antigens but must remain tolerant of (that is, must not respond to) autoantigens. We now know, particularly through experiments with transgenic mice, that the individual mechanisms for ensuring self-tolerance (Table 99–3) are practically never completely successful: a few autoreactive T cells are present in all healthy individuals, although in various states of nonreactivity. Failure of the control mechanisms for ensuring nonreactivity allows clonal expansion of these cells, with subsequent autoimmune disease if the response is sufficiently vigorous.

During development the thymus is mainly responsible for eliminating autoreactive T cells (clonal deletion) and for positively selecting appropriate T cells to constitute the immune repertoire.[25, 26] These processes depend on the interaction of endogenous peptides, presented by thymic APCs, with the naive TCR repertoire. Inevitably, a few T cells escape tolerance, which is particularly likely if specific endogenous antigens are unavailable for presentation in the thymus because of low abundance outside a developing organ, for example. For these antigens, peripheral tolerance, including both deletion and anergy (see Fig. 102–3), may be very important for regulation of self-reactivity.

As well as deletion and anergy, clonal ignorance is effective protection against autoreactivity. Simply put, autoantigen-specific lymphocytes are harmless unless they become activated by autoantigen, and therefore autoimmune disease will not result from such cells if they do not come into contact with autoantigen or if the necessary costimulatory signals are not provided. Autoreactive $CD8^+$ T cells and B cells remain harmless or "ignorant" of self-antigens unless activated by helper T cells, and therefore, provided that the latter are controlled, autoimmune disease will not result. However, it should be noted that $CD8^+$ T cells and B cells are subject to central tolerance mechanisms in the fetal thymus or bone marrow and liver, respectively.[27] Another mechanism for conferring immunologic privilege at an anatomic site, whereby it becomes protected from recognition, is localized expression of FasL, which will induce apoptosis in potentially autoaggressive lymphocytes entering the site; examples of such FasL expression are Sertoli cells, corneal cells, and the placental trophoblast.[20]

Subsidiary control over autoreactive T cells is provided by a number of suppressor mechanisms that remain to be fully characterized. Inhibitory cytokines, such as those producing reciprocal inhibition of T_H1 and T_H2 subset responses, provide one means of suppression of harmful autoimmune responses,[18] but antigen-specific suppressor phenomena have apparently been defined in many situations, especially in animal cell transfer experiments.[28, 29] Potential mechanisms include killing of autoreactive $CD4^+$ cells by $CD8^+$ cells or an inhibitory interaction between part of a self-reactive TCR (the idiotype) on a helper cell and a TCR on a suppressor cell with specificity for the idiotype (called an anti-idiotype).

Tolerance to self-antigens can be broken at one or more of the levels at which it operates (see Table 102–3) and may involve both genetic and environmental factors:

1. Autoreactive T cells may not be deleted or rendered anergic in the thymus (e.g., through inheritance of particular MHC genes or, in animals, after neonatal thymectomy).
2. T cells escaping thymic tolerance may fail to be deleted or rendered anergic in the periphery (e.g., because of abnormal provision of costimulatory signals; see Fig. 102–3).
3. Failure of immunologic tolerance may occur (e.g., because of altered FasL expression).
4. Cross-reactive exogenous antigens induce a response against a normally "silent" autoantigen (e.g., myocarditis after streptococcal infections).
5. Suppressor mechanisms may fail to occur (e.g., provision of high concentrations of endogenous or exogenous cytokines).

EXPERIMENTAL AUTOIMMUNE THYROIDITIS

The development of animal models of experimental autoimmune thyroiditis (EAT) (Table 99–4) has allowed profound insight into the development of thyroid autoimmunity; for example, Figure 99–6 show how autoimmune thyroid disease can arise in mice through modulation at the different stages of T cell tolerance, some of the principles of which were described in the last section. Several different types of EAT have been described,[30] and these types more or less resemble

TABLE 99–4. Summary of the Main Animal Models of Experimental Autoimmune Thyroiditis

Model	Antigen	Comments
Immunization, usually with adjuvant (mouse, rat, rabbit, guinea pig)	TG, TPO, TSH-R	Strain dependent, transient, and transferable via T cells; TSH-R does not induce a Graves' disease–like model because the TSH-R antibodies are without stimulatory action
Thymectomy induced (mouse, rat)	TG	Depends on time of thymectomy and strain; may need sublethal irradiation transferable with T cells
T cell manipulations (mouse)	TG	Cyclosporine A and transfer of specific T cells to T cell–depleted animals induce thyroiditis
Spontaneous (chicken, dog, rat)	TG + other autoantigens	Thyroiditis occurs in OS chickens, beagles, NOD mice, and BB and Buffalo strain rats (NOD and BB animals also have autoimmune diabetes)
Virus induced (mouse)	TG + polyendocrine autoantigens	Reovirus infection of certain strains of mice
SCID mouse	TG, TPO, TSH-R	SCID mice allow long-term study of transplanted thyroid tissue from patients with Graves' and Hashimoto's diseases; disease does not develop in the mice themselves
cDNA immunization (mouse)	TSH-R	Allows production of monoclonal TSH-R antibodies
Immunization with fibroblasts transfected with TSH-R and MHC class II (mouse)	TSH-R	Hyperthyroidism and histologic features of Graves' disease develop, but without lymphocytic infiltration

MHC, major histocompatibility complex; SCID, severe combined immunodeficiency disease; TG, thyroglobulin; TPO, thyroid peroxidase; TSH-R, thyroid-stimulating hormone receptor.

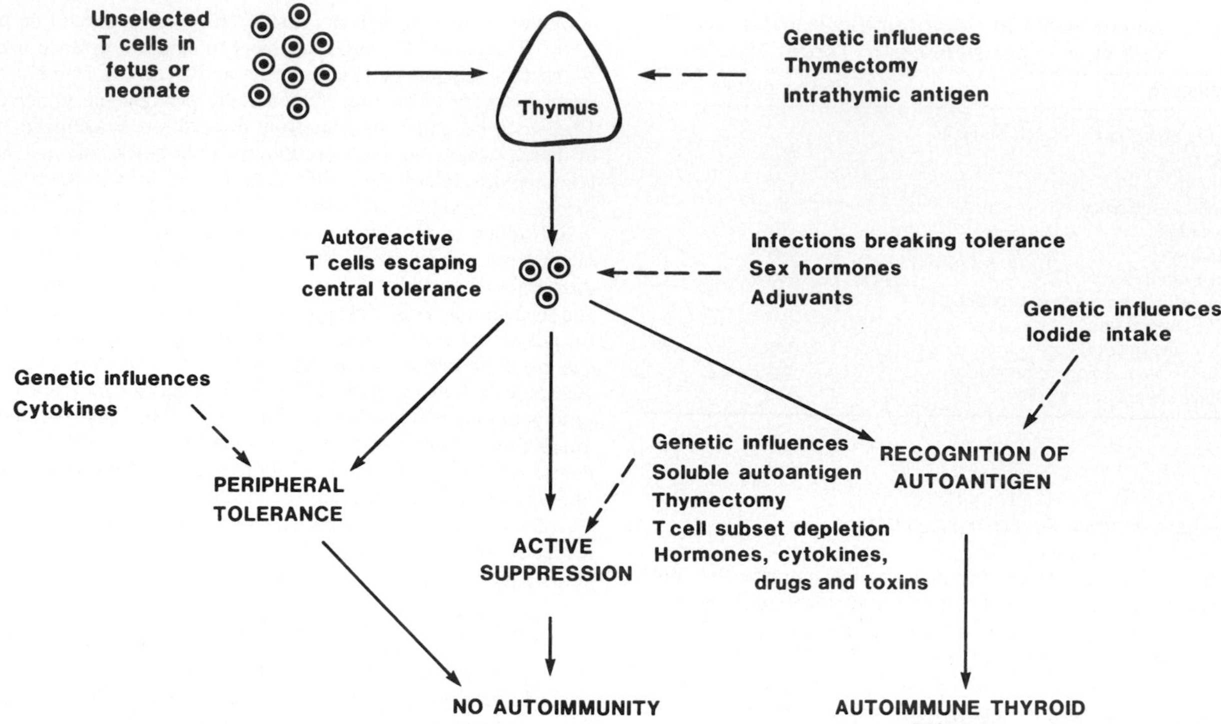

FIGURE 99–6. Control of autoreactive T cells in experimental autoimmune thyroiditis in mice. The sites at which genetic and other factors act are shown as *dotted lines*; the development of autoimmune thyroid disease depends on the balance between these multiple influences. (From Weetman AP, McGregor AM: Autoimmune thyroid disease: Further developments in our understanding. Endocr Rev 15:788–830, © 1994, The Endocrine Society.)

Hashimoto's thyroiditis, with lymphocytic infiltration of the thyroid, TG antibodies, and variable degrees of hypothyroidism.[30] Most recently, attempts to produce animal models of Graves' disease[31, 32] have had some success, although they remain incompletely characterized. The key lessons from these animal models can be summarized as follows.

A strong genetic tendency is apparent in all models such that manipulations that readily induce EAT in one strain may induce either no disease or a different autoimmune disease (such as oophoritis or gastritis) in a different strain. In both the spontaneous and immunization-induced models, the MHC makes a contribution to genetic susceptibility, but it is clear that other non-MHC loci are also involved; in the OS chicken, for example, these loci control T cell responsiveness, glucocorticoid tonus, and intrinsic properties of the thyroid, which makes the OS chicken more susceptible to autoimmunity.[33] Perhaps the most elegant demonstration of susceptibility is the creation of HLA-DRB1*0301 (DR3) transgenic mice; HLA-DR3 is an MHC specificity known to confer susceptibility to autoimmune disease in humans (see below). Thyroiditis develops in HLA-DR3, but not HLA-DR2 transgenic mice after TG immunization, thereby confirming that this HLA-DRB1 polymorphism determines, at least in part, susceptibility to autoimmune thyroiditis.[34]

In addition, a number of environmental and endogenous factors contribute to susceptibility, and more must await discovery. Excess iodine exacerbates spontaneous thyroiditis, possibly through the generation of toxic metabolites formed with oxygen in the thyroid, but it is also known that a major T cell epitope on TG requires iodination for recognition by autoreactive T cells.[35] Antithyroid drugs suppress EAT without any reduction in thyroid hormone levels, which confirms the direct immunomodulatory effects of these drugs.[36]

The potential adverse effects of infection are illustrated by the absence of EAT in suitably thymectomized rats reared under germ-free conditions; transfer of normal gut microflora will induce disease.[37] It is possible that this result is due to the nonspecific effects of gut microflora, such as polyclonal lymphocytic activation or release of cytokines, or to some thyroid cross-reactive antigen. Environmental toxins, such as 3-methylcholanthrene, can induce EAT in genetically susceptible strains of rats.[30] As in humans, female animals generally have more severe EAT than males; this difference is dependent on sex hormones, for estrogen administration worsens thyroiditis whereas testosterone has the opposite effect.[38]

In all models, the role of T cells is paramount, as illustrated by the effects of T cell manipulation on disease induction (see Table 102–4), and disease is only transferred poorly, if at all, by thyroid antibodies. In general, transfer of both $CD4^+$ and $CD8^+$ autoreactive T cells from a donor with EAT is needed to induce EAT in a recipient. The $CD4^+$ T cell population in mice and rats also contains an important regulatory subset that suppresses the activity of those TG-reactive T cells that escape thymic and peripheral tolerance mechanisms.[39] The activity of this regulatory subset can be modified by different concentrations of TG (see Fig. 99–6) or by presenting it in a different form. For instance, oral administration of TG to mice with EAT induces amelioration of thyroiditis, and this type of tolerance induction may depend on the effects of antigen presentation in the gut to such regulatory T cells.[40] Intravenous administration of deaggregated TG will produce tolerance in both the T_H1 and T_H2 subsets of effector cells and suppress induction of EAT, and $CD8^+$ T cells are not involved, so it is clear that tolerance can be induced at multiple levels by TG.[41]

No correlation has been found between the level of TG antibodies and the severity of EAT,[30] further demonstrating the uncertain pathologic role for these autoantibodies in EAT. Indeed, in transgenic mice it has been shown that tolerance is not induced in B cells by membrane-bound antigen expressed on thyroid cells, presumably because the pre-immune B cells are sequestered from the antigen by basement membrane and endothelium.[42] Because tolerance is induced in T cells in this model, it appears that somehow thyroid surface antigens can affect the development of these cells, either by transport to the thymus or by some type of peripheral tolerance. This observation is important and implies that thyroid autoreactive B cells will be frequent but remain ignorant; the frequent appearance of thyroid autoantibodies in otherwise healthy populations could be explained by the activation of these B cells if T cell tolerance breaks down or is bypassed.

THYROID AUTOANTIGENS

Thyroglobulin

TG is a 660-kDa glycoprotein composed of two identical subunits and secreted by thyroid follicular cells into the follicular lumen, where it is stored as colloid. Each TG molecule has around 100 tyrosine residues, a quarter of which are iodinated; at four to eight so-called hormonogenic sites these residues couple to form the thyroid hormones triiodothyronine (T_3) and thyroxin (T_4). The sequence of human TG has been determined.[43] Despite considerable work, the exact location of T and B cell epitopes within TG is still uncertain, even in EAT, in which it is possible to immunize animals with defined peptides.[44] A key T cell epitope in the spontaneous thyroiditis of OS chickens contains iodine, and poorly iodinated TG is only weakly immunogenic.[35]

It has long been recognized that each 330-kDa TG subunit has two major B cell epitopes and a minor epitope.[45] However, as the titer of TG antibodies rises in Hashimoto's thyroiditis with time, other regions of the molecule become targets for autoantibodies, a process reflected in mice immunized with human TG, in which an array of epitopes subsequently develop in these mice.[46] The two major B cell epitopes on TG are conformational,[47] although linear epitopes have also been identified that react with a small proportion of Hashimoto sera.[48]

Thyroid Peroxidase

TPO is the key enzyme in thyroid hormone synthesis, an apical 100- to 105-kDa protein responsible for tyrosine iodination and coupling. Many studies have confirmed the identity of the previously defined thyroid microsomal antigen as TPO.[49] Multiple T cell epitopes exist within the molecule, and individual patients respond to different sets of epitopes without any obvious clinical correlations.[50, 51]

It is also apparent that multiple B cell epitopes are present, some conformational and some linear, because TPO antibodies can recognize native, denatured, or denatured and reduced antigen.[52] As reviewed extensively elsewhere,[53] studies using human and murine monoclonal TPO antibodies have defined two neighboring major domains, A and B, that constitute the antibody reactivity of over 80% of Hashimoto sera (Fig. 99-7). Some sera bind to epitopes overlapping the two domains. It is striking that the antibody response to TPO is restricted at the level of the germline heavy and light chain variable (V) regions.[53, 54] Cocrystallization of TPO with monoclonal TPO antibody

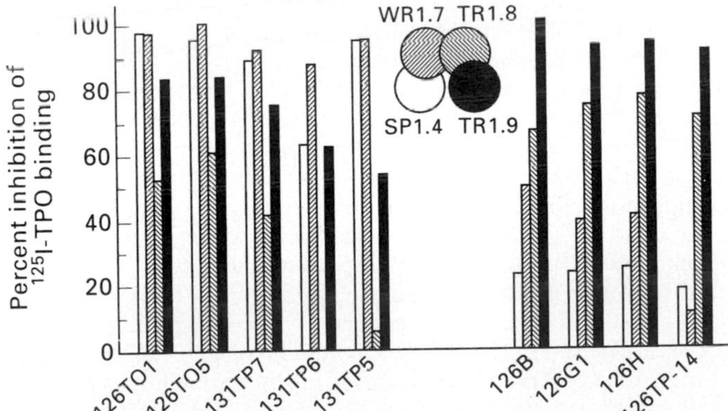

FIGURE 99–7. Epitopic domains on thyroid peroxidase (TPO). Domains A1, A2, B1, and B2 have been defined by the recombinant monoclonal TPO antibodies SP1.4, WR1.7, TR1.8, and TR1.9, respectively (center of diagram), and the *bars* represent the inhibition of binding of these four monoclonal reagents (shading of *bars* corresponds to the shading of the domains) by a separate panel of TPO monoclonal antibodies. Those binding predominantly to domain A are shown on the left and to domain B on the right. (From Guo J, McIntosh RS, Czarnocka B, et al: Relationship between autoantibody epitopic recognition and immunoglobulin gene usage. Clin Exp Immunol 111:408–414, 1998.)

TABLE 99–5. Classification of Main Thyroid-Stimulating Hormone Receptor Antibodies

Antibody	Assay
TSAbs	Bioassay; usually measurement of cAMP production by primary cultures of thyroid cells, thyroid cell lines (e.g., FRTL-5), or cells transfected with TSH-R
Thyroid-blocking antibodies	Bioassay; measurement of inhibition of cAMP production after TSH-mediated stimulation of the TSH-R; may operate at the level of TSH binding or receptor signaling
TSH binding–inhibiting immunoglobulins	Measurement of inhibition of radiolabeled TSH binding to TSH-R by antibodies; unable to distinguish function
Long-acting thyroid stimulator	Original description of TSAb; used bioassay in whole mouse to assess effects of antibodies on radioiodine release

cAMP, cyclic adenosine monophosphate; TSAb, thyroid-stimulating antibody; TSH-R, thyroid-stimulating hormone receptor.

fragments will be required for further elucidation of the epitopes within the main domains of this autoantigen.

Thyroid-Stimulating Hormone Receptor

TSH-R is a member of the G protein–coupled receptor family; activation of TSH-R by TSH or that subset of TSH-R antibodies with stimulatory activity leads to intracellular signaling by the cyclic adenosine monophosphate (cAMP) pathway, although other signaling pathways operate at high ligand concentrations. TSH-R has a 398-amino acid extracellular domain, a 266–amino acid transmembrane domain (organized in seven loops), and an 83–amino acid intracellular domain.[55] Variants of TSH-R have been described, in particular a form that does not include the transmembrane region.[56] This potentially shed form may have immunologic activity, as may the extrathyroidal expression of TSH-R, particularly in the orbit, where it could serve as a cross-reactive autoantigen in the ophthalmopathy associated with Graves' disease.[57]

As with TPO, multiple T cell epitopes have been defined, including TSH-R sequences recognized by 10% to 20% of healthy individuals.[58, 59] B cell epitopes are generally conformational, and it is clear that the response is heterogeneous both within and between patients because some antibodies can stimulate via the receptor in several ways and other TSH-R antibodies bind to the receptor without stimulating it, a proportion of these antibodies interfering with TSH-mediated stimulation (Table 99–5). Antibodies binding to the amino terminal area are stimulatory, whereas those binding to amino acids 261 to 370 or 388 to 403, near the cell surface, have blocking activity.[60] Further characterization of these B cell epitopes awaits the development of human TSH-R monoclonal antibodies, a daunting task given the low frequency of TSH-R antibody–secreting B cells and the difficulty of expressing the receptor in vitro in its native form.[53, 61]

Other Autoantigens

Cloning and sequencing of the Na^+/I^- symporter (NIS) has allowed confirmation of NIS as a fourth major thyroid autoantigen, first demonstrated using cultured dog thyroid cells.[62] Around a third of Graves' disease sera and 15% of Hashimoto sera contain antibodies that inhibit NIS-mediated iodide uptake in vitro.[63] Further work is needed to clarify the role of these antibodies in vivo. Antibodies to thyroid hormones can be found in 10% to 25% of patients with autoimmune thyroid disease,[64] and nonspecific autoantibodies against DNA, tubulin, and other cytoskeletal proteins can also be detected in a small proportion of patients.

GENETIC FACTORS

The role of heredity in autoimmune thyroid disease has been illustrated by numerous studies showing a higher frequency of autoimmune thyroid disease or thyroid antibodies in family members of patients with autoimmune hypothyroidism and Graves' disease.[30] That both types of thyroid disease cluster together in families provides additional support for the notion that these conditions share etiologic and pathogenic features. A number of patterns of inheritance and candidate genes have been suggested, but ascertainment artifacts and the drawbacks of genetic association studies have produced many inconsistencies in the results. For instance, transmission of thyroid autoantibodies is now known to be more complex than the dominant inheritance originally proposed,[65] and meticulous twin studies have shown a concordance rate of only 22% for Graves' disease, much lower than previously thought.[66]

The most important susceptibility factor thus far recognized is the association with particular HLA-DR alleles; the role that these MHC class II genes play in the immune response makes them excellent candidates. HLA-DR3 is associated with both Graves' disease and Hashimoto's thyroiditis in whites and gives a relative risk of between 2 and 6, whereas HLA-DR4 and HLA-DR5 have been associated with goitrous but not atrophic thyroiditis in some white populations.[67] Postpartum thyroiditis has only a weak association with HLA-DR5. It should be noted that nonwhite populations have very different HLA associations.[68]

Recently, detailed family studies have been undertaken and have found only weak evidence of linkage between the HLA region and autoimmune thyroid disease.[69, 70] These results imply the existence of other susceptibility loci. Of the candidates tested, which include genes encoding immunoglobulins, TCR, TSH-R, and various cytokines, the most robust association has been with two linked polymorphisms of the CTLA-4 gene, which exists in both Graves' disease and autoimmune hypothyroidism and confers a relative risk of around 2.[71, 72] This association is apparently independent of ethnic origin[73] but is weak; it can be detected by association but not linkage analysis.[70] Moreover, the same polymorphism confers susceptibility for type 1 diabetes mellitus and therefore presumably reflects some generalized effect on autoreactive T cell regulation. Further progress will undoubtedly be made by the large-scale multiplex family studies now under way in several centers that entail the use of a genome-wide series of polymorphic markers to identify previously unsuspected susceptibility loci.

ENVIRONMENTAL FACTORS

Work in EAT has identified several environmental influences on thyroiditis (see earlier), and epidemiologic evidence supports a role for some of these environmental factors in humans. An excess of thyroid autoantibodies and thyroiditis occurs after iodination programs, reviewed in detail elsewhere[74]; as in EAT, iodine may increase the immunogenicity of thyroid autoantigens or have a role in the generation of toxic metabolites. Radioiodine given therapeutically can rarely induce autoimmune responses in patients with nodular goiters.[75] The mechanism is obscure but could relate to the release of thyroid autoantigens (possibly altered by radiation damage and therefore more immunogenic) or to the effect of ^{131}I on radiation-sensitive regulatory T cell subsets. Support for the latter comes from the changes in circulating T cell subsets reported after ^{131}I administration and the higher than expected frequency of autoimmune thyroid disease in children exposed to radiation fallout.[76] Similar increases in thyroid autoimmunity occur after mantle irradiation for Hodgkin's disease.[77]

No convincing evidence has indicated a role for infection in autoimmune hypothyroidism, except for the high frequency of this condition in patients with congenital rubella syndrome; however, an association has been proposed between *Yersinia* infection and Graves' disease, and *Yersinia* contains proteins that mimic TSH-R immunologically.[78] The relative importance of this association has not been established but seems low given the relative frequencies of Graves' disease and *Yersinia* infection. Attempts to implicate retroviruses in Graves' disease also remain to be confirmed.[79] Autoimmune thyroid disease only occurs rarely, if at all, after subacute thyroiditis.[80]

A number of retrospective surveys have identified stress during the year before the initial evaluation as an important risk factor for Graves' disease, but these surveys suffer from potential flaws in their dependence on recall and other sources of bias.[81] Any such effect presumably results from the neuroendocrine response to stress altering the regulation of autoreactive lymphocytes. Attacks of allergic rhinitis are associated with an increased risk of relapse in those with Graves' disease, most likely because of the nonspecific effects of cytokines produced during the attack.[82] Exogenous cytokines given therapeutically, particularly interferon-α (IFN-α), exacerbate preexisting thyroid and other types of autoimmunity and lead to the development of autoimmune hypothyroidism in predisposed individuals.[83] The role of toxins and pollutants remains underexplored, although the adverse effects of smoking on Graves' disease and ophthalmopathy provide a clear example that these factors could be important.[84]

T CELL–MEDIATED RESPONSES

Many studies have been performed to characterize the circulating T cell population in autoimmune thyroid disease, but because the functional consequences of alterations in T cell phenotype are still not clear, particularly within this lymphocyte compartment, the meaning of any changes is open to debate. Although complete consensus has not been achieved, it seems that CD8$^+$ T cell numbers are decreased in active Hashimoto's thyroiditis and in Graves' disease, with an increase in activated T cells expressing markers such as HLA-DR.[85, 86] Both CD4$^+$ and CD8$^+$ T cells occur in the thyroid lymphocytic infiltrate, with a preponderance of activated CD4$^+$ cells.[87, 88]

More recently, attention has focused on possible clonal restriction of intrathyroidal T cells, as shown by limited usage of the V gene families encoding the α chain of the TCR.[89] Although this concept seems plausible in the earliest stages of an autoimmune response, by the time that disease is recognizable clinically, multiple antigens and epitopes are responsible for T cell autoreactivity (so-called spreading of the immune response) and such restriction would therefore not be expected; little evidence of TCR restriction is apparent when IL-2 receptor–positive (and hence recently activated) intrathyroidal T cells in Graves' disease are analyzed.[90] However, restricted V gene usage by CD8$^+$ T cells is seen in Hashimoto's thyroiditis, which could reflect clonal expansion of cytotoxic populations.[91] Certainly, cytotoxic T cells have been cloned from this population.[92] These cells have the αβ TCR, but a second cytotoxic population with γδ TCRs has also been identified in Graves' disease; the nature of the thyroid surface autoantigen and mode of its presentation to these T cells is unknown.[93]

A wide array of cytokines, including IL-2, IFN-γ, tumor necrosis factor-α (TNF-α), IL-4, IL-6, IL-10, IL-12, IL-13, and IL-15, are produced by the lymphocytic infiltrate in autoimmune thyroid disease, with some variations between patients and yet no predominance of a T_H1 or T_H2 response.[94] Once again, this situation could reflect the late stage of disease and the mixed cell populations that have been analyzed in such studies. Ideally, one would wish to examine only thyroid autoantigen-specific CD4$^+$ T cells to determine the pattern of helper T cell cytokine production, but establishing such clones has been difficult, and the very process of expanding these cells in vitro may well distort their behavior. Weak in vitro responses to TG, TPO, and TSH-R, used either as whole antigen or putative peptide epitopes, have been detected in circulating and intrathyroidal T cell populations in assays of proliferation, secretion of migration inhibition factor, or B cell helper activity as readouts.[30, 50, 51, 58, 59, 95] Attempts to define thyroid antigen-specific suppressor T cells with such systems have also been made, but the suppressor cell defects suggested in autoimmune thyroid disease by such assays[95] have been disputed on grounds of specificity and the nonphysiologic nature of the assay systems.[96]

B CELL RESPONSES

TG and TPO antibodies occur, often in very high concentrations, in patients with Hashimoto's thyroiditis and primary myxedema (see Fig.

99–8); in patients without circulating antibodies, they can be detected by culture of intrathyroidal lymphocytes.[97] These antibodies are less common, but still frequent in Graves' disease, whereas TPO rather than TG antibodies are frequent in postpartum thyroiditis.[6] Both antibodies show partial restriction to the IgG1 and IgG4 subclass and κ light chain restriction of TPO antibodies.[53, 98] The pathogenic role of TG antibodies is unclear because the epitopes on the antigen are too widely spaced to allow bound autoantigen to cross-link and thus fix complement, but these antibodies can mediate ADCC, at least in vitro.[98] In contrast, TPO antibodies do fix complement, and immunohistochemical evidence has established the formation of terminal complement complexes within the thyroid in autoimmune thyroid disease.[99] Because TPO is located at the apical surface and within the thyroid cell cytoplasm, it seems that under normal circumstances, TPO antibodies do not gain access to their autoantigen, which accounts for the euthyroidism in healthy individuals with TPO antibodies and in neonates born to mothers with high levels of TPO antibodies. Cell-mediated injury may be necessary for TPO antibodies to gain access to their antigen and become pathogenic; for instance, cytokines such as IL-1α could induce dissociation of the junctional complexes between thyroid cells in a follicle (see Fig. 99–8).[100]

Thyroid-stimulating antibodies (TSAbs) directed against the TSH-R are the hallmark of Graves' disease and would presumably be detected in 100% of patients with sensitive enough assays; currently, around 95% positivity is attainable. These antibodies are often κ chain restricted and of the IgG1 subclass,[101, 102] which suggests origin from a small number of B cell clones. It is now established that TSAbs also occur in a small proportion of patients with autoimmune hypothyroidism, but their effects are obscured by TSH-R–blocking antibodies and destructive processes.[60, 103] In some patients, fluctuation in the relative proportion of the two types of TSH-R antibody may produce a confusing clinical picture of alternating hyperthyroidism and hypothyroidism, and such fluctuation may also occur after pregnancy.[104] Blocking antibodies have been found in 10% to 20% of patients with autoimmune hypothyroidism, and in Asian populations it seems to be most closely associated with atrophic rather than goitrous thyroiditis.[105] In whites, however, they appear in Hashimoto's thyroiditis as well, and in such patients the goiter is most likely to be the result of lymphocytic infiltration.[106] The existence of separate populations of growth-stimulating and growth-inhibiting immunoglobulins, operating independently of the TSH-R, remains disputed.[107, 108] In Graves' disease, at least it is TSAbs that mediate goitrogenesis.

PATHOGENIC MECHANISMS

Graves' disease clearly results from the action of TSAbs, primarily via the cAMP pathway, although other signaling pathways may be used by TSH-R antibodies in some patients, which suggests a subdivision based on the effector function of these antibodies.[109] TSAbs also increase the vascularity of the Graves thyroid by enhancing local expression of vascular endothelial growth factor and its receptor.[110] In around 15% of patients with Graves' disease treated with antithyroid drugs, hypothyroidism supervenes years later, thus indicating that similar destructive mechanisms operate in Graves' disease and autoimmune hypothyroidism. These shared pathogenic mechanisms will be detailed after considering the role of thyroid follicular cells as APCs.

The discovery that thyroid cells express MHC class II molecules in autoimmune thyroid disease, but not under normal circumstances, led to the suggestion that such expression could permit thyroid autoantigen presentation, which in turn could initiate or exacerbate disease.[111] It is now clear that thyroid cells generally express class II molecules only after stimulation with IFN-γ, which implies that a T cell infiltrate must precede such expression, so class II expression is a secondary event.[112] Furthermore, thyroid cells do not express B7 1 or B7-2 costimulatory molecules and can therefore act as APCs only for T cells that no longer require such costimulation, in general those that have previously been activated. In vitro experiments confirm that thyroid cells can act as APCs under such circumstances, but they are also able to induce anergy in naive T cells that require costimulation[113] (see Fig. 102–3). Teleologically, MHC class II expression is likely to be an important means of ensuring peripheral T cell tolerance under normal circumstances, but such expression is damaging under conditions of thyroid autoimmunity (Fig. 99–9). Class II expression is more readily induced by IFN-γ in Graves' thyroid cells than those from multinodular goiter, thus suggesting a genetically regulated component to this response.[114]

Cytokines have a large number of other effects on thyroid cells that may be of pathogenic relevance. As well as adversely affecting thyroid growth and function, a number of immunologically important mole-

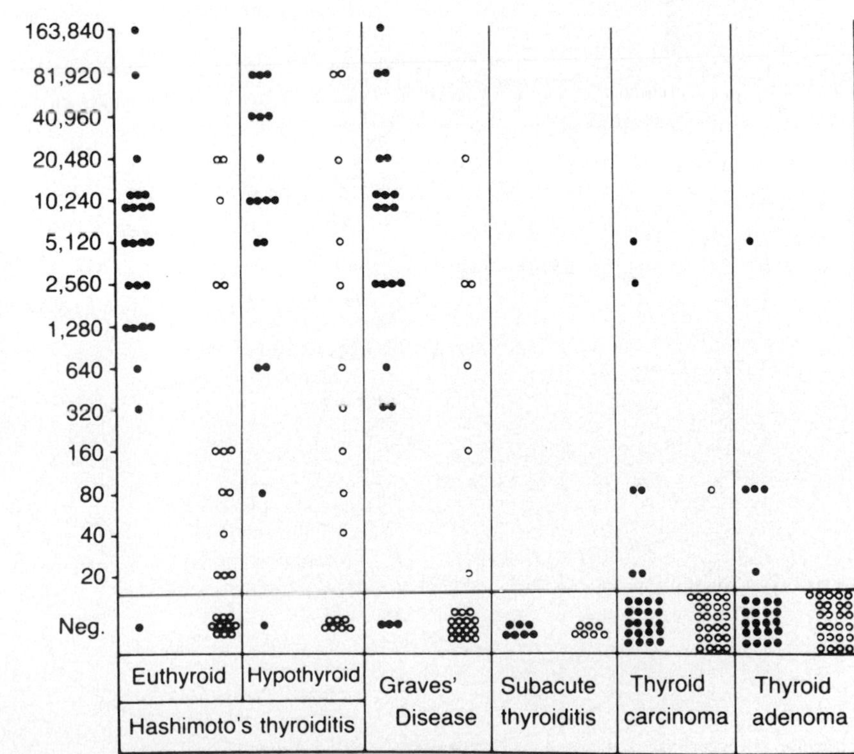

FIGURE 99–8. Titers of microsomal/thyroid peroxidase (TPO) hemagglutination antibodies (MCHAs), shown as *solid circles,* and thyroglobulin hemagglutination antibodies (TGHAs) in various thyroid diseases. (From Amino N, Hagan SR, Yamada N, Refetoff S: Measurement of circulating thyroid microsomal antibodies by the tanned red cell haemagglutination technique: Its usefulness in the diagnosis of autoimmune thyroid disease. Clin Endocrinol 5:115–126, 1976.)

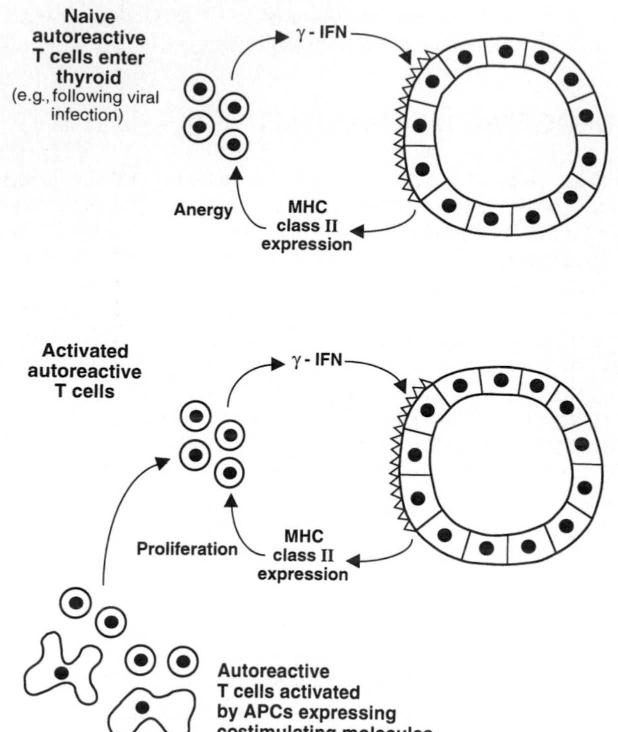

FIGURE 99–9. Alternative outcomes after major histocompatibility complex (MHC) class II expression by thyroid cells. Naive T cells require costimulation for activation, and anergy can be induced by interaction with the MHC class II molecule/antigenic epitope alone *(upper panel, peripheral tolerance)*. If T cells receive costimulation from classic antigen-presenting cells (APCs), class II expression by thyroid cells can enhance the T cell response *(lower panel)*.

cules are expressed by thyroid cells in response to cytokines known to be produced locally by the infiltrating leukocytes in Graves' disease and autoimmune hypothyroidism[94] (Fig. 99–10). Expression of ICAM-1, LFA-3, and MHC class I molecules is enhanced by IL-1, TNF, and IFN-γ, and this response increases the ability of cytotoxic T cells to mediate lysis.[115] Thyroid cell destruction is mediated both by perforin-containing T cells, which accumulate in the thyroid,[116] and by Fas-dependent mechanisms.[117] A unique type of suicide has also been suggested by reports that IL-1β–stimulated thyroid cells in Hashimoto's thyroiditis express FasL, which could lead to self-ligation with Fas and thus cell death,[117] but these findings have not been consistently reproduced.[118] Cytokines and other toxic molecules such as nitric oxide and reactive oxygen metabolites probably also contribute directly to cell-mediated tissue injury.

Humoral immunity most likely exacerbates cell-mediated damage in a secondary fashion, both by direct complement fixation (for TPO antibodies) and by ADCC.[98, 119] These effects are in addition to the inhibitory effects of NIS and TSH-R–blocking antibodies on thyroid cell function. Thyroid cells increase their expression of a number of regulatory proteins (CD46, CD55, CD59) in response to cytokines, and these proteins prevent cell death in the face of widespread complement damage in autoimmune thyroid disease.[59, 120] Nonetheless, sublethal complement attack, initiated via the classic or alternative pathway, impairs the metabolic function of thyroid cells and induces them to secrete IL-1, IL-6, reactive oxygen metabolites, and prostaglandins, all of which could enhance the autoimmune response.[121]

As well as T and B cells, dendritic cells and monocytes/macrophages accumulate in the thyroid, where they presumably play a major role as APCs capable of providing costimulatory signals. Thyroid cell–derived monocyte chemoattractant-1, produced after TNF, IFN-γ, or IL-1 stimulation, is likely to be responsible for the accumulation of monocytes.[122] Besides acting as APCs, these cells are important sources of cytokines, as shown by the inhibition of thyroid cell growth by IL-1 and IL-6 derived from dendritic cells.[123]

NATURAL HISTORY AND RESPONSE TO TREATMENT

The natural history of subclinical hypothyroidism, present in many cases of focal thyroiditis, is now well established from epidemiologic surveys: the presence of thyroid autoantibodies in addition to this biochemical picture confers a considerable future risk of permanent hypothyroidism, much greater than the presence of autoantibodies alone.[124] Around a quarter of patients with postpartum thyroiditis progress to permanent hypothyroidism,[6] but as in the case of subclinical hypothyroidism, it is unclear which factors predispose to this

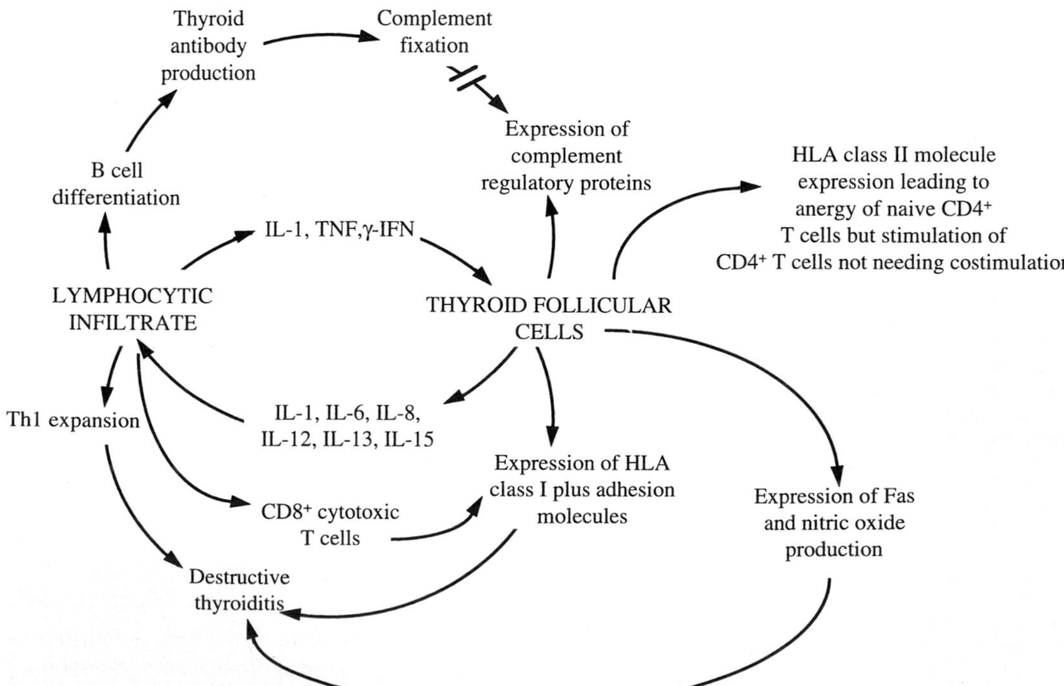

FIGURE 99–10. Interaction between thyroid cells and the immune system via cytokines. Expression of complement regulatory proteins in response to interleukin-1 (IL-1), tumor necrosis factor (TNF), and interferon-γ (IFN-γ) will protect against complement-mediated injury, and class II expression may induce T cell anergy under appropriate conditions; the other cytokine-induced events will amplify the autoimmune process. (From Weetman AP, Ajjan RA, Watson PF: Cytokines and Graves' disease. Baillieres Clin Endocrinol Metab 11:481–497, 1997.)

outcome. One speculation is that maternal microchimerism, caused by the transfer of fetal cells bearing paternal antigens at delivery, leads to the enhancement of any ongoing autoimmune response, and the most severe disease would therefore accompany the greatest cell transfer.[125]

Spontaneous resolution of Graves' disease and autoimmune hypothyroidism does occur but seems unusual, and thus far no prospective study has fully established whether any remission is permanent rather than temporary. However, patients with autoimmune hypothyroidism and TSH-R–blocking antibodies seem particularly likely to enter remission after T_4 treatment, although no consensus has been reached on whether this remission is associated with decreases in antibody levels.[105, 126] Intermittent exposure to a crucial environmental agent could explain some remissions, and it is noteworthy that many animal models of EAT spontaneously remit. This finding is compatible with the idea that thyroid autoreactivity is controlled at several different levels (see Table 102–3), so it may well be possible to manipulate the immune system therapeutically to restore tolerance.

Treatment with antithyroid drugs (carbimazole, methimazole, propylthiouracil) for Graves' disease leads to a decline in TSAbs and other thyroid antibodies and a decline in the severity of thyroiditis, as well as other immunologic changes (Table 99–6). These effects have been explained by the fall in thyroid hormone levels produced by antithyroid drugs exerting a beneficial effect on the immune system,[127] but this reasoning seems unlikely because the same drugs inhibit EAT in the presence of euthyroidism.[36] An alternative explanation is the inhibitory effects of antithyroid drugs on the release of proinflammatory molecules by thyroid cells, which would explain both the altered immune response during treatment and its thyroid specificity.[121]

Radioiodine therapy is followed after 3 to 6 months by a striking rise in thyroid autoantibodies, and the possibility of differential effects on TSAbs and TSH-R–blocking antibodies could explain transient thyroid dysfunction at this time.[128] Thyroid-associated ophthalmopathy may also worsen transiently after radioiodine treatment in some patients.[129] Both events may be related to the release of thyroid autoantigens or radiation effects on T cell subpopulations inasmuch as activated T cells increase in the circulation weeks after ^{131}I administration.[130]

Undoubtedly, further understanding of the immunologic basis of Graves' disease will ultimately lead to immunologically based treatment aimed at reinducing tolerance to TSH-R. Already, pilot studies have been performed to assess the potential for oral tolerance with the use of TG,[131] and it is possible that any such treatment might have benefit for ophthalmopathy as well. On the other hand, T_4 is such simple treatment for autoimmune hypothyroidism that at present, novel treatments are most unlikely.

RELATION TO OTHER DISEASES

Thyroiditis and thyroid antibodies are found in a quarter to a third of patients with thyroid cancer, and such patients have an improved prognosis.[132] Preexisting Hashimoto's thyroiditis is the major risk factor for the development of primary thyroid lymphoma.[133] Other novel associations have been suggested by studies showing an increased frequency of autoimmune thyroiditis in women with breast cancer,[134] persistent miscarriages,[135] and depression.[136] In all these examples, the reasons for the links with thyroid autoimmunity are presently unclear. Finally, autoimmune thyroid disease is a well-recognized component of autoimmune polyglandular syndrome type 2 and a minor component of the type 1 syndrome.[137, 138] In both cases, a common genetic origin for the immunologic defects leading to autoimmune endocrinopathies forms the basis for the association.

TABLE 99–6. Immunologic Effects of Antithyroid Drugs

In vivo
- Reduction in levels of TSH-R, TG, and TPO antibodies but not nonthyroid autoantibodies
- Reduction in thyroid lymphocytic infiltration in Graves' disease and experimental/spontaneous autoimmune thyroiditis in animals
- Reversal of thymic hyperplasia
- Restoration of elevated circulating levels of activated and $CD69^+$ T cells and increased CD4/CD8 ratio
- Reduction in circulating levels of soluble markers of immune response (terminal complement complexes, CD8, ICAM-1)

In vitro
- Suppression of immunoglobulin synthesis
- Oxygen metabolite scavenger
- Enhanced IL-2 production and T cell proliferation
- Suppression of IL-1, IL-6, and prostaglandin synthesis by thyroid cells
- Variable effects on thyroid cell surface expression of MHC molecules

ICAM-1, intercellular adhesion molecule-1; IL-2, interleukin-2; MHC, major histocompatibility complex; TG, thyroglobulin; TPO, thyroid peroxidase; TSH-R, thyroid-stimulating hormone receptor.

SUMMARY

Autoimmune thyroid disease is the result of a complex interaction between genetic and environmental factors, many of which remain to be defined, that leads to a failure of one or more mechanisms responsible for controlling thyroid-reactive T and B cells. Such cells are probably present, to a greater or lesser extent, in all individuals, with disease only resulting when the autoreactive lymphocytes are able to escape tolerance or ignorance. Both cell-mediated and humoral immune responses contribute to tissue injury in autoimmune hypothyroidism; in Graves' disease, production of TSAbs leads to hyperthyroidism. The thyroid cell interacts with the immune system at a number of points in the development of autoimmunity, and many of these interactions appear to exacerbate the disease process. The multistep development of disease suggests that it will be possible to restore normal tolerance and treat Graves' disease immunologically with novel agents directed at the interaction between T cells and APCs or at immunoregulatory T cell subsets.

REFERENCES

1. Rose NR, Witebsky E: Changes in the thyroid glands of rabbits following active immunization with rabbit thyroid extracts. J Immunol 76:417–427, 1956.
2. Roitt IM, Doniach D, Campbell PN, et al: Autoantibodies in Hashimoto's disease (lymphadenoid goitre). Lancet 2:820–821, 1956.
3. Adams DD: The presence of an abnormal thyroid-stimulating hormone in the serum of some thyrotoxic patients. J Clin Endocrinol Metab 18:699–712, 1958.
4. Okayasu I, Hara Y, Nakamura K, et al: Racial and age-related differences in incidence and severity of focal autoimmune thyroiditis. Anat Pathol 101:698–702, 1993.
5. Jacobson DL, Gange SJ, Rose NR, et al: Epidemiology and estimated population burden of selected autoimmune diseases in the United States. Clin Immunol Immunopathol 84:223–243, 1997.
6. Smallridge RC: Postpartum thyroid dysfunction: A frequently undiagnosed endocrine disorder. Endocrinologist 6:44–50, 1996.
7. LiVolsi VA: Pathology of thyroid disease. *In* Falk SA (ed): Thyroid Disease: Endocrinology, Surgery, Nuclear Medicine and Radiotherapy. New York, Raven Press, 1990, pp 127–175.
8. Mizukami Y, Michigishi T, Kawato M, et al: Thyroid function and histologic correlations in 601 cases. Hum Pathol 23:980–988, 1991.
9. Hayashi Y, Tamai H, Fukata S, et al: A long term clinical, immunological, and histological follow-up study of patients with goitrous chronic lymphocytic thyroiditis. J Clin Endocrinol Metab 61:1172–1177, 1985.
10. Weetman AP, McGregor AM, Wheeler MH, et al: Extrathyroidal sites of autoantibody synthesis in Graves' disease. Clin Exp Immunol 56:330–336, 1984.
11. Van Parijs L, Abbas AK: Homeostasis and self-tolerance in the immune system: Turning lymphocytes off. Science 280:243–248, 1998.
12. Germain RN: MHC-dependent antigen processing and peptide presentation: Providing ligands for T lymphocyte activation. Cell 76:287–299, 1994.
13. Nepom GT, Erlich H: MHC class II molecules and autoimmunity. Annu Rev Immunol 9:493–525, 1991.
14. Reiser H, Stadecker MJ: Costimulatory B7 molecules in the pathogenesis of infectious and autoimmune diseases. N Engl J Med 33:1369–1377, 1996.
15. Clark LB, Foy TM, Noelle RJ: CD40 and its ligand. Adv Immunol 63:43–78, 1996.
16. Mosmann TR, Sad S: The expanding universe of T-cell subsets: Th1, Th2 and more. Immunol Today 17:139–145, 1996.
17. Coffman RL, von der Weid T: Multiple pathways for the initiation of T helper 2 (Th2) responses. J Exp Med 185:373–375, 1997.
18. Murray JS: How the MHC selects Th1/Th2 immunity. Immunol Today 19:157–163, 1998.
19. Epstein FH: Lymphocyte-mediated cytolysis and disease. N Engl J Med 335:1651–1659, 1996.
20. De Maria R, Testi R: Fas-FasL interactions: A common pathogenetic mechanism in organ-specific autoimmunity. Immunol Today 19:121–125, 1998.
21. Malissen M, Trucy J, Jourin-Marche E, et al: Regulation of TCRα and β gene allelic exclusion during T-cell development. Immunol Today 13:315–322, 1992.
22. Born WK, O'Brien R, Modlin RL: Antigen specificity of γδ T lymphocytes. FASEB J 5:2699–2705, 1991.

23. Matsuda F, Honjo T: Organization of the human immunoglobulin heavy-chain locus. Adv Immunol 62:1–29, 1996.
24. Laver WG, Air GM, Webster RG, et al: Epitopes on protein antigens: Misconceptions and realities. Cell 61:553–556, 1990.
25. Ramsdell F, Fowlkes BJ: Clonal deletion versus clonal anergy: The role of the thymus in inducing self tolerance. Science 248:1342–1348, 1990.
26. Mondino A, Khoruts A, Jenkins MK: The anatomy of T-cell activation and tolerance. Proc Natl Acad Sci U S A 93:2245–2252, 1996.
27. Goodnow CC: Balancing immunity and tolerance: Deleting and tuning lymphocyte repertoires. Proc Natl Acad Sci U S A 93:2264–2271, 1996.
28. Cone RE, Malley A: Soluble, antigen-specific T-cell proteins: T-cell–based humoral immunity? Immunol Today 17:318–322, 1996.
29. Bloom BR, Salgame P, Diamond B: Revisiting and revising suppressor T cells. Immunol Today 13:131–136, 1992.
30. Weetman AP, McGregor AM: Autoimmune thyroid disease: Further developments in our understanding. Endocr Rev 15:788–830, 1994.
31. Yamaguchi K-I, Shimojo N, Kikuoka S, et al: Genetic control of anti-thyrotropin receptor antibody generation in H-2^k mice immunized with thyrotropin receptor–transfected fibroblasts. J Clin Endocrinol Metab 82:4266–4272, 1997.
32. Costagliola S, Rodien P, Many M-C, et al: Genetic immunization against the human thyrotropin receptor causes thyroiditis and allows production of monoclonal antibodies recognizing the native receptor. J Immunol 160:1458–1465, 1998.
33. Wick G, Cole R, Dietrich H, et al: The obese strain of chickens with spontaneous thyroiditis as a model for Hashimoto disease. *In* Cohen IR, Miller A (eds): Autoimmune Disease Models. San Diego, CA, Academic Press, 1994, pp 107–122.
34. Kong Y-C, Lomo LC, Mott RW, et al: HLA-DRB1 polymorphism determines susceptibility to autoimmune thyroiditis in transgenic mice: Definitive association with HLA-DRB1*0301 (DR3) gene. J Exp Med 184:1167–1172, 1996.
35. Brown TR, Zhao G, Palmer KC, et al: Thyroid injury, autoantigen availability, and the initiation of autoimmune thyroiditis. Autoimmunity 27:1–12, 1997.
36. Rennie DP, McGregor AM, Keast D, et al: The influence of methimazole on thyroglobulin-induced autoimmune thyroiditis in the rat. Endocrinology 112:326–330, 1983.
37. Penhale WJ, Young PR: The influence of the normal microbial flora on the susceptibility of rats to experimental autoimmune thyroiditis. Clin Exp Immunol 72:288–292, 1988.
38. Okayasu I, Kong YM, Rose NR: Effect of castration and sex hormones on experimental autoimmune thyroiditis. Clin Immunol Immunopathol 20:240–245, 1981.
39. Taguchi O, Takahashi T: Mouse models of autoimmune disease suggest that self-tolerance is maintained by unresponsive autoreactive T cells. Immunology 89:13–19, 1996.
40. Guimaraes VC, Quintans J, Fisfalen M-E, et al: Suppression of development of experimental autoimmune thyroiditis by oral administration of thyroglobulin. Endocrinology 136:3353–3359, 1995.
41. Tang H, Braley-Mullen H: Intravenous administration of deaggregated mouse thyroglobulin suppresses induction of experimental autoimmune thyroiditis and expression of both Th1 and Th2 cytokines. Int Immunol 9:679–687, 1997.
42. Akkaraju S, Canaan K, Goodnow CC: Self-reactive B cells are not eliminated or inactivated by autoantigen expressed on thyroid epithelial cells. J Exp Med 186:2005–2012, 1997.
43. Malthiery Y, Lissitzky S: Primary structure of human thyroglobulin deduced from the sequence of its 8848-base complementary DNA. Eur J Biochem 105:491–498, 1987.
44. Carayanniotis G, Rao VP: Searching for pathogenic epitopes in thyroglobulin: Parameters and caveats. Immunol Today 18:83–88, 1997.
45. Nye L, Pontes de Carvalho L, Roitt I: Restriction in the response to autologous thyroglobulin in the human. Clin Exp Immunol 41:252–263, 1980.
46. Bresler HS, Burek CL, Hoffman WH, et al: Autoantigenic determinants on human thyroglobulin. II. Determinants recognized by autoantibodies from patients with chronic autoimmune thyroiditis compared to autoantibodies from healthy subjects. Clin Immunol Immunopathol 54:76–86, 1990.
47. Prentice L, Kiso Y, Fukuma N, et al: Monoclonal thyroglobulin autoantibodies: Variable region analysis and epitope recognition. J Clin Endocrinol Metab 80:977–986, 1995.
48. Tomer Y: Anti-thyroglobulin autoantibodies in autoimmune thyroid diseases: Cross-reactive or pathogenic? Clin Immunol Immunopathol 82:3–11, 1997.
49. McLachlan SM, Rapoport B: The molecular biology of thyroid peroxidase: Cloning, expression, and role as autoantigen in autoimmune thyroid disease. Endocr Rev 13:192–206, 1992.
50. Tandon N, Freeman M, Weetman AP: T cell responses to synthetic thyroid peroxidase peptides in autoimmune thyroid disease. Clin Exp Immunol 86:56–60, 1991.
51. Fisfalen M-E, Soliman M, Okamoto Y, et al: Proliferative responses of T cells to thyroid antigens and synthetic thyroid peroxidase peptides in autoimmune thyroid disease. J Clin Endocrinol Metab 80:1597–1604, 1995.
52. Hamada N, Jaeduck N, Portman L, et al: Antibodies against denatured and reduced thyroid microsomal antigen in autoimmune thyroid disease. J Clin Endocrinol Metab 64:230–238, 1987.
53. McIntosh R, Watson P, Weetman A: Somatic hypermutation in autoimmune thyroid disease. Immunol Rev 162:219–231, 1998.
54. Chazenbalk GD, Portolano S, Russo D, et al: Human organ-specific autoimmune disease. Molecular cloning and expression of an autoantibody gene repertoire for a major autoantigen reveals an antigenic immunodominant region and restricted immunoglobulin gene usage in the target organ. J Clin Invest 92:62–74, 1993.
55. Vassart G, Dumont JE: The thyrotropin receptor and the regulation of thyrocyte function and growth. Endocr Rev 13:596–611, 1992.
56. Graves PN, Tomer Y, Davies TF: Cloning and sequencing of a 1.3kb variant of human thyrotropin receptor mRNA lacking the transmembrane domain. Biochem Biophys Res Commun 187:1135–1143, 1992.
57. Bahn RS, Dutton CM, Natt N, et al: Thyrotropin receptor expression in Graves' orbital adipose/connective tissues: Potential autoantigen in Graves' ophthalmopathy. J Clin Endocrinol Metab 83:998–1002, 1998.
58. Tandon N, Freeman MA, Weetman AP: T cell responses to synthetic TSH receptor peptides in Graves' disease. Clin Exp Immunol 89:468–473, 1992.
59. Martin A, Nakashima M, Zhou A, et al: Detection of major T cell epitopes on human thyroid stimulating hormone receptor by overriding immune heterogeneity in patients with Graves' disease. J Clin Endocrinol Metab 82:3361–3366, 1997.
60. Prabhakar BS, Fan J-L, Seetharamaiah GS: Thyrotropin-receptor–mediated diseases: A paradigm for receptor autoimmunity. Immunol Today 18:437–442, 1997.
61. McLachlan SM, Rapoport B: Monoclonal, human autoantibodies to the TSH receptor—The Holy Grail and why are we looking for it. J Clin Endocrinol Metab 81:3152–3154, 1996.
62. Raspé E, Costagliola S, Ruf J, et al: Identification of the thyroid Na^+/I^- symporter in the sera of patients with autoimmune thyroid disease. Biochem Biophys Res Commun 224:399–405, 1996.
63. Ajjan RA, Findlay C, Metcalfe RA, et al: The modulation of the human sodium iodide symporter activity by Graves' disease sera. J Clin Endocrinol Metab 83:1217–1221, 1998.
64. Benvenga S, Trimarchi F, Robbins J: Circulating thyroid hormone autoantibodies. J Endocrinol Invest 10:605–610, 1987.
65. Phillips DIW, Shields DC, Dougoujon JM, et al: Complex segregation analysis of thyroid autoantibodies: Are they inherited as an autosomal dominant trait? Hum Hered 43:141–146, 1993.
66. Brix TH, Kyvik KO, Hegedüs L: What is the evidence of genetic factors in the etiology of Graves' disease? A brief review. Thyroid 8:627–635, 1998.
67. Weetman AP: Endocrinology. *In* Lechler RI, Warrens A (eds): Handbook of HLA and Disease, ed 2. London, Academic Press, 2000 (in press).
68. Parkes AB, Darke C, Othman S, et al: Major histocompatibility complex class II and complement polymorphisms in postpartum thyroiditis. Eur J Endocrinol 134:449–453, 1996.
69. Shields DC, Ratanachaiyavong S, McGregor AM, et al: Combined segregation and linkage analysis of Graves' disease with a thyroid autoantibody diathesis. Am J Hum Genet 55:540–554, 1994.
70. Tomer Y, Barbesino G, Kedache M, et al: Mapping of a major susceptibility locus for Graves' disease (GD-1) to chromosome 14q31. J Clin Endocrinol Metab 82:1645–1648, 1997.
71. Yanagawa T, Hidaka Y, Guimaraes V, et al: CTLA-4 gene polymorphism associated with Graves' disease in Caucasian population. J Clin Endocrinol Metab 80:41–45, 1995.
72. Kotsa K, Watson PF, Weetman AP: A CTLA-4 gene polymorphism is associated with both Graves' disease and autoimmune hypothyroidism. Clin Endocrinol 46:551–554, 1997.
73. Yanagawa T, Taniyama M, Enomoto S, et al: CTLA-4 gene polymorphism confers susceptibility to Graves' disease in Japanese. Thyroid 7:843–846, 1997.
74. McGregor AM, Weetman AP, Ratanachaiyavong S, et al: Iodine: An influence on the development of autoimmune thyroid disease? *In* Hall R, Köbberling J (eds): Thyroid Disorders Associated with Iodine Deficiency and Excess. New York, Raven Press, 1985, pp 209–216.
75. Huysmans DAKC, Hermus ADRMM, Edelbroek MAL, et al: Autoimmune hyperthyroidism occurring late after radioiodine treatment for volume reduction of large multinodular goiters. Thyroid 7:535–538, 1997.
76. Vykhovanets EV, Chernyshov VP, Slukvin II, et al: ^{131}I dose-dependent thyroid autoimmune disorders in children living around Chernobyl. Clin Immunol Immunopathol 84:251–259, 1997.
77. Hancock SL, Cox RS, McDougall IR: Thyroid diseases after treatment of Hodgkin's disease. N Engl J Med 325:599–605, 1991.
78. Tomer Y, Davies TF: Infection, thyroid disease, and autoimmunity. Endocr Rev 14:107–120, 1993.
79. Jaspan JB, Sullivan K, Garry RF, et al: The interaction of a type A retroviral particle and class II human leukocyte antigen susceptibility genes in the pathogenesis of Graves' disease. J Clin Endocrinol Metab 81:2271–2279, 1996.
80. Bartalena L, Bogazzi F, Percori F, et al: Graves' disease occurring after subacute thyroiditis: Report of a case and review of the literature. Thyroid 6:345–348, 1996.
81. Bartalena L, Bogazzi F, Tanda ML, et al: Cigarette smoking and the thyroid. Eur J Immunol 133:507–512, 1995.
82. Chiovato L, Pinchera A: Stressful life events and Graves' disease. Eur J Endocrinol 134:680–682, 1996.
83. Marazuela M, Garcia-Buey L, González-Fernández B, et al: Thyroid autoimmune disorders in patients with chronic hepatitis C before and during interferon-α therapy. Clin Endocrinol 44:635–642, 1996.
84. Hidaka Y, Amino N, Iwatani Y, et al: Recurrence of thyrotoxicosis after attack of allergic rhinitis in patients with Graves' disease. J Clin Endocrinol Metab 77:1667–1670, 1993.
85. Ludgate ME, McGregor AM, Weetman AP, et al: Analysis of T cell subsets in Graves' disease: Alterations associated with carbimazole. BMJ 288:526–530, 1984.
86. Iwatani Y, Amino N, Hidaka Y, et al: Decreases in $\alpha\beta$ T cell receptor negative T cells and $CD8^+$ cells, and an increase in $CD4^+$, $CD8^+$ cells in active Hashimoto's disease and subacute thyroiditis. Clin Exp Immunol 87:444–449, 1992.
87. Aichinger G, Fill H, Wick G: In situ immune complexes, lymphocyte subpopulations, and HLA-DR positive epithelial cells in Hashimoto's thyroiditis. Lab Invest 52:132–140, 1985.
88. Ueki YM, Eguchi K, Otsubo T, et al: Phenotypic analysis of concanavalin-A–induced suppressor cell dysfunction of thyroidal lymphocytes from patients with Graves' disease. J Clin Endocrinol Metab 67:1018–1024, 1988.
89. Davies TF, Martin A, Concepcion ES, et al: Evidence for selective accumulation of intrathyroidal T lymphocytes in human autoimmune thyroid disease based on T cell receptor V gene usage. J Clin Invest 89:157–162, 1992.
90. McIntosh RS, Tandon N, Pickerill AP, et al: IL-2 receptor positive intrathyroidal

lymphocytes in Graves' disease: Analysis of Vα transcript microheterogeneity. J Immunol 91:3884–3893, 1993.
91. McIntosh RS, Watson PF, Weetman AP: Analysis of T cell receptor Vα repertoire in Hashimoto's thyroiditis: Evidence for the restricted accumulation of CD8+ T cells in the absence of CD4+ T cell restriction. J Clin Endocrinol Metab 82:1140–1146, 1997.
92. MacKenzie WA, Davies TF: An intrathyroidal T-cell clone specifically cytotoxic for human thyroid cells. Immunology 61:101–103, 1987.
93. Catálfamo M, Roura-Mir C, Sospedra M, et al: Self-reactive cytotoxic γδ T lymphocytes in Graves' disease specifically recognize thyroid epithelial cells. J Immunol 156:804–811, 1996.
94. Weetman AP, Ajjan RA, Watson PF: Cytokines and Graves' disease. Baillieres Clin Endocrinol Metab 11:481–497, 1997.
95. Volpé R: Immunoregulation in autoimmune thyroid disease. Thyroid 4:373–377, 1994.
96. Martin A, Davies TF: T cells in human autoimmune thyroid disease. Emerging data shows lack of need to invoke suppressor T cell problems. Thyroid 2:247–261, 1992.
97. Baker JR, Saunders NB, Tseng YC, et al: Seronegative Hashimoto thyroiditis with thyroid autoantibody production localized to the thyroid. Ann Intern Med 108:26–30, 1988.
98. Weetman AP, Black CM, Cohen SB, et al: Affinity purification of IgG subclasses and the distribution of thyroid autoantibody reactivity in Hashimoto's thyroiditis. Scand J Immunol 30:73–82, 1989.
99. Weetman AP, Cohen SB, Oleesky DA, et al: Terminal complement complexes and C1/C1 inhibitor complexes in autoimmune thyroid disease. Clin Exp Immunol 77:25–30, 1989.
100. Nilsson M, Husmark J, Björkman U, Ericson LE: Cytokines and thyroid epithelial integrity: Interleukin-1α induces dissociation of the junctional complex and paracellular leakage in filter-cultured human thyrocytes. J Clin Endocrinol Metab 83:945–952, 1998.
101. Williams RC, Marshall NJ, Kilpatrick K, et al: Kappa/lambda immunoglobulin distribution of Graves' thyroid stimulating antibodies. Simultaneous analysis of Cλ gene polymorphisms. J Clin Invest 82:1306–1312, 1988.
102. Weetman AP, Yateman ME, Ealey PA, et al: Thyroid-stimulating antibody activity between different immunoglobulin G subclasses. J Clin Invest 86:723–727, 1990.
103. Kohn LD, Suzuki K, Hoffman WH, et al: Characterization of monoclonal thyroid-stimulating and thyrotropin binding–inhibiting autoantibodies from a Hashimoto's patient whose children had intrauterine and neonatal thyroid disease. J Clin Endocrinol Metab 82:3998–4009, 1997.
104. Kung AWC, Jones BM: A change from stimulatory to blocking antibody activity in Graves' disease during pregnancy. J Clin Endocrinol Metab 83:514–518, 1998.
105. Cho BY, Kim WB, Chung JH, et al: High prevalence and little change in TSH receptor blocking antibody titres with thyroxine and antithyroid drug therapy in patients with non-goitrous autoimmune thyroiditis. Clin Endocrinol 43:465–471, 1995.
106. Kraiem Z, Lahat N, Glaser B, et al: Thyrotrophin receptor blocking antibodies: Incidence, characterization and in vivo synthesis. Clin Endocrinol 27:409–421, 1987.
107. Drexhage HA: Autoimmunity and thyroid growth. Where do we stand? Eur J Immunol 135:39–45, 1996.
108. Vitti P, Chiovato L, Tonacchera M, et al: Failure to detect thyroid growth-promoting activity in immunoglobulin G of patients with endemic goiter. J Clin Endocrinol Metab 78:1020–1025, 1994.
109. Di Cerbo A, Di Paola R, Bonati M, et al: Subgroups of Graves' patients identified on the basis of the biochemical activities of their immunoglobulins. J Clin Endocrinol Metab 80:2785–2790, 1995.
110. Sato K, Yamazaki K, Shizume K, et al: Stimulation by thyroid-stimulating hormone and Graves' immunoglobulin G of vascular endothelial growth factor mRNA expression in human thyroid follicles in vitro and *flt* mRNA expression in the rat thyroid in vivo. J Clin Invest 96:1295–1302, 1995.
111. Bottazzo GF, Pujol-Borrell R, Hanafusa T, et al: Role of aberrant HLA-DR expression and antigen presentation in induction of endocrine autoimmunity. Lancet 2:1115–1119, 1983.
112. Hamilton F, Black M, Farquharson MA, et al: Spatial correlation between thyroid epithelial cells expressing class II MHC molecules and interferon-gamma–containing lymphocytes in human thyroid autoimmune disease. Clin Exp Immunol 83:64–68, 1991.
113. Marelli-Berg F, Weetman AP, Frasca L, et al: Antigen presentation by epithelial cells induces anergic immunoregulatory CD45R0+ T cells and deletion of CD45RA+ T cells. J Immunol 159:5853–5861, 1997.
114. Sospedra M, Obiols G, Babi LFS, et al: Hyperinducibility of HLA class II expression of thyroid follicular cells from Graves' disease. J Immunol 154:4213–4222, 1995.
115. Weetman AP, Freeman MA, Borysiewicz LK, et al: Functional analysis of intercellular adhesion molecule-1 expressing human thyroid cells. Eur J Immunol 20:271–275, 1990.
116. Wu Z, Podack ER, McKenzie JM, et al: Perforin expression by thyroid-infiltrating T cells in autoimmune thyroid disease. Clin Exp Immunol 98:470–477, 1994.
117. Giordano C, Stassi G, De Maria R, et al: Potential involvement of Fas and its ligand on the pathogenesis of Hashimoto's thyroiditis. Science 275:960–963, 1997.
118. Arscott PL, Baker JR Jr: Apoptosis and thyroiditis. Clin Immunol Immunopathol 87:207–217, 1998.
119. Chiovato L, Bassi P, Santini F, et al: Antibodies producing complement-mediated thyroid cytotoxicity in patients with atrophic or goitrous autoimmune thyroiditis. J Clin Endocrinol Metab 77:1700–1705, 1993.
120. Tandon N, Yan SL, Morgan BP, et al: Expression and function of multiple regulators of complement activation in autoimmune thyroid disease. Immunology 84:643–647, 1994.
121. Weetman AP, Tandon N, Morgan BP: Antithyroid drugs and release of inflammatory mediators by complement-attacked thyroid cells. Lancet 340:633–636, 1992.
122. Kasai K, Banba N, Motohashi S, et al: Expression of monocyte chemoattractant protein-1 mRNA and protein in cultured human thyrocytes. FEBS Lett 394:137–140, 1996.
123. Simons PJ, Delemarre FGA, Drexhage HA: Antigen-presenting dendritic cells as regulators of the growth of thyrocytes: A role of interleukin-1β and interleukin-6. Endocrinology 139:3148–3156, 1998.
124. Vanderpump MPJ, Tunbridge WMG, French JM, et al: The incidence of thyroid disorders in the community: A twenty-year follow-up of the Whickham survey. Clin Endocrinol 43:55–68, 1995.
125. Nelson JL: Microchimerism and autoimmune disease. N Engl J Med 338:1224–1225, 1998.
126. Takasu N, Yamada Y, Takasu M, et al: Disappearance of thyrotropin-blocking antibodies and spontaneous recovery from hypothyroidism in autoimmune thyroiditis. N Engl J Med 326:513–518, 1992.
127. Volpé R: Evidence that the immunosuppressive effects of antithyroid drugs are mediated through actions on the thyroid cell, modulating thyrocyte-immunocyte signalling. Thyroid 4:217–221, 1994.
128. Michelangeli VP, Poon C, Topliss DJ, et al: Specific effects of radioiodine treatment on TSAb and TSAb levels in patients with Graves' disease. Thyroid 5:171–176, 1995.
129. Bartalena L, Marcocci C, Bogazzi F, et al: Relation between therapy for hyperthyroidism and the course of Graves' ophthalmopathy. N Engl J Med 338:73–78, 1998.
130. Teng WP, Stark R, Munro AJ, et al: Peripheral blood T cell activation after radioiodine treatment for Graves' disease. Acta Endocrinol 122:233–240, 1990.
131. Lee S, Scherberg N, DeGroot LJ: Induction of oral tolerance in human autoimmune thyroid disease. Thyroid 8:229–234, 1998.
132. Baker JR Jr, Fosso CK: Immunological aspects of cancers arising from thyroid follicular cells. Endocr Rev 13:729–746, 1993.
133. Matsuzuka F, Miyauchi A, Katayama S, et al: Clinical aspects of primary thyroid lymphoma: Diagnosis and treatment based on our experience of 119 cases. Thyroid 3:93–99, 1993.
134. Pratt DE, Kaberlein G, Dudkiewicz A, et al: The association of antithyroid antibodies in euthyroid nonpregnant women with recurrent first trimester abortions in the next pregnancy. Fertil Steril 60:1001–1005, 1993.
135. Giani C, Fierabracci P, Bonacci R, et al: Relationship between breast cancer and thyroid disease: Relevance of autoimmune thyroid disorders in breast malignancy. J Clin Endocrinol Metab 81:990–994, 1996.
136. Pop VJ, Maartens LH, Leusink G, et al: Are autoimmune thyroid dysfunction and depression related? J Clin Endocrinol Metab 83:3194–3197, 1998.
137. Muir A, Maclaren NK: Autoimmune diseases of the adrenal glands, parathyroid glands, gonads, and hypothalamic-pituitary axis. Endocrinol Metab Clin North Am 20:619–644, 1991.
138. Betterle C, Greggio NA, Volpato M: Autoimmune polyglandular syndrome type 1. J Clin Endocrinol Metab 83:1049–1055, 1998.

Chapter 100

Graves' Disease

Luca Chiovato ▪ Giuseppe Barbesino ▪ Aldo Pinchera

Toxic diffuse goiter, commonly referred to as Graves' disease, is a uniquely human disease and since its first descriptions has stimulated and puzzled clinicians and scientists. In its classic form it is characterized by excessive production of thyroid hormones by the thyroid gland (hyperthyroidism) and by diffuse enlargement of the thyroid. Graves' disease is often (but not always) associated with a unique eye inflammatory disorder termed Graves' ophthalmopathy. When present, Graves' ophthalmopathy makes the diagnosis of Graves' disease almost unmistakable. Other more rarely associated features are a localized infiltrative dermopathy (pretibial myxedema) and Graves' acropachy. Graves' disease is now universally classified among the autoimmune organ-specific diseases because it fulfills all the criteria required for this definition (Table 100–1). Circulating antibodies directed to the thyroid-stimulating hormone receptor (TSHR) that mimic the effect of pituitary TSH on the thyroid gland cause Graves' hyperthyroidism. TSHR is therefore the main antigen of Graves' disease. After cloning of TSHR, the structure-function relationship of TSHR and its mode of interaction with thyroid-stimulating antibodies (TSAbs) have been clarified to a large extent.

On the clinical side, the clinician can take advantage of several available options when treatment is being planned. The decision-making process is now supported by the experience derived from evaluating the large body of clinical data.

In spite of these major advancements, the ultimate cause of Graves' disease has not been unveiled. We have only begun to understand the influence of genetic background and environmental factors leading to disruption of tolerance and eventually to expansion of the immune response to TSHR. Also, the mechanisms that link Graves' disease to Graves' ophthalmopathy remain largely unclear, and treatment of the ocular manifestations of the disease (probably its most disabling feature) is still controversial and to some extent unsatisfactory.

TABLE 100–1. Criteria for Organ-Specific Autoimmune Diseases and Their Presence in Graves' Disease

Criteria	Present in Graves' Disease
Lymphocytic infiltration of the target organ	Yes
Identification of the specific antigen(s)	Yes
Production of humoral and/or cellular autoimmune responses (or both) in animals sensitized by autologous antigen	Yes
Presence of organ-specific lesions in autosensitized animals	Yes
Association with other autoimmune diseases	Yes

HISTORICAL NOTES

Graves' disease is the eponym by which a syndrome characterized by diffuse goiter and hyperthyroidism is recognized in English-speaking countries. Robert James Graves (Fig. 100–1) was a brilliant and productive Irish physician who contributed in many ways to the medical science of his time.[1] Credit for his prominent position is probably due to his description in 1835 of ". . . three cases of violent and long palpitations in females, in each of which the same peculiarity presented...enlargement of the thyroid gland, . . ." which was the first report of toxic diffuse goiter.[2] However, Caleb Hillier Parry, a less renowned physician of Bath, England, had described a similar syndrome earlier, in 1825: "There is one malady which I have in five cases seen coincident with what appears to be enlargement of the heart, and which, so far as I know has not been noticed in that connection by medical writers. This malady to which I allude is enlargement of the thyroid gland."[3] He also described protrusion of the eyes as a feature of the syndrome. Even earlier than that, in 1805, the Italian Giuseppe Flajani in Rome had reported two cases of diffuse swelling of the neck accompanied by palpitations.[4] He failed to recognize the thyroidal origin of the swelling and named it "*bronchocele.*" In 1840 in Germany, Carl A. von Basedow described "*Exophthalmos durch Hypertrophie del Zellgewebes in der Augenhohle*," or exophthalmos caused by hypertrophy of the cellular tissue of the orbit; this first description of the complete syndrome included the triad of exophthalmos, struma, and palpitations of the heart. He was struck

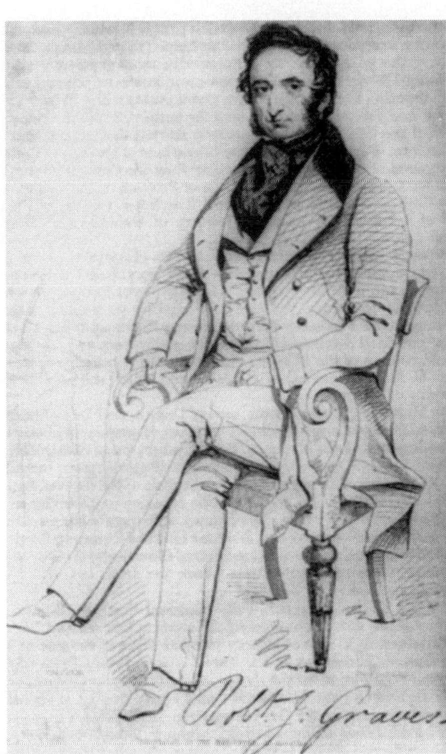

FIGURE 100–1. Portrait of Dr. Robert J. Graves. (From Taylor S: Robert Graves[1]. The Golden Years of Irish Medicine. New York, Royal Society of Medicine Services, 1989.)

by the prominence of the eye changes and made exophthalmos the hallmark of the disease.[5] His descriptions were widely disseminated at the time, so in most non–English-speaking European countries the disease is called "Basedow's disease." In 1880 Ludwig Rehn performed the first thyroidectomy for toxic diffuse goiter, and in 1909 Kocher was awarded the Nobel Prize for his innovations in thyroid surgery. In 1886 Moebius proposed that exophthalmic goiter was due to excessive function of the thyroid gland.[6] In 1911 Marine proposed treatment of Graves' disease with iodine in the form of Lugol's solution.[7] In the early 1940s the antithyroid drugs thioureas were described,[8] and Astwood introduced them into clinical use for the control of thyrotoxicosis.[9] At the same time, physicists and physicians in Boston and in Berkeley started to treat thyrotoxic patients with radioiodine (^{131}I).[10] Therefore, in the space of a few years the two mainstays of modern treatment of Graves' disease were initiated. The following decade was marked by the discovery in 1956 of the long-acting thyroid stimulator (LATS) by Adams and Purves[11] and by the subsequent identification of this stimulator as an antibody, thus forming the basis of our current understanding of the pathogenesis of Graves' disease. Cloning of TSHR,[12, 13] the main autoantigen of Graves' disease, is only the most recent and will certainly not be the last memorable event in the uncovering of a disease that has paralleled the development of modern medicine across two centuries.

EPIDEMIOLOGY

Graves' disease is a relatively prevalent disorder. It is the most frequent cause of thyrotoxicosis in iodine-sufficient countries.[14] Comparison of historical surveys is made difficult by the use of different criteria in population sampling. Moreover, diagnostic tools for distinguishing among different causes of hyperthyroidism have changed over the years. For example, in the Unites States a large survey performed in the 1970s estimated the prevalence of Graves' disease to be 0.4%.[15] The Whickham survey in the United Kingdom suggested a prevalence of 1.1% to 1.6% (i.e., about threefold to fourfold higher) for thyrotoxicosis of all causes, of which Graves' disease was presumably the most frequent.[16] A recent meta-analysis of various studies has estimated the general prevalence of the disorder to be about 1%,[17] which makes it one of the most frequent clinically relevant autoimmune disorders. The iodine alimentary supply of populations appears to be a major determinant of the prevalence of autoimmune thyroid disease in general and Graves' disease in particular. Iodine supplementation of previously iodine-deficient Tasmania induced a sharp (threefold) increase in the incidence of hyperthyroidism in the 3 years after initiation of the program.[18] This increase was attributed to iodine-induced thyrotoxicosis in patients with previously iodine-deprived autonomously functioning nodules or goiters. However, subsequent studies have shown that LATSs or LATS protectors were present in a number of cases of thyrotoxicosis in the early supplementation period,[19] thus suggesting that some of the iodine-induced cases of hyperthyroidism may have been due to the unveiling of preexisting subclinical Graves' disease, also previously iodine deprived. Since the Tasmanian report, outbursts of iodine-induced thyrotoxicosis have been reported in many countries after the implementation of extensive iodine supplementation programs.[20] Thyrotoxicosis occurred primarily in older people with preexisting nodular goiter, when severely iodine-deficient populations acutely increased their iodine intake. A modest and transient increase in the incidence of Graves' disease has also been noted in Switzerland after stepwise, full iodine supplementation of the population[21] (Fig. 100–2). In the latter report, the increase in the overall rate of thyrotoxicosis (detectable only in the first 2 to 3 years after supplementation) was transient and mostly caused by cases of toxic multinodular goiter. The net result 10 years later was a sharp decrease in the overall incidence of thyrotoxicosis, mainly as a result of a reduction in the frequency of toxic nodular goiter. Similar increases in the prevalence of thyrotoxicosis have been reported in Sweden (16.6/100,000),[22] New Zealand (15/100,000),[23] and Britain (23/100,000).[24] Population-based studies also show differences in the incidence of Graves' disease in populations with different, but relatively constant iodine intake. In a comparison between two genetically identical populations that differed with regard to iodine intake, the annual incidence of Graves' disease hyperthyroidism was about 20 per 100,000 inhabitants in iodine-sufficient Iceland, with the incidence of thyrotoxicosis of all causes being 23 per 100,000. In contrast, the incidence of Graves' disease was 15 per 100,000 inhabitants of iodine-deficient East Jutland, but the overall incidence of thyrotoxicosis was distinctly higher (39/100,000).[14] These data clearly show that fear of an increased incidence of Graves' disease should not prevent the implementation of iodine supplementation programs because the end result will be a decrease in the number of new cases of thyrotoxicosis caused by toxic nodular goiter after a relatively short time.

Although ethnic differences in susceptibility to Graves' disease are likely to exist, they have not been consistently investigated in comparative studies. Previous reports of a low incidence of Graves' disease

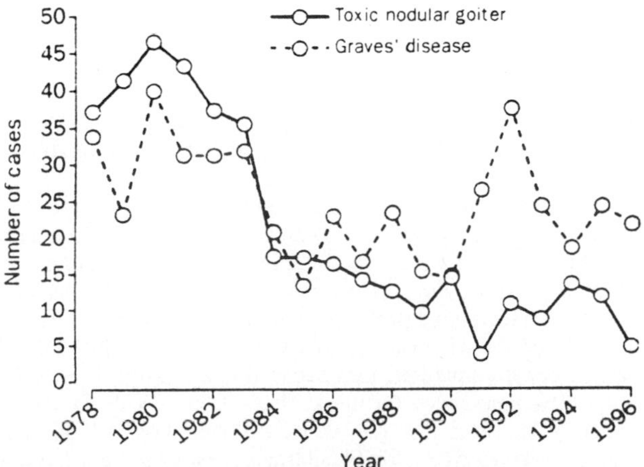

FIGURE 100–2. Increased incidence of hyperthyroidism from Graves' disease and toxic nodular goiter in Switzerland after the introduction of iodine supplementation. (From Burgi H, Kohler M, Morselli B: Thyrotoxicosis incidence in Switzerland and benefit of improved iodine supply. Lancet 352:1034, 1998, © by The Lancet, 1998.)

in African natives have been criticized because of possible referral bias in mixed native rural and immigrant urban populations.[25]

As with many other autoimmune disorders, Graves' disease is about fivefold more prevalent in women than men. The reasons for this observation are only partially understood, but some hypotheses will be discussed later. The annual incidence is clearly and consistently related to age, with peaks in the fourth to sixth decades of life,[23] although Graves' disease can be observed in people of any age, including children.

ETIOLOGY

Much of the immune pathology of Graves' disease has been clarified in the more than 40 years since the first description of LATS.[11] Graves' disease has been characterized as an organ-specific autoimmune disorder with T cell– and B cell–mediated autoimmunity to thyroid and eye antigens. Among the thyroid antigens, TSHR is the main one. Circulating autoantibodies against TSHR that are capable of stimulating the receptor (TSH receptor antibodies [TRAbs]) are responsible for the most distinctive features of the disease, hyperthyroidism and goiter. In spite of advancements in understanding these pathogenic mechanisms, the ultimate cause of the disease remains elusive. Most investigators share the opinion that Graves' disease is a multifactorial disease caused by a complex interplay of genetic, hormonal, and environmental influences leading to the loss of tolerance to thyroid antigens and the initiation of a sustained immune reaction directed at thyroid and still unidentified orbital antigens.

Genetics of Graves' Disease

It is common for endocrinologists to observe familial clustering of Graves' disease by simply eliciting the family history of patients. Besides this practical knowledge, a body of evidence indicates the existence of a genetic predisposition to Graves' disease.

Twin studies are very important tools for studying the genetics of a disease. Dizygotic twins share on average 50% of their genome, whereas monozygotic twins share 100%. Moreover, twins are likely to share environmental factor more so than any other kind of siblings. Large twin studies are not available for Graves' disease. Older studies suggested a concordance rate of 76% in monozygotic[26] and 11% in dizygotic twins. More recent data obtained with modern diagnostic tools, but in a small sample, have shown a lower, but still significant concordance (30%) in monozygotic twins, as opposed to a lack of concordance in dizygotic twins.[27] These findings clearly show a genetic influence, possibly characterized by low penetrance of the involved genes.

Another tool widely used to establish the existence of a genetic predisposition to any condition is family studies, in which the prevalence of the disease in relatives of index cases is compared with the general or expected prevalence. Early family studies showed a high prevalence of Graves' disease and other thyroid abnormalities in first-degree relatives of patients with Graves' disease and Hashimoto's thyroiditis.[28] The prevalence of circulating thyroid autoantibodies in siblings of patients was as high as 50% in some studies,[29] which suggested a dominant mode of inheritance for these markers. This observation has been consistently confirmed in highly selected populations,[30–33] but the results may not be applicable to the general population because of ascertainment bias. In an extensive segregation analysis with randomly ascertained probands, circulating antibodies were found in only 25% of the offspring of positive parents and in 14% of the offspring of negative parents, thus suggesting a multigenic model with less than 100% penetrance for the antibody trait.[34] With the exception of very early studies,[35] the prevalence of overt Graves' disease has been found to be relatively low in siblings of patients. In a large study with a follow-up of 5 years, Graves' disease developed in only 3 of 69 (4.3%) relatives of patients with Graves' disease. Many others (24%), however, showed initial abnormalities in thyroid function compatible with subclinical hyperthyroidism or hypothyroidism.[36] Hashimoto's thyroiditis is frequently observed in families in which the proband has Graves' disease, and occasionally one of two identical twins has Graves' disease whereas the other has Hashimoto's thyroiditis,[37] thus indicating that the two diseases may share at least part of the susceptibility genes. Other organ-specific autoimmune phenomena such as circulating gastric parietal cell autoantibodies and adrenal autoantibodies may also be more prevalent in relatives of patients with Graves' disease.[38]

These data and those obtained in twin studies are indicative of a complex multigenic pattern of inheritance of Graves' disease. Some of the components of the phenotype, such as the presence of circulating antithyroglobulin and antithyroperoxidase antibodies, may be inherited in a dominant fashion with high penetrance.[29, 39] However, these genetic determinants do not appear to be sufficient for full expression of the disease. Clearly, other genes must be involved, which is in line with the complexity of the inheritance observed. Also, it appears from epidemiologic and experimental data that environmental factors (reviewed in other sections of this chapter) play an important role in genesis of the disease by modulating the effect of the inherited predisposition. Based on the above evidence, a number of genes or loci have been investigated as candidates for predisposing factors. The genes studied so far can be grouped into three categories: the HLA complex, non-HLA immunoregulatory genes, and thyroid autoantigen genes.

In the absence of spontaneous animal models, two major methods are available to clinical geneticists to identify and map genetic determinants of inherited disorders: association studies and linkage analysis. In most studies involving complex diseases showing positive associations (including the study of Graves' disease), the "associated" allele is also present in a relevant percentage of the control population, and many patients (often the majority) do not carry the allele. This observation suggests that in most cases association studies only detect risk factors and not the presence of the major genes necessary for manifestation of the disease. On the other hand, these methods are very sensitive and may detect minor determinants of genetic susceptibility.[40] In linkage analysis, cosegregation of any allele of the marker with the disease in families is analyzed with sophisticated statistical tools. Positive linkage indicates the presence of a major susceptibility gene in the chromosomal region where the marker is located.[41] Linkage analysis allows screening of the whole genome and can detect genes without any prior knowledge of their function.[41] Susceptibility to Graves' disease has been studied by both methods, and some of the results available are summarized in the following sections.

HLA Complex and Genetic Predisposition to Graves' Disease

The HLA complex, which is located on the short arm of human chromosome 6, contains the sequence encoding for about a hundred genes, most of which are involved in regulation of the immune response. The HLA genes are classically grouped into three major classes. Class I includes histocompatibility genes expressed on the surface of most cells (HLA-A, HLA-B, and HLA-C determinants). Class II includes histocompatibility genes expressed exclusively on the surface of leukocytes and immune cells (HLA-DR determinants). Class III includes a heterogeneous group of genes coding for factors involved in the immune response but not directly involved in histocompatibility reactions, such as a number of complement factors, cytokines (tumor necrosis factor-α), and lymphocyte surface molecules (TAP-1 and TAP-2). Other genes included in this class are genes localized within the complex but without a clear relationship to immunity, such as the 21-hydroxylase gene and the hemochromatosis gene. Most genes of the HLA complex are highly polymorphic, which makes them excellent candidates for disease susceptibility genes.

Experimental thyroiditis in the mouse was the first autoimmune disease to be associated with HLA.[42] In these studies, expression of experimental thyroiditis was related to alleles of the H locus in congenic mice and was largely independent of the strains' genetic background. Early population studies in humans first indicated an association of Graves' disease with HLA-B8 and a relative risk of 3.9 in white patients.[43] Subsequent studies also suggested an influence of that haplotype on the clinical course of the disease by showing that HLA-

TABLE 100–2. Polymorphisms in the CTLA-4 Gene Associated with Graves' Disease in Different Studies

Author, Year	Associated Allele	Number of Patients (% Positive)	Number of Controls (% Positive)	Relative Risk
Yanagawa, 1994	106 bp	266 (26.7)	170 (13.5)	2.82
Nistico', 1996	49 A/G	94 (73.0)	77 (62.0)	1.7
Donner, 1997	49 A/G	305 (74.0)	325 (59.0)	2.0
Kotsa, 1997	106 bp	312 (23.4)	182 (12.6)	2.2
*Sale, 1997	106 bp	150 (37.6)	194 (30.4)	NS
Yanagawa, 1997	49 A/G	153 (93.0)	200 (83.0)	2.6
*Heward, 1998	−318 C/T	188 (10)	355 (8)	NS

*Negative studies.

B8–positive patients were more prone to relapses and more resistant to treatment.[44] HLA-DR3 was later shown to increase the risk to a greater extent and was considered to be the true determinants of the disease because it was in linkage dysequilibrium with the B8 allele.[45] Further refinements in HLA typing methods eventually led to identification of DQA1*0501 as the major risk-determining allele within DR3 itself.[46] This allele is in linkage dysequilibrium with both B8 and DR3 and gives a relative risk of 3 to 4 for Graves' disease in the white population. In the male Graves' disease population, DQA1*0501 seems to be a stronger determinant and is associated with a relative risk of 9.[47] This difference has been attributed to a stronger genetic predisposition in subgroups of patients with a lower absolute risk for the disease. The consistent association of DQA1*0501 with Graves' disease observed in population-based studies has also been confirmed in family-based association studies,[48] thus establishing this haplotype as a true risk factor for Graves' disease, at least in the white population. In fact, different haplotypes seem to be involved in different ethnic groups: DQ3 in patients of African descent[49] and Bw46 in those of Asian descent,[50] although the data available are limited and have not always been reproducible.[51] In general, HLA associations have been shown to confer comparatively low relative risk, even with alleles that have a relatively high prevalence in the general population. Linkage analysis, a powerful tool for mapping essential predisposition genes, has been negative when the HLA region was examined using different polymorphisms at the same locus.[52, 53] These findings indicate that the HLA locus explains only a small fraction of the total genetic predisposition. It therefore seems that the HLA locus is neither the major nor the only determinant of genetic predisposition to Graves' disease, although it certainly represents an established risk-increasing factor.

Non-HLA Genes and Graves' Disease

In the search for other genetic determinants of Graves' disease, a number of loci other than the HLA loci have been studied. Two categories of genes have been analyzed: genes involved in the immune response and genes coding for the major thyroid autoantigens. The immunoglobulin genes were among the first to be studied. Conflicting results were observed in association studies. Initially, an association with IgG heavy-chain Gm allotypes and Graves' disease was reported.[54, 55] However, these results were not confirmed in other studies.[56] Similarly, the T cell receptor α and β loci have produced conflicting results in a number of studies.[56–59] Other candidate immunoregulatory genes studied include interleukin-1 (IL-1) and IL-1 receptor antagonist,[60] tumor necrosis factor receptor-2,[61] and interferon-γ (INF-γ).[62] None of these candidate genes showed significant associations with Graves' disease. More recently, polymorphisms of the cytotoxic T lymphocyte–associated-4 (CTLA-4) gene have consistently been found to be associated with Graves' disease in a number of studies in white[63–66] (Table 100–2) and Japanese[67] populations. CTLA-4 is a T lymphocyte surface protein with a major role in downregulation of the immune response.[68] Similar to the HLA locus, however, the observed relative risk for Graves' disease was quite low, thus indicating a small contribution to genetic predisposition. Linkage analysis of several of these immunoregulatory genes in a subset of informative Graves' disease families has yielded negative results for the T cell receptor, immunoglobulin, and CTLA-4 genes, which excludes these genes as major susceptibility determinants,[69] at least in the large data set studied. More recent data, however, have suggested linkage of CTLA-4 to Graves' disease[70] in another data set, a finding that is difficult to reconcile with the comparatively low relative risk observed in association studies. It has been suggested that the combined influence of the HLA-DR and CTLA-4 alleles accounts for half of the genetic influence in Graves' disease. The genes for thyroid autoantigens, such as thyroid peroxidase, thyroglobulin, and TSHR, have also been studied as potential candidates but excluded in both association studies[59, 71] and linkage analysis.[72, 53]

Progress in the human genome mapping projects in the past few years has provided investigators in genetics the precise genomic location for an extremely large number of polymorphic markers, and genetic disorders can be mapped with the powerful tool of linkage analysis through whole genome scanning. In an ongoing project aiming at identification of the susceptibility genes for autoimmune thyroid disease, three loci have shown results suggesting linkage in families with Graves' disease: one locus on chromosome 14q31 (GD-1), a locus on chromosome 20 (GD-2), and a locus on chromosome Xq21-22 (GD-3).[73–75] Although these results must be considered preliminary until replicated in different data sets, they suggest the presence of Graves' disease susceptibility genes in these chromosomal locations.

In summary, Graves' disease is a genetic disorder with a complex mode of inheritance. The genetic factors involved have only started to be unraveled (Table 100–3). Established risk factors include the HLA and CTLA-4 loci, but they cannot completely explain the genetic susceptibility observed in epidemiologic studies.

Environmental Factors in Graves' Disease

Studies in twins have indicated low penetrance (<50%) for predisposition factors to Graves' disease,[76] and this finding has also been confirmed in family studies.[77, 78] It is therefore evident that environmental factors play a major role in inducing the disease in susceptible individuals.

Infection

Over the years, both experimental and epidemiologic evidence has suggested that infection could play a role in the pathogenesis of Graves' disease.[79] Seasonal and geographic variation in incidence of the disease has been reported.[80, 81] Blood group nonsecretors, who are more prone than secretors to infection, are more frequently found

TABLE 100–3. Known Genetic Determinants of Graves' Disease and Their Chromosomal Locations

Gene/Locus	Chromosomal Location	Identification Method	Possible Mechanism
HLA-DR*	6p21.3	Association	Impaired antigen presentation
CTLA-4*	2q33	Association/linkage analysis	Impaired antigen presentation
GD-1	14q31	Linkage analysis	Unknown
GD-2	20q11	Linkage analysis	Unknown
GD-3	Xq21-22	Linkage analysis	Unknown

*Factors that have been confirmed in multiple studies.

among patients with Graves' disease than controls.[82] This observation has been interpreted as indirect evidence that infectious pathogens may be involved in the etiology of Graves' disease, although a direct genetic effect of the secretor status could also explain these results. Evidence of a recent viral infection has been observed in a high percentage of patients with Graves' disease,[83] and an increased frequency of anti–influenza B virus antibodies was found in thyrotoxic patients.[84]

Molecular mimicry has been invoked to explain the association between infection and Graves' disease. Molecular mimicry is based on the hypothesis that cross-reaction of some microbial antigens with a self-antigen may cause an immune response to the autoantigenic structure itself upon infection. In Graves' disease, the pathogen *Yersinia enterocolitica* has been thoroughly studied after reports of association of this microbe with the disease. A high prevalence of circulating antibodies against *Y. enterocolitica*, strain O:3, has been observed in patients with Graves' disease,[85–87] and *Yersinia* antibodies were found to interact with thyroid structures.[88–90] Saturable binding sites for TSH have been found in *Yersinia* and were also recognized by TRAbs from patients with Graves' disease.[91, 92] *Yersinia* cDNA fragments could also be amplified with human TSHR primers.[93] In animals immunized with *Yersinia* proteins, antibodies developed against human thyroid epithelial cells and TSHR.[94, 95] Overall, the affinity of these cross-reactive antibodies to the thyroid was low, and immune responses were transient.[90] Low-affinity binding sites for TSH have also been found in other bacteria, for example, species of *Leishmania* and *Mycoplasma*.[96] However, it must be noted that thyroid autoimmune disease does not develop in most patients with *Yersinia* infection.[97] Thus the evidence in favor of *Yersinia* infection as a precipitating cause of Graves' disease remains circumstantial and awaits confirmation.

Viruses could theoretically trigger autoimmunity through several mechanisms, including interactions with autoantigens, permanent expression of viral proteins on the surface of epithelial cells, aberrant induction of HLA antigens on epithelial cells (see later), and molecular mimicry.[79] In 1989 the presence of retroviral (HIV-1 glycosaminoglycan protein) sequences in the thyroid and peripheral mononuclear cells of patients with Graves' disease was reported,[98] but viral sequences were not found in control thyroids. This finding, however, remained isolated and was not confirmed in subsequent studies.[99, 100] More recently, human foamy virus antigens were shown by immunofluorescence to be present in the thyroids of patients with Graves' disease.[101] Again, further studies using more specific and sensitive techniques failed to identify foamy virus DNA and antiviral antibodies in the blood of affected subjects.[102, 103] Homology between another HIV-1 protein (Nef) and human TSHR has also been reported,[104] although sera from patients with Graves' disease did not react with the peptide bearing the highest degree of homology. Another retroviral protein, p15E, has been isolated from the thyroids of patients with Graves' disease but not from control glands.[105] In this regard it is worthwhile emphasizing that retroviral-like proteins, including p15E, are encoded by the normal human genome. Although their function is unclear, they may be expressed in many epithelial tissues under certain conditions, including inflammation, and may modulate but not initiate the immune response.[106] The finding of retroviral sequences or proteins in the glands of patients with Graves' disease may therefore represent a secondary rather than a causative phenomenon. Recently, circulating antibodies against another retroviral particle termed HIAP-1 have been found in as many as 87.5% of patients with Graves' disease as compared with 10% to 15% of controls, which included patients with other thyroid diseases or other autoimmune diseases and healthy individuals.[107] The possibility of cross-reactivity between thyroid autoantigens and the retroviral particle was not examined in this work, which awaits confirmation. Finally, a highly speculative hypothesis has been raised that involves superantigens. Superantigens are endogenous or exogenous proteins capable of stimulating a strong immune response through molecular interactions with nonvariant parts of the T cell receptor and the HLA class II proteins. Through this mechanism, superantigens are in theory capable of stimulating the expansion of autoreactive T cells and therefore capable of driving an autoimmune response.[79] Such a mechanism has been suggested in rheumatoid arthritis.[108] Recently, a similar mechanism has been proposed for Graves' disease. In vitro superantigen stimulation of glands with autoimmune thyroid disease induced expression of HLA class II molecules on thyrocytes, and this phenomenon was IFN-γ dependent.[109] The interpretation of this observation is that superantigen-reactive T cells exist among the lymphocytes infiltrating the thyroid in autoimmune thyroid disease and that these lymphocytes may have been activated after exposure to extrinsic superantigens.

In summary, although epidemiologic evidence indicates that infection may play an important role as a causative factor in Graves' disease, we are still lacking definitive identification of the etiologic organism(s) and a reasonable explanation for the mechanism by which it could precipitate the disorder.

Stress

The suggestion that psychologic stress may be a precipitating factor in Graves' disease has been made as early as the first description of the disease.[3] The occurrence of stressful events before the onset of Graves' disease is a recurrent impression among clinicians, and by the end of the 19th century Graves' disease was considered to be a result of prolonged emotional disturbances. In recent cross-sectional studies some investigators have shown an increased prevalence of stressful life events in the months preceding the onset of Graves' disease.[110–114] These studies were all based on questionnaires regarding the occurrence of a number of life events in the months preceding the onset of Graves' disease in patients and compared the occurrence of these events in matched control populations. A number of the recorded events (such as arguments with spouses and in the workplace) could have been influenced by the behavior of patients with still undetected hyperthyroidism and therefore be a consequence rather than the cause of the disease. Other events, however, were largely independent of patient behavior (unemployment, financial difficulties). In some studies patients were asked to rate the stressfulness of life events, and patients with Graves' disease ranked such events more stressful than did controls.[114] It is possible that the perception of the impact of life events is different in hyperthyroid patients. In cross-sectional studies, an increase in the prevalence of Graves' disease was reported during World War II in Germany, but not during the civil unrest in Ireland[115] or during the German occupation of Belgium, which suggests that the stressful events of personal life may be more important than "social stress." Stress is associated with increased adrenocorticotropic hormone (ACTH) and cortisol secretion, which can in turn determine immune suppression,[116] but additional non–ACTH-related immunosuppressive phenomena also occur.[117] Recovery from such immune suppression can be associated with rebound immune hyperactivity, which could precipitate autoimmunity. The best example of such a phenomenon is perhaps the well-documented immune suppression of pregnancy,[118] often followed by new or recurrent onset of Graves' disease[119, 120] (see below). In summary, limited but significant evidence indicates that stress may be a contributing factor in the etiology of Graves' disease, probably in connection with other predisposing factors. The available studies are all retrospective and therefore carry a number of possible biases. Worried patients sick with hyperthyroidism may be more prone to recall upsetting events, and subclinical undetected thyrotoxicosis present before clinical diagnosis may have altered the perception of life events and even the behavior of patients. Unfortunately, prospective studies addressing the problem of stress and Graves' disease and its interplay with genetic factors are not available to date.[121]

Gender

Graves' disease is typically, but not exclusively a disease of women. In most series the female-to-male ratio ranges from 5 to 10 at any age,[16, 17] although the difference may be smaller during childhood.[122] The reason for the disproportionate prevalence of Graves' disease in women is not known, but genetic and nongenetic factors must play a role. A number of studies indicate a stronger immune system in women.[123] Autoimmune phenomena and diseases are in general more prevalent in women.[124] A large body of evidence clearly indicates the existence of sexual dimorphism in normal and abnormal immune responses in spontaneous and experimental animal models, including models of autoimmune thyroiditis (see Chiovato et al.[125] for an extensive review). In these models, male hormones appear to downregulate immunity and therefore protect animals from autoimmunity, whereas the effect of estrogen is not always unequivocal. In spite of the evidence obtained from animal studies, little evidence in the literature supports a role for sex hormones in the high prevalence of Graves' disease in women. Women with normal baseline levels of estrogen, but with an increased sensitivity to the hormone as shown by the presence of melasma, had a higher prevalence of thyroid autoimmune disorders.[126] A clear association between exogenous estrogen administration and Graves' disease has never been reported. Moreover, thyroid autoimmunity is often found in patients with Turner's syndrome, who typically have low estrogen levels.[127–129] Conversely, male patients with primary hypogonadism such as in Klinefelter's syndrome do not show a higher incidence of Graves' disease or Hashimoto's thyroiditis.[128] In these human conditions, however, the chromosomal abnormality probably plays an important role that is largely independent of sex hormone levels (see below).

Pregnancy is an important risk factor, and it is well recognized that in any woman the risk of development of Graves' disease increases fourfold to eightfold in the postpartum year.[130] The abrupt fall in the level of pregnancy-associated immunosuppressive factors immediately after delivery (rebound immunity) is likely to be the mechanism responsible for the precipitation of Graves' disease. These factors may include but are not limited to estrogen and progestin.[131]

Besides sex hormones, factors on the X chromosome could explain the epidemiologic evidence of a female preponderance in Graves' disease. Recent linkage analysis in families with Graves' disease has located a putative Graves' disease susceptibility locus on the long arm of the X chromosome.[73] Although most X-linked disorders are expressed phenotypically only in men, it is possible that a gene with a dose-dependent effect may determine more relevant clinical effects in women. This finding could help explain the higher incidence of Graves' disease observed in women and, possibly, in patients with Turner's syndrome.[129]

PATHOLOGY

It is now rare to observe the full pathologic changes that occur in the thyroid glands of untreated patients. On gross pathology the gland is very significantly enlarged, with a smooth and hyperemic surface. A prominent pyramidal lobe is often visible, and the contour of the gland is irregular with multiple lobulations. Microscopically, both hypertrophy and hyperplasia are found. Follicles are small, with scanty colloid as a result of ongoing thyroid hormone secretion. The follicular epithelium presents a columnar aspect, with even a pseudopapillary appearance. Blood vessels are large and congested. Various degrees of lymphocytic infiltration can be found between the follicles. T cells predominate in the interstitium, whereas B cells and plasma cells predominate in the occasional lymphoid follicles. On electronic microscopy, the cellular hyperactivity is demonstrated by an increase in the Golgi reticulum and the number of mitochondria and by the presence of prominent microvilli. With long-standing Graves' disease, distinct nodularities with an adenomatous appearance may develop, and the lymphocytic infiltrate may become more prominent and resemble chronic thyroiditis.

This pathologic picture of active Graves' disease is dramatically changed by antithyroid drugs and iodine treatment, which is now universally performed before surgery. Vascularity and vascular congestion are much less pronounced, and the follicles are enlarged with abundant colloid.

PATHOGENESIS OF GRAVES' DISEASE

Although the ultimate cause of Graves' disease is still unknown, over the years a large body of evidence has accumulated and provided important insight into the immune mechanisms that eventually lead to the clinical manifestations of the disease. Since their first description in 1956,[11] much attention has been devoted to the study of TRAbs. It has also been recognized that although TRAbs are the ultimate cause of both goiter and hyperthyroidism, the nature of the immune dysfunction involves many aspects of the immune system, including changes in both B cell and T cell function. The follicular cell per se may also play an independent role.

Role of TSH Receptor Antibodies

Nomenclature

The nomenclature of TRAbs is complex and largely dependent on the assay used to detect these antibodies in serum.[132] Assays measuring displacement of radiolabeled TSH from its receptor by the immunoglobulin fraction of sera detect TRAbs regardless of their functional activity. These antibodies have been termed TSH-binding inhibitory immunoglobulins (TBIIs). Assays for TSAbs use cellular systems carrying a functional TSHR and detect the release of cyclic adenosine monophosphate (cAMP) in the culture medium upon challenge with serum or purified immunoglobulins.[133, 134] These antibodies are essentially the cause of hyperthyroidism in Graves' disease. In the same bioassay system, antibodies with blocking activity on the TSHR (TBAbs) can be detected.[135] These antibodies characterize a subset of patients with autoimmune hypothyroidism caused by atrophic thyroiditis, but they can also occasionally be found in patients with Graves' disease,[133] in combination with TSAbs.

Major Autoantigen in Graves' Disease: Structure-Function Relationship of the TSHR

Definitive proof that TSHR is the target of TSAbs came from the cloning of this protein in the late 1980s.[12, 13, 136] The receptor is a member of the G protein–coupled receptor superfamily. Its structure includes seven hydrophobic transmembrane domains, an extracellular N-terminal domain (ectodomain), and an intracellular C-terminal domain. Heavy glycosylation of the extracellular domain accounts for about 20% of its molecular weight of 84 kDa. The primary structure of the protein consists of 744 residues.[137] The gene is located on chromosome 14q31 and is formed by 10 exons[138] that yield a single polypeptide. It is unclear whether the mature receptor maintains its primary structure on the membrane or it is spliced in two or more subunits at the posttranslational level.[139–141] Site-directed mutation analysis has shown that high-affinity TSH binding requires multiple residues discontinuously distributed in the primary structure and located in the extracellular and transmembrane domains.[142] Correct folding and glycosylation of the receptor are also required.[143]

The observation of TRAbs with different biologic activity on the TSHR has prompted a search for epitopes responsible for the stimulatory activity observed in Graves' disease sera. As with many other autoantigens and at odds with T cell–dependent epitopes, TSHR epitopes are tridimensional; that is, they involve residues that may be distant from one another on the primary structure of the protein but come close to each other in the tertiary structure. In keeping with this concept, the use of small linear peptides of the TSHR in the immunization of animals has rarely yielded antibodies with affinity comparable to the one observed in humans.[141] The reactivity of chimeric receptors (in which parts of the TSHR ectodomain were replaced by homologous, but nonidentical parts of the luteinizing hormone–chorionic gonadotropin receptor) with human sera was also analyzed with the expectation that such a change would maintain the tridimensional structure of the receptor and help clarify the residues that are crucial for specific TSH and TRAb binding. These studies support the notion that TSH- and TSAb-binding sites largely overlap but do not coincide and occupy the N-terminal end of the extracellular portion of the TSHR.[144, 145] The binding site for TBAb, although largely overlapping with that of TSAb, appears to be located at the C-terminal end of the receptor ectodomain.[146–148]

Assays for TSH Receptor Antibody

The pioneering era of in vivo bioassays for TRAb[11, 149] has been superseded by the present period, in which a number of in vitro assays are more readily performed by many laboratories and provide more reproducible and reliable measures of TRAb levels in the serum of patients. The radioreceptor assay uses TSHR from various sources: porcine[150, 151] or human recombinant TSHR from transfected cell lines.[152–155] Although assay design varies in all these methods, they all rely on displacement of labeled TSH from solubilized TSHR in the serum of patients. Studies in hyperthyroid patients with Graves' disease show positive TBII tests with these methods in 75% to 95% of patients.[151, 156, 157] The recently designed second-generation radioreceptor assay attains even higher sensitivity while maintaining high specificity (99%).[155] Because these assays do not require permanent cell cultures, they are the most readily available (also commercially) and are therefore the most frequently used in clinical practice. The TBII test, however, does not give information on the functional properties of the antibody detected and can be positive in the presence of TBAb.

The functional properties of TSAb can be studied in in vitro bioassays based on the measurement of cAMP production from cells with a functional TSHR. Human thyroid follicular cells,[158–160] a rat thyroid cell strain (FRTL-5),[161–163] and Chinese hamster ovary cells stably transfected with human TSHR (CHO-R)[156, 157, 164] have all been used for this purpose. With these assays TSAb can be detected in 90% and more of patients with untreated Graves' disease (Fig. 100–3). The system using CHO-R cells has some advantages over the others: it is slightly more sensitive than the FRTL-5 cell method and relies on easier culture conditions, which also makes it more reproducible in different laboratories. As stated above, the bioassays have the advantage of giving information on the functional properties of TRAb and, in a modification of the assay, can also identify TBAb. However, they require permanent cell culture equipment and prepurification of the immunoglobulin fraction of serum, which makes these assays not readily available to routine endocrine laboratories. The latter problem has recently been overcome by very sensitive assays in which activation of a transfected firefly luciferase gene produces chemiluminescence in response to TSHR stimulation by whole serum.[165, 166]

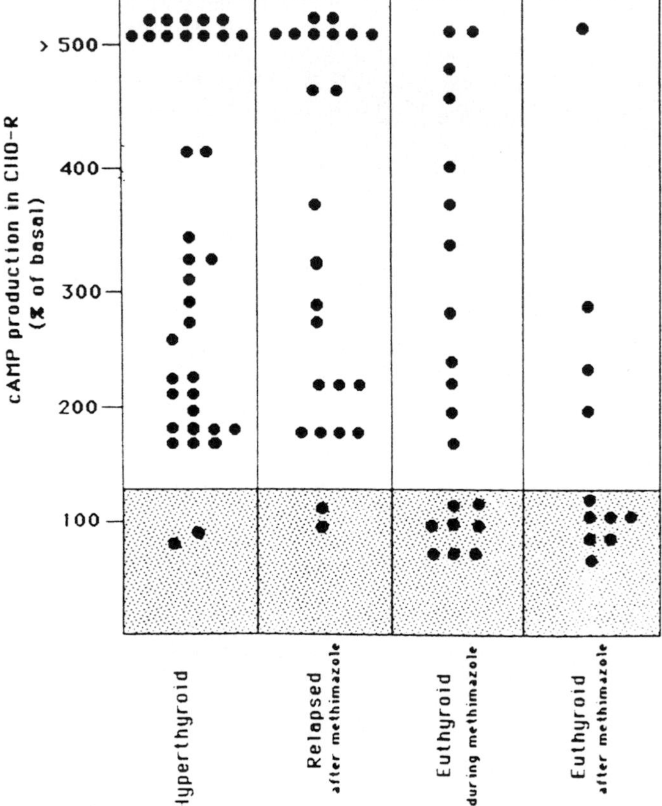

FIGURE 100–3. Prevalence of positive serum thyroid-stimulating antibody tests in Chinese hamster ovary cells transfected with recombinant human thyroid-stimulating hormone (TSH) receptor (CHO-R). Serum IgG was purified from untreated and treated patients with Graves' disease. Cyclic adenosine monophosphate (cAMP) release in the cells' supernatants is expressed as a percentage of basal values obtained with normal serum IgG. The *shaded area* indicates the mean plus 2 SD of results obtained with normal IgG.[156]

Thyroid-Stimulating Antibody in the Pathogenesis and Natural History of Graves' Disease

Historically, identification of TSAb as the cause of hyperthyroidism and goiter in Graves' disease came from the demonstration of a stimulating factor in the sera of hyperthyroid patients with a half-life much longer than that of TSH (LATS).[11] Subsequently, this factor was shown to be an autoantibody.[167–169] TSAbs were shown to interact with TSHR in that they act as a potent agonist and thus cause hyperfunction of the thyroid gland.[132] Definitive proof that TRAbs interact with TSHR eventually came from studies with the cloned protein.[142, 170, 171] A clear-cut demonstration of the role of TSAb in the pathogenesis of hyperthyroidism is provided by the observation that the transplacental transfer of antibodies from TSAb-positive pregnant mothers to the fetus may cause a form of transient neonatal thyrotoxicosis that vanishes with the disappearance of TSAb from the serum of the newborn.[172, 173]

TSAbs are of oligoclonal origin,[174–177] and this observation has suggested a primary defect at the B cell level. TSAb appears to be produced mainly by thyroid-infiltrating lymphocytes and lymphocytes in the draining lymph nodes.[178] Synthesis by peripheral blood lymphocytes has been documented as well.[179–181] By sensitive in vitro bioassays, TSAb can be detected in more than 90% of patients with untreated Graves' disease hyperthyroidism.[156, 158, 159, 182] The observation of a small proportion of patients with undetectable TBIIs or TSAbs has been attributed to the occurrence of these autoantibodies at a serum level too low to be detected by current methods. Alternatively, restricted intrathyroidal production of TRAbs has been hypothesized.[183] A positive correlation between TSAb levels and serum triiodothyronine (T_3) levels,[184] serum thyroglobulin levels,[185] and goiter size[184] has been observed.

TRAb levels usually fall during long-term treatment with antithyroid drugs.[186–189] This phenomenon has been attributed to an immunosuppressive effect of methimazole (or propylthiouracil) itself,[190] but it could also result from the correction of thyrotoxicosis or even reflect the natural history of the disease (see the section on antithyroid drug treatment).

Role of Cellular Immunity

The primary requirement for a specific autoimmune (either humoral or cell-mediated) response is an antigen-specific T cell. Activation of T cells requires presentation of antigenic peptides in the context of HLA molecules. This task is accomplished by a specialized subset of immune cells called professional antigen-presenting cells. Once activated, helper ($CD4^+$) T cells can be subdivided into two functional subtypes according to their cytokine production pattern[191, 192]: the T_H1 subset, mainly involved in delayed-type hypersensitivity reactions, and the T_H2 subset, prominently involved in humoral immune responses. T_H1 cells produce tumor necrosis factor-β, IFN-γ, and IL-2; T_H2 cells secrete mainly IL-4, IL-5, IL-6, and IL-13. T_H1 cells have been implicated in organ-specific, chronic destructive autoimmune diseases,[193] such as experimental allergic encephalitis and spontaneous type 1 diabetes in the mouse.[194, 195] The subset of T lymphocytes primarily activated by specific antigens and the cytokine milieu produced by antigen-presenting cells determine the direction of the immune response toward a T_H1 cell-mediated tissue-damaging reaction, a more prominent humoral reaction (T_H2 mediated), or a balance of the two.[192]

Studies of patients with Graves' disease showed activated T cells both in the peripheral circulation and in the thyroid gland.[196–198] T cells infiltrating the thyroid gland in Graves' disease have been studied by surface monoclonal antibody phenotyping. The percentage of $CD8^+$ (suppressor/cytotoxic) T cells was found to be much lower in Graves' disease than in Hashimoto's thyroiditis.[199–202] The phenotype of the $CD4^+$ (helper/inducer) T cell population was predominantly composed of memory cells.[203, 204] Further studies involved cloning of infiltrating T cells. Most of the resulting T cell lines belonged to the memory ($CD4^+$, $CD29^+$) subtype and responded with significant growth and/or cytokine production to challenge with autologous thyroid follicular cells or thyroid antigens.[201, 205–209]

As assessed by their cytokine profile, intrathyroidal T cells were found to be predominantly of the T_H1 subtype,[201, 210] and this pattern was also true for TSHR-responsive clones.[211] This finding is somewhat unexpected in a disease such as Graves' disease, which is mainly characterized by the action of TSAbs producing thyroid hyperfunction and follicular cell growth. However, it is worthwhile noting that T_H1 cells may also induce antibody production through secretion of IL-10,[192] which in turn activates B cells. In keeping with this sequence of events, TRAbs of Graves' disease are more often of the IgG1 subclass,[212] which is selectively induced by T_H1 cells. A significant proportion of T_H0 (uncommitted) cells were also detected among TSHR autoreactive T cells.[211]

The basis for an organ-specific autoimmune process is the interaction of antigen-specific T cells with the target tissue itself in a way that leads to selection and clonal expansion of autoreactive cells. The specificity of this interaction is provided by the immense variability in mature T cell antigen receptors caused by the somatic rearrangement of their variable (V) chain with the constant (C) and the junction (J) regions.[213, 214] When an immune response is initiated, T cells carrying the individual receptor specific for the antigen involved are stimulated and clonally expanded. In keeping with this concept, restricted use of T cell receptor V_α and V_β genes was observed in T lymphocytes obtained by fine-needle aspiration of Graves' disease thyroids.[215] When surgically obtained specimens of thyroids with Graves' disease have been examined, selective use of T cell receptor V_α or V_β genes has been confirmed in some,[216–219] but not all studies.[220, 221] These observations indicate that a highly selective response to thyroid autoantigens is elicited in the thyroid glands of patients with Graves' disease during the initial phase of the disease. Afterward, spreading of the autoimmune response occurs and leads to less restricted T cell receptor gene usage.

The antigen specificity of autoreactive T cells has also been tested. Initial studies with thyroid follicular cells in culture or with their subcellular fractions suffered from contamination with thyroid autoantigens other than TSHR, so the antigen specificity of T cells was questionable. Indeed, thyroid peroxidase– and thyroglobulin-specific T cells also exist within the thyroid gland of patients with Graves' disease.[211] Since the cloning of TSHR cDNA, however, a number of laboratories have searched for TSHR-specific T cell clones and investigated their role in thyroid autoimmunity and Graves' disease. Studies using TSHR peptides identified specific responses and showed positive stimulation indexes of peripheral blood mononuclear cells from patients with Graves' disease, as well as from healthy controls.[217] Considerable effort has also been expended in identifying immunodominant epitopes on the TSHR. Four distinct peptides were recognized by lymphocytes from most patients with Graves' disease in one study.[222] The response to one of the above epitopes was also found to be associated with the development of thyroid autoimmune disease in an extended family.[223] More recently, another set of immunodominant peptides has been described that are only partially overlapping with the previous ones.[211] It is possible that HLA haplotypes and other poorly understood factors play a role in determining which epitope is immunodominant in individual patients. Overall, these observations show that immunodominant T cell–dependent epitopes exist within the TSHR and that these epitopes may be at least partially shared by different patients. Identification of T cell–dependent epitopes would be important in efforts to design immunologic approaches to the treatment of Graves' disease, such as tolerizing vaccines or antigen-specific lymphocyte deletion.

Role of Thyroid Follicular Cells

The question of whether primary defects in the thyroid gland could be contributing to the pathogenesis of thyroid autoimmunity has been pondered since the mid-1980s.[224–226] The observation that thyroid cells from patients with Hashimoto's thyroiditis and Graves' disease express HLA class II antigen (DR), which is usually expressed by professional antigen-presenting cells,[227] led to the hypothesis that aberrant expression of these molecules on thyroid cells could initiate thyroid autoimmunity via direct thyroid autoantigen presentation.[227, 228] It was later suggested that expression of HLA class II molecules on thyroid cells is a secondary rather than a primary phenomenon, as determined by the cytokines released by the lymphocytic infiltrate.[229–231] Thyroidal HLA-DR expression can be induced by cytokines such as IFN-γ, which was able to induce thyroiditis when administered to susceptible mice in one study.[232] IFN-γ, however, may not be the sole determinant inasmuch as interference with its action by blocking antibodies[233] or by genetic disruption[234] reduced the severity of experimental thyroiditis but did not abrogate it. Moreover, in experimental models of thyroiditis, HLA class II expression appeared to be a late phenomenon that was present only after the infiltrate had appeared, although such observations may depend on the sensitivity of the detecting system used.[235] Thus it would appear that HLA class II antigen expression is probably not the primary mechanism leading to Graves' disease, but rather it is important for perpetuation and enhancement of the autoimmune reaction.[226, 236] In this regard, thyroid cells have been shown to be capable of stimulating T lymphocytes both in the presence[236–238] and in the absence of professional antigen-presenting cells.[239] Co-culture of peripheral blood mononuclear cells from Graves' disease patients with homologous thyrocytes induced T cell activation[225] as well as IFN-γ production and HLA class II antigen expression on thyroid cells.[240] Professional antigen-presenting cells, such as dendritic cells, macrophages, and even B cells, also exist within the thyroid lymphocytic infiltrate in close relationship with thyrocytes and are involved in thyroid autoantigen presentation.[241, 242]

Professional antigen-presenting cells express a family of costimulatory proteins named B7 on their surface that interact with molecules (CD28 and CTLA-4) on the surface of helper ($CD4^+$) T cells during antigen presentation.[243] This costimulatory process is critical for determining the direction of the immune response because its absence may result in anergy and/or deletion of antigen-specific T cells. The B7-1 and B7-2 molecules are not expressed on thyroid cells derived from patients with Graves' disease,[244] which suggests that these cells must rely on other costimulatory factors, perhaps from professional antigen-presenting cells.[245] Costimulatory molecules may also influence the resulting T_H1 or T_H2 T cell phenotype.[192] In this regard, recent studies on antigen presentation indicate that in the absence of costimulatory signals, such as those provided by B7 molecules, HLA class II expression by thyroid cells will lead to continued activation of T cells if the immune response has already been established by professional antigen-presenting cells, whereas it will induce peripheral tolerance of naive, not previously stimulated T cells.[246]

Animal Model of Graves' Disease

No spontaneous models mimicking human Graves' disease have been reported, and the absence of such an animal model has slowed the acquisition of knowledge on processes leading to this disease. Experimental immunization with soluble forms of TSHR was reviewed above and has led only to antibodies deprived of stimulating activity that did not cause hyperthyroidism in the immunized animals. More recently, a different approach has been used. Mice are immunized with fibroblasts that after transfection with full-length human TSHR receptor DNA, are capable of expressing the native protein on their surface and also expressing the appropriate DR molecules. In about one-fourth of the mice so immunized, hyperthyroidism and goiter developed without prominent thyroidal infiltration.[247] This model shows that the entire receptor, properly expressed on the cell surface, is necessary to provide the conformational epitopes needed to generate stimulating antibodies. Most recently, direct immunization with TSHR DNA has been used to successfully produce a model of Graves' disease in which inflammatory involvement of the animals' eyes is also present.[248] In BALB/c mice immunized by this procedure, TSHR antibodies (although not of the stimulatory type) developed in addition to thyroiditis and, most remarkably, some eye changes resembling those of Graves' ophthalmopathy in humans, thus indicating that TSHR is indeed the common antigen involved in the thyroidal and orbital features of Graves' disease.

CLINICAL ASPECTS OF GRAVES' DISEASE

The hallmarks of Graves' disease are a diffuse goiter associated with the symptoms and signs of thyrotoxicosis and the typical ophthalmopathy. More rarely, pretibial myxedema may be present. The onset of symptoms is usually gradual over a period of weeks to months, but it may be abrupt in some cases. In other cases mild symptoms may exist for years before a diagnosis is made.

Although some symptoms of the syndrome are almost unique to Graves' disease, many are entirely due to thyrotoxicosis and are therefore common to other thyroid disorders but are usually more prominent and severe. Among the distinctive symptoms, ophthalmopathy and pretibial myxedema are most helpful in establishing the correct diagnosis.

Clinical Manifestations of Graves' Hyperthyroidism

Thyrotoxic symptoms of Graves' disease do not differ from those seen in thyrotoxicosis of other causes (Table 100–4). Most organs are sensitive to thyroid hormone action and are therefore altered by thyroid hormone excess. Symptoms of thyrotoxicosis consequently encompass a wide range of manifestations, each contributing to a clinical picture that can rarely be mistaken when all its components are present. However, the spectrum of manifestations of thyrotoxicosis may range widely from the classic picture to more subtle signs and symptoms that depend on many variables, including age at onset, duration of thyrotoxicosis, severity of thyrotoxicosis, and possibly, poorly understood individual factors.

Thyroid

The thyroid gland is usually symmetrically enlarged (Fig. 100–4), although nodular glands may be seen mainly in geographic areas of iodine deficiency, where nodular goiter often preexisted. Sometimes true nodules are difficult to distinguish from the lobulations typical of a hyperplastic gland. Goiter size is widely variable, and a minority (3%) of patients may even have a gland of normal size. Large goiters can be associated with engorgement of the jugular veins and a positive Pemberton sign (swelling of the jugular veins upon elevation of the arms). By palpation the consistency of the gland is generally firm, although softer than in Hashimoto's thyroiditis. Thrills and bruits resulting from increased blood flow may be present on the gland, especially in the early phases of the disease and with a large goiter.

TABLE 100–4. Symptoms of Hyperthyroidism and Their Frequency

Symptom	Frequency (%)
Nervousness	80–95
Fatigue	50–80
Palpitations	65–95
Dyspnea	65–80
Weight loss	50–85
Heat intolerance	40–90
Fatigability	45–85
Oligomenorrhea	45–80
Increased appetite	10–65
Sweating	50–90
Diarrhea	8–33
Eye signs	50–60

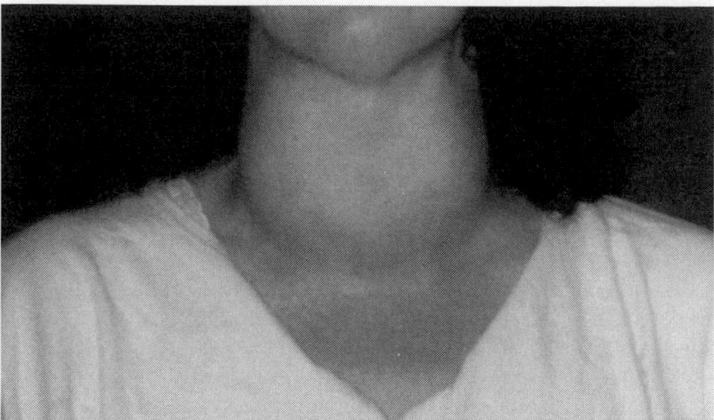

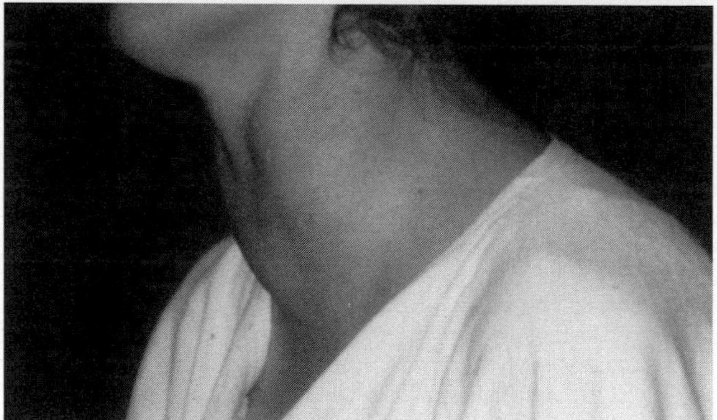

FIGURE 100–4. Large, diffuse symmetrical goiter in a patient with Graves' disease.

Skin and Appendages

The skin of a thyrotoxic patient is warm, thin, and moist; palmar erythema is common. Dermatographism and pruritus are often reported, but their significance is unclear.[249] Urticaria may be associated. Vitiligo is frequent and not a consequence of thyrotoxicosis, but rather an associated autoimmunity to skin melanocytes.[250] The hair is friable, diffuse alopecia of mild degree is often observed, but alopecia areata is rare. Nails are soft and friable with longitudinal striations, and onycholysis (detachment of the nail from the ungual bed) is observed in long-lasting cases. Pretibial myxedema and thyroid acropachy, described elsewhere in this chapter, may also be seen.

Cardiovascular System

Heart-related symptoms are a frequent initial complaint in patients with Graves' disease. The most common are tachycardia and palpitations. Signs and symptoms of heart failure may also develop, and edema of the lower extremities is often found in elderly patients. The heart and vascular system are major targets of thyroid hormone action, which explains the high prevalence of cardiovascular symptoms in thyrotoxic patients with Graves' disease. Cardiac complications may be a major concern in the care of these patients. Thyrotoxicosis causes an increase in both inotropism and chronotropism of the heart. Overall vascular resistance is decreased because of peripheral vasodilation. The net effect of these changes is increased cardiac output,[251] which is the major pathophysiologic event. Increased cardiac workload causes increased oxygen consumption, which in turn can precipitate angina pectoris in the presence of preexisting coronary artery disease. Peripheral edema can be observed in the absence of overt heart failure. Dyspnea on exertion or at rest and chest pain may also be present and are prominent features of thyrotoxic heart disease.

On physical examination, the heart of a thyrotoxic patient is characterized by resting tachycardia. Heart sounds are accentuated. A systolic murmur may be heard on the precordium, sometimes related to associated mitral valve prolapse. Arrhythmias can range from sporadic premature beats to atrial fibrillation.

Electrocardiographic findings are nonspecific and include sinus tachycardia with ST elevation, QT shortening, and PR prolongation. Atrial fibrillation or flutter can occur in up to 10% to 15% of patients, especially the elderly. Ischemic changes can be found when underlying coronary artery disease is present. The observation of reversible heart failure in younger patients with thyrotoxicosis[252] has raised the question of whether a distinct thyrotoxic cardiomyopathy exists in the absence of preexisting detectable heart disease.[251] Technically, the high-output heart failure typically observed in these cases may not be due to "failure" of the heart pump, but instead only to the changes in the peripheral circulation induced by vasodilation and sodium-water retention. However, long-lasting tachyarrhythmias have been shown to impair the contractility of cardiac myocytes, and this mechanism has been proposed for thyrotoxicosis-induced heart failure in young patients.[251] In most cases, however, cardiac complications occur in elderly patients, in whom underlying heart disease is likely to exist. In this setting, heart failure occurs mainly in the presence of atrial fibrillation or ischemic heart disease.[253]

Gastrointestinal Tract

Increased appetite associated with weight loss is a very common complaint and is due to increased catabolism. Increased gastrointestinal motility of the bowel leads to frequent bowel movements and, less often, to diarrhea.[254] This symptom can be associated with some degree of malabsorption and steatorrhea, which can contribute to the weight loss.[255] Atrophic gastritis of autoimmune origin may be associated with Graves' disease. Major toxic effects of thyroid hormone on the liver have not been reported. Nonetheless, mild elevations of liver enzymes are often detected in thyrotoxic patients.[256] Thyrotoxicosis-induced liver function abnormalities can last for months and need to be taken into account when examining patients during treatment with antithyroid drugs because they can be mistaken for adverse reactions to thionamides.

Nervous System

Psychic and nervous symptoms are a prominent and relevant part of the clinical picture. Insomnia and irritability are the most frequent complaints. The patient appears restless and agitated, and logorrhea is often present and becomes evident during history taking. Concentration ability is also decreased. This picture may sometimes confound the physician, and manic disorders have initially been diagnosed in many patients with Graves' disease. Fatigability and asthenia are often present and are important in differentiation from true manic or bipolar disorders. In some cases, nervous signs take the form of "apathetic thyrotoxicosis" with severe apathy, lethargy, and pseudodementia.[257] This profile is more common in elderly patients. In rare cases, true psychoses can be precipitated by thyrotoxicosis[258] and improve with restoration of euthyroidism.

The peripheral nervous system is also deeply affected. Fine distal tremor is an almost universal finding and can also be observed on protrusion of the tongue or at the eyelids. Deep tendon reflexes are brisk, with a shortened relaxation time. Clonus can be sometimes elicited. The characteristic stare of a thyrotoxic patient is due to autonomic hyperstimulation of the elevator muscle of the lid and can also be found in the absence of Graves' ophthalmopathy. True thyrotoxic neuropathy has occasionally been reported and is characterized by areflexic flaccid quadriparesis.[259, 260]

Muscles

Thyrotoxic patients frequently report muscle weakness and easy exhaustion. In more severe cases, atrophy of variable degree can occur in the setting of a more general wasting syndrome. Specific diseases of the muscle can be associated with Graves' disease. Less than 1% of patients with Graves' disease have classic myasthenia gravis,[261, 262] although ocular myasthenia gravis may be more frequent in these patients.[263] Conversely, about 3% of patients with myasthenia gravis have Graves' disease.[264] The pathogenic significance of this association is not known, but it is interesting that the two prototypic diseases characterized by cell surface receptor autoimmunity can occur together. Recognition of this association is clinically important because thyrotoxic myopathy can worsen the muscular symptoms of myasthenia. Moreover, it is important to correctly distinguish the ocular manifestations of the two disorders (they both cause diplopia) because the treatment is different. Therefore, when the degree of ocular muscle dysfunction in a patient with Graves' disease is disproportionate to the degree of proptosis and inflammatory changes, a test for anti–acetylcholine receptor antibodies and a Tensilon (edrophonium chloride) test are warranted.

In some patients, Graves' disease thyrotoxicosis can precipitate crises of periodic hypokalemic paralysis. The syndrome is in all regards identical to familial periodic paralysis, but thyrotoxicosis of various causes is invariably present.[265] The reason for the more frequent association with Graves' disease may merely be that Graves' disease is the most frequent cause of severe and long-lasting thyrotoxicosis in susceptible populations. Periodic hypokalemic paralysis is much more frequent in Asian subjects, in whom an association with certain HLA haplotypes has been observed,[266] but it has also been reported in white and Native American patients.[265] The mechanism leading to the disorder is unknown, but it is likely that intracellular processing of potassium is impaired in these patients. Effective treatments include potassium replacement, β-blocking agents, and rapid correction of thyrotoxicosis. Relapse of the hypokalemic crisis has occasionally been reported in patients after definitive treatment of the thyrotoxicosis, but it is rare.[267, 268]

Skeletal System

Thyroid hormone excess causes an increased rate of bone remodeling. The disproportionate increase in bone resorption over new bone formation leads to net bone loss.[269] Accordingly, hyperthyroid patients have reduced bone mass.[270] Bone density improves after attainment of euthyroidism, but it often remains below the normal range.[271] The degree of osteoporosis depends on the duration of hyperthyroidism and the coexistence of other risk factors for osteoporosis. Hence postmenopausal women with a history of hyperthyroidism have an increased risk of fractures,[272, 273] and hyperthyroid women are found more frequently among women with fractures.[274] The consequences of this effect of thyrotoxicosis on public health have been demonstrated in a large recent epidemiologic survey showing that fracture-related mortality is significantly increased among women with a history of hyperthyroidism.[275] Hypercalcemia and increased alkaline phosphatase occur in a significant proportion of thyrotoxic patients as a consequence of thyroid hormone action on bone metabolism. Bone turnover markers such as osteocalcin and collagen degradation products are increased and closely correlated with the thyroid hormone level,[276, 277] but they return to normal after correction of the thyrotoxicosis.

Hematopoietic System

Mild leukopenia with relative lymphocytosis is a common finding in patients with thyrotoxic Graves' disease. Normocytic anemia is rare, but can occur.[278] Pernicious anemia occurs in a small minority of patients with Graves' disease, but circulating autoantibodies to gastric parietal cells are found in a much higher percentage of cases[279] and are a sign of associated gastric autoimmunity. Graves' disease is occasionally associated with autoimmune thrombocytopenic purpura, but nonimmunologic alterations in hemostasis have also been reported. Increases in factor VIII levels and fibrinogen[280, 281] have been reported most consistently, but the clinical relevance of these findings is unknown.

Reproductive System

FEMALES. In severe thyrotoxicosis the menstrual cycle is often deranged and characterized by oligomenorrhea or amenorrhea.[282] As a consequence of impaired ovulation, fertility is decreased, but pregnancy can still occur. The mechanisms for these alterations are poorly understood, but they almost exclusively occur in women with severe weight loss. In women (and in men) with thyrotoxicosis, sex hormone–binding globulin (SHBG) is increased,[283] but the physiologic consequences of this increase are unclear. Thyrotoxicosis in pregnancy is associated with an increased incidence of low-birth-weight infants and preeclampsia (see below).

MALES. Gynecomastia may develop in men,[284] and erectile dysfunction and reduced sperm count are not infrequent. Other features suggesting estrogenic excess include spider angiomas and reduced libido.[284] Total testosterone is increased as a result of increased SHBG concentrations,[283] but unbound and bioavailable testosterone levels remain in the normal range. The circulating estradiol level is increased, probably because of increased peripheral aromatization of testosterone.[285] All these changes are fully reversible with treatment of the thyrotoxicosis and require no other specific treatment. Treatment of reduced libido with testosterone may result in worsening of gynecomastia.

Metabolic Changes

Significant weight loss with normal or increased caloric intake is a hallmark of thyrotoxicosis. It is explained by an increased metabolic rate, with increased heat production as a net result. Mitochondrial oxygen consumption is increased by thyroid hormone in almost every tissue. Increased mitochondrial activity and numbers were also shown in several tissues in experimental thyrotoxicosis. The use of oxygen by mitochondria is inefficient in experimental thyrotoxicosis in that fewer molecules of high-energy substrates are produced per molecule of oxygen used. However, this mechanism (mitochondrial uncoupling) does not seem to be significant in vivo. A widespread increase in the use of ATP by cation transporters in tissues has been proposed to explain the increased energy use, although this point is still controversial. Whatever the mechanism, increased heat production and dispersion are manifested as a moderate rise in body temperature that is partially compensated for by increased sweating, heat intolerance, and weight loss.[286–288]

Peripheral utilization of carbohydrates is increased in thyrotoxicosis, in keeping with the enhanced energy consumption, and the primary mechanism seems to be an increased cellular transport of glucose.[289] Thyrotoxicosis, however, also causes some degree of insulin resistance.[290] Consequently, diabetes mellitus may be exacerbated by thyrotoxicosis.

Serum cholesterol and triglyceride levels are decreased in thyrotoxicosis, mainly because of a decrease in low-density lipoproteins (LDLs).[291] This reduction in lipids can result from the decrease in total body fat as a consequence of the weight loss, but specific actions of thyroid hormone on lipid metabolism have also been described. Cholesterol conversion to bile acid in the liver is enhanced, and LDL receptor number on adipocytes is increased as well.[292] These phenomena may account for the increased turnover of cholesterol and triglycerides.

Protein metabolism is altered during thyrotoxicosis, with both increased protein synthesis and degradation. In most cases, however, degradation predominates and causes negative nitrogen balance. This imbalance can be partly controlled by adequate calorie and protein intake.

Distinctive Manifestations of Graves' Disease

Graves' Ophthalmopathy

Graves' ophthalmopathy is the clinical manifestation of an inflammatory disorder of the orbit and is almost exclusively associated with Graves' disease. The many aspects of this puzzling disorder are examined in detail elsewhere in this book. The prominence of the signs of Graves' ophthalmopathy makes this feature the most striking physical finding in some patients (Fig. 100–5). Most of the manifestations of Graves' ophthalmopathy are related to its central pathophysiologic event, an increase in the volume of retro-orbital tissue because of inflammation. As a consequence, the eye bulb is pushed forward and proptosis or exophthalmos results. Venous congestion causes swelling and edema of the periorbital tissue. Inflammatory changes also involve the extraocular muscles and may cause diplopia.[293] The eyes are protruding, often asymmetrically. Lid retraction is seen and can be worsened by the concurrent thyrotoxicosis. Edema and swelling of the lids are also typical. The conjunctival mucosa is injected and edematous (chemosis). Lagophthalmos (incomplete palpebral closure) and lacrimal gland dysfunction may combine to cause drying of the mucosal and corneal surfaces and consequently irritation and (less often) corneal ulceration. Photophobia, burning sensation, retrobulbar pain, tearing, and a sandy sensation are common symptoms and may initially mislead clinicians into making a diagnosis of conjunctivitis. Optic neuropathy resulting from optic nerve compression by inflamed and swollen extraocular muscles at the orbital apex may occur in the most severe cases and cause permanent loss of vision. When the proptosis is extremely severe, subluxation of the bulb outside the orbit may occur and pose an immediate threat to visual function. The onset of Graves' ophthalmopathy coincides with the onset of thyrotoxicosis in about 40% of cases, follows it in another 40%, and precedes it in 20%.[293] Even when the onset of the two disorders does not coincide, each occurs within 18 months from the onset of the first manifestation.[294]

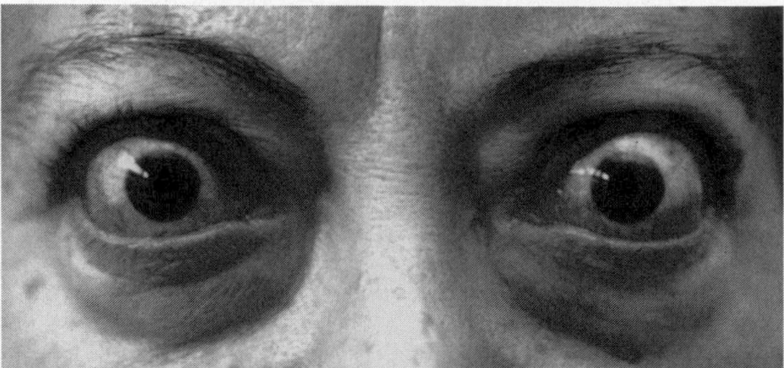

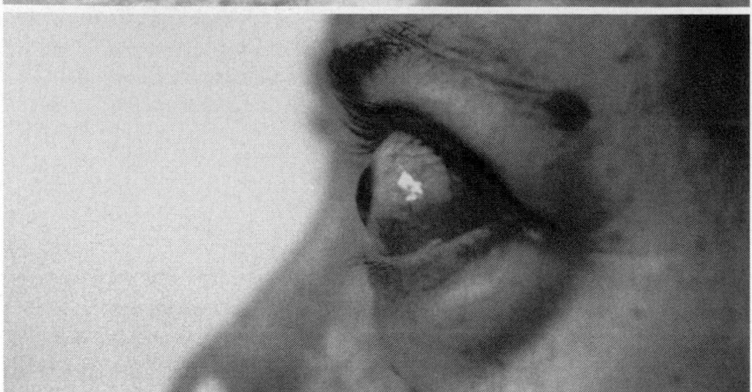

FIGURE 100–5. Typical ophthalmopathy in a patient with Graves' disease. Inflammatory signs such as conjunctival injection and palpebral edema are quite evident. The upper eyelid is retracted, with a positive Graefe sign. On the lateral view, marked proptosis is also visible.

Pretibial (or Localized) Myxedema and Thyroid Acropachy

When von Basedow first described his cases of Graves' disease,[5] he also reported a puzzling manifestation of the skin characterized by a nonpitting swelling of the pretibial areas, brownish and reddish in color, well delimited, and containing little free fluid. The skin surface appears wrinkled around the hair follicles and has the typical appearance of "orange skin" (Fig. 100–6). This manifestation of unknown pathogenesis is relatively rare in patients with Graves' disease,[262] but it never occurs alone and is so typically associated with moderate to severe Graves' ophthalmopathy that it is almost pathognomonic of the disorder.[295] Although most frequently localized to the pretibial regions, it has also been observed on the forearms and other areas.[296, 297] Different degrees of severity have been described. Diffuse pretibial myxedema refers to the mildest form, with only superficial diffuse edema. Localized areas of more prominent infiltration that assume a papular aspect characterize the nodular form. In the most severe forms,

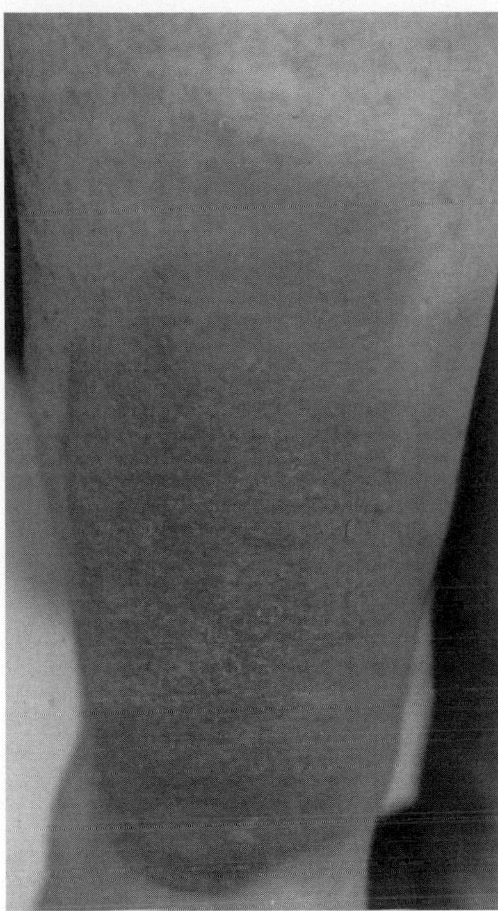

FIGURE 100–6. Pretibial myxedema in a patient with Graves' disease. The skin of the pretibial area appears swollen, reddened, and typically wrinkled and takes the appearance of orange skin.

elephantiasis occurs with extensive swelling and sometimes ulceration. Histopathologic studies have shown that the swelling is caused by the inordinate accumulation of hyaluronic acid in the subcutaneous layers of the involved areas,[298] strikingly similar to the diffuse myxedematous changes of hypothyroidism. A lymphocytic infiltrate may be observed, but it is by no means a constant finding.[299] The cause of pretibial myxedema is unknown, as is its relationship to the pathogenetic events causing thyrotoxicosis in Graves' disease. The origin of the mucinous material (hyaluronic acid) appears to be the skin fibroblast.[300] Activated fibroblasts are found at the involved sites[299, 301] and have been shown to produce excess glycosaminoglycans in vitro in both normal controls and patients.[302] Pretibial fibroblasts appear to respond with increased glycosaminoglycan production to serum components that are not immunoglobulins.[303] Serum IgG from patients with pretibial myxedema was apparently devoid of effect on pretibial fibroblasts in two studies.[304, 305] In vitro experiments suggest that thyroid hormone might be responsible for the increased synthesis of glycosaminoglycan,[306] although it remains unclear why thyrotoxicosis of other causes is not associated with localized myxedema. A line of studies supports the concept that pretibial myxedema is another autoimmune manifestation of Graves' disease. Indeed, T cell receptor V chain restriction has been observed in the lymphocytic infiltration of patients with early pretibial myxedema and suggests the presence of an ongoing antigen-specific immune response.[307] TSHR is an obvious candidate antigen. Using patients' serum as a tool, one group detected putative TSH-binding sites on pretibial fibroblasts,[308] whereas another group showed expression of TSHR mRNA[309] and detected TSHR immunoreactivity in human fibroblasts from the pretibial region.[310] However, these studies failed to explain the specific location of the clinical disease because control fibroblasts from other areas were not investigated.[308, 309] In summary, the pathogenesis of pretibial myxedema, similar to that of Graves' ophthalmopathy, remains obscure, although most studies support the hypothesis of an autoimmune disorder because of the ectopic expression of thyroidal antigens or the presence of cross-reacting antigens localized to restricted regions of the human skin.[311]

Thyroid acropachy refers to a rare manifestation of Graves' disease that is observed most often in long-lasting forms and usually with severe Graves' ophthalmopathy and pretibial myxedema. It is characterized by clubbing and soft tissue swelling of the last phalanx of the fingers and toes.[312] These changes are similar to those observed in chronic respiratory insufficiency. The overlying skin is often discolored and thickened. Microscopically, increased glycosaminoglycan deposition in the skin is observed. Subperiosteal new bone formation is also present.[312] The disease develops without symptoms over a period of years, and it often goes unnoticed by the patient. This manifestation of Graves' disease is harmless and asymptomatic and requires no treatment.

Clinical Diagnosis

The typical patient with Graves' disease is a woman in her late reproductive years with complaints of palpitations, nervousness, weight loss, and increased appetite. The patient appears restless, anxious, and logorrheic. On physical examination the eye signs of Graves' ophthalmopathy, proptosis and lid lag, are often immediately detected and contribute to the "frightened" appearance of the patient. A symmetrical goiter is often present on inspection and almost always palpable. The skin is moist and warm, thin and smooth. The typical fine distal tremor is easily observed and readily distinguished from other forms of tremor. Examination of the cardiovascular system shows tachycardia with loud heart sounds. Premature beats are frequent, and complete arrhythmia from atrial fibrillation is sometime present. In its classic form the diagnosis of Graves' disease is readily made on clinical grounds, before any laboratory test is performed. Infrequent, but significant exceptions to this rule include the coexistence of nodules, which may suggest toxic nodular goiter, or nonthyroidal diseases, which may blunt or confuse the clinical picture. Graves' disease at its very beginning may produce a mild clinical picture and can be difficult to recognize in otherwise healthy people. In some cases the thyroid may not be enlarged and ophthalmopathy may be absent or clinically undetectable. Symptoms of hyperthyroidism may be less evident in elderly people, who often have the apathetic variant of the disease. For these reasons and to establish a thorough baseline assessment of the patient, the clinical diagnosis must be supported by an accurate laboratory workup.

Laboratory Diagnosis

Hormone Measurements

Although laboratory assessment of thyroid function is treated in detail elsewhere in this book, it seems appropriate to review in this section the mainstays of the diagnosis of Graves' hyperthyroidism. Suspicion of hyperthyroidism can be confirmed by thyroid hormone measurements. TSH is the single most useful test in confirming the presence of thyrotoxicosis. By sensitive third-generation assays, TSH should be undetectable or low (<0.3 mU/L) in all patients with thyrotoxicosis of thyroidal origin. Low TSH levels can also be observed in a number of conditions such as nonthyroidal illnesses or endogenous or exogenous corticosteroid excess. Therefore, parallel measurement of thyroid hormone levels is recommended in all patients for a correct interpretation of a low TSH level. Total thyroxine (TT_4) and triiodothyronine (TT_3) measurements are relatively inexpensive and reliable but can yield high values in otherwise euthyroid subjects with conditions characterized by increased levels of serum thyroxine-binding globulin (TBG), most commonly pregnancy, oral contraceptive use, and chronic liver disease. Familial excess of TBG and familial dysalbuminemic hyperthyroxinemia are rare disorders that also cause elevated TT_4 levels.[313] Free thyroid hormone measurements, although not completely devoid of flaws, are therefore more satisfactory, but more expensive.[314] In most iodine-sufficient countries a single free thyroxine (FT_4) measurement is sufficient to confirm or reject the suspicion of thyrotoxicosis. After the TSH level, FT_4 is the test most often used in North America for thyroid function screening[315, 316] and therefore the one that most clinicians are familiar with. However, in iodine-deficient countries, a significant proportion of hyperthyroid patients (up to 12%) may have normal FT_4 levels with elevated free T_3 (FT_3) levels,[317, 318] a condition termed T_3 toxicosis. Conversely, FT_4 can be falsely elevated in conditions causing reduced peripheral conversion of T_4 to T_3, such as amiodarone administration or high-dose propranolol treatment. In our practice we initially measure both FT_4 and FT_3 levels together with TSH with little additional expense to obtain a complete baseline assessment of thyroid function status.[316] Circulating thyroglobulin concentrations are high in hyperthyroidism and low in factitious thyrotoxicosis. Measurement of thyroglobulin in serum is therefore useful in the differential diagnosis of thyrotoxicosis in patients with no goiter or ophthalmopathy.[319]

Circulating Autoantibodies

Although by no means necessary, tests for circulating thyroglobulin (TgAb) and thyroid peroxidase (TPOAb) antibodies may be useful in confirming the presence of thyroid autoimmunity. TPOAbs can be detected by commercial radioimmunoassays in up to 90% of patients with untreated Graves' disease,[320] whereas TgAbs are less frequently positive, in about 50% to 60% of cases, depending on the sensitivity of the method used.[279, 321] Both antibodies can be detected in a relatively high percentage (up to 25%) of normal subjects, especially elderly women, or in patients with other nonautoimmune thyroid disorders such as nodular goiter or thyroid carcinoma.[322] Tests for TPOAb and TgAb therefore have limited diagnostic value and must be considered complementary to the diagnosis.

TRAb assay is very specific and sensitive for hyperthyroid Graves' disease. More than 90% of untreated patients are positive with second-generation radioreceptor assays,[155] with very few false-positive results. The radioreceptor test for TRAb is widely available in commercial laboratories, but quite expensive. It is needed in selected situations in which confirmation of the nature of the thyrotoxicosis is required or when the clinical picture or thyroid function tests are not clear. These situations include the differential diagnosis of thyrotoxicosis in pregnancy; the nodular variants of Graves' disease, which must be differentiated from toxic nodular goiter[323]; and patients with exophthalmos without thyrotoxicosis (euthyroid Graves' disease).[293]

Thyroid Radioiodine Uptake and Scanning

Before the introduction of accurate thyroid hormone and TSH measurements, a radioactive iodine uptake (RAIU) test was always required for the evaluation of thyrotoxicosis. Normal ranges for RAIU vary according to the status of iodine supply in the population.[324, 325] In iodine-replete countries, the upper limit of normal RAIU 24 hours after the administration of a tracer dose of radioiodine is around 25%, whereas it may reach 40% in areas with mild to moderate iodine deficiency. In patients with Graves' disease a high value is always found after 24 hours, and in some cases the value after 3 or 6 hours can be even higher as a consequence of the rapid iodine turnover typical of Graves' disease glands. The RAIU test is not readily available as an office-based approach and is not always required. It can be very useful, however, to rule out destructive thyrotoxicosis secondary to silent or subacute thyroiditis, factitious thyrotoxicosis, and type II amiodarone-induced thyrotoxicosis[326] (Table 100–5). RAIU results are also required before radioiodine treatment of hyperthyroidism to calculate the dose needed (see below). RAIU, like any other radioisotopic in vivo procedure, is absolutely contraindicated during pregnancy.

Thyroid imaging with radioisotopes can be performed with radioiodine at the time that RAIU is performed or by using pertechnetate 99m (Fig. 100–7A). Thyroid scanning in Graves' disease is useful when coexisting nodules are detected by palpation and their functional status needs to be evaluated.

TABLE 100–5. Causes of Thyrotoxicosis and Aspects Different from Graves' Disease

Cause	Distinctive Feature
Toxic nodular goiter	Thyroid scan, ultrasound
Subacute thyroiditis	Low thyroid RAIU, neck pain
Painless thyroiditis	Low thyroid RAIU
Factitious thyrotoxicosis	Low serum thyroglobulin, low thyroid RAIU
Struma ovarii	Low thyroid RAIU, positive abdominal RAIU
Amiodarone-induced thyrotoxicosis	Low RAIU, high urinary iodine

RAIU, radioactive iodine uptake.

Thyroid Ultrasound

The thyroid gland is an excellent candidate for ultrasound studies given its superficial anatomic location and the presence of a high number of liquid-solid interfaces (virtually one at every follicle/colloid-lining surface), which in normal conditions produce high reflectivity. Although the equipment is still quite costly, it is now affordable at the office level and requires little maintenance. Thyroid ultrasound is an invaluable tool in the diagnosis of thyroid nodular disorders and has become more and more an extension of the physical examination for many endocrinologists. Its application to nonnodular disorders of the thyroid has come from early observations of typical changes of the gland's echoic structure in thyroid autoimmune diseases.[327] In hyperthyroid Graves' disease, the echoic pattern undergoes diffuse changes. The tissue, possibly because of the reduction in colloid content, the increase in thyroid vascularity, and the lymphocytic infiltrate, becomes typically hypoechoic (Fig. 100–7B). This pattern is similar to the one observed in chronic thyroiditis and, when diffuse, is almost pathognomonic of thyroid autoimmunity.[328] Therefore, thyroid ultrasound can be useful during the evaluation of thyrotoxicosis to confirm the suspicion of thyroid autoimmunity. Thyroid ultrasound also allows accurate measurement of thyroid size,[329] information that can help in the decision-making process when definitive treatment is being planned (see below). Moreover, careful definition of coexisting nodules can be obtained when needed. Therefore, thyroid ultrasonography provides very useful information in the initial evaluation of patients with Graves' disease, although it is seldom strictly required for purely diagnostic purposes.

Color flow Doppler (CFD) techniques have been applied to the study of glands with Graves' disease. CFD allows semiquantitative measurement of blood flow to the thyroid gland. In untreated Graves' disease, a distinct CFD pattern characterized by markedly increased signals with a patchy distribution[330] is usually observed (Fig. 100–7C). This pattern was observed in 17 of 18 patients with untreated Graves' disease, a feature that in conjunction with a hypoechoic pattern allowed distinction from Hashimoto's thyroiditis.[331] In this setting, CFD studies of the thyroid gland can be useful in distinguishing hyperthyroidism of Graves' disease from thyrotoxicosis of other causes, such as amiodarone-induced thyrotoxicosis, subacute thyroiditis,[332] and possibly, painless thyroiditis and factitious thyrotoxicosis. For this reason, CFD evaluation may become a valid substitute for RAIU when these conditions are included in the differential diagnosis.

Treatment of Graves' Disease

Etiologic treatment of Graves' disease is not available at present. Therefore, the major aim of current methods of treating Graves' disease is correction of thyrotoxicosis in all cases and treatment of Graves' ophthalmopathy when present and severe (detailed elsewhere in this textbook). Additional goals include relief of compressive symptoms from large goiters.

Correction of thyroid hormone overproduction can be obtained by inhibition of its synthesis or release or by ablation of thyroid tissue via surgery or radioiodine. In addition, the peripheral metabolism of thyroid hormone can be altered in a favorable way by available drugs.

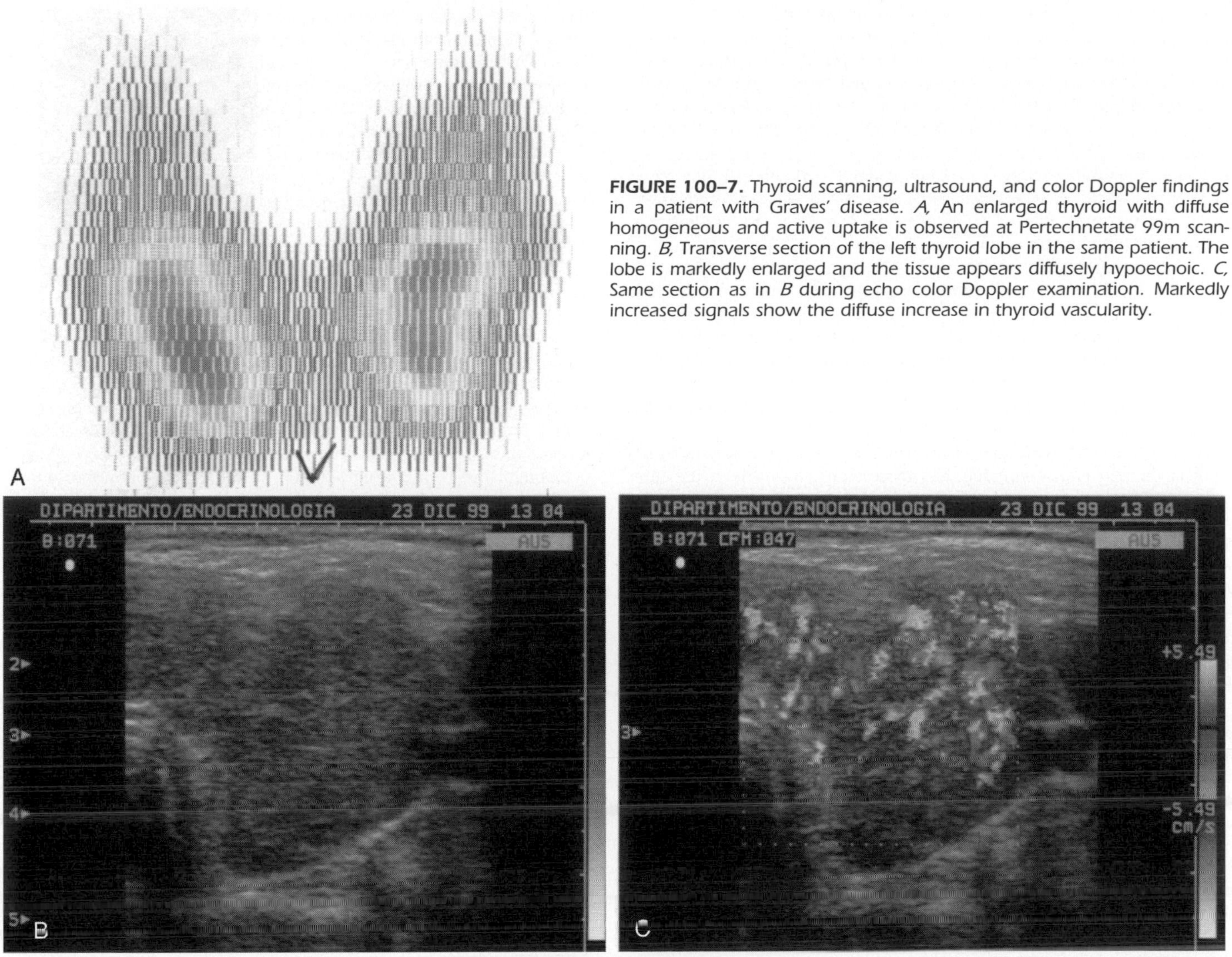

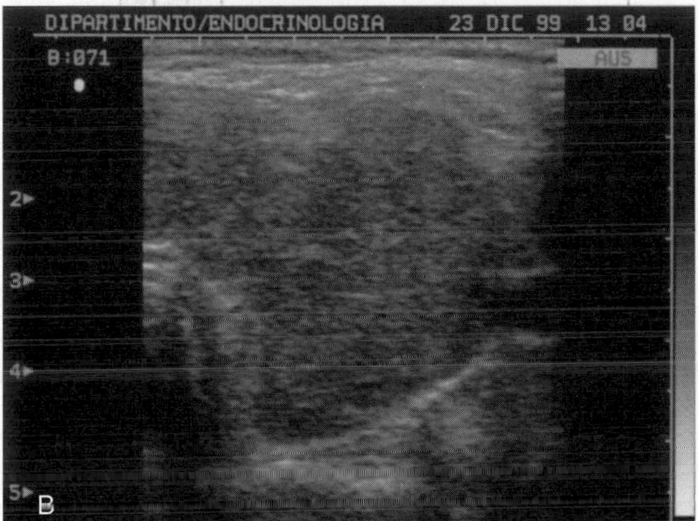

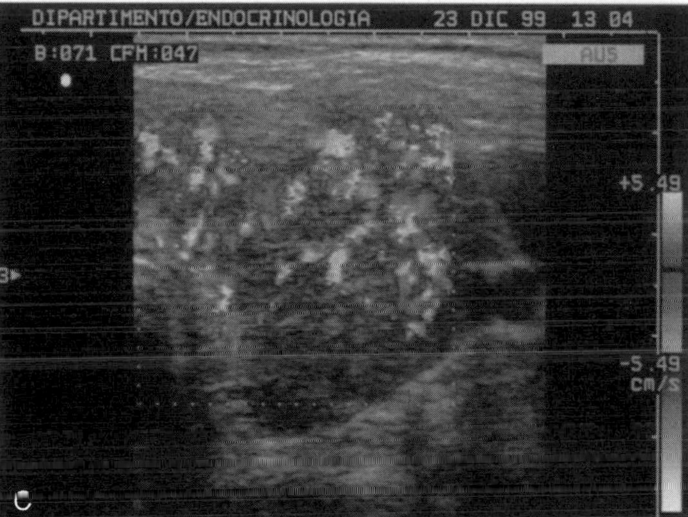

FIGURE 100–7. Thyroid scanning, ultrasound, and color Doppler findings in a patient with Graves' disease. *A,* An enlarged thyroid with diffuse homogeneous and active uptake is observed at Pertechnetate 99m scanning. *B,* Transverse section of the left thyroid lobe in the same patient. The lobe is markedly enlarged and the tissue appears diffusely hypoechoic. *C,* Same section as in *B* during echo color Doppler examination. Markedly increased signals show the diffuse increase in thyroid vascularity.

Selection of the treatment option from among those available should be made after careful consideration of the many variables inherent in any given patient, but there is room for the patient's choice in most cases. The patient should therefore participate in the choice of treatment, after thorough information on the therapeutic alternatives.

Overview of Therapeutic Tools in Graves' Disease Thyrotoxicosis

THIONAMIDES

Clinical Pharmacology. Thionamides (methimazole, carbimazole, and propylthiouracil) were first described and introduced into clinical practice in the early 1940s.[9] The major action of thionamides is to inhibit the organification of iodide and coupling of iodotyrosines, thus blocking the synthesis of thyroid hormones.[333] Carbimazole is not active as it is, but it is almost completely converted to methimazole in the body and their effects are comparable. Propylthiouracil has the additional effect of partially inhibiting the conversion of T_4 to T_3 in peripheral tissues,[334] but this effect is of limited clinical value.[335] Methimazole is at least 10 times more potent than propylthiouracil. The pharmacologic properties of the two major thionamides are compared in Table 100–6.

Both methimazole and propylthiouracil are very effective in controlling hyperthyroidism, and their side effect record is quite similar, thus making the choice between the two drugs largely a matter of personal preference and local availability. Antithyroid drugs do not block the release of preformed thyroid hormones, so euthyroidism is not obtained until intrathyroidal hormone and iodine stores are depleted. This process requires 1 to 6 weeks,[336] depending on factors such as disease activity, initial levels of circulating thyroid hormones, and intrathyroidal hormone and iodine stores. Large goiters with abundant deposits of thyroid hormone, especially when iodine excess is present, often show a delayed response to thionamides.

The main problem with thionamide treatment is the high relapse rate of thyrotoxicosis after discontinuation of even long-term treatment. Although remission rates on the order of 50% to 60% within 1 year after withdrawal of thionamides have been reported in a few series,[337] in most studies hyperthyroidism recurred in 50% to 80% of patients,

TABLE 100–6. Pharmacologic Properties of Thionamides: Comparison between Methimazole and Propylthiouracil

Property	Methimazole	Propylthiouracil
Relative potency	>10 (up to 50)	1
Administration route	PO	PO
Absorption	Almost complete	Almost complete
Binding to serum proteins	Negligible	75%
Serum half-life (hr)	4–6	1–2
Duration of action (hr)	>24	12–24
Transplacental passage	Low	Lower
Levels in breast milk	Low	Lower
Inhibition of deiodinase	No	Yes

depending on the duration of the follow-up period.[338–340] Remission rates have been decreasing in the last decades, possibly as a result of increased iodine supply in the diet.[341, 342] A practical problem is that no single test or combination of tests will accurately separate patients who will relapse from those who will not. Size of the goiter before or during antithyroid drug treatment, HLA-DR3 typing, TRAb or TPOAb levels, serum thyroglobulin concentrations, thyroid echogenicity by ultrasound, circulating activated T cells, and T cell subset ratios have all been indicated as significant pretreatment risk factors for relapse, but none has the required sensitivity or specificity to predict the outcome in individual patients. The presence of a large goiter seems to be the most significant predictor of future hyperthyroidism relapse[340] (Fig. 100–8). Similar considerations apply to such parameters during treatment as T_3 suppression of ^{99m}Tc uptake, the thyrotropin-releasing hormone test, and the T_3/T_4 ratio at the time of discontinuation of thionamide therapy.[339, 340, 343–349] The best predictor of relapse of hyperthyroidism is a positive TSAb test before discontinuation of medical treatment. However, even when TSAbs disappear, the chances of relapse are still high, 20% to 50%.[348]

Most relapses of hyperthyroidism occur within 3 to 6 months after medical therapy is discontinued, and more than two-thirds of patients who relapse will do so within 2 years. However, hyperthyroidism can also recur much later. Late evolution to primary hypothyroidism can be observed as well, mainly in patients who remain euthyroid after discontinuation of therapy.[350, 351] Relapse of hyperthyroidism after a full cycle of thionamides is a strong indication for alternative treatments such as radioiodine or thyroidectomy, but a second course of the drug can be given, for example, to adolescents, while bearing in mind that people who have relapsed once are more likely to do so after the second cycle.

Minor side effects of thionamides have been reported in 1% to 15% of patients, but the average appears to be 6%. Pruritus, skin rash, and much less commonly, urticaria are the most prominent manifestations.[333] Arthralgias have also been reported often. These side effects frequently resolve spontaneously despite continued therapy. However, when any of them occur, it is generally advisable to replace one thionamide with the other, although cross-sensitivity to these drugs may occur. Antihistamine drugs can be used to control mild side effects. Slight elevations in liver enzyme levels have often been reported,[352] and sometimes it is difficult to distinguish this effect of thionamides from the effect of thyrotoxicosis itself. When detected, serious alterations in liver function test results must be monitored closely because toxic hepatitis may develop suddenly.

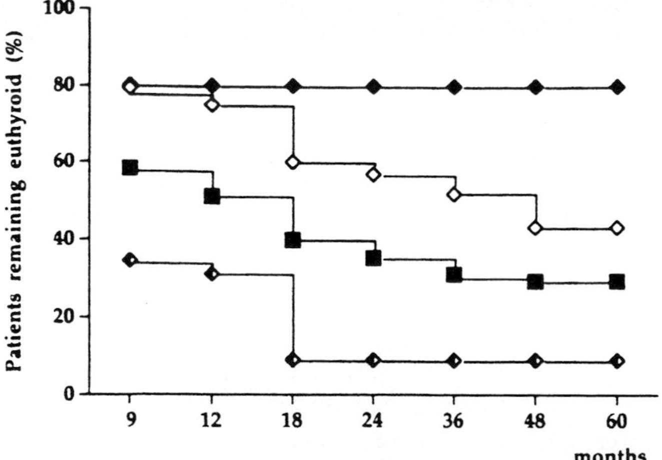

■ whole group.

◇ goiter ≤40 mL/TRAb ≤ 30 U/L (34% of all patients).

◆ goiter >40 mL/TRAb >30 U/L (19% of all patients).

◆ goiter ≤40 mL/TRAb ≤ 30 U/L/age >40 yr (6.5% of all patients).

FIGURE 100–8. Effect of goiter size and thyroid-stimulating hormone receptor antibody (TRAb) level at the time of antithyroid drug discontinuation on the incidence of relapses of hyperthyroidism in a cohort of patients with Graves' disease. (From Vitti P, Rago T, Chiovato L, et al: Clinical features of patients with Graves' disease undergoing remission after antithyroid drug treatment. Thyroid 7:369–375, 1997.)

Serious side effects are uncommon with thionamides and are observed in approximately 3 of every 1000 patients.[353] Agranulocytosis (granulocyte count <500/mm³) may be observed with both methimazole and propylthiouracil. Agranulocytosis has been reported more frequently in elderly patients but can occur at any age. It is most often detected within the first 3 to 4 months after starting therapy. Agranulocytosis may develop so suddenly that even weekly white blood cell counts may not detect it. Agranulocytosis is typically initially manifested by fever and evidence of infection, most often in the upper respiratory tract. Instructing all patients taking antithyroid drugs to report these symptoms immediately is probably the safest measure for immediate detection of this complication. Routine white blood cell counts should be performed in all patients before initiation of treatment because mild leukopenia is common in Graves' disease and needs to be distinguished from a drug reaction. In addition to prompt discontinuation of the antithyroid drug, treatment of agranulocytosis includes the administration of broad-spectrum antibiotics and growth factors to stimulate bone marrow recovery. Patients usually recover within 2 to 3 weeks, but some deaths have been reported from this complication.

Cholestatic or necrotic hepatitis is another rare, but severe complication of thionamide treatment with significant mortality that sometimes requires liver transplantation.[354] Vasculitis and lupus-like syndromes are even rarer. In the presence of a major adverse reaction to thionamides such as agranulocytosis, hepatitis, or vasculitis, prompt withdrawal of therapy with the drug is mandatory.[355] The risk of cross-reactivity is such that switching from methimazole to propylthiouracil or vice versa is not recommended when side effects are severe, so alternative treatments of thyrotoxicosis must be sought.

Treatment Strategies. The purpose of treatment of Graves' disease hyperthyroidism with antithyroid drugs is to achieve stable euthyroidism. Antithyroid drugs can be used either as preparatory treatment before surgery or radioiodine treatment or as a primary management tool of the disease in an attempt to induce long-term remission of thyrotoxicosis. A direct effect of methimazole and propylthiouracil on the immune system has been proposed to explain the observation that a minority of patients experience long-lasting remissions of Graves' disease thyrotoxicosis after withdrawal of these drugs.[190] This view is suggested by the following lines of evidence. In some follow-up studies patients treated with antithyroid drugs had a higher remission rate than did those to whom β-blockers alone were administered,[190] but randomized studies have never been performed. Treatment of Graves' disease with antithyroid drugs is followed by a fall in the levels of circulating TRAb, AbTg, and AbTPO,[186, 356–358] although this effect is not dose dependent.[337] In vitro experiments have suggested a downregulating effect of methimazole on antigen presentation,[359] and in vivo studies have shown that the drug is able to reduce the severity of experimental thyroiditis.[360, 361] Despite these observations, the immunosuppressive effect of thionamides remains controversial. A decrease in circulating thyroid antibody titer has also been observed in hyperthyroid patients treated with perchlorate, a drug with different pharmacologic properties.[362] Restoration of euthyroidism per se might be responsible for the decrease in thyroid autoantibodies through a direct effect of thyroid hormone on the immune system.[363] The natural history of the disease, which like that of many other autoimmune disorders is characterized by cycles of spontaneous relapse and remission, could also explain the reduction in thyroid autoantibody titer. In other words, a course of 12 to 24 months of thionamides would merely be a way of keeping the patient euthyroid while waiting for the autoimmune process to subside or even vanish.

Thionamide treatment is usually started with high doses (20–40 mg/day of methimazole or 200–400 mg/day of propylthiouracil). Doses of methimazole above 40 mg/day are rarely necessary. When long-term thionamide treatment is planned, one of two treatment strategies is currently used:

1. Maintenance of euthyroidism with the minimum effective dose

throughout the trial period, with thyroid function tests performed every 3 to 6 months. The minimum dose capable of maintaining euthyroidism is derived by "back-titration" every 4 to 6 weeks.

2. Administration of fixed, relatively high doses of thionamide in combination with levothyroxine to prevent iatrogenic hypothyroidism, the so-called block-and-replace regimen.

With both schemes, patients should be kept completely euthyroid, with serum TSH levels within the normal range.

The second protocol was proposed because of the supposed immunosuppressive effect of higher doses of thionamides and because of studies suggesting a greater remission rate of hyperthyroidism in Graves' patients treated with high doses of thionamides (60 vs. 15 mg of methimazole per day).[364] The addition of levothyroxine supposedly provides an extra advantage, and very high remission rates have been reported in Japanese patients treated with methimazole for 6 months and then given a combination of methimazole and levothyroxine for an additional year, followed by levothyroxine alone for 3 years.[364, 365] However, the latter results have not been reproduced by a number of subsequent studies.[366–370] In a prospective randomized trial of low (10 mg/day) vs. moderately high (40 mg/day) doses of methimazole, no advantages were observed in terms of a decrease in TRAb titer or the rate of relapse of hyperthyroidism.[337] The rate of adverse reactions was greater in the group of patients receiving methimazole at 40 mg/day. Thus at present the block-and-replace regimen has no proven advantage, although one point in favor of it is that it probably requires less testing. The block-and-replacement strategy can also be useful in rare patients who experience changes from hyperthyroidism to hypothyroidism and vice versa after minimal changes in the dosage of antithyroid drugs ("brittle hyperthyroidism"). In these unusual patients, maintenance of euthyroidism is difficult with antithyroid drugs alone.

Regardless of the chosen regimen, treatment is maintained for 12 to 24 months, after which thionamide therapy is usually discontinued. Indefinite treatment even with low doses of thionamides is not a common practice.

In summary, thionamide treatment of Graves' disease thyrotoxicosis has the major advantages of not causing permanent hypothyroidism and of limiting exposure to radiation. It is, however, associated with a very high failure rate, and in many cases it is only a way to delay thyroid ablation by radioiodine or surgery.

IODIDE AND IODIDE-CONTAINING COMPOUNDS. Inorganic iodide given in pharmacologic doses (as Lugol's solution or as saturated solution of potassium iodide [SSKI]) decreases its own transport into the thyroid, inhibits iodide organification (the Wolff-Chaikoff effect), and blocks the release of T_4 and T_3 from the gland.[371] As an additional advantage, iodide sharply decreases the vascularity of the thyroid in Graves' disease.[372, 373] These effects are, however, transient and last a few days or weeks, after which the antithyroid action of pharmacologic iodide is lost and thyrotoxicosis recurs or may worsen. Therefore, iodide therapy is now used only for short periods in the preparation of patients for surgery, after euthyroidism has already been achieved and maintained with thionamides. Iodide is also used in the management of severe thyrotoxicosis (thyroid storm) because of its ability to inhibit thyroid hormone release acutely. The usual dose of Lugol's solution is 3 to 5 drops three times a day, and that of SSKI is 1 to 3 drops three times daily.

Oral cholecystographic agents (iopanoic acid and sodium ipodate) produce a very rapid fall in the serum concentration of thyroid hormones.[374–377] These agents act through a dual mechanism: virtually complete inhibition of the peripheral conversion of T_4 to T_3 and prevention of thyroid hormone secretion because of the inorganic iodide released from the drug.[378] The first action is the predominant one and makes these drugs highly effective when rapid management of thyrotoxicosis is needed. The rate of fall in T_3 levels after treatment is started approaches the physiologic half-life of the hormone, approximately 1 day. Although early reports suggested that these iodinated compounds could be successfully used as primary therapy for hyperthyroidism in doses of 0.5 to 1 g/day, they proved to be of limited value in long-term treatment because of the escape of thyroid hormone synthesis from the blocking effect of iodide.[379–381] Moreover, they provide the thyroid with a load of iodine, which may make the use of radioiodine unfeasible for some weeks. Therefore, these agents are ideally used in emergency situations when rapid control of thyrotoxicosis is needed, in preparation for thyroid surgery, or while waiting for the effect of radioiodine therapy. In the latter case they may also be used to prevent or correct the transient thyrotoxicosis caused by the release of preformed thyroid hormone, such as may follow radioiodine treatment.

PERCHLORATE. Perchlorate inhibits active transport of iodide into the thyroid.[382] Side effects (gastric irritation) and adverse effects (aplastic anemia) are not infrequent and preclude the use of perchlorate in the long-term management of Graves' disease thyrotoxicosis.[383] In conjunction with thionamides, perchlorate has been successfully used as a tool for depleting the thyroidal iodine overload in amiodarone-induced hyperthyroidism.[384]

β-ADRENERGIC ANTAGONIST DRUGS. Many of the manifestations of thyrotoxicosis, especially those in the cardiovascular system, are due to hyperactivity or hypersensitivity of the sympathetic nervous system.[385, 386] Blockade of β-adrenergic receptors thus ameliorates manifestations of thyrotoxicosis that are related to sympathetic action, such as tachycardia, palpitation, tremor, and anxiety.[387] This effect is much faster than that obtained with thionamides, and for this reason β-blockers are important in the early management of thyrotoxicosis. β-Adrenergic antagonists do not affect thyroid hormone synthesis and release or their action at the level of many tissues, such as bone. These drugs should not be used alone in Graves' disease thyrotoxicosis, except for short periods before and/or after radioiodine therapy. Since the introduction of propranolol, a number of new agents became available with a longer duration (atenolol, metoprolol, and nadolol) or with greater cardioselectivity (atenolol, metoprolol, bisoprolol). None of these drugs have been proved to have an advantage over the others, and the choice largely depends on the personal experience of the physician. Propranolol has the additional advantage of mild inhibition of the peripheral conversion of T_4 to T_3,[388] but the real clinical advantage provided by this pharmacologic property is unclear. The usual contraindications to β-adrenergic antagonists, such as asthma, should be taken into account. β-Blocker use can be rapidly tapered and discontinued once stable euthyroidism is obtained with thionamides, radioiodine, or surgery.

GLUCOCORTICOIDS. Glucocorticoids in high doses inhibit the peripheral conversion of T_4 to T_3. In Graves' disease thyrotoxicosis, glucocorticoids appear to decrease T_4 secretion by the thyroid, possibly by immune suppression, but the efficiency and duration of this effect are unknown. Because of the significant side effects associated with the long-term use of glucocorticoids and the effectiveness of alternative treatments, use of these drugs in the management of Graves' hyperthyroidism is not justified. On the contrary, the immunosuppressive effect of glucocorticoids in high doses is commonly exploited in the treatment of ophthalmopathy and dermopathy of Graves' disease. In severe thyrotoxicosis or thyroid storm, short-term glucocorticoid administration may be used as a general supportive treatment.

RADIOIODINE. Radioactive isotopes of iodine were initially used in the treatment of Graves' disease in the 1940s.[10] Among different radioactive isotopes of iodine, ^{131}I is the agent of choice in the treatment of thyroid hyperfunction because of its half-life and its favorable emission profile. After oral administration, radioiodine is completely absorbed, rapidly concentrated, oxidized, and organified by thyroid follicular cells—exactly the same fate as occurs with ^{127}I (the stable isotope). Thyroid cells are destroyed by the ionizing effects of β particles with an average path length of 1 to 2 mm. One microcurie of ^{131}I retained per gram of thyroid tissue delivers approximately 70 to 90 rad. The early biologic effects of radioiodine include necrosis of follicular cells and vascular occlusion, which fully develop over a period of weeks to months after a single dose of radioiodine. As a consequence, control of hyperthyroidism requires at least weeks or months to be achieved. Long-term effects include shorter survival, impaired replication of surviving cells with atrophy and fibrosis, and a chronic inflammatory response resembling Hashimoto's thyroiditis. These later effects account for the development of hypothyroidism even years after treatment.[389]

Treatment Strategies. In Graves' disease, the goal of radioiodine therapy is to destroy enough thyroid tissue to cure thyrotoxicosis with one dose of ^{131}I, possibly given in a single session. Three outcomes of radioiodine treatment are possible: (1) the patient is rendered stably euthyroid. Achievement of euthyroidism was once considered the "success" situation, but it might not be the ideal outcome in patients with coexistent Graves' ophthalmopathy, in whom greater thyroid antigen ablation may be desirable; (2) The patient remains thyrotoxic. This result is, of course, a failure and requires a second treatment; and (3) The patient becomes permanently hypothyroid. This outcome is now considered an acceptable consequence of radioiodine treatment because correction of hypothyroidism with levothyroxine is easy, safe, and inexpensive. In any patient with Graves' disease who receives radioiodine, the likelihood of these possible outcomes depends on the amount of radioiodine that is delivered and retained by the thyroid tissue and on other incompletely understood individual factors. The latter make it impossible to predict a successful dose in every single patient. The dose of radioiodine to be administered is most often calculated on the basis of thyroid size and uptake of ^{131}I and is determined by using the following equation[390]:

$$\text{Dose (mCi)} = \frac{\text{estimated thyroid weight (g)} \times \text{planned dose } (\mu\text{Ci/g})}{\text{Fractional 24-hour radioiodine uptake} \times 1000}$$

The planned dose varies according to the aim of treatment and ranges from 80 to 200 μCi/g in different centers. In some centers, standard fixed doses are given. Lower doses result in a lower rate of early (within 1 year) hypothyroidism, but at the expense of a higher rate of recurrent or persistent thyrotoxicosis and thus the necessity of a second or, less frequently, a third dose. Even patients given a lower dose and remaining euthyroid in the first year have a high incidence of late-onset hypothyroidism. The cumulative incidence of postradioiodine hypothyroidism steadily increases at a rate of 2% to 3% new cases per year. The overall incidence of postradioiodine hypothyroidism approaches a total of 40% at 5 years and 60% or more at 10 years.[391] Therefore, in many centers, including our own, the strategy of radioiodine treatment is to give a dose of radioiodine that ensures cure in the highest number of patients while being aware that most of the "cured" patients will eventually become hypothyroid. Hypothyroidism should be regarded as a common outcome of radioiodine treatment rather than a true complication, and it can be easily and economically controlled with levothyroxine substitution treatment. Further arguments can be made in favor of this approach. Recurrence of thyrotoxicosis can rarely occur even in patients who were euthyroid after the first dose of radioiodine. These recurrences are psychologically disturbing for the patient and may carry additional cardiovascular risk, especially in the elderly. Moreover, in some centers, treatment of moderate to severe Graves' ophthalmopathy, when needed, is delayed until permanent correction of thyrotoxicosis is achieved, so rapid attainment of this goal is desirable.

With the use of relatively high delivered doses of ^{131}I, 150 to 200 μCi/g of estimated thyroid weight, nearly 70% of patients are cured after one dose of ^{131}I, 25% require a second dose, and rare patients need a third or fourth dose. Large goiter size, rapid iodine turnover, and adjunctive therapy with antithyroid drugs too soon after radioiodine are associated with a higher rate of persistence of hyperthyroidism, but other individual factors are also likely to exist. The decision to give a second dose of ^{131}I is not usually made before 6 to 12 months after the first one, when firm demonstration of persistence of thyrotoxicosis can be obtained. Transient hypothyroidism may be observed in the first 6 months after ^{131}I therapy. To correctly detect these cases, levothyroxine substitution should be initiated at submaximal doses so that TSH can be rechecked 2 to 4 months later; if high, the hypothyroidism is very likely to be permanent.

Short-Term Adverse Effects of Radioiodine. Transient exacerbation of mild to moderate preexisting Graves' ophthalmopathy may occur in the few months after radioiodine therapy,[392] although this experience is not shared by all investigators. Because worsening of ophthalmopathy is transient and effectively controlled with a short course of oral corticosteroids,[392] the presence of mild to moderate ophthalmopathy is not a contraindication to the use of radioiodine. When severe Graves' ophthalmopathy is present, specific treatment with high-dose oral or intravenous corticosteroids and/or external radiation therapy should be started soon after radioiodine treatment.

Radioiodine treatment causes a radiation-induced acute thyroiditis that can rarely be clinically manifested 3 or 4 days after administration of the isotope by pain and swelling in the neck. This side effect is benign and self-limited and can be treated with a short course of anti-inflammatory drugs. The destruction of thyroid tissue after radioiodine treatment also induces the release of preformed thyroid hormone from the gland, which can result in re-exacerbation of thyrotoxicosis in the weeks after the procedure. To prevent this phenomenon by depleting intrathyroidal stores of hormones, a few months' course of thionamide is often given and discontinued 3 to 8 days before radioiodine administration. True relapses of hyperthyroidism after thionamide withdrawal in preparation for ^{131}I administration may also occur and account for the increase in thyroid hormone levels observed after radioiodine administration.[393] Because the effect of radioiodine is relatively delayed, several months may be required for complete control of the thyrotoxicosis. While waiting for the effect of radioiodine, a short course of antithyroid drugs can be initiated 2 weeks after treatment and the dose smoothly tapered in the following months. Earlier thionamide treatment has been associated with a higher rate of radioiodine failure. Alternatively, iopanoic acid or sodium ipodate can be administered a few days after the administration of radioiodine. This form of treatment has the advantage of rapidly controlling both thyrotoxicosis from radiation thyroiditis and transient relapse of hyperthyroidism.

Potential Long-Term Risks of Radioiodine. Radioisotope treatment of a benign disorder such as Graves' disease may raise concern regarding possible carcinogenic effects and the risk of genetic damage (i.e., the risk of causing germline mutations in the offspring of patients treated during the child-bearing years). Although external head and neck irradiation is undoubtedly associated with an increased rate of thyroid carcinoma,[394, 395] no association between radioiodine treatment of hyperthyroidism and thyroid cancer was found in large epidemiologic studies.[275] Similarly, no evidence has indicated that radioiodine therapy for hyperthyroidism increases the patient's risk for leukemia or solid tumors.[275] A minimal increase in the risk of gastric cancer 10 years or more after treatment was found in a survey in Sweden,[396] but not in a large epidemiologic study in the United Kingdom[275] and in the United States.[397] No association between radioiodine treatment of hyperthyroidism and congenital abnormalities in subsequent offspring has been observed.[398] A rough estimate of the dose to the ovaries is about 0.2 rad/mCi of administered ^{131}I. Thus the dose to the ovaries in a patient receiving 10 mCi of radioiodine is similar to that received from a barium enema or intravenous pyelography. It has been calculated that if a genetic risk induced by ^{131}I really does exist, the risk would be only 0.003% per rad of parental gonadal exposure and therefore a very small fraction of the spontaneous incidence of genetic disorders.[399] Thus the experience accumulated in more than 50 years of radioiodine treatment of hyperthyroidism has shown that potential long-term risks are absent or negligible in the adult population. Unfortunately, no large studies are available on such risks in the pediatric population. Data from populations exposed to radioactive isotopes after the Chernobyl accident indicate that in infancy the thyroid is much more susceptible to radioiodine-induced carcinogenesis.[400–402] These observations are based on data that are very skewed with regard to the amount and duration of exposure to the radioactive fallout and therefore cannot be extrapolated to the therapeutic use of radioiodine; most authorities do not currently recommend radioiodine treatment for persons younger than 16 to 18 years.

Surgery. The aim of surgical treatment in Graves' hyperthyroidism is to reduce the excessive secretion of thyroid hormones and prevent relapse of thyrotoxicosis by removal of enough thyroid tissue. Subtotal thyroidectomy has for a long time been the choice of surgery for Graves' disease. The classic procedure consists of removing the bulk of the gland, with a few grams of tissue left in both lobes. With subtotal thyroidectomy many patients remain euthyroid but are exposed to the risk of future relapse of thyrotoxicosis. A significant number of patients treated with subtotal thyroidectomy also become hypothyroid[403, 404] (Fig. 100–9). Therefore, lifelong surveillance is needed after subtotal thyroidectomy. Near-total thyroidectomy consists of the removal of most thyroid tissue, with only subcentimeter frag-

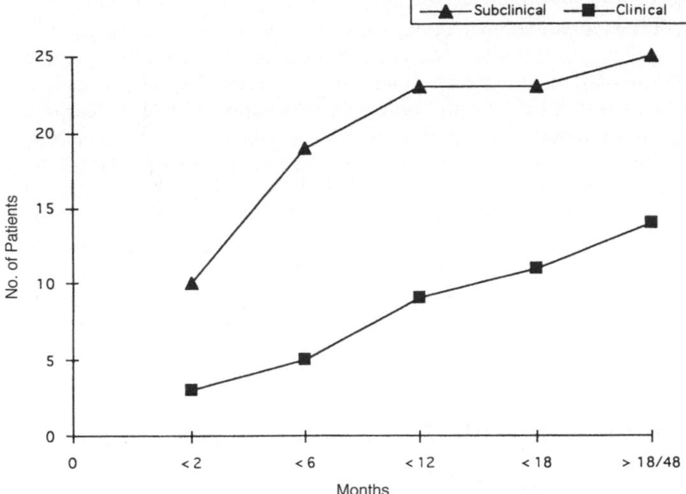

FIGURE 100–9. Prevalence of subclinical and clinical hypothyroidism in a cohort of patients with Graves' disease treated by subtotal thyroidectomy. (From Miccoli P, Vitti P, Rago T, et al: Surgical treatment of Graves' disease: Subtotal or total thyroidectomy? Surgery 120:1020–1025, 1996.)

ments left in sensitive regions, such as around the laryngeal recurrent nerve or the parathyroid glands. Near-total thyroidectomy has more recently been performed in patients with Graves' disease and results in a higher rate of hypothyroidism, but a much smaller incidence of recurrent hyperthyroidism.[403, 405] Because of the very low risk of relapse of thyrotoxicosis, near-total thyroidectomy has become the preferred operation in specialized centers.[404] Total thyroidectomy (e.g., removal of all visible thyroid tissue) may have the additional advantage of removing virtually all thyroidal autoantigens, and thus it might have a positive influence on the course of Graves' ophthalmopathy when present, but this issue is still under study.

Preparation of the patient for thyroid surgery is of paramount importance. A course of thionamide treatment is recommended to restore and maintain euthyroidism and to deplete intrathyroidal stores of hormones that could be released during surgery. The preoperative administration (10 days) of inorganic iodide induces involution of the gland and a reduction in vascularity.[372] Another approach has been proposed, namely, preparation with propranolol and iodide alone, which allows earlier surgery. In the absence of a real need for rapid surgery, however, this approach should be discouraged because it exposes patients to unnecessary risks. When emergency surgery is needed, oral cholecystographic agents represent the fastest way to obtain euthyroidism.[406, 407]

Besides the common nonspecific complications of surgery and anesthesia, thyroid surgery exposes patients to certain specific complications, including thyroid storm, which is now extremely rare, bleeding, injury to the recurrent laryngeal nerve, and hypoparathyroidism. In particular, the risk of laryngeal nerve injury and hypoparathyroidism cannot be disregarded. The incidence of these complications depends on the skill and experience of the surgeon and may range from 2% in specialized centers with wide experience in thyroid surgery up to 10% to 15% in some series.[408–411]

As stated before, these two potential complications need to be carefully explained to the patient when the discussion of treatment options is started. Postoperative thyroid function largely depends on the extent of thyroidectomy and duration of follow-up. Insufficient tissue removal results in persistent hyperthyroidism or in later relapse of hyperthyroidism, which may occur in 5% to 10% of patients within 5 years and in up to 40% within 30 years after limited thyroidectomy. Recurrence of hyperthyroidism is particularly undesirable because a second operation is technically more difficult than the first one and involves a higher risk of complications. With few exceptions, therefore, such patients should be treated with radioiodine. Extensive thyroidectomy results in postoperative thyroid failure, which always occurs after total and near-total thyroidectomy and often after subtotal thyroidectomy. In the first year after surgery, hypothyroidism has been reported in percentages of patients ranging from 5% to 60%.[391, 403, 405, 412] Late-onset cases develop in an additional 1% to 3% per year. Hypothyroidism is easily and economically treated with levothyroxine replacement therapy, so thyroid failure after thyroidectomy for Graves' hyperthyroidism should not be considered a real complication.

Making the Choice of Treatment

In the above paragraphs, the possible therapeutic tools for Graves' disease thyrotoxicosis (antithyroid drugs, radioiodine, and surgery) have been examined. Some of them represent alternatives to the others. It is therefore important to discuss the relevant variables that will guide both the patient and the clinician in the choice of the best option for the particular case. General advantages and disadvantages of three major tools for the treatment of Graves' disease hyperthyroidism are listed in Table 100–7. Scientific evidence collected over the past 50 years or so is of invaluable help in making the correct decision. In many cases the choice is in fact guided by preference, by personal experience of both the patient and the physician, or by environmental conditions (for example, the lack of an experienced surgeon or a well-equipped nuclear medicine facility). In 1987 a survey of practice in Europe showed that a large majority of European endocrinologists still preferred medical treatment with thionamides in many cases of Graves' hyperthyroidism, including the most typical one, a woman in her forties with a medium-sized goiter. Ninety-five percent of European endocrinologists would have chosen this approach in a younger patient (e.g., a 19-year-old woman).[413] In contrast, when the same questionnaire was given to North American endocrinologists, 69% selected radioiodine for the older patient and 27% chose it for the 19-year-old hyperthyroid female.[414] In both groups, thyroidectomy was not considered adequate in small to medium-sized goiters. Such wide differences in the perception of the best option for the treatment of Graves' disease not only reflect different traditions and experiences worldwide but also the fact that none of the available options has a clear-cut advantage over the others.

In a typical uncomplicated Graves' disease case, for example, a middle-aged woman with a medium-sized goiter and mild Graves' ophthalmopathy, it is therefore reasonable to offer the patient a trial of antithyroid drugs in an attempt to obtain persistent remission of hyperthyroidism, with the knowledge that this result will be obtained in a small, albeit significant minority of cases. At the same time, the patient can also be presented with the possibility of definitive treatment

TABLE 100–7. Advantages and Disadvantages of Available Treatment Modalities for Graves' Disease Thyrotoxicosis

Treatment Modality	Advantages	Disadvantages
Radioiodine	Definitive treatment of thyrotoxicosis	Delayed control of thyrotoxicosis
	Rare, mild, and transient side effects	Lower efficacy in large goiters
	No surgical risks	Radiation hazard (?)
	Easy to perform, fast	Transient worsening of preexisting eye disease
	Low cost	
Thyroidectomy	Definitive treatment of thyrotoxicosis	Hypoparathyroidism (0.9%–2%)
	No radiation hazards	Recurrent laryngeal nerve damage (0.1%–2%)
	Fast correction of thyrotoxicosis	
	Removal of large goiters	Bleeding/infection/anesthesia
		Scarring
		High cost
Thionamides	No radiation hazards	Frequent relapses
	No surgical risks	Requires frequent testing
	Almost no permanent hypothyroidism	Side effects and adverse reactions

of hyperthyroidism with radioiodine and should receive an explanation regarding the fact that the most likely result will be permanent hypothyroidism. In many cases, however, this basic approach to the treatment of hyperthyroidism must be modified in light of other factors, which makes the choice of treatment somewhat less optional.

AGE. Although radioiodine has been effectively used in adolescents and young adults with no adverse effects,[415, 416] because of the lack of studies on the long-term effects of radioiodine, we usually exert caution in this situation and our primary choice for treatment is antithyroid drugs, at least until the patient is 20 years old or so. Thyroidectomy may also be advised in children and adolescents who are allergic or noncompliant with antithyroid drugs. However, subtotal thyroidectomy may be more hazardous in children, in whom acute complications are reported in 16% to 35% and permanent complications in up to 8%.[417, 418]

In women in the reproductive age, pregnancy must be delayed for at least 4 months after radioiodine administration and possibly for 1 year.[419] Therefore, the treatment plan should be designed with the patient according to her family plans, with antithyroid drug treatment being safe and effective during pregnancy (see below).

Opposite considerations can be made in elderly subjects, in whom faster definitive correction of hyperthyroidism may be warranted. Relapse of hyperthyroidism after antithyroid drug treatment increases the cardiovascular risk in elderly patients, and surgery may present excessive risks in these patients. Therefore, radioiodine can be considered the best choice in the elderly.

GOITER SIZE AND ASSOCIATED NODULAR THYROID DISEASE. Large goiters are relatively resistant to ^{131}I and often require multiple treatments before correction of hyperthyroidism.[340] Moreover, radioiodine only induces partial and slow shrinkage of the goiter. Therefore, when the patient has a large goiter, especially if compressive symptoms are present, surgery is the best choice of treatment, provided that an experienced surgeon is available.

Surgery is also recommended when Graves' disease is superimposed on endemic goiters with multiple cold nodules, which are not expected to respond with shrinkage to radioiodine. Finally, surgery is mandatory when a suspicion of malignancy cannot be ruled out in an associated single cold nodule, regardless of the size of the goiter.

GRAVES' OPHTHALMOPATHY. The possible untoward effects of radioiodine on preexisting mild or moderate Graves' ophthalmopathy have been considered above. The presence of severe Graves' ophthalmopathy requiring active treatment may modify the clinical approach. In a recent survey most European thyroidologists chose antithyroid drug treatment in an index case with severe ophthalmopathy,[420] which implies that most of them were concerned with a possible worsening of Graves' ophthalmopathy after radioiodine treatment. The fact that thionamide treatment does not appear to be associated with worsening of ophthalmopathy was also responsible for this choice.[421] As an alternative option, prompt definitive treatment of thyrotoxicosis by radioiodine or surgery may be warranted in the hope that the ongoing autoimmune process in the thyroid gland may drive the one in the orbit and that removal of possible cross-reacting thyroidal antigen(s) may improve orbital autoimmunity. Relapses of thyrotoxicosis after discontinuation of treatment with antithyroid drugs are also frequent and may result in exacerbation of the orbital inflammatory process. Therefore, in these cases we usually advise rapid ablation of the thyroid with radioiodine or surgery, closely followed by the appropriate treatment of Graves' ophthalmopathy.

CONCURRENT NONTHYROIDAL ILLNESSES. The presence of nonthyroidal illnesses, especially heart disease, requires special attention in the choice of treatment of Graves' thyrotoxicosis. In these patients surgery may be contraindicated or involve excessive risk, and relapses of thyrotoxicosis can worsen the concurrent heart disease. For these reasons, radioiodine is the therapeutic tool of choice, preceded by accurate short-term antithyroid drug preparation and followed by protection from postradioiodine thyrotoxicosis by thionamides or iopanoic acid (see below). A similar approach can be taken with other nonthyroidal disorders that can be affected by thyroid function status, such as diabetes and severe psychiatric diseases, although in the latter conditions thyroidectomy can be advised as well.

PATIENT'S CHOICE AND ENVIRONMENTAL FACTORS. From the preceding it is apparent that only rarely is the choice of one treatment modality mandatory. As a consequence, the patient can often be directly involved in the decision-making process after complete information on advantages and disadvantages. For example, some patients may have a disproportionate perception and fear of the meaning of "treatment with radioactive compounds." In other cases, the presence of a goiter is perceived as disfiguring, and the patient may require surgery for aesthetic purposes. Yet other patients may be reluctant to submit to long-term drug therapy or may wish to solve the problem quickly. Other considerations that must be taken into account when selecting the treatment modality are the availability of an experienced surgeon and/or an experienced nuclear medicine facility. In some countries, restrictive legislation makes administration of sufficient doses of radioiodine more difficult.

Special Situations

Graves' Disease and Pregnancy

A higher incidence of abortion, preterm delivery, low-birth-weight infants, and neonatal mortality is seen in pregnancies complicated by maternal hyperthyroidism.[422] Besides fetal complications, hyperthyroidism may also cause maternal complications such as heart failure and thyroid storm during delivery. Recognition of thyrotoxicosis during gestation or before a planned pregnancy warrants immediate and appropriate treatment inasmuch as pregnancies in which hyperthyroidism is fully controlled have excellent outcomes in mothers with Graves' disease.[423] It should also be added that for this reason pregnancy is not contraindicated in patients with Graves' disease, and conversely, thyrotoxicosis is not a reason for recommending abortion.

When Graves' disease is diagnosed in a woman planning pregnancy, pregnancy can be allowed after restoration of euthyroidism with thionamide drugs and treatment continued during pregnancy (see later). Alternatively, the radioiodine option can be offered because of a lack of evidence of an association between ^{131}I treatment of hyperthyroidism and congenital abnormalities in subsequent offspring. Current guidelines recommend that pregnancy be delayed for at least 4 months after radioiodine therapy,[424] but in a conservative approach, we usually advise the patient to wait for 1 year, when thyroid function is fully normalized and the outcome of treatment is clear. Thyroidectomy may also be considered as an alternative because of more rapid restoration of euthyroidism.

Radioiodine therapy is absolutely contraindicated during pregnancy because it may result in congenital hypothyroidism and may cause malformations. Surgery is restricted to exceptional cases. Thionamides are the first choice for treatment in a pregnant woman with Graves' disease. Clinical improvement with thionamides occurs after the first week, and euthyroidism may be reached after 2 to 4 weeks of therapy. Both propylthiouracil and methimazole cross the placenta[425] and in excessive doses may cause hypothyroidism and goiter in the fetus and in the neonate.[426, 427] Because propylthiouracil is less lipid soluble and more highly protein bound, its placental transfer appears to be lower, so preferential use of this drug in pregnancy has been advocated by some experts, mainly in the United States. However, a study at term showed no difference between propylthiouracil and methimazole in suppressing fetal thyroid function.[428] Also, methimazole has been anecdotally associated with aplasia cutis (a reversible malformation of the scalp) in a few neonates, but epidemiologic studies have not been able to provide evidence for a causal relationship.[429] In practice, none of the two drugs appears to be clearly advantageous over the other. Treatment should be monitored so that maternal FT_4 is kept in the high normal range. This level will ensure fetal euthyroidism inasmuch as FT_4 levels in the mother's serum are correlated with fetal FT_4 levels, as assessed in cord blood.[423] A low TSH level is not a reliable index to judge the adequacy of treatment because it may not reflect changes in thyroid function as promptly as FT_4 does, but it is very important to test it because a high level always indicates overtreatment and should prompt adjustment of the thionamide dose. Because of the immunosuppressive effect of pregnancy, partial and transient remission of Graves' disease may occur in the second and third trimesters and

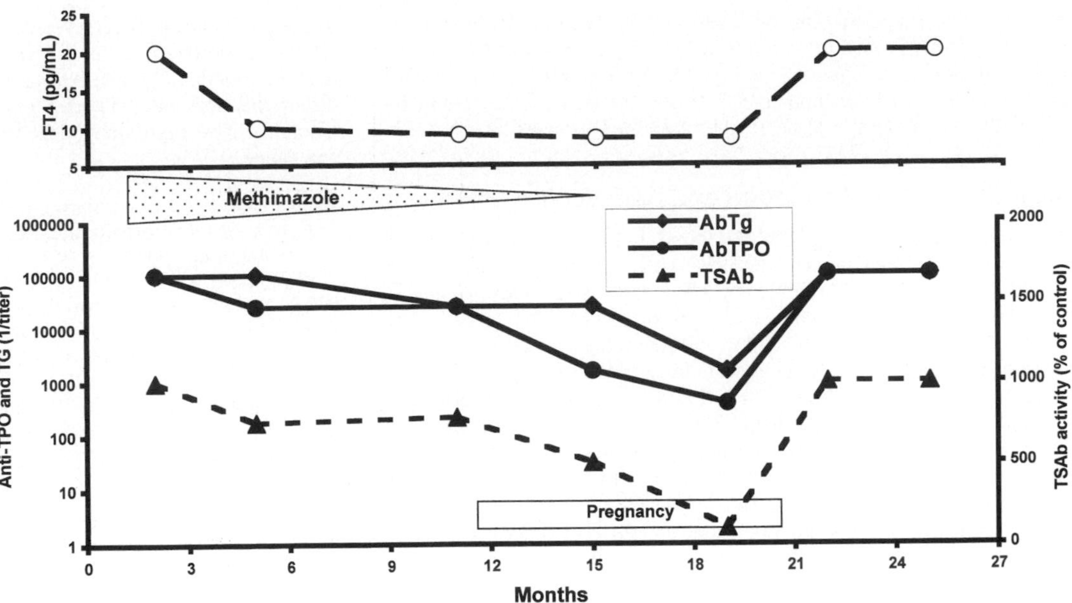

FIGURE 100–10. Course of hyperthyroidism in a patient with Graves' disease before, during, and after pregnancy. The immunosuppressive effect of pregnancy is shown by the reduction in serum antithyroid peroxidase (AbTPO) and antithyroglobulin (AbTg) titers and by the disappearance of serum anti–thyroid-stimulating hormone receptor antibodies (TSAb) during the third trimester of pregnancy, which allowed discontinuation of methimazole treatment *(lower panel)*. Serum free thyroxine (FT4) remained within the normal range without treatment *(upper panel)*, until a relapse of the autoimmune process (shown by an increase in the titer of the three antibodies) caused a relapse of thyrotoxicosis shortly after the end of pregnancy.

allow a reduction and even discontinuation of thionamide treatment (Fig. 100–10). On the other hand, relapse of hyperthyroidism is frequent postpartum.[430]

The block-and-replace regimen is contraindicated in pregnancy because much more thionamide than levothyroxine will cross the placenta and cause fetal hypothyroidism. Iodide is avoided because of the risk of fetal hypothyroidism and goiter caused by the greater sensitivity of the fetal thyroid to the Wolff-Chaikoff effect. The use of β-blockers is controversial in pregnancy, but most authorities will not recommend them, at least for prolonged periods.

Both methimazole and propylthiouracil are secreted in breast milk (methimazole more than propylthiouracil) in small amounts.[431] Low to medium doses of thionamides (up to 10 mg of methimazole or 150 mg of propylthiouracil) given to the mother during breast-feeding have been shown to not affect thyroid function in the infant.[432, 433] Under these conditions breast-feeding can be allowed. It has been calculated that even higher doses might be safely administered, but neonatal thyroid function should be monitored in such cases.

Surgical treatment is only occasionally indicated and may be considered in cases of poor compliance, severe drug allergy, very large goiter, associated thyroid malignancy, or the necessity of using high doses of thionamides to maintain euthyroidism. When needed, thyroidectomy is most safely performed in the second trimester. Complications of surgery, such as vocal cord paralysis or hypoparathyroidism, are both disabling, and the latter may be difficult to treat during pregnancy. Levothyroxine therapy for the mother should be promptly initiated postoperatively.

Neonatal and Fetal Transfer Thyrotoxicosis

Immunoglobulins cross the placenta and maternal TSAbs can also do so (Fig. 100–11). Because of this phenomenon, neonatal thyrotoxicosis may occur in association with maternal Graves' disease.[172] Mothers who have had Graves' disease and are euthyroid after thyroidectomy or radioiodine treatment may still have circulating TSAbs capable of causing neonatal thyrotoxicosis. Therefore, this possibility should be considered in all pregnant women with a current or past history of Graves' disease. Because of its pathogenesis, neonatal transfer thyrotoxicosis is always transient and spontaneously remits once maternal TSAbs disappear from the circulation, but it can cause acceleration of growth and craniosynostosis. Tachycardia, jaundice, heart failure, and failure to thrive characterize neonatal thyrotoxicosis.[434] Onset may be delayed for a few days after delivery, until maternal thionamides clear, or rarely, for a few weeks when an admixture of TBAbs and TSAbs is present in the serum. In mothers with high-titer TRAb in serum, testing for these antibodies in fetal cord blood can be performed at the time of delivery to predict the onset of neonatal thyrotoxicosis.[435]

Neonatal transfer thyrotoxicosis requires prompt treatment in close collaboration with a neonatologist. Thionamides, methimazole (0.5–1 mg/kg/day) or propylthiouracil (5–10 mg/kg/day), must be administered every 8 hours. Propranolol may be added to slow the heart rate and reduce hyperactivity. Iodine (1 drop of Lugol's solution, equivalent to 8 mg of iodine every 8 hours) is also used in addition to thionamides to inhibit the release of preformed thyroid hormones. As an alternative form of treatment, sodium ipodate alone, 0.5-g doses every 3 days, has been reported to rapidly normalize serum T_4 and T_3 in thyrotoxic neonates. In severely ill infants, glucocorticoids may be added as a general supportive measure and to block conversion of T_4 to T_3.[436]

When hyperthyroidism occurs during fetal life, the diagnosis is suggested by a heart rate over 160 beats per minute after 22 weeks of

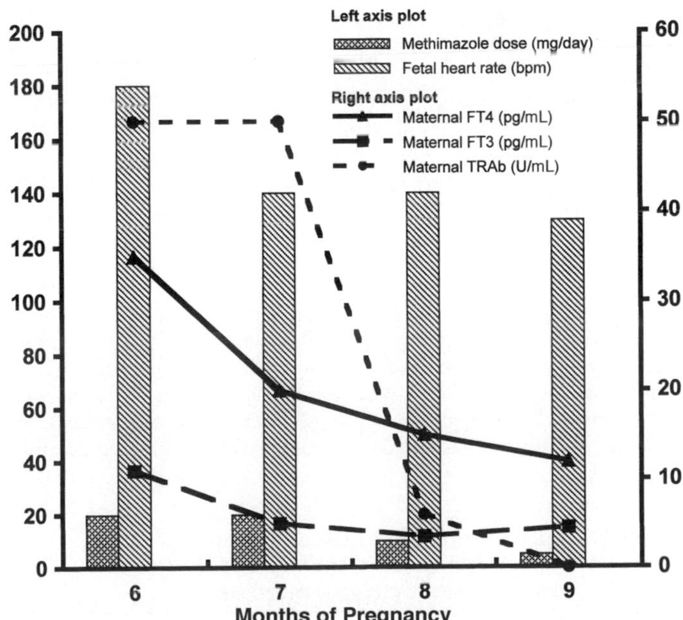

FIGURE 100–11. Fetal heart rate, maternal thyroid hormone, and maternal serum thyroid-stimulating hormone receptor antibodies (TRAb) during methimazole treatment in a woman in whom Graves' disease was diagnosed at the sixth month of pregnancy. FT3, Free triiodothyronine; FT4, free thyroxine.

gestation. The diagnosis can be confirmed by fetal cord blood sampling,[437] but this procedure is risky, with a 1% chance of fetal loss.[436] In utero treatment of hyperthyroidism may be accomplished by giving antithyroid drugs to the mother.[438] The dose of thionamide should be adjusted to maintain a fetal heart rate of about 140 beats/min.

Graves' Disease in Childhood and Adolescence

Graves' disease may occur in childhood, but it is rarely seen before 10 years of age. Most cases occur around puberty, between the ages of 11 and 15. The clinical findings are often impressive, with prominent neuropsychologic manifestations and an acceleration of growth that can result in premature ossification of bone end plates and reduced final height. Antithyroid drugs, radioiodine, and surgery have all been successfully used in children.[416] Radioiodine has proved to be effective in children with hyperthyroidism,[415] but its long-range potential for radiation oncogenesis and gonadal damage remains to be established. Long-term follow-up studies of radioiodine therapy in children, that is, in patients who have a 60- to 70-year life expectancy, are still limited, although some authors consider this form of treatment safe.[416] Given the above considerations, most children are treated with thionamides for long periods (3–4 years) in an attempt to induce stable remission or until they reach an age when radioiodine treatment or surgery is more suitable (usually 18 to 20 years of age). Long-term courses of therapy imply close medical supervision and parental involvement because compliance may be low in this age group.

Thyroidectomy is rarely performed in children and adolescents because permanent complications occur at a relatively higher rate in this age group and have a greater impact on developmental age. Nevertheless, very large goiters or poor compliance with antithyroid drug therapy may be an indication for surgical treatment.

Hyperthyroidism in the Elderly with Heart Disease

In the elderly, hyperthyroidism and cardiac disease are often associated. Hyperthyroid symptoms may be quite different in aged patients, and symptoms related to adrenergic hyperactivity such as hyperactive reflexes, increased sweating, heat intolerance, tremor, nervousness, and increased appetite are found less frequently than in younger patients[439] (Table 100–8). Weight loss is more often associated with anorexia, depression, and lethargy than with decreased appetite.[440] Overall, these findings justify the expression "apathetic thyrotoxicosis." Graves' ophthalmopathy has been reported to be more severe in the elderly, when present.[441]

Hyperthyroidism may precipitate heart failure or may worsen preexisting heart conditions, and atrial fibrillation is found in 30% to 60% of patients at diagnosis.[440, 439] Therefore, special attention should be put into rapidly controlling hyperthyroidism, avoiding relapses, and preventing additional heart complications. When heart disease is already present at the time of diagnosis, the treatment plan should be particularly cautious and include (1) prompt restoration of euthyroidism with antithyroid drugs while independently addressing the heart disease, (2) administration of β-adrenergic antagonists, (3) definitive, ablative treatment of hyperthyroidism with high doses of radioiodine, (4) protection of the heart from the possible radioiodine-induced transient thyrotoxicosis with β-adrenergic antagonists (immediately) and/or oral cholecystographic agents (2 weeks after radioiodine), (5) resumption of thionamide therapy 2 weeks after radioiodine administration to control hyperthyroidism while waiting for the complete effect of radioiodine, (6) strict control of thyroid function in the next 12 months, (7) cautious tapering of antithyroid drug doses until discontinuation, and (8) correction of hypothyroidism with the minimal amount of levothyroxine needed to maintain serum TSH in the normal range.

TABLE 100–8. Distinctive Initial Symptoms of Hyperthyroidism in the Elderly (Apathetic Hyperthyroidism)

Tachycardia	Depression
Congestive heart failure	Lethargy
Atrial fibrillation	Agitation and anxiety
Weight loss associated with anorexia	Confusion and dementia
Muscle wasting and weakness	Osteoporosis and bone fracture

Treatment of Pretibial Myxedema

In most cases pretibial myxedema causes little discomfort, but it can be disfiguring in others. Itching may also be a dominant symptom. Application of occlusive dressings with topical high-potency corticosteroids appears to be an effective treatment,[295, 442] as shown by the only available study including a sufficient cohort of patients.[295] Alternative treatment modalities include local injections of corticosteroids or hyaluronidase.[443] The treatment needs to be repeated from time to time because the disease is characterized by a course of remissions and relapses. Eventually, stable remissions are obtained in most cases. In more severe cases, surgical excision of pseudotumorous or polypous forms has been performed with success.[444, 445] Systemic treatment has included plasmapheresis[446] and high-dose corticosteroids.[447] Plasmapheresis is effective, but its favorable effects are transient when used alone without long-term immunosuppression. High-dose intravenous immunoglobulins have been used as well in uncontrolled studies, but this treatment is very expensive and offers no advantages over corticosteroids.

Thyroid Storm

Thyroid storm is an acute and severe life-threatening complication of thyrotoxicosis characterized by manifestations of severe hypermetabolism with high fever, tachyarrhythmias, profuse sweating, diarrhea and vomiting, confusion, delirium, and coma.[448] Congestive heart failure is often a relevant part of the picture. Thyroid storm occurs in patients with poor nutritional status and long-standing thyrotoxicosis, most often Graves' disease, either not recognized or not adequately treated. Although the cause is thought to be an abrupt release of large quantities of stored thyroid hormones into the circulation, in many cases the mechanism cannot be found. Before the use of antithyroid drugs, thyroid surgery and radioiodine therapy were relatively common causes of thyroid storm. Infections, trauma, surgical distress, metabolic disorders, and pulmonary and cardiovascular diseases are among the other factors that may precipitate a thyroid storm. Thyroid storm used to be much more frequent in the past and was associated with very high mortality, up to 75%.[449]

True thyroid storm is an extremely rare event now. However, less severe forms of thyrotoxic crisis are not exceptional and may be a medical emergency requiring prompt recognition and adequate treatment. Underlying nonthyroidal illnesses should be promptly recognized and specifically treated. Normalization of body temperature may require the use of cooling blankets and/or pharmacologic agents such as acetaminophen, chlorpromazine, or meperidine. Intravenous corticosteroids are beneficial in sustaining the peripheral circulation and preventing shock. Supportive measures such as oxygen and intravenous fluids should be given in case of hypoxia or dehydration. All means should be used to reduce the level of circulating thyroid hormone. Inhibition of the synthesis and release of thyroid hormones can be achieved with the use of thionamides and iodides, but this effect is delayed and therefore not sufficient, although necessary. Inhibition of the peripheral conversion of T_4 to T_3 by iodinated contrast agents is probably the fastest way to obtain a significant reduction in circulating T_3. Block of the peripheral effects of thyroid hormones by β-adrenergic antagonists (propranolol, metoprolol, atenolol) is also indicated. Removal of excess thyroid hormones from the circulation by plasmapheresis, peritoneal dialysis, extracorporeal resin perfusion, or charcoal plasma perfusion have all been reported in extreme situations. All drugs should be used in maximal doses. Patients require continuous monitoring of the electrocardiogram and an intravenous line to administer fluids and drugs. Alternatively, drugs can be delivered by nasogastric tube.

REFERENCES

1. Taylor S: Robert Graves. The Golden Years of Irish Medicine. New York, Royal Society of Medicine Services, 1989.
2. Graves RJ: Newly observed affection of the thyroid. London Med Surg J 7:515–523, 1835.
3. Parry CH: Collections from the Unpublished Medical Writings of the Late Caleb Hillier Parry. London, Underwood, 1825.
4. Flajani G: Sopra un tumor freddo nell'anterior parte del collo detto broncocele. [Collezione d'osservazioni e riflessioni di chirurgia.] 3:270–273, 1802.
5. von Basedow KA: Exophthalmos durch hypertrophie des zellgewebes in der Augenhole. Wochenschr Ges Heilk Berl 6:197, 1840.
6. Hennemannn G: Historical aspects about the development of our knowledge of morbus Basedow. J Endocrinol Invest 14:617–624, 1991.
7. Medvei VC: History of Clinical Endocrinology. New York, Parthenon, 1992.
8. MacKenzie JB, MacKenzie CG, McCollum EV: The effect of sulfanylguanidine on the thyroid in the rat. Science 94:518–519, 1941.
9. Astwood EB: Treatment of of hyperthyroidism with thiourea and thiouracil. JAMA 122:78, 1943.
10. Sawin CT, Becker DV: Radioiodine and the treatment of hyperthyroidism: The early history. Thyroid 7:163–176, 1997.
11. Adams DD, Purves HD: Abnormal responses in the assay of thyrotropin. Proc Univ Otago Med Sch 34:11–12, 1956.
12. Nagayama Y Kaufman KD, Seto P, Rapoport B: Molecular cloning, sequence and functional expression of the cDNA for the human thyrotropin receptor. Biochem Biophys Res Commun 165:1184–1190, 1989.
13. Parmentier M, Libert F, Maenhaut C, et al: Molecular cloning of the thyrotropin receptor. Science 246:1620–1622, 1989.
14. Laurberg P, Pedersen KM, Vestergaard H, Sigurdsson G: High incidence of multinodular toxic goitre in the elderly population in a low iodine intake area vs. high incidence of Graves' disease in the young in a high iodine intake area: Comparative surveys of thyrotoxicosis epidemiology in East-Jutland Denmark and Iceland. J Intern Med 229:415–420, 1991.
15. Furszyfer J, Kurland LT, McConahey WM, et al: Epidemiologic aspects of Hashimoto's thyroiditis and Graves' disease in Rochester Minnesota (1935–1967), with special reference to temporal trends. Metabolism 21:197–204, 1972.
16. Tunbridge W, Evered DC, Hall R, et al: The spectrum of thyroid disease in a community: The Whickham survey. Clin Endocrinol (Oxf) 7:481–493, 1977.
17. Jacobson DL, Gange SJ, Rose NR, Graham NM: Epidemiology and estimated population burden of selected autoimmune diseases in the United States. Clin Immunol Immunopathol 84:223–243, 1997.
18. Connolly RJ, Vidor GI, Stewart JC: Increase in thyrotoxicosis in endemic goitre area after iodination of bread. Lancet 1:500–502, 1970.
19. Adams DD, Fastier FN, Howie JB, et al: Stimulation of the human thyroid by infusions of plasma containing LATS protector. J Clin Endocrinol Metab 39:826–832, 1974.
20. Stanbury JB, Ermans AE, Bourdoux P, et al: Iodine-induced hyperthyroidism: Occurrence and epidemiology. Thyroid 8:83–100, 1998.
21. Burgi H, Kohler M, Morselli B: Thyrotoxicosis incidence in Switzerland and benefit of improved iodine supply. Lancet 352:1034, 1998.
22. Lundgren E, Christensen Borup S: Decreasing incidence of thyrotoxicosis in an endemic goitre inland area of Sweden. Clin Endocrinol 33:133–138, 1990.
23. Brownlie BE, Wells JE: The epidemiology of thyrotoxicosis in New Zealand: Incidence and geographical distribution in north Canterbury, 1983–1985. Clin Endocrinol (Oxf) 33:249–259, 1990.
24. Barker DJP, Phillips DIW: Current incidence of thyrotoxicosis and past prevalence of goitre in 12 British towns. Lancet 2:567–570, 1984.
25. Hoffenberg R: Aetiology of hyperthyroidism. BMJ 3:452–455, 1974.
26. Harvald B, Hauge M: A catamnestic investigation of Danish twins. Dan Med Bull 3:150–158, 1956.
27. Brix TH, Christensen K, Holm NV, et al: A population-based study of Graves' disease in Danish twins. Clin Endocrinol (Oxf) 48:397–400, 1998.
28. Hall R, Stanbury JB: Familial studies of autoimmune thyroiditis. Clin Exp Immunol 2:719–725, 1967.
29. Hall RO, Owen SG, Smart GA: Evidence for a genetic predisposition to formation of thyroid autoantibodies. Lancet ii:187–190, 1960.
30. Phillips D, McLachlan S, Stephenson A, et al: Autosomal dominant transmission of autoantibodies to thyroglobulin and thyroid peroxidase. J Clin Endocrinol Metab 70:742–746, 1990.
31. Phillips D, Prentice L, McLachlan SM, et al: Autosomal dominant inheritance of the tendency to develop thyroid autoantibodies. Exp Clin Endocrinol 97:170–172, 1991.
32. Pauls DL, Zakarija M, McKenzie JM, Egeland JA: Complex segregation analysis of antibodies to thyroid peroxidase in Old Order Amish families. Am J Med Genet 47:375–379, 1993.
33. Shields DC, Ratanachaiyavong S, McGregor AM, et al: Combined segregation and linkage analysis of Graves' disease with a thyroid autoantibody diathesis. Am J Hum Genet 55:540–554, 1994.
34. Hall R, Dingle PR, Roberts DF: Thyroid antibodies: A study of first degree relatives. Clin Genet 3:319–324, 1972.
35. Bartels ED: Twin examinations: Heredity in Graves' disease. Munksgaad, Copenhagen, 1941.
36. Tamai H, Ohsako N, Takeno K, et al: Changes in thyroid function in euthyroid subjects with family history of Graves' disease; a followup study of 69 patients. J Clin Endocrinol Metab 51:1123–1128, 1980.
37. Chertow BS, Fidler WJ, Fariss BL: Graves' disease and Hashimoto's thyroiditis in monozygotic twins. Acta Endocrinol 72:18–24, 1973.
38. Howell Evans AW, Woodrow JC, McDougall CDM, et al: Antibodies in the families of thyrotoxic patients. Lancet 1:636–641, 1967.
39. Jaume JC, Guo J, Pauls DL, et al: Evidence for genetic transmission of thyroid peroxidase autoantibody epitopic "fingerprints." J Clin Endocrinol Metab 84:1424–1431, 1999.
40. Risch N, Merikangas K: The future of genetic studies of complex human diseases. Science 273:1516–1517, 1996.
41. Greenberg DA: Linkage analysis of "necessary" loci versus "susceptibility" loci. Am J Hum Genet 52:135–143, 1993.
42. Vladutiu AO, Rose NR: Autoimmune murine thyroiditis: Relation to histocompatibility (H-2) type. Science 174:1137–1139, 1971.
43. Farid NR, Barnard JM, Marshall WH: The association of HLA with autoimmune thyroid disease in Newfoundland. The influence of HLA homozygosity in Graves' disease. Tissue Antigens 8:181–189, 1976.
44. Irvine WJ, Gray RS, Morris PJ, Ting A: Correlation of HLA and thyroid antibodies with clinical course of thyrotoxicosis treated with antithyroid drugs. Lancet 2:898–900, 1977.
45. Allannic H, Fauchet R, Lorcy Y, et al: HLA and Graves' disease: An association with HLA-DRw3. J Clin Endocrinol Metab 51:863–867, 1980.
46. Yanagawa T, Mangklabruks A, Chang YB, et al: Human histocompatibility leukocyte antigen-DQA1*0501 allele associated with genetic susceptibility to Graves' disease in a Caucasian population. J Clin Endocrinol Metab 76:1569–1574, 1993.
47. Yanagawa T, Mangklabruks A, DeGroot LJ: Strong association between HLA-DQA1*0501 and Graves' disease in a male Caucasian population. J Clin Endocrinol Metab 79:227–229, 1994.
48. Heward JM, Allahabadia A, Daykin J, et al: Linkage disequilibrium between the human leukocyte antigen class II region of the major histocompatibility complex and Graves' disease: Replication using a population case control and family-based study. J Clin Endocrinol Metab 83:3394–3397, 1998.
49. Ofosu MH, Dunston G, Henry L, et al: HLA-DQ3 is associated with Graves' disease in African-Americans. Immunol Invest 25:103–110, 1996.
50. Chan SH, Yeo PP, Lui KF, et al: HLA and thyrotoxicosis (Graves' disease) in Chinese. Tissue Antigens 12:109–114, 1978.
51. Yanagawa T, DeGroot LJ: HLA class II associations in African-American female patients with Graves' disease. Thyroid 6:37–39, 1996.
52. Roman SH, Greenberg D, Rubinstein P, et al: Genetics of autoimmune thyroid disease: Lack of evidence for linkage to HLA within families. J Clin Endocrinol Metab 74:496–503, 1992.
53. Tomer Y, Barbesino G, Keddache M, et al: Mapping of a major susceptibility locus for Graves' disease (GD-1) to chromosome 14q31. J Clin Endocrinol Metab 82:1645–1648, 1997.
54. Farid NR, Newton RM, Noel EP, Marshall WH: Gm phenotypes in autoimmune thyroid disease. J Immunogenet 4:429–432, 1977.
55. Kozma L, Stenszky V, Kraszits E, et al: The association of IgG heavy-chain allotypes (Gm) with Graves' disease in Hungary. Exp Clin Immunogenet 2:154–157, 1985.
56. Demaine AG, Ratanachaviyavong S, Pope R, et al: Thyroglobulin antibodies in Graves' disease are associated with T-cell receptor beta chain and major histocompatibility complex loci. Clin Exp Immunol 77:21–24, 1989.
57. Demaine A, Welsh KI, Hawe BS, Farid NR: Polymorphism of the T cell receptor beta-chain in Graves' disease. J Clin Endocrinol Metab 65:643–646, 1987.
58. Weetman AP, So AK, Roe C, et al: T-cell receptor alpha chain V region polymorphism linked to primary autoimmune hypothyroidism but not Graves' disease. Hum Immunol 20:167–173, 1987.
59. Mangklabruks A, Cox N, DeGroot LJ: Genetic factors in autoimmune thyroid disease analyzed by restriction fragment length polymorphisms of candidate genes. J Clin Endocrinol Metab 73:236–244, 1991.
60. Cuddihy RM, Bahn RS: Lack of an association between alleles of interleukin-1 alpha and interleukin-1 receptor antagonist genes and Graves' disease in a North American Caucasian population. J Clin Endocrinol Metab 81:4476–4478, 1996.
61. Rau H, Donner H, Usadel KH, Badenhoop K: Polymorphisms of tumor necrosis factor receptor 2 are not associated with insulin-dependent diabetes mellitus or Graves' disease. Tissue Antigens 49:535–536, 1997.
62. Siegmund T, Usadel KH, Donner H, et al: Interferon-gamma gene microsatellite polymorphisms in patients with Graves' disease. Thyroid 8:1013–1017, 1998.
63. Yanagawa T, Hidaka Y, Guimaraes V, et al: CTLA-4 gene polymorphism associated with Graves' disease in a Caucasian population. J Clin Endocrinol Metab 80:41–45, 1995.
64. Nistico L, Buzzetti R, Pritchard LE, et al: The CTLA-4 gene region of chromosome 2q33 is linked to, and associated with, type 1 diabetes. Belgial Diabetes Registry Hum Mol Genet 5:1075–1080, 1996.
65. Donner H, Rau H, Walfish PG, et al: CTLA4 alanine-17 confers genetic susceptibility to Graves' disease and to type 1 diabetes mellitus. J Clin Endocrinol Metab 82:143–146, 1997.
66. Kotsa K, Watson PF, Weetman AP: A CTLA-4 gene polymorphism is associated with both Graves disease and autoimmune hypothyroidism. Clin Endocrinol (Oxf) 46:551–554, 1997.
67. Awata T, Kurihara S, Iitaka M, et al: Association of CTLA-4 gene A-G polymorphism (IDDM12 locus) with acute-onset and insulin-depleted IDDM as well as autoimmune thyroid disease (Graves' disease and Hashimoto's thyroiditis) in the Japanese population. Diabetes 47:128–129, 1998.
68. Thompson CB, Allison JP: The emerging role of CTLA-4 as an immune attenuator. Immunity 7:445–450, 1997.
69. Barbesino G, Tomer Y, Concepcion E, et al: Linkage analysis of candidate genes in autoimmune thyroid disease: 1. Selected immunoregulatory genes. International Consortium for the Genetics of Autoimmune Thyroid Disease. J Clin Endocrinol Metab 83:1580–1584, 1998.
70. Vaidya B, Imrie H, Perros P, et al: The cytotoxic T lymphocyte antigen-4 is a major Graves' disease locus. Hum Mol Genet 8:1195–1199, 1999.
71. Cuddihy RM, Dutton CM, Bahn RS: A polymorphism in the extracellular domain of the thyrotropin receptor is highly associated with autoimmune thyroid disease in females. Thyroid 5:89–95, 1995.

72. De Roux N, Shields DC, Misrahi M, et al: Analysis of the thyrotropin receptor as a candidate gene in familial Graves' disease. J Clin Endocrinol Metab 81:3483–3486, 1996.
73. Barbesino G, Tomer Y, Concepcion ES, et al: Linkage analysis of candidate genes in autoimmune thyroid disease. II. Selected gender-related genes and the X-chromosome. International Consortium for the Genetics of Autoimmune Thyroid Disease. J Clin Endocrinol Metab 83:3290–3295, 1998.
74. Tomer Y, Barbesino G, Greenberg DA, et al: A new Graves disease-susceptibility locus maps to chromosome 20q11.2. International Consortium for the Genetics of Autoimmune Thyroid Disease. Am J Hum Genet 63:1749–1756, 1998.
75. Tomer Y, Barbesino G, Greenberg DA, et al: Linkage analysis of candidate genes in autoimmune thyroid disease. III: Detailed analysis of chromosome 14 localizes Graves' disease-1 (GD-1) close to multinodular goiter-1 (MNG-1). International Consortium for the Genetics of Autoimmune Thyroid Disease. J Clin Endocrinol Metab 83:4321–4327, 1998.
76. Brix TH, Christensen K, Niels VH, et al: Genetic versus environment in Graves' disease—a population based twin study. Thyroid 7(suppl):13, 1997.
77. Chopra IJ, Solomon DH, Chopra U, et al: Abnormalities in thyroid function in relatives of patients with Graves' disease and Hashimoto's thyroiditis: Lack of correlation with inheritance of HLA-B8. J Clin Endocrinol Metab 45:45–54, 1977.
78. Stenszky V, Kozma L, Balazs C, et al: The genetics of Graves' disease: HLA and disease susceptibility. J Clin Endocrinol Metab 61:735–740, 1985.
79. Tomer Y, Davies TF: Infection, thyroid disease and autoimmunity. Endocr Rev 14:107–120, 1993.
80. Phillips DI, Barker DJ, Rees SB, et al: The geographical distribution of thyrotoxicosis in England according to the presence or absence of TSH-receptor antibodies. Clin Endocrinol (Oxf) 23:283–287, 1985.
81. Cox SP, Phillips DIW, Osmond C: Does infection initiate Graves disease? A population based 10 year study. Autoimmunity 4:43–49, 1989.
82. Toft AD, Blackwell CC, Saadi AT, et al: Secretor status and infection in patients with Grave's disease. Autoimmunity 7:279–289, 1990.
83. Valtonen VV, Ruutu P, Varis K, et al: Serological evidence for the role of bacterial infections in the pathogenesis of thyroid diseases. Acta Med Scand 219:105–111, 1986.
84. Joasoo A, Robertson P, Murray I: Letter: Viral antibodies and thyrotoxicosis. Lancet 2:125, 1975.
85. Shenkman L, Bottone EJ: Antibodies to *Yersinia enterocolitica* in thyroid disease. Ann Intern Med 85:735–739, 1976.
86. Bech K, Clemmensen O, Larsen JH, Bendixen G: Thyroid disease and *Yersinia*. Lancet 1:1060–1061, 1977.
87. Takuno H, Sakata S, Miura K: Antibodies to *Yersinia enterocolitica* serotype 3 in autoimmune thyroid disease. Endocrinol Jpn 37:489–500, 1990.
88. Lidman K, Eriksson U, Norberg R, Fagraeus A: Indirect immunofluorescence staining of human thyroid by antibodies occurring in *Yersinia enterocolitica* infections. Clin Exp Immunol 23:429–435, 1976.
89. Gripenberg M, Miettinen A, Kurki P, Linder E: Humoral immune stimulation and anti-epithelial antibodies in yersinial infections. Arthritis Rheum 21:904–908, 1978.
90. Ingbar SH: A possible role for bacterial antigens in the pathogenesis of autoimmune thyroid disease. In Pincheta A, Ingbar SH, McKenzie JM, Fewor GF (eds): Thyroid Immunity. New York, Plenum, 1987, pp 35–44.
91. Weiss M, Ingbar SH, Winblad S, Kasper DL: Demonstration of a saturable binding site for thyrotropin in *Yersinia enterocolitica*. Science 219:1331–1333, 1983.
92. Heyma P, Harrison LC, Robinsk-Browne R: Thyrotrophin (TSH) binding sites on *Yersinia enterocolitica* recognized by immunoglobulins from humans with Graves' disease. Clin Exp Immunol 64:249–254, 1986.
93. Burman KD, Lukes YG, Gemiski P: Molecular homology between the human TSH receptor and *Yersinia enterocolitica* (abstract). Thyroid 1(suppl):62, 1991.
94. Wenzel BE, Heesemann J, Heufelder A, et al: Enteropathogenic *Yersinia enterocolitica* and organ-specific autoimmune diseases in man. Contrib Microbiol Immunol 12:80–88, 1991.
95. Luo G, Fan JL, Seetharamaiah GS, et al: Immunization of mice with *Yersinia enterocolitica* leads to the induction of antithyrotropin receptor antibodies. J Immunol 151:922–928, 1993.
96. Safran M, Paul TL, Roti E, Braverman LE: Environmental factors affecting autoimmune thyroid disease. Endocrinol Metab Clin North Am 16:327–342, 1987.
97. Lindholm H, Visakorpi R: Late complications after a *Yersinia enterocolitica* epidemic: A follow up study. Ann Rheum Dis 50:694–696, 1991.
98. Ciampolillo A, Mirakian R, Schulz T, et al: Retrovirus-like sequences in Graves' disease: Implications for human autoimmunity. Lancet 1:1096–1099, 1989.
99. Humphrey M, Baker JJ, Carr FE, et al: Absence of retroviral sequences in Graves' disease. Lancet 337:17–18, 1991.
100. Tominaga T, Katamine S, Namba H, et al: Lack of evidence for the presence of human immunodeficiency virus type 1–related sequences in patients with Graves' disease. Thyroid 1:307–314, 1991.
101. Wick G, Grubeck-Loebenstein B, Trieb K, et al: Human foamy virus antigens in thyroid tissue of Graves' disease patients. Int Arch Allergy Immunol 99:153–156, 1992.
102. Schweizer M, Turek R, Reinhardt M, Neumann HD: Absence of foamy virus DNA in Graves' disease. AIDS Res Hum Retroviruses 10:601–605, 1994.
103. Schweizer M, Turek R, Hahn H, et al: Markers of foamy virus infections in monkeys, apes, and accidentally infected humans: Appropriate testing fails to confirm suspected foamy virus prevalence in humans. AIDS Res Hum Retroviruses 11:161–170, 1995.
104. Burch HB, Nagy EV, Lukes YG, et al: Nucleotide and amino acid homology between the human thyrotropin receptor and HIV-1 nef protein: Identification and functional analysis. Biochem Biophys Res Commun 181:498–505, 1991.
105. Tas M, de Haan-Meulman M, Kabel PJ, Drexhage HA: Defects in monocyte polarization and dendritic cell clustering in patients with Graves' disease. A putative role for a non-specific immunoregulatory factor related to retroviral p15E. Clin Endocrinol 34:441–448, 1991.
106. Leib-Mosch C, Bachmann M, Brack-Werner R, et al: Expression and biological significance of human endogenous retroviral sequences. Leukemia 6(suppl):72–75, 1992.
107. Jaspan JB, Luo H, Ahmed B, et al: Evidence for a retroviral trigger in Graves' disease. Autoimmunity 20:135–142, 1995.
108. Pallard X, West SG, Lafferty JA, et al: Evidence for the effects of a superantigen in rheumatoid arthritis. Science 253:325–329, 1991.
109. Fierabracci A, Hammond L, Lowdell M, et al: The effect of staphylococcal enterotoxin B on thyrocyte HLA molecule expression. J Autoimmun 12:305–314, 1999.
110. Leclere J, Germain M, Weryha G, et al: Role of stressful life-events in the onset of Graves' disease. *In* Proceedings of the 10th International Thyroid Conference. The Hague, Netherlands, 1991.
111. Winsa B, Adami H, Bergstrom R, et al: Stressful life events and Graves' disease. Lancet 338:1475–1479, 1991.
112. Sonino N, Girelli M, Boscaro M, et al: Life events in the pathogenesis of Graves' disease. A controlled study. Acta Endocrinol 128:293–296, 1993.
113. Radosavljevic VR, Jankovic SM, Marinkovic JM: Stressful life events in the pathogenesis of Graves' disease. Eur J Endocrinol 134:699–701, 1996.
114. Yoshiuchi K, Kumano H, Nomura S, et al: Stressful life events and smoking were associated with Graves' disease in women, but not in men. Psychosom Med 60:182–185, 1998.
115. Hadden DR, McDevitt DG: Environmental stress and thyrotoxicosis. Absence of association. Lancet 2:577–578, 1974.
116. Locke S, Ader R, Besedovsky H, et al: Foundations of Psychoneuroimmunology. New York, Aldine, 1985.
117. Stein SP, Keller SE, Schleifer SJ: Stress and immunomodulation: The role of depression and neuroendocrine function. J Immunol 135(suppl):827–833, 1985.
118. Amino N: Postpartum thyroid disease. *In* Bercu BB, Shulman DI (eds): Advances in Perinatal Thyroidology. New York, Plenum, 1991, p 167.
119. Amino N, Miyai K: Postpartum Autoimmune Endocrine Syndromes. New York, Wiley, 1983.
120. Stagnaro GA, Roman SH, Cobin RH, et al: A prospective study of lymphocyte-initiated immunosuppression in normal pregnancy: Evidence of a T-cell etiology for postpartum thyroid dysfunction. J Clin Endocrinol Metab 74:645–653, 1992.
121. Chiovato L, Pinchera A: Stressful life events and Graves' disease. Eur J Endocrinol 134:680–682, 1996.
122. Wong GW, Kwok MY, Ou Y: High incidence of juvenile Graves' disease in Hong Kong. Clin Endocrinol (Oxf) 43:697–700, 1995.
123. Grossman CJ: Regulation of the immune system by sex steroids. Endocr Rev 5:435, 1984.
124. Beeson PB: Age and sex associations of 40 autoimmune diseases. Am J Med 96:457–462, 1994.
125. Chiovato L, Lapi P, Fiore E, et al: Thyroid autoimmunity and female gender. J Endocrinol Invest 16:384–391, 1993.
126. Lutfi RJ, Fridmanis M, Misiunas AL, et al: Association of melasma with thyroid autoimmunity and other thyroidal abnormalities and their relationship to the origin of the melasma. J Clin Endocrinol Metab 61:28–31, 1985.
127. Williams ED, Engel E, Forbes AP: Thyroiditis and gonadal dysgenesis. N Engl J Med 270:805, 1964.
128. Vallotton MB, Forbes AP: Autoimmunity in gonadal dysgenesis and Klinefelter's syndrome. Lancet 1:648–651, 1967.
129. Chiovato L, Larizza D, Bendinelli G, et al: Autoimmune hypothyroidism and hyperthyroidism in patients with Turner's syndrome. Eur J Endocrinol 134:568–575, 1996.
130. Jansson R, Dahlberg PA, Winsa B, et al: The postpartum period constitutes an important risk for the development of clinical Graves' disease in young women. Acta Endocrinol (Copenh) 116:321–325, 1987.
131. Pope RM: Immunoregulatory mechanisms present in the maternal circulation during pregnancy. Baillieres Clin Rheumatol 4:33–52, 1990.
132. Rees Smith B, McLachlan SM, Furmaniak J: Autoantibodies to the thyrotropin receptor. Endocr Rev 9:106–121, 1988.
133. McKenzie JM, Zakarija M: Clinical review 3: The clinical use of thyrotropin receptor antibody measurements. J Clin Endocrinol Metab 69:1093–1096, 1989.
134. Vitti P, Chiovato L, Fiore E, et al: Use of cells expressing the human thyrotropin (TSH) receptor for the measurement of thyroid stimulating and TSH-blocking antibodies. Acta Med Austriaca 23:52–56, 1996.
135. Chiovato L, Vitti P, Bendinelli G, et al: Detection of antibodies blocking thyrotropin effect using Chinese hamster ovary cells transfected with the cloned human TSH receptor. J Endocrinol Invest 17:809–816, 1994.
136. Libert F, Ruel J, Ludgate M, et al: Complete nucleotide sequence of the human thyroperoxidase-microsomal antigen cDNA: Nucleic Acids Res 15:6735, 1987.
137. Tonacchera M, Van Sande J, Parma J, et al: TSH receptor and disease. Clin Endocrinol 44:621–633, 1996.
138. Libert F, Passage E, Lefort A, et al: Localization of human thyrotropin receptor gene to chromosome 14q31 by in situ hybridization. Cytogenet Cell Genet 54:82–83, 1991.
139. Ban T, Kosugi S, Kohn LD: Specific antibody to the thyrotropin receptor identifies multiple receptor forms in membranes of cells transfected with wild-type receptor complementary deoxyribonucleic acid: Characterization of their relevance to receptor synthesis, processing, structure, and function. Endocrinology 131:815–829, 1992.
140. Loosfelt H, Pichon C, Jolivet A, et al: Two-subunit structure of the human thyrotropin receptor. Proc Natl Acad Sci U S A 89:3765–3769, 1992.
141. Sanders J, Oda Y, Roberts SA, et al: Understanding the thyrotropin receptor function-structure relationship. Baillieres Clin Endocrinol Metab 11:451–479, 1997.
142. Nagayama Y, Rapoport B: The thyrotropin receptor 25 years after its discovery: New insight after its molecular cloning. Mol Endocrinol 6:145–156, 1992.
143. Prentice L, Sanders JF, Perez M, et al: Thyrotropin (TSH) receptor autoantibodies do not appear to bind to the TSH receptor produced in an in vitro transcription/translation system. J Clin Endocrinol Metab 82:1288–1292, 1997.
144. Nagayama Y, Wadsworth HL, Russo D, et al: Binding domains of stimulatory

and inhibitory TSH receptor autoantibodies determined with chimeric TSH-LH/CG receptors. J Clin Invest 88:336–340, 1991.

145. Watanabe Y, Tahara K, Hirai A, et al: Subtypes of anti-TSH receptor antibodies classified by various assays using CHO cells expressing wild-type or chimeric human TSH receptor. Thyroid 7:13–19, 1997.

146. Murakami M, Mori M: Identification of immunogenic regions in human thyrotropin receptor for immunoglobulin G of patients with Graves' disease. Biochem Biophys Res Commun 171:512–518, 1990.

147. Kosugi S, Ban T, Akamizu T, Kohn LD: Identification of separate determinants on the thyrotropin receptor reactive with Graves' thyroid-stimulating antibodies and with thyroid-stimulating blocking antibodies in idiopathic myxedema: These determinants have no homologous sequence on gonadotropin receptors. Mol Endocrinol 6:168–180, 1992.

148. Dallas JS, Seetharamaiah GS, Cunningham SJ, et al: A region on the human thyrotropin receptor which can induce antibodies that inhibit thyrotropin-mediated activation of in vitro thyroid cell function also contains a highly immunogenic epitope. J Autoimmun 7:469–483, 1994.

149. McKenzie JM: Delayed thyroid response to serum from thyrotoxic patients. Endocrinology 62:865–868, 1958.

150. Shewring G, Smith BR: An improved radioreceptor assay for TSH receptor antibodies. Clin Endocrinol (Oxf) 17:409–417, 1982.

151. Southgate K, Creagh F, Teece M, et al: A receptor assay for the measurement of TSH receptor antibodies in unextracted serum. Clin Endocrinol (Oxf) 20:539–548, 1984.

152. Filetti S, Foti D, Costante G, Rapoport B: Recombinant human TSH receptor in a radioreceptor assay for the measurement of TSH receptor autoantibodies. J Clin Endocrinol Metab 72:1096–1101, 1991.

153. Costagliola S, Swillens S, Niccoli P, et al: Binding assay for thyrotropin receptor autoantibodies using the recombinant receptor protein. J Clin Endocrinol Metab 75:1540–1544, 1992.

154. Ludgate M, Costagliola S, Danguy D, et al: Recombinant TSH-receptor for determination of TSH-receptor-antibodies. Exp Clin Endocrinol 100:73–74, 1992.

155. Costagliola S, Morgenthaler NG, Hoermann R, et al: Second generation assay for thyrotropin receptor antibodies has superior diagnostic sensitivity for Graves' disease. J Clin Endocrinol Metab 84:90–97, 1999.

156. Vitti P, Elisei R, Tonacchera M, et al: Detection of thyroid-stimulating antibody using Chinese hamster ovary cells transfected with cloned human thyrotropin receptor. J Clin Endocrinol Metab 76:499–503, 1993.

157. Morgenthaler NG, Pampel I, Aust G, et al: Application of a bioassay with CHO cells for the routine detection of stimulating and blocking autoantibodies to the TSH-receptor. Horm Metab Res 30:162–168, 1998.

158. Toccafondi RS, Aterini S, Medici MA, et al: Thyroid-stimulating antibody (TSab) detected in sera of Graves' patients using human thyroid cell cultures. Clin Exp Immunol 40:532–539, 1980.

159. Bidey SP, Marshall NJ, Ekins RP: Bioassay of thyroid-stimulating immunoglobulins using human thyroid cell cultures: Optimization and clinical assessment. Clin Endocrinol (Oxf) 19:193–206, 1983.

160. Rapoport B, Greenspan FS, Filetti S, Pepitone M: Clinical experience with a human thyroid cell bioassay for thyroid-stimulating immunoglobulin. J Clin Endocrinol Metab 58:332–338, 1984.

161. Vitti P, Valente WA, Ambesi-Impiombato FS, et al: Graves' IgG stimulation of continuously cultured rat thyroid cells: A sensitive and potentially useful clinical assay. J Endocrinol Invest 5:179–182, 1982.

162. Vitti P, Rotella CM, Valente WA, et al: Characterization of the optimal stimulatory effects of Graves' monoclonal and serum immunoglobulin G on adenosine 3′,5′-monophosphate production in fRTL-5 thyroid cells: A potential clinical assay. J Clin Endocrinol Metab 57:782–791, 1983.

163. Kasagi K, Konishi J, Iida Y, et al: A sensitive and practical assay for thyroid stimulating antibodies using FRTL-5 thyroid cells. Acta Endocrinol (Copenh) 115:30–36, 1987.

164. Ludgate M, Perret J, Parmentier M, et al: Use of the recombinant human thyrotropin receptor (TSH-R) expressed in mammalian cell lines to assay TSH-R autoantibodies. Mol Cell Endocrinol 73:R13–R18, 1990.

165. Watson PF, Ajjan RA, Phipps J, et al: A new chemiluminescent assay for the rapid detection of thyroid stimulating antibodies in Graves' disease. Clin Endocrinol (Oxf) 49:577–581, 1998.

166. Evans C, Morgenthaler NG, Lee S, et al: Development of a luminescent bioassay for thyroid stimulating antibodies. J Clin Endocrinol Metab 84:374–377, 1999.

167. McKenzie JM: The gamma globulin of Graves' disease: Thyroid stimulation by fraction and fragment. Trans Assoc Am Physicians 78:174–186, 1965.

168. Kriss JP, Pleshakov V, Rosenblum AL, et al: Studies on the pathogenesis of the ophthalmopathy of Graves' disease. J Clin Endocrinol Metab 27:582–593, 1967.

169. Pinchera A, Liberti P, De Santis R, et al: Relationship between the long-acting thyroid stimulator and circulating thyroid antibodies in Graves' disease. J Clin Endocrinol Metab 27:1758–1760, 1967.

170. Vassart G, Dumont JE: The thyrotropin receptor and the regulation of thyrocyte function and growth. Endocr Rev 13:596–611, 1992.

171. Vassart G, Parma J, Van Sande J, Dumont JE: The thyrotropin receptor and the regulation of thyroid function and growth: Update 1994. Endocr Rev Monogr 3:77–115, 1994.

172. Zakarija M, McKenzie JM: Pregnancy-associated changes in thyroid-stimulating antibody of Graves' disease and the relationship to neonatal hyperthyroidism. J Clin Endocrinol Metab 57:1036–1040, 1983.

173. McKenzie JM, Zakarija M: Fetal and neonatal hyperthyroidism and hypothyroidism due to maternal TSH receptor antibodies. Thyroid 2:155–159, 1992.

174. Zakarija M: Immunochemical characterization of the thyroid-stimulating antibody (TSAb) of Graves' disease: Evidence for restricted heterogeneity. J Clin Lab Immunol 10:77–85, 1983.

175. Williams RC: Molecular mimicry and rheumatic fever. Clin Rheum Dis 11:573–590, 1985.

176. Knight J, Laing P, Knight A, et al: Thyroid-stimulating autoantibodies usually contain only lambda-light chains: Evidence for the "forbidden clone" theory. J Clin Endocrinol Metab 62:342–347, 1986.

177. Weetman AP, Yateman ME, Ealey PA, et al: Thyroid-stimulating antibody activity between different immunoglobulin G subclasses. J Clin Invest 86:723–727, 1990.

178. Leovey A, Nagy E, Balazs G, Bako G: Lymphocytes resided in the thyroid are the main source of TSH-receptor antibodies in Basedow's-Graves' disease? Exp Clin Endocrinol 99:147–150, 1992.

179. McLachlan SM, Dickinson AM, Malcolm A, et al: Thyroid autoantibody synthesis by cultures of thyroid and peripheral blood lymphocytes. I: Lymphocyte markers and response to pokeweed mitogen. Isr J Med Sci 52:45–53, 1983.

180. Okuda J, Akamizu T, Sugawa H, et al: Preparation and characterization of monoclonal antithyrotropin receptor antibodies obtained from peripheral lymphocytes of hypothyroid patients with primary myxedema. J Clin Endocrinol Metab 79:1600–1604, 1994.

181. Morgenthaler NG, Kim MR, Tremble J, et al: Human immunoglobulin G autoantibodies to the thyrotropin receptor from Epstein-Barr virus–transformed B lymphocytes: Characterization by immunoprecipitation with recombinant antigen and biological activity. J Clin Endocrinol Metab 81:3155–3161, 1996.

182. Botero D, Brown RS: Bioassay of thyrotropin receptor antibodies with Chinese hamster ovary cells transfected with recombinant human thyrotropin receptor: Clinical utility in children and adolescents with Graves disease. J Pediatr 132:612–618, 1998.

183. Sugenoya A, Kobayashi S, Kasuga Y, et al: Evidence of intrathyroidal accumulation of TSH receptor antibody in Graves' disease. Acta Endocrinol (Copenh) 126:416–418, 1992.

184. Bliddal H, Bech K, Kirkegaard C, et al: Evidence of correlation between thyrotropin receptor binding inhibition and thyroid adenylate cyclase activation by immunoglobulins in Graves' disease before and during long-term antithyroid treatment. Acta Endocrinol 101:35–40, 1982.

185. Aizawa T, Ishihara M, Koizumi Y, et al: Serum thyroglobulin concentration as an indicator for assessing thyroid stimulation in patients with Graves' disease during antithyroid drug therapy. Am J Med 89:175–180, 1990.

186. Pinchera A, Liberti P, Martino E, et al: Effects of antithyroid therapy on the long-acting thyroid stimulator and the antithyroglobulin antibodies. J Clin Endocrinol 29:231–289, 1969.

187. Schleusener H, Finke R, Kotulla P, et al: Determination of thyroid stimulating immunoglobulins (TSI) during the course of Graves' disease. A reliable indicator for remission and persistence of Graves' disease? J Endocrinol Invest 1:155–160, 1978

188. Fenzi GF, Hashizume K, Roudeboush CP, DeGroot LJ: Changes in thyroid-stimulating immunoglobulins during antithyroid therapy. J Clin Endocrinol Metab 48:572–576, 1979.

189. Bliddal H, Kirkegaard C, Siersbaek-Nielsen K, Friis T: Prognostic value of thyrotropin binding inhibiting immunoglobulins (TBII) in long-term antithyroid treatment, 131-I therapy given in combination with carbimazole and in euthyroid ophthalmopathy. Acta Endocrinol 98:364–370, 1981.

190. Weetman AP, McGregor AM, Hall R: Evidence for an effect of antithyroid drugs on the natural history of Graves' disease. Clin Endocrinol 21:163–172, 1984.

191. Romagnani S: Human TH1 and TH2 subsets: Doubt no more. Immunol Today 12:256–257, 1991.

192. Abbas AK, Murphy KM, Sher A: Functional diversity of T lymphocytes. Nature 383:787–793, 1996.

193. Charlton B, Lafferty KJ: The Th1/Th2 balance in autoimmunity. Curr Opin Immunol 7:793–798, 1995.

194. Renno T, Zeine R, Girard JM, et al: Selective enrichment of Th1 CD45RBlow CD4+ T cells in autoimmune infiltrates in experimental allergic encephalomyelitis. Int Immunol 6:347–354, 1994.

195. Rabinovitch A, Suarez PW, Sorensen O, et al: IFN-gamma gene expression in pancreatic islet-infiltrating mononuclear cells correlates with autoimmune diabetes in nonobese diabetic mice. J Immunol 154:4874–4882, 1995.

196. Jackson RA, Haynes BF, Burch WM, et al: Ia+ T cells in new onset Graves' disease. J Clin Endocrinol Metab 59:187–190, 1984.

197. Matsunaga M, Eguchi K, Fukuda T, et al: Class II major histocompatibility complex antigen expression and cellular interactions in thyroid glands of Graves' disease. J Clin Endocrinol Metab 62:723–728, 1986.

198. Zeki K, Fujihira T, Shirakawa F, et al: Existence and immunological significance of circulating Ia+ T cells in autoimmune thyroid diseases. Acta Endocrinol (Copenh) 115:282–288, 1987.

199. McLachlan SM, Pegg CA, Atherton MC, et al: Subpopulations of thyroid autoantibody secreting lymphocytes in Graves' and Hashimoto thyroid glands. Clin Exp Immunol 65:319–328, 1986.

200. Aozasa M, Amino N, Iwatani Y, et al: Separation and analysis of mononuclear cells infiltrating the thyroid of patients with Graves' disease. Clin Immunol Immunopathol 43:343–353, 1987.

201. Mariotti S, del Prete GF, Mastromauro C, et al: The autoimmune infiltrate of Basedow's disease: Analysis of clonal level and comparison with Hashimoto's thyroiditis. Exp Clin Endocrinol 97:139–146, 1991.

202. Martin A, Davies TF: T cells and human autoimmune thyroid disease: Emerging data show lack of need to invoke suppressor T-cell problems. Thyroid 2:247–261, 1992.

203. Ueki Y, Eguchi K, Otsubo T, et al: Phenotypic analyses and concanavalin-A–induced suppressor cell dysfunction of intrathyroidal lymphocytes from patients with Graves' disease. J Clin Endocrinol Metab 67:1018–1024, 1988.

204. Martin A, Goldsmith NK, Friedman EW, et al: Intrathyroidal accumulation of T cell phenotypes in autoimmune thyroid disease. Autoimmunity 6:269–281, 1990.

205. Londei M, Bottazzo GF, Feldmann M: Human T-cell clones from autoimmune thyroid glands: Specific recognition of autologous thyroid cells. Science 228:85–89, 1985.

206. Mackenzie WA, Davies TF: An intrathyroidal T-cell clone specifically cytotoxic for human thyroid cells. Immunology 61:101–103, 1987.

207. Mackenzie WA, Schwartz AE, Friedman EW, Davies TF: Intrathyroidal T cell clones from patients with autoimmune thyroid disease. J Clin Endocrinol Metab 64:818–824, 1987.
208. Fisfalen ME, DeGroot LJ, Quintans J, et al: Microsomal antigen–reactive lymphocyte lines and clones derived from thyroid tissue of patients with Graves' disease. J Clin Endocrinol Metab 66:776–784, 1988.
209. Dayan CM, Londei M, Corcoran AE, et al: Autoantigen recognition by thyroid-infiltrating T cells in Graves' disease. Proc Natl Acad Sci U S A 88:7415–7419, 1991.
210. Watson PF, Pickerill AP, Davies R, Weetman AP: Analysis of cytokine gene expression in Graves' disease and multinodular goiter. J Clin Endocrinol Metab 79:355–360, 1994.
211. Fisfalen ME, Palmer EM, Van Seventer GA, et al: Thyrotropin-receptor and thyroid peroxidase–specific T cell clones and their cytokine profile in autoimmune thyroid disease. J Clin Endocrinol Metab 82:3655–3663, 1997.
212. Weetman AP, Yateman ME, Ealey PA, et al: Thyroid-stimulating antibody activity between different immunoglobulin G subclasses. J Clin Invest 86:723–727, 1990.
213. Davis MM, Bjorkman PJ: T-cell antigen receptor genes and T-cell recognition. Nature 334:395–402, 1988.
214. Weiss A: Structure and function of the T cell antigen receptor. J Clin Invest 86:1015–1022, 1990.
215. Davies TF, Concepcion ES, Ben-Nun A, et al: T-cell receptor V gene use in autoimmune thyroid disease: Direct assessment by thyroid aspiration. J Clin Endocrinol Metab 76:660–666, 1993.
216. Davies TF, Martin A, Concepcion ES, et al: Evidence of limited variability of antigen receptors on intrathyroidal T cells in autoimmune thyroid disease. N Engl J Med 325:238–244, 1991.
217. Tandon N, Freeman MA, Weetman AP: T cell response to synthetic TSH receptor peptides in Graves' disease. Clin Exp Immunol 89:468–473, 1992.
218. Heufelder AE, Wenzel BE, Scriba PC: Antigen receptor variable region repertoires expressed by T cells infiltrating thyroid, retroorbital, and pretibial tissue in Graves' disease. J Clin Endocrinol Metab 81:3733–3739, 1996.
219. Nakashima M, Kong YM, Davies TF: The role of T cells expressing TcR V beta 13 in autoimmune thyroiditis induced by transfer of mouse thyroglobulin-activated lymphocytes: Identification of two common CDR3 motifs. Clin Immunol Immunopathol 80:204–210, 1996.
220. McIntosh RS, Watson PF, Pickerill AP, et al: No restriction of intrathyroidal T cell receptor V alpha families in the thyroid of Graves' disease. Clin Exp Immunol 91:147–152, 1993.
221. Caso-Pelaez E, McGregor AM, Banga JP: A polyclonal T cell repertoire of V-alpha and V-beta T cell receptor gene families in intrathyroidal T lymphocytes of Graves' disease patients. Scand J Immunol 41:141–147, 1995.
222. Martin A, Nakashima M, Zhou A, et al: Detection of major T cell epitopes on human thyroid stimulating hormone receptor by overriding immune heterogeneity in patients with Graves' disease. J Clin Endocrinol Metab 82:3361–3366, 1997.
223. Soliman M, Kaplan E, Guimaraes V, et al: T-cell recognition of residue 158–176 in thyrotropin receptor confers risk for development of thyroid autoimmunity in siblings in a family with Graves' disease. Thyroid 6:545–551, 1996.
224. Bottazzo GF, Todd I, Pujol BR: Hypotheses on genetic contributions to the etiology of diabetes mellitus. Immunol Today 5:230, 1984.
225. Davies TF: Co-culture of human thyroid monolayer cells and autologous T cells: Impact of HLA class II antigen expression. J Clin Endocrinol Metab 61:418–422, 1985.
226. Weetman AP: The potential immunological role of the thyroid cell in autoimmune thyroid disease. Thyroid 4:493–499, 1994.
227. Hanafusa T, Pujol BR, Chiovato L, et al: Aberrant expression of HLA-DR antigen on thyrocytes in Graves' disease: Relevance for autoimmunity. Lancet 2:1111–1115, 1983.
228. Bottazzo GF, Pujol BR, Hanafusa T, Feldmann M: Role of aberrant HLA-DR expression and antigen presentation in induction of endocrine autoimmunity. Lancet 2:1115–1119, 1983.
229. Jansson R, Karlsson A, Forsum U: Intrathyroidal HLA-DR expression and T lymphocyte phenotypes in Graves' thyrotoxicosis, Hashimoto's thyroiditis and nodular colloid goiter. Clin Exp Immunol 58:264–272, 1984.
230. Aichinger G, Fill H, Wick G: In situ immune complexes, lymphocyte subpopulations, and HLA-DR–positive epithelial cells in Hashimoto thyroiditis. Lab Invest 52:132–140, 1985.
231. Roman SH, Martin A, Goldsmith NK, Davies TF: Do CD8+ T cells home to the thyroid gland in Graves' disease (abstract)? *In* Proceedings of the 71st Annual Meeting of the Endocrine Society, Seattle, 1989.
232. Kawakami Y, Kuzuya N, Watanabe T, et al: Induction of experimental thyroiditis in mice by recombinant interferon gamma administration. Acta Endocrinol (Copenh) 122:41–48, 1990.
233. Tang H, Mignon-Godefroy K, Meroni PL, et al: The effects of a monoclonal antibody to interferon-gamma on experimental autoimmune thyroiditis (EAT): Prevention of disease and decrease of EAT-specific T cells. Eur J Immunol 23:275–278, 1993.
234. Alimi E, Huang S, Brazillet MP, Charreire J: Experimental autoimmune thyroiditis (EAT) in mice lacking the IFN-gamma receptor gene. Eur J Immunol 28:201–208, 1998.
235. Voorby HAM, Kabel PJ, De Haan M, et al: Dendritic cells and class II MHC expression on thyrocytes during the autoimmune thyroid disease of the BB rat. Clin Immunol Immunopathol 55:9–22, 1990.
236. Davies TF: The complex role of epithelial cell MHC class II antigen expression in autoimmune thyroid disease. Autoimmunity 8:87–89, 1990.
237. Londei M, Lamb JR, Bottazzo GF, Feldmann M: Epithelial cells expressing aberrant MHC class II determinants can present antigen to cloned human T cells. Nature 312:639–641, 1984.
238. Weetman AP, Volkman DJ, Burman KD, et al: The production and characterization of thyroid-derived T-cell lines in Graves' disease and Hashimoto's thyroiditis. Clin Immunol Immunopathol 39:139–150, 1986.
239. Kimura H, Davies TF: Thyroid-specific T cells in the normal Wistar rat. II: T cell clones interact with cloned Wistar rat thyroid cells and provide direct evidence for autoantigen presentation by thyroid epithelial cells. Clin Immunol Immunopathol 58:195–206, 1991.
240. Eguchi K, Otsubo T, Kawabe K, et al: The remarkable proliferation of helper T cell subset in response to autologous thyrocytes and intrathyroidal T cells from patients with Graves' disease. Isr J Med Sci 70:403–410, 1987.
241. Hutchings P, Rayner DC, Champion BR, et al: High efficiency antigen presentation by thyroglobulin-primed murine spleen B cells. Eur J Immunol 17:393–398, 1987.
242. Kabel PJ, Voorbij HA, De Haan M, et al: Intrathyroidal dendritic cells. J Clin Endocrinol Metab 66:199–207, 1988.
243. Reiser H, Stadecker MJ: Costimulatory B7 molecules in the pathogenesis of infectious and autoimmune diseases. N Engl J Med 335:1369–1377, 1996.
244. Battifora M, Pesce G, Paolieri F, et al: B7.1 costimulatory molecule is expressed on thyroid follicular cells in Hashimoto's thyroiditis, but not in Graves' disease. J Clin Endocrinol Metab 83:4130–4139, 1998.
245. Tandon N, Metcalfe RA, Barnett D, Weetman AP: Expression of the costimulatory molecule B7/BB1 in autoimmune thyroid disease. Q J Med 87:231–236, 1994.
246. Weetman AP, McGregor AM: Autoimmune thyroid disease: Further developments in our understanding. Endocr Rev 15:788–830, 1994.
247. Shimojo N, Kohno Y, Yagamuchi K, et al: Induction of Graves-like disease in mice by immunization with fibroblasts transfected with the thyrotropin receptor and a class II molecule. Proc Natl Acad Sci U S A 93:11074–11079, 1996.
248. Many MC, Costagliola S, Detrait M, et al: Development of an animal model of autoimmune thyroid eye disease. J Immunol 162:4966–4974, 1999.
249. Leznoff A, Sussman GL: Syndrome of idiopathic chronic urticaria and angioedema with thyroid autoimmunity: A study of 90 patients. J Allergy Clin Immunol 84:66–71, 1989.
250. Hegedus L, Heidenheim M, Gervil M, et al: High frequency of thyroid dysfunction in patients with vitiligo. Acta Derm Venereol 74:120–123, 1994.
251. Klein I, Ojamaa K: Thyrotoxicosis and the heart. Endocrinol Metab Clin North Am 27:51–62, 1998.
252. Cavallo A, Joseph CJ, Casta A: Cardiac complications in juvenile hyperthyroidism. Am J Dis Child 138:479–482, 1984.
253. Polikar R, Burger AG, Scherrer U, Nicod P: The thyroid and the heart. Circulation 87:1435–1441, 1993.
254. Shafer RB, Prentiss RA, Bond JH: Gastrointestinal transit in thyroid disease. Gastroenterology 86:852–855, 1984.
255. Thomas FB, Caldwell JH, Greenberger NJ: Steatorrhea in thyrotoxicosis. Relation to hypermotility and excessive dietary fat. Ann Intern Med 78:669–675, 1973.
256. Gurlek A, Cobankara V, Bayraktar M: Liver tests in hyperthyroidism: Effect of antithyroid therapy. J Clin Gastroenterol 24:180–183, 1997.
257. Palacios A, Cohen MA, Cobbs R: Apathetic hyperthyroidism in middle age. Int J Psychiatry Med 21:393–400, 1991.
258. Lazarus A, Jaffe R: Resolution of thyroid-induced schizophreniform disorder following subtotal thyroidectomy: Case report. Gen Hosp Psychiatry 8:29–31, 1986.
259. Feibel JH, Campa JF: Thyrotoxic neuropathy (Basedow's paraplegia). J Neurol Neurosurg Psychiatry 39:491–497, 1976.
260. Pandit L, Shankar SK, Gayathri N, Pandit A: Acute thyrotoxic neuropathy—Basedow's paraplegia revisited. J Neurol Sci 155:211–214, 1998.
261. Ohno M, Hamada N, Yamakawa J, et al: Myasthenia gravis associated with Graves' disease in Japan. Jpn J Med 26:2–6, 1987.
262. Bartley GB: The epidemiologic characteristics and clinical course of ophthalmopathy associated with autoimmune thyroid disease in Olmsted County Minnesota. Trans Am Ophthalmol Soc 92:477–588, 1994.
263. Marino M, Ricciardi R Pinchera A, et al: Mild clinical expression of myasthenia gravis associated with autoimmune thyroid diseases. J Clin Endocrinol Metab 82:438–443, 1997.
264. Marino M, Barbesino G, Manetti L, et al: Mild clinical expression of myasthenia gravis associated with autoimmune thyroid disease (letter). J Clin Endocrinol Metab 82:3905–3906, 1997.
265. Ober KP: Thyrotoxic periodic paralysis in the United States. Report of 7 cases and review of the literature. Medicine (Baltimore) 71:109–120, 1992.
266. Tamai H, Tanaka K, Komaki G, et al: HLA and thyrotoxic periodic paralysis in Japanese patients. J Clin Endocrinol Metab 64:1075–1078, 1987.
267. Coates JT, Mirick MJ, Rubino FJ: Thyrotoxic periodic paralysis with relapse during the euthyroid state. Wis Med J 86:20–22, 1987.
268. Gonzalez-Trevino O, Rosas-Guzman J: Normokalemic thyrotoxic periodic paralysis: A new therapeutic strategy. Thyroid 9:61–63, 1999.
269. Mosekilde L, Eriksen EF, Charles P: Effects of thyroid hormones on bone and mineral metabolism. Endocrinol Metab Clin North Am 19:35–63, 1990.
270. Toh SH, Claunch BC, Brown PH: Effect of hyperthyroidism and its treatment on bone mineral content. Arch Intern Med 145:883–886, 1985.
271. Wakasugi M, Wakao R, Tawata M, et al: Change in bone mineral density in patients with hyperthyroidism after attainment of euthyroidism by dual energy x-ray absorptiometry. Thyroid 4:179–182, 1994.
272. Solomon BL, Wartofsky L, Burman KD: Prevalence of fractures in postmenopausal women with thyroid disease. Thyroid 3:17–23, 1993.
273. Cummings SR, Nevitt MC, Browner WS, et al: Risk factors for hip fracture in white women. Study of Osteoporotic Fractures Research Group. N Engl J Med 332:767–773, 1995.
274. Wejda B, Hintze G, Katschinski B, et al: Hip fractures and the thyroid: A case-control study. J Intern Med 237:241–247, 1995.
275. Franklyn JA, Maisonneuve P, Sheppard MC, et al: Mortality after the treatment of hyperthyroidism with radioactive iodine. N Engl J Med 338:712–718, 1998.
276. Garnero P, Vassy V, Bertholin A, et al: Markers of bone turnover in hyperthyroidism and the effects of treatment. J Clin Endocrinol Metab 78:955–959, 1994.
277. Loviselli A, Mastinu R, Rizzolo E, et al: Circulating telopeptide type I is a peripheral

marker of thyroid hormone action in hyperthyroidism and during levothyroxine suppressive therapy. Thyroid 7:561–566, 1997.

278. Fein HG, Rivlin RS: Anemia in thyroid diseases. Med Clin North Am 59:1133–1145, 1975.
279. Mariotti S, Pisani S, Russova A, et al: A solid phase immunoradiometric assay for gastric parietal cell antibodies. Clin Exp Immunol 58:745–753, 1984.
280. Farid NR, Griffiths BL, Collins JR, et al: Blood coagulation and fibrinolysis in thyroid disease. Thromb Haemost 35:415–422, 1976.
281. Marongiu F, Conti M, Murtas ML, et al: Activation of blood coagulation and fibrinolysis in Graves' disease. Horm Metab Res 23:609–611, 1991.
282. Koutras DA: Disturbances of menstruation in thyroid disease. Ann N Y Acad Sci 816:280–284, 1997.
283. Selby C: Sex hormone binding globulin: Origin, function and clinical significance. Ann Clin Biochem 27:532–541, 1990.
284. Kidd GS, Glass AR, Vigersky RA: The hypothalamic-pituitary-testicular axis in thyrotoxicosis. J Clin Endocrinol Metab 48:798–802, 1979.
285. Chopra IJ, Tulchinsky D: Status of estrogen-androgen balance in hyperthyroid men with Graves' disease. J Clin Endocrinol Metab 38:269–277, 1974.
286. Nolte J, Blumenstein J, Scriba PC: The effect of thyrotoxicosis on the energy providing metabolism. *In* von zur Muhlen A, Schleusener H (eds): Biochemical Basis of Thyroid Stimulation and Thyroid Hormone. Stuttgart, Germany, Thieme, 1976, pp 196–203.
287. Muller MJ, Seitz HJ: Thyroid hormone action on intermediary metabolism. Part I: Respiration, thermogenesis and carbohydrate metabolism. Klin Wochenschr 62:11–18, 1984.
288. Luvisetto S: Hyperthyroidism and mitochondrial uncoupling. Biosci Rep 17:17–21, 1997.
289. Weinstein SP, Watts J, Haber RS: Thyroid hormone increases muscle/fat glucose transporter gene expression in rat skeletal muscle. Endocrinology 129:455–464, 1991.
290. Mouradian M, Abourizk N: Diabetes mellitus and thyroid disease. Diabetes Care 6:512–520, 1983.
291. Boberg J, Dahlberg PA, Vessby B, Lithell H: Serum lipoprotein and apolipoprotein concentrations in patients with hyperthyroidism and the effect of treatment with carbimazole. Acta Med Scand 215:453–459, 1984.
292. Engler H, Riesen WF: Effect of thyroid function on concentrations of lipoprotein(a). Clin Chem 39:2466–2469, 1993.
293. Burch HB, Wartofsky L: Graves' ophthalmopathy: Current concepts regarding pathogenesis and management. Endocr Rev 14:747–793, 1993.
294. Marcocci C, Bartalena L, Bogazzi F, et al: Studies on the occurrence of ophthalmopathy in Graves' disease. Clin Endcocrinol (Oxf) 120:473–478, 1989.
295. Fatourechi V, Pranswav AF: Dermopathy of Graves' disease (pretibial myxedema). Medicine (Baltimore) 73:1–7, 1994.
296. Wortsman J, Dietrich J, Traycoff RB, Stone S: Preradial myxedema in thyroid disease. Arch Dermatol 117:635–638, 1981.
297. Noppakun N, Bancheun K, Chandraprasert S: Unusual locations of localized myxedema in Graves' disease. Report of three cases. Arch Dermatol 122:85–88, 1986.
298. Sisson JC: Hyaluronic acid in localized myxedema. J Clin Endocrinol Metab 28:433–436, 1968.
299. Peacey SR, Flemming L, Messenger A, Weetman AP: Is Graves' dermopathy a generalized disorder? Thyroid 6:41–45, 1996.
300. Weetman AP: Extrathyroidal complications of Graves' disease. Q J Med 86:473–477, 1993.
301. Ishii M, Nakagawa K, Hamada T: An ultrastructural study of pretibial myxedema utilizing improved ruthenium red stain. J Cutan Pathol 11:125–131, 1984.
302. Shishiba Y, Tanaka T, Ozawa Y, et al: Chemical characterization of high buoyant density proteoglycan accumulated in the affected skin of pretibial myxedema of Graves' disease. Endocrinol Jpn 33:395–403, 1986.
303. Cheung HS, Nicoloff JT, Kamiel MB, et al: Stimulation of fibroblast biosynthetic activity by serum of patients with pretibial myxedema. J Invest Dermatol 71:12–17, 1978.
304. Tao TW, Leu SL, Kriss JP: Biological activity of autoantibodies associated with Graves' dermopathy. J Clin Endocrinol Metab 69:90–99, 1989.
305. Metcalfe RA, Davies R, Weetman AP: Analysis of fibroblast-stimulating activity in IgG from patients with Graves' dermopathy. Thyroid 3:207–212, 1993.
306. Shishiba Y, Takeuchi Y, Yokoi N, et al: Thyroid hormone excess stimulates the synthesis of proteoglycan in human skin fibroblasts in culture. Acta Endocrinol (Copenh) 123:541–549, 1990.
307. Heufelder AE, Bahn RS, Scriba PC: Analysis of T-cell antigen receptor variable region gene usage in patients with thyroid-related pretibial dermopathy. J Invest Dermatol 105:372–378, 1995.
308. Chang TC, Wu SL, Hsiao YL, et al: TSH and TSH receptor antibody–binding sites in fibroblasts of pretibial myxedema are related to the extracellular domain of entire TSH receptor. Clin Immunol Immunopathol 71:113–120, 1994.
309. Heufelder AE, Dutton CM, Sarkar G, et al: Detection of TSH receptor RNA in cultured fibroblasts from patients with Graves' ophthalmopathy and pretibial dermopathy. Thyroid 3:297–300, 1993.
310. Stadlmayr W, Spitzweg C, Bichlmair AM, Heufelder AE: TSH receptor transcripts and TSH receptor–like immunoreactivity in orbital and pretibial fibroblasts of patients with Graves' ophthalmopathy and pretibial myxedema. Thyroid 7:3–12, 1997.
311. Heufelder AE: Involvement of the orbital fibroblast and TSH receptor in the pathogenesis of Graves' ophthalmopathy. Thyroid 5:331–340, 1995.
312. Winkler A, Wilson D: Thyroid acropachy. Case report and literature review. Mo Med 82:756–761, 1985.
313. Refetoff S: Inherited thyroxine-binding globulin abnormalities in man. Endocr Rev 10:275–293, 1989.
314. Ekins R: Measurement of free hormones in blood. Endocr Rev 11:5–46, 1990.
315. Singer PA, Cooper DS, Levy E, et al: Treatment guidelines for patients with hyperthyroidism and hypothyroidism. JAMA 273:808–812, 1995.
316. Bartalena L, Bogazzi F, Brogioni S, et al: Measurement of serum free thyroid hormone concentrations: An essential tool for the diagnosis of thyroid dysfunction. Horm Res 45:142–147, 1996.
317. Sterling K, Refetoff S, Selenkow HA: T_3 thyrotoxicosis. Thyrotoxicosis due to elevated serum triiodothyronine levels. JAMA 213:571–575, 1970.
318. Hollander CS, Mitsuma T, Nihei N, et al: Clinical and laboratory observations in cases of triiodothyronine toxicosis confirmed by radioimmunoassay. Lancet 1:609–611, 1972.
319. Mariotti S, Martino E, Cupini C, et al: Low serum thyroglobulin as a clue to the diagnosis of thyrotoxicosis factitia. N Engl J Med 307:410–412, 1982.
320. Mariotti S, Caturegli P, Piccolo P, et al: Antithyroid peroxidase autoantibodies in thyroid diseases. J Clin Endocrinol Metab 71:661–669, 1990.
321. Ericsson UB, Christensen SB, Thorell JI: A high prevalence of thyroglobulin autoantibodies in adults with and without thyroid disease as measured with a sensitive solid-phase immunosorbent radioassay. Clin Immunol Immunopathol 37:154–162, 1985.
322. Mariotti S, Sansoni P, Barbesino G, et al: Thyroid and other organ-specific autoantibodies in healthy centenarians. Lancet 339:1506–1508, 1992.
323. Macchia E, Concetti R, Borgoni F, et al: Assays of TSH-receptor antibodies in 576 patients with various thyroid disorders: Their incidence, significance and clinical usefulness. Autoimmunity 3:103–112, 1989.
324. Pittman JA Jr, Dailey GE 3d, Beschi RJ: Changing normal values for thyroidal radioiodine uptake. N Engl J Med 280:1431–1434, 1969.
325. O'Hare NJ, Murphy D, Malone JF: Thyroid dosimetry of adult European populations. Br J Radiol 71:535–543, 1998.
326. Martino E, Bartalena L, Mariotti S, et al: Radioactive iodine thyroid uptake in patients with amiodarone-iodine–induced thyroid dysfunction. Acta Endocrinol (Copenh) 119:167–173, 1988.
327. Gutekunst R, Hafermann W, Mansky T, Scriba PC: Ultrasonography related to clinical and laboratory findings in lymphocytic thyroiditis. Acta Endocrinol (Copenh) 121:129–135, 1989.
328. Vitti P, Lampis M, Piga M, et al: Diagnostic usefulness of thyroid ultrasonography in atrophic thyroiditis. J Clin Ultrasound 22:375–379, 1994.
329. Vitti P, Martino E, Aghini-Lombardi F, et al: Thyroid volume measurement by ultrasound in children as a tool for the assessment of mild iodine deficiency. J Clin Endocrinol Metab 79:600–603, 1994.
330. Ralls PW, Mayekawa DS, Lee KP, et al: Color-flow Doppler sonography in Graves' disease: "Thyroid inferno." AJR 150:781–784, 1988.
331. Vitti P, Rago T, Mazzeo S, et al: Thyroid blood flow evaluation by color-flow Doppler sonography distinguishes Graves' disease from Hashimoto's thyroiditis. J Endocrinol Invest 18:857–861, 1995.
332. Bogazzi F, Bartalena L, Brogioni S, et al: Color flow Doppler sonography rapidly differentiates type I and type II amiodarone-induced thyrotoxicosis. Thyroid 7:541–545, 1997.
333. Cooper DS: Antithyroid drugs for the treatment of hyperthyroidism caused by Graves' disease. Endocrinol Metab Clin North Am 27:225–247, 1998.
334. Furth ED, Rives K, Becker DV: Nonthyroidal action of propylthiouracil in euthyroid, hypothyroid and hyperthyroid man. J Clin Endocrinol Metab 26:239–246, 1966.
335. Cooper DS, Saxe VC, Meskell M, et al: Acute effects of propylthiouracil (PTU) on thyroidal iodide organification and peripheral iodothyronine deiodination: Correlation with serum PTU levels measured by radioimmunoassay. J Clin Endocrinol Metab 54:101–107, 1982.
336. Okamura K, Ikenoue H, Shiroozu A, et al: Reevaluation of the effects of methylmercaptoimidazole and propylthiouracil in patients with Graves' hyperthyroidism. J Clin Endocrinol Metab 65:719–723, 1987.
337. Reinwein D, Benker G, Lazarus JH, Alexander WD: A prospective randomized trial of antithyroid drug dose in Graves' disease therapy. European Multicenter Study Group on Antithyroid Drug Treatment. J Clin Endocrinol Metab 76:1516–1521, 1993.
338. Hedley AJ, Young RE, Jones SJ, et al: Antithyroid drugs in the treatment of hyperthyroidism of Graves' disease: Long-term follow-up of 434 patients. Scottish Automated Follow-Up Register Group. Clin Endocrinol (Oxf) 31:209–218, 1989.
339. Schleusener H, Schwander J, Fischer C, et al: Prospective multicentre study on the prediction of relapse after antithyroid drug treatment in patients with Graves' disease [published erratum appears in Acta Endocrinol (Copenh) 1989 Aug;121(2):304]. Acta Endocrinol (Copenh) 120:689–701, 1989.
340. Vitti P, Rago T, Chiovato L, et al: Clinical features of patients with Graves' disease undergoing remission after antithyroid drug treatment. Thyroid 7:369–375, 1997.
341. Wartofsky L: Low remission after therapy for Graves disease. Possible relation of dietary iodine with antithyroid therapy results. JAMA 226:1083–1088, 1973.
342. Solomon BL, Evaul JE, Burman KD, Wartofsky L: Remission rates with antithyroid drug therapy: Continuing influence of iodine intake? Ann Intern Med 107:510–512, 1987.
343. Davies TF, Yeo PP, Evered DC, et al: Value of thyroid-stimulating-antibody determinations in predicting short-term thyrotoxic relapse in Graves' disease. Lancet 1:1181–1182, 1977.
344. Eshoj O, Kvetny J, Mogensen EF, et al: Prediction of the course of Graves' disease after medical antithyroid treatment. Acta Med Scand 217:225–228, 1985.
345. Nagataki S: Prediction of relapse in Graves' disease. Ann Acad Med Singapore 15:486–491, 1986.
346. Weetman AP, Ratanachaiyavong S, Middleton GW, et al: Prediction of outcome in Graves' disease after carbimazole treatment. Q J Med 59:409–419, 1986.
347. Wilson R, McKillop JH, Henderson N, et al: The ability of the serum thyrotrophin receptor antibody (TRAb) index and HLA status to predict long-term remission of thyrotoxicosis following medical therapy for Graves' disease. Clin Endocrinol (Oxf) 25:151–156, 1986.
348. Talbot JN, Duron F, Feron R, et al: Thyroglobulin, thyrotropin and thyrotropin binding inhibiting immunoglobulins assayed at the withdrawal of antithyroid drug therapy as predictors of relapse of Graves' disease within one year. J Endocrinol Invest 12:589–595, 1989.

349. Ikenoue H, Okamura K, Sato K, et al: Prediction of relapse in drug-treated Graves' disease using thyroid stimulation indices. Acta Endocrinol (Copenh) 125:643–650, 1991.
350. Lamberg BA, Salmi J, Wagar G, Makinen T: Spontaneous hypothyroidism after antithyroid treatment of hyperthyroid Graves' disease. J Endocrinol Invest 4:399–402, 1981.
351. Feldt-Rasmussen U, Schleusener H, Carayon P: Meta-analysis evaluation of the impact of thyrotropin receptor antibodies on long term remission after medical therapy of Graves' disease. J Clin Endocrinol Metab 78:98–102, 1994.
352. Liaw YF, Huang MJ, Fan KD, et al: Hepatic injury during propylthiouracil therapy in patients with hyperthyroidism. A cohort study. Ann Intern Med 118:424–428, 1993.
353. Romaldini JH, Werner MC, Bromberg N, Werner RS: Adverse effects related to antithyroid drugs and their dose regimen. Exp Clin Endocrinol 97:261–264, 1991.
354. Levy M: Propylthiouracil hepatotoxicity. A review and case presentation. Clin Pediatr (Phila) 32:25–29, 1993.
355. Bartalena L, Bogazzi F, Martino E: Adverse effects of thyroid hormone preparations and antithyroid drugs. Drug Saf 15:53–63, 1996.
356. Davies TF, Yeo PP, Evered DC, et al: Value of thyroid-stimulating-antibody determinations in predicting short-term thyrotoxic relapse in Graves' disease. Lancet 1:1181–1182, 1977.
357. McGregor AM, Petersen MM, McLachlan SM, et al: Carbimazole and the autoimmune response in Graves' disease. N Engl J Med 303:302–304, 1980.
358. Marcocci C, Chiovato L, Mariotti S, Pinchera A: Changes of circulating thyroid autoantibody levels during and after the therapy with methimazole in patients with Graves' disease. J Endocrinol Invest 5:13–19, 1982.
359. Weetman AP, McGregor AP, Hall R: Methimazole inhibits thyroid autoantibody production by an action on accessory cells. Clin Immunol Immunopathol 28:39–45, 1983.
360. Weiss I, Davies TF: Inhibition of immunoglobulin-secreting cells by antithyroid drugs. J Clin Endocrinol Metab 53:1223–1228, 1981.
361. Rennie DP, McGregor AM, Keats D, et al: The influence of methimazole on thyroglobulin-induced autoimmune thyroiditis in the rat. Endocrinology 112:326–330, 1983.
362. Wenzel KW, Lente JR: Similar effects of thionamide drugs and perchlorate on thyroid-stimulating immunoglobulins in Graves' disease: Evidence against an immunosuppressive action of thionamide drugs. J Clin Endocrinol Metab 58:62–69, 1984.
363. Mariotti S, Pinchera A: Role of the immune system in the control of thyroid function. *In* Greer MA (eds): The Thyroid Gland. New York, Raven, 1990, pp 147–218.
364. Hashizume K, Ichikawa K, Sakurai A, et al: Administration of thyroxine in treated Graves' disease—effects on the level of antibodies to thyroid stimulating hormone receptors and on the risk of recurrence of hyperthyroidism. N Engl J Med 324:947–953, 1991.
365. Romaldini JH, Bromberg N, Werner RS, et al: Comparison of effects of high and low dosage regimens of antithyroid drugs in the management of Graves' hyperthyroidism. J Clin Endocrinol Metab 57:563–570, 1983.
366. Weetman AP, Pickerill AP, Watson P, et al: Treatment of Graves' disease with the block-replace regimen of antithyroid drugs: The effect of treatment duration and immunogenetic susceptibility on relapse. Q J Med 87:337–341, 1994.
367. Tamai H, Hayaki I, Kawai K, et al: Lack of effect of thyroxine administration on elevated thyroid stimulating hormone receptor antibody levels in treated Graves' disease patients. J Clin Endocrinol Metab 80:1481–1484, 1995.
368. Rittmaster RS, Zwicker H, Abbott EC, et al: Effect of methimazole with or without exogenous L-thyroxine on serum concentrations of thyrotropin (TSH) receptor antibodies in patients with Graves' disease. J Clin Endocrinol Metab 81:3283–3288, 1996.
369. Rizvi A, Crapo LM: Failure of thyroxine therapy for Graves disease (letter). Ann Intern Med 124:694, 1996.
370. Rittmaster RS, Abbott EC, Douglas R, et al: Effect of methimazole, with or without L-thyroxine, on remission rates in Graves' disease. J Clin Endocrinol Metab 83:814–818, 1998.
371. Emerson CH, Anderson AJ, Howard WJ, Utiger RD: Serum thyroxine and triiodothyronine concentrations during iodide treatment of hyperthyroidism. J Clin Endocrinol Metab 40:33–36, 1975.
372. Marigold JH, Morgan AK, Earle DJ, et al: Lugol's iodine: Its effect on thyroid blood flow in patients with thyrotoxicosis. Br J Surg 72:45–47, 1985.
373. Chang DC, Wheeler MH, Woodcock JP, et al: The effect of preoperative Lugol's iodine on thyroid blood flow in patients with Graves' hyperthyroidism. Surgery 102:1055–1061, 1987.
374. Burgi H, Wimpfheimer C, Burger A, et al: Changes of circulating thyroxine, triiodothyronine and reverse triiodothyronine after radiographic contrast agents. J Clin Endocrinol Metab 43:1203–1210, 1976.
375. Wu SY, Chopra IJ, Solomon DH, Bennett LR: Changes in circulating iodothyronines in euthyroid and hyperthyroid subjects given ipodate (Oragrafin), an agent for oral cholecystography. J Clin Endocrinol Metab 46:691–697, 1978.
376. Costa A: The use of x-ray contrast media in the treatment of hyperthyroidism. J Endocrinol Invest 2:461–462, 1979.
377. Robuschi G, Manfredi A, Salvi M, et al: Effect of sodium ipodate and iodide on free T_4 and free T_3 concentrations in patients with Graves' disease. J Endocrinol Invest 9:287–291, 1986.
378. Laurberg P, Boye N: Inhibitory effect of various radiographic contrast agents on secretion of thyroxine by the dog thyroid and on peripheral and thyroidal deiodination of thyroxine to tri-iodothyronine. J Endocrinol 112:387–390, 1987.
379. Wu SY, Shyh TP, Chopra IJ, et al: Comparison of sodium ipodate (Oragrafin) and propylthiouracil in early treatment of hyperthyroidism. J Clin Endocrinol Metab 54:630–634, 1982.
380. Shen DC, Wu SY, Chopra IJ, et al: Long term treatment of Graves' hyperthyroidism with sodium ipodate. J Clin Endocrinol Metab 61:723–727, 1985.
381. Martino E, Balzano S, Bartalena L, et al: Therapy of Graves' disease with sodium ipodate is associated with a high recurrence rate of hyperthyroidism. J Endocrinol Invest 14:847–851, 1991.
382. DeGroot LJ, Buhler U: Effect of perchlorate and methimazole on iodine metabolism. Acta Endocrinol (Copenh) 68:696–706, 1971.
383. Barzilai D, Sheinfeld M: Fatal complications following use of potassium perchlorate in thyrotoxicosis. Report of two cases and a review of the literature. Isr J Med Sci 2:453–456, 1966.
384. Bartalena L, Brogioni S, Grasso L, et al: Treatment of amiodarone-induced thyrotoxicosis, a difficult challenge: Results of a prospective study. J Clin Endocrinol Metab 81:2930–2933, 1996.
385. Pimstone BL: Beta-adrenergic blockade in thyrotoxicosis. S Afr Med J 43(suppl):27–30, 1969.
386. Wiener L, Stout BD, Cox JW: Influence of beta sympathetic blockade (propranolol) on the hemodynamics of hyperthyroidism. Am J Med 46:227–233, 1969.
387. Henderson JM, Portmann L, Van Melle G, et al: Propranolol as an adjunct therapy for hyperthyroid tremor. Eur Neurol 37:182–185, 1997.
388. Wiersinga WM: Propranolol and thyroid hormone metabolism. Thyroid 1:273–277, 1991.
389. Dobyns BM, Vickery AL, Maloof F, Chapman EM: Functional and histologic effects of therapeutic doses of radioiodine therapy for hyperthyroidism. J Clin Endcrinol Metab 13:548, 1953.
390. Beierwaltes WH: The treatment of hyperthyroidism with iodine-131. Semin Nucl Med 8:95–103, 1978.
391. Franklyn JA, Daykin J, Drolc Z, et al: Long-term follow-up of treatment of thyrotoxicosis by three different methods. Clin Endocrinol (Oxf) 34:71–76, 1991.
392. Bartalena L, Marcocci C, Bogazzi F, et al: Relation between therapy for hyperthyroidism and the course of Graves' ophthalmopathy. N Engl J Med 338:73–78, 1998.
393. Burch HB, Solomon BL, Wartofsky L, Burman KD: Discontinuing antithyroid drug therapy before ablation with radioiodine in Graves' disease. Ann Intern Med 121:553–559, 1994.
394. Block MA, Miller MJ, Horn RC Jr: Carcinoma of the thyroid after external radiation to the neck in adults. Am J Surg 118:764–769, 1969.
395. Ron E, Saftlas AF: Head and neck radiation carcinogenesis: Epidemiologic evidence. Otolaryngol Head Neck Surg 115:403–408, 1996.
396. Hall P, Holm LE: Late consequences of radioiodine for diagnosis and therapy in Sweden. Thyroid 7:205–208, 1997.
397. Ron E, Doody MM, Becker DV, et al: Cancer mortality following treatment for adult hyperthyroidism. Cooperative Thyrotoxicosis Therapy Follow-up Study Group. JAMA 280:347–355, 1998.
398. Graham GD, Burman KD: Radioiodine treatment of Graves' disease. An assessment of its potential risks. Ann Intern Med 105:900–905, 1986.
399. Hennemann G, Krenning EP, Sankaranarayanan K: Place of radioactive iodine in treatment of thyrotoxicosis. Lancet 1:1369–1372, 1986.
400. Baverstock K, Egloff B, Pinchera A, et al: Thyroid cancer after Chernobyl. Nature 359:21–22, 1992.
401. Baverstock KF: Thyroid cancer in children in Belarus after Chernobyl. World Health Stat Q 46:204–208, 1993.
402. Pacini F, Vorontsova T, Demidchik EP, et al: Post-Chernobyl thyroid carcinoma in Belarus children and adolescents: Comparison with naturally occurring thyroid carcinoma in Italy and France. J Clin Endocrinol Metab 82:3563–3569, 1997.
403. Cusick EL, Krukowski ZH, Matheson NA: Outcome of surgery for Graves' disease re-examined. Br J Surg 74:780–783, 1987.
404. Miccoli P, Vitti P, Rago T, et al: Surgical treatment of Graves' disease: Subtotal or total thyroidectomy? Surgery 120:1020–1025, 1996.
405. Kasuga Y, Sugenoya A, Kobayashi S, et al: Clinical evaluation of the response to surgical treatment of Graves' disease. Surg Gynecol Obstet 170:327–330, 1990.
406. Baeza A, Aguayo J, Barria M, Pineda G: Rapid preoperative preparation in hyperthyroidism. Clin Endocrinol (Oxf) 35:439–442, 1991.
407. Tomaski SM, Mahoney EM, Burgess LP, et al: Sodium ipodate (Oragrafin) in the preoperative preparation of Graves' hyperthyroidism. Laryngoscope 107:1066–1070, 1997.
408. Max MH, Scherm M, Bland KI: Early and late complications after thyroid operations. South Med J 76:977–980, 1983.
409. Kasemsuwan L, Nubthuenetr S: Recurrent laryngeal nerve paralysis: A complication of thyroidectomy. J Otolaryngol 26:365–367, 1997.
410. Pattou F, Combemale F, Fabre S, et al: Hypocalcemia following thyroid surgery: Incidence and prediction of outcome. World J Surg 22:718–724, 1998.
411. Sosa JA, Bowman HM, Tielsch JM, et al: The importance of surgeon experience for clinical and economic outcomes from thyroidectomy. Ann Surg 228:320–330, 1998.
412. Sugino K, Mimura T, Toshima K, et al: Follow-up evaluation of patients with Graves' disease treated by subtotal thyroidectomy and risk factor analysis for post-operative thyroid dysfunction. J Endocrinol Invest 16:195–199, 1993.
413. Glinoer D, Hesch D, Lagasse R, Laurberg P: The management of hyperthyroidism due to Graves' disease in Europe in 1986. Results of an international survey. Acta Endocrinol Suppl 285:3–23, 1987.
414. Wartofsky L, Glinoer D, Solomon B, Lagasse R: Differences and similarities in the treatment of diffuse goiter in Europe and the United States. Exp Clin Endocrinol 97:243–251, 1991.
415. Freitas JE, Swanson DP, Gross MD, Sisson JC: Iodine-131: Optimal therapy for hyperthyroidism in children and adolescents? J Nucl Med 20:847–850, 1979.
416. Rivkees SA, Sklar C, Freemark M: Clinical review 99: The management of Graves' disease in children, with special emphasis on radioiodine treatment. J Clin Endocrinol Metab 83:3767–3776, 1998.
417. Waldhausen JH: Controversies related to the medical and surgical management of hyperthyroidism in children. Semin Pediatr Surg 6:121–127, 1997.
418. Witte J, Goretzki PE, Roher HD: Surgery for Graves' disease in childhood and adolescence. Exp Clin Endocrinol Diabetes 105:58–60, 1997.
419. Lazarus JH: Guidelines for the use of radioiodine in the management of hyperthyroid-

ism: A summary. Prepared by the Radioiodine Audit Subcommittee of the Royal College of Physicians Committee on Diabetes and Endocrinology, and the Research Unit of the Royal College of Physicians. J R Coll Physicians Lond 29:464–469, 1995.

420. Weetman AP, Wiersinga WM: Current management of thyroid-associated ophthalmopathy in Europe. Results of an international survey. Clin Endocrinol (Oxf) 49:21–28, 1998.
421. Wiersinga WM: Preventing Graves' ophthalmopathy. N Engl J Med 338:121–122, 1998.
422. Millar LK, Wing DA, Leung AS, et al: Low birth weight and preeclampsia in pregnancies complicated by hyperthyroidism. Obstet Gynecol 84:946–949, 1994.
423. Momotani N, Ito K, Hamada N, et al: Maternal hyperthyroidism and congenital malformation in the offspring. Clin Endocrinol (Oxf) 20:695–700, 1984.
424. Gittoes NJ, Franklyn JA: Hyperthyroidism. Current treatment guidelines. Drugs 55:543–553, 1998.
425. Marchant B, Brownlie BE, Hart DM, et al: The placental transfer of propylthiouracil, methimazole and carbimazole. J Clin Endocrinol Metab 45:1187–1193, 1977.
426. Refetoff S, Ochi Y, Selenkow HA, Rosenfield RL: Neonatal hypothyroidism and goiter in one infant of each of two sets of twins due to maternal therapy with antithyroid drugs. J Pediatr 85:240–244, 1974.
427. Cheron RG, Kaplan MM, Larsen PR, et al: Neonatal thyroid function after propylthiouracil therapy for maternal Graves' disease. N Engl J Med 304:525–528, 1981.
428. Wing DA, Millar LK, Koonings PP, et al: A comparison of propylthiouracil versus methimazole in the treatment of hyperthyroidism in pregnancy. Am J Obstet Gynecol 170:90–95, 1994.
429. Mandel SJ, Brent GA, Larsen PR: Review of antithyroid drug use during pregnancy and report of a case of aplasia cutis. Thyroid 4:129–133, 1994.
430. Stagnaro GA: Pregnancy and thyroid disease. Immunol Allergy Clin North Am 14:865–878, 1994.
431. Johansen K, Andersen AN, Kampmann JP, et al: Excretion of methimazole in human milk. Eur J Clin Pharmacol 23:339–341, 1982.
432. Kampmann JP, Johansen K, Hansen JM, Helweg J: Propylthiouracil in human milk. Revision of a dogma. Lancet 1:736–737, 1980.
433. Lamberg BA, Ikonen E, Osterlund K, et al: Antithyroid treatment of maternal hyperthyroidism during lactation. Clin Endocrinol (Oxf) 21:81–87, 1984.
434. Polak M: Hyperthyroidism in early infancy: Pathogenesis, clinical features and diagnosis with a focus on neonatal hyperthyroidism. Thyroid 8:1171–1177, 1998.
435. Tamaki H, Amino N, Takeoka K, et al: Prediction of later development of thyrotoxicosis or central hypothyroidism from the cord serum thyroid-stimulating hormone level in neonates born to mothers with Graves' disease. J Pediatr 115:318–321, 1989.
436. Zimmerman D: Fetal and neonatal hyperthyroidism. Thyroid 9:727–733, 1999.
437. Polak M, Leger J, Luton D, et al: Fetal cord blood sampling in the diagnosis and the treatment of fetal hyperthyroidism in the offsprings of a euthyroid mother, producing thyroid stimulating immunoglobulins. Ann Endocrinol 58:338–342, 1997.
438. Masiukiewicz US, Burrow GN: Hyperthyroidism in pregnancy: Diagnosis and treatment. Thyroid 9:647–652, 1999.
439. Trivalle C, Doucet J, Chassagne P, et al: Differences in the signs and symptoms of hyperthyroidism in older and younger patients. J Am Geriatr Soc 44:50–53, 1996.
440. Martin FI, Deam DR: Hyperthyroidism in elderly hospitalised patients. Clinical features and treatment outcomes. Med J Aust 164:200–203, 1996.
441. Perros P, Crombie AL, Matthews JN, Kendall TP: Age and gender influence the severity of thyroid-associated ophthalmopathy: A study of 101 patients attending a combined thyroid-eye clinic. Clin Endocrinol (Oxf) 38:367–372, 1993.
442. Kriss JP, Pleshakov V, Rosenblum A, Sharp G: Therapy with occlusive dressings of pretibial myxedema with fluocinolone acetonide. J Clin Endocrinol Metab 27:595–604, 1967.
443. Lang PG, Sisson JC, Lynch PJ: Intralesional triamcinolone therapy for pretibial myxedema. Arch Dermatol 111:197–202, 1975.
444. Derrick EK, Tanner B, Price ML: Successful surgical treatment of severe pretibial myxoedema. Br J Dermatol 133:317–318, 1995.
445. Pingsmann A, Ockenfels HM, Patsalis T: Surgical excision of pseudotumorous pretibial myxedema. Foot Ankle Int 17:107–110, 1996.
446. Noppen M, Velkeniers B, Steenssens L, Vanhaelst L: Beneficial effects of plasmapheresis followed by immunosuppressive therapy in pretibial myxedema. Acta Clin Belg 43:381–383, 1988.
447. Koshiyama H, Mori S, Fujiwara K, et al: Successful treatment of hypothyroid Graves' disease with a combination of levothyroxine replacement, intravenous high-dose steroid and irradiation to the orbit. Intern Med 32:421–423, 1993.
448. Tietgens ST, Leinung MC: Thyroid storm. Med Clin North Am 79:169–184, 1995.
449. Wartofsky L: Treatment options for hyperthyroidism. Hosp Pract 31:69–73, 76–78, 81–84, 1996.

Chapter 101

Ophthalmopathy

Henry B. Burch ▪ Colum A. Gorman ▪ George B. Bartley

Graves' ophthalmopathy occurs as a spectrum of disease ranging from subclinical enlargement of the extraocular muscles in most patients to disfiguring and vision-threatening involvement of the entire orbit in an unfortunate few. Although the diagnosis of ophthalmopathy in patients with Graves' disease may precede, accompany, or follow that of hyperthyroidism, eye involvement is generally diagnosed concurrently or after the diagnosis of thyrotoxicosis[1–5] (Fig. 101–1A and B).

The link between the thyroid and the eye in Graves' disease has been challenged on the basis of the existence of patients with euthyroid ophthalmopathy or unilateral eye disease and a poor numerical correlation between thyroid-stimulating antibody levels and the presence of eye disease. However, these arguments have been superseded by the demonstration of subtle thyroid abnormalities in most "euthyroid" ophthalmopathy patients,[6, 7] the finding of contralateral eye muscle abnormality in most patients with apparent unilateral disease,[1] and the demonstration of a definite qualitative association between the severity of ophthalmopathy and other peripheral manifestations of Graves' disease and thyroid-stimulating antibody titers.[8, 9]

Studies investigating the pathogenesis of Graves' ophthalmopathy have served to expand the understanding of ophthalmopathy beyond a purely mechanical description.[10] These efforts have focused on the identification of orbital cells actively participating in the retrobulbar immune response, elucidation of immune mechanisms responsible for the activation of these cells, and attempts to demonstrate expression of autoantigenic target proteins within the orbit, such as the thyrotropin (thyroid-stimulating hormone [TSH]) receptor. Despite this progress, a number of important limitations remain in the understanding of these processes.

Management of Graves' ophthalmopathy requires a carefully integrated approach involving the endocrinologist and ophthalmologist, with the goal of preserving the patient's vision and restoring favorable self-perception and quality of life.[11] In this chapter we provide an examination of the present state of knowledge regarding the pathogenesis of Graves' ophthalmopathy and an up-to-date review of current methods in the diagnosis and management of this disorder.

EPIDEMIOLOGY

Clinically evident ophthalmopathy occurs in 10% to 25% of unselected patients with Graves' disease if lid signs are excluded, in 30% to 45% if lid signs are included,[1, 12] and in approximately 70% of patients without overt eye disease if computed tomography (CT) or increased intraocular pressure on upgaze is used to establish the diagnosis.[13–16] Magnetic resonance imaging (MRI) was recently shown to disclose extraocular muscle enlargement in 71% of patients without overt findings on physical examination.[17] Fortunately, less than 5% of patients with Graves' disease have severe ophthalmopathy.[18] The age-adjusted incidence of Graves' ophthalmopathy in the population of Olmsted County, Minnesota, was found to be 16 cases per 100,000 population per year for women and 2.9 for men.[19] A bimodal distribution was noted, with peak incidence in the age groups 40 to 44 and 60 to 64 years in women and 45 to 49 and 65 to 69 years in men. Additional peripheral manifestations of Graves' disease such as dermopathy and acropachy occur with lower frequency. Thyroid dermopathy is found in 4% to 15% of patients with Graves' ophthalmopathy, and 7% of dermopathy patients will also have thyroid acropachy.[4]

PATHOGENESIS

Mechanical Factors

The bones of the orbit are unyielding in response to increases in intraorbital tissue bulk, with only forward displacement left as a natural means of orbital decompression. After varying degrees of proptosis, forward displacement is itself limited by the orbital septum and tethering action of the extraocular muscles on the globe. Cadaveric studies have shown that a 1.0-mm increase in proptosis occurs with every 0.67-mL increase in orbital volume. In this model, 6 mm of proptosis was observed after as little as a 4-mL increase in orbital contents.[10] CT studies have shown that the mean volume of extraocular muscle increases by as much as 81% and the mean volume of fat and connective tissue increases by as much as 22% in patients with ophthalmopathy.[13] Therefore, considerable increases in orbital pressure and proptosis are anticipated under these circumstances.

Predisposing Influences

Genetic Influence

Genetic predisposition to Graves' hyperthyroidism and ophthalmopathy, although extensively studied, remains poorly characterized. Graves' disease has been associated with HLA-DR3 and HLA-B8 in whites; the correlation is weak, however, with HLA-DR3 positivity conferring a relative disease risk of only 2.1 to 5.7.[1] Ethnic variability is characteristic of this association, with HLA-DRw6 positivity found with increased prevalence in blacks with Graves' disease,[20] HLA-Bw46 in the Chinese, and HLA-B35 in the Japanese.[21] Inconsistent susceptibility patterns have been found between HLA loci and Graves' ophthalmopathy.[21–25] A recent study found that European patients have a 6.4-fold higher risk of eye disease developing than do Asians living in the same region.[26] Molecular analysis of the DPβ2.1/8 locus identified a significantly reduced occurrence of this allele in patients with Graves' ophthalmopathy when compared with those without eye disease and a group of normal controls.[27] Additional minor genetic associations between Graves' ophthalmopathy and non-HLA gene

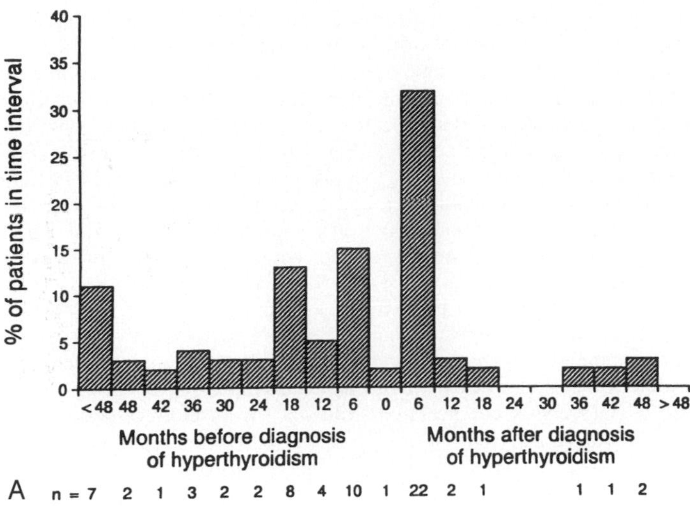

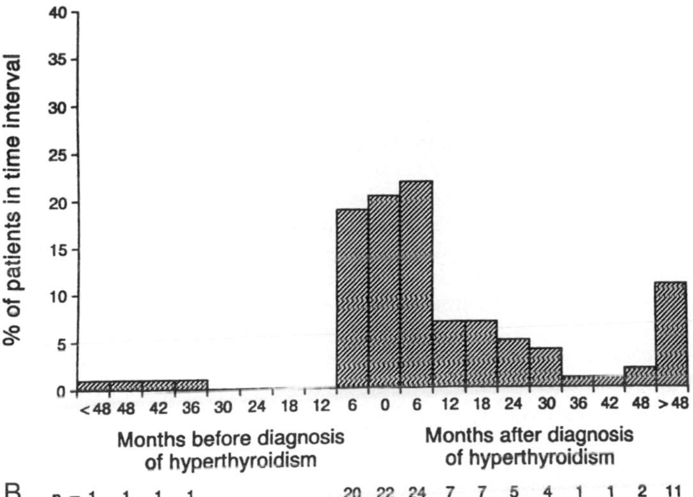

FIGURE 101-1. Onset of eye symptoms and diagnosis of Graves' ophthalmopathy relative to the time of diagnosis of hyperthyroidism (0 on the horizontal axis). *A,* The number of patients who first experienced eye symptoms within a given 6-month period is expressed as a percentage of the entire group. *B,* Number of patients in whom Graves' ophthalmopathy was first diagnosed within a given 6-month period. (From Bartley GB, Fatourechi V, Kadrmas EF, et al: The chronology of Graves' ophthalmopathy in an incidence cohort. Am J Ophthalmol 121:426–434, 1996. Published with permission from the American Journal of Ophthalmology. Copyright by the Ophthalmic Publishing Company.)

products have been found, including immunoglobulin heavy chain markers[28] and blood group antigens,[29] which further illustrates the complexity of the polygenic influences on this disorder. Other new genetic associations with Graves' disease were uninformative with respect to the presence of ophthalmopathy.[30, 31] The concordance rate of only 22% for the development of Graves' disease in identical twins underscores the importance of nongenetic influences in the pathogenesis of this disorder.[32, 33]

Tobacco Smoking

A striking association between cigarette smoking and Graves' ophthalmopathy has been noted in several studies. One group of researchers found that current smokers or ex-smokers represented 64% of patients with Graves' disease and ophthalmopathy as compared with 47.9% of those without overt ophthalmopathy, 23.6% of patients with toxic nodular goiter, 30.4% of individuals with nontoxic goiter, 33.5% of patients with Hashimoto's thyroiditis, and 27.8% of normal controls[34] (Fig. 101–2). These effects do not appear to be related to behavioral changes associated with thyrotoxicosis, nor do they seem to be due to differences in the age, gender, or educational background of the study patients and their controls.[35] Although the mechanisms underlying this association remain unknown, smokers have larger thyroids and higher thyroglobulin levels than nonsmokers do, which suggests that thyroid damage may be involved. Other contributors may include the effect of orbital hypoxia[36] or the action of free radicals contained in tobacco smoke on orbital fibroblast proliferation.[37] Smokers have lower levels of interleukin-1 receptor antagonists than nonsmokers do,[38] which could lead to enhanced negative effects of interleukin-1 on the orbital inflammatory process.[39] Finally, smokers in one study were more likely to experience aggravation of ophthalmopathy after radioiodine therapy than nonsmokers were.[40] The strong association between smoking and ophthalmopathy may provide important clues to the pathogenesis of this disorder in at least a subset of patients.

Age and Gender

Patient age and gender may also affect the prevalence and severity of Graves' ophthalmopathy. Female-to-male ratios in series of ophthalmopathy patients have ranged from 1.8:1 to 2.8:1, which is considerably lower than the ratio of 8:1 generally cited for Graves' disease in general.[41] Men also appear to be disproportionately represented among patients with severe ophthalmopathy. One study found a female-to-male ratio of 9.3:1 in patients with mild disease, 3.2:1 in patients with moderate disease, and 1.4:1 in patients with severe ophthalmopathy.[42]

Therapy for Thyrotoxicosis

An area of considerable controversy concerns the impact of the choice of therapy for hyperthyroidism on the subsequent course of ophthalmopathy in Graves' disease.[43–46] Until recently, only retrospective studies had examined this issue, often with conflicting results (reviewed by Burch and Wartofsky[1]). Prospective trials have now focused on this area.[47–51] Two recent studies allow a direct comparison between the effects of radioiodine and either thyroidectomy or antithyroid drug therapy alone.[48, 51] In the first of these studies, 114 patients aged 35 to 55 years were randomized to receive radioiodine, thyroidectomy, or methimazole alone.[48] As assessed with an ophthalmopathy index, new or worsened eye involvement occurred in 10% of patients treated medically, 16% of those treated surgically, and 33% of those treated with ^{131}I. Interpretation of this small study was hampered by a higher prevalence of cigarette smokers in the radioiodine-treated pa-

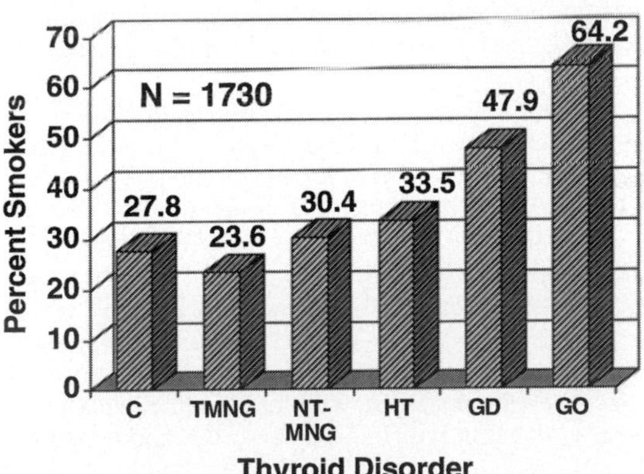

FIGURE 101–2. The prevalence of past and present cigarette smokers among patients with various thyroid disorders. Percentages shown (on the vertical axis) represent the prevalence of cigarette smokers in the group. Normal controls (NC), toxic nodular goiter (TG), nontoxic goiter (NTG), Hashimoto's thyroiditis (HT), Graves' disease without eye involvement (GD), and Graves' disease with ophthalmopathy (GO) are shown. Smokers represented significantly increased proportions among patients with diagnoses of Graves' disease and Graves' ophthalmopathy. (From Burch HB, Wartofsky L: Graves' ophthalmopathy: Current concepts regarding pathogenesis and management. Endocr Rev 14:747–793, © 1993, The Endocrine Society.)

tients, a period of hypothyroidism before starting thyroid hormone therapy in patients treated with radioiodine, and a requirement for multiple doses of radioiodine in nearly half the patients receiving this therapy, which suggests both refractory disease and a mechanism by which repeated release of thyroid antigen may have contributed to the autoimmune response.[1, 52] However, these authors later showed that elevated TSH levels after ^{131}I treatment did not correlate with worsening eye status[53, 54] and that eye changes in smokers were no more frequent than eye changes in nonsmokers. Finally, the authors noted that most patients receiving multiple doses of ^{131}I had worsening of eye status before the second dose of radioiodine was given.[55]

Another recent randomized trial compared eye changes in 150 patients treated with radioiodine, 148 patients receiving methimazole alone, and a third group of 145 patients receiving both radioiodine and prophylactic prednisone.[51] Patients were monitored for 1 year and assessed for change by largely objective criteria, as well as an activity score and patient self-assessment. The groups were similar with regard to percentages of smokers or patients with preexisting ophthalmopathy. Hypothyroidism or persistent hyperthyroidism was corrected within 2 to 3 weeks of testing performed every 1 to 2 months. Worsening of eye disease occurred within 6 months after radioiodine therapy in 15% of patients vs. 2.7% of patients receiving antithyroid drugs alone. Seventy-four percent of patients experiencing worsening eye status after radioiodine therapy had preexisting ophthalmopathy. The eye changes that occurred were largely mild and returned to baseline within 2 to 3 months in 65% of cases. However, 8 patients (5%) in the radioiodine group required orbital radiation or high-dose corticosteroids as compared with 1 patient in the methimazole group and no patients in the combined prednisone and radioiodine group. Patients who had preexisting ophthalmopathy and those who were smokers were more likely to have progression after radioiodine administration.

Is this issue settled? The statistical methods used in the latter study have been challenged,[56] and although the authors followed largely objective measurement, it was possible to qualify for worsening of disease by subjective criteria alone. Furthermore, one might question whether it is possible to fully mask a skilled observer to the rapid effects of radioiodine on a patient's goiter size or the severity of thyrotoxicosis. Are alternate explanations for these results possible? A beneficial effect of antithyroid drugs[57] rather than harmful effects of radioiodine might yield similar findings.[58] Despite the continuing controversy, these studies appear to have influenced management practices in patients with Graves' hyperthyroidism and overt eye involvement. A recent survey of members of the European Thyroid Association revealed that 60% of respondents believed that their choice of therapy would be influenced by the presence of ophthalmopathy, two-thirds of whom would avoid radioiodine in the presence of severe eye disease.[59] However, many members of this organization would not chose radioiodine as the first therapy even in the absence of eye disease.[60]

A cautious interpretation of the two controlled studies in this area is that patients with Graves' disease treated with radioiodine therapy may have a slightly increased risk for worsening eye status in comparison to those treated with antithyroid drugs alone. These effects are generally mild and reversible. Patients with preexisting eye disease or those who smoke or have severe thyrotoxicosis may be more likely to experience this complication, but concurrent use of corticosteroids appears to negate this risk.[61, 62] The authors use an approach tailored to the individual patient. Thyrotoxicosis in patients with mild ophthalmopathy is generally managed with radioiodine without concurrent corticosteroids. Patients with more severe ophthalmopathy are managed with antithyroid drugs alone or the combined use of radioiodine and corticosteroids. Near-total thyroidectomy is occasionally the treatment of choice, such as in a patient who is allergic to thionamides and has progressive ophthalmopathy. Thyroidectomy and total thyroid ablation share the theoretic advantage of removing thyroid antigen, such as the TSH receptor, which might otherwise bolster the autoimmune response.[43]

The Retrobulbar Autoimmune Response

The retrobulbar autoimmune response can be dissected into contributions from constituent cells of the inflamed orbit, including extraocular myocytes, connective tissue (fibroblasts, adipocytes, and intercellular matrix), and "professional" immune effector cells and their products.[1, 63] Histologic analysis has revealed largely intact muscle fibers, an expanded extracellular compartment, and infiltration by macrophages, activated T lymphocytes and to a lesser extent B lymphocytes, and natural killer cells[64, 65] (Fig. 101–3). Further characterization of the activated retro-ocular T lymphocytes reveals increases in both $CD4^+$ and $CD8^+$ lymphocytes and restriction in the T cell receptor repertoire.[66] T cell phenotyping has shown both Th1[67] and Th2[68] profiles for cytokine gene expression, without a clear preponderance of either phenotype in recent studies.[69, 70] Expansion of the connective tissue compartment can be ascribed to a proliferation of retro-ocular fibroblasts and an attendant increase in the secretion of hydrophilic glycosaminoglycans by these cells. The resultant edema leads to retro-ocular tissue expansion, which causes forward displacement of the globe and venous compression, followed by orbital congestion and further edema.

Orbital Immune Targets

Although extraocular muscle enlargement and subsequent fibrosis occupy a central role in the mechanics of Graves' ophthalmopathy, the retro-ocular fibroblast and the embryologically related preadipocyte may have a greater role in the molecular events contributing to orbital autoimmunity. Retro-ocular $CD8^+$ T cells proliferate in response to autologous retro-ocular fibroblasts but not eye muscle extracts, which suggests that fibroblasts may contain antigenic targets for activated T lymphocytes.[71] Similar results were recently found with the use of retro-ocular $CD4^+$ T cells against autologous orbital fibroblast protein.[72] Retro-ocular fibroblasts respond to various cytokines with proliferation, release of glycosaminoglycan, and expression of several immunomodulatory proteins, including HLA class II molecules (Fig. 101–4), lymphocyte adhesion molecules such as intercellular adhesion molecule-1 (Fig. 101–5), and heat shock proteins.[1, 63, 64] Orbital fibroblasts also appear to have unique characteristics and responses to cytokines that facilitate their participation in the autoimmune response, as opposed to fibroblasts derived from other sources.[36, 73–75]

Coexpression of thyroid autoantigen in the retro-ocular tissue has received considerable attention in studies investigating the pathogenesis of Graves' ophthalmopathy. Studies of this sort have difficulty distinguishing a secondary immune response against previously sequestered antigens released during tissue damage from a primary autoimmune response. It is now generally believed that antibodies against such retro-ocular proteins as the 64-kDa extraocular muscle protein,[76] protein 1D,[77] and the 23-kDa fibroblast protein[78] are secondary phenomena.

Because the autoimmune response against the thyrotropin receptor (hTSH-R) is responsible for the hyperthyroidism of Graves' disease, a

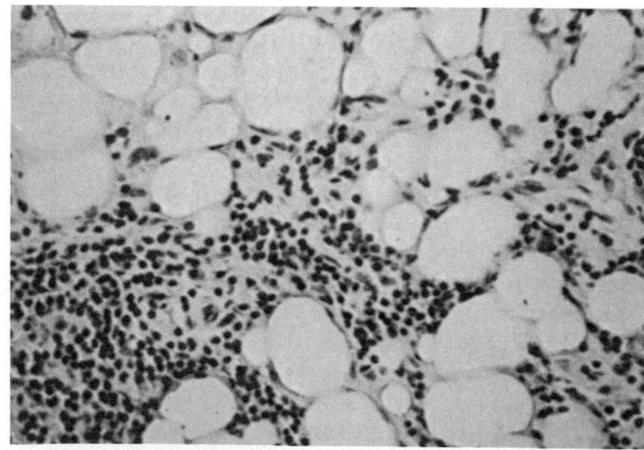

FIGURE 101–3. Hematoxylin-eosin–stained, formalin-fixed retro-ocular connective tissue (obtained from a patient with severe Graves' ophthalmopathy during orbital decompression surgery). Mononuclear cell infiltration is present throughout the retro-ocular connective tissue (×160).

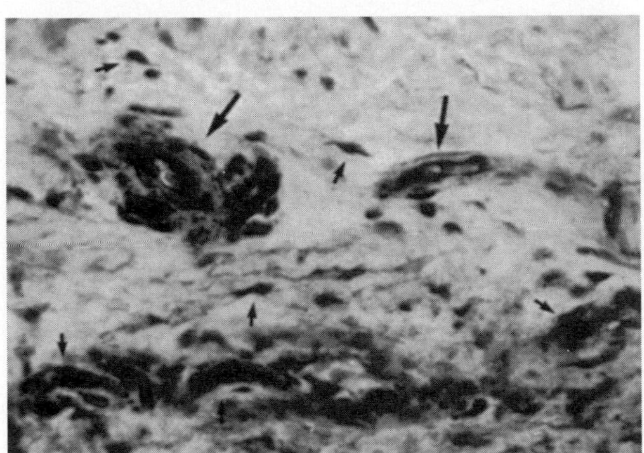

FIGURE 101–4. Immunoperoxidase staining of a cryostat section of retro-ocular connective tissue (obtained from a patient with severe Graves' ophthalmopathy during orbital decompression). A monoclonal antibody directed against the HLA-DR antigen was used. Strong HLA-DR immunoreactivity is present throughout the retro-ocular connective tissue and is detected in blood vessels and perivascular areas *(large arrows)*, as well as in connective tissue cells *(small arrows)* and their surrounding extracellular matrix (×320).

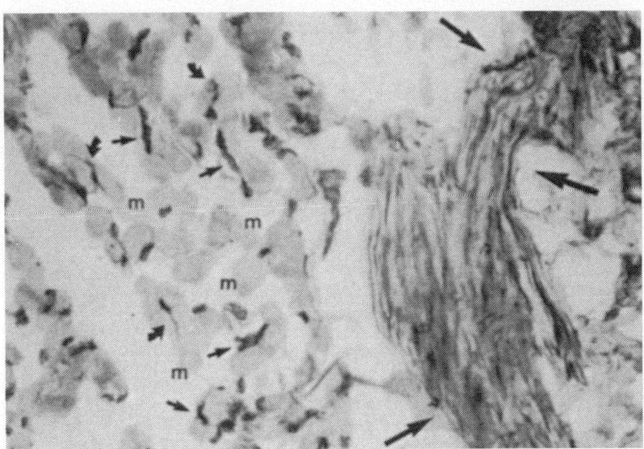

FIGURE 101–5. Immunoperoxidase staining of a cryostat section through the belly of the inferior rectus muscle derived at autopsy from a patient with severe Graves' ophthalmopathy. A monoclonal antibody directed against intercellular adhesion molecule-1 (ICAM-1) was used. ICAM-1 immunoreactivity is detected in cells residing in the retro-ocular connective tissue *(large arrows)*, in the extraocular muscle interstitium *(straight small arrows)*, and in the perimysial connective tissue *(curved small arrows)* surrounding extraocular muscle fibers (m). No ICAM-1 immunoreactivity is detected in extraocular muscle tissue itself (×160).

number of studies have examined retro-ocular tissue for expression of the TSH-R or antigenically related proteins. Although this matter remains to be settled, most studies show at least a low level of TSH-R gene expression in retro-ocular fibroblasts,[79, 80] preadipocytes,[81] or retro-orbital fat[82] and a suggestion of either TSH-R or antigenically related protein[74, 75, 83, 84] in these cells. The challenge in interpreting RNA studies is discerning physiologic TSH-R gene expression from that caused by illegitimate transcription, as detected with ultrasensitive polymerase chain reaction techniques. For protein studies, the challenge is to determine whether it is TSH-R or an antigenically related substance being detected and, if it is TSH-R, whether it is present to an extent that would allow participation in the retro-ocular immune response. A more complete understanding of the pathogenesis of Graves' ophthalmopathy awaits answers to these key questions. A current model for the pathogenesis of Graves' ophthalmopathy is shown in Figure 101–6.

HISTORY AND EXAMINATION

To diagnose the clinical features of Graves' ophthalmopathy, it is helpful for the physician to be familiar with a problem-focused ophthalmic history and examination.[85, 86]

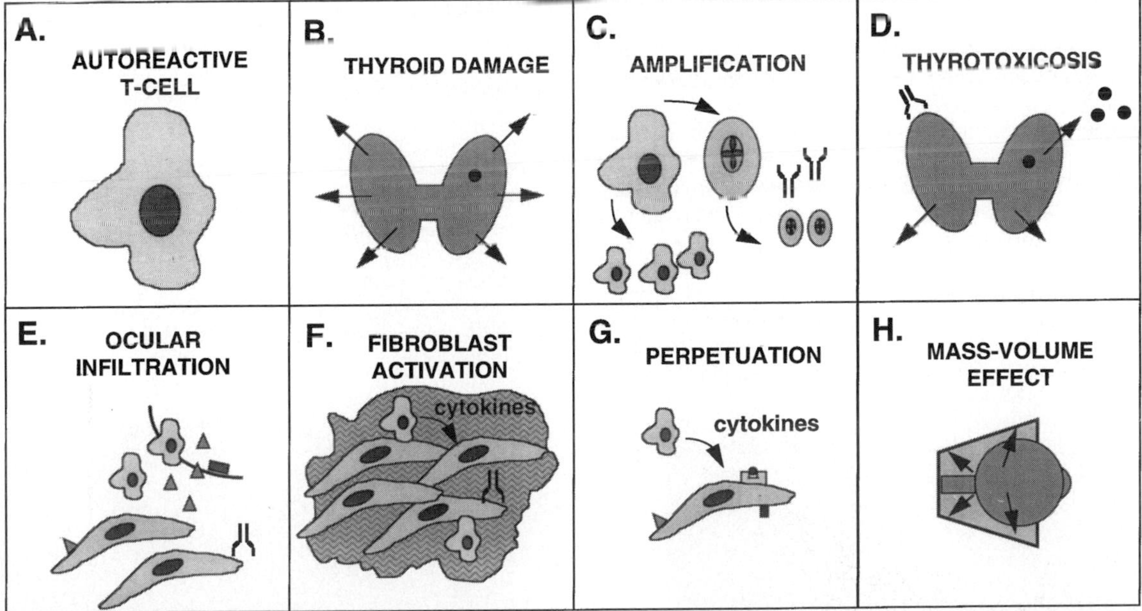

FIGURE 101–6. The authors' current concept of the pathogenesis of Graves' ophthalmopathy (GO). *A,* In the presence of a permissive immunogenetic milieu, thyroid damage leads to activation of autoimmune thyroid disease *(B)*. *C,* Release of thyroid antigen leads to activation of autoreactive T lymphocytes, which results in an amplification of both the cellular and humoral immune response against thyroid antigens such as the thyroid-stimulating hormone receptor (TSH-R), thyroglobulin, and thyroid peroxidase. *D,* Thyrotoxicosis results from activation of the TSH-R by circulating antibodies against this receptor. *E,* Circulating activated T lymphocytes infiltrate the orbit in response to the elaboration of specific lymphocyte adhesion molecules by retro-ocular connective tissue cells. *F,* Activated T lymphocytes synthesize and release cytokines that stimulate fibroblasts to proliferate and release glycosaminoglycans. *G,* Presentation of thyroid-eye cross-reactive antigens, such as hTSH-R, leads to further activation of the local autoimmune response. *H,* Increases in the retro-ocular connective tissue compartment and increased edema caused by glycosaminoglycan-associated hydrophilic forces result in progressive edema and orbital mass-volume mismatch.

History of the Present Illness

A complete eye history should be taken for each new patient with Graves' disease at the initial evaluation and periodically thereafter. Does the patient have frequent injection, tearing, foreign body sensation, or photophobia from exposure keratitis? Is diplopia present, and if so, is it intermittent or constant? Has the patient experienced visual blurring or blind spots (scotomas)? If visual blurring is present, is it relieved with blinking, such as occurs with dryness, or by covering one eye, as occurs with unilateral neuropathy or extraocular muscle dysfunction? Is pain or a sense of pressure felt behind the eyes?

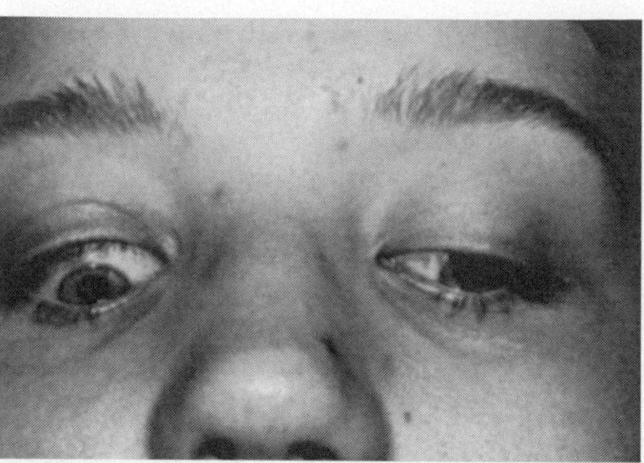

FIGURE 101–8. Lid lag of the right upper eyelid, a common sign of Graves' ophthalmopathy.

The Past Ophthalmic History

Patients should be questioned about previous ophthalmic surgical procedures or treatments to help determine whether recent eye complaints are related to previous disorders. Specifically, has the patient undergone cataract extraction, strabismus operations, retinal detachment repair, or laser surgery? Some patients with a history of strabismus may not recall that they had crossed eyes during childhood or had extraocular muscle surgery; this historical detail may imply the presence of amblyopia (lazy eye), of which many patients are surprisingly unaware until unrelated ophthalmic problems develop in adulthood. A history of ocular trauma or treatment of glaucoma is of obvious importance, and the past or present use of topical ophthalmic medications, several of which have systemic side effects, should be recorded.

Examination of the Eye

An Ophthalmic Evaluation for the Nonophthalmologist

Objective measurement and recording of eye findings are essential for assessing both the severity of ophthalmopathy and the response to therapy.[87] In addition, an assessment of disease activity and the patient's self-assessment of the disease state are important.[88] The following eight areas should be included in the eye evaluation.

VISUAL ACUITY. Visual acuity is usually measured as a Snellen fraction (e.g., 20/30) for distance vision. During bedside or office examinations, however, one may use a near-vision acuity card, several of which are commercially available. In the absence of a standardized card, the patient may be asked to read any available printed material, for example, the smallest type possible in a newspaper; the size of the print can be recorded, or the material itself can be taped in the patient's record. Of course, patients should wear their glasses when visual acuity is being checked. Because loss of color perception may be an early sign of optic neuropathy, color vision evaluation is an important diagnostic test.[89, 90] One simple method for detecting possible early optic neuropathy is to check whether the patient perceives a difference between the two eyes in the color intensity of a red object; the top of a bottle of mydriatic eye drops is commonly used for this purpose. More advanced color vision testing should be performed by an ophthalmologist.

PUPILS. Direct and consensual pupillary responses should be checked. An afferent pupillary defect (Marcus Gunn pupil) may indicate optic neuropathy.

EYELIDS. Upper eyelid retraction is a common finding in patients with Graves' ophthalmopathy.[5, 91–93] Early in the course of Graves' disease, eyelid malpositions may result from increased sympathetic activity. With chronicity, the eyelid retractors (levator palpebrae superioris and Müller's muscle) become hypertrophic, eventually fibrotic, and adherent to orbital tissues.[94] Lid retraction may be unilateral or bilateral and may be subtle in some instances. The upper lid usually rests 1 to 2 mm below the junction of the cornea and sclera; therefore, if the white of the eye is seen above the corneoscleral limbus, eyelid retraction of at least 1.5 mm is present. The level of the lower eyelid is typically at the inferior corneoscleral limbus. Lower eyelid retraction is a less constant and specific finding and is not usually seen in patients with Graves' ophthalmopathy without concomitant retraction of the upper lids. Lid lag (Figs. 101–7 and 101–8), which is diagnosed by asking the patient to look down and then observing delayed or restricted excursion of the upper eyelids as they follow the globes, and lagophthalmos (Fig. 101–9), which is an inability to close the eyelids completely, are also stigmata of Graves' ophthalmopathy. Eyelid retraction, lid lag, and lagophthalmos frequently interfere with the maintenance of an adequate tear film on the eye. The result is ocular irritation and dryness, reflex tearing, photophobia, and corneal scarring or even ulceration in severe cases.

CONJUNCTIVA AND CORNEA. The conjunctiva is the clear, thin tissue that covers the sclera. It is normally transparent, except for the small blood vessels that course within it. In Graves' ophthalmopathy, the conjunctiva may become hyperemic (usually termed injection) or edematous (chemosis) from exposure or from decreased venous drainage secondary to orbital suffusion. A characteristic conjunctival finding in patients with Graves' eyes is focal injection over the inser-

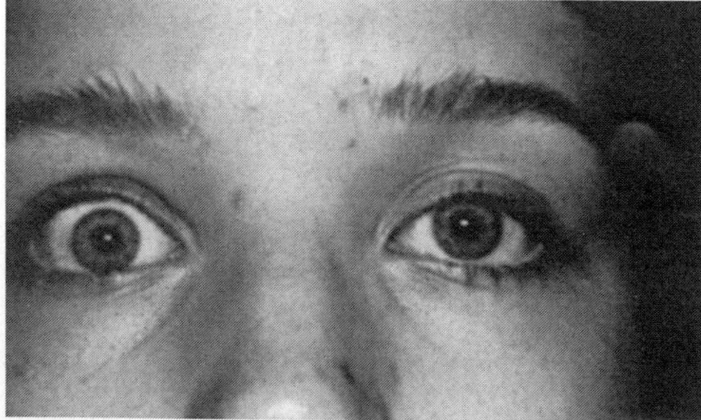

FIGURE 101–7. Right upper eyelid retraction in a patient with Graves' ophthalmopathy.

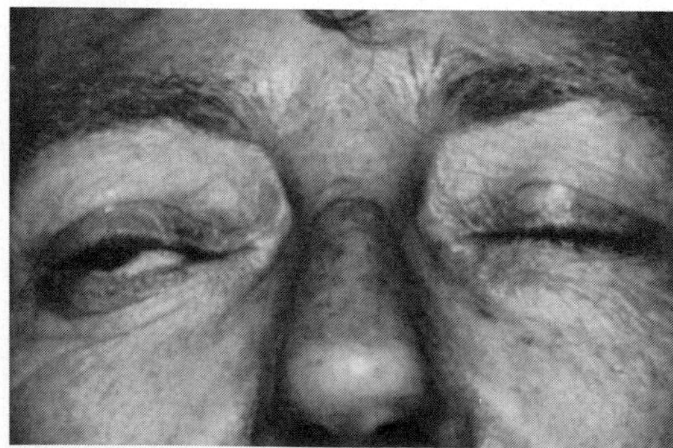

FIGURE 101–9. Lagophthalmos (an inability to close the eyelids completely) often causes exposure keratopathy (dryness of the cornea and conjunctiva).

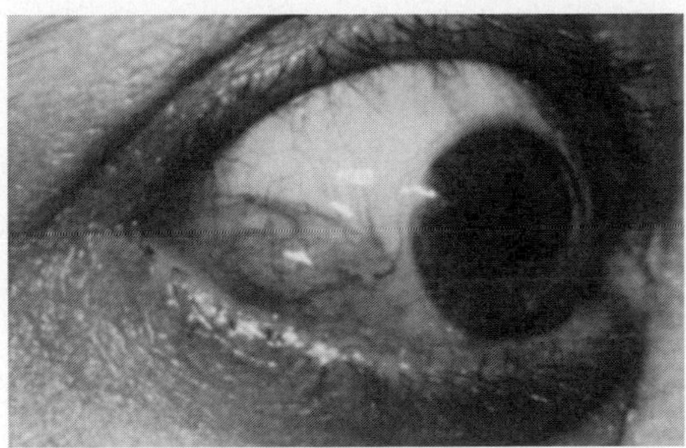

FIGURE 101–10. Chemosis (conjunctival edema) and focal injection (conjunctival blood vessel dilation) over the lateral rectus muscle insertion in a patient with Graves' ophthalmopathy.

tions of the lateral or medial rectus muscles (Fig. 101–10). The engorged blood vessels do not extend to the corneoscleral limbus.

The cornea should normally appear transparent and lustrous. Dryness resulting from exposure is difficult to detect without slit-lamp biomicroscopy. Corneal ulceration, which is an ophthalmic emergency, can usually be seen grossly with a penlight and is typically accompanied by severe pain.[95]

EXOPHTHALMOMETRY. Proptosis may be quantitated with an exophthalmometer, an instrument that measures the position of the globes in relation to the lateral orbital rim. The device is easy to use and is helpful in documenting the results of treatment. Exophthalmometry measurements in most adult eyes are 22 mm or less, and the difference between the patient's two eyes does not usually exceed 2 mm.[96] Whites tend to have Hertel exophthalmometry measurements of less than 18 to 20 mm, which is higher than that of Asians (16–18 mm) and lower than those seen in many blacks (20–22 mm).[97–99]

OCULAR MOTILITY. The range of movement should be evaluated for each eye separately and then with the eyes together, during which time the patient should be asked to state whether double vision is noted. Diplopia is most likely to occur in upgaze or in the extremes of lateral gaze because of restriction of the inferior or medial recti. Any or all of the extraocular muscles may be involved in Graves' ophthalmopathy, however, and unusual patterns of strabismus may occur (Fig. 101–11).

VISUAL FIELDS. As noted above, scotomas may appear in the visual field from optic neuropathy. Gross visual field defects may be detected with careful confrontation testing. An Amsler grid, a handheld card with a pattern of perpendicular crossed lines, may be used in the office or at the bedside as a simple screening tool. Formal perimetry testing should be performed by an ophthalmologist.

OPHTHALMOSCOPY. Examination of the posterior pole of the retina may show a swollen optic disk from the compressive optic neuropathy or choroidal folds (a slatlike, corrugated pattern) that occasionally accompany mechanical orbital processes. Visually significant disorders such as opacities of the ocular media (corneal irregularities or cataracts) or macular degeneration may also be easily noted with the direct ophthalmoscope.

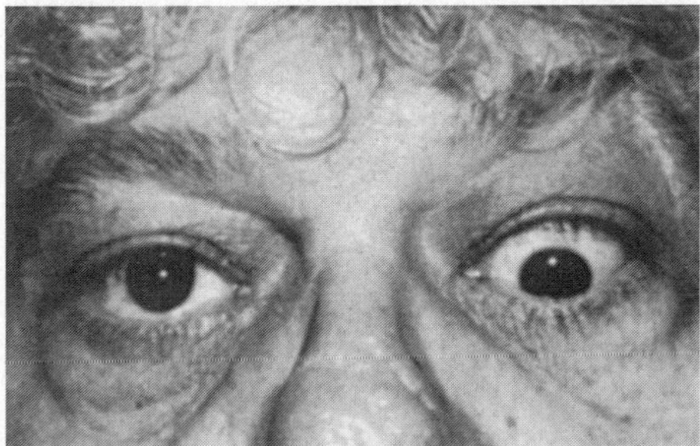

FIGURE 101–11. Hypotropia of the left eye secondary to contraction of the left inferior rectus muscle in Graves' ophthalmopathy. Unusual patterns of strabismus are characteristic of both Graves' ophthalmopathy and myasthenia gravis, diseases that may occur concomitantly.

Formal Ophthalmology Testing

Patients with positive findings in any of the above areas should be referred to an ophthalmologist for additional testing, which may include color vision testing, perimetry (visual fields), measurement of intraocular pressure, and slit-lamp biomicroscopy.

Subtle evidence of optic neuropathy may be assessed with visual evoked potentials,[100] color vision testing, or automated perimetry. A Farnsworth-Munsell panel detects subtle acquired color vision defects better than do most pseudoisochromatic color plate systems, which are designed to evince congenital color vision abnormalities.[101] It is important to remember that approximately 7% to 8% of the male population has some degree of congenital red-green color "blindness." Measurement of extraocular muscle dysfunction relies on the Maddox rod test, the alternate cover test, the Hess chart, or the Lancaster red-green test. Exposure keratitis may be detected by slit-lamp examination with rose bengal or fluorescein staining.

DIFFERENTIAL DIAGNOSIS

Each major manifestation of Graves' ophthalmopathy has an associated differential diagnosis. The combination of more than one finding, such as lid retraction and proptosis, or the finding of biochemical thyroid dysfunction increases the likelihood that one is dealing with a manifestation of Graves' disease.[102]

Visual loss caused by optic neuropathy in Graves' ophthalmopathy needs to be distinguished from that resulting from exposure keratitis, cataracts, macular degeneration, intracranial or orbital tumors, diabetic retinopathy, or psychogenic causes.

The differential diagnosis for eyelid retraction includes neurogenic, myogenic, and mechanical etiologies.[103] Pseudoretraction of an eyelid may occur in response to aponeurogenic ptosis in the normal-appearing contralateral eye.[103, 104]

Proptosis measurements may be affected by systemic nonthyroidal illness, with recession of the orbit in wasting disorders and forward protrusion in obesity. Proptosis of up to 25 mm has been described as a familial trait.[105] The differential diagnosis for proptosis is reviewed in Table 101–1.

Extraocular muscle enlargement may be seen with orbital malignancies, orbital "pseudotumor," and other inflammatory conditions, including sarcoidosis and Wegener's granulomatosis.[1]

TABLE 101–1. Differential Diagnosis of Proptosis

Endocrine	Granulomatous
Graves' ophthalmopathy	Sarcoidosis
Cushing's syndrome	Wegener's granulomatosis
Orbital neoplasms	Infectious
Primary neoplasms	Orbital cellulitis
Hemangioma	Syphilis
Lymphoma	Mucormycosis
Optic nerve glioma	Parasitic
Choroidal melanoma	Vascular
Lacrimal gland tumors	Carotid-cavernous fistula
Meningioma	Miscellaneous
Rhabdomyosarcoma	Lithium therapy
Extension of paranasal sinus tumors	Cirrhosis
Metastatic disease	Obesity
Melanoma	Amyloidosis
Breast carcinoma	Dermoid and epidermoid cysts
Lung carcinoma	Foreign body
Kidney	
Prostate	
Inflammatory	
Orbital pseudotumor	
Orbital myositis	

Vascular anomalies of the orbit that may simulate the clinical features of Graves' ophthalmopathy include dural–cavernous sinus fistulas (low-flow shunts), carotid–cavernous sinus fistulas (high-flow shunts),[106] and orbital varices. Historical features and appropriate radiographic studies usually facilitate proper diagnosis.

Myasthenia gravis may cause both eyelid malposition and extraocular muscle dysfunction and be confused with or add to the severity of Graves' ophthalmopathy. Patients with ocular myasthenia are more likely to have an associated autoimmune thyroid disease and less likely to be anticholinesterase antibody positive than are patients with generalized myasthenia.[107]

NATURAL HISTORY

The natural history of Graves' ophthalmopathy is characterized by a period of progression over a span of 3 to 6 months, a plateau phase, and then gradual improvement. Individual components of ophthalmopathy have differing natural histories. Lid retraction is unlikely to be present at long-term follow-up, and soft tissue changes such as chemosis and lid edema improve or resolve in the vast majority of patients over short-term follow-up. Strabismus regresses spontaneously in only 30% to 40% of patients without specific therapy, and proptosis persists to some degree in up to 90% of carefully monitored individuals.[1] A recent follow-up survey of an incidence cohort of patients with Graves' ophthalmopathy at a mean of 9.4 years after initial eye examination revealed that 10% had experienced diplopia within the preceding 4 weeks and 32.6% experienced ocular discomfort within the prior 4 weeks. Sixty-one percent of patients believed that their eyes had not returned to baseline, and 37.9% were dissatisfied with the appearance of their eyes.[108] Another study found that among 59 patients with mild Graves' ophthalmopathy not receiving disease-modifying eye therapy and monitored for a median of 12 months, 64% showed spontaneous improvement, 22% showed no change, and 13.5% showed deterioration.[109]

THERAPY

The vast majority of patients experiencing Graves' ophthalmopathy will have a self-limited disease course requiring only local measures for symptomatic relief. For patients with more advanced disease, early attention is directed toward protection of the cornea, relief of discomfort, and shrinkage of orbital soft tissues by immunosuppressive drugs. Later in the course, surgical expansion of the bony orbital space is occasionally necessary. Correction of extraocular muscle dysfunction and restoration of normal eyelid position may complete the patient's rehabilitation. In all patients it is important to restore thyroid hormone levels to normal before any type of orbital surgery is performed. The single exception to this rule is when very severe ophthalmopathy threatens vision and requires urgent orbital decompression. The effect of ophthalmopathy on the selection of therapy for thyrotoxicosis is discussed under the heading Therapy for Thyrotoxicosis.

Local Measures

Symptoms resulting from corneal drying are effectively treated with instillation of methylcellulose-containing eye drops and taping the eyelids shut at night to prevent nocturnal corneal drying.[110] Worsening of diplopia and soft tissue changes at night results from dependent edema, which may respond to elevation of the head. The use of sunglasses or tinted lenses may assist in decreasing photophobia. Prisms are occasionally useful for the correction of mild diplopia. In a recent survey of members of the European Thyroid Association on management of an index case of ophthalmopathy, 76% of respondents recommended methylcellulose eye drops, 21% would use diuretics to decrease ocular edema, and 18% would recommend prisms to correct diplopia.[111] The topical use of guanethidine eye drops to correct lid retraction has been associated with local irritation and variable effectiveness[112] and is rarely encouraged today.

Immunomodulatory Therapy

Corticosteroids

Corticosteroids have been used for nearly 50 years in the treatment of Graves' ophthalmopathy. These agents have both anti-inflammatory and immunomodulatory effects and may inhibit the synthesis and release of glycosaminoglycan by fibroblasts.[113–115] In general, corticosteroid therapy provides rapid relief from the pain, injection, and conjunctival edema associated with the inflammatory soft tissue changes in Graves' ophthalmopathy. Corticosteroid therapy is also highly effective in the treatment of compressive optic neuropathy, with most patients showing at least some improvement.[1] Regression in proptosis and ophthalmoplegia has been reported, but such regression occurs to a lesser extent and with a higher likelihood of exacerbation after drug withdrawal.[1]

Corticosteroid therapy is generally initiated with a relatively high dose, such as 40 to 80 mg of prednisone per day.[1] After 2 to 4 weeks, the daily dose is tapered by 2.5 to 10.0 mg every 2 to 4 weeks. In many instances, drug withdrawal results in exacerbation, which requires increases in dosage and a slowing of the rate of subsequent taper.[116, 117] Improvement in soft tissue inflammation begins within 1 to 2 days, and typical courses range from 3 to 12 months. Side effects associated with high-dose corticosteroid therapy may include gastrointestinal irritation, weight gain, psychosis, osteoporosis, and glucose intolerance.[1]

The use of depot subconjunctival or retrobulbar corticosteroid injections has been advocated as a means of attaining a high local concentration of drug and minimizing systemic side effects.[119, 120] However, the risk,[121] patient discomfort, and lack of benefit beyond conventional regimens[119] limit the practical utility of this approach.

Pulse therapy with intravenous methylprednisolone has been studied in patients with Graves' ophthalmopathy.[122–124] Using 3 doses of 500 mg on alternate days intravenously, followed by an oral regimen, one study found clinical improvement in 83% of the patients studied.[125] Similar results have been found by others,[122] including one study consisting of five patients with optic neuropathy.[124]

Predictors of clinical response to corticosteroids include high scores on a disease activity scale,[126] signal intensity on T1-weighted MRI,[127, 128] orbital uptake of radiolabeled somatostatin analogues,[129, 130] and duration of disease.[1]

Combined use of corticosteroids with other forms of immunomodulatory therapy such as orbital radiation or cyclosporine is detailed in the relevant sections below.

Cyclosporine

Cyclosporine inhibits helper T cell proliferation and cytokine production, prevents cytotoxic T cell activation, and suppresses immunoglobulin production by B lymphocytes.[131] Two prospective randomized trials have examined the efficacy of cyclosporine in Graves' ophthalmopathy.[132, 133] In one study,[132] patients receiving prednisone alone were compared with those given both prednisone and cyclosporine, with changes in an activity score used to monitor therapy. Combined therapy resulted in a more rapid fall in activity score and a greater decrease in extraocular muscle thickness by CT. Recurrences were seen after stopping corticosteroid therapy in nearly half the patients in the prednisone-alone group as compared with only 5% in the combined treatment group. In a second study,[133] cyclosporine and prednisone were directly compared as single-agent therapies, and patients failing either drug alone were given combination therapy. Prednisone was superior to cyclosporine as single-agent therapy, but nearly 60% of patients not responding to either drug alone subsequently improved with combined therapy. Despite this apparent efficacy, the high cost of cyclosporine and the requirement for frequent drug monitoring together with an extensive side effect profile limit the utility of this drug in clinical practice.

Somatostatin Analogue Therapy

The presence of somatostatin receptors on the surface of activated lymphocytes has been suggested as the explanation for orbital uptake of radiolabeled somatostatin analogues[130] and has provided a rationale for the therapeutic use of octreotide and lanreotide in Graves' ophthalmopathy.[134, 135] In an early uncontrolled study, 6 ophthalmopathy patients treated with octreotide, 100 μg three times daily for 3 months, experienced amelioration of soft tissue changes or improvement in extraocular muscle function.[136] In a nonrandomized trial, 7 of 12 patients with active Graves' ophthalmopathy experienced improvement in an eye index score after treatment with octreotide for 3 months as compared with none of 8 patients not receiving therapy.[134] Five of 7 patients showing improvement with octreotide had positive orbital uptake of labeled analogue vs. only 1 of 5 patients with no response.[134] Similar results were obtained with the long-acting somatostatin analogue lanreotide[135] in 5 patients when compared with matched controls. Interestingly, orbital uptake of labeled octreotide diminished after therapy in all patients. Larger, randomized trials are needed to confirm these interesting results.

Plasmapheresis

The utility of removal of circulating immunoglobulins by plasmapheresis in ophthalmopathy patients has been examined in several small studies (reviewed elsewhere[1]). However, interpretation of the results of these studies is hampered by a lack of controls and the concurrent use of immunosuppressive therapy.

Orbital Radiotherapy

The rationale for the use of orbital radiation therapy in Graves' ophthalmopathy involves the marked radiosensitivity of the lymphocyte, thought to be a primary effector in this disorder. Radiation to the orbits is generally administered at 20 Gy (2000 rad) calculated at the midline and delivered by lateral ports angled 5 degrees posteriorly to prevent inclusion of the anterior chamber and retina. Therapy is delivered in 10 fractions over a 2-week period. Several European centers have used a lower total dosage effectively.[137, 138] A beneficial effect has been reported within 1 to 4 weeks after starting therapy[139, 140] and may continue for as long as 12 months after completion.

In a review of 14 uncontrolled studies of orbital radiotherapy in Graves' ophthalmopathy, orbital radiation appeared to be well tolerated and seemed to provide benefit in approximately two-thirds of the patients treated.[1] The largest single-center experience involved more than 300 patients treated with megavoltage irradiation, one-third of whom received concurrent corticosteroid therapy.[141, 142] After orbital irradiation, 80% of patients had improvement in soft tissue changes, 51% had recession of proptosis, 56% had improvement in eye muscle function, and 67% had improvement in vision. Despite this improvement, 29% of patients required one or more eye surgeries after orbital irradiation, most of which were performed to correct strabismus. Similar results were recently reported elsewhere.[143] It has been suggested that rather than obviating the need for corrective surgery, radiation may shorten the interval until stabilization of disease, thereby allowing earlier surgical intervention.[144]

Despite the apparent beneficial effects of radiation therapy for Graves' ophthalmopathy, a true measure of its effectiveness requires a randomized trial comparing irradiated and nonirradiated (and otherwise untreated) eyes. Results from these ongoing trials await publication. In a randomized double-blind trial comparing orbital irradiation with prednisone in patients with Graves' ophthalmopathy, these two therapies yielded similar results, but orbital irradiation had fewer side effects.[145] In another study, a combination of orbital irradiation and corticosteroid therapy was deemed to be superior to medical therapy alone.[146] These authors found that 26 of 36 (72%) patients treated with concurrent corticosteroids and orbital irradiation experienced a good or excellent response as compared with only 3 of 12 (25%) patients treated with steroids alone.[146]

Side effects of orbital irradiation include temporary hair loss at the temples and transient worsening of soft tissue changes. Rare cases of retinopathy and cataracts have been described after orbital irradiation, which underscores the importance of reliance on a center having expertise with this application.[147, 148] Diabetic retinopathy is considered a contraindication to orbital irradiation because this condition increases vascular susceptibility to radiation damage.[144]

Other Immunomodulatory Therapy

Additional immune therapy for active Graves' ophthalmopathy has included azathioprine, cyclophosphamide, ciamexon, and intravenous immunoglobulin, all with either no benefit or no clear improvement over conventional therapy.[1] A recent trial compared patients randomized to receive intravenous immunoglobulins or prednisolone for 20 weeks and found no difference in efficacy, although fewer side effects occurred with immunoglobulin therapy.[149] Pentoxifylline, a phosphodiesterase inhibitor with anti–tumor necrosis factor-α (TNFA) properties, was recently shown to reduce soft tissue changes but not proptosis or ophthalmoplegia in 8 of 10 patients with severe ophthalmopathy who received this medication for 12 weeks.[150] Patients experiencing improvement with pentoxifylline had concurrent reductions in TNFA and serum glycosaminoglycan levels.

Nonimmunomodulatory Therapy

Nonimmunomodulatory therapy for Graves' ophthalmopathy has been tested with varying results, including local injection of botulinum toxin,[151] bromocriptine,[152] metronidazole,[153] and acupuncture.[154, 155]

Surgical Treatment of Graves' Ophthalmopathy

A tripartite approach is most commonly used in the surgical treatment of Graves' ophthalmopathy: orbital decompression to relieve optic neuropathy or proptosis, extraocular muscle surgery to reduce diplopia, and eyelid procedures to treat retraction and cosmetic disfigurement. Although only a small fraction of patients with Graves' disease require operative intervention, some patients with severe ophthalmopathy need multiple procedures to achieve satisfactory functional and aesthetic results.[156]

ORBITAL DECOMPRESSION. The orbit is decompressed by removing one or more of its bony walls, which expands the eye socket and increases the potential space for the orbital contents. Indications for the procedure include optic neuropathy, severe proptosis (which in some patients may cause subluxation of the globe anterior to the lids), vision-threatening ocular exposure, debilitating retrobulbar and periorbital pain, or intolerable corticosteroid side effects.[157] Additionally, because some extraocular muscle procedures used in patients with Graves' ophthalmopathy may worsen exophthalmos, preliminary orbital decompression may be useful in those with severe proptosis. Finally, orbital expansion may be considered in some of these patients who do not have functional ocular disease but desire enhanced cosmesis.[158]

Optic neuropathy is the most common indication for orbital decompression. In most instances, the optic nerve is compressed by the enlarged or noncompliant extraocular muscles at the crowded orbital apex[159, 160] (Fig. 101–12); in some patients, however, the muscles are of essentially normal size.[161] By removing one or more walls of the bony orbit, pressure on the nerve is reduced. Numerous approaches to orbital decompression have been described; variations include the number of walls removed (one, two, three, or four) and the avenue for surgical access—lateral, medial, transpalpebral, transantral, transcranial, through a bicoronal incision, endoscopically, or with a combination of procedures.[162, 163] Transantral orbital decompression with removal of a portion of the medial wall and the orbital floor has been the preferred method at the Mayo Clinic over the past 25 years.[164–167] Potential complications of orbital decompression include worsened diplopia, hypoglobus, numbness in the distribution of the infraorbital nerve, eyelid malposition, nasolacrimal duct obstruction, cerebrospinal fluid leakage, meningitis, and even death in rare instances.

It is important to recognize that patients with optic neuropathy often have less exophthalmos than do patients without optic nerve compromise because proptosis may function as the body's way of "autodecompressing" the orbit.[168] Needle aspiration of the orbital contents, previously recommended as a preliminary adjunct to orbital decompression, should be avoided.

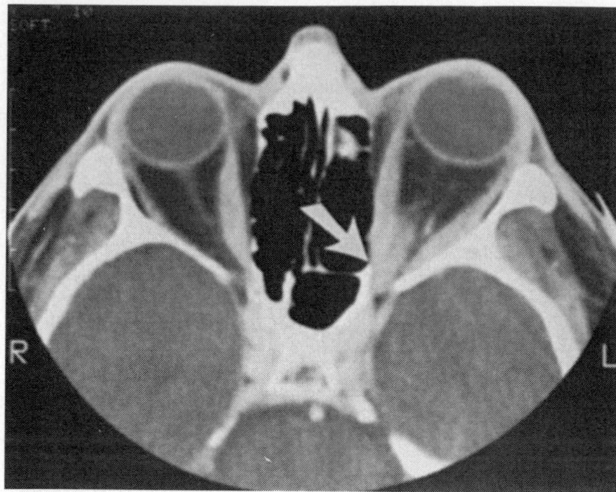

FIGURE 101–12. Computed tomography is useful to demonstrate fusiform enlargement of the extraocular muscles in Graves' ophthalmopathy. In the left orbital apex, the optic nerve is compressed by the hypertrophied muscles *(arrow)*.

EXTRAOCULAR MUSCLE SURGERY. Diplopia resulting from extraocular muscle involvement in Graves' ophthalmopathy is often difficult to treat. When the disease is active, ocular alignment may vary from hour to hour and preclude prism spectacle correction or surgical repair. If the inflammation has stabilized and double vision cannot be corrected with glasses, strabismus surgery is indicated.[169] Because the underlying problem is usually a restrictive myopathy (not paralysis, as suggested in older reports) from tight, hypertrophied, and eventually fibrotic muscles, strabismus procedures for Graves' ophthalmopathy most frequently involve weakening the muscles by recessing their insertions onto the globe. The goal of surgery is to allow single vision in primary (straight ahead) gaze, as well as in the reading position; postoperative diplopia in the extremes of lateral gaze or in upgaze is common and does not signify an unsuccessful procedure.

EYELID SURGERY. Eyelid surgery for Graves' ophthalmopathy is typically performed after orbital decompression and strabismus procedures, if either or both are needed[170] (Figs. 101–13 and 101–14). The retractors of the upper eyelid, the levator palpebrae superioris and Müller's muscle, undergo pathologic changes similar to those seen in the extraocular muscles. Upper lid retraction is relieved by weakening (recessing) the muscles; lower lid retraction is treated with analogous procedures, although spacers of hard palate mucosa, tarsus, donor sclera, or cartilage are often grafted into the lids to counteract the tendency of gravity to pull the lids inferiorly during the postoperative period. Blepharoplasty (removal of excess eyelid and orbital tissue that prolapses anteriorly from the increase in orbital volume) may be helpful in selected patients to reduce the unappealing aesthetic sequelae of Graves' ophthalmopathy.

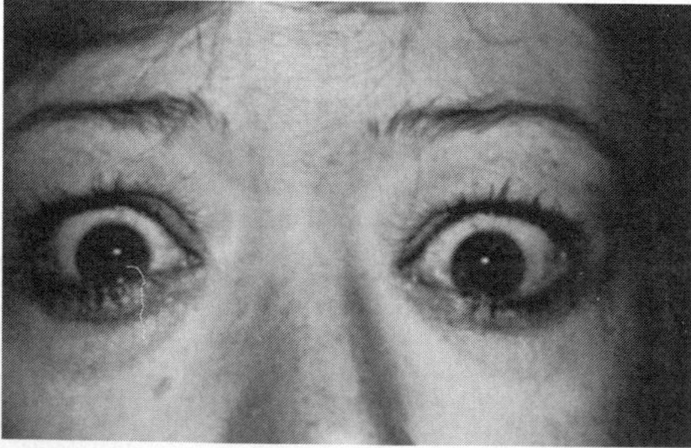

FIGURE 101–13. A patient with Graves' ophthalmopathy who has undergone bilateral transantral orbital decompression and strabismus surgery. Treatment for upper eyelid retraction is indicated both to reduce ocular exposure and to enhance cosmesis.

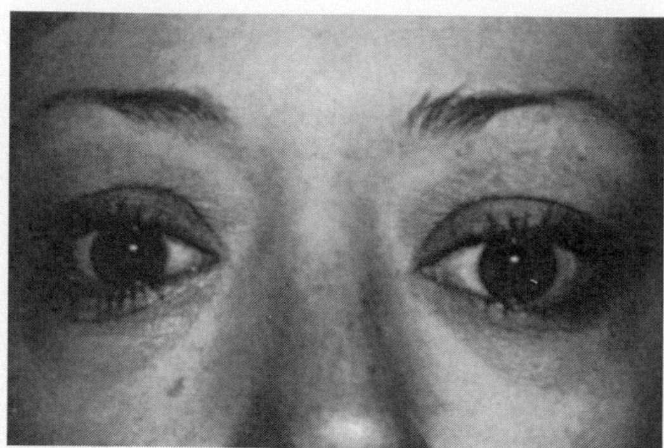

FIGURE 101–14. Same patient as in Figure 101–13 after recession of Müller's muscle and the levator palpebrae superioris muscle in each upper eyelid.

SUMMARY

Through judicious application of the diagnostic and multidisciplinary therapeutic measures outlined in this chapter, most patients with severe Graves' ophthalmopathy will be given comfortable functional eyes and achieve satisfactory cosmesis. Early assessment of the patient's priorities and expectations forms a key element in the alignment of patient and physician goals for successful therapy.

REFERENCES

1. Burch HB, Wartofsky L: Graves' ophthalmopathy: Current concepts regarding pathogenesis and management. Endocr Rev 14:747–793, 1993.
2. Gorman CA: Temporal relationship between onset of Graves' ophthalmopathy and diagnosis of thyrotoxicosis. Mayo Clin Proc 58:515–519, 1983.
3. Bartels EC, Irie M: Thyroid function in patients with progressive exophthalmos: Study of 117 cases requiring orbital decompression. *In* Pitt-Rivers R (ed): Advances in Thyroid Research, Transactions of the Fourth International Goiter Conference. London, Pergamon, 1961, pp 163–170.
4. Fatourechi V, Fransway AF, Pajouhi M: Dermopathy of Graves disease (pretibial myxedema). Review of 150 cases. Medicine (Baltimore) 73:1–7, 1994.
5. Bartley GB, Fatourechi V, Kadrmas EF, et al: The chronology of Graves' ophthalmopathy in an incidence cohort. Am J Ophthalmol 121:426–434, 1996.
6. Salvi M, Zhang Z-G, Haegert D, et al: Patients with endocrine ophthalmopathy not associated with overt thyroid disease have multiple thyroid immunological abnormalities. J Clin Endocrinol Metab 70:89–94, 1990.
7. Kasagi K, Konishi J, Iida Y, et al: Scintigraphic findings of the thyroid in euthyroid ophthalmic Graves' disease. J Nucl Med 35:811–817, 1994.
8. Morris JC, Hay ID, Nelson RE, Jiang NS: Clinical utility of thyrotropin receptor antibody assays: Comparison of radioreceptor and bioassay methods. Mayo Clin Proc 63:707, 1988.
9. Chang TC, Chang TJ, Change CC, et al: TSH and TSH receptor antibody-binding sites in fibroblasts of pretibial myxedema are related to the extracellular domain of entire TSH receptor. Clin Immunol Immunopathol 71:113–120, 1994.
10. Rundle FF, Pochin EE: The orbital tissues in thyrotoxicosis: A quantitative analysis relating to exophthalmos. Clin Sci 5:51–74, 1944.
11. Gerding MN, Terwee CB, Dekker FW, et al: Quality of life in patients with Graves' ophthalmopathy is markedly decreased: Measurement by the medical outcomes study instrument. Thyroid 7:885–889, 1997.
12. Werner SC, Coelho B, Quimby EH: Ten year results of I-131 therapy in hyperthyroidism. Bull N Y Acad Med 33:783–806, 1957.
13. Forbes G, Gorman CA, Brennan MD, et al: Ophthalmopathy of Graves' disease: Computerized volume measurements of the orbital fat and muscle. Am J Neuroradiol 7:651–656, 1986.
14. Chang TC, Huang KM, Chang TJ, Lin SL: Correlation of orbital computed tomography and antibodies in patients with hyperthyroid Graves' disease. Clin Endocrinol 32:551–558, 1990.
15. Gamblin GT, Harper DG, Galentine P, et al: Prevalence of increased intraocular pressure in Graves' disease—evidence of frequent subclinical ophthalmopathy. N Engl J Med 308:420–424, 1983.
16. Gamblin GT, Galentine PG, Eil C: Intraocular pressure and thyroid disease. *In* Gorman CA, Campbell RJ, Dyer JA (eds): The Eye and Orbit in Thyroid Disease. New York, Raven Press, 1984, pp 155–166.
17. Villadolid MC, Nagataki S, Uetani M, et al: Untreated Graves' disease patients without clinical ophthalmopathy demonstrate a high frequency of extraocular muscle (EOM) enlargement by magnetic resonance. J Clin Endocrinol Metab 80:2830–2833, 1995.

18. Bartley GB, Fatourechi V, Kadrmas EF, et al: Clinical features of Graves' ophthalmopathy in an incidence cohort. Am J Ophthalmol 121:284–290, 1996.
19. Bartley GB, Fatourechi V, Kadrmas EF, et al: The incidence of Graves' ophthalmopathy in Olmsted Countly, Minnesota. Am J Ophthalmol 120:511–517, 1995.
20. Sridama V, Hara Y, Fauchet R, DeGroot LJ: HLA immunogenic heterogeneity in black American patients with Graves' disease. Arch Intern Med 147:229–231, 1987.
21. Kawa A, Nakamura S, Nakazawa M, et al: HLA-B35 and B5 in Japanese patients with Graves' disease. Acta Endocrinol (Copenh) 86:754–757, 1977.
22. Bech K, Lumholtz B, Nerup J, et al: HLA antigens in Graves' disease. Acta Endocrinol (Copenh) 86:510–516, 1977.
23. Kendall-Taylor P, Stephenson A, Stratton A, et al: Differentiation of autoimmune ophthalmopathy from Graves' hyperthyroidism by analysis of genetic markers. Clin Endocrinol 28:601–610, 1988.
24. Schleusener H, Peters H, Bogner U, et al: Immunogenetics in Graves' disease. An overview. Acta Endocrinol (Copenh) 121(suppl 2):123–129, 1989.
25. Weetman AP, So AK, Warner CA, et al: Immunogenetics of Graves' ophthalmopathy. Clin Endocrinol 28:619–628, 1988.
26. Tellez M, Cooper J, Edmonds C: Graves' ophthalmopathy in relation to cigarette smoking and ethnic origin. Clin Endocrinol 36:291–294, 1992.
27. Weetman AP, Zhang L, Webb S, Shine B: Analysis of HLA-DQB and HLA-DPB alleles in Graves' disease by oligonucleotide probing of enzymatically amplified DNA. Clin Endocrinol 33:65–71, 1990.
28. Frecker M, Stenszky V, Balazs C, et al: Genetic factors in Graves' ophthalmopathy. Clin Endocrinol 25:479–485, 1986.
29. Kendall-Taylor P, Stephenson A, Stratton A, et al: Differentiation of autoimmune ophthalmopathy from Graves' hyperthyroidism by analysis of genetic markers. Clin Endocrinol 28:601–610, 1988.
30. Kotsa K, Weetman AP, Watson PF: A CTLA-4 gene polymorphism is associated with both Graves disease and autoimmune hypothyroidism. Clin Endocrinol (Oxf) 46:551–554, 1997.
31. Blakemore AI, Duff GW, Weetman AP, Watson PF: Association of Graves' disease with an allele of the interleukin-1 receptor antagonist gene. J Clin Endocrinol Metab 80:111–115, 1995.
32. Brix TH, Kyvik KO, Hegedus L: What is the evidence of genetic factors in the etiology of Graves' disease? A brief review. Thyroid 8:727–734, 1998.
33. Farid NR, Balazs C: The genetics of thyroid associated ophthalmopathy. Thyroid 8:407–409, 1998.
34. Bartalena L, Martino E, Marcocci C, et al: More on smoking habits and Graves' ophthalmopathy. J Endocrinol Invest 12:733–737, 1989.
35. Prummel MF, Wiersinga WM: Smoking and risk of Graves' disease. JAMA 269:479–482, 1993.
36. Metcalfe RA, Weetman AP: Stimulation of extraocular muscle fibroblasts by cytokines and hypoxia: Possible role in thyroid associated ophthalmopathy. Clin Endocrinol (Oxf) 40:67–72, 1994.
37. Burch HB, Lahiri S, Bahn R, Barnes SG: Superoxide radical production stimulates human retroocular fibroblast proliferation in Graves' ophthalmopathy. Exp Eye Res 65:311–316, 1997.
38. Hofbauer LC, Muhlberg T, Konig A, et al: Soluble interleukin-1 receptor antagonist serum levels in smokers and nonsmokers with Graves' ophthalmopathy undergoing orbital radiotherapy. J Clin Endocrinol Metab 82:2244–2247, 1997.
39. Tan GH, Dutton CM, Bahn RS: Interleukin-1 (IL-1) receptor antagonist and soluble IL-1 receptor inhibit IL-1–induced glycosaminoglycan production in cultured human orbital fibroblasts from patients with Graves' ophthalmopathy. J Clin Endocrinol Metab 81:449–452, 1996.
40. Bartalena L, Marcocci C, Tanda ML, et al: Cigarette smoking and treatment outcomes in Graves ophthalmopathy. Ann Intern Med 129:632–635, 1998.
41. Vanderpump MP, Tunbridge WM, French JM, et al: The incidence of thyroid disorders in the community: A twenty-year follow up of the Whickham survey. Clin Endocrinol (Oxf) 43:55–68, 1995.
42. Perros P, Kendall-Taylor P: Pathogenetic mechanisms in thyroid-associated ophthalmopathy. J Intern Med 231:205–211, 1992.
43. DeGroot LJ, Gorman CA, Pinchera A, Bartalena L, et al: Therapeutic controversies. Retro-orbital radiation and radioactive iodide ablation of the thyroid may be good for Graves' ophthalmopathy. J Clin Endocrinol Metab 80:339–340, 1995.
44. Gorman CA: Therapeutic controversies. Radioiodine therapy does not aggravate Graves' ophthalmopathy. J Clin Endocrinol Metab 80:340–342, 1995.
45. Pinchera A, Bartalena L, Marcocci C: Therapeutic controversies. Radioiodine may be bad for Graves' ophthalmopathy, but.... J Clin Endocrinol Metab 80:342–345, 1995.
46. Wartofsky L: Therapeutic controversies. Summation, commentary, and overview: Concerns over aggravation of Graves' ophthalmopathy by radioactive iodine treatment and the use of retrobulbar radiation therapy. J Clin Endocrinol Metab 80:347–349, 1995.
47. Bartalena L, Marcocci C, Bogazzi F, et al: Use of corticosteroids to prevent progression of Graves' ophthalmopathy after radioiodine therapy for hyperthyroidism. N Engl J Med 321:1349–1352, 1989.
48. Tallstedt L, Lundell G, Tørring O, et al: Occurrence of ophthalmopathy after treatment for Graves' hyperthyroidism. N Engl J Med 326:1733–1738, 1992.
49. Kung AW, Cheng A, Yau CC: The incidence of ophthalmopathy after radioiodine therapy for Graves' disease: Prognostic factors and the role of methimazole. J Clin Endocrinol Metab 79:542–546, 1994.
50. Fernandez-Sanchez JR, Vara-Thorbeck R, Garbin-Fuentes I, et al: Graves' ophthalmopathy after subtotal thyroidectomy and radioiodine therapy. Br J Surg 80:1134–1136, 1993.
51. Bartalena L, Pinchera A, Martino E, et al: Relation between therapy for hyperthyroidism and the course of Graves' ophthalmopathy. N Engl J Med 338:73–78, 1998.
52. Mendlovic DB, Saeed Zafar M: Ophthalmopathy after treatment for Graves' hyperthyroidism. N Engl J Med 327:1320, 1992.
53. Torring O, Hamberger B, Saaf M, et al: Graves' hyperthyroidism: Treatment with antithyroid drugs, surgery, or radioiodine—a prospective, randomized study. Thyroid Study Group. J Clin Endocrinol Metab 81:2986–2993, 1996.
54. Tallstedt L, Lundell G: Radioiodine treatment, ablation, and ophthalmopathy: A balanced perspective. Thyroid 7:241–245, 1997.
55. Tallstedt L: Ophthalmopathy after treatment for Graves' hyperthyroidism. N Engl J Med 327:1321, 1992.
56. Gorman CA, Offord K: Therapy for hyperthyroidism and Graves' ophthalmopathy. N Engl J Med 338:1546–1547, 1998.
57. Wartofsky L: Has the use of antithyroid drugs for Graves' disease become obsolete? Thyroid 3:335–344, 1993.
58. Wiersinga WM: Preventing Graves' ophthalmopathy. N Engl J Med 338:121–122, 1998.
59. Weetman AP, Wiersinga WM: Current management of thyroid-associated ophthalmopathy in Europe. Results of an international survey. Clin Endocrinol (Oxf) 49:21–28, 1998.
60. Wartofsky L, Glinoer D, Solomon B, et al: Differences and similarities in the diagnosis and treatment of Graves' disease in Europe, Japan, and the United States. Thyroid 1:129–135, 1991.
61. Bartalena L, Marcocci C, Bogazzi F, et al: Use of corticosteroids to prevent progression of Graves' ophthalmopathy after radioiodine therapy for hyperthyroidism. N Engl J Med 321:1349–1352, 1989.
62. Bartalena L, Pinchera A, Martino E, et al: Relation between therapy for hyperthyroidism and the course of Graves' ophthalmopathy. N Engl J Med 338:73–78, 1998.
63. Bahn RS, Heufelder AE: Pathogenesis of Graves' ophthalmopathy. N Engl J Med 329:1468–1475, 1993.
64. Heufelder AE: Pathogenesis of Graves' ophthalmopathy: Recent controversies and progress. Eur J Endocrinol 132:532–541, 1995.
65. Delemarre FG, Drexhage HA, Simons PJ: Histomorphological aspects of the development of thyroid autoimmune diseases: Consequences for our understanding of endocrine ophthalmopathy. Thyroid 6:369–377, 1996.
66. Heufelder AE, Scriba PC, Wenzel BE: Antigen receptor variable region repertoires expressed by T cells infiltrating thyroid, retroorbital, and pretibial tissue in Graves' disease. J Clin Endocrinol Metab 81:3733–3739, 1996.
67. de Carli M, del Prete G, Romagnani S, et al: Cytolytic T cells with Th1-like cytokine profile predominate in retroorbital lymphocytic infiltrates of Graves' ophthalmopathy. J Clin Endocrinol Metab 77:1120–1121, 1993.
68. McLachlan SM, Rapoport B, Prummel MF: Cell-mediated or humoral immunity in Graves' ophthalmopathy? Profiles of T-cell cytokines amplified by polymerase chain reaction from orbital tissue. J Clin Endocrinol Metab 78:1070–1074, 1994.
69. Forster G, Kahaly G, Ochs K, et al: Analysis of orbital T cells in thyroid-associated ophthalmopathy. Clin Exp Immunol 112:427–434, 1998.
70. Pappa A, Lightman S, Weetman AP, et al: Analysis of extraocular muscle-infiltrating T cells in thyroid-associated ophthalmopathy (TAO). Clin Exp Immunol 109:362–369, 1997.
71. Riley FC: Orbital pathology in Graves' disease. Mayo Clin Proc 47:975–979, 1972.
72. Otto EA, Kahaly GJ, Wall JR, et al: Orbital tissue–derived T lymphocytes from patients with Graves' ophthalmopathy recognize autologous orbital antigens. J Clin Endocrinol Metab 81:3045–3050, 1996.
73. Smith TJ, Bahn RS, Gorman CA, Cheavens M: Stimulation of glycosaminoglycan accumulation by interferon gamma in human cultured retroocular fibroblasts. J Clin Endocrinol Metab 72:1169–1171, 1991.
74. Burch HB, Sellitti D, Barnes SG, et al: TSH receptor antisera for the detection of immunoreactive protein species in retroocular fibroblasts obtained from patients with Graves' ophthalmopathy. J Clin Endocrinol Metab 78:1384–1391, 1994.
75. Heufelder AE: Involvement of the orbital fibroblast and TSH receptor in the pathogenesis of Graves' ophthalmopathy. Thyroid 5:331–340, 1995.
76. Kubota S, Wall J, Hiromatsu Y, et al: The 64-kilodalton eye muscle protein is the flavoprotein subunit of mitochondrial succinate dehydrogenase: The corresponding serum antibodies are good markers of an immune-mediated damage to the eye muscle in patients with Graves' hyperthyroidism. J Clin Endocrinol Metab 83:443–447, 1998.
77. Bernard NF, Nygen TN, Tyutyunikov A, et al: Antibodies against 1D, a recombinant 64-kDa membrane protein, are associated with ophthalmopathy in patients with thyroid autoimmunity. Clin Immunol Immunopathol 70:225–233, 1994.
78. Bahn RS, Gorman CA, Johnson CM, Smith TJ: Presence of antibodies in the sera of patients of patients with Graves' disease recognizing a 23 kilodalton fibroblast protein. J Clin Endocrinol Metab 69:622–628, 1989.
79. Mengistu M, Lukes YG, Nagy EV, et al: TSH receptor gene expression in retroocular fibroblasts. J Endocrinol Invest 17:437–441, 1994.
80. Heufelder AE, Dutton CM, Sarkar G, et al: Detection of TSH receptor RNA in cultured fibroblasts from patients with Graves' ophthalmopathy and pretibial dermopathy. Thyroid 3:297–300, 1993.
81. Bahn RS, Heufelder AE, Spitzweg C, et al: Thyrotropin receptor expression in Graves' orbital adipose/connective tissues: Potential autoantigen in Graves' ophthalmopathy. J Clin Endocrinol Metab 83:998–1002, 1998.
82. Feliciello A, Fenzi G, Avvedimento EV, et al: Expression of thyrotropin-receptor mRNA in healthy and Graves' disease retro-orbital tissue. Lancet 342:337–338, 1993.
83. Stadlmayr W, Heufelder AE, Bichlmair AM, Spitzweg C: TSH receptor transcripts and TSH receptor–like immunoreactivity in orbital and pretibial fibroblasts of patients with Graves' ophthalmopathy and pretibial myxedema. Thyroid 7:3–12, 1997.
84. Perros P, Kendall-Taylor P: Demonstration of thyrotropin binding sites in orbital connective tissue: Possible role in the pathogenesis of thyroid-associated ophthalmopathy. J Endocrinol Invest 17:163–170, 1994.
85. Erie JC: Ophthalmic history and examination. *In* Bartley BG, Liesegang TJ (eds): Essentials of Ophthalmology. Philadelphia, JB Lippincott, 1992, pp 3–25.
86. Bartley GB, Waller RR: Graves' ophthalmopathy. *In* van Heerden JA (ed): Common Problems in Endocrine Surgery. Chicago, Year Book, 1989, pp 25–29.
87. Gorman CA: The measurement of change in Graves' ophthalmopathy. Thyroid 8:539–543, 1998.

88. Anonymous: Classification of eye changes of Graves' disease. Thyroid 2:235–236, 1992.
89. Fells P: Management of dysthyroid eye disease. Br J Ophthalmol 75:245–246, 1991.
90. Neigel JM, Rootman J, Belkin RI, et al: Dysthyroid optic neuropathy. The crowded orbital apex syndrome. Ophthalmology 95:1515–1521, 1988.
91. Bahn RS, Garrity JA, Bartley GB, Gorman CA: Diagnostic evaluation of Graves' ophthalmopathy. Endocrinol Metab Clin North Am 17:527–545, 1988.
92. Bartley GB, Gorman CA: Diagnostic criteria for Graves' ophthalmopathy. Am J Ophthalmol 119:792–795, 1995.
93. Bartley GB, Fatourechi V, Kadrmas EF, et al: Clinical features of Graves' ophthalmopathy in an incidence cohort. Am J Ophthalmol 121:284–290, 1996.
94. Feldon SE, Levin L: Graves' ophthalmopathy: V. Etiology of upper eyelid retraction in Graves' ophthalmopathy. Br J Ophthalmol 74:484–485, 1991.
95. Bahn RS, Bartley GB, Gorman CA: Emergency treatment of Graves' ophthalmopathy. Ballieres Clin Endocrinol Metab 6:95–105, 1992.
96. Bogren HG, Franti CE, Wilmarth SS: Normal variations of the position of the eye in the orbit. Ophthalmology 93:1072–1077, 1986.
97. Werner SC: Modification of the classification of the eye changes of Graves' disease: Recommendations of the ad hoc committee of the American Thyroid Association. J Clin Endocrinol Metab 44:203–204, 1977.
98. Migliori ME, Gladstone GJ: Determination of the normal range of exophthalmometric values for black and white adults. Am J Ophthalmol 98:438–442, 1984.
99. Amino N, Yuasa T, Yabu Y, et al: Exophthalmos in autoimmune thyroid disease. J Clin Endocrinol Metab 51:1232–1234, 1980.
100. Salvi M, Zhang Z-G, Haegert D, et al: Patients with endocrine ophthalmopathy not associated with overt thyroid disease have multiple thyroid immunological abnormalities. J Clin Endocrinol Metab 70:89–94, 1990.
101. Mourits MPH, Koornneef L, Wiersinga WM, et al: Clinical criteria for the assessment of disease activity in Graves' ophthalmopathy: A novel approach. Br J Ophthalmol 73:639–644, 1989.
102. Waller RR, Jacobson DH: Endocrine ophthalmopathy: Differential diagnosis. *In* Gorman CA, Campbell RJ, Dyer JA (eds): The Eye and Orbit in Thyroid Disease. New York, Raven Press, 1984, pp 213–220.
103. Bartley GB: The differential diagnosis and classification of eyelid retraction. Ophthalmology 103:168–176, 1996.
104. Gonnering RS: Pseudoretraction of the eyelid in thyroid-associated orbitopathy. Arch Ophthalmol 106:1078–1080, 1988.
105. Werner SC, Coleman DJ, Frazen LA: Ultrasonographic evidence of a consistent orbital involvement in Graves' disease. N Engl J Med 290:1447–1450, 1974.
106. Merlis AL, Schaiberger CL, Adler R: External carotid-cavernous sinus fistula simulating unilateral Graves' ophthalmopathy. J Comput Assist Tomogr 6:1006–1009, 1982.
107. Marino M, Mariotti S, Muratorio A, et al: Mild clinical expression of myasthenia gravis associated with autoimmune thyroid diseases. J Clin Endocrinol Metab 82:438–443, 1997.
108. Bartley GB, Fatourechi V, Kadrmas EF, et al: Long-term follow-up of Graves ophthalmopathy in an incidence cohort. Ophthalmology 103:958–962, 1996.
109. Perros P, Kendall-Taylor P, Crombie AL: Natural history of thyroid associated ophthalmopathy. Clin Endocrinol (Oxf) 42:45–50, 1995.
110. Jacobson DH, Gorman CA: Diagnosis and management of Graves' ophthalmopathy. Med Clin North Am 69:973 988, 1985.
111. Weetman AP, Wiersinga WM: Current management of thyroid-associated ophthalmopathy in Europe. Results of an international study. Clin Endocrinol 49:21–28, 1998.
112. Martin B, Jay B: Use of guanethidine eye drops in dysthyroid lid retraction. Proc R Soc Med 62:18–19, 1969.
113. Sisson JC: Stimulation of glucose utilization and glycosaminoglycan production by fibroblasts derived from retrobulbar tissue. Exp Eye Res 12:285–292, 1971.
114. Smith TJ, Bahn RS, Gorman CA: Connective tissue, glycosaminoglycans, and diseases of the thyroid. Endocr Rev 10:366–391, 1989.
115. Smith TJ: Dexamethasone regulation of glycosaminoglycan synthesis in cultured human skin fibroblasts: Similar effects of glucocorticoid and thyroid hormone therapy. J Clin Invest 74:2157–2163, 1984.
116. Wiersinga WM: Immunosuppressive treatment of Graves' ophthalmopathy. Trends Endocrinol Metab 1:377–381, 1990.
117. Burman KD: Treatment of autoimmune ophthalmopathy. Endocrinologist 1:102–110, 1991.
118. Reference deleted.
119. Marcocci C, Bartalena L, Panicucci M, et al: Orbital cobalt irradiation combined with retrobulbar or systemic corticosteroids for Graves' ophthalmopathy: A comparative study. Clin Endocrinol 27:33–42, 1987.
120. Yamamoto K, Saito K, Takai T, Yoshida S: Treatment of Graves' ophthalmopathy by steroid therapy, orbital radiation therapy, plasmapheresis, and thyroxine replacement. Endocrinol Jpn 29:495–501, 1982.
121. Kahaly G, Beyer J: Immunosuppressant therapy of thyroid eye disease. Klin Wochenschr 66:1049–1059, 1988.
122. Nagayama Y, Izumi M, Kiriyama T, et al: Treatment of Graves' ophthalmopathy with high-dose intravenous methylprednisolone pulse therapy. Acta Endocrinol (Copenh) 116:513–518, 1987.
123. Kendall-Taylor P, Crombie AL, Stephenson AM, et al: Intravenous methylprednisolone in the treatment of Graves' ophthalmopathy. BMJ 297:1574–1578, 1988.
124. Guy JR, Fagien S, Donovan JP, Rubin ML: Methylprednisolone pulse therapy in severe dysthyroid optic neuropathy. Ophthalmology 96:1048–1053, 1989.
125. Kendall-Taylor P, Crombie AL, Perros P: High-dose intravenous methylprednisolone pulse therapy in severe thyroid-associated ophthalmopathy (abstract). Thyroid 2(suppl 1):29, 1992.
126. Mourits MP, Koornneef L, Wiersinga WM, et al: Clinical criteria for the assessment of disease activity in Graves' ophthalmopathy: A novel approach. Br J Ophthalmol 73:639–644, 1989.
127. Laitt RD, Hoh B, Wakeley C, et al: The value of short tau inversion recovery sequence in magnetic resonance imaging of thyroid eye disease. Br J Radiol 67:244–247, 1994.
128. Hiromatsu Y, Kojima K, Ishisaka N, et al: Role of magnetic resonance imaging in thyroid-associated ophthalmopathy: Its predictive value for therapeutic outcome of immunosuppressive therapy. Thyroid 2:299–305, 1992.
129. Moncayo R, Donnemiller E, Kendler D, et al: Evaluation of immunological mechanisms mediating thyroid-associated ophthalmopathy by radionuclide imaging using the somatostatin analog ^{111}In-octreotide. Thyroid 7:21–29, 1997.
130. Kahaly G, Bockisch A, Hommel G, et al: Indium-111-pentetreotide in Graves' disease. J Nucl Med 39:533–536, 1998.
131. Wiersinga WM: Novel drugs for the therapy of Graves' ophthalmopathy. *In* Wall JR, How J (eds): Graves' Ophthalmopathy. Cambridge, Blackwell, 1990, pp 111–126.
132. Kahaly G, Schrezenmeir J, Krause U, et al: Ciclosporin and prednisone in treatment of Graves' ophthalmopathy: A controlled, randomized and prospective study. Eur J Clin Invest 16:415–422, 1986.
133. Prummel MF, Mourits MP, Berghout A, et al: Prednisone and cyclosporine in the treatment of severe Graves' ophthalmopathy. N Engl J Med 321:1353–1359, 1989.
134. Krassas GE, Kaltsas T, Pontikides N, Dumas A: Somatostatin receptor scintigraphy and octreotide treatment in patients with thyroid eye disease. Clin Endocrinol (Oxf) 42:571–580, 1995.
135. Krassas GE, Tolis G, Pontikides N, et al: Lanreotide in the treatment of patients with thyroid eye disease. Eur J Endocrinol 136:416–422, 1997.
136. Chang TC, Kao SCS, Huang KM: Octreotide and Graves' ophthalmopathy and pretibial myxoedema. BMJ 304:158, 1992.
137. Sautter-Bihl M-L: Orbital radiotherapy: Recent experience in Europe. *In* Wall JR, How J (eds): Graves' Ophthalmopathy. Cambridge, Blackwell, 1990, pp 145–157.
138. Sautter-Bihl M-L, Heinze HG: Radiotherapy of Graves' ophthalmopathy. Dev Ophthalmol 20:139–154, 1989.
139. Palmer D, Greenberg P, Cornwell P, Parker RG: Radiation therapy for Graves' ophthalmopathy: A retrospective analysis. Int J Radiat Oncol Biol Phys 13:1815–1820, 1987.
140. Pigeon P, Orgiazzi J, Berthezene F, et al: High voltage orbital radiotherapy and surgical orbital decompression in the management of Graves' ophthalmopathy. Horm Res 26:172–176, 1987.
141. Kriss JP, Peterson IA, Donaldson SS, McDougall IR: Supervoltage orbital radiotherapy for progressive Graves' ophthalmopathy: Results of a twenty year experience. Acta Endocrinol (Copenh) 121(suppl 2):154, 1989.
142. Peterson IA, Kriss JP, McDougall IR, Donaldson SS: Prognostic factors in the radiotherapy of Graves' ophthalmopathy. Int J Radiat Oncol Biol Phys 19:259–264, 1990.
143. Wilson WB, Prochoda M: Radiotherapy for thyroid orbitopathy. Effects on extraocular muscle balance. Arch Ophthalmol 113:1420–1425, 1995.
144. Wiersinga W, Prummel MF: Therapeutic controversies. Retrobulbar radiation in Graves' ophthalmopathy. J Clin Endocrinol Metab 80:345–347, 1995.
145. Prummel MF, Mourits MP, Blank L, et al: Randomized double-blind trial of prednisone versus radiotherapy in Graves' ophthalmopathy. Lancet 342:949–954, 1993.
146. Bartalena L, Marcocci C, Chiovato L, et al: Orbital cobalt irradiation combined with systemic corticosteroids for Graves' ophthalmopathy: Comparison with systemic corticosteroids alone. J Clin Endocrinol Metab 56:1139–1144, 1983.
147. Kinyoun JL, Kalina RE, Brower SA, et al: Radiation retinopathy following orbital irradiation for Graves' ophthalmopathy. Arch Ophthalmol 102:1473–1476, 1984.
148. Parsons JT, Fitzgerald CR, Hood CI, et al: The effects of irradiation on the eye and optic nerve. Int J Radiat Oncol Biol Phys 9:609–622, 1983.
149. Kahaly G, Hommel G, Muller-Forell W, Pitz S: Randomized trial of intravenous immunoglobulins versus prednisolone in Graves' ophthalmopathy. Clin Exp Immunol 106:197–202, 1996.
150. Balazs C, Farid NR, Molnar I, et al: Beneficial effect of pentoxifylline on thyroid associated ophthalmopathy: A pilot study. J Clin Endocrinol Metab 82:1999–2002, 1997.
151. Lyons CJ, Vickers SF, Lee JP: Botulinum toxin therapy in dysthyroid strabismus. Eye 4:538–540, 1990.
152. Lopatynsky MO, Krohel GB: Bromocriptine therapy for thyroid ophthalmopathy. Am J Ophthalmol 107:680–681, 1989.
153. Harden RM, Chisholm CJS, Cant JS: The effect of metronidazole on thyroid function and exophthalmos in man. Metabolism 16:890–898, 1967.
154. Zesen W, Shubai J, Zutong Z: The effect of acupuncture in 40 cases of endocrine ophthalmopathy. J Trad Chin Med 5:19–21, 1985.
155. Rogvi-Hansen B, Perrild H, Christensen T, et al: Acupuncture in the treatment of Graves' ophthalmopathy. A blinded randomized study. Acta Endocrinol (Copenh) 124:143–145, 1991.
156. Bartley GB, Fatourechi V, Kadrmas EF, et al: The treatment of Graves' ophthalmopathy in an incidence cohort. Am J Ophthalmol 121:200–206, 1996.
157. Kazim M, Trokel S, Moore S: Treatment of acute Graves' orbitopathy. Ophthalmology 98:1443–1448, 1991.
158. Fatourechi V, Garrity JA, Bartley GB, et al: Graves' ophthalmopathy. Results of transantral orbital decompression performed primarily for cosmetic indications. Ophthalmology 101:938–942, 1994.
159. Hallin ES, Feldon SE: Graves' ophthalmopathy: I. Simple CT estimates of extraocular muscle volume. Br J Ophthalmol 72:674–677, 1988.
160. Hallin ES, Feldon SE: Graves' ophthalmopathy: II. Correlation of clinical signs with measures derived from computed tomography. Br J Ophthalmol 72:678–682, 1988.
161. Anderson RL, Tweeten JP, Patrinely JR, et al: Dysthyroid optic neuropathy without extraocular muscle involvement. Ophthalmic Surg 20:568–574, 1989.
162. Wilson WB, Manke WF: Orbital decompression in Graves' disease. The predictability of reduction of proptosis. Arch Ophthalmol 109:334–345, 1991.
163. Mourits MPH, Koornneef L, Wiersinga WM, et al: Orbital decompression for Graves' ophthalmopathy by inferomedial, by inferomedial plus lateral, and by coronal approach. Ophthalmology 97:636–641, 1990.

164. DeSanto LW, Gorman CA: Selection of patients and choice of operation for orbital decompression in Graves' ophthalmopathy. Laryngoscope 83:945–959, 1973.
165. DeSanto LW: The total rehabilitation of Graves' ophthalmopathy. Laryngoscope 90:1652–1678, 1980.
166. Gorman CA, DeSanto LW, MacCarty CS, Riley FC: Optic neuropathy of Graves's disease. Treatment by transantral or transfrontal orbital decompression. N Engl J Med 290:70–75, 1974.
167. Garrity JA, Fatourechi V, Bergstralh EJ, et al: Results of transantral orbital decompression in 428 patients with severe Graves' ophthalmopathy. Am J Ophthalmol 116:533–547, 1993.
168. Frueh BR, Musch DC, Garber FW: Exophthalmometer readings in patients with Graves' eye disease. Ophthalmic Surg 17:37–40, 1986.
169. Dyer JA: Ocular muscle surgery. *In* Gorman CA, Campbell RJ, Dyer JA (eds): The Eye and Orbit in Thyroid Disease. New York, Raven Press, 1984, pp 253–262.
170. Bartley GB: The eyelids in Graves' ophthalmopathy. *In* Bosniak S (ed): Principles and Practice of Ophthalmic Plastic Reconstructive Surgery. Philadelphia, WB Saunders, 1997, pp 514–524.

Chapter 102

Autonomously Functioning Thyroid Nodules and Other Causes of Thyrotoxicosis

Georg Hennemann

Thyrotoxicosis literally means poisoning by thyroid hormone. The term includes any situation in a patient who shows clinical and/or biochemical characteristics of overactivity of thyroid hormone. Thus it involves not only hyperfunction of the thyroid gland, termed hyperthyroidism, but also any other condition with elevated thyroid hormone levels in combination with characteristics of overactivity of thyroid hormones. For instance, when thyroid hormones leak from the thyroid gland because of infectious or other damaging processes or is produced outside the thyroid gland in toxic amounts (struma ovarii, thyroid carcinoma metastasis) or ingested in overdose, thyrotoxicosis may ensue. In thyrotoxicosis, free hormone levels are invariably increased. The reverse is not true in that increased free thyroid hormone levels do not always point to thyrotoxicosis. In resistance to thyroid hormones (see Chapter 114), increased free hormone levels are present while the patients are clinically euthyroid or even sometimes hypothyroid.

The following causes of thyrotoxicosis are distinguished and will be discussed in this chapter in so far they are not dealt with in other chapters.

Graves' disease: see Chapter 100
Toxic multinodular goiter: see Chapter 107
Subacute (de Quervain's) thyroiditis: see Chapter 104
Hashimoto's thyroiditis: see Chapter 103
Congenital hyperthyroidism: see Chapters 111–114
Autonomously functioning thyroid nodules (AFTNs)
Silent or painless thyroiditis
Thyrotoxicosis factitia
Thyrotoxicosis caused by pregnancy and trophoblastic disease
Iodine-induced thyrotoxicosis (IIT)
Hyperthyroidism caused by inappropriate thyroid-stimulating hormone (TSH) secretion
Thyrotoxicosis caused by metastatic thyroid carcinoma
Struma ovarii

AUTONOMOUSLY FUNCTIONING THYROID NODULES

AFTNs are defined as (mostly) single nodules present in the thyroid gland that produce and secrete thyroid hormone independent of stimulation by TSH. On statistical grounds, these nodules are almost always adenoma and seldom carcinoma (see below). For that reason the term autonomously functioning adenoma is often used synonymously. From a functional point of view, three types of AFTN are differentiated: a toxic, hot, and warm nodule. Both toxic and hot nodules accumulate more radioactivity on scintiscan than the surrounding (normal) tissue. The patient is thyrotoxic in the first case, but euthyroid in the latter. When the nodule is warm, radioactivity in the nodule is similar to that in the surrounding tissue, in a euthyroid patient.

Epidemiology and Natural History

About 5% to 10% of solitary thyroid nodules are toxic. This figure varies from country to country and is higher in Europe.[1, 2] In nodules with a diameter of less than 2.5 cm, the percentage that are toxic is only 1.9, whereas in nodules of 2.5 cm or greater, this figure is 42.6%. In a study of patients 60 years and older with AFTNs, 57% were thyrotoxic. In patients younger than 60 years, thyrotoxicity was noted in only 13%. In patients younger than 40 years, only 19.5% had AFTNs with a diameter of 3 cm or larger, but in older patients this figure was 45.9%.[1] The proportion of AFTNs that are responsible for the hyperthyroidism of referred patients varies geographically between 1.5% and 44.5% (Table 102–1). About five times more women than men suffer from this disorder.[3] The natural history of the growth of AFTNs varies. They may stay the same over the years, grow, or shrink. In a group of 159 patients observed for 1 to 15 years, an increase in size was seen in 10% and a decrease in 4%.[1] Changes in function of the nodule over the years also occur. In an observation period of 6 years, 10% of patients with AFTNs became toxic, and loss of function because of degeneration was observed in 4%.[1] Development of hyperthyroidism predominantly occurred in nodules greater than 3 cm in diameter,[1] with a minimal volume of 16 mL by ultrasound.[4]

Pathogenesis

From a histologic point of view, two types of nodules (Figs. 102–1 and 102–2) may be discerned: a monoclonal and a polyclonal type.[5, 6] Studer and his group developed the concept that even if monoclonal at the molecular level, nodules may become polyclonal from a functional and histologic aspect during evolution. They suggest that individual follicular cells may acquire new qualities that were not present

TABLE 102–1. Frequency of Toxic Adenoma in Various Countries

Location	Period	No. of Toxic Patients	% of Toxic Adenomas
Europe			
Austria	1966–1968	821	44.5
England	1948	107	3.7
Finland	1996	125	18
France			
Paris	1962	24	11.7
Marseilles	1964	537	
Montpellier	1965–1967	240	24
Germany	1965	350	19.7
Greece	1968	686	9.5
Italy	1968	1121	11.4
Switzerland	1967	—	33
General survey	1968	924	27.9*
North America			
Cleveland	1962	2846†	1.6
New York	1944	2431‡	1.5
Rochester	1912	1627	23.9
Rochester	1954–1965	215	15.8
Southfield, MI	1961–1979	—	2
Australia			
Tasmania	1973§	88	17

*Patients younger than 50 years.
†Graves' disease plus toxic adenoma.
‡Thyrotoxicosis submitted to surgery.
§Six years after bread iodination.
From Orgiazzi JJ, Mornex R: Hyperthyroidism. *In* Greer MA (ed): The Thyroid Gland. New York, Raven, 1990, p 442.

in the mother cells but become inheritable during further replication. Obviously, this change supposes some sort of genetic event. This sequence of events may lead to loss of anatomic and functional integrity of the follicular cells. The process may be accelerated by stimulatory factors such as TSH (e.g., in iodine deficiency, by goitrogens) and by local stimulatory and growth factors.[7]

At the genetic level, two types of monoclonal autonomously functioning nodules have been reported. Both are somatic mutations. One involves the TSH receptor (TSH-R) gene and the other involves the $G_s\alpha$ protein gene. Both mutations lead to constitutive activation of the adenylate cyclase system, probably also activation of the inositol phosphates pathways[8] in the follicular cell, and to autonomy of the follicle. Mutations of the TSH-R gene have thus far been found more frequently than mutations of the $G_s\alpha$ gene. When 13 AFTNs were screened for somatic mutations in the $G_s\alpha$ gene at codons 201 and 227, constitutive activating mutations were found in 5. None was found in 16 nonfunctioning adenomas.[8] Thirty-three toxic adenomas from 31 Belgian patients were analyzed for mutations in the TSH-R and $G_s\alpha$ genes. In 27 toxic adenomas, 12 different mutations were detected in the TSH-R gene and 2 in the $G_s\alpha$ gene, and in 4 toxic adenomas no mutations were found.[9] In a Japanese study investigating mutations in the "hot spots" of the TSH-R gene (i.e., coding for the third cytoplasmic loop and the sixth transmembrane segment) in 38 patients with AFTNs, only 1 nonfunctional mutation was found.[10] Apparently, racial differences are present in the frequency of TSH-R gene mutations, at least with regard to the nucleotide loci investigated. In Austria, mutations were found in 18% of AFTNs, in these same locations of the TSH-R gene.[11] Because 16 different activating mutations were identified in the TSH-R gene, Van der Sande et al. hypothesized that the wild-type TSH-R is in a constrained conformation.[12] The authors concluded that the C-terminal portion of the large extracellular domain plays a role in maintenance of this constraint. Further studies from the same group indicated that the first and second extracellular loops contributed to silencing of the non–ligand-bound receptor and that the activating mutations are distributed over the first and second extracellular loops, the third intracellular loop, and the third, sixth, and seventh transmembrane segments.[9] Apart from these gain of function TSH-R and $G_s\alpha$ gene mutations causing toxic adenoma, the natural heterogeneity of thyrocytes responding to these mutations may play a role in the phenotypic expression of the abnormality, which may affect the degree of (hyper)function and histomorphology in the sense of monoclonal or polyclonal outgrowth of the nodule.[5, 6, 13]

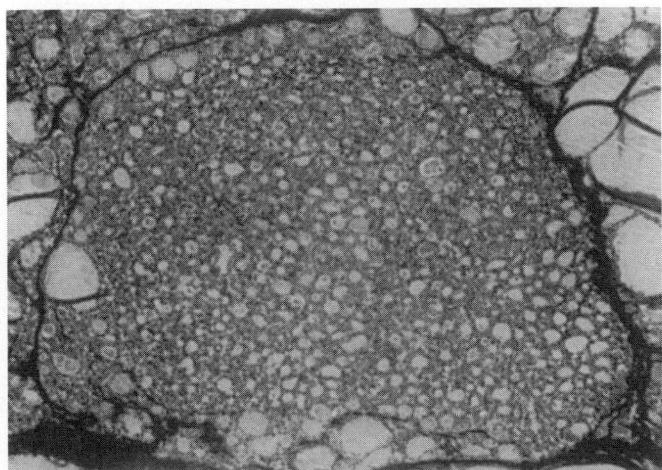

FIGURE 102–1. Uniform nature of cells formed in a nodule by proliferation of only one or a few clones of epithelial cells. (From Studer H, Ramelli F: Simple goiter and its variants: Euthyroid and hyperthyroid multinodular goiters. Endocr Rev 3:40, © 1982, The Endocrine Society.)

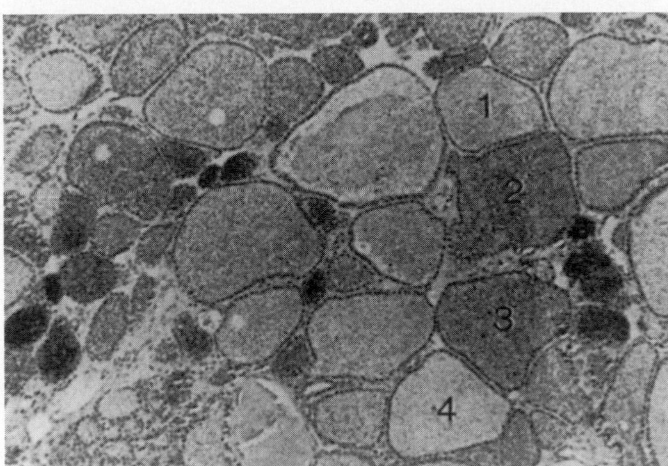

FIGURE 102–2. Autoradiograph of a hot nodule illustrating areas with different capacity of uptake of radioiodine. (From Studer H, Gerber H, Peter HJ: Multinodular goiter. *In* DeGroot LJ (ed): Endocrinology, vol 1, ed 2. Philadelphia, WB Saunders, 1989, p 722.)

Pathology

On macroscopic examination, a solitary toxic nodule is surrounded by normal thyroid tissue that is functionally suppressed. Rarely, a microscopically monotonous picture is seen that consists of uniform follicular cells without signs of malignancy. Usually the picture is heterogeneous with cells of different size, sometimes with signs of fresh and old hemorrhage and calcification. This picture, however, does not exclude a monoclonal origin of the nodule but may be the result of stimulatory local growth factors (see Pathogenesis). No information is available at present on the exact ratio between primarily monoclonal and polyclonal AFTNs of the thyroid. Sometimes, autonomously functioning micronodules are present in the surrounding thyroid tissue. This finding is in agreement with the thesis of Studer et al. that the true adenoma is one end of a large spectrum of thyroid nodules growing from single thyrocytes or tiny cell families, each replicating with an individual growth rate, whereas the grossly abnormal multinodular goiter is at the other end of the scale.[5, 6]

Clinical Features

The signs and symptoms of patients with toxic adenoma are those of thyrotoxicosis, without the specific signs of Graves' disease, such as eye signs, pretibial myxedema, and acropachy (see Chapter 100). On palpation of the thyroid region, a nodule is found in one of the lobes, with a diameter of usually 3 cm or larger.[1] The thyroid tissue surrounding the nodule and the thyroid lobe on the other side are not usually palpable because of TSH suppression.

Laboratory Diagnosis

When a single nodule is found in the thyroid, and the patient is clinically thyrotoxic, estimation of serum TSH is sufficient for the diagnosis of toxic adenoma. To have an idea about the severity of the thyrotoxicosis, estimation of serum free thyroxine (T_4) is sufficient. If this parameter is normal, serum triiodothyronine (T_3) or free T_3 should be determined because it may be solely elevated in minimal thyrotoxicosis, that is, T_3 toxicosis. If findings on palpation are inconclusive, it is wise to perform a scintiscan of the thyroid. In the case of a toxic nodule, activity is seen in the nodule with minimal or no activity anywhere else in the thyroid region (Fig. 102–3). The presence of a thyroid carcinoma in an AFTN is rare.[14] Although some authors are of the opinion that the occurrence of carcinoma in an AFTN may be more than coincidental,[15] most thyroidologists believe that such is not the case. The differential diagnosis of a toxic nodule includes relapse of hyperthyroid Graves' disease in remnant thyroid tissue after thyroid surgery or in thyroid dysgenesis. The latter possibility is especially remote. Theoretically, a TSH stimulation test would distinguish between an AFTN and the two other possibilities, but this test is hardly ever necessary in clinical practice. It is of no value to perform fine-needle aspiration cytology of an AFTN because differentiation between a follicular adenoma and carcinoma is difficult if not impossible with this technique. When a hot nodule is present, that is, prominent uptake in the nodule but less in the surrounding tissue while serum TSH is normal, autonomous function can be tested by performing a T_3 or T_4 suppression test. In the case of autonomous function, uptake in the nodule is still present after the administration of 25 μg T_3 three times daily for 10 days or 125 μg T_4 for 14 days, whereas uptake is suppressed in the surrounding tissue. Sometimes uptake in a single nodule is indistinguishable from uptake in the surrounding tissue, a situation described as a "warm" nodule. This picture may be generated either by normal affinity of the nodular tissue for the isotope or because a nonfunctioning nodule is surrounded by normal thyroid tissue. Thus the possibility of the presence of a carcinoma in a warm nodule is certainly not excluded, which means that it should be evaluated as though it were a cold nodule (see Chapter 109).

Treatment

No treatment of a hot nodule is necessary as long as the patient remains euthyroid. Regular TSH measurement at intervals of a half to 1 year suffices. Most patients remain euthyroid. Occasionally, a hemorrhage in the nodule leads to spontaneous resolution. Treatment of toxic nodules with antithyroid drugs is useless because after discontinuation of medication, relapse invariably occurs. Three modes of treatment of toxic nodules include nodulectomy, administration of radioactive iodine, and percutaneous injection of alcohol into the nodule. Nodulectomy is very effective in rendering the patient euthyroid and has a low surgical complication rate. Surprisingly, permanent hypothyroidism develops in about 5% of patients, perhaps because of coexistent thyroid disease.[2, 16] Obviously, the disadvantages of surgery are its operative risks, the residual scar, and its cost, which is high relative to the other two forms of treatment.

Treatment with radioactive iodine is safe, cheap, and effective. Two reports indicate no risk of posttreatment hypothyroidism 6 months after treatment in a total of 93 patients.[17, 18] However, when a longer period of follow-up was taken into account in 23 patients, such as 4 to 16.5 years after treatment, hypothyroidism developed in up to 36%.[19] In another study of 126 patients with autonomously functioning nodules, the percentage of hypothyroidism after a mean period of 10 years was 9.7% when the nodules were hot and 1.5% when toxic.[20] In this and the previous study no relationship was found between the total dose administered, the size of the nodule, and the development of hypothyroidism. However, if thyroid autoantibodies were present, hypothyroidism occurred in 18% of patients and, when absent, in 1.4%.[20] It is important that when ^{131}I is administered, uptake be present only in the nodule and not in the surrounding tissue or in the other lobe, which could occur after pretreatment with antithyroid drugs. To avoid this complication, pretreatment with T_3 or T_4 might be considered. In some patients typical Graves' disease has developed months after treatment of a toxic nodule with ^{131}I. Possibly antigens released by the ^{131}I therapy induce or exacerbate an autoimmune response.

The third treatment modality is of rather recent date and involves percutaneous alcohol injection into the nodule. Euthyroidism is achieved in 65% to 85% of patients by 12 months after treatment. Injections are repeated 2 to 12 times at weekly intervals. The treatment is usually well tolerated, with few side effects. When nodule volume exceeds 15 mL, results are less favorable.[21, 22] All three treatment

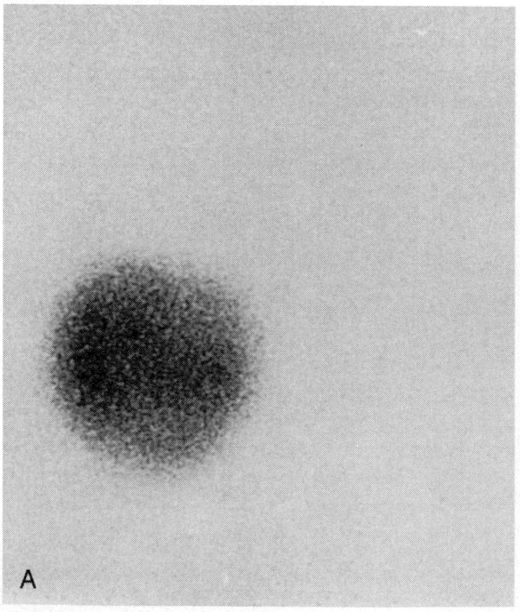

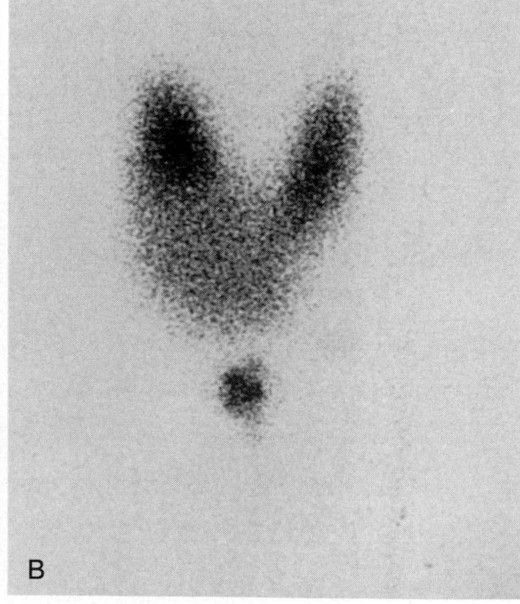

FIGURE 102–3. Thyroid with toxic nodule before *(A)* and after *(B)* treatment with ^{131}I.

modalities are acceptable, with the choice depending on local circumstances and the patient's preference.

SILENT OR PAINLESS THYROIDITIS

Silent thyroiditis is an autoimmune thyroiditis that usually comes to clinical attention because of symptoms of thyrotoxicosis caused by leakage of thyroid hormone from a painless thyroid gland. The condition often occurs in the postpartum period.

Incidence

The incidence varies geographically. In 1980 this syndrome accounted for 10% of cases of thyrotoxicosis in Japan, but only 3% to 4% in New York City.[23, 24] A random poll showed that silent thyroiditis was uncommon in Argentina, Europe, and the east and the west coast of the United States, but it occurred more frequently around the Great Lakes and in Canada.[25] Patients are usually between 30 and 60 years old, and the female-to-male ratio is 1.5 to 1. Apart from its association with pregnancy, known then as postpartum thyroiditis, the condition is currently rarely diagnosed. Postpartum thyroiditis occurs in 5% to 9% of women in the first year after delivery, especially in those who have circulating autoantibodies against thyroperoxidase.[26]

Etiology

Silent thyroiditis is an autoimmune lymphocytic thyroiditis, and many patients with this disease have a family history of thyroid disease. Postpartum thyroiditis has been significantly associated with HLA-D3 and HLA-D5.[27] Exposure to iodine, such as in the form of amiodarone, or to lithium, interleukin-2, and interferon has been suggested as an initiating event.[28–30] Silent thyroiditis is associated with other autoimmune diseases such as rheumatoid arthritis, systemic sclerosis, Graves' disease, primary adrenal insufficiency, and systemic lupus erythematosus.[31–35]

Pathology

Microscopically, follicles are disrupted and infiltration of lymphocytes and plasma cells occurs. The infiltration may be focal or diffuse, and sometimes formation of lymphoid follicles is seen. Follicular cells may be cuboidal or, when stimulated by TSH in the hypothyroid phase, columnar. Sometimes Hürthle or Askanazy cells are present. These cells are large and oxyphilic and contain many mitochondria. Thyroid tissue obtained during hypothyroidism or the recovery phase shows regenerating follicles with little colloid. Occasionally, persistent lymphocytic infiltration is observed. Extensive fibrosis may ultimately develop. A few multinucleated giant cells are regularly present.[36]

Clinical Features

The initial symptoms in 112 patients with 122 episodes of silent thyroiditis have been reviewed.[37] Characteristically, thyroid pain was absent in all cases. The female-to-male ratio was 1.3:1. The mean age (±SD) in females and males was 32 ± 8.5 and 24.9 ± 8.2 years, respectively. Recurrences were uncommon. The symptoms are similar to other causes of thyrotoxicosis and varied from mild to severe. Specific signs characteristic of Graves' disease, such as eye signs, pretibial myxedema, and acropachy, were absent. The mean duration of the toxic phase in these patients was 3.6 ± 2.0 months. In most reports the thyroid gland had a firm consistency. In about half the patients a goiter was present. The course of the disease follows four sequential stages (Fig. 102–4): thyrotoxicosis, euthyroidism, hypothyroidism, and euthyroidism. These stages need not necessarily to be present in all patients. In this series, 57 of 112 patients became euthyroid and hypothyroidism did not develop. In only 32 patients

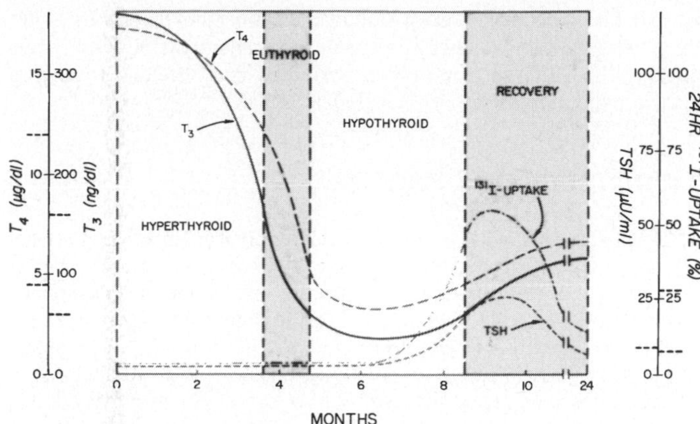

FIGURE 102–4. Schematic representation of the four phases of silent thyroiditis. (From Gegick CG, Harring WB: Painless subacute thyroiditis: A report of two cases. N C Med J 38:387, 1977.)

was clinical hypothyroidism present. Hypothyroidism was transient in 24 patients, but permanent in 8, who required thyroid hormone substitution. Ultimately, about half of the patients with silent thyroiditis become permanently hypothyroid.[38]

Laboratory Findings

The acute (first) phase of the disease is characterized by leakage of thyroid hormone and thyroglobulin from the damaged thyroid. This leakage results in elevated serum concentrations of thyroid hormones and thyroglobulin and suppression of serum TSH. Uptake of radioactive iodine by the thyroid is absent in this stage. The erythrocyte sedimentation rate (ESR) is mostly, but not always, slightly elevated. The ESR was elevated in 34 of 53 episodes but higher than 40 mm only in 8.[37] This result contrasts with subacute thyroiditis, in which the ESR is invariably much more elevated. T_4 and T_3 start to decline in the first phase and reach normal levels in the second (euthyroid) phase, but TSH remains suppressed. In the third (hypothyroid) phase, thyroid hormone levels are subnormal and serum TSH starts to rise at the end of this stage. Because of TSH stimulation, the fourth stage is characterized by normalization of serum T_4 and T_3. Serum TSH ultimately normalizes, but normalization may take several months, so temporary subclinical hypothyroidism intervenes. For the mean period of the different phases see Figure 102–4.

Treatment

The degree of thyrotoxicosis is usually mild in silent thyroiditis and treatment is not usually necessary. Prescription of β-adrenergic blocking agents may be considered. Antithyroid drugs have a very limited role because the thyrotoxicosis is not the result of increased thyroid hormone synthesis. Propylthiouracil or ipodate to block peripheral conversion of T_4 to T_3 may be of some value. In more serious cases, prednisone in a dose between 30 and 60 mg/day has a rapid ameliorating effect. The dose should be continued for 1 to 2 weeks and than slowly tapered.[39] In case of relapsing thyroiditis, prednisone can be reinstituted. It is seldom necessary to perform thyroidectomy. If necessary, radiochemical "thyroidectomy" may be contemplated during remission when sufficient thyroid uptake of radioactive iodine is present for effective treatment, often in the presence of prednisone administration. As stated, thyrotoxicosis is usually mild and "definitive" treatment seldom necessary. After the thyrotoxic phase, temporary hypothyroidism develops in about 40% of patients. If needed, thyroid hormone treatment can be instituted in a dose that allows TSH to remain mildly elevated to promote resumption of thyroid hormone synthesis in the recovery phase. Only a small proportion of patients (see above) need permanent and full-dose substitution at this stage. Finally, however, permanent hypothyroidism develops in about half of the patients. This result is in contrast to subacute thyroiditis, after which patients almost always become permanently euthyroid. Thus patients who suffered from silent thyroiditis need lifelong follow-up because hypothyroidism may develop years later.[40]

THYROTOXICOSIS FACTITIA

Thyrotoxicosis factitia is primarily a psychiatric disorder. Patients surreptitiously ingest thyroid hormone in excessive amounts. When confronted with the situation, they usually deny doing so. Physicians should be aware of the phenomenon or the diagnosis may be missed. Patients are usually overtly thyrotoxic but do not show eye signs, except those of sympathetic overactivity, such as eyelid retraction.

Other signs of Graves' disease such as eye signs, pretibial edema, acropachy, and goiter are also absent. Differentiation from Graves' disease is also feasible by color Doppler sonography, which shows absent thyroid vascularity and low-normal peak velocity, whereas these signs are increased in Graves' disease.[41] Because of TSH suppression, the thyroid shrinks and is often not palpable. Thyroid uptake of radioactive iodine is absent. Serum thyroglobulin is low or below detection limits in thyrotoxicosis factitia but elevated in silent thyroiditis. Factitious thyrotoxicosis is not difficult to distinguish from toxic multinodular goiter or toxic adenoma. Differentiation from subacute thyroiditis is easy on clinical grounds because these patients suffer from frequent severe pain in the thyroid region. Furthermore, the ESR and serum thyroglobulin concentration are elevated in subacute thyroiditis. The diagnosis of thyrotoxicosis factitia should be considered when laboratory results are contradictory. Psychiatric help is urgently needed for such patients.

Thyrotoxicosis caused by accidental intake of excessive amounts of thyroid hormone has been observed in the "hamburger toxicosis patients." Two epidemics were caused by the inclusion of bovine thyroid in hamburger.[42, 43]

THYROTOXICOSIS CAUSED BY PREGNANCY AND TROPHOBLASTIC DISEASE

Human chorionic gonadotropin (hCG) has intrinsic TSH-like activity. In about 2% to 3% of normal pregnancies, gestational transient thyrotoxicosis (GTT) is present because of elevated hCG serum concentrations. Familial gestational hyperthyroidism has recently been described and is caused by a missense mutation in the TSH-R that renders it hypersensitive to hCG. Thyrotoxicosis may also be induced by molar pregnancy and by trophoblastic disease in men and women.

TSH-like Activity of Human Chorionic Gonadotropin

The hCG from concentrated human pregnant urine has weak TSH-like activity when tested in a mouse bioassay.[44] The hCG purified from molar tissue has intrinsic TSH bioactivity in the same bioassay, although 4000 times less than that of human TSH on a molar basis.[45] However, when produced in sufficient amounts, it may induce clinical hyperthyroidism in humans as shown in 2 of 20 patients with gestational trophoblastic neoplasia.[46] These patients had extremely high serum (3,220,000 and 6,720,000 IU/L) and urine concentrations of hCG that correlated closely with TSH-like bioactivity. Other patients with moderately elevated serum hCG levels, between 110,000 and 310,000 IU/L, were euthyroid. When tested on human thyroid cell membranes, 1.0 IU hCG is biologically roughly equivalent to 0.27 μIU hTSH.[47] Both hCG and human luteinizing hormone (hLH) compete with TSH for the TSH-R, and hLH also has weak (10 to 100 times higher than hCG) TSH-like activity.[47–49] The β subunit of hCG and hLH share 85% sequence identity in the first 114 amino acids but differ in the carboxyl-terminal peptide because hCG-β contains an extension of 31 amino acids.[50] Carboxypeptidase digestion of hCG, with amino acid residues 142 to 145 cleaved from the β subunit, leads to an increase in its capacity to stimulate adenylate cyclase in human thyroid membranes.[51] A variant of hCG lacking the C-terminus of the β subunit because of enzymatic cleavage has been identified in pregnancy serum and molar tissue.[52] In studies using human thyroid membranes[53] or a cell line transfected with human TSH-R,[54] desialylated forms of hCG exhibited stronger inhibition of TSH-mediated cyclic adenosine monophosphate responses than did native hCG. Both TSH binding and TSH-induced adenylate cyclase stimulation were found to be more effectively inhibited by desialylated variants of hCG than unmodified hCG was.[55] From these and other studies it seems that the biologic effect of hCG is predominantly confined to hCG containing little or no sialic acid. In cultured FRTL-5 cells, hCG has been found to increase iodide uptake, and it also causes a dose-related increment in adenylate cyclase activity and thymidine uptake.[56, 57]

Gestational Transient Thyrotoxicosis

GTT occurs in 2% to 3% of pregnant women.[58, 59] It is mostly diagnosed between the 8th and the 14th weeks, when hCG levels peak. Levels are usually above 75,000 and 100,000 U/L and of sufficient duration to cause hyperthyroidism. About half of patients with GTT have clinical symptoms of hyperthyroidism. Differential diagnosis from Graves' disease is important. GTT is a nonautoimmune type of hyperthyroidism, which means that circulating thyroid autoantibodies and the characteristic symptoms of Graves' disease, such as eye signs, pretibial myxedema, and acropachy, are absent. Hyperthyroidism disappears spontaneously when serum hCG levels decrease. Treatment with antithyroid drugs is necessary only when hyperthyroidism is severe. In severe cases, hyperemesis is invariably present and hospital admission is pertinent. In patients with hyperemesis, the β subunit of hCG, but not the α subunit is elevated in serum.[60] If treatment is necessary in milder cases, administration of β-adrenergic blocking agents is sufficient to suppress symptoms.

Familial Gestational Hyperthyroidism

Recently, a mother and a daughter were described who suffered from recurrent gestational hyperthyroidism but hCG serum levels were normal during pregnancy. Both patients were heterozygous for a missense mutation, guanine for adenine, at codon 183 in exon 7 in the TSH-R gene. This mutation resulted in replacement of a lysine residue by arginine at position 138 of the receptor, which is in the middle of its extracellular N-terminal domain. Because the mutant receptor was about 3.5 times more sensitive to hCG than the wild type, hyperthyroidism developed in these women during pregnancy. Both women had concomitant hyperemesis as well.[61] No information is as yet available about the frequency of this syndrome.

Molar Pregnancy and Trophoblastic Disease

Several early reports describe molar pregnancy in combination with hyperthyroidism and disappearance of thyrotoxicosis after removal of a hydatidiform mole.[62–65] Bioassayable serum TSH was decreased in parallel with normalization of thyroid function parameters and a decrease in serum hCG. From the parallelism of thyroid-stimulating and hCG activity, it was suggested that both are caused by the same molecule, hCG.[65] The thyroid stimulator extracted from the serum of a patient with hyperthyroidism caused by a mole differed biologically and immunologically from TSH, from hCG found in normal placentas, and from thyroid-stimulating immunoglobulins. It contained less sialic acid and was biologically more active than normal pregnancy hCG.[62, 66] In patients with chorionic carcinoma, a similar relationship is present between thyroid-stimulating activity in serum and hCG serum concentrations, the β subunit of human hCG, and quantitation of tumor burden.[67] Choriocarcinoma associated with hyperthyroidism in males is exceedingly rare. About four cases have been reported in the literature.[68] The clinical picture of patients with trophoblastic hyperthyroidism is that of Graves' disease without the specific features of the latter.

Therapeutically, removal of the mole resolves the problem. In the case of choriocarcinoma, total removal of the tumor should be undertaken if possible. If necessary because of the hyperthyroidism, preoperative treatment with β-adrenergic blocking drugs or, in more serious cases, combined with iodide and antithyroid drugs, should be initiated. In patients not suitable for surgery, antithyroid drug treatment or administration of radioactive iodine in combination with chemotherapy is the best treatment available.

IODINE-INDUCED THYROTOXICOSIS

IIT may be subdivided into different groups: (1) patients from endemic goiter areas, (2) patients with previous nonendemic goiter, (3) patients with previous or with actual Graves' disease, and (4) patients without apparent previous thyroid disease.[69]

One of the best known studies on IIT is that by Connolly et al.[70] They found a steep rise in the incidence of thyrotoxicosis in the late months of 1966 in Tasmania (Australia), an area of iodine deficiency with a high prevalence of goiter. This increase was due to the addition of potassium iodide to bread in early 1966. The increased incidence occurred predominantly in subjects older than 40 years, in whom a rise in incidence from 50 to a maximum of 130 cases per 100,000 was seen in 1967 to 1968. By 1974 the incidence decreased to about the pre-epidemic level. Most thyrotoxic patients had nodular goiter and few patients had Graves' disease. Later it was recognized that a pre-epidemic increase in the incidence of thyrotoxicosis had been caused by the use of iodophor disinfectants on dairy farms.[71] Despite the continued increase in the iodide supply, the prevalence of IIT decreased after its peak in 1967–1968. It was argued that this increase in thyrotoxicosis starting from 1964, in this area of relative iodine deficiency with a high prevalence of goiter, was due to autonomy in the nodular goiters. For a review of IIT caused by iodine prophylaxis in Tasmania and other countries see Stanbury et al.[72]

Many substances such as iodinated drugs, radiographic contrast agents, iodochloroxyquinoline, iodine containing contrast agents, disinfectants, and iodine-containing drugs may also cause IIT.[69, 74] Precipitation of thyroid storm is rare. Subjects with long standing goiter are especially susceptible to IIT. In a study of 85 consecutive patients with IIT, a preexisting thyroid disorder was present in at least 20%. Spontaneous reversal to euthyroidism occurred after a mean period of 6 months in 50 of 85 patients. Return to euthyroidism may be preceded by subclinical hypothyroidism.[74] The recently developed nonionic contrast media do not prevent the development of IIT in elderly subjects.[75]

Evidence from human and animal studies suggests that chronic excess iodine intake may modulate thyroid autoimmunity and lead to thyrotoxicosis in genetically susceptible individuals. Although some studies report IIT in subjects without (apparent) preexisting thyroid disorders, it is still doubtful whether iodide can on its own merit induce thyroid autoimmunity.[76] A necrotic effect of iodide excess has been demonstrated in vivo in various animal species and also in human thyroid follicles in vitro.[77]

The antiarrhythmic drug amiodarone is currently widely used. Because of its high iodine content (37.2%), it has been the cause of IIT in many patients from all parts of the world. Its basic molecular structure has some similarity to that of the iodothyronines. Amiodarone may also interfere with thyroid hormone transport into cells and with pathways of intracellular thyroid hormone metabolism and action. It interferes with 5′-monodeiodination of thyroid hormones, which leads to a decrease in intracellularly derived T_3 from T_4, thus inducing tissue hypothyroidism. An exceptional case of myxedema coma leading to death despite intervention with T_4 and T_3 occurred in a patient after long-term amiodarone therapy.[78] Hypothyroidism occurs predominantly in patients with preexisting thyroid autoimmune disease and was recognized in 6% of 467 patients chronically treated with amiodarone.[79] It is being used in many cardiac patients, particularly in France. The reported incidence of IIT caused by amiodarone varies between 0.003% and 11.5%.[60] Estimation of serum total or free T_4 in patients using amiodarone is not specific because they may be elevated in hyperthyroid, euthyroid, and even hypothyroid patients. The two latter conditions are explained by a decrease in T_4 metabolic clearance by amiodarone because of inhibition of T_4 transport into tissues and subsequent T_4 deiodination. This process results in high T_4 plasma levels and may lead to subnormal tissue T_3 concentrations. To differentiate between these possibilities, determination of serum TSH and T_3 is useful.

Of the two forms of amiodarone-induced thyrotoxicosis, type 1 is due to an iodine-induced increase in thyroid hormone synthesis and type 2 involves iodine- or amiodarone-induced cytotoxic damage of the thyroid gland, with subsequent leakage of iodothyronines into the circulation. The picture of type 2 on electron microscopy characteristically shows two types of damage: multilamellar lysosomal inclusions and intramitochondrial glycogen inclusions with a morphologic picture of thyrocyte hyperfunction.[80] Thyroid radioactive uptake is usually low to normal in type 1 but low to suppressed in type 2. Serum interleukin-6 levels are normal to slightly elevated in type 1 and markedly elevated in type 2. Color flow sonography has been shown to differentiate between the two conditions. Type 1 shows normal vascularity (pattern 1) or increased vascularity (pattern 2) with a patchy distribution, whereas type 2 shows no vascularity (pattern 0).[81] Amiodarone-associated IIT type 1 is a serious problem in many instances because of the coexisting heart disease of these patients, and treatment may often be difficult.[82] Administration of a combination of methimazole and potassium perchlorate is reported to be effective in type 1.[83, 84] Treatment of type 2 thyrotoxicosis consists of administration of prednisone starting at a dose of 40 mg/day, for example. Normalization of thyroid hormone levels is achieved in about 1 week.[82] Patients with previous type 2 thyrotoxicosis are at risk for hypothyroidism when given excessive iodine.[85]

Radiographic contrast agents contain between 30% and 50% iodine and may also induce IIT. Patients who have multinodular goiter or live in countries where iodine intake is low are especially at risk.[86] IIT often develops several weeks after the administration of radiographic contrast agents, so follow-up of such patients is advisable. In some instances, prophylactic administration of methimazole may be necessary. In view of the wide use of radiographic contrast agents, the probability of inducing IIT by these substances is probably low, but it may be inversely related to the iodine intake of the population.

HYPERTHYROIDISM CAUSED BY INAPPROPRIATE TSH SECRETION

These situations are typified by increased production of thyroid hormone with clinical and/or biochemical characteristics of thyrotoxicosis in combination with nonsuppressed or even supranormal serum TSH concentrations. This picture may be seen in the presence of a TSH-secreting pituitary tumor or be the result of selective partial pituitary resistance to thyroid hormone.

Selective Partial Tissue Resistance of the Pituitary to Thyroid Hormone

This syndrome is described in Chapter 114 and is probably part of the spectrum of the syndromes of thyroid hormone resistance, with resistance predominant at the pituitary level. Because only the pituitary is partially resistant to thyroid hormone, the set-point of the pituitary, that is, the specific TSH/thyroid hormone ratio needed to ensure normal thyroid gland activation, is set at a higher level of serum thyroid hormone concentration. Because the other body tissues appear to have a sensitivity to thyroid hormone that is at least higher than that of the pituitary but may be even normal, the clinical picture of thyrotoxicosis is present, although without eye symptoms and other characteristics specific for Graves' disease. This syndrome may be inherited in an autosomal dominant mode.[87–89] Because no pituitary tumor is present, the ratio of TSH α subunits to total TSH is less than

1, whereas in the case of a TSH-producing pituitary tumor (see below), this ratio is usually above 1.

Hyperthyroidism Caused by a TSH-Secreting Pituitary Adenoma

A TSH-secreting pituitary tumor is a rare condition, although since the use of ultrasensitive TSH measurements, its detection has increased. In a 1993 publication, 2.8% of all pituitary tumors consisted of TSH-producing adenomas.[90] More than 70% of these tumors are macroadenomas.[91] Patients are usually mildly hyperthyroid, and specific symptoms of Graves' disease are lacking. Serum levels of free T_4 and/or free T_3 are elevated, with a normal or increased serum TSH concentration. Visualization of the pituitary by magnetic resonance imaging shows a pituitary tumor. The concentration of TSH α subunits in blood is above normal, as is the ratio of TSH-α/TSH.[92] Pituitary TSH-secreting adenomas produce normal forms of TSH but secrete them in variable amounts with variable biologic activity, which explains the variable degree of hyperthyroidism in these patients.[93] Treatment consists of surgery and postsurgical pituitary irradiation. About two-thirds of patients have normal serum TSH after surgery alone or in combination with irradiation, but only one-third of the patients are considered cured.[91] Treatment with somatostatin analogues such as octreotide returns TSH levels to normal in 80% of patients, and tumor size shrinks in 50%. Vision improves in 75% and euthyroidism returns in almost all patients.[94] Recent results with long-acting somatostatin analogues have shown them to be effective as well.[95] Somatostatin treatment is also effective in surgical failures.

THYROTOXICOSIS CAUSED BY METASTATIC DIFFERENTIATED THYROID CARCINOMA

Thyrotoxicosis resulting from functioning metastasis of differentiated thyroid carcinoma is rare. Recently, 54 cases reported in the literature were analyzed.[96] The age and sex distribution of these patients is no different from that of other patients with differentiated carcinoma but without thyrotoxicosis. About 85% of patients are older than 40 years, and the female-to-male ratio is 3:1. The clinical picture of this type of thyrotoxicosis is no different from other causes of thyrotoxicosis. Iodine uptake and thyroid hormone synthesis by the tumor are generally poor, and excessive hormone production is due to the large mass of metastatic tissue.[97] The inefficient thyroid hormone synthesis is at least partly due to relative iodine deficiency in tumor tissue and the presence of abnormal thyroglobulin.[98] Other deficiencies and abnormalities in the complicated process of thyroid hormone synthesis may, however, be present in carcinomatous tissue. For instance, evidence suggests that expression of the TSH receptor and Na^+/I^- symporter may be absent or low in carcinomatous thyroid tissue.[99] In many cases, clinical symptoms are caused by T_3 toxicosis with suppressed serum TSH and normal, sometimes even low serum T_4.[97, 98, 100] Uptake of radioactive iodine in metastatic tissue is often absent when the thyroid gland is still present. The metastatic pattern of this type of adenocarcinoma is the same as usually found in patients with thyroid adenocarcinoma, predominantly to bone, lung, and the mediastinum.

Treatment of metastatic functioning thyroid carcinoma consists of the administration of radioactive iodine. The usual dose ranges between 3700 and 7400 MBq (100–200 mCi). Exacerbation of thyrotoxicosis, even precipitating thyroid storm, has been reported.[101] For this reason, radioactive iodine for treatment of a functioning metastatic thyroid carcinoma should be administered with caution and only after adequate preparation of elderly patients with cardiovascular disease. If normal thyroid tissue is still present, it is appropriate to eradicate this tissue either by surgery or by radioactive iodine to ensure more efficient uptake of therapeutic doses of radioactive iodine in the metastatic tissue. Furthermore, it is dangerous to administer the above-mentioned doses of radioiodine in the presence of a normal thyroid gland because severe radiation thyroiditis may ensue. The combination of Graves' disease and follicular carcinoma may not be a coincidence[102–104] because recent knowledge suggests an association between Graves' disease and thyroid carcinoma, possibly as a result of long-standing thyroid stimulation by immunoglobulins.[105] Although it has been postulated that thyroid carcinoma in patients with Graves' disease behaves more aggressively,[106] this statement has recently been denied.[107]

STRUMA OVARII

Struma ovarii is a rare tumor occurring in a teratoma or dermoid of the ovary. It constitutes about 1% of all ovarian tumors.[108] Often admixed with a carcinoid tumor,[109] it has also been reported to occur in association with multiple endocrine neoplasia type IIA.[110] Ovarian strumal carcinoid tumors have been found to synthesize different peptide hormones, including calcitonin, adrenocorticotropic hormone, somatotropin release–inhibiting factor, neuron-specific enolase, chromogranin, synaptophysin, serotonin, and other peptides.[109–111] Struma ovarii is unilaterally localized in about 90% of patients, and about 80% or more are benign.[112, 113] Because differentiation between carcinoid and struma tissue is sometimes difficult, electron microscopic studies in combination with specific immunochemistry are sometimes necessary. Struma ovarii seldom causes hyperthyroidism. In thyrotoxicosis caused by struma ovarii, uptake of radioactive iodine by the thyroid gland is low in the presence of elevated serum thyroid hormones and suppressed TSH. Uptake of radioactive iodine over the ovarian tumor confirms the diagnosis.[114] Although in thyrotoxic cases resulting from struma ovarii one would suspect that the thyroid gland would be reduced in size, in several reports the thyroid was enlarged.[112–115]

The pathogenesis of hyperthyroidism caused by struma ovarii is not clear. It has been suggested that thyroid-stimulating immunoglobulins stimulate ovarian strumal tissue or that struma ovarii may become autonomous.[116] Treatment of struma ovarii, either with euthyroidism or thyrotoxicosis, should be effected by removal of the ovarian tumor. In the case of coexistent thyrotoxicosis, preparation for surgery should be done by administration of antithyroid drugs, sometimes in combination with β-adrenergic blocking agents. Because of the coexisting teratoma, it is sometimes difficult to determine whether the thyroid tissue in the tumor is benign or malignant. It is not advised that patients with thyrotoxic struma ovarii be treated with radioiodine because of the possibility that the tumor is malignant, which cannot be determined on clinical grounds, and because of the unknown radiation effects on the other ovarian elements.

REFERENCES

1. Hamburger JI: Evolution of toxicity in solitary non-functioning thyroid nodules. J Clin Endocrinol Metab 50:1089, 1980.
2. Bransom CJ, Talbot CH, Henry J, et al: Solitary toxic adenoma of the thyroid gland. Br J Surg 66:590, 1997.
3. Horst W, Rosler H, Schneider C, et al: 306 Cases of toxic adenoma: Clinical aspects, findings in radioiodine diagnostics, radiochromatography and histology; results of 131-I and surgical treatment. J Nucl Med 8:515, 1967.
4. Emrich D, Erlenmaier U, Pohl M, et al: Determination of the autonomously functioning volume of the thyroid. Eur J Nucl Med 20:410, 1993.
5. Studer H, Gerber H, Peter HJ: Multinodular goiter. *In* DeGroot LJ (ed): Endocrinology, vol 1, ed 2. Philadelphia, WB Saunders, 1989, p 722.
6. Studer H, Ramelli F: Simple goiter and its variants: Euthyroid and hyperthyroid multinodular goiters. Endocr Rev 3:40, 1982.
7. Studer H, Peter HJ, Gerber H: Natural heterogeneity of thyroid cells: The basis for understanding thyroid function and nodular goiter growth. Endocr Rev 10:125, 1989.
8. O'Sullivan C, Barton CM, Staddon SI, et al: Activation point mutations of the GSP oncogene in human thyroid adenomas. Mol Carcinog 4:345, 1992.
9. Parma J, van de Sande J, Swillens S, et al: Somatic mutations causing constitutive activation of the thyrotropin receptor are the mayor cause of hyperfunctioning thyroid adenomas: Identification of additional mutations indicating both the cyclic 3′,5′-monophosphate and inositol phosphate Ca^{2+} cascades. Mol Endocrinol 9:725, 1995.
10. Takeshita A, Nagayama Y, Yokoyama N, et al: Rarity of oncogenic mutations in the thyrotropin receptor of autonomously functioning thyroid nodules in Japan. J Clin Endocrinol Metab 80:2607, 1995.
11. Lax SF, Semlitsch G, Schauer S, et al: Point mutations of the thyrotropin receptor gene in autonomously functioning thyroid gland nodules: Correlation with clinical findings and morphology. Verh Dtsch Ges Pathol 81:145, 1997.

12. Van Sande J, Massart C, Costagliola S, et al: Specific activation of the thyrotropin receptor by trypsin. Moll Cell Endocrinol 119:161, 1996.
13. Derwahl M: TSH receptor and Gs-alpha gene mutations in the pathogenesis of toxic thyroid adenoma—a note of caution (editorial). J Clin Endocrinol Metab 81:1783, 1996.
14. Sandler MP, Fellmeth B, Salhany KE, Patton JA: Thyroid carcinoma masquerading as a solitary benign hyperfunctioning nodule. Clin Nucl Med 30:410, 1988.
15. Hamburger JI: Solitary autonomously functioning thyroid lesions: Diagnosis, clinical features and pathogenetic considerations. Am J Med 58:740, 1975.
16. Eyre-Brook IA, Talbot CH: The treatment of autonomous functioning thyroid nodules. Br J Surg 69:577, 1982.
17. Ratcliffe GE, Cooke S, Fogelman I, Maisey MN: Radioiodine treatment of solitary functioning thyroid nodules. Br J Radiol 59:385, 1986.
18. Ross DS, Ridgway EC, Daniels GH: Successful treatment of solitary toxic nodules with relatively low-dose ^{131}I with low prevalence of hypothyroidism. Ann Intern Med 101:488, 1984.
19. Goldstein R, Hart IR: Follow-up of solitary autonomous thyroid nodules treated with ^{131}I. N Engl J Med 309:1473, 1983.
20. Mariotti S, Martino E, Francesconi M, et al: Serum thyroid auto-antibodies as a risk factor for development of hypothyroidism after radioactive iodine therapy for single thyroid "hot" nodule. Acta Endocrinol (Copenh) 113:500, 1986.
21. Lippi F, Ferrari C, Manetti L, et al: Treatment of solitary autonomous thyroid nodules by percutaneous ethanol injection: Results of an Italian multicenter study. The Multicenter Study Group. J Clin Endocrinol Metab 81:3261, 1996.
22. Paracchi A, Reschini E, Ferrari C, et al: Changes in radioiodine turnover in patients with autonomous thyroid adenoma treated with percutaneous ethanol injection. J Nucl Med 39:1012, 1998.
23. Tokuda Y, Kasagi K, Lida Y, et al: Sonography of subacute thyroiditis: Changes in the findings during the cause of the disease. J Clin Ultrasound 18:21, 1990.
24. Vitug AC, Goldman JM: Silent (painless) thyroiditis. Evidence of a geographic variation in frequency. Arch Intern Med 145:437, 1985.
25. Schneeberg NG: Silent thyroiditis. Arch Intern Med 143:2214, 1983.
26. Lazarus JH, Ammari F, Oretti R, et al: Clinical aspects of recurrent postpartum thyroiditis. Br J Gen Pract 47:305, 1997.
27. Farid NR, Hawe BS, Walfish PG: Increased frequency of HLA D3 and 5 in the syndromes of painless thyroiditis with transient thyrotoxicosis: Evidence for an auto immune etiology. Clin Endocrinol 19:669, 1983.
28. Gudbjornsson B, Kistinsson A, Geirsson G, et al: Painless autoimmune thyroiditis occurring in amiodarone therapy. Acta Med Scand 221:229, 1987.
29. Chow CC, Lee S, Shek CC, et al: Lithium associated transient thyrotoxicosis in 4 Chinese women with autoimmune thyroiditis. Aust N Z J Psychiatry 27:246, 1993.
30. Sauter MP, Atkins MB, Meir JW, Lechan RM: Transient thyrotoxicosis and persistent hypothyroidism during acute autoimmune thyroiditis after interleukin 2 and interferon-alpha therapy for metastatic carcinoma: A case report. Am J Med 92:441, 1992.
31. Sakata S, Nagai K, Shibata T, et al: A case of rheumatoid arthritis associated with silent thyroiditis. J Endocrinol Invest 15:377, 1992.
32. Yamamoto M, Fuwa Y, Chimori K, et al: A case of progressive systemic sclerosis (PSS) with silent thyroiditis and anti-bovine thyrotropin antibodies. Endocrinol Jpn 38:265, 1991.
33. Itaka M, Ishii J, Ishikaea N, et al: A case with Graves' disease with false hyperthyrotropinemia who developed silent thyroiditis. Endocrinol Jpn 38:667, 1991.
34. Parker Klien I, Fishman LM, Levey GS: Silent thyrotoxic thyroiditis in association with chronic adrenocortical insufficiency. Arch Intern Med 143:2214, 1983.
35. Magaro M, Zoli A, Altomonte L, et al: The association with silent thyroiditis and active systemic lupus erythematosus. Clin Exp Rheumatol 10:67, 1992.
36. Mizukami Y, Michigishi T, Hashimoto T, et al: Silent thyroiditis: A histologic and immunohistochemical study. Hum Pathol 19:423, 1988.
37. Wolff PD: Transient painless thyroiditis with hyperthyroidism: A variant of lymphocytic thyroiditis? Endocr Rev 1:411, 1980.
38. Gegick CG, Harring WB: Painless subacute thyroiditis: A report of two cases. N C Med J 38:387, 1977.
39. Nicolai TF, Coombs GJ, McKenzie AK, et al: Treatment of lymphocytic thyroiditis with spontaneously resolving hyperthyroidism (silent thyroiditis). Arch Intern Med 142:2281, 1982.
40. Nicolai TF, Coombs GJ, McKenzie AK: Lymphocytic thyroiditis with spontaneously resolving hyperthyroidism and subacute thyroiditis. Long-term follow-up. Arch Intern Med 141:1455, 1981.
41. Bogazzi F, Bartalena LA, Vitti P, et al: Color flow Doppler sonography in thyrotoxicosis factitia. J Endocrinol Invest 19:603, 1996.
42. Kinney JS, Hurwitz ES, Fishbein DB, et al: Community outbreak of thyrotoxicosis: Epidemiology, immunogenetic characteristics and long-term outcome. Am J Med 84:10, 1988.
43. Hedberg CW, Fishbein DB, Janssen RS, et al: An outbreak of thyrotoxicosis caused by the consumption of bovine thyroid gland in ground beef. N Engl J Med 316:993, 1987.
44. Nisula BC, Ketelslegers J-M: Thyroid-stimulating activity and chorionic gonadotropin. J Clin Invest 54:494, 1974.
45. Kenimer JG, Hershman JM, Higgins HP: The thyrotropin in hydatiform moles is human chorionic gonadotropin. J Clin Endocrinol Metab 40:482, 1975.
46. Nisula BC, Taliadouros GS: Thyroid function in gestational trophoblastic neoplasia: Evidence that the thyrotropic activity of chorion gonadotropin mediates the thyrotoxicosis of choriocarcinoma. Am J Obstet Gynecol 77:138, 1980.
47. Carayon P, Lefort G, Nisula BC: Interaction of human chorionic gonadotropin and human luteinizing hormone with human thyroid membranes. Endocrinology 106:1907, 1980.
48. Williams JF, Davies TF, Catt KJ, et al: Receptor-binding activity of highly purified bovine luteinizing hormone and thyrotropin, and their subunits. Endocrinology 106:1353, 1980.
49. Yoshimura M, Hershman JM, Pang XP, et al: Activation of the thyrotropin (TSH) receptor by human chorionic gonadotropin and luteinizing hormone in Chinese hamster cells expressing human TSH receptors. J Clin Endocrinol Metab 77:1009, 1993.
50. Yoshimura M, Hershman JM: Thyrotropic action of human chorionic gonadotropin. Thyroid 5:425, 1995.
51. Carayon P, Amir S, Nisula B, et al: Effect of carboxypeptidase digestion of the human choriogonadotropin molecule on its thyrotropic activity. Endocrinology 108:1891, 1981.
52. Cole LA, Kardana A: Discordant results in human chorionic gonadotropin assays. Clin Chem 38:263, 1992.
53. Ouchimura H, Nagataki S, Ito K, et al: Inhibition of the thyroid adenylate cyclase response to thyroid-stimulating immunoglobulin G and asialo-chorionic gonadotropin. J Clin Endocrinol Metab 55:347, 1982.
54. Hoerman R, Broecker M, Grossmann M, et al: Interaction of human chorionic gonadotropin (hCG) and asialo-hCG with recombinant human thyrotropin receptor. J Clin Endocrinol Metab 78:933, 1994.
55. Hoerman R, Amir SM, Ingbar SH: Evidence that partially desialylated variants of human chorionic gonadotropin (hCG) are the factors in crude hCG that inhibit the response to thyrotropin in human thyroid membranes. Endocrinology 123:1535, 1988.
56. Davies TF, Platzer M: hCG-induced TSH receptor activation and growth acceleration in FRTL-thyroid cells. Endocrinology 118:2149, 1986.
57. Hershman JM, Lee H-Y, Sugawara M, et al: Human chorionic gonadotropin stimulates iodide uptake, adenylate cyclase, and deoxyribonucleic acid synthesis in cultured rat thyroid cells. J Clin Endocrinol Metab 67:74, 1988.
58. Glinoer D: The regulation of thyroid function in pregnancy: Pathways of endocrine adaptation from physiology to pathology. Endocr Rev 18:404, 1997.
59. Glinoer D: Thyroid hyperfunction during pregnancy. Thyroid 8:859, 1998.
60. Goodwin TM, Hershman JM, Cole L: Increased concentration of the free beta-subunit of human chorionic gonadotropin in hyperemesis gravidarum. Acta Obstet Gynecol Scand 73:770, 1994.
61. Rodien P, Bremont C, Rafin Sanson M-L, et al: Familial gestational hyperthyroidism caused by a mutant thyrotropin receptor hypersensitive to human chorionic gonadotropin. N Engl J Med 339:1823, 1998.
62. Hershman JM, Higgins P: Hydatidiform mole—a cause of clinical hyperthyroidism. N Engl J Med 284:573, 1971.
63. Dowling JT, Ingbar SH, Frenkel N: Iodine metabolism in hydatidiform mole and choriocarcinoma. J Clin Endocrinol Metab 20:1, 1960.
64. Kock H, Vessel HV, Stolte L, et al: Thyroid function in molar pregnancy. J Clin Endocrinol Metab 26:1128, 1966.
65. Higgins HP, Hershman JM, Kenimer JG, et al: The thyrotoxicosis of hydatidiform mole. Ann Intern Med 83:307, 1975.
66. Yoshimura M, Pekary AE, Pang XP, et al: Thyrotropic activity of basic isoelectric forms of human chorionic gonadotropin extracted from hydatidiform mole tissues. J Clin Endocrinol Metab 78:862, 1994.
67. Anderson NR, Lockich JJ, McDermott WV Jr, et al: Gestational choriocarcinoma and thyrotoxicosis. Cancer 44:304, 1979.
68. Orgiazzi JJ, Rousset D, Cosentino C, et al: Plasma thyrotropic activity in a man with choriocarcinoma. J Clin Endocrinol Metab 39:653, 1974.
69. Fradkin JE, Wolff J: Iodine-induced thyrotoxicosis. Medicine (Baltimore) 62:1, 1983.
70. Connolly RJ, Vidor GI, Stewart JC: Increase in thyrotoxicosis in endemic goitre area after iodination of bread. Lancet 1:500, 1970.
71. Stewart JC, Vidor GI: Thyrotoxicosis induced by iodine contamination of food—a common unrecognized condition? BMJ 1:372, 1976.
72. Stanbury JB, Ermans AE, Pourdiux P, et al: Iodine-induced hyperthyroidism: Occurrence and epidemiology. Thyroid 8:83, 1998.
73. Herrmann J, Krüskemper HL: Gefardung von Patienten mit latenter und manifester Hyperthyreose durch jodhaltige Röntgenkontrastmittel und Medikamente. Dtsch Med Wochenschr 103:1437, 1978.
74. Leger AF, Massin JP, Laurent MF, et al: Iodine-induced thyrotoxicosis: Analysis of eighty-five consecutive cases. Eur J Clin Invest 14:449, 1984.
75. Martin FIR, Tress BW, Colman P, Deam DR: Iodine-induced hyperthyroidism due to nonionic contrast radiography in the elderly. Am J Med 95:78, 1933.
76. Mariotti S, Pinchera A: Role of the immune system in the control of thyroid function. *In* Greer MA (ed): The Thyroid Gland. New York, Raven, 1990, p 147.
77. Many M-C, Mestdagh C, van den Hove M-F, et al: In vitro study of acute toxic effects of high iodide doses in human thyroid follicles. Endocrinology 131:621, 1992.
78. Mazson PD, Williams ML, Cantley LK, et al: Myxedema coma during long-term amiodarone therapy. Am J Med 77:751, 1984.
79. Martino E, Aghini-Lombardi F, Bartalena L, et al: Enhanced susceptibility to amiodarone-induced hypothyroidism in patients with thyroid autoimmune disease. Arch Intern Med 154:12, 1994.
80. Cappiello E, Boldorini R, Tosoni A, et al: Ultrastructural evidence of thyroid damage in amiodarone-induced thyrotoxicosis. J Endocrinol Invest 18:862, 1995.
81. Bogazzi F, Bartalena L, Brogioni S, et al: Color flow Doppler sonography differentiates type 1 and type 2 amiodarone-induced thyrotoxicosis. Thyroid 7:541, 1997.
82. Bartalena L, Brogioni S, Grasso L, et al: Treatment of amiodarone-induced thyrotoxicosis, a difficult challenge: Results of a prospective study. J Endocrinol Metab 81:2930, 1996.
83. Martino E, Aghini-Lombardi F, Mariotti S, et al: Treatment of amiodarone-associated thyrotoxicosis by simultaneous administration of potassium perchlorate and methimazole. J Endocrinol Invest 5:201, 1986.
84. Reichert LJ, de Rooy HA: Treatment of amiodarone induced hyperthyroidism with potassium perchlorate and methimazole during amiodarone treatment. BMJ 298:1547, 1989.
85. Roti E, Minelli R, Gardini E, et al: Iodine-induced subclinical hypothyroidism in euthyroid subjects with a previous episode of amiodarone-induced thyrotoxicosis. J Clin Endocrinol Metab 75:1273, 1992.

86. Martino E, Aghini-Lombardi F, Mariotti S, et al: Amiodarone: A common source of iodine-induced thyrotoxicosis. Horm Res 26:158, 1987.
87. Emerson CH, Utiger RD: Hyperthyroidism and excessive thyrotropin secretion. N Engl J Med 287:328, 1972.
88. Gershengorn MC, Weintraub BD: Thyrotropin-induced hyperthyroidism caused by selective pituitary resistance to thyroid hormone. J Clin Invest 56:633, 1975.
89. Rösler A, Litvin Y, Hage C, et al: Familial hyperthyroidism due to inappropriate thyrotropin secretion successfully treated with triiodothyronine. J Clin Endocrinol Metab 54:76, 1982.
90. Mindermann T, Wilson CB: Thyrotropin-producing pituitary adenomas. J Neurosurg 79:521, 1993.
91. Beck-Peccoz P, Brucker-Davis F, Persani L, et al: Thyrotropin-secreting pituitary tumors. Endocr Rev 17:610, 1996.
92. McDermott MT, Ridgway EC: Central hyperthyroidism. Endocrinol Metab Clin North Am 27:187, 1998.
93. Sergi E, Medri G, Papandreou MJ, et al: Polymorphism of thyrotropin and alpha subunit in human pituitary adenomas. J Endocrinol Invest 16:45–55, 1993.
94. Shimon I, Melmed S: Management of pituitary tumors. Ann Intern Med 129:472, 1998.
95. Cancel A, Vuillermet P, Legrand A, et al: Effects of a slow release formulation of the new somatostatin analogue lanreotide in TSH-secreting pituitary adenomas. Clin Endocrinol (Oxf) 40:421, 1994.
96. Salvatori M, Saletnich I, Rufini V, et al: Severe thyrotoxicosis due to functioning pulmonary metastasis of well-differentiated cancer. J Nucl Med 39:1202, 1998.
97. Paul SJ, Sisson JC: Thyrotoxicosis caused by thyroid cancer. Endocrinol Metab Clin North Am 19:593, 1990.
98. Nakashima T, Enue K, Shiro-osu A, et al: Predominant T_3 synthesis in the metastatic thyroid carcinoma in a patient with T_3-toxicosis. Metabolism 30:327, 1981.
99. Caillou B, Troalen F, Baudin E, et al: NA^+/I^- symporter distribution in human thyroid tissues: An immunohistochemical study. J Clin Endocrinol Metab 83:4102, 1998.
100. Sung LC, Cavalieri RR: T_3 toxicosis due to metastatic thyroid carcinoma. J Clin Endocrinol Metab 36:215, 1973.
101. Cerletty JM, Listwan WJ: Hyperthyroidism due to functioning metastatic thyroid carcinoma. Precipitation of thyroid storm with therapeutic radioactive iodine. JAMA 242:269, 1979.
102. Grayzel EF, Bennett B: Graves' disease, follicular thyroid carcinoma and functioning pulmonary metastases. Cancer 43:1885, 1979.
103. Kasagi K, Takeichi R, Miyamoto S, et al: Metastatic thyroid cancer presenting as thyrotoxicosis: Report of three cases. Clin Endocrinol 40:429, 1994.
104. Steffensen FH, Aunsholt NA: Hyperthyroidism associated with metastatic thyroid carcinoma. Clin Endocrinol 41:685, 1994.
105. Mazzaferri EL: Thyroid cancer and Graves' disease (editorial). J Clin Endocrinol Metab 70:826, 1990.
106. Belfiore A, Charofalo MR, Giuffrida D: Increased aggressiveness of thyroid cancer in patients with Graves' disease. J Clin Endocrinol Metab 70:830, 1990.
107. Hales IB, McElduff A, Crummer P, et al: Does Graves' disease or thyrotoxicosis affect the prognosis of thyroid cancer. J Clin Endocrinol Metab 75:886, 1992.
108. Ayhan A, Yanik F, Tuncer R, et al: Struma ovarii. Int J Gynaecol Obstet 42:143, 1993.
109. Tamsen A, Mazur MT: Ovarian strumal carcinoid in association with multiple endocrine neoplasia, type IIA. Arch Pathol Lab Med 116:200, 1992.
110. Sakura H, Fujii T, Okamoto K: A study of human calcitonin in an ovarian carcinoid and ovarian cancers. Exp Clin Endocrinol 97:91, 1991.
111. Ozerwenka KF, Schon HJ, Bock P: Immunochemical and ultrastructural studies of an ovarian strumal carcinoid. Wien Klin Wochenschr 102:687, 1990.
112. Kempers RD, Dockerty MB, Hoffman DL, et al: Struma ovarii—ascitic, hyperthyroid and asymptomatic syndromes. Ann Intern Med 72:883, 1970.
113. Devaney K, Snyder R, Norris HJ, et al: Proliferative and histologically malignant struma ovarii: A clinicopathologic study of 54 cases. Int J Gynaecol Pathol 12:333, 1993.
114. Pardo-Mindan FJ, Vazquez JJ: Malignant struma ovarii. Light and electron microscopic study. Cancer 51:337, 1983.
115. Ross DS: Syndromes of thyrotoxicosis with low radioactive iodine uptake. Endocrinol Metab Clin North Am 27:169, 1998.
116. Bayot MR, Chopra IJ: Coexistence of struma ovarii and Graves' disease. Thyroid 5:469, 1995.

Chapter 103

Chronic (Hashimoto's) Thyroiditis

Nobuyuki Amino ▪ Hisato Tada ▪ Yoh Hidaka

Among the inflammatory diseases in the thyroid gland, chronic thyroiditis is the most common disorder. It is also called autoimmune thyroiditis or Hashimoto's thyroiditis. Autoimmune thyroiditis is a lifelong autoimmune disease of the thyroid gland. The enlarged thyroid gland gradually atrophies in association with the development of hypothyroidism in typical patients.

CHRONIC THYROIDITIS: CURRENT CONCEPTS

The first variety of chronic thyroiditis, struma lymphomatosa, was described by Hakaru Hashimoto in 1912.[1] Hashimoto reported four patients with diffuse goiter and clarified the four histologic characteristics: diffuse lymphocytic infiltration, formation of lymphoid follicles, destruction of epithelial cells, and proliferation of fibrous tissue. The term Hashimoto's disease or Hashimoto's thyroiditis is sometimes used to refer only to goitrous thyroiditis, but it may usually be considered, in a broad sense, a synonym of chronic thyroiditis or autoimmune thyroiditis, including atrophic and nongoitrous thyroiditis.

Chronic thyroiditis can be classified into four subgroups according to clinical stage (Table 103–1). In the early stage, patients are euthyroid and have no or a very small goiter. Chronic thyroiditis is subclinical, and the only evidence of autoimmune thyroiditis is a positive reaction for antithyroid antibodies. Postmortem histologic examination has revealed that positive tests for serum antithyroid antibodies, especially antithyroid microsomal antibodies (MCAbs), in subjects without overt thyroid disease indicate the presence of lymphocytic infiltration into the thyroid.[2] As the disease progresses, patients show a firm, diffuse goiter of small to moderate size and are generally said to have chronic autoimmune thyroiditis. Their thyroid function is variable, from euthyroidism to thyrotoxicosis. A large, firm goiter develops when the disease is more advanced, and this type is the classic or goitrous Hashimoto's disease. When a cytotoxic autoimmune reaction is predominant, atrophic thyroiditis eventually develops in association with hypothyroidism. This combination is the final stage of Hashimoto's disease.

In the general population, MCAbs are found in 10.0% of women and 5.3% of men.[3] Subclinical autoimmune thyroiditis is further evidenced by the fact that thyroid dysfunction develops after delivery in about half of these MCAb-positive women.[4] Therefore, when subclinical autoimmune thyroiditis is included, chronic thyroiditis is a very common disease. One in 10 to 30 women in the general population has autoimmune thyroiditis.

PATHOLOGY

Hashimoto's Thyroiditis

In the classic form of Hashimoto's thyroiditis (struma lymphomatosa) with a firm, enlarged thyroid, the normal follicular structure is extensively replaced by lymphocytic and plasma cell infiltrates with the formation of lymphoid germinal centers[1] (Fig. 103–1A). Thyroid follicles remain isolated or in small clusters, are small or atrophic, and are empty or contain sparse colloid. Some persistent follicular epithelial cells are transformed into Askanazy cells, which have an eosinophilic granular cytoplasm. These cells are found in many other thyroid diseases and probably represent a damaged state of epithelial cells. Fibrosis of variable extent and lymphocytic infiltration are found in the interstitial tissue.

Focal Thyroiditis

Focal thyroiditis was first recognized by Woolner et al.[5] as a mild form of Hashimoto's disease. In focal thyroiditis, destruction of normal thyroid structure is mild, and lymphocytes infiltrate focally into the disrupted follicles and interstitial tissue. Many follicles are preserved intact and are viable. Fibrosis may exist to some extent. Focal thyroiditis is common and is found in association with various thyroid

TABLE 103–1. Classification of Chronic (Autoimmune or Hashimoto's) Thyroiditis

Characteristic	Subclinical Autoimmune Thyroiditis	Chronic Autoimmune Thyroiditis	Classic Hashimoto's Thyroiditis	Atrophic Thyroiditis
Stage	Early	Mild	Advanced	Final
Antithyroid antibodies (agglutination methods)	Positive	Positive	Positive	Positive
Goiter	None or very small Soft to firm	Small or moderate Firm	Large Firm	None
Thyroid function	Euthyroid	Euthyroid Hypothyroid Destructive thyrotoxicosis	Euthyroid Hypothyroid Destructive thyrotoxicosis	Hypothyroid

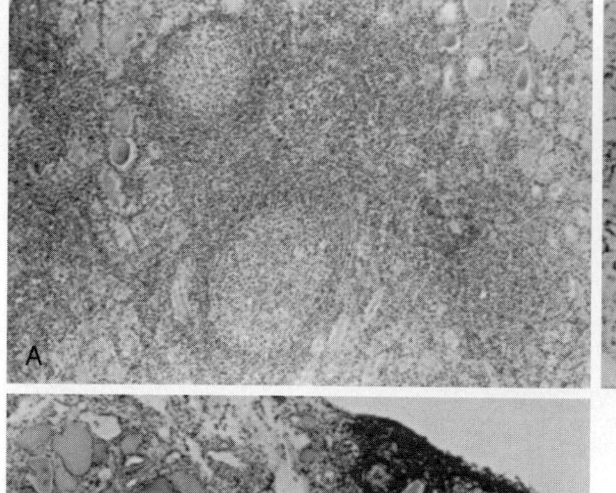

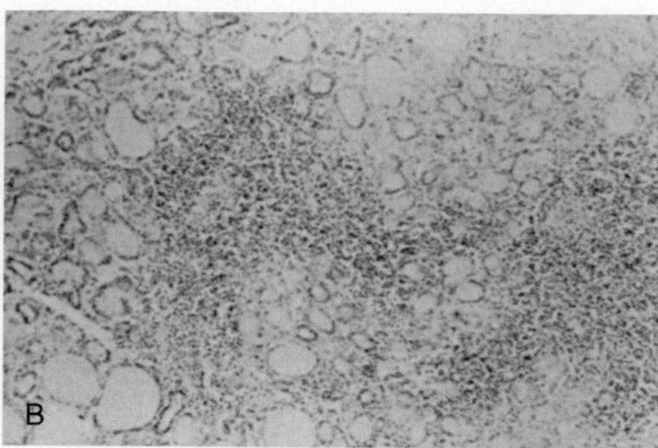

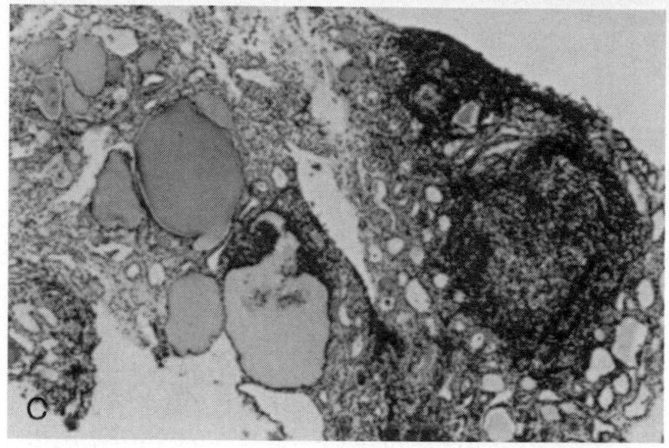

FIGURE 103–1. *A,* Hashimoto's thyroiditis with destruction of normal follicular architecture by lymphocytic and plasma cell infiltration and the formation of lymphoid germinal centers. A few atrophic thyroid follicles are seen (hematoxylin-eosin, ×100). *B,* Focal thyroiditis. Lymphocytic infiltration is less extensive and is observed focally in the area of disrupted follicles and interstitial tissues. Many follicles are preserved (hematoxylin-eosin, ×100). *C,* Silent thyroiditis. Lymphocytic infiltration with the formation of a lymphoid follicle surrounded by atrophic or disrupted thyroid follicles is seen. A few thyroid follicles are persistent with slight damage (hematoxylin-eosin, ×25). (Courtesy of Dr. F. Matsuzuka, Kuma Hospital, Kobe, Japan.)

diseases. This type of thyroiditis is also seen in many cases of subclinical autoimmune thyroiditis (see Fig. 103–1B).

Silent (Painless) Thyroiditis

The histologic characteristics of silent or painless thyroiditis are similar to those of chronic thyroiditis. Although lymphocytic infiltration and fibrosis may be less prominent in silent thyroiditis, one cannot distinguish it from chronic thyroiditis histologically,[6] which is one of the reasons to consider this type of thyroiditis to be autoimmune in nature. Histologic examination of needle biopsy specimens reveals focal or diffuse infiltration of lymphocytes and collapsed thyroid follicles (see Fig. 103–1C). Fibrosis may be minimal. In contrast to subacute thyroiditis, a granulomatous reaction is not noted. After recovery from the acute inflammation, the histologic findings spontaneously improve, with well-preserved thyroid follicles and slight focal lymphocytic infiltration.[7]

AUTOIMMUNE ABNORMALITIES

Initiation of Thyroid Autoimmunity

Similar to other autoimmune diseases, autoimmune thyroiditis may arise from a breakdown of self-tolerance to thyroid antigens. Immunologic self-tolerance is thought to be induced during the perinatal period when immature lymphocytes are exposed to self-antigens.[8] At this critical point, clonal deletion or induced anergy of autoreactive T cells in the thymus provides self-tolerance to autoantigens. If an abnormality occurs during this period, self-tolerance may not be induced[8] and autoimmune thyroiditis may develop. A possible abnormality is that a genetically induced organ-specific suppressor T lymphocyte defect may deregulate a thyroid-specific helper T cell population,[9] although this assumption is not widely accepted.[10] Environmental factors may also cause additional effects.[11] Further breakdown in self-tolerance may be induced by altered self-antigen, exposure to environmental antigens that mimic a self-antigen, polyclonal immune activation, or idiotypic cross-reaction of self-antigens. These factors may augment low levels of autoimmune thyroiditis. For example, infection, drugs, or other factors may activate autoreactive helper T lymphocytes. Locally produced interferon-γ (IFN-γ) may induce major histocompatibility complex (MHC) class II antigen expression on thyroid cell surfaces, which may promote autoimmunity.[12]

Antibodies to Thyroid Antigens

Thyroglobulin

A classic experimental autoimmune thyroiditis with histologic findings similar to those of Hashimoto's thyroiditis can be induced in animals by immunization with human thyroglobulin in an adjuvant. However, thyroglobulin is not isolated from the immune system in thyroid follicles, but it is normally present in the circulation of humans.[13] Thyroglobulin-binding lymphocytes can also be detected in the fetus.[14]

At least seven epitopes are present on human thyroglobulin, most of which are located in the middle part (in the region of amino acids 1097–1560) of thyroglobulin. Antithyroglobulin antibodies found in the sera of patients with autoimmune thyroiditis most frequently recognize a particular epitope in the region of amino acids 1149 to 1250, whereas antibodies from healthy subjects more frequently recognize another region.[15–17] Little evidence has been presented that antithyroglobulin antibodies are directly related to tissue damage, especially since they rarely have complement-fixing cytotoxicity.

Figure 103–2 shows antithyroglobulin antibody titers measured with hemagglutination (TGHAs) in various thyroid diseases. The frequency of positive TGHAs in Hashimoto's thyroiditis is 56%, which is lower than the frequency of positive microsomal antibodies (MCAbs) (Table 103–2). However, when a more sensitive radioimmunoassay is used, 70% of TGHA-negative patients with Hashimoto's disease were found to have positive antithyroglobulin antibody titers.[18]

Thyroid Peroxidase

Thyroid peroxidase (TPO) is the major antigen of the thyroid microsomal fraction recognized by MCAbs.[19] The thyroid microsomal fraction also includes thyroglobulin and other proteins in the membrane.

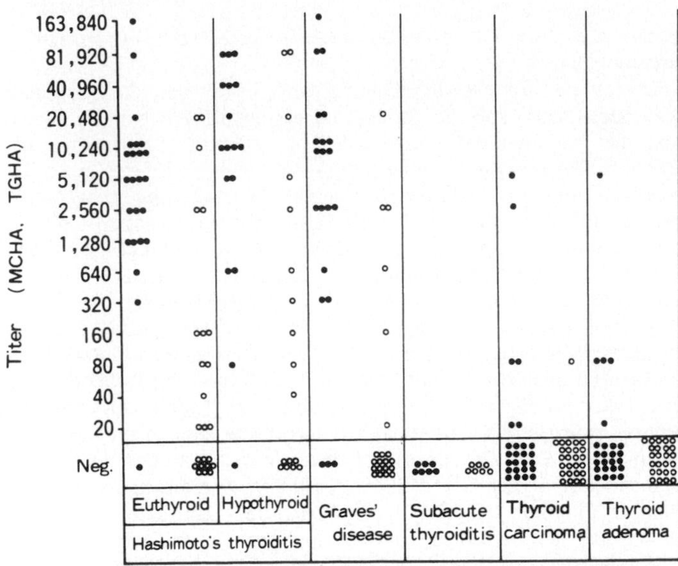

FIGURE 103–2. Titers of microsomal hemagglutination (MCHA) and thyroglobulin hemagglutination (TGHA) antibodies in patients with various thyroid diseases. (From Amino N, Hagan SR, Yamada N, Refetoff S: Measurement of circulating thyroid microsomal antibodies by the tanned red cell haemagglutination technique: Its usefulness in the diagnosis of autoimmune thyroid diseases. Clin Endocrinol 5:115–125, 1976.)

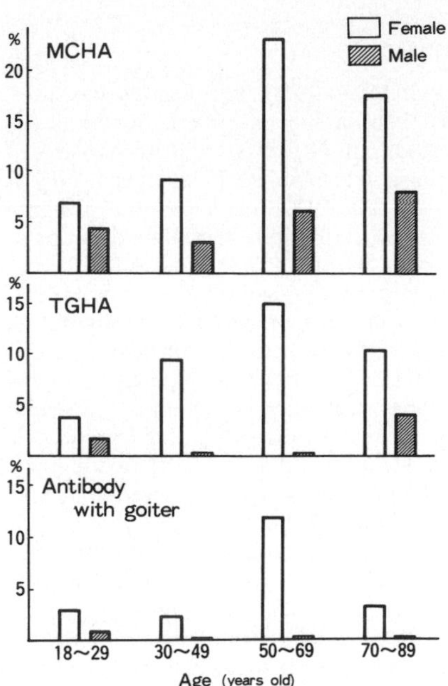

FIGURE 103–3. Incidence of antithyroid microsomal hemagglutination (MCHA) and antithyroglobulin hemagglutination (TGHA) antibodies in 1015 subjects from the general population shown in relation to age, sex, and thyroid enlargement. (From Amino N: Antithyroid antibodies. *In* Ingbar SH, Braverman LE (eds): The Thyroid, ed 5. Philadelphia, JB Lippincott, 1986, pp 546–559.)

We can consider anti-TPO antibodies to be effectively identical to MCAbs.

Anti-TPO antibodies are reported to be able to induce complement dependent cytotoxicity.[20] Anti-idiotypic antibodies against antimicrosomal antibodies are occasionally found in the sera of patients with autoimmune thyroid disease and might be involved in the regulation of autoimmunity.[21] However, the significance of anti TPO antibody in vivo is not certain. Microsomal antibodies transferred passively from mothers with Hashimoto's thyroiditis do not seem to affect thyroid function in the fetus or neonate.[22] Presently, the clinical importance of anti-TPO antibodies lies in the diagnosis of thyroid autoimmunity.

Figure 103–2 shows titers of antithyroid microsomal antibodies measured with hemagglutination (MCHAs) in various thyroid diseases. MCHA is positive in more than 90% of patients with Hashimoto's thyroiditis regardless of the presence of hypothyroidism or euthyroidism. Ten percent of women in the general population have positive MCHA titers and are thought to have subclinical autoimmune thyroiditis (Fig. 103–3). A more sensitive radioimmunoassay for the measurement of anti-TPO antibodies with human TPO used as an antigen is presently available.[18]

Thyroid-Stimulating Hormone Receptor

Thyroid-stimulating hormone (TSH) stimulation–blocking antibody (TSBAb) can inhibit TSH action on the thyroid and cause atrophic hypothyroidism in autoimmune thyroiditis.[23] Although the specific epitopes for thyroid-stimulating antibody (TSAb) or TSBAb are still uncertain, the major epitope of TSBAb seems to be in the C-terminal part of the extracellular domain (around 300–400 amino acids),[24, 25] whereas the N-terminal region of the TSH receptor (TSH-R) may be important in TSAb action.[26, 27] However, in vitro conversion from TSBAb to TSAb after the addition of antihuman IgG antibody suggests that TSAb and TSBAb are not determined solely by their epitopes, and the same TSH-R antibody may act as a stimulator or a blocker depending on the influence of other factors.[28]

TABLE 103–2. Incidence of Thyroid Autoantibodies in Different Thyroid Disorders

	Antithyroglobulin			Antimicrosomal			Antibodies to Thyroid Hormones	
Disorder	*TGHA*	*RIA*	Anti-CA2	*MCHA*	*RIA*	Anti-TSH Receptor Antibody (TBII)	T_4	T_3
Grave's disease	29	89	41	86	98	95	5.9	20.5
Hashimoto's disease	56	100	74	95	100	7*		
Primary hypothyroidism	59	94	16	94	100	14	14	34.9
Subacute thyroiditis	0	33†	33†	0		0		
Thyroid adenoma	0			20		0		
Thyroid carcinoma	3.8			23		0		
Normal population								
Male	1.8	4.2	3	6.0	8.4	0	0	0
Female	5.3			10.0			0	0

Values are percentages and are cited from reports described in the text.
*Incidence in hypothyroid Hashimoto's disease with goiter.
†One of three patients.
CA2, colloid antigen-2; MCHA, antithyroid microsomal hemagglutination antibody; RIA, radioimmunoassay; TBII, TSH-binding inhibitor immunoglobulin; TGHA, antithyroglobulin hemagglutination antibody; TSH, thyroid-stimulating hormone.
Modified from Amino N: Antithyroid antibodies. *In* Ingbar SH, Braverman LE (eds): The Thyroid, ed 5. Philadelphia, JB Lippincott, 1986, pp 546–559.

Other Antigens

The Na^+/I^- symporter (NIS) was recently cloned,[29] and Northern analysis revealed it as a specific protein in thyrocytes. Endo et al. reported that antibody to NIS was found in the sera of patients with Hashimoto's disease and inhibited I^- uptake in NIS-expressing Chinese hamster ovary cells.[30] However, the clinical importance of anti-NIS antibodies is modest because the antibodies are positive in only 15% of patients with Hashimoto's thyroiditis.[31]

Antibodies to thyroxine (T_4) and triiodothyronine (T_3) are sometimes found in patients with autoimmune or other thyroid diseases.[32] They are seen in 14% and 35% of patients with primary hypothyroidism, in most of whom TGHAs are found in high titer.[3, 33] The pathogenetic significance of these antibodies is not known. Probably they are of little importance as long as the thyroid can produce enough thyroid hormone to keep adequate serum levels of free hormone. These antibodies interfere with the measurements of serum T_4 and T_3, especially in assays of free T_4 and free T_3.[34]

Anti-bovine TSH autoantibodies, occasionally found in Graves' disease, are also reported in Hashimoto's thyroiditis.[35] Their pathogenetic significance is unclear. They are speculated to be anti-idiotypic antibodies to anti-TSH receptor antibodies (TRAbs) in Graves' disease. They may interfere with the measurement of TRAbs and give unusually high or negative titers.

Autoantibodies against several other thyroid components have been reported. Antibodies to colloid antigen-2 are detected by diffuse immunofluorescence of colloid. This antigen is distinct from thyroglobulin. Antibodies to cell surface antigen are detected by the patchy immunofluorescent staining of the cell surface or by mixed hemabsorption. The antigen is distinct from TPO. Antibodies that promote or reduce thyroid cell growth directly (i.e., not via TSH-R stimulation) are called growth-stimulating antibodies or growth-blocking antibodies. The former were found in the sera of patients with goitrous Hashimoto's thyroiditis and may cause goiter formation. Growth-blocking antibodies, found in primary myxedema, may cause thyroid atrophy. The presence of such antibodies has been controversial because of lack of reproducibility of the detection methods.[36] Recently, a sensitive bioassay for growth-stimulating antibody that uses cytochalasin B was developed[37] and may settle the controversy.

Autoantibodies against other cellular components (not always thyroid cell specific) are also reported. Anti-DNA antibodies in patients with Hashimoto's thyroiditis increase during postpartum exacerbation.[38] Antibodies to tubulin and calmodulin,[39] to the ganglioside asialo-GM_1 present in the plasma membrane of human thyroid,[40] and to the α-galactosylcarbohydrate structure Galα1 → 3Galβ1 → 4GlcNAcR, which is not expressed on the surface of normal human thyroid cells, may bind if aberrant expression of this epitope occurs, as in cancer.[41] Antibodies to other organs (e.g., islet cells, adrenal cortex, gastric mucosa, parathyroid) are found in autoimmune thyroiditis in higher incidence than in the general population.[39]

MECHANISM OF DEVELOPMENT OF HYPOTHYROIDISM

It is important to understand the mechanism of the development of hypothyroidism in patients with Hashimoto's disease. Recently, Fas–Fas ligand interactions among thyrocytes were suggested to contribute to clinical hypothyroidism in Hashimoto's disease.[42] Fas is an apoptosis-signaling receptor molecule found on the surface of a number of cell types.[43] Interaction of Fas with its ligand regulates a number of physiologic and pathologic processes involved in cell death.[44] Fas ligand was expressed in thyrocytes from both normal controls and patients with Hashimoto's thyroiditis, but Fas was expressed in thyrocytes from patients with Hashimoto's thyroiditis but not those from normal controls.[42] Interleukin-1β (IL-1β), abundantly produced by the glands of patients with Hashimoto's thyroiditis, induced Fas expression in normal thyrocytes, and cross-linking of Fas resulted in massive thyrocyte apoptosis. Soluble Fas molecule lacks the transmembrane domain because of alternative splicing and blocks Fas-mediated apoptosis.[45] Decreased serum levels of soluble Fas in Hashimoto's disease may also induce destruction of thyroid cells by promoting their apoptosis.[46]

Several in vitro cytotoxic mechanisms have been demonstrated. Cytotoxic T cells specific for thyroid epithelial cells can be cloned from the intrathyroidal lymphocytes of patients with Hashimoto's disease.[47] The proportion of intrathyroidal $CD8^+$, $CD11b^-$ cytotoxic T cells is high in Hashimoto's disease.[48] These findings suggest a potential role for cytotoxic T cells in the thyroid damage of Hashimoto's disease. Complement-dependent cytotoxic antibodies are found in almost all sera from patients with Hashimoto's disease[49] and are thought to be identical to microsomal antibody. However, these antibodies do not act on intact thyroid cells in vitro.[50] Microsomal antibodies passively transferred from mothers with Hashimoto's disease have no effect on neonatal thyroid function.[22] Therefore, this antibody may have little cytotoxic effect in vivo. Antibody-dependent cell-mediated cytotoxicity (ADCC) activity was found in the sera of patients with Hashimoto's disease,[51] and the cytotoxic effect was correlated with microsomal antibody titers.[52] Increased killer lymphocyte counts were found at the time of thyroid destruction in Hashimoto's disease.[53] Furthermore, the percentage and absolute count of killer lymphocytes were inversely correlated with serum thyroid hormone levels in autoimmune thyroid disease. Thus the higher number of killer cells and increased ADCC activity may lead to reduced thyroid function in autoimmune thyroid disease.

Cellular Abnormalities

Differentiated human $CD4^+$ T lymphocytes can be subdivided into functionally distinct subsets based on their cytokine secretion profiles.[54] Type 1 helper T cells (T_H1) produce IL-2, IFN-γ, and lymphotoxin and induce cellular responses. T_H2 cells secrete IL-4, IL-5, IL-6, IL-10, and IL-13 and promote the production of antibodies. The T cell clones from patients with Hashimoto's disease were preferentially T_H1 cells, whereas in Graves' disease, both T_H0 cells and T_H1 cells were present.[55] By reverse transcriptase polymerase chain reaction, increased mRNA levels of T_H1 cytokines were found in Hashimoto's thyroid glands, although both T_H1 cytokines and T_H2 cytokines were detected.[56–58] More recently, activated intrathyroidal T lymphocytes were found to produce predominantly IFN-γ in Hashimoto's disease by single-cell analysis of cytokines with intracellular labeling techniques.[59] Moreover, serum levels of IL-12, which is critical for development of the T_H1 phenotype, were increased in patients with active Hashimoto's thyroiditis (silent thyroiditis).[60] These findings suggest that a T_H1-type immune response is important in the pathogenesis of Hashimoto's disease.

B7-1 (CD80) molecule preferentially acts as a costimulator for the generation of T_H1 cells and has been recognized on thyrocytes in Hashimoto's disease, but not in Graves' disease.[61] This phenomenon, together with expression of MHC class II and intercellular adhesion molecule-1,[62] might lead to T cell differentiation to T_H1 cells and maintenance of thyroid autoimmunity. Thyroid cells in autoimmune thyroid disease are also reported to produce several cytokines (e.g., IL-1, IL-6, tumor necrosis factor-β [TNF-β]) that might influence lymphocytic responses.

In studies of intrathyroid infiltrating lymphocyte populations, T lymphocytes predominate over B cells, and $CD8^+$ T lymphocytes are increased[10] in Hashimoto's thyroiditis. Analysis of the gene for the variable region of the α chain (Vα gene) of the T cell receptor (TCR) suggests that the infiltrating T cells are a highly restricted population,[63] although this notion has been disputed. Among these cells, activated ($HLA\text{-}DR^+$) cells are increased when compared with those in the peripheral blood, especially DR^+, $CD8^+$, and natural killer (NK)/killer cells ($CD57^+/Leu7^+$)].[64] Some reports suggest an antigen-specific defect in suppressor T lymphocyte function in these cells,[9] although this mechanism is not always accepted.[10]

In lymphocytic populations in the peripheral circulation, activated T cells ($HLA\text{-}DR^+$, $CD3^+$) are increased,[65] and ordinary αβ TCR^+ T cells are decreased in Hashimoto's thyroiditis. The most prominent changes are observed at the time of exacerbation of Hashimoto's thyroiditis. $CD8^+$ cells decrease, unusual subsets such as γδ TCR^+ T cells (Tγδ) are decreased, and CD4+, CD8+ cells are increased during this thyrotoxic period.[66] The decrease in CD8+ and Tγδ cells may reflect their accumulation in the thyroid with subsequent cell lysis. An increase in CD5+ B cells,[67] which produce autoantibodies and have immunoregulatory functions, has been reported, but a more obvious increase is observed in Graves' disease.[68] NK/killer cells (CD57+) are also increased at the time of exacerbation in Hashimoto's disease. NK cells are found to change in number and activity in the course of a normal pregnancy,[69] and such change may influence the clinical course during pregnancy and the postpartum period.

Cytokines

Cytokines are known to have a wide variety of inflammatory and immunomodulatory effects, and thus it might be thought that many steps in thyroid autoimmunity are mediated and/or modulated by cytokines.[70] Indeed, administration of IL-2 or IFN-γ to animals can induce thyroid autoimmunity, and autoimmunity occurs in humans who received IL-2 or IFN for the treatment of cancer or viral hepatitis.[71, 72]

IFN-γ, which is produced by T lymphocytes and NK cells that have infiltrated into the thyroid, is reported to have several effects on thyrocytes and lymphocytes. Acting directly on thyrocytes, it stimulates both HLA class I and class II expression on their surface. In cultured thyroid cells, IFN-γ reduces the content of TPO[73] and thyroglobulin mRNA and the secretion of thyroglobulin[74] and thyroid hormones in response to TSH. IFN-γ also causes morphologic changes in thyrocytes, which are thought to represent dedifferentiation.[72]

TNF-α, which is mainly produced by monocytes, has cytotoxic and cytostatic effects on many kinds of cultured cells, including thyrocytes. It can induce HLA class I antigen expression on thyrocytes. It cannot activate HLA class II expression alone, but by acting synergistically with IFN-γ, TNF-α enhances HLA class II expression.

IL-1 and IL-6 are produced by thyrocytes as well as by lymphocytes. Thus interleukins produced by thyrocytes would stimulate intrathyroidal lymphocytes. IL-1 stimulates T cells to release lymphokines and has many other inflammatory effects. Moreover, as described earlier, IL-1 can induce thyrocyte apoptosis through Fas–Fas ligand interaction.

IL-6 is known as a B cell stimulatory factor. Antithyroid drugs are reported to reduce the production of these interleukins by thyrocytes attacked by complement and may have immunomodulatory effects.[75] Table 103–3 summarizes the effect of these cytokines on thyroid cells.[70]

GENETIC FACTORS

It is widely known that autoimmune thyroid diseases (both Hashimoto's thyroiditis and Graves' disease) occur in families. This tendency could be due to genetic predisposition, as well as environmental influences. Studies of genetic predisposition have revealed that autoimmune thyroid diseases are often associated with particular genetic markers. These markers include histocompatibility lymphocytic antigens, allotypes of immunoglobulin heavy chains, variations in the TCR and TPO, and so on. The associations have been examined serologically and recently by analysis of restriction fragment length polymorphisms (RFLPs), which allow more direct DNA-defined typing of genetic markers. The reports are not always consistent with each other, probably because of the subjects chosen and the small sizes of some studies.

The association of HLA genes, especially class II HLA (DR, DQ, DX, etc.) genes, has been examined extensively. In whites,[39] goitrous Hashimoto's thyroiditis is associated with HLA-DR3 and HLA-DR5 and atrophic autoimmune thyroiditis with HLA-DR3 and HLA-B8. HLA-DR3 is also associated with Graves' disease, which might reflect genetic effects in common with Hashimoto's thyroiditis. Association with HLA-DQw2 was detected by RFLP analysis, probably because of its linkage disequilibrium with HLA-DR3.[76] In further analysis, Shi et al. reported an association of Hashimoto's thyroiditis with HLA-DQA0301, which is in linkage disequilibrium with HLA-DR4, and HLA-DQB0201, which is in linkage disequilibrium with HLA-DR3.[77] Postpartum thyroid dysfunction is reported to be associated with HLA-DR5.[78] In Japanese, Hashimoto's thyroiditis is reported to be associated with HLA-DRw53[79] and HLA-B51,[80] and in Shanghai Chinese, with HLA-DR9 and HLA-Bw46,[81] thus indicating racial differences. In Japanese, permanent hypothyroidism is likely to develop in patients with postpartum hypothyroidism when they have the HLA-DRw9 and/or HLA-B51 genotypes, and thus HLA typing is helpful during the observation of patients.[82]

Linkage of specific TCR genes to inheritance of Hashimoto's thyroiditis is also reported. A specific TCR β subunit RFLP was increased in Hashimoto's thyroiditis, as well as in Graves' disease,[80] and a TaqI RFLP for the Vα gene of TCR was also increased.[83] These findings were not reproduced in another report.[76] In an analysis of polymorphism in codon 17 (Thr/Ala) in cytotoxic T lymphocyte antigen type 4 (CTLA-4) (Ala alleles were reported to confer genetic susceptibility to Graves' disease and type 1 diabetes mellitus), Ala alleles were found more frequently in patients with Hashimoto's disease.[84] The inheritance of specific allotypes of IgG heavy chain is also reported to relate to autoimmune thyroiditis,[85] as in Graves' disease.[86] These associations may not prove that the genes examined are causative because another gene near the locus examined may actually be causative. To settle this matter, further studies are necessary.

CLINICAL FEATURES

Thyroid Dysfunction

Autoimmune thyroiditis progresses slowly and is not self-limited. Therefore, the development of thyroid dysfunction depends on age. With time, some patients progress from the metabolically normal stage to hypothyroidism, often associated with disappearance of the goiter. The prevalence of hypothyroidism is therefore higher in the elderly[87] (Fig. 103–4). Approximately 10% of patients with Hashimoto's disease who visited a clinic showed overt hypothyroidism.[87] An important recent finding is that about 5% of patients have an associated destruc-

TABLE 103–3. Effect of Cytokines on the Function and Growth of Thyroid Cells

Cytokine	Secretion		Gene Expression		DNA Synthesis	MHC Class II Antigen Expression
	T_3	*TG*	*TPO*	*TG*		
INF-α	→	→	→	→	→	→
β	→	→	→	→	→	→
γ	↓	↓	↓	↓	→	↑
IL-1 α/β	↓	↓	↓	↓	↑	→
2	→	→	→	→	→	→
6	↓	?	↓	?	→	→
TNF-α	↓	↓	↓	↓	→	→

IFN, interferon; IL, interleukin; MHC, major histocompatibility complex; T_3, triiodothyronine; TG, thyroglobulin; TNF, tumor necrosis factor; TPO, thyroid peroxidase; →, no change; ↑, increase; ↓, decrease.

Data from Nagataki S, Eguchi K: Cytokines and immune regulation in thyroid autoimmunity. Autoimmunity 13:27–34, 1992.

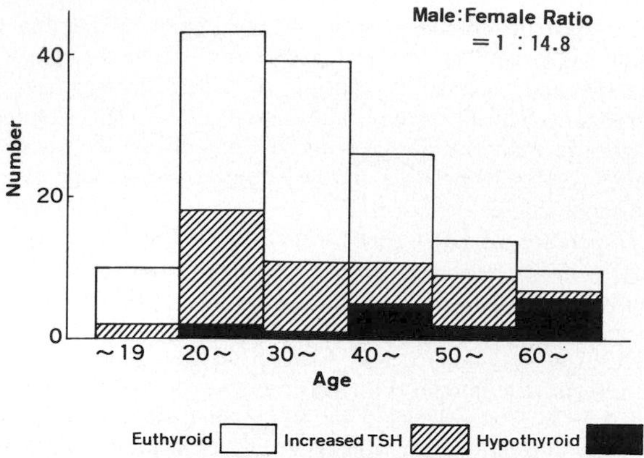

FIGURE 103–4. Age distribution and thyroid functional state in patients with Hashimoto's disease. (From Amino N: Autoimmunity and hypothyroidism. Baillieres Clin Endocrinol Metab 2:591–617, 1988.)

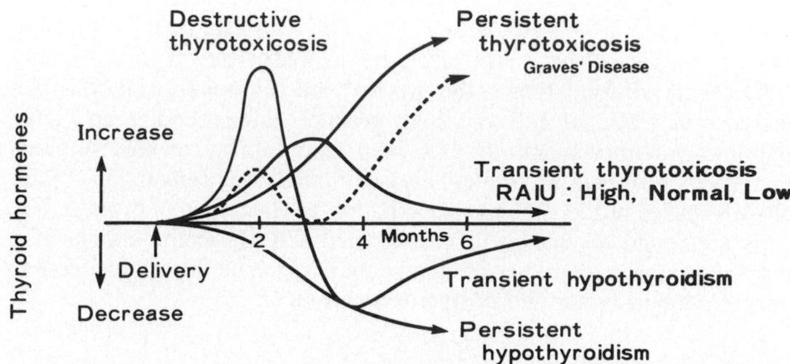

FIGURE 103–5. Various types of postpartum thyroid dysfunction. (From Amino N, Miyai K: Postpartum autoimmune endocrine syndromes. *In* Davies TF (ed): Autoimmune Endocrine Disease. New York, John Wiley & Sons, 1983, pp 247–272.)

tive thyrotoxicosis. This condition is otherwise called silent or painless thyroiditis (see below).

Hawkins et al.[88] reported that thyroid microsomal antibodies provide a useful diagnostic test given the high predictive value of a raised serum TSH concentration in a randomly selected population. They found increased TSH levels in 36% to 44% of subjects who were positive for MCHAs. With the use of a hemagglutination method, we found positive MCHAs in 64 (10.2%) of 629 women and in 24 (6.1%) of 395 men in the general population in Japan, but a raised serum TSH concentration (>6 μIU/mL) was found in only 9.1% of subjects with positive MCHAs.[89] In subjects with MCHAs who were younger than 50 years, the prevalence of increased TSH was only 2.2%, and the mean serum TSH concentration was not significantly different from that of age- and sex-matched controls without MCHAs. High TSH levels, however, were found in 16.2% of older subjects with positive MCHAs. Thus an age effect should be considered when assessing the predictive value of MCHAs for a raised serum TSH. About 90% of patients with Hashimoto's disease have positive MCHAs, but no difference is seen in titers and the prevalence of antibodies between euthyroid and hypothyroid patients.

Patients with an acute aggravation of thyroid autoimmunity are subject to destruction-induced thyrotoxicosis. These episodes are usually followed by transient hypothyroidism (see the next section). High iodine ingestion may aggravate autoimmune thyroiditis and thus induce hypothyroidism. Therefore, whenever we examine patients, it is important to consider recent excessive iodine ingestion. In children, Hashimoto's disease is less common, and titers of antithyroid antibodies are usually lower than those in adult patients. Children usually have a small symptomless goiter, and hypothyroidism is uncommon.

Silent and Postpartum Thyroiditis

Silent (painless) thyroiditis is a syndrome that has a clinical course of thyroid dysfunction similar to that of subacute thyroiditis but with no anterior neck pain and no tenderness of the thyroid.[90] Initially, patients have a thyrotoxic phase, later passing through euthyroidism to hypothyroidism and, finally, a return to euthyroidism. Postpartum thyroiditis occurs within 6 months after delivery and runs an identical clinical course.[4] Postpartum thyroiditis is now considered to be identical to silent thyroiditis, and this term is used for patients in whom silent thyroiditis develops in the postpartum period.[4] After delivery, other forms of autoimmune thyroid dysfunction also occur, including Graves' disease, transient hypothyroidism without preceding destructive thyrotoxicosis, and persistent hypothyroidism (Fig. 103–5). To include all these conditions, the term postpartum autoimmune thyroid syndrome is often used.[91]

In recent years, the term painless thyroiditis has also been used frequently, and the same disorder has been described with different names, such as thyrotoxicosis with painless thyroiditis,[92] occult subacute thyroiditis,[93] hyperthyroiditis,[94] lymphocytic thyroiditis with spontaneously resolving hyperthyroidism,[95] and transient hyperthyroidism with lymphocytic thyroiditis.[96] The thyrotoxicosis is induced by leakage of intrathyroidal hormones into the circulation after damage to thyroid epithelial cells from inflammation. Thus thyroid radioactive iodine uptake is low. Therefore, the early phase of thyrotoxicosis in silent thyroiditis, postpartum thyroiditis, and subacute thyroiditis can be grouped together as destruction-induced thyrotoxicosis or simply as destructive thyrotoxicosis.[97]

Much evidence, including histopathologic and immunologic studies, indicates that this disorder is an autoimmune thyroid disease. During the clinical course of subclinical[2] or very mild autoimmune thyroiditis, aggravating factors cause exacerbation of the destructive process. Ta-

TABLE 103–4. Clinical Data on Patients with Destruction-Induced Thyrotoxicosis

	Silent Thyroiditis		Subacute Thyroiditis
	Postpartum	*Spontaneous*	
No. of patients examined	29	27	57
No. (%) of female patients	29 (100)	25 (93)	52 (91)
Age <30 y, No. (%)	24 (83)†	7 (26)*	2 (4)
Antibodies			
Positive TGHA‡, No. (%)	11 (38)*	11 (41)†	0 (0)
Positive MCHA‡, No. (%)	24 (83)†	23 (85)†	0 (0)
Goiter			
Palpable at thyrotoxic state, No. (%)	26 (90)	27 (100)	57 (100)
Persistence, No. (%)	26 (90)†	26 (96)†	0 (0)

*Significantly different from subacute thyroiditis ($P < 0.01$, χ-square test).
†Significantly different from subacute thyroiditis ($P < 0.001$, χ-square test).
‡TGHA, antithyroglobulin hemagglutination antibody; MCHA, antithyroid microsomal hemagglutination antibody.
From Amino N: Postpartum and silent thyroiditis. *In* Monaco F, Satta MA, Shapiro B, Troncone L (eds): Thyroid Diseases: Clinical Fundamentals and Therapy. Boca Raton, FL, CRC Press, 1993, pp 239–249.

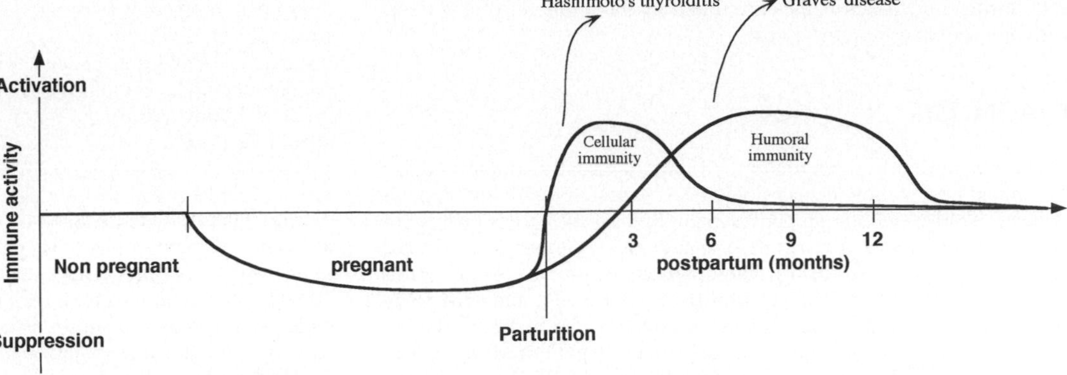

FIGURE 103–6. Immune rebound hypothesis regarding the onset of postpartum thyroiditis. Possible immunosuppression in pregnancy may disappear at delivery, and "transient enhancement" of the immune reactions may occur after delivery. (From Amino N, Tada H, Hidaka Y: Autoimmune thyroid disease and pregnancy. J Endocrinol Invest 19:59–70, 1996.)

ble 103–4 summarizes clinical data on patients with destruction-induced thyrotoxicosis.[98] We find that postpartum thyroiditis develops in all women with subclinical autoimmune thyroiditis and an MCAb titer of greater than 1:5120 before pregnancy.[4] A significant percentage of patients with silent thyroiditis have personal or family histories of autoimmune thyroid disease. Most patients have a complete remission, but persistent hypothyroidism develops in some.[99, 100] Recurrence of disease is common in silent thyroiditis but very rare in subacute thyroiditis. In view of all these data, we assume that silent thyroiditis is caused by the exacerbation of autoimmune thyroiditis induced by aggravating factors. Thyroiditis frequently recurs, and seasonal allergic rhinitis is reported to be an initiating factor.[101] Physically vigorous massage on the neck was also reported to be a contributing factor for silent thyroiditis.[102] Silent thyroiditis, including postpartum disease, accounts for 4.9% of all types of thyrotoxicosis. Spontaneous silent thyroiditis is three times more frequent than postpartum thyroiditis.

An immune rebound mechanism (Fig. 103–6) has been established for the induction of postpartum thyroiditis.[4] Postpartum thyroid destruction is associated with an increase in NK cell counts and activity.[103] Cessation of steroid therapy has initiated silent thyroiditis in a patient with autoimmune thyroiditis and rheumatoid arthritis,[104] presumably because of immune rebound. In patients with Cushing's syndrome who have associated subclinical autoimmune thyroiditis, silent thyroiditis has occurred after unilateral adrenalectomy.[105] Typically, painless thyroiditis or destructive thyrotoxicosis occurs 1 to 3 months postpartum. Painless transient thyrotoxicosis was found in 20 (2.9%) of 680 consecutive postpartum women. When patients with transient hypothyroidism were included, the incidence increased to 4.1%. The range of incidence of postpartum thyroiditis was reported to be 1.2% to 16.7%. The reason for the variability is not clear but may be attributed to differences in analytic methods, ethnic groups, or environmental or genetic risk factors. Most probably, the prevalence of postpartum thyroiditis ranges from 3% to 6%.

Relation to Graves' Disease

After treatment, patients with Graves' disease often progress to hypothyroidism,[106] possibly because of the autoimmune tissue destruction described above. Another mechanism for the appearance of hypothyroidism is an increase in TSBAbs. Macchia et al. found that 15 of 135 thyrotoxic patients with Graves' disease (11.1%) had blocking activity after TSH-induced adenylate cyclase stimulation but no TSAb activity.[107] That is, some patients with Graves' disease have both stimulating and blocking antibodies. When they have predominantly stimulating antibodies, hyperthyroidism develops, and when blocking antibodies becomes predominant, they progress to hypothyroidism. The clinical features of patients depend on the balance between the stimulating, blocking, and destructive aspects of humoral and cellular immunity.[87] When stimulating factors are predominant, Graves' thyrotoxicosis develops. A predominance of destructive factors, such as ADCC, T lymphocyte cytotoxicity, lymphotoxin (TNF), and cytotoxic antibody, may produce Hashimoto's disease or myxedema. Blocking factors such as TSBAb also cause a reduction in thyroid function. Once thyroid cells are destroyed completely, stimulating factors are ineffective.[108]

Relation to Other Autoimmune Diseases

Patients with other autoimmune diseases are often found to be positive for MCHAs and/or TGHAs, and these disorders are thus associated with autoimmune thyroid diseases.[1] The incidence is higher than in the general population (Table 103–5). Autoimmune thyroid disease is found in association with both organ-specific autoimmune diseases (e.g., vitiligo, myasthenia gravis, thrombocytopenic purpura, alopecia, Sjögren's syndrome[109]) and systemic autoimmune diseases (e.g., rheumatoid arthritis, systemic lupus erythematosus, and progressive systemic sclerosis). An association with other endocrine autoimmune diseases (such as insulin-dependent diabetes mellitus, autoimmune adrenalitis, autoimmune hypoparathyroidism, autoimmune hypophysitis) is also found in autoimmune thyroiditis. Such autoimmunity may occur simultaneously in multiple organs (polyendocrine autoimmune disease).

On the other hand, the frequency with which patients with autoimmune thyroid disease suffer from another autoimmune disease is low, except for autoimmune gastritis.[110] Anti–parietal cell antibodies and/or

TABLE 103–5. Incidence of Antithyroglobulin and Antithyroid Microsomal Hemagglutination Antibodies in Other Autoimmune Diseases

Disease	Number Examined	TGHA Titer		MCHA Titer	
		20 and Over	*More than 10^4*	*20 and Over*	*More than 10^4*
Systemic lupus erythematosus	104	19* (18)†	4 (4)	43 (41)	5 (5)
Rheumatoid arthritis	38	8 (21)	2 (5)	15 (39)	5 (13)
Progressive systemic sclerosis	37	4 (11)	0 (0)	13 (35)	3 (8)
Sjögren's syndrome	19	4 (21)	0 (0)	10 (53)	4 (21)
Myasthenia gravis	183	18 (10)	2 (1)	52 (28)	5 (3)
Idiopathic thrombocytopenic purpura	64	9 (14)	5 (8)	26 (41)	11 (17)

*Indicates number of patients.
†Indicates percentage of patients.
MCHA, antithyroid microsomal hemagglutination antibody; TGHA, antithyroglobulin hemagglutination antibody.
From Amino N: Antithyroid antibodies. *In* Ingbar SH, Braverman LE (eds): The Thyroid, ed 5. Philadelphia, JB Lippincott, 1986, pp 546–559.

anti–intrinsic factor antibodies are found in about one-third of patients with autoimmune thyroid disease.

DIAGNOSIS

The diagnosis of autoimmune thyroiditis is usually simple to make by clinical observation and serologic tests, especially in overt hypothyroidism. A diffuse goiter and positive antithyroid antibodies (antithyroglobulin antibodies and/or anti-TPO antibodies) without any evidence of other thyroid disease lead to the diagnosis of goitrous Hashimoto's thyroiditis. Tests of thyroid function (free T_4, free T_3, and TSH) may not be helpful because thyroiditis is subclinical in about 90% of patients. In patients who seem to have primary hypothyroidism with an atrophic thyroid, the existence of blocking-type anti–TSH-R antibodies (TSBAbs) can be assessed, although their prevalence is low.[111]

Histologic examination is confirmative but not necessary for diagnosis and management of the thyroiditis because lymphocytic infiltration into the thyroid is observed in all seropositive patients.[2] Conversely, either TGHA or MCHA is detectable in more than 95% of histologically confirmed cases of Hashimoto's disease. Indeed, detection of the antibodies is sufficient for a diagnosis of autoimmune thyroid disease. Antibodies are also found in about 10% of individuals in the general population without any clinical manifestation, and these patients should be considered to have subclinical autoimmune thyroiditis. For the small number of seronegative patients who have overt or latent hypothyroidism, the diagnosis of Hashimoto's thyroiditis is likely, but histologic examination is the only way to prove its existence. Thyroid biopsy will be necessary if the goiter is rapidly increasing and is very hard or fixed, that is, when thyroid tumors are suspected.

During the thyrotoxic phase of acute exacerbations of Hashimoto's thyroiditis and in silent thyroiditis, it is necessary to rule out Graves' disease, subacute thyroiditis, and toxic nodular goiter. As shown in Table 103–6, Graves' thyrotoxicosis lasts for more than 3 months, but the increased thyroid hormone levels in silent thyroiditis usually disappear within 3 months. Patients with Graves' disease have anti–TSH-R antibody, and TSH-binding inhibitory immunoglobulin, measured by radioreceptor assay, is positive in about 90% of patients. These antibodies are usually negative in silent thyroiditis, although some exceptions may be found.[112] The serum T_3/T_4 ratio (nanogram per microgram) is a simple indicator for differentiation between the two types of thyrotoxicosis. Eighty percent of patients with Graves' thyrotoxicosis show a ratio of more than 20, but it is less than 20 in destructive thyrotoxicosis, including silent thyroiditis. After complete remission of Graves' disease, silent thyroiditis sometimes develops in the same patients. Therefore, the previous history is not useful for differentiation.

TREATMENT

No practical way has been found to manipulate the autoimmune abnormality itself. The major approach is to treat the associated hypothyroidism or attempt to shrink the goiter to release pressure symptoms or simply for cosmetic reasons. T_4 replacement therapy is not usually necessary in euthyroid patients with small or moderate goiters. These patients should be examined once a year to recognize the later development of hypothyroidism. When hypothyroidism develops, patients should be treated with T_4. The daily replacement dose is 100 to 200 μg/day (about 2 μg/kg/day). In patients with long-standing hypothyroidism, replacement therapy should be initiated with a small dose of T_4 and built up gradually until a satisfactory maintenance dose is achieved. Hypothyroidism in patients with large goiters and high iodine uptake is often transient,[113] especially in patients younger than 30 years. Restriction of high iodine ingestion may be effective in these patients. Hypothyroidism in patients with postpartum thyroiditis is usually transient. In these patients, lifelong T_4 therapy is not necessary. T_3 therapy rather than T_4 is useful for a short period to quickly relieve the hypothyroid symptoms.

In patients with silent and postpartum thyroiditis, the thyrotoxicosis is usually mild and self-limited, and special treatment may not be required. To relieve thyrotoxic symptoms, β-adrenergic antagonists are sometimes effective. Steroid therapy reduces the inflammatory process,[90] but the optimal starting dose and duration of therapy have not been established. Painful subacute exacerbation of goitrous Hashimoto's disease is rare, and corticosteroid therapy is useful in these cases. About 10% to 20% of patients have recurrent episodes of destructive thyroiditis, but thyroid suppression therapy is not effective for prevention. In rare patients who have frequent recurrences, surgical removal of the gland or ^{131}I therapy has been recommended.[90, 96]

TABLE 103–6. Differential Diagnosis of Thyrotoxicosis between Silent Thyroiditis and Graves' Disease

Feature	Silent Thyroiditis	Graves' Disease
Duration of symptoms (mo)	<3	>3
Eye signs	No	30% yes
Radioactive iodine uptake	Low	High
Anti-TSH receptor antibody	Negative	Positive
T_3/T_4 ratio (ng/μg)	<20	80% >20
Thyrotoxicosis	Transient	Persistent

T_3, triiodothyronine; T_4, thyroxine; TSH, thyroid-stimulating hormone.

From Amino N: Postpartum and silent thyroiditis. *In* Monaco F. Satta MA, Shapiro B, Toncone L (eds): Thyroid Diseases. Clinical Fundamentals and Therapy. Boca Raton, FL, CRC Press, 1993, pp 239–249.

NATURAL HISTORY

Most patients with Hashimoto's thyroiditis are either euthyroid or have latent hypothyroidism with goiter in their youth. As time passes, some progress to overt hypothyroidism. The goiter becomes smaller and occasionally atrophies. Histologically, fibrosis spreads, and few thyroid follicles remain in this stage of thyroiditis. Thus elderly patients with Hashimoto's thyroiditis are more likely to be hypothyroid. It is appropriate for patients with subclinical autoimmune thyroiditis to be examined periodically (once or twice a year), although the incidence of hypothyroidism is not high.

Patients may experience periods of transient hypothyroidism under certain conditions. In some cases of Hashimoto's thyroiditis, the hypothyroidism seems to be reversible.[113] This transient hypothyroidism may occur in the course of Hashimoto's thyroiditis when destruction of the thyroid is slow. The hypothyroidism is often transient when a goiter is present and the serum thyroglobulin concentration is high.[114] The thyroid response to TSH after the administration of thyrotropin releasing hormone can be used to evaluate potential recovery from hypothyroidism in patients undergoing T_4 therapy.[115] Of patients with postpartum hypothyroidism, about 70% recover in several months, whereas permanent hypothyroidism develops in 30%.[82]

About 5% of patients experience destructive thyrotoxicosis.[97] Acute inflammatory symptoms (such as high fever and spontaneous pain in the thyroid) may be present. After the thyrotoxic phase, a period of transient hypothyroidism follows, and then such patients usually recover to euthyroidism.

In a region where iodine-containing food (such as seaweed) is common, as in Japan, excessive dietary iodine intake (1000 μg/day or more) may cause transient hypothyroidism in patients with subclinical autoimmune thyroiditis. This condition is easily reversible with a reduction in iodine intake.[116]

A rare but important complication of Hashimoto's thyroiditis is malignant lymphoma. The frequency of malignant lymphoma of thyroid origin is increased in patients with Hashimoto's thyroiditis.[117]

REFERENCES

1. Hashimoto H: Zur Kenntniss der lymphomatösen Veränderung der Schilddrüse (Struma lymphomatosa). Arch Klin Chir 97:219, 1912.
2. Yoshida H, Amino N, Yagawa K, et al: Association of serum antithyroid antibodies with lymphocytic infiltration of the thyroid gland: Studies of seventy autopsied cases. J Clin Endocrinol Metab 46:859, 1978.

3. Amino N: Antithyroid antibodies. *In* Ingber SH, Braverman LE (eds): The Thyroid, ed 5. Philadelphia, JB Lippincott, 1986, p 546.
4. Amino N, Miyai K: Postpartum autoimmune endocrine syndromes. *In* Davies TF (ed): Autoimmune Endocrine Disease. New York, John Wiley & Sons, 1983, p 247.
5. Woolner LB, McConahey WM, Beahrs OH: Struma lymphomatosa (Hashimoto's thyroiditis and related thyroidal disorders). J Clin Endocrinol 19:53, 1959.
6. Gluck FB, Nusynowitz ML, Plymate S: Chronic lymphocytic thyroiditis, thyrotoxicosis, and low radioactive iodine uptake. Report of four cases. N Engl J Med 293:624, 1975.
7. Inada M, Nishikawa M, Oishi M, et al: Transient thyrotoxicosis associated with painless thyroiditis and low radioactive iodine uptake. Arch Intern Med 139:597, 1979.
8. Nossal GJ, Pike BL: Evidence for the clonal abortion theory of B-lymphocyte tolerance. J Exp Med 141:904, 1975.
9. Volpe R, Iitaka M: Evidence for an antigen-specific defect in suppressor T-lymphocytes in autoimmune thyroid disease. Exp Clin Endocrinol 97:133, 1991.
10. Martin A, Davies TF: T cells and human autoimmune thyroid disease: Emerging data show lack of need to invoke suppressor T cell problems. Thyroid 2:247, 1992.
11. Volpe R: Immunology of human thyroid disease. *In* Volpe R (ed): Autoimmunity in Endocrine Diseases. Boca Raton, FL, CRC Press, 1990, p 73.
12. Bottazzo GF, Pujol-Borrell R, Hanafusa T, et al: Role of aberrant HLA-DR expression and antigen presentation in induction of endocrine autoimmunity. Lancet 2:1115, 1983.
13. Roitt IM, Torrigiani G: Identification and estimation of undegraded thyroglobulin in human serum. Endocrinology 81:421, 1967.
14. Roberts IM, Whittingham S, Mackay IR: Tolerance to an autoantigen-thyroglobulin. Antigen-binding lymphocytes in thymus and blood in health and autoimmune disease. Lancet 2:936, 1973.
15. Piechaczyk M, Bouanani M, Salhi SL, et al: Antigenic domains on the human thyroglobulin molecule recognized by autoantibodies in patients' sera and by natural autoantibodies isolated from the sera of healthy subjects. Clin Immunol Immunopathol 45:114, 1987.
16. Bouanani M, Piechaczyk M, Pau B, et al: Significance of the recognition of certain antigenic regions on the human thyroglobulin molecule by natural autoantibodies from healthy subjects. J Immunol 143:1129, 1989.
17. Henry M, Zanelli E, Piechaczyk M, et al: A major human thyroglobulin epitope defined with monoclonal antibodies is mainly recognized by human autoantibodies. Eur J Immunol 22:315, 1992.
18. Tamaki H, Amino N, Iwatani Y, et al: Detection of thyroid microsomal and thyroglobulin antibodies by new sensitive radioimmunoassay in Hashimoto's disease; comparison with conventional hemagglutination assay. Endocrinol Jpn 38:97, 1991.
19. Portmann L, Hamada N, Heinrich G, et al: Anti-thyroid peroxidase antibody in patients with autoimmune thyroid disease: Possible identity with anti microsomal antibody. J Clin Endocrinol Metab 61:1001, 1985.
20. Khoury EL, Hammond L, Bottazzo GF, et al: Presence of the organ-specific 'microsomal' autoantigen on the surface of human thyroid cells in culture: Its involvement in complement-mediated cytotoxicity. Clin Exp Immunol 45:316, 1981.
21. Tandon N, Jayne DR, McGregor AM, et al: Analysis of anti-idiotypic antibodies against anti-microsomal antibodies in patients with thyroid autoimmunity. J Autoimmun 5:557, 1992.
22. Tamaki H, Amino N, Aozasa M, et al: Effective method for prediction of transient hypothyroidism in neonates born to mothers with chronic thyroiditis. Am J Perinatol 6:296, 1989.
23. Konishi J, Iida Y, Kasagi K, et al: Primary myxedema with thyrotrophin-binding inhibitor immunoglobulins. Clinical and laboratory findings in 15 patients. Ann Intern Med 103:26, 1985.
24. Dallas JS, Desai RK, Cunningham SJ, et al: Thyrotropin (TSH) interacts with multiple discrete regions of the TSH receptor: Polyclonal rabbit antibodies to one or more of these regions can inhibit TSH binding and function. Endocrinology 134:1437, 1994.
25. Kosugi S, Ban T, Akamizu T, et al: Use of thyrotropin receptor (TSHR) mutants to detect stimulating TSHR antibodies in hypothyroid patients with idiopathic myxedema, who have blocking TSHR antibodies. J Clin Endocrinol Metab 77:19, 1993.
26. Nagayama Y, Wadworth HL, Chazenbalk GD, et al: Thyrotropin–luteinizing hormone/chorionic gonadotropin receptor extracellular domain chimeras as probes for thyrotropin receptor function. Proc Natl Acad Sci USA 88:902, 1991.
27. Tahara K, Ban T, Minegishi T, et al: Immunoglobulins from Graves' disease patients interact with different sites on TSH receptor/LH-CG receptor chimeras than either TSH or immunoglobulins from idiopathic myxedema patients. Biochem Biophys Res Commun 179:70, 1991.
28. Amino N, Watanabe Y, Tamaki H, et al: In-vitro conversion of blocking type anti-TSH receptor antibody to the stimulating type by anti-human IgG antibodies. Clin Endocrinol (Oxf) 27:615, 1987.
29. Dai G, Levy O, Carrasco N: Cloning and characterization of the thyroid iodine transporter. Nature 379:458, 1996.
30. Endo T, Kaneshige M, Nakazato M, et al: Autoantibody against thyroid iodine transporter in the sera from patients with Hashimoto's thyroiditis possesses iodide transport activity. Biochem Biophys Res Commun 228:199, 1996.
31. Endo T, Kogai T, Nakazato M, et al: Autoantibody against Na^+/I^- symporter in the sera of patients with autoimmune thyroid disease. Biochem Biophys Res Commun 224:92, 1996.
32. Sakata S, Nakamura S, Miura K: Autoantibodies against thyroid hormones or iodothyronine. Implications in diagnosis, thyroid function, treatment, and pathogenesis. Ann Intern Med 103:579, 1985.
33. Staeheli V, Vallotton MB, Burger A: Detection of human anti-thyroxine and anti-triiodothyronine antibodies in different thyroid conditions. J Clin Endocrinol Metab 41:669, 1975.
34. Konishi J, Iida Y, Kousaka T, et al: Effect of anti-thyroxin autoantibodies on radioimmunoassay of free thyroxin in serum. Clin Chem 28:1389, 1982.
35. Sakata S, Takuno H, Nagai K, et al: Anti-bovine thyrotropin autoantibodies in patients with Hashimoto's thyroiditis, subacute thyroiditis, and systemic lupus erythematosus. J Endocrinol Invest 14:123–130, 1991.
36. Zakaria M, MacKenzie J: Do thyroid growth-promoting immunoglobulins exist? J Clin Endocrinol Metab 70:308, 1990.
37. Miyamoto S, Kasagi K, Alam MS, et al: Assessment of thyroid growth stimulating activity of immunoglobulins from patients with autoimmune thyroid diseases by cytokinesis arrest assay. Eur J Endocrinol 136:499, 1997.
38. Tachi J, Amino N, Iwatani Y, et al: Increase in antideoxyribonucleic acid antibody titer in postpartum aggravation of autoimmune thyroid disease. J Clin Endocrinol Metab 67:1049, 1988.
39. DeGroot LJ, Quintans J: The causes of autoimmune thyroid disease. Endocr Rev 10:537, 1989.
40. Sawada K, Sakurami T, Imura H, et al: Anti–asialo-GM_1 antibody in sera from patients with Graves' disease and Hashimoto's thyroiditis (letter). Lancet 2:198, 1980.
41. Thall A, Etienne-Decerf J, Winand RJ, et al: The alpha-galactosyl epitope on mammalian thyroid cells. Acta Endocrinol (Copenh) 124:692, 1991.
42. Giordano C, Stassi G, De Maria R, et al: Potential involvement of Fas and its ligand in the pathogenesis of Hashimoto's thyroiditis. Science 275:960, 1997.
43. Itoh N, Yonehara S, Ishii A, et al: The polypeptide encoded by the cDNA for human cell surface antigen Fas can mediate apoptosis. Cell 66:233, 1991.
44. Suda T, Takahashi T, Golstein P, et al: Molecular cloning and expression of the Fas ligand, a novel member of the tumor necrosis factor family. Cell 75:1169, 1993.
45. Cheng J, Zhou T, Liu C, et al: Protection from Fas-mediated apoptosis by a soluble form of the Fas molecule. Science 263:1759, 1994.
46. Shimaoka Y, Hidaka Y, Okumura M, et al: Serum concentration of soluble Fas in patients with autoimmune thyroid diseases. Thyroid 8:43, 1998.
47. MacKenzie WA, Schwartz AE, Friedman EW, et al: Intrathyroidal T cell clones from patients with autoimmune thyroid disease. J Clin Endocrinol Metab 64:818, 1987.
48. Iwatani Y, Hidaka Y, Matsuzuka F, et al: Intrathyroidal lymphocyte subsets, including unusual $CD4^+$ $CD8^+$ cells and CD3loTCR alpha beta lo/-$CD4^-CD8^-$ cells, in autoimmune thyroid disease. Clin Exp Immunol 93:430, 1993.
49. Iwatani Y, Amino N, Mori H, et al: A microcytotoxicity assay for thyroid-specific cytotoxic antibody, antibody-dependent cell-mediated cytotoxicity and direct lymphocyte cytotoxicity using human thyroid cells. J Immunol Methods 48:241, 1982.
50. Pulvertaft RJV, Doniach D, Roitt IM: The cytotoxic factor in Hashimoto's disease and its incidence in other thyroid diseases. Br J Exp Pathol 42:496, 1961.
51. Calder EA, McLeman D, Irvine WJ: Lymphocyte cytotoxicity induced by pre-incubation with serum from patients with Hashimoto thyroiditis. Clin Exp Immunol 15:467, 1973.
52. Bogner U, Schleusener H, Wall JR: Antibody-dependent cell mediated cytotoxicity against human thyroid cells in Hashimoto's thyroiditis but not Graves' disease. J Clin Endocrinol Metab 59:734, 1984.
53. Amino N, Mori H, Iwatani Y, et al: Peripheral K lymphocytes in autoimmune thyroid disease: Decrease in Graves' disease and increase in Hashimoto's disease. J Clin Endocrinol Metab 54:587, 1982.
54. Mosmann TR, Sad S: The expanding universe of T-cell subsets: Th1, Th2 and more. Immunol Today 17:138, 1996.
55. Fisfalen ME, Palmer EM, Van Seventer GA, et al: Thyrotropin-receptor and thyroid peroxidase–specific T cell clones and their cytokine profile in autoimmune thyroid disease. J Clin Endocrinol Metab 82:3655, 1997.
56. Heuer M, Aust G, Ode-Hakim S, et al: Different cytokine mRNA profiles in Graves' disease, Hashimoto's thyroiditis, and nonautoimmune thyroid disorders determined by quantitative reverse transcriptase polymerase chain reaction (RT-PCR). Thyroid 6:97, 1996.
57. Ajjan RA, Watson PF, McIntosh RS, et al: Intrathyroidal cytokine gene expression in Hashimoto's thyroiditis. Clin Exp Immunol 105:523, 1996.
58. Paschke R, Schuppert F, Taton M, et al: Intrathyroidal cytokine gene expression profiles in autoimmune thyroiditis. J Endocrinol 141:309, 1994.
59. Roura-Mir C, Catalfamo M, Sospedra M, et al: Single cell analysis of intrathyroidal lymphocytes shows differential cytokine expression in Hashimoto's and Graves' disease. Eur J Immunol 27:3290, 1997.
60. Hidaka Y, Okumura M, Fukata S, et al: Increased serum concentration of interleukin-12 in patients with silent thyroiditis and Graves' disease. Thyroid 9:149–153, 1999.
61. Battifora M, Pesce G, Paolieri F, et al: B7.1 costimulatory molecule is expressed on thyroid follicular cells in Hashimoto's thyroiditis, but not in Graves' disease. J Clin Endocrinol Metab 83:4130, 1998.
62. Weetman AP, Freeman M, Borysiewicz LK, et al: Functional analysis of intercellular adhesion molecule-1–expressing human thyroid cells. Eur J Immunol 20:271, 1990.
63. Davies TF, Martin A, Concepcion ES, et al: Evidence of limited variability of antigen receptors on intrathyroidal T cells in autoimmune thyroid disease. N Engl J Med 325:238, 1991.
64. Aozasa M, Amino N, Iwatani Y, et al: Intrathyroidal HLA-DR–positive lymphocytes in Hashimoto's disease: Increases in CD8 and Leu7 cells. Clin Immunol Immunopathol 52:516, 1989.
65. Ohashi H, Okugawa T, Itoh M: Circulating activated T cell subsets in autoimmune thyroid diseases: Differences between untreated and treated patients. Acta Endocrinol (Copenh) 125:502, 1991.
66. Iwatani Y, Amino N, Hidaka Y, et al: Decreases in alpha beta T cell receptor negative T cells and CD8 cells, and an increase in $CD4^+$ $CD8^+$ cells in active Hashimoto's disease and subacute thyroiditis. Clin Exp Immunol 87:444, 1992.
67. Suranyi P, Szegedi G, Damjanovich S, et al: B lymphocyte subsets in Hashimoto's thyroiditis. Immunol Lett 22:147, 1989.
68. Iwatani Y, Amino N, Kaneda T: Marked increase of $CD5^+$ B cells in hyperthyroid Graves' disease. Clin Exp Immunol 78:196, 1989.
69. Hidaka Y, Amino N, Iwatani Y, et al: Changes in natural killer cell activity in normal pregnant and postpartum women: Increases in the first trimester and postpartum period and decrease in late pregnancy. J Reprod Immunol 20:73, 1991.

70. Nagataki S, Eguchi K: Cytokines and immune regulation in thyroid autoimmunity. Autoimmunity 13:27, 1992.
71. Kaplan MM: Hypothyroidism after treatment with interleukin-2 and lymphokine-activated killer cells. N Engl J Med 318:1157, 1988.
72. Nagayama Y, Ohta K, Tsuruta M, et al: Exacerbation of thyroid autoimmunity by interferon alpha treatment in patients with chronic viral hepatitis: Our studies and review of the literature. Endocr J 41:565, 1994.
73. Asakawa H, Hanafusa T, Kobayashi T, et al: Interferon-gamma reduces the thyroid peroxidase content of cultured human thyrocytes and inhibits its increase induced by thyrotropin. J Clin Endocrinol Metab 74:1331, 1992.
74. Kung AW, Ma L, Lau KS: The role of interferon-gamma in lymphocytic thyroiditis: Its functional and pathological effect on human thyrocytes in culture. Clin Exp Immunol 87:261, 1992.
75. Weetman AP, Tandon N, Morgan BP: Antithyroid drugs and release of inflammatory mediators by complement-attacked thyroid cells. Lancet 340:633, 1992.
76. Mangklabruks A, Cox N, DeGroot LJ: Genetic factors in autoimmune thyroid disease analyzed by restriction fragment length polymorphisms of candidate genes. J Clin Endocrinol Metab 73:236, 1991.
77. Shi Y, Zou M, Robb D, et al: Typing for major histocompatibility complex class II antigens in thyroid tissue blocks: Association of Hashimoto's thyroiditis with HLA-DQA0301 and DQB0201 alleles. J Clin Endocrinol Metab 75:943, 1992.
78. Vargas MT, Briones-Urbina R, Gladman D, et al: Antithyroid microsomal autoantibodies and HLA-DR5 are associated with postpartum thyroid dysfunction: Evidence supporting an autoimmune pathogenesis. J Clin Endocrinol Metab 67:327, 1988.
79. Honda K, Tamai H, Morita T, et al: Hashimoto's thyroiditis and HLA in Japanese. J Clin Endocrinol Metab 69:1268, 1989.
80. Ito M, Tanimoto M, Kamura H, et al: Association of HLA antigen and restriction fragment length polymorphism of T cell receptor beta-chain gene with Graves' disease and Hashimoto's thyroiditis. J Clin Endocrinol Metab 69:100, 1989.
81. Wang FW, Yu ZQ, Xy JJ, et al: HLA and hypertrophic Hashimoto's thyroiditis in Shanghai Chinese. Tissue Antigens 32:235, 1988.
82. Tachi J, Amino N, Tamaki H, et al: Long term follow-up and HLA association in patients with postpartum hypothyroidism. J Clin Endocrinol Metab 66:480, 1988.
83. Weetman AP, So AK, Roe C, et al: T-cell receptor alpha chain V region polymorphism linked to primary autoimmune hypothyroidism but not Graves' disease. Hum Immunol 20:167, 1987.
84. Donner H, Braun J, Seidl C, et al: Codon 17 polymorphism of the cytotoxic T lymphocyte antigen 4 gene in Hashimoto's thyroiditis and Addison's disease. J Clin Endocrinol Metab 82:4130, 1997.
85. Tamai H, Uno H, Hirota Y, et al: Immunogenetics of Hashimoto's and Graves' diseases. J Clin Endocrinol Metab 60:62, 1985.
86. Uno H, Sasazuki T, Tamai H, et al: Two major genes, linked to HLA and Gm, control susceptibility to Graves' disease. Nature 292:768, 1981.
87. Amino N: Autoimmunity and hypothyroidism. Baillieres Clin Endocrinol Metab 2:591, 1988.
88. Hawkins BR, Cheah PS, Dawkins RL, et al: Diagnostic significance of thyroid microsomal antibodies in randomly selected population. Lancet 2:1057, 1980.
89. Amino N, Mori H, Iwatani Y, et al: Significance of thyroid microsomal antibodies (letter). Lancet 2:1369, 1980.
90. Nikolai TF, Coombs GJ, McKenzie AK, et al: Treatment of lymphocytic thyroiditis with spontaneously resolving hyperthyroidism (silent thyroiditis). Arch Intern Med 142:2281, 1982.
91. Amino N, Iwatani Y, Tamaki H: Postpartum autoimmune thyroid syndromes. *In* Walfish PG, Wall RV Jr (eds): Autoimmunity and Thyroid. New York, Academic Press, 1985, p 89.
92. Woolf PD, Daly R: Thyrotoxicosis with painless thyroiditis. Am J Med 60:73, 1976.
93. Hamburger JI: Occult subacute thyroiditis: Diagnostic challenge. Mich Med 70:1125, 1976.
94. Woolf PD: Transient painless thyroiditis with hyperthyroidism: A variant of lymphocytic thyroiditis? Endocr Rev 1:11, 1980.
95. Nikolai TF, Brosseau J, Kettrick MA, et al: Lymphocytic thyroiditis with spontaneously resolving hyperthyroidism (silent thyroiditis). Arch Intern Med 140:478, 1980.
96. Gorman CA, Duick DS, Woolner LB, et al: Transient hyperthyroidism in patients with lymphocytic thyroiditis. Mayo Clin Proc 53:359, 1978.
97. Amino N, Yabu Y, Miyai K, et al: Differentiation of thyrotoxicosis induced by thyroid destruction from Graves' disease. Lancet 2:344, 1978.
98. Amino N: Postpartum and silent thyroiditis. *In* Monaco F, Satta MA, Shapiro B, et al (eds): Thyroid Diseases. Clinical Fundamentals and Therapy. Boca Raton, FL, CRC Press, 1993, p 239.
99. Amino N, Mori H, Iwatani Y, et al: High prevalence of transient post-partum thyrotoxicosis and hypothyroidism. N Engl J Med 306:849, 1982.
100. Nikolai TF, Coombs GJ, McKenzie AK: Lymphocytic thyroiditis with spontaneously resolving hyperthyroidism and subacute thyroiditis. Long-term follow-up. Arch Intern Med 141:1455, 1981.
101. Yamamoto M, Shibuya N, Chen LC, et al: Seasonal recurrence of transient hypothyroidism in a patient with autoimmune thyroiditis. Endocrinol Jpn 35:135, 1988.
102. Tachi J, Amino N, Miyai K: Massage therapy on neck: A contributing factor for destructive thyrotoxicosis? Thyroidology 2:25, 1990.
103. Hidaka Y, Amino N, Iwatani Y, et al: Increase in peripheral natural killer cell activity in patients with autoimmune thyroid disease. Autoimmunity 11:239, 1992.
104. Maruyama H, Kato M, Mizuno O, et al: Transient thyrotoxicosis occurred after cessation of steroid therapy in a patient with autoimmune thyroiditis and rheumatoid arthritis. Endocrinol Jpn 29:583, 1982.
105. Takasu N, Komiya I, Nagasawa Y, et al: Exacerbation of autoimmune thyroid dysfunction after unilateral adrenalectomy in patients with Cushing's syndrome due to an adrenocortical adenoma. N Engl J Med 322:1708, 1990.
106. Wood LC, Ingbar SH: Hypothyroidism as a late sequela in patient with Graves' disease treated with antithyroid agents. J Clin Invest 64:1429, 1979.
107. Macchia E, Concetti R, Carone G, et al: Demonstration of blocking immunoglobulins G, having a heterogeneous behaviour, in sera of patients with Graves' disease: Possible coexistence of different autoantibodies directed to the TSH receptor. Clin Endocrinol (Oxf) 28:147, 1988.
108. Tamaki H, Amino N, Iwatani Y, et al: Improvement of infiltrative ophthalmopathy in parallel with decrease of thyroid-stimulating antibody (TSAb) activity in two patients with hypothyroid Graves' disease. J Endocrinol Invest 12:47, 1989.
109. Karsh J, Pavlidis N, Weintraub BD, et al: Thyroid disease in Sjögren's syndrome. Arthritis Rheum 23:1326, 1980.
110. Irvine WJ, Sumerling MD, Davies SH: Immunologic aspects of pernicious anaemia. N Engl J Med 273:432, 1965.
111. Tamaki H, Amino N, Kimura M, et al: Low prevalence of thyrotropin receptor antibody in primary hypothyroidism in Japan. J Clin Endocrinol Metab 71:1382, 1990.
112. Morita T, Tamai H, Oshima A, et al: The occurrence of thyrotropin binding-inhibiting immunoglobulins and thyroid-stimulating antibodies in patients with silent thyroiditis. J Clin Endocrinol Metab 71:1051, 1990.
113. Yoshinari M, Okamura K, Tokuyama T, et al: Clinical importance of reversibility in primary goitrous hypothyroidism. BMJ 287:720, 1983.
114. Sato K, Okamura K, Ikenoue H, et al: TSH dependent elevation of serum thyroglobulin in reversible primary hypothyroidism. Clin Endocrinol (Oxf) 29:231, 1988.
115. Takasu N, Komiya I, Asawa T, et al: Test for recovery from hypothyroidism during thyroxine therapy in Hashimoto's thyroiditis. Lancet 336:1084, 1990.
116. Tajiri J, Higashi K, Morita M, et al: Studies of hypothyroidism in patients with high iodine intake. J Clin Endocrinol Metab 63:412, 1986.
117. Hamburger JI, Miller JM, Kini SR: Lymphoma of the thyroid. Ann Intern Med 99:685, 1983.

Chapter 104

Infectious, Subacute, and Sclerosing Thyroiditis

Robert Volpé

INFECTIOUS (SUPPURATIVE) THYROIDITIS

Infectious thyroiditis comprises (usually acute) inflammations of the thyroid gland caused by microorganisms. By convention, viruses are excluded, as these are considered the likely cause of subacute (de Quervain's) thyroiditis (see below).

Infections of the thyroid gland by bacteria are rare; however, parasitic or fungal infections of the thyroid are so extremely rare as to be considered medical oddities. These infections may be suppurative or nonsuppurative. Generally, the illness is acute, but it may be chronic and indolent, particularly in the case of fungal thyroiditis. In this chapter, emphasis is on bacterial infections of the thyroid.

Bauchet[1] first described acute inflammation of the thyroid in five patients in 1857. Perhaps the most useful review of this topic was that of Berger et al.[2] in 1983 who reviewed 224 reported cases culled from the literature between 1900 and 1980. The disease was more common in women than in men, and there was no particular age incidence.

Etiology and Pathogenesis

The organisms most commonly cultured from these lesions include *Streptococcus haemolyticus*, *Staphylococcus aureus*, *Pneumococcus*, and coliform bacilli.[2–4] A variety of other organisms have also been reported, including *Salmonella*, *Mycobacterium* (including *M. tuberculosis*), *Treponema* (including *T. pallidum*), *Actinomyces*, and various fungi and parasites.[2, 3] Acute suppurative thyroiditis may occur as a complication of nearby bacterial infections by extension or may occasionally result from bacteremia secondary to a distant focus. The routes by which infection can reach the thyroid gland include the blood stream, direct invasion from adjacent structures, direct trauma, lymphatics, and persistent thyroglossal duct. Often, some abnormality of the thyroid gland is found to be the focus upon which the infection develops. While the gland has shown itself to be resistant to infection by the hematogenous route, it is exceedingly difficult to implicate any other mechanism in many cases. In some patients, the source of the thyroid infection cannot be determined.[2–6]

Pathology

Pathologic examination reveals the characteristic changes of acute inflammation with a heavy polymorphonuclear and lymphocytic cellular infiltrate in the initial phase, often associated with necrosis and abscess formation. Once this happens, the pus usually dissects anteriorly through the ribbon muscles toward the skin. Occasionally, the abscess may move into the mediastinum or even rupture into the trachea or esophagus. Fibrosis is prominent as healing occurs.[3, 4]

In other instances, no abscess develops and spontaneous subsidence has been reported. Thrombophlebitis of the internal jugular vein may also occur. As mentioned previously, the process may involve the normal gland or may occur in a focal thyroid abnormality, such as a cyst.[2–4, 6]

Symptoms and Signs

The chief symptom is pain, usually severe, in the region of the thyroid gland, which may become enlarged, warm, and tender. The patient is usually unable to extend the neck backward and sits with the neck flexed to avoid pressure on the thyroid gland. There is considerable dysphagia in association with the lesion because of the painful swelling. The pain is often referred to the ear, the mandible, or the occiput on the side of the lesion. Moving the head also elicits severe pain. There are often signs of infection in structures adjacent to the thyroid, and lymphadenopathy in adjacent lymph nodes is common.

These local symptoms may be preceded by the sudden onset of malaise, fever, chills, and tachycardia. On examination, temperatures often vary from 38° to 40.5°C. The pulse rate is constantly elevated. There is swelling in the region of the thyroid, usually confined to one lobe and associated with extreme tenderness. On occasion, the whole gland may be involved. In later stages, there may be redness over the involved area, and lymphadenopathy can be demonstrated. Fluctuation generally cannot be elicited because of the induration of the overlying tissues.[2–4, 6]

Laboratory Findings

There is usually a polymorphonuclear leukocytosis of moderate or marked degree. The patient usually remains euthyroid, with normal values of thyroxine and triiodothyronine throughout the illness, although occasionally there may be a mild increase in serum thyroid hormone concentrations consequent to the release of stored hormone from the inflamed region into the systemic circulation. While the radioactive thyroidal uptake is generally within normal limits, the involved area may not pick up the radionuclide well and thus appears as a "cold" area on scanning. An ultrasonographic examination may show what appears to be a cystic lesion or may appear "complex." Thyroid antibodies do not appear during the course of the illness.

Diagnosis

The diagnosis requires an index of suspicion in the early phases. It is not difficult to establish when all of the aforementioned manifestations are present. If signs of inflammation of the thyroid are associated with local redness, exquisite tenderness, lymph node enlargement, a flexed neck, marked hyperpyrexia, and leukocytosis, the diagnosis would appear to be obvious. The condition must be differentiated from subacute thyroditis (SAT), which does not involve the neck structures, and is usually associated with less pain. Moreover, thyroid function is characteristically altered in SAT (see below). Nevertheless these conditions may be difficult to differentiate from one another prior to the development of suppuration.

At times, malignant neoplasms may develop focal necrosis and can mimic quite closely a primary pyogenic infection. Conversely, when the manifestations of infectious thyroiditis are more insidious, it in turn can mimic thyroid carcinoma. Infectious thyroiditis also can be mistaken for hemorrhage into a thyroid cyst, or chronic thyroiditis. Usually the passage of time serves to make the correct diagnosis obvious, particularly with the progression of pain, the appearance of or advance in swelling and redness in the thyroid region, and the onset and persistence of fever and leukocytosis. A lateral radiograph may also be useful in localizing the area of inflammation within the thyroid, and an ultrasonogram is similarly useful.[3, 4, 6]

Course and Management

The course is generally progressive, with complications of rupture of the abscess, septicemia, and thrombophlebitis apt to develop unless adequate treatment is instituted. Occasionally, the infection may subside spontaneously.

Conservative measures include rest, local heat, and antibiotics. These may be successful, but much depends on the identification of the infecting microorganisms. Gram-positive cocci are common offenders, and appropriate antibiotics have often proved to be effective.

If an abscess develops, and prompt response to antibiotics does not occur, surgical incision and drainage are necessary. Sometimes subtotal lobectomy must be performed for recurrent disease.

Currently the prognosis is usually excellent when a patient is treated appropriately with antibiotic therapy as well as surgery when required. The lesions generally heal with reasonable speed, and recurrences are uncommon. Function of the thyroid remains intact if treatment is adequate and begun promptly.[2–4, 6]

Chronic Infection

Chronic infection of the thyroid may result from a variety of organisms, although this occurrence is exceedingly rare. Chronic pyogenic thyroiditis caused by *Salmonella typhi* has been reported, but often chronic infections of the thyroid do not suppurate. Cases of syphilis, tuberculosis, and echinococcosis fall into this category. *Actinomyces* has also been reported several times as the organism responsible for an indolent and frequently suppurative form of thyroiditis, and these cases have generally responded to drainage and antibiotic therapy.

SUBACUTE THYROIDITIS

The term *subacute thyroiditis* now describes a well-defined clinical entity, characterized by a generally self-limiting, usually painful inflammatory lesion of the thyroid gland, probably of viral origin.[7–11] It is generally distinguishable from a somewhat similar disorder, namely, *painless* or *silent thyroiditis*, which disturbs thyroid function in a manner similar to SAT, but without pain or tenderness, and with a different pathologic appearance. Of course, the term *subacute thyroiditis* connotes a temporal quality that could apply to any thyroidal inflammatory process of intermediate duration and severity. However, the term is accepted currently as referring specifically to those patients showing a pseudogranulomatous pathologic appearance in the thyroid gland (which is virtually specific for the disease) and a characteristic clinical syndrome in which there is (usually) a painful tender goiter, malaise, fever, and evidence of thyroid dysfunction, to be described more fully below.[7–11] There is a strong preponderance of females over males in this condition.[7–11]

The first description of this disorder appears to be that of Mygind[12] who reported 18 cases of "thyroiditis akuta simplex" in 1895. However, the publications of de Quervain, who described this condition very thoroughly in 1904, and again in 1936, are generally given precedence.[13, 14] Subacute thyroiditis has several synonyms, some reflecting misconceptions regarding the etiology or pathology of the condition. These include acute simple thyroiditis, noninfectious thyroiditis, de Quervain's thyroiditis, acute or subacute diffuse thyroiditis, granulomatous thyroiditis, struma granulomatosa, pseudogranulomatous thyroiditis, giant cell thyroiditis, pseudo–giant cell thyroiditis, migratory "creeping" thyroiditis, pseudotuberculous thyroiditis, and viral thyroiditis. As noted below, the "giant cells" or "granulomas" actually only simulate such structures.[6, 7]

Incidence

Compared to other thyroid diseases, SAT is uncommon, occurring at the rate of about 1 case per 5 cases of Graves' disease (GD) and 1 case per 15 or 20 cases of Hashimoto's thyroiditis.[15] It has been reported most commonly from the temperate zone; it occurs most commonly between the second and fifth decades, is rare in children, seems to occur seasonally, and the female-male ratio is 3 to 6:1.[15]

Etiology

Considerable indirect evidence suggests that SAT represents a viral infection of the thyroid gland. In keeping with this theory, the condition is often preceded by a prodromal phase characterized by musculoskeletal aches and pains, malaise and fatigue, or a frank upper respiratory tract infection.[7–11] In some instances, the illness has occurred at the time of the outbreak of a specific viral infection, and its highest seasonal occurrence coincides with peaks of summer enterovirus infections.[15] After some weeks or months, complete recovery is the rule. The leukocyte count may sometimes be moderately elevated. Moreover, epidemics of SAT have been reported.[15]

SAT has been reported in association with mumps in several reports.[7] Still other reports associate SAT with measles,[7] influenza,[7] the common cold,[7] adenovirus,[7] infectious mononucleosis,[7] coxsackievirus,[7] myocarditis,[7] cat-scratch fever,[7] St. Louis encephalitis,[7] hepatitis A,[16] and the parvovirus B19 infection.[17] A virologic study in 28 patients with this disease performed in 1975 resulted in the isolation of a cytopathic virus of possible pathogenic significance from the thyroid glands of five patients of this group.[18–20] However, viral inclusion bodies have not been observed within sections of thyroid tissue in this disorder.[8]

In one study in Toronto, antibodies to some common viruses such as coxsackievirus, adenovirus, and influenza and mumps viruses were detected in the convalescent phase of this disease.[21] However, in a later study of 10 patients in Singapore, no such antibodies were observed.[22] Of course, the presence of such antibodies may not reflect pathogenic significance, but may instead result from an anamnestic response to the inflammatory process within the thyroid.

Certain nonviral infections such as Q fever and malaria have been associated with a clinical syndrome that at least simulates SAT.[7] The significance of these observations remains to be determined. In addition, a case of SAT occurring simultaneously with giant cell arteritis has been reported.[23] Another case of SAT developed during interferon-alfa treatment for hepatitis C.[24]

Although immunologic phenomena are seen during the course of SAT, the fact that they are transitory, arising after the onset, and disappearing with recovery, marks them as secondary.[25] These include the appearance of antibodies in some cases, T lymphocyte sensitization to thyroidal antigen,[25] and thyrocyte HLA-DR expression.[25] Significant titers of antibodies to thyroperoxidase and thyroglobulin appear transiently in only a small minority of patients,[79, 21, 25–28] and in one study the former antibodies correlated with the phase of transient hypothyroidism.[27] Antibodies to an unpurified thyroid preparation can be detected for up to 4 years after a course of SAT.[28]

Antibodies to the thyrotropin or thyroid-stimulating hormone (TSH) receptor have been detected in some patients by several workers during the course of SAT.[29–32] In most of these reported studies, the radioreceptor assay was employed, in which the antibody prevents the binding of TSH to thyroid cell membranes (thyrotropin-binding inhibitory immunoglobulin, TBII, TBIAb). This assay does not measure the ability of the antibody to stimulate thyroid cells (thyroid-stimulating antibody, TSAb). In most studies, there has been no correlation between the presence of the TBII and the hyperthyroid phase of the thyroiditis,[29–31] although one report did suggest such a relationship.[32] In the majority of reports, TBII was positive in some patients in the hypothyroid phase and negative in others; when positive, it ultimately became negative without respect to the status of thyroid function. When TSAb was studied instead of TBII, once again a good correlation with thyroid functional status did not exist.[33] On the other hand, when thyroid-blocking antibody was determined, there was some correlation with the development of hypothyroidism.[31] It would seem that the appearance of these TSH receptor antibodies, as with the other thyroid antibodies that occur in this condition, result from damage to the thyrocytes, with desquamation of their membranes, and an immune response thereto.

Following recovery from the inflammatory process, all immunologic phenomena disappear, in contrast to the continuing presence of these abnormalities in autoimmune thyroid disease (AITD).[25, 34] This difference helps to illuminate the pathogenesis of AITD; the transitory immunologic markers observed during the course of subacute thyroiditis appear to be secondary to the release of antigenic material from the thyroid and thus appear to be a normal, physiologic response to the inflammatory destruction of the gland.[25] The appearance of TSH receptor antibodies, both TSAb and thyroid-blocking antibody, would fit into this concept.[25, 34] The corollary is consistent with the view that antigen-driven events can produce a transient immunologic disturbance, but does not, or is most unlikely to, culminate in chronic AITD. This constitutes evidence against a purely antigen-driven causation for AITD, and is consistent with the concept that AITD results primarily from dysfunction of the immune system.[25] This concept has relevance in relation to the proposal that microbial antigens, which might have homology with thyroid antigens, might have a pathogenic role in AITD.[35] In the light of the above observations, and the lack of any direct evidence,[36, 37] this seems unlikely. Moreover, since many patients with subacute thyroiditis do manifest TSH receptor antibodies, it follows that many normal persons have the genes to produce such antibodies (and do so under the circumstances of this condition), but are ordinarily prevented from doing so by normal immunoregulation.[25, 37]

There is no direct association with AITD, and it is rare for SAT to progress to either GD or Hashimoto's disease, although this has been reported in a few cases. Werner[38] reported a case of painful thyroiditis that progressed to GD and reviewed the literature in 1979. He argued that such inflammatory lesions of the thyroid gland could liberate sufficient antigen to induce GD. Wartofsky and Schaaf[39] presented similar arguments in 1987. This sequence was reviewed in 1996.[40] However, because this development occurs so rarely, and GD usually occurs de novo, the possibility that excessive TSH receptor antigenic release has precipitated GD does not seem likely, and at least would have to be superimposed on genetic susceptibility. It is possible that the illness of SAT might act as a nonspecific stress acting on the immune system to precipitate GD.[25]

About 72% of patients with SAT, no matter what their ethnic background, are positive for HLA-Bw35.[41–44] The significance of this finding is not yet clear, but may reflect a genetic susceptibility of the thyroid to (certain) viral infections.

Pathology[7–12, 45, 46]

The thyroid gland is enlarged and somewhat edematous and may be slightly adherent to adjacent structures, although it can be freed from these without difficulty. Microscopically, the process may be diffuse or irregular in its involvement, with various stages of the disease sometimes present within the same specimen. The follicular cells sometimes virtually disappear, leaving a fragile and fine follicular lining. The initial phase is characterized by the appearance of neutrophils, followed by large mononuclear cells and lymphocytes (Fig. 104–1). The follicles appear much larger than normal with disruption of the epithelial lining and hyperplasia of the surviving follicular cells. Histiocytes congregate around masses of colloid both within the follicles and in the interstitial tissues, producing "giant cells"; because often these giant cells actually consist of masses of colloid surrounded by large numbers of individual histiocytes, they should in such cases be termed "pseudo–giant cells." The term "granulomatous thyroiditis," another synonym for SAT, should likewise in such circumstances be changed to "pseudo–granulomatous thyroiditis." However, true giant cells and granulomas do appear also in this disease.[47] There is considerable edema, with histiocytes and lymphocytes in the interstitial tissue.

The inflammatory process is often irregularly distributed in either or both lobes. With recovery, the inflammatory reaction recedes, and a variable amount of fibrosis may then appear. Areas of follicular regeneration are seen, but there is no caseation, hemorrhage, or calcification. The degree of recovery is generally virtually complete, aside from the residual fibrosis already mentioned. Only in rare instances is there complete destruction of the thyroid parenchyma leading to permanent hypothyroidism. Viral inclusion bodies have not been demonstrated in the few electron microscopic studies that have been reported.[8] There is marked thickening of the basement membrane and some evidence to suggest increased cellular activity, although no apical pseudopods with colloid droplets are seen after TSH stimulation.[8]

Fine-needle aspiration biopsies often show large numbers of histio-

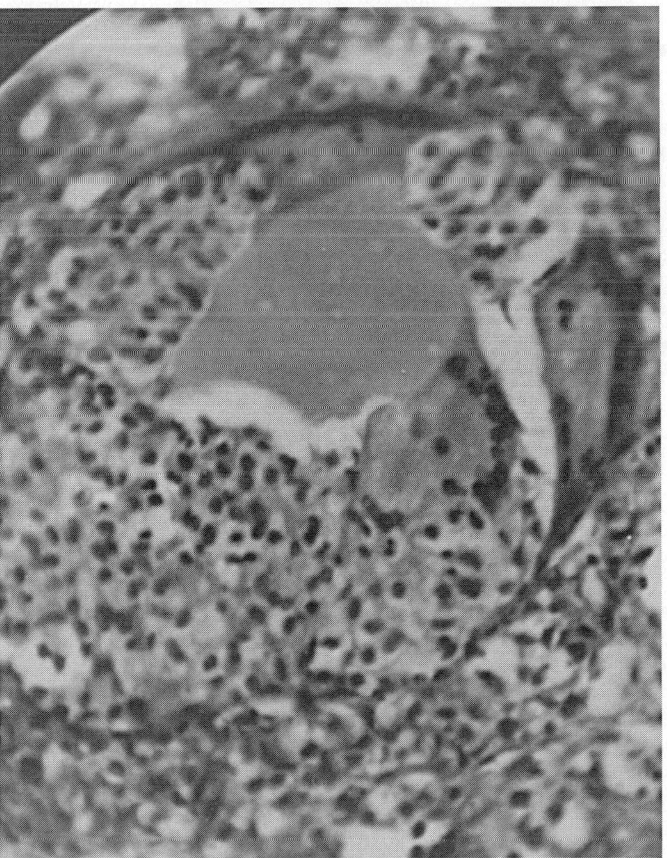

FIGURE 104–1. Pathologic findings in subacute thyroiditis. Note the severe destruction of the thyroid follicle, with the remaining colloid being surrounded by large numbers of histiocytes, giving the appearance of a giant cell (pseudo–giant cell). Marked interstitial edema is noted, with cellular infiltration and considerable destruction of the thyroid parenchyma.

cytes, which can be misinterpreted. The features of SAT, namely epithelioid granulomas, multinucleated giant cells, and follicular cells with intravacuolar granules can be identified.[47, 48]

Clinical Features

The mode of onset and severity of the disorder vary widely. The manifestations may be preceded by upper respiratory tract symptoms, or a prodromal phase of malaise, musculoskeletal aches and pains, and feverishness.[7–11, 49] Pain in the region of the thyroid gland may be moderate or severe but in a few cases is entirely lacking. Similarly, tenderness may be moderate or severe (or even exquisite), or, conversely, may also be lacking. Either one or both lobes may be initially involved, or the disorder may commence in one lobe, and later spread to the opposite lobe (creeping thyroiditis) or may involve both lobes from the outset. The systemic reaction may be minimal or severe, and fever may reach as high as 40°C. Although patients without pain may often be categorized as having "silent thyroiditis," surgical thyroidectomy or biopsy has demonstrated the typical granulomatous picture in some of such specimens.

Patients can generally localize the pain to the region of the thyroid gland over one or both lobes. They may refer to their symptoms as a "sore throat," but with appropriate questioning, it should become apparent that the pain is in the neck, not within the pharynx.[49] Typically, the pain radiates from the region of the thyroid up to the angle of the jaw, to the ear on the affected side or sides. The pain may also radiate to the anterior chest or may be centered only over the thyroid. Moving the head, swallowing, or coughing may aggravate the pain. Many patients become aware of their goiters, as swelling in the neck.

Although some patients have no systemic symptoms, most complain of myalgia, malaise, fatigue, and mild feverishness. The malaise can sometimes be extreme, and can be associated with arthralgia. Symptoms of mild to moderate hyperthyroidism occur in the early phase in most patients, with nervousness, tremulousness, some weight loss, heat intolerance, and rapid heartbeat.[7–11, 49, 50]

Most patients appear uncomfortable and flushed on inspection, with variable fever, occasionally as high as 40°C. The thyroid gland may be only slightly to moderately enlarged, with one lobe larger than the other. Indeed, if the thyroid gland is much larger than this, a diagnosis of subacute thyroiditis would be suspect. The consistency of the involved area is usually quite firm to almost hard, and there is tenderness of moderate to severe magnitude. When the tenderness subsides, the gland may maintain its size and consistency for several weeks. Cervical lymphadenopathy is rare. Physical signs of mild to moderate hyperthyroidism are often demonstrable. About 8% to 16% of patients with this condition are noted to have a preexistent goiter.

Course of the Disease

The duration of subacute thyroiditis is quite variable; it may last 2 to 5 months without treatment. Recurrences after recovery have been reported, but are unusual, on the order of 2.3% per year.[32]

The initial phase is characterized by hyperthyroidism in over half of the patients.[50] This is due to a disruptive process within the thyroid gland with continuous leakage of colloid into the interstitial spaces, where it is broken down into its component parts, liberating thyroid hormones, thyroglobulin, and other iodoamino acids into the circulation.[32, 50–56] The thyroid cells during this phase are virtually incapable of producing new thyroid hormone; thus the stored follicular colloid is depleted within 2 to 3 months, resulting thereafter in a phase of transient hypothyroidism in patients in whom the process has persisted over the interval.[27] Because disruption of the thyroid parenchyma can continue for months, the hypothyroidism may then also last for months. With recovery, the thyroid is reconstituted, repleted with colloid, thyroid function is restored, and a variable amount of interstitial fibrosis persists.[7–11, 27, 32, 50–56] This transient hypothyroidism may be subclinical or overt and occurs in about two thirds of patients.

While minimal degrees of subclinical hypothyroidism (i.e., slight TSH elevations, coupled with normal levels of thyroid hormones) may persist permanently in some patients, only rarely does SAT progress to permanent overt hypothyroidism.[7–11, 27, 57] In these cases, progression may be due to total destruction of the thyroid, with consequent fibrosis; in even more rare instances, the disorder may seem to culminate in autoimmune thyroiditis with hypothyroidism. Indeed, as mentioned above, a few patients have developed GD following recovery from SAT.[38–40, 58]

Thyroid Function Studies

Studies of thyroid function show dynamic changes consequent to the evolution of the pathologic process[7–11, 50, 56] The initial inflammatory destruction of the thyroid results in leakage and breakdown of the colloid from the damaged follicles into the interstices and thence into the circulation, with delivery thereto of iodinated materials—protein, proteases, peptides, and amino acids. Increased serum thyroxine (T_4) and triiodothyronine (T_3) in this phase result from cleavage of thyroid hormones from the discharged colloid, reflected by clinical hyperthyroidism (Fig. 104–2). In contrast to GD, in which the serum T_3 is usually disproportionately elevated when compared to the serum T_4, in SAT the increased serum T_3 is only *proportionate* to the amount of T_4 released into the circulation. This undoubtedly accounts for the mildness of the clinical manifestations in SAT, because the severity of the clinical manifestations of GD relates closely to levels of circulating T_3. This phase of hyperthyroidism can continue only until the gland is depleted of its preformed colloid. When the ultimate fall in serum T_4 begins, it may be exponential at that time.[55]

During the active phase, the damaged thyroid follicular cells cannot function adequately and cannot trap iodide; the 24-hour radioactive iodine uptake is characteristically suppressed to 0% to 1%.[7–11, 50, 51] Even if only part of the gland is actually involved, the uptake may be similarly depressed as a result of suppression of pituitary TSH owing to the elevated levels of thyroid hormone.[54–56] Thus SAT is one of the hyperthyroid conditions associated with high levels of thyroid hormones but a very low radioactive iodine uptake, characteristic of the early phase. Under these circumstances, only very minute new thyroid hormone biosynthesis is sustained, and what is produced leaks out.[51] In addition, iodoproteins such as thyroglobulin and iodoalbumin are discharged from the gland into the circulation.[51] Indeed, plasma thyroglobulin may remain elevated long after all other evidence of the inflammatory process has subsided.[53]

Isotope scans of the thyroid gland in the early phases of this malady reveal a patchy and irregular distribution of the tracer or no uptake whatsoever.[59, 60] Ultrasound examinations show hypoechoic focal areas, and can be used for guided fine-needle cytology.[48, 58, 61–63] The TSH is usually undetectable in the hyperthyroid phase[54, 55] and the TSH response to thyrotropin-releasing hormone (TRH) is, as expected, diminished at this time.[64–67] Perchlorate or thyocyanate administration generally does not cause release of excessive amounts of iodine from the gland.[61, 62, 67] Likewise, large doses of TSH generally do not cause a rise in the radioactive iodine uptake, except when some parts of the gland are uninvolved.[59] This lack of response to exogenous TSH administration persists during the first weeks of the disease, reflecting continuing thyroid cell impairment and failure of the iodide-concentrating mechanism. Indeed, the radioactive iodine uptake may, for similar reasons, remain suppressed for several weeks after the onset of the disorder.[50–52] There is complete suppression of the various stages of intrathyroidal iodine metabolism during this interval.[7–10] As mentioned earlier, when recovery of cellular function is delayed, a consequent phase of transient hypothyroidism may last for months.[7, 10, 50–52] This phase is, of course, associated with an elevated TSH.[54–56] Ultimate recovery is the general rule; conversely, permanent overt hypothyroidism is unusual.[7–11] In my own experience, such permanent hypothyroidism occurs in about 1% of patients, although other reports put it as high as 5%. However, minimal degrees of subclinical, compensated hypothyroidism (with slight elevations of TSH) may be noted somewhat more frequently. Moreover, recovered patients are more prone to iodide-induced hypothyroidism than otherwise normal persons.[68] There is often a lag between the reestablishment of the iodide-

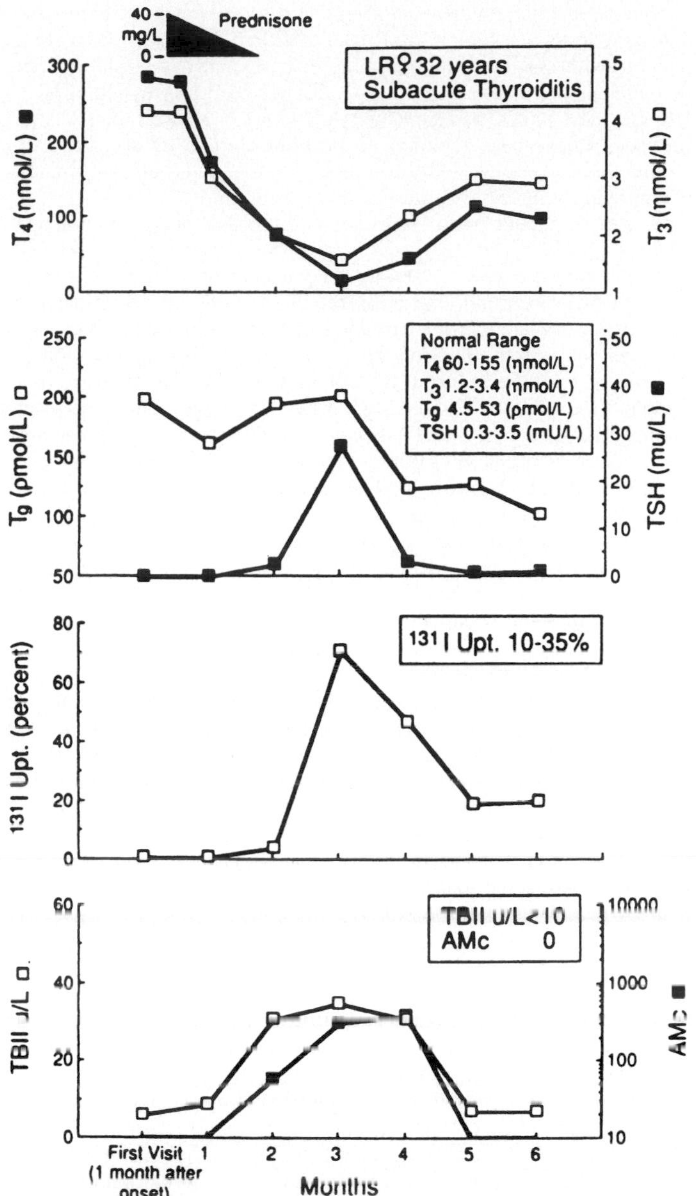

FIGURE 104–2. Salient laboratory features during the course of subacute thyroiditis. TBII, thyrotropin-binding inhibitory immunoglobulin; AMc, antimicrosomal (antithyroperoxidase) antibody; Tg, thyroglobulin; T_4, thyroxine; T_3, triiodothyronine.

concentrating process within the thyroid gland and the resumption of hormone synthesis, secretion, and repletion within the gland.[69]

The erythrocyte sedimentation rate (ESR) is characteristically markedly elevated in SAT, often to values of 80 to 100 mm/hour.[7–11, 70] Indeed, if the ESR is normal, the diagnosis should be suspect. The leukocyte count is normal in about half the patients, elevated in the remainder,[7–11, 14, 70] and has been reported as high as 18×10^9/L in this illness. The leukocyte counts correlate with serum concentrations of granulocyte colony-stimulating factor.[71] There may be a mild normochromic anemia, and an increase in α_2-globulin is frequently seen as a nonspecific inflammatory response.[72] Alkaline phosphatase and other hepatic enzymes may be elevated in the early phase. It has been suggested that SAT actually represents a multisystem disease also affecting the thyroid gland.[73] There are also increases in serum ferritin,[74] soluble intercellular adhesion molecule-1 (sICAM-1),[75] selectin,[76] and interleukin-6[77] levels during the inflammatory phase.

Tests of thyroid antibodies are positive in a minority of cases; these develop several weeks after the onset and tend to decline and disappear thereafter.[21, 22, 26] However, as previously mentioned, an antibody against an unpurified thyroid antigen persists for years after clinical features have subsided.[28] Also, as mentioned above, antibodies to the TSH receptor, either of the stimulating or blocking variety, may appear transiently without relationship to the thyroid functional state.[29–32]

Diagnosis

The diagnosis of SAT should present no difficulties in patients with fairly typical manifestations. Because "sore throat" is a frequent complaint, however, many patients are initially misdiagnosed with pharyngitis.[50] It is thus important that the thyroid gland be carefully palpated in patients presenting with upper respiratory infections or complaints of sore neck or throat or earache.

Occasionally patients with Hashimoto's thyroiditis have painful, tender thyroid enlargement that is virtually indistinguishable initially from SAT.[78] The radioactive iodine uptake is rarely as completely suppressed in Hashimoto's thyroiditis as it is in SAT, and the titers of thyroid autoantibodies are usually high enough to suggest lymphocytic thyroiditis. Rarely, thyroid lymphoma (which generally emanates from Hashimoto's thyroiditis) may present with similar symptoms and signs.

Acute suppurative thyroiditis may be initially difficult to distinguish from SAT. However, when clinical signs of suppuration appear, the diagnosis should become evident. In globus hystericus, patients complain of a sense of pressure or a feeling of a "ball" in the throat, and this may be associated with mild diffuse neck tenderness. However, there is no specific thyroid enlargement or tenderness.

Severe pain and tenderness may occur in a rapidly growing anaplastic thyroid carcinoma,[79] but this lesion is usually obvious by virtue of its large size, adherence to adjacent structures, lymphadenopathy, and characteristic progressive course. Hemorrhage into a thyroid nodule may also cause thyroid pain and tenderness, but its very localized nature, and the obvious nodule, usually lead to the correct diagnosis.

As mentioned above, the most important laboratory tests consistent with SAT include a high ESR, increased serum T_4 and T_3 levels, and a low radioactive iodine uptake. The serum thyroglobulin is also elevated. Fine-needle aspiration biopsies may be useful, but may show large numbers of histiocytes and thus may be misleading. Occasionally, a large-needle biopsy may be required for a definitive diagnosis.

Other possible erroneous diagnoses include hyperthyroidism and hypothyroidism, respectively, but a careful history should suffice to place the thyroid function in its proper context.

Therapy

Although the pathogenesis of SAT is not fully understood, treatment (while empiric) is highly effective.[7–11] The use of corticosteroids has proved to be valuable in the vast majority of patients.[7–11] Relief of symptoms occurs often within 24 hours. The basic disease process may not be altered, but the inflammatory response is clearly suppressed, allowing the pathologic process to run its now subclinical course.

Generally, prednisone or a similar analog of cortisol is prescribed. The treatment is initiated with pharmacologic dosages (e.g., 10 mg four times daily). The dosage levels are gradually diminished over 4 to 6 weeks and can then be discontinued altogether in most instances. In about 20% of patients, however, as the dosage is reduced, recrudescence of the manifestations necessitates the restoration of a higher dose once again. It is sometimes necessary to provide repeated courses of treatment before recovery ultimately occurs. In most instances, exacerbations do not occur, and patients go on to full recovery.

There have been reports that T_3 can bring about rapid relief in the acute phase.[54, 80] In my own experience, it has not been of benefit when patients are chemically hyperthyroid at the time of therapy. However, after repeated exacerbations, the addition of T_4 or T_3 may often result in amelioration of the condition and appear to prevent further recurrences.[7–11] Endogenous TSH may play some role in maintaining the disorder under these circumstances; indeed, exogenous TSH may aggravate or precipitate thyroiditis.[10]

In the past generation, radiation therapy was employed effectively for SAT. Dosages varied between 200 and 2000 rad of external radiation.[7–9, 49] There was a failure rate of about 25%, and the response was considerably slower and less predictable than with corticosteroids. Perhaps because of the major concern about the effects of low-dose radiation in inducing late thyroid carcinoma,[81] such therapy is no longer used.

Sodium ipodate has recently been employed in the management of the hyperthyroidism of SAT.[82] The treatment was quite effective in causing normalization of thyroid function, although the inflammatory state persisted for up to 6 weeks thereafter.

In milder cases of this malady, salicylates and other nonsteroidal anti-inflammatory drugs have been administered with some success.[7–10, 52] For more severe cases, however, corticosteroids are far more rapid in their effect, and are dramatically more effective.

Thiouracil and TSH have been reported to be beneficial, but such drugs have not found general favor.[10] Antibiotics are of no value. The high incidence of postoperative hypothyroidism has discouraged thyroidectomy as treatment for SAT, and because recovery is almost certain, thyroidectomy almost never needs to be recommended. Only in the unusual situation of a very prolonged course, with malaise and local distress continuing almost indefinitely, should thyroidectomy be considered.[9, 10]

After complete recovery, late recurrences are unusual, as noted above. As also previously mentioned, permanent clinically significant hypothyroidism is a rare complication.

SCLEROSING THYROIDITIS

Background and Definition

Sclerosing thyroiditis (invasive fibrous thyroiditis, Riedel's struma) is a rare disorder of unknown cause, characterized pathologically by dense fibrous tissue, which replaces the normal thyroid parenchyma, and extends into adjacent tissues, such as muscles, blood vessels, and nerves.[7, 83–85] The first description was by Riedel in 1896 who described cases of chronic sclerosing thyroiditis primarily affecting women, which frequently caused pressure symptoms in the neck, and tended to progress ultimately to complete destruction of the thyroid gland.[86–88] Riedel's interesting description was that of a "specific inflammation of mysterious nature producing an iron-hard *[eisenharte]* tumefaction of the thyroid." Synonyms for the term *chronic invasive fibrous thyroiditis* include Riedel's struma, struma fibrosa, ligneous struma, chronic fibrous thyroiditis, and chronic productive thyroiditis.

Incidence

This condition is quite rare. In thyroidectomies performed for all disorders, an incidence between 0.03% and 0.98% has been reported from a small group of centers.[89, 90] At the Mayo Clinic, the operative incidence over 64 years was 0.06%, and the overall incidence in outpatients was 1.06 per 100,000.[91–94] Because the manifestations associated with this disorder are likely to lead to surgery, the incidence of Riedel's thyroiditis among patients undergoing thyroidectomy is much greater than the incidence in patients with goiters in general.

Etiology

The cause of this disorder remains unknown. A generation ago, chronic lymphocytic thyroiditis was considered to be an earlier stage of invasive fibrous thyroiditis. Although this view was not supported for several years, several cases of Riedel's struma have been reported that emanated from Hashimoto's thyroiditis.[95–105] Five patients with Riedel's struma with antecedent GD have also been reported.[106–108] In the past, thyroid autoantibodies were thought to be unusual in Riedel's struma, but a 1985 report stated that significant titers of thyroid autoantibodies could be found in 45% of patients, again suggesting a possible relationship between autoimmune thyroid disease and Riedel's struma.[92] Moreover, one patient with Riedel's struma coexisting with pernicious anemia, another autoimmune disease, has been reported,[109] and an overrepresentation of Riedel's struma has been observed in patients with still other autoimmune diseases, such as insulin-dependent diabetes mellitus and Addison's disease.[110–111] Expression of HLA-DR and heat shock protein (HSP—72 kDa),[112] as well as sICAM-1 receptor,[113] have been reported in the fibrosclerotic tissue of Riedel's struma and have suggested a role for an active cell-mediated immune response early in the evolution of this condition.

Of course, patients with Hashimoto's thyroiditis, a common disease, when followed for many years, almost never progress to Riedel's struma, which is a very rare entity. The aforementioned evidence does not confirm an autoimmune basis for the disease, and most cases of Riedel's struma are clearly unrelated to such autoimmune disease. It has been suggested that the key event might be proliferation by fibroblasts, in turn induced by cytokine production from B or T lymphocytes, or both.[109] Consistent with this suggestion is the recent finding by Many et al.[114] of histologic modifications similar to those observed in Riedel's thyroiditis in nonobese diabetic (NOD) mice during the development of iodine-induced thyroditis, in the presence of T helper 2 (T_H2) cytokines favoring autoantibody production.

The recent observations of Heufelder et al.[115] of marked tissue eosinophilia and eosinophil degranulation in Riedel's struma have suggested another possibility, namely that these elements may represent an important fibrogenic stimulus, possibly via the release of eosinophil-derived products. The nature of such products is as yet unknown.

While SAT has also been suggested as a possible precursor to Riedel's thyroiditis, there is no convincing evidence to link these two entities.[116–118] Whatever the ultimate explanation proves to be, it will have to take into account the extracervical fibrosclerosis, first noted as early as 1885, as a common accompaniment of Riedel's struma.[119] These associations include salivary gland fibrosis, sclerosing cholangitis, pseudotumors of the orbits, fibrous mediastinitis, retroperitoneal fibrosis, and lacrimal gland fibrosis.[7, 83–85, 106] Long-term follow-up of patients with Riedel's thyroiditis (follow-up time 10 years) has shown that one third develop fibrosing disorders of the retroperitoneal space (often leading to ureteral obstruction), chest, or orbits.[100] DeLange et al.[106] have cited all of the available literature on this point. On the other hand, two-thirds of patients with Riedel's struma do not develop extracervical fibrosis within the ensuing 10 years, and it is rare for one patient to have extracervical fibrosis in more than one site. Conversely, less than 1% of patients with retroperitoneal fibrosis have Riedel's struma. It is considered likely that these apparently disparate fibrotic lesions may be different manifestations of the same generalized fibrosing disease; however, the thyroid fibrosis seems common, central, and integral to this disease complex, implying an important role for it in the pathogenesis.

The established association of certain drugs with retroperitoneal fibrosis has not been observed with Riedel's struma.[106] Aside from one example of two brothers, children of consanguineous parents, who developed fibrosclerosis in multiple sites (including Riedel's struma in one of the brothers),[114, 120] there does not seem to be a genetic predisposition to this condition.

Clinical Features

The age of onset has varied between 23 and 78 years, although most cases are diagnosed in the fourth to sixth decades.[7, 83–85, 92, 93] The female-male ratio has been reported to be between 2:1 and 4:1 (Table 104–1).

A gradually or rapidly enlarging goiter is a constant feature of this condition, precipitating the local symptoms within the neck. These include a marked sense of pressure or severe dyspnea, with symptoms out of proportion to the size of the goiter.[107–110] Sensations of suffocation, cough, dysphagia, and a sense of heaviness in the neck are common. Recurrent laryngeal nerve palsy with hoarseness is described. Pain is unusual, although the sense of pressure may be inappropriately described as pain by the patient. The presence or degree of obstruction varies with the extent to which the surrounding structures have been invaded. Some patients have only mild and infrequent symptoms with

TABLE 104–1. Clinical Features: Riedel's vs. Hashimoto's Thyroiditis

	Riedel's	Hashimoto's
Age	23–70 yr (mostly > 50 yr)	Any age (mostly >20 yr, gradually increasing with age)
Sex (F/M)	2–4:1	4–10:1
Symptoms	Pressure goiter	Often goiter
Thyroid involvement	Unilateral or diffuse	Generally diffuse, occasionally goiter quite large
Thyroid status	Occasionally hypothyroid, rarely hypoparathyroid	Commonly hypothyroid, but may be euthyroid or hyperthyroid
Thyroid antibodies	Up to 45%	Almost invariably
Follow-up	Often regresses	Usually proceeds to hypothyroidism

minimal dysphagia and dyspnea. Others may have stridor, severe dyspnea, or attacks of suffocation. In some patients, the entire gland is involved with the fibrotic process and hypothyroidism develops with a recorded prevalence rate of 25% to 29%.[93, 94, 104, 106, 118] Occasionally tetany due to hypoparathyroidism may be observed.[104, 118]

On examination, the thyroid gland is variable in size, from small to very large.[7, 83–85] The lesion may be limited to one lobe, may be present in both, or (as mentioned above) may involve the entire gland. The goiter is rock-hard, densely adherent to adjacent cervical structures (such as muscles, blood vessels, and nerves), and may thus move scarcely upon swallowing. It has a harder consistency than carcinoma, and is only rarely tender. Although adjacent lymph nodes are occasionally enlarged, when they are present and associated with a hard thyroid mass, a diagnosis of carcinoma is often suspected.[7, 83–85]

As previously mentioned, hypothyroidism, or, occasionally, hypoparathyroidism also, may occur, due to involvement of the gland and its surroundings by fibrosis.[93, 94, 103, 104, 118] Because of the frequency of fibrotic lesions elsewhere, the examination must include a careful search for such disorders associated with retroperitoneal fibrosis causing ureteral obstruction, a not unusual feature.[7, 83–85, 104, 106]

Laboratory Findings

Most commonly, the patient is clinically euthyroid, and thyroid function tests provide correspondingly normal values. As mentioned above, however, some patients develop hypothyroidism due to complete fibrosis of the entire thyroid gland. Thyroid autoantibodies may be detected in up to 45% of these patients.[94] Indeed, as described above, AITD seems to have preceded Riedel's struma in a small number of cases. Additionally, as also noted above, fibrosis of the whole gland can occasionally result in hypoparathyroidism, with consequent low serum calcium, and high serum phosphorus values.[103, 104, 118] Thus thyroid and parathyroid function should be measured in all cases. Thyroid scintiscans may show "cold" areas, corresponding to the extent of the lesions.[7, 83–85] Axial computed tomography (CT) and ultrasound examinations can also be helpful.[104] The white blood cell count may be normal or elevated, and the ESR is usually moderately elevated.[7, 83–85] Antinuclear factor was once reported as present.[104]

Pathology

Pathologic findings consist of an exuberant fibrosing process involving part or all of the thyroid gland.[7, 83–85, 93, 94] It may be unilateral or bilateral, and has been described as woody or very hard. The German *eisenharte* applied to the lesion signifies its "iron-hard" quality. Extension of the fibrosis beyond the capsule of the thyroid into adjacent structures such as nerves, blood vessels, and muscles is a characteristic feature, and also accounts for the occasional instance in which the parathyroid glands have been obliterated by this fibrosing process. There are no tissue planes, making surgical extirpation virtually impossible.[7, 83–85] An adenoma may occur in the midst of the fibrous mass. Isolated thyroid amyloidosis has been described in one case of Riedel's struma.

Woolner and coworkers have described microscopy findings for this condition.[93, 94] These include complete destruction of involved thyroid tissue with absence of normal lobulation; lack of a granulomatous reaction; and extension of the fibrosis beyond the thyroid into adjacent structures, such as skeletal muscle, nerves, blood vessels, and fat. Lymphocytes and Hürthle cells are sparse, in contrast to the findings in Hashimoto's thyroiditis, although occasionally a few foci of lymphocytes may be observed. An associated arteritis and phlebitis with intimal proliferation, medial destruction, adventitial inflammation, and frequent thrombosis may also occur.[7, 83–85, 93, 94] Heufelder et al.[115] have recently taken note that eosinophilia and eosinophilic degranulation are also common and probably crucial features, as mentioned above.

Similar features are also observed in the extracervical fibrosclerotic lesions in the retroperitoneal or mediastinal regions, in the orbit or lacrimal glands, or in cholangitis.

Diagnosis and Treatment

Invasive fibrous thyroiditis may appear as a painless, fixed, hard goiter, with either slow or rapid growth. Whether it is associated with local lymphadenopathy or not, it may be impossible to distinguish this lesion from carcinoma or lymphoma of the thyroid on the basis of clinical findings alone.[7, 83–85] The disorder can usually be differentiated from classic Hashimoto's thyroiditis or subacute thyroiditis, as indicated in Table 104–1. Hashimoto's thyroiditis is not associated with any extension of the lesion beyond the capsule; the goiters are usually large and lobulated, although goiters in Riedel's thyroiditis may sometimes be quite large. The thyroid antibodies are generally markedly elevated in Hashimoto's thyroiditis, and are usually not as elevated, or may be negative, in Riedel's struma.[7, 83–85] Subacute thyroiditis is associated with severe pain and tenderness, frequent fever, and a rapidly evolving course. There is also no extension of the lesion beyond the capsule. Needle biopsy findings in Riedel's struma may be difficult to interpret, although open surgical biopsies are quite useful.

There have been reports of improvement during glucocorticoid therapy, and relapses reversed by the reinstitution of steroids[102, 103, 117]; thus glucocorticoids should be considered in appropriate situations. However, glucocorticoid treatment has not been helpful in all instances.[104, 106] Thyroid hormone suppressive therapy has also been recommended; although adequate assessment has not been carried out, this therapy does not add much to the management of this rare disease in the absence of hypothyroidism.[7, 103, 104] Of course, T_4 therapy is necessary in cases in which hypothyroidism has resulted from the disorder.[104] In addition, calcium and vitamin D therapy is indicated in those cases with associated hypoparathyroidism.[104]

When surgical intervention is under consideration for pressure symptoms or for the diagnosis or treatment of a hard goiter, the possibility of Riedel's struma must be kept in mind so as to limit the extent of the surgery if no malignancy is found. Surgical intervention is indicated on two grounds: (1) to exclude malignancy and (2) to relieve tracheal compression. Operation is confined to excising a wedge of thyroid isthmus when the process is diffuse.[7, 83–85] Extensive resection is not indicated, particularly because the course of Riedel's struma often tends to be benign and self-limiting. Moreover, an extensive procedure may add considerable risk of injury to adjacent involved vital structures within the neck, such as the carotid artery and the recurrent laryngeal nerve. Indeed, without actual impingement by the surgeon on the recurrent laryngeal nerve, the edema occurring with the surgery acting upon an already partially compromised structure can result in transient palsies, and occult hypoparathyroidism may be converted into overt hypoparathyroidism by this means. Subtotal lobectomy may be performed, however, if the process is localized to one thyroid lobe.

Occasionally, more extensive resection is justified in a patient whose thyroid is diffusely painful and tender. The extrathyroidal fibrotic lesions, if present, will also require appropriate treatment, including possible surgical correction.

Prognosis

The course of the lesion may be slowly progressive, may stabilize, or may remit. Following surgery, the disease sometimes subsides, or takes a benign, self-limiting course. Spontaneous remissions without surgery may occur, and secondary surgery is only rarely required.[7, 83–85] The mortality rate has been reported to range from 6% to 10%, with deaths usually attributed to asphyxia secondary to tracheal compression or laryngospasm.[7, 83–85] However, the mortality rates mentioned are derived from the older literature, and may not reflect the (presumably lower) current rates. As mentioned, hypothyroidism is relatively uncommon, and hypoparathyroidism is unusual. In many instances, the condition is self-limiting, and improvement often persists after an isthmic wedge resection. As also mentioned above, the disorder is often further complicated by fibrotic lesions elsewhere in the body, and these require appropriate treatment, including the possibility of surgical management.

REFERENCES

Infectious Thyroiditis

1. Bauchet JL: De la thyroïdite (goitre aigu) et du goitre enflammé (goitre chronique enflammé). Gazette Hebdomadaire Med Chir 4:19–23, 1857.
2. Berger SA, Zonszein J, Villamena P, Mittman N: Infectious diseases of the thyroid gland. Rev Infect Dis 5:108–122, 1983.
3. Edwards H: Acute thyroiditis. *In* LiVolsi VA, LoGerfo P (eds): Thyroiditis. Boca Raton, FL, CRC Press, 1981, pp 6–19.
4. Hazard JB: Thyroiditis: A review. Am J Clin Pathol 25:289–298, 399–426, 1955.
5. LiVolsi VA, LoGerfo P (eds): Thyroiditis. Boca Raton, FL, CRC Press, 1981, pp 5–20.
6. Volpé R: Suppurative thyroiditis. *In* Werner SC, Ingbar SH (eds): The Thyroid, a Fundamental and Clinical Text, ed 4. New York, Harper & Row, 1978, pp 983–985.

Subacute and Sclerosing Thyroiditis

7. Volpé R: Subacute and sclerosing thyroiditis. *In* DeGroot LG(ed): Endocrinology, (ed 3). Philadelphia, WB Saunders, 1995, pp 742–751.
8. Bastenie PA, Ermans AM: Thyroiditis and thyroid function. Clinical, morphological and physiological studies. International Series of Monographs in Pure and Applied Biology. Modern Trends in Physiological Sciences, vol. 36. New York, Pergamon Press, 1972.
9. LiVolsi VA, LoGerfo P (eds): Thyroiditis. Boca Raton, FL, CRC Press, 1981, pp 21–42.
10. Greene JN: Subacute thyroiditis. Am J Med 1971; 51:97–108.
11. Steinberg FU: Subacute granulomatous thyroiditis: A review. Ann Intern Med 52:1014–1025, 1960.
12. Mygind H: Thyroiditis akuta simplex. J Laryngol 91:181–193, 1895.
13. de Quervain F: Die akute nicht eiterige Thyreoiditis und die Beteiligung der Schilddrüse und akuten Intoxikationen und Infectionen überhaupt. Mitt Grenzgebieiten Med Chir 2(Suppl):1–165, 1904.
14. de Quervain F, Giordandengo G: Die akute und subakute nicht eiterige Thyreoiditis. Mitt Grenzgeheiten Med Chir 44:538–590, 1936.
15. Nikolai TF: Silent thyroiditis and subacute thyroiditis. *In* Braverman LE, Utiger R (eds): Werner and Ingbar's The Thyroid, A Fundamental and Clinical Text, ed 6. Philadelphia, JB Lippincott, 1991, pp 720–727.
16. Wesenfelder L, Raynard B, Eugene C, et al: Thyroïdite subaiquë de de Quervain rélévant une hepatite à virus A. Gastroenterol Clin Biol 18:905–909, 1994.
17. Vejlgaard TB, Nielsen OB: Subacute thyroiditis in parvovirus B19 infection. Ugeskr Laeger 156:6039–6040, 1994.
18. Stancek D, Gressnerova M: A viral agent isolated from a patient with subacute de Quervain type thyroiditis. Acta Virol 18:365, 1974.
19. Stancek D, Stancekova M, Gressnerova M, et al: Isolation and some serological and epidemiological data on viruses recovered from patients with subacute thyroiditis of de Quervain. Med Microbiol Immunol 161:133–144, 1975.
20. Stancek D, Ciampor E, Mucha V, et al: Morphological, cytological and biological observations on viruses isolated from patients with subacute thyroiditis of de Quervain. Acta Virol 20:183, 1976.
21. Volpé R, Row VV, Ezrin C: Circulating viral and thyroid antibodies in subacute thyroiditis. J Clin Endocrinol Metab 27:1275–1284, 1967.
22. Yeo PPB, Rauff A, Chan SW, et al: Subacute (de Quervain's) thyroiditis in the tropics. *In* Stockigt JR, Nagataki S (eds): Thyroid Research VIII. Canberra, Australian Academy of Science, 1980, pp 570–574.
23. Arend SM, Westedt ML: Simultaneous onset of giant cell arteritis and subacute thyroiditis. Ann Rheum Dis 52:839–840, 1993.
24. Falaschi P, Martocchia A, D'Urso R, Proietti A: Subacute thyroiditis during interferon-alpha therapy for chronic hepatitis C. J Endocrinol Invest 20:24–28, 1997.
25. Volpé R: Immunology of the thyroid. *In* Volpé R (ed): Autoimmune Diseases of the Endocrine System. Boca Raton, FL, CRC Press, 1990, pp 73–240.
26. Bech K, Feldt-Rasmussen U, Bliddal H, et al: Persistence of autoimmune reactions during recovery of subacute thyroiditis. *In* Pinchera A, Ingbar SH, McKenzie JM, Fenzi GF (eds): Thyroid Autoimmunity. New York, Plenum Press, 1987, pp 623–625.
27. Lio S, Pontecorvi A, Caruso M, et al: Transitory subclinical and permanent hypothyroidism in the course of subacute thyroiditis (de Quervain). Acta Endocrinol 106:67–70, 1984.
28. Weetman AP, Smallridge RC, Nutman TB, Burman KD: Persistent thyroid autoimmunity after subacute thyroiditis. J Lab Clin Immunol 23:1–6, 1987.
29. Strakosch CR, Joyner D, Wall JR: Thyroid stimulating antibodies in subacute thyroiditis. J Clin Endocrinol Metab 46:345–348, 1978.
30. Wall JR, Strakosch CR, Brandy P, Bayly R: Nature of thyrotropin displacement activity in subacute thyroiditis. J Clin Endocrinol Metab 54:349–353, 1982.
31. Tamai H, Nozaki T, Mukuta T, et al: The incidence of thyroid stimulating blocking antibodies during the hypothyroid phase in patients with subacute thyroiditis. J Clin Endocrinol Metab 73:245–250, 1991.
32. Iitaka M, Momotani N, Ishii J, Ito K: Incidence of subacute thyroiditis recurrences after a prolonged latency: 24 year survey. J Clin Endocrinol Metab 81:466–469, 1996.
33. Hashizume K, Roudebush CP, Fenzi GF, DeGroot LJ: Effect of antithyroid therapy and thyroid stimulating immunoglobulin phase in Graves' disease. *In* Proceedings of the 53rd Meeting of the American Thyroid Association, Cleveland, Sept 7–10, 1977.
34. Volpé R: Autoimmunity causing thyroid dysfunction. Endocrinol Metab Clin North Am 20:565–578, 1991.
35. Tomer Y, Davies TF: Infection, thyroid disease, and autoimmunity. Endocr Rev 14:107–120, 1993.
36. Volpé R: A perspective on human autoimmune thyroid disease: Is there an abnormality of the target cell which predisposes to the disorder? Autoimmunity 12:3–9, 1992.
37. Volpé R: The immunology of human autoimmune thyroid disease. *In* Volpé R (ed): The Autoimmune Endocrinopathies, Contemporary Endocrinology Series, Totowa NJ, Humana Press 1999, pp 217–244.
38. Werner SC: Graves' disease following subacute thyroiditis. Arch Intern Med 139:1313–1315, 1979.
39. Wartofsky L, Schaaf M: Graves' disease with thyrotoxicosis following subacute thyroiditis. Am J Med 83:761–764, 1987.
40. Bartalena L, Bogazzi F, Pecori F, Martino E: Graves' disease occurring after subacute thyroiditis: Report of a case and review of the literature. Thyroid 6:345–348, 1996.
41. Bech K, Nerup J, Thomsen M, et al: Subacute thyroiditis de Quervain: A disease associated with HLA-B antigen. Acta Endocrinol 86:504–509, 1977.
42. Nyulassy S, Hnilica P, Buc M, et al: Subacute (de Quervain's) thyroiditis: Association with HLA-Bw35 antigen, and abnormalities of the complement system, immunoglobulins and other serum proteins. J Clin Endocrinol Metab 45:270–274, 1977.
43. Tamai H, Goto H, Uno H, et al: HLA in Japanese patients with subacute (de Quervain's) thyroiditis. Tissue Antigens 24:58–59, 1984.
44. Yeo PPB, Chan SH, Aw TC, et al: HLA and Chinese patients with subacute (de Quervain's) thyroiditis. Tissue Antigens 17:249–250, 1981.
45. Hazard JB: Thyroiditis: A review. Am J Clin Pathol 25:289–298, 399–426, 1955.
46. Harland WA, Frantz VK: Clinicopathologic study of 261 surgical cases of so-called thyroiditis. J Clin Endocrinol Metab 16:1433–1437, 1956.
47. Solano JC, Bascunana AG, Perez JS, et al: Fine-needle aspiration of subacute granulomatous thyroiditis (de Quervain's thyroiditis): A clinico-cytologic review of 36 cases. Diagn Cytopathol 16:214–220, 1997.
48. Lu CP, Chang TC, Wang CY, Hsiao YL: Serial changes in ultrasound-guided fine needle aspiration cytology in subacute thyroiditis. Acta Cytol 41:238–243, 1997.
49. Volpé R, Johnston MW: Subacute thyroiditis: A disease commonly mistaken for pharyngitis. Can Med Assoc J 77:297–307, 1957.
50. Volpé R, Johnston MW, Huber N: Thyroid function in subacute thyroiditis. J Clin Endocrinol Metab 18:65–78, 1958.
51. Ingbar SH, Freinkel N: Thyroid function and metabolism of iodine in patients with subacute thyroiditis. Arch Intern Med 101:339–346, 1958.
52. Dorta T, Beraud T: New investigations on subacute thyroiditis. Helv Med Acta 28:19–41, 1961.
53. Izumi M, Larsen PR: Correlation of sequential change in serum thyroglobulin, triiodothyronine, and thyroxine in patients with Graves' disease and subacute thyroiditis. Metabolism 27:449–460, 1978.
54. Larsen PR: Serum triiodothyronine and thyrotropin during hyperthyroid and recovery phases of subacute non-suppurative thyroiditis. Metabolism 23:467–471, 1974.
55. Weihl AC, Daniels GH, Ridgeway ED, Maloof F: Thyroid function during the early days of subacute thyroiditis. J Clin Endocrinol Metab 44:1107–1114, 1977.
56. Glinoer D, Puttemans N, Van Herle AJ, et al: Sequential study of the impairment of thyroid function in the early stage of subacute thyroiditis. Acta Endocrinol 77:26–39, 1974.
57. Jay HK: Permanent myxedema: An unusual complication of granulomatous thyroiditis. J Clin Endocrinol Metab 21:1384–1387, 1961.
58. Bennedbaek FN, Gram J, Hegedus L: The transition of subacute thyroiditis to Graves' disease as evidenced by diagnostic imaging. Thyroid 6:457–459, 1996.
59. Lewitus W, Rechnic J, Lubin E: Sequential scanning of the thyroid as an aid to the diagnosis of subacute thyroiditis. Isr J Med Sci 3:847–854, 1967.
60. Hamburger JL, Kadian G, Rossin HW: Subacute thyroiditis—evaluations depicted by serial ^{131}I scintigrams. J Nucl Med 6:560–565, 1965.
61. Bennedbaek FN, Hegedus L: The value of ultrasonography in the diagnosis and follow-up of subacute thyroiditis. Thyroid 7:45–50, 1997.
62. Benker G, Olbricht TH, Windeck R, et al: The sonographic and functional sequelae of de Quervain's subacute thyroiditis. Acta Endocrinol 117:435–441, 1988.
63. Tokuda Y, Kasagi K, Iida Y, et al: Sonography of subacute thyroiditis: Changes in the findings during the course of the disease. J Clin Ultrasound 18:21–26, 1990.
64. Berthezine F, Kressman J, Olivier J, Fournier M: Le fonctionnement de l'axe hypophyso-thyroïdien au cours de thyroïdites subaiguës. Ann Endocrinol 36:169–170, 1975.
65. Demeester-Mirkine N, Brauman H, Corvilain J: Delayed adjustment of the pituitary response in circulating thyroid hormones in a case of subacute thyroiditis. Clin Endocrinol 5:9–14, 1976.
66. Lebacq EG, Therasse G, Schmitz A, et al: Subacute thyroiditis. Acta Endocrinol 82:705–715, 1976.

67. Staub JJ: The TRH test in subacute thyroiditis. Lancet 1:868–870, 1975.
68. Roti E, Minelli R, Gardini E, et al: Iodine induced hypothyroidism in euthyroid subjects with a previous episode of subacute thyroiditis. J Clin Endocrinol Metab 70:1581–1586, 1990.
69. Kamio N, Kobayashi I, Mori M, et al: Permissive role of thyrotrophin in thyroid radioiodine uptake during the recovery phase of subacute thyroiditis. Metabolism 26:295–299, 1977.
70. Nicklaus Muller E, Mullhaupt B, Perschak H: Steroid therapy and course of blood sedimentation rate in de Quervain's thyroiditis. Schweiz Rundsch Med Prax 83:95–100, 1994.
71. Sakane S, Murakami Y, Sasaki M, et al: Serum concentrations of granulocyte colony-stimulating factor (G-CSF) determined by a highly-sensitive chemiluminescent immunoassay during the clinical course of subacute thyroiditis. Endocr J 42:391–396, 1995.
72. Skillern PG, Lewis LA: Fractional plasma protein values in subacute thyroiditis. J Clin Invest 36:780–783, 1957.
73. Hamada S, Yagura T, Ishii H, et al: Subacute thyroiditis as a systemic multisystem disease. *In* Nagataki S, Torizuka K (eds): The Thyroid 1988. Excerpta Medica International Congress Series 796. Amsterdam, Elsevier, 1988, pp 521–525.
74. Sakata S, Nagai K, Maekawa H, et al: Serum ferritin concentrations in subacute thyroiditis. Metabolism 40:682–688, 1991.
75. Ozata M, Bolu E, Sengul A, et al: Soluble intercellular adhesion molecule-1 concentrations in patients with subacute thyroiditis and in patients with Graves' disease with or without ophthalmopathy. Endocr J 43:517–525, 1996.
76. Hara H, Sugita E, Sato R, Ban Y: Plasma selectin levels in patients with Graves' disease. Endocr J 43:709–713, 1996.
77. Yamada T, Sato A, Aizawa T: Dissociation between serum interleukin-6 rise and other parameters of disease activity in subacute thyroiditis during treatment with corticosteroid. J Clin Endocrinol Metab 81:577–579, 1996.
78. Volpé R: Autoimmune thyroiditis. *In* Braverman LE, Utiger R (eds): Werner and Ingbar's The Thyroid, A Fundamental and Clinical Text, ed 6. Philadelphia, JB Lippincott, 1991, pp 921–933.
79. Rosen F, Row VV, Volpé R, Ezrin C: Anaplastic carcinoma of thyroid with abnormal circulating iodoprotein. A case simulating subacute thyroiditis. Can Med Assoc J 95:1039–1041, 1966.
80. Higgins HP, Bayley TA, Diosy A: Suppression of endogenous TSH: A treatment of subacute thyroiditis. J Clin Endocrinol Metab 23:235–242, 1963.
81. Walfish PG, Volpé R: Irradiation related thyroid cancer. Ann Intern Med 88:261–262, 1978.
82. Chopra IJ, Van Herle AJ, Korenman SG, et al: Use of sodium iodate in management of hyperthyroidism in subacute thyroiditis. J Clin Endocrinol Metab 80:2178–2180, 1995.
83. Bastenie PA: Invasive fibrous thyroiditis (Riedel). *In* Bastenie PA, Ermans AM: Thyroiditis and Thyroid Function. International Series of Monographs in Pure and Applied Biology, Modern Trends in Physiological Sciences, vol. 36. Oxford, Pergamon Press, 1972, pp 99–108.
84. Livolsi VA: Riedel's struma. *In* LiVolsi VA, LoGerfo PA (eds): Thyroiditis. Boca Raton, FL, CRC Press, 1981, pp 133–146.
85. Schwaegerle SM, Bauer TW, Esselstyn CB: Riedel's thyroiditis. Am J Clin Pathol 90:715–722, 1988.
86. Riedel BM: Ueber Verlauf and Ausgang der chronischer Strumitis. Munch Med Wochenschr 57:1946–1947, 1910.
87. Riedel BM: Vorstellung eines Kranken mit chronischer Strumitis. Verh Ges Chir 26:127–129, 1896.
88. Riedel BM: Die chronische zur Bildung eisenharter Tumoren führende Entzündung der Schilddrüse. Verh Ges Chir 25:101–105, 1896.
89. DeCourcey JL: A new theory concerning the etiology of Riedel's struma. Surgery 12:754–762, 1942.
90. Goodman HI: Riedel's thyroiditis: Review and report of two cases. Am J Surg 54:472–478, 1941.
91. Hay ID, McConahey WM, Carney JA, Woolner LB: Invasive fibrous thyroiditis (Riedel's struma) and associated extracervical fibrosclerosis: Bowlby's disease revisited (abstract). Ann Endocrinol 43:29A, 1982.
92. Hay ID: Thyroiditis: A clinical update. Mayo Clin Proc 60:836–843, 1985.
93. Woolner LB, McConahey WM, Beahrs O: Invasive fibrous thyroiditis (Riedel's struma). J Clin Endocrinol Metab 17:201–220, 1957.
94. Woolner LB: Thyroiditis: Classification and clinicopathologic correlations. *In* Hazard JB, Smith DE (eds): The Thyroid. Baltimore, Williams & Wilkins, 1964, pp 123–142.
95. Ewing J: Neoplastic Diseases: A Treatise on Tumors. Philadelphia, WB Saunders, 1922, pp 908–909.
96. Goetsch E, Kammer M: Chronic thyroiditis and Riedel's struma: Etiology and pathogenesis. J Clin Endocrinol Metab 15:1010–1034, 1955.
97. Reist A: Über chronische Thyroiditis. Frankfurter Z Pathol 28:141–200, 1922.
98. Williamson GS, Pearse IH: Lymphadenoid goitre and its clinical significance. BMJ 1:4–8, 1929.
99. Beierwaltes W: Thyroiditis. Ann N Y Acad Sci 124:586–604, 1965.
100. Merrington WR: Chronic thyroiditis: A case showing features of both Riedel's and Hashimoto's thyroiditis. Br J Surg 35:423–426, 1948.
101. Baker TJ: Riedel's struma and struma lymphomatosa (Hashimoto). South Med J 46:1168–1171, 1953.
102. Baloch ZW, Saberi M, Livolsi VA: Simultaneous involvement of thyroid by Riedel's disease and fibrosing Hashimoto's thyroiditis: A case report. Thyroid 8:337–341, 1998.
103. Thomson JA, Jackson IMD, Duguid WP: The effect of steroid therapy on Riedel's thyroiditis. Scott Med J 13:13–16, 1968.
104. Best TB, Munro RE, Burwell S, Volpé R: Riedel's thyroiditis associated with Hashimoto's thyroiditis, hypoparathyroidism, and retroperitoneal fibrosis. J Endocrinol Invest 14:767–772, 1991.
105. Taubenberger JK, Merino MJ, Medeiros LJ: A thyroid biopsy with histologic features of both Riedel's thyroiditis and the fibrosing variant of Hashimoto's thyroiditis. Hum Pathol 23:1072–1075, 1992.
106. DeLange WE, Freling NJM, Molenaar WM, Doarenbos H: Invasive fibrous thyroiditis (Riedel's struma): A case report with review of the literature. Q J Med 268:709–717, 1989.
107. Heufelder AE, Hay ID, Carney JA, Gorman CA: Coexistence of Graves' disease and Riedel's (invasive fibrous) thyroiditis: Further evidence of a link between Riedel's thyroiditis and organ-specific autoimmunity. Clin Invest 72:788–793, 1994.
108. Heufelder AE, Hay ID: Further evidence for autoimmune mechanisms in the pathogenesis of Riedel's invasive thyroiditis. J Intern Med 238:85–86, 1995.
109. Zimmermann-Belsing T, Feldt-Rasmussen U: Riedel's thyroiditis: An autoimmune or primary fibrotic disease? J Intern Med 235:271–274, 1994.
110. Shaw AFB, Smith RP: Riedel's chronic thyroiditis: With a report of six cases and a contribution to the pathology. Br J Surg 13:93–108, 1925.
111. Drury ME, Sweeney EC, Heffernan SJ: Invasive fibrous thyroiditis. Ir Med J 67:388–390, 1974.
112. Heufelder AE, Hays ID: Expression of HLA-DR and heat shock protein 72 in Riedel's invasive thyroiditis (abstract). Clin Res 40:49A, 1992.
113. Heufelder AE, Bahn RS: Soluble intercellular adhesion molecule-1 in sera of patients with Graves' ophthalmopathy and thyroid diseases. Clin Exp Immunol 92:296–302, 1993.
114. Many MC, Carpentier S, Eggermont J, et al: Towards an experimental model for Riedel's fibrous thyroiditis (abstract). J Endocrinol Invest 4 (Suppl):92, 1998.
115. Heufelder AE, Goellner JR, Bahn RS, et al: Tissue eosinophilia and eosinophil degranulation in Riedel's invasive fibrous thyroiditis. J Clin Endocrinol Metab 81:977–984, 1996.
116. Rose E, Rayster HP: Invasive fibrous thyroiditis (Riedel's struma). JAMA 176:224–226, 1961.
117. Katsikas D, Shorthouse AJ, Taylor S: Riedel's thyroiditis: Br J Surg 63:929–931, 1976.
118. Chopra D, Wool MS, Crosson A, Sawin CT: Riedel's struma associated with subacute thyroiditis, hypothyroidism and hypoparathyroidism. J Clin Endocrinol Metab 46:869–871, 1978.
119. Bowlby AA: Diseases of the ductless glands. I. Infiltrating fibroma (?sarcoma) of the thyroid gland. Trans Pathol Soc (Lond) 36:420–423, 1885.
120. Comings DS, Skubi KB, Van Eyes J, Motulsky AG: Familial multifocal fibrosclerosis. Ann Intern Med 66:884–892, 1967.

Chapter 105

Hypothyroidism and Myxedema Coma

Wilmar M. Wiersinga

DEFINITION AND EPIDEMIOLOGY OF HYPOTHYROIDISM

Hypothyroidism can be defined as a syndrome characterized by the clinical and biochemical manifestations of thyroid hormone deficiency in the target tissues of thyroid hormone. Strictly speaking, hypothyroidism denotes deficient thyroid gland production of thyroid hormone. This deficiency may be caused by an abnormality in the thyroid gland itself (primary hypothyroidism) or by insufficient thyroid-stimulating hormone (TSH) stimulation of the thyroid gland because of an abnormality in the pituitary or hypothalamus (secondary and tertiary, or central, hypothyroidism). The vast majority of patients with thyroid hormone deficiency have primary hypothyroidism. Symptoms and signs of thyroid hormone deficiency in a small number of patients are caused by mutations in the thyroid hormone receptor TRβ; the condition, known as resistance to thyroid hormone (see Chapter 114), is associated with increased production of thyroid hormone by the thyroid gland. The term hypothyroidism may therefore be used in a broader sense to indicate deficient thyroid hormone action in target tissues, irrespective of its cause.

The first step in the spontaneous development of primary hypothyroidism is a slight fall in thyroid secretion of thyroxine (T_4), which causes increased release of TSH. The decreased T_4 secretion results in a modest decrease in the serum concentration of free thyroxine (FT_4), which still remains within the normal reference range, but serum TSH increases to values above the upper normal limit because of the exquisite sensitivity of the pituitary thyrotroph for circulating thyroid hormone (thereby giving rise to the log-linear relationship between serum TSH and FT_4). The condition is known as subclinical hypothyroidism. The hypersecretion of TSH may sometimes restore thyroid secretion of T_4 by stimulating thyroid hyperplasia and hypertrophy. The increase in TSH furthermore induces preferential thyroid secretion of triiodothyronine (T_3) by stimulating the synthesis of T_3 more than T_4 and by increasing thyroidal 5′-monodeiodination of T_4 into T_3.[1, 2] The fractional conversion rate of T_4 into T_3 in extrathyroidal tissues (notably the brain) increases. These mechanisms result in a relative overproduction of T_3 in comparison to T_4 and serve—in view of the greater biologic potency of T_3 than T_4—to restrict the impact of thyroid hormone deficiency in peripheral tissues. This preferential T_3 production explains why in subclinical hypothyroidism the serum concentration of T_3 sometimes exceeds the upper normal limit. Progression of the thyroid disease will cause a greater decline in thyroidal secretion of T_4 and result in serum FT_4 levels below the normal reference range and a further rise in serum TSH; serum T_3 remains within normal limits because of maintenance of T_3 production. Finally, when serum T_4 has decreased even more, serum T_3 values fall into the subnormal range. Hypothyroidism is thus a graded phenomenon[3] (Fig. 105–1) that ranges from subclinical hypothyroidism to myxedema coma, the most severe manifestation of the syndrome.

Primary hypothyroidism is a common disease worldwide, especially in iodine-deficient areas (see Chapter 108). It is also a very prevalent disease in iodine-replete regions. The most extensive epidemiologic data have been obtained from a population-based study of subjects 18 years and older in Whickham County in northeast England[4, 5] (Table 105–1). The initial survey was done between 1972 and 1974, with a follow-up 20 years later. The data seem representative of other countries inasmuch as similar figures have been reported from Sweden, Japan, and the United States.[6–10] Most striking are the high prevalence (especially of subclinical hypothyroidism), the marked female preponderance, and the increasing occurrence with advancing age. The mean age at diagnosis of hypothyroidism in women is 60 years. Most cases are due to chronic autoimmune thyroiditis (incidence of 3.5 per 1000 women per year), followed by destructive treatment for thyrotoxicosis (incidence of 0.6 per 1000 women per year). The probability of spontaneous hypothyroidism developing in women at a particular time increases with age: from 1.4 to 14 per 1000 per year at ages 20 to 25 and 75 to 80 years, respectively. Risk factors for progression to overt hypothyroidism are the presence of thyroid autoantibodies and an already elevated TSH (Table 105–2). The risk correlates with the strength of the titer of thyroid antimicrosomal autoantibodies and with the extent of the TSH increase. Interestingly, the probability of hypothyroidism developing rises even at TSH levels in the high normal range of 2 to 5 mU/L, independent of age or antibody status.[5, 11]

CAUSES OF HYPOTHYROIDISM

The various causes of hypothyroidism can be classified according to their site of interference (in the hypothalamus-pituitary, in the thyroid gland, or in the peripheral target tissues) and their nature (organic lesions resulting in loss of functional tissue or functional disturbances resulting in deficient hormone biosynthesis and release) (Table 105–3). Most cases of hypothyroidism are acquired and permanent; congenital hypothyroidism and transient forms of hypothyroidism are in the minority.

Central Hypothyroidism

The reduced T_4 secretion in central hypothyroidism is due to insufficient stimulation of the thyroid gland by TSH, which is caused by

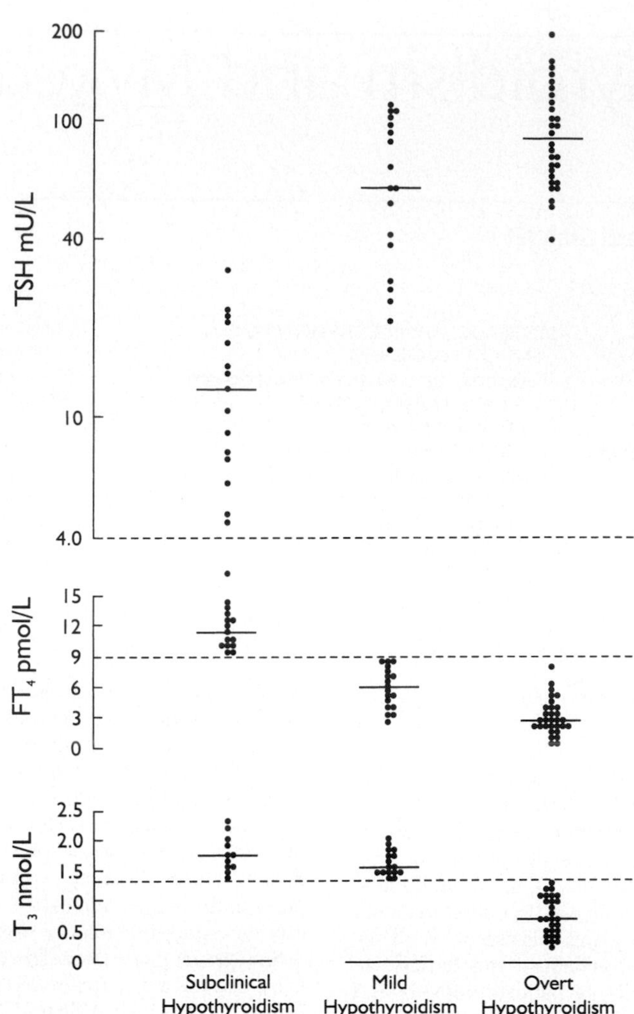

FIGURE 105–1. Individual and median values of thyroid function tests in various grades of primary hypothyroidism. *Interrupted horizontal lines* indicate upper (thyroid-stimulating hormone [TSH]) and lower (free thyroxin [FT_4] and triiodothyronine [T_3]) limits of the normal reference range. Progression from grade I to III can be observed in the transition from the euthyroid to the severely hypothyroid state, and vice versa upon treatment of hypothyroidism.

Grade I	Subclinical hypothyroidism	TSH slightly elevated	FT_4 normal	T_3 normal or slightly elevated
Grade II	Mild hypothyroidism	TSH moderately high	FT_4 low	T_3 normal
Grade III	Overt hypothyroidism	TSH very high	FT_4 low	T_3 low

lesions in the pituitary (secondary hypothyroidism) or the hypothalamus (tertiary hypothyroidism resulting from deficient thyrotropin-releasing hormone [TRH] release). The term central hypothyroidism is preferred because lesions sometimes involve both sites and thus prevent clear-cut distinction. Furthermore, although an absent TSH response to exogenous TRH would suggest a pituitary cause and a delayed response would suggest a hypothalamic cause,[12] the TSH profiles after TRH are not very well correlated to the anatomic site of the lesion. Basal serum TSH values in central hypothyroidism can be low, normal, or even slightly elevated up to 10 mU/L.[13] The apparent paradox of central hypothyroidism in the presence of a normal or even increased serum TSH concentration is explained by the reduced biologic activity of TSH in these patients related to abnormal TSH glycosylation.[13–15] Chronic treatment with oral TRH restores the biologic activity of TSH, thus suggesting that deficient hypothalamic TRH release induces both quantitative and qualitative abnormalities in

TABLE 105–1. Prevalence and Incidence of Primary Hypothyroidism in the Adult Population as Established in the Whickham Survey

		Women	Men
Prevalence	Hypothyroidism	18/1000	1/1000
	Unsuspected	3/1000	0/1000
	Known	15/1000	1/1000
	Subclinical hypothyroidism	75/1000	28/1000
Incidence	Hypothyroidism	4.1/1000/yr	0.6/1000/yr

Data from Tunbridge et al.[4] and Vanderpump et al.[5]

TABLE 105–2. Percentage of Women Acquiring Spontaneous Primary Hypothyroidism during 20 Years of Follow-up in the Whickham Survey

	Initial Thyroid Autoantibodies	
Initial Serum TSH	***Negative***	***Positive***
Normal	4%	27%
Elevated	33%	55%

TSH, thyroid-stimulating hormone.
Data from Vanderpump et al.[5] and Wang and Crapo.[10]

TABLE 105–3. Causes of Hypothyroidism

Central (hypothalamic/pituitary) hypothyroidism
Loss of functional tissue
Tumors (pituitary adenoma, craniopharyngioma, meningioma, dysgerminoma, glioma, metastases)
Trauma (surgery, irradiation, head injury)
Vascular (ischemic necrosis, hemorrhage, stalk interruption, aneurysm of internal carotid artery)
Infections (abscess, tuberculosis, syphilis, toxoplasmosis)
Infiltrative (sarcoidosis, histiocytosis, hemochromatosis)
Chronic lymphocytic hypophysitis
Congenital (pituitary hypoplasia, septo-optic dysplasia, basal encephalocele)
Functional defects in TSH biosynthesis and release
Mutations in genes encoding for TRH receptor, TSH-β, or Pit-1
Drugs: dopamine, glucocorticoids, L-thyroxine withdrawal
Primary (thyroidal) hypothyroidism
Loss of functional thyroid tissue
Chronic autoimmune thyroiditis
Reversible autoimmune hypothyroidism (silent and postpartum thyroiditis, cytokine-induced thyroiditis)
Surgery and irradiation (^{131}I or external irradiation)
Infiltrative and infectious diseases, subacute thyroiditis
Thyroid dysgenesis
Functional defects in thyroid hormone biosynthesis and release
Congenital defects in thyroid hormone biosynthesis
Iodine deficiency and iodine excess
Drugs: antithyroid agents, lithium, natural and synthetic goitrogenic chemicals
"Peripheral" (extrathyroidal) hypothyroidism
Thyroid hormone resistance

TRH, thyrotropin-releasing hormone; TSH, thyroid-stimulating hormone.

TSH secretion.[16] Central hypothyroidism is also associated with a decreased nocturnal TSH surge (because of loss of the usual nocturnal increase in TSH pulse amplitude but not TSH pulse frequency), which might further hamper maintenance of normal thyroid function.[17, 18]

The prevalence of central hypothyroidism in the general population is unknown; a rough estimate is 0.005%. The sex distribution is about equal, and central hypothyroidism occurs with peaks in childhood and in adults 30 to 60 years of age. TSH deficiency caused by loss of functional tissue usually becomes manifested after the development of growth hormone and gonadotropin deficiency.[19]

Congenital cases are due to pituitary hypoplasia, midline defects such as septo-optic dysplasia (TSH deficiency in 20%), Rathke's pouch cysts, or rare "loss of function" mutations in the TRH receptor gene,[20] TSH-β subunit gene,[21] or Pit-1 gene.[22] Pit-1 is a pituitary-specific transcription factor confined to the nuclei of somatotropes, lactotropes, and thyrotropes in the anterior pituitary; Pit-1 deficiency results in growth hormone and prolactin deficiency and variable hypothyroidism because of TSH deficiency. Childhood cases are mostly caused by craniopharyngioma (TSH deficiency in 53%) or cranial irradiation (e.g., for dysgerminoma or hematologic malignancies). Adult cases are most frequently due to pituitary macroadenomas (hypothyroidism in 10%–25%) and pituitary surgery or irradiation. TSH deficiency may sometimes disappear after selective adenomectomy.[23] Cranial radiotherapy for brain tumors causes hypothyroidism in 65%, depending on the radiation dose; the onset varies between 1 and 26 years after irradiation.[24] Radiotherapy for pituitary tumors is followed by hypothyroidism in at least 15% (up to 55% when combined with surgery).[25] Less common causes are head injury (TSH deficiency in 85%),[26] ischemic necrosis from postpartum hemorrhage (Sheehan's syndrome) or severe shock, pituitary apoplexy (hemorrhage in a pituitary adenoma), infiltrative diseases, and lymphocytic hypophysitis.[27] Lymphocytic hypophysitis is most likely an autoimmune disease that occurs predominantly in women during pregnancy and the postpartum period and is characterized by a pituitary mass and hypopituitarism.[27] Despite the many known causes of central hypothyroidism, idiopathic cases are still encountered.

In critically ill patients receiving dopamine, serum TSH and the T_4 production rate decrease by 60% and 56%, respectively, as a result of direct inhibition of pituitary TSH.[28] Transient functional inhibition of TSH release is observed after withdrawal of long-term levothyroxine suppressive therapy, which may last up to 6 weeks.[29] A similar pattern can be seen after the treatment of thyrotoxicosis: serum TSH may remain suppressed despite restoration of the euthyroid state.[30] Finally, glucocorticoid excess dampens pulsatile TSH release, which rarely results in decreased serum FT_4.[31] Likewise, octreotide therapy does not cause hypothyroidism despite decreasing TSH secretion.

Chronic Autoimmune Thyroiditis

Hypothyroidism secondary to chronic autoimmune thyroiditis is caused mainly by destruction of thyrocytes. The goitrous variant (hypothyroid Hashimoto's goiter) is characterized by massive lymphocytic infiltration of the thyroid with the formation of germinal centers, oxyphilic changes in thyrocytes called Hürthle or Askanazy cells, and some fibrosis. In the atrophic variant (atrophic myxedema), fibrosis is the predominant feature, along with lymphocytic infiltration. The less common goitrous variant is characterized by a diffuse goiter of firm "rubbery" consistence; the histology remained essentially unaltered after 20 years, and the goiter did not regress despite T_4 treatment in 43%.[32] The more prevalent atrophic variant is thus not simply the end stage of the goitrous variant. Many patients with chronic autoimmune thyroiditis are euthyroid (see Chapter 103), and a few have an initial transient hyperthyroid stage (labeled as "Hashitoxicosis"). Hashimoto's disease is used by many as an umbrella term to indicate autoimmune-mediated destruction of thyrocytes, frequently but not always resulting in hypothyroidism, as opposed to Graves' disease, in which TSH receptor–stimulating antibodies usually result in hyperthyroidism. The two disease entities overlap and can be viewed as opposite ends of a continuous spectrum of thyroid autoimmunity. Destruction of thyrocytes and development of hypothyroidism in Hashimoto's disease are mediated by cytotoxic T cells and cytokines (especially interferon-γ and tumor necrosis factor) released by infiltrating T cells and macrophages. Humoral immunity appears less important in this respect, but (a subset of) thyroid peroxidase (TPO) antibodies may contribute via antibody-dependent cell-mediated cytotoxicity, complement-mediated cytotoxicity, and inhibition of TPO enzymatic activity (see Chapter 103). TSH receptor–blocking antibodies will enhance thyroid atrophy and hypothyroidism, possibly also by inducing apoptosis. Whereas the presence of TPO antibodies in serum is a hallmark of chronic autoimmune thyroiditis, TSH receptor–blocking antibodies are less prevalent. They occur more often in Japanese patients[33] than white patients.[34] TSH receptor antibodies (but not TSH) are negatively correlated with serum FT_4 and thyroid size, both in euthyroid and hypothyroid patients.[35]

The diversity in the clinical features of Hashimoto's disease with respect to thyroid function and thyroid growth is best explained as being the net result of the various immunologic effector mechanisms involved in chronic autoimmune thyroiditis. Genetic and environmental factors enhance the susceptibility of individuals to development of the disease and may determine the direction of the evolving autoimmune reaction. Autoimmune thyroid disease runs in families (80% of patients have a positive family history) and is 4 to 10 times more common in women. Autoimmune hypothyroidism in whites is weakly associated with HLA-DR3; other still unidentified genes are probably involved. Iodine intake has been identified as an environmental factor because the prevalence of autoimmune hypothyroidism is higher in iodine-replete than in iodine-deficient areas[36, 37] and the incidence increases after supplemental iodine is introduced.

Reversible Autoimmune Hypothyroidism

CHRONIC AUTOIMMUNE THYROIDITIS. Autoimmune hypothyroidism may spontaneously revert into euthyroidism in connection with the disappearance of TSH receptor–blocking antibodies.[38] The presence of a goiter and high thyroidal radioiodine uptake increase the likelihood of spontaneous recovery,[39, 40] just like an increase in serum T_3 in response to TRH during T_4 treatment.[41] The incidence of spontaneous recovery is about 5%,[42] but possibly higher in Japan where—in the face of a high ambient iodine intake—iodide restriction alone may induce a remission.[39] Autoimmune hypothyroidism is, however, permanent in most patients, and it remains doubtful whether withdrawal of thyroid hormone therapy or specific tests to assess recovery of thyroid function are indicated. Peculiar cases of alternating hypothyroidism and hyperthyroidism are explained by changes in coexisting TSH receptor–blocking and TSH receptor–stimulating antibodies.[43]

SILENT AND POSTPARTUM THYROIDITIS. Silent or painless thyroiditis and postpartum thyroiditis are variant forms of chronic autoimmune thyroiditis. Thyroid histology shows lymphocytic infiltration but no germinal centers or fibrosis. The autoimmune attack is rather intense (resulting in mainly T cell–mediated destructive thyroiditis) but transient, which explains the characteristic pattern of transient thyrotoxicosis followed by transient hypothyroidism in the recovery stage. Each stage lasts from 2 to 8 weeks. Most patients remain asymptomatic and revert spontaneously to euthyroidism. Occurrence is very common in the first year after delivery: the incidence of postpartum thyroiditis is 4% to 6% and up to 25% in patients with type 1 diabetes mellitus.[44–46] Several patterns are recognized: thyrotoxicosis alone occurs in 38%, thyrotoxicosis followed by hypothyroidism in 26%, and hypothyroidism alone in 36%. TPO antibodies in serum of 100 kU/L or greater at 12 weeks' gestation predict to a certain extent postpartum thyroiditis (positive predictive value, 0.50; negative predictive value, 0.98).[45] Thyroid antibody titers decrease in the second and third trimesters and increase postpartum. Women with postpartum thyroiditis are at risk for recurrent postpartum thyroiditis after delivery (about 40%) and for permanent hypothyroidism (20%–30% after 5 years) related to higher antibody titers and absence of a thyrotoxic phase.[47, 48] TPO antibodies are associated with depression[49] and impaired child development.[50]

CYTOKINE-INDUCED THYROIDITIS. Treatment of malignant tumors or hepatitis C or B with interleukin-2 or interferon-α is causally related to the de novo occurrence of TPO antibodies and development of thyroid dysfunction.[51–53] Typical features are similar to those of silent and postpartum thyroiditis and include sudden onset, biphasic pattern of thyrotoxicosis followed by hypothyroidism (although hypothyroidism alone is most frequent), and spontaneous resolution after discontinuation of treatment. The incidence is 5% to 20%; risk factors are female sex and preexistent thyroid antibodies. Induction of autoantibodies directed against nonthyroidal antigens occurs less often.

Postoperative and Postradiation Hypothyroidism

SURGERY. Total thyroidectomy results in overt hypothyroidism within 1 month. Subtotal thyroidectomy for Graves' hyperthyroidism is followed by hypothyroidism in 40% after 10 years[54]; risk factors are a small thyroid remnant, lymphocytic infiltration, and subsequent exposure to iodine. Most patients become hypothyroid in the first year after surgery; thereafter, the cumulative incidence of hypothyroidism increases by only 1% to 2% per year. Immediate postoperative hypothyroidism does not always indicate permanent hypothyroidism; it may resolve spontaneously by 6 months. Subtotal thyroidectomy for (toxic) nodular goiter carries a much lower risk (about 15%) for postoperative hypothyroidism.

RADIOIODINE. ^{131}I treatment of Graves' hyperthyroidism results in a cumulative incidence of hypothyroidism of up to 70% after 10 years,[54] depending on the dose of ^{131}I administered. Most cases occur in the first year (spontaneous return to euthyroidism is observed in some patients); thereafter, the annual incidence of hypothyroidism is 0.5% to 2%, also related to persisting chronic autoimmune thyroiditis. Hypothyroidism after ^{131}I treatment of toxic nodular goiter is less common (6%–13%).[55] ^{131}I treatment of nontoxic goiter to reduce goiter size carries a cumulative risk of 58% for the development of hypothyroidism in 8 years, the risk being related to the (relatively high) dose of ^{131}I and the presence of TPO antibodies.[56] Hypothyroidism caused by ionizing radiation has been reported in subjects exposed to atomic or hydrogen bomb explosions. A high prevalence of serum TPO antibodies is found in children exposed to the Chernobyl radioactive fallout[57]; they seem to be at risk for future development of hypothyroidism.

EXTERNAL IRRADIATION. External radiotherapy of the neck for Hodgkin's or non-Hodgkin's lymphomas causes hypothyroidism in 25% to 50% of patients; the risk is related to the radiation dose, the use of iodine-containing contrast agents before radiotherapy,[58] and the duration of follow-up. The risk decreases by shielding of the thyroid during mantle field irradiation. External radiotherapy for head and neck cancer has an actuarial risk of 40% for the development of subclinical hypothyroidism and 15% for overt hypothyroidism 3 years after treatment.[59] Total body irradiation with subsequent bone marrow transplantation for acute leukemia or aplastic anemia is associated with (mainly subclinical) hypothyroidism in about 25%, which usually occurs after 1 year; it is transient in half the patients.[60]

Infiltrative and Infectious Diseases

A rare cause of hypothyroidism is thyroidal infiltration by systemic disease. Hypothyroidism is observed in the course of invasive fibrous thyroiditis of Riedel (in 30%–40%, see Chapter 104), cystinosis (up to 86% in adults), progressive systemic sclerosis, and amyloidosis.[61] Infections of the thyroid gland are rare and associated with preexistent thyroid disease and immunocompromising conditions. Occasionally, damage to the thyroid causes hypothyroidism. Hypothyroidism in the recovery phase of subacute thyroiditis of de Quervain (related to previous viral infections) is, in contrast, a very common event (see Chapter 104).

Congenital Hypothyroidism

Congenital hypothyroidism can be permanent (incidence, 1 in 3100 newborns) or transient. Causes include loss of functional thyroid tissue (thyroid dysgenesis), functional defects in thyroid hormone biosynthesis (related to loss-of-function mutations in genes encoding for the TSH receptor, Na^+/I^- symporter, thyroglobulin, or TPO), and thyroid hormone resistance (mutated TRβ) (see Chapters 111 through 114).

Iodine Deficiency and Iodine Excess

Hypothyroidism can be caused by either iodine deficiency (see Chapter 108) or iodine excess. Inorganic iodide in excess of daily doses of 500 to 1000 μg inhibits organification of iodide, known as the Wolff-Chaikoff effect. Usually the thyroid gland escapes the Wolff-Chaikoff effect after several weeks, because autoregulatory mechanisms inhibit thyroid iodide transport and the intrathyroidal iodine concentration consequently falls below the level required for inhibition of organification[62] (Fig. 105–2). Failure to escape results in hypothyroidism, which occurs in the presence of underlying thyroid disease such as chronic autoimmune thyroiditis, previous subacute or postpartum thyroiditis, and ^{131}I or surgical therapy.[63] Iodide-induced hypothyroidism may be due to inorganic iodide or organic iodine compounds that are deiodinated in vivo. Sources of iodine excess are an iodine-rich diet (such as in Japan with a high consumption of seaweed[39]), iodine-containing medications such as potassium iodide, vitamins, kelp, topical antiseptics, radiographic contrast agents, and amiodarone.[63] The incidence of amiodarone-induced hypothyroidism in areas with high environmental iodine intake is higher than in areas with low iodine intake (22% and 5%, respectively)[64]; cases occur predominantly in the first 18 months of amiodarone treatment, especially in females with preexistent thyroid antibodies.[65]

Drug-Induced Hypothyroidism

Drugs on rare occasion cause hypothyroidism by inhibition of TSH secretion (see Central Hypothyroidism) or by decreasing the absorption, transport, or metabolism of thyroid hormone[66] (see Table 105–5).

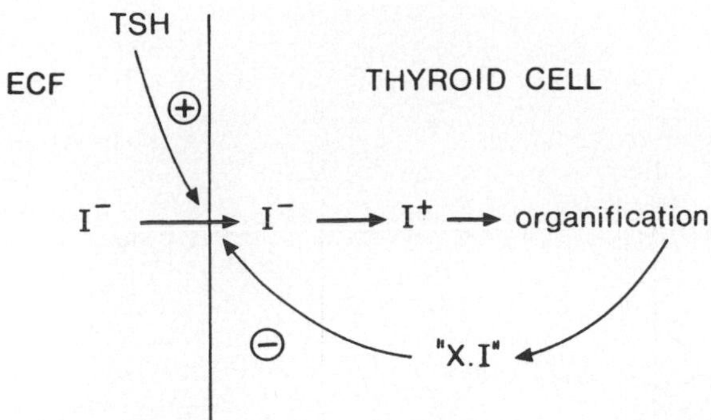

FIGURE 105–2. Inhibition of thyroid iodide transport by iodine excess requires organification of the administered iodide; it is mediated by a specific iodinated compound X.I, presumably an iodinated lipid. This autoregulatory mechanism for iodine excess may fail because of preexistent subtle organification defects that result via decreased X.I in uninhibited iodide uptake and persistence of the Wolff-Chaikoff effect. (From Wiersinga WM, Touber JL, Trip MD, van Royen EA: Uninhibited thyroidal uptake of radioiodine despite iodine excess in amiodarone-induced hypothyroidism. J Clin Endocrinol Metab 63:485–491, © 1986, The Endocrine Society.)

Drugs causing hypothyroidism by interference with thyroid hormone production and/or release in the thyroid gland include the thiouracils and imidazoles (used in the treatment of thyrotoxicosis), lithium, cytokines (see Reversible Autoimmune Hypothyroidism), iodine (see Iodine Deficiency and Iodine Excess), and a variety of environmental and industrial goitrogenic chemicals.[61] Examples of the latter group are naturally occurring goitrogens, such as flavonoids and resorcinol (present in watersheds of the coal- and shale-rich regions of Colombia and Kentucky[67]), and industrial pollution with polychlorinated biphenyls.[68] Lithium inhibits thyroidal iodide transport and release of T_4 and T_3. Long-term lithium treatment results in goiter in up to 50%, subclinical hypothyroidism in about 20%, and hypothyroidism in about 20%[66, 69]; goiter and hypothyroidism usually occur in the first 2 years of treatment, especially in patients with preexisting thyroid antibodies.

SYSTEMIC MANIFESTATIONS OF HYPOTHYROIDISM

Systemic manifestations vary considerably, depending on the cause, duration, and severity of the hypothyroid state. The characteristic clinical finding is slowing of physical and mental activity and many organ functions. The characteristic pathologic finding is accumulation of hyaluronic acid and other glycosaminoglycans in interstitial tissue, which is related to loss of the inhibitory effects of thyroid hormone on the synthesis of hyaluronate, fibronectin, and collagen by fibroblasts.[70] The hydrophilic properties of glycosaminoglycans lead to a peculiar mucinous nonpitting edema (myxedema) that is most obvious in the dermis but can be present in many organs.

Energy and Nutrient Metabolism

Thyroid hormone deficiency causes slowing of a wide variety of metabolic processes, which results in decreased resting energy expenditure, oxygen consumption, and utilization of substrates. Reduced thermogenesis is related to the characteristic cold intolerance of hypothyroid patients. The fall in metabolic rate and substrate utilization contributes to decreased appetite and food intake. Body weight increases on average by 10% because of an increase in body fat and retention of water and salt.[71] Hypothyroidism delays glucose absorption from the intestine. Insulin secretion in response to oral glucose is appropriate for the slightly flattened oral glucose tolerance curve. Hepatic gluconeogenesis and glucose utilization usually remain normal, and blood glucose levels are maintained within normal limits. The occurrence of hypoglycemia in hypothyroid patients should alert the physician to concomitant diseases (such as hypopituitarism). The development of hypothyroidism in patients with insulin-dependent diabetes mellitus may require lowering of the insulin dose to counteract the decreased rate of insulin degradation. Synthesis and degradation of proteins are reduced in hypothyroidism; one of the obvious consequences during childhood is impaired growth. Biosynthesis of fatty acids and lipolysis are also reduced. The changes in fat metabolism result in an increase in plasma lipid concentrations in hypothyroid patients, which are reversible, however, upon thyroid hormone replacement. Plasma triglycerides do not change or increase slightly because of a reduced fractional removal rate, which is related to decreased lipoprotein lipase activity in postheparin plasma.[72, 73] The elevation in total cholesterol in plasma is quantitatively related to the decrease in serum thyroid hormones and fractional nuclear T_3 receptor occupancy in the liver.[74] The increase in plasma cholesterol is largely accounted for by an increase in low-density lipoprotein (LDL) cholesterol (associated with an increase in apolipoprotein B) because of decreased expression of the T_3-responsive LDL receptor gene in the liver, which is involved in LDL clearance. Recent studies also indicate increased oxidizability of LDL particles in hypothyroidism.[75] A modest increase in high-density lipoprotein-2 (HDL_2) cholesterol is seen, but not in HDL_3 cholesterol (associated with an increase in apolipoprotein AI but not AII)[72, 76]; this finding has been explained by decreased activity of the cholesteryl ester transfer protein[77, 78] (which redistributes cholesteryl esters in HDL to the less dense apolipoprotein B–containing lipoproteins) and hepatic lipase[73] (which is involved in the conversion of HDL_2 to HDL_3). The ratios of total cholesterol/HDL cholesterol and LDL/HDL cholesterol both decrease with treatment of hypothyroidism.[76] Lipoprotein(a) is increased in hypothyroidism in some but not all studies.[72, 73] Taken together, the changes in plasma lipids in hypothyroidism result in an atherogenic lipid profile.

Skin and Appendages

Skin changes are very prevalent among hypothyroid patients. The skin is dry, pale, thick, and rough with scales, and it feels cold. Dryness is related to decreased function of sebaceous and sweat glands. Pallor is related to decreased skin blood flow and anemia. Yellowish discoloration of the skin can be present, especially on the palms and soles, because of the deposition of carotene, which is converted to a lesser extent to vitamin A. The thick rough skin with scales is caused by mucinous swelling of the dermis and hyperkeratosis of the stratum corneum in the epidermis. The nonpitting swelling is most marked in the extremities and the face and gives rise to the so called myxedema face (Fig. 105 3). This classic appearance of primary hypothyroidism is nowadays less often seen, probably because of earlier diagnosis by widespread use of the TSH assay. The hair becomes dull, coarse, and brittle. Hair loss occurs in 50%; it is usually diffuse and involves the scalp, beard, and genital hair, less often the eyebrows. Nail deformities are also very common: the nails become thin and brittle, have grooves, and grow more slowly.

Nervous System

Thyroid hormones are essential for normal brain development; congenital hypothyroidism, if left untreated, results in mental retardation and neurologic abnormalities (see Chapters 108, 180, and 184). In adult hypothyroid patients, decreased cerebral blood flow and increased cerebral vascular resistance have been demonstrated, but no alterations in brain glucose or oxygen use.[79] Recent studies using ^{32}P nuclear magnetic resonance spectroscopy of the frontal lobe of adult hypothyroid patients report reversible alterations in phosphate metabolism, which suggests impairment of mitochondrial metabolism.[80] Thyroid hormone receptors are present in the human brain. The low-voltage electroencephalogram, prolonged central motor conduction time, and reduced visual and somatosensory evoked potential amplitude with longer latency in adult hypothyroid patients are reversible with T_4 treatment. These findings indicate the adult human brain as a thyroid hormone–responsive organ and provide a biologic basis for the

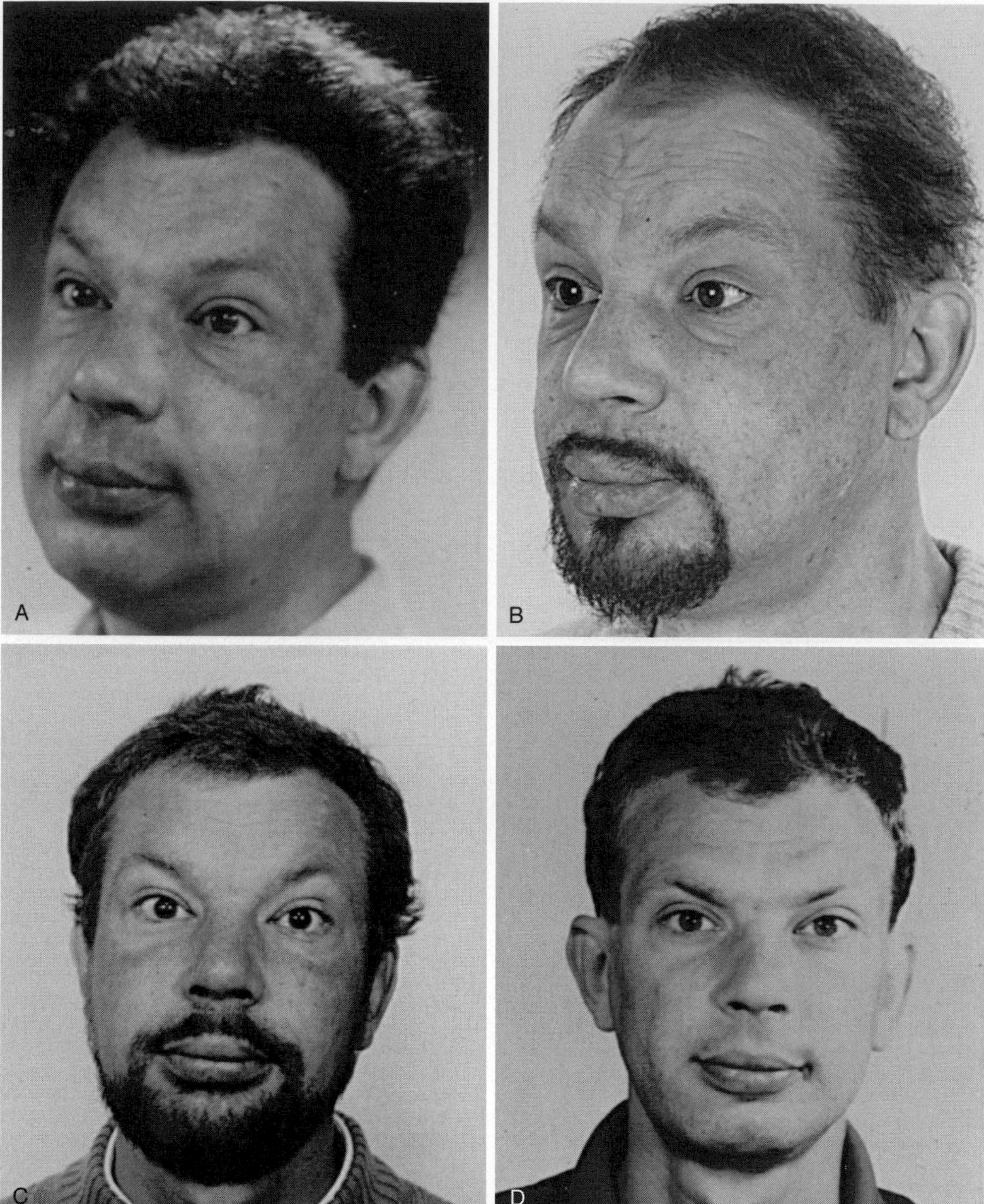

FIGURE 105–3. Appearance of a 47-year-old man 12 years *(A)*, 5 years *(B)*, and 3 years *(C)* before hypothyroidism secondary to atrophic myxedema *(D)* was diagnosed. Note the typical myxedema face characterized by puffy nonpitting swelling of the skin and coarse facial features. (Reproduced with permission of the patient.)

very prevalent neurobehavioral symptoms and cognitive impairment associated with adult hypothyroidism.[81]

Typically, a hypothyroid patient is slow in movement and thought, is less alert, and is less able to concentrate and memorize. Speech becomes slow, often hoarse. Hearing can be impaired. The patient sleeps longer and may fall asleep during the daytime. Hypothyroidism is listed as one of the treatable causes of dementia, although complete reversibility seems to be rare.[82] Patients may accept the limitations in physical and mental activity as part of the unavoidable aging process, but many become anxious or depressed. Rarely, severe anxiety and agitation occur, a condition known as myxedematous madness. Depression develops in over 40%,[83] most likely related to reduced synthesis and turnover of brain 5-hydroxytryptamine; indeed, central 5-hydroxytryptamine activity is reduced in hypothyroid patients,[84] and T_3 supplementation might increase the efficacy of antidepressant drugs.[85]

Thyroid hormone deficiency may give rise to several reversible neurologic syndromes. Cerebellar ataxia may occur, especially in elderly people, and is associated with an unsteady gait and intention tremor. More common is the carpal tunnel syndrome, which is linked to entrapment of the median nerve by thickening of the connective tissue of tendon sheaths. Complaints of paresthesias occur in 64%; objective findings of polyneuropathy are observed in 33%.[86]

Musculoskeletal System

MUSCLES. Muscle symptoms are very prevalent in hypothyroid patients and include myalgia, weakness, stiffness, cramps, and easy fatigability. The biochemical substrate of these complaints is partly provided by a rise in the inorganic phosphate–to-ATP ratio in resting muscle and an important decrease in phosphocreatine in working hypothyroid muscle with a greater fall in intracellular pH than in controls.[87] Impairment of mitochondrial oxidative metabolism has also been demonstrated in subclinical hypothyroidism.[88] Transition from white fast type II to red slow type I muscle fibers is involved in the change in muscle bioenergetics, which is probably multifactorial. The histopathology varies; most common is type II fiber atrophy, but fiber hypertrophy may be present along with interstitial edema and sarcoplasmic degeneration. Rarely, chronic hypothyroid myopathy results in increased volume of muscles (notably in the tongue and extremities), which may cause entrapment syndromes.[89] Serum creatine kinase (MM fraction derived from skeletal muscle) is often elevated and correlates with the severity of hypothyroidism. The decreased rate of muscle contractility in hypothyroidism is evident from slow deep tendon reflexes. The half-relaxation time of the Achilles reflex is prolonged in many hypothyroid patients, but substantial overlap is seen in euthyroid subjects.

JOINTS. Arthralgia and joint stiffness are common complaints. Synovial effusions (usually of the knee) are rare.

BONES. Hypothyroidism leads to decreased bone formation and bone resorption, but bone mineral density is comparable to that of matched controls. Urinary excretion of hydroxyproline and serum alkaline phosphatase and osteocalcin levels can be decreased; serum calcium is usually normal.

Cardiovascular System

Changes in cardiovascular dynamics in hypothyroidism include an increase (of 50%–60%) in peripheral vascular resistance and a decrease (of 30%–50%) in cardiac output.[90] As a result, mean blood pressure is largely unaltered, although systolic pressure may fall and diastolic pressure may rise. The mechanism of the increase in systemic vascular resistance is incompletely understood; T_3 acts as a vasodilator, and thyroid hormone deficiency increases vascular smooth muscle tone, possibly by interference with ion fluxes. The decrease in cardiac output is due to a decrease in stroke volume and heart rate. The preejection time and isovolumic contraction time are prolonged, and the ventricular relaxation rate during diastole is slower. The mechanism of the reduced cardiac contractility with subnormal systolic and diastolic performance is multifactorial. Changes in T_3-dependent myocardial gene expression are involved, especially in genes coding for calcium regulatory proteins.[91] Blood volume is decreased. Edema may develop by albumin extravasation as a result of increased capillary permeability; it may give rise to pericardial, pleural, or peritoneal effusions.

Cardiovascular symptoms of hypothyroid patients are dyspnea and decreased exercise tolerance; the hemodynamic response to exercise is usually preserved. Physical examination may reveal a slow pulse rate, diastolic hypertension (in 20%), weak heart sounds, occasionally cardiac enlargement (caused by pericardial effusion or, rarely, by T_4-reversible cardiomyopathy[91]), and peripheral nonpitting or pitting edema (rarely caused by heart failure except when the cardiac disease is preexisting). The electrocardiogram may demonstrate bradycardia, low-voltage conduction disturbances, and nonspecific ST-T changes. Asymmetrical septal hypertrophy in hypothyroid patients occurs less frequently than previously thought.[92] Silent myocardial ischemia in the absence of coronary artery disease has been described.[93] Symptomatic ischemic heart disease with anginal complaints occurs in about 3%[94]; the reduced need for oxygen in view of the hypometabolic state might give some protection. The atherogenic profile of serum lipids and the hyperhomocysteinemia[95] in hypothyroidism would suggest a greater prevalence of coronary atherosclerosis in these patients; coronary disease in autopsy studies was indeed more prevalent in hypothyroid patients with coexistent hypertension than in normotensive hypothyroidism.[96] A 20-year population-based follow-up study, however, did not find an association between thyroid antibodies or hypothyroidism and ischemic heart disease.[97]

Respiratory System

Respiratory symptoms of hypothyroidism are shortness of breath and sleep apnea. Shortness of breath can be caused by the cardiac effects of thyroid hormone deficiency, by weakness of respiratory muscles, by pleural effusion, or by impaired pulmonary function. In most nonobese hypothyroid patients, pulmonary function is nearly normal. Reduced ventilatory drive is observed in 34%; the depressed response to hypercapnia and/or hypoxia is usually rapidly restored upon T_4 treatment.[98] Severe obstructive sleep apnea occurs in 7.7%,[99] partly as a result of increased size of the tongue and pharyngeal muscles with a slow and sustained muscle contraction; the contribution of reduced ventilatory drive to sleep apnea is less marked but can be substantial in obese patients.

Urogenital System

KIDNEYS AND FLUID METABOLISM. Renal plasma flow and the glomerular filtration rate are reduced in hypothyroidism in accordance with the changes in cardiovascular hemodynamics. Serum creatinine is raised by 10% to 20%,[95] and hyponatremia occurs in one third of patients.[100] Hyponatremia is associated with the increased total body water and sodium content in hypothyroidism, which is a result of the increased vascular permeability and extravascular accumulation of hydrophilic glycosaminoglycans. Free water clearance in hypothyroidism is diminished, irrespective of the presence of hyponatremia. Plasma arginine vasopressin is frequently raised in hypothyroid patients; arginine vasopressin levels rise normally in response to hypertonic saline, but they are not suppressed normally after water ingestion. The syndrome of inappropriate antidiuresis in hypothyroidism is thus not fully understood.[101] The significance of low serum antinuclear factor concentrations in hypothyroidism is presently unclear.[102]

REPRODUCTIVE SYSTEM. Juvenile hypothyroidism results in delay in sexual maturation, seldom in precocious puberty (explained by spillover of the action of TRH on gonadotropes and the action of TSH on follicle-stimulating hormone receptors[103, 104]). In adult hypothyroid men, semen analysis is usually normal; loss of libido and potency do occur but may be nonspecific. Serum free testosterone, follicle-stimulating hormone, and luteinizing hormone levels are mostly normal. In adult hypothyroid women, pulsatile gonadotropin release in the follicular phase is normal,[105] but the ovulatory surge may not occur. Irregular, anovulatory cycles with menorrhagia are common. Some patients are initially seen with the galactorrhea-amenorrhea syndrome, which is due to hyperprolactinemia induced by thyroid hormone deficiency. Despite restricted fertility, conception may occur with successful pregnancy outcome. Pregnancy-induced hypertension is two to three times more common in hypothyroid women[106]; low birth weight is secondary to premature delivery for gestational hypertension. Recent studies do not report an increased risk of fetal death or congenital anomalies.

Gastrointestinal System

Hypothyroidism causes a decrease in electrical and motor activity of the esophagus, stomach, small intestine, and colon. Gastric emptying and intestinal transit time are prolonged.[107] The decreased motility explains the common complaint of constipation, which may range from mild to very severe (with rarely paralytic ileus and intestinal pseudo-obstruction). Intestinal absorption is mostly normal. Malabsorption may be due to pernicious anemia or celiac sprue, which are frequently associated with autoimmune hypothyroidism. About 25%

of patients with chronic autoimmune thyroiditis have parietal cell antibodies; some of them have achlorhydria and vitamin B_{12} malabsorption. Myxedematous ascites is rare.[108]

Slightly abnormal liver function test results are common, but usually fully reversible (except when caused by associated autoimmune liver disease such as chronic active hepatitis and primary biliary cirrhosis). Hypotonia of the gallbladder may occur.

Hematopoietic System

ERYTHROCYTES. Anemia occurs in about 30% and is usually mild and normocytic normochromic. It develops as a normal response to the decreased oxygen requirement and results in a decrease in erythropoietin and erythropoiesis with slight bone marrow hypoplasia. Because of the concomitant fall in plasma volume, the anemia is less marked than it would otherwise be. The anemia disappears slowly with T_4 treatment. Microcytic hypochromic anemia is seen in 2% to 15% and is mostly due to iron deficiency caused by excessive menstrual bleeding or by reduced iron absorption in the case of hypochlorhydria; both conditions are common in hypothyroid women. Macrocytic hyperchromic anemia indicates vitamin B_{12} or folic acid deficiency and is caused by either the hypothyroid state itself or pernicious anemia associated with chronic autoimmune thyroiditis.

LEUKOCYTES AND THROMBOCYTES. Granulocyte, lymphocyte, and platelet counts are usually normal in hypothyroidism. Leukopenia might indicate associated vitamin B_{12} or folic acid deficiency. Mean platelet volume can be decreased.

HEMOSTASIS. Hypothyroid patients may have bleeding symptoms such as easy bruising, menorrhagia, or prolonged bleeding after tooth extraction. The most frequent defects in hemostasis are a prolonged bleeding time, decreased platelet adhesiveness, and low plasma concentrations of factor VIII and von Willebrand factor.[109] Desmopressin rapidly reduces these abnormalities[110] and may be of value for the acute treatment of bleeding or as cover for surgery. Fibrinolytic activity in hypothyroidism is increased. Usually the clinical relevance of these abnormalities is limited, as illustrated by no excess blood loss or bleeding complications during and after surgery in a large series of hypothyroid patients.[111]

Endocrine System

PITUITARY. The decrease in growth hormone secretion in hypothyroidism is related to an increase in hypothalamic somatostatinergic tone[112] and results in low insulin-like growth factor (IGF-I) serum concentrations. It may cause dramatic growth retardation in hypothyroid children. Serum IGF-II, IGF-binding protein-1 (IGFBP-1), and IGFBP-3 also fall, whereas IGFBP-2 rises; these changes reverse with T_4 treatment.[113]

Moderate hyperprolactinemia is frequently observed in hypothyroid patients, especially in young women. It may cause galactorrhea and amenorrhea, particularly in long-standing hypothyroidism.[114] The prolactin response to TRH is increased in hypothyroidism. Increased expression of hypothalamic TRH because of diminished negative feedback exerted by T_3 might explain the (reversible) hyperprolactinemia in hypothyroidism.

Hypothyroidism in the presence of a pituitary mass does not always indicate central hypothyroidism. The hypersecretion of TSH in primary hypothyroidism is accompanied by hyperplasia and hypertrophy of pituitary thyrotrophs. Rarely, this alteration may cause a distinct pituitary macroadenoma in severely hypothyroid patients with very high TSH levels (even with impaired vision) that shrinks after thyroid hormone therapy.[115]

PARATHYROID. Thyroid hormone deficiency reduces the activity of osteoclasts and osteoblasts (only the latter possess nuclear T_3 receptors), which results in a slow rate of bone resorption and formation in the bone structural unit. Because of decreased bone resorption, serum calcium levels fall slightly, followed by an increase in parathyroid hormone and 1,25-dihydroxyvitamin D and a rise in intestinal calcium absorption. Calcium losses in urine and feces decrease.

ADRENAL CORTEX. Metabolic clearance and, to a lesser extent, production of cortisol are decreased in hypothyroidism[116]; serum cortisol and 24-hour urinary cortisol remain within normal limits. The adrenal response to exogenous adrenocorticotropic hormone and the pituitary response to hypoglycemia or metyrapone is usually maintained or slightly decreased. Some patients with chronic autoimmune thyroiditis have associated autoimmune adrenalitis. Hypocortisolemia by itself may cause slightly elevated TSH levels that return to normal with glucocorticoid replacement, thus illustrating the negative feedback of cortisol on TSH secretion.[117]

Hypothyroidism decreases angiotensinogen production in the liver, serum angiotensin-converting enzyme, and plasma renin activity. Serum aldosterone remains normal: the decrease in clearance is neutralized by a decrease in secretion. The effects of these changes in the renin-angiotensin-aldosterone system are minimal and are not responsible for the hypertension in hypothyroid patients.

SYMPATHOADRENAL SYSTEM. Serum norepinephrine concentrations are increased in hypothyroid patients because of an increased production rate[118]; epinephrine production is not affected. The increased central sympathetic output seems to be compensatory for the reduced response to catecholamines in target tissues such as the heart.[119] Mechanisms involved include a decreased number of β-adrenergic receptors. Defects in the β-adrenergic–cyclic adenosine mono-

TABLE 105–4. Accuracy of 12 Symptoms and Signs in the Diagnosis of Primary Hypothyroidism

Symptoms and Signs	Sensitivity (%)	Specificity (%)	Positive Predictive Value (%)	Negative Predictive Value (%)	Score if Present
Symptoms					
Hearing impairment	22	98	90	53	1
Diminished sweating	54	86	80	65	1
Constipation	48	85	76	62	1
Paresthesia	52	83	75	63	1
Hoarseness	34	88	73	57	1
Weight increase	54	78	71	63	1
Dry skin	76	64	68	73	1
Physical signs					
Slow movements	36	99	97	61	1
Periorbital puffiness	60	96	94	71	1
Delayed ankle reflex	77	94	92	80	1
Coarse skin	60	81	76	67	1
Cold skin	50	80	71	62	1
Sum of all symptoms and signs present*					12†

*Add 1 point for women younger than 55 years.

†Hypothyroid, ≥6 points; intermediate, 3–5 points; euthyroid, ≤2 points.

From Zulewski H, Müller B, Exer P, et al: Estimation of tissue hypothyroidism by a new clinical score: Evaluation of patients with various grades of hypothyroidism and controls. J Clin Endocrinol Metab 82:771–776, © 1997, The Endocrine Society.

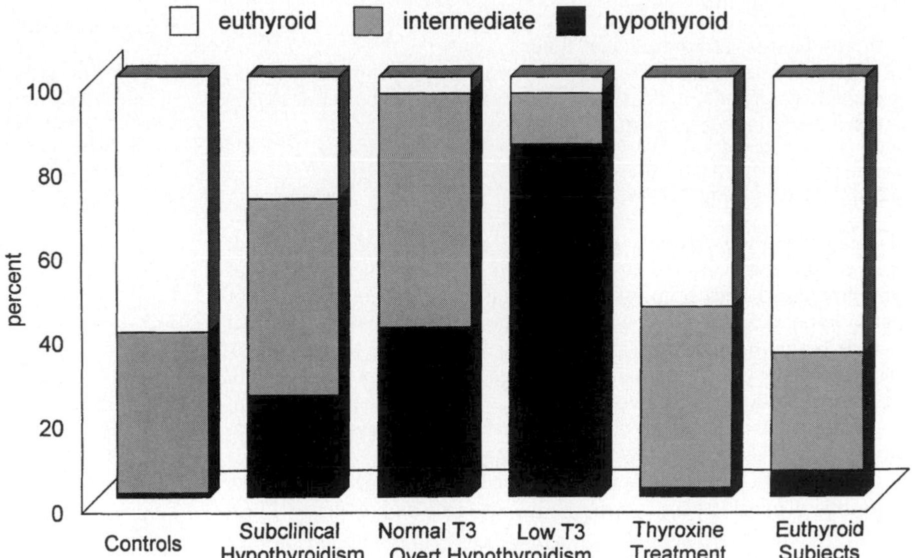

FIGURE 105–4. Assessment of hypothyroidism by a clinical score in 50 patients with overt hypothyroidism, 80 age-matched controls, 93 patients with subclinical hypothyroidism, 67 hypothyroid patients treated with thyroxine (T_4), and an additional 109 euthyroid subjects. (From Zulewski H, Müller B, Exer P, et al: Estimation of tissue hypothyroidism by a new clinical score: Evaluation of patients with various grades of hypothyroidism and controls. J Clin Endocrinol Metab 82:771–776, © 1997, The Endocrine Society.)

phosphate pathway and Ca^{2+} mobilization contribute to impaired lipolysis, glycogenolysis, and gluconeogenesis in hypothyroidism.

DIAGNOSIS OF HYPOTHYROIDISM

Two phases can be distinguished in the diagnosis of hypothyroidism. First, it should be ascertained whether a thyroid hormone deficiency exists (syndromal diagnosis). Thereafter, the cause of the demonstrated thyroid hormone deficiency should be looked for (nosologic diagnosis). Diagnosis of the hypothyroid syndrome starts with the history and physical examination and ends—in the case of sufficient clinical suspicion—with an assay of TSH and FT_4 in serum. One of the rationales for clinical examination is to increase the pretest likelihood of hypothyroidism so that fewer patients need hormone tests; because of the higher prevalence of hypothyroidism in the remaining patients, the diagnostic accuracy of hormone tests will increase. The rationale for a nosologic diagnosis is to look for cases of potentially reversible hypothyroidism and increase awareness of the possible existence of other conditions associated with a specific cause.

Syndromal Diagnosis

CLINICAL ASSESSMENT. Statistical methods based on the frequency of symptoms and signs in patients and controls have been applied to the clinical diagnosis of hypothyroidism. The Billewicz score consists of points given in a weighted manner for the presence or absence of 17 symptoms and signs.[120] Application of this score to patients suspected of hypothyroidism increases the pretest probability of hypothyroidism by 15% to 19%.[121] A recently introduced, simpler score is derived by awarding 1 point each for the presence of 12 symptoms and signs[122] (Table 105–4 and Fig. 105–4); because of a high frequency in euthyroid controls, cold intolerance and pulse rate had predictive values below 70% and were excluded from the score. The score was higher in older than younger control women; correction for age is done by adding 1 point for subjects younger than 55 years. The positive predictive value for hypothyroidism is 96.9% with a score of 6 or more points; the negative predictive value for exclusion of hypothyroidism is 94.2% with a score of 2 points or less. Sixty-two percent of all overt hypothyroid and 24% of subclinical hypothyroid patients are classified as clinically hypothyroid by this new score; the corresponding figures with the Billewicz score are 42% and 6%. Receiver operating curves of both scores are, however, very similar.

The clinical diagnosis of hypothyroidism can be very easy but also very difficult because of the nonspecific nature of the symptoms and signs and the marked diversity of findings.[123] It is incompletely understood why the clinical manifestations of thyroid hormone deficiency vary considerably between patients. Age and smoking have been identified as factors that modify clinical expression of the disease. Chilliness, paresthesias, weight gain, and muscle cramps occur less frequently in elderly patients, who also have a smaller number of clinical signs than younger patients.[124] Smokers have more severe manifestations of hypothyroidism (as assessed by the Billewicz score, serum LDL cholesterol, and creatine kinase) than nonsmokers do.[125]

BIOCHEMICAL ASSESSMENT. The ideal diagnostic test for hypothyroidism would be one that accurately measures the effect of thyroid hormone deficiency in target tissues. Peripheral tissue function tests such as serum cholesterol and creatine kinase, however, lack sufficient sensitivity and specificity to be of much use. Without a doubt, serum TSH is the single best assay for detection of hypothyroidism. By using the flow diagram presented in Figure 105–5, the following results can be obtained:

1. TSH normal. Euthyroidism is almost certain, and no further tests are necessary. The only exception is central hypothyroidism; usually, clinical examination offers sufficient clues to suspect hypothalamic/pituitary disease because isolated TSH deficiency is very rare.
2. TSH elevated, FT_4 decreased. Primary hypothyroidism is almost always present. In a few cases, TSH values of 5 to 15 mU/L are associated with central hypothyroidism.
3. TSH elevated, FT_4 normal. The results indicate subclinical hypothyroidism, sometimes nonthyroidal illness.
4. TSH elevated, FT_4 increased. This peculiar combination of test results indicates one of the rare patients with thyroid hormone resistance or thyrotoxicosis caused by a TSH-producing adenoma.
5. TSH decreased, FT_4 decreased. These results are compatible with

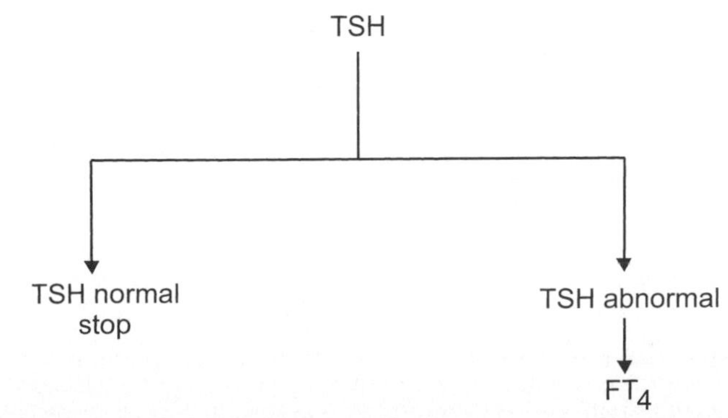

FIGURE 105–5. Flow diagram for the biochemical diagnosis of hypothyroidism.

central hypothyroidism, hypothyroidism after recent therapy for thyrotoxicosis, or nonthyroidal illness.

6. TSH decreased, FT_4 increased or normal. Hypothyroidism is excluded. The results indicate overt thyrotoxicosis, subclinical hyperthyroidism, or rarely, nonthyroidal illness.

Nosologic Diagnosis

The history and physical examination usually provide important clues to the cause of the hypothyroidism. Symptoms and signs of hypopituitarism and pituitary mass effects suggest the presence of central hypothyroidism. Physical examination may reveal a goiter, but many if not most hypothyroid patients have no palpable thyroid gland. Goitrous hypothyroidism occurs in goitrous Hashimoto's disease (with the characteristic firm rubbery consistency), in postpartum and subacute thyroiditis, in iodine deficiency, in iodine excess (small firm goiter), and in drug-induced cases. The most useful laboratory test is the assay of TPO antibodies: high titers indicate chronic autoimmune thyroiditis. Thyroid scans usually show low and inhomogeneous uptake of the radioisotope.

Clues for potential reversible hypothyroidism can be obtained from the history (recent delivery? exposure to iodine excess? use of antithyroid drugs? recent thyroid surgery or ^{131}I therapy?). In patients with chronic autoimmune thyroiditis, the presence of a goiter, preserved thyroidal radioiodine uptake, and homogeneous distribution of the tracer increases the likelihood of reversible hypothyroidism[39, 40]; it may also indicate iodine excess.[62]

Recovery of hypothyroidism by eliminating its cause is possible in cases secondary to (antithyroid) drugs or iodine excess. Spontaneous recovery from hypothyroidism in the natural course of the disease is the rule in subacute thyroiditis; it is common in postpartum thyroiditis, occurs less frequently in hypothyroidism developing in the first 6 months after surgery or ^{131}I therapy for thyrotoxicosis, and is exceptional (5%) in chronic autoimmune thyroiditis.

TREATMENT OF HYPOTHYROIDISM

The vast majority of hypothyroid patients need lifelong replacement therapy with T_4.[126] In the small minority of patients with a high likelihood of reversible hypothyroidism, one may refrain from treatment or—if symptoms and signs are severe—prescribe T_4 for a few months. The goal of treatment is restoration of the euthyroid state in all tissues. Gradual disappearance of the systemic manifestations of hypothyroidism can be expected several weeks to months after initiation of therapy; symptoms and signs related to the skin, appendages, and nervous system resolve rather slowly. Treatment of hypothyroid patients is very gratifying because the symptoms and signs are usually fully reversible. For the treatment of infants, see Chapter 180.

Replacement with Thyroxine

T_4 is prescribed as levothyroxine sodium, which comes in tablets of different strength. The sodium salt increases the absorption of levothyroxine, which is greater in the fasting than in the fed state. Gastrointestinal absorption of oral levothyroxine sodium is on average 80%.[127] Generic and brand name levothyroxine preparations are mostly bioequivalent,[128] but altered bioavailability from changes in the formulation of preparations has been reported.[129] About 25% of the exogenous T_4 is converted into T_3 and provides 80% of the circulating T_3 pool.[127] The half-life of serum T_4 is approximately 7 days, which allows a single daily dose of levothyroxine sodium. Omission of an occasional tablet has little or no clinical relevance.

The initial daily dose of levothyroxine sodium will depend on the severity and the duration of the hypothyroid state, the age of the patient, and the coexistence of cardiac disease. In the case of mild hypothyroidism, short duration of hypothyroidism, young age, and no heart disease, the initial dose can be rather high, on the order of 50 to 100 μg daily. In the case of severe long-standing hypothyroidism, older age, and especially the presence of ischemic heart disease, it is prudent to start with a low dose, on the order of 25 to 50 μg daily. Too high a starting dose under these circumstances may be poorly tolerated by the patient, who is accustomed to a low metabolic rate, which is now reversed. The patient may experience agitation, palpitations, and worsening or development of anginal complaints because of the increased need for oxygen. Individualization of the initial dose is thus recommended, and the same holds true for the rate at which the initial dose is raised until the full replacement dose (on average, 1.6 μg/kg/day, but with large interindividual variation) has been reached.[130–133] In mild low-risk cases, the daily levothyroxine sodium dose can be increased by 50 μg every 4 weeks and, in severe high-risk cases, by 25 to 50 μg every 4 to 6 weeks. It usually takes 3 to 6 months before the euthyroid state is restored. The mean replacement dose of levothyroxine sodium is 125 μg daily, in line with the daily production rate of 100 μg of thyroxine in normal subjects; it varies, however, widely between 50 and 200 μg (Fig. 105–6). The final dose required is a function of body weight (especially lean body mass[134]) and initial TSH value,[135] but it is not always predictable. The dose should be titrated against serum TSH and FT_4 concentrations. These assays should be done not earlier than 4 to 6 weeks after a change in T_4 dose, when a new steady state has been established. One aims for TSH values in the low normal range, which results in FT_4 values that are significantly higher than those in controls (see Fig. 105–6) and often slightly above the upper normal limit.[127] The high T_4 levels under these circumstances serve to maintain serum T_3 (predominantly derived from 5′-deiodination of T_4) in the midnormal range. In patients with central hypothyroidism, one should rely primarily on serum FT_4 and T_3.

Some patients feel better with a slightly higher dose of levothyrox-

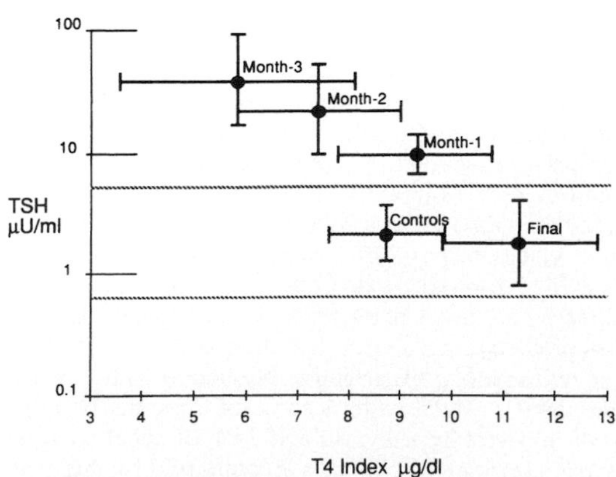

FIGURE 105–6. Dosage titration of levothyroxine *(left panel)* and the free thyroxine index *(right panel)* as a function of serum thyroid-stimulating hormone (TSH). Values are expressed by month, counting backward from the final dose. The bars represent 1 SD from the mean. (Reprinted, by permission, from Fish LH, Schwartz HL, Cavanaugh J, et al: Replacement dose, metabolism, and bioavailability of levothyroxine in the treatment of hypothyroidism. Role of triiodothyronine in pituitary feedback in humans. N Engl J Med 316:764–770, 1987. Copyright © 1987 Massachusetts Medical Society. All rights reserved.)

ine sodium and, consequently, suppressed TSH. This dose can be accepted as long as serum T_3 is still within the normal range and serum TSH is (arbitrarily) not lower than 0.2 mU/L.[131] TSH values of 0.1 mU/L or less carry a risk of atrial fibrillation[136] and bone loss[137] (especially in postmenopausal women). Indeed, long-term levothyroxine therapy at TSH-suppressive doses markedly affects cardiac function[138] and increases the risk of ischemic heart disease in patients younger than 65 years.[139] However, no excess of fractures has been observed in patients maintained with levothyroxine even if TSH is suppressed.[139, 140]

Lifelong treatment with levothyroxine sodium, when properly monitored, seems to be free of complications. Long-term morbidity and mortality are normal. Cutaneous allergy to the dye used to color the tablets is very rarely observed. The replacement dose required for hypothyroidism after surgical or radioiodine treatment of Graves' hyperthyroidism may increase with time because of the disappearance of TSH receptor–stimulating antibodies. The converse situation in patients with chronic autoimmune thyroiditis is exceptional and related to a switch from blocking to stimulating TSH receptor antibodies.[43]

Factors Requiring Dose Adjustment

When euthyroidism has been restored by the full replacement dose of levothyroxine, it usually suffices to check the patient's thyroid state once a year.[132, 133] The main reason for the annual follow-up visit is to enhance compliance with lifelong levothyroxine sodium treatment. Some patients will need adjustment of the levothyroxine sodium dose for reasons outlined in Table 105–5.

INCREASED DOSE REQUIREMENT. T_4 is mainly absorbed from the small intestine, which explains the higher dose requirements in malabsorption and short-bowel syndromes.[141] Nonspecific absorption of T_4 by dietary fibers decreases the bioavailability of T_4 and necessitates a higher dose in patients with high intake of dietary fiber (whole wheat bread, granola, bran).[142] T_4 and T_3 conjugates are excreted in bile and partially deconjugated in the intestine, with the release of small amounts of T_4 and T_3 for reabsorption.[143] Interference with this enterohepatic circulation of thyroid hormone by bile acid sequestering agents may cause a slight increase in TSH in levothyroxine-treated patients but not in normal subjects.[144, 145] Other drugs such as sucralfate,[146] aluminum hydroxide,[147] and ferrous sulfate[148] also decrease the absorption of T_4; serum TSH rises in some but not all levothyroxine-treated patients. The effect of these drug interactions is modest and can largely be avoided by taking levothyroxine sodium and the other drug several hours apart.[143]

TABLE 105–5. Conditions Requiring Adjustment of the Replacement Dose of Thyroxine for Hypothyroidism

Increased dose requirement
- Decreased intestinal absorption of T_4
  - Malabsorption (e.g., celiac disease) and short-bowel syndrome[141]
  - Dietary fiber supplements[142]
  - Drugs: bile acid sequestering agents (colestipol,[144] cholestyramine[145]), sucralfate,[146] aluminum hydroxide,[147] ferrous sulfate[148]
- Increased need for T_4
  - Weight gain
  - Pregnancy[150, 151]
- Increased clearance of T_4
  - Phenobarbital, phenytoin, carbamazepine, rifampicin[152]
- Precise mechanism unknown
  - Amiodarone,[153] sertraline,[154] chloroquine[155]
- Noncompliance[156]

Decreased dose requirement
- Decreased need for T_4
  - Weight loss
  - Androgens[158]
- Decreased clearance of T_4
  - Old age[134, 159, 160]

T_4, thyroxine.

Considerable weight gain may increase the need for T_4. Pregnancy also requires more thyroid hormone, probably related to increased lean body mass and increased serum concentrations of T_4-binding globulin.[149] In up to 75% of women who received adequate treatment with levothyroxine sodium before pregnancy, serum TSH becomes elevated as early as 4 weeks' gestation; to restore a normal TSH concentration, a mean increment in the daily levothyroxine sodium dose of 50 μg is required.[150, 151] It is prudent to anticipate these events, and assessment of thyroid function in each trimester is recommended. After delivery, the dose used before pregnancy can be reinstituted.

Several antiepileptic and tuberculostatic drugs increase the clearance of T_4 by stimulating the mixed-function oxygenases responsible for hepatic drug oxidation.[143, 152] Serum TSH increases in levothyroxine-treated hypothyroid patients when amiodarone is administered,[153] possibly related to inhibition of T_4 conversion into T_3. The mechanism by which other drugs such as sertraline[154] and chloroquine[155] increase T_4 requirements is unknown. The most common reason, however, for persistently elevated TSH values despite apparently adequate replacement doses is poor compliance of the patient with intake of levothyroxine tablets.[126, 156] Noncompliance is a challenge to the treating physician to solve this difficult management problem; in the process it is important to not lose the patient's confidence. One option is to administer levothyroxine under supervision once weekly.[157] A slightly larger dose than seven times the normal daily dose may be required; a single weekly dose of 1000 μg of levothyroxine sodium orally seems to be effective and well tolerated.

DECREASED DOSE REQUIREMENT. Considerable weight loss may decrease the need for levothyroxine. In women receiving long-term levothyroxine replacement therapy, administration of androgens for breast cancer may result—via a decrease in serum T_4-binding globulin—in thyrotoxicosis within 4 weeks; the levothyroxine dose has to be reduced by 25% to 50%.[158] Production and metabolic clearance rates of T_4 are slightly decreased in old age; the net result is no change in the serum FT_4 concentration. The levothyroxine replacement dose decreases in elderly people by about 25% in association with the decrease in lean body mass with age.[134, 159, 160]

Other Thyroid Hormone Preparations

ANIMAL THYROID EXTRACT. Extracts of animal thyroid glands (primarily cattle) were the first thyroid hormone preparations available. Desiccated thyroid, although effective, is no longer used in view of the lack of precise standardization and the availability of synthetic levothyroxine. After the ingestion of desiccated thyroid, elevated serum concentrations of T_3 can occur in the postabsorptive period and cause transient thyrotoxic symptoms such as palpitations.[161] Such effects do not occur after a dose of levothyroxine, which is gradually converted into T_3.

LIOTHYRONINE SODIUM. After oral liothyronine (L-T_3) administration, serum T_3 concentrations reach elevated values within hours, with a decline to basal levels in the next couple of hours.[130] The half-life of liothyronine is approximately 1 day. Liothyronine preparations are useful in the management of patients with thyroid cancer: after abrupt withdrawal of liothyronine, the period of hypothyroidism before ^{131}I whole-body scan and ^{131}I therapy is shorter than after withdrawal of levothyroxine.

COMBINATION OF LEVOTHYROXINE AND LIOTHYRONINE. Synthetic levothyroxine and liothyronine have been combined in a single tablet in a ratio of 4:1. New interest in this kind of formula has been inspired by animal studies demonstrating that the euthyroid state of thyroidectomized rats could be restored in all tissues only by the combination of levothyroxine and liothyronine and not by levothyroxine alone.[162] A recent study indeed reports that treatment of hypothyroid patients with the combination of levothyroxine and liothyronine improves mood and neuropsychologic function when compared with higher doses of levothyroxine alone, without suppressing serum TSH levels.[163] Combining levothyroxine and liothyronine in the same ratio as their respective thyroidal secretion rates, preferably in a slow-release pharmaceutical form to avoid unwanted cardiac effects, might theoretically be ideal, but such formulas are not currently available for further clinical studies.

Interference with Coexistent Conditions

CORTISOL DEFICIENCY. Treatment of hypothyroidism in patients with glucocorticoid deficiency may provoke adrenal insufficiency because the adrenal is incapable of meeting the increasing demand for cortisol caused by the increased metabolic rate. Glucocorticoids should be given before starting levothyroxine therapy.

ISCHEMIC HEART DISEASE. Levothyroxine increases the need for oxygen in the myocardium. In a large series of hypothyroid patients, new-onset angina developed in 2% upon levothyroxine treatment. Preexisting angina disappeared or improved in 38%, did not change in 46%, and worsened in 16%.[94] Worsening or de novo development of anginal complaints should call for tempering of the levothyroxine dose or institution of antianginal drugs. Alternatively, coronary artery bypass surgery or angioplasty is a rather safe procedure, even when euthyroidism has not yet been restored.[111, 164]

SURGERY. Surgery in hypothyroid patients is associated with an increased risk of several minor perioperative complications.[111] A higher incidence of heart failure and gastrointestinal and neuropsychiatric complications has been reported. Patients have fever less frequently during infections.

DRUGS. The metabolism of many drugs is slowed in hypothyroidism, which results in higher sensitivity to a loading dose and a lower maintenance dose. Hypothyroid patients can experience marked respiratory depression after a single small dose of morphine. Restoration of the euthyroid state may require dose adjustments, for example, an increase in the dose of digoxin or insulin.

MYXEDEMA COMA

Myxedema coma is a rare, life-threatening clinical condition in patients with long-standing severe untreated hypothyroidism. The term is largely a misnomer because most patients are not comatose. Rather, the entity represents a form of decompensated hypothyroidism in which a precipitating event leads to functional disorders of the cardiovascular and central nervous system that if not recognized and reversed, frequently have a fatal outcome.[165]

PATHOGENESIS. A normal body core temperature is preserved in compensated hypothyroidism because of neurovascular adaptations, including chronic peripheral vasoconstriction, mild diastolic hypertension, and diminished blood volume. The hypothyroid heart also compensates by performing more work at a given amount of oxygen by better coupling of ATP to contractile events.[165] These adaptations to thyroid hormone deficiency maintain homeostasis, albeit at a precarious balance. A further reduction in blood volume (e.g., secondary to gastrointestinal bleeding or the use of diuretics) may disrupt this precarious balance that homeostatic mechanisms are no longer able to restore. Likewise, the already compromised ventilatory drive may progress to respiratory failure by intercurrent pulmonary infections. Impairment in central nervous system function can be further provoked by stroke, the use of sedatives, and hyponatremia (a common phenomenon in severe hypothyroidism).[166]

DIAGNOSIS. The three key diagnostic features of myxedema coma are[165]

1. Altered mental status: from disorientation and lethargy to psychosis and coma
2. Defective thermoregulation: hypothermia or the absence of fever despite infectious disease
3. Precipitating event: cold exposure, infection, drugs (diuretics, sedatives, tranquilizers), trauma, stroke, heart failure, gastrointestinal bleeding

Most cases of myxedema coma occur in elderly women in wintertime. Early recognition is of prime importance, but in many cases the condition is diagnosed rather late, often after inadequate response to treatment of the precipitating event. The presence of cool pale skin and the absence of mild diastolic hypertension are warning signs of impending myxedema coma.[165] Serum FT_4 is low; serum TSH is usually very high but is sometimes only slightly elevated because of the effect of intercurrent nonthyroidal illness. Serum creatine phosphokinase is mostly very high.

TREATMENT. Rapid institution of thyroid hormone replacement therapy and supportive measures (Table 105–6) are essential for a successful outcome; the prognosis remains poor, however, with a mortality of about 20%.[167] Patients should be closely monitored for vital signs.

No consensus has been reached regarding the most appropriate dose, route of administration, and form (liothyronine or levothyroxine) of thyroid hormone replacement.[130] Too high a dose may provoke cardiac ischemia and arrhythmias. Oral administration may be less efficacious because of reduced gastrointestinal absorption. T_3 abruptly increases the metabolism, which carries a risk of cardiac complications, but T_4 may be converted less well into T_3 because of nonthyroidal illness. The severity of the patient's condition might be considered, but clinical experience is that too conservative an approach worsens the outcome. Current recommendations are a starting dose of 300 to 500 μg of levothyroxine intravenously, followed by 50 to 100 μg of levothyroxine intravenously daily until oral medication can be taken.[130, 165–167] If no improvement is seen within 24 to 48 hours, liothyronine might be given (e.g., 10 μg given intravenously every 4 hours or 25 μg given intravenously every 8 hours).

Hypothermia is treated just with blankets; active rewarming is dangerous because the peripheral vasodilatation induced may provoke vascular collapse. Mechanical respiratory assistance is indicated at the first signs of respiratory failure, and one should not delay endotracheal intubation. Hypoxia is worsened by anemia, a common finding in hypothyroidism. In case of hypotension, transfusion of whole blood may restore blood volume and oxygen-carrying capacity. Digoxin and diuretics should be used cautiously for congestive heart failure. Hypoglycemia might indicate hypopituitarism or primary adrenal insufficiency; however, also in the absence of hypoglycemia or hypocortisolemia, all patients should receive intravenous hydrocortisone (200–400 mg daily in divided doses) in view of the blunted cortisol response to stress in severe hypothyroidism. Last but not least, one should try to identify precipitating factors and eliminate them if possible. Infections (pneumonia or urosepsis) are present in 35%,[167] but less easily detected because fever, tachycardia, and leukocytosis are usually absent. A differential count of leukocytes and cultures should be ordered, and broad-spectrum antibiotics are indicated even if the suspicion of infection is modest.

SUBCLINICAL HYPOTHYROIDISM AND SCREENING

Subclinical hypothyroidism is defined as an elevated serum TSH concentration in the presence of normal serum FT_4 and T_3. It is a very prevalent condition (see Table 105–1) that occurs especially in women and elderly people.[4] The causes can be endogenous (chronic autoimmune thyroiditis, subacute or postpartum thyroiditis) or exogenous (^{131}I therapy, thyroidectomy, antithyroid drugs).

The natural course of subclinical hypothyroidism secondary to chronic autoimmune thyroiditis is reasonably well known.[5] Spontane-

TABLE 105–6. Characteristics and Treatment of Myxedema Coma

Hypothyroxinemia	Large doses of intravenous levothyroxine
Hypothermia	Blankets, no active rewarming
Hypoventilation	Mechanical ventilation
Hypotension	Cautious volume expansion with crystalloid or whole blood
Hyponatremia	Mild fluid restoration
Hypoglycemia	Glucose administration
Hypocortisolemia	Glucocorticoid administration
Precipitating event	Identification and elimination by specific treatment

ous return to normal TSH values occurs in 5% to 6%. Progression to overt hypothyroidism is a common event, especially if thyroid antibodies are present (see Table 105–2); the annual incidence is about 5%.

SYSTEMIC MANIFESTATIONS. The term "subclinical" hypothyroidism suggests the absence of symptoms and signs of thyroid hormone deficiency, but clinical experience tells otherwise.[168, 169] Nonspecific complaints such as fatigue and weight gain can be present, as well as depressive feelings and mild cognitive disturbances (poor ability to concentrate, poor memory). Subjects score higher on a clinical scale for hypothyroidism[122] (see Fig. 105–4). Peripheral tissue function tests rather frequently indicate a limited degree of thyroid hormone deficiency; examples are prolongation of the Achilles tendon reflex relaxation time, prolongation of systolic time intervals, decrease in cardiac contractility, impairment of muscle energy metabolism, and an increase in LDL cholesterol.

TREATMENT. Treatment of subclinical hypothyroidism is still debated. However, randomized clinical trials have demonstrated improvement in symptom scores and psychometric performance in about one-third of levothyroxine-treated subjects, which was significantly better than the outcome in control subjects.[170–173] A meta-analysis concludes that normalization of serum TSH decreases serum cholesterol by 0.4 mmol/L (95% confidence interval, 0.2–0.6 mmol/L), independent of the starting value.[174] Taken together, the findings (especially the high rate of progression toward overt hypothyroidism) argue against a "wait and see" policy and favor early T_4 replacement therapy. When in doubt because of nonspecific complaints, a trial of T_4 treatment for at least 3 months can be considered; such therapy seems especially worthwhile in the case of mood disturbances or cognitive impairment.

SET-POINT. Subclinical hypothyroidism seems to be a misnomer, but how to explain that some subjects with subclinical thyroid dysfunction experience clinical symptoms and signs whereas other subjects are really asymptomatic despite similar serum FT_4 concentrations remains an unanswered question. Repeated measurements of thyroid function tests in the same individual over time demonstrate a rather narrow fluctuation around the mean value.[175] Apparently, each individual is characterized by a rather fixed relationship between serum TSH and FT_4 concentrations; this point can be called the working point of the pituitary-thyroid axis of that individual. From longitudinal observations in subjects in whom abnormal thyroid function develops, it can be deduced that an intraindividual log-linear relationship exists between TSH and FT_4, as depicted by a straight line[127, 176]; the working point moves along this line, upward in the case of hypothyroidism (Fig. 105–7). The position of the working point of an individual determines the maximally allowed changes in thyroid function test results within the conventional reference range before they are labeled

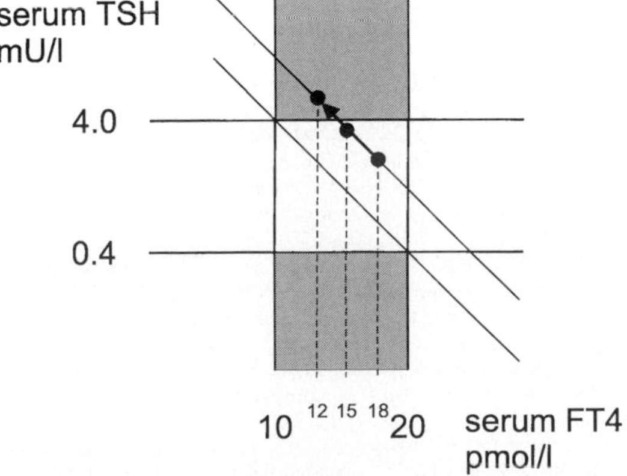

FIGURE 105–7. The log-linear relationship between thyroid-stimulating hormone (TSH) and free thyroxine (FT_4) of a particular individual is depicted by a *straight line;* the working point of that individual moves upward along this line if hypothyroidism develops. Variation between individuals is given by the different location of the working point on the same or parallel lines. The upper *hatched area* represents subclinical hypothyroidism, and the central area encompasses the normal range of both TSH and FT_4. For further explanation, see the text.

abnormal. In the example depicted in Figure 105–7, the subject with subclinical hypothyroidism and a serum FT_4 of 12 pmol/L might have an original working point at 18 pmol/L (indicating a decrease in serum FT_4 by 33%) or at 15 pmol/L (indicating a decrease in serum FT_4 by 20%). It is conceivable that symptoms and signs are present in the former but not in the latter situation.

SCREENING. In view of the high prevalence of thyroid disease in the general population, the question arises of whether a screening program in adults is justified.[10, 168] A simple, inexpensive, and accurate screening test is available: the sensitive TSH assay. The disease to be screened (hypothyroidism and thyrotoxicosis) has a high prevalence and can be treated effectively. However, the burden of disease is limited, and it has not been proved that clinical outcome is improved by early diagnosis and treatment in the asymptomatic stage. Nevertheless, a computer-derived decision model concludes that it is cost-effective to screen persons in the general community for mild hypothyroidism with a serum TSH combined with a serum cholesterol every 5 years after the age of 35 years.[177, 178] Screening of elderly women is especially cost-effective. For the time being, case finding is a suitable alternative, that is, determination of serum TSH in patients (especially women older than 40 years) who consult the physician because of unrelated problems. A high degree of suspicion of thyroid function disorders is warranted in patients with nonspecific complaints.

REFERENCES

1. Ishii H, Inada M, Tanaka K, et al: Induction of outer and inner ring monodeiodinases in human thyroid gland by thyrotropin. J Clin Endocrinol Metab 57:500–505, 1983.
2. Lum SM, Nicoloff JT, Spencer CA, Kaptein EM: Peripheral tissue mechanism for maintenance of serum triiodothyronine values in a thyroxine-deficient state in man. J Clin Invest 73:570–575, 1984.
3. Evered DC, Ormston BJ, Smith PA, et al: Grades of hypothyroidism. BMJ 1:657–662, 1973.
4. Tunbridge WMG, Evered DC, Hall R, et al: The spectrum of thyroid disease in the community. The Whickham survey. Clin Endocrinol 7:481–493, 1977.
5. Vanderpump MPJ, Tunbridge WMG, French JM, et al: The incidence of thyroid disorders in the community: A twenty-year follow-up of the Whickham survey. Clin Endocrinol 43:55–68, 1995.
6. Dos Remedios LV, Weber PM, Feldman R, et al: Detecting unsuspected thyroid dysfunction by the free thyroxine index. Arch Intern Med 140:1045–1049, 1980.
7. Sawin CT, Castelli WP, Hershman JM, et al: The aging thyroid. Thyroid deficiency in the Framingham study. Arch Intern Med 145:1386–1388, 1985.
8. Okamura K, Ueda K, Sone H, et al: A sensitive TSH assay for screening of thyroid functional disorder in elderly Japanese. J Am Geriatr Soc 37:317–322, 1989.
9. Sundbeck G, Lundberg PA, Lindstedt G, et al: Incidence and prevalence of thyroid disease in elderly women: Results from the longitudinal population study of elderly people in Gothenburg, Sweden. Age Ageing 20:291–298, 1991.
10. Wang C, Crapo LM: The epidemiology of thyroid disease and implication for screening. Endocrinol Metab Clin North Am 26:189–218, 1997.
11. Geul KW, van Sluisveld ILL, Grobbee DE, et al: The importance of thyroid microsomal antibodies in the development of elevated serum TSH in middle-aged women: Associations with serum lipids. Clin Endocrinol 39:275–280, 1993.
12. Faglia G: The clinical impact of the thyrotropin-releasing hormone test. Thyroid 8:903–908, 1998.
13. Faglia G, Bitensky L, Pinchera A, et al: Thyrotropin secretion in patients with central hypothyroidism: Evidence for reduced biological activity of immunoreactive thyrotropin. J Clin Endocrinol Metab 48:989–998, 1979.
14. Miura Y, Perkel VS, Papenberg KA, et al: Concanavalin-A, lentil, and ricin lectin affinity binding characteristic of human thyrotropin: Differences in the sialylation of thyrotropin in sera of euthyroid, primary, and central hypothyroid patients. J Clin Endocrinol Metab 69:985–995, 1989.
15. Horimoto M, Nishikawa M, Ishihara T, et al: Bioactivity of thyrotropin (TSH) in patients with central hypothyroidism: Comparison between in vivo 3,5,3′-triiodothyronine response to TSH and in vitro bioactivity of TSH. J Clin Endocrinol Metab 80:1124–1128, 1995.
16. Beck-Peccoz P, Amr S, Menezes-Ferreira NM, et al: Decreased receptor binding of biologically inactive thyrotropin in central hypothyroidism: Effect of treatment with thyrotropin-releasing hormone. N Engl J Med 312:1085–1090, 1985.
17. Samuels MH, Lillehei K, Kleinschmidt-Demasters BK, et al: Patterns of pulsatile glycoprotein secretion in central hypothyroidism and hypogonadism. J Clin Endocrinol Metab 70:391–395, 1990.
18. Adriaanse R, Brabant G, Endert E, Wiersinga WM: Pulsatile TSH release in patients with untreated pituitary disease. J Clin Endocrinol Metab 77:205–209, 1993.
19. Vance ML: Hypopituitarism. N Engl J Med 330:1651–1662, 1994.
20. Collu R, Tang J, Castagné J, et al: A novel mechanism for isolated central hypothyroidism: Inactivating mutations in the thyrotropin-releasing hormone receptor gene. J Clin Endocrinol Metab 82:1361–1365, 1997.
21. Dacou-Voutetakis C, Feltquate DM, Drakopoulo M, et al: Familial hypothyroidism caused by a nonsense mutation in the thyroid-stimulating hormone β-subunit gene. Am J Hum Genet 46:988–993, 1990.
22. de Zegher F, Pernasetti F, Vanhole C, et al: The prenatal role of thyroid hormone

evidenced by fetomaternal Pit-1 deficiency. J Clin Endocrinol Metab 80:3127–3130, 1995.
23. Arafah BM: Reversible hypopituitarism in patients with large non-functioning pituitary adenomas. J Clin Endocrinol Metab 62:1173–1179, 1986.
24. Constine LS, Woolf PD, Cann D, et al: Hypothalamic-pituitary dysfunction after radiation for brain tumors. N Engl J Med 328:87–94, 1993.
25. Snijder PJ, Fowble BF, Schatz NJ, et al: Hypopituitarism following radiation therapy of pituitary adenomas. Am J Med 81:457–462, 1986.
26. Edwards BM, Clark JDA: Post-traumatic hypopituitarism: Six cases and a review of the literature. Medicine (Baltimore) 65:281–290, 1986.
27. Cosman F, Post KD, Holub D, et al: Lymphocytic hypophysitis. Report of 3 new cases and review of the literature. Medicine (Baltimore) 68:240–256, 1989.
28. Kaptein EM, Spencer CA, Kamile MB, Nicoloff JT: Prolonged dopamine administration and thyroid hormone economy in normal and critically ill subjects. J Clin Endocrinol Metab 51:387–393, 1980.
29. Vagenakis AG, Braverman LE, Azizi F, et al: Recovery of pituitary thyrotropic function after withdrawal of prolonged thyroid suppression therapy. N Engl J Med 293:681–684, 1975.
30. Davis JRE, Black EG, Sheppard MC: Evaluation of a sensitive chemiluminescent assay for TSH in the follow-up of treated thyrotoxicosis. Clin Endocrinol 27:563–570, 1987.
31. Adriaanse R, Brabant G, Endert E, Wiersinga WM: Pulsatile thyrotropin secretion in patients with Cushing's syndrome. Metabolism 43:782–786, 1994.
32. Hayashi Y, Tamai H, Fukata S, et al: A long-term clinical, immunological, and histological follow-up study of patients with goitrous chronic lymphocytic thyroiditis. J Clin Endocrinol Metab 61:1172–1178, 1985.
33. Arikawa K, Ichikawa Y, Yoshida T, et al: Blocking type antithyrotropin receptor antibody in patients with nongoitrous hypothyroidism: Its incidence and characteristics of action. J Clin Endocrinol Metab 60:953–959, 1985.
34. Kraiem Z, Lahat N, Glaser B, et al: Thyrotropin receptor blocking antibodies: Incidence, characterization and in vivo synthesis. Clin Endocrinol 27:409–421, 1987.
35. Rieu M, Portos C, Lissak B, et al: Relationship of antibodies to thyrotropin receptors and to thyroid ultrasonographic volume in euthyroid and hypothyroid patients with autoimmune thyroiditis. J Clin Endocrinol Metab 80:641–645, 1996.
36. Laurberg P, Pedersen KM, Hreidarsson A, et al: Iodine intake and the pattern of thyroid disorders: A comparative epidemiological study of thyroid abnormalities in the elderly in Iceland and in Jutland, Denmark. J Clin Endocrinol Metab 83:765–769, 1998.
37. Sundrick RS, Bagchi N, Brown TR: The role of iodine in thyroid autoimmunity: From chickens to humans: A review. Autoimmunity 13:61–68, 1992.
38. Takasu N, Yamada T, Takasu M, et al: Disappearance of thyrotropin-blocking antibodies and spontaneous recovery from hypothyroidism in autoimmune thyroiditis. N Eng J Med 326:513–518, 1992.
39. Okamura K, Sato K, Ikenoue H, et al: Reevaluation of thyroidal radioactive iodine uptake test, with special reference to reversible primary hypothyroidism with elevated thyroid radioiodine uptake. J Clin Endocrinol Metab 67:720–726, 1988.
40. Comtois R, Faucher L, Laflèche L: Outcome of hypothyroidism caused by Hashimoto's thyroiditis. Arch Intern Med 155:1404–1408, 1995.
41. Takasu N, Komiya I, Asawa T, et al: Test for recovery from hypothyroidism during thyroxine therapy in Hashimoto's thyroiditis. Lancet 336:1084–1086, 1990.
42. Nikolai TF: Recovery of thyroid function in primary hypothyroidism. Am J Med Sci 297:18–21, 1989.
43. Kraiem Z, Baron E, Kahana L, et al: Changes in stimulating and blocking TSH receptor antibodies in a patient undergoing three cycles of transition from hypo- to hyperthyroidism and back to hypothyroidism. Clin Endocrinol 36:211–216, 1992.
44. Gerstein HC: How common is postpartum thyroiditis? A methodologic overview of the literature. Arch Intern Med 150:1397–1400, 1990.
45. Kuypens JL, Pop VJ, Vader HL, et al: Prediction of postpartum thyroid dysfunction: Can it be improved? Eur J Endocrinol 139:36–43, 1998.
46. Alvarez-Marfany M, Roman SH, Drexler AJ, et al: Long-term prospective study of postpartum thyroid function in women with insulin dependent diabetes mellitus. J Clin Endocrinol Metab 79:10–16, 1994.
47. Othman S, Phillips DI, Parkes AB, et al: A long-term follow-up of postpartum thyroiditis. Clin Endocrinol 32:559–564, 1990.
48. Kuypens JL, de Haan-Meulman M, Vader HL, et al: Cell-mediated immunity and postpartum thyroid dysfunction: A possibility for the prediction of disease? J Clin Endocrinol Metab 83:1959–1966, 1998.
49. Harris B, Othman S, Davies JA, et al: Association between postpartum thyroid dysfunction and thyroid antibodies and depression. BMJ 305:152–156, 1992.
50. Pop VJ, de Vries E, van Baar A, et al: Maternal thyroid peroxidase antibodies during pregnancy: A marker of impaired child development? J Clin Endocrinol Metab 80:3561–3566, 1995.
51. Vialettes B, Guillerand MA, Viens P, et al: Incidence rate and risk factors for thyroid dysfunction during recombinant interleukin-2 therapy in advanced malignancies. Acta Endocrinol 129:31–38, 1993.
52. Preziati D, La Rosa L, Covini G, et al: Autoimmunity and thyroid function in patients with chronic active hepatitis treated with recombinant interferon alpha-2a. Eur J Endocrinol 132:587–593, 1995.
53. Marazuela M, Garcia-Buey L, Gonzalez-Fernandez B, et al: Thyroid autoimmune disorders in patients with chronic hepatitis C before and during interferon-therapy. Clin Endocrinol 44:635–642, 1996.
54. Nofal MN, Beierwaltes WH, Patno ME: Treatment of hyperthyroidism with sodium iodide I-131, a 16-year experience. JAMA 197:605–610, 1966.
55. Huysmans DA, Corstens FH, Kloppenborg PW: Long-term follow-up in toxic solitary autonomous thyroid nodules treated with radioactive iodine. J Nucl Med 32:27–30, 1991.
56. Le Moli R, Wesche MFT, Tiel-van Buul MMC, Wiersinga WM: Determinants of long-term outcome of radioiodine therapy of sporadic non-toxic goitre. Clin Endocrinol 50:783–789, 1999.
57. Pacini F, Vorontsova T, Molinaro E, et al: Prevalence of thyroid autoantibodies in children and adolescents from Belarus exposed to the Chernobyl radioactive fallout. Lancet 352:763–766, 1998.
58. Smith RE, Adler RA, Clark P, et al: Thyroid function after mantle irradiation in Hodgkin's disease. JAMA 245:46–49, 1981.
59. Tell R, Sjödin H, Lundell G, et al: Hypothyroidism after external radiotherapy for head and neck cancer. Int J Radiat Oncol Biol Phys 39:303–308, 1997.
60. Katsanis E, Shapiro RS, Robison LL, et al: Thyroid dysfunction following bone marrow transplantation: Long-term follow-up of 80 pediatric patients. Bone Marrow Transplant 5:335–340, 1990.
61. Barsano CP: Other forms of hypothyroidism. *In* Braverman LE, Utiger RD (eds): The Thyroid: A Fundamental and Clinical Text, ed 7. Philadelphia, JB Lippincott, 1996, pp 768–778.
62. Wiersinga WM, Touber JL, Trip MD, van Royen EA: Uninhibited thyroidal uptake of radioiodine despite iodine excess in amiodarone-induced hypothyroidism. J Clin Endocrinol Metab 63:485–491, 1986.
63. Braverman LE: Iodine and the thyroid: 33 years of study. Thyroid 4:351–356, 1994.
64. Martino E, Safran M, Aghini-Lombardi F, et al: Environmental iodine intake and thyroid dysfunction during chronic amiodarone therapy. Ann Intern Med 101:28–34, 1984.
65. Trip MD, Wiersinga WM, Plomp TA: Incidence, predictability, and pathogenesis of amiodarone-induced thyrotoxicosis and hypothyroidism. Am J Med 91:507–511, 1991.
66. Surks MI, Sievert R: Drugs and thyroid function. N Engl J Med 333:1688–1694, 1995.
67. Gaitan E, Cooksey RC, Legan J, et al: Antithyroid and goitrogenic effects of coal-water extracts from iodine-sufficient goiter areas. Thyroid 3:49–53, 1993.
68. Langer P, Tajtakova M, Fodor G, et al: Increased thyroid volume and prevalence of thyroid disorders in an area heavily polluted by polychlorinated biphenyls. Eur J Endocrinol 139:402–409, 1998.
69. Perrild H, Hegedüs L, Baastrup PC, et al: Thyroid function and ultrasonically determined thyroid size in patients receiving long-term lithium treatment. Am J Psychiatry 147:1508–1521, 1990.
70. Smith TJ, Bahn RS, Gorman CA: Connective tissue, glycosaminoglycans, and diseases of the thyroid. Endocr Rev 10:366–391, 1989.
71. Seppel T, Kosel A, Schlaghecke R: Bioelectrical impedance assessment of body composition in thyroid disease. Eur J Endocrinol 136:493–498, 1997.
72. Pazos F, Alvarez JJ, Rubies-Prat J, et al: Long term thyroid replacement therapy and levels of lipoprotein (a) and other lipoproteins. J Clin Endocrinol Metab 80:562–566, 1995.
73. Martinez-Triguero ML, Hernandez-Myares A, Nguyen TT, et al: Effect of thyroid hormone replacement on lipoprotein (a), lipids, and apolipoproteins in subjects with hypothyroidism. Mayo Clin Proc 73:837–841, 1998.
74. Bantle JP, Dillman WH, Oppenheimer JH, et al: Common clinical indices of thyroid hormone action: Relationship of serum free 3,5,3′-triiodothyronine concentration and estimated nuclear occupancy. J Clin Endocrinol Metab 50:286–293, 1980.
75. Diekman T, Demacker PNM, Kastelein JJP, et al: Increased oxidizability of low-density lipoproteins in hypothyroidism. J Clin Endocrinol Metab 83:1752–1755, 1998.
76. O'Brien T, Katz K, Hodge D, et al: The effect of treatment of hypothyroidism and hyperthyroidism on plasma lipids and apolipoproteins AI, AII and E. Clin Endocrinol 46:17–20, 1997.
77. Dullaart RPF, Hoogenberg K, Groener JEM, et al: The activity of cholesterol ester transfer protein is decreased in hypothyroidism: A possible contribution to alterations in high-density lipoproteins. Eur J Clin Invest 20:581–587, 1990.
78. Tan KCB, Shiu SWM, Kung AWC: Plasma cholesteryl ester transfer protein activity in hyper- and hypothyroidism. J Clin Endocrinol Metab 83:140–143, 1998.
79. Sensenbach W, Madison L, Eisenberg S, Ochs L: The cerebral circulation and metabolism in hyperthyroidism and myxedema. J Clin Invest 33:1434–1440, 1954.
80. Smith CD, Ain KB: Brain metabolism in hypothyroidism studied with ^{31}P magnetic-resonance spectroscopy. Lancet 345:619–620, 1995.
81. Dugbartey AT: Neurocognitive aspects of hypothyroidism. Arch Intern Med 158:1413–1418, 1998.
82. Clarnette RM, Peterson CJ: Hypothyroidism: Does treatment cure dementia? J Geriatr Psychiatry Neurol 7:23–27, 1994.
83. Whybrow P, Prange A, Treadway C: Mental changes accompanying thyroid gland dysfunction. Arch Gen Psychiatry 20:48–62, 1969.
84. Cleare AJ, McGregor A, O'Keane V: Neuroendocrine evidence for an association between hypothyroidism, reduced central 5-HT activity and depression. Clin Endocrinol 43:713–719, 1995.
85. Aronson R, Offman HJ, Joffe RT, Naylor CD: Triiodothyronine augmentation in the treatment of refractory depression. Arch Gen Psychiatry 53:842–848, 1996.
86. Beghi E, Delodovici ML, Bogliun G, et al: Hypothyroidism and polyneuropathy. J Neurol Neurosurg Psychiatry 52:1420–1423, 1989.
87. Kaminsky P, Robin-Lherbier B, Brunotte F, et al: Energetic metabolism in hypothyroid skeletal muscle, as studied by phosphorus magnetic resonance spectroscopy. J Clin Endocrinol Metab 74:124–129, 1992.
88. Monzani F, Caraccio N, Siciliano G, et al: Clinical and biochemical features of muscle dysfunction in subclinical hypothyroidism. J Clin Endocrinol Metab 82:3315–3318, 1997.
89. Hsu I-H, Thadhani RI, Daniels GH: Acute compartment syndrome in a hypothyroid patient. Thyroid 5:305–308, 1995.
90. Klein I, Ojamaa K: The cardiovascular system in hypothyroidism. *In* Braverman LE, Utiger RD (eds): The Thyroid: A Fundamental and Clinical Text, ed 7. Philadelphia, JB Lippincott, 1996, pp 799–804.
91. Ladenson PW, Sherman SI, Baughman KL, et al: Reversible alterations in myocardial gene expression in a young man with dilated cardiomyopathy and hypothyroidism. Proc Natl Acad Sci U S A 89:5251–5255, 1992.

92. Bernstein R, Midtbø K, Smith G, et al: Incidence of hypertrophic cardiomyopathy in hypothyroidism. Thyroid 5:277–281, 1995.
93. Bernstein R, Müller C, Midtbø K, et al: Silent myocardial ischemia in hypothyroidism. Thyroid 5:443–447, 1995.
94. Keating FR, Parkin TW, Selby J, Dickinson LS: Treatment of heart disease associated with myxedema. Prog Cardiovasc Dis 3:364–381, 1961.
95. Nedrebø BG, Ericsson U B, Nygård O, et al: Plasma total homocysteine levels in hyperthyroid and hypothyroid patients. Metabolism 47:89–93, 1998.
96. Steinberg AD: Myxedema and coronary artery disease—a comparative autopsy study. Ann Intern Med 68:338–344, 1968.
97. Vanderpump MPJ, Tunbridge WMG, French JM, et al: The development of ischemic heart disease in relation to autoimmune thyroid disease in a 20-year follow-up study of an English community. Thyroid 6:155–160, 1996.
98. Ladenson PW, Goldenheim PD, Ridgway EC: Prediction and reversal of blunted ventilatory responsiveness in patients with hypothyroidism. Am J Med 84:877–883, 1988.
99. Pelttari L, Rauhala E, Polo O, et al: Upper airway obstruction in hypothyroidism. J Intern Med 236:177–181, 1994.
100. Montenegro J, Gonzalez O, Saracho R, et al: Changes in renal function in primary hypothyroidism. Am J Kidney Dis 27:195–198, 1996.
101. Hanna FWF, Scanlon MF: Hyponatraemia, hypothyroidism and role of arginine-vasopressin. Lancet 350:755–756, 1997.
102. Bernstein R, Midtbø K, Urdal P, et al: Serum N-terminal pro-atrial natriuretic factor 1–98 before and during thyroxine replacement therapy in severe hypothyroidism. Thyroid 7:415–419, 1997.
103. Bruder JM, Samuels MH, Bremner WJ, et al: Hypothyroidism-induced macroorchidism: Use of a gonadotropin-releasing hormone agonist to understand its mechanism and augment adult stature. J Clin Endocrinol Metab 80:11–16, 1995.
104. Anasti JN, Flack MR, Froehlich J, et al: A potential novel mechanism for precocious puberty in juvenile hypothyroidism. J Clin Endocrinol Metab 80:276–279, 1995.
105. Samuels MH, Veldhuis JD, Henry P, Ridgway EC: Pathophysiology of pulsatile and copulsatile release of thyroid-stimulating hormone, luteinizing hormone, follicle-stimulating hormone, and alpha-subunit. J Clin Endocrinol Metab 71:425–432, 1990.
106. Leung AS, Millar LK, Koonings PP, et al: Perinatal outcome in hypothyroid pregnancies. Obstet Gynecol 81:349–353, 1993.
107. Rahman Q, Haboubi NY, Hudson PR, et al: The effect of thyroxine on small intestinal motility in the elderly. Clin Endocrinol 35:443–446, 1991.
108. Depczynski B, Ward R, Eisman J: The association between myxedematous ascites and extreme elevation of serum tumor markers. J Clin Endocrinol Metab 81:4175, 1996.
109. Ford HC, Carter JM: Haemostasis in hypothyroidism. Postgrad Med J 66:280–284, 1990.
110. Erfurth EM, Ericsson U-BC, Egervalh K, Lethagen SR: Effect of acute desmopressin and of long-term thyroxine replacement on haemostasis in hypothyroidism. Clin Endocrinol 42:373–378, 1995.
111. Ladenson PW, Levin AA, Ridgway EC, Daniels GH: Complications of surgery in hypothyroid patients. Am J Med 77:261–266, 1984.
112. Valcavi R, Valente F, Dieguez C, et al: Evidence against depletion of the growth hormone (GH)-releasable pool in human primary hypothyroidism. Studies with GH releasing hormone, pyridostigmine, and arginine. J Clin Endocrinol Metab 77:616–620, 1993.
113. Miell JP, Zini M, Quin JD, et al: Reversible effects of cessation and recommencement of thyroxine treatment on insulin-like growth factors (IGFs) and IGF-binding proteins in patients with total thyroidectomy. J Clin Endocrinol Metab 79:1507–1512, 1994.
114. Contreras P, Generini G, Michelsen H, et al: Hyperprolactinemia and galactorrhea: Spontaneous versus iatrogenic hypothyroidism. J Clin Endocrinol Metab 53:1036–1039, 1981.
115. Sarlis NJ, Brucker-Davis F, Doppman JL, Skarulis MC: MRI-demonstrable regression of a pituitary mass in a case of primary hypothyroidism after a week of acute thyroid hormone therapy. J Clin Endocrinol Metab 82:808–811, 1997.
116. Iranmanesh A, Lizarralde G, Johnson ML, Veldhuis JD: Dynamics of 24-hour endogenous cortisol secretion and clearance in primary hypothyroidism assessed before and after partial thyroid hormone replacement. J Clin Endocrinol Metab 70:155–161, 1990.
117. Topliss DJ, White EL, Stockigt JR: Significance of thyrotropin excess in untreated primary adrenal insufficiency. J Clin Endocrinol Metab 50:52–56, 1980.
118. Coulombe P, Dussault JH: Catecholamine metabolism in thyroid disease. II. Norepinephrine secretion rate in hyperthyroidism and hypothyroidism. J Clin Endocrinol Metab 44:1185–1189, 1977.
119. Polikar R, Kennedy B, Maisel A, et al: Decreased adrenergic sensitivity in patients with hypothyroidism. J Am Coll Cardiol 15:94–98, 1990.
120. Billewicz WL, Chapman RS, Crooks J, et al: Statistical methods applied to the diagnosis of hypothyroidism. Q J Med 38:255–266, 1969.
121. Seshadri MS, Samuel BU, Kanagasabapathy AS, Cherian AM: Clinical scoring system for hypothyroidism: Is it useful? J Gen Intern Med 4:490–492, 1989.
122. Zulewski H, Müller B, Exer P, et al: Estimation of tissue hypothyroidism by a new clinical score: Evaluation of patients with various grades of hypothyroidism and controls. J Clin Endocrinol Metab 82:771–776, 1997.
123. Tachman ML, Guthrie GP: Hypothyroidism: Diversity of presentation. Endocr Rev 5:456–465, 1984.
124. Doucet J, Trivalle C, Chassagne P, et al: Does age play a role in clinical presentation of hypothyroidism? J Am Geriatr Soc 42:984–986, 1994.
125. Müller B, Zulewski H, Huber P, et al: Impaired action of thyroid hormone associated with smoking in women with hypothyroidism. N Engl J Med 333:964–969, 1995.
126. Toft AD: Thyroxine therapy. N Engl J Med 331:174–180, 1994.
127. Fish LH, Schwartz HL, Cavanaugh J, et al: Replacement dose, metabolism, and bioavailability of levothyroxine in the treatment of hypothyroidism. Role of triiodothyronine in pituitary feedback in humans. N Engl J Med 316:764–770, 1987.
128. Dong BJ, Hauck WW, Gambertoglio JG, et al: Bioequivalence of generic and brand-name levothyroxine products in the treatment of hypothyroidism. JAMA 227:1205–1213, 1997.
129. Olveira G, Almaraz MC, Soriguer F, et al: Altered bioavailability due to changes in the formulation of a commercial preparation of levothyroxine in patients with differentiated carcinoma. Clin Endocrinol 46:707–711, 1997.
130. Roti E, Minelli R, Gardini E, Braverman LE: The use and misuse of thyroid hormone. Endocr Rev 14:401–423, 1993.
131. Oppenheimer JH, Braverman LE, Toft A, et al: Thyroid hormone treatment: When and what? J Clin Endocrinol Metab 80:2875–2883, 1995.
132. Singer PA, Cooper DS, Levy EG, et al: Treatment guidelines for patients with hyperthyroidism and hypothyroidism. JAMA 273:808–812, 1995.
133. Vanderpump MPJ, Ahlquist JAO, Franklyn JA, Clayton RN: Consensus statement for good practice and audit measures in the management of hypothyroidism and hyperthyroidism. BMJ 313:539–544, 1996.
134. Cunningham JJ, Barzel NS: Lean body mass is a predictor of the daily requirement of thyroid hormone in older men and women. J Am Geriatr Soc 32:204–207, 1984.
135. Kabadi UM, Jackson T: Serum thyrotropin in primary hypothyroidism. A possible predictor of optimal daily levothyroxine dose. Arch Intern Med 155:1046–1048, 1995.
136. Sawin CT, Geller A, Wolf PA, et al: Low serum thyrotropin concentrations as a risk factor for atrial fibrillation in older persons. N Engl J Med 331:1249–1252, 1994.
137. Uzzan B, Campos J, Cucherat M, et al: Effects on bone mass of long term treatment with thyroid hormones: A meta-analysis. J Clin Endocrinol Metab 81:4278–4289, 1996.
138. Biondi B, Fazio S, Carella C, et al: Cardiac effects of long term thyrotropin-suppressive therapy with levothyroxine. J Clin Endocrinol Metab 77:334–338, 1993.
139. Leese GP, Jung RT, Guthrie C, et al: Morbidity in patients on L-thyroxine: A comparison of those with a normal TSH to those with a suppressed TSH. Clin Endocrinol 37:500–503, 1992.
140. Solomon BL, Wartofsky L, Burman KD: Prevalence of fractures in postmenopausal women with thyroid disease. Thyroid 3:17–23, 1993.
141. Topliss DJ, Wright JA, Volpe R: Increased requirement for thyroid hormone after a jejunal bypass operation. Can Med Assoc J 123:765–766, 1980.
142. Liel Y, Harman-Boehm I, Shany S: Evidence for a clinically important adverse effect of fiber-enriched diet on the availability of levothyroxine in adult hypothyroid patients. J Clin Endocrinol Metab 81:857–859, 1996.
143. Surks MI, Sievert R: Drugs and thyroid function. N Engl J Med 333:1688–1694, 1995.
144. Witztum JL, Jacobs LS, Schonfeld G: Thyroid hormone and thyrotropin levels in patients placed on colestipol hydrochloride. J Clin Endocrinol Metab 46:838–840, 1978.
145. Harmon SM, Seifert CF: Levothyroxine-cholestyramine interaction reemphasized. Ann Intern Med 115:658–659, 1991.
146. Havrankova J, Lahaie R: Levothyroxine binding by sucralfate. Ann Intern Med 147:445–446, 1992 [Erratum 118:398, 1993].
147. Sperber AD, Liel Y: Evidence for interference with the intestinal absorption of levothyroxine sodium by aluminium hydroxide. Arch Intern Med 152:183–184, 1992.
148. Campbell NRC, Hasinoff BB, Stalts H, et al: Ferrous sulfate reduces thyroxine efficacy in patients with hypothyroidism. Ann Intern Med 117:1010–1013, 1992.
149. Glinoer D, De Nayer P, Bourdoux P, et al: Regulation of maternal thyroid function during pregnancy. J Clin Endocrinol Metab 71:276–287, 1990.
150. Mandell SJ, Larson PR, Seely EW, Brent GA: Increased need for thyroxine during pregnancy in women with primary hypothyroidism. N Engl J Med 323:91–96, 1990.
151. Kaplan MM: Monitoring thyroxine treatment during pregnancy. Thyroid 2:147–152, 1992.
152. Isley WL: Effect of rifampin therapy on thyroid function tests in a hypothyroid patient on replacement L-thyroxine. Ann Intern Med 107:517–518, 1987.
153. Figge J, Dluhy RG: Amiodarone-induced elevation of thyroid stimulating hormone in patients receiving levothyroxine for primary hypothyroidism. Ann Intern Med 113:553–555, 1990.
154. McCowen KC, Garber JR, Spark R: Elevated serum thyrotropin in thyroxine-treated patients with hypothyroidism given sertraline. N Engl J Med 337:1010–1011, 1997.
155. Munera Y, Hugues FC, Le Jeunne C, Pays IF: Interaction of thyroxine sodium with antimalarial drugs. BMJ 314:1593, 1997.
156. Ain KB, Refetoff S, Fein HG, Weintraub BD: Pseudomalabsorption of levothyroxine. JAMA 266:2118–2120, 1991.
157. Grebe SKG, Cooke RR, Ford HC, et al: Treatment of hypothyroidism with once weekly thyroxine. J Clin Endocrinol Metab 82:870–875, 1997.
158. Arafah BM: Decreased levothyroxine requirement in women with hypothyroidism during androgen therapy for breast cancer. Ann Intern Med 121:247–251, 1994.
159. Rosenbaum RL, Barzel US: Levothyroxine replacement dose for primary hypothyroidism decreases with age. Ann Intern Med 96:53–55, 1982.
160. Griffin JE: Hypothyroidism in the elderly. Am J Med Sci 299:334–345, 1990.
161. Jackson S, William E, Cobb E: Why does anyone still use desiccated thyroid USP? Am J Med 64:284–288, 1978.
162. Escobar-Morreale HF, Escobar del Ray F, Obregon MJ, Morreale de Escobar G: Only the combined treatment with thyroxine and triiodothyronine ensures euthyroidism in all tissues of the thyroidectomized rat. Endocrinology 137:2490–2502, 1996.
163. Bunevicius R, Kazanavicius G, Zalinkevicius R, Prange AJ: Effects of thyroxine as compared with thyroxine plus triiodothyronine in patients with hypothyroidism. N Engl J Med 340:424–429, 1999.
164. Sherman SI, Ladenson PW: Percutaneous transluminal coronary angioplasty in hypothyroidism. Am J Med 90:367–370, 1991.
165. Nicoloff JT, LoPresti JS: Myxedema coma. A form of decompensated hypothyroidism. Endocrinol Metab Clin North Am 22:279–290, 1993.
166. Jordan RM: Myxedema coma. Pathophysiology, therapy, and factors affecting prognosis. Med Clin North Am 79:185–194, 1995.

167. Arlot S, Debussche X, Lalaw JD, et al: Myxedema coma: Response of thyroid hormone with oral intravenous high-dose L-thyroxine treatment. Intens Care Med 19:16–18, 1991.
168. Weetman AP: Hypothyroidism: Screening and subclinical disease. BMJ 314:1175–1178, 1997.
169. Woeber KA: Subclinical thyroid dysfunction. Arch Intern Med 157:1065–1068, 1997.
170. Cooper DS, Alpern R, Wood LC, et al: L-Thyroxine therapy in subclinical hypothyroidism. A double-blind, placebo-controlled trial. Ann Intern Med 101:18–24, 1984.
171. Nyström E, Caidahl K, Fager G, et al: A double-blind cross-over 12-month study of L-thyroxine treatment of women with 'subclinical' hypothyroidism. Clin Endocrinol 29:63–76, 1988.
172. Monzani F, Del Guerra P, Caraccio N, et al: Subclinical hypothyroidism: Neurobehavioral features and beneficial effect of L-thyroxine treatment. Clin Invest 71:367–371, 1993.
173. Jaeschke R, Guyatt G, Gerstein H, et al: Does treatment with L-thyroxine influence health status in middle aged and older adults with subclinical hypothyroidism? J Geriatr Intern Med 11:744–749, 1996.
174. Tavis BC, Westendorp RGJ, Smelt AHM: Effect of thyroid substitution on hypercholesterolaemia in patients with subclinical hypothyroidism: A reanalysis of intervention studies. Clin Endocrinol 44:643–649, 1996.
175. Nagayama I, Yamamoto K, Saito K, et al: Subject-based reference values in thyroid function test. Endocr J 40:557–562, 1993.
176. Spencer CA, LoPresti JS, Guttler RB, et al: Application of a new chemiluminescent thyrotropin assay to subnormal measurements. J Clin Endocrinol Metab 70:453–460, 1990.
177. Danese MD, Powe NR, Sawin CT, Ladenson PW: Screening for mild thyroid failure at the periodic health examination: A decision and cost-effectiveness analysis. JAMA 276:285–292, 1996.
178. Powe NR, Danese MD, Ladenson PW: Decision analysis in endocrinology and metabolism. Endocrinol Metab Clin North Am 26:89–112, 1997.

Chapter 106

Nonthyroidal Illness Syndrome

Leslie J. DeGroot

During starvation and in illness, thyroid hormones in blood are reduced to levels typical of hypothyroidism. This response has been interpreted over several decades as an adaptive response causing serum total hormone levels to drop while metabolism remains "normal." For this reason it has been described as the "euthyroid sick syndrome." However, in severe illness, the changes in thyroid hormone supply are associated with a dramatically increased chance of death. Whether the changes are adaptive or maladaptive remains uncertain.[1, 2] The noncommittal term "nonthyroidal illness syndrome" (NTIS) seems more suitable.

LOW SERUM T_3 IN STARVATION

Serum triiodothyronine (T_3) drops during starvation in animals and humans. Serum thyroid hormone–binding proteins are typically reduced,[3, 4] but a more important cause is the reduced generation of T_3. "Reducing equivalents" available for the deiodination of thyroxine (T_4) to T_3 are diminished in the liver and presumably elsewhere, thus lowering the function of type I iodothyronine deiodinase.[5, 6] Animals (and probably humans) also have a drop in the level of deiodinase enzyme,[7] apparently resulting from hypothyroidism because it can be reversed by giving T_3. Low serum T_3 is also found at birth as a result low fetal generation of T_3, is encountered in old age, and is induced by the action of a variety of drugs, including steroids, propranolol, and amiodarone.[1, 8]

The starvation-induced drop in serum T_3 is associated with an approximately 10% decline in basal metabolic rate (BMR)[9] and, in some studies, reduced nitrogen excretion[10, 11] and evidence of tissue hypothyroidism,[12] as examined by timing of arterial sounds and other imprecise indicators of thyroid hormone action on cells. Administering T_3 in supraphysiologic amounts during starvation can elevate the BMR and nitrogen excretion and return the cardiac indices toward normal.[9, 10–12] However, in some studies, the BMR has not been altered by replacement doses of T_3, and nitrogen excretion has not been augmented.[13] Thus correlation between the drop in T_3 and the metabolic changes associated with starvation remains uncertain. In any event, the drop in T_3, in parallel with a reduced BMR, is considered, based on teleologic thinking, to provide protection against prolonged starvation. It may be an adaptive response built into our genes over countless millennia as a protection against periodic episodes of starvation. No apparent association exists between a drop in serum T_3 (alone) and adverse outcome, and thus the clinical importance of this change is limited.

NONTHYROIDAL ILLNESS SYNDROME WITH LOW SERUM T_3 AND T_4

As starvation and illness together continue and worsen, in addition to low T_3, total serum T_4 drops below normal. This change is associated with (typically) normal or reduced serum thyroid-stimulating hormone (TSH), in contrast to the expected elevation. These changes define NTIS. NTIS is found in most patients in any hospital intensive care unit (ICU), especially those who have been in intensive care for more than a week.[1] Typically, all patients with severe adult respiratory distress syndrome, those who are wasting from tumors, and patients with severe infections, renal failure, liver failure, or cardiac failure have evidence of NTIS.[13–19] Although clinically the low T_3 syndrome seems to shade imperceptibly into the worse NTIS syndrome, it is uncertain that the pathophysiology is the same. Clearly, the clinical importance is different. In individuals in an ICU setting, the drop in serum T_4 is directly correlated with the probability of death. Several studies have shown that when serum T_4 is below 4 μg/dL, the probability of death is approximately 50%, and when the serum T_4 is below 2 μg/dL, the probability of death is nearly 80%.[20–22] Obviously, this relationship does not prove cause and effect, but it does point out the association of this syndrome with an adverse medical outcome. If individuals recover, serum T_3 and T_4 levels return toward normal, and TSH often transiently rises above normal, thus suggesting prior hypothyroidism.[23] In individuals who progressively get sicker and die, the serum hormone levels drop further, and TSH progressively drops.[23]

SERUM HORMONE MEASUREMENTS

The exact state of tissue hormone supplies and the response to thyroid hormone remain imperfectly defined. Evidence is most compatible with a state of acquired central hypothyroidism. Although total T_4 is universally reduced, reported values for free T_4 have shown much variability. Most disagreement relates to free hormone values in patients with serum T_4 above 4 μg/dL. When patients with a serum T_4 concentration below this level are considered separately, results of free T_4 and free T_3 levels are more uniformly reduced. As shown in Table 106–1, estimates of free T_4 that depend on measurement of serum T_4 or T_3 binding to "correct" the total T_4 level characteristically report a low free T_4 level. Studies using ultrafiltration or dialysis indicate that free T_4 is low, normal, or even elevated in NTIS.[24, 29, 30, 34, 35] It must be noted that in one important study showing elevated values, there is reason to question the "normal" range because other individuals in the hospital studied at the same time, who did not have NTIS, had on average hormone levels in the thyrotoxic range.[29] Data based on ultrafiltration of free T_4 have also been variable, some values indicating high free T_4 and some indicating low levels.[36, 37] Similar confusion exists with regard to free T_3. Most reported data suggest that the values are low, although one recent study indicates that free T_3 levels are normal[33, 38, 39] (Fig. 106–1). This later study was performed with a direct dialysis and radioimmunoassay technique, but in a system in which unlabeled T_3 was added to the dialysate. Overall, the measured values of free T_4 and T_3 are still a source of confusion, and several reasons, discussed below, may explain these discrepancies.

TABLE 106–1. Thyroid Hormone Assays in Patients with Nonthyroidal Illness and Thyroxine Less than 5 μg/dL

Reference	No. of Cases	Ft_4, Dialysis, RIA	FT_4 Index (Talc)	FT_4-TBG (TBG RIA), Corning	FT_4 "Gamma Coat" Clinical Assays	FT_4 "Immuno-Phase," Corning (Method 1)	FT_4 "Liquisol," Damon	FT_4 "Immuno-Phase," Corning (Method 2)	FT_4 Amerlex	rT_3	T_3 Resin Uptake Ratio (A)	FT_4 Index B, Bermudez Method	FT_4, Abbott "Tetrazyme"	Ultra-filtration	FT_4 by RIA	FT_3, Dialysis	Serum T_4	Serum T_3, RIA	FT_3 Ultra-filtration
Melmed et al.[24]	14	36% ↓	71% ↓	36% ↓	27% ↓	100% ↓	29% ↓			64% ↑									
Chopra et al.[25]	11	55% ↑ 18% ↓	64% ↓			18% ↑		55% ↓			64% ↑	55% ↓			18% ↑				
Kaplan et al.[26]	17		53% ↓ (charcoal)																
Wood et al.[27]	18		43% ↓																
Kaptein et al.[28]	6		100% ↓							100% ↑	100% ↑								
Chopra et al.[29]	18	44% ↑ 17% ↓	100% ↓							61% ↑						66% ↓		100% ↓ 89% ↓	
Kaptein et al.[30]	16	13% ↑ 19% ↓	100% ↓	69% ↓	44% ↑ 13% ↓	94% ↓	87% ↓					81% ↓	13% ↑ 13% ↓						
Slag et al.[21]	20	45% ↓		45% ↓	15% ↑ 15% ↓	70% ↓	10% ↑ 0% ↓					25% ↓							
Wang et al.[31]	20		Mean, ↓ 36%						Mean, ↓ 54%					Mean, ↓ 32%				Mean, ↓ 70%	Mean, ↓ 31%
Braverman et al.[32]	17	Average, ↓ 7%				Average, ↓ 19%													
Chopra[33]	7	Average, ↑ 21%														Average, ↓ 17%	Average, <3.5 μg/dL	100% ↓	

Values are approximated from published studies.

FT_3, free triiodothyronine; FT_4, free thyroxine; RIA, radioimmunoassay; rT_3, reverse T_3; TBG, thyroxine-binding globulin.

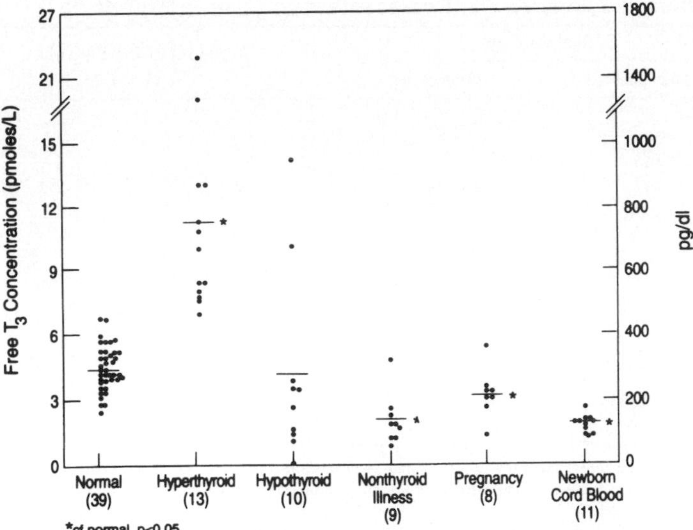

FIGURE 106–1. Free triiodothyronine (T_3) concentrations in different groups of patients, as reported by Chopra.[33] In this report, patients with nonthyroidal illness syndrome have significantly lowered free T_3 levels than normal subjects do. (From Chopra IJ: Simultaneous measurement of free thyroxine and free 3,5,3′-triiodothyronine in undiluted serum by direct equilibrium dialysis/radioimmunoassay: Evidence that free triiodothyronine and free thyroxine are normal in many patients with the low triiodothyronine syndrome. Thyroid 8:249–257, 1998.)

THYROID HORMONE TURNOVER STUDIES

The supply of thyroid hormone to tissues has been measured by Kaptein et al. and others in elegant studies using tracer kinetics.[38, 40, 41] These studies clearly show that in patients with NTIS, degradation of T_4 each day is reduced by about 35% (Table 106–2) and degradation of T_3 is reduced by nearly 75%[38, 40] (Table 106–3). Tracer turnover kinetics have long been considered the most exact method for analyzing tissue hormone availability, and the data clearly suggest a radical drop in supply of thyroid hormones. Thyroid production of T_3 has not been directly measured[41] and is not known with precision (Table 106–4). Presumably, the drop in degradation is caused by a drop in supply. If the degradation rate were primarily reduced, the result would be elevated serum hormone levels, not reduced T_3 and T_4.

TABLE 106–2. T_4 Kinetics in the Low T_4 State of Nonthyroidal Illness

Case Number	TT_4 (μg/dL)	Free T_4 (ng/dL)	PR (μg/day/m²)
Normal subjects (n = 19)			
Mean	7.1	2.21	50.3
±SE	0.4	0.13	3.4
Sick patients			
1	2.7	2.05	32.4
2	3.0	1.23	51.1
3	1.2	0.48	39.0
4	1.4	1.04	23.7
5	1.3	0.75	22.2
6	3.0	1.35	34.6
7	1.9	1.33	36.6
8	2.0	1.88	25.3
9*	0.4	0.28	10.0
10*	1.5	1.50	13.7
11*	1.6	1.70	18.4
Mean	1.8	1.24	27.9
±SE	0.2	0.17	3.7
P†	<.001	<.001	<.001

*Patients receiving dopamine.
†All *P* values are for unpaired *t*-tests.
PR, production rate; TT_4, total thyroxine.
Data from Kaptein EM, Grieb DA, Spencer CA, et al: Thyroxine metabolism in the low thyroxine state of critical nonthyroidal illnesses. J Clin Endocrinol Metab 53:764–771, © 1981, The Endocrine Society.

TABLE 106–3. T_3 Kinetics in the Low T_4 State of Nonthyroidal Illness

Case Number	Total T_3 (ng/dL)	Free T_3 (pg/dL)	PR (μg/day/m²)
Normal subjects (n = 12)			
Mean	162	503	23.47
±SE	5	46	2.12
Sick patients			
3	30	272	6.18
5	42	247	5.67
6	25	151	5.41
7	34	266	8.39
12*	45	282	6.07
Mean	35	244	6.34
±SE	4	24	0.53
P†	<.001	<.001	<.005

*Patients receiving dopamine.
†All *P* values are for unpaired *t*-tests.
PR, production rate; T_3, triiodothyronine.
Data from Kaptein EM, Robinson WJ, Greib DA, Nicoloff JT: Peripheral serum thyroxine, triiodothyronine and reverse triiodothyronine kinetics in the low thyroxine state of acute nonthyroidal illnesses. A noncompartmental analysis. J Clin Invest 69:526–535, 1982.

ENTRY OF T_4 AND T_3 INTO CELLS

Uptake of T_4 into tissues is probably blunted. Patients with NTIS appear to have substances in blood that inhibit uptake of T_4 into cells.[42–45] Kinetic analysis in animals and humans indicates reduced uptake of T_4 into tissues leading to reduced availability of T_4 for deiodination to T_3.[40] Tissue uptake is an energy-dependent process.[46] There is evidence for a drop in tissue ATP levels, in both animals and humans, during starvation.[46, 47] The diminution in tissue uptake is probably related to low ATP levels in tissues, including the liver.

Tissue hormone levels have been examined extensively in only one study, by Arem et al.[48] These authors found levels of T_3 and T_4 generally reduced to about 50% of normal (Table 106–5). However, unaccountably high levels of T_3 and T_4 were noted in some tissues in occasional patients. These important observations have not been confirmed or explained as of this time. Nevertheless, the general result of this study was that tissue levels of hormones were very low in NTIS. Thyroid hormone receptor levels in humans during NTIS are not known with certainty. One study suggests that levels are normal.[49] In animals, starvation and illness are associated with a reduction in thyroid hormone receptor levels.[50–52]

THYROTROPIN-RELEASING AND THYROID-STIMULATING HORMONE PRODUCTION

Hypothalamic thyrotropin-releasing hormone (TRH) is diminished in NTIS in humans and in animals[53, 54] (Fig. 106–2). Pituitary TSH has not been directly measured in NTIS in humans, but it is radically reduced by starvation in animals.[55] As previously noted, serum TSH levels in patients with NTIS are either low or "inappropriately" normal, based on the usual relation to serum T_4 levels. In addition, the circulating TSH probably has low bioactivity because the reduction in TRH leads to poorly glycosylated TSH. The response of TSH to TRH is variable, sometimes reduced but still present.[56] Patients with NTIS respond to infusions of TRH with a dramatic increase in production of TSH and elevation of serum T_4 and T_3[57] (Fig. 106–3). TSH may become transiently elevated if patients recover and, in contrast, progressively drops in patients who succumb to their illness (Fig. 106–4).

TABLE 106–4. Turnover Rate of T_4 and T_3 and Thyroidal Secretion of T_3 before L-T_4 Replacement in Uremic Patients*

Group and Patient	T_4 Metabolism		T_3 Metabolism		T_3 Secreted by Thyroid (% of DT_3)	
	TT_4 (ng/100 mL)	D (µg/day)	*TT_3* (µg/100 mL)	D (µg/day)		
Normal						
Patient 1	6.0	88	136	31.8	1.1	3.5
Patient 2	6.7	66	146	22.5	1.1	4.9
Patient 3	5.6	77	142	24.6	0.6	2.5
Patient 4	6.5	87	130	28.0	3.5	12.5
Patient 5	8.0	82	145	22.5	2.4	10.7
Mean ± SD	6.6 ± 0.9	80 ± 9	140 ± 7	25.9 ± 4.0	1.8 ± 1.2	6.9 ± 4.4
Before HD						
Patient 6	5.4	59	72	12.2	5.2	42.6
Patient 7	4.3	43	55	5.6	1.2	21.4
Patient 8	5.2	53	88	13.7	5.8	42.3
Patient 9	3.4	41	58	9.0	2.5	27.8
Mean ± SD	4.6 ± 0.9	49 ± 9	68 ± 15	10.1 ± 3.6	3.7 ± 2.2	33.5 ± 10.5
P†	NS	NS	<0.01	<0.01	NS	<0.01

*The turnover rates (D) of T_4 and T_3 were calculated from the respective metabolic clearance rate determined during L-T_4 replacement and the total T_4 and T_3 concentrations measured before L-T_4 treatment. The amount of T_3 secreted by the thyroid gland was derived from turnover rates of T_4 and T_3 and the percentage of T_4 converted to T_3. Individual values from all four groups were analyzed by analysis of variance and summarized as F ratio, degree-of-freedom, and *P* values.

†The significance of the difference between the means of each patient group and the controls (*P*) was derived by using the mean square within value.

DT_3, Turnover rate of triiodothyronine (T_3), HD, hemodialysis; NS, not significant; TT_3, total T_3; TT_4, total thyroxine.

Data from Lim VS, Fang VS, Katz AI, Refetoff S: Thyroid dysfunction in chronic renal failure. A study of the pituitary-thyroid axis and peripheral turnover kinetics of thyroxine and triiodothyronine. J Clin Invest 60:522–534, 1977.

EVIDENCE FOR ALTERED TISSUE METABOLISM

Tissue markers of clinical hypothyroidism are at best imprecise, but available data can be reviewed. For example, patients with NTIS are reported to have reduced angiotensin-converting enzyme[58] but normal testosterone-estradiol–binding globulin and osteocalcin.[59] Because of starvation and other illnesses, cholesterol and liver enzyme levels are probably not representative of metabolic status. In a uremic model of NTIS in animals, liver enzyme activity was diminished,[51] and thyroid hormone replacement brought the levels back to normal. In human subjects with NTIS caused by uremia, administration of T_3 in replacement doses augments urea nitrogen excretion.[60] This result was interpreted by the authors as a disadvantageous response. However, these studies are compatible with the idea that tissue responses are typical of hypothyroidism and that provision of thyroid hormone returned metabolism toward normal. Whether augmented nitrogen turnover would prove derogatory or beneficial for these patients is unknown.

EXPLANATIONS THAT HAVE BEEN OFFERED FOR THYROID HORMONE ALTERATIONS IN NONTHYROIDAL ILLNESS SYNDROME

Inhibition of Serum Hormone Binding

Numerous explanations have been proposed for the changes in thyroid hormone parameters described above. One explanation offered is that inhibitors of binding of thyroid hormone to plasma proteins cause the alleged discrepancy between low total T_4 and "normal" serum free hormone levels.[61, 62] Substances (which appear to be lipids) that inhibit binding of T_3 to serum proteins have been extracted from the serum of patients with NTIS.[61, 63–65] Similar material has been demonstrated in tissues and could possibly alter the cellular uptake of hormone.[65] The presence of nondialyzable inhibitors of hormone binding to thyronine-binding globulin (TBG) would tend to cause elevation of both the free T_4 index (FTI) and free hormone levels. It has been

TABLE 106–5. Tissue T_3 Concentrations in Nonthyroidal Illness Syndrome (nmol of T_3/kg of Wet Weight)

Tissue	Control Group			NTI Group	
	Mean	*SD*	*P*	*Mean*	*SD*
Cerebral cortex	2.2	0.9	<.05	1.2	1.1
Hypothalamus	3.9	2.2	<.01	1.4	1.2
Anterior pituitary	6.8	2.5	<.005	3.7	1.1
Liver	3.7	2.3	<.01	0.9	0.9
Kidney	12.9	4.3	<.001	3.7	2.8
Lung	1.8	0.8	<.01	0.8	0.5
Skeletal muscle	2.3	1.2	NS	>10.9	
Heart	4.5	1.5	NS	>16.3	

NS, not significantly different; NTI, nonthyroidal illness; T_3, triiodothyronine.

Data from Arem R, Wiener GJ, Kaplan SG, et al: Reduced tissue thyroid hormone levels in fatal illness. Metabolism 42:1102–1108, 1993.

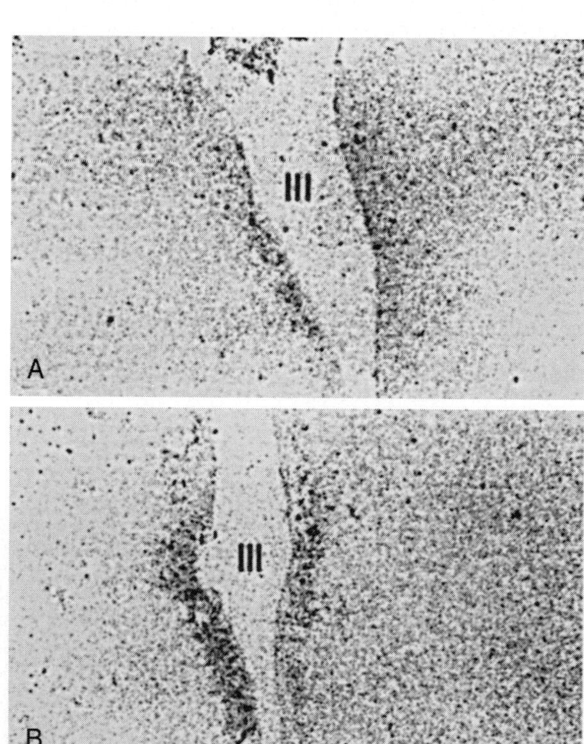

FIGURE 106–2. In situ hybridization study demonstrating mRNA for thyrotropin-releasing hormone (TRH) in the periventricular nuclei of a subject who died with nonthyroidal illness syndrome (NTIS) (panel *A*) and a subject who died accidentally (panel *B*). mRNA for TRH is significantly reduced in patients with NTIS. (From Mendel CM, Laughton CW, McMahon FA, Cavalieri RR: Inability to detect an inhibitor of thyroxine-serum protein binding in sera from patients with nonthyroidal illness. Metabolism 40:491–502, 1991.)

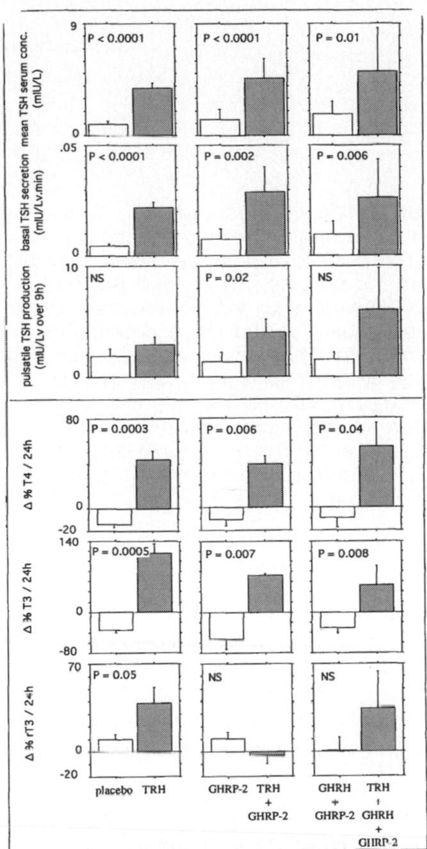

FIGURE 106–3. Study demonstrating the effect of a 1-μg/kg/hour infusion of thyrotropin-releasing hormone (TRH) vs. placebo, TRH plus growth hormone–releasing peptide (GHRP)-2 (1 μg/kg/hr) vs. GHRP-2, and growth hormone–releasing hormone (GHRH) plus GHRP-2 vs. TRH, GHRH, and GHRP-2. Values for mean serum thyroid-stimulating hormone (TSH) and basal and pulsatile TSH secretion are shown in the *upper panel*, and 24-hour changes in peripheral thyroid hormone levels in the three study groups are shown in the *lower panel*. TRH infusion increased TSH secretion, TSH concentration, thyroxine (T_4), triiodothyronine (T_3), and reverse T_3 (rT_3). (From Van den Berghe G, De Zegher F, Baxter KRC, et al: Neuroendocrinology of prolonged critical illness: Effects of exogenous thyrotropin-releasing hormone and its combination with growth hormone secretagogues. J Clin Endocrinol Metab 83:309–319, © 1998, The Endocrine Society.)

suggested that elevated free fatty acids may be present in serum in vivo and alter hormone binding.[61] However, it is unlikely that even during starvation or exercise will free fatty acid levels ever reach a level (5 mM/L) that could significantly inhibit binding of thyroid hormone to albumin and thus alter free hormone levels.[62, 66] In contrast, it seems quite possible that the liberation of free fatty acids during dialysis of serum samples in vitro may falsely elevate apparent free hormone levels. When patients are given even low doses of heparin (0.08 U/kg intravenously or 5,000 U subcutaneously), as is common among ICU patients, serum lipase is elevated.[67] If serum samples from these patients are incubated over a prolonged period during dialysis in vitro, free fatty acids are generated. Free fatty acids bind to albumin, displace T_4 and T_3, and can alter the apparent free hormone levels.[67, 68] Thus heparin treatment may produce artifactually high, or apparently normal, free hormone in dialysis assays unless this artifact is excluded. Substances present in the serum of patients with uremia (indoxyl sulfate and others) and bilirubin in patients with liver disease can also inhibit T_4 entry into cells.[42, 55] Dialyzable inhibitors would presumably be lost from a serum sample during dialysis, and this loss would produce falsely reduced levels of free hormone. Dialyzable inhibitors of hormone binding to cells should in theory cause tissue hypothyroidism in the presence of elevated serum hormone levels—a combination not typical of NTIS. Inhibition of T_4 and T_3 binding to TBG by dialyzable factors would tend to cause an elevated FTI and reduced free T_4 by dialysis, again not typical of observations in NTIS. In analysis of 100 sera from patients with NTIS, Mendel et al. found no evidence of inhibitors of serum hormone binding.[69] Perhaps the most telling argument against the importance of inhibition of binding in the serum of patients with NTIS is the clinical observation offered by Brent and Hershman[70] (Fig. 106–5). These authors treated 12 patients with NTIS by administration of 1.5 μg T_4 per kilogram body weight intravenously daily. Within 2 days of treatment, serum T_4 levels had returned to normal. In these individuals, it was clearly a reduced hormone supply that caused the low serum T_4 and not inhibition of hormone binding to serum proteins.

Reduced Cell Uptake of Hormone

As described above, evidence is strong for reduced cell uptake of T_4, which would result in reduced availability of T_4 for deiodination to T_3. Severe illness and starvation with low cellular ATP may (as noted above) be a cause for this reduced cell uptake. Concomitantly, because of starvation, a drop is seen in the function of intracellular type 1 iodothyronine deiodinase, and there may well be a drop in supply of the deiodinase enzyme as well. These factors would tend to keep T_4 levels elevated and reduce T_3 levels. Although these phenomena may play a role in NTIS, they do not offer a unitary explanation for the changes observed in hormone supply and serum hormone levels.

The Pituitary Response Is "Normal"

One interpretation offered for reduced TSH in NTIS is that the hormone supply is actually normal or elevated as suggested by some free T_4 assays. However, no author appears to suggest that these patients are actually hyperthyroid. It has also been suggested that intracellular production of T_3 or triiodothyroacetic acid may be augmented and cause euthyroidism despite a low T_4 supply and that these levels may not be reflected in serum values.[71]

Another "explanation" is that T_4 to T_3 deiodination is augmented in the pituitary in NTIS, so pituitary T_3 levels remain normal and the pituitary is "euthyroid" and thus secretes low levels of TSH, even though the rest of the body is hypothyroid. Experimental support for this response has been found in animals with induced uremia.[72] In this explanation the body would be hypothyroid.

Induced Hypothyroidism: A Beneficial Response

A common point of view is that the changes are those of hypothyroidism and are beneficial to the individual by reducing caloric consumption or in other ill-defined ways. Obviously, this explanation is teleologic and has no basis in factual observations. Quite the contrary, the observed correlation of the drop in hormone levels with death suggests that the changes are not beneficial to ill patients. The concept of a potential beneficial induced reduction in caloric requirement seems quite irrelevant in view of the fact that all patients with severe illness are provided caloric supplementation, if at all possible. It cannot be denied that hypothyroidism could have other benefits, but no data support this contention.

Central Hypothyroidism: A Potentially Disadvantageous Response

A last, and perhaps most logical explanation is that NTIS represents physiology gone wrong. It is quite possible that the initial alterations in thyroid hormone supply, with a drop in serum T_3, represent an induced change designed to save calories. However, it is unlikely that evolutionarily we have developed an adaptation beneficial for survival

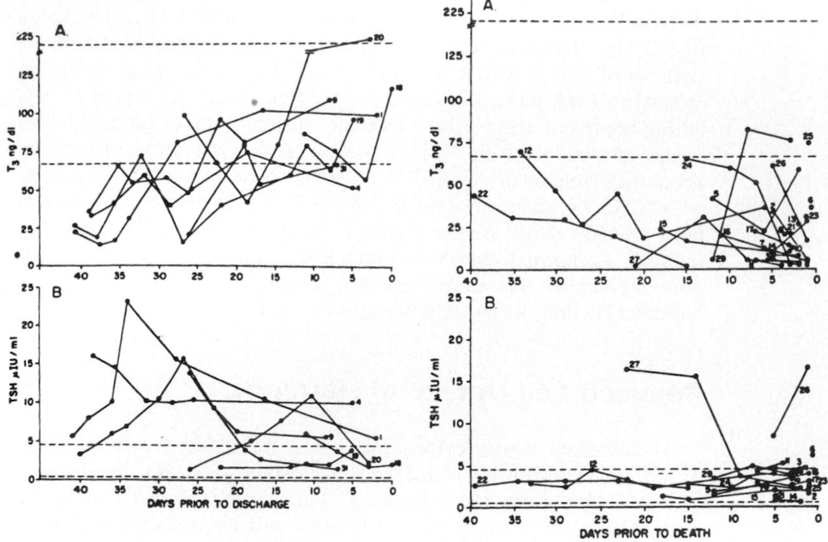

FIGURE 106–4. Triiodothyronine (T_3) and thyroid-stimulating hormone (TSH) concentrations are shown in patients with nonthyroidal illness who were eventually discharged from the hospital *(left panels)*. The *broken line* indicates ±2 SD of the mean value in the normal subjects. The *right panel* displays T_3 and TSH concentrations in patients with nonthyroidal illness syndrome who died. Subjects are indicated by numbers. Note the elevated TSH in some patients who recovered and the generally dropping T_3 and low TSH levels in patients who died. (From Bacci V, Schussler GC, Kaplan TB: The relationship between serum triiodothyronine and thyrotropin during systemic illness. J Clin Endocrinol Metab 54:1229–1235, © 1982, The Endocrine Society.)

in the ICU. Possibly, although we are currently able by all sorts of supportive treatment to maintain the life of individuals who are severely ill, the metabolic changes that go on during prolonged illness are disadvantageous. Van den Berghe and coworkers reached this conclusion after carefully analyzing the endocrine changes that differ between short-term and long-term illness.[73] These changes include, in long-term illness, a drop in thyroid hormone supply, a drop in growth hormone and insulin-like growth factor type I levels, first elevated and then sometimes diminished cortisol responses, and a wasting syndrome.[73] These authors believe that provision of multiple hormonal support, including thyroid hormone, growth hormone, and androgens, may be beneficial.[57, 73]

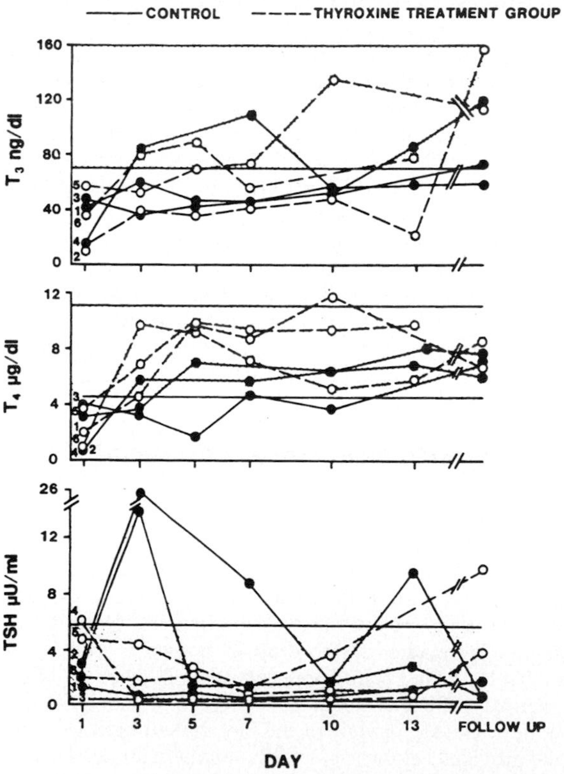

FIGURE 106–5. Patients with severe nonthyroidal illness syndrome were randomized and left untreated or given thyroxine (T_4) intravenously over a 2-week period. Serum triiodothyronine (T_3), T_4, and thyroid-stimulating hormone (TSH) concentrations are shown for the survivors of the control (*filled circles*, 1–3), and T_4-treated (*open circles*, 4–6) groups during the study period and at the time of follow-up. The *shaded area* designates the normal range. Note the prompt recovery of T_4 values to the normal range immediately after intravenous treatment with T_4. Also note the elevated TSH levels in some patients. T_3 levels did not return to normal after T_4 treatment for up to 2 weeks. (From Brent GA, Hershman JM: Thyroxine therapy in patients with severe nonthyroidal illnesses and lower serum thyroxine concentration. J Clin Endocrinol Metab 63:1–8, © 1986, The Endocrine Society.)

FACTORS POSSIBLY CAUSING HYPOTHYROIDISM

Cytokines

How are the metabolic changes in NTIS orchestrated? Much interest has been centered on the role of cytokines, which are often altered in acute illness. No clear evidence has been presented that levels of tumor necrosis factor-α correlate with serum hormone values.[74, 75] Interleukin-1 (IL-1) is often elevated in experimental nonthyroidal illness in animals. However, blockade of IL-1 action does not alter NTIS.[76–79] IL-6 is also frequently elevated. Administration of IL-6 to animals can cause an NTIS-like syndrome. However, administration of IL-6 over several weeks to human subjects did not cause sustained alterations in thyroid hormone levels[80] (Fig. 106–6). Blockade of IL-6 function did not prevent development of the syndrome.[81, 82] Thus although a correlation is seen with the levels of some cytokines, especially IL-6 and NTIS, there is no evidence as yet for a causal relationship.[83, 84] Presumably, if these cytokines are involved, it could be through altering the metabolism of thyroid hormone in peripheral tissues or by an inhibitory effect on the brain and hypothalamic centers.

Leptin

Leptin is diminished in starvation. Associated with this decreased leptin in experimental animals is a drop in hypothalamic TRH and TSH production and thyroid hormone levels.[85] Treating starving rats with leptin restores hormone levels by approximately 50%[85] and restores paraventricular TRH mRNA toward normal.[86] The effect of leptin is thought to be via the arcuate nucleus,[87] which by secondary signals affects the feedback sensitivity of paraventricular TRH-secreting nuclei. In clinical trials, stimulation of growth hormone secretion by growth hormone secretogogues increased insulin and leptin levels in severely ill ICU patients.[57]

Although the studies with leptin are highly suggestive, it seems probable that more than one signal is involved. A likely explanation is that multiple factors, possibly including cytokines, leptin, and other

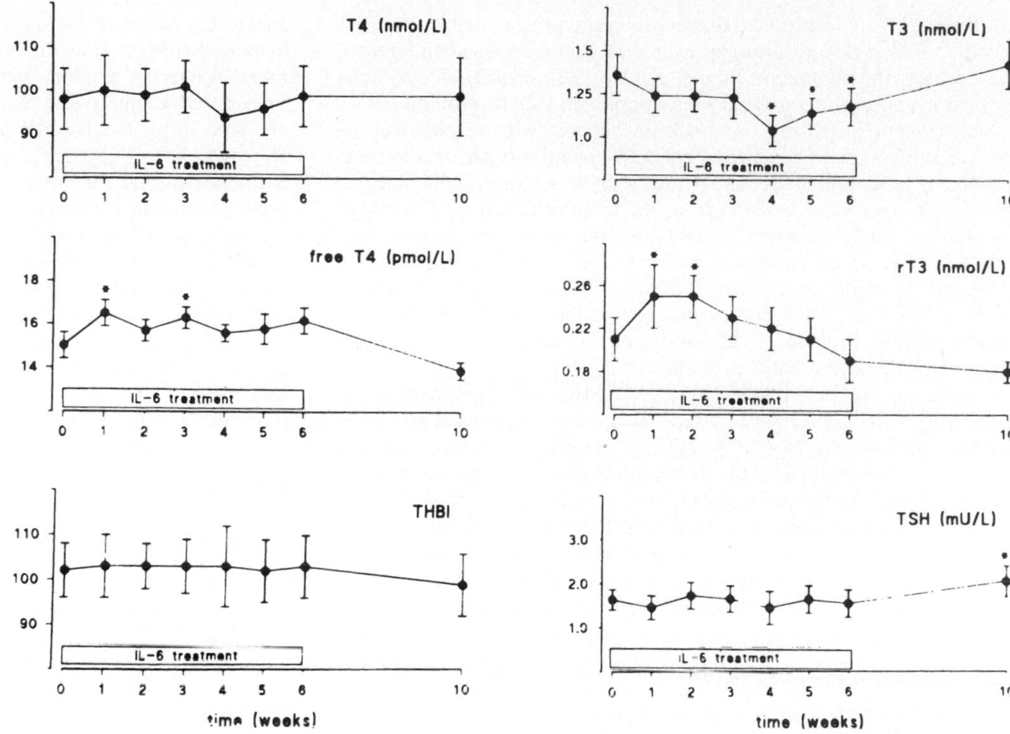

FIGURE 106–6. Interleukin-6 (IL-6) was administered for 6 weeks, and changes in thyroid hormone levels and thyroid-stimulating hormone (TSH) were recorded. Except for a transient elevation in reverse triiodothyronine (rT_3) and minimal suppression of T_3, no significant alteration in hormone levels was produced. (From Stouthard JML, van der Poll T, Endert E, et al: Effects of acute and chronic interleukin-6 administration on thyroid hormone metabolism in humans. J Clin Endocrinol Metab 79:1342–1346, © 1994, The Endocrine Society.)

factors, alter the set-point for feedback control in the hypothalamus and thereby allow a reduction in TRH generation and thus induce central hypothyroidism. For example, cortisol is often elevated in stress and may feed back to suppress TRH and TSH secretion.[88, 89] Glucagon levels are inversely related to the changes in serum hormones seen in NTIS[90] and may also play a role.

DIAGNOSIS OF NONTHYROIDAL ILLNESS SYNDROME

The diagnosis of NTIS is not generally difficult. The hallmarks of the syndrome are the low serum total T_4, low FTI values, low serum total T_3, and usually normal or suppressed TSH. Patients characteristically do not display signs of hypothyroidism that match the reduced serum hormone levels, possibly because of coincident illness masking the symptomatology or because the duration of hypothyroidism is brief.[91] Three to 4 weeks of complete T_4 deprivation is necessary before clinical signs of hypothyroidism develop. (Alternatively, of course, it may be that the patients are actually not hypothyroid because of some undescribed compensatory mechanisms that allow a diminished hormone supply to provide normal metabolic responses.) Acetylsalicylic acid, phenytoin (Dilantin), and carbamazepine can "falsely" lower serum T_4 and the FTI but do not chronically suppress TSH. TSH and serum hormone levels can be suppressed by dopamine and less so by steroids. In NTIS, TSH can be below 0.01 μU/mL and suggest the presence of hyperthyroidism.[92, 93] However, it is difficult to believe that clinically significant hyperthyroidism could actually occur with the combination of serum values and TSH that are observed in NTIS. Reverse T_3 is often normal but can be elevated or low. Production of reverse T_3 is reduced by the reduction in T_4 substrate, and its metabolism is slowed.[38] Thus serum rT_3 levels may remain in the normal range.[94] TSH is elevated in some patients, which suggests a pituitary response to hypothyroidism, and is often transiently elevated during recovery (if indeed recovery occurs). Patients with untreated hypothyroidism can have a reduction in serum TSH levels to nearly normal during NTIS, and thus the possibility of hypothyroidism being present before the illness should always be kept in mind. Some agents used in treating patients with NTIS may compound the problem (especially dopamine) by depressing TRH production and TSH release. Dopamine appears to induce severe hypothyroidism in some individuals with NTIS.[95]

Hypopituitarism needs to be considered in the differential diagnosis. NTIS is most likely a form of acquired central hypopituitarism.[96, 97] It is useful to measure serum cortisol levels, which should be above 20 μg/dL in individuals with severe illness in an ICU.[98] The presence of "normal" levels of prolactin and detectable follicle-stimulating and luteinizing hormone can suggest that the pituitary is functional and that the main problem is the lowering of serum thyroid hormone levels. However, it should be recognized that individuals with serious illness have generalized hypothalamic suppression and that follicle-stimulating and luteinizing hormone levels drop by more than 50% in these patients, along with a similar decrease in testosterone levels.[96, 97] Although it is true that patients may have elevated TSH levels during NTIS, especially if they are in the recovery phase, a clear elevation in TSH suggests the presence of primary hypothyroidism, which may be coincidental and should be analyzed by checking thyroid antibodies, past history, and physical signs.

RESULTS OF TREATMENT

Two valuable studies are available on thyroid hormone replacement therapy in patients with NTIS. Brent and Hershman treated half of 24 patients suffering from severe NTIS with 1.5 μg T_4 intravenously per kilogram body weight daily.[70] Eighty percent of both the treated and untreated group died, thus indicating the seriousness of their illnesses. In this study, which used T_4 for therapy, serum T_4 levels returned to normal immediately, but serum T_3 did not reach normal levels during 2 weeks of therapy. This result is expected because of diminished T_3 generation. This study clearly shows that treatment should be with T_3, if it is to be done, but does not indicate a benefit or adverse effect of the treatment.

Becker et al. studied Air Force members who were severely burned. Treatment with 200 μg of T_3 daily failed to alter the outcome.[99] This study is most interesting because it used T_3, but it is possible that the very high dosage may have induced hyperthyroidism and negatively affected outcome. Nevertheless, this study does show that even high levels of T_3 can be given without apparent adverse effects. Treatment of patients with NTIS associated with uremia induced an increase in nitrogen excretion, which was considered by the investigators to be disadvantageous.[60] However, dialysis is generally available, so it is uncertain that increased nitrogen excretion would be disadvantageous, and perhaps the treatment should actually be considered beneficial because it appeared to reverse hypothyroidism. Short-term studies of T_3 replacement in patients in shock, in patients with respiratory disease, in subjects who are brain dead and potential organ donors, and in patients undergoing coronary artery bypass grafting all suggest modest cardiovascular benefits from the administration of T_3 through augmenting cardiac output or reducing the need for pressor support.[99–108] One study reported benefit by replacing T_3 to elevate the depressed T_3 levels in premature infants.[109] A few studies found no apparent effects.[110] The general outcome of these studies is that they weakly support the use of T_3, and none of the studies have found evidence of damage caused by treatment.

Similar studies in animals have shown that administration of T_3 augments cardiac performance after induction of myocardial infarction in pigs[111] or shock in dogs[112, 113] and that treatment of uremic rats with T_3 restores liver enzyme levels to normal.[51] In two studies of NTIS in animals, thyroid hormone treatment failed to alter outcome.[114, 115]

From all of the studies it is clear that there is no evidence of any damaging effect of replacement therapy. There is weak support for a benefit, although not in terms of prolongation of life or prevention of death. It must be acknowledged that treatment with thyroid hormone alone may be inappropriate. It may be that provision of other hormones, including growth hormone and anabolic steroids such as testosterone, may be equally important. No data are available to analyze these possible beneficial responses, although administration of TRH and a growth hormone secretogogue to ICU patients was shown by Van den Berghe et al. to result in a definite increase in TSH, T_4, and T_3.[57] Unfortunately, for present evaluation, it is clear that a large prospective study will be needed to prove the benefit or adverse effects of treatment. One may presume that if thyroid hormone treatment is beneficial, it will not be in terms of curing all patients with NTIS but rather in terms of increasing the possibility of survival by 5%, 10%, or 20%. One may make an analogy to the use of β-blockers after myocardial infarction. Studies on thousands of patients showed that mortality was reduced by approximately 14% when these drugs were continuously administered.[116] Such a study is needed among ICU patients.

At the present time, a decision has to be made by the physician caring for the ICU patient regarding whether the evidence supports the presence of hypothyroidism and whether treatment is beneficial (Table 106–6). There is strong evidence that hormone supply and function in tissues are diminished in these patients. There is no evidence that providing replacement doses of thyroid hormone is disadvantageous and weak evidence that it is advantageous. There is evidence that levels of serum T_4 below 4 ng/dL are associated with an increased risk of death. It is appropriate to at least consider replacement therapy in patients with serum T_4 at or below this level. Thus for some, including this author, replacement by administering T_3 in doses of 30 μg twice daily and starting replacement with thyroxine at 50 μg/day seems appropriate. Serum hormone levels should be assayed frequently during the course of replacement therapy. There is also no proven reason to withhold treatment from patients with cardiac disease, including arrhythmias and cardiac failure.[117]

Whether it is theoretically best to "do no evil" by leaving the apparent hypothyroidism untreated or to "do no evil" by treating the apparent hypothyroidism remains a philosophical question in the absence of clear physiologic answers. Many authors either deny the presence of hypothyroidism in patients with NTIS or accept the dogma that even if present, it should be left untreated. Several reviews offering this analysis are available.[1–3, 118]

TABLE 106–6. Summary of Observations in Nonthyroidal Illness Syndrome

1. Hypothalmic mRNA for TRH is reduced, and cytokines may be involved.
2. TSH levels are inappropriately low for serum hormone levels, presumably because of reduced secretion.
3. TRH injection causes an elevation in TSH, T_4, and T_3, thereby reversing many aspects of the syndrome and suggesting that low TRH secretion may be a primary problem.
4. Measured serum levels of apparent free T_4 and T_3 may be low or normal and, in some assays, even elevated, *but no assay can be certified to be free of artifact.*
5. Inhibitors of T_4 and T_3 binding to serum proteins and possibly receptors have been postulated but remain of unproven significance.
6. T_4 and T_3 production rates have been clearly demonstrated to be markedly reduced.
7. Based on scant data, levels of hormone in most tissues are *greatly reduced.*
8. Replacement hormone therapy has not been shown to be disadvantageous and in some studies appears to be beneficial.
9. Serum hormone was, in the one study available, restored by administration of physiologic doses of hormone.

T_3, triiodothyronine; T_4, thyroxine; TRH, thyrotropin-releasing hormone; TSH, thyroid-stimulating hormone.

REFERENCES

1. McIver B, Gorman CA: Euthyroid sick syndrome: An overview. Thyroid 7:125–132, 1997.
2. Hennemann G, Docter R, Krenning EP: Causes and effects of the low T_3 syndrome during caloric deprivation and non-thyroidal illness: An overview. Acta Med Kaust 15:42–45, 1988.
3. Docter R, Krenning EP, Jong M de, Hennemann G: The sick euthyroid syndrome: Changes in thyroid hormone serum parameters and hormone metabolism. Clin Endocrinol 39:499–518, 1993.
4. Tamai H, Mori K, Matsubayashi S, et al: Hypothalamic-pituitary-thyroidal dysfunctions in anorexia nervosa. Psychother Psychosom 46:127–131, 1986.
5. Visser TJ: Role of glutathione and other thiols in thyroid hormone metabolism. *In* Dolphin D, Poulson R, Avramovic O (eds): Glutathione: Chemical, Biochemical, and Medical Aspects. New York, John Wiley & Sons, 1989, pp 572–612.
6. Visser TJ, Kaptein E, Terpstra OT, Krenning EP: Deiodination of thyroid hormone by human liver. J Clin Endocrinol Metab 67:17–24, 1988.
7. Kaplan MM: Regulatory influences on iodothyronine deiodination in animal tissues. *In* Hennemann G (ed): Thyroid Hormone Metabolism. New York, Marcel Dekker, 1986, pp 231–253.
8. Docter R, Krenning EP, de Jong M, Hennemann G: The sick euthyroid syndrome: Changes in thyroid hormone serum parameters and hormone metabolism. Clin Endocrinol 39:499–518, 1993.
9. Welle SL, Campbell RG: Decrease in resting metabolic rate during rapid weight loss is reversed by low dose thyroid hormone treatment. Metabolism 35:289–291, 1986.
10. Gardner DF, Kaplan MM, Stanley CA, Utiger RD: Effect of triiodothyronine replacement on the metabolic and pituitary responses to starvation. N Engl J Med 300:579–584, 1979.
11. Burman KD, Wartofsky L, Dinterman RE, et al: The effect of T_3 and reverse T_3 administration on muscle protein catabolism during fasting as measured by 3-methylhistidine excretion. Metabolism 28:805–813, 1979.
12. Osburne RC, Myers EA, Rodbard D, et al: Adaptation to hypocaloric feeding: Physiologic significance of the fall in serum T_3 as measured by the pulse wave arrival time. Metabolism 32:9–13, 1983.
13. Byerley LO, Heber D: Metabolic effects of triiodothyronine replacement during fasting in obese subjects. J Clin Endocrinol Metab 81:968–976, 1996.
14. Phillips RH, Valente WA, Caplan ES, et al: Circulating thyroid hormone changes in acute trauma: Prognostic implications for clinical outcome. J Trauma 24:116–119, 1984.
15. Cherem HJ, Nellen HH, Barabejski FG, et al: Thyroid function and abdominal surgery. A longitudinal study. Arch Med Res 23:143–147, 1992.
16. Vardarli I, Schmidt R, Wdowinski JM, et al: The hypothalamo-hypophyseal thyroid axis, plasma protein concentrations and the hypophyseogonadal axis in low T_3 syndrome following acute myocardial infarct. Klin Wochenschr 65:129–133, 1987.
17. Eber B, Schumacher M, Langsteger W, et al: Changes in thyroid hormone parameters after acute myocardial infarction. Cardiology 86:152–156, 1995.
18. Holland FW, Brown PS, Weintraub BD, Clark RE: Cardiopulmonary bypass and thyroid function: A "euthyroid sick syndrome." Ann Thorac Surg 52:46–50, 1991.
19. Vexiau P, Perez-Castiglioni P, Socie G, et al: The 'euthyroid sick syndrome': Incidence, risk factors and prognostic value soon after allogeneic bone marrow transplantation. Br J Haematol 85:778–782, 1993.
20. Maldonado LS, Murata GH, Hershman JM, Braunstein GD: Do thyroid function tests independently predict survival in the critically ill? Thyroid 2:119, 1992.
21. Slag MF, Morley JE, Elson MK, et al: Hypothyroxinemia in critically ill patients as a predictor of high mortality. JAMA 245:43–45, 1981.
22. Kaptein EM, Weiner JM, Robinson WJ, et al: Relationship of altered thyroid hormone indices to survival in nonthyroidal illnesses. Clin Endocrinol 16:565–574, 1982.
23. Bacci V, Schussler GC, Kaplan TB: The relationship between serum triiodothyronine and thyrotropin during systemic illness. J Clin Endocrinol Metab 54:1229–1235, 1982.
24. Melmed S, Geola FL, Reed AW, et al: A comparison of methods for assessing thyroid function in nonthyroidal illness. J Clin Endocrinol Metab 54:300–306, 1982.
25. Chopra IJ, Van Herle AJ, Chua Teco GN, Nguyen AH: Serum free thyroxine in thyroidal and nonthyroidal illnesses: A comparison of measurements by radioimmunoassay equilibrium dialysis, and free thyroxine index. J Clin Endocrinol Metab 51:135, 1980.

26. Kaplan MM, Larsen PR, Crantz FR, et al: Prevalence of abnormal thyroid function test results in patients with acute medical illnesses. Am J Med 72:9, 1982.
27. Wood DG, Cyrus J, Samols E: Low T_4 and low FT_4I in seriously ill patients: Concise communication. J Nucl Med 21:432, 1980.
28. Kaptein EM, Levitan D, Feinstein EI, et al: Alterations of thyroid hormone indices in acute renal failure and in acute critical illness with and without acute renal failure. Am J Nephrol 1:138, 1981.
29. Chopra IJ, Solomon DH, Hepner GW, Morgenstein AA: Misleadingly low free thyroxine index and usefulness of reverse triiodothyronine measurement in nonthyroidal illnesses. Ann Intern Med 90:905–912, 1979.
30. Kaptein EM, MacIntyre SS, Weiner JM, et al: Free thyroxine estimates in nonthyroidal illness: Comparison of eight methods. J Clin Endocrinol Metab 52:1073–1077, 1981.
31. Wang Y-S, Pekary AE, England ML, Hershman JM: Comparison of a new ultrafiltration method for serum free T_4 and free T_3 with two RIA kits in eight groups of patients. J Endocrinol Invest 8:495, 1985.
32. Braverman LE, Abreau CM, Brock P, et al: Measurement of serum free thyroxine by RIA in various clinical states. J Nucl Med 21:233, 1980.
33. Chopra IJ: Simultaneous measurement of free thyroxine and free 3,5,3′-triiodothyronine in undiluted serum by direct equilibrium dialysis/radioimmunoassay: Evidence that free triiodothyronine and free thyroxine are normal in many patients with the low triiodothyronine syndrome. Thyroid 8:249–257, 1998.
34. Faber J, Sierbaek-Nielsen K: Serum free 3,5,3′-triiodothyronine (T_3) in nonthyroidal somatic illness, as measured by ultrafiltration and immunoextraction. Clin Chim Acta 256:115–123, 1996.
35. Sapin R, Schlienger JL, Kaltenbach G, et al: Determination of free triiodothyronine by six different methods in patients with nonthyroidal illness and in patients treated with amiodarone. Ann Clin Biochem 32:314–324, 1995.
36. Surks MI, Hupart KH, Pan C, Shapiro LE: Normal free thyroxine in critical nonthyroidal illnesses measured by ultrafiltration of undiluted serum and equilibrium dialysis. J Clin Endocrinol Metab 67:1031–1039, 1988.
37. Wang Y-S, Hershman JM, Pekary AE: Improved ultrafiltration method for simultaneous measurement of free thyroxine and free triiodothyronine in serum. Clin Chem 31:517–522, 1985.
38. Kaptein EM, Robinson WJ, Grieb DA, Nicoloff JT: Peripheral serum thyroxine, triiodothyronine and reverse triiodothyronine kinetics in the low thyroxine state of acute nonthyroidal illnesses. A noncompartmental analysis. J Clin Invest 69:526–535, 1982.
39. Chopra IJ, Taing P, Mikus L: Direct determination of free triiodothyronine (T_3) in undiluted serum by equilibrium dialysis/radioimmunoassay. Thyroid 6:255–259, 1996.
40. Kaptein EM, Grieb DA, Spencer CA, et al: Thyroxine metabolism in the low thyroxine state of critical nonthyroidal illnesses. J Clin Endocrinol Metab 53:764–771, 1981.
41. Lim VS, Fang VS, Katz AI, Refetoff S: Thyroid dysfunction in chronic renal failure. A study of the pituitary thyroid axis and peripheral turnover kinetics of thyroxine and triiodothyronine. J Clin Invest 60:522–534, 1977.
42. Lim C-F, Docter R, Visser TJ, et al: Inhibition of thyronine transport into cultured rat hepatocytes by serum of nonuremic critically ill patients: Effects of bilirubin and nonesterified fatty acids. J Clin Endocrinol Metab 76:1165–1172, 1993.
43. Vos RA, de Jong M, Bernard BF, et al: Impaired thyroxine and 3,5,3′-triiodothyronine handling by rat hepatocytes in the presence of serum of patients with nonthyroidal illness. J Clin Endocrinol Metab 80:2364–2370, 1995.
44. Lim C-F, Docter R, Krenning EP, et al: Transport of thyroxine into cultured hepatocytes. Effects of mild nonthyroidal illness and calorie restriction in obese subjects. Clinical Endocrinol 40:79–85, 1994.
45. Sarne DH, Refetoff S: Measurement of thyroxine uptake from serum by cultured human hepatocytes as an index of thyroid status: Reduced thyroxine uptake from serum of patients with nonthyroidal illness. J Clin Endocrinol Metab 61:1046–1052, 1985.
46. Krenning DP, Docter R, Bernard HF, et al: Decreased transport of thyroxine (T_4), 3,3′,5-triiodothyronine (T_3) and 3,3′,5′-triiodothyronine (rT_3) into rat hepatocytes in primary culture due to a decrease of cellular ATP content and various drugs. FEBS Lett 140:229–233, 1982.
47. Masson S, Henriksen O, Stengaard A, et al: Hepatic metabolism during constant infusion of fructose: Comparative studies with 31-P-magnetic resonance spectroscopy in men and rats. Biochim Biophys Acta 119:166–174, 1994.
48. Arem R, Wiener GJ, Kaplan SG, et al: Reduced tissue thyroid hormone levels in fatal illness. Metabolism 42:1102–1108, 1993.
49. Williams GR, Franklyn JA, Neuberger JM, Sheppard MC: Thyroid hormone receptor expression in the "sick euthyroid" syndrome. Lancet 2:1477–1481, 1989.
50. DeGroot LJ, Coleoni AH, Rue PA, et al: Reduced nuclear triiodothyronine receptors in starvation-induced hypothyroidism. Biochem Biophys Res Commun 79:173–178, 1977.
51. Lim VS, Henriquez C, Seo H, et al: Thyroid function in a uremic rat model. Evidence suggesting tissue hypothyroidism. J Clin Invest 66:946–954, 1980.
52. Sanchez B, Jolin T: Triiodothyronine-receptor complex in rat brain: Effects of thyroidectomy, fasting, food restriction, and diabetes. Endocrinology 129:361–367, 1991.
53. Fliers E, Guldenaar SEF, Wiersinga WM, Swaab DF: Decreased hypothalamic thyrotropin-releasing hormone gene expression in patients with nonthyroidal illness. J Clin Endocrinol Metab 82:4032–4036, 1997.
54. Blake NG, Eckland JA, Foster OJF, Lightman SL: Inhibition of hypothalamic thyrotropin-releasing hormone messenger ribonucleic acid during food deprivation. Endocrinology 129:2714–2718, 1991.
55. Lim C-F, Bernard HF, de Jong M, et al: A furan fatty acid and indoxyl sulphate are the putative inhibitors of thyroxine hepatocyte transport in uremia. J Clin Endocrinol Metab 76:318–324, 1993.
56. Vierhapper H, Laggner A, Waldhausl W, et al: Impaired secretion of TSH in critically ill patients with 'low T_4-syndrome.' Acta Endocrinol 101:542–549, 1982.
57. Van den Berghe G, De Zegher F, Baxter KRC, et al: Neuroendocrinology of prolonged critical illness: Effects of exogenous thyrotropin-releasing hormone and its combination with growth hormone secretagogues. J Clin Endocrinol Metab 83:309–319, 1998.
58. Brent GA, Hershman JM, Reed AW, et al: Serum angiotensin converting enzyme in severe nonthyroidal illness associated with low serum thyroxine concentration. Ann Intern Med 100:680–683, 1986.
59. Seppel T, Becker A, Lippert F, Schlaghecke R: Serum sex hormone–binding globulin and osteocalcin in systemic nonthyroidal illness associated with low thyroid hormone concentrations. J Clin Endocrinol Metab 81:1663–1665, 1996.
60. Lim VS, Tsalikian E, Flanigan MJ: Augmentation of protein degradation by l-triiodothyronine in uremia. Metabolism 38:1210–1215, 1989.
61. Chopra IJ, Chua Teco GN, Mead JF, et al: Relationship between serum free fatty acids and thyroid hormone binding inhibitor in nonthyroid illnesses. J Clin Endocrinol Metab 60:980–984, 1985.
62. Liewendahl K, Helenius T, Naveri H, Tikkanen H: Fatty acid–induced increase in serum dialyzable free thyroxine after physical exercise: Implication for nonthyroidal illness. J Clin Endocrinol Metab 74:1361–1365, 1992.
63. Chopra IJ, Huang TS, Beredo A, et al: Serum thyroid hormone binding inhibitor in nonthyroidal illnesses. Metabolism 35:152–159, 1986.
64. Chopra IJ, Huang TS, Beredo A, et al: Serum thyroid hormone binding inhibitor in nonthyroidal illnesses. Metabolism 35:152–159, 1986.
65. Chopra IJ, Solomon DH, Chua-Teco GN, Eisenberg JB: The presence of an inhibitor of serum binding of thyroid hormones in extrathyroidal tissues. Science 215:407–409, 1982.
66. Mendel CM, Frost PH, Cavalieri RR: Effect of free fatty acids on the concentration of free thyroxine in human serum: The role of albumin. J Clin Endocrinol Metab 63:1394–1399, 1986.
67. Jaume JC, Mendel CM, Frost PH, et al: Extremely low doses of heparin release lipase activity into the plasma and can thereby cause artifactual elevations in the serum-free thyroxine concentration as measured by equilibrium dialysis. Thyroid 6:79, 1996.
68. Csako G, Zweig MH, Benson C, Ruddel M: On the albumin-dependence of the measurement of free thyroxine. II. Patients with nonthyroidal illness. Clin Chem 33:87–92, 1987.
69. Mendel CM, Laughton CW, McMahon FA, Cavalieri RR: Inability to detect an inhibitor of thyroxine-serum protein binding in sera from patients with nonthyroidal illness. Metabolism 40:491–502, 1991.
70. Brent GA, Hershman JM: Thyroxine therapy in patients with severe nonthyroidal illnesses and lower serum thyroxine concentration. J Clin Endocrinol Metab 63:1–8, 1986.
71. Beale E, Srivastava P, Liang H, et al: Triiodothyroacetic acid (T_3AC)—is it an intracellular autocrine acting form of thyroid hormone (abstract OR1-1)? *In* Proceedings of the 79th Annual Meeting of the Endocrine Society. Minneapolis, MN, 1997.
72. Lim VS, Passo C, Murata Y, et al: Reduced triiodothyronine content in liver but not pituitary of the uremic rat model: Demonstration of changes compatible with thyroid hormone deficiency in liver only. Endocrinology 114:280–286, 1984.
73. Van den Berghe G, De Zegher F, Bouillon R: Acute and prolonged critical illness as different neuroendocrine paradigms. J Clin Endocrinol Metab 83:1827–1834, 1998.
74. van der Poll T, Romijn JA, Wiersinga WM, Saurwein HP: Tumor necrosis factor: A putative mediator of the sick euthyroid syndrome in man. J Clin Endocrinol Metab 71:1567–1572, 1990.
75. Chopra IJ, Sakane S, Chua Teco GN: A study of the serum concentration of tumor necrosis factor-α in thyroidal and nonthyroidal illnesses. J Clin Endocrinol Metab 72:1113–1116, 1991.
76. Hermus ARMM, Sweep CGJ, van der Meer MJM, et al: Continuous infusion of interleukin-1 induces a nonthyroidal illness syndrome in the rat. Endocrinology 131:2139–2146, 1992.
77. Cannon JG, Tompkins RG, Gelfand JA, et al: Circulating interleukin-1 and tumor necrosis factor in septic shock and experimental endotoxin fever. J Infect Dis 161:79–84, 1990.
78. van der Poll T, Van Zee KJ, Endert E, et al: Interleukin-1 receptor blockade does not affect endotoxin-induced changes in plasma thyroid hormone and thyrotropin concentrations in man. J Clin Endocrinol Metab 80:1341–1346, 1995.
79. Boelen A, Platvoet-ter Schiphorst MC, Wiersinga WM: Immunoneutralization of interleukin-1, tumor necrosis factor, interleukin-6 or interferon does not prevent the LPS-induced sick euthyroid syndrome in mice. J Endocrinol 153:115–122, 1997.
80. Stouthard JML, van der Poll T, Endert E, et al: Effects of acute and chronic interleukin-6 administration on thyroid hormone metabolism in humans. J Clin Endocrinol Metab 79:1342–1346, 1994.
81. Bartalena L, Brogioni S, Grasso L, et al: Relationship of the increased serum interleukin-6 concentration to changes of thyroid function in nonthyroidal illness. J Endocrinol Invest 17:269–274, 1994.
82. Boelen A, Platvoet-ter Schiphorst MC, Wiersinga WM: Association between serum interleukin-6 and serum 3,5,3′-triiodothyronine in nonthyroidal illness. J Clin Endocrinol Metab 77:1695–1699, 1993.
83. Boelen A, Platvoet-ter Schiphorst MC, Wiersinga WM: Relationship between serum 3,5,3′-triiodothyronine and serum interleukin-8, interleukin-10 or interferon-gamma in patients with nonthyroidal illness. J Endocrinol Invest 19:480–483, 1996.
84. Boelen A, Platvoet-ter Schiphorst MC, Wiersinga WM: Soluble cytokine receptors and the low 3,5,3′-triiodothyronine syndrome in patients with nonthyroidal disease. J Clin Endocrinol Metab 80:971–976, 1995.
85. Ahima RS, Prabakaran D, Mantzoros C, et al: Role of leptin in the neuroendocrine response to fasting. Nature 382:250–252, 1996.
86. Legradi G, Emerson CH, Ahima RS, et al: Leptin prevents fasting-induced suppression of prothyrotropin-releasing hormone messenger ribonucleic acid in neurons of the hypothalamic paraventricular nucleus. Endocrinology 138:2569–2576, 1997.

87. Legradi G, Emerson CH, Ahima RS, et al: Arcuate nucleus ablation prevents fasting-induced suppression of proTRH mRNA in the hypothalamic paraventricular nucleus. Neuroendocrinology 68:89–97, 1998.
88. Nicoloff JT, Fisher DA, Appleman MD Jr: The role of glucocorticoids in the regulation of thyroid function in man. J Clin Invest 49:1922, 1970.
89. Bianco AC, Nunes MT, Hell NS, Maciel RMB: The role of glucocorticoids in the stress-induced reduction of extrathyroidal 3,5,3′-triiodothyronine generation in rats. Endocrinology 120:1033–1038, 1987.
90. Custro N, Scafidi V, Costanzo G, Calanni S: Role of high blood glucagon in the reduction of serum levels of triiodothyronine in severe nonthyroid diseases. Minerva Endocrinol 14:221–226, 1989.
91. DeGroot LJ, Manowitz N, Chait L, Mayor G: Differential end organ responsiveness to suboptimal thyroid hormone concentrations as assessed by short-term withdrawal of levothyroxine sodium in athyreotic patients (abstract). *In* Proceedings of the 70th Annual Meeting of the American Thyroid Association. Colorado Springs, CO, 1997.
92. Chopra IJ, Chopra U, Smith Sr, et al: Reciprocal changes in serum concentrations of 3,3′,5′-triiodothyronine (reverse T_3) and 3,3′,5-triiodothyronine (T_3) in systemic illnesses. J Clin Endocrinol Metab 41:1043–1049, 1975.
93. Franklyn JA, Black EG, Betteridge J, Sheppard MC: Comparison of second and third generation methods for measurement of serum thyrotropin in patients with overt hyperthyroidism, patients receiving thyroxine therapy, and those with nonthyroidal illness. J Clin Endocrinol Metab 78:1368–1371, 1994.
94. Burmeister LA: Reverse T_3 does not reliably differentiate hypothyroid sick syndrome from euthyroid sick syndrome. Thyroid 5:435–442, 1995.
95. Van den Berghe G, de Zegher F, Lauwers P: Dopamine and the sick euthyroid syndrome in critical illness. Clin Endocrinol 41:731–737, 1994.
96. Spratt DI, Bigos ST, Beitins I, et al: Both hyper- and hypogonadotropic hypogonadism occur transiently in acute illness: Bio- and immunoactive gonadotropins. J Clin Endocrinol Metab 75:1562–1570, 1992.
97. Spratt DI, Cox P, Orav J, et al: Reproductive axis suppression in acute illness is related to disease severity. J Clin Endocrinol Metab 76:1548–1554, 1993.
98. Faber J, Kirkegaard C, Rasmussen B, et al: Pituitary-thyroid axis in critical illness. J Clin Endocrinol Metab 65:315–320, 1987.
99. Becker RA, Vaughan GM, Ziegler MG, et al: Hypermetabolic low triiodothyronine syndrome of burn injury. Crit Care Med 10:870–875, 1982.
100. Hesch RD, Husch M, Kodding R, et al: Treatment of dopamine-dependent shock with triiodothyronine. Endocr Res Commun 8:299–301, 1981.
101. Meyer T, Husch M, van den Berg E, et al: Treatment of dopamine-dependent shock with triiodothyronine: Preliminary results. Dtsch Med Wochenschr 104:1711–1714, 1979.
102. Dulchavsky SA, Maitra SR, Maurer J, et al: Beneficial effects of thyroid hormone administration on metabolic and hemodynamic function in hemorrhagic shock (abstract). FASEB J 4:952, 1990.
103. Novitzky D, Cooper DK, Reichart B: Hemodynamic and metabolic responses to hormonal therapy in brain-dead potential organ donors. Transplantation 43:852–855, 1987.
104. Dulchavsky SA, Hendrick SR, Dutta S: Pulmonary biophysical effects of triiodothyronine (T_3) augmentation during sepsis-induced hypothyroidism. Trauma 35:104–109, 1993.
105. Dulchavsky SA, Kennedy PR, Geller ER, et al: T_3 preserves respiratory function in sepsis. J Trauma 31:753–759, 1991.
106. Novitzky D, Cooper DKC, Zuhdi N: Triiodothyronine therapy in the cardiac transplant recipient. Transplant Proc 20:65–88, 1986.
107. Novitzky D, Cooper DKC, Chaffin JS, et al: Improved cardiac allograft function following triiodothyronine therapy to both donor and recipient. Transplantation 49:311–316, 1990.
108. Klemperer JD, Klein I, Gomez M, et al: Thyroid hormone treatment after coronary-artery bypass surgery. N Engl J Med 333:1522–1527, 1995.
109. Schoenberger W, Grimm W, Emmrich P, Gempp W: Thyroid administration lowers mortality in premature infants. Lancet 2:1181, 1979.
110. Bennett-Guerro E, Jimenez JL, White WD, et al: Cardiovascular effects of intravenous triiodothyronine in patients undergoing coronary artery bypass graft surgery. A randomized, double-blind, placebo-controlled trial. Duke T_3 Study Group. JAMA 275:687–692, 1996.
111. Hsu R-B, Huang T-S, Chen Y-S, Chu S-H: Effect of triiodothyronine administration in experimental myocardial injury. J Endocrinol Invest 18:702–709, 1995.
112. Shigematsu H, Shatney CH: The effect of triiodothyronine and reverse triiodothyronine on canine hemorrhagic shock. Nippon Geka Gakkai Zasshi 89:1587–1593, 1988.
113. Facktor MA, Mayor GH, Nachreiner RF, D'Alecy LG: Thyroid hormone loss and replacement during resuscitation from cardiac arrest in dogs. Resuscitation 26:141–162, 1993.
114. Chopra IJ, Huang TS, Boado R, et al: Evidence against benefit from replacement doses of thyroid hormones in nonthyroidal illness: Studies using turpentine oil–injected rat. J Endocrinol Invest 10:559–564, 1987.
115. Little JS: Effect of thyroid hormone supplementation on survival after bacterial infection. Endocrinology 117:1431–1435, 1985.
116. Yusuf S, Peto R, Lewis J, et al: Beta blockade during and after myocardial infarction: An overview of the randomized trials. Prog Cardiovasc Dis 27:335–371, 1985.
117. Hamilton MA, Stevenson LW: Thyroid hormone abnormalities in heart failure: Possibilities for therapy. Thyroid 6:527–529, 1996.
118. Chopra IJ: Nonthyroidal illness syndrome or euthyroid sick syndrome? Endocr Pract 2:45–52, 1996.

Chapter 107

Multinodular Goiter

Laszlo Hegedüs ▪ Hans Gerber

BASIC ASPECTS

Definition

Multinodular goiters are clinically recognizable enlargements of the thyroid gland characterized by excessive growth and structural and/or functional transformation of one or several areas within the normal thyroid tissue. Together with diffuse goiter and in the absence of thyroid dysfunction, autoimmune thyroid disease, thyroiditis, and thyroid malignancy, they constitute an entity described as "simple goiter." When associated with clinical and laboratory evidence of thyroid hyperfunction, it is called toxic multinodular goiter.

Clinical Manifestations

Multinodular goiter is very prevalent, especially in iodine-deficient areas. Most goiters are relatively small and produce few or no clinical symptoms (Table 107–1). When present, the clinical manifestations of multinodular goiter are related to those of the following:

- *Growth.* An anterior cervical or retrosternal/intrathoracic space-occupying mass is present. Symptoms and signs range from none (incidental finding) to varying degrees of pressure symptoms and signs: from a sensation of fullness to grotesque disfiguration with inspiratory stridor, disturbances in swallowing, cava-superior obstruction (rarely), and Horner's syndrome (rarely)—caused by pressure on the trachea, esophagus, cervical veins, and sympathetic nerves, respectively. Hoarseness is a rare symptom, but when present, the possibility of thyroid malignancy should be contemplated.
- *Function.* Patients with nontoxic multinodular goiter by definition do not have any symptoms or signs of thyroid dysfunction. However, many such goiters have a growth potential and, with that, the potential for increasing autonomy and hypersecretion of thyroid hormone. Because the condition is slowly evolving and most often seen in the elderly, the symptoms of hyperfunction are at variance with those seen in Graves' disease. Often, cardiovascular (congestive heart failure, atrial fibrillation) and gastrointestinal symptoms are dominant. Frequently, overt hyperthyroidism is preceded by a lengthy period of subclinical hyperthyroidism that may, when looked for, be associated with a number of organ manifestations in the central nervous system, heart, bone, and musculoskeletal system.

TABLE 107–1. Clinical Signs and Symptoms of Multinodular Goiter

Slowly growing nodular anterior neck mass
Enlargement during pregnancy
Tracheal deviation or compression, upper airway obstruction, dyspnea
Sudden pain or enlargement secondary to hemorrhage
Occasional cough and dysphagia
Gradually developing hyperthyroidism
Iodide-induced thyrotoxicosis
Superior vena cava obstruction syndrome
Recurrent nerve palsy (rare)
Horner's syndrome (rare)

Morphology

Macroscopic and Microscopic Aspects

The macroscopic, histologic, autoradiographic, and immunohistochemical aspects of simple goiters are extremely variable. At one end of the large spectrum are scattered areas consisting of small clusters of morphologically normal, but functionally abnormal follicles that take up iodide at a slower or faster rate than surrounding normal tissue does. At the other end of the spectrum is a grossly enlarged thyroid containing numerous nodules of widely differing size, structure, and function. In fact, a considerable degree of regional heterogeneity, structural as well as functional, is—together with the invariably present nodule formation—the most characteristic hallmark of simple goiters[1–10] (Fig. 107–1).

The microscopic appearance of thyroid nodules has been well known since the early days of thyroid histology.[11] A nodule may consist of either small follicles with little stored colloid and high cuboidal cells or large follicles containing huge amounts of colloid held together by a thin layer of flat cells. Many nodules contain small and large follicles side by side. In nodular and extranodular goiter tissue, varying amounts of extracellular matrix may separate individual follicles or groups of follicles.[12] Cyst formation, hemorrhage, fibrosis, and calcification are also common findings.[1, 2, 12]

The classic morphologic criteria of "thyroid activity," such as columnar epithelium, low follicular diameter, and thin colloid, may be a sign of functional activity in some cases. However, autoradiographic studies have clearly shown that very quiescent-appearing tissue with flat thyrocytes surrounding large follicles may have considerable radioiodine or thymidine incorporation.[1–4, 7, 8] These and other experiments[13] have definitely challenged the classic concepts of regulation of follicular size and morphology. For example, iodine depletion and repletion have very considerable effects on thyroid morphology and in particular on follicular size.[14] Therefore, general histologic criteria are not valid for the unequivocal and reliable identification of thyroid functional and proliferative activity.

Immunohistochemistry and Autoradiography

Immunohistochemical studies have contributed to the understanding of goiter pathogenesis, but a note of caution should be made at this point. A number of growth factors such as epidermal growth factor (EGF), insulin-like growth factor type I (IGF-I), and fibroblast growth

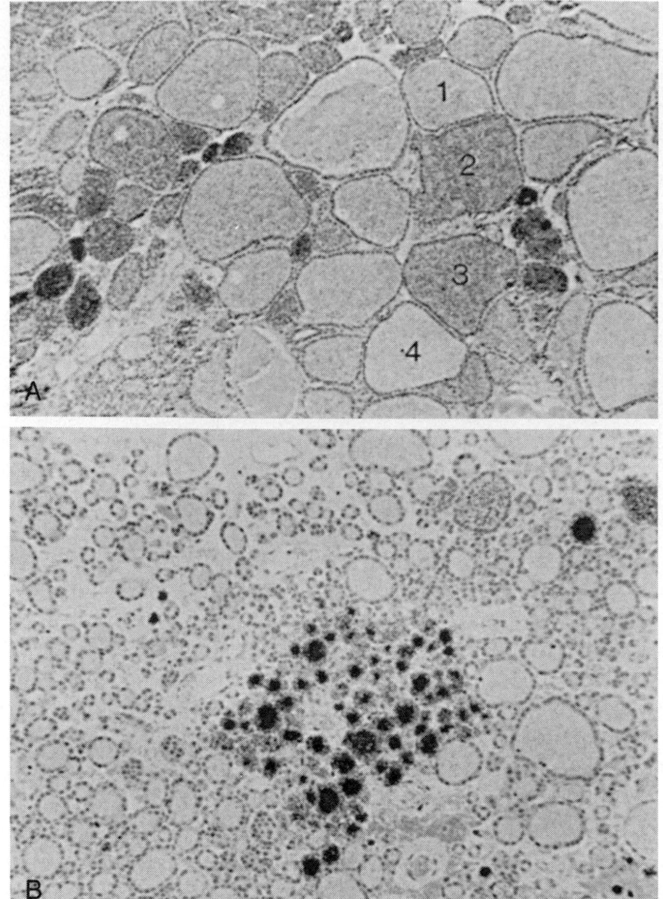

FIGURE 107–1. Autoradiograph of nodular goiters illustrating interfollicular heterogeneity in iodine metabolism. *A,* Hot nodule. ^{125}I was given 14 days before surgery (hematoxylin-eosin ×88; exposure time, 45 days). Many follicles of this active nodule escape the law of an inverse correlation between follicular size and relative velocity of intrafollicular iodine turnover that is characteristic of normal thyroid glands. For example, follicles numbered 1 to 4 are morphologically similar. Nevertheless, grain density is considerably higher in follicles 2 and 3 than in the adjacent follicles 1 and 4. This example is but one illustration of the fundamental functional difference between normal and goiter follicles. In addition, the autoradiograph demonstrates the nearly total lack of correlation between the morphology of a follicle and the intensity of its iodine turnover. *B,* Hyperthyroid nodular goiter. ^{125}I was given 17 hours before surgery (nuclear fast red, ×110; exposure time, 24 days). A cohort of tiny follicles with intense iodine metabolism has grown amidst morphologically identical follicles with very little iodine turnover. Additional hot and intermediately active follicles are scattered all over. No capsule of connective tissue delimiting hot from cold follicles is present. Here, a large number of morphologically identical, but functionally very heterogeneous, microfollicles have been generated in the process of goitrogenesis.

factor types 1 and 2 (FGF-1 and FGF-2) are involved in thyroid growth regulation and can easily be stained with immunohistochemical methods.[10, 15–18] Because these growth factors are expressed in variable and probably episodic patterns in thyroid tissue in many different disease entities, their presence has to be interpreted with caution and cannot be used directly to identify autonomous areas. The same holds true for proto-oncogene products such as p21ras and proliferation markers such as Ki-67 and proliferating cell nuclear antigen. It may be misleading to draw any conclusions on thyrocyte or follicular proliferation or autonomy from the spatially and temporarily variable expression pattern of growth factors, growth factor receptors, and proto-oncogene products, and actual proliferation as the endpoint of all regulatory mechanisms has in fact to be studied and documented.

Autoradiography offers a very elegant and reliable way to study thyroid-stimulating hormone (TSH)-dependent and autonomous follicular function and proliferation. The classic way of studying autonomous function by autoradiography is to label the human or animal thyroid gland with radioiodine after suppressing the individual's TSH, be it an experimental animal,[19] a nude mouse bearing human or animal transplants,[8, 20–23] or a human patient.[1–6] Under these conditions, autoradiography reveals autonomous iodine incorporation and therefore allows identification of autonomously functioning areas. With the same technique it is also possible to demonstrate thymidine incorporation in thyroid cells, follicles, or tissue in vivo and in vitro after labeling with ^{3}H-thymidine.[1–3, 7, 8, 20–23] To prove functional and proliferative autonomy of thyroid tissue, autoradiography is therefore a very helpful method, and simple morphology and immunohistochemistry do not substantially contribute to this end.

Circumscribed areas of tissue with definite proliferative or functional autonomy—as proved by autoradiography after labeling with ^{3}H-thymidine or radioiodine in the absence of TSH—can be identified, cut out from autoradiographs, and processed for molecular biologic studies. We have recently reported TSH receptor mutations in hot areas of multinodular goiters labeled with ^{125}I preoperatively in patients with endogenously or exogenously suppressed TSH.[24] It must be emphasized that for meaningful studies of the molecular aspects of thyroid autonomy, the scientist has to be certain that the tissue investigated really is autonomous. This issue is particularly important in view of the well-known heterogeneity of human goiter tissue (see below). An impressive autoradiographic illustration of functional heterogeneity is provided by the coexistence, within the same goiter, of cold follicles caused by a trapping defect along with morphologically identical follicles that are unable to organify the normally trapped iodide.[9] The unique heterogeneity of size, shape, and iodine turnover among the individual follicles is one of the most characteristic hallmarks of nodular goiter.[1–4] The heterogeneity of iodine trapping and incorporation reflects the striking heterogeneity of Na^+/I^- symporter (NIS) expression in human goiter tissue, as demonstrated recently by Jhiang et al.[25] (Fig. 107–2).

The autoradiographic findings explain why a scintiscan of a nodular goiter with ^{131}I or ^{99m}Tc-pertechnetate invariably shows a mottled aspect. This appearance may be caused by different mechanisms: (1) smaller or larger clusters of hot follicles may be scattered throughout the entire goiter, (2) the goiter may contain hot nodules embedded within normal or suppressed paranodular tissue, and (3) the goiter may contain cysts and/or connective tissue in various states of degeneration. In view of the differences in iodide clearance and iodine discharge from one nodule to another or even from one follicle to its neighbor, the appearance of a ^{131}I scintiscan is expected to vary considerably in accordance with the time elapsed since administration of the tracer. In view of the autoradiographic findings and the fact that roughly half of all benign thyroid nodules are completely cold, scintigraphy is of little help in deciding whether a growing nodule should be surgically explored. Moreover, although in single autonomous adenomas the degree of suppression of surrounding tissue is believed to be inversely correlated with the amount of hormone produced by the nodule, this rule does not apply to goiters containing autonomously functioning micronodules scattered all over the gland.

Biochemistry

In this section, only some findings regarding thyroglobulin and iodine are briefly discussed. For a review of biochemical studies on the regulation of thyroid growth and function in normal and goitrous tissue, see Chapter 96.

Thyroglobulin in endemic or sporadic nodular goiters is often poorly iodinated but can be readily iodinated in vitro (see Chapter 92). The simplest explanation for the pathogenesis of poorly iodinated thyroglobulin in the absence of iodine shortage is the loss of normal synchronization in goiter follicles between the cellular process of thyroglobulin synthesis and endocytosis on the one hand and iodide transport and organification on the other hand. Low iodination of thyroglobulin is a very serious handicap for hormone synthesis and has a profound impact on thyroidal iodine turnover.[26] Indeed, iodine content is the most decisive single factor regulating the iodothyronine content of thyroglobulin. The ratio of iodothyronine to iodotyrosine

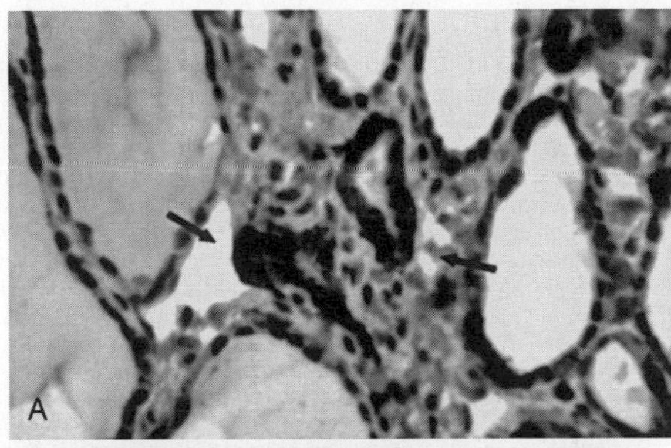

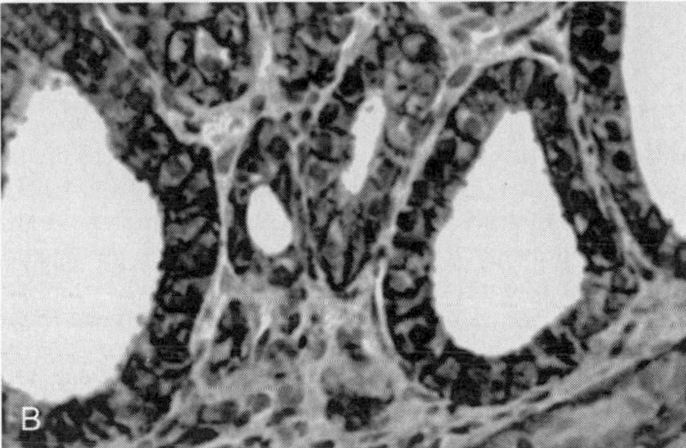

FIGURE 107–2. Immunohistochemical staining for the human Na^+/I^- symporter (hNIS) in human thyroid tissues. *A,* Only a minority of thyrocytes in normal thyroid tissues were stained by anti-hNIS (indicated by *arrows*) when the thyroid tissues are not stimulated by elevated thyroid-stimulating hormone (TSH). *B,* Most thyrocytes in Graves' thyroid tissues were strongly stained by anti-hNIS at the basal and lateral membranes. Note the complete absence of hNIS staining in the fibroblasts of connective tissues. The tissue sections were counterstained with hematoxylin. Panels *A* and *B* were taken under the same magnification. (From Jhiang SM, Cho JY, Ryu KY, et al: An immunohistochemical study of Na^+/I^- symporter in human thyroid tissues and salivary gland tissues. Endocrinology 139:4416–4419, 1998, © 1998, The Endocrine Society.)

residues is severely depressed in poorly iodinated thyroglobulin.[26] Consequently, a larger fraction of poorly iodinated thyroglobulin must be broken down to produce the same amount of hormone.

The concentration of total iodine per gram of wet tissue is low in most multinodular goiters, although this finding is not true for every single area within a goiter.[26] The total amount of iodine per goiter is, surprisingly enough, as high as or even higher than that in normal glands, but not all iodine stores may be available for hormone synthesis.[26] The existence of different iodine compartments in human and experimental animal goiters has been known for a long time. They may well be of functional relevance, for example, in the adaptation of thyroid hormone secretion to antithyroid drugs or in severe and prolonged iodine deficiency when very slow compartments may become an important source of minimal quantities of iodine and thyroid hormone.[26, 27] Colloid inclusions, for example, may well explain the surprisingly large total iodine store in human endemic goiters, even in the presence of severe iodine deficiency. Up to 70% of the total iodine can be found, for example, in the particulate fraction of human nodular goiters in Switzerland.[26] In any case, "total thyroidal iodine" is a very crude measure. It is evident that the existence of multiple iodine compartments and, in particular, the existence of particulate slow-turnover pools complicate the interpretation of total glandular iodine measurements with modern techniques such as x-ray fluorescence, positron emission tomography, and others.

Pathogenesis

Goiter Growth

Nodular goiters result from focal hyperplasia of follicular cells at one or multiple sites within the thyroid gland. The basic process in goitrogenesis is the generation of new follicular cells, which are used either to form new follicles or to enlarge the size of the newly formed follicles.[1–4] The driving force behind multinodular goiter growth is the intrinsically abnormal growth potential of a small fraction of the thyroid cells,[1–4] in much the same way as in other benign tumors. Extrathyroidal and intrathyroidal growth factors may act on this basic process and thereby accelerate goiter growth.

Regulation of thyroid growth and function is amply discussed in Chapters 93 and 96. In our chapter, this section is therefore only briefly addressed, with a focus on nodular goiter growth.

A number of growth factors such as TSH, IGF-I, FGF-1 and FGF-2, EGF, and others are involved in thyroid growth regulation. TSH is undoubtedly the most important stimulator of thyroid growth and function under physiologic in vivo conditions.[28] However, experimental results, obtained mostly with cell cultures, have clearly established the growth-promoting effect of some ubiquitous growth factors such as EGF, IGF-I, FGF-1, and FGF-2[1–4, 28–31] and the growth-inhibiting action of others such as transforming growth factor-β[32] (see also Chapters 93 and 96). Their role in in vivo growth remains to be clarified, but undoubtedly the local production of such growth factors, including proto-oncogene products, is severely altered in nodular goiters. Such alteration has been shown for IGF-I, FGF-1, and FGF-2, which are produced in loco by autonomously growing thyroid nodules.[15–17] Although few authors doubt the decisive role of TSH—together with autoregulatory mechanisms triggered by thyroidal iodine depletion—in endemic goiter caused by iodine deficiency (see Chapter 108), multinodular goiter has a different pathogenesis in nonendemic areas. In this case, it is an intrinsic disease of the thyroid gland. To put it in simple terms, multinodular goiter is a multifocally growing benign tumor of the thyroid gland.[1–4] Indeed, it has recently been demonstrated that growth of nodular goiter proceeds by episodic, autonomous replication of a multitude of cell cohorts scattered all over the single nodules and even over presumably normal extranodular tissue.[10]

It is on this substrate that extrathyroidal growth-stimulating agents such as TSH (in the case of iodine deficiency) or thyroid-stimulating immunoglobulin (in the case of Graves' disease) may come to act. Some authors have described "growth-stimulating immunoglobulins" in patients with nodular goiters, but their existence is still controversial[33] (see Chapter 100). Whatever extrathyroidal stimulus may be present, the inevitable nodularity of a long-standing goiter can be understood only if the constitutive heterogeneity of the growth response between individual cells is taken into account.[1–4] If thyroid-stimulating agents are present in the blood stream in high concentration, diffuse hyperplastic goiters result. This point is illustrated, on the one hand, by Graves' disease (see Chapter 100) and, on the other, by the TSH-induced thyroid hyperplasia in severe endemic goiter or in experimentally induced goiters in laboratory animals.[13] However, the evolution of an entirely different intrinsic thyroid disease, namely, simple nodular goiter, may be promoted if only small amounts of stimulating agents are circulating in the blood, as in the case of slightly increased TSH or other growth factors. In this event, response is seen in only the most sensitive of all follicular functions, which is the replication of a few cells with an unusually high growth potential.[1–4] Because proliferation of these particular cells is stimulated without concomitant hypertrophy (which is produced by different mechanisms), gentle growth promotion acting for a long enough period produces nodules consisting of a large number of new follicles lacking the morphologic signs of acute hyperstimulation.

Over the years, ample evidence for an important role of iodine as a moderator of thyroid growth and function has accumulated (see also Chapter 108). The mechanisms through which thyroid growth is induced in iodine deficiency are still somewhat controversial. The classic concept states that any shortage in iodide supply decreases thyroid hormone secretion by intrathyroidal autoregulation, thereby increasing TSH long before the thyroid becomes markedly depleted of iodine. In recent years, the direct growth-inducing effect of iodine depletion through intrathyroidal mechanisms irrespective of increased TSH has been postulated mainly by Gärtner.[29] In our view, both mechanisms are at play in iodine depletion–induced goitrogenesis. Depending on the degree of iodine deficiency, one of them may prevail: In heavy iodine deficiency, probably TSH increases, whereas in moderate iodine

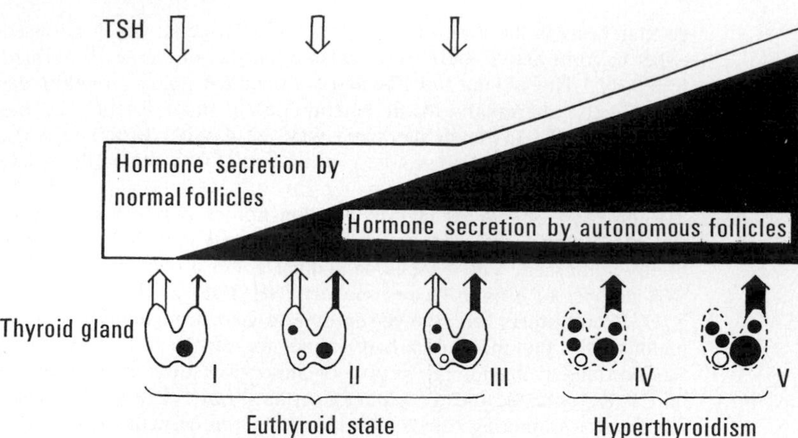

FIGURE 107–3. Evolution of hyperthyroidism in multinodular goiter. As the goiter progresses in the course of many years or decades from stage I to stage V, an increasing number of follicles with high rates of autonomous iodine turnover are generated. Some hot follicles form large clusters and mimic hot adenomas *(black areas)*, whereas others are scattered throughout the gland. Their joint hormone production insidiously rises and eventually (stage III) exceeds the needs of the organism. At this point, endogenous thyroid-stimulating hormone (TSH) secretion is shut off, and hormone production in normal follicles is thereby set at its lowest possible level (which is always somewhat above zero). Simultaneously, nodules that consist of cold follicles *(white area)* may also develop but do not contribute to hormone synthesis. (From Braverman LE, Utiger R (eds): Werner's and Ingbar's The Thyroid, ed 7. Philadelphia, JB Lippincott, 1996.)

deficiency, the autoregulatory mechanism prevails. In addition, the relationship between dietary iodide intake and its availability to the thyroid is influenced by a number of factors such as thiocyanate and other goitrogens (see below).

Goiter Function

Because most follicles have at least some degree of nonsuppressible iodine turnover and many of the newly formed hot follicles have a much higher than average autonomous iodine turnover, overall hormone production by any nodular goiter depends on the number of new follicles on the one hand and on the relative fraction of cold and hot follicles on the other. Because follicle neogeneration is a slow process, most nodular goiters are euthyroid, and thyrotoxicosis insidiously appears only in the course of many years.[1–6, 34, 35] This pattern is in sharp contrast to the stormy onset of Graves' thyrotoxicosis (see Chapter 100). The pathogenetic concept of Plummer's disease (i.e., thyrotoxicosis caused by multinodular goiters) is, in essence, that originally proposed by Miller and Block[5] some 30 years ago[1–6] (Fig. 107–3).

Generation of Heterogeneity

In addition to somatic mutations leading to clonal tumor growth (see Chapters 102 and 109), three basically different phenomena are involved in generation of the tremendous regional heterogeneity in growth, structure, and function of multinodular human goiters.[1–10, 18, 25]

CONSTITUTIVE HETEROGENEITY OF NORMAL FOLLICULAR CELLS. A normal follicle consists of a number of cell subsets with widely differing qualities. For instance, some normal follicular cells have a very high capacity to iodinate thyroglobulin, whereas others almost completely lack this quality.[1–4, 19] Similarly, large differences in the expression of peroxidase, thyroglobulin, and NIS may exist between different cells within the same follicle.[1–4, 25] Perhaps most impressive is the enormous variation in growth potential among the many cell families building up a single follicle.[1–4, 7–9] Some of the cells may have constitutively active growth mechanisms enabling them to proliferate autonomously in much the same way as the cells of other benign tumors[1–4] (Fig. 107–4). This type of intercellular heterogeneity is probably not due to somatic mutations but to a number of epigenetic mechanisms whose ability to change the phenotype and function of daughter cells and their progeny is becoming increasingly known. Somatic mutations may, of course, occur in dividing cells, in addition to their diversity caused by epigenetic events.

ACQUISITION OF NEW INHERITABLE QUALITIES BY REPLICATING EPITHELIAL CELLS. Modern molecular biology has recognized that the gene expression of a cell is less uniform and immutable than hitherto thought and that newly generated cells may well acquire qualities not previously present in the mother cells by mechanisms that do not involve genomic mutations.[36] New qualities may also be passed on from mother to daughter cells by extrachromosomal mechanisms. Although the appearance of entirely new cell qualities acquired by mechanisms operating in addition to somatic mutation is well known in malignant tumors,[36] intercellular heterogeneity has rather recently been recognized to be a feature of normal cells as well.[1–4, 19, 37] Growing, simple goiters provide unique examples of the acquisition of new inheritable properties by some cell sublines of autonomously replicating benign human tissue.[1–4] The most impressive example of this process is the abnormal growth pattern of all or part of human and animal goiter tissue that is faithfully reproduced when a tiny sample grows as a transplant in a nude mouse.[8, 20–22] Other regionally variable functional properties of human goitrous tissue, such as responsiveness to TSH,[37] may arise in the same way.

SECONDARY FUNCTIONAL AND STRUCTURAL ABNORMALITIES IN GROWING GOITERS. New follicles produced during goitrogenesis may have widely differing qualities depending on the individual mother cells from which they originate. Replicating follicular cells with a high thyroglobulin and colloid production rate but low capacity for endocytosis produce large follicles. In addition, morphologic and histochemical evidence indicates that follicles of the second and subsequent generations, formed during goiter growth, are less perfectly built than their mother follicles and therefore the multiple coordinated function of a single follicle, such as iodide transport, thyroglobulin synthesis, storage, endocytosis, and deiodination, may become desynchronized.[1–4] A striking example of the impact of secondary failure of a particular cell function comes from the conversion,

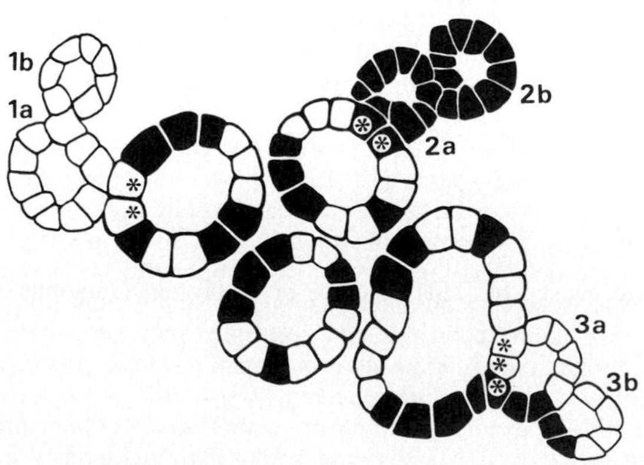

FIGURE 107–4. Generation of two consecutive progenies of heterogeneous daughter follicles from normal polyclonal mother follicles. *Asterisks* indicate normal follicular cells with a high intrinsic growth potential that is transmissible to the offspring. The whole progeny therefore divides at a higher than average rate, either autonomously or in response to an extrathyroidal stimulus such as thyroid-stimulating hormone (TSH). *Solid black,* high peroxidase content; *solid white,* low peroxidase content; *1,* cold follicle; *2,* hot follicle; *3,* mixed follicle. (From Gerber H, Peter HJ, Ramelli F, et al: Autonomie und Heterogenität der Follikel in der euthyreoten und hyperthyreoten menschlichen Knotenstruma: Die Lösung alter Rätsel? Schweiz Med Wochenschr 113:1178, 1983.)

in the aging mouse and hamster thyroid, of an ever-increasing number of follicles into oversized, colloid-stuffed, and functionless units.[38, 39]

Autonomy

Most people will agree that in clinical thyroidology, autonomy means "autonomy from TSH," that is, growth or function of the thyroid gland or part of it in the absence of TSH. We should keep in mind that autonomous growth or function in the absence of TSH in no way precludes the further stimulation of growth or function by TSH. It is also important to realize that autonomous function and autonomous growth may be entirely unrelated qualities of individual thyroid cells.[1–4, 7, 8] This concept explains the common clinical observation that cold areas of nodular goiter have exactly the same growth potential as hot ones. Similarly, they may both respond or be refractory to TSH-suppressing thyroxine (T_4) treatment.

AUTONOMY OF GROWTH. Normal thyroid glands contain subpopulations of follicular cells with a constitutively high growth potential.[1–4, 7, 8] In thyroid tissue destined to become a goiter, a fraction of these cells may replicate autonomously, that is, by constitutive activation of the cell's own growth machinery. Some molecular mechanisms, such as, for example, activating TSH receptor and G protein mutations causing accelerated cell growth, have been unraveled in toxic nodules[40, 41] (see Chapter 102). Recently, TSH receptor mutations have also been demonstrated in some multinodular goiters.[24, 40, 41] The autonomous cells, scattered in multiple small foci all over the gland, divide at variable individual rates even in the absence of TSH. Autonomously growing cells steadily take a larger share of the entire follicular cell population. This process results in the growth of clinically apparent nodules and may evolve at such a rate that rapidly growing polyclonal and even monoclonal nodules appear even in children and young adults. Once the autonomously growing and rapidly dividing cells are present in large enough numbers, the whole thyroid or parts thereof may autonomously grow in the absence of any further extrathyroidal stimulation.[1–4, 7, 8, 23]

Autonomously growing cells in the adult thyroid behave very much like the thyrocytes of fetal glands. Indeed, evidence suggests that these cells have failed to develop the control system transforming autonomously growing fetal cells into TSH-dependent adult cells.[21] The largely autonomous, that is, TSH-independent, nature of nonendemic goiter is demonstrated by the common failure of TSH-suppressing doses of T_4 to stop progression of nodular growth,[42] let alone revert a nodular goiter into normal thyroid tissue. However, because TSH, even in low concentrations, is still one of many growth factors, a certain growth-retarding effect is often observed even in largely autonomous goiters.

AUTONOMY OF FUNCTION. It has been mentioned before that the normal thyroid contains subsets of cells with constitutively higher than average iodinating capacity. If new follicles happen to arise from these cells, they have high iodine turnover as well[1–4] (see Fig. 107–4). Their intrinsic metabolism is less suppressible by abolition of TSH secretion than that of their genuinely less active sister cells, although some degree of residual autonomous iodine turnover is present in most follicular cells.[1–9, 19] Not discussed in detail here is the functional autonomy caused by TSH receptor or G protein mutations[24, 40, 41, 43] (see Chapters 102 and 109).

Nodule Formation

It is a common observation that nearly every long-standing goiter and even most normal thyroids of aged individuals become nodular with time.[1–4, 34, 44, 45] In most cases, no morphologic, functional, or biochemical characteristic clearly distinguishes these nodules from extranodular tissue. Thyroidal nodule formation can be explained by three mechanisms[1–4]: (1) The presence of thyrocyte subpopulations and their tendency to remain clustered cause uneven proliferation within the thyroid gland and lead to focal hyperplasia or nodular transformation over the years. The chronic growth stimulation can be caused by a number of different agents such as TSH—raised by goitrogens or iodine deficiency—or any other growth factor. (2) Another mechanism is somatic mutation conferring a heritable growth advantage to a single cell and finally resulting in the formation of a clonal tumor. (3) A third mechanism is the nodular growth pattern caused by the network of fibrous strands resulting from the scarring necrosis and hemorrhage that occur in most growing goiters.

CLONALITY OF THYROID NODULES. The question whether thyroid nodules are monoclonal or polyclonal has been addressed by several groups in recent years.[46–51] Thomas et al.[46] studied X-linked isoenzyme expression in the thyroid nodules of heterozygous individuals, whereas other authors have made use of the methylation patterns of X-linked restriction fragment polymorphisms as clonal markers. Our group has introduced the highly informative polymorphic X chromosome probe M27β in the thyroid field and performed clonal analysis of thyroid nodules.[49] Using the same probe, Kopp et al.[50] and Bamberger et al.[51] have more recently demonstrated the coexistence of polyclonal and monoclonal nodules within nonendemic and endemic multinodular goiters. The coexistence of polyclonal and monoclonal nodules within individual goiters is in accord with the concepts of goitrogenesis outlined above. Cells with an intrinsically high proliferation rate have a higher chance of acquiring somatic mutations such as activating point mutations in oncogenes or allelic deletions of tumor suppressor genes. Any single cell undergoing such a mutation will then clonally outgrow the other thyroid cells.[1–4, 24]

Etiology

Worldwide, the most frequent single cause of endemic multinodular goiter is still iodine deficiency (see Chapter 108). In areas where the iodine supply is scarce, TSH-mediated and autoregulatory intrathyroid compensatory mechanisms are set into motion.[1–4, 29, 52] As a consequence, the thyroid gland diffusely enlarges and, as time passes, gradually becomes nodular by the mechanisms described above.

Iodine deficiency, however, is not the only cause of endemic goiter because a high prevalence of goiter has been reported from areas where the iodine supply is abundant and because multinodular goiter continues to prevail, although at a low prevalence, in areas such as Switzerland, where iodine deficiency has long been eradicated.[1–4, 53]

Goitrogenic environmental and dietary factors besides iodine deficiency have been discussed in some areas,[51, 55] but they do not seem to be involved in the vast majority of sporadic and endemic goiters. Thiocyanate, for example, is a goitrogen generated from cigarette smoke[53, 56] and produced metabolically from such components as glucosinolates and glucosides found in vegetable foods such as cassava.[54, 55]

The role of circulating growth factors such as growth hormone and IGF-I in goitrogenesis is well illustrated by the development of goiter in many patients with acromegaly[57] and the low goiter prevalence in pygmies.[4, 58]

The foregoing section on pathogenesis should make it clear that nonendemic nodular goiters are, just as in other clonal and polyclonal benign tumors, the late results of intrinsic disorders of intracellular growth control mechanisms. The goitrogenic process is induced or in some cases speeded by environmental, dietary, endocrine, and other factors. In clonal thyroid nodules, a somatic cell mutation activating an intrinsic growth control cascade is thought to be the initial culprit (see Chapters 102 and 109).

Heredity

The clustering of thyroid diseases, including simple goiters, in some families has prompted a host of investigations on the possible role of hereditary factors in the genesis of euthyroid goiter. Existing evidence indicates that genetic factors help determine the development of goiter, but no simple mode of inheritance has been identified up to now.

Since the discovery of inherited disorders of thyroid hormone synthesis (see Chapter 112), the suspicion has arisen that in sporadic and possibly even endemic goiter, such a disorder could be at least an ancillary causative factor. However, none of the inherited disorders of thyroid hormone synthesis or action has been convincingly demonstrated to be responsible for the bulk of sporadic or endemic multinodular goiters. All abnormalities of iodine metabolism found in this disease may be explained as secondary events. Very recently, a historical cohort study of 5479 twin pairs in Denmark has provided evidence that genetic factors play a major role in the etiology of simple goiter in women living in nonendemic goiter areas with borderline iodine deficiency,[59] but unraveling the hereditary basis of nonendemic multinodular goiter still remains a rather remote goal.

CLINICAL ASPECTS

Occurrence

Epidemiologic studies of multinodular goiter are hampered by problems such as selection criteria (age, sex), influence of environmental factors (e.g., iodine intake and smoking habits), evaluation of size and morphology (palpation, ultrasound, scintigraphy), and determination of thyroid function and whether subjects with subclinical hyperthyroidism are categorized as euthyroid or hyperthyroid. Most studies have focused on middle-aged women and the elderly, whereas only few have documented the prevalence of multinodular thyroid disease in a cross-sectional investigation of the adult population in a community. Longitudinal studies covering many years are necessary to give valid figures on incidence, etiologic risk factors, and the natural history. Such studies that take the above-mentioned problems into consideration are not available. These limitations should therefore be borne in mind when considering the available data.

Iodine deficiency is still the most frequent single cause of multinodular endemic goiter worldwide (see Chapter 108). Considerable regional variation exists even in nonendemic goiter areas. In the Whickham survey, 16% of the cohort had simple goiter.[60, 61] In men, the prevalence declined with age from 7% in those younger than 25 years to 4% in those older than 65 years. Among women, the frequency declined from 31% in those younger than 45 years to 12% in those older than 75 years. No man older than 75 years had goiter. In view of the well-known relation of thyroid volume to age and body weight,[62] it is interesting that cross-sectional surveys seem to indicate a decline in the prevalence of goiter with age.[63] Because lean body mass decreases with age, this finding is compatible with lean body mass being the major determinant of thyroid size.[64]

As an illustration of the influence of iodine intake on the epidemiology of sporadic goiter as well, 31 of 423 (7.3%) 68-year-olds had goiter in Jutland, Denmark (low iodine intake area), vs. 2 of 100 (2%) in Reykjavik, Iceland (high iodine intake area).[65]

A cross-sectional study of the community in Whickham found a prevalence of hyperthyroidism of 25 per 1000 women and 2 per 1000 men in an adult population.[61] Others have found similar figures.[61] The yearly incidence of hyperthyroidism (all types) varies between 0.1 and 0.2 per 1000 men and 0.3 and 1.3 per 1000 women. As with nontoxic goiter, iodine intake is of paramount importance inasmuch as countries with low iodine intake have a high proportion of multinodular toxic goiter (Denmark, 50%)[66] whereas countries with high or sufficient iodine intake have a lower proportion of multinodular goiter (Iceland, 6%)[67] and more cases of Graves' disease.

Natural History

The natural history of multinodular goiter, with respect to goiter growth and function, varies and is difficult to predict in a given patient. The goiter can remain stable in size or grow very slowly over many years. The spontaneous growth rate in selected populations has been estimated to be up to 20% yearly[68] but is usually much lower. Rapid growth of one or several nodules is also possible. No specific parameter exists that can accurately predict the growth potential of multinodular goiter. This potential can be accurately assessed by serial yearly measurements of the size of the goiter and individual nodules by ultrasonography.[62]

Painful nodules are usually the result of hemorrhage into a nodule or a cyst in the goiter. The diagnosis is readily made by ultrasonographic examination and fine-needle aspiration biopsy. Such a growing painful nodule may represent thyroid malignancy and should be investigated accordingly.

Multinodular goiter is not usually associated with a significantly increased risk for the development of thyroid malignancy. However, any fast-growing goiter or thyroid nodule is capable of harboring a malignancy and should undergo biopsy or be removed.[69, 70]

Patients with nontoxic multinodular goiter can become hyperthyroid or, less commonly, hypothyroid. However, thyroid dysfunction usually develops only after the nontoxic goiter has existed for many years. Hyperthyroidism in such patients often develops insidiously, in contrast to that of Graves' disease. It often begins with a prolonged period of subclinical hyperthyroidism characterized by low serum TSH and normal serum free T_4 and triiodothyronine (T_3) concentrations.[71, 72] This hyperthyroid state is the consequence of goiter growth and an associated increase in the mass of autonomously hormone-producing thyroid cells.[34, 35] Hyperthyroidism can also be the result of an increase in iodine intake from iodine-containing drugs such as disinfectants and amiodarone or from radiographic contrast agents, which, in a goiter with increased autonomous iodine metabolism, leads to the production of excessive amounts of thyroid hormone.

Development of hypothyroidism in a patient with multinodular nontoxic goiter is rarer. This observation is difficult to explain because goiters in such patients usually contain considerable amounts of iodine.[26]

Diagnosis

Clinical Examination

With practice, the thyroid gland can also be palpated when of normal size, but to most the thyroid gland does not become palpable until the volume has doubled. A visibly diffusely enlarged goiter has often reached a volume of 30 to 40 mL. Detection of nodules depends on their size, morphology, location within the thyroid parenchyma, anatomy of the patient's neck, and most of all, the training of the physician. The patient is usually unaware of the presence of nodules smaller than 2 cm in diameter. Awareness may, however, depend on localization, speed of growth, and the possible pain or discomfort related to hemorrhage into a nodule (Table 107–2).

Inspection and palpation of the neck, preferably done with the patient swallowing gulps of water and the head tilted slightly backward, may disclose anything from a single nodule in an otherwise normal nonpalpable thyroid to a large compressive multinodular gland extending retroclavicularly or into the mediastinum. In young thin subjects, most nodules 1 cm in diameter or larger can be palpated. If anteriorly located, even smaller nodules may be detected. Nevertheless, it seems that clinical examination of the thyroid is a lost or unlearned art for many physicians as demonstrated by considerable interobserver and intraobserver variation regarding size and morphology of the thyroid.[73]

Although clinical diagnosis of nodular goiter is usually considered to be straightforward, differential diagnostic considerations include goitrous autoimmune thyroiditis, thyroid cancer, and rarely, long-standing Graves' disease, in which the gland may become firm and irregular. It should be borne in mind that physical examination of the thyroid

TABLE 107–2. Diagnosis of Multinodular Goiter

Multinodularity on examination
Asymmetry, tracheal deviation
No adenopathy
Thyroid-stimulating hormone normal or decreased, free thyroxine and free triiodothyronine normal or increased, thyroglobulin elevated
Calcitonin normal
Thyroid antibodies negative in approximately 90%
Scintigraphy with hot and cold areas
Ultrasound finding of nodularity (nonhomogeneity)
Computed tomography and magnetic resonance imaging demonstrating a nonhomogeneous mass
Fine-needle aspiration of dominant nodules—benign cytology

includes examination of the neck, as well as the regional lymph nodes and the trachea, but also that glands harboring malignancy are in many cases indistinguishable from those that are not.

Laboratory Investigations

Because transition from nontoxic to toxic goiter is part of the natural history of this disease[34, 35, 71, 72] and because detection of borderline, but clinically relevant hyperthyroidism requires laboratory tests, annual screening with a sensitive TSH assay is recommended. The possibility of hyperthyroidism must be considered in any goitrous patient with otherwise unexplained illness. This point is particularly true for patients with cardiac failure or arrhythmias. Subnormal serum TSH values should lead to a determination of free T_4 and free T_3. Even in the presence of normal serum thyroid hormone levels, suppressed serum TSH should lead to treatment, especially in the elderly.[74]

Thyroglobulin in serum is positively correlated with thyroid size,[75] but in our opinion it has no place in the routine investigation or in the follow-up of patients with multinodular goiter.

Calcitonin, a marker of medullary thyroid cancer (see Chapters 109 and 189) when elevated in serum, can aid in the early detection of sporadic cases of this disease. Routine determination in nodular thyroid disease has been suggested.[76, 77] This view is, however, disputed,[78] and the test is recommended only by 43% of European thyroidologists in the absence of a family history of thyroid malignancy.[79]

Antithyroid antibodies (thyroid peroxidase [TPO] and thyroglobulin antibodies) in serum should in our opinion be routinely determined in the work-up of these patients. This recommendation is based mainly on the fact that Hashimoto's thyroiditis may be mistaken for simple multinodular goiter and the recent recognition of these antibodies as being markers of an increased risk for radioiodine-induced hypothyroidism, as well as Graves' disease, in patients with toxic[80] and nontoxic multinodular goiter.[81]

Determination of *^{131}I uptake* aids in the diagnosis of iodine contamination, ensures that uptake is adequate, and allows calculation of the ^{131}I dose before ^{131}I therapy. It is, however, used routinely in the work-up of such patients only by a minority of clinical European Thyroid Association members.[79]

Diagnostic Imaging

Although not adequately investigated, it has repeatedly been stated that imaging rarely provides information decisive in clinical management in individual cases (see Chapter 97). The clinical diagnosis of nodular goiter is generally considered uncomplicated, but it can in fact be difficult even when scintigraphy[82] or ultrasound[83] is used to determine whether the gland is diffuse, uninodular, or multinodular and to accurately determine its size.[73] Recognition of this difficulty may be the main reason for such an overwhelming majority of European thyroidologists (88%) using either scintigraphy (66%), ultrasound (80%), or both (58%) in the evaluation of patients with nodular thyroid disease.[79]

Scintigraphy aids in verification of the clinical diagnosis and allows a determination of the relative mass of hyperfunctioning (hot) and nonfunctioning (cold) thyroid areas. Imaging can be performed with ^{123}I, ^{131}I, or ^{99m}Tc-pertechnetate, the latter being preferred (86%) among European thyroidologists,[79] although the first two should be used if the aim is to also reduce the risk of overlooking malignancy. If a clinically dominant nodule is cold on scintigraphy, it should be treated as a solitary cold nodule—the risk of malignancy being the same[84]—and fine-needle biopsy should be performed on euthyroid patients.[69] In the case of hyperthyroidism, the risk of malignancy is thought to be much lower, as is the need for fine-needle biopsy, which is not necessary in the vast majority of cases.

Ultrasound, which is often used in Europe[79] and less so in the United States,[85] allows a determination of total thyroid volume and individual nodule size and an evaluation of regional lymph nodes, regional blood flow, and nodule vascularity. It aids in performing accurate biopsies and cyst punctures. It is of great help in therapeutic procedures such as cyst punctures and alcohol sclerosis of solid or cystic nodules.[86] In the vast majority of patients, ultrasound can neither confirm nor exclude malignancy.[85] For an objective determination of thyroid size, whether before therapy, such as in the dose calculation of ^{131}I, or for follow-up posttherapy, it is the technique of choice.

Computed tomography and *magnetic resonance imaging* are generally of little value except for evaluation of a retroclavicular or intrathoracic goiter and for evaluation and follow-up of malignant thyroid disease. Routine radiography of the trachea has no place in these patients. Tracheal diameter can be evaluated by computed tomography[87] and upper airway obstruction by flow-volume loops,[87, 88] which may give additional information in selected patients, mainly those with large compressive goiters.

Fine-Needle Aspiration Biopsy

This procedure may be helpful when carcinoma is suspected, but it can never exclude carcinoma.[85, 89] The examination should focus on the dominant nodule or nodules or on those that have a different consistency from other nodules within the gland.[85, 87, 89] If malignancy is clinically suspected (see Chapter 109), a benign cytology should naturally be disregarded and the patient offered surgery. In subjects referred for evaluation of symptomatic multinodular nontoxic goiter and offered surgery, the incidence of carcinoma was 1% to 4%.[90] This figure included small papillary carcinomas of dubious clinical significance. In unselected patients with multinodular goiter, the prevalence of clinically important malignancy is probably less than 1%, lower in toxic than in nontoxic patients. Fine-needle biopsy cannot rule out malignancy but can probably reduce the risk of overlooking malignancy to below 1% and, in the worst case, could lead to delay in making the correct diagnosis.

In our opinion, neither diagnostic imaging nor fine-needle aspiration biopsy is necessary in most patients with nodular thyroid disease if the preferred treatment is surgery. However, an increasing number of centers—including ours—are offering nonsurgical treatment not only to toxic but also to nontoxic patients.[69, 87, 91] We support the more liberal use of diagnostic imaging and fine-needle aspiration biopsy in this setting.

Treatment

Nodular thyroid disease is very common, but most of these goiters do not cause significant symptoms and are best left untreated. Treatment is indicated in the case of

1. Progressive growth of the entire gland or individual nodules
2. Compression of the trachea or esophagus, recurrent laryngeal nerve damage, or cervical veins causing inspiratory stridor, disturbances in deglutition, hoarseness, or marked venous outflow obstruction
3. Overt or subclinical hyperthyroidism
4. Marked neck disfigurement

In a number of clinical situations a discrepancy is seen between clinical findings and complaints of the patients. In this context, the decision whether to treat can be more difficult. In the following, treatment of nontoxic and toxic multinodular goiter will be dealt with separately.

Multinodular Nontoxic Goiter

Surgery

Bilateral subtotal thyroidectomy is still regarded as standard therapy for patients with nontoxic multinodular goiter (Table 107–3; see also Chapter 110). The goal is removal of all thyroid tissue with a nodular appearance. Further resection is not usually recommended if final pathologic evaluation reveals an incidental cancer less than 1 cm in size. This not uncommon finding accounts for most cancers found in surgical series, and such cancers are mostly of little if any clinical significance. Macroscopically normal perinodular tissue often harbors microscopic growth foci, which explains the relatively high risk of recurrence in these patients.[42]

TABLE 107–3. Treatment Options for Patients with Nontoxic Multinodular Goiters

Treatment	Advantages	Disadvantages	Comments
Surgery	Rapid decompression of vital structures. Allows pathologic examination	Not all patients eligible. Surgical mortality (<1%). Postoperative tracheal obstruction. Reoperation because of hemorrhage (1%). Recurrent laryngeal nerve injury (1%–2%). Hypoparathyroidism (0.5%–5%). Hypothyroidism* and goiter recurrence.* Cosmetic problems (1%–2%). All figures related to side effects higher in reoperations	Until recently, standard therapy in most centers, especially for large goiters when rapid decompression is required
Thyroxine	Possibly hinders formation of new nodules. Questionable goiter size reduction	Small decrease in mainly perinodular volume. Clinically relevant effect only in small goiters. Treatment should be lifelong and aimed at TSH suppression, which induces side effects caused by subclinical hyperthyroidism and inadvertent effects on bone and the heart	Its role on the wane. Possible alternative for a period in young patients with small goiters
Radioiodine	Halving of thyroid volume within 1 yr. Can be repeated. Preferred by patients	Only gradual decrease in volume and seldom normalization. Side effects increasingly recognized: radiation thyroiditis (3%), Graves' disease (4%), hypothyroidism (20% within 5 yr). Treatment needs to be repeated in some. Theoretic risk of radiation-induced malignancy and ophthalmopathy	Has replaced surgery as the standard therapy in most patients in Danish centers, for example. Should be contemplated instead of reoperation and in those not fit for surgery

*The percentage of patients affected depends on the extent of surgery.
TSH, thyroid-stimulating hormone.

Surgery leads to rapid decompression and only extremely rarely is a thoracic approach necessary. Not all patients are surgical candidates, but among those undergoing surgery, the surgical mortality rate is less than 1% in experienced centers. Surgical morbidity is highest in patients with large goiters and in those who undergo a reoperation because of recurrent goiter. Disadvantages include the general risks and side effects of a surgical procedure. More specific risks include recurrent laryngeal nerve damage, including voice changes caused by superior laryngeal nerve damage (1%–2%). Permanent hypoparathyroidism is seen in 1% to 2% and postoperative tracheal obstruction from hemorrhage or tracheomalacia in 1%. Hypothyroidism and goiter recurrence are inversely related in that the more radical the surgery, the higher the risk of hypothyroidism and the lower the risk of goiter recurrence. Although hypothyroidism is easily treated, the recurrence seen in up to 10% to 20% of patients within 10 years of thyroidectomy[42] carries a high risk of surgical morbidity if a reoperation is necessary. Although levothyroxine is frequently prescribed postoperatively to hinder recurrence, the only randomized long-term prospective study, which monitored 206 patients for a median of 10 years and used an objective ultrasonic evaluation of recurrence, could not demonstrate a clinically significant effect of prophylactic postoperative levothyroxine treatment.[42] It cannot be excluded that this therapy or iodine may prove beneficial in iodine-deficient areas.[92]

Thyroid Hormone Treatment

Both T_4 and T_3 suppress pituitary TSH secretion but do not affect the TSH-independent autonomous growth of goiter nodules. It is therefore not surprising that the treatment, provided that TSH is suppressed, is effective in reducing the volume of diffuse nontoxic goiters by up to 30%.[93] Based on a number of inadequately controlled trials with inhomogeneous patient populations and lack of objective thyroid size measurements, this treatment has been used by a number of centers also in multinodular nontoxic goiters (reviewed elsewhere[70]). Only one randomized, placebo-controlled trial using ultrasonic follow-up of thyroid size has been reported.[68] In that study, 58% of patients had a significant (>13%) decrease in thyroid volume. In those with a response, the mean decrease was 25% after 9 months of TSH suppression and was followed by regrowth after discontinuation of therapy. The fact that T_4 has little or no effect on goiter recurrence after thyroidectomy[42] or on solitary nodule volume but decreases perinodular volume[94] suggests that T_4 treatment, at least in non–iodine-deficient areas, has little or very marginal influence on the natural history of nontoxic multinodular goiter.

A high proportion of patients are ineligible for this therapy because they have autonomous function with decreased serum TSH.[95] If given, such treatment may lead to overt hyperthyroidism without any likelihood of thyroid volume reduction. Subclinical hyperthyroidism, which is the aim of T_4 therapy, is associated with substantial side effects. Thus a recent meta-analysis demonstrated a 5% to 9% decrease in bone mineral density in postmenopausal women, whereas no adverse effects could be demonstrated in premenopausal women or men.[96] Loss of bone in postmenopausal women is prevented by concomitant estrogen therapy. This increased loss of bone is normalized by antithyroid drugs,[97] as well as by ^{131}I therapy.[98] The possible cardiac side effects of subclinical hyperthyroidism have also received increasing attention.[72, 95]

Because it is necessary to disregard: (1) patients with moderate to large goiters, (2) those with decreased serum TSH, and (3) those older than 60 years—and in view of the very questionable effect on thyroid size—we find little room for this treatment. In fact, we do not use it. In our view, patients with multinodular goiter and well-documented subclinical hyperthyroidism should be treated as those with overt hyperthyroidism.[91]

Radioiodine Therapy

During the last decade, ^{131}I therapy for symptomatic multinodular nontoxic goiter has been introduced in a number of mainly European centers as a nonsurgical alternative to levothyroxine therapy.[87, 91] From the relatively few and small studies the following conclusions can be drawn: Thyroid volume can be reduced by approximately 40% after 1 year[87, 99–102] and by approximately 50% to 60% after 2 years, without further reduction.[87, 100] Sixty percent of this decrease is seen within 3 months of therapy.[100] No significant early increase in thyroid volume or obstructive symptoms is noted.[103] In fact, relief of compressive symptoms, a decrease in upper airway obstruction—as estimated by pulmonary function testing and flow-volume loops—and an increase in cross-sectional area of the tracheal lumen can be expected in most patients.[88, 102] Also, patients with monstrous, partly intrathoracic goiters have been treated with beneficial results.[102] The treatment can be repeated with an expected additional volume reduction.[100] It is likely that a reduction in scintigraphically cold areas occurs. Because of the often large goiters, normalization of thyroid volume, as seen in diffuse toxic[104] and nontoxic goiters,[105] can rarely be achieved. A secondary increase in thyroid volume has been seen, although uncommon, and should raise the suspicion of malignancy.[106] Generally, ^{131}I doses of

100 μCi (3.7 MBq) per gram of thyroid tissue corrected for 100% 24-hour ^{131}I uptake, have been given.[91, 99–102]

Radiation thyroiditis is seen in 3% within the first months of ^{131}I therapy[81] and is easily treated with salicylates or corticosteroids. Another complication is a Graves'-like autoimmune hyperthyroidism, which is seen in 5% (9 of 191 patients).[81] This abnormality is most likely triggered by ^{131}I-related release of thyroid antigens and is associated with the appearance of TSH receptor antibody. It can also be seen after surgical manipulation of the thyroid[107] or after subacute thyroiditis.[108] It typically occurs 3 months after treatment. The development of postradioiodine thyroid-associated ophthalmopathy in one patient lends further support to this suggested chain of events.[109] The risk of hypothyroidism, including subclinical cases, is approximately 20% after 5 years.[100] The pretreatment presence of anti-TPO antibody seems to confer an increased risk for Graves'-like hyperthyroidism (22%), hypothyroidism (29%), and radiation thyroiditis (11%), as compared with 2%, 13%, and 2%, respectively, in anti-TPO antibody–negative subjects.[81]

No data are available on the risk of overlooking or inducing carcinoma, but it is thought to be lower than the risk of serious side effects of surgery in the elderly and in those requiring a reoperation.[87, 110] In Denmark, this therapy has replaced surgery as the treatment of choice in most patients.[91] Whether this swing of the pendulum is justified remains to be established.

Alcohol Sclerotherapy

In use for the last few years, mainly in Italian centers, in solitary hot or toxic nodules and solitary cysts (for review see Bennedbæk et al.[86] and Chapters 102 and 109), alcohol sclerotherapy could theoretically be used in multinodular nontoxic goiter. Drawbacks are related to pain, risk of recurrent laryngeal nerve damage, and the possibility of extrathyroidal fibrosis complicating subsequent surgery. At present, this treatment should be considered experimental.

Multinodular Toxic Goiter

Surgery

The optimum treatment of multinodular toxic goiter continues to be controversial, and regional differences are to a high degree influenced by local tradition and practical conditions such as lack of alternatives (Table 107–4). Surgery leads to rapid decompression, and only extremely rarely is a thoracic approach necessary (see also Chapter 110). The aim of surgery for multinodular toxic goiter does not differ from that for multinodular nontoxic goiter. Because this disorder is seen mainly in the elderly, not all patients are surgical candidates. Among those undergoing surgery, the surgical mortality, in experienced centers, is no higher (<1%) than that seen in multinodular nontoxic goiter, given adequate pretreatment of the hyperthyroidism.[87, 111] Surgical morbidity is highest in patients with large goiters and in those undergoing reoperation because of recurrent goiter. Although the clinical importance of an incidental finding of thyroid malignancy, as evidenced by five cancers (four papillary and one follicular) in a series of 174 patients (3%) from the Mayo Clinic in Rochester,[112] remains unclarified, it is important to stress that surgery does allow pathologic examination. Fine-needle biopsy is not generally recommended in hyperthyroid patients and rarely performed in our institutions. On the assumption that antithyroid drugs are not used postoperatively, thyroid function is more rapidly normalized after surgery than after radioiodine therapy.[112] No consensus has been reached on whether preoperative iodine has a beneficial effect.[113]

Specific risks include transient (6%) or permanent (2%) vocal cord paralysis, transient (6%) or permanent (5%) hypoparathyroidism, and postoperative bleeding (1%), as reported from the Mayo Clinic.[112] Others have found lower figures (see Chapter 109). Other complications from that series, including various cardiovascular complications, were seen in approximately 10%.[112] Because the aim of surgery is to avoid persistence or recurrence of hyperthyroidism and goiter, the operation is often radical and a small remnant is left. Therefore, a high frequency (80%–90%) of hypothyroidism should be expected.[112] Postoperative levothyroxine therapy should be given in the case of hypothyroidism, but no evidence has shown that prophylactic routine administration hinders recurrence.[42,70]

Antithyroid Drugs

Hyperthyroidism is easily treated with antithyroid drugs. Remission is, however, extremely rare and lifelong treatment should be anticipated.[87, 113] Antithyroid drugs are indicated before thyroid surgery to lower the operative risk and can be stopped in the immediate postoperative period.[113] If used before and after radioiodine treatment to achieve euthyroidism more quickly and to reduce the risk of exacerbation of hyperthyroidism, respectively, use of the antithyroid drug should be discontinued at least 4 days before and resumed no sooner than 3 days afterward.[113] It has been suggested that pretreatment[114] and postradioiodine treatment with antithyroid drugs[115] decrease its effect, but this hypothesis is at present unclarified. No evidence of antithyroid drugs reducing thyroid size has been demonstrated.

Radioiodine Therapy

Radioiodine treatment is considered safe and appropriate in nearly all types of hyperthyroidism, especially in elderly patients.[113] Generally, radioiodine is thought to carry a lower rate of complications

TABLE 107–4. Treatment Options for Patients with Toxic Multinodular Goiters

Treatment	Advantages	Disadvantages	Comments
Surgery	Rapid decompression of vital structures. Rapid achievement of euthyroidism. Allows pathologic examination	Not all patients eligible. Surgical mortality and morbidity a little higher than in nontoxic goiter.* Persistence or recurrence of hyperthyroidism.* All side effects more common in reoperations	Recommended in patients with large goiters when rapid decompression is required.
Antithyroid drugs	Easiest treatment option	Lifelong treatment needed, no chance of remission; risk of adverse effects, approximately 5%. Continuous goiter growth	Major indications are before thyroid surgery and before and after radioiodine in elderly patients and those with concurrent health problems. Long-term treatment recommended only when surgery or radioiodine cannot be used
Radioiodine	Effective in rendering patients euthyroid and in reducing thyroid volume. Can be repeated. Preferred by patients	Only gradual reversal of hyperthyroidism. Gradual reduction in thyroid volume, which is rarely normalized. Side effects increasingly recognized: Graves' disease (4%), hypothyroidism (14% within 5 yr). Treatment needs to be repeated in some. Theoretic risk of radiation-induced malignancy and ophthalmopathy	Has replaced surgery as the standard therapy in most patients in Danish centers, for example. Should be preferred instead of reoperation and in those not fit for surgery

*The percentage of patients affected depends on the extent of surgery.

and have a lower cost than surgery.[113] The fact that remission of hyperthyroidism cannot be expected and surgery is associated with a relatively high risk of complications,[112] even in eligible patients, has led a number of centers to offer radioiodine as the first choice of therapy in the vast majority of patients. When compared with Graves' disease (see Chapter 100), surprisingly few data are available regarding the effects and side effects of radioiodine therapy in multinodular toxic goiter.

In contrast to surgery, which cures nearly all patients and normalizes hyperthyroidism within a few days,[112] only 50% become euthyroid within 3 months of radioiodine therapy, given that antithyroid drugs are not administered.[106, 112] Twenty percent to 40% need additional radioiodine therapy, and even up to five treatment sessions will not cure all patients[106]; in contrast, persistence of hyperthyroidism after surgery is rare.[112]

Thyroid volume can be reduced by approximately 40% to 50% within 2 years of radioiodine therapy, with approximately two-thirds of this reduction evident within 3 months of therapy.[106, 116] This reduction is independent of pretreatment with antithyroid drugs.[106] Thereafter, no further reduction is seen.[106] This volume reduction is very similar to that obtained in multinodular nontoxic goiter.[99, 100] No significant early increase is seen in thyroid volume or obstructive symptoms. [106] Even radioiodine doses that do not cure the patient will reduce thyroid volume by 25% on average.[106] Because of the often large goiters, normalization of thyroid volume, as seen in diffuse toxic[104] and nontoxic goiter,[105] can rarely be achieved. The treatment can be repeated both in the case of persistent hyperthyroidism and to reduce thyroid volume in a euthyroid patient.[100, 106] In most centers, the ^{131}I dose is calculated on the basis of ^{131}I uptake and thyroid size. However, whether such dosage adjustment is worthwhile has been questioned,[117] and fixed doses are given in a number of centers.

None of 130 consecutive patients treated with radioiodine had thyroiditis, which therefore seems to be a rare complication.[106] Graves'-like hyperthyroidism was seen in 6 of 149 patients (4%) with nodular toxic goiter,[80] similar to that described for nontoxic multinodular goiter.[81] The condition is related to the appearance of TSH receptor antibodies and typically occurs 3 to 6 months after radioiodine therapy. In the only long-term (median of 6 years) follow-up of a large population (130 subjects), the risk of hypothyroidism was found to be 14% after 5 years,[106] similar to that found in nontoxic multinodular goiter.[81] Pretreatment presence of anti-TPO antibody seems to confer an increased risk for both Graves'-like hyperthyroidism (10%) and hypothyroidism (30%) when compared with these conditions (0.8% and 5%, respectively) in anti-TPO antibody–negative subjects.[80]

No data are available on the risk of overlooking or inducing carcinoma of the thyroid or the theoretic possibility of radioiodine-induced ophthalmopathy, but it is generally believed to be lower than the risk of serious side effects of surgery in the elderly and in those requiring a reoperation.[87, 113]

Acknowledgments

The contribution of professor Hugo Studer to this work is gratefully acknowledged—in particular, his agreement to include in this chapter passages of his contribution with H. G. to the last edition of this textbook. The work of H. G. has generously been supported by the Swiss National Science Foundation and that of L. H. by the Agnes and Knut Mørks Foundation. Mrs. Pia Vogn is thanked for excellent secretarial help.

REFERENCES

1. Studer H, Peter HJ, Gerber H: Natural heterogeneity of thyroid cells: The basis for understanding thyroid function and nodular goiter growth. Endocr Rev 10:125–135, 1989.
2. Studer H, Gerber H: Non-toxic goiter. *In* Greer MA (ed): The Thyroid Gland. Comprehensive Endocrinology. New York, Raven, 1990, pp 391–404.
3. Studer H, Derwahl M: Mechanisms of nonneoplastic endocrine hyperplasia—a changing concept: A review focused on the thyroid gland. Endocr Rev 16:411–426, 1995.
4. Peter HJ, Bürgi U, Gerber H: Pathogenesis of nontoxic diffuse and nodular goiter. *In* Braverman LE, Utiger R (eds): Werner's and Ingbar's The Thyroid, ed 7. Philadelphia, JB Lippincott, 1996, pp 890–895.
5. Miller JM, Block MA: Relative function of the "hot" autonomous thyroid nodule: Double and single isotope autoradiographic studies. J Nucl Med 10:691–696 1969.
6. Studer H, Hunziker HR, Ruchti C: Morphologic and functional substrate of thyrotoxicosis caused by nodular goiters. Am J Med 65:227–234, 1978.
7. Peter HJ, Studer H, Forster R, Gerber H: The pathogenesis of "hot" and "cold" follicles in multinodular goiters. J Clin Endocrinol Metab 55:941–946, 1982.
8. Peter HJ, Gerber H, Studer H, Smeds S: Pathogenesis of heterogeneity in human multinodular goiter: A study on growth and function of thyroid tissue transplanted onto nude mice. J Clin Invest 76:1990–2002, 1985.
9. Schürch M, Peter HJ, Gerber H, Studer H: Cold follicles in a multinodular human goiter arise partly from a failing iodide pump and partly from deficient iodine organification. J Clin Endocrinol Metab 71:1224–1229, 1990.
10. Studer H, Gerber H, Zbären J, Peter HJ: Histomorphological and immunohistochemical evidence that human nodular goiters grow by episodic replication of multiple clusters of thyroid follicular cells. J Clin Endocrinol Metab 75:1151–1158, 1992.
11. LiVolsi VA: Surgical pathology of the thyroid. *In* Major Problems in Pathology, vol 22. Philadelphia, WB Saunders, 1990.
12. Bürgi-Saville ME, Gerber H, Peter HJ, et al: Expression patterns of extracellular matrix components in native and cultured human thyroid tissue and in human toxic adenoma tissue. Thyroid 7:347–356, 1997.
13. Gerber H, Huber G, Peter HJ, et al: Transformation of normal thyroids into colloid goiters in rats and mice by diphenylthiohydantoin. Endocrinology 135:2688–2699, 1994.
14. Gerber H, Bürgi U, Peter HJ, Wagner HE: The transformation of normal thyroid cells to goiter: The role of iodine depletion and repletion. *In* Naumann J, Glinoer D, Braverman LE, Hostalek U (eds): The Thyroid and Iodine. New York, Schattauer, 1996, pp 65–74.
15. Williams DW, Williams ED, Wynford-Thomas D: Evidence for autocrine production of IGF-1 in human thyroid adenomas. Mol Cell Endocrinol 61:139–143, 1989.
16. Minuto F, Barreca A, Del Monte P, et al: Immunoreactive insulin-like growth factor I (IGF-I) and IGF-I–binding protein content in human thyroid tissue. J Clin Endocrinol Metab 68:621–626, 1989.
17. Thompson SD, Franklyn JA, Watkinson JC, et al: Fibroblast growth factors 1 and 2 and fibroblast growth factor receptor 1 are elevated in thyroid hyperplasia. J Clin Endocrinol Metab 83:1336–1341, 1998.
18. Marti U, Ruchti C, Kämpf J, et al: Nuclear expression of epidermal growth factor (EGF) and its receptor (EGFR) in normal and pathologically altered human thyroid tissue (abstract 101). J Endocrinol Invest 20(suppl 5):51, 1997.
19. Gerber H, Studer H, von Grünigen C: Paradoxical effects of thyrotropin on diffusion of thyroglobulin in the colloid of rat thyroid follicles after long term thyroxine treatment. Endocrinology 116:303–310, 1985.
20. Peter HJ, Gerber H, Studer H, et al: Autonomy of growth and of iodine metabolism in hyperthyroid feline goiters transplanted onto nude mice. J Clin Invest 80:491–498, 1987.
21. Peter HJ, Studer H, Groscurth P: Autonomous growth, but not autonomous function, in embryonic human thyroids: A clue to understanding autonomous goiter growth. J Clin Endocrinol Metab 66:968–973, 1988.
22. Teuscher J, Peter HJ, Gerber H, et al: Pathogenesis of nodular goiter and its implications for surgical management. Surgery 103:87–93, 1988.
23. Gerber H, Peter HJ, Peterson ME, Ferguson DC: Etiopathology of feline toxic nodular goiter. Vet Clin North Am Small Anim Pract 24:541–565, 1994.
24. Wohlgemuth S, Krohn K, Gerber H, Paschke R: Identification of constitutively activating TSH receptor mutations in scintigraphically hot areas of euthyroid goiters (abstract v069). Exp Clin Endocrinol 106(suppl 1):18, 1998.
25. Jhiang SM, Cho JY, Ryu KY, et al: Immunohistochemical study of Na^+/I^- symporter in human thyroid tissues and salivary gland tissues. Endocrinology 139:4416–4419, 1998.
26. Studer H, Gerber H: Intrathyroidal iodine: Heterogeneity of iodocompounds and kinetic compartmentalization. Trends Endocrinol Metab 2:29–34, 1991.
27. Gerber H, Peter HJ, Bürgi U, et al: Colloidal aggregates of insoluble inclusions in human goiters. Biochimie 81:441–445, 1999.
28. Dumont JE, Lamy F, Roger P, Maenhaut C: Physiological and pathological regulation of thyroid cell proliferation and differentiation by thyrotropin and other factors. Physiol Rev 72:667–697, 1992.
29. Gärtner R: Growth factors of the thyroid. Exp Clin Endocrinol 101:83–91, 1993.
30. Eggo MC, Sheppard MC: Autocrine growth factors produced in the thyroid. Mol Cell Endocrinol 100:97–102, 1994.
31. Nilsson M: Actions of epidermal growth factor and its receptor in the thyroid. Trends Endocrinol Metab 6:175–182, 1995.
32. Grubeck-Loebenstein B, Buchan G, Sadeghi R, et al: Transforming growth factor beta regulates thyroid growth. J Clin Invest 83:764–770, 1989.
33. Brown RS: Immunoglobulins affecting thyroid growth: A continuing controversy (editorial). J Clin Endocrinol Metab 80:1506–1508, 1995.
34. Berghout A, Wiersinga WM, Smits NJ, et al: Interrelationships between age, thyroid volume, thyroid nodularity, and thyroid function in patients with sporadic non-toxic goiter. Am J Med 89:602–608, 1990.
35. Fenzi GF, Ceccarelli C, Macchia E, et al: Reciprocal changes of serum thyroglobulin and TSH in residents of a moderate endemic goiter area. Clin Endocrinol 23:115–122, 1985.
36. Gruenert DC, Cozens AL: Inheritance of phenotype in mammalian cells: Genetic vs. epigenetic mechanisms. Am J Physiol 260:386–394, 1991.
37. Gerber H, Peter HJ, Bachmeier C, et al: Progressive recruitment of follicular cells with graded secretory responsiveness during stimulation of the thyroid gland by thyrotropin. Endocrinology 120:91–96, 1987.
38. Gerber H, Peter HJ, Studer H: Age-related failure of endocytosis may be the pathogenetic mechanism responsible for "cold" follicle formation in the aging mouse thyroid. Endocrinology 120:1758–1764, 1987.

39. Mestdagh C, Many MC, Halpern S, et al: Correlated autoradiographic and ion-microscopic study of the role of iodine in the formation of "cold" follicles in young and old mice. Cell Tissue Res 260:449–457, 1990.
40. Ledent C, Parma J, Dumont J, et al: Molecular genetics of thyroid diseases. Mini-review. Eur J Endocrinol 130:8–14, 1994.
41. Paschke R, Ludgate M: The thyrotropin receptor in thyroid diseases. N Engl J Med 337:1675–1681, 1997.
42. Hegedüs L, Nygaard B, Hansen JM: Is routine thyroxine treatment to hinder postoperative recurrence of nontoxic goiter justified? J Clin Endocrinol Metab 84:756–760, 1999.
43. Kopp P, van Sande J, Parma J, et al: Congenital hyperthyroidism caused by a neomutation in the thyrotropin receptor gene. N Engl J Med 332:150–154, 1995.
44. Mortensen JD, Woolner LB, Bennet WA: Gross and microscopic findings in clinically normal thyroid glands. J Clin Endocrinol Metab 15:1270–1280, 1955.
45. Horlocker TT, Hay JE, James EM, et al: Prevalence of incidental nodular thyroid disease detected during high-resolution parathyroid ultrasonography. *In* Medeiros-Neto GA, Gaitan E (eds): New Frontiers in Thyroidology. New York, Plenum, 1986, pp 1309–1312.
46. Thomas GA, Williams D, Williams ED: The clonal origin of thyroid nodules and adenomas. Am J Pathol 134:141–147, 1989.
47. Namba H, Matsuo K, Fagin JA: Clonal composition of benign and malignant human thyroid tumors. J Clin Invest 86:120–125, 1990.
48. Hicks DG, LiVolsi VA, Neidich JA, et al: Clonal analysis of solitary follicular nodules in the thyroid. Am J Pathol 137:553–562, 1990.
49. Fey M, Peter HJ, Hinds HL, et al: Clonal analysis of human tumours with M27, a highly informative polymorphic X-chromosomal probe. J Clin Invest 89:1438–1444, 1992.
50. Kopp P, Aeschimann S, Asmis L, et al: Polyclonal and clonal nodules may coexist within multinodular goiters. J Clin Endocrinol Metab 79:134–139, 1994.
51. Bamberger AM, Bamberger CM, Barth J, et al: Clonal analysis of thyroid nodules from patients with multinodular goiters: Determination by X chromosome inactivation analysis using the highly polymorphic M27beta probe (abstract). *In* Proceedings of the 75th Annual Meeting of the Endocrine Society. Las Vegas, NV, June 1993, p 157.
52. Bürgi U, Gerber H, Studer H: Goitrogenesis in iodine deficiency. *In* Delange F, Dunn J, Glinoer D (eds): Iodine Deficiency in Europe. A Continuing Concern. New York, Plenum, 1993, pp 61–67.
53. Bürgi H, Supersaxo Z, Selz B: Iodine deficiency diseases in Switzerland one hundred years after Theodor Kocher's survey: A historical review with some new goitre prevalence data. Acta Endocrinol (Copenh) 123:577–590, 1990.
54. Gaitan E (ed): Environmental Goitrogenesis. Boca Raton, FL, CRC Press, 1989, pp 1–250.
55. Green WL: Antithyroid compounds. *In* Braverman LE, Utiger R (eds): Werner's and Ingbar's The Thyroid, ed 7. Philadelphia, JB Lippincott, 1996, pp 266–276.
56. Bertelsen JB, Hegedüs L: Cigarette smoking and the thyroid. Thyroid 4:327–331, 1994.
57. Cheung NW, Boyages SC: The thyroid gland in acromegaly: An ultrasonographic study. Clin Endocrinol 46:545–549, 1997.
58. Dormitzer PR, Ellison PT, Bode HH: Anomalously low endemic goiter prevalence among Efe pygmies. Am J Phys Anthropol 78:527–531, 1989.
59. Brix T, Kyvik KO, Hegedüs L: Modelling genetic and environmental influences in the etiology of nontoxic goiter—a study of female twins living in an area of borderline iodine deficiency (abstract 44). *In* Proceedings of the 71st Annual Meeting of the American Thyroid Association. September 1998, p 22.
60. Tunbridge WMG, Evered DC, Hall R, et al: The spectrum of thyroid disease in the community: The Whickham survey. Clin Endocrinol 7:481–493, 1977.
61. Vanderpump MPJ, Tunbridge WMG, French JM, et al: The incidence of thyroid disorders in the community: A twenty-year follow-up of the Whickham survey. Clin Endocrinol 43:55–68, 1995.
62. Hegedüs L: Thyroid size determined by ultrasound. Influence of physiological factors and non-thyroidal disease. Thesis. Dan Med Bull 37:249–263, 1990.
63. Kilpatrick R, Milne JS, Rushbrooke M, et al: A survey of thyroid enlargement in two general practices in Great Britain. BMJ 1:29–32, 1963.
64. Wesche MFT, Wiersinga WM, Smits NJ: Lean body mass as a determinant of thyroid size. Clin Endocrinol 48:701–706, 1998.
65. Laurberg P, Pedersen KM, Hreidarsson A, et al: Iodine intake and the pattern of thyroid disorders: A comparative epidemiological study of thyroid abnormalities in the elderly in Iceland and in Jutland, Denmark. J Clin Endocrinol Metab 83:765–769, 1998.
66. Laurberg P, Pedersen KM, Vestergaard H, et al: High incidence of multinodular toxic goiter in the elderly population in a low iodine intake area vs. high incidence of Graves' disease in the young in a high iodine intake area: Comparative surveys of thyrotoxicosis epidemiology in East-Jutland, Denmark and Iceland. J Intern Med 229:415–420, 1991.
67. Haraldsson A, Gudmundsson ST, Larusson G, et al: Thyrotoxicosis in Iceland 1980–1982. An epidemiological survey. Acta Med Scand 217:253–258, 1985.
68. Berghout A, Wiersinga WM, Drexhage HA, et al: Comparison of placebo with L-thyroxine alone or with carbimazole for treatment of sporadic non-toxic goitre. Lancet 336:193–197, 1990.
69. Gharib H: Management of thyroid nodules: Another look. Thyroid Today 20:1–11, 1997.
70. Gharib H, Mazzaferri EL: Thyroxine suppressive therapy in patients with nodular thyroid disease. Ann Intern Med 128:386–394, 1998.
71. Gemsenjæger E, Staub JJ, Girard J, et al: Preclinical hyperthyroidism in multinodular goiter. J Clin Endocrinol Metab 43:810–816, 1976.
72. Sawin CT, Geller A, Wolf PA, et al: Low serum thyrotropin concentrations as a risk factor for atrial fibrillation in older persons. N Engl J Med 331:1249–1252, 1994.
73. Jarløv AE, Nygaard B, Hegedüs L, et al: Observer variation in the clinical evaluation of patients with suspected thyroid disease. Thyroid 8:393–398, 1998.
74. Jayme JJ, Ladenson PW: Subclinical thyroid dysfunction in the elderly. TEM 5:79–86, 1994.
75. Date J, Feldt-Rasmussen U, Blichert-Toft M, et al: Increased serum thyroglobulin 10 years after partial resection of nontoxic goiter and relation to ultrasonographically demonstrated relapse. World J Surg 20:351–357, 1996.
76. Niccoli P, Wion-Barbot N, Caron P, et al: Interest of routine measurement of serum calcitonin: Study in a large series of thyroidectomized patients. J Clin Endocrinol Metab 82:338–341, 1997.
77. Vierhapper H, Raber W, Bieglmayer C, et al: Routine measurement of plasma calcitonin in nodular thyroid disease. J Clin Endocrinol Metab 82:1589–1593, 1997.
78. Feld S: AACE Clinical Practice Guidelines for the Diagnosis and Management of Thyroid Nodules: AACE Thyroid Guidelines. AACE, 1996, pp 1–16.
79. Bennedbæk FN, Perrild H, Hegedüs L: Diagnosis and treatment of the solitary thyroid nodule. Results of a European survey. Clin Endocrinol (Oxf) 50:357–363, 1999.
80. Nygaard B, Faber J, Veje A, et al: Pretreatment presence of anti-TPOab as a risk marker of ^{131}I induced Graves' disease and hypothyroidism in nodular toxic goiter. Thyroid (submitted for publication).
81. Nygaard B, Knudsen JH, Hegedüs L, et al: Thyrotropin receptor antibodies and Graves' disease, a side-effect of ^{131}I treatment in patients with nontoxic goiter. J Clin Endocrinol Metab 82:2926–2930, 1997.
82. Jarløv AE, Gjørup T, Hegedüs L, et al: Observer variation in the scintigraphic diagnosis of solitary cold thyroid lesions. Clin Endocrinol 33:1–11, 1990.
83. Jarløv AE, Nygaard B, Hegedüs L, et al: Observer variation in ultrasound examination of the thyroid gland. Br J Radiol 66:625–627, 1993.
84. Belfiore A, La Rosa GL, La Porta GA, et al: Cancer risk in patients with cold thyroid nodules: Relevance of iodine intake, sex, age, and multinodularity. Am J Med 93:363–369, 1992.
85. Blum M, Yee J: Advances in thyroid imaging: Thyroid sonography—when and how should it be used? Thyroid Today 20:1–13, 1997.
86. Bennedbæk FN, Karstrup S, Hegedüs L: Percutaneous ethanol injection therapy in the treatment of thyroid and parathyroid diseases. Eur J Endocrinol 136:240–250, 1997.
87. Hermus AR, Huysmans DA: Treatment of benign nodular thyroid disease. N Engl J Med 338:1438–1447, 1998.
88. Nygaard B, Søes-Petersen U, Høilund-Carlsen PF, et al: Improvement of upper airway obstruction after ^{131}I treatment of multinodular nontoxic goiter evaluated by flow volume loop curves. J Endocrinol Invest 19:71–75, 1996.
89. Giuffrida D, Gharib H. Controversies in the management of cold, hot, and occult thyroid nodules. Am J Med 99:642–650, 1995.
90. Franklyn JA, Daykin J, Young J, et al: Fine-needle aspiration cytology in diffuse or multinodular goitre compared with solitary thyroid nodules. BMJ 307:240, 1993.
91. Nygaard B, Faber J, Hegedüs L, et al: ^{131}I treatment of nodular, non-toxic goitre. Eur J Endocrinol 134:15–20, 1996.
92. Miccoli P, Antonelli A, Iacconi P, et al: Prospective, randomized, double-blind study about effectiveness of levothyroxine suppressive therapy in prevention of recurrence after operation: Result at the third year of follow-up. Surgery 114:1097–1101, 1993.
93. Perrild H, Hansen JM, Hegedüs L, et al: Triiodothyronine and thyroxine treatment of diffuse non-toxic goitre evaluated by ultrasonic scanning. Acta Endocrinol 100:382–387, 1982.
94. Bennedbæk FN, Nielsen LK, Hegedüs L: Effect of percutaneous ethanol injection therapy versus suppressive doses of L thyroxine on benign solitary solid cold thyroid nodules: A randomized trial. J Clin Endocrinol Metab 83:830–835, 1998.
95. Woeber KA: Subclinical thyroid dysfunction. Arch Intern Med 157:1065–1068, 1997.
96. Uzzan B, Campos J, Cucherat M, et al: Effects on bone mass of long term treatment with thyroid hormones: A meta-analysis. J Clin Endocrinol Metab 81:4278–4289, 1996.
97. Mudde AH, Hauben AJHM, Kurseman ACN: Bone metabolism during anti-thyroid drug treatment of endogenous subclinical hyperthyroidism. Clin Endocrinol 41:421–424, 1994.
98. Faber J, Jensen IW, Petersen L, et al: Normalization of serum thyrotrophin by means of radioiodine treatment in subclinical hyperthyroidism: Effect on bone loss in postmenopausal women. Clin Endocrinol 48:285–290, 1998.
99. Hegedüs L, Hansen BM, Knudsen N, et al: Reduction of size of thyroid with radioactive iodine in multinodular non-toxic goitre. BMJ 297:661–662, 1988.
100. Nygaard B, Hegedüs L, Gervil M, et al: Radioiodine treatment of multinodular non-toxic goitre. BMJ 307:828–832, 1993.
101. de Klerk JMH, van Isselt JW, van Dijk A, et al: Iodine-131 therapy in sporadic non-toxic goiter. J Nucl Med 38:372–376, 1997.
102. Huysmans DAKC, Hermus ARMM, Corstens FHM, et al: Large, compressive goiters treated with radioiodine. Ann Intern Med 121:757–762, 1994.
103. Nygaard B, Faber J, Hegedüs L: Acute changes in thyroid volume and function following ^{131}I therapy of multinodular goitre. Clin Endocrinol 41:715–718, 1994.
104. Nygaard B, Hegedüs L, Gervil M, et al: Influence of compensated radioiodine therapy on thyroid volume and incidence of hypothyroidism in Graves' disease. J Intern Med 238:491–497, 1995.
105. Hegedüs L, Bennedbæk FN: Radioiodine for non-toxic diffuse goitre. Lancet 350:409–410, 1997.
106. Nygaard B, Hegedüs L, Ulriksen P, et al: Radioiodine therapy for multinodular toxic goiter. Arch Intern Med 159:1364–1368, 1999.
107. Walfish PG, Caplan D, Rosen IB: Postparathyroidectomy transient thyrotoxicosis. J Clin Endocrinol Metab 75:224–227, 1992.
108. Bennedbæk FN, Gram J, Hegedüs L: The transition of subacute thyroiditis to Graves' disease as evidenced by diagnostic imaging. Thyroid 6:457–459, 1996.
109. Nygaard B, Metcalfe RA, Phipps J, et al: Graves' disease and thyroid-associated ophthalmopathy triggered by ^{131}I treatment of non-toxic goiter. J Endocrinol Invest 22:481–485, 1999.

110. Huysmans DAKC, Buijs WCAM, van de Ven MTJ, et al: Dosimetry and risk estimates of radioiodine therapy for large, multinodular goiters. J Nucl Med 37:2072–2079, 1996.
111. Jensen MD, Gharib H, Naessens JM, et al: Treatment of toxic multinodular goiter (Plummer's disease): Surgery or radioiodine? World J Surg 10:673–680, 1986.
112. Erickson D, Gharib H, Li H, et al: Treatment of patients with toxic multinodular goiter. Thyroid 8:277–282, 1998.
113. Vanderpump MPJ, Ahlquist JAO, Franklyn JA, et al: Consensus statement for good practice and audit measures in the management of hypothyroidism and hyperthyroidism. BMJ 313:539–544, 1996.
114. Imseis RE, Van Middlesworth L, Massie JD, et al: Pretreatment with propylthiouracil but not methimazole reduces the therapeutic efficacy of iodine-131 in hyperthyroidism. J Clin Endocrinol Metab 83:685–687, 1998.
115. Velkeniers B, Cytryn R, Van Haelst L, et al: Treatment of hyperthyroidism with radioiodine: Adjunctive therapy with antithyroid drugs reconsidered. Lancet 1:1127–1129, 1988.
116. Hegedüs L, Hansen JM: Radioactive iodine for thyrotoxicosis. Lancet 2:339–340, 876, 1986.
117. Jarløv AE, Hegedüs L, Kristensen LØ, et al: Is calculation of the dose in radioiodine therapy of hyperthyroidism worthwhile? Clin Endocrinol 43:325–329, 1995.

Chapter 108

Iodine Deficiency Disorders

Geraldo Medeiros-Neto

Iodine deficiency is the world's most common endocrine problem, the easiest of the major nutritional deficiencies to correct, and the most preventable cause of mental retardation in many underdeveloped countries. Given these facts, it is remarkable that iodine deficiency continues to be a major public health problem. It is best known for causing endemic goiter, but its manifestations and consequences reach much deeper into human pathology (Table 108–1). Goiter, although frequently the most obvious feature, is much less important than the adverse effects of iodine deficiency on normal development, particularly normal development of the brain. To emphasize the more severe consequences, this health problem is now described as iodine deficiency disorders instead of endemic goiter.

For many years it has been recognized that a close and inverse relationship usually, if not always, exists between iodine in the soil and water and the appearance of endemic goiter and allied diseases. Nevertheless, it cannot be said as of this writing that the cause of iodine deficiency disorders has been completely determined in all cases, or even in any case, because nutritional, constitutional, genetic, or immunologic factors may be additive in the sum total of causes that lead to the appearance of these diseases. Therefore, iodine deficiency is a *necessary* cause, although it may not always be a *sufficient* cause. The role of iodine deficiency as the main etiologic factor in endemic goiter and cretinism has been extensively confirmed by the success of iodine prophylaxis programs in several countries, although iodine deficiency has persisted despite readily available means of supplementation, such as iodized salt and iodized oil.[1–14]

TABLE 108–1. The Spectrum of Iodine Deficiency Disorders

Fetus	Abortions
	Stillbirths
	Congenital anomalies
	Increased perinatal mortality
	Increased infant mortality
	Neurologic cretinism: mental deficiency, deaf-mutism, spastic diplegia
	Myxedematous cretinism: dwarfism, mental deficiency
	Psychomotor defects
Neonate	Neonatal goiter
	Neonatal hypothyroidism
Child and adolescent	Goitrous juvenile hypothyroidism
	Impaired mental function
	Retarded physical development
Adult	Goiter with its complications
	Hypothyroidism
	Impaired mental function

Adapted from Hetzel BS, Dunn JT, Stanbury JB (eds): The Prevention and Control of Iodine Deficiency Disorders. Amsterdam, Elsevier, 1987.

IODINE SUPPLY

Iodine is found in relative abundance in marine plants and animals, in the thyroid gland of vertebrates, in deposits of organic origin, in certain natural mineral water, in sedimentary phosphate rock, and in association with certain mineral deposits. Most of the iodine ingested by humans comes from food of animal and plant origin. This iodine, in turn, is derived from the soil. Only a relatively small fraction is derived from drinking water. A most important factor in the depletion of iodine has been glaciation, which removes old soil and scrapes bare the virgin rocks, which have iodine concentrations far lower than those of the covering soil. This situation is found in regions that remained longest under Quaternary glaciers and lost their iodine when the ice thawed.

OPTIMAL IODINE INTAKE

Iodine is an essential component of the thyroid hormones thyroxin (T_4) and triiodothyronine (T_3) and contributes 65% and 59% of their respective molecular weights. To meet the demand for adequate hormone, the thyroid has developed an elaborate mechanism for concentrating iodine from the circulation and converting it into hormone, which it then stores and releases into the circulation as needed. The recommended intake of iodine is 150 μg/day for adults, 200 μg for pregnant or lactating women, and lower amounts for children.[12, 13] About 90% of iodine is eventually excreted in urine. The median urinary iodine concentration in casual samples, expressed as micrograms per deciliter, is currently the most practical biochemical laboratory marker of community iodine nutrition.[15] It is more useful and much simpler than measuring 24-hour samples or calculating urinary iodine-creatinine ratios. Recommendations by the International Council for the Control of Iodine Deficiency Disorders, the World Health Organization, and the United Nations International Children's Emergency Fund set 10 μg/dL as the minimal urinary iodine concentration for iodine sufficiency.[13] This figure roughly corresponds to a daily intake of 150 μg iodine. A recent paper on iodine nutrition in the United States indicated adequate iodine intake for the overall U.S. population,[16] but the median concentration decreased more than 50% between 1971 and 1974 (32.0 ± 0.6 μg/dL) and 1988 and 1994 (14.5 ± 0.3 μg/dL). Low urinary iodine concentrations (<5 μg/dL) were found in 11.7% of the 1988–1994 population, a 4.5-fold increase over the proportion on the 1971–1974 study. Possible reasons for this decline include changes in national food consumption patterns (lower salt intake) and food industry practices. Another point is that the use of iodinated salt has remained voluntary. A current estimate is that only 50% of the U.S. population uses iodized table salt.[17] Adequate monitoring of urinary iodine levels in future national nutrition surveys will probably detect further trends in iodine intake by the U.S. population.

PREVALENCE

It is much easier to list the iodine-sufficient countries than those with different degrees of iodine deficiency. In the beginning of the 1990s it was estimated that 29% of the global population lived in areas of iodine deficiency. It is remarkable that large segments of Europe (including affluent countries such as Germany, France, Italy, and Belgium) continue to have significant iodine deficiency. In one recent informal assessment of the 137 most populous countries, iodine deficiency was regarded as severe in 29, moderate in 54, mild in 24, uncertain in 17, and absent in only 13.[12] Significant iodine deficiency is present in 45 countries in Africa, 16 in the Americas, 24 in Europe and the Central Asian Republic, 11 in Southeast Asia, 10 in the Middle East, and 8 in the Far East. Recent reports on goiter and iodine deficiency in Europe[14, 18] have indicated, however, that goiter persists in adults (but is seldom seen in children) in Bulgaria, Czechoslovakia, The Netherlands, Switzerland, and Belgium. Substantial areas of high goiter prevalence persist in Austria, Hungary, Romania, Poland, Yugoslavia, and western Russia. In other countries (southwestern Germany, Greece, Italy, Portugal, Romania, Spain, and Turkey), iodine prophylaxis is not mandatory, and goiter and even endemic cretinism continue to be major problems, either nationally or regionally (goiter prevalence rates of 18%–22%). The overall results of this study give grounds for concern and point to the need for a comprehensive iodination program in Europe.

Goiter prevalence is high in some South American countries, especially in the mountainous ranges of the Andes (Ecuador, Peru, and Bolivia), as well as in the central part of South America (Paraguay).[8] In these countries goiter prevalence is still high in school children.[9–11] In Brazil, an effective salt iodination program has eliminated iodine deficiency disorders in most areas of the country, but 8.9% of schoolchildren living in the western part of the country still had goiter (Fig. 108–1). In the sub-Himalayan area of Pakistan, the overall prevalence of goiter is 39.7%, and endemic cretinism is common.[19] The Himalayas of India, Nepal, Buthan, and southern China, as well as the mountains extending into northern Burma, Thailand, Laos, and Vietnam, have long been known as goitrous areas. The Philippines and Indonesia are also severely iodine deficient. Worse conditions persist in the remote regions of African countries,[20–23] some with relatively recent statehood (Zaire, Nigeria, Senegal, Tanzania), where pioneering surveys and experimental investigation of endemic goiter and cretinism have been carried out by investigators from Belgium.[22] In Papua New Guinea, goiter and cretinism are as severe as in some provinces of the Republic of Zaire.[24] It is estimated that 30 million Chinese have goiter and possibly 200,000 suffer from the consequences of endemic cretinism.[25] An intensive program of salt iodination and administration of iodized oil (orally and intramuscularly), however, has reduced the prevalence of goiter and endemic cretinism in China.[13] With the increase in the world population, iodine deficiency disorders may become worse and spread further unless a program of world public health and welfare is established to eliminate iodine deficiency.

TABLE 108–2. Goitrogenic Factors Associated with Endemic Goiter

Factor	Agent	Action
Bacterial pollution	Progoitrin	Inhibits organification
	Thyroid-stimulating factor	Promotes growth
Millet	Thiocyanate phenolics	Inhibit I^- uptake
Cassava	Thiocyanate	Inhibits iodine transport
Babassu coconut	Flavonoids	Inhibit thyroperoxidase
Brassica genus	Goitrin (VTO)	Inhibits organification
Water borne	Disulfides	Inhibit organification
Soybean	Unknown	Fecal loss of T_4
Seaweed (kelp)	Iodine excess	Inhibits release of hormones
Malnutrition	Vitamin A deficiency	Abnormal Tg structure

T_4, thyroxine; Tg, thyroglobulin; VTO, 1,5-vinyl-2-thiooxazolidone. Data from Oginsky EL, Stein AE, Greer MA: Myrosinase activity in bacteria as demonstrated by the conversion of progoitrin into goitrin. Proc Soc Exp Biol Med 119:360–364, 1965.

ETIOLOGY

Absolute and chronic iodine deficiency is the principal cause of endemic goiter and allied disorders. It is entirely possible that in certain limited situations other etiologic factors such as genetic predisposition in highly inbred and isolated groups, the presence of effective goitrogens in unusual dietary situations (Table 108–2), and autoimmune phenomena may be considered factors contributing to local

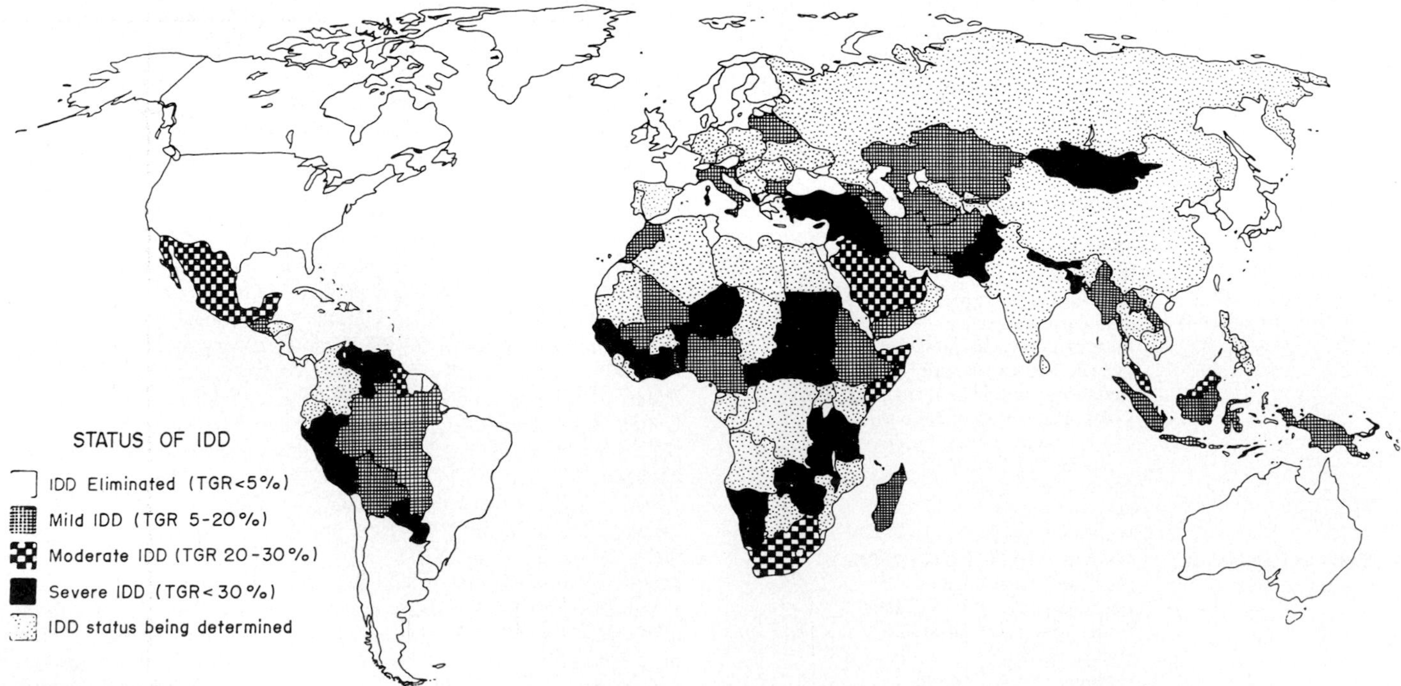

FIGURE 108–1. Current status of iodine deficiency disorders based on the total goiter rate in school children. (Based on data from Dunn[12] and WHO et al.,[13] actualized to 1997.)

endemic conditions. The argument supporting iodine deficiency as the cause of endemic goiter is threefold:

1. An association between low iodine content in the soil and water and the appearance of the disease in the population has been recognized.
2. A reduction in goiter incidence occurs when iodine is added to the diet.
3. It has been demonstrated that the metabolism of iodine by patients with endemic goiter fits the pattern that is produced in animals subjected to a low iodine diet.

Some observations, however, suggest that iodine deficiency may be present in populations (notably Indians from the upper part of the Orinoco River in Venezuela) in which no abnormal prevalence of goiter was noticed.[26] A more recent study, however, indicated that most Yanomano children have enlarged thyroid glands with predictable higher serum T_3 and thyroid-stimulating hormone (TSH) concentrations.[27] Another example is the wide prevalence of goiter on a Lake Kivu island in Zaire.[22] Here, northern villages show a prevalence of more than 60%, but the incidence of goiter is limited to 10% in the southwest part of the island. The degree of iodine deficiency, as assessed by iodine urinary excretion and ^{131}I thyroid uptake, was found to be nearly identical in the two populations. The areas also have very homogeneous ethnic, nutritional, and socioeconomic patterns. The *geologic nature of soils* might be responsible for the difference in goiter prevalence between the two populations, or geologic differences, soil characteristics, trace elements in drinking water, and bacterial pollution could act in association with iodine deficiency to increase the prevalence of goiter in a population.[28] A possible connection between *bacterial pollution* in drinking water and endemic prevalence has been raised by several investigators.[29, 30] Supporting evidence for this concept is available. Cultures of *Escherichia coli* contain an antithyroid compound that diminishes iodine uptake in the murine thyroid.[29] *Paracolobactrum* bacteria produce myrosinase, an enzyme that converts the naturally occurring progoitrin into the active thyroid blocker goitrin.[30] *Natural goitrogens* (i.e., organic and microbial water pollutants) (see Table 108–2) may be considered significant determinants of the prevalence of endemic goiter, either in iodine-deficient areas or in localities where iodine intake is abundant. This finding was very well documented in studies conducted by Gaitan in Colombia[31] and, more recently, in the coal-rich Appalachian area of eastern Kentucky.[32] Goitrogenic effects[31–38] may be related to the consumption of certain foodstuffs (cassava, millet, babassu coconut, piñon, and vegetables from the genus *Brassica*). The goitrogenic factor in cassava is related to the hydrocyanic acid liberated from the cyanogenetic glucoside (linamarin) and endogenously changed to thiocyanate, which competitively inhibits trapping and promotes the efflux of intrathyroidal iodine.[33] *Pearl millet* is one of the most important food crops in the semiarid tropics (large portions of Africa and Asia). Millet porridge is rich in C-glucosylflavones and also contains thiocyanate.[38] Both are additive in their antithyroid effects. *Babassu coconut* is largely consumed in northern Brazil, and studies have demonstrated the possible presence of flavonoids in the edible part of the nut.[35] Thus in areas where millet and babassu coconut are a major component of the diet, their ingestion may contribute to the genesis of goiter. Furthermore, flavonoids, besides being potent inhibitors of thyroid peroxidase, also interact with thyroid hormone at the peripheral level.[31] From turnips the compound 1-5-vinyl-2-thiooxazolidone (VTO, goitrin) was isolated; it is similar in action and potency to synthetic antithyroid drugs.[36] Soybean-based foods and soybean milk formulas increase the loss of T_4 from the blood via bile into the gut.[37] Disulfides of aliphatic hydrocarbons from sedimentary rock drained by water into deep wells are believed to be the cause of the incomplete reduction of endemic goiter after the use of iodized salt in Colombia.[32]

Excess consumption of iodine-rich kelp (dry seaweed, 80–200 mg iodine per day) has caused sporadic and even endemic goiter in humans.[39] In this case, goiter is common in some families and more frequent in girls at puberty, which suggests possible influences of additional genetic and hormonal factors. The organification of iodine and, consequently, the synthesis of T_4 and T_3 were lower than normal, and iodine-rich colloid goiter was observed in patients from the goiter endemic coast of Hokkaido, Japan, after thyroidectomy.[39]

Generalized malnutrition (protein-calorie deprivation) has been recognized as an additive factor in the prevalence of endemic goiter in afflicted populations.[40] On the basis of epidemiologic data recorded in goitrous patients living in Senegal, it was recently observed that goiter correlated with vitamin A deficiency.[41] Also, vitamin A deficiency was reported to alter thyroglobulin (Tg) structure, with poorly mannosylated Tg and abnormal spatial rearrangement of tyrosyl residues. This incorrect alignment increases the distance separating tyrosyl residues and hampers normal closure of several disulfide linkages, thereby rendering tyrosine-to-thyronine coupling reactions less efficient. Thus the hormonogenic potency of Tg is severely depressed and, in combination with iodine deficiency, could be considered one explanation for the additional effects of prolonged malnutrition in areas of endemic goiter. *Abnormal immunologic phenomena* have been associated with sporadic and endemic goiter.[42–58] Thyrotropin (TSH) receptor autoantibodies have been described in multinodular euthyroid goiters, either as TSH-binding inhibiting immunoglobulins or as thyroid-stimulating immunoglobulins.[42, 43] Later, it was reported that patients with endemic goiter showed high IgA levels and positive responses to thyroid antigen in the leukocyte migration inhibition test.[44] It was also found that IgG isolated from patients with large goiters (some recurring after partial thyroidectomy) increases DNA synthesis in guinea pig thyroid cell cultures.[45] This finding was interpreted as the effect of a distinct type of autoantibody (thyroid growth–promoting IgG [TGI]) that promotes thyroid cell growth without stimulation of function.[43] The same group of investigators reported that 67% of euthyroid patients with nonendemic goiter had a positive cytochemical bioassay for thyroid growth–stimulating immunoglobulins, and values tended to be high in diffuse goiters, nodular goiters recurring after partial thyroidectomy, and those with recent growth.[46] These studies were confirmed by observing ^3H-thymidine incorporation in cultivated porcine thyroid follicles[47] and raised the question of whether thyroid growth in sporadic and endemic goiter could be partially dependent on an autoimmune mechanism.[42] Growth-promoting activity was found in IgGs prepared from the sera of 24 of 42 goitrous subjects from a region of severe iodine deficiency in northern Brazil.[48] In the latter patients, treatment with iodized oil injection resulted in loss of positive growth in every case after 1 year, simultaneously with a considerable reduction in goiter size.

Some doubt has been raised about the value of TGI studies. In particular, methods of measuring cell growth and preparing IgG have been criticized.[49, 50] TGI activity was also evaluated in purified IgG preparations by measuring thyrocyte replication as the endpoint.[51] A positive growth stimulation index was found in IgG preparations from 65 of 71 patients with endemic goiter and in 9 of 14 IgG preparations from patients with sporadic goiter. Cultured cell (FRTL-5 cells) growth stimulation with those IgGs could be detected only when IgG was tested in combination with a small concentration of TSH.

More recently, studies of subjects in the sub-Himalayan region of India and in the Alpine region associated with endemic goitrous areas in northern Italy were unable to detect thyroid growth–promoting immunoglobulins in goitrous patients vs. indigenous controls in two different assays of thyroid cell growth.[52, 53] These results fail to support a role for autoimmunity in endemic goiter.[54, 55]

Another stimulator of follicular cell growth that acts synergistically with endogenous TSH is the anti-GAL antibody.[56] This human polyclonal antibody was found to mimic the in vitro TSH effects of stimulation of cyclic adenosine monophosphate synthesis, ^{125}I uptake, and cellular proliferation of cultured porcine thyrocytes. Anti-GAL antibodies were found to be higher in goitrous individuals and positively correlated with the size of goiter.[56] Whether these antibodies contribute to the pathogenesis of the disease needs further clarification.

Increased oral iodine intake may cause the development of autoimmune thyroid disease in patients with endemic goiter.[57, 58] This finding was not verified in patients who received an injection of iodized oil.[59]

PATHOPHYSIOLOGY

The theoretic basis for human adaptation to iodine deficiency was surmised by Stanbury and Hetzel in classic field studies in Mendoza,

Argentina.[3] Goiter was regarded as an obligatory response to prolonged and severe iodine deficiency, and an increase in thyroid iodine clearance was shown to be the basic mechanism of iodine conservation. Subsequently, a shift in thyroid hormone synthesis in favor of T_3 indicated an additional mechanism.[60, 61] These concepts have improved our understanding of how humans cope with low iodine intake, as well as the effects that both lack of iodine and adaptation mechanisms have on thyroid physiology.[61–74] Thus adaptation to iodine deficiency involves a number of biochemical and physiologic adjustments that ultimately result in maintenance of the intracellular concentration of T_3 within normal limits. These mechanisms are listed in Table 108–3.

Increase in Thyroid Clearance of Plasma Inorganic Iodine

An increase in thyroid clearance of plasma inorganic iodine is the fundamental adaptive mechanism by which the thyroid gland maintains a constant concentration of accumulated iodine in the presence of chronic iodine deficiency. A clear inverse relationship between the plasma inorganic iodine concentration and thyroid clearance was found by several authors.[60, 61] The relationship is such that the product of thyroid clearance and iodine concentration is constant within the observed range of serum iodine concentrations. This product represents absolute iodine uptake, which is the mass of iodine available to the gland per unit of time. Despite the elevated clearance, absolute iodine uptake tends to be lower in iodine-deficient areas, thus indicating that the compensatory mechanism is neither perfect nor complete.[60] An inability to fully compensate for the low plasma inorganic iodine with an appropriate increase in thyroid clearance probably accounts for the fall in iodine concentration in endemic goiter. The increased iodine trapping reflects TSH stimulation, as well as an intrinsic autoregulatory mechanism dependent on the intrathyroidal iodine concentration.

Hyperplasia of the Thyroid

Although thyroid clearance may be increased without a demonstrable goiter, the anatomic accompaniment of functional activity is an increase in gland mass.[62] Another interesting point is that iodine-concentrating ability is not uniformly distributed among follicular cells, even in normal glands. A certain level of TSH-dependent, autonomous iodine trapping is a feature of normal thyroid follicles, and the generation of new follicles from mother cells with an inherently high capacity for iodine trapping could well explain the heterogeneity in iodine metabolism among the follicles of glands affected by endemic goiter.[63] Also, partial autonomy of iodine trapping could account for the persistently high uptake after the administration of iodine supplements.[62] Deficiency of cytosolic superoxide dismutase in endemic goitrous tissue has been claimed to cause more prolonged exposure to oxygen free radicals and contribute to the degenerative changes found in these tissues.[64]

Changes in Iodine Stores and Thyroglobulin Synthesis

A constant finding reported in endemic goiter is a drastic reduction in iodine concentration expressed in iodine per gram of tissue. The amount of organic iodine in a thyroid affected by endemic goiter may range from 1.0 to 2.5 mg, in contrast with values of 10 mg obtained in normal control glands.[65] Concomitantly, thyroid iodine turns over much faster, as shown by an increase in the rate of release of ^{131}I from the gland. Ermans postulated the presence of two compartments of organic iodine in an iodine-deficient gland: a slow- and a fast-releasing compartment with different sizes.[60] The fast-release pattern is seen in children and adolescents with small, diffuse goiters and is associated with a rapid rise in plasma-bound ^{131}I. Most adult goitrous patients have a slow-release pattern with normal or low protein-bound ^{131}I and a prolonged biologic half-life of thyroid ^{131}I. Such observations suggest that intrathyroidal iodine in these long-standing multinodular glands is turning over at a subnormal rate. Slow secretion of the tracer is apparently due to dilution in a large endogenous pool of stable iodine, largely as monoiodotyrosine (MIT) and diiodotyrosine (DIT), which are present to an excessive degree in the poorly iodinated Tg.

TABLE 108–3. Mechanisms Involved in the Adaptation to Iodine Deficiency

Increased thyroid clearance of plasma inorganic iodine
Hyperplasia of the thyroid and morphologic abnormalities
Changes in iodine stores and thyroglobulin synthesis
Modifications of the iodoamino acid content of the gland
Enrichment of thyroid secretion in triiodothyronine
Enhanced peripheral conversion of T_4 to T_3 in some tissues
Increased thyroid-stimulating hormone production

T_3, triiodothyronine; T_4, thyroxine.

Modification of the Iodoamino Acid Content of the Gland

Experimental studies in the rat show that thyroid hyperplasia induced by iodine deficiency is associated with an altered pattern of iodine distribution within the gland.[66–68] An increase in labeled MIT and a decrease in the concentration of DIT, as well as a progressive increase in the ratio of T_3 to T_4, are the main changes in the thyroid gland occurring during prolonged iodine deficiency and are directly related to the degree of iodine depletion of the gland. These alterations caused by iodine deficiency appear to be associated with a structural change in Tg. Experimental studies have shown a greater degree of heterogeneity in the Tg molecule. Its altered sedimentation peak, significantly lower than 19 S, indicates failure of Tg maturation.[60] In large human goiters, as the concentration of iodine is reduced, the MIT/DIT ratio increases and the fraction of tracer found in the form of T_4 and T_3 is markedly reduced. Possibly, many of the iodotyrosyl groups do not have the spatial configuration that favors the normal coupling process, and therefore only a small fraction of the iodine accumulated is actually incorporated into the normal pathway of hormone synthesis and secretion. A significant amount of iodine seems to be wasted by incorporation into iodo compounds that are clearly different from Tg, that are resistant to hydrolysis, and that have a very long half-life and low molecular weight. These iodo compounds are, at least in part, fragments of Tg.

Preferential Secretion of Triiodothyronine

The enhanced synthesis and release of T_3 at the expense of T_4 constitute an additional adaptive mechanism entirely different from those described above. T_3 contains one iodine atom less than T_4 does, and its biologic activity is greater. Therefore, increasing the T_3/T_4 ratio of the hormones actually secreted by the thyroid makes the secretion biologically more active although it contains less iodine. Data on thyroidal and extrathyroidal iodine kinetics obtained from experimental models and in humans with goiter have suggested preferential T_3 release.[66–71] Coupling of MIT and DIT seems to be favored over that of two DIT molecules and is directly related to the decreasing levels of Tg iodination.[60] A low level of Tg iodination and intense TSH stimulation are necessary conditions for increasing T_3 biosynthesis and release.

Enhanced Peripheral Conversion of Thyroxine to Triiodothyronine

A compensatory increase in the peripheral conversion of T_4 to T_3 can occur in those with chronic iodine deficiency. It has been demonstrated in iodine-deficient animals that a striking increase in the conversion of T_4 to T_3 is observed in the cerebral cortex, whereas the liver shows a change in the opposite direction.[61, 69] Thus tissues highly dependent on T_4 for their intracellular content of T_3, such as the brain, undergo a significant increase in conversion of T_4 to T_3 in the presence of chronic deficiency of iodine, and this adaptation may prevent harmful consequences on brain development in the early stages of life.[69, 72]

Increased Thyrotropin Production

In iodine deficiency, as in other thyroid conditions with a limited glandular reserve, subjects with normal serum T_3 and low T_4 levels may have elevated levels of serum TSH, although they are clinically euthyroid. A clear-cut increase in the mean level of serum TSH was found in subjects living in areas where the iodine supply was reduced, and no difference was evident between individuals with and without goiter.[73–78] Also, it has been demonstrated that serum TSH levels correlate much better with serum T_4 than with serum T_3. When T_4 is low, the pituitary seems to be hypothyroid, whereas most other tissues are not metabolically affected, provided that the serum T_3 level is normal or elevated.[61] The most elevated TSH values have been observed in newborns and young adults living in areas with severe endemic goiter, whereas in long-standing multinodular goiter the increased thyroid mass and the presence of autonomous areas may bring serum TSH levels toward the normal range.[73] An increased sensitivity of endemic goiter tissue to TSH has been proposed as an additional factor for continuous goiter growth.[75] Both thyroid peroxidase activity and 5′-deiodinase activity are elevated in the presence of normal serum TSH, and this increased activity has been claimed to be related to increased tissue sensitivity to TSH. In an attempt to further delineate the role of TSH in the pathogenesis of goiter, various investigators have administered thyrotropin-releasing hormone (TRH) to goitrous patients.[74–77] The exaggerated and sustained TSH response to TRH observed in most studies indicates an increase in pituitary TSH reserve and less than optimal T_4-induced TSH suppression at the pituitary level. This finding further documents the role in the pituitary of intracellular T_3 generated from T_4 in suppressing TSH (Fig. 108–2).

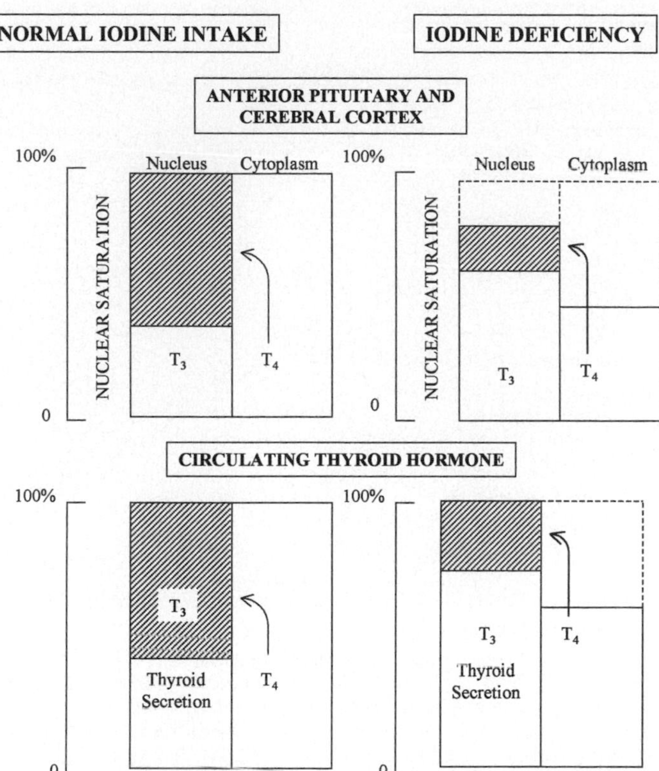

FIGURE 108–2. Normally, half of the pituitary nuclear triiodothyronine (T_3) is produced locally from thyroxine (T_4) deiodination, and the remainder is from the blood (via plasma as shown in the *upper panel, left side*). Plasma T_3 is mostly produced (~75%) from T_4 *(lower panel, left side)*. In iodine deficiency, as a consequence of stimulation by thyroid-stimulating hormone and a low iodide concentration, thyroid secretion preferentially shifts to T_3 secretion *(lower panel, right side)*. The pituitary is significantly depleted of T_3 because of the shortage of T_4, and diminished nuclear saturation results *(upper panel, right side)*.

Associated Pathology

In most regions of the globe in which selenium deficiency is endemic, iodine deficiency is also endemic, but the converse is not true.[79, 80] Selenium deficiency is more severe in China and Tibet than in central Africa[79] and could affect many organs, including the thyroid gland. Selenium, as selenocysteine, is an integral component of two important enzymes: glutathione peroxidase and iodothyronine deiodinase.[81] The former catalyzes the breakdown of hydrogen peroxide, thereby protecting against oxidative damage. The later catalyzes the deiodination of T_4 to T_3. Selenium and iodine are thus linked biochemically because both are involved in thyroid hormone production. The clinical consequences of selenium deficiency include cardiomyopathy (Keshan disease), hypothyroid cretinism (some regions of central Africa) and Kashin-Beck disease, an osteoarthropathy of the hands, fingers, elbows, knees, and ankles in children and adolescents.[82] Recent studies in Tibet have suggested that this disorder results from a combination of selenium and iodine deficiency[83] (Fig. 108–3). One possibility is that necrosis of the growth plate and epiphyseal chondrocytes is dependent on locally produced T_3 and sensitive to oxidative damage. Thus deficiency of iodothyronine deiodinase and glutathione peroxidase might result in local thyroid hormone deficiency and cellular injury, a combination that causes chondronecrosis.

CLINICAL AND LABORATORY DIAGNOSIS

The clinical picture of endemic goiter is identical to that of sporadic or simple goiter, the difference being only an epidemiologic one. Classically, infants and children up to school age have only diffuse enlargement of the thyroid gland. Further thyroid growth is often observed, mostly in girls, until puberty and constitutes what is commonly called *diffuse colloid goiter.* After adolescence the gland becomes more nodular and grows in size as the adult ages. A few patients (less than 15% of the adult goitrous population) may exhibit very large multinodular glands, with the total mass estimated to be over 150 g. Age and gender influence the prevalence of goiter, females being more often affected than males.[84]

The presence of endemic goiter does not cause any other recognized changes in the body, unless the patient is hypothyroid, which is unusual. Goitrous individuals in areas of endemic goiter seem to feel perfectly good, are able to perform hard work, and show no signs of intellectual or physical impairment. A few patients with very large goiters may show symptoms of tracheal compression, with dyspnea or other symptoms caused by compression of the jugular veins. The intensity of the symptoms and signs resulting from compression on structures surrounding the goiter is not necessarily dependent on goiter size. Large, pendulous goiters can be seen in patients who do not have any other complaint. On the other hand, relatively small goiters enclosed in the upper thoracic region can generate signs of tracheal obstruction.

A frequent complication in large multinodular goiters is hemorrhage or infarction of a thyroid nodule, often accompanied by an inflammatory reaction and an abrupt rise in serum Tg concentration. Hyperthyroidism, often caused by an autonomously functioning adenoma, is frequently observed if patients have access to even a small iodine load.[85] Thyroiditis, a rare complication, is often subacute and sometimes focal. The pathologic features of endemic goiter do not materially differ from those of simple nodular goiter. These pathologic changes have been described in detail in an excellent review by Studer and Ramelli.[62] Follicular and anaplastic carcinomas and especially

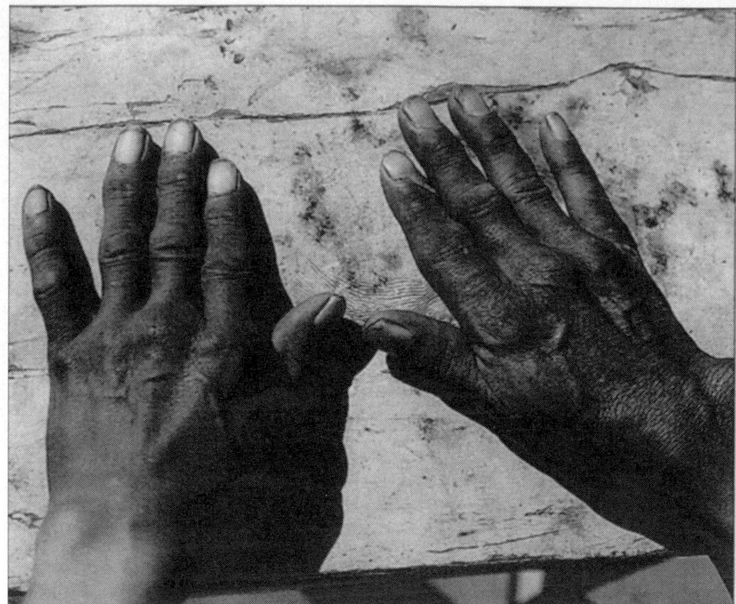

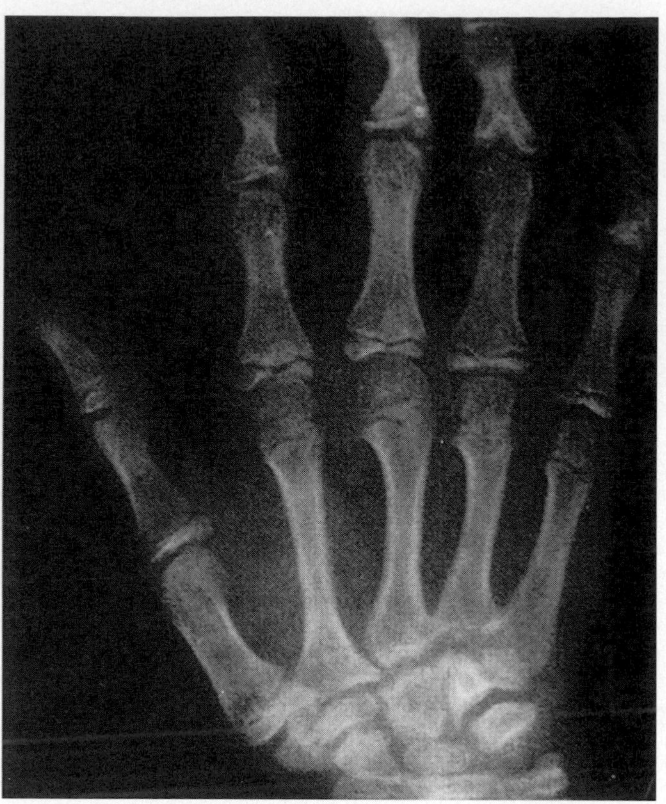

FIGURE 108–3. Affected subjects with Kashin-Beck disease (associated with selenium deficiency) have varying degrees of joint deformation, with necrosis of growth plates and joint cartilage. Iodine deficiency and Kashin-Beck disease are linked in Tibet. (Reprinted, by permission, from Moreno Reyes R, Suetens C, Mathieuw F, et al: Kashin-Beck osteoarthropathy in rural Tibet in relation to selenium and iodine status. N Engl J Med 339:1112–1120, 1998. Copyright © 1998 Massachusetts Medical Society. All rights reserved.)

sarcomas are more frequent in regions of endemic goiter. The prevalence of these tumor types means that highly aggressive thyroid cancer prevails in countries with endemic goiter whereas relatively benign forms (papillary carcinomas) are less frequently recognized.[86] The prognosis of thyroid cancer in regions of endemic goiter is worse than in goiter-free areas because most patients are first seen with a tumor stage in which no cure by surgery can be expected.[86, 87] Highly aggressive, prognostically poor types of thyroid malignancy prevail in patients with endemic goiter. Iodine supplementation results in a relative decrease in these tumor types and hence forms of thyroid cancer with a better prognosis.

A large number of laboratory tests have been applied to the study and evaluation of chronic iodine deficiency and its consequences.[88, 89] Test results are substantially altered after iodine supplementation (iodized salt or iodized oil).[88] Radioiodine uptake is usually high (>50% per 24 hours), but some subjects may have normal uptake. An inverse correlation is found between urinary ^{127}I excretion (micrograms of iodine per 24 hours) and ^{131}I uptake. An appreciable number of subjects have high radioactive iodine uptake, low levels of protein-bound ^{131}I, and a long biologic half-life of tracer within the gland. This finding suggests that some glands affected by endemic goiter may retain incoming iodine in compartments with slowly labeled pools.[60]

Serum T_3 levels in inhabitants of regions where goiter is endemic are typically normal or moderately elevated at a time when serum T_4 is below normal or low.[67–71] Elevated serum T_3 levels provide an explanation for the apparent paradox of clinical euthyroidism despite subnormal T_4 levels. Serum TSH is elevated in goitrous patients with low T_4 and correlates better with serum T_4 than with serum T_3 levels. The serum T_3/T_4 ratio is commonly used to express the adaptive processes that are described above. Euthyroid subjects living in areas where iodine is abundant have a mean ratio of 15:1, whereas in areas of endemic goiter, mean T_3/T_4 ratios reach values of 29 to 34:1.[66] Treatment with iodized oil causes a progressive fall in this ratio.[88] Serum reverse T_3 (rT_3) tends to follow the direction of serum T_4, but in the serum of pregnant women from areas of endemic goiter, rT_3 is significantly higher than rT_3 levels in nonpregnant subjects from the same region.[70] An increased binding capacity of thyroxine-binding globulin is observed and may be related to the elevated serum T_3 concentrations. This increased capacity could play an important role in the maintenance of a normal level of free T_3.[89]

Subjects with goiter have significantly higher peak TSH values than do normal individuals without goiter after a provocative test with TRH. The exaggerated and sustained TSH response to TRH may be seen in spite of a normal serum T_4 concentration and normal or elevated serum T_3 levels.[74–77] When goitrous patients move to an urban area where iodine supply is more abundant, a blunted TSH response to TRH is often observed[85, 90] and has been attributed to significantly higher production of both T_3 and T_4 from autonomous nodules within the multinodular gland. A third of these patients may also show signs of a mild, transient form of thyrotoxicosis.

Serum Tg levels are often elevated in patients with endemic goiter.[91–96] Serum Tg correlates positively with log TSH, but factors other than TSH might also be operative in the release of Tg. Other investigators have concluded that circulating Tg values, although elevated, are not dependent on TSH stimulation but rather correlate significantly with goiter size.[94] Varying elevated concentrations of Tg in the serum of patients with endemic goiter may result from leakage via intercellular junctions and from episodic necrosis of follicles, which allows Tg to be taken up by the lymph channels.[95] Others have reported that the increased serum Tg concentrations in endemic goiter could be partly related to the reduced concentration of iodine in goitrous tissue and the intrathyroidal metabolic changes secondary to persistent and chronic iodine deficiency.[96] Thyroid peroxidase activity has been shown to be decreased in endemic goitrous glands, and this decreased activity may affect the relative concentrations of T_3 and T_4 in the Tg molecule.[97]

Serum basal and peak Tg responses to bovine TSH are elevated in untreated endemic goiter, and it was found that both values slowly return to the normal range 30 months after treatment with iodized oil.[93]

PRINCIPLES OF TREATMENT

Treatment of endemic goiter can be carried out by oral administration of L-thyroxine (0.15–0.20 mg/day) for a prolonged period. This suppressive therapy induces, through a decrease in TSH and the TSH response to TRH, functional atrophy of the goiter. Results are often satisfactory in relatively small colloid goiters but less effective in large multinodular glands. Iodine administration is equally effective when introduced as adjunctive therapy with L-thyroxine or intramuscularly as iodized oil. The increased thyroidal secretion of thyroid hormones suppresses pituitary TSH, and more than half of the treated population experiences a remarkable reduction in goiter size. Surgery should be considered when the goiter is very large, when more than one-third of the normal width of the tracheal lumen is affected, and when malignancy is suspected. In patients who have previously had thyroid surgery, the possibility of shrinking the gland with radioiodine should be considered. Also, ^{131}I treatment can be used in patients in whom surgery is not an option because of increased risk.[98, 99] The goal of ^{131}I treatment is to reduce thyroid size, which can be achieved only by relatively large doses of the isotope. A rather high percentage (32%) of patients will become hypothyroid years after treatment, as also noted in subjects treated with radioiodine for Graves' disease.[98, 99] Prophylactic L-thyroxine treatment in these patients could be instituted to prevent recurrence of the goiter and/or hypothyroidism.

ENDEMIC CRETINISM

Endemic cretinism is now largely a disease in remote, underdeveloped areas of the Third World (Fig. 108–4). It occurs when iodine intake is below a critical level of 25 μg/day and may affect up to 10% of populations living in conditions of severe iodine deficiency.[100, 101] The disorder is found in India, Indonesia, China, Oceania (Papua New Guinea), Africa (Zaire), and South America (Ecuador, Peru, Bolivia). In all these locations, with the exception of Zaire, neurologic features are predominant.[101, 102] Endemic cretinism may be defined as irreversible changes in mental development in individuals born in an area of endemic goiter; such individuals exhibit a combination of some of the following characteristics not explained by other causes: (1) a predominantly neurologic syndrome consisting of defects of hearing and speech associated or not with characteristic disorders of stance and gait of varying degree, (2) stunted growth, (3) mental deficiency, and (4) hypothyroidism. In its most common form, mental deficiency, deaf-mutism, and spastic diplegia are associated with or without goiter. This condition is referred to as the *neurologic form* of endemic cretinism, in contrast to the *myxedematous* form[101, 103] (see Fig. 108–4). It should be made clear, however, that the two types of endemic cretinism represent polar opposites of a wide spectrum of clinical abnormalities.[101–119] Although the myxedematous type is more common in Zaire, the condition may be found in the Himalayas, the Hetian and Luopu districts of Xing-Jiang (China), Sicily (Italy), and South America (Bolivia and Peru).

In central Africa (Zaire), the severity of cretinism was found to be proportional to the degree of hypothyroidism; the severity was also shown to correlate with selenium deficiency.[120–123] The hypothesis was put forth that defective glutathione peroxidase caused by selenium deficiency results in a lack of protection against peroxidative damage induced by high levels of H_2O_2 in the thyroid cell. Glutathione peroxidase activity was found to be decreased in selenium-deficient areas in Zaire and Ubangi, and the enzyme activity in cretins was half the level in normal subjects.[121] The same observation on serum glutathione peroxidase activity was recently made in a selenium-deficient population in the Lhasa district in central Tibet.[82, 83] Selenium supplementation for 2 months corrected the enzyme levels in both normal subjects and endemic cretins.[122] However, this treatment also produced decreases in serum T_4 and T_3 and an increase in TSH.[123] In view of these findings it is advisable to provide iodine supplementation before administration of selenium in populations deficient in both these elements.

Thyroid growth–inhibiting immunoglobulins have been found in myxedematous endemic cretins with thyroid atrophy.[124–126] In these patients, purified IgG fractions inhibited thyrotropin-induced DNA synthesis in guinea pig thyroid segments in a sensitive cytochemical bioassay[124] and also had an inhibiting effect on cellular growth expressed by diminished incorporation of ^{3}H-thymidine into the DNA of TSH-stimulated FRTL-5 cells.[125, 126] The thyroid-blocking antibodies are believed to be directed against the thyrotropin receptor and may inhibit thyroid cell growth. In patients from the Andean region (Peru) and in Italy, humoral thyroid autoimmunity was not confirmed.[127] The subject has been considered controversial and probably associated with racial and environmental differences between the groups studied.[128, 129]

Deaf-Mutism and Endemic Cretinism

An endemic cretin is frequently partially or completely deaf. The cause of the deafness is uncertain. Lesions can be produced experimentally in the organ of Corti in the chick by injecting an antithyroid drug into the yolk sac.[109] Also, antithyroid drug (propylthiouracil) administered to pregnant mice or to pups after birth causes abnormalities in the tectorial membrane of the organ of Corti and results in deafness.[110, 111] These experiments strongly suggest that intrauterine hypothyroidism somehow damages the developing auditory system and causes deafness and other neurologic defects. The absence of deafness in severely hypothyroid endemic cretins from central Africa remains unexplained. Its absence in sporadic congenital hypothyroidism may be a result of the protective action of thyroid hormone passing to the fetus from the mother.

Diagnosis of Endemic Cretinism

Differentiation between sporadic congenital hypothyroidism and endemic cretinism is important both clinically and etiologically. The

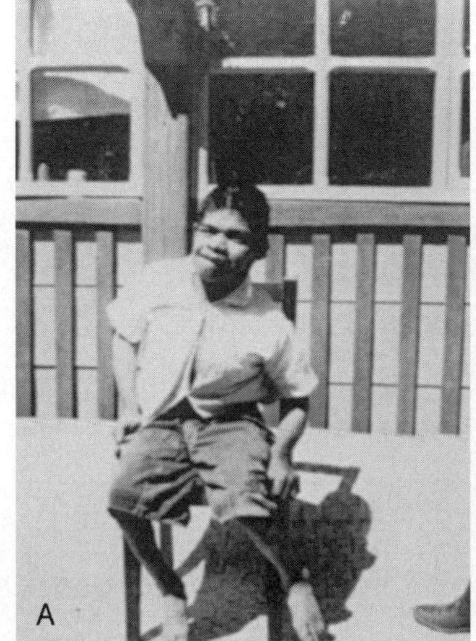

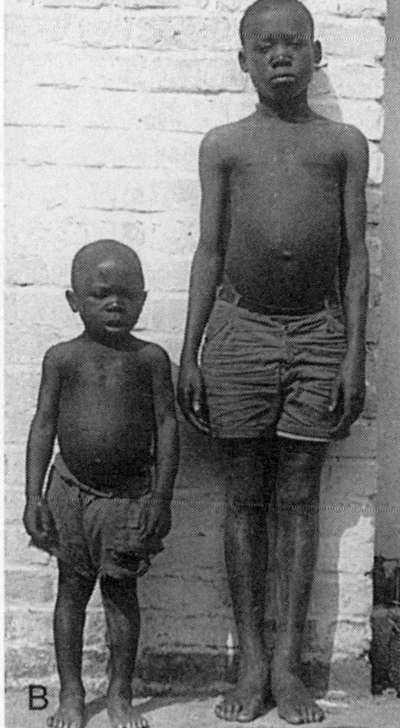

FIGURE 108–4. *A,* A typical *neurologic* endemic cretin from South America with deaf-mutism, spastic diplegia, goiter, and mental retardation. Although thyroid hormone levels are usually normal, an exaggerated and sustained thyroid-stimulating hormone response to thyrotropin-releasing hormone is frequently observed and suggests a low thyroid reserve. *B,* Two boys of the same age in Zaire (central Africa). The boy on the left is a myxedematous cretin with severe thyroid insufficiency and dwarfism. Thyroid atrophy is commonly found later in life in myxedematous cretins and has been attributed to environmental agents and/or blocking autoantibodies.

former is a result of hypothyroidism caused by developmental anomalies or metabolic defects, whereas the latter is associated with severe iodine deficiency in the maternal-fetal unit. Thus the common form of endemic cretinism during childhood or in adults, unlike untreated sporadic congenital hypothyroidism, is often not associated with severe clinical hypothyroidism,[103, 107] although a decreased thyroid reserve, an enlarged sella turcica, and an exaggerated TSH response to TRH are often found in neurologic cretins.[113] Mixed forms with both neurologic and myxedematous features occur. Important studies from South America, Papua New Guinea, and Indonesia reveal subnormal coordination in otherwise normal children whose mothers were iodine deficient during pregnancy.[114–116] This neurologic defect indicates that the effect of fetal iodine deficiency extends beyond the full clinical picture of endemic cretinism and has been described as endemic mental retardation.[114]

Neonatal Hypothyroidism in Iodine-Deficient Areas

A serious consequence of chronic iodine deficiency is a higher incidence of neonatal hypothyroidism. In India and Zaire it has been reported that this condition is 200- to 500-fold more frequent than in countries with adequate iodine intake.[117–119] In iodine-deficient areas of India, as many as 4% of newborn babies have a cord blood serum T_4 level below 2 μg/dL,[117] and in Zaire, low T_4 concentrations have been observed in up to 10%.[118] Further deterioration in thyroid function occurred in Zaire children between 2 and 4 years of age, followed by a pronounced prevalence of hypothyroidism between 5 and 7 years of age. This pattern is linked to persistent iodine deficiency accompanied by an increased thiocyanate load originating from very high consumption of cassava.[119]

Experimental work has confirmed that severe iodine deficiency affects brain development by reducing both maternal and fetal thyroid function. When sheep or marmosets are maintained on a severely iodine-deficient diet for 6 to 12 months before pregnancy and also during pregnancy, reduced brain weight and low DNA content of the fetal cerebral cortex occur as early as day 70 of gestation.[130]

Similarly, the number of spines on the shafts of pyramidal neurons from the visual cortex of iodine-deficient rats is lower than in animals supplemented with iodine.[131] This finding supports the concept that thyroid hormone affects brain maturation through specific effects on cell differentiation. The severe neurologic damage found in endemic cretinism is probably due to thyroid hormone deficiency early in pregnancy (first trimester), and it might have become irreversible by birth, at which time thyroid hormones reverse the hypothyroidism, if present, but not the neurologic deficits. Both forms of the syndrome, however, can be prevented by correction of the severe iodine deficiency before pregnancy by iodized oil injections. When given in the first trimester, however, iodized oil does not prevent the syndrome of endemic cretinism, which suggests that these effects of maternal iodine deficiency arise very early.[130] Thus elemental iodine, apart from its hormonal role, may be essential for normal neural tube development, but the mechanism responsible for this action is not known.

PROPHYLAXIS AND TREATMENT OF IODINE DEFICIENCY DISORDERS

Prevention of endemic goiter and cretinism by the addition of iodine supplements to the daily diet has been accepted and widely used since the beginning of the 20th century. The main resources for mass correction of iodine deficiency are iodized salt and iodized oil.

Iodized Salt

The sources of most common salt are solar evaporation of sea water and salt mines. Sea salt, as usually produced, does not contain enough iodine to meet minimal human needs because the average iodine content of ocean salts is approximately 2 ppm. Human salt consumption (5–15 g/day) varies widely among cultures and with climatic conditions. Thus the level of iodination of salt may be varied to conform to regional conditions (1:25,000 to 1:100,000). It is accepted that 30 ppm (30 mg of potassium iodate per kilogram of salt) is the lowest level that will ensure the provision of 100 μg of iodine per day. Many local problems confound the program of iodination of salt for the many millions of people at risk.[132] Inadequate iodinate of the salt, difficulties in importing potassium iodate, problems of transportation and coordination of distribution efforts, and the consumption of poorly iodinated "cattle" salt by the rural population are the main problems that have obstructed effective iodination prophylaxis. Successful salt iodination programs have been implemented in many countries and are highly dependent on continuous surveillance of the iodized salt produced and consumed.[132]

An increase in the incidence of thyrotoxicosis has been reported after the institution of iodized salt programs in Europe and South America and after the introduction of iodized bread in Holland and Tasmania.[133] Thyrotoxicosis was more frequently seen in patients older than 40 years and was closely associated with increasing weight and nodularity of the goiter and with the existence of nonhomogeneity on thyroid scans.[134] A mild and transient form of thyrotoxicosis or a prethyrotoxic state characterized by a blunted TSH response to TRH is frequently observed in endemic goiter patients moving to urban areas, where iodized salt is commonly used.[85, 135–138] These large multinodular goiters, adapted to chronic iodine deficiency, have autonomous areas particularly susceptible to small loads of iodine and produce excessive amounts of T_3 or T_4.

A new outbreak of iodine-induced hyperthyroidism (IIH) was recently reported in two African countries after the introduction of salt with a higher level of iodination. In a severely iodine-deficient area of Kivu in Zaire,[139–141] 25% of 200 unselected adult subjects with visible goiter had an undetectable serum level of thyrotropin (TSH). In half of the TSH-suppressed patients, serum thyroid hormones reached the level of overt hyperthyroidism. High serum thyroid hormone levels remained unchanged at a 1-year interval, which suggests that the thyrotoxicosis was not transient. The urinary iodide concentrations of these patients did not differ from the levels observed in euthyroid patients, 24 μg/dL. In most of these patients, the clinical picture was not characteristic of thyrotoxicosis.

In Zimbabwe, all cases of hyperthyroidism detected by laboratory tests in the main Hospital of Harare from 1991 to 1995 were reviewed.[142] Since 1993, a threefold increase was demonstrated after the consumption of salt iodinated at a level of 30 to 90 ppm. Fatal outcomes occurred mainly from cardiac complications. The median concentration of urinary iodide in the population was 28 μg/dL.

The biologic basis for IIH appears most often to be mutational events in thyroid cells that lead to autonomy of function.[135] When the mass of cells with such mutations becomes sufficient and the iodine supply is increased, the subject may become thyrotoxic. These changes may occur in localized foci within the gland or in the process of nodule formation. IIH may also occur with an increase in iodine intake in those whose hyperthyroidism (Graves' disease) is not expressed because of iodine deficiency.[134] The risks of IIH are principally to the elderly, who may have heart disease, and to those who live in regions with limited access to medical care. The same situation is also found in endemic goiter areas when iodized oil injections are introduced.[138] This hyperthyroidism is often transient, and hormone production will eventually decrease in 6 to 12 months without a need for therapy unless cardiovascular disease and related complications are present.

Water Iodination

A reduction in the goiter rate from 61% to 30%, with 70% of goiters showing visible reduction, has been demonstrated after water iodination.[143, 144] The introduction of an iodine filter in the wells used in small villages provided an accessible and simple method for control of iodine deficiency disorders. It was also suggested that iodinated water may be more convenient than iodized salt, with less likelihood of iodine-induced thyrotoxicosis, but this method is appropriate at the village level only if a specific source of drinking water can be identified.

Iodized Oil

Intramuscular injection or oral administration of the iodized ethyl esters of fatty acids of poppy seed, walnut, and soybean oil (475–540 mg iodine per milliliter) has been used for the prevention of endemic goiter and cretinism.[145–151] Doses have varied from 0.5 to 1.0 mL in infants and young children to 0.5 to 2.0 mL for adults. The oil is stored in the muscle and intermuscular fibrous tissue. This mode of administration was started in Papua New Guinea and extended to South America, Zaire, Nepal, Sudan, Indonesia, India, and China. Oral administration of iodized soybean oil was extensively studied in China and reported to be effective in a mass population program to control endemic goiter.[146–150]

A large breakdown in iodinated compounds occurs during the first few months (1–5 mg iodine excreted per day), and the urine may contain more than 50 μg iodine per day for 2 to 5 years. Although oral administration of iodized oil is cheaper, safer, and simpler, its effective duration is considerably shorter than that of the injected form. From data on urinary iodine, levels were always satisfactory 6 months after oral administration and frequently for 2 years.[147] After the injection of iodized oil, serum T_4 and T_3 increase to normal or elevated levels, with a concomitant decrease in serum TSH and the TSH peak response to TRH and a sharp decline in the previously elevated serum Tg levels.[148] A 1992 report mentions the reversibility of severe hypothyroidism after treatment with iodized oil in children with endemic cretinism. Such reversibility was more evident in younger children than in older groups.[147] In a few patients, the lowering of serum thyroid hormones and an increase in TSH suggest an acute Wolff-Chaikoff effect.

A few cases of thyrotoxicosis have been reported in South America after the administration of iodized oil,[138] but none so far in Papua New Guinea, India, or Zaire.[148] This condition, called IIH, is largely confined to people older than 40 years, who constitute a relatively small proportion of the population in developing countries. This complication may be minimized by restricting the administration of iodized oil to those younger than 40 years. An autoimmune reaction characterized by the development of anti-Tg and mainly antimicrosomal antibodies was reported in 42.8% of patients treated with iodized oil and was associated with glandular necrosis caused by the large dose of iodine. This finding was not confirmed, however, in other studies in Indonesia and China involving a larger number of patients.[148, 150] Also, a controlled study reported that anti-Tg or antimicrosomal antibodies were not found in a group of individuals who received iodized oil during the following 5 years of observation.[59]

The use of iodized oil has proved to be effective not only in reducing the frequency of endemic goiter but also in reducing the size of established goiters and in preventing the major neuromotor, physical, and mental deficits that are found in association with endemic goiter and endemic cretinism.[137] Iodized oil provides effective, safe, and economically sound prophylaxis against endemic goiter and related disabilities in situations in which salt iodination is not feasible for economic or political reasons.

REFERENCES

1. Dunn JT, Medeiros-Neto GA: Endemic Goiter and Cretinism: Continuing Threats to World Health. Washington, DC, Pan American Health Organization, 1974, Publication 292.
2. Ibbertson HK: Endemic goitre and cretinism. Clin Endocrinol Metab 8:97–128, 1979.
3. Stanbury JB, Hetzel BS: Endemic Goiter and Endemic Cretinism. New York, John Wiley, 1980.
4. Dunn JT, Pretell EA, Daza CH, Viteri FE (eds): Towards Eradication of Endemic Goiter, Cretinism and Iodine Deficiency. Washington, DC, Pan American Health Organization, 1986, Publication 502.
5. Matovinovic J: Endemic goiter and cretinism at the dawn of the Third Millennium. Annu Rev Nutr 3:341–412, 1983.
6. Hetzel BS: Iodine deficiency disorders (IDD) and their eradication. Lancet 2:1126–1129, 1983.
7. Hetzel BS, Dunn JT, Stanbury JB (eds): The Prevention and Control of Iodine Deficiency Disorders. Amsterdam, Elsevier, 1987.
8. Medeiros-Neto GA: Iodine deficiency disorders. Thyroid 1:73–82, 1990.
9. Gaitan E, Nelson NC, Poole GV: Endemic goiter and endemic thyroid disorders. World J Surg 15:205–215, 1991.
10. Gaitan E, Dunn JT: Epidemiology of iodine deficiency. Trends Endocrinol Metab 3:170–175, 1992.
11. Boyages SC: Iodine deficiency disorders. J Clin Endocrinol Metab 77:587–591, 1993.
12. Dunn JT: Iodine deficiency: Consequences and prevention. Thyroid Today 20:1–9, 1997.
13. WHO, UNICEF, ICCIDD: Indicators for Assessing Iodine Deficiency Disorders and Their Control through Salt Iodination. Geneva, World Health Organization, 1994.
14. Delange F, Dunn JT, Glinoer D (eds): Iodine Deficiency in Europe: A Continuing Concern. Brussels, NATO ASI Series A, Life Sciences, vol 241, 1993.
15. Dunn JT, Crutschfield HE, Gutekunst R, Dunn AD: Two simple methods for measuring iodine in urine. Thyroid 3:119–123, 1993.
16. Hollowell JG, Staehling NW, Hannon WH, et al: Iodine nutrition in the United States. Trends and public health implications. Iodine excretion data from National Health and Nutrition Examination Surveys I and III (1971–1974 and 1988–1994). J Clin Endocrinol Metab 83:3401–3408, 1998.
17. Dunn JT: What's happening to our iodine (editorial)? J Clin Endocrinol Metab 83:3398–3400, 1998.
18. Burgi H, Supersaxo Z, Selz B: Iodine deficiency diseases in Switzerland one hundred years after Theodor Kocher's survey: A historical review with some new goitre prevalence data. Acta Endocrinol (Copenh) 123:577–590, 1990.
19. Subramian P: Goiter and iodine deficiency disorders control through universal iodination of salt in India. IDD Newslett 3:12–16, 1987.
20. Wachter W, Mvungi MG, Triebel E, et al: Iodine deficiency, hypothyroidism and endemic goiter in Southern Tanzania. J Epidemiol Community Health 39:263–270, 1985.
21. Aquaron R, Zarrouck K, El Jarabi M, et al: Endemic goiter in Morocco: Skoura-Toundoute areas in the high Atlas. J Endocrinol Invest 16:9–13, 1993.
22. Delange F: Endemic Goiter and Thyroid Function in Central Africa. Monographs in Pediatrics 2. Basel, Karger, 1974.
23. Das SS, Isichei UP: The fetomaternal thyroid function inter-relationships in an iodine-deficient region in Africa: The role of T3 in possible fetal defense. Acta Endocrinol 128:116–120, 1993.
24. Buttfield IH, Hetzel BS: Endemic goiter in eastern New Guinea with special reference to the use of iodized oil in prophylaxis and treatment. Bull World Health Organ 36:243–262, 1967.
25. Ma T, Lu TZ: Iodine deficiency disorders in China: Current state, control measures, and future strategy. IDD Newslett 1:4–5, 1985.
26. Roche M: Elevated thyroidal ^{131}I uptake in the absence of goiter in isolated Venezuelan Indians. J Clin Endocrinol Metab 19:1440–1446, 1959.
27. Cooper DS, Cevallos JL, Houston R, et al: The thyroid status of the Yanomano Indians of southern Venezuela: 1992 update. J Clin Endocrinol Metab 77:878–880, 1993.
28. Koutras DA: Trace elements, genetic and other factors. *In* Stanbury JB, Hetzel BS (eds): Endemic Goiter and Endemic Cretinism. New York, John Wiley, 1980, pp 255–268.
29. Vought RL, Brown FA, Sibinovic KH: Antithyroid compound(s) produced by *E. coli*: Preliminary report. J Clin Endocrinol Metab 38:861–865, 1974.
30. Oginsky EL, Stein AE, Greer MA: Myrosinase activity in bacteria as demonstrated by the conversion of progoitrin into goitrin. Proc Soc Exp Biol Med 119:360–364, 1965.
31. Gaitan E: Goitrogens in the etiology of endemic goiter. *In* Stanbury JB, Hetzel BS (eds): Endemic Goiter and Endemic Cretinism. New York, John Wiley, 1980, pp 219–236.
32. Gaitan E: Iodine-sufficient goiter and autoimmune thyroiditis: The Kentucky and Colombian experience. *In* Medeiros-Neto G, Gaitan E (eds): Frontiers in Thyroidology. New York, Plenum, 1986, pp 19–26.
33. Bourdoux P, Delange F, Gerard M, et al: Evidence that cassava ingestion increases thiocyanate formation: A possible etiologic factor in endemic goiter. J Clin Endocrinol Metab 46:613–621, 1978.
34. Osman AK, Basu TK, Dickerson JWT: A goitrogenic agent from millet in Darfur province, Western Sudan. Ann Nutr Metab 27:14–18, 1983.
35. Gaitan E, Cooksey RC, Legan J, et al: Antithyroid effects in vivo of babassu and mandioca: A staple food in endemic goiter areas of Brazil. Eur J Endocrinol 131:138–144, 1994.
36. Eltom M, Salih MAM, Bostrom H, Dahlberg PA: Differences in etiology and thyroid function in endemic goitre between rural and urban areas of the Darfur region of the Sudan. Acta Endocrinol (Copenh) 108:356–360, 1985.
37. Krusius FE, Reltola P: The goitrogenic effect of naturally occurring L-5-vinyl and L-5-phenyl-l2-thiooxazolidone in rats. Acta Endocrinol 53:342–347, 1966.
38. Von Wykj J, Arnold MB, Wynn J, Pepper F: The effects of a soybean product on thyroid function in humans. Pediatrics 24:752–760, 1959.
39. Suzuki H: Etiology of endemic goiter and iodine excess. *In* Stanbury JB, Hetzel BS (eds): Endemic Goiter and Endemic Cretinism. New York, John Wiley, 1980, pp 237–253.
40. Medeiros-Neto GA: General nutrition and endemic goiter. *In* Stanbury JB, Hetzel BS (eds): Endemic Goiter and Endemic Cretinism. New York, John Wiley, 1980, pp 269–283.
41. Ingenbleek Y: Vitamin A deficiency impairs the normal mannosylation conformation and iodination of thyroglobulin: A new etiological approach to endemic goitre. *In* Mauron J (ed): Nutritional Adequacy, Nutrient Availability and Needs. Basel, Birkhauser, 1983, pp 264–297.
42. Brown RS, Jackson IMD, Pohl S, Reichlin S: Do thyroid stimulating immunoglobulins cause nontoxic and toxic multinodular goitre? Lancet 1:904–906, 1978.
43. Smyth PPA, McMullan NM, Grubeck-Loebenstein B, O'Donovan DK: Thyroid growth-stimulating immunoglobulins in goitrous disease: Relationship to thyroid-stimulating immunoglobulins. Acta Endocrinol 111:321–330, 1986.

44. Moto NGS, Kiy Y, Iwasso MTR, Peracoli MTS: Tumoral and cell-mediated immunity in large nontoxic multinodular goitre. Clin Endocrinol (Oxf) 13:173–180, 1980.
45. Drexhage H, Botazzo GF, Doniach D: Evidence for thyroid growth stimulating immunoglobulins in some goitrous thyroid diseases. Lancet 2:287–292, 1980.
46. Van der Gaag RD, Drexhage HA, Wiersinga WM, et al: Further studies on thyroid growth stimulating immunoglobulins in euthyroid nonendemic goiter. J Clin Endocrinol Metab 60:972–979, 1985.
47. Schatz H, Pschierer-Berg K, Nickel JA, et al: Assay for thyroid growth stimulating immunoglobulins: Stimulation of (3H) thymidine incorporation into isolated thyroid follicles by TSH, EGF, and immunoglobulins from goitrous patients in an iodine-deficient region. Acta Endocrinol 112:523–530, 1986.
48. Medeiros-Neto GA, Halpern A, Cozzi Z, et al: Thyroid growth immunoglobulins (TGI) in large multinodular endemic goiter. Effect of iodized oil. J Clin Endocrinol Metab 63:644–650, 1986.
49. Dumont JE, Roger PP, Ludgate M: Assays for thyroid growth immunoglobulins and their clinical implications, methods, concepts, and misconceptions. Endocr Rev 8:448–452, 1987.
50. Zakarija M, McKenzie JM: Do thyroid growth-promoting immunoglobulins exist? J Clin Endocrinol Metab 70:308–310, 1990.
51. Wilders-Truschmig MM, Drexhage HA, Leb G, et al: Chromatographically purified immunoglobulin G of endemic and sporadic goiter patients stimulates FRTL 5 cell growth in a mitotic arrest assay. J Clin Endocrinol Metab 70:444–452, 1990.
52. Vitti P, Chiovato L, Tonacchera M, et al: Failure to detect thyroid growth promoting activity in immunoglobulin G of patients with endemic goiter. J Clin Endocrinol Metab 78:1020–1025, 1994.
53. Davies R, Lawry J, Bhatia V, Weetman AP: Growth stimulating antibodies in endemic goitre: A reappraisal. Clin Endocrinol 43:189–195, 1995.
54. Brown RS: Immunoglobulins affecting thyroid growth: A continuing controversy. J Clin Endocrinol Metab 80:1506–1508, 1995.
55. Drexhage HA: Autoimmunity and thyroid growth. Where do we stand? Eur J Endocrinol 135:39–45, 1996.
56. Knobel M, Umezawa ES, Cardia MS, et al: Elevated anti-galactosyl antibody titers in endemic goiter. Thyroid 9:493–498, 1999.
57. Boukis MA, Koutras DA, Souvatzoglou A, et al: Thyroid hormones and immunological studies in endemic goiter. J Clin Endocrinol Metab 57:859–862, 1983.
58. Kahaly GJ, Dienes HP, Beyer J, Hommel G: Iodine induces thyroid autoimmunity in patients with endemic goitre: A randomised, double-blind, placebo-controlled trial. Eur J Endocrinol 139:290–297, 1998.
59. Knobel M, Medeiros-Neto G: Iodized oil treatment for endemic goiter does not induce the surge of positive serum concentrations of antithyroglobulin or antimicrosomal autoantibodies. J Endocrinol Invest 9:321–324, 1986.
60. Ermans AM: Etiopathogenesis of endemic goiter. *In* Stanbury JB, Hetzel BS (eds): Endemic Goiter and Endemic Cretinism. New York, John Wiley, 1980, pp 287–301.
61. Silva JE: Adaptation to iodine deficiency in the light of some newer concepts of thyroid physiology. *In* Soto R, Sartorio E, Forteza J (eds): New Concepts in Thyroid Disease. New York, Alan R Liss, 1983, pp 75–104.
62. Studer H, Ramelli F: Simple goiter and its variants: Euthyroid and hyperthyroid multinodular goiters. Endocr Rev 3:40–61, 1982.
63. Knobel M, Bisi H, Peres CA, Medeiros-Neto GA: Correlated functional and morphological aspects in human multinodular simple goiter tissues. Endocr Pathol 4:205–214, 1993.
64. Sugawara M, Kita T, Lee ED, et al: Deficiency of superoxide dismutase in endemic goiter tissues. J Clin Endocrinol Metab 67:1156–1161, 1988.
65. Riesco G, Taurog A, Larsen PR, Krulich L: Acute and chronic responses to iodine deficiency in rats. Endocrinology 100:303–308, 1977.
66. Silva JE, Larsen PR: Contributions of plasma triiodothyronine and local thyroxine monodeiodination to triiodothyronine to nuclear triiodothyronine receptor saturation in pituitary, liver and kidney of hypothyroid rats. J Clin Invest 61:1247–1259, 1978.
67. Vagenakis AG, Koutras DA, Burger A, et al: Studies of serum triiodothyronine, thyroxine and thyrotropin concentrations in endemic goiter in Greece. J Clin Endocrinol Metab 37:485–489, 1973.
68. Patel YC, Pharoah POD, Hornabrook RW, Hetzel BS: Serum triiodothyronine, thyroxine, and thyroid-stimulating hormone in endemic goitre: A comparison of goitrous and nongoitrous subjects in New Guinea. J Clin Endocrinol Metab 37:783–789, 1973.
69. Larsen PR, Silva JE, Kaplan MM: Relationship between circulating and intracellular thyroid hormones: Physiological and clinical implications. Endocr Rev 2:87–102, 1981.
70. Medeiros-Neto GA, Walfish PH, Almeida F, et al: 3,3′,5′-Triiodothyronine, thyroxine, triiodothyronine, and thyrotropin levels in maternal and cord blood sera from endemic goiter regions of Brazil. J Clin Endocrinol Metab 47:508–511, 1978.
71. Hershman JM, Due DT, Sharp B, et al: Endemic goiter in Vietnam. J Clin Endocrinol Metab 57:243–249, 1983.
72. Morreale de Escobar G, Escobar del Rey F, Ruiz-Marcos A: Thyroid hormone and the developing brain. *In* Dussault JH, Walker P (eds): Congenital Hypothyroidism. New York, Marcel Dekker, 1983.
73. Delange F, Hershman JM, Ermans AM: Relationship between the serum thyrotropin level, the prevalence of goiter and the pattern of iodine metabolism in Idjwi Island. J Clin Endocrinol Metab 33:261–268, 1971.
74. Kochupillai N, Karmakar MC, Weightman D, et al: Pituitary-thyroid axis in Himalayan endemic goiter. Lancet 1:1021–1024, 1973.
75. Bachtarzi H, Benmiloud M: TSH-regulation and goitrogenesis in severe iodine deficiency. Acta Endocrinol (Copenh) 103:21–29, 1983.
76. Rothenbuchner G, Koutras DA, Raptis S, et al: The effect of TRH on serum TSH levels in nontoxic goiter. Horm Metab Res 6:501–505, 1974.
77. Medeiros-Neto GA, Penna M, Monteiro K, et al: The effect of iodized oil on the TSH responses to TRH in endemic goiter patients. J Clin Endocrinol Metab 41:504–510, 1975.
78. Weber P, Krause U, Gaffga G, et al: Unaltered pulsatile and circadian TSH release in euthyroid patients with endemic goitre. Acta Endocrinol 124:386–390, 1991.
79. Ge K, Yang G: The epidemiology of selenium deficiency in the etiological study of endemic diseases in China. Am J Clin Nutr 57(suppl):259–263, 1993.
80. Ma T, Guo J, Wang F: The epidemiology of iodine-deficiency diseases in China. Am J Clin Nutr 57(suppl):264–266, 1993.
81. St Germain DL, Galton VA: The deiodinase family of selenoproteins. Thyroid 7:655–668, 1997.
82. Utiger RD: Kashin-Beck disease: Expanding the spectrum of iodine-deficiency disorders. N Engl J Med 339:1156–1158, 1998.
83. Moreno Reyes R, Suetens C, Mathieuw F, et al: Kashin-Beck osteoarthropathy in rural Tibet in relation to selenium and iodine status. N Engl J Med 339:1112–1120, 1998.
84. Freire Maia DV, Freire Maia A: Sex and age prevalence of endemic goitre: An epidemiological study. J Hyg Epidemiol Microbiol Immunol 25:401–406, 1981.
85. Lima N, Medeiros-Neto GA: Transient thyrotoxicosis in endemic goiter patients following exposure to a normal iodine intake. Clin Endocrinol (Oxf) 21:631–637, 1984.
86. Riccabona G: Thyroid cancer and endemic goiter. *In* Stanbury JB, Hetzel BS (eds): Endemic Goiter and Endemic Cretinism. New York, John Wiley, 1980, p 333.
87. Harach HR, Escalante DA, Onativia A, et al: Thyroid carcinoma and thyroiditis in an endemic goiter region before and after iodine prophylaxis. Acta Endocrinol (Copenh) 108:55–60, 1985.
88. Medeiros-Neto G: Laboratory evaluation in iodine deficiency disorders. Arq Bras Endocrinol Metab 29:100–113, 1984.
89. Glinoer D, Fernandez-Deville M, Ermans AM: Use of direct TBG measurements in the evaluation of thyroid function. J Endocrinol Invest 1:329–335, 1978.
90. Kiy Y, Lima N, Medeiros-Neto GA: Effective salt iodination changes in the pattern of the TSH response to TRH in endemic goiter patients. Med Sci Res 15:849–850, 1987.
91. Van Herle AJ, Chopra IJ, Hershman JM, Hornabrook RW: Serum thyroglobulin in inhabitants of an endemic goiter region of New Guinea. J Clin Endocrinol Metab 43:512–516, 1976.
92. Pezzino V, Vigneri R, Squatrito S, et al: Increased serum thyroglobulin levels in patients with nontoxic goiter. J Clin Endocrinol Metab 46:653–657, 1978.
93. Lima N, Knobel M, Medeiros-Neto GA: Long term effect of iodized oil on serum thyroglobulin levels in endemic goitre patients. Clin Endocrinol 24:635–641, 1986.
94. Macchia E, Fenzi GF, Monzani F, et al: Relationship between serum thyroglobulin, serum TSH and goiter size in an endemic area (abstract). Ann Endocrinol (Paris) 44:53, 1983.
95. Gebel F, Ramelli F, Burgi U, et al: The site of leakage of intrafollicular thyroglobulin into the blood stream in simple human goiter. J Clin Endocrinol Metab 57:915–919, 1983.
96. Unger J, de Maertelaer V, Golstein J, et al: Relationship between serum thyroglobulin and intrathyroidal stable iodine in human simple goiter. Clin Endocrinol (Oxf) 23:16, 1985.
97. Sugawara M, Summer CN, Kobayashi A, et al: Thyroid peroxidase in endemic goiter tissue. J Endocrinol Invest 13:893–899, 1990.
98. Nygaard B, Hegedüs L, Gervil M et al: Radioiodine treatment of multinodular non-toxic goitre. BMJ 307:828–832, 1993.
99. Huysmans DAKC, Hermus RMM, Corstens FHM, et al: Large, compressive goiters treated with radioiodine. Ann Intern Med 121:757–762, 1994.
100. Hetzel BS, Potter BJ: Iodine deficiency and the role of thyroid hormones in brain development. *In* Dreosti JE, Smith RM (eds): Neurobiology of the Trace Elements. Clifton, NJ, Humana, 1983, pp 83–133.
101. Stanbury JB, Kroc RL: Human Development and the Thyroid Gland: Relation to Endemic Cretinism. New York, Plenum, 1972.
102. Halpern JP, Boyages SC, Maberly GF, et al: The neurology of endemic cretinism: A study of two endemias. Brain 114:825–841, 1991.
103. Boyages SC, Halpern JP: Endemic cretinism: Toward a unifying hypothesis. Thyroid 3:59–71, 1993.
104. Delong GR: The effect of iodine deficiency on neuromuscular development. IDD Newslett 6:19, 1990.
105. Shenkman L, Medeiros-Neto GA, Mitsuma T, et al: Evidence for hypothyroidism in endemic cretinism in Brazil. Lancet 2:67–70, 1973.
106. Fierro-Benitez R, Penafiel W, DeGroot LJ, Ramirez I: Endemic goiter and endemic cretinism in the Andean region. N Engl J Med 280:296–302, 1969.
107. Squatrito S, Delange F, Trimarchi F, et al: Endemic cretinism in Sicily. J Endocrinol Invest 4:295–302, 1981.
108. Boyages SC, Halpern JP, Maberly GF, et al: A comparative study of neurological and myxedematous endemic cretinism in western China. J Clin Endocrinol Metab 67:1262–1271, 1988.
109. Doel MS: An experimental approach to the understanding and treatment of hereditary syndrome with congenital deafness and hypothyroidism. J Med Genet 10:235–243, 1973.
110. Van Middleworth L, Norris CH: Audiogenic seizures and cochlear damage in rats after perinatal antithyroid treatment. Endocrinology 106:1686–1690, 1980.
111. Uziel A, Legrand C, Ohresser M, Marot M: Maturational and degenerative processes in the organ of Corti after neonatal hypothyroidism. Horm Res 11:203–218, 1983.
112. Medeiros-Neto GA, Hollander CS, Knobel M, et al: Effects of iodines on the hypothalamic-pituitary-thyroid axis in neurological endemic cretinism: Evidence for compensated thyroidal failure in adult life. Clin Endocrinol (Oxf) 8:213–218, 1978.
113. Medeiros-Neto GA, Kourides IA, Almeida F, et al: Enlargement of the sella turcica in some patients with longstanding untreated endemic cretinism: Serum TSH-alpha, TSH-beta, and prolactin responses to TRH. J Endocrinol Invest 4:303–307, 1981.
114. Fierro-Benitez R, Cazar R, Stanbury JB: The effect of iodine deficiency correction by iodized oil on endemic mental retardation of the Andean rural communities endemized by goiter. *In* Medeiros-Neto G, Gaitan E (eds): Frontiers in Thyroidology. New York, Plenum, 1986, pp 1051–1054.
115. Connolly KC, Pharoah POD, Hetzel BS: Fetal iodine deficiency and motor performance during childhood. Lancet 2:1149–1151, 1979.

116. Bleichrodt N, Drenth PJD, Querido A: Effects of iodine deficiency on mental and psychomotor abilities. Am J Phys Anthropol 53:55–67, 1980.
117. Pandav CS, Kochupillai N, Godbole MM, Karmakar MC: Iodine deficiency and neonatal hypothyroidism in India (abstract). Ann Endocrinol (Paris) 44:20, 1983.
118. Vanderpass J, Bourdoux P, Lagasse R, et al: Endemic infantile hypothyroidism in severe endemic goitre area of central Africa. Clin Endocrinol 20:327–340, 1984.
119. Sava L, Delange F, Belfiore A, et al: Transient impairment of thyroid function in newborn from an area of endemic goiter. J Clin Endocrinol Metab 59:90–95, 1984.
120. Goyens P, Golstein J, Nsombola B, et al: Selenium deficiency as a possible factor in the pathogenesis of myxedematous endemic cretinism. Acta Endocrinol (Copenh) 114:497–502, 1987.
121. Vanderpas JB, Contempre B, Duale NL, et al: Iodine and selenium deficiency associated with cretinism in northern Zaire. Am J Clin Nutr 52:1087–1093, 1990.
122. Contempre B, Dumont J, Bebe N, et al: Effect of selenium supplementation in hypothyroid subjects of an iodine and selenium deficient area: The possible danger of indiscriminate supplementation of iodine-deficient subjects with selenium. J Clin Endocrinol Metab 73:213–215, 1991.
123. Berry MJ, Reed Larsen P: The role of selenium in thyroid hormone action. Endocr Rev 13:207–219, 1992.
124. Boyages SC, Maberly GF, Chen J, et al: Endemic cretinism: Possible role for thyroid autoimmunity. Lancet 2:529–531, 1989.
125. Medeiros-Neto GA, Tsuboi K, Lima N: Thyroid autoimmunity and endemic cretinism. Lancet 335:111, 1990.
126. Tsuboi K, Lima N, Ingbar SH, Medeiros-Neto G: Thyroid atrophy in myxedematous endemic cretinism: Possible role for growth blocking immunoglobulins. Autoimmunity 9:201–206, 1991.
127. Chiovato L, Vitti P, Bendinelli G, et al: Humoral thyroid autoimmunity is not involved in the pathogenesis of myxedematous endemic cretinism. J Clin Endocrinol Metab 80:1509–1514, 1995.
128. Boyages SC, Medeiros-Neto G: Pathogenesis of myxedematous endemic cretinism. J Clin Endocrinol Metab 81:1671–1672, 1996.
129. Chiovato L, Vitti P, Bendinelli G, et al: Pathogenesis of myxedematous endemic cretinism (reply). J Clin Endocrinol Metab 81:1673–1674, 1996.
130. Pharoah POD, Buttfield IH, Hetzel BS: Neurological damage to the fetus resulting from severe iodine deficiency during pregnancy. Lancet 1:308–310, 1971.
131. Obregon MJ, Santisteban P, Rodriquez-Pena A, et al: Cerebral hypothyroidism in rats with adult-onset iodine deficiency. Endocrinology 115:614–624, 1984.
132. Dunn JT: Seven deadly sins in confronting endemic iodine deficiency and how to avoid them. J Clin Endocrinol Metab 81:1332–1335, 1996.
133. Delange F: Correction of iodine deficiency: Benefits and possible side effects. Eur J Endocrinol 132:542–543, 1995.
134. Stanbury JB, Ermans AE, Bourdoux P, et al: Iodine induced hyperthyroidism: Occurrence and epidemiology. Thyroid 8:83–99, 1998.
135. Corvilain B, van Sande J, Dumont J, et al: Autonomy in endemic goiter. Thyroid 8:107–113, 1998.
136. Van Leewen E: Eon vorm van genuine hyperthyreose (M. Basedow zonder exophthalmus) na Gebruik van geojodeerd brood. Tijdschr Geneeskd 98:81–85, 1954.
137. Vidor CI, Stewart JC, Wall JR, et al: Pathogenesis of iodine induced thyrotoxicosis studies in northern Tasmania. J Clin Endocrinol Metab 37:901–909, 1973.
138. Martins MC, Lima N, Knobel M, Medeiros-Neto GA: Natural course of iodine-induced thyrotoxicosis (Jod-Basedow) in endemic goiter area: A 5 year follow-up. J Endocrinol Invest 12:239–244, 1989.
139. Ermans AM, Mugisho S, Tonglet R, et al: Thyrotoxicosis by the consumption of highly iodinated salt in a severely deficient population in Kivu. J Endocrinol Invest 17:71–75, 1994.
140. Ermans AM, Gullo D, Mugisho SG, et al: Iodine supplementation must be monitored at the population level in iodine deficient areas. Thyroid 5:272–276, 1995.
141. Bourdoux P, Ermans AM, Makalay WA, et al: Iodine-induced thyrotoxicosis in Kivu, Zaire. Lancet 347:552–553, 1996.
142. Todd CH, Allain T, Gomo ZAR, et al: Increase in thyrotoxicosis associated with iodine supplements in Zimbabwe. Lancet 346:1563–1565, 1995.
143. Maberly G, Eastman CJ, Corcoran J: Effect of iodination of a village water-supply on goitre size and thyroid function. Lancet 2:1270–1272, 1981.
144. Squatrito S, Vigneri R, Runelo F, et al: Prevention and treatment of endemic iodine deficiency goiter by iodination of a municipal water supply. J Clin Endocrinol Metab 63:368–375, 1986.
145. Pretell E, Moncloa F, Salinas R, et al: Prophylaxis and treatment of endemic goiter in Peru with iodized oil. J Clin Endocrinol Metab 29:1586–1594, 1969.
146. Lu TZ, Ma T: A clinical investigation in China on the use of oral versus intramuscular iodized oil in the treatment of endemic goiter. *In* Medeiros-Neto G, Maciel RMB, Halpern A (eds): Iodine Deficiency Disorders and Congenital Hypothyroidism. São Paulo, Brazil, Aché, 1986.
147. Tonglet R, Bourdoux P, Munga T, Ermans AM: Efficacy of low oral doses of iodized oil in the control of iodine deficiency in Zaire. N Engl J Med 326:236–241, 1992.
148. Thilly CH, Delange F, Coldstein-Golaire J, Ermans AM: Endemic goiter prevention by iodized oil: A reassessment. J Clin Endocrinol Metab 36:1196–1203, 1973.
149. Djokomoeljanto R, Tarwotjo IG, Maspaitella F: Goiter control program in Indonesia. *In* Ui N, Torizuka K, Nagataki S, Miyai K (eds): Current Problems in Thyroid Research, ICS 605. Amsterdam, Excerpta Medica, 1984, pp 403–405.
150. Ouyang A, Wang O, Liu ZT, et al: Progress in the prevention and treatment of endemic goiter with iodized oil in China. *In* Ui N, Torizuka K, Nagataki S, Miyai K (eds): Current Problems in Thyroid Research, ICS 605. Amsterdam, Excerpta Medica, 1984, pp 403–405.
151. Lazarus JH, Parkes AB, John R, et al: Endemic goitre in Senegal, thyroid function, etiological factors and treatment with oral iodized oil. Acta Endocrinol (Copenh) 126:149–154, 1992.

Chapter 109

Thyroid Neoplasia

Furio Pacini ▪ Leslie J. DeGroot

Thyroid cancer is statistically a minor health problem that accounts for 0.4% of all cancer deaths and kills only 8 in 1 million people per year in the United States. Its clinical importance, however, is much greater because up to 4% of the population harbor clinically detectable thyroid nodules, which must raise the possible diagnosis of thyroid cancer. This discussion evaluates the problem of the thyroid nodule and, subsequently, the management of diagnosed thyroid cancer.

THYROID NODULES

Incidence and Prevalence of Nodules

Thyroid nodules are the most common endocrine lesions, particularly in countries where dietary iodine intake is low. The main problem posed by the discovery of a thyroid nodule is the distinction between its benign or malignant nature and, consequently, its appropriate treatment.

In recent years the problem has been largely solved by the introduction in clinical practice of fine-needle aspiration cytology (FNAC), which has allowed diagnosis of the nature of thyroid nodules with great sensitivity and specificity. FNAC has resulted in a significant reduction in the number of nodules sent to the surgeon and, if surgery is needed, in better planning of the surgery to be performed.

In countries where iodine deficiency has been corrected by iodine prophylaxis, palpable thyroid nodules are present in about 4% to 5% of the general population.[1–5] Data on prevalence come from the population sampled in Framingham, Massachusetts,[1] where 4% were found to have a palpable thyroid nodule (or nodules). Half the lesions were considered multinodular and half solitary. New nodules appeared with an incidence of 1 per 1000 per year.[2] A study from Connecticut indicates a prevalence of 2% of nodular glands in an adult population.[6] Of all the thyroid glands that on surgical resection prove to contain solitary nodules, 70% to 80% are benign adenomas and about 10% to 30% are malignant growths.[3, 4]

In autopsy series, the incidence of thyroid nodules in apparently normal thyroid glands is also very high. In a report from the Mayo Clinic[5] on 1000 consecutive autopsies in individuals with clinically normal thyroid glands, an age-related increase in thyroid weight and nodularity was noted. Fifty percent had one or more nodules, and 12% had a solitary nodule. The prevalence of thyroid carcinoma was 2.1%. If we also consider nonpalpable nodules, which are more and more frequently discovered during ultrasound exploration for nonthyroidal diseases, such as carotid exploration, hypercalcemia, and cervical adenopathies (Table 109–1), the prevalence of thyroid nodules can be as high as 20% to 30% in unselected population and even higher in older age groups.[7, 8]

A higher prevalence of thyroid nodules is usually reported in countries affected by moderate or severe iodine deficiency, where diffuse goiter is frequent and evolves with time to multinodular goiter. The problem of whether thyroid cancer is more common in this environment is still debated. In a prospective study performed by Belfiore et al. in an iodine-deficient area of Sicily (Italy), the prevalence of thyroid nodules was higher with respect to a control area with sufficient iodine intake.[9] The number of thyroid cancers was not increased when express as percentage of the nodules, but it was higher in absolute numbers because of the higher prevalence of thyroid nodules.

Most thyroid nodules are benign, particularly in multinodular goiters, although great variation is observed between clinical and surgical series. The incidence of thyroid carcinoma is around 3% to 4% of all thyroid nodules, and its mortality accounts for only 0.4% of all cancer deaths. The above findings justify a conservative therapeutic approach, whenever possible, because surgical treatment of all clinical thyroid nodules, without any selection, would expose an extraordinary number

TABLE 109–1. Prevalence of Nonpalpable Thyroid Nodules Detected on Ultrasound

Series	Purpose of Examination	Prevalence (%)
Harlocker et al.	Hyperparathyroidism	46
Stark et al.	Hyperparathyroidism	40
Carroll et al.	Carotid examination	13
Ezzat et al.	Prospective	67
Brander et al.	Prospective	27
Woestyn et al.	Prospective	19
Tomimori et al.	Prospective	17

Reproduced with permission from Tan GH, Gharib H: Thyroid incidentalomas: Management approaches to nonpalpable nodules discovered incidentally on thyroid imaging. Ann Intern Med 126:226, 1997.

of people to surgical treatment. Furthermore, considering that only few of them will have thyroid carcinoma, that many, especially if operated on by inexperienced surgeons, will have surgical complications, and that the financial cost will be high, one must realize that surgical treatment of thyroid nodules must be rigorously based on a rational diagnostic protocol.

Nature and Pathology of Nodules

Thyroid nodules are not a unique disease, but the clinical manifestation of several different thyroid diseases. They may be single or multiple and may be found in the context of a normal gland or a diffuse goiter. In multinodular goiter one of the nodules may become clinically dominant in terms of growth, dimension, and functional character. A clinical-pathologic classification of thyroid nodules is presented in Table 109–2.

Benign Neoplasia

The first distinction to be made among benign nodules is between functioning ("hot" on thyroid scan) and nonfunctioning ("cold"). Whereas a "hot" nodule is almost synonymous with a benign nodule, a "cold" nodule is not synonymous with a malignant nodule because only a minority will turn out to be thyroid carcinomas. Cold nodules can also be distinguished as solid or cystic (around 10%–20% of the total). However, mixed, solid-cystic forms are also frequent and should be considered solid in terms of frequency of malignancy. As a general rule, thyroid carcinoma is more frequent among solid, single cold nodules.

Most adenomas are follicular and have a histologic appearance characteristic of thyroid tissue. The adenomas usually exhibit a uniform orderly architecture and few mitoses and show no lymphatic or blood vessel invasion. They are characteristically enveloped by a discrete fibrous capsule or a thin zone of compressed surrounding thyroid tissue. Fetal and embryonal adenomas show a progressively less "adult" structure. Whether papillary adenoma is a real entity is debatable; most observers believe that all papillary tumors should be considered carcinomas. Others believe that some papillary tumors are benign adenomas. It is our impression that papillary tumors are best thought of as carcinomas, although the degree of invasive potential may be very slight in some instances. The same confusion extends to Hürthle cell adenomas. Many pathologists consider all these tumors low-grade carcinomas in view of their frequent late recurrence. For this reason, the nondefinitive term *Hürthle cell tumor* is commonly used. Hürthle cell tumors are found on electron microscopy to be packed with mitochondria, which accounts for their special eosinophilic staining quality.

Nearly half of all single nodules have on gross inspection a gelatinous appearance, are composed of large colloid-filled follicles, and are not completely surrounded by a well-defined fibrous capsule. These nodules are listed as colloid variants of follicular adenomas in our classification. Many pathologists report them as colloid nodules and suggest that each is a focal process perhaps related to multinodular goiter rather than a true adenoma. These tumors are not usually surrounded by a capsule of compressed normal tissue and often show degeneration of parenchyma, hemosiderosis, and colloid phagocytosis. The histologic pattern of various benign tumors of the thyroid is shown in Figure 109–1.

Thyroid adenomas are usually monoclonal "new growths"[10] that are formed in response to the same sort of stimuli as carcinomas are. Heredity does not appear to play a major role in their appearance. One clue to their origin is that they are four times more frequent in women than in men, although no definitive relationship of estrogen to cell growth has been demonstrated. Thyroid radiation, chronic thyroid-stimulating hormone (TSH) stimulation, and oncogenes (see below) believed to be related to the origin of these lesions are discussed below in the section on thyroid cancer. Of specific interest in relation to benign nodules is the frequent involvement of *ras* gene mutations found in follicular adenomas[11] and the observation by Parma and colleagues that activating mutations of the TSH receptor are the specific cause of most hyperfunctioning adenomas.[12]

TABLE 109–2. Clinical and Pathologic Classification of Thyroid Nodules

- Non-neoplastic nodules
  - Hyperplastic
    - Spontaneous
    - Thyroid hemiagenesis
    - Compensatory after partial thyroidectomy
  - Inflammatory
    - Acute bacterial thyroiditis
    - Subacute thyroiditis
    - Hashimoto's thyroiditis
- Benign neoplasia
  - Nonfunctioning
    - Adenoma
    - Cyst
    - Thyroglossal cyst
  - Functioning
    - Toxic (or pretoxic) adenoma
- Malignant neoplasia
  - Primary carcinomas
    - Papillary
    - Follicular
    - Anaplastic
    - Medullary
  - Lymphomas
  - Thyroid metastasis from other primaries
- Nonthyroidal lesions
  - Cystic hygroma
  - Aneurysm
  - Parathyroid adenoma or cyst

Non-Neoplastic Nodules

These lesions are not true nodules but represent focal areas of glandular hyperplasia arising spontaneously or, more frequently, as a consequence of previous partial thyroidectomies. Also, thyroid hemiagenesis may rarely be manifested as hyperplasia of the existing lobe and mimic a thyroid nodule. Nodule(s) associated with Hashimoto's thyroiditis are the expression of lymphocytic infiltration. The nodules seen during the initial phase of subacute thyroiditis are a result of the inflammatory process giving origin to typical granulomas.

Micronodules

Micronodules are nodules 1 cm or less in diameter. With the routine use of neck ultrasound, the discovery of micronodules is increasing, and nearly 50% of women older than 60 years have such nodularities. One view is that micronodules are in general not clinically relevant and, in absence of other clinically suspicious findings, do not require any investigation or treatment. The usual advice is to repeat thyroid ultrasound at regular intervals and reconsider therapy if growth is seen. An alternative view is that such nodules are as frequently malignant as larger nodules and should be evaluated by FNAC under ultrasound guidance.

Course and Symptomatology

Adenomas grow slowly, remain dormant for years, must reach a size of 0.5 to 1 cm before they can be palpated, and are typically asymptomatic. Thus they are often discovered accidentally by the patient or physician and rarely produce local symptoms. Occasionally, bleeding into a tumor causes local pain and tenderness and, very rarely, transient thyrotoxicosis. Such bleeding may be followed by spontaneous regression of the nodule but more often results in cyst formation.

About 70% of thyroid nodules or adenomas are hypofunctional in terms of accumulation of radioactive iodide and are "cold" on isotope scans. About 20% may be borderline in function and on isotope scan

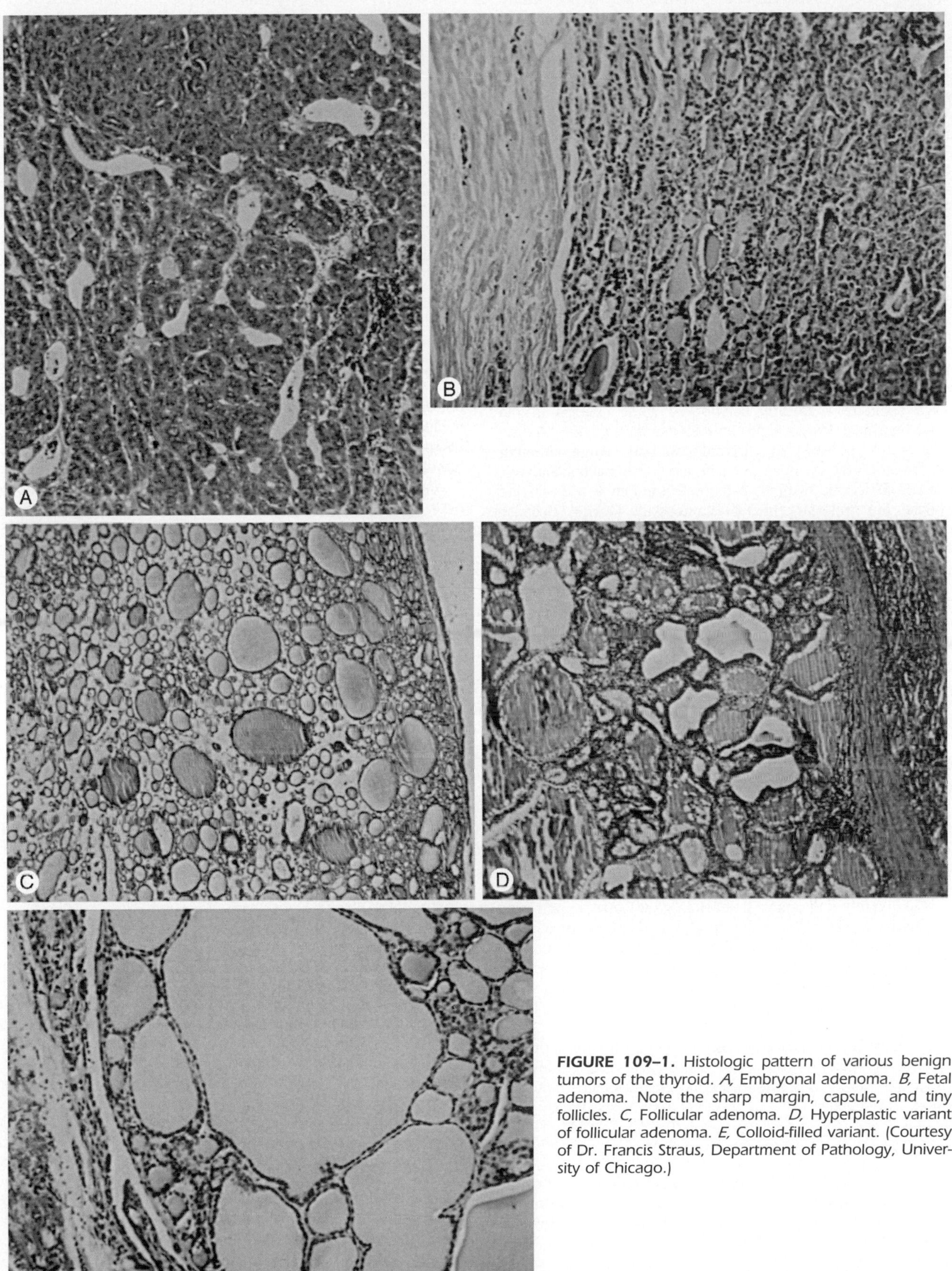

FIGURE 109–1. Histologic pattern of various benign tumors of the thyroid. *A,* Embryonal adenoma. *B,* Fetal adenoma. Note the sharp margin, capsule, and tiny follicles. *C,* Follicular adenoma. *D,* Hyperplastic variant of follicular adenoma. *E,* Colloid-filled variant. (Courtesy of Dr. Francis Straus, Department of Pathology, University of Chicago.)

appear to have uptake similar to that of the remainder of the thyroid. One in 10 (or less) is hyperfunctional, concentrates iodide avidly, may suppress function of the normal gland, and may even produce thyrotoxicosis. This process typically occurs when the functioning nodule has grown larger than 3 cm in diameter and in older patients. Activating TSH receptor mutations have been found by Parma and coworkers to be the cause of most hyperfunctional adenomas[12] and are also common in "hot" nodules in patients with multinodular goiter.[13, 14] These mutations involve the extracellular loops of the transmembrane domain and the transmembrane segments and have been proved to induce hyperfunction of the TSH receptor by transfection studies. Mutations of the stimulatory guanosine triphosphate–binding protein subunit are also present in some patients with hyperfunctioning thyroid adenomas.[15]

Usually an adenoma, once formed, seems to be committed to this "life-style" indefinitely, although, rarely, pathologic evidence suggests that adenomas can transform into invasive carcinoma. Sequential change from hyperplasia to adenoma formation to invasive carcinoma has been found in patients with congenital goitrous hypothyroidism and can be produced experimentally in animals.

Interesting studies have been reported on the metabolic function of nodules. Cold nodules are typically unable to transport iodide into the thyroid as a result of a specific deletion of some element of the transport mechanism.[16] They are not able to maintain a concentration gradient for iodide between the thyroid cell and serum, although peroxidase function may be intact in the tissue.[17, 18] In such adenomas, thyrotropin (TSH) is able to bind to the cell membrane and activate adenyl cyclase, but subsequent metabolic steps are lacking. Because other factors related to transport are normal, such as Na^+,K^+-ATPase levels, a specific deletion in elements of the iodide transport mechanism appears to be present. Other "cold nodules" have been shown to lack peroxidase enzyme.[19] These studies suggest that adenoma formation is associated with genetic mutational events causing loss or dysfunction of specific enzymes in the iodide metabolic pathway. Recent cloning of the Na^+-I^- symporter gene,[20] the gene responsible for iodine uptake by the follicular cell, has opened a new field of research that might give new insight into the mechanism underlying the lack of iodine uptake of cold nodules.

Clinical Evaluation and Management of Nodules

The aim of clinical evaluation is to detect nodules that should be referred to a surgeon. Among benign lesions, the aim is to differentiate between adenomas (functioning or nonfunctioning), cysts, and nodules in the context of an underlying benign thyroid disease. This differential diagnosis is extremely important in deciding the most appropriate therapy. Similarly important in benign lesions is detection of clinical symptoms or signs that per se could suggest a need for surgical therapy, such as compression of the trachea and/or the esophagus or a recurrent nerve deficit. A schematic list of the clinical and laboratory features associated with a high risk for cancer is reported in Table 109–3.

Factors that must be considered while reaching a decision on management include the history of the lesion; age, sex, and family history of the patient; physical characteristics of the gland; local symptoms; and laboratory evaluation.

Personal History

The age of the patient is an important consideration because the ratio of malignant to benign nodules is higher in youth and lower in older age. In a study involving nonirradiated children with cold thyroid nodules, a twofold increased risk of thyroid cancer, regardless of sex,[21] was found when compared with that for adults.[2] In adult men, nodules are less frequent, and a greater proportion are malignant.

Rarely, the family history may be helpful in making a decision regarding surgery. Patients with the heritable multiple endocrine neoplasia (MEN) syndrome, type 1, may have thyroid adenomas, parathyroid adenomas, islet cell tumors, and adrenal tumors, whereas patients with MEN type 2 have pheochromocytomas, medullary thyroid carcinomas, hyperparathyroidism, and mucosal neuromas.[22–24] Familial medullary cancer (without MEN) is also possible. Furthermore, we have noted that 6% of our patients with differentiated thyroid carcinoma have other family members with a history of malignant (nonmedullary) thyroid neoplasm. Familial papillary thyroid tumors occur independently and in Cowden's disease, Gardner's syndrome, and familial polyposis coli.[25]

TABLE 109–3. Clinical Features Suggesting Malignancy of a Thyroid Nodule

History
External irradiation during childhood
Familial history of medullary cancer
Age <20 or >60 yr
Male sex
Thyroid nodule
Rapidly growing (especially during L-thyroxine therapy)
Firm or hard or pain
Fixed to soft tissue
Local symptoms
Other
Lymphadenopathy
Dysphagia, hoarseness

As discussed below, a history of prior irradiation to the head or neck during infancy or childhood is strongly associated with the subsequent occurrence of carcinoma.[26] A history of such radiation exposure and the presence of a palpable nodule or nodules must raise the possibility of thyroid cancer, which requires a cytologic diagnosis.

The epidemic of childhood papillary thyroid cancer observed in Belarus and Ukraine after the Chernobyl nuclear accident[27] is believed to be the result of contamination from radioactive fallout, mainly iodine isotopes, which were released in huge amounts into the atmosphere. No increase in the risk of thyroid cancer has been reported after diagnostic or therapeutic exposure to ^{131}I. However, the possibility that many naturally occurring thyroid carcinomas may be due to fallout radiation after nuclear tests, other radiation sources, or natural background must be seriously considered.

The history of the neck lump itself is important. Recent onset, growth, hoarseness, pain, regional nodes, symptoms of brachial plexus irritation, and local tenderness all suggest malignancy but, of course, do not prove it. The usual cause of sudden swelling and tenderness in a nodule is hemorrhage into a benign lesion. Although the presence of a nodule for many years suggests a benign process, some cancers grow slowly. In our series, the average time from recognition of a nodule to the diagnosis of cancer was 3 years.

Coexisting benign thyroid disease is important in evaluating the cancer risk associated with a thyroid nodule. A history of residence in an endemic goiter zone during the first decades of life is also relevant and must raise the possibility of multinodular goiter as the true diagnosis. Hashimoto's thyroiditis is frequently associated with discrete nodules, which are an expression of the autoimmune process. The frequency of thyroid carcinoma is not increased in patients with Hashimoto's thyroiditis. However, Hashimoto's thyroiditis is a frequent preexisting condition in patients in whom thyroid lymphoma develops.[28] A higher risk of differentiated thyroid cancer has been found in patients with Graves' disease and cold thyroid nodules,[28–31] and increased aggressiveness of such Graves' disease–associated thyroid cancer has been proposed.[32] In the authors' experience and that of other groups,[33, 34] the response to traditional therapy and the final outcome of patients with thyroid cancer and Graves' disease are not different with respect to thyroid cancer patients without Graves' disease.

Physical Examination Findings

Accurate palpation of the thyroid gland and the cervical node chains is of paramount importance in the evaluation of thyroid nodular pathology. It gives an idea of the number and size of the nodule(s), their consistency and motility, and the status of the rest of the thyroid gland, as well as the presence and the importance of lymph node involvement.

The adenoma is typically felt as a discrete lump in an otherwise normal gland, and it moves with the thyroid. Enlarged lymph nodes should be carefully sought, particularly in the area above the isthmus, in the cervical chains, and in the supraclavicular areas. Their presence suggests malignant disease unless a good alternative diagnosis is apparent, such as recent oropharyngeal sepsis or viral infection. Fixation of the nodule to strap muscles or the trachea is alarming. Characteristically, a benign thyroid adenoma is part of the thyroid and moves with deglutition, but it can be moved in relation to the strap muscles and within the gland substance to some extent. Pain, tenderness, or sudden swelling of the nodule usually indicates hemorrhage into the nodule but can also indicate invasive malignancy. Hoarseness may arise from pressure or by infiltration of a recurrent laryngeal nerve by a neoplasm. Obviously, the presence of a firm, fixed lesion associated with pain, hoarseness, or any one of these features should signal some degree of alarm. It is worth noting that these signs are not specific for the diagnosis of malignancy. In a study correlating suspicious clinical features with the histologic diagnosis, the authors found benign disease in 29% of patients with palpable cervical adenopathy, 50% of patients with hard nodules, 29% of patients with apparent nodule fixation, and 17% of patients with true vocal cord paralysis.[35] The converse situation, the absence of such characteristics, suggests but does not prove benignity. Fluctuance in the lesion suggests the presence of a cyst that is usually benign.

The presence of a diffusely multinodular gland, ascertained on the basis of palpation, ultrasound, or scanning, is generally interpreted as a sign of safety. Multinodular goiters coming to surgery have a significant prevalence of carcinoma (4%–17%), but this finding is believed to be due largely to selection of patients for surgery and not to be typical of multinodular goiter in the general population.[36] If one area within a multinodular goiter seems different from the remainder of the gland on the basis of palpation or function or has demonstrated rapid growth or if two discrete nodules are found in a gland that is otherwise normal, one should consider malignant change rather than a benign multinodular goiter.

Occasionally the gland has, in addition to a nodule, the diffuse enlargement and firm consistency of chronic thyroiditis, a palpable pyramidal lobe, and antibody test results that may be positive. These findings strongly suggest thyroiditis but do not disclose the nature of the nodule, which must be evaluated independently. It should be remembered that 14% to 20%[37, 38] of thyroid cancer specimens contain diffuse or focal thyroiditis.

Thyroid Function Tests

Unless a toxic adenoma is present, the patient is usually euthyroid, and this impression is supported by normal values for serum free thyroxine (FT_4), free triiodothyronine (FT_3), and TSH. Low thyroid hormones or elevated TSH results should raise the question of thyroiditis. Measurement of serum antithyroid autoantibodies (antithyroglobulin [anti-Tg] and antithyroperoxidase [anti-TPO]) in every new patient in search of an underlying autoimmune thyroid disease is advocated by several centers. The serum Tg concentration may be elevated, as in all other goitrous conditions, and is therefore not a valuable tool in the differential diagnosis. On the contrary, elevation of circulating calcitonin levels in a patient with a thyroid nodule is almost always diagnostic of medullary thyroid cancer. Several prospective studies have shown that routine measurement of circulating calcitonin in thyroid nodules allows the preoperative diagnosis of medullary thyroid carcinoma with better accuracy than seen with FNAC and without false-positive results[39–42] (Table 109–4). Such screening offers the possibility of finding tumors before they have metastasized, thus increasing the chance of definitive cure. According to these authors, measurement of serum calcitonin should be considered in the diagnostic evaluation of thyroid nodules. Whether the considerable expense is justified cannot be determined yet; routine screening has been adopted in several European clinics, but not in the United States. Calcitonin assay is of course indicated in the presence of a suggestive family history or coincident features of the MEN-2 syndromes.

TABLE 109–4. Medullary Thyroid Cancer Diagnosed by Routine Measurement of Serum Calcitonin and by Fine-Needle Aspiration Cytology in Nodular Thyroid Diseases

Authors	Patients	MTC Detected by CT	MTC Detected by FNAC
Pacini, 1994	1385	8 (0.57%)	2 (0.14%)
Rieu, 1995	469	4 (0.85%)	1 (0.21%)
Vierhapper, 1997	1062	13 (1.22%)	—
Niccoli, 1977	1167	12 (1.02%)	3 (0.25%)

Routine measurement of serum calcium is also advocated by several centers. The aim is not directly related to the diagnosis of thyroid nodules, but to detect undiagnosed parathyroid adenomas.

Imaging

THYROID ULTRASOUND. Thyroid ultrasound is becoming more and more popular in the first-line evaluation of thyroid nodules. Good technique demonstrates nodules if larger than 3 mm, indicates cystic areas, and may demonstrate a capsule around the nodule and the size of the lobes. It often displays multiple nodules when only one is noted clinically. The technique is more sensitive than scintiscanning, is noninvasive, involves less time, allows serial examination, and is usually less expensive. From 3% to 20% of lesions are found to be totally or partially cystic. Purely cystic lesions are reported to have a lower incidence of malignancy than solid tumors (3% vs. 10%), and diagnosis of a cyst raises the possibility of aspiration therapy.[43] Mixed solid and cystic lesions allegedly have a higher frequency of malignant change than do either pure cysts or solid lesions.

ISOTOPE SCANS AND OTHER IMAGING TECHNIQUES. Isotope scintiscans provide some help but are relatively less important if a cytologic study is done.[44, 45] Nodules that are hyperfunctional and produce hyperthyroidism are rarely malignant, and those that accumulate iodide in concentrations equal to the surrounding normal thyroid tissue are usually, but not always benign[46, 47] (Fig. 109–2). Cold nodules are also typically benign, but when viewed the other way, most thyroid cancers are seen as inactive areas on thyroid scan. In practice, except for the specific case of a toxic nodule, scans are probably of little help in the differential diagnosis, and the tendency to omit scanning from diagnostic maneuvers is growing. Scintiscans can confirm the diagnosis of multinodular goiter and can show the presence of diffuse disease (such as Hashimoto's thyroiditis) in some patients when nodularity is suspected.

Newer scanning techniques have been developed that show promise

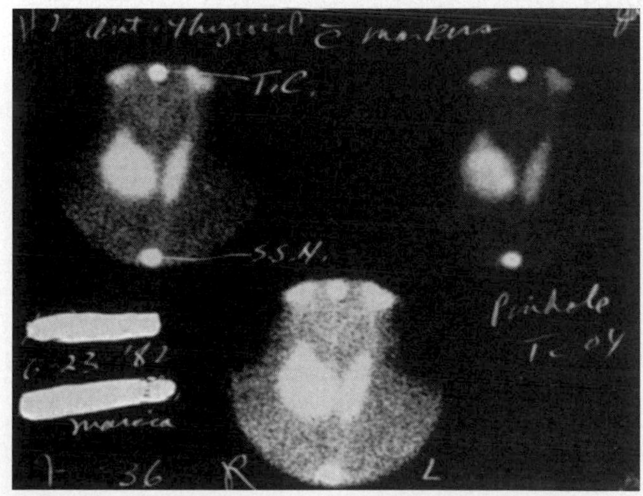

FIGURE 109–2. Scintillation scan view of a functioning nodule in a 36-year-old woman. At surgery the nodule proved to be a mixed papillary-follicular neoplasm.

for differential diagnosis. Lesions that concentrate radioactive phosphorus or selenomethionine but do not concentrate iodide are said to usually be malignant. Differentiated cancers can generally be visualized by ^{201}Th chloride scanning, and anaplastic cancers usually accumulate ^{67}Ga citrate. However, these techniques have not found a place in routine preoperative evaluation. Fluorescent thyroid scanning allows quantitation of the distribution of stable iodide in thyroid nodules[48] and has been reported to allow differentiation of benign from malignant lesions.[49] Our own studies do not support this contention. Echo imaging using ultrasound can delineate cystic structures, which are usually associated with a benign process[50] (Fig. 109–3). Unfortunately, this fact is of little assistance in managing an individual patient. Thyroid thermography, thyroidography using injections of contrast media directly into the substance of the gland, and thyroid arteriography have also been used. Computed tomography (CT) is expensive but occasionally useful, especially in unusually large substernal glands. Magnetic resonance imaging (MRI) is rarely necessary but is useful for identifying abnormal nodes.

A chest radiograph should be taken if a normal film has not been reported in the prior 6 months. Soft tissue x-ray films of the neck may disclose indentation or deviation of the trachea if the tumor is more than 3 or 4 cm in diameter. Fine, stippled calcifications through the tumor (psammoma bodies) are virtually pathognomonic of papillary cancer. Patchy or "signet ring" calcification occurs in old cysts and degenerating adenomas and has no such connotation.

Fine-Needle Aspiration Cytology

Although all the above-mentioned procedures may give some indication, only the result of FNAC can give a definitive answer regarding the nature of a thyroid nodule. FNAC has now been widely adopted after the initial favorable reports by Walfish et al.[51] and Gershengorn et al.[52] It has replaced the core needle biopsy previously used to provide a histologic diagnosis.[53] In expert hands, adequate specimens can be obtained in over 90% of patients, with a diagnostic sensitivity and specificity near or superior to 95%. Willems and Lowhagen, in reviewing a collected series of nearly 4000 surgically proven fine-needle aspiration (FNA) studies, found that 11.8% were considered malignant lesions.[54] False-negative diagnoses of cancer were made in 6.6% to 27.5% and false-positive diagnoses in only 0% to 2%. Currently, the results of FNAC are viewed as the "gold standard" for diagnosis in most cases and play a crucial role in the selection of patients for surgery. Gharib and coworkers analyzed data on 10,000 FNA procedures and found it to be the preferred first step in diagnosis.[55] The diagnostic accuracy was nearly 98%, with fewer than 2% false positives and false negatives. Miller et al. compared FNA, large-needle aspiration, and cutting needle biopsy.[56] They found that FNAC examination was able to detect almost all carcinomas but believe that cutting needle biopsy is a useful additional procedure, especially in larger (over 2–3 cm) nodules.

In our practice, 5% to 8% of aspirates are diagnostic of malignancy, 10% to 20% are considered suspicious but not diagnostic, 2% to 5% fail to provide an adequate specimen, and the remainder are considered benign, usually suggestive of a "colloid nodule" or thyroiditis. With respect to pre-FNAC years, various centers using the results of FNAC for therapeutic decisions have observed a 35% to 75% reduction in the number of patients sent to surgery, a twofold to threefold increase in the percentage of cancers found at surgery, and a variable, but constant reduction in the cost of thyroid nodule management.

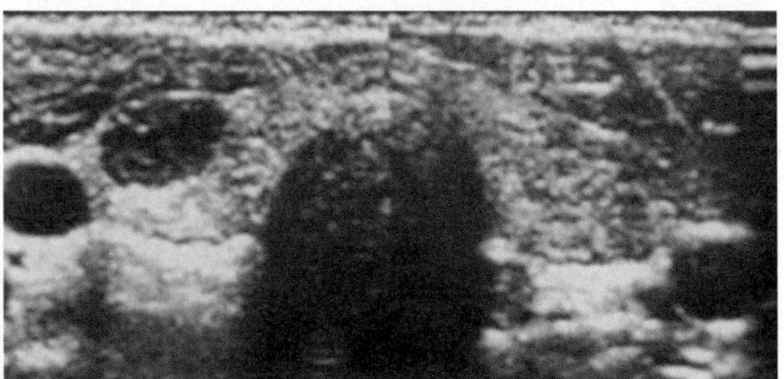

FIGURE 109–3. Sagittal echo scan of a palpable 2-cm single nodule showing a lesion in the R lobe. On aspiration, 2 mL of brownish colloid was obtained. The few cells present showed Hürthle cell changes.

FNAC is performed with a 22- to 25-gauge needle. Specimen adequacy requires a minimum of two slides (from separate aspirates) showing at least six to eight cell clusters.[57] The method is simple, inexpensive, and very well tolerated and, if necessary, may be repeated several times. Complications are very rare and consist mainly of hematomas. In several large series it has been found that around 70% (range, 53%–90%) of aspirates are classified as benign, 4.0% (1%–10%) as malignant, 10% (5%–23%) as suspicious (including follicular proliferation), and 17% (15%–20%) as inadequate for diagnosis.[58–61] When the sample obtained is of good quality (i.e., high cellularity), the cytologic diagnosis of thyroid carcinoma, especially in the case of a papillary histotype, is highly reliable and false-negative or false-positive results are very rare. Medullary thyroid carcinoma is easily diagnosed by cytology in classic cases, but sometimes the cellular pattern is atypical and can be interpreted as follicular and even papillary proliferation. Problems may also arise in the case of thyroid lymphoma because the smear may be composed of follicular cells mixed with lymphocytes, which can mimic chronic lymphocytic thyroiditis or may be confused with anaplastic carcinoma. Cytology of cystic nodules shows the presence of colloid, necrotic material, macrophages, and rare epithelial cells. In most cases these lesions are benign, but the possibility of cystadenocarcinoma must be considered.

A particular problem is represented by cases in which cytology is indicative of follicular proliferation or Hürthle cell proliferation. In this case, cytology is not able to distinguish between follicular adenoma or follicular carcinoma because the distinction is based mainly on the presence of capsular or vascular invasion, which cannot be seen on a cytologic smear. Therefore, histologic evaluation of the lesion is mandatory, and 10% to 20% of these nodules will prove to be malignant.

The major limitation of FNAC is inadequate specimens. The rate of inadequacy is variable among different centers, with a realistic estimation of between 15% and 25%.[58, 59] Inadequacy raises the question of therapy for the nodule with nondiagnostic FNAC. Some authors recommend surgical treatment for all these nodules, whereas others select for surgery only those suspicious by other clinical or laboratory features. Even if only the most suspicious nodules with inadequate FNAC are selected for surgery, the yield of malignancy at histology is relatively low and ranges from 8% to 19%.[57, 62, 63] In any case, these patients should be carefully monitored by repeated FNAC and referred to a surgeon in case of an increase in size.

An additional indication for FNAC is the diagnostic evaluation of cervical nodes, both at initial evaluation and when a diagnosis of thyroid cancer has already been established. In the case of lymph nodes suspected of being of thyroid metastatic origin, FNAC may be integrated with the measurement of Tg in the liquid recovered from washing the needle used for the aspiration. As shown in Figure 109–4, in case of a metastatic lesion from differentiated thyroid carcinoma, this technique demonstrates the presence of high levels of Tg.[64]

In conclusion, FNAC should be performed on any thyroid nodule. In case of multinodular goiter, FNAC should be performed on as many nodules as possible. In dubious cases, FNAC may be repeated immediately or over the years if the final decision is to not operate on the patient. It is worth mentioning that the preoperative diagnosis of thyroid carcinoma is useful not only to select the patients to be operated on but also to plan in advance the most appropriate surgical procedure.

A variety of techniques have been applied to improve the accuracy of interpretation of FNA histology or cytology. Staining with antibodies to TPO and Tg or to T cell antigens is fairly routine. Currently, demonstration of increased expression of the *MUC1* gene and telomerase activity in carcinomas rather than in adenomas has aroused interest, but these techniques have thus far been applied only to operative specimens.[65, 66]

Diagnostic Protocol

A possible practical diagnostic approach to patients with thyroid nodules is schematically represented in Figure 109–5.

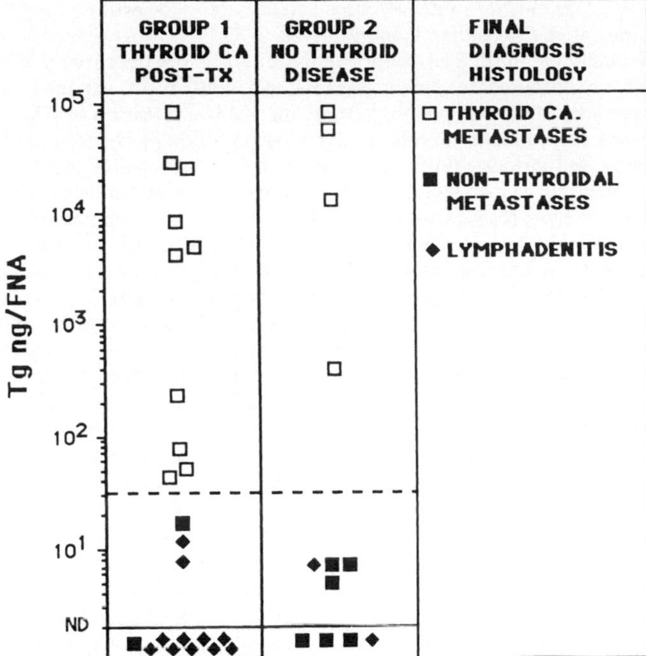

FIGURE 109–4. Concentration of thyroglobulin (Tg) in fine-needle aspirates of neck masses from patients with (group 1) or without (group 2) known thyroid cancer, according to the final diagnosis at histology. (From Pacini F, Fugazzola L, Lippi F, et al: Detection of thyroglobulin in fine needle aspirates of nonthyroidal neck masses: A clue to the diagnosis of metastatic thyroid cancer. J Clin Endocrinol Metab 74:1401, © 1992, The Endocrine Society.)

Serum thyroid hormone and TSH measurement and thyroid ultrasound are performed as the first-line exploration. Determination of antithyroid antibodies and calcitonin may also be performed.

If TSH is suppressed or low, a thyroid scan is performed to confirm the presence of an autonomously functioning nodule; the subsequent approach will depend on the presence of clinical or subclinical thyrotoxicosis and the size of the nodule.

If the nodule is cold and cystic, FNAC will be performed both as a therapeutic technique (evacuation) and as a diagnostic tool to detect the small percentage of cystic adenocarcinomas.

If the nodule is cold and totally or partially solid, the therapeutic decision will depend on the results of FNAC.

Therapy

A complete diagnostic evaluation, as outlined above, is a prerequisite to determine the choice of treatment for thyroid nodules. Then the problem is whether the nodule requires any therapy and, if so, whether it is manageable by medical or surgical therapy.

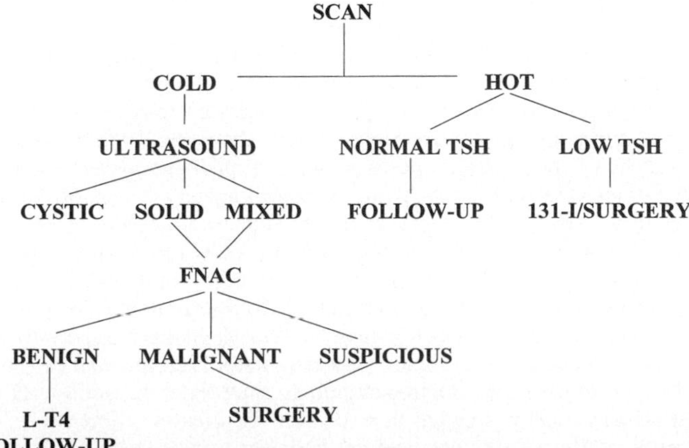

FIGURE 109–5. Flow chart for the diagnostic evaluation of thyroid nodules. FNAC, fine-needle aspiration cytology; L-T4, levothyroxine; TSH, thyroid-stimulating hormone.

Surgical Therapy

We favor selecting the malignant nodules for surgery and suggest medical therapy or follow-up for the others. However, surgical treatment should also be suggested for some benign lesions, either single or associated with multinodular goiter, when the size is large enough to give symptoms and signs of discomfort or aesthetic concern. Another surgical indication is for questionable nodules, including follicular proliferation on FNAC.

If surgery is selected, we believe that it is crucial to work in conjunction with a surgeon who has frequent and continuous experience in thyroid surgery to obtain good results. This is not to say that resection of a thyroid lobe for a nodule is a difficult procedure. However, if more extensive surgery is required, especially if total or near-total thyroidectomy and lymph node resection are indicated, it is imperative that the surgeon have the proper knowledge and experience to reduce the possibility of damage to the recurrent laryngeal nerves and parathyroid glands. The usual procedure is lobectomy, which is relatively harmless and has an incidence of complications approaching zero. Usually patients are discharged within 2 to 3 days. Complications are more common if more extensive dissection is done, as discussed below. The thyroid specimen itself, any abnormal areas in the gland, and any abnormal-appearing lymph nodes should be immediately examined by frozen section. Differentiating benign from malignant thyroid lesions is admittedly difficult, especially with frozen sections, but experienced pathologists can make the distinction with a high degree of reliability. Occasionally, follicular lesions are believed by the pathologist to be benign at surgery, but permanent sections reveal changes that indicate malignancy. Reoperation with near-total thyroidectomy is probably desirable in these patients because up to one-third can be expected to have residual tumor in the contralateral lobe.[67] To avoid these second operations, we recommend lobectomy and contralateral subtotal resection for very cellular follicular lesions as the initial procedure. Occasionally, a small papillary or follicular cancer is found in the pathologic specimen after conclusion of the operation. If this cancer is less than 1 cm and has a well-demarcated single focus and the patient is younger than 45 years, nothing further need be done. After surgery, all patients are maintained on replacement levothyroxine therapy in the hope of preventing the recurrence of other nodules.

Medical Therapy

BENIGN SOLID COLD NODULE. Appropriate management of these nodules is strongly debated. A recent meta-analysis[67a] has indicated that about 25% respond to thyroxine treatment with a decrease in size whereas the remainder are unchanged, at least over several months. Some physicians believe that once malignancy has been ruled out, medical therapy is indicated for solid cold nodules with normal or subnormal thyroid function, especially when associated with thyroid enlargement. The drug of choice is levothyroxine. Some physicians advocate a dose sufficient to suppress pituitary TSH secretion as demonstrated by a serum TSH level less than 0.1 μU/mL. The rationale for this therapy is the unequivocal observation that TSH is to some extent a growth factor not only for the normal thyroid but also for thyroid nodules. Experimental and clinical evidence has shown that even mild iodine deficiency elicits subminimal increases in TSH levels, which leads first to glandular hyperplasia and later to multinodular goiter. On the other hand, the functional heterogeneity and the variable degree of mitogenicity of follicular cells upon stimulation by TSH are an explanation for the appearance of a nodule without diffuse goiter. When the nodule and/or the goiter are of recent origin, suppression of TSH stimulation by levothyroxine is often sufficient to eliminate the nodule or to at least reduce its size and that of the thyroid gland. In long-standing cases, both the nodules and the goiter are seldom cured, but a significant reduction in size and arrest of the progression are likely to occur.

Once instituted, levothyroxine therapy must go on for years to be effective. Age is very important in the selection of patients to be treated. Treatment is always indicated in young patients and adults up to about 50 years of age. In older patients the opportunity to initiate suppressive therapy must be considered on an individual basis after excluding other underlying diseases such as heart problems. However, if a patient is already receiving levothyroxine treatment and has good compliance and no side effects, the treatment can be continued after 50 and even 60 years of age with the daily dosage slightly decreased.

An alternative approach is to aim for a TSH of 0.3 to 1 μU/mL because this level will have some suppressive effect, perhaps inhibit the growth of nodules over subsequent years, and is free of the minimal risks of mild thyrotoxicosis.

At the other end of the spectrum of opinion are physicians who believe that thyroxin therapy is useless and who simply offer continued observation without treatment.

Another aspect to be considered is functional thyroid status. Before instituting levothyroxine therapy, to avoid iatrogenic thyrotoxicosis one must be certain that the patient is perfectly euthyroid and that serum TSH, measured with an ultrasensitive assay, is not already suppressed, as so often can happen in multinodular goiters with areas of functional autonomy.

The last important aspect is the dose to be given. The usual suppressive dose is between 1.5 and 2 μg/kg/day, administered in the morning. The dose is checked after 3 to 4 months by measuring FT_3, which should stay in the normal range, and TSH, which should be in the range selected, with an FT_4 value usually in the upper limit of the normal range.[68] If the results show that TSH is not suppressed or that the patient has been overtreated, an appropriate dosage modification will be made, with another hormonal control determined 3 to 4 months later and then yearly.

Once the few precautions described above are observed, levothyroxine treatment is generally useful and safe. Our own experience and data from the literature indicate that significant shrinkage is obtained in 15% to 50% of the nodules and that many others do not progress. Side effects on the heart and bone, described by some authors, are not observed when careful avoidance of subclinical thyrotoxicosis is maintained.[69]

When clinical signs of hyperthyroidism suddenly develop during levothyroxine therapy, one must suspect the occurrence of functional autonomy of the nodule(s) and levothyroxine treatment must be immediately withdrawn. An indication for referring the patient to a surgeon is an increase in size of the nodule during levothyroxine therapy. Such a situation is not unusual and, although regarded as suspicious, does not constitute definite evidence of malignancy.

AUTONOMOUSLY FUNCTIONING THYROID NODULE. The incidence of cancer in an autonomously functioning thyroid nodule (AFTN) (hot nodule) is so low that the therapeutic approach is mainly dictated by the presence of thyrotoxicosis and/or the size of the nodule. Sometimes hot nodules are found in the presence of detectable TSH, the extranodular uptake being reduced but not suppressed. Many AFTNs are associated with subclinical thyrotoxicosis, the only abnormality being a low or undetectable serum TSH. Overt thyrotoxicosis is present in the remaining cases. AFTNs tend to occur in young adults, and their size is usually smaller than 3 cm.

AFTNs of small dimension (<3 cm), without thyrotoxicosis, can be left untreated and observed. About 20% to 30% of the nodules, more frequently when they are larger than 3 cm, evolve to thyrotoxicosis, sometimes decades after discovery. In the case of thyrotoxicosis, three therapeutic options are available: surgery, radioiodine, and ethanol injection. Radioiodine is a very effective therapy and is the treatment of choice in many patients with AFTNs. Euthyroidism and a variable degree of tumor shrinkage are always obtained after ^{131}I treatment, but a hard nodule usually persists for life. The activity of ^{131}I to be administered depends on the size of the nodule and ranges between 7 and 40 mCi. Surgery is an acceptable alternative therapy and is indicated for large nodules (>3 cm) and for patients who refuse to be treated with radioiodine. Surgery consists of total lobectomy and, in the case of thyrotoxicosis, must be performed after restoration of normal thyroid function by adequate preparation with antithyroid drugs (methimazole or propylthiouracil). The development of hypothyroidism after treatment is unusual after surgery and occurs in about 10% of cases after radioiodine therapy.

Recently, a third therapeutic option for the treatment of AFTN has been proposed by Italian authors and consists of percutaneous intranodular ethanol injection.[70, 71] The mechanism of action of ethanol is based on induction of cellular dehydration followed by coagulative necrosis and vascular thrombosis and occlusion. The technique, when performed by well-trained staff, is effective and safe. Transient local pain is the most frequent side effect. Percutaneous intranodular ethanol injection may be considered a possible alternative to surgery and radioiodine in selected cases (small nodules easily accessible to palpation). This method has now been used for several years, and so far evaluation has not revealed long-term complications. Use of the technique has thus far been confined largely to Europe.

THYROID CYSTS. Thyroid cysts are easily managed by aspiration, but recurrence of the cyst is very frequent. Suppressive therapy with levothyroxine may reduce the risk of relapse, especially if aspiration is performed after a few months of levothyroxine treatment, but the risk of relapse remains significantly high. An emerging alternative therapy is cyst sclerotherapy by ethanol injection into the nodule after complete aspiration of the cystic fluid.[72] The technique appears to be effective and safe. It might become the treatment of choice for thyroid cysts. When the above-mentioned therapy fails to avoid cyst recurrence or when the size of the nodule is too large, surgery is necessary.

A small proportion (about 3%) of cystic nodules diagnosed as thyroid cysts do not originate from the follicular epithelium, but rather from the parathyroids. These cysts may be suspected from the color of the cystic fluid, which usually, but not always, is transparent like water. The final diagnosis is easily achieved by finding high concentrations of parathyroid hormone and low or undetectable concentrations of Tg in the fluid aspirate.[73] Most of the time calcemia is normal. The differential diagnosis between thyroid and parathyroid cysts has important therapeutic implications in that parathyroid cysts do not tend to recur after FNA and, of course, do not respond to levothyroxine treatment.

THYROID CARCINOMA

Epidemiology

Thyroid cancer accounts for under 1% of all cases of malignant neoplasia. It is rare in children and increases in frequency with age, and it is among the five most frequent cancers in the second, third, and forth decades of life. Differentiated thyroid cancers are two to four times as frequent in females as in males. However, the female preponderance decreases in prepubertal and postmenopausal ages, which suggests that sex hormones might play some role in the pathogenesis.

The estimated incidence rate of thyroid nodules is about 1 per 1000 persons per year, and that of thyroid carcinoma in various part of the world ranges from 0.5 to 10 cases per 100,000 persons per year. Thus 0.5% to 10% of patients with thyroid nodules have thyroid cancer. It is not certain that carcinoma occurs with increased frequency in areas of endemic goiter, although a clear increase is seen in the relative proportion of follicular and anaplastic neoplasms. Thyroid carcinoma has occurred in the United States during the past 20 years with an incidence of about 40 new cases per million people per year[74] and has been associated with a death rate of approximately 8 per million per year (Fig. 109–6). This figure seems to reflect the incidence of clinically important thyroid carcinomas well; however, continuous improvement in diagnostic methods, mainly ultrasound and FNAC, is increasing the discovery of minimal thyroid carcinomas that might have been biologically unimportant. Studies by Sampson and coworkers[75] and Fukunaga and Yatani[76] indicate that a high prevalence (up to 5.7%) of unsuspected microcarcinomas may exist in adults. These lesions are mostly smaller than 0.5 cm in greatest dimension, are usually papillary in nature, and are believed to behave in a relatively benign manner. They are, effectively, detected only by a pathologist. Recognition of such "minimal thyroid cancers" does not demand the same therapeutic response as does the discovery of a larger tumor,

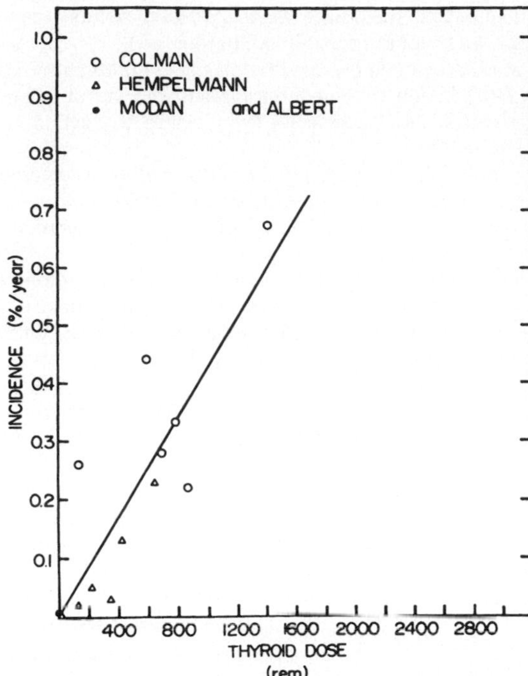

FIGURE 109–6. Estimated dose response for thyroid cancer in humans from external irradiation. The incidence of carcinoma each year is plotted against the original thyroid radiation dose. (From Maxon H, Thomas SR, Saenger EL, et al: Ionizing irradiation and the induction of clinically significant disease in the human thyroid gland. Am J Med 63:967, 1977.)

although small tumors can certainly metastasize and are occasionally fatal. Studies from the Mayo Clinic suggest that the incidence of thyroid cancer is about 36 per million cases per year but increases to 60 per million if small, occult tumors are included in the statistics.[77] A significant proportion of thyroid cancers are not diagnosed during life and are not the cause of death of the patient. The prevalence of neoplasm at autopsy is highly variable, depending on the population selected and the care of the survey. Prevalence ranges from 0.1% to 2.7%.[78, 79] Two studies of consecutive autopsies of patients dying in hospitals found that 2.7% of thyroids harbored unsuspected thyroid cancer and that an equivalent percentage had metastatic carcinoma in the gland.[79, 80] Accurate pathologic examination of resected multinodular goiters, so frequent in areas of iodine deficiency, is able to detect many occult tumors, which again might be of no relevance from the clinical point of view. All these data are evidence for leisurely growth of most thyroid tumors.

When compared with other malignancies, thyroid cancer is probably the most curable cancer, with very high long-term survival rates, at least in the well-differentiated histotypes. However, some patients are at high risk for recurrent disease or even death. Most of these patients can be identified at the time of diagnosis by using well-defined prognostic indicators.

Pathology

Histologic diagnosis of malignancy is usually very simple, but in some tumors it is difficult. Pathologic examination of thyroid tumors is organized to differentiate between *benign* and *malignant* lesion, to define pathologic *prognostic factors* among variants of papillary and follicular carcinoma, and to detect large cell *anaplastic cancer, medullary cancer,* and *rare forms* of thyroid cancer. A schematic classification and definition of thyroid tumors are presented in Table 109–5.

Papillary and *follicular* carcinomas are the two most frequent entities, usually referred to as differentiated thyroid cancer. The diagnosis of papillary carcinoma is based on the presence of typical features. The diagnosis of follicular carcinoma is based on the presence of follicular differentiation without the features typical of papillary cancer.[81] Immunostaining for Tg is almost always positive in both papillary and follicular tumors and may serve to confirm the thyroid origin of a metastasis.

Papillary Thyroid Carcinoma: Classic Type

According to their size and extension, papillary carcinomas may be classified as *microcarcinomas*, carcinomas *limited to the thyroid gland*, and carcinomas *extending outside the thyroid*.

Microcarcinomas refer to tumors smaller than 1 cm in diameter and are also called "occult." They may have the features of a classic papillary carcinoma of small size, or they may appear as unencapsulated sclerotic nodules of a few millimeters infiltrating the surrounding thyroid. Microcarcinomas are found in 5% to 35% at autopsy, depending on the geographic area and the methodology,[5, 82] but they are very rare in childhood. As a result of the general improvement in diagnostic techniques, the number of microcarcinomas selected for surgery is increasing. Their prognosis is very good.[83, 84]

Larger, clinically detectable tumors represent nearly 70% of all papillary cancers. They appear as firm nonencapsulated or partly encapsulated tumors.[81, 85] A few papillary cancers may be partly necrotic or cystic. Papillary cancer is often *multicentric* in one lobe and bilateral, with a frequency varying between 20% and 80% in different series.[86, 87]

Microscopically, papillary carcinomas contain papillary areas either with a focal distribution or with a diffuse pattern. The papillae consist of a stromal-vascular axis lined by characteristic cells. The presence of true papillae is a peculiar feature of papillary thyroid cancer, and these papillae must be differentiated from the pseudopapillae and the macropapillae seen in Graves' disease, in benign nodules, or in goiter with hypothyroidism.

Other aspects may be associated with the papillae. *Follicles* filled with colloid or a *trabecular* or *lobular* aspect, *squamous metaplasia*, and *psammoma bodies* are other distinguishing features present in 40%

TABLE 109–5. Classification and Definition of Thyroid Tumors

Epithelial Thyroid Tumors	Definition
Benign	
Follicular adenoma	A benign encapsulated tumor with evidence of follicular cell differentiation
Malignant	
Papillary carcinoma	A malignant epithelial tumor with evidence of follicular differentiation, alterations in papillary and follicular structure, and characteristic nuclear changes
Follicular carcinoma	A malignant epithelial tumor showing follicular cell differentiation without the diagnostic features of papillary carcinoma
Undifferentiated carcinoma	A highly malignant tumor composed in part or wholly of undifferentiated cells
Medullary carcinoma	A malignant tumor showing evidence of C cell differentiation
Malignant nonepithelial tumors	
Sarcoma	A malignant tumor lacking all evidence of epithelial differentiation and showing definite evidence of specific sarcomatous differentiation
Hemangioendothelioma	A highly malignant tumor with extensive necrosis or hemorrhage and a vascular-like cleft lined by cells displaying features of endothelial cells
Malignant lymphoma	A malignant tumor with positive staining for leukocyte common antigen or similar antigens
Secondary tumors	Pathologic features depend on the primary tumor

Modified from Hedinger C, Williams ED, Sobin LH: Histologic typing of thyroid tumors, vol II. *In* International Histological Classification of Tumors, ed 2. Berlin, Springer-Verlag, 1988.

to 50% of the tumors. Also typical of papillary lesions are areas of sclerosis found either in the central portion of the tumor or at the periphery.

Nuclei are characteristic. They are larger than those found in normal follicular cells when superimposed on one another, are pale and transparent at the center, and contain hypodense chromatin and prominent nuclear membranes. The shape is irregular and may be "fissured" like "coffee grains." Large, circular, well-delimited intranuclear inclusions, an expression of cytoplasmic invagination, are present.[88] In the absence of other features of the tumor, the diagnosis of papillary cancer is based on typical feature of the nuclei.[81]

Scattered lymphocytes are frequently found at the invasive periphery of the tumor. More rarely, a true *lymphocyte infiltrate* resembling chronic lymphocytic thyroiditis is seen in the tumor and is associated with a favorable prognosis.[89]

Frequently and early in the disease, papillary carcinoma invades lymphatic vessels. The invasion progresses from the perithyroid chains to more distant chains. Nodes along the recurrent nerve are most frequently involved. Lymphatic spread within the thyroid is probably the reason for the high frequency of multifocality of the tumor.[86, 87] Venous invasion and distant metastases (mostly to the lung and bone) are rare and account for 5% to 7% of cases.[90]

VARIANTS OF PAPILLARY THYROID CARCINOMA. The *follicular variant* is grossly encapsulated[91, 92] and shows a diffuse pattern of follicular growth with colloid-containing follicles. The papillary nature of this tumor can be recognized by the finding of clear nuclei, psammoma bodies, desmoplastic reaction, and lymphocytic infiltration. Lung metastases are frequent and respond well to conventional treatment. The prognosis is similar to that of the classic variants. They are frequently found in young subjects, and 21% of the post-Chernobyl childhood thyroid cancers in Belarus were classified as follicular variants.[93]

The rare *diffuse sclerosing variant* is mostly found in children and young adults.[94] Its characteristics are those of diffuse thyroid enlargement as seen in goiter, but with both lobes replaced by a very firm and calcified tumor. At microscopy this form is almost always multicentric. Tumor papillae are associated with squamous metaplasia without keratinization and abundant psammoma bodies. Extensive lymphocytic infiltration of the gland is often found, and lymph node metastases are present in 100% of cases. Also, distant metastases are frequent. The prognosis is less favorable than for classic papillary cancer, although the response to treatment may be excellent.

In the *tall cell* variant[95] and the *columnar cell* variant,[96] the tumor is usually large and extends outside the thyroid gland. These tumors have a papillary pattern, and the cells are tall and have a granular, eosinophilic cytoplasm. Frequent vascular invasion is seen, and they are typical of older patients. A poor prognosis has been reported with this variant.

The *encapsulated variant* is characterized by a capsule similar to an adenoma, but focally invaded. Microscopically, the typical cytologic and nuclear features of papillary tumor and psammoma bodies are found. This variant represents 8% to 13% of cases.[97]

In subjects affected by *polyposis coli*, papillary thyroid cancer has typical features: frequent multifocality with classic papillary aspects associated with solid areas and elongated cells.

Follicular Thyroid Carcinoma

At variance with the papillary histotype, *follicular carcinoma* is usually seen as a *solitary*, more or less encapsulated *nodule* in the thyroid. Depending on the degree of invasiveness, the tumor is classified as *minimally invasive* (encapsulated) or *widely invasive*.[81] The distinction has great prognostic impact because the prognosis is more severe when more vascular invasion is present.[98]

Minimally invasive carcinomas represent more than 50% of cases. The diagnosis of malignancy is totally based on the demonstration of unequivocal vascular invasion and/or invasion of the full thickness of the capsule. Examination of multiple blocks, including the periphery of the nodule, is often necessary to exclude or confirm the presence of invasion. Cytologically, they cannot be distinguished from benign adenomas. Thus FNAC is of no help in the differential diagnosis between benign and malignant lesions. Frozen section may lead to misdiagnosis and should probably be discouraged.

Widely invasive tumors present few diagnostic problems. They show widespread infiltration of blood vessels and the surrounding thyroid tissue. The capsule, when present, is infiltrated in several areas and grossly disrupted.

In both minimally and widely invasive follicular carcinoma the morphology is variable and ranges from *well differentiated* with well-formed follicles full of colloid *to poorly differentiated* with a solid, cellular growth pattern.

Follicular cancer invades blood vessels but rarely lymphatics. The metastases are spread hematogenously to the lungs, bones, and less frequently the brain and liver.[90] Metastases are very frequent with the widely invasive variant, less frequent with the minimally invasive variant.

VARIANTS OF FOLLICULAR CARCINOMA. *Clear cell* tumor is a rare variant, with architectural and clinical features similar to those of the usual follicular carcinomas. The cells are clear because of the formation of intracytoplasmic vesicles, glycogen or fat accumulation, or intracellular Tg deposition. These tumors must be distinguished from clear cell adenoma, from parathyroid adenoma or carcinoma, and particularly from metastatic clear cell renal carcinoma.

The *oxyphilic cell type* (or *Hürthle cell type*) is composed of cells derived from the follicular epithelium and characterized by large size with abundant granular, eosinophilic cytoplasm, large nuclei, and prominent nucleoli. The granular appearance of the cytoplasm is conferred by the large number of mitochondria inside the cell.

Because Hürthle cells can be found in papillary carcinomas and in a number of benign conditions, including nodular goiter, hyperthyroidism, Hashimoto's thyroiditis, and benign nodules, the same criteria of malignancy mentioned for follicular tumors (i.e., invasion) also apply to oxyphilic cell tumors. As with follicular carcinoma, macroscopically the oxyphilic variant is seen as a solitary thyroid nodule with complete or partial encapsulation. In several series the prognosis of this variant has been reported as less favorable than that of the follicular cell type.[99]

Insular carcinoma is also a rare variant.[100] It is a poorly differentiated, invasive follicular cancer with a solid aspect and follicular differentiation represented by small vesicles with very little colloid. The cells are very homogeneous in shape and smaller and more dense than in typical follicular cancer. The general picture may resemble that of carcinoid tumors. Metastases, very frequent, are found in lymph nodes and in distant organs. The prognosis is poor.

Other Tumors

Anaplastic cancer originates from the follicular epithelium, but its high degree of undifferentiation does not allow the recognition of any feature of the thyroid gland. It represents 5% to 15% of all thyroid cancers and is one of the most aggressive human cancers. Local extension at diagnosis and distant metastases are almost the rule.

Medullary tumors derive from the calcitonin-secreting parafollicular C cells of the thyroid. They occur as solid masses of spindle or rounded cells with large nuclei, much fibrosis, and deposits of amyloid. In the familial syndromes MEN-2A and MEN-2B, C cell hyperplasia precedes the cancer and is typically present in the gland. Immunochemical staining for calcitonin is useful for differentiating medullary thyroid tumors from other histologic types, especially when the origin of metastatic adenocarcinoma is being considered.

Other rare tumors include primary thyroid lymphoma or tumor arising from other cell types.

Etiology

Oncogenes

The most interesting new concept in tumor etiology relates to the role played by oncogenes and tumor suppressor genes. Recent advances in molecular biology have resulted in significant improvement in our understanding of the pathogenesis of thyroid carcinoma.[101] Gene rearrangements involving the *RET* and *TRK* proto-oncogenes have been demonstrated as causative events specific for a subset of the papillary histotype. Oncogenic activation of these genes is accomplished by fusion of their tyrosine kinase domain with the N-terminal promoter sequences of other genes in the same or other chromosomes. *TRK* oncogenes are created by rearrangement of the *NTK1* gene, which encodes a receptor for nerve growth factor and is linked to at least three different activating genes.[99] In the case of *RET* rearrangements, the resulting chimeric oncogenes have been called *PTC*, an acronym for papillary thyroid cancer.[102, 103] Several chimeric forms have been identified, the most frequent being *RET/PTC 1*, *2*, and *3*. Although strictly associated with papillary thyroid carcinoma, *RET/PTC* is found in less than half of cases unassociated with irradiation.[103–106] In papillary thyroid carcinomas occurring after irradiation, the frequency of *RET/PTC* activation is between 60% and 80%, either in Belarus children heavily exposed to radiation after the Chernobyl nuclear disaster[107–110] or in patients who received external radiation treatment during childhood.[111] Worthy of note, these radiation-induced tumors are frequently of the solid variant of papillary cancer and the oncogene involved is mainly *RET/PTC 3*. In spontaneous tumors or in the classic papillary variant of radiation-induced cancers, *RET/PTC 1* is the predominant rearrangement.[112] Based on this finding, one can speculate that *RET/PTC 3* is specifically linked to radiation as a mutagenic event. The other possibility is that *RET/PTC* activation, particularly type 3, is a distinctive characteristic of solid papillary tumors arising in patients of young age (most Belarus cancers were diagnosed in children) with or without the cooperation of radiation. This second hypothesis is supported by data showing a significant correlation between high rates of *RET/PTC* activation and lower age at diagnosis in Italian patients not exposed to radiation.[113]

Mutated forms of the H-*ras*, K-*ras*, and N-*ras* oncogenes are found in differentiated thyroid cancer. However, in this case the mutations are not specifically restricted to malignant lesions because the same mutations have also been found in benign thyroid nodules.[114] It is conceivable that mutations of the *ras* gene family may represent early events in thyroid tumorigenesis. Activating mutations of the genes encoding the thyrotropin receptor and the α subunit of the G_s protein, similar to those found in toxic adenomas and probably of irrelevant pathogenic importance, have been reported in a few follicular carcinomas.[115] Inactivating mutations of the p53 tumor suppressor gene are rare in patients with differentiated thyroid carcinoma but common in those with undifferentiated thyroid carcinoma.[107, 116] Recently, simian virus 40–like DNA sequences have been found integrated in the genome of tumor samples of patients with papillary thyroid carcinoma,[117] but the pathogenic role of this finding has not been established.

Expression of C-*myc* and C-*fos* is stimulated in normal thyroid tissue by TSH and occurs in adenomas and carcinomas,[118] perhaps as a consequence of the neoplastic phenotype. The tumor suppressor gene at the 11q13 locus is lost in some follicular adenomas and carcinomas.[119] Farid and coworkers have found that the *RB* tumor suppressor gene is also mutated or deleted in a high proportion of thyroid tumors.[120]

Based on the gene defects discovered in the different types of thyroid carcinoma, a hypothetic model of the sequential changes involved in the tumorigenesis of follicular thyroid cells is offered in Figure 109–7.

Ionizing Radiation

External irradiation of the neck during childhood increases the risk of papillary thyroid carcinoma.[26, 37, 121–123] The latency period between exposure and diagnosis is at least 5 years, is maximal at about 20 years, remains high for about 20 years, and then decreases gradually. A linear dose-response relationship is found between external irradiation and thyroid cancer, starting with radiation doses as low as 10 cGy up to 1500 cGy. Beyond this point the risk of thyroid cancer decreases, probably because of thyroid cell killing. A major risk factor is young age at the time of irradiation; after the age of 15 or 20 years, the risk is not increased. In children exposed to a dose of 1 Gy (100 rad) to the thyroid, the excess risk of thyroid cancer is 7.7-fold.[121]

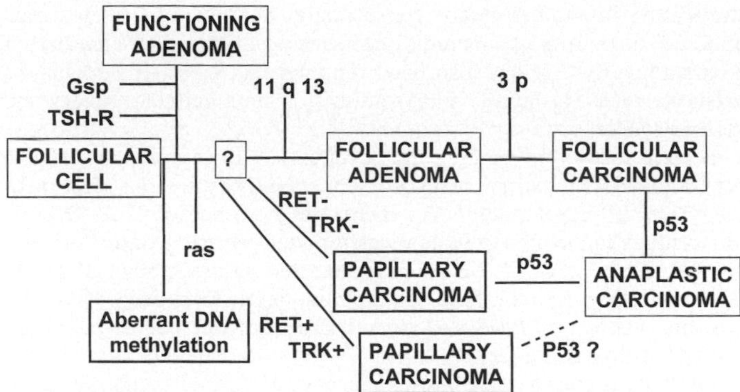

FIGURE 109–7. Proposed model of molecular events in thyroid tumorigenesis. TSH-R, thyroid-stimulating hormone receptor.

Diagnostic or therapeutic administration of radioactive iodine (^{131}I) does not seem to be associated with an increased risk for thyroid cancer.[122–124] However, the increased incidence of papillary thyroid cancer in children in the Marshall Islands after atomic bomb testing and, more recently, in Belarus and Ukraine after the Chernobyl nuclear reactor accident[27, 125–128] suggests a direct carcinogenic effect of radioactive isotopes, both ^{131}I and/or short-lived isotopes, on the thyroid gland. At variance with the cancers observed after external irradiation, the post-Chernobyl cancers diagnosed in Belarus and Ukrainian children and young adults (Table 109–6) developed after a very short mean latency period (6.5 years on average) from exposure to diagnosis.[125] Whether these discrepancies are due to different radiation doses to the thyroid, to the very young age of the patients, when the growing thyroid is particularly sensitive to radiation, or to a combination of these and other environmental (iodine deficiency) factors is still a matter of discussion.

Other Factors

In countries where iodine intake is adequate, differentiated thyroid cancers account for more than 80% of all thyroid carcinomas, with the papillary histotype being the more frequent form (60%–80%). In areas with nutritional iodine deficiency, a relative increase in follicular and anaplastic cancer with respect to papillary tumors is the rule, but no definite demonstration of an increased prevalence of thyroid cancer has been made in such countries.[122, 124] Chronic stimulation by slightly elevated TSH levels may be the underlying mechanism for thyroid hyperplasia and possibly carcinomatous degeneration in iodine-deficient countries. In thyroid hyperplasia in humans, whether induced by congenital metabolic defects or other causes, the resultant elevation in TSH levels can lead to carcinomatous degeneration if the hypothyroidism is unrecognized and untreated for decades.[129]

Abnormalities in TSH receptors have been sought in tumor cells. It appears that differentiated tumors have normal receptors, presumably explaining their TSH-dependent growth, whereas anaplastic cancers lack high-affinity receptors and thus respond poorly to TSH.[130] The thyroid-stimulating immunoglobulins present in the sera of patients who have coincident autoimmune thyroid disease may cause tumor growth and occasionally appear to make the tumors behave more aggressively, but usually concurrence of Graves' disease does not worsen the prognosis.[33] Although no evidence indicates that thyroid-

TABLE 109–6. Thyroid Cancer in Belarus Before and After the Chernobyl Accident

Age (yr)	1974–1985	1986–1998	Fold Increase
3–14	8	600	75.0
15–18	13	132	10.1
19–29	117	438	3.7
>29	1254	4279	3.4
All	1392	5449	3.9

stimulating immunoglobulins cause malignancy, it is of interest that up to 6% of thyroid glands removed because of Graves' disease harbor a carcinoma.[30, 131] It has also been reported that positive associations exist between Hashimoto's thyroiditis (or multinodular goiter) and thyroid cancer.

Genetic factors influencing the development of thyroid cancer have been reported, including chromosome instability in patients with medullary thyroid carcinoma.[132] An increased incidence of HLA-DR1 in differentiated thyroid carcinoma was reported by one group[133] but was not found by others.[134] We recently detected an association of HLA-DR7 with differentiated follicular thyroid cancer in patients without a previous history of head and neck irradiation, but not in radiation-associated thyroid cancer.[135]

Thyroid carcinomas are present in several familial syndromes, including Cowden's disease (hamartomas, multinodular goiters, and thyroid, breast, colon, and lung cancer),[136] familial adenomatous polyposis,[137, 138] Gardner's syndrome,[139] and familial chemodectomas.[140] The incidence of thyroid cancer is estimated to be increased 100-fold above baseline in patients with intestinal polyposis.[137, 138] Cases of familial papillary thyroid cancer have been reported in about 3% of patients.[141]

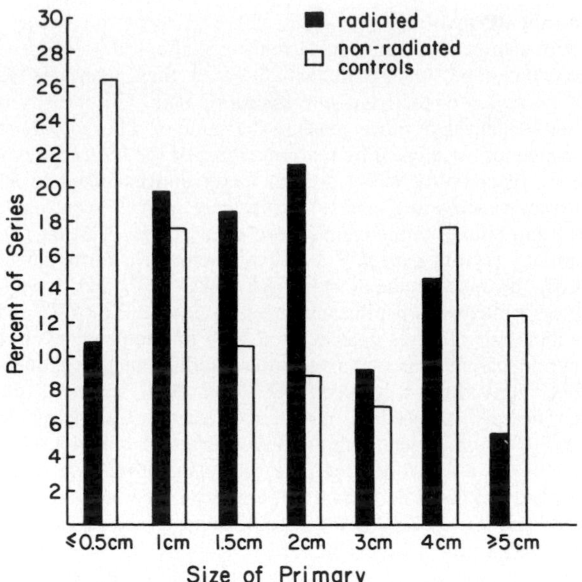

FIGURE 109–8. Comparison of the distribution of the size of primary tumors among 100 non–radiation-associated thyroid malignancies and an equal number of radiation-associated tumors. All were differentiated thyroid carcinomas. The distribution of sizes was not statistically different, although the radiation-associated tumors were slightly larger on average in this comparison than the tumors lacking association with prior x-ray treatment.

Diagnosis, Clinical Features, and Course

The initial feature of differentiated (papillary and follicular) and frequently of medullary thyroid carcinomas is the discovery, often fortuitous, of an asymptomatic thyroid nodule. Sometimes, particularly in children, one or more metastatic lymph nodes may be the first sign of the disease. More rarely, distant metastases in the lung or bone from follicular carcinoma may be the initial symptom. Hoarseness, dysphagia, and/or dyspnea are seldom a hallmark of the tumor; this finding is suggestive of advanced stages of the disease. At physical examination the nodule, usually single, is firm, movable during swelling, and often not distinguishable from a benign lesion. Carcinoma should be suspected when the nodule is single in an otherwise normal thyroid; when it is found in children or adolescents, in the male sex, or in association with ipsilateral enlarged lymph nodes; and particularly when a history of previous exposure to external radiation is present. Whatever the manifestation, the final diagnosis of malignancy must rely on the results of FNAC, which should be performed on any palpable nodule. Provided that an adequate specimen is obtained, three cytologic results are possible: benign, malignant, or indeterminate (or suspicious). False-negative and false-positive results are rare. Other diagnostic procedures are seldom useful in the diagnostic evaluation of thyroid nodules. Measurement of thyroid hormones and TSH may help in revealing the small proportion of "hot," almost invariably benign nodules. Positive thyroid autoantibodies suggest the presence of an underlying autoimmune disease, which reduces but does not extinguish the possibility of an association with thyroid malignancy. Thyroid ultrasonography, although not able to differentiate benign and malignant lesions, is useful for assessing the number and size of the nodule(s) and the structure of the extranodular thyroid and for guiding the aspiration of poorly palpable nodules.

Papillary carcinomas occur at any age. They are found in children and increase in frequency to have highest incidence in the third and fourth decades.[142] Papillary carcinomas remain in the thyroid gland for a long time, and multicentric lesions are present in half the patients. One-third are initially found to have nodal metastases, about 10% have extrathyroidal invasion, and 7.5% have distant metastasis.[34, 143] These tumors may exist for decades without producing serious symptoms or causing death.[144] The tumors tend to metastasize to cervical lymph nodes and ultimately to the lungs. It is an especially benign process in young adults and rarely causes death in persons younger than 40 years. In older patients the disease is more invasive and behaves in some instances like undifferentiated carcinoma.[145] Positive cervical nodes do not seem to carry an adverse risk in young individuals, but they do imply a worse prognosis in patients older than 40 (Fig. 109–8). Pulmonary metastasis may be manifested as large "snowballs" or may give a diffuse mottling appearance on chest radiography. Almost all papillary cancer metastases have some ability to take up ^{131}I when first diagnosed. Occasionally, these lesions produce large amounts of thyroid hormone. Obstructive pulmonary disease, arteriovenous shunting, hypoxia, and cyanosis tend to gradually develop in patients with extensive pulmonary metastases. The primary lesions are, as noted above, commonly found to have areas with both papillary and follicular patterns, and the metastatic deposits may be of either variety. Lesions with mixed papillary and follicular elements in the primary tumor behave more or less like papillary cancers, but in our experience they tend to be more malignant, with a greater incidence of recurrence, invasion, and death than seen in lesions with a purely papillary histology. The mortality from papillary cancer is 8% to 20%, mainly among older patients who have fixed or invasive cervical lesions or distant metastases at the time of diagnosis[83] (Fig. 109–9). About half the patients dying of this disease succumb because of local invasion.

Papillary carcinoma tends to be aggressive in preteenagers. Children have lymph node or pulmonary metastases more frequently than adults do,[146] and the tumor causes death in 10% or more of the patients. Treatment is essentially as outlined for adults, but long-term follow-up is stressed because of the continued occurrence of relapses.

Follicular cancers occur in an older age group, with the peak incidence in the fifth decade of life. They are frequently manifested as a slowly growing thyroid mass, with extrathyroidal invasion in 25%, involvement of local nodes in 5% to 10%, and distant metastases in 10% to 20%. The histologic pattern ranges from almost normal-appearing thyroid tissue to rather anaplastic-looking sheets of cells. Direct invasion of strap muscles and the trachea is characteristic, and resectability depends on this feature. These lesions tend to metastasize to the lungs and bone. The bone metastases are usually osteolytic. Commonly, the lesions retain the ability to accumulate radioactive iodide and are thus theoretically susceptible to ^{131}I treatment. The results, which are not so satisfactory, are discussed below. Follicular cancers are more lethal than papillary tumors, and the mortality, over 10 or 15 years after diagnosis, is 10% to 50%, again primarily in patients with fixed or invasive disease or distant metastases at the time of initial diagnosis.[83]

Hürthle cell carcinomas behave much like the other follicular tumors.[98] They have a pronounced tendency to recur in the neck many years after the original resection and to cause death by local invasion. Hürthle cell carcinomas usually accumulate ^{131}I poorly and are infrequently amenable to this therapy.

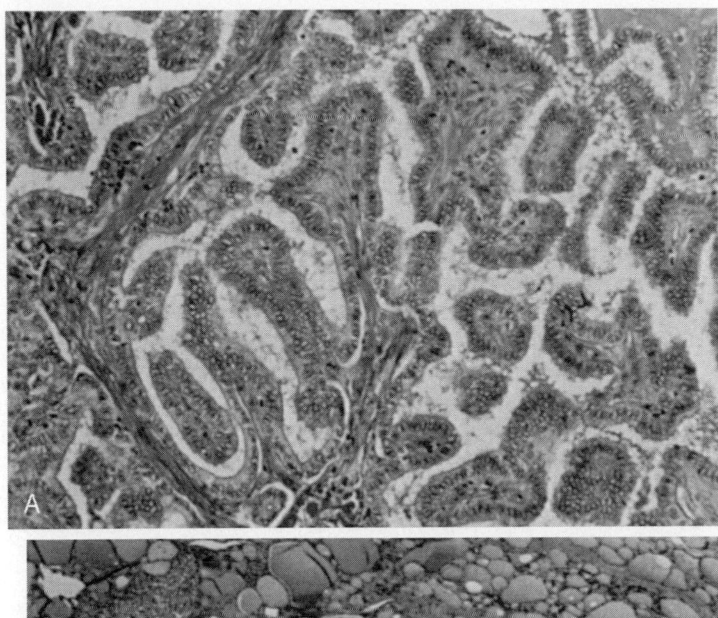

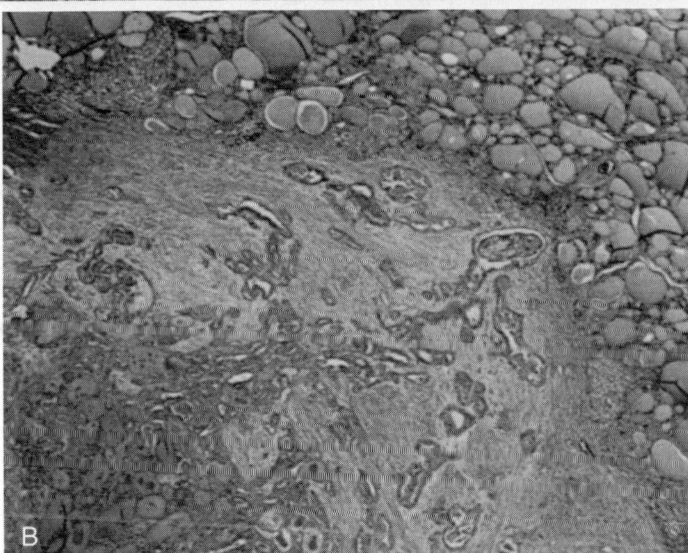

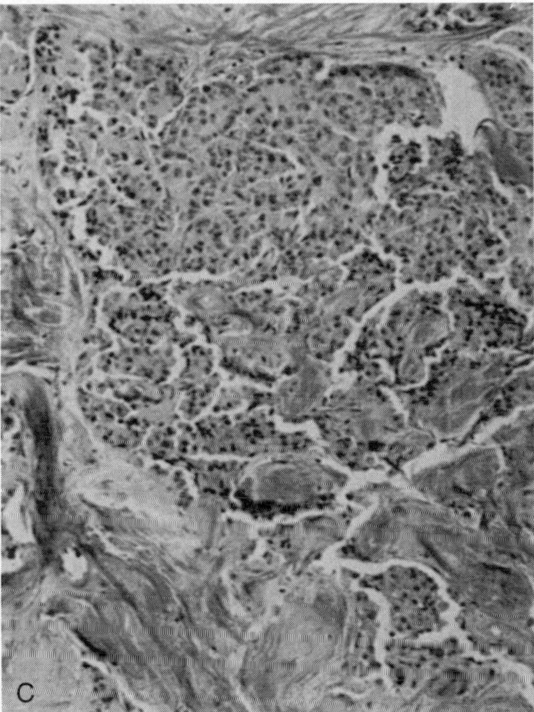

FIGURE 109–9. *A*, Histologic pattern of malignant tumors of the thyroid—papillary carcinoma. Note the tall cells and the fibrovascular core of the papillae. *B*, Follicular adenocarcinoma showing fair preservation of architecture, active colloid resorption, and vesicular nuclei. *C*, Medullary carcinoma with sheets of large cells, fibrosis, and amyloid visible by Congo red staining. (Courtesy of Dr. Francis Straus.)

Medullary thyroid cancer was first described as a unique tumor of the thyroid characterized by sheets of cells with large nuclei, fibrosis, multicentricity, and extensive amyloid deposits with an unexpectedly benign course.[86] These tumors account for 4% to 10% of thyroid cancers and are now known to be derived from the C cells, or parafollicular cells, which are of ultimobranchial origin. About 70% occur alone and 30% as part of MEN-2A in association with pheochromocytoma, parathyroid adenoma, and cutaneous lichen amyloidosis or as part of MEN-2B in association with unilateral or bilateral pheochromocytomas, mucosal neuromas, neurofibromas, café au lait spots, and possibly Gardner's syndrome.[22, 148] Hyperplasia of the C cells precedes the development of cancer.[148] Medullary tumors secrete calcitonin and carcinoembryonic antigen, which allows for their diagnosis, and in addition can produce serotonin, prostaglandins, adrenocorticotropic hormone, histaminase, and other peptides.[149–151] Calcitonin is produced in excess, but the patients are typically eucalcemic. In sporadic cases, the diagnosis can be achieved by measuring calcitonin levels in the basal condition[39] or after a provocative stimulus with calcium infusion or pentagastrin stimulation.[152, 153] In familial cases, the recent discovery that germline point mutations of the *ret* proto-oncogene are specific causative events in almost 100% of affected kindreds[154] has allowed the development of genetic screening tests for the early diagnosis and preventive treatment of familial medullary thyroid cancer.[155] The tumors follow a course almost like that of follicular cancer and can often be controlled by surgery.

Undifferentiated tumors occur with various configurations, which has given rise to terms such as giant cell carcinoma, carcinosarcoma, and epidermoid carcinoma. They behave much as invasive tumors elsewhere and tend to cause local invasion and compression of structures in the neck, and they metastasize to the lymph nodes and lungs. Perhaps no more than 10% are resectable when first discovered; the remainder are rapidly and uniformly lethal within 6 months to 1 year. A variety of evidence suggests that some anaplastic cancers originate from long-existing differentiated thyroid cancer.[156] A subgroup of tumors previously classified as anaplastic, with characteristic islands of cells, have been designated as the *insular variant of follicular carcinoma*. These tumors are less aggressive than the usual anaplastic cancer; because they often collect therapeutically useful quantities of ^{131}I, their recognition is important.[157]

Lymphoma may originate in the thyroid gland. In 30% to 80% of these cases the thyroid gland is also extensively involved with Hashimoto's thyroiditis, and hypothyroidism may be present as well. It appears probable that the lymphomas arise from the lymphocytes associated with thyroiditis. The lymphomas are typically of the diffuse, large cell variety. The clinical picture is usually that of a rapidly enlarging neck mass producing symptoms from pressure on contiguous structures in an adult. The lesion spreads to adjacent lymph node clusters, enlarges rapidly, and is often painful. Confusion with thyroiditis or small cell carcinoma is common on biopsy unless appropriate tumor cell markers are identified. Although the incidence is low, Hashimoto's disease is definitely a risk factor for lymphoma.

Metastatic carcinomas occur in a significant proportion of patients dying of other malignancies. These come from melanomas, breast tumors, pulmonary carcinomas, gastric, pancreatic, and intestinal carci-

TABLE 109–7. Prognostic Factors for Differentiated Thyroid Carcinoma

Patient-related factors
Age
Sex
Autoimmune thyroid diseases
Histopathologic factors
Tumor histotype and its variants
Tumor grade and DNA ploidy
Tumor burden
Primary tumor
Multicentric tumor
Extrathyroidal invasion
Lymph node metastases
Distant metastases
Molecular factors
Oncogenes, antioncogenes, and oncogene-encoded proteins
Treatment-related factors
Extent of primary surgery
^{131}I ablation of thyroid residue
Tumor markers
Serum thyroglobulin
Prognostic scoring systems
EORTC
Institute Gustave-Roussy
TNM
AMES
Clinical class
AGES-MACIS
Ohio State University

AGES, age, grade (Broders'), tumor extent, size of primary; AMES, age, distant metastases, extent and size of primary tumor; EORTC, European Organization for Research on Treatment of Cancer; TNM, primary tumor, lymph node status, distant metastases; MACIS, distant metastases, age, completeness of surgery, invasion of extrathyroidal tissue, size.

nomas, lymphomas, cervical carcinomas, and renal cancers. It is sometimes difficult to differentiate these lesions from primary thyroid cancer. Rarely, thyroidectomy is needed for this purpose.

Prognostic Factors and Selection of Therapy

Most patients, particularly those with differentiated histotypes, have high cure rates after initial treatment, but some are at risk of recurrence or death. Univariate analysis of the risk of recurrence or death has considered several potential prognostic factors that are based on epidemiologic, biologic, clinical, pathologic, and more recently, molecular features of the tumor, as listed in Table 109–7. Those more frequently associated with an adverse prognosis are reported in Table 109–8.

Age and Sex

In the papillary and follicular histotypes the risk of recurrence and cancer-related death increases linearly with age at diagnosis.[34, 83, 85, 158–165] In older patients, clinical relapses occur more rapidly after initial treatment, and the interval between the detection of recurrence and death is shorter.[160] Older patients tend to have more locally aggressive tumor and a higher incidence of distant metastases at diagnosis and more aggressive histologic variants. Their metastases frequently lack ^{131}I uptake. On the other hand, children and adolescents have an excellent long-term prognosis and a very low mortality rate even when affected by metastatic disease.[146, 166–168] Male sex has been reported as an independent risk factor in some series[34, 160, 164, 169] but not in others. Its importance as a prognostic factor is always less than that of age.

TABLE 109–8. Factors Associated with Adverse Prognosis

Older age
Distant metastases
Less well differentiated histologic variant
Follicular widely invasive, tall cells, columnar cells, oxyphilic cells, Hürthle cells, insular
Large tumor size
Extrathyroidal invasion
Multicentricity
Lymph node metastases
High tumor grade and DNA aploidy
Male sex

Associated Autoimmune Phenomena

With the exception of one report,[32] no major differences have been found in several series of differentiated thyroid cancer patients with or without Graves' disease with regard to clinical features and response to therapy[29, 31, 33, 131, 170–172] or to tumor-related mortality.[173] On the contrary, the association of Hashimoto's thyroiditis[174] or lymphocytic infiltration[89] with papillary thyroid cancer seems to confer a better prognosis. In a series from Italy,[175] circulating thyroid autoantibodies were found in 23% of patients with differentiated thyroid cancer. No difference in the final outcome was found between antibody-positive and antibody-negative patients. The disappearance of circulating antibodies was correlated with effective treatment of the disease, whereas their persistence was associated with stable or progressive disease (Fig. 109–10).

Histopathologic Factors

A poor prognosis has been reported with the tall cell variant,[95, 176] the columnar cell variant,[177] and the oxyphilic variant[178, 179] of papillary thyroid cancer. A good prognosis is found with the encapsulated[97, 180, 181] and the follicular variants.[85, 91, 92] An intermediate prognosis has been reported for the diffuse sclerosing variant.[94, 182]

Widely invasive follicular cancers have a less favorable prognosis than do minimally invasive tumors. Other follicular variants, such as the Hürthle cell, insular, and trabecular variants, are frequently associated with a poor prognosis.[160, 183, 184]

Tumor Grade and DNA Ploidy

Tumor grade was a significant prognostic factor both by univariate analysis and by multivariate analysis in papillary thyroid carcinoma studied at the Mayo Clinic[174] and in three European series.[159, 185, 186]

In the report by Joensuu et al., DNA aneuploidy was an adverse factor in univariate analysis but was not an independent prognostic factor.[187] In the Mayo Clinic's series, abnormal DNA content was associated with higher cancer mortality in high-risk tumors.[34]

Size of the Primary Tumor and Multicentricity

Microcarcinomas (or minimal or occult) have an excellent prognosis in terms of both survival and relapse-free survival, whatever the extent

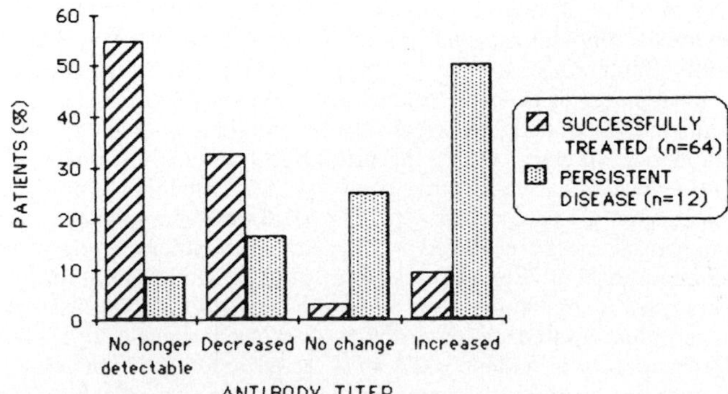

FIGURE 109–10. Changes in antithyroid autoantibody titers in relation to tumor outcome in differentiated thyroid cancer. (From Pacini F, Mariotti S, Formica N, et al: Thyroid autoantibodies in thyroid cancer: Incidence and relationship with tumour outcome. Acta Endocrinol (Copenh) 119:373, 1988.)

of the primary surgical treatment. Several series have reported a progressive increase in the risk of recurrence and tumor-specific mortality with increasing size of the primary tumor.[34, 143, 165, 183, 188] Tumor size seems to be more predictive in papillary than in follicular tumors.

Multicentricity, whether an expression of intrathyroidal metastases or of multiple primary tumoral foci,[180] has been associated with significantly higher rates of lymph node metastases,[180, 190, 191] locally persistent disease and distant metastases,[180] and 30-year mortality.[188]

Extrathyroidal Invasion

Extrathyroidal invasion is present in 5% to 10% of papillary tumors and in 3% to 5% of follicular tumors and exposes the patient to higher rates of local recurrence or distant metastases, as well as to a higher percentage of tumor-related death.[143, 159, 34, 180, 188, 192, 193] Invasion limited to the thyroid capsule, without infiltration of soft tissues, carries the same adverse prognosis seen with overt extrathyroidal invasion.[170]

Lymph Node Metastases

Lymph node metastases are present in 37% to 65% in different series of papillary carcinoma[85, 34, 83, 143, 183, 194, 195] and much less frequent (nearly 17%) in the follicular histotype.[196] Local node involvement is found both with microcarcinomas and with large tumors and may be bilateral in case of bilateral tumors. Some authors have shown that regional lymph node metastases are associated with higher rates of tumor recurrence and cancer-specific mortality,[143, 160, 169, 188, 193, 197–199] whereas others have found that cumulative survival is not significantly affected.[34, 90, 177, 200] In the series of The Ohio State University,[188] the presence of lymph node metastases was an important independent prognostic factor that predicted cancer death. Bilateral cervical and mediastinal nodes were particularly likely to be associated with cancer deaths. In the series of the Department of Endocrinology in Pisa, of 304 patients with lymph node metastases, 253 (83.2%) were cured after surgery and ^{131}I therapy, 37 had persistent progressive disease, and 14 (4.6%) died of their disease during a mean follow-up period of 12 years. All together, these data indicate that lymph node metastases are a potential cause of death and underscore the importance of early and thorough treatment.

Distant Metastases

Distant metastases at diagnosis confer the poorest prognosis in patients with papillary, follicular, or medullary thyroid carcinoma. The tumor-specific mortality of patients with distant metastases ranges from 36% to 47% at 5 years and reaches approximately 70% at 15 years.[34, 184, 201–203] Univariate analysis has shown the following factors to be associated with better prognosis in the case of distant metastases: young age, well-differentiated histotype, localization in the lung rather than in bone, small size, and the presence of ^{131}I uptake. However, multivariate analysis has shown that the extent of metastatic involvement rather than the site (lung or bone) has prognostic value.[184, 204, 205] The best outcome is found with micronodular metastases visible with radioiodine whole body scanning (WBS) but not visible with standard radiographs.[90, 146, 184, 201, 204–207]

Oncogenes, Antioncogenes, and Oncogene-Encoded Proteins

The presence of gene alterations or of oncogene-encoded proteins has been correlated with prognosis. Loss of expression of thyroid-specific differentiation genes, such as the TSH receptor and the Tg and TPO genes, is associated with a poor outcome of poorly differentiated or undifferentiated tumors.[208] Somatic mutations of the *p53* oncogene or hyperexpression of its encoded protein is found exclusively in poorly differentiated and anaplastic tumors.[116, 209] Point mutations of the *ras* gene and overexpression of p21 protein have been found in papillary thyroid carcinoma and have been correlated with poor survival rates.[210] Likewise, c-*myc* expression has been correlated with more aggressive thyroid carcinomas.[211]

The prognostic value of *RET/PTC* rearrangements in papillary thyroid carcinoma needs to be addressed in large series of patients, but its activation has been correlated with a favorable prognosis. Somatic *RET* proto-oncogene mutations, found in 50% of cases of sporadic medullary thyroid carcinoma, have been associated with metastatic progression and a worse outcome than that of tumors not carrying the mutation.[212]

The above findings are only the beginning of a new way to look into tumor biology and indicate that exploration of oncogenes and oncogene products may give new insight with regard to the prognosis of thyroid tumors.

Extent of Primary Surgery

Total (or near-total) thyroidectomy is associated with fewer cancer recurrences and tumor-related deaths.[213–216] In the Mayo Clinic's series the extent of surgery significantly affected the risk of local recurrence.[83] Data from the University of Chicago reported that when compared with lobectomy or bilateral subtotal resection, near-total thyroidectomy decreased the risk of death in papillary tumors larger than 1 cm and decreased the risk of recurrence among all patients.[143] A much higher frequency of recurrent cancer in the form of lung metastases has been reported with subtotal thyroidectomy.[217] In another series, patients with tumors 1.5 cm or larger, multicentric tumors, local invasion, or cervical metastases had significantly fewer recurrences after total (11.3%) than after subtotal (22.0%) thyroidectomy.[218] Similar results have been observed in the series of the Institute of Endocrinology in Pisa.

^{131}I Ablation of Thyroid Residue

Postsurgical radioiodine ablation of the thyroid residue may destroy microscopic neoplastic foci and reduce the risk of relapse. Whereas some authors have found no significant effect of ^{131}I ablation on the rate of recurrence or tumor-related death,[34, 159] others have shown beneficial effects in terms of both recurrence and long-term survival,[143, 188] at least in patients with tumors larger than 1.5 cm. However, no randomized study is available, and the retrospective studies suffer from the comparison of groups of patients (ablated vs. not ablated) not always accurately matched with regard to other important clinicopathologic factors. Ablation also increases the sensitivity of subsequent ^{131}I WBS and the specificity of serum Tg determination and provides reassurance to the patient when these tests are negative on subsequent examination.

Serum Thyroglobulin Measurement

Serum Tg measured after initial treatment gives valuable predictive information on subsequent disease evolution. After surgical treatment and when ^{131}I imaging is negative, the finding of undetectable serum Tg in the absence of thyroid hormone administration is an excellent indicator of definitive cure.[219–221] On the contrary, persistence of elevated serum Tg concentrations requires extensive clinical evaluation, including WBS after the administration of therapeutic doses of ^{131}I as well as imaging studies, to detect the site of Tg production and to plan the most appropriate treatment.[184, 222]

Prognostic Scoring Systems

Prognostic scoring systems based on multiple regression analysis of prognostic factors are intended to distinguish between low-risk patients to be treated with less aggressive protocols and high-risk patients to be treated with the most aggressive therapy.

Several scoring systems are available (Table 109–9). The *EORTC (European Organization for the Research and Treatment of Cancer)* system considers age at diagnosis, sex, principal histotype, extrathyroidal invasion, and distant metastases.[223, 224] The *IGR (Institut Gustave-Roussy)* system is based on age at diagnosis and histotype.[160] The *TNM (by the International Union Against Cancer)* system is based on the extent of the primary tumor (T), lymph node status (N), the presence of distant metastases (M), and since the last version, age (younger or older than 45 years) and capsule (encapsulated or nonen-

TABLE 109–9. Variables Considered in Different Prognostic Scoring Systems for Differentiated Thyroid Cancer

Variable	EORTC	TNM	AMES	AGES	MACIS	Clinical Class	Ohio University	IGR
Age	Yes	Yes	Yes	Yes	Yes			Yes
Sex	Yes							
Histology	Yes							Yes
Extrathyroid invasion	Yes	Yes	Yes	Yes	Yes	Yes	Yes	
Extent of primary tumor	Yes	Yes	Yes	Yes	Yes	Yes		
Lymph node metastases	Yes				Yes	Yes		
Distant metastases	Yes	Yes	Yes	Yes	Yes	Yes	Yes	
Tumor capsule	Yes							
Histologic grade			Yes					
Completeness of surgery					Yes			

IGR, Institut Gustave-Roussy; other acronyms as listed in Table 109–7.

capsulated).[225, 226] *AMES,* an acronym for age, distant metastases, and extent and size of the primary tumor,[227] was subsequently modified to DAMES by adding DNA ploidy to AMES.[228] *AGES* includes age, grade (by Broders' classification), tumor extent (local invasion and distant metastases), and size of the primary tumor.[34] In 1993, AGES was revised to *MACIS,* which includes distant metastases, age, completeness of surgery, invasion of extrathyroidal tissues, and size.[173] *Ohio State University* considers tumor size, the presence or absence of cervical metastases, multiple tumors, local tumor invasion, and distant metastases.[188] *Clinical Class,* a very simple and effective staging system developed at the University of Chicago,[143] consists of four classes that depend on the extent of tumor tissue: class I includes patients with single or multiple intrathyroidal foci, class II patients have lymph node metastases, in class III are patients whose tumor (or unresectable lymph nodes) has invaded outside the thyroid gland, and class IV patients have distant metastases. This classification is primarily anatomic but correlates well with prognosis.

Initial Treatment of Thyroid Cancer

In differentiated thyroid cancer, each prognostic system defines low- and high-risk patients. We find that the distinction between low- and high-risk groups is clearly reflected in the simple Clinical Class staging just described. High-risk patients are mainly those with invasive or metastatic disease. However, in most instances it is impossible to correctly stage cancer at the time of surgery because final pathologic review, node status, and results of ^{131}I scanning are unavailable. Some "low-risk" tumors unfortunately behave as though they were "high risk," and this difference cannot be predicted.[229] Complications of surgery are minimal in the hands of an experienced surgeon.[143, 230] Thyroxin replacement is probably indicated in every patient who has had thyroid cancer, regardless of the extent of surgery. The radiation exposure from ^{131}I scanning and ablation is equal to that of one CT scan and is probably inconsequential. More complete thyroid surgery (at least a lobectomy plus contralateral subtotal thyroidectomy or near-total thyroidectomy) improves the overall prognosis even for low-risk patients with tumors larger than 1 cm in clinical classes I and II.[84, 143] Ablation with ^{131}I decreases recurrence and may[84, 143, 231] or may not[34] decrease deaths, but it clearly improves the value of postablation WBS and makes serial Tg measurements useful. Further study is needed to prove the value of routine postoperative ^{131}I ablation.[232] For these reasons, we believe that the patient's best interest is served in most cases by more complete surgery, postoperative ^{131}I ablation, T_4 replacement, and careful follow-up, as described below.

Class I Differentiated (Papillary and Follicular) Carcinoma

Intrathyroidal lesions are treated by lobectomy and contralateral subtotal lobectomy by many surgeons, and this operation is probably appropriate, especially if the surgeon is not a specialist in this area. If the lesion is larger than a "minimal" 1-cm lesion, we usually prefer near-total thyroidectomy and biopsy of nodes in the adjacent tracheo-esophageal groove (see Table 109–4). This operation is a planned attempt to take out most of the thyroid without damaging the recurrent laryngeal nerves or parathyroid glands. These structures are carefully identified, and portions of the thyroid (especially the posterior capsule on the contralateral side) are left behind, if necessary, to prevent damage. No attempt is made to remove every piece of thyroid tissue. The value of near-total thyroidectomy for low-risk patients has been confirmed by the results of second "completion" thyroidectomy performed in the centers of the two authors of this chapter. The percentage of patients with detectable tumor in the reoperative specimens was 31% at the University of Chicago[67] and 44% at the University of Pisa. In the last series no difference in the rate of second tumors was found between patients defined as low risk or high risk at the time of the first operation (Fig. 109–11).

In lesions that are found to be multicentric on the basis of observations by the surgeon or pathologist, greater effort is made to perform total thyroidectomy, as long as it can be done without compromise of the parathyroid glands. After surgery, residual thyroid tissue is ablated by ^{131}I administration in most cases, especially in patients who have either multicentric foci or a history of irradiation. All patients are given suppressive therapy with thyroid hormone.

Our own experience[143] and long-term follow-up of 576 cases of papillary thyroid cancer by Mazzaferri and Young[214, 231] appear to support this approach. Patients with near-total thyroidectomy and postoperative ablation had a significantly improved prognosis, especially when follow-up extended over 10 to 15 years. Massin and coworkers also found that "complete thyroidectomy" and ^{131}I ablation gave the lowest incidence of late metastatic recurrence,[217] as did Samaan et al.,[84] who found that ^{131}I treatment was the most important influence on recurrence and survival.

It must be noted that different opinions exist with regard to the appropriate operation for this lesion. Perhaps the most common alter-

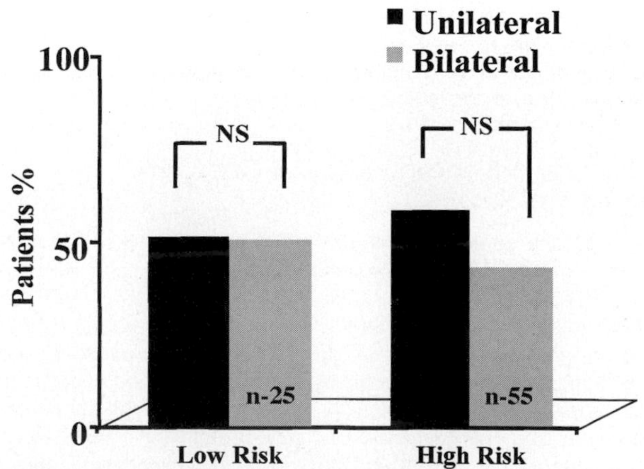

FIGURE 109–11. Percentage of contralateral tumor involvement in low- or high-risk patients who underwent completion thyroidectomy for differentiated thyroid cancer.

native is to perform a lobectomy on the involved side if no evidence of multicentricity can be found.[224, 233, 234] Several surgical studies support this position and indicate that a more limited operation minimizes damage to the parathyroid glands and recurrent laryngeal nerves and that survival after lobectomy is nearly equal to that for the general population and comparable to results obtained by more extensive surgical procedures.[235] Most series reporting on the results of total or near-total thyroidectomy indicate that hypoparathyroidism occurs in 1% to 15% of patients and recurrent unilateral nerve damage in 2% to 5%, but fortunately, bilateral nerve injury is rare.[236] It is because of these complications and the apparently satisfactory results with lobectomy that some investigators prefer the simpler procedure. On the other hand, 20% to 80% of stage I thyroid cancers are multicentric.[86, 237] It is clear that not all these foci are of clinical importance, but the recurrence rate of cancer in the contralateral lobe after unilateral lobectomy is at least 6%, and some patients with recurrence eventually die of their lesion.[217, 238, 239] Because of known multicentricity, the ability of our collaborating surgeons to avoid hypoparathyroidism, and the associated improved prognosis,[143] we prefer the more extensive resection. Surgeons who are especially skilled in performing thyroidectomies can hold the incidence of hypoparathyroidism to about 1% and have an equally low incidence of recurrent nerve damage.

In past years, more radical procedures, including prophylactic radical neck dissection, were advocated for thyroid carcinomas. Forty-six percent of patients with presumed stage I disease were in fact found to have lymph node involvement when specimens were thoroughly studied after prophylactic neck dissection.[240] Apparently, however, these lymph node metastases, when not clinically detectable, are in some way controlled by the body's defense mechanisms and rarely lead to death of the patient. Thus recent opinion is strongly against prophylactic node dissection and against radical or en bloc neck dissection.

Because follicular lesions tend to be more directly invasive and lethal than papillary lesions,[98] many surgeons pursue a more aggressive operative approach with stage I follicular cancer than with papillary cancer and perform routine near-total thyroidectomies in patients with the former lesion.[241] Postoperative ^{131}I thyroid ablation and continuous thyroid hormone administration are considered essential.[242]

Up to 20% of low-grade follicular neoplasms are misdiagnosed on operative frozen sections as benign, with the diagnosis achieved 1 to 3 days later after review of permanent sections. If the lesion is smaller than 1 cm, unicentric, and intrathyroidal and the patient is younger than 45 years, no further surgery is required, and as indicated before, some physicians accept lobectomy as a definitive procedure. In general, in patients with lesions larger than 1 cm who are older than 45 years or with multifocality, we prefer reoperation to achieve near-total thyroidectomy and subsequent ^{131}I therapy. As already mentioned, in an analysis of patients who have undergone a second operation, we found that in 31% of the operations residual cancer was recovered on the remaining lobe.[67] This problem is best avoided by performing at least a lobectomy plus contralateral subtotal thyroidectomy if any question at surgery about the benignity of the "adenoma" is still unanswered.

The use of radioactive iodide, as described above, can also be questioned because the ablative dosage exposes these patients, who are frequently young, to 10 or 15 rad of whole body radiation. Although the genetic and carcinogenic risk of this radiation dosage cannot be completely ignored, it is minimally different from the average background whole body radiation exposure that individuals normally receive by age 30 and is most likely not a significant hazard.

Ten percent to 20% of patients who undergo an initial near-total thyroidectomy for stage I cancer will later have cervical lymph node recurrence. These patients ultimately require neck dissection or simple node removal.

Class II Differentiated Carcinoma

Less disagreement surrounds the management of class II disease. The usual procedure is a near-total or total thyroidectomy.[217, 235, 243] Small portions of the gland may be left in situ (for later radioiodide ablation), if necessary, to preserve the recurrent laryngeal nerves or viability of the parathyroid glands. A modified neck dissection is also performed to remove involved nodes. An attempt is made to retain the jugular vein and sternocleidomastoid muscles, and an en bloc resection is not attempted, except occasionally in patients with metastatic follicular cancer. If both sides of the neck are involved, resections are usually staged because otherwise the incidence of tracheal edema requiring tracheotomy is significant. Radical neck dissection with removal of the jugular vein and sternocleidomastoid muscle is not favored because the disease can usually be managed by the less mutilating procedure and uninvolved nodes that become apparent at a later date can generally be successfully resected. Patients are given ^{131}I to ablate residual thyroid tissue after surgery and to treat functioning metastases found on scanning.

Class III Differentiated Carcinoma

Patients with class III disease should receive a near-total or total thyroidectomy, appropriate lymph node dissection, and resection of all possible invading neoplasm. The tendency at present is to avoid mutilating surgery in patients younger than 45 years in an effort to resect all cancerous tissue because less extensive surgery, ^{131}I treatment, and suppressive thyroid hormone therapy usually lead to prolonged survival or cure, even if complete excision of the tumor is impossible.[244] ^{131}I therapy is given as discussed below. External irradiation may be useful in preventing recurrence.[245] However, because most cases appear to be controlled by surgery and ^{131}I and definitive experience with supplemental prophylactic irradiation is not available, the usual course is to withhold irradiation until recurrence is seen in younger patients but to advise prophylactic treatment in patients older than 45 to 50 years who have known residual disease.

Class IV Differentiated Disease

Patients with a thyroid mass and solitary metastasis to the lung or bone should probably have thyroidectomy and excision of the single metastasis because cure or prolonged survival may be obtained. If multiple metastases are present, thyroidectomy is probably the quickest way to achieve hypothyroidism so that uptake of radioactive iodide in the metastases and possible therapies can be evaluated.

Hürthle Cell Carcinoma

It is clear that Hürthle cell tumors range in invasiveness from zero to an aggressively locally invading lesion or a tumor with rapidly growing pulmonary metastases. These variations result in a wide range of opinion on therapy. We advocate treatment as described for follicular cancer, of which these are a subgroup. Postoperative ^{131}I ablation is carried out, although its value may be restricted because many Hürthle cell tumors fail to accumulate ^{131}I. Invasive tumors (class III) should be treated by mantle irradiation. ^{131}I treatment is attempted for class III or IV tumors but is not usually possible despite the presence of functioning metastases as proved by elevated Tg levels.

Lymphoma

Staging should include neck, chest, and abdominal CT scans and bone marrow biopsy. If the disease appears to be limited to the thyroid gland and contiguous lymph nodes, thyroidectomy is advised, although occasionally only biopsy is possible. Patients with intrathyroidal lymphoma or disease limited to the neck and upper part of the mediastinum have conventionally been treated by mantle irradiation to about 45 Gy over a 3- to 4-week period.[246] Because the overall survival rate at 5 years has been about 50%,[246–248] patients are increasingly being treated primarily by chemotherapy followed by radiotherapy. Patients with more extensive disease and those who relapse are given chemotherapy.

Undifferentiated Thyroid Carcinoma

Undifferentiated thyroid carcinoma is among the most aggressive malignant tumors in humans. Management of this type of cancer is cause for major concern because its poor prognosis is not ameliorated by surgery, chemotherapy, or radiotherapy. As soon as a diagnosis of undifferentiated thyroid cancer has been made, total thyroidectomy should be attempted. Unfortunately, infiltration of the soft tissues of the neck, almost invariably present at surgery, makes radical surgery impossible. External radiotherapy is used after surgery to control local disease, but this treatment is also generally unsatisfactory.[249] Several chemotherapeutic protocols, including single (doxorubicin) and combination (doxorubicin plus cisplatin) drugs, have been totally disappointing.[250, 251] The combination of radiotherapy and chemotherapy has been used with very modest advantage.[252–254] With any form of treatment, mean survival ranges between 3 and 12 months after diagnosis,[252–255] although individual survival exceeding 2 to 3 years has been reported.[256]

Because radical surgery, as mentioned above, is rarely feasible, a novel approach is to use hyperfractionated radiotherapy in combination with chemotherapy as initial treatment, with surgery left as a second step.[257] The idea is to control and reduce the primary tumor with medical therapy, thus giving the surgeon more chance to perform a radical thyroidectomy. Further radiotherapy and chemotherapy may be added after surgery to stabilize the results of treatment. With this integrated therapeutic approach, complete local control has been obtained in 5 of 16 patients, and 3 patients survived more than 20 months in one study.[258] Other schemes based on the same combination of radiotherapy and chemotherapy have been used with similar results.[259, 260]

In perspective, the discovery of point mutations of the p53 tumor suppressor gene specifically associated with undifferentiated thyroid carcinoma[116, 261] have open a new field of research aimed at the development of more effective treatment strategies at the molecular level.

Radioiodine Ablation of Postsurgical Thyroid Remnants

Any postsurgical thyroid remnant should be ablated by therapeutic doses of radioiodine based on the following considerations. Destroying any residual thyroid cell will facilitate subsequent follow-up and therapy based on serum Tg measurement and diagnostic radioiodine WBS and ^{131}I therapy; furthermore, ^{131}I may destroy microscopic foci of multicentric papillary carcinoma, thus decreasing subsequent tumor recurrence.

Postoperative ^{131}I therapy is performed 4 to 6 weeks after surgery, without thyroid hormone administration in the interim, or it may be performed later after discontinuing replacement therapy. Two different strategies may be used. Some centers measure thyroid bed uptake by using a tracer dose of ^{131}I and then give a standard therapeutic dose of ^{131}I (between 30 and 100 mCi), followed by the institution of levothyroxine suppressive therapy. WBS is performed again 7 to 10 days after treatment depending on ^{131}I uptake. In patients who have undergone total or near-total thyroidectomy, total ablation is achieved in 60% to 80% of patients after either 30- or 100-mCi doses.[262] Thus the use of lower (30 mCi) doses is probably to be preferred. Other centers prefer to start with a diagnostic ^{131}I WBS with a 1- to 2-mCi tracer dose and then treat the patients with therapeutic doses according to the results of the diagnostic scan. A post-therapy scan is also performed.

Diagnostic and Therapeutic Follow-up After Surgery and Thyroid Ablation

It is well known that the great majority of local recurrence or distant metastases develop or are detected in the first 2 to 3 years after diagnosis. However, in a minority of cases, distant metastases may develop in late follow-up, even as late as 20 years after the initial treatment,[90] which suggests that follow-up of differentiated thyroid cancer should go on throughout the patient's life.

Five percent to 20% of patients with differentiated thyroid cancer have local or regional recurrence, which is usually due to persistent or recurrent disease in thyroid remnants or lymph nodes after incomplete initial treatment or is the expression of aggressive tumors. Local or regional disease may be easily detected by palpation, ultrasonography, or CT scan. WBS performed after either a diagnostic or a therapeutic dose of ^{131}I is most important in revealing disease.

According to several large series, the frequency of distant metastases in differentiated thyroid carcinoma ranges between 10% and 18% of cases.[90, 201, 217, 263–266] Sometimes, distant metastases, particularly in bone, may be the initial symptom of the disease, but usually (two-thirds of cases) they are discovered at the time of the primary diagnosis or soon after thyroidectomy when performing the first WBS with ^{131}I.[90] However, distant metastases may develop later in the course of follow-up, even as late as 20 years after initial treatment.[90]

Lung metastases are the most common site of distant metastases, followed by bone metastases. The combination of lung and bone disease is found in about one-third of patients with distant metastases. Other less common localization is to the brain, the liver, and the skin, all of which are more likely to occur in association with lung or bone metastases. The pattern of metastatic lung involvement may vary from one or more macronodules (>1 cm in diameter) to a diffuse micronodular spread.[90, 263, 264] The latter are not usually detected by chest radiography and sometimes not even by CT scanning, but they can easily be diagnosed with ^{131}I WBS. Not infrequently, especially in papillary tumors, enlarged lymph nodes in the mediastinum may also be present.[206, 217] Bone metastases are mainly associated with the follicular histotype and tend to occur in older patients. The vertebrae, pelvis, and ribs are the sites more frequently affected, but occasionally any skeletal segment may be affected. Single lesions are present in one-third of patients. Most metastases are detectable by both WBS and radiography, but a minority (about 25%) are visible only by WBS.[90, 267] This latter group is the one more likely to respond to ^{131}I therapy.

Diagnostic and therapeutic strategies for monitoring patients with differentiated thyroid carcinoma are both well established and very effective in detecting and treating most of the patients who are not cured after initial treatment. Basically, after total thyroidectomy and radioiodine ablation of thyroid residue, two powerful tools are available to raise the suspicious of local or distant metastases and to localize them: serum Tg measurement and ^{131}I WBS, respectively. On the other hand, radioiodine therapy and reoperation are very effective modalities of treatment for metastatic patients with well-differentiated carcinoma.

Diagnostic Procedures

CLINICAL, ULTRASONOGRAPHIC, AND RADIOGRAPHIC EXAMINATION. Clinical examination with accurate palpation of the thyroid bed and lymph node chains of the neck is performed every 6 to 12 months in any patient being monitored for thyroid carcinoma.

Ultrasonography of the neck may complement the clinical examination. Small, thin, oval lymph nodes detected either by palpation or by ultrasound may be a normal finding in the neck and should not create unnecessary concern. If lymph node metastases are suspected, ultrasonographically guided FNA for cytology and for Tg measurement should be performed.[64]

Routine chest and bone radiographs are of little diagnostic value in the early discovery of distant metastases to the lungs or bones, particularly in patients who have undetectable levels of serum Tg. These tests are useful in patients with known metastatic disease for monitoring the evolution of the lesions and for patients with negative ^{131}I WBS but elevated serum Tg levels suggestive of metastases that do not take up radioiodine.

SERUM THYROGLOBULIN MEASUREMENT. Tg, the principal iodoprotein of the thyroid gland, is produced and released into the circulation by normal and neoplastic follicular cells, but not by other cell systems in the body. Thus serum Tg measurement can be used in clinical practice as a specific and sensitive tumor marker of differentiated thyroid cancer.[268] After total thyroid ablation, undetectable serum Tg levels are found in patients free of disease, whereas detectable and often elevated serum Tg concentrations are found in patients with persistent or recurrent disease.[220, 269, 270] Two important factors must be considered when interpreting a serum Tg value: the level of serum TSH and the presence of circulating anti-Tg autoantibodies. Tg production by neoplastic cells is, at least partially, under TSH control. As a consequence, serum Tg concentrations are lowered, even to undetectable levels, during TSH suppression by thyroid hormone administration and are increased after withdrawal of therapy.[219, 252, 271] Serum Tg results may be artifactually altered by circulating anti-Tg antibodies, which are present in about 15% of patients.[175] Antibodies interfere with the Tg assay by producing false-positive or false-negative results, depending on the assay used.[272] After thyroid ablation and in the absence of tumor, serum Tg should be less than 2 ng/mL when measured in a sensitive assay using the World Health Organization standard.

As a rule, patients with undetectable serum Tg levels who are not receiving levothyroxine therapy may be considered free of disease.[220, 269, 270] On the contrary, in patients with distant metastases, serum Tg concentrations are elevated when measured after withdrawal of levothyroxine therapy and are reduced, but still detectable during levothyroxine treatment with respect to "off therapy" values. In the case of lymph node metastases, serum Tg may be low or undetectable during levothyroxine therapy but becomes elevated after levothyroxine withdrawal.[220, 263] A comparison of the results of serum Tg measurement and ^{131}I WBS shows good agreement between these two techniques.[273, 274] Detectable serum Tg levels are usually associated with positive WBS and indicate the presence of residual or metastatic disease. Undetectable serum Tg levels are found in patients with a negative scan and indicate that the patient is in complete remission. However, as shown in Figure 109–12, serum Tg assay is superior to WBS in predicting the presence of metastases in a significant proportion of patients (about 13%) who have increased serum Tg levels but negative basal WBS, as demonstrated by the presence in these patients of abnormal foci of ^{131}I uptake after the administration of therapeutic doses of ^{131}I.[222, 275, 276] A representative example of this possibility is shown in Figure 109–13.

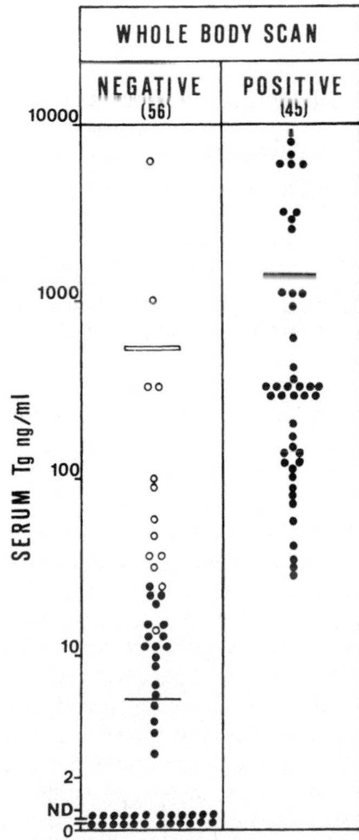

FIGURE 109–12. Relationship between serum thyroglobulin (Tg) and ^{131}I uptake at whole body scanning in patients with differentiated thyroid cancer (after total thyroidectomy). *Open symbols* in the left column indicate patients with proven nonfunctioning metastases. (From Pacini F, Pinchera A, Giani C, et al: Serum thyroglobulin concentrations and 131-I whole body scans in the diagnosis of metastases from differentiated thyroid carcinoma (after thyroidectomy). Clin Endocrinol (Oxf) 13:107, 1980.)

^{131}I WHOLE BODY SCAN. Many metastatic well-differentiated thyroid cancers retain the ability to concentrate iodine, which is the rationale for the traditional diagnostic and therapeutic use of ^{131}I in metastatic thyroid cancer. Radioiodine uptake by metastatic tissue is dependent on TSH stimulation, thus requiring (until recently) a state of hypothyroidism. For this reason, total thyroidectomy and ablation of postsurgical thyroid remnants are the fundamental prerequisites for radioactive imaging. The other important point is withdrawal of levothyroxine therapy for a period long enough to induce high serum levels of endogenous TSH.[277, 278] The minimum level of serum TSH required for adequate incorporation of ^{131}I in neoplastic tissues is around 30 μU/mL, a level usually achieved after 30 to 45 days without levothyroxine and 2 weeks without L-triiodothyronine. Unfortunately, this period of hypothyroidism may be very uncomfortable for many patients.

Alternatively, moderate hypothyroidism can be induced by reducing the patient's daily dose by 50%. In patients who have previously been ablated and who are not receiving excessive doses of thyroxine, TSH will be raised to an average value of 50 μU/mL after 6 weeks. In practice, it is useful to measure serum TSH in the fifth week, and if it is above 20 μU/mL, satisfactory elevation (>30 μU/mL) will be anticipated in the sixth week at the time of the scan. It may take a longer period to elevate the TSH to a satisfactory level if patients have an on-treatment TSH value less than 0.1 μU/mL.

Recombinant human TSH (rhTSH) has recently been approved in the United States for use in humans and will alter for the better the postoperative management of patients with thyroid carcinoma. In clinical trials the drug has been very effective[279]; in patients with suppressed TSH levels (<0.1 μU/mL), two daily 0.9-mg injections stimulate thyroidal ^{131}I uptake and Tg secretion to a degree equal to 2 to 3 weeks of hormone withdrawal. The results of WBS performed after rhTSH and after levothyroxine withdrawal have shown very good but not perfect concordance between the two techniques. Side effects are minimal, and no anti-TSH antibody formation has been detected, at least in the short term. Thus it will be possible to stimulate ^{131}I uptake and Tg secretion without induction of hypothyroidism, which will make ^{131}I WBS and Tg testing more acceptable to patients and doctors. It is not exactly clear how the pattern of scanning or testing during follow-up will be altered, but it is likely that ^{131}I postoperative ablation will be more routine, that scans will be somewhat more frequent, that yearly stimulated Tg testing will be able to dictate the need for WBS or therapy, and that ^{131}I therapy may be more effective (a tentative flow chart for the use of rhTSH in differentiated thyroid cancer is presented in Fig. 109–14).

Another requirement for effective ^{131}I uptake is that the patient not be contaminated by recent ingestion of stable iodine, which would prevent the uptake of radioactive iodine by the metastases. Because serum TSH not sufficiently high and contamination by iodine are the most frequent causes of false-negative ^{131}I WBS, it is necessary to check the serum TSH concentration before ^{131}I WBS and ^{131}I therapy and to measure urinary iodine excretion if uptake is low.

WBS is performed 48 to 72 hours after the administration of ^{131}I by either rectilinear scan or a gamma camera. ^{131}I doses of 2 to 5 mCi are generally used as tracer; higher doses are not indicated because of the possibility that they will produce a sublethal radiation effect in the metastatic cells (stunning effect) that prevents uptake of the therapeutic dose of ^{131}I to be administered after a few days.[280]

If no abnormal ^{131}I uptake is found despite elevation of serum Tg while not receiving levothyroxine, a therapeutic dose of ^{131}I (100 mCi) can be administered and a post-therapy scan obtained 5 to 7 days later. This procedure will allow the identification of small foci of ^{131}I in more than 80% of the patients with a negative basal scan and elevated serum Tg concentrations.[222, 275, 276] If no localization is found, the search for metastases should include chest radiography, CT, MRI of the neck, bone scintigraphy, and liver echography.

Whenever a metastasis has been localized by WBS, a complete radiologic assessment should also be obtained. In bone metastases the aim is to assess whether the location is accessible to radical surgical therapy, which in the case of a single location may be curative.[267, 281]

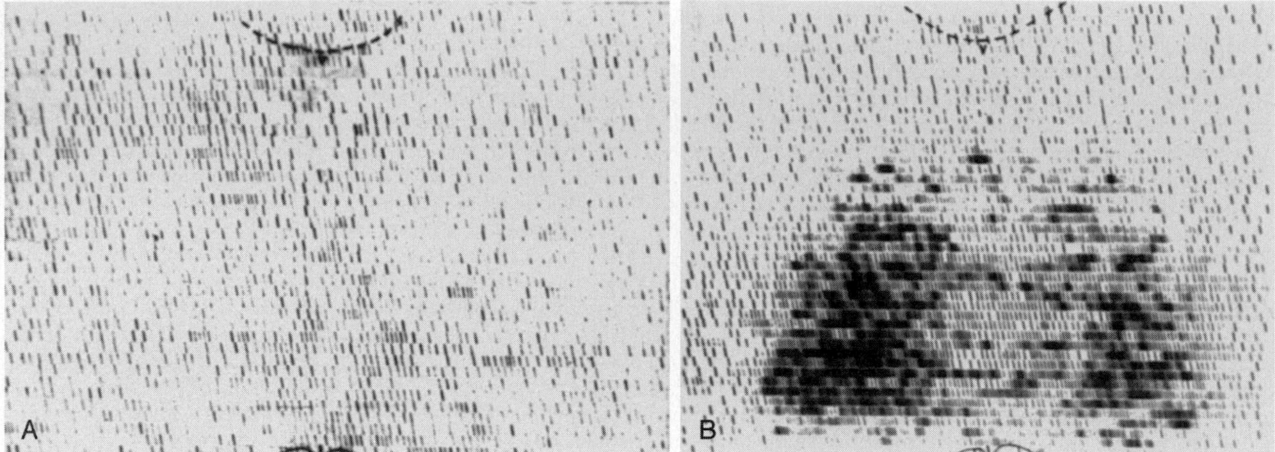

FIGURE 109–13. Representative example of a patient with negative diagnostic whole body scanning *(A)* that becomes positive for diffuse lung metastases in the posttherapy (100 mCi of ^{131}I) scan *(B)*.

In the case of lung metastases, it is extremely important to establish the presence of one or more macronodular lesions or multiple micronodules not visible on the plain chest film but only on CT scan. This point is of relevant prognostic utility because diffuse lung metastases not detectable by radiography but able to take up radioiodine (such as those frequently encountered in children) are highly responsive to ^{131}I treatment.[166, 262, 276]

Clinical, biochemical, and scintigraphic evaluations and radioiodine therapy, if needed, should be performed every 6 to 12 months in patients with persistent disease. Patients considered disease-free (i.e., negative scan and undetectable serum Tg without levothyroxine therapy) on two occasions may be monitored annually with a clinical examination and serum TSH and Tg measurements. Any other tests are unnecessary as long as serum Tg remains undetectable. If serum Tg becomes detectable during levothyroxine therapy, ^{131}I WBS should be immediately planned.

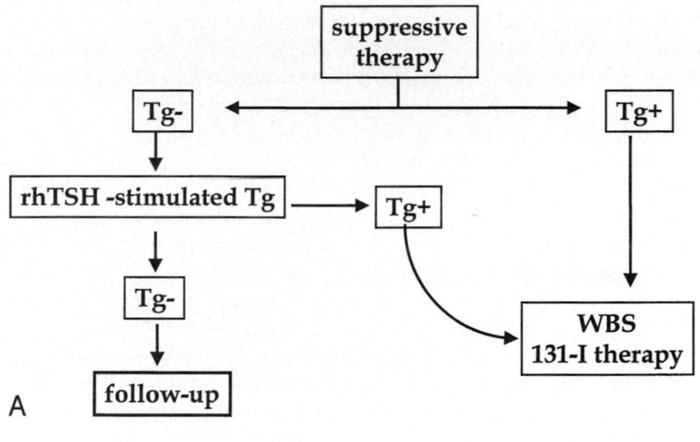

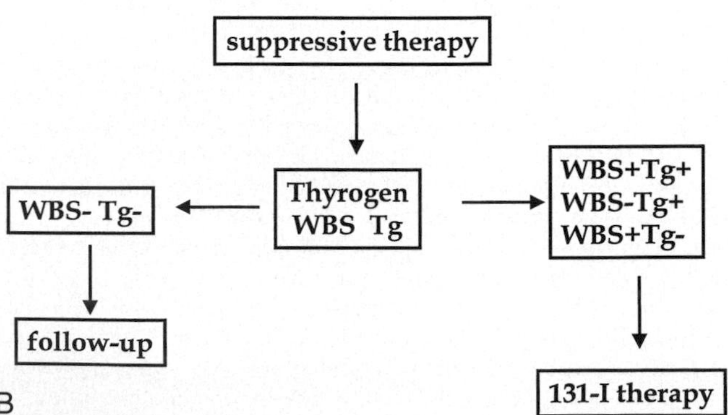

FIGURE 109–14. Tentative flow chart for the use of recombinant human thyroid-stimulating hormone (rhTSH) in the diagnostic follow-up of differentiated thyroid cancer after thyroidectomy. Panel *A* applies to centers that will base their decision mainly on thyroglobulin (Tg) evaluation and panel *B* to those using the combination of Tg and whole body scanning (WBS).

Treatment

LOCAL AND REGIONAL RECURRENCE. After primary surgery, recurrences in the neck may develop in the thyroid bed and the surrounding soft tissues or in the regional lymph nodes. They carry an unfavorable prognosis, and most patients dying of differentiated thyroid cancer are in this group.[200, 282, 283] The prognosis is better when the recurrent cancer is diagnosed by ^{131}I scintigraphy rather than clinically and when it is able to concentrate iodine.[90, 282, 284] Any clinically detectable local recurrence should be treated by surgery if possible, although radical reoperation involving central dissection is difficult and risks complications to the parathyroid glands and recurrent laryngeal nerve.

Recurrent disease in the lateral cervical nodes is easier to treat surgically because the operative field has not been previously dissected. The preferred surgical procedure is a modified radical neck dissection. When lymph nodes concentrate iodine, treatment with ^{131}I is an effective adjunct to reoperation. Two or three therapeutic courses of ^{131}I are effective in treating more than 60% of patients.[90] If nodal disease persists after ^{131}I, reoperation with the use of an intraoperative probe[285] may be considered.

Local recurrences that cannot be completely excised and do not take up ^{131}I can benefit from external radiotherapy.[286]

TREATMENT OF DISTANT METASTASES. Effective treatment of distant metastases depends largely on the size, location, number of metastatic lesions, and their ability to take up radioiodine. Micronodular diffuse lung metastases and, to a lesser extent, small metastatic bone foci revealed by WBS in the absence of radiographic changes have the greatest chance of cure. This observation is particularly true in children, who often have a diffuse pattern of metastatic pulmonary spread and do exceptionally well with radioiodine therapy.[90, 146, 166] Macronodules in the lung and large bone metastases carry a poor prognosis. Loss of radioiodine uptake is also a prognostic indicator of poor outcome. All together, these findings emphasize the concept that early recognition and early treatment of distant metastases are of paramount importance to the final outcome.

Surgical Treatment. The decision to treat distant metastases by surgery depends on their location, spread, ability to concentrate radioiodine, and radiologic pattern.

Lung metastases are typically treatable by radioiodine therapy, with the choice of surgical therapy left to a minority of selected cases. Patients eligible for surgery are those with a single macronodular lesion or more than one in the same lobe, with or without mediastinal lymph node involvement, particularly when they are devoid of radioiodine uptake. Too few patients have undergone surgery for lung metastases to allow a statistical conclusion to be made on their outcome. However, some appear to achieve long-term remission and, in less advanced cases (one single pulmonary nodule), even definitive cure.[287]

The surgical approach to bone metastases is gaining support because of their relative insensitivity to radioiodine therapy.[267, 281, 287, 288] The intent of bone surgery may be palliative or curative. Palliation is required for pathologic fractures or to ameliorate neurologic symptoms resulting from spinal cord compression by vertebral metastases. Curative surgery is possible in single, localized metastases. For large metastases not radically resectable, surgery may be of help in reducing the tumor mass to allow more effective action of radioiodine therapy.

Brain metastases are extremely rare and range from 0.15% to 1.3% in different series.[288–292] They carry a very poor prognosis. Although they usually demonstrate ^{131}I uptake, the therapy of choice, whenever feasible, is surgery because of severe neurologic symptoms.

RADIOIODINE TREATMENT. The role and the indications for ^{131}I therapy in the management of distant metastases from differentiated thyroid carcinoma are well established. Results are reproducible in large series of patients and indicate complete responses in 35% to 45% of patients.[90, 262–265] Lung metastases, particularly when micronodular, respond better than bone metastases. The poor prognosis of patients with bone metastases is usually linked to the bulkiness of the lesions and the presence of tumor cells that do not concentrate ^{131}I.[267, 284] In adult patients the treatment dose is usually 100 to 200 mCi, repeated every 6 to 8 months. Lower doses (empirically 1 mCi/kg body weight) should be used in children with lung metastases, particularly of the diffuse type, to avoid the risk of radiation-induced pulmonary fibrosis.[166, 293]

An alternative method is to adjust the dosage of ^{131}I to a maximally tolerable level based on dosimetric analysis of a tracer dose. With this method, doses of 200 to 500 mCi are sometimes given. Because it is cumbersome, expensive, and of unproven benefit, the protocol is currently used in only a few institutions.

In a review of 118 patients with distant metastases treated with ^{131}I therapy,[90] 43 patients (36.4%) were cured (defined as negative WBS and undetectable serum Tg while not receiving levothyroxine), 28 (23.7%) died of their disease, and the others had persistent disease. Metastases from papillary tumors had better response than did follicular tumors. The risk of dying was higher if lung metastases were macronodular and detectable by chest radiography, if bone metastases were multiple, and if both lung and bone metastases were present. The mean cumulative dose of ^{131}I used in cured patients was 233 mCi delivered in 2.2 treatment courses over a 3.4-year period. Loss of radioiodine uptake was seen in 5.2% of the patients after a mean cumulative dose of 161 mCi. Six patients with single bone metastases and one with a macronodular lung metastasis were given surgical therapy.

As previously mentioned, some patients (15%–20%) have elevated serum Tg levels and no uptake detected by diagnostic WBS.[273, 274] The site of metastatic involvement in such patients, usually the lung or mediastinal lymph nodes, may be detected by WBS performed 5 to 7 days after the administration of high doses of ^{131}I (100 mCi).[222, 275, 276] This procedure is also of possible therapeutic value. A few days after the administration of ^{131}I therapy a transient increase in serum Tg concentration occurs and can be explained by release into the circulation of stored Tg by radiation-damaged tumor cells. Furthermore, progressive normalization of WBS and serum Tg levels over years[222, 275, 276] and normalization of chest CT scans in patients with radiographic evidence of micronodular lung metastases[275] have been observed in patients periodically treated with this treatment modality. This treatment does expose patients to significant radiation, and as of this time there is no proof that it alters outcome or prolongs life.

Side effects after the administration of therapeutic ^{131}I doses are usually very mild and reversible in few days. They consist mainly of gastrointestinal symptoms, nausea and occasionally vomiting, and acute sialoadenitis. More serious complications affect the blood and bone marrow. An increased risk of leukemia on the order of 5 cases per 1000 treated patients has been documented by several published series, especially in patients who have received more than 600 mCi total dosage.[262] The risk increases with increasing cumulative doses, reduction of the interval between each treatment, and administration of total doses per treatment greater than 2 Gy.[294] Pancytopenia has been reported in 4.4% of patients treated with mean ^{131}I doses of 536 mCi.[295] In the same study anemia was found in about 25% of patients and thrombocytopenia in one-third. In patients given more than 100 mCi, dry mouth often develops and salivary obstruction or loss of saliva leading to dental problems may develop.

Another rare complication of radioiodine therapy is radiation-induced pulmonary fibrosis, which may develop in patients repeatedly treated for lung metastases, particularly of the diffuse type. Children seem to be particularly prone to this complication.

Finally, transient and permanent testicular damage limited to the germinal epithelium has been reported in men, as well as transient ovarian failure in women, after treatment with high levels of ^{131}I.[296, 297] ^{131}I-induced genetic damage in the offspring of patients treated with ^{131}I has not been documented in recent series addressing this issue.[298, 299] The only anomaly reported was an increased frequency of miscarriage in women treated with ^{131}I during the year before conception.

LEVOTHYROXINE SUPPRESSIVE THERAPY. Both the function and the growth of metastatic thyroid cells are under TSH control. It is a common observation that bone or lung metastases increase in size and take up radioiodine during a period of levothyroxine withdrawal, whereas a reduction in size and depressed uptake is observed with levothyroxine administration. Serum Tg, a marker of cell function, increases dramatically during hypothyroidism, whereas it returns to low levels during hormone therapy. Suppression of endogenous TSH to low or undetectable levels is a true antineoplastic therapy and should never be omitted in patients with active disease.

The drug of choice is levothyroxine and the effective dosage is between 2.2 and 2.8 μg/kg body weight. A higher dosage is usually

TABLE 109–10. Indications for Radiation Therapy

Tumor	Stage	Treatment (15–20 MV Electrons or ^{60}Co)
Papillary or follicular	Invasive, patient younger than 45 yr	Possibly 4000 rad at 2- to 3-cm depth to thyroid bed after RAI treatment; value uncertain in this instance
	Invasive or possible residual, patient older than 45 yr	5000 rad* to the thyroid bed after RAI treatment
	Recurrent, patient of any age	5000 rad* to the thyroid bed after RAI treatment
	Isolated lesion in bone	5000–6000 rad, as required for symptoms after RAI treatment
Medullary	Stage III	4000–5000 rad† to the thyroid bed
	Abnormal or increasing thyrocalcitonin	5000 rad† to the mantle
	Recurrent tumor, isolated metastasis	5000–6000 rad* to area
		5000–6000 rad for symptoms
Lymphoma	All	5000 rad† to the thyroid and mantle
Anaplastic	All	4500–5500 rad† to the thyroid and mantle

Note: Spinal cord dosage does not exceed 3000* or 3500† rad.
RAI, radioactive iodine.

TABLE 109–11. Chemotherapy for Thyroid Carcinoma

Primary tumor
- Progressive differentiated thyroid cancer, symptomatic medullary cancer, anaplastic cancer; two programs have been proposed:
  - Doxorubicin (Adriamycin) + *cis*-diamminedichloroplatinum + VP-16
  - Doxorubicin (Adriamycin) + *cis*-diamminedichloroplatinum

Secondary therapy for failure of primary treatment
- Differentiated cancer: bleomycin + cyclophosphamide
- Medullary cancer: fluorouracil + streptozocin
- Anaplastic cancer: bleomycin + hydroxyurea

required in children. In every patient an attempt should be made to use the smallest dose necessary to suppress TSH secretion. Adequacy of therapy is monitored by measurement of serum TSH. Serum TSH should theoretically be undetectable with an ultrasensitive assay, but levels less than 0.1 μU/mL are probably acceptable. FT_3 should be in the normal range to avoid iatrogenic thyrotoxicosis. When these guidelines are followed, levothyroxine suppressive therapy is safe and devoid of long-term side effects on the heart or bone.[69]

A shift from suppressive therapy to replacement therapy is appropriate in patients who have well-documented stable and complete remission, as assessed by a negative ^{131}I WBS and undetectable serum Tg in the absence of levothyroxine therapy.

Radiation Therapy

Radiation therapy is appropriate for any class III differentiated tumor not responding to ^{131}I therapy or hormone suppression, for class III Hürthle cell tumors and follicular cancers in older patients, for any expanding class IV lesion, for painful osseous metastases, and for lymphomas and undifferentiated tumors.[300] Unfortunately, no adequate studies are available to assess the value of prophylactic radiation after resection of class III tumors. Prophylactic mantle radiotherapy may be useful in medullary thyroid cancer patients who have residual hypercalcitoninemia after surgery in the absence of detectable lesions (Table 109–10), but the value of this treatment is debated.[301]

Chemotherapy

A variety of chemotherapeutic approaches have been attempted with uncertain success. The overall response rate of thyroid cancer to various chemotherapeutic agents, including the alkylating agents 5-fluorouracil and methotrexate, is estimated to be 10% to 15%, which is comparable to that for other solid tumors.[302] Bleomycin and especially doxorubicin (Adriamycin) have been reported to provide a higher percentage of remission (20%–33%).[260, 302–307] However, the response to these chemotherapeutic agents is partial and of short duration, with limitation imposed by toxicity of the medication. Chemotherapeutic agents given in combination appear to be slightly more effective than doxorubicin alone.[260, 302–307] Chemotherapy in differentiated thyroid carcinoma, preferably doxorubicin, is warranted in class III and IV lesions after other modalities of therapy have been exhausted and tumor growth is certain (Table 109–11). As already mentioned, chemotherapy may be used for the treatment of anaplastic thyroid carcinoma after surgery in combination with external irradiation.

REFERENCES

1. Vander JB, Gaston EA, Dawber TR: Significance of solitary non-toxic thyroid nodules. N Engl J Med 251:970, 1954.
2. Vander JB, Gaston EA, Dawber TR: The significance of nontoxic thyroid nodules. Final report of a 15-year study of the incidence of thyroid malignancy. Ann Intern Med 69:537, 1968.
3. Tunbridge WM, Evered DC, Hall R, et al: The spectrum of thyroid disease in an English community: The Wickham survey. Clin Endocrinol 7:481, 1977.
4. Liechty RD, Stoffel PT, Zimmerman DE, Silverberg SG: Solitary thyroid nodules. Arch Surg 112:59, 1977.
5. Mortensen JD, Woolner LB, Bennett WA: Gross and microscopic findings in clinically normal thyroid glands. J Clin Endocrinol Metab 15:1270, 1955.
6. Baldwin DB, Rowett D: Incidence of thyroid disorders in Connecticut. JAMA 239:742, 1978.
7. Tan GH, Gharib H: Thyroid incidentalomas: Management approaches to nonpalpable nodules discovered incidentally on thyroid imaging. Ann Intern Med 126:226, 1997.
8. Brander A, Viikinkoski P, Nickels J, Kivisaari L: Thyroid gland: US screening in a random adult population. Radiology 181:683, 1991.
9. Belfiore A, LaRosa GL, LaPorta GA, et al: Cancer risk in patients with cold thyroid nodules: Relevance of iodine intake, sex, age, and multinodularity. Am J Med 93:363, 1992.
10. Namba H, Matsuo K, Fagin JA: Clonal composition of benign and malignant human thyroid tumors. J Clin Invest 86:120–125, 1990.
11. Namba H, Rubin SA, Fagin JA: Point mutations of Ras oncogenes are an early event in thyroid tumorigenesis. Mol Endocrinol 4:1474, 1990.
12. Parma J, Duprez L, Van Sande J, et al: Somatic mutations in the thyrotropin receptor gene cause hyperfunctioning thyroid adenomas. Nature 365:649–651, 1993.
13. Tonacchera M, Chiovato L, Pinchera A, et al: Hyperfunctioning thyroid nodules in toxic multinodular goiter share activating thyrotropin receptor mutations with solitary toxic adenoma. J Clin Endocrinol Metab 83:492, 1998.
14. Tonacchera M, Vitti P, Agretti P, et al: Activating thyrotropin receptor mutations in histologically heterogeneous hyperfunctioning nodules of multinodular goiter. Thyroid 8:559, 1998.
15. Suarez HG, du Villard JA, Caillou B, et al: Gsp mutations in human thyroid tumors. Oncogene 6:677–679, 1991.
16. DeGroot LJ: Lack of iodide trapping in "cold" thyroid nodules. Acta Endocrinol Panam 1:27, 1970.
17. Field JB, Larsen PR, Yamashita K, et al: Demonstration of iodide transport defect but normal iodide organification in nonfunctioning nodules of human thyroid glands. J Clin Invest 52:2404, 1973.
18. Fragu P, Nataf BM: Human thyroid peroxidase activity in benign and malign thyroid disorders. J Clin Endocrinol Metab 45:1089, 1977.
19. Demeester-Mirkine N, Van Sande J, Corvilain H, Dumont JE: Benign thyroid nodule with normal iodide trap and defective organification. J Clin Endocrinol Metab 41:1169, 1975.
20. Morris JC: Mutations and disorders involving the thyroid iodide transporter—The next wave in thyroid diseases. J Clin Endocrinol Metab 82:3964, 1997.
21. Miller JM, Zafar SU, Karo JJ: The cystic thyroid nodule: Recognition and management. Radiology 110:257–261, 1974.
22. Sipple JH: Association of pheochromocytoma with carcinoma of thyroid gland. Am J Med 31:163, 1961.
23. Schimke RN, Hartmann WH, Prout TE, Rimoin DL: Syndrome of bilateral pheochromocytoma, medullary thyroid carcinoma, and multiple neuromas. N Engl J Med 279:1, 1968.
24. Sapira JD, Altman M, Vandyk K, Shapiro AP: Bilateral adrenal pheo-chromocytoma and medullary thyroid carcinoma. N Engl J Med 273:140, 1965.
25. Loh K-C: Familial nonmedullary thyroid carcinoma: A meta-review of case series. Thyroid 7:107, 1997.
26. Refetoff S, Harrison J, Karanfilski BT, et al: Continuing occurrence of thyroid carcinoma after irradiation to the neck in infancy and childhood. N Engl J Med 292:171, 1975.
27. Kazakov VS, Demidchik EP, Astakhova LN: Thyroid cancer after Chernobyl. Nature 359:21, 1992.
28. Compagno J, Oertel JE: Malignant lymphoma and other lymphoproliferative disorders of the thyroid gland. Am J Clin Pathol 74:1–11, 1980.
29. Farbota LM, Calandra DB, Lawrence AM, et al: Thyroid carcinoma in Graves' disease. Surgery 98:1148–1152, 1985.
30. Pacini F, Elisei R, DiCoscio GC, et al: Thyroid carcinoma in thyrotoxic patients treated by surgery. J Endocrinol Invest 11:107–112, 1988.
31. Shapiro SJ, Friedmen NB, Perzik SL, et al: Incidence of thyroid carcinoma in Graves' disease. Cancer 26:1261–1270, 1970.
32. Belfiore A, Garofalo MR, Giuffrida D, et al: Increased aggressiveness of thyroid cancer in patients with Graves' disease. J Clin Endocrinol Metab 70:830, 1990.
33. Hales JB, McElduff A, Crummer P, et al: Does Graves' disease or thyrotoxicosis affect the prognosis of thyroid cancer? J Clin Endocrinol Metab 75:886–889, 1992.
34. Hay ID: Papillary thyroid carcinoma. Endocrinol Metab Clin North Am 19:545, 1990.
35. Hamming JF, Goslings BM, Van Steenis GJ, et al: The value of fine-needle aspiration biopsy in patients with nodular thyroid disease divided into groups of suspicion of malignant neoplasms on clinical grounds. Arch Intern Med 150:113–1088, 1990.
36. Veith FJ, Brooks JR, Grigsby WP, Selenkow HA: The nodular thyroid gland and cancer. N Engl J Med 270:431, 1964.
37. DeGroot LJ, Paloyan E: Thyroid carcinoma and radiation. A Chicago endemic. JAMA 225:487, 1973.
38. Hoffman GL, Thompson NW, Heffron C: The solitary thyroid nodule. Arch Surg 105:379, 1972.
39. Pacini F, Fontanelli M, Fugazzola L, et al: Routine measurement of serum calcitonin in nodular thyroid diseases allows the preoperative diagnosis of unsuspected sporadic medullary thyroid carcinoma. J Clin Endocrinol Metab 78:826–829, 1994.
40. Rieu M, Lame MC, Richard A, et al: Prevalence of sporadic medullary thyroid carcinoma: The importance of routine measurement of serum calcitonin in the diagnostic evaluation of thyroid nodules. Clin Endocrinol (Oxf) 42:453–457, 1995.
41. Niccoli P, Wion-Barbot N, Caron P, et al: Interest of routine measurement of serum calcitonin: Study in a large series of thyroidectomized patients. J Clin Endocrinol Metab 82:338–341, 1997.
42. Vierhapper H, Raber W, Bieglmayer C, et al: Routine measurement of plasma calcitonin in nodular thyroid diseases. J Clin Endocrinol Metab, 82:1589, 1997.
43. Clark OH, Okerlund MD, Cavalieri RR, Greenspan FS: Diagnosis and treatment of thyroid, parathyroid, and thyroglossal duct cysts. J Clin Endocrinol Metab 48:983, 1979.
44. Rojeski MT, Gharib H: Nodular thyroid disease: Evaluation and management. N Engl J Med 313:428–436, 1985.

45. Sokal JE: The problem of malignancy in nodular goiter—recapitulation and a challenge. JAMA 170:61, 1959.
46. Van Herle AJ, Rich P, Ljung BM, et al: The thyroid nodule. Ann Intern Med 96:221–232, 1982.
47. Kendall LW, Condon RE: Prediction of malignancy in solitary thyroid nodules. Lancet 1:1071, 1969.
48. Hoffer PB, Gottschalk A, Refetoff S: Thyroid scanning techniques: The old and the new. Curr Probl Radiol 2:5, 1972.
49. Hollifield JW, Patton JA, Lee GS, Brill AB: Differentiation of malignant from benign thyroid nodules by fluorescent thyroid scanning. J Nucl Med 17:1721, 1976.
50. Thijs LJ: Diagnostic ultrasound in clinical thyroid investigation. J Clin Endocrinol Metab 32:709, 1971.
51. Walfish PG, Hazani E, Strawbridge HTG, et al: Combined ultrasound and needle aspiration cytology in the assessment and management of hypofunctioning thyroid nodule. Ann Intern Med 87:270, 1977.
52. Gershengorn MC, McClung MR, Chu WE, et al: Fine-needle aspiration cytology in the preoperative diagnosis of thyroid nodules. Ann Intern Med 87:265, 1977.
53. Hamlin E, Vickery AL: Needle biopsy of the thyroid gland. N Engl J Med 254:742, 1956.
54. Willems J-S, Lowhagen T: Fine needle aspiration cytology in thyroid disease. Clin Endocrinol Metab 2:247–256, 1981.
55. Gharib H, Goellner JR, Johnson DA: Fine needle aspiration cytology of the thyroid. A 12-year experience with 11,000 biopsies. Clin Lab Med 13:699–709, 1993.
56. Miller JM, Hamburger JI, Kini S: Diagnosis of thyroid nodules. Use of fine needle aspiration and needle biopsy. JAMA 241:481, 1979.
57. Hamburger JL, Husain M, Nishiyama R, et al: Increasing the accuracy of fine-needle biopsy for thyroid nodules. Arch Pathol Lab Med 113:1035–1041, 1989.
58. Caruso D, Mazzaferri EL: Fine-needle aspiration in the management of thyroid nodules. Endocrinologist 1:194–202, 1991.
59. Gharib H, Goellner JR: Fine-needle aspiration of the thyroid: An appraisal. Ann Intern Med 118:282–289, 1993.
60. Giuffrida D, Gharib H: Controversies in the management of cold, hot, and occult thyroid nodules. Am J Med 99:642–650, 1995.
61. Ridgway EC: Clinician's evaluation of a solitary thyroid nodule. J Clin Endocrinol Metab 74:231–235, 1992.
62. Caplan RH, Kisken WA, Strutt PJ, et al: Fine-needle aspiration biopsy of thyroid nodules: A cost-effective diagnostic plan. Postgrad Med 90:183–190, 1991.
63. Gollner JR, Gharib H, Grant CS, et al: Fine-needle aspiration cytology of the thyroid, 1980 to 1986. Acta Cytol 31:587–590, 1987.
64. Pacini F, Fugazzola L, Lippi F, et al: Detection of thyroglobulin in fine needle aspirates of nonthyroidal neck masses: A clue to the diagnosis of metastatic thyroid cancer. J Clin Endocrinol Metab 74:1401–1404, 1992.
65. Bieche I, Ruffet E, Zweibaum A, et al: MUC1 mucin gene, transcripts, and protein in adenomas and papillary carcinomas of the thyroid. Thyroid 7:725, 1997.
66. Brousset P, Chaouche N, Leprat F, et al: Telomerase activity in human thyroid carcinomas originating from the follicular cells. J Clin Endocrinol Metab 82:4214–4216, 1997.
67. DeGroot LJ, Kaplan EL: Second operations for "completion" of thyroidectomy in treatment of differentiated thyroid cancer. Surgery 110:936–940, 1991.
67a. Zelmanovits F, Genro S, Gross JL: Suppressive therapy with levothyroxine for solitary thyroid nodules: A double-blind controlled clinical study and cumulative meta-analyses. J Clin Endocrinol Metab 83:3881–3885, 1998.
68. Bartalena L, Martino E, Pacchiarotti I, et al: Factors affecting suppression of endogenous thyrotropin secretion by thyroxine treatment: Retrospective analysis in athyreotic and goitrous patients. J Clin Endocrinol Metab 64:849–855, 1987.
69. Marcocci C, Golia F, Bruno-Bossio G, et al: Carefully monitored levothyroxine suppressive therapy is not associated with bone loss in premenopausal women. J Clin Endocrinol Metab 78:818, 1994.
70. Lippi F, Ferrari C, Manetti L, et al: Treatment of solitary autonomous thyroid nodules by percutaneous ethanol injection: Results of an Italian multicenter study. The Multicenter Study Group. J Clin Endocrinol Metab 81:3261–3264, 1996.
71. Martino E, Murtas ML, Loviselli A, et al: Percutaneous intranodular ethanol injection for treatment of autonomously functioning thyroid nodules. Surgery 112:1161–1165, 1992.
72. Monzani F, Lippi F, Goletti O, et al: Percutaneous aspiration and ethanol sclerotherapy for the thyroid cysts. J Clin Endocrinol Metab 78:800–804, 1994.
73. Pacini F, Antonelli A, Lari R, et al: Unsuspected parathyroid cysts diagnosed by measurement of thyroglobulin and parathyroid hormone concentrations in fluid aspirates. Ann Intern Med 102:793, 1985.
74. Annual Cancer Statistical Review. National Institutes of Health Publication No. 882789, 1987.
75. Sampson RJ, Woolner LB, Bahn RC, Kurland LT: Occult thyroid carcinoma in Olmsted County, Minnesota: Prevalence at autopsy compared with that in Hiroshima and Nagasaki, Japan. Cancer 34:2072, 1974.
76. Fukunaga FH, Yatani R: Geographic pathology of occult thyroid carcinomas. Cancer 36:1095, 1975.
77. Verby JE, Woolner LB, Nobrega FT, et al: Thyroid cancer in Olmsted County, 1935–1965. J Natl Cancer Inst 43:813, 1969.
78. Vanderlaan WP: The occurrence of carcinoma of the thyroid gland in autopsy material. N Engl J Med 237:221, 1947.
79. Silverberg SG, Vidone RA: Carcinoma of the thyroid in surgical and postmortem material. Ann Surg 164:291, 1966.
80. Bisi H, Fernandes VSO, Asato de Camargo RY, et al: The prevalence of unsuspected thyroid pathology in 300 sequential autopsies, with special reference to the incidental carcinoma. Cancer 64:1888–1893, 1989.
81. Hedinger C, Williams ED, Sobin LH: Histological typing of thyroid tumours, vol 11. *In* International Histological Classification of Tumors, ed 2. Berlin, Springer-Verlag, 1988.
82. Lang W, Borrush H, Bauer L: Occult carcinoma of the thyroid. Evaluation of 1020 sequential autopsies. Am J Clin Pathol 90:72, 1988.
83. McConahey WM, Hay ID, Woolner LB, et al: Papillary thyroid cancer treated at the Mayo Clinic, 1946 through 1970: Initial manifestation, pathologic findings, therapy, and outcome. Mayo Clin Proc 61:978–996, 1986.
84. Samaan NA, Schultz PN, Hickey RC, et al: The results of various modalities of treatment of well differentiated thyroid carcinoma: A retrospective review of 1,599 patients. J Clin Endocrinol Metab 75:714–720, 1992.
85. Carcangiu ML, Zampi G, Pupi A, et al: Papillary carcinoma of the thyroid: A clinicopathologic study of 241 cases treated at the University of Florence, Italy. Cancer 55:805, 1985.
86. Iida F, Yonekura M, Miyakawa M: Study of intraglandular dissemination of thyroid cancer. Cancer 24:764, 1969.
87. Katoh R, Sasaki J, Kurihara H, et al: Multiple thyroid involvement (intraglandular metastasis) in papillary thyroid carcinoma: A clinicopathologic study of 105 consecutive patients. Cancer 70:1585, 1992.
88. Chan JKC, Saw D: The grooved nucleus: A useful diagnostic criterion of papillary carcinoma of the thyroid. Am J Surg Pathol 10:672, 1986.
89. Matsubayashi S, Kawai K, Matsumoto Y, et al: The correlation between papillary thyroid carcinoma and lymphocytic infiltration in the thyroid gland. J Clin Endocrinol Metab 80:3421–3424, 1995.
90. Pacini F, Cetani F, Miccoli P, et al: Outcome of 309 patients with metastatic differentiated thyroid carcinoma treated with radioiodine. World J Surg 18:600–604, 1994.
91. Rosai J, Zampi G, Carcangiu ML: Papillary carcinoma of the thyroid: A discussion of its several morphologic expressions, with particular emphasis on the follicular variant. Am J Surg Pathol 7:809, 1983.
92. Tielens ET, Sherman SI, Hruban RH, et al: Follicular variant of papillary thyroid carcinoma. Cancer 73:424, 1994.
93. Furmanchuk AW, Averkin JI, Egloff B, et al: Pathomorphological findings in thyroid cancers of children from the Republic of Belarus: A study of 86 cases occurring between 1986 (post Tchernobyl) and 1991. Histopathology 21:401, 1992.
94. Carcangiu ML, Bianchi S: Diffuse sclerosing variant of papillary thyroid carcinoma: Clinicopathologic study of 15 cases. Am J Surg Pathol 13:1041, 1989.
95. Johnson TL, Lloyd RV, Thompson NW, et al: Prognostic implications of the tall cell variant of papillary thyroid carcinoma. Am J Surg Pathol 12:22, 1988.
96. Sobrinho-Simoes M, Nesland JM, Johannessen JV: Columnar cell carcinoma: Another variant of poorly differentiated carcinoma of the thyroid. Am J Clin Pathol 89:264, 1988.
97. Schroder S, Bocker W, Dralle H, et al: The encapsulated papillary carcinoma of the thyroid: A morphologic subtype of the papillary thyroid carcinoma. Cancer 54:90, 1984.
98. Lang W, Choritz H, Hundeshagen H: Risk factors in follicular thyroid carcinomas. A retrospective follow-up study covering a 14 year period with emphasis on morphological findings. Am J Surg Pathol 10:246–255, 1986.
99. Bronner MP, Livolsi VA: Oxyphilic (Askanazy/Hürthle cell) tumors of the thyroid: Microscopic features predict biologic behaviour. Surg Pathol 1:137, 1988.
100. Carcangiu ML, Zampi G, Rosai J: Poorly differentiated "insular" thyroid carcinoma. A reinterpretation of Langhans "wuchernde Struma." Am J Surg Pathol 8:655, 1984.
101. Schlumberger M, Suarez H, Caillou B, Bressac B: Thyroid oncogenes and antioncogenes. J Endocrinol Invest 15:35, 1992.
102. Fusco A, Grieco M, Santoro M, et al: A new oncogene in human thyroid papillary carcinomas and their lymph-nodal metastases. Nature 328:170–172, 1987.
103. Santoro M, Carlomagno F, Hay ID, et al: Ret oncogene activation in human thyroid neoplasms is restricted to the papillary cancer subtype. J Clin Invest 89:1517–1522, 1992.
104. Zou M, Shi Y, Farid NR: Low rate of ret proto-oncogene activation (PTC/ret TPC) in papillary thyroid carcinomas from Saudi Arabia. Cancer 73:176–180, 1994.
105. Wajjwalku W, Nakamura S, Hasegawa Y, et al: Low frequency of rearrangements of the ret and trk proto-oncogenes in Japanese thyroid papillary carcinomas. Jpn J Cancer Res 83:671–675, 1992.
106. Namba H, Yamashita S, Pei HC, et al: Lack of PTC gene (ret proto-oncogene rearrangement) in human thyroid tumors. Endocrinol Jpn 38:627–632, 1991.
107. Ito T, Seyama T, Iwamoto KS, et al: Activated RET oncogene in thyroid cancers of children from areas contaminated by Chernobyl accident. Lancet 344:259, 1994.
108. Fugazzola L, Pilotti S, Pinchera A, et al: Oncogenic rearrangements of the RET proto-oncogene in papillary thyroid carcinomas from children exposed to the Chernobyl nuclear accident. Cancer Res 55:5617, 1995.
109. Klugbauer S, Lengfelder E, Demidchik EP, Rabes HM: High prevalence of RET rearrangement in thyroid tumors of children from Belarus after the Chernobyl reactor accident. Oncogene 11:2459, 1995.
110. Elisei R, Romei C, Capezzone M, et al: Ret protooncogene rearrangements (RET/PTC) in malignant and benign thyroid nodular diseases, both spontaneous and radioinduced (abstract). J Endocrinol Invest 21:76, 1998.
111. Bounacer A, Wicker R, Caillou B, et al: High prevalence of activating ret protooncogene rearrangements, in thyroid tumors from patients who had received external radiation. Oncogene 15:1263, 1997.
112. Nikiforov YE, Rowland JM, Bove KE, et al: Distinct pattern of ret oncogene rearrangements in morphological variants of radiation-induced and sporadic thyroid papillary carcinomas in children. Cancer Res 57:1690, 1997.
113. Bongarzone I, Fugazzola L, Vigneri P, et al: Age-related activation of the tyrosine kinase receptor protooncogenes RET and NTRK1 in papillary thyroid carcinoma. J Clin Endocrinol Metab 81:2006–2009, 1996.
114. Challeton C, Bounacer A, Du Villard JA, et al: Pattern of ras and gsp oncogene mutations in radiation-associated human thyroid tumors. Oncogene 11:601–603, 1995.
115. Russo D, Arturi F, Schlumberger M, et al: Activating mutations of the TSH receptor in differentiated thyroid carcinomas. Oncogene 11:1907–1911, 1995.

116. Fagin JA, Matsuo K, Karmakar A, et al: High prevalence of mutations of the p53 gene in poorly differentiated human thyroid carcinomas. J Clin Invest 91:179–184, 1993.
117. Pacini F, Vivaldi A, Santoro M, et al: Simian virus 40–like DNA sequences in human papillary thyroid carcinoma. Oncogene 16:665, 1998.
118. Yamashita S, Ong J, Fagin JA, Melmed S: Expression of the myc cellular protooncogene in human thyroid tissue. J Clin Endocrinol Metab 63:1170, 1986.
119. Matsuo K, Tang SH, Fagin JA: Allelotype of human thyroid tumors: Loss of chromosome 11q13 sequences in follicular neoplasms. Mol Endocrinol 5:1873–1879, 1991.
120. Farid NR, Shi Y, Zou M: Molecular basis of thyroid cancer. Endocr Rev 15:202–228, 1994.
121. Ron E, Lubin JH, Shore RE, et al: Thyroid cancer after exposure to external radiation: A pooled analysis of seven studies. Radiat Res 141:259–277, 1995.
122. Schneider AB, Ron E: Pathogenesis. *In* Braverman LE, Utiger RD (eds): Werner and Ingbar's The thyroid: A Fundamental and Clinical Text, ed 7. Philadelphia, Lippincott-Raven, 1996, pp 902–909.
123. Favus MJ, Schneider AB, Stachyra ME: Thyroid cancer occurring as a late consequence of head-and-neck irradiation. N Engl J Med 294:1019, 1976.
124. Franceschi S, Boyle P, Maissonneuve P: The epidemiology of thyroid carcinoma. Crit Rev Oncog 4:25–52, 1993.
125. Pacini F, Vorontsova T, Demidchik EP, et al: Post-Chernobyl thyroid carcinoma in Belarus children and adolescents: Comparison with naturally occurring thyroid carcinoma in Italy and France. J Clin Endocrinol Metab 82:3563–3569, 1997.
126. Tronko N, Bogdanova T, Kommisarenko I, et al: Thyroid cancer in children and adolescents in Ukraine after the Chernobyl accident (1986–1995). *In* Karaoglou A, Desmet G, Kelly GN, Menzel HG (eds): The Radiological Consequences of the Chernobyl Accident. ERU 16544 EN, European Union, Luxembourg, 1996, p 683.
127. Dobyns BM, Hyrmer BA: The surgical management of benign and malignant thyroid neoplasms in Marshall Islanders exposed to hydrogen bomb fallout. World J Surg 16:126–140, 1992.
128. Baverstock K, Egloff B, Pinchera A, et al: Thyroid cancer after Chernobyl. Nature 359:21, 1992.
129. Cooper DS, Axelrod L, DeGroot LJ, et al: Congenital goiter and the development of metastatic follicular carcinoma with evidence for a leak of nonhormonal iodide: Clinical, pathological, kinetic, and biochemical studies and a review of the literature. J Clin Endocrinol Metab 52:294–303, 1981.
130. Abe Y, Ichikawa Y, Muraki T, et al: Thyrotropin (TSH) receptor and adenylate cyclase activity in human thyroid tumors: Absence of high affinity receptor and loss of TSH responsiveness in undifferentiated thyroid carcinoma. J Clin Endocrinol Metab 52:23–28, 1981.
131. Behar R, Arganini M, Wu TC, et al: Graves' disease and thyroid cancer. Surgery 100:1121–1127, 1986.
132. Hsu TC, Pathak S, Samaan N, Hickey RC: Chromosome instability in patients with medullary carcinoma of the thyroid. JAMA 246:2046–2048, 1981.
133. Panza N, Vecchio LD, Maio M, et al: Strong association between an HLA-DR antigen and thyroid carcinoma. Tissue Antigen 20:155–158, 1982.
134. Weissel M, Kainz H, Hoefer R, Mayr WR: HLA-DR and differentiated thyroid cancer. Lack of association with the nonmedullary types and possible association with the medullary type. Cancer 62:2486–2488, 1988.
135. Sridama V, Hara Y, Fauchet R, DeGroot LJ: Association of differentiated thyroid carcinoma with HLA-DR7 antigen (abstract 24). *In* Proceedings of the 59th Meeting of the American Thyroid Association. New Orleans, October 1983.
136. Lloyd KM II, Dennis M: Cowden's disease. A possible new symptom complex with multiple system involvement. Ann Intern Med 58:136–142, 1963.
137. de Mestier P: Thyroid cancer and familial rectocolonic polyposis. Chirurgie 116:514–516, 1990.
138. Plail RO, Bussey HJ, Glazer G, Thomson JP: Adenomatous polyposis: An association with carcinoma of the thyroid. Br J Surg 74:377–380, 1987.
139. Camiel MR, Mule JE, Alexander LL, Benninghoff DL: Association of thyroid carcinoma with Gardner's syndrome in siblings. N Engl J Med 278:1056, 1968.
140. Albores-Saavedra J, Duran ME: Association of thyroid carcinoma in chemodectoma. Am J Surg 116:887–890, 1968.
141. Godgar DE, Easton DF, Cannon-Albright LA, Skolnick MH: Systematic population-based assessment of cancer risk in first-degree relatives of cancer probands. J Natl Cancer Inst 86:1600–1608, 1994.
142. McDermott WV Jr, Morgan WS, Hamlin E Jr, Cope O: Cancer of the thyroid. J Clin Endocrinol Metab 14:1336, 1954.
143. DeGroot LJ, Kaplan EL, McCormick M, Straus FH: Natural history, treatment, and course of papillary thyroid carcinoma. J Clin Endocrinol Metab 71:414–424, 1990.
144. Woolner LB, Lemmon ML, Beahrs OH, et al: Occult papillary carcinoma of the thyroid: Study of 140 cases observed in a 30-year period. J Clin Endocrinol Metab 20:89, 1960.
145. Franssila K: Value of histologic classification of thyroid cancer. Acta Pathol Microbiol Scand [A] 225(suppl):1–76, 1971.
146. Schlumberger M, De Vathaire F, Travagli JP, et al: Differentiated thyroid carcinoma in childhood: Long-term follow-up of 72 patients. J Clin Endocrinol Metab 65:1088–1094, 1987.
147. Hazard JB, Hawk WA, Crile G Jr: Medullary (solid) carcinoma of the thyroid: A clinicopathologic entity. J Clin Endocrinol Metab 19:152, 1959.
148. Wolfe HJ, Melvin KEW, Cervi-Skinner SJ, et al: C-cell hyperplasia preceding medullary thyroid carcinoma. N Engl J Med 289:437, 1973.
149. Donahower GF, Schumacher OP, Hazard JB: Medullary carcinoma of the thyroid. A cause of Cushing's syndrome: Report of two cases. J Clin Endocrinol Metab 28:1199, 1968.
150. Pacini F, Basolo F, Elisei R, et al: Medullary thyroid cancer. An immunohistochemical and humoral study using six separate antigens. Am J Clin Pathol 95:300, 1991.
151. Graze K, Spiler IJ, Tashjian AH Jr, et al: Natural history of familial medullary thyroid carcinoma. Effect of a program for early diagnosis. N Engl J Med 299:980–985, 1978.
152. Melvin KEW, Miller HH, Tashjian AH: Early diagnosis of medullary carcinoma of the thyroid gland by means of calcitonin assay. N Engl J Med 285:1115–1120, 1971.
153. Wells SA Jr, Baylin SB, Linehan WM, et al: Provocative agents and the diagnosis of medullary carcinoma of the thyroid gland. Ann Surg 188:139, 1978.
154. Eng C, Clayton D, Schuffenecker I, et al: The relationship between specific RET proto-oncogene mutation and disease phenotype in multiple endocrine neoplasia type 2: International RET Mutation Consortium Analysis. JAMA 276:1575–1579, 1996.
155. Pacini F, Romei C, Miccolo P, et al: Early treatment of hereditary medullary thyroid carcinoma after attribution of multiple endocrine neoplasia type 2 gene carrier status by screening for ret gene mutations. Surgery 118:1031–1035, 1995.
156. Harada T, Ito K, Shimaoka K, et al: Fatal thyroid carcinoma. Anaplastic transformation of adenocarcinoma. Cancer 39:2588–2596, 1977.
157. Justin EP, Seabold JE, Robinson RA, et al: Insular carcinoma: A distinct thyroid carcinoma with associated iodine-131 localization. J Nucl Med 32:1358–1363, 1991.
158. Casara D, Rubello D, Saladini G, et al: Differentiated thyroid carcinoma in the elderly. Aging Clin Exp Res 4:333, 1992.
159. Simpson WJ, McKinney SE, Carruthers JS, et al: Papillary and follicular thyroid cancer: Prognostic factors in 1578 patients. Am J Med 83:479, 1987.
160. Tubiana M, Schlumberger M, Rougier P, et al: Long-term results and prognostic factors in patients with differentiated thyroid carcinoma. Cancer 55:794, 1985.
161. Akslen LA, Haldorsen T, Thoresen SO, Glattre E: Survival and causes of death in thyroid cancer: A population-based study of 2479 cases from Norway. Cancer Res 51:1234–1241, 1991.
162. DeGroot LJ, Kaplan EL, Shukla MS, et al: Morbidity and mortality in follicular thyroid cancer. J Clin Endocrinol Metab 80:2946–2953, 1995.
163. Joensuu H, Klemi PJ, Paul R, et al: Survival and prognostic factors in thyroid carcinoma. Acta Radiol Oncol 25:243, 1986.
164. Mizukami Y, Noguchi M, Michigishi T, et al: Papillary thyroid carcinoma in Kanazawa, Japan: Prognostic significance of histological subtypes. Histopathology 20:243, 1992.
165. Shah JP, Loree TR, Dharker D, et al: Prognostic factors in differentiated carcinoma of the thyroid gland. Am J Med 164:658, 1992.
166. Ceccarelli C, Pacini F, Lippi F, et al: Thyroid cancer in children and adolescents. Surgery 104:1143, 1988.
167. La Quaglia MP, Corbally MT, Heller G, et al: Recurrence and morbidity in differentiated thyroid carcinoma in children. Surgery 104:1149, 1988.
168. Thoresen S, Akslen LA, Glattre E, et al: Thyroid cancer in children in Norway, 1953–1987. Eur J Cancer 29A:365, 1993.
169. Akslen LA, Myking AO, Salvesen H, et al: Prognostic importance of various clinicopathological features in papillary thyroid carcinoma. Eur J Cancer 29A:44, 1993.
170. Ahuja S, Ernst H: Hyperthyroidism and thyroid carcinoma. Acta Endocrinol (Copenh) 124:146, 1991.
171. Dobyns BM, Sheline GE, Workman JB, et al: Malignant and benign neoplasms of the thyroid in patients treated for hyperthyroidism: A report of the Cooperative Thyrotoxicosis Therapy Follow-up Study. J Clin Endocrinol Metab 38:976, 1974.
172. Soh EY, Park CS: Diagnostic approach to thyroid carcinoma in Graves' disease. Yonsei Med J 34:191, 1993.
173. Hay ID, Bergstralh EJ, Goellner JR, et al: Predicting outcome in papillary thyroid carcinoma: Development of a reliable prognostic scoring system in a cohort of 1779 patients surgically treated at one institution during 1940 through 1989. Surgery 114:1050, 1993.
174. Segal K, Ben-Bassat M, Avraham A, et al: Hashimoto's thyroiditis and carcinoma of the thyroid gland. Int Surg 70:205–209, 1985.
175. Pacini F, Mariotti S, Formica N, et al: Thyroid autoantibodies in thyroid cancer: Incidence and relationship with tumour outcome. Acta Endocrinol (Copenh) 119:373–380, 1988.
176. Hawk WA, Hazard JB: The many appearances of papillary carcinoma of the thyroid. Clev Clin Q 43:207, 1976.
177. Evans HL: Columnar-cell carcinoma of the thyroid: A report of two cases of an aggressive variant of thyroid carcinoma. Am J Clin Pathol 85:77, 1986.
178. Herrera MF, Hay ID, Wu PS-C, et al: Hürthle cell (oxyphilic) papillary thyroid carcinoma: A variant with more aggressive biologic behaviour. World J Surg 16:669, 1992.
179. Sobrinho-Simoes MA, Nesland JM, Holm R, et al: Hürthle cell and mitochondrion-rich papillary carcinomas of the thyroid gland: An ultrastructural and immunocytochemical study. Ultrastruct Pathol 8:131, 1985.
180. Carcangiu ML, Zampi G, Rosai J: Papillary thyroid carcinoma: A study of its many morphologic expressions and clinical correlates. Pathol Ann 20:1, 1985.
181. Evans HL: Encapsulated papillary neoplasms of the thyroid: A study of 14 cases followed for a minimum of 10 years. Am J Surg Pathol 11:592, 1987.
182. Soares J, Limbert E, Sobrinho-Simoes M: Diffuse sclerosing variant of papillary thyroid carcinoma: A clinicopathologic study of 10 cases. Pathol Res Pract 185:200, 1989.
183. Akslen LA, Myking AO: Differentiated thyroid carcinomas: The relevance of various pathological features for tumour classification and prediction of tumour progress. Virchows Arch 421:17, 1992.
184. Schlumberger M, Challeton C, De Vathaire F, et al: Radioactive iodine treatment and external radiotherapy for lung and bone metastases from thyroid carcinoma. J Nucl Med 37:598, 1996.
185. Schelfhout LJDM, Creuzberg CL, Hamming JF, et al: Multivariate analysis of survival in differentiated thyroid cancer: The prognostic significance of the age factor. Eur J Cancer Clin Oncol 24:331, 1988.
186. Schroder S, Dralle H, Rehpenning W, et al: Prognostic criteria in papillary thyroid carcinoma. Langenbecks Arch Chir 371:263, 1987.
187. Joensuu H, Klemi PJ, Eerola E, Tuominen J: Influence of cellular DNA content on survival in differentiated thyroid cancer. Cancer 58:2462–2467, 1986.

188. Mazzaferri EL: Impact of initial tumor features and treatment selected on the long-term course of differentiated thyroid cancer. Thyroid Today, vol 18, No 3, p 1, 1995.
189. Schindler AM, van Melle G, Evequoz B, et al: Prognostic factors in papillary carcinoma of the thyroid. Cancer 68:324, 1991.
190. Katoh R, Sasaki J, Kurihara H, et al: Multiple thyroid involvement (intraglandular metastasis) in papillary thyroid carcinoma: A clinicopathologic study of 105 consecutive patients. Cancer 70:1585, 1992.
191. Tscholl-Ducommun J, Hedinger CE: Papillary thyroid carcinomas: Morphology and prognosis. Virchows Arch 396:19, 1982.
192. Cody HS III, Shah JP: Locally invasive, well differentiated thyroid cancer: 22 years' experience at Memorial Sloan-Kettering Cancer Center. Am J Surg 142:480, 1981.
193. Salvesen H, Njolstad PR, Akslen LA, et al: Papillary thyroid carcinoma: A multivariate analysis of prognostic factors including an evaluation of the p-TNM staging system. Eur J Surg 158:583, 1992.
194. Noguchi M, Kinami S, Kinoshita K, et al: Risk of bilateral cervical lymph node metastases in papillary thyroid cancer. J Surg Oncol 52:155, 1993.
195. Rossi RL: Lymph node metastasis in thyroid carcinoma: Incidence, patterns of progression, and significance. Lahey Clin Found Bull 32:168, 1983.
196. Mazzaferri EL: Thyroid carcinoma: Papillary and follicular. *In* Mazzaferri EL, Samaan N (eds): Endocrine Tumors. Cambridge, Blackwell, 1993, pp 278–804.
197. Coburn M, Wanebo HJ: Prognostic factors and management considerations in patients with cervical metastases of thyroid cancer. Am J Surg 164:671, 1992.
198. Scheumann GFW, Gimm O, Wegener G, et al: Prognostic significance and surgical management of locoregional lymph node metastases in papillary thyroid cancer. World J Surg 18:559–568, 1994.
199. Sellers M, Beenken S, Blankenship A, et al: Prognostic significance of lymph node metastases in differentiated thyroid cancer. Am J Surg 164:578, 1992.
200. Coburn M, Teates D, Wanebo HJ: Recurrent thyroid cancer: Role of surgery versus radioactive iodine (I^{131}). Ann Surg 219:587, 1994.
201. Hoie J, Stenwig AE, Kullmann G, et al: Distant metastases in papillary thyroid cancer: A review of 91 patients. Cancer 61:1, 1988.
202. Ozaki O, Ito K, Sugino K: Clinico-pathologic study of pulmonary metastasis of differentiated thyroid carcinoma: Age-, sex-, and histology-matched case-control study. Int Surg 78:218, 1993.
203. Rodriquez-Cuevas S, Almendaro SL, Cardoso JMR, et al: Papillary thyroid cancer in Mexico: Review of 409 cases. Head Neck 15:537, 1993.
204. Casara D, Rubello D, Saladini G, et al: Distant metastases in differentiated thyroid cancer: Long-term results of radioiodine treatment and statistical analysis of prognostic factors in 214 patients. Tumori 77:432, 1991.
205. Casara D, Rubello D, Saladini G, et al: Different features of pulmonary metastases in differentiated thyroid cancer: Natural history and multivariate analysis of prognostic variables. J Nucl Med 34:1626, 1993.
206. Beierwaltes WH, Nishiyama RH, Thompson NW, et al: Survival time and "cure" in papillary and follicular thyroid carcinoma with distant metastases: Statistics following University of Michigan therapy. J Nucl Med 23:561, 1982.
207. Rossi RL, Cady B, Silverman ML, et al: Surgically incurable well-differentiated thyroid carcinoma: Prognostic factors and results of therapy. Arch Surg 123:569, 1988.
208. Elisei R, Pinchera A, Romei C, et al: Expression of thyrotropin receptor (TSH-R), thyroglobulin, thyroperoxidase, and calcitonin messenger ribonucleic acids in thyroid carcinomas: Evidence of TSH-R gene transcript in medullary histotype. J Clin Endocrinol Metab 78:867–871, 1994.
209. Pollina L, Pacini F, Fontanini G, et al: bcl-2, p53 and proliferating cell nuclear antigen expression is related to the degree of differentiation in thyroid carcinomas. Br J Cancer 73:139–143, 1996.
210. Basolo F, Pinchera A, Fugazzola L, et al: Expression of the p21 ras protein as a prognostic factor in papillary thyroid cancer. Eur J Cancer 30A:171–174, 1994.
211. Romano MI, Grattone M, Karner MP, et al: Relationship between the level of c-myc mRNA and histologic aggressiveness in thyroid tumors. Horm Res 39:161, 1993.
212. Romei C, Elisei E, Pinchera A, et al: Somatic mutation of the ret protooncogene in sporadic medullary thyroid carcinoma are not restricted to exon 16 and are associated with tumor recurrence. J Clin Endocrinol Metab 81:1619–1622, 1996.
213. Halnan KE: Influence of age and sex on incidence and prognosis of thyroid cancer: 344 cases followed for ten years. Cancer 19:1534–1541, 1966.
214. Mazzaferri EL, Young RL: Papillary thyroid carcinoma: A 10 year follow-up report of the impact of therapy in 576 patients. Am J Med 70:511–518, 1981.
215. Mazzaferri EL, Young RL, Oertel JE, et al: Papillary thyroid carcinoma: The impact of therapy in 576 patients. Medicine (Baltimore) 56:171–196, 1977.
216. Samaan NA, Mageshwari YK, Nadal S, et al: Impact of therapy for differentiated carcinoma of the thyroid: An analysis of 706 cases. J Clin Endocrinol Metab 56:1131–1138, 1983.
217. Massin JP, Savoie JP, Garnier H, et al: Pulmonary metastases in differentiated thyroid carcinoma: Study of 58 cases with implications for the primary treatment. Cancer 53:982–987, 1984.
218. Mazzaferri EL: Papillary thyroid carcinoma: Factors affecting prognosis and current therapy. Semin Oncol 14:315, 1987.
219. Pacini F, Ceccarelli C, Elisei R, et al: Serum thyroglobulin determination in thyroid cancer: A ten years experience. *In* Nagataki S, Torizuka K (eds): The Thyroid. New York, Elsevier, 1988, p 685.
220. Pacini F, Mari R, Mazzeo S, et al: Diagnostic value of a single serum tg determination on and off thyroid suppressive therapy in the follow-up of differentiated thyroid cancer. Clin Endocrinol (Oxf) 23:405, 1985.
221. Schlumberger M, Parmentier C, de Vathaire F, Tubiana M: 131-I and external radiation in the treatment of local and metastatic thyroid cancer. *In* Falk S (ed): Thyroid Disease. New York, Raven, 1990, p 537.
222. Pacini F, Lippi F, Formica N, et al: Therapeutic doses of iodine-131 reveal undiagnosed metastases in thyroid cancer patients with detectable serum thyroglobulin levels. J Nucl Med 28:1888, 1987.
223. Byar DP, Green SB, Dor P, et al: A prognostic index for thyroid carcinoma: A study of the EORTC Thyroid Cancer Cooperative Group. Eur J Cancer 15:1033, 1979.
224. Tennvall J, Biorklund A, Moller T, et al: Is the EORTC prognostic index of thyroid cancer valid in differentiated thyroid carcinoma? Retrospective multivariate analysis of differentiated thyroid carcinoma with long follow-up. Cancer 57:1405, 1986.
225. Hermanek P, Henson DE, Hutter RVP, et al: TNM Supplement 1993: A Commentary on Uniform Use, International Union Against Cancer. Berlin, Springer-Verlag, 1993.
226. Hermanek P, Sobin LH: TNM Classification of Malignant Tumors: International Union Against Cancer, ed 4. New York, Springer-Verlag, 1987.
227. Cady B, Rossi R: An expanded view of risk-group definition in differentiated thyroid carcinoma. Surgery 104:947, 1988.
228. Pasieka JL, Zedenius J, Azuer G, et al: Addition of nuclear DNA content to the AMES risk-group classification for papillary thyroid cancer. Surgery 112:1154, 1992.
229. Allo MD, Christianson W, Koivunen D: Not all "occult" papillary carcinomas are "minimal." Surgery 104:971–976, 1988.
230. Clark OH, Levin K, Zeng QH, et al: Thyroid cancer: The case for total thyroidectomy. Eur J Cancer Clin Oncol 24:305–313, 1988.
231. Mazzaferri EL: Treating differentiated thyroid carcinoma: Where do we draw the line? Mayo Clin Proc 66:105–111, 1991.
232. Snyder J, Gorman C, Scanlon P: Thyroid remnant ablation: Questionable pursuit of an ill-defined goal. J Nucl Med 24:659–665, 1983.
233. Andry G, Chantrain G, Van Glabbeke M, Dor P: Papillary and follicular thyroid carcinoma. Individualization of the treatment according to the prognosis of the disease. Eur J Cancer Clin Oncol 24:1641–1646, 1988.
234. Brennan MD, Bergstralh EJ, van Heerden JA, McConahey WM: Follicular thyroid cancer treated at the Mayo Clinic, 1946 through 1970: Initial manifestations, pathologic findings, therapy, and outcome. Mayo Clin Proc 66:11–22, 1991.
235. Buckwalter JA, Thomas CG: Selection of surgical treatment for well-differentiated thyroid carcinomas. Ann Surg 176:565, 1972.
236. Rustad WH, Lindsay S, Dailey ME: Comparison of the incidence of complications following total and subtotal thyroidectomy for thyroid carcinoma. Surg Gynecol Obstet 116:109, 1963.
237. Black B, Yadeau R, Woolner L: Surgical treatment of thyroid carcinomas. Arch Surg 88:610, 1964.
238. Shands WC, Gatling RR: Cancer of the thyroid: Review of 109 cases. Ann Surg 171:735, 1970.
239. Tollefsen HR, Shah JP, Huvos AG: Papillary carcinoma of the thyroid. Recurrence in the thyroid gland after initial surgical treatment. Am J Surg 124:468, 1972.
240. Tollefson H, DeCosse J: Papillary carcinoma of the thyroid: The case for radical neck dissection. Am J Surg 108:547, 1964.
241. Duffield RGM, Lowe D, Burnand KG: Treatment of well differentiated carcinoma of the thyroid based on initial staging. Br J Surg 69:426–428, 1982.
242. Young RL, Mazzaferri EL, Rahe AJ, Dorfman SG: Pure follicular thyroid carcinoma: Impact of therapy in 214 patients. J Nucl Med 21:733–737, 1980.
243. Block GE, Wilson SM: A modified neck dissection for carcinoma of the thyroid. Surg Clin North Am 51:139, 1971.
244. Mustard RA: Treatment of papillary carcinoma of the thyroid with emphasis on conservative neck dissection. Am J Surg 120:697, 1970.
245. Simpson WJ, Panzarella T, Carruthers JS, et al: Papillary and follicular thyroid cancer: Impact of treatment in 1578 patients. Int J Radiat Oncol Biol Phys 14:1063–1075, 1988.
246. Devine RM, Edis AJ, Banks PM: Primary lymphoma of the thyroid: A review of the Mayo Clinic experience through 1978. World J Surg 5:33–38, 1981.
247. Butler JS Jr, Brady LW, Amendola BE: Lymphoma of the thyroid. Report of five cases and review. Am J Clin Oncol 13:64–69, 1990.
248. Leedman PJ, Sheridan WP, Downey WF, et al: Combination chemotherapy as single modality therapy for stage IE and IIE thyroid lymphoma. Med J Aust 152:40–43, 1990.
249. Smedal MI, Messner WA: The results of x-ray treatment in undifferentiated carcinoma of the thyroid. Radiology 76:927, 1961.
250. Shimaoka K, Schoenfeld DA, DeWys WD: A randomized trial of doxorubicin versus doxorubicin plus cisplatin in patients with advanced thyroid carcinoma. Cancer 56:2155, 1985.
251. Sokal M, Harmer GI: Chemotherapy for anaplastic carcinoma of the thyroid. Clin Oncol 4:3, 1978.
252. Pacini F, Pinchera A, Mancusi F, et al: Anaplastic thyroid carcinoma: A retrospective clinical and immunohistochemical study. Oncol Rep 1:921, 1994.
253. Tallroth E, Wallin G, Lundell G, et al: Multimodality treatment in anaplastic giant cell thyroid carcinoma. Cancer 60:1428, 1987.
254. Werner B, Abele J, Alveryd A, et al: Multimodal therapy in anaplastic giant cell thyroid carcinoma. J World Surg 8:64, 1984.
255. Nel CJ, van Heerden JA, Goellner JR: Anaplastic carcinoma of the thyroid: A clinicopathological study of eighty-two cases. Mayo Clin Proc 60:51, 1985.
256. Venkatesh YSS, Ordonez NG, Schultz PN, et al: Anaplastic carcinoma of the thyroid: A clinicopathological study of 121 cases. Cancer 66:321, 1990.
257. Tenvall J, Tallroth E, El Hassan A, et al: Anaplastic thyroid carcinoma. Doxorubicin, hyperfractionated radiotherapy and surgery. Acta Oncol 29:1025, 1990.
258. Tennvall J, Lundell G, Hallquist A, et al: Combined doxorubicin, hyperfractionated radiotherapy, and surgery in anaplastic thyroid carcinoma. Cancer 74:1348–1354, 1994.
259. Schlumberger M, Parmentier C, Delisle MJ, et al: Combination therapy for anaplastic giant cell thyroid carcinoma. Cancer 67:564–566, 1991.
260. Kim JH, Leeper RD: Treatment of anaplastic giant and spindle cell carcinoma of the thyroid gland with combination Adriamycin and radiation therapy: A new approach. Cancer 52:954, 1983.
261. Ito T, Seyama T, Mizuno T, et al: Unique association of p53 mutations with undifferentiated but not with differentiated carcinomas of the thyroid gland. Cancer Res 52:1369–1371, 1992.
262. Maxon HR III, Smith HS: Radioiodine-131 in the diagnosis and treatment of meta-

static well differentiated thyroid cancer. Endocrinol Metab Clin North Am 19:685–718, 1990.
263. Schlumberger M, Tubiana M, De Vathaire F, et al: Long-term results of treatment of 238 patients with lung and bone metastases from differentiated thyroid carcinoma. J Clin Endocrinol Metab 63:960, 1986.
264. Brown AP, Greening WP, McCready VR, et al: Radioiodine treatment of metastatic thyroid carcinoma: The Royal Marsden Hospital Experience. Br J Radiol 57:323, 1984.
265. Samaan NA, Schultz PN, Haynie TP, Ordonez NG: Pulmonary metastasis of differentiated thyroid carcinoma: Treatment results in 101 patients. J Clin Endocrinol Metab 60:376, 1985.
266. Ruegemer JJ, Hay ID, Bergstralh EJ, et al: Distant metastases in differentiated thyroid carcinoma: A multivariate analysis of prognostic variables. J Clin Endocrinol Metab 67:501, 1988.
267. Marcocci C, Pacini F, Elisei R, et al: Clinical and biological behaviour of bone metastases from differentiated thyroid carcinoma. Surgery 106:960, 1989.
268. Van Herle AJ, Uller RP: Elevated serum thyroglobulin. A marker of metastases in differentiated thyroid carcinomas. J Clin Invest 56:272–277, 1975.
269. Schlumberger M, Fragu P, Parmentier C, Tubiana M: Thyroglobulin assay in the follow-up of patients with differentiated thyroid carcinomas: Comparison of its value in patients with or without normal residual tissue. Acta Endocrinol (Copenh) 98:215–221, 1981.
270. Ozata M, Suzuki S, Miyamoto T, et al: Serum thyroglobulin in the follow-up of patients with treated differentiated thyroid cancer. J Clin Endocrinol Metab 79:98–105, 1994.
271. Edmonds CJ, Smith T: The long-term hazard of the treatment of thyroid cancer with radioiodine. Br J Radiol 59:45, 1986.
272. Mariotti S, Barbesino G, Caturegli P, et al: Assay of thyroglobulin in serum with thyroglobulin autoantibodies: An unobtainable goal? J Clin Endocrinol Metab 80:468–472, 1995.
273. Pacini F, Pinchera A, Giani C, et al: Serum thyroglobulin concentrations and 131-I whole body scans in the diagnosis of metastases from differentiated thyroid carcinoma (after thyroidectomy). Clin Endocrinol (Oxf) 13:107, 1980.
274. Ashcraft MW, Van Herle AJ: The comparative value of serum thyroglobulin measurements and iodine-131 total body scans in the follow-up study of patients with treated differentiated thyroid cancer. Am J Med 71:806, 1981.
275. Schlumberger M, Arcangioli O, Piekarski JD, et al: Detection and treatment of lung metastases of differentiated thyroid carcinoma in patients with normal chest x-rays. J Nucl Med 29:1790–1794, 1988.
276. Pineda JD, Lee T, Ain K, et al: Iodine-131 therapy for thyroid cancer patients with elevated thyroglobulin and negative diagnostic scan. J Clin Endocrinol Metab 80:1488–1492, 1995.
277. Schlumberger M, Charbord P, Fragu P, et al: Circulating thyroglobulin and thyroid hormones in patients with metastases of differentiated thyroid carcinoma: Relationship to serum thyrotropin levels. J Clin Endocrinol Metab 51:513, 1980.
278. Schneider AB, Line BR, Goldman JM, Robbins J: Sequential serum thyroglobulin determinations, ^{131}I scans, and ^{131}I uptakes after triiodothyronine withdrawal in patients with thyroid cancer. J Clin Endocrinol Metab 53:1199–1206, 1981.
279. Ladenson PW, Braverman LE, Mazzaferri EL, et al: Comparison of administration of recombinant human thyrotropin with withdrawal of thyroid hormone for radioactive iodine scanning in patients with thyroid carcinoma. N Engl J Med 337:888–896, 1997.
280. Jeevanram RK, Shah DH, Sharma SM, et al: Influence of initial large dose on subsequent uptake of therapeutic radioiodine in thyroid cancer patients. Nucl Med Biol 13:277, 1986.
281. Roy-Camille R, Leger FA, Merland JJ, et al: Perspectives actuelles dans le traitement des metastases osseuses des cancers thyroidiens. Chirurgie 106:32, 1980.
282. Rossi RL, Cady B, Silverman ML, et al: Current results of conservative surgery of differentiated thyroid carcinoma. World J Surg 10:612, 1986.
283. Kukkonen ST, Reijo KH, Kaarle OF, et al: Papillary thyroid carcinoma: The new, age-related TNM classification system in a retrospective analysis of 199 patients. World J Surg 14:837, 1990.
284. Grant MD, Hay MB, Gough IR, et al: Local recurrence in papillary thyroid carcinoma: Is extent of surgical resection important? Surgery 104:654, 1988.
285. Ricard M, Tenenbaum F, Schlumberger M, et al: Intraoperative detection of pheochromocytoma with iodine-125 labelled meta-iodobenzylguanidine: A feasibility study. Eur J Nucl Med 20:426–430, 1993.
286. Tubiana M, Haddad E, Schlumberger M, et al: External radiotherapy in thyroid cancers. Cancer 55(suppl):2062–2071, 1985.
287. Niederle B, Roka R, Schemper M, et al: Surgical treatment of distant metastases in differentiated thyroid cancer: Indication and results. Surgery 100:1088, 1986.
288. Proye CAG, Dromer DHR, Carnaille BM, et al: It is still worthwhile to treat bone metastases from differentiated thyroid carcinoma with radioactive iodine? World J Surg 16:640, 1992.
289. Mazzaferri EL: Papillary and follicular thyroid cancer: A selective approach to diagnosis and treatment. Annu Rev Med 32:73, 1981.
290. Parker LN, Wu SY, Kim DD, et al: Recurrence of papillary thyroid carcinoma presenting as a focal neurological deficit. Arch Intern Med 146:1985, 1986.
291. Hay ID: Brain metastases from papillary thyroid carcinoma. Arch Intern Med 147:607, 1987.
292. Venkatesh A, Leavens ME, Samaan NA: Brain metastases in patients with well-differentiated thyroid carcinoma: Study of 11 cases. Eur J Surg Oncol 16:448, 1990.
293. Rall JE, Alpers JB, Lewallen CG, et al: Radiation pneumonitis and fibrosis: A complication of radioiodine treatment of pulmonary metastases from cancer of the thyroid. J Clin Endocrinol Metab 17:1263, 1957.
294. Leeper R: Controversies in the treatment of thyroid cancer: The New York Memorial Hospital approach. Thyroid Today 5:1, 1982.
295. Schober O, Gunter HH, Schwarzrock R, et al: Hamatologische langzeitveranderungen bei der schilddrusenkarzinoms. Strahlenther Onkol 163:464, 1987.
296. Pacini F, Gasperi M, Fugazzola L, et al: Testicular function in patients with differentiated thyroid carcinoma treated with radioiodine. J Nucl Med 35:1418, 1994.
297. Raymond JP, Izembart M, Marliac V, et al: Temporary ovarian failure in thyroid cancer patients after thyroid remnant ablation with radioactive iodine. J Clin Endocrinol Metab 69:186–190, 1989.
298. Dottorini ME, Lomuscio G, Mazzucchelli L, et al: Assessment of female fertility and carcinogenesis after iodine-131 therapy for differentiated thyroid carcinoma. J Nucl Med 36:21–27, 1995.
299. Schlumberger M, De Vathaire F, Ceccarelli C, et al: Exposure to radioactive iodine-131 for scintigraphy or therapy does not preclude pregnancy in thyroid cancer patients. J Nucl Med 37:606–612, 1996.
300. Simpson WJ, Carruthers JS: The role of external radiation in the management of papillary and follicular thyroid cancer. Am J Surg 136:457–460, 1978.
301. Grauer A, Raue F, Gagel RF: Changing concepts in the management of hereditary and sporadic medullary thyroid carcinoma. Endocrinol Metab Clin North Am 19:613–635, 1990.
302. Shimaoka K: Adjunctive management of thyroid cancer: Chemotherapy. J Surg Oncol 15:283–286, 1980.
303. Bukowski RM, Brown L, Weick JK, et al: Combination chemotherapy of metastatic thyroid cancer. Phase II study. Am J Clin Oncol 6:579–581, 1983.
304. De Besi P, Busnardo B, Toso S, et al: Combined chemotherapy with bleomycin, Adriamycin, and platinum in advanced thyroid cancer. J Endocrinol Invest 14:475–480, 1991.
305. Droz JP, Schlumberger M, Rougier P, et al: Chemotherapy in metastatic nonanaplastic thyroid cancer: Experience at the Institut Gustave-Roussy. Tumori 76:480–483, 1990.
306. Gottlieb JA, Hill CS: Adriamycin (NSC123127) therapy in thyroid carcinoma. Cancer Chemother Rep 6:283–296, 1975.
307. Hill CS: Chemotherapy of thyroid cancer. *In* Kaplan EL (ed): Surgery of the Thyroid and Parathyroid Glands. Edinburgh, Churchill Livingstone, 1983, pp 120–126.

Chapter 110

Surgery of the Thyroid

Edwin L. Kaplan ▪ Sonia L. Sugg

Modern thyroid surgery, as we know it today, began in the 1860s in Vienna with the school of Billroth.[1] The mortality associated with thyroidectomy was high, recurrent laryngeal nerve injuries were common, and tetany was thought to be due to "hysteria." The parathyroid glands in humans were not discovered until 1880 by Sandstrom,[2] and the fact that hypocalcemia was the definitive cause of tetany was not wholly accepted until several decades into the 20th century. Kocher, a master thyroid surgeon who operated in the late 19th and early 20th centuries in Bern, practiced meticulous surgical technique and greatly reduced the mortality and operative morbidity of thyroidectomy for goiter. He described "cachexia strumipriva" in patients years after thyroidectomy[3] (Fig. 110–1). Kocher recognized that this dreaded syndrome developed only in patients who had total thyroidectomy. As a result, he stopped performing total resection of the thyroid. We now know, of course, that cachexia strumipriva was surgical hypothyroidism. Kocher received the Nobel Prize for this very important contribution, which proved beyond a doubt the physiologic importance of the thyroid gland.

By 1920, advances in thyroid surgery had reached the point that Halsted referred to this operation as a "feat which today can be accomplished by any competent operator without danger of mishap."[1] Unfortunately, decades later complications still occur. In the best of hands, however, thyroid surgery can be performed today with a mortality that varies little from the risk of general anesthesia alone, as well as with low morbidity. To obtain such enviable results, however, surgeons must have a thorough understanding of the pathophysiology

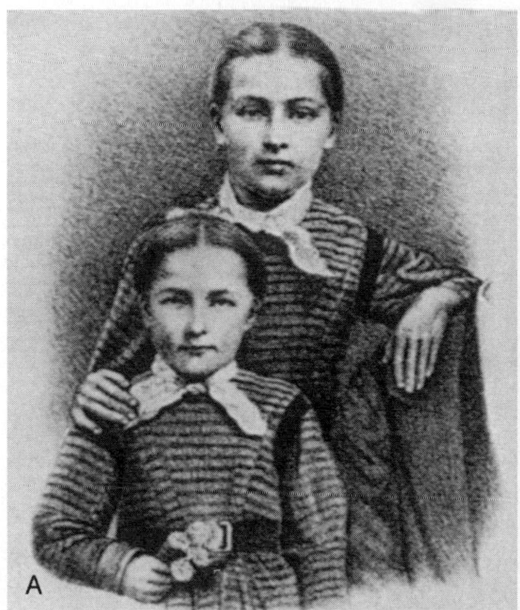

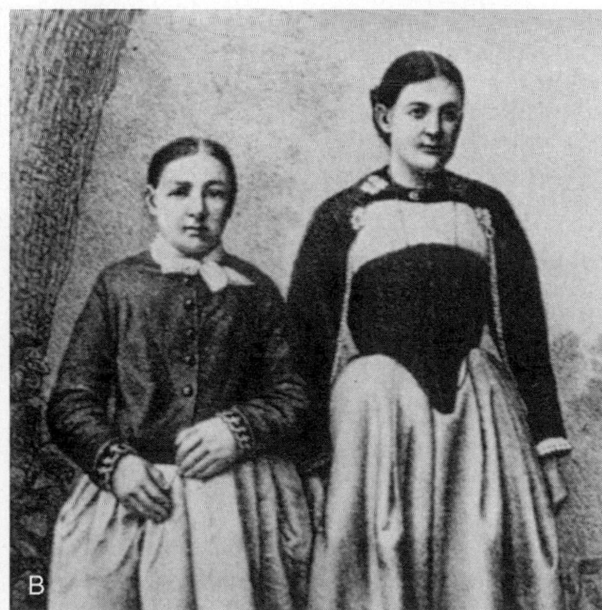

FIGURE 110–1. The dramatic case of Maria Richsel, the first patient with postoperative myxedema to have come to Kocher's attention. *A,* The child and her younger sister before the operation. *B,* Changes 9 years after the operation. The younger sister, now fully grown, contrasts vividly with the dwarfed and stunted patient. Also note Maria's thickened face and fingers, which are typical of myxedema. (From Kocher T: Uber Kropfextirpation und ihre Folgen. Arch Klin Chir 29:254, 1883.)

of thyroid disorders, be versed in the preoperative and postoperative care of patients, have a clear knowledge of the anatomy of the neck region, and finally, use an unhurried, careful, meticulous operative technique.

IMPORTANT SURGICAL ANATOMY

The thyroid gland, which means "shield," is composed of two lobes connected by an isthmus that lies on the trachea approximately at the level of the second tracheal ring (Fig. 110–2). The gland is enveloped by the deep cervical fascia and is attached firmly to the trachea by the ligament of Berry. Each lobe resides in a bed between the trachea and larynx medially and the carotid sheath and sternocleidomastoid muscles laterally. The strap muscles are anterior to the thyroid lobes, and the parathyroid glands and recurrent laryngeal nerves are associated with the posterior surface of each lobe. A pyramidal lobe is often present. This structure is a long, narrow projection of thyroid tissue extending upward from the isthmus and lying on the surface of the thyroid cartilage. It represents a vestige of the embryonic thyroglossal duct and often becomes palpable in cases of thyroiditis or Graves' disease. The normal thyroid varies in size in different parts of the world, depending on the iodine content in the diet. In the United States it weighs about 15 g.

Vascular Supply

The thyroid has an abundant blood supply. The arterial supply to each thyroid lobe is twofold. The *superior thyroid artery* arises from the external carotid artery on each side and descends several centimeters in the neck to reach the upper poles of each thyroid lobe, where they branch. The *inferior thyroid arteries*, each of which arises from the thyrocervical trunk of the subclavian artery, cross beneath the carotid sheath and enter the lower or midpart of the thyroid lobe. The *thyroidea ima* is sometimes present; it arises from the arch of the aorta and enters the thyroid in the midline. A venous plexus forms under the thyroid capsule. Each lobe is drained by the *superior thyroid vein* at the upper pole, which flows into the internal jugular vein, and the *middle thyroid vein* at the middle part of the lobe, which enters either the internal jugular or the innominate vein. Arising from each lower pole is the *inferior thyroid vein*, which drains directly into the innominate vein.

Nerves

The thyroid gland's relationship to the *recurrent laryngeal nerve* and to the *external branch of the superior laryngeal nerve* is of major surgical significance because damage to these nerves leads to disability in phonation or to difficulty breathing.[4] Both nerves are branches of the vagus nerve.

Recurrent Laryngeal Nerve

The *right recurrent laryngeal nerve* arises from the vagus nerve, loops posteriorly around the subclavian artery, and ascends behind the right lobe of the thyroid (Fig. 110–3). It enters the larynx behind the cricothyroid muscle and the inferior cornu of the thyroid cartilage and innervates all the intrinsic laryngeal muscles except the cricothyroid. The left recurrent laryngeal nerve comes from the left vagus nerve, loops posteriorly around the arch of the aorta, and ascends in the tracheoesophageal groove posterior to the left lobe of the thyroid, where it enters the larynx and innervates the musculature in a similar fashion as the right nerve. Several factors make the recurrent laryngeal nerve vulnerable to injury, especially in the hands of inexperienced surgeons.[4]

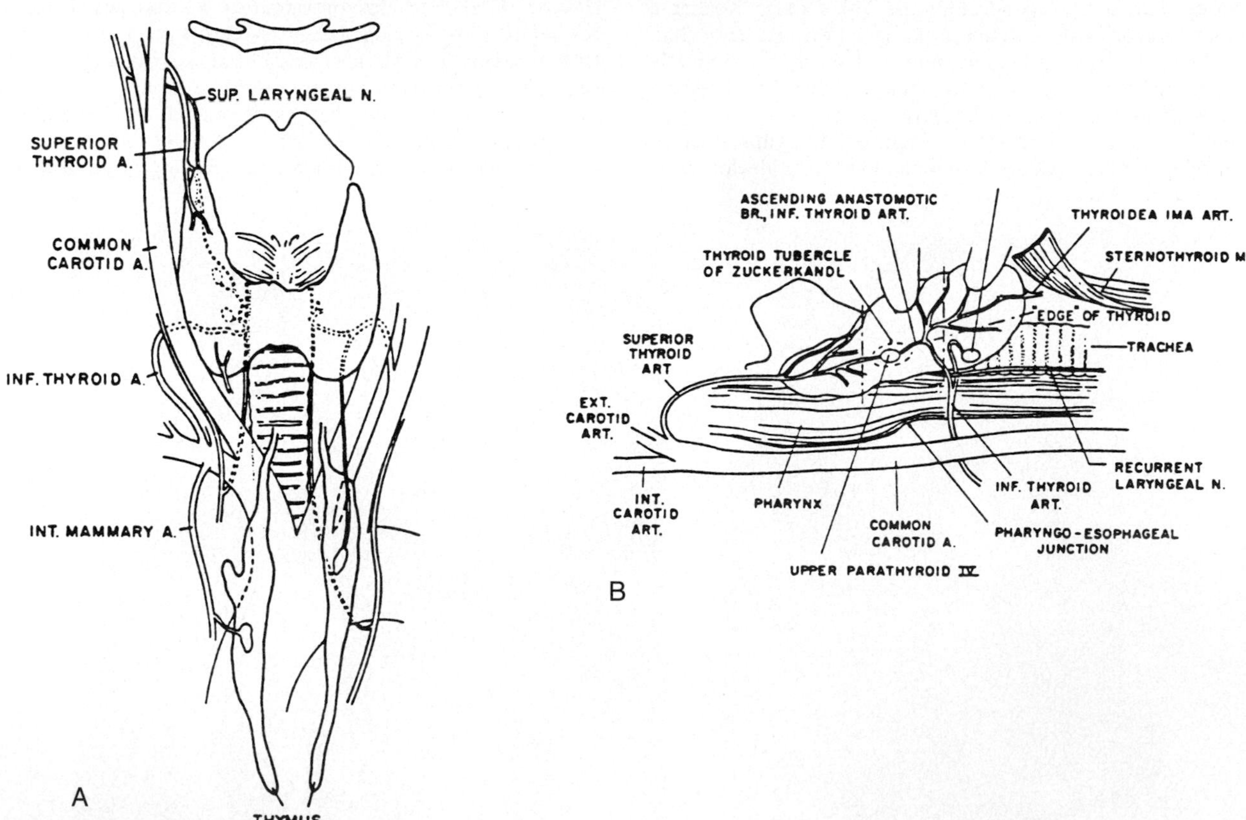

FIGURE 110–2. Anatomy of the thyroid and parathyroid glands. *A,* Anterior view. *B,* Lateral view with the thyroid retracted anteriorly and medially to show the surgical landmarks (the head of the patient is to the left). (From Kaplan EL: Thyroid and parathyroid. *In* Schwartz SI (ed): Principles of Surgery, ed 5. New York, McGraw-Hill, 1989, pp 1613–1685. Copyright © by McGraw-Hill, Inc. Used by permission of McGraw-Hill Book Company.)

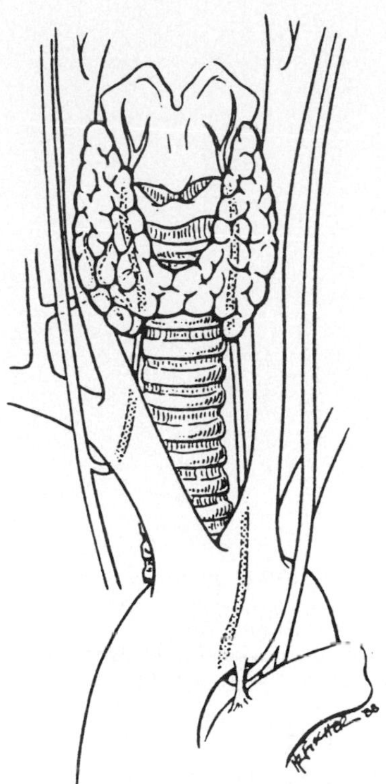

FIGURE 110–3. Anatomy of the recurrent laryngeal nerves. (From Thompson NW, Demers M: Exposure is not necessary to avoid the recurrent laryngeal nerve during thyroid operations. *In* Simmons RL, Udekwu AO (eds): Debates in Clinical Surgery. Chicago, Year Book, 1990.)

1. The presence of a nonrecurrent laryngeal nerve (Fig. 110–4). Nonrecurrent nerves occur more on the right side (0.6%) than on the left (0.04%).[5] They are associated with vascular anomalies, an aberrant takeoff of the right subclavian artery from the descending aorta (on the right), or a right-sided aortic arch (on the left). In these abnormal position, each is at greater risk of being divided.

2. Proximity of the recurrent nerve to the thyroid gland (Fig. 110–5). The recurrent nerve is not always in the tracheoesophageal groove where it is expected to be. It can often be posterior or anterior to this position or may even be surrounded by thyroid parenchyma. Thus the nerve is vulnerable to injury if it is not visualized and traced up to the larynx during thyroidectomy.

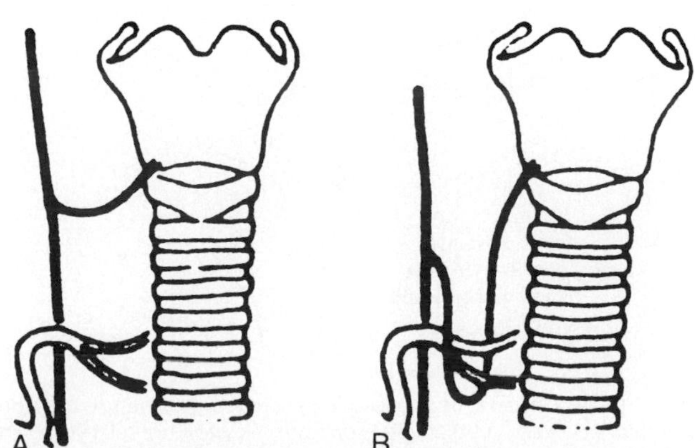

FIGURE 110–4. "Nonrecurrent" right laryngeal nerves coursing near the superior pole vessels *(A)* or around the inferior thyroid artery *(B)*. Because of the abnormal location of "nonrecurrent" nerves, they are much more likely to be damaged during surgery. (From Skandalakis JE, Droulis C, Harlaftis N, et al: The recurrent laryngeal nerve. Am Surg 42:629–634, 1976.)

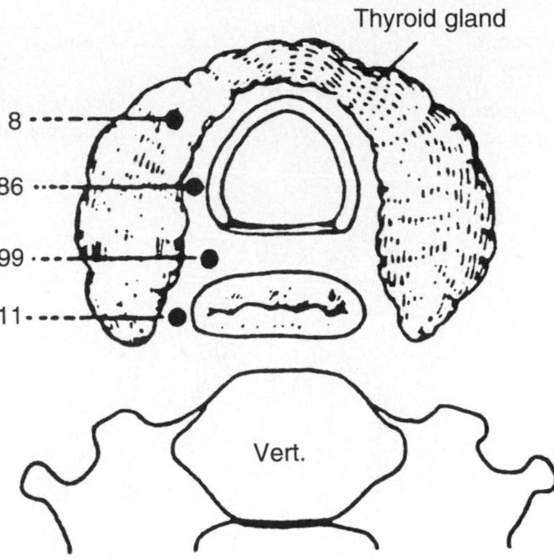

FIGURE 110–5. The location of 204 recurrent laryngeal nerves in dissections from 102 cadavers. (From Skandalakis JE, Droulis C, Harlaftis N, et al: The recurrent laryngeal nerve. Am Surg 42:629–634, 1976.)

3. Relationship of the nerve to the inferior thyroid artery. The nerve frequently passes anterior, posterior, or through the branches of the inferior thyroid artery. Medial traction of the lobe often lifts the nerve anteriorly, thereby making it more vulnerable. Likewise, ligation of this artery, practiced by many surgeons, may be dangerous if the nerve is not identified first.

4. Deformities from large thyroid nodules.[6] In the presence of large nodules the laryngeal nerves may not be anatomically in their "correct" location but may be found even anterior to the thyroid (Fig. 110–6). Once more, there is no substitute for identification of the nerve in a gentle and careful manner.

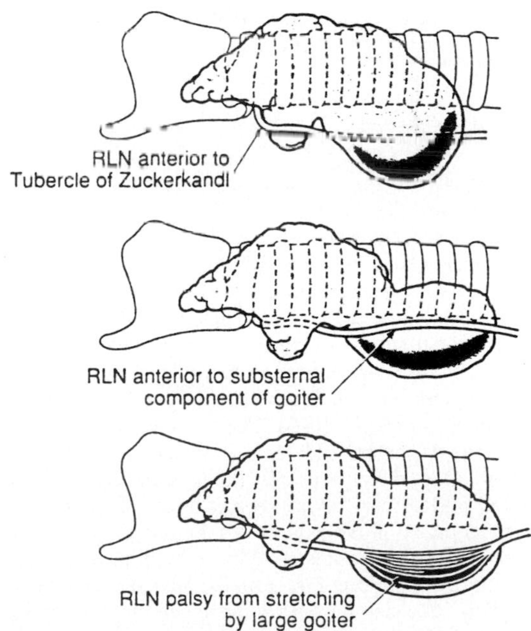

FIGURE 110–6. Recurrent laryngeal nerve (RLN) displacements by cervical and substernal goiters. Such nerves are at risk during lobectomy unless anticipated at possible locations. Rarely the nerves are so stretched that spontaneous palsy results. After careful dissection and preservation, functional recovery may occur postoperatively. (From Thompson NW, Demers M: Exposure is not necessary to avoid the recurrent laryngeal nerve during thyroid operations. *In* Simmons RL, Udekwu AO (eds): Debates in Clinical Surgery. Chicago, Year Book, 1990.)

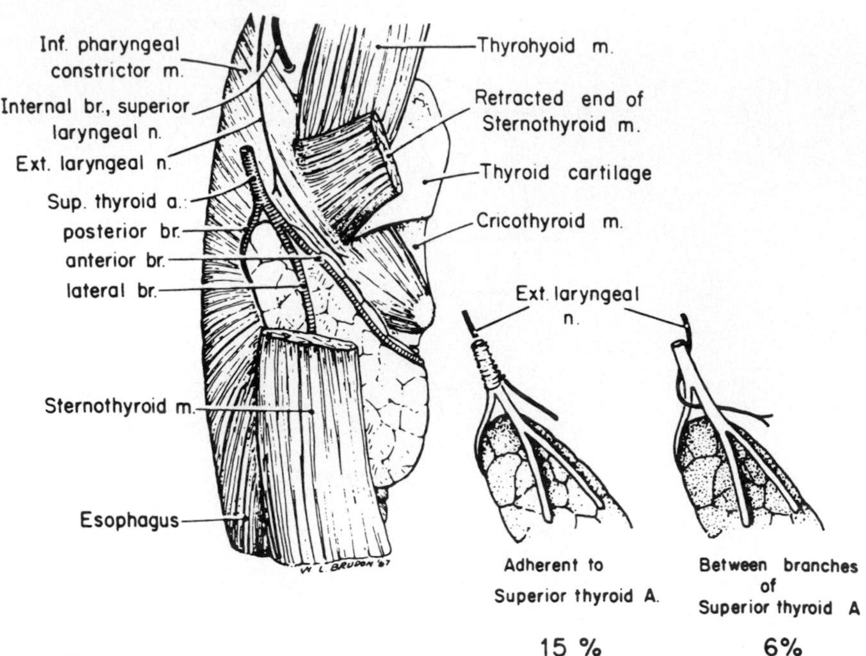

FIGURE 110–7. Proximity of the external branch of the superior laryngeal nerve to the superior thyroid vessels. (From Moosman DA, DeWeese MS: The external laryngeal nerve as related to thyroidectomy. Surg Gynecol Obstet 127:1101, 1968.)

External Branch of the Superior Laryngeal Nerve

On each side, the *external branch of the superior laryngeal nerve* innervates the cricothyroid muscle. In most cases these nerves lie close to the vascular pedicles of the superior poles of the thyroid glands,[7] which requires that the vessels be ligated with care to avoid injury to them (Fig. 110–7). In 21% these nerves are intimately associated with the superior thyroid vessels. In only 15% of cases is the superior laryngeal nerve sufficiently distant from the superior pole vessels to be protected from manipulation by the surgeon. Unfortunately, many surgeons do not even attempt to identify this nerve before ligation of the upper pole of the thyroid.[8]

Parathyroid Glands

The parathyroids are small glands that secrete parathyroid hormone, the major hormone that controls serum calcium homeostasis in humans. Usually four glands are present, but three to six glands have been found. Each gland normally weighs 30 to 40 mg but may be heavier if more fat is present. Because of their small size, their delicate blood supply, and their usual anatomic position adjacent to the thyroid gland, these structures are at risk of being accidentally removed, traumatized, or devascularized during thyroidectomy.[9]

The upper parathyroid glands arise embryologically from the fourth pharyngeal pouch (see Fig. 110–3). They descend only slightly during embryologic development, and their position in adult life remains quite constant. This gland is usually found adjacent to the posterior surface of the middle part of the thyroid lobe, often just anterior to the recurrent laryngeal nerve as it enters the larynx.

The lower parathyroid glands arise from the third pharyngeal pouch along with the thymus (see Fig. 110–3). Hence they often descend with the thymus. Because they travel so far in embryologic life, they have a wide range of distribution in adults, from just beneath the mandible to the anterior mediastinum[10] (Fig. 110–8). Usually, however, these glands are found on the lateral or posterior surface of the lower part of the thyroid gland or within several centimeters of the lower thyroid pole within the thymic tongue.

Parathyroid glands can be recognized by their tan appearance, their small vascular pedicle, the fact that they bleed freely when a biopsy is performed, as opposed to fatty tissue, and their darkening color of hematoma formation when they are traumatized. With experience, one becomes much more adept at recognizing these very important structures and in differentiating them from either lymph nodes or fat. Frozen section examination during surgery can be helpful in their identification.

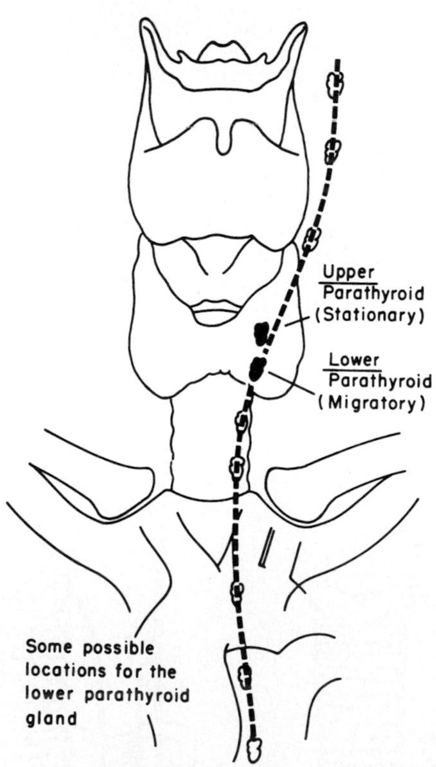

FIGURE 110–8. Descent of the lower parathyroid. Whereas the upper parathyroid occupies a relatively constant position in relation to the middle or upper third of the lateral thyroid lobe, the lower parathyroid normally migrates in embryonic life and may end up anywhere along the course of the *dotted line*. When this gland is in the chest, it is nearly always in the anterior mediastinum. (From Kaplan EL: Thyroid and parathyroid. *In* Schwartz SI (ed): Principles of Surgery, ed 5. New York, McGraw-Hill, 1989, pp 1613–1685. Copyright © by McGraw-Hill, Inc. Used by permission of McGraw-Hill Book Company.)

Lymphatics

A practical description of the lymphatic drainage of the thyroid gland for the thyroid surgeon has been proposed by Taylor.[11] The results of his studies, which are clinically very relevant to the lymphatic spread of thyroid carcinoma, are summarized below.

Central Compartment of the Neck

1. The most constant site to which dye goes when injected into the thyroid is the trachea, the wall of which contains a rich network of lymphatics. This fact probably accounts for the frequency with which the trachea is involved by thyroid carcinoma, especially when it is anaplastic. This involvement is sometimes the limiting factor in surgical excision.
2. A chain of lymph nodes lies in the groove between the trachea and the esophagus.
3. Lymph can always be shown to drain toward the mediastinum and to the nodes intimately associated with the thymus.
4. One or more nodes lying above the isthmus and therefore in front of the larynx are sometimes involved. These nodes have been called the *Delphian nodes* (named for the oracle of Delphi) because it has been said that if palpable, they are diagnostic of carcinoma. However, this clinical sign is often misleading.
5. Central lymph node dissection clears out all these lymph nodes from one carotid artery to the other carotid artery and down into the superior mediastinum as far as possible.

Lateral Compartment of the Neck

A constant group of nodes lies along the jugular vein on each side of the neck. The lymph glands found in the supraclavicular fossae may also be involved in more distant spread of malignant disease from the thyroid gland. Finally, it should not be forgotten that the thoracic duct on the left side of the neck, a lymph vessel of considerable size, arches up out of the mediastinum and passes forward and laterally to drain into the left subclavian vein, usually just lateral to its junction with the internal jugular vein. If the thoracic duct is damaged, the wound is likely to fill with lymph; in such cases the duct should always be sought and tied. A wound that discharges lymph postoperatively should always raise suspicion of damage to the thoracic duct or a major tributary. A *lateral lymph node dissection* encompasses removal of these lateral lymph nodes. Rarely, the submental nodes are involved by metastatic thyroid cancer as well.

INDICATIONS FOR THYROIDECTOMY

Thyroidectomy is usually performed for the following reasons:

1. As therapy for some individuals with thyrotoxicosis, both those with Graves' disease and others with hot nodules
2. To establish a definitive diagnosis of a mass within the thyroid gland, especially when cytologic analysis after fine-needle aspiration (FNA) is either nondiagnostic or equivocal
3. To treat benign and malignant thyroid tumors
4. To alleviate pressure symptoms or respiratory difficulties associated with a benign or malignant process
5. To remove an unsightly goiter

SOLITARY THYROID NODULES

Solitary thyroid nodules are present in 4% to 9% of patients by clinical examination and in 22% of patients by ultrasound in the United States, and most are benign.[12] Therefore, rather than operating on every patient with a thyroid nodule, the physician or surgeon should *select patients for surgery who are at high risk for thyroid cancer.* Furthermore, each surgeon must know the complications of thyroidectomy and be able to perform a proper operation for thyroid cancer in a safe and effective manner or refer the patient to a center where it can be done.

Low-Dose External Irradiation of the Head and Neck

A history of *low-dose external irradiation* of the head or neck is probably the most important historical fact that can be obtained because it indicates that cancer of the thyroid is more likely (about 35% of cases), even if the gland is multinodular.[13, 14] Low-dose irradiation and its implications are discussed in Chapter 109.

High-Dose External Irradiation Therapy

High-dose external irradiation therapy, that is, more than 2000 rad, does not confer safety from thyroid carcinoma, as was previously thought.[15] Rather, an increased prevalence of thyroid carcinoma, usually papillary cancer, has been found, particularly in patients with Hodgkin's disease and other lymphomas who received upper mantle irradiation that included the thyroid gland. Usually a dose of about 4000 to 5000 rad was given. Both benign and malignant thyroid nodules are being recognized now that these persons survive for longer periods.[16] If a thyroid mass appears, it should be treated aggressively. These patients should also be observed carefully for the development of hypothyroidism.

Diagnosis of Thyroid Nodules

A number of diagnostic modalities have been used in the past, but currently most have been superseded by FNA of the mass with *cytologic analysis.*[17] In the hands of a good thyroid cytologist, more than 90% of nodules can be categorized histologically. Approximately 65% to 70% are found to be compatible with a colloid nodule. Twenty percent demonstrated sheets of follicular cells with little or no colloid. Five percent to 10% are malignant, and less than 10% are nondiagnostic.

All patients who have *malignant* cytologic results should be operated on. False-positive diagnoses are rare. All patients with sheets of follicular cells with little or no colloid should also undergo surgery because their findings are compatible with a follicular neoplasm. Most prove to be benign, that is, up to 90%. However, follicular carcinomas exhibit the same cytologic characteristics and cannot be differentiated by this technique. Only by careful histologic examination after operative removal can follicular carcinoma and adenoma be differentiated. Follicular cancers exhibit capsular and/or vascular invasion.

When the diagnosis of *colloid nodule* is made cytologically, the patient should be observed and not operated upon unless tracheal compression or a substernal goiter is present or unless the patient desires the benign mass to be removed. Finally, if an *inadequate specimen* is obtained, FNA with cytologic examination should be repeated. With small, nonpalpable masses, FNA should be performed under ultrasound guidance. Thus FNA with cytologic assessment is the most powerful tool in our armamentarium for the diagnosis of a thyroid nodule.[18]

In summary, the algorithm for the diagnosis of a thyroid nodule with isotope scintigraphy and ultrasonography as initial steps (Fig. 110–9) has been replaced in most hospitals, including our own, by emphasizing the importance of early cytologic examination of the needle aspirate (Fig. 110–10). Far fewer isotope scans are currently being done because carcinomas represent only 5% to 10% of all cold nodules.

PREPARATION FOR SURGERY

Most patients undergoing a thyroid operation are euthyroid and require no specific preoperative preparation related to their thyroid gland. Determination of the serum calcium level may be helpful, and indirect laryngoscopy should definitely be performed in those who are hoarse and in others who have had a prior thyroid or parathyroid operation in order to detect the possibility of a recurrent laryngeal nerve injury.

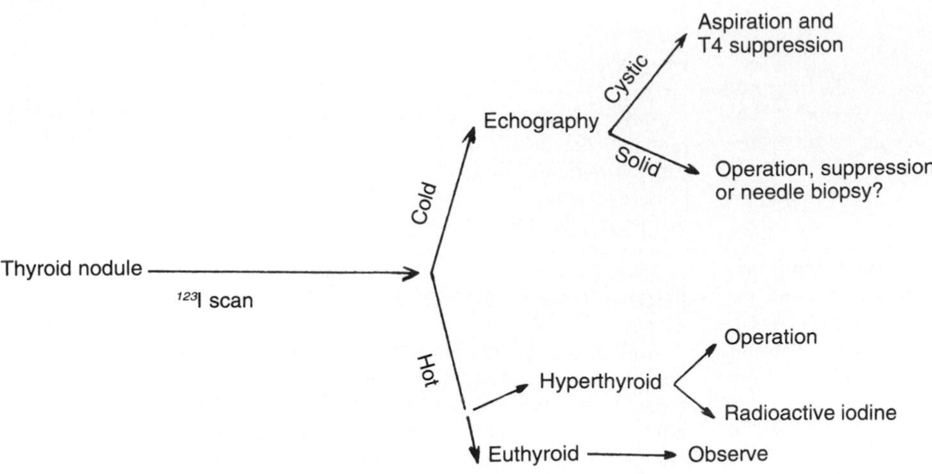

FIGURE 110–9. Algorithm for the diagnosis of a thyroid nodule with isotope scanning and ultrasound examination (echography) as primary modalities. Needle aspiration with cytologic examination is performed on selected nodules.

Hypothyroidism

Modest hypothyroidism is of little concern when treating a surgical patient; however, severe hypothyroidism can be a significant risk factor. Severe hypothyroidism can be diagnosed clinically by myxedema, as well as slowness of affect, speech, and reflexes.[19] Circulating total thyroxine and free thyroxine index values are low. The serum thyroid-stimulating hormone (TSH) level is high in all cases of hypothyroidism that are not due to pituitary insufficiency and is the best test of thyroid function. In the presence of severe hypothyroidism, both the morbidity and the mortality of surgery are increased as a result of the effects of both the anesthesia and the operation. Such patients have a higher incidence of perioperative hypotension, cardiovascular problems, gastrointestinal hypomotility, prolonged anesthetic recovery, and neuropsychiatric disturbances. They metabolize drugs slowly and are very sensitive to all medications. Therefore, when severe myxedema is present, it is preferable to defer elective surgery until a euthyroid state is achieved.

If urgent surgery is necessary, it should not be postponed simply for repletion of thyroid hormone. Endocrine consultation is imperative, and an excellent anesthesiologist is mandatory for success. In most cases, intravenous thyroxine can be started preoperatively and continued thereafter. In general, small doses of thyroxine are initially given to patients who are severely hypothyroid, and then the dose is gradually increased.

Hyperthyroidism

In the United States, most patients with thyrotoxicosis have Graves' disease. Persons with Graves' disease or other thyrotoxic states should be treated preoperatively to restore a euthyroid state and prevent *thyroid storm*, a severe accentuation of the symptoms and signs of hyperthyroidism that can occur during or after surgery. Thyroid storm results in tachycardia or cardiac arrhythmias, fever, disorientation, coma, and even death. In the early days of thyroid surgery, operations on the toxic gland were among the most dangerous surgical procedures because of the frequent occurrence of severe bleeding, as well as all the symptoms and signs of thyroid storm. Now, with proper preoperative preparation,[20] operations on the thyroid gland in Graves' disease can be performed with about the same degree of safety as operations for other thyroid conditions.

In mild cases of Graves' disease with thyrotoxicosis, iodine therapy alone has been used for preoperative preparation, although we do not recommend this approach routinely.[19] Lugol's solution or a saturated solution of potassium iodide is given for several weeks. Although only several drops per day is needed to block the release of thyroxine from the toxic thyroid gland, it is our practice to administer three drops two or three times daily. This medication is taken in milk or orange juice to make it more palatable.

Most of our patients with Graves' disease are treated initially with the antithyroid drugs propylthiouracil or methimazole (Tapazole) until they approach a euthyroid state. Then iodine is added to the regimen for 10 to 14 days before surgery. The iodine decreases the vascularity and increases the firmness of the gland. Sometimes thyroxine is added to this regimen to prevent hypothyroidism and to decrease the size of the gland. β-Adrenergic blockers such as propranolol (Inderal) have increased the safety of thyroidectomy for patients with Graves' disease.[20] We use them frequently with antithyroid drugs to block β-adrenergic receptors and ameliorate the major signs of Graves' disease by decreasing the patient's pulse rate and eliminating the tremor. Some surgeons recommend preoperative use of propranolol alone or with iodine.[21] These regimens, they believe, shorten the preparation time of patients with Graves' disease for surgery and make the operation easier because the thyroid gland is smaller and less friable than it would otherwise be.[21] We do not favor these regimens for routine preparation because they do not appear to offer the same degree of safety as do preoperative programs that restore a euthyroid state before surgery. Instances of fever and tachycardia have been reported in persons with Graves' disease who were taking only propranolol. We have used propranolol therapy alone or with iodine without difficulty in some patients who are allergic to antithyroid medications. In such patients it is essential to continue the propranolol for 1 to 2 weeks

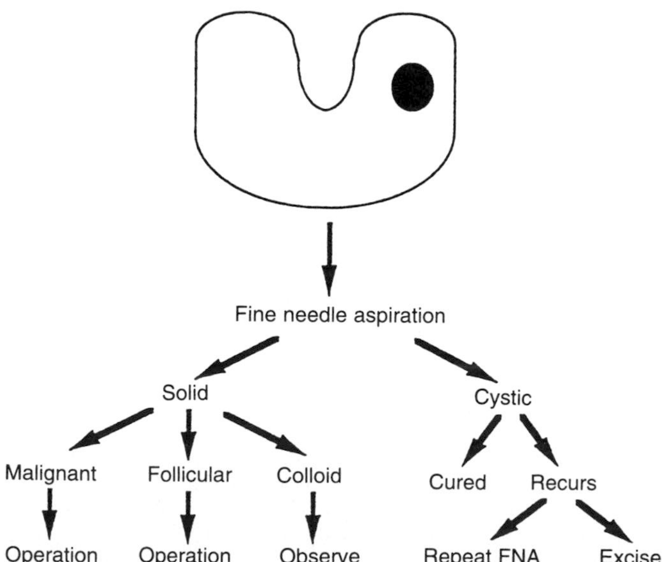

FIGURE 110–10. Algorithm for the diagnosis of a thyroid nodule with fine-needle aspiration (FNA) and cytologic examination of each nodule. Greater accuracy is obtained by using this diagnostic scheme. (Courtesy of Dr. Jon van Heerden.)

TABLE 110–1. Ablative Treatment of Graves' Disease with Thyrotoxicosis

Method	Dose or Extent of Surgery	Onset of Response	Complications	Remarks
Surgery	Subtotal (90%–95%) excision of gland	Immediate	Mortality: <1% Permanent hypothyroidism: 20%–30% Recurrent hyperthyroidism: <15% Vocal cord paralysis: ~1% Hypoparathyroidism: ~1%	Applicable in younger patients and pregnant women
Radioiodine	5–10 mCi	Several weeks to months	Permanent hypothyroidism: 50%–70%, often with delayed onset; multiple treatments sometimes necessary; recurrence possible	Potential risks require ongoing study; close long-term follow-up needed; avoid in children or pregnant women

postoperatively. Remember that they are still in a thyrotoxic state immediately after surgery, although the peripheral manifestations of their disease have been blocked.

The advantages and disadvantages of radioiodine vs. thyroidectomy as definitive treatment of Graves' disease are listed in Table 110–1. In our patients we have never had a death from thyroidectomy in close to 30 years. Surgical resection involves either subtotal thyroidectomy (Fig. 110–11) or lobectomy with contralateral subtotal lobectomy. Currently we leave about 3 to 4 g of thyroid tissue in the neck at the end of the operative procedure. Leaving more leads to a higher rate of recurrence.[22] In children and adolescents, one should consider leaving smaller remnants because the incidence of recurrence of thyrotoxicosis appears to be greater in this group. Finally, when operating for severe ophthalmopathy we try to perform near-total or total thyroidectomy. The major benefits of thyroidectomy appear to be the speed with which normalization is achieved and the lower rate of hypothyroidism than after radioiodine therapy.

SURGICAL APPROACH TO THYROID NODULES

Nonirradiated Patients

Any nodule suspected of being a carcinoma should be completely removed, along with surrounding tissue, which means that a total lobectomy (or lobectomy with isthmectomy) is the initial operation of choice in most patients (see Fig. 110–11). A frozen section should be obtained intraoperatively. If a *colloid nodule* is diagnosed, the operation is terminated. If a follicular *adenoma* is diagnosed, treatment is more controversial. Differentiating follicular adenoma from follicular carcinoma or a benign Hürthle cell tumor from Hürthle cell carcinoma on frozen section is usually very difficult. These diagnoses require careful assessment of cellular morphology, as well as capsular and vascular invasion, which are often difficult to evaluate on frozen section. To aid in the diagnosis, enlarged lymph nodes of the central

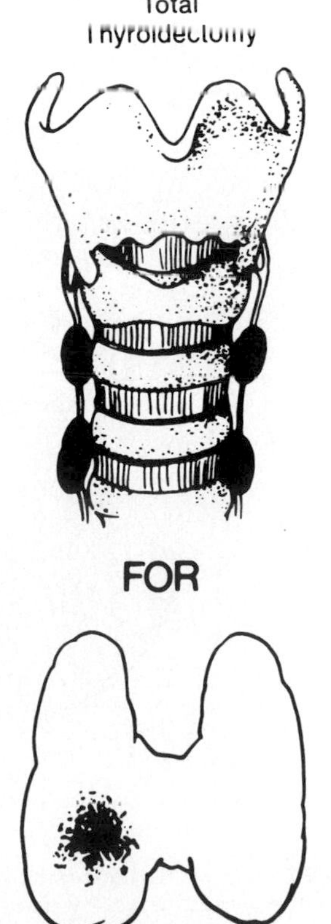

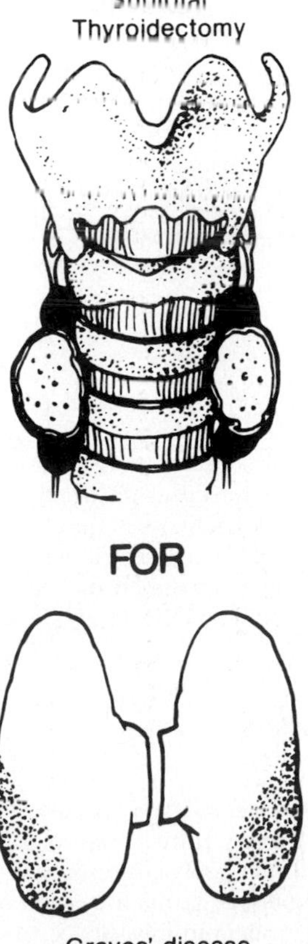

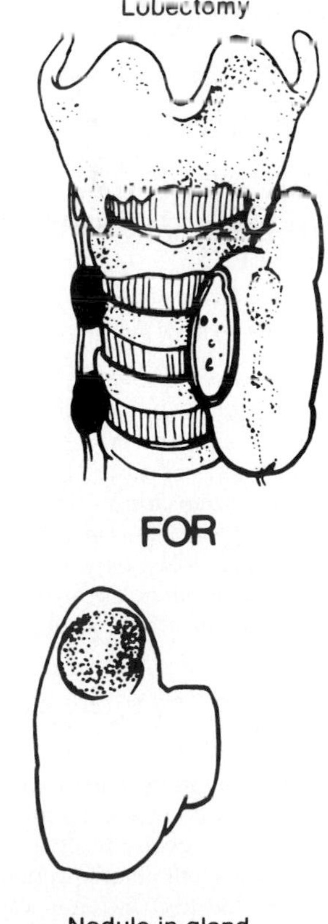

FIGURE 110–11. Common operations on the thyroid. In near-total thyroidectomy a small amount of thyroid tissue is left to protect the recurrent laryngeal nerve and upper parathyroid gland. (From Kaplan EL: Surgical endocrinology. *In* Polk HC, Stone HH, Gardner B (eds): Basic Surgery, ed 4. St Louis, Quality Medical Publishing, 1993, pp 162–195.)

compartment are sampled, and a biopsy of the jugular nodes is also performed. If the result is negative, two options are available: stopping the operation after lobectomy, with the understanding that a second operation may be necessary to complete the thyroidectomy if a carcinoma is ultimately diagnosed, or performing a subtotal resection on the contralateral side. We favor the latter approach if the patient consents, particularly when preoperative needle aspiration suggests that a follicular lesion will be encountered intraoperatively or if examination of frozen sections identifies a follicular neoplasm. We treat most patient with benign neoplasms with thyroxine replacement anyway, even if only one lobe has been removed. Furthermore, a second operation is usually eliminated if the lesion is later diagnosed as malignant because the remaining small thyroid remnant can be ablated with radioiodine therapy.

Irradiated Patients

In patients who have been exposed to low-dose, external irradiation of the head and neck during infancy, childhood, or adolescence, because of the frequency of bilaterality of the disease, the known coincidence of benign and malignant nodules in the same gland, and the prevalence of papillary carcinoma in 35% to 40% of such patients, near-total resection of the thyroid gland with biopsy of the jugular nodes is usually performed, even if a frozen section of the dominant nodule is benign.[14] This therapy is thought to be advantageous because small cancers can be present in the same gland and the remaining thyroid remnant of these patients can usually be ablated with radioiodine if a carcinoma is found on permanent section analysis. In any event, these patients require therapy with thyroid hormone.

Patients who have received high-dose radiation to their thyroid bed, such as those treated with mantle irradiation for Hodgkin's disease, are also at greater risk for the development of thyroid carcinoma years later and should be monitored carefully.[15] Once more, if they are operated on for nodular disease, most of the thyroid tissue should be removed even if the dominant mass is thought to be benign.

SURGICAL APPROACH TO THYROID CANCER

Papillary Carcinoma

The surgical treatment of papillary carcinoma is best divided into two groups based on the clinical characteristics and virulence of these lesions.

Treatment of Minimal Papillary Carcinoma

The term *minimal papillary carcinoma* refers to a small papillary cancer, less than 1 cm in diameter, that demonstrates no local invasiveness through the thyroid capsule, is not associated with lymph node metastases, and is often found in a young person as an occult lesion when thyroidectomy has been performed for another benign condition. In such instances, especially when the cancer is unicentric and 5 mm or smaller, lobectomy is sufficient and reoperations are unnecessary. Thyroid hormone is given to suppress serum TSH levels, and the patient is monitored at regular intervals.

Standard Treatment of Most Papillary Carcinomas

Most papillary carcinomas are neither minimal nor occult. These tumors are known to be microscopically multicentric in up to 80% of cases, occasionally to invade locally into the trachea or esophagus, to metastasize commonly to lymph nodes and later to the lungs and other tissues, and to recur clinically in the other thyroid lobe in 7% to 18% of patients if treated only by thyroid lobectomy.[23]

The authors firmly believe that the best treatment of papillary cancer is near-total or total thyroidectomy (see Fig 110–11), with appropriate central and lateral neck dissection when nodes are involved. The so-called cherry-picking operations, which remove only the enlarged lymph nodes, should not be performed. Rather, when tumor is found in the lateral triangle, a modified radical neck dissection should be performed[24] (Fig. 110–12). At the conclusion of a modified radical neck dissection, the lymph node–bearing tissue from the lateral triangle is removed while the carotid artery, jugular vein, phrenic nerve, sympathetic ganglia, brachial plexus, and spinal accessory nerve are spared and left in place. Many times sensory nerves can be retained as well. Prophylactic neck dissection of the lateral triangle should not be performed for papillary cancer. Such dissections should be done only when enlarged nodes with tumor are found.

Surgeons with limited experience should probably not perform total or near-total thyroidectomy unless capable of doing so with a low incidence of recurrent laryngeal nerve injuries and permanent hypoparathyroidism because these complications are serious. Otherwise, it may be advisable to refer such patients to a major medical center where such expertise is available.

After surgery, radioiodine scanning and treatment are frequently used.[25] ^{131}I is taken up by most metastatic papillary cancers, but only if the TSH level is very high and normal thyroid tissue has been removed or ablated. If all or most of a lobe of normal thyroid remains, radioiodine scanning and treatment of metastases cannot be performed effectively.

Controversies

Because no randomized prospective study has ever been performed, controversy still exists over the proper treatment of papillary cancer in some patients. Many clinicians now accept that patients with this disease can be separated into different risk groups according to a set of prognostic factors. Using the AGES,[26] AMES,[27] or MACIS[28] criteria, which evaluate risk by age, distant metastases, extent of local involvement, and size (MACIS adds completeness of excision), almost 80% of patients fall into a low-risk group. Treatment of this low-risk group is most controversial. Should a lobectomy be done, or is bilateral thyroid resection more beneficial?

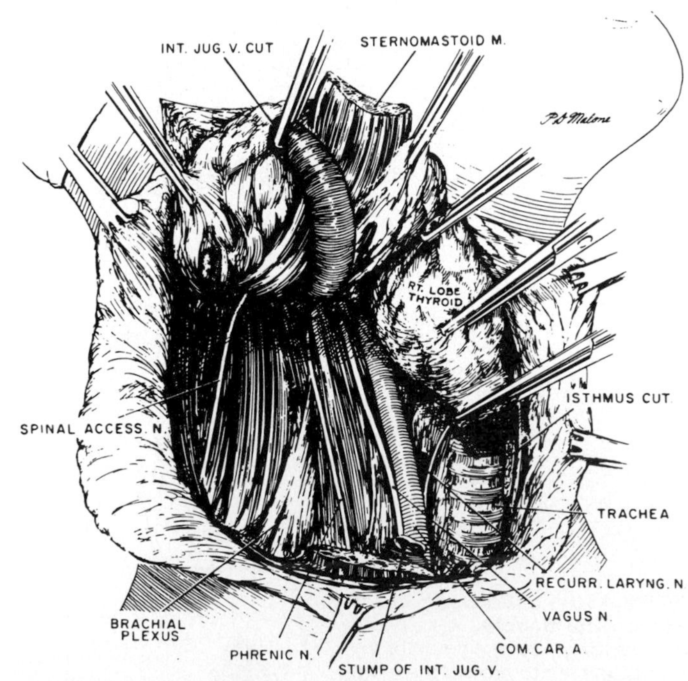

FIGURE 110–12. Lateral neck dissection. Note that during this procedure the vagus nerve, sympathetic ganglia, phrenic nerve, brachial plexus, and spinal accessory nerve are preserved. In a modified neck dissection the sternocleidomastoid muscle is not usually divided and the jugular vein is not removed unless lymph nodes with tumor are adherent to it. (From Sedgwick CE, Cady B: *In* Surgery of the Thyroid and Parathyroid Glands. Philadelphia, WB Saunders, 1980, p 180.)

LOW-RISK PAPILLARY CANCER. Hay and associates studied 1685 patients treated at the Mayo Clinic between 1940 and 1991; the mean follow-up period was 18 years.[29] Of the total, 98% had complete tumor resection and 38% had initial nodal involvement. Twelve percent had unilateral lobectomy whereas 88% had bilateral lobar resection—total thyroidectomy, 18%; near-total thyroidectomy, 60%. Cause-specific mortality at 30 years was 2%, and distant metastases occurred in 3%. These indices did not differ between surgical groups. However, local recurrence and nodal metastases in the lobectomy group (14% and 19%, respectively) were significantly higher than the 2% and 6% rates seen after near-total or total thyroidectomy.

This study is excellent. Although no differences in mortality were reported, a threefold difference in recurrence rates in the thyroid bed and lymph nodes was reported. In addition, this study recognizes patients' anxiety about tumor recurrence and their strong desire to face an operation only once and to be cured of their disease. It appears that if the operation can be done safely with low morbidity, this study supports the use of near-total or total thyroidectomy for patients with low-risk papillary cancer.

HIGH-RISK PAPILLARY CANCER. For high-risk patients, it is generally agreed that bilateral thyroid resection improves survival[26] and reduces recurrence rates[30] when compared with unilateral resection. At the University of Chicago such patients also receive radioiodine scanning along with ablation or treatment with radioiodine as indicated.[31]

In general, our studies[31, 32] and those of Mazzaferri and Jhiang[33] have demonstrated a decrease in mortality and in recurrence after near-total or total thyroidectomy followed by radioiodine ablation or therapy.

Follicular Carcinoma

True follicular carcinomas are far less common than papillary cancer and are now rather uncommon. Remember that the "follicular variant" of papillary cancer should be classified and treated as a papillary carcinoma. Patients with follicular carcinoma are usually older than those with papillary cancer, and once more, females predominate. Microscopically, the diagnosis of follicular cancer is made when vascular and/or capsular invasion is present. Tumor multicentricity and lymph node metastases are far less common than in papillary carcinoma. Metastatic spread of tumor often occurs by hematogenous dissemination to the lungs, bones, and other peripheral tissues.

A follicular cancer that demonstrates only *microinvasion* of the capsule has a very good prognosis.[34] In this situation, ipsilateral lobectomy is probably sufficient. However, for most patients with follicular cancer that demonstrates gross capsular invasion or vascular invasion, the ideal operation is similar to that for papillary cancer, although the rationale for its performance differs. Near-total or total thyroidectomy should be performed not because of multicentricity but rather to facilitate a later total body scan with radioiodine.[33] Remnants of normal thyroid in the neck are ablated by radioiodine, and if peripheral metastases are detected (Fig. 110–13), they should be treated with high-dose radioiodine therapy. Although lymph node metastases in the lateral region of the neck are not commonly found, a modified radical neck dissection should be performed if they are present.

Finally, regardless of the operation, all patients with papillary or follicular cancer should be treated with levothyroxine therapy for life in sufficient doses to suppress the TSH level.[33] Care should be taken to not cause cardiac or other problems from thyrotoxicosis, however.

Hürthle Cell Tumors and Cancer

Hürthle cell tumors are thought to be variants of follicular neoplasms. They are more difficult to treat than the usual follicular neoplasms, however, for several reasons.[35] (1) The incidence of carcinoma varies from 5.3% to 62% in different clinical series. (2) Benign-appearing tumors later metastasize in up to 2.5% of patients. (3) Hürthle cell cancers are far less likely to concentrate radioiodine than the usual follicular carcinomas are, which makes treatment of metastatic disease particularly difficult.

Of 54 patients with Hürthle cell tumors whom we treated,[35] 4 had grossly malignant lesions, 10 had questionable diagnoses ("intermediate" lesions) because of partial penetration of their capsule by tumor, and 40 (74%) had lesions that were thought to be benign. About half the patients had a history of low-dose external irradiation. Many had separate papillary or follicular cancers in the same thyroid gland

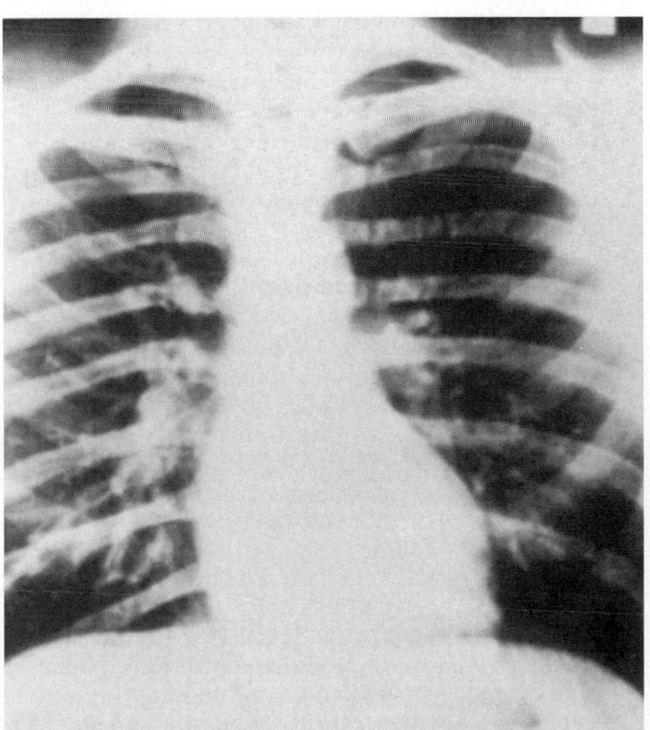

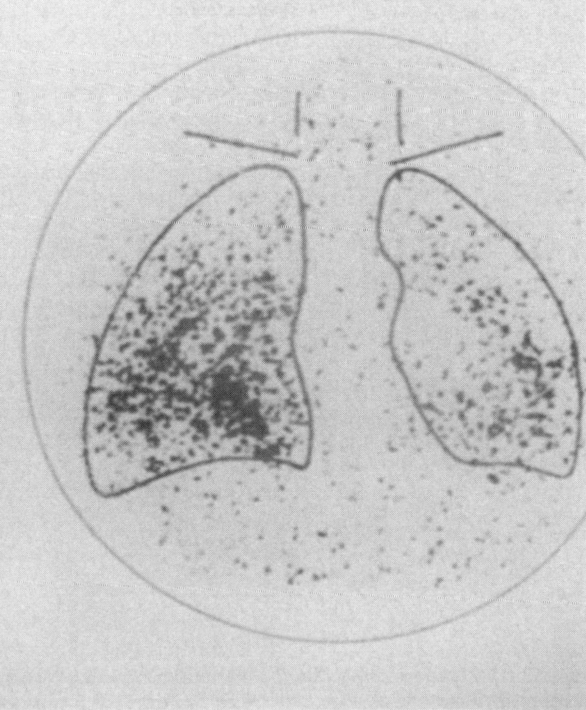

FIGURE 110–13. Despite the fact that the chest radiograph was read as normal, a total body scan using radioiodine demonstrated uptake in both lung fields, thus signifying the presence of unknown metastatic disease. Note that the thyroid has been removed surgically because no uptake of isotope is present in the neck.

During a mean follow-up period of 8.4 years, three additional Hürthle cell tumors were recognized as malignant after metastases were discovered: two were originally classified as intermediate lesions, and one was in the benign-appearing group. Thus 7 of 54 (13%) of our patients who had a Hürthle cell tumor had Hürthle cell carcinoma. One of the 7 patients with Hürthle cell cancer died of widespread metastases after 35 years, and the other 6 are currently free of disease.

We believe that treatment of these lesions should be individualized.[35, 36] Total thyroid ablation is appropriate for frankly malignant Hürthle cell cancers, for all Hürthle cell tumors in patients who received low-dose childhood irradiation, for patients with associated papillary or follicular carcinomas, for all large tumors, and for patients whose tumors exhibit partial capsular invasion. On the other hand, single, well-encapsulated, benign-appearing Hürthle cell tumors that are small may be treated by lobectomy and careful follow-up because the chance that they will later exhibit malignant behavior is low (2.5% in our series and 1.5% among patients described in the literature).[35] Nuclear DNA analysis may aid the surgeon in recognizing tumors that are potentially aggressive because such tumors usually demonstrate aneuploidy.[37] Furthermore, increased genetic abnormalities have been shown in Hürthle cell carcinomas when compared with Hürthle cell adenomas.[38]

In a review of follicular cancers at the University of Chicago,[36] the overall mortality was 16%, twice that of papillary carcinomas. However, in non–Hürthle cell follicular cancers the mortality was 12%, whereas in Hürthle cell cancers it was 24%, thus demonstrating the difficulty in treating metastatic disease, which cannot be resected in the latter group.

Anaplastic Carcinoma

Anaplastic thyroid carcinoma remains one of the most virulent of all cancers in humans. The tumor grows very rapidly, and systemic symptoms are common. Survival for most patients is measured in months. The previously so-called small cell type is now known to be a lymphoma and is most often treated by a combination of external radiation and chemotherapy. The "large cell type" may be manifested as a solitary thyroid nodule early in its clinical course. If it is operated on at that time, near-total or total thyroidectomy should be performed, with appropriate central and lateral neck dissection. However, anaplastic cancer is almost always advanced when the patient is first evaluated. In such patients, surgical cure is unlikely no matter how aggressively it is pursued. In particularly advanced cases, diagnosis by needle biopsy or by small open biopsy may be all that is appropriate. Sometimes the isthmus must be divided to relieve tracheal compression, or a tracheostomy might be beneficial. Most treatment, however, has been by external radiation therapy, chemotherapy, or both. Hyperfractionated external radiation therapy that uses several treatments per day has some enthusiasts, but complications may be high.[39] Radioiodine treatment is almost always ineffective because tumor uptake is absent. Although some success has been observed with doxorubicin, prolonged remissions are rarely achieved, and multidrug regimens and combinations of chemotherapy with radiation therapy are being tried.[40, 41] Although remissions do occur, cures have rarely if ever been achieved in advanced cases. Our most recent regimen includes preoperative external radiation therapy with 7500 rad to the neck and courses of aggressive chemotherapy with cisplatin, hydroxyurea, and paclitaxel (Taxol).[42] Total thyroidectomy and neck dissection follow only if no metastatic disease outside the neck is present after this regimen.

Medullary Thyroid Carcinoma

Medullary thyroid carcinoma is a C cell, calcitonin-producing tumor that contains amyloid or an amyloid-like substance. In addition to calcitonin, it may elaborate or secrete other peptides and amines such as carcinoembryonic antigen, serotonin, neurotensin, and a high-molecular-weight adrenocorticotropic hormone–like peptide. These substances may result in a carcinoid-like syndrome with diarrhea, as well as Cushing's syndrome, especially when widely metastatic tumor is present. Most medullary cancer of the thyroid is sporadic (about 70%–80%), but it can also be transmitted in a familial pattern. This tumor or its precursor, C cell hyperplasia, occurs as a part of the multiple endocrine neoplasia type 2A (MEN-2A) and MEN-2B syndromes[43] (Table 110–2 and Fig. 110–14) or rarely as part of the familial medullary thyroid cancer syndrome. The MEN-2 syndromes are transmitted as an autosomal dominant trait, so 50% of the offspring would be expected to have this disease. Recently, mutations of the *ret* oncogene on chromosome 10 have been found to be the cause of the MEN-2 syndromes.[44] These defects are germline mutations and can therefore be found in blood samples. All patients with medullary thyroid carcinoma should be screened for hyperparathyroidism and pheochromocytoma.[45] If a pheochromocytoma (or its precursor, adrenal medullary hyperplasia) is present, this growth should be operated upon *first* because it has the greatest immediate risk to the patient. Family members, including children, of a patient with medullary cancer of the thyroid should also be screened for medullary cancer of the thyroid, especially if the tumor is bilateral or if C cell hyperplasia is present. Genetic testing for *ret* mutations has largely replaced screening by calcitonin in family members. However, calcitonin measurement is still useful for screening patients with a thyroid mass when FNA analysis raises the possibility of medullary thyroid cancer.

Medullary cancer spreads to the lymph nodes of the neck and mediastinum and later disseminates to the lungs, bone, liver, and elsewhere. The tumor is relatively radioresistant, does not take up radioiodine, and is not responsive to thyroid hormone suppression. *Hence an aggressive surgical approach is mandatory.* The operation of choice for medullary cancer is total thyroidectomy coupled with *aggressive* resection of the central and mediastinal lymph nodes.[46] If lymph nodes of the lateral neck area contain tumor, careful and extensive modified radical neck dissection is required. Reoperations for metastatic tumor were rarely considered to be rewarding until the work of Tisell and Jansson.[46] Their work and that of others demonstrated that 25% to 35% of patients with elevated circulating calcitonin levels could be rendered eucalcitoninemic after extensive, meticulous, *reoperative* neck dissection under magnification to remove all the tiny lymph nodes. In other patients, computed tomography (CT) and magnetic resonance imaging (MRI) have localized some sites of tumor recurrence, whereas thallium and meta-iodobenzylguanidine scanning have sometimes been helpful. Recently, technetium-labeled sestamibi scanning and positron emission tomography have been successful in some patients.

Cure is most likely in young children who are found by genetic screening to have a mutated *ret* oncogene. One hopes to operate on them when C cell hyperplasia is present and before medullary cancer has started. Patients with MEN-2A syndrome have a better prognosis than do those with sporadic tumor.[43] Patients with MEN-2B syndrome have very aggressive tumors and rarely survive to middle age. Thus in recent years, prophylactic thyroidectomy has been practiced in children by 5 years of age who are found to have MEN-2A to prevent the development of medullary cancer. In children with MEN-2B and with a mutated *ret* oncogene, total thyroidectomy should be done at an earlier age, often by age 2 because this cancer develops at a younger age than MEN-2A does.[47] With these prophylactic operations, cures are expected.

Long-term studies of medullary cancer from the Mayo Clinic group have shown that in patients without initial distant metastatic involvement and with complete resection of their medullary cancer, the 20-

TABLE 110–2. Diseases Included in the MEN Type 2 Syndromes

MEN-2A	MEN-2B
Medullary carcinoma	Medullary carcinoma
Pheochromocytoma	Pheochromocytoma
Hyperparathyroidism	Hyperparathyrodism
	Ganglioneuroma phenotype

MEN, multiple endocrine neoplasia.

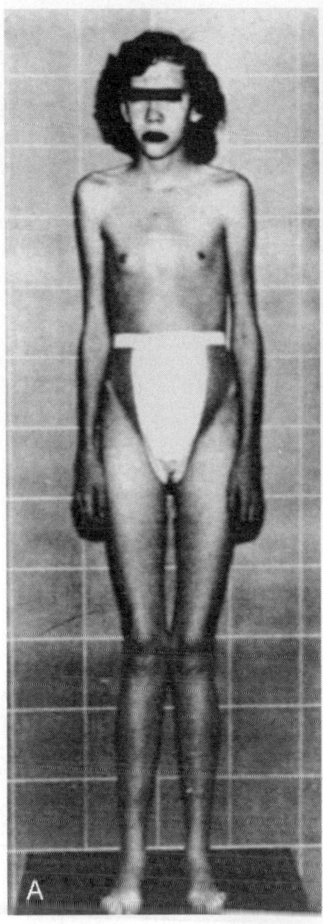

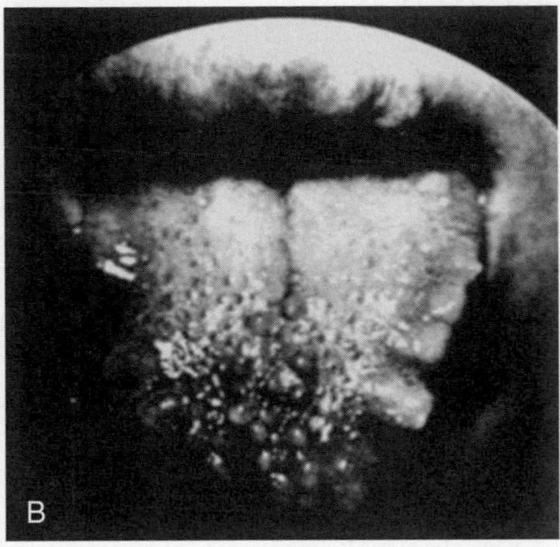

FIGURE 110–14. An 18-year-old girl who demonstrates the appearance typically associated with multiple endocrine neoplasial type 2B (MEN-2B) was found to have bilateral medullary carcinoma of the thyroid gland at surgery. *A*, The Marfan-like body habitus and facial features typically present in patients with MEN-2B are clearly seen. *B*, Multiple neuromas of the tongue and lips are demonstrated. (Courtesy of Glen W. Sizemore.)

year survival rate free of distant metastatic lesions was 81%.[48] Overall 10- and 20-year survival rates were 63% and 44%, respectively. Thus early diagnosis and complete initial resection of tumor are very important. Treatment of pheochromocytoma and hyperparathyroidism is discussed elsewhere.

OPERATIVE TECHNIQUE FOR THYROIDECTOMY

Under general endotracheal anesthesia, the patient is placed in a supine position with the neck extended. A low collar incision is made and carried down through the subcutaneous tissue and platysma muscle (Fig. 110–15). Superior and inferior subplatysmal flaps are developed, and the strap muscles are divided vertically in the midline and retracted laterally.

Lobectomy or Total Thyroidectomy

The thyroid isthmus is usually divided early in the course of the operation. The thyroid lobe is bluntly dissected free from its investing fascia and rotated medially. The middle thyroid vein is ligated. The superior pole of the thyroid is dissected free, and care is taken to identify and preserve the external branch of the superior laryngeal nerve (see Fig. 110–7). The superior pole vessels are ligated adjacent to the thyroid lobe rather than cephalic to it to prevent damage to this nerve. The inferior thyroid artery and recurrent laryngeal nerve are identified. To preserve blood supply to the parathyroid glands, the inferior thyroid artery should not be ligated laterally; rather, its branches should be ligated individually on the capsule of the lobe after they have supplied the parathyroid glands (Fig. 110–16). The parathyroid glands are identified, and an attempt is made to leave each with an adequate blood supply. Any parathyroid gland that appears to be devascularized can be minced and implanted into the sternocleidomastoid muscle after a frozen section biopsy confirms that it is in fact a parathyroid gland. Care is taken to try to identify the recurrent laryngeal nerve along its course if a total lobectomy is to be done. The nerve is gently unroofed from surrounding tissue, with care taken to avoid trauma to it. The nerve is in greatest danger near the junction of the trachea with the larynx, where it is adjacent to the thyroid gland. Once the nerve and parathyroid glands have been identified and preserved, the thyroid lobe can be removed from its tracheal attachments by dividing the ligament of Berry. The contralateral thyroid lobe is removed in a similar manner when total thyroidectomy is performed. A near-total thyroidectomy means that a small amount of thyroid tissue is left on the contralateral side to protect the parathyroid glands and recurrent nerve. Careful hemostasis and visualization of all important anatomic structures are mandatory for success.

When closing, we do not tightly approximate the strap muscles in

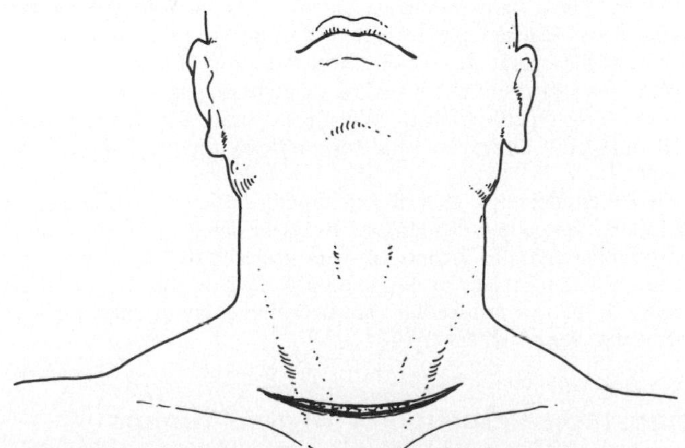

FIGURE 110–15. Incision for thyroidectomy. The neck is extended and a symmetrical, gently curved incision is made 1 to 2 cm above the clavicle.

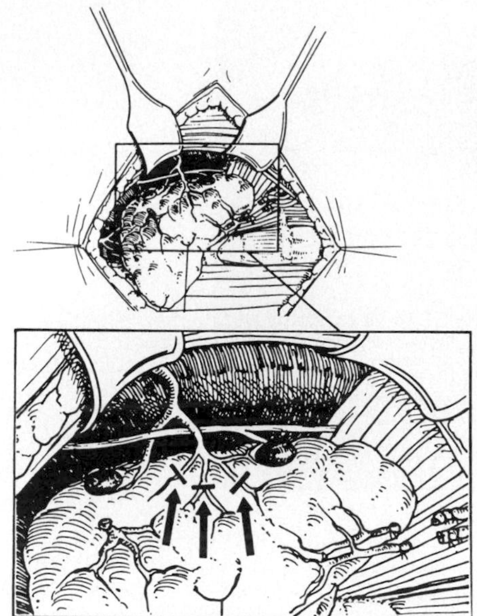

FIGURE 110–16. The thyroid lobe is retracted medially, and by careful blunt dissection, the recurrent laryngeal nerve, the inferior thyroid artery, and the parathyroid glands are identified. The inferior thyroid artery is not ligated laterally as a single trunk. Rather, each small branch is ligated and divided at a point distal to the parathyroid glands *(arrows)* to preserve their blood supply. Then the thyroid lobe can be removed from its tracheal attachments if a lobectomy is to be performed. (From Kaplan EL: Surgery of the thyroid glands. *In* DeGroot LS, Larsen PR, Refetoff S, Stanbury JB (eds): The Thyroid and its Diseases. New York, John Wiley & Sons, p 851, Copyright © 1984. Reprinted by permission of John Wiley & Sons, Inc.)

the midline to allow drainage of blood superficially and thus prevent a hematoma in the closed deep space. Furthermore, we obtain better cosmesis by not approximating the platysmal muscle. Rather, the dermis is approximated by interrupted 4-0 sutures, and the epithelial edges are approximated with a running 5-0 absorbable suture. Sterile paper tapes (Steri-strips) are then applied and left in place for about a week. A small suction catheter is often inserted through a small stab wound and is generally removed within 12 hours.

Subtotal Thyroidectomy

Bilateral subtotal lobectomy is the usual operation for Graves' disease. An alternative operation, which is equally good, is lobectomy on one side and subtotal lobectomy on the other side. Once more, the parathyroid glands and recurrent nerves should be identified and preserved. Great care should be taken to not damage the recurrent laryngeal nerve when cutting across or suturing the thyroid lobe. At the end of the operation several grams of thyroid tissue is usually left in place. The aim is to try to achieve an euthyroid state without a high recurrence of hyperthyroidism. When the operation is done for severe ophthalmopathy, however, near-total or total thyroidectomy is performed.

After thyroidectomy, even if a modified neck dissection is done for carcinoma, the patient can almost always be safely discharged on the first postoperative day. Others are kept longer if the need arises. I do not think that it is safe to discharge a patient on the day of surgery because of the risk of bleeding; however, same-day discharge is being practiced at some centers.[49]

Endoscopic Resection of Thyroid Tumors

Video-assisted thyroidectomy or endoscopic thyroidectomy is being pioneered in several centers.[50–52] Its aim is to minimize the length of incisions in the neck or to hide the incisions by placing them below the clavicle or far lateral in the neck. In the hands of very skilled operators, the recurrent laryngeal nerve and parathyroid glands can be seen and a lobectomy performed. Other groups have performed mainly nodulectomy. This operative method may have merit for small lesions; however, the results and complications must be carefully assessed. Is proper thyroid resection still being performed when this technique is used for thyroid cancer? Will there be a learning curve (as occurs with most new procedures) with increased rates of bleeding, nerve injury, or hypoparathyroidism? Finally, do the "improved cosmetic results" justify the possibility of greater morbidity? Careful assessment of these new procedures seems warranted.

POSTOPERATIVE COMPLICATIONS

Many authors have reported large series of thyroidectomies with no deaths. In other reports, mortality does not differ greatly from that of anesthesia alone. Four major complications are associated with thyroid surgery: thyroid storm, wound hemorrhage, recurrent laryngeal nerve injury, and hypoparathyroidism.

Thyroid Storm

Thyroid storm reflects an exacerbation of a thyrotoxic state and is seen most often in Graves' disease, but it can occur less commonly in patients with toxic adenoma or toxic multinodular goiter. Clinical manifestations and management of thyroid storm are discussed elsewhere in this text.

Wound Hemorrhage

Wound hemorrhage with hematoma is an uncommon complication reported in 0.3% to 1.0% of patients in most large series. However, it is a well-recognized and potentially lethal complication. A small hematoma deep to the strap muscles can compress the trachea and cause respiratory distress. A small suction drain placed in the wound is not usually adequate for decompression if bleeding occurs from an arterial vessel. Swelling of the neck and bulging of the wound can be quickly followed by respiratory impairment.

Wound hemorrhage is an emergency situation. Treatment consists of immediately opening the wound and evacuating the clot, even at the bedside. Pressure should be applied with a sterile sponge and the patient returned to the operating room. Later, the bleeding vessel can be ligated in a careful and more leisurely manner under optimal conditions with good lighting in the operating room. The urgency of treating this condition as soon as it occurs cannot be overemphasized.

Injury to the Recurrent Laryngeal Nerve

Injuries to the recurrent laryngeal nerve occur in 1% to 2% of thyroid operations when performed by experienced neck surgeons and at a higher prevalence when thyroidectomy is done by less experienced surgeons. They occur more frequently when thyroidectomy is done for malignant disease. Nerve injuries can be unilateral or bilateral and temporary or permanent, and they can be deliberate or accidental. Loss of function can be caused by transection, ligation, traction, or handling of the nerve. Tumor invasion can also involve the nerve. Occasionally, vocal cord impairment occurs as a result of pressure from the balloon of an endotracheal tube. In *unilateral* recurrent nerve injuries, the voice becomes husky because the vocal cords do not approximate one another. Usually, vocal cord function returns within several months but certainly within 6 to 9 months if it is to return. If no function returns by that time, the voice can be improved by operative means. The choice is insertion of a piece of Silastic to move the paralyzed cord to the midline.

Bilateral recurrent laryngeal nerve damage is much more serious because both vocal cords may assume a median or paramedian position and cause airway obstruction and difficulty with respiratory toilet.

Most often, tracheostomy is required. In the authors' experience, permanent injuries to the recurrent laryngeal nerve are best avoided by identifying and carefully tracing the path of the recurrent nerve. Accidental transection occurs most often at the level of the upper two tracheal rings, where the nerve closely approximates the thyroid lobe in the area of Berry's ligament. If recognized, the transected nerve should be reapproximated by microsurgical techniques. A number of procedures to reinnervate the laryngeal muscles have been attempted with only limited success.[53]

Injury to the *external branch of the superior laryngeal nerve* may occur when the upper pole vessels are divided (see Fig. 110–7) if the nerve is not visualized.[8] This injury results in an inability to forcefully project one's voice or to sing high notes. Often, this disability improves during the first 3 months after surgery.

Hypoparathyroidism

The incidence of hypoparathyroidism has been reported to be as high as 20% when total thyroidectomy and radical neck dissection are performed and as low as 0.9% for subtotal thyroidectomy. Other excellent neck surgeons have reported a lower incidence of permanent hypoparathyroidism.[54] Postoperative hypoparathyroidism is rarely the result of inadvertent removal of all of the parathyroid glands but, more commonly, is due to disruption of their delicate blood supply. Devascularization can be minimized during thyroid lobectomy by carefully ligating the branches of the inferior thyroid artery on the thyroid capsule distal to their supply of the parathyroid glands (see Fig. 110–16) and by treating the parathyroids with great care. If a parathyroid gland is recognized to be nonviable during surgery, after identification by frozen section it can be autotransplanted at that time. The gland is minced into 1- to 2-mm cubes and placed into pockets in the sternocleidomastoid muscle.

Postoperative hypoparathyroidism results in hypocalcemia and hyperphosphatemia and is manifested by circumoral numbness, tingling of the fingers and toes, and intense anxiety occurring soon after surgery. Chvostek's sign appears early, and carpopedal spasm can occur. Symptoms develop in most patients when the serum calcium level is less than 7.5 to 8 mg/dL.

Routinely we measure the serum calcium level every 12 hours while the patient is in the hospital. Most patients are able to leave the hospital on the day after surgery if they are asymptomatic and their serum calcium level is 7.8 mg/dL or above. Oral calcium pills are used liberally. Patients with symptomatic hypocalcemia are treated in the hospital with 1 g (10 mL) of 10% calcium gluconate infused intravenously over a period of several minutes, and then 2 to 5 g of this calcium solution should be placed in each 500-mL intravenous bottle to run continuously during each 8-hour period. Oral calcium, usually as calcium carbonate (3 to 4 g in divided doses), should be started. With this treatment regimen most patients become asymptomatic. The intravenous therapy is stopped as soon as possible and the patient is sent home and told to take oral calcium pills. This condition is referred to as *transient* hypocalcemia or transient hypoparathyroidism.

Management of more persistent severe hypocalcemia requires the addition of a vitamin D preparation to facilitate the absorption of oral calcium. We prefer the use of 1,25-dihydroxyvitamin D (Rocaltrol) because it is the active metabolite of vitamin D and has a more rapid action. Rocaltrol (0.5 μg) with oral calcium carbonate therapy is given four times daily for the first several days. Then this priming dose of vitamin D is reduced. The usual maintenance dose for most patients with permanent hypoparathyroidism is Rocaltrol, 0.25–0.5 μg daily, along with calcium carbonate, 500 mg Ca^{2+} once or twice daily, although some patients require larger doses. Serum calcium levels must be monitored carefully after discharge, and the dosage of the medications is adjusted promptly to prevent hypercalcemia as well as hypocalcemia. Finally, the serum parathyroid hormone level should be analyzed periodically to determine whether *permanent* hypoparathyroidism is truly present because we and others have seen cases of postoperative tetany, perhaps caused by "bone hunger," that later resolved completely. In such cases, circulating parathyroid hormone is normal and all therapy could be stopped. Remember that in bone hunger, both the serum calcium and phosphorus values are low, whereas in hypoparathyroidism, the serum calcium value is low but the phosphorus level is elevated.

DEVELOPMENTAL ABNORMALITIES OF THE THYROID

To understand the different thyroid anomalies, it is important to briefly review normal development of this gland. The thyroid is embryologically an offshoot of the primitive alimentary tract, from which it later becomes separated[55–58] (Figs. 110–17 and 110–18). During the third to fourth week in utero, a median anlage of epithelium arises from the pharyngeal floor in the region of the foramen cecum of the tongue, that is, at the junction of the anterior two-thirds and the posterior third of the tongue. The main body of the thyroid, referred to as the median lobe or median thyroid component, follows the descent of the heart and great vessels and moves caudally into the neck from this origin. It divides into an isthmus and two lobes, and by 7 weeks it forms a "shield" over the front of the trachea and thyroid cartilage. It is joined by a pair of lateral thyroid lobes originating from the fourth and fifth branchial pouches[3, 4] (Fig. 110–19). From these lateral thyroid components, now frequently called the ultimobranchial bodies, C cells (parafollicular cells) enter the thyroid lobes. C cells contain and secrete calcitonin and are the cells that give rise to medullary carcinoma of the thyroid gland. Williams and associates have described cystic structures in the neck near the upper parathyroid glands in cases in which thyroid tissue was totally lingual in location.[59] These cysts contained both cells staining for calcitonin and others staining for thyroglobulin. This study, they believe, offers evidence that the ultimobranchial body contributes both C cells and follicular cells to the thyroid gland of humans.

As the gland moves downward, it leaves behind a trace of epithelial cells known as the thyroglossal tract. From this structure both thyroglossal duct cysts and the pyramidal lobe of the thyroid develop. The eventual mature thyroid gland may take on many different configurations depending on the embryologic development of the thyroid and its descent (Fig. 110–20).

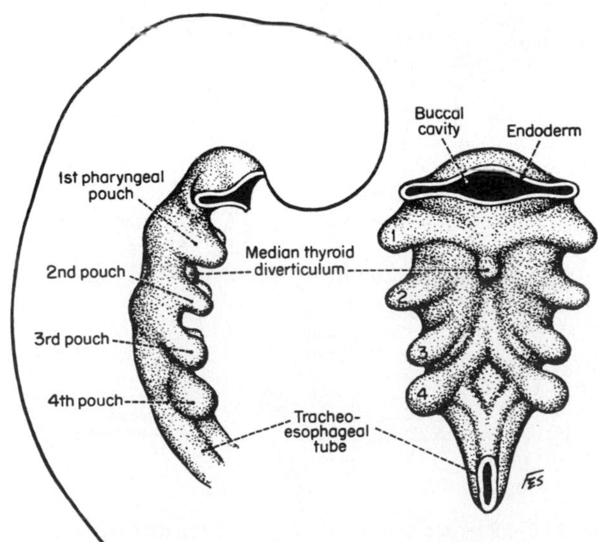

FIGURE 110–17. Early embryologic development of the pharyngeal anlage in a 4-mm embryo. Note the beginning of thyroid development in the median thyroid diverticulum. (From Sedgwick CE, Cady B: Surgery of the Thyroid and Parathyroid Glands, ed 2. Philadelphia, WB Saunders, 1980, p 7; adapted from Weller GL: Development of the thyroid, parathyroid and thymus glands in man. Contrib Embryol Carnegie Inst Wash 24:93–142, 1933.)

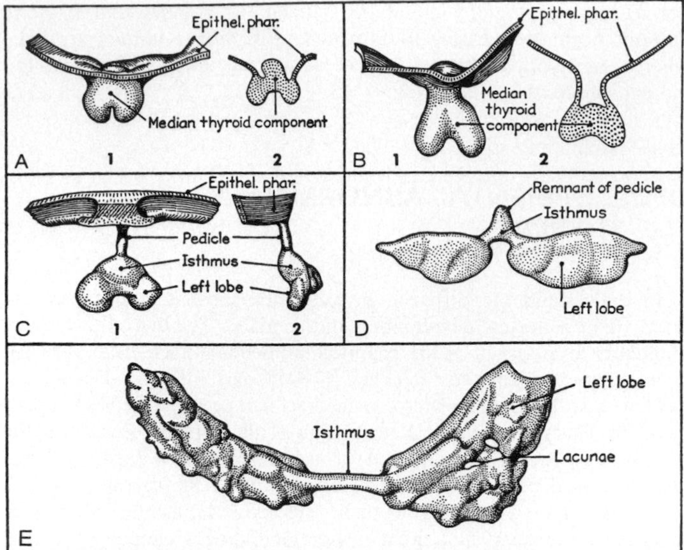

FIGURE 110–18. Stages in the development of the thyroid gland. *A, 1,* Thyroid primordium and pharyngeal epithelium of a 4.5-mm human embryo; *2,* section through the same structure showing a raised central portion. *B, 1,* Thyroid primordium of a 6.5-mm embryo; *2,* section through the same structure. *C, 1,* Thyroid primordium of an 8.2-mm embryo beginning to descend; *2,* lateral view of the same structure. *D,* Thyroid primordium of an 11-mm embryo. The connection with the pharynx is broken, and the lobes are beginning to grow laterad. *E,* Thyroid gland of a 13.5-mm embryo. The lobes are thin sheets curving around the carotid arteries. Several lacunae, which are not to be confused with follicles, are present in the sheets. (From Weller GL: Development of the thyroid, parathyroid and thymus glands in man. Contrib Embryol Carnegie Inst Wash 24:93–142, 1933.)

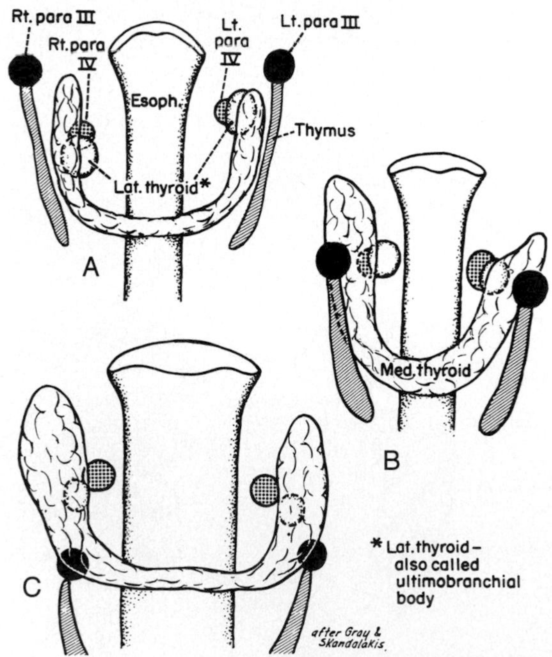

FIGURE 110–19. *A* and *B,* Shifts in location of the thyroid, parafollicular, and parathyroid tissues. *C* approximates the adult location. Note that what has been called the lateral thyroid is now commonly referred to as the ultimobranchial body, which contains both C cells and follicular elements. (From Sedgwick CE, Cady B: Surgery of the Thyroid and Parathyroid Gland, ed 2. Philadelphia, WB Saunders, 1980; adapted from Norris EH: Parathyroid glands and lateral thyroid in man: Their morphogenesis, histogenesis, topographic anatomy and prenatal growth. Contrib Embryol Carnegie Inst Wash 26:247–294, 1937.)

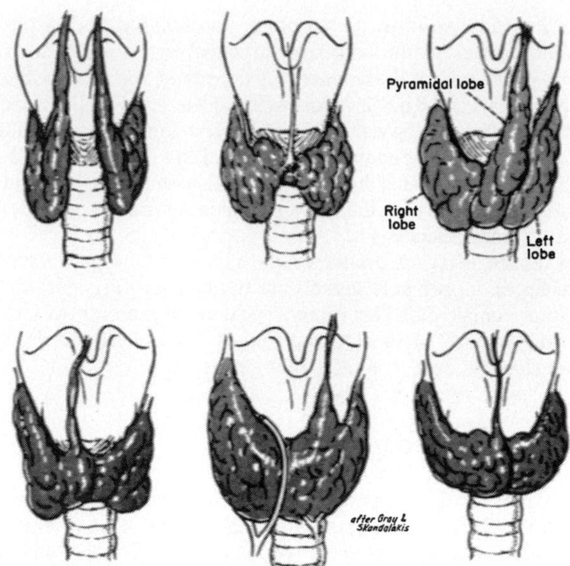

FIGURE 110–20. Variations of normal adult thyroid anatomy resulting from embryologic descent and division of the thyroid gland. (From Sedgwick CE, Cady B: Surgery of the Thyroid and Parathyroid Glands, ed 2. Philadelphia, WB Saunders, 1980; adapted from Gray SW, Skandalakis JE: Embryology for Surgeons. Philadelphia, WB Saunders, 1972.)

Thyroid Abnormalities

The median thyroid anlage may on rare occasion fail to develop. The resultant *athyrosis*, or absence of the thyroid gland, is associated with cretinism, or it may differentiate in locations other than the isthmus and lateral lobes. The most common developmental abnormality, if looked on as such, is the *pyramidal lobe*, which has been reported to be present in as many as 80% of patients in whom the gland was surgically exposed. Usually the pyramidal lobe is small; however, in Graves' disease or lymphocytic thyroiditis, it is often enlarged and is frequently clinically palpable. The pyramidal lobe generally lies in the midline but can arise from either lobe. Origin from the left lobe is more common than origin from the right lobe.[60]

Thyroid Hemiagenesis

More than 100 cases have been reported in which only one lobe of the thyroid is present.[61] The left lobe is absent in 80% of cases. Often the thyroid lobe that is present is enlarged, and both hyperthyroidism and hypothyroidism have been reported at times. Females are affected three times as often as males. Both benign and malignant nodules have been reported in this condition.[62]

Other variations involving the median thyroid anlage represent an arrest in the usual descent of part or all of the thyroid-forming material along the normal pathway. *Ectopic thyroid development* can result in a lingual thyroid or in thyroid tissue in a suprahyoid, infrahyoid, or intratracheal location. Persistence of the thyroglossal duct as a sinus tract or cyst called a *thyroglossal duct cyst* is the most common of the clinically important anomalies of thyroid development. Finally, the entire gland or part of it may descend more caudally, which results in thyroid tissue located in the superior mediastinum behind the sternum, adjacent to the aortic arch or between the aorta and pulmonary trunk, within the upper portion of the pericardium, and even within the interventricular septum of the heart. Most *intrathoracic goiters*, however, are not true anomalies, but rather extensions of pathologic elements of a normally situated gland into the anterior or posterior mediastinum. Each of these abnormalities is discussed in greater depth.

Ectopic Thyroid

Lingual Thyroid

A lingual thyroid is relatively rare and estimated to occur in 1 in 3000 cases of thyroid disease. However, it represents the most common location for functioning ectopic thyroid tissue. Lingual thyroid tissue is associated with an absence of the normal cervical thyroid in 70% of cases. It occurs much more commonly in women than in men.

The diagnosis is usually made by the discovery of an incidental mass on the back of the tongue in an asymptomatic patient (Fig. 110–21). The mass may enlarge and cause dysphagia, dysphonia, dyspnea, or a sensation of choking.[63] Hypothyroidism is frequently present and may cause the mass to enlarge and become symptomatic, but hyperthyroidism is very unusual. In women, symptomatic lingual thyroid glands develop during puberty or early adulthood in most cases. Buckman, in his review of 140 cases of symptomatic lingual thyroids in females, reported that 30% occurred in puberty, 55% between the ages of 18 and 40 years, 10% at menopause, and 5% in old age.[64] He attributed this distribution to hormonal disturbances, which are more apparent in female subjects during puberty and may be precipitated by pregnancy. The incidence of malignancy in lingual thyroid glands is low.[65] The diagnosis of a lingual thyroid should be suspected when a mass is detected in the region of the foramen cecum of the tongue and is definitively established by radioisotope scanning (see Fig. 110–21).

The usual treatment of this condition is thyroid hormone therapy to suppress the lingual thyroid and reduce its size. Only rarely is surgical excision necessary. Indications for extirpation are failure of suppressive therapy to reduce the size, ulceration, hemorrhage, or suspicion of malignancy.[66] Autotransplantation of thyroid tissue has been tried on rare occasion when no other thyroid tissue is present and has apparently been successful. Recently, a lingual thyroid was reported in two natural brothers, which suggests that this condition may be inherited.[67]

Suprahyoid and Infrahyoid Thyroid

In these cases thyroid tissue is present in a midline position above or below the hyoid bone. Hypothyroidism with elevation of thyrotropin (TSH) secretion is commonly present because of the absence of a normal thyroid gland in most instances. An enlarging mass commonly occurs during infancy, childhood, or later life. Often this mass is mistaken for a thyroglossal duct cyst, for it is usually located in the same anatomic position.[68] If it is removed, all thyroid tissue may be ablated, a consequence that has definite physiologic as well as possible medicolegal implications. To prevent total thyroid ablation, many recommend that a thyroid scan be performed in all cases of thyroglossal duct cyst before its removal to be certain that a normal thyroid gland is present. Furthermore, before removing what appears to be a thyroglossal duct cyst, a prudent surgeon should be certain that no solid areas are present. If any doubt exists, the normal thyroid gland should be explored and palpated. Finally, if ectopic thyroid tissue rather than a thyroglossal duct cyst is encountered at surgery, its blood supply should be preserved, the ectopic gland divided vertically, and each half translocated laterally, deep to the strap muscles, where it is no longer manifested as a mass. If normal thyroid tissue is demonstrated to be present elsewhere, it may be better to remove the ectopic tissue rather than transplant it because carcinoma arising from these developmental abnormalities, although rare, has been reported.

Thyroglossal Duct Cysts

Both cysts and fistulas can develop along the course of the thyroglossal duct[69] (Fig. 110–22). These cysts are the most common anomaly in thyroid development seen in clinical practice.[70] Normally the thyroglossal duct becomes obliterated early in embryonic life, but occasionally it persists as a cyst. Such lesions occur equally in males and females. They are seen at birth in about 25% of cases, most appear in early childhood, and the final third become apparent only after age 30.[71] Cysts usually appear in the midline or just off the midline between the isthmus of the thyroid and the hyoid bone. They frequently become repeatedly infected and may rupture spontaneously. When this complication occurs, a sinus tract or fistula persists. Removal of a thyroglossal cyst or fistula requires excision of the central part of the hyoid bone and dissection of the thyroglossal tract to the base of the tongue if recurrence is to be minimized (the Sistrunk procedure). This procedure is necessary because the thyroglossal duct is intimately associated with the central part of the hyoid bone (Fig. 110–23). Recurrent cysts are very common if this operative procedure is not followed.

At least 115 cases of thyroid carcinoma have been reported to originate from the thyroglossal duct.[70] Not infrequently, an association is noted with low-dose external irradiation of the head and neck in infancy or childhood in such cases. Almost all carcinomas have been papillary, and their prognosis is excellent. If a carcinoma is recognized, at the time of surgery the thyroid gland should be inspected for evidence of other tumor nodules, and the lateral lymph nodes should be sampled. Our practice and that of many others is to perform near-total or total thyroidectomy with appropriate nodal resection when a thyroglossal duct carcinoma is found and resected. In one series of 35 patients with papillary carcinoma arising in a thyroglossal duct cyst, the thyroid gland of 4 patients (11.4%) also contained papillary cancer.[70]

In addition to papillary cancer, about 5% of all carcinomas arising from a thyroglossal duct cyst are squamous; rare cases of Hürthle cell and anaplastic cancer have also been reported. Finally, three families have been reported in which a total of 11 members had a thyroglossal duct cyst.[72]

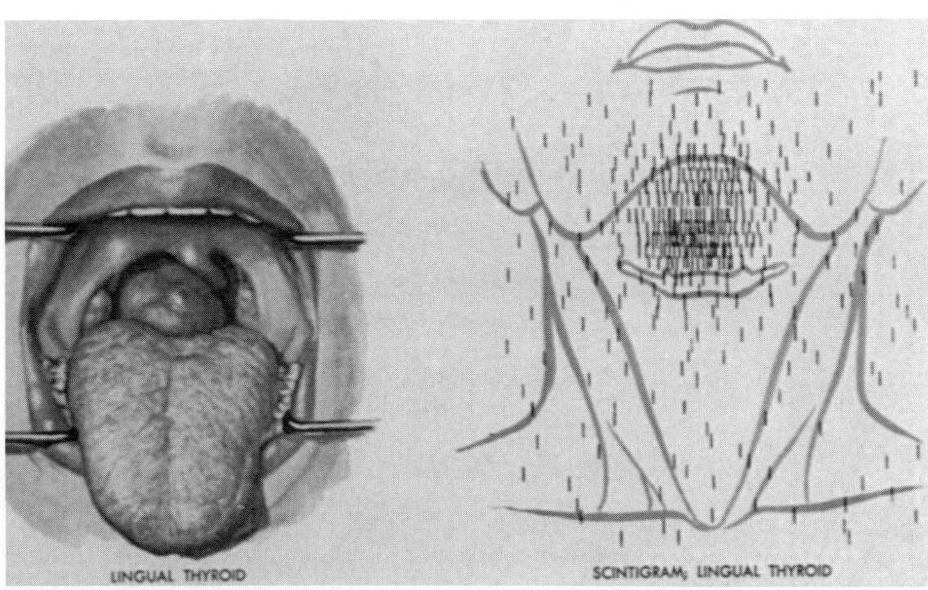

FIGURE 110–21. *Left,* The appearance of a large lingual thyroid. *Right,* A radioiodine scan demonstrating all activity to be above the hyoid bone, with no evidence of the presence of normally placed thyroid issue. (From Netter RA: Endocrine system and selected metabolic diseases. *In* Ciba Collection of Medical Illustrations. Summit, NJ, Ciba-Geigy, 1974, p 45.)

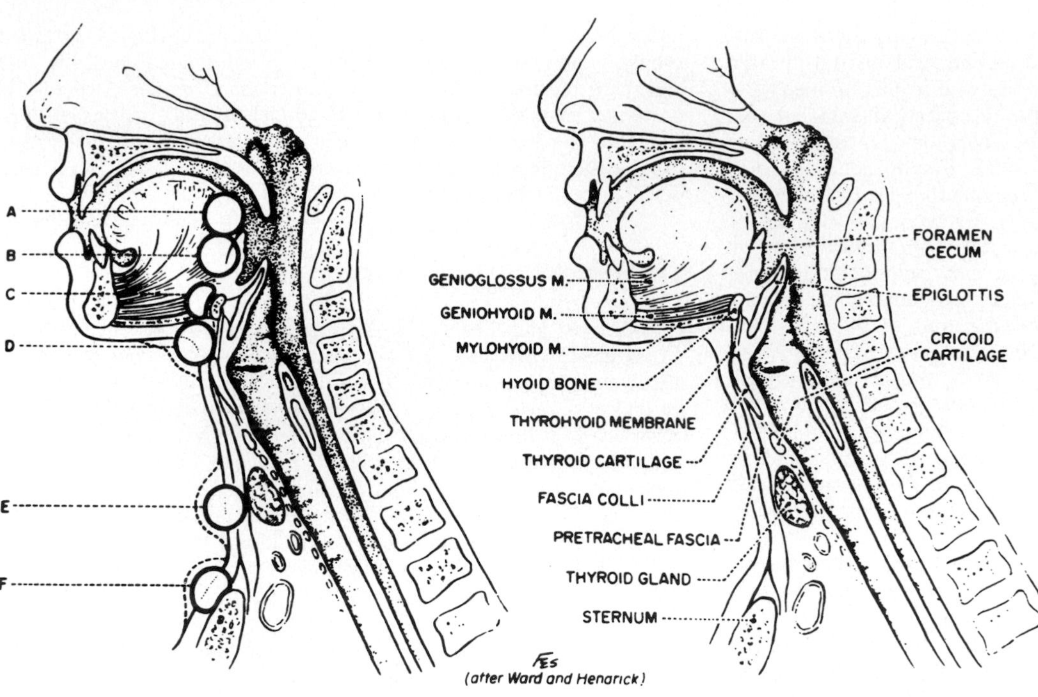

FIGURE 110–22. Location of thyroglossal cysts. A, In front of the foramen cecum; B, at the foramen cecum; C, suprahyoid; D, infrahyoid; E, area of the thyroid gland; F, suprasternal. (From Sedgwick CE, Cady B: Surgery of the Thyroid and Parathyroid Glands, ed 2. Philadelphia, WB Saunders, 1980.)

Lateral Aberrant Thyroid

Small amounts of histologically normal thyroid tissue are occasionally found separate from the thyroid. If these tissue elements are near the thyroid, not in lymph nodes, and entirely normal histologically, it is possible that they represent developmental abnormalities. True lateral aberrant thyroid tissue or embryonic rests of thyroid tissue in the lymph nodes of the lateral neck region are very rare. Most agree that the overwhelming number of cases of what in the past was called "lateral aberrant thyroid" actually represented well-differentiated, metastatic thyroid cancer within cervical lymph nodes or replacing them rather than an embryonic rest. In such cases, we favor near-total or total thyroidectomy with a modified radical neck dissection on the side of the lymph node, probably followed by radioiodine therapy.

Several lateral thyroid masses have been reported that are said to be benign adenomas in lateral ectopic sites.[73, 74] The authors of these studies suggest that they may develop ectopically because of failure of fusion of the lateral thyroid component with the median thyroid. However, before accepting this explanation, it is important to be certain that each of these lesions does not represent a well-differentiated metastasis that has totally replaced a lymph node and in which the primary thyroid carcinoma is small or even microscopic and was not recognized.

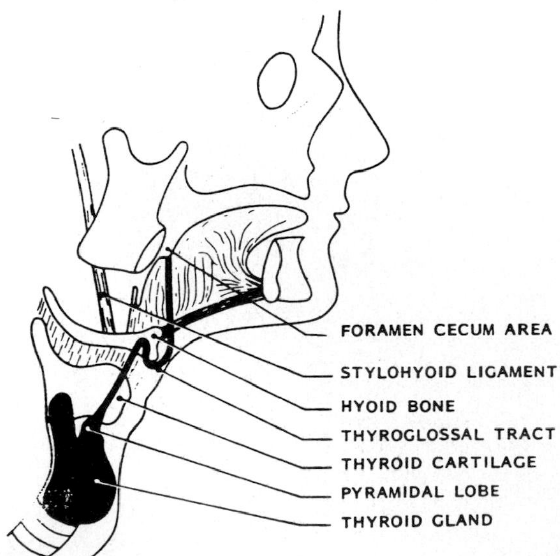

FIGURE 110–23. Diagram of the course of the thyroglossal tract. Note its proximity to the hyoid bone. (From Allard RHB: The thyroglossal cyst. Head Neck Surg 5:134–146, 1982.)

Substernal Goiters

Developmental abnormalities may lead to the finding of thyroid tissue in the mediastinum, rarely even within the tracheal or esophageal wall. However, most substernal goiters undoubtedly originate in the neck and then "fall" or are "swallowed" into the mediastinum and are not embryologically determined at all.

Intrathoracic goiters have been reported to occur in 0.1% to 21% of patients in whom thyroidectomies were performed. This large variability is undoubtedly due partly to a difference in classification among the authors but may also be due to the incidence of endemic goiter. More recent series report an incidence of 2% or less.[75]

Many substernal goiters are found on routine chest radiography in patients who are completely asymptomatic. Other patients may have dyspnea or dysphagia from tracheal or esophageal compression or displacement. Superior vena caval obstruction can occasionally occur with edema and cyanosis of the face,[76] and venous engorgement of the arms and face is present (Fig. 110–24). Most individuals with substernal goiters are euthyroid or hypothyroid; however, hyperthyroidism is possible. Although the goiters of Graves' disease are rarely intrathoracic, single or multiple "hot" nodules may occur within an intrathoracic goiter and result in hyperthyroidism as part of a toxic nodular goiter.

Intrathoracic goiters are usually found in the anterior mediastinum and less commonly in the posterior mediastinum. In either instance the diagnosis is suggested if a goiter can be palpated in the neck and appears to continue below the sternum. Rarely, however, no thyroid enlargement in the cervical area is present, and instead of being in continuity, the intrathoracic component may be attached to the cervical thyroid only by a narrow bridge of thyroid or fibrous tissue. The diagnosis of an intrathoracic thyroid mass can be made with certainty by the use of a thyroid isotope scan; however, CT or MRI may also be helpful.

Regarding therapy, we generally agree with the recommendation made by Lahey and Swinton more than 50 years ago that goiters that

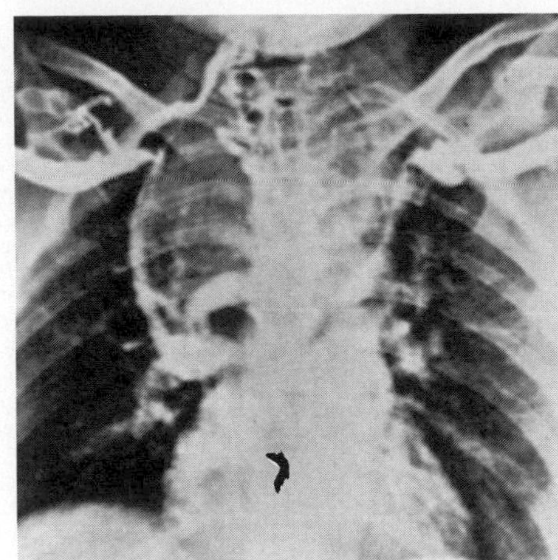

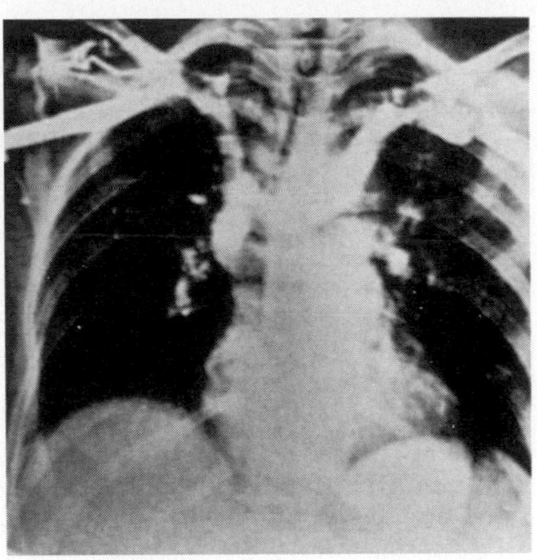

FIGURE 110–24. Large substernal goiter resulting in superior vena caval syndrome. *Left,* A venogram demonstrated complete obstruction of the superior vena cava, displacement of the innominate veins, and marked collateral circulation. *Right,* Three weeks after thyroidectomy, patency of the vena cava was restored. Some displacement of the innominate veins remained at that time. (From Lesavoy MA, Norberg HP, Kaplan EL: Substernal goiter with superior vena caval obstruction. Surgery 77:325–329, 1975.)

are definitely intrathoracic should usually be removed if the patient is a good operative risk.[77] Because of the cone-shaped anatomy of the upper thoracic outlet, once part of a thyroid goiter has passed into the superior mediastinum, it can increase its size only by descending further into the chest. Thus delay in surgical management may lead to increased size of the lesion, a greater degree of symptoms, and perhaps a more difficult or hazardous operative procedure.

Substernal goiters should be operated on initially through a cervical incision because the blood supply to the substernal thyroid almost always originates in the neck and can be readily controlled in this area. Only rarely does an intrathoracic goiter receive its blood supply from mediastinal vessels; however, such a finding favors a developmental cause. Thus in most instances, good hemostasis can be obtained by control of the superior and inferior thyroid arteries in the neck. The thyroid gland is carefully dissected along its capsule by blunt dissection into the superior mediastinum. While gentle traction is exerted from above, the mass is elevated by the surgeon's fingers or blunt, curved clamps (Fig. 110–25). Frequently, these maneuvers suffice to permit extraction of a mass from the mediastinum and into the neck area. Any fluid-filled cysts may be aspirated to reduce the size of the mass and permit its egress through the thoracic outlet. Piecemeal morcellation of the thyroid gland should not be practiced, for this occasionally has led to severe bleeding. Furthermore, several substernal goiters have been found to contain carcinoma, and this technique violates all principles of cancer surgery.

With the use of this method, the great majority of substernal thyroid glands can be removed transcervically. If the thyroid gland cannot be easily extracted from the mediastinum, however, a partial or complete sternotomy should be performed. This procedure affords direct control of any mediastinal vessels and permits resection of the thyroid gland to be carried out safely.

As in all thyroid surgery, the recurrent laryngeal nerves must be preserved and treated with care. The parathyroid glands should be identified and preserved, and the inferior thyroid artery's branches should be ligated close to the thyroid capsule to prevent ischemia of the parathyroid glands, which might result in hypoparathyroidism.

Struma Ovarii

Ectopic development of thyroid tissue far from the neck area can also lead to difficulties in rare instances. Dermoid cysts or teratomas, which are uncommon ovarian germ cell tumors, occur in female subjects of all age groups. About 3% can be classified as an *ovarian struma*, for they contain functionally significant thyroid tissue or thyroid tissue occupying more than 50% of the volume of the tumor. Many more such tumors contain small amounts of thyroid tissue. Some strumae ovarii are associated with carcinoid-appearing tissue. These strumal-carcinoid tumors secrete or contain thyroid hormones as well as somatostatin, chromogranin, serotonin, glucagon, insulin, gastrin, or calcitonin.[78] Some are associated with carcinoid syndromes.

Struma ovarii is sometimes manifested as an abdominal mass lesion, often with peritoneal or pleural effusion, which may be bloody. Most of these lesions synthesize and iodinate thyroglobulin poorly, and thus despite growth of the mass, thyrotoxicosis does not develop. However, perhaps one-fourth to one-third of ovarian strumae are associated with thyrotoxicosis.[79, 80] Many of these lesions may be contributing to autoimmune hyperthyroidism in response to a common stimulator such as long-acting thyroid stimulator or thyroid-stimulating immunoglobulins. In other instances, the struma alone is clearly responsible for the thyrotoxicity. An elevated free thyroxine index, a suppressed TSH value, and uptake of radioiodine in a mass in the pelvis are the obvious prerequisites for making the diagnosis.[81] Often in ovarian struma, symptoms and findings of thyrotoxicosis are present in patients who

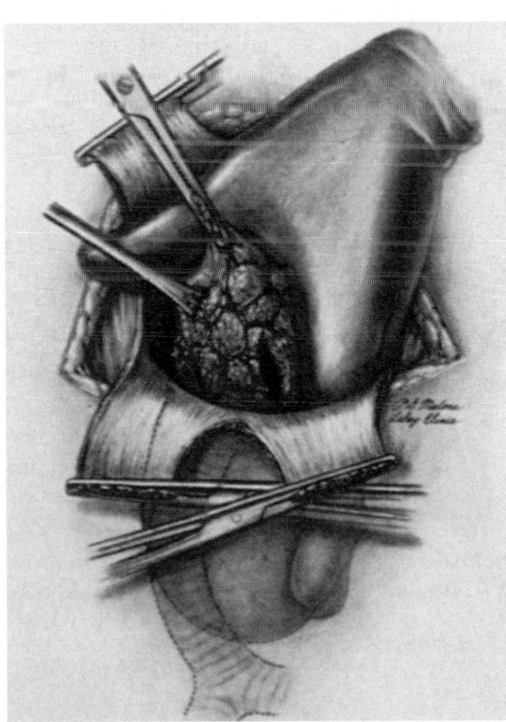

FIGURE 110–25. Finger dissection of a substernal goiter. Note that the index finger is inserted into the mediastinum outside the thyroid capsule and is swept around until the gland is freed from the pleura and other tissue in the mediastinum. Occasionally, despite traction a substernal goiter does not pass out through the superior thoracic outlet because of its size. In such cases, it may be necessary to evacuate some of the colloid material from within the goiter. Then with gentle upward traction on the capsule the mass can be elevated into the neck wound and resected. (From Sedgwick CE, Cady B: Surgery of the Thyroid and Parathyroid Glands, ed 2. Philadelphia, WB Saunders, 1980.)

have *low uptake of radioiodine in their thyroid gland.* Thus a "high index of suspicion" is most important. Usually, operative resection of an ovarian tumor is indicated. After surgery, transient postoperative hypothyroidism and "thyroid storm" have occasionally been reported.

Benign thyroid adenomas in strumae are common, and about 5% manifest evidence of carcinoma.[82] Usually these lesions are resectable, but radiation therapy and/or ^{131}I ablation has been advised after resection of the tumors to avoid the tendency for late recurrence or metastatic disease, which has sometimes been fatal. Metastatic disease occurs in about 5% of these malignant tumors. It is best treated with ^{131}I therapy, and TSH suppression should be given as for thyroid cancer originating in the usual location.

Struma Cordis

Functioning, apparently "normal" intracardiac thyroid tissue has been reported a few times and has been visualized by radioiodine imaging.[83] The clinical finding is usually a right ventricular mass, and the diagnosis has typically been made after operative removal.

ACKNOWLEDGMENT

Supported in part by a generous grant from the Nathan and Frances Goldblatt Society for Cancer Research. We thank Kim Maddy for her assistance in preparation of this manuscript.

REFERENCES

1. Halsted WS: The operative story of goitre. Johns Hopkins Hosp Rep 19:71, 1920.
2. Thompson NW: The history of hyperparathyroidism. Acta Chir Scand 156:5–21, 1990.
3. Kocher T: Uber Kropfextirpation und ihre Folgen. Arch Klin Chirurgie 29:254, 1883.
4. Kaplan EL, Kadowaki MH, Schark C: Routine exposure of the recurrent laryngeal nerve is important during thyroidectomy. *In* Simmons RL, Udekwu AO (eds): Debates in Clinical Surgery, vol 1. Chicago, Year Book, 1990, pp 191–206.
5. Henry JF, Audriffe J, Denizot A, et al: The non-recurrent inferior laryngeal nerve: Review of 33 cases including 2 on the left side. Surgery 104:977–984, 1988.
6. Thompson NW, Demers M: Exposure is not necessary to avoid the recurrent laryngeal nerve during thyroid operations. *In* Simmons RL, Udekwu AO (eds): Debates in Clinical Surgery, vol 1. Chicago, Year Book, 1990, pp 207–219.
7. Moosman DA, DeWeese JS: The external laryngeal nerve as related to thyroidectomy. Surg Gynecol Obstet 127:1011, 1968.
8. Lennquist S, Cahlin C, Smeds S: The superior laryngeal nerve in thyroid surgery. Surgery 102:999, 1987.
9. Kaplan EL, Sugimoto J, Yang H, Fredland A: Postoperative hypoparathyroidism: Diagnosis and management. *In* Kaplan EL (ed): Surgery of the Thyroid and Parathyroid Glands. New York, Churchill Livingstone, 1983, pp 262–274.
10. Gilmour JR: The embryology of the parathyroid glands, the thymus and certain associated rudiments. J Pathol 45:507, 1937.
11. Taylor S: Surgery of the thyroid gland. *In* DeGroot LJ, Stanbury JB: The Thyroid and Its Diseases, ed 4. New York, John Wiley & Sons, 1975, pp 776–779.
12. Ezzat S, Sarti DA, Cain DR, Braunstein GD: Thyroid incidentalomas. Prevalence by palpation and ultrasonography. Arch Intern Med 154:1838–1840, 1994.
13. DeGroot LJ: Clinical features and management of radiation-associated thyroid carcinoma. *In* Kaplan EL (ed): Surgery of the Thyroid and Parathyroid Glands. Edinburgh, Churchill Livingstone, 1983, p 940.
14. Kaplan EL: An operative approach to the irradiated thyroid gland with possible carcinoma: Criteria technique and results. *In* DeGroot LJ, Frohman LA, Kaplan EL, Refetoff S (eds): Radiation Associated Carcinoma of the Thyroid. New York, Grune & Stratton, 1977, p 371.
15. Naunheim KS, Kaplan EL, Straus FH II, et al: High dose external radiation to the neck and subsequent thyroid carcinoma. *In* Kaplan EL (ed): Surgery of the Thyroid and Parathyroid Glands. New York, Churchill Livingstone, 1983, pp 51–62.
16. Shafford EA, Kingston JE, Healy JC, et al: Thyroid nodular disease after radiotherapy to the neck for childhood Hodgkin's disease. Br J Cancer 80:808–814, 1999.
17. Backdahl M, Wallin G, Lowhagen T, et al: Fine needle biopsy cytology and DNA analysis. Surg Clin North Am 67:197, 1987.
18. Grant CS, van Heerden JA, Goellner JR: New diagnostic techniques in endocrine surgery. Probl Gen Surg 1:141–153, 1984.
19. Becker C: Hypothyroidism and atherosclerotic heart disease: Pathogenesis, medical management, and the role of coronary artery bypass surgery. Endocr Rev 6:432, 1985.
20. Klementschitsch P, Shen K-L, Kaplan EL: Reemergence of thyroidectomy as treatment for Graves' disease. Surg Clin North Am 59:35, 1979.
21. Lennquist S, Jortso E, Anderberg B, Smeds S: Beta-blockers compared with antithyroid drugs as preoperative treatment of hyperthyroidism: Drug tolerance, complications and postoperative thyroid function. Surgery 98:1141, 1985.
22. Sridama V, Reilly M, Kaplan EL, et al: Long term follow up study of compensated low dose ^{131}I therapy for Graves' disease. N Engl J Med 311:426, 1984.
23. Clark OH: Total thyroidectomy: The treatment of choice for patients with differentiated thyroid cancer. Ann Surg 196:361–370, 1982.
24. Attie JN: Modified neck dissection in treatment of thyroid cancer: A safe procedure. Eur J Cancer Clin Oncol 2:315–324, 1988.
25. Beierwaltes WH: Treatment of metastatic thyroid cancer with radioiodine and external radiation therapy. *In* Kaplan EL (ed): Surgery of the Thyroid and Parathyroid Glands, Clinical Surgery International, vol 4. Edinburgh, Churchill Livingstone, 1983, p 103.
26. Hay ID, Grant CS, Taylor WF, et al: Ipsilateral lobectomy versus bilateral lobar resection in papillary thyroid carcinoma: A retrospective analysis of surgical outcome using a novel prognostic scoring system. Surgery 102:1088, 1988.
27. Cady B, Rossi R: An expanded view of risk-group definition in differentiated thyroid carcinoma. Surgery 104:947, 1988.
28. Hay ID, Bergstralh EJ, Goellner JR, et al: Predicting outcome in papillary thyroid carcinoma: Development of a reliable scoring system in a cohort of 1779 patients surgically treated at one institution during 1940 through 1989. Surgery 114:1050–1058, 1993.
29. Hay ID, Grant CS, Bergstralh MS, et al: Unilateral lobectomy: Is it sufficient surgical treatment for patients with AMES low-risk papillary thyroid carcinoma? Surgery 124:958–964, 1998.
30. Grant CS, Hay ID, Gough IR, et al: Local recurrence in papillary thyroid carcinoma. Is extent of surgical resection important? Surgery 104:954–962, 1988.
31. DeGroot LJ, Kaplan EL, McCormick M, Straus FH II: Natural history, treatment and course of papillary thyroid carcinoma. J Clin Endocrinol Metab 71:414–424, 1990.
32. DeGroot LJ, Kaplan EL, Straus FH II, Shukla MS: Does the method of management of papillary thyroid carcinoma make a difference in outcome? World J Surg 18:123–130, 1994.
33. Mazzaferri EL, Jhiang SM: Long-term impact of initial surgical and medical therapy on papillary and follicular thyroid cancer. Am J Med 97:418–428, 1994.
34. van Heerden JA, Hay ID, Goellner JR, et al: Follicular thyroid carcinoma with capsular invasion alone: A non-threatening malignancy. Surgery 112:1130–1136, 1992.
35. Arganini M, Behar R, Wu FL, et al: Hürthle cell tumors: A twenty five year experience. Surgery 100:1108, 1986.
36. DeGroot LJ, Kaplan EL, McCormick M, Straus FH II: Morbidity and mortality in follicular thyroid cancer. J Clin Endocrinol Metab 80:2946–2952, 1995.
37. Schark C, Fulton N, Yashiro T, et al: The value of measurement of ras oncogenes and nuclear DNA analysis in the diagnosis of Hürthle cell tumors of the thyroid. World J Surg 16:745–752, 1992.
38. Segev DL, Saji M, Phillips GS, et al: Polymerase chain reaction-based microsatellite polymorphism analysis of follicular and Hurthle cell neoplasms of the thyroid. J Clin Endocrinol Metab 83:2036–2042, 1998.
39. Mitchell G, Huddart R, Harmer C: Phase II evaluation of high dose accelerated radiotherapy for anaplastic thyroid carcinoma. Radiother Oncol 50:33–38, 1999.
40. Hill SC Jr: Chemotherapy of thyroid cancer. *In* Kaplan EL (ed): Surgery of the Thyroid and Parathyroid Glands, Clinical Surgery International, vol 4. Edinburgh, Churchill Livingstone, 1983, p 103.
41. Tennvall J, Lundell G, Hallquist A, et al: Combined doxorubicin, hyperfractionated radiotherapy and surgery in anaplastic thyroid carcinoma. Report on two protocols. The Swedish Anaplastic Thyroid Cancer Group. Cancer 74:1348–1354, 1994.
42. Sweeney PJ, Haraf DJ, Recant W, et al: Clinical case: Anaplastic carcinoma of the thyroid. Ann Oncol 7:739–744, 1996.
43. Sizemore GW, van Heerden JA, Carney JA: Medullary carcinoma of the thyroid gland and the multiple endocrine neoplasia type 2 syndrome. *In* Kaplan EL (ed): Surgery of the Thyroid and Parathyroid Glands, Clinical Surgery International, vol 4, Edinburgh, Churchill Livingstone, 1983, p 75.
44. Hofstra RM, Landsvater RM, Ceccherini I, et al: A mutation in the RET proto oncogene associated with multiple endocrine neoplasia type 2B and sporadic medullary thyroid carcinoma. Nature 367:375–376, 1994.
45. Goretzki PE, Hoppner W, Dotzenrath C, et al: Genetic and biochemical screening for endocrine disease. World J Surg 22:1202–1207, 1998.
46. Tisell LE, Jansson S: Recent results of reoperative surgery in medullary carcinoma of the thyroid. Wien Klin Wochenschr 100:347–348, 1988.
47. Skinner MA, DeBenedetti MK, Moley JF, et al: Medullary thyroid carcinoma in children with multiple endocrine neoplasia types 2A and 2B. J Pediatr Surg 31:177–181, 1996.
48. Gharib H, McConahey WM, Tiego RD, et al: Medullary thyroid carcinoma: Clinicopathologic features and long term follow up of 65 patients treated during 1946 through 1970. Mayo Clin Proc 67:934–940, 1992.
49. Schwartz AE, Clark O, Ituarte P, LoGerfo P: Therapeutic controversy. Thyroid surgery—the choice. J Clin Endocrinol Metab 83:1097–1105, 1998.
50. Iacconi P, Bendinelli C, Miccoli P: Endoscopic thyroid and parathyroid surgery. Surg Endosc 13:314, 1999.
51. Shimizu K, Akira S, Tanaka S: Video assisted neck surgery: Endoscopic resection of benign thyroid tumor aiming at scarless surgery of the neck. J Surg Oncol 69:178–180, 1998.
52. Yeung GH: Endoscopic surgery of the neck: A new frontier. Surg Laparosc Endosc 8:227–232, 1998.
53. Miyauchi A, Matsusaka K, Kihara M, et al: The role of ansa to recurrent laryngeal nerve anastomosis in operations for thyroid cancer. Eur J Surg 164:927–933, 1998.
54. Pattou F, Combemale F, Fabre S, et al: Hypocalcemia following thyroid surgery: Incidence and prediction of outcome. World J Surg 22:718–724, 1998.
55. Sedgwick CE, Cady B: Surgery of the Thyroid and Parathyroid Glands, ed 2. Philadelphia, WB Saunders, 1980.
56. Weller GL: Development of the thyroid, parathyroid and thymus glands in man. Contrib Embryol Carnegie Inst Wash 24:93–142, 1933.
57. Gray SW, Skandalakis JE: Embryology for Surgeons. Philadelphia, WB Saunders, 1972.
58. Norris EH: Parathyroid glands and lateral thyroid in man: Their morphogenesis, histogenesis, topographic anatomy and prenatal growth. Contrib Embryol Carnegie Inst Wash 26:247–294, 1937.
59. Williams ED, Toyn CE, Harach HR: The ultimobranchial gland and congenital thyroid abnormalities in man. J Pathol 159:135–141, 1989.

60. Siraj QH, Aleem N, Inam-Ur-Rehman A, et al: The pyramidal lobe: A scintigraphic assessment. Nucl Med Commun 10:685–693, 1989.
61. Vasquez-Chavez C, Acevedo-Rivera K, Sartorius C, Espinosa-Said L: Thyroid hemiagenesis: Report of 3 cases and review of the literature. Gac Med Mex 125:395–399, 1989.
62. Khatri VP, Espinosa MH, Harada WA: Papillary adenocarcinoma in thyroid hemiagenesis. Head Neck 14:312–315, 1992.
63. Netter RA: Endocrine system and selected metabolic diseases. *In* Ciba Collection of Medical Illustrations. Summit, NJ, Ciba Pharmaceutical Company, 1974, p 45.
64. Buckman LT: Lingual thyroid. Laryngoscope 46:765–784, 878–897, 935–955, 1936.
65. Zink A, Rave F, Hoffmann R, Ziegler R: Papillary carcinoma in ectopic thyroid. Horm Res 35:86–88, 1991.
66. Elprana D, Manni JJ, Smals AGH: Lingual thyroid. ORL J Otorhinolaryngol Relat Spec 46:147–152, 1984.
67. Defoer FY, Mahler C: Lingual thyroid in two natural brothers. J Endocrinol Invest 13:65–67, 1990.
68. Conklin WT, Davis RM, Dabb RW, Reilly CM: Hypothyroidism following removal of a "thyroglossal duct cyst." Plast Reconstr Surg 68:930–932, 1981.
69. Allard RHB: The thyroglossal cyst. Head Neck 5:134–146, 1982.
70. Weiss SD, Orlich CC: Primary papillary carcinoma of a thyroglossal duct cyst: Report of a case and review of the literature. Br J Surg 78:87–89, 1991.
71. Katz AD, Hachigian M: Thyroglossal duct cysts: A thirty year experience with emphasis on occurrence in older patients. Am J Surg 155:741–744, 1988.
72. Issa MM, de Vries P: Familial occurrence of thyroglossal duct cyst. J Pediatr Surg 26:30–31, 1991.
73. Helidonis E, Dokianakis G, Papazoglou G, et al: Ectopic thyroid gland in the submandibular region. J Laryngol Otol 94:219–224, 1980.
74. Stanton A, Allen-Mersh TG: Is laterally situated ectopic thyroid tissue always malignant? J R Soc Med 77:333–334, 1984.
75. Wychulis AR, Payne WS, Clagett OT, et al: Surgical treatment of mediastinal tumors. J Thorac Cardiovasc Surg 62:379, 1971.
76. Lesavoy MA, Norberg HP, Kaplan EL: Substernal goiter with superior vena caval obstruction. Surgery 77:325–329, 1975.
77. Lahey FH, Swinton NW: Intrathoracic goiter. Surg Gynecol Obstet 59:627, 1934.
78. Stagno PA, Petras RE, Hart WR: Strumal carcinoids of the ovary: An immunohistologic and ultrastructural study. Arch Pathol Lab Med 111:440–446, 1987.
79. Ramagopal E, Stanbury JB: Studies of the distribution of iodine and protein in a struma ovarii. J Clin Endocrinol Metab 25:526, 1965.
80. Kempers RD, Dockerty MB, Hoffman DL, Bartholomew LG: Struma ovarii–ascitic, hyperthyroid, and asymptomatic syndromes. Ann Intern Med 72:883, 1970.
81. March DE, Desai AG, Park CH, et al: Struma ovarii: Hyperthyroidism in a postmenopausal woman. J Nucl Med 29:263–265, 1988.
82. Thomas RD, Batty VB: Metastatic malignant struma ovarii: Two case reports. Clin Nucl Med 17:577–578, 1992.
83. Rieser GD, Ober KP, Cowan RJ, Cordell AR: Radioiodide imaging of struma cordis. Clin Nucl Med 13:421, 1988.

Chapter 111

Thyroid-Stimulating Hormone Receptor Mutations

Gilbert Vassart

GAIN-OF-FUNCTION MUTATIONS

For a hormone receptor, "gain of function" may have three meanings: activation in the absence of ligand (constitutivity), increased sensitivity to its normal agonist, or broadening of its specificity. When the receptor is part of a chemostat, as is the case for the thyroid-stimulating hormone (TSH) receptor, the first situation is expected to lead to tissue "autonomy" whereas the second would be expected to simply cause adjustment of the agonist concentration to a lower value. In the third case, inappropriate stimulation of the gland is expected to occur because the promiscuous agonist is not expected to be subjected to the normal negative feedback. If a gain-of-function mutation of the first category occurs in a single cell normally expressing the receptor (somatic mutation), it will become symptomatic only if the regulatory cascade controlled by the receptor is mitogenic in this particular cell type. Autonomous activity of the receptor will cause clonal expansion of the mutated cell. If the regulatory cascade also positively controls function, the resulting tumor will progressively take over function of the normal tissue and ultimately result in autonomous hyperfunction. If the mutation is present in all cells of an organism (germline mutation), autonomy will be displayed by the whole tissue expressing the receptor. In cases in which the regulatory cascade is both mitogenic and activates function, the expected result is hyperplasia associated with hyperfunction.

From what we know of thyroid cell physiology it is easy to predict the phenotypes associated with gain-of-function mutations of the cyclic adenosine monophosphate (cAMP)-dependent regulatory cascade. Two observations provide pertinent models of this situation. Transgenic mice made to ectopically express the adenosine A2a receptor in their thyroid display severe hyperthyroidism associated with thyroid hyperplasia.[1] Because the A2a adenosine receptor is coupled to G_s and displays constitutive activity as a result of continuous stimulation by ambient adenosine,[2] this model closely mimics the situation expected for a gain-of-function germline mutation of the TSH receptor. Patients with the McCune-Albright syndrome are mosaic for mutations in G_s (*gsp* mutations), which also leads to constitutive stimulation of adenylyl cyclase.[3] Hyperfunctioning thyroid adenomas develop in these patients from cells harboring the mutation, which makes them a model for gain-of-function somatic mutations of the TSH receptor. A transgenic model in which *gsp* mutations are targeted for expression in the mouse thyroid has been constructed.[4]

Familial Nonautoimmune Hyperthyroidism or Hereditary Toxic Thyroid Hyperplasia

The major cause of hyperthyroidism in adults is Graves' disease, in which an autoimmune reaction is mounted against the thyroid gland and autoantibodies are produced that recognize and stimulate the TSH receptor. This etiology may explain why the initial description by the group of Leclère of a family showing segregation of thyrotoxicosis as an autosomal dominant trait in the absence of signs of autoimmunity was met with skepticism.[5] Reinvestigation of this family together with another family from Reims identified two mutations of the TSH receptor gene that segregated in perfect linkage with the disease.[6] A series of additional families have been studied since, and surprisingly, they each showed a different mutation of the TSH receptor gene.[7, 8] The functional characteristics of these mutant receptors confirm that they are constitutively stimulated (see below). This new nosologic entity, hereditary toxic thyroid hyperplasia (HTTH), sometimes called Leclère's disease, is characterized by the following clinical characteristics: autosomal dominant transmission; hyperthyroidism with a variable age of onset (from infancy to adulthood, even within a given family); hyperplastic goiter of variable size, but with steady growth; and absence of clinical or biologic stigmata of autoimmunity. An observation common to the cases described to date is the need for drastic ablative therapy (surgery or radioiodine) to control the disease once the patient has become hyperthyroid. The autonomous nature of the thyroid tissue from these patients has been elegantly demonstrated by grafting in nude mice.[9] In contrast to tissue from patients with Graves' disease, HTTH cells continue to grow in the absence of stimulation by TSH or thyroid-stimulating antibody.

The prevalence of HTTH is difficult to estimate at the present time. It is likely that many cases have been (and still are) mistaken for Graves' disease. This confusion may be explained by the relative insensitivity and lack of specificity of thyroid-stimulating antibody assays, together with the high frequency of the other thyroid autoantibodies (antithyroglobulin, antithyroperoxidase) in the general population. It is expected that wider knowledge of the existence of the disease will lead to better diagnosis. This problem is not purely academic because presymptomatic diagnosis in children of affected families may prevent the developmental or psychologic complications associated with infantile or juvenile hyperthyroidism.

Sporadic Toxic Thyroid Hyperplasia

Cases of toxic thyroid hyperplasia have been described in children of unaffected parents.[10–16] Conspicuously, congenital hyperthyroidism was present in most of the patients and required aggressive treatment. Mutations of one TSH receptor allele were identified in the children but were absent in the parents. Because paternity was confirmed by minisatellite or microsatellite testing, these cases qualify as true neomutations. When comparing the amino acid substitutions implicated in hereditary and sporadic cases, for the majority, they do not overlap (Fig. 111–1). Although most of the sporadic cases harbor mutations that are also found in toxic adenomas, most of the hereditary cases have "private" mutations. Analysis of the functional characteristics of the individual mutant receptors in COS cells and the clinical course of individual patients suggests an explanation for this observation: "sporadic" mutations seem to have a stronger activating effect

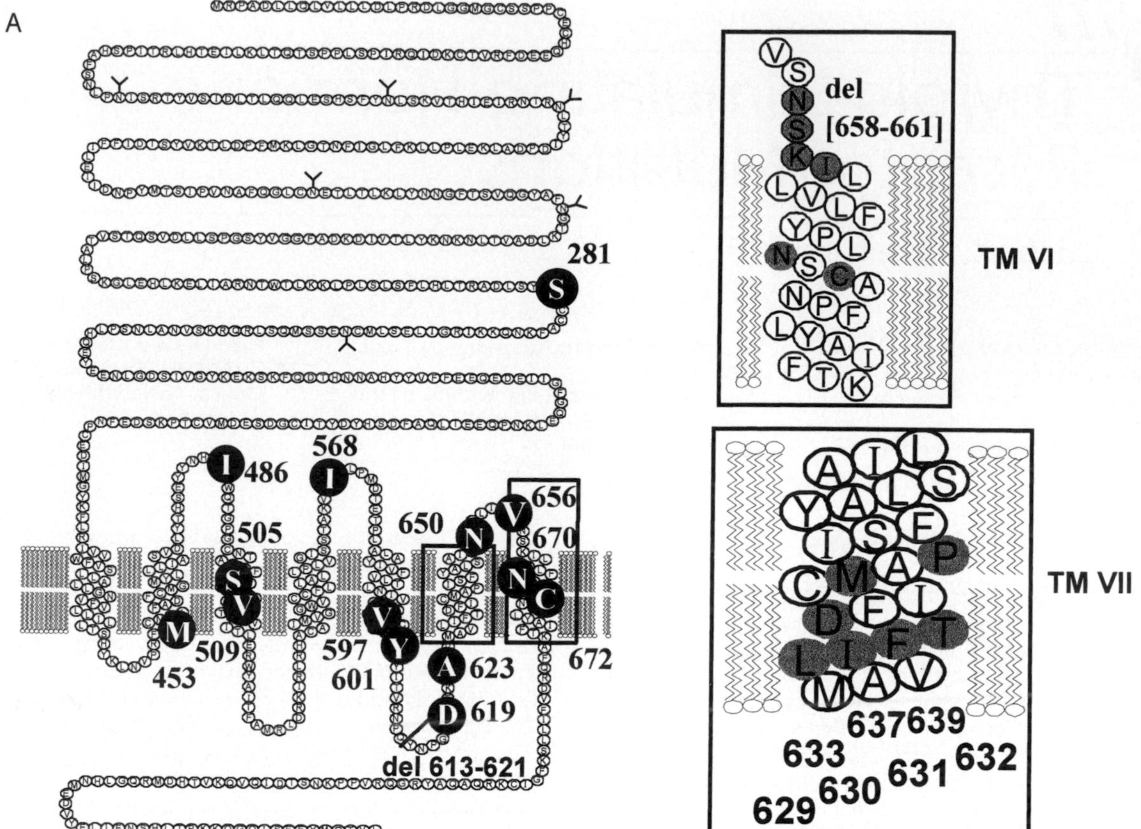

B

CODON	Substitution	Somatic mutation	Germline Neomutation	Germline Familial	Stimulation of [cAMP]	Stimulation of [IP]	References
Ser 281	Asn	+			+	-	31
	Thr	+	+		+	-	28,13
	Ile		+		+	-	16
Met453	Thr	+	+		+	-	12,31
Ile 486	Phe	+			+	+	25
	Met	+			+	+/-	25
Ser505	Arg			+	+	-	7
	Asn		+		+	-	
Val509	Ala			+	+	-	6
Ile568	Thr	+			+	+/-	25
Del613-631		+			+	-	26
Asp619	Gly	+			+	-	22
Ala623	Ile	+			+	+/-	22
	Val	+			+	-	27
	Ser	+			+	-	34
Leu629	Phe	+		+	+	-	31,8, 34
Ile630	Leu	+			+	-	34
Phe631	Leu	+	+		+	-	10
	Cys	+					23
Thr632	Ile	+	+		+	-	24,23
	Ala	+					37
Asp633	Tyr	+			+	-	23,31
	Glu	+			+	-	23,27,31,34
	His	+			+	-	36
	Ala	+			+	-	31
Pro639	Ser	+		+	+	+	34
Asn650	Tyr			+	+	-	7
Val656	Phe	+			+	-	27
Del658-661		+			+	-	31
Asn670	Ser			+	+	-	7
Cys672	Tyr			+	+	-	6

FIGURE 111–1. Schematic representation of the thyroid-stimulating hormone (TSH) receptor. *A*, The locations of known activating mutations are indicated. *B*, The nature of the mutations is indicated with their origins (somatic, germline sporadic, germline familial), effects on intracellular regulatory cascades, and the original references.

than "hereditary" mutations do. From their severe phenotypes, it is likely that newborns with neomutations would not have survived if not treated efficiently. On the contrary, from inspection of the available pedigrees, it seems that the milder phenotype of patients with "hereditary" mutations has only a limited effect on reproductive fitness. The fact that "hereditary" mutations are rarely observed in toxic adenomas is compatible with the suggestion that they would cause extremely slow tissue growth and, accordingly, would rarely cause thyrotoxicosis. If this explanation holds true, one may predict that mutations of the hereditary type may be found in older patients with toxic adenoma.

Somatic Mutations: Autonomous Toxic Adenomas

Soon after mutations of $G_s\alpha$ had been found in adenomas of the pituitary somatotrophs,[3] similar mutations (also called *gsp* mutations) were found in some toxic thyroid adenomas and follicular carcinomas.[17–20] The mutated residues (Arg201, Glu227) are homologous to those found mutated in the *ras* proto-oncogenes; that is, the mutations decrease the endogenous guanine triphosphatase activity of the G protein, thereby resulting in a constitutively active molecule.

Toxic adenoma was found to be a fruitful source of somatic mutations activating the TSH receptor, probably because the phenotype is very conspicuous and easy to diagnose. Most of the mutations are located in the third cytoplasmic loop or in the adjacent sixth transmembrane segment of the receptor (see Fig. 111–1). The clustering reflects the pivotal role of this portion of the molecule in activation mechanisms.[21] However, amino acid substitutions were found over most of the serpentine portion of the receptor[22–27] and even in the extracellular amino-terminal domain.[28]

Despite some dispute about the prevalence of TSH receptor mutations in toxic adenomas, which may be due to different origin of the patients[29, 30] or different sensitivity of the methodology, we conclude that in countries with a moderate shortage of iodine, activating mutations of the TSH receptor are the major cause of solitary toxic adenomas and account for about 80% of cases.[27, 31] In some patients with multinodular goiter and two zones of autonomy at scintigraphy, a different mutation of the TSH receptor was identified in each nodule.[32–35] This finding indicates that the pathophysiologic mechanism responsible for solitary toxic adenomas can be at work on a background of multinodular goiter and may be responsible for some of the autonomous zones appearing late in the evolution of these patients. The independent occurrence of two activating mutations in a patient may seem highly improbable at first. However, the multiplicity of the possible targets for activating mutations within the TSH receptor (at least 20 different residues) makes this event less unlikely. It is also possible that a mutagenic environment is created in glands exposed to chronic stimulation by TSH in which H_2O_2 is produced. Finally, involvement of TSH receptor mutations in thyroid cancer has been implicated in a limited proportion of follicular thyroid carcinomas selected for their high basal activity of adenylyl cyclase.[36, 37]

Structure-Function Relationships of the TSH Receptor, as Deduced from Activating Mutations

Most of the activating mutations of the TSH receptor have been studied by transient expression in COS cells. By the built-in amplification of the transfected construct, this system makes it possible to detect even slight increases in constitutive activity of the TSH receptor. An important observation has been that the wild-type receptor itself displays significant constitutive activity.[6, 38] This characteristic is not unique to the TSH receptor,[39–41] but interestingly, it is not shared by its close relative, the luteinizing hormone/chorionic gonadotropin (LH/CG) receptor. The effect of activating mutations must accordingly be interpreted in terms of "increase in constitutive activity." Most amino acid substitutions found in toxic adenomas and/or toxic thyroid hyperplasia share common characteristics: (1) they increase the constitutive activity of the receptor toward stimulation of adenylyl cyclase; (2) with a few notable exceptions,[25] they do not display constitutive activity toward the inositol phosphate/diacylglycerol pathway; (3) their expression at the cell surface is decreased (from slightly to severely); (4) most, but not all of them keep responding to TSH for stimulation of cAMP and inositol phosphate generation, with a tendency to do so at decreased median effective concentrations; and (5) they bind ^{125}I-labeled bovine TSH with an apparent affinity higher than that of the wild-type receptor.

No simple relationship exists between the position of the mutations or the nature of the amino acid substitution and their functional characteristics. Mutations found in transmembrane segments 2, 3, 6, and 7 and the third cytoplasmic loop all have similar phenotypes; they involve amino acids belonging to all classes (charged, polar, hydrophobic), with substitutions not necessarily involving a shift to another class. Mutations involving Ile486 and Ile568 in the first and second extracellular loops, respectively, and Pro639 in transmembrane segment 6 are exceptional in that in addition to stimulating adenylyl cyclase, they cause constitutive activation of the inositol phosphate pathway.[25] Three additional mutations deserve special mention because of their unexpected nature or location: the four amino acid deletion (residues 658–661) in the third extracellular loop,[37] the nine–amino acid deletion in the third intracellular loop,[37] and the substitutions at serine 281 in the amino-terminal extracellular domain.[28]

No direct relationship is found between the level of cAMP achieved by different mutants in transfected COS cells and their level of expression at the cell membrane,[42] which means that individual mutants have widely different "specific constitutive activity" (measured as the stimulation of cAMP accumulation/receptor number at the cell surface). Although this specific activity may tell us something about the mechanisms of receptor activation, it is not a measure of the actual phenotypic effect of the mutation in vivo. Indeed, one of the relatively mild mutations, observed up to now only in a family with HTTH (Cys672Tyr), is among the strongest according to this criterion. It would be logical to expect the best correlation to be found between the phenotype and the actual level of cAMP achieved, irrespective of the level of receptor expression. However, differences between the effects of the mutants in COS cells and thyrocytes in vivo may render these correlations a difficult exercise.

According to a current model of G protein–coupled receptor (GPCR) activation, the receptor would exist under at least two interconverting conformations: R (silent conformation) and R* (the active forms).[43] The unliganded receptor would shuttle between both forms, the equilibrium being in favor of R. Binding of the ligand, to the slit between the transmembrane segments (for biogenic amines) and/or residues of the N-terminal segment or extracellular loops (for neuropeptides), is believed to stabilize the R* conformation. The resulting R-to-R* transition is supposed to involve a conformational change that modifies the relative position of transmembrane helices, which in turn would translate into conformational changes in the cytoplasmic domains interacting with trimeric G proteins. Seminal studies with the adrenergic receptor α_{1b} have shown that a variety of amino acid substitutions in the C-terminal portion of the third intracellular loop lead to their constitutive activation.[44] The observation that all amino acid substitutions at Ala293 were effective in activating the receptor led to the concept that the silent form of GPCRs would be submitted to a structural constraint requiring the wild-type primary structure of the third intracellular loop. This constraint could be released by a wide spectrum of amino acid substitutions in this segment.[43–46]

The observation that amino acid substitutions in a large number of residues scattered over the serpentine portion of the TSH receptor cause an increase in its constitutive activity is fully compatible with the above model and provides arguments for its extension. The fact that mutations in residues distributed over most of the serpentine portion of the receptor are equally effective in activating it (which does not seem to be a general characteristic in all GPCRs) suggests that the unliganded TSH receptor might be less constrained than others. The readily measurable constitutive activity of the wild-type receptor is compatible with this contention. Being already "noisy," the TSH receptor would be more prone to further destabilization by a variety of mutations.

The precise effects of individual mutations in structural terms are difficult to predict: the sixth transmembrane segment and its continuation in the C-terminal portion of the third cytoplasmic loop is clearly a hot segment (see Fig. 111–1), with a series of contiguous residues potentially implicated in keeping the receptor inactive. The fact that consecutive residues in the sixth transmembrane helix are implicated (residues 631, 632, and 633) is at odds with a simple model in which activation would simply result from the rupture of an interaction with specific residues in another transmembrane helix (e.g., segment 3). Nevertheless, it is likely that the common consequence of activating mutations is stabilization of a conformation of the serpentine portion of the receptor with individual helices in a different relative position. The identification of activating amino acid substitutions in transmembrane domains 2, 3, and 7 also fits well with this notion. The deletion of nine residues in the third cytoplasmic loop is believed to activate the receptor by facilitating binding of $G_s\alpha$ to portions of the transmembrane domains.[26]

The activating mutations identified in the extracellular loops and the amino-terminal extracellular domain are more difficult to interpret in terms of a simple model based on constraint involving only the serpentine portion of the receptor. They are compatible with an extension of this model in which the unliganded amino-terminal domain would contribute to the constraint by keeping the serpentine portion silent. According to this model, activation would result from the release of a silencing interaction between the extracellular loops and the amino-terminal domain.

Familial Gestational Hyperthyroidism

Some degree of stimulation of the thyroid gland by human chorionic gonadotropin (hCG) is commonly observed during early pregnancy. It is usually responsible for a decrease in serum thyrotropin with increases in the concentration of free thyroxine (T_4), which remains within the normal range (for references see elsewhere[47, 48]). When concentrations of hCG are abnormally high, such as in molar pregnancy, true hyperthyroidism may ensue. The pathophysiologic mechanism is believed to be promiscuous stimulation of the TSH receptor by excess hCG, as suggested by the rough correlation between serum hCG and free T_4 concentrations.[49, 50] A convincing rationale is provided by the close structural relationships of the glycoprotein hormones and their receptors.[51]

A new syndrome was described in 1998 in a family with dominant transmission of hyperthyroidism limited to pregnancy.[52] The proposita and her mother had severe thyrotoxicosis together with hyperemesis gravidarum during the course of each of their pregnancies (Fig. 111–2). When nonpregnant, they were clinically and biologically euthyroid. Both patients were heterozygous for a Lys183Arg mutation in the extracellular amino-terminal domain of the TSH receptor. When tested by transient transfection in COS cells, the mutant receptor displayed normal characteristics toward TSH. However, a convincing explanation for the phenotype was provided in that it showed higher sensitivity to stimulation by hCG than the wild-type TSH receptor (see Fig. 111–2).

The amino acid substitution responsible for promiscuous stimulation of the TSH receptor by hCG is surprisingly conservative. Also surprising is the observation that residue 183 is a lysine in both the TSH and LH/CG receptors. When placed on the available three-dimensional model of the hormone-binding domain of the TSH receptor,[53] residue 183 belongs to one of the β sheets that constitute the putative surface of interaction with the hormones.[54] It is likely that an arginine in position 183 would confer a slight increase in stability to the illegitimate hCG/TSH receptor complex.[55] This increase in stability would be enough to cause signal transduction by the hCG concentrations achieved in pregnancy, but not by the LH concentrations observed after menopause. Indeed, the mother of the proposita remained euthyroid after menopause. This finding is compatible with a relatively modest gain of function of the Lys183Arg mutant upon stimulation by hCG.

In contrast to other mammals, humans and primates rely on CG for maintenance of the corpus luteum in early pregnancy.[56] The frequent

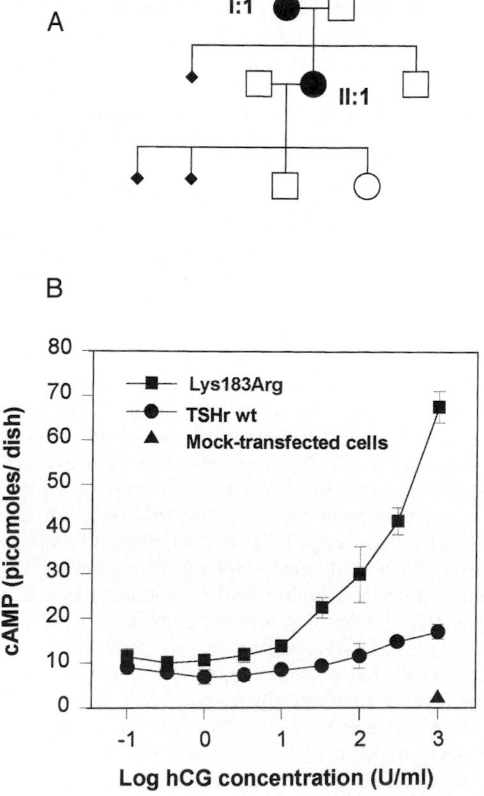

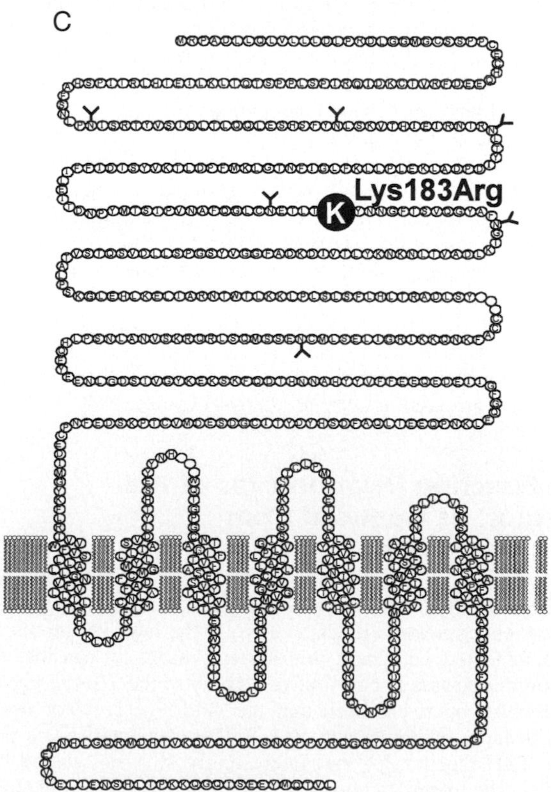

FIGURE 111–2. Familial gestational hyperthyroidism. *A*, The pedigree is indicated with *large black circles* pointing to the affected subjects (I.1 and II.1) and *small black diamonds* pointing to early fetal losses. *B*, Functional characteristics of the mutant receptor from patient II.1 after transient transfection of its cDNA in COS cells. *C*, Location of the mutation on a schematic representation of thyroid-stimulating hormone (TSH) receptor (for details see Rodien et al.[52]).

partial suppression of TSH observed at peak hCG levels during normal pregnancy indicates that evolution has selected physiologic mechanisms operating very close to the border of thyrotoxicosis. This finding may provide a rationale for the observation that in comparison to other species, the glycoprotein hormones of primates display lower biologic activity because of positive evolutionary selection of specific amino acid substitutions in their α subunits.[51] If this reasoning is correct, it is likely that further cases of hereditary gestational thyrotoxicosis will be identified with mutations in the α or β subunits of the hCG genes of the fetus.

LOSS-OF-FUNCTION MUTATIONS

Loss-of-function mutations in the TSH receptor gene are expected to cause a syndrome of "resistance to TSH." The expected phenotype is likely to resemble that of patients with mutations in TSH itself. These mutations have been described earlier because of the prior availability of information on TSH α and β genes.[57–59] A mouse model of resistance to TSH is available in the *hyt/hyt* line. Homozygous *hyt/hyt* mice are hypothyroid as a result of a developmental anomaly of their thyroid glands, which remain hypoplastic.[60] The cause has been traced to a mutation of the TSH receptor gene (Pro556Leu).[61] From this information one would expect patients with two mutated alleles to exhibit a degree of hypothyroidism in accordance with the extent of the loss of function. Heterozygous carriers are expected to be normal or display minimal increase in plasma TSH.

Clinical Cases with the Mutations Identified

A few patients with convincing resistance to TSH have been described before molecular genetics permitted identification of the mutations.[62, 63] Another family has been described more recently, but no mutation was found in the receptor gene.[64] The first cases described in molecular terms were euthyroid siblings with elevated TSH.[65] Sequencing of the TSH receptor gene identified a different mutation in each allele of the affected individuals, which made them compound heterozygotes. The substitutions were in the extracellular amino-terminal portion of the receptor (maternal allele, Pro162Ala; paternal allele, Ile167Asn). The functional characteristics of the mutant receptors were studied by transient expression in COS cells: the paternal allele was virtually completely nonfunctional, whereas the maternal allele displayed an increase in the median effective concentration for stimulation of cAMP production by TSH. Recent additional experiments have shown that the paternal allele is expressed in normal amounts in COS cells, but that it remains trapped intracellularly and does not reach the

A

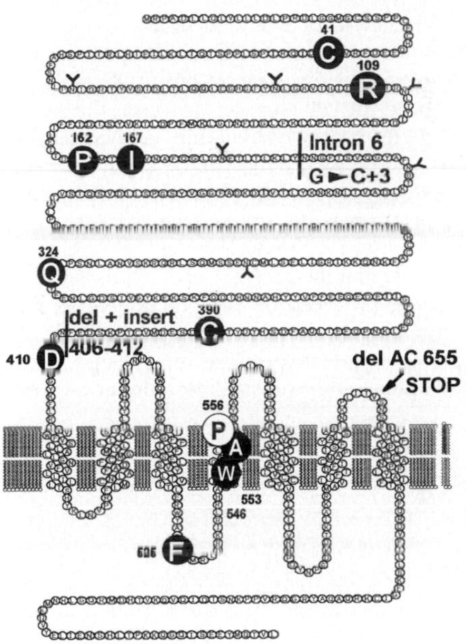

B

Position	Substitution	Loss-of-function	References
Cys 41	Ser	partial (?)	68
Arg 109	Gln	partial	69
Pro 162	Ala	partial	65
Ile 167	Asn	complete	65
Gln 324	Stop	complete	68
Cys 390	Trp	partial (?)	66,68
406 - 412	del + insert	complete	66
Asp 410	Asn	partial	68
Phe 525	Leu	partial (?)	68
Trp 546	Stop	complete	68,69
Ala 553	Thr	complete	67
655 del AC		complete	70
+3 IVS 6	G > C	complete	70
Pro 556 (hyt/hyt mouse)	Leu	complete	61

FIGURE 111–3. Loss-of-function mutations of the thyroid-stimulating hormone (TSH) receptor depicted by schematic representation. *A*, The locations of known loss-of-function mutations are indicated. *B*, The nature of the mutations is indicated together with the extent of their effects and the original references.

cell surface. However, even when assayed on cell membranes, the paternal allele does not bind TSH, which suggests that the mutations have profound structural consequences affecting both the routing of the receptor to the plasma membrane and its ability to bind TSH. When both mutations are displayed on a tentative model of the extracellular domain, their location is compatible with the observed phenotype: the Pro162Ala mutation affects a residue predicted to be at the surface of the molecule, which may explain its interference with the effects of TSH. The Ile167Asn mutation affects a residue protruding within the hydrophobic tunnel between the α helices and the β sheets of the doughnut-shaped model.[53] It is expected that a polar residue would be incompatible with such a position and result in severe misfolding of the whole extracellular domain. Coexpression in COS cells of the wild-type and mutated receptors did not show evidence of dominant negative effects of the mutants.

Recently, familial cases with loss-of-function mutations of the TSH receptor have been identified in the course of screening programs for congenital hypothyroidism[66–70] (Fig. 111–3). Some of the patients displayed the usual criteria for congenital hypothyroidism, including high TSH, low free T_4, and undetectable trapping of ^{99}Tc. The thyroids were small and normally located at ultrasonography. Surprisingly, plasma thyroglobulin levels were normal or high. In one case,[66] the patient was a compound heterozygote for mutations situated in the extracellular domain (Cys390Trp and an insertion/deletion causing a frameshift). The functional characteristics have not been published yet. In another case with familial occurrence,[67] the patients were siblings born to consanguineous parents and were homozygous for a mutation in transmembrane segment 4 (Ala553Thr), close to the *hyt* mutation of the mouse. When transiently expressed in COS cells, the mutants were barely expressed at the cell surface. However, the residual expression was compatible with some TSH binding and stimulation of cAMP production by TSH. When the phenotype of these cases is known in more detail, they will provide a means of understanding the role of the receptor in thyroid organogenesis. Indeed, the difference in phenotype between people with mutations knocking out the hormone and those with mutations knocking out the receptor will tell us whether the mere expression of a functional receptor (and its constitutive activity on adenylyl cyclase stimulation, see above) plays a role in the development of a structurally normal thyroid. The relationship, if any, of these cases with the pathophysiology of sporadic athyreosis remains to be established.

REFERENCES

1. Ledent C, Dumont JE, Vassart G, Parmentier M: Thyroid expression of an A2 adenosine receptor transgene induces thyroid hyperplasia and hyperthyroidism. EMBO J 11:537–542, 1992.
2. Maenhaut C, Van Sande J, Libert F, et al: RDC8 codes for an adenosine A2 receptor with physiological constitutive activity. Biochem Biophys Res Commun 173:1169–1178, 1990.
3. Weinstein LS, Shenker A, Gejman PV, et al: Activating mutations of the stimulatory G protein in the McCune-Albright syndrome. N Engl J Med 325:1688–1695, 1991.
4. Michiels FM, Caillou B, Talbot M, et al: Oncogenic potential of guanine nucleotide stimulatory factor alpha subunit in thyroid glands of transgenic mice. Proc Natl Acad Sci U S A 91:10488–10492, 1994.
5. Thomas JS, Leclere J, Hartemann P, et al: Familial hyperthyroidism without evidence of autoimmunity. Acta Endocrinol (Copenh) 100:512–518, 1982.
6. Duprez L, Parma J, Van Sande J, et al: Germline mutations in the thyrotropin receptor gene cause non autoimmune autosomal dominant hyperthyroidism. Nat Genet 7:396–401, 1994.
7. Tonacchera M, Van Sande J, Cetani F, et al: Functional characteristics of three new germline mutations of the thyrotropin receptor gene causing autosomal dominant toxic thyroid hyperplasia. J Clin Endocrinol Metab 81:547–554, 1996.
8. Fuhrer D, Wonerow P, Willgerodt H, Paschke R: Identification of a new thyrotropin receptor germline mutation (Leu629Phe) in a family with neonatal onset of autosomal dominant nonautoimmune hyperthyroidism. J Clin Endocrinol Metab 82:4234–4238, 1997.
9. Leclere J, Béné M, Duprez A, et al: Behavior of thyroid tissue from patients with Graves' disease in nude mice. J Clin Endocrinol Metab 59:175–177, 1984.
10. Kopp P, Van Sande J, Parma J, et al: Congenital non-autoimmune hyperthyroidism caused by a neomutation in the thyrotropin receptor gene. N Engl J Med 332:150–154, 1995.
11. Kohler B, Biebermann H, Krohn HP, et al: A novel germline mutation in the TSH receptor gene causing nonautoimmune congenital hyperthyroidism (abstract). *In* Proceedings of the International Congress of Endocrinology. San Francisco, 1996, p 946.
12. De Roux N, Polak M, Couet J, et al: A neomutation of the thyroid-stimulating hormone receptor in a severe neonatal hyperthyroidism. J Clin Endocrinol Metab 81:2023–2026, 1996.
13. Gruters A, Schoneberg T, Biebermann H, et al: Severe congenital hyperthyroidism caused by a germ-line neo mutation in the extracellular portion of the thyrotropin receptor. J Clin Endocrinol Metab 83:1431–1436, 1998.
14. Kopp P, Jameson JL, Roe TF: Congenital nonautoimmune hyperthyroidism in a nonidentical twin caused by a sporadic germline mutation in the thyrotropin receptor gene. Thyroid 7:765–770, 1997.
15. Holzapfel HP, Wonerow P, von Petrykowski W, et al: Sporadic congenital hyperthyroidism due to a spontaneous germline mutation in the thyrotropin receptor gene. J Clin Endocrinol Metab 82:3879–3884, 1997.
16. Kopp P, Muirhead S, Jourdain N, et al: Congenital hyperthyroidism caused by a solitary toxic adenoma harboring a novel somatic mutation (serine281→isoleucine) in the extracellular domain of the thyrotropin receptor. J Clin Invest 100:1634–1639, 1997.
17. Lyons J, Landis CA, Harsh G, et al: Two G protein oncogenes in human endocrine tumors. Science 249:655–659, 1990.
18. Goretzki PE, Lyons J, Stacy Phipps S, et al: Mutational activation of RAS and GSP oncogenes in differentiated thyroid cancer and their biological implications. World J Surg 16:576–581, 1992.
19. Suarez HG, du Villard JA, Caillou B, et al: *gsp* mutations in human thyroid tumours. Oncogene 6:677–679, 1991.
20. O'Sullivan C, Barton CM, Staddon SL, et al: Activating point mutations of the *gsp* oncogene in human thyroid adenomas. Mol Carcinog 4:345–349, 1991.
21. Gether U, Lin S, Ghanouni P, et al: Agonists induce conformational changes in transmembrane domains III and VI of the beta2 adrenoceptor. EMBO J 16:6737–6747, 1997.
22. Parma J, Duprez L, Van Sande J, et al: Somatic mutations in the thyrotropin receptor gene cause hyperfunctioning thyroid adenomas. Nature 365:649–651, 1993.
23. Porcellini A, Ciullo I, Laviola L, et al: Novel mutations of thyrotropin receptor gene in thyroid hyperfunctioning adenomas. J Clin Endocrinol Metab 79:657–661, 1994.
24. Paschke R, Tonacchera M, Van Sande J, et al: Identification and functional characterization of two new somatic mutations causing constitutive activation of the TSH receptor in hyperfunctioning autonomous adenomas of the thyroid. J Clin Endocrinol Metab 79:1785–1789, 1994.
25. Parma J, Van Sande J, Swillens S, et al: Somatic mutations causing constitutive activity of the TSH receptor are the major cause of hyperfunctional thyroid adenomas: Identification of additional mutations activating both the cAMP and inisitolphosphate-Ca^{++} cascades. Mol Endocrinol 9:725–733, 1995.
26. Wonerow P, Schoneberg T, Schultz G, et al: Deletions in the third intracellular loop of the thyrotropin receptor. A new mechanism for constitutive activation. J Biol Chem 273:7900–7905, 1998.
27. Fuhrer D, Holzapfel HP, Wonerow P, et al: Somatic mutations in the thyrotropin receptor gene and not in the Gs alpha protein gene in 31 toxic thyroid nodules. J Clin Endocrinol Metab 82:3885–3891, 1997.
28. Duprez L, Parma J, Costagliola S, et al: Constitutive activation of the TSH receptor by spontaneous mutations affecting the N-terminal extracellular domain. FEBS Lett 409:469–474, 1997.
29. Takeshita A, Nagayama Y, Yokoyama N, et al: Rarity of oncogenic mutations in the thyrotropin receptor of autonomously functioning thyroid nodules in Japan. J Clin Endocrinol Metab 80:2607–2611, 1995.
30. Russo D, Arturi F, Wicker R, et al: Genetic alterations in thyroid hyperfunctioning adenomas. J Clin Endocrinol Metab 80:1347–1351, 1995.
31. Parma J, Duprez L, Van Sande J, et al: Diversity and prevalence of somatic mutations in the TSH receptor and Gs alpha genes as a cause of toxic thyroid adenomas. J Clin Endocrinol Metab 82:2695–2701, 1997.
32. Duprez L, Hermans J, Van Sande J, et al: Two autonomous nodules of a patient with multinodular goiter harbor different activating mutations of the thyrotropin receptor gene. J Clin Endocrinol Metab 82:306–308, 1997.
33. Tonacchera M, Vitti P, Agretti P, et al: Activating thyrotropin receptor mutations in histologically heterogeneous hyperfunctioning nodules of multinodular goiter. Thyroid 8:559–564, 1998.
34. Tonacchera M, Chiovato L, Pinchera A, et al: Hyperfunctioning thyroid nodules in toxic multinodular goiter share activating thyrotropin receptor mutations with solitary toxic adenoma. J Clin Endocrinol Metab 83:492–498, 1998.
35. Holzapfel HP, Fuhrer D, Wonerow P, et al: Identification of constitutively activating somatic thyrotropin receptor mutations in a subset of toxic multinodular goiters. J Clin Endocrinol Metab 82:4229–4233, 1997.
36. Russo D, Arturi F, Schlumberger M, et al: Activating mutations of the TSH receptor in differentiated thyroid carcinomas. Oncogene 11:1907–1911, 1995.
37. Spambalg D, Sharifi N, Elisei R, et al: Structural studies of the TSH receptor and G_{sa} in human thyroid cancers: Low prevalence of mutations predicts infrequent involvement in malignant transformation. J Clin Endocrinol Metab 81:3898–3901, 1996.
38. Kosugi S, Okajima F, Ban T, et al: Mutation of alanine 623 in the third cytoplasmic loop of the rat TSH receptor results in a loss in the phosphoinositide but not cAMP signal induced by TSH and receptor autoantibodies. J Biol Chem 267:24153–24156, 1992.
39. Eggerickx D, Denef JF, Labbe O, et al: Molecular cloning of an orphan G-protein–coupled receptor that constitutively activates adenylate cyclase. Biochem J 309:837–843, 1995.
40. Westphal RS, Backstrom JR, Sanders Bush E: Increased basal phosphorylation of the constitutively active serotonin 2C receptor accompanies agonist-mediated desensitization. Mol Pharmacol 48:200–205, 1995.
41. Tiberi M, Caron MG: High agonist-independent activity is a distinguishing feature of the dopamine D1B receptor subtype. J Biol Chem 269:27925–27931, 1994.
42. Van Sande J, Parma J, Tonacchera M, et al: Somatic and germline mutations of the TSH receptor gene in thyroid diseases. J Clin Endocrinol Metab 80:2577–2585, 1995.
43. Samama P, Cotecchia S, Costa T, et al: A mutation-induced activated state of the beta 2-adrenergic receptor. Extending the ternary complex model. J Biol Chem 268:4625–4636, 1993.

44. Kjelsberg MA, Cotecchia S, Ostrowski J, et al: Constitutive activation of the alpha 1B-adrenergic receptor by all amino acid substitutions at a single site. Evidence for a region which constrains receptor activation. J Biol Chem 267:1430–1433, 1992.
45. Ren Q, Kurose H, Lefkowitz RJ, et al: Constitutively active mutants of the α2-adrenergic receptor. J Biol Chem 268:16483–16487, 1993.
46. Lefkowitz RJ, Cotecchia S, Samama P, et al: Constitutive activity of receptors coupled to guanine nucleotide regulatory proteins. Trends Pharmacol Sci 14:303–307, 1994.
47. Glinoer D: The regulation of thyroid function in pregnancy: Pathways of endocrine adaptation from physiology to pathology. Endocr Rev 18:404–433, 1997.
48. Burrow GN: Thyroid function and hyperfunction during gestation. Endocr Rev 14:194–202, 1993.
49. Goodwin TM, Montoro M, Mestman JH, et al: The role of chorionic gonadotropin in transient hyperthyroidism of hyperemesis gravidarum. J Clin Endocrinol Metab 75:1333–1337, 1992.
50. Swaminathan R, Chin RK, Lao TT, et al: Thyroid function in hyperemesis gravidarum. Acta Endocrinol (Copenh) 120:155–160, 1989.
51. Grossmann M, Weintraub BD, Szkudlinski MW: Novel insights into the molecular mechanisms of human thyrotropin action: Structural, physiological, and therapeutic implications for the glycoprotein hormone family. Endocr Rev 18:476–501, 1997.
52. Rodien P, Bremont C, Sanson ML, et al: Familial gestational hyperthyroidism caused by a mutant thyrotropin receptor hypersensitive to human chorionic gonadotropin. N Engl J Med 339:1823–1826, 1998.
53. Kajava AV, Vassart G, Wodak SJ: Modeling of the three-dimensional structure of proteins with the typical leucine-rich repeats. Structure 3:867–877, 1995.
54. Nagayama Y, Russo D, Chazenbalk GD, et al: Extracellular domain chimeras of the TSH and LH/CG receptors reveal the mid-region (amino acids 171–260) to play a vital role in high affinity TSH binding. Biochem Biophys Res Commun 173:1150–1156, 1990.
55. Mrabet NT, Van den Broeck A, Van den Brande I, et al: Arginine residues as stabilizing elements in proteins. Biochemistry 31:2239–2253, 1992.
56. Stewart HJ, Jones DSC, Pascall JC, et al: The contribution of recombinant DNA technology to reproductive biology. J Reprod Fertil 83:1–57, 1988.
57. Miyai K, Azukizawa M, Kumahara Y: Familial isolated thyrotropin deficiency with cretinism. N Engl J Med 285:1043–1048, 1971.
58. Hayashizaki Y, Hiraoka Y, Endo Y, et al: Thyroid-stimulating hormone (TSH) deficiency caused by a single base substitution in the CAGYC region of the beta-subunit [published erratum appears in EMBO J 1989 Nov 8(11):3542]. EMBO J 8:2291–2296, 1989.
59. Hayashizaki Y, Hiraoka Y, Tatsumi K, et al: Deoxyribonucleic acid analyses of five families with familial inherited thyroid stimulating hormone deficiency. J Clin Endocrinol Metab 71:792–796, 1990.
60. Stein SA, Shanklin DR, Krulich L, et al: Evaluation and characterization of the hyt/hyt hypothyroid mouse. II. Abnormalities of TSH and the thyroid gland. Neuroendocrinology 49:509–519, 1989.
61. Stein S, Oates E, Hall C, et al: Identification of a point mutation in the thyrotropin receptor of the hyt/hyt hypothyroid mouse. Mol Endocrinol 8:129–138, 1994.
62. Stanbury JB, Rocmans P, Buhler UK, Ochi Y: Congenital hypothyroidism with impaired thyroid response to thyrotropin. N Engl J Med 279:1132–1136, 1968.
63. Codaccioni JL, Carayon P, Michel Bechet M, et al: Congenital hypothyroidism associated with thyrotropin unresponsiveness and thyroid cell membrane alterations. J Clin Endocrinol Metab 50:932–937, 1980.
64. Takeshita A, Nagayama Y, Yamashita S, et al: Sequence analysis of the TSH receptor gene in congenital primary hypothyroidism associated with TSH unresponsiveness. Thyroid 4:255–259, 1994.
65. Sunthornthepvarakul T, Gottschalk M, Hayashi Y, et al: Resistance to thyrotropin caused by mutations in the thyrotropin-receptor gene. N Engl J Med 332:155–160, 1995.
66. Biebermann H, Schoneberg T, Krude H, et al: Mutations of the human thyrotropin receptor gene causing thyroid hypoplasia and persistent congenital hypothyroidism. J Clin Endocrinol Metab 82:3471–3480, 1997.
67. Abramowicz MJ, Duprez L, Parma J, et al: Familial congenital hypothyroidism due to inactivating mutation of the thyrotropin receptor causing profound hypoplasia of the thyroid gland. J Clin Invest 99:3018–3024, 1997.
68. De Roux N, Misrahi M, Brauner R, et al: Four families with loss of function mutations of the thyrotropin receptor. J Clin Endocrinol Metab 81:4229–4235, 1996.
69. Clifton-Bligh RJ, Gregory JW, Ludgate M, et al: Two novel mutations in the thyrotropin (TSH) receptor gene in a child with resistance to TSH. J Clin Endocrinol Metab 82:1094–1100, 1997.
70. Gagne N, Parma J, Deal C, et al: Apparent congenital athyreosis contrasting with normal plasma thyroglobulin levels and associated with inactivating mutations in the thyrotropin receptor gene: Are athyreosis and ectopic thyroid distinct entities? J Clin Endocrinol Metab 83:1771–1775, 1998.

Chapter 112

Genetic Defects in Thyroid Hormone Synthesis and Action: Defects in Thyroid Hormone Synthesis

Jan J.M. de Vijlder ▪ Thomas Vulsma

Thyroid hormone production is elaborated exclusively by the thyroid gland. Its synthesis, storage, and secretion require a sequence of precisely tuned reactions in which a large number of proteins and factors are involved.[1] Disturbances may lead to abnormalities in thyroid development or metabolic defects in thyroid hormone synthesis. Thyroid metabolism is closely linked to the action of the hypothalamus and pituitary gland. Metabolic disorders along the thyrotropic axis also come under the rubric of genetic thyroid diseases.[2] Although the great majority of patients with genetic thyroid disease suffer from the consequences of impaired thyroid hormone production, the spectrum of genetic defects can result in a wide range of clinical manifestations, from severe hypo- to severe hyperthyroidism.

Both the absence of thyroid tissue leading to sporadic cretinism and myxedema and the occurrence of endemic cretinism due to iodine deficiency have been described since the middle of the 19th century. The first descriptions of inherited defects causing hypothyroidism and goiter are from Pendred[3] and Osler[4] just over a century ago. The major problem in both congenital hypothyroidism (CH) and in iodine deficiency is the disturbance of brain development, expressed as lifelong cognitive and motor problems. Their extent depends on the severity and duration of the hypothyroid condition.

Since these initial descriptions of inherited goiter, our understanding of inborn errors of thyroid metabolism has grown tremendously (Fig. 112–1, Table 112–1). To date several inherited defects have been elucidated at the molecular level. With the development and application of sensitive and rapid techniques, our knowledge of this field will certainly increase in coming years. The disorders of hormonogenesis are mostly autosomal recessive, indicating single protein defects. Disturbances in the ontogeny of the thyroid and pituitary gland appear to be more complex in etiology and, since mutated transcription factors have been found, the involvement of genetic factors is indicated.

In this chapter we review defects in thyroid hormone synthesis as listed in Table 112–1. A general approach to clinical and biochemical investigations of the inherited disorders is presented.

CLINICAL MANIFESTATIONS

In its natural course, CH results in serious mental and motor handicaps, sometimes to such an extent that the patient is unable to function independently and sooner or later needs institutionalization. Because of the protective effects of a substantial maternal-fetal transfer of thyroxine (T_4),[5] the delay in cerebral developmental is mainly the result of lack of thyroid hormone after birth. Prevention by timely administration of T_4 is easy if the diagnosis can be made immediately after birth.

The clinically detectable consequences of CH are strongly dependent on the extent and duration of the lack of thyroid hormone, but there is also a large interindividual variability in expression. At a very young age only the patients with severe types of CH have clinical manifestations. Milder types can remain unnoticed for years. The only characteristic sign of CH is goiter, but a minority of patients have a defect that includes the risk of goitrogenesis. So, most characteristic of young infants with CH is the absence of specific signs.

Even among patients with genetic defects in thyroid hormone synthesis, in only a minority is the thyroid clearly visible or easily palpable in the first weeks after birth, and at that time there appears to be no clear correlation between the extent of the defect (represented by the plasma free T_4 concentration) and the degree of goitrogenesis. Rarely goitrogenesis results in airway obstruction. If T_4 administration is started in the first weeks of life, and normal thyroid-stimulating hormone (TSH) concentrations are maintained, the tendency to develop a goiter can be suppressed permanently.

NEONATAL SCREENING

Because in early infancy CH is hardly detectable clinically, often several months of precious time for cerebral development may be wasted. It became possible in 1974 to measure T_4 and TSH relatively easily, inexpensively, on a large scale, and with just a few drops of blood absorbed in filter paper. Many countries introduced neonatal mass screening procedures. Since this introduction, the apparent overall incidence of CH has increased considerably as a consequence of the detection of very mild disorders that either formerly remained undetected or were not recognized as congenital problems.

Results from a number of recent international studies show that the incidence of permanent primary CH is approximately 1 in 3500 newborn children (in areas without iodine deficiency). There is considerable ethnic variation in incidence, ranging between the 1 in 30,000 in blacks in the United States[6] and 1 in 900 in Asian populations in the United Kingdom.[7] It is noteworthy that with few exceptions the international screening data ignore patients with permanent CH due to pituitary and hypothalamic disorders, which have an estimated inci-

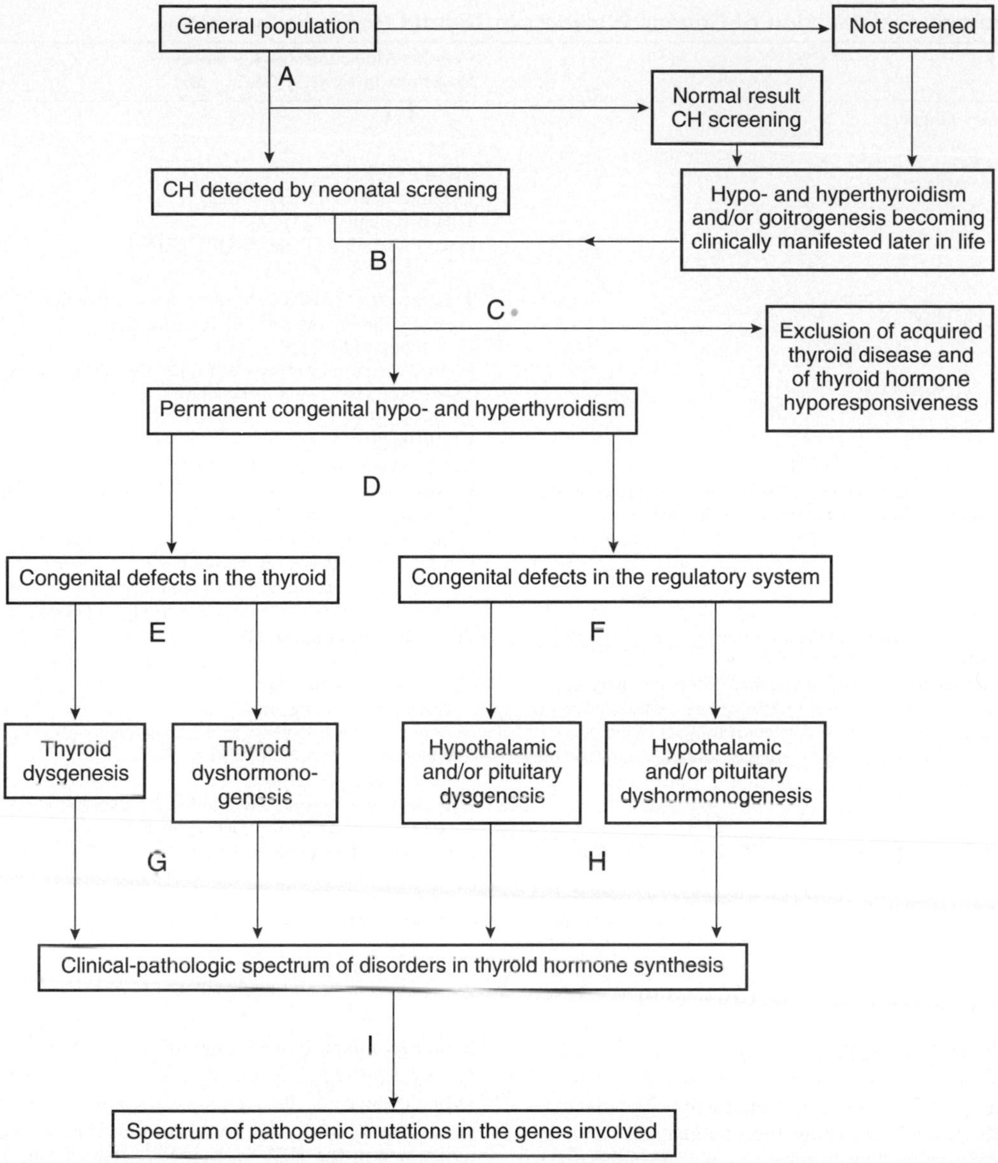

FIGURE 112–1. Flow chart for the etiologic classification of disorders of thyroid hormone synthesis. *A,* Screening by measuring thyroid-stimulating hormone (TSH) or thyroxine (T_4) + thyroxine-binding globulin + TSH in filter paper blood spots. *B,* Confirmation by plasma free T_4 and TSH. *C,* Clinical data, auto- or maternal antithyroid immunoglobulins, urinary iodine excretion; increased plasma free T_4 in relation to the plasma TSH level. *D,* Inappropriate plasma free T_4 in relation to the plasma TSH level. *E,* Ultrasound or radioiodide imaging of the neck. *F,* Magnetic resonance imaging of the brain. *G,* Measuring plasma thyroglobulin, radioiodide uptake in the thyroid, perchlorate effect, and urinary excretion of abnormal iodopeptides or iodotyrosines. *H,* Testing of the various hypothalamic-pituitary axes with thyrotropin-releasing hormone and other releasing hormones. *I,* Investigation of genes with DNA mutation analysis techniques.

dence of roughly 1 in 25,000.[8, 9] These types of CH also harbor interesting genetic defects, most of which result in multiple pituitary hormone deficiencies.

ETIOLOGIC CLASSIFICATION

With regard to the etiologic classification of CH, we follow primarily a clinicopathologic approach, this to make the diagnostic process as efficient as possible, aiming to realize optimal treatment, an adequate estimation of the risk of recurrence, the risk of other endocrine defects or nonendocrine complications, and estimation of the consequences of CH for later cognitive and motor development. For each patient the clinical relevance of diagnostic evidence has to be balanced against the burden of the necessary investigations. For obvious reasons only diagnostic tools adapted for use in very young children are suitable.

We developed a set of diagnostic profiles for the currently known causes.[10] Each of the available determinants (plasma concentrations of free T_4, TSH, thyroglobulin [Tg], urinary excretion of iodinated peptides, ultrasound or radioiodide imaging of thyroid tissue, and uptake studies with radioiodide and sodium perchlorate) has a low specificity, but by combining the test results it is possible to classify the causes of CH unequivocally. The final goal is to assign a specific cause to every case of CH. Especially in cases with borderline plasma free T_4 and TSH concentrations, only a specific etiologic diagnosis provides conclusive evidence for the diagnosis of CH (see Table 112–1).

Although DNA diagnostics has great advantages, it has to be kept in mind that demonstrating mutations in one of the genes involved in thyroid hormone synthesis does not automatically mean that the ultimate cause of the patient's CH is elucidated. It has to be established by in vitro expression of the mutated DNA whether the detected mutations actually lead to impaired production or activity of the protein in question. Currently, in only a minority of the cases is it possible to establish the ultimate cause, so usually one is confined to a global clinicopathologic description.

TABLE 112–1. Etiologic Classification of Genetic Disorders in Thyroid Hormone Synthesis

Clinicopathologic Entity *Defects in:*	**Cellular-Molecular Backgrounds** *Mutations in Gene(s) Coding for:*
Hypothalamus and Pituitary Gland	
1. Pituitary gland	
Ontogeny*	HESX1[11] [3p21]
Function	TRH receptor (TRHR)[12] [8q23][13]
	TSH β subunit[14–16] [1p22][17]
	POU1F1[18–20] [3p11] and PROP1[21–23][5q]
Thyroid Gland	
2. Thyroid stimulation:	TSH receptor (TSHR) [14q31][24] "loss of function"[25–27]
Hyporesponsiveness to TSH	Transcription factors for TSHR expression
	G_s α subunit [20q13][28]
	Factors† or proteins† involved more distally in the signaling complex[29]
Hyperresponsiveness to TSH	TSHR [14q31][24] "gain of function"[30]
3. Thyroid ontogeny*	PAX8 [2q12-q14][31]
	TTF2 [9q22][32, 33]
4. Iodide transport	Na^+/I^- symporter (NIS) [19p13][34–37]
5. Iodide organification defects, characterized by substantial release of iodide from the thyroid after administration of (sodium) perchlorate.	Promoter or structural TPO gene[38, 39] [2p24-p25][40, 41] leading to:
	Partial or total inactivation[42, 43]
	Impaired heme binding[44]
	Impaired anchorage in membrane[42, 45]
	Abnormal intracellular localization[42, 46]
	Thyroid oxidase(s)†[73a] involved in H_2O_2 generation[47]
6. Pendred's syndrome: partial iodide organification defect combined with sensorineural hearing loss	PDS (pendrin) [7q22-q31][48–50]
7. Thyroglobulin (Tg) synthesis defect: any aberration occurring along the whole pathway from Tg gene transcription to endocytosis; characterized by decreased release of Tg from the thyroid in relation to TSH stimulation and the presence of circulating iodoproteins (mainly iodoalbumin) and the urinary excretion of iodinated peptides	Tg [8q24][1, 51] leading to:
	Truncated Tg molecule[52, 53]
	Abnormal Tg fragments and alternatively spliced products[54–56]
	Endoplasmic reticulum storage disease[57, 58]
	Abnormal glycosylation
	Enzymes† and factors† involved in Tg expression pathway,[59] transcription factors; deficiency of TTF1[60] [14q12]
8. Iodide recycling defect: presence of mono- and diiodotyrosine in plasma and urine.	Iodotyrosine dehalogenase,†[61] or other involved enzymes

TRH, thyrotropin-releasing hormone; TSH, thyroid-stimulating hormone; TTF, thyroid-specific transcription factor; TPO, thyroid peroxidase; Tg, thyroglobulin.
*Entities until now restricted to subgroups of patients with pituitary or thyroid dysgenesis.
†Not yet elucidated.

CENTRAL HYPOTHYROIDISM

Congenital CH might be caused by a dysfunctioning hypothalamus, pituitary gland, or both. Knowledge about the ontogeny of the hypothalamus and the mechanism of thyrotropin-releasing hormone (TRH) production and secretion is limited. Moreover TRH production is not restricted to hypothalamic tissue, indicating that TRH is not exclusively involved in the regulation and synthesis of thyroid hormone. Central CH might be caused by a distorted development of the thyroid regulatory system or a failure in TSH synthesis due to structural or regulatory gene defects.

Ontogeny of the Hypothalamus and Pituitary Gland

The pituitary gland is formed from an invagination of the floor of the third ventricle and from Rathke's pouch, an invagination of oral ectoderm, developing into the thyrotropic cell line and the four other neuroendocrine cell types, each defined by the hormone produced: adrenocorticotropic hormone (ACTH), growth hormone (GH), prolactin (PRL), and luteinizing hormone (LH) or follicle-stimulating hormone (FSH). A number of homeobox genes are implicated in pituitary gland development, including HESX1, PROP-1, and POU1F1 (pituitary-specific transcription factor-1, Pit-1).

In mice, the transcription factor *hesx1* has been described to be necessary for the normal development of forebrain, eyes, and other anterior structures, such as the hypothalamus, the pituitary gland, and olfactory placodes. Defects in the gene coding for HESX1 cause disorders that are comparable to septo-optic dysplasia in humans. This entity is characterized by hypoplasia of the optic nerve, various types of forebrain defects, and pituitary hormone deficiencies, including hypothyroidism. Indeed, Dattani et al.[11] showed that among 38 patients having septo-optic dysplasia, 2 siblings, from a consanguineous family, with agenesis of the corpus callosum, optic nerve hypoplasia, and panhypopituitarism, harbored a homozygous Arg53Cys missense mutation within the HESX1 homeodomain, destroying the protein's ability to bind DNA. Heterozygous family members were phenotypically normal. Whether this gene plays a role in the more frequently occurring sporadic form of septo-optic dysplasia remains to be proved. In the near future defects in other genes responsible for regulation and development of the pituitary and hypothalamus will be elucidated.

Defects in the TRH Receptor

Isolated central hypothyroidism with complete absence of TSH and PRL responses to TRH has been described by Collu et al.[12] They found inactivating mutations in the G protein–coupled TRH receptor linked to the phospholipase C second messenger pathway. A 9-year-old boy was a compound heterozygote, having inherited parental TRH alleles, both differently mutated at the 5′ part of the gene. Both mutated genes gave rise to biologically inactive receptors, unable to bind TRH.

Defects in Regulation of TSH Synthesis

TSH is synthesized in the pituitary gland, regulated by local thyroid hormone and TRH concentration. Transcription of the β subunit is under control of several transcription factors. The transcription factors POU1F1 and PROP-1 act as main stimulators of GH, TSH, and PRL synthesis by means of cell-specific *cis*-acting elements of these gene promoters. Indeed, TSH deficiency combined with a lack of GH and

PRL has been described[18–23] (see Table 112–1). Aberrations in the human POU1 domain, class 1 transcription factor gene (POU1F1) have been found to cause this type of hereditary hypothyroidism. Patients who are compound heterozygotes for a POU1F1 deletion and for an Ala158Pro mutation have been described,[18] as well as patients with nonsense and missense mutations.[19, 20] Usually the GH deficiency dominates the clinical manifestations.

Combined pituitary hormone deficiency has also been described in families with homozygosity or compound heterozygosity for inactivating point mutations in the PROP-1 gene. Moreover Wu et al.[21] described an A301G302 deletion in the PROP-1 gene. This 2-bp deletion results in a frameshift in the second α-helix of the DNA-binding domain predicting a truncated protein of 108 amino acids. This study established that defects in PROP-1 are responsible for subtypes of a combined pituitary hormone deficiency syndrome that includes GH, TSH, PRL, and gonadotropin deficiency. These results were confirmed by a study of Rosenbloom et al.[23] of a large family in which two sibships with possibly related mothers but no parental consanguinity are described. Eight affected patients are homozygous for a 2-bp deletion in an AG-rich region in exon 2 of the PROP-1 gene. The severity of the hormone deficiency phenotype is compatible with the complete loss of PROP-1 activity. All patients were extremely small and sexually immature; their intelligence was normal, probably reflecting the relatively mild hypothyroid state, while none received hormonal therapy. Three of them had a markedly increased sella turcica area, determined from lateral skull films.

Structural TSH Defects

TSH stimulates the function and growth of the thyroid gland via interaction with a specific plasma membrane receptor. TSH consists of two different (α and β) noncovalently linked subunits. The amino acid sequence for the α subunit has TSH in common with LH, FSH, and chorionic gonadotropin (CG). The β subunit is different for each of these hormones and carries specific information about receptor binding and expression of hormonal action. For biologic activity the heterodimer is required, as the free β subunit is inactive.[62]

Both CH due to lack of TSH and to abnormalities in the TSH molecule are reported. Patients even have high plasma TSH concentrations compensating for the impaired biologic activity of the TSH molecule; other patients had plasma TSH concentrations below detection level, while other pituitary glycoprotein hormones were present.[63] Hayashizaki et al.[14] described three hypothyroid patients from different families. TSH was totally inactive as a consequence of a Gly(CGA)29Arg(AGA) mutation in the Cys-Ala-Gly-Tyr-Cys region of the TSH-β subunit, presumably involved in association with the α subunit, preventing dimerization. Other severely hypothyroid patients harbored single base mutations or a deletion in the genes coding for the β subunit. Both mutations introduce premature termination signals, giving inactive TSH fragments.[15, 16]

HYPORESPONSIVENESS TO THYROID-STIMULATING HORMONE

Hyporesponsiveness to TSH may occur because of abnormalities in the TSH molecule (see preceding section) or because of lesions in specific parts of the TSH stimulation pathway, that is, in the receptor molecule or in modulating proteins downstream in the signaling pathway, such as G proteins, adenylate cyclase, or the various kinases.

Defects in the TSH Receptor

The TSH receptor belongs to the superfamily of G protein–coupled receptors. It contains an extracellular N-terminal domain with a repetitive leu-rich motif, seven transmembrane helixes, three intra- and three extracellular loops, and an intracellular C-terminal part.[1]

The activated TSH receptor is coupled to regulatory transducing proteins, G_s and G_p, which in turn bind GTP (guanosine triphosphate). Activated G_s binds to and activates adenylate cyclase, catalyzing adenosine triphosphate (ATP) conversion to cyclic adenosine monophosphate (cAMP). Via an activated G_p protein, TSH activates a phospholipase C that specifically hydrolyzes PIP_2 (phosphatidylinositol 4,5-biphosphate) into IP_3 (inositol 1,4,5-triphosphate) and DAG (diacylglycerol). DAG stimulates specific protein kinases and IP_3 causes release of Ca^{2+}. Each intracellular signal molecule (cAMP, DAG, Ca^{2+}) induces phosphorylation of specific proteins. Although the relation of phosphorylation to the physiologic effects of the hormone are still largely unknown, TSH exerts its effects via many metabolic steps in hormonogenesis, including iodide transport, iodination and endocytosis of Tg, and release and secretion of thyroid hormone.

Somatic,[64] germline,[65] and de novo[66] mutations in the TSH receptor mostly cause constitutive activation of the receptor or "gain of function" (see Table 112–1), resulting in toxic adenomas, nonautoimmune hyperthyroidism, and congenital hyperthyroidism. After the first publication of a mutation in the extracellular domain causing hypothyroidism[25] that could be compensated by high TSH concentrations, 13 other deactivating or inactivating mutations have been described.[27] The diagnostic criterion for these disorders is CH with a thyroid in the normal position. When the binding of TSH to its receptor is diminished, the effect can be compensated by high TSH plasma concentrations. The high TSH level does not result in exaggerated stimulation of thyroid metabolism and consequently goitrogenesis is not observed. In case of a total failure of the TSH receptor the patient is severely hypothyroid, since the complete lack of TSH stimulation represses almost completely the metabolic activity of the thyroid gland.[26]

Abnormalities in the G_s Protein Subunit

A related type of TSH hyporesponsiveness is found in patients with pseudohypoparathyroidism type 1a (Albright's hereditary osteodystrophy),[67] a variably expressed disorder with autosomal dominant inheritance. The cause is a defect in the expression of the α subunit of the G_s protein. Several mutations have been found.[28] The patients tend to have mild manifestations of hypothyroidism with slightly decreased plasma free T_4 levels. Detection of patients with pseudohypoparathyroidism type 1a by neonatal thyroid screening has been reported, but it is likely that most affected newborns will be missed because their blood TSH and T_4 concentrations will not reach the cutoff levels used in the screening programs.[10] Otherwise, the mild hypothyroidism is just a minor component of this disease.

Other Causes

That hyporesponsiveness to TSH may also be caused by factors other than mutations in TSH, G_s, or TSH receptor was shown by Xie et al.[29] who found TSH hyporesponsiveness in members of three families in which no mutations could be found in one of the mentioned proteins. Defects more distal in the signal pathway may occur in thyroid-specific disorders.

THYROID DYSGENESIS

Dysgenesis caused by inactivation of the TSH receptor has been described (see preceding section). Since thyroid transcription factors TTF1, TTF2, and PAX8 are crucial for thyroid development they also might be involved in thyroid dysgenesis. In a study[31] done in a screening population of 145 patients with CH in Italy, 2 patients were found to harbor monoallelic mutations in the PAX8 gene. One patient with a dystopic thyroid remnant showed a de novo C→T mutation in exon 3 creating an Arg108 stop transition. The other patient with a dysgenic eutopic thyroid showed an Arg(CGC)31His(CAC) mutation. The authors describe three other affected persons (mother and two children) in a Berlin family, all having dysgenic eutopic thyroids. These patients harbored a monoallelic Leu(CTT)63Arg(CGT) mutation. The father appeared to be unaffected.[31]

PAX8 transcription factor is known to recognize DNA via the conserved paired domain. Inserting the mutations into a normal PAX8 sequence followed by in vitro translation showed that the mutated PAX8 molecules were unable to bind to or to activate a thyroid peroxidase (TPO) promoter coupled to a luciferase gene, giving evidence that these mutations were indeed causing a severe loss of PAX8 function as a consequence of decreased DNA binding.

A mutation in TTF2 associated with congenital hypothyroidism, cleft palate, and choanal atresia has been described by Clifton-Bligh et al.[33] in two siblings with a homozygous missense mutation (Ala65-Val) within the forkhead domain of TTF2.

When we consider patients with CH, for which the molecular background is unknown, it is clear that a large proportion of these cases await a molecular explanation.

That monoallelic PAX8 mutations can give rise to CH has been discussed.[68] Possibly reduction of Pax8 protein, synthesized only by one allele, would result in insufficient thyroid hormone production, a phenomenon called haploinsufficiency. This reduction in the amount of Pax8 protein would perturb the binding equilibrium with competitors or cofactors. In that case the phenotype would not only depend on the mutations in the PAX gene but also on mutations in competitor or cofactor genes, as was recently demonstrated with Ref-1 nuclear protein,[69] a factor controlling the DNA-binding capacity of Pax8. These findings are broadening the pathogenic mechanisms possibly involved in CH.

IODIDE TRANSPORT DEFECT

The first step in thyroidal iodine metabolism is cellular iodide uptake from the extracellular fluid. Iodide is transported against a chemical and electrical gradient. Iodide uptake is followed by rapid oxidation and protein binding, mainly to Tg, a process also called iodide organification. This organification process occurs most likely on the outside of the cell at the apical border. Under normal conditions the iodide uptake is the rate-limiting step in this process. Iodide transport over the plasma membrane is performed by an Na^+ iodide symporter (NIS).[70] The efflux of iodide over the apical membrane, as shown by autographic and compartmental studies, also needs an active transporter. The nature of this transporter is unknown. Active iodide transport is not confined to the thyroid gland. It also occurs in the salivary glands, gastric mucosa, small intestinal mucosa, lacrimal gland, nasopharynx, thymus, skin, lung tissue, choroid plexus, ciliary body, uterus, lactating mammary tissue, and placenta.[71] Only in the thyroid is iodide transport regulated by TSH.

The active transport process is catalyzed by NIS. In 1996 this symporter messenger RNA (mRNA) from rat[70] and human[34] was isolated. The complementary DNA (cDNA) was cloned, sequenced, and expressed in oocytes.[70] The gene coding for the human NIS was mapped to chromosome 19 and appeared to have 15 exons with an open reading frame of 1926 nucleotides. The sequence codes for 643 amino acids. Presumably, NIS with an estimated molecular mass of 68,700 has 12 transmembrane domains with intracellular N-terminal and C-terminal parts.[34] Thyroidal iodide transport defects were already postulated for patients with goiters that could not be visualized with radioiodide. To date about 40 patients, originating from 28 families in which an iodide transport defect was observed, have been reported.[42]

In three patients with iodide transport defects the aberration at the molecular level has been elucidated (see Table 112–1). One patient appeared to be homozygous for a Thr354Pro mutation[35] giving an inactive symporter; another patient harbored a homozygous Cys272 stop mutation.[36] The Thr354Pro appeared to be a recurrent mutation. The substituted threonine lies in the midst of a well-conserved putative transmembrane segment. The hydroxyl group near the β carbon of the residue at position 354 is essential for NIS function, most likely for Na^+ binding and translocation, a function performed together with the cluster of hydroxyl groups originating with the serine and threonine residues present in the ninth transmembrane helix.[72]

Another patient with an iodide transport defect, described by Pohlenz et al.,[37] appeared to be heterozygous for two different mutations in the NIS gene. The aberrant protein, paternally derived, showed an amino acid substitution in which Gln at position 267 was replaced by Glu, resulting in an inactive symporter. The maternally derived allele showed a C1940G transversion. The mutation creates a downstream cryptic 3′ splice acceptor site in exon 13 of the NIS gene, resulting in a 67-bp deletion and a frameshift giving an unstable mRNA. The predicted transcript would code for a truncated NIS, lacking 129 amino acids.

In the neonatal period infants with a transport defect are found to have a normal-sized or sowewhat enlarged thyroid gland by ultrasonography and very elevated serum Tg levels.[73] The radioactive iodide uptake is absent. Measurement of the saliva-to-plasma ^{123}I ratio is around unity. With normal amounts of iodine in the diet the children described are severely hypothyroid.

DEFECTS IN IODINATION AND COUPLING

Iodide transported into the thyroid gland is oxidized by hydrogen peroxide (H_2O_2), catalyzed by thyroid-specific NADPH oxidase,[73a] and bound to tyrosine residues in Tg. Subsequently, iodinated tyrosine residues couple to form iodothyronine residues, mainly T_4.[74] Both iodination and coupling are catalyzed extracellularly by TPO at the apical border of the thyrocyte. Normally, iodide entering the thyroid is rapidly oxidized and bound to protein, mainly Tg. Accumulation of iodide in the thyroid gland reaches a steady state between active influx, protein binding, and efflux, resulting in a relatively low free intracellular iodide concentration under normal conditions. The kinetics of iodide uptake and release can be traced by administration of radioiodide. Complete inhibition of iodide uptake after radioiodide administration by anions of similar molecular size and charge, such as perchlorate or thiocyanate, gives an impression of the thyroidal iodide concentration in relation to that in serum and the degree of iodine bound to protein. Depending on the degree to which iodide can be organified, the iodination defect will be partial or total. Total iodide organification defects are characterized by discharge of more than 90% of the (radio)iodide taken up by the gland within 1 hour after administration of sodium perchlorate, usually given 2 hours after the radioiodide. A complete loss of the thyroid's image of the scintiscan is observed. Partial iodide organification defects are characterized by discharge of more than 20% of the accumulated radioiodide. The main metabolic pathways needed for iodination and thyroid hormonogenesis are H_2O_2 generation catalyzed by thyroid oxidase,[73a] iodination of Tg, and coupling of iodotyrosine residues catalyzed by TPO.[1, 74] Iodide organification defects, caused by various cellular or molecular disorders, are given in Table 112–1.

From studies in thyroid tissue and from DNA linkage studies a number of iodide organification defects, transmitted as autosomal recessive traits, have been related to abnormalities in the TPO gene.[75] The human TPO gene is located on chromosome 2p24→p25 and spans about 150 kb of DNA; the coding sequence of 3048 bp is divided over 17 exons.[38]

Inactivating mutations in both TPO alleles have been found in patients from 18 unrelated families. Of these families 11 were homozygous and 7 were compound heterozygous. The 13 different mutants consist of 6 frameshifts, 4 missense mutations, 1 nonsense mutation, and 2 mutations possibly related to alternative splicing. From these results it might be concluded that total inability to oxidize iodide can almost completely be explained by mutations in TPO. The most frequent mutation (14 of 36 alleles) appeared to be the duplication of GGCC in exon 8.[43] The little research done on partial organification defects does not give an indication that these defects are caused by mutations in the gene coding for TPO.

PENDRED'S SYNDROME

A remarkable variant of a partial iodide organification defect is Pendred's syndrome.[3] The syndrome is characterized by overt or subclinical hypothyroidism, goiter, and moderate to severe sensorineural hearing impairment. The prevalence of Pendred's syndrome varies between 1 in 15,000 and 1 in 100,000, and it may be the most common hereditary metabolic disorder causing hypothyroidism. Thyroid hormone synthesis is only mildly impaired and not surprisingly, therefore, few patients with Pendred's syndrome are detected by neonatal thyroid screening.[10] In general, the discharge of (radio)iodide after administration of sodium perchlorate is moderately increased (>20%). Recently Everett et al.[48] reported the identification of the PDS gene (see Table 112–1). The transcript of about 5 kb, with an open reading frame at 2243 bp, encodes a protein, called pendrin, that is predicted to contain 780 amino acids (86 kDa). The amino acid sequence reveals 11 putative transmembrane domains and shows homology to a class of sulfate transporters or a chloride-iodide transporter.[48a] Its function in thyroid hormone synthesis and hearing is still unknown. The PDS mRNA is significantly expressed in the thyroid.

Mutation analysis has been performed up till now in 18 families in which the Pendred's syndrome occurs. The 18 mutations consist of 4 frameshift mutations, 2 mutations leading to aberrant splicing processes, and 12 different missense mutations. The 18 mutations are most probably disease-causing. Since the function of pendrin is unknown, a structure-function analysis is not yet possible. The Leu236Pro and the Thr416Pro proved to be recurrent mutations, found in 9 of the 18 families. Mutations could not be found in controls.[49] The occurrence of frequent mutations in the PDS gene will facilitate the diagnosis of Pendred's syndrome.

DEFECTS IN THYROGLOBULIN SYNTHESIS

Tg synthesis occurs exclusively in the thyroid gland. The human Tg gene codes for a polypeptide of 300 kDa. The gene contains 8307 coding sequences,[76] divided over 48 exons.[76a] Following a signal peptide of 19 amino acids, the polypeptide chain is composed of 2750 amino acids containing 66 tyrosine residues. Tg is a dimer with identical 330-kDa subunits containing 10% carbohydrate residues. The polypeptide chain contains four domains, each having its own characteristic repeats, except domain 4.[77]

To obtain a Tg molecule of intact tertiary and quaternary structure, many processes have to be passed through. After entering the endoplasmic reticulum, Tg synthesis proceeds according to general principles with proper carbohydrate attachment and folding with the aid of chaperone molecules. In the Golgi complex carbohydrate attachment is completed. Phosphorylation and sulfatation have been described as part of the processing. Iodination and coupling of iodotyrosine residues are the last post-translational processes.

Specific tyrosine residues are involved in preferential iodination and thyroid hormone formation. Tyrosine residue 5 (acceptor) is considered as the preferential site where thyroid hormone is formed by coupling with another iodotyrosine residue (donor), most likely tyrosine residue 130. Other acceptor and donor residues have been described. After formation of thyroid hormone residues in Tg, a process that occurs at the apical border of the cell, thyroid hormone is freed from Tg after endocytosis and lysosomal proteolysis. Disorders in all these steps have to be included in the diagnosis of Tg synthesis defects. The term must not be restricted to defects in the coding, splicing, or regulating part of the Tg gene itself (see Table 112–1).

Up till the 1960s it was believed that leakage of Tg out of the thyroidal follicles was completely prevented by the tight junctions connecting the thyrocytes. However with the introduction of radioimmunoassays, it became clear that besides thyroid hormone, also small amounts of Tg and other (iodinated) proteins are released into the circulation by the thyroid.[78] Various mechanisms underlying the enhanced release of Tg and other iodinated proteins under the influence of TSH or thyroid-stimulating antibodies have been described.[79]

Patients suffering from disorders in the synthesis of Tg are moderately to severely hypothyroid.[1] Usually the plasma Tg concentration is low, especially in relation to the TSH concentrations. Treatment with T_4 does not decrease[10, 80] and injection of TSH does not increase the plasma Tg concentration. However, there are exceptions, as, for example, in a patient with a high plasma concentration of a Tg antigen of low molecular weight.[81] Patients classified in the category "Tg synthesis defects" often have abnormal iodoproteins, mainly iodinated plasma albumin,[82] and they excrete iodopeptides of low molecular weight in the urine.[83]

In Afrikander cattle homozygous nonsense mutation, Arg697stop (exon 9), resulted in truncated Tg of 75 kDa. In this case also an alternatively spliced mRNA lacking exon 9 sequence was observed, encoding a Tg protein of 250 kDa.[54, 84] In Dutch goats a homozygous nonsense mutation, Tyr296stop, resulted in truncated Tg (40 kDa in vivo), causing hypothyroidism with goiter.[52, 85] Administration of extra iodine restored euthyroidism, but the goiter remained.[86] Furthermore, in a mouse model (cog/cog mouse), congenital goiter is linked to the Tg locus and is caused by a Leu2366Pro transition in the Tg molecule.[57] This defect resulted in an endoplasmic reticulum storage disease.

To date, mutations in the Tg gene have been elucidated only in four humans with CH and goiter. A homozygous mutation at the acceptor splice site of intron 3 gives an "in-frame" deletion in exon 4 (nc 275–478) from the Tg mRNA, resulting in an aberrant Tg protein lacking hormonogenic site Tyr130 and a Cys-Trp-Cys repeat.[55] Another patient with a homozygous in-frame mRNA deletion of 138 bp (nc 5552–5789) has been described.[58] The preferential accumulation of a Tg mRNA alternative splice product with an in-frame deletion of 171 bp (nc 4529–4699, exon 22) has also been reported, linked to a homozygous nonsense mutation at position 1510,[56] resulting in an endoplasmic reticulum storage disease as in the cog/cog mice.

Furthermore a homozygous nonsense mutation in the Tg mRNA of moderately hypothyroid patients with goiter has been described. A homozygous nonsense mutation, Arg277stop, resulted in a truncated Tg of 30 kDa. As in the Dutch goats the truncated Tg glycoprotein was still able to be iodinated and to synthesize thyroid hormone.[53]

Six CH patients[59] with the clinicopathologic characteristics of a Tg synthesis defect did not show any major mutations in the Tg mRNA, indicating that the clinicopathologic classification is not sufficiently specific to point out a particular molecular defect. Therefore we suggest defining the entity "Tg synthesis defect" in a broad sense so that defects along the whole process from transcription to exocytosis are included. In this way deficiency of essential factors for processing will also cause Tg synthesis defects. For example, deficiency of TTF1[60] can be classified under this denomination.

DEFECTS IN RECYCLING OF IODINE

Tg, internalized by (micro)pinocytosis from the follicular lumen, has been found to be present in the early and late endosomes. In these organelles, containing proteolytic enzymes, thyroid hormones are freed. The hydrolysate contains amino acids, including monoiodotyrosine (MIT) and diiodotyrosine (DIT). Subsequently MIT and DIT are deiodinated by a specific dehalogenase(s) found not only in the thyroid but also in many peripheral tissues. Hereditary disorders in this deiodinating system lead to excessive renal loss of iodine, in the form of MIT and DIT, mimicking hypothyroidism due to iodine deficiency.[61, 87] Patients with iodotyrosine dehalogenase deficiency have a high to very high initial radioiodide uptake, followed by a relatively rapid decline in the radioiodine content. Administration of perchlorate does not result in discharge, and much of the radioiodine is found in the form of radiolabeled MIT and DIT. The MIT and DIT formed by hydrolysis of Tg are not deiodinated, but released into the circulation. The wasting of tyrosine-bound iodine from the thyroid, enhanced by increased TSH secretion, may lead to an extremely low thyroidal iodine content. Since the enzyme(s) is also deficient in peripheral tissues (especially liver and kidney), the MIT and DIT are excreted as such in the urine.

Although the inheritance must be considered as autosomal recessive, some features of the disorder are expressed in heterozygous relatives. For example, in goiter, a relatively high radioiodide uptake and increased urinary DIT excretion are seen. The clinical expression strongly depends on the iodine content of the diet, which might explain why autosomal dominant inheritance has been suggested[88] in some families.

DIAGNOSIS

The great majority of patients with congenital hypothyroidism detected by neonatal screening have a thyroid malformation. Therefore, the first step in classification should be an imaging procedure, either ultrasonography or ^{123}I scintigraphy. If the infant has a normally shaped and located thyroid gland, irrespective of its size, further studies with ^{123}I will provide information about the thyroidal uptake of iodide, the response to perchlorate, and the saliva-blood ratio of radioiodine.

Measurements of serum Tg and low-molecular-weight iodopeptides in the urine help to discriminate between the various types of defects, and measurement of the total urinary iodine excretion helps to differentiate inborn errors from acquired, transient forms of hypothyroidism due to iodine deficiency or iodine excess. Because it is essential to treat the affected newborn infant without delay, blood and urine samples must be obtained immediately after referral. In an infant with severe hypothyroidism the radioiodide study may be done after T_4 therapy is started, so long as the patient's serum TSH concentration is high. However, if the infant has only a slightly low serum free T_4 concentration, the ^{123}I study should be performed either before the start of the treatment or several years later after interruption of T_4 therapy for at least 4 weeks. A definite determination of the underlying cause depends on elucidation of the responsible mutation in the genetic code.

TREATMENT

In general, treatment of a patient with a genetic defect in thyroid hormone secretion is the same as for any other hypothyroid patient of the same age and sex. Irrespective of the cause of congenital hypothyroidism, early treatment is mandatory to prevent cerebral damage. Therefore, the patient should be given sufficient T_4 to maintain normal plasma TSH concentrations[89] so that not only growth and development will be normal but also goiter will be prevented. In most of the genetic disorders the thyroid will eventually become hyperplastic and nodular if plasma TSH concentrations are even only slightly elevated for a longer period. However, if T_4 therapy is started at a very young age, and plasma TSH concentrations are maintained within the normal range, goiter should not occur. In patients who have elevated plasma Tg concentrations initially, maintaining them within the normal range will help to minimize thyroid growth. In patients with TSH deficiency, the optimal dose of T_4 must be based on determinations of the serum (free) T_4 concentration. In exceptional patients, like those with partial TSH hyporesponsiveness, hypothyroidism may be completely compensated and goiter does not occur. Yet, because establishing the correct etiologic diagnosis will take several weeks or longer, initially these patients should be treated immediately like any infant with CH.

REFERENCES

1. Vassart G, Dumont JE, Refetoff S. Thyroid disorders. *In* Scriver CR, Beaudet AL, Sly WS, Valle D (eds): The Metabolic and Molecular Bases of Inherited Disease, ed 7. New York, McGraw-Hill, 1995, pp 2883–2926.
2. Martino E, Bartalena L, Faglia G, Pinchera A: Central hypothyroidism. *In* Braverman LE, Utiger RD (eds): Werner and Ingbar's The Thyroid, ed 7. Philadelphia, Lippincott-Raven, 1996, pp 220–241.
3. Pendred V: Deaf mutism and goitre. Lancet 2:532, 1896.
4. Osler W: Sporadic cretinism in America. Trans Congress Am Physicians Surg 4:169–206, 1896.
5. Vulsma T, Gons MH, De Vijlder JJM: Maternal-fetal transfer of thyroxine in congenital hypothyroidism due to a total organification defect or thyroid agenesis. N Engl J Med 321:13, 1989.
6. Brown AL, Fernhoff PM, Milner J, et al: Racial differences in the incidence of congenital hypothyroidism. J Pediatr 99:934–936, 1981.
7. Rosenthal M, Addison GM, Price DA: Congenital hypothyroidism: Increased incidence in Asian families. Arch Dis Child 63:790–793, 1988.
8. LaFranchi SH, Hanna CE, Krainz PL, et al: Screening for congenital hypothyroidism with specimen collection at two time periods: Results of the Northwest Regional Screening program. Pediatrics 76:734–740, 1985.
9. Vulsma T, Delemarre HA, de Muinck Keizer SMPF, et al: Detection and classification of congenital thyrotropin deficiency in the Netherlands. *In* Drexhage HA, De Vijlder JJM, Wiersinga WM (eds): The Thyroid Gland, Environment and Autoimmunity. Amsterdam, Elsevier Science V, 1990, pp 343–346.
10. De Vijlder JJM, Vulsma T: Hereditary metabolic disorders causing hypothyroidism. *In* Braverman LE, Utiger RD (eds): Werner and Ingbar's The Thyroid, ed 7. Philadelphia, Lippincott-Raven, 1996, pp 749–755.
11. Dattani MT, Martinez-Barbera JP, Thomas PQ, et al: Mutations in the homeobox gene HESX1/hesx1 associated with septo-optic dysplasia in human and mouse. Nat Genet 19:125–133, 1998.
12. Collu R, Tang J, Castagne J, et al: A novel mechanism for isolated central hypothyroidism: Inactivating mutations in the thyrotropin-releasing hormone receptor gene. J Clin Endocrinol Metab 82:1561–1565, 1997.
13. Hinuma S, Hosoya M, Ogi K, et al: Molecular cloning and functional expression of a human thyrotropin-releasing hormone (TRH) receptor gene. Biochim Biophys Acta 1219:251–259, 1994.
14. Hayashizaki Y, Hiraoka Y, Tatsumi K, et al: Deoxyribonucleic acid analyses of five families with familial inherited thyroid stimulating hormone deficiency. J Clin Endocrinol Metab 71:792, 1990.
15. Dacou-Voutetakis C, Feltquate DM, Drakopoulou M, et al: Familial hypothyroidism caused by a nonsense mutation in the thyroid stimulating hormone beta-subunit gene. Am J Hum Genet 46:988, 1990.
16. Medeiros-Neto G, Herodotou DT, Rajan S, et al: A circulating biologically inactive thyrotropin caused by a mutation in the beta subunit gene. J Clin Invest 97:1250–1256, 1996.
17. Dracopoli NC, Retting WJ, Whitfield GK, et al: Assignment of the gene for the β-subunit of thyroid stimulating hormone to the short arm of human chromosome 1. Proc Natl Acad Sci U S A 83:1822, 1986.
18. Pfäffle RW, DiMattia GE, Parks JS, et al: Mutation of the POU-specific domain of Pit-1 and hypopituitarism without pituitary hypoplasia. Science 257:1118–1121, 1992.
19. Radovick S, Nations M, Du Y, Berg LA, et al: A mutation in the POU-homeodomain of Pit-1 responsible for combined pituitary hormone deficiency. Science 292:1115–1121, 1992.
20. Fofanova OV, Takamura N, Kinoshita E, et al: Rarity of PIT 1 involvement in children from Russia with combined pituitary hormone deficiency. Am J Med Genet 77:360–365, 1998.
21. Wu W, Cogan JD, Pfäffle RW, et al: Mutations in PROP1 cause familial combined pituitary hormone deficiency. Nat Genet 18:147–149, 1998.
22. Fofanova O, Takamura N, Kinoshita E, et al: Compound heterozygous deletion of the PROP-1 gene children with combined pituitary hormone deficiency. J Clin Endocrinol Metab 83:2601–2604, 1998.
23. Rosenbloom AL, Selman Almonte A, Brown MR, et al: Clinical and biochemical phenotype of familial anterior hypopituitarism from mutation of the PROP1 gene. J Clin Endocrinol Metab 84:50–57, 1999.
24. Rousseau-Merck MF, Misrahi M, Loosfelt H, et al: Assignment of the human TSH receptor gene to chromosome 14q31. Genomics 8:233–236, 1990.
25. Sunthornthepvarakul T, Gottschalk ME, Hayashi Y, Refetoff S: Resistance to thyrotropin caused by mutations in the thyrotropin receptor gene. N Engl J Med 332:155–160, 1995.
26. Biebermann H. Schöneberg T, Krude H, et al: Mutations of the human thyrotropin receptor gene causing thyroid hypoplasia and persistent congenital hypothyroidism. J Clin Endocrinol Metab 82:3471–3480, 1997.
27. Gagné N, Parma J, Deal G, et al: Apparent congenital athyreosis contrasting with normal plasma thyroglobulin levels and associated with inactivating mutations in the thyrotropin receptor gene: Are athyreosis and ectopic thyroid distinct entities? J Clin Endocrinol Metab 83:1771–1775, 1998.
28. Spiegel AM, Shenker A, Weinstein LS: Receptor-effector coupling by G proteins: Implications for normal and abnormal signal transduction. Endocr Rev 13:536–565, 1992.
29. Xie J, Pannain S, Pohlenz J, et al: Resistance to thyrotropin (TSH) in three families is not associated with mutations in the TSH receptor or TSH. J Clin Endocrinol Metab 82:3933–3940, 1997.
30. Kopp P, van Sande J, Parma J, et al: Congenital hyperthyroidism caused by a mutation in the thyrotropin receptor gene. N Engl J Med 332:150, 1995.
31. Macchia PE, Lapi P, Krude H, et al: PAX8 mutations associated with congenital hypothyroidism caused by thyroid dysgenesis. Nat Genet 19:83–86, 1998.
32. Chadwick BP, Obermayr F, Frischauf A-M: FKHL15, a new human member of the forkhead gene family located on chromosome 9q22. Genomics 41:390–396, 1997.
33. Clifton-Bligh RJ, Wentworth JM, Heinz P, et al: Mutation of the gene encoding human TTF-2 associated with thyroid agenesis, cleft palate and choanal atresia. Nat Genet 19:399–401, 1998.
34. Smanik PA, Ryu KY, Theil KS, et al: Expression, exon-intron organization and chromosome mapping of the human sodium iodide symporter. Endocrinology 138:3555–3558, 1997.
35. Fujiwara H, Tatsumi K, Miki K, et al: Congenital hypothyroidism caused by a missense mutation in the Na^+/I^- symporter. [erratum Nat Genet 17:122, 1997]. Nat Genet 16:124–125, 1997.
36. Pohlenz J, Medeiros-Neto G, Gross JL, et al: Hypothyroidism in a Brazilian kindred due to iodide trapping defect caused by a homozygous mutation in the sodium/iodide symporter gene. Biochem Biophys Res Commun. 240:488–491, 1997.
37. Pohlenz J, Rosenthal IM, Weiss RE, et al: Congenital hypothyroidism due to mutations in the sodium/iodide symporter. J Clin Invest 101:1028–1035, 1998.
38. Kimura S, Hong US, Kotani T, et al: Structure of the human thyroid peroxidase gene: Comparison and relationship to the human myeloperoxidase gene. Biochemistry 28:4481, 1989.
39. Libert F, Ruel J, Ludgate M, et al: Thyroperoxidase, an autogen with a mosaic structure made of nuclear and mitochondrial gene modules. EMBO J 6:4193, 1987.
40. De Vijlder JJM, Dinsart C, Libert F, et al: Regional localization of the gene for thyroid peroxidase to human chromosome 2pter-p12. Cytogenet Cell Genet 47:170, 1988.
41. Barnett PS, Jones TA, McGregor AM, et al: Regional sublocalization of the human thyroid peroxidase gene (TPO) by tritium and fluorescence in situ hybridization to chromosome 2p25p24. Cytogenet Cell Genet 62:88, 1993.

42. Medeiros-Neto G, Stanbury JB: Inherited Disorders of the Thyroid System. Boca Raton, FL, CRC Press, 1994, pp 1–22.
43. Bikker H, Bakker E, Vulsma T, De Vijlder JJM: Identification of two novel mutations in the TPO gene of patients with severe congenital hypothyroidism due to a total iodide organification defect.—Frequency of TPO inactivating mutations. J Endocrinol Invest 21:82, 1998.
44. Niepomiszcze H, Rosenbloom AL, DeGroot LJ, et al: Differentiation defect of two abnormalities in thyroid peroxidase causing organification defect and goitrous hypothyroidism. Metabolism 24:57, 1975.
45. Sjollema BE, Den Hartog MT, De Vijlder JJM, et al: Congenital hypothyroidism in two cats due to defective organification: Data suggesting loosely anchored thyroperoxidase. Acta Endocrinol 125:435–440, 1991.
46. Niepomiszcze H, Castells S, DeGroot LE, et al: Peroxidase defect in congenital goiter with complete organification block. J Clin Endocrinol Metab 36:347, 1973.
47. Niepomiszcze H, Targovnik HM, Gluzman BE, et al: Abnormal H_2O_2 supply in the thyroid of a patient with goiter and iodine organification defect. J Clin Endocrinol Metab 65:344, 1987.
48. Everett LA, Glaser B, Beck JC, et al: Pendred syndrome is caused by mutations in a putative sulphate transporter gene (PDS). Nat Genet 17:411–422, 1997.
48a. Scott DA, Wang R, Kreman TM, et al: The Pendred syndrome gene encodes a chloride-iodide transporter protein. Nat Genet 21:440–443, 1999.
49. Van Hauwe P, Everett LA, Coucke P, et al: Two frequent missense mutations in Pendred syndrome. Hum Mol Genet 7:1099–1104, 1998.
50. Li XC, Everett LA, Lalwani AK, et al: A mutation on PDS causes non-syndromic recessive deafness. Nat Genet 18:215–217, 1998.
51. Baas F, Bikker H, Geurts van Kessel A, et al: The human thyroglobulin gene: A polymorphic marker localized distal to c myc on chromosome 8 band q24. Hum Genet 67:301–305, 1985.
52. Veenboer GJM, De Vijlder JJM: Molecular basis of the thyroglobulin synthesis defect in Dutch goats. Endocrinology 132:377–381, 1993.
53. Van de Graaf SAR, Ris-Stalpers C, Veenboer GJM, et al: A premature stopcodon in thyroglobulin mRNA results in familial goiter and moderate hypothyroidism. J Clin Endocrinol Metab 84:2537–2542, 1999.
54. Ricketts MH, Simons MJ, Parma J, et al: A nonsense mutation caused hereditary goitre in the Afrikander cattle and unmasks alternative splicing of thyroglobulin transcripts. Proc Natl Acad Sci U S A 84:3181–3184, 1987.
55. Ieiri T, Cochaux R, Targovnik HM, et al: A 3′ splice site mutation in the thyroglobulin gene responsible for congenital goiter with hypothyroidism. J Clin Invest 88:1901–1905, 1991.
56. Targovnik HM, Medeiros-Neto G, Varela V, et al: A nonsense mutation causes human hereditary congenital goiter with preferential production of a 171-nucleotide-deleted thyroglobulin ribonucleic acid messenger. J Clin Endocrinol Metab 77:210–215, 1993.
57. Kim PS, Hossain SA, Park YN, et al: A single amino acid change in the acetylcholesterase-like domain of thyroglobulin causes congenital goiter with hypothyroidism in the cog/cog mouse, a model of human endoplasmatic storage diseases. Proc Natl Acad Sci U S A 95:9909–9912, 1998.
58. Targovnik HM, Vono J, Billerbeck AEC, et al: A 138-nucleotide-deletion in the thyroglobulin ribonucleic acid messenger in a congenital goiter with defective thyroglobulin synthesis. J Clin Endocrinol Metab 80:3356–3360, 1995.
59. Van de Graaf SAR, Cammenga C, Ponne NH, et al: The screening for mutations in the thyroglobulin cDNA from six patients with congenital hypothyroidism. Biochimie 81:425–532, 1999.
60. Acebron A, Aza-Blanc P, Rossi DL, et al: Congenital human thyroglobulin defect due to low expression of thyroid-specific transcription factor. J Clin Invest 96:781, 1995.
61. Choufour JC, Kassenaar AAH, Querido A: The syndrome of congenital hypothyroidism with defective dehalogenation of iodotyrosines. Further observations and a discussion of the pathophysiology. J Clin Endocrinol Metab 20:983, 1960.
62. Wondisford F, Magner JA, Weintraub BD: Thyrotropin: Chemistry and biosynthesis of thyrotropin. *In* Braverman LE, Utiger RD (eds): Werner and Ingbar's The Thyroid ed 7. Philadelphia, Lippincott-Raven, 1996, pp 190–207.
63. Miyai K, Azukizawa M, Kumahara Y: Familial isolated thyrotropin deficiency with cretinism. N Engl J Med 285:1043–1048, 1971.
64. Parma J, Duprez L, Van Sande J, et al: Somatic mutations in the thyrotropin receptor gene cause hyperfunctioning thyroid ademoma. Nature 365:649–651, 1993.
65. Duprez L, Parma J, Van Sande J, et al: Germline mutations in the thyrotropin receptor gene cause non-autosomal dominant hyperthyroidism. Nat Genet 7:396–401, 1994.
66. Kopp P, Van Sande J, Parma J, et al: Congenital hyperthyroidism caused by a mutation in the thyrotropin-receptor gene. N Engl J Med 332:150–154, 1995.
67. Albright F, Burnett CH, Smith PH, Parson W: Pseudohypoparathyroidism: An example of "Seabright-Bantam syndrome." Report of three cases. Endocrinology 30:922, 1942.
68. Damante G. Thyroid defects due to Pax8 gene mutations. Eur J Endocrinol. 139:563–566, 1998.
69. Tell G, Pellizarri L, Cimarosti D, et al: Ref-1 controls Pax-8 DNA-binding activity. Biochem Biophys Res Com 252:178–183, 1998.
70. Dai G, Levy O, Carrasco N: Cloning and characterisation of the thyroid iodide symporter. Nature 379:458–460, 1996.
71. Caillou B, Troalen F, Baudin E, et al: Na^+/I^- symporter distribution in human thyroid tissues: An immunohistochemical study. J Clin Endocrinol Metab 83:4101–4106, 1998.
72. Levy O, Ginter CS, De la Vieja A, et al: Identification of a structural requirement for thyroid $Na^+/I-$symporter (NIS) junction from analysis of a mutation that causes human congenital hypothyroidism. FEBS Lett 429:36–40, 1998.
73. Vulsma T, Rammeloo JA, Gons MH, De Vijlder JJM: The role of serum thyroglobulin concentration and thyroid ultrasound imaging in the detection of iodide transport defects in infants. Acta Endocrinol 124:405–410, 1991.
73a. Dupuy C, Ohayon R, Valent A, et al: Purification of a novel flavoprotein involved in the thyroid NADPH oxidase. Cloning of the porcine and human cDNAs. J Biol Chem 274:37265–37269, 1999.
74. De Vijlder JJM, Den Hartog MT: Anionic iodotyrosine residues are required for iodothyronine synthesis. Eur J Endocrinol 138:227–231, 1998.
75. Bikker H, Baas F, De Vijlder JJM: Molecular analysis of mutated thyroid peroxidase detected in patients with total iodide organification defects. J Clin Endocrinol Metab 82:649–653, 1997.
76. Van de Graaf SAR, Pauws E, De Vijlder JJM, Ris-Stalpers C: The revised 8307 base pair coding sequence of human thyroglobulin transiently expressed in eukaryotic cells. Eur J Endocrinol 136:508–515, 1997.
76a. Mendive FM, Rivolta CM, Vassart G, Targovnik HM: Genomic organization of the 3′ region of the human thyroglobulin gene. Thyroid 9:903–912, 1999.
77. Malthièry Y, Lissitzky S: The primary structure of human thyroglobulin deduced from the sequence of its 8448 base complementary DNA. Eur J Biochem 165:491–498, 1987.
78. Spencer CA: Thyroglobulin. *In* Braverman LE, Utiger RD (eds): Werner and Ingbar's The Thyroid, ed 7. Philadelphia, Lippincott-Raven; 1996, pp 406–415.
79. De Vijlder JJM, Ris-Stalpers C, Vulsma T: On the origin of circulating thyroglobulin. Eur J Endocrinol 140:7–8, 1999.
80. Medeiros-Neto GA, Marcondes JA, Cavaliere H, et al: Serum thyroglobulin (Tg) stimulation with bovine TSH: A useful test for diagnosis for congenital goitrous hypothyroidism due to defective Tg synthesis. Acta Endocrinol 110:61–65, 1985.
81. Enrique J, Santelices R, Hishihara M, Schneider A: Low molecular weight thyroglobulin leading to a goiter in a 12 year old girl. J Clin Endocrinol Metab 58:526, 1984.
82. De Vijlder JJM, Veenboer GJM, van Dijk JE: Thyroid albumin originates from blood. Endocrinology 131:578, 1992.
83. Gons MH, Kok JH, Tegelaers WHH, De Vijlder JJM: Concentration of plasma thyroglobulin and urinary excretion of iodinated material in the diagnosis of thyroid disorders in congenital hypothyroidism. Acta Endocrinol 104:27, 1983.
84. Tassi VPN, Di Lauro R, van Jaarsveld P, Alvino CG: Two abnormal thyroglobulin-like polypeptides are produced from Afrikander cattle congenital goiter mRNA. J Biol Chem 259:10507–10510, 1984.
85. Sterk A, van Dijk JE, Veenboer GJM, et al: Normal sized thyroglobulin mRNA in Dutch goats with a thyroglobulin synthesis defect is translated into a 35,000 molecular weight N-terminal fragment. Endocrinology 124:477–183, 1989.
86. Van Voorthuizen WF, De Vijlder JJM, van Dijk JE, Tegelaers WHH: Euthyroidism via iodide supplementation in hereditary congenital goiter with thyroglobulin deficiency. Endocrinology 103:2105, 1978.
87. Stanbury JB, Kassenaar AAH, Meijer JWA, Terpstra J: The occurrence of mono- and di-iodotyrosine in the blood of a patient with congenital goiter. J Clin Endocrinol Metab 15: 1216, 1955.
88. Ismail-Beigi F, Rahimifar M: A variant of iodotyrosine-dehalogenase deficiency. J Clin Endocrinol Metab 44:499, 1977.
89. Alemzadeh R, Friedman S, Fort P, et al: Is there compensated hypothyroidism in infancy? Pediatrics 90:70, 1992.

Chapter 113

Transport Protein Variants

Jan R. Stockigt

It was shown almost 60 years ago that circulating thyroid hormones bind noncovalently to plasma proteins.[1] As discussed in Chapter 94, well over 99% of circulating thyroxine (T_4) and triiodothyronine (T_3) is protein bound in normal plasma. At a normal total T_4 concentration of 60 to 140 nmol/L, only 10 to 25 pmol/L exists in the free state at equilibrium, which yields an unbound fraction of 1:3000 to 1:4000. The free fraction of T_3 is approximately 10-fold higher. About 70% of the circulating T_4 is normally bound to thyroxine-binding globulin (TBG), with the rest distributed about equally between transthyretin (TTR, or prealbumin) and albumin. It should be noted that the bound and free moieties are in constant rapid equilibrium, with the bound portion serving as a reservoir to almost instantaneously replenish the free hormone concentration as this fraction enters cells or is irreversibly cleared.

Numerous important structural variants of the three major thyroid hormone-binding proteins have been described (Table 113–1). These proteins were initially recognized from the investigation of euthyroid subjects who showed markedly abnormal levels of total serum T_4 or T_3, but more recently, variants have been identified from population screening and genetic studies. The total concentrations of serum T_4 and T_3 range widely in association with variant binding proteins, but none of the multiple hereditary binding alterations has been shown to confer any advantage or disadvantage or to produce any disturbance in thyroid hormone action, unless associated thyroid disease is present. Plasma thyroid-stimulating hormone (TSH) concentrations remain normal, as do free T_4 and T_3 concentrations, provided that the method of estimation is free of artifact. In general, TBG abnormalities tend to affect T_4 and T_3 similarly; by contrast, some albumin variants lead to selective abnormalities in T_4 or T_3 binding.

The estimated proportion of total circulating T_4 carried on the three major binding proteins in the various binding anomalies reported to date in euthyroid subjects is consistent with the hypothesis that each class of binding protein is in separate reversible equilibrium with the free moiety of plasma T_4. Proportional carriage of T_4 is determined by the concentration and affinity of each class of binding site. In contrast, the *occupancy* of each binding site at a normal free hormone concentration relates solely to affinity. (The equilibrium dissociation constant, K_d, is defined as the free hormone concentration that would result in half-occupancy of that binding site.) The proportional carriage of T_4 on normal and variant binding proteins is summarized in Figure 113–1.

Variants of iodothyronine-binding proteins have attracted the attention of clinicians and basic scientists for numerous reasons:

1. Effect on diagnostic tests. In euthyroid subjects, abnormal total T_4 or T_3 concentrations occur in association with normal free hormone concentrations. Particularly with the albumin variants, method-dependent artifacts may compromise measurements of free and occasionally total T_4 or T_3.
2. Modes of inheritance. TBG variants are X-linked, whereas TTR and albumin variants show autosomal dominant inheritance.
3. Structure-function relationships of specific hormone-binding sites can be studied by using the large amount of material available in

TABLE 113–1. Known Human Variants of Thyroid Hormone-Binding Proteins

Protein	Circulating Protein Concentration	T_4-Binding Affinity	Number of Variants
TBG	Undetectable	—	6
	Low	Low	6
	Normal	Normal	1
	Normal	Undetectable	1
	High	Normal	1
TTR*	?Normal	Undetectable	1
	?Normal	Low	5
	?Normal	Normal	3
	Normal/high	Increased	4
Albumin	Normal	Increased	3†
	Undetectable	—	1

*The T_4-binding affinity of over 30 additional variants remains undefined.

†One variant has selective affinity for triiodothyronine. T_4, thyroxine; TBG, thyroxine-binding globulin; TTR, transthyretin. Data from Refetoff et al.,[4] Carvalho et al.,[9] Sunthornthepvarakul et al.,[26] and Rosen et al.[41]

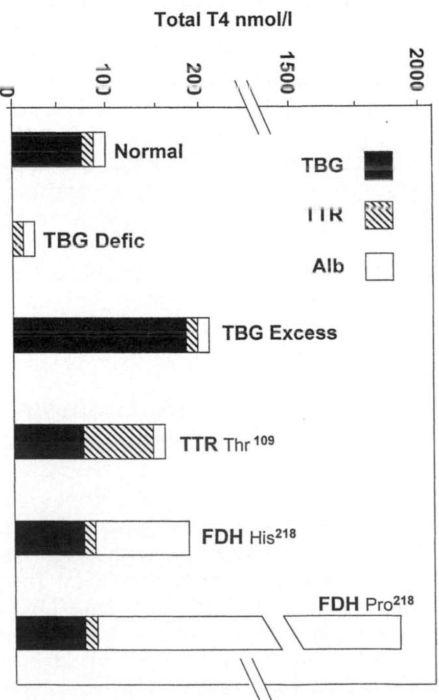

FIGURE 113–1. Estimated proportional carriage of thyroxin (T_4) on the three major plasma binding proteins is shown for euthyroid subjects with normal or variant T_4-binding proteins. In the face of normal free T_4 and thyroid-stimulating hormone (TSH) concentrations, the concentration of total T_4 can vary from about 25 nmol/L in total thyroxine-binding globulin (TBG) deficiency to about 1800 nmol/L in the Pro218 variant of familial dysalbuminemic hyperthyroxinemia described in several Japanese kindreds.

serum. Albumin variants have shown how structural changes can *increase* the binding affinity for a particular ligand. In contrast, TBG mutants show either normal or diminished binding affinity, often associated with abnormal heat lability of the protein.

4. The effects of variant binding proteins on T_4 and T_3 distribution, clearance, and delivery to tissues can test whether it is the free hormone concentration, as determined at equilibrium, that determines hormone clearance and action.

5. Other associated pathology, for example, familial amyloidosis with some TTR variants, can elucidate the tissue effects of abnormal proteins.

In contrast to the multitude of clearly defined plasma protein-binding variants, the possibility of genetically determined abnormalities in cell membrane transport, cytoplasmic binding, or deiodination of iodothyronines remains ill defined and speculative (see below).

THYROXINE-BINDING GLOBULIN

TBG is a single polypeptide chain α-globulin with a molecular weight of about 54 kDa synthesized as a 415–amino acid protein.[2–4] The first 20 amino acid residues of the TBG peptide are hydrophobic and probably represent the signal peptide removed in the endoplasmic reticulum, with a mature protein of 395 amino acids in a single chain having a molecular weight of about 44 kDa remaining. Multiple glycosylation sites allow an average of 10 terminal sialic acid moieties. The carbohydrate moieties of TBG influence protein half-life in blood, stability in vitro, and microheterogeneity on electrophoresis, with only minor effects on immunoreactivity or T_4-binding capacity. Although TBG is stable in stored serum at 4°C, it gradually loses its binding affinity for T_4 at 37°C or above. Differences in the rate of loss of binding affinity at raised temperature have been important in identifying TBG variants.

The amino acid sequence of human TBG shows homology with rat TBG (70%), human cortisol-binding globulin (55%), and members of the serum protease inhibitor family (SERPINS), which includes α-antitrypsin (53% homology) and α_1-antichymotrypsin (58% homology).[5] The significance of the structural similarity between human TBG, cortisol-binding globulin, and the SERPINS remains unclear; the hormone-binding proteins appear to be devoid of antiprotease activity.

The normal concentration of human plasma TBG as measured by radioimmunoassay is between 10 and 30 mg/L (0.2–0.6 μmol/L). TBG is normally 20% to 40% occupied by T_4 and less than 1% occupied by T_3. Occupancy may increase markedly in hyperthyroidism as a result of both an increase in total T_4 and a decrease in TBG concentration, which leads to a disproportionate rise in free T_4 relative to total T_4. T_4-binding affinity (K_d) is about 50 pmol/L at 37°C, consistent with the estimate that TBG is approximately 30% occupied by T_4 at the normal free T_4 concentration of about 20 pmol/L.[6]

Hereditary Thyroxine-Binding Globulin Variants

The single 8-kb human TBG gene has been localized to the X chromosome at site Xq22.2.[7] Male hemizygotes, who express only the mutant allele, can show one of three variant phenotypes for T_4 binding to TBG: increase, decrease, or absolute deficiency. Despite the presence of two X chromosomes, normal females have TBG levels similar to the levels in males. Females heterozygous for complete TBG deficiency usually show less than the anticipated 50% reduction in serum TBG, a phenomenon attributed to selective inactivation of the mutant allele.[4] However, selective inactivation of the normal allele may occasionally result in females showing complete deficiency of TBG.[8]

Multiple inherited TBG variants, often designated geographically, can result in partial or complete deficiency of immunoreactive TBG in serum. Of at least 15 known X-linked TBG mutants, 6 cause complete TBG deficiency and at least 6 other types are associated with reduced affinity for T_4, often in connection with subnormal concentrations of immunoreactive serum TBG.[2–4, 9] The structural basis

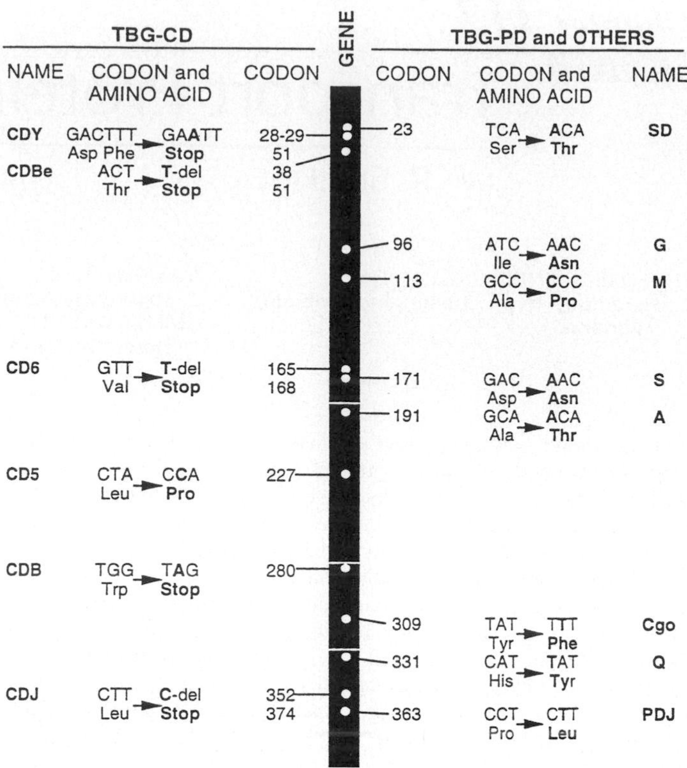

FIGURE 113–2. Locations on the thyroxine-binding globulin (TBG) gene of mutations that cause either complete deficiency *(left)* or partial deficiency *(right)* of TBG in plasma. Mutations are distributed throughout the TBG gene with no "hot spots" and no correlation between the site of the mutation and the phenotype. CD, complete deficiency; PD, partial deficiency. Nucleotide and amino acid mutations are shown in *bold type*. TBG variants are designated as follows: Y, Yonago; Be, Bedouin; B, Buffalo; J, Japan; SD, San Diego; G, Gary: M. Montreal; S, Slow; A, Aborigine; Cgo, Chicago; Q, Quebec variants. (From Carvalho GA, Weiss RE, Refetoff S: Complete thyroxine-binding globulin (TBG) deficiency produced by a mutation in acceptor splice site causing frameshift and early termination of translation (TBG-Kanakee). J Clin Endocrinol Metab 83:3604–3608, © 1998, The Endocrine Society.)

of these variants is summarized in Figure 113–2. In numerous instances, variants of TBG show increased heat lability in vitro, which generally correlates with accelerated clearance in vivo. Classifications based on heat lability and T_4-binding affinity and on DNA sequencing have replaced earlier distinctions made on the basis of electrophoretic mobility. In general, the various methods of serum free T_4 estimation, as well as binding corrections based on T_3 uptake measurements, give a useful semiquantitative correction for TBG abnormalities, whether hereditary or acquired.

In total TBG deficiency, total T_4 is about 25 nmol/L (see Fig. 113–1), with normal free T_4 and TSH concentrations. By contrast, in hemizygous TBG excess, the total T_4 concentration is typically greater than 200 nmol/L, over 80% of which is carried on TBG (see Fig. 113–1). The amount of T_4 that is bound to TBG (relative to normal) and the concentrations of immunoreactive normal and denatured TBG in several mutants are shown in Figure 113–3.[4] TBG deficiency (complete or partial) can be attributed to single nucleotide deletions or substitutions that lead to a frameshift and premature termination of translation to produce a truncated protein that is retained and degraded intracellularly.[2–4]

From newborn screening studies, the prevalence of partial TBG deficiency in males is about 1 in 5000, with 1 in 15,000 showing complete deficiency.[4] Hereditary TBG excess, probably caused by gene duplication,[10] appears to have a prevalence of about 1 in 25,000 in newborn males.[4] The binding of T_4 to TBG with inherited X-linked TBG excess is indistinguishable from T_4 binding to the common type of TBG. In contrast to the albumin variants, no known TBG mutant shows increased T_4-binding affinity.

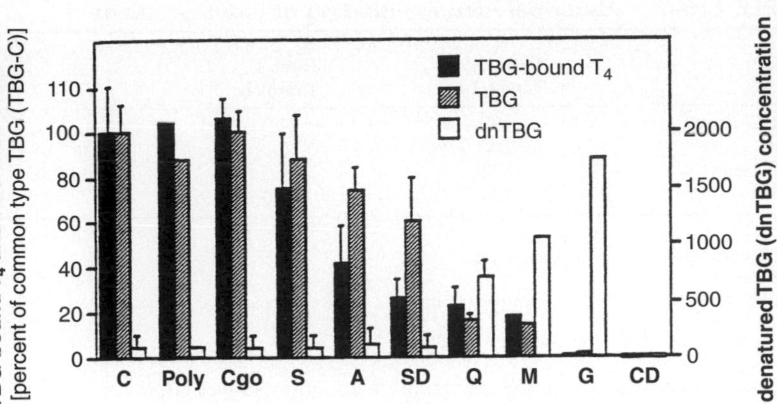

FIGURE 113–3. Serum thyroxine (T_4) bound to thyroxine-binding globulin (TBG) expressed as a percentage of normal binding, together with serum concentrations of immunoreactive TBG and denatured TBG found in hemizygous subjects with various TBG mutants. Abbreviations are as in Figure 113–2. Poly, polymorphic. (From Refetoff S, Murata Y, Mori Y, et al: Thyroxine-binding globulin: Organisation of the gene and variants. Horm Res 45:128–138, 1996.)

Diminished TBG binding of T_4 is especially prevalent in some ethnic groups, for example, among Australian aborigines, up to 30% of whom have subnormal serum concentrations of total T_4 associated with subnormal serum concentrations of an abnormally heat-labile TBG that shows subnormal affinity for T_4.[11] Because of a very high gene frequency in this population, the pattern of inheritance was initially thought to be autosomal dominant.[12] Abnormal heat lability at 37°C was found in both male and female subjects from affected families, but the pattern of intermediate heat lability was found exclusively in female subjects,[13] thus demonstrating that inheritance must be X-linked (Fig. 113–4). Of particular interest are a variant with markedly increased heat stability (TBG-Chicago)[14] and a variant with an extremely heat-labile protein having an abnormally high concentration of denatured TBG and subnormal total T_4 (TBG-Gary).[15]

ALBUMIN

Human serum albumin, a highly conserved 66-kDa nonglycoprotein,[16] has a molar plasma concentration of approximately 600 μmol/L, which corresponds to about 40 g/L. As well as being the principal carrier of numerous hydrophobic compounds in serum, albumin binds T_4 in its region 2, with an affinity about four orders of magnitude less than that of normal TBG. Albumin normally carries 10% to 15% of the circulating T_4, but the proportion of albumin occupied by T_4 is less than 0.002%.

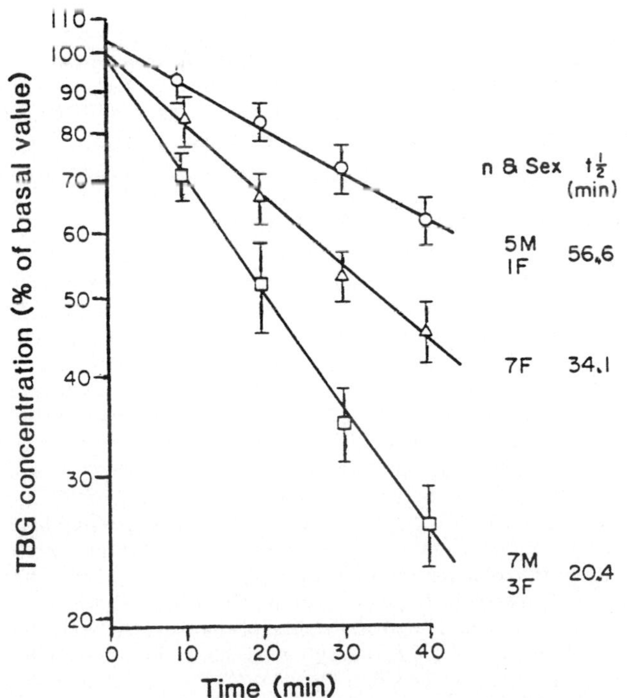

FIGURE 113–4. Heat stability of thyroxine-binding globulin (TBG) at 56°C in sera from Australian aborigines. Both male and female subjects showed either normal *(upper line)* or markedly reduced *(lower line)* stability. No male subject showed the intermediate affinity *(middle line)* which demonstrates the heterozygous state, thereby confirming X-linked inheritance. (From Refetoff S, Murata Y: X-chromosome–linked inheritance of the variant thyroxine-binding globulin in Australian aborigines. J Clin Endocrinol Metal 60:356–360, © 1985, The Endocrine Society.)

Hereditary Albumin Variants

Hyperthyroxinemia results from variant albumin with increased affinity for T_4 or T_3, the total albumin concentration being normal (Table 113–2). In familial dysalbuminemic hyperthyroxinemia (FDH), the total T_4 concentration in affected individuals is about 200 nM,[17, 18] with over 50% of T_4 carried on the variant albumin (see Fig. 113–1). FDH appears to be the most common hereditary T_4-binding abnormality, with a prevalence as high as 1 in 1000 in some Latin-American populations.[19] As with other variants that show enhanced binding affinity or capacity, the increased concentration of total circulating T_4 appears to be an appropriate response to maintain a normal free T_4 concentration in a feedback relationship with TSH.[18]

In FDH, Scatchard analysis of albumin binding shows two T_4-binding sites, a normal site with a K_d 4.3 mmol/L and an abnormal site with 50- to 100-fold higher affinity and a K_d of 50 mmol/L.[20] The capacity of the higher-affinity T_4-binding site is approximately 200 mmol/L, which suggests that relative to the molar concentration of albumin, at least one-third of albumin molecules have the abnormal binding site.[20] As a result, the occupancy of albumin by T_4 increases fivefold to about 0.01%. This variant is due to an Arg-His substitution at position 218 of human albumin.[21] The recombinant His218 protein has a T_4 affinity 65-fold greater than normal,[22] similar to the affinity reported for the natural protein more than a decade before.[20]

In FDH, because of a markedly increased affinity of the variant protein for numerous T_4 analogue tracers (Fig. 113–5), serum free T_4 measured by analogue-based methods gives results suggestive of thyrotoxicosis.[23] Greater albumin binding of tracer in samples than in standards makes less tracer available for binding to the assay antibody and thereby leads to spuriously high free T_4 estimates.

Kinetic studies in vivo show altered distribution of T_4 in favor of the extracellular compartment and a reduced metabolic clearance rate of T_4. However, the intracellular T_4 pool size and T_4 disposal rate are normal in patients with FDH, consistent with the normal serum free T_4 in these euthyroid subjects.[24]

A related autosomal dominant albumin variant at the same site (Arg218Pro), thus far reported only in Japanese,[25] shows an even higher selective affinity for T_4 than the common FDH phenotype found in whites. In euthyroid subjects with normal TSH, total T_4 is almost 20-fold elevated at about 1800 nmol/L (see Fig. 113–1), whereas total T_3 is only about 2-fold elevated. Free T_4 estimates using an analogue tracer also show spurious elevations in this variant.[25]

To explain the mechanism of increased T_4 affinity in both types of FDH it has been suggested that the guanidino group of arginine 218 may normally give an unfavorable binding interaction with T_4. Histi-

TABLE 113–2. Abnormal Albumin Binding of Iodothyronines

	Total T_4* (mmol/L)	Total T_3 (mmol/L)	Relative Affinity T_4	Relative Affinity T_3	Mutation	References
Normal serum	100	2.0	1	1	—	
FDH	200	2.2	50	1.5	Arg218His	17–22
FDH Japan†	1800	4.0	>1000‡	?	Arg218Pro	25
FDH T_3	120	5.0	1.5	40	Leu66Pro	26

*Free T_4 is normal by valid methods.
†FDH type described in Japanese kindreds.[25]
‡Predicted.
FDH, familial dysalbuminemic hyperthyroxinemia; T_3, triiodothyronine; T_4, thyroxine.

dine or proline, which lack the guanidino group, allow higher-affinity binding than is found with wild-type albumin.[25]

A recent report has described a mutation of the albumin gene at a different site (Leu66Pro) with selective affinity for T_3 rather than T_4.[26] Eight euthyroid members of a Thai family showed total T_3 levels of 4 to 8 nmol/L (normal, 1.0–2.6) when measured by radioimmunoassay with I^{125}-labeled T_3. Free T_3 and free T_4 were normal. This mutant albumin was estimated to have 40-fold higher T_3 affinity than normal albumin, but only 1.5-fold higher affinity for T_4. In this variant, spuriously *low* total T_3 values were found when T_3 conjugates were used as a tracer in enzyme-linked immunosorbent assays.[26] These anomalous results probably occur because conjugate tracers, linked to either alkaline phosphatase or peroxidase, showed *less* binding to the variant albumin than to the normal protein, which makes *more* tracer available for binding to antibody in samples than in the standard, thereby giving spuriously low assay values. This artifact is the inverse of that found with analogue-based free T_4 estimates in the common type of FDH.

Only a few cases of total hereditary analbuminemia have been described in humans, but one kindred was reported to have evidence of mild TSH excess,[27] consistent with impaired thyroid hormone delivery. In contrast, the Nagase strain of analbuminemic rat showed no evidence of any abnormality of thyroid hormone action or distribution.[28]

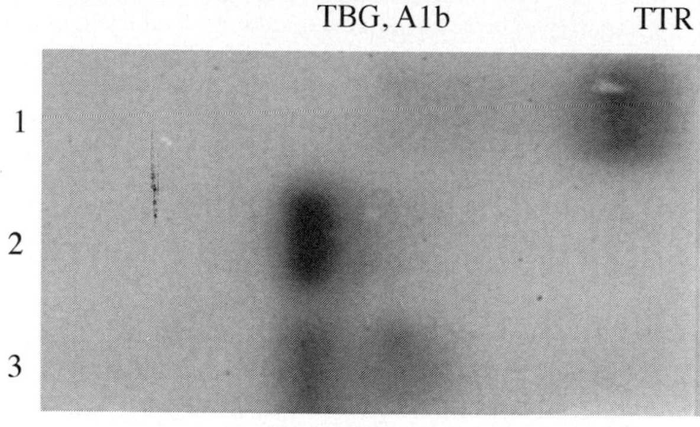

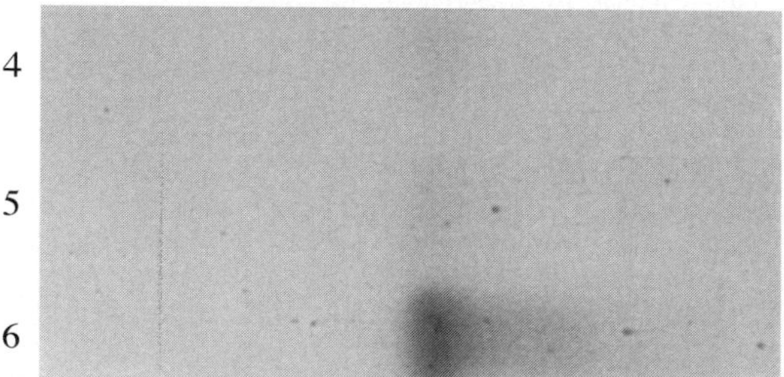

FIGURE 113–5. Autoradiography after polyacrylamide gel electrophoresis of serum containing either ^{125}I-labeled thyroxine (T_4) (1, 2, 3) or an ^{125}I-labeled T_4 analogue tracer from a commercial one-step free T_4 assay (4, 5, 6). Sera were from thyroxine-binding globulin (TBG)-deficient (1, 4), normal (2, 5), and familial dysalbuminemic hyperthyroxinemia (FDH) subjects (3, 6). ^{125}I-labeled T_4 shows increased binding to albumin in FDH His218. The labeled analogue shows weak binding to normal albumin and much increased albumin binding in FDH serum, thus explaining the spuriously high free T_4 values found in FDH with analogue tracers.

TRANSTHYRETIN

TTR (previously known as prealbumin), a protein of approximately 55 kDa that circulates in the serum of a wide range of vertebrates, is a tetramer consisting of four identical polypeptide chains held together by noncovalent bonds. Each monomer is a 127–amino acid chain regulated by a single gene on chromosome 18. The tetramer is symmetric about a central cavity, which completely penetrates the molecule and contains two T_4-binding sites, one at each end of the central cavity.[29]

The normal serum concentration of TTR in healthy humans (2–8 μmol/L, 100–400 mg/L) can decrease rapidly during acute illness or malnutrition as a result of reduced hepatic synthesis.[30] At normal concentrations, TTR is less than 1% occupied by T_4, with an affinity for T_4 intermediate between that of TBG and albumin ($K_d \sim 10$ nmol/L) and about 10-fold lower affinity for T_3. The liver is the principal site of synthesis of TTR, but the choroid plexus[31] and the pancreatic islets[32] are additional sites of TTR synthesis. In evolutionary terms, TTR synthesis at the choroid plexus long preceded the ontogeny of TTR synthesis in the liver.[33] The T_4-binding domain of TTR appears to have been conserved over the past 350 million years.[33]

Hereditary Transthyretin Variants

Many autosomal dominant TTR variants characterized by single–amino acid substitutions have been described in humans, some found in association with familial amyloidosis.[34] Mutant forms of TTR can accumulate in the extracellular space as aggregates of insoluble fibrillar protein and cause familial amyloid polyneuropathy or cardiomyopathy.[34] Complete deficiency of TTR has never been described in humans, which suggests that a deficiency of this protein might be lethal. However, TTR-null mice produced by gene knockout show no obvious abnormality in thyroid hormone metabolism or action.[35]

The Thr109 TTR variant[36] can give rise to mild hyperthyroxinemia with a total T_4 concentration of 160 to 200 nmol/L,[37] along with some increase in the total concentration of TTR.[37] Kinetic studies with this variant protein show a T_4-binding affinity about sevenfold higher than that found in normal TTR.[38] In the face of normal TBG and albumin concentrations, Thr109 TTR probably binds about 50% of the circulating T_4 in euthyroid subjects (see Fig. 113–1). The Val109 and Met119 variants of TTR also have increased affinity for T_4, but serum total T_4 is outside the reference range only in the former.[39, 40] TTR variants are not known to cause spurious assay values for total or free T_4.

Of at least 50 mutations described for TTR, many have now been examined for T_4 affinity. In a study comparing the interaction of T_4 with 10 different naturally occurring human TTR variants, a wide spectrum of T_4 affinity was observed.[41] Relative to the wild-type TTR, 3 show increased affinity for T_4, the Thr109 and Val109 variants being of sufficient affinity to cause euthyroid hyperthyroxinemia, whereas 3 have approximately normal affinity and 5 TTR variants show reduced affinity for T_4.[42]

DETECTION OF BINDING PROTEIN VARIANTS

Binding protein variants are usually suspected when T_4 or T_3 measurements, free or total, are out of line with clinical assessment and plasma TSH concentrations. In euthyroid subjects, abnormal total hormone values generally reflect a physiologic response to the altered binding protein so that normal free T_4 concentrations are maintained. Electrophoretic techniques, immunoprecipitation, and estimates of binding capacity and affinity are generally used to identify new variants. Most techniques of free T_4 estimation give a useful correction for the hereditary TBG anomalies. If the T_3 resin uptake test is used for binding correction, it is important to perform the calculation as resin/serum rather than resin/total counts to better correct for samples at the high and low extremes of TBG concentration.[43]

Whereas a normal level of TSH usually rules out thyrotoxicosis, the distinction between unusual binding abnormalities and hormone resistance syndromes can be difficult. Spurious method-dependent abnormal free T_4 results are common with albumin variants. High-capacity T_4 binding of abnormal affinity can be readily detected by loading the sample with an excess of unlabeled T_4 to saturate the low-capacity sites of TBG. FDH is associated with a unique persistence of increased ^{125}I-labeled T_4 binding as the concentration of unlabeled T_4 is progressively increased[44] (Fig. 113–6).

OTHER TRANSPORT ABNORMALITIES IN HUMANS

Several reports have described persistent excess of circulating T_4 in euthyroid subjects without an identifiable plasma protein-binding abnormality.[45, 46]

Defective type I deiodinase was suggested, although subsequent studies appear to have ruled this possibility out.[47] The findings are consistent with abnormal cell membrane transport of T_4,[46] but no definite mechanism has been identified. In addition, no pattern of inheritance has been determined.

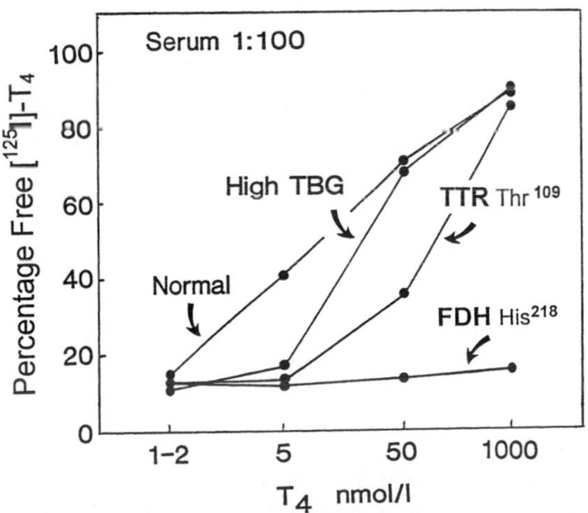

FIGURE 113–6. Effect of a progressive increase in the load of unlabeled thyroxine (T_4) on dextran-charcoal uptake of ^{125}I-labeled T_4 at 4°C in sera (diluted in phosphate buffer) from normal, thyroxine-binding globulin (TBG) excess, transthyretin (TTR) Thr109, and familial dysalbuminemic hyperthyroxinemia (FDH) His218 subjects. In the presence of 1000-fold T_4 excess, FDH shows unique persistence of ^{125}I-labeled T_4 binding at 4°C (low charcoal uptake) characteristic of a high-capacity site of increased affinity. (Data from Stockigt JR, Dyer SA, Mohr VS, et al: Specific methods to identify plasma binding abnormalities in euthyroid hyperthyroxinemia. J Clin Endocrinol Metab 62:230–233, 1986. Illustration modified from Stockigt JR: Serum TSH and thyroid hormone measurements and assessment of thyroid hormone transport. *In* Braverman LE, Utiger RD (eds): Werner and Ingbar's The Thyroid, ed 7. Philadelphia, JB Lippincott, 1996, pp 377–396.)

REFERENCES

1. Trevorrow V: Studies on the nature of the iodine in blood. J Biol Chem 127:737–750, 1939.
2. Refetoff S: Inherited thyroxine-binding globulin abnormalities in man. Endocr Rev 10:275–293, 1989.
3. Refetoff S: Inherited thyroxine-binding globulin abnormalities in man: Update 1994. *In* Braverman LE, Refetoff S (eds): Endocrine Reviews Monographs, vol 3, Clinical and Molecular Aspects of Diseases of the Thyroid. Bethesda, MD, The Endocrine Society, 1994, pp 162–164.
4. Refetoff S, Murata Y, Mori Y, et al: Thyroxine-binding globulin: Organisation of the gene and variants. Horm Res 45:128–138, 1996.
5. Flink IL, Bailey TJ, Gustafson TA, et al: Complete amino acid sequence of human thyroxine-binding globulin deduced from cloned DNA: Close homology to the serine antiproteases. Proc Natl Acad Sci USA 83:7708–7712, 1986.
6. Robbins J, Bartalena L: Plasma transport of thyroid hormones. *In* Hennemann G (ed): Thyroid Hormone Metabolism. New York, Marcel Dekker, 1986, pp 3–38.
7. Mori Y, Miura Y, Oiso Y, et al: Precise localization of the human thyroxine-binding globulin gene to chromosome Xq22.2 by fluorescence in situ hybridization. Hum Genet 96:481–482, 1995.
8. Okamoto H, Mori Y, Tani Y et al: Molecular analysis of females manifesting thyroxine-binding globulin (TBG) deficiency: Selective X-chromosome inactivation responsible for the difference between phenotype and genotype in TBG-deficient females. J Clin Endocrinol Metab 81:2204–2208, 1996.
9. Carvalho GA, Weiss RE, Refetoff S: Complete thyroxine-binding globulin (TBG) deficiency produced by a mutation in acceptor splice site causing frameshift and early termination of translation (TBG-Kankakee). J Clin Endocrinol Metab 83:3604–3608, 1998.
10. Mori Y, Miura Y, Takeuchi H, et al: Gene amplification as a cause of inherited thyroxine-binding globulin excess in two Japanese families. J Clin Endocrinol Metab 80:3758–3762, 1995.
11. Murata Y, Refetoff S, Sarne DH, et al: Variant thyroxine-binding globulin in serum of Australian aborigines: Its physical, chemical and biological properties. J Endocrinol Invest 8:225–232, 1985.
12. Watson F, Dick M: Distribution and inheritance of low serum thyroxine-binding globulin levels in Australian aborigines. Med J Aust 2:385–387, 1980.
13. Refetoff S, Murata Y: X-chromosome-linked inheritance of the variant thyroxine-binding globulin in Australian aborigines. J Clin Endocrinol Metab 60:356–360, 1985.
14. Janssen OE, Chen B, Büttner C, et al: Molecular and structural characterization of the heat-resistant thyroxine-binding globulin-Chicago. J Biol Chem 270:28234–28238, 1995.
15. Murata Y, Takamatsu J, Refetoff S: Inherited abnormality of thyroxine-binding globulin with no demonstrable thyroxine-binding activity and high serum levels of denatured thyroxine-binding globulin. N Engl J Med 314:694–699, 1986.
16. Peters T Jr: Serum albumin. Adv Protein Chem 37:161–245, 1985.
17. Hennemann G, Docter R, Krenning EP, et al: Raised total thyroxine and free thyroxine index but normal free thyroxine. Lancet 1:639–642, 1979.
18. Stockigt JR, Topliss DJ, Barlow JW, et al: Familial euthyroid thyroxine excess: An appropriate response to abnormal thyroxine binding associated with albumin. J Clin Endocrinol Metab 53:353–359, 1981.
19. Arevalo G: Prevalence of familial dysalbuminemic hyperthyroxinemia in serum samples received for thyroid testing. Clin Chem 37:1430–1431, 1991.
20. Barlow JW, Csicsmann JM, White EL, et al: Familial euthyroid thyroxine excess: Characterisation of abnormal intermediate-affinity thyroxine binding to albumin. J Clin Endocrinol Metab 55:244–250, 1982.
21. Petersen CE, Scottolini AG, Cody LR, et al: A point mutation in the human serum albumin gene results in familial dysalbuminaemic hyperthyroxinaemia. J Med Genet 31:355–359, 1994.
22. Petersen CE, Ha CE, Mandel M, et al: Expression of a human serum albumin variant with high affinity for thyroxine. Biochem Biophys Res Commun 214:1121–1129, 1995.
23. Stockigt JR, Stevens V, White EL, et al: "Unbound analog" radioimmunoassays for free thyroxin measure the albumin-bound hormone fraction. Clin Chem 29:1408–1410, 1983.
24. Mendel CM, Cavalieri RR: Thyroxine distribution and metabolism in familial dysalbuminemic hyperthyroxinemia. J Clin Endocrinol Metab 59:499–504, 1984.
25. Wada N, Chiba H, Shimizu C, et al: A novel missense mutation in codon 218 of the albumin gene in a distinct phenotype of familial dysalbuminemic hyperthyroxinemia in a Japanese kindred. J Clin Endocrinol Metab 82:3246–3250, 1997.
26. Sunthornthepvarakul T, Likitmaskul S, Ngowngarmratana S, et al: Familial dysalbuminemic hypertriiodothyroninemia: A new, dominantly inherited albumin defect. J Clin Endocrinol Metab 83:1448–1454, 1998.
27. Kallee E: Bennhold's analbuminemia: A follow-up study of the first two cases (1953–1992). J Lab Clin Med 127:470–480, 1996.
28. Mendel CM, Cavalieri RR, Gavin LA, et al: Thyroxine transport and distribution in Nagase analbuminemic rats. J Clin Invest 83:143–148, 1989.
29. Robbins J, Cheng S-Y, Gershengorn MC, et al: Thyroxine transport proteins of plasma, molecular properties and biosynthesis. Rec Prog Horm Res 34:477–519, 1978.
30. Schreiber G: Synthesis, processing and secretion of plasma proteins by the liver and other organs and their regulation. *In* Putnam PW (ed): The Plasma Proteins: Structure, Function and Genetic Control, vol 5, ed 2. Orlando, FL, Academic Press, 1987, pp 293–363.

31. Schreiber G, Aldred AR, Jaworowski A, et al: Thyroxine transport from blood to brain via transthyretin synthesis in choroid plexus. Am J Physiol 258:R338–R345, 1990.
32. Jacobsson B, Carlstrom A, Plotz A, et al: Transthyretin messenger ribonucleic acid expression in the pancreas and in endocrine tumors of the pancreas and gut. J Clin Endocrinol Metab 71:875–880, 1990.
33. Richardson SJ, Bradley AJ, Duan W, et al: Evolution of marsupial and other vertebrate thyroxine-binding plasma proteins. Am J Physiol 266:R1359–R1370, 1994.
34. Saraiva MJM: Transthyretin mutations in health and disease. Hum Mutat 5:191–196, 1995.
35. Palha JA, Episkopou V, Maede S, et al: Thyroid hormone metabolism in a transthyretin-null mouse strain. J Biol Chem 269:33135–33139, 1994.
36. Moses AC, Rosen HN, Moller DE, et al: A point mutation in transthyretin increases affinity for thyroxine and produces euthyroid hyperthyroxinaemia. J Clin Invest 86:2025–2033, 1990.
37. Moses AC, Lawlor J, Haddow J, et al: Familial euthyroid hyperthyroxinemia resulting from increased thyroxine binding to thyroxine-binding prealbumin. N Engl J Med 306:966–969, 1982.
38. Lalloz MRA, Byfield PGH, Himsworth RL: A prealbumin variant with an increased affinity for T_4 and reverse-T_3. Clin Endocrinol 21:331–338, 1984.
39. Refetoff S, Marinov VSZ, Tunca H, et al: A new family with hyperthyroxinemia caused by transthyretin Val^{109} misdiagnosed as thyrotoxicosis and resistance to thyroid hormone—a clinical research centre study. J Clin Endocrinol Metab 81:3335–3340, 1996.
40. Curtis AJ, Scrimshaw BJ, Topliss DJ, et al: Thyroxine binding by human transthyretin variants: Mutations at position 119, but not position 54, increase thyroxine binding affinity. J Clin Endocrinol Metab 78:459–462, 1994.
41. Rosen HN, Moses AC, Murrell JR, et al: Thyroxine interactions with transthyretin: A comparison of 10 different naturally occurring human transthyretin variants. J Clin Endocrinol Metab 77:370–374, 1993.
42. Bartalena L: Thyroid hormone-binding proteins: Update 1994. *In* Braverman LE, Refetoff S (eds): Endocrine Review Monographs, vol 3, Clinical and Molecular Aspects of Diseases of the Thyroid. Bethesda, MD, The Endocrine Society, 1994, pp 140–142.
43. Larsen PR, Alexander NM, Chopra IJ, et al: Revised nomenclature for tests of thyroid hormones and thyroid-related proteins in serum. J Clin Endocrinol Metab 64:1089–1092, 1987.
44. Stockigt JR, Dyer SA, Mohr VS, et al: Specific methods to identify plasma binding abnormalities in euthyroid hyperthyroxinemia. J Clin Endocrinol Metab 62:230–233, 1986.
45. Kleinhaus N, Faber J, Kahana L, et al: Euthyroid hyperthyroxinemia due to a generalized 5′-deiodinase defect. J Clin Endocrinol Metab 66:684–688, 1988.
46. Hennemann G, Vos RA, de Jong M et al: Decreased peripheral 3,5,3′-triiodothyronine (T_3) production from thyroxine (T_4): A syndrome of impaired thyroid hormone activation due to transport inhibition of T_4 into T_3-producing tissues. J Clin Endocrinol Metab 77:1431–1435, 1993.
47. Toyoda N, Kleinhaus N, Larsen PR: The structure of the coding and 5′-flanking region of the type 1 iodothyronine deiodinase (*dio1)* gene is normal in a patient with suspected congenital *dio1* deficiency. J Clin Endocrinol Metab 81:2121–2124, 1996.

Chapter 114

Resistance to Thyroid Hormone

V. Krishna Chatterjee ▪ Paolo Beck-Peccoz

CLINICAL FEATURES
DIFFERENTIAL DIAGNOSIS
MOLECULAR GENETICS
PROPERTIES OF MUTANT RECEPTORS
PATHOGENESIS OF VARIABLE RESISTANCE
ANIMAL MODELS OF RESISTANCE
MANAGEMENT

The effects of thyroid hormones on physiologic processes are mediated principally by a receptor protein (TR), belonging to the steroid/nuclear receptor superfamily of ligand-inducible transcription factors that modulates target gene expression in different tissues. TR binds preferentially to promoter regulatory DNA sequences (thyroid response elements [TREs]) as a heterodimer with the retinoid X receptor (RXR). In the absence of hormone, unliganded receptor recruits corepressors (nuclear receptor corepressor, N-CoR; silencing mediator for RAR/TR, SMRT) to repress or "silence" gene transcription; hormone binding results in corepressor dissociation and relief of repression together with ligand-dependent transcriptional activation, mediated by a complex of coactivators (steroid receptor-coactivator 1 [SRC-1], CREB-binding protein [CBP], and CBP-associated factor [pCAF]).[1] In humans, two receptor genes (TRα and TRβ) on chromosomes 17 and 3, respectively, are alternately spliced to generate three highly homologous receptor isoforms—TRα_1, TRβ_1, and TRβ_2 with differing tissue distributions: TRα_1 is most abundant in the central nervous system, myocardium, and skeletal muscle; TRβ_1 is present in the liver and kidney; and TRβ_2 is most highly expressed in the pituitary and hypothalamus.[2]

The syndrome of resistance to thyroid hormone (RTH) is an uncommon disorder characterized by reduced responsiveness of target tissues to circulating thyroid hormones. The biochemical hallmark of RTH, elevated circulating levels of free thyroid hormones together with a nonsuppressed pituitary thyroid-stimulating hormone (TSH) secretion, reflects resistance to thyroid hormone action in the hypothalamic-pituitary-thyroid axis and is accompanied by variable refractoriness in peripheral tissues.

CLINICAL FEATURES

Resistance to thyroid hormone was first described in 1967 in two siblings who were clinically euthyroid despite high circulating thyroid hormone levels. These siblings exhibited several other abnormalities, including deaf-mutism, stippled femoral epiphyses with delayed bone maturation, and short stature as well as dysmorphic facies and winging of the scapulae and pectus carinatum.[3] It is now clear that some of these features are unique to this kindred in which the disorder was recessively inherited. The majority of RTH cases that have been described since then are dominantly inherited with highly variable clinical features. Many patients with RTH are either asymptomatic or have nonspecific symptoms and may be noted to have a goiter, prompting thyroid function tests that suggest the diagnosis. In these individuals, classified as exhibiting generalized resistance (GRTH), the high thyroid hormone levels are thought to compensate for ubiquitous tissue resistance, resulting in a euthyroid state. In contrast, several individuals with the same biochemical abnormalities exhibit clinical features of thyrotoxicosis. In adults, these can include weight loss, tremor, palpitations, insomnia, and heat intolerance; in children, failure to thrive, accelerated growth, and hyperkinetic behavior have also been noted. When this clinical entity was first described, patients were thought to have "selective" pituitary resistance to thyroid hormone action (PRTH) with preservation of normal hormonal responses in peripheral tissues.[4] Hypothyroid features, such as growth retardation, delayed dentition, and bone age in children or asthenia and hypercholesterolemia in adults have also been observed in RTH and may coexist with thyrotoxic symptoms in the same individual.[5]

The incidence of RTH is probably about 1 in 50,000, and the disorder can be diagnosed neonatally by screening with both TSH and T_4 measurements.[6] More than 400 cases of RTH have now been described worldwide, enabling the clinical features of this disorder to be progressively delineated.

GOITER. The commonest presenting feature—a palpable goiter—has been documented in 65% of individuals, particularly women. The enlargement is usually diffuse, with multinodular glands being typical of recurrent goiters after a partial thyroidectomy. Interestingly, fewer children with RTH born to affected mothers exhibited thyroid enlargement (35%) compared with offspring of unaffected mothers (87%), suggesting that maternal hyperthyroxinemia with transplacental passage of thyroid hormones during development might protect against goitrogenesis.[7] The bioactivity of circulating TSH has been shown to be significantly enhanced in RTH, perhaps accounting for the goiter and greatly elevated serum thyroid hormones despite the normal immunoreactive TSH levels, observed in some cases.[8]

CARDIOVASCULAR. Before the advent of sensitive TSH assays, the combination of cardiovascular symptoms with goiter often led to misdiagnosis of Graves' disease in RTH. The incidence of palpitations and resting tachycardia is much higher than that found in the general population, occurring in 75% of patients with GRTH and almost all cases of PRTH, with a predisposition to atrial fibrillation in older subjects. Although the resting heart rate in affected and unaffected family members with RTH is similar,[7] approximately 30% of patients showed echocardiographic features of increased myocardial contractility and impaired diastolic relaxation with mitral valve prolapse in seven cases.[7]

MUSCULOSKELETAL SYSTEM. Growth retardation and delayed skeletal maturation is commoner in childhood in patients with RTH, with a height below the 5th centile in 18% and delayed bone age (>2 standard deviations) in 29%[7] and no significant differences between GRTH and PRTH cases. Despite these abnormalities, the final adult height is often not affected.[9] With the known adverse effects of hyperthyroidism on bone mineralization, we conducted a cross-sectional survey of 39 adult RTH patients, and observed a reduction in bone mineral density that is more marked in the femoral neck (mean Z score of −0.41) than in the lumbar spine (mean Z score of −0.24).

The basal metabolic rate (BMR) is variably affected in RTH, being normal in some cases.[10] In keeping with others,[7] we have observed an elevated BMR particularly in childhood RTH, which may account for the abnormally low body mass index seen in approximately one-third of children.

CENTRAL NERVOUS SYSTEM. Two studies have documented neuropsychological abnormalities in RTH. First, a history of attention deficit hyperactivity disorder (ADHD) in childhood was elicited more frequently (75%) in patients with RTH compared with their unaffected relatives (15%).[11] A second study showed that both children and adults with RTH exhibited problems with language development, manifested by poor reading skills and problems with articulation including speech delay and stuttering.[12] However, frank mental retardation (IQ <60) is relatively uncommon (3%), but 30% of patients show mild learning disability (IQ <85), probably owing to uncompensated central nervous system hypothyroidism.[10] A direct comparison of individuals with

ADHD and RTH versus ADHD alone indicates an association with lower nonverbal intelligence and academic achievement in the former group.[13] In detailed analysis of one family, RTH cosegregated with lower IQ rather than ADHD.[14] However, two different surveys of unselected children with ADHD failed to detect any cases of RTH by biochemical screening, suggesting that the latter disorder is unlikely to be a common cause of hyperactivity.[15, 16] Although magnetic resonance imaging shows that anomalies of the sylvian fissure or Heschl's gyri are more frequent in RTH, these features do not correlate with ADHD.[17]

Significant hearing loss has been documented in 21% of RTH cases, similar to the prevalence reported in congenital hypothyroidism.[7] In the majority, audiometric tests indicated a conductive defect, probably related to the increased incidence of recurrent ear infections in childhood RTH (67% in RTH versus 28% in normal controls). Abnormal otoacoustic emissions, consistent with cochlear dysfunction, were also documented in those with hearing deficit.[7]

OTHER FEATURES. A greater frequency of recurrent upper respiratory tract and pulmonary infections has been reported in RTH, and affected individuals have reduced serum immunoglobulin levels.[7] Intrauterine growth retardation has only been documented in two neonates with RTH. Pubertal development, fertility, and overall survival are not adversely affected by the disorder.

DIFFERENTIAL DIAGNOSIS

Several conditions other than RTH are associated with hyperthyroxinemia and a nonsuppressed TSH (Table 114–1). The first step in making a diagnosis of RTH is to verify the validity of hormone measurements. Elevated free thyroid hormones in equilibrium dialysis or two-step assays that exclude dysalbuminemic or anti-iodothyronine antibodies and preservation of linearity when TSH is assayed in dilution suggests the latter measurement is not artifactual. Other causes (e.g., nonthyroidal illness, psychiatric disorder, neonatal period, drugs) can be excluded by clinical context. Differentiation of RTH, particularly the form associated with hyperthyroid features, from a TSH-secreting pituitary tumor can be difficult. Similar abnormalities in thyroid function in first-degree relatives strongly suggest RTH together with normal pituitary imaging and serum glycoprotein α-subunit levels. Other factors that are helpful in making this differential diagnosis, such as dynamic testing and clinical/biochemical features, are discussed in greater detail in Chapter 102.

The rare and probably coincidental association of RTH and autoimmune thyroid disease has been described.[18] Development of Graves' disease in RTH is suggested by atypical features such as ophthalmopathy, severe thyrotoxic symptoms, and a further rise in thyroid hormones leading to a subnormal or suppressed TSH. After antithyroid drug treatment, TSH levels become elevated despite normalization of thyroid hormones. Similarly, normalization of TSH but with elevated thyroid hormones, following supraphysiologic doses of thyroxine replacement in primary hypothyroidism, suggests coexistent RTH.

In addition to clinical features, the measurement of various tissue markers of thyroid hormone action is useful in evaluating the differing responses of various target organs and tissues to elevated circulating thyroid hormones (Table 114–2). Whereas these measurements are most useful in assessing the tissue effects of marked thyroid hormone excess as in overt thyrotoxicosis, they may be less discriminatory in borderline hyperthyroidism or in hypothyroidism. In order to improve the sensitivity and specificity of these parameters, it has been suggested to assess individuals with RTH by measuring tissue responses dynamically, following the administration of graded supraphysiologic doses of T_3 (50, 100, and 200 μg/day, each given for 3 days) with comparison of any change in indices from baseline values to the hormone responses in normal subjects.[19]

TABLE 114–1. Causes of Hyperthyroxinemia with Detectable TSH

Raised serum-binding proteins
Familial dysalbuminemic hyperthyroxinemia
Anti-iodothyronine antibodies
Anti-TSH antibodies
Nonthyroidal illness
Acute psychiatric disorders
Neonatal period
Drugs (e.g., amiodarone)
Thyroxine replacement therapy
TSH–secreting pituitary tumor
Resistance to thyroid hormone

TSH, thyroid-stimulating hormone.

TABLE 114–2. Measurement of Tissue Resistance in RTH

Pituitary: TSH
General: Basal metabolic rate
Hepatic: Sex hormone–binding globulin, ferritin, cholesterol
Muscle: Creatine kinase, ankle jerk relaxation time
Cardiac: Sleeping pulse rate; systolic time interval; diastolic isovolumic relaxation time
Bone: Height, bone age; bone density; osteocalcin; alkaline phosphatase; pyridinium cross-links; type 1 collagen telopeptide
Hematologic: soluble interleukin-2 receptor
Lung: Angiotensin-converting enzyme

RTH, resistance to thyroid hormone; TSH, thyroid-stimulating hormone.

MOLECULAR GENETICS

Following the cloning of thyroid hormone receptors, resistance to thyroid hormone (RTH), was shown to be tightly linked to the TRβ gene locus in a single family.[20] This prompted analysis of the TRβ gene in other cases, and since then a large number of receptor defects have been associated with this disorder. Ninety percent of RTH is familial, dominantly inherited, and associated with heterozygous mutations in the TRβ gene[10, 21–23] with de novo receptor mutations occurring in the remaining 10% of sporadic cases. More than 80 different defects, including point mutations, inframe deletions, and frameshift insertions have been documented to date, which all localize to three mutation clusters within the ligand binding domain of the receptor (Fig. 114–1). Within each cluster, some codon changes (e.g., R243W, R338W, R438H), representing transitions in mutation-prone CpG dinucleotides, occur more frequently and are overrepresented.[24]

Based on the supposition that PRTH was associated with selective pituitary resistance, it had been hypothesized that this disorder might be associated with defects in the pituitary type II 5′-deiodinase enzyme or the $TR\beta_2$ receptor isoform. However, several reports have documented TRβ mutations in PRTH.[22, 25, 26] Receptor mutations found in individuals with PRTH have also been associated with GRTH in unrelated kindreds. Furthermore, even within a single family, the same receptor mutation can be associated with abnormal thyroid function and thyrotoxic features consistent with PRTH in some individuals, but similar biochemical abnormalities and a lack of symptoms indicative of GRTH in other members. Overall, these findings indicate that GRTH and PRTH represent differing phenotypic manifestations of a single genetic entity.

In a few cases, clear-cut biochemical evidence of RTH is not associated with a mutation in the coding region of $TR\beta_1$. Possible theoretical explanations in such individuals include a somatic $TR\beta_1$ mutation whose tissue expression is limited and not detectable in peripheral blood leukocyte DNA. Alternatively, the possibility of defects in non-TR pathways disrupting thyroid hormone action should also be considered. This hypothesis is supported by reports of families or sporadic cases, with thyroid function tests and resistance to exogenous T_3 similar to RTH, not associated with mutations in $TR\beta_2$ or $TR\beta_1$, and defects at the TRα gene locus excluded by linkage.[27] In one case, TRβ showed aberrant binding to a unique 84-kDa protein from a patient but not control fibroblast nuclear extracts, suggesting abnormal receptor interaction with a cofactor.[28] It is known that patients with Rubinstein-Taybi syndrome, a disorder associated with defects in the nuclear receptor coactivator CBP, exhibit a number of somatic abnormalities (broad thumbs, mental retardation, short stat-

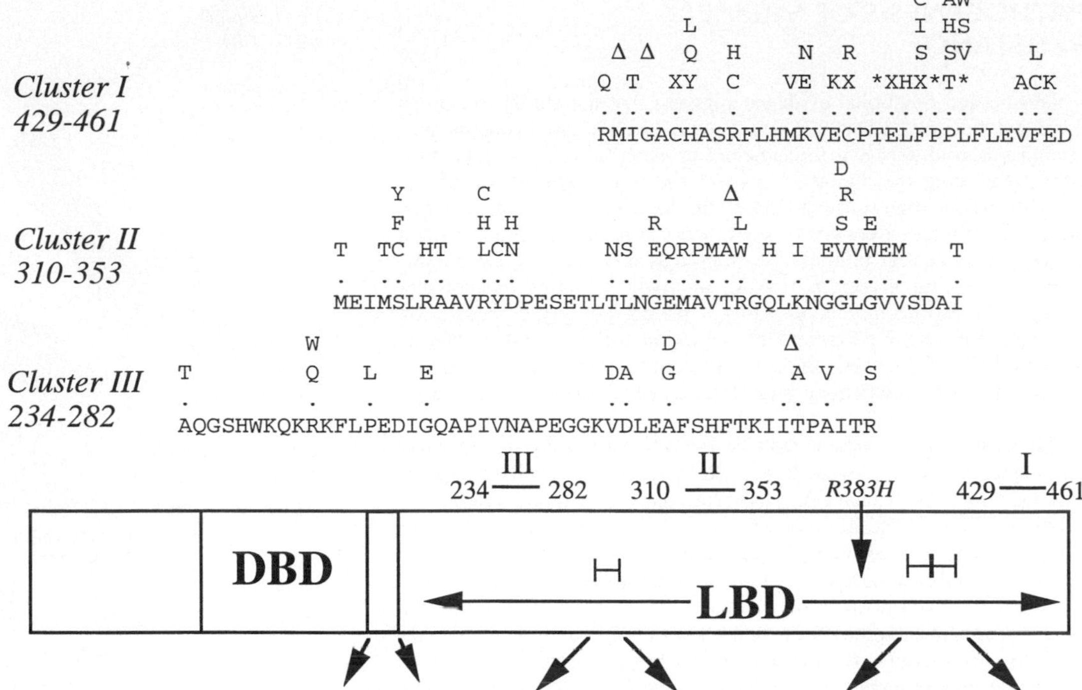

FIGURE 114–1. A schematic representation of the domains of TRβ showing that, with one exception (R383H), RTH receptor mutations localize to three clusters within the ligand-binding domain (LBD). The receptor defects described hitherto include different missense substitutions at each codon, inframe codon deletions (Δ), premature termination codons (X) and frameshift mutations (*). The mutations shown include published information together with some of our unpublished data. No RTH receptor mutations have been described in the zinc finger DNA binding domain (DBD) or its carboxyterminal extension (CTE), which together mediate interaction with DNA, or regions in the LBD that are important for corepressor binding or dimerization with RXR.

ure), yet have normal circulating free T_4 and TSH levels.[29] However, disruption of the steroid receptor coactivator 1 (SRC-1) gene in mice results in resistance to thyroid and steroid hormones,[30] raising the possibility of a homologous human defect. Finally, the administration of RXR-selective agonists inhibits pituitary TSH secretion, which results in central hypothyroidism[31] and raises the possibility that defects in pituitary-expressed RXR might also impair negative feedback in the pituitary-thyroid axis and manifest as RTH.

PROPERTIES OF MUTANT RECEPTORS

Consonant with their location in the hormone-binding domain, most receptor mutants identified in RTH exhibit moderate or greatly reduced T_3 binding, and consequently their ability to activate or repress target gene expression is impaired.[32, 33] More recently, a subset of RTH mutations, associated with markedly abnormal thyroid function in vivo and altered transcriptional function in vitro but little impairment in ligand binding have been described. Such natural mutations involve residues that mediate receptor interaction with transcriptional coactivators.[23, 34] In the first RTH family described, with the recessively inherited form of the disorder, the two affected siblings were found to be homozygous for a complete deletion of both alleles of the TRβ receptor gene.[35] Importantly, the obligate heterozygotes in this family, harboring a deletion of one TRβ allele, were completely normal with no evidence of thyroid dysfunction. This suggested that simple deficiency of functional β-receptor, as a consequence of the single deleted TRβ allele, was insufficient to generate the resistance phenotype. This led to the hypothesis that the heterozygous mutant receptors in RTH were not simply functionally impaired but also capable of inhibiting wild-type receptor action. Studies confirmed that when coexpressed, the mutant proteins are able to inhibit the function of their wild-type counterparts in a dominant negative manner.[36, 37] Further clinical and genetic evidence supporting this notion was provided by a childhood case, in which severe resistance with marked developmental delay and growth retardation associated with cardiac hyperthyroidism was ultimately fatal owing to heart failure following septicemia. This individual was homozygous for a mutation in both alleles of the TRβ gene, and the extreme phenotype presumably reflected the compound effect of two dominant negative mutant β-receptors.[38]

Functional studies of mutant receptors indicate that although they are transcriptionally impaired and dominant negative inhibitors, their ability to bind DNA and form heterodimers with RXR is preserved.[32, 33] Conversely, it has been shown that the introduction of additional artificial mutations that abolish DNA binding or heterodimer formation abrogates the dominant negative activity of mutant receptors.[33, 39, 40] It has also been suggested that the ability of mutant receptors in RTH to repress or "silence" basal gene transcription is likely to be an important factor contributing to their dominant negative potency. Non–T_3-binding mutants exhibit constitutive silencing function, particularly when bound to DNA as homodimers, which cannot be relieved by ligand and conversely, RTH mutants with impaired homodimerization properties are weaker dominant negative inhibitors.[41] With the identification of corepressors, these observations have been extended to show that some RTH mutants either bind corepressor more avidly when unliganded or fail to dissociate fully from corepressor upon T_3 binding.[42] Furthermore, artificial mutations that abolish corepressor binding abrogate the dominant negative activity of RTH receptor mutants.[42] Most recently, it has been suggested that corepressors mediate basal activation of negatively regulated gene promoters (e.g., TRH, TSHα, TSHβ) by TR.[43] An unusual RTH receptor mutant (R383H) exhibits both delayed corepressor release and impaired negative transcriptional regulation.[44] Given the pivotal role of negatively regulated target genes in the pathogenesis of RTH, aberrant corepressor recruitment or release may well prove to be the critical receptor abnormality in this disorder.

Together, these observations allow a model to be constructed (Fig. 114–2) in which occupancy of target gene–binding sites by mutant receptor-corepressor complexes mediates dominant negative inhibition by RTH mutants. Mapping of the three clusters of RTH receptor mutations identified hitherto, on the crystal structure of the ligand-binding domain (LBD) of TRβ, provides insights into structure-function relationships in TR (Fig. 114–3).[45] As expected from their impaired ligand-binding properties, most mutations are located around the hormone-binding cavity, and receptor regions mediating DNA binding, dimerization, and corepressor interaction are devoid of naturally occurring mutations, possibly because they lack dominant negative activity and therefore elude discovery because they are clinically and biochemically silent.

PATHOGENESIS OF VARIABLE RESISTANCE

Genetic and functional evidence suggests that the ability to exert a dominant negative effect on target genes within the hypothalamic-pituitary-thyroid axis is a fundamental property of RTH receptor mutants, generating the abnormal thyroid function characteristic of the disorder. Indeed, one study indicates that, for a subset of RTH mutants, there is a correlation between their functional impairment in vitro and the degree of central pituitary resistance, as measured by the magnitude of elevation in serum free T_4 in vivo.[46] On this biochemical background, the heterogeneous clinical phenotype may be caused by differing degrees of peripheral resistance in different individuals as well as by variable resistance in different tissues within a single subject. Several factors may contribute to such variable tissue resistance.

One contributory element may be the differing tissue distributions of receptor isoforms. As the hypothalamus/pituitary and liver express predominantly $TR\beta_2$ and $TR\beta_1$ receptors respectively and $TR\alpha$ is the major species detected in myocardium, mutations in the $TR\beta$ gene are likely to be associated with pituitary and liver resistance, as exemplified by normal sex hormone–binding globulin (SHBG) and nonsuppressed TSH levels seen in patients, whereas tachycardia and cardiac hyperthyroidism in some cases may represent retention of myocardial sensitivity to thyroid hormones acting via a normal α-receptor. Another factor that may influence the degree of tissue resistance is the relative expression of mutant versus wild-type $TR\beta$ alleles. Whereas one study has suggested that both alleles are equally expressed,[47] another showed marked differences in the relative levels of wild-type and mutant receptor messenger RNA in skin fibroblasts from two RTH cases.[48] In one of these individuals, a temporal variation in expression of the mutant allele in fibroblasts appeared to correlate with the degree of skeletal tissue resistance. The dominant negative inhibitory potency of mutant receptors has been shown to differ depending on target gene promoter context[33, 49] and is a further variable that may influence the degree of resistance. Finally, non-$TR\beta$ gene–related factors might influence the phenotype. For example, a deleterious R316H mutation was associated with normal thyroid hormone levels in some members of one kindred,[50] but clearly abnormal thyroid function in an unrelated family,[22] suggesting that other genetic variables can modulate the effect of receptor mutations.

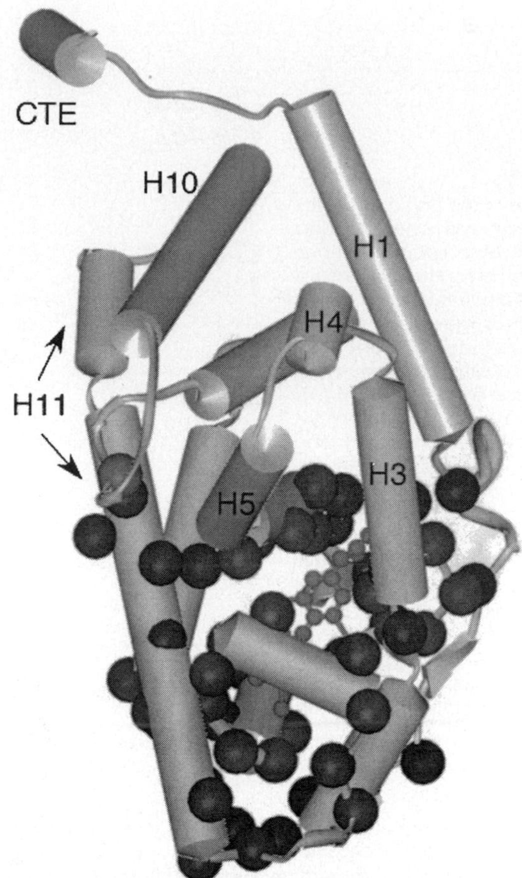

FIGURE 114–3. The crystal structure of the $TR\beta$ ligand-binding domain (LBD), composed of 12 α-helices, is shown, with the location of missense mutations associated with RTH superimposed. As anticipated from their functional properties, most mutations involve residues that surround the hydrophobic ligand-binding cavity. Helices that mediate DNA binding (carboxyterminal extension of DNA binding domain, CTE), corepressor interaction (H1, H3, H4, H5), or dimerization (H10, H11), are devoid of natural receptor mutations.

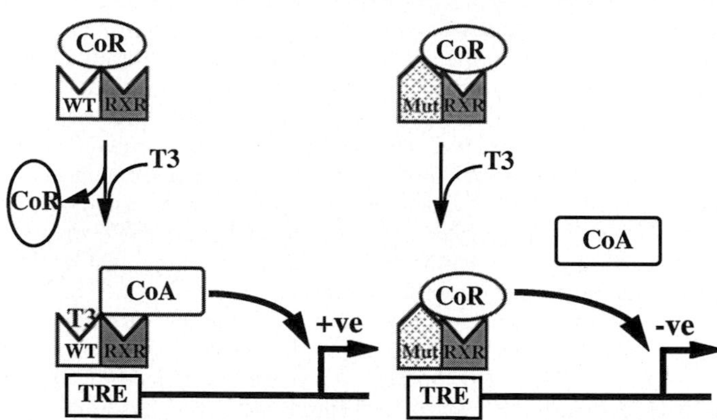

FIGURE 114–2. A model for dominant negative inhibition by mutant receptors in RTH. The *left panel* depicts current understanding of wild-type TR action on target genes. The unliganded TR-RXR heterodimer or homodimer (not shown) recruits a corepressor complex (CoR) to inhibit or silence basal gene transcription. Receptor occupancy by T_3 promotes corepressor dissociation and derepression, followed by binding of coactivators (CoA), which leads to target gene activation. The *right panel* shows RTH receptor mutant action. In comparison to wild-type TR, the primary defect in mutant receptors may be impaired hormone-dependent corepressor dissociation and coactivator recruitment. For most receptor mutants, this functional alteration is a consequence of their reduced ability to bind ligand. However, a subset of mutants exhibit enhanced corepressor binding or delayed corepressor release or impaired coactivator recruitment per se, with relative preservation of hormone binding. Mutant receptor-CoR complexes compete with their wild type counterparts for occupancy of promoter thyroid response elements (TREs), resulting in inhibition of target gene expression. In this model DNA binding, dimerization, and corepressor interaction are functional properties that are preserved in mutant receptors and required for their dominant negative activity.

Whereas the absence or presence of overt thyrotoxic features allows patients to be classified as either GRTH or PRTH (a clinical definition that will probably remain useful as a guide to the most appropriate form of treatment), studies indicate that there is some overlap of features between the two forms of the disorder. For example, there are no significant differences in age, sex ratio, frequency of goiter, thyroid function or clinical features among patients with GRTH or PRTH (Table 114–3). Importantly, features such as tachycardia, hyperkinetic behavior, and emotional disturbance have been documented in individuals with GRTH.[51] Conversely, serum SHBG, a hepatic index of thyroid hormone action, is almost invariably normal in patients with PRTH, suggesting that tissue resistance is not solely confined to the hypothalamic-pituitary-thyroid axis in this group of patients.[52]

Attempts to correlate the phenotype of RTH with the nature of the underlying $TR\beta$ mutation have been confounded by three factors: (1) the relative imprecision of clinical criteria used to define GRTH and PRTH; (2) the apparent temporal variation in hyperthyroid features in some RTH cases, such that thyrotoxic symptoms and signs can develop and disappear spontaneously when individuals are followed for several years[51]; and (3) the relatively small number of patients with any given mutation that have been identified hitherto. Nevertheless, some interesting correlations are emerging from the published literature. The

TABLE 114–3. Clinical Features of Patients with GRTH and PRTH

Features	PRTH (No. = 52)	GRTH (No. = 387)	RTH (No. = 439)
Sex (M:F)	24:28	183:204	207:232
Age (yr)	1.3–80	0.1–75	0.1–80
Familial cases (%)	80	90	82
Tachycardia (%)	94	75	80
Cardiac diseases (%)	—	—	30
Goiter (%)	96	95	95
Thyroid ablation (%)	69	45	48
Hyperkinetic behavior (%)	88	68	72
ADHD (%)	6	12	11
Emotional disturbance (%)	84	60	65
Learning disabilities (%)	22	30	28
Mental retardation (%) (IQ = <60)	1	3	2.7
Speech impediment (%)	—	—	28
Hearing loss (%)	—	—	8
Growth retardation (%)	16	20	19

ADHD, attention deficit hyperactivity disorder; GRTH, generalized resistance to thyroid hormone; PRTH, pituitary resistance to thyroid hormone.

first patient reported to have PRTH[4] was found to harbor an R338W receptor mutation,[25] and the same phenotype has been described in most individuals with this or similar substitutions at this codon.[22, 26] Interestingly, when tested in vitro, this mutant exhibits dominant negative activity with the negatively regulated pituitary TSHα subunit gene promoter but is a relatively poor inhibitor of wild-type receptor action in other promoter contexts.[33] Furthermore, when introduced into other RTH receptor mutant backgrounds, this mutation weakens their dominant negative potency on positively regulated reporter genes.[53] A patient with the R383H receptor defect, which is impaired mainly in regulation of TRH and TSH genes, exhibited predominant central resistance following T_3 administration.[54] The R429Q mutation, with similar functional properties, may also occur more frequently in association with PRTH. Safer et al. have studied some receptor mutants (R338W or L, V349M, R429Q, I431T) associated with PRTH and shown that they exert a greater dominant negative inhibitory effect in a $TR\beta_2$ setting than a $TR\beta_1$ context.[55]

ANIMAL MODELS OF RESISTANCE

Many of the features in the recessively inherited cases of RTH associated with a deletion encompassing the TRβ gene have been recapitulated by an animal model with targeted disruption of the mouse TRβ locus.[56] Homozygous TRβ knockout mice had elevated serum thyroid hormones and an inappropriately elevated TSH analogous to RTH. Importantly heterozygous animals were biochemically normal, thus corroborating findings in their human counterparts. The homozygous mice also exhibited profound sensorineural deafness without obvious cochlear malformation, indicating that the deaf-mutism in recessive human RTH is also related to a defect in TRβ, rather than to the deletion of a contiguous gene. Together with the hearing abnormalities found in patients with dominantly inherited RTH, these findings emphasize the importance of TRβ in auditory development and function.

RTH receptor mutant expression has also been selectively targeted to the pituitary using a tissue-specific promoter.[57] Interestingly, such transgenic mice showed elevated TSH but only marginally raised T_4 levels, suggesting that the additional dominant negative effect of mutant receptors on the hypothalamic TRH gene might be required to produce the full biochemical phenotype. Ubiquitous, transgenic mutant TRβ expression results in an animal model with more generalized tissue resistance.[58] Such mice displayed decreased body weight, hyperactivity, and learning deficit, which are recognized features of the human syndrome.

The introduction of point mutations into $TR\alpha_1$, homologous to the TRβ defects in RTH, generates mutant receptor proteins with dominant negative activity in vitro,[49] raising the possibility that naturally occurring defects in the human TRα gene might also be associated with some form of RTH. However, mice with a selective knockout of $TR\alpha_1$ exhibit low or normal serum thyroid hormones, a decreased heart rate, and lower body temperature—a phenotype quite dissimilar to RTH,[59] suggesting that human $TR\alpha_1$ mutations are not likely to manifest in this manner.

MANAGEMENT

The management of RTH is difficult, because variable resistance makes it difficult to maintain euthyroidism in all tissues. However, in general, the presence or absence of hyperthyroid features is a useful guide to the need for therapy. In most individuals, the receptor defect is compensated by high circulating thyroid hormone levels, leading to euthyroid state not associated with abnormalities other than a small goiter. Attempts to treat the biochemical abnormality with surgery or radioiodine are often unsuccessful, with recrudescence of the goiter and disruption of the thyroid axis. Certain circumstances, such as hypercholesterolemia in adults or developmental delay and growth retardation in young children, may warrant the administration of supraphysiologic doses of L-T_4 to overcome a higher degree of resistance in certain tissues. Although successful in some cases,[10] such therapy requires careful monitoring of indices of thyroid hormone action (e.g., SHBG, heart rate, BMR, bone markers) to avoid the adverse cardiac effects or excess catabolism associated with thyroxine overtreatment. Inappropriate thyroid ablation also renders the RTH patient hypothyroid, with elevated TSH levels and risk of thyrotroph hyperplasia,[60] and is another context in which supraphysiologic thyroxine replacement is indicated.

In contrast, a general reduction in thyroid hormone levels may be beneficial in the management of patients with thyrotoxic symptoms. However, the administration of conventional antithyroid drugs usually causes a further rise in serum TSH levels, which stimulates thyroid enlargement and may also induce thyrotroph hyperplasia with a theoretical risk of developing autonomous neoplasms at either site. Accordingly, agents that inhibit pituitary TSH secretion, yet are devoid of peripheral thyromimetic effects, are used to reduce thyroid hormone levels. The most widely used example is the thyroid hormone analogue 3,5,3′-triiodothyroacetic acid (TRIAC), which has been shown to be beneficial in both childhood and adult cases.[61–63] This compound has several interesting properties that make it an attractive therapeutic option in RTH: (1) it exerts predominantly pituitary and hepatic thyromimetic effects in vivo[64]—target tissues that are relatively refractory to thyroid hormones in RTH; and (2) it exhibits a higher affinity for TRβ than TRα in vitro.[65] A daily dose of 1.4 to 2.8 mg is generally used, and one study suggested that twice daily administration might be optimal in inhibiting TSH secretion.[66] The use of TRIAC in pregnancy successfully controlled maternal thyrotoxic symptoms but may have induced fetal goiter.[67] Treatment with TRIAC is not always effective[68] and dextro-thyroxine (D-T_4) is another agent that has been shown to be useful in some cases.[69, 70] If these compounds fail, the dopaminergic agent bromocriptine[71] or the somatostatin analogue octreotide[72] may be administered. However, past experience indicates that TSH secretion escapes from the inhibitory effects of bromocriptine[61, 70] as well as octreotide.[73] In view of the spontaneous variation in thyrotoxic symptoms in RTH, periodic cessation of thyroid hormone–lowering therapy and re-evaluation of the clinical status of the patient is advisable. In rare cases, such as severe thyrotoxic cardiac failure associated with RTH, thyroid ablation followed by subphysiologic thyroxine replacement could be used.

The treatment of thyrotoxic features (e.g., failure to thrive) in childhood RTH also requires careful monitoring to ensure that any reduction in thyroid hormone levels is not associated with growth retardation or adverse neurologic sequelae. Indeed, control of cardiac and sympathomimetic manifestations with β-blockade may be the safest course in this context. One study showed that L-T_3 therapy improved hyperactivity in nine children with ADHD and RTH, including three individuals who did not respond to treatment with methylphenidate.[74]

The recent identification of a thyroid hormone analogue with selective thyromimetic action on $TR\beta_1$ versus $TR\alpha_1$[75] or the future development of receptor-isoform specific antagonists might represent a more rational therapeutic approach.

REFERENCES

1. Horlein AJ, Heinzel T, Rosenfeld MG: Gene regulation by thyroid hormone receptors. Curr Opin Endocrinol Diabetes 3:412–416, 1996.
2. Lazar MA: Thyroid hormone receptors: Multiple forms, multiple possibilities. Endocr Rev 14:184–193, 1993.
3. Refetoff S, De Wind LT, De Groot LJ: Familial syndrome combining deaf-mutism, stippled epiphyses, goiter and abnormally high PBI: Possible target organ refractoriness to thyroid hormone. J Clin Endocrinol Metab 27:279–294, 1967.
4. Gershengorn MC, Weintraub BD: Thyrotropin-induced hyperthyroidism caused by selective pituitary resistance to thyroid hormone: A new syndrome of inappropriate secretion of TSH. J Clin Invest 56:633–642, 1975.
5. Magner JA, Petrick P, Menezes-Ferreira M, et al: Familial generalized resistance of thyroid hormones: a report of three kindreds and correlation of patterns of affected tissues with the binding of [^{125}I]triiodothyronine to fibroblast nuclei. J Endocrinol Invest 9:459–469, 1986.
6. Snyder D, Sesser D, Skeels M, et al: Thyroid disorders in newborn infants with elevated screening T_4 (abstract). Thyroid 2(suppl 1):S–29, 1997.
7. Brucker-Davis F, Skarulis MC, Grace MB, et al: Genetic and clinical features of 42 kindreds with resistance to thyroid hormone. Ann Intern Med 123:572–583, 1995.
8. Persani L, Asteria C, Tonacchera M et al: Evidence for the secretion of thyrotopin with enhanced bioactivity in syndromes of thyroid hormone resistance. J Clin Endocrinol Metab 78:1034–1039, 1994.
9. Weiss RE, Refetoff S: Effect of thyroid hormone on growth: Lessons from the syndrome of resistance to thyroid hormone. Endocrinol Metab Clin North Am 25:719–730, 1996.
10. Refetoff S, Weiss RE, Usala SJ: The syndromes of resistance to thyroid hormone. Endocr Rev 14:348–399, 1993.
11. Hauser P, Zametkin AJ, Martinez P, et al: Attention deficit-hyperactivity disorder in people with generalized resistance to thyroid hormone. N Engl J Med 328:997–1001, 1993.
12. Mixson AJ, Parrilla R, Ransom SC, et al: Correlation of language abnormalities with localization of mutations in the β-thyroid hormone receptor in 13 kindreds with generalized resistance to thyroid hormone: Identification of four new mutations. J Clin Endocrinol Metab 75:1039–1045, 1992.
13. Stein MA, Weiss RE, Refetoff S: Neurocognitive characteristics of individuals with resistance to thyroid hormone: Comparisons with individuals with attention-deficit hyperactivity disorder. J Dev Behav Pediatr 16:406–411, 1995.
14. Weiss RE, Stein MA, Duck SC, et al: Low intelligence but not attention deficit hyperactivity disorder is associated with resistance to thyroid hormone caused by mutation R316H in the thyroid hormone receptor β gene. J Clin Endocrinol Metab 78:1525–1528, 1994.
15. Weiss RE, Stein MA, Trommer B, et al: Attention-deficit hyperactivity disorder and thyroid function. J Paediatr 123:539–545, 1993.
16. Valentine J, Rossi E, O'Leary P, et al: Thyroid function in a population of children with attention deficit hyperactivity disorder. J Paediatr Child Health 33:117–120, 1997.
17. Leonard CM, Martinez P, Weintraub BD, et al: Magnetic resonance imaging of cerebral anomalies in subjects with resistance to thyroid hormone. Am J Med Genet 60:238–243, 1995.
18. Wang TWM, Chatterjee VKK: Clinical Case: Case No. 29—Answer. The Association of Clinical Biochemists News Sheet 398:22, 1996.
19. Sarne DH, Refetoff S, Rosenfield RL, et al: Sex hormone-binding globulin in the diagnosis of peripheral tissue resistance to thyroid hormone: The value of changes after short term triiodothyronine administration. J Clin Endocrinol Metab 66:740–746, 1988.
20. Usala SJ, Bale AE, Gesundheit N, et al: Tight linkage between the syndrome of generalized thyroid hormone resistance and the human c-erbA β gene. Mol Endocrinol 2:1217–1220, 1988.
21. Parrilla R, Mixson AJ, McPherson JA, et al: Characterization of seven novel mutations of the c-erbA β gene in unrelated kindreds with generalized thyroid hormone resistance: Evidence for two "hot spot" regions of the ligand binding domain. J Clin Invest 88:2123–2130, 1991.
22. Adams M, Matthews CH, Collingwood TN, et al: Genetic analysis of twenty-nine kindreds with generalized and pituitary resistance to thyroid hormone. J Clin Invest 94:506–515, 1994.
23. Collingwood TN, Wagner R, Matthews CH, et al: A role of helix 3 of the TRβ ligand binding domain in coactivator recruitment identified by characterization of a third cluster of mutations in resistance to thyroid hormone. EMBO J 17:4760–4770, 1998.
24. Weiss RE, Weinberg M, Refetoff S: Identical mutations in unrelated families with generalized resistance to thyroid hormone occur in cytosine-guanine-rich areas of the thyroid hormone receptor β gene. J Clin Invest 91:2408–2415, 1993.
25. Mixson AJ, Renault JC, Ransom S, et al: Identification of a novel mutation in the gene encoding the β-triiodothyronine receptor in a patient with apparent selective pituitary resistance to thyroid hormone. Clin Endocrinol 38:227–234, 1993.
26. Sasaki S, Nakamura H, Tagami T, et al: Pituitary resistance to thyroid hormone associated with a base mutation in the hormone-binding domain of the human 3,5,3′-triiodothyronine receptor β. J Clin Endocrinol Metab 76:1254–1258, 1993.
27. Pohlenz J, Weiss RE, Macchia PE, et al: Five new families with resistance to thyroid hormone not caused by mutations in the thyroid hormone receptor β gene. J Clin Endocrinol Metab 84:3919–3928, 1999.
28. Weiss RE, Hayashi Y, Nagaya T, et al: Dominant inheritance of resistance to thyroid hormone not linked to defects in the thyroid hormone receptor α or β genes may be due to a defective cofactor. J Clin Endocrinol Metab 81:4196–4203, 1996.
29. Olson DP, Koenig RJ: Thyroid function in Rubinstein-Taybi syndrome. J Clin Endocrinol Metab 82:3264–3266, 1997.
30. Weiss RE, Xu J, Ning G, et al: Mice deficient in the steroid receptor coactivator 1 (SRC-1) are resistant to thyroid hormone. EMBO J 18:1900–1904, 1999.
31. Sherman SI, Gopal J, Haugen BR, et al: Central hypothyroidism associated with retinoid X receptor-selective ligands. N Engl J Med 340:1075–1079, 1999.
32. Meier CA, Dickstein BM, Ashizawa K, et al: Variable transcriptional activity and ligand binding of mutant 1 3,5,3′-triiodothyronine receptors from four families with generalized resistance to thyroid hormone. Mol Endocrinol 6:248–258, 1992.
33. Collingwood TN, Adams M, Tone Y, et al: Spectrum of transcriptional dimerization and dominant negative properties of twenty different mutant thyroid hormone β receptors in thyroid hormone resistance syndrome. Mol Endocrinol 8:1262–1277, 1994.
34. Collingwood TN, Rajanayagam O, Adams M, et al: A natural transactivation mutation in the thyroid hormone β receptor: Impaired interaction with putative transcriptional mediators. Proc Natl Acad Sci U S A 94:248–253, 1997.
35. Takeda K, Sakurai A, De Groot LJ, et al: Recessive inheritance of thyroid hormone resistance caused by complete deletion of the protein-coding region of the thyroid hormone receptor-β gene. J Clin Endocrinol Metab 74:49–55, 1992.
36. Sakurai A, Miyamoto T, Refetoff S, et al: Dominant negative transcriptional regulation by a mutant thyroid hormone receptor β in a family with generalized resistance to thyroid hormone. Mol Endocrinol 4:1988–1994, 1990.
37. Chatterjee VKK, Nagaya T, Madison LD, et al: Thyroid hormone resistance syndrome: Inhibition of normal receptor function by mutant thyroid receptors. J Clin Invest 87:1977–1984, 1991.
38. Ono S, Schwartz ID, Mueller OT, et al: Homozygosity for a dominant negative thyroid hormone receptor gene responsible for generalized resistance to thyroid hormone. J Clin Endocrinol Metab 73:990–994, 1991.
39. Nagaya T, Madison LD, Jameson JL: Thyroid hormone receptor mutants that cause resistance to thyroid hormone: Evidence for receptor competition for DNA sequences in target genes. J Biol Chem 267:13014–13019, 1992.
40. Nagaya T, Jameson JL: Thyroid hormone receptor dimerization is required for dominant negative inhibition by mutations that cause thyroid hormone resistance. J Biol Chem 268:15766–15771, 1993.
41. Kitajima K, Nagaya T, Jameson JL: Dominant negative and DNA-binding properties of mutant thyroid hormone receptors that are defective in homodimerization but not heterodimerization. Thyroid 5:343–353, 1995.
42. Yoh SM, Chatterjee VKK, Privalsky ML: Thyroid hormone resistance syndrome manifests as an aberrant interaction between mutant T_3 receptors and transcriptional corepressors. Mol Endocrinol 11:470–480, 1997.
43. Tagami T, Madison LD, Nagaya T, et al: Nuclear receptor corepressors activate rather than suppress basal transcription of genes that are negatively regulated by thyroid hormone. Mol Cell Biol 17:2642–2648, 1997.
44. Clifton-Bligh RJ, de Zegher F, Wagner RL, et al: A novel TRβ mutation (R383H) in resistance to thyroid hormone predominantly impairs corepressor release and negative transcriptional regulation. Mol Endocrinol 12:609–621, 1998.
45. Wagner RL, Apriletti JW, McGrath ME, et al: A structural role for hormone in the thyroid hormone receptor. Nature 378:690–697, 1995.
46. Hayashi Y, Weiss RE, Sarne DH, et al: Do clinical manifestations of resistance to thyroid hormone correlate with the functional alteration of the corresponding mutant thyroid hormone β receptors? J Clin Endocrinol Metab 80:3246–3256, 1995.
47. Hayashi Y, Janssen OE, Weiss RE, et al: The relative expression of mutant and normal thyroid hormone receptor genes in patients with generalized resistance to thyroid hormone determined by estimation of their specific messenger ribonucleic acid products. J Clin Endocrinol Metab 76:64–69, 1993.
48. Mixson AJ, Hauser P, Tennyson G, et al: Differential expression of mutant and normal β T_3 receptor alleles in kindreds with generalized resistance to thyroid hormone. J Clin Invest 91:2296–2300, 1993.
49. Zavacki AM, Harney JW, Brent GA, et al: Dominant negative inhibition by mutant thyroid hormone receptors is thyroid response element and receptor isoform specific. Mol Endocrinol 7:1319–1330, 1993.
50. Geffner ME, Su F, Ross NS, et al: An arginine to histidine mutation in codon 311 of the *c-erb*A β gene results in a mutant thyroid hormone receptor that does not mediate a dominant negative phenotype. J Clin Invest 91:538–546, 1993.
51. Beck Peccoz P, Chatterjee VKK: The variable clinical phenotype in thyroid hormone resistance syndrome. Thyroid 4:225–232, 1994.
52. Beck Peccoz P, Roncoroni R, Mariotti S, et al: Sex hormone-binding globulin measurement in patients with inappropriate secretion of thyrotropin (IST): Evidence against selective pituitary thyroid hormone resistance in nonneoplastic IST. J Clin Endocrinol Metab 71:19–25, 1990.
53. Ando S, Nakamura H, Sasaki S, et al: Introducing a point mutation identified in a patient with pituitary resistance to thyroid hormone (Arg 338 to Trp) into other mutant thyroid hormone receptors weakens their dominant negative activities. J Endocrinol 151:293–300, 1996.
54. Safer JD, O'Connor MG, Colan SD, et al: The thyroid hormone receptor-β gene mutation R383H is associated with isolated central resistance to thyroid hormone. J Clin Endocrinol Metab 84:3099–3109, 1999.
55. Safer JD, Langlois MF, Cohen R, et al: Isoform variable action among thyroid hormone receptor mutants provides insight into pituitary resistance to thyroid hormone. Mol Endocrinol 11:16–26, 1997.
56. Forrest D, Hanebuth E, Smeyne RJ, et al: Recessive resistance to thyroid hormone in mice lacking thyroid hormone receptor β: Evidence for tissue-specific modulation of receptor function. EMBO J 15:3006–3015, 1996.
57. Abel ED, Kaulbach HC, Campos-Barros A, et al: Novel insight from transgenic mice into thyroid hormone resistance and the regulation of thyrotropin. J Clin Invest 103:271–279, 1999.
58. Wong R, Vasilyev VV, Ting Y-T, et al: Transgenic mice bearing a human mutant thyroid hormone β_1 receptor manifest thyroid function anomalies, weight reduction and hyperactivity. Mol Med 3:303–314, 1997.

59. Wikstrom L, Johansson C, Salto C, et al: Abnormal heart rate and body temperature in mice lacking thyroid hormone receptor α_1. EMBO J 17:455–461, 1998.
60. Gurnell M, Rajanayagam O, Barbar I, et al: Reversible pituitary enlargement in the syndrome of resistance to thyroid hormone. Thyroid 8:679–682, 1998.
61. Beck Peccoz P, Piscitelli G, Cattaneo MG, et al: Successful treatment of hyperthyroidism due to nonneoplastic pituitary TSH hypersecretion with 3,5,3′-triiodothyroacetic acid (TRIAC). J Endocrinol Invest 6:217–223, 1983.
62. Crino A, Borrelli P, Salvatori R, et al: Anti-iodothyronine autoantibodies in a girl with hyperthyroidism due to pituitary resistance to thyroid hormones. J Endocrinol Invest 15:113–120, 1992.
63. Radetti G, Persani L, Molinaro G, et al: Clinical and hormonal outcome after two years of TRIAC treatment in a child with thyroid hormone resistance. Thyroid 7:775–778, 1997.
64. Bracco D, Morin O, Schutz Y, et al: Comparison of the metabolic and endocrine effects of 3,5,3′-triiodothyroacetic acid and thyroxine. J Clin Endocrinol Metab 77:221–228, 1993.
65. Takeda T, Suzuki S, Liu R-T, et al: Triiodothyroacetic acid has unique potential for therapy of resistance to thyroid hormone. J Clin Endocrinol Metab 80:2033–2040, 1995.
66. Ueda S, Takamatsu J, Fukata S, et al: Differences in response of thyrotropin to 3,5,3′-triiodothyronine and 3,5,3′-triiodothyroacetic acid in patients with resistance to thyroid hormone. Thyroid 6:563–570, 1996.
67. Asteria C, Rajanayagam O, Collingwood TN, et al: Prenatal diagnosis of thyroid hormone resistance. J Clin Endocrinol Metab 84:405–410, 1999.
68. Kunitake JM, Hartman N, Henson LC, et al: 3,5,3′-Triiodothyroacetic acid therapy for thyroid hormone resistance. J Clin Endocrinol Metab 69:461–466, 1989.
69. Hamon P, Bovier-LaPierre M, Robert M, et al: Hyperthyroidism due to selective pituitary resistance to thyroid hormones in 15-month-old boy: Efficacy of D-thyroxine therapy. J Clin Endocrinol Metab 67:1089–1093, 1988.
70. Dorey F, Strauch G, Gayno JP: Thyrotoxicosis due to pituitary resistance to thyroid hormones: Successful control with D-thyroxine: A study in three patients. Clin Endocrinol 32:221–227, 1990.
71. Dulgeroff AJ, Geffner ME, Koyal SN, et al: Bromocriptine and TRIAC therapy for hyperthyroidism due to pituitary resistance to thyroid hormone. J Clin Endocrinol Metab 75:1071–1075, 1992.
72. Williams G, Kraenzlin M, Sandler L, et al: Hyperthyroidism due to non-tumoral inappropriate TSH secretion: Effect of long-acting somatostatin analogue (SMS 201–995). Acta Endocr (Copenh) 113:42–46, 1986.
73. Beck Peccoz P, Mariotti S, Guillausseau PJ, et al: Treatment of hyperthyroidism due to inappropriate secretion of thyrotropin with the somatostatin analog SMS 201–995. J Clin Endocrinol Metab 68:208–214, 1989.
74. Weiss RE, Stein MA, Refetoff S: Behavioral effects of liothyronine (L-T_3) in children with attention deficit hyperactivity disorder in the presence and absence of resistance to thyroid hormone. Thyroid 7:389–393, 1997.
75. Chiellini G, Apriletti JW, Yoshihara HA, et al: A high-affinity subtype-selective agonist ligand for the thyroid hormone receptor. Chem Biol 5:299–306, 1998.

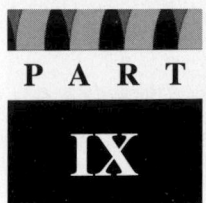

PART IX Adrenal Gland and Glucocorticoids

Editor: D. Lynn Loriaux

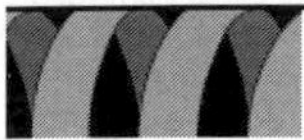

BASIC PHYSIOLOGY

Chapter 115

The Principles, Pathways, and Enzymes of Human Steroidogenesis

Richard J. Auchus ▪ Walter L. Miller

OVERVIEW OF THE HUMAN STEROIDOGENIC ENZYMES AND STEROIDOGENESIS

All steroid hormones derive from cholesterol in a process that can be conceptualized as having five components:

1. The conversion of cholesterol to pregnenolone. Although viewed superficially as a single chemical transformation, the mobilization of cholesterol into the steroidogenic pathways is a complex event that not only serves as a key locus of regulation but also conventionally defines a tissue as "steroidogenic." In humans, only the adrenal cortex, ovarian theca cells, trophoblast cells of the placenta, and glial cells of the brain possess the capacity to cleave cholesterol into pregnenolone (the C_{21} precursor of all active steroid hormones) and isocaprialdehyde. It is the differences both in how this process is regulated and in how pregnenolone is subsequently metabolized that defines the roles of the various steroidogenic cells and tissues in human physiology. Unlike peptide-secreting glands, steroidogenic cells do not store steroid hormones and intermediates, and it is the activation of this first step that enables the rapid production of steroids in response to hormonal and environmental stimuli.

2. The transformation of pregnenolone to active hormones, intermediates, and exported steroid derivatives. The repertoire of enzymes and cofactor proteins present in a given steroidogenic cell generates the characteristic steroid profile of that cell type, and the coordinate regulation of their expression promotes the completion of all steps of a given pathway. Thus, these enzymes determine qualitatively *what* steroids are made, but since these steps are not kinetically limiting, it is step 1 that quantitatively regulates *how much* steroids are made at a given moment. Steroids diffuse into the bloodstream, although the sulfation of Δ^5 steroids helps to promote their solubility and to prolong their half-lives in the circulation.

3. Peripheral metabolism of hormones and precursors. Although not "steroidogenic" as defined earlier, some organs, such as the liver and skin, possess tremendous capacity to transform various steroids. For example, 70% to 80% of circulating testosterone in normal cycling women derives from the conversion of adrenal DHEA.[1]

4. Target tissue metabolism. Steroids can be activated in target tissues, such as the conversion of testosterone by steroid 5α-reductase type II to dihydrotestosterone in the prostate.[2] In contrast, active androgens and estrogens are inactivated in the uterus[3] and other peripheral tissues by 17βHSD type II.[4]

5. Catabolism and unproductive metabolism. A panopoly of steroids can be isolated from human plasma and tissues, many of which have negligible biologic activity. Most inactive by-products derive from hepatic transformations, such as 6α/6β-hydroxylation of C_{19} steroids and 4-hydroxylation of estrogens, which promote renal excretion of these steroids.

Steroids are biomolecules derived from the cyclopentanoperhydrophenanthrene four-ring hydrocarbon nucleus (Fig. 115–1). As such a relatively inert structure, the enzymes involved in their biosynthetic metabolism are relatively limited (Fig. 115–2). Note that all of these reactions are essentially unidirectional. All P450-mediated hydroxylations and carbon-carbon bond cleavage reactions are mechanistically and physiologically irreversible, and although some hydroxysteroid dehydrogenase reactions can run "backwards" in vitro under certain conditions, each hydroxysteroid dehydrogenase functions essentially only in either the oxidative or reductive mode in vivo. However, some pairs of hydroxysteroid dehydrogenases catalyze opposite reactions, such as 11β-hydroxysteroid dehydrogenases type I (reductive) and type II (oxidative).

P450s. Mammalian cytochromes P450 fall into two broad classes, the type I and type II enzymes. Type I enzymes and their electron transfer proteins reside in the mitochondria (Table 115–1) of eukaryotes; almost all bacterial P450s are also type I enzymes. Type I enzymes receive electrons from the reduced form of nicotinamide-adenine dinucleotide phosphate (NADPH) via adrenodoxin, a small, soluble iron-sulfur protein. Adrenodoxin does not oxidize NADPH directly, however, but receives the two electrons from NADPH via the flavoprotein adrenodoxin reductase (Fig. 115–3). Type II enzymes, in contrast, receive electrons from NADPH via the flavin adenine dinucleotide (FAD)-flavin mononucleotide (FMN) two-flavin protein, P450 oxidoreductase (OR). Type II enzymes are exclusively located in the smooth endoplasmic reticulum and constitute the majority of the human P450 enzymes.[5]

P450 enzymes activate molecular oxygen using their heme center and electrons from NADPH. Substrate binding is required prior to

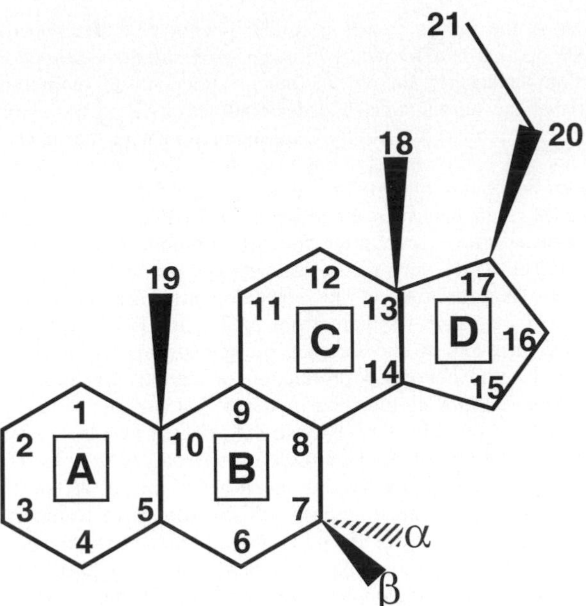

FIGURE 115–1. Perhydrophenanthrene steroid nucleus. Steroid rings are identified with *boxed capital letters,* and carbon atoms are numbered. Substituents and hydrogens are labeled as α or β if they are positioned behind or in front of the plane of the page, respectively.

heme reduction, and the bound substrate is subsequently attacked by the active oxygenating species, which is generally considered to be an iron oxene (Fig. 115–4). Thus, P450 reactions on steroids are limited to oxygen insertion (hydroxylation) reactions and, in a few notable cases, oxidative carbon-carbon bond cleavage reactions (Table 115–2).

Hydroxysteroid Dehydrogenases (HSDs) and Reductases. All HSDs and related enzymes use nicotinamide cofactors either to reduce or to oxidize the steroid by two electrons. Most examples involve the conversion of a secondary alcohol to a ketone or vice versa, and in the case of the 3β-hydroxysteroid dehydrogenase/$\Delta^{5/4}$-isomerases, the dehydrogenation is accompanied by the isomerization of the adjacent carbon-carbon double bond from the Δ^5 (between carbons 5 and 6) to the Δ^4 positions (see Figs. 115–1 and 115–2). A few members of this family, such as the human steroid 5α-reductases types I and II, reduce olefinic carbon-carbon double bonds to the saturated state rather than acting on oxygenated carbon centers.

TABLE 115–1. Intracellular Location of Steroidogenic Proteins

Mitochondria	Cytoplasm	Endoplasmic Reticulum
P450scc		P450c17
P450c11β		P450c21
P450c11AS		P450aro
Adrenodoxin reductase	Adrenodoxin	P450-oxidoreductase
StAR	StAR	Cytochrome b_5
3β-HSDII	3β-HSDII	3β-HSDII
	17β-HSDI	17β-HSDI–III*
	17β-HSDV	5α-Reductase I and II
	3α-HSD	11β-HSD I and II

*17β-HSDIV is located in peroxisomes.
HSD, hydroxysteroid dehydrogenase.

The HSDs can be broadly dichotomized according to either structural or functional classification schemes. *Structurally,* HSDs are members of either the short-chain dehydrogenase reductase (SDR) or aldo-keto reductase (AKR) families. The SDR enzymes, as first described for glyceralde 3-phosphate dehydrogenase[6] and later observed in x-ray structures of bacterial 3α,20β-HSD[7] and human 17β-HSDI,[8] are β-α-β proteins where up to seven parallel β-strands fan across the center of the molecule (Fig. 115–5A, see also color plate), forming the "Rossman fold" characteristic of oxidation/reduction enzymes that use nicotinamide cofactors. The AKR enzymes are soluble proteins that contain the TIM barrel motif, named after the prototypical structure of triosephosphate isomerase in which this fold was first observed.[9] The TIM barrel fold also comprises a continuous α-β-pattern, but the eight parallel β-strands lie in a circular distribution like the staves of a barrel, the fold observed in rat liver 3α-HSD[10] (see Fig. 115–5B). In both cases, the active site contains a critical tyrosine and lysine pair of residues involved in proton transfer from or to the steroid alcohol during catalysis (see Fig. 115–5). *Functionally,* HSDs act either as true dehydrogenases, using NAD^+ as a cofactor to convert hydroxysteroids to ketosteroids, or as ketosteroid reductases, utilizing predominantly NADPH to reduce ketosteroids. Although some HSDs can run in either direction in vitro by adjusting the pH and cofactor concentrations,[11] these enzymes, when expressed in mammalian cells, drive steroid flux in only a single direction. Although the details of this in vivo catalytic selectivity have not been elucidated fully, cofactor utilization is undoubtedly the crucial parameter in determining the direction of the reaction, because cofactor concentrations can exceed steroid concentrations by many orders of magnitude.

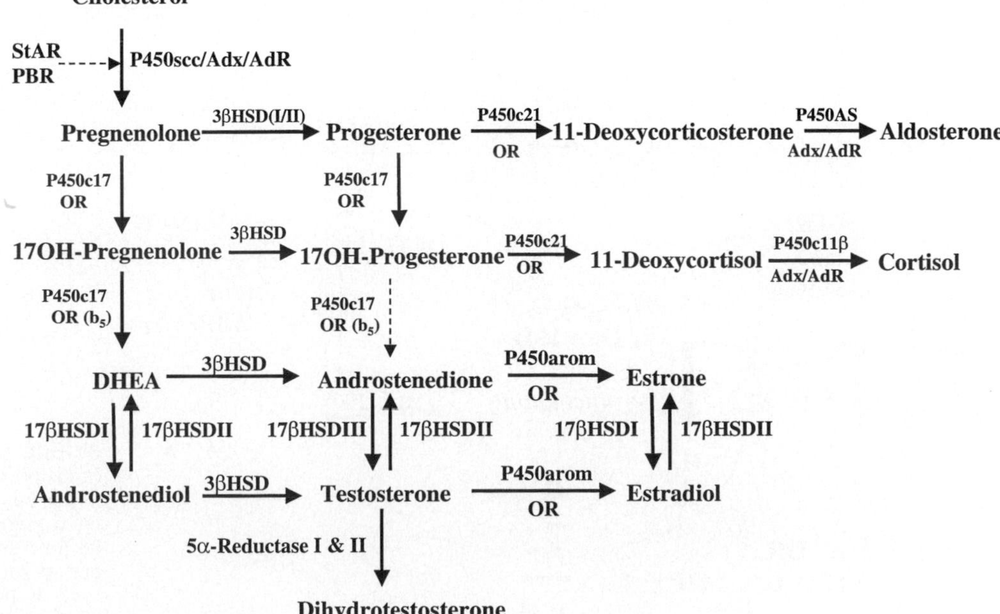

FIGURE 115–2. Major human steroidogenic pathways. Key enzymes and cofactor proteins are shown near *arrows.* Not all intermediate steroids or enzymes (i.e., 11β-hydroxysteroid dehydrogenase [HSD] and 3α-HSDs) are shown.

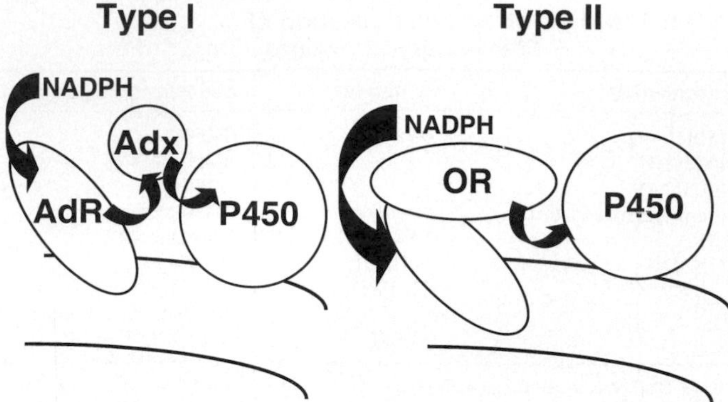

FIGURE 115–3. Electron transfer pathways for steroidogenic cytochrome P450 enzymes. In type I enzymes, the two electrons from the reduced form of nicotinamide adenine dinucleotide phosphate (NADPH) pass from adrenodoxin reductase (AdR) to adrenodoxin (Adx) and then to the P450. In type II enzymes, the flavoprotein P450 oxidoreductase (OR) both receives electrons from NADPH and directly transfers the two electrons to the P450.

Acute Regulation of Steroidogenesis. Every time that a pulse of ACTH reaches the adrenal cortex or a pulse of luteinizing hormone (LH) reaches the gonad, a subsequent pulse of steroid hormone production is observed within minutes. Although it has long been known that the loss of trophic hormones from the pituitary gland leads to adrenal and gonadal atrophy,[12, 13] the action of ACTH and LH to promote organ survival and to maintain steroidogenic capacity occurs at the level of gene expression, which requires hours to days. This paradox suggested that a second, cyclic adenosine monophosphate (cAMP)-mediated process allowed the rapid mobilization of cholesterol for steroidogenesis. This acute response, however, is abrogated by the protein synthesis inhibitor cycloheximide, which suggested that a short-lived protein species mediated this process.[14] Although other proteins are undoubtedly involved, particularly in the chronic replenishment of mitochondrial cholesterol, abundant biochemical and genetic evidence implicates the steroidogenic acute regulatory protein (StAR) as this labile protein mediator.[15]

StAR is a unique 37-kDa phosphoprotein that is cleaved to a 30-kDa form upon entering the mitochondria. Overexpression of mouse StAR in mouse Leydig MA-10 cells increased their basal steroidogenesis rate,[16] and co-transfection of expression vectors for both StAR and the P450scc system in nonsteroidogenic COS-1 cells augmented pregnenolone synthesis above that obtained with the P450scc system alone.[17] Finally, mutations in StAR cause congenital lipoid adrenal hyperplasia[17, 18] in which no steroids are made, and targeted disruption of StAR in the mouse causes a similar phenotype.[19] The mechanism of StAR's action is unknown. Although StAR enters the mitochondria, its action appears to be on the outer mitochondrial membrane, as deletion of the mitochondrial leader confines StAR to the cytoplasm but does not reduce its activity.[20] Its interaction with the outer membrane appears to involve changes in protein conformation of StAR.[21] Although StAR is required for the acute steroidogenic response, steroidogenesis will persist in the absence of StAR at about 14% of the StAR-induced rate,[22] accounting for the steroidogenic capacity of tissues that lack StAR, such as the placenta and the brain.

Chronic Maintenance of the Steroidogenic Machinery. The episodic bursts of cAMP resultant from ACTH and LH binding to their respective receptors on the adrenals and gonads are necessary but not sufficient for the continued production of steroids by these glands. Patients with inactivating mutations in the ACTH receptor[23] or LH receptor[24, 25] make negligible steroids from the affected glands. Conversely, activating mutations of the $G_s\alpha$ protein that couples receptor binding to cAMP generation and activating mutations of the LH receptor cause hypersecretion of steroids.[26] Indeed, cAMP-responsive elements have been identified in the genes for most of the human steroidogenic P450 enzymes, but it is obvious that this mechanism alone does not allow for the diversity of steroid production observed in the various zones of the adrenal cortex, the gonads of both sexes, the placenta, and the brain.

Other transcription factors, such as AP-2 and SP-1, aid in defining the basal- and cAMP-stimulated transcription of each gene, which is also regulated in a tissue-specific manner by the regulatory elements unique to each gene. Among these factors, steroidogenic factor-1 (SF-1), an orphan nuclear receptor also known as Ad4BP, appears central to the coordinate expression of steroidogenic enzymes in adrenal and gonadal cells.[27] By contrast, steroidogenesis in the brain[28] and placenta[29] is independent of SF-1. Targeted disruption of SF-1 in the mouse not only disrupts steroid biosynthesis but also blocks the development of the adrenal glands, gonads, and some areas of the hypothalamus in homozygous animals.[30] Furthermore, SF-1 does not act in isolation, but its action is modified by other transcription factors such as WT-1 and DAX-1[31] or by phosphorylation.[32] Thus the development of steroidogenic organs is intimately related to the capacity to produce steroids, and multiple factors acting on the genes for steroidogenic enzymes yield both common features and diversity among the steroidogenic tissues.

Unlike some modular proteins, such as the estrogen receptor, in which alternate splicing generates variant proteins with a spectrum of biologic activities,[33] most steroidogenic enzymes derive from a single mRNA species. The most prominent exception to this paradigm is aromatase, whose gene has four different promoters that enable vastly different regulation of expression of the same aromatase protein in

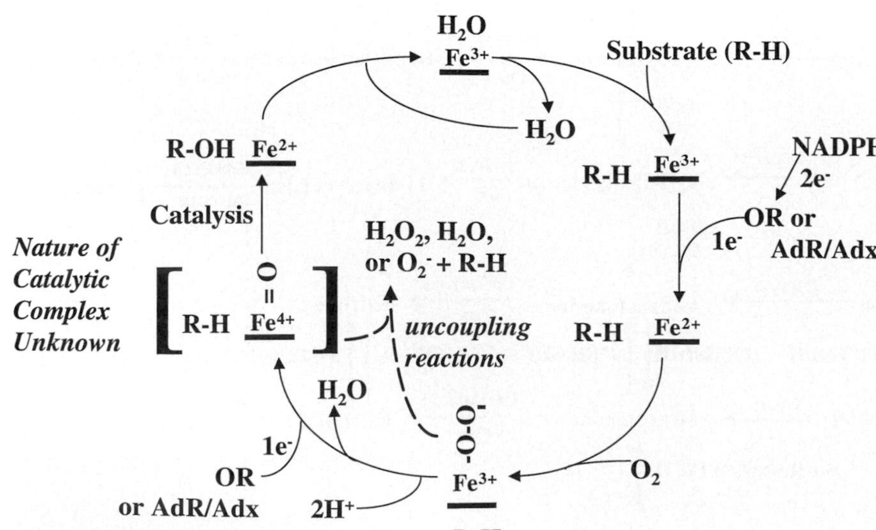

FIGURE 115–4. The P450 reaction cycle. Inorganic reductants can supply the first of two electrons to the P450, but a redox partner protein (Adx, OR, or possibly b_5) must be involved in the second electron transfer for a successful catalytic cycle. A typical hydroxylation product is shown, but a similar if not identical cycle is believed to occur for carbon-carbon bond cleavage steps.

TABLE 115–2. Key Human Steroidogenic Enzymes and Cofactor Proteins

Protein	Gene	Gene Size	Chromosomal Locus	Location	Substrates	Activities	Deficiency Syndromes
P450scc	*CYP11A1*	>20	15q23–q24	ZG/ZF/ZR Gonads (L,T), placenta, brain	Cholesterol Hydroxysterols	22R-Hydroxylase 20R-Hydroxylase 20,22-Lyase	Not described (presumed lethal)
P450c17	*CYP17*	6.6	10q24.3	ZF/ZR Gonads (L,T)	Preg, 17OH-Preg Prog, [17OH-Prog] DHEA	17α-Hydroxylase [16α-Hydroxylase] 17,20-Lyase [Δ^{16}-Synthase]	17-Hydroxylase deficiency Isolated 17,20-Lyase deficiency
P450c21	*CYP21B*	3.4	6p21.1	ZG/ZF/ZR	Prog, 17OH-Prog	21-Hydroxylase	21-Hydroxylase deficiency
P450c11β	*CYP11B1*	9.5	8q21–q22	ZF/ZR	11-Deoxycortisol 11-DOC	11-Hydroxylase	11-Hydroxylase deficiency
P450c11AS	*CYP11B2*	9.5	8q21–q22	ZG	Corticosterone 11-DOC 18OH-Corticosterone	11-Hydroxylase 18-Hydroxylase 18-Oxidase	CMO I deficiency CMO II deficiency
P450aro	*CYP19*	>52	15q21.1	Gonads (L,G), placenta, brain, fat	Androstenedione Testosterone	19-Hydroxylase 19-Oxidase, aromatization	Aromatase deficiency
3β-HSDI	*HSD3B1*	7.8	1p13	Placenta, liver, brain	Preg, 17OH-Preg DHEA, Adiol	3β-Dehydrogenase $\Delta^{5/4}$-Isomerase	Not described (presumed lethal)
3β-HSDII	*HSD3B2*	7.8	1p13	ZG/ZF>ZR Gonad (L,T)	Preg, 17OH-Preg DHEA, Adiol	3β-Dehydrogenase $\Delta^{5/4}$-Isomerase	3β-HSD deficiency
17β-HSDI	*HSD17B1*	3.3	17q21	Gonad (G), placenta, etc.	Estrone, [DHEA]	17β-Ketosteroid reductase	Not described
17β-HSDII	*HSD17B2*	>40	16q24	Endometrium, broadly	Testosterone, Estradiol, DHT	17β-Hydroxysteroid dehydrogenase	Not described
17β-HSDIII	*HSD17B3*	>60	9q22	Gonad (L)	Androstenedione [Estrone, DHEA]	17β-Ketosteroid reductase	Male 17-ketosteroid Reductase deficiency
17β-HSDV†	*HSD17B5*	—	10p14–15	Prostate broadly	Androstenedione DHT, 3α-Asdiol 3α-Androstanediol Asone, Asdione	17β-Ketosteroid reductase* 3α-Hydroxysteroid dehydrogenase*	Not described
5α-Reductase type I	*SRD5A1*	>35	5p15	Liver, brain, skin	Testosterone, C_{21}-steroids	5α-Reduction	Not described
5α-Reductase type II	*SRD5A2*	>35	2p23	Prostate, genital skin	Testosterone, C_{21}-steroids	5α-Reduction	5α-Reductase deficiency
11β-HSDI	*HSD11B1*	9	1	Liver, brain, placenta, etc.	Cortisol, cortisone, corticosterone, 11-DehydroB	11β-Ketosteroid reductase*	Not described
11β-HSDII	*HSD11B2*	6.2	16p22	Kidney, gut, placenta	Cortisol, corticosterone	11β-Hydroxysteroid dehydrogenase	Syndrome of apparent mineralocorticoid excess
Adrenodoxin	*ADX*	>30	11q22	Ubiquitous	Mitochondrial P450s	Electron transfer	Not described (presumed lethal)
Adrenodoxin reductase	*ADR*	11	17q24–q25	Ubiquitous	Mitochondrial P450s	Electron transfer	Not described (presumed lethal)
StAR	*STAR*	8	8p11.2	Adrenals, gonad	Cholesterol flux within mitochondria	Sterol delivery to P450scc	Lipoid CAH
P450-OR	*CPR*	22	7p15–q35	Ubiquitous	Microsomal P450s	Electron transfer	Not described
Cytochrome b_5	*CYB5*	32	18q23	ZR>ZG/ZF, gonads, etc.	Aids P450c17	Augments 17,20-lyase activity	?17,20-Lyase deficiency with methemoglobinemia

*Reversible reactions.

†The nomenclature for the 3α-HSD and 17β-HSD type V enzyme(s) is currently evolving.

ZG/ZF/ZR = adrenal zona glomerulosa/fasciculata/reticularis, respectively; L, Leydig cells; T, theca cells; G, granulosa cells; 17OH-Preg, 17α-hydroxypregnenolone; 17OH-Prog, 17α-hydroxyprogesterone; 11-DehydroB, 11-dehydrocorticosterone; CAH, congenital adrenal hyperplasia; CMO, corticosterone methyl oxidase.

Minor substrates and activities peripheral to the main steroidogenic pathways are in brackets; Adiol, Δ^5-3β-androstanediol; DHEA, dehydroepiandrosterone; DHT, dihydrotestosterone; DOC, deoxycorticosterone; 3α-Asdiol, 3α-androstanediol; Asdione, androstanedione; Asone, androsterone; steroids in brackets are weak substrates.

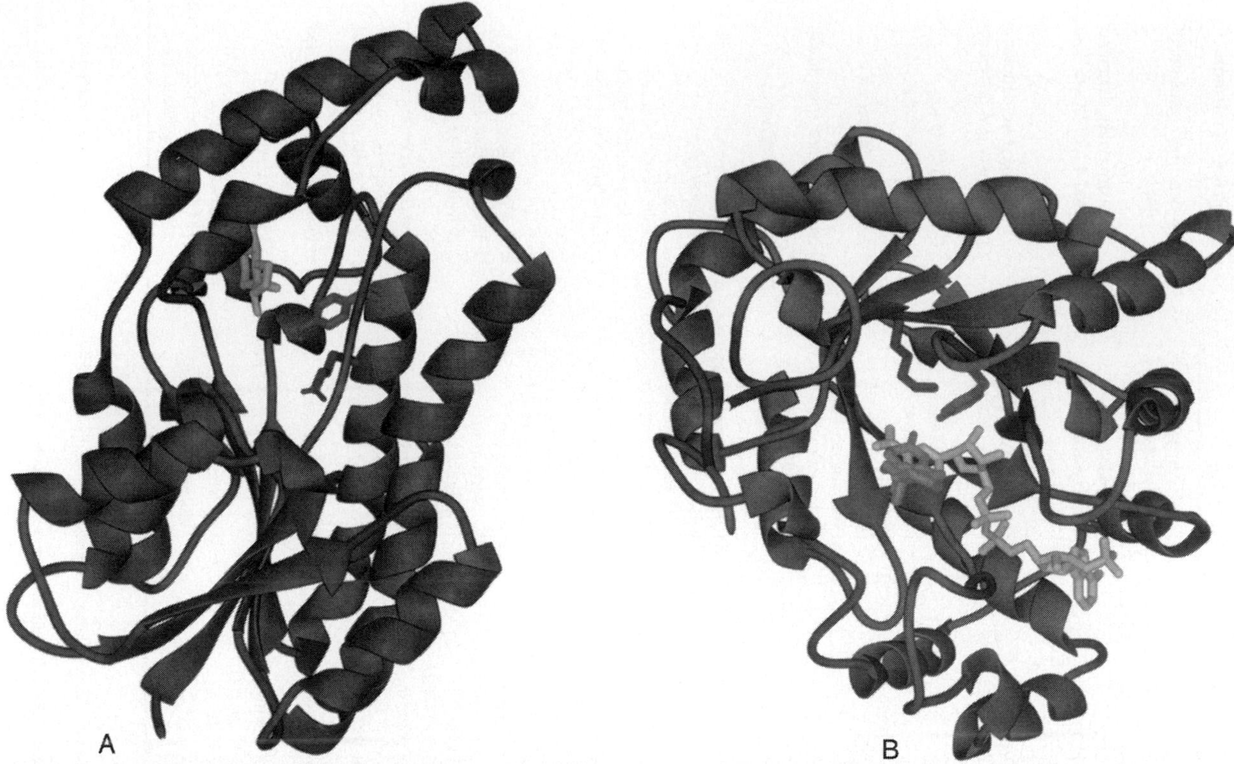

FIGURE 115–5. The two types of hydroxysteroid dehydrogenase (HSD) structures. The representative structure shown for the short-chain dehydrogenase reductase (SDR) class is human 17β-HSDI (Research Collaboratory for Structural Bioinformatics [rcsb, website http://www.rcsb.org] PDB ID No. 1IOL, panel *A*), with bound estradiol in yellow and the Tyr and Lys residues critical for catalysis are shown in magenta and blue, respectively. The basic SDR structure contains the strands of a β-sheet core (upward *arrows* at the bottom of the figure) plus helices on the top and sides of the molecule. The representative structure for the aldo-keto reductase (AKR) class is rat liver 3α-HSD (rcsb PDB No.1AFS, panel *B*). The bound substrate testosterone is in green; cofactor $NADP^+$ is in yellow; and the Tyr and Lys residues that are critical for catalysis are shown in magenta and blue, respectively. The TIM barrel structure of the AKR enzymes is the circular array of β-sheets *(arrows)* with the active site at the "hole" in the barrel and helices at the periphery of the molecule. Note that the Tyr and Lys occupy similar juxtaposition in three-dimensional space in both structures, although the two residues lie on adjacent turns of the same helix in 17β-HSDI but on adjacent β-sheet strands in 3α-HSD. See color plate.

many different tissues.[34] Although different transcripts of several genes including 17β-HSDs types I to III have been described,[4, 35, 36] the encoded proteins derived from "exon skipping" are inactive if translated.[37]

HUMAN STEROIDOGENIC P450s

P450scc. Encoded by the *CYP11A1* gene, P450scc consumes three equivalents of NADPH and molecular oxygen during the conversion of cholesterol to pregnenolone. Although the enzyme is named for the cleavage of the cholesterol side chain, this process consists of three discrete steps: (1) the 22-hydroxylation of cholesterol; (2) the 20-hydroxylation of 22(R)-hydroxycholesterol; and (3) the oxidative scission of the C20-C22 bond of 20(R), 22(R)-dihydroxycholesterol—the side chain cleavage event.[38] The enzyme will utilize free hydroxysterol intermediates as substrates for the side-chain cleavage reaction, a tool that is used experimentally because the hydroxysterols are much more soluble than cholesterol and because their access to P450scc is independent of StAR.[17] In vivo, however, little free intermediates accumulate because their k_{cat}/K_m ratios are much higher than that for cholesterol. The K_m of P450scc for cholesterol is estimated to be 5000 nM, which is roughly the solubility limit for cholesterol in water. In contrast, the affinity of P450scc for the more soluble hydroxysterol intermediates is up to 300-fold greater than that for cholesterol.[39] In addition, the high K_D for pregnenolone (about 3000 nM) drives product dissociation.[40] This complex process is the rate-limiting step in steroidogenesis, with turnover numbers of less than 1 molecule of cholesterol per molecule P450scc per minute.[41]

The single human gene for P450scc[42, 43] encodes a mRNA of 2 kb. A 39-amino acid mitochondrial leader peptide that targets P450scc to the mitochondria is then proteolytically removed to yield a 482 amino acid protein.[43, 44] Forms of P450scc engineered to lack the mitochondrial leader are inactive,[45] demonstrating that the mitochondrial environment is required for activity. Expression of P450scc is induced in the adrenal zona fasciculata/reticularis, testis, and ovary by cAMP[46–50] and in the zona glomerulosa by intracellular calcium/protein kinase C.[48, 51] In contrast, placental P450scc expression is constitutive[52] and is caused at least in part by a transcription factor called LBP-1, which participates in HIV infection.[29] Side chain cleavage activity and pregnenolone biosynthesis have been demonstrated in the rat[53] and human brain,[54] and abundant P450scc expression is found in the rodent brain, especially in fetal life.[55] Deletion of the rabbit P450scc gene has been described, abrogating all steroidogenesis and thus proving that P450scc is the only enzyme that can convert cholesterol to pregnenolone.[56] However, mutations in human P450scc have never been found, because this would prevent placental synthesis of progesterone, causing spontaneous abortion.[57]

P450c17. For investigators unraveling the enzymology and genetics of the steroidogenic pathways, P450c17 proved to be a stumbling block for many years. Clinical observations showed that adrenal 17α-hydroxylase activity (reflected by cortisol production rates) was fairly constant throughout life, whereas adrenal 17,20-lyase activity was low in early childhood but rose abruptly during adrenarche at ages 8 to 10.[58, 59] This dichotomy between adrenal 17α-hydroxylase products (cortisol) and 17,20-lyase products (DHEA) suggested that distinct enzymes performed the two transformations, a hypothesis that was reinforced by the description of patients with putative isolated 17,20-lyase deficiency.[60, 61] Consequently, the reports from Peter Hall's laboratory, which claimed that the 17α-hydroxylase and 17,20-lyase activities of neonatal pig testes co-purified were received initially with great skepticism.[62] This controversy of "one enzyme or two" persisted until the cDNA for bovine P450c17 was cloned and shown to confer both 17-hydroxylase and 17,20-lyase activities when expressed in nonsteroidogenic COS-1 cells.[63] In humans, there is one gene for P450c17, which is expressed in the adrenals and gonads[64] (not two tissue-specific isozymes as had been thought). A single 2.1-kb mRNA species yields a 57-kDa protein in these tissues, and mutations in this gene produce a spectrum of deficiencies in 17-hydroxysteroids and C_{19} steroids.

Human P450c17 17-hydroxylates both pregnenolone and progesterone with approximately equal efficiency,[65, 66] but all other reactions show prominent differences between Δ^4 and Δ^5 substrates. The 17,20-lyase activity is about 50 times faster for the 17α-hydroxypregnenolone-to-DHEA reaction than for the 17α-hydroxyprogesterone-to-androstenedione reaction.[65, 66] Although the rate of the lyase reaction can be increased over 10-fold by the addition of a molar excess of cytochrome b_5,[65–67] the Δ^5 preference persists, and the lyase rate never quite reaches the rate of the hydroxylase reactions. In addition, human P450c17 16α-hydroxylates progesterone but not pregnenolone,[66, 68, 69] and in the presence of cytochrome b_5, diverts about 10% of pregnenolone metabolism to a Δ^{16} andiene product[65] that is also formed by this pathway in pigs and acts as a pheromone in that species.[70] Although experiments to study the chemistry of human P450c17 often require certain manipulations that could be considered nonphysiologic, the remarkable consistency for substrate preferences and kinetic constants observed for the modified, solubilized P450c17 expressed in *E. coli*[65, 67] and native P450c17 expressed in yeast microsomes[66] or intact COS-1 cells[69, 71] or that obtained from human tissues and cells[66, 68] serve to verify these conclusions.

The chemistry of P450c17-mediated hydroxylations is believed to proceed via the common iron oxene species and "oxygen rebound" mechanism proposed for prototypical P450 hydroxylations.[72] The mechanism of the 17,20-lyase reaction involving a carbon-carbon bond cleavage, however, is not immediately obvious. Although this reaction could also proceed via the ferryl oxene species, the most parsimonious proposal, alternative mechanisms that exploit a ferryl peroxide analogous to the Bayer-Villager reaction, cannot be excluded.[73] Recent computer modeling studies suggest that the active site cannot accommodate both a ferryl peroxide and substrate in the correct geometry for such catalysis, and the failure of hydrogen peroxide alone to support catalysis[74] as has been shown for some other P450-mediated deacylation reactions[75] argue against the peroxide mechanism. Nonetheless, no isotopic labeling studies that definitively exclude either mechanism have been performed, thus this controversy persists.

One consequence of the Δ^5 preference of the human enzyme for the 17,20-lyase reaction is that most human sex steroids derive from DHEA as an intermediate. This Δ^5 preference allows for the phenomenon of adrenarche to occur in humans, an event that cannot take place in animals whose adrenal glands do not express P450c17 (e.g., rodents) or whose P450c17 enzyme lacks 17,20-lyase activity for Δ^5 steroids (e.g., the guinea pig). Yet Δ^5-lyase activity is not sufficient for adrenarche, because some monkeys such as rhesus macaques produce high amounts of DHEA throughout life, and lower species such as cows never produce much DHEA.[75a] The biochemistry of P450c17, with the differential regulation of the 17α-hydroxylase and 17,20-lyase activities, provides clues to the genesis of this enigmatic process of adrenarche. P450c17 is a phosphoprotein, and phosphorylation selectively enhances the 17,20-lyase activity.[76] As mentioned, cytochrome b_5 augments the 17,20-lyase activity, and high expression of b_5 in the zona reticularis of monkeys[77] and humans[78] suggests that the developmentally regulated expression of b_5 might be a key event. Finally, limiting steroid flux to the Δ^5 pathway by lowering 3β-HSD activity in the zona reticularis (where most DHEA derives) should potentiate the effect of increased 17,20-lyase activity.[79, 80]

The initial description of 17α-hydroxylase deficiency was a case in which both 17α-hydroxylase and 17,20-lyase products were absent.[81] When the gene for human P450c17 was cloned, patients with 17α-hydroxylase deficiency were found to harbor mutations in the *CYP17* gene,[82, 83] but molecular techniques and subsequent clinical evaluations failed to implicate *CYP17* mutations as the cause of isolated 17,20-lyase deficiency. Three cases of isolated 17,20-lyase deficiency have been confirmed by molecular genetics, identifying homozygous mutations R347H,[84] R358Q,[84] and F417C.[85] Computer modeling studies demonstrate that R347H and R358Q neutralize positive charges in the redox partner-binding site,[74, 84] whereas F417C lies on the edge of that surface.[74] Biochemical studies confirm that mutations R347H and R358Q impair interactions of P450c17 with its electron donor P450-OR and with cytochrome b_5.[86] Therefore, isolated 17,20-lyase deficiency is not caused by an inability of the mutant enzymes to bind the intermediate 17α-hydroxypregnenolone[84, 86] but rather is due to subtle disturbances in interactions with redox partners.[74]

P450c21. Microsomal P450c21 performs the 21-hydroxylation of the Δ^4 steroids progesterone and 17α-hydroxyprogesterone, an essential step in the biosynthesis of both mineralocorticoids and glucocorticoids (see Fig. 115–4). This hydroxylation is unusual in that, from a thermodynamic perspective, the hydroxylation of a methyl group adjacent to a carbonyl is highly unfavorable because the resultant electron-deficient C21 carbon radical is quite unstable. The human P450c21 protein is found only in the adrenal glands; the extra-adrenal 21-hydroxylase activity found in other organs such as the liver and the aorta[87] is not catalyzed by P450c21.[88]

The locus containing the *CYP21* genes is among the most complex in the human genome and explains why 21-hydroxylase deficiency (affecting 1 of 14,000 live births) is one of the most common autosomal recessive diseases. The *CYP21B* gene and the *CYP21A* pseudogene lie on chromosomal locus 6p21.1 in the midst of the HLA locus. Because the HLA locus is highly recombinogenic, exchange between the *CYP21A* and *CYP21B* loci is common. Thus, 85% of cases of 21-hydroxylase deficiency derive from micro- or macro-gene conversion events where some or all of the *CYP21A* pseudogene replaces the corresponding area of the *CYP21B* gene, thus reducing the expression of the encoded P450c21 protein or impairing its activity.[89] In addition, at least eight additional genes lie in this locus (Fig. 115–6), including the liver-specific C4A and C4B genes, the adrenal-specific "ZA" and "ZB" genes, and the ubiquitously expressed tenascin X or XB gene.[90] Occasionally, a patient with 21-hydroxylase deficiency and Ehlers-Danlos syndrome will have a contiguous gene syndrome with tenascin X deficiency as well.[91]

Much less is known about the enzymology of P450c21 than P450c17, in part due to difficulty in the expression of P450c21 in *E. coli*. The available evidence suggests that P450c21 is not very sensitive to the abundance of OR or b_5, but detailed structure-function studies have not been published. It is clear that genotype consistently predicts phenotype in very severe and very mild cases of 21-hydroxylase deficiency. In contrast, patients with P450c21 variants (e.g., the Ile172Asn and Val281Leu substitutions), which have 3% to 10% of wild type activity,[92, 93] can have various phenotypes, implicating that additional factors can modify the clinical manifestations of 21-hydroxylase deficiency.

P450c11β and P450c11AS. The classical descriptions of distinct deficiencies in 11β-hydroxylase, 18-hydroxylase (also called corticosterone methyl oxidase I or CMOI), and 18-oxidase (CMOII) suggested that three enzymes executed these three respective transformations.[94, 95] Analogous to the scenario for P450c17, an enzyme[96] and corresponding gene[97] were found in bovine adrenals that possessed all three activities. In contrast, humans have two genes named *CYP11B1* and *CYP11B2*[98–101] that encode the mitochondrial enzymes 11β-hydroxylase (P450c11β) and aldosterone synthase (P450c11AS), respectively. Although P450c11β and P450c11AS both possess 11β-hydroxylase activities, P450c11AS also performs the two oxygenations at C18 required for aldosterone biosynthesis.[102, 103] Mutations in *CYP11B1* cause 11β-hydroxylase deficiency,[104] whereas defects in *CYP11B2* cause either CMOI or CMOII deficiencies.[105] Thus, severe defects can impair all P450c11AS activities, leading to the clinical phenotype of CMOI deficiency[102] with P450c11β providing 11β-hydroxylase activity. Analogous to the biochemistry of isolated 17,20-lyase activity, fortuitous site-directed mutagenesis experiments of nature have found amino acid substitutions such as Arg181Trp plus Val386Ala, which mainly impair 18-oxidase activity and lead to CMOII deficiency.[106]

The coding regions of the *CYP11B1* and *CYP11B2* genes share 93% amino acid identity and the same exonic gene structure found in all mitochondrial P450 genes.[107] Despite the sequence similarities of these tandem genes, located within 40 kb on chromosome 8q24.3, the expression of P450c11AS is restricted to the adrenal zona glomerulosa, whereas P450c11β is found in the zona fasciculata and zona reticularis.

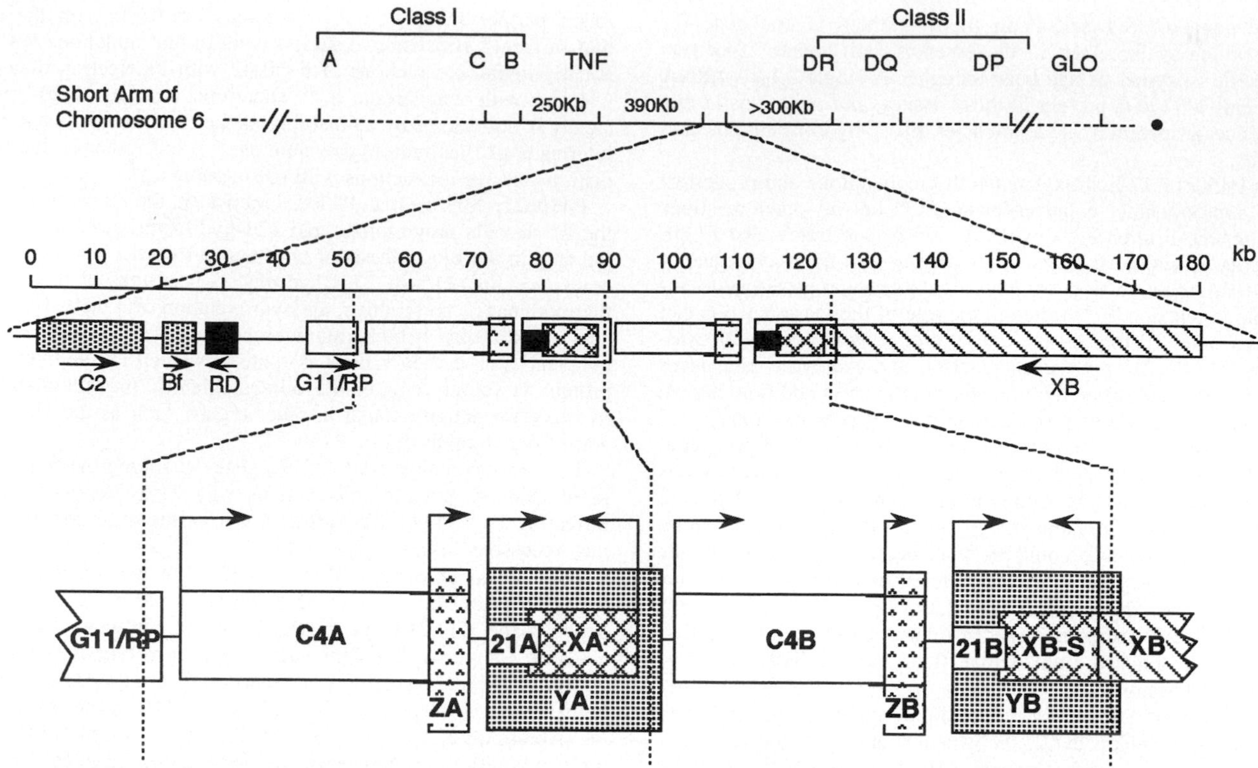

FIGURE 115–6. Genetic map of the human leukocyte antigen (HLA) locus containing the genes for P450c21. The top line shows the p21.1 region of chromosome 6, with the telomere to the left and the centromere to the right. Most HLA genes are found in the class I and class II regions; the class III region containing the *CYP21* genes lies between these two. The second line shows the scale (in kb) for the diagram immediately below, showing (from left to right) the genes for complement factor C2, properdin factor Bf, and the RD and G11/RP genes of unknown function; *arrows* indicate transcriptional orientation. The bottom line shows the 21-hydroxylase locus on an expanded scale, including the C4A and C4B genes for the fourth component of complement, the inactive *CYP21A* gene (21A) and the active *CYP21B* gene (21B) that encodes P450c21. XA, YA, and YB are adrenal-specific transcripts that lack open reading frames. The XB gene encodes the extracellular matrix protein tenascin-X; XB-S encodes a truncated adrenal-specific form of the tenascin-X protein whose function is unknown. ZA and ZB are adrenal-specific transcripts that arise within the C4 genes and have open reading frames, but it is not known if they are translated into protein; however, the promoter elements of these transcripts are essential components of the *CYP21A* and *CYP21B* promoters. The *arrows* indicate transcriptional orientation. The *vertical dotted lines* designate the boundaries of the genetic duplication event that led to the presence of A and B regions.

The regulation of P450c11β is driven mainly by cAMP elevations in response to ACTH, whereas P450c11AS expression derives from angiotensin II activation of the protein kinase C pathway.[108] Thus, under normal circumstances, 18-hydroxylase and 18-oxidase activities are restricted to the zona glomerulosa where 17-hydroxylase activity is low, limiting the repertoire of steroids that can undergo 18-oxygenation.

Although the organization of two highly homologous, adjacent *CYP11B1* and *CYP11B2* genes on chromosome 8 is reminiscent of the genetics of the *CYP21A* and *CYP21B*, gene conversion in the *CYP11B* locus occurs rarely.[109] Instead, a clinical entity called glucocorticoid remediable aldosteronism (GRA) arises when an unequal crossing over of the *CYP11B1* and *CYP11B2* genes creates a third, hybrid gene in which the ACTH-regulated promoter of *CYP11B1* drives expression of a chimeric protein with aldosterone synthase activity.[110–112] As a result, 18-hydroxylase and 18-oxidase activities are ectopically expressed in the zona fasciculata, leading to elevated renin-independent production of aldosterone as well as 18-oxygenated metabolites of cortisol. The expression of this gene is suppressed by blunting ACTH production with glucocorticoids such as dexamethasone, leading to logical albeit suboptimal diagnostic and treatment strategies[113] and to the coining of additional names (e.g., dexamethasone suppressible aldosteronism) for this condition. Although formerly considered a rare disease, genetic testing has shown this disease to be more common than was previously thought, perhaps accounting for 5% of referred patients with hypertension.[114]

The genetics of GRA has assisted in the precise identification of residues in P450c11AS that enable 18-oxygenase activities. Residues 288, 296, 301, 302, 325, and perhaps most importantly 320 are critical for 18-oxygenase activities.[115–117] Therefore, crossovers 3′ to codon 320 do not enable aldosterone synthase activity. These key residue lie in or near the I-helix, which contains the catalytically important threonine residue implicated in oxygen activation for almost all P450s, and thus these mutations would be expected to alter active site geometry.

P450aro (aromatase). The oxidative demethylation of C_{19} steroids such as androstenedione consumes three equivalents of molecular oxygen and NADPH, yielding formic acid and C_{18}, A-ring aromatized estranes. As is the case for P450scc, each subsequent oxygenation proceeds with greater efficiency, aiding in the completion of this transformation that is essential for estrogen biosynthesis in all animals.[118] Although there are many similarities between this transformation and that of lanosterol demethylase, which removes a 14α-methyl group during the biosynthesis of cholesterol,[119] P450aro products contain an aromatic A-ring, hence the common name for this enzyme, aromatase. The mechanism of this aromatization must account for the incorporation of the final oxygen atom from molecular oxygen in the formic acid by-product. The weight of evidence favors a hydroxylation at C2 of 19-oxo-androstenedione, followed by an enzyme-assisted rearrangement and tautomerization of the intermediate dienone to the phenolic A-ring.[120, 121]

Unlike most human steroidogenic P450s, P450aro is expressed both in steroidogenic tissues (ovarian granuloma cells, placenta) and widely in nonsteroidogenic adipose tissue and brain.[118] The *CYP19* gene for P450aro spans over 75 kb[122] and contains five different transcriptional start sites[123] with individual promoters that permit the tissue-specific regulation of expression in diverse tissues. P450aro is a glycoprotein, but glycosylation per se does not appear to affect activity.[124] Recent reports of patients with aromatase deficiency confirm that biologically significant estrogen synthesis derives entirely from this enzyme,[125, 126] although some estrogenic effect in animals with aromatase deficiency can derive from dietary phytoestrogens.[127]

REDOX PARTNER PROTEINS

The proteins collectively referred to as "redox partners" channel reducing equivalents from NADPH to the heme centers of P450 enzymes. Recent studies, however, suggest that these proteins act to promote catalysis by more than just their electron transfer properties.[128] In this way, the precise nature of the interactions of the P450s with their redox partners is of considerable importance, and our understanding of these interactions has been greatly advanced by the x-ray crystal structures of these four proteins, all of which have been solved by mid-1999.

Adrenodoxin (Adx). Adx is a member of the ferredoxin family of iron-sulfur proteins. The gene for Adx on chromosome 11q22 spans over 30 kb, producing a small (14 kDa), soluble Fe_2S_2 electron shuttle protein that resides either free in the mitochondrial matrix or loosely bound to the inner mitochondrial membrane.[129, 130] Adx is expressed in many tissues,[131] and its expression in steroidogenic tissues is induced by cAMP in parallel with P450scc.[132, 133]

Bovine Adx consists of two domains,[134] a core region and an interaction domain (Fig. 115–7A, see also color plate). The core region contains residues 1–55 and 91-end (bovine numbering), including the four cysteines whose sulfur atoms tether the Fe_2S_2 cluster to the

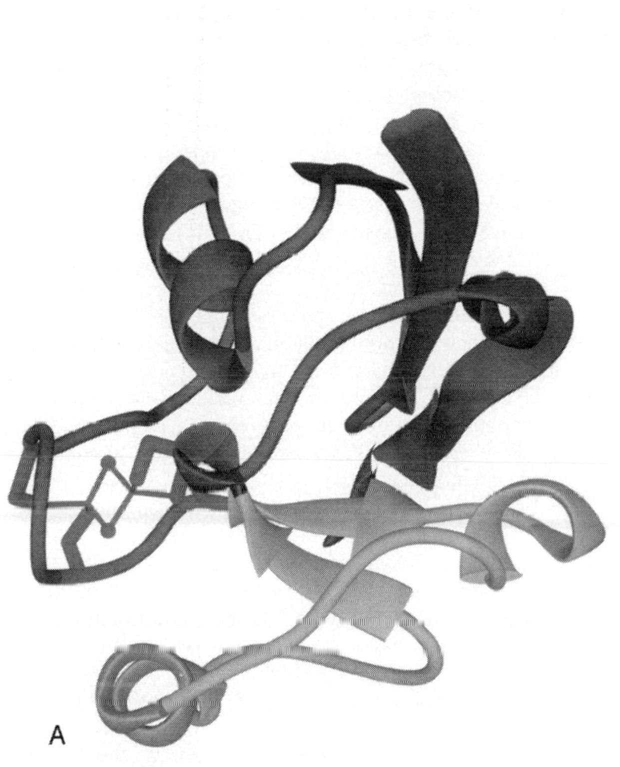

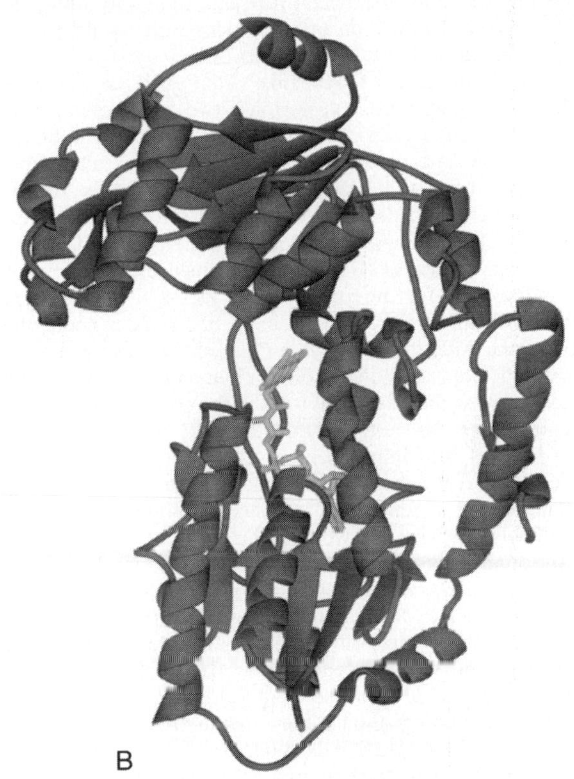

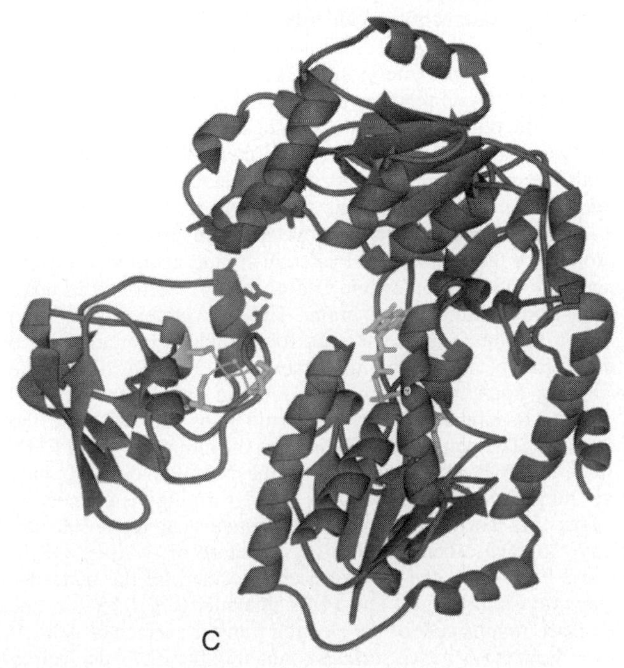

FIGURE 115–7. Mitochondrial electron transport proteins. The backbone atoms of bovine adrenodoxin (Adx, rcsb PDB ID No. 1AYF) are shown in panel *A* with the interaction domain in yellow, the core domain in gray, and the Fe_2S_2 cluster in red. The backbone atoms of bovine adrenodoxin reductase (AdR, rcsb PDB ID No. 1CJC) appear in panel *B* with the flavin shown in yellow. A model of the docked Adx-AdR complex is shown in panel *C*, with prosthetic groups in yellow, key negative charges on Adx in red, and key positive charges on AdR in blue. Note the pairing of positive charges on AdR with negative charges on Adx in this model. See color plate.

protein. Residues 56 to 90 form the interaction domain, which is a hairpin containing at its periphery a helix on which acidic residues known to be critical for the interaction of Adx with P450scc reside,[135] specifically aspartates 72, 76, and 79, plus glutamate 73 (see Fig. 115–7C). The Fe_2S_2 cluster lies in a protuberance in the molecule at the junction of its two domains. The charged residues of Adx cluster in the interaction domain, giving the molecule a highly negatively charged surface above the Fe_2S_2 cluster. This description of the Adx molecule concurs with earlier studies that showed that overlapping sets of negative charges on Adx drive Adx interactions with positive charges on both P450scc and adrenodoxin reductase (AdR).[136–139] Because a preponderance of the evidence favors a model in which the same surface of Adx shuttles between AdR and the P450 to transport electrons,[138] a model of how Adx interacts with AdR would approximate how mitochondrial P450s interact with Adx.

Adrenodoxin Reductase (AdR). Like Adx, AdR is widely expressed in human tissues, but its expression is two orders of magnitude higher in steroidogenic tissues.[140] The primary RNA transcript from the 11-kb AdR gene on chromosome 17q24–q25[141, 142] is alternatively spliced, generating two mRNA species that differ by only 18 bp,[143] but only the protein encoded by the shorter mRNA is active in steroidogenesis.[144] Unlike most steroidogenic genes, the promoter for AdR contains six copies of GGGCGGG sequences, which is the canonical binding site for the transcription factor SP-1[141] typically found in "housekeeping genes." Accordingly, cAMP does not regulate transcription of the AdR gene, as is the case for Adx and P450scc,[140] implying that AdR holds additional roles in human physiology beyond steroidogenesis. Given their essential roles in the conversion of cholesterol to pregnenolone, no null mutations in AdR or Adx have been described in humans, and impairment of the *Drosophila* AdR homologue *dare* causes developmental arrest and degeneration of the adult nervous system owing to the loss of ecdysteroid production.[145]

Bovine AdR also consists of two domains, each comprised of a β-sheet core surrounded by α-helices.[146] The NADP(H)-binding domain is a compact region comprised of residues 106 to 331 (bovine numbering), and the more open FAD domain, formed by the remaining amino- and carboxy-terminal residues, binds the dinucleotide portion of FAD across a Rossman fold with the redox-active flavin isoalloxazine ring abutting the NADP(H) domain (see Fig. 115–7B). By analogy to related structures including glutathione- and thioredoxin reductases, the nicotinamide ring of NADPH is modeled to lie adjacent to the flavin ring in position to transfer its two electrons to the FAD. Thus, intramolecular electron transfer occurs in the cleft formed by the angled apposition of these two domains. Within this cleft, basic residues abound, including arginines 240 and 244, which have been shown to be important for interactions with Adx.[138, 147] Hypothetical docking of the two structures (see Fig. 115–7C) shows that the negative surface of Adx fits elegantly into the positive surface of AdR, even with NADP(H) bound.[146] Basic residues have also been shown to be critical for the interaction of P450scc with the negative surface charges on Adx,[135] so that AdR-Adx docking is expected to share some key features with the mitochondrial P450-Adx interaction.

P450 oxidoreductase (OR). The flavoprotein OR is expressed widely in human tissues and serves as the sole essential electron transfer protein for all microsomal P450s, including xenobiotic-metabolizing hepatic P450s, steroidogenic P450s, and P450s found in other tissues such as the kidney and brain. The OR protein contains a flexible amino terminus that tethers its four domains containing two flavins to the endoplasmic reticulum membrane. The NADPH in the cofactor-binding domain lies above the FAD in a β-sheet-rich FAD domain, and an α-helical connecting domain joins the FAD and the FMN domains.[148] The polypeptide chain exits the amino-terminal FMN domain (that has a β-α-β structure like the NADPH domain) in a disordered "hinge" of about 25 residues before forming the connecting domain, suggesting that the FMN and FAD domains can move substantially relative to each other. In the x-ray structure of rat liver OR,[148] the FMN and FAD lie at the base of a cleft formed by the butterfly-shaped apposition of the FAD and FMN domains (Fig. 115–8A, see also color plate), reminiscent of the electron transfer surface of AdR.[146] It is not clear how the concave surface containing the FMN docks into the redox partner-binding surface of the P450 (which is also concave), but the flexible hinge region on which the FMN domain resides suggests that the FMN domain can reorient itself significantly to accommodate docking to the P450.[66, 128]

In this regard, the x-ray structure of the complex between the P450 and flavoprotein domains of the bacterial protein $P450_{BM3}$ serves as a model of this flavoprotein-P450 interaction.[149] Although some differences in the redox properties of the FMN domains of OR and $P450_{BM3}$ exist, this structure demonstrates how negative charges of the FMN domain guide interactions with positive charges on the P450 (see Fig. 115–8B), mirroring the electrostatic forces driving Adx-P450 interactions. The FMN approaches no closer than 18 Å from the heme,[149] similar to the 16 Å distance of FAD from the Fe_2S_2 cluster in the modeled AdR-Adx complex and presumably similar to the distance of the heme from the Fe_2S_2 cluster in the P450-Adx complex.[146] These distances are much too far for electrons to "jump" directly to the heme. Rather, the FMN and an adjacent tryptophan indole ring lie about 4 Å from atoms 13 to 18 residues from the heme-liganding cysteine, suggesting that electron transfer uses the polypeptide chain as a conduit.[149] Basic residues in the redox-partner binding surface have been shown to be crucial for interactions with OR and for electron transfer,[150–154] and these positive charges in human P450c17 have been shown to be critical for maximal 17,20-lyase activity.[74, 84, 86] Thus, these structures demonstrate several key principles of the electron transfer proteins involved in human steroidogenesis: NADPH and prosthetic groups lie at the interfaces of protein domains in which electron transfers occur; the electron transfer surfaces are negatively charged to pair with positive charges on the P450s; the terminal electron transfer moiety (FMN domain or Adx) must be mobile or soluble to pass electrons on to the P450; and electrons flow from the FMN or Fe_2S_2 cluster along the adjacent polypeptide chain to the heme.

Cytochrome b_5 (b_5). The small (12–17 kDa) hemoprotein b_5 is found in many tissues, as a membrane-bound cytochrome in liver and as a soluble protein lacking the C-terminal membrane anchor in erythrocytes. Importantly, b_5 is expressed in both the adrenals and gonads where it can interact with P450c17, and recent evidence demonstrates that adrenal expression is zone-specific and may contribute to the genesis of adrenarche.[78] Much evidence has shown that b_5 can augment some activities of certain P450 enzymes, and the mechanism of this effect has been presumed to involve electron transfer from b_5 to the P450 for at least the second electron during the P450 cycle (see Fig. 115–3).[155, 156] Although b_5 can certainly receive electrons from flavoproteins like OR,[157] the redox potentials of b_5 and one electron reduced P450 are unfavorable for b_5-to-P450 electron transfer.[158] Indeed, some of the actions of b_5 in experimental systems can be observed with apo-b_5[159] or Mn^{2+}-b_5 (which does not transfer electrons),[160] including the stimulation of 17,20-lyase activity of human P450c17.[66] These experiments suggest that b_5 acts not alone as an electron donor but rather in concert with OR to somehow aid catalysis.

The soluble form of bovine b_5 was one of the first proteins studied by x-ray crystallography,[161] and a wealth of structural data for b_5 have been acquired using molecular dynamics[162] and nuclear magnetic resonance (NMR) spectroscopy for both the holo-[163] and apo-[164] forms of b_5. Analogous to Adx, b_5 consists of two domains, a heme-liganding core 1 domain (residues 40–65, bovine numbering) and a structural core 2 domain from which the C-terminal membrane-anchoring helix extends (see Fig. 115–8C). The heme extends more to the periphery of b_5 than does the Fe_2S_2 cluster of Adx, but there is no cluster of negative charges surrounding the heme. In addition, the core 1 domain acquires considerable conformational flexibility in apo-b_5, whereas the core 2 domain remains folded as in holo-b_5.[164] Finally, the C-terminal membrane-spanning helix (exiting the core 2 domain) is required to stimulate the 17,20-lyase activity of human P450c17, but the signal peptide is not.[165] These results suggest that the core 2 domain is the active region of cytochrome b_5 in stimulating C_{19} steroid biosynthesis. Efforts to map the interaction of b_5 with P450c17 implicate basic residues in P450c17 as important for this action,[74, 86, 160] but a complete picture of the b_5-P450c17-OR complex in which 17,20-lyase activity is optimized is not yet known.

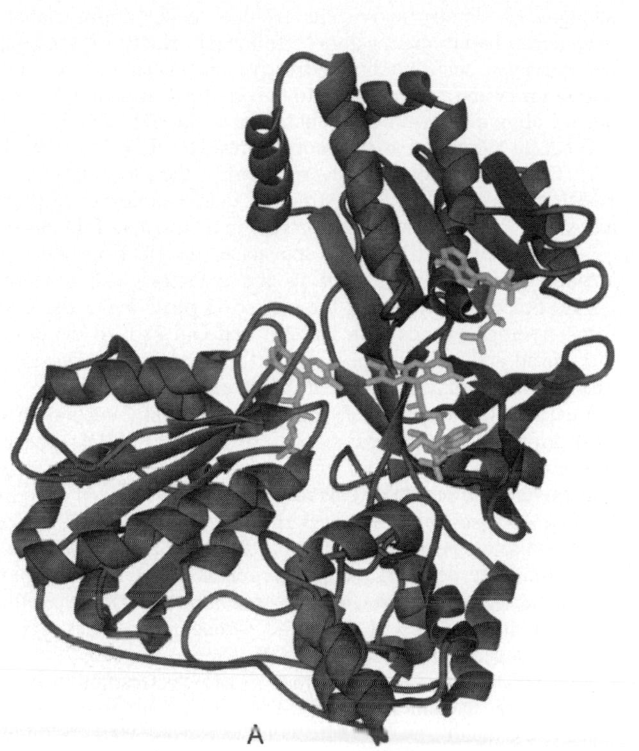

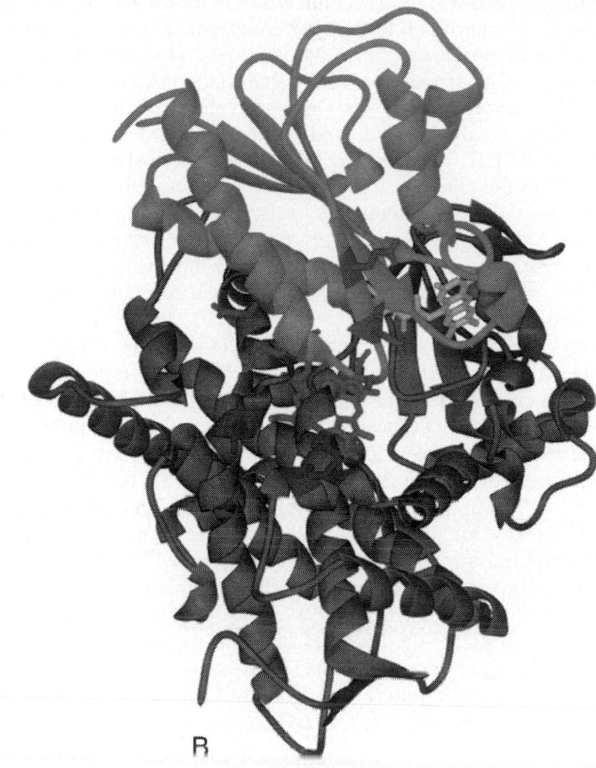

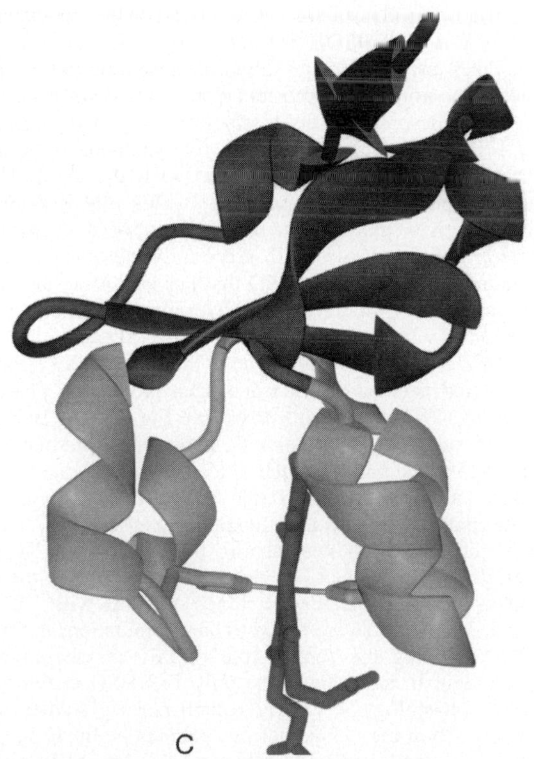

FIGURE 115–8. Flavoproteins and hemoproteins that interact with type II P450 enzymes. Panel *A* shows a ribbon diagram of rat liver P450-OR structure (rcsb PDB ID No. 1AMO), with (clockwise from lower right) bound nicotinamide adenine dinucleotide phosphate, reduced form (NADPH), flavin adenine dinucleotide (FAD), and flavin mononucleotide (FMN) cofactors in yellow. Panel *B* shows the structure of the complex between the FMN domain (green) and P450 domain (gray) of $P450_{BM3}$ (rcsb PDB ID No. 1BVY). The flavin is shown in yellow; the heme is shown in magenta; and positive and negative charges in the interaction surface are highlighted with blue and red, respectively. The hemoprotein cytochrome b_5 is shown in panel *C*, with the heme-binding core 1 domain in yellow and the core 2 domain in gray; the heme is shown red. See color plate.

STEROIDOGENIC DEHYDROGENASES AND REDUCTASES

3β-Hydroxysteroid dehydrogenase/$\Delta^{5/4}$-isomerases (3β-HSDs). Conversion of Δ^5 steroids into their Δ^4 congeners, a step required for the production of progestins, mineralocorticoids, glucocorticoids, and sex steroids, consists of two chemical transformations, both performed by the 3β-HSD enzymes. The first reaction is the oxidation of the 3β-hydroxyl group to the ketone, and during this process NAD^+ is converted to NADH. The intermediate Δ^5, 3β-ketosteroid remains tightly bound to the enzyme with nascent NADH, and the presence of NADH in the cofactor–binding site activates the enzyme's second activity, the $\Delta^{5/4}$-isomerase activity.[166] Competition experiments have shown that the dehydrogenase and isomerase activities reside in a single active site,[167] yet these enzymes are often referred to by their dehydrogenase activity alone.

Although rodents contain multiple 3β-HSD isoforms,[168] only two active genes have been identified in humans.[169, 170] The type I enzyme (3β-HSDI) is expressed in the placenta, liver, brain, and some other peripheral tissues.[170] This placental isoform is required for progesterone production during pregnancy, which may explain why a deficiency of 3β-HSDI has never been described. In contrast, the type II enzyme (3β-HSDII) is by far the principal isoform in the adrenals and gonads.[170] Deficiency of 3β-HSDII causes the rare form of congenital adrenal hyperplasia known as "3β-HSD deficiency."[171] The presence of the type I isozyme in these patients helps to explain the paradox of why 46,XX individuals born with severe 3β-HSDII deficiency can virilize slightly in utero: the 3β-HSD block in the adrenal diverts Δ^5 away from cortisol and toward DHEA; extra-adrenal 3β-HSDI enables testosterone synthesis despite (adrenal) 3-HSD deficiency.

Types I and II enzymes share 93.5% amino acid identity, and all biochemical studies comparing the two enzymes yield very similar results. The enzymes are strongly inhibited by Δ^4 products[167] and by synthetic Δ^4 steroids such as medroxyprogesterone acetate.[172] Both enzymes have very similar affinities for all three Δ^5 steroid substrates, about 5 μM.[172, 173] The enzymes are primarily membrane-bound and are found both in the microsomal and mitochondrial fractions during subcellular fractionation.[173, 174] Ultrastructural studies using immunogold labeling confirm that, at least in bovine adrenal zona glomerulosa cells, 3-HSD immunoreactivity is indeed found not only in mitochondria and the endoplasmic reticulum but also in the cytoplasm.[175]

Considerable evidence suggests that 3β-HSD activity is an important factor in regulating adrenal dehydroepiandrosterone sulfate (DHEAS) production. The human fetal adrenal, which produces vast amounts of DHEAS, contains little 3β-HSD immunoreactivity.[176] Furthermore, the expression of 3β-HSD in the innermost regions of the adrenal cortex declines as the zona reticularis develops in childhood,[79, 80, 177] and 3β-HSD immunoreactivity is low in the zona reticularis of the adult rhesus macaque.[77] Thus, the development of an adrenal cell type (reticularis) relatively deficient in 3β-HSD activity coincides with and may contribute substantially to the genesis of adrenarche, in which adrenal production of the Δ^5 steroids DHEA and DHEAS rises dramatically.

17β-Hydroxysteroid Dehydrogenases (17β-HSDs). There are at least five human 17β-HSD isoforms; these isoforms differ widely in size, structure, substrate specificity, cofactor utilization, and physiologic functions.[178, 179] This section focuses on the human isoforms that possess significant, rather than gratuitous, 17-HSD activity.

17β-HSD Type I. The interconversion of estrone and estradiol in human tissues was described almost 50 years ago,[180] and the study of this "estradiol dehydrogenase" activity was fueled by the abundance of a soluble form of this enzyme in human term placenta[181] that was easily purified.[182] Consequently, 17β-HSDI has been studied more extensively than any other human steroidogenic enzyme. Three groups reported the cloning of the cDNA for this enzyme almost simultaneously.[183–185] Located on chromosome 17q25[186] adjacent to a pseudogene,[35] the *HSD17B1* gene encodes a 34-kDa protein subunit that is expressed primarily in the placenta and in ovarian granulosa cells of developing follicles.[186] The enzyme, which is active only as a dimer, accepts mainly steroids with aromatic A-rings such as estrone and estradiol. Although the enzyme can oxidize 17β-hydroxysteroids in the presence of NAD^+ in vitro at a high pH,[11] the enzyme functions in vivo to reduce estrone to estradiol and 16α-hydroxyestrone to estriol.[187]

Detailed kinetic analyses of 17β-HSDI began in the late 1960s, and attempts to identify active site residues using affinity labels[182] and mechanism-based inactivators[188] followed. NMR experiments using an acetylenic secoestradiol derivative suggested that a catalytically important lysine residue was found in the active site,[189, 190] and sequence alignments with other members of the SDR family[191] identified a Tyr-X-X-X-Lys active-site motif in residues 155–159 (see Fig. 115–5A). These predictions were verified when the x-ray structure of 17β-HSDI was solved.[8, 192] The structure demonstrates that cofactor lies across the β-sheet core of the protein in a Rossman fold characteristic of all SDR enzymes. Steroid appears to dangle from the top of the enzyme almost perpendicular to the cofactor, with a hydrophobic pocket holding the body of the steroid in place while the 3-hydroxyl forms hydrogen bonds with His 221 and Glu 282. At the place where the steroid and cofactor meet, Ser 142, Tyr 155, and Lys 159 help to form a charge-relay system that drives catalysis.

Because steroid flux to estrogens preferentially occurs via the aromatization of androstenedione to estrone, 17β-HSDI appears to be required for the conversion of estrone to biologically active estradiol in the ovary and placenta. This role has not been proved unequivocally, because no cases of human 17β-HSDI deficiency have been reported. Such a disease is theoretically compatible with life, because fetuses with aromatase deficiency and estrogen insensitivity (ER_α mutations) are viable.[126] Nevertheless, this enzyme is probably critical for ovulation and may be important in the pathogenesis and progression of estrogen-dependent breast cancers.[193]

17β-HSD Type II. In contrast to the "activating" role of 17β-HSDI in the placenta and ovary, human endometrium was known to inactivate estradiol by the conversion to estrone.[3] This activity, which was induced by progestins, was not 17β-HSDI, because 17β-HSDI mRNA was not detected in the human uterus.[186] Instead, a microsomal *HSD17B2* cDNA was cloned[4] and found to be expressed not only in endometrium but also in the placenta and widely in other tissues as well.[194] In fact, 17β-HSDII not only converts estradiol to estrone but also oxidizes testosterone and dihydrotestosterone to their inactive 17-ketosteroid homologues androstenedione and androstanedione, respectively. The widespread tissue distribution and broad substrate specificity of 17β-HSDII suggests that its role in human physiology is to protect tissues from excessive exposure to active steroid hormones by oxidation to inactive 17-ketosteroids.[179] This role is again somewhat speculative given that a human deficiency of this enzyme has not been described, but 17β-HSDII is certainly the most prevalent human inactivating (oxidizing) 17β-HSD that has been described to date. The type II enzyme also oxidizes 20α-dihydroprogesterone to progesterone, but this activity is low relative to the 17β-HSD activity.

17β-HSDIII. The Δ^5 preference of human P450c17 for the 17,20-lyase reaction necessitates that androgen production proceeds principally through DHEA as a precursor (see Fig. 115-2). Because the 3β-HSD reactions are unidirectional, human testosterone biosynthesis mainly follows the pathway DHEA to androstenedione to testosterone. Therefore, it was recognized that a 17β-HSD enzyme capable of reducing androstenedione to testosterone had to exist, and reports of male pseudohermaphrodites lacking this androgenic "17-ketosteroid reductase" activity surfaced in the 1970s.[195, 196] When the large, complex gene for 17β-HSDIII was cloned, patients with "17-ketosteroid reductase deficiency" were found to harbor mutations in this *HSD17B3* gene,[36, 197] proving the central role of this enzyme in male sexual differentiation. In fact, this is the only 17β-HSD enzyme whose role in human physiology is clearly established by studies of a human deficiency syndrome. Nonetheless, patients with 17β-HSDIII deficiency make small amounts of testosterone, suggesting that at least one additional 17β-HSD enzyme in humans can convert androstenedione to testosterone. Similarly, the human ovary exports some testosterone despite an absence of 17β-HSDIII expression, and women with 17β-HSDIII deficiency are asymptomatic.[198]

Unlike 17β-HSDI, which has been the subject of intense biochemical study, relatively little is known about 17β-HSDIII enzymology.

This knowledge gap is at least in part due to the relatively recent cloning of the gene for this enzyme, as well as the very hydrophobic nature of the encoded 310 amino acid protein. The type III enzyme also converts dehydroepiandrosterone to 5-androstenediol and estrone to estradiol.

17β-HSD Types IV and V. Additional HSD isoforms have been described in rodents and in humans, but the activities of these isoforms for steroids are generally poor. For example, the type IV enzyme is a trifunctional protein located in peroxisomes,[199] but its (oxidative) HSD activity toward estradiol is 10^6 times slower than its 3-hydroxyacyl-coenzyme A dehydrogenase activity.[200] Deficiency of the type IV enzyme causes Zellweger syndrome, in which bile acid synthesis is disturbed but steroidogenesis is not affected.[201, 202] Thus, these enzymes, which are variably present in different species, have 17β-HSD activity as one of their repertoire of transformations, but at least in humans, steroidogenesis is probably not their principal physiologic function.

Unlike 17β-HSDs types I to IV, the type V enzyme is an AKR enzyme expressed both in steroidogenic and nonsteroidogenic tissues.[203] There has been some confusion about the nature of the type V enzyme because of inconsistent results of sequencing and enzymology experiments from different laboratories. Originally described as hepatic 3α-HSD type II for its ability to reduce dihydrotestosterone to 3α-androstanediol,[204] this protein was later found to also have 17β-HSD activity towards androstenedione.[205] Another cDNA that differs from the initially described cDNA by two codons was later isolated, but these differences appear to be allelic variants of the same protein.[179] The 17β-HSD activity of this enzyme is rather labile and is mostly lost during homogenization, whereas 3α-HSD activity persists.[206] Thus, the type V enzyme can reduce androstenedione to testosterone in vivo, and this enzyme may account for most of the extratesticular androstenedione-to-testosterone conversion.

Steroid 5α-Reductases. The conversion of testosterone to 5α dihydrotestosterone (DHT) in target tissues was described in the 1960s,[207] and studies using fibroblasts suggested that at least two enzymes with different pH optima and genetics performed these transformations in humans.[208] These initial results were confirmed when the genes encoding the type I and type II enzymes were cloned,[209, 210] and patients with clinical 5α-reductase deficiency were found to have mutations in the type II gene. The two isoforms are very hydrophobic 30-kDa microsomal proteins that share 50% identity. The type I enzyme is limited to the nongenital skin and liver, and it is not expressed significantly in the fetus, which explains why a deficiency of the type II enzyme is not compensated by the type I enzyme.[211] The type II enzyme remains the predominant enzyme in genital skin, male accessory sex glands, and prostate, and the type II enzyme accounts for most of the hepatic 5α-reduction.[209]

Although 5α-reductase activity is generally discussed in the context of male genital differentiation and androgen action, both isozymes reduce a variety of steroids in what are believed to be degradative pathways in humans. In fact, progesterone is the best substrate for both 5α-reductases, and cortisol, cortisone, and corticosterone and its derivatives are also good substrates. The 5α- (and 5β-) reduced steroids may be metabolized further or glucuronidated for excretion in the urine. Given the importance of 5α-reductase type II in prostate growth, inhibitors of the type II enzyme have been developed for the treatment of prostatic hyperplasia[212] and the prevention of its recurrence after surgery.[213] Finasteride is currently the only such drug approved for these uses in the United States.

3α-Hydroxysteroid Dehydrogenases (3α-HSDs). The 3α-HSD enzymes function in pathways involving the 5α- and 5β-reductases to produce tetrahydrosteroids. As examples, prostatic 3α-HSD reduces the potent androgen dihydrotestosterone to 3α-androstanediol, which is not an androgen; conversely, brain 3α-HSD reduces 5α-dihydroprogesterone to tetrahydroprogesterone (allopregnanolone), which is an allosteric activator of the $GABA_A$ receptor-chloride channel complex with a nanomolar affinity. The nomenclature of the 3α-HSD isoforms is currently in a state of flux, but there are at least types I to III enzymes in humans, with a liver-specific type I[214]; a type II enzyme cloned from liver,[214] prostate,[205] and brain[215]; and a type III enzyme found in the prostate[216] and brain.[215] Furthermore, the amino acid compositions of the type II and III enzymes found in various tissues differ by a few residues, leaving open the question of whether their cDNAs derive from different genes or result from allelic variation or RNA processing differences. These minor differences in composition, however, cannot be neglected, because these differences can greatly change substrate utilization.

Recent studies have indicated an important role for 3α-HSDs in the nervous system. Antidepressant drugs in the selective serotonin reuptake inhibitor class, such as fluoxetine and paroxetine, directly lower the K_m of brain type II 3α-HSD for 5α-dihydroprogesterone by almost 10-fold,[215] which explains why these drugs augment brain allopregnanolone concentrations and perhaps contribute to their antidepressant activity. In addition, x-ray crystallography has shown that the β-subunit of the mammalian voltage-gated potassium channel is a tetrameric structure[217] in which each subunit closely resembles rat liver 3α-HSD[10] and even contains bound $NADP^+$ with high occupancy. Although the broader implications of this work is not yet known, these studies suggest a role of HSDs in coupling intracellular redox chemistry to membrane excitability.

The 3α-HSDs differ from the 11β-HSDs, 3β-HSDs, and 17β-HSDs types I to IV in several respects, because all 3α-HSDs are AKR enzymes rather than SDR enzymes.[218] As AKR enzymes, they function as monomers with a TIM-barrel structure (see Fig. 115–5B); they bind cofactor with the nicotinamide ring draped across the mouth of the "barrel" and have a salt bridge to the pyrophosphate (rather than lying in a Rossman fold); and their kinetic mechanisms allow for reversible equilibria in vivo at physiologic pH ranges rather than unidirectional steroid flux.[219] As shown in the structure of rat 3α-HSD,[10, 220] their active sites also contain tyrosine and lysine residues to facilitate proton transfers during catalysis (see Fig. 115–5B), but these residues are distantly located in linear sequence rather than confined to the Tyr-X-X-X-Lys motif as in SDR enzymes.[221]

11β-Hydroxysteroid Dehydrogenases (11β-HSDs). Although the 11β-HSD enzymes are not components of the major biosynthetic pathways, the two human isoforms deserve a brief discussion because they play an important role in regulating the bioactivity of endogenous and synthetic glucocorticoids and because they exemplify some key principles of HSD enzymology (Table 115–3). Both enzymes are hydrophobic, membrane-bound proteins that bind cortisol/cortisone and corticosterone/11-dehydrocorticosterone, but otherwise their properties and physiologic roles differ substantially[222] (see Table 115–3). The type II enzyme shares only 21% sequence identity with 11β-HSD type I, but it shares 37% identity with 17β-HSD type II, which is also an oxidative enzyme in vivo. Thus, the types I and II enzymes are only distantly related members of the SDR family, yet they perform opposite functions in specific tissues in human physiology and pharmacology.

The 34-kDa type I enzyme (11β-HSDI)[223] is expressed in the liver, testis, lung, and proximal convoluted tubule. The type I enzyme catalyzes both the oxidation of cortisol using $NADP^+$ as cofactor (K_m 1–2 μM) and the reduction of cortisone using NADPH cofactor (K_m 0.1–0.3 μM). The net flux of steroid driven by 11β-HSDI depends on

TABLE 115–3. Comparison of 11β-Hydroxysteroid Dehydrogenases Types I and II

Property	Type I	Type II
Size	34 kDa	41 kDa
Orientation in ER	Luminal	Cytoplasmic
Expression	Liver, decidua, lung, gonad, pituitary, brain	Kidney, placenta, colon, salivary gland
Function	Reductive	Oxidative
Cofactor usage	NADPH	NAD^+
Substrate binding	Low affinity (K_m 0.2–2 μM)	High affinity (K_m 0.01–0.1 μM)
Inhibition by carbenoxolone	++	++++

ER, endoplasmic reticulum; NADPH, nicotinamide adenine dinucleotide phosphate, reduced form.

the relative concentrations of NADPH and $NADP^+$, which usually favors reduction, especially given the high K_m of the enzyme for cortisol.[224, 225] In contrast, the 41-kDa type II enzyme[226] catalyzes only the oxidation of cortisol and corticosterone using NAD^+, and this enzyme has a high affinity for its steroid substrates (K_m 0.01–0.1 μM).[227, 228] Many synthetic glucocorticoid drugs such as prednisone and cortisone are 11-ketosteroids that must be reduced to their 11β-hydroxy derivatives to attain biologic activity, and given the kinetic parameters of the 11β-HSD enzymes, these transformations are performed mainly in the liver by the type I enzyme.

Cortisol is a potent agonist at the mineralocorticoid (glucocorticoid type II) receptor in the distal nephron,[229] but its oxidized 11-keto derivative, cortisone, is not a mineralocorticoid. The reason why cortisol does not act as a mineralocorticoid in vivo, even though cortisol concentrations can exceed aldosterone concentrations by three orders of magnitude, is because cortisol is enzymatically converted to cortisone in the cells lining the cortical and medullary collecting ducts. Thus, the type II enzyme inactivates the mineralocorticoid activity of cortisol in the kidney tubule,[230] and inactivating mutations in the type II enzyme cause a syndrome of apparent mineralocorticoid excess.[231] The presence of the type II enzyme in the placenta[232, 233] also inactivates endogenous and synthetic corticosteroids such as prednisolone, allowing the use of these agents during pregnancy without affecting the fetus. In contrast, 9-fluorinated steroids such as dexamethasone are minimally inactivated by the type II enzyme, primarily because of a shift in the oxidation/reduction equilibrium rather than a reduction in affinity for the enzyme.[234] It is this resistance to inactivation by placental 11β-HSD type II that is essential for synthetic glucocorticoids to "cross the placenta" and to exert a pharmacologic effect on the fetus. Furthermore, the relatively high placental concentrations of $NADP^+$ favor the oxidative action of 11β-HSDI, so that both placental enzymes protect the fetus from high maternal concentrations of cortisol that occur during pregnancy.[222]

REFERENCES

1. Arlt W, Justl H-G, Callies F, et al: Oral dehydroepiandrosterone for adrenal androgen replacement: Pharmacokinetics and peripheral conversion to androgens and estrogens in young healthy females after dexamethasone suppression. J Clin Endocrinol Metab 83:1928–1934, 1998.
2. Russell DW, Wilson JD: Steroid 5 alpha-reductase: Two genes/two enzymes. Annu Rev Biochem 63:25–61, 1994.
3. Tseng L, Gurpide E: Estradiol and 20-dihydroprogesterone dehydrogenase activities in human endometrium during the menstrual cycle. Endocrinology 94:419–423, 1974.
4. Wu L, Einstein M, Geissler WM, et al: Expression cloning and characterization of human 17β-hydrosteroid dehydrogenase type 2, a microsomal enzyme possessing 20α-hydroxysteroid dehydrogenase activity. J Biol Chem 268:12964, 1993.
5. Nelson DR, Kamataki T, Waxman DJ, et al: The P450 superfamily: Update on new sequences, gene mapping, accession numbers, early trivial names of enzymes, and nomenclature. DNA Cell Biol 12:1–51, 1993.
6. Rossmann MG, Ford GC, Watson HC, Banaszak LJ: Molecular symmetry of glyceraldehyde-3-phosphate dehydrogenase. J Mol Biol 64:237–245, 1972.
7. Ghosh D, Wawrzak Z, Weeks CM, et al: The refined three-dimensional structure of 3α, 20β-hydroxysteroid dehydrogenase and possible roles of the residues conserved in short-chain dehydrogenases. Structure 2:629–640, 1994.
8. Ghosh D, Pletnev VZ, Zhu DW, et al: Structure of human estrogenic 17β-hydroxysteroid dehydrogenase at 2.20 Å resolution. Structure 3:503–513, 1995.
9. Banner DW, Bloomer AC, Petsko GA, et al: Structure of chicken muscle triose phosphate isomerase determined crystallographically at 2.5 angstrom resolution using amino acid sequence data. Nature 255:609–614, 1975.
10. Hoog SS, Pawlowski JE, Alzari PM, et al: Three-dimensional structure of rat liver 3α-hydroxysteroid/dihydrodiol dehydrogenase: A member of the aldo-keto reductase superfamily. Proc Natl Acad Sci U S A 91:2517–2521, 1994.
11. Auchus RJ, Covey DF: Mechanism-based inactivation of 17β,20α-hydroxysteroid dehydrogenase by an acetylenic secoestradiol. Biochemistry 25:7295–7300, 1986.
12. Gaunt R: History of the adrenal cortex. *In* Greep RO, Astwood EB (eds): Handbook of Physiology: Endocrinology, section 7, vol 6. Washington, DC, American Physiological Society, 1975, p 1.
13. Baxter JD: Cortisone and the adrenal cortex. Trans Assoc Am Physicians 100:clxvii, 1987.
14. Simpson ER: Cholesterol side-chain cleavage, cytochrome P450, and the control of steroidogenesis. Mol Cell Endocrinol 13:213–227, 1979.
15. Stocco DM, Clark BJ: Regulation of the acute production of steroids in steroidogenic cells. Endocr Rev 17:221–244, 1996.
16. Clark BJ, Wells J, King SR, Stocco DM: The purification, cloning and expression of a novel luteinizing hormone-induced mitochondrial protein in MA-10 mouse Leydig tumor cells: Characterization of the steroidogenic acute regulatory protein (StAR). J Biol Chem 269:28314–28322, 1994.
17. Lin D, Sugawara T, Strauss JF III, et al: Role of steroidogenic acute regulatory protein in adrenal and gonadal steroidogenesis. Science 267:1828–1831, 1995.
18. Bose HS, Sugawara T, Strauss JF III, Miller WL: The pathophysiology and genetics of congenital lipoid adrenal hyperplasia. N Engl J Med 335:1870–1878, 1996.
19. Caron K, Soo S-C, Wetsel W, et al: Targeted disruption of the mouse gene encoding steroidogenic acute regulatory protein provides insights into congenital lipoid adrenal hyperplasia. Proc Natl Acad Sci U S A 94:11540–11545, 1997.
20. Arakane F, Sugawara T, Nishino H, et al: Steroidogenic acute regulatory protein (StAR) retains activity in the absence of its mitochondrial targeting sequence: Implications for the mechanism of StAR action. Proc Natl Acad Sci U S A 93:13731–13736, 1996.
21. Bose HS, Whittal RM, Baldwin MA, Miller WL: The active form of the steroidogenic acute regulatory protein, StAR, appears to be a molten globule. Proc Natl Acad Sci U S A 96:7250–7255, 1999.
22. Miller WL, Strauss JF III: Molecular pathology and mechanism of action of the steroidogenic acute regulatory protein, StAR. J Steroid Biochem Mol Biol 69:131–141, 1999.
23. Tsigos C, Arai K, Hung W, Chrousos GP: Hereditary isolated glucocorticoid deficiency is associated with abnormalities of the adrenocorticotropin receptor gene. J Clin Invest 92:2458–2461, 1993.
24. Martens JW, Verhoef-Post M, Abelin N, et al: A homozygous mutation in the luteinizing hormone receptor causes partial Leydig cell hypoplasia: Correlation between receptor activity and phenotype. Mol Endocrinol 12:775–784, 1998.
25. Tapanainen JS, Aittomaki K, Min J, et al: Men homozygous for an inactivating mutation of the follicle-stimulating hormone (FSH) receptor gene present variable suppression of spermatogenesis and fertility. Nat Genet 15:205–206, 1997.
26. Shenker A: G protein-coupled receptor structure and function: The impact of disease-causing mutations. Baillieres Clin Endocrinol Metab 9:427–451, 1995.
27. Parker KL, Schimmer BP: Steroidogenic factor 1: A key determinant of endocrine development and function. Endocr Rev 18:361–377, 1997.
28. Zhang P, Rodriguez H, Mellon SH: Transcriptional regulation of P450scc gene expression in neural and in steroidogenic cells: Implications for regulation of neurosteroidogenesis. Mol Endocrinol 9:1571–1582, 1995.
29. Huang N, Miller WL: Cloning of factors related to HIV-inducible LBP proteins that regulate steroidogenic factor-1-independent human placental transcription of the cholesterol side-chain cleavage enzyme, P450scc. J Biol Chem 275:2852–2858, 2000.
30. Luo X, Ikeda Y, Parker KL: A cell-specific nuclear receptor is essential for adrenal and gonadal development and sexual differentiation. Cell 77:481–490, 1994.
31. Nachtigal MW, Hirokawa Y, Enyeart-VanHouten DL, et al: Wilms' tumor 1 and Dax-1 modulate the orphan nuclear receptor SF-1 in sex-specific gene expression. Cell 93:445–454, 1998.
32. Hammer GD, Krylova I, Zhang Y, et al: Phosphorylation of the nuclear receptor SF-1 modulates cofactor recruitment: Integration of hormone signaling in reproduction and stress. Mol Cell 3:521–526, 1999.
33. Auchus RJ, Fuqua SA: Hormone-nuclear receptor interactions in health and disease. The oestrogen receptor. Baillieres Clin Endocrinol Metab 8:433–449, 1994.
34. Simpson ER, Zhao Y, Agarwal VR, et al: Aromatase expression in health and disease. Recent Prog Horm Res 52:185–214, 1997.
35. Luu-The V, Labrie C, Simard J, et al: Structure of two in tandem human 17β-hydroxysteroid dehydrogenase genes. Mol Endocrinol 4:268 275, 1990.
36. Geissler WM, Davis DL, Wu L, et al: Male pseudohermaphroditism caused by mutations of testicular 17β-hydroxysteroid dehydrogenase 3. Nat Genet 7:34–39, 1994.
37. Labrie Y, Durocher F, Lachance Y, et al: The human type II 17β-hydroxysteroid dehydrogenase gene encodes two alternatively spliced mRNA species. DNA Cell Biol 14:849–861, 1995.
38. Shimizu K, Hayano M, Gut M, Dorfman RI: The transformation of 20α-hydroxycholesterol to isocaproic acid and C_{21} steroids. J Biol Chem 236:695–699, 1961.
39. Lambeth JD, Kitchen SE, Farooqui AA, et al: Cytochrome P-450scc-substrate interactions: Studies of binding and catalytic activity using hydroxycholesterols. J Biol Chem 257:1876–1884, 1982.
40. Hall PF: Cytochromes P450 and the regulation of steroid synthesis. Steroids 48:131, 1986.
41. Morisaki M, Duque C, Ikekawa H, Shikita M: Substrate specificity of adrenocortical cytochrome P450. I: Effect of structural modification of cholesterol side chain on pregnenolone production. J Steroid Biochem Mol Biol 13:545–550, 1980.
42. Matteson KJ, Chung B, Urdea MS, Miller WL: Study of cholesterol side chain cleavage (20,22 desmolase) deficiency causing congenital lipoid adrenal hyperplasia using bovine-sequence P450scc oligodeoxyribonucleotide probes. Endocrinology 118:1296–1305, 1986.
43. Chung B, Matteson KJ, Voutilainen R, et al: Human cholesterol side-chain cleavage enzyme, P450scc: cDNA cloning, assignment of the gene to chromosome 15, and expression in the placenta. Proc Natl Acad Sci U S A 83:8962–8966, 1986.
44. Matocha M, Waterman MR: Synthesis and processing of mitochondrial steroid hydroxylases: In vivo maturation of the precursor of cytochrome P450scc, cytochrome P450 and adrenodoxin. J Biol Chem 260:12259, 1985.
45. Black SM, Harikrishna JA, Szklarz GD, Miller WL: The mitochondrial environment is required for activity of the cholesterol side-chain cleavage enzyme, cytochrome P450scc. Proc Natl Acad Sci U S A 91:7247–7251, 1994.
46. John ME, John MC, Boggaram V, et al: Transcriptional regulation of steroid hydroxylase genes by corticotropin. Proc Natl Acad Sci U S A 83:4715–4719, 1986.
47. Mellon SH, Vaisse C: cAMP regulates P450scc gene expression by a cycloheximide-insensitive mechanism in cultured mouse Leydig MA-10 cells. Proc Natl Acad Sci U S A 86:7775–7779, 1989.
48. Moore CCD, Brentano ST, Miller WL: Human P450scc gene transcription is induced by cyclic AMP and repressed by 12-*O*-tetradecanolyphorbol-13-acetate and A23187 by independent *cis*-elements. Mol Cell Biol 10:6013–6023, 1990.
49. Moore CCD, Hum DW, Miller WL: Identification of positive and negative placental-specific basal elements, a transcriptional repressor, and a cAMP response element in the human gene for P450scc. Mol Endocrinol 6:2045–2058, 1992.

50. Ahlgren R, Simpson ER, Waterman MR, Lund J: Characterization of the promoter/regulatory region of the bovine CYP11A (P450scc) gene. J Biol Chem 265:3313–3319, 1990.
51. Barrett PQ, Bollag WB, Isales CM, et al: The role of calcium in angiotensin II-mediated aldosterone secretion. Endocr Rev 10:496–518, 1989.
52. Hum DW, Aza-Blanc P, Miller WL: Characterization of placental-specific transcription of the human gene for P450scc. DNA Cell Biol 14:451–463, 1995.
53. Mellon SH, Deschepper CF: Neurosteroid biosynthesis: Genes for adrenal steroidogenic enzymes are expressed in the brain. Brain Res 629:283–292, 1993.
54. Baulieu EE: Neurosteroids of the nervous system, by the nervous system, for the nervous system. Recent Prog Horm Res 52:1–32, 1997.
55. Compagnone NA, Bulfone A, Rubenstein JLR, Mellon SH: Expression of the steroidogenic enzyme P450scc in the central and peripheral nervous systems during rodent embryogenesis. Endocrinology 136:2689–2696, 1995.
56. Yang X, Iwamoto K, Wang M, et al: Inherited congenital adrenal hyperplasia in the rabbit is caused by a deletion in the gene encoding cytochrome P450 cholesterol side-chain cleavage enzyme. Endocrinology 132:1977–1982, 1993.
57. Miller WL: Why nobody has P450scc (20, 22 desmolase) deficiency (letter). J Clin Endocrinol Metab 83:1399–1400, 1998.
58. Orentreich N, Brind JL, Rizer RL, Vogelman JH: Age changes and sex differences in serum dehydroepiandrosterone sulfate concentrations throughout adulthood. J Clin Endocrinol Metab 59:551–555, 1984.
59. Sklar CA, Kaplan SL, Grumbach MM: Evidence for dissociation between adrenarche and gonadarche: Studies in patients with idiopathic precocious puberty, gonadal dysgenesis, isolated gonadotropin deficiency, and constitutionally delayed growth and adolescence. J Clin Endocrinol Metab 51:548–556, 1980.
60. Zachmann M, Vollmin JA, Hamilton W, Prader A: Steroid 17,20 desmolase deficiency: A new cause of male pseudohermaphroditism. Clin Endocrinol 1:369–385, 1972.
61. Goebelsmann U, Zachmann M, Davajan V, et al: Male pseudohermaphroditism consistent with 17,20-desmolase deficiency. Gynecol Invest 7:138–156, 1976.
62. Nakajin S, Shively JE, Yuan P, Hall PF: Microsomal cytochrome P450 from neonatal pig testis: Two enzymatic activities (17α-hydroxylase and C17,20-lyase) associated with one protein. Biochemistry 20:4037–4042, 1981.
63. Zuber MX, Simpson ER, Waterman MR: Expression of bovine 17α-hydroxylase cytochrome P450 cDNA in non-steroidogenic (COS-1) cells. Science 234:1258–1261, 1986.
64. Chung B, Picado-Leonard J, Haniu M, et al: Cytochrome P450c17 (steroid 17α-hydroxylase/17,20 lyase): Cloning of human adrenal and testis cDNAs indicates the same gene is expressed in both tissues. Proc Natl Acad Sci U S A 84:407–411, 1987.
65. Lee-Robichaud P, Wright JN, Akhtar ME, Akhtar M: Modulation of the activity of human 17α-hydroxylase-17,20-lyase (CYP17) by cytochrome b_5: endocrinologic and mechanistic implications. Biochem J 308:901–908, 1995.
66. Auchus RJ, Lee TC, Miller WL: Cytochrome b_5 augments the 17,20 lyase activity of human P450c17 without direct electron transfer. J Biol Chem 273:3158–3165, 1998.
67. Katagiri M, Kagawa N, Waterman MR: The role of cytochrome b_5 in the biosynthesis of androgens by human P450c17. Arch Biochem Biophys 317:343–347, 1995.
68. Swart P, Swart AC, Waterman MR, et al: Progesterone 16-hydroxylase activity is catalyzed by human cytochrome P450 17α-hydroxylase. J Clin Endocrinol Metab 77:98–102, 1993.
69. Lin D, Black SM, Nagahama Y, Miller WL: Steroid 17α-hydroxylase and 17,20 lyase activities of P450c17: Contributions of serine 106 and P450 reductase. Endocrinology 132:2498–2506, 1993.
70. Nakajin S, Takahashi M, Shinoda M, Hall PF: Cytochrome b_5 promotes the synthesis of Δ^{16}-C_{19} steroids by homogeneous cytochrome P-450 C21 side-chain cleavage from pig testis. Biochem Biophys Res Commun 132:708–713, 1985.
71. Lin D, Harikrishna JA, Moore CCD, et al: Missense mutation Ser[106] Ø Pro causes 17-hydroxylase deficiency. J Biol Chem 266:15992–15998, 1991.
72. Ortiz de Montellano PR: Oxygen activation and reactivity. *In* Ortiz de Montellano PR (ed): Cytochrome P-450: Structure, Mechanism and Biochemistry, 2nd ed. New York, Plenum Press, 1995, pp 245–303.
73. Akhtar M, Corina D, Miller S, et al: Mechanism of the acyl-carbon cleavage and related reactions catalyzed by multifunctional P-450s: Studies on cytochrome P-450(17α). Biochemistry 33:4410–4418, 1994.
74. Auchus RJ, Miller WL: Molecular modeling of human P450c17 (17α-hydroxylase/17,20-lyase): Insights into reaction mechanisms and effects of mutations. Mol Endocrinol 13:1169–1182, 1999.
75. Vaz ADN, Roberts ES, Coon MJ: Olefin formation in the oxidative deformylation of aldehydes by cytochrome P-450: Mechanistic implications for catalysis by oxygen-derived peroxide. J Am Chem Soc 113:5886–5887, 1991.
75a. Cutler GB, Glenn M, Bush M, et al: Adrenarche: A survey of rodents, domestic animals and primates. Endocrinology 103:2112–2118, 1978.
76. Zhang L, Rodriguez H, Ohno S, Miller WL: Serine phosphorylation of human P450c17 increases 17,20 lyase activity: Implications for adrenarche and for the polycystic ovary syndrome. Proc Natl Acad Sci U S A 92:10619–10623, 1995.
77. Mapes S, Corbin C, Tarantal A, Conley A: The primate adrenal zona reticularis is defined by expression of cytochrome b_5, 17α-hydroxylase/17,20-lyase cytochrome P450 (P450c17) and NADPH-cytochrome P450 reductase (reductase) but not 3β-hydroxysteroid dehydrogenase/Δ5–4 isomerase (3β-HSD). J Clin Endocrinol Metab 84:3382–3385, 1999.
78. Yanase T, Sasano H, Yubisui T, et al: Immunohistochemical study of cytochrome b_5 in human adrenal gland and in adrenocortical adenomas from patients with Cushing's syndrome. Endocr J 45:89–95, 1998.
79. Gell JS, Carr BR, Sasano H, et al: Adrenarche results from development of a 3β-hydroxysteroid dehydrogenase-deficient adrenal reticularis. J Clin Endocrinol Metab 83:3695–3701, 1998.
80. Dardis A, Saraco N, Rivarola MA, Belgorosky A: Decrease in the expression of the 3β-hydroxysteroid dehydrogenase gene in human adrenal tissue during prepuberty and early puberty: Implications for the mechanism of adrenarche. Pediatr Res 45:384–388, 1999.
81. Biglieri EG, Herron MA, Brust N: 17-Hydroxylation deficiency in man. J Clin Invest 45:1946–1954, 1966.
82. Yanase T: 17α-Hydroxylase/17,20 lyase defects. J Steroid Biochem Mol Biol 53:153–157, 1995.
83. Auchus RJ, Miller WL: Genetics and biochemistry of defects in human P450c17. *In* Mason JI (ed): Modern Genetics. Philadelphia, Harwood Academic Publishers (in press).
84. Geller DH, Auchus RJ, Mendonca BB, Miller WL: The genetic and functional basis of isolated 17,20 lyase deficiency. Nature Genet 17:201–205, 1997.
85. Biason-Lauber A, Leiberman E, Zachmann M: A single amino acid substitution in the putative redox partner-binding site of P450c17 as cause of isolated 17,20 lyase deficiency. J Clin Endocrinol Metab 82:3807–3812, 1997.
86. Geller DH, Auchus RJ, Miller WL: P450c17 mutations R347H and R358Q selectively disrupt 17,20-lyase activity by disrupting interactions with P450 oxidoreductase and cytochrome b_5. Mol Endocrinol 13:167–175, 1999.
87. Casey ML, MacDonald PC: Extra-adrenal formation of a mineralocorticoid: Deoxycorticosterone and deoxycorticosterone sulfate biosynthesis and metabolism. Endocr Rev 3:396–403, 1982.
88. Mellon SH, Miller WL: Extra-adrenal steroid 21-hydroxylation is not mediated by P450c21. J Clin Invest 84:1497–1502, 1989.
89. Morel Y, Miller WL: Clinical and molecular genetics of congenital adrenal hyperplasia due to 21-hydroxylase deficiency. Adv Hum Genet 20:1–68, 1991.
90. Bristow J, Tee MK, Gitelman SE, et al: Tenascin-X. A novel extracellular matrix protein encoded by the human XB gene overlapping P450c21B. J Cell Biol 122:265–278, 1993.
91. Burch GH, Gong Y, Liu W, et al: Tenascin-X deficiency is associated with Ehlers-Danlos syndrome. Nat Genet 17:104–108, 1997.
92. Chiou SH, Hu MC, Chung B-C: A missense mutation of Ile[172] → Asn or Arg[356] → Trp causes steroid 21-hydroxylase deficiency. J Biol Chem 256:3549–3552, 1990.
93. Wu DA, Chung B: Mutations of P450c21 (steroid 21-hydroxylase) at Cys 428, Val 281, or Ser 268 result in complete, partial, or no loss of enzymatic activity. J Clin Invest 88:519–523, 1991.
94. Ulick S: Diagnosis and nomenclature of the disorders of the terminal portion of aldosterone biosynthetic pathway. J Clin Endocrinol Metab 43:92–96, 1976.
95. Veldhuis JD, Kulin HE, Santen RJ, et al: Inborn error in the terminal step of aldosterone biosynthesis: Corticosterone methyl oxidase type II deficiency in a North American pedigree. N Engl J Med 303:118, 1980.
96. Yanagibashi K, Haniu M, Shively JE, et al: The synthesis of aldosterone by the adrenal cortex: Two zones (fasciculata and glomerulosa) possess one enzyme for 11-, 18-hydroxylation, and aldehyde synthesis. J Biol Chem 261:3556–3562, 1986.
97. Morohashi K, Yoshioka H, Gotoh O, et al: Molecular cloning and nucleotide sequences of DNA of mitochondrial P-450 (11β-) of bovine adrenal cortex. J Biochem 102:559, 1986.
98. Mornet E, Dupont J, Vitek A, White PC: Characterization of two genes encoding human steroid 11β-hydroxylase (P45011β). J Biol Chem 264:20961–20967, 1989.
99. Chua SC, Szabo P, Vitek A, et al: Cloning of cDNA encoding steroid 11β-hydroxylase, P450c11. Proc Natl Acad Sci U S A 84:7193–7197, 1987.
100. Kawamoto T, Mitsuuchi Y, Toda K, et al: Cloning of cDNA and genomic DNA for human cytochrome P-45011β. FEBS Lett 269:345–349, 1990.
101. Kawamoto T, Mitsuuchi Y, Ohnishi T, et al: Cloning and expression of a cDNA for human cytochrome P450aldo as related to primary aldosteronism. Biochem Biophys Res Commun 173:309–316, 1990.
102. Carnow KM, Tusie-Lung M, Pascoe L, et al: The product of the CYP11B2 gene is required for aldosterone biosynthesis in the human adrenal cortex. Mol Endocrinol 5:1513–1522, 1991.
103. Kawamoto T, Mitsuuchi Y, Toda K, et al: Role of steroid 11β-hydroxylase and 18-hydroxylase in the biosynthesis of glucocorticoids and mineralocorticoids in humans. Proc Natl Acad Sci U S A 89:1458–1462, 1992.
104. White PC, Dupont J, New MI, et al: A mutation in CYP11B1 (Arg 448 → His) associated with steroid 11β-hydroxylase deficiency in Jews of Moroccan origin. J Clin Invest 87:1664–1667, 1991.
105. White PC, Curnow KM, Pascoe L: Disorders of steroid 11 beta-hydroxylase isozymes. Endocr Rev 15:421–438, 1994.
106. Pascoe L, Curnow K, Slutsker L, et al: Mutations in the human CYP11B2 (aldosterone synthase) gene causing corticosterone methyloxidase II deficiency. Proc Natl Acad Sci U S A 89:4996–5000, 1992.
107. Fu GK, Portale AA, Miller WL: Complete structure of the human gene for the vitamin D 1α-hydroxylase, P450c1α. DNA Cell Biol 16:1499–1507, 1997.
108. Malee MP, Mellon SH: Zone-specific regulation of two distinct messenger RNAs for P450c11 (11/18-hydroxylase) in the adrenals of pregnant and non-pregnant rats. Proc Natl Acad Sci U S A 88:4731–4735, 1991.
109. Fardella CE, Hum DW, Rodriguez H, et al: Gene conversion in the CYP11B2 gene encoding aldosterone synthase (P450c11AS) is associated with, but does not cause, the syndrome of corticosterone methyl oxidase II deficiency. J Clin Endocrinol Metab 81:321–326, 1996.
110. Lifton R, Dluhy RG, Powers M, et al: A chimeric 11β-hydroxylase/aldosterone synthase gene causes glucocorticoid-remediable aldosteronism and human hypertension. Nature 335:262–265, 1992.
111. Pascoe L, Curnow K, Slutsker L, et al: Glucocorticoid-suppressible hyperaldosteronism results from hybrid genes created by unequal crossover between CYP11B1 and CYP11B2. Proc Natl Acad Sci U S A 89:8327–8331, 1992.
112. Ulick S, Wang JZ, Morton H: The biochemical phenotypes of two inborn errors in the biosynthesis of aldosterone. J Clin Endocrinol Metab 74:1415–1420, 1992.
113. Peter M, Fawaz L, Drop SL, et al: Hereditary defect in biosynthesis of aldosterone: Aldosterone synthase deficiency 1964–1997. J Clin Endocrinol Metab 82:3525–3528, 1997.

114. Gordon RD, Zlesak MD, Tunny J, et al: Evidence that primary aldosteronism may not be uncommon: 12% incidence among antihypertensive drug trial volunteers. Clin Exp Pharmacol Physiol 20:296–298, 1993.

114a. Fardella CE, Mosso L, Gomez-Sanchez C, et al: Primary hyperaldosteronism in essential hypertensives: Prevalence, biochemical profile and molecular biology. J Clin Endocrinol Metab 85:1863–1867, 2000.

115. Bottner B, Schrauber H, Bernhardt R: Engineering a mineralocorticoid- to a glucocorticoid-synthesizing cytochrome P450. J Biol Chem 271:8028–8033, 1996.

116. Bottner B, Denner K, Bernhardt R: Conferring aldosterone synthesis to human CYP11B1 by replacing key amino acid residues with CYP11B2-specific ones. Eur J Biochem 252:458–466, 1998.

117. Curnow KM, Mulatero P, Emeric-Blanchouin N, et al: The amino acid substitutions Ser288Gly and Val320Ala convert the cortisol producing enzyme, CYP11B1, into an aldosterone producing enzyme (letter). Nat Struct Biol 4:32–35, 1997.

118. Simpson ER, Mahendroo MS, Means GD, et al: Aromatase cytochrome P450, the enzyme responsible for estrogen biosynthesis. Endocr Rev 15:342–355, 1994.

119. Shyadehi AZ, Lamb DC, Kelly SL, et al: The mechanism of the acyl-carbon bond cleavage reaction catalyzed by recombinant sterol 14 alpha-demethylase of *Candida albicans* (other names are: lanosterol 14 alpha-demethylase, P-45014DM, and CYP51). J Biol Chem 271:12445–12450, 1996.

120. Fishman J, Raju MS: Mechanism of estrogen biosynthesis: Stereochemistry of C-1 hydrogen elimination in the aromatization of 2β-hydroxy-19-oxoandrostenedione. J Biol Chem 256:4472–4477, 1981.

121. Beusen DD, Carrell HL, Covey DF: Metabolism of 19-methyl-substituted steroids by human placental aromatase. Biochemistry 26:7833–7841, 1987.

122. Mahendroo MS, Means GD, Mendelson CR, Simpson ER: Tissue-specific expression of human P-450AROM: The promoter responsible for expression in adipose tissue is different from that utilized in placenta. J Biol Chem 266:11276–11281, 1991.

123. Simpson ER, Mahendroo MS, Means GD, et al: Tissue-specific promoters regulate aromatase cytochrome P450 expression. J Steroid Biochem Mol Biol 44:321–330, 1993.

124. Shimozawa O, Sakaguchi M, Ogawa H, et al: Core glycosylation of cytochrome P-450(arom): Evidence for localization of N terminus of microsomal cytochrome P-450 in the lumen. J Biol Chem 268:21399–21402, 1993.

125. Conte FA, Grumbach MM, Ito Y, et al: A syndrome of female pseudohermaphrodism, hypergonadotropic hypogonadism, and multicystic ovaries associated with missense mutations in the gene encoding aromatase (P450arom). J Clin Endocrinol Metab 78:1287–1292, 1994.

126. Grumbach MM, Auchus RJ: Estrogen: Consequences and implications of human mutations in synthesis and action. J Clin Endocrinol Metab 84:4677–4694, 1999.

127. Fisher CR, Graves KH, Parlow AF, Simpson ER: Characterization of mice deficient in aromatase (ArKO) because of targeted disruption of the cyp19 gene. Proc Natl Acad Sci U S A 95:6965–6970, 1998.

128. Auchus RJ, Geller DH, Lee TC, Miller WL: The regulation of human P450c17 activity: Relationship to premature adrenarche and the polycystic ovary syndrome. Trends Endocrinol Metab 9:47–50, 1998.

129. Omura T, Sanders S, Estabrook RW, et al: Isolation from adrenal cortex of a nonheme iron protein and a flavoprotein functional as a reduced triphosphopyridine nucleotide-cytochrome P-450 reductase. Arch Biochem Biophys 117:660–673, 1966.

130. Hanukoglu I, Suh BS, Himmelhoch S, Amsterdam A: Induction and mitochondrial localization of cytochrome P450scc system enzymes in normal and transformed ovarian granulosa cells. J Cell Biol 111:1373–1381, 1990.

131. Picado-Leonard J, Voutilainen R, Kao L, et al: Human adrenodoxin: Cloning of three cDNAs and cycloheximide enhancement in JEG-3 cells. J Biol Chem 263:3240–3244, corrected 11016, 1988.

132. Voutilainen R, Picado-Leonard J, DiBlasio AM, Miller WL: Hormonal and developmental regulation of human adrenodoxin mRNA in steroidogenic tissues. J Clin Endocrinol Metab 66:383–388, 1988.

133. Mellon SH, Kushner JA, Vaisse C: Expression and regulation of adrenodoxin and P450scc mRNAs in rodent tissues. DNA Cell Biol 10:339–347, 1991.

134. Muller A, Muller JJ, Muller YA, et al: New aspects of electron transfer revealed by the crystal structure of a truncated bovine adrenodoxin, Adx(4–108). Structure 6:269–280, 1998.

135. Coghlan VM, Vickery LE: Site-specific mutations in human ferredoxin that affect binding to ferredoxin reductase and cytochrome P450scc. J Biol Chem 266:18606–18612, 1991.

136. Geren LM, O'Brien P, Stonehuerner J, Millett F: Identification of specific carboxylate groups on adrenodoxin that are involved in the interaction with adrenodoxin reductase. J Biol Chem 259:2155–2160, 1984.

137. Wada A, Waterman MR: Identification by site-directed mutagenesis of two lysine residues in cholesterol side chain cleavage cytochrome P450 that are essential for adrenodoxin binding. J Biol Chem 267:22877–22882, 1992.

138. Vickery LE: Molecular recognition and electron transfer in mitochondrial steroid hydroxylase systems. Steroids 62:124–127, 1997.

139. Beckert V, Bernhardt R: Specific aspects of electron transfer from adrenodoxin to cytochromes p450scc and p45011β. J Biol Chem 272:4883–4888, 1997.

140. Brentano ST, Black SM, Lin D, Miller WL: cAMP post-transcriptionally diminishes the abundance of adrenodoxin reductase in mRNA. Proc Natl Acad Sci U S A 89:4099–4103, 1992.

141. Lin D, Shi Y, Miller WL: Cloning and sequence of the human adrenodoxin reductase gene. Proc Natl Acad Sci U S A 87:8516–8520, 1990.

142. Sparkes RS, Klisak I, Miller WL: Regional mapping of genes encoding human steroidogenic enzymes: P450scc to 15q23–q24, adrenodoxin to 11q22; adrenodoxin reductase to 17q24–q25; and P450c17 to 10q24–q25. DNA Cell Biol 10:359–365, 1991.

143. Solish SB, Picado-Leonard J, Morel Y, et al: Human adrenodoxin reductase: Two mRNAs encoded by a single gene of chromosome 17cenqØ25 are expressed in steroidogenic tissues. Proc Natl Acad Sci U S A 71:7104–7108, 1988.

144. Brandt ME, Vickery LE: Expression and characterization of human mitochondrial ferredoxin reductase in *Escherichia coli*. Arch Biochem Biophys 294:735, 1992.

145. Freeman MR, Dobritsa A, Gaines P, et al: The dare gene: Steroid hormone production, olfactory behavior, and neural degeneration in Drosophila. Development 126:4591–4602, 1999.

146. Ziegler GA, Vonrhein C, Hanukoglu I, Schulz GE: The structure of adrenodoxin reductase of mitochondrial P450 systems: Electron transfer for steroid biosynthesis. J Mol Biol 289:981–990, 1999.

147. Brandt ME, Vickery LE: Charge pair interactions stabilizing ferredoxin-ferredoxin reductase complexes: Identification by complementary site-specific mutations. J Biol Chem 268:17126–17130, 1993.

148. Wang M, Roberts DL, Paschke R, et al: Three-dimensional structure of NADPH-cytochrome P450 reductase: Prototype for FMN- and FAD-containing enzymes. Proc Natl Acad Sci U S A 94:8411–8416, 1997.

149. Sevrioukova I, Huiying L, Zhong H, et al: Structure of a cytochrome P450-redox partner electron-transfer complex. Proc Natl Acad Sci U S A 96:1863–1868, 1999.

150. Stayton PS, Poulos TL, Sligar SG: Putidaredoxin competitively inhibits cytochrome b5-cytochrome P-450cam association: A proposed molecular model for a cytochrome P-450cam electron-transfer complex. Biochemistry 28:8201–8205, 1989.

151. Stayton PS, Sligar SG: The cytochrome P-450 cam binding surface as defined by site-directed mutagenesis and electrostatic modeling. Biochemistry 29:7381–7386, 1990.

152. Shimizu T, Tateishi T, Hatano M, Fujii-Kuriyama Y: Probing the role of lysines and arginines in the catalytic function of cytochrome P450d by site-directed mutagenesis: Interaction with NADPH-cytochrome P450 reductase. J Biol Chem 266:3372–3375, 1991.

153. Hasemann CA, Kurumbail RG, Boddupalli SS, et al: Structure and function of cytochromes P450: A comparative analysis of three crystal structures. Structure 2:41–62, 1995.

154. Bridges A, Gruenke L, Chang YT, et al: Identification of the binding site on cytochrome P450 2B4 for cytochrome b_5 and cytochrome P450 reductase. J Biol Chem 273:17036–17049, 1998.

155. Hildebrandt A, Estabrook RW: Evidence for the participation of cytochrome b_5 in hepatic microsomal mixed-function oxidation reactions. Arch Biochem Biophys 143:66–79, 1971.

156. Hall PF: Role of cytochromes P-450 in the biosynthesis of steroid hormones. Vitam Horm 42:315–368, 1985.

157. Enoch HG, Strittmatter P: Cytochrome b_5 reduction by NADPH-cytochrome P-450 reductase. J Biol Chem 254:8976–8981, 1979.

158. Pompon D, Coon MJ: On the mechanism of action of cytochrome P-450: Oxidation and reduction of the ferrous dioxygen complex of liver microsomal cytochrome P-450 by cytochrome b_5. J Biol Chem 259:15377–15385, 1984.

159. Yamazaki H, Johnson WW, Ueng YF, et al: Lack of electron transfer from cytochrome b_5 in stimulation of catalytic activities of cytochrome P450 3A4: Characterization of a reconstituted cytochrome P450 3A4/NADPH-cytochrome P450 reductase system and studies with apo-cytochrome b_5. J Biol Chem 271:27438–27444, 1996.

160. Lee-Robichaud P, Akhtar ME, Akhtar M: Control of androgen biosynthesis in the human through the interaction of Arg 347 and Arg 358 of CYP17 with cytochrome b_5. Biochem J 332:293–296, 1998.

161. Mathews FS, Strittmatter P: Crystallographic study of calf liver cytochrome b_5. J Mol Biol 41:295–297, 1969.

162. Storch EM, Daggett V: Structural consequences of heme removal: Molecular dynamics simulations of rat and bovine apocytochrome b_5. Biochemistry 35:11596–11604, 1996.

163. Muskett FW, Kelly GP, Whitford D: The solution structure of bovine ferricytochrome b_5 determined using heteronuclear NMR methods. J Mol Biol 258:172–189, 1996.

164. Falzone CJ, Mayer MR, Whiteman EL, et al: Design challenges for hemoproteins: the solution structure of apocytochrome b_5. Biochemistry 35:6519–6526, 1996.

165. Lee-Robichaud P, Kaderbhai MA, Kaderbhai N, et al: Interaction of human CYP17 (P-$450_{17\alpha}$, 17α-hydroxylase-17,20-lyase) with cytochrome b_5: Importance of the orientation of the hydrophobic domain of cytochrome b_5. Biochem J 321:857–863, 1997.

166. Thomas JL, Frieden C, Nash WE, Strickler RC: An NADH-induced conformational change that mediates the sequential 3β-hydroxysteroid dehydrogenase/isomerase activities is supported by affinity labeling and the time-dependent activation of isomerase. J Biol Chem 270:21003–21008, 1995.

167. Thomas JL, Berko EA, Faustino A, et al: Human placental 3β-hydroxy-5-ene-steroid dehydrogenase and steroid 5/4-ene-isomerase: Purification from microsomes, substrate kinetics, and inhibition by product steroids. J Steroid Biochem 31:785–793, 1988.

168. Payne AH, Abbaszade IG, Clarke TR, et al: The multiple murine 3β-hydroxysteroid dehydrogenase isoforms: Structure, function, and tissue- and developmentally specific expression. Steroids 62:169–175, 1997.

169. Lachance Y, Luu-The V, Labrie C, et al: Characterization of human 3β-hydroxysteroid dehydrogenase/Δ^5-Δ^4-isomerase gene and its expression in mammalian cells. J Biol Chem 265:20469–20475, 1990.

170. Rhéaume E, Lachance Y, Zhao HL, et al: Structure and expression of a new complementary DNA encoding the almost exclusive 3β-hydroxysteroid dehydrogenase/Δ^5-Δ^4-isomerase in human adrenals and gonads. Mol Endocrinol 5:1147–1157, 1991.

171. Moisan AM, Ricketts ML, Tardy V, et al: New insight into the molecular basis of 3β-hydroxysteroid dehydrogenase deficiency: Identification of eight mutations in the HSD3B2 gene—eleven patients from seven new families and comparison of the functional properties of twenty-five mutant enzymes. J Clin Endocrinol Metab 84:4410–4425, 1999.

172. Lee TC, Miller WL, Auchus RJ: Medroxyprogesterone acetate and dexamethasone are competitive inhibitors of different human steroidogenic enzymes. J Clin Endocrinol Metab 84:2104–2110, 1999.

173. Thomas JL, Myers RP, Strickler RC: Human placental 3β-hydroxy-5-ene-steroid dehydrogenase and steroid 5/4-ene-isomerase: Purification from mitochondria and kinetic profiles, biophysical characterization of the purified mitochondrial and microsomal enzymes. J Steroid Biochem 33:209–217, 1989.

174. Cherradi N, Defaye G, Chambaz EM: Dual subcellular localization of the 3β-hydroxysteroid dehydrogenase isomerase: Characterization of the mitochondrial enzyme in the bovine adrenal cortex. J Steroid Biochem Mol Biol 46:773–779, 1993.
175. Cherradi N, Rossier MF, Vallotton MB, et al: Submitochondrial distribution of three key steroidogenic proteins (steroidogenic acute regulatory protein and cytochrome P450scc and 3β-hydroxysteroid dehydrogenase isomerase enzymes) upon stimulation by intracellular calcium in adrenal glomerulosa cells. J Biol Chem 272:7899–7907, 1997.
176. Mesiano S, Coulter CL, Jaffe RB: Localization of cytochrome P450 cholesterol side-chain cleavage, cytochrome P450 17α-hydroxylase/17,20 lyase, and 3β-hydroxysteroid dehydrogenase-isomerase steroidogenic enzymes in human and rhesus monkey fetal adrenal glands: Reappraisal of functional zonation. J Clin Endocrinol Metab 77:1184–1189, 1993.
177. Endoh A, Kristiansen SB, Casson PR, et al: The zona reticularis is the site of biosynthesis of dehydroepiandrosterone and dehydroepiandrosterone sulfate in the adult human adrenal cortex resulting from its low expression of 3β-hydroxysteroid dehydrogenase. J Clin Endocrinol Metab 81:3558–3565, 1996.
178. Labrie F, Luu-The V, Lin SX, et al: The key role of 17β-hydroxysteroid dehydrogenases in sex steroid biology. Steroids 62:148–158, 1997.
179. Peltoketo H, Luu-The V, Simard J, Adamski J: 17β-Hydroxysteroid dehydrogenase (HSD)/17-ketosteroid reductase (KSR) family; nomenclature and main characteristics of the 17HSD/KSR enzymes. J Mol Endocrinol 23:1–11, 1999.
180. Ryan K, Engel LL: The interconversion of estrone and estradiol by human tissue slices. Endocrinology 52:287–291, 1953.
181. Jarabak J, Sack GH: A soluble 17β-hydroxysteroid dehydrogenase from human placenta. Biochemistry 8:2203–2212, 1969.
182. Murdock GL, Chin CC, Warren JC: Human placental estradiol 17β-dehydrogenase: sequence of a histidine-bearing peptide in the catalytic region. Biochemistry 25:641–646, 1986.
183. Peltoketo H, Isomaa V, Mäenlavsta O, Vihko R: Complete amino acid sequence of human placental 17β-hydroxysteroid dehydrogenase deduced from cDNA. FEBS Lett 239:73–77, 1988.
184. Luu-The V, Lechance Y, Labrie C, et al: Full length cDNA structure and deduced amino acid sequence of human 3β-hydroxy-5-ene steroid dehydrogenase. Mol Endocrinol 3:1310–1312, 1989.
185. Gast MJ, Sims HF, Murdock GL, et al: Isolation and sequencing of a complementary deoxyribonucleic acid clone encoding human placental 17β-estradiol dehydrogenase. Identification of the putative cofactor binding site. Am J Obstet Gynecol 161:1726–1731, 1989.
186. Tremblay Y, Ringler GE, Morel Y, et al: Regulation of the gene for estrogenic 17-ketosteroid reductase lying on chromosome 17cenq 25. J Biol Chem 264.20458–20462, 1989.
187. Dumont M, Luu-The V, de Launoit Y, Labrie F: Expression of human 17β-hydroxysteroid dehydrogenase in mammalian cells. J Steroid Biochem Mol Biol 41:605–608, 1992.
188. Thomas JL, LaRochelle MC, Covey DF, Strickler RC: Inactivation of human placental 17β,20α-hydroxysteroid dehydrogenase by 16-methylene estrone, an affinity alkylator enzymatically generated from 16-methylene estradiol-17β. J Biol Chem 258:11500–11504, 1983.
189. Auchus RJ, Covey DF: Dehydrogenase inactivation by an enzyme-generated acetylenic ketone: Identification of a lysyl enaminone by ^{13}C NMR. J Am Chem Soc 109:280–282, 1987.
190. Auchus RJ, Covey DF, Bork V, Schaefer J: Solid-state NMR observation of cysteine and lysine Michael adducts of inactivated estradiol dehydrogenase. J Biol Chem 263.11640–11645, 1988.
191. Jornvall H, Persson B, Krook M, et al: Short-chain dehydrogenases/reductases (SDR). Biochemistry 34:6003–6013, 1995.
192. Azzi A, Rehse PH, Zhu DW, et al: Crystal structure of human estrogenic 17β-hydroxysteroid dehydrogenase complexed with 17β-estradiol. Nat Struct Biol 3:665–668, 1996.
193. Sasano H, Frost AR, Saitoh R, et al: Aromatase and 17β-hydroxysteroid dehydrogenase type 1 in human breast carcinoma. J Clin Endocrinol Metab 81:4042–4046, 1996.
194. Casey ML, MacDonald PC, Andersson S: 17β-Hydroxysteroid dehydrogenase type 2: Chromosomal assignment and progestin regulation of gene expression in human endometrium. J Clin Invest 94:2135–2141, 1994.
195. Saez JM, De Peretti E, Morera AM, et al: Familial male pseudohermaphroditism with gynecomastia due to a testicular 17-ketosteroid reductase defect. I: Studies in vivo. J Clin Endocrinol Metab 32:604–610, 1971.
196. Ademola Akesode F, Meyer WJd, Migeon CJ: Male pseudohermaphroditism with gynecomastia due to testicular 17-ketosteroid reductase deficiency. Clin Endocrinol (Oxf) 7:443–452, 1977.
197. Andersson S, Geissler WM, Wu L, et al: Molecular genetics and pathophysiology of 17β-hydroxysteroid dehydrogenase 3 deficiency. J Clin Endocrinol Metab 81:130–136, 1996.
198. Mendonca BB, Arnhold IJ, Bloise W, et al: 17β-Hydroxysteroid dehydrogenase 3 deficiency in women. J Clin Endocrinol Metab 84:802–804, 1999.
199. Adamski J, Normand T, Leenders F, et al: Molecular cloning of a novel widely expressed human 80 kDa 17β-Hydroxysteroid dehydrogenase IV. Biochem J 311:437–443, 1995.
200. Qin YM, Poutanen MH, Helander HM, et al: Peroxisomal multifunctional enzyme of beta-oxidation metabolizing D-3-hydroxyacyl-CoA esters in rat liver: Molecular cloning, expression and characterization. Biochem J 321:21–28, 1997.
201. Novikov D, Dieuaide-Noubhani M, Vermeesch JR, et al: The human peroxisomal multifunctional protein involved in bile acid synthesis: Activity measurement, deficiency in Zellweger syndrome and chromosome mapping. Biochim Biophys Acta 1360:229–240, 1997.
202. van Grunsven EG, van Berkel E, Ijlst L, et al: Peroxisomal D-hydroxyacyl-CoA dehydrogenase deficiency: Resolution of the enzyme defect and its molecular basis in bifunctional protein deficiency. Proc Natl Acad Sci U S A 95:2128–2133, 1998.
203. El-Alfy M, Luu-The V, Huang XF, et al: Localization of type 5 17β-hydroxysteroid dehydrogenase, 3β-hydroxysteroid dehydrogenase, and androgen receptor in the human prostate by in situ hybridization and immunocytochemistry. Endocrinology 140:1481–1491, 1999.
204. Deyashiki Y, Ogasawara A, Nakayama T, et al: Molecular cloning of two human liver 3α-hydroxysteroid/dihydrodiol dehydrogenase isoenzymes that are identical with chlordecone reductase and bile-acid binder. Biochem J 299:545–552, 1994.
205. Lin HK, Jez JM, Schlegel BP, et al: Expression and characterization of recombinant type 2 3α-hydroxysteroid dehydrogenase (HSD) from human prostate: Demonstration of bifunctional 3α/17-HSD activity and cellular distribution. Mol Endocrinol 11:1971–1984, 1997.
206. Dufort I, Rheault P, Huang XF, et al: Characteristics of a highly labile human type 5 17β-hydroxysteroid dehydrogenase. Endocrinology 140:568–574, 1999.
207. Bruchovsky N, Wilson JD: The intranuclear binding of testosterone and 5α-androstan-17-β ol-3-one by rat prostate. J Biol Chem 243:5953–5960, 1968.
208. Moore RJ, Wilson JD: Steroid 5-reductase in cultured human fibroblasts. Biochemical and genetic evidence for two distinct enzyme activities. J Biol Chem 251:5895–5900, 1976.
209. Jenkins EP, Andersson S, Imperato-McGinley J, et al: Genetic and pharmacologic evidence for more than one human steroid 5α-reductase. J Clin Invest 89:293–300, 1992.
210. Andersson S, Berman DM, Jenkins EP, Russell DW: Deletion of a steroid 5α-reductase 2 gene in male pseudohermaphroditism. Nature 354:159–161, 1991.
211. Thigpen AE, Silver RI, Guileyardo JM, et al: Tissue distribution and ontogeny of steroid 5α-reductase isozyme expression. J Clin Invest 92:903–910, 1993.
212. Rittmaster RS: 5α-reductase inhibitors. J Androl 18:582–587, 1997.
213. McConnell JD, Bruskewitz R, Walsh P, et al: The effect of finasteride on the risk of acute urinary retention and the need for surgical treatment among men with benign prostatic hyperplasia: Finasteride Long-Term Efficacy and Safety Study Group. N Engl J Med 338:557–563, 1998.
214. Khanna M, Qin KN, Wang RW, Cheng KC: Substrate specificity, gene structure and tissue-specific distribution of multiple human 3α-hydroxysteroid dehydrogenases. J Biol Chem 270:20162–20168, 1995.
215. Griffin LD, Mellon SH: Selective serotonin reuptake inhibitors directly alter activity of neurosteroidogenic enzymes. Proc Natl Acad Sci U S A 96:13512–13517, 1999.
216. Dufort I, Soucy P, Labrie F, Luu-The V: Molecular cloning of human type 3 3α-hydroxysteroid dehydrogenase that differs from 20α-hydroxysteroid dehydrogenase by seven amino acids. Biochem Biophys Res Commun 228:474–479, 1996.
217. Gulbis JM, Mann S, MacKinnon R: Structure of a voltage-dependent K^+ channel beta subunit. Cell 97:943–952, 1999.
218. Penning TM, Bennett MJ, Smith-Hoog S, et al: Structure and function of 3α-hydroxysteroid dehydrogenase. Steroids 62:101–111, 1997.
219. Askonas LJ, Ricigliano JW, Penning TM: The kinetic mechanism catalysed by homogeneous rat liver 3α-hydroxysteroid dehydrogenase: Evidence for binary and ternary dead-end complexes containing non-steroidal anti-inflammatory drugs. Biochem J 278:835–841, 1991.
220. Bennett MJ, Albert RH, Jez JM, et al: Steroid recognition and regulation of hormone action: crystal structure of testosterone and $NADP^+$ bound to 3α-hydroxysteroid/dihydrodiol dehydrogenase. Structure 5:799–812, 1997.
221. Duax WL, Ghosh D: Structure and function of steroid dehydrogenases involved in hypertension, fertility, and cancer. Steroids 62:95–100, 1997.
222. White PC, Mune T, Agarwal AK: 11β-Hydroxysteroid dehydrogenase and the syndrome of apparent mineralocorticoid excess. Endocr Rev 18:135–156, 1997.
223. Tannin GM, Agarwal AK, Monder C, et al: The human gene for 11β-hydroxysteroid dehydrogenase: Structure, tissue distribution, and chromosomal localization. J Biol Chem 266:16653–16658, 1991.
224. Agarwal AK, Tusie-Luna M-T, Monder C, White PC: Expression of 11β-hydroxysteroid dehydrogenase using recombinant vaccinia virus. Mol Endocrinol 4:1827–1832, 1990.
225. Moore CCD, Mellon SH, Murai J, et al: Structure and function of the hepatic form of 11β-hydroxysteroid dehydrogenase in the squirrel monkey, an animal model of glucocorticoid resistance. Endocrinology 133:368–375, 1993.
226. Albiston AL, Obeyesekere VR, Smith RE, Krozowski ZS: Cloning and tissue distribution of the human 11-hydroxysteroid dehydrogenase type II enzyme. Mol Cell Endocrinol 105:R11–R17, 1994.
227. Brown RW, Chapman KE, Edwards CRW, Seckl JR: Human placental 11 beta-hydroxysteroid dehydrogenase: Evidence for and partial purification of a distinct NAD^+-dependent isoform. Endocrinology 132:2614–2621, 1993.
228. Rusvai E, Náray-Fejes-Tóth A: A new isoform of 11β-hydroxysteroid dehydrogenase in aldosterone target cells. J Biol Chem 268:10717–10720, 1993.
229. Arriza JL, Weinberger C, Cerelli G, et al: Cloning of human mineralocorticoid receptor DNA: Structural and functional kinship with the glucocorticoid receptor. Science 237:268–275, 1987.
230. Funder JW, Pearce PT, Smith R, Smith I: Mineralocorticoid action: Target tissue specificity is enzyme, not receptor, mediated. Science 242:583–585, 1988.
231. Mune T, Rogerson FM, Nikkila H, et al: Human hypertension caused by mutations in the kidney isozyme of 11 beta-hydroxysteroid dehydrogenase. Nat Genet 10:394–399, 1995.
232. Krozowski Z, MacGuire JA, Stein-Oakley AN, et al: Immunohistochemical localization of the 11β-hydroxysteroid dehydrogenase type II enzyme in human kidney and placenta. J Clin Endocrinol Metab 80:2203–2209, 1995.
233. Hirasawa G, Sasano H, Suzuki T, et al: 11β-Hydroxysteroid dehydrogenase type 2 and mineralocorticoid receptor in human fetal development. J Clin Endocrinol Metab 84:1453–1458, 1999.
234. Li KX, Obeyesekere VR, Krozowski ZS, Ferrari P: Oxoreductase and dehydrogenase activities of the human and rat 11β-hydroxysteroid dehydrogenase type 2 enzyme. Endocrinology 138:2948–2952, 1997.

Chapter 116

Glucocorticoid Action: Physiology

Allan Munck ▪ Anikó Náray-Fejes-Tóth

HISTORICAL DEVELOPMENTS AND BACKGROUND

Glucocorticoid physiology has at times occupied the mainstream of endocrinology, at other times, a backwater. In this chapter we describe some of these ebbs and flows, up to the critical events around 1950 that set glucocorticoid physiology and pharmacology on divergent courses.

The Adrenal Cortex and Survival: Role of Glucocorticoids and Mineralocorticoids

Thomas Addison's discovery in the mid-1800s that the adrenal cortex was essential to survival[1, 2] preceded by nearly a century the demonstration with pure steroids that this gland produced at least two distinct hormones—eventually called glucocorticoids and mineralocorticoids[3]—that were necessary for normal life.[4, 5] During the intervening years many of the actions on glucose metabolism that would characterize glucocorticoids, and on salt and water balance that would characterize mineralocorticoids, were foreshadowed in the symptoms of addisonian patients[2] and adrenalectomized animals,[6] and in the effects of lipid extracts from the adrenal cortex.[7–10] First ascribed to a single hormone, those actions stirred debate as to which were the most critical for survival.[5, 11]

Abnormalities of electrolyte and water balance in addisonian patients and adrenalectomized animals, and reversal of the abnormalities by administration of salt or adrenal extracts, favored primacy of control of electrolytes.[5] But the accompanying abnormalities of carbohydrate metabolism and their reversal by adrenal extracts[12–14] led to the proposal in 1932 that the "prepotent function" of the adrenal cortex was control of carbohydrate metabolism, accounting for all actions, including maintenance of life.[14] This sweeping view soon became untenable, and by 1940 the controversies had been settled by studies with pure glucocorticoids and mineralocorticoids. Each hormone was essential to life. Mineralocorticoids sustained life by maintaining electrolyte balance. How glucocorticoids sustained life remained obscure for decades.

Carbohydrate Metabolism

Glucocorticoids were named for their hyperglycemic effect.[3] Low blood glucose in addisonian patients and adrenalectomized animals and low liver glycogen in the latter were described in the early 1900s.[15–18] The 1930s saw the use of adrenal extracts to restore normal glucose levels,[12–14] as well as the striking discovery that adrenalectomy,[19] like hypophysectomy,[20] ameliorated symptoms of diabetes. A landmark paper by Long et al.[11] in 1940 demonstrated that glucocorticoids stimulate gluconeogenesis from amino acids derived from protein catabolism, decrease glucose oxidation, and can elicit steroid diabetes. Ingle showed that glucocorticoids decrease glucose utilization[21] and cause insulin resistance.[22] These papers set the stage for most later work in this area.[23]

Glucocorticoid-Induced Apoptosis of Lymphoid Cells

Lymphoid tissue as a target for glucocorticoids was perhaps first noted by Addison, who observed "a considerable excess of white corpuscles" in the blood of one of his patients.[2] By 1900 thymus enlargement had been described in addisonian patients[24] and adrenalectomized rats.[25] Around that time pathologists, using as norms for lymphoid tissues specimens—actually atrophied—from victims of prolonged illness, pronounced the resounding diagnosis of "status thymico-lymphaticus" in cases of sudden death where the thymus and other lymphoid tissues—actually normal—were judged to be enlarged.[26] Hans Selye[27] found that through mediation of the adrenals any illness or other source of stress can atrophy the thymus, an effect later reproduced with adrenal extracts and pure glucocorticoids[4, 28, 29] and noted in other lymphoid tissues.[30] Glucocorticoids were eventually shown to induce lymphocytolysis by apoptosis, a mechanism that underlies death of many other types of cells and plays an essential role in tissue remodeling.[31–33]

"Regulatory" and "Permissive" Glucocorticoid Actions in Stress

Evidence for an intimate connection between stress and hormones of the adrenal cortex began to appear in the 1930s with observations that stress stimulates adrenocortical secretion and adrenal extracts protect against stress.[27, 34–36] Eventually the protective role was ascribed to glucocorticoids.[36] Selye, a major contributor to this subject and its renowned popularizer,[37] demonstrated that a broad range of noxious and other stimuli activated the adrenal cortex.[27] His unified theory of stress introduced such concepts as the "alarm reaction," the "general adaptation syndrome," "adaptation energy," and the much-disputed idea that through increased levels of adrenocortical hormones stress could cause "diseases of adaptation" such as diffuse collagen disease and allergy.[35] As to how glucocorticoids might protect against stress, Selye suggested that they supply an increased need for sugar[35]; White and Dougherty proposed that through lymphocytolysis they enhance immune responses by releasing preformed antibodies.[38] Neither of these ideas survived. Glucose could not replace glucocorticoid,[39, 40] and antibody release from lymphocytes was not confirmed.[36, 41]

Ingle[39, 42] described a protective role for glucocorticoids distinct from the "regulatory" one of high, stress-induced levels. Observing that adrenalectomized animals respond normally to certain forms of stress if administered glucocorticoids at basal levels, he concluded that stress-induced levels are not required for all stress-induced responses, and proposed that basal levels exert "permissive" effects necessary to maintain the capacity of some homeostatic functions to respond to stress. He recognized, though, that stress-induced levels contribute to maintaining homeostasis in severe stress.[39]

Feedback Regulation

Regulation of glucocorticoid secretion began to be understood in the 1930s. Smith[43] found that hypophysectomy in rats caused atrophy of the adrenal cortex that could be reversed by implanted pituitaries. Adrenocorticotropic hormone (ACTH), the factor responsible, was later purified from pituitaries.[44, 45] Negative feedback control of ACTH by a hormone from the adrenal cortex was described in a remarkable half-page article by Ingle and Kendall,[46] who showed that administration of adrenal extracts to rats caused atrophy of the adrenal cortex that was countered by simultaneous administration of a pituitary extract. Stress of normal but not of hypophysectomized animals was found to lead to hypertrophy of the adrenal cortex, implying that stress stimulated secretion of ACTH.[47] Harris's 1937 proposal that control of secretion of ACTH resides in the hypothalamus,[48] followed by evidence that this control is mediated by a hormone via the hypophysial portal vessels,[49] led eventually to identification of the corticotropin-releasing hormone (CRH).[50]

Anti-inflammatory Effects and Glucocorticoid Physiology

By the late 1940s the main outlines of glucocorticoid physiology appeared to be firmly drawn. Then 1949 brought a watershed event that was to cast a long shadow over this discipline. Hench et al.[51] reported that cortisone had powerful anti-inflammatory activity that dramatically improved the condition of patients with rheumatoid arthritis.[52] This unexpected discovery threw glucocorticoid physiology into turmoil.[5] Adrenal physiologists were quick to point out that anti-inflammatory actions were at odds with Selye's idea of diseases of adaptation.[36, 52] They were unable, however, to provide a physiologic explanation for those actions, which were completely inconsistent with the conventional view that glucocorticoids protected against stress by enhancing—not suppressing—defense mechanisms.[53] Despite a rare voice to the contrary,[53] physiologists concluded that anti-inflammatory actions were pharmacologic rather than physiologic in nature.[5, 36]

That view persisted for decades: for example, neither in a 1952 review by Ingle[39] nor in a 1971 review by Hoffman[54] on the role of the adrenal cortex in homeostasis are anti-inflammatory actions even mentioned. Consequently, the spectacular rise in therapeutic applications of these hormones, the "miracle drugs" of the 1950s, and the development of synthetic glucocorticoid analogs such as prednisone, prednisolone, and dexamethasone, proceeded largely without a base in physiology, a situation probably unique in endocrinology. A central but unrealized goal in the early development of synthetic analogs was to separate anti-inflammatory activity from the "side effects" caused by physiologic glucocorticoid actions such as feedback suppression.[55] As we shall see, anti-inflammatory actions are in fact physiologic, and glucocorticoids administered to produce one physiologic effect generally produce others. Some progress in separating anti-inflammatory from other effects has been achieved recently with hormone analogs selected on the basis of molecular mechanisms underlying physiologic actions. Steroids that preferentially induce gene repression over activation exhibit relatively enhanced anti-inflammatory activity.[56]

GENERAL MOLECULAR ASPECTS OF GLUCOCORTICOID PHYSIOLOGY

Glucocorticoids initiate most of their known effects by binding to glucocorticoid receptors (GRs) or mineralocorticoid receptors (MRs), intracellular receptors of the steroid-thyroid-retinoid nuclear receptor superfamily that regulate transcription of particular genes in a cell-specific manner. These effects are generally slow, taking one or several hours to be manifested in the whole organism. Nongenomic glucocorticoid effects,[57–63] in some cases rapid and mediated through putative plasma membrane receptors, have also been observed in various systems. They may be important, but at present their physiologic significance is unclear and will not be discussed. Similarly, the roles of several variants of GRs and MRs remain unsettled[64–68] and will not be dealt with.

GRs, originally identified in thymocytes,[69–71] are found in almost all nucleated cells. When activated by a ligand they can regulate target genes in various ways. By binding as dimers to glucocorticoid response elements (GREs) (short palindromic sequences of nucleotides in the target gene) they can activate transcription of the gene. Similarly, they can repress transcription by binding as dimers to negative GREs (nGREs). They can also repress transcription through a third general mechanism, the so-called transcriptional crosstalk via tethering,[72, 73] that does not require binding to DNA or even the presence of GREs in the regulated gene. Hormone-activated receptors bind, apparently as monomers, to transcription factors such as the AP-1 proteins (cJun/cFos), the cyclic adenosine monophosphate (cAMP) response element binding protein (CREB), and nuclear factor κB (NF-κB), generally inhibiting transcription of genes activated by those factors. Such cases include many genes involved in immune and inflammatory reactions. The physiologic relevance of these molecular mechanisms will become evident when we describe recent results with transgenic animals. Selection of the steroids with relatively enhanced anti-inflammatory activity mentioned in the preceding section depended on the ability to repress AP-1–regulated gene transcription while inducing little gene activation.[56]

Since the discovery that the natural glucocorticoids, cortisol and corticosterone, have much higher affinity for MRs than GRs[74, 75] much evidence has indicated that under physiologic conditions some glucocorticoid effects, notably in the hippocampus,[68] are mediated through MRs. Whereas MRs in mineralocorticoid target tissues are "protected" by 11β-hydroxysteroid dehydrogenase type 2 (11β-HSD2), which inactivates cortisol and corticosterone by oxidizing them respectively to cortisone and 11-dehydrocorticosterone,[76] in the hippocampus the enzyme is absent.[68] In Leydig's,[77, 78] uterine,[79] and placental[80] cells, 11β-HSD2 may protect GRs from excessive glucocorticoid levels. Another isoform of the enzyme, 11β-HSD1, is found in liver and other tissues. In contrast to 11β-HSD2, which functions exclusively as an oxidase, 11β-HSD1 functions primarily (not exclusively) as a reductase, thus activating cortisone and 11-dehydrocorticosterone to cortisol and corticosterone. In 11β-HSD1 knockout mice, stress-induced glucocorticoid responses are weakened.[81]

Because natural glucocorticoids have higher affinity for MRs than GRs, at low basal levels they occupy mainly unprotected MRs. As levels increase during the circadian cycle, MRs approach saturation and a substantial fraction of GRs become occupied. After stress, glucocorticoid levels may rise sufficiently to nearly saturate the GRs.[68] As we shall see, some permissive actions of glucocorticoids are mediated by MRs and suppressive actions by GRs.

FEEDBACK REGULATION OF GLUCOCORTICOID PRODUCTION

Although glucocorticoids are essential to the response to stress and to survival, normally they exert major control over few physiologic processes other than their own feedback mechanisms. For example, while they are important regulators of blood glucose, the dominant regulators are clearly insulin and glucagon. Reflecting this role, and contrasting with hormones such as insulin and aldosterone, plasma levels of glucocorticoids are controlled mainly by negative feedback from the hormones themselves rather than from their physiologic effects, a design common to hormones with widely dispersed homeostatic functions that are not tightly coupled to a few essential variables. This scheme is outlined in Figure 116–1, which emphasizes a theme we pursue throughout this chapter, namely, the broad physiologic function of glucocorticoids in protecting the organism against stress.

Glucocorticoid levels are regulated in ways that reflect these varying physiologic needs, as well as the vulnerability of the organism to harm from overexposure to the hormones. Basal hormone levels, which follow a circadian rhythm and reach peak values before the period of daily activity,[82–84] exert actions required to maintain or "prime" many homeostatic mechanisms and protect against moderate stress.[85] Stress-induced levels, which can far exceed peak basal levels, appear to be necessary to cope with severe stress.[86–87a] Peak basal levels can cause Cushing's syndrome if maintained indefinitely, so the circadian lowering of glucocorticoid concentrations may be a physiologic necessity.

Synthesis and secretion of glucocorticoids are controlled by neural and humoral signals that change throughout the day and respond to stress and to negative feedback from the hormones themselves.[84, 88–90] The main components of this system (see Fig. 116–1) are the adrenal cortex, where glucocorticoid secretion is stimulated by ACTH; the anterior pituitary, where ACTH secretion is stimulated by CRH, vasopressin (VP), and other secretagogues, and inhibited by glucocorticoids; and the central nervous system (CNS), where CRH and VP synthesis in the hypothalamus is stimulated by stress and other influences, and inhibited by glucocorticoids.

Sites through which glucocorticoids exert feedback control include the pituitary corticotrophs, the paraventricular nucleus (PVN) of the hypothalamus, and probably the hippocampus.[68, 84, 89, 91, 92] Synthetic analogs like dexamethasone penetrate the brain poorly, acting predominantly on the pituitary.[68] At basal levels the natural glucocorticoids may affect the pituitary less than the brain, because pituitary cells contain corticosteroid-binding globulin (CBG)–like molecules that compete for hormone with the GRs.[68] There is evidence that glucocorticoid regulation is mediated by both GRs, which are found throughout the brain with high concentrations in the PVN, and by MRs, which are located mainly in the hippocampus and lateral septum.[68, 89, 93] Broadly speaking, actions on the brain via MRs permissively maintain the basal capacity of the hypothalamic-pituitary-adrenal (HPA) axis to respond to stress, whereas actions through GRs suppress activated responses.[68] In the hippocampus, however, which in rats appears to exert a tonic inhibitory influence on HPA activity, glucocorticoids maintain this inhibitory influence through MRs and abrogate it through GRs.[68]

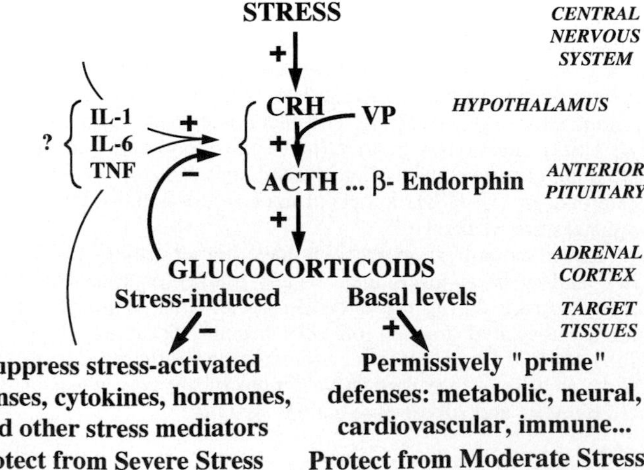

FIGURE 116–1. Outline of regulation and actions of glucocorticoids. See text for details. IL, interleukin; TNF, tumor necrosis factor; CRH, corticotropin releasing hormone; VP, vasopressin; ACTH, adrenocorticotropic hormone.

As indicated in Figure 116–1, cytokines such as interleukin-1 (IL-1) and IL-6, which are generated peripherally mainly by activated cells of the immune system but also within the brain, can stimulate the HPA axis.[94, 95] Regulation at each stage of the HPA feedback loop will now be considered.

Adrenal Cortex: Glucocorticoids

Synthesis of glucocorticoids in the adrenal cortex[96–98] is closely tied to plasma levels of ACTH, which exhibit episodic peaks and circadian rhythm similar to plasma levels of glucocorticoids.[82, 84] In rats the sensitivity of the adrenals to ACTH increases at the height of basal secretion.[84] ACTH stimulates steroidogenesis by binding to membrane receptors[99] on adrenal cells, which activates adenylate cyclase and also causes hypertrophy and hyperplasia of the adrenal cortex.[84, 88]

Pituitary: ACTH

Both synthesis and secretion of ACTH in anterior pituitary corticotrophs are stimulated by CRH and VP, modulated by catecholamines, and inhibited by glucocorticoids.[100–104] CRH binds to receptors on pituitary cell membranes and activates adenylate cyclase; cAMP mediates the effects of CRH on both secretion and synthesis of ACTH.[102, 105] Activity of CRH is strongly potentiated by VP,[101, 106] and these two hormones interact at several levels within the cell.[102] Whereas CRH increases the amount of ACTH secreted from each responsive corticotroph, it appears that VP, probably through the phosphoinositide pathway, increases the number of CRH-responsive corticotrophs.[107, 108] Regulation of ACTH may exhibit considerable plasticity, as shown by studies with mice defective in the type 1 CRH receptor. Those mice respond to inflammatory stress with pronounced increases in ACTH and corticosterone that do not depend critically on CRH or VP.[109]

Glucocorticoids inhibit ACTH secretion directly by suppressing POMC (proopiomelanocortin) expression in pituitary corticotrophs, and indirectly by inhibiting secretion of CRH and VP.[84, 88, 91] After adrenalectomy ACTH secretion rises, retaining its circadian rhythm.[89] CRH and VP levels in the PVN also rise. These and other changes are reversed by glucocorticoids.[84] It has been proposed that lipocortin 1, a glucocorticoid-induced protein that may be responsible for some anti-inflammatory actions of glucocorticoids, mediates glucocorticoid inhibition of secretion of ACTH from the pituitary.[110]

Feedback has been classified according to how rapidly it inhibits ACTH secretion: fast (within 30 minutes of hormone administration), delayed (minutes to hours), and slow (hours to days).[84, 88, 111] The first two are expected to operate physiologically after moderate or intermittent stress, the third, in pathologic conditions or following therapy with sustained high glucocorticoid levels for days.[88] All three types inhibit stimulated ACTH secretion: slow feedback also inhibits basal secretion, and is associated with decreased messenger RNA (mRNA) for POMC in the pituitary.[84] All types of feedback appear to require both RNA and protein synthesis.[111]

Sensitivity to feedback depends on many factors, including the time of day.[89, 92] Basal ACTH release is less sensitive than stimulated release. Furthermore, a stressful stimulus in some way "facilitates" the response to a subsequent stress, so that the magnitude of the ACTH response to the second stimulus is undiminished despite the feedback inhibition due to the elevated glucocorticoid levels produced by the first stress.[92] Regulation of basal activity of the HPA axis requires binding to both MRs and GRs.[84, 89, 91] Inhibition of basal secretion of ACTH by corticosterone in rats at the low point of diurnal HPA activity (the morning) appears to be mediated through MRs, whereas inhibition at peak activity (evening) is through GRs potentiated by MRs.[112, 113] Suppression of stimulated ACTH secretion, which prevents overactivity of the stress-induced HPA axis, is through binding to GRs in pituitary corticotrophs and hypothalamic CRH neurons.[84, 89, 91, 111] Feedback also differs qualitatively with the kind of stress. For example in sheep, dexamethasone blocks the response to hypoglycemia at both pituitary and hypothalamic levels, but blocks the response to an audiovisual stress only at the pituitary level.[114] Not all feedback to the pituitary is negative. Some can be seen as facilitative or permissive. For example, glucocorticoids increase the coupling of the VP VIb receptor to phospholipase C,[115] which may facilitate VP stimulation of ACTH secretion in the face of stress-elevated glucocorticoid levels.

ACTH is produced as part of a larger precursor protein, POMC, which is also the progenitor of β-endorphin and the lipoproteins.[102, 116] Synthesis of POMC in pituitary corticotrophs is stimulated by CRH[117, 118] and inhibited by glucocorticoids,[88, 89] at least partly at the level of transcription of the POMC gene. The gene has promoter elements required for high basal transcription. Direct repression by glucocorticoids is through nGREs, which may repress by disrupting interactions that maintain basal transcription.[102, 103, 119, 120] Indirect repression is via the hypothalamus.

Corticotrophs are also directly influenced by other hormones, including angiotensin II, paracrine secretions from neighboring pituitary cells,[100–102, 104, 108] and probably cytokines such as IL-1, IL-6, and TNF-α (tumor necrosis factor-α).[94, 108]

Hypothalamus: Corticotropin-Releasing Hormone and Vasopressin

CRH and VP secretion from the PVN, along with other ACTH secretagogues, are subject to both humoral and neural regulation.[68, 89, 91] They increase following adrenalectomy, are stimulated in a stress-specific manner by hemorrhage, injury, hypoglycemia, hypoxia, pain, fear, and other kinds of stress, and inhibited by glucocorticoids[68, 84, 114, 118, 121] (see Fig. 116–1). CRH output can be modulated by catecholamines[104] and cytokines.[94, 122] Acute hemorrhage raises levels in hypothalamic neurons of mRNA for CRH but not VP.[123] Release of CRH, VP, and oxytocin from hypothalamic cells in culture can be stimulated by activators of the cAMP and phosphoinositide pathways and inhibited by dexamethasone.[124]

Here again, not all effects of glucocorticoids are negative. Whereas high levels of glucocorticoids in rats were found to suppress basal or stress-activated CRH gene expression in rat PVN, in adrenalectomized animals there was no stress activation of CRH gene expression unless the animals were treated prior to stress with low levels of glucocorticoids.[125] The low, facilitative, or permissive levels were thought to act through MRs and the high, suppressive levels through GRs.[125]

Cytokine Feedback

Physiologic roles for cytokines in control of the HPA axis, for which there is now substantial evidence, were first proposed by Besedovsky and Sorkin[126] to account for the observation that a challenge with an antigen is followed after several days by a rise in glucocorticoid levels coincident with activation of the immune response. Immune and nervous systems were envisioned as linked in a negative feedback loop, in which activated immune cells produce cytokines that signal increased immune activity to the brain, thereby stimulating the HPA axis which, through glucocorticoids, suppresses the immune reactions.[126] (In Fig. 116–1 the question mark indicates uncertainty about which cytokines are most important and how their message is conveyed.) These and related studies[127] have given rise to the new discipline of neuroimmunoendocrinology.[94, 95, 128]

IL-1 has been shown to mediate HPA stimulation by endotoxin.[129] IL-1α, IL-1β, IL-6, and TNF-α administered peripherally increase HPA activity, manifested as increased levels of glucocorticoids, ACTH or POMC mRNA, and CRH or CRH mRNA.[94, 95, 130, 131] IL-1 causes release of both CRH and VP from neurosecretory cells.[122] The brain has receptors for IL-1, IL-2, IL-6, and other cytokines, and produces IL-1.[94, 95, 132, 133] Transgenic knockout mice lacking IL-1β fail to respond to the inflammatory stress of subcutaneous turpentine injection with increased plasma corticosterone, whereas mice lacking IL-1α respond normally, suggesting that IL-1β but not IL-1α is crucial to the neuroimmunoendocrine response.[134] An unsettled issue is whether peripherally released cytokines like IL-1 enter the brain in physiologically significant amounts, and if they do not, how their message reaches the hypothalamus.[95, 132] Adding to the complexity of this issue is the fact that one cytokine may induce production of another; for example, IL-1 induces IL-6. A number of hypotheses have been proposed, such as that cytokine messages are transmitted via the vagus or through specialized brain regions like the OVLT (organum vascularis laminae terminalis), or via mediators such as eicosanoids, catecholamines, nitric oxide, or cytokines generated in the brain.[95, 135–137]

Cytokines may also directly affect the pituitary and the adrenal cortex: IL-1α, IL-1β, IL-6, and TNF-α stimulate ACTH secretion from cultured pituitary preparations[94, 95, 132]; and IL-1α, IL-1β, and IL-6 stimulate glucocorticoid production in cultured adrenal preparations.[94, 95, 138, 139] Whether these effects occur in intact organisms is not known.

PHYSIOLOGIC ACTIONS OF GLUCOCORTICOIDS

Metabolism

Control of Blood Glucose

Glucocorticoids are among the hormones that maintain blood glucose levels, facilitating stress responses requiring rapid and intense physical exertion such as the encounter of prey and predator. From the standpoint of evolution, that may be their main role in metabolism.[87a] From a clinical standpoint, however, glucocorticoids are usually considered "counterregulatory" hormones that protect the body from insulin-induced hypoglycemia. These functions, which manifest different facets of the same endocrine mechanisms, are shared with the much more rapidly acting glucagon and epinephrine[140–142] and to some extent with growth hormone. In addition, glucocorticoids interact with insulin during feeding and fasting in complex ways that not only maintain blood glucose but influence appetite, feeding patterns, disposal of foodstuffs, and body composition.[143] Antagonism with insulin on both glucose synthesis and utilization presumably accounts at least partly for the diabetogenic actions of excessive glucocorticoids.

Glucocorticoids maintain or raise blood glucose by (1) stimulating hepatic gluconeogenesis, supported by release of gluconeogenic substrates from peripheral tissues; (2) permissively enhancing and prolonging the effects of glucagon and epinephrine on gluconeogenesis and glycogenolysis; (3) inhibiting peripheral glucose utilization; and (4) promoting liver glycogen synthesis, storing substrate in preparation for acute responses to glycogenolytic agents such as glucagon and epinephrine.

Gluconeogenesis

Hepatic gluconeogenesis is stimulated by glucocorticoids mainly through the increased activities of phosphoenolpyruvate carboxykinase (PEPCK) and glucose-6-phosphatase. These enzymes catalyze the conversion of oxaloacetate to phosphoenolpyruvate and of glucose-6-phosphate to glucose, both rate-limiting steps in gluconeogenesis.[144–147] Glucocorticoids can also regulate expression of 6-phosphofructo-2-kinase/fructose-2, 6-biphosphatase, a bifunctional enzyme that controls the level of fructose-2, 6-biphosphate. Fructose-2, 6-biphosphate is an allosteric regulator of gluconeogenic and glycolytic enzymes.[146] PEPCK activity is controlled principally through synthesis of the enzyme.[145, 146] At the molecular level the PEPCK gene displays some of the complexity of regulation of gluconeogenesis in the body that, besides glucocorticoids, involves insulin, glucagon, and catecholamines.[146, 148–151] The gene has a complex glucocorticoid response unit (GRU) spanning 110 bps. There are two GR-binding sites and two accessory factor–binding sites, all of which are required for glucocorticoid regulation. Within the GRU are insulin-responsive and retinoic acid–responsive sequences.[146, 152] Control of the activity of 6-phosphofructo-2-kinase/fructose-2, 6-biphosphatase by glucocorticoids also occurs through increased transcription of the gene. This gene has a complex GRE in the first intron which bears some resemblance to the

GRU of the PEPCK gene.[153] Substrates for gluconeogenesis are increased by glucocorticoids through release of amino acids from muscle and other peripheral tissues[145] and release of glycerol concomitantly with lipolysis.[145, 154]

Permissive actions of glucocorticoids on gluconeogenesis by glucagon and epinephrine, possibly due to enhanced responsiveness to cAMP or other intracellular mediators, are evidenced by the impairment of gluconeogenesis caused by adrenalectomy and its normalization by glucocorticoids.[145, 154, 155] Permissive actions are also seen on glycogenolysis in muscle and liver, which are similarly impaired by adrenalectomy.[155, 156]

Glucose Utilization

Glucocorticoid inhibition of peripheral glucose utilization can be demonstrated both in intact organisms and with isolated cells.[23, 157] It probably accounts for significant insulin antagonism and for the early rise in blood glucose seen after glucocorticoid treatment,[23, 142, 158] and may play a role in releasing gluconeogenic substrates from peripheral tissues.[23, 154] Glucose uptake is inhibited by direct glucocorticoid actions on normal skin,[159] fibroblasts,[160] adipose tissue,[161] adipocytes,[154, 162] lymphoid cells,[163] and polymorphonuclear leukocytes.[164] This inhibition, which requires RNA and protein synthesis, has been postulated to be mediated by a glucocorticoid-induced protein[162, 165, 166]; it results mainly from translocation of glucose transporters from the plasma membrane to intracellular sites.[160, 167] Glucose uptake by muscle is inhibited in intact organisms treated with glucocorticoids.[157] This action is apparently indirect, perhaps via the glucose–fatty acid cycle.[23, 168]

Glycogen Synthesis

Stimulation of glycogen synthesis by glucocorticoids takes place in the fetus and the adult.[169] It is not a consequence of the rise in blood glucose and insulin,[170, 171] and can be elicited directly by glucocorticoids in fetal liver explants.[172, 173] The stimulation depends on increased synthesis of hepatic glycogen synthase and activation by dephosphorylation of its inactive form, as well as on inactivation by dephosphorylation of phosphorylase *a*.[169, 171, 174, 175] Some of these changes can be accounted for by increases in glycogen-bound phosphatase activity, possibly mediated by a glucocorticoid-induced protein.[171]

Fat Metabolism

Glucocorticoids not only inhibit glucose transport by adipose cells but stimulate free fatty acid release, which in humans results in an increase in plasma free fatty acids within 1 to 2 hours of administration of hormone.[154] Increased release of fatty acids also occurs after incubation of adipose tissue with glucocorticoids, an effect due partly to decreased re-esterification resulting from the decrease in glucose uptake and partly to increased lipolysis. Stimulation of lipolysis is largely a permissive effect seen in the presence of growth hormone and other lipolytic agents.[154]

In rats with adequate food intake, high levels of glucocorticoids interact with insulin in such a way as to promote lipogenesis and fat deposition, much as in Cushing's syndrome.[143]

Glucocorticoids are known to be permissive for the obesity syndrome in mutant rodents, which is ameliorated by adrenalectomy. This permissive effect may be due to inhibition of the action of leptin, the hormone secreted from adipose tissue that restricts body fat deposition.[176, 177] Glucocorticoid levels in adipose tissue may be partly controlled by 11β-HSD1.[177a]

Catabolic Effects

Chronic high levels of glucocorticoids lead to massive catabolic effects on proteins and other components of peripheral tissues, and redistribution of fat. These pathologic changes are not well understood, but as already noted in the case of fat metabolism, may result from interactions with insulin and other hormones.[143, 145, 154]

Bone

Bone and cartilage are targets for complex glucocorticoid actions. Under physiologic conditions glucocorticoids may exert permissive effects by increasing levels of receptors and sensitivity to parathyroid hormone, vitamin D, and insulin-like growth factor-1 (IGF-1), whereas during anti-inflammatory or immunosuppressive therapy they can accelerate osteoporosis and impair skeletal growth.[178, 179] Underlying mechanisms are unclear, but probably they involve local modulation by glucocorticoids of the actions or concentrations of IL-1, growth hormone, IGF-1, and IGF-binding protein.[178–182, 182a]

Immune and Inflammatory Reactions

Anti-inflammatory and Immunosuppressive Actions

Among the major applications of hormones in therapy is the use of glucocorticoids for suppression of inflammatory and immune reactions and for treatment of cancers of the lymphoid system.[183] Immunosuppression emerged as an unwanted side effect of glucocorticoid therapy shortly after the discovery of the anti-inflammatory actions, when patients treated with large doses of glucocorticoids for inflammatory conditions became immunosuppressed and less resistant to infection.[53] Anti-inflammatory and immunosuppressive actions are now known to be closely related, sharing cellular and molecular mechanisms involving control of cytokines and other mediators.

For years these actions were assumed to be pharmacologic. Strong evidence, however, points to their physiologic nature.[86, 87] They are elicited through the same receptor-mediated, genomic mechanisms as established physiologic effects, with similar dose-response relations.[184, 185] Adrenalectomy[186, 187] or administration of the glucocorticoid antagonist RU 486[187] enhances the response to inflammatory agents, showing that endogenous glucocorticoids control inflammation. There is similar endogenous control of autoimmune reactions.[188] A striking example is the susceptibility of Lewis rats to arthritis after challenge with streptococcal cell wall (SCW) polysaccharide,[189, 190] and to experimental allergic encephalomyelitis (EAE) after injection of guinea pig myelin basic protein.[191] Lewis rats have a defect in biosynthesis of CRH that curtails the glucocorticoid response to a challenge.[192] Injection of Lewis rats with dexamethasone protects them from SCW polysaccharide, whereas pretreatment of normally resistant Fischer rats with RU 486 makes them susceptible to SCW polysaccharide, showing that in this case glucocorticoids are the principal endogenous immunosuppressive agents.[189] Other factors are probably also important, and in certain rat strains no genetic linkage was found between resistance to development of EAE and high corticosterone levels.[193] Perhaps as an adaptive compensation for insufficient CRH and glucocorticoids Lewis rats have high plasma levels of VP, which may contribute to the excessive inflammatory response.[194] These and other observations suggest that defective HPA functions may play an etiologic role in rheumatoid arthritis.[195, 196] In addition to their suppressive actions on the immune system, glucocorticoids also exert permissive actions, as will be described below.

Immunoregulatory agents besides glucocorticoids may be mobilized by stimulation of the HPA axis.[197–199] For example, stress of adrenalectomized or hypophysectomized rats causes inhibition of mitogen-stimulated lymphocyte proliferation (but not lymphopenia).[200] One such ent may be CRH,[201–203] which paradoxically has been found to act locally as a proinflammatory agent.[204] What role such glucocorticoid-independent phenomena normally play in the immune response to stress is uncertain.

Effects on Leukocytes

Glucocorticoids influence most cells that participate in immune and inflammatory reactions, including lymphocytes,[128, 205, 206] natural killer (NK) cells,[207] monocytes and macrophages,[205, 208] eosinophils, neutrophils,[209] mast cells, and basophils.[210] There is decreased accumulation of most of these cells at inflammatory sites, an effect that can be induced by local application of the hormones.[208–210] Blood counts of lymphocytes, monocytes, eosinophils, and basophils drop within 1 to 3 hours of glucocorticoid administration, generally recovering in 12 to 48 hours. NK cells are unaffected,[211] and neutrophil counts rise.[209] CD4 or helper T cells are more sensitive to lymphopenia than B cells, and CD8 or cytotoxic T cells are relatively insensitive.[211] Increased neutrophil number is thought to reflect increased release of marginated cells to the circulation and increased half-life.[209] These alterations in cell traffic to and from various sites probably depend on changes in surface molecules such as endothelial cell leukocyte adhesion molecule-1 (ELAM-1) and intercellular adhesion molecule-1 (ICAM-1)[212–215] that control adhesion of leukocytes to endothelial and other cells. They may be mediated through both GRs and MRs.[216]

Glucocorticoid administration usually reduces antigen- or lectin-induced mitogenesis measured with peripheral lymphocytes,[211] an effect also observed with lymphocytes in culture.[217] T cells are more sensitive than B cells,[211] and helper T cells more sensitive than cytotoxic T cells.[218] Glucocorticoids also directly inhibit T and B cell proliferation, early B cell differentiation,[211] NK activity,[207, 211] differentiation and function of macrophages[219, 220] and antigen presentation by monocytes, expression of major histocompatibility (MHC) class II proteins, and shift responses from T helper 1 (T_h1) cells to T_h2 cells.[208, 221, 222] Although stimulatory effects of glucocorticoids have long been reported on immunoglobulin synthesis in cell culture,[223, 224] in whole organisms glucocorticoids usually inhibit B cell function.[225]

Permissive glucocorticoid actions on T cell function have been observed in human volunteers treated with endotoxin: when administered within 6 hours of endotoxin, cortisol hemisuccinate suppressed the endotoxin-induced increase in TNF, but if given 12 to 144 hours before endotoxin it magnified the TNF response.[226] Both in rats and in cultured splenic lymphocytes, glucocorticoids at low concentrations, presumably acting through MRs, can enhance T cell responses to concanavalin A, whereas at higher concentrations, through GRs, they are suppressive.[227–230] Hormone concentration and timing appear to be important for these actions to be displayed separately from the usually dominant suppressive effects.

Lymphocyte Apoptosis

The ability of glucocorticoids to kill thymocytes and other lymphocytes by apoptosis is one of the most striking and widely studied effects of these hormones, but its physiologic significance and underlying mechanism is still unknown.[32, 231–233] It has been invoked to account for immunosuppression which, however, is better explained by the actions on cytokines to be described below. In some cases apoptosis might serve to eliminate toxic or otherwise dangerous activated lymphocytes.[234, 235] Glucocorticoids can also protect lymphocytes from apoptosis,[236, 237] and several plausible ideas, as yet unverified, have been proposed for glucocorticoid involvement in positive or negative thymic selection of the T cell repertoire.[231, 236, 238, 239]

Effects via Cytokines and Other Mediators, and via Their Receptors

Many suppressive effects of glucocorticoids on immune and inflammatory reactions appear to be consequences of suppression of the production or activity of cytokines and other mediators that are released during stress responses. Table 116–1 lists the mediators that have been shown to be suppressed by glucocorticoids. They are not as neatly classified as the headings imply; for example, cytokines like IL-1 and IL-6 could be listed as inflammatory agents or neurotransmitters. Neutral proteases like collagenase are included in Table 116–1 as mediators because they contribute to initiation and progression of normal inflammatory processes and some of the peptides they release, like the kinins, mediate chemotactic and other activities.

These mediators constitute communication networks within defense mechanisms that respond to stress-induced challenges to homeostasis. Thus, neurotransmitters respond to a sudden "fight or flight" encounter; pressor agents respond to hemorrhage; inflammatory agents, to tissue damage; cytokines and chemokines, to infection, and so on. By blocking communication via such mediators glucocorticoids can limit propagation of the stress response, preventing it from overshooting and damaging the organism. Furthermore, since most mediators in excess can be toxic and even lethal,[240, 241] the glucocorticoids also prevent such toxicity. For example, glucocorticoids apparently protect against endotoxic shock by blocking both the secretion and lethal effects[242] of TNF-α, and induce tolerance to endotoxin by attenuating the induction of inducible nitric oxide synthase.[243]

Chemokines, or chemotactic cytokines as they are also known, are a family of mediators that are produced locally in tissues, influencing traffic and homing of leukocytes by binding to G protein–coupled cell surface receptors.[244, 245] Their secretion, probably stimulated by such proinflammatory cytokines as IL-1 and TNF-α, is dramatically increased during inflammation, resulting in recruitment of leukocytes to the inflamed site. Significant glucocorticoid effects on cell traffic may be due to inhibition of chemokine secretion.

Molecular mechanisms by which glucocorticoids control mediator production vary. Among the peptides, IL-1 is blocked at the level of transcription, translation, and secretion.[247, 300, 301] TNF-α[268] and granulocyte-macrophage colony-stimulating factor (GM-CSF)[272] appear to be blocked through increased degradation of their mRNAs. IL-2,[258, 264] IL-3,[277] and possibly interferon-γ (IFN-γ)[264] are blocked at the transcriptional level. Some, like nitric oxide,[243] may be suppressed because induction of the enzyme that synthesizes them is blocked. Glucocorticoids also inhibit certain effects of mediators, such as the response of lymphocytes to IL-2[218] and of eosinophils to IL-3, IL-5, GM-CSF, and IFN-γ.[302]

Not all mediators are suppressed by glucocorticoids. Some, like IL-4, IL-10, and epinephrine, which in Table 116–1 are marked with (±), are suppressed under some conditions and stimulated under others. Transforming growth factor-β (TGF-β) may be stimulated.[303] Nerve growth factor (NGF) may be increased in the spinal cord.[304] Macrophage colony-stimulating factor (M-CSF) has been found not to be

TABLE 116–1. Mediators Suppressed by Glucocorticoids

Cytokines	Chemokines	Inflammatory Agents	Hormones and Neurotransmitters
IL-1*[246–248]	IL-8[249–251]	Eicosanoids[252–254]	CRH*[114,125,255]
IL-2*[256–259]	MCP-1[260]	Bradykinin[185,261]	VP*[40,262,263]
IFN-γ*[221,264,265]	RANTES[266]	5-HT*[185]	Oxytocin[267]
TNF-α[226,268,269]	MIP-1α[270]	Histamine[271]	ACTH[84,88,111]
GM-CSF*[218,250,272]	CINC/gro[273]	Plasminogen activator[274,275]	β-Endorphin[276]
IL-3[277]	LIX[278]	Collagenase[275,279]	LH[280]
IL-4*(±)[221,281]		Elastase[275]	Insulin*[282,283]
IL-5[221,284]			Norepinephrine*[40,285,286]
IL-6*[226,250,287,288]			Epinephrine(±)[226,289,290]
IL-10(±)[221,291]			Nitric oxide[243,292–295]
IL-12[296,297]			Substance P[298]

*Receptors induced by glucocorticoids (reviewed in references 87, 230, and 299).

IL, interleukin; IFN, interferon; TNF, tumor necrosis factor, GM-CSF, granulocyte-macrophage colony-stimulating factor; MIP, macrophage inflammatory protein; CINC, cytokine-induced neutrophil chemoattractant; 5-HT, 5-hydroxytryptamine; CRH, corticotropin-releasing hormone; VP, vasopressin; ACTH, adrenocorticotropic hormone; LH, luteinizing hormone.

suppressed in fibroblasts.[250] A mediator that is induced by glucocorticoids is lipocortin 1 (annexin 1), which belongs to the family of annexin proteins.[305, 306] It was first identified as a mediator of glucocorticoid inhibition of eicosanoid production, but that role has since been ascribed to glucocorticoid suppression of transcription of the inducible form of cyclooxygenase.[252, 253, 307, 308] Other results, however, including identification of specific binding sites for lipocortin 1 on leukocytes[305] and demonstration of anti-inflammatory activity of lipocortin 1 in a number of systems[295, 306, 309] have revived the possibility that lipocortin 1 contributes to glucocorticoid actions on inflammation. As mentioned, it may also mediate inhibitory effects of glucocorticoids on release of ACTH from the pituitary.[110]

Table 116–1 indicates with asterisks several mediators that are suppressed by glucocorticoids but have receptors that, paradoxically, are induced by glucocorticoids. As discussed later, glucocorticoid induction of mediator receptors is a possible mechanism for some permissive effects.

Cardiovascular System

Glucocorticoids have complex—sometimes opposing—effects on the cardiovascular system and on electrolyte balance. The most significant of these is the regulation of vascular reactivity and blood pressure. Glucocorticoid effects are exerted on a number of target cells (epithelia, vascular smooth muscle and endothelium, cardiocytes) and can be both direct and indirect.

Under normal physiologic conditions perhaps the most important cardiovascular action of glucocorticoids is permissive enhancement of vascular reactivity to other vasoactive agents (angiotensin II, norepinephrine), which contributes to maintenance of normal blood pressure. This action is best appreciated in patients with glucocorticoid deficiency or in adrenalectomized animals, which are generally hypotensive and exhibit reduced reactivity to vasoconstrictors.[40, 310, 311] In normal rats, the GR antagonist RU 486 blunts vascular reactivity to norepinephrine and angiotensin II.[312] Loss of permissive effects can contribute to cardiovascular collapse in addisonian patients. Although the exact mechanisms of these permissive actions remain to be determined, increased numbers of receptors for vasoactive hormones may play a significant role. Glucocorticoids induce transcription and expression of α_{1B}- and β_2-receptors in smooth muscle cells.[313, 314] They also have direct effects on the heart, such as induction of Na^+,K^+-ATPase in cardiocytes[315] and enhanced cardiac epinephrine synthesis.[290] These effects could be responsible for the positive inotropic effect of glucocorticoids which leads to an increased cardiac output.[316] Increased uptake of Ca^{2+} due to induction of voltage-dependent Ca^{2+} channels is observed in isolated vascular smooth muscle cells[317] and might also contribute to increased vascular contractility.

Chronic exposure to high levels of glucocorticoids (as in Cushing's disease) frequently leads to hypertension. The mechanism(s) of glucocorticoid-induced hypertension is still unknown. It is also not clear how much of this effect is mediated through glucocorticoids and how much through MRs.[74, 75] Elevated blood pressure in glucocorticoid excess is probably due to several factors.[318, 319] When endogenous glucocorticoids are not inactivated by 11β-HSD2 in the kidney, severe hypertension develops due to the mineralocorticoid-like effects of glucocorticoids.[320–322] Chronically elevated levels of glucocorticoids are also likely to have direct effects on the heart[290] and on vascular smooth muscle cells,[317] and may increase responses to vasoconstrictor agents through their permissive action.[85, 311] The renin-angiotensin system is probably not of major significance in glucocorticoid-induced hypertension, as plasma renin activity is often normal or low in Cushing's syndrome.[323] Furthermore, although glucocorticoids induce angiotensinogen (i.e., renin substrate) production by the liver,[323, 324] this action is unlikely to affect blood pressure since the only rate-limiting step in the activity of the renin-angiotensin system is renin release. Atrial natriuretic factor (ANF) is also unlikely to play a role, as its synthesis is increased by glucocorticoids (see below), which would decrease rather than increase blood pressure. On the other hand, glucocorticoids coordinately inhibit the expression of both cyclooxygenase 2[252, 253, 307] and inducible nitric oxide synthetase.[293, 325] Since prostaglandins and nitric oxide are powerful vasodilators, inhibition of their synthesis could be responsible for part of the hypertensive effect of glucocorticoids. Finally, the CNS may have a role because intraventricular administration of glucocorticoids was found to cause hypertension.[326, 327] In summary, glucocorticoid-induced hypertension is probably due to complex interactions at peripheral (kidney, vasculature) and central (CNS) levels.

Electrolyte Homeostasis

Direct Epithelial Effects

Glucocorticoids directly increase epithelial Na^+ absorption and K^+ secretion both in cultured collecting duct cells[328] and in the colon.[329, 330] These effects are mediated through GRs. Cortisol and corticosterone can also induce salt retention via MRs, but these effects are rarely observed under physiologic conditions because endogenous glucocorticoids are rapidly inactivated by the enzyme 11β-HSD2 in aldosterone target cells.[76, 331, 332] If the enzyme is congenitally defective, however, as in the syndrome of apparent mineralocorticoid excess,[320, 321] or inhibited as after licorice consumption,[322] cortisol can occupy both renal MRs and GRs and induce salt retention and hypertension. Cortisol can also bind to MRs if the capacity of 11β-HSD2 is overwhelmed by large amounts of glucocorticoids, as might occur in Cushing's disease. Inhibition of 11β-HSD2 in pregnant rats produces elevated blood pressure in the adult offspring, suggesting that excessive exposure of the fetus to maternal glucocorticoids programs subsequent hypertension.[333]

Glucocorticoids increase renal tubular acid secretion, most likely through increased activity of Na^+-H^+ exchanger in the proximal tubule.[334] They can also induce phosphaturia by inhibiting sodium-dependent phosphate uptake in brush border membrane vesicles.[334]

Indirect Effects

Glucocorticoid deficiency is associated with a decreased ability to excrete water, which appears to be the consequence of decreased glomerular filtration rate (GFR), and increased synthesis of VP. Administration of glucocorticoids increases GFR and thus urine flow both in humans and experimental animals,[335] and produces kaliuresis and natriuresis.[336–338] The mechanism of the diuretic and natriuretic action of glucocorticoids is still unknown, but recent data indicate the involvement of ANF. Glucocorticoids increase the rate of transcription of ANF mRNA in cardiocytes,[339, 340] stimulate ANF secretion,[341–343] and upregulate ANF receptors on endothelial cells.[344] Plasma concentrations of ANF were found to be elevated in patients with Cushing's disease,[345] and exogenous glucocorticoids seem to have a permissive effect on ANF-mediated natriuresis and diuresis in patients with adrenocortical insufficiency.[346]

Suppression of synthesis of VP[263] by glucocorticoids, which is part of the negative feedback mechanism by which glucocorticoids regulate their own concentration (see Fig. 116–1), leads to increased free water clearance. Patients with adrenal insufficiency have reduced free water clearance and increased plasma VP levels, probably due to increased rate of transcription of VP mRNAs.[262]

Glucocorticoids and the Central Nervous System

Glucocorticoids influence behavior, mood, excitability, and electrical activity of neurons. Behavioral changes are frequently observed with both excess and deficiency of glucocorticoids, and sleep disorders are a common feature of glucocorticoid therapy.[347] High HPA activity and plasma cortisol levels are found in many patients with depression.[68] Stress and glucocorticoids impair retrieval of long-term memory.[348] Either glucocorticoid excess or deficiency can damage neurons: adrenalectomy may result in the loss of neurons of the dentate gyrus and pyramidal neurons[349]; extremely high levels of glucocorticoids can cause death of CA3 neurons in the hippocampus and potentiate neuronal death evoked by toxic substances.[304, 350–353]

Both GRs and MRs are present in the brain and other parts of the CNS, including the spinal cord.[68, 304] MRs, though not identified as such, were implicated early as potential brain mediators of glucocorticoid actions.[354] MRs are particularly abundant in the dentate gyrus and pyramidal cells of the hippocampus and other regions of the limbic system, whereas GRs are found widely dispersed in neurons and glial cells. MRs that are protected from glucocorticoids by 11β-HSD2, and are consequently aldosterone-selective, are present only in the anterior hypothalamus and circumventricular organs. There is no detectable 11β-HSD2 in the hippocampus, although there is 11β-HSD1.[68] Other MRs in limbic structures, however, are unprotected and mediate glucocorticoid effects. Electrophysiologic studies with isolated hippocampal tissue from adrenalectomized rats demonstrate that low concentrations of corticosterone, which mainly activate MRs, diminish afterhyperpolarization of neuronal membranes and enhance neuronal excitability. High concentrations of corticosterone or specific glucocorticoid agonists activate GRs, and suppress hippocampal excitability.[68] Thus, glucocorticoids at basal levels acting via MRs maintain neuronal excitability. Stress-induced levels of glucocorticoids acting via GRs suppress stimulated neuronal activity.[68]

A number of enzymes and transport processes in the CNS are influenced by glucocorticoids, with physiologic consequences that are not yet clear.[304] Glucocorticoids induce glycerophosphate dehydrogenase[355] and glutamine synthetase in cultured astrocytes,[356] potassium channels in pituitary cells,[357] and Na^+,K^+-ATPase subunit mRNA in the spinal cord.[304] They inhibit glucose transport in hippocampal neurons and glia.[358]

STUDIES WITH TRANSGENIC MICE

Results of potentially great physiologic significance are emerging from studies with transgenic mice in which some element of the HPA system is impaired. Transgenic mice lacking CRH[359] or GRs,[360] expressing dimerization-defective GRs in place of normal GRs,[361] and with a gene for GR antisense mRNA[362, 364] have been tested for various functions. With MR knockout mice[365, 366] only defects in mineralocorticoid functions and the renin-angiotensin systems have been described so far, and are not discussed here.

CRH knockout mice homozygous for the defective gene were viable as long as they received glucocorticoids during the period from a week before birth till 2 weeks after birth. Without glucocorticoids they died within 12 hours of gestation due to inadequate lung development. Glucocorticoids are known to be important for lung development, particularly for synthesis of surfactant.[367, 368] Compared to normal mice, the CRH knockout mice gave a drastically diminished rise in corticosterone levels in response to stress.[359]

Homozygous GR knockout mice, very few of which survived beyond birth, also failed to develop normal lungs. They had enlarged and disorganized adrenal cortices, atrophied adrenal medullae lacking phenylethanolamine-*N*-methyltransferase (PNMT), and impaired activation of genes for hepatic gluconeogenic enzymes like PEPCK. Their ACTH and corticosterone levels were high, as would be expected.[360]

Glucocorticoids in transgenic mice with dimerization-defective GRs should be unable to regulate genes via GRE-dependent transactivation, which, as described earlier, apparently requires GR dimerization. Via transcriptional crosstalk, however, which does not require dimerization and DNA binding, the defective GRs could repress genes activated by transcription factors such as AP-1 and NF-κB. Studies on cells from the mutant mice supported these inferences. For example, in immortalized fibroblasts from these mice, glucocorticoids suppressed the phorbol ester–activated collagenase-3 gene, known to be mediated through AP-1, but barely activated a transfected reporter under control of the MMTV (mouse mammary tumor virus) promoter, which requires GR binding to GREs. The homozygous offspring were viable, suggesting that normal lung development depends on repression of gene expression. The adrenal medulla and PNMT levels were also normal. As expected, treatment of the mice with glucocorticoids failed to induce such liver enzymes as PEPCK. CRH expression and plasma ACTH levels were normal, but concentrations of ACTH and POMC mRNA in the anterior pituitary were high, suggesting that glucocorticoids regulate ACTH secretion without GR dimerization and binding to GREs. Thymus cells from the mice were insensitive to dexamethasone-mediated apoptosis.[361]

Mice heterozygous or homozygous for a GR antisense gene had low expression of GR mRNA. Their most striking abnormality was an increase in fat deposition which could double their weight compared to normal mice. Since they ate less than normal they are presumed to have increased energy efficiency. They had high ACTH and low corticosterone serum levels. Their immune system was relatively insensitive to glucocorticoids since high corticosterone levels did not reduce thymus weight.[362–364]

Failure of lung development is the only fatal defect reported so far for any of these transgenic mice. Their viability after this hurdle has been passed despite drastically impaired glucocorticoid functions is not surprising, since under laboratory conditions adrenalectomized rats and mice can thrive without glucocorticoids as long as they are given salt to compensate for lack of aldosterone and are not stressed. How well the transgenic mice can tolerate stressors of various kinds remains to be determined.

GLUCOCORTICOID PHYSIOLOGY IN RELATION TO STRESS

Stress and the Hypothalamic-Pituitary-Adrenal Axis

An intimate association between stress and glucocorticoids is manifested in several ways.[35, 39, 54, 84, 86, 87a] Stress from many sources—cold, infection, trauma, hypoglycemia, emotional distress, inflammatory agents, pain, heavy exercise, hemorrhage, and other challenges to homeostasis—stimulates the HPA axis with increased secretion of glucocorticoids. Untreated addisonian patients and adrenalectomized animals can succumb to even mild stress, but are protected by glucocorticoids. Stressed organisms with basal levels of glucocorticoids but unable to increase the levels in response to stress—patients or animals with suppressed or otherwise compromised HPA functions—can tolerate mild stress but succumb to severe stress. The question of what levels of glucocorticoids are needed for protection is still open.[369, 370] As Ingle suggested,[39] a graded response seems likely, basal levels sufficing for mild stress but progressively higher levels being required for more severe stress.[40]

Possible Physiologic Mechanisms of Glucocorticoid Protection in Stress: Permissive and Suppressive Actions

How glucocorticoids protect against stress may be traced to two common threads linking many otherwise disparate effects of glucocorticoids.[85, 86] One is the need for permissive effects of glucocorticoids to maintain or "prime" many homeostatic defense mechanisms so that they can be called into action when necessary. In the preceding sections we have described such permissive actions on gluconeogenesis, glycogenolysis, and lipolysis; on several immune reactions; on pressor activities of vasoactive agents; on the hypothalamic response to stress and the pituitary response to CRH; on bone; and on neural processes. Without glucocorticoids—usually required at low levels, in advance of a stressor—those defenses cannot respond adequately to a challenge.

The second thread is the need for glucocorticoids—usually at higher, stress-induced levels—to suppress activated defense mechanisms, preventing them from overshooting and damaging the organism. Among the most striking suppressive actions are those exerted through inhibition of production or activities of the numerous mediators listed in Table 116–1. Substantial evidence indicates that when an impaired HPA axis cannot increase glucocorticoid activity in response to stress, activated but unrestrained defense mechanisms do overshoot and damage or kill the organism.[86] As described earlier, Lewis rats injected with an inflammatory agent or antigen, and similarly injected Fischer rats that have been treated with RU 486, are overwhelmed by the inflammatory response.[189, 190] We have also mentioned the role of glucocorticoids in protecting against endotoxic shock by suppressing TNF-α-inducible nitric oxide synthase.[242, 243] Glucocorticoids also protect against hemorrhagic shock. Among adrenalectomized rats treated with corticosterone in various ways and subjected to the stress of hemorrhage, those that succumbed (probably from ischemia) had much higher plasma levels of VP and norepinephrine than those that survived. Untreated adrenalectomized rats had the highest levels and control rats (sham-adrenalectomized) the lowest, suggesting that glucocorticoids were protective by restraining the pressor response to hemorrhage transmitted by VP and norepinephrine.[40] Glucocorticoids have also been shown to inhibit catecholamine synthesis and release in rats at rest and during immobilization stress.[285]

In the acute phase response, which involves IL-1, IL-6, and TNF, glucocorticoids both potentiate induction by cytokines of certain acute phase proteins, and suppress production of the cytokines.[371, 372]

Combined Effects

Glucocorticoids can be viewed as sustaining life through two different but related mechanisms: on the one hand they are required to activate some homeostatic defense mechanisms, and on the other to prevent such mechanisms from overshooting. In the course of normal diurnal variation they probably exert both these influences to varying degrees; under stress, the second may predominate. If glucocorticoid regulation is defective, an organism may succumb either because its defense mechanisms cannot react or because they overreact. These are extremes; there are probably intermediate states. Not all defense mechanisms controlled by glucocorticoids are under dual regulation. Inflammation, for example, does not appear to require permissive effects, since it is usually exacerbated by lack of glucocorticoids.

Permissive actions protect against stress much as originally envisioned by Ingle.[39, 42] The role of suppressive actions in physiology has been more controversial. That such actions might protect against stress was proposed in germinal form by Tausk[53] in the context of glucocorticoid therapy soon after the discovery of anti-inflammatory effects. Physiologists, however, had concluded that anti-inflammatory effects were not physiologic. Tausk's idea, published in a pharmaceutical company house organ, never entered the regular endocrine literature. It was proposed anew in 1984 in a general physiologic context,[86] as we have presented it here.

How the apparently opposing permissive and suppressive actions might complement each other can be illustrated with a simple model based on molecular mechanisms by which glucocorticoids regulate certain mediators of defense mechanisms.[85] As shown in Table 116–1, in several cases (e.g., IFN-γ and IL-6), glucocorticoids can both permissively enhance activity of a mediator by inducing its receptors on target cells, and suppress its activity by inhibiting its synthesis. The outcomes predicted from the model are illustrated in Figure 116–2 for two different circumstances. In one (solid lines), both permissive and suppressive actions are assumed to be exerted via binding to GRs, with identical dose-response relationships; in the other (dotted lines), permissive actions are assumed to be via MRs and suppressive actions via GRs, as may occur in several cases described earlier. Since the affinity of cortisol for MRs is much higher than for GRs, the dotted dose-response curves are shifted toward lower cortisol concentrations.

In the upper panel of Figure 116–2, dose-response curves for concentrations of mediator and mediator receptor are plotted on arbitrary vertical scales over a range of cortisol concentrations. The bell-shaped curves in the lower panel of Figure 116–2 represent "mediator activity," assumed to be proportionate to the concentration of mediator-receptor complexes formed at each cortisol concentration. Mediator activity can be thought of more generally as the activity of any defense mechanism regulated by glucocorticoids through permissive and suppressive actions: as cortisol concentrations increase from low levels, activity first increases permissively, reaches a peak value, and at high cortisol levels is suppressed. Similar bell-shaped curves would be generated by almost any combination of permissive and suppressive actions, regardless of the specific mechanisms underlying those actions.

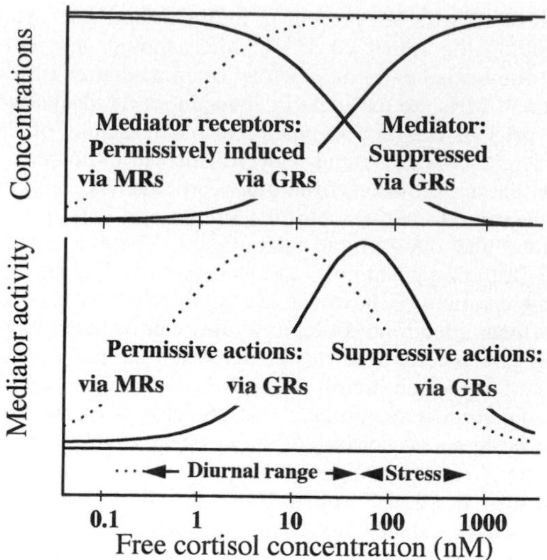

FIGURE 116–2. Model of cortisol-regulated mediator system. *Upper panel* (arbitrary linear vertical scale): Cortisol is assumed to permissively increase the concentration of mediator receptors and to suppress the concentration of the mediator. Solid curves depict effects via binding of cortisol to glucocorticoid receptors (GRs) with dissociation constant $K_d = 30$ nM, the effects being proportionate to the concentration of cortisol-GR complex. The *dotted curve* depicts the effect on mediator receptors through binding of cortisol to mineralocorticoid receptors (MRs) with $K_d = 0.5$ nM, the effect being proportionate to the concentration of cortisol-MR complex. *Lower panel* (arbitrary linear vertical scale): Mediator activity for each cortisol concentration is calculated to be proportionate to the concentration of mediator-receptor complex formed by binding of mediator to mediator receptor, using the concentrations of mediator and mediator receptor in the upper panel.[85] The *solid bell-shaped curve* shows how mediator activity varies with cortisol concentration when mediator receptors are permissively induced via GRs and mediator is suppressed via GRs. The *dotted curve* shows mediator activity when mediator receptors are induced via MRs and mediator is suppressed via GRs. See text for further details.

Under normal unstressed conditions, basal levels of free glucocorticoids vary diurnally over a range (indicated roughly below the lower panel of Fig. 116–2) that corresponds to what might be called the "permissive" left slope of the solid bell-shaped curve, up to about the peak. Stress-induced levels (also shown in Fig. 116–2) can increase well beyond the peak, to the suppressive slope on the right. Thus, basal glucocorticoid levels can be viewed as varying diurnally in such a way as to permissively "prime" homeostatic defenses to a state of peak readiness for the activities of the day. Even at basal levels, however, as seen in the upper panel, glucocorticoids can exert suppressive activity and control responses to moderate stress. Stress-induced levels, on the other hand, are summoned for emergencies to prevent activated defense mechanisms from overshooting. The conclusions that emerge from the model can be extended to other mechanisms for permissive and suppressive glucocorticoid actions, and correspond well with the physiologic roles of glucocorticoids we have sketched earlier.

REFERENCES

1. Addison T: Anaemia—disease of the supra-renal capsules. London Medical Gazette 43:517–518, 1849.
2. Addison T: On the Constitutional and Local Effects of Disease of the Suprarenal Capsules. London, Highley, 1855.
3. Selye H: Textbook of Endocrinology. Montreal, Acta Endocrinologica, 1947.
4. Wells BB, Kendall EC: A qualitative difference in the effect of compounds separated from the adrenal cortex on distribution of electrolytes and on atrophy of the adrenal and thymus glands of rats. Proc Mayo Clinic 15:133–139, 1940.
5. Gaunt R: History of the adrenal cortex. *In* Blaschko H, Sayers G, Smith AD (eds): Handbook of Physiology, Section 7: Endocrinology; Volume VI: Adrenal Gland. Washington, DC, American Physiological Society, 1975, pp 1–12.
6. Brown-Séquard CE: Recherches expérimentales sur la physiologie et la pathologie des capsules surrénales. Arch Gen Med Ser 5, No.8:385–401, 1856.
7. Hartman FA, Brownell KA: The hormone of the adrenal cortex. Science 72:76, 1930.

8. Hartman FA, Brownell KA, Hartman WE: A further study of the hormone of the adrenal cortex. Am J Physiol 95:670–680, 1930.
9. Swingle WW, Pfiffner JJ: An aqueous extract of the suprarenal cortex which maintains the life of bilaterally adrenalectomized cats. Science 71:321–322, 1930.
10. Swingle WW, Pfiffner JJ: Studies on the adrenal cortex. I. The effect of a lipid fraction upon the life-span of adrenalectomized cats. Am J Physiol 96:153–163, 1931.
11. Long CNH, Katzin B, Fry EG: The adrenal cortex and carbohydrate metabolism. Endocrinology 26:309–344, 1940.
12. Britton SW, Silvette H: Some effects of cortico-adrenal extract and other substances on adrenalectomized animals. Am J Physiol 99:15–32, 1931.
13. Britton SW, Silvette H: Effects of cortico-adrenal extract on carbohydrate metabolism in normal animals. Am J Physiol 100:693–700, 1932.
14. Britton SW, Silvette H: The apparent prepotent function of the adrenal glands. Am J Physiol 100:701–713, 1932.
15. Bierry H, Malloizel L: Hypoglycémie après décapsulation. Effets de l'injection d'adrénaline sur les animaux décapsulés. Ct R Soc Biol 65:232–234, 1908.
16. Porges O: Ueber Hypoglykämie bei Morbus Addison sowie bei nebennierenlosen Hunden. Z Klin Med 69:341–349, 1909.
17. Porges O: Zur Pathologie des Morbus Addison. II. Ueber Glycogenschwund nach doppelseitiger Nebennieren-extirpation bei Hunden. Z Klin Med 70:244–250, 1910.
18. Cori CF, Cori GT: The fate of sugar in the animal body. VII. The carbohydrate metabolism of adrenalectomized rats and mice. J Biol Chem 74:473–494, 1927.
19. Long CNH, Lukens FDW: The effects of adrenalectomy and hypophysectomy upon experimental diabetes in the cat. J Exp Med 63:465–490, 1936.
20. Houssay BA, Biasotti A: The hypophysis, carbohydrate metabolism and diabetes. Endocrinology 15:511–523, 1931.
21. Ingle DJ: The production of glycosuria in the normal rat by means of 17-hydroxy-11-dehydrocorticosterone. Endocrinology 29:649–652, 1941.
22. Ingle DJ, Sheppard R, Evans JS, Kuizenga MH: A comparison of adrenal steroid diabetes and pancreatic diabetes in the rat. Endocrinology 37:341–356, 1945.
23. Munck A: Glucocorticoid inhibition of glucose uptake by peripheral tissues: Old and new evidence, molecular mechanisms, and physiological significance. Perspect Biol Med 14:265–289, 1971.
24. Star P: An unusual case of Addison's disease; sudden death; remarks. Lancet 284, 1895.
25. Boinet E: Recherches expérimentales sur les fonctions des capsules surrénales. Ct R Soc Biol 51:671–672, 1899.
26. Greenwood M, Woods HM: "Status thymico-lymphaticus" considered in the light of recent work on the thymus. J Hygiene 26:305–326, 1927.
27. Selye H: Thymus and adrenals in the response of the organism to injuries and intoxications. Br J Exp Pathol 17:234–248, 1936.
28. Ingle DJ: Atrophy of the thymus in normal and hypophysectomized rats following administration of cortin. Proc Soc Exp Biol Med 38:443–444, 1938.
29. Ingle DJ: Effect of two steroid compounds on weight of thymus of adrenalectomized rats. Proc Soc Exp Biol Med 44:174–175, 1940.
30. Dougherty TF, White A: Functional alterations in lymphoid tissue induced by adrenal cortical secretion. Am J Anat 77:81–116, 1945.
31. Kerr JFR, Wyllie AH, Currie AR: Apoptosis: A basic biological phenomenon with wide-ranging implications in tissue kinetics. Br J Cancer 26:239–257, 1972.
32. Wyllie AH: Glucocorticoid-induced thymocyte apoptosis is associated with endogenous endonuclease activation. Nature 284:555–556, 1980.
33. Vaux DL, Korsmeyer SJ: Cell death in development. Cell 96:245–254, 1999.
34. Selye H: The significance of the adrenals for adaptation. Science 85:247–248, 1937.
35. Selye H: The general adaptation syndrome and the diseases of adaptation. J Clin Endocrinol Metab 6:117–230, 1946.
36. Sayers G: The adrenal cortex and homeostasis. Physiol Rev 30:241–320, 1950.
37. Selye H: The Stress of Life. New York, McGraw-Hill, 1956.
38. White A, Dougherty TF: The pituitary adrenotrophic hormone control of the rate of release of serum globulins from lymphoid tissue. Endocrinology 36:207–217, 1945.
39. Ingle DJ: The role of the adrenal cortex in homeostasis. J Endocrinol 8:xxiii–xxxvii, 1952.
40. Darlington DN, Chew G, Ha T, et al: Corticosterone, but not glucose, treatment enables fasted adrenalectomized rats to survive moderate hemorrhage. Endocrinology 127:766–772, 1990.
41. Waksman BH: Neuroimmunomodulation of homeostasis and host defense. J Immunol 135:862s, 1985.
42. Ingle DJ: Permissibility of hormone action. A review. Acta Endocrinol 17:172–186, 1954.
43. Smith PE: Hypophysectomy and a replacement therapy in the rat. Am J Anat 45:205–273, 1930.
44. Li CH, Evans HM, Simpson ME: Adrenocorticotropic hormone. J Biol Chem 149:413–424, 1943.
45. Sayers G, White A, Long CNH: Preparation and properties of adrenotropic hormone. J Biol Chem 149:425–436, 1943.
46. Ingle DJ, Kendall EC: Atrophy of the adrenal cortex of the rat produced by the administration of large amounts of cortin. Science 86:245, 1937.
47. Ingle DJ: The time for the occurrence of cortico-adrenal hypertrophy in rats during continued work. Am J Physiol 124:627–630, 1938.
48. Harris GW: The induction of ovulation in the rabbit, by electrical stimulation of the hypothalamo-hypophysial mechanism. Proc Ry Soc Lond B Biol Sci 122:374–394, 1937.
49. Harris GW: Neural control of the pituitary gland. Physiol Rev 28:139–179, 1948.
50. Vale W, Spiess J, Rivier C, Rivier J: Characterization of a 41-residue ovine hypothalamic peptide that stimulates secretion of corticotropin and β-endorphin. Science 213:1394, 1981.
51. Hench PS, Kendall EC, Slocumb CH, Polley HF: The effect of a hormone of the adrenal cortex (17-hydroxy-11-dehydrocorticosterone: compound E) and of pituitary adrenocorticotropic hormone on rheumatoid arthritis. Proc Mayo Clin 24:181–197, 1949.
52. Kendall EC: Cortisone. New York, Scribner's, 1971.
53. Tausk M: Hat die Nebenniere tatsächlich eine Verteidigungsfunktion? Das Hormon 3:1–24, 1951.
54. Hoffman FG: Role of the adrenal cortex in homeostasis and growth. *In* Christy NP (ed): The Human Adrenal Cortex. New York, Harper & Row, 1971, pp 303–316.
55. Fried J, Borman A: Synthetic derivatives of cortical hormones. Vitam Horm 16:303–374, 1958.
56. Vayssièrre BM, Dupont S, Choquart A, et al: Synthetic glucocorticoids that dissociate transactivation and AP-1 transrepression exhibit antiinflammatory activity *in vivo*. Mol Endocrinol 11:1245–1255, 1997.
57. Bucala R, Fishman J, Cerami A: Formation of covalent adducts between cortisol and 16α-hydroxyestrone and protein: Possible role in the pathogenesis of cortisol toxicity and systemic lupus erythematosus. Proc Natl Acad Sci U S A 79:3320–3324, 1982.
58. Gametchu B: Glucocorticoid receptor–like antigen in lymphoma cell membranes: Correlation to cell lysis. Science 235:456–461, 1987.
59. Hua H-Y, Chen Y-Z: Membrane receptor–mediated electrophysiological effects of glucocorticoid on mammalian neurons. Endocrinology 124:687–691, 1989.
60. Orchinik M, Murray TF, Moore FL: A corticosteroid receptor in neuronal membranes. Science 252:1848–1851, 1991.
61. Orchinik M, McEwen BS: Rapid steroid actions in the brain: a critique of genomic and nongenomic mechanisms. *In* Wehling M (ed): Genomic and Non-Genomic Effects of Aldosterone. Boca Raton, FL, CRC Press, 1995, pp 77–108.
62. Brann DW, Hendry LB, Mahesh VB: Emerging diversities in the mechanism of action of steroid hormones. J Steroid Biochem Mol Biol 52:113–133, 1995.
63. Wehling H: Specific, nongenomic actions of steroid hormones. Annu Rev Physiol 59:365–393, 1997.
64. de Castro M, Elliot S, Kino T, et al: The non-ligand binding β-isoform of the human glucocorticoid receptor (hGRβ): Tissue levels, mechanism of action, and potential physiologic role. Mol Med 2:597–607, 1996.
65. Oakley RH, Webster JC, Sar M, et al: Expression and subcellular distribution of the β-isoform of the human glucocorticoid receptor. Endocrinology 138:5028–5038, 1997.
66. Hecht K, Carlstedt-Duke J, Stierna P, et al: Evidence that the β-isoform of the human glucocorticoid receptor does not act as a physiologically significant repressor. J Biol Chem 272:26659–26664, 1997.
67. Otto C, Reichardt HA, Schütz G: Absence of glucocorticoid receptor-β in mice. J Biol Chem 272:26665–26668, 1997.
68. De Kloet ER, Vreugdenhil E, Oitzl MS, Joëls M: Brain corticosteroid receptor balance in health and disease. Endoc Rev 19:269–301, 1998.
69. Munck A, Brinck-Johnsen T: Specific metabolic and physicochemical interactions of glucocorticoids in vivo and in vitro with rat adipose tissue and thymus cells. Excerpta Medica Int Congress Ser 132:472–481, 1967.
70. Munck A, Brinck-Johnsen T: Specific and nonspecific physicochemical interactions of glucocorticoids and related steroids with rat thymus cells *in vitro*. J Biol Chem 243:5556–5565, 1968.
71. Schaumburg BP, Bojesen E: Specificity and thermodynamic properties of the corticosteroid binding to a receptor of rat thymocytes *in vitro*. Biochim Biophys Acta 170:172–188, 1968.
72. Miner JN, Diamond MI, Yamamoto KR: Joints in the regulatory lattice: Composite regulation by steroid receptor-AP1 complexes. Cell Growth Differ 2:525–530, 1991.
73. Göttlicher M, Heck S, Herrlich P: Transcriptional cross-talk, the second mode of steroid receptor action. J Mol Med 76:480–489, 1998.
74. Krozowski ZS, Funder JW: Renal mineralocorticoid receptors and hippocampal corticosterone-binding species have identical steroid specificity. Proc Natl Acad Sci U S A 80:6056–6060, 1983.
75. Beaumont K, Fanestil DD: Characterization of rat brain aldosterone receptors reveals high affinity for corticosterone. Endocrinology 113:2043–2051, 1983.
76. Rusvai E, Náray-Fejes-Tóth A: A new isoform of 11β-hydroxysteroid dehydrogenase in aldosterone target cells. J Biol Chem 268:10717–10720, 1993.
77. Gao H-B, Shan L-X, Monder C, Hardy MP: Suppression of endogenous corticosterone levels *in vivo* increases the steroidogenic capacity of rat Leydig cells *in vitro*. Endocrinology 137:1714–1718, 1996.
78. Ge R-S, Hardy DO, Catterall JF, Hardy MP: Developmental changes in glucocorticoid receptor and 11β-hydroxysteroid dehydrogenase oxidative and reductive activities in rat Leydig cells. Endocrinology 138:5089–5095, 1997.
79. Burton PJ, Krozowski ZS, Waddel BJ: Immunolocalization of 11β-hydroxysteroid dehydrogenase types 1 and 2 in rat uterus: Variation across the estrous cycle and regulation by estrogen and progesterone. Endocrinology 139:376–382, 1998.
80. Waddell BJ, Benediktsson R, Brown RW, Sekl JR: Tissue-specific messenger ribonucleic acid expression of 11β-hydroxysteroid dehydrogenase types 1 and 2 and the glucocorticoid receptor within rat placenta suggests exquisite local control of glucocorticoid action. Endocrinology 139:1517–1523, 1998.
81. Kotelevtsev Y, Holmes MC, Burchell A, et al: 11β-hydroxysteroid dehydrogenase type 1 knockout mice show attenuated glucocorticoid-inducible responses and resist hyperglycemia on obesity or stress. Proc Natl Acad Sci U S A 94:14924–14929, 1997.
82. Krieger DT, Allen W, Rizzo F, Krieger HP: Characterization of the normal temporal pattern of plasma corticosteroid levels. J Clin Endocrinol 32:266–284, 1970.
83. Hellman L, Nakada F, Curti J, et al: Cortisol is secreted episodically by normal man. J Clin Endocrinol 30:411–422, 1970.
84. Dallman MF, Akana SF, Cascio CS, et al: Regulation of ACTH secretion: Variations on a theme of B. Recent Prog Horm Res 43:113–173, 1987.
85. Munck A, Náray-Fejes-Tóth A: The ups and downs of glucocorticoid physiology. Permissive and suppressive effects revisited. Mol Cell Endocrinol 90:C1–C4, 1992.
86. Munck A, Guyre PM, Holbrook NJ: Physiological functions of glucocorticoids in stress and their relation to pharmacological actions. Endocr Rev 5:25–44, 1984.
87. Munck A, Náray-Fejes-Tóth A: Glucocorticoids and stress: Permissive and suppressive actions. Ann N Y Acad Sci 746:115–130, 1994.

87a. Sapolsky RM, Romero LM, Munck AU: How do glucocorticoids influence stress responses? Integrating permissive, suppressive, stimulatory and preparative actions. Endocr Rev 21:55–89, 2000.
88. Keller-Wood ME, Dallman MF: Corticosteroid inhibition of ACTH secretion. Endocr Rev 5:1–24, 1984.
89. Bradbury MJ, Akana SF, Cascio CS, et al: Regulation of basal ACTH secretion by corticosterone is mediated by both Type I (MR) and Type II (GR) receptors in the brain. J Steroid Biochem Mol Biol 40:133–142, 1991.
90. Windle RJ, Wood SA, Shanks N, et al: Ultradian rhythm of basal corticosterone release in the female rat: Dynamic interaction with the acute response to stress. Endocrinology 139:443–450, 1998.
91. De Kloet ER, Rosenfeld P, Van Eekelen JAM, et al: Stress, glucocorticoids and development. Prog Brain Res 73:101–120, 1988.
92. Akana SF, Dallman MF, Bradbury MJ, et al: Feedback and facilitation in the adrenocortical system: Unmasking facilitation by partial inhibition of the glucocorticoid response to prior stress. Endocrinology 131:57–68, 1992.
93. Joëls M, De Kloet ER: Control of neuronal excitability by corticosteroid hormones. Trends Neurosci 15:25–30, 1992.
94. Besedovsky HO, del Rey A: Immuno-neuro-endocrine interactions: Facts and hypotheses. Endocr Rev 17:64–102, 1996.
95. Turnbull AV, Rivier CL: Regulation of the hypothalamic-pituitary-adrenal axis by cytokines: Actions and mechanisms of action. Physiol Rev 79:1–71, 1999.
96. Miller WL: Molecular biology of steroid hormone synthesis. Endocr Rev 9:295–318, 1988.
97. Simpson ER, Waterman MR: Regulation of the synthesis of steroidogenic enzymes in adrenal cortical cells by ACTH. Annu Rev Physiol 50:427–440, 1988.
98. Hanukoglu I: Steroidogenic enzymes: Structure, function, and role in regulation of steroid hormone biosynthesis. J Steroid Biochem Mol Biol 43:779–804, 1992.
99. Ramachandran J, Tsubokawa M, Gohil K: Corticotropin receptors. Ann N Y Acad Sci 512:415–425, 1987.
100. Rivier C, Vale W: Modulation of stress-induced ACTH release by corticotrophin-releasing factor, catecholamines and vasopressin. Nature 305:325–327, 1983.
101. Abou-Samra A-B, Harwood JP, Catt K, Aguilera G: Mechanisms of action of CRF and other regulators of ACTH release in pituitary corticotrophs. Ann N Y Acad Sci 512:67–84, 1987.
102. Lundblad JR, Roberts JL: Regulation of proopiomelanocortin gene expression in pituitary. Endocr Rev 9:135–158, 1988.
103. Drouin J, Sun YL, Nemer M: Glucocorticoid repression of proopiomelanocortin gene transcription. J Steroid Biochem Mol Biol 34:63–69, 1989.
104. Plotsky PM, Cunningham ET Jr, Widmaier EP: Catecholaminergic modulation of corticotropin-releasing factor and adrenocorticotropin secretion. Endocr Rev 10:437–458, 1989.
105. Aguilera G, Millan MA, Hauger RL, Catt KJ: Corticotropin-releasing factor receptors: Distribution and regulation in brain, pituitary, and peripheral tissues. Ann N Y Acad Sci 512:48–66, 1987.
106. Bilezikjian LM, Vale WW: Regulation of ACTH secretion from corticotrophs: the interaction of vasopressin and CRF. Ann N Y Acad Sci 512:85–96, 1987.
107. Canny BJ, Jia L-G, Leong DA: Corticotropin-releasing factor, but not arginine vasopressin, stimulates concentration-dependent increases in ACTH secretion from a single corticotrope. Implications for intracellular signals in stimulus-secretion coupling. J Biol Chem 267:8325–8329, 1992.
108. Schwartz J, Cherny R: Intercellular communication within the anterior pituitary influencing the secretion of hypophysial hormones. Endocr Rev 13:453–475, 1992.
109. Turnbull AV, Smith GW, Lee S, et al: CRF type I receptor-deficient mice exhibit a pronounced pituitary-adrenal response to local inflammation. Endocrinology 140:1013–1017, 1999.
110. Taylor AD, Christian HC, Morris JF, et al: An antisense oligodeoxynucleotide to lipocortin 1 reverses the inhibitory actions of dexamethasone on the release of adrenocorticotropin from rat pituitary tissue *in vitro*. Endocrinology 138:2909–2918, 1997.
111. Dayanithi G, Antoni FA: Rapid as well as delayed inhibitory effects of glucocorticoid hormones on pituitary adrenocorticotropic hormone release are mediated by type II glucocorticoid receptors and require newly synthesized messenger ribonucleic acid as well as protein. Endocrinology 125:308–313, 1989.
112. Dallman MF, Levin N, Cascio CS, et al: Pharmacological evidence that the inhibition of diurnal adrenocorticotropin secretion by corticosteroids is mediated via type I corticosterone-preferring receptors. Endocrinology 124:2844–2850, 1989.
113. Bradbury MJ, Akana SF, Dallman MF: Role of Type I and Type II corticosteroid receptors in regulation of basal activity in the hypothalamo-pituitary-adrenal axis during the diurnal trough and the peak: Evidence for a nonadditive effect of combined receptor occupancy. Endocrinology 134:1286–1296, 1994.
114. Canny BJ, Funder JW, Clarke IJ: Glucocorticoids regulate ovine hypophysial portal levels of corticotropin-releasing factor and arginine vasopressin in a stress-specific manner. Endocrinology 125:2532–2539, 1989.
115. Rabadan-Diehl C, Aguilera G: Glucocorticoids increase vasopressin V1b receptor coupling to phospholipase C. Endocrinology 139:3220–3226, 1998.
116. Nakanishi S: Nucleotide sequence of cloned cDNA for bovine corticotropin–β-lipotropin precursor. Nature 278:423–427, 1979.
117. Taylor AL, Fishman LM: Corticotropin-releasing hormone. N Engl J Med 319:213–222, 1988.
118. Orth DN: Corticotropin-releasing hormone in humans. Endocr Rev 13:164–191, 1992.
119. Riegel AT, Lu Y, Remenick J, et al: Proopiomelanocortin gene promoter elements required for constitutive and glucocorticoid-repressed transcription. Mol Endocrinol 5:1973–1982, 1991.
120. Drouin J, Sun YL, Chamberland M, et al: Novel glucocorticoid receptor complex with DNA element of the hormone-repressed POMC gene. EMBO J 12:145–156, 1993.
121. Swanson LW, Sawchenko PE, Lind RW, Rho J-H: The CRH motoneuron: Differential peptide regulation in neurons with possible synaptic, paracrine, and endocrine outputs. Ann N Y Acad Sci 512:12–23, 1987.
122. Whitnall MH, Perlstein RS, Mougey EH, Neta R: Effects of interleukin-1 on the stress-responsive and -nonresponsive subtypes of corticotropin-releasing neurosecretory axons. Endocrinology 131:37–44, 1992.
123. Darlington DN, Barraclough CA, Gann DS: Hypotensive hemorrhage elevates corticotropin-releasing hormone messenger ribonucleic acid (mRNA) but not vasopressin mRNA in the rat hypothalamus. Endocrinology 130:1281–1288, 1992.
124. Hu S-B, Tannahill LA, Biswas S, Lightman SL: Release of corticotrophin-releasing factor-41, arginine vasopressin and oxytocin from rat fetal hypothalamic cells in culture: Response to activation of intracellular second mesengers and to corticosteroids. J Endocrinol 132:57–65, 1992.
125. Tanimura SM, Watts AG: Corticosterone can facilitate as well as inhibit corticotropin-releasing hormone gene expression in the rat hypothalamic paraventricular nucleus. Endocrinology 139:3830–3836, 1998.
126. Besedovsky H, Sorkin E: Network of immune-neuroendocrine interactions. Clin Exp Immunol 27:1–12, 1977.
127. Blalock JE, Smith EM: The immune system: Our mobile brain. Immunol Today 6:115–117, 1985.
128. Wick G, Schwarz S, Kroemer G: Immunoendocrine communication via the hypothalamo-pituitary-adrenal axis in autoimmune diseases. Endocr Rev 14:539–563, 1993.
129. Rivier C, Chizzonite R, Vale W: In the mouse, the activation of the hypothalamic-pituitary-adrenal axis by a lipopolysaccharide (endotoxin) is mediated through interleukin-1. Endocrinology 125:2800–2805, 1989.
130. Besedovsky HO, del Rey A, Klusman I, et al: Cytokines as modulators of the hypothalamus-pituitary-adrenal axis. J Steroid Biochem Mol Biol 40:613–618, 1991.
131. Sweep CGJ, van der Meer MJM, Hermus ARMM, et al: Chronic stimulation of the pituitary-adrenal axis in rats by interleukin-1β infusion: *In vivo* and *in vitro* studies. Endocrinology 130:1153–1164, 1992.
132. Koenig JI: Presence of cytokines in the hypothalamic-pituitary axis. Prog Neuroendocrinimmun 4:143–153, 1991.
133. Schneider H, Pitossi F, Balschun D, et al: A neuromodulatory role of interleukin-1β in the hippocampus. Proc Natl Acad Sci U S A 95:7778–7793, 1998.
134. Horai R, Asano M, Sudo K, et al: Production of mice deficient in genes for interleukin (IL)-1α, IL-1β, IL-1α/β, and IL-1 receptor antagonist shows that IL-1β is crucial in turpentine-induced fever development and glucocorticoid secretion. J Exp Med 187:1463–1475, 1998.
135. Navarra P, Tsagarakis S, Faria MS, et al: Interleukins-1 and -6 stimulate the release of corticotropin-releasing hormone-41 from rat hypothalamus *in vitro* via the eicosanoid cyclooxygenase pathway. Endocrinology 128:37–44, 1991.
136. Dinarello CA: Role of interleukin-1 in infectious diseases. Immunol Rev 127:119–146, 1992.
137. Blatteis CM, Sehic E: Fever: How may circulating pyrogens signal the brain? News Physiol Sci 12:1–9, 1997.
138. Andreis PG, Neri G, Belloni AS, et al: Interleukin-1β enhances corticosterone secretion by acting directly on the rat adrenal gland. Endocrinology 129:53–57, 1991.
139. Tominaga T, Fukata J, Naito Y, et al: Prostaglandin-dependent *in vitro* stimulation of adrenocortical steroidogenesis by interleukins. Endocrinology 128:526–531, 1991.
140. Cryer PE, White NH, Santiago JV: The relevance of glucose counterregulatory systems to patients with insulin-dependent diabetes mellitus. Endocr Rev 7:131–139, 1986.
141. Saccà L: Role of counterregulatory hormones in the regulation of hepatic glucose metabolism. Diabetes Metab Rev 3:207–229, 1987.
142. McMahon M, Gerich J, Rizza R: Effects of glucocorticoids on carbohydrate metabolism. Diabetes Metab Rev 4:17–30, 1988.
143. Dallman MF, Strack AM, Akana SF, et al: Feast and famine: Critical role of glucocorticoids with insulin in daily energy flow. Front Neuroendocrinol 14:303–347, 1993.
144. Shrago E, Lardy HA, Nordlie RC, Foster DO: Metabolic and hormonal control of phosphoenolpyruvate carboxykinase and malic enzyme in rat liver. J Biol Chem 238:3188–3192, 1963.
145. Exton JH: Regulation of gluconeogenesis by glucocorticoids. *In* Baxter JD, Rousseau GG (eds): Glucocorticoid Hormone Action. Berlin, Springer-Verlag, 1979, pp 535–546.
146. Pilkis SJ, Granner DK: Molecular physiology of the regulation of hepatic gluconeogenesis and glycolysis. Annu Rev Physiol 54:885–909, 1992.
147. Croniger C, Leahy P, Reshef L, Hanson RW: C/EBP and the control of phosphoenolpyruvate carboxykinase gene transcription in the liver. J Biol Chem 273:31629–31632, 1998.
148. Wynshaw-Boris A, Short JM, Loose DS, Hanson RW: Characterization of the phosphoenolpyruvate carboxykinase (GTP) promoter-regulatory region. 1. Multiple hormone regulatory elements and the effects of enhancers. J Biol Chem 261:9714–9720, 1986.
149. Lucas PC, Granner DK: Hormone response domains in gene transcription. Annu Rev Biochem 61:1131–1173, 1992.
150. Imai E, Miner JN, Mitchell JA, et al: Glucocorticoid receptor-cAMP response element-binding protein interaction and the response of the phosphoenolpyruvate carboxykinase gene to glucocorticoids. J Biol Chem 268:5353–5356, 1993.
151. Friedman JE, Yun JS, Patel YM, et al: Glucocorticoids regulate the induction of phosphoenolpyruvate carboxykinase (GTP) gene transcription during diabetes. J Biol Chem 268:12952–12957, 1993.
152. Sugiyama T, Scott DK, Wang J-C, Granner DK: Structural requirements of the glucocorticoid and retinoic acid response units in the phosphoenolpyruvate carboxykinase gene promoter. Mol Endocrinol 12:1487–1498, 1998.
153. Lange AJ, Espinet C, Hall R, et al: Regulation of gene expression of rat skeletal muscle/liver 6-phosphofructo-2-kinase/fructose-2,6-biphosphatase. Isolation and characterization of a glucocorticoid response element in the first intron of the gene. J Biol Chem 267:15673–15680, 1992.

154. Fain JN: Inhibition of glucose transport in fat cells and activation of lipolysis by glucocorticoids. *In* Baxter JD, Rousseau GG (eds): Glucocorticoid Hormone Action. Berlin, Springer-Verlag, 1979, pp 547–560.
155. Exton JH: Mechanisms of hormonal regulation of hepatic glucose metabolism. Diabetes Metab Rev 3:163–183, 1987.
156. Miller TB, Exton JH, Park CR: A block in epinephrine-induced glycogenolysis in hearts from adrenalectomized rats. J Biol Chem 246:3672–3678, 1971.
157. Riddick FA, Reisler DM, Kipnis DM: The sugar transport system in striated muscle. Effect of growth hormone, hydrocortisone and alloxan diabetes. Diabetes 11:171–178, 1962.
158. Shamoon H, Soman V, Sherwin RS: The influence of acute physiological increments of cortisol on fuel metabolism and insulin binding to monocytes in normal humans. J Clin Endocrinol Metab 50:495–501, 1980.
159. Overell BG, Condon SE, Petrow V: The effect of hormones and their analogues upon the uptake of glucose by mouse skin *in vitro*. J Pharm Pharmacol 12:150–153, 1960.
160. Horner HC, Munck A, Lienhard GE: Dexamethasone causes translocation of glucose transporters from the plasma membrane to an intracellular site in human fibroblasts. J Biol Chem 262:17696–17702, 1987.
161. Munck A: The effect *in vitro* of glucocorticoids on net glucose uptake by rat epididymal adipose tissue. Biochim Biophys Acta 48:618–620, 1961.
162. Czech MP, Fain JN: Dactinomycin inhibition of dexamethasone action on glucose metabolism in white fat cells. Biochim Biophys Acta 230:185–193, 1971.
163. Morita Y, Munck A: Effect of glucocorticoids *in vivo* and *in vitro* on net glucose uptake and amino acid incorporation by rat-thymus cells. Biochim Biophys Acta 93:150–157, 1964.
164. Simonsson B: Depression of ^{3}H-glucose uptake into rabbit polymorphonuclear leukocytes by glucocorticoids in concentrations partly saturating the specific glucocorticoid uptake. Evidence for a glucocorticoid receptor. Acta Physiol Scand 86:398–409, 1972.
165. Mosher KM, Young DA, Munck A: Evidence for irreversible, actinomycin D-sensitive, and temperature-sensitive steps following binding of cortisol to glucocorticoid receptors and preceding effects on glucose metabolism in rat thymus cells. J Biol Chem 246:654–659, 1971.
166. Carter-Su C, Okamoto K: Inhibition of hexose transport in adipocytes by dexamethasone: Role of protein synthesis. Am J Physiol 248:E215–E223, 1985.
167. Carter-Su C, Okamoto K: Effect of glucocorticoids on hexose transport in rat adipocytes: Evidence for decreased transporters in the plasma membrane. J Biol Chem 260:11091–11098, 1985.
168. Randle PJ, Garland PB, Hales CN, Newsholme EA: The glucose fatty-acid cycle. Its role in insulin sensitivity and the metabolic disturbances of diabetes mellitus. Lancet 1:785–789, 1963.
169. Stalmans W, Laloux M. Glucocorticoids and hepatic glycogen metabolism. *In* Baxter JD, Rousseau GG (eds): Glucocorticoid Hormone Action. Berlin, Springer-Verlag, 1979, pp 517–533.
170. Dorsey JL, Munck A: Studies on the mode of action of glucocorticoids in rats: A comparison of the effects of cortisol and glucose on the formation of liver glycogen. Endocrinology 71:605–608, 1962.
171. Bollen M, Stalmans W: The structure, role, and regulation of type 1 protein phosphatases. Crit Rev Biochem Mol Biol 27:227–281, 1992.
172. Monder C, Coufalik A: Influence of cortisol on glycogen synthesis and gluconeogenesis in fetal rat liver in organ culture. J Biol Chem 247:3608–3617, 1972.
173. Eisen HJ, Goldfine ID, Glinsmann WH: Regulation of hepatic glycogen synthesis during fetal development: Role of hydrocortisone, insulin, and insulin receptors. Proc Natl Acad Sci U S A 70:3454–3457, 1973.
174. Hornbrook KR, Burch HB, Lowry OH: The effects of adrenalectomy and hydrocortisone on rat liver metabolites and glycogen synthetase activity. Mol Pharmacol 2:106–116, 1966.
175. von Holt C, Fister J: The effect of cortisol on synthesis and degradation of liver glycogen. Biochim Biophys Acta 90:232–238, 1964.
176. Zakrzewska KE, Cusin I, Sainsbury A, et al: Glucocorticoids as counterregulatory hormones of leptin. Toward an understanding of leptin resistance. Diabetes 46:717–719, 1997.
177. Arvaniti K, Ricquier D, Champigny O, Richard D: Leptin and corticosterone have opposite effects on food intake and the expression of UCP1 mRNA in brown adipose tissue of *lep^{ob}/lep^{ob}* mice. Endocrinology 139:4000–4003, 1998.
177a. Livingstone DEW, Jones CC, Smith K, et al: Understanding the role of glucocorticoids in obesity: Tissue-specific alterations of corticosterone metabolism in obese Zucker rats. Endocrinology 141:560–563, 2000.
178. Marusic A, Raisz LG: Cortisol modulates the actions of interleukin-1α on bone formation, resorption, and prostaglandin production in cultured mouse parietal bones. Endocrinology 129:2699–2706, 1991.
179. Canalis E: Inhibitory actions of glucocorticoids on skeletal growth. Is local insulin-like growth factor to blame? (editorial). Endocrinology 139:3041–3042, 1998.
180. Delany AM, Canalis E: Transcriptional repression of insulin-like growth factor I by glucocorticoids in rat bone cells. Endocrinology 136:4776–4781, 1995.
181. Conover CA, Lee PDK, Riggs BL, Powell DR: Insulin-like growth factor–binding protein-1 expression in cultured human bone cells: Regulation by insulin and glucocorticoid. Endocrinology 137:3295–3301, 1996.
182. Jux C, Leiber K, Hügel U, et al: Dexamethasone impairs growth hormone (GH)-stimulated growth by suppression of local insulin-like growth factor (IGF)-I production and expression of GH- and IGF-I-receptor in cultured rat chondrocytes. Endocrinology 139:3296–3305, 1998.
182a. McCarthy TL, Ji C, Chen Y, et al: Time- and dose-related interactions between glucocorticoid and cyclic adenosine 3′,5′-monophosphate on CCAAT/enhancer-binding protein-dependent insulin-like growth factor I expression of osteoblasts. Endocrinology 141:127–137, 2000.
183. Akana SF, Dallman MF: Chronic cold in adrenalectomized, corticosterone (B)-treated rats: Facilitated corticotropin responses to acute restraint emerge as B increases. Endocrinology 138:3249–3258, 1997.
184. Fahey JV, Guyre PM, Munck A: Mechanisms of antiinflammatory actions of glucocorticoids. Adv Inflamm Res 2:21–51, 1981.
185. Tsurufuji S, Ohuchi K: In vivo models of inflammation: A review with special reference to the mechanisms of action of glucocorticoids. *In* Schleimer RP, Claman HN, Oronsky AL (eds): Anti-inflammatory Steroid Action. Basic and Clinical Aspects. New York, Academic Press, 1989, pp 259–279.
186. Flower RJ, Parente L, Persico P, Salmon JA: A comparison of the acute inflammatory response in adrenalectomised and sham-operated rats. Br J Pharmacol 87:57–62, 1986.
187. Laue L, Kawai S, Brandon DD, et al: Receptor-mediated effects of glucocorticoids on inflammation: Enhancement of the inflammatory response with a glucocorticoid antagonist. J Steroid Biochem Mol Biol 29:591–598, 1988.
188. Derijk R, Berkenbosch F: The immune-hypothalamo-pituitary-adrenal axis and autoimmunity. Int J Neurosci 59:91–100, 1991.
189. Sternberg EM, Hill JM, Chrousos GP, et al: Inflammatory mediator-induced hypothalamic-pituitary-adrenal axis activation is defective in streptococcal cell wall arthritis–susceptible Lewis rats. Proc Natl Acad Sci U S A 86:2374–2378, 1989.
190. Karalis K, Crofford L, Wilder RL, Chrousos GP: Glucocorticoid and/or glucocorticoid antagonist effects in inflammatory disease–susceptible Lewis rats and inflammatory disease–resistant Fischer rats. Endocrinology 136:3107–3112, 1995.
191. Mason D: Genetic variation in the stress response: Susceptibility to experimental allergic encephalomyelitis and implications for human inflammatory disease. Immunol Today 12:57–60, 1991.
192. Sternberg EM, Young SW III, Bernardini R, et al: A central nervous system defect in biosynthesis of corticotropin-releasing hormone is associated with susceptibility to streptococcal cell wall-induced arthritis in Lewis rats. Proc Natl Acad Sci U S A 86:4771–4775, 1989.
193. Villas PA, Dronsfield MJ, Blankenhorn EP: Experimental allergic encephalomyelitis and corticosterone studies in resistant and susceptible rat strains. Clin Immunol Immunopathol 61:29–40, 1991.
194. Patchev VK, Kalogeras KT, Zelazowski P, et al: Increased plasma concentrations, hypothalamic content, and *in vitro* release of arginine vasopressin in inflammatory disease-prone, hypothalamic corticotropin-releasing hormone-deficient Lewis rats. Endocrinology 131:1453–1457, 1992.
195. Neeck G, Federlin K, Graef V, et al: Adrenal secretion of patients with rheumatoid arthritis. J Rheumatol 17:24–29, 1990.
196. Chikanza IC, Petrou P, Kingsley G, et al:Defective hypothalamic response to immune and inflammatory stimuli in patients with rheumatoid arthritis. Arthritis Rheum 35:1281–1288, 1992.
197. Shavit Y: Stress-induced immune modulation in animals: opiates and endogenous opioid peptides. *In* Ader R, Felten DL, Cohen N (eds): Psychoneuroimmunology. New York, Academic Press, 1991, pp 789–806.
198. Heijnen CJ, Kavelaars A, Ballieux RE: Corticotropin-releasing hormone and proopiomelanocortin-derived peptides in the modulation of immune function. *In* Ader R, Felten DL, Cohen N (eds): Psychoneuroimmunology. New York, Academic Press, 1991, pp 429–446.
199. Vamvakopoulos NC, Chrousos GP: Hormonal regulation of human corticotropin-releasing hormone gene expression: Implications for the stress response and immune/inflammatory reaction. Endocr Rev 15:409–430, 1994.
200. Keller SE, Schleifer SJ, Demetrikopoulos MK: Stress-induced changes in immune function in animals: Hypothalamo-pituitary-adrenal influences. *In* Ader R, Felten DL, Cohen N (eds): Psychoneuroimmunology. New York, Academic Press, 1991, pp 771–787.
201. Jain R, Zwickler D, Hollander CS, et al: Corticotropin-releasing factor modulates the immune response to stress in the rat. Endocrinology 128:1329–1336, 1991.
202. Berkenbosch F, Wolvers DAW, Derijk R: Neuroendocrine and immunological mechanisms in stress-induced immunomodulation. J Steroid Biochem Mol Biol 40:639–647, 1991.
203. Webster EL, Torpy DJ, Elenkov IJ, Chrousos GP: Corticotropin-releasing hormone and inflammation. Ann N Y Acad Sci 840:21–32, 1998.
204. Karalis K, Sano H, Redwine J, et al: Autocrine or paracrine inflammatory actions of corticotropin-releasing hormone *in vivo*. Science 254:421–423, 1991.
205. Munck A, Guyre PM: Glucocorticoids and immune function. *In* Ader R, Felten DL, Cohen N (eds): Psychoneuroimmunology. New York, Academic Press, 1991, pp 447–474.
206. Gonzalo JA, González-García A, Martínez AC, Kroemer G: Glucocorticoid-mediated control of the activation and clonal deletion of peripheral T cells in vivo. J Exp Med 177:1239–1246, 1993.
207. Holbrook NJ, Cox WI, Horner HC: Direct suppression of natural killer activity in human peripheral blood leukocyte cultures by glucocorticoids and its modulation by interferon. Cancer Res 43:4019–4025, 1983.
208. Guyre PM, Munck A: Glucocorticoid actions on monocytes and macrophages. *In* Schleimer RP, Claman HN, Oronsky A (eds): Anti-inflammatory Steroid Action. Basic and Clinical Aspects. New York, Academic Press, 1989, pp 199–225.
209. Butterfield JH, Gleich GJ: Anti-inflammatory effects of glucocorticoids on eosinophils and neutrophils. *In* Schleimer RP, Claman HN, Oronsky AL (eds): Anti-inflammatory Steroid Action. Basic and Clinical Aspects. New York, Academic Press, 1989, pp 151–225.
210. Schleimer RP: The effects of glucocorticoids on mast cells and basophils. *In* Schleimer RP, Claman HN, Oronsky AL (eds): Anti-inflammatory Steroid Action. Basic and Clinical Aspects. New York, Academic Press, 1989, pp 226–258.
211. Cupps TR: Effects of glucocorticoids on lymphocyte function. *In* Schleimer RP, Claman HN, Oronsky AL (eds): Anti-inflammatory Steroid Action. Basic and Clinical Aspects. New York, Academic Press, 1989, pp 132–150.
212. Cronstein BN, Kimmel SC, Levin RI, et al: A mechanism for the antiinflammatory effects of corticosteroids: The glucocorticoid receptor regulates leukocyte adhesion to endothelial cells and expression of endothelial-leukocyte adhesion molecule 1 and intercellular adhesion molecule 1. Proc Natl Acad Sci U S A 89:9991–9995, 1992.

213. van de Stolpe A, Caldenhoven E, Raaijmakers JAM, et al: Glucocorticoid-mediated repression of intercellular adhesion molecule-1 expression in human monocytic and bronchial epithelial cell lines. Am J Respir Cell Mol Biol 8:340–347, 1993.
214. van de Stolpe A, Caldenhoven E, Stade BG, et al: 12-*O*-tetradecanoylphorbol-13-acetate– and tumor necrosis factor α–mediated induction of intercellular adhesion molecule 1 is inhibited by dexamethasone. J Biol Chem 269:6185–6192, 1994.
215. Caldenhoven E, Liden J, Wissink S, et al: Negative cross-talk between RelA and the glucocorticoid receptor: A possible mechanism for the antiinflammatory action of glucocorticoids. Mol Endocrinol 9:401–412, 1995.
216. Miller AH, Spencer RL, Hassett J, et al: Effects of selective type I and II adrenal steroid agonists on immune cell distribution. Endocrinology 135:1934–1944, 1994.
217. Nowell PC: Inhibition of human leukocyte mitosis by prednisolone *in vitro*. Cancer Res 21:1518–1521, 1961.
218. Kelso A, Munck A: Glucocorticoid inhibition of lymphokine secretion by alloreactive T lymphocyte clones. J Immunol 133:784–791, 1984.
219. Norton JM, Munck A: In vitro actions of glucocorticoids on murine macrophages: Effects on glucose transport and metabolism, growth in culture, and protein synthesis. J Immunol 125:259–266, 1980.
220. Baybutt HN, Holsboer F: Inhibition of macrophage differentiation and function by cortisol. Endocrinology 127:476–480, 1990.
221. Brinkmann V, Kristofic C: Regulation by corticosteroids of Th1 and Th2 cytokine production in human $CD4^+$ effector T cells generated from $CD45RO^-$ and $CD45RO^+$ subsets. J Immunol 155:3322–3328, 1995.
222. Ramírez F, Fowell DJ, Puclavec M, et al: Glucocorticoids promote a Th2 cytokine response by $CD4^+$ T cells in vitro. J Immunol 156:2406–2412, 1996.
223. Ambrose CT: The essential role of corticosteroids in the induction of the immune response *in vitro*. *In* Wolstenholme GEW, Knights J (eds): Hormones and the Immune Response. CIBA Foundation Study Group No. 36. London, Churchill Livingstone, 1970, pp 100–125.
224. Wu CY, Sarfati M, Heusser C, et al: Glucocorticoids increase the synthesis of immunoglobulin E by interleukin 4-stimulated human lymphocytes. J Clin Invest 87:870–877, 1991.
225. Goldstein RA, Bowen DL, Fauci AS: Adrenal corticosteroids. *In* Gallin JI, Goldstein IM, Snyderman R (eds): Inflammation. Basic Principles and Clinical Correlates. New York, Raven Press, 1992, pp 1061–1081.
226. Barber AE, Coyle SM, Marano MA, et al: Glucocorticoid therapy alters hormonal and cytokine responses to endotoxin in man. J Immunol 150:1999–2006, 1993.
227. Wiegers GJ, Croiset G, Reul JMHM, et al: Differential effects of corticosteroids on rat peripheral blood T-lymphocyte mitogenesis in vivo and in vitro. Am J Physiol 265:E825–E830, 1993.
228. Wiegers GJ, Reul JMHM, Holsboer F, De Kloet ER: Enhancement of rat splenic lymphocyte mitogenesis after short term preexposure to corticosteroids *in vitro*. Endocrinology 135:2351–2357, 1994.
229. Wiegers GJ, Labeur MS, Stec IEM, et al: Glucocorticoids accelerate anti-T cell receptor-induced T cell growth. J Immunol 155:1893–1902, 1995.
230. Wiegers GJ, Reul JMHM: Induction of cytokine receptors by glucocorticoids: Functional and pathological significance. Trends Pharmacol Sci 19:317–321, 1998.
231. Cohen JJ: Glucocorticoid-induced apoptosis in the thymus. Semin Immunol 4:363–369, 1992.
232. Thompson EB: Apoptosis and steroid hormones. Mol Endocrinol 8:665–673, 1994.
233. Hughes FM Jr, Cidlowski JA: Glucocorticoid-induced thymocyte apoptosis: Protease-dependent activation of cell shrinkage and DNA degradation. J Steroid Biochem Mol Biol 65:207–217, 1998.
234. Strasser A: Death of a T cell. Nature 373:385–386, 1995.
235. Abbas AK: Die and let live: Eliminating dangerous lymphocytes. Cell 84:655–657, 1996.
236. Ashwell JD, King LB, Vacchio MS: Cross talk between the T cell antigen receptor and the glucocorticoid receptor regulates thymocyte development. Stem Cells 14:490–500, 1996.
237. D'Adamio F, Zollo O, Moraca R, et al: A new dexamethasone-induced gene of the leucine zipper family protects T lymphocytes from TCR/CD3-activated cell death. Immunity 7:803–812, 1997.
238. Iwata M, Hanaoka S, Sato K: Rescue of thymocytes and T cell hybridomas from glucocorticoid-induced apoptosis by stimulation via the T cell receptor/CD3 complex: A possible *in vitro* model for positive selection of the T cell repertoire. Eur J Immunol 21:643–648, 1991.
239. Vacchio MS, Ashwell JD, King LB: A positive role for thymus-derived steroids in formation of the T-cell repertoire. Ann N Y Acad Sci 840:317–327, 1998.
240. Lowry SF: Cytokine mediators of immunity and inflammation. Arch Surg 128:1235–1241, 1993.
241. McEwen BS: Protective and damaging effects of stress mediators. N Engl J Med 338:171–179, 1998.
242. Bertini R, Bianchi M, Ghezzi P: Adrenalectomy sensitizes mice to the lethal effects of interleukin 1 and tumor necrosis factor. J Exp Med 167:1708–1712, 1988.
243. Szabó C, Thiemermann C, Wu C-C, et al: Attenuation of induction of nitric oxide synthase by endogenous glucocorticoids accounts for endotoxin tolerance *in vivo*. Proc Natl Acad Sci U S A 91:271–275, 1994.
244. Baggiolini M: Chemokines and leukocyte traffic. Nature 392:565–568, 1988.
245. Luster AD: Chemokines—chemotactic cytokines that mediate inflammation. N Engl J Med 338:436–445, 1998.
246. Snyder DS, Unanue ER: Corticosteroids inhibit murine macrophage Ia expression and interleukin 1 production. J Immunol 129:1803–1805, 1982.
247. Kern JA, Lamb RJ, Reed JC, et al: Dexamethasone inhibition of interleukin 1 beta production by human monocytes: Posttranscriptional mechanisms. J Clin Invest 81:237–244, 1988.
248. Lane SJ, Wilkinson JRW, Cochrane GM, et al: Differential *in vitro* regulation by glucocorticoids of monocyte-derived cytokine generation in glucocorticoid-resistant bronchial asthma. Am Rev Respir Dis 147:690–696, 1993.
249. Standiford TJ, Kunkel SL, Rolfe MW, et al: Regulation of human alveolar macrophage– and blood monocyte–derived interleukin-8 by prostaglandin E_2 and dexamethasone. Am J Respir Cell Mol Biol 6:75–81, 1992.
250. Tobler A, Meier R, Seitz M, et al: Glucocorticoids downregulate gene expression of GM-CSF, NAP-1/IL-8, and IL-6, but not M-CSF in human fibroblasts. Blood 79:45–51, 1992.
251. Wertheim WA, Kunkel SL, Standiford TJ, et al: Regulation of neutrophil-derived IL-8: The role of prostaglandin E_2, dexamethasone, and IL-4. J Immunol 151:2166–2175, 1993.
252. O'Banion MK, Sadowski HB, Winn V, Young DA: A serum- and glucocorticoid-regulated 4-kilobase mRNA encodes a cyclooxygenase-related protein. J Biol Chem 266:23261–23267, 1991.
253. O'Banion MK, Winn VD, Young DA: cDNA cloning and functional activity of a glucocorticoid-regulated inflammatory cyclooxygenase. Proc Natl Acad Sci U S A 89:4888–4892, 1992.
254. Coyne DW, Nickols M, Bertrand W, Morrison AR: Regulation of mesangial cell cyclooxygenase synthesis by cytokines and glucocorticoids. Am J Physiol 263:F97–F102, 1992.
255. Wynn PC, Harwood JP, Catt KJ, Aguilera G: Regulation of corticotropin-releasing-factor (CRF) receptors in the rat pituitary gland: Effects of adrenalectomy on CRF receptors and corticotroph responses. Endocrinology 116:1653–1659, 1985.
256. Gillis S, Crabtree GR, Smith KA: Glucocorticoid-induced inhibition of T-cell growth factor production. I. The effect on mitogen-induced lymphocyte proliferation. J Immunol 123:1624–1631, 1979.
257. Gillis S, Crabtree GR, Smith KA: Glucocorticoid-induced inhibition of T-cell growth factor production. II. The effect on the in vitro generation of cytolytic T cells. J Immunol 123:1632–1638, 1979.
258. Vacca A, Martinotti S, Screpanti I, et al: Transcriptional regulation of the interleukin 2 gene by glucocorticoid hormones. J Biol Chem 265:8075–8080, 1990.
259. Vacca A, Felli MP, Farina AR, et al: Glucocorticoid receptor–mediated suppression of the interleukin 2 gene expression through impairment of the cooperativity between nuclear factor of activated T cells and AP-1 enhancer elements. J Exp Med 175:637–646, 1992.
260. Kawahara RS, Deng Z-W, Deuel TF: Glucocorticoids inhibit the transcriptional induction of JE, a platelet-derived growth factor–inducible gene. J Biol Chem 266:13261–13266, 1991.
261. Newcombe DS, Fahey JV, Ishikawa Y: Hydrocortisone inhibition of the bradykinin activation of human synovial fibroblasts. Prostaglandins 13:235–244, 1977.
262. Davies LG, Arentzen R, Reid JM, et al: Glucocorticoid sensitivity of vasopressin mRNA levels in the paraventricular nucleus of the rat. Proc Natl Acad Sci U S A 83:1145–1149, 1986.
263. Raff H: Glucocorticoid inhibition of neurohypophysial vasopressin secretion. Am J Physiol 252:R635–R644, 1987.
264. Arya SK, Wong-Staal F, Gallo RC: Dexamethasone-mediated inhibition of human T cell growth factor and γ-interferon messenger RNA. J Immunol 133:273–276, 1984.
265. Cipitelli M, Sica A, Viggiano V, et al: Negative transcriptional regulation of the interferon-γ promoter by glucocorticoids and dominant negative mutants of c-Jun. J Biol Chem 270:12548–12556, 1995.
266. Stellato C, Beck LA, Gorgone GA, et al: Expression of the chemokine RANTES by a human bronchial epithelial cell line. Modulation by cytokines and glucocorticoids. J Immunol 155:410–418, 1995.
267. Harbuz MS, Chover-Gonzalez AJ, Conde GL, et al: Interleukin-1β-induced effects on plasma oxytocin and arginine vasopressin: Role of adrenal steroids and route of administration. Neuroimmunomodulation 3:358–363, 1996.
268. Beutler B, Cerami A: Cachectin (tumor necrosis factor): A macrophage hormone governing cellular metabolism and inflammatory response. Endocr Rev 9:57–66, 1988.
269. Brenner T, Yamin A, Abramsky O, Gallily R: Stimulation of tumor necrosis factor-α production by mycoplasmas and inhibition by dexamethasone in cultured astrocytes. Brain Res 608:273–279, 1993.
270. VanOtteren GM, Standiford TJ, Kunkel SL, et al: Expression and regulation of macrophage inflammatory protein-1α by murine alveolar and peritoneal macrophages. Am J Respir Cell Mol Biol 10:8–15, 1994.
271. Daëron M, Sterk AR, Hirata F, Ishizaka T: Biochemical analysis of glucocorticoid-induced inhibition of IgE-mediated histamine release from mouse mast cells. J Immunol 129:1212–1220, 1982.
272. Shaw G, Kamen R: A conserved AU sequence from the 3′ untranslated region of GM-CSF mRNA mediates selective mRNA degradation. Cell 46:659–667, 1986.
273. Ohtsuka T, Kubota A, Hirano T, et al: Glucocorticoid-mediated gene suppression of rat cytokine-induced neutrophil chemoattractant CINC/gro, a member of the IL-8 family, through impairment of NF-κB activation. J Biol Chem 271:1651–1659, 1996.
274. Cwikel BJ, Barouski-Miller PA, Coleman PL, Gelehrter TD: Dexamethasone induction of an inhibitor of plasminogen activator on HTC hepatoma cells. J Biol Chem 259:6847–6851, 1984.
275. Werb Z: Biochemical actions of glucocorticoids on macrophages in culture. Specific inhibition of elastase, collagenase and plasminogen activator secretion and effects on other metabolic functions. J Exp Med 147:1695–1712, 1978.
276. Simantov R: Glucocorticoids inhibit endorphin synthesis by pituitary cells. Nature 280:684–687, 1979.
277. Culpepper JA, Lee F: Regulation of IL 3 expression by glucocorticoids in cloned murine T lymphocytes. J Immunol 135:3191–3197, 1985.
278. Smith JB, Herschman HR: Glucocorticoid-attenuated response genes encode intercellular mediators, including a new C-X-C chemokine. J Biol Chem 270:16756–16765, 1995.
279. Koob TJ, Jeffrey JJ, Eisen AZ: Regulation of human skin collagenase activity by hydrocortisone and dexamethasone in organ culture. Biochem Biophys Res Commun 61:1083–1088, 1974.
280. Suter DE, Schwartz NB: Effects of glucocorticoids on secretion of luteinizing

hormone and follicle-stimulating hormone by female rat pituitary cells *in vitro*. Endocrinology 117:849–854, 1985.

281. Wu CY, Fargeas C, Nakajima Y, Delespesse G: Glucocorticoids suppress the production of interleukin 4 by human lymphocytes. Eur J Immunol 21:2645–2647, 1991.
282. McDonald AR, Goldfine ID: Glucocorticoid regulation of insulin receptor gene transcription in IM 9 cultured lymphocytes. J Clin Invest 81:499–504, 1988.
283. Philippe J, Missotten M: Dexamethasone inhibits insulin biosynthesis by destabilizing insulin messenger ribonucleic acid in hamster insulinoma cells. Endocrinology 127:1640–1645, 1990.
284. Wang Y, Campbell HD, Young IG: Sex hormones and dexamethasone modulate interleukin-5 gene expression in T lymphocytes. J Steroid Biochem Mol Biol 44:203–210, 1993.
285. Kvetnansky R, Fukuhara K, Pacák K, et al: Endogenous glucocorticoids restrain catecholamine synthesis and release at rest and during immobilization stress in rats. Endocrinology 133:1411–1419, 1993.
286. Pacak K, Kvetnansky R, Palkovits M, et al: Adrenalectomy augments in vivo release of norepinephrine in the paraventricular nucleus during immobilization stress. Endocrinology 133:1404–1410, 1993.
287. Guerne P-A, Carson DA, Lotz M: IL-6 production by human articular chondrocytes. Modulation of its synthesis by cytokines, growth factors, and hormones *in vitro*. J Immunol 144:499–505, 1990.
288. Schöbitz B, van den Dobbelsteen M, Holsboer F, et al: Regulation of interleukin 6 gene expression in rat. Endocrinology 132:1569–1576, 1993.
289. Romanoff PA, Funder JW: Differential glucocorticoid effects on catecholamine responses to stress. Am J Physiol 266:E118–E128, 1994.
290. Kennedy B, Ziegler MG: Cardiac epinephrine synthesis. Regulation by a glucocorticoid. Circulation 84:891–895, 1991.
291. Wan S, LeClerc J-L, Vincent J-L: Cytokine responses to cardiopulmonary bypass: Lessons learned from cardiac transplantation. Ann Thorac Surg 63:269–276, 1997.
292. Radomski MW, Palmer RMJ, Moncada S: Glucocorticoids inhibit the expression of an inducible, but not the constitutive, nitric oxide synthase in vascular endothelial cells. Proc Natl Acad Sci U S A 87:10043–10047, 1990.
293. Geller DA, Nussler AK, Di Silvio M, et al: Cytokines, endotoxin, and glucocorticoids regulate the expression of inducible nitric oxide synthase in hepatocytes. Proc Natl Acad Sci U S A 90:522–526, 1993.
294. Singh K, Balligand J-L, Fischer TA, et al: Glucocorticoids increase osteopontin expression in cardiac myocytes and microvascular endothelial cells. Role in regulation of inducible nitrogen oxide synthetase. J Biol Chem 270:28471–28478, 1995.
295. Wu C-C, Croxtall JD, Perretti M, et al: Lipocortin 1 mediates the inhibition by dexamethasone of the induction by endotoxin of nitric oxide synthase in the rat. Proc Natl Acad Sci U S A 92:3473–3477, 1995.
296. Elenkov IJ, Papanicolaou DA, Wilder RL, Chrousos GP: Modulatory effects of glucocorticoids and catecholamines on human interleukin-12 and interleukin-10 production. Clinical implications. Proc Assoc Am Physicians 108:374–381, 1996.
297. Kubin M, Chow JM, Trinchieri G: Differential regulation of interleukin 12 (IL-12), tumor necrosis factor α, and IL-1β production in human myeloid leukemia cell lines and peripheral blood mononuclear cells. Blood 83:1847–1855, 1994.
298. Freidin M, Kessler JA: Cytokine regulation of substance P expression in sympathetic neurons. Proc Natl Acad Sci U S A 88:3200–3203, 1991.
299. Almawi WY, Beyhum HN, Rahme AA, Rieder MJ: Regulation of cytokine and cytokine receptor expression by glucocorticoids. J Leukoc Biol 60:563–572, 1996.
300. Knudsen PJ, Dinarello CA, Strom TB: Glucocorticoids inhibit transcriptional and post-transcriptional expression of interleukin 1 in U937 cells. J Immunol 139:4129–4134, 1987.
301. Lew W, Oppenheim JJ, Matsushima K: Analysis of the suppression of IL-1α and IL-1β production in human peripheral blood mononuclear adherent cells by a glucocorticoid hormone. J Immunol 140:1895–1902, 1988.
302. Wallen N, Kita H, Weiler D, Gleich GJ: Glucocorticoids inhibit cytokine-mediated eosinophil survival. J Immunol 147:3490–3495, 1991.
303. Oursler MJ, Riggs BL, Spelsberg TC: Glucocorticoid-induced activation of latent transforming growth factor-β by normal human osteoblast-like cells. Endocrinology 133:2187–2196, 1993.
304. De Nicola AF, Ferrini M, Gonzalez SL, et al: Regulation of gene expression by corticoid hormones in the brain and spinal cord. J Steroid Biochem Mol Biol 65:253–272, 1998.
305. Goulding NJ, Guyre PM: Regulation of inflammation by lipocortin 1. Immunol Today 13:295–297, 1992.
306. Goulding NJ: Corticosteroids — a case of mistaken identity. Br J Rheumatol 37:477–483, 1998.
307. Han J-W, Sadowski H, Young DA, Macara IG: Persistent induction of cyclooxygenase in p60^{v-src}-transformed 3T3 fibroblasts. Proc Natl Acad Sci U S A 87:3373–3377, 1990.
308. Lukiw WJ, Pelaez RP, Martinez J, Bazan NG: Budesonide epimer R or dexamethasone selectively inhibit platelet-activating factor–induced or interleukin 1β–induced DNA binding activity of *cis*-acting transcription factors and cyclooxygenase-2 gene expression in human epidermal keratinocytes. Proc Natl Acad Sci U S A 95:3914–3919, 1998.
309. Perretti M, Croxtall JD, Wheller SK, et al: Mobilizing lipocortin 1 in adherent human leukocytes downregulates their transmigration. Nat Med 2:1259–1262, 1996.
310. Christy NP: Adrenal cortical steroids in various types of hypertension. *In* Manger MW (ed): Hormones and Hypertension. Springfield, IL, Charles C Thomas, 1966, p 169.
311. Saruta T, Suzuki H, Handa M, et al: Multiple factors contribute to the pathogenesis of hypertension in Cushing's syndrome. J Clin Endocrinol Metab 62:275–279, 1986.
312. Grünfeld J-P, Eloy L, Moura A-M, et al: Effects of antiglucocorticoids on glucocorticoid hypertension in the rat. Hypertension 7:292–299, 1985.
313. Sakaue M, Hoffman BB: Glucocorticoids induce transcription and expression of the α1B adrenergic receptor gene in DTT1 MF-2 smooth muscle cells. J Clin Invest 88:385–389, 1991.
314. Collins S, Caron MG, Lefkowitz RJ: β_2-Adrenergic receptors in hamster smooth muscle cells are transcriptionally regulated by glucocorticoids. J Biol Chem 263:9067–9070, 1988.
315. Orlowski J, Lingrel JB: Thyroid and glucocorticoid hormones regulate the expression of multiple Na,K-ATPase genes in cultured neonatal rat cardiac myocytes. J Biol Chem 265:3462–3470, 1990.
316. Sambhi MP, Weil MH, Udhoji VN: Acute pharmacological effects of glucocorticoids: Cardiac output and related hemodynamic changes in normal subjects and patients with shock. Circulation 31:523–530, 1965.
317. Hayashi T, Nakai T, Miyabo S: Glucocorticoids increase Ca^{2+} uptake and [^{3}H]dihydropyridine binding in A7r5 vascular smooth muscle cells. Am J Physiol 261:C106–C114, 1991.
318. Whitworth JA, Brown MA, Kelly JJ, Williamson PM: Mechanisms of cortisol-induced hypertension in humans. Steroids 60:76–80, 1995.
319. Saruta T: Mechanism of glucocorticoid-induced hypertension. Hypertension Res 19:1–8, 1996.
320. Stewart PM, Corrie JET, Shackleton CHL, Edwards CRW: Syndrome of apparent mineralocorticoid excess: A defect in the cortisol-cortisone shuttle. J Clin Invest 82:340–349, 1988.
321. Edwards CRW, Stewart PM, Burt D, et al: Localization of 11β-hydroxysteroid dehydrogenase–tissue specific protector of the mineralocorticoid receptor. Lancet 2:986–989, 1988.
322. Stewart PM, Wallace AM, Valentino R, et al: Mineralocorticoid activity of licorice: 11-Beta-hydroxysteroid dehydrogenase deficiency comes of age. Lancet 2:821–824, 1987.
323. Mantero F, Armanini D, Boscaro M, et al: Steroids and hypertension. J Steroid Biochem Mol Biol 40:35–44, 1991.
324. Krakoff LR, Elijovich F: Cushing's syndrome and exogenous glucocorticoid hypertension. Clin Endocrinol Metab 10:479–487, 1981.
325. Walker G, Pfeilschifter J, Kunz D: Mechanisms of suppression of inducible nitric-oxide synthase (iNOS) expression in interferon (IFN)-gamma–stimulated RAW 264.7 cells by dexamethasone. Evidence for glucocorticoid-induced degradation of iNOS protein by calpain as a key step in post-transcriptional regulation. J Biol Chem 272:16679–16687, 1997.
326. Scoggins BA, Coghlan JP, Denton DA, et al: Understanding the mechanism of adrenocortical steroid hypertension. J Steroid Biochem 32:205–208, 1989.
327. Grünfeld J-P: Glucocorticoids and blood pressure regulation. Horm Res 34:111–113, 1990.
328. Náray-Fejes-Tóth A, Fejes-Tóth G: Glucocorticoid receptors mediate mineralocorticoid-like effects in cultured collecting duct cells. Am J Physiol 259:F672–F678, 1990.
329. Bastl CP, Binder HJ, Hayslett JP: Role of glucocorticoids and aldosterone in maintenance of colonic cation transport. Am J Physiol 238:F181–F186, 1980.
330. Bastl CP: Effect of spironolactone on glucocorticoid-induced colonic cation transport. Am J Physiol 25:F1235–F1242, 1988.
331. Funder JW, Pearce PT, Smith R, Smith AI: Mineralocorticoid action: Target tissue specificity is enzyme, not receptor, mediated. Science 242:583–585, 1988.
332. Náray-Fejes-Tóth A, Watlington CO, Fejes-Tóth G: 11β-Hydroxysteroid dehydrogenase activity in the renal target cells of aldosterone. Endocrinology 129:17–21, 1991.
333. Lindsay RM, Edwards CR, Seckl JR: Inhibition of 11-beta hydroxysteroid dehydrogenase in pregnant rats and the programming of blood pressure in the offspring. Hypertension 27:1200–1204, 1996.
334. Freiberg JM, Kinsella J, Sacktor B: Glucocorticoids increase the Na^+-H^+ exchange and decrease the Na^+ gradient–dependent phosphate-uptake systems in renal brush border membrane vesicles. Proc Natl Acad Sci U S A 79:4932–4936, 1982.
335. Kurokawa K, Fukagawa M, Hayashi M, Saruta T: Renal receptors and cellular mechanisms of hormone action in the kidney. *In* Seldin DW, Giebisch G (eds): The Kidney. New York, Raven Press, 1992, pp 1339–1372.
336. Bia MJ, Tyler K, DeFronzo RA: The effect of dexamethasone on renal electrolyte excretion in the adrenalectomized rat. Endocrinology 111:882–888, 1982.
337. Campen TJ, Vaughn DA, Fanestil DD: Mineralo- and glucocorticoid effects on renal excretion of electrolytes. Pflugers Arch 399:93–101, 1983.
338. Clore JN, Estep H, Ross-Clunis H, Watlington CO: Adrenocorticotropin and cortisol-induced changes in urinary sodium and potassium excretion in man: Effects of spironolactone and RU 486. J Clin Endocrinol Metab 67:824–831, 1988.
339. Gardner DG, Gertz BJ, Deschepper CF, Kim DY: Gene for the atrial natriuretic peptide is regulated by glucocorticoids in vitro. J Clin Invest 82:1275–1281, 1988.
340. Argentin S, Sun YL, Lihrmann I, et al: Distal *cis*-acting promotor sequences mediate glucocorticoid stimulation of cardiac atrial natriuretic factor gene transcription. J Biol Chem 266:23315–23322, 1991.
341. Shields PP, Dixon JE, Glembotski CC: The secretion of atrial natriuretic factor-(99–126) by cultured cardiac myocytes is regulated by glucocorticoids. J Biol Chem 263:12619–12628, 1988.
342. Fullerton MJ, Krozowski ZS, Funder JW: Adrenalectomy and dexamethasone administration: Effect on atrial natriuretic peptide synthesis and circulating forms. Mol Cell Endocrinol 82:33–40, 1991.
343. Weidmann P, Matter DR, Matter EE, et al: Glucocorticoid and mineralocorticoid stimulation of atrial natriuretic peptide release in man. J Clin Endocrinol Metab 66:1233–1239, 1988.
344. Lanier-Smith KL, Currie MG: Glucocorticoid regulation of atrial natriuretic peptide receptors on cultured endothelial cells. Endocrinology 129:2311–2317, 1991.
345. Yamaji T, Ishibashi M, Yamada A, et al: Plasma levels of atrial natriuretic hormone in Cushing's syndrome. J Clin Endocrinol Metab 67:348–352, 1988.
346. Damjancic P, Vierhapper H: Permissive action of glucocorticoid substitution therapy on the effects of atrial natriuretic peptide (hANP) in patients with adrenocortical insufficiency. Exp Clin Endocrinol 95:315–321, 1990.
347. McEwen BS, Sakai RR, Spencer RL: Adrenal steroid effects on the brain: Versatile hormones with good and bad effects. *In* Schulkin J (ed): Hormonally Induced Changes in Mind and Brain. New York, Academic Press, 1993, pp 157–189.

348. de Quervan DJ-F, Roozendaal B, McGaugh JL: Stress and glucocorticoids impair retrieval of long-term memory. Nature 394:787–790, 1998.
349. Sapolsky RM, Stein-Behrens BA, Armanini MP: Long-term adrenalectomy causes loss of dentate gyrus and pyramidal neurons in the adult hippocampus. Exp Neurol 114:246–249, 1991.
350. Stein-Behrens BA, Elliott EM, Miller CA, et al: Glucocorticoids exacerbate kainic acid–induced extracellular accumulation of excitatory amino acids in the rat hippocampus. J Neurochem 58: 1730–1735, 1992.
351. Packan DR, Sapolsky RM: Glucocorticoid endangerment of the hippocampus: Tissue, steroid and receptor specificity. Neuroendocrinology 51:613–618, 1990.
352. Scully JL, Otten U: Glucocorticoids, neurotrophins and neurodegeneration. J Steroid Biochem Mol Biol 52:391–401, 1995.
353. McEwen BS: Re-examination of the glucocorticoid hypothesis of stress and aging. Prog Brain Res 93:365–383, 1992.
354. McEwen BS, Weiss JM, Schwartz LS: Selective retention of corticosterone by limbic structures in rat brain. Nature 220:911–912, 1968.
355. McCarthy KD, de Vellis J: Preparation of separate astroglial and oligodendral glial cell cultures from rat cerebral tissue. J Cell Biol 85:890–902, 1980.
356. Hallermayer K, Harmening C, Hamprecht B: Cellular localization and regulation of glutamine synthetase in primary cultures of brain cells from newborn mice. J Neurochem 37:43–52, 1981.
357. Levitan ES, Hemmick LM, Birnberg NC, Kaczmarek LK: Dexamethasone increases potassium channel messenger RNA and activity in clonal pituitary cells. Mol Endocrinol 5:1903–1908, 1991.
358. Horner HC, Packan DR, Sapolsky RM: Glucocorticoids inhibit glucose transport in cultured hippocampal neurons and glia. Neuroendocrinology 52:57–64, 1990.
359. Muglia L, Jacobson L, Dikkes P, Majzoub JA: Corticotropin-releasing hormone deficiency reveals major fetal but not adult glucocorticoid need. Nature 373:427–432, 1995.
360. Cole TJ, Blendy JA, Monaghan AP, et al: Targeted disruption of the glucocorticoid receptor gene blocks adrenergic chromaffin development and severely retards lung maturation. Genes Dev 9:1608–1625, 1995.
361. Reichardt HM, Kaestner KH, Tuckermann J, et al: DNA binding of the glucocorticoid receptor is not essential for survival. Cell 93:531–541, 1998.
362. Pepin M-C, Pothier F, Barden N: Impaired type II glucocorticoid-receptor function in mice bearing antisense RNA transgene. Nature 355:725–728, 1992.
363. Morale MC, Batticane N, Gallo F, et al: Disruption of hypothalamic-pituitary-adrenocortical system in transgenic mice expressing Type II glucocorticoid receptor antisense ribonucleic acid permanently impairs T cell function: Effects on T cell trafficking and T cell responsiveness during postnatal development. Endocrinology 136:3949–3960, 1995.
364. Richard D, Chapdelaine S, Deshaies Y, et al: Energy balance and lipid metabolism in transgenic mice bearing an antisense CGR construct. Am J Physiol 265:R146–R150, 1993.
365. Berger S, Bleich M, Schmid W, et al: Mineralocorticoid receptor knockout mice: Pathophysiology of Na^+ metabolism. Proc Natl Acad Sci U S A 95:9424–9429, 1998.
366. Hubert C, Gasc J-M, Berger S, et al: Effects of mineralocorticoid receptor gene disruption on the components of the renin-angiotensin system in 8-day-old mice. Mol Endocrinol 13:297–306, 1999.
367. Ballard PL, Ballard RA: Glucocorticoid receptors and the role of glucocorticoids in fetal lung development. Proc Natl Acad Sci U S A 69:2668, 1972.
368. Wang J, Kuliszewski M, Yee W, et al: Cloning and expression of glucocorticoid-induced genes in fetal rat lung fibroblasts. J Biol Chem 270:2722–2728, 1995.
369. Udelsman R, Ramp J, Gallucci WT, et al: Adaptation during surgical stress: A reevaluation of the role of glucocorticoids. J Clin Invest 77:1377–1381, 1986.
370. Giuffre KA, Udelsman R, Listwak S, Chrousos GP: Effects of immune neutralization of corticotropin-releasing hormone, adrenocorticotropin, and β-endorphin in the surgically stressed rat. Endocrinology 122:306–310, 1988.
371. Akira S, Taga T, Kishimoto T: Interleukin-6 in biology and medicine. Adv Immunol 54:1–78, 1993.
372. Jensen LE, Whitehead AS: Regulation of serum amyloid A protein expression during the acute-phase response. Biochem J 334:489–503, 1998.

Chapter **117**

Glucocorticoid Action: Biochemistry

Roger L. Miesfeld

OVERVIEW OF GLUCOCORTICOID ACTION

Glucocorticoids (GCs) exert their effects on responsive cells by binding to and activating a 90-kDa intracellular glucocorticoid receptor (GR) protein. Molecular studies using cloned GR cDNA have mapped the human *GR* gene to chromosome 5[1] and the mouse *GR* gene to chromosome 18.[2] In situ hybridization techniques and genomic sequencing have shown that the human *GR* gene is located within chromosome bands 5q31-q32.[3,4] The *GR* gene is relatively large, contains nine exons, and spans more than 80 kb in humans[5] and more than 110 kb in mice.[6] The molecular mechanism of GC action has been shown to result from GR-mediated transcriptional regulation of specific genes. Two primary modes of transcriptional regulation by GR are direct binding to DNA sequences in target genes and protein-protein interactions between GR and other transcription factors. Unlike endocrine systems, which display tightly regulated temporal and spatial production of steroidal ligands and cell-specific expression of receptor proteins, GC production in mammals is continuous throughout life and GR is expressed in essentially all cell types. One of the central questions in molecular endocrinology has been to understand the basis for cell-specific GC action. The theme of this chapter is to give a broad overview of GR structure and function, followed by a brief description of nonreceptor proteins that interact with GR and modulate its transcriptional regulatory function.

Figure 117–1 depicts a simplified model of GC action at the cellular level. Numerous studies have shown that GR is localized in the cytoplasm of the cell and only upon ligand binding does it become tightly associated with the nuclear compartment.[7–10] In the absence of hormone, cytoplasmic GR is associated with a large protein complex of approximately 330 kDa.[11] The components of this inactive complex have been shown to include various chaperonin proteins that function to maintain GR in an inactive conformation that is competent for GC binding.[12,13] Although somewhat controversial because of differences between experimental systems, the most abundant cytoplasmic GR complex appears to include two subunits of the 90-kDa heat shock protein hsp90,[14] a 52-kDa immunophilin protein (FK506-binding protein-52 [FKBP52]/hsp56),[15] and a 23-kDa protein.[16] Some evidence also indicates that other proteins transiently associate with GR to facilitate formation of the inactive complex, most likely as components of a multistep "refolding" process after GC dissociation. These assembly proteins include members of the hsp70 family,[17,18] the 48-kDa Hip protein,[19] a p60 protein,[20] and a DnaJ-like protein called p40.[21] Several steps in the proposed GR assembly pathway appear to require ATP hydrolysis.[7] A central role for hsp90 in stabilizing the inactive GR complex in a ligand binding–competent conformation has been demonstrated by treating cells with geldanamycin, a benzoquinone ansamycin inhibitor of hsp90. Geldanamycin treatment has been shown to block GR activation in intact cells.[22–24]

As shown in Figure 117–1, GC binding to the GR stimulates hsp90 complex disassembly and localization of GR to the nucleus. In vivo studies using a GR fusion protein containing the coding sequence of the green fluorescent protein GFP have indicated that GC binding promotes rapid nuclear localization (half-maximal accumulation, 10

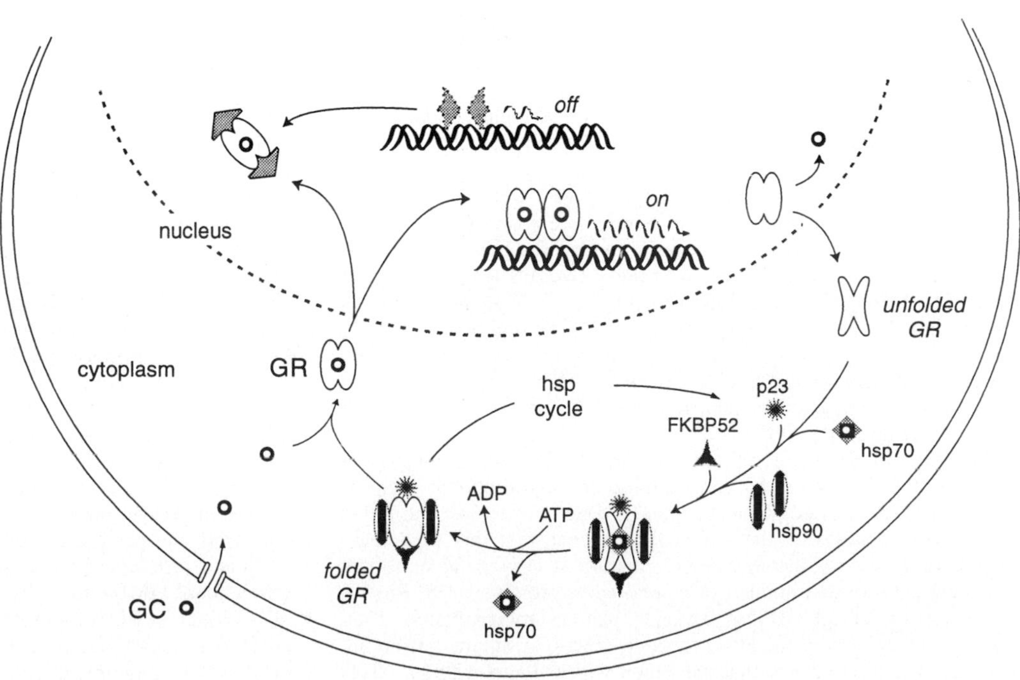

FIGURE 117–1. Glucocorticoid receptor (GR) cytoplasmic-nuclear shuttling. In the absence of glucocorticoids (GCs), inactive GR is primarily localized to the cytoplasm and is complexed with chaperonin proteins such as the heat shock protein hsp90. Hormone binding converts GR to the active form and stimulates nuclear translocation. Transcriptional regulation by the ligand-activated GR involves both DNA-dependent and DNA-independent mechanisms leading to gene induction (on) and gene repression (off), respectively. Ligand dissociation from GR reinitiates the hsp folding cycle. ADP, adenosine diphosphate; ATP, adenosine triphosphate; FKBP52, FK506-binding protein-52.

minutes)[25, 26] and is dependent on intact cytoskeletal structures.[26] Ligand-activated GR binds to specific DNA sequences in the regulatory region of target genes and interacts with other transcription factors in a DNA-independent manner. The functional consequences of these protein-DNA and protein-protein interactions are transcriptional induction or repression of gene expression.[27]

GR is a very stable protein with an in vivo half-life of more than 10 hours in most cells that have been studied.[28, 29] One advantage of a long half-life for GR is that it provides a mechanism for rapid cycling between the inactive and active state. Using a variety of approaches, DeFranco and colleagues have shown that GR is actively transported out of the nucleus in an ATP-dependent manner.[30–33] Based on in vitro studies using digitonin-permeabilized cells, they proposed that phosphorylation of unliganded GR on tyrosine residues may be a stimulus for nuclear export.[32] The GR cycling model proposes that newly exported unliganded GR associates with chaperonin proteins, which initiates an ATP-driven refolding process culminating in assembly of the cytoplasmic GR complex (GR-hsp90-FKBP52-p23).[21]

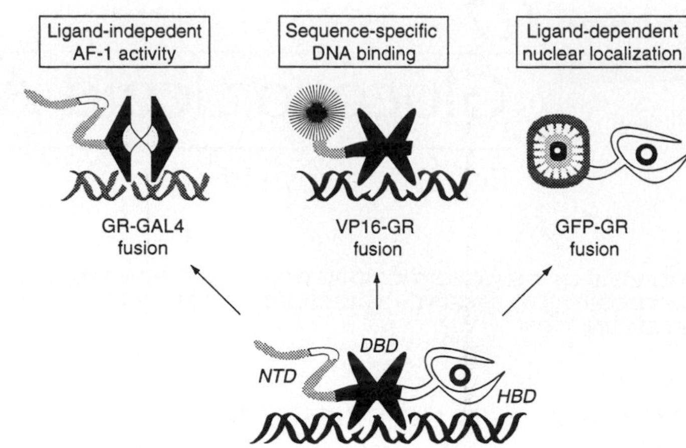

FIGURE 117–2. Functional subdomains of glucocorticoid receptor (GR). Molecular genetic studies have shown that GR can essentially be divided into three subdomains: the N-terminal domain (NTD), the DNA-binding domain (DBD), and the hormone-binding domain (HBD). The functional integrity of these three GR subdomains has been demonstrated in gene fusion experiments with heterologous proteins such as the yeast GAL4 DBD, the herpes simplex virus VP16 activation protein, and the jellyfish green fluorescent protein (GFP). AF-1, activation function-1.

GLUCOCORTICOID RECEPTOR STRUCTURE AND FUNCTION

Through a combination of biochemical,[34, 35] immunologic,[36–38] and ultimately molecular biologic approaches,[39, 40] the complete coding sequence of GR from the rat,[41] mouse,[42] human,[1] marmoset,[43] guinea pig,[44] frog,[45] and trout[46] has been elucidated. Sequence comparisons of GR between these vertebrate species have revealed that the GR coding sequences are greater than 80% identical, with the majority of differences being localized to the variable N-terminal domain.[47] The most abundant GR protein in human cells is the α isoform, which represents the fully functional hormone-activated receptor species.[1] A second GR protein called the β isoform is expressed in some cell types as a result of alternative splicing.[1] GR-β has been proposed to play a role in modulating the transcriptional regulatory activities of GR-α by competing for rate-limiting protein determinants[48, 49] or by forming nonfunctional GR-α/GR-β heterodimers.[50] The physiologic relevance of the GR-β form is somewhat controversial, however, because of its very low level of expression in most cell types.[51, 52]

Biochemical studies using partial proteolysis treatment have shown that GR consists of several protein subdomains that coincide with three discrete GR functions: (1) transcriptional transactivation, (2) specific DNA binding, and (3) GC binding.[53–55] Deletion and site-directed mutagenesis analyses of GR cDNA within these three regions have confirmed the earlier biochemical studies and, surprisingly, have shown that GR subdomains can function somewhat independently of one another.[56–59] Figure 117–2 graphically illustrates the structural relationship between the three major protein domains: the DNA-binding domain (DBD), the hormone-binding domain (HBD), and the N-terminal domain (NTD), which contains the ligand-independent transcriptional activation function (AF-1). The functional integrity of these three domains has been demonstrated via protein fusions between the GR DBD, HBD, and AF-1 sequences and heterologous gene sequences from viral, bacterial, and invertebrate sources.[7, 25, 60–68] Numerous other GR activities have also been mapped within the receptor-coding sequence. These activities include two nuclear localization signals (NL1 and NL2),[69] an hsp90-binding site,[70–72] ligand-dependent transcriptional regulatory sequences (AF-2),[68, 73, 74] and residues likely to be involved in transcriptional repression[75–77] and receptor dimerization.[78, 79] Phosphorylation studies of GR have indicated that several of these receptor functions are modulated by serine and threonine phosphorylation in the GR NTD.[80–83]

The C-terminal end of GR encodes the HBD, which consists of around 300 amino acids that constitute a very hydrophobic segment having an isoelectric point greater than 9. One of the most intriguing findings from studies on the GR HBD has been that this subdomain can function as a regulatory module capable of conferring hormone-dependent activity to a number of heterologous proteins.[66, 84–86] Proteolytic digestion of rat GR has revealed that an approximately 135–amino acid fragment of the HBD (residues 536–673) retains the ability to specifically bind dexamethasone, albeit with reduced affinity.[87] This core region contains within it 2 amino acids (Met622 and Cys656) that have been identified by electrophilic[88] and photoaffinity[89] labeling as ligand contact residues with dexamethasone. Similar studies have identified analogous residues in the mouse GR HBD.[90] Point mutations in the mouse GR HBD that define additional residues that appear to influence dexamethasone binding have been described.[42, 91] Some of these mutations cause complete loss of hormone binding (Glu546 → Gly and Cys742 → Gly), whereas others only decrease hormone-binding affinity (Tyr770 → Asn and Pro547 → Ala). The results of these and other studies suggest that ligand binding by the GR HBD may require a few critical residues within the regions already identified, as well as a number of other amino acids spread across the HBD that may contribute weaker interactions with the hormone. Interestingly, if Cys656 of rat GR is mutated to either a Gly or Ser residue, the ligand-binding affinity of these receptors is actually increased, and "super" GRs are created.[92]

Another approach to investigating receptor-ligand interactions has been to study the effects of hormone antagonists on GR function. One of the best characterized GR antagonists is RU 486 (mifepristone).[93] This potent antagonist [17β-hydroxy-11α-(4-dimethylaminophenyl)-17α-1-propynyl-estra-4,9-dien-3-one] was discovered by scientists at the French pharmaceutical company Roussel UCLAF in 1981; it was first described as an antiprogestin and is best known for its abortifacient action.[94] Mifepristone has also been used clinically to treat symptoms of hypercortisolism and Cushing's syndrome.[95] Because of its strong antiglucocorticoid activity, a number of studies have sought to determine the mechanism of mifepristone action in the hope of identifying important structure-function relationships between GR and GC ligands. Purified GR has been found to bind to specific DNA sequences in vitro, even when bound by mifepristone.[96, 97] However, GR bound by mifepristone in vivo is inefficiently translocated to the nucleus.[98, 99] Moreover, in vivo DNA footprinting fails to detect GR binding of these mifepristone complexes to regulatory regions within the tyrosine aminotransferase gene.[100] Taken together, these data suggest that mifepristone inhibits GR function by interfering with the conversion of GR to the activated state.

Specific DNA binding by GR has been extensively characterized both from the perspective of amino acid residues in GR that contact DNA and with regard to the identification of nucleotides that constitute a functional GR-binding site (for reviews see Freedman[101] and Dahlman-Wright et al.[102]). Figure 117–3 shows the structure of the GR DBD bound to DNA as determined by x-ray crystallography.[78] The most striking feature of this structure is the requirement for zinc as

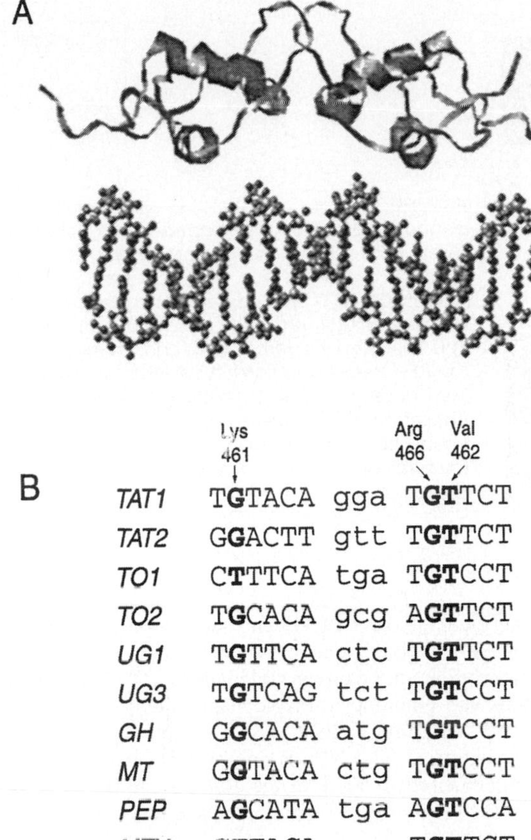

A
B
Lys
461
Arg
466
Val
462
TAT1 TGTACA gga TGTTCT
TAT2 GGACTT gtt TGTTCT
TO1 CTTTCA tga TGTCCT
TO2 TGCACA gcg AGTTCT
UG1 TGTTCA ctc TGTTCT
UG3 TGTCAG tct TGTCCT
GH GGCACA atg TGTCCT
MT GGTACA ctg TGTCCT
PEP AGCATA tga AGTCCA
MTV GTTACA aac TGTTCT
Con GGTACA nnn TGTTCT

FIGURE 117–3. Molecular determinants of sequence-specific DNA binding by glucocorticoid receptor (GR). *A,* Structure of the rat GR DNA-binding zinc finger domain as determined by Luisi et al.[78] The protein structure is shown above the DNA strand to illustrate alignment of GR α helical regions with the major groove of DNA. *B,* DNA sequences from functionally defined glucocorticoid response elements (GREs). The conserved protein-DNA contact points between the GR dimer and one strand of the DNA are shown. Note that Lys461 and Arg466/Val462 are the three amino acids from each GR monomer that together make six contacts with the double-stranded DNA. The GREs listed are from the tyrosine aminotransferase (TAT), tryptophan oxygenase (TO), uteroglobin (UG), growth hormone (GH), metallothionein (MT), phosphoenolpyruvate carboxykinase (PEP), and mouse mammary tumor virus (MTV) genes. Con refers to the consensus GRE sequence.

the coordinating group to stabilize the helical regions of each subdomain.[103] This evolutionarily conserved protein structure is called a "zinc finger," [104] and GR has two such zinc fingers.[105, 106] As can be seen in Figure 117–3, the GR DBD binds to DNA in the form of a head-to-head homodimer at sites containing an inverted repeat DNA sequence. The GR-specific DNA sequence recognition site is called a glucocorticoid response element (GRE). Examples of natural functionally defined GRE sequences are shown in Figure 117–3.

Luisi et al. used multiple isomorphous replacement to solve the crystal structure of an 86–amino acid fragment of the rat GR that encompasses the DBD[78] (amino acids 440–525, see Fig. 117–3). This fragment was cocrystallized with a self-complementary oligonucleotide that differs from the palindromic GRE by insertion of a single nucleotide between the two half-sites. This DNA molecule (GRE_s4) contains four nucleotides between the two GRE half-sites and is unlike known functional GREs, which have been found to contain a three-nucleotide spacer between the two half-sites. Based on high-resolution data from GR/GRE_s4 complexes (2.9 Å) and data from GR/GRE_s3 complexes (resolution of 4.0 Å), it has been determined that GR amino acids Lys461, Val462, and Arg466 make contact with at least three different bases in the GRE-binding site. In addition, analysis of the crystal structure of the GR DBD revealed that receptor dimerization, mediated through amino acids in the DBD, most likely accounts for the observed cooperative binding of GR to a GRE.[107]

With purified GR it was determined by in vitro DNA-binding experiments that the relative affinity of GR for specific sites is approximately 2×10^3 times higher than it is for nonspecific DNA sequences.[108] Several components contribute to this very high affinity for specific DNA sequences. First, amino acid residues in the DBD of GR make contacts with specific nucleotides in the GRE sequence. Second, GR is known to bind cooperatively to DNA such that a fully occupied GRE contains two monomers of GR.[78, 109, 110] Third, many functional GREs exist in tandem or are located near binding sites for other transcription factors.[111] This arrangement facilitates synergistic protein-protein interactions between GR homodimers[110, 112] and between GR and various coreceptor proteins.[113]

Functional analysis of transcriptional regulation by GR has revealed as many as three and possibly four distinct regions within GR that may be capable of regulating target gene expression. This mechanism has been evolutionarily conserved, as evidenced by the finding that GR transactivation regions can function in transfected yeast,[114] *Drosophila,*[115] and plant cells.[116] Most studies of GR transcriptional regulatory activities have used an in vivo transient expression assay incorporating a GR expression plasmid and a GRE containing reporter plasmid.[41, 56, 57, 59] Functional mapping of the GR NTD has identified a subregion called AF-1 (also called tau 1 or enh 2), which if deleted results in a 90% decrease in transactivation activity.[65, 76, 117]

The physiologic importance of the NTD has been confirmed by molecular analysis of the S49 nt^i GR mutation. Dieken et al. showed that as a result of aberrant RNA splicing, the NTD is deleted from the defective nt^i GR protein.[118] Because chimeric nt^i GR proteins containing potent transactivation regions from either the herpes simplex virus VP16 or the adenovirus E1A proteins are capable of inducing apoptosis in stably transfected S49 cells,[illegible] it is likely that AF-1 functions are similar to those of other acidic activating sequences.[119, 120] Figure 117–4 compares the amino acid sequences of the GR AF-1 core regions from five different vertebrate species. It can be seen that the spacing of hydrophobic and hydrophilic residues within AF-1 is conserved between humans and teleost. Two putative α helices have been identified in this region of the NTD,[121, 122] and three of the major serine phosphorylation sites in GR are contained within the AF-1 domain.[83, 123]

MECHANISMS OF GLUCOCORTICOID RECEPTOR–REGULATED TRANSCRIPTION

The molecular basis of GR-regulated transcription relies on specific protein-protein interactions between GR and other gene regulatory proteins.[124, 125] Together, the assembly of large protein complexes ultimately results in altered rates of transcriptional initiation by RNA polymerase II at target promoters. In the context of transcriptional activation, many of these interactions occur while GR is bound to DNA, whereas GR-mediated transcriptional repression often involves DNA-independent events. Initial characterization of GC-induced transcription relied on simple gene paradigms in which one or more canonic GR-binding sites were positioned upstream of relatively weak promoters. The best-studied GR target promoter in this regard is from the long terminal repeat (LTR) of the mouse mammary tumor virus (MMTV).[126–128] GR binding to the four primary GRE sequences found in the MMTV LTR results in greater than 100-fold induction of basal transcription.[129] It has been shown that in the absence of GR binding, the MMTV promoter is functionally inactive because of the presence of inhibitory chromatin structures that partially block the binding of basal transcription factors such as nuclear factor 1 (NF-1).[130–132] In the presence of GCs, GR complexes bind with high affinity to the MMTV GREs, thus promoting chromatin remodeling and promoter activation.

Perhaps one of the best-understood natural GR target genes in mammals is the hepatic phosphoenolpyruvate carboxykinase (*PEPCK*) gene, which encodes a rate-limiting enzyme required for gluconeogen-

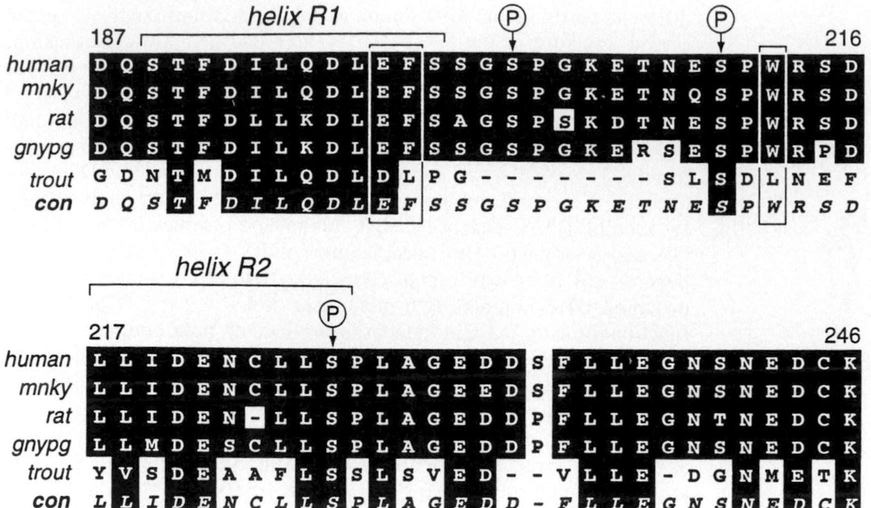

FIGURE 117–4. Evolutionary conservation of the ligand-independent transcriptional activation function (AF-1) sequences in the glucocorticoid receptor (GR) N-terminal domain (NTD). Amino acids 187–246 of the human GR NTD are compared with the same region in monkey (mnky), rat, guinea pig (gnypg), and trout GR. The spacing of hydrophobic and charged residues in the AF-1 region are conserved across these five species. Two putative α helical regions (R1 and R2) and three phosphorylation sites (P) have been identified in AF-1. Amino acids found to be required for AF-1 function on the basis of site-directed mutagenesis studies are shown by *boxes.*

esis. Granner and colleagues have performed extensive molecular genetic analysis of the rat *PEPCK* gene promoter to understand how GR binding mediates the observed 10-fold induction of *PEPCK* transcription.[133–137] Figure 117–5 shows the DNA sequence architecture of the *PEPCK* gene regulatory region and illustrates the proposed binding of cellular transcription factors in GC-treated hepatocytes. Recent data suggest that GR binding to the GR1 and GR2 sequence elements in the distal *PEPCK* regulatory region (approximately −350 bp from the start site of transcription) facilitates interactions with C/enhancer binding protein (EBP)-β protein bound at the proximal promoter.[137] The formation of GR-C/EBP-β interactions within the larger *PEPCK* transcriptosome leads to increased rates of transcriptional initiation by RNA polymerase II. Based on what is known about general mechanisms of transcriptional activation in eukaryotic cells,[138–140] GC induction of *PEPCK* expression most likely involves GR-mediated remodeling of chromatin by histone deacetylation, conformational changes in the transcriptosome complex, and possibly, phosphorylation of the RNA polymerase II C-terminal domain.

Transcriptional repression by GR may be the most important function of GC action based on the finding that transgenic mice expressing a DNA-binding mutant form of GR are viable.[141] Because this mutant GR retains transcriptional repression functions but lacks transactivation activity, it is suggested that DNA binding and transactivation by GR are not absolutely required for life.[142] Two general types of GR-mediated transcriptional repression have been described. In the first type, GR binds to "negative" GRE sequences (nGREs), which results in decreased rates of transcriptional initiation.[143] GR-mediated repression at nGREs appears to be due to exclusion of transcriptional activators.[144] A variation of this theme is transcriptional repression by GR at composite (or complex) GREs. The best-studied example of this type is GC-regulated repression of proliferin gene expression by GR through interactions with members of the activator protein-1 (AP-1) family of transcription factors.[145–148]

The second general class of GR-mediated repression results from inhibition of NF-κB activity, a well-characterized component of the proinflammatory signaling pathways in mammals.[149, 150] Cytokines such as interleukins and granulocyte-macrophage colony-stimulating factor activate the NF-κB pathway in a variety of cell types by binding to membrane receptors.[151] The NF-κB complex is made up of a family of transcription factors related to the Rel protein.[152] After cytokine stimulation, the cytoplasmic NF-κB complex is activated by phosphorylation and subsequent degradation of the inhibitory IκB subunit. The functional p65-p50 dimer of NF-κB is translocated to the nucleus, where it binds to specific DNA sequences located in the regulatory region of NF-κB target genes. GC treatment of cytokine-stimulated cells has been found to blunt this NF-κB–mediated cytokine response.[153, 154] It has been proposed that GR-mediated inhibition of cytokine signaling through NF-κB accounts for the anti-inflammatory and immunosuppressive effects of GCs.[155]

Figure 117–6 illustrates two mechanisms that have been proposed to account for GR inhibition of NF-κB activation. First, GR can interfere with transcriptional transactivation functions of the p65 NF-κB subunit either by direct protein-protein binding or by indirectly sequestering a shared coactivator protein. Second, GR can induce synthesis of the inhibitory IκB protein by stimulating transcription of the IκB gene. Elevated intracellular levels of IκB would result in inhibition of NF-κB activation. Although it is possible that GR may interfere with NF-κB function by both mechanisms,[157] most data support a role of inhibitory protein-protein interactions between GR and p65 as the most predominant mechanism.[156] Evidence supporting this conclusion comes from the finding that GR and p65 form stable complexes in vitro[158, 159] and that GR inhibits the p65-mediated transactivation functions of GAL4-p65 fusion proteins.[160] Moreover, many cell types in which GC treatment inhibits NF-κB function do not show GC-induced expression of IκB protein.[160–163] Finally, NF-κB transcriptional regulatory functions can be inhibited by treating cells

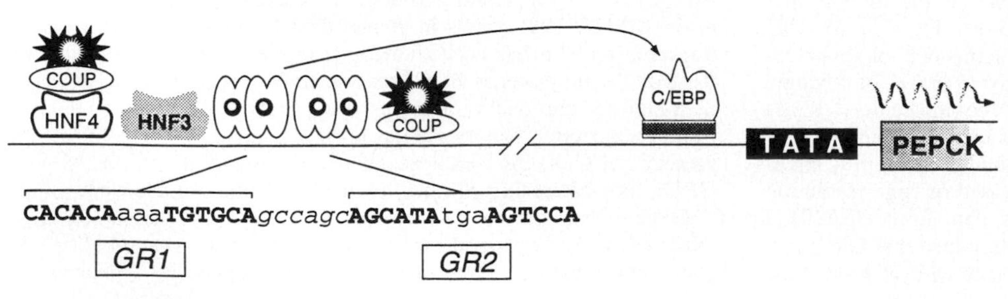

FIGURE 117–5. Proposed promoter architecture of the rat phosphoenolpyruvate carboxykinase *(PEPCK)* gene. Studies by Granner and colleagues[133–137] have identified a complex arrangement of glucocorticoid response elements (GR1 and GR2) and binding sites for auxiliary transcription factors (COUP, HNF4, HNF3, and C/EBP), which together control glucocorticoid responsiveness of the *PEPCK* gene. *PEPCK* is thought to represent a typical glucocorticoid receptor–regulated gene in mammals.

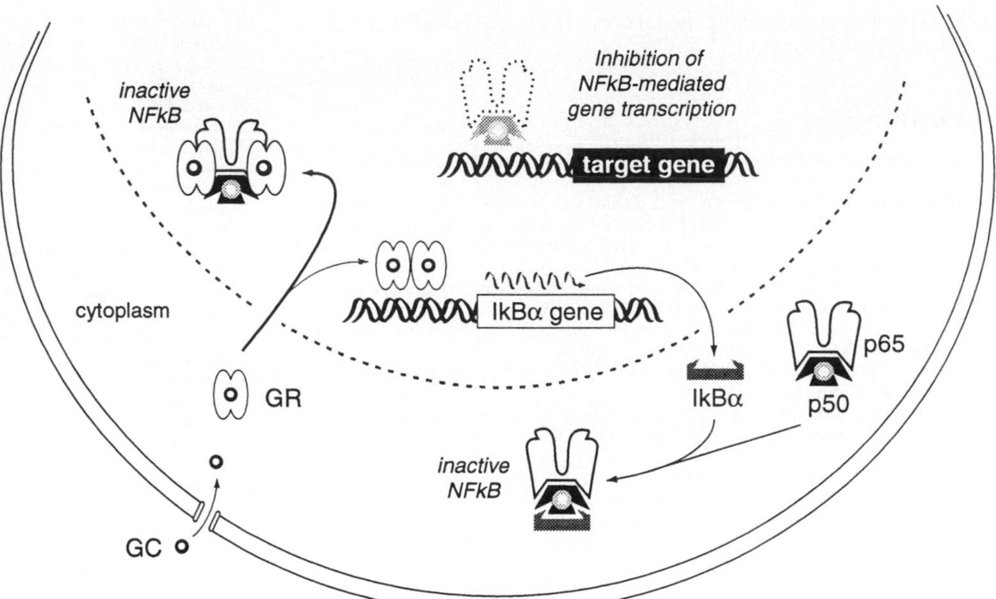

FIGURE 117–6. Proposed mechanisms of glucocorticoid receptor–mediated inhibition of nuclear factor NF-κB signaling in mammalian cells. Glucocorticoid (GC) treatment of cytokine-stimulated cells appears to inhibit NF-κB signaling by sequestering active p65-p50 complexes away from NF-κB target genes and by upregulating expression of the NF-κB inhibitory protein I-κB. Current data suggest that GR–NF-κB protein-protein interactions may be the most important of these two inhibitory mechanisms. (Reprinted from Dumont A, Hehner SP, Schmitz ML, et al: Cross-talk between steroids and NF-kB: What language? Trends Biochem Sci 23:233–235, 1998 with permission from Elsevier Science.)

with the steroid antagonist mifepristone,[164] which suggests that DNA-independent GR functions are the most relevant.

CORECEPTOR PROTEINS MODULATE GLUCOCORTICOID RECEPTOR ACTIVITY

One of the features that sets GC action apart from other types of steroid-regulated pathways is that most, if not all cell-types express appreciable levels of GR. The molecular basis of cell-specific GC responsiveness is therefore not due to cell-specific GR expression, as is often the case for androgen, estrogen, and progesterone effects. For example, the *PEPCK* gene is induced by GCs in the liver and kidney, but PEPCK expression is repressed by GCs in adipose tissue.[165] Analysis of GR-regulated transcription of PEPCK in liver and adipocyte cells has revealed that the same promoter is used in both cell types.[166] Additional examples of cell-specific GC responses include control of the tyrosine aminotransferase gene in the liver but not in pituitary cells[167, 168] and GR regulation of the growth hormone gene in pituitary cells but not liver cells.[169]

Given the fact that GR protein levels and GC bioavailability are fairly similar in most all cell types, what accounts for these observed cell-specific GC responses? The answer probably involves cell-specific differences in the expression of coreceptor proteins that function as coactivators and corepressors of transcription.[124] Other factors contributing to cell-specific GC responsiveness include the chromatin structure and DNA methylation status of GR target genes; however, much less is understood about the selective role of these two important molecular determinants.

The most abundant GR coreceptor proteins identified to date belong to three distinct gene families. The first coreceptor protein to be described was steroid receptor coactivator-1 (SRC-1),[170] which is a member of the p160 family of coactivator proteins that interact with the HBD of ligand-bound nuclear receptors.[171, 172] SRC-1 is ubiquitously expressed and interacts equally well with most all members of the nuclear receptor superfamily. A second p160 coreceptor protein called GR-interacting protein-1 (GRIP-1) was isolated in a yeast two-hybrid screen with the GR HBD domain used as bait in a ligand dependent assay.[173, 174] SRC-1 and GRIP-1 are related proteins that share 43% sequence identity at the amino acid level. A third GR coactivator protein is p/CIP, which is a 152-kDa protein that interacts with the CBP/p300 family of histone acetylase coactivators and mediates nuclear receptor function.[175]

Figure 117–7 summarizes the conserved nuclear receptor–interacting motifs present in SRC-1, GRIP-1, and p/CIP that have been found to associate in vitro with amino acid residues in the GR HBD. Although it is not yet clear what role, if any, these three members of the p160 family of nuclear receptor coactivators play in specifying the *cell-specific* effects of GC action, it is reasonable to propose that similar coreceptor proteins may be selectively expressed in cell types exhibiting differential GC responsiveness. Moreover, various inhibitory GR corepressor proteins, only some of which have been identified, are

A. GR HBD residues that interact with p160 coreceptor proteins

helix H3 — helix H4 — helix H5 — helix H12

568 GRQVIAA**VKWAK** AI **PGFR** NLH **LDDQMLLLQ** . . . . EFP **EMLAEII** *759*

B. p160 coreceptor protein residues that interact with the GR HBD

	NR BOX I		NR BOX II		NR BOX III
GRIP 1	SKGQTK **L** LQ **LL** TT	...	LKEKHKI **L** HR **LL** Q	...	KKKE---NAL **L** RY **LL** DKDD
P/CIP	SKGHKK **L** LQ **LL** TC	...	LQEKHRI **L** HK **LL** Q	...	KKKE--NNAL **L** RY **LL** EKDD
SRC-1	SQTSHK **L** VQ **LL** TT	...	LTERHKI **L** HR **LL** Q	...	KKKESKDHQL **L** RY **LL** DKDE

FIGURE 117–7. Protein-protein interactions between glucocorticoid receptor (GR) and coreceptor proteins modulate ligand-dependent activation functions. *A,* AF-2 activator function in the GR hormone-binding domain (HBD) has been mapped to several putative α helical regions (H3, H4, H5, H12) that are thought to make direct contacts with p160 coreceptor proteins. *B,* Nuclear receptor–interacting sequences (NR BOXI, II, III) are conserved among the three primary GR coreceptor proteins in the p160 family (GRIP-1, p/CIP, and SRC-1).

likely to provide counteracting modulatory effects that could contribute to cell-specific GC action.

REFERENCES

1. Hollenberg SM, Weinberger C, Ong ES, et al: Primary structure and expression of a functional human glucocorticoid receptor cDNA. Nature 318:635–641, 1985.
2. Miesfeld RL, Rusconi S, Okret S, et al: Preliminary analyses of the glucocorticoid receptor gene and its expression: A DNA-binding protein essential for hormone-dependent transcriptional enhancement. *In* UCLA Symposium on Molecular Cellular Biology. Los Angeles, 1985, pp 535–545.
3. Theriault A, Boyd E, Harrap SB, et al: Regional chromosomal assignment of the human glucocorticoid receptor gene to 5q31. Hum Genet 83:289–291, 1989.
4. Francke U, Foellmer BE: The glucocorticoid receptor gene is in 5q31-q32. Genomics 4:610–612, 1989.
5. Encio IJ, Detera-Wadleigh SD: The genomic structure of the human glucocorticoid receptor. J Biol Chem 266:7182–7188, 1991.
6. Strahle U, Schmidt A, Kelsey G, et al: At least three promoters for direct expression of the mouse glucocorticoid receptor gene. Proc Natl Acad Sci U S A 89:6731–6735, 1992.
7. Picard D, Yamamoto KR: Two signals mediate hormone-dependent nuclear localization of the glucocorticoid receptor. EMBO J 6:3333–3340, 1987.
8. Picard D, Kumar V, Chambon P, et al: Signal transduction by steroid hormones: Nuclear localization is differentially regulated in estrogen and glucocorticoid receptors. Cell Regul 1:291–299, 1990.
9. Yang J, DeFranco DB: Assessment of glucocorticoid receptor heat shock protein 90 interactions in vivo during nucleocytoplasmic trafficking. Mol Endocrinol 10:3–13, 1996.
10. Pratt WB: The role of the hsp90-based chaperone system in signal transduction by nuclear receptors and receptors signaling via MAP kinase. Annu Rev Pharmacol Toxicol 37:297–326, 1997.
11. Rexin M, Busch W, Segnitz B, et al: Structure of the glucocorticoid receptor in intact cells in the absence of hormone. J Biol Chem 267:9619–9621, 1992.
12. Pratt WB: The role of heat shock proteins in regulating the function, folding, and trafficking of the glucocorticoid receptor. J Biol Chem 268:21455–21458, 1993.
13. Smith DF, Toft DO: Steroid receptors and their associated proteins. Mol Endocrinol 7:4–11, 1993.
14. Sanchez ER, Meshinchi S, Tienrungroj W, et al: Relationship of the 90-kDa murine heat shock protein to the untransformed and transformed states of the L cell glucocorticoid receptor. J Biol Chem 262:6986–6991, 1987.
15. Tai P-KK, Albers MW, Chang H, et al: Association of a 59-kilodalton immunophilin with the glucocorticoid receptor complex. Science 256:1315–1318, 1992.
16. Hutchison KA, Stancato LF, Owens-Grillo JK, et al: The 23-kDa acidic protein in reticulocyte lysate is the weakly bound component of the hsp foldosome that is required for assembly of the glucocorticoid receptor into a functional heterocomplex with hsp90. J Biol Chem 270:18841–18847, 1995.
17. Hutchison KA, Dittmar KD, Stancato LF, et al: Ability of various members of the hsp70 family of chaperones to promote assembly of the glucocorticoid receptor into a functional heterocomplex with hsp90. J Steroid Biochem Mol Biol 58:251–258, 1996.
18. Hutchison KA, Dittmar KD, Czar MJ, et al: Proof that hsp70 is required for assembly of the glucocorticoid receptor into a heterocomplex with hsp90. J Biol Chem 269:5043–5049, 1994.
19. Prapapanich V, Chen SY, Nair SC, et al: Molecular cloning of human p48, a transient component of progesterone receptor complexes and an hsp70-binding protein. Mol Endocrinol 10:420–431, 1996.
20. Dittmar KD, Hutchison KA, Owens-Grillo JK, et al: Reconstitution of the steroid receptor•hsp90 heterocomplex assembly system of rabbit reticulocyte lysate. J Biol Chem 271:12833–12839, 1996.
21. Dittmar KD, Banach M, Galigniana MD, et al: The role of DnaJ-like proteins in glucocorticoid receptor•hsp90 heterocomplex assembly by the reconstituted hsp90•p60•hsp70 foldosome complex. J Biol Chem 273:7358–7366, 1998.
22. Whitesell L, Cook P: Stable and specific binding of heat shock protein 90 by geldanamycin disrupts glucocorticoid receptor function in intact cells. Mol Endocrinol 10:705–712, 1996.
23. Czar MJ, Galigniana MD, Silverstein AM, et al: Geldanamycin, a heat shock protein 90–binding steroid-dependent translocation of the glucocorticoid receptor from the cytoplasm to the nucleus. Biochemistry 36:7776–7785, 1997.
24. Galigniana MD, Scruggs JL, Herrington J, et al: Heat shock protein 90–dependent (geldanamycin-inhibited) movement of the glucocorticoid receptor through the cytoplasm to the nucleus requires intact cytoskeleton. Mol Endocrinol 12:1903–1913, 1998.
25. Htun H, Barsony J, Renyi I, et al: Visualization of glucocorticoid receptor translocation and intranuclear organization in living cells with a green fluorescent protein chimera. Proc Natl Acad Sci U S A 93:4845–4850, 1996.
26. Galigniana MD, Scruggs JL, Herrington J, et al: Heat shock protein 90–dependent movement of the glucocorticoid receptor through the cytoplasm to the nucleus requires intact cytoskeleton. Mol Endocrinol 12:1903–1913, 1998.
27. Geley S, Fiegl M, Hartmann BL, et al: Genes mediating glucocorticoid effects and mechanisms of their regulation. Rev Physiol Biochem Pharmacol 128:1–97, 1996.
28. McIntyre WR, Samuels HH: Triamcinolone acetonide regulates glucocorticoid-receptor levels by decreasing the half-life of the activated nuclear-receptor form. J Biol Chem 260:418–427, 1985.
29. Distelhorst CW, Howard KJ: Kinetic pulse-chase labeling study of the glucocorticoid receptor in mouse lymphoma cells. Effect of glucocorticoid and antiglucocorticoid hormones on intracellular receptor half-life. J Biol Chem 264:13080–13085, 1989.
30. Madan AP, DeFranco DB: Bidirectional transport of glucocorticoid receptors across the nuclear envelope. Proc Natl Acad Sci U S A 90:3588–3592, 1993.
31. Tang YT, DeFranco DB: ATP-dependent release of glucocorticoid receptors from the nuclear matrix. Mol Cell Biol 16:1989–2001, 1996.
32. Yang J, Liu JM, DeFranco DB: Subnuclear trafficking of glucocorticoid receptors in vitro: Chromatin recycling and nuclear export. J Cell Biol 137:523–538, 1997.
33. Liu J, DeFranco DB: Chromatin recycling of glucocorticoid receptors: Implications for multiple roles of heat shock protein 90. Mol Endocrinol 13:355–365, 1999.
34. Wrange, Okret S, Radojcic M, et al: Characterization of the purified activated glucocorticoid receptor from rat liver cytosol. J Biol Chem 259:4534–4541, 1984.
35. Govindan MV, Gronemeyer H: Characterization of the rat liver glucocorticoid receptor purified by DNA-cellulose and ligand affinity chromatography. J Biol Chem 259:12915–12924, 1984.
36. Westphal HM, Moldenhauer G, Beato M: Monoclonal antibodies to the rat liver glucocorticoid receptor. EMBO J 1:1467–1471, 1982.
37. Okret S, Wikström AC, Wrange O, et al: Monoclonal antibodies against the rat liver glucocorticoid receptor. Proc Natl Acad Sci U S A 81:1609–1613, 1984.
38. Gametchu B, Harrison R: Characterization of a monoclonal antibody to the rat liver glucocorticoid receptor. Endocrinology 114:274–279, 1984.
39. Miesfeld RL, Okret S, Wikström A-C, et al: Characterization of a steroid hormone receptor gene and mRNA in wild-type and mutant cells. Nature 312:779–781, 1984.
40. Weinberger C, Hollenberg SM, Ong WS, et al: Identification of human glucocorticoid receptor complementary DNA clones by epitope selection. Science 228:740–742, 1985.
41. Miesfeld RL, Rusconi S, Godowski PJ, et al: Genetic complementation of a glucocorticoid receptor deficiency by expression of cloned receptor cDNA. Cell 46:389–399, 1986.
42. Danielsen M, Northrop JP, Ringold GM: The mouse glucocorticoid receptor: Mapping of functional domains by cloning, sequencing and expression of wild-type and mutant receptor proteins. EMBO J 5:2513–2522, 1986.
43. Brandon DD, Markwick AJ, Flores M, et al: Genetic variation of the glucocorticoid receptor from a steroid-resistant primate. J Mol Endocrinol 7:89–96, 1991.
44. Keightley MC, Fuller PJ: Cortisol resistance and the guinea pig glucocorticoid receptor. Steroids 60:87–92, 1995.
45. Gao X, Kalkhoven E, Peterson-Maduro J, et al: Expression of the glucocorticoid receptor gene is regulated during early embryogenesis of *Xenopus laevis*. Biochim Biophys Acta 1218:194–198, 1994.
46. Ducouret B, Tujague M, Ashraf J, et al: Cloning of a teleost fish glucocorticoid receptor shows that it contains a deoxyribonucleic acid–binding domain different from that of mammals. Endocrinology 136:3774–3783, 1995.
47. Martinez E, Moore DD, Keller E, et al: The nuclear receptor resource: a growing family. Nucleic Acids Res 26:239–241, 1998.
48. Oakley RH, Sar M, Cidlowski JA: The human glucocorticoid receptor β isoform—expression, biochemical properties, and putative function. J Biol Chem 271:9550–9559, 1996.
49. Oakley RH, Webster JC, Sar M, et al: Expression and subcellular distribution of the β-isoform of the human glucocorticoid receptor. Endocrinology 138:5028–5038, 1997.
50. Leung DYM, Hamid Q, Vottero A, et al: Association of glucocorticoid insensitivity with increased expression of glucocorticoid receptor β. J Exp Med 186:1567–1574, 1997.
51. Otto C, Reichardt HM, Schütz G: Absence of glucocorticoid receptor-β in mice. J Biol Chem 272:26665–26668, 1997.
52. Hecht K, Carlstedt-Duke J, Stierna P, et al: Evidence that the β-isoform of the human glucocorticoid receptor does not act as a physiologically significant repressor. J Biol Chem 272:26659–26664, 1997.
53. Reichman ME, Foster CM, Eisen LP, et al: Limited proteolysis of covalently labeled glucocorticoid receptors as a probe of receptor structure. Biochemistry 23:5376–5384, 1984.
54. Rehmus EH, Howard KJ, Janiga KE, et al: Immunochemical comparison of mutant glucocorticoid receptors and wild type receptor fragments produced by neutrophil elastase and chymotrypsin. J Steroid Biochem 28:167–177, 1987.
55. Carlstedt-Duke J, Stromstedt PE, Wrange O, et al: Domain structure of the glucocorticoid receptor protein. Proc Natl Acad Sci U S A 84:4437–4440, 1987.
56. Giguère V, Hollenberg SM, Rosenfeld MG, et al: Functional domains of the human glucocorticoid receptor. Cell 46:645–652, 1986.
57. Danielsen M, Northrop JP, Jonklaas J, et al: Domains of the glucocorticoid receptor involved in specific and non specific deoxyribonucleic acid binding, hormone activation, and transcriptional enhancement. Mol Endocrinol 1:816–822, 1987.
58. Rusconi S, Yamamoto KR: Functional dissection of the hormone and DNA binding activities of the glucocorticoid receptor. EMBO J 6:1309–1315, 1987.
59. Miesfeld RL, Godowski PJ, Maler BA, et al: Glucocorticoid receptor mutants that define a small region sufficient for enhancer activation. Science 236:423–427, 1987.
60. Godowski PJ, Picard D, Yamamoto KR: Signal transduction and transcriptional regulation by glucocorticoid receptor–lexA fusion proteins. Science 241:812–816, 1988.
61. Oro AE, Hollenberg SM, Evans RM: Transcriptional inhibition by a glucocorticoid receptor β-galactosidase fusion protein. Cell 55:1109–1114, 1988.
62. Rosenthal D, Hong T, Cherney B, et al: Expression and characterization of a fusion protein between the catalytic domain of poly(ADP-ribose) polymerase and the DNA binding domain of the glucocorticoid receptor. Biochem Biophys Res Commun 202:880–887, 1994.
63. Scherrer LC, Picard D, Massa E, et al: Evidence that the hormone binding domain of steroid receptors confers hormonal control on chimeric proteins by determining their hormone-regulated binding to heat-shock protein 90. Biochemistry 32:5381–5386, 1993.
64. Dieken ES, Miesfeld RL: Transcriptional transactivation functions localized to the glucocorticoid receptor N terminus are necessary for steroid induction of lymphocyte apoptosis. Mol Cell Biol 12:589–597, 1992.
65. Chapman MS, Askew DJ, Kuscuoglu U, et al: Transcriptional control of steroid-regulated apoptosis in murine thymoma cells. Mol Endocrinol 10:967–978, 1996.

66. Brocard J, Feil R, Chambon P, et al: A chimeric Cre recombinase inducible by synthetic, but not by natural ligands of the glucocorticoid receptor. Nucleic Acids Res 26:4086–4090, 1998.
67. Muller M, Baniahmad C, Kaltschmidt C, et al: Multiple domains of the glucocorticoid receptor involved in synergism with the CACCC box factor(s). Mol Endocrinol 5:1498–1503, 1991.
68. Webster NJ, Green S, Jin JR, et al: The hormone-binding domains of the estrogen and glucocorticoid receptors contain an inducible transcription activation function. Cell 54:199–207, 1988.
69. Savory JG, Hsu B, Laquian IR, et al: Discrimination between NL1- and NL2-mediated nuclear localization of the glucocorticoid receptor. Mol Cell Biol 19:1025–1037, 1999.
70. Dalman FC, Scherrer LC, Taylor LP, et al: Localization of the 90-kDa heat shock protein–binding site within the hormone-binding domain of the glucocorticoid receptor by peptide competition. J Biol Chem 266:3482–3490, 1991.
71. Cadepond F, Schweizer-Groyer G, Segard-Maurel I, et al: Heat shock protein 90 as a critical factor in maintaining glucocorticosteroid receptor in a nonfunctional state. J Biol Chem 266:5834–5841, 1991.
72. Xu M, Dittmar KD, Giannoukos G, et al: Binding of hsp90 to the glucocorticoid receptor requires a specific 7–amino acid sequence at the amino terminus of the hormone-binding domain. J Biol Chem 273:13918–13924, 1998.
73. Feng W, Ribeiro RC, Wagner RL, et al: Hormone-dependent coactivator binding to a hydrophobic cleft on nuclear receptors. Science 280:1747–1749, 1998.
74. Boruk M, Savory JG, Hache RJ: AF-2–dependent potentiation of CCAAT enhancer binding protein beta–mediated transcriptional activation by glucocorticoid receptor. Mol Endocrinol 12:1749–1763, 1998.
75. Sakai DD, Helms S, Carlstedt-Duke J, et al: Hormone-mediated repression: A negative glucocorticoid response element from the bovine prolactin gene. Genes Dev 2:1144–1154, 1988.
76. Iñiguez-Lluhí JA, Lou DY, Yamamoto KR: Three amino acid substitutions selectively disrupt the activation but not the repression function of the glucocorticoid receptor N terminus. J Biol Chem 272:4149–4156, 1997.
77. Heck S, Kullmann M, Gast A, et al: A distinct modulating domain in glucocorticoid receptor monomers in the repression of activity of the transcription factor AP-1. EMBO J 13:4087–4095, 1994.
78. Luisi BF, Xu WX, Otwinowski Z, et al: Crystallographic analysis of the interaction of the glucocorticoid receptor with DNA. Nature 352:497–505, 1991.
79. Segard-Maurel I, Rajkowski K, Jibard N, et al: Glucocorticosteroid receptor dimerization investigated by analysis of receptor binding to glucocorticosteroid responsive elements using a monomer-dimer equilibrium model. Biochemistry 35:1634–1642, 1996.
80. DeFranco DB, Qi M, Borror KC, et al: Protein phosphatase types 1 and/or 2A regulate nucleocytoplasmic shuttling of glucocorticoid receptors. Mol Endocrinol 5:1215–1228, 1991.
81. Borror KC, Garabedian MJ, DeFranco DB: Glucocorticoid receptor phosphorylation in v-mos–transformed cells. Steroids 60:375–382, 1995.
82. Krstic MD, Rogatsky I, Yamamoto KR, et al: Mitogen-activated and cyclin-dependent protein kinases selectively and differentially modulate transcriptional enhancement by the glucocorticoid receptor. Mol Cell Biol 17:3947–3954, 1997.
83. Rogatsky I, Waase CLM, Garabedian MJ: Phosphorylation and inhibition of rat glucocorticoid receptor transcriptional activation by glycogen synthase kinase-3 (GSK-3)—species-specific differences between human and rat glucocorticoid receptor signaling as revealed through GSK-3 phosphorylation. J Biol Chem 273:14315–14321, 1998.
84. Picard D, Salser SJ, Yamamoto KR: A movable and regulable inactivation function within the steroid binding domain of the glucocorticoid receptor. Cell 54:1073–1080, 1988.
85. Spanjaard RA, Chin WW: Reconstitution of ligand-mediated glucocorticoid receptor activity by *trans*-acting functional domains. Mol Endocrinol 7:12–16, 1993.
86. Carey KL, Richards SA, Lounsbury KM, et al: Evidence using a green fluorescent protein–glucocorticoid receptor chimera that the Ran/TC4 GTPase mediates an essential function independent of nuclear protein import. J Cell Biol 133:985–996, 1996.
87. Simons SS Jr, Sistare FD, Chakraborti PK: Steroid binding activity is retained in a 16-kDa fragment of the steroid binding domain of rat glucocorticoid receptors. J Biol Chem 264:14493–14497, 1989.
88. Simons SS Jr, Pumphrey JG, Rudikoff S, et al: Identification of cysteine 656 as the amino acid of hepatoma tissue culture cell glucocorticoid receptors that is covalently labeled by dexamethasone 21-mesylate. J Biol Chem 262:9676–9680, 1987.
89. Carlstedt-Duke J, Strömstedt P-E, Persson B, et al: Identification of hormone-interacting amino acid residues within the steroid-binding domain of the glucocorticoid receptor in relation to other steroid hormone receptors. J Biol Chem 263:6842–6846, 1988.
90. Smith LI, Bodwell JE, Mendel DB, et al: Identification of cysteine-644 as the covalent site of attachment of dexamethasone 21-mesylate to murine glucocorticoid receptors in WEHI-7 cells. Biochemistry 27:3747–3753, 1988.
91. Byravan S, Milhon J, Rabindran SK, et al: Two point mutations in the hormone-binding domain of the mouse glucocorticoid receptor that dramatically reduce its function. Mol Endocrinol 5:752–758, 1991.
92. Chakraborti PK, Garabedian MJ, Yamamoto KR, et al: Creation of "super" glucocorticoid receptors by point mutations in the steroid binding domain. J Biol Chem 266:22075–22078, 1991.
93. Mao J, Regelson W, Kalimi M: Molecular mechanism of RU 486 action: A review. Mol Cell Biochem 109:1–8, 1992.
94. Cadepond F, Ulmann A, Baulieu EE: RU486 (mifepristone): Mechanisms of action and clinical uses. Annu Rev Med 48:129–156, 1997.
95. Nieman L, Loriaux D: Clinical applications of the glucocorticoid and progestin antagonist RU 486. *In* Agarwal MK (ed): Receptor Mediated Anti-steroid Action. New York, Walter de Gruyter, 1987, pp 77–97.
96. Willmann T, Beato M: Steroid-free glucocorticoid receptor binds specifically to mouse mammary tumour virus DNA. Nature 324:688–691, 1986.
97. Rajpert EJ, Lemaigre FP, Eliard PH, et al: Glucocorticoid receptors bound to the antagonist RU 486 are not downregulated despite their capacity to interact in vitro with defined gene regions. J Steroid Biochem 26:513–520, 1987.
98. Rajpert EJ, Lemaigre FP, Eliard PH, et al: Glucocorticoid receptors bound to the antagonist RU486 are not downregulated despite their capacity to interact in vitro with defined gene regions. J Steroid Biochem 26:513–520, 1987.
99. Groyer A, Schweizer-Groyer G, Cadepond F, et al: Antiglucocorticosteroid effects suggest why steroid hormone is required for receptors to bind DNA in vivo but not in vitro. Nature 328:624–626, 1987.
100. Becker PB, Gloss B, Schmid W, et al: In vivo protein-DNA interactions in a glucocorticoid response element require the presence of the hormone. Nature 324:686–688, 1986.
101. Freedman LP: Anatomy of the steroid receptor zinc finger region. Endocr Rev 13:129–145, 1992.
102. Dahlman-Wright K, Wright A, Carlstedt-Duke J, et al: DNA-binding by the glucocorticoid receptor: A structural and functional analysis. J Steroid Biochem Mol Biol 41:249–272, 1992.
103. Berg JM: Zinc finger domains: Hypotheses and current knowledge. Annu Rev Biophys Biophys Chem 19:405–421, 1990.
104. Churchill ME, Tullius TD, Klug A: Mode of interaction of the zinc finger protein TFIIIA with a 5S RNA gene of *Xenopus*. Proc Natl Acad Sci U S A 87:5528–5532, 1990.
105. Schena M, Freedman LP, Yamamoto KR: Mutations in the glucocorticoid receptor zinc finger region that distinguish interdigitated DNA binding and transcriptional enhancement activities. Genes Dev 3:1590–1601, 1989.
106. La Baer J, Yamamoto KR: Analysis of the DNA-binding affinity, sequence specificity and context dependence of the glucocorticoid receptor zinc finger region. J Mol Biol 239:664–688, 1994.
107. Baniahmad C, Muller M, Altschmied J, et al: Co-operative binding of the glucocorticoid receptor DNA binding domain is one of at least two mechanisms for synergism. J Mol Biol 222:155–165, 1991.
108. Perlmann T, Eriksson P, Wrange O: Quantitative analysis of the glucocorticoid receptor–DNA interaction at the mouse mammary tumor virus glucocorticoid response element. J Biol Chem 265:17222–17229, 1990.
109. Schmid W, Strahle U, Schütz G, et al: Glucocorticoid receptor binds cooperatively to adjacent recognition sites. EMBO J 8:2257–2263, 1989.
110. Dahlman-Wright K, Siltala-Roos H, Carlstedt-Duke J, et al: Protein-protein interactions facilitate DNA binding by the glucocorticoid receptor DNA-binding domain. J Biol Chem 265:14030–14035, 1990.
111. Tsai MJ, O'Malley BW: Molecular mechanisms of action of steroid/thyroid receptor superfamily members. Annu Rev Biochem 63:451–486, 1994.
112. Eriksson P, Wrange O: Protein-protein contacts in the glucocorticoid receptor homodimer influence its DNA binding properties. J Biol Chem 265:3535–3542, 1990.
113. Shibata H, Spencer TE, Onate SA, et al: Role of co-activators and co-repressors in the mechanism of steroid/thyroid receptor action. Recent Prog Horm Res 52:141–164, 1997.
114. Schena M, Yamamoto KR: Mammalian glucocorticoid receptor derivatives enhance transcription in yeast. Science 241:965–967, 1988.
115. Yoshinaga SK, Yamamoto KR: Signaling and regulation by a mammalian glucocorticoid receptor in *Drosophila* cells. Mol Endocrinol 5:844–853, 1991.
116. Schena M, Lloyd AM, Davis RW: A steroid-inducible gene expression system for plant cells. Proc Natl Acad Sci U S A 88:10421–10425, 1991.
117. Almlöf T, Gustafsson J, Wright APH: Role of hydrophobic amino acid clusters in the transactivation activity of the human glucocorticoid receptor. Mol Cell Biol 17:934–945, 1997.
118. Dieken ES, Meese EU, Miesfeld RL: nt[i] glucocorticoid receptor transcripts lack sequences encoding the amino-terminal transcriptional modulatory domain. Mol Cell Biol 10:4574–4581, 1990.
119. Carey M: The enhanceosome and transcriptional synergy. Cell 92:5–8, 1998.
120. Lee TI, Young RA: Regulation of gene expression by TBP-associated proteins. Genes Dev 12:1398–1408, 1998.
121. Dahlman-Wright K, Baumann H, McEwan IJ, et al: Structural characterization of a minimal functional transactivation domain from the human glucocorticoid receptor. Proc Natl Acad Sci U S A 92:1699–1703, 1995.
122. Dahlman-Wright K, McEwan IJ: Structural studies of mutant glucocorticoid receptor transactivation domains establish a link between transactivation activity in vivo and α-helix–forming potential in vitro. Biochemistry 35:1323–1327, 1996.
123. Webster JC, Jewell CM, Bodwell JE, et al: Mouse glucocorticoid receptor phosphorylation status influences multiple functions of the receptor protein. J Biol Chem 272:9287–9293, 1997.
124. Horwitz KB, Jackson TA, Rain DL, et al: Nuclear receptor coactivators and corepressors. Mol Endocrinol 10:1167–1177, 1996.
125. Perlmann T, Evans RM: Nuclear receptors in Sicily: All in the famiglia. Cell 90:391–397, 1997.
126. Ringold GM, Yamamoto KR, Tomkins GM, et al: Dexamethasone-mediated induction of mouse mammary tumor virus RNA: A system for studying glucocorticoid action. Cell 6:299–305, 1975.
127. Payvar F, DeFranco D, Firestone GL, et al: Sequence-specific binding of glucocorticoid receptor to MTV DNA at sites within and upstream of the transcribed region. Cell 35:381–392, 1983.
128. Chandler VL, Maler BA, Yamamoto KR: DNA sequences bound specifically by glucocorticoid receptor in vitro render a heterologous promoter hormone responsive in vivo. Cell 33:489–499, 1983.
129. Ucker DS, Ross SR, Yamamoto KR: Mammary tumor virus DNA contains sequences required for its hormone-regulated transcription. Cell 27:257–266, 1981.
130. Archer TK, Lefebvre P, Wolford RG, et al: Transcription factor loading on the

MMTV promoter: A bimodal mechanism for promoter activation [published erratum appears in Science 1992. Apr 10;256(5054):161]. Science 255:1573–1576, 1992.
131. Ostlund Farrants AK, Blomquist P, Kwon H, et al: Glucocorticoid receptor–glucocorticoid response element binding stimulates nucleosome disruption by the SWI/SNF complex. Mol Cell Biol 17:895–905, 1997.
132. Blomquist P, Li Q, Wrange O: The affinity of nuclear factor 1 for its DNA site is drastically reduced by nucleosome organization irrespective of its rotational or translational position. J Biol Chem 271:153–159, 1996.
133. Petersen DD, Magnuson MA, Granner DK: Location and characterization of two widely separated glucocorticoid response elements in the phosphoenolpyruvate carboxykinase gene. Mol Cell Biol 8:96–104, 1988.
134. Imai E, Stromstedt PE, Quinn PG, et al: Characterization of a complex glucocorticoid response unit in the phosphoenolpyruvate carboxykinase gene. Mol Cell Biol 10:4712–4719, 1990.
135. Hall RK, Sladek FM, Granner DK: The orphan receptors COUP-TF and HNF-4 serve as accessory factors required for induction of phosphoenolpyruvate carboxykinase gene transcription by glucocorticoids. Proc Natl Acad Sci U S A 92:412–416, 1995.
136. Scott DK, Stromstedt PE, Wang JC, et al: Further characterization of the glucocorticoid response unit in the phosphoenolpyruvate carboxykinase gene. The role of the glucocorticoid receptor–binding sites. Mol Endocrinol 12:482–491, 1998.
137. Yamada K, Duong DT, Scott DK, et al: CCAAT/enhancer-binding protein beta is an accessory factor for the glucocorticoid response from the cAMP response element in the rat phosphoenolpyruvate carboxykinase gene promoter. J Biol Chem 274:5880–5887, 1999.
138. Tjian R, Maniatis T: Transcriptional activation: A complex puzzle with few easy pieces. Cell 77:5–8, 1994.
139. Sauer F, Tjian R: Mechanisms of transcriptional activation: Differences and similarities between yeast, *Drosophila*, and man. Curr Opin Genet Dev 7:176–181, 1997.
140. Jenster G, Spencer TE, Burcin MM, et al: Steroid receptor induction of gene transcription: A two-step model. Proc Natl Acad Sci U S A 94:7879–7884, 1997.
141. Reichardt HM, Kaestner KH, Tuckermann J, et al: DNA binding of the glucocorticoid receptor is not essential for survival. Cell 93:531–541, 1998.
142. Karin M: New twists in gene regulation by glucocorticoid receptor: Is DNA binding dispensable? Cell 93:487–490, 1998.
143. Sakai DD, Helms S, Carlstedt-Duke J, et al: Hormone-mediated repression: A negative glucocorticoid response element from the bovine prolactin gene. Genes Dev 2:1144–1154, 1988.
144. Chatterjee VK, Madison LD, Mayo S, et al: Repression of the human glycoprotein hormone alpha-subunit gene by glucocorticoids: Evidence for receptor interactions with limiting transcriptional activators. Mol Endocrinol 5:100–110, 1991.
145. Mordacq JC, Linzer DI: Co-localization of elements required for phorbol ester stimulation and glucocorticoid repression of proliferin gene expression. Genes Dev 3:760–769, 1989.
146. Diamond MI, Miner JN, Yoshinaga SK, et al: Transcription factor interactions: Selectors of positive or negative regulation from a single DNA element. Science 249:1266–1272, 1990.
147. Miner JN, Yamamoto KR: The basic region of AP-1 specifies glucocorticoid receptor activity at a composite response element. Genes Dev 6:2491–2501, 1992.
148. Pearce D, Matsui W, Miner JN, et al: Glucocorticoid receptor transcriptional activity determined by spacing of receptor and nonreceptor DNA sites. J Biol Chem 273:30081–30085, 1998.
149. Baeuerle P: Pro-inflammatory signaling: Last pieces in the nf-kb puzzle? Curr Biol 8:R19–R22, 1998.
150. Baeuerle PA: IκB–NF-κB structures: At the interface of inflammation control. Cell 95:729–731, 1998.
151. Baeuerle PA, Baltimore D: NF-κB: Ten years after. Cell 87:13–20, 1996.
152. Verma IM, Stevenson JK, Schwarz EM, et al: Rel/NF-kappa B/I kappa B family: Intimate tales of association and dissociation. Genes Dev 9:2723–2735, 1995.
153. Scheinman RI, Gualberto A, Jewell CM, et al: Characterization of mechanisms involved in transrepression of NF-κB by activated glucocorticoid receptors. Mol Cell Biol 15:943–953, 1995.
154. Scheinman RI, Cogswell PC, Lofquist AK, et al: Role of transcriptional activation of IκB in mediation of immunosuppression by glucocorticoids. Science 270:283–286, 1995.
155. Caldenhoven E, Liden J, Wissink S, et al: Negative cross-talk between RelA and the glucocorticoid receptor: A possible mechanism for the antiinflammatory action of glucocorticoids. Mol Endocrinol 9:401–412, 1995.
156. Dumont A, Hehner SP, Schmitz ML, et al: Cross-talk between steroids and NF-κB: What language? Trends Biochem Sci 23:233–235, 1998.
157. Wissink S, Van Heerde EC, Van der Burg B, et al: A dual mechanism mediates repression of NF-κB activity by glucocorticoids. Mol Endocrinol 12:355–363, 1998.
158. Ray A, Siegel MD, Prefontaine KE, et al: Anti-inflammation: Direct physical association and functional antagonism between transcription factor NF-κB and the glucocorticoid receptor. Chest 107(suppl):139, 1995.
159. Auphan N, DiDonato JA, Rosette C, et al: Immunosuppression by glucocorticoids: Inhibition of NF-κB activity through induction of IκB synthesis. Science 270:286–290, 1995.
160. De Bosscher K, Schmitz ML, Vanden Berghe W, et al: Glucocorticoid-mediated repression of nuclear factor-κB–dependent transcription involves direct interference with transactivation. Proc Natl Acad Sci U S A 94:13504–13509, 1997.
161. Brostjan C, Anrather J, Csizmadia V, et al: Glucocorticoid-mediated repression of NFκB activity in endothelial cells does not involve induction of IκB synthesis. J Biol Chem 271:19612–19616, 1996.
162. Palvimo JJ, Reinikainen P, Ikonen T, et al: Mutual transcriptional interference between RelA and androgen receptor. J Biol Chem 271:24151–24156, 1996.
163. Wissink S, Van Heerde EC, Schmitz ML, et al: Distinct domains of the RelA NF-κB subunit are required for negative cross-talk and direct interaction with the glucocorticoid receptor. J Biol Chem 272:22278–22284, 1997.
164. Heck S, Bender K, Kullmann M, et al: IκB-independent downregulation of NF-κB activity by glucocorticoid receptor. EMBO J 16:4698–4707, 1997.
165. Nechushtan H, Benvenisty N, Brandeis R, et al: Glucocorticoids control phosphoenolpyruvate carboxykinase gene expression in a tissue specific manner. Nucleic Acids Res 15:6405–6417, 1987.
166. Eisenberger CL, Nechushtan H, Cohen H, et al: Differential regulation of the rat phosphoenolpyruvate carboxykinase gene expression in several tissues of transgenic mice. Mol Cell Biol 12:1396–1403, 1992.
167. Grange T, Roux J, Rigaud G, et al: Two remote glucocorticoid responsive units interact cooperatively to promote glucocorticoid induction of rat tyrosine aminotransferase gene expression. Nucleic Acids Res 17:8695–8709, 1989.
168. Grange T, Roux J, Rigaud G, et al: Cell-type specific activity of two glucocorticoid responsive units of rat tyrosine aminotransferase gene is associated with multiple binding sites for C/EBP and a novel liver-specific nuclear factor. Nucleic Acids Res 19:131–139, 1991.
169. Ivarie RD, Schacter BS, O'Farrell PH: The level of expression of the rat growth hormone gene in liver tumor cells is at least eight orders of magnitude less than that in anterior pituitary cells. Mol Cell Biol 3:1460–1467, 1983.
170. Onate SA, Tsai SY, Tsai MJ, et al: Sequence and characterization of a coactivator for the steroid hormone receptor superfamily. Science 270:1354–1357, 1995.
171. Kamei Y, Xu L, Heinzel T, et al: A CBP integrator complex mediates transcriptional activation and AP-1 inhibition by nuclear receptors. Cell 85:403–414, 1996.
172. Hong H, Darimont BD, Ma H, et al: An additional region of coactivator GRIP1 required for interaction with the hormone-binding domains of a subset of nuclear receptors. J Biol Chem 274:3496–3502, 1999.
173. Hong H, Kohli K, Trivedi A, et al: GRIP1, a novel mouse protein that serves as a transcriptional coactivator in yeast for the hormone binding domains of steroid receptors. Proc Natl Acad Sci U S A 93:4948–4952, 1996.
174. Hong H, Kohli K, Garabedian MJ, et al: GRIP1, a transcriptional coactivator for the AF-2 transactivation domain of steroid, thyroid, retinoid, and vitamin D receptors. Mol Cell Biol 17:2735–2744, 1997.
175. Torchia J, Rose DW, Inostroza J, et al: The transcriptional co-activator p/CIP binds CBP and mediates nuclear-receptor function. Nature 387:677–684, 1997.

Chapter 118

Diagnostic Implications of Adrenal Physiology and Clinical Epidemiology for Evaluation of Glucocorticoid Excess and Deficiency

David C. Aron

The evaluation of adrenal function, although dependent upon clinical judgment, also relies to a large extent on biochemical testing. This chapter is introduced by general considerations to be taken into account in laboratory testing of the CRH-ACTH-cortisol axis and then is organized by the questions a clinician might ask in the course of an evaluation of a patient's adrenal function. For the patient in whom the diagnosis of Cushing's syndrome is being considered, the questions include: (1) Does the patient have glucocorticoid excess? (2) Has the patient who has been treated for glucocorticoid excess been "cured" or "controlled?" For a patient in whom the diagnosis of adrenal insufficiency is being considered, the questions include: (1) Does the patient in an unstressed state have glucocorticoid deficiency now? (2) Can the patient respond to stress? (3) Is the patient taking the appropriate replacement dose of cortisol? Questions of determining the cause of Cushing's syndrome and adrenal insufficiency are left to Chapters 124 and 125.

BASIC PHYSIOLOGIC PRINCIPLES AND THEIR IMPLICATIONS FOR ASSESSMENT OF GLUCOCORTICOID FUNCTION

Episodic Secretion and Diurnal Rhythm

Normally, cortisol is secreted episodically from the zona fasciculata of the adrenal cortex with a diurnal rhythm paralleling the secretion of adrenocorticotropic hormone (ACTH) (Fig. 118–1).[1–5] Each secretory episode of cortisol release results in a sharp rise in plasma concentration, followed by a slower decline. These discrete episodes occur at somewhat irregular intervals ranging from a half-hour to several hours. Consequently, normal levels of plasma cortisol cover a broad range; the levels found in both adrenal insufficiency and in Cushing's syndrome may at any given time fall within the "normal" range. The secretory episodes occur most frequently in the late evening and early morning hours, resulting in a circadian rhythm in which plasma cortisol levels are usually highest early in the morning, decrease gradually throughout the day, and reach a nadir in the late evening. About half of the total daily cortisol output is secreted during the period of highest secretory activity. In fact, at the usual nadir of secretory activity in the first few hours of sleep, plasma cortisol levels may be undetectable. When assessed with a typical radioimmunoassay (RIA, the most commonly used method), basal values and responses to stimuli vary from assay to assay, but cortisol concentrations range from about 275 to 555 nmol/L (10 to 20 μg/dL) in the early morning (within 1 hour of the usual time of awakening), from 85 to 275 nmol/L (3 to 10 μg/dL) at 4 PM, and are usually less than 140 nmol/L (5 μg/dL) after the usual bedtime. In addition to the underlying circadian rhythm, there is an increase in cortisol secretion in response to eating and exercise. Although this general pattern is consistent, individuals vary from day to day and there is considerable interindividual variation.[6] The circadian rhythm may be altered by changes in sleep pattern, light-dark exposure, and feeding times. The rhythm is also changed by physical stresses such as major illness, surgery, trauma, or starvation; psychological stress, including severe anxiety, endogenous depression, and the manic phase of manic-depressive disorder; central nervous system and pituitary disorders; Cushing's syndrome; liver disease and other conditions that affect cortisol metabolism; chronic renal failure; and alcoholism. Consequently, documenting the presence or absence of diurnal rhythm in a simple fashion is difficult; single plasma cortisol determinations obtained in the morning or evening may be uninterpretable because of the pulsatility of pathologic and physiologic ACTH and cortisol secretion. Of note, cortisol is secreted episodically not only in normal persons but also in patients with Cushing's syndrome, whether caused by pituitary tumors, adrenal tumors, or the ectopic ACTH syndrome.

Cortisol Secretory Rate

Cortisol secretion (or production) rates have been assessed by isotopic and nonisotopic dilution methods. These methods have little practi-

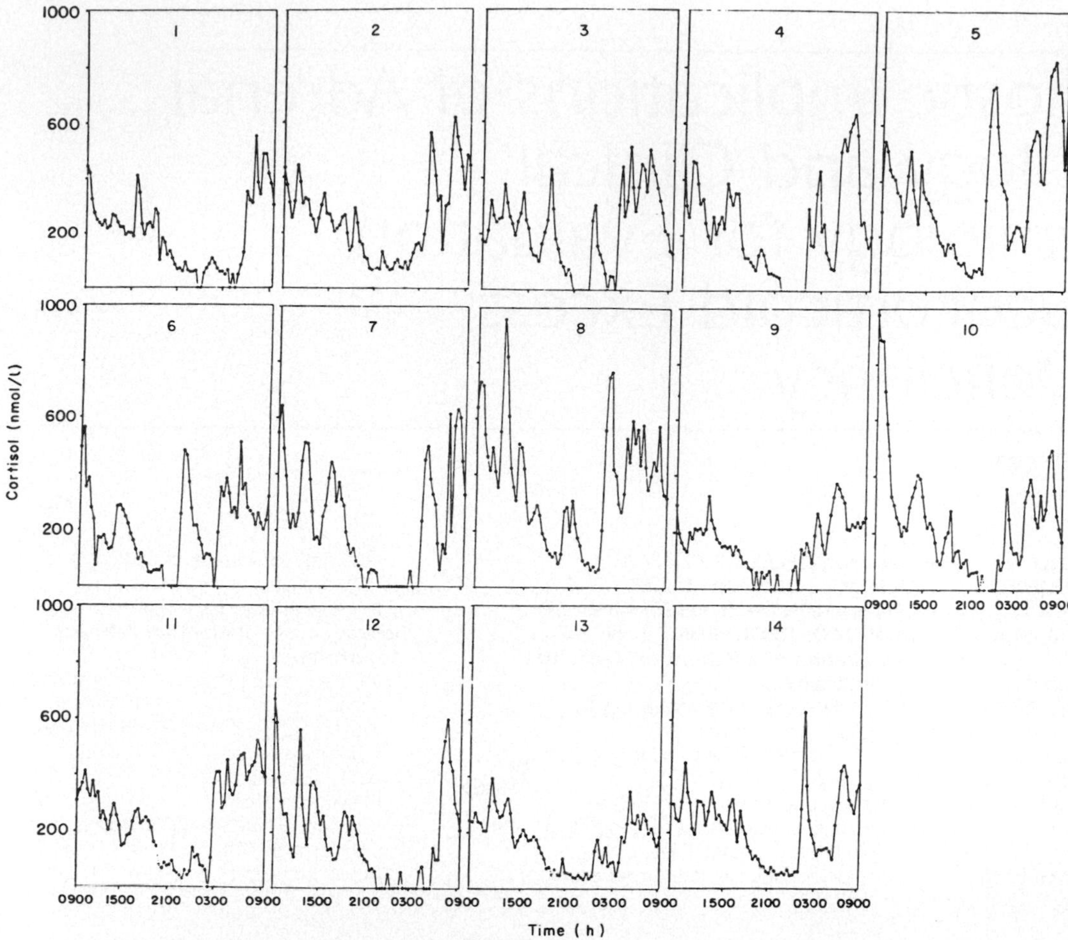

FIGURE 118–1. Episodic secretion and circadian rhythm of cortisol. The 24-hour profiles for cortisol are displayed for 14 normal children. The profiles are labeled with the subject's number. Results in adults are similar.[1, 3, 5] (From Wallace WHB, Crowne EC, Shalet SM, et al: Episodic ACTH and cortisol secretion in normal children. Clin Endocrinol 34:218, 1991.)

cal clinical utility. In addition, while an increased cortisol secretion rate is the hallmark of naturally occurring Cushing's syndrome, rates higher than those observed under normal basal conditions may be seen in a variety of circumstances. Furthermore, although frank adrenal insufficiency is associated with decreased cortisol secretory rates, there is also a state of decreased adrenal reserve in which the basal cortisol secretion rate remains normal while there is decreased ability to respond to stress. Even for research purposes, assessment of the cortisol secretion rate has some serious methodologic limitations, for example, the absence of a unique urinary metabolite for cortisol and the different secretion rate estimates depending upon the method used. However, the results of such studies have important implications for the determination of the appropriate dose of glucocorticoid replacement therapy. Cortisol secretion under basal (i.e., nonstressed) conditions ranges from 8 to 25 mg/day (22 to 69 μmol/day) with a mean of about 9.2 mg/day (25 μmol/day).[7, 8] More recent studies have estimated daily cortisol secretion at rates considerably lower than most previous calculations.[9–12] There is also seasonal variation.[6, 13]

The Hypothalamic-Pituitary-Adrenal Axis: Regulation of Cortisol and ACTH Secretion

Negative Feedback and Response to Stress

Cortisol secretion is regulated by feed-forward stimulation and feedback inhibition of corticotropin-releasing hormone (CRH) and ACTH. Glucocorticoid negative feedback inhibition occurs at both the pituitary and hypothalamus. There are two distinct mechanisms: fast and delayed feedback inhibition. Delayed feedback inhibition involves both time- and dose-dependent effects and has major implications for diagnostic testing. Glucocorticoid administration will result in suppression of endogenous cortisol secretion in normal persons, but not in most patients with Cushing's syndrome. This is the basis of the low-dose dexamethasone suppression test (see below). In addition, chronic pharmacologic doses of glucocorticoids will result in suppression of corticotropin-releasing hormone (CRH) and ACTH release and atrophy of the zona fasciculata and reticularis. Thus, in many, but not all cases of secondary adrenal insufficiency, there is an impaired response of the zona fasciculata to acute administration of ACTH (see below).

The hypothalamic-pituitary-adrenal axis responds to "stress" with an increase in CRH secretion, followed by an increase in ACTH secretion, followed in turn by an increase in cortisol secretion. Such stress includes hypotension, hypoglycemia, and a variety of serious illnesses.[14–18] In addition to the predictable cortisol response to severe stress, there is a somewhat more variable response to stresses as "mild" as the anticipation of a university examination or athletic event or venipuncture. Consequently, persons *without* Cushing's syndrome subjected to stress may have plasma cortisol levels that equal or even exceed those found in a typical case of Cushing's syndrome.[2, 15, 18, 19] For example, one study of 28 critically ill patients in an intensive care unit found a mean plasma cortisol value of 40.1 μg/dL, far in excess of the usual "normal" range that typically applies to morning levels in healthy subjects in the outpatient setting.[20] We can take advantage of the response to stress and negative feedback to assist in interpretation of hormone levels. For example, a plasma cortisol sample obtained from a hypotensive patient should be elevated. In fact, if it is not high, it is "low," even if the level falls into the "normal" (i.e., reference) range. The "normal" range is not applicable to persons in shock because it would be inappropriately low for the circumstances. Similarly, a plasma cortisol level obtained in a normal subject following administration of dexamethasone (a synthetic glucocorticoid not measured in cortisol assays) should be low, that is, suppressed. In fact, if it is not low, it is high, even if the level falls into the "normal" range; the normal range for healthy persons not taking dexamethasone does not apply.

Cortisol Transport and Metabolism

Cortisol, although secreted in the unbound state, binds to plasma proteins, corticosteroid-binding globulin (CBG, transcortin) and, to a lesser extent, to albumin.[21] Under basal conditions, about 5% to 10% of the circulating cortisol is free, about 75% is bound to CBG, and the remainder is bound to albumin. However, it is the free cortisol in plasma that is biologically active and it is the free level that is sensed and regulated by the CRH-ACTH axis. Plasma free cortisol cannot be readily measured in clinical practice; we rely on measurement of total plasma cortisol. Normal CBG has a cortisol-binding capacity of about 25 μg/dL; increases in total plasma cortisol concentrations above this level result in rapid increases in levels of free cortisol concentration. In otherwise normal individuals with states of high CBG levels, for example, high-estrogen states (pregnancy; estrogen or oral contraceptive use), hyperthyroidism, diabetes, and hereditary CBG excess, plasma free cortisol is maintained at normal levels, but total plasma cortisol levels are increased. This situation is analogous to the levels of free thyroxine, total thyroxine, and thyroxine-binding globulin in the euthyroid individual taking estrogen. Since it is the free cortisol that is regulated by CRH-ACTH, interpretation of the total plasma cortisol response to dexamethasone may be difficult in a patient with CBG excess. Similarly, in states of low CBG levels, for example, familial CBG deficiency, hypothyroidism, and protein deficiency states such as severe liver disease or nephrotic syndrome, normal plasma free cortisol levels are maintained with lower total plasma cortisol concentrations. The cortisol-binding capacity of albumin is greater than that of CBG, but its affinity is lower.

Relatively little cortisol is excreted in the urine unchanged—less than 1%. Over 95% of cortisol and the metabolites of cortisol and its 11-dehydrogenated form—cortisone—are conjugated in the liver and then excreted in the urine. Alteration in cortisol metabolism occurs in a variety of circumstances. However, now that we rely primarily on urine free cortisol measurements rather than measurements of metabolites of cortisol, for example, 17-hydroxycorticosteroids (17-OHCS) and 17-ketogenic steroids, there are relatively few implications for such alterations for routine biochemical testing. Although pharmacologic inducers of hepatic microsomal enzymes, for example, phenytoin and rifampin, increase cortisol metabolism, normal plasma levels of cortisol in otherwise normal individuals are maintained. In contrast, these drugs have a greater effect on the metabolism of dexamethasone and other synthetic glucocorticoids. This fact has implications for the interpretation of dexamethasone suppression tests; patients taking phenytoin may achieve relatively low levels of dexamethasone. In the kidney, cortisol is converted to cortisone by the enzyme 11-hydroxysteroid dehydrogenase. Reduction in the activity of this enzyme by ingestion of licorice or in the setting of familial enzyme deficiency may result in elevated urine free cortisol levels.[22] However, normal plasma cortisol levels are maintained.

Assays and Assay Methodology

PLASMA CORTISOL. Older methods of measurement of plasma (or serum) cortisol such as Porter-Silber chromogens which measure 17-OHCS, fluorimetric assays, and competitive protein-binding assays have been replaced almost entirely by RIA and its variants. Interpretation of the older literature will require some familiarity with these methods and their shortcomings—steroid cross-reactivity and drug interference.[23–25] Readers are referred to Chapters 119 and 123 and to other text.[26, 27] Other assays with good performance characteristics have been developed, for example, high-performance liquid chromatography (HPLC) and radioreceptor assay, but practical considerations have limited their clinical utility.[28] Antibody-based assays are the preferred method for measurement of plasma cortisol. RIA is the most commonly used method, although other antibody-based methods have been developed. Because each antibody, whether polyclonal or monoclonal, has its own particular affinity and cross-reactivity with other plasma steroids, results vary from one assay to another (Table 118–1). However, all these assays measure total plasma cortisol. Because assays for plasma free cortisol, the biologically active fraction of total plasma cortisol, are not readily available for clinical use, measurement of salivary cortisol by RIA or competitive protein-binding assay has been suggested as an alternative procedure.[29, 30] Free cortisol diffuses freely from plasma into saliva and this process is relatively independent of the salivary flow rate.[31] Thus, salivary cortisol levels reflect plasma free cortisol better than do total plasma cortisol levels. Although initial studies are very promising and salivary cortisol measurements may be particularly useful in certain circumstances, for example, diurnal rhythm assessment, this method has not yet been adopted into routine clinical practice. In addition, intraindividual variation of baseline salivary cortisols and their response to low doses of dexamethasone may exceed that of plasma cortisol, raising concerns about test repeatability.[32, 33]

URINARY CORTISOL. The complex pattern of cortisol secretion has necessitated assessment of the cortisol secretory rate by means of measurement of urinary excretion of cortisol and its metabolites. Plasma free cortisol is filtered by the glomerulus and there is some tubular resorption. Although urinary cortisol constitutes less than 1% of daily cortisol secretion, it does integrate the day's serum free cortisol concentration and thus reflects the cortisol secretory rate. Measurement of urinary cortisol excretion by immunoassay or HPLC has replaced older methods.[34] Some older RIAs have higher normal ranges (20 to 90 to 100 μg/day; 55 to 250 to 285 nmol/day) than newer RIAs or HPLC because of cross-reactivity. The better immunoassays and HPLC typically have normal ranges of about 10 to 55 μg/day (27 to 150 nmol/day). However, even these assays are subject to artifacts; falsely high urinary cortisol results in the HPLC assay are observed in patients taking carbamazepine.[35] Because urinary cortisol reflects plasma free cortisol concentration and because the binding

TABLE 118–1. Serum Cortisol Response to Cosyntropin (Synacthen) in Healthy Volunteers According to Sex

		Method*			
Time (min)	Sex	*TDX*	*ACS*	*Delfia*	*DPC*
0	M	313 [166–527]	326 [186–578]	309 [164–475]	356 [203–573]
	F	368 [150–884]	352 [194–691]	309 [162–632]	424 [200–935]
30	M	750 [585–909]	705 [554–876]	689 [501–900]	786 [605–1040]
	F	871† [629–1456]	786‡ [543–1193]	729 [510–1383]	920‡ [586–1571]
60	M	888 [676–1077]	830 [624–998]	814 [553–956]	990 [632–1282]
	F	1066† [880–1879]	927‡ [662–1354]	897‡ [631–1317]	1057‡ [778–1834]
30–0	M	404 [238–552]	350 [120–509]	376 [218–533]	423 [219–698]
	F	509† [295–808]	406§ [193–607]	417 [216–673]	511 [206–773]
60–0	M	540 [344–716]	468 [254–660]	481 [221–657]	547 [255–864]
	F	681‡ [488–1037]	539‡ [351–742]	582‡ [337–830]	676§ [375–1037]

TDX (Abbott Diagnostics, Maidenhead, UK); ACS180 (Chiron Diagnostics, Halstead, UK); Delfia (Pharmacia Wallac, Milton Keynes, UK); Coat-a-Count (Diagnostic Products Corp. DRC, Llanveris, UK).

*Values are given as median [5th–95th percentiles], nmol/L.

†$P < .001$ vs. males.

‡$P < .01$ vs. males.

§$P < .05$ vs. males.

Modified from Clark PM, Neylon I, Raggatt PR, et al: Defining the normal cortisol response to the short Synacthen test: Implications for the investigation of hypothalamic-pituitary disorders. Clin Endocrinol 49:289, 1998.

capacity of CBG is nearly saturated at the peak episodes in a normal cortisol secretory rate, urinary cortisol levels increase rapidly when serum total cortisol concentrations exceed the binding capacity of CBG at about 25 μg/dL (690 nmol/L). Therefore, urinary cortisol excretion is a better indicator of endogenous cortisol secretory rate than it is an indicator of the adequacy of cortisol (hydrocortisone) replacement therapy (see below).

Measurement of cortisol precursors and cortisol metabolites is now limited to a few specific circumstances in clinical practice. For example, the plasma 11-deoxycortisol concentration, which is normally undetectable (i.e., <1 μg/dL or ~30 nmol/L at 8 AM) by current RIAs under basal conditions, is used to assess the CRH-ACTH-cortisol axis in the metyrapone test (see below).[35a] The 17-hydroxyprogesterone response to ACTH is used in the diagnosis of 21-hydroxylase (CYP21A2, P450c_{21}) deficiency. This cortisol precursor is usually measured by RIA. Assessment of urinary cortisone levels measured by HPLC may be useful in distinguishing factitious Cushing's syndrome due to ingestion of hydrocortisone from endogenous ACTH-independent Cushing's syndrome.[36, 37]

PLASMA ACTH. Measurement of ACTH is most readily accomplished with immunoassays, especially the two-site immunoradiometric assay (IRMA).[38] The episodic secretion, short plasma half-life (<10 minutes), rapid response to stress, and diurnal rhythm limit the utility of single samples, except under defined circumstances. Interpretation of plasma ACTH levels must be done in the context of simultaneous plasma cortisol levels (Fig. 118–2).[39] The reliability of ACTH measurements is also limited by the instability of ACTH in blood at room temperature and by its adherence to glass. Careful attention to sample collection and storage is essential, but these problems have been reduced with the use of plastic tubes and appropriate preservatives (e.g., ethylenediaminetetraacetic acid, EDTA). Normal ranges for ACTH are fairly broad and, like cortisol levels, are time-dependent. They also vary from assay to assay. A typical normal range for an 8 AM sample using an IRMA is from 10 to 50 pg/mL (2.2 and 12 pmol/L); levels are usually less than 20 pg/mL (4.5 pmol/L) at 4 PM and less than 5 to 10 pg/mL (1.1 to 2.2 pmol/L) at midnight. Older RIAs have somewhat wider ranges. Assays also vary in their cross-reactivity and interference by ACTH precursors and fragments (see Chapters 121 and 193). CRH can also be measured by RIA, but its clinical utility is limited.[40–42]

Dynamic Testing

Because the characteristics of the CRH-ACTH-cortisol axis limit the utility of single measurements of plasma cortisol, dynamic testing must be used. Both synthetic CRH and ACTH are available to assess the cortisol response to stimulation. In addition, other agents can be used to test the integrity of the system, for example, insulin-induced hypoglycemia, metyrapone, and dexamethasone. The uses of these agents are detailed in the context of the clinical questions below.

Avoiding Laboratory Errors and Getting Good Results

Even the endocrinologist who orders the appropriate tests relies on the tests to be performed correctly and measurements to be made accurately by the clinical laboratory. The most common sources of error in test performance relate to the difficulty in collecting 24-hour urine specimens properly; compliance with taking medication faithfully; and obtaining samples at the proper time. As diagnosis has shifted to the ambulatory setting, these difficulties, never trivial, have been compounded. Patients' and staff adherence to instructions requires careful education and reinforcement. Obtaining complete urine collections is particularly problematic. Although the completeness of the collection can be estimated based on measurement of creatinine excretion, the normal diurnal variation of cortisol secretion precludes accurate extrapolation of 24-hour cortisol excretion from an incomplete collection. Still, measurement of creatinine excretion is useful. As a rule of thumb, in adults under the age of 50 years, daily creatinine excretion should be 20 to 25 mg/kg (177 to 221 mmol/kg) lean body weight in men and 15 to 20 mg/kg (133 to 177 mmol/kg) lean body weight in women. From the ages of 50 to 90 years, there is a progressive 50% decline in creatinine excretion (to about 10 mg/kg in men), due primarily to a loss of muscle mass.[27]

Laboratories also vary in their reliability, quality-control procedures notwithstanding. In addition, some assays tend to be more reliable than others. Finally, interference with assays by drugs and other factors may produce misleading results. Rules of thumb have been suggested for detecting inconsistencies in the laboratory data. For example, 24-hour urinary steroid excretion reflects the integrated 24-hour plasma steroid concentration. The mean plasma cortisol concentration during the course of a day is about 220 nmol/L (8 μg/dL). Average daily urinary free cortisol is about 75 nmol (27 μg). Thus, multiplying the mean plasma cortisol (in nanomoles per liter) by 0.35 approximates 24-hour urinary excretion of free cortisol (in nanomoles) and multiplying the mean plasma cortisol (in micrograms per deciliter) by 3.5 approximates 24-hour urinary free cortisol (in micrograms).[27]

BASIC PRINCIPLES OF CLINICAL EPIDEMIOLOGY AND THEIR IMPLICATIONS FOR ASSESSMENT OF GLUCOCORTICOID FUNCTION

The evaluation of adrenal function begins with a clinical question. The more vague the question, the more difficult it is to obtain a clear

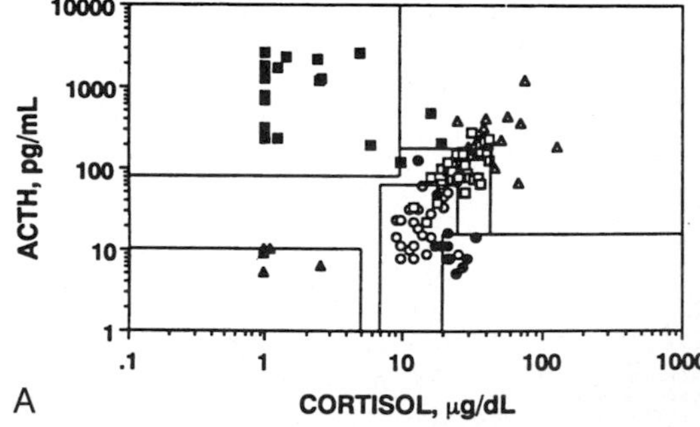

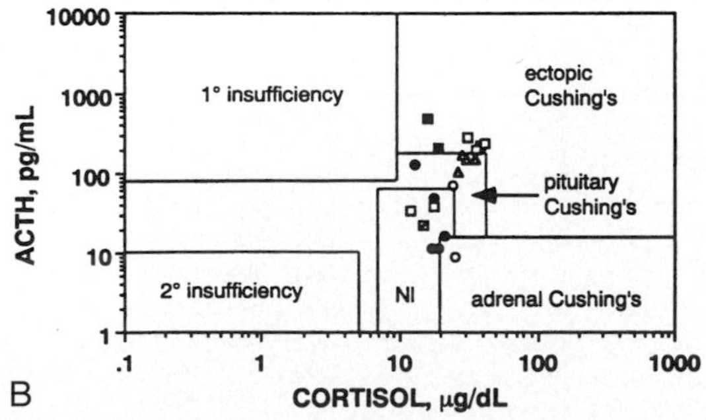

FIGURE 118–2. Plasma AM adrenocorticotropic hormone (ACTH, corticotropin) and AM cortisol values in adrenal dysfunction. *A,* Values from healthy normal subjects and from patients with adrenal dysfunction. Boundaries shown *(solid lines)* provide the best distinction among disease groups. *B,* Laboratory results that overlap into areas inconsistent with diagnosed disease. The crosshatched square was a repeat testing from a patient with pituitary-dependent Cushing's syndrome; the other value was within the range for pituitary-based Cushing's syndrome. Nl, normal; ○, healthy subjects; □, pituitary-dependent Cushing's syndrome; △, ectopic Cushing's syndrome; ●, adrenal-dependent Cushing's syndrome; ■, primary adrenal insufficiency; ▲, secondary adrenal insufficiency. (From Snow K, Jiang N, Kao P, Scheithauer B: Biochemical evaluation of adrenal dysfunction: The laboratory perspective. Mayo Clin Proc 67:1060, 1992.)

answer. Part of this step involves a clinical judgment about the likelihood of the disease prior to obtaining a test and its results. This pretest probability will be combined with the performance characteristics of the test and its use—sensitivity and specificity, receiver operating characteristic (ROC) curves, likelihood ratios, predictive values, and diagnostic accuracy—for proper interpretation.[43, 44] Use of diagnostic tests must take into account several types of variation: variability of the test itself; variability in the disease-free population; and variability in the population with disease. Clinicians must be aware of the distinction between efficacy and effectiveness when translating published results into practice. As applied to diagnostic testing, efficacy refers to the degree to which the test has been shown scientifically to accomplish the desired outcome. In contrast, effectiveness refers to the degree to which the test achieves this outcome in actual clinical practice. Most large studies have been performed in research venues and thus are efficacy studies, while the effectiveness of tests in practice has not been extensively evaluated. For example, in comparing one's own results with a published report or laboratory normal range, it is important to take into account those conditions, for example, tests done in hospital, clinical research center, or as an outpatient; accuracy in the clinical setting may not equal that in the experimental setting where many extraneous influences are controlled. This is a particular problem when evaluating the CRH-ACTH-cortisol axis.

There have also been relatively few studies on the reliability of measurements, that is, the degree of intraindividual variation. One study found that the minimum number of replicate measurements necessary to achieve satisfactory reliability of the mean (intraclass correlation coefficient = 0.8) of basal levels was 3 for plasma cortisol and 18 for salivary cortisol.[42] Responses to dynamic tests required fewer replicates to achieve the same reliability (one or two samples). In interpreting a test, the patient's result is usually compared with a normal range. In establishing a normal range, whether using parametric or nonparametric methods, some normal subjects will have values outside the limits of normal. For example, if the normal range is defined as encompassing the mean ±2 SD, 5% of disease-free subjects will have a result outside the limits of normal. Thus, a result outside normal limits is not equivalent to disease. Moreover, values within the normal range do not necessarily exclude disease. Frequently, that normal range is developed by using a reference group of people assumed (or shown) to be disease-free. Ideally, when using a test to exclude the diagnosis of Cushing's syndrome, the reference group should be made up of individuals who look like they have the disease, but do not. However, reference groups are usually made up of subjects who are readily accessible (medical students, laboratory technicians) and not more appropriate comparisons. In theory, sensitivity and specificity are characteristics of the test itself and not of the patients to whom the test is applied. However, this may not be correct in practice. The sensitivity of a test may be affected by the stage or severity of the disease and the specificity may depend upon the characteristics of the reference population. Sensitivity and specificity might be higher in a research study population than in a heterogeneous clinical setting. The nature of the groups used to establish the cut points that differentiate normal from abnormal must be appropriate and should be specified in any report of a diagnostic test. The value chosen for a cutoff point will also affect the sensitivity and specificity (see below).

In addition to the limitations on the operating characteristics based on the samples from which the data are derived, sensitivity and specificity are not independent of each other. They vary with the cutoff level chosen to represent positive and negative test results. In general, as sensitivity increases, specificity decreases, and as specificity increases, sensitivity decreases. This phenomenon is depicted graphically in an ROC curve.[45] In an ROC curve the true-positive rate (sensitivity) is plotted on the vertical axis and the false-positive rate (specificity) is plotted on the horizontal axis for different cutoff points for the test. A straight line is drawn (at 45 degrees when the axes are on the same scale) representing the hypothetical results of a test in which the true-positive rate equals the false-positive rate. Such a test provides no useful information. Ideally, a test would provide results that could be plotted on one point in the top left corner—a 100% true-positive rate and a 100% true-negative rate. Analysis of the area between the actual results and this straight line indicates how good the test is. The greater the area under the curve, the better the test. The curves may be used to decide an optimal cutoff level for a single test. ROC curves may also be used to compare two or more tests by comparing the areas under the curves, which represent the inherent accuracy of each test. It is important to remember, however, that ROC curves are only as good as the operating characteristics from which they are generated.

Tests can be combined in the hope that diagnostic accuracy is enhanced. Two tests can be performed in parallel (simultaneously) or in series (sequentially). When two tests are performed in parallel, a positive result in either test would establish the diagnosis; when two tests are performed in series, positive results in both tests are required to make the diagnosis. Thus, parallel testing increases sensitivity at the cost of specificity, while series testing increases specificity at the cost of sensitivity. For this approach to be better than one test alone, the second test has to provide information not provided by the first test. A common practice is to repeat the same test. This approach may be quite logical when the disorder is intermittently active, for example, periodic hormonogenesis in Cushing's syndrome, or when there is concern about the way the first test was performed. However, too often the same test is repeated until the desired results are obtained. When tests are performed in series, the first test is usually the one with the higher sensitivity so that many patients with the disease are picked up. False positives are then identified by a second test with higher specificity. Another approach to sequential testing uses as the first test the one with highest specificity so that fewer patients without the disease go on to further testing. This approach makes sense when the second test is associated with more morbidity. Adjusting cut points for the first test can make it 100% specific (at the cost of some sensitivity). This approach has been used frequently in tests related to Cushing's syndrome.[43, 46] One caveat applies to the method of choosing the cutoff point. In addition to considering whether the patients without the disease are an appropriate control group, attention should be paid to sample size. When the sample size is small, it cannot be assumed that the chosen cut point for 100% specificity will produce the same specificity when it is applied to other cases. For example, 95% confidence intervals for the sample are calculated by the formula mean ±1.96 SD. This formula will provide an estimate of results for the population as a whole. However, as the sample size decreases, the extent of the underestimation of the population value increases, and this underestimation increases faster when sample sizes are very small, for example, less than 10. The likelihood ratio, which is derived from sensitivity and specificity, is an expression of the odds that a sign, symptom, or test result would be expected in a patient with a given disease as opposed to one without. Finally, determining cost-effective diagnostic strategies requires careful evaluation not only of a test in isolation but also in the context of the other information available and the likelihood of disease. Consideration must be given to the question of the value added by a test or procedure. For example, traditionally, high-dose dexamethasone suppression testing has been utilized in the differential diagnosis of Cushing's syndrome. In one study, this test had a sensitivity and specificity of 81.0% and 66.7%, respectively.[47] However, using statistical models, this test added nothing to overall diagnostic accuracy after taking into account other clinical factors, including age, sex, duration of illness, serum potassium, plasma ACTH, and 24-hour urinary cortisol (Table 118–2).

Evaluation of a Patient for Cushing's Syndrome

Does the Patient Have Endogenous Glucocorticoid Excess?

The clinical suspicion of Cushing's syndrome must be confirmed with biochemical studies. Initially, a general assessment of the patient regarding the presence of other illnesses, drugs, alcohol, or psychiatric problems must be done since these factors may confound the evaluation. The use of exogenous glucocorticoids must be excluded. In addition to oral glucocorticoid therapy, most commonly prednisone, Cushing's syndrome can also be caused by intra-articular, epidural, topical, and inhaled glucocorticoids and by medroxyprogesterone acetate, a progestational agent with some intrinsic glucocorticoid activity.

TABLE 118–2. Logistic Regression Modeling of Probability of Cushing's Disease in Patients Who Underwent High-Dose Dexamethasone Test

Model	Variables	Sensitivity (%)	Specificity (%)	Diagnostic Accuracy (%)
1	Age, sex, duration, hypokalemia, urine free cortisol, plasma ACTH, suppression by ≥50%	100	80	95.6
2	Age, sex, duration, hypokalemia, urine free cortisol, plasma ACTH, % suppression	98.1	80	94.1
3	Age, sex, duration, hypokalemia, urine free cortisol, plasma ACTH	98.1	78.3	92.7
4	Duration, hypokalemia, plasma ACTH	98.1	66.7	91.2
5	Suppression by ≥50%			77.9
6	% Suppression			77.9

ACTH, adrenocorticotropic hormone.

Adapted from Aron DC, Raff H, Findling JW: Effectiveness versus efficacy: The limited value in clinical practice of high dose dexamethasone suppression testing in the differential diagnosis of adrenocorticotropin-dependent Cushing's syndrome. J Clin Endocrinol Metab 82:1784, 1997. © The Endocrine Society.

Surreptitious glucocorticoid intake or factitious Cushing's syndrome is rare, but it can be difficult to diagnose, especially if the patient is taking hydrocortisone.

In the majority of cases, the biochemical diagnosis of Cushing's syndrome can be easily performed in the ambulatory setting. The two most commonly used approaches to establishing the diagnosis of Cushing's syndrome are low-dose dexamethasone suppression testing and assessment of 24-hour urinary free cortisol. Other tests have been used, for example, assessment of diurnal rhythm and combined CRH-dexamethasone testing. Because none of the tests is perfect, and because the disorder is rare, there is little agreement about the most appropriate protocol to be used.[48] Some start with low-dose dexamethasone and confirm with urinary cortisol. Others start with urinary cortisol and confirm with assessment of diurnal rhythm. Parenthetically, recent studies in patients with adrenal incidentalomas and with diabetes suggest that the frequency of Cushing's syndrome, at least as defined by nonsuppressible cortisol secretion, is more common than previously thought.[48–50] As with most conditions, if the diagnosis is obvious clinically, then biochemical confirmation is usually simple; if the diagnosis is not clear, then biochemical confirmation or exclusion of the diagnosis is often much more difficult. A variety of strategies emerge. In fact, several attempts over a period of weeks or months may be necessary to establish or exclude the diagnosis in particularly difficult cases. Even then, the possibility of error will remain.[51]

Dexamethasone Suppression Test

RATIONALE. Cortisol secretion is regulated by feedback inhibition by glucocorticoids of CRH and ACTH. Glucocorticoid administration in supraphysiologic doses will result in suppression of endogenous cortisol secretion in normal individuals, but not in most patients with Cushing's syndrome.[52] Dexamethasone, which is not detected in the assay for cortisol, is used in doses three to four times the usual replacement dosage for the test period. This relatively high dose should consistently suppress normal pituitary ACTH secretion leading to reduction of cortisol secretion. Although the dexamethasone dose is higher than physiologic replacement, adverse effects are unusual, because only one or a few doses are necessary.

PROTOCOL 1. Overnight test: 1.0 mg of dexamethasone at 11 PM midnight and measurement of serum cortisol at 8 AM the next morning. A dose of 0.3 mg/m^2 body surface area can be used in children.

INTERPRETATION. A normal response is an 8 AM serum cortisol concentration of less than 5 μg/dL (<138 nmol/L). Serum cortisol concentrations greater than 275 nmol/L (10 μg/mL) are strongly suggestive of Cushing's syndrome, while levels between 5 and 10 μg/dL are equivocal.

PITFALLS. The overnight dexamethasone suppression test is commonly used as a screening test in the diagnosis of Cushing's syndrome.[48, 53–57] However, there are a large number of pitfalls in its interpretation.

TABLE 118–3. Single-Dose Overnight Dexamethasone Suppression Test*

	Normal Controls	Obese Controls†	Other Controls†	Cushing's Syndrome	Cortisol Assay‡	Morning Cortisol Upper Limit of Normal (μg/dL)
	119/120	19/19	—	0/9	PS	10
	16/16	20/20	10/20	0/17	PS	5.0
	44/44	33/40	—	1/10	DID	5.0
	30/30	18/18	33/42	0/3	F	10
	16/16	16/17	13/15	0/9	F	6.0
	39/39	—	45/71	—	F	7.0
	72/76	—	—	1/6	PS	10
	31/31	20/21	24/26	0/5	F	4.5
	7/7	2/2	—	0/20	PS	4.0
	50/50	7/15	—	1/24	F	7.0
	37/37	16/21	33/40	0/5	CPB	3.5
	—	—	—	0/13	F	3.8
	—	—	88/114	0/33	F	6.0
Totals (%)	461/466 (99)	151/173 (87)	246/320 (77)	3/154 (1.9)		

*The data are expressed as n/N where n is the number of subjects whose morning (8–9 AM) plasma cortisol levels are less than or equal to the indicated upper limit of normal following 1 mg (2 mg[85] and 1.5 mg[86]) of oral dexamethasone at 11 PM or midnight, and N is the total number of patients in each designated category.

†Obese controls include subjects with generalized and central obesity. Other controls include hospitalized and nonhospitalized patients with nonacute illnesses, except in reference 12 where other controls include normal and obese subjects and subjects with nonacute illnesses.

‡Details of these plasma cortisol assays are discussed in the text.

§Reference 2 is a review of the literature combined with a presentation of the authors' own data.

PS, Porter-Silber colorimetric reactions; DID, double-isotope derivative; F, fluorimetric reaction; CPB, competitive protein binding.

Adapted from Crapo L: Cushing's syndrome: A review of diagnostic tests. Metabolism 28:958, 1979.

What is the right cutoff for diagnosis? Crapo[53] reviewed a number of reports on this test and combined their results (Table 118–3). The sensitivity and specificity of the test were 98.1% and 98.9%, respectively. In the individual studies cited, sensitivity ranged from 83% to 100% and specificity from 77% to 100%. It is important to note that the data come from studies that differed in the cortisol assays, doses of dexamethasone, and criteria for a positive test. Caution must be exercised in drawing conclusions from such combined data. In order to apply the sensitivity and specificity of a test derived from one study sample to a different population, the test cannot deviate from the methods used (e.g., dose of dexamethasone, type of cortisol assay, timing of dexamethasone administration, and cortisol assay) when the optimal cutoff was determined, and the sample studied must be similar to the new population to be tested. To meet this last prerequisite, the sample studied must have accounted for the variability of diseased individuals, that is, defined subjects with disease using the best available gold standard (independent of the test in question) and included a broad-enough cross-section of those with disease (e.g., mild vs. severe disease, different causes of disease, as well as age, sex, and race) to establish a reliable range of measurements. The characteristics of the reference sample of subjects without the disease are equally important. Although the 1-mg overnight dexamethasone suppression test is still believed to have reasonably good sensitivity, it has serious problems with specificity, and false-positive results have been described with a variety of drugs as well as under medical, surgical, and psychiatric conditions. This is illustrated by the data in Crapo's review (Table 118–4). If the controls, that is, individuals without Cushing's syndrome, include, in addition to normals, the "obese" and "other controls," that is, hospitalized and nonhospitalized patients with nonacute illnesses, then the specificity falls to 89.5%. In fact, if only results from the "obese" and "other controls" are used, then the specificity is only 80.5%. Because of the relatively high false-positive rate, other criteria for suppression of plasma cortisol have been proposed; a cutoff point of 200 nmol/L (7.2 μg/dL) reduces the false-positive rate to 7.3% from 12% to 15%. However, by necessity, the false-negative rate increases. Similarly, because test sensitivity is less than 100% and this is a serious disease whose diagnosis one would like not to miss, cutoff points of 1.8 and 2.5 μg/dL have been proposed.[55, 57] However, such cutoff points, while missing fewer patients who really have the disease, will falsely identify more patients as having the disease (decreased specificity). Since total rather than free plasma cortisol is measured, false-positive results are observed in states of high CBG. For example, false-positive rates as high as 50% have been observed in women taking oral contraceptives.[58]

TABLE 118–4 Diagnosis of Cushing's Syndrome with the 1-mg Overnight Dexamethasone Suppression Test

Test Characteristics with Normal Controls

		Cushing's Syndrome	
		Present	*Absent*
1-mg overnight dexamethasone suppression test	No suppression	151	5
	Suppression	3	461

Sensitivity = 151/(151 + 3) = 98.1%; specificity = 461/(5 + 461) = 98.9%.

Test Characteristics with All Controls

		Cushing's Syndrome	
		Present	*Absent*
1-mg overnight dexamethasone suppression test	No suppression	151	101
	Suppression	3	858

Specificity = 858/(101 + 858) = 89.5%.

Test Characteristics with "Obese" and "Other" Controls

		Cushing's Syndrome	
		Present	*Absent*
1-mg overnight dexamethasone suppression test	No suppression	151	96
	Suppression	3	397

Specificity = 397/(96 + 397) = 80.5%.
Based on data from Crapo.[53]
From Danese RD, Aron DC: Principles of epidemiology and their application to the diagnosis of Cushing's syndrome: Rev. Bayes meets Dr. Cushing. Endocrinologist 5:342, 1999.

What are the sources of false negatives? Although a level of less than 5 μg/dL has been used in the past, several false-negative results have been discovered using this test criterion, presumably due to the exquisite sensitivity of glucocorticoid negative feedback in some patients with pituitary ACTH–dependent Cushing's syndrome (Cushing's disease), as well the occasional intermittent nature of the hypercortisolism (cyclic Cushing's syndrome and periodic hormonogenesis), that is, day-to-day variation.[48, 59, 60] This appears to be a particular problem in patients with mild hypercortisolism in whom the sensitivity of the test is as low as 55%. Thus, its use as a screening test in mild cases may be quite limited.

What are the sources of false positives? False-positive results of the overnight 1-mg dexamethasone suppression test may be caused by malabsorption, patients receiving drugs that accelerate dexamethasone metabolism (phenytoin, phenobarbital, rifampin) or drugs with estrogen action (hormone replacement therapy, oral contraceptives, tamoxifen), in patients with renal failure, in severe alcoholism, in patients suffering from endogenous depression, or in any patient undergoing a stressful event or serious illness.[61–67] The last may result in diagnostic difficulty because patients with Cushing's syndrome have a relatively high frequency of depression and are susceptible to infection. Patients who have the clinical features of Cushing's syndrome, but who lack biochemical confirmation are termed "pseudo–Cushing's syndrome."

Naturally, failure to take the dexamethasone will result in a false-positive test. Assuming that the patient has actually taken the dexamethasone, the drug must be absorbed properly and appropriate plasma levels achieved. Acceleration of dexamethasone degradation occurs in patients taking inducers of hepatic cytochrome P450 enzymes, such as barbiturates, phenytoin, rifampin, and aminoglutethimide.[68] Measurement of plasma dexamethasone may uncover this problem. Nomograms for cortisol and dexamethasone levels have been developed, although their use has been limited.[69] An alternative approach has been to use cortisol itself as the exogenous agent. The metabolism of cortisol is less affected by these drugs than that of dexamethasone. Corticosterone, a cortisol precursor, can be measured by RIA as an index of endogenous cortisol secretion.[70]

Chronic alcoholism may result in the clinical and biochemical features of Cushing's syndrome, including resistance to suppression with dexamethasone.[71] Abstinence is followed by resolution of the hormonal abnormalities. Abnormalities (hyperactivity) of hypothalamic-pituitary-adrenal function have been demonstrated in some psychiatric patients, particularly those with affective disorders.[72] These abnormalities in cortisol dynamics tend to mimic those of Cushing's syndrome. Cortisol secretion is increased (usually modestly). Diurnal variation may be absent because of the persistence of active cortisol secretion during the evening hours. Normally, because of its long half-life, 1 mg of dexamethasone will suppress ACTH and hence cortisol secretion for 24 hours. In some patients with depression, early escape from dexamethasone suppression is observed, that is, normally suppressed levels are found at 8 AM, but plasma cortisol levels are abnormally high at 4 PM. Although the dexamethasone suppression test has been advocated as a test for endogenous depression, the low specificity of the test limits its utility. The hormonal abnormalities disappear after remission of depression. Whether it has any role in clinical practice is not certain. However, depression is a common cause of a false-positive dexamethasone suppression test when looking for Cushing's syndrome. Because of the problems associated with this test, it should only be employed as a screening tool for the consideration of Cushing's syndrome; biochemical confirmation must rely on other studies.

PROTOCOL 2. Two-day test: First, at least one basal 24-hour urine collection is obtained for urinary cortisol and creatinine (usually 8 AM to 8 AM). Some also measure cortisol metabolites (17-OHCS). Immediately following, dexamethasone 0.5 mg is administered orally every 6 hours, usually at 8 AM, 2 PM, 8 PM, and 2 AM, for a total of eight doses, while the urine collection is continued. Dose modifications for children weighing less than 45 kg have been reported. Six hours after the last dexamethasone dose, the last urine collection is completed and blood can be drawn for measurement of cortisol and, if desired, plasma ACTH and dexamethasone.

INTERPRETATION. A normal response is a urine cortisol less than 10 μg (27 nmol)/24 hours on the second day of dexamethasone administration. In addition, urinary 17-OHCS excretion should fall to less than 2.5 mg (6.9 nmol)/day. The plasma cortisol level should be less than 5 μg/dL (140 nmol/L). Parenthetically, one would expect a plasma ACTH concentration of less than 5 pg/mL (1.1 pmol/L) and a plasma dexamethasone level of 2.0 to 6.5 ng/mL (5 to 17 nmol/L).

PITFALLS. Although it would seem that the 2-day test would be more reliable, it suffers from similar limitations as the overnight test. In addition, the risk of improper urine collection is added. Patients with mild hypercortisolism due to pituitary ACTH–dependent Cushing's syndrome may suppress urine steroid secretion to undetectable ranges with even low doses of dexamethasone. In addition, 15% to 25% of patients with a pseudo-Cushing's state (such as depression or alcoholism) may have false-positive tests. In patients with mild hypercortisolism, in whom one would hope that the test would be most helpful, the test has an accuracy of only 70% and a sensitivity of only 55%. However, in fairness, others have had better results even in this subset of patients.[48]

PROTOCOL 3. Intravenous tests: Dexamethasone 5 μg/kg/hour is administered from 10 AM to 3 PM. Plasma cortisol is obtained at 7 PM and at 8 AM the following morning.[73] Other protocols have been proposed.[74, 75]

INTERPRETATION. Obese patients had suppression of plasma cortisol to less than 1.4 μg/dL by 7 PM, while patients with Cushing's syndrome failed to suppress to less than 2.5 μg/dL at 7 PM and had levels exceeding 5 μg/dL at 8 AM the following morning.[73]

PITFALLS. Although intravenous administration of dexamethasone ensures that patients actually receive the drug and mitigates against the problems of malabsorption, the utility of this test relative to other protocols has not been confirmed.

Urine Free Cortisol

RATIONALE. Urinary cortisol secretion integrates the serum free cortisol concentration over 24 hours and thus reflects the cortisol secretory rate, particularly under normal circumstances, that is, when cortisol concentrations do not exceed the binding capacity of CBG.

PROTOCOL. A 24 hour urine collection is obtained (usually from 8 AM to 8 AM) for measurement of cortisol and creatinine.

INTERPRETATION. The normal range for urine cortisol is 20 to 90 μg (50 to 250 nmol)/24 hours when older RIAs are used. With newer and more specific RIAs or HPLC, the normal ranges typically are about 10 to 55 μg (27 to 150 nmol)/day.

PITFALLS. Essential to the performance of this test is an accurate and complete urine collection and measurement of cortisol by a good clinical laboratory. Assay artifacts are much less common with measurement of urine cortisol than with 17-OHCS. However, even with the best assays in the best hands, there are potential artifacts; falsely high urinary cortisol results in the HPLC assay are observed in patients taking carbamazepine.

What is the right cutoff for diagnosis? Sensitivity and specificity vary according to the urine free cortisol level chosen as the cutoff point (or operating position) to determine a positive test. An ROC curve can be used to assist in determining the optimal cutoff point. An example, based on data from Streeten et al.,[76] is shown in Figure 118–3. The optimal cutoff point may be chosen depending upon the purpose of the test; for purposes of screening, high sensitivity is required and therefore point A would be the appropriate operating position. The optimal cutoff may also be chosen depending upon health costs (morbidity and mortality associated with an error in diagnosis), financial costs, or the need for maximal information (the operating position giving the greatest increase in post-test probability).

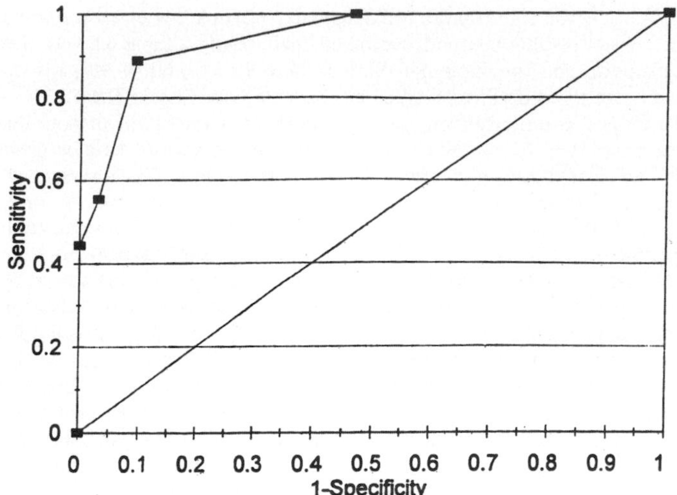

FIGURE 118–3. Receiver operating characteristic curve for urinary free cortisol based on data from Streeten et al.[76] DST, dexamethasone suppression test. (From Danese RD, Aron DC: Principles of epidemiology and their application to the diagnosis of Cushing's syndrome: Rev. Bayes meets Dr. Cushing. Endocrinologist 5:343, 1999.)

What are the sources of false negatives? Because there is a spectrum of normal CRH-ACTH-cortisol function, patients with early or mild Cushing's syndrome may have degrees of abnormality that overlap normal function. In addition, false negatives may be observed in patients with periodic hormonogenesis and cyclic Cushing's syndrome.[59, 60] Of note, in one series of 146 patients, 11% had at least one of four 24-hour collections with values within the normal range.[77] Patients with factitious Cushing's syndrome due to synthetic glucocorticoid ingestion may have low urine cortisol levels.

What are the sources of false positives? The cortisol production rate of obese patients may be increased and elevated levels of urinary 17-OHCS may lead to an erroneous diagnosis of Cushing's syndrome. Less than 5% of obese subjects will have mild elevations of urine free cortisol, although as many as 10% to 15% will have elevations of 17-OHCS excretion. False-positive results can be seen in patients with chronic alcoholism, depression, the syndrome of apparent mineralocorticoid excess, or any serious illness.[22, 62, 64, 71, 72, 78] Factitious Cushing's syndrome in a patient taking hydrocortisone will give a false-positive test, at least false in the sense of diagnosing endogenous Cushing's syndrome.[36]

Diurnal Rhythm and Midnight Cortisol Levels

RATIONALE. Normally, cortisol is secreted episodically with a diurnal rhythm paralleling the secretion of ACTH. Levels are usually highest early in the morning and decrease gradually throughout the day, reaching a nadir in the late evening. This normal nadir is maintained in obese and depressed patients, but usually not in those with Cushing's syndrome; the absence of a normal diurnal rhythm has been considered the hallmark of the diagnosis of Cushing's syndrome, although rare patients with the disease actually maintain a diurnal rhythm, albeit with a high cortisol set-point.[79, 80]

PROTOCOL. Plasma cortisol is measured at 8 AM, 4 PM, and midnight. More extensive day curves may be constructed by obtaining more plasma cortisol samples.

INTERPRETATION AND PITFALLS. Documenting the presence or absence of diurnal rhythm is difficult because single determinations obtained in the morning or evening are usually uninterpretable because of the pulsatility of pathologic and physiologic ACTH and cortisol secretion. Nonetheless, midnight serum cortisol levels in nonstressed patients provide good sensitivity and specificity for the diagnosis of Cushing's syndrome. In a study of 240 patients with Cushing's syndrome of different types and 23 patients with pseudo–Cushing's syndrome, a single midnight serum cortisol concentration greater than 7.5 μg/dL (207 nmol/L) had 96% sensitivity and 100% specificity.[81] This study was performed on sleeping patients in whom an intravenous line for blood sampling had been placed previously. Other studies have achieved similar or better diagnostic accuracy using an even lower cutoff point—less than 2 μg/dL (50 nmol/L).[82] Still others use a cutoff point of 5 μg/dL (138 nmol/L). However, these studies have been limited to research institutions and performed in hospital. Comparison of cortisol levels obtained in the sleeping state with those obtained in awake patients has not been performed. False positives may be observed in patients with severe illness of any type.[64] In addition, the degree of day-to-day variation in a given individual has not been evaluated. The stress of venipuncture may be sufficient to raise plasma cortisol levels in normal subjects, necessitating placement of an indwelling catheter prior to sampling. Having patients drive to the hospital at night to get a blood test is not likely to provide useful data. Until there are studies showing otherwise, this test should be performed only in sleeping patients. False-negative results can be seen in patients with cyclic or intermittent Cushing's syndrome. Since cortisol is secreted as free cortisol, the measurement of salivary cortisol may provide a simple more convenient means of probing nighttime cortisol secretion in a practical fashion. Studies have shown that patients with Cushing's syndrome have midnight salivary cortisol levels that usually exceed 0.4 μg/dL (normal range, 0.1 to 0.2 μg/dL).[83, 84] However, confirmation of the clinical effectiveness of this procedure is necessary. Timed urine collections from 10 PM to 11 PM or from 8 PM to midnight have been able to distinguish patients with Cushing's syndrome from normal subjects.[85, 86] Although a urine collection obviates the stress of venipuncture, proper collection remains an issue. Moreover, these studies did not include patients with pseudo–Cushing's syndrome, raising concern about their clinical utility.

Corticotropin-Releasing Hormone–Low-Dose Dexamethasone Suppression Test

RATIONALE. The hypercortisolism associated with pseudo Cushing's syndrome appears to be mediated via increased CRH secretion, although negative feedback of cortisol restrains the degree of endogenous cortisol secretion. In patients with Cushing's syndrome, CRH is suppressed due to the hypercortisolism. In general, Cushing's disease is more resistant to dexamethasone than in pseudo Cushing's syndrome and more sensitive to the stimulatory effect of exogenous CRH. This combined test takes advantage of these different responses to distinguish true Cushing's disease from a pseudo-Cushing's state.

PROTOCOL. The CRH test is performed 2 hours after the last 0.5-mg dose of dexamethasone in the standard 2-day low-dose dexamethasone suppression test. Synthetic ovine CRH 1 μg (200 nmol)/kg body weight is injected as an intravenous bolus. Blood samples for ACTH and cortisol are drawn 15 and 0 minutes before and 5, 10, 15, 30, 45, and 60 minutes after CRH injection.

INTERPRETATION. In one report, the serum cortisol concentration was less than 1.4 μg/dL (38 nmol/L) 15 minutes after CRH (given 2 hours after the last 0.5-dexamethasone dose in the standard 2-day low-dose dexamethasone test) in all 19 patients with pseudo–Cushing's syndrome vs. none of 35 patients with Cushing's disease, in none of 2 patients with ectopic ACTH secretion, and in none of 2 patients with primary adrenal disease (100% sensitivity and 100% specificity for Cushing's syndrome).[46] Similar low values were observed in a second study involving 20 normal subjects.[87] Comparison of this test with the dexamethasone suppression tests and CRH stimulation tests performed individually is shown in Table 118–5.

PITFALLS. Relatively few studies have been performed and the total number of patients studied is small. This test also requires a very sensitive plasma cortisol assay that is accurate at low levels. Such assay performance may not be readily achieved in routine clinical laboratory practice.

The Asymptomatic Patient with an Incidentally Discovered Adrenal Mass

The appropriate biochemical evaluation with an incidental adrenal mass and no clinical features of Cushing's syndrome is controversial. The most common functioning lesion in patients with an incidentally discovered adrenal mass appears to be the autonomous secretion of cortisol.[49, 88–90] Approximately 6% to 12% of patients with adrenal incidentalomas (and perhaps even more) ranging from 2 to 5 cm in diameter have pathologic cortisol secretion. These benign adrenal adenomas secrete small amounts of cortisol that are often not sufficient to elevate urine cortisol excretion, but are able to cause some suppression of the hypothalamic-pituitary axis.[49, 88–90] These patients may be identified by their failure to suppress cortisol to less than 3 μg/dL following an overnight 1-mg dexamethasone suppression test. As noted above, dexamethasone suppression testing has limited specificity, especially when a low dose is utilized. In one report, the investigators found that 15% of those with adrenal incidentalomas had decreased suppression of cortisol in response to dexamethasone 1 mg compared

TABLE 118–5. Comparison of Criteria Chosen to Yield 100% Specificity for Diagnosis of Cushing's Syndrome in 58 Patients with Mild Hypercortisolism

Test Variable*	Criterion	Specificity (%)	Sensitivity (%)	Positive Predictive Value (%)	Negative Predictive Value (%)	Diagnostic Accuracy (%)
Low-Dose Dexamethasone Test						
17-OHCS day 4	>11.0 μmol/d	74	69	84	54	71
17-OHCS day 4	>14.6 μmol/d	100	54	100	51	69
Urine free cortisol day 4	>100 nmol/d	100	56	100	53	71
CRH Test without Dexamethasone Pretreatment						
Cortisol sum of post-CRH levels	>3450 nmol/L	100	64	100	58	76
CRH test peak corticotropin	>35.0 pmol/L	100	13	100	36	41
Dexamethasone-CRH Test						
Basal cortisol (before CRH)	>38.0 nmol/L	100	90	100	84	91
Cortisol 15 min after CRH	>38.0 nmol/L	100	100†‡	100	100†‡	100†‡
Corticotropin 30 min after CRH	>3.5 pmol/L	100	74	100	66	83

*Criteria for each test variable were derived from receiver operating characteristic analysis.[24] Results are given for the standard low-dose dexamethasone criterion of 17-hydroxycorticosteroid (17-OHCS) excretion levels greater than 11 μmol/day and for criteria chosen to yield 100% specificity for the diagnosis of Cushing's syndrome. When the tests are compared under these conditions, the dexamethasone–corticotropin-releasing hormone (CRH) test, 15-minute cortisol value has a significantly greater sensitivity and diagnostic accuracy than any of the other tests.

†$P < .01$, dexamethasone–CRH test 15-minute cortisol vs. low-dose dexamethasone suppression test, or CRH test performed without dexamethasone pretreatment.

‡$P < .05$, dexamethasone–CRH test 15-minute cortisol vs. dexamethasone–CRH test basal cortisol or dexamethasone–CRH corticotropin.

Modified from Yanovski JA, Cutler GB Jr, Chrousos GP, Nieman LK: Corticotropin-releasing hormone stimulation following low-dose dexamethasone administration. A new test to distinguish Cushing's syndrome from pseudo-Cushing's states. JAMA 269:2235, 1993. Reproduced with permission.

with 8% of controls, a specificity of only 92%, assuming the controls truly did not have the disease. In another study, clinically euadrenal controls suppressed plasma cortisol levels to less than 28 nmol/L, while 57 patients with adrenal incidentalomas had postdexamethasone cortisol levels ranging from undetectable to 216 nmol; 12% had cortisol levels less than 140 nmol/L and 67% had cortisol levels between 28 and 140 nmol/L.[49] However, since the diagnosis of ACTH-dependent Cushing's syndrome is not a consideration, only a high-dose test (discussed in Chapter 121), such as the overnight 8-mg test, needs to be employed. This test has high sensitivity for Cushing's syndrome resulting from adrenal tumors and is likely to have higher specificity than the 1-mg test. Some have suggested an intermediate dose, for example, 3 mg, which would be expected to be equally sensitive to, but more specific than, the 1-mg test. In addition, the basal levels of ACTH in these patients tend to be subnormal or frankly suppressed. CRH by itself has had limited use in distinguishing mild Cushing's syndrome from the pseudo-Cushing's state, but may be useful to distinguish adrenal autonomy from normal. Blunted responses to CRH have been observed in 20% to more than 70% of cases of "preclinical" Cushing's syndrome.[49, 91, 92]

Response to Therapy of Cushing's Syndrome

Has the patient who has been treated for glucocorticoid excess been "cured" or "controlled"?

Following successful surgical therapy of Cushing's syndrome, most patients will develop a period of secondary adrenal insufficiency. A period of hypocortisolemia (low, especially undetectable, morning plasma cortisol and low urine cortisol) predicts remission, although not with 100% accuracy.[93] In addition, in some successfully treated patients, there is a postoperative reduction in cortisol levels, but not actual hypocortisolemia. There should also be a return to normal dexamethasone suppressibility. However, exceptions to every test have been reported. Other tests have been proposed, for example, the cortisol response to metyrapone (see below).[94]

Differential Diagnosis

The epidemiologic considerations for diagnosis of Cushing's syndrome also apply to the determination of the cause of the disorder. The differential diagnosis of Cushing's syndrome is often difficult and should always be performed in consultation with, or by an endocrinologist experienced with this disorder. The introduction of several technological advances over the past 10 to 15 years, including a specific and sensitive immunometric assay for ACTH, the CRH stimulation test, inferior petrosal sinus sampling, and computed tomography (CT) and magnetic resonance imaging (MRI) of the pituitary and adrenal glands have all provided means for an accurate differential diagnosis.

Evaluation of a Patient for Adrenal Insufficiency

Does the Patient Have Glucocorticoid Deficiency Now?

The biochemical confirmation of adrenal insufficiency requires the demonstration of inappropriately low cortisol production.[95] The diagnostic approach varies depending upon the clinical state of the patient; different questions demand different strategies.

Basal Hormone Levels in the Unstressed State

PLASMA CORTISOL. Because of the nature of episodic secretion, single randomly drawn cortisol levels in the unstressed state are of limited utility. Because plasma cortisol levels are usually low in the late afternoon and evening, reflecting the normal diurnal rhythm, samples drawn at these times are of virtually no value for this diagnosis. Plasma cortisol levels are usually highest in the early morning. Although samples drawn in the morning may provide more information, there is considerable overlap between adrenal insufficiency and normal. A plasma cortisol level less than 138 nmol/L (5 μg/dL) at 8 AM strongly suggests the diagnosis; the lower the level, the more likely the diagnosis. Conversely, a plasma cortisol level greater than 20 μg/dL (550 nmol/L) virtually excludes the diagnosis. Similarly, a salivary cortisol level less than 5 nmol/L (1.8 ng/mL) at 8 AM strongly suggests adrenal insufficiency, while levels in excess of 16 nmol/L (5.8 ng/mL) greatly reduce the probability of the diagnosis. Plasma cortisol levels between 5 and 10 μg/dL at least raise the possibility of adrenal insufficiency, but intermediate levels (10 to 20 μg/dL) are less helpful. Basal plasma cortisol levels in excess of 275 nmol/L (10 μg/dL) generally predict normal cortisol responsiveness to administration of ACTH or to insulin-induced hypoglycemia, but do not exclude the possibility of secondary adrenal insufficiency.[96] Even here there are exceptions. In a study of 21 patients with Addison's disease, the baseline cortisol levels ranged from less than 20 nmol/L to 410 nmol/L.[96a] Of the three patients with baseline cortisol levels greater than 275 nmol/L, none had an adequate response to ACTH.

URINE CORTISOL. In frank adrenal insufficiency, the cortisol secretory rate is decreased even under basal unstressed conditions. In this circumstance, basal 24-hour urinary cortisol levels (and levels of cortisol metabolites, e.g., 17-OHCS) will be low. However, in patients with partial adrenal insufficiency, basal urine cortisol levels may overlap the normal range, albeit usually at the lower extreme. Thus, this test is of limited diagnostic use.

PLASMA ACTH. In patients with untreated *primary* adrenal insufficiency, plasma ACTH levels exceed the upper limit of the normal range (>50 pg/mL) and usually exceed 200 pg/mL (44 pmol/L). Plasma ACTH concentration is usually less than 30 pg/mL (6.8 pmol/L) in patients with secondary adrenal insufficiency. However, the basal ACTH level must always be interpreted in light of the clinical situation, especially because of the episodic nature of ACTH secretion and its short plasma half-life. For example, ACTH levels will frequently exceed the normal range during recovery of the CRH-ACTH-cortisol axis from secondary adrenal insufficiency and may be confused with levels seen in primary adrenal insufficiency. Patients with untreated primary adrenal insufficiency *consistently* have elevated ACTH levels. In fact, the ACTH concentration will be elevated early in the course of adrenal insufficiency even before a significant reduction in the basal cortisol level or its response to exogenous ACTH occurs. Therefore, plasma ACTH measurements may serve as a valuable screening study for *primary* adrenal insufficiency. Parenthetically, in a patient with established adrenal insufficiency, plasma ACTH will localize the cause—adrenal vs. pituitary or hypothalamus (see Chapter 120). In treated primary adrenal insufficiency, plasma ACTH levels fall toward the normal range. Because of the dose and timing of physiologic replacement, plasma ACTH levels usually remain in the high-normal to modestly elevated range.[97–100]

Hormone Levels in the Stressed State

When a patient presents with signs and symptoms consistent with acute adrenal insufficiency (adrenal or "addisonian" crisis), then the clinician's priority shifts from diagnosis to treatment. The most expeditious diagnostic strategy consists of obtaining plasma cortisol and ACTH samples and then immediately treating the patient for adrenal insufficiency while awaiting the results. Under conditions such as hypotension and sepsis, one would expect the plasma cortisol concentration to be elevated, that is, greater than 20 μg/dL. Some have suggested the performance of a short ACTH stimulation test (see below) with the administration of dexamethasone after the baseline cortisol and ACTH samples are obtained. The degree to which this strategy improves overall diagnostic accuracy is unknown. When the patient is not acutely ill and there is time to safely perform an ACTH stimulation test without concomitant glucocorticoid replacement, then this approach is preferred. However, even under these circumstances, a single plasma cortisol level may be predictive. In one study of hospitalized patients basal plasma cortisol levels that ranged from 288 to 1585 nmol/L (mean, 706 nmol/L) correlated with cortisol response to ACTH administration.[2] It is essential that the plasma ACTH sample be obtained prior to initiation of glucocorticoid therapy because the latter will suppress ACTH levels. If a patient has been treated with glucocorticoids, time must elapse before a valid assessment of the ACTH level can be made—24 hours after the last dose of hydrocortisone and even longer after the last dose of prednisone or dexamethasone. When necessary and only if safe to do so, the 8 AM plasma ACTH concentration can be assessed after the patient has been switched to physiologic replacement with hydrocortisone. Since assessment of the plasma ACTH level under these circumstances assists only in differentiating primary from secondary adrenal insufficiency and not in establishing the diagnosis of adrenal insufficiency, and since this differentiation can be accomplished by other means, it may be unnecessary to discontinue glucocorticoid therapy. In contrast to measurement of plasma cortisol, there is no role for measurement of baseline urine cortisol or its metabolites in the setting of an acutely ill patient.

Dynamic and Stimulation Testing

For the reasons noted above and because of the need to establish the diagnosis of adrenal insufficiency before the patient presents in acute distress, dynamic testing has been favored over baseline measurements. Dynamic testing of different portions of the CRH-ACTH-cortisol axis allows for greater diagnostic accuracy, with both greater sensitivity and specificity. When cortisol response to stimulation is combined with measurement of ACTH concentration, differentiation between primary and secondary adrenal insufficiency can be made. In addition, the CRH stimulation test can differentiate pituitary from hypothalamic causes. Besides the standard tests—ACTH stimulation, metyrapone test, CRH infusion, and insulin-induced hypoglycemia—other tests have been proposed, for example, vasopressin infusion and naloxone tests.[101] The role of these other tests in clinical practice is uncertain.

ACTH Stimulation Test

RATIONALE. ACTH administration will stimulate the zona fasciculata to synthesize and secrete cortisol. A variety of doses and durations have been proposed. In theory, at least, patients with both primary and secondary insufficiency would fail to demonstrate an appropriate cortisol response to a brief infusion of ACTH; in primary adrenal insufficiency, there is inadequate adrenal tissue to respond, while in secondary adrenal insufficiency, the loss of the trophic action of ACTH results in adrenal atrophy. In contrast, with long infusions, patients with secondary adrenal insufficiency respond. In this chapter, we limit the discussion to short infusion tests because of their greater practicality. The prolonged ACTH stimulation tests are seldom performed because sensitive assays of plasma ACTH used in conjunction with the 30-minute ACTH test provide the necessary information. A short ACTH stimulation test using the currently available synthetic peptide can be performed in virtually anyone. Synthetic ACTH (1–24) (cosyntropin, Cortrosyn, Synacthen) has the full biologic potency of native ACTH (1–39) and side effects of administration are exceedingly rare. Because the zona glomerulosa responds acutely to ACTH, the assessment of the aldosterone response to ACTH has been proposed as a method to detect primary adrenal insufficiency (see Chapter 120).[102, 103]

PROTOCOL 1. High-dose test: A 250-μg bolus is given intravenously or intramuscularly. With such a dose, the peak concentration of ACTH achieves a pharmacologic level exceeding 10,000 pg/mL; this study assesses maximal adrenocortical capacity. Samples for plasma cortisol are obtained at time 0 and at 30 and 60 minutes.

PROTOCOL 2. Low-dose test: A 1-μg or 0.5-μg/1.73 m^2 body surface area bolus is administered intravenously. With such a dose, the peak concentration of ACTH achieves a level of about 450 to 1900 pg/mL which still exceeds, but more closely approximates, the levels observed in metyrapone testing or acute illness.[104, 105] Samples for plasma cortisol are obtained at time 0 and at 30 minutes.

INTERPRETATION. In general, the peak cortisol response, 30 to 60 minutes later, should exceed 18 to 20 μg/dL (>500 to 550 nm/L), but there is considerable variation among assays[53, 54, 104, 106–112] (see Table 118–1). Criteria involving minimum increments in cortisol secretion lack validity; a stressed patient may be maximally stimulated at baseline. In fact, a cortisol level of greater than 20 μg/dL at any time during the test effectively excludes primary adrenal insufficiency. A normal response excludes the diagnosis of primary adrenal insufficiency, while a subnormal response establishes the presence of adrenal insufficiency but does not establish the cause, that is, primary vs. secondary.

PITFALLS. The major problem associated with short ACTH tests is the sensitivity for secondary adrenal insufficiency.[104, 113–121] The high-dose test has relatively low sensitivity for secondary adrenal insufficiency, especially if it is partial or of recent onset, for example, following pituitary surgery. In these circumstances, the degree of atrophy of the zona fasciculata is limited so that some responsiveness to ACTH is maintained. The more physiologic dose administered in the 1-μg test is designed to improve this sensitivity.[104, 122–125] The cortisol response to 1 μg of ACTH correlates better with the cortisol response to insulin-induced hypoglycemia in patients with chronic secondary adrenal insufficiency. However, the results in secondary adrenal insufficiency of recent onset are less reliable.[126] Performance of the 1-μg test is also associated with some technical problems. Currently available vials of ACTH contain 250 μg; there are no ready-to-use vials containing 1 μg. Consequently, appropriate dilutions must be prepared and special care must be taken because doses lower than 1 μg will produce significantly lower responses and the established criteria will not apply.[127] In contrast to the 250-μg test, the 1-μg test has been evaluated only after intravenous injection; criteria for response to intramuscular administration have not been established and this mode of administration should not be used. In addition criteria for aldosterone response to ACTH have not been established with the 1-μg dose. Finally, there is controversy about the diagnostic criteria for the 1-μg test.[105, 128–131] Even should this issue be resolved, clinicians must be wary of comparisons of different cortisol assays (see above). These problems notwithstanding, the low-dose (1-μg) ACTH stimulation test is gaining greater acceptance and may emerge as the diagnostic procedure of choice in suspected secondary adrenal insufficiency (unless the cost of CRH is greatly reduced).

Metyrapone Test

RATIONALE. The metyrapone stimulation test assesses the entire CRH-ACTH-cortisol axis. Metyrapone inhibits the enzyme CYP11B1 (11β-hydroxylase, P450c_{11}) and thus blocks the last step in the synthesis of cortisol, the conversion of 11-deoxycortisol to cortisol. The decreased levels of cortisol reduce the negative feedback inhibition of CRH and ACTH secretion. Consequently, the levels of these two peptide hormones rise and steroid synthesis up to the point of the blockade is increased. The level of 11-deoxycortisol (along with ACTH) can be measured. This test is particularly sensitive, even for partial pituitary ACTH deficiency, because reduction in the level of negative feedback by cortisol is less of a stimulus to CRH secretion than is hypoglycemia. There are several protocols for this test. Only the overnight test, which relies on measurements of plasma and not urine, is presented. The overnight test appears to be as reliable as the multiday tests. Because this test depends on reduction in negative feedback, it is essential that the patient not be taking any glucocorticoid.

PROTOCOL. Overnight single-dose metyrapone test: A single dose of metyrapone based on the patient's weight is administered orally at midnight with a snack (to reduce gastrointestinal upset). The dose of metyrapone is as follows: 30 mg/kg body weight, or 2 g for patients weighing less than 70 kg, 2.5 g for patients 70 to 90 kg, and 3 g for patients greater than 90 kg body weight.[132, 133] Plasma 11-deoxycortisol and cortisol levels are measured at 8 AM the following morning. A sample for plasma ACTH level can also be obtained.

INTERPRETATION. The test requires adequate blockade of cortisol synthesis; the plasma cortisol level at 8 AM should be less than 138 nmol/L (5 μg/dL). Assuming this to be the case, the plasma 11-deoxycortisol concentration should exceed 210 nmol/L (7 μg/dL). Measurement of ACTH will distinguish primary from secondary adrenal insufficiency; a normal ACTH response consists of a level exceeding about 17 pmol/L (75 pg/mL).[134–137]

PITFALLS. This test is not without some risk and should probably not be performed in a patient who is already symptomatic from glucocorticoid deficiency. Because metyrapone administration will reduce cortisol synthesis, symptoms of glucocorticoid deficiency (nausea, vomiting, and hypotension) may develop during the test. Symptomatic treatment, that is, volume repletion, is usually adequate to permit completion of the test. This test should not be performed in the outpatient setting in a patient in whom there is a high pretest probability of adrenal insufficiency. Although the sensitivity of the metyrapone test is excellent, its specificity is less well established.[134–138] For example, an abnormal response to metyrapone with a normal response to hypoglycemia has been observed in steroid-treated patients.[109, 135] False-positive tests are observed in patients taking glucocorticoids. Particularly problematic would be a patient taking dexamethasone; the 8 AM cortisol level would be low, suggesting adequate blockade. The clearance of metyrapone is increased by inducers of hepatic cytochrome P450 enzymes (e.g., phenytoin, phenobarbital, rifampin, and mitotane). In addition, some people, as many as 4% of the population, normally exhibit rapid metyrapone clearance. In this case, there will be inadequate blockade of cortisol synthesis. Plasma 11-deoxycortisol levels may be high in a variety of conditions: oral contraceptive use, hypothyroidism, congestive heart failure, chronic renal failure, diabetes, and obesity.[136] The availability of metyrapone itself is quite variable.

Corticotropin-Releasing Hormone Stimulation Test

RATIONALE. CRH will stimulate the pituitary corticotrophs to secrete ACTH which in turn will stimulate the zona fasciculata to synthesize and secrete cortisol. CRH is expensive and this test is not generally used to establish a diagnosis of adrenal insufficiency. It can be used to distinguish between CRH deficiency and ACTH deficiency and thus it is most useful as a test of pituitary function, although the clinical utility of such a biochemical distinction is limited.[139, 140]

PROTOCOL. The test is performed with the patient in a fasting state, preferably an overnight fast. An intravenous line is placed at least 15 minutes prior to collection of the first sample. Baseline samples for ACTH and cortisol are obtained 15 minutes and just prior to the administration of synthetic ovine CRH. (Ovine CRH has a similar potency to human CRH, but has a longer duration of action.[141]) CRH 100 μg or 1 μg (200 nmol)/kg body weight is injected as an intravenous bolus. Blood samples are then obtained at 5, 10, 15, 30, 45, 60, 90, and 120 minutes following the injection. Protocols with less extensive sampling have been proposed, for example, plasma ACTH at 0, 15, and 30 minutes and cortisol at −15, 0, 45, and 60 minutes. Mild side effects, especially facial flushing and dyspnea, are common, so the patient should be warned.

INTERPRETATION AND PITFALLS. The normal ACTH and cortisol responses to ovine CRH have been defined as a 35% increase in the basal plasma ACTH level and a 20% increase in the basal plasma cortisol level. The responses in normal persons are quite variable both between individuals and within a single individual tested on multiple occasions. Patients with secondary adrenal insufficiency due to pituitary ACTH deficiency have decreased plasma ACTH and cortisol responses to CRH, while patients with hypothalamic CRH deficiency tend to have exaggerated and prolonged plasma ACTH responses with subnormal plasma cortisol responses. In contrast, patients with primary adrenal deficiency have high baseline ACTH levels and exaggerated responses to CRH; the plasma cortisol concentrations are low before and after CRH injection. Naturally, subnormal cortisol responses are observed. Because the differentiation between primary and secondary adrenal insufficiency can be made by measurement of baseline ACTH levels alone, the CRH test is not necessary. The CRH test may be useful in the assessment of recovery of the CRH-ACTH-cortisol axis in patients who have received chronic glucocorticoid therapy.[142]

Insulin-Induced Hypoglycemia Test

RATIONALE. Insulin-induced hypoglycemia assesses the entire CRH-ACTH-cortisol axis. Normally, hypoglycemia is a potent stimulator of CRH secretion, which will in turn increase ACTH secretion and then cortisol secretion.

PROTOCOL. This test is associated with significant risk and is contraindicated in the presence of ischemic heart disease, cerebrovascular disease, or seizure disorder. It is rarely necessary in any patient in whom the pretest probability of adrenal insufficiency is reasonably high. It should not be performed in patients in whom the baseline morning cortisol is less than 3 to 5 μg/dL. The test is performed under constant medical supervision with ready availability of intravenous dextrose. The patient should be in a fasting state, preferably an overnight fast. An intravenous line is placed at least 15 minutes prior to collection of the first sample. Insulin is administered intravenously. Although the standard dose is 0.1 μg/kg, the dose should depend on the pretest probability of adrenal insufficiency. If the probability is high, then a low initial dose should be used, for example, 0.5 μg/kg. Cortisol samples should be obtained at 0, 30, 45, 60, 90, and 120 minutes following the injection. ACTH samples may also be obtained. A valid test requires documented blood glucose less than 40 mg/dL and symptoms and signs of hypoglycemia (e.g., diaphoresis and tachycardia). If there is severe or prolonged (>20 minutes) hypoglycemia or a decline in mental status, it may be necessary to administer intravenous glucose, but sampling should be continued. Following completion of the test, the patient should receive food.

INTERPRETATION AND PITFALLS. A normal cortisol response is a peak greater than 20 μg/dL. The normal rise in cortisol level is usually greater than 6 μg/dL. The major drawback of this test relates to safety concerns in patients with a high pretest probability of disease. Its use outside the research or academic practice setting has been reduced greatly, if not eliminated entirely, as attractive alternatives have been developed.

Can the Patient Respond to Stress?

The clinical presentation of glucocorticoid deficiency depends upon the rate and degree of adrenocortical destruction or atrophy plus those extra-adrenal factors which may precipitate an acute crisis. Frank adrenal insufficiency requires the destruction of 80% to 90% of both adrenal glands. Destruction is gradual in most cases. As the destruction of the adrenal glands progresses, compensatory increases in ACTH and angiotensin II stimulate the failing adrenals and adequate basal secretion may be maintained. Therefore, before complete insufficiency occurs, there is a phase characterized by normal basal steroid secretion but with inability to respond to stress, that is, decreased adrenal reserve. However, when stressed with an infection, surgery, or trauma, the adrenals are unable to respond normally. An analogous situation pertains to the patient who has received chronic glucocorticoid therapy. The gold standard assessment of a patient's ability to respond to stress can be accomplished by measuring the response to insulin-induced hypoglycemia. However, this whole area is controversial for several reasons. First, it is not clear that a maximal adrenal response to stress is necessary for survival in the acute situation.[64, 143, 144] Second, while in most cases the cortisol response to other stimulation tests (e.g., the short ACTH stimulation test) correlate with the response to insulin-induced hypoglycemia, even in patients with discordant results, the clinical sequelae are not clear. As a general rule, patients with normal responses to ACTH stimulation do not require glucocorticoid supplementation for stress. However, an exception should be made and special caution taken in patients with ACTH deficiency of recent onset, for example, post pituitary surgery. They may have normal responses to ACTH stimulation because adrenal atrophy has not occurred yet, but be utterly unable to increase their endogenous ACTH secretion. Such patients will require glucocorticoid supplementation for stress and surgery. Similar caution may be necessary in patients who have received potent inhaled glucocorticoids.

Is the Patient in the Unstressed State Taking the Appropriate Replacement Dose of Cortisol?

Traditionally, assessment of the adequacy of glucocorticoid replacement has involved clinical, but not biochemical measures.[145] Plasma cortisol day curves, that is, multiple samples for plasma cortisol concentration, have been proposed, but not widely adopted. Two major factors have prompted a reassessment of this issue. First, there is a greater appreciation of the potential risks of over- or under treatment. Recent evidence suggests that subclinical Cushing's syndrome associated with adrenal incidentalomas contributes to poor control of blood sugar and blood pressure in diabetic patients, decreased bone turnover, and increased serum lipid levels.[88, 146–148] The levels of cortisol secretion by many incidentalomas are similar to those observed in patients with adrenal insufficiency receiving mild cortisol overreplacement. In addition, studies in patients on glucocorticoid replacement demonstrate an inverse relationship between dose and bone mineral density and a positive correlation between dose and markers of bone resorption. Second, there is recognition that there is considerable variation among individuals in terms of the plasma levels of cortisol achieved with orally administered hydrocortisone or cortisol[149] (Fig. 118–4). Using a simplified protocol for plasma cortisol day curves (cortisol levels at 9 AM, 12:30 PM (prior to any lunchtime dose), and 5:30 PM (prior to the evening), Howlett[149] found that an optimal replacement regimen would require thrice-daily dosing with an appropriate starting dose of 10 mg on rising, 5 mg at lunch, and 5 mg in the evening (Fig. 118–5). Although use of 24-hour urinary cortisol levels might seem an attractive method for following such patients, there are serious limitations. In one study, a significant correlation was found between *peak* plasma cortisol levels and 24-hour urine cortisol or creatinine levels.[150] However, in addition to the problems inherent in obtaining complete urine collections, there is considerable variation among individuals.[149] Moreover, the correlation between the mean cortisol and the urine results was less strong, probably related to the modulating effects of CBG. A very high level of urinary cortisol would suggest overreplacement, but by no means confirm it. There are still problems with plasma cortisol day curves. For example, the criteria for appropriate replacement are somewhat arbitrary. Management of patients with abnormally high (or low) concentrations of CBG would be problematic. This discussion has been predicated on the use of hydrocortisone as replacement therapy. The use of other glucocorticoids, for example, prednisone, could not be assessed with these measures. In addition, there is no easy way to account for differential sensitivity to glucocorticoids. It is clear that what are lacking are good, that is, sensitive, specific, and practical, measures of glucocorticoid action.

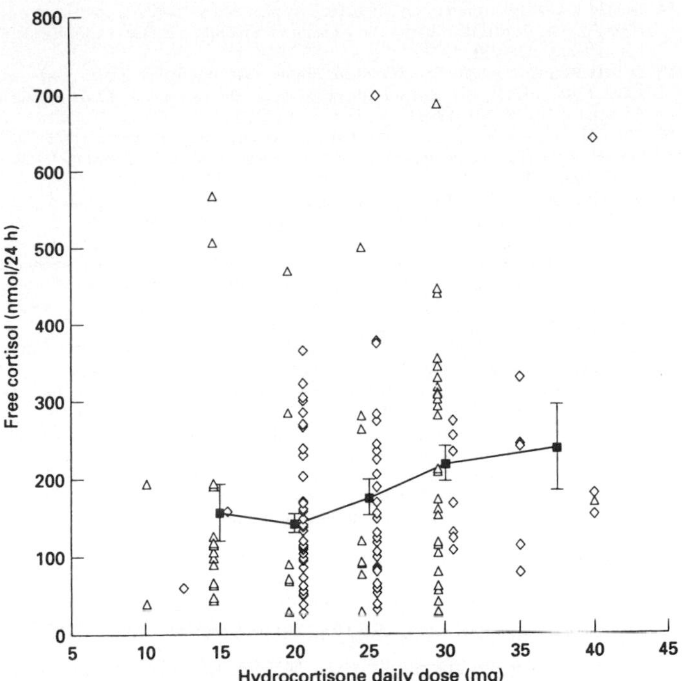

FIGURE 118–5. Comparison of urine free cortisol (UFC) with total daily dose of hydrocortisone. △, individual values in patients on twice-daily regimens; ◇, individual values in patients on thrice-daily regimens; ■, mean value for each hydrocortisone dose (error bars represent SEM). Mean UFC was significantly higher after 30 mg than after 20 mg total daily dose of hydrocortisone ($P < .001$ by t-test). Reference range for the normal population, 28–200 nmol/24 hours. (From Howlett TA: An assessment of optimal hydrocortisone replacement therapy. Clin Endocrinol 46:266, 1997.)

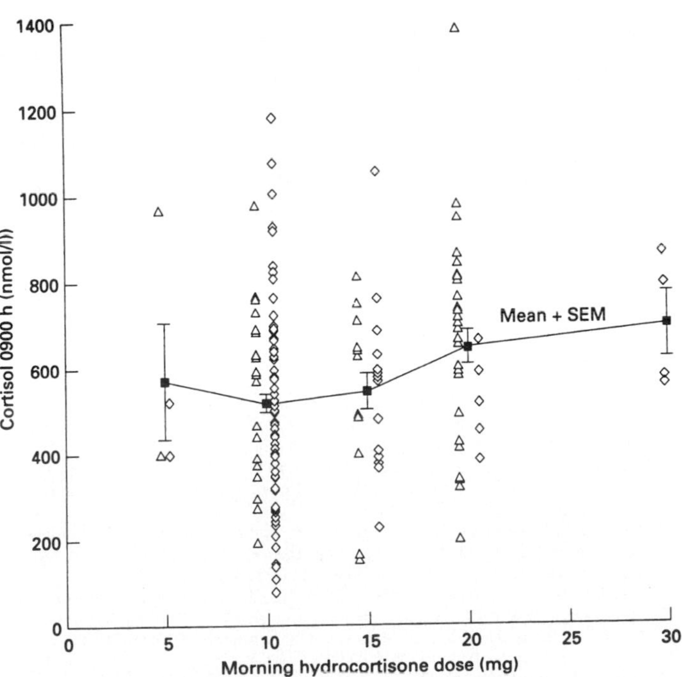

FIGURE 118–4. Comparison of 9 AM serum cortisol level with morning dose of hydrocortisone. △, individual values in patients on twice-daily regimens; ◇, individual values in patients on thrice-daily regimens; ■, mean value for each hydrocortisone dose (error bars represent SEM). Mean 9 AM cortisol was significantly higher after 20 mg than after 10 mg total daily dose of hydrocortisone ($P < .01$ by t-test). Reference range for the normal population, 100–700 nmol/L. (From Howlett TA: An assessment of optimal hydrocortisone replacement therapy. Clin Endocrinol 46:265, 1997.)

REFERENCES

1. Krieger DT, Allen W, Rizzo F, Krieger HP: Characterization of the normal temporal pattern of plasma corticosteroid levels. J Clin Endocrinol Metab 32:266–284, 1971.
2. Patel S, Selby C, Jeffcoate W: The short synacthen test in acute hospital admissions. Clin Endocrinol 35:259–261, 1991.
3. Veldhuis JD, Iranmanesh A, Johnson ML, Lizarralde G: Amplitude, but not frequency, modulation of adrenocorticotropin secretory bursts gives rise to nyctohemeral rhythm of the corticotropic axis in man. J Clin Endocrinol Metab 71:452–463, 1990.
4. Wallace WHB, Crowne EC, Shalet SM, et al: Episodic ACTH and cortisol secretion in normal children. Clin Endocrinol 34:215–221, 1991.
5. Weitzman ED, Fukushima D, Nogeire C, et al: Twenty-four hour pattern of the episodic secretion of cortisol in normal subjects. J Clin Endocrinol Metab 33:14–22, 1971.
6. Maes M, Mommen K, Hendrick D, et al: Components of biological variation, including seasonality, in blood concentrations of TSH, TT3, FT4, PRL, cortisol and testosterone in healthy volunteers. Clin Endocrinol 46:587–598, 1997.
7. de Lacerda L, Kowarski A, Migeon CJ: Diurnal variation of the metabolic clearance rate of cortisol. Effect on measurement of cortisol production rate. J Clin Endocrinol Metab 36:1043–1049, 1973.
8. Gallagher TF, Fukushima DK, Hellman L: The clarification of discrepancies in cortisol secretion rate. J Clin Endocrinol Metab 31:625–631, 1970.
9. Esteban NV, Loughlin T, Yergey AL, et al: Daily cortisol production rate in man determined by stable isotope dilution/mass spectrometry. J Clin Endocrinol Metab 72:39–45, 1991.
10. Kraan GP, Dullaart RP, Pratt JH, et al: Kinetics of intravenously dosed cortisol in four men. Consequences for calculation of the plasma cortisol production rate. J Steroid Biochem Mol Biol 63:139–146, 1997.
11. Kraan GP, Dullaart RP, Pratt JJ, et al: The daily cortisol production reinvestigated in healthy men. The serum and urinary cortisol production rates are not significantly different. J Clin Endocrinol Metab 83:1247–1252, 1998.
12. Linder BL, Esteban NV, Yergey AL, et al: Cortisol production rate in childhood and adolescence. J Pediatr 117:892–896, 1990.
13. Walker BR, Best R, Noon JP, et al: Seasonal variation in glucocorticoid activity in healthy men. J Clin Endocrinol Metab 82:4015–4019, 1997.

14. Donald RA: Plasma immunoreactive corticotrophin and cortisol response to insulin hypoglycemia in normal subjects and patients with pituitary disease. J Clin Endocrinol Metab 32:225–231, 1971.
15. Donald RA, Crozier IG, Foy SG, et al: Plasma corticotrophin releasing hormone, vasopressin, ACTH and cortisol responses to acute myocardial infarction. Clin Endocrinol 40:499–504, 1994.
16. Ellis MJ, Schmidli RS, Donald RA, et al: Plasma corticotrophin-releasing factor and vasopressin responses to hypoglycaemia in normal man. Clin Endocrinol (Oxf) 32:93–100, 1990.
17. Fish HR, Chernow B, O'Brian JT: Endocrine and neurophysiologic responses of the pituitary to insulin-induced hypoglycemia: A review. Metab Clin Exp 35:763–780, 1986.
18. Ross R, Miell J, Holly J, et al: Levels of GH binding activity, IGFBP-1, insulin, blood glucose and cortisol in intensive care patients. Clin Endocrinol 35:361–367, 1991.
19. Post F, Soule S, Willcox P, Levitt N: The spectrum of endocrine dysfunction in active pulmonary tuberculosis. Clin Endocrinol 40:367–371, 1994.
20. Zipser RD, Davenport MW, Martin KL, et al: Hyperreninemic hypoaldosteronism in the critically ill: A new entity. J Clin Endocrinol Metab 53:867–873, 1981.
21. Hammond GL: Molecular properties of corticosteroid binding globulin and the sex-steroid binding proteins. Endocr Rev 11:65–79, 1990.
22. White PC, Mune T, Agarwal AK: 11 Beta-hydroxysteroid dehydrogenase and the syndrome of apparent mineralocorticoid excess. Endocr Rev 18:135–156, 1997.
23. Borushek S, Gold JJ: Commonly used medications that interfere with routine endocrine laboratory procedures. Clin Chem 10:41–52, 1964.
24. Young DS, Pestaner LC, Gibberman V: Effects of drugs on clinical laboratory tests. Clin Chem 21:1D–432D, 1975.
25. Young DS: Effects of drugs on clinical laboratory tests. Ann Clin Biochem 34:579–581, 1997.
26. Miller WL, Tyrrell JB: The adrenal cortex. *In* Felig P, Baxter JD, Frohman LA (eds): Endocrinology and Metabolism, ed 3. New York, McGraw-Hill, 1995, pp 555–712.
27. Orth DN, Kovacs WJ: The adrenal cortex. *In* Wilson JD, Foster BW, Kronenberg HM, Larsen PR (eds): Williams Textbook of Endocrinology, ed 9. Philadelphia, WB Saunders, 1998, pp 517–664.
28. Samaan GJ, Porquet D, Demelier JF, Biou D: Determination of cortisol and associated glucocorticoids in serum and urine by an automated liquid chromatographic assay. Clin Biochem 26:153–158, 1993.
29. Robin P, Predine J, Milgrom E: Assay of unbound cortisol in plasma. J Clin Endocrinol Metab 46:277–283, 1978.
30. Vining RF, McGinley RA, Maksvytis JJ, Ho KY: Salivary cortisol: A better measure of adrenal cortical function than serum cortisol. Ann Clin Biochem 20:329–335, 1983.
31. Vining RF, McGinley RA, Symons RG: Hormones in saliva: Mode of entry and consequent implications for clinical interpretation. Clin Chem 29:1752–1756, 1983.
32. Coste J, Strauch G, Letrait M, Bertagna X: Reliability of hormonal levels for assessing the hypothalamic-pituitary-adrenocortical system in clinical pharmacology. Br J Clin Pharmacol 38:474–479, 1994.
33. Reynolds RM, Bendall HE, Whorwood CB, et al: Reproducibility of the low dose dexamethasone suppression test: Comparison between direct plasma and salivary cortisol assays. Clin Endocrinol 49:307–310, 1998.
34. Nahoul K, Patricot MC, Moatti JP, Revol A: Determination of urinary cortisol with three commercial immunoassays. J Steroid Biochem Mol Biol 43:573–580, 1992.
35. Findling JW, Pinkstaff SM, Shaker JL, et al: Pseudohypercortisoluria: Spurious elevation of urinary cortisol due to carbamazepine. Endocrinologist 8:51–54, 1998.
35a. Mahajan DK, Wahlen JD, Tyler FH, West CD: Plasma 11-deoxycortisol radioimmunoassay for metyrapone tests. Steroids 20:609–620, 1972.
36. Cizza G, Nieman LK, Doppman JL, et al: Factitious Cushing syndrome. J Clin Endocrinol Metab 81:3573–3577, 1996.
37. Lin CL, Wu TJ, Machacek DA, et al: Urinary free cortisol and cortisone determined by high performance liquid chromatography in the diagnosis of Cushing's syndrome. J Clin Endocrinol Metab 82:151–155, 1997.
38. Findling JW: Clinical application of a new immunoradiometric assay for ACTH. Endocrinologist 2:360–365, 1992.
39. Snow K, Jiang N, Kao P, Scheithauer B: Biochemical evaluation of adrenal dysfunction: The laboratory perspective. Mayo Clin Proc 67:1055–1065, 1992.
40. Cunnah D, Jessop DS, Besser GM, Rees LH: Measurement of circulating corticotrophin-releasing factor in man. J Endocrinol 113:123–131, 1987.
41. Orth DN: Corticotropin-releasing hormone in humans. Endocr Rev 13:164–191, 1992.
42. Yanovski JA, Nieman LK, Doppman JL, et al: Plasma levels of corticotropin-releasing hormone in the inferior petrosal sinuses of healthy volunteers, patients with Cushing's syndrome, and patients with pseudo-Cushing states. J Clin Endocrinol Metab 83:1485–1488, 1998.
43. Danese RD, Aron DC: Principles of epidemiology and their application to the diagnosis of Cushing's syndrome: Rev. Bayes meets Dr. Cushing. Endocrinologist 5:339–346, 1999.
44. Kraemer HC. Evaluating Medical Tests: Objective and Quantitative Guidelines. Newbury Park, CA, Sage, 1992.
45. Zweig MH, Campbell G: Receiver-operating characteristic (ROC) plots: A fundamental evaluation tool in clinical medicine. Clin Chem 39:561–577, 1993.
46. Yanovski JA, Cutler GB Jr, Chrousos GP, Nieman LK: Corticotropin-releasing hormone stimulation following low-dose dexamethasone administration. A new test to distinguish Cushing's syndrome from pseudo-Cushing's states. JAMA 269:2232–2238, 1993.
47. Aron DC, Raff H, Findling JW: Effectiveness versus efficacy: The limited value in clinical practice of high dose dexamethasone suppression testing in the differential diagnosis of adrenocorticotropin-dependent Cushing's Syndrome. J Clin Endocrinol Metab 82:1780–1785, 1997.
48. Newell-Price J, Trainer P, Besser M, Grossman A: The diagnosis and differential diagnosis of Cushing's syndrome and pseudo-Cushing's states. Endocr Rev 19:647–672, 1998.
49. Tsagarakis S, Kokkoris P, Roboti C, et al: The low-dose dexamethasone suppression test in patients with adrenal incidentalomas: Comparisons with clinically euadrenal subjects and patients with Cushing's syndrome. Clin Endocrinol 48:627–633, 1998.
50. Leibowitz G, Tsur A, Chayen SD, Salameh M, et al: Pre-clinical Cushing's syndrome: An unexpected frequent cause of poor glycaemic control in obese diabetic patients. Clin Endocrinol 44:722, 1996.
51. Jeffcoate W: Probability in practice in the diagnosis of Cushing's syndrome. Clin Endocrinol 47:271–272, 1997.
52. Liddle GW: Tests of pituitary-adrenal suppressibility in the diagnosis of Cushing's syndrome. J Clin Endocrinol Metab 20:1539–1560, 1960.
53. Crapo L: Cushing's Syndrome: A review of diagnostic tests. Metabolism 28:955–977, 1979.
54. Cronin C, Igoe D, Duffy MJ, et al: The overnight dexamethasone test is a worthwhile screening procedure. Clin Endocrinol 33:27–33, 1990.
55. Fok ACK, Tan KT, Jacob E, Sum CF: Overnight (1 mg) dexamethasone suppression testing reliably distinguishes non-Cushingoid obesity from Cushing's syndrome. Steroids 56:549–551, 1991.
56. Montwill J, Igoe D, McKenna TJ: The overnight dexamethasone test is the procedure of choice in screening for Cushing's syndrome. Steroids 59:296–298, 1994.
57. Wood PJ, Barth JH, Freedman DB, et al: Evidence for the low dose dexamethasone suppression test to screen for Cushing's syndrome—recommendations for a protocol for biochemistry laboratories. Ann Clin Biochem 34:222–229, 1997.
58. Tiller JW, Maguire KP, Schweitzer I, et al: The dexamethasone suppression test: A study in a normal population. Psychoneuroendocrinology 13:377–384, 1988.
59. Atkinson AB, McCance DR, Kennedy L, Sheridan B: Cyclical Cushing's syndrome first diagnosed after pituitary surgery: A trap for the unwary. Clin Endocrinol 36:297–299, 1992.
60. Hermus AR, Pieters GF, Borm GF, et al: Unpredictable hypersecretion of cortisol in Cushing's disease: Detection by daily salivary cortisol measurements. Acta Endocrinol 128:428–432, 1993.
61. Arana GW, Reichlin S, Workman R, et al: The dexamethasone suppression index: Enhancement of DST diagnostic utility for depression by expressing serum cortisol as a function of serum dexamethasone. Am J Psychiatry 145:707–711, 1988.
62. Aron DC, Tyrrell JB, Fitzgerald PA, et al: Cushing's syndrome: Problems in diagnosis. Medicine (Baltimore) 60:25–35, 1981.
63. Fink RS, Short F, Marjot DH, James VH: Abnormal suppression of plasma cortisol during the intravenous infusion of dexamethasone to alcoholic patients. Clin Endocrinol 15:97–102, 1981.
64. Lamberts SW, Bruining HA, de Jong FH: Corticosteroid therapy in severe illness. N Engl J Med 337:1285–1292, 1997.
65. Ramirez G, Gomez-Sanchez C, Meikle AW, Jubiz W: Evaluation of the hypothalamic hypophyseal adrenal axis in patients receiving long-term hemodialysis. Arch Intern Med 142:1448–1458, 1982.
66. Sharp NA, Devlin JT, Rimmer JM: Renal failure obfuscates the diagnosis of Cushing's disease. JAMA 256:2564–2565, 1986.
67. Workman RJ, Vaughn WK, Stone WJ: Dexamethasone suppression testing in chronic renal failure: Pharmacokinetics of dexamethasone and demonstration of a normal hypothalamic-pituitary-adrenal axis. J Clin Endocrinol Metab 63:741–746, 1986.
68. Meikle AW, Lagerquist LG, Tyler FH: Apparently normal pituitary-adrenal suppressibility in Cushing's syndrome: Dexamethasone metabolism and plasma levels. J Lab Clin Med 86:472–478, 1975.
69. Meikle AW: Dexamethasone suppression tests: Usefulness of simultaneous measurement of plasma cortisol and dexamethasone. Clin Endocrinol 16:401–408, 1982.
70. Meikle AW, Stanchfield JB, West CD, Tyler FH: Hydrocortisone suppression test for Cushing syndrome therapy with anticonvulsants. Arch Intern Med 134:1068–1071, 1974.
71. Groote Veldman R, Meinders AE: On the mechanism of alcohol-induced pseudo-Cushing's syndrome. Endocr Rev 17:262–268, 1996.
72. Gold PW, Loriaux DL, Roy A, et al: Response to corticotropin-releasing hormone in the hypercortisolism of depression and Cushing's disease. N Engl J Med 314:1329–1335, 1986.
73. Atkinson AB, McAteer EJ, Hadden DR, et al: A weight-related intravenous dexamethasone suppression test distinguishes obese controls from patients with Cushing's syndrome. Acta Endocrinol (Copenh) 120:753–759, 1989.
74. Biemond P, de Jong FH, Lamberts SW: Continuous dexamethasone infusion for seven hours in patients with the Cushing syndrome. A superior differential diagnostic test. Ann Intern Med 112:738–742, 1990.
75. Streeten DH, Anderson GH Jr, Brennan S, Jones C: Suppressibility of plasma adrenocorticotropin by hydrocortisone: Potential usefulness in the diagnosis of Cushing's disease. J Clin Endocrinol Metab 83:1114–1120, 1998.
76. Streeten DH, Stevenson CT, Dalakos TG, et al: The diagnosis of hypercortisolism. Biochemical criteria differentiating patients from lean and obese normal subjects and from females on oral contraceptives. J Clin Endocrinol Metab 29:1191–1211, 1969.
77. Nieman LK, Cutler GB Jr: The sensitivity of the urine free cortisol measurement as a screening test for Cushing's syndrome. Presented at 72nd Annual Meeting of the Endocrinology Society, Atlanta, GA, 1990, abstract P-822.
78. Carroll BJ, Curtis GC, Davies BM, et al: Urinary free cortisol excretion in depression. Psychol Med 6:43–50, 1976.
79. Glass AR, Zavadil AP III, Halberg F, et al: Circadian rhythm of serum cortisol in Cushing's disease. J Clin Endocrinol Metab 59:161–165, 1984.
80. Van Cauter E, Refetoff S: Evidence for two subtypes of Cushing's disease based on the analysis of episodic cortisol secretion. N Engl J Med 312:1343–1349, 1985.
81. Papanicolaou DA, Yanovski JA, Cutler GB, et al: A single midnight cortisol measurement discriminates Cushing syndrome from pseudo-Cushing states. Presented at 76th

Annual Meeting of the Endocrinology Society, Anaheim, Cal, June 15–18, 1994, abstract 1270.

82. Newell-Price J, Trainer P, Perry L, et al: A single sleeping midnight cortisol has 100% sensitivity for the diagnosis of Cushing's syndrome. Clin Endocrinol 43:545–550, 1995.
83. Laudat MH, Cerdas S, Fournier C, et al: Salivary cortisol measurement: A practical approach to assess pituitary-adrenal function. J Clin Endocrinol Metab 66:343–348, 1988.
84. Raff H, Raff JL, Findling JW: Late-night salivary cortisol as a screening test for Cushing's Syndrome. J Clin Endocrinol Metab 83:2681–2686, 1998.
85. Contreras LN, Hane S, Tyrrell JB: Urinary cortisol in the assessment of pituitary-adrenal function: Utility of 24-hour and spot determinations. J Clin Endocrinol Metab 62:965–969, 1986.
86. Laudat MH, Billaud L, Thomopoulos P, et al: Evening urinary free corticoids: A screening test in Cushing's syndrome and incidentally discovered adrenal tumours. Acta Endocrinol 119:459–464, 1988.
87. Yanovski JA, Cutler GB Jr, Chrousos GP, Nieman LK: The dexamethasone-suppressed corticotropin-releasing hormone stimulation test differentiates mild Cushing's disease from normal physiology. J Clin Endocrinol Metab 83:348–352, 1998.
88. Ambrosi B, Peverelli S, Passini E, et al: Abnormalities of endocrine function in patients with clinically "silent" adrenal masses. Eur J Endocrinol 132:422–428, 1995.
89. Aron DC: Adrenal incidentalomas and glucocorticoid autonomy. Clin Endocrinol 449:157–158, 1998.
90. Terzolo M, Osella G, Ali A, et al: Subclinical Cushing's syndrome in adrenal incidentaloma. Clin Endocrinol 48:89–97, 1998.
91. Mantero F, Masini AM, Opocher G, et al, on behalf of the National Italian Study Group on Adrenal Tumor: Adrenal incidentaloma: An overview of hormonal data from the National Italian Study Group. Horm Res 47:284–289, 1997.
92. Reincke M, Nieke J, Krestin GP, et al: Preclinical Cushing's syndrome in adrenal "incidentalomas": Comparison with adrenal Cushing's syndrome. J Clin Endocrinol Metab 75:826–832, 1992.
93. Hermus AR: Early assessment of outcome of pituitary surgery for Cushing's disease. Clin Endocrinol 47:151–152, 1997.
94. Aken M, van Herder W, den Lely AJ, et al: Postoperative metyrapone test in the early assessment of outcome of pituitary surgery for Cushing's disease. Clin Endocrinol 47:145–149, 1997.
95. Grinspoon SK, Biller BM: Clinical review 62: Laboratory assessment of adrenal insufficiency. J Clin Endocrinol Metab 79:923–931, 1994.
96. Hagg E, Asplund K, Lithner F: Value of basal plasma cortisol assays in the assessment of pituitary-adrenal insufficiency. Clin Endocrinol 26:221–226, 1987.
96a. Kong MF, Jeffcoate W: Eighty-six cases of Addison's disease. Clin Endocrinol 41:757–761, 1994.
97. Aanderud S, Myking OL, Bassoe HH: ACTH suppression after oral administration of cortisone in Addisonian and adrenalectomized patients. Acta Endocrinol 100:588–594, 1982.
98. Feek CM, Ratcliffe JG, Seth J, et al: Patterns of plasma cortisol and ACTH concentrations in patients with Addison's disease treated with conventional corticosteroid replacement. Clin Endocrinol 14:451–458, 1981.
99. Oelkers W, Diederich S, Bahr V: Diagnosis and therapy surveillance in Addison's disease: Rapid adrenocorticotropin (ACTH) test and measurement of plasma ACTH, renin activity, and aldosterone. J Clin Endocrinol Metab 75:259–264, 1992.
100. Scott RS, Donald RA, Espiner EA: Plasma ACTH and cortisol profiles in Addisonian patients receiving conventional substitution therapy. Clin Endocrinol 9:571–576, 1978.
101. Inder WJ, Ellis MJ, Evans MJ, Donald RA: A comparison of the naloxone test with ovine CRH and insulin hypoglycaemia in the evaluation of the hypothalamic-pituitary-adrenal axis in normal man. Clin Endocrinol 43:425–431, 1995.
102. Daidoh H, Morita H, Mune T, et al: Responses of plasma adrenocortical steroids to low dose ACTH in normal subjects. Clin Endocrinol 43:311–315, 1995.
103. Dluhy RG, Himathongkam T, Greenfield M: Rapid ACTH test with plasma aldosterone levels: Improved diagnostic discrimination. Ann Intern Med 80:693–696, 1974.
104. Dickstein G, Arad E, Shechner C: Low-dose ACTH stimulation test. Endocrinologist 7:285–293, 1997.
105. Mayenknecht J, Diedrich S, Bahr V, et al: Comparison of low and high dose corticotropin stimulation tests in patients with pituitary disease. J Clin Endocrinol Metab 83:1558–1562, 1998.
106. Barth J, Seth J, Howlett TA, Freedman DB: A survey of endocrine function testing by clinical biochemistry laboratories in the UK. Ann Clin Biochem 32:442–449, 1995.
107. Clark PM, Neylon I, Raggatt PR, et al: Defining the normal cortisol response to the short Synacthen test: Implications for the investigation of hypothalamic-pituitary disorders. Clin Endocrinol 49:287–292, 1998.
108. Clayton RN: Short Synacthen test versus insulin stress test for assessment of the hypothalmo-pituitary-adrenal axis: Controversy revisited. Clin Endocrinol 44:147–149, 1996.
109. Hartzband PI, Van Herle AJ, Sorger L, Cope D: Assessment of hypothalmic-pituitary-adrenal dysfunction: A comparison of ACTH stimulation, insulin-hypoglycaemia and metyrapone. J Endocrinol Invest 11:769–776, 1988.
110. Hurel SJ, Thompson CJ, Watson MJ, et al: The short Synacthen and insulin stress tests in the assessment of the hypothalamic-pituitary-adrenal axis. Clin Endocrinol 44:141–146, 1996.
111. Lindholm J, Kehlet H: Re-evaluation of the clinical value of the 30 min ACTH test in assessing the hypothalamic-pituitary-adrenocortical function. Clin Endocrinol 26:53–59, 1987.
112. May ME, Carey RM: Rapid adrenocorticotropic hormone test in practice. Retrospective review. Am J Med 79:679–684, 1985.
113. Ammari F, Issa BG, Milward E, Scanlon MF: A comparison between short ACTH and insulin stress tests for assessing hypothalamo-pituitary-adrenal function. Clin Endocrinol 44:473–476, 1996.
114. Borst GC, Michenfelder HJ, O'Brian JT: Discordant cortisol response to exogenous ACTH and insulin-induced hypoglycemia in patients with pituitary disease. N Engl J Med 306:1462–1464, 1982.
115. Crowley S, Hindmarsh PC, Holownia P, et al: The use of low doses of ACTH in the investigation of adrenal function in man. J Endocrinol 130:475–479, 1991.
116. Cunningham SK, Moore A, McKenna TJ: Normal cortisol response to corticotropin in patients with secondary adrenal failure. Arch Intern Med 143:2276–2279, 1983.
117. Erturk E, Jaffe CA, Barkan AL: Evaluation of the integrity of the hypothalamic-pituitary-adrenal axis by insulin hypoglycemia test. J Clin Endocrinol Metab 83:2350–2354, 1998.
118. Kane KF, Emery P, Sheppard MC, Stewart PM: Assessing the hypothalamo-pituitary-adrenal axis in patients on long-term glucocorticoid therapy: The short Synacthen versus the insulin tolerance test. Q J Med 88:263–267, 1999.
119. Orme SM, Peacey SR, Barth JH, Belchetz PE: Comparison of tests of stress-released cortisol secretion in pituitary disease. Clin Endocrinol 45:135–140, 1996.
120. Soule S, Fahie-Wilson M, Tomlinson S: Failure of the short ACTH test to unequivocally diagnose long-standing symptomatic secondary hypoadrenalism. Clin Endocrinol 44:137–140, 1996.
121. Weintrob N, Sprecher E, Josefsberg Z, et al: Standard and low-dose short adrenocorticotropin test compared with insulin-induced hypoglycemia for assessment of the hypothalamic-pituitary-adrenal axis in children with idopathic multiple pituitary hormone deficiencies. J Clin Endocrinol Metab 83:88–92, 1998.
122. Rasmusson S, Olsson T, Hagg E: A low dose ACTH test to assess the function of the hypothalamic-pituitary-adrenal axis. Clin Endocrinol 44:151–156, 1996.
123. Talwar V, Lodha S, Dash RJ: Assessing the hypothalamo-pituitary-adrenocortical axis using physiological doses of adrenocorticotropic hormone. Q J Med 91:285–290, 1998.
124. Thaler LM, Blevins LS Jr: The low dose (1-μg) adrenocorticotropin stimulation test in the evaluation of patients with suspected central adrenal insufficiency. J Clin Endocrinol Metab 83:2726–2729, 1998.
125. Tordjman K, Jaffe A, Grazas N, et al: The role of the low dose (1 microgram) adrenocorticotropin test in the evaluation of patients with pituitary diseases. J Clin Endocrinol Metab 80:1301–1305, 1995.
126. Mukherjee JJ, de Castro JJ, Afshar KF, et al: A comparison of the insulin tolerance/glucagon test with the short ACTH stimulation test in the assessment of the hypothalamo-pituitary adrenal axis in the early post-operative period after hypophysectomy. Clin Endocrinol 47:51–60, 1997.
127. Dickstein G, Spigel D, Arad E, Shechner C. One microgram is the lowest ACTH dose to cause a maximal cortisol response. There is no diurnal variation of cortisol response to submaximal ACTH stimulation. Eur J Endocrinol 137:172–175, 1997.
128. Dickstein G: Commentary to the article: Comparison of low and high dose corticotropin stimulation tests in patients with pituitary disease. J Clin Endocrinol Metab 83:4531–4532, 1998.
129. Oelkers W: Comparison of low- and high-dose corticotropin stimulation tests in patients with pituitary disease-Author's response. J Clin Endocrinol Metab 83:4532–4533, 1998.
130. Thaler LM: Comment on the low-dose corticotropin stimulation test is more sensitive than the high dose test. J Clin Endocrinol Metab 83:4530–4531, 1998.
131. Tordjman K, Jaffe A, Greenman Y, Stern N: Comments on the comparison of low and high dose corticotropin stimulation tests in patients with pituitary disease. J Clin Endocrinol Metab 83:4530, 1998.
132. Jubiz W, Matsukura S, Meikle AW, et al: Plasma metyrapone, adrenocorticotropic hormone, cortisol, and deoxycortisol levels. Sequential changes during oral and intravenous metyrapone administration. Arch Intern Med 125:468–471, 1970.
133. Jubiz W, Meikle AW, West CD, Tyler FH: Single-dose metyrapone test. Arch Intern Med 125:472–474, 1970.
134. Dolman LI, Nolan G, Jubiz W: Metyrapone test with adrenocorticotrophic levels. Separating primary from secondary adrenal insufficiency. JAMA 241:1251–1253, 1979.
135. Feek CM, Bevan JS, Ratcliffe JG, et al: The short metyrapone test: Comparison of the plasma ACTH response to metyrapone with the cortisol response to insulin-induced hypoglycaemia in patients with pituitary disease. Clin Endocrinol 15:75–80, 1981.
136. Spiger M, Jubiz W, Meikle AW, et al: Single-dose metyrapone test: Review of a four-year experience. Arch Intern Med 135:698–700, 1975.
137. Staub JJ, Noelpp B, Girard J, et al: The short metyrapone test: Comparison of the plasma ACTH response to metyrapone and insulin-induced hypoglycaemia. Clin Endocrinol 10:595–601, 1979.
138. Flad TM, Kirby JM, Cunningham SK, McKenna TJ: The overnight single-dose metyrapone test is a simple and reliable index of the hypothalamic-pituitary-adrenal axis. Clin Endocrinol 40:603–609, 1994.
139. Schulte HM, Chrousos GP, Avgerinos P, et al: The corticotropin-releasing hormone stimulation test: A possible aid in the evaluation of patients with adrenal insufficiency. J Clin Endocrinol Metab 58:1064–1067, 1984.
140. Sheldon WR Jr, DeBold CR, Evans WS, et al: Rapid sequential intravenous administration of four hypothalamic releasing hormones as a combined anterior pituitary function test in normal subjects. J Clin Endocrinol Metab 60:623–630, 1985.
141. Trainer PJ, Faria M, Newell-Price J, et al: A comparison of the effects of human and ovine corticotropin-releasing hormone on the pituitary-adrenal axis. J Clin Endocrinol Metab 80:412–417, 1995.
142. Schlaghecke R, Kornely E, Santen RT, Ridderskamp P: The effect of long-term glucocorticoid therapy on pituitary-adrenal responses to exogenous corticotropin-releasing hormone. N Engl J Med 326:226–230, 1992.
143. Glowniak JV, Loriaux DL: A double-blind study of perioperative steroid requirements in secondary adrenal insufficiency. Surgery 121:123–129, 1997.
144. Munck A, Guyre PM, Holbrook NJ: Physiological functions of glucocorticoids in stress and their relation to pharmacological actions. Endocr Rev 5:25–44, 1984.

145. Monson JP: The assessment of glucocorticoid replacement therapy. Clin Endocrinol 46:269–270, 1997.
146. Fernandez-Real JM, Engel WR, Simos R, et al, and the Study Group of Incidental Adrenal Adenoma: Study of glucose tolerance in consecutive patients harbouring incidental adrenal tumours. Clin Endocrinol 49:53–61, 1998.
147. Osella G, Terzolo M, Reimondo G, et al: Serum markers of bone and collagen turnover in patients with Cushing's syndrome and in subjects with adrenal incidentalomas. J Clin Endocrinol Metab 82:3303–3307, 1997.
148. Tsagarakis S, Roboti C, Kokkoris P, et al: Elevated post–dexamethasone suppression cortisol concentrations correlate with hormonal alterations of the hypothalamo-pituitary adrenal axis in patients with adrenal incidentalomas. Clin Endocrinol 49:165–171, 1998.
149. Howlett TA: An assessment of optimal hydrocortisone replacement therapy. Clin Endocrinol 46:263–268, 1997.
150. Peacey SR, Guo C-Y, Robinson AM, et al: Glucocorticoid replacement therapy: Are patients overtreated and does it matter? Clin Endocrinol 46:255–261, 1997.

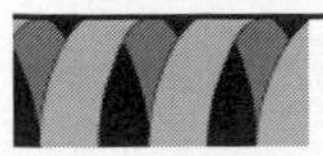

CLINICAL DISORDERS

Chapter 119

Glucocorticoid Therapy

Lloyd Axelrod

This chapter examines the risks associated with the use of glucocorticoids as anti-inflammatory or immunosuppressive agents and provides guidelines for the administration of these commonly prescribed substances.

STRUCTURE OF COMMONLY USED GLUCOCORTICOIDS

Figure 119–1 presents the structures of several commonly used glucocorticoids.[1, 2] *Cortisol (hydrocortisone)* is the principal circulating glucocorticoid in humans. The presence of a hydroxyl group at carbon 11 of the steroid molecule is an absolute requirement for glucocorticoid activity. Cortisone and prednisone, which are 11-keto compounds, lack glucocorticoid activity until they are converted in vivo to cortisol and prednisolone, the corresponding 11β-hydroxyl compounds.[3, 4] This conversion occurs predominantly in the liver. Thus, topical application of cortisone is ineffective in the treatment of dermatologic diseases that respond to topical application of cortisol.[4] Similarly, the anti-inflammatory action of cortisone injected into joints is minimal compared with the effect of cortisol administered in the same manner.[3] Cortisone and prednisone are used only for systemic therapy. All glucocorticoid preparations marketed for topical or local use are 11β-hydroxyl compounds, obviating the need for biotransformation.

PHARMACODYNAMICS

Half-Life, Potency, and Duration of Action

The important differences among the systemically used glucocorticoid compounds are duration of action, relative glucocorticoid potency, and relative mineralocorticoid potency[1, 2] (Table 119–1). The commonly used glucocorticoids are classified as *short-acting, intermediate-acting,* and *long-acting* on the basis of the duration of adrenocorticotropic hormone (ACTH) suppression after a single dose, equivalent in anti-inflammatory activity to 50 mg of prednisone[5] (see Table 119–1). The relative potencies of the glucocorticoids correlate with their affinities for the glucocorticoid receptor.[6] The observed potency of a glucocorticoid, however, is determined not only by the intrinsic biologic potency but also by the duration of action.[6, 7] The relative potency of two glucocorticoids varies as a function of the time interval between the administration of the two steroids and the determination of the potency. In particular, failure to consider the duration of action may lead to a marked underestimation of the potency of dexamethasone.[7]

There is little correlation between the *circulating half-life* ($T_{1/2}$) of a glucocorticoid and its *potency.* The $T_{1/2}$ of cortisol in the circulation is 80 to 115 minutes.[1] The $T_{1/2}$s of other commonly used agents are as follows: cortisone, 0.5 hour; prednisone, 3.4 to 3.8 hours; prednisolone, 2.1 to 3.5 hours; methylprednisolone, 1.3 to 3.1 hours; and dexamethasone, 1.8 to 4.7 hours.[1, 7, 8] While prednisolone and dexamethasone have comparable $T_{1/2}$s, dexamethasone is clearly more potent. Similarly, there is little correlation between the $T_{1/2}$ of a glucocorticoid and its *duration of action.* The many actions of glucocorticoids do not have an equal duration.

The duration of action is also a function of the dose. The duration of ACTH suppression is not simply a function of the level of anti-inflammatory activity because variations in the duration of ACTH suppression are achieved by doses of glucocorticoids with comparable anti-inflammatory activity. The duration of ACTH suppression produced by an individual glucocorticoid, however, probably is dose-related.[5]

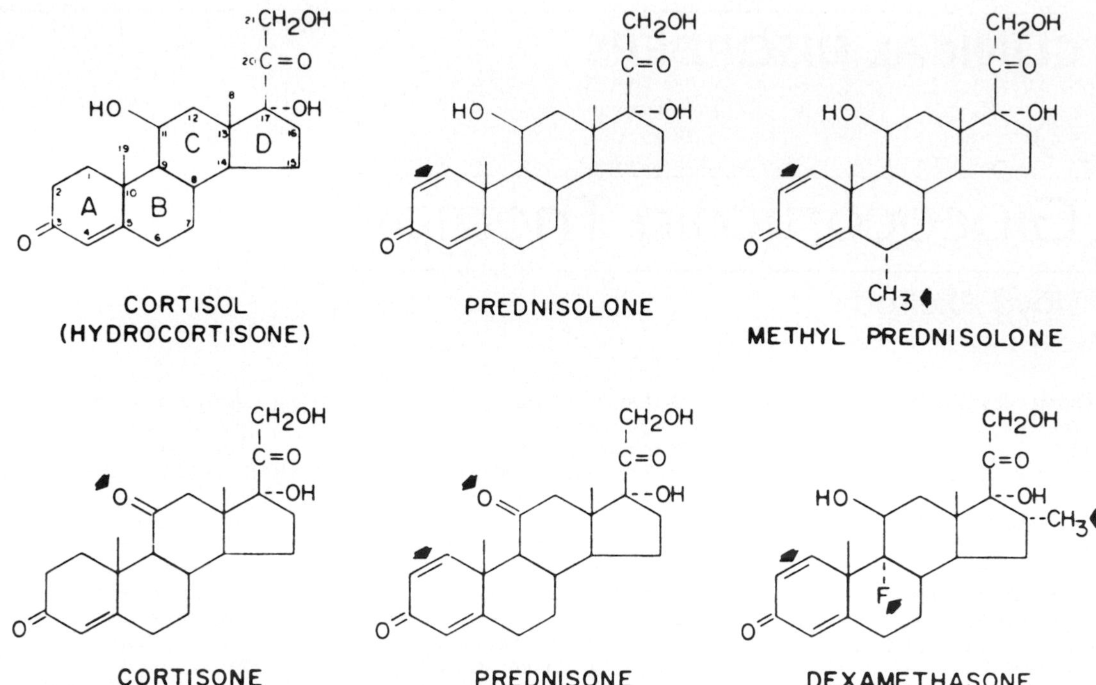

FIGURE 119–1. The structures of commonly used glucocorticoids. In the depiction of cortisol, the 21 carbon atoms of the glucocorticoid skeleton are indicated by numbers and the four rings are designated by letters. The *arrow heads* indicate the structural differences between cortisol and each of the other molecules. (Data from Axelrod L: Glucocorticoid therapy. Medicine (Baltimore) 55:39–65, 1976; Axelrod L: Glucocorticoids. *In* Kelley WN, Harris ED Jr, Ruddy S, Sledge CB (eds): Textbook of Rheumatology, ed 4. Philadelphia, WB Saunders, 1993; and Axelrod L: Corticosteroid therapy. *In* Becker KL (ed): Principles and Practice of Endocrinology and Metabolism, ed 2. Philadelphia, JB Lippincott, 1995.)

In short, the slight differences in the $T_{1/2}$s of the glucocorticoids contrast with their marked differences in potency and duration of ACTH suppression. Thus, the duration of action of a glucocorticoid is not determined by its presence in the circulation. This is consistent with the mechanism of action of steroid hormones. Steroid molecules bind to a specific intracellular receptor protein. The steroid-receptor complex modifies the process of transcription by which RNA is transcribed from the DNA template. This process alters the rate of synthesis of specific proteins. The steroid thereby modifies the phenotypic expression of the genetic information. Thus, a glucocorticoid *continues* to act inside the cell after it has disappeared from the circulation. Moreover, the events initiated by a glucocorticoid may continue to occur, or a product of these events (such as a specific protein) may be present, after the disappearance of the glucocorticoid from the circulation.

TABLE 119–1. Commonly Used Glucocorticoids

Duration of Action*	Glucocorticoid Potency†	Equivalent Glucocorticoid Dose (mg)	Mineralocorticoid Activity
Short-Acting			
Cortisol (hydrocortisone)	1.0	20	Yes‡
Cortisone	0.8	25	Yes‡
Prednisone	4.0	5.0	No
Prednisolone	4.0	5.0	No
Methylprednisolone	5.0	4.0	No
Intermediate-Acting			
Triamcinolone	5.0	4.0	No
Long-Acting			
Betamethasone	25	0.60	No
Dexamethasone	30	0.75	No

*The classification by duration of action is based on Harter JG: Corticosteroids. NY State J Med 66:827–840, 1966.

†The values given for glucocorticoid potency are relative. Cortisol is arbitrarily assigned a value of 1.

‡Mineralocorticoid effects are dose-related. At doses close to or within the basal physiologic range for glucocorticoid activity, no such effect may be detectable.

Data from Axelrod L: Glucocorticoid therapy. Medicine (Baltimore); 55:39–65, 1976; Axelrod L: Adrenal corticosteroids. *In* Miller RR, Greenblatt DJ (eds): Handbook of Drug Therapy. New York, Elsevier North-Holland, 1979; Axelrod L: Glucocorticoids. *In* Kelley WN, Harris ED Jr, Ruddy S, Sledge CB (eds): Textbook of Rheumatology, ed 4. Philadelphia, WB Saunders, 1993; and Axelrod L: Corticosteroid therapy. *In* Becker KL (ed): Principles and Practice of Endocrinology and Metabolism, ed 2. Philadelphia, JB Lippincott, 1995.

Bioavailability, Absorption, and Biotransformation

Normally, the plasma cortisol level is much lower after oral administration of cortisone than after an equal dose of cortisol.[9] Although oral cortisone may be adequate replacement therapy in chronic adrenal insufficiency, the oral form of this agent should not be used when pharmacologic effects are sought. Comparable plasma prednisolone levels are achieved in normal persons after equivalent oral doses of prednisone and prednisolone.[8, 10] After the administration of either of these substances, there is wide variation in individual prednisolone concentrations, which may reflect variability in absorption.[8]

In contrast to the marked increase in the plasma cortisol level that follows the intramuscular injection of hydrocortisone, the plasma cortisol level increases little, or not at all, after an intramuscular injection of cortisone acetate. When given intramuscularly, cortisone acetate does not provide an adequate plasma cortisol level and offers no advantage over hydrocortisone delivered by the same route. The explanation for the failure of intramuscular cortisone acetate to provide adequate plasma cortisol levels is not known. It may reflect poor absorption from the site of injection. Also, intramuscular cortisone acetate, which reaches the liver through the systemic circulation, may be metabolically inactivated before it can be converted to cortisol in the liver, in contrast to oral cortisone acetate, which reaches the liver through the portal circulation.

Plasma Transport Proteins

In normal people, circadian fluctuations occur in the capacity of corticosteroid-binding globulin (transcortin) to bind cortisol and prednisolone. Patients who have received prednisone for a prolonged period have no diurnal variation in the binding capacity of corticosteroid-binding globulin for cortisol or prednisolone, and both capacities are reduced in comparison with normal persons. Thus, long-term glucocorticoid therapy not only changes the endogenous secretion of steroids but also affects the transport of some glucocorticoids in the circulation. This may explain why the disappearance of prednisolone from the circulation is more rapid in those persons who have previously received glucocorticoids.

GLUCOCORTICOID THERAPY IN THE PRESENCE OF LIVER DISEASE

Plasma cortisol levels are normal in patients with liver disease. Although the clearance of cortisol is reduced in patients with cirrhosis, the hypothalamic-pituitary-adrenal (HPA) homeostatic mechanism remains intact. Consequently, the decreased clearance rate is accompanied by decreased synthesis of cortisol.

The conversion of prednisone to prednisolone is impaired in patients with active liver disease.[11] This is offset in large part by a decreased rate of elimination of prednisolone from the plasma.[11] In patients with liver disease, the plasma availability of prednisolone is quite variable after oral doses of either prednisone or prednisolone.[12] The percentage of plasma prednisolone that is bound to protein is reduced in patients with active liver disease; the unbound fraction is inversely related to the serum albumin concentration. The frequency of prednisone side effects is increased at low serum albumin levels.[12] Both findings may reflect impaired hepatic function. Because the impairment of conversion of prednisone to prednisolone is quantitatively small in patients with liver disease and is offset by the decreased clearance rate of prednisolone, and because of the marked variability in plasma prednisolone levels after the administration of either corticosteroid, there is no clear mandate to use prednisolone rather than prednisone in patients with active liver disease or cirrhosis.[8] If prednisone or prednisolone is used, however, a dose somewhat lower than usual should be given if the serum albumin level is low.[8]

GLUCOCORTICOID THERAPY AND THE NEPHROTIC SYNDROME

When hypoalbuminemia is caused by the nephrotic syndrome, the fraction of prednisolone that is protein-bound is decreased. The unbound fraction is inversely related to the serum albumin concentration. The unbound prednisolone concentration remains normal, however.[13, 14] Because the pharmacologic effect is determined by the unbound concentration, altered prednisolone kinetics do not explain the increased frequency of prednisolone-related side effects in patients with the nephrotic syndrome.

GLUCOCORTICOID THERAPY AND HYPERTHYROIDISM

The bioavailability of prednisolone after an oral dose of prednisone is reduced in patients with hyperthyroidism because of decreased absorption of prednisone and increased hepatic clearance of prednisolone.[15]

GLUCOCORTICOIDS DURING PREGNANCY

Glucocorticoid therapy is well tolerated in pregnancy.[16] Glucocorticoids cross the placenta, but there is no compelling evidence that this produces clinically significant HPA suppression or Cushing's syndrome in the neonate, although subnormal responsiveness to exogenous ACTH may occur.[16] Similarly, there is no evidence that glucocorticoids increase the incidence of congenital defects in humans.[16] Glucocorticoids do appear to decrease the birth weight of full-term infants; the long-term consequences of this are unknown. Because the concentrations of prednisone and prednisolone in breast milk are low, the administration of these drugs to the mother of a nursing infant is unlikely to produce deleterious effects in the infant.

GLUCOCORTICOID THERAPY AND AGE

The clearance of prednisolone and methylprednisolone decreases with age.[17, 18] Although prednisolone levels are higher in elderly subjects than in young subjects after comparable doses, endogenous plasma cortisol levels are suppressed to a lesser extent in the elderly.[17] These findings may be associated with an increased incidence of side effects and suggest the need to use smaller doses in the elderly than in young patients.

DRUG INTERACTIONS

The concomitant use of other medications can alter the effectiveness of glucocorticoids; the reverse also is true.[19]

Effects of Other Medications on Glucocorticoids

The metabolism of glucocorticoids is accelerated by substances that induce hepatic microsomal enzyme activity, such as phenytoin, barbiturates, and rifampin. The administration of these medications can increase the corticosteroid requirements of patients with adrenal insufficiency or lead to deterioration in the condition of patients whose underlying disorders are well controlled by glucocorticoid therapy. These substances should be avoided if possible in patients receiving corticosteroids. Diazepam does not alter the metabolism of glucocorticoids and is preferable to barbiturates in this setting. If drugs that induce hepatic microsomal enzyme activity must be used in patients taking corticosteroids, an increase in the required dose of corticosteroids should be anticipated.

Conversely, ketoconazole increases the bioavailability of large doses of prednisolone (0.8 mg/kg) because of inhibition of hepatic microsomal enzyme activity.[20] Oral contraceptive use decreases the clearance of prednisone and increases its bioavailability.[21]

The bioavailability of prednisone is decreased by antacids in doses comparable to those used clinically.[22] The bioavailability of prednisolone is not impaired by sucralfate, H_2-receptor blockade, or cholestyramine.

Effects of Glucocorticoids on Other Medications

The concurrent administration of a glucocorticoid and a salicylate may reduce the serum salicylate level. Conversely, reduction of the glucocorticoid dose during the administration of a fixed dose of salicylate may produce a higher and possibly toxic serum salicylate level. This interaction may reflect the induction of salicylate metabolism by glucocorticoids.[23]

Glucocorticoids may increase the required dose of insulin or oral hypoglycemic agents, blood pressure medications, or glaucoma medications. They also may alter the required dose of sedative-hypnotic or antidepressant therapy. Digitalis toxicity can result from hypokalemia caused by glucocorticoids, as from hypokalemia of any cause. Glucocorticoids can reverse the neuromuscular blockade induced by pancuronium.

CONSIDERATIONS BEFORE INITIATING THE USE OF GLUCOCORTICOIDS AS PHARMACOLOGIC AGENTS

Cushing's syndrome is a life-threatening disorder. The 5-year mortality rate was over 50% at the beginning of the era of glucocorticoid and ACTH therapy.[24] Infections and cardiovascular complications were frequent causes of death. High-dose exogenous glucocorticoid therapy is similarly hazardous.

Table 119–2 presents the important questions to consider before initiating glucocorticoid therapy.[25] These questions enable the physician to assess the potential risks of treatment that must be weighed against the possible benefits. The more severe the underlying disorder, the more readily systemic glucocorticoid therapy can be justified. Thus, corticosteroids are commonly used in patients with severe forms of systemic lupus erythematosus, sarcoidosis, active vasculitis, asthma, transplantation rejection, pemphigus, or diseases of comparable severity. Systemic corticosteroids should not be administered to patients with mild rheumatoid arthritis or mild bronchial asthma, who should receive more conservative therapy first. Although these patients may experience symptomatic relief from glucocorticoids, it may prove difficult to withdraw the drugs. Consequently, they may unnecessarily experience Cushing's syndrome and HPA suppression.

Duration of Therapy

The anticipated duration of glucocorticoid therapy is a critical consideration. The use of glucocorticoids for 1 to 2 weeks for a condition such as poison ivy or allergic rhinitis is unlikely to be associated with serious side effects in the absence of a contraindication. An exception to this rule is a corticosteroid-induced psychosis, which may occur after only a few days of high-dose glucocorticoid therapy, even in patients with no previous history of psychiatric disease.[26, 27] Because the risk of so many complications is related to the dose and duration of therapy, one should prescribe the smallest possible dose for the shortest possible period. If hypoalbuminemia is present, the dose should be reduced. If long-term treatment is indicated, the use of alternate-day glucocorticoid therapy should be considered (see below).

Local Use

A local corticosteroid preparation should be employed whenever possible because systemic effects are minimal when these substances are used correctly. Examples include topical therapy in dermatologic disorders, corticosteroid aerosols in bronchial asthma and allergic rhinitis, and corticosteroid enemas in ulcerative proctitis. Systemic absorption of inhaled glucocorticoids leading to Cushing's syndrome and HPA suppression is a rare occurrence when these agents are administered correctly at prescribed doses.[28, 29] The intra-articular injection of corticosteroids may be of value in carefully selected patients if strict aseptic techniques are employed and if frequent injections are avoided.

TABLE 119–2. Considerations Before the Use of Glucocorticoids as Pharmacologic Agents

1. How serious is the underlying disorder?
2. How long will therapy be required?
3. What is the anticipated effective corticosteroid dose?
4. Is the patient predisposed to any of the potential hazards of glucocorticoid therapy?
   - Diabetes mellitus
   - Osteoporosis
   - Peptic ulcer, gastritis, or esophagitis
   - Tuberculosis or other chronic infections
   - Hypertension and cardiovascular disease
   - Psychological difficulties
5. Which glucocorticoid preparation should be used?
6. Have other modes of therapy been used to minimize the glucocorticoid dose and to minimize the side effects of glucocorticoid therapy?
7. Is an alternate-day regimen indicated?

Modified from Thorn GW: Clinical considerations in the use of corticosteroids. N Engl J Med 274:775–781, 1966.

Selecting a Systemic Preparation

Agents with no mineralocorticoid activity should be used when a glucocorticoid is prescribed for pharmacologic purposes. If the dosage is to be tapered over a few days, a long-acting agent should be avoided. For alternate-day therapy, one should use a short-acting agent that generally does not cause sodium retention (e.g., prednisone, prednisolone, or methylprednisolone). There is no indication for glucocorticoid conjugates designed to achieve a prolonged duration of action (several days or several weeks) after a single intramuscular injection. The bioavailability of such preparations cannot be regulated precisely, the duration of action cannot be estimated reliably, and it is not possible to taper the dosage rapidly in the event of an adverse reaction such as a corticosteroid-induced psychosis. Such preparations may cause HPA suppression more frequently than comparable doses of the same glucocorticoid given orally. The use of supplemental medications to minimize the systemic corticosteroid dose and to reduce the side effects of systemic glucocorticoids should always be considered. In asthma, for example, treatment should include inhaled glucocorticoids and bronchodilators, such as β-adrenergic agonists and theophylline, and may include cromolyn.

EFFECTS OF EXOGENOUS GLUCOCORTICOIDS

Anti-inflammatory and Immunosuppressive Effects

Endogenous glucocorticoids protect the organism from damage caused by its own defense reactions and the products of these reactions during stress.[30] Consequently, the use of glucocorticoids as anti-inflammatory and immunosuppressive agents represents an application of the physiologic effects of glucocorticoids to the treatment of disease.[30]

Glucocorticoids inhibit synthesis of almost all known cytokines and of several cell surface molecules required for immune function.[31–33] When an immune stimulus such as tumor necrosis factor binds to its receptor, nuclear factor kappa B (NF-κB) moves to the nucleus, where it activates many immunoregulatory genes. This activation of NF-κB involves the degradation of its cytoplasmic inhibitor IκBα and the translocation of NF-κB to the nucleus. Glucocorticoids are potent inhibitors of NF-κB activation. This inhibition is mediated by the induction of the IκBα inhibitory protein, which traps activated NF-κB in inactive cytoplasmic complexes.[31–33] This reduction in NF-κB activity appears to explain the ability of glucocorticoids to inhibit the production of cytokines and cell surface molecules and to suppress the immune response.

Influence on Blood Cells and on the Microvasculature

Glucocorticoid effects on inflammatory and immune phenomena include effects on leukocyte movement, leukocyte function, and humoral factors. In general, glucocorticoids have a greater effect on leukocyte traffic than on function and more effect on cellular than on humoral processes.[34, 35] Glucocorticoids alter the traffic of all the major leukocyte populations in the circulation.

Perhaps the most important anti-inflammatory effect of glucocorticoids is the ability to inhibit the recruitment of neutrophils and monocyte-macrophages to an inflammatory site.[35] Glucocorticoids modify the increased capillary and membrane permeability that occurs in an area of inflammation. By decreasing the dilation of the microvasculature and the increased capillary permeability that occur during an inflammatory response, the exudation of fluid and the formation of edema may be reduced and the migration of leukocytes may be impaired.[2, 35, 36] The decrease in the accumulation of inflammatory cells is also related to decreased adherence of inflammatory cells to the vascular endothelium. It is not possible to determine the relative contributions of the direct vascular effect, the effect on inflammatory cell adherence to the vascular wall, and the effect on chemotaxis to the reduction in inflammation caused by glucocorticoids.

Glucocorticoids have many effects on leukocyte function.[35] Glucocorticoids suppress cutaneous delayed hypersensitivity responses. Monocyte-macrophage traffic and function are sensitive to glucocorticoids. Glucocorticoids in divided daily doses depress the bactericidal activity of monocytes. The sensitivity of monocytes to glucocorticoids may explain the effectiveness of these agents in many granulomatous diseases because the monocyte is the principal cell involved in granuloma formation.[35] Although neutrophil traffic is sensitive to glucocorticoids, neutrophil function appears to be relatively resistant to these agents.[35] Whereas most in vivo studies of neutrophil phagocytosis have found no evidence for impairment of phagocytosis or bacterial killing,[35] other studies suggest that glucocorticoids induce a generalized phagocytic defect, affecting both granulocytes and monocytes.

Glucocorticoid therapy retards the disappearance of sensitized erythrocytes, platelets, and artificial particles from the circulation.[35] This may account for the efficacy of glucocorticoids in the treatment of idiopathic thrombocytopenic purpura and autoimmune hemolytic anemia.

Influence on Arachidonic Acid Derivatives

Glucocorticoids inhibit prostaglandin (PG) and leukotriene synthesis by inhibiting the release of arachidonic acid from phospholipids.[37] The inhibition of arachidonic acid release appears to be mediated by the induction of lipocortins, a family of related proteins that inhibit phospholipase A_2, an enzyme that liberates arachidonic acid from phospholipids.[38, 39] This mechanism is distinct from the mechanism of action of the nonsteroidal anti-inflammatory agents, such as salicylates and indomethacin, which inhibit the cyclooxygenase that converts arachidonic acid to the cyclic endoperoxide intermediates in the PG synthetic pathway; in some tissues, glucocorticoids inhibit cyclooxygenase activity. Thus, the glucocorticoids and the nonsteroidal anti-inflammatory agents exert their anti-inflammatory effects at two distinct, but adjacent, loci in the pathway of arachidonic acid metabolism. Glucocorticoids and nonsteroidal anti-inflammatory agents have different therapeutic effects. Some of the therapeutic effects of glucocorticoids that are not produced by the nonsteroidal anti-inflammatory agents may be related to the inhibition of leukotriene formation.[37]

Side Effects

The side effects of glucocorticoids include the diverse manifestations of Cushing's syndrome and HPA suppression.[40] (Table 119–3) Iatrogenic Cushing's syndrome differs from endogenous Cushing's syndrome in several respects. Hypertension, acne, menstrual disturbances, male erectile dysfunction, hirsutism or virilism, striae, purpura, and plethora are more common in endogenous Cushing's syndrome. Benign intracranial hypertension, glaucoma, posterior subcapsular cataract, pancreatitis, and avascular necrosis of bone are virtually unique to iatrogenic Cushing's syndrome. Obesity, psychiatric symptoms, and poor wound healing have nearly equal frequency in endogenous and exogenous Cushing's syndrome.[40, 41] These differences may be explained as follows. When Cushing's syndrome is caused by exogenous glucocorticoids, ACTH secretion is suppressed. In spontaneous, ACTH-dependent Cushing's syndrome, the elevated ACTH output causes bilateral adrenal hyperplasia. In the former circumstance, the secretion of adrenocortical androgens and mineralocorticoids is not increased. Conversely, when ACTH output is elevated, the secretion of adrenal androgens and mineralocorticoids may be increased.[1] The augmented secretion of adrenal androgens may account for the higher prevalence of virilism, acne, and menstrual irregularities in the endogenous form of Cushing's syndrome, and the enhanced production of mineralocorticoids may explain the higher prevalence of hypertension.[1] Some of the complications that are virtually unique to exogenous Cushing's syndrome arise after the prolonged use of large doses of glucocorticoids. Examples are benign intracranial hypertension, posterior subcapsular cataract, and avascular necrosis of bone.[1]

TABLE 119–3. Adverse Reactions to Glucocorticoids

Ophthalmic

Posterior subcapsular cataracts, increased intraocular pressure and glaucoma, exophthalmos

Cardiovascular

Hypertension
Congestive heart failure in predisposed patients

Gastrointestinal

Peptic ulcer disease, pancreatitis

Endocrine-Metabolic

Truncal obesity, moon facies, supraclavicular fat deposition, posterior cervical fat deposition (buffalo hump), mediastinal widening (lipomatosis), hepatomegaly caused by fatty liver
Acne, hirsutism or virilism, erectile dysfunction, menstrual irregularities
Suppression of growth in children
Hyperglycemia; diabetic ketoacidosis; hyperosmolar, nonketotic diabetic coma; hyperlipoproteinemia
Negative balance of nitrogen, potassium, and calcium
Sodium retention, hypokalemia, metabolic alkalosis
Secondary adrenal insufficiency

Musculoskeletal

Myopathy
Osteoporosis, vertebral compression fractures, spontaneous fractures
Avascular necrosis of femoral and humeral heads and other bones

Neuropsychiatric

Convulsions
Benign intracranial hypertension (pseudotumor cerebri)
Alterations in mood or personality
Psychosis

Dermatologic

Facial erythema, thin fragile skin, petechiae and ecchymoses, violaceous striae, impaired wound healing

Immune, Infectious

Suppression of delayed hypersensitivity
Neutrophilia, monocytopenia, lymphocytopenia, decreased inflammatory responses
Susceptibility to infections

Data from Axelrod L: Adrenal corticosteroids. *In* Miller RR, Greenblatt DJ (eds): Handbook of Drug Therapy. New York, Elsevier North-Holland, 1979; Axelrod L: Glucocorticoids. *In* Kelley WN, Harris ED Jr, Ruddy S, Sledge CB (eds): Textbook of Rheumatology, ed 4. Philadelphia, WB Saunders, 1993; and Axelrod L: Corticosteroid Therapy. *In* Becker KL (ed): Principles and Practice of Endocrinology and Metabolism, ed 2. Philadelphia, JB Lippincott, 1995.

Although the association of glucocorticoid therapy and peptic ulcer disease is controversial,[42–47] glucocorticoids appear to increase the risk of peptic ulcer disease and also gastrointestinal hemorrhage.[45] The magnitude of the association between glucocorticoid therapy and these complications is small and is related to the total dose and duration of therapy.[42, 45] The risk of peptic ulcer disease and related gastrointestinal problems is increased by the concurrent use of glucocorticoids and nonsteroidal anti-inflammatory drugs.[48, 49]

Glucocorticoid therapy, especially daily therapy, may suppress the immune response to skin tests for tuberculosis. When possible, tuberculin skin testing should be performed before the initiation of glucocorticoid therapy. Routine isoniazid prophylaxis is not indicated for corticosteroid-treated patients, even for those with positive tuberculin skin test results.[50]

Some patients respond to, and experience side effects of, glucocorticoids more readily than others at comparable doses. Variations in responsiveness to glucocorticoids may be a consequence of drug interactions or of variations in the severity of the underlying disease. Alterations in bioavailability probably do not account for variations in the therapeutic response to glucocorticoids. In patients who experience side effects, the metabolic clearance rate of prednisolone and the volume of distribution are lower,[10, 51] and the $T_{1/2}$ is longer than in those who do not.[51] Impaired renal function may contribute to a decrease in the clearance of prednisolone and an increase in the prevalence of cushingoid features.[52] Patients who have a cushingoid habitus while taking prednisolone have higher endogenous plasma cortisol levels than those without this complication, perhaps because of resistance of the HPA axis to suppression by exogenous glucocorticoids.[53]

Variations in the effectiveness of corticosteroids may be the result of altered cellular responsiveness to the drugs.[54–57] In patients with primary open-angle glaucoma, exogenous glucocorticoids produce a more pronounced rise of intraocular pressure[54]; a greater suppression of the 8 AM plasma cortisol level when dexamethasone 0.25 mg is administered the previous evening at 11 PM[56]; and greater suppression of phytohemagglutinin-induced lymphocyte transformation[55, 57] than in normal persons. Primary open-angle glaucoma is relatively common. These findings suggest that a distinct subpopulation of patients are hyperresponsive to glucocorticoids and that this sensitivity is genetically determined.

Prevention of Side Effects

More and more, the issues of concern to physicians and patients with respect to glucocorticoid therapy are not only HPA suppression but long-term complications such as glucocorticoid-induced osteoporosis and *Pneumocystis carinii* pneumonia. Of course, the risk of many complications can be reduced by the use of the lowest possible dose of a glucocorticoid for the shortest possible period, by the use of regional or topical rather than systemic steroids, and by the use of alternate-day steroid therapy. In addition, pharmacologic interventions to prevent specific complications such as bone disease and *P. carinii* pneumonia are now widely used.

Osteoporosis

The majority of patients who receive long-term glucocorticoid therapy will develop low bone mineral density. By some estimates, more than one-fourth of patients on long-term therapy will sustain osteoporotic fractures.[58] The prevalence of vertebral fractures in asthmatic patients on glucocorticoid therapy for at least a year is 11%.[58] Patients with rheumatoid arthritis who are treated with glucocorticoids have an increased incidence of fractures of the hip, ribs, spine, leg, ankle, and foot.[58] Skeletal wasting occurs most rapidly during the first year of therapy. Trabecular bone is affected more than cortical bone. The effects on the skeleton are related to the cumulative dose and duration of treatment.[58] Alternate-day glucocorticoid therapy does not reduce the risk of osteopenia. Inhaled steroids have been associated with bone loss.

The pathogenesis of glucocorticoid-induced osteoporosis involves several different mechanisms.[58] Glucocorticoids decrease intestinal absorption of calcium and phosphate by vitamin D–independent mechanisms. Urinary calcium excretion is increased, possibly as a result of direct effects on renal tubular calcium reabsorption. These changes may lead to secondary hyperparathyroidism in at least some patients. Glucocorticoids reduce sex hormone production. This may be a direct effect by decreasing gonadal hormone release. It may also be indirect by reducing ACTH secretion and adrenal androgen production. Also, inhibition of luteinizing hormone secretion can result in decreased estrogen and testosterone production by the gonads. Glucocorticoids also have an inhibitory effect on the proliferation of osteoblasts, the attachment of osteoblasts to matrix, and the synthesis of type I collagen and noncollagenous proteins by osteoblasts.

The evaluation of the patient should emphasize risk factors for osteoporosis, including inadequate dietary calcium and vitamin D intake, alcohol consumption, smoking, menopause, and any history of infertility or erectile dysfunction suggesting hypogonadism in males. Attention should also be devoted to the possibility of thyrotoxicosis, overtreatment with thyroid hormone medication, renal osteodystrophy, multiple myeloma, osteomalacia, or hyperparathyroidism. In selected patients, laboratory studies should be ordered for evaluation of these disorders. When glucocorticoid therapy will be administered for more than a few months, it is reasonable to obtain a baseline measurement of bone mineral density using dual energy x-ray absorptiometry.

All patients should receive calcium and vitamin D supplementation to correct any nutritional deficiency. Calcium therapy alone is associated with rapid rates of spinal bone loss and offers only partial protection from this loss. There is no evidence that the combination of calcium and vitamin D prevents bone loss due to glucocorticoids.[59] Bisphosphonates, specifically alendronate and etidronate, and calcitriol are effective in the prevention of bone loss.[60–63] If calcitriol is used, careful follow-up of serum calcium levels is necessary. Postmenopausal women should receive hormone replacement therapy unless contraindicated; hypogonadotropic men should receive testosterone therapy unless contraindicated. The patient should be educated about the risks and the consequences of osteoporosis and the factors in their own lives that may contribute thereto. Since steroids also affect muscle mass and function, the patient should be advised about exercises to maintain muscle strength.

Pneumocystis carinii Pneumonia

Glucocorticoids predispose patients to many different infections. Until recently, prophylaxis against infections for patients treated with glucocorticoids was limited to patients receiving transplantation of organs, who also receive other forms of immunosuppression. Currently, prophylaxis for patients with other disorders who are treated with glucocorticoids is often used, particularly for *P. carinii* pneumonia.[64, 65]

In a series of 116 patients without AIDS who experienced a first episode of *P. carinii* pneumonia between 1985 and 1991, 105 (90.5%) had received glucocorticoids within 1 month before the diagnosis of *P. carinii* pneumonia was established.[64] The median daily dose was equivalent to 30 mg of prednisone; 25% of the patients had received as little as 16 mg/day. The median duration of glucocorticoid therapy was 12 weeks before the development of the pneumonia. In 25% of the patients, *P. carinii* pneumonia developed after 8 weeks or less of glucocorticoid therapy. However, the attack rate in patients with primary or metastatic central nervous system tumors who receive glucocorticoid therapy is about 1.3% and may be lower in other conditions.[65] Also, prophylactic therapy may produce side effects.

Some physicians recommend prophylaxis (e.g., with trimethoprim-sulfamethoxazole one double-strength tablet a day) for patients with impaired immunocompetence conferred by chemotherapy, transplantation, or an inflammatory disease who have received prednisone 20 mg or more per day for more than 1 month. Controlled studies with such prophylaxis in steroid-treated patients are not available. Physicians at the Mayo Clinic have detected no cases of *P. carinii* pneumonia in patients who received adequate chemoprophylaxis when not contraindicated in recipients of bone marrow or organ transplantation from 1989 to 1995.[64]

Withdrawal from Glucocorticoids

The symptoms associated with glucocorticoid withdrawal include anorexia, myalgia, nausea, emesis, lethargy, headache, fever, desquamation, arthralgia, weight loss, and postural hypotension. Many of these symptoms can occur with normal plasma glucocorticoid levels and in patients with normal responsiveness to conventional tests of HPA function.[66, 67] These patients may have abnormal responses to a low-dose ACTH test using 1 μg of α1-24 ACTH rather than the conventional 250-μg dose.[68, 69] Because glucocorticoids inhibit PG production and because many of the features of the glucocorticoid withdrawal syndrome can be produced by PGs such as PGE_2 and PGI_2, this syndrome may be caused by a sudden increase in PG production after the withdrawal of exogenous corticosteroids. The glucocorticoid withdrawal syndrome may contribute to psychological dependence on glucocorticoid treatment and to difficulties in withdrawing such therapy.

SUPPRESSION OF THE HYPOTHALAMIC-PITUITARY-ADRENAL SYSTEM

The Development of Hypothalamic-Pituitary-Adrenal Suppression

Few well-documented cases of acute adrenocortical insufficiency after prolonged glucocorticoid therapy have been reported and none after ACTH therapy.[1] After ACTH and glucocorticoids were introduced into clinical practice in the late 1940s, patients were reported in whom shock was attributed to adrenocortical insufficiency caused by these agents, but biochemical evidence of adrenocortical insufficiency was not available to substantiate the diagnosis.[1] Prolonged hypotension or an apparent response of hypotension to intravenous hydrocortisone is not a reliable means of assessing adrenocortical function. One must demonstrate simultaneously that the plasma cortisol level is lower than the values found in normal persons experiencing a comparable degree of stress. When measurement of plasma cortisol levels became available in the early 1960s, three cases were described that met these criteria. The paucity of reports may be due to the facts that acute adrenocortical insufficiency after glucocorticoid therapy is uncommon in properly treated patients, and that physicians are reluctant to report such events.

The minimal duration of glucocorticoid therapy that can produce HPA suppression must be determined from studies of adrenocortical weight and adrenocortical responsiveness to provocative tests.[1, 2] Any patient who has received a glucocorticoid in a dose equivalent to 20 to 30 mg/day of prednisone for more than 5 days should be suspected of having HPA suppression.[1, 2] If the dose is closer to, but above, the physiologic range, 1 month is probably the minimal interval.[1, 2]

The stress of general anesthesia and surgery is not hazardous to patients who have received only replacement doses (no more than 25 mg of hydrocortisone, 5 mg of prednisone, 4 mg of triamcinolone, or 0.75 mg of dexamethasone), as long as the corticosteroid is given early in the day. If doses of this size are given late in the day, suppression may occur due to inhibition of the diurnal surge of ACTH release.

Assessment of Hypothalamic-Pituitary-Adrenal Function

When HPA suppression is suspected, it may be helpful to assess the integrity of the HPA system. A test of HPA reserve is required only when the result will modify therapy. In practice, this applies to patients who may need an increase in the glucocorticoid dosage to cover a stressful event (such as general anesthesia and surgery) and to patients in whom withdrawal of glucocorticoid therapy is contemplated. In the latter group, a test of the HPA axis is indicated only when the glucocorticoid dosage has been reduced to replacement levels, for example, prednisone 5 mg/day (or an equivalent dose of another glucocorticoid). In stable patients receiving prolonged glucocorticoid therapy, frequent tests of HPA reserve function are not indicated. For example, it is not necessary to test before each reduction in dose during tapering of the steroid regimen. The responsiveness of the HPA system may change as glucocorticoid therapy continues, and repeated testing is costly.

The short ACTH test is a valuable guide to the presence or absence of HPA suppression in glucocorticoid-treated patients (Table 119–4). Although this test assesses directly only the adrenocortical response to ACTH, it is an effective measure of the integrity of the entire HPA axis. Because hypothalamic-pituitary function returns before adrenocortical function during recovery from HPA suppression, a normal adrenocortical response to ACTH in this setting implies that hypothalamic-pituitary function also is normal. This rationale is supported by clinical studies. Thus, the maximal response of the plasma cortisol level to ACTH corresponds to the maximal plasma cortisol level observed during the induction of general anesthesia and surgery in patients who have received glucocorticoid therapy.[1, 2] A normal response to ACTH before surgery is not likely to be followed by impaired secretion of cortisol during anesthesia and surgery in glucocorticoid-treated patients. An abnormal response to ACTH is a necessary but not a sufficient condition for the occurrence of adrenal insufficiency in a steroid-treated patient who undergoes surgery because some patients with an abnormal response to ACTH tolerate surgery without steroid treatment.[70] Furthermore, hypotension in the operative or postoperative period in a patient who has been treated previously with glucocorticoid therapy is often due to another cause, such as volume depletion or a reaction to anesthetic medication. The hypotension often responds to treatment of these other factors.

TABLE 119–4. Assessment of Hypothalamic-Pituitary-Adrenal (HPA) Function in Patients Treated with Glucocorticoids

Method

Withhold exogenous glucocorticoids for 24 hr

Give cosyntropin (synthetic α1-24 ACTH) 250 μg as intravenous bolus or intramuscular injection

Obtain plasma cortisol level 30 or 60 min after administration of ACTH

Performance of the test in the morning is customary but not essential

Interpretation

Normal response: plasma cortisol level > 18 μg/dL at 30 or 60 min after ACTH administration

Note: Traditional recommendations also specify an increment above baseline of 7 μg/dL at 30 min or 11 μg/dL at 60 min and a doubling of the baseline value at 60 min. There values are valid in normal, unstressed subjects but are frequently misleading in ill patients with a normal HPA axis, in whom stress may raise the baseline plasma cortisol level by an increase in *endogenous* ACTH levels.

From Axelrod L: Glucocorticoids. *In* Kelley WN, Harris ED Jr, Ruddy S, Sledge CB (eds): Textbook of Rheumatology, ed 4. Philadelphia: WB Saunders, 1993; and Axelrod L: Corticosteroid therapy. *In* Becker KL (ed): Principles and Practice of Endocrinology and Metabolism, ed 2. Philadelphia, JB Lippincott, 1995.

Other tests of HPA function generally are not indicated. The low-dose (1-μg) short ACTH test is more sensitive than the conventional ACTH test in patients treated with glucocorticoids.[68] The conventional dose of ACTH used in the short ACTH test (and other ACTH tests) produces circulating ACTH levels that are well above the physiologic range. These supraphysiologic levels may result in a normal plasma cortisol level in patients with partial adrenocortical insufficiency. Nevertheless, the low-dose short ACTH test has not yet replaced the conventional-dose short ACTH test in clinical practice. The lower limit of the normal range for the low-dose ACTH test has not been defined.[69] Also, there are no commercial preparations of ACTH available for use in the low-dose short ACTH test. The injection for the low-dose short ACTH test must be prepared by dilution, a source of inconvenience and potential error. Insulin-induced hypoglycemia may be dangerous (especially in patients with cardiac or neurologic disease) and the symptoms may be uncomfortable. This procedure is more time-consuming and expensive than the ACTH test because more cortisol values must be obtained. The measurement of plasma cortisol levels before and after the administration of corticotropin-releasing hormone also has been proposed.[71] This test also is longer and more expensive than the ACTH test and has not been compared to a physiologic stress such as anesthesia and surgery. It offers no advantage over the short ACTH test.

ACTH and the Hypothalamic-Pituitary-Adrenal System

Pharmacologic doses of ACTH produce elevated cortisol secretory rates and increased plasma cortisol levels. The elevated plasma cortisol levels might be expected to suppress ACTH secretion. In fact, there is no evidence that ACTH therapy causes significant hypothalamic-pituitary suppression in patients.[1] The failure of ACTH therapy to suppress hypothalamic-pituitary function is not explained by the dose of ACTH used, the frequency of injection, the time of administration, or the plasma cortisol pattern after ACTH administration. Alternatively, the hyperplastic and overactive adrenal cortex that results from ACTH therapy may compensate for hypothalamic-pituitary suppression. Although the threshold adrenocortical sensitivity to ACTH is not changed in patients who have received daily ACTH therapy, adrenocortical responsiveness to ACTH in the physiologic range may be enhanced. Also, the normal response of the plasma cortisol level in patients treated with ACTH may be preserved, at least in part, because ACTH treatment reduces the rate of endogenous ACTH secretion but not the total amount secreted, while glucocorticoids reduce both the rate of secretion and the total amount secreted.[72]

Recovery from Hypothalamic-Pituitary-Adrenal Suppression

During recovery from HPA suppression, hypothalamic-pituitary function returns before adrenocortical function.[1, 2, 73] Twelve months must elapse after the withdrawal of large glucocorticoid doses given for a prolonged period before HPA function, including responsiveness to stress, returns to normal.[1, 2, 73] Conversely, recovery from HPA suppression induced by a brief course of glucocorticoids (i.e., prednisone, 25 mg, twice daily for 5 days) occurs within 5 days.[74] Patients with mild suppression of the HPA axis (i.e., normal basal plasma and urine corticosteroid levels but impaired responses to ACTH and insulin-induced hypoglycemia) resume normal HPA function more rapidly than do those with severe depression of the HPA axis (i.e., low basal plasma and urine corticosteroid levels and impaired responses to ACTH and insulin-induced hypoglycemia).[75] The time course of recovery correlates with the total duration of previous glucocorticoid therapy and the total previous glucocorticoid dose.[75–77] However, in an individual patient, one cannot predict the duration of recovery from a course of glucocorticoid therapy at supraphysiologic doses lasting more than a few weeks. Therefore, the physician should suspect persistence of HPA suppression for 12 months after such treatment. The recovery interval after suppression of the contralateral adrenal cortex by the products of an adrenocortical tumor may exceed 12 months. The recovery from HPA suppression induced by glucocorticoid therapy may be more rapid in children than in adults.

WITHDRAWAL OF PATIENTS FROM GLUCOCORTICOID THERAPY

Risks of Withdrawal

The decision to discontinue glucocorticoid therapy provokes apprehension among physicians. The potentially harmful consequences of such an action include precipitation of adrenocortical insufficiency, development of the glucocorticoid withdrawal syndrome, and exacerbation of the underlying disease. Adrenocortical insufficiency after the withdrawal of glucocorticoids is an appropriate concern. The probability of precipitating the underlying disease depends on the activity and natural history of the condition under treatment. When there is any possibility of an exacerbation of the underlying illness, the glucocorticoid should be withdrawn gradually, over an interval of weeks to months, with frequent reassessment of the patient.

Treatment of Patients with Hypothalamic-Pituitary-Adrenal Suppression

There is no proven method for hastening a return to normal HPA function once inhibition has resulted from glucocorticoid therapy. The administration of ACTH does not prevent or reverse the development of glucocorticoid-induced adrenal insufficiency. Conversion to an alternate-day schedule permits recovery to occur but does not accelerate it. In children, alternate-day glucocorticoid therapy may delay recovery.

The recovery from glucocorticoid-induced adrenal insufficiency is time-dependent and spontaneous. The rate of recovery is determined not only by the doses given when the glucocorticoid is being tapered but also by the doses administered during the initial phase of treatment, before tapering is commenced. During the course of recovery a small dose of hydrocortisone (10 to 20 mg) or prednisone (2.5 to 5.0 mg) given in the morning may alleviate the withdrawal symptoms. Recovery of HPA function continues to occur when a small dose of a glucocorticoid is administered in the morning. The possibility cannot be excluded, however, that a small dose of a glucocorticoid given in the morning retards the rate of recovery from HPA suppression.

ALTERNATE-DAY GLUCOCORTICOID THERAPY

Alternate-day glucocorticoid therapy is defined as the administration of a short-acting glucocorticoid with no appreciable mineralocorticoid effect (i.e., prednisone, prednisolone, or methylprednisolone) once every 48 hours in the morning at about 8 AM. The purpose of this approach is to minimize the adverse effects of glucocorticoids while retaining the therapeutic benefits. The original basis for this schedule was the hypothesis that the anti-inflammatory effects of glucocorticoids persist longer than the undesirable metabolic effects.[78–80] This hypothesis is not supported by observations of the duration of glucocorticoid effects. A second hypothesis emphasizes that intermittent, rather than continuous, administration produces a cyclic, although not diurnal, pattern of glucocorticoid levels in the circulation and within the target cells that simulates the normal diurnal cycle.[34] This may prevent the development of Cushing's syndrome and HPA suppression and provide therapeutic benefit. Because the full expression of a disease frequently occurs only when the level of inflammatory activity is elevated over a protracted period, the intermittent administration of a glucocorticoid may be sufficient to shorten the interval during which the disorder develops without interruption and thereby prevent the level of disease activity from becoming apparent clinically[34] (Fig. 119–2). The duration of action of the glucocorticoid is an important consideration. The selection of prednisone, prednisolone, and methylprednisolone as the agents of choice for alternate-day therapy and of 48 hours as the appropriate interval between doses has an empiric basis. It has been found that intervals of 36, 24, and 12 hours are accompanied by adrenal suppression, and that an interval of 72 hours is therapeutically ineffective when prednisone is used.[80] An interval of 48 hours is optimal.

Alternate-Day Glucocorticoid Therapy and Manifestations of Cushing's Syndrome

An alternate-day regimen can prevent or ameliorate the manifestations of Cushing's syndrome.[1, 2] The susceptibility to infections that characterizes Cushing's syndrome may be diminished. Patients have been described in whom refractory infections cleared after conversion from daily to alternate-day regimens. In addition, the frequency of infections is low in patients receiving alternate-day therapy. Children treated with alternate-day steroid therapy regain or retain tonsillar and peripheral lymphoid tissue. The available information strongly suggests that alternate-day regimens are associated with a lower incidence of infections than are daily regimens, but does not firmly establish this point.

Host defense mechanisms have been studied in patients receiving alternate-day therapy. Patients maintained on such schedules have normal blood neutrophil and monocyte counts, normal cutaneous inflammatory responses, and normal neutrophil $T_{1/2}$s on the days they do not take the glucocorticoid. Patients receiving daily therapy, however, demonstrate neutrophilia, monocytopenia, decreased cutaneous neutrophil and monocyte inflammatory responses, and prolongation of the neutrophil $T_{1/2}$. Patients studied on the days they do not receive treatment do not have the lymphocytopenia observed in patients who receive daily therapy. Monocyte cellular function is normal in patients receiving alternate-day therapy at 4 hours and at 24 hours after a

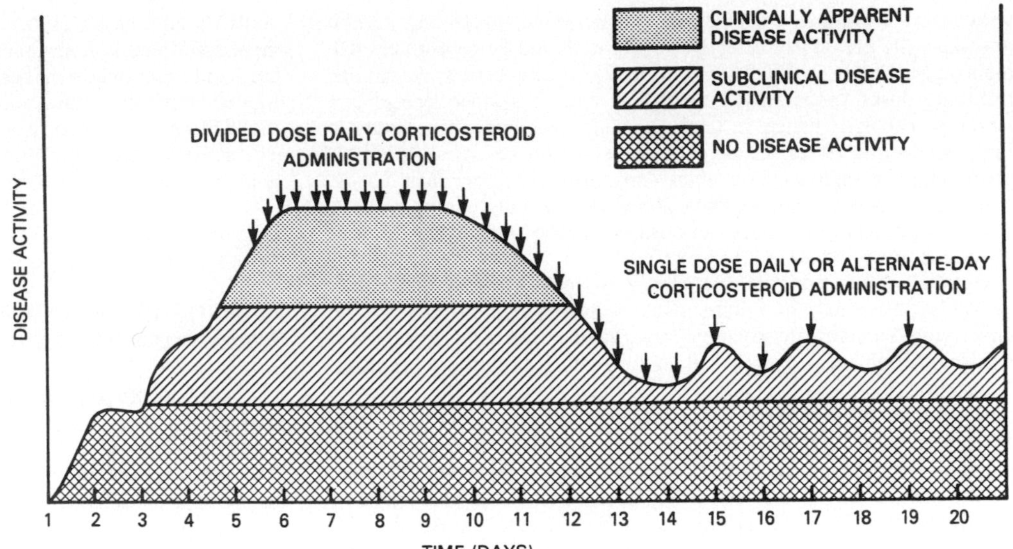

FIGURE 119–2. The effect of glucocorticoid administration on the activity of the underlying disease. A divided daily dose schedule may be necessary initially in some disorders. When the disease is controlled, or from the start of therapy in certain diseases, alternate-day therapy may be effective. (From Fauci AS, Dale DC, Balow JE: Glucocorticosteroid therapy: Mechanisms of action and clinical considerations. Ann Intern Med 84:304–315, 1976.)

dose. Intermittently normal leukocyte kinetics, preservation of delayed hypersensitivity, and preservation of monocyte cellular function may explain the apparently reduced susceptibility to infection in patients receiving alternate-day therapy.[81–83]

Effects of Alternate-Day Glucocorticoid Therapy on Hypothalamic-Pituitary-Adrenal Responsiveness

Patients receiving alternate-day glucocorticoid therapy may have some suppression of basal corticosteroid levels, but they have normal or nearly normal responsiveness to provocative tests such as the corticotropin-releasing hormone stimulation test, the ACTH stimulation test, insulin-induced hypoglycemia, and the metyrapone test.[1, 2, 84] They have less suppression of HPA function than have patients receiving daily therapy.

Effects of Alternate-Day Therapy on the Underlying Disease

Alternate-day glucocorticoid therapy is as effective, or nearly as effective, in controlling diverse disorders as daily therapy in divided doses.[1, 2] This approach has provided apparent benefit in patients with the following disorders: childhood nephrotic syndrome, adult nephrotic syndrome, membranous nephropathy, renal transplantation, mesangiocapillary glomerulonephritis, lupus nephritis, ulcerative colitis, rheumatoid arthritis, acute rheumatic fever, myasthenia gravis, Duchenne's muscular dystrophy, dermatomyositis, idiopathic polyneuropathy, asthma, Sjögren's syndrome, sarcoidosis, alopecia areata and other chronic dermatoses, and pemphigus vulgaris. Prospective, controlled studies demonstrate the efficacy of alternate-day therapy in membranous nephropathy and renal transplantation. The role of alternate-day therapy in giant cell arteritis is controversial.[85–87]

Use of Alternate-Day Therapy

Because alternate-day therapy can prevent or ameliorate the manifestations of Cushing's syndrome, can avert or permit recovery from HPA suppression, and is as effective (or nearly as effective) as continuous therapy, patients for whom long-term glucocorticoid administration is indicated should receive such therapy whenever possible. Nevertheless physicians sometimes are reluctant to use alternate-day schedules often because of an unsuccessful experience. Many efforts fail because of lack of familiarity with the indications for, and use of, such therapy.

The benefits of alternate-day glucocorticoid therapy are demonstrable only when corticosteroids are used for a prolonged period. There is no need to use an alternate-day schedule when the anticipated duration of therapy is a few weeks or less.

Alternate-day glucocorticoid therapy may not be necessary or appropriate during the initial stages of therapy or during exacerbation of the underlying disease. On the other hand, patients with many chronic disorders have been treated with an alternate-day regimen as initial therapy with apparent benefit.[1, 2] In patients with rheumatoid arthritis, it may be easier to establish treatment with alternate-day corticosteroids than to convert from daily therapy. Physicians treating recipients of renal transplants initially use daily therapy and then convert to an alternate-day schedule.

Alternate-day therapy may be hazardous in the presence of adrenocortical insufficiency of any cause because patients are not protected against glucocorticoid insufficiency during the last 12 hours of the 48-hour cycle. In patients who have been taking glucocorticoids for more than a brief period, or in those who may have adrenal insufficiency on another basis, the adequacy of HPA function should be determined before the initiation of an alternate-day program. It may be possible to address this issue by giving a small dose of a short-acting glucocorticoid (i.e., 10 mg of hydrocortisone) during the afternoon of the second day; this approach has not been studied systematically.

Alternate-day glucocorticoid therapy may fail to prevent or ameliorate the manifestations of Cushing's syndrome or HPA suppression if a short-acting glucocorticoid is not used, or if it is used incorrectly. For example, the use of prednisone four times a day on alternate days may be less successful than the use of the same total dose once every 48 hours.

An abrupt alteration from daily to alternate-day therapy should be avoided. First, the prolonged use of daily-dose glucocorticoids may have caused HPA suppression. In addition, patients with normal HPA function may experience withdrawal symptoms and have an exacerbation of the underlying disease.

No schedule of conversion from daily therapy in divided doses to alternate-day therapy has been shown to be optimal. One approach is to reduce the frequency of drug administration until the total dose for each day is given in the morning, and then to increase the dose gradually on the first day of each 2-day period and to decrease the dose on the second day. Another approach is to double the dose on the first day of each 2-day cycle, to give this as a single morning dose if possible and then to taper the dose gradually on the second day.[88] It is not clear how often changes in dosage should be made with any approach. This depends on many variables, including the disease under treatment, the duration of previous glucocorticoid therapy, the personality of the patient, and the physician's ability to use adjunctive therapy. Nonetheless, the conversion should be made as quickly as the patient can tolerate it. If adrenal insufficiency, the glucocorticoid withdrawal syndrome, or an exacerbation of the underlying disease develops, the previously effective regimen should be reinstituted and then tapered more gradually. Occasionally, it is necessary to resume full daily doses temporarily. An absolute change in dose represents a larger percentage change in dose at small total daily doses than at large total daily doses. Changes in dose should be about 10 mg of prednisone (or equivalent) at total daily doses of more than 30 mg, 5 mg at total doses of more than 20 mg, and 2.5 mg at lower doses. The interval between changes in dosage may be as short as 1 day or as long as many weeks.

Optimal results from alternate-day glucocorticoid therapy may not be achieved because of failure to use supplemental therapy for the underlying disorder. Conservative (nonglucocorticoid) therapy often is used until a glucocorticoid is initiated, at which time these less toxic therapeutic measures are ignored. Adjunctive therapeutic measures may facilitate the use of the lowest possible glucocorticoid dose. With alternate-day therapy, these measures should be used especially during the end of the second day, when symptoms may be prominent. Supplemental therapy may be especially helpful in disorders in which patients are likely to experience symptoms of the disease on the day off therapy, such as asthma and rheumatoid arthritis. In illnesses in which disabling symptoms are less likely to appear on the alternate day, such as the childhood nephrotic syndrome, less difficulty may be encountered.

Alternate-day therapy may be unsuccessful because of failure to inform patients about the purposes of this regimen. Because glucocorticoids may induce euphoria, patients may be reluctant to accept modification of a schedule of frequent doses. A careful explanation about the risks of glucocorticoid excess, attuned to each patients's intellectual and emotional ability to comprehend, enhances the prospects of success.

DAILY SINGLE-DOSE GLUCOCORTICOID THERAPY

Sometimes, alternate-day therapy fails because the patient experiences symptoms of the underlying disease during the last few hours of the second day. In these situations, single-dose glucocorticoid therapy may be of value.[1, 2] This regimen appears to be as effective as divided daily doses in controlling such underlying diseases as rheumatoid arthritis, systemic lupus erythematosus, polyarteritis, and proctocolitis. In giant cell arteritis, a daily dose in the morning is nearly as effective as daily therapy in divided doses.[85] Daily single-dose therapy reduces the likelihood that HPA suppression will develop. The manifestations of Cushing's syndrome probably are not prevented or ameliorated by a daily single-dose schedule.

GLUCOCORTICOIDS OR ACTH?

Disorders that respond to glucocorticoid therapy also respond to ACTH therapy if the adrenal cortex is normal. There is no evidence, however, that ACTH is superior to glucocorticoids for the treatment of any disorder when comparable doses are used.[1, 2, 89] Hydrocortisone and ACTH given intravenously in pharmacologically equivalent doses (determined by plasma cortisol levels and urinary corticosteroid excretion rates) are equally effective in the treatment of inflammatory bowel disease.[90] Similarly, there is no difference in the effectiveness of prednisone and ACTH in the treatment of infantile spasms.[91] Because ACTH does not appear to offer any therapeutic advantage, glucocorticoids are preferable for therapeutic purposes: they can be administered orally, the dose can be regulated precisely, their effectiveness does not depend on adrenocortical responsiveness (an important consideration in patients who have been treated with glucocorticoids), and they produce a lower frequency of certain side effects such as acne, hypertension, and increased pigmentation.[1, 2] If alternate-day therapy cannot be used, ACTH might appear to be preferable because it does not suppress the HPA axis. This benefit usually is outweighed by the advantages of glucocorticoids and by the fact that daily injections of ACTH are not superior to single daily doses of short-acting glucocorticoids; in both cases, HPA suppression is unlikely to result, but Cushing's syndrome is not prevented. In life-threatening situations, glucocorticoids are indicated because maximal blood levels are obtained immediately after intravenous administration, whereas with ACTH infusion, the plasma cortisol level rises to a plateau over several hours. The principal indication for ACTH continues to be the assessment of adrenocortical function.

DOSAGE

Anti-inflammatory or Immunosuppressive Therapy

The glucocorticoid dose required for anti-inflammatory or immunosuppressive therapy is variable, and depends on the disease under treatment. In general, the dose ranges from just above that needed for long-term replacement therapy up to 60 to 80 mg of prednisone or its equivalent daily. Although much larger dosages sometimes are recommended for diseases such as asthma, systemic lupus erythematosus, and cerebral edema, controlled studies have not shown the need for such large amounts of medication. The role of massive doses of corticosteroids in asthma is controversial.[92, 93] Most studies report no advantage of high-dose therapy (e.g., more than 60 to 80 mg of prednisone per day). Many physicians use intravenous pulse therapy (e.g., 1 g/day of methylprednisolone intravenously for 3 consecutive days) for severe manifestations of systemic lupus erythematosus, rapidly progressive glomerulonephritis, or other entities. There are no controlled studies that compare pulse therapy with a dose of 60 to 80 mg/day of prednisone. Thus, the superiority of pulse therapy has not been demonstrated.[94, 95]

Whcn alternate-day therapy is used, the dose is variable and depends upon the disease under treatment. It may range from just above that needed for long-term replacement therapy, to 150 mg of prednisone every other day.

Perioperative Management

Traditional doses of glucocorticoids recommended for perioperative coverage in glucocorticoid-treated patients, for example, hydrocortisone 100 mg intravenously every 8 hours or methylprednisolone 20 mg intravenously every 8 hours on the day of surgery, with a gradual taper over the ensuing days, are arbitrary and have no empiric basis.[70] A study in cynomolgus monkeys explored the doses required to prevent postoperative hypotension.[96] Bilateral adrenalectomies were performed in the experimental animals and replacement doses of steroids were given for 4 months. The animals were then divided into three groups, given normal, one-tenth normal, or 10 times thc normal replacement doses of glucocorticoids. A cholecystectomy was performed on each animal under these conditions. The animals that received one-tenth the normal replacement dose had an increased mortality rate, decreased peripheral vascular resistance, and hypotension. The group that received a normal replacement dose of steroids had no more hypotension or postoperative complications than did the group receiving 10 times the replacement dose. A double-blind study in patients provided similar results.[97] The investigators studied patients who had taken at least 7.5 mg of prednisone a day for several months and had an abnormal response to an ACTH test. All patients received their usual daily dose of prednisone on the day of surgery. One group of 12 patients received perioperative injections of saline. The other group of 6 patients received hydrocortisone in saline. There was no significant difference in outcome between the groups in this small study. It appears that patients with secondary adrenal insufficiency due to glucocorticoid therapy do not experience hypotension or tachycardia when given only their usual daily dose of steroids for surgical procedures such as joint replacements and abdominal operations.

Based on an analysis of the literature, an interdisciplinary group suggests the use of variable doses, depending on the magnitude of the surgical stress.[70] For *minor surgical stress* (e.g., an inguinal herniorrhaphy), the glucocorticoid target dose is 25 mg of hydrocortisone or equivalent. For *moderate surgical stress* (e.g., a lower extremity revascularization or total joint replacement), the target is 50 to 75 mg of hydrocortisone or equivalent. This might constitute continuation of the patient's usual dose of prednisone such as 10 mg/day and 50 mg of hydrocortisone intravenously intraoperatively. For *major surgical stress* (e.g., esophagogastrectomy or cardiopulmonary bypass), the patient might receive his or her usual steroid dose, for example, prednisone 40 mg, and 50 mg of hydrocortisone intravenously every 8 hours after the initial dose for the first 48 to 72 hours.

Glucocorticoid therapy should not be tapered inadvertently to a dosage below that known to control the underlying disease.

Other Considerations

The glucocorticoid dose may have to be modified in patients with certain diseases, in the setting of hypoalbuminemia, in elderly patients, and in patients receiving certain other medications. These considerations are addressed elsewhere in this chapter.

REFERENCES

1. Axelrod L: Glucocorticoid therapy. Medicine (Baltimore) 55:39–65, 1976.
2. Axelrod L: Glucocorticoids. *In* Kelley WN, Harris ED Jr, Ruddy S, Sledge CB (eds): Textbook of Rheumatology, ed 4. Philadelphia: WB Saunders, 1993.
3. Hollander JL, Brown EM Jr, Jessar RA, Brown CY. Hydrocortisone and cortisone injected into arthritic joints. JAMA 147:1629–1635, 1951.
4. Robinson RCV, Robinson HM Jr: Topical treatment of dermatoses with steroids. South Med J 49:260–266, 1956.
5. Harter JG: Corticosteroids: Their physiologic use in allergic disease. NY State J Med 66:827–840, 1966.
6. Ballard PL, Carter JP, Graham BS, Baxter JD: A radioreceptor assay for evaluation of the plasma glucocorticoid activity of natural and synthetic steroids in man. J Clin Endocrinol Metab 41:290–304, 1975.
7. Meikle AW, Tyler FH: Potency and duration of action of glucocorticoids: Effects of hydrocortisone, prednisone and dexamethasone on human pituitary-adrenal function. Am J Med 63:200–207, 1977.
8. Pickup ME: Clinical pharmacokinetics of prednisone and prednisolone. Clin Pharmacokinet 4:111–128, 1979.
9. Jenkins JS, Sampson PA: Conversion of cortisone to cortisol and prednisone to prednisolone. BMJ 2:205–207, 1967.
10. Gambertoglio JG, Amend WJC Jr, Benet LZ: Pharmacokinetics and bioavailability of prednisone and prednisolone in healthy volunteers and patients: A review. J Pharmacokinet Biopharm 8:1–52, 1980.
11. Davis M, Williams R, Chakraborty J, et al: Prednisone or prednisolone for the treatment of chronic active hepatitis? A comparison of plasma availability. Br J Clin Pharmacol 5:501–505, 1978.
12. Lewis GP, Jusko WJ, Burke CW, et al: Prednisone side-effects and serum-protein levels. A collaborative study. Lancet 2:778–781, 1971.
13. Frey FJ, Frey BM: Altered prednisolone kinetics in patients with the nephrotic syndrome. Nephron 32:45–48, 1982.
14. Gatti G, Perucca E, Frigo GM, et al: Pharmacokinetics of prednisone and its metabolite prednisolone in children with nephrotic syndrome during the active phase and in remission. Br J Clin Pharmacol 17:423–431, 1984.
15. Frey FJ, Horber FF, Frey BM: Altered metabolism and decreased efficacy of prednisolone and prednisone in patients with hyperthyroidism. Clin Pharmacol Ther 44:510–521, 1988.
16. Schatz M, Patterson R, Zeitz S, et al: Corticosteroid therapy for the pregnant asthmatic patient. JAMA 233:804–807, 1975.
17. Stuck AE, Frey BM, Frey FJ: Kinetics of prednisolone and endogenous cortisol suppression in the elderly. Clin Pharmacol Ther 43:354–362, 1988.
18. Tornatore KM, Logue G, Venuto RC, Davis PJ: Pharmacokinetics of methylprednisolone in elderly and young healthy males. J Am Geriatr Soc 42:1118–1122, 1994.
19. Jubiz W, Meikle AW: Alterations of glucocorticoid actions by other drugs and disease states. Drugs 18:113–121, 1979.
20. Zürcher RM, Frey BM, Frey FJ: Impact of ketoconazole on the metabolism of prednisolone. Clin Pharmacol Ther 45:366–372, 1989.
21. Legler UF, Benet LZ: Marked alterations in dose-dependent prednisolone kinetics in women taking oral contraceptives. Clin Pharmacol Ther 39:425–429, 1986.
22. Uribe M, Casian C, Rojas S, et al: Decreased bioavailability of prednisone due to antacids in patients with chronic active liver disease and in healthy volunteers. Gastroenterology 80:661–665, 1981.
23. Graham GG, Champion GD, Day RO, Paull PD: Patterns of plasma concentrations and urinary excretion of salicylate in rheumatoid arthritis. Clin Pharmacol Ther 22:410–420, 1977.
24. Plotz CM, Knowlton AI, Ragan C: The natural history of Cushing's syndrome. Am J Med 13:597–614, 1952.
25. Thorn GW: Clinical considerations in the use of corticosteroids. N Engl J Med 274:775–781, 1966.
26. Boston Collaborative Drug Surveillance Program: Acute adverse reactions to prednisone in relation to dosage. Clin Pharmacol Ther 13:694–698, 1972.
27. Perry PJ, Tsuang MT, Hwang MH: Prednisolone psychosis: Clinical observations. Drug Intell Clin Pharm 18:603–609, 1984.
28. Hollman GA, Allen DB: Overt glucocorticoid excess due to inhaled corticosteroid therapy. Pediatrics 81:452–455, 1988.
29. Stead RJ, Cooke NJ: Adverse effects of inhaled corticosteroids. BMJ 298:403–404, 1989.
30. Munck A, Guyre PM: Glucocorticoid physiology and homeostasis in relation to anti-inflammatory actions. *In* Schleimer RP, Claman HN, Oronsky A (eds): Anti-inflammatory Steroid Action: Basic and Clinical Aspects. San Diego, Academic Press, 1989.
31. Scheinman RI, Cogswell PC, Lofquist AK, Baldwin AS Jr: Role of transcriptional activation of IκBα in mediation of immunosuppression by glucocorticoids. Science 270:283–286, 1995.
32. Auphan N, DiDonato JA, Rosette C, et al: Immunosuppression by glucocorticoids: Inhibition of NF-κB activity through induction of IκB synthesis. Science 270:286–290, 1995.
33. Marx J: How the glucocorticoids suppress immunity. Science 270:232–233, 1995.
34. Fauci AS, Dale DC, Balow JE: Glucocorticosteroid therapy: Mechanisms of action and clinical considerations. Ann Intern Med 84:304–315, 1976.
35. Parrillo JE, Fauci AS: Mechanisms of glucocorticoid action on immune processes. Annu Rev Pharmacol Toxicol 19:179–201, 1979.
36. Cupps TR, Fauci AS: Corticosteroid-mediated immunoregulation in man. Immunol Rev 65:133–155, 1982.
37. Samuelsson B: Leukotrienes: Mediators of immediate hypersensitivity reactions and inflammation. Science 220:568–575, 1983.
38. DiRosa M, Flower RJ, Hirata F, et al: Anti-phospholipase proteins. Prostaglandins 28:441–442, 1984.
39. Parente L, DiRosa M, Flower RJ, et al: Relationship between the anti-phospholipase and anti-inflammatory effects of glucocorticoid-induced proteins. Eur J Pharmacol 99:233–239, 1984.
40. Axelrod L: Side effects of glucocorticoid therapy. *In* Schleimer RP, Claman H, Oronsky A (eds): Antiinflammatory Steroid Action: Basic and Clinical Aspects. San Diego, Academic Press, 1989.
41. Ragan C: Corticotropin, cortisone and related steroids in clinical medicine: Practical considerations. Bull N Y Acad Med 29:355–376, 1953.
42. Conn HO, Blitzer BL: Nonassociation of adrenocorticosteroid therapy and peptic ulcer. N Engl J Med 294: 473–479, 1976.
43. Langman MJS, Cooke AR: Gastric and duodenal ulcer and their associated diseases. Lancet 1:680–683, 1976.
44. Jick H, Porter J: Drug-induced gastrointestinal bleeding. Lancet 2:87–89, 1978.
45. Messer J, Reitman D, Sacks HS, et al: Association of adrenocorticosteroid therapy and peptic-ulcer disease. N Engl J Med 309:21–24, 1983.
46. Spiro HM: Is the steroid ulcer a myth? N Engl J Med 309:45–47, 1983.
47. Conn HO, Poynard T: Adrenocorticosteroid administration and peptic ulcer: A critical analysis. J Chronic Dis 38:457–468, 1985.
48. Piper JM, Ray WA, Daugherty JR, Griffin MR: Corticosteroid use and peptic ulcer disease: Role of nonsteroidal anti-inflammatory drugs. Ann Intern Med 114:735–740, 1991.
49. Gabriel SE, Jaakkimainen L, Bombardier C: Risk for serious gastrointestinal complications related to use of nonsteroidal anti-inflammatory drugs. A meta-analysis. Ann Intern Med 115:787–796, 1991.
50. Schatz M, Patterson R, Kloner R, Falk J: The prevalence of tuberculosis and positive tuberculin skin tests in a steroid-treated asthmatic population. Ann Intern Med 84:261–265, 1976.
51. Kozower M, Veatch L, Kaplan MM: Decreased clearance of prednisolone, a factor in the development of corticosteroid side effects. J Clin Endocrinol Metab 38:407–412, 1974.
52. Bergrem H, Jervell J, Flatmark A: Prednisolone pharmacokinetics in cushingoid and non-cushingoid kidney transplant patients. Kidney Int 27:459–464, 1985.
53. Frey FJ, Amend WJC Jr, Lozada F, et al: Endogenous hydrocortisone, a possible factor contributing to the genesis of cushingoid habitus in patients on prednisone. J Clin Endocrinol Metab 53:1076–1080, 1981.
54. Becker B: Intraocular pressure response to topical corticosteroids. Invest Ophthalmol 4:198–205, 1965.
55. Bigger JF, Palmberg PF, Becker B: Increased cellular sensitivity to glucocorticoids in primary open angle glaucoma. Invest Ophthalmol 11:832–837, 1972.
56. Becker B, Podos SM, Asseff CF, Cooper DG: Plasma cortisol suppression in glaucoma. Am J Ophthalmol 75:73–76, 1973.
57. Becker B, Shin DH, Palmberg PF, Waltman SR: HLA antigens and corticosteroid response. Science 194:1427–1428, 1976.
58. American College of Rheumatology Task Force on Osteoporosis Guidelines: Recommendations for the prevention and treatment of glucocorticoid-induced osteoporosis. Arthritis Rheum 39:1791–1801, 1996.
59. Sambrook PN: Calcium and vitamin D therapy in corticosteroid bone loss: What is the evidence? J Rheumatol 23:963–964, 1996.
60. Sambrook P, Birmingham J, Kelly P, et al: Prevention of corticosteroid osteoporosis. A comparison of calcium, calcitriol, and calcitonin. N Engl J Med 328:1747–1752, 1993.
61. Adachi JD, Bensen WG, Brown J, et al: Intermittent etidronate therapy to prevent corticosteroid-induced osteoporosis. N Engl J Med 337:382–387, 1997.
62. Reid IR: Preventing glucocorticoid-induced osteoporosis. N Engl J Med 337:420–421, 1997.
63. Saag KG, Emkey R, Schnitzer TJ, et al: Alendronate for the prevention and treatment of glucocorticoid-induced osteoporosis. N Engl J Med 339:292–299, 1998.
64. Yale SH, Limper AH: *Pneumocystis carinii* pneumonia in patients without acquired immunodeficiency syndrome: Associated illnesses and prior corticosteroid therapy. Mayo Clinic Proc 71:5–13, 1996.
65. Sepkowitz KA: *Pneumocystis carinii* pneumonia without acquired immunodeficiency syndrome: Who should receive prophylaxis? Mayo Clinic Proc 71:102–103, 1996.
66. Amatruda TT Jr, Hollingsworth DR, D'Esopo ND, et al: A study of the mechanism of the steroid withdrawal syndrome: Evidence for integrity of the hypothalamic-pituitary-adrenal system. J Clin Endocrinol Metab 20:339–354, 1960.

67. Amatruda TT Jr, Hurst MM, D'Esopo ND: Certain endocrine and metabolic facets of the steroid withdrawal syndrome. J Clin Endocrinol Metab 25:1207–1217, 1965.
68. Dickstein G, Shechner C, Nicholson WE, et al: Adrenocorticotropin stimulation test: Effects of basal cortisol level, time of day, and suggested new sensitive low-dose test. J Clin Endocrinol Metab 72:773–778, 1991.
69. Streeten DHP: Shortcomings in the low-dose (1 μg) ACTH test for the diagnosis of ACTH deficiency states. J Clin Endocrinol Metab 84:835–837, 1999.
70. Salem M, Tainsh RE Jr, Bromberg J, et al: Perioperative glucocorticoid coverage. A reassessment 42 years after emergence of a problem. Ann Surg 219:416–425, 1994.
71. Schlaghecke R, Kornely E, Santen RT, Ridderskamp P: The effect of long-term glucocorticoid therapy on pituitary-adrenal responses to exogenous corticotropin-releasing hormone. N Engl J Med 326:226–230, 1992.
72. Daly JR, Fletcher MR, Glass D, et al: Comparison of effects of long-term corticotropin and corticosteroid treatment on responses of plasma growth hormone, ACTH, and corticosteroid to hypoglycaemia. BMJ 2:521–524, 1974.
73. Graber AL, Ney RL, Nicholson WE, et al: Natural history of pituitary-adrenal recovery following long-term suppression with corticosteroids. J Clin Endocrinol Metab 25:11–16, 1965.
74. Streck WF, Lockwood DH: Pituitary adrenal recovery following short-term suppression with corticosteroids. Am J Med 66:910–914, 1979.
75. Spitzer SA, Kaufman H, Koplovitz A, et al: Beclomethasone dipropionate and chronic asthma. The effect of long-term aerosol administration on the hypothalamic-pituitary-adrenal axis after substitution for oral therapy with corticosteroids. Chest 70:38–42, 1976.
76. Westerhof L, Van Ditmars MJ, DerKinderen PJ, et al: Recovery of adrenocortical function during long-term treatment with corticosteroids. BMJ 4:534–537, 1970.
77. Westerhof L, Van Ditmars MJ, DerKinderen PJ, et al: Recovery of adrenocortical function during long-term treatment with corticosteroids. BMJ 2:195–197, 1972.
78. Haugen HN, Reddy WJ, Harter JG: Intermittent steroid therapy in bronchial asthma. Nord Med 63:15–18, 1960.
79. Reichling GH, Kligman AM: Alternate-day corticosteroid therapy. Arch Dermatol 83:980–983, 1961.
80. Harter JG, Reddy WJ, Thorn GW: Studies on an intermittent corticosteroid dosage regimen. N Engl J Med 269:591–596, 1963.
81. MacGregor RR, Sheagren JN, Lipsett MB, Wolff SM: Alternate-day prednisone therapy: Evaluation of delayed hypersensitivity responses, control of disease and steroid side effects. N Engl J Med 280:1427–1431, 1969.
82. Dale DC, Fauci AS, Wolff SM: Alternate-day prednisone: Leukocyte kinetics and susceptibility to infections. N Engl J Med 291:1154–1158, 1974.
83. Fauci AS, Dale DC: Alternate-day therapy and human lymphocyte sub-populations. J Clin Invest 55:22–32, 1975.
84. Schürmeyer TH, Tsokos GC, Avgerinos PC, et al: Pituitary-adrenal responsiveness to corticotropin-releasing hormone in patients receiving chronic, alternate day glucocorticoid therapy. J Clin Endocrinol Metab 61:22–27, 1985.
85. Hunder GG, Sheps SG, Allen GL, Joyce JW: Daily and alternate day corticosteroid regimens in treatment of giant cell arteritis: Comparison in a prospective study. Ann Intern Med 82:613–618, 1975.
86. Abruzzo JL: Alternate-day prednisone therapy. Ann Intern Med 82:714, 1975.
87. Bengtsson B-A, Malmvall B-E: An alternate-day corticosteroid regimen in maintenance therapy of giant cell arteritis. Acta Med Scand 209:347–350, 1981.
88. Fauci AS: Alternate-day corticosteroid therapy. Am J Med 64:729–731, 1978.
89. Allander E: ACTH or corticosteroids? A critical review of results and possibilities in the treatment of severe chronic disease. Acta Rheum Scand 15:277–296, 1969.
90. Kaplan HP, Portnoy B, Binder HJ, et al: A controlled evaluation of intravenous adrenocorticotropic hormone and hydrocortisone in the treatment of acute colitis. Gastroenterology 69:91–95, 1975.
91. Hrachovy RA, Frost JD Jr, Kellaway P, Zion TE: Double-blind study of ACTH vs prednisone therapy in infantile spasms. J Pediatr 103:641–645, 1983.
92. Steroids in acute severe asthma (editorial). Lancet 340:1384–1386, 1992.
93. McFadden ER Jr: Dosages of corticosteroids in asthma. Am Rev Respir Dis 147:1306–1310, 1993.
94. Elenbaas J: Steroid pulse therapy in systemic lupus erythematosus. Drug Intell Clin Pharm 17:342–344, 1983.
95. Kurki P (ed): High dose intravenous corticosteroid therapy of systemic lupus erythematosus and primary crescenteric rapidly progressive glomerulonephritis. Proceedings of a symposium. Scand J Rheumatol Suppl 54:1–34, 1984.
96. Udelsman R, Ramp J, Gallucci WT, et al: Adaptation during surgical stress: A reevaluation of the role of glucocorticoids. J Clin Invest 77:1377–1381, 1986.
97. Glowniak JV, Loriaux DL: A double-blind study of perioperative steroid requirements in secondary adrenal insufficiency. Surgery 121:123–129, 1997.

Chapter 120

Adrenal Insufficiency

D. Lynn Loriaux ▪ Walter J. McDonald

BACKGROUND

Adrenal insufficiency is the first clinical disorder that was linked unequivocally to pathologic changes in an endocrine organ. The recognition of this disease by Addison is generally accepted as the beginning of clinical endocrinology as a specialty. The adrenal glands were first recognized as organs distinct from the kidneys by Bartolomeo Eustachi in 1563[1] (Fig. 120–1). Three hundred years passed before the clinical importance of the adrenal glands was recognized by Addison[2] and described in one of the classic papers in medicine. He showed that destruction of the adrenal glands in humans was associated with a fatal outcome. Of the 11 patients described, 5 had bilateral and 1 had unilateral adrenal tuberculosis, 3 had carcinomatous adrenal involvement, 1 had adrenal hemorrhage, and 1 showed atrophy and fibrosis. Addison's findings were quickly confirmed by Brown-Sequard,[3] who verified Addison's hypothesis in several laboratory animals and showed that bilateral adrenalectomy was a uniformly fatal intervention. The clinical syndrome was named for Addison by Trousseau in 1856.[4] Osler[5] attempted unsuccessfully to treat a young patient with Addison's disease, employing a glycerine extract of fresh pig adrenals given orally. The effects were inconclusive. Wintersteiner and Pfiffner,[6] Kendall,[7] de Fremery et al.,[8] and Grollman[9] isolated and characterized cortisone and cortisol in the 1930s, and Sarett[10] devised a partial synthesis for cortisone from deoxycholic acid in 1945. The clinical effects of cortisone were soon made apparent by the work of Hench et al.[11] in the treatment of rheumatoid arthritis and by Thorn and Forsham[12] in the treatment of adrenal insufficiency. The role of the pituitary gland in regulating adrenal function was clarified largely by Cushing,[13] and the role of the hypothalamus in regulating pituitary function was clarified by Harris[14] in the 1950s. Adrenocorticotropic hormone (ACTH) was isolated and characterized by Li et al.[15] in 1958, and corticotropin-releasing hormone (CRH), in turn, was characterized by Vale et al.[16] in 1983. Finally, the syndrome of acute adrenal insufficiency was recognized in a surgical patient who had atrophic adrenal glands secondary to long-standing glucocorticoid treatment in 1961.[17]

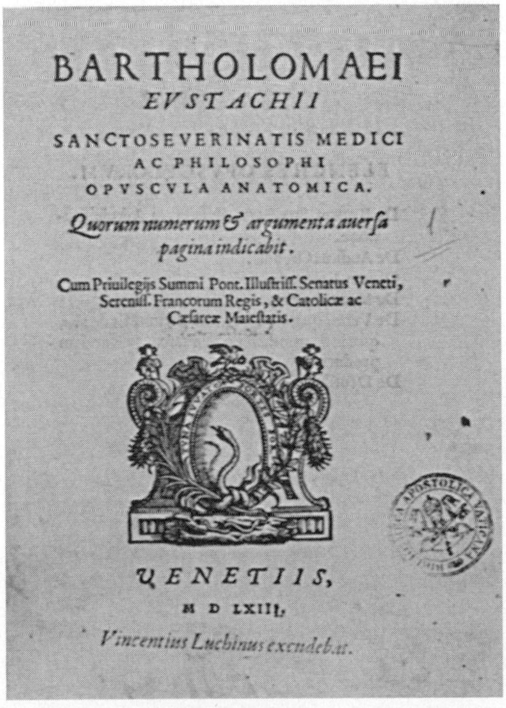

FIGURE 120–1. The frontispiece page from the 1563 edition of *Opuscula Anatomica* by Eustachi and Fallopio.

CLINICAL FEATURES

Adrenal insufficiency can be categorized into two types depending on the locus of the pathologic lesion causing the disorder. *Primary adrenal insufficiency* (Addison's disease) is caused by disordered adrenal function. It is characterized by a low cortisol production rate and a high plasma ACTH concentration. *Secondary adrenal insufficiency* is caused by disordered function of the hypothalamus and pituitary gland. It is characterized by a low cortisol production rate and a normal or low plasma ACTH concentration.

The adrenal steroids that play an important role in the syndromes of adrenal insufficiency are cortisol and aldosterone. Both are deficient in primary adrenal insufficiency. In secondary adrenal insufficiency, however, only cortisol is deficient, because the adrenal gland is normal in this condition, and aldosterone is regulated primarily by the renin-angiotensin system, which is independent of the hypothalamus and the pituitary gland. This difference underlies the very different clinical "presentations" of primary and secondary adrenal insufficiency.

The actions and mechanisms of action of glucocorticoid and mineralocorticoid are treated extensively elsewhere in this text. The actions of each class of steroid that have a role in the clinical syndromes of adrenal insufficiency, however, are limited in number. Glucocorticoid modulates ACTH secretion,[18, 19] maintains inotropy of the cardiac muscle,[20–23] modulates vascular response to the β agonists,[24] and antagonizes insulin action.[19, 25] Mineralocorticoid modulates the renal handling of sodium, potassium, and hydrogen ions, in effect promoting sodium retention at the expense of potassium and hydrogen excretion.[26] Thus, glucocorticoid deficiency is clinically manifested as ACTH-mediated hyperpigmentation (if the hypothalamic-pituitary unit is normal), hypotension characterized by tachycardia, reduced stroke volume, decreased peripheral vascular resistance, and in some cases, hypoglycemia. Mineralocorticoid deficiency is clinically manifested through isosmotic dehydration leading to hyponatremia, hyperkalemia,

TABLE 120–1. Primary Adrenal Insufficiency in Industrialized Countries

Idiopathic (including polyendocrine deficiency syndrome)	65%
Tuberculosis	20%
Other causes	15%
Fungi	
Adrenal hemorrhage	
Metastases	
Sarcoidosis	
Amyloidosis	
Adrenoleukodystrophy	
Adrenomyeloneuropathy	
Acquired immunodeficiency syndrome	
Congenital adrenal hyperplasia	
Congenital adrenal hypoplasia	
Congenital unresponsiveness to ACTH	
Medications	

ACTH, adrenocorticotropic hormone.

and metabolic acidosis. In primary adrenal insufficiency, the combined effects of glucocorticoid and mineralocorticoid deficiency lead to hyperpigmentation, orthostatic hypotension, hyponatremia, hyperkalemia, and a mild metabolic acidosis. In secondary adrenal insufficiency, the isolated effects of glucocorticoid insufficiency in association with ACTH deficiency lead to hypotension, hyponatremia secondary to antidiuretic hormone (ADH)–mediated water retention, normal potassium and hydrogen ion concentrations, and the absence of ACTH-mediated hyperpigmentation.

The causes of primary adrenal insufficiency are listed in Table 120–1. The most common cause worldwide is still tuberculosis. Tuberculosis causes adrenal insufficiency by replacing the adrenal cortex with caseating granulomas. Initially enlarged in most cases, the adrenal glands eventually fibrose and shrink, calcifying in 50% of cases.[27] The most common cause of adrenal insufficiency in the industrialized West is idiopathic adrenal insufficiency, also known as *autoimmune adrenal insufficiency* or the *polyendocrine deficiency syndrome.* There is evidence of both cell-mediated and humoral immune activity directed against all layers of the adrenal cortex. About 50% of these patients show evidence of other autoimmune endocrine disorders. These patients are classified as having polyendocrine autoimmune syndrome. In this disorder, an autoimmune "adrenalitis" leads to destruction of the adrenal cortex. This syndrome has two forms, designated types I and II[28] (Table 120–2). Type I is a rare disease of childhood, having a mean age of onset of 12 years. Type II, which is more common, has a mean age of onset of 24 years. The dominant features of type I disease are adrenal insufficiency, hypoparathyroidism, and mucocutaneous candidiasis. The dominant features of type II disease are adrenal insufficiency, autoimmune thyroid disease, and diabetes mellitus. Other important differences include the patterns of inheritance; type I is transmitted in an autosomal recessive pattern, occurring only across sibships,[29] whereas type II has a "dominant" pattern of inheritance, appearing in multiple generations of an affected family.[30] Finally, type I disease has no HLA association, while type II is associated with the DR3/DR4 haplotypes. Both disorders appear to be mediated by an autoimmune process. For example, circulating antibodies to one or more endocrine organs are found in most patients,[31] and defects in T lymphocyte function such as a decrease in "suppressor" activity are described.[32–42]

TABLE 120–2. Polyendocrine System

Manifestation	Type I	Type II
Mean age of onset	12 yr	24 yr
Adrenal insufficiency	+	+
Diabetes mellitus	−	+
Autoimmune thyroid disease	−	+
Hypoparathyroidism	+	−
Mucocutaneous candidiasis	+	−
Hypogonadism	+	±
Chronic active hepatitis	+	−
Pernicious anemia	+	−
Vitiligo	+	+

All the clinically important fungi except *Candida* can cause adrenal insufficiency. The most common is histoplasmosis, particularly prominent in the Ohio and Tennessee River Valleys and along the Piedmont Plateau of the Middle Atlantic States.[35, 36] South American blastomycosis is the next most common fungal cause of adrenal insufficiency,[37] followed by North American blastomycosis,[38] coccidioidomycosis, and cryptococcosis, all rare causes of adrenal destruction. The pathophysiology of this process is much like that of tuberculosis, with adrenal enlargement due to caseating granuloma formation. If there is healing, the adrenal glands can shrink and sometimes resume a relatively normal volume. This healing process is often accompanied by calcification.

With the advent of the abdominal computed tomography (CT) scan, adrenal hemorrhage is much more frequently recognized as a cause of adrenal insufficiency than in years past. The usual setting is a stressed individual anticoagulated for the prevention of pulmonary emboli or other thrombotic phenomena. Other scenarios include sepsis, trauma, and hypertension.[39] Another, more frequently recognized relationship is that of adrenal hemorrhage and the antiphospholipid syndrome.[40] Typically, the patient will complain of back pain, followed in a few days by the onset of the first signs and symptoms of adrenal insufficiency.[41–43] Rarely, patients may recover adrenal functions.[44]

Metastases to the adrenal gland are common, as high as 60% in patients with disseminated breast or lung cancer. Adrenal insufficiency as a result of metastases, however, is uncommon,[45] although abnormalities in adrenal function in patients with bilateral adrenal metastases can be demonstrated with higher frequency.[46] Tumors commonly associated with adrenal insufficiency are cancers of the breast, lung, stomach, and colon, melanoma, and some lymphomas.

Acquired immunodeficiency syndrome (AIDS) can be associated with adrenal insufficiency in its late stages. The adrenals are involved with infection or tumor in well over half the autopsy cases, although less than 50% of the adrenal gland is destroyed in 97% of cases.[47] This explains the rarity of overt symptoms. Cytomegalovirus infection of the adrenal glands is common in this condition, as is infection with *Mycobacterium avium-intracellulare* and the various fungi that can colonize and destroy the adrenal glands. The plasma cortisol response to ACTH administration, however, is abnormal in only 10% to 15% of these patients.[48]

Adrenoleukodystrophy and adrenomyeloneuropathy appear to be two clinical presentations of the same disorder. Adrenoleukodystrophy, also known as *brown Schilder's disease* (*brown* being an adjective describing the hyperpigmentation of the skin) or *sudanophilic leukodystrophy* is a disease of children characterized by rapidly progressive central demyelination eventuating in seizures, dementia, cortical blindness, coma, and death. Death usually occurs before puberty is complete.[49, 50] Adrenomyeloneuropathy is a disease of young adults that is characterized by a slowly progressive mixed motor and sensory peripheral neuropathy associated with an upper motor neuropathy leading to an ascending spastic paraparesis. Both forms of the disease are associated with progressive failure of the steroid-secreting cells leading to adrenal and gonadal failure.[51, 52] The metabolic marker for these diseases is an elevated circulating level of very long chain fatty acids (VLCFAs), C_{26} and greater in length. The cause of this abnormality seems to be an abnormal peroxisomal transporter protein that prevents the appropriate metabolism of the VLCFAs.[53] How this abnormality leads to the associated clinical manifestations remains unknown. Several treatments have been tried, but only autologous bone marrow transplantation appears to be successful.[54–56]

Other rare causes of primary adrenal insufficiency include amyloidosis,[57] congenital unresponsiveness to ACTH,[58] congenital adrenal hypoplasia,[59] and familial glucocorticoid insufficiency.[60] Although medications may precipitate adrenal insufficiency, they are rarely the cause (fluconazole, ketoconazole, phenytoin sodium, rifampin, barbiturate).

The causes of secondary adrenal insufficiency are listed in Table

TABLE 120–3. Causes of Secondary Adrenal Insufficiency

1. Hypothalamic-pituitary-adrenal suppression
   A. Exogenous
      i. Glucocorticoids
      ii. ACTH
   B. Endogenous: Cushing's syndrome, ACTH-dependent or ACTH-independent
2. Lesions of the hypothalamus or pituitary gland
   A. Neoplasm
      i. Pituitary tumor
      ii. Metastatic tumor
   B. Craniopharyngioma
   C. Infection
      i. Tuberculosis
      ii. Actinomycosis
      iii. Nocardia
3. Sarcoid
4. Head trauma
5. Isolated deficiency of ACTH

ACTH, adrenocorticotropic hormone.

120–3. The most common cause of secondary adrenal insufficiency is the suppression of CRH and ACTH synthesis and secretion that occurs as a result of exogenous steroid administration. If the exogenous steroids are discontinued for any reason, a period of absolute or relative adrenal insufficiency will ensue. Symptoms usually begin in the first 48 hours after discontinuation of the steroid medication. The likelihood of adrenal suppression in this situation, its magnitude, and its duration all depend on the dose of steroid given, its administration schedule, and the duration of administration. The least suppressive regimen is a dose of glucocorticoid that is less than the replacement dose given once a day in the morning for 2 weeks or less. In this case, meaningful adrenal suppression is unlikely.[18] At the other extreme is the administration of supraphysiologic doses of glucocorticoid given in divided doses around the clock for a period long enough to allow early signs of Cushing's syndrome to develop. In this case, the chance of meaningful adrenal suppression is almost a certainty, and its duration can be as long as 1 year.[61] Although rare, topical steroid cream can cause adrenal suppression, as can large-dose progesterone therapy such as is employed for treatment of breast carcinoma.[62, 63]

Suppression of hypothalamic and pituitary function also can result from endogenous glucocorticoid overproduction, as seen in Cushing's syndrome caused by an ACTH secretion, pituitary microadenoma, or cortisol-secreting adrenal carcinoma. Therapeutic interventions that eliminate the glucocorticoid excess unmask the secondary adrenal insufficiency.

Tumors and other destructive processes in the region of the sella turcica can lead to secondary adrenal insufficiency. Examples include pituitary tumor,[64] metastatic tumors to the region, sarcoid,[65] amyloid,[66] craniopharyngioma, and Rathke's pouch cyst. Infections such as actinomycosis and nocardiosis and vascular accidents such as Sheehan's syndrome can also lead to adrenal insufficiency. Finally, isolated ACTH deficiency can occur. In most cases, this appears to result from an autoimmune lymphocytic hypophysitis.[67]

SIGNS AND SYMPTOMS

The symptoms of adrenal insufficiency are the same for primary and secondary disease (Table 120–4). Addison's description of the clinical presentation remains as accurate today as it was in 1855: "anemia, general languor and debility, remarkable weakness of the heart's action, irritability of the stomach, and a peculiar change of color in the skin."[5] The usual complaints center around weakness, fatigue, loss of appetite, and weight loss. There are frequent gastrointestinal complaints that range from nausea to severe pain, possibly related to loss of gut mobility.[67] Some patients complain of dizziness on standing, and some complain of darkening of the skin, hair, and nails.

The signs of adrenal insufficiency characteristic of both primary and secondary disease include weight loss and orthostatic hypotension (Table 120–5). Signs specific to primary disease include hyperpigmentation, vitiligo, and adrenal calcification (Figs. 120–2 to 120–5).

Acute adrenal insufficiency is usually clinically manifested as shock poorly responsive to volume expansion and pressor agents. Supraventricular tachycardia, reduced stroke volume, and decreased peripheral resistance are usual.[68]

TABLE 120–4. Symptoms of Adrenal Insufficiency

Manifestation	Incidence
Weakness and fatigue	100%
Anorexia	~100%
Nausea, diarrhea	~ 50%
Muscle, joint, and abdominal pain	~ 10%
Postural dizziness	~ 10%

TABLE 120–5. Signs of Adrenal Insufficiency

Manifestation	Incidence
Weight loss	~100%
Orthostatic hypotension	~ 90%
Hyperpigmentation (primary)	~ 90%
Adrenal calcification (primary)	~ 10%
Vitiligo (primary)	~ 5%

LABORATORY FINDINGS

The traditional laboratory abnormalities associated with adrenal insufficiency include normochromic, normocytic anemia, relative lymphocytosis with increased eosinophil count, a mild metabolic acidosis, and some degree of prerenal azotemia. Electrolyte abnormalities include hyponatremia and hyperkalemia in primary disease and hyponatremia alone in secondary disease.[69] In the former case, the electrolyte abnormalities are attributable primarily to mineralocorticoid deficiency with its attendant salt wasting,[70] whereas in the second case, the abnormalities can be attributed primarily to free water retention mediated by vasopressin secreted to defend the "relative" volume deficiency caused by glucocorticoid deficiency.[71]

DIAGNOSIS

Traditional Tests of Adrenal Function

PORTER-SILBER CHROMOGENS. The 17-, 20-, and 21-carbon configuration of cortisol is the same as that of dihydroxyacetone (Fig. 120–6). Other adrenal steroids that have this configuration in the D ring side chain include cortisone, 11-deoxycortisol, tetrahydrocortisone, tetrahydro 11-deoxycortisol, and tetrahydrocortisol (Fig. 120–7). Dihydroxyacetone reacts with *meta*-dinitrobenzene to form a colored adduct with an absorption maximum at 410 μm. Steroids containing this reactive group do the same, a reaction that provides the chemical basis for the measurement of this group of steroids, as first described by Porter and Silber.[72] Because the urinary representatives of these steroids are, for the most part, conjugated to glucuronic and sulfuric acid (to provide water solubility), measurement of the Porter-Silber chromogens first involves an acid hydrolysis to clear the conjugates, followed by a lipid extraction with a solvent such a dichloromethane. The Porter-Silber reaction is then performed on the steroids in the lipid extract. The absorption maximum is quantitated spectrophotometrically. The normal range for Porter-Silber excretion is 2 to 12 mg/day. The excretion of these steroids is greatly affected by body size, and the normal range can be considerably tightened by normalizing

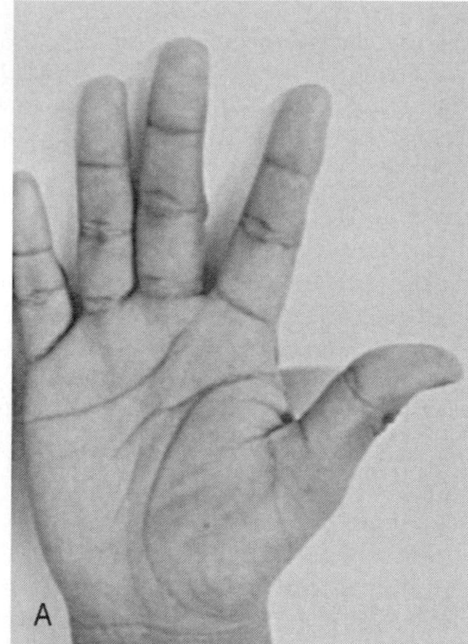

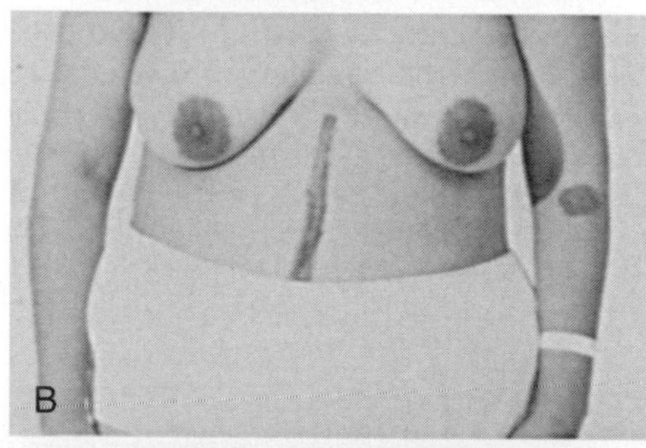

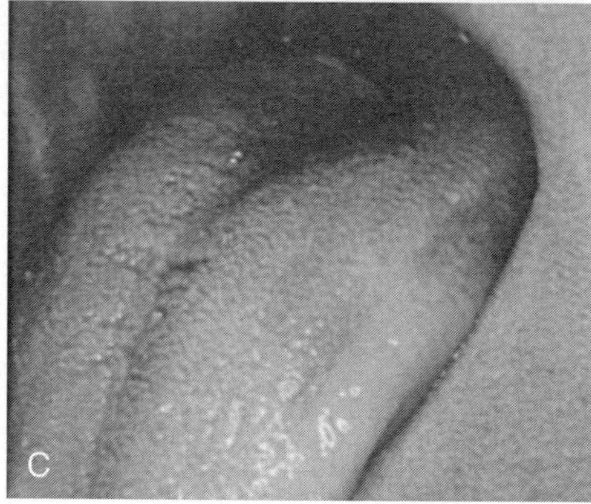

FIGURE 120–2. Hyperpigmented hand, scar, areolae, and buccal mucosa. (From Loriaux L, Cutler G Jr: Diseases of the adrenal gland. *In* Kohler P (ed): Clinical Endocrinology. New York, Churchill-Livingstone, 1986, p 211.)

the measurement with the urinary creatinine excretion.[73] With this correction, the normal range is the same for all ages, 4.5 ± (SD) mg/g creatinine/day.[74] The normal range includes the extinction point for the assay, rendering the measurement of values below the normal range impossible with this assay.

17-KETOSTEROIDS. 17-Ketosteroids react with *para*-aminobenzoic acid to yield a colored adduct with an absorption maximum at 520 μm.[75] Steroids of adrenal origin having the 17-ketosteroid configuration include dehydroepiandrosterone, androstenedione, etiocholanolone, androsterone, and their reduced metabolites (Fig. 120–8). This group of steroids is referred to, collectively, as the *adrenal androgens.* The normal range for 17-ketosteroid excretion is sex- and age-dependent and reflects the process of adrenarche.[76] The production rate of glucocorticoid is only indirectly reflected by this assay. Suppression of adrenal androgen secretion by exogenous glucocorticoid and recovery of adrenal androgen secretion from suppression by exogenous glucocorticoid both have a different pattern from that for cortisol secretion.[77, 78]

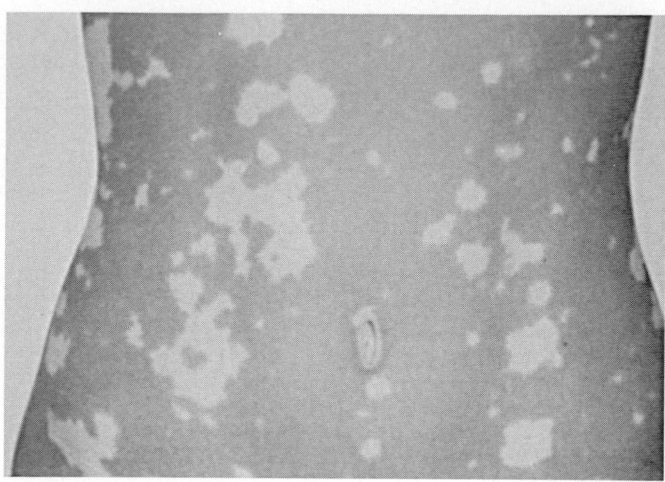

FIGURE 120–3. Vitiligo. (From Loriaux L, Cutler G Jr: Diseases of the adrenal gland. *In* Kohler P (ed): Clinical Endocrinology. New York, Churchill-Livingstone, 1986, p 211.)

17-KETOGENIC STEROIDS. The 17-ketogenic steroid measurement quantitates those urinary steroids that can be oxidized with periodic acid to yield the 17-keto configuration.[79, 80] In the usual measurement of the 17-ketogenic steroids, extant 17-ketosteroids are first reduced with sodium or lithium borohydride. Newly produced 17-ketosteroids can then be measured without interference from these pre-existing steroids that primarily reflect adrenal androgen production. Steroids that form 17-ketosteroids when oxidized by periodic acid are primarily the C-21 steroids with a 17-hydroxyl group (see Fig. 120–8). The 17-ketogenic steroid measurement had its greatest utility in measuring pregnanetriol, a metabolite of 17-hydroxy progesterone, the "marker" steroid for 21-hydroxylase deficiency. It is a complex assay that is now rarely used.

URINARY FREE CORTISOL. Urinary free cortisol is the fraction of urinary cortisol that is unconjugated to glucuronic acid or sulfate.[81] It can be extracted from urine with a lipid solvent such a dichloromethane. It represents that fraction of plasma protein unbound cortisol

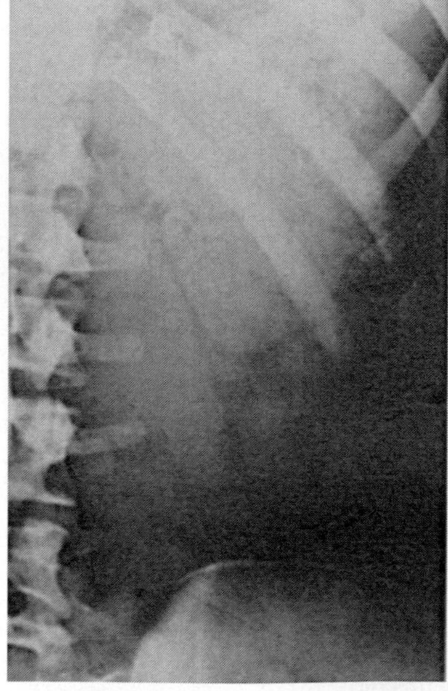

FIGURE 120–4. Adrenal calcification on "flat plate" of the abdomen. (From Loriaux L, Cutler G Jr: Diseases of the adrenal gland. *In* Kohler P (ed): Clinical Endocrinology. New York, Churchill-Livingstone, 1986, p 211.)

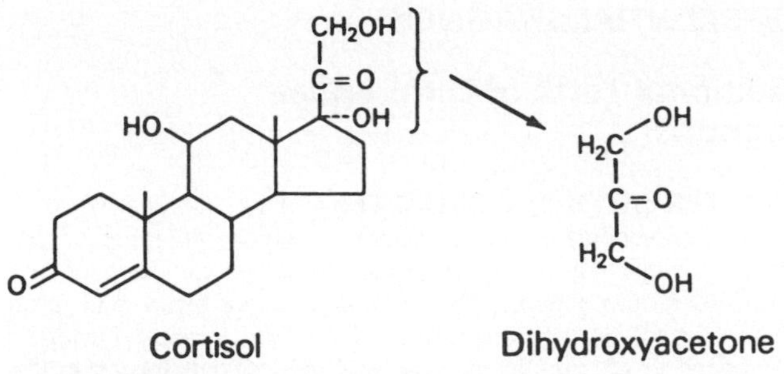

FIGURE 120–5. The dihydroxyacetone side chain of cortisol.

that is filtered by the glomerulus and not reabsorbed by the nephron. This varies between 1% and 5% of the filtered cortisol. The detection limit of this assay is usually in the normal range of cortisol excretion and is thus not a reliable test for the diagnosis of adrenal insufficiency.

METYRAPONE TEST. Metyrapone is a competitive inhibitor of the 11-hydroxylase enzyme that is responsible for the conversion of 11-deoxycortisol into cortisol. In the presence of metyrapone, the plasma cortisol concentration falls. To restore this to normal, ACTH secretion is increased and cortisol is restored to the normal range. This adjustment occurs until the enzyme is completely blocked. At that point, all steroid precursor shunted into the synthesis of cortisol is released into the general circulation as 11-deoxycortisol. 11-Deoxycortisol is cleared from the plasma at twice the rate of cortisol because of its reduced affinity for the cortisol-binding globulin (CBG). Thus, if plasma cortisol should reach a level of 20 μg/dL under maximal ACTH stimulation, 11-deoxycortisol should achieve a plasma concentration of at least 10 μg/dL in the presence of "blocking" concentrations of metyrapone if the feedback axis is intact. The traditional test is performed by administering 750 g metyrapone four times a day, orally, for 48 hours.[82] At the end of the test, plasma cortisol should be less than 5 μg/dL, documenting the completeness of the enzyme blockade, and 11-deoxycortisol should be greater than 10 μg/dL if the feedback axis is normally functional. If the plasma cortisol level is greater than 5 μg/dL, the test cannot be interpreted. If it is an interpretable test, 11 deoxycortisol concentrations higher than 10 μg/dL signify a normally functioning hypothalamic-pituitary-adrenal "axis." Lesser values imply a failure of feedback regulation.

The test has some value in the differential diagnosis of adrenal hyperfunction, identifying patients with Cushing's disease.[83] The test is frequently employed in the diagnosis of adrenal insufficiency, but in all forms of this disorder the test is abnormal and gives no useful diagnostic or differential diagnostic information. Untoward side effects are common.[84] In addition, the standard 2-day test can be hazardous in that marginally adequate cortisol concentrations are further impaired as a result of the examination. In the opinion of the authors, this test is no longer indicated for the diagnosis and differential diagnosis of adrenal insufficiency.

INSULIN TOLERANCE TEST. Insulin-induced hypoglycemia is a powerful stimulus for the secretion of cortisol. This stimulus depends on an intact hypothalamic stimulation of pituitary ACTH secretion and on the ability of the adrenal gland to respond to ACTH with the secretion of cortisol. Thus, a normal test indicates a normally functioning "adrenal" axis. An abnormal test implies a lesion in this system that can be anywhere between the hypothalamus and the adrenal gland. The usual test is done by administering 0.15 units/kg of regular insulin intravenously as a bolus and measuring blood sugar and cortisol at 15-minute intervals over the subsequent hour. The blood glucose

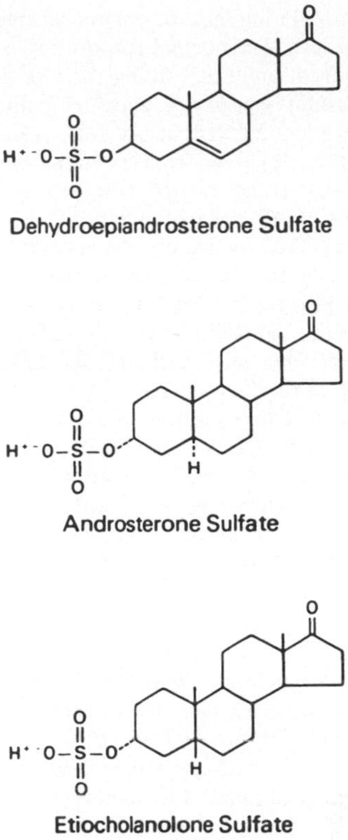

FIGURE 120–7. The major urinary 17-ketosteroids.

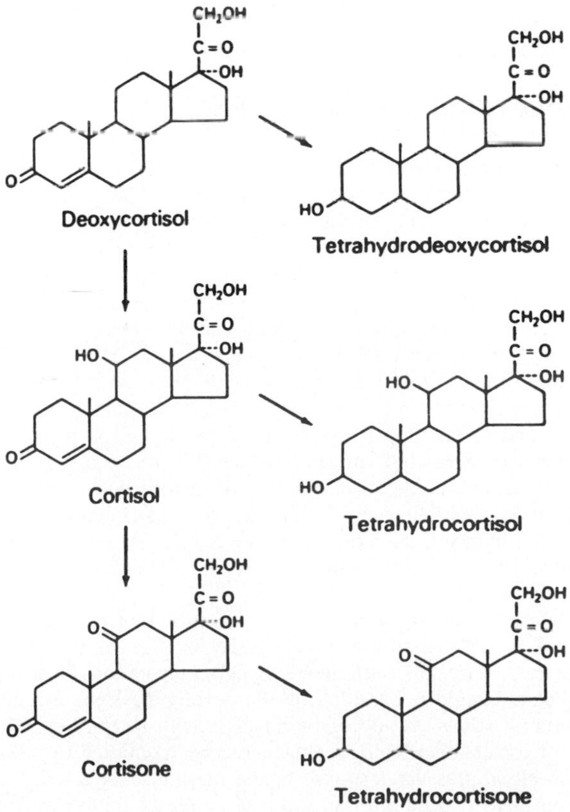

FIGURE 120–6. Adrenal products having the dihydroxyacetone side chain.

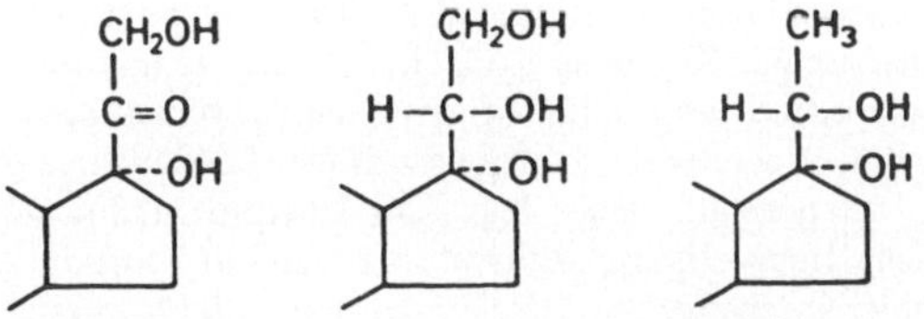

FIGURE 120–8. D-ring configurations susceptible to sodium bismuthate oxidation.

level must fall below 45 mg/mL to ensure adequate stimulation for interpretation of the test. The normal response is a plasma cortisol of greater than 20 μg/dL at any time during the test. The test is complex and depends on insulin sensitivity and the rapidity of the fall in glucose. The test is plagued with many false-negative results and is uncomfortable for the subject as well as hazardous. This test, in the opinion of the authors, is no longer indicated for the diagnosis and differential diagnosis of adrenal insufficiency.[85, 86]

PLASMA CORTISOL. Intuitively, the measurement of circulating plasma cortisol should provide the most direct assessment of adrenal cortisol secretion. Plasma cortisol has been measured fluorometrically,[87] with a binding globulin,[88] and by radioimmunoassay.[81] The normal range provided by each technique is roughly equivalent and depends on the time of day the plasma is sampled and the sleep-wake pattern of the subject. The secretion of cortisol is pulsatile, with a steady frequency of about 1 pulse an hour in adults. The amplitude of these pulses, however, varies greatly with about 8 to 10 high-amplitude pulses clustering in the early morning hours.[89] This pattern creates a diurnal secretory rhythm in plasma cortisol concentration.[90] Cortisol circulates predominately bound to a glycosylated 59-kDa α_2-globulin, CBG, or transcortin.[91] This binding globulin protects circulating cortisol from hepatic clearance, giving cortisol a relatively long plasma half-life of between 60 and 80 minutes. Normal plasma cortisol concentrations range between 5 and 20 μg/dL, but most normal subjects, at some time each day, have plasma concentrations of cortisol that cannot be differentiated from zero. These biologic complexities render hazardous the interpretation of any single plasma cortisol. If cortisol is measured at frequent intervals (30 minutes) over a 24-hour period and the values are averaged, the mean plasma cortisol concentration has a value of 7.5 μg/dL and a standard deviation of 1 μg/dL.[92] To work within this narrow confidence interval, however, requires the measurement of a large number of plasma cortisol concentrations—prohibitive except in extraordinary circumstances.

ACTH STIMULATION TESTS. To circumvent the problems that the pulsatile secretion of cortisol presents to an evaluation of adrenal function using plasma measurements of cortisol and the analogous problems that variability in the hepatic metabolism of cortisol and its metabolites presents to an evaluation of adrenal function using urinary measurements of adrenal steroid metabolites, tests of maximum adrenal function were devised using ACTH as a stimulus. Early tests employed ACTH extracted from bovine pituitary glands. This material was contaminated with antidiuretic hormone, and its administration often resulted in transient water intoxication.[93] This shortcoming was rectified with the availability of synthetic ACTH (1–24). This material is synthesized chemically, is pure, and is essentially free of serious side effects. Many ACTH stimulation tests have been devised, generally entailing different doses of ACTH, different preparations, and different routes of administration. Of these, one has become preeminent in the diagnosis of adrenal insufficiency, and this test constitutes the mainstay of the current approach to the diagnosis of this disorder.

Contemporary Tests for the Diagnosis of Adrenal Insufficiency

CORTROSYN TEST. This test has become the standard screening test for the diagnosis of adrenal insufficiency. The test depends on the fact that the normal adrenal gland, under maximal and acute ACTH stimulation, has at the lower bound of the normal range a plasma cortisol concentration of 20 μg/dL.[94] The test is simply done and simply interpreted. Synthetic ACTH, 250 μg, is administered as an intravenous bolus, any time of day, and a blood sample for the measurement of cortisol is drawn 45 minutes later. Values greater than 20 μg/dL are normal; values less than 20 μg/dL (18 μg/dL in some laboratories) imply dysfunction of the adrenal "axis." The test is quick, stable, insensitive to interference from diet or medication, simple to interpret, reliable, and can be applied to people of all ages without fear of untoward effect.

DIFFERENTIAL DIAGNOSIS

Traditional Tests of Differential Diagnosis

48-HOUR ACTH INFUSION TEST. This test is performed by infusing intravenously, in a continuous fashion, 80 units of ACTH daily for 2 days. The response parameter is the excretion of urinary Porter-Silber chromogens. The normal adrenal gland will produce enough cortisol during this test to elevate the urinary Porter-Silber chromogens to 45 mg/day or greater. Subjects with primary adrenal insufficiency are unable to increase the excretion of urinary Porter-Silber chromogens, and patients with secondary adrenal insufficiency fall in between.[95] This test requires hospitalization to perform and, mainly for that reason, has become obsolete in the differential diagnosis of adrenal insufficiency.

ALDOSTERONE RESPONSE TO ACTH STIMULATION. Normally, both cortisol and aldosterone respond to ACTH stimulation.[96] In primary adrenal insufficiency, neither cortisol nor aldosterone responds to an ACTH challenge, the adrenal glands being destroyed. Thus, the response of aldosterone to an acute ACTH challenge can often distinguish primary from secondary adrenal insufficiency.[97, 98]

Contemporary Tests of Differential Diagnosis

PLASMA ACTH CONCENTRATION. The development of the two-site IRMA assay for ACTH has simplified considerably the differential diagnosis of adrenal insufficiency. The normal range of plasma ACTH extends up to 100 pg/mL. Adrenal insufficiency in association with low or normal plasma concentrations of ACTH is secondary in nature; adrenal insufficiency in association with high plasma ACTH concentrations is primary. The test is simple, reliable, inexpensive, and compatible with the outpatient nature of the contemporary evaluation of this disorder.[99]

TREATMENT

Chronic Adrenal Insufficiency

The treatment of adrenal insufficiency consists of the replacement of the missing steroid hormones: cortisol in secondary adrenal insufficiency and cortisol and aldosterone in primary adrenal insufficiency. Many glucocorticoid preparations are available for this use. Only one, hydrocortisone itself, is appropriate for this purpose. Most of the synthetic steroids such as prednisone and dexamethasone are longer-acting and have no mineralocorticoid activity. Hence, these steroids are ideally suited for pharmacologic intervention in diseases of inflammation and as probes for differential diagnosis, but not for physiologic replacement. Cortisone acetate has a reputation for reduced efficacy and is no longer frequently used.[100, 101] The usual dose of hydrocortisone (cortisol) ranges between 12 and 15 mg/m^2 of body surface area.[13, 69] Hydrocortisone can be given as a "once a day" oral dose, and compliance is enhanced with this regimen. The only preparation available to replace mineralocorticoid activity is florinef. The usual dose is 100 μg/day by mouth. There is no parenteral preparation of florinef.

Response to therapy is monitored clinically. Glucocorticoid undertreatment is evidenced by weight loss, hyponatremia, and, in patients with primary adrenal insufficiency, hyperpigmentation. Overtreatment with glucocorticoid is heralded by the developing signs of Cushing's syndrome in adults and deceleration of growth in children. The adequacy of mineralocorticoid treatment can be monitored by measuring postural blood pressure response or the plasma renin activity. Undertreatment is associated with an increased renin activity; overtreatment with a plasma renin activity resistant to stimulation by 4 hours of upright posture.

Chronic Adrenal Suppression

The goal in treating chronic adrenal suppression is to replace glucocorticoid in a fashion that will permit a reasonable quality of life and at the same time encourage recovery of normal hypothalamic-pituitary-adrenal function. This is usually accomplished by prescribing a dose of hydrocortisone in the range of 12 mg/m^2 as a "once every morning" dose. Recovery can be gauged by the response of plasma cortisol to an intravenous injection of cosyntropin (Cortrosyn), recovery being indicated by a plasma cortisol level of greater than 20 μg/dL. This test can reasonably be done at 6 months and every 3 months thereafter until recovery is documented. When recovery is documented, hydrocortisone replacement therapy can be discontinued safely.

Acute Adrenal Insufficiency

Acute adrenal insufficiency should be considered in any ill patient who has been taking glucocorticoids or has a systemic disease associated with adrenal insufficiency such as metastatic cancer, AIDS, or tuberculosis. At one extreme is unexplained fever, abdominal pain, and orthostatic hypotension. At the other extreme is shock unresponsive to pressors and volume replacement. In this case, a blood sample should be drawn for the measurement of cortisol, after the administration of ACTH if time permits. Depending on the severity of the illness and the availability of rapid cortisol measurements, the physician may elect to treat on the assumption that the illness is acute adrenal insufficiency or to hold treatment pending the results of the diagnostic evaluation. Obviously, in cases of shock or "pending" shock, waiting is imprudent. Treatment consists of replacing intravascular volume, sodium chloride, and glucocorticoid. Volume and sodium chloride can be replaced together in the form of normal saline infused as quickly as the cardiovascular status will permit. Infusions of 2 to 3 L/hr are not unusual. As the hypotension improves, the rate of infusion should be metered back to 3 to 4 L/day of normal saline. Glucocorticoid should be given intravenously if possible, 100 mg hydrocortisone every 6 hours. If adrenal insufficiency is the sole cause of the clinical picture, clear improvement can be expected within 12 hours. This regimen should be maintained until the results of the blood tests return. If the diagnosis is confirmed, the hydrocortisone dose can be "tapered" into the normal range over the next 2 or 3 days. If the diagnosis is not confirmed, the regimen should be discontinued.

Stress

The adjustment of glucocorticoid dose with "stress" remains a problematic issue. The standard of practice is to double the dose with minor stresses such as upper respiratory infections, low-grade febrile illnesses, and minor surgical procedures such as dental work and minor trauma such as small lacerations and contusions. The general practice is to increase the daily dose of hydrocortisone to about 400 mg/day for major stresses such as intracavitary surgical procedures. There are few data to support this practice other than the early observations that cortisol excretory products rise with stress,[102] and there is recent laboratory evidence suggesting that cortisol supplementation may not be necessary.[103] Nonetheless, until it is convincingly demonstrated that the practice has no value, the prudent course is to conform.

REFERENCES

1. Eustachi B, Fallopio G: Opuscula Anatomica. Venice, 1563.
2. Addison T: On the Constitutional and Local Effects of Disease of the Suprarenal Capsules. London, Highly, 1855.
3. Brown-Sequard CE: Recherches Experimentales sur la Physiologie et la Pathologie des Capsules Surrenales. Acad Sci Paris 43:422–425, 1856.
4. Trousseau A: Bronze Addison's disease. Arch Gen Med 8:478, 1856.
5. Osler W: Case of Addison's disease: Death during treatment with the supravital extra. Bull Johns Hopkins Hosp 7:208–209, 1896.
6. Wintersteiner OP, Pfiffner J: Chemical studies on the adrenal cortex, part II. J Biol Chem 111:599–612, 1935.
7. Kendall EC: A chemical and physiological investigation of the suprarenal cortex. Symp Quant Biol 5:299, 1937.
8. de Fremery P, Laquer E, Reichstein T, et al: Corticosterone: A crystalloid compound with biological activity of the adrenal-cortical hormone. Nature 139:26–27, 1937.
9. Grollman A: Physiological and chemical studies on the adrenal cortical hormone. Symp Quant Biol 5:313, 1937.
10. Sarett L: The synthesis of hydrocortisone from desoxycholic acid. J Biol Chem 162:601, 1946.
11. Hench PS, Slocumb CH, Barnes AR, et al: The effects of the adrenal cortical hormone, compound E, on the acute phase of rheumatic fever: A preliminary report. Proc Mayo Clin 24:277–297, 1949.
12. Thorn GW, Forsham PH: The treatment of adrenal insufficiency. Rec Prog Horm Res 4:229, 1949.
13. Cushing HW: The Pituitary Body and Its Disorders. Philadelphia, JB Lippincott, 1912.
14. Harris GW: Neural control of the pituitary gland. Physiol Rev 28:139, 1948.
15. Li CH, Dixon JS, Chung D: The structure of bovine corticotropin. J Am Chem Soc 80:2587–2596, 1958.
16. Vale W, Spiers J, Rivier C, Rivier J: Characterization of a 41-residue ovine hypothalamic peptide that stimulates secretion of corticotropin and beta-endorphin. Science 213:585–587, 1981.
17. Sampson PA, Brooke BN, Winstone NE: Biochemical confirmation of collapse due to adrenal failure. Lancet 1:1377, 1961.
18. Speigel RJ, Vigersky RA, Oliff AI: Adrenal suppression after short term corticosteroid therapy. Lancet 1:630–632, 1979.
19. Olefsky JM: The effect of dexamethasone on insulin binding, glucose transport, and glucose oxidation of isolated rat adipocytes. J Clin Invest 56:1499–1508, 1975.
20. Reidenberg MM, Ohler EA, Seuy RW, Harakal C: Hemodynamic changes in adrenalectomized dogs. Endocrinology 72:918–923, 1963.
21. Clarke APW, Cleghorn RA, Ferguson JKW, Fowler JLA: Factors concerned in the circulatory failure of adrenal insufficiency. J Clin Invest 26:359–363, 1947.
22. Lefer AM, Verrier RL, Carson WW: Cardiac performance in experimental adrenal insufficiency. Circ Res 22:817–827, 1968.
23. Lefer AM: Influence of corticosteroids on mechanical performance of isolated rat papillary muscles. Am J Physiol 214:518–524, 1968.
24. Rodan SB, Rodan GA: Dexamethasone effects on beta-adrenergic receptors and adenylate cyclase regulatory proteins Gs and Gi in ROS 17/2.8 cells. Endocrinology 118:2510–2518, 1986.
25. Livingstone JN, Lockwood DH: Effect of glucocorticoids on the glucose transport system of isolated fat cells. J Biol Chem 250:8353–8360, 1975.
26. [illegible] Miner Electrolyte Metab 9:1–32, 1983.
27. Vita JA, Silverberg SJ, Goland RS, et al: Clinical clues to the cause of Addison's disease. Am J Med 78:461–466, 1985.
28. Neufeld M, Maclaren NK, Blizzard RM: Two types of autoimmune Addison's disease associated with different polyglandular autoimmune syndromes. Medicine 60:355–362, 1981.
29. Eisenbarth GS, Jackson RA: The immunoendocrinopathy syndromes. *In* Wilson JD, Foster DW (eds): Williams Textbook of Endocrinology, ed 8. Philadelphia, WB Saunders, 1992, p 1561.
30. Eisenbarth GS, Wilson P, Ward F: HLA type and occurrence of disease in familial polyglandular failure. N Engl J Med 298:92–94, 1978.
31. Nerup J: Addison's disease: Serological studies. Acta Endocrinol (Copenh) 76:142–153, 1974.
32. Arulanantham K, Dwyer JM, Genel M: Evidence of defective immunoregulation in the syndrome of familial candidiasis endocrinopathy. N Engl J Med 300:164–170, 1979.
33. Fairchild RS, Schimke RN, Abdou NI: Immunoregulation abnormalities in familial Addison's disease. J Clin Endocrinol Metab 51:1074–1077, 1980.
34. Rabinowe SL, Jackson RA, Dluhy RG: Ia-positive lymphocytes in recently diagnosed idiopathic Addison's disease. Am J Med 77:597–601, 1984.
35. Sarosi GA, Voth DW, Dahl BA, et al: Disseminated histoplasmosis: Results of long term follow-up. Ann Intern Med 75:511–516, 1971.
36. Levine E: CT evaluation of active adrenal histoplasmosis. Urol Radiol 13:103–106, 1991.
37. Osa SR, Peterson RE, Roberts RB: Recovery of adrenal reserve following treatment of South American blastomycosis. Am J Med 71:298–301, 1981.
38. Abernathy RS, Melby JC: Addison's disease in North American blastomycosis. N Engl J Med 266:552–554, 1962.
39. Dahlberg PJ, Goellner MH, Pehling GB: Adrenal insufficiency secondary to adrenal hemorrhage. Arch Intern Med 150:905–909, 1990.
40. Levy EN, Ramsey-Goldman R, Kahl LE: Adrenal insufficiency in two women with anticardiolipin antibodies: cause and effect? Arthritis Rheum 35:1842–1846, 1990.
41. Jain CU, Gudi K, Giovanniello J: ACTH-induced bilateral adrenal hemorrhage. AJR 154:424–425, 1990.
42. Siu SC, Kitzman DW, Sheedy PF, Northcutt RC: Adrenal insufficiency from bilateral adrenal hemorrhage. Mayo Clin Proc 65:664–670, 1990.
43. Chin R: Adrenal crisis. Crit Care Clin 7:23–42, 1991.
44. Feurstein B, Streeten DHF: Recovery of adrenal function after failure resulting from traumatic bilateral adrenal hemorrhages. Ann Intern Med 115:785–786, 1991.
45. Hasan RI, Yonan NA, Lawson RA: Adrenal insufficiency due to bilateral metastases from oat cell carcinoma of the esophagus. Eur J Cardiothorac Surg 5:336–337, 1991.
46. Ihde JK, Turnbull AD, Bajorunas DR: Adrenal insufficiency in the cancer patient: Implications for the surgeon. Br J Surg 77:1335–1337, 1990.
47. Glasgow BJ, Steinsapir BS, Anders K, et al: Adrenal pathology in the acquired immunodeficiency syndrome. Am J Clin Pathol 84:594–597, 1985.
48. Guerra I, Kimmel PL: Hypokalemic adrenal crisis in a patient with AIDS. South Med J 84:1265–1267, 1991.

49. Schaumberg H, Powers JM, Raine CS, et al: Adrenoleukodystrophy: A clinical and pathological study of 17 cases. Arch Neurol 32:577–585, 1975.
50. Johnson AB, Ascauhberg HH, Powers TM: Histochemical characteristics of the striated inclusions of adrenoleukodystrophy. J Histochem Cytochem 24:725–730, 1976.
51. Griffen JW, Goren E, Schaumberg H: Adrenomyelopathy: A probable variant of adrenoleukodystrophy. Neurology 27:1107–1111, 1977.
52. Schaumberg H, Powers JM, Raine CS: Adrenomyeloneuropathy: General, pathologic, neuropathologic, and biochemical aspects. Neurology 27:1114–1120, 1977.
53. Mosser J, Douar AM, Sarde CO, et al: Putative X-linked adrenoleukodystrophy gene shares unexpected homology with ABC transporters. Nature 361:726–730, 1993.
54. Moser HW, Moser AB, Smith KD, et al: Adrenoleukodystrophy: Phenotypic variability and implications for therapy. J Inherit Metab Dis 15:645–664, 1992. (Published erratum appears in J Inherit Metab Dis 15(6):918, 1992.)
55. Hoogerbrugge PM, Brouwer OF, Fischer A: Bone marrow transplantation for metabolic diseases with severe neurological symptoms. Bone Marrow Transplant 7(suppl 2):71, 1991.
56. Aubourg P, Blanche S, Jambaquë I, et al: Reversal of early neurologic and neuroradiologic manifestations of X-linked adrenoleukodystrophy by bone marrow transplantation. N Engl J Med 322:1860–1866, 1990.
57. Arik N, Tasdemir I, Karaaslan Y, et al: Subclinical adrenocortical insufficiency in renal amyloidosis. Nephron 56:246–248, 1990.
58. Migeon CJ, Kenney FM, Kowarsky A: The syndrome of congenital adrenocortical unresponsiveness. Pediatr Res 2:501–509, 1968.
59. Wise JE, Matalon R, Morgan AM, et al: Phenotypic features of patients with congenital adrenal hypoplasia and glycerol kinase deficiency. J Dis Child 141:744–747, 1987.
60. Moshang T, Rosenfield RL, Bongiovanni AM, et al: Familial glucocorticoid insufficiency. J Pediatr 82:821–827, 1973.
61. Graber AL, Ney RL, Nicholson WE, et al: Natural history of pituitary-adrenal recovery following long-term suppression with corticosteroids. J Clin Endocrinol Metab 25:11–17, 1965.
62. Staughten RCD, August PJ: Cushing's syndrome and pituitary-adrenal suppression due to clobetasol propionate. BMJ 2:419–421, 1975.
63. Hug V, Kau S, Hertobagi GN, et al: Adrenal failure in patients with breast carcinoma after long-term treatment of cyclic alternating oestrogen progesterone. Br J Cancer 63:454–456, 1991.
64. Comtois R, Beauregard H, Somma M, et al: The clinical and endocrine outcome to transsphenoidal microsurgery of non-secreting pituitary adenomas. Cancer 68:860–866, 1991.
65. Verhage TL, Godfried MH, Alberts C: Hypothalamic-pituitary dysfunction with adrenal insufficiency and hyperprolactinemia in sarcoidosis. Sarcoidosis 7:139–141, 1990.
66. Erdkamp FL, Gams RO, Hoorntje SJ: Endocrine organ failure due to systemic AA-amyloidosis. Neth J Med 38:24–28, 1991.
67. Sugiura M, Hashimoto A, Shizawa M, et al: Heterogeneity of anterior pituitary cell antibodies detected in insulin-dependent diabetes mellitus and ACTH deficiency. Diabetes Res 3:111–114, 1986.
68. Claussen MS, Landercasper J, Cogbill TH: Acute adrenal insufficiency presenting as shock after trauma and surgery: Three cases and a review of the literature. J Trauma 32:94–100, 1992.
69. Pearson OH, Whitmore WF, West CD: Clinical and metabolic studies of bilateral adrenalectomy for advanced cancer in man. Surgery 34:543–552, 1953.
70. Lipsett MB, Pearson OH: Pathophysiology and treatment of adrenal crisis. N Engl J Med 254:511–515, 1956.
71. Boykin T, DeTorrente A, Erikson A: The role of plasma vasopressin in impaired water excretion of glucocorticoid deficiency. J Clin Invest 62:738–746, 1978.
72. Silber RH, Porter CC: The determination of 17,21-dihydroxy-20-ketosteroids in urine and plasma. J Biol Chem 210:923–930, 1954.
73. Streeten DHP, Stephenson CT, Dalakos TG, et al: The diagnosis of hypercortisolism: Biochemical criteria differentiating patients from lean and obese normal subjects and from females on oral contraceptives. J Clin Endocrinol Metab 29:1191–1211, 1969.
74. Franks RC: 17-Hydroxy corticosteroid and cortisol excretion in childhood. J Clin Endocrinol Metab 36:702–710, 1973.
75. Zimmerman W: Eine Farbreaktion der Sexualhormone und ihre Anwendung zur Quantitativen Colorimetrischen Bestimmung. Z Physiol Chem 233:257–273, 1935.
76. Humburger C: Normal urinary excretion of neutral 17-ketosteroids with special reference to age and sex variations. Acta Endocrinol (Copenh) 1:19–29, 1948.
77. Cutler GB, Davis SE, Johnsonbaugh RE, Loriaux DL: Dissociation of cortisol and adrenal androgen secretion in patients with secondary adrenal insufficiency. J Clin Endocrinol Metab 49:604–609, 1979.
78. Rittmaster RS, Loriaux DL, Cutler GB Jr: Sensitivity of cortisol and adrenal androgens to dexamethasone suppression in hirsute women. J Clin Endocrinol Metab 61:462–466, 1985.
79. Appleby JI, Gibson G, Norynbersky JK, et al: Indirect analysis of corticosteroids. Biochem J 60:453–460, 1955.
80. Few JD: A method for analysis of urinary 17-hydroxycorticosteroids. J Endocrinol 22:31–39, 1961.
81. Ruder HJ, Guy RL, Lipsett MB: A radioimmunoassay for cortisol in plasma and urine. J Clin Endocrinol Metab 35:219–223, 1972.
82. Liddle GW, Estep HL, Kendall TW, et al: Clinical application of a new test of pituitary reserve. J Clin Endocrinol Metab 19:875–880, 1959.
83. Tucci TR: Metyrapone test in Cushing's disease. J Clin Endocrinol Metab 40:521–526, 1975.
84. Nelson TC, Tindall DJ: A comparison of the adrenal responses to hypoglycemia, metyrapone, and ACTH. Am J Med Sci 275:165–170, 1978.
85. Plumpton FS, Besser GM: The adrenocortical response to surgery and insulin-induced hypoglycemia in corticosteroid treated and normal subjects. Br J Surg 56:216–220, 1969.
86. Lindholm J, Kehlet H, Blichert-Toft M, et al: Reliability of the 30-minute ACTH test in assessing hypothalamic-pituitary-adrenal function. J Clin Endocrinol Metab 47:272–279, 1978.
87. Espiner EA: The relationship between free cortisol in urine and urinary free 11-hydroxysteroids as measured by fluorescence. J Endocrinol 33:233–240, 1965.
88. Murphy BEP: Clinical evaluation of urinary cortisol determinations by competitive protein binding radioassay. J Clin Endocrinol Metab 28:343–350, 1968.
89. Veldhuis JD, Iranmanesh A, Johnson ML, et al: Amplitude, but not frequency, modulation of ACTH secretory bursts gives rise to the nyctohemeral rhythm of the corticotropic axis in man. J Clin Endocrinol Metab 71:452–463, 1990.
90. Kreiger DT, Allen W, Rizzo F: Characterization of the normal temporal pattern of plasma corticosteroid levels. J Clin Endocrinol Metab 32:266–270, 1971.
91. Hammond GL, Smith CL, Goping IS, et al: Primary structure of human corticosteroid binding globulin, deduced from hepatic and pulmonary cDNA's, exhibits homology with serine protease inhibitors. Proc Natl Acad Sci U S A 84:5153–5157, 1987.
92. Chrousos GP, Vingerhoeds A, Brandon D, et al: Primary cortisol resistance in man: A glucocorticoid receptor-mediated disease. J Clin Invest 69:1261–1269, 1982.
93. Baumann G, Rayfield RJ, Rose LI, et al: "Trace" contamination of corticotropin and human growth hormone with vasopressin: Clinical significance. J Clin Endocrinol Metab 34:801–804, 1972.
94. Kehlet H, Binder C: Value of an ACTH test in assessing hypothalamic-pituitary-adrenocortical function in glucocorticoid-treated patients. BMJ 2:147–152, 1973.
95. Rose LI, Williams GH, Jagger PI: The 48-hour ACTH infusion test for adrenocortical insufficiency. Ann Intern Med 73:49–59, 1970.
96. Quinn SJ, Williams GH: Regulation of aldosterone secretion. Annu Rev Physiol 50:409–426, 1988.
97. Underwood RH, Williams GH: The simultaneous measurement of aldosterone, cortisol, and corticosterone in human peripheral plasma by displacement analysis. J Lab Clin Med 79:848–862, 1972.
98. Williams GH, Rose LI, Dluhy RG, et al: Aldosterone response to sodium restriction and ACTH stimulation in panhypopituitarism. J Clin Endocrinol Metab 32:27–35, 1971.
99. Schulte HM, Chrousos GP, Avgerinos P, et al: The CRH test: A possible aid in the evaluation of patients with adrenal insufficiency. J Clin Endocrinol Metab 58:1064–1068, 1984.
100. Kehlet H, Madsen SN, Binder C: Cortisol and cortisone acetate in parenteral glucocorticoid therapy. Acta Med Scand 195:421–425, 1974.
101. Fariss BL, Hane S, Shinsako H: Comparison of absorption of cortisone acetate and hydrocortisone hemisuccinate. J Clin Endocrinol Metab 47:1137–1140, 1978.
102. Beisel WR, Bruton J, Anderson KD, et al: Adrenocortical responses during tularemia in human subjects. J Clin Endocrinol Metab 27:61–68, 1967.
103. Udelsman R, Chrousos GP, Loriaux DL: Adaptation during surgical stress. J Clin Invest 77:1377–1381, 1986.

Chapter 121

Cushing's Syndrome

Lynnette K. Nieman

BACKGROUND AND HISTORICAL INFORMATION

Harvey Cushing was the first to codify the symptom complex of obesity, diabetes, hirsutism, and adrenal hyperplasia[1] and to postulate that the basophilic adenomas found at autopsy in six of eight patients caused the disease that now bears his name.[2] Shortly thereafter, Walters and associates[3] identified the etiologic contribution of adrenal tumors and the therapeutic role of adrenalectomy. Over the ensuing 66 years, understanding of the pathogenesis of Cushing's syndrome has expanded to include ectopic production of adrenocorticotropic hormone (ACTH)[4] and corticotropin-releasing hormone (CRH)[5] and recognition of bilateral adrenal stimulation by factors other than corticotropin.[6–9] The treatment options for Cushing's syndrome have increased to include medical agents that decrease the secretion or bioactivity of cortisol, as well as surgical resection of eutopic and ectopic ACTH-producing tumors. Because full-blown Cushing's syndrome is ultimately fatal, early diagnosis and treatment have always been important. The variety of causes and the specific therapies now available dictate that correct diagnosis is also crucial. This chapter reviews the manifestations, etiologies, approaches to diagnosis, and treatment of this complicated and multifaceted syndrome.

DEFINITIONS

Cushing's syndrome is a symptom complex that reflects excessive tissue exposure to cortisol. The diagnosis cannot be made unless both clinical features and biochemical abnormalities are present.

Symptoms and Physical Findings

Excessive cortisol production has widespread systemic effects[10–14] (Table 121–1). Although the full-blown cushingoid phenotype is unmistakable, the clinical diagnosis may be equivocal for patients with few of the typical characteristics (Fig. 121–1). Some features consistent with the diagnosis of Cushing's syndrome, such as obesity, are common in the general population and may provoke unwarranted and costly screening tests for patients not likely to be affected.

One useful strategy when considering the diagnosis of Cushing's syndrome is to look for evidence of progressive physical changes by examination of serial photographs, especially of individuals photographed at annual events such as holidays, birthdays, or school milestones (Fig. 121–2). Another approach relies on identification of signs and symptoms that correctly classify patients suspected of having the disorder. Central obesity, ecchymoses, plethora, proximal muscle weakness, osteopenia, hypertension, and a white blood cell (WBC) count of at least 11,000/ mm^3 are good discriminant indices for Cushing's syndrome.[10, 15]

Increased deposition of fat, one of the earliest signs, occurs in almost all patients and is reported as increasing weight or difficulty in maintaining weight. The distribution of fat is altered also, with increased amounts in the peritoneal cavity, mediastinum, and subcutaneous sites on the face and neck. Increased intra-abdominal fat results in the truncal obesity described by Cushing in about 50% of patients. Increased fat in the face ("moon facies"), supraclavicular or temporal fossae, and the dorsocervical area ("buffalo hump") is uncommon in normal people. When extreme, the supraclavicular fat may present as a "collar" rising above the clavicles (Fig. 121–3); filling of the temporal fossae may prevent eyeglass frames from seating properly.

Abnormal fat deposition may occur in the epidural space. Spinal epidural lipomatosis causing neurologic deficit, a rare complication of long-term exogenous steroid use, has been reported in a few patients with endogenous Cushing's syndrome.[16, 17] Lumbosacral findings were seen in both men and women, whereas thoracic obstruction was restricted to men. The condition can be diagnosed by magnetic resonance imaging (MRI), avoiding the technical problems associated with myelography.[18]

Loss of subcutaneous tissue results in a variety of skin abnormalities that are unusual in the general population and suggest hypercortisolism. Ecchymoses, often after minimal trauma, and cutaneous atrophy, seen as a fine "cigarette paper" wrinkling or tenting over the dorsum of the hand and elbows, are typical. Cutaneous atrophy is influenced by gender and age, with men and the young having greater skin thickness. Two maxims follow. First, it is useful to compare the patient's skin with that of a near age- and sex-matched healthy person. Second, skin thickness is relatively preserved in cushingoid women with increased androgen production or preservation of ovarian function (Fig. 121–4).

Facial plethora, especially over the cheeks, also reflects loss of

TABLE 121–1. The Percentage Frequency of Clinical Signs and Symptoms of Cushing's Syndrome as Described in Five Large Studies from 1952 to 1982

Signs and Symptoms	Ross & Linch,[10] 1982 (n = 70)	Urbanic & George,[11] 1981 (n = 31)	Soffer et al.,[12] 1961 (n = 50)	Sprague et al.,[13] 1956 (n = 100)	Plotz et al.,[14] 1952 (n = 33)
Obesity or weight gain	97	79	86	84	97
Hypertension	74	77	88	90	84
Plethora	94		78	81	89
Round face	88		92	92	89
Hirsutism	81	64	84	74	73
Thin skin		84			
Abnormal glucose tolerance	50	39	84		94
Ecchymoses	62	77	68	62	60
Weakness	56	90	58		83
Osteopenia/fracture	50	48	56		83
ECG changes/atherosclerosis	55		34		66/89
Menstrual changes	84	69	72	35	86
Decreased libido, men/women	100	55	100/33		86
Lethargy, depression	62	48	40		67
Headache	47				58
Backache	43	39			83
Striae	56	51	50	64	60
Edema	50	48	66		60
Acne	21	35		64	82
Dorsal fat pad	54		34	67	
Female balding	13		51		
Lipid abnormalities					39
Recurrent infections	25		14		
Poor wound healing/severe infection					42
Abdominal pain	21				
Renal calculi					15

subcutaneous tissue. While plethora is more obvious in pale whites, it may be present and should be sought in darker-skinned persons. Because erythema may be induced in normal persons by ultraviolet radiation from lamps or sunlight, wind, or medications (including topical drying agents, glucocorticoids, and antipsoriatic treatments), exposure to these agents should be ascertained before plethora is ascribed to endogenous hypercortisolism. A demarcation line, representing collar, sleeve, or shoulder straps, may differentiate exogenous from endogenous causes. Flushing caused by other conditions (e.g., mastocytosis, hyperthyroidism, vasomotor instability or estrogen insufficiency in women, and the carcinoid syndrome) should be considered.

Purple striae more than 1 cm in diameter are virtually pathogno-

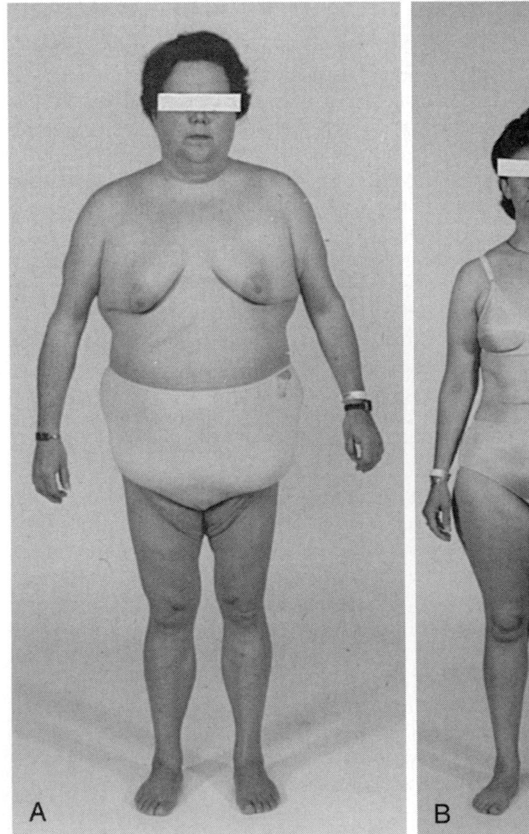

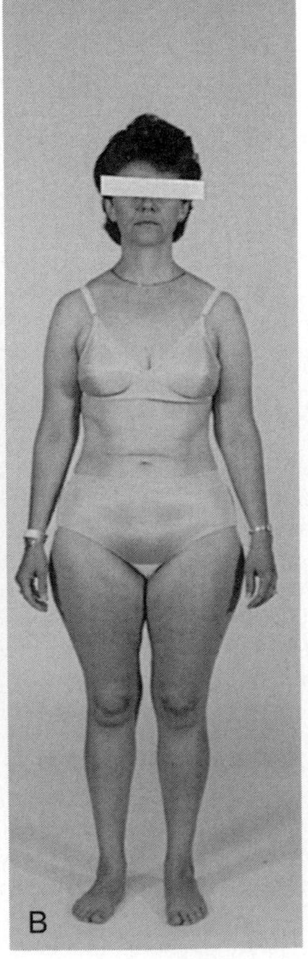

FIGURE 121–1. Body habitus of two patients with proven Cushing's syndrome. Features typical of the syndrome—central obesity, round face and supraclavicular fat pads—are present in patient A but not in patient B, illustrating that the diagnosis is not always apparent from the initial physical examination.

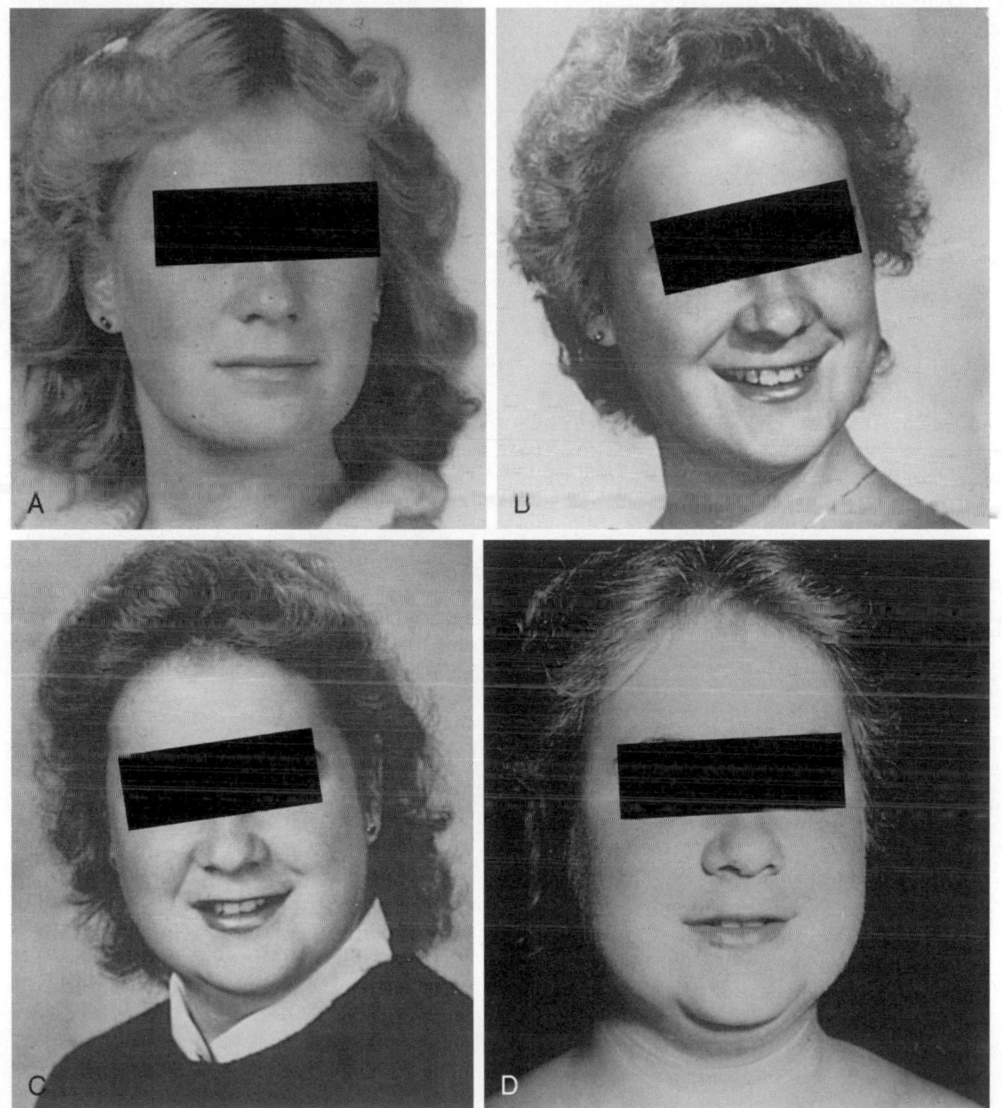

FIGURE 121–2. Progression of cushingoid features as shown in photographs taken at 1-year intervals (*A–D,* progress from earliest to latest).

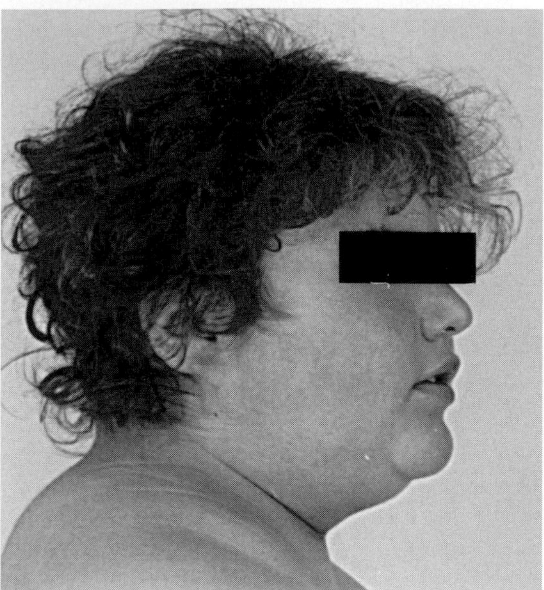

FIGURE 121–3. Fat may fill, or in this case rise above, the supraclavicular fossa of Cushing's syndrome patients.

monic for Cushing's syndrome (Fig. 121–5). Although the silvery, healed striae that are typical post partum are not caused by active Cushing's syndrome, other pink, less-pigmented, and thinner striae are seen. While most common over the abdomen, striae occur also over the hips, buttocks, thighs, breasts, and upper arms. The tear in the subcutaneous tissue may be best appreciated by indirect (side) lighting, which throws the striae into relief, or by light stroking of the skin.

Proximal muscle weakness with preservation of distal strength is a hallmark of Cushing's syndrome. Histologically, this is reflected in profound atrophy of fibers without necrosis.[19–21] Weakness is best assessed historically by questions related to use of these muscles: Is there difficulty or weakness in climbing stairs; in getting up from a chair or bed without using hand propulsion; in caring for the hair; in reaching objects in overhead cabinets; or in performing activities using the shoulders (changing ceiling light bulbs, painting, shooting baskets, throwing a ball)? Formal muscle testing is useful. Assess the strength of the hip flexors by asking the patient to get out of a chair without using his or her arms. If this can be done, the patient is asked to rise from a squat. Inability to perform either task, in the absence of hip or lower extremity arthropathy or other myopathic processes, is suggestive of Cushing's syndrome. Leg extension while seated is a quantifiable test of proximal muscle strength. The number of seconds for which this position is held can be used to judge deterioration or progress after treatment.

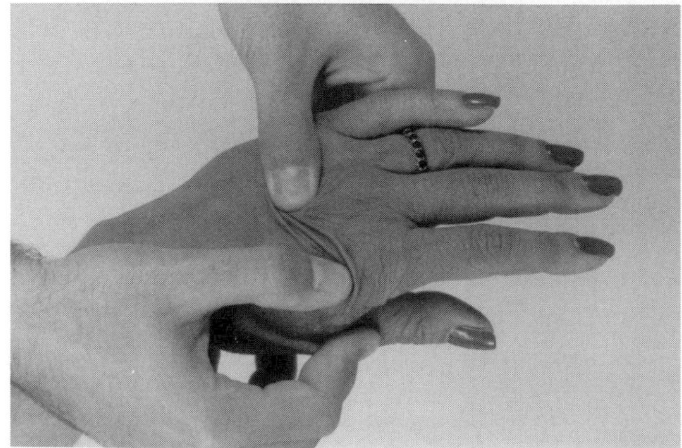

FIGURE 121–4. Thinning of the skin may be demonstrated by twisting the skin on the dorsum of the hand.

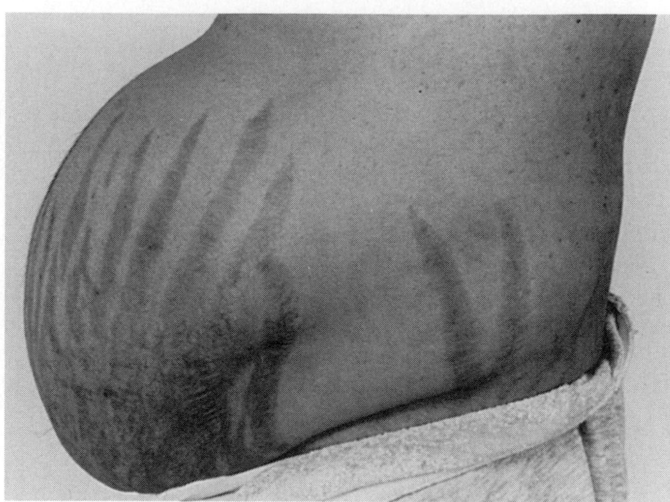

FIGURE 121–5. Typical abdominal striae of a patient with hypercortisolism. These are greater than 1 cm in width and violaceous.

Osteopenia is common. A history of fractures, typically of the feet, ribs, and vertebrae, may be one of the only signs of Cushing's syndrome, especially in men.[11, 12, 22] Avascular necrosis of bone, a rare complication of endogenous hypercortisolism, is more common in iatrogenic hypercortisolism.[23, 24]

Vellus hypertrichosis of the forehead or upper cheeks distinguishes Cushing's syndrome from the more common causes of hirsutism and may be appreciated only by careful visual and tactile inspection (Fig. 121–6). Excessive terminal hair on the face and body, and acne, either pustular, reflecting increased androgens, or papular, reflecting pure glucocorticoid excess, may be present.[25] Frank virilization is uncommon and suggests adrenal carcinoma.

Most patients experience emotional and cognitive changes (including increased fatigue, irritability, crying, and restlessness), depressed mood; decreased libido; insomnia; anxiety; impaired memory, concentration, and verbal communication; and changes in appetite. These changes correlate with the degree of hypercortisolism.[26] Irritability, characterized as a decreased threshold for uncontrollable verbal outbursts, may be one of the earliest symptoms. The global impairment in neuropsychological function correlates well with performance of serial 7 subtractions and recall of the names of three cities, bedside

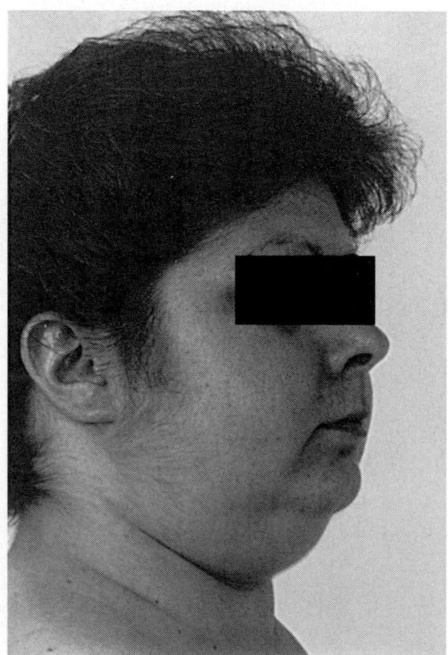

FIGURE 121–6. Vellus hirsutism, especially on the cheeks, is often present in women with Cushing's syndrome.

tests that can be used by the clinician to quantify this symptom complex.[27]

About 80% of patients meet strict criteria for a major affective disorder, 50% with unipolar depression and 30% with bipolar illness.[28, 29] While the quality of the depressed mood ranges from suicide attempts to sadness, the time course is characteristically intermittent, rarely lasting more than 3 days, in contrast with the constant dysphoria reported by depressed patients without Cushing's syndrome.[26] A minority of patients are manic. The improvement in neuropsychiatric findings after cure of Cushing's syndrome, coupled with similar features in patients treated with exogenous steroids, and the association of hypercortisolism with poor cognitive performance in depressed patients both suggest glucocorticoid excess as a cause.[30, 31]

Additional signs that may indicate significant hypercortisolism are hypertension, opportunistic and fungal infections, and altered reproductive function. Although hypertension is common in the general population, its presence in patients less than 40 years of age, especially if difficult to control, may herald the syndrome. The lipid abnormalities, hypertension, and diabetes common in Cushing's syndrome predispose these patients to atherosclerotic cardiac disease.[32]

The association of hypercortisolism and fungal infections of the skin, such as mucocutaneous candidiasis, tinea versicolor, and pityriasis, and poor wound healing are common features. Wound dehiscence occurs less often.

Patients with marked hypercortisolism (plasma cortisol >70 μg/dL) are at risk for two potentially catastrophic events: perforation of the viscera and opportunistic and fungal infections such as *Pneumocystis carinii* infection, aspergillosis, nocardiosis, cryptococcosis, histoplasmosis, and *Candida* infection.[33–35] In my experience, these complications occur only if the daily urine free cortisol (UFC) excretion is greater than 2000 μg. Classic clinical signs, such as loss of bowel sounds and fever, may be absent, and the typical leukocytosis of hypercortisolism may not increase further. Thus, the threshold of suspicion for opportunistic infections and surgical abdomen must be low in patients with severe hypercortisolism.

Libido is decreased uniformly in men and to a lesser extent (44%) in women,[11] in whom increased libido may indicate excess androgen production by an adrenocortical carcinoma. Menstrual irregularities, amenorrhea, and infertility are common and may be the presenting complaints.[36] Impotence is common.

Laboratory Findings

The seminal laboratory findings in endogenous Cushing's syndrome reflect overproduction of glucocorticoids. While morning plasma cortisol values may be normal, an increased nighttime nadir blunts or obliterates the normal diurnal rhythm.[37–39] This increase in mean 24-hour plasma values is reflected in increased levels of free, or unbound, cortisol in urine[40] and saliva.[41] The capacity of corticosteroid-binding globulin (CBG) for cortisol is exceeded at a serum cortisol value of about 25 μg/dL. At this point, the excretion of free cortisol increases dramatically in direct proportion to the increased unbound circulating cortisol values.

Hypokalemic metabolic alkalosis is observed, usually when daily urine cortisol excretion is greater than 1500 μg.[42] This probably represents a mineralocorticoid action of cortisol at the renal tubule due to incomplete 11β-hydroxysteroid dehydrogenase.[43] Very-low-density lipoprotein (VLDL), low-density lipoprotein (LDL), high-density lipoprotein (HDL), and triglyceride levels increase as a result of increased hepatic synthesis without altered clearance.[44] Frank diabetes or glucose intolerance occurs in up to 70% of patients, probably because of cortisol-induced postreceptor blockade of insulin action. Hypercortisolism suppresses the thyroidal and gonadal axes so that the nocturnal surge of thyroid-stimulating hormone (TSH)[45] and plasma levels of triiodothyronine (T_3), thyroxine (T_4), thyroxine-binding globulin (TBG), luteinizing hormone (LH), follicle-stimulating hormone (FSH), and gonadal steroids are reduced.[36, 46, 47]

INCIDENCE AND DISTRIBUTION

While the true incidence of Cushing's syndrome is not known, iatrogenic cases account for the majority because of the common therapeutic use of high-dose glucocorticoids. The annual incidence of endogenous Cushing's syndrome per million population in the United States can be estimated based on the relative proportion of patients with adrenal adenoma and carcinoma (15%), ectopic ACTH secretion (15%), and pituitary disease (70%). The incidence of adrenal cancer was estimated in 1975 to be 1 in 1 million, yielding an annual incidence of Cushing's syndrome of about 3000 per year. Similar calculations based on the incidence of small cell carcinoma indicate that the annual incidence of ectopic ACTH syndrome is vastly underestimated in the endocrine literature. The incidence of ectopic ACTH secretion would be about 528 per million using a conservative estimate of recognized ACTH secretion from small cell cancer of 264 patients per million, based on a 1% to 8% incidence of Cushing's syndrome in this condition[48] and an incidence of small cell carcinoma of 33,000 per million population.

Sex and age distribution vary with the cause of Cushing's syndrome. Adrenal adenoma, carcinoma, and corticotroph adenomas (Cushing's disease) occur four to six times more commonly in women than in men.[14, 32, 49] Ectopic ACTH secretion is the only cause of the syndrome that is more common in men,[50] although this is expected to change as more women develop lung cancer, the most common cause of ectopic ACTH secretion. Lung cancer is more common after age 40, and this accounts for the increased mean age of patients with ectopic ACTH secretion as compared with Cushing's disease, which occurs between 25 and 40 years of age.[14] The other major cause of ectopic ACTH secretion, intrathoracic carcinoids, has a peak incidence around 40 years and only a slightly increased male-to-female ratio.[51] The age distribution of adrenal cancer is bimodal, with peaks in childhood and adolescence and late in life, while adrenal adenoma occurs most often around 35 years of age.

DIFFERENTIAL DIAGNOSIS

The diagnosis of Cushing's syndrome rests on the demonstration of both physical and biochemical features of glucocorticoid excess. Thus, the diagnosis is unequivocal in a typical patient with many of the physical features discussed above in the setting of fourfold normal cortisol excretion. However, many of the signs of hypercortisolism, such as obesity, hypertension, mood changes, menstrual irregularities, and hirsutism, are common in the general population. Similarly, mild glucocorticoid excess (urine cortisol up to threefold normal) is seen in affective disorders,[52] strenuous exercise,[53] chronic alcoholism and withdrawal from alcohol,[54, 55] renal failure,[56, 57] and hypoglycemia. Diagnostic strategies for distinguishing between these pseudo-Cushing's states and true Cushing's syndrome are discussed below.

Glucocorticoid resistance is characterized by abnormal glucocorticoid receptor number or binding, causing compensatory increases in ACTH and excessive glucocorticoid production to maintain normal glucocorticoid-mediated effects at the target tissues. The diagnosis should be considered in the hypokalemic, hypertensive, hypercortisolemic patient without typical glucocorticoid-mediated signs of Cushing's syndrome.[58]

ETIOLOGY AND PATHOPHYSIOLOGY

Pseudo–Cushing's Syndrome

Unlike most forms of Cushing's syndrome, the pathophysiology of pseudo-Cushing's states has not been established. One hypothesis is that these stressful conditions increase the activity of the CRH neuron, resulting in excessive ACTH secretion, adrenal hyperplasia, and increased cortisol production.[59] The model predicts only intermittent and modest hypercortisolism because of appropriate corticotroph reduction in ACTH secretion in response to negative feedback by cortisol (Fig. 121–7). This construct presumes also that the hypertrophied adrenal glands produce excessive glucocorticoids in response to normal ACTH levels, an assumption that is supported by the blunted ACTH, but not cortisol, response to exogenous CRH in anorexia nervosa,[60] depression,[61] and obligate athleticism.[53]

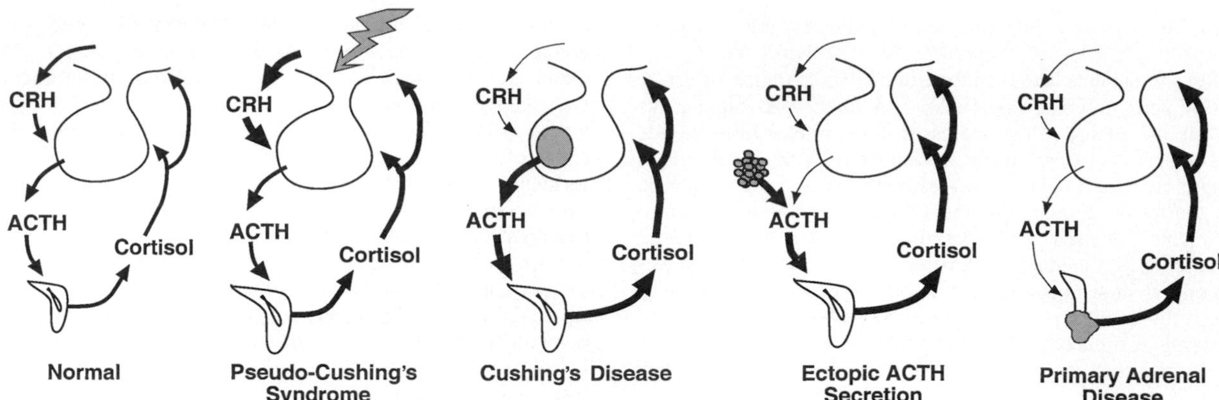

FIGURE 121–7. Physiology of the hypothalamic-pituitary-adrenal axis in normal individuals and hypercortisolemic states. Corticotropin-releasing hormone (CRH) secretion from the hypothalamus normally stimulates adrenocorticotropic hormone (ACTH) secretion from the pituitary gland. This in turn results in increased cortisol production from the adrenal glands. The system is modulated by negative feedback inhibition by cortisol of both CRH and ACTH secretion. In pseudo–Cushing's syndrome the CRH neuron is activated by central input *(large shaded arrow)* resulting in increased CRH output which eventuates in hypercortisolism. Increased cortisol production restrains corticotroph activation but does not completely reverse the activation of the CRH neuron, so that mild to moderate hypercortisolism may persist. In Cushing's disease a corticotroph adenoma secretes ACTH in excess and is only partially inhibited by rising cortisol levels. In this setting and that of ectopic ACTH secretion and primary adrenal disease, the CRH neuron is suppressed by hypercortisolism. In ectopic ACTH secretion, excessive secretion of ACTH from a nonpituitary tumor is not inhibited by glucocorticoid feedback. In this setting and that of autonomous production of cortisol by the adrenal gland, ACTH secretion by normal corticotrophs is suppressed by hypercortisolism.

Cushing's Syndrome

The causes of Cushing's syndrome can be divided into ACTH-dependent and -independent (Table 121–2). The ACTH-dependent forms are characterized by excessive ACTH production from a corticotroph adenoma (known as *pituitary-dependent Cushing's syndrome* or *Cushing's disease*), from an ectopic tumoral source (the *syndrome of ectopic ACTH secretion*), or from normal corticotrophs under the influence of excessive CRH production *(ectopic CRH secretion)*. ACTH stimulates all layers of the adrenal glands to grow and secrete steroids. When excessive, this results in histologic hyperplasia and increased adrenal weight. Micronodules and macronodules (>1 cm) may be seen. Plasma values of androgens, as well as glucocorticoids, are increased.

ACTH-independent forms, apart from exogenous administration of glucocorticoids, represent adrenal activation by mechanisms other than trophic ACTH support. This enlarging group includes unilateral disease (adenoma and carcinoma), bilateral disease (primary pigmented nodular adrenal disease, McCune-Albright syndrome, and macronodular adrenal disease of unknown cause or caused by ectopic expression of receptors for ligands such as gastric inhibitory polypeptide [GIP], β-adrenergic agents, and vasopressin), and hyperfunction of adrenal rest tissue.

Adrenal adenomas, composed of zona fasciculata cells, produce only glucocorticoids, in contrast to activation of the entire adrenal cortex seen in other causes of Cushing's syndrome. ACTH levels are suppressed by hypercortisolism, and the nonadenomatous tissue atrophies because of lack of this trophic factor. As a result, androgenic signs, such as pustular acne and hirsutism, are uncommon, and dehydroepiandrosterone sulfate (DHEAS) levels are low.

TABLE 121–2. Etiology of Cushing's Syndrome

Exogenous—most common cause of Cushing's syndrome, glucocorticoid- or ACTH-driven
Endogenous
- ACTH-independent—adrenal activation apart from ACTH
  - Adrenal adenoma (40%–50%)
  - Adrenal carcinoma (40%–50%)
  - Primary pigmented nodular adrenal disease (uncommon)
  - McCune-Albright syndrome (rare)
  - Idiopathic massive macronodular adrenal disease, MMAD (rare)
  - MMAD caused by ectopic/increased receptors (rare)
- ACTH-dependent—adrenal activation caused by excessive ACTH
  - Corticotroph adenoma (80%)
  - Ectopic ACTH secretion by noncorticotroph tumor (20%)
  - Ectopic CRH secretion/corticotroph hyperplasia (rare)

ACTH, adrenocorticotropic hormone; CRH, corticotropin-releasing hormone.

Pituitary-Dependent Cushing's Syndrome

Cushing's disease is almost always caused by a solitary monoclonal corticotroph adenoma.[62] While these are usually intrasellar microadenomas (<1 cm in diameter), macroadenomas and extrasellar extension or invasion may occur. This heterogeneity may reflect differences in etiology; the cause(s) of Cushing's disease is not known. Plasma pro-opiomelanocortin (POMC) and pro-ACTH levels usually are not elevated, except in macroadenomas, suggesting that microadenomas do not arise because of aberrent processing of ACTH precursors.[63, 64] Although a hypothalamic factor(s) has been proposed to stimulate corticotrophs and cause adenoma formation,[65] the uncommon incidence of clinical features predicted by this theory, such as corticotroph hyperplasia, multiple adenomas, and frequent recurrence after adenoma resection, mitigates against it. While nodular corticotroph hyperplasia without evidence of a CRH-producing neoplasm does occur, it represents 2% or less of large surgical series.[66, 67]

Others have postulated two distinct causes based on an intermediate lobe rather than anterior lobe origin, as identified by the presence of argyrophilic neural tissue in the tumor, relative resistance to dexamethasone, elevated prolactin values, and suppression of ACTH by bromocriptine.[68] This was not substantiated by a subsequent study that showed argyrophil staining in 50% of anterior lobe tumors and no correlation with dexamethasone suppressibility.[69]

Ectopic ACTH Secretion

The *syndrome of ectopic hormone secretion* was first codified by Liddle and coworkers, who defined it as "any hormone produced by a neoplasm which is derived from tissue not normally engaged in the production of the hormone in question."[4] ACTH and other POMC products were subsequently identified in many noncorticotroph tumors, although not all were associated with increased circulating levels or the development of Cushing's syndrome.[4, 70]

The variable distribution of the causes of ectopic ACTH secretion in larger series probably represents differences in referral patterns (Table 121–3). An intrathoracic neoplasm (carcinoma of the lung or carcinoid of the bronchus or thymus) accounts for about 60% of ectopic ACTH secretion, followed by pancreatic tumors (islet cell or carcinoid) and pheochromocytoma (about 5% to 10%), and medullary

TABLE 121–3. The Incidence and Types of Tumors Causing the Syndrome of Ectopic ACTH Secretion

Tumor	Incidence (%)
Carcinoma of lung (small cell or oat cell)	19–50
Carcinoid of bronchus	2–37
Carcinoid of thymus	8–12
Pancreatic tumors, carcinoid and islet cell	4–12
Pheochromocytoma, neuroblastoma, ganglioma, paraganglioma[324]	5–12
Medullary carcinoma of the thyroid	0–5
Miscellaneous*	<1

*Miscellaneous tumors reported to secrete ACTH in 1 to 10 cases include ovary, prostate, breast, thyroid, kidney, salivary glands, testes, gastric carcinoid, gallbladder, esophagus, appendix, acute myeloblastoma in leukemia, melanoma, cloacogenic cancer of the anal canal.

Data from Odell,[72] Howlett et al.,[188] and Jex et al.[323]

carcinoma of the thyroid (about 0% to 5%). Up to 2% of all patients with lung cancer[71] and up to 8% of those with small cell carcinoma have ectopic ACTH secretion.[48] The high incidence of these tumors in the general population makes this the most common cause of ectopic ACTH secretion, accounting for about 50% of the cases.[72] Small cell carcinoma may be the most common cause of Cushing's syndrome, if, as reported by Gilby et al.,[73] the majority of patients lack suppressibility to dexamethasone but are not referred to endocrinologists because typical cushingoid features are absent.

The mechanism whereby the POMC gene becomes derepressed in noncorticotroph tumors is not understood. One hypothesis is that these cells are derived from a common multipotential progenitor cell capable of producing peptide hormones so that ACTH production is a reversion to a less differentiated state.[71] The observation that many ACTH-producing tumors are derived from neural crest amine precursor uptake and decarboxylation (APUD) cells may support this view.[75] However, because endodermally derived tumors also produce ACTH, the acquisition of APUD characteristics may be but one manifestation of dedifferentiation and may not represent the cause of ectopic ACTH production.

Although the mechanism of gene derepression is not understood, the regulation of POMC production and processing has been investigated. POMC, corticotropin-like intermediate lobe protein (CLIP), and larger forms of ACTH ("big" or pro-ACTH) that are not usually secreted may circulate, and the intracellular ratio of the POMC products may be abnormal.[76, 77] Investigation of cell lines of small cell carcinoma of the lung that synthesize POMC and pro-ACTH showed that only ACTH precursors were secreted, suggesting that processing to ACTH is defective.[78] The pattern of POMC messenger RNA (mRNA) species in ACTH-producing tumors has been characterized. A 1200-bp transcript similar to that of a corticotroph adenoma,[79] a shorter-than-normal 800-bp mRNA lacking a signal sequence for secretion,[79, 80] and a larger 1400- to 1500-bp POMC transcript have been identified. The larger species appears to originate upstream of the usual pituitary promoter, with preservation of the normal translation start site.[81, 82] It is possible that the promoters that initiate this transcription are not regulated by glucocorticoids, and this may explain, in part, the lack of responsiveness to glucocorticoid suppression noted clinically in these patients. In vitro investigation of human small cell cancer cell lines and pancreatic islet cell tumors with normal glucocorticoid receptor binding has found, for the most part, no regulation of POMC, tyrosine aminotransferase, or the glucocorticoid receptor mRNA at doses of hydrocortisone that would normally suppress pituitary production.[83–85] However, clinical observation of suppression of ACTH production by some bronchial carcinoids during glucocorticoid administration suggests retention of a functional glucocorticoid response element that regulates POMC production.[86]

Ectopic Corticotropin-Releasing Hormone Secretion

Tumor secretion of CRH with or without ACTH secretion is a rare cause of Cushing's syndrome. Although many tumors contain CRH, its secretion is less common, and most patients do not develop cushingoid features.[87] Thus, the diagnosis rests on demonstration of elevated plasma CRH levels. The literature includes fewer than 20 patients who fit this criterion. Their tumors include ACTH-secreting bronchial and thymic carcinoids, ACTH- and CRH-secreting pheochromocytoma, gangliocytoma, and paraganglioma.[88–92] Other patients with small cell carcinoma of the lung, metastatic prostate cancer, and Ewing's sarcoma had suggestive but not definitive evidence for CRH secretion.[90] The biochemical responses to diagnostic tests can be similar to those seen in ectopic ACTH secretion.[92]

Primary Adrenal Disease

The primary adrenal forms of Cushing's syndrome do not share a common cause. The cause of adrenocortical neoplasia is not known, although allelic loss on chromosomes 11p, 13q, and 17p has been found in adrenal cancer but not in adenomas or hyperplasia.[93] Adenomas and carcinomas tend to be monoclonal, while the nodular hyperplasias are often polyclonal.[94] Adrenal adenomas are encapsulated benign tumors, usually less than 40 g in weight. Adrenal carcinomas are usually encapsulated, usually weigh more than 100 g, and may lack histologic features of malignancy, although nuclear pleomorphism, necrosis, mitotic figures, and vascular or lymphatic invasion suggest the diagnosis.[95] The adjacent adrenal tissue is atrophic in both conditions.

Primary pigmented nodular adrenal disease (PPNAD), also known as *micronodular adrenal disease*, is a rare form of Cushing's syndrome characterized histologically by small to normal-sized glands (combined weight <12 g) with cortical micronodules (average, 2 to 3 mm) that may be dark or black in color. The intervening cortex is almost always atrophic.[96] About half of the cases of PPNAD are sporadic. The remainder occur as part of the Carney complex in association with a variety of other abnormalities, including myxomatous masses of the heart, skin, or breast; blue nevi or lentigenes; and other endocrine disorders (sexual precocity; Sertoli cell, Leydig's cell, or adrenal rest tumor; and acromegaly). The Carney complex is inherited as a mendelian dominant; the gene has been mapped to chromosome 2 in some but not all kindreds.[97, 98]

Macronodular adrenal disease is a rare non–ACTH-dependent form of Cushing's syndrome that involves huge adrenal glands, causing confusion with Cushing's disease, and biochemical tests that are consistent with a nonpituitary form of the disorder. Feminization has been reported.[9] While the cause remains unclear in most cases, some nodules express increased numbers of receptors normally found on the adrenal gland, or ectopic receptors for circulating ligands that then can stimulate cortisol production. For example, normal postprandial increase in GIP appeared to cause Cushing's syndrome in two middle-aged women with bilateral multinodular adrenal enlargement, mildly elevated UFC values, and undetectable plasma ACTH values. Fasting morning serum cortisol values were low or normal. Cortisol values increased dramatically after meals and after in vivo or in vitro exposure to GIP.[7, 8] In one patient, curative bilateral adrenalectomy revealed multinodular adrenal glands weighing 20 and 35 g.[8] In the other, treatment with octreotide ameliorated the syndrome.[7] Ectopic expression of GIP receptors was found in these patients, while in others eutopic increased expression of vasopressin receptors, or ectopic expression of β-adrenergic receptors appeared to stimulate cortisol production.[99]

Adrenal rest tissue in the liver, in the adrenal beds, or in association with the gonads may rarely cause Cushing's syndrome, usually in the setting of ACTH-dependent disease after adrenalectomy.[100–103] Ectopic cortisol production by an ovarian carcinoma has been reported.[104]

CLINICAL SPECTRUM

The typical patient with Cushing's disease presents at midlife complaining of gradual development of symptoms. Hypokalemia, virilization, and extremely high cortisol excretion (>10-fold normal) are distinctly uncommon. Pituitary macroadenomas account for up to 10% of corticotropinomas. Their clinical presentation, apart from visual field changes caused by suprasellar expansion, is not unique. By contrast, invasive pituitary adenomas present at a slightly younger age; cavernous sinus and dural involvement may result in cranial neuropathies and facial neuralgia.[105, 106] Only a few case reports attest to cerebrospinal or extracranial metastasis of ACTH-producing pituitary adenomas.[107]

Nelson's syndrome is characterized by the development of hyperpigmentation and high ACTH levels after bilateral adrenalectomy for Cushing's disease. The unresolved role of "prophylactic" radiation of the pituitary in patients undergoing adrenalectomy remains an important question because of the risk of Nelson's syndrome (8% to 45%). When given after development of the syndrome, radiation therapy does not always ameliorate the locally invasive nature of these tumors.[108–111] The tumor growth after adrenalectomy has been explained by the relative resistance of these tumors to glucocorticoid suppression.

An abrupt onset of severe Cushing's syndrome should prompt an evaluation for ectopic ACTH secretion. This variant of ectopic ACTH secretion classically presents as a paraneoplastic syndrome in the context of a known malignancy. The features were captured in the initial formulation of Liddle et al.[4]: weight loss, hypokalemia, weakness, and diabetes. Cushing's syndrome caused by ectopic ACTH secretion also may present with weight gain and striae but without a clinically apparent tumor. This presentation has been referred to as "occult," in reference to the unknown nature of the tumor, which may elude localization for many years. It is patients with this syndrome who most often present a diagnostic dilemma. They tend to have UFC excretion in the range seen in pituitary disease, and they tend not to show hypokalemia, hyperpigmentation, or the other findings typical of severe ectopic ACTH secretion.

Adrenocortical carcinomas are inefficient producers of cortisol and tend to evidence Cushing's syndrome when the tumor is large (>6 cm), if at all. Abdominal pain or a palpable mass suggests this cause. Feminization in a man or virilization and increased libido in a woman, indicating involvement of the zona reticularis, suggests adrenal cancer or the more rare macronodular adrenal disease. The typical patient with PPNAD is a child or young adult who may present with an intermittent course or a family history of associated signs. Lentigenes may be the initial clue to this cause. By contrast, patients with the massive macronodular variant of ACTH-independent Cushing's syndrome tend to be more than 40 years old.

Special Clinical Presentations and Problems

Periodic and Spontaneously Remitting Cushing's Syndrome

Most patients with Cushing's syndrome demonstrate consistently elevated glucocorticoid values. A small subset show significant variability in glucocorticoid secretion, alternating normal and elevated values on a regular or irregular basis.[112] The few cases of spontaneous remission of Cushing's syndrome, including Cushing's first patient, may fit into this category.[2, 113, 114] The clinical course of patients with this type of intermittent, cyclic, or periodic Cushing's syndrome may be invariant, usually with mild signs and cushingoid symptoms, or it may parallel the biochemical abnormalities, with exacerbation of cushingoid features that parallels increased glucocorticoid production.

The etiologic distribution is altered; in one report, Cushing's disease, ectopic ACTH secretion, and primary adrenal causes accounted for 50%, 40%, and 10%, respectively, of 30 cases.[112] Carcinoid tumors of thymus, lung, stomach, and kidney accounted for all but one case of ectopic ACTH secretion.

Patients with periodic Cushing's syndrome often show conflicting or "inappropriate" responses to standard diagnostic tests, particularly dexamethasone suppression.[115] Since up to 50% of carcinoid tumors may suppress ACTH and thus glucocorticoid secretion during dexamethasone administration,[116, 117] it is possible that increasing ACTH and cortisol levels in turn may inhibit POMC production in these tumors and in pituitary corticotrophs. Some patients with Cushing's disease show suppressed glucocorticoid production with hydrocortisone but not with dexamethasone.[118] In others, the "response" may reflect increasing or decreasing endogenous activity, without relationship to the action of the agent administered.[119, 120] This may be deduced if a patient has conflicting patterns of response to multiple administrations of the test agent. Discrepant urine tests have been reported in these patients, with elevated 17-hydroxysteroids and normal UFC excretion.[121] If studied during a quiescent period, patients with nonpituitary disease may be misclassified as having Cushing's disease, and those with "normal" responses to low-dose dexamethasone may be incorrectly diagnosed as not having Cushing's syndrome.[122] Dynamic testing is best interpreted if performed during a sustained period of hypercortisolism, as documented by failure to suppress serum cortisol to 1 mg dexamethasone, concurrent increased evening plasma cortisol, and elevated urine cortisol excretion.

Macronodular Cushing's Syndrome

The presence of macronodules (>1 cm) on one or both adrenal glands presents a large differential diagnosis. A unilateral mass usually indicates Cushing's disease if a normal-sized or enlarged contralateral gland has uptake with iodocholesterol scanning[123, 124] and if both plasma ACTH and DHEAS levels are normal. The converse pertains to patients with adrenal adenoma; the contralateral gland is atrophic, without iodocholesterol uptake, and ACTH and DHEAS values are suppressed.

Although Cushing's disease is the most common cause of bilateral *macronodular adrenal disease*, the terms cannot be equated. Bilateral adrenal masses occur also in ectopic ACTH secretion and the recently described massive macronodular adrenal disease; very rarely they represent single bilateral adenomas.[125–128]

Patients with the macronodular subset of Cushing's disease tend to be older, and have a longer duration of symptoms and a greater incidence of nonsuppression with dexamethasone compared with Cushing's disease patients without adrenal nodules.[129, 130] The failure to suppress glucocorticoid excretion during dexamethasone administration implies either a failure to suppress ACTH or autonomy of adrenal function when ACTH values decrease.

Factitious and Iatrogenic Cushing's Syndrome

Appropriate therapeutic but supraphysiologic doses of glucocorticoids given for a medical condition cause most cases of iatrogenic Cushing's syndrome, which is usually an expected, unavoidable adverse effect of therapy. Exogenous hypercortisolism may result also when a prescribed dose of glucocorticoid is increased inappropriately by the patient.[131] While most common with oral agents, Cushing's syndrome may result from glucocorticoids administered to the nasal or rectal mucosa, tracheobronchial tree, or the skin, especially if it is broken or covered by an occlusive dressing.[132–134] The use of prescription and over-the-counter medications, including nasal drops, inhalants, and topical agents, should be assessed in all cushingoid patients. Agents not given for their glucocorticoid activity, such as fludrocortisone acetate (Florinef Acetate) and megestrol,[135] also may produce cushingoid features.

Factitious Cushing's syndrome, which may be a form of Münchausen's syndrome, is rare. The typical suppression of plasma ACTH and DHEAS may lead to a mistaken diagnosis of primary adrenal disease.[136] Plasma and urine cortisol values vary, depending on the route, schedule, and type of glucocorticoid ingested. For example, intravenous (IV) injection of hydrocortisone may suppress ACTH values and increase UFC levels without increasing single random plasma cortisol values.[137] If basal urine or plasma cortisol values are low, it may be useful to screen the urine for synthetic glucocorticoids such as prednisone.[136]

The Anephric Patient

Plasma levels of cortisol are normal in chronic renal failure when assessed with radioimmunoassays using an organic extraction procedure[138, 139] but may be increased if other assay techniques are used[140];

ACTH levels are increased.[138] The ACTH and cortisol responses to ovine CRH may be suppressed in renal failure patients except for those undergoing continuous ambulatory peritoneal dialysis.[139] Relative "resistance" to dexamethasone has been described in which plasma cortisol levels decrease after administration of 8 mg, but not 1 mg, of dexamethasone by mouth.[57, 141] The metabolism and, in general, the bioavailability of dexamethasone are normal, but the increased time interval to suppression of cortisol suggests a prolonged half-life of cortisol. Occasional reports of impaired absorption of oral dexamethasone[141, 142] indicate that plasma dexamethasone levels are needed to facilitate interpretation of the test if protocols using IV administration of dexamethasone are not used.[143] The cortisol response to insulin-induced hypoglycemia is normal or absent.[142, 144] Cushing's syndrome has been recognized in the setting of chronic renal failure only rarely.[56, 145]

Children

The most common presentation of Cushing's syndrome in children is growth retardation, often with a decrease in height percentile over time as the weight percentile increases.[146, 147] However, hypercortisolemic patients with virilizing adrenal carcinoma may show growth acceleration; thus, the absence of growth failure does not exclude the diagnosis of Cushing's syndrome.[148] Thin skin and striae have been alleged to be less[149] and more common, respectively, in younger (<30 years) than in older patients.[11] Muscle weakness may be less common in the pediatric patient.[11] This may reflect the effect of exercise rather than age, because older patients who follow an exercise program tend to maintain strength. In addition to the spectrum of psychiatric and cognitive changes seen in adults, children may show "compulsive diligence" and do quite well in school.[146] Depression is less common in children than in adults.

ACTH-independent causes of Cushing's syndrome are more common in children, especially before the age of 8 years. Signs of virilization or feminization with hypercortisolism suggest adrenal carcinoma in this age group.[150–152] Two primary adrenal causes of Cushing's syndrome, McCune-Albright syndrome and PPNAD, deserve special consideration. Cushing's syndrome resulting from bilateral nodular adrenal disease is an uncommon feature of McCune-Albright syndrome.[153, 154] The molecular basis of this disease is a substitution of other amino acids for an arginine residue at position 201 of the α subunit of the G protein that stimulates cyclic adenosine monophosphate (cAMP) formation. This apparently results in constitutive activation of the gene in affected tissues, including gonads, adrenal, thyroid, and pituitary gland.[155] PPNAD, either as a sporadic case or as part of the Carney syndrome, is a disease of children and young adults.

In children older than 8 years of age, pituitary disease accounts for about 50% of cases. There is no sex predilection in prepubertal children, in contrast to the female predominance in adults.[149, 151, 156] Ectopic secretion of ACTH occurs at a lesser frequency than in adults. Sources of ectopic ACTH production in children include Wilms' tumor,[157] neuroblastoma, pheochromocytoma, pancreatic islet cell tumor,[158] bronchial carcinoid,[147] and carcinoid tumor of the kidney.[159]

Cushing's Syndrome in Pregnancy

The pregnant woman with possible Cushing's syndrome presents a diagnostic challenge to the physician because of the physical and biochemical changes that are common to both conditions, including weight gain, fatigue, striae, hypertension, and glucose intolerance.[160] Total serum cortisol levels increase in pregnancy, beginning in the first trimester and peaking at 6 months, with a decline only after delivery,[161] probably reflecting increased induction of hepatic corticosteroid-binding globulin (CBG) production by estrogen. The diurnal pattern of serum cortisol is preserved, albeit at a higher level, so that nadir values range between 5 and 10 μg/dL and peak levels between 32 and 56 μg/dL.[162] Free cortisol levels in blood and urine increase to overlap those seen in Cushing's syndrome.[162] The set-point for dexamethasone suppression of urine cortisol excretion increases progressively.[163] Since no normative values are available for interpretation of the 1-mg overnight dexamethasone test, UFC is most commonly used as a screening test, with allowance for a higher upper limit of normal.

Diagnostic Protocols

Establishing the Diagnosis of Cushing's Syndrome

The diagnosis of Cushing's syndrome is usually considered when a careful history and physical examination reveal clinical features that are consistent with the syndrome. These patients should undergo the biochemical screening tests for Cushing's syndrome detailed below and in Table 121–4. Screening for Cushing's syndrome is probably not cost-effective in patients with obesity, hypertension, or menstrual irregularity unless there are additional features of the syndrome. It is important to remember that the urgency for diagnosis and treatment of Cushing's syndrome is greatest when the symptoms are severe. In milder cases, the patient is best served by waiting until the diagnosis is clear. Periodic reevaluation with urine screening tests and documentation of body habitus with photographs may reveal progression.

The biochemical diagnosis of Cushing's syndrome rests on documentation of excessive glucocorticoid levels in urine or blood. Measurement of urinary steroids began in 1935 with description of an assay for 17-ketosteroids, which measures metabolites of androstenedione, dehydroepiandrosterone (DHEA), and DHEAS in women, and also testosterone in men.[164] This test is largely of historical interest, since it was supplanted by assessment of urinary 17-hydroxycorticosteroids (17-OHCS, the Porter-Silber chromogens), which reflect about 50% of cortisol production and the cortisone metabolites tetrahydrocortisol (THF) and tetrahydrocortisone (THE), as well as the reduced metabolite of 11β-deoxycortisol (compound S), THS.[165, 166] There are three major problems associated with the measurement of 17-OHCS, 17-ketosteroids, and ketogenic steroids for the detection of Cushing's syndrome. First, a significant proportion of the material in a 24-hour sample does not represent cortisol metabolites. Second, the colorimetric and fluorimetric assay methods are often affected by medications and other substances so that the assay cannot be performed or the

TABLE 121–4. Evaluation of Suspected Cushing's Syndrome

- Look for signs of hypercortisolism at the initial history and physical examination:
  - History: fatigue, change in libido, impotence, irregular or no menses, weakness, increased weight, easy bruising, stretch marks, poor wound healing, fracture, irritability, change in mood
  - Physical examination
    - General: hypertension, weight, fat distribution (moon facies; dorsocervical, supraclavicular, temporal fat; central obesity)
    - Skin: acne, hirsutism, thin skin, bruises, plethora, striae
    - Neurologic: proximal muscle strength
  - Laboratory findings:
    - WBC >11,000/mm^3
    - Glucose intolerance
    - Hypokalemia
- If the patient has findings consistent with hypercortisolism, screen for hypercortisolism: 24-hour urine for creatinine, free cortisol on 3 days, or overnight 1-mg dexamethasone suppression test
- If abnormal, get UFC
- If UFC is up to fourfold elevated, exclude pseudo-Cushing's states:
  - History of depression, affective disorder, exercise, "stress," alcohol use
  - If present, remove or treat and remeasure UFC
- If UFC is normal, pseudo-Cushing's state is probable; follow up at intervals
- If UFC remains elevated and physical features are specific for Cushing's syndrome, especially if progression is documented, Cushing's syndrome is probably present
- If UFC remains mildly elevated and physical features are not convincing, or if UFC is intermittently normal, continue to elevate at intervals; this may be either pseudo–Cushing's syndrome or intermittent Cushing's syndrome
- If UFC is greater than fourfold elevated (>400 μg/day in most assays), Cushing's syndrome is present

WBC, white blood cell count; UFC, urine free cortisol.

result is not accurate. Third, 17-OHCS measurement is affected by hepatic and renal disease and is increased in many obese individuals relative to normal-weight subjects. If 17-OHCS excretion is expressed as milligrams per day per milligram creatinine excretion, there is no difference between obese individuals and normal controls, however.[167] Based on these observations, it is recommended that 17-OHCS excretion be "corrected" by creatinine excretion when screening for excess glucocorticoid production to avoid false-positive results in obese individuals. 17-Ketosteroids and 17-ketogenic steroids represent both glucocorticoid and androgenic pathways and thus are not a good choice for discrimination of glucocorticoid excess.

Measurement of UFC by immunoassay or by high-pressure liquid chromatography (HPLC) is the best urine screening test for Cushing's syndrome.[168, 169] These assays measure unbound urine cortisol (HPLC) and closely related metabolites (immunoassays) and are not affected by medications, obesity, or other medical conditions. Other, usually structurally similar steroids may cross-react in an immunoassay, depending on the antibody used, which accounts for the twofold difference in the upper limit of normal of the antibody-based assays compared with HPLC. These differences are important to note because they change the normal reference range.

The UFC value is useful only when the patient has collected the entire 24-hour urine output. Under- or overcollection of urine yields spuriously low or high results. The urine creatinine value may be used to assess the completeness of the collection, since this value does not vary by more than approximately 15% from day to day.[167] It cannot be used to correct for incomplete collection, however, because the rates of cortisol and creatinine excretion are not parallel over the 24-hour period. In contrast to measurement of 17-OHCS, which is rendered more reliable when divided by the urine creatinine, the UFC value may be interpreted without correction in adults.[170] In children, standard urinary screening with 17-OHCS should be interpreted after adjustment for urinary creatinine,[146] and UFC should be corrected for body surface area.[171]

If the previous caveats have been satisfied, the UFC measurement can be interpreted. Values greater than fourfold normal (around 400 μg/day in most radioimmunoassays) are rare except in Cushing's syndrome. Lesser values are compatible with either Cushing's syndrome or pseudo-Cushing's states so that one must exclude the latter diagnosis. If conditions associated with pseudo-Cushing's states are found, treatment or avoidance should result in eucortisolism. Conversely, when biochemical evidence of Cushing's syndrome is not obtained in the setting of clinical features that suggest the diagnosis, repeated measurement of urine cortisol may demonstrate cyclicity or progression.

Up to 11% of patients with proven Cushing's syndrome may have a UFC value within the normal range on one of four samples.[172] Thus, documentation of three or four normal UFC values may be required to exclude the diagnosis.

The normal diurnal rhythm of plasma cortisol is blunted or absent in Cushing's syndrome,[37–39] with normal or increased morning values and an increase in the nighttime nadir. Meal-related and stress-related increases in plasma cortisol may result in apparently elevated values in normal persons. As a result, plasma levels of cortisol discriminate patients with Cushing's syndrome best when obtained around midnight, either through an indwelling line for awake patients[173] or by direct venipuncture of sleeping patients.[174] In these studies, normal sleeping subjects had values less than 1.8 μg/dL, pseudo-Cushing's patients had values less than 7.5 μg/dL, and most patients with Cushing's syndrome had values greater than 7.5μg/dL.[39, 167, 173, 174] However, patients with severe medical illness, depression, and mania may have cortisol values one to three times normal, so this test may not always help distinguish between these states and Cushing's syndrome.[52, 170] In-home collection of saliva in the late evening or at midnight, with subsequent measurement of cortisol, is more convenient and offers good diagnostic accuracy, but few commercial laboratories have validated this test.[175]

Dexamethasone suppression has been used to evaluate whether the normal mechanisms of negative feedback are operative. A 1-mg dose is given at 11 PM or midnight, and plasma cortisol is measured at 8 AM.[176] When the test was reviewed by Crapo,[170] normal subjects suppressed morning cortisol from 3.5 to 10 μg/dL, depending on the assay, while patients with Cushing's syndrome generally had higher values. Crapo's meta-analysis found a 98% sensitivity but a specificity of 77% to 87% for obese individuals and patients with acute and chronic illnesses. Many patients with pseudo-Cushing's states and up to 13% of normal subjects also fail to suppress serum cortisol after this dexamethasone test, especially when current assays and conservative cut points (3.6 μg/dL) are used.[177, 178] A number of medications increase or decrease dexamethasone metabolism (Table 121–5) and may cause a spuriously elevated result in a normal individual who is a "fast" metabolizer, or an inappropriately suppressed value in a patient with Cushing's syndrome who is a "slow" metabolizer.[179, 180] The use and interpretation of this test should consider these issues.

The low-dose dexamethasone suppression test, in which 17-OHCS excretion is measured daily for 2 days during the administration of dexamethasone 500 μg every 6 hours, has been used to exclude the diagnosis of Cushing's syndrome since its introduction in 1960.[181] 17-OHCS excretion greater than 4 mg/day is considered to indicate Cushing's syndrome. The test fails to identify up to 6% of patients with Cushing's syndrome and inappropriately diagnoses up to 15% of patients with pseudo-Cushing's states.[52, 167, 170] It has not been standardized for the use of UFC as an endpoint. Measurement of serum cortisol, using a discriminant of 1.8 μg/dL or more for the detection of Cushing's syndrome, yielded a sensitivity of 98%, but a comparison group was not tested.[174]

More recently, a combined dexamethasone-CRH test has been evaluated for the differential diagnosis of Cushing's syndrome.[182] Dexamethasone 500 μg every 6 hours was given for eight doses, ending 2 hours before administration of ovine CRH (1 μg/kg IV), to 58 adults with mild hypercortisolism (UFC <360 μg/day). Subsequent evaluation proved 39 to have Cushing's syndrome and 19 to have a pseudo-Cushing's state. The plasma cortisol value 15 minutes after CRH was less than 1.4 μg/dL in all patients with pseudo-Cushing's states and greater in all patients with Cushing's syndrome. This test may prove to be a major advance in the ability to distinguish between Cushing's syndrome and pseudo-Cushing's states.

The insulin tolerance test may be a useful adjunct to distinguish Cushing's syndrome from pseudo-Cushing's states. Plasma cortisol values increase in normal people after acute hypoglycemia, presumably because of central stimulation of CRH. The sustained hypercortisolism of Cushing's syndrome suppresses CRH secretion and so blunts this response. The CRH neuron is presumed to be overactive in pseudo-Cushing's states, so a normal response to hypoglycemia should be maintained. Unfortunately, up to 40% of normal individuals and patients with affective disorders fail to respond normally,[183] and up to 18% of patients with Cushing's syndrome, especially those with minimal hypercortisolism, show a normal response to adequate hypoglycemia (blood glucose <40 mg/dL).[52] Thus, the test has a poor diagnostic accuracy in the patients most likely to be evaluated.

Excluding ACTH-Independent Causes of Cushing's Syndrome

Having made the diagnosis of Cushing's syndrome, its cause must be determined. The strategy for the differential diagnosis of Cushing's

TABLE 121–5. Spurious Causes of Abnormal Dexamethasone Suppression

Spurious suppression because of reduced metabolism:
- High-dose benzodiazepines
- Increased estrogens: oral estrogens, combination progestin pills

Spurious lack of suppression due to accelerated clearance:
- Barbiturates, phenytoin, meprobamate, methaqualone, glutethimide, carbamazepine, rifampin

Spurious lack of suppression due to pseudo-Cushing's states:
- Alcoholism, especially during withdrawal[325]
- Exercise, mild or moderate[326,327]
- Affective disorders: mania, schizophrenia, obsessive-compulsive neurosis, dementia[328]
- Liver disease[329]

syndrome (Fig. 121–8) begins with measurement of plasma ACTH by radioimmunoassay to distinguish between ACTH-dependent and ACTH-independent causes. Only assays that can reliably detect values below 10 pg/mL should be used, because this is the range seen in patients with non–ACTH-dependent disorders. Commercially available assays use either polyclonal antibodies, which detect fragments of ACTH as well as the intact molecule, or monoclonal antibodies to each end of the ACTH molecule so that only the intact 1–39 molecule is recognized by the antibody "sandwich."[184] Although the latter assay is more precise at the lower ranges of detection, it may fail to detect unusual circulating forms of ACTH in some patients with ectopic ACTH secretion. It has been argued, therefore, that only a polyclonal assay should be used for detection of ACTH-dependent Cushing's syndrome,[185] but no large-scale comparison of these assays has been made. Regardless of the assay methodology, ACTH is susceptible to degradation by peptidases so that the sample must be kept in an ice water bath and centrifuged, aliquoted, and frozen within a few hours to avoid a spuriously low result. If the sample has been handled appropriately and the plasma ACTH value is less than 10 pg/mL, the patient has an ACTH-independent cause of Cushing's syndrome. When the basal ACTH level is indeterminate (in our laboratory, corresponding to values of 10 to 20 pg/mL), further measurements should be obtained. The response to CRH may be useful in this setting. Patients with primary adrenal disease rarely show maximal ACTH values greater than 20 pg/mL, while patients with Cushing's disease almost always exceed this value (L. Nieman, unpublished observations, 1982–1999).

Radiologic tests are a mainstay in differentiating between the various types of ACTH-independent Cushing's syndrome. High-resolution computed tomography (CT) scanning of the adrenal glands has excellent diagnostic accuracy for masses greater than 1 cm; the contralateral gland must be evaluated if a mass is seen.[126] With this approach, adrenal tumors present as a unilateral mass with an atrophic contralateral gland. If the mass is smaller than 4 cm, it is likely to be a benign adenoma; conversely, carcinoma is more likely if the mass is larger than 6 cm. The adrenal glands in PPNAD appear normal or slightly lumpy but are not enlarged.[186] Massive macronodular adrenal disease is characterized by bilaterally huge (>5 cm) nodular or hyperplastic glands.[9, 128] The CT appearance of the adrenals in this disorder may be similar to the appearance in other forms of bilateral ACTH-independent adrenal disease and the ACTH-dependent forms of Cushing's syndrome, so that further tests are required. Exogenous administration of glucocorticoids results in adrenal atrophy; very small glands may be a clue as to this entity.

Structural details are better assessed by CT than MRI, so CT is the initial radiologic procedure of choice. However, MRI may be used for the differential diagnosis of adrenal masses; the T2-weighted signal is progressively darker in pheochromocytoma, carcinoma, adenoma, and finally normal tissue.[187]

Iodocholesterol scintigraphy identifies functional adrenal tissue capable of taking up a radioactively tagged cholesterol analog. It may distinguish adrenal adenoma from carcinoma, because the latter does not usually accumulate the tracer. Iodocholesterol scanning may be especially valuable in patients with unilateral adrenal masses. In ACTH-dependent cases, the contralateral gland as well as the mass is visualized, whereas the contralateral gland is not metabolically active (due to lack of ACTH support) in patients with adrenal adenoma.[126]

Differentiating Between ACTH-Dependent Causes of Cushing's Syndrome

Plasma ACTH values of greater than 20 pg/mL indicate ACTH-dependent Cushing's syndrome. While some patients with ectopic ACTH secretion, often those with overt tumors, have extremely elevated values of plasma ACTH (>100 pg/mL), ACTH values alone cannot differentiate reliably the ACTH-dependent forms of Cushing's

Plasma ACTH × 2

ACTH <10 pg/mL
ACTH-Independent Causes

ACTH 10–20 pg/mL
Indeterminate

ACTH >20 pg/mL
ACTH-Dependent Causes

Remeasure ACTH, or
measure ACTH after CRH

ACTH <20 pg/mL

ACTH >20 pg/mL

Adrenal CT Scan

Bilaterally Small Glands
PPNAD
Exogenous steroids

Unilateral Mass
Contralateral Gland Small
Adrenal adenoma
Adrenal carcinoma

Bilateral Masses
Idiopathic massive macronodular adrenal disease
Massive macronodular adrenal disease/abnormal receptors
McCune-Albright syndrome
Bilateral adenomas
(Consider iodocholesterol scan to determine functional state of masses)
(Reconsider ACTH-dependent forms)

Biochemical Tests

IPSS with CRH
Central:Peripheral ACTH Gradient

<2	2–3	>3
Cushing's Disease	Indeterminate	Ectopic ACTH

CRH Stimulation Test
ACTH Response[1]

>34%	<34%
Cushing's disease	Indeterminate

Dexamethasone Suppression Test
UFC or 17-OHCS Response[2]

Present	Absent
Cushing's disease	Indeterminate

Metyrapone Stimulation Test
17-OHCS or Compound S Response[3]

Present	Absent
Cushing's disease	Indeterminate

Congruent responses on ≥2 tests required to identify Cushing's disease (responses present) or ectopic ACTH secretion (responses absent). IPSS and CRH are preferred tests. Consider IPSS if responses are not consistent.

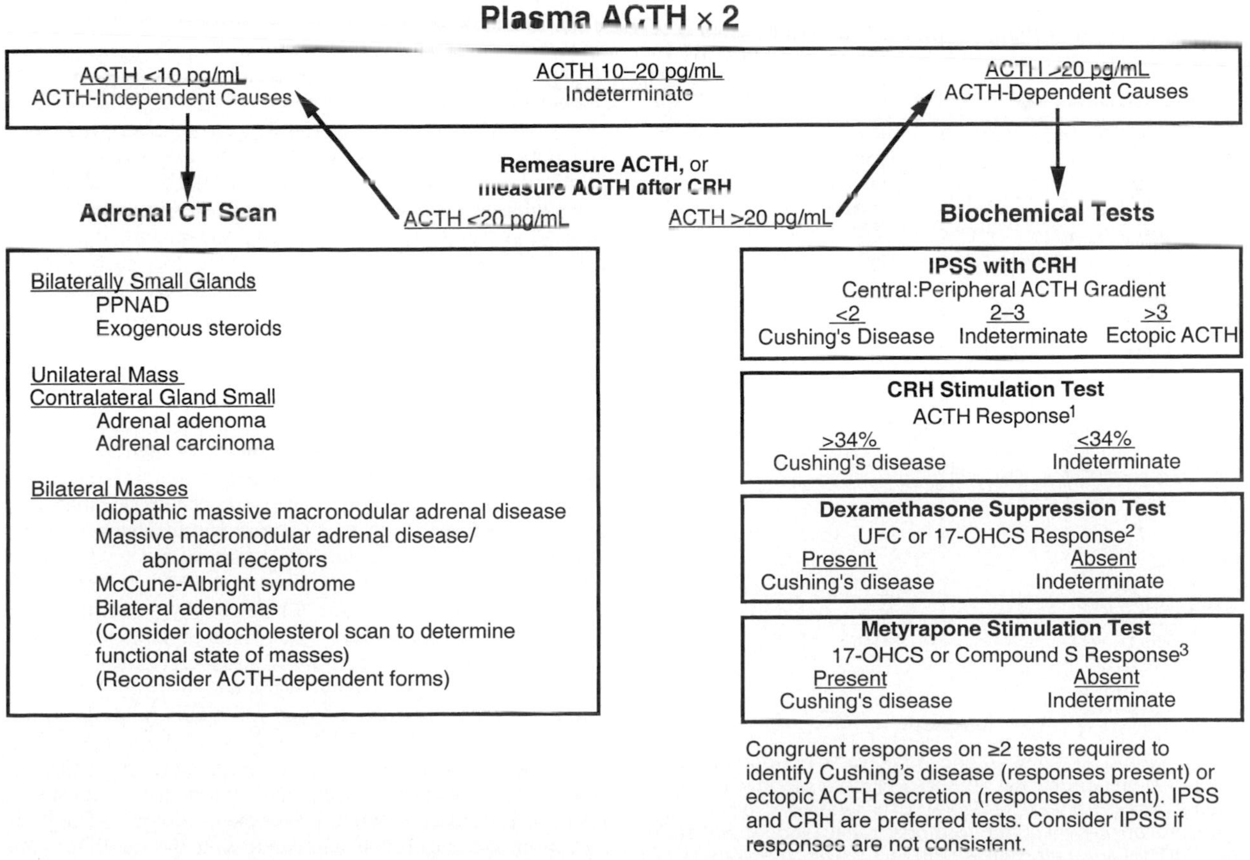

FIGURE 121–8. Diagnostic strategy for the evaluation of Cushing's syndrome. *1,* from reference 208; *2,* urinary free cortisol greater than 90% suppression or 17-hydroxycorticosteroid (17-OHCS) greater than 69% suppression = Cushing's disease, from reference 199; *3,* plasma deoxycortisol increase 400-fold or urine 17-OHCS increase of 70% = Cushing's disease, from reference 204. (ACTH, adrenocorticotropic hormone; CRH, corticotropin-releasing hormone; IPSS, inferior petrosal sinus sampling; PPNAD, primary pigmented nodular adrenal disease.)

syndrome. Howlett and coworkers[188] further refined this point by comparing ACTH levels in patients with overt and occult tumors secreting ACTH ectopically and patients with Cushing's disease. There was a complete overlap between values in occult ectopic ACTH secretion and Cushing's disease.[188]

The ACTH-dependent forms of Cushing's syndrome present the greatest diagnostic challenge. We have taken the stance that diagnostic protocols must maximize the ability to identify ectopic ACTH secretion so that these patients will not be misdiagnosed and suffer either from inappropriate treatment or from the lack of aggressive evaluation of potentially fatal tumors.[51] Since within the ACTH-dependent etiologies the incidence of Cushing's disease is about four times that of ectopic ACTH secretion, a test must have better than 80% sensitivity to perform better than chance alone.

A variety of functional tests of the hypothalamic-pituitary-adrenal axis have been developed to take advantage of the differences in pathophysiology between the ACTH-dependent causes of Cushing's syndrome.

BILATERAL INFERIOR PETROSAL SINUS SAMPLING. Bilateral inferior petrosal sinus sampling (IPSS) is the best test for distinguishing ACTH-dependent forms of Cushing's syndrome, if performed in the setting of prolonged hypercortisolism.[189–191] The test exploits the normal venous drainage of each half of the pituitary gland into the corresponding petrosal sinus. Each petrosal sinus is catheterized separately via a femoral approach, and blood for measurement of ACTH is obtained simultaneously from each sinus and a peripheral vein at two time points before and 3, 5, and 10 minutes after the administration of ovine CRH (1 μg/kg IV)[192] (Fig. 121–9).

ACTH concentrations are greater in the central samples in Cushing's disease and increase after CRH administration, reflecting ACTH secretion by the corticotroph adenoma. In contrast, ACTH values in the central and peripheral specimens are similar in ectopic ACTH secretion and do not increase after CRH. A ratio of the central (i.e., petrosal) to

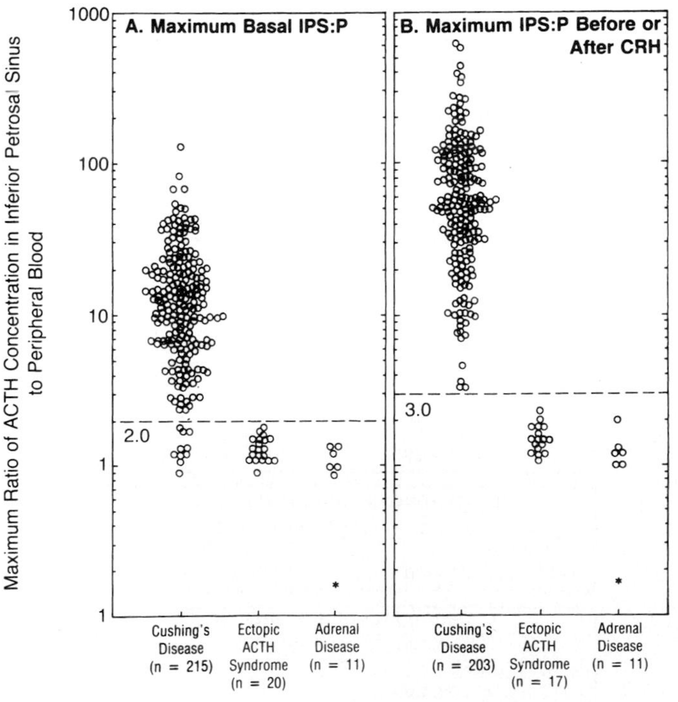

FIGURE 121–9. Maximum ratio of adrenocorticotropic hormone (ACTH) concentration in the inferior petrosal sinus to peripheral blood in patients with confirmed Cushing's disease, ectopic ACTH syndrome, or adrenal disease before corticotropin-releasing hormone (CRH) *(A)* or at any time before or after CRH administration *(B)*. A ratio of 3.0 had 100% sensitivity and specificity. (Data from Oldfield EH, Doppman JL, Nieman LK, et al: Petrosal sinus sampling with and without corticotropin-releasing hormone for the differential diagnosis of Cushing's syndrome. N Engl J Med 325:897–905, 1991.)

peripheral ACTH values is calculated. Pre-CRH gradients of up to 2.0 have been reported in both Cushing's disease and ectopic ACTH secretion; maximal post-CRH gradients in ectopic ACTH secretion (1.5, 1.7, and 2.3) were below the respective minimal post-CRH gradients in Cushing's disease (2.4, 3.2, and 3.2).[189–191] Although a cut point of 2.3 or 2.4 would identify correctly all patients in these studies, it is likely that overlap will occur. Thus, a maximal petrosal-to-peripheral gradient between 2 and 3 should be interpreted with caution.

An additional advantage of IPSS is its potential ability to localize the tumor to the right or left side of the pituitary gland. An interpetrosal sinus (i.e., maximal-to-minimal right or left petrosal) gradient of more than 1.4 has been proposed for this purpose and has correlated with the operative outcome in 47% to 75% of cases.[191]

What are the problems with this procedure? Five cases of transient (n = 2) or permanent (n = 3) neurologic complications, including pontine cerebrovascular accident, have been reported with the use of a specific type of catheter for an incidence of less than 0.5%. The radiologist must be vigilant for early symptoms that may herald a more serious problem.[193] Three additional considerations pertain. First, the success of the test relies on adequate cannulation of both petrosal sinuses, since the diagnostic accuracy decreases significantly when only one petrosal sinus result is considered.[189–191] Thus, technique is paramount: the radiologist must be facile with catheterization, must have sufficient opportunity to perform the procedure, and must confirm the venous anatomy and catheter placement before and after sampling. Abnormal venous anatomy can give false-negative results. Second, optimal results are obtained only when CRH is administered during the sampling. The agent is available commercially in the United States, but not worldwide, for peripheral testing. Substitution of other agents such as desmopressin has not been evaluated formally in a large number of patients and cannot be endorsed at this time. Third, the test is not reliable in mild or intermittent hypercortisolism. We and others have observed IPSS results consistent with Cushing's disease in normal individuals, those with mild ACTH-induced forms of Cushing's syndrome, and patients with ectopic ACTH secretion recently treated with adrenal blockade.[194, 195] For this reason, I recommend determination of midnight plasma cortisol or UFC excretion immediately prior to petrosal sinus sampling to confirm hypercortisolism.

Some have advocated sampling of the cavernous sinus, located closer to the pituitary gland than the petrosal sinus, but others found a 20% false-negative rate.[196] The technique requires insertion of smaller "tracker" catheters into the cavernous sinuses and might be more susceptible to occlusive events. Jugular venous sampling has the advantage of being easier to perform, and potentially more available, than IPSS. Its sensitivity (88%) is less than that of IPSS, but its specificity is 100%, using the same criteria for interpretation as IPSS.[197] Thus, it may be a reasonable initial procedure if referral for IPSS can be obtained when results are negative.

DEXAMETHASONE SUPPRESSION TEST. Since its inception in 1960 the high-dose (8-mg) dexamethasone suppression test has been used to identify patients with Cushing's disease.[181] As originally conceived, 17-hydroxysteroid excretion was used to evaluate the ability of a potent glucocorticoid to suppress ACTH secretion and hence adrenal steroid production. Because corticotropinomas retain some, albeit reduced, sensitivity to glucocorticoid feedback, they would show suppression after dexamethasone administration, while patients with other causes of Cushing's syndrome would not show a decrease in glucocorticoid excretion. The test is usually performed by collecting urine on two baseline days when no glucocorticoid is administered and during subsequent glucocorticoid administration. Dexamethasone is given at doses of 0.5 mg every 6 hours for 2 days (low dose) followed by 2.0 mg every 6 hours for 2 days (high dose). In children, these doses are weight-adjusted to 20 and 80 μg/kg, respectively.[146]

In Liddle's initial study,[181] 23 of 24 patients with Cushing's disease and 0 of 7 patients with adrenal tumors had a greater than 50% decrease in urinary 17-OHCS excretion on day 2 of high-dose dexamethasone administration compared with the baseline value. Subsequent reports, including patients with ectopic ACTH secretion, have shown that the sensitivity (75% to 85%) and specificity (75% to 90%) of this test vary widely.[170, 185] A variety of factors account for this variability. As reviewed earlier, slow or fast metabolism of dexamethasone may alter the response, and the measurement of 17-OHCS may be influenced by medications and medical disease. Additionally, patients with endogenous variability in glucocorticoid excretion may have an inappropriate response. Finally, some patients with ectopic ACTH secretion from carcinoid tumors show reproducible suppression by 50% or more during high-dose dexamethasone administration.

UFC has been evaluated as an alternative endpoint to the test[198] (Fig. 121–10). In this study, suppression of UFC by more than 90% of the mean basal values or suppression of 17-OHCS excretion by more than 64% on the second day of high-dose dexamethasone was associated with 100% specificity in 118 patients. The sensitivity of the test (86%) was higher using a combination of the two criteria than that achieved using either criterion alone (75%) and was higher than that obtained using the traditional criterion of 50% suppression for 17-OHCS excretion (80%).[198] However, subsequent experience showed that a criterion of 69% suppression was necessary to maintain 100% specificity.[199] This emphasizes that values close to any cut point must be viewed with skepticism.

An overnight single 8-mg dexamethasone suppression test has been evaluated. In the original test schedule, dexamethasone 8 mg was administered at 11 PM, and plasma cortisol was measured between 7 and 8 AM that morning and the next morning; a decrease in plasma cortisol of 50% or more was the criterion for Cushing's disease. Two such studies with a total of 93 patients (albeit few with ectopic ACTH secretion) showed a sensitivity of 89% and a specificity of 100%.[200, 201] A subsequent evaluation including 7 patients with ectopic ACTH secretion showed 71% sensitivity and 100% specificity using sampling times of 8:30 AM before and 9:00 AM after dexamethasone, and a criterion of at least 68% suppression for Cushing's disease. Although the sensitivity of the test is not high, dexamethasone is widely available and inexpensive and the test is relatively convenient, so that it is widely used.

METYRAPONE STIMULATION TEST. The metyrapone stimulation test was originally developed in 1959 to distinguish pituitary from primary adrenal causes of Cushing's syndrome.[202] As currently performed, metyrapone 750 mg is given orally every 4 hours for six doses. The agent blocks 11 hydroxylation of deoxycortisol. As a result, plasma levels of 11-deoxycortisol (compound S) increase, and plasma and urine concentrations of cortisol fall. In patients with pituitary-dependent Cushing's syndrome, ACTH levels increase in response to decreased cortisol feedback, plasma compound S increases to greater than 10 μg/dL after 24 hours, and its urinary metabolites (17-OHCS or 17-oxygenic steroids) increase one- to twofold on the day of or after metyrapone administration.[203] By contrast, ACTH values do not increase in patients with primary adrenal disease, and 17-OHCS excretion remains the same or may decrease.

Meta-analysis of multiple studies confirmed that the metyrapone stimulation test works well to discriminate between pituitary disease and adrenal causes of Cushing's syndrome.[170] However, this discrimination is more easily made by determination of basal plasma ACTH. The little available data comparing responses in the ACTH-dependent forms of the syndrome suggest that neither measurements of plasma levels of ACTH nor measurements of urinary 17-oxygenic or 17-hydroxysteroids are useful in making this distinction, since responses of one of these outcome parameters are seen in up to 60% of patients with ectopic ACTH secretion and 90% of those with Cushing's disease.[170, 188] A recent reevaluation of the test in 155 patients with ACTH-dependent Cushing's syndrome yielded 100% specificity and 67% sensitivity for Cushing's disease using criteria of a greater than 400-fold increase in plasma compound S or an increase in urine 17-OHCS of greater than 70%.[204]

A short overnight metyrapone stimulation test using a single weight-adjusted dose (2 g for body weight <70 kg, 2.5 g for 70 to 90 kg, and 3 g for >90 kg) administered at midnight, with measurement of cortisol and 11-deoxycortisol at 9 AM on both days was evaluated in 57 patients with Cushing's disease and 6 patients with ectopic ACTH secretion. One hundred percent specificity and 65% sensitivity were achieved using an increase in plasma 11-deoxycortisol of more than 220-fold or a suppression of plasma cortisol of more than 40% for the diagnosis of Cushing's disease.[205] A test using IV administration lacks extensive evaluation in hypercortisolemic patients.[170] A pediatric test using a dose of 1 g/m^2 at 8 AM with measurement of plasma deoxycortisol 3 hours later correlated well with the standard longer test in normal children and adolescents but has had limited application in patients with Cushing's syndrome.[206]

CRH STIMULATION TEST. The use of ovine CRH stimulation for the differential diagnosis of ACTH-dependent Cushing's syndrome relies on these assumptions: (1) that corticotropinomas retain responsivity to CRH, while noncorticotroph tumors lack CRH receptors and cannot respond to the agent, and (2) that hypercortisolism has been sufficient to inhibit the normal corticotroph response. Most patients with Cushing's disease respond to ovine CRH, either 1 μg/kg or 100 μg IV, with increases in plasma ACTH or cortisol, while patients

with ectopic ACTH secretion do not.[110, 207, 209] Results are similar after morning (8 to 9 AM) and evening (8 PM) administration. Controversy exists as to the specificity of the test, in part because few centers have developed and validated criteria for response. We demonstrated 100% specificity and 93% sensitivity using an increase in mean post-CRH ACTH values (at 15 and 30 minutes) of at least 34% to indicate Cushing's disease[208] (Fig. 121–11). A cortisol criterion of an increase of at least 20% in the mean post-CRH value (at 30 and 45 minutes) to indicate Cushing's disease yielded an 88% specificity and 91%

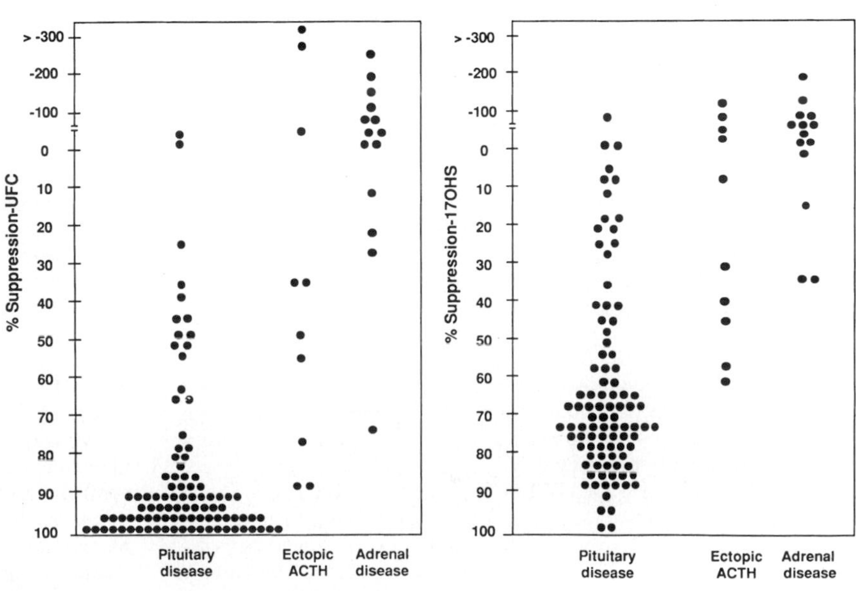

FIGURE 121–10. Suppression of urine free cortisol (UFC) and 17-hydroxycorticosteroid (17-OHCS) excretion during a standard high-dose dexamethasone suppression test in 118 patients with surgically confirmed cases of Cushing's syndrome. Percent suppression represents the ratio of urine excretion on the second day of dexamethasone, 2 mg every 6 hours, divided by the mean of urine excretion on 2 baseline days, expressed as a percentage. The criterion of UFC greater than 90% suppression or 17-OHCS greater than 64% suppression for the diagnosis of Cushing's disease yielded 86% sensitivity and 100% specificity. The criterion of 64% suppression was later increased to 69% suppression to maintain 100% sensitivity. (Data from Flack MR, Oldfield EH, Cutler GB Jr, et al: Urine free cortisol in the high-dose dexamethasone suppression test for the differential diagnosis of the Cushing syndrome. Ann Intern Med 116:211–217, 1992; and Dichek HL, Nieman LK, Oldfield EH, et al: A comparison of the standard high-dose dexamethasone suppression test and the overnight 8-mg dexamethasone suppression test for the differential diagnosis of Cushing's syndrome. J Clin Endocrinol Metab 78:418–422, 1994.)

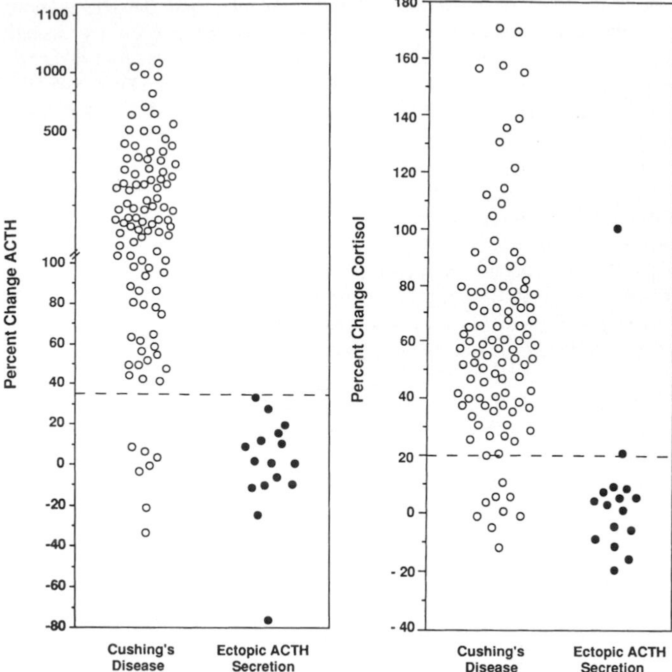

FIGURE 121–11. Response of adrenocorticotropic hormone (ACTH) and cortisol to ovine corticotropin-releasing hormone (oCRH) in patients with Cushing's disease and ectopic ACTH secretion. ACTH responses are expressed as the percent change in mean concentration 15 and 30 minutes after oCRH from the mean basal value 1 and 5 minutes before the injection. The *dashed line* indicates a response of 35%, representing a diagnostic criterion with 100% specificity and 93% sensitivity. Cortisol responses are expressed as the percent change in mean cortisol concentration 30 and 45 minutes after oCRH from the mean basal value 1 and 5 minutes before the injection. The *dashed line* indicates a response of 20%, representing a diagnostic criterion with 88% specificity and 91% sensitivity. (Data from Nieman LK, Oldfield EH, Wesley R, et al: A simplified morning ovine corticotropin-releasing hormone stimulation test for the differential diagnosis of ACTH-dependent Cushing syndrome. J Clin Endocrinol Metab 77:1308–1312, 1993.)

sensitivity. A recent meta-analysis of 10 studies suggested criteria for the diagnosis of Cushing's disease: increase in peak cortisol of 20% or more above baseline, and an increase in peak ACTH of 50% or more above baseline.[185] As different time points were used in the various studies, no test protocol could be recommended. However, the large number of patients (126 Cushing's disease, 21 ectopic ACTH secretion, 19 adrenal disease) provides robust evidence for the general diagnostic utility of the test. Human CRH was found not as useful as ovine CRH for the differential diagnosis of ACTH-dependent Cushing's syndrome in one study,[210] but to be similar in another.[211]

VASOPRESSIN STIMULATION. Newell-Price and colleagues[212] recently reviewed the diagnostic performance of lysine and arginine vasopressin, and desmopressin, a long-acting vasopressin analog, for the differential diagnosis of Cushing's syndrome. These agents are thought to stimulate ACTH release through the specific corticotroph receptor, V3 (or V1b), an effect that is separate from the V1-mediated pressor activity of vasopressin, and the V2-mediated renal effects of desmopressin. These agents seem inferior to CRH for the differential diagnosis of Cushing's syndrome. This meta-analysis of three studies of 63 patients (50 Cushing's disease, 7 ectopic ACTH, 6 adrenal), showed a sensitivity of 84% and a specificity of 83%, using cortisol as an endpoint, while diagnostic accuracy using ACTH was less. Thus, if CRH is available, it is a better choice.[212] Desmopressin is the analog of choice, if this class of compounds is used, to avoid the hypertension and nausea seen with the vasopressins.

COMBINED TEST STRATEGIES. Since none of the noninvasive tests has 100% diagnostic accuracy, a number of investigators have evaluated the utility of combined test strategies. A diagnosis is assigned if at least two tests give a concordant result. Alternatively, criteria may be set to maximize specificity (100%) so that a positive result to any test would be considered indicative of Cushing's disease. The CRH and high-dose dexamethasone test have been paired in this way, yielding a 79% concordance,[213] a 98% to 100% sensitivity, and an 88% to 100% specificity.[208, 209, 214] Taken together, these data suggest that a combined test strategy using stringent criteria for response may yield excellent diagnostic accuracy.

There is no consensus on the correct test strategy for the differential diagnosis of Cushing's syndrome. I recommend that at least two tests be done to differentiate between the ACTH-dependent forms of Cushing's syndrome, that conservative criteria be used to interpret the tests, and that a diagnosis not be assigned unless the test results are congruent. Ideally, IPSS would be performed in all patients because of its high diagnostic accuracy and lateralization information, and CRH would be the other test. In centers in which these tests are not available, the combination of dexamethasone and metyrapone can be used with jugular venous sampling, with referral of the patient for IPSS if the test results do not agree. While some investigators with extensive experience in the evaluation of these patients follow a similar approach,[212] others do not rely on IPSS, and prefer noninvasive tests,[215] and others favor IPSS as the primary test.[216]

LOCALIZATION OF ACTH-SECRETING TUMORS. A number of tests have been used to localize or identify the source of ACTH. MRI of the sella obtained on a 1.5-T scanner with 3-mm contiguous slices before and after administration of gadolinium contrast material identifies a tumor in about two thirds of patients with Cushing's disease and about 5% of normal individuals.[217] Thus, MRI yields improved sensitivity for a pituitary tumor compared with CT, but specificity for Cushing's disease is only about 95%.[185] Despite the low sensitivity for detection of tumor, pituitary MRI should be obtained when the diagnosis of Cushing's disease is considered likely (e.g., if noninvasive tests suggest the diagnosis), when IPSS may be performed (because if there is a large tumor and a positive noninvasive test, IPSS would not be needed), or when surgery is scheduled (to aid in tumor localization and to assess the anatomy of the sphenoid sinus and carotid arteries).

Biochemical and radiologic tests may identify the source of ectopic ACTH production. Both CT and MRI of the chest should be obtained—the information is complementary, and the likelihood of an intrathoracic tumor is high.[218] Thymic rebound hyperplasia is common when eucortisolism has been restored by glucocorticoid blockade or adrenalectomy, especially in the younger patients, and is part of the differential diagnosis of a new anterior mediastinal mass in patients with an occult ectopic ACTH-producing tumor. CT and MRI (T2-weighted or stir sequence) of the pancreas, adrenal glands, and neck, and measurement of marker peptides, such as calcitonin, gastrin, 5-hydroxyindoleacetic acid (HIAA), serotonin, catecholamines, and human CRH, may identify a neuroendocrine tumor. Neither venous sampling[219] nor bronchoscopy[220] localizes these tumors, but CT-guided aspiration of masses for measurement of ACTH may provide useful functional information.[221] Octreotide scintigraphy has been recommended for localization or identification of neuroendocrine tumors having somatostatin receptors, including pancreatic tumors, carcinoids, glomus tumors, and small cell cancer of the lung.[215] A recent evaluation of the utility of this approach in 18 consecutive patients with ectopic ACTH secretion showed that octreoscan did not detect tumor in any patient when MRI or CT scan was negative. Octreoscan was falsely positive in 6 patients, falsely negative in 5, but confirmed a lesion seen on CT or MRI in 7 patients. Thus, while CT and MR represent the best initial screening examinations, octreotide may be a useful adjunctive imaging modality.[222]

THERAPY

Optimal treatment for Cushing's syndrome renders the patient eucortisolemic with minimal morbidity and mortality. With the advent of synthetic glucocorticoid therapy, adrenalectomy became the treatment of choice because it conferred rapid and, in most cases, permanent resolution of Cushing's syndrome.[223] Improvements in neurosurgical techniques and appreciation of the sources of ectopic ACTH secretion have changed the therapeutic approach to Cushing's syndrome so that surgery now is directed toward resection of abnormal tissue, whether ACTH- or cortisol-producing. This optimal approach cannot be realized if the patient cannot safely undergo surgery or if the tumor is occult or metastatic. Other second-line therapies that are less specific, and may have greater morbidity, must be chosen in these settings.

Medical Treatment

The medical treatments for hypercortisolism have two broad mechanisms of action. One class of compounds modulates ACTH release from a pituitary tumor and is restricted to the treatment of Cushing's disease. The second class of agents reduces cortisol levels or action through adrenolytic activity, inhibition of steroidogenesis, or antagonism of cortisol action at the level of the receptor. These compounds are used in the treatment of all forms of Cushing's syndrome.

Agents That Modulate ACTH Release

Compounds that affect CRH or ACTH synthesis or release, including cyproheptadine, bromocriptine, somatostatin, and valproic acid, have been examined as therapeutic agents for Cushing's disease, but no large-scale, placebo-controlled trials have been reported.

Dopamine agonist therapy normalizes cortisol levels in a small percentage of patients with Cushing's disease.[224–226] Pituitary histology, the response to dexamethasone, the basal prolactin levels, and the ACTH response to acute challenge with bromocriptine do not predict the long-term response to therapy. Postural hypotension and nausea at the usual doses of bromocriptine, 3 to 30 mg/day, may limit this approach.

The antiserotonergic agent cyproheptadine inhibits ACTH secretion in normal persons.[227] An efficacy of up to 50% has been reported if treatment is continued for at least 3 weeks at a daily dose of 24 mg.[65, 228, 229] Because of its long onset of action and the high incidence of relapse on discontinuation, cyproheptadine is not a good choice for a patient who requires rapid control of hypercortisolism or for long-term treatment. Ritanserin, a more selective type 2 serotonin receptor antagonist, normalized UFC values in two of three patients.[230]

Valproic acid decreases ACTH levels in patients receiving the agent for its antiseizure effects,[231] an action probably mediated by inhibition of CRH release through blockade of hypothalamic γ-aminobutyric acid (GABA) reuptake. Despite reports of ACTH inhibition with short-term infusion, chronic therapy did not normalize cortisol or ACTH values in one small study of patients with Cushing's disease.[226]

The availability of the potent somatostatin analog octreotide has allowed investigation of its utility in decreasing both ectopic and eutopic production of ACTH. Although octreotide failed to alter plasma ACTH values in seven patients with Cushing's disease, a few case reports attest to its efficacy in reducing ACTH secretion in Nelson's syndrome, from tumors producing ACTH ectopically, and in one patient with GIP-responsive macronodular adrenal disease.[232]

Agents Inhibiting Steroidogenesis

Mitotane, trilostane, ketoconazole, aminoglutethimide, and metyrapone decrease cortisol production by inhibiting steroidogenesis at one or more enzymatic steps. There is little clinical experience with other agents, such as etomidate and other imidazole derivatives with a similar mechanism of action. Unfortunately, apart from etomidate (see below), no available agent can be given parenterally.

Steroidogenesis blockade can be titrated to complete or partial inhibition of cortisol production.[233] Patients receiving full adrenal blockade require glucocorticoid replacement to avoid symptoms of adrenal insufficiency. Partial inhibition of cortisol production ("adjusted adrenal blockade") aims to render the patient eucortisolemic and does not require additional exogenous hydrocortisone. Both approaches, if properly monitored and managed, can render the patient effectively eucortisolemic. Full adrenal blockade with hydrocortisone replacement is often advocated so as to avoid potential adrenal insufficiency with adjusted adrenal blockade in a patient with variable cortisol production. However, the converse often pertains with this approach; complete inhibition of cortisol production is not achieved, and the additive effects of exogenous and endogenous cortisol render the patient hypercortisolemic. Another disadvantage of full compared with adjusted adrenal blockade is the necessity for a greater number of drugs in larger amounts, with resultant increase in toxicity and cost. For these reasons, I recommend adjusted adrenal blockade with frequent monitoring to identify a dose that maintains eucortisolism while avoiding adrenal insufficiency or excess. Patients and their physicians must be alert to the signs and symptoms of adrenal insufficiency.

Mitotane, or *o,p'*-DDD, inhibits steroidogenesis catalyzed by cholesterol desmolase,[234] 11- and 18-hydroxylase, and 3β-hydroxysteroid dehydrogenase.[235] Its additional adrenolytic action has led to its chemotherapeutic use in the treatment of adrenal cancer,[236–238] but the contribution of the agent to improved survival of these patients remains somewhat controversial. High serum levels enhanced the likelihood of measurable tumor regression and increased survival in one of two studies.[239, 240]

Mitotane alone, 12 g/day, can achieve remission in up to 83% of patients with Cushing's disease, but only about a third have a sustained remission after discontinuation of treatment.[241] More commonly, mitotane is used with radiation therapy for the treatment of Cushing's disease. Mitotane is useful also in the treatment of hypercortisolism associated with ectopic secretion of ACTH, alone or in combination with metyrapone or aminoglutethimide.[242]

Mitotane therapy begins at a dose of 0.5 to 1.0 g/day, which is increased gradually, by 0.5 to 1.0 g, every 1 to 4 weeks. The agent has a long half-life (18 to 159 days), due in part to its lipophilic properties, and has been detected in adipose tissue as long as 22 months after discontinuation of therapy.[243] The utility of mitotane is limited by its gastrointestinal and neurologic toxicity. Nausea is common at doses up to 2 g/day (used with radiation therapy) and is ubiquitous at more than 4 g/day (used for adrenal carcinoma).[236] Diarrhea is common. These side effects may be avoided by very gradual increases in dose and by administration of the agent with meals or at bedtime with food. They may be alleviated by changing the schedule of administration of the agent to once-daily or alternate day administration. At the higher doses, neurologic findings are common and include gait disturbances, dizziness or vertigo, confusion, and problems with language expression, including anomia. Fatigue (perhaps due to decreased cortisol levels), gynecomastia, skin rash, hyperlipidemia, hypouricemia, and elevated serum liver enzymes also occur. Adrenal insufficiency is rare and should be treated with hydrocortisone. If adrenal crisis or gastrointestinal symptoms occur, the drug should be stopped. Usually, symptoms improve within a week, and mitotane can be restarted at a previously tolerated lower dose.

Mitotane is relatively contraindicated in women desiring fertility within 2 to 5 years. It may induce spontaneous abortion and act as a teratogen, effects that may persist for a number of years after discontinuation due to deposition in fat.[243]

Mitotane increases the metabolic clearance of exogenously administered steroids.[244] For example, the replacement dose of hydrocortisone must be increased by about a third, to around 30 mg/day. The proportion of fewer polar metabolites of cortisol increases; because these are not extracted by the Porter-Silber chromogen procedure, a factitiously low value for urinary 17-OHCS is obtained.[245] Also, since hepatic CBG production is induced by mitotane, total plasma cortisol values increase. For these reasons, UFC excretion should be used to monitor the efficacy of mitotane therapy.

A number of agents reduce cortisol production by competitive inhibition of steroidogenic enzymes. Some, such as trilostane (3β-hydroxysteroid dehydrogenase)[246] and metyrapone (11β-hydroxylase),[247] block primarily a single enzyme; others, such as aminoglutethimide[248] and ketoconazole,[249] act at a number of sites. The clinical experience with aminoglutethimide and metyrapone in the treatment of nonpituitary causes of Cushing's syndrome is more extensive, spanning almost 40 years.[4, 250] A disadvantage of these agents in the treatment of Cushing's disease is the need to increase the dose to maintain eucortisolism. This must be done because corticotroph tumors increase ACTH production to overcome the block in cortisol production. It is unusual for patients to remain in remission when medical therapy is discontinued, unless radiation therapy to decrease ACTH production has been given.[251–255]

Trilostane is a relatively weak inhibitor of steroidogenesis. Even at maximal daily doses of 980 mg, only a minority of patients achieve remission.[256] Although its use in combination therapy has not been reported, trilostane may prove to be a useful addition to such a therapeutic strategy. Side effects include abdominal discomfort, diarrhea, and paresthesias. Trilostane is detected in fluorometric assays for 11-hydroxycorticoids, including cortisol, and in radioimmunoassays for estrogen and testosterone, probably because of structural similarities to the steroids of interest. Radioimmunoassay of UFC should be used to monitor treatment.

Metyrapone and aminoglutethimide may be useful as sole treatment for ectopic ACTH secretion or adrenal adenoma or in combination with radiation therapy of the pituitary for Cushing's disease.[251, 253, 257–259] Metyrapone is begun at a daily dose of 1.0 g (in four divided doses) and increased every few days to a maximal daily dose of 4.5 g, although often no further gain is obtained beyond a daily dose of 2.0 g. Inhibition of 11β-hydroxylase by metyrapone increases androgenic and mineralocorticoid precursors, resulting in hypertension, acne, and hirsutism during long-term treatment.[260] These effects are dose-dependent, being nearly universal at 3 g/day but decreasing to 33% at a daily dose of less than 2 g.[261] Nausea and dizziness also may limit its use. Metyrapone induces hepatic mixed function oxidases so that doses of agents metabolized in this way may require adjustment. The increase in 11-deoxycortisol induced by metyrapone is reflected in the urine 17-OHCS. For this reason, UFC, and not 17-OHCS, should be used to monitor metyrapone therapy.

Aminoglutethimide is begun at a dose of 500 mg/day in four divided doses and can be increased by 250 to 500 mg every 3 to 4 days to a total dose of 2 g. Neurologic complaints, including somnolence, dizziness, depression, and blurred vision, are common (30%), especially at daily doses greater than 1 g.[253] A transient morbiliform rash and fever are seen in about one fifth of patients within the first 2 weeks of therapy, but the agent need not be discontinued. Aminoglutethimide blocks thyroid hormone synthesis. While thyroid-stimulating hormone (TSH) levels usually increase to maintain euthyroidism, goiter and hypothyroidism may result.

Ketoconazole, a more recent addition to this class of compounds, inhibits cytochrome P450 enzymes, including side-chain cleavage, 17,20-lyase, 11β-hydroxylase, and 17β-hydroxylase.[249, 262] It effectively reduces plasma cortisol levels at doses of 400 to 1600 mg/day given every 6 to 8 hours. Side effects of gastrointestinal distress and gynecomastia occur in less than 15% of patients. Irregular menses may develop in menstruating women. Reversible hepatic dysfunction, manifested by increased serum hepatocellular enzymes, is common and need not result in discontinuation of the agent if levels remain below two- to threefold the upper normal range. While reports of idiosyncratic hepatic dyscrasia, occurring in about 1 in 15,000 cases, have diminished enthusiasm for its use somewhat,[263] a relatively benign spectrum of side effects and the potential for single-agent therapy make ketoconazole a first choice for many patients.[264] Because gastric acidity is necessary to metabolize it into the active compound, ketoconazole is not an option in patients treated with histamine H_2 receptor antagonists, unless it is formulated locally in an acidic vehicle.

The anesthetic etomidate is an imidazole derivative that inhibits cholesterol side-chain cleavage and 11β-hydroxylase. At a nonsedating continuous IV dose of 0.3 mg/kg/hour, it reduced plasma cortisol within 12 hours in six patients.[265] While experience is limited, it represents a potentially life-saving approach in patients who cannot take oral medications.[266] It is important to recognize that the etomidate preparations available in Europe are dissolved in an alcohol-based vehicle, while the currently available preparation in the United States uses propylene glycol, which may have additional side effects.

RU 486 is a steroid that binds competitively to the glucocorticoid and progestin receptors and inhibits the action of the endogenous ligands. Its use in Cushing's syndrome has been limited to a few investigational studies of patients with ectopic ACTH secretion.[267] In nonpituitary causes of hypercortisolism, the effects of cortisol are antagonized effectively at doses of 10 to 20 mg/kg/day. Because efficacy must be judged by glucocorticoid-sensitive parameters rather than by ACTH or cortisol concentrations, assessment of response and dose adjustment is difficult, especially in patients with variable glucocorticoid production. The increase in plasma ACTH values after RU 486 administration in normal individuals and patients with Cushing's disease[268] would likely limit its use in the latter condition. Unfortunately, the agent remains investigational in the United States and is not available commercially for this purpose in Europe.

Transsphenoidal Resection of Corticotropinoma

At this time, transsphenoidal resection is the preferred treatment of corticotropinomas with minimal suprasellar extension.[269] The procedure is usually performed using a gingival approach, as originally devised by Kanavel and Halsted and later popularized by Cushing.[270] The development of the operating microscope led to the introduction of transsphenoidal resection of pituitary microadenomas by Hardy in 1968.

The goal of surgery is to remove the adenoma selectively and so preserve as much normal pituitary tissue as possible. If a tumor cannot be identified, the surgeon may elect to end the procedure or remove a part or all of the gland. Hemihypophysectomy of the side of the gland with an ACTH gradient on petrosal sinus sampling may induce remission in up to 80% of patients (E. H. Oldfield, unpublished observations, 1982–1997), but the incidence of hypopituitarism and long-term remission has not been evaluated in a large series of patients. When performed by an experienced neurosurgeon, initial cure ranges from 66% to 89% but may be much lower in less experienced hands or after repeat surgery.[271–277] The success of surgery also depends on the correct diagnosis; retrospective analysis from a number of centers revealed that incorrect diagnosis accounts for up to 12% of patients with surgical failure.[278] The procedure works equally well in children; early studies suggesting an unacceptably high recurrence rate have not been confirmed by subsequent analysis of a larger number of patients.[147, 279–282]

The success of transsphenoidal or transcranial resection of macroadenomas or tumors invading the cavernous sinus decreases dramatically to between 50% and 70%, and surgical therapy has not been clearly established as superior to treatment with radiation therapy and adrenolytic agents in these settings.[273–275]

The mortality of transsphenoidal surgery is 1% or less.[274] Perioperative morbidity, transient diabetes insipidus, cerebrospinal fluid leak, and meningitis respond to medical management and occur in less than 10% of patients. Permanent complications include diabetes insipidus; injury to the carotid arteries, nose, optic nerve, or nerves of the cavernous sinus (causing ptosis or diplopia); and partial or complete hypopituitarism. These occur in less than 5% of patients after initial resection of a microadenoma but are more common after resection of larger tumors or larger amounts of normal pituitary tissue (or stalk) or after repeat surgery.[273, 274, 283]

After surgery, most patients who achieve long-term remission are hypocortisolemic and require glucocorticoid replacement until the hypothalamic-pituitary-adrenal axis is normalized, usually within the first postoperative year (see Therapeutic Protocols, below). The recurrence rate after initial surgery is probably 10% or less.[284, 285] However, because relatively few patients have been followed for more than 5 years, the true long-term recurrence rate is unknown.

Radiation Therapy

As currently administered, radiation therapy is delivered at a total dose of 4500 cGy (rad) in 25 fractional doses over 35 days using a three-field technique. This approach ensures that the daily dose to neural tissue does not exceed 180 cGy and avoids the complications of optic neuritis and cortical necrosis associated with larger total and fractional doses.[286] When radiation therapy is used alone, only a minority of adults achieve normal (20%) or improved (33%) glucocorticoid excretion.[287] By contrast, similar regimens achieve remission in 80% of children treated before the age of 18 years.[288] The reason for this difference is not known. The response of adults to radiation therapy is improved to between 53% and 83% by the adjuvant use of metyrapone, aminoglutethimide, ketoconazole, or mitotane.[109, 241, 257, 289] Medical therapy is initiated at the onset of radiation therapy and increased as needed to normalize cortisol values; subsequent monitoring is necessary to reduce the dose and if possible discontinue the medication. When the UFC value is around 50 μg/day (mid-normal) or plasma cortisol is around 10 μg/dL, the dose of adrenal blockade should be reduced and biochemical parameters monitored frequently to avoid hypocortisolism. If symptoms of adrenal insufficiency occur, the agent(s) should be discontinued and hydrocortisone should be given until cortisol values are normal. Radiation therapy inhibits the secretion of ACTH without normalizing its diurnal variation. Thus, when medication can be discontinued, usually after 0.7 to 10 years, the mean 24-hour serum cortisol level is normal at the expense of elevated evening values. Some patients require adrenolytic agents (mitotane 250 mg to 4 g/day or on alternate days) for up to 15 years after radiation therapy. Since remission has not been reported with discontinuation of medical therapy beyond 11 years after radiation, it may be reasonable to consider bilateral adrenalectomy in patients requiring adrenal blockade at that time.

The side effects of current radiation therapy regimens include temporal hair loss at the time of therapy, and hypopituitarism, which may develop many years later. The incidence of endocrine abnormalities following radiation therapy varies widely depending on the series, probably as a function of the length of follow-up and techniques used to assess endocrine function. TSH deficiency is seen in 10% to 20% and gonadotropin deficiency in 33% to 50% of patients evaluated 6 to 15 years after treatment with 4500 cGy for Cushing's disease or acromegaly.[109, 290] Although "catch-up" growth of 3 to 20 cm may occur after successful radiation therapy at bone ages of 7 to 18 years, final adult height is less than predicted, either because of irreparable loss of time to grow or possibly because basal and stimulated growth hormone values are suppressed by radiation therapy.[288]

Radiosurgery

Radiosurgery of the pituitary gland using heavy charged particles from proton or helium beams has been available at a few centers since the 1950s. When radiosurgery was delivered in three or four fractionated doses (60 to 150 cGy) over 5 days using a stereotactic system for dose localization within 0.3 mm,[291] 40 of 42 patients achieved normal cortisol levels.[292] When given over alternate days, the same dose was effective in 15 of 22 patients. With this, as with conventional forms of radiation therapy, it appears that younger patients have a better response, as 5 of 5 teenagers responded as compared with 50 of 59 adults. Three patients in this series were reported to have visual-field defects or transient partial third cranial nerve palsies. About a third were reported to have endocrine deficiency. More recently, stereotactic administration of gamma or linear accelerator radiation, in one or a few sessions, has become available. The scant data available suggest that this technique, like the others above, has a shorter response time compared to conventional radiation therapy.[293] Additional advantages would be the small number of visits and the ability to target a small volume accurately. However, the overall effectiveness and long-term adverse effects remain unclear, so that many clinicians do not recommend this as a primary modality.

Adrenalectomy

Resection of the affected adrenal gland(s) is the treatment of choice only for non–ACTH-dependent hypercortisolism of adrenal origin or when a specific surgical approach to the ACTH-dependent causes is not feasible. Bilateral adrenalectomy as a second line of treatment has the advantage of providing rapid resolution of hypercortisolism and has no risk of hypopituitarism, in contrast to radiation therapy. Its disadvantages include perioperative morbidity and mortality and the lifelong requirement for glucocorticoid and mineralocorticoid replacement therapy.

The mortality and morbidity of traditional open adrenalectomy via an anterior or posterior incision range from 1% to 20% in various series, probably reflecting differences in the severity of Cushing's syndrome and the presence of associated conditions, such as cardiovascular disease.[187, 223] Apart from resection of suspected carcinoma, these approaches have been supplanted by laparoscopic resection, which has a low mortality and morbidity when done by an experienced surgeon. Glands as large as 7.5 cm may be removed using this approach.[294]

Plasma cortisol levels decrease to the limit of detection of the assay (1 μg/dL) after successful adrenalectomy. Early failure to achieve hypocortisolism is usually related to incomplete resection of the gland(s). Recurrence, especially in the ACTH-dependent forms of Cushing's syndrome, may be related to regrowth of adrenal cells in the surgical bed or to growth of adrenal rest tissue.

Special Therapeutic Problems

Persistent or Recurrent Cushing's Disease

Cushing's disease persisting after transsphenoidal exploration should prompt reevaluation of the diagnosis, especially if previous diagnostic test results were indeterminate or conflicting or if no tumor was found on pathologic examination. Petrosal sinus sampling after transsphenoidal surgery can confirm a pituitary source of ACTH, but the rate of correct lateralization decreases, probably because of alterations in venous anatomy caused by the prior surgery; so the procedure cannot be used to direct a second operative search or decision for hemihypophysectomy.

The treatment options for patients with recurrent or persistent Cushing's disease include repeat surgery, radiation therapy, and adrenalectomy. Limited evaluations of repeat surgery performed 2 weeks to 10 years after the initial operation for persistent or recurrent hypercortisolism demonstrated a success rate of about 70%.[277, 295] The likelihood of remission after repeat surgery is greatest when some or all of the following outcome parameters are present: the diagnosis is correct, as evidenced by previous curative surgery with pathologic confirmation of an ACTH-staining adenoma; the initial exposure or resection was incomplete; or residual tumor is seen on CT or MRI scan without evidence of cavernous sinus invasion. Repeat sellar exploration is less likely to be helpful in patients with empty sella syndrome or very little pituitary tissue on CT or MRI images. Patients with cavernous sinus or dural invasion identified at the initial procedure are not candidates for repeat surgery to treat hypercortisolism and should receive radiation therapy.

There are no data to indicate whether the risk of Nelson's syndrome is increased after bilateral adrenalectomy for recurrent Cushing's disease. Adrenalectomy or radiation therapy may be equivalent options except for patients with rapid tumor growth, who probably should undergo radiation therapy.

Pregnancy

Maternal hypercortisolism is associated with a poor pregnancy outcome, including an increased rate of premature delivery and stillbirth.[160] It is unclear whether this is a toxic effect of hypercortisolism on the fetus or placenta or is related to associated medical conditions such as hypertension and diabetes. However, pregnancy outcome has been slightly better in women with adrenal causes of Cushing's syndrome who received surgical treatment while pregnant. An additional reason for early resection of adrenal masses is the significant incidence of adrenal carcinoma in pregnancy. Although anesthesia increases the risk of premature labor, both maternal and fetal outcome are improved by resolution of hypercortisolism, and surgery should not be delayed because of this concern.[296] Many patients with Cushing's disease have not been treated during the pregnancy; metyrapone, cyproheptadine, radiation therapy, and transsphenoidal surgery[297] have all been used in a few cases.[160] Since ketoconazole is teratogenic in animals and blocks steroidogenesis, its use is contraindicated.[262]

Therapeutic Protocols

Preoperative Evaluation and Treatment

I recommend routine preoperative adrenal blockade only if wound healing would be compromised by severe hypercortisolism. The empiric goal in this setting is a minimum of 1 month of eucortisolism prior to surgery. If this cannot be achieved by medical therapy (i.e., if cortisol values are reduced but remain elevated), the patient should proceed to surgery. Additionally, any patient awaiting surgery who develops a life-threatening infection should receive antibiotics as well as steroidogenesis inhibitors.

Since nearly all patients will be hypercortisolemic at the time of surgery, the associated medical conditions of hypercortisolism, especially hypertension and cardiovascular disease, should be assessed and treated so as to decrease perioperative morbidity and mortality. Spironolactone blockade of mineralocorticoid action, a good theoretical choice for blood pressure reduction, is often insufficient. β-Adrenergic blockers and angiotensin-converting enzyme inhibitors may be more effective. Glucose tolerance should be addressed in the usual fashion.

Postoperative Evaluation and Treatment

Patients typically receive supraphysiologic doses of glucocorticoids after all surgical procedures, at initial daily doses of up to 300 mg hydrocortisone (4 mg dexamethasone), tapering off within 3 or 4 days (after transsphenoidal surgery) or when the patient can take oral medication (after abdominal or thoracic procedures). Ideally, morning serum cortisol and daily UFC measurements are then obtained for 3 days without glucocorticoid administration, during which time the patient should be observed for development of signs of adrenal insufficiency. This approach allows for prompt classification of remission or persistent hypercortisolism, but may not be practical in settings where the patient must be discharged within a day or two of surgery.

Plasma cortisol values that remain unchanged from preoperative values reflect surgical failure. Eucortisolemic patients with morning cortisol values of 6 to 9 μg/dL are at risk of recurrence compared with hypocortisolemic patients.[271, 298–300]

Postoperative hypocortisolism reflects adequate removal of the cause of hypercortisolism, which then unmasks the underlying suppression of the entire hypothalamic-pituitary-adrenal axis: inactivity of the CRH neuron, inability of the pituitary to release ACTH in response to exogenous CRH, and adrenal atrophy and inability to respond to ACTH.[298, 301] Morning plasma cortisol values of less than 3.6 μg/dL and daily UFC excretion less than 20 μg suggest cure.[298] If cortisol values are consistently below 5 μg/dL, dexamethasone replacement, usually 0.5 mg/day in the morning, is started. This allows continued assessment of cortisol secretion. Prior to discharge, hydrocortisone, at a physiologic replacement dose of 12 to 15 mg/m^2, is substituted for dexamethasone.[302] This agent, in contrast to prednisone, hydrocortisone acetate, or dexamethasone, is consistently absorbed and has biologic effects identical to those of cortisol. Additionally, the available tablet formulations provide great flexibility in dose adjustment and scheduling. Most patients do well with a single morning dose of steroids taken before getting out of bed; a split-dose strategy in which one third of the total daily dose is taken between 3 and 6 PM may be effective for those complaining of extreme evening fatigue. Later administration of glucocorticoids may result in disordered sleep and nightmares.

Patients with preoperative adrenal steroidogenesis blockade or episodic Cushing's syndrome may have had partial recovery of the hypothalamic-pituitary-adrenal axis so that postoperative cortisol values may be normal and cannot be used to assess surgical efficacy. The diurnal cortisol rhythm can be used for this purpose, however, since it will be normal after successful surgery, with a midnight nadir of less than 5 μg/dL. By contrast, patients who are not cured after surgery continue to show a loss of diurnal rhythm.

The response to ovine CRH in the second postoperative week may provide a useful index of the risk of recurrence of Cushing's disease. The ACTH and cortisol responses to CRH are blunted or subnormal at this time.[272, 298–300, 303] Patients with subsequent recurrence tend to have higher responses. A recent study of postoperative responses to CRH in 221 patients suggested that a cortisol response greater than 5 μg/dL at 60 minutes had a positive predictive value of 42% and a negative predictive value of 94% for recurrence of disease.[303] Since patients with partial recovery of the axis would be expected to have a normal response, regardless of risk of recurrence, the CRH test cannot be interpreted and should not be used in this setting. Some glucocorticoid-induced abnormalities, including hypokalemia, hypertension, and glucose intolerance, are normalized during the postoperative period so that preoperative treatments may not be required.

A triphasic pattern of diuresis, water intoxication, and permanent diabetes insipidus seen in some patients during the 3 weeks after transsphenoidal surgery has been ascribed to surgical manipulation of the posterior pituitary and stalk, with initial inability to secrete vasopressin, followed by wallerian degeneration and leakage of vasopressin from injured nerves and, finally, by cell death and permanent loss of vasopressin secretion.[304] Although the clinical features and response to therapy are consistent with a syndrome of vasopressin deficiency and excess, vasopressin levels have not been reported in these patients, and the potential contributions of glucocorticoid withdrawal and atrial natriuretic peptide to the disordered fluid economy have not been assessed.

Although many patients lack the second and third components, diuresis is common after transsphenoidal surgery and may result from intraoperative or glucocorticoid-induced fluid overload in addition to the mechanism postulated above. For these reasons, it is advisable to withhold vasopressin therapy unless the serum osmolality is greater than 295 mOsmol/mL, the serum sodium is greater than 145 mEq/L, and the urine output is greater than 200 mL/hour. Vasopressin (5 to 10 U) is given by vein or subcutaneously only as needed. The agent is discontinued and fluids arc restricted to about 2 L/day when the serum sodium concentration is normal. If patients enter the second phase, characterized by hyponatremia, fluid intake is restricted to 1 L or less each day. Menstruant women and patients who had extensive gland exploration are most likely to demonstrate such hyponatremia, usually around a week after surgery.[305] Usually, the serum sodium concentration does not fall below 125 mEq/L, and symptoms are restricted to nausea and headache. Hypertonic saline is required only rarely.

A small minority of patients proceed to (apparently) permanent diabetes insipidus, requiring long-term treatment with a vasopressin analog. A dose and schedule of administration should be chosen to provide unbroken sleep but allow for a period of "breakthrough" urination each day. This goal is often achieved using desmopressin 100 μL intranasally in the evening.

After bilateral adrenalectomy, a modified regimen is followed. The postoperative hydrocortisone dose is maintained at about twice the replacement dose, and saline 0.9% is given IV until the patient can take oral medications. This provides sodium and sufficient mineralocorticoid activity until fludrocortisone 100 μg/day can be given by mouth. Cortisol secretion to confirm adequacy of resection is then assessed while the patient receives dexamethasone and fludrocortisone. Discharge orders should substitute hydrocortisone and retain fludrocortisone. The dose of fludrocortisone is adjusted according to the patient's blood pressure, exposure to heat, and salt intake; the usual dose is 100 μg/day but ranges from 50 to 400 μg. A normal plasma renin activity measurement provides evidence for adequate mineralocorticoid replacement and can be used to gauge therapy. Adjustments in daily hydrocortisone dosage above 15 mg/m^2 are rarely necessary if mineralocorticoid replacement is adequate.

The components of the hypothalamic-pituitary-adrenal axis gradually recover after surgical cure of Cushing's syndrome, provided that at least one adrenal gland remains. The time until recovery may be as short as 3 months and as long as 2 years.[298, 306] The duration of recovery may be shorter in patients with mild hypercortisolism and those with recurrence, and longer after resection of an adrenal adenoma.

All patients receiving chronic glucocorticoid replacement therapy should be instructed that they are "dependent" on taking glucocorticoids as prescribed, and that failure to take or absorb the medication will lead to adrenal crisis and possibly death. They should also obtain a medical information bracelet or necklace that identifies this requirement (Medic Alert Foundation, 2323 Colorado Ave, Turlock, CA 95382; telephone 1-800-432-5378). Education should stress the effects of glucocorticoid withdrawal[307]; the need for compliance with the daily dose of glucocorticoid; the need to double the oral dose for nausea, diarrhea, and fever; and the need for parenteral administration and medical evaluation during emesis, trauma, or severe medical stress.

The patient should be told to expect flulike symptoms (malaise, joint aching, anorexia, and nausea) during the postoperative months and that these are signs that indicate remission. Most patients tolerate these symptoms of glucocorticoid withdrawal much better if they are forewarned and alerted to their positive nature. Physicians should not increase the glucocorticoid dose in the absence of intercurrent illness based on these symptoms alone but should seek signs of adrenal insufficiency, such as vomiting, electrolyte abnormalities, or postural hypotension.[308]

Recovery of the adrenal axis can be monitored by the cortisol response to synthetic ACTH (cosyntropin 250 μg) administered at intervals during the expected time of recovery.[307, 309] Since recovery after transsphenoidal surgery rarely occurs before 3 to 6 months and is common at 1 year, initial testing at 6 to 9 months is cost-effective. Glucocorticoid replacement can be discontinued abruptly when the cortisol response at 30 to 60 minutes exceeds 18 μg/dL. The cortisol response to ovine CRH parallels that seen after cosyntropin, so ovine CRH testing does not provide a superior evaluation of the recovery of the axis.[298]

Glucocorticoid replacement during recovery of the axis may be managed in a variety of ways, as long as adrenal insufficiency and iatrogenic Cushing's syndrome are avoided. The cosyntropin test and clinical assessment of the patient's sense of well-being, blood pressure, weight, and regression of cushingoid features provide useful measures of recovery. The hydrocortisone dose should be recalculated and adjusted as the patient loses weight. The patient also may be weaned from hydrocortisone, beginning at around 6 months postoperatively, if the cortisol response to cosyntropin exceeds 9 μg/dL, by reducing the total daily dose by 5 mg every 4 to 8 weeks. For the typical patient receiving 20 to 25 mg/day, glucocorticoids would be discontinued 11 to 15 months after surgery. This strategy avoids deleterious effects from subtle excessive glucocorticoid replacement as the axis is recovering. The potential role of weaning in accelerating the recovery of the axis has not been evaluated formally, but the timing of glucocorticoid discontinuation using this strategy is similar to the pattern of spontaneous recovery. One disadvantage of weaning is that patients may complain of intolerable symptoms of glucocorticoid withdrawal. If this occurs, the daily dose of hydrocortisone may be increased by 2.5 or 5.0 mg, and the steroid taper may be reinitiated 2 months later. Other approaches to weaning include administration of double the daily dose on alternate days or adjustment of the dose based on the response to cosyntropin. There are no published data to evaluate the utility of these strategies, however.

Two late but unrelated conundrums may arise: the questions of recurrence and permanent lack of recovery of the axis. Patients who articulate that the Cushing's syndrome has returned are often correct, even before physical and biochemical evidence are unequivocal. Measurement of UFC is warranted in a patient with these complaints or with recurrent physical signs characteristic of the hypercortisolemic phase. This should be done initially on dexamethasone 0.5 mg/day if the patient is not yet weaned from glucocorticoids. If the UFC result is increased, evaluation of hypercortisolism should proceed. If the result is subnormal or low, the patient should be questioned about the actual dose of glucocorticoid that has been taken. Often patients take additional hydrocortisone, either because they discover that this decreases the symptoms of glucocorticoid withdrawal or because they have increased the dose "for stress," often without following strict guidelines. These patients have a suppressed axis and very slow regression of cushingoid features because of exogenous hypercortisolism. They require education and support along with reduction in the daily dose of hydrocortisone to recommended levels. The rare patient who has a subnormal cortisol response to ACTH 2 years after transsphenoidal surgery (in the absence of overreplacement) will usually have lifelong ACTH deficiency; deficiencies of other pituitary hormones should be sought, since this may result from previous surgical trauma to the stalk or nontumorous portions of the pituitary gland.

Cushing's Disease

Transsphenoidal resection of a microadenoma is the optimal therapy for the patient with Cushing's disease, with up to a 90% chance of postoperative cure for patients operated on by an experienced neurosurgeon. As reviewed earlier, the likelihood of a successful outcome decreases if the initial surgery was not curative, in recurrence, and in macroadenomas. Alternative therapy should be considered for these patients.

Radiation therapy to the pituitary gland with adjunctive medical therapy to normalize cortisol levels is a good option for patients who cannot undergo surgery and for those in whom the risk of Nelson's syndrome is deemed great. Adrenalectomy may be chosen over radiation therapy by young patients desiring fertility who have concerns about radiation-induced hypopituitarism and loss of reproductive function, despite the disadvantage of lifelong glucocorticoid and mineralocorticoid replacement. Laparoscopic adrenalectomy is preferred also if rapid normalization of hypercortisolism is needed. Medical therapy alone is rarely appropriate, because it requires close monitoring and adjustment of dose and has low long-term efficacy. When this approach is chosen, mitotane may be the best agent if an adrenolytic dose can be tolerated.

Ectopic ACTH and Corticotropin-Releasing Hormone Secretion

Patients with ACTH or CRH secretion from an ectopic source can be cured if the tumor is not metastatic and if it can be found and removed. This is the optimal approach; it preserves normal function of the hypothalamic-pituitary-adrenal axis and removes a potentially malignant tumor. If the source of ACTH cannot be localized, or if metastatic disease precludes surgery, alternative treatment of hypercortisolism must be chosen. Intermittent surveillance for occult tumors must continue because of their malignant potential.

For the patient with occult disease, medical therapy allows for interval tumor surveillance with the goal of eventual tumor resection. Because some tumors remain occult for up to 20 years, this may not prove practical for all patients, and adrenalectomy is appropriate when the patient cannot tolerate the cost, medical side effects, or psychological effects of long-term medical therapy and monitoring. Long-term medical therapy also may be the treatment of choice for the patient with widely disseminated disease who is not a good surgical candidate for adrenalectomy. Short-term medical therapy may be used to prepare a patient for adrenalectomy.

Somatostatin reduces ACTH secretion from some neuroendocrine islet cell tumors, but the molecular concomitants of this phenomenon are unknown, and experience with these agents is limited.[232, 310]

Bilateral adrenalectomy is the treatment of choice for any patient requiring rapid correction of hypercortisolism or when hypercortisolism cannot be controlled with medical therapy. I choose adrenalectomy when maximal daily doses of ketoconazole (1600 mg), aminoglutethimide (2 g), and metyrapone (2 g) given in combination do not render the patient eucortisolemic, when previously effective medical therapy must be discontinued because of significant medical side effects or intolerance, or when a severely hypercortisolemic patient is unable to take oral medications or etomidate.

Additional consideration and treatment should be given based on the type of tumor producing ACTH. It is not clear if nodal resection, radiation, or combined therapy to the mediastinum is warranted for intrathoracic carcinoids.[311]

Primary Adrenal Disease

Nonmalignant causes of Cushing's syndrome deriving from the adrenal gland(s) are cured by resection of the abnormal tissue, whether unilateral or bilateral. ACTH-independent bilateral macronodular disease requires bilateral adrenalectomy, as does PPNAD, even though some patients have done relatively well with unilateral adrenalectomy.

Surgery is the mainstay of treatment of adrenal cancer; more aggressive surgical approaches probably account for the increase in life span reported in this disease.[25, 312] This approach may require multiple operations to resect primary lesions, local recurrences, and hepatic, thoracic, and occasionally intracranial metastases. Adjuvant treatment with suramin,[313] ketoconazole,[314, 315] gossypol,[316] and combination chemotherapy[317] have been reported in small series, with variable responses. The role of adjunctive adrenolytic therapy with mitotane has been discussed already.[236] It is the treatment of choice for patients requiring control of hypercortisolism after surgery, since it may provide chemotherapeutic benefit.

Exogenous Cushing's Syndrome

The treatment of exogenous Cushing's syndrome is to discontinue glucocorticoid ingestion. If this is possible, a weaning schedule should be followed until a replacement dose of hydrocortisone is reached, at which point the patient may be weaned gradually as discussed earlier for postoperative treatment. If the degree of suppression of the axis cannot be estimated from the medication and dose received, the response to cosyntropin can be used as a rough gauge of adrenal suppression.

For the patient in whom glucocorticoids cannot be discontinued, a change in dose or schedule may ameliorate symptoms of Cushing's syndrome. Patients requiring supraphysiologic glucocorticoid therapy should undergo measurement of bone density and be counseled to maintain adequate calcium intake and to exercise.

PROGNOSIS

The life expectancy of patients with nonmalignant causes of Cushing's syndrome, once a uniformly fatal illness, has improved dramatically with effective surgical and medical treatments and the availability of antibiotics, antihypertensive agents, and glucocorticoids. In a 1952 review, Plotz et al.[14] reported a 5-year mortality of 50% in hypercortisolemic patients, with 46% caused by bacterial infection and 40% due to cardiovascular complications (cardiac failure, cardiovascular accidents, or renal insufficiency). In 1961, the mortality rate was similar, but the causes had changed: two thirds were due to postoperative adrenal crisis before cortisone was available or from metastatic adrenal cancer.[12] Cardiovascular events related to hypertension (stroke, heart failure, renal failure, myocardial infarction) led to death in about 20%; infectious causes had decreased to about 15%.[12] Ten years later, in 1971, 30% of patients with benign causes of Cushing's syndrome died within 5 years of diagnosis, most from cardiovascular disease or infection, despite decreased postoperative mortality.[32] In 1979, a lower incidence of death, 6%, was noted within 2 to 10 years of radiation therapy, mitotane, or combination treatment of Cushing's disease.[241] The improvement may reflect earlier detection of Cushing's syndrome, better treatment of hypercortisolism and the associated medical complications, such as hypertension, or lower perioperative mortality. The assertion in 1982 that the mortality rate of patients with Cushing's syndrome is four times that of the general population matched for age and sex, even after curative surgery, likely reflects earlier data.[10] Large-scale assessment of mortality in the current era of transsphenoidal surgery and cardiovascular treatment is not available.

Although limited data suggest a modest improvement in osteopenia after cure of hypercortisolism, or with alendronate treatment,[318] the long-term morbidity associated with this complication of hypercortisolism has not been assessed.[319–321]

The prognosis of the neoplastic causes of Cushing's syndrome is variable, reflecting the malignant potential of the disease. Adrenal cancer, as reviewed earlier, has an extremely poor prognosis. Tumors that produce ACTH ectopically tend to have a poor prognosis, particularly when compared with tumors from the same tissue that do not produce ACTH. Islet cell tumors and thymic carcinoids[322] illustrate this phenomenon. Among the causes of ectopic ACTH secretion, pheochromocytoma and bronchial carcinoid appear to offer the best prognosis after tumor resection, but this is not universal.

Recurrence of Cushing's syndrome after surgical cure varies depending on the cause; it is rare in patients with adrenal adenoma, occurs in about 10% of patients with Cushing's disease, and is extremely common in patients with adrenal cancer. The incidence of recurrent hypercortisolism after apparent surgical cure of a tumor producing ectopic ACTH is variable, depending on the tumor type. When it occurs, it is an ominous sign that usually indicates metastatic, and often unresectable, disease.

REFERENCES

1. Cushing H: The Pituitary Body and Its Disorders: Clinical States Produced by Disorders of the Hypophysis Cerebri. Philadelphia, JB Lippincott, 1912.
2. Cushing H: The basophil adenomas of the pituitary body and their clinical manifestations (pituitary basophilism). Bull John Hopkins Hosp 50:137–195, 1932.
3. Walters W, Wilder RM, Kepler EJ: The suprarenal cortical syndrome with presentation of ten cases. Ann Surg 100:670–688, 1934.
4. Liddle GW, Nicholson WE, Island DP, et al: Clinical and laboratory studies of ectopic humoral syndromes. Recent Prog Horm Res 25:283–314, 1969.
5. Howlett TA, Rees LH, Besser GM: Cushing's syndrome. Clin Endocrinol Metab 14:911–945, 1985.
6. Bertagna X: New causes of Cushing's syndrome. N Engl J Med 327:1024–1025, 1992.
7. Reznik Y, Allali-Zerah V, Chayvialle JA, et al: Food-dependent Cushing's syndrome mediated by aberrant adrenal sensitivity to gastric inhibitory polypeptide. N Engl J Med 327:981–986, 1992.
8. Lacroix A, Bolte E, Tremblay J, et al: Gastric inhibitory polypeptide-dependent cortisol hypersecretion: A new cause of Cushing's syndrome. N Engl J Med 327:974–980, 1992.
9. Malchoff DC, Rosa J, DeBold CR, et al: Adrenocorticotropin-independent bilateral macronodular adrenal hyperplasia: An unusual cause of Cushing's syndrome. J Clin Endocrinol Metab 68:855–860, 1989.
10. Ross EJ, Linch DC: Cushing's syndrome—Killing disease: Discriminatory value of signs and symptoms aiding early diagnosis. Lancet 2:646–649, 1982.
11. Urbanic RC, George JM: Cushing's disease—18 years' experience. Medicine (Baltimore) 60:14–24, 1981.
12. Soffer LJ, Iannaccone A, Gabrilove JL: Cushing's syndrome: A study of fifty patients. Am J Med 300:129–135, 1961.
13. Sprague RG, Randall RV, Salassa RM, et al: Cushing's syndrome: A progressive and often fatal disease. Arch Intern Med 98:389–398, 1956.
14. Plotz CM, Knowlton AI, Ragan C: The natural history of Cushing's syndrome. Am J Med 13:597–614, 1952.
15. Nugent CA, Warner HR, Dunn JT, Tyler FH: Probability theory in the diagnosis of Cushing's syndrome. J Clin Endocrinol 24:621–627, 1974.
16. Roy-Camille R, Mazel C, Husson JL, Saillant G: Symptomatic spinal epidural lipomatosis induced by a long-term steroid treatment. Spine 16:1365–1371, 1991.
17. Noel P, Pepersack T, Vanbinst A, Alle J-L: Spinal epidural lipomatosis in Cushing's syndrome secondary to an adrenal tumor. Neurology 42:1250–1251, 1992.
18. Healy ME, Hesselink JR, Ostrup RC, Alksne JF: Demonstration by magnetic resonance of symptomatic spinal epidural lipomatosis. Neurosurgery 21:414–415, 1987.
19. Pleasure DE, Engel WK: Atrophy of skeletal muscle in patients with Cushing's syndrome. Arch Neurol 22:118–125, 1970.
20. Muller R, Kugelberg E: Myopathy in Cushing's syndrome. J Neurol Neurosurg Psychiatry 222:314–321, 1959.
21. Afifi AK, Bergman RA, Harvey JC: Steroid myopathy. Johns Hopkins Med J 123:158–174, 1968.
22. Vertebral compression fractures with accelerated bone turnover in a patient with Cushing's disease (clinicopathologic conference). Am J Med 68:932–940, 1980.
23. Kingsley GH, Hickling P: Polyarthropathy associated with Cushing's disease. BMJ 292:1363, 1986.
24. Phillips KA, Nance AP, Rodriguez RM, Kaye JJ: Avascular necrosis of bone: A manifestation of Cushing's disease. South Med J 79:825–829, 1986.
25. Bertagna C, Orth DN: Clinical and laboratory findings and results of therapy in 58 patients with adrenocortical tumors admitted to a single medical center (1951 to 1978). Am J Med 71:855–875, 1981.
26. Starkman MN, Schteingart DE: Neuropsychiatric manifestations of patients with Cushing's syndrome: Relationship to cortisol and adrenocorticotropic hormone levels. Arch Intern Med 141:215–219, 1981.
27. Starkman MN, Schteingart DE, Schork MA: Correlation of bedside cognitive and neuropsychological tests in patients with Cushing's syndrome. Psychosomatics 27:508–511, 1986.
28. Haskett RF: Diagnostic categorization of psychiatric disturbance in Cushing's syndrome. Am J Psychiatry 142:911–916, 1985.
29. Hudson JI, Hudson MS, Griffing GT, et al: Phenomenology and family history of affective disorder in Cushing's disease. Am J Psychiatry 144:951–953, 1987.
30. Rubinow DR, Post RM, Savard R, et al: Cortisol hypersecretion and cognitive impairment in depression. Arch Gen Psychiatry 41:279–283, 1984.
31. Kathol RG: Etiologic implications of corticosteroid changes in affective disorder. Psychiatr Med 3:135–162, 1985.
32. Welbourn RB, Montgomery DA, Kennedy TL: The natural history of treated Cushing's syndrome. Br J Surg 58:1–16, 1971.
33. Bakker RC, Gallas PR, Romijn JA, Wiersinga WM: Cushing's syndrome complicated by multiple opportunistic infections. J Endocrinol Invest 21:329–333, 1998.

34. Graham BS, Tucker WJ: Opportunistic infections in endogenous Cushing's syndrome. Ann Intern Med 101:334–338, 1984.
35. Sarlis NJ, Chanock SJ, Nieman LK: Cortisolemic indices predict severe infections in Cushing syndrome due to ectopic production of adrenocorticotropin. J Clin Endocrinol Metab 85:42–47, 2000.
36. Iannacone A, Gabrilove JL, Sohval AR, et al: The ovaries in Cushing's syndrome. N Engl J Med 261:775, 1959.
37. Halbreich U, Zumoff B, Kream J, Fukushima D: The mean 1300–1600 plasma cortisol concentration as a diagnostic test for hypercortisolism. J Clin Endocrinol Metab 54:1262–1264, 1982.
38. Liu JH, Kazer RR, Rasmussen DD: Characterization of the twenty-four hour secretion patterns of adrenocorticotropin and cortisol in normal women and patients with Cushing's disease. J Clin Endocrinol Metab 64:1027–1035, 1987.
39. Refetoff S, Van Cauter E, Fang VS, et al: The effect of dexamethasone on the 24-hour profiles of adrenocorticotropin and cortisol in Cushing's syndrome. J Clin Endocrinol Metab 60:527–535, 1985.
40. Mengden T, Hubmann P, Muller J, et al: Urinary free cortisol versus 17-hydroxycorticosteroids: A comparative study of their diagnostic value in Cushing's syndrome. J Clin Invest 70:545–548, 1992.
41. Evans PJ, Peters JR, Dyas J, et al: Salivary cortisol levels in true and apparent hypercortisolism. Clin Endocrinol 20:709–715, 1984.
42. Christy NP, Laragh JH: Pathogenesis of hypokalemic alkalosis in Cushing's syndrome. N Engl J Med 265:1083, 1961.
43. Stewart PM, Walker BR, Holder G, et al: 11β-Hydroxysteroid dehydrogenase activity in Cushing's syndrome: Explaining the mineralocorticoid excess state of the ectopic adrenocorticotropin syndrome. J Clin Endocrinol Metab 80:3617–3620, 1995.
44. Taskinen MR, Nikkila EA, Pelkonen R, Sane T: Plasma lipoproteins, lipolytic enzymes, and very low density lipoprotein triglyceride turnover in Cushing's syndrome. J Clin Endocrinol Metab 57:619–626, 1983.
45. Caron PC, Nieman LK, Rose S, Nisula BC: Deficient nocturnal surge of TSH in central hypothyroidism. J Clin Endocrinol Metab 62:960–964, 1986.
46. Luton J-P, Thieblot P, Valcke J-C, et al: Reversible gonadotropin deficiency in male Cushing's disease. J Clin Endocrinol Metab 45:488–495, 1977.
47. Lado AJ, Rodriguez AJ, Newell PJ, et al: Menstrual abnormalities in women with Cushing's disease are correlated with hypercortisolemia rather than raised circulating androgen levels. J Clin Endocrinol Metab 83:3083–3088, 1998.
48. Abeloff MD, Trump DL, Baylin SP: Ectopic adrenocorticotrophic (ACTH) syndrome and small cell carcinoma of the lung: Assessment of clinical implications in patients on combination chemotherapy. Cancer 48:1082–1087, 1981.
49. Bay JW, Sheeler LR: Results of transsphenoidal surgery for Cushing's disease. Cleve Clin J Med 55:357–364, 1988.
50. Howanitz PJ, Howanitz JH: Hypercortisolism. Clin Lab Med 4:683–702, 1984.
51. Leinung MC, Young WFJ, Whitaker MD, et al: Diagnosis of corticotropin producing bronchial carcinoid tumors causing Cushing's syndrome. Mayo Clin Proc 65:1377–1430, 1990.
52. Besser GM, Edwards CRW: Cushing's syndrome. Clin Endocrinol Metab 1:451–490, 1972.
53. Luger A, Deuster P, Kyle S, et al: Acute hypothalamic-pituitary-adrenal responses to the stress of treadmill exercise: Physiologic adaptations to physical training. N Engl J Med 316:1309–1315, 1987.
54. Lamberts SW, Klijn JG, de Jong FH, Birkenhager JC: Hormone secretion in alcohol-induced pseudo-Cushing's syndrome: Differential diagnosis with Cushing disease. JAMA 242:1640–1643, 1979.
55. Wand GS, Dobs A: Alterations in the hypothalamic-pituitary-adrenal axis in actively drinking alcoholics. J Clin Endocrinol Metab 72:1290–1295, 1991.
56. Sharp NA, Devlin JT, Rimmer JM: Renal failure obfuscates the diagnosis of Cushing's disease. JAMA 256:2564–2565, 1986.
57. Wallace EZ, Rosman P, Toshav N, et al: Pituitary-adrenocortical function in chronic renal failure: Studies of episodic secretion of cortisol and dexamethasone suppressibility. J Clin Endocrinol Metab 50:46–51, 1980.
58. Werner S, Thoren M, Gustafsson J, Bronnegard M: Glucocorticoid receptor abnormalities in fibroblasts from patients with idiopathic resistance to dexamethasone diagnosed when evaluated for adrenocortical disorders. J Clin Endocrinol Metab 75:1005–1009, 1992.
59. Chrousos GP, Schuermeyer TH, Doppman J, et al: NIH conference: Clinical applications of corticotropin-releasing factor. Ann Intern Med 102:344–358, 1985.
60. Gold P, Gwirtzman H, Avgerinos P, et al: Abnormal hypothalamic-pituitary adrenal function in anorexia nervosa: Pathophysiologic mechanisms in underweight and weight corrected patients. N Engl J Med 314:1335–1342, 1986.
61. Gold PW, Loriaux DL, Roy A, et al: Responses to corticotropin-releasing hormone in the hypercortisolism of depression and Cushing's disease: Pathophysiologic and diagnostic implications. N Engl J Med 314:1329–1335, 1986.
62. Biller BM, Alexander JM, Zervas NT, et al: Clonal origins of adrenocorticotropin-secreting pituitary tissue in Cushing's disease. J Clin Endocrinol Metab 75:1303–1309, 1992.
63. Crosby SR, Stewart MF, Ratcliffe GC, White A: Direct measurement of the precursors of adrenocorticotropin in human plasma by two-site immunoradiometric assay. J Clin Endocrinol Metab 67:1271–1277, 1988.
64. Hale AC, Millar JBG, Ratter SJ: A case of pituitary-dependent Cushing's disease with clinical and biochemical features of the ectopic ACTH syndrome. Clin Endocrinol (Oxf) 22:479–488, 1985.
65. Krieger DT: Physiopathology of Cushing's disease. Endocr Rev 4:22–43, 1983.
66. Mampalam TJ, Tyrrell JB, Wilson CB: Transsphenoidal microsurgery for Cushing disease: A report of 216 cases. Ann Intern Med 109:487–493, 1988.
67. Young WF, Scheithauer BW, Gharib H, et al: Cushing's syndrome due to primary multinodular corticotrope hyperplasia. Mayo Clin Proc 63:256–262, 1988.
68. Lamberts SWJ, deLange SA, Stefanko SZ: Adrenocorticotropin secreting pituitary adenomas originate from the anterior or the intermediate lobe in Cushing's disease: Differences in the regulation of hormone secretion. J Clin Endocrinol Metab 54:286–291, 1982.
69. McNicol AM, Teasdale GM, Beastall GH: A study of corticotroph adenomas in Cushing's disease: No evidence of intermediate lobe origin. Clin Endocrinol (Oxf) 24:715–722, 1986.
70. Imura H: Ectopic hormone syndromes. J Clin Endocrinol Metab 9:235–260, 1980.
71. Rees L: The biosynthesis of hormones by non-endocrine tumors: A review. J Endocrinol 67:143–175, 1975.
72. Odell WD: Ectopic ACTH secretion: A misnomer. Endocrinol Metab Clin North Am 20:371–379, 1991.
73. Gilby ED, Rees LH, Bardy PK: Ectopic Hormones as Markers of Response to Therapy in Cancer. Excerpta Medical International Congress Series No. 375. Amsterdam, Excerpta Medica, 1975, p 132.
74. de Bustros A, Baylin SB: Hormone production by tumours: Biological and clinical aspects. Clin Endocrinol Metab 14:221–256, 1985.
75. Pearse AGE: Common cytochemical and ultrastructural characteristics of cells producing polypeptide hormones (the APUD series) and their relevance to thyroid and ultimobranchial C cells and calcitonin. Proc R Soc Lond B Biol Sci 170:71–80, 1968.
76. Pullan PT, Clement-Jones V, Corder R, et al: ACTH, LPH and related peptides in the ectopic ACTH syndrome. Clin Endocrinol (Oxf) 13:437–445, 1980.
77. Rees LH, Bloomfield GA, Gilkes JJ, et al: ACTH as a tumor marker. Ann N Y Acad Sci 297:603–620, 1977.
78. Stewart MF, Crosby SR, Gibson S, et al: Small cell lung cancer cell lines secrete predominantly ACTH precursor peptides not ACTH. Br J Cancer 60:20–24, 1989.
79. White A, Clark AJL, Stewart MF: The synthesis of ACTH and related peptides by tumours. Ballieres Clin Endocrinol Metab 4:1–27, 1990.
80. DeBold CR, Menefee JK, Nicholson WE, Orth DN: Pro-opiomelanocortin gene is expressed in many normal human tissues and in tumours not associated with ectopic ACTH syndrome. Mol Endocrinol 2:862–870, 1988.
81. de Keyzer Y, Bertagna X, Luton JP, Kahn A: Variable modes of pro-opiomelanocortin gene transcription in human tumours. Mol Endocrinol 3:215–223, 1989.
82. Clark AJL, Lavender PM, Besser GM, Rees LH: Pro-opiomelanocortin in ACTH-dependent Cushing's syndrome. J Mol Endocrinol 2:3–9, 1989.
83. Clark AJL, Stewart MF, Lavender PM, et al: Defective glucocorticoid regulation of proopiomelanocortin gene expression and peptide secretion in a small cell lung cancer cell line. J Clin Endocrinol Metab 70:485–490, 1990.
84. Roth KA, Newell DC, Dorin RI, et al: Aberrant production and regulation of proopiomelanocortin-derived peptides in ectopic Cushing's syndrome. Horm Metab Res 20:225–229, 1988.
85. Melmed S, Yamashita S, Kovacs K, et al: Cushing's syndrome due to ectopic pro-opiomelanocortin gene expression by islet cell carcinoma of the pancreas. Cancer 59:772–778, 1987.
86. Limper AH, Carpenter PC, Scheithauer B, Staats BA: The Cushing syndrome induced by bronchial carcinoid tumors. Ann Intern Med 117:209–214, 1992.
87. Asa SL, Kovacs K, Vale W, et al: Immunohistologic localization of corticotrophin-releasing hormone in human tumors. Am J Clin Pathol 87:327–333, 1987.
88. Schteingart DE, Lloyd RV, Akil H, et al: Cushing's syndrome secondary to ectopic corticotropin releasing hormone-adrenocorticotropin secretion. J Clin Endocrinol Metab 63:770–775, 1986.
89. Ishikawa T, Inoue C, Sasaki H, et al: Thymic carcinoid associated with ectopic ACTH syndrome (in Japanese). Nihon Kyobu Shikkan Gakkai Zasshi 34:471–476, 1996.
90. Wajchenberg BL, Mendonca B, Liberman B, et al: Ectopic ACTH syndrome [erratum appears in J Steroid Biochem Mol Biol 54:287, 1995]. J Steroid Biochem Mol Biol 53:139–151, 1995.
91. Asa SL, Kovacs K, Tindall GT, et al: Cushing's disease associated with an intrasellar gangliocytoma producing corticotrophin-releasing factor. Ann Intern Med 101:789–793, 1984.
92. Belsky JL, Cuello B, Swanson LW, et al: Cushing's syndrome due to ectopic production of corticotropin-releasing factor. J Clin Endocrin Metab 60:496–500, 1985.
93. Yano T, Linehan M, Anglard P, et al: Genetic changes in human adrenocortical carcinomas. J Natl Cancer Inst 81:518–523, 1989.
94. Beuschlein F, Reincke M, Karl M, et al: Clonal composition of human adrenocortical neoplasms. Cancer Res 54:4927–4932, 1994.
95. Weiss LM, Medeiros J, Vickery AL: Pathologic features of prognostic significance in adrenocortical carcinoma. Am J Surg Pathol 13:202–206, 1989.
96. Travis WD, Tsokos M, Doppman JL, et al: Primary pigmented nodular adrenocortical disease. Am J Surg Pathol 13:921–930, 1989.
97. Stratakis CA, Carney JA, Lin JP, et al: Carney complex, a familial multiple neoplasia and lentiginosis syndrome. Analysis of 11 kindreds and linkage to the short arm of chromosome 2. J Clin Invest 97:699–705, 1996.
98. Milunsky J, Huang XL, Baldwin CT, et al: Evidence for genetic heterogeneity of the Carney complex (familial atrial myxoma syndromes). Cancer Genet Cytogenet 106:173–176, 1998.
99. N'Diaye N, Tremblay J, Hamet P, Lacroix A: Hormone receptor abnormalities in adrenal Cushing's syndrome. Horm Metab Res 30:440–446, 1998.
100. Maschler I, Rosenmann E, Ehrenfeld EN: Ectopic functioning adrenocorticomyelolipoma in long-standing Nelson's syndrome. Clin Endocrinol (Oxf) 10:494–497, 1979.
101. Lalau JD, Vieau D, Tenenbaum F, et al: A case of pseudo-Nelson's syndrome: Cure of ACTH hypersecretion by removal of a bronchial carcinoid tumor responsible for Cushing's syndrome. J Endocrinol Invest 13:531–537, 1990.
102. Adeyemi SD, Grange AO, Giwa-Osagie OF, Elesha SO: Adrenal rest tumour of the ovary associated with isosexual precocious pseudopuberty and cushingoid features. Eur J Pediatr 145:236–238, 1986.
103. Contreras P, Altieri E, Liberman C, et al: Adrenal rest tumor of the liver causing Cushing's syndrome: Treatment with ketoconazole preceding an apparent surgical cure. J Clin Endocrinol Metab 60:21–28, 1985.
104. Marieb NJ, Spangler S, Kashgarian M, et al: Cushing's syndrome secondary to

ectopic cortisol production by an ovarian carcinoma. J Clin Endocrinol Metab 57:737–740, 1983.
105. King AB: The diagnosis of cancer of the pituitary gland. Bull J Hopkins Hosp 89:339, 1951.
106. Martins AN, Hayes GJ, Kempe LG: Invasive pituitary adenomas. J Neurosurg 22:268, 1965.
107. Della CS, Corsello SM, Satta MA, et al: Intracranial and spinal dissemination of an ACTH secreting pituitary neoplasia. Case report and review of the literature. Ann Endocrinol (Paris) 58:503–509, 1997.
108. Hopwood NJ, Kenny FM: Incidence of Nelson's syndrome after adrenalectomy for Cushing's disease in children: Results of a nationwide survey. Am J Dis Child 131:1353–1356, 1977.
109. Howlett TA, Plowman PN, Wass JA, et al: Megavoltage pituitary irradiation in the management of Cushing's disease and Nelson's syndrome: Long-term follow-up. Clin Endocrinol (Oxf) 31:309–323, 1989.
110. Wild W, Nicolis GL, Gabrilove JL: Appearance of Nelson's syndrome despite pituitary irradiation prior to bilateral adrenalectomy for Cushing's syndrome. Mt Sinai J Med 40:68–71, 1973.
111. Young LW, Lim GH, Forbes GB, Bryson MF: Postadrenalectomy pituitary adenoma (Nelson's syndrome) in childhood: Clinical and roentgenologic detection. AJR 126:550–559, 1976.
112. Shapiro MS, Shenkman L: Variable hormonogenesis in Cushing's syndrome. Q J Med 79:351–363, 1990.
113. Kramer H, Barter M: Spontaneous remission of Cushing's disease. Am J Med 67:519–523, 1979.
114. Hayslett JP, Cohn GL: Spontaneous remission of Cushing's disease. N Engl J Med 276:968–970, 1967.
115. Brown RD, VanLoon GR, Orth DN, Liddle GW: Cushing's disease with periodic hormonogenesis: One explanation for paradoxical response to dexamethasone. J Clin Endocrinol Metab 36:445–451, 1973.
116. Malchoff CD, Orth DN, Abboud C, et al: Ectopic ACTH syndrome caused by a bronchial carcinoid tumor responsive to dexamethasone, metyrapone and corticotropin-releasing factor. Am J Med 84:760–764, 1989.
117. Strott CA, Nugent CA, Tyler FH: Cushing's syndrome caused by bronchial adenomas. Am J Med 44:97–104, 1968.
118. Schweikert H-U, Fehm HL, Fahlbusch R, et al: Cyclic Cushing's syndrome combined with cortisol suppressible, dexamethasone non-suppressible ACTH secretion: A new variant of Cushing's syndrome. Acta Endocrinol (Copenh) 110:289–295, 1985.
119. Kendall JW, Sloop PRJ: Dexamethasone-suppressible adrenocortical tumor. N Engl J Med 279:532–535, 1968.
120. Braverman LE, Woeber KA, lngbar SH: An unusual case of Cushing's syndrome. N Engl J Med 273:1018–1020, 1965.
121. Vagnucci AH, Evans E: Cushing's disease with intermittent hypercortisolism. Am J Med 80:83–88, 1986.
122. Kreze A, Veleminsky J, Spirova E: A follow-up of the "low dose suppressible" hypercortisolism. Endocrinol Exp 17:119–123, 1983.
123. Leiba S, Shindel B, Weinberger I, et al: Cushing's disease coexisting with a single macronodule simulating adenoma of the adrenal cortex. Acta Endocrinol (Copenh) 112:323–328, 1986.
124. Schteingart DE, Tsao HS: Coexistence of pituitary adrenocorticotropin-dependent Cushing's syndrome with a solitary adrenal adenoma. J Clin Endocrinol Metab 50:961–966, 1980.
125. Mimou N, Sakato S, Nakabayashi H, et al: Cushing's syndrome associated with bilateral adrenal adenomas. Acta Endocrinol (Copenh) 108:245–254, 1985.
126. Fig LM, Gross MD, Shapiro B, et al: Adrenal localization in the adrenocorticotropic hormone–independent Cushing syndrome. Ann Intern Med 109:547–553, 1988.
127. Doppman JL, Miller DL, Dwyer AJ, et al: Macronodular adrenal hyperplasia in Cushing disease. Radiology 166:347–352, 1988.
128. Doppman JL, Nieman LK, Travis WD, et al: CT and MR imaging of massive macronodular adrenocortical disease: A rare cause of autonomous primary adrenal hypercortisolism. J Comput Assist Tomogr 15:773–779, 1991.
129. Aron DC, Findling JW, Fitzgerald PA, et al: Pituitary ACTH dependency of nodular adrenal hyperplasia in Cushing's syndrome: Report of two cases and review of the literature. Am J Med 71:302–306, 1981.
130. Smals AGH, Pieters GFFM, van Haelst UJG, Kloppenborg PWC: Macronodular adrenocortical hyperplasia in long-standing Cushing's disease. J Clin Endocrinol Metab 58:25–31, 1984.
131. Dixon RB, Christy NP: On the various forms of corticosteroid withdrawal syndrome. Am J Med 68:224–230, 1980.
132. Tsuruoka S, Sugimoto K, Fujimura A: Drug-induced Cushing syndrome in a patient with ulcerative colitis after betamethasone enema: Evaluation of plasma drug concentration. Ther Drug Monit 20:387–389, 1998.
133. Findlay CA, Macdonald JF, Wallace AM, et al: Childhood Cushing's syndrome induced by betamethasone nose drops, and repeat prescriptions. BMJ 317:739–740, 1998.
134. Quddusi S, Browne P, Toivola B, Hirsch IB: Cushing syndrome due to surreptitious glucocorticoid administration. Arch Intern Med 158:294–296, 1998.
135. Mann M, Koller E, Murgo A, et al: Glucocorticoidlike activity of megestrol. A summary of Food and Drug Administration experience and a review of the literature. Arch Intern Med 157:1651–1656, 1997.
136. Cizza G, Nieman LK, Doppman JL, et al: Factitious Cushing syndrome. J Clin Endocrinol Metab 81:3573–3577, 1996.
137. O'Hare JP, Vale JA, Wood S, Corrall RJ: Factitious Cushing's syndrome. Acta Endocrinol (Copenh) 111:165–167, 1986.
138. Luger A, Lang I, Kovarik J, et al: Abnormalities in the hypothalamic-pituitary-adrenocortical axis in patients with chronic renal failure. Am J Kidney Dis 9:51–54, 1987.
139. Siamopoulos KC, Dardamanis M, Kyriaki D, et al: Pituitary adrenal responsiveness to corticotropin-releasing hormone in chronic uremic patients. Perit Dial Int 10:153–156, 1990.
140. Nolan GE, Smith JB, Chavre VJ, Jubiz W: Spurious overestimation of plasma cortisol in patients with chronic renal failure. J Clin Endocrinol Metab 52:1242–1245, 1981.
141. Workman RJ, Vaughn WK, Stone WJ: Dexamethasone suppression testing in chronic renal failure: Pharmacokinetics of dexamethasone and demonstration of a normal hypothalamic-pituitary-adrenal axis. J Clin Endocrinol Metab 63:741–746, 1986.
142. Ramirez G, Gomez-Sanchez C, Meikle WA, Jubiz W: Evaluation of the hypothalamic hypophyseal adrenal axis in patients receiving long-term hemodialysis. Arch Intern Med 142:1448–1452, 1982.
143. Rosman PM, Farag A, Peckham R, et al: Pituitary-adrenocortical function in chronic renal failure: Blunted suppression and early escape of plasma cortisol levels after intravenous dexamethasone. J Clin Endocrinol Metab 54:528–533, 1982.
144. Rodger RS, Dewar JH, Turner SJ, et al: Anterior pituitary dysfunction in patients with chronic renal failure treated by hemodialysis or continuous ambulatory peritoneal dialysis. Nephron 43:169–172, 1986.
145. Otokida K, Fujiwara T, Oriso S, Kato M: Cortisol and its metabolites in the plasma and urine in Cushing's syndrome with chronic renal failure (CRF), compared to Cushing's syndrome without CRF. Nippon Jinzo Gakkai Shi 31:651–656, 1989.
146. Streeten DHP, Faas FH, Elders MJ, et al: Hypercortisolism in childhood: Shortcomings of conventional diagnostic criteria. Pediatrics 56:797–803, 1975.
147. Magiakou MA, Mastorakos G, Oldfield EH, et al: Cushing's syndrome in children and adolescents. Presentation, diagnosis, and therapy. N Engl J Med 331:629–636, 1994.
148. Lee PD, Winter RJ, Green OC: Virilizing adrenocortical tumors in childhood: Eight cases and a review of the literature. Pediatrics 76:437–444, 1985.
149. Jones KL: The Cushing syndromes. Pediatr Clin North Am 37:1313–1332, 1990.
150. Neblett WW, Frexes-Steed M, Scott HWJ: Experience with adrenocortical neoplasms in childhood. Am Surg 53:117–125, 1987.
151. Thomas CJ, Smith AT, Griffith JM, Askin FB: Hyperadrenalism in childhood and adolescence. Ann Surg 199:538–548, 1984.
152. Jones GS, Shah KJ, Mann JR: Adreno-cortical carcinoma in infancy and childhood: A radiological report of ten cases. Clin Radiol 36:257–262, 1985.
153. Yoshimoto M, Nakayama M, Baba T, et al: A case of neonatal McCune-Albright syndrome with Cushing syndrome and hyperthyroidism. Acta Pediatr Scand 80:984–987, 1991.
154. Danon M, Robboy SJ, Kim S, et al: Cushing syndrome, sexual precocity, and polyostotic fibrous dysplasia (Albright syndrome) in infancy. J Pediatr 87:917–921, 1975.
155. Weinstein LS, Shenker A, Gejman PV, et al: Activating mutations of the stimulatory G protein in the McCune-Albright syndrome. N Engl J Med 325:1688–1695, 1991.
156. McArthur RG, Hayles AB, Salassa RM: Childhood Cushing's disease: Results of bilateral adrenalectomy. J Pediatr 95:214–219, 1979.
157. Pombo M, Alvez F, Varela-Cives R, et al: Ectopic production of ACTH by Wilms' tumor. Horm Res 16:160–163, 1982.
158. Styne DM, Isaac R, Miller WL, et al: Endocrine, histological, and biochemical studies of adrenocorticotropin-producing islet cell carcinoma of the pancreas in childhood with characterization of proopiomelanocortin. J Clin Endocrinol Metab 5:723–731, 1983.
159. Hannah J, Lippe B, Lai-Goldman M, Bhuta S: Oncocytic carcinoid of the kidney associated with periodic Cushing's syndrome. Cancer 61:2136–2140, 1988.
160. Sheeler LR: Cushing's syndrome and pregnancy. Endocrinol Metab Clin North Am 23:619–627, 1994.
161. Brien TG: Human corticosteroid binding globulin. Clin Endocrinol (Oxf) 14:193–212, 1981.
162. Nolten WE, Lindheimer MD, Rueckert PA, et al: Diurnal patterns and regulation of cortisol secretion in pregnancy. J Clin Endocrinol Metab 51:466–472, 1980.
163. Odagiri E, Ishiwatari N, Abe Y, et al: Hypercortisolism and the resistance to dexamethasone suppression during gestation. Endocrinol J 35:685–690, 1988.
164. Zimmerman W: Eine Farbreaktion der sexual Hormone und ihre Anwendung zur quantitoven colorimetrischen Bestimmung. Hoppe Seylers Z Physiol Chem 233:257–264, 1935.
165. Porter CC, Silber RH: A quantitative color reaction for cortisone and related 17,21-dihydroxy-20-ketosteroids. J Biol Chem 185:201–207, 1950.
166. Fukushima DK, Bradlow HL, Hellman L, et al: Metabolic transformation of hydrocortisone-4-C14 in normal men. J Biol Chem 235:2246–2252, 1969.
167. Streeten DH, Stevenson CT, Dalakos TG, et al: The diagnosis of hypercortisolism: Biochemical criteria differentiating patients from lean and obese normal subjects and from females on oral contraceptives. J Clin Endocrinol Metab 29:1191–1211, 1969.
168. Burke CW, Beardwell CG: Cushing's syndrome: An evaluation of the clinical usefulness of urinary free cortisol and other urinary steroid measurements in diagnosis. Q J Med 42:175–204, 1973.
169. Turpeinen U, Markkanen H, Valimaki M, Stenman UH: Determination of urinary free cortisol by HPLC. Clin Chem 43:1386–1391, 1997.
170. Crapo L: Cushing's syndrome: A review of diagnostic tests. Metabolism 28:955–977, 1979.
171. Carpenter PC: Diagnostic evaluation of Cushing's syndrome. Endocrinol Metab Clin North Am 17:445–472, 1988.
172. Nieman L, Cutler GB Jr: The sensitivity of the urine free cortisol measurement as a screening test for Cushing's syndrome. Presented at the 72nd Annual Meeting of the Endocrine Society, New Orleans, 1990.
173. Papanicolaou DA, Yanovski JA, Cutler GJ, et al: A single midnight serum cortisol measurement distinguishes Cushing's syndrome from pseudo-Cushing states. J Clin Endocrinol Metab 83:1163–1167, 1998.
174. Newell PJ, Trainer P, Perry L, et al: A single sleeping midnight cortisol has 100% sensitivity for the diagnosis of Cushing's syndrome. Clin Endocrinol (Oxf) 43:545–550, 1995.
175. Raff H, Raff JL, Findling JW: Late-night salivary cortisol as a screening test for Cushing's syndrome. J Clin Endocrinol Metab 83:2681–2686, 1998.

176. Nugent CA, Nichols T, Tyler FH: Diagnosis of Cushing's syndrome—single-dose dexamethasone suppression test. Arch Intern Med 116:172–176, 1965.
177. Stokes PE, Stoll PM, Koslow SH, et al: Pretreatment DST and hypothalamic-pituitary-adrenocortical function in depressed patients and comparison groups: A multicenter study. Arch Gen Psychiatry 41:257–267, 1984.
178. Barrou Z, Guiban D, Maroufi A, et al: Overnight dexamethasone suppression test: comparison of plasma and salivary cortisol measurement for the screening of Cushing's syndrome. Eur J Endocrinol 134:93–96, 1996.
179. Caro JF, Meikle AW, Check JH, Cohen SN: "Normal suppression" to dexamethasone in Cushing's disease: An expression of decreased metabolic clearance for dexamethasone. J Clin Endocrinol Metab 47:667–670, 1978.
180. Meikle AW, Lagerquist LG, Tyler FH: Apparently normal pituitary-adrenal suppressibility in Cushing's syndrome: Dexamethasone metabolism and plasma levels. J Lab Clin Med 86:472–478, 1975.
181. Liddle GW: Tests of pituitary-adrenal suppressibility in the diagnosis of Cushing's syndrome. J Clin Endocrinol 20:1539–1561, 1960.
182. Yanovski JA, Cutler GB Jr, Chrousos GP, Nieman LK: Corticotropin-releasing hormone stimulation following low-dose dexamethasone administration: A new test to distinguish Cushing syndrome from pseudo-Cushing states. JAMA 269:2232–2238, 1993.
183. Butler PW, Besser GM: Pituitary-adrenal function in severe depressive illness. Lancet 1:1234–1236, 1968.
184. White A, Smith H, Hoadley M, et al: Clinical evaluation of a two-site immunoradiometric assay for adrenocorticotrophin in unextracted human plasma using monoclonal antibodies. Clin Endocrinol (Oxf) 26:41–52, 1987.
185. Kaye TB, Crapo L: The Cushing syndrome: An update on diagnostic tests. Ann Intern Med 112:434–444, 1990.
186. Doppman JL, Travis WD, Nieman L, et al: Cushing syndrome due to primary pigmented nodular adrenocortical disease: Findings at CT and MR imaging. Radiology 172:415–420, 1989.
187. Perry RR, Nieman LK, Cutler GB Jr, et al: Primary adrenal causes of Cushing's syndrome: Diagnosis and surgical management. Ann Surg 210:59–68, 1989.
188. Howlett TA, Drury PL, Perry L, et al: Diagnosis and management of ACTH-dependent Cushing's syndrome: Comparison of the features in ectopic and pituitary ACTH production. Clin Endocrinol (Oxf) 24:699–713, 1986.
189. Oldfield EH, Doppman JL, Nieman LK, et al: Petrosal sinus sampling with and without corticotropin-releasing hormone for the differential diagnosis of Cushing's syndrome. N Engl J Med 325:897–905, 1991.
190. Findling JW, Kehoe ME, Shaker JL, Raff H: Routine inferior petrosal sinus sampling in the differential diagnosis of adrenocorticotropin (ACTH)-dependent Cushing's syndrome: Early recognition of the occult ectopic ACTH syndrome. J Clin Endocrinol Metab 73:408–413, 1991.
191. Tabarin A, Greselle JF, San-Galli F, et al: Usefulness of the corticotropin-releasing hormone test during bilateral inferior petrosal sinus sampling for the diagnosis of Cushing disease. J Clin Endocrinol Metab 73:53–59, 1991.
192. Miller DL, Doppman JL: Petrosal sinus sampling: Technique and rationale. Radiology 178:37–47, 1991.
193. Sturrock ND, Jeffcoate WJ: A neurological complication of inferior petrosal sinus sampling during investigation for Cushing's disease: A case report. J Neurol Neurosurg Psychiatry 62:527–528, 1997.
194. Yanovski J, Cutler GB Jr, Doppman JL, et al: The limited ability of inferior petrosal sinus sampling with corticotropin-releasing hormone to distinguish ACTH-dependent Cushing disease from pseudo-Cushing states or normal physiology. J Clin Endocrinol Metab 77:503–509, 1993.
195. Yamamoto Y, Davis DH, Nippoldt TB, et al: False-positive inferior petrosal sinus sampling in the diagnosis of Cushing's disease. Report of two cases. J Neurosurg 83:1087–1091, 1995.
196. Doppman JL, Nieman LK, Chang R, et al: Selective venous sampling from the cavernous sinuses is not a more reliable technique than sampling from the inferior petrosal sinuses in Cushing's syndrome. J Clin Endocrinol Metab 80:2485–2489, 1995.
197. Doppman JL, Oldfield EH, Nieman LK: Bilateral sampling of the internal jugular vein to distinguish between mechanisms of adrenocorticotropic hormone-dependent Cushing syndrome. Ann Intern Med 128:33–36, 1998.
198. Flack MR, Oldfield EH, Cutler GB Jr, et al: Urine free cortisol in the high-dose dexamethasone suppression test for the differential diagnosis of the Cushing syndrome. Ann Intern Med 116:211–217, 1992.
199. Dichek HL, Nieman LK, Oldfield EH, et al: A comparison of the standard high-dose dexamethasone suppression test and the overnight 8-mg dexamethasone suppression test for the differential diagnosis of Cushing's syndrome. J Clin Endocrinol Metab 78:418–422, 1994.
200. Tyrrell JB, Findling JW, Aron DC, et al: An overnight high-dose dexamethasone suppression test for rapid differential diagnosis of Cushing's syndrome. Ann Intern Med 104:180–186, 1986.
201. Bruno OD, Rossi MA, Contreras LN, et al: Nocturnal high-dose dexamethasone suppression test in the aetiological diagnosis of Cushing's syndrome. Acta Endocrinol (Copenh) 109:158–162, 1985.
202. Liddle GW, Estep HL, Kendall JW, et al: Clinical application of a new test of pituitary reserve. J Clin Endocrinol Metab 19:875–894, 1959.
203. Sindler BH, Griffin GT, Melby JC: The superiority of the metyrapone test versus the high-dose dexamethasone test in the differential diagnosis of Cushing's syndrome. Am J Med 74:657–662, 1983.
204. Avgerinos PC, Yanovski JA, Oldfield EH, et al: The metyrapone and dexamethasone suppression tests for the differential diagnosis of the adrenocorticotropin-dependent Cushing syndrome: A comparison [see comments]. Ann Intern Med 121:318–327, 1994.
205. Avgerinos PC, Nieman LK, Oldfield EH, Cutler GB Jr: A comparison of the overnight and the standard metyrapone test for the differential diagnosis of adrenocorticotrophin-dependent Cushing's syndrome. Clin Endocrinol (Oxf) 45:483–491, 1996.
206. Leisti S: Evaluation of 3 hour metyrapone test in children and adolescents. Clin Endocrinol (Oxf) 6:305–320, 1977.
207. Nieman LK, Chrousos GP, Oldfield EH, et al: The ovine corticotropin-releasing hormone stimulation test and the dexamethasone suppression test in the differential diagnosis of Cushing's syndrome. Ann Intern Med 105:862–867, 1986.
208. Nieman LK, Oldfield EH, Wesley R, et al: A simplified morning ovine corticotropin-releasing hormone stimulation test for the differential diagnosis of ACTH-dependent Cushing syndrome. J Clin Endocrinol Metab 77:1308–1312, 1993.
209. Hermus AR, Pieters GF, Pesman GJ, et al: The corticotropin-releasing-hormone test versus the high-dose dexamethasone test in the differential diagnosis of Cushing's syndrome. Lancet 2:540–544, 1986.
210. Nieman LK, Cutler GB Jr, Oldfield EH, et al: The ovine corticotropin-releasing hormone (CRH) stimulation test is superior to the human CRH stimulation test for the diagnosis of Cushing's disease. J Clin Endocrinol Metab 69:165–169, 1989.
211. Trainer PJ, Faria M, Newell PJ, et al: A comparison of the effects of human and ovine corticotropin-releasing hormone on the pituitary-adrenal axis. J Clin Endocrinol Metab 80:412–417, 1995.
212. Newell-Price J, Trainer P, Besser M, Grossman A: The diagnosis and differential diagnosis of Cushing's syndrome and pseudo-Cushing's states. Endocr Rev 19:647–672, 1998.
213. Tabarin A, San-Galli F, Dezou S, et al: The corticotropin-releasing factor test in the differential diagnosis of Cushing's syndrome: A comparison with the lysine-vasopressin test. Acta Endocrinol (Copenh) 123:331–338, 1990.
214. Grossman AB, Howlett TA, Perry L, et al: CRF in the differential diagnosis of Cushing's syndrome: A comparison with the dexamethasone suppression test. Clin Endocrinol (Oxf) 29:167–178, 1988.
215. Orth DN: Cushing's syndrome [erratum appears in N Engl J Med 332:1527, 1995]. N Engl J Med 332:791–803, 1995.
216. Findling JW, Doppman JL: Biochemical and radiologic diagnosis of Cushing's syndrome. Endocrinol Metab Clin North Am 23:511–537, 1994.
217. Doppman JL, Frank JA, Dwyer AJ, et al: Gadolinium DTPA enhanced imaging of ACTH-secreting microadenomas of the pituitary gland. J Comput Assist Tomogr 12:728–735, 1988.
218. Doppman JL, Pass HI, Nieman LK, et al: Detection of ACTH-producing bronchial carcinoid tumors: MR imaging vs CT. AJR 156:39–43, 1991.
219. Doppman JL, Pass HI, Nieman LK, et al: Corticotropin-secreting carcinoid tumors of the thymus: Diagnostic unreliability of thymic venous sampling. Radiology 184:71–74, 1992.
220. Doppman JL, Pass HI, Nieman LK, et al: Failure of bronchial lavage to detect elevated levels of ACTH in patients with ACTH-producing bronchial carcinoids. J Clin Endocrinol Metab 69:1302–1304, 1989.
221. Doppman JL, Nieman LK, Miller DL, et al: The ectopic ACTH syndrome: Localizing studies in 28 patients. Radiology 172:115–124, 1989.
222. Torpy D, Chen C, Mullen N, et al: Lack of utility of ^{111}In-pentetreotide scintigraphy in localizing ectopic ACTH producing tumors: Follow-up of 18 patients. J Clin Endocrinol Metab 84:1186–1192, 1999.
223. Sarkar R, Thompson NW, McLeod MK: The role of adrenalectomy in Cushing's syndrome. Surgery 108:1079–1084, 1990.
224. Hayashi H, Mercado AL, Murayama M, et al: Reduction of pituitary tumor size with clinical and biochemical improvement with bromocriptine in a normoprolactinemic Cushing's disease. Endocr J 37:875–882, 1990.
225. McKenna MJ, Linares M, Mellinger RC: Prolonged remission of Cushing's disease following bromocriptine therapy. Henry Ford Hosp Med J 35:188–191, 1987.
226. Koppeschaar HPF, Croughs RJM, Thijssen JHH, Schwarz F: Response to neurotransmitter modulating drugs in patients with Cushing's disease. Clin Endocrinol (Oxf) 25:661–667, 1986.
227. Cavagnini F, Panerai AE, Valentini F, et al: Inhibition of ACTH response to oral and intravenous metyrapone by antiserotonergic treatment in man. J Clin Endocrinol Metab 41:143–148, 1975.
228. Krieger DT, Amorosa L, Linick F: Cyproheptadine-induced remission of Cushing's disease. N Engl J Med 293:893–896, 1975.
229. Krieger DT: Cyproheptadine for pituitary disorders (letter). N Engl J Med 295:394–395, 1976.
230. Sonino N, Boscaro M, Fallo F, Fava G: Potential therapeutic effects of ritanserin in Cushing's disease. JAMA 267:1073, 1992.
231. Kritzler RK, Vining EPG, Plotnick LP: Sodium valproate and corticotropin suppression in the child treated for seizures. J Pediatr 102:142–143, 1983.
232. de Herder WW, Lamberts SW: Is there a role for somatostatin and its analogs in Cushing's syndrome? Metabolism 83–85, 1996.
233. Yanovski J, Cutler GB Jr: Cushing's disease: Medical treatment. *In* Cooper P (ed): Contemporary Diagnosis and Management of Pituitary Adenomas. Park Ridge, IL, American Association of Neurological Surgeons, 1991, pp 125–138.
234. Hart MM, Swackhamer ES, Straw JA: Studies on the site of action of *o,p'*-DDD in the dog adrenal cortex: TNPH and corticosteroid precursor stimulation of *o,p'*-DDD inhibited steroidogenesis. Steroids 17:575–586, 1971.
235. Ojima M, Saitoh M, Itoh N, et al: The effects of *o,p'*-DDD on adrenal steroidogenesis and hepatic steroid metabolism. Nippon Naibunpi Gakkai Zasshi Folia Endocrinol Jpn 61:168–178, 1985.
236. Hutter AM, Kayhoe DE: Adrenal cortical carcinoma: Results of treatment with *o,p'*-DDD in 138 patients. Am J Med 41:581–592, 1966.
237. Lubitz JA, Freeman L, Okun R: Mitotane use in inoperable adrenal cortical carcinoma. JAMA 223:1109–1112, 1973.
238. Guttierrez ML, Crooke ST: Mitotane (*o,p'*-DDD) in inoperable adrenocortical carcinoma. Cancer Treat Rev 7:49–55, 1980.
239. van Slooten H, Moolenaar AJ, van Seters AP, Smeenk D: The treatment of adrenocortical carcinoma with *o,p'*-DDD: The prognostic implications of serum level monitoring. Eur J Cancer Clin Oncol 20:47–53, 1984.
240. Touitou Y, Moolenaar AJ, Bogdan A, et al: *o,p'*-DDD (mitotane) treatment for

Cushing's syndrome: Adrenal drug concentration and inhibition in vitro of steroid synthesis. Eur J Clin Pharmacol 29:483–487, 1985.
241. Luton JP, Mahoudeau JA, Bouchard P, et al: Treatment of Cushing's disease by *o,p'*-DDD: Survey of 62 cases. N Engl J Med 300:459–464, 1979.
242. Carey RM, Orth DN, Hartmann WH: Malignant melanoma with ectopic production of adrenocorticotropic hormone: Palliative treatment with inhibitors of adrenal steroid biosynthesis. J Clin Endocrinol Metab 36:482–487, 1973.
243. Leiba S, Weinstein R, Shindel B, et al: The protracted effect of *o,p'*-DDD in Cushing's disease and its impact on adrenal morphogenesis of young human embryo. Ann Endocrinol 50:49–53, 1989.
244. Hague RV, May W, Cullen DR: Hepatic microsomal enzyme induction and adrenal crisis due to *o,p'*-DDD therapy for metastatic adrenocortical carcinoma. Clin Endocrinol 31:51–57, 1989.
245. Bledsoe T, Island DP, Ney RL, Liddle GW: The effect of *o,p'*-DDD on cortisol and 6 beta hydroxycortisol secretion and metabolism in man. J Clin Endocrinol Metab 24:1303–1311, 1971.
246. Potts GO, Creange JE, Harding HR, Schane HP: Trilostane, an orally active inhibitor of steroid biosynthesis. Steroids 32:257–267, 1978.
247. Gower DB: Modifiers of steroid hormone metabolism: A review of their chemistry, biochemistry and clinical applications. J Steroid Biochem 5:501–523, 1974.
248. Santen RJ, Misbin RI: Aminoglutethimide: Review of pharmacology and clinical use. Pharmacotherapy 1:95–120, 1981.
249. Feldman D: Ketoconazole and other imidazole derivatives as inhibitors of steroidogenesis. Endocr Rev 7:409–420, 1986.
250. Daniels H, van Amstel WJ, Schopman W, van Dommelen C: Effect of metopirone in a patient with adrenocortical carcinoma. Acta Endocrinol (Copenh) 44:346–354, 1963.
251. Verhelst JA, Trainer PJ, Howlett TA, et al: Short- and long-term responses to metyrapone in the medical management of 91 patients with Cushing's syndrome. Clin Endocrinol (Oxf) 35:169–178, 1991.
252. Orth DN: Metyrapone is useful only as adjunctive therapy in Cushing's disease (editorial). Ann Intern Med 89:128–130, 1978.
253. Misbin R, Canary J, Willard D: Aminoglutethimide in the treatment of Cushing's syndrome. J Clin Pharmacol 16:645–651, 1976.
254. Zachman M, Gitzelman RP, Zagalak M, Prader A: Effect of aminoglutethimide on urinary cortisol and cortisol metabolites in adolescents with Cushing's syndrome. Clin Endocrinol (Oxf) 7:63–71, 1977.
255. Horky K, Kuchel O, Gregvoria I, Starka L: Qualitative alterations in urinary 17-ketosteroid excretion during aminoglutethimide administration. J Clin Endocrinol Metab 29:297–301, 1969.
256. Dewis DC, Bullock DE, Earnshaw R, Kelly WF: Experience with trilostane in the treatment of Cushing's syndrome. Clin Endocrinol (Oxf) 18:533–540, 1983.
257. Ross WM, Evered DC, Hunter P, et al: Treatment of Cushing's disease with adrenal blocking drugs and megavoltage therapy to the pituitary. Clin Radiol 30:149–153, 1979.
258. Fishman LM, Liddle GW, Island DP, et al: Effects of aminoglutethimide on adrenal function in man. J Clin Endocrinol Metab 27:481–490, 1967.
259. Gorden P, Becker C, Levey GS, Roth J: Efficacy of aminoglutethimide in the ectopic ACTH syndrome. J Clin Endocrinol 28:921–923, 1968.
260. Jeffcoate WJ, Rees LH, Tomlin S, et al: Metyrapone in long-term management of Cushing's disease. Br J Med 2:215–217, 1977.
261. Child DF, Burke CW, Burley DM, et al: Drug control of Cushing's syndrome: Combined aminoglutethimide and metyrapone therapy. Acta Endocrinol (Copenh) 82:330–341, 1976.
262. Sonino N: The use of ketoconazole as an inhibitor of steroid production. N Engl J Med 317:812–818, 1987.
263. Lewis JH, Hyman JZ, Benson GD, Ishak KG: Hepatic injury associated with ketoconazole therapy. Gastroenterology 86:503–513, 1984.
264. Winquist EW, Laskey J, Crump M, et al: Ketoconazole in the management of paraneoplastic Cushing's syndrome secondary to ectopic adrenocorticotropin production. J Clin Oncol 13:157–164, 1995.
265. Schulte HM, Benker G, Reinwein D, et al: Infusion of low dose etomidate: Correction of hypercortisolemia in patients with Cushing's syndrome and dose-response relationship in normal subjects. J Clin Endocrinol Metab 70:1426–1430, 1990.
266. Drake WM, Perry LA, Hinds CJ, et al: Emergency and prolonged use of intravenous etomidate to control hypercortisolemia in a patient with Cushing's syndrome and peritonitis. J Clin Endocrinol Metab 83:3542–3544, 1998.
267. Nieman L, Chrousos G, Kellner C, et al: Successful treatment of Cushing's syndrome with the glucocorticoid antagonist RU 486. J Clin Endocrinol Metab 61:536–540, 1985.
268. Gaillard RC, Riondel A, Muller AF, et al: RU 486: A steroid with antiglucocorticosteroid activity that only disinhibits the human pituitary-adrenal system at a specific time of day. Proc Natl Acad Sci U S A 81:3879–3882, 1984.
269. Melby JC: Therapy of Cushing disease: A consensus for pituitary microsurgery. Ann Intern Med 109:445–446, 1988.
270. Welbourn RB: The evolution of transsphenoidal pituitary microsurgery. Surgery 100:1185–1189, 1986.
271. Pieters GF, Hermus AR, Meijer E, et al: Predictive factors for initial cure and relapse rate after pituitary surgery for Cushing's disease. J Clin Endocrinol Metab 69:1122–1126, 1989.
272. Nakane T, Kuwayama A, Watanabe M, et al: Long-term results of transsphenoidal adenomectomy in patients with Cushing's disease. Neurosurgery 21:218–222, 1987.
273. Mapalam TJ, Tyrrell JB, Wilson CB: Transsphenoidal microsurgery for Cushing's disease: A report of 216 cases. Ann Intern Med 109:487–493, 1988.
274. Burke CW, Adams CBT, Esiri MM, et al: Transsphenoidal surgery for Cushing's disease: Does what is removed determine the endocrine outcome? Clin Endocrinol (Oxf) 33:525–537, 1990.
275. Burch W: A survey of results with transsphenoidal surgery in Cushing's disease. N Engl J Med 308:103–104, 1983.
276. Boggan JE, Tyrrell JB, Wilson CB: Transsphenoidal microsurgical management of Cushing's disease. J Neurosurg 59:195–200, 1983.
277. Friedman RB, Oldfield EH, Nieman LK, et al: Repeat transsphenoidal surgery for Cushing's disease. J Neurosurg 71:520–527, 1989.
278. Chandler WF, Schteingart DE, Lloyd RV, et al: Surgical treatment of Cushing's disease. J Neurosurg 66:204–212, 1987.
279. Knappe UJ, Ludecke DK: Transnasal microsurgery in children and adolescents with Cushing's disease. Neurosurgery 39:484–492; discussion 492–493, 1996.
280. Buchfelder M, Fahlbusch R: Neurosurgical treatment of Cushing's disease in children and adolescents. Acta Neurochir Suppl (Wien) 35:101–105, 1985.
281. Haddad SF, VanGilder JC, Menezes AH: Pediatric pituitary tumors. Neurosurgery 29:509–514, 1991.
282. Blevins LJ, Christy JH, Khajavi M, Tindall GT: Outcomes of therapy for Cushing's disease due to adrenocorticotropin-secreting pituitary macroadenomas. J Clin Endocrinol Metab 83:63–67, 1998.
283. Wilson CB, Dempsey LC: Transsphenoidal microsurgical removal of 250 pituitary adenomas. J Neurosurg 48:13–22, 1978.
284. Knappe UJ, Ludecke DK: Persistent and recurrent hypercortisolism after transsphenoidal surgery for Cushing's disease. Acta Neurochir Suppl (Wien) 65:31–34, 1996.
285. Guilhaume B, Bertagna X, Thomsen M, et al: Transsphenoidal pituitary surgery for the treatment of Cushing's disease: Results in 64 patients and long term follow-up studies. J Clin Endocrinol Metab 66:1056–1064, 1988.
286. Sheline GE, Wara WM, Smith V: Therapeutic irradiation and brain injury. Int J Radiat Oncol Biol Phys 6:1215–1228, 1980.
287. Orth DN, Liddle GW: Results of treatment in 108 patients with Cushing's syndrome. N Engl J Med 285:243–247, 1971.
288. Jennings AS, Liddle GW, Orth DN: Results of treating childhood Cushing's disease with pituitary irradiation. N Engl J Med 297:957–962, 1977.
289. Schteingart DE, Tsao HS, Taylor CI, et al: Sustained remission of Cushing's disease with mitotane and pituitary irradiation. Ann Intern Med 92:613–619, 1980.
290. Estrada J, Boronat M, Mielgo M, et al: The long-term outcome of pituitary irradiation after unsuccessful transsphenoidal surgery in Cushing's disease [see comments]. N Engl J Med 336:172–177, 1997.
291. Levy RP, Fabrikant JI, Frankel KA, et al: Heavy-charged-particle radiosurgery of the pituitary gland: Clinical results of 840 patients. Stereotact Funct Neurosurg 57:22–35, 1991.
292. Linfoot JA, Nakagawa JS, Wiedemann E, et al: Heavy particle therapy: Pituitary tumors. Bull Los Angeles Neurol Soc 42:175–189, 1977.
293. Martinez R, Bravo G, Burzaco J, Rey G: Pituitary tumors and gamma knife surgery. Clinical experience with more than two years of follow-up. Stereotact Funct Neurosurg 1:110–118, 1998.
294. Wells SA, Merke DP, Cutler GJ, et al: Therapeutic controversy. The role of laparoscopic surgery in adrenal disease. J Clin Endocrinol Metab 83:3041–3049, 1998.
295. Ram Z, Doppman J, Oldfield EH: Immediate repeat transsphenoidal surgery for persistent Cushing's disease: Results and prediction of outcome. J Neurosurg 80:37–45, 1994.
296. Bevan JS, Gough MH, Gillmer M, et al: Cushing's syndrome in pregnancy: The timing of definitive treatment. Clin Endocrinol (Oxf) 27:225–233, 1987.
297. Casson IF, Davis JC, Jeffreys RV, et al: Successful management of Cushing's disease during pregnancy by transsphenoidal adenectomy. Clin Endocrinol (Oxf) 27:423–428, 1987.
298. Avgerinos PC, Chrousos GP, Nieman LK, et al: The corticotropin-releasing hormone test in the postoperative evaluation of patients with Cushing's syndrome. J Clin Endocrinol Metab 65:906–913, 1987.
299. Bochicchio D, Losa M, Buchfelder M: Factors influencing the immediate and late outcome of Cushing's disease treated by transsphenoidal surgery: A retrospective study by the European Cushing's Disease Survey Group [see comments]. J Clin Endocrinol Metab 80:3114–3120, 1995.
300. Lamberts SW, Klijn GJ, de Jong FH: The definition of true recurrence of pituitary-dependent Cushing's syndrome after transsphenoidal operation. Clin Endocrinol (Oxf) 26:707–712, 1987.
301. Fraser GG, Preuss FS, Bigford WD: Adrenal atrophy and irreversible shock associated with cortisone therapy. JAMA 149:1542–1543, 1952.
302. Kehlet H, Binder C, Blichert-Toft M: Glucocorticoid maintenance therapy following adrenalectomy: Assessment of dosage and preparation. Clin Endocrinol (Oxf) 5:37–41, 1976.
303. Nieman LK, Gumowski J, DeVroom H, Ram Z, Oldfield EH: Prediction of long-term remission of Cushing's disease after successful transsphenoidal resection of ACTH-secreting tumor. Presented at the 80th Annual Meeting of the Endocrine Society, New Orleans, 1998, p 345.
304. Hollinshead WH: The interphase of diabetes insipidus. Mayo Clin Proc 39:95–100, 1964.
305. Olson BR, Rubino D, Gumowski J, Oldfield EH: Isolated hyponatremia after transsphenoidal pituitary surgery. J Clin Endocrinol Metab 80:85–91, 1995.
306. Doherty GM, Nieman LK, Cutler GB Jr, et al: Time to recovery of the hypothalamic-pituitary-adrenal axis after curative resection of adrenal tumors in patients with Cushing's syndrome. Surgery 108:1085–1090, 1990.
307. Byyny RL: Withdrawal from glucocorticoid therapy. N Engl J Med 295:30–33, 1976.
308. Leshin M: Acute adrenal insufficiency: Recognition, management and prevention. Urol Clin North Am 9:229–235, 1982.
309. Kehlet H, Lindhold J, Bjerre P: Value of the 30-min ACTH test in assessing hypothalamic-pituitary adrenocortical function after pituitary surgery in Cushing's disease. Clin Endocrinol 20:349–353, 1984.
310. Lamberts SWJ, Tilanus KHW, Klooswijk AIJ, et al: Successful treatment with SMS 201–995 of Cushing syndrome caused by ectopic adrenocorticotropin secretion for a metastatic gastrin-secreting pancreatic islet cell carcinoma. J Clin Endocrinol Metab 67:1080–1083, 1988.
311. Pass HI, Doppman JL, Nieman L, et al: Management of the ectopic ACTH syndrome due to thoracic carcinoids. Ann Thorac Surg 50:52–57, 1990.

312. Bellantone R, Ferrante A, Boscherini M, et al: Role of reoperation in recurrence of adrenal cortical carcinoma: Results from 188 cases collected in the Italian National Registry for Adrenal Cortical Carcinoma. Surgery 122:1212–1218, 1997.
313. Allolio B, Reincke M, Arlt W, et al: Suramin for treatment of adrenocortical carcinoma. Lancet 2:277, 1989.
314. Contreras P, Rojas A, Biagini L, et al: Regression of metastatic adrenal carcinoma during palliative ketoconazole treatment (letter). Lancet 2:151–152, 1985.
315. Verhelst JA, Druwe P, van Erps P, et al: Use of ketoconazole in the treatment of a virilizing adrenocortical carcinoma. Acta Endocrinol (Copenh) 121:229–234, 1989.
316. Flack MR, Pyle RG, Mullen NM, et al: Oral gossypol in the treatment of metastatic adrenal cancer. J Clin Endocrinol Metab 76:1019–1024, 1993.
317. Berruti A, Terzolo M, Pia A, et al: Mitotane associated with etoposide, doxorubicin, and cisplatin in the treatment of advanced adrenocortical carcinoma. Italian Group for the Study of Adrenal Cancer. Cancer 83:2194–2200, 1998.
318. DiSomma C, Colao A, Pivonello R, et al: Effectiveness of chronic treatment with alendronate in the osteoporosis of Cushing's disease. Clin Endocrinol (Oxf) 48:655–662, 1998.
319. Hough S, Teitelbaum SL, Bergfeld MA, Avioli LV: Isolated skeletal involvement in Cushing's syndrome: Response to therapy. J Clin Endocrinol Metab 52:1033–1038, 1981.
320. Manning PJ, Evans MC, Reid IR: Normal bone mineral density following cure of Cushing's syndrome. Clin Endocrinol (Oxf) 36:229–234, 1992.
321. Pocock NA, Eisman JA, Dunstan CR, et al: Recovery from steroid-induced osteoporosis. Ann Intern Med 107:319–323, 1987.
322. Wick MR, Rosai J: Neuroendocrine tumors of the thymus. Pathol Res Pract 183:188–199, 1988.
323. Jex RK, van Heerden J, Carpenter PC, Grant CS: Ectopic ACTH syndrome. Am J Surg 149:276–282, 1985.
324. Grizzle WE, Tolbert L, Pittman CS, et al: Corticotropin production by tumors of the autonomic nervous system. Arch Pathol Lab Med 108:545–550, 1984.
325. Ravi SD, Dorus W, Park YN, et al: The dexamethasone suppression test and depressive symptoms in early and late withdrawal from alcohol. Am J Psychiatry 141:1445–1448, 1984.
326. Hirschfeld RM, Koslow SH, Kupfer DJ: The clinical utility of the dexamethasone suppression test in psychiatry: Summary of a National Institute of Mental Health workshop. JAMA 250:2172–2174, 1983.
327. Blumenfield M, Rose LI, Richmond LH, Beering SC: Dexamethasone suppression in basic trainees under stress. Arch Gen Psychiatry 23:299–304, 1970.
328. Lamberts SW: Neuroendocrine aspects of the dexamethasone suppression test in psychiatry. Life Sci 39:91–95, 1986.
329. Kapcala LP, Hamilton SM, Meikle AW: Cushing's disease with "normal suppression" due to decreased dexamethasone clearance. Arch Intern Med 144:636–637, 1984.

Chapter 122

Generalized Glucocorticoid Resistance

Diana M. Malchoff ▪ Carl D. Malchoff

BACKGROUND

Generalized glucocorticoid resistance, also known as primary cortisol resistance, was first described by Vingerhoeds et al. in 1976.[1] It is quite rare.

Fewer than 15 separate probands have been reported.[1–9] In the largest kindred studied, 15 affected subjects were identified.[10] It is characterized by hypercortisolism without clinical features of glucocorticoid excess and is sometimes caused by functionally abnormal human glucocorticoid receptors (hGRs). The hypothalamic-pituitary-adrenal (HPA) axis is reset, so that circulating adrenal hormone concentrations are higher than normal. The clinical presentation of glucocorticoid resistance varies from asymptomatic hypercortisolism to clinical syndromes of mineralocorticoid or adrenal androgen excess, or both. Some of the hGR mutations which cause this disorder have been elucidated. However, in some subjects the hGR primary structure is normal, and the cause remains unknown.

ENDOCRINE PHYSIOLOGY AND PATHOPHYSIOLOGY

Generalized glucocorticoid resistance is caused by functionally abnormal hGR. This was first demonstrated in assays of hGR function.[4–9, 11] More recent studies have validated this expectation by identifying mutant hGRs.[12–16] In this way resistance to glucocorticoids is similar to syndromes of resistance to vitamin D, thyroid hormone, androgens, and estrogens. Receptors for these hormones are very similar in structure to the hGR,[17] and mutations of each receptor cause resistance to its respective hormone.[18–22] This is in contrast to the hormone resistance of pseudohypoparathyroidism; in this disorder the signal transduction proteins, and not the receptors, are functionally and structurally abnormal, and there is resistance to multiple hormones.

The clinical findings of glucocorticoid resistance are a consequence of the functional abnormality of the hGR. The HPA axis and its negative feedback regulation of cortisol production are described elsewhere. The glucocorticoid sensitivity of all tissues is decreased in glucocorticoid resistance. The entire HPA axis is reset (Fig. 122–1). At the pituitary and hypothalamus, serum cortisol concentrations, which otherwise would be considered normal, are insufficient to suppress corticotropin-releasing hormone (CRH) and adrenocorticotropic hormone (ACTH) secretion. Therefore, secretion of CRH and ACTH hormones is increased. Since ACTH secretion is increased, the adrenal glands are stimulated to produce greater than normal amounts of cortisol, adrenal androgens, and mineralocorticoids. In the peripheral tissues the glucocorticoid resistance is equal to that of the pituitary and hypothalamus; however, sensitivity to androgens and mineralocorticoids is normal. Hence, the clinical findings are not those of glucocorticoid excess, but rather those of mineralocorticoid or androgen excess.

Although the HPA axis is reset so that each gland secretes greater than normal amounts of its respective hormone, the normal circadian rhythm and the response to stress are maintained. In the cases that have been described, the resistance to cortisol is partial, and plasma ACTH concentrations can be suppressed by high doses of exogenous glucocorticoids. Complete glucocorticoid resistance may be incompatible with life, as suggested by animal models.[23]

FEATURES AND CHARACTERISTICS

Clinical Features and Characteristics

The clinical characteristics of glucocorticoid resistance are based on the rare cases reported in the literature. Therefore, the impression of the relative frequency of the different clinical presentations may change as more affected individuals are evaluated more completely.

The most common characteristic is hypercortisolism without features of glucocorticoid excess. It was this finding that led to the first

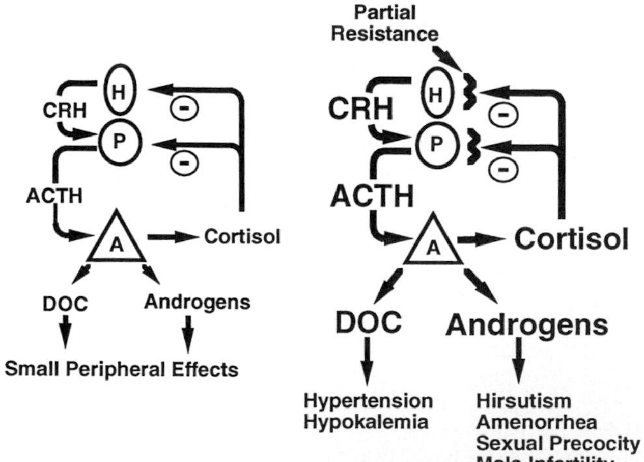

FIGURE 122–1. Hypothalamic-pituitary-adrenal (HPA) axis in normal and in glucocorticoid-resistant subjects. Normally, corticotropin-releasing hormone (CRH) from the hypothalamus (H) stimulates the pituitary (P) to produce adrenocorticotropic hormone (ACTH). ACTH stimulates production of mineralocorticoids, cortisol, and adrenal androgens by the adrenal gland (A). Cortisol inhibits (−) secretion of CRH and ACTH from the hypothalamus and pituitary, respectively. In generalized glucocorticoid resistance there is partial blockade of the negative feedback at the pituitary and hypothalamus. This causes increased secretion of CRH and ACTH. ACTH stimulates the adrenal gland to make excess glucocorticoids, mineralocorticoids, and androgens. The HPA axis is qualitatively normal, but quantitatively reset at higher hormone concentrations than normal. (Adapted from Javier EC, et al: Endocrinologist 1:141–148, 1991.)

description of the syndrome,[1] and occasionally it is discovered in the investigation of other problems unrelated to glucocorticoid resistance.[6] Hypercortisolism is usually identified by an elevated urinary cortisol excretion or cortisol secretion rate. However, this may not be a universal finding.[11] Many features of glucocorticoid excess are nonspecific or subtle. Therefore, it may be difficult to establish that the features of glucocorticoid excess are completely absent. For instance, the triad of obesity, hypertension, and diabetes is relatively common in the general population and also is caused by Cushing's syndrome. A patient with this triad and glucocorticoid resistance could be mistakenly diagnosed to have Cushing's syndrome. Alternatively, early in Cushing's syndrome, the clinical features can be very subtle, so that a patient with early mild Cushing's syndrome could be mistaken to have glucocorticoid resistance. In summary, hypercortisolism without features of glucocorticoid excess is often present, but exceptions to this rule may occur.

Although hypercortisolism without cushingoid features usually suggests the diagnosis, this constellation of features usually does not bring the patient to clinical attention. The presenting clinical features are secondary to excess androgens or mineralocorticoids. The most common clinical presentation is evidence of increased androgens in women. This was the presentation in four of the six probands described by Lamberts et al.,[11] and the characteristics include hirsutism, acne, and menstrual irregularities. This presentation is caused by the increased adrenal androgens. Isosexual precocious pseudopuberty was the clinical presentation in a 6½-year-old boy,[4] but has not been described in others. The reasons that this presentation is not more common is unclear. It may have been overlooked in many of the initial patients. Infertility in men has been reported and is secondary to the increased adrenal androgen production and subsequent suppression of the hypothalamic-pituitary-testicular axis.[15]

Hypertension and hypokalemia were the presenting clinical findings of the first subject described by Vingerhoeds et al.[1] Hypertension with severe thiazide-induced hypokalemia occurred in another patient.[11] Other subjects have been found to be hypertensive without hypokalemia.[6, 7, 11] In these the contribution of glucocorticoid resistance to the hypertension is less clear, since essential hypertension is common. Thus, hypertension and hypokalemia occurred in only two of the probands described.

At least one subject with glucocorticoid resistance developed nodular adrenal hyperplasia.[11] The frequency of this event in all affected subjects has not been ascertained. Anticipated clinical presentations that have not yet been described include heterosexual precocious pseudopuberty in a girl and adrenal hyperplasia as an incidental finding on abdominal imaging.

In general, individuals with the greatest degree of hypercortisolism produce the most androgens and mineralocorticoids and subsequently have the most clinical findings. Variability of clinical characteristics within a kindred may be due in part to a gene dosage effect. Homozygotes are affected to a greater degree than heterozygotes. Women seem to be affected more frequently than men. This is probably because they are more likely to present with features of increased adrenal androgens. It is not entirely clear why androgen effects seem to predominate in some patients, while the mineralocorticoid effects seem to predominate in others.

One subject with severe glucocorticoid resistance and a missense hGR mutation developed Cushing's syndrome due to an ACTH-secreting pituitary adenoma.[15] Presumably, the hGR mutation was a primary genomic abnormality which combined with necessary somatic pituitary gene mutations to affect the adenoma phenotype.

The possibility of tissue-specific or localized glucocorticoid resistance is in early stages of investigation. It does occur in some neoplasms. In ACTH-dependent Cushing's syndrome the pituitary or the ectopic ACTH source is well known to be more resistant to glucocorticoids than are the normal tissues. The molecular basis of this resistance is being probed, and hGR mutations, gene deletions, or both, occur in some circumstances.[15, 24–26] Some neoplasms of hematopoietic origin demonstrate glucocorticoid resistance to apoptosis, and in some cell lines derived from these neoplasms hGR mutations have been shown to cause glucocorticoid resistance.[27, 28] It is attractive to speculate that differences in tissue sensitivity to glucocorticoids could contribute to the development of clinical disorders such as glucocorticoid-resistant asthma,[29] rheumatoid arthritis,[30] obesity,[31] hypertension,[32] insulin resistance, and diabetes.[33] It is also possible that infection with the HIV virus may increase[34, 35] or decrease[36] glucocorticoid sensitivity. Studies of these possible relationships and their mechanisms are evolving.

Inheritance Pattern

Initial studies suggested an autosomal dominant transmission of glucocorticoid resistance. With the application of molecular biology and determination of the exact hGR mutations responsible for this disorder, the patterns of inheritance are becoming more clear. The inheritance pattern may vary depending upon the exact hGR mutation. It is clearly autosomal dominant in the kindred with a splice site microdeletion of one allele.[14] In the kindred described by Vingerhoeds et al.[1] and investigated further in collaboration with Loriaux and Chrousos and coworkers,[5, 10] the proband, who is most severely affected, is homozygous for a mutation of the hGR ligand-binding domain. The son and nephew, who are mildly affected, are both heterozygous.[1, 5, 10, 12] Therefore, this seems to be either a recessive disorder or a disorder dependent upon a gene dosage effect. The hGR mutation in one family arose as a new mutation, so that both parents were unaffected.[15] However, this individual had more severe glucocorticoid resistance than would be expected from an abnormality of a single allele and subsequent in vitro studies suggested that the mutant receptor had a dominant negative effect. Extensive family studies noting genotype-phenotype correlations have not been performed. In summary, inheritance patterns vary, and biochemical investigation of familial members may not necessarily identify all the subjects carrying the mutant hGR allele.

Biochemical Characteristics

Hypercortisolism, usually measured as increased urinary cortisol excretion, was found in all affected individuals in the initial studies.[1, 5–7, 9, 10] However, more recent evaluations demonstrate that this may not be invariant; urinary cortisol excretion is occasionally normal.[11] In contrast, in the most severely affected patients, urinary cortisol excretion may exceed the upper normal limit by 200-fold.[1, 11] This considerable variability suggests heterogeneity in the degree of resistance and in the pathogenetic receptor abnormality.

Hypercortisolism of glucocorticoid resistance is distinguished from that of Cushing's syndrome by the presence of a diurnal variation in serum cortisol. As discussed before, the HPA axis is qualitatively normal, but quantitatively reset with higher than normal hormone concentrations. Serum cortisol concentrations usually decrease by at least 50% from 8 AM to 8 PM in normal subjects[37] and in glucocorticoid-resistant subjects,[4, 5, 11] whereas in Cushing's syndrome there is loss of the diurnal variation.[38] An example of the diurnal variation of serum cortisol reset at higher than normal concentrations in a subject with generalized glucocorticoid resistance is shown in Figure 122–2.

Serum cortisol concentrations can be increased up to eightfold above normal, but may be normal if the resistance is mild.[1, 5, 11] Comparison of cortisol concentrations must be made with controls from the same time of day. The 8 AM serum cortisol is usually not suppressed normally by 1 mg of dexamethasone given orally at 11 PM the previous evening.[11] As expected, cortisol production is ACTH-dependent, and ACTH concentrations can be suppressed by supraphysiologic doses of glucocorticoids.[4, 5] Plasma ACTH concentrations are less frequently increased than are cortisol concentrations, but tend to be the highest in individuals with the greatest resistance.

Adrenal androgens (androstenedione, dehydroepiandrosterone, and dehydroepiandrosterone sulfate) are increased in most children and women.[1, 4–7, 9, 11] These increases range from mild to fivefold above the upper normal limit, and they can be suppressed by high doses of glucocorticoids. It is these hormones that produce the clinical features that bring women to clinical attention and cause precocious pseudopuberty.

The mineralocorticoids have been less extensively studied. How-

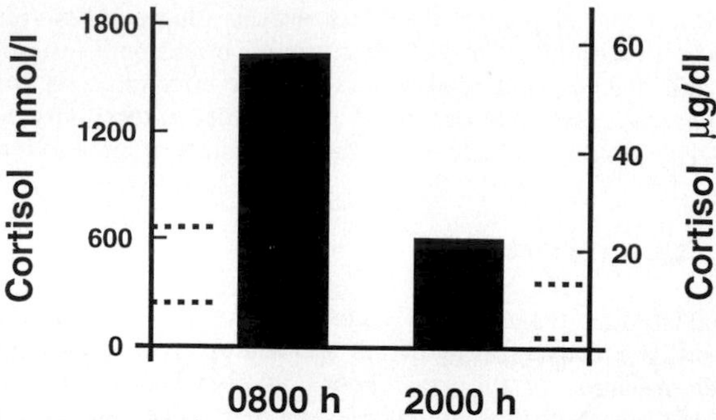

FIGURE 122–2. Diurnal variation of serum cortisol in a subject with generalized glucocorticoid resistance. Serum cortisol concentrations are represented in nanomoles per liter on the left ordinate and in micrograms per deciliter on the right ordinate. The 8 AM and 8 PM serum cortisol concentrations from a patient with glucocorticoid resistance are shown. The results are the mean of three separate determinations. The normal range of serum cortisol at 8 AM is shown by the dotted lines on the left ordinate, and the normal range at 8 PM is shown by the dotted lines on the right ordinate. (Adapted from Malchoff C, Javier E, Malchoff D, et al: Primary cortisol resistance presenting as isosexual precocity. J Clin Endocrinol Metab 70:503–507, 1990. © The Endocrine Society.)

ever, when they have been measured, deoxycorticosterone (DOC) and corticosterone are usually increased by two- to fivefold above the upper normal limit, while aldosterone concentrations are low and plasma renin activity is suppressed.[4–7] Production of DOC and corticosterone is ACTH-dependent, since serum concentrations can be suppressed by supraphysiologic doses of dexamethasone.[39] DOC or cortisol causes hypokalemia and volume-dependent hypertension by activating the aldosterone receptor. Volume expansion suppresses plasma renin activity, and subsequently angiotensin II and aldosterone are also decreased.

Glucocorticoid Receptor Abnormalities

Functionally abnormal hGRs cause glucocorticoid resistance. However, this has not been conclusively proved for all cases. The hGR has two major functional domains; the ligand-binding domain which is in the C-terminus and the DNA-binding domain which is near the mid-portion of the molecule and contains the zinc fingers.[17] Functional changes include decreased receptor number,[6, 11] decreased receptor affinity for glucocorticoids,[4, 5, 11] decreased binding to DNA,[7] and thermolability.[8]

There is no assay that is completely sensitive and specific for all hGR functional abnormalities. Binding of [^{3}H] dexamethasone is used most commonly, but this is normal in some subjects.[11] A number of possibilities could account for this finding. These include mutations in the hGR DNA-binding domain or mutations in an accessory protein necessary for glucocorticoid action. In isolated cases dexamethasone induction of aromatase in cultured skin fibroblasts[40] and dexamethasone suppression of mitogen-stimulated thymidine incorporation into mononuclear leukocytes[11] have been used to identify decreased glucocorticoid responsiveness.

Pathogenetic mutations of the hGR gene have been found in some, but not all, subjects. These mutations can cause glucocorticoid resistance by decreasing the number of expressed hGRs or by expressing an hGR carrying a functionally significant missense mutation. A splice-site microdeletion, which interferes with hGR messenger RNA (mRNA) processing and reduces the hGR number by 50%, is the likely cause of glucocorticoid resistance in one kindred.[14] Figure 122–3 summarizes the three missense point mutations that have been identified. The original subject of Vingerhoeds et al., who presented with hypertension and hypokalemia, is homozygous for an aspartate-to-valine change at amino acid 641.[12] A boy presenting with isosexual precocious pseudopuberty is homozygous for a valine-to-isoleucine mutation at amino acid 729.[4] Both of these mutations decrease the affinity of the hGR for dexamethasone and impair dexamethasone-stimulated gene transcription.[12, 16] It is of interest that both of these mutations are in parts of the ligand-binding domain that are homologous to the regions of the ligand-binding domain of the androgen receptor which are mutated in androgen resistance.[41] The apparent hGR number is reduced in a subject with the isoleucine-to-asparagine mutation at amino acid 559.[15] It is likely that different mutations will be identified in other affected individuals. These early results also suggest that homozygous individuals may be more clinically affected than heterozygous individuals. Some hGR mutations are silent polymorphisms.[42] Therefore, identification of an hGR mutation is not conclusive evidence of hGR resistance.

DIFFERENTIAL DIAGNOSIS

It is essential to distinguish glucocorticoid resistance from ACTH-dependent Cushing's syndrome. This can be difficult, since no single test is completely discriminatory. The physical examination is the initial clue to the diagnosis, since individuals with glucocorticoid resistance lack features of glucocorticoid excess. However, as discussed earlier, the features of glucocorticoid excess may be subtle, and some are nonspecific. For example, the ectopic ACTH syndrome, which presents predominantly with hypertension, hypokalemia, and ACTH-dependent hypercortisolism, may mimic glucocorticoid resistance. Therefore, the physical examination may be misleading or indeterminate. Studies which demonstrate the qualitative integrity of the HPA axis are useful. A normal circadian rhythm is found in glucocorticoid resistance, but is absent in Cushing's syndrome. As mentioned previously, serum cortisol concentrations are elevated, but are expected to fall by at least 50% from 8 AM to 8 PM. An insulin tolerance test has also been used to test the functional integrity of the axis. There is a normal response to hypoglycemic stress in glucocorticoid resistance,[4] but not in Cushing's syndrome.[43] Although these tests have been useful in a limited number of patients, they may not be perfect. In Cushing's syndrome, cortisol concentrations may vary throughout the day[38] and mimic a diurnal variation. Therefore, there is no single clinical test that can be expected to unambiguously distinguish ACTH-dependent Cushing's syndrome from glucocorticoid resistance. Clinical judgment and repeated evaluations over time are essential.

In children with glucocorticoid resistance, the growth curves may help to distinguish patients with glucocorticoid resistance from those with Cushing's syndrome. In Cushing's syndrome growth is slowed. Although the growth curves in most patients with glucocorticoid resistance have not been carefully examined, it seems unlikely that growth would be slowed. In the child presenting with isosexual precocious pseudopuberty, growth was accelerated compared to the expected normal rate and was much greater than that expected for a child with

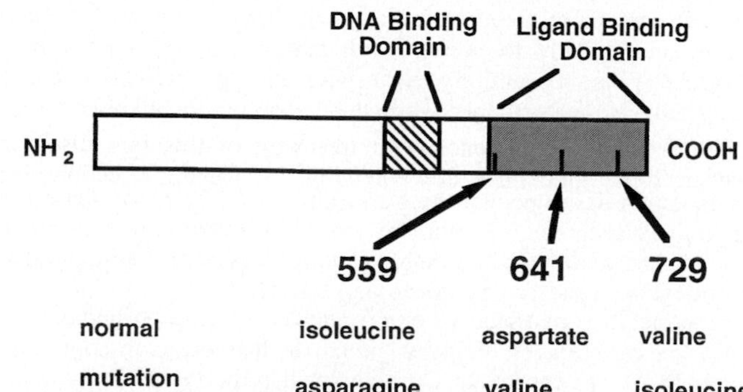

FIGURE 122–3. Diagrammatic representation of the human glucocorticoid receptor (hGR) point mutations in generalized glucocorticoid resistance. The DNA-binding domain *(diagonal lines)* and ligand-binding domain *(shaded area)* are two of the major functional units of the receptor. Point mutations have been identified at amino acids (aa) 559, 641, and 729. Not shown is a splice-site microdeletion which disrupts processing of the hGR messenger RNA (mRNA). (Adapted from Javier EC, et al: Endocrinologist 1:141–148, 1991.)

Cushing's syndrome. This accelerated growth was presumably due to increased adrenal androgens.[4]

Other diagnostic considerations include increased cortisol-binding globulin (CBG) and administration of carbamazepine. Increased CBG may imitate glucocorticoid resistance, since it causes high serum cortisol concentrations with a diurnal variation. Radioimmunoassays for CBG are commercially available, and CBG is normal in glucocorticoid resistance.[4, 5] Carbamazepine interferes with testing of the HPA axis in multiple ways. It increases the rate of dexamethasone metabolism, so that patients may appear resistant to this glucocorticoid. Patients taking carbamazepine demonstrate increased circulating cortisol concentrations and increased urinary cortisol excretion, although usually not out of the normal range.[44] Finally, carbamazepine or its metabolites may interfere with some of the commercial high-performance liquid chromatography (HPLC) assays for cortisol.

Subjects with hypertension and hypokalemia, but without increased aldosterone, should be evaluated for glucocorticoid resistance, so that they are not mistaken for other rare causes of volume-dependent hypertension. In this situation a serum cortisol or 24-hour urinary excretion of cortisol is probably sufficient to detect individuals with possible glucocorticoid resistance. Naturally, the diagnosis of Cushing's syndrome would also be considered in such a situation.

Since the most common clinical presentation is hyperandrogenism in women, then the polycystic ovary syndrome and idiopathic hirsutism should be considered in the differential diagnosis. These disorders are much more common than glucocorticoid resistance. No studies have been done to try and ascertain the frequency of glucocorticoid resistance in the population of women carrying these diagnoses. It is anticipated that the yield of glucocorticoid resistance would be quite low. However, it can be argued that appropriate investigation may be indicated, since it is a treatable inherited disorder. Similarly, the frequency of this disorder in those children with early adrenarche is unknown. However, it can be argued that the diagnosis of glucocorticoid resistance should be considered, since it would be likely to alter therapy. The frequency of glucocorticoid resistance in this clinical presentation may be greater than anticipated from the current literature, which has identified only one child presenting with evidence of increased androgens.[4]

If the clinical and biochemical studies suggest the diagnosis of glucocorticoid resistance, then direct hGR functional studies may be confirmatory. As discussed, a number of functional receptor abnormalities have been reported.[4–9, 11] Unfortunately, this testing requires fresh or cultured mononuclear leukocytes and is not commercially available. In addition, there may be other causes of abnormal ligand binding. The apparent receptor number may be slightly decreased in Cushing's syndrome,[45] and in patients with AIDS the hGR may have a decreased affinity for glucocorticoids.[46] Finally, there may be some subjects with glucocorticoid resistance with normal primary sequence of the hGRs.[47] Therefore, even this research tool is not completely sensitive or specific, and the diagnosis can be difficult to establish unambiguously.

THERAPY

There is limited experience with treatment of this rare disorder. However, some guidelines are emerging for patient selection and treatment protocols. Therapy is reserved for those with significant clinical features.

The most common approach to therapy is the use of exogenous glucocorticoids (Fig. 122–4A). It has been used for patients with hypertension and hypokalemia,[11, 48] with sexual precocity,[39] and for women with hirsutism.[9, 11] The goal is to suppress adrenal androgen and mineralocorticoid concentrations without using so much dexamethasone as to cause Cushing's syndrome. Dexamethasone, which does not interfere with radioimmunoassays for cortisol, is chosen so that serum cortisol concentrations can be monitored and titrated into the normal range.[9, 11, 39] These doses will vary from patient to patient. If cortisol is not suppressed below the normal range, then it seems unlikely that Cushing's syndrome will develop as a side effect. With this therapy androgens and mineralocorticoids fall and the clinical features improve.[9, 11, 39, 48]

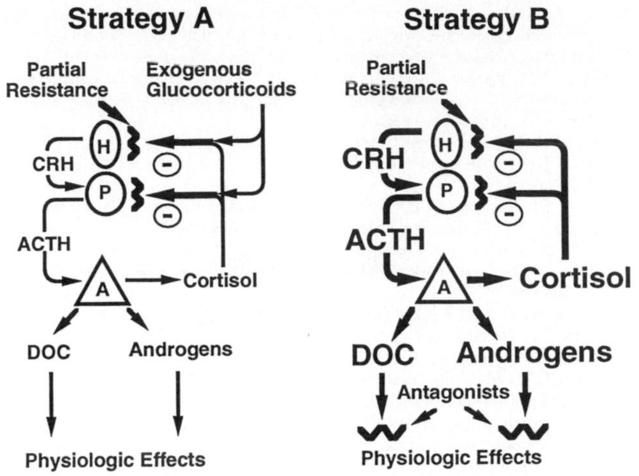

FIGURE 122–4. Treatment strategies for generalized glucocorticoid resistance. Two strategies have been proposed. In the first strategy *(A)*, exogenous glucocorticoids (usually dexamethasone) are administered to decrease adrenocorticotropic hormone (ACTH) secretion and subsequently decrease the secretion of adrenal steroids. The dose is adjusted to titrate cortisol into the normal range. In the second *(B)*, mineralocorticoid and androgen antagonists are used to block the peripheral effects of the hormones producing clinical effects. (CRH, corticotropin-releasing hormone; H, hypothalamus; P, pituitary; A, adrenal gland.) (Adapted from Malchoff EC, et al: Current Therapy in Endocrinology and Metabolism, ed 5. St. Louis, MO, Mosby-Year Book, 1994, pp 167–171.)

An alternative approach (Fig. 122–4B) is to use mineralocorticoid or androgen antagonists or both. For example, if the only clinical features are hypertension and hypokalemia, then this should be treatable with spironolactone, which blocks the mineralocorticoid receptor, or with amiloride, which blocks the sodium-potassium exchange in the distal tubule.

No therapy is indicated for biochemically affected subjects who are otherwise asymptomatic. Adrenal insufficiency is not a common feature of this disease, since the block of glucocorticoid effects is partial, and there is considerable reserve for increased cortisol production by the adrenal gland. No patient has been described who requires exogenous glucocorticoids during stress. However, glucocorticoids should not be withheld from a resistant subject if adrenal insufficiency is suspected during a significant physical stress.

SUMMARY

Glucocorticoid resistance is a rare disorder characterized by hypercortisolism, and the absence of the clinical features caused by glucocorticoid excess. ACTH-mediated overproduction of adrenal androgens and mineralocorticoids produces a clinical syndrome in some individuals. The disorder is receptor-mediated, and four distinct hGR mutations have been described. Therapy is reserved for those patients with significant clinical abnormalities, and two different treatment strategies are presented.

REFERENCES

1. Vingerhoeds A, Thijssen J, Shwarz F: Spontaneous hypercortisolism without Cushing's syndrome. J Clin Endocrinol Metab 43:1128–1133, 1976.
2. Karl M, von Wichert G, Kempter E, et al. Nelson's syndrome associated with a defect in the glucocorticoid receptor gene. Presented at the 76th Annual Meeting of the Endocrine Society, Anaheim, CA, June 15–18, 1994.
3. Lamberts SW, Koper JW, de Jong FH: Familial and iatrogenic cortisol receptor resistance. J Steroid Biochem Mol Biol 43:385–388, 1992.
4. Malchoff C, Javier E, Malchoff D, et al: Primary cortisol resistance presenting as isosexual precocity. J Clin Endocrinol Metab 70:503–507, 1990.
5. Chrousos GP, Vingerhoeds ACM, Brandon D, et al: Primary cortisol resistance in man: A glucocorticoid receptor-mediated disease. J Clin Invest 69:1261–1269, 1982.
6. Iida S, Gomi M, Moriwaki K, et al: Primary cortisol resistance accompanied by a reduction in glucocorticoid receptors in two members of the same family. J Clin Endocrinol Metab 60:967–971, 1985.

7. Nawata H, Sekiya K, Higuchi K, et al: Decreased deoxyribonucleic acid binding of glucocorticoid-receptor complex in cultured skin fibroblasts from a patient with glucocorticoid resistance syndrome. J Clin Endocrinol Metab 65:219–226, 1987.
8. Bronnegard M, Werner S, Gustafsson J: Primary cortisol resistance associated with a thermolabile glucocorticoid receptor in a patient with fatigue as the only symptom. J Clin Invest 78:1270–1278, 1986.
9. Lamberts SWJ, Poldermans D, Zweens M, de Jong FH: Familial cortisol resistance: Differential diagnostic and therapeutic aspects. J Clin Endocrinol Metab 63:1328–1333, 1986.
10. Chrousos G, Vingerhoeds A, Loriaux D, Lipsett M: Primary cortisol resistance: A family study. J Clin Endocrinol Metab 56:1243–1245, 1983.
11. Lamberts SWJ, Koper JW, Biemond P, et al: Cortisol receptor resistance: The variability of its clinical presentation and response to treatment. J Clin Endocrinol Metab 74:313–321, 1992.
12. Hurley D, Accili D, Stratakis C, et al: Point mutation causing a single amino acid substitution in the hormone binding domain of the glucocorticoid receptor in familial glucocorticoid resistance. J Clin Invest. 87:680–686, 1991.
13. Brufsky A, Malchoff D, Javier E, et al: A glucocorticoid receptor mutation in a subject with primary cortisol resistance. Trans Assoc Am Physicians 103:53–63, 1990.
14. Karl M, Lamberts SWJ, Detera-Wadleigh SD, et al: Familial glucocorticoid resistance caused by a splice site deletion in the human glucocorticoid receptor gene. J Clin Endocrinol Metab 76:683–689, 1993.
15. Karl M, Lamberts SW, Koper JW, et al: Cushing's disease preceded by generalized glucocorticoid resistance: Clinical consequences of a novel, dominant-negative glucocorticoid receptor mutation. Proc Assoc Am Physicians 108:296–307, 1996.
16. Malchoff DM, Brufsky A, Reardon G, et al: A point mutation of the human glucocorticoid receptor in primary cortisol resistance. J Clin Invest 91:1918–1925, 1993.
17. Evans R: The steroid and thyroid hormone receptor superfamily. Science 240:889–895, 1988.
18. French F, Lubahn D, Brown T, et al: Molecular basis of androgen insensitivity. Recent Prog Hormone Res 46:1, 1990.
19. Hughes M, Malloy P, Kieback D, et al: Point mutations in the human vitamin D receptor gene associated with hypocalcemic rickets. Science 242:1702–1705, 1988.
20. Marcelli M, Tiley W, Wilson C, et al: A single nucleotide substitution introduces a premature termination codon into the androgen receptor gene of a patient with receptor-negative androgen resistance. J Clin Invest 85:1522–1528, 1990.
21. Sakurai A, Takeda K, Ain K, et al: Generalized resistance to thyroid hormone associated with a mutation in the ligand-binding domain of the human thyroid hormone receptor b. Proc Natl Acad Sci U S A 86:8977–8981, 1989.
22. Usala SJ, Tennyson GE, Bale AE, et al: A base mutation of the c-*erb*Ab thyroid hormone receptor in a kindred with generalized thyroid hormone resistance. J Clin Invest 85:93–100, 1990.
23. Cole TJ, Blendy JA, Monaghan AP, et al: Targeted disruption of the glucocorticoid receptor gene blocks adrenergic chromaffin cell development and severely retards lung maturation. Genes Dev 9:1608–1621, 1995.
24. Karl M, von Wichert G, Kempter E, et al: Nelson's syndrome associated with a somatic frame shift mutation in the glucocorticoid receptor gene. J Clin Endocrinol Metab 81:124–129, 1996.
25. Huizenga NA, de Lange P, Koper JW, et al: Human adrenocorticotropin-secreting pituitary adenomas show frequent loss of heterozygosity at the glucocorticoid receptor gene locus. J Clin Endocrinol Metab 83:917–921, 1998.
26. Dahia PL, Honegger J, Reincke M, et al: Expression of glucocorticoid receptor gene isoforms in corticotropin-secreting tumors. J Clin Endocrinol Metab 82:1088–1093, 1997.
27. Strasser-Wozak EM, Hattmannstorfer R, Hala M, et al: Splice site mutation in the glucocorticoid receptor gene causes resistance to glucocorticoid-induced apoptosis in a human acute leukemic cell line. Cancer Res 55:348–353, 1995.
28. Hala M, Hartmann BL, Bock G, et al: Glucocorticoid-receptor-gene defects and resistance to glucocorticoid-induced apoptosis in human leukemic cell lines. Int J Cancer 68:663–668, 1996.
29. Sher ER, Leung DY, Surs W, et al: Steroid resistant asthma. Cellular mechanisms contributing to inadequate response to glucocorticoid therapy. J Clin Invest 93:33–39, 1994.
30. Schlaghecke R, Kornely E, Wollenhaupt J, Specker C: Glucocorticoid receptors in rheumatoid arthritis. Arthritis Rheum 35:740–744, 1992.
31. Huizenga NA, Koper JW, de Lange P, et al: A polymorphism in the glucocorticoid receptor gene may be associated with an increased sensitivity to glucocorticoids in vivo. J Clin Endocrinol Metab 83:144–151, 1998.
32. Panarelli M, Holloway CD, Fraser R, et al: Glucocorticoid receptor polymorphism, skin vasoconstriction, and other metabolic intermediate phenotypes in normal human subjects. J Clin Endocrinol Metab 83:1846–1852, 1998.
33. Nyirenda MJ, Lindsay RS, Kenyon CJ, et al: Glucocorticoid exposure in late gestation permanently programs rat hepatic phosphoenolpyruvate carboxykinase and glucocorticoid receptor expression and causes glucose intolerance in adult offspring. J Clin Invest 101:2174–2181, 1998.
34. Guo WX, Antakly T, Cadotte M, et al: Expression and cytokine regulation of glucocorticoid receptors in Kaposi's sarcoma. Am J Pathol 148:1999–2008, 1996.
35. Refaeli Y, Levy DN, Weiner DB: The glucocorticoid receptor type II complex is a target of the HIV-1 *vpr* gene product. Proc Natl Acad Sci U S A 92:3621–3625, 1995.
36. Norbiato G, Bevilacqua M, Vago T, Clerici M: Glucocorticoids and interferon-alpha in the acquired immunodeficiency syndrome. J Clin Endocrinol Metab 81:2601–2606, 1996.
37. Rivest R, Schulz P, Lustenberger S, Sizonenko P: Differences between circadian and ultradian organization of cortisol and melatonin rhythms during activity and rest. J Clin Endocrinol Metab 68:721–729, 1989.
38. Van Cauter E, Refetoff S: Evidence for two subtypes of Cushing's disease based on the analysis of episodic cortisol secretion. N Engl J Med 312:1343–1349, 1985.
39. Malchoff CD, Reardon G, Javier EC, et al: Dexamethasone therapy for isosexual precocious pseudopuberty caused by generalized glucocorticoid resistance. J Clin Endocrinol Metab 79:1632–1636, 1994.
40. Berkovitz GD, Carter KM, Levine MA, Migeon CJ: Abnormal induction of aromatase activity by dexamethasone in fibroblasts from a patient with cortisol resistance. J Clin Endocrinol Metab 70:1608–1611, 1990.
41. McPhaul M, Marcelli M, Zoppi S, et al: Mutations in the ligand-binding domain of the androgen receptor gene cluster in two regions of the gene. J Clin Invest 90:2097–2101, 1992.
42. Koper JW, Stolk RP, de Lange P, et al: Lack of association between five polymorphisms in the human glucocorticoid receptor gene and glucocorticoid resistance. Hum Genet 99:663–668, 1997.
43. Besser G, Edwards C: Cushing's Syndrome. Clin Endocrinol Metab 1:451–490, 1972.
44. Perini G, Devinsky O, Hauser P, et al: Effects of carbamazepine on pituitary-adrenal function in health volunteers. J Clin Endocrinol Metab 74:406–412, 1992.
45. Kontula K, Pelkonen R, Andersson L, Sivula A: Glucocorticoid receptors in adrenocorticoid disorders. J Clin Endocrinol Metab 51:654–657, 1980.
46. Norbiato G, Bevilacqua M, Vago T, et al: Cortisol resistance in acquired immunodeficiency syndrome. J Clin Endocrinol Metab 74:608–613, 1992.
47. Karl M, Arai K, Stratakis CA, et al: Molecular studies of the glucocorticoid receptor in patients with generalized glucocorticoid resistance and steroid resistant asthma. Presented at the 77th Annual Meeting of the Endocrine Society, Washington, DC, pp 3–55.
48. Lipsett M, Tomita M, Brandon D, et al: Cortisol resistance in man. Adv Exp Med Biol 196:97–110, 1986.

Chapter 123

Defects of Adrenal Steroidogenesis

Michael P. Wajnrajch ▪ Maria I. New

The human adrenal gland is composed of the cortex and the medulla. Whereas the medulla produces bioamines, the adrenal cortex secretes several classes of steroids (corticosteroids). The adrenal cortex can be considered to be made up of three distinct subunits, each having a characteristic steroid profile. The outermost unit, the zona glomerulosa, produces mineralocorticoids, principally aldosterone, that serve to maintain sodium and fluid balance. Glucocorticoids, primarily cortisol, arise from the central zona fasciculata and maintain glucose homeostasis and vascular integrity. The innermost subunit, the zona reticularis, secretes sex steroids (androgens). Disorders of adrenal steroidogenesis may involve overproduction, underproduction, or simultaneous overproduction and underproduction of corticosteroids (Fig. 123–1). The following conditions will be discussed:

1. Disorders of P-450c21 resulting in the 21-hydroxylase deficiency form of congenital adrenal hyperplasia (CAH) (salt-wasting, simple virilizing, and nonclassic forms)
2. Disorders of P-450c11, including
   A. 11β-Hydroxylase deficiency form of CAH (classic and nonclassic forms)
   B. Corticosterone methyl oxidase type I and type II (CMOI/CMOII) deficiency
   C. Dexamethasone-suppressible hyperaldosteronism (DSH)
3. 3β-Hydroxysteroid dehydogenase (3β-HSD) deficiency form of CAH (classic and nonclassic forms)
4. Disorders of P-450c17 activity, including
   A. Isolated 17α-hydroxylase deficiency
   B. Isolated 17,20-lyase deficiency
   C. Combined 17α-hydroxylase deficiency/17,20-lyase deficiency
5. Lipoid CAH

A summary of the clinical and hormonal features of these steroidogenic defects appears in Table 123–1.

The most common adrenal steroidogenic defects are those related to cortisol production and are collectively referred to as the *congenital adrenal hyperplasias*. These defects are transmitted as autosomal recessive traits, and the genetic errors causing them have been described. Loss of negative feedback inhibition of the hypothalamic-pituitary-adrenal axis by cortisol induces oversecretion of adrenocorticotropic hormone (ACTH) by the anterior pituitary and subsequent adrenocortical hyperplasia. The specific forms of CAH are defined by the abnormal patterns of glucocorticoid, mineralocorticoid, and sex steroid secretion and accompanying clinical manifestations, including abnormal fetal genital development, disturbances in sodium and potassium homeostasis and blood pressure regulation, and postnatal consequences of sex steroid imbalance affecting somatic growth and fertility. Lifelong, carefully monitored treatment with glucocorticoids and salt-retaining steroids can afford many patients with CAH relatively normal lives despite their potentially life-threatening metabolic defects. However, it is not yet possible to ensure normal hormonal levels throughout the day, ultimate normal stature, and fertility. Prenatal diagnosis can be of significant importance in case management by allowing the opportunity for prenatal treatment.

Distinction is made between classic forms of disease, defined by significantly reduced enzyme activity manifested clinically at birth, and nonclassic forms, in which the enzyme defect is less severe, symptoms are not present at birth, and when they do appear, the symptoms are generally milder. The classification of CAH subtypes has significant clinical implications for treatment and prenatal diagnosis, but it should be appreciated that patients exist on a clinical spectrum rather than within absolute, distinct, easily defined conditions. By far the greatest number of cases of classic CAH are due to 21-hydroxylase deficiency,[1] and defects in the enzymes 11β-hydroxylase and 3β-HSD account for almost all the rest. 17α-Hydroxylase deficiency and lipoid CAH are very rare.

The 21-hydroxylase and 11β-hydroxylase deficiencies, which occur late in cortisol synthesis, cause a shunting of accumulated precursor steroids into the pathways of androgen biosynthesis, which do not require these enzymes. Because the external genitalia of the fetus are sensitive to androgens,[2] the excess androgen secretion of the adrenal masculinizes the female genitalia and causes genital ambiguity in affected females, but no genital alterations in affected males. Postnatal hyperandrogenism affects both sexes.

Imbalances in salt metabolism and fluid volume are part of what differentiates one form from another. In 21-hydroxylase deficiency, deficient aldosterone synthesis causes salt-wasting and hypovolemia, whereas in 11β-hydroxylase deficiency, excess of mineralocorticoids (e.g., deoxycorticosterone [DOC]) causes expanded fluid volume and hypertension. The nonclassic forms of 21-hydroxylase and 11β-hydroxylase deficiency do not cause severe hypertension or masculinized genitalia in newborn females.

The 3β-HSD defect is characterized by poor conversion of Δ^5 to Δ^4 steroids. The Δ^5 steroid precursors are relatively inactive, but the

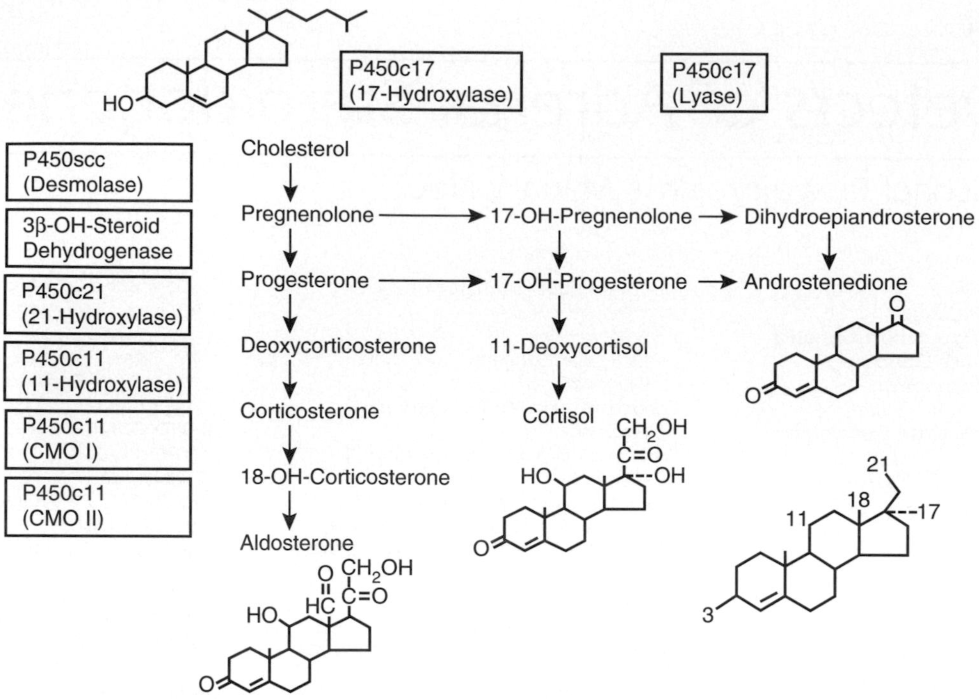

P450c17 (17-Hydroxylase)
P450c17 (Lyase)
P450scc (Desmolase)
3β-OH-Steroid Dehydrogenase
P450c21 (21-Hydroxylase)
P450c11 (11-Hydroxylase)
P450c11 (CMO I)
P450c11 (CMO II)
Cholesterol
Pregnenolone → 17-OH-Pregnenolone → Dihydroepiandrosterone
Progesterone → 17-OH-Progesterone → Androstenedione
Deoxycorticosterone
11-Deoxycortisol
Corticosterone
Cortisol
18-OH-Corticosterone
Aldosterone

FIGURE 123–1. Adrenal steroidogenesis. Biosynthetic pathways from cholesterol to mineralocorticoids (aldosterone), glucocorticoids (cortisol), and androgens (androstenedione) are shown and the cellular location of enzyme activities indicated. HSD, hydroxysteroid dehydrogenase; OH, hydroxylase. (Reprinted, by permission, from White PC, New MI, Dupont B: Medical progress: Congenital adrenal hyperplasia. N Engl J Med 316:1519–1524, 1987. Copyright © 1987 Massachusetts Medical Society. All rights reserved.)

defective cortisol and aldosterone synthesis causes profound salt-wasting. Whereas lack of potent Δ^4 androgens produces hypovirilization in males, enormously high levels of relatively inactive Δ^5 androgens, which are converted peripherally to active Δ^4 steroids, may cause masculinization of the external genitalia in females.

The nonclassic forms of 21-hydroxylase, 11β-hydroxylase, and 3β-HSD deficiencies may be extremely common (and treatable) causes of hyperandrogenism.

In 17α-hydroxylase/17,20-lyase deficiency, blocked production of both 17α-hydroxy (glucocorticoid) and C-19/C-18 (sex) steroids causes pseudohermaphroditism in males and sexual infantilism in females. Shunting of 17α-hydroxylase precursor steroids into the 17-deoxy pathway produces excess mineralocorticoids (e.g., DOC) and hypertension. Isolated 17α-hydroxylase deficiency prevents the conversion of mineralocorticoids to glucocorticoids, whereas isolated 17,20-lyase deficiency is a variant of 17α-hydroxylase deficiency in which only androgen synthesis is disturbed and glucocorticoid and mineralocorticoid levels are relatively unaffected.

Lipoid CAH is manifested as an inability to produce any of the steroid products of cholesterol. Accordingly, affected individuals are aldosterone, cortisol, and sex steroid deficient. All affected individuals are phenotypic females, regardless of the genetic sex.

HISTORY

The observation of hyperplastic adrenal glands in association with internal female gonads and ductal structures in a phenotypic male appeared in the anatomic literature in 1865 with De Crecchio's description of his autopsy of a Neapolitan pseudohermaphrodite.[3] Fibiger,[4] Apert,[5] and Gallais[6] amassed case histories involving precocious puberty, hirsutism, pseudohermaphroditism, and obesity early in this century and attempted to classify them. The term *adrenogenital syndrome* was used for many years to describe conditions characterized by elevated adrenal androgens caused by either virilizing adrenal tumors or CAH.

The first comprehensive view of CAH was based on the biochemical discoveries of the 1940s and 1950s.[7] Among the pioneers who subsequently characterized the variants of CAH in the late 1950s and early 1960s were Bongiovanni and Eberlein,[8–10] Prader and Siebenmann,[11] Biglieri et al.,[12] and New.[13] CAH is now more appropriately referred to by the names of the specific deficiencies that characterize them.

In 1977, discovery of the association between the well-studied human leukocyte antigens (HLA) and 21-hydroxylase trait opened a window to a new form of definition of CAH through molecular genetics.[14] Since isolation of the gene responsible for classic 21-hydroxylase deficiency (found within the HLA complex) in 1984,[15] knowledge of the specific mutations that cause the different forms of CAH has grown rapidly, much the way that the biochemical discoveries of the earlier era led to construction of the scheme for steroidogenesis. Mutations in the genes encoding the steroidogenic enzymes have been confirmed as the basis of all but one of the forms of CAH. The sole exception, congenital lipoid adrenal hyperplasia, has been shown to be due to mutations in the steroidogenic acute regulatory (StAR) protein[16] and not, as previously believed, the cholesterol desmolase enzyme (also known as the cholesterol side chain cleavage enzyme, P-450scc). Notably, in rabbits, congenital lipoid adrenal hyperplasia has been shown to be due to mutations in the cholesterol desmolase gene.[16]

Evidence is accumulating that correlation between clinical expression of endocrine disease and mutations of the primary structural gene is not perfect. Thus, the role of the clinician in ascertaining physiologic facts remains central to the prospect of future growth in our understanding of the pathogenesis of CAH and the basis for its treatment.

21-HYDROXYLASE DEFICIENCY

The three clinically identified expressions of 21-hydroxylase deficiency are classic simple virilizing with manifestations of excess androgen secretion; classic salt-wasting, which is characterized by aldosterone deficiency in addition to excess androgen secretion because of the 21-hydroxylase defect in the parallel mineralocorticoid pathway in the zona glomerulosa; and nonclassic simple virilizing, a less severe hyperandrogenic, variably expressed, and allelically distinct form of the disease.

TABLE 123–1. Clinical and Hormonal Features of Certain Steroidogenic Defects

Condition	Onset	Abnormality	Genitalia	Mineralocorticoid Effect	Typical Features	Gene
Lipoid CAH	Congenital	StAR protein	Female, with no future sexual development	Salt-wasting	All steroid products low	*StAR,* 8p11.2
3β-HSD deficiency, classic	Congenital	3β-HSD	Females virilized, males hypovirilized	Salt-wasting	Elevated DHEA, 17-pregnenolone; low androstenedione, testosterone; elevated K; low Na, CO_2	*HSD3B2,* 1p13.1
3β-HSD deficiency, nonclassic	Postnatal	3β-HSD	Normal genitalia with mild to moderate hyperandrogenism postnatally	None	Elevated DHEA, 17-pregnenolone; low androstenedione, testosterone	—
17α-OH deficiency	Congenital	P-450c17	All phenotypic female, with no future sexual development	Low-renin hypertension	Absent androgens and estrogen; elevated DOC, corticosterone	*CYP17,* 10q24.3
17,20-Lyase deficiency	Congenital	P-450c17	All phenotypic female, with no future sexual development	None	Decreased androgens and estrogen	*CYP17,* 10q24.3
21-OH deficiency, classic, salt-wasting	Congenital	P-450c21	Females prenatally virilized, males unchanged	Salt-wasting	Elevated 17-OHP, DHEA, and androstenedione; elevated K; low Na, CO_2	*CYP21,* 6p21.3
21-OH deficiency, classic, simple, virilizing	Congenital	P-450c21	Females prenatally virilized, males unchanged	None	Elevated 17-OHP, DHEA, and androstenedione; normal electrolytes	*CYP21,* 6p21.3
21-OH deficiency, nonclassic	Postnatal	P-450c21	All with normal genitalia at birth, hyperandrogenism postnatally	None	Elevated 17-OHP, DHEA, and androstenedione upon ACTH stimulation	*CYP21,* 6p21.3
11β-OH deficiency, classic CAH	Congenital	P-450c11B1	Females virilized, males unchanged	Low-renin hypertension	Elevated DOC, 11-deoxycortisol (S) and androgens; low K; elevated Na, CO_2	*CYP11B1,* 8q24.3
11β-OH deficiency, nonclassic CAH	Postnatal	P-450c11B1	All with normal genitalia at birth, hyperandrogenism postnatally	Normal	Elevated 11-deoxycortisol ± DOC, elevated androgens	*CYP11B1,* 8q24.3
CMO I deficiency	Congenital	P-450c11B2	All normal	Severe salt-wasting	No aldosterone, low-normal 18-OH-corticosterone, elevated K, low Na and CO_2	*CYP11B2,* 8q24.3
CMO II deficiency	Congenital	P-450c11B2	All normal	Mild salt-wasting, especially in infancy with spontaneous resolution	Low-normal aldosterone, very elevated 18-OH-corticosterone, elevated K, low Na and CO_2	*CYP11B2,* 8q24.3
Dexamethasone-suppressible hyper-aldosteronism	Congenital	Chimeric P-450c11B1/P-450c11B2	All normal	Low-renin hypertension	Elevated aldosterone; elevated NA, CO_2; low K	*CYP11B1/CYP11B2,* 8q24.3

ACTH, adrenocorticotropic hormone; CAH, congenital adrenal hyperplasia; CMO, corticosterone methyl oxidase; DHEA, dehydroepiandrosterone; DOC, deoxycorticosterone; HSD, hydroxysteroid dehydroxylase; OHP, hydroxyprogesterone; StAR, steroidogenic acute regulatory protein.

The result of 21-hydroxylase deficiency is that 17-hydroxyprogesterone (17-OHP) is not converted to 11-deoxycortisol (compound S) in the pathway of cortisol synthesis, which results in (1) deficiency of the essential glucocorticoid cortisol (compound F) and (2) overproduction and accumulation of cortisol precursors proximal to the 21-hydroxylation step (17-OHP, progesterone, 17-hydroxypregnenolone, and pregnenolone) as a result of the loss of normal feedback regulation on the hypothalamus and pituitary. The 17-hydroxylated precursors are converted to the adrenal androgens dehydroepiandrosterone (DHEA), Δ^4-androstenedione, and testosterone in the zona fasciculata.

Epidemiology and Population Genetics

The results of newborn screening in a number of localities around the world yield a worldwide incidence of classic 21-hydroxylase deficiency of approximately 1 in 14,500 live births.[17–21] It has been estimated that 75% have the salt-wasting phenotype.[22] Applying the Hardy-Weinberg formula for a population at equilibrium gives a computed heterozygote frequency for classic 21-hydroxylase deficiency of 1 in 61 persons.

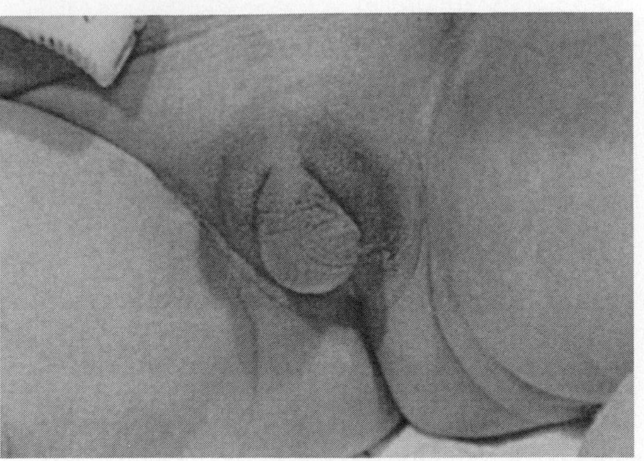

FIGURE 123–2. Ambiguous genitalia in a newborn female with congenital adrenal hyperplasia caused by 21-hydroxylase deficiency. Note the enlarged clitoris, single orifice on the perineum, and scrotalization of the labia majora. (From New MI, Levine LS: Congenital adrenal hyperplasia. *In* Harris H, Hirschhorn K (eds): Advances in Human Genetics, vol 4. New York, Plenum, 1973, pp 251–326.)

Nonclassic 21-hydroxylase deficiency is one of the most common autosomal recessive diseases, more frequent than cystic fibrosis. The frequency is ethnic specific, as first determined by Speiser et al.[23] Incidences are 1 in 27 Ashkenazi Jews, 1 in 40 Hispanics, 1 in 50 Yugoslavs, 1 in 300 Italians, and 1 in 100 in a heterogeneous New York population.[23–25] In an attempt to determine the earliest date of appearance of a founder mutation within the Ashkenazi Jewish population, DNA analysis was undertaken in representative individuals from the Roman Jewish ghetto, a community already established by the time of the second Diaspora (70 Common Era [CE]). No evidence of the B14-related nonclassic 21-hydroxylase deficiency mutation was seen in the Roman Jews, thus suggesting a date after 70 CE for the appearance of this mutation among Ashkenazi Jews.[26] Further genetic characterization of this population concerning its affinity to both the general European population and other Jewish groups continues.[27] The nonclassic 21-hydroxylase deficiency mutation can be dated to between 70 CE and the second millennium based on a high frequency in Ashkenazi Jews that is not found in Sephardic Jews.

Classic 21-Hydroxylase Deficiency

Effects of Hyperandrogenism

EXTERNAL GENITALIA. Adrenocortical cell differentiation occurs early in embryogenesis, and although the biochemical schedule of steroid synthesis has not been completely elucidated, it is clear that genital development in the fetus takes place in the setting of active fetal adrenal steroid synthesis. Because differentiation of the external genitalia is sensitive to androgen, excess adrenal androgen produces genital ambiguity in females affected with classic 21-hydroxylase deficiency. In utero masculinization consists of mild to pronounced clitoral enlargement, varying degrees of labioscrotal fusion, and a urogenital sinus with the type and degree of virilization proportional to the onset and degree of hyperandrogenism (Figs. 123–2 and 123–3). The 21-hydroxylase form of congenital adrenal hyperplasia is the most common cause of genital ambiguity in females. **Every phenotypic male with hypospadias and bilateral cryptorchidism should be considered a female with CAH and immediately evaluated for classic 21-hydroxylase deficiency.**

Although differentiation of male genitalia in utero is not affected, the genitalia of infants of both sexes undergo androgen-stimulated growth postnatally. High testosterone levels—of adrenal origin—cause gonadotropin suppression, which results in the characteristic finding of a large penis and small testes in older boys. Hyperpigmentation of the genitalia of both males and females can also result from high ACTH secretion.

INTERNAL GENITALIA. Gonadal differentiation and internal genital morphogenesis are not affected by the enzyme abnormalities of classic steroid 21-hydroxylase deficiency. Because anomalous secretion of antimüllerian hormone (which is synthesized by the Sertoli cells of the fetal testis) is not a factor, müllerian duct development in the female proceeds normally into the uterus and fallopian tubes.[28] Thus, high normal child-bearing capacity exists in females. Wolffian duct stabilization and differentiation normally take place in the context of *local* testosterone levels in the male, and this process appears to be unaffected by elevated prenatal adrenal androgens.

GROWTH. Postnatal somatic growth in both sexes is markedly affected by the chronic hyperandrogenism of untreated 21-hydroxylase deficiency. High levels of androgens cause accelerated growth in early childhood and produce an unusually tall and often quite muscular child, an "infant Hercules" (Fig. 123–4). This early growth spurt, however, is followed by premature epiphyseal maturation and closure and ultimately a final height that is short relative to that expected on the basis of the midparental target height. Exposure to glucocorticoids used in replacement therapy at dosages that may exceed the physiologic requirement has been postulated to be another important factor in the poor growth of these patients.[29]

We have previously shown that final height is one of the features of CAH least amenable to replacement therapy.[30] Analysis of 47 patients with classic CAH separated into two groups defined by the degree of hormonal control failed to show a significant difference in height outcome with standard treatment.[31] We have recently initiated a pilot study at the New York Presbyterian Hospital–Weill Medical

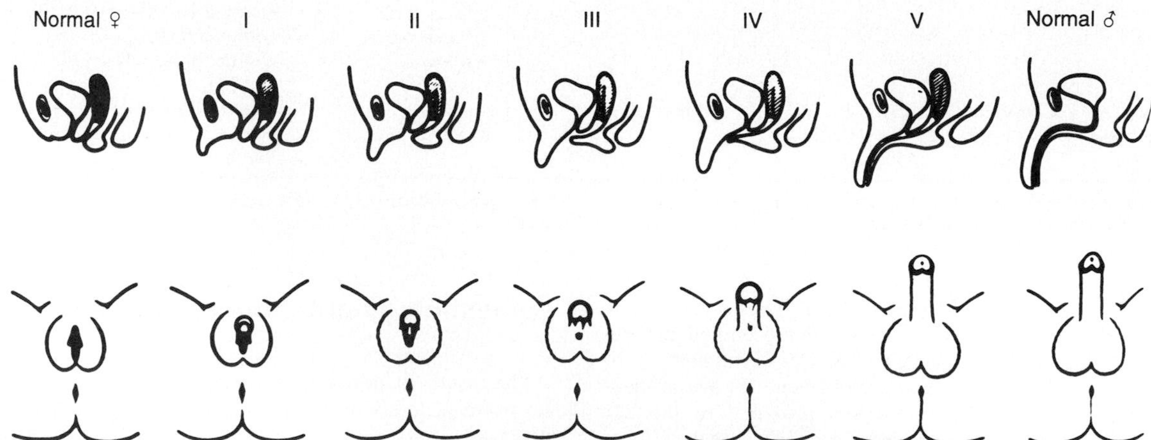

FIGURE 123–3. Prader characterization of the range of genital malformations found in females with classic 21-hydroxylase deficiency. In type I the only abnormality is enlargement of the clitoris, type II is characterized by partial labioscrotal fusion, in type III a funnel-shaped urogenital sinus is seen at the posterior end of a small vulva, in type IV a very small urogenital sinus is found at the base of an enlarged phallus, and in type V is seen a penile urethra. (From Prader A: Die haufigkeit der kongenitalen adrenogenitalen syndromes. Helv Paediatr Acta 13:5, 1958.)

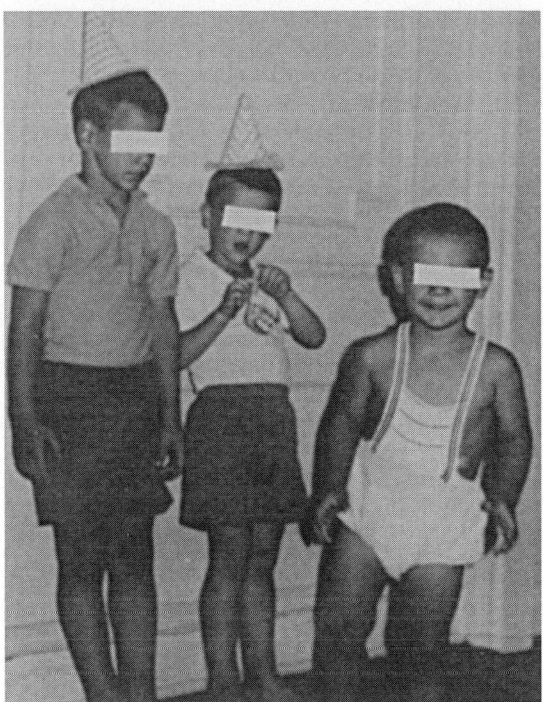

FIGURE 123–4. Untreated congenital adrenal hyperplasia in two brothers: a 4-year-old on the left and a 2-year-old on the right. In the center is their normal 6-year-old brother. (From New MI, Levine LS: Congenital adrenal hyperplasia. *In* Harris H, Hirschhorn K (eds): Advances in Human Genetics, vol 4. New York, Plenum, 1973, pp 251–326.)

College of Cornell University in which growth hormone is being combined with a gonadotropin releasing hormone superagonist to improve final height in patients with CAH, advanced skeletal maturation, and poor predicted final adult height; preliminary results are very encouraging.

HAIR AND SKIN GLAND ABNORMALITIES. Facial, axillary, and pubic hair appear very early; pubarche sometimes occurs in infancy. Adult body odor in children, temporal balding, and severe acne are other typical features reversible with treatment.

FERTILITY. Excess adrenal sex steroids inhibit the pubertal changes in gonadotropin secretion directed by the hypothalamic-pituitary axis, probably via a negative feedback effect at the hypothalamus or the pituitary. This inhibition is reversible by suppression of adrenal androgen production. In most untreated or poorly treated adolescent girls and in some adolescent boys, spontaneous pubertal development does not occur until proper glucocorticoid treatment is instituted. Menstrual irregularity and secondary or even primary amenorrhea with or without hirsutism can occur in poorly treated women. Virilizing CAH has also been associated with polycystic ovary syndrome.[32] Poor control of the disease in males with classic CAH has been associated with small testes and azoospermia. Cases of normal testicular maturation, spermatogenesis, and fertility in untreated men, however, have also been reported.[33]

In most well-treated patients, the onset of puberty occurs at the expected chronologic age. The gonadotropin response to gonadotropin-releasing hormone (or luteinizing hormone–releasing hormone) is appropriate for age in well-controlled prepubertal and pubertal female patients unless ovarian disease is present. Treated males are normally fertile and have normal pubertal development, spermatogenesis, and testicular function. Later in life, nodular hyperplasia of adrenal rest tissue may develop and cause enlargement of the testes. This enlargement may respond to high-dose glucocorticoid treatment.

The limits of reproductive capacity in females with classic CAH are not fully known. Fertility is reduced in women with salt-wasting CAH,[34] with only rare reports of pregnancy.[35, 36]

Salt-Wasting

Salt-wasting is characterized by hyponatremia and hyperkalemia, inappropriate sodium excretion in the urine, and low serum aldosterone with concomitantly high plasma renin activity (PRA).

Salt-wasting results from inadequate secretion of salt-retaining steroids, especially aldosterone. In addition, hormone precursors elevated in 21-hydroxylase deficiency may act as mineralocorticoid antagonists (e.g., 17-OHP). Newborns are especially prone to the development of salt-wasting crisis because the sodium-conserving mechanism of their renal tubules is only marginally competent.

Current understanding is that a single enzyme is responsible for 21-hydroxylation in both the zona fasciculata and zona glomerulosa. The pathogenetic difference between salt-wasting and simple virilizing 21-hydroxylase deficiency may merely be the result of a quantitative difference in enzyme activity caused by conformational changes induced by the specific mutations. In vitro expression studies show that as little as 1% of the normal activity of 21-hydroxylase allows adequate aldosterone synthesis to prevent significant salt-wasting.[37, 38] The issue is complicated by the occasional finding of discordance in salt-wasting expression among siblings with identical mutations in their inherited 21-hydroxylase genes and by observed improvement in salt-wasting in some individuals over time.[39–42] In one case, a girl born with male genitalia and salt-wasting, presumably with severe enzyme deficiency, was no longer a salt-waster by age 4. Another important case finding was that of a girl with homozygous deletion of the 21-hydroxylase gene and a history of multiple salt-wasting crises in infancy who discontinued her therapy in adolescence and was found at that time to be secreting aldosterone.[43]

SALT-WASTING CRISIS. Infants of both sexes with classic CAH are at risk for a hypovolemic and hypoglycemic adrenal crisis, typically occurring within the first 4 to 6 weeks of life. Undiagnosed males, who lack the genital ambiguity that usually calls attention to the condition in a newborn female, are at added risk for shock and death, as evidenced by the higher female-to-male ratio of salt-wasting adults. In females, the degree of genital ambiguity in a newborn does not indicate the likelihood or potential for salt-wasting. Thus, surveillance of infants of both sexes in the newborn period for incipient adrenal crisis is essential, and it should continue on a close basis after discharge from the hospital. Infants should remain in the hospital after birth for about 7 days or until the aldosterone/sodium balance status has been established, although it should be stressed that the first salt-wasting crisis may not occur for several months. In older children and adults, acute adrenal insufficiency can be precipitated by physical exertion or emotional stress, undertreatment, or noncompliance with therapy or be a result of immunization, infection, trauma, or surgery. The salt-wasting crisis of the newborn period associated with CAH is often confused with pyloric stenosis, which may occur at the same age and is also often manifested as an ill-appearing newborn with vomiting and dehydration. The salt-wasting crisis associated with CAH (manifested as hyponatremia, hyperkalemia, and metabolic acidosis) should immediately be differentiated from that of pyloric stenosis (hypokalemia, hypochloremia, and metabolic alkalosis) by routine biochemical tests.

Nonclassic 21-Hydroxylase Deficiency

Nonclassic 21-hydroxylase deficiency is distinguished from the classic form symptomatically by its age of onset and biochemically by its less severe impairment of steroid 21-hydroxylation; because of these two factors, it does not result in ambiguous genitalia in newborn females. It is often initially manifested just before the age of normal puberty, although it may appear at any age after birth. Patients may be homozygous for a mild genetic defect or be compound heterozygous for one severe mutation and one mild mutation. Nonclassic 21-hydroxylase deficiency was first defined in the course of family studies of patients with classic CAH. Family members who should have been carriers for 21-hydroxylase deficiency were found to have overt hormonal disturbances that were associated with distinct alleles at the

21-hydroxylase locus. These alleles were determined to be in linkage disequilibrium with the HLA locus on chromosome 6. It was found through these studies that the gene locus for 21-hydroxylase lies between HLA-B and HLA-DR.[44]

In addition to linkage of the 21-hydroxylase locus with the neighboring HLA-B and HLA-DR antigen loci, 21-hydroxylase deficiency alleles are found in linkage disequilibrium with other HLA genes or haplotypic combinations that may include specific alleles of the neighboring genes *C4A* and *C4B* encoding the fourth component of serum complement.[45] The two most prominent such cases are linkage disequilibrium of the extended haplotype HLA-A3, Bw47, DR7 with the classic salt-wasting form and HLA-B14, DR1 with nonclassic 21-hydroxylase deficiency.[46]

Clinical Features

The clinical features of nonclassic 21-hydroxylase deficiency vary widely, begin at any age, and commonly wax and wane over time. Although genital ambiguity in the newborn period is never a feature of this disorder, appearance of any of the other signs and symptoms of hyperandrogenism can prompt the patient to seek medical attention, or patients may be identified through family or population screening. Individuals are commonly evaluated for the first time just before the time of expected pubarche. Underlying biochemical abnormalities are always demonstrable by ACTH stimulation testing, regardless of whether symptoms are evident.[47]

Nonclassic 21-hydroxylase deficiency can result in premature development of pubic hair (pubarche), which has occurred as early as 6 months of age.[48] In one study, nonclassic 21-hydroxylase deficiency was found in 30% of children with premature pubarche,[49] whereas a lower prevalence was reported by another group.[50] Severe cystic acne refractory to oral antibiotics and retinoic acid has been associated with nonclassic 21-hydroxylase deficiency by some.[51, 52] In one young woman, male pattern baldness was the sole initial symptom. Menarche in females can be normal or delayed, and secondary amenorrhea or oligomenorrhea is frequent. Final height, as in classic 21-hydroxylase deficiency, is less than predicted on the basis of midparental target height and linear growth percentiles, even though excess androgen secretion may not have been apparent.[31]

A number of women with polycystic ovary disease are found, upon ACTH testing, to have a primary adrenal defect such as nonclassic 21-hydroxylase deficiency, 3β-HSD deficiency, or 11β-hydroxylase deficiency.[53–57] The reported prevalence of nonclassic 21-hydroxylase deficiency as an etiology of these endocrine symptoms in women ranges from 1.2% to 30%. The scope of the range may relate to differences in the ethnic makeup of the groups studied.

In boys, initial signs include early beard growth, pubarche, acne, and an accelerated growth spurt. In men, signs of androgen excess are difficult to perceive, and the manifestations of adrenal androgen excess may be limited to short stature or oligospermia and diminished fertility from adrenal sex steroid–induced gonadal suppression.

Fertility in Nonclassic 21-Hydroxylase Deficiency

It has been recognized for some 30 years that infertility in women may be reversed by glucocorticoid therapy. In one report, 5 patients with irregular menses and high 17-keto(oxo)steroid levels resumed regular menses and demonstrated adequate suppression of 17-ketosteroids and pregnanetriol within 2 months of beginning therapy with glucocorticoids alone, thus suggesting the presence of an adrenal 21-hydroxylating defect.[58] In another report of 18 infertile women with acne and/or facial hirsutism and hormonal criteria consistent with 21-hydroxylase deficiency, 7 conceived shortly after initiating prednisone treatment alone; an additional 4 women conceived within 2 months of the addition of clomiphene to the therapeutic regimen.[59] Hormonal profiles after the initiation of therapy were not reported in this study. As mentioned earlier, oligospermia and subfertility have been reported in men with nonclassic 21-hydroxylase deficiency.[60] We recommend screening for nonclassic 21-hydroxylase deficiency in the evaluation of infertility.

Molecular Genetics

The molecular genetic basis of 21-hydroxylase deficiency has been studied extensively. The 21-hydroxylase enzyme is a microsomal cytochrome P-450 enzyme termed P-450c21. The structural gene encoding P-450c21, *CYP21*, and a pseudogene, *CYP21P*, are located on chromosome 6p21.3, adjacent to the genes *C4B* and *C4A*, which encode the two isoforms of the fourth component of serum complement in the class III region of the HLA complex.[61, 62] *CYP21* and *CYP21P* each contain 10 exons. Their nucleotide sequences are 98% identical in exons and about 96% identical in introns.[63]

Many of the mutations known to cause 21-hydroxylase deficiency are apparently the result of either of two types of recombination between *CYP21* and *CYP21P*: (1) chromatid misalignment and unequal crossing over resulting in large-scale DNA deletions and (2) gene conversion events that result in the transfer to *CYP21* of smaller-scale deleterious mutations normally present in the *CYP21P* pseudogene. Seven of the 8 possible exonic differences between *CYP21* and *CYP21P* have been observed and confirmed to be causative of 21-hydroxylase deficiency. At least 25 mutations causing 21-hydroxylase have been identified; 1 single nucleotide mutation altering the splicing of an intron is particularly common and is associated with both the simple virilizing and salt-wasting phenotypes (Fig. 123–5).

Correlation of Genotype with Phenotype

In general, the functional consequence of each DNA alteration corresponds with the clinical severity of the inherited disease: total deletion of the functional gene, stop codon (nonsense) mutations, frameshifts, and several amino acid substitutions (missense mutations) have been shown to result in salt-wasting classic alleles; one nonconservative amino acid substitution has been exclusively associated with simple virilizing disease; and a single conservative amino acid substitution (V281L) is the mutation associated with the HLA-B14, DR1 haplotype found so frequently in nonclassic disease.[64]

However, comparison of the clinical characteristics and molecular genetic data at the New York Presbyterian Hospital–Weill Medical College of Cornell University in 532 affected individuals reveals that the genotype correctly predicts the phenotype in 89% of cases—a high figure but significantly shy of the 100% that might be expected. This analysis underlines the need for careful ongoing clinical assessment of all persons affected with 21-hydroxylase deficiency (unpublished data from Weill Medical College Children's Clinical Research Center).

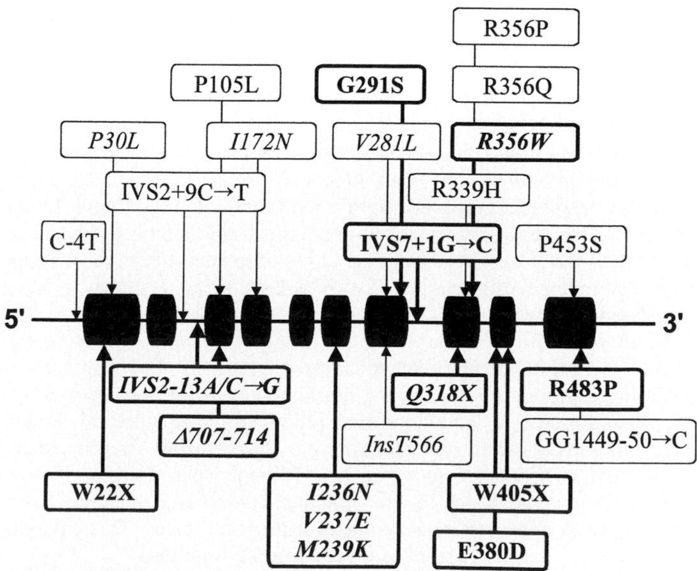

FIGURE 123–5. Mutations in the *CYP21* gene causing the 21-hydroxylase deficiency form of congenital adrenal hyperplasia. Classic alleles are printed in bold and nonclassic in standard print, whereas mutations arising from conversion events are printed in italics.

Diagnosis

Differential Diagnosis

The differential diagnosis of steroidogenic enzyme defects in CAH is made on the basis of (1) clinical findings, (2) biochemical and hormonal values, and (3) molecular genetic analysis of mutations. Hormonal values will establish the diagnosis of an enzyme defect by demonstrating an increased precursor-product ratio. The substrate of the enzyme will be markedly increased, whereas the product will be normal or slightly decreased. Molecular genetic analysis of the DNA will demonstrate the specific mutations.

Biochemical Characterization

In classic CAH, baseline serum cortisol levels are at the lower limits of detection or in the low-normal range. Baseline concentrations of serum 17-OHP and adrenal androgens are elevated, with serum 17-OHP levels often several hundred times normal.[65] In nonclassically affected persons, because of pulsatile and diurnal variations in 17-OHP secretion, midmorning and afternoon concentrations may be normal.[66] Of all single measurements, early morning measurement of the serum 17-OHP concentration is the most likely to show an elevation. However, we caution against relying on baseline 17-OHP levels to exclude nonclassic 21-hydroxylase deficiency; mild defects may be associated with only minimally elevated levels—especially in the afternoon—and lead to many false-negative diagnoses.

The standard procedure for diagnosing all forms of CAH is the 60-minute (synthetic) ACTH stimulation test. At 8 AM, when cortisol secretion is at its normal diurnal peak, blood is drawn before and then 60 minutes after intravenous injection of a 0.25-mg bolus of ACTH. A nomogram (Fig. 123–6) that relates baseline to ACTH-stimulated serum concentrations of 17-OHP has been constructed and can be used to identify individuals with classic and nonclassic as well as heterozygote carriers of the 21-hydroxylase deficiency form of CAH.

Neonatal screening via heel-stick capillary blood has been available since 1977[67] and is mandated in several states. The 17-OHP content of the dried blood, which is sampled on filter paper, analogous to the phenylketonuria test standard for all newborns, can be determined by a qualified laboratory.

The 8 AM salivary level of 17-OHP correlates extremely well with serum assays and is highly recommended as a screening test.[66] It is especially useful when venipuncture is difficult.

Diagnosis at Birth

The following data should be collected when evaluating a newborn with possible CAH:

1. Karyotype or other genetic analysis to establish the genetic sex in cases of ambiguous genitalia.
2. ACTH stimulation test with the serum 17-OHP concentration measured before and after ACTH stimulation. *This test should* **not** *be performed during the initial 24 hours of life* because samples from this period are typically elevated in all infants and may yield false-positive results.
3. Aldosterone and plasma renin levels during the ACTH test.
4. Urinary sodium and potassium to assess salt-preserving ability.
5. Evidence of suppression of steroid secretion by glucocorticoid administration.

Further characterization of DNA by molecular genetic analysis is desirable where available.

DISORDERS OF 11β-HYDROXYLASE ACTIVITY

Steroid 11β-hydroxylase activity in the adrenal cortex is required for the synthesis of both glucocorticoids and mineralocorticoids. It has been shown that distinct isozymes of P-450c11 participate in cortisol and aldosterone synthesis in humans. The two isozymes of 11β-hydroxylase, P-450c11B1 and P-450c11B2, are 93% identical in predicted amino acid sequence and are encoded by two vicinal genes[68] on chromosome 8q24.3.[69, 70] Although highly homologous in their coding sequence, significant differences in the regulatory regions of these two genes result in quite distinct expression patterns. Disorders of 11β-hydroxylase enzymes may be manifested as hypocortisolism (i.e., CAH), hypoaldosteronism, or hyperaldosteronism.

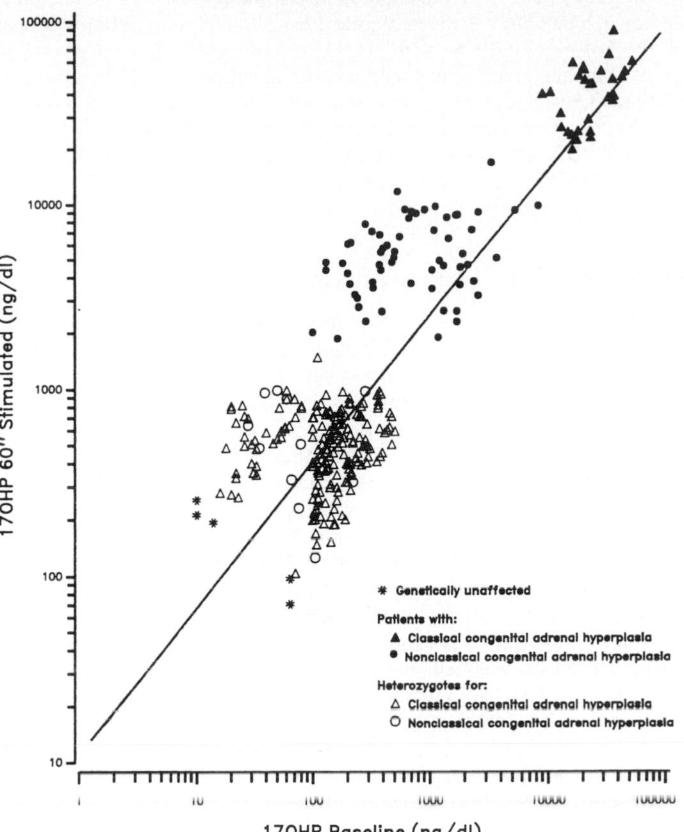

FIGURE 123–6. Nomogram relating baseline to adrenocorticotropic hormone (ACTH)-stimulated serum concentrations of 17-hydroxyprogesterone. Scales are logarithmic. The regression line shown is for all data points. Data points cluster as shown into three nonoverlapping groups: classic (congenital adrenal hyperplasia [CAH]) and nonclassic forms of 21-hydroxylase deficiency are readily distinguished from each other and from the heterozygote/unaffected state. Distinguishing unaffected from heterozygote responses is difficult.

11β-Hydroxylase Deficiency Form of Congenital Adrenal Hyperplasia

Abnormal steroid secretion attributed to impeded 11β-hydroxylation was first described by Eberlein and Bongiovanni in 1955.[10] It has proved to be the second most common form of CAH (5%–8% of all cases in the general population).[71] In the cortisol pathway, conversion of 11-deoxycortisol to cortisol is reduced. As a result, 11-deoxysteroids (11-deoxycortisol and 11-DOC) accumulate. The hyperandrogenism resulting from shunting of cortisol precursors is similar to that of 21-hydroxylase deficiency, including genital ambiguity in classically affected females.

About two-thirds of patients with 11β-hydroxylase deficiency become hypertensive, with or without hypokalemic alkalosis, sometimes early in life. Hypertension does not correlate with the presence or degree of hypokalemia or with the extent of virilization.[72]

In addition to the classic form (i.e., present at birth), milder nonclassic forms of 11β-hydroxylase deficiency have been reported[73–77] and may represent allelic variants, analogous to 21-hydroxylase deficiency. Investigators have been unable to demonstrate a consistent biochemical defect in the obligate heterozygote parents of classic patients, either in the baseline state or with ACTH stimulation.[78] As noted earlier, such a biochemical defect can be demonstrated in 21-hydroxylase heterozygotes. As in 21-hydroxylase deficiency, persons with identical 11β-hydroxylase mutations may differ in the severity of their signs and symptoms of androgen and mineralocorticoid excess, which suggests a role for other epigenetic or nongenetic factors in the expression of clinical phenotype.[79]

Hypertension in 11β-Hydroxylase Deficiency

The hypertension in the 11β-hydroxylase deficiency form of CAH is commonly attributed to DOC-induced sodium retention, which results in volume expansion. However, it has not been consistently proved that DOC causes hypertension.[80] In 1970, New and Seaman showed that the large amounts of DOC produced in 11β-hydroxylase deficiency are glucocorticoid (dexamethasone) suppressible and therefore originate in the zona fasciculata rather than in the zona glomerulosa.[81] When DOC is suppressed with dexamethasone treatment, renin levels rise and cause secretion of aldosterone in the zona glomerulosa, where the 11β-hydroxylase enzyme (P-450c11B2) is normal.

Suppression of DOC by glucocorticoid treatment, however, may not lower blood pressure in hypertensive 11β-hydroxylase–deficient patients. Normotensive patients with markedly elevated DOC levels,[82, 83] hypertensive patients with normal or only mildly elevated DOC,[84, 85] and atypical 11β-hydroxylase–deficient patients with normal PRA[86] present a challenge to the DOC-centered explanation of hypertension. Of course, lack of response to treatment is a feature of long-standing hypertension of many causes.

Epidemiology

The classic 11β-hydroxylase deficiency form of CAH (caused by defects in the *CYP11B1* gene) occurs in about 1 in 100,000 births in the general white population.[87] A large number of cases have been reported in Israel. The incidence there is now estimated to be 1 in 5000 to 1 in 7000 births, with a gene frequency of between 1 in 71 and 1 in 83.[88] This unexpected clustering of cases was traced to Jewish families of North African origin, particularly from Morocco and Tunisia. Turkish Jews have also been found to carry the identical 11β-hydroxylase gene mutation with high frequency.[72, 87] The incidence of the nonclassic form is not known at present but would be predicted to be considerably higher than that of the classic form, as in 21-hydroxylase deficiency.

Molecular Genetics

One of the 11β-hydroxylase genes, *CYP11B1*, is expressed at high levels in normal adrenal glands.[68] Transcription of this gene is regulated by cyclic adenosine monophosphate (cAMP) (the second messenger for ACTH). Low levels of transcripts of the second gene, *CYP11B2*, have been detected in normal adrenal gland by reverse-transcription polymerase chain reaction (RT-PCR). The enzymes encoded by the *CYP11B1* and *CYP11B2* genes have been studied by expressing the corresponding complementary DNA (cDNA) in cultured cells and after actual purification from aldosterone-secreting tumors.[89–91]

The isozyme encoded by *CYP11B2*, termed P-450c11B2, 11β-hydroxylates 11-DOC to corticosterone and is capable of 11β-hydroxylating 11-deoxycortisol to cortisol. It also 18-hydroxylates corticosterone and further oxidizes 18-hydroxycorticosterone to aldosterone, the latter steps referred to as CMO I and CMO II activity, respectively. The *CYP11B2* promoter is sensitive to renin/angiotensin. P-450c11B2 is also referred to as CMO I/CMO II, as well as P-450c18 and aldosterone synthase.

In contrast, the product of *CYP11B1*, termed P-450c11B1, has strong 11β-hydroxylase activity but 18-hydroxylates only about one-tenth as well as P-450c11B2. P-450c11B1 does not synthesize detectable amounts of aldosterone from 18-hydroxycorticosterone. The *CYP11B1* promoter is responsive to ACTH/cAMP.

These data suggest that P-450c11B1 predominantly synthesizes cortisol in the zona fasciculata whereas P-450c11B2 predominantly synthesizes aldosterone in the zona glomerulosa. This hypothesis has been confirmed by studying individuals with defective cortisol or aldosterone synthesis caused by deficiencies in 11β-hydroxylase and CMO II activities, respectively.

Mutations in the zona fasciculata enzyme (P-450c11B1) result in defective synthesis of cortisol and produce hypertension from precursor (e.g., DOC) accumulation. Mutations in the zona glomerulosa gene product (P-450c11B2) result in defective synthesis of aldosterone and consequent salt-wasting. An interesting molecular defect of the 11β-hydroxylase genes results in glucocorticoid-responsive hyperaldosteronism and resultant hypertension.

Almost all affected alleles in the Moroccan-Israeli population carry the same mutation, substitution of histidine for arginine at codon 448 (R448H) in the *CYP11B1* gene.[92] This mutation is incompatible with normal enzymatic activity[93] and appears to represent a founder effect. At least 31 mutations causing the 11β-hydroxylase deficiency form of CAH have been identified and are shown in Figure 123–7.

Diagnosis

Elevated 11-deoxycortisol (compound S) and DOC in serum confirmed by marked urinary elevation of their tetrahydro metabolites is diagnostic. Further confirmation can be found by complete absence of any 11-oxygenated C-19 or C-21 steroids in blood or urine.[94] Determination of PRA is the standard test for mineralocorticoid excess.

Diagnosis is made as for 21-hydroxylase deficiency, with the addition of baseline and ACTH-stimulated levels of serum 11-deoxycortisol (compound S) and DOC. Further characterization by molecular genetic analysis should be pursued in families anticipating additional children, with prenatal diagnosis now also available. Diagnosis in a newborn is quite difficult because the characteristic hypertension does not generally appear during the newborn period and distinction from 21-hydroxylase deficiency on the basis of steroid patterns is also problematic at this age since 17-OHP levels will typically also be elevated in cases of 11β-OH deficiency. However, in 21-OH deficiency, deoxycortisol and DOC are *not* elevated.[95]

Corticosterone Methyl Oxidase I Deficiency

The conversion of corticosterone to 18-hydroxycorticosterone is referred to as CMO I activity, whereas the subsequent 18-oxidation to aldosterone is known as CMO II activity. In the zona glomerulosa these steps are catalyzed by distinct domains within a single enzyme, P-450c11B2, also referred to as P-450c18, aldosterone synthase, or P-450aldo. Deficient CMO I activity typically results in (practically) no aldosterone production and is phenotypically more severe than CMO II deficiency. Defects in CMO I activity have been reported but appear to be less common than those of CMO II.[96, 97] Defects in both CMO I and CMO II activity are inherited as autosomal recessive conditions, and because cortisol synthesis is not affected in either condition, defects of P-450aldo are not considered to be forms of CAH.

Corticosterone Methyl Oxidase II Deficiency

Infants with CMO II deficiency are subject to potentially fatal electrolyte abnormalities; in childhood, however, a variable degree of hyponatremia and hyperkalemia and poor growth are characteristic.[98] Adults may be asymptomatic, their affected status coming to light only in the course of family studies of a symptomatic child. This disorder is characterized by an elevated ratio of serum 18-hydroxycorticosterone to aldosterone or the major metabolites of these steroids (tetrahydro-18-hydroxy-11-dehydrocorticosterone and tetrahydroaldo-

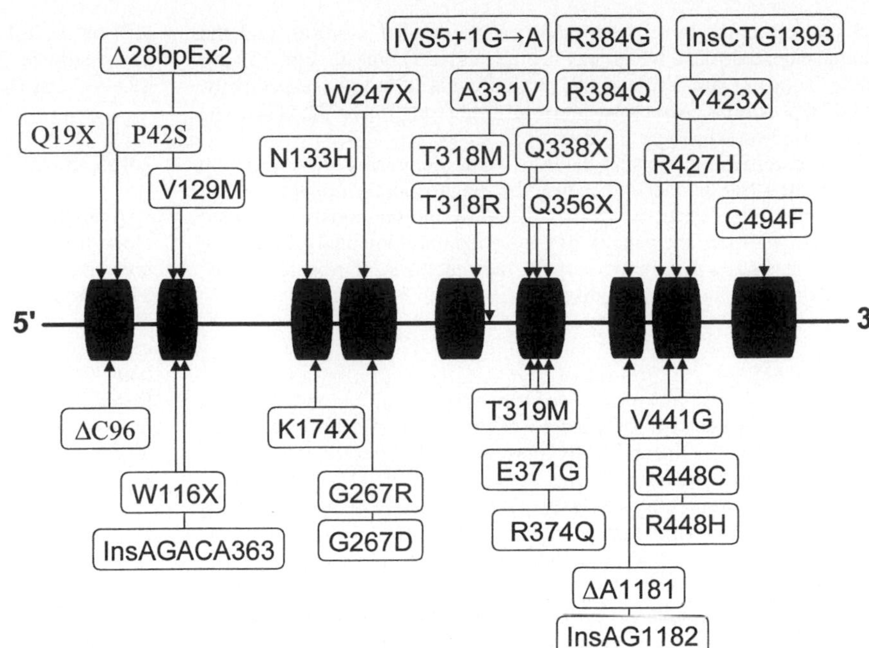

FIGURE 123–7. Mutations in the *CYP11B1* gene causing the 11β-hydroxylase deficiency form of congenital adrenal hyperplasia.

sterone) in urine. CMO II deficiency has been found at an increased frequency among Jews of Iranian origin, some of whose pedigrees have been studied.[99] Molecular analyses have demonstrated two missense mutations in the *CYP11B2* genes of affected individuals: replacement of arginine by tryptophan at position 181 (R181W) and replacement of valine by alanine at position 386 (V386A).[100]

Dexamethasone (Glucocorticoid)-Suppressible Hyperaldosteronism

DSH (also known as glucocorticoid-remediable aldosteronism) is a rare form of hypertension[101, 102] in which aldosterone synthesis appears to be abnormally regulated by ACTH.[103] DSH is characterized by (1) rapid and complete suppression of aldosterone when dexamethasone is administered, (2) continued rise in aldosterone with chronic administration of ACTH, (3) suppressed PRA, and (4) a dominant mode of inheritance.[104] Urinary excretion of 18-hydroxycortisol and 18-oxocortisol is increased.[105, 106]

Individuals with DSH have been shown to have an intergenic recombination juxtaposing the promoter of *CYP11B1* with the coding sequence of *CYP11B2*.[107, 108] The fusion or chimeric gene creates an alteration in regulation of the synthesis of aldosterone that makes the zona glomerulosa sensitive to ACTH rather than renin-angiotensin and thereby results in glucocorticoid-responsive hyperaldosteronism and hypertension.

3β-HYDROXYSTEROID DEHYDROGENASE DEFICIENCY

The enzyme 3β-HSD is necessary for the synthesis of bioactive Δ^4 adrenal and gonadal steroids from the relatively inactive Δ^5 precursors. In addition to 3β-hydroxysteroid dehydrogenation, this enzyme also performs 3-oxosteroid isomerization, thereby giving rise to the alternate term Δ^5/Δ^4 isomerase. 3β-HSD is present not only in the adrenal cortex, gonads, and placenta but also in the liver and in nearly all peripheral tissues. The placental form is distinct from the adrenal/gonadal form. Differences in the level of 3β-HSD activity in different tissues suggest tissue-specific forms or tissue-specific regulation of one or more shared forms of this protein.[109–112]

Classic 3β-HSD Deficiency

3β-HSD deficiency is an autosomal recessive form of CAH and was first described by Bongiovanni in 1962.[113] The exact frequency of this rare disorder is unknown. It has been postulated that individuals with defects early in the pathway of steroidogenesis, which severely impair cortisol synthesis (i.e., 3β-HSD and StAR), have poor survival rates.

Because of reduced 3β-HSD enzyme activity in the gonads, genetic males are incompletely masculinized and exhibit genital ambiguity at birth, with hypospadias. In affected females, on the other hand, very high levels of circulating DHEA converted peripherally to active androgens produce a limited androgen effect. Clitoral enlargement and, rarely, labial fusion are seen. As with the 21-hydroxylase and 11β-hydroxylase enzymes, the severity of the enzyme defect may not be determined on the basis of the appearance of the external genitalia at birth. Deficient steroid production in 3β-HSD deficiency may result in salt-wasting, although such is clearly not true in every case.[114, 115]

Nonclassic 3β-HSD Deficiency

As with nonclassic 21-hydroxylase deficiency, nonclassic 3β-HSD deficiency is an attenuated enzyme defect with no major developmental abnormalities.[54, 116] Signs of virilization appear in females after adrenarche or at the time of puberty.

The possibility that nonclassic 3β-HSD deficiency may be a significantly underdiagnosed cause of excess androgen symptoms, including hirsutism and infertility, has been suggested.[117] Review of clinical data from over 700 women with signs of androgen excess demonstrated decreased 3β-HSD activity in 16%.[118] It has been suggested that nonclassic 3β-HSD deficiency may be more frequent than nonclassic 21-hydroxylase deficiency in women with androgen excess syndrome.[118] In a group of 25 menarchal women with 3β-HSD deficiency, an improvement in regulation of menses and in acne was observed to result from glucocorticoid therapy of at least 3 months' duration.[117] Hirsutism was less well reversed by treatment, and polycystic ovary disease was noted in 50% of these women.

Biochemistry and Molecular Genetics

Two genes encoding 3β-HSD have been localized to chromosome 1p13.1 and cloned.[111, 119] These genes, *HSD3B1* and *HSD3B2*, encode the skin-placental form, referred to as the type I isoform, and the adrenal-gonadal form, which has been designated type II (Fig. 123–8). These isozymes are 372 and 371 amino acids in length, respectively, and 93.5% similar. A representation of mutations in the 3β-HSD type II gene is shown in Figure 123–8.[120–122]

We recommend exercising caution when diagnosing the nonclassic form of 3β-HSD deficiency because the diagnostic hormonal profile in this condition has been shown to "disappear" in previously confirmed cases.[54] In addition, the paucity of confirmed mutation analysis/enzyme expression studies has made suspect the diagnosis of nonclassic 3β-HSD deficiency as a genetic disorder.

Diagnosis

The external genitalia of affected newborn males with classic 3β-HSD deficiency are incompletely masculinized, whereas females are masculinized to a variable degree. A high ratio of Δ^5 to Δ^4 steroids, characterized specifically by elevated serum levels of the Δ^5 steroids pregnenolone, 17-hydroxypregnenolone, and DHEA, along with increased excretion of the Δ^5 metabolites pregnenetriol and 16-pregnenetriol in the urine, are diagnostic for this enzyme disorder. These criteria should not be used during the newborn period when Δ^5 steroids are universally elevated and represent a "physiologic 3β-HSD deficiency."[114] The 3β-HSD defect is diagnosed by 60-minute ACTH testing with elevations of 2 SD or greater above the mean in all of the following: (1) serum Δ^5-17-hydroxypregnenolone, (2) DHEA concentration, and serum ratios of (3) Δ^5-17-hydroxypregnenolone/17-OH-progesterone and (4) Δ^5-17-hydroxypregnenolone/cortisol.[115] Findings limited to elevated Δ^5-17-hydroxypregnenolone and/or DHEA are nonspecific and do not establish the diagnosis of "partial" or "mild" 3β-HSD deficiency. Although this condition may represent a true abnormality in endocrine physiology, it has not been shown to have a genetic basis.

To rule out an adrenal or ovarian steroid-producing tumor, a dexamethasone suppression test (0.5 mg every 6 hours for 3 days) is routinely performed with subsequent measurement of serum hormone concentrations. An ovarian source of the androgens is excluded by addition of the progestogen norethindrone acetate (5 mg every 8 hours for 3 days) to the dexamethasone. Both adrenal and ovarian hormones should be suppressed with this regimen. Ovarian sonography and either adrenal computed tomography or magnetic resonance imaging may be performed when a high index of suspicion for an adrenal or ovarian tumor exists, such as rapid progression or failure to suppress steroid production with dexamethasone or with dexamethasone and norethindrone. As an aid to diagnosis, one can use published nomograms (Fig. 123–9A and B). Reference data established by Temeck et al.[49] on ACTH-stimulated hormonal values are used for the diagnosis of nonclassic 3β-HSD in children with precocious adrenarche (Fig. 123–9C and D).

DISORDERS OF P-450c17

A single enzyme (P-450c17) catalyzes both the conversion of mineralocorticoids to glucocorticoids (17α-hydroxylase activity) and the conversion of glucocorticoids to sex steroids (17,20-lyase activity). The enzyme P-450c17 is encoded by the gene *CYP17*, located on chromosome 10q24-25. Abnormal enzyme function can, however, be manifested as isolated 17α-hydroxylase deficiency, isolated 17,20-lyase deficiency, or combined 17α-hydroxylase/17,20-lyase deficiency. Based on the total number of reported cases (in both sexes), 17α-hydroxylase/17,20-lyase deficiency appears to be a rare steroidogenic defect.[123]

Isolated 17α-Hydroxylase Deficiency

The enzyme domain that performs the 17α-hydroxylase activity is functionally distinct from the domain that performs the 17,20-lyase function. It is therefore reasonable to expect that isolated deficiency of either function may be found. However, because the product of 17α-hydroxylation is the precursor for 17,20-lyase action, isolated 17α-hydroxylase deficiency may be difficult to identify inasmuch as it should occur as the more common combined 17α-hydroxylase/17,20-lyase deficiency. Individuals with "pure 17α-hydroxylase deficiency" would be expected to have hypokalemic hypertension with alkalosis, possibly with normal sexual development. These individuals could be identified by expression studies of mutant enzymes in cell culture, and it has been suggested that 20% or greater residual 17,20-lyase function would not be apparent. Clinically, at least one such description has been reported,[124] but in reality these cases represent a quantitative rather than qualitative difference. Such individuals would be phenocopies of patients with DSH, as is the case with the patient reported in the literature.

Isolated 17,20-Lyase Deficiency

Deficiency of 17,20-lyase activity impedes the synthesis of C-19 sex steroids in the adrenals and gonads[125] without affecting cortisol synthesis in the adrenal gland and is therefore not a form of CAH but a potential cause of abnormal sexual development. Urinary pregnenetriolone, a metabolite of 17-OHP, is increased and increases further

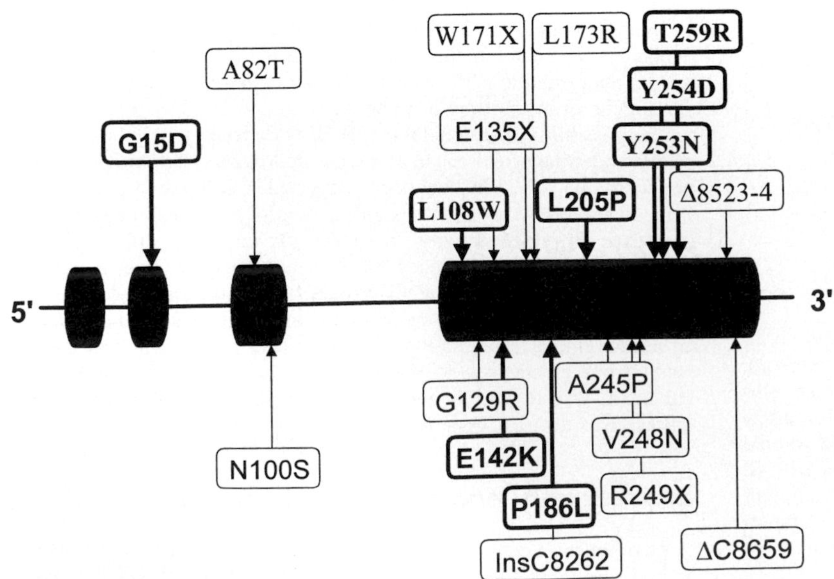

FIGURE 123–8. Mutations in the *HSD3B2* gene causing the 3β-hydroxysteroid dehydrogenase/Δ^5-Δ^4 isomerase deficiency form of congenital adrenal hyperplasia. Alleles associated with salt-wasting are printed in bold; non–salt-wasting alleles are in standard print.

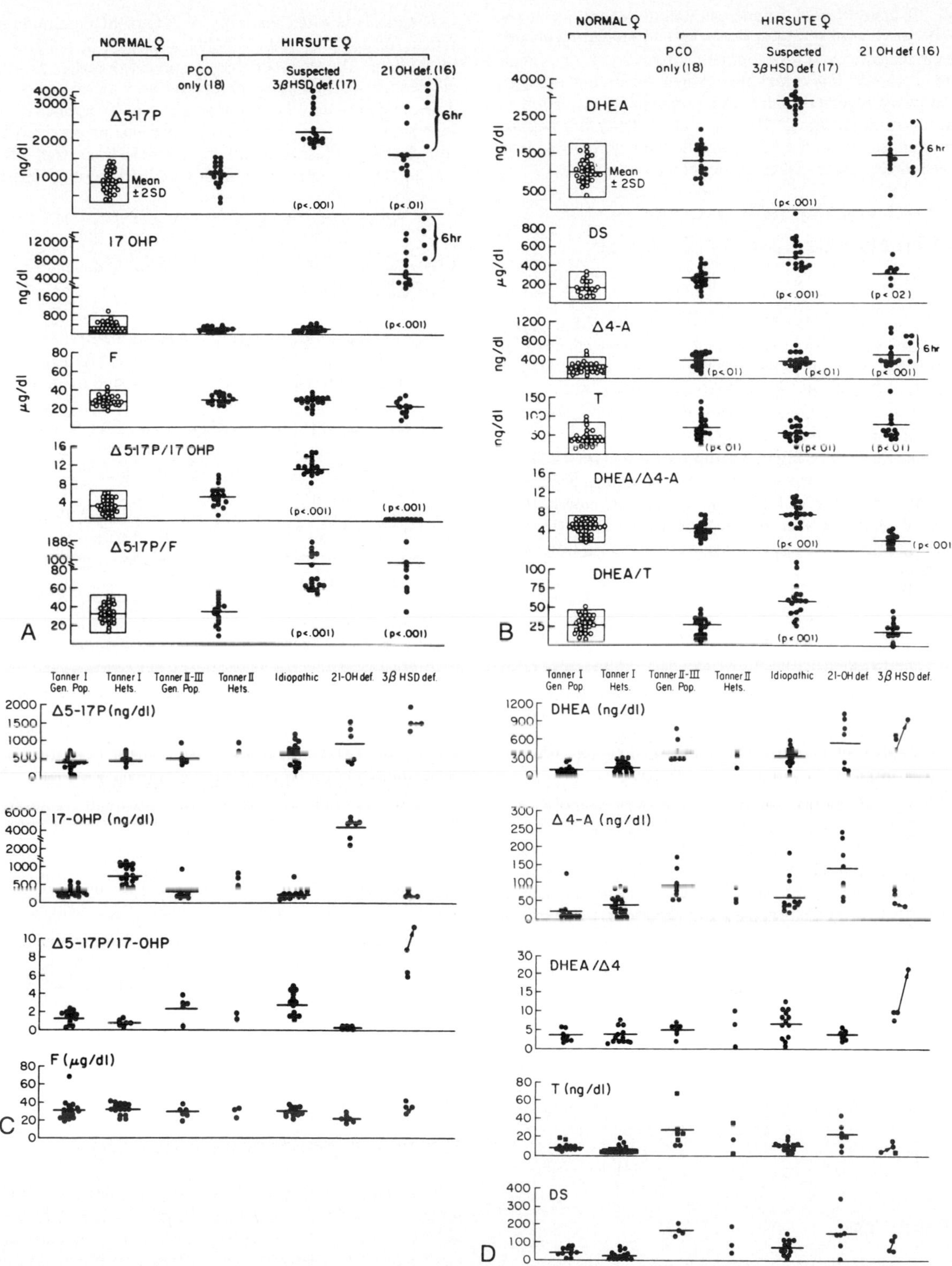

FIGURE 123–9. *A,* Serum 17-hydroxysteroid responses to adrenocorticotropic hormone (ACTH) stimulation (1 hour after a 0.25-mg intravenous bolus dose) in normal women and women with hirsutism. *B,* Serum androgen levels after ACTH stimulation in normal women and women with hirsutism. (From Pang S, Lerner AJ, Stoner E, et al: Late-onset adrenal steroid 3β-hydroxysteroid dehydrogenase deficiency: A cause of hirsutism in pubertal and postpubertal women. J Clin Endocrinol Metab 60:428, copyright © 1985, The Endocrine Society.) *C,* ACTH-stimulated serum 17-hydroxysteroid levels in normal children from the general population, from proven heterozygotes for 21-hydroxylase deficiency, and in children with premature pubarche. The children with premature pubarche are classified as idiopathic (no steroidogenic defect) or as patients with 21-hydroxylase deficiency or 3β-hydroxysteroid dehydrogenase (3β-HSD) deficiency. *D,* ACTH-stimulated serum androgen levels in normal children from the general population, from proven heterozygotes for 21-hydroxylase deficiency, and in children with premature pubarche. The children with premature pubarche are classified as idiopathic (no steroidogenic defect) or as patients with 21-hydroxylase deficiency or 3β-HSD deficiency. The testosterone (T) levels in males are represented by *filled squares.* (From Temeck JW, Pang S, Nelson C, New MI: Genetic defects of steroidogenesis in premature pubarche. J Clin Endocrinol Metab 64:609–617, copyright © 1987, The Endocrine Society.)

after ACTH and human chorionic gonadotropin (hCG) stimulation. DHEA and testosterone excretion do not rise appreciably. At birth, such individuals all have normal female genitalia—regardless of the genetic sex—and are generally initially seen at adolescence with primary amenorrhea/lack of sexual development. Importantly, one longitudinal study of a 46,XY individual who began receiving estrogen replacement at puberty revealed apparently progressive extinction of 17α-hydroxylating activity from age 20 to age 26.[126] Thus, this patient, who started life with an isolated 17,20-lyase deficiency, converted to a combined 17α-hydroxylase/17,20-lyase deficiency at puberty.

Combined 17α-Hydroxylase/17,20-Lyase Deficiency

A defect in 17α-hydroxylase/17,20-lyase will result in diminished production of cortisol as well as sex steroids, whose production requires the 17,20-lyase function. The enzyme defect affects steroid synthesis in both the adrenals and the gonads and reduces production of all androgens and estrogens. Genetic males have pseudohermaphroditism, whereas in females, infantile genitalia are present.[127] At puberty, gonadotropins rise to very high concentrations, the very low sex steroid production failing to provide adequate regulatory feedback. Breast development may occur in males. In females at pubertal age, no secondary sexual characteristics develop, and they have primary amenorrhea. Other oversecreted steroids (e.g., corticosterone) subserve glucocorticoid function.

Hypertension

Hypertension is observed in the 17α-hydroxylase deficiency form of CAH. The serum concentration of DOC is markedly elevated (30–60 times normal), but as in 11β-hydroxylase deficiency,[87] circulating levels of DOC do not entirely correlate with blood pressure values, thus suggesting that other factors contribute to the hypertension in this condition.[128, 129] The serum aldosterone level in some individuals is also elevated, although the aldosterone concentration is **usually** very low—secondary to the volume expansion caused by the excess mineralcorticoid (e.g., DOC) secretion and the resultant suppressed renin. Hypertension may develop in childhood.

As in 21-hydroxylase deficiency, sibling pairs expected to have a common genetic defect do not always exhibit the same biochemical findings.[123]

Partial Defects

The heterozygous state has been identified by ACTH stimulation testing[130]; however, a nonclassic form has not been identified. The steroid pattern of some cases of low-renin hypertension without sexual abnormalities[131] raises the possibility that an isolated 17α-hydroxylase deficiency may be a more common cause of low-renin hypertension than is currently recognized.[123]

Molecular Genetics

Human cDNA corresponding to P-450c17 has been characterized,[132] and the single-copy *CYP17* gene locus is situated on chromosome 10q24-25.[133] Many structural and gene-regulatory mutations in *CYP17* have been identified in patients with combined 17α-hydroxylase/17,20-lyase deficiency (Fig. 123–10). An interesting finding reported by Imai et al. is the discovery of a mutation (a four-base duplication) common to two "unrelated" Canadian Mennonite pedigrees and six families (eight individuals) living in the Friesland region of The Netherlands. This mutation almost certainly represents a "founder" effect inasmuch as a branch of this religious sect is known to have settled in the Ukraine, which is the country of origin of both Canadian families before their immigration.[134]

Diagnosis

Diagnosis is often made by ACTH or hCG stimulation testing in a female or apparent female being evaluated at pubertal age for sexual infantilism. The disorder may be revealed earlier in 46,XY karyotype cases seen in infancy or childhood with hernia or an inguinal mass. These patients may be hypokalemic and hypertensive at diagnosis. In long-standing untreated cases, hypertension of considerable severity can develop. Plasma levels of corticosterone and 18-hydroxy-DOC and an elevated ratio of 18-hydroxycorticosterone/aldosterone are used in diagnosis.[135]

LIPOID CONGENITAL ADRENAL HYPERPLASIA

Lipoid CAH, a rare form of CAH originally described by Prader in 1955,[11, 136] is the most extreme form of CAH. Limited conversion of cholesterol to pregnenolone at the initial step in steroid synthesis leads to negligible production of all steroids. Massive accumulations of cholesterol in the adrenocortical tissue (but interestingly not in the Leydig cells of the testis, where the enzyme is also active) lead to the characteristic fatty appearance of the glands and the descriptive name used for the disorder.

Cholesterol side chain cleavage enzyme (P-450scc, also known as cholesterol desmolase and encoded by the *CYP11A* gene) catalyzes the conversion of cholesterol to pregnenolone—the first and rate-limiting step in the production of corticosteroids—and was therefore the most logical candidate as the cause of lipoid CAH. Nevertheless, to date, no mutations have been found in the *CYP11A* gene of affected individuals.[137] Mutations have been found, however, in the gene encoding for the steroidogenic acute regulator (StAR) protein on chromosome 8p11.2. StAR serves to shuttle cholesterol to the inner mitochondrial membrane, where the P-450scc enzyme is located.[16]

Affected individuals exhibit hypogonadism, severe fluid and electrolyte disturbances, hyperpigmentation, and susceptibility to infection. They often do not survive infancy. Lipoid CAH seems to occur with less severity and somewhat more frequency among Japanese and Koreans.[138]

Diagnosis

In addition to the absence of any steroids in plasma or urine, high basal concentrations of ACTH and high PRA are found. In 46,XY patients the genitalia are ambiguous, whereas 46,XX females have infantile female genitalia.

TREATMENT OF CONGENITAL ADRENAL HYPERPLASIA

Hormone Replacement Therapy

The fundamental aim of endocrine therapy for CAH is to provide replacement of the deficient hormones. Since 1949 when Wilkins et al.[139] and Bartter[140] discovered the efficacy of cortisone therapy for CAH caused by 21-hydroxylase deficiency, glucocorticoid therapy has been the cornerstone of treatment for this disorder. Glucocorticoid administration replaces the deficient cortisol and suppresses ACTH overproduction; a concomitant reduction in adrenal cortex activity takes place, thereby reducing the production of other adrenal steroids (i.e., "precursor by-products") and resulting in remission of (most) symptoms over time.

Adrenal suppression in 21-hydroxylase, 11β-hydroxylase, and 3β-HSD deficiency reduces the production of androgens, which averts further virilization, slows the accelerated growth and bone age advancement to a more normal rate, and allows a normal onset of puberty. An improved body habitus is seen with progressively earlier start of treatment (Fig. 123–11). Individuals with the salt-wasting type

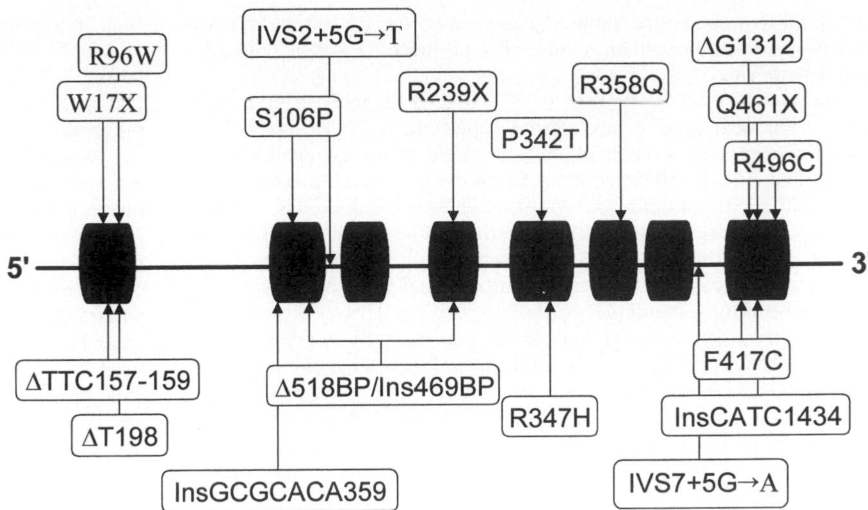

FIGURE 123–10. Mutations in the *CYP17* gene causing 17α-hydroxylase/17,20-lyase deficiency.

of 21-hydroxylase or 3β-HSD deficiency require the administration of a salt-retaining steroid to maintain adequate sodium balance. Suppression of adrenal activity in 11β-hydroxylase and 17α-hydroxylase deficiency normalizes DOC secretion and often results in remission of hypertension. In lipoid CAH, total hormone replacement is required.

Excessive glucocorticoid administration should be avoided because such treatment produces cushingoid facies, growth retardation, and inhibition of epiphyseal maturation.

Hydrocortisone (cortisol) is the corticosteroid of choice for children with all forms of CAH. It is the physiologic hormone and is most often used in the treatment of children because of easy dose adjustment. Oral administration is the preferred and usual mode of treatment and is conventionally given in two divided doses: 10 to 15 mg/m² hydrocortisone divided as one-third in the morning and two-thirds in the evening. We prefer to use the tablet form of hydrocortisone, even in young

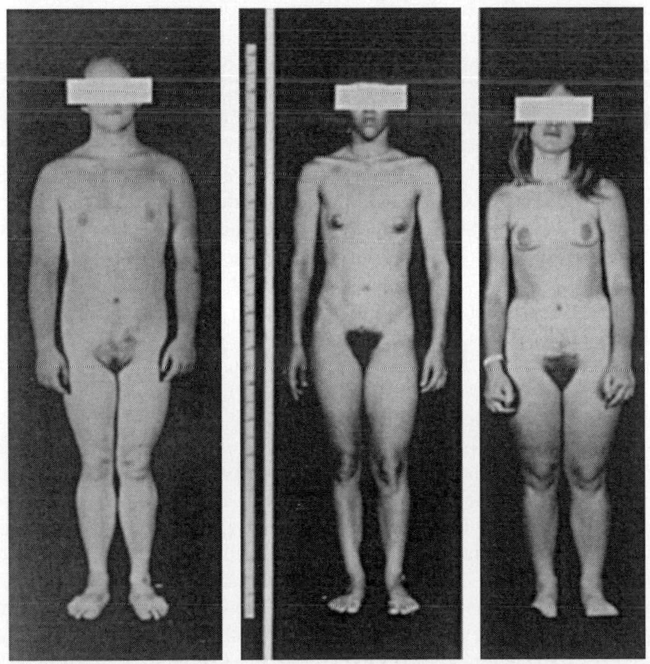

FIGURE 123–11. Habitus of pubertal girls with congenital adrenal hyperplasia caused by 21-hydroxylase deficiency. The patient on the *left* was untreated until 16 years of age, the patient in the *center* was started on treatment when 9 years old, and the patient on the *right* was treated from 4 years of age. Note the progressively more feminine habitus with earlier treatment. (After New MI, Levine LS: Congenital adrenal hyperplasia. *In* Harris H, Hirschhorn K (eds): Advances in Human Genetics, vol 4. New York, Plenum, 1973, pp 251–326.)

infants, because liquid formulations have been found to have inconsistent concentrations stemming from difficulties in solubilizing hydrocortisone. As noted above, excessive replacement with glucocorticoids will be detrimental, and although some children may (temporarily) require greater than 15 mg/m²/day, individuals' cushingoid features have been reported to develop with as little as 16 mg/m²/day of hydrocortisone.

If hormonal control is poor with hydrocortisone at the standard dose, the dosage may be temporarily increased to 20 (or even 30) mg/m²/day, or the regimen may be changed to a synthetic hormone analogue such as prednisone or dexamethasone. These agents are more potent and longer acting, although their relative glucocorticoid and mineralocorticoid effects differ and the smaller amounts used make dosage adjustment more crucial. Because of individual variations in the activity of hepatic enzymes metabolizing 11-oxosteroids and thus differences in plasma clearance and half-life, prednisolone (the 11β-hydroxy analogue of prednisone, also called Δ¹-cortisol) is more effective than prednisone (Δ¹-cortisone) as glucocorticoid replacement in some patients. Individuals without overt salt-wasting have been shown to have elevated renin levels,[141–147] and fluctuation of these levels may correlate with ACTH. Addition of a mineralocorticoid to the therapeutic regimen in individuals with the simple virilizing form of 21-hydroxylase deficiency has been shown to result in improved hormonal control at the same glucocorticoid dose. A longer-term benefit of a reduced glucocorticoid requirement is improved statural growth.[146, 147]

In non–life-threatening illness or stress, the glucocorticoid dosage should be increased to two or three times the maintenance regimen for the duration of the stress. Each family must be given injection kits of hydrocortisone for emergency use (25 mg for infants, 50 mg for young children, and 100 mg for older patients). In the event of a surgical procedure, a total of 5 to 10 times the daily maintenance dose (depending on the nature of the operative procedure) may be required over the first 24 hours. For elective surgery, we recommend hydrocortisone, 100 mg/m² orally at midnight preceding the operation, followed by 100 mg/m² intramuscularly on call to the operating room and then another 100 mg/m² by intravenous drip for every 6 hours of surgery. During the first 24 hours after surgery, the patient should receive 100 mg/m²/day divided into four doses. Beginning the second postoperative day, in cases without complications the dose can be tapered rapidly, dropping to 50 mg/m²/day for the second day and then on the following day resuming the normal preoperative corticosteroid schedule. Stress doses should not be given in the form of dexamethasone because of the delayed onset of action. Mineralocorticoid doses need not be increased in response to stress.

Patients with the salt-wasting forms of CAH (21-hydroxylase and 3β-HSD deficiency) require mineralocorticoid replacement. The cortisol analogue 9α-fluorohydrocortisone (Florinef) is used because of its potent mineralocorticoid activity. Additionally, salt should be allowed ad libitum. In an adrenal crisis, liberal infusions of isotonic saline and parenteral hydrocortisone should be used at a dose of 100 mg/m^2/day. At this dose, hydrocortisone subserves all necessary mineralocorticoid function.

Patients with StAR, 3β-HSD, or 17α-hydroxylase/17,20-lyase deficiency will also require sex steroid replacement, regardless of the sex of rearing. Sex steroids should be added at the developmentally appropriate time to allow children to optimally resemble their peers. CMO I/CMO II (aldosterone synthase)-deficient individuals will require salt and mineralocorticoid replacement, whereas the hypertension seen in 11β-hydroxylase and 17α-hydroxylase deficiency may not resolve with glucocorticoid replacement, especially when the hypertension has been long-standing.

It is of the utmost importance for all patients with adrenal insufficiency or those receiving steroid replacement/suppressive therapy (e.g., for CAH) *to wear a "Medic-Alert" bracelet or medallion listing the medical condition, chronic medications, and standard emergency procedures for the particular diagnosis* (e.g., administration of fluids and hydrocortisone). *In addition, the patient and family members must be trained in the intramuscular administration of hydrocortisone.*

Monitoring Treatment

Glucocorticoid doses should be titrated to optimize biochemical control balanced against physiologic parameters (e.g., in a growing child with 21-hydroxylase deficiency, a 17-OHP concentration of between 500 and 1000 ng/dL and suppressed androgens while maintaining good growth velocity). The goal, with respect to corticosteroid replacement, is to give the minimal dose required for optimal control. Serum 17-OHP and Δ^4-androstenedione concentrations determined by radioimmunoassay can be used to monitor biochemical control in patients with 21-hydroxylase deficiency.[148–150] In females and prepubertal males (but not in newborn and pubertal males) the serum testosterone level is also a useful index.[149] Combined determinations of PRA, 17-OHP, and serum androgens, as well as clinical assessment of growth and pubertal status, must all be considered when adjusting the dose of glucocorticoid and salt-retaining steroid for optimal therapeutic control. A combination of hydrocortisone and 9α-fluorohydrocortisone has proved to be a highly effective treatment modality.[148] Measurement of PRA can be used to monitor the efficacy of treatment in all forms of CAH. PRA is elevated in the "salt-losing" state and suppressed in the "volume-overloaded" state. Its normalization will indicate improved hormonal control.

Although glucocorticoid treatment has been available since 1950, which regimen gives the best outcome in terms of height has not been agreed upon. Recent studies suggest that even the most compliant patient may not achieve a final height compatible with parental stature. It is not known whether this deficiency is due to overtreatment or the failure of oral glucocorticoid therapy given twice or even three times daily to suppress excess androgen production—or due to simultaneous overtreatment and undertreatment. A simple home-based system to monitor the hormonal status of patients at frequent intervals may improve hormonal control and final growth. A recent report using salivary 17-OHP concentrations may provide an easy means for monitoring hormone levels on a daily basis.[66] Similar considerations may apply to the preservation of fertility.

Management of Ambiguous Genitalia

A newborn with ambiguous genitalia represents a medical emergency. Determination of genetic sex by karyotype and accurate diagnosis of the specific underlying defect are essential for initial management, but these factors do not address the questions of gender identity and sexual orientation, questions that are often raised by confused parents at an extremely vulnerable time. It is well established that steroids influence aspects of central nervous system development,[151, 152] but data are controversial regarding specific androgen effects resulting from CAH.[153–155] It has been proposed that a masculinized gender role in girls, with behavioral manifestations such as "tomboyishness," results from prenatal androgen excess in CAH. Similarly considered, behavior changes resulting from alterations in the androgen milieu are seen in studies of male pseudohermaphrodites with 5α-reductase or 17α-HSD deficiency, who often elect a male gender identity at puberty.[156, 157] A great body of psychologic studies, however, indicates that in humans, unlike other mammals, the sex of rearing overrides prenatal hormonal effects.[158, 159]

In assigning a sex of rearing to a pseudohermaphrodite, the genetic sex is of less consideration than the physiologic and anatomic character of the genitalia, their potential for development and function, and the psychosocial milieu of the infant. Sex assignment of female pseudohermaphrodites with 21- or 11β-hydroxylase deficiency or 3β-HSD deficiency in the newborn period should be as a female. Wide individual variability is seen in the manifestation of ambiguous genitalia in these patients. When medical treatment is begun early in life, the initially large and prominent clitoris may shrink slightly. As the surrounding structures grow normally, the clitoris becomes much less prominent, and surgical revision may not be required. When the clitoral enlargement is conspicuous enough to interfere with parent-child bonding or the formation of female gender identity in the patient raises doubts in the parents about the "true sex" of the infant, corrective surgery on the genitalia should be carried out as early as possible and certainly when the child is younger than 2 years.[159] Psychoendocrinologically trained psychologists and/or psychiatrists provide a vital component of the treatment regimen inasmuch as one of the major goals of therapy is to ensure that gender role, gender behavior, and gender identity are isosexual with the sex of assignment.[160, 161]

Clitoral recession (*not* resection) is the current recommended surgical procedure, with preservation of erectile tissue along with the dorsal neurovascular bundle and thus clitoral erotic sensation. It must be determined before menarche that the vaginal formation permits adequate outflow of blood, and an early procedure to ensure outflow may have to be performed in rare cases. Vaginoplasty performed before regular sexual intercourse may require continual mechanical dilatation of the vagina. Surgery before the patient is able to take responsibility for the mechanical dilatation risks recurrent stenosis, formation of adhesions, and scarring, with a need for further surgery and permanent harm to the vaginal orifice. Too long a delay, on the other hand, risks harm to the patient's sense of self as a normal female. All these factors are taken into account when choosing the age for the necessary procedure(s), which is generally in the patient's early to middle adolescence. In some patients, mechanical dilatation may be sufficient. In the hands of an experienced surgeon, vaginoplasty can yield excellent results.[162] Because of the normal internal genitalia and gonads in these patients, normal puberty, fertility, and child-bearing are possible when early and proper therapeutic intervention is achieved.

The rare cases of late diagnosis of classic 21-hydroxylase, 11β-hydroxylase, and 3β-HSD deficiency with interim misassignment as a male must be dealt with on an individual basis. Corrective surgery to change the sex of assignment is not recommended in a child older than 2 years. Primary responsibility should be taken by a psychoendocrinologist in consultation with the family.

For male pseudohermaphrodites, a male sex assignment is by no means always best. The basic questions to ask are (1) will the child be able to urinate standing and (2) will sexual intercourse as a man be possible? If a male pseudohermaphrodite is to be raised as a female, surgical correction of the genitalia and gonadectomy are required. With appropriate therapeutic measures, relatively normal, albeit infertile female sexual development and activity usually ensue in adolescence and adulthood if the parents and patient are well managed medically and psychologically. Administration of sex steroids is required to induce the development of appropriate sexual characteristics at puberty. Assigned males who have impaired androgen synthesis will require androgen replacement. Almost all male pseudohermaphrodites to be raised as males require surgery for correction of the birth defects of the external genitalia caused by inadequate prenatal masculinization.

The process of assigning and accepting a sex of rearing for a child with ambiguous genitalia is extremely complicated. A team approach combining the insights of a pediatrician, endocrinologist, psychoendocrinologist, surgeon, and the child's parents or guardian is essential. Moreover, it should be anticipated that ongoing counseling will be helpful to most families.

PRENATAL DIAGNOSIS

21-Hydroxylase Deficiency

A pregnancy occurring in a family in which steroid 21-hydroxylase deficiency has been identified has a 25% chance of resulting in an affected newborn. Since 1965, when Jeffcoate et al. correlated a clearly elevated value of amniotic fluid pregnenetriol with the diagnosis of an affected child (confirmed at term), amniotic fluid steroid hormone assay has been performed in pregnancies at risk.[163–166] Radioimmunoassay of amniotic fluid for 17-OHP has shown that in all cases affected with the salt-wasting form, the amniotic fluid 17-OHP concentration is unambiguously elevated[167–171]; however, in simple virilizing 21-hydroxylase deficiency, the 17-OHP value may not be elevated above normal.[172] Amniotic fluid Δ^4-androstenedione and testosterone levels also have been measured, but the latter is less useful because testosterone is normally high in the amniotic fluid of a male fetus.[170, 173]

Fetal cells (mostly fibroblasts) in the amniotic fluid may be cultured for DNA analysis. HLA serotyping in conjunction with hormonal assay has been used since 1979 but is less sensitive than direct mutation analysis.[174] Specific probes for 21-hydroxylase mutations allow for rapid identification of known mutations directly by using PCR—i.e., allele-specific PCR. One panel of oligonucleotide probes currently available for use in prenatal diagnosis[175] is expected to identify well over 95% of current 21-hydroxylase mutations.

According to the population studied, deletions of the active 21-hydroxylase gene (*CYP21*) occur in anywhere from 20% to over 40% of patients (northwest United Kingdom)[176, 177]; the remaining 60% to 80% of cases represent missense and nonsense mutations, as well as small deletions—sometimes even complicated noncontiguous deletions. These mutations are commonly the result of gene conversions, or nonreciprocal transfers of the nucleotide sequence of longer or shorter segments of the pseudogene (*CYP21P*) to the active gene, with deleterious results.

11β-Hydroxylase Deficiency

Levels of 11-deoxysteroids and metabolites in amniotic fluid and maternal urine have been found to be increased in pregnancies with a fetus affected with 11β-hydroxylase deficiency,[178, 179] which suggests that prenatal diagnosis of this disorder by hormonal measurement may be feasible,[180] although the reliability of this method has not been reported by other groups. However, the 11β-hydroxylase genes have been cloned and many such mutations have been described. When the mutations are known, prenatal diagnosis by DNA analysis of material obtained by chorionic villus sampling (CVS) is possible and recommended. Experience with prenatal diagnosis in the 11β-hydroxylase deficiency form of CAH is limited.

PRENATAL TREATMENT

Dexamethasone crosses the placenta without undergoing significant metabolism and has therefore been used in the treatment of various fetal abnormalities. For a fetus at risk for 21- or 11β-hydroxylase deficiency, prophylactic treatment should be started as soon as pregnancy is confirmed.[181–186] CVS is currently advocated to permit diagno-

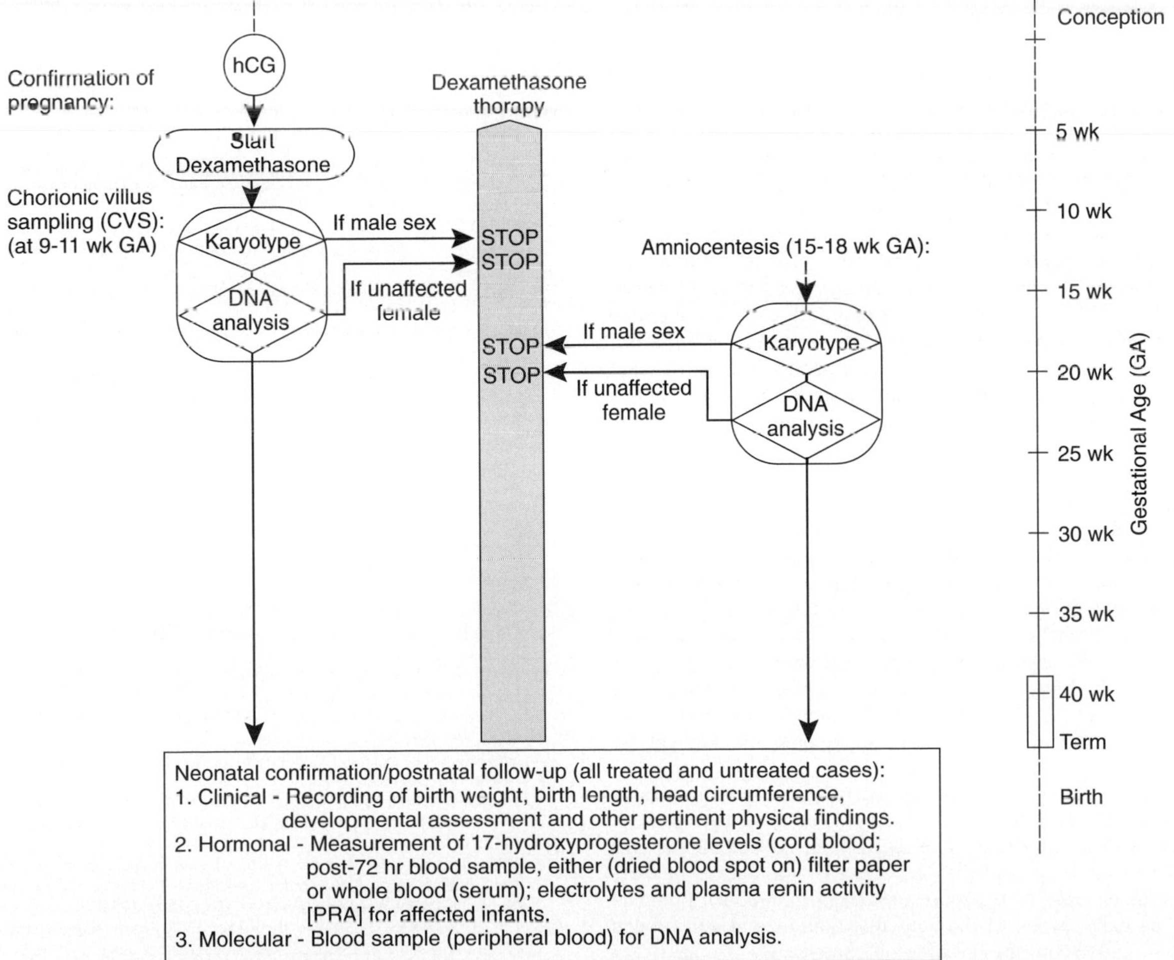

FIGURE 123–12. Protocol for prenatal diagnosis and treatment. (From Mercado AB, Wilson RC, Cheng KC, et al: Extensive personal experience: Prenatal treatment and diagnosis of congenital adrenal hyperplasia owing to 21-hydroxylase deficiency. J Clin Endocrinol Metab 80:2014–2020, copyright © 1995, The Endocrine Society.)

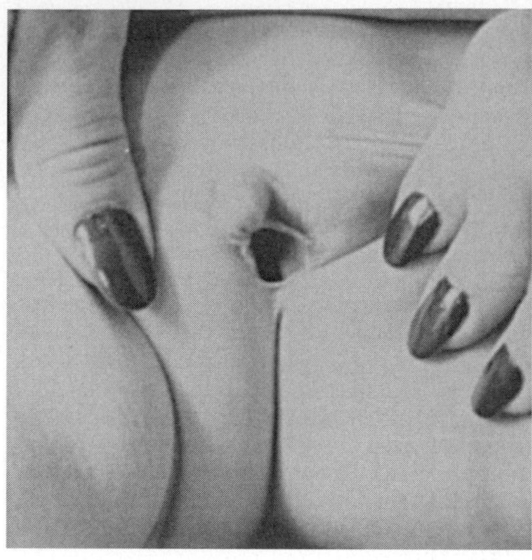
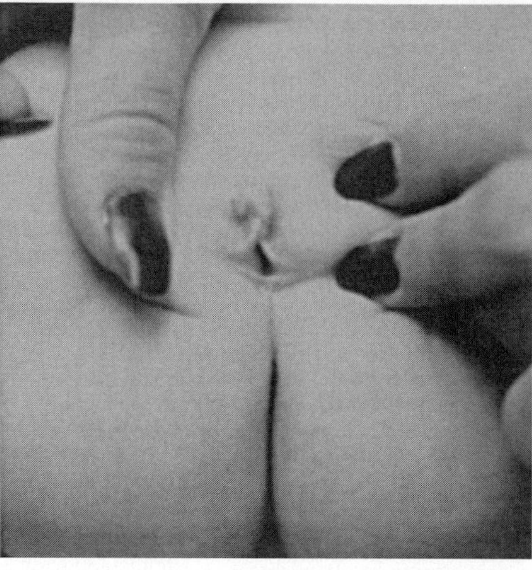

FIGURE 123–13. Untreated and prenatally treated female newborns. (From Speiser PW, Laforgia N, Kato K, et al: First trimester prenatal treatment and molecular genetic diagnosis of congenital adrenal hyperplasia (21-hydroxylase deficiency). J Clin Endocrinol Metab 70:838–848, copyright © 1990, The Endocrine Society.)

sis in the first trimester and to allow discontinuation of unnecessary steroid treatment in the case of a male fetus or an unaffected female fetus (Fig. 123–12). Initiation of steroid therapy by the sixth or seventh week of gestation should effectively suppress fetal adrenal androgen production in time to allow for normal separation of the vaginal and urethral orifices and continued suppression through gestation to prevent or reduce the degree of clitoromegaly (Fig. 123–13). The current dosage recommendation is 20 μg of dexamethasone per kilogram of maternal (prepregnant) weight per day in three divided doses. To date, no fetus of a mother treated with dexamethasone in low dose has been found to have any congenital malformations other than genital ambiguity. Specifically, there are no reports of increases in the number of cases of cleft palate, placental degeneration, or fetal death, all of which are observed in rodent models of in utero exposure to *high-dose* glucocorticoids.[187] We have recently completed a study of all prenatal diagnoses between 1978 and 1998 that confirms the safety and efficacy of this treatment protocol. Of 403 pregnancies evaluated, 84 were found to be affected, 52 of which were females. In 16 of these cases, the families declined dexamethasone treatment. The girls in this cohort were highly virilized at birth, with a mean Prader score of 3.9. Of the 36 pregnancies receiving treatment, 23 began dexamethasone early (before 6 weeks' gestation) and continued to term. The girls in this group were only mildly virilized, with a mean Prader score of 1.17. In the remaining 13 pregnancies, either treatment was begun late or the treatment was only partial. The girls in this group had an intermediate degree of virilization, with a mean Prader score of 2.75. The only statistically significant adverse effect of dexamethasone treatment was an excess (maternal) weight gain of 8 lb relative to the untreated group. No correlation was found between prenatal dexamethasone treatment and fetal demise, birth weight, hypertension, gestational diabetes mellitus, edema, or striae.[188] Normal birth weight and length as well as normal physical and psychologic development were reported for all 21 treated fetuses (affected and unaffected) in the French multicenter study[189] and in our series.[190] These studies reflect the experience with prenatal treatment of pregnancies at risk for 21-hydroxylase deficiency, but prenatal treatment for pregnancies at risk for 11β-hydroxylase deficiency has been similarly successful and is predicted to have the same outcome and degree of safety.

Dexamethasone treatment is initiated early in all pregnancies at risk and maintained until diagnosis after CVS at 8 to 10 weeks or amniocentesis at 15 to 18 weeks. The increase in risk of miscarriage after CVS is very low[190, 191] and may be offset by the benefit of early diagnosis (shortened time of exposure to steroid treatment). Pregnant women must be made aware of the available options and led through these options to understand the possible outcomes.

The prognosis for individuals with disorders of adrenal steroidogenesis has improved remarkably over the last 50 years since the introduction of cortisone therapy. Improved glucocorticoid and mineralocorticoid replacement has had a tremendous impact on both the quantity and quality of life of affected individuals and their families. Early research into gene therapy for some of these disorders—most importantly the 21-hydroxylase form of CAH—is quite promising and may become the new standard treatment in the years to come.

Acknowledgment

The authors would like to thank Laurie Vandermolen for her insightful advice and extensive editorial assistance. We would also like to thank Drs. Barbara Cerame and Robert Wilson for their helpful discussion of 11β-hydroxylase activity.

REFERENCES

1. New MI, White PC, Pang S, et al: The adrenal hyperplasias. *In* Scriver CR, Beaudet AL, Sly WS, et al (eds): The Metabolic Basis of Inherited Disease, ed 6. New York, McGraw-Hill, 1989, pp 1881–1917.
2. Grumbach MM, Conte FA: Disorders of sex differentiation. *In* Wilson JD, Foster DW (eds): Williams' Textbook of Endocrinology, ed 8. Philadelphia, WB Saunders, 1992, pp 853–951.
3. De Crecchio L: Sopra un caso di apparenze virile in una donna. Morgagni 7:1951, 1865.
4. Fibiger J: Beiträge zur Kenntnis des weiblichen Scheinzwittertums. Virchows Arch Pathol Anat 181:1–51, 1905.
5. Apert A: Dystrophies en relation avec des lésions de capsules surrénales. Hirsutisme et progeria. Bull Soc Pediatr (Paris) 12:501–518, 1910.
6. Migeon CJ: Diagnosis and treatment of adrenogenital disorders. *In* DeGroot L, et al (eds): Endocrinology, ed 2. Philadelphia, WB Saunders, 1989, pp 1676–1704.
7. Wilkins L: The Diagnosis and Treatment of Endocrine Disorders, ed 3. Springfield, IL, Charles C Thomas, 1965, pp 368–381.
8. Bongiovanni AM: Detection of pregnanediol and pregnanetriol in urine of patients with adrenal hyperplasia: Suppression with cortisone: A preliminary report. Bull Johns Hopkins Hosp 92:244–251, 1953.
9. Bongiovanni AM, Root AW: The adrenogenital syndrome. N Engl J Med 268:1283–1289, 1342–1351, 1391–1399, 1963.
10. Eberlein WR, Bongiovanni AM: Congenital adrenal hyperplasia with hypertension: Unusual steroid pattern in blood and urine. J Clin Endocrinol Metab 15:1531–1534, 1955.
11. Prader A, Siebenmann RE: Nebenniereninsuffizienz bei kongenitaler Lipoid hyperplasie der Nebennieren. Helv Paediatr Acta 12:569–595, 1957.
12. Biglieri EG, Herron MA, Brust N: 17-Hydroxylation deficiency in man. J Clin Invest 45:1946–1954, 1966.
13. New MI: Male pseudohermaphroditism due to 17α-hydroxylase deficiency. J Clin Invest 49:1930–1941, 1970.
14. Dupont B, Oberfield SE, Smithwick EM, et al: Close genetic linkage between HLA and congenital adrenal hyperplasia (21-hydroxylase deficiency). Lancet 2:1309–1312, 1977.
15. White PC, New MI, Dupont B: HLA-linked congenital adrenal hyperplasia results from a defective gene encoding a cytochrome P-450 specific for steroid 21-hydroxylation. Proc Natl Acad Sci U S A 81:7505–7509, 1984.
16. Lin D, Sugawara T, Strauss JF 3rd, et al: Role of steroidogenic acute regulatory protein in adrenal and gonadal steroidogenesis. Science 267:1828–1831, 1995.
17. Suwa S, Shimozawa K, Kitagawa T, et al: Collaborative study on regional neonatal screening for congenital adrenal hyperplasia in Japan. *In* Therell BL Jr (ed): Advances in Neonatal Screening. New York, Elsevier, 1987, pp 279–286.
18. Wallace AM, Beastall GH, Kennedy R, Girdwood RWA: Congenital adrenal hyper-

plasia screening in 120,000 Scottish neonates. *In* Therell BL Jr (ed): Advances in Neonatal Screening. New York, Elsevier, 1987, pp 293–295.
19. Sólyom J, Hughes IA: Value of selective screening for congenital adrenal hyperplasia in Hungary. Arch Dis Child 64:338–342, 1989.
20. Pang SP, Wallace MA, Hofman L, et al: Worldwide experience in newborn screening for classical congenital adrenal hyperplasia due to 21-hydroxylase deficiency. Pediatrics 81:866–874, 1988.
21. Cutfield WS, Webster D: Newborn screening for congenital adrenal hyperplasia in New Zealand. J Pediatr 126:118–121, 1995.
22. Allen DB, Hoffman GL, Fitzpatrick P, et al: Improved precision of newborn screening for congenital adrenal hyperplasia using weight-adjusted criteria for 17-hydroxyprogesterone levels. J Pediatr 130:128–133, 1997.
23. Speiser PW, Dupont B, Rubinstein P, et al: High frequency of nonclassical steroid 21-hydroxylase deficiency. Am J Hum Genet 37:650–667, 1985.
24. Sherman SL, Aston CE, Morton NE, et al: A segregation and linkage study of classical and nonclassical 21-hydroxylase deficiency. Am J Hum Genet 42:830–838, 1988.
25. Dumic M, Brkljacic L, Speiser PW, et al: An update on the frequency of nonclassic deficiency of adrenal 21-hydroxylase in the Yugoslav population. Acta Endocrinol 122:703–710, 1990.
26. Bonné-Tamir B, Bodmer JG, Bodmer WF, et al: HLA polymorphism in Israel: 9. An overall comparative analysis: Tissue Antigens 11:235–250, 1978.
27. Kidd KK, Kidd JR, Bonné-Tamir B, New MI: Nuclear DNA polymorphisms and population relationships. *In* Bonné-Tamir B, Adam A (eds): Genetic Diversity Among Jews. New York, Oxford University Press, 1992, pp 33–44.
28. Josso N: Antimüllerian hormone: New perspectives for a sexist molecule. Endocr Rev 7:421–433, 1986.
29. Klingensmith GJ, Garcia SC, Jones HW Jr, et al: Glucocorticoid treatment of girls with congenital adrenal hyperplasia: Effects on height, sexual maturation, and fertility. J Pediatr 90:996–1004, 1977.
30. DiMartino-Nardi J, Stoner E, O'Connell A, New MI: The effect of treatment of final height in classical congenital adrenal hyperplasia (CAH). Acta Endocrinol Suppl 279:305–314, 1986.
31. New MI, Gertner JM, Speiser PW, del Balzo P: Growth and final height in classical and nonclassical 21-hydroxylase deficiency. Acta Paediatr Jpn 30(suppl):79–88, 1988.
32. Futterweit W: Polycystic Ovarian Disease. New York, Springer-Verlag, 1984, pp 118–129.
33. Prader A, Zachmann M, Illig R: Normal spermatogenesis in adult males with congenital adrenal hyperplasia after discontinuation of therapy. *In* Lee PA, Plotnick LP, Kowarski AA, et al (eds): Congenital Adrenal Hyperplasia. Baltimore, University Park Press, 1977, p 397.
34. Mulaikal RM, Migeon CJ, Rock JA: Fertility rates in female patients with CAH due to 21-hydroxylase deficiency. N Engl J Med 316:178–182, 1987.
35. Thibaud E, Rappaport R, Salamon BJ, et al: Fertilité normale chez 2 femmes traitées pour hyperplasie congénitale des surrénales (HCS) avec syndrome de perte de sel (SPS) et ambiguité génitale Prader III et IV (abstract). *In* Proceedings of Sexual Differentiation: Basic and Clinical Aspects. Montpellier, France, March 17–19, 1989.
36. Blumberg DL, Reggiardo D, Sklar C, David R: Congenital adrenal hyperplasia and fertility (letter). N Engl J Med 319:951, 1988.
37. Tusie-Luna M-T, Traktman P, White PC: Determination of functional effects of mutations in the steroid 21-hydroxylase gene (*CYP21*) using recombinant vaccinia virus. J Biol Chem 265:20916–20922, 1990.
38. Chiou S-H, Hu M C, Chung B-C: A missense mutation at Ile172-Asn or Arg356-Trp causes steroid 21-hydroxylase deficiency. J Biol Chem 265:3549–3552, 1990.
39. Prader A: Vollkommen männliche äussere Genitalentwicklung und Salzverlustsyndrom bei Madchen mit kongenitalem adrenogenitalem Syndrom. Helv Paediatr Acta 13:5–14, 1958.
40. Horner JM, Hintz RL, Luetscher JA: The role of plasma renin and angiotensin in salt-losing 21-hydroxylase deficiency: Amniotic fluid steroid analysis. Prenat Diagn 2:97, 1982.
41. Stoner E, DiMartino J, Kuhnle U, et al: Is salt wasting in congenital adrenal hyperplasia due to the same gene as the fasciculata defect? Clin Endocrinol 24:9–20, 1986.
42. Morel Y, David M, Forest MGH, et al: Gene conversions and rearrangements cause discordance between inheritance of forms of 21-hydroxylase deficiency and HLA types. J Clin Endocrinol Metab 68:592–599, 1989.
43. Speiser PW, Agdere L, Ueshiba H, et al: Aldosterone synthesis in salt-wasting congenital adrenal hyperplasia with complete absence of adrenal 21-hydroxylase. N Engl J Med 324:145–149, 1991.
44. Dupont B, Pollack MS, Levine LS, et al: Congenital adrenal hyperplasia and HLA: Joint report from the Eighth International Histocompatibility Workshop. *In* Terasaki PI (ed): Histocompatibility Testing 1980. Los Angeles, UCLA Tissue Typing Laboratory, 1981, pp 693–706.
45. Trowsdale J, Ragoussis J, Campbell RD: Map of the human MHC. Immunol Today 12:443–446, 1991.
46. Dupont B, Virdis R, Lerner AJ, et al: Distinct HLA B antigen associations for the salt-wasting and simple virilizing forms of congenital adrenal hyperplasia due to 21-hydroxylase deficiency. *In* Albert ED, Baur MP, Mayr WR (eds): Histocompatibility Testing 1984. Berlin, Springer-Verlag, 1984, p 660.
47. Levine LS, Dupont B, Lorenzen F, et al: Cryptic 21-hydroxylase deficiency in families of patients with classical congenital adrenal hyperplasia. J Clin Endocrinol Metab 51:1316–1324, 1980.
48. Kohn B, Levine LS, Pollack MS, et al: Late-onset steroid 21-hydroxylase deficiency: A variant of classical congenital adrenal hyperplasia. J Clin Endocrinol Metab 55:817–827, 1988.
49. Temeck JW, Pang S, Nelson C, New MI: Genetic defects of steroidogenesis in premature pubarche. J Clin Endocrinol Metab 64:609–617, 1987.
50. Granoff AB, Chasalow FI, Blethen SL: 17-Hydroxyprogesterone responses to adrenocorticotropin in children with premature adrenarche. J Clin Endocrinol Metab 60:409–415, 1985.
51. Lucky AW, Rosenfield RL, McGuire J, et al: Adrenal androgen hyperresponsiveness to adrenocorticotropin in women with acne and/or hirsutism: Adrenal enzyme defects and exaggerated adrenarche. J Clin Endocrinol Metab 62:840–848, 1986.
52. Rose LI, Newmark SR, Strauss JS, Pochi PE: Adrenocortical hydroxylase deficiencies in acne vulgaris. J Invest Dermatol 66:324–326, 1976.
53. Lobo RA, Goebelsmann U: Adult manifestations of congenital adrenal hyperplasia due to incomplete 21-hydroxylase deficiency mimicking polycystic ovarian disease. Am J Obstet Gynecol 138:720–726, 1980.
54. Pang S, Lerner AJ, Stoner E, et al: Late-onset adrenal steroid 3β-hydroxysteroid dehydrogenase deficiency: A cause of hirsutism in pubertal and postpubertal women. J Clin Endocrinol Metab 60:428–439, 1985.
55. Child DF, Bullock DE, Anderson DC: Adrenal steroidogenesis in hirsute women. Clin Endocrinol 12:595–601, 1980.
56. Gibson M, Lackritz R, Schiff I, Tulchinsky D: Abnormal adrenal responses to adrenocorticotropic hormone in hyperandrogenic women. Fertil Steril 33:43–48, 1980.
57. Chrousos GP, Loriaux DL, Mann DL, Cutler GB: Late-onset 21-hydroxylase deficiency mimicking idiopathic hirsutism or polycystic ovarian disease: An allelic variant of congenital virilizing adrenal hyperplasia with a milder enzymatic defect. Ann Intern Med 96:143–148, 1982.
58. Riddick DH, Hammond CB: Adrenal virilism due to 21-hydroxylase deficiency in the postmenarchial female. Obstet Gynecol 45:21–24, 1975.
59. Birnbaum MD, Rose LI: The partial adrenocortical hydroxylase deficiency syndrome in infertile women. Fertil Steril 32:536–541, 1979.
60. Chrousos GP, Loriaux DL, Sherins RJ, Cutler GH Jr: Bilateral testicular enlargement resulting from inapparent 21 hydroxylase deficiency. J Urol 126:127–128, 1981.
61. White PC, Grossberger D, Onufer BJ, et al: Two genes encoding steroid 21-hydroxylase are located near the genes encoding the fourth component of complement in man. Proc Natl Acad Sci U S A 82:1089–1093, 1985.
62. Carroll MC, Campbell RD, Porter RR: The mapping of 21-hydroxylase genes adjacent to complement component C4 genes in HLA, the major histocompatibility complex in man. Proc Natl Acad Sci U S A 82:521–525, 1985.
63. White PC, New MI, Dupont B: Structure of the human steroid 21-hydroxylase genes. Proc Natl Acad Sci U S A 83:5111 5115, 1986.
64. Speiser PW, New MI, White PC: Molecular genetic analysis of nonclassic steroid 21-hydroxylase deficiency associated with HLA B14; DR1. N Engl J Med 319:19–23, 1988.
65. Bongiovanni AM, Eberlein WR, Goldman AS, New MI: Disorders of adrenal steroid biogenesis. Recent Prog Horm Res 23:375–449, 1967.
66. Zerah M, Pang S, New MI: Morning salivary 17-hydroxyprogesterone is a useful screening test for nonclassical 21-hydroxylase deficiency. J Clin Endocrinol Metab 65:227–232, 1987.
67. Pang S, Hotchkiss J, Drash AL, et al: Microfilter paper method for 17α-hydroxyprogesterone radioimmunoassay: Its application for rapid screening for congenital adrenal hyperplasia. J Clin Endocrinol Metab 45:1003–1008, 1977.
68. Mornet E, Dupont J, Vitek A, White PC: Characterization of two genes encoding human steroid 11β-hydroxylase (P 450 11β). J Biol Chem 264:20961–20967, 1989.
69. Chua SC, Szabo P, Vitek A, et al: Cloning of cDNA encoding steroid 11β-hydroxylase (P450c11). Proc Natl Acad Sci U S A 84:7193–7197, 1987.
70. Taymans SE, Pack S, Pak E, et al: Human *CYP11B2* (aldosterone synthase) maps to chromosome 8q24.3. J Clin Endocrinol Metab 83:1033–1036, 1998.
71. Rösler A, Leiberman E: Enzymatic defects of steroidogenesis: 11β-Hydroxylase deficiency congenital adrenal hyperplasia. *In* New MI, Levine LS (eds): Adrenal Diseases in Childhood. Basel, Karger, 1984, pp 47–71.
72. Rösler A, Leiberman E, Sack J, et al: Clinical variability of congenital adrenal hyperplasia due to 11β-hydroxylase deficiency. Horm Res 16:133–141, 1982.
73. Gabrilove JL, Sharma DC, Dorfman R: Adrenocortical 11β-hydroxylase deficiency first manifest in the adult woman. N Engl J Med 272:1189–1194, 1965.
74. Newmark S, Dluhy RG, Williams GH, et al: Partial 11- and 21-hydroxylase deficiencies in hirsute women. Am J Obstet Gynecol 127:594–598, 1977.
75. Cathelineau G, Brerault JL, Fiet J, et al: Adrenocortical 11β-hydroxylation defect in adult women with postmenarchial onset of symptoms. J Clin Endocrinol Metab 51:287–291, 1980.
76. Birnbaum MD, Rose LI: Late onset adrenocortical hydroxylase deficiencies associated with menstrual dysfunction. Obstet Gynecol 63:445–451, 1984.
77. Hurwitz A, Brautbar C, Milwidsky A, et al: Combined 21- and 11β-hydroxylase deficiency in familial congenital adrenal hyperplasia. J Clin Endocrinol Metab 60:631–638, 1985.
78. Pang S, Levine LS, Lorenzen F, et al: Hormonal studies in obligate heterozygotes and siblings of patients with 11β-hydroxylase deficiency congenital adrenal hyperplasia. J Clin Endocrinol Metab 50:586–589, 1980.
79. White PC, Pascoe L: Disorders of steroid 11β-hydroxylase isozymes. Trends Endocrinol 3:229–234, 1992.
80. Levine LS, Rauh W, Gottesdiener K, et al: New studies of the 11β-hydroxylase and 18-hydroxylase enzymes in the hypertensive form of congenital adrenal hyperplasia. J Clin Endocrinol Metab 51:258–263, 1980.
81. New MI, Seaman MP: Secretion rates of cortisol and aldosterone precursors in various forms of congenital adrenal hyperplasia. J Clin Endocrinol Metab 30:361–371, 1970.
82. Gandy HLM, Keutmann EH, Isso AJ: Characterization of urinary steroids in adrenal hyperplasia: Isolation of metabolites of cortisol, compound S, and deoxycorticosterone from a normotensive patient with adrenogenital syndrome. J Clin Invest 39:364–377, 1960.
83. Blunck W: Die β-ketolischen Cortisol und Corticosteronmetaboliten sowie die 11-Oxy- und 11-Desoxy-17-ketosteroide im Urin von Kindern. Acta Endocrinol 59(suppl 134):9–112, 1968.

84. Green OC, Migeon CJ, Wilkins L: Urinary steroids in the hypertensive form of congenital adrenal hyperplasia. J Clin Endocrinol Metab 30:929–946, 1960.
85. Glenthoj A, Nielsen MD, Starup J: Congenital adrenal hyperplasia due to 11β-hydroxylase deficiency: Final diagnosis in adult age in three patients. Acta Endocrinol 93:94–99, 1980.
86. New MI, Nemery RL, Chow DM, et al: Low-renin hypertension of childhood. *In* Mantero F (ed): Adrenal Hypertension: From Cloning to Clinic (Serono Symposia, Tokyo, July 25–26, 1988). New York, Raven, 1988, pp 323–343.
87. Zachmann M, Tassinari D, Prader A: Clinical and biochemical variability of congenital adrenal hyperplasia due to 11β-hydroxylase deficiency. J Clin Endocrinol Metab 56:222–229, 1983.
88. Rösler A: Classic and nonclassic congenital adrenal hyperplasia among non-Ashkenazi Jews. *In* Bonne-Tamir B (ed): New Perspectives on Genetic Markers and Diseases among the Jewish People. Oxford, Oxford University Press, 1992.
89. Kawamoto T, Mitsuuchi Y, Ohnishi T, et al: Cloning and expression of a cDNA for human cytochrome P450aldo as related to primary aldosteronism. Biochem Biophys Res Commun 173:309–316, 1990.
90. Curnow KM, Tusie-Luna MT, Pascoe L, et al: The product of the *CYP11B* gene is required for aldosterone biosynthesis in the human adrenal cortex. Mol Endocrinol 5:1513–1522, 1991.
91. Ogishima T, Shibata H, Shimada H, et al: Aldosterone synthase cytochrome P-450 expressed in the adrenals of patients with primary aldosteronism. J Biol Chem 266:10731–10734, 1991.
92. White PC, Dupont J, New MI, et al: A mutation in *CYP11B1* (Arg-448-His) associated with steroid 11β-hydroxylase deficiency in Jews of Moroccan origin. J Clin Invest 87:1664–1667, 1991.
93. Curnow KM, Slutsker L, Vitek J, et al: Mutations in the *CYP11B1* gene causing congenital adrenal hyperplasia and hypertension cluster in exons 6, 7, and 8. Proc Natl Acad Sci U S A 90:4552–4556, 1993.
94. Eberlein WR, Bongiovanni AM: Plasma and urinary corticosteroids in the hypertensive form of congenital adrenal hyperplasia. J Biol Chem 223:85–94, 1956.
95. Mimouni M, Kaufman H, Roitman A, et al: Hypertension in a neonate with 11β-hydroxylase deficiency. Eur J Pediatr 143:231–233, 1985.
96. Mitsuuchi Y, Kawamoto K, Ulick S, et al: Congenitally defective aldosterone biosynthesis in humans: Inactivation of the P450c18 gene *CYP11B2* due to nucleotide deletion in CMO I deficient patients. Biochem Biophys Res Commun 190:864–869, 1993.
97. Portrat-Doyen S, Tourniaire J, Richard O, et al: Isolated aldosterone synthetase deficiency caused by simultaneous E98D and V386A mutations in the *CYP11B2* gene. J Clin Endocrinol Metab 83:4156–4161, 1998.
98. Hauffa BP, Sólyom J, Gláz E, et al: Severe hypoaldosteronism due to corticosterone methyl oxidase type II deficiency in two boys: Metabolic and gas chromatography–mass spectrometry studies. Eur J Pediatr 150:149–153, 1991.
99. Globerman H, Rösler A, Theodor R, et al: An inherited defect in aldosterone biosynthesis caused by a mutation in or near the gene for steroid 11-hydroxylase. N Engl J Med 319:1193–1197, 1988.
100. Pascoe L, Curnow KM, Slutzker L, et al: Mutations in the human *CYP11B2* (aldosterone synthase) gene causing corticosterone methyloxidase II deficiency. Proc Natl Acad Sci U S A 89:4996–5000, 1992.
101. New MI, Petersen RE: A new form of congenital adrenal hyperplasia (letter). J Clin Endocrinol Metab 27:300–305, 1967.
102. Sutherland DJA, Ruse JL, Laidlaw LC: Hypertension, increased aldosterone secretion and low plasma renin activity relieved by dexamethasone. Can Med Assoc J 95:1109–1119, 1966.
103. Oberfield SE, Levine LS, Stoner E, et al: Adrenal glomerulosa function in patients with dexamethasone-suppressible hyperaldosteronism. J Clin Endocrinol Metab 53:158–163, 1981.
104. New MI, Oberfield SE, Levine LS, et al: Autosomal dominant transmission and absence of HLA linkage in dexamethasone-suppressible hyperaldosteronism (letter). Lancet 1:550–551, 1980.
105. Ulick S, Chu MD: Hypersecretion of a new corticosteroid, 18-hydroxycortisol, in two types of adrenocortical hypertension. Clin Exp Hypertens 10(suppl 9):1771–1777, 1982.
106. Gomez-Sanchez CE, Montgomery M, Ganguly A, et al: Elevated urinary secretion of 18-oxocortisol in glucocorticoid-suppressible aldosteronism. J Clin Endocrinol Metab 59:1022–1024, 1984.
107. Lifton RP, Dluhy RG, Powers M, et al: A chimaeric 11β-hydroxylase/aldosterone synthase gene causes glucocorticoid-remediable aldosteronism and human hypertension. Nature 355:262–265, 1992.
108. Pascoe L, Curnow KM, Slutsker L, et al: Glucocorticoid suppressible hyperaldosteronism results from hybrid genes created by unequal crossovers between *CYP11B1* and *CYP11B2*. Proc Natl Acad Sci U S A 89:8327–8331, 1992.
109. Lachance Y, Luu-The V, Verreault H, et al: Structure of the human type II 3β-hydroxysteroid dehydrogenase deficiency gene: Adrenal and gonadal specificity. DNA Cell Biol 10:701, 1991.
110. Lachance Y, Luu-The V, Labrie C, et al: Characterization of human 3β-hydroxysteroid dehydrogenase/Δ^5-Δ^4 isomerase gene and its expression in mammalian cells. J Biol Chem 265:20469–20475, 1990.
111. Simard J, Rhéaume E, van Seters AP, et al: Molecular basis of classical 3β-hydroxysteroid dehydrogenase/Δ-5/Δ-4 isomerase deficiency (abstract). The Endocrine Society, San Antonio, TX, 1992.
112. Rhéaume E, Simard J, Morel Y, et al: Congenital adrenal hyperplasia due to point mutations in the type II 3β-hydroxysteroid dehydrogenase gene. Nat Genet 1:239–245, 1992.
113. Bongiovanni AM: The adrenogenital syndrome with deficiency of 3β-hydroxysteroid dehydrogenase. J Clin Invest 41:2086–2092, 1962.
114. Bongiovanni AM: Congenital adrenal hyperplasia due to 3β-hydroxysteroid deficiency. *In* New MI, Levine LS (eds): Pediatric and Adolescent Endocrinology, vol 13, Adrenal Diseases in Childhood. Basel, Karger, 1984, pp 72–82.
115. Pang S, Levine LS, Stoner E, et al: Non–salt-losing congenital adrenal hyperplasia due to 3β-hydroxysteroid dehydrogenase activity with normal glomerulosa function. J Clin Endocrinol Metab 56:808–818, 1983.
116. Rosenfield RL, Rich BH, Wolfsdorf JI, et al: Pubertal presentation of congenital (Δ^5-3β-hydroxysteroid dehydrogenase deficiency. J Clin Endocrinol Metab 51:345–353, 1980.
117. Schram P, Zerah M, Mani P, et al: Nonclassical 3β-hydroxysteroid dehydrogenase deficiency: A review of our experience with 25 female patients. Fertil Steril 58:129–136, 1992.
118. Zerah M, Schram P, New MI: The diagnosis and treatment of nonclassical 3β-HSD deficiency. Endocrinologist 1(2):75–81, 1991.
119. Lorence MC, Corbin CJ, Kamimura N, et al: Structural analysis of the gene encoding human 3β-hydroxysteroid dehydrogenase/$\Delta^{5,4}$-isomerase. Mol Endocrinol 4:1850–1855, 1990.
120. Katsumata N, Tanae A, Yasunaga T, et al: A novel missense mutation in the type II 3β-hydroxysteroid dehydrogenase gene in a family with classical salt-wasting congenital adrenal hyperplasia due to 3β-hydroxysteroid dehydrogenase deficiency. Hum Mol Genet 4:745–746, 1995.
121. Tajima T, Fujieda K, Nakae J, et al: Molecular analysis of type II 3b-hydroxysteroid dehydrogenase gene in Japanese patients with classical 3β-hydroxysteroid dehydrogenase deficiency. Hum Mol Genet 4:969–971, 1995.
122. Morel Y, Mebarki F, Rheaume E, et al: 3β-Hydroxysteroid dehydrogenase: Contribution made by the molecular genetics of 3β-hydroxysteroid dehydrogenase deficiency. Steroids 62:176–184, 1997.
123. Yanase T, Simpson ER, Waterman MR: 17α-Hydroxylase/17,20-lyase deficiency: From clinical investigation to molecular definition. Endocr Rev 12:91–108, 1991.
124. Miura K, Yasuda K, Yanase T, et al: Mutation of cytochrome P-45017α gene (*CYP17*) in a Japanese patient previously reported as having glucocorticoid-responsive hyperaldosteronism: With a review of Japanese patients with mutations of *CYP17*. J Clin Endocrinol Metab 81:3797–3801, 1996.
125. Zachmann M, Prader A: 17,20-Desmolase deficiency. *In* New MI, Levine LS (eds): Pediatric and Adolescent Endocrinology, vol 13, Adrenal Diseases in Childhood. Basel, Karger, 1984, p 95.
126. Zachmann M, Kempken B, Manella B, Navarro E: Conversion from pure 17,20-desmolase- to combined 17,20-desmolase/17alpha-hydroxylase deficiency with age. Acta Endocrinol 127:97–99, 1992.
127. Mantero F, Scaroni C, Pasini CV, Fajiolo U: No linkage between HLA and congenital adrenal hyperplasia due to 17α-hydroxylase deficiency (letter). N Engl J Med 303:530, 1980.
128. Ulick S: Diagnosis and nomenclature of the disorders of the terminal portion of the aldosterone biosynthetic pathway. J Clin Endocrinol Metab 43:92–96, 1976.
129. Griffing GT, Wilson TE, Holbrook MM, et al: Plasma and urinary 19-nor-DOC in 17-hydroxylase deficiency syndrome. J Clin Endocrinol Metab 59:1011–1015, 1984.
130. Wit JM, van Roermund HPC, Oostdik W, et al: Heterozygotes for 17α-hydroxylase deficiency can be detected with a short ACTH test. Clin Endocrinol 28:657–664, 1988.
131. Miura K, Yoshinaga K, Goto K, et al: A case of glucocorticoid-responsive hyperaldosteronism. J Clin Endocrinol Metab 28:1807–1815, 1968.
132. Chung BC, Picado-Leonard J, Haniu M, et al: Cytochrome P450c17 (steroid 17α-hydroxylase/17,20-lyase): Cloning of human adrenal and testis cDNAs indicates the same gene is expressed in both tissues. Proc Natl Acad Sci U S A 84:407–411, 1987.
133. Matteson KJ, Picado-Leonard J, Chung B-C, et al: Assignment of the gene for adrenal $P\text{-}450_{17\alpha}$- (steroid 17α-hydroxylase/17,20 lyase) to human chromosome 10. J Clin Endocrinol Metab 63:789–791, 1986.
134. Imai T, Yanase T, Waterman MR, et al: Canadian Mennonites and individuals residing in the Friesland region of the Netherlands share the same molecular basis of 17α-hydroxylase deficiency. Hum Genet 89:95–96, 1992.
135. D'Armiento M, Reda G, Kater C, et al: 17α-Hydroxylase deficiency: Mineralocorticoid hormone profiles in an affected family. J Clin Endocrinol Metab 56:697–701, 1983.
136. Prader A, Gurtner HP: Das syndrom des Pseudohermaphroditismus masculinus bei kongenitaler Nebennierenrinden ohne Androgenüberproduktion (Adrenaler Pseudohermaphroditismus masculinus)-hyperplasie. Helv Paediatr Acta 10:397–412, 1955.
137. Lin D, Gitelman SE, Saenger P, Miller WL: Normal genes for the cholesterol side chain cleavage enzyme, P450scc, in congenital lipoid adrenal hyperplasia. J Clin Invest 88:1955–1962, 1991.
138. Yoo HW, Kim GH: Molecular and clinical characterization of Korean patients with congenital lipoid adrenal hyperplasia. J Pediatr Endocrinol Metab 11:707–711, 1998.
139. Wilkins L, Lewis RA, Klein R, Rosemberg E: The suppression of androgen secretion by cortisone in a case of congenital adrenal hyperplasia. Bull Johns Hopkins Hosp 86:249–252, 1950.
140. Bartter FC: Adrenogenital syndromes: From physiology to chemistry (1950–1975). *In* Lee PA, Plotnick LP, Lowarski AA, Migeon CJ (eds): Congenital Adrenal Hyperplasia. Baltimore, University Park Press, 1977, pp 9–18.
141. Godard C, Riondel AM, Veyrat R, et al: Plasma renin activity and aldosterone secretion in congenital adrenal hyperplasia. Pediatrics 41:883–896, 1968.
142. Simopoulos AP, Marshall JR, Delea CS, Bartter FC: Studies on the deficiency of 21-hydroxylation in patients with congenital adrenal hyperplasia. J Clin Endocrinol Metab 32:438–443, 1971.
143. Strickland AL, Kotchen TA: A study of the renin-aldosterone system in congenital adrenal hyperplasia. J Pediatr 81:962–969, 1972.
144. Dillon MJ, Ryness J: Proceedings: Plasma renin activity and aldosterone concentrations in children: Results in salt-wasting states. Arch Dis Child 50:330, 1975.
145. Edwin C, Lanes R, Migeon CJ, et al: Persistence of the enzymatic block in adolescent patients with salt-losing congenital adrenal hyperplasia. J Pediatr 95:534–537, 1979.
146. Rösler A, Levine LS, Schneider B, et al: The interrelationship of sodium balance, plasma renin activity and ACTH in congenital adrenal hyperplasia. J Clin Endocrinol Metab 45:500–512, 1977.

147. Kuhnle U, Rösler A, Pareira JA, et al: The effects of long term normalization of sodium balance on linear growth in disorders with aldosterone deficiency. Acta Endocrinol 102:577–582, 1983.
148. Winter JSD: Maximal comment: Current approaches to the treatment of congenital adrenal hyperplasia. J Pediatr 97:81–82, 1980.
149. Korth-Schutz S, Virdis R, Saenger P, et al: Serum androgens as a continuing index of adequacy of treatment of congenital adrenal hyperplasia. J Clin Endocrinol Metab 46:452–458, 1978.
150. Golden MP, Lippe BM, Kaplan SA, et al: Management of congenital adrenal hyperplasia using serum dehydroepiandrosterone sulfate and 17-hydroxyprogesterone concentrations. Pediatrics 61:867–871, 1978.
151. Döhler K-D: The special case of hormonal imprinting, the neonatal influence of sex. Experientia (Basel) 42:759–769, 1986.
152. Döhler K-D, Hancke JL, Srivastava SS, et al: Participation of estrogens in female sexual differentiation of the brain; neuroanatomical, neuroendocrine and behavioral evidence. Prog Brain Res 61:99–117, 1984.
153. Berenbaum SA: Congenital adrenal hyperplasia: Intellectual and psychosexual functioning. *In* Holmes CPS (ed): Psychoneuroendocrinology: Brain, Behavioral, and Hormonal Interactions. New York, Springer-Verlag, 1990, pp 227–260.
154. Nass R, Baker S: Learning disabilities in children with congenital adrenal hyperplasia. J Child Neurol 6:306–312, 1991.
155. Nass R, Heier L, Moshang T, et al: Magnetic resonance imaging in the congenital adrenal hyperplasia population: Increased frequency of white-matter abnormalities and temporal lobe atrophy. J Child Neurol 12:181–186, 1997.
156. Herdt GH, Davidson J: The Sambia "Turnim-man": Sociocultural and clinical aspects of gender formation in male pseudohermaphrodites with 5α-reductase deficiency in Papua New Guinea. Arch Sex Behav 17:33–56, 1988.
157. Price P, Wass JAH, Griffin JE, et al: High dose androgen therapy in male pseudohermaphroditism due to 5α-reductase deficiency and disorders of the androgen receptor. J Clin Invest 74:1496–1508, 1984.
158. Money J, Hampson JG, Hampson JL: Hermaphroditism: Recommendations concerning assignment of sex, change of sex, and psychologic management. Bull Johns Hopkins Hosp 96:284–300, 1955.
159. Money J, Ehrhardt AA: Man and Woman, Boy and Girl: Differentiation and Dimorphism of Gender Identity. Baltimore, Johns Hopkins University Press, 1972, pp 89, 152.
160. Baker SW: Psychological management of intersex children. *In* Josso N (ed): Pediatric Adolescent Endocrinology, vol 8, The Intersex Child. Basel, Karger, 1981, p 261.
161. Meyer-Bahlburg HFL: Gender identity: Development in intersex patients. Child Adolesc Psychiatr Clin North Am 2:501–512, 1993.
162. Nihoul-Fekete C: Feminizing genitoplasty in the intersex child. *In* Josso N (ed): Pediatric Adolescent Endocrinology, vol 8, The Intersex Child. Basel, Karger, 1981, p 247.
163. Jeffcoate TN, Fleigner JR, Russell SH, et al: Diagnosis of the adrenogenital syndrome before birth. Lancet 2:553–555, 1965.
164. Merkatz IR, New MI, Seaman MP: Prenatal diagnosis of adrenogenital syndrome by amniocentesis. J Pediatr 75:977–982, 1969.
165. New MI, Levine LS: Congenital adrenal hyperplasia. *In* Harris H, Hirschhorn K (eds): Advances in Human Genetics. New York, Plenum, 1973, pp 251–326.
166. Levine LS: Prenatal detection of congenital adrenal hyperplasia. *In* Milunsky A (ed): Genetic Disorders and the Fetus. New York, Plenum, 1986, pp 369–385.
167. Frasier SD, Thorneycroft IH, Weill DA, Horton R: Elevated amniotic fluid concentration of 17-hydroxyprogesterone in congenital adrenal hyperplasia. J Pediatr 86:310, 1975.
168. Nagamani M, McDonough PG, Ellegood JO, Mahesh VB: Maternal and amniotic fluid 17-hydroxyprogesterone levels during pregnancy: Diagnosis of congenital adrenal hyperplasia in utero. Am J Obstet Gynecol 130:791–794, 1978.
169. Hughes IA, Laurence KM: Antenatal diagnosis of congenital adrenal hyperplasia. Lancet 2:7–9, 1979.
170. Pang S, Levine LS, Cederqvist LL, et al: Amniotic fluid concentration of Δ^5 and Δ^4 steroids in fetuses with congenital adrenal hyperplasia due to 21-hydroxylase deficiency and in anencephalic fetuses. J Clin Endocrinol Metab 51:223–229, 1980.
171. Hughes IA, Laurence KM: Prenatal diagnosis of congenital adrenal hyperplasia due to 21-hydroxylase deficiency: Amniotic fluid steroid analysis. Prenat Diagn 2:97, 1982.
172. Pang S, Pollack MS, Loo M, et al: Pitfalls of prenatal diagnosis of 21-hydroxylase deficiency congenital adrenal hyperplasia. J Clin Endocrinol Metab 61:89–97, 1985.
173. Frasier SD, Weiss BA, Horton R: Amniotic fluid testosterone: Implications for the prenatal diagnosis of congenital adrenal hyperplasia. J Pediatr 84:738–741, 1974.
174. Pollack MS, Levine LS, Pang S, et al: Prenatal diagnosis of congenital adrenal hyperplasia (21-hydroxylase deficiency) by HLA typing. Lancet 1:1107–1108, 1979.
175. Speiser PW, Dupont J, Zhu D, et al: Disease expression and molecular genotype in congenital adrenal hyperplasia due to 21-hydroxylase deficiency. J Clin Invest 90:584–595, 1992.
176. Werkmeister JW, New MI, Dupont B, White PC: Frequent deletion and duplication of the steroid 21-hydroxylase genes. Am J Hum Genet 39:461–469, 1986.
177. Collier S, Sinnott PJ, Dyer PA, et al: Pulsed field gel electrophoresis identifies a high degree of variability in the number of tandem 21-hydroxylase and complement C4 gene repeats in 21-hydroxylase deficiency. EMBO J 8:1393–1402, 1989.
178. Rösler A, Leiberman E, Rosenmann A, et al: Prenatal diagnosis of 11β-hydroxylase deficiency congenital adrenal hyperplasia. J Clin Endocrinol Metab 49:546–551, 1979.
179. Schumert Z, Rosenmann A, Landau H, Rösler A: 11-Deoxycortisol in amniotic fluid: Prenatal diagnosis of congenital adrenal hyperplasia due to 11β-hydroxylase deficiency. Clin Endocrinol 12:257–260, 1980.
180. Rösler A, Weshler N, Leiberman E, et al: 11β-Hydroxylase deficiency congenital adrenal hyperplasia: Update of prenatal diagnosis. J Clin Endocrinol Metab 66:830–838, 1988.
181. David M, Forest MG: Prenatal treatment of congenital adrenal hyperplasia resulting from 21-hydroxylase deficiency. J Pediatr 105:799–803, 1984.
182. Evans MI, Chrousos GP, Mann DW, et al: Pharmacologic suppression of the fetal adrenal gland in utero. JAMA 253:1015–1020, 1985.
183. Dörr HG, Sippell WG, Haack D, et al: Pitfalls of prenatal treatment of congenital adrenal hyperplasia (CAH) due to 21-hydroxylase deficiency. *In* Proceedings of the 25th Annual Meeting of the European Society for Paediatric Endocrinology. Zurich, August 1986.
184. Petersen KE, Damkjaer Nielsen M, Buus O, Couillin P: Congenital adrenal hyperplasia (CAH): Prenatal treatment. Pediatr Res 20:1201, 1986.
185. Forest MG, Betuel H, David M: Traitement antenatal de l'hyperplasie congenitale des surrenales par deficit en 21-hydroxylase: Etude multicentrique. Ann Endocrinol (Paris) 48:31–34, 1987.
186. Speiser PW, Laforgia N, Kato K, et al: First trimester prenatal treatment and molecular genetic diagnosis of congenital adrenal hyperplasia (21-hydroxylase deficiency). J Clin Endocrinol Metab 70:838–848, 1990.
187. Goldman AS, Shapiro BH, Katsumata M: Human foetal palatal corticoid receptors and teratogens for cleft palate. Nature 272:464–466, 1978.
188. Carlson AD, Obeid JS, Kanellopoulou N, et al: Congenital adrenal hyperplasia: Update on prenatal diagnosis and treatment. J Steroid Biochem Mol Biol 69:19–29, 1999.
189. Forest MG, Betuel H, David M: Prenatal treatment in congenital adrenal hyperplasia due to 21-hydroxylase deficiency: Update 88 of the French multicentric study. Endocr Res 15:277–301, 1989.
190. Wilson D, McGillivray B, Kalousek D, et al: Multicentre randomised clinical trial of chorion villus sampling and amniocentesis: First report. Lancet 1:1–6, 1989.
191. Simpson JL: Chorionic villus sampling. Semin Perinatol 14:446–455, 1990.

Chapter 124

Adrenarche

Lawrence N. Parker

Adrenarche is the overall term for the striking series of adrenal gland maturational changes which occur in humans and some animal species well before the onset of puberty. In children of both sexes, this process is characterized clinically by the pubarche, the appearance of axillary and pubic hair between 6 and 8 years of age. With respect to the secretion of adrenocortical steroid hormones during this time, there is an increase in the secretion of a variety of adrenal androgens, in the absence of corresponding increases in the secretion of adrenocorticotropic hormone (ACTH), cortisol, or mineralocorticoids.

ADRENAL ANDROGEN METABOLISM

The human adrenal gland secretes glucocorticoids, androgens, and mineralocorticoids, all derived from the common precursor pregnenolone, which is derived from cholesterol esters. An overview of adrenal steroidogenic pathways is shown in Figure 124–1.

The initial and rate-limiting step in adrenal steroidogenesis is the conversion of cholesterol to pregnenolone, which is regulated by ACTH, and mediated by the heme-containing cytochrome P450 side-chain cleavage enzyme cytochrome (P450*scc*). Other cytochrome P450 steroidogenic enzymes are 17α-hydroxylase and 17,20-lyase or 17,20-desmolase ($P450c_{17}$), which constitute a single enzyme with two activities; 21-hydroxylase ($P450c_{21}$), 11β-hydroxylase ($P450c_{11}\beta$), and the enzyme closely related to $P450c_{11}$, $P450c_{11AS}$ (aldosterone synthase), which has combined 11β-hydroxylase, 18-hydroxylase, and 18-methyloxidase activities.

Conversion of steroids of the Δ^5 conformation, such as pregnenolone and dehydroepiandrosterone, to those of the Δ^4 conformation, such as androstenedione and progesterone, is mediated by the microsomal non-P450 enzyme 3β-hydroxysteroid dehydrogenase/isomerase. There are two isozymes of this enzyme. The type II enzyme is found in the adrenal, ovary, and testis, while the type I enzyme is located in brain, placenta, and other tissues.

Dehydroepiandrosterone sulfate is the steroid hormone found in greatest concentration in the human circulation. It is formed by the action of steroid sulfotransferase on dehydroepiandrosterone, or from conversion of sulfated cholesterol or pregnenolone. The reverse reaction is catalyzed by the enzyme steroid sulfatase.

Androstenedione is a central hormone with respect to sexual differentiation. Reversible reduction of the 17-keto group of androstenedione to testosterone is mediated by the non-P450 enzyme 17β-hydroxysteroid dehydrogenase (17β-hydroxysteroid oxidoreductase; 17-ketosteroid reductase), which exists in several forms, and is necessary for virilization. The same enzymatic activity is necessary for the reduction of estrone to estradiol, which is necessary for feminization, both mainly gonadal functions. Androstenedione is also converted by the adrenal gland to 11β-hydroxyandrostenedione.

Dehydroepiandrosterone is also converted to androstenediol, an adrenal steroid which is unusual in that it has intrinsic estrogenic bioactivity, due to its ability to bind to estrogen receptors. Many of these steroidal hormones have been measured in preadrenarchal and adrenarchal children.

ADRENAL ANDROGEN SECRETION BEFORE THE ADRENARCHE

In the neonatal period, plasma concentrations of cortisol are highly variable and demonstrate no sex difference, a finding which persists during early childhood. Cortisol production rates after the first 5 days of life are similar in infants, children, adolescents, and young and middle-aged adults when corrected for body surface area. In contrast, as shown in Figure 124–2, plasma concentrations of dehydroepiandrosterone sulfate fall sharply during the first month of life due to involution of the fetal zone of the adrenal cortex. A similar pattern occurs with dehydroepiandrosterone in both sexes. Androstenedione levels also decrease during the neonatal period, although they remain higher in boys due to transient activity of the testes during the first 3 months of life.

After the neonatal period and during early childhood, circulating concentrations of cortisol, dehydroepiandrostenedione, androstenedione, dehydroepiandrostenedione sulfate, and 11β-hydroxyandrostenedione are constant. Until 6 years of age, levels of adrenal androgens in normal children are at their lifetime minimum. Patterns of adrenal androgen secretion in preadrenarchal and adrenarchal children have been reviewed in detail.[1]

ADRENAL ANDROGEN SECRETION DURING THE ADRENARCHE

In children 6 to 8 years of age, while cortisol concentrations remain constant, and before pubertal increases of gonadotropins are noted, circulating levels of adrenal androgens increase. As shown in Figure 124–2, plasma concentrations of dehydroepiandrosterone demonstrate some variability, but undergo a definite increase in both sexes. Concentrations of dexamethasone-suppressible androstenedione and 11β-hydroxyandrostenedione also increase during this time. Adrenal androgen levels continue to increase during adolescence, and peak concentrations are noted during the third decade of life, with a continuous and variable decrease during aging. During late adrenarche, and throughout puberty, as shown in Figure 124–3, circulating concentrations of ACTH and cortisol are constant.

ADRENARCHE IN ANIMALS

Circulating steroid concentrations have been measured in various animals to ascertain whether nonhuman species also demonstrate an adrenarche. Concentrations of dehydroepiandrosterone, androstenedione, and dehydroepiandrosterone sulfate were measured in the rat, guinea pig, hamster, rabbit, dog, sheep, pig, goat, horse, cow, chicken, rhesus monkey, chimpanzee, gorilla, orangutan, colobus monkey, baboon, Barbary ape, and langur.[2] In animals studied before sexual maturation, the only ones that had dehydroepiandrosterone concentrations above the assay detection limit were the rhesus monkey, chimpanzee, and other primates. The only species that had detectable

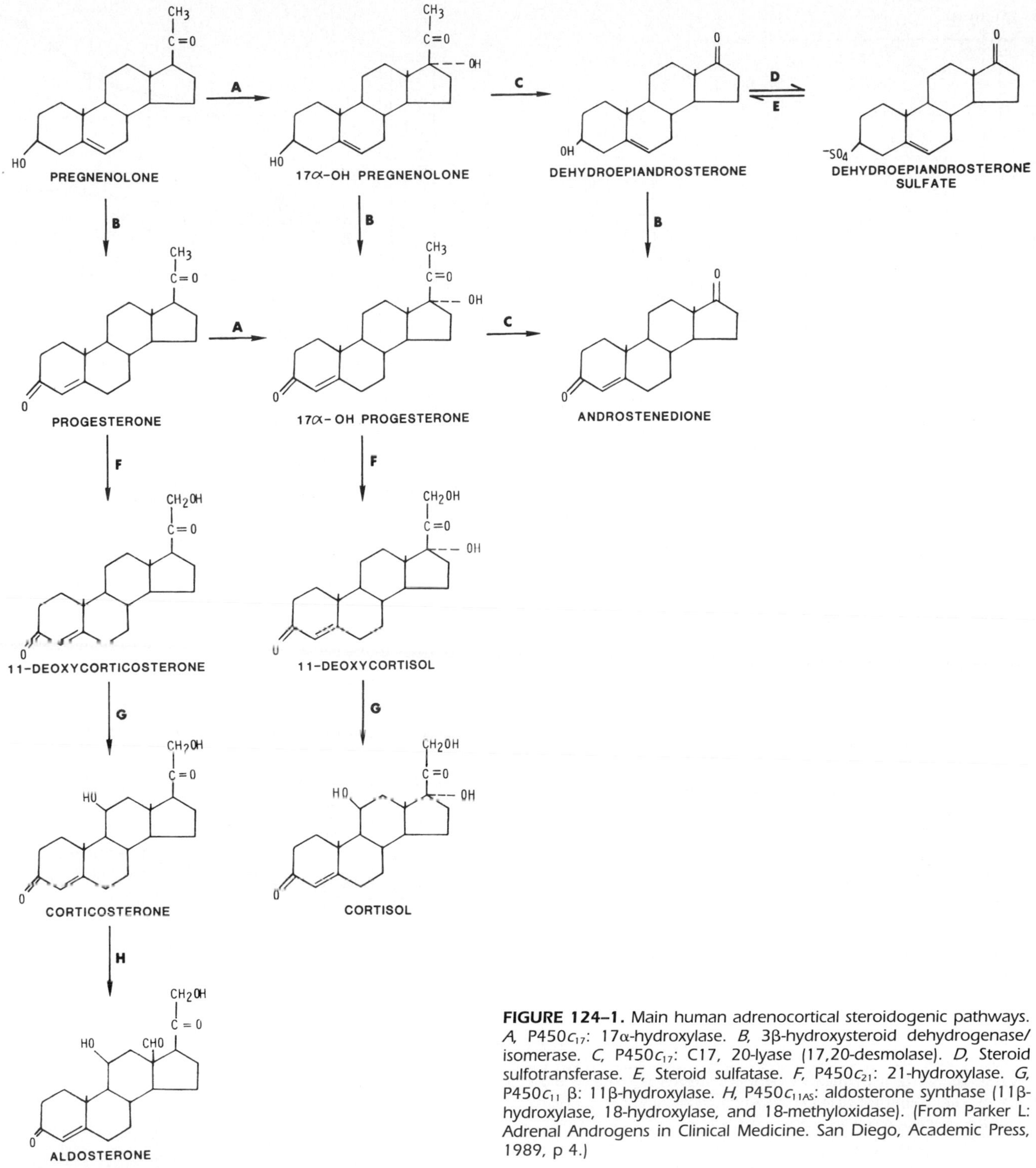

FIGURE 124–1. Main human adrenocortical steroidogenic pathways. *A*, $P450_{C17}$: 17α-hydroxylase. *B*, 3β-hydroxysteroid dehydrogenase/isomerase. *C*, $P450_{C17}$: C17, 20-lyase (17,20-desmolase). *D*, Steroid sulfotransferase. *E*, Steroid sulfatase. *F*, $P450_{C21}$: 21-hydroxylase. *G*, $P450_{C11}$ β: 11β-hydroxylase. *H*, $P450_{C11AS}$: aldosterone synthase (11β-hydroxylase, 18-hydroxylase, and 18-methyloxidase). (From Parker L: Adrenal Androgens in Clinical Medicine. San Diego, Academic Press, 1989, p 4.)

dehydroepiandrosterone sulfate levels were the rhesus monkey, chimpanzee, gorilla, colobus monkey, and baboon. Of these species, the chimpanzee was found to have an age-related increase in concentrations of dehydroepiandrosterone, androstenedione, and dehydroepiandrosterone sulfate before puberty. As in humans, simultaneous concentrations of cortisol were unchanged, so the chimpanzee appears to have an adrenarche analogous to that found in humans.

THEORIES ABOUT THE ETIOLOGY OF ADRENARCHE

The hypothalamic-pituitary axis exerts a major influence on cortisol secretion via the actions of ACTH. However, it is not clear what constitutes a specific stimulus for secretion of dehydroepiandrosterone and other adrenal androgens.

Genetic Factors

In a study of monozygotic and dizygotic twins, serum androstenedione concentrations were measured during pubertal development. In this age-matched population, serum androstenedione concentrations showed significantly higher intrapair similarity in monozygotic twins than in dizygotic twins.[3] In another study of 178 individuals drawn from 26 families, when the effect of age was factored out, a genetic component to the variation of serum levels of dehydroepiandrosterone

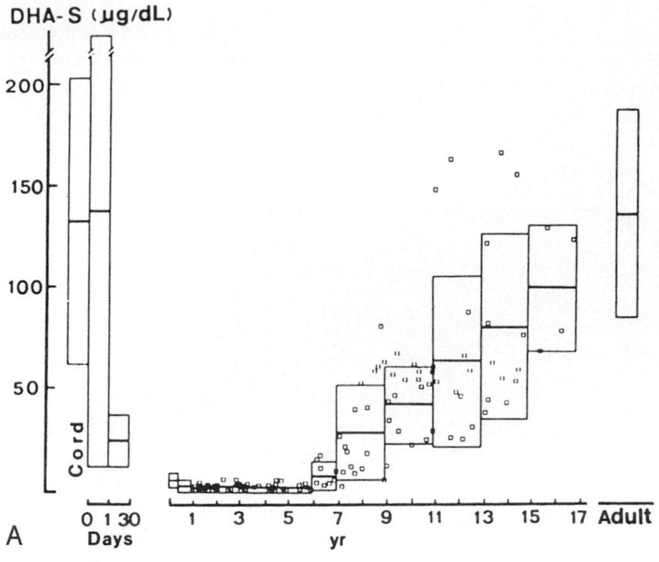

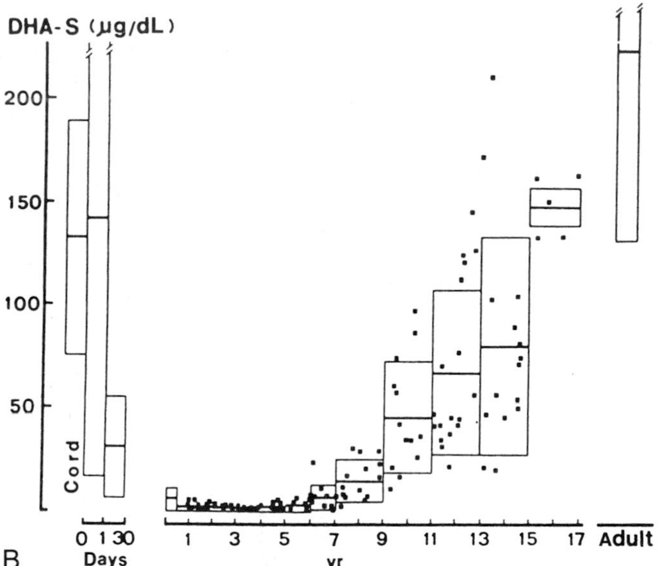

FIGURE 124–2. Plasma concentrations of dehydroepiandrosterone sulfate in *(A)* girls and *(B)* boys from 1 to 17 years of age. (From dePeretti E, Forest A: Pattern of plasma dehydroepiandrosterone sulfate levels in humans from birth to adulthood. J Clin Endocrinol Metab 47:572, 1978. © The Endocrine Society.)

sulfate was found, with a heritability of 65%,[4] which is close to the heritability of 58% found for urinary dehydroepiandrosterone reported in twins during adrenarche.[5]

Control by ACTH

ACTH is a regulating factor for secretion of dehydroepiandrosterone sulfate under certain physiologic and pharmacologic conditions, as inferred from studies of ACTH stimulation and suppression. However, whereas ACTH stimulation causes an acute and chronic increase in cortisol secretion, it has little acute effect on dehydroepiandrosterone sulfate, and a variable chronic effect. ACTH stimulation causes an acute increase in dehydroepiandrosterone secretion, but also a variable chronic effect.[6] Acute dexamethasone administration has been found to cause a decrease in cortisol and dehydroepiandrosterone sulfate concentrations, but often to a dissimilar degree. As shown in Figure 124–4, when chronic glucocorticoid suppression is discontinued in adults, cortisol concentrations have been found to return to normal values more quickly than those of dehydroepiandrosterone or its sulfate.[7] In addition, in children under the age of adrenarche, glucocorticoids have not had the same suppressive effects on dehydroepiandrosterone sulfate which they exert after adrenarche.[8]

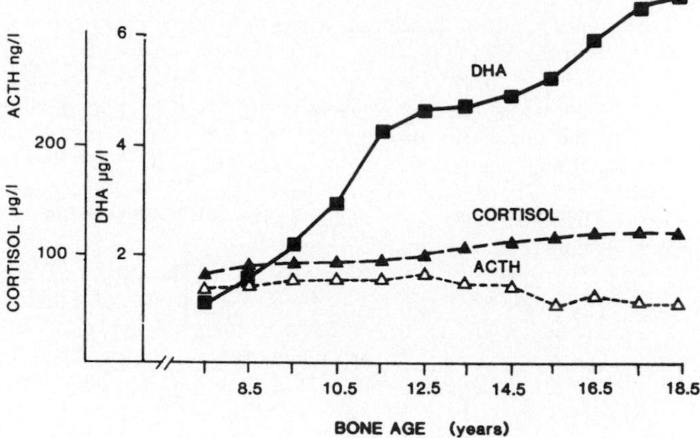

FIGURE 124–3. Serum adrenocorticotropic hormone, dehydroepiandrosterone, and cortisol concentrations in prepubertal and pubertal girls. (From Apter D, Pakkerinen A, Hammond G, et al: Adrenocortical function in puberty. Acta Paediatr Scand 68:599, 1979.)

In additional to pharmacologic studies of the effects of ACTH and glucocorticoids on adrenal androgens, there are a number of physiologic and pathologic situations reported in which there is a dissociation of ACTH and adrenal androgen secretion, as measured by cortisol and dehydroepiandrosterone concentrations. Adrenarche and puberty, as mentioned previously, are two examples. Another condition with an increase of dehydroepiandrosterone and its sulfate occurs without an increase in cortisol is in the polycystic ovarian syndrome.[9, 10]

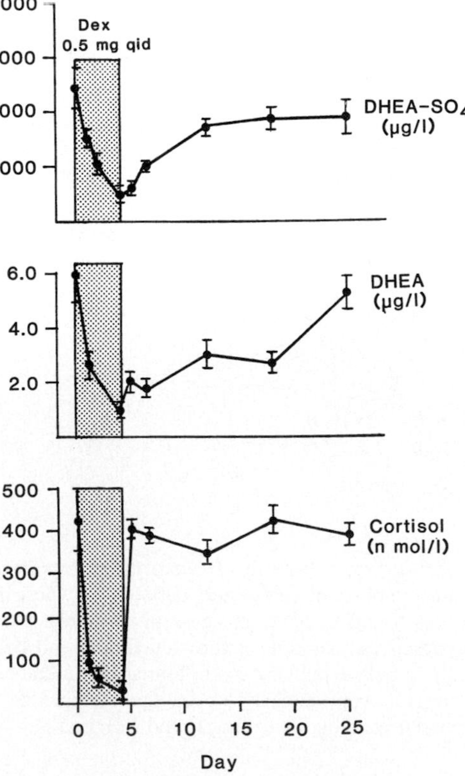

FIGURE 124–4. Serum concentrations of dehydroepiandrosterone sulfate (DHAS), dehydroepiandrosterone (DHA), and cortisol in adults before, during, and after dexamethasone administration. (From Dunn P, Mahood C, Speed J, et al: Dehydroepiandrosterone sulfate concentrations in asthmatic patients. N Z Med J 97:805, 1984.)

The opposite type of dissociation occurs with normal aging, and with many types of stress or illness. Instead of an increased ratio of dehydroepiandrosterone to cortisol, as in adrenarche, puberty, and early adulthood, the opposite ratio is found. In the case of numerous physical stressors and anorexia nervosa, the ratio corrects itself with treatment of the underlying disorder.[11–13] However, in spite of these observations of dissociation of cortisol and adrenal androgen secretion, it has been noted that children with 21-hydroxylase deficiency congenital adrenal hyperplasia (CAH) treated with nonsuppressive doses of glucocorticoids do not exhibit typical adrenarchal increases of dehydroepiandrosterone sulfate.[14] In addition, a lack of adrenarche has been reported in the rare autosomal recessive disorder of familial glucocorticoid deficiency, in which there are defects in the ACTH receptor or postreceptor mechanisms, which would indicate at least a partial role for ACTH in adrenarche, either by itself, or as a factor which "primes" the adrenal, or coordinates its action with that of another adrenal stimulating factor.[15–17]

Control by Intrinsic Adrenal Factors

Mechanisms intrinsic to the adrenal gland have also been investigated with respect to the shift of pregnenolone metabolism to adrenal androgen rather than cortisol production. Some of these studies have focused on differences in adrenal histology. Lipid-rich cells of the adrenal cortex contain large amounts of cholesterol and cholesterol esters, and constitute the zona fasciculata. Lipid-poor compact cells compose the inner zona reticularis. The relative widths of these zones are variable. After ACTH stimulation, the zona reticularis widens, sometimes sufficiently to obliterate the adjacent zona fasciculata. The zona reticularis has been reported to appear as a focally recognizable structure at age 5 years, and as a continuous layer by 8 years of age.

Studies of the zona reticularis have shown that it is rich in dehydroepiandrosterone sulfotransferase activity by immunoperoxidase staining.[18] The zona reticularis of the fetal and adult adrenal has also been shown to express decreased messenger RNA (mRNA) for 3β-hydroxysteroid dehydrogenase, which would have the effect of shifting pregnenolone metabolism to dehydroepiandrosterone.[19] In a study of autopsy and surgical adrenal specimens, a decrease was found in immunohistochemical staining for 3β-hydroxysteroid dehydrogenase from subjects 8 to 13 years of age, as compared with those 5 to 7 years of age, which would correspond to the adrenarche.[20] As mentioned previously, there is a marked decrease in adrenal androgen concentrations with age, so by this mechanism a corresponding increase in enzyme activity would be expected, which was not observed in subjects 25 to 56 years of age. However, it is possible that mechanisms of altered adrenal androgen metabolism in adrenarche are different from those involved in aging, or in chronic illness. A potential confounding factor in studies of only dehydroepiandrosterone in adrenarche is that explanations other than simply decreased activity of 3β-hydroxysteroid dehydrogenase would have to be invoked to explain adrenarchal increases in other steroids, such as androstenedione and 11β-hydroxyandrostenedione, which are produced by this enzyme.

Another line of inquiry has focused on the enzyme P450c_{17}, which although coded by one gene, has two activities. The 17α-hydroxylase component hydroxylates pregnenolone and progesterone, while the 17,20-lyase (desmolase) component synthesizes dehydroepiandrosterone and androstenedione. Studies of this enzyme have shown that activity can be regulated differentially by electron donors.[21] A shortage of electron donors favors 17α-hydroxylase activity, while an abundance of electron donors increases 17,20-lyase activity, and therefore adrenal androgen formation. Two possible mechanisms to influence the concentration of electron donors are the availability of cytochrome b_5, and the degree of serine or threonine phosphorylation of the enzyme in response to a cyclic adenosine monophosphate (cAMP)–dependent mechanism.[21] This enzymatic mechanism could theoretically underlie changes of adrenal androgen-to-cortisol ratios in adrenarche, aging, and other situations, presumably in response to more proximal stimuli acting on the adrenal.

Immunostaining of the human adrenal has shown considerable interweaving of adrenal medullary and cortical cells, which might allow for paracrine control of the inner zones of the adrenal cortex by the medulla.[22] This type of mechanism would also theoretically allow for extra-adrenal control of adrenal androgen secretion, since the adrenal medulla is part of the sympathetic nervous system. In isolated perfused porcine adrenals with an intact nerve supply, electrical stimulation of the splanchnic nerves has been shown to cause increased androstenedione secretion.[23] It has also been reported that urinary adrenal androgen metabolite excretion in adrenarchal children is higher, inversely proportional to birth weight.[24] It is not clear if this would involve an intrinsic or extrinsic regulation of the adrenal.

Control by Extrinsic Adrenal Factors

ACTH, as discussed above, has a definite but limited effect on adrenal androgen secretion, which has led to investigation of a number of other possible modulating factors. These factors could theoretically function by themselves or modify other control mechanisms.

Estrogens have been found to cause inhibition of 3β-hydroxysteroid dehydrogenase in some in vitro systems, but this effect has not been noted in vivo.[25] Among groups of people studied, patients with gonadal dysgenesis have shown unchanged concentrations of dehydroepiandrosterone and androstenedione after estrogen therapy. Since some patients with hyperprolactinemia also have elevated adrenal androgen concentrations, and prolactin receptors have been described in human adrenal glands,[26] prolactin has been studied. However, stimulatory effects in vitro have been variable, and prolactin levels have been found to be unchanged during adrenarche.[27] Melatonin receptors have been reported in rat adrenal, and melatonin has been found to stimulate dehydroepiandrosterone secretions in mouse adrenals,[28] but a lack of temporal relation of concentrations to normal or premature adrenarche has been observed.[29]

Although epidermal growth factor (EGF) has been found to stimulate secretion of dehydroepiandrosterone sulfate by human fetal adrenal in vitro, a study of normal children revealed a decrease in urinary excretion of EGF after 2 years of age.[30] In animal studies, fibroblast growth factor (FGF) has stimulated androgen secretion in gonadal cells,[31] but adrenal effects have not been reported. In the human fetal adrenal, angiotensin II has been found to stimulate secretion of dehydroepiandrosterone sulfate, but in a nonselective manner, as it also stimulated cortisol secretion.[32] A decrease in dehydroepiandrosterone secretion in response to angiotensin II stimulation has been found in vitro in human adrenocortical H295R carcinoma cells.[33]

The endothelins, a family of endothelially derived vasoconstrictor peptides, have been shown to stimulate secretion of aldosterone in bovine adrenal cells, and testosterone in rat Leydig cells. In humans, an infusion of endothelin-1 did not alter basal or ACTH-stimulated cortisol secretion.[34] However, human adrenal cells have been found to express the genes to synthesize endothelin-1 and its receptor subtypes ET_A and ET_B, and to respond to endothelin stimulation with increased secretion of cortisol and aldosterone.[35] In these studies, adrenal androgens were not measured. If stimulation by endothelins is physiologically important, it might occur via an autocrine or paracrine mechanism in vivo.

Other potential endocrine or paracrine influences on adrenal androgen secretion include the heterodimeric glycoproteins, activins and inhibins, of the transforming growth factor-β (TGF-β) family. In cultured human fetal adrenal cells, TGF-β has been shown to inhibit dehydroepiandrosterone sulfate production and decrease immunoreactive steroid sulfotransferase.[36] In women with polycystic ovarian syndrome a correlation has been found between serum levels of α-inhibin and androstenedione,[37] probably reflecting an effect of inhibin on ovarian function, which could be paracrine as well. In human adult adrenal cell suspensions, both activin and inhibin decreased ACTH-stimulated production of dehydroepiandrosterone and androstenedione, while having no effect on cortisol production.[38] Expression of activin and inhibin subunits has been shown in rat adrenal,[39] and the above effect could potentially explain at least some instances of dissociation of cortisol and adrenal androgen secretion.

The cytokines tumor necrosis factor-α (TNF-α) and interleukin-6 (IL-6), secreted by macrophages and monocytes, respectively, are often increased in inflammatory states, and stimulate ACTH and cortisol secretion. Cortisol, in turn, feeds back to decrease TNF-α and IL-6 secretion in a dose-related manner.[40] With respect to adrenal androgens, TNF-α has caused a reduction in secretion of dehydroepiandrosterone sulfate in human fetal adrenal cells.[41] IL-6 and IL-6 receptors have been demonstrated to be expressed in human adrenal, and IL-6 has stimulated cortisol, dehydroepiandrosterone, and aldosterone secretion by macrophage-depleted adrenal cells.[42] These findings indicate the possibilty of an autocrine adrenal glucocorticoid, androgen, and mineralocorticoid control mechanism. In a study using pharmacologic doses of IL-6 in cancer patients, ACTH and cortisol concentrations were increased initially, with a decreased response after 1 week.[43] Adrenal androgens were not measured. A negative correlation has been found between IL-6 and dehydroepiandrosterone sulfate concentrations in aging, and it has been theorized that there might be a causative relationship,[44, 45] but IL-6 was not reported in children of adrenarchal age.

Insulin, insulin-like growth factors (IGFs), and leptin, all of which have adrenal gland receptors,[46, 47] have been studied as possible modulators of adrenal androgen secretion. In human fetal adrenal cells, IGF-1 and IGF-2 stimulated dehydroepiandrosterone sulfate and cortisol secretion, and expression of P450c_{17}.[48] In human adult adrenal cells, insulin and IGF-1 induced expression of mRNA for both 17α-hydroxylase and 3β-hydroxysteroid dehydrogenase, with the net effect of decreasing the molar ratio of synthesized dehydroepiandrosterone to cortisol.[49] However, in vivo, although insulin and IGF-1 levels were correlated in boys and girls of adrenarchal age, insulin and dehydroepiandrosterone sulfate concentrations were not correlated.[50] Similarly, in a study of aging, older men had decreased concentrations of dehydroepiandrosterone sulfate, IGF-1 and IGF binding protein-3, as compared with younger men, but a correlation was not found.[51] Leptin has been shown to inhibit ACTH-stimulated dehydroepiandrosterone, cortisol, and aldosterone secretion by human adrenal in vitro, and cause a decrease in ACTH-stimulated P450c_{17} mRNA expression.[47] However, in a longitudinal study of prepubertal boys, although leptin levels increased transiently just before the onset of puberty, concentrations of this adipocyte-derived hormone did not correlate with adrenarche.[52]

Decreased concentrations of dehydroepiandrosterone and dehydroepiandrosterone sulfate are often found in children with growth hormone deficiency. These levels are not fully restorable by growth hormone treatment, and are often lowest in children with multiple noncorticotropin pituitary hormonal deficiencies, rather than isolated growth hormone deficiency,[53] which has prompted investigation of adrenal control by noncorticotropic pituitary factors. In one study, chimpanzees, which, as mentioned above, undergo an adrenarche, were hypophysectomized or sham-hypophysectomized. In the hypophysectomized animals, it was found that ACTH and thyroxine replacement was adequate for maintenance of cortisol, but not dehydroepiandrosterone secretion.[54]

A noncorticotropin human fetal pituitary factor has been found to stimulate dehydroepiandrosterone sulfate secretion in human fetal adrenal glands.[55] Similar findings have been reported in human adult pituitary, tested in human adult and fetal adrenal glands, in which a proopiomelanocortin (POMC) fragment, joining peptide (JP), has been found to bind to human adrenal and synergize with ACTH in stimulation of adrenal androgen secretion.[56] In related studies of the bioactivity of monomeric JP in human adrenal in vitro, adrenal androgen secretion relative to cortisol secretion was shown by JP alone or in coordination with ACTH.[57, 58] In other studies, the effect was small[59] or not observed.[60] At present it is not clear if the monomeric or dimeric form of JP is more potent, or if amidation of the peptide is essential. JP was also found to stimulate aldosterone secretion in coordination with ACTH, as was β-endorphin.[61] Receptors for β-endorphin have been demonstrated on bovine adrenal cells.[62] Adrenarchal and pubertal children have increased circulating concentrations of β-lipotropin and β-endorphin,[63] which may indicate differential processing of POMC, possibly due to age, or the local concentration of androgens.[64]

POMC can be synthesized in the adrenal, as well as the pituitary; and JP has been shown to synergize with histamine, which can also be synthesized in the adrenal, so it has been theorized that JP might have a paracrine role.[58] In animal studies, rat and bovine JP have been shown to possess sodium pump inhibitor activity, and cause cardiovascular effects when given intracisternally.[65] Since many POMC derivatives, including γ_3-melanocortin-stimulating hormone (γ_3-MSH)[66] and those mentioned previously, have been shown to have a role in modulating adrenal glucocorticoid, androgen, or mineralocorticoid secretion, it is possible that the ratio of ACTH to another POMC peptide may be a factor controlling adrenocortical secretion. Further research will be needed to evaluate the relative physiologic importance of the various POMC peptides. Another factor may be corticotropin-releasing hormone (CRH), which has been shown to directly stimulate dehydroepiandrosterone sulfate secretion by human fetal adrenal cells,[67] as well as stimulate synthesis of POMC.

CLINICAL SIGNIFICANCE OF THE ADRENARCHE

A small but significant growth spurt has been found in boys and girls between 6.5 and 8.5 years of age. This growth spurt is due to a transient increase in long bone growth,[68] and correlates partially with increases in adrenal androgen concentrations, but may terminate while adrenal androgen concentrations continue to increase. In children with precocious puberty in whom gonadotropin secretion is suppressed with a gonadotropin-releasing hormone (GnRH) analog, serum dehydroepiandrosterone sulfate concentrations have been found to correlate with the rate of skeletal maturation.[69]

A decrease in sex hormone–binding globulin (SHBG) has been found in adrenarchal boys, which may represent an androgenic effect of adrenal androgens and cause an increase in concentrations of unbound testosterone.[70] Other clinical manifestations of adrenarche include an increase in sebum secretion and blood pressure, and a decrease in circulating concentrations of the protease α_2-macroglobulin.[71–73]

Adrenarche may also have a relationship to diabetes. It was found that women who develop type 1 diabetes before 8 years of age have a 20-year risk of 13.9% of transmitting this disease to their offspring, whereas after 8 years of age the risk drops to 2.4%. This has been theorized to result from androgen-induced T cell suppressor activity.[74]

Relationship to Puberty

Adrenarchal increases in adrenal androgen concentrations precede puberty, and it has been suggested that adrenarche may have an effect on GnRH secretion and the pubertal process. Consistent with this theory is the observation that some children with oversecretion of adrenal androgens due to undertreatment of CAH develop true precocious puberty. Adrenarche and puberty, however, can occur independently. For example, boys treated for primary adrenal insufficiency have been found to begin puberty at the normal age.[75]

Abnormalities of Adrenarche

A clinical variant of adrenarche is premature adrenarche, a common cause of premature pubarche. This occurs in the absence of puberty or virilization, and is characterized by mild hyperandrogenism. It is more common in girls and in children with central nervous system abnormalities. Bone age and height may be advanced for chronologic age, but adult height is generally normal, and although age of puberty is generally normal, a slightly earlier menarche has been noted.[76] Other causes of premature pubarche include CAH and adrenal and gonadal tumors.[77] *Exaggerated adrenarche* has been the term used to describe the clinical situation of abnormally elevated concentrations of androstenedione and dehydroepiandrosterone in the absence of CAH. In girls it has been associated with an increased frequency of insulin resistance, and ovarian androgen hypersecretion, including functional ovarian hyperandrogenism or polycystic ovarian syndrome, the latter possibly linked to genetic factors that cause low birth weight or a familial pattern of premature male pattern baldness.[78–80] The opposite situation, delayed adrenarche, has been observed in conditions including hypogonadotropic hypogonadism and thalassemia.[81] As in the cases of premature and exaggerated adrenarche, the cause is unclear, and theoretically could be related to factors that regulate normal adrenarche.

REFERENCES

1. Parker L: Adrenarche and puberty. *In* Parker L: Adrenal Androgens in Clinical Medicine. San Diego, Academic Press, 1989, p 98.
2. Cutler G, Glenn M, Bush M, et al: Adrenarche: A survey of rodents, domestic animals and primates. Endocrinology 103:2112, 1978.
3. Akamine Y, Kato K, Ibayashi H: Studies on changes in the concentration of serum adrenal androgens in pubertal twins. Acta Endocrinol 93:356, 1980.
4. Rotter J, Wong F, Lifrak E, et al: A genetic component to the variation of dehydroepiandrosterone sulfate. Metabolism 34:371, 1985.
5. Pratt J, Manatunga A, Li W: Familial influences on the adrenal androgen excretion rate during the adrenarche. Metabolism 43:186, 1994.
6. Nieschlag E, Loriaux D, Ruder H, et al: The secretion of dehydroepiandrosterone in man. J Endocrinol 57:123, 1973.
7. Dunn P, Mahood C, Speed J, et al: Dehydroepiandrosterone sulfate concentrations in asthmatic patients. N Z Med J 97:805, 1984.
8. Kreitzer P, Blethen S, Chasalow F: Dehydroepiandrosterone sulfate levels are not suppressible by glucocorticoids before adrenarche. J Clin Endocrinol Metab 69:1309, 1989.
9. Gonzalez F: Adrenal involvement in polycystic ovarian syndrome. Semin Reprod Endocrinol 15:137, 1997.
10. Chang R, Wolfsen A, Judd H: Circulating levels of plasma ACTH in polycystic ovarian disease. J Clin Endocrinol Metab 54:1265, 1982.
11. Parker L, Levin E, Lifrak E: Evidence for adrenocortical adaptation to severe illness. J Clin Endocrinol Metab 60:947, 1985.
12. Treasure J, Wheeler M, Saeich B, et al: Anorexia nervosa and the adrenal: The effect of weight gain. J Psychiatr Res 19:221, 1985.
13. Luppa P, Munker R, Nagel D, et al: Serum androgens in intensive care patients: Correlation with clinical findings. Clin Endocrinol 34:305, 1991.
14. Brunelli V, Chiumello G, David M, et al: Adrenarche does not occur in treated patients with congenital adrenal hyperplasia resulting from 21-hydroxylase deficiency. Clin Endocrinol 42:461, 1995.
15. Weber A, Clark A, Perry L, et al: Diminished adrenal androgen secretion in familial glucocorticoid deficiency implicates a significant role for ACTH in the induction of adrenarche. Clin Endocrinol 46:431, 1997.
16. Grumbach M, Richards, Kaplan S: Clinical disorders of adrenal function and puberty: An assessment of the role of the adrenal cortex in puberty and evidence for an ACTH-like pituitary adrenal androgen stimulating hormone. *In* James V (ed): The Endocrine Function of the Human Adrenal Cortex. London, Academic Press, 1978, p 583.
17. Cutler G, Johnsonbaugh R, Loriaux D: Dissociation of cortisol and adrenal androgen secretion in patients with secondary adrenal insufficiency. J Clin Endocrinol Metab 49:604, 1979.
18. Kennerson A, McDonald D, Adams J: Dehydroepiandrosterone sulfotransferase localization in human adrenal glands: A light and electron microscopic study. J Clin Endocrinol Metab 56:786, 1983.
19. Endoh A, Kristiansen S, Casson P, et al: The zona reticularis is the site of biosynthesis of dehydroepiandrosterone and dehydroepiandrosterone sulfate in the adult human adrenal cortex resulting from its low expression of 3β-hydroxysteroid dehydrogenase. J Clin Endocrinol Metab 81:3558, 1996.
20. Gell J, Carr B, Sasano H, et al: Adrenarche results from development of a 3β-hydroxysteroid dehydrogenase–deficient adrenal reticularis. J Clin Endocrinol Metab 83:3695, 1998.
21. Geller D, Auchus R, Miller W: The role of P450c_{17} in androgen biosynthesis. *In* Azziz R, Nestler J, Dewailly D (eds): Androgen Excess Disorders in Women. Philadelphia, Lippincott-Raven, 1997, p 315.
22. Bornstein S, Gonzalez-Hernandez J, Ehrhart-Bornstein M, et al: Intimate contact of cortical and chromaffin cells within the human adrenal gland forms the cellular basis for important intra-adrenal interactions. J Clin Endocrinol Metab 78:225, 1994.
23. Ehrhart-Bornstein M, Bornstein S, Guse-Behling H, et al: Sympathoadrenal regulation of adrenal androstenedione release. Neuroendocrinology 59:406, 1994.
24. Clark P, Hindmarsh P, Shiell A, et al: Size at birth and adrenocortical function in childhood. Clin Endocrinol 45:721, 1996.
25. Ditkoff E, Fruzzeti F, Chang L, et al: Impact of estrogen on adrenal androgen sensitivity in PCOS. J Clin Endocrinol Metab 80:603, 1995.
26. Glasow A, Matthias B, Haidan A, et al: Functional aspects of the effect of prolactin on adrenal steroidogenesis and distribution of the prolactin receptor in the human adrenal gland. J Clin Endocrinol Metab 81:3103, 1996.
27. Parker L, Sack J, Fisher D, Odell W: The adrenarche: Prolactin, gonadotropins, adrenal androgens and cortisol. J Clin Endocrinol Metab 46:396, 1978.
28. Haus E, Nicolau G, Ghinea E, et al: Stimulation of dehydroepiandrosterone secretion by melatonin in mouse adrenals *in vitro*. Life Sci 58:263, 1996.
29. Cavallo A: Melatonin secretion during adrenarche in normal human puberty and in pubertal disorders. J Pineal Res 12:71, 1992.
30. Mattila A, Perheentupa J, Personen K, et al: Epidermal growth factor in human urine from birth to puberty. J Clin Endocrinol Metab 61:997, 1985.
31. Sordoillet C, Savona C, Chauvin M, et al: Basic FGF enhances testosterone secretion in cultured porcine Leydig cells. Mol Cell Endocrinol 89:163, 1992.
32. Rainey W, Bird I, Mason J, Carr B: Angiotensin II receptors on human fetal adrenal cells. Am J Obstet Gynecol 167:1679, 1992.
33. Bird I, Pasquarette M, Rainey W, Mason J: Differential control of 17α-hydroxylase and 3β-hydroxysteroid dehydrogenase expression in human adrenocortical H295R cells. J Clin Endocrinol Metab 81:2171, 1996.
34. Vierhapper H, Nowotny P, Waldhausl W: Effect of endothelin-1 in man. J Clin Endocrinol Metab 80:948, 1995.
35. Rossi G, Albertin G, Neri G, et al: Endothelin-1 stimulates steroid secretion of human adrenocortical cells *ex vivo* via both ET_A and ET_B receptor subtypes. J Clin Endocrinol Metab 82:3445, 1997.
36. Parker C, Stankovic A, Falany C, et al: Effect of TGF on dehydroepiandrosterone sulfotransferase in cultured human fetal adrenal cells. Ann N Y Acad Sci 774:326, 1995.
37. Pigny P, Desailloud R, Cortet-Rudelli C, et al: Serum-inhibin levels in polycystic ovarian syndrome: Relationship to the serum androstenedione level. J Clin Endocrinol Metab 82:1939, 1997.
38. Clarke D, Fearon U, Cunningham T, McKenna T: Activin and inhibin modulate human adrenal steroidogenesis *in vitro*. Presented at the 77th Annual Meeting of the Endocrine Society, Washington, DC, 1997, p 608.
39. Meunier H, Rivier C, Vale W: Gonadal and extragonadal expression of inhibin α, βA, and βB subunits in various tissues predicts diverse functions. Proc Natl Acad Sci U S A 85:247, 1988.
40. DeRijk R, Michelson D, Karp B, et al: Exercise and circadian rhythm-induced variations in plasma cortisol differentially regulate interleukin-1β, IL-6, and TNFα production in humans: High sensitivity of TNFα and resistance of IL-6. J Clin Endocrinol Metab 82:2182, 1997.
41. Jaattela M, Ilvesmaki V, Voutilainen R, et al: Tumor necrosis factor as a potent inhibitor of ACTH-induced cortisol production and steroidogenic P450 enzyme gene expression in cultured human fetal adrenal cells. Endocrinology 128:623, 1991.
42. Path G, Bornstein S, Ehrhart-Bornstein M, et al: IL-6 and the IL-6 receptor in the human adrenal gland: Expression and effects on steroidogenesis. J Clin Endocrinol Metab 82:2343, 1997.
43. Mastorakos G, Chrousos G, Weber J: Recombinant IL-6 activates the hypothalamic-pituitary-adrenal axis in humans. J Clin Endocrinol Metab 77:1690, 1993.
44. Daynes R, Araneo B, Ershler W, et al: Altered regulation of IL-6 production with normal aging. J Immunol 150:5219, 1993.
45. Straub R, Konecna L, Hrach S, et al: Serum dehydroepiandrosterone (DHEA) and DHEA sulfate are negatively correlated with serum IL-6, and DHEA inhibits IL-6 secretion from mononuclear cells in man *in vitro*: Possible link between endocrinosenescence and immunosenescence. J Clin Endocrinol Metab 83:2012, 1998.
46. Pillion D, Arnold P, Yang M, et al: Receptors for insulin and IGF-1 in the human adrenal gland. Biochem Biophys Res Commun 165:204, 1989.
47. Glasow A, Haidan A, Hilbers U, et al: Expression of Ob receptor in normal human adrenals: Differential regulation of adrenocortical and adrenomedullary function by leptin. J Clin Endocrinol Metab 83:4459, 1998.
48. Mesiano S, Katz S, Lee J, Jaffe R: IGF augments steroid production and expression of steroidogenic enzymes in human fetal adrenal cortical cells: Implications for adrenal androgen regulation. J Clin Endocrinol Metab 82:1390, 1997.
49. Kristiansen S, Endoh A, Casson P, et al: Induction of steroidogenic enzyme genes by insulin and IGF-1 in cultured human adrenocortical cells and resultant changes in the dehydroepiandrosterone/cortisol synthesis ratio. Steroids 62:258, 1997.
50. Smith C, Dunger D, Williams A, et al: Relationship between insulin, IGF and DHAS concentrations during childhood, puberty and adult life. J Clin Endocrinol Metab 68:932, 1989.
51. Benbassat C, Maki K, Unterman T: Circulating levels of IGFBP1 and 3 in aging men: Relationships to insulin, glucose, IGF and DHAS levels and anthropometric measures. J Clin Endocrinol Metab 82:1484, 1997.
52. Mantzoros C, Flier J, Rogol A: A longitudinal assessment of hormonal and physical alterations during normal puberty in boys. V. Rising leptin levels may signal the onset of puberty. J Clin Endocrinol Metab 82:1066, 1997.
53. Ilondo M, Vanderschueren M, Pizarro M, et al: Plasma androgens in children and adolescents. Horm Res 16:78, 1982.
54. Albertson B, Hobson W, Burnett B, et al: Dissociation of cortisol and adrenal androgen secretion in the hypophysectomized, ACTH-replaced chimpanzee. J Clin Endocrinol Metab 59:13, 1984.
55. Brubaker P, Baird A, Bennett H, et al: Corticotropic peptides in the human fetal pituitary. Endocrinology 111:1150, 1982.
56. Parker L, Lifrak E, Gelfand R, et al: Isolation, purification synthesis and binding of human adrenal gland cortical androgen stimulating hormone. Endocrine J 1:441, 1993.
57. Clarke D, Fearon U, Cunningham S, McKenna T: The steroidogenic effects of β-endorphin and joining peptide: A potential role in the modulation of adrenal androgen production. J Endocrinol 151:301, 1996.
58. Orso E, Szalay K, Szabo D, et al: Effects of joining peptide (1–18) and histamine on DHEA and DHEAS production of human adrenocortical cells *in vitro*. J Steroid Biochem 58:207, 1996.
59. Penhoat A, Sanchez P, Jaillard C, et al: Human POMC 79–96 does not affect steroidogenesis in cultured human adult adrenal cells. J Clin Endocrinol Metab 72:23, 1991.
60. Mellon S, Shively J, Miller W, et al: Human POMC 79–96, a proposed androgen stimulatory hormone, does not affect steroidogenesis in cultured human fetal adrenal cells. J Clin Endocrinol Metab 72:19, 1991.
61. Molloy E, Clarke D, Fearon U, et al: Non-ACTH POMC fragments stimulate aldosterone production by human adrenal cells *in vitro*. Steroids 63:459, 1998.
62. Gelfand R, Bobrow A, Young C, Parker L: β-Endorphin binding in cultured adrenal cortical cells. Endocrine 3:201, 1995.

63. Genazzani A, Facchinetti F, Petraglia F, et al: Correlation between plasma levels of opioid peptides and adrenal androgens in prepuberty and puberty. J Steroid Biochem 19:891, 1983.
64. Joshi D, Miller M, Seidah N, et al: Age-regulated alterations in the expression of prohormone convertase mRNA levels in hypothalamic POMC mRNA neurons in the female C57BL/6J mouse. Endocrinology 136:2721, 1995.
65. Hamakubo T, Yoshida M, Nakajima K, et al: Central cardiovascular effects of joining peptide in genetically hypertensive rats. Am J Physiol 265:R1184, 1993.
66. Pedersen R, Brownie A: Gamma$_3$-melanocortin promotes mitochondrial cholesterol accumulation in the rat adrenal cortex. Mol Cell Endocrinol 50:149, 1987.
67. Smith R, Mesiano S, Eng-Cheng C, et al: CRH directly and preferentially stimulates dehydroepiandrosterone sulfate secretion by human fetal adrenal cortical cells. J Clin Endocrinol Metab 83:2916, 1998.
68. Molinari L, Largo R, Prader A: Analysis of the growth spurt at age seven. Helv Paediatr Acta 35:325, 1980.
69. Wierman M, Beardsworth D, Crawford J, et al: Adrenarche and skeletal maturation during GnRH hormone analog suppression of gonadarche. J Clin Invest 77:121, 1986.
70. Belgorosky A, Rivarola M: Progressive increase in non–SHBG-bound testosterone from infancy to late prepuberty in boys. J Clin Endocrinol Metab 64:482, 1987.
71. Stewart M, Downing D, Cook J, et al: Sebaceous gland activity and serum DHAS levels in boys and girls. Arch Dermatol 128:1345, 1992.
72. Pratt J, Manatunga A, Wagner M, et al: Adrenal androgen excretion during adrenarche: Relation to race and blood pressure. Hypertension 16:462, 1990.
73. Levine J, Chasalow F, Udall J, et al: The relationship between biochemical adrenarche and decreasing α-2 macroglobulin levels in children. Steroids 53:219, 1989.
74. Bleich D, Polak M, Eisenbarth G, Jackson R: Decreased risk of Type I diabetes in offspring of mothers who acquire diabetes during adrenarche. Diabetes 42:1433, 1993.
75. Urban M, Lee P, Migeon C: Androgens in pubertal males with Addison's disease. J Clin Endocrinol Metab 51:925, 1980.
76. Pere A, Perheentupa J, Peter M, Voutilainen R: Followup of growth and steroids in premature adrenarche. Eur J Pediatr 154:346, 1995.
77. Toscano V, Balducci R, Mangiantini A, et al: Hyperandrogenism in the adolescent female. Steroids 63:308, 1998.
78. Likitmaskul S, Cowell C, Donaghue K, et al: Exaggerated adrenarche in children presenting with premature adrenarche. Clin Endocrinol 42:265, 1995.
79. Carey A, Chan K, Short F, et al: Evidence for a single gene effect causing PCOS and male pattern baldness. Clin Endocrinol 38:653, 1993.
80. Ibanez L, Potau N, Francois I, deZegher F: Precocious pubarche, hyperinsulinism and ovarian hyperandrogenism in girls: Relation to reduced fetal growth. J Clin Endocrinol Metab 83:3558, 1998.
81. Filosa A, DiMaio S, Saviano A, et al: Can adrenarche influence the degree of osteopenia in thalassemic children? J Pediatr Endocrinol Metab 9:401, 1996.

Chapter 125

Adrenal Imaging

John L. Doppman

Cross-sectional imaging techniques, especially computed tomography (CT) and magnetic resonance imaging (MRI), visualize the adrenal glands with a resolution and clarity unimagined even 20 years ago.[1–3] Although the anatomic resolution of modern scanners is impressive—even breathtaking—such images provide no information about excessive (or insufficient) elaboration of steroidal or catecholamine hormones, which is the basis of all diagnostic and therapeutic decisions in adrenal endocrinologic problems. Interpretation of adrenal images should never be attempted without knowledge of the patient's hormonal status and other pertinent clinical information.

In this chapter, adrenal imaging is considered from two perspectives: (1) a directed study of the adrenal glands initiated by the presence of an established endocrinologic abnormality, such as hypercortisolism, hyperaldosteronism, adrenal cortical insufficiency, or catecholamine excess, and (2) differential diagnostic workup initiated by the demonstration of an incidental abnormality of the adrenal gland, such as a mass, calcification, or bilateral hyperplasia.

ANATOMY OF THE ADRENAL GLANDS

The adrenal glands consist of two hormonally active and embryologically distinct components: the steroid-producing, mesodermally derived adrenal cortex enveloping the catecholamine-producing, neuroectodermally derived adrenal medulla. The cortex forms the larger component, with the medullary tissue confined principally to the caudal half of the gland.[4]

Both glands lie in the upper retroperitoneal region on either side of the spine and consist of medial and lateral limbs that tend to diverge inferiorly.[5, 6] The right gland lies above the upper pole of the right kidney; its medial and lateral limbs join anteriorly in the configuration of an inverted V (Fig. 125–1A). The medial limb lies lateral and parallel to the right crus of the diaphragm; the more inferior lateral limb extends horizontally, often parallel to the posterior surface of the inferior vena cava. Proximity to the cava accounts for the short course of the right adrenal vein, which drains directly into the posterior wall of the inferior vena cava and always presents a challenge to angiographers seeking selective samples. The medial limb of a normal right adrenal gland averages 3 to 4 mm in thickness and never exceeds 5 mm. It can be conveniently compared with the adjacent right diaphragmatic crus, which provides a reasonable standard for the presence of hyperplasia. It is easier to assess minimal degrees of hyperplasia in the right rather than the left adrenal gland. Measurements of normal adrenal glands on CT have been reported, but the range is wide. An estimate of hyperplasia or hypoplasia by an experienced radiologist is probably as reliable.

The left adrenal gland lies at a lower level than the right gland, medial to the upper pole of the left kidney. Its medial and lateral limbs are shorter and their confluence thicker, which gives the gland an arrowhead configuration (see Fig. 125–1B). Venous drainage from the

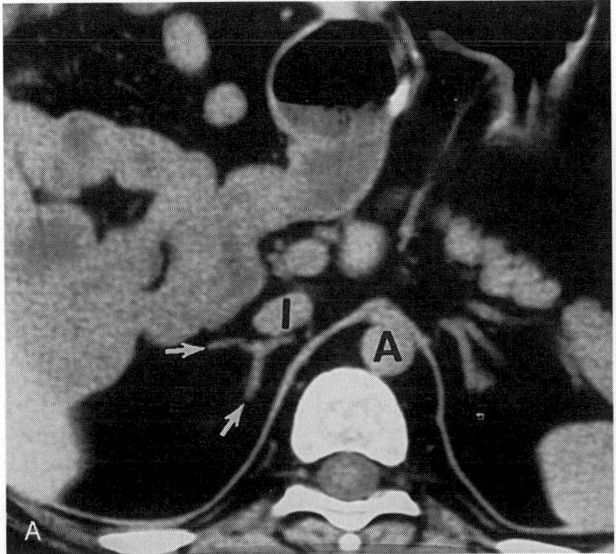

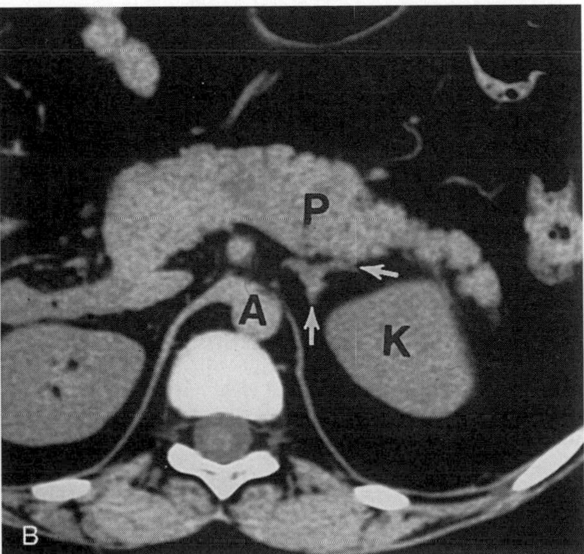

FIGURE 125–1. *A,* Computed tomographic scan of a typical right adrenal gland. The medial limb *(arrow)* curves posteriorly, parallel to the right crus of the diaphragm. The lateral limb *(arrow)* extends horizontally. Both limbs converge behind the inferior vena cava, which accounts for the short course of the right adrenal vein. A, aorta; I, inferior vena cava. *B,* The left adrenal gland lies at a lower level medial to the upper pole of the kidney (K). Note its chunkier triangular shape *(arrows)*. Immediately anterior is the pancreas (P) and medial is the aorta (A).

left adrenal gland descends to the left renal vein; the left adrenal vein is a longer vessel in which a catheter can be easily and securely positioned for selective sampling. Anomalous venous drainage is extremely rare on the left side. On the right side, venous drainage into an adjacent hepatic vein occurs in 3% to 5% of patients and may render selective catheterization impossible.

Unlike the venous drainage, the arterial blood supply to both adrenal glands is symmetrical and derived from three sources: the inferior adrenal arteries ascend from the ipsilateral renal arteries, the middle adrenal arteries arise directly from the aorta, and the superior adrenal arteries descend from the inferior phrenic arteries on each side. Adrenal arteriography requires multiple selective catheterizations of small arteries and is seldom indicated except for the preoperative evaluation of a large mass such as an adrenocortical carcinoma.

Normal adrenal glands are richly vascularized, delicate organs with abundant stores of catecholamine. These glands have limited tolerance to the invasive tactics of interventional radiologists. Vigorous retrograde injection of contrast material into an adrenal vein during sampling procedures produces severe localized back pain and may result in staining of the gland or hemorrhage. With modern cross-sectional imaging techniques, there is never an indication for performing diagnostic retrograde venography. Fine-needle aspiration of adrenal masses is usually safe but has resulted in hemorrhage and, especially in the case of unsuspected pheochromocytomas, severe catecholamine reactions.[7, 8] Careful evaluation of the size and imaging characteristics (radiodensity on CT or changes in signal intensity on in-phase/out-of-phase MRI) of an incidental adrenal mass, coupled with the patient's clinical and biochemical findings, should precede aspiration biopsy and often justifies follow-up by serial imaging.

IMAGING TECHNIQUES

Computed Tomography

CT has revolutionized imaging of the adrenal glands and is the modality of choice. Before its introduction, intravenous urography and the retroperitoneal injection of air, both in conjunction with x-ray tomography, were the only available methods for imaging the adrenal glands but were limited to the demonstration of large adrenal masses. With modern CT scanners, normal adrenal glands are imaged in practically 100% of patients.[9–11] Sections 5 or 3 mm in thickness are optimal when searching for small masses such as aldosteronomas. The CT examination should always extend several centimeters above and below the visualized limits of both glands because exophytic masses arising from the medial or lateral limbs of the gland are not unusual (Fig. 125–2). Oral or intravenous contrast material is not routinely required. Structures adjacent to the right and left adrenal glands, however, may be misinterpreted as adrenal masses (so-called pseudotumors)[12] and could necessitate the use of oral or intravenous contrast material. Adrenal pseudotumors are most common on the left. The superior tip of the spleen, which angulates medially, may appear separate from its parent organ and resemble a left adrenal mass. A tortuous splenic artery adjacent to the lateral limb of the left adrenal gland may simulate a mass but can usually be distinguished by tracing its course on serial images. Intravenous contrast can help make this distinction. A gastric diverticulum arising from the posterior wall of the fundus of the stomach can be distinguished by repeating the scan with oral contrast[13] (Fig. 125–3). Fewer pseudotumors occur on the right, but a steeply ascending right renal vein adjacent to the confluence of the medial and lateral limbs may simulate a right adrenal mass. Retroperitoneal portosystemic collateral veins, even in the absence of portal hypertension, may cluster about both adrenal glands and give an appearance of multinodularity.[14]

Adrenal masses larger than 10 cm can be difficult to distinguish from masses of the upper pole of the kidney (bilateral) or masses of hepatic origin (right side). Such difficulty is particularly true for adrenal carcinomas and cysts. Renal and hepatic arteriography cannot be relied on to make this distinction because large adrenal masses often parasitize the blood supply from both the adjacent kidney and the liver, even though no direct invasion has occurred into these

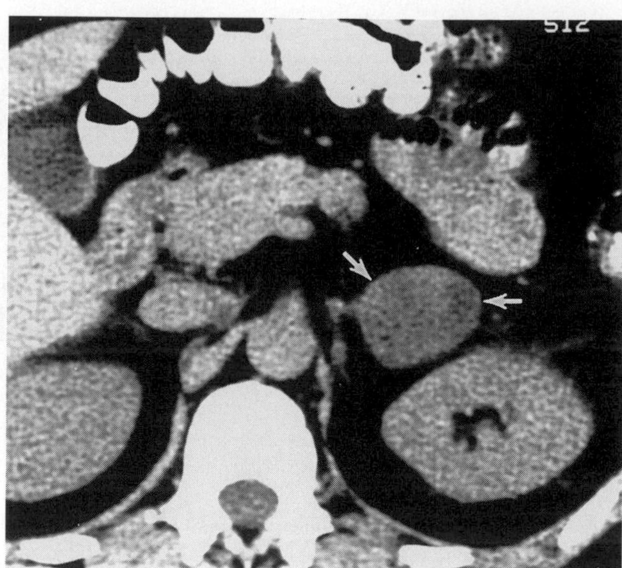

FIGURE 125–2. Adenoma *(arrows)* arising from the tip of the lateral limb of the left adrenal gland, which appeared normal on the more cranial sections.

organs. It is crucial under such circumstances to detect the connective tissue planes separating the adrenal mass from the upper pole of the kidney or from the undersurface of the liver because adrenal cancers seldom invade these adjacent organs directly. Ultrasonography and MRI, with their capability for coronal and sagittal imaging, are often better than CT in demonstrating planes between large adrenal masses and adjacent organs.

CT can distinguish nonhyperfunctional adrenal adenomas (incidentalomas) from metastases by measuring decreased signal intensity (Hounsfield units [HU]) in adenomas as a result of their lipid content.[15] With HU values of 10 or less, an adrenal mass is adrenocortical in origin and can be monitored by serial imaging.[16, 17] Adrenal masses with density measurement over 20 HU are usually metastatic and should undergo biopsy if confirmation is critical to patient care. In many cancer patients, only contrast-enhanced studies of the abdomen are performed. Korobkin et al.[18] demonstrated that if unenhanced studies are not available to measure lipid content, tracking the clearance of contrast (from adenomas faster than from metastases) by taking a post–30-minute scan successfully discriminates adenomas from metastases.[19]

Magnetic Resonance Imaging

MRI, despite spatial resolution inferior to that of CT, makes a definite contribution to adrenal imaging by virtue of its improved tissue contrast and its ability to image in multiple planes. In addition, analysis of MRI signal intensities may provide a clue to the histology of an adrenal mass.[20] On spin-echo T1-weighted MRI the adrenal glands have low signal intensity in comparison to the liver and are clearly outlined by bright retroperitoneal fat. On T2-weighted images, normal and hyperplastic adrenal glands tend to remain of low signal intensity, similar to the liver, as do masses composed of benign cortical tissue, such as the nonhyperfunctioning adenoma, or so-called incidentaloma (Fig. 125–4). In this respect, adrenocortical adenomas differ from all other endocrine adenomas (e.g., parathyroid, islet cell, and pituitary), which are bright on T2-weighted MRI. Adrenocortical carcinomas and metastases show increased signal intensity relative to the liver, and pheochromocytomas have a bright or "light bulb" appearance (Fig. 125–5).

A more sensitive MRI technique for distinguishing incidentalomas from metastases is based on the fact that most adrenocortical adenomas contain lipid and metastases never do. Conventional MRI pulse sequences produce images by summing the signal from protons in fat

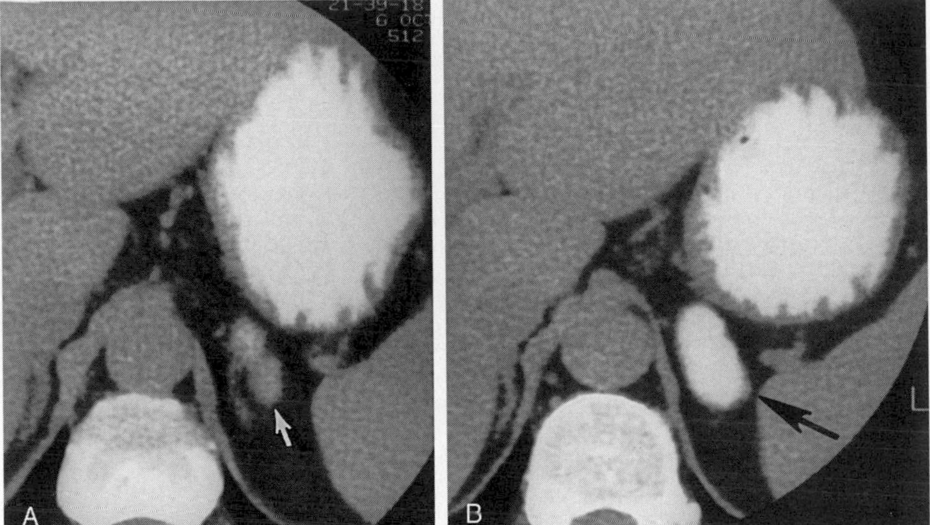

FIGURE 125–3. A mass contiguous with the lateral limb of the left adrenal gland *(arrow, A)* was originally interpreted as an adenoma on computed tomography and magnetic resonance imaging. After distention of the stomach with an oral contrast agent, the adrenal pseudotumor proved to be a posterior gastric diverticulum *(arrow, B)*.

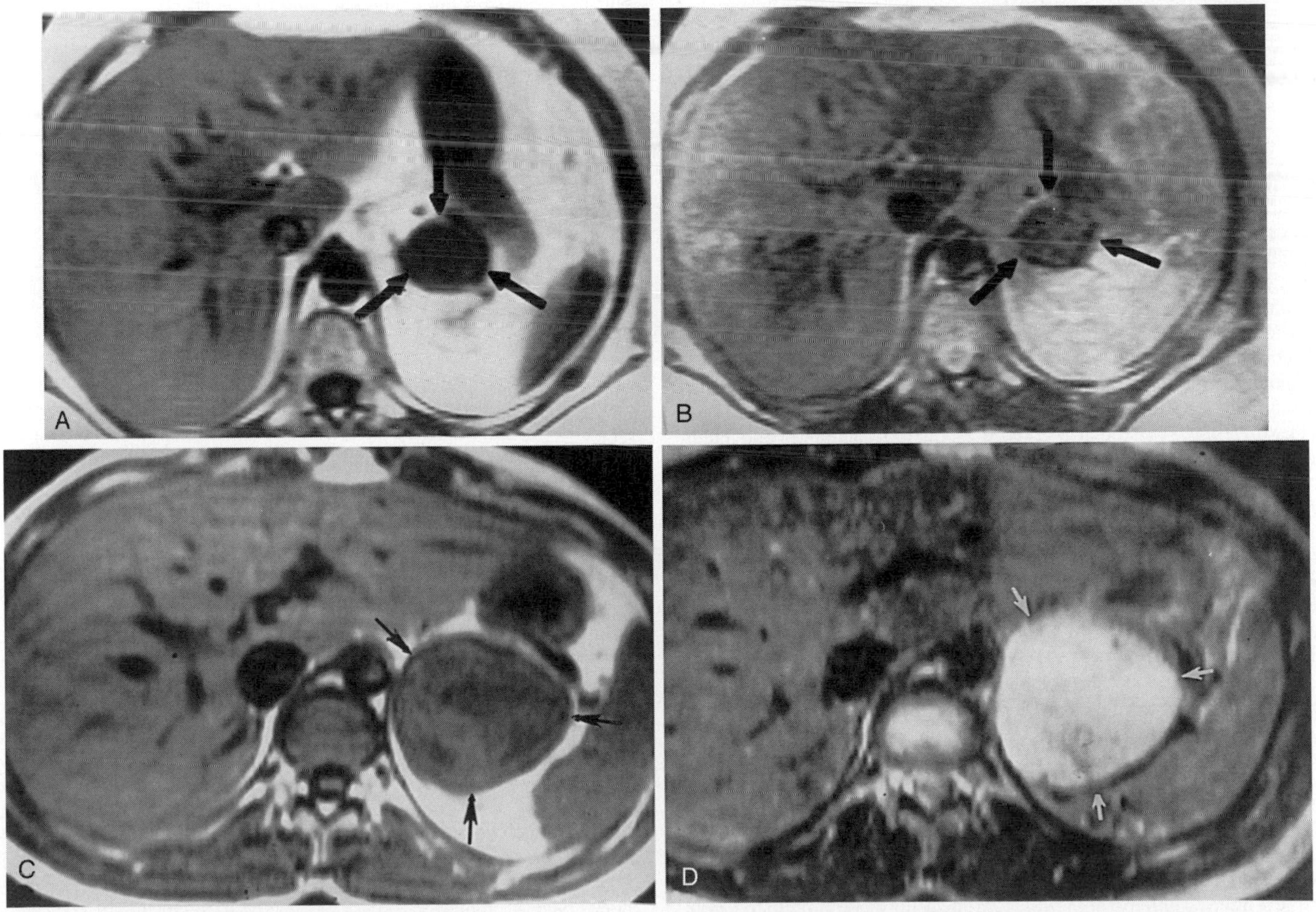

FIGURE 125–4. An adrenocortical adenoma shows low signal intensity comparable to the liver on both T1-weighted *(arrows, A)* and T2-weighted *(arrows, B)* images. An adrenocortical carcinoma has low signal intensity on a T1-weighted image *(arrows, C)* but appears bright or of high signal intensity on a T2-weighted image *(arrows, D)*.

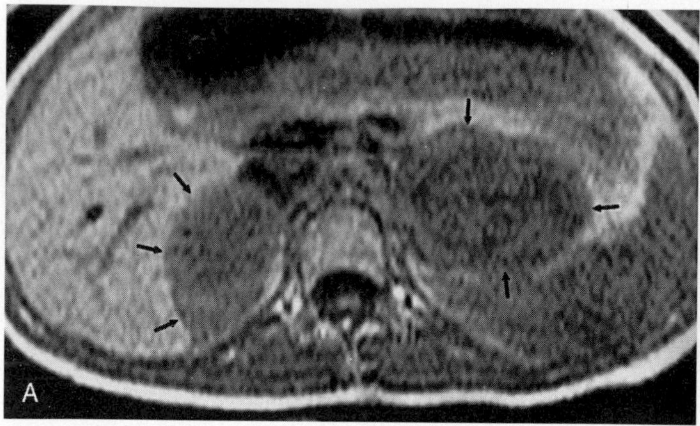

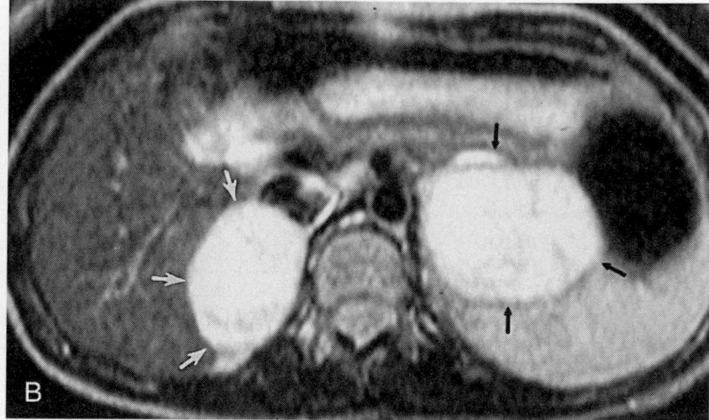

FIGURE 125–5. Note the low signal intensity of bilateral pheochromocytomas on a T1-weighted image *(arrows, A)* and their brightness on a T2-weighted image *(arrows, B)* in a patient with multiple endocrine neoplasia type IIa.

and water (in-phase imaging). However, the protons in fat and water precess at slightly different Larmour frequencies and can be separated by gradient echo pulse sequences using two different times to echo (TE). With out-of-phase MRI pulse sequences, signal from fat protons cancels signal from an equivalent number of water protons, which results in a reduction in signal intensity from a mass containing lipid. Therefore, an adrenal mass that loses signal intensity in out-of-phase vs. in-phase images is an adrenocortical adenoma.[21–25] This technique is often called chemical shift MRI.

Arteriography and Venous Sampling

Arteriography is seldom indicated in the investigation of adrenal masses. The complex arterial supply that arises from three sources (renal artery, aorta, and inferior phrenic artery), the nonspecificity of arteriographic appearances (cortical adenomas, carcinomas, and pheochromocytomas are all hypervascular masses), the risk of catecholamine release during arteriography of pheochromocytomas, and the development of superior cross-sectional imaging techniques have eliminated any role for arteriography, save to define the blood supply to adrenal carcinomas before resection[26] or, rarely, to search for extra-adrenal pheochromocytomas.

Venous sampling is performed not to define anatomy but to lateralize functioning tumors by measuring differential hormone levels in both adrenal veins. Symptomatic cortisol-producing adenomas and pheochromocytomas are almost always larger than 1.5 cm and easily visualized by CT. Adrenal venous sampling is not indicated in Cushing's syndrome or pheochromocytomas. Aldosteronomas are small tumors (the average size of 143 tumors was 1.8 cm; 20% were less than 1 cm),[27] and because of the importance of distinguishing a unilateral adenoma from bilateral hyperplasia as the cause of primary hyperaldosteronism, venous sampling is indicated when CT fails to reveal an adenoma or when bilateral nodules are present but postural studies and 18-hydroxycorticosterone levels suggest an aldosteronoma.

It is critical that venous samples be obtained simultaneously from the right and left adrenal veins because of the periodicity of hormone secretion.[28] Therefore, catheters are introduced under local anesthesia into both femoral veins. The left adrenal vein can be successfully catheterized in nearly all patients because of its greater length and predictable drainage into the left renal vein. The left inferior phrenic vein usually joins the left adrenal vein just below the adrenal gland. Samples should be obtained below the confluence of both veins or by selectively catheterizing the left adrenal branch because samples from the left inferior phrenic vein will not reflect hormone production from the left adrenal gland. When selectively engaging the left adrenal vein, care must be taken to not become wedged in this vessel because venous stasis can lead to hemorrhage or thrombosis of the intraglandular venous system. Unilateral adrenal injury and even Addison's disease[29] have been reported as complications of adrenal venous sampling and venography.

The right adrenal vein is more difficult to catheterize because of its short course, variable drainage into the posterior wall of the inferior vena cava between the right renal vein and the diaphragm, and occasional drainage into hepatic veins. Success rates for right adrenal vein catheterization vary between 20% and 80%,[27] although in our recent review of 40 consecutive cases of primary hyperaldosteronism, right adrenal vein sampling was successfully performed in 40 patients (100%).[30] A common frustration when attempting to sample the right adrenal vein is an inability to aspirate blood despite successful catheterization of the vein. A side hole proximal to the catheter tip permits aspiration without excessive dilution of the sample with blood from the inferior vena cava.[28] Measurement of an elevated cortisol level in such a sample as compared with cortisol levels in a peripheral vein indicates that one is sampling gland effluent despite dilution by caval blood. A corrected level of aldosterone can be obtained by computing an aldosterone-cortisol ratio to compensate for the dilution from caval blood.[31] Calculation of aldosterone-cortisol ratios and stimulation with adrenocorticotropic hormone (ACTH) are discussed more fully in the section on hyperaldosteronism.

Retrograde venography should never be performed in association with adrenal venous sampling because of the risk of extravasation of contrast agent and injury to the adrenal gland. Lateralization of adrenal pathology should be based on gradients of hormone production, not on faintly imaged intraglandular tumors. Injections of 0.5 to 1 mL of contrast material are performed during the placement of catheters and at the conclusion of the study to verify catheter position during sampling, but forceful retrograde venography should be abandoned as a diagnostic study or as a component of adrenal venous sampling.

In addition to the possibility of clot formation at the femoral vein puncture sites (all patients should receive 50 U/kg of heparin during the procedure), the major risks of adrenal venous sampling are extravasation of contrast material and adrenocortical insufficiency, if bilateral.[29] In a review of complications of adrenal vein sampling, Hessel et al. reported extravasation in 48 of 604 cases (8%), with 2 instances of adrenal insufficiency.[32] Extravasation is usually associated with severe loin pain lasting up to 24 hours and requiring narcotics for relief. Percutaneous adrenal ablation in patients with breast carcinoma[33–35] or Cushing's disease[36] has been attempted by deliberate extravasation of contrast material or another agent into the gland. In our experience with a small series of proven aldosteronomas, deliberate extravasation of contrast agent failed to cure a single patient.[37] Similarly, efforts at bilateral adrenal ablation using transcatheter techniques have been ineffective and associated with considerable morbidity. Particular care must be taken with the use of alcohol on either the arterial[38] or the venous[39] side because it produces a massive release of catecholamine from normal medullary tissue. In our experience, bilateral adrenalectomy is the only acceptable technique for adrenal ablation. Bilateral adrenalectomy using laparoscopic techniques is replacing conventional surgical techniques.[40, 41]

Ultrasonography

Although the adrenal glands can be visualized with ultrasonographic techniques, CT and MRI have largely replaced ultrasonography in the evaluation of functional adrenal disease. Ultrasonography can be used to demonstrate planes between the adrenocortical carcinoma and the ipsilateral kidney and liver preoperatively to evaluate resectability. Otherwise, ultrasonography plays a minor role in the imaging of adrenal disease.

Scintigraphy

Scintigraphy, like adrenal venous sampling, evaluates gland function rather than anatomy. Radionuclide tracers have been developed for imaging both the adrenal cortex and the adrenal medulla, and although not routinely required, they can be extremely helpful in evaluating functional adrenal disease. Scintigraphic imaging of the adrenal cortex is based on the administration of 6β-^{131}I-iodomethyl-19-norcholesterol (NP-59), which is incorporated into the intraglandular biosynthesis of cholesterol.[42] This activity occurs over a period of several days, so repeated scintigraphic studies must be obtained from days 2 to 6 after administration to allow radioactive background counts to decline. Normal glands are not imaged. In Cushing's syndrome, bilateral uptake suggests an ACTH-dependent disease or, less commonly, an ACTH-independent bilateral adrenal cause, such as primary pigmented nodular adrenal disease (PPNAD) or ACTH-independent macronodular adrenal hyperplasia (AIMAH). Unilateral uptake is seen with autonomous cortisol-producing adenomas[42] (Fig. 125–6). In primary hyperaldosteronism, dexamethasone suppression should precede scanning. Unilateral uptake indicates an aldosteronoma, and bilateral uptake indicates idiopathic hyperplasia. The thyroid gland should be blocked by administering iodide solution several days before and continuing throughout the study. Incorporation of the radioisotope tracer into the steroid pool causes a significant radiation dose to the adrenal glands (range, 15–30 rad/mCi of tracer), as well as to the ovaries.[43] This radiation dose, coupled with the 3- to 5-day duration of the study, has led us to limit the use of radioiodinated cholesterol imaging to specific problems (e.g., hypercortisolemic children with normal glands by CT and suppressed ACTH levels). In our experience, adrenocortical scintigraphy is seldom necessary in the differential diagnosis of adult Cushing's syndrome or primary hyperaldosteronism.

^{131}I-metaiodobenzylguanidine (^{131}I-MIBG), an analogue of guanethidine, localizes in adrenergic vesicles and can be used to image intra-adrenal or extra-adrenal pheochromocytomas.[44] After intravenous administration of 0.5 mCi ^{131}I-MIBG, normal adrenal medullary tissue is not visualized, but the isotope is retained in pheochromocytomas for several days. Although most intra-adrenal pheochromocytomas are successfully imaged by ^{131}I-MIBG scanning, CT is a less expensive, simpler technique for the localization of intra-adrenal pheochromocytomas. ^{131}I-MIBG is useful for screening for ectopic pheochromocytomas and for detecting metastatic disease.

DISEASES OF THE ADRENAL CORTEX

Cushing's Syndrome

The initial goal in the workup of a patient with Cushing's syndrome is to separate ACTH-dependent from ACTH-independent hypercortisolemia. If ACTH levels are elevated, CT usually demonstrates diffusely enlarged glands (Fig. 125–7). Adrenal imaging has little impact on the workup of a patient with ACTH-dependent hypercortisolemia. In such patients, MRI of the pituitary gland[45] and inferior petrosal sinus sampling[46] are the critical imaging studies used in separating pituitary from ectopic sources of ACTH overproduction.

The most common cause of ACTH-independent hypercortisolemia is an adrenocortical adenoma.[47] Such tumors are invariably 1.5 cm or larger in diameter and are readily visualized in a fat-filled retroperitoneum. Fig et al. reviewed the CT findings in 89 patients with ACTH-independent Cushing's syndrome[48]: all 70 adenomas and 19 carcinomas were visualized by CT. On CT, cortisol-producing adenomas may be of soft tissue density or have Hounsfield values in the negative range. They seldom approach the radiolucency of retroperitoneal fat. When an adrenal mass measures more than 6 cm in diameter, when it is inhomogeneous (suggesting necrosis), or when it contains calcification, a functioning adrenal carcinoma must be considered. When carcinoma is suspected, T2 weighted MRI may demonstrate increased signal intensity in comparison to a benign adenoma (see Fig. 125–4). Adenomas demonstrate unilateral uptake on NP-59 scintigraphy, but radionuclide studies are seldom necessary. Steroidogenesis is less efficient in carcinomas, and they may not demonstrate uptake on NP-59 scintigraphy.

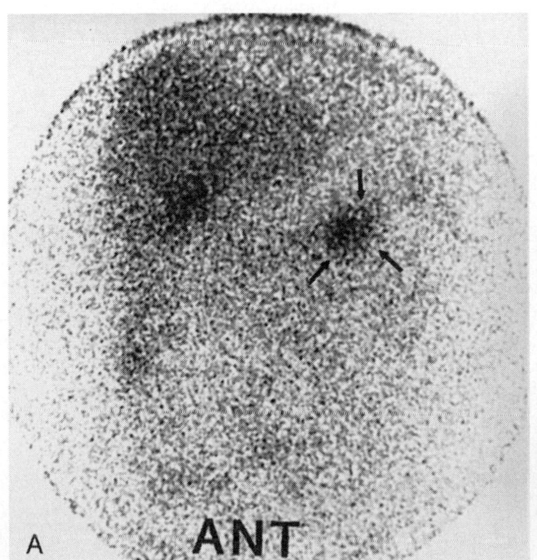

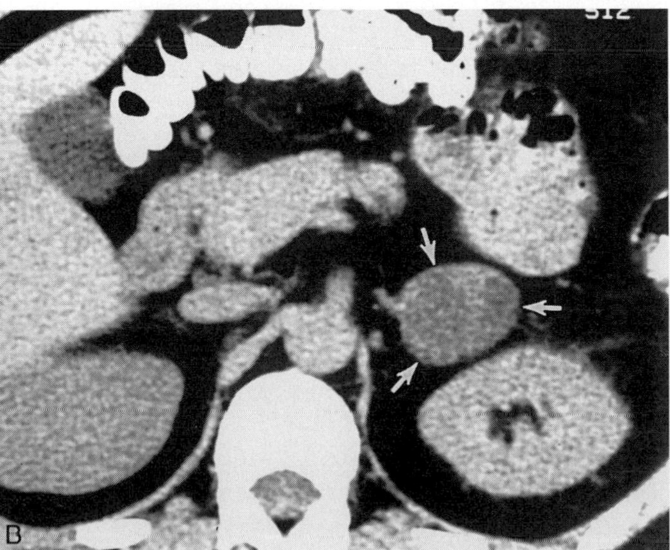

FIGURE 125–6. An NP-59 radionuclide scan in a patient with adrenocorticotropic hormone–independent hypercortisolemia shows uptake in a left adrenal mass *(arrows, A)*. Computed tomography shows the hyperfunctioning left adenoma *(arrows, B)* with reduced radiation exposure, especially to the gonads, and reduced cost.

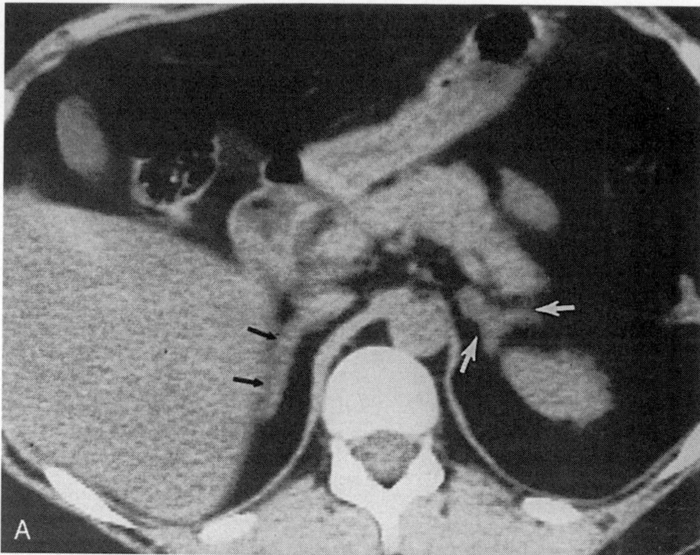

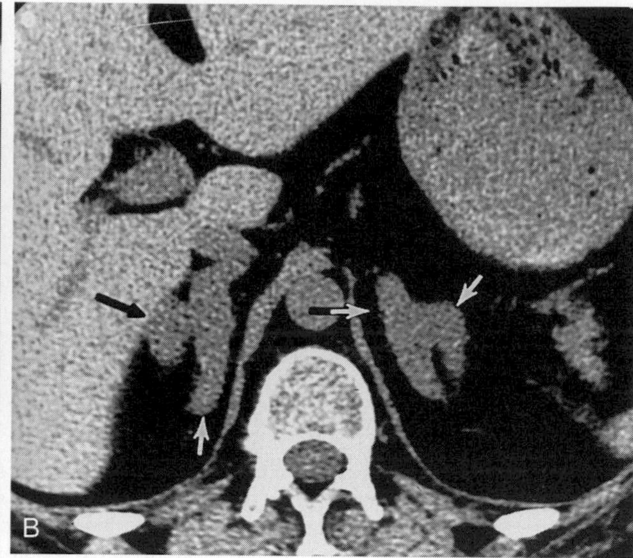

FIGURE 125–7. Computed tomography of the adrenal glands in a patient with Cushing's disease shows moderate enlargement of both glands *(arrows, A)*, but 50% of patients with proven adrenocorticotropic hormone (ACTH)-secreting pituitary adenomas have normal-sized adrenal glands. *B,* Marked hyperplasia *(arrows)* in ACTH-dependent hypercortisolism suggests ectopic ACTH production.

In the presence of an obvious unilateral adrenal tumor, it is essential to carefully inspect the ipsilateral uninvolved and contralateral glands. The limbs of the adrenal gland that contain an autonomous adenoma should be of normal thickness or atrophic (Fig. 125–8). Similarly, the contralateral gland should appear normal or, less commonly, atrophic, a reflection of suppressed ACTH levels. If the ipsilateral uninvolved or contralateral gland is hyperplastic, the possibility of ACTH-dependent macronodular hyperplasia[49–51] with a unilaterally dominant nodule should be considered. Older patients with ACTH-dependent Cushing's syndrome caused by a pituitary or ectopic source of ACTH may develop multiple adrenocortical nodules in addition to diffusely enlarged glands (Fig. 125–9). When this process is unilateral (Fig. 125–10), confusion with an autonomously functioning adrenal adenoma is possible,[52, 53] particularly since many of these patients display atypical suppression and stimulation tests (Fig. 125–11). In all instances, careful inspection reveals hyperplasia of the uninvolved adrenal cortex, which is indicative of an ACTH-dependent process. The nodules decrease in size after transsphenoidal resection of an ACTH-secreting pituitary adenoma but seldom disappear.

Two additional, less common causes of autonomous adrenal hypercortisolism can demonstrate pathognomonic CT findings.[54, 55] PPNAD affects children and adolescents, many of whom have short stature or severe osteoporosis rather than the classic signs of Cushing's syndrome.[56, 57] PPNAD is usually associated with Carney's complex, which consists of such elements as lentigines, cardiac and soft tissue myxomas, pituitary tumors that cause acromegaly, fibrolamellar hepatomas, and calcified Sertoli cell tumors of the testes.[58–62] The hypercortisolism in PPNAD is ACTH independent and caused by multiple autonomously functioning pigmented adrenocortical nodules[63] ranging in size from submicroscopic to 10 mm in diameter. The total adrenal gland weight is usually normal (<12 g). In the past, imaging studies were noncontributory. CT sections 3 mm thick, however, can detect subtle nodularity or lumpiness in affected glands even in the presence of subcentimeter nodules (Fig. 125–12). This unique and pathognomonic finding results from atrophy of the internodular adrenocortical tissue, which leads to a "string-of-beads" appearance that is normally never seen in the adrenal glands of patients younger than 20 years. In our series of six patients with surgically proven PPNAD,[64] CT demonstrated nodularity in all five patients older than 10 years. When

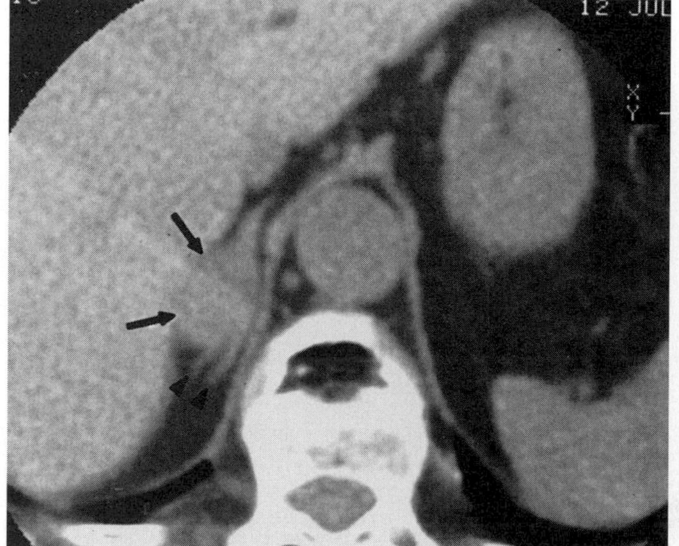

FIGURE 125–8. Adrenocorticotropic hormone–independent hypercortisolemia caused by an autonomously functioning right adrenal adenoma *(arrows)*. Note that the medial and lateral limbs of this gland *(arrowheads)* appear atrophic. The left gland showed no signs of hyperplasia.

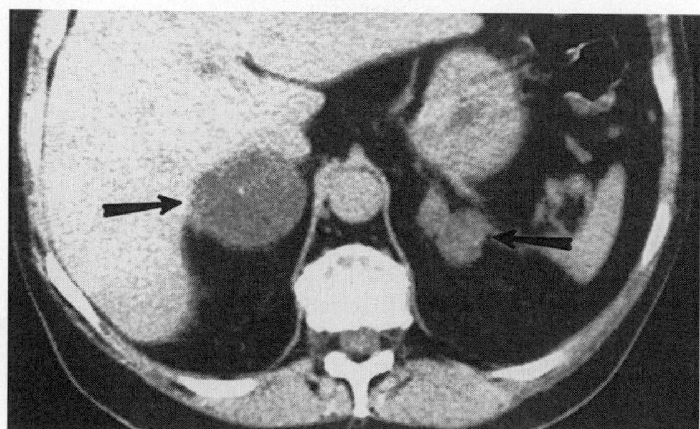

FIGURE 125–9. Note the bilaterally hyperplastic nodules *(arrows)*. This finding represents macronodular hyperplasia in a patient with an adrenocorticotropic hormone–secreting pituitary adenoma.

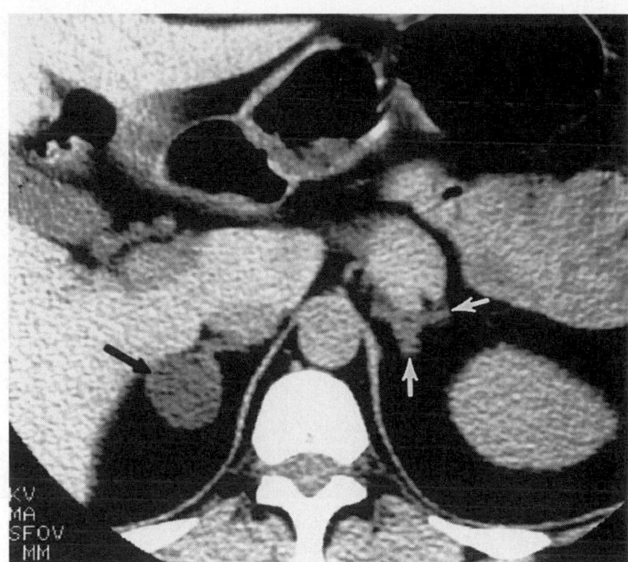

FIGURE 125–10. Note the 2-cm nodule *(black arrow)* involving the lateral limb of the right adrenal gland. The remaining right gland and the left gland *(white arrows)* appear hyperplastic and suggest adrenocorticotropic hormone–dependent macronodular hyperplasia with a right-sided dominant nodule. Petrosal sinus sampling revealed the presence of a right-sided corticotropic adenoma, and Cushing's syndrome remitted completely after removal of a pituitary adenoma by transsphenoidal surgery.

hypercortisolemia secondary to PPNAD occurs in infancy or early childhood, CT reveals small to normal-sized glands without nodularity. Under these conditions, bilateral uptake on NP-59 scintigraphy in the presence of depressed ACTH levels is diagnostic. With longer survival, macronodules may develop in patients with PPNAD. Two older patients (ages 28 and 32 years) with Carney's complex had 2- and 3-cm unilateral adrenal masses that in conjunction with suppressed ACTH levels could not be distinguished from the much more common autonomous adrenal adenoma[65] (Fig. 125–13). Surgeons should understand the significance of multiple pigmented micronodules or macronodules and be prepared under such circumstances to remove the contralateral adrenal gland. Bilateral adrenalectomy is the only treatment of PPNAD.[66] All such patients should undergo periodic echocardiography because the first symptom of an intracardiac myxoma may be a major embolic episode.

Twelve patients have been seen at the National Institutes of Health with AIMAH (combined adrenal weights of 60–150 g).[67, 68] CT demonstrated multiple bilateral adrenocortical nodules (Figs. 125–14 and 125–15) ranging up to 5 cm in diameter and totally obliterating the normal adrenal contours.[68] This finding is unlike that in ACTH-dependent macronodular hyperplasia, in which the nodules are less numerous and a normal adrenal configuration persists. The adrenal glands in AIMAH often extend from above the superior pole of the kidney to the level of the hilar vessels. The uninvolved adrenal cortex in these patients is impossible to recognize on CT but appears normal or atrophic histologically.

Most patients with AIMAH are older than patients with ACTH-dependent Cushing's syndrome, and the female preponderance is lacking.[69] The CT appearance is so distinctive that confusion with ACTH-dependent macronodular hyperplasia is usually not a problem. The combined weight of normal adrenal glands is 8 to 10 g, and the combined weight of hyperplastic glands in ACTH-dependent Cushing's syndrome seldom exceeds 25 g.[70] In AIMAH, combined gland weights of more than 300 g have been reported.

It has been speculated that AIMAH represents progression of ACTH-dependent hyperplasia to autonomous adrenal function with suppression of the pituitary corticotroph adenoma. Hermus et al. presented data that support such an evolution from pituitary-dependent to adrenal-dependent Cushing's syndrome.[71] None of the patients with AIMAH in our series or in the literature have shown unmasking of a pituitary adenoma after bilateral adrenalectomy. The original patient reported from the National Institutes of Health in 1964 underwent MRI of her pituitary gland 28 years after bilateral adrenalectomy[72]; no evidence of an emerging corticotroph adenoma was seen.[67] For these reasons, we believe that AIMAH represents a distinct and uncommon cause of ACTH-independent adrenal hypercortisolism with bilateral involvement. A subset of patients with AIMAH show ectopic expression and/or increased responsiveness to gastric inhibitory polypeptide

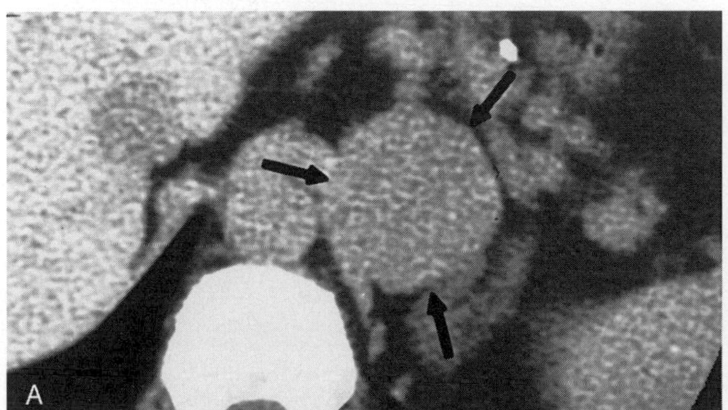

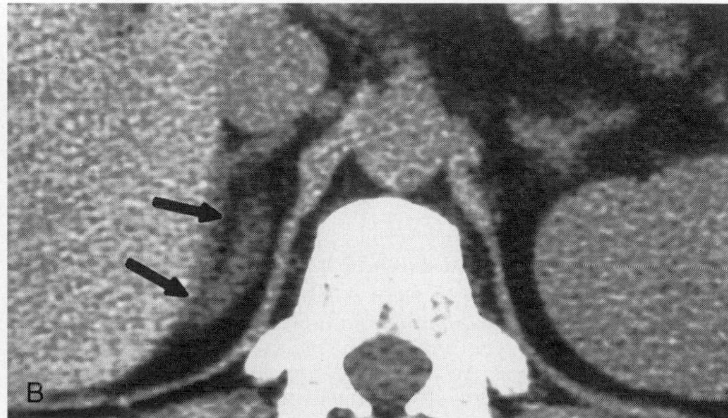

FIGURE 125–11. A 6-cm mass *(arrows, A)* replaces the left adrenal gland. The right adrenal gland is free of nodules, but the medial limb *(arrows, B)* shows marked hyperplasia indicative of an adrenocorticotropic hormone (ACTH)-dependent state. Petrosal sinus sampling demonstrated an ACTH gradient in the right petrosal sinus, and remission followed transsphenoidal surgery.

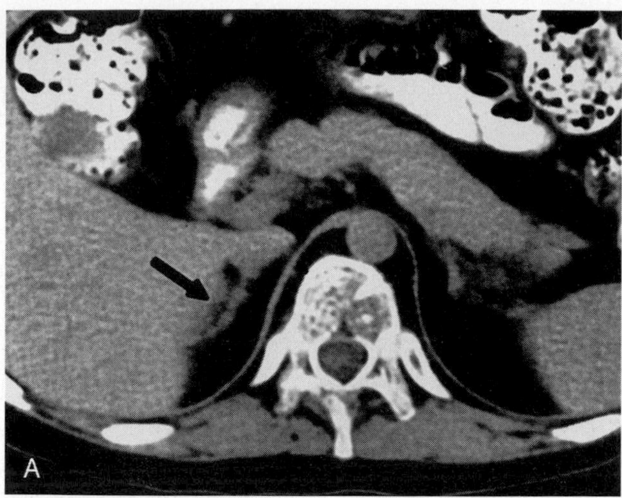

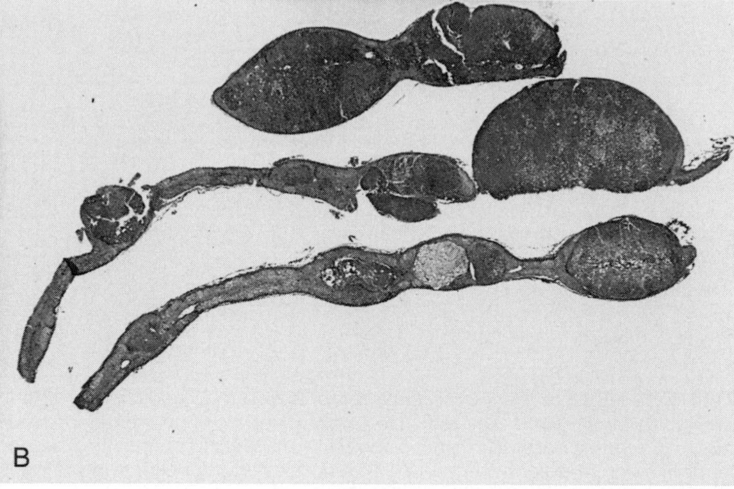

FIGURE 125–12. Multiple nodules with a "string-of-beads" appearance *(arrow, A)* in a right adrenal gland of normal size suggested the diagnosis of primary pigmented nodular adrenal disease in this 14-year-old patient with Carney's complex. *B,* A sectioned adrenal gland from another patient demonstrates the atrophic cortex between nodules that is responsible for the "string-of-beads" appearance. (From Doppman JL, Travis WD, Nieman L, et al: Cushing's syndrome due to primary pigmented nodular adrenocortical disease: Findings at CT and MR imaging. Radiology 172:415–420, 1989.)

receptors[73] (food-dependent hypercortisolism), vasopressin receptors,[74] and β-adrenergic receptors,[75] which suggests that the massive adrenocortical hyperplasia may be secondary to abnormalities of receptors for various non-ACTH hormones or growth factors.[76] The treatment is bilateral adrenalectomy.[77]

Table 125–1 summarizes the preferred imaging modalities in the hypercortisolemic syndromes of adrenal origin.

Primary Aldosteronism

The role of adrenal imaging in primary hyperaldosteronism is to separate the surgically remediable unilateral aldosteronoma from bilateral hyperplasia.[78, 79] Once the clinical diagnosis of primary hyperaldosteronism is established, CT should be the first imaging study. Most aldosteronomas are smaller than cortisol-secreting tumors; in a recent review of 143 surgically treated aldosteronomas, the average diameter was 1.8 cm and 20% of the tumors were smaller than 10 mm.[27] CT sections 3 mm thick should be obtained and particular care taken to avoid "geographic misses." Spiral CT scanners can image 3-mm-thick sections of both adrenal glands in a single breath hold. Thus geographic misses resulting from irregular depth of respiration are avoided and intra-adrenal masses as small as 5 to 7 mm are resolved.

Aldosteronomas tend to have lower CT density than do cortisol-producing adenomas, their density often approaching that of retroperitoneal fat[80] (Fig. 125–16). Care must be taken to not misinterpret an adenoma as an angiolipoma.

The improved resolution of modern CT scanners has created a tendency to abandon adrenal venous sampling and rely on CT to distinguish aldosteronoma from hyperplasia.[27, 81] When a unilateral adrenal tumor and a normal contralateral gland are demonstrated by CT in a patient whose postural tests and 18-hydroxycorticosterone levels support the diagnosis of aldosteronoma, adrenal venous sam-

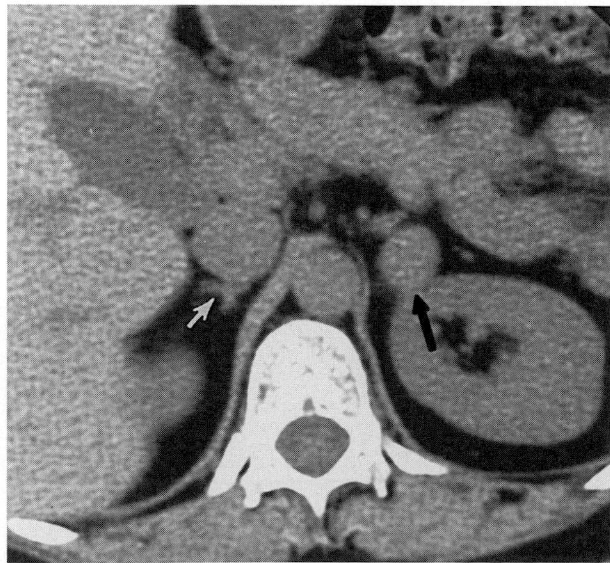

FIGURE 125–13. Left adrenal gland containing a 2-cm nodule *(black arrow)* in a 27-year-old woman with adrenocorticotropic hormone–independent Cushing's syndrome and the stigmata of Carney's complex. The right adrenal gland *(white arrow)* appears normal. At bilateral adrenalectomy, a 2-cm pigmented nodule was present in the left gland with multiple subcentimeter pigmented nodules found bilaterally. (From Doppman JL, Travis WD, Nieman L, et al: Cushing's syndrome due to primary pigmented nodular adrenocortical disease. Findings at CT and MR imaging. Radiology 172:301–307, 1989.)

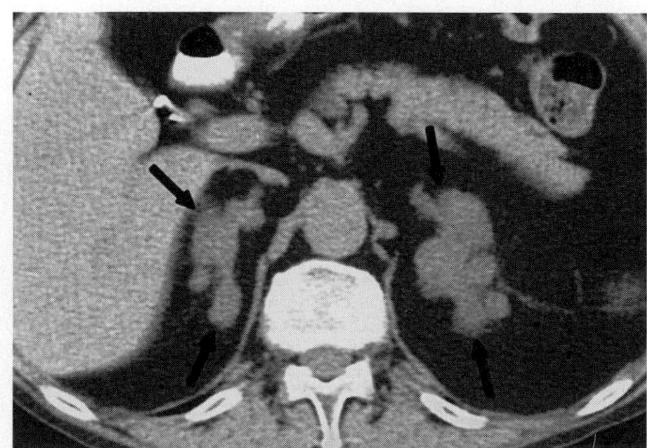

FIGURE 125–14. Note the multiple macronodules *(arrows)* involving both adrenal glands. The combined adrenal weight was 120 g. (From Doppman JL, Nieman LK, Travis WD, et al: CT and MR imaging of massive macronodular adrenocortical disease: A rare cause of autonomous primary adrenal hypercortisolism. J Comput Assist Tomogr 15:773–779, 1991.)

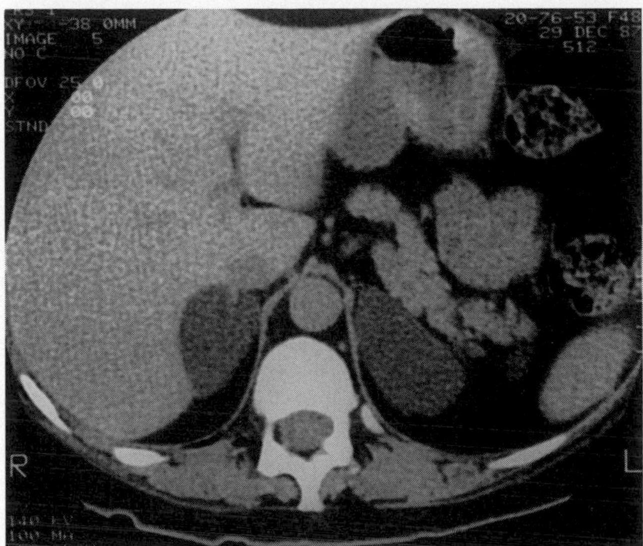

FIGURE 125–15. Massively enlarged hyperplastic adrenal glands (combined weight of 160 g) in a patient with adrenocorticotropic hormone–independent hypercortisolemia. At surgery the glands contained multiple microscopic nodules. (From Doppman JL, Nieman LK, Travis WD, et al: CT and MR imaging of massive macronodular adrenocortical disease: A rare cause of autonomous primary adrenal hypercortisolism. J Comput Assist Tomogr 15:773–779, 1991.)

pling is not indicated (Fig. 125–17). Most patients with hyperaldosteronism are in the 40- to 60-year-old age range and have a significant incidence of incidental adrenal nodules. Institutions that rely on CT to distinguish a unilateral aldosteronoma from hyperplasia have reported an increasing incidence of hyperplasia. Before the introduction of CT, most series of patients with primary hyperaldosteronism reported 75% caused by unilateral aldosteronomas and 25% caused by hyperplasia. Investigators who relied on imaging techniques reported hyperplasias in up to 45% of their total patient population.[27, 81, 82] We reviewed 24 consecutive patients with primary hyperaldosteronism, all of whom underwent bilateral adrenal venous sampling regardless of the CT findings. Six of 24 patients (25%) with a CT diagnosis of hyperplasia based on the demonstration of bilateral nodularity were proved by adrenal venous sampling and subsequent surgery to have aldosteronomas. All patients with a dominant unilateral nodule and normal contralateral gland proved to have aldosteronomas at surgery. A diagnosis of hyperplasia based on the CT demonstration of bilateral nodularity or enlarged glands was incorrect, however, in a significant number of patients who proved to have aldosteronomas. As imaging techniques improve, the demonstration of small, incidental adrenal nodules in the middle-aged population has increased and is compromising the diagnosis of primary hyperaldosteronism secondary to hyperplasia based on imaging findings alone.[83] Figures 125–18 and 125–19 show bilateral nodules or hyperplastic glands in two patients who were proved by adrenal venous sampling and surgery to have aldosteronomas. Other investigators have recently recommended adrenal venous sampling as a critical study in hyperaldosteronism.[84–86]

TABLE 125–1. Imaging Modalities for Demonstrating Adrenal Pathology in ACTH-Independent Hypercortisolemia*

Cause	Preferred Imaging Modality
Adrenal adenoma	CT
Adrenal carcinoma	CT or MRI
Primary pigmented nodular adrenal disease	
>10 yr	CT
<10 yr	Adrenal scintigraphy
ACTH-independent macronodular adrenal disease	CT

*Beware of asymmetrical ACTH-dependent macronodular hyperplasia.

NP-59 scintigraphy, preceded by 6 days of dexamethasone suppression, demonstrates unilateral uptake in 75% to 80% of patients with surgically proven aldosteronomas,[87] a performance not significantly better than that achieved with CT. The relative unavailability of NP-59, the 3 to 5 days required for the study, and the general reluctance to use radionuclides because of the high radiation dose to the adrenal glands and gonads have led most investigators to perform CT as the initial study. If results are equivocal, adrenal venous sampling is the preferred second study because it is almost 100% reliable when correctly performed.

Adrenal Insufficiency

Adrenal insufficiency is most commonly due to autoimmune atrophy, which may be part of the polyendocrine deficiency syndrome. CT demonstrates minuscule glands bilaterally[88] (Fig. 125–20). When

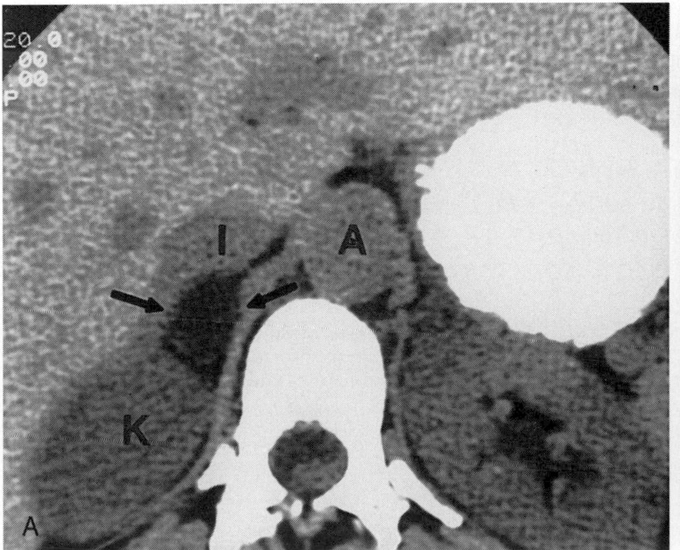

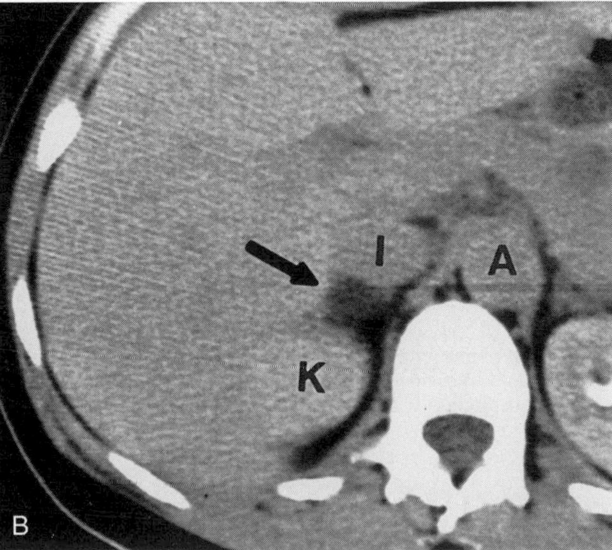

FIGURE 125–16. Note the low density, approaching that of fat, of two aldosterone-secreting adenomas *(arrows, A* and *B)*. A, aorta; I, inferior vena cava; K, kidney.

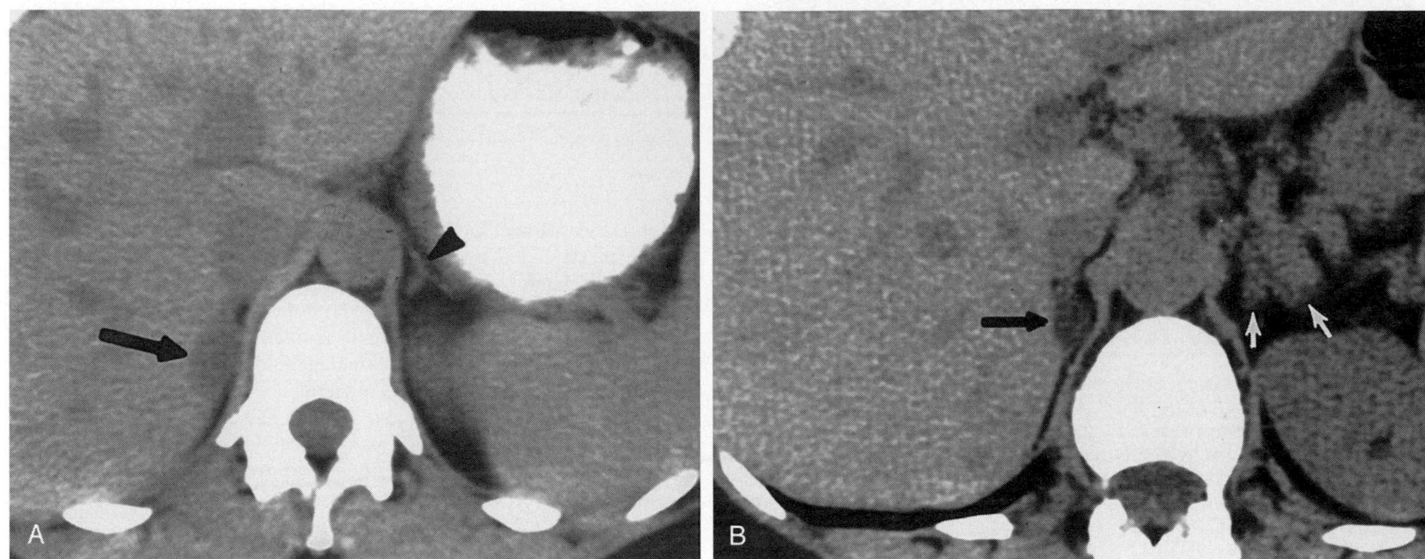

FIGURE 125–17. *A,* Note the low-density right adrenal mass *(arrow)* and the normal left adrenal gland *(arrowhead)*. If postural tests and 18-hydroxycorticosterone levels support a diagnosis of aldosteronoma, no further workup is indicated. *B,* The left adrenal gland appears hyperplastic *(white arrows)*, in addition to a focal hypodense mass in the right gland *(black arrow)*. Under such circumstances the diagnosis of hyperplasia cannot be presumed. Venous sampling demonstrated a right-sided aldosteronoma that was confirmed by surgery, with subsequent complete remission of the patient's hyperaldosteronism after right adrenalectomy.

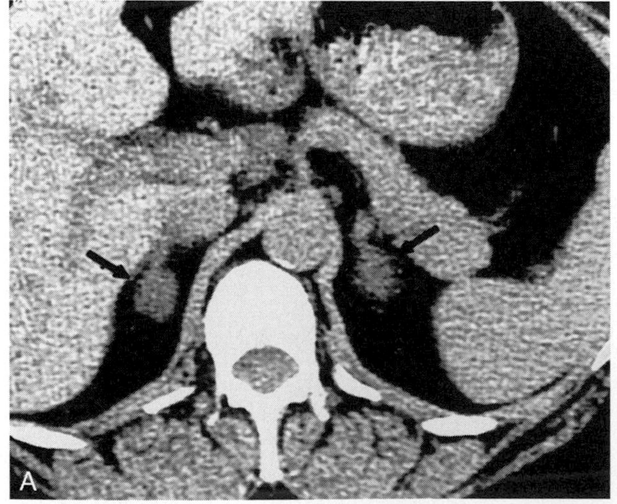

Adrenal Venous Samples

Location	Aldosterone ng/dl	Cortisol μg/dL	Aldosterone/Cortisol Ratio
Basal			
Right adrenal vein	1970	16	126
Left adrenal vein	67	54	1
Peripheral vein	53	5.1	10.4
After ACTH			
Right adrenal vein	6980	299	23.3
Left adrenal vein	316	546	0.6
Peripheral vein	118	12	10

B

FIGURE 125–18. *A,* Bilateral adrenal nodules are demonstrated *(arrows)* in a patient with hyperaldosteronism. Adrenal venous sampling with adrenocorticotropic hormone (ACTH) stimulation reveals evidence *(B)* of a right aldosteronoma which was confirmed by surgery. Note that the more dilute right-sided samples (lower cortisol levels) show a marked response to ACTH whereas the aldosterone-cortisol ratio on the left shows nonresponse of aldosterone production with an aldosterone-cortisol ratio below peripheral levels.

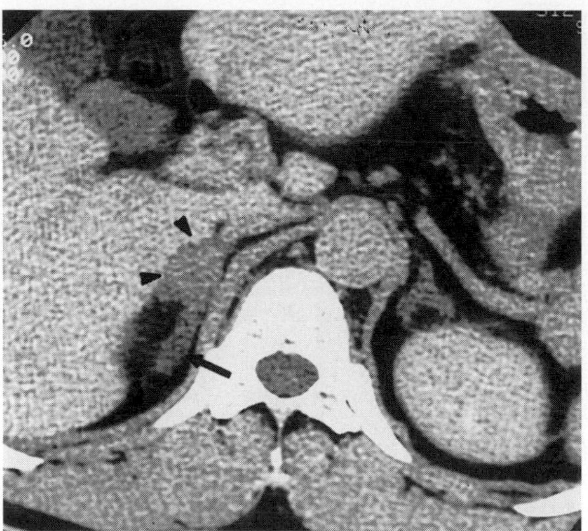

FIGURE 125–19. Note the right adrenal mass *(arrowheads)*, as well as the hyperplastic medial limb of the right adrenal gland *(arrow)*, in a patient with hyperaldosteronism. At a lower level, both adrenal glands appeared hyperplastic. Adrenal venous sampling revealed evidence of a right-sided aldosteronoma, which was confirmed by surgery.

granulomatous diseases such as tuberculosis and histoplasmosis are suspected as causes of adrenal insufficiency, CT provides clinically useful information. Within a few months of the onset of adrenal insufficiency from granulomatous adrenalitis, large glands are usually demonstrated bilaterally, often with an inhomogeneous texture indicating caseous necrosis[89] (Fig. 125–21). The glands retain their triangular shape as opposed to cases of adrenal insufficiency from bilateral metastases, in which the glands are more often replaced by round masses.[90, 91] Adrenal insufficiency of recent onset associated with enlarged glands from active granulomatous adrenalitis should be recognized because antibacterial therapy may restore some adrenal function.[92, 93]

Adrenal insufficiency caused by granulomatous disease of greater than 1 year in duration demonstrates atrophic glands associated with calcification and no visible uninvolved glandular tissue[88] (Fig. 125–22A). Similar adrenal calcification may be encountered in patients without adrenal insufficiency; such calcification is probably due to perinatal intra-adrenal hemorrhage. Thin-slice high-resolution CT always demonstrates uninvolved noncalcified adrenal tissue in patients with normal adrenal function (see Fig. 125–22B).

Primary or secondary hemochromatosis can produce mild adrenal insufficiency from iron deposition in the pituitary gland, as well as in the adrenal glands.[94] Adrenal imaging demonstrates small, dense glands of normal configuration. Although these patients may not have overt adrenal insufficiency, the demonstration of dense glands suggests that they may be subject to stress-induced addisonian crisis (Fig. 125–23). Bilateral adrenal masses caused by metastatic disease seldom lead to adrenal insufficiency. Adrenal insufficiency has been reported in association with AIDS.[95–97] Adrenal insufficiency may also complicate antiphospholipid antibody syndrome secondary to bilateral infarction.[98, 99] The imaging findings in adrenal insufficiency associated with AIDS and the antiphospholipid antibody syndrome are nonspecific (i.e., enlarged, normal, or atrophic glands).

The demonstration of bilaterally dense adrenal masses in the presence of acute adrenal insufficiency is diagnostic of hemorrhage[100–102] (Fig. 125–24). Sepsis, anticoagulant therapy, collagen vascular disease, and the "postpartum state" are the most common associated conditions. Idiopathic adrenal apoplexy also occurs. Recognition of bilateral adrenal hemorrhage by CT in patients with nonspecific symptoms of hypotension, lethargy, and vomiting is critical because replacement therapy must be instituted immediately.

Adrenal imaging is not indicated in congenital adrenal hyperplasia. Depending on the adequacy of steroid replacement, normal to diffusely hyperplastic glands are found.[103, 104] Because of chronically elevated levels of ACTH, congenital rests of adrenal tissue in the testis may undergo hyperplasia and lead to testicular masses, pain, and infertility.[105–107] Histologically, these masses cannot be distinguished from Leydig cell tumors. Hyperplastic adrenal rests appear as low-intensity foci within the bright testis with MRI (Fig. 125–25). Ultrasonography usually demonstrates bilateral masses. Orchiectomy is not indicated.

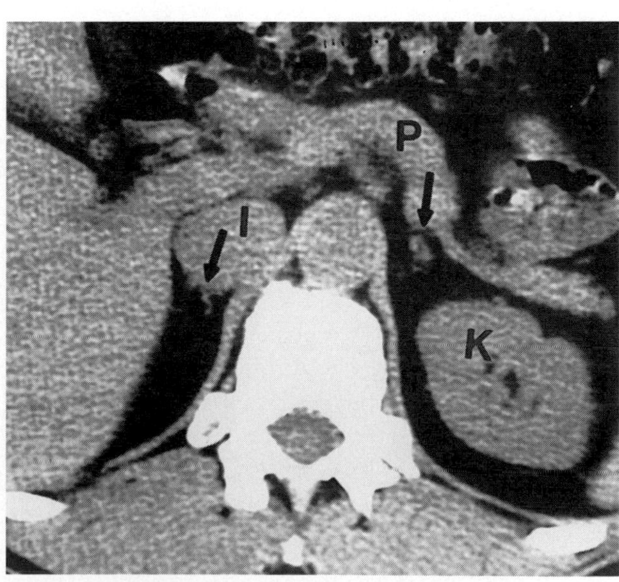

FIGURE 125–20. Note the bilateral minuscule adrenal glands *(arrows)* in a patient with autoimmune adrenal insufficiency. I, inferior vena cava; K, kidney; P, pancreas.

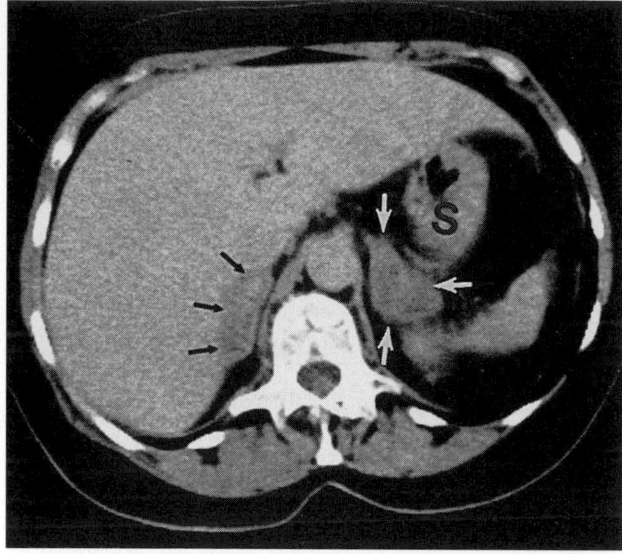

FIGURE 125–21. In a 59-year-old woman with a long-standing history of breast carcinoma and recent onset of adrenal insufficiency, both adrenal glands *(arrows)* are enlarged with preserved adrenal contours. Inhomogeneity indicates caseous necrosis. Preservation of adrenal shape suggests granulomatous adrenalitis rather than metastases. Needle aspiration yielded histoplasmosis. The glands decreased in size after antibiotic therapy. S, stomach. (From Doppman JL, Gill JR Jr, Nienhuis AW, et al: CT findings in Addison's disease. J Comput Assist Tomogr 6:757–761, 1982.)

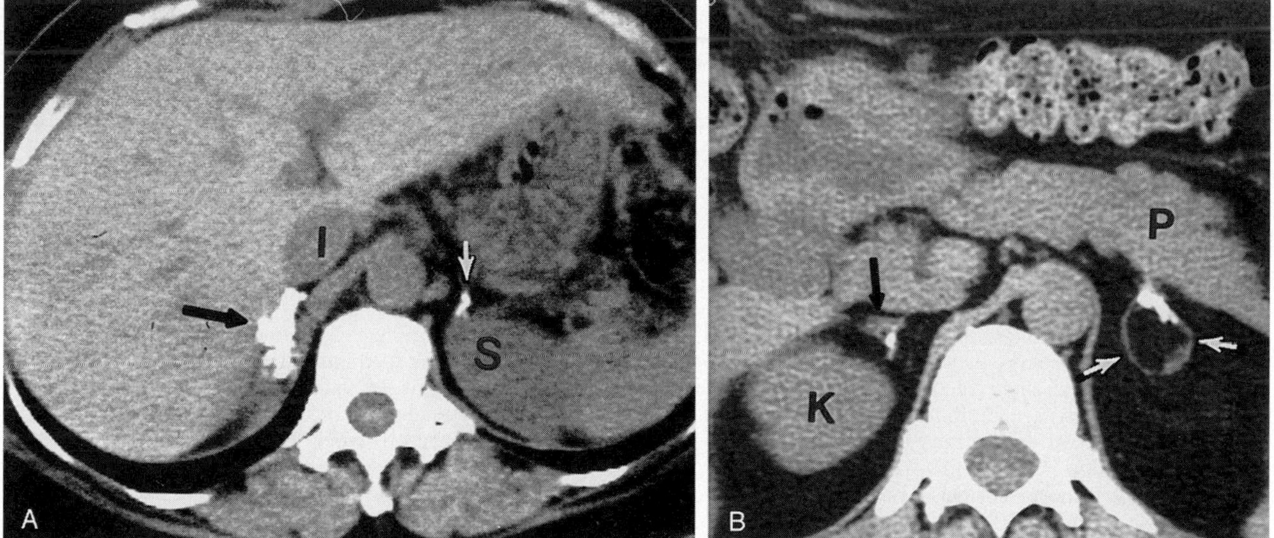

FIGURE 125–22. *A,* A patient with long-standing adrenal insufficiency caused by tuberculosis has bilateral calcification *(arrows)* with no uncalcified adrenal remnant. I, inferior vena cava; S, spleen. *B,* Idiopathic adrenal calcification in a patient with normal adrenocortical function shows uncalcified adrenal remnants *(black and white arrows)*. K, kidney; P, pancreas.

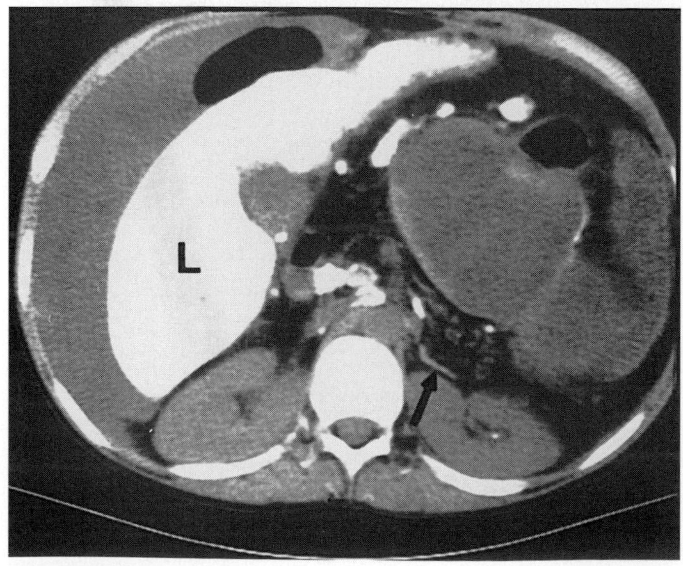

FIGURE 125–23. Note the very dense left adrenal gland *(arrow)* in a patient with secondary hemochromatosis resulting from multiple transfusions for chronic anemia (thalassemia). Dense liver (L) and para-aortic lymph nodes are present, as well as ascites secondary to hemochromatotic cirrhosis.

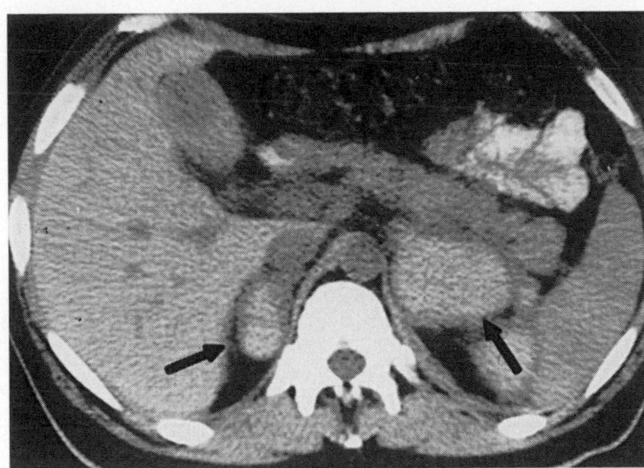

FIGURE 125–24. Bilateral dense adrenal masses *(arrows)* in a man with acute adrenal insufficiency caused by bilateral adrenal hemorrhage. (From Doppman JL, Gill JR Jr, Nienhuis AW, et al: CT findings in Addison's disease. J Comput Assist Tomogr 6:757–761, 1982.)

Selective testicular venous sampling reveals cortisol production from such intratesticular masses[107] (Table 125–2).

DISEASES OF THE ADRENAL MEDULLA

Pheochromocytomas

Because 85% of pheochromocytomas are intra-adrenal, radiologic investigation of patients with symptoms of catecholamine excess should begin with CT of the adrenal glands. Symptomatic pheochromocytomas are almost always 2 cm or larger, and CT identifies more than 90%.[108–111] Many pheochromocytomas are inhomogeneous on CT because of areas of necrosis. They may also contain calcification (Fig. 125–26). A patient with typical clinical symptoms supported by appropriate laboratory tests needs only CT of the adrenal area for localization. Pheochromocytomas are extremely bright on T2-weighted MRI,[112] but MRI adds little to a CT diagnosis of an intra-adrenal pheochromocytoma.

Unlike adrenocortical carcinomas, the size of pheochromocytomas does not always determine their malignant potential. Tumors less than 5 cm may be malignant and metastasize, whereas some of the largest pheochromocytomas have been benign and totally resectable[113] (Fig. 125–27). MRI does not distinguish benign from malignant pheochromocytomas because both are bright on T2-weighted images.

TABLE 125–2. Testicular Vein Samples in Infertile Male with Congenital Adrenal Hyperplasia and Intratesticular Adrenal Rests

	Right Testicular Vein	Peripheral Vein
Cortisol (g/dL)	9.1	<1.0
Testosterone (ng/dL)	270	260

A number of hereditary disorders are associated with bilateral pheochromocytomas, including multiple endocrine neoplasia (MEN) type 2a (Sipple's syndrome) and 2b, familial paragangliomatosis, neurofibromatosis, and von Hippel–Lindau syndrome.[114] Asymptomatic lesions frequently smaller than 2 cm can be identified in this group of patients. In such circumstances, the high signal intensity of such intra-adrenal lesions on T2-weighted images may indicate the presence of asymptomatic pheochromocytomas. The medullary hyperplasia associated with MEN-2a and MEN-2b cannot be diagnosed by CT or MRI. Extra-adrenal pheochromocytomas are also more common in the hereditary pheochromocytoma syndromes.

MRI has the advantage of scanning in the coronal plane. Because most ectopic pheochromocytomas occur in the infrarenal paravertebral region, T2-weighted coronal MRI of the abdomen and pelvis is helpful in screening for ectopic pheochromocytomas (Fig. 125–28). Many ectopic paravertebral pheochromocytomas are embedded in retroperitoneal fat, so an MRI sequence that suppresses fat makes these tumors even more conspicuous. The use of gadolinium-enhanced diethylenetriamine pentaacetic acid (Gd-DTPA) contrast material provides little additional information when scanning for ectopic pheochromocytomas with T2-weighted images. With fat-suppressed T1-weighted sequences, Gd-DTPA can be helpful. Pheochromocytomas of the urinary bladder can be obscured on enhanced CT studies by contrast-laden urine, but such tumors are readily imaged by ultrasonography when the bladder is distended (Fig. 125–29).

The cause of the high signal intensity of pheochromocytomas on T2-weighted MRI remains unexplained. Although many of these tumors are necrotic or cystic (both conditions confer high signal intensity on T2-weighted images), even a small homogeneously cellular pheochromocytoma displays characteristic MRI brightness on T2-weighted images. Only necrotic adrenal metastases and adrenal cysts have comparably high signal intensity on T2-weighted imaging and could not be differentiated from pheochromocytomas on MRI.

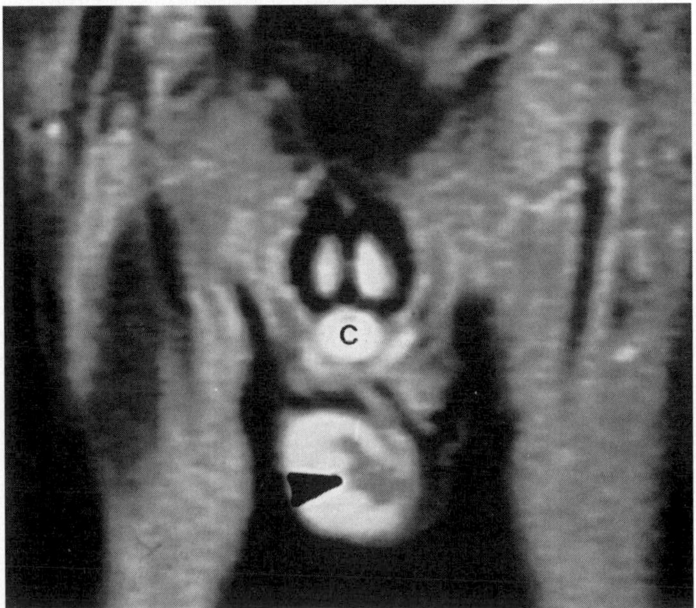

FIGURE 125–25. Note the area of low signal intensity *(arrowhead)* within the right testis compatible with an intratesticular tumor. C, corpus spongiosum. Left orchiectomy was previously performed for "Leydig cell" tumor, which in retrospect probably represented hyperplastic adrenal rests. Magnetic resonance imaging of the adrenal glands demonstrated bilaterally enlarged glands compatible with congenital adrenal dysplasia. Testicular vein samples (see Table 125–2) demonstrated insignificant testosterone production from the right testis (the patient was examined because of pain, as well as infertility) but definite cortisol production.

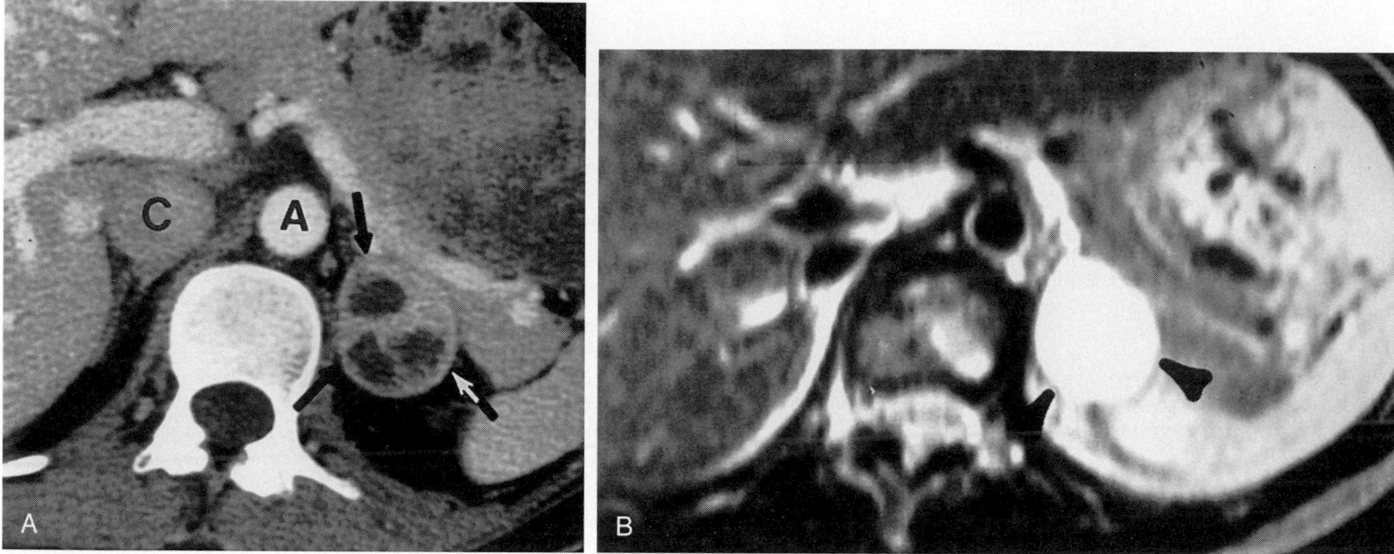

FIGURE 125–26. *A,* Contrast-enhanced computed tomography (CT) reveals an enhancing left adrenal pheochromocytoma *(arrows)* containing areas of decreased signal intensity indicative of necrosis. A, aorta; C, inferior vena cava. On T1-weighted coronal magnetic resonance imaging (MRI), the pheochromocytoma lying above the upper pole of the left kidney had low signal intensity. *B,* On a T2-weighted axial scan the pheochromocytoma *(arrowheads)* is extremely bright. MRI adds little to the CT diagnosis of intra-adrenal pheochromocytoma. Neither T1- nor T2-weighted images demonstrate areas of necrosis as well as the dynamic CT study does.

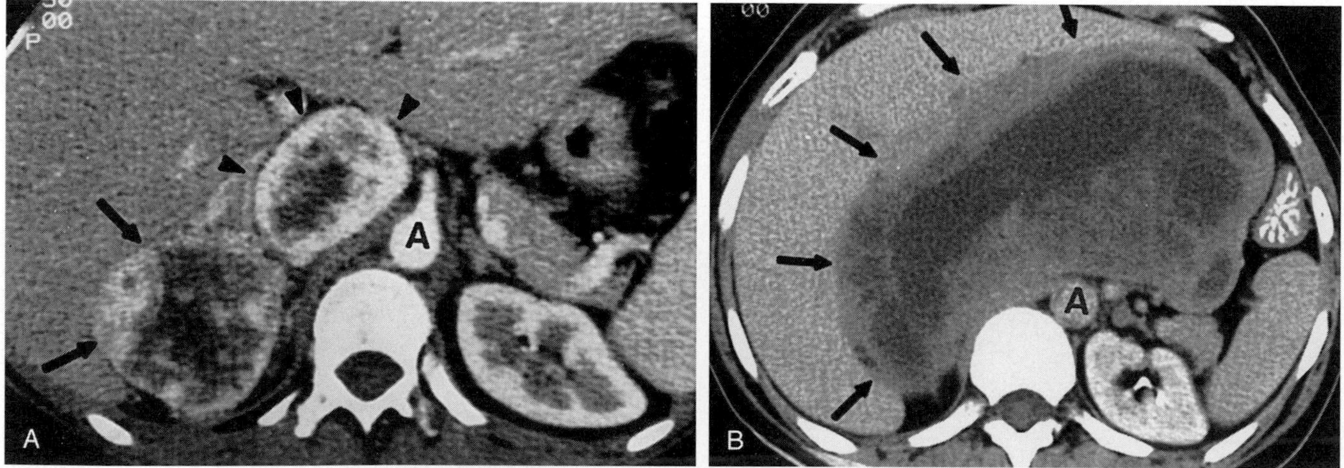

FIGURE 125–27. *A,* A 7-cm right adrenal pheochromocytoma with central cavitation *(arrows)* has already metastasized to a paracaval lymph node *(arrowheads)*. A, aorta. *B,* A huge necrotic tumor *(arrows)* arising from the right adrenal gland and extending into the left epigastric area was benign and completely resected for cure. Ultrasonography and coronal magnetic resonance imaging demonstrated a plane between the adrenal mass and the liver.

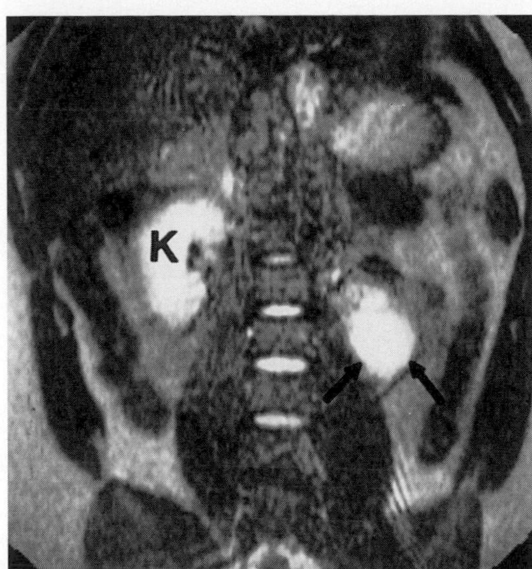

FIGURE 125–28. Note the bright paravertebral pheochromocytoma *(arrows)* lying below the left kidney, which is not imaged on this slice. Computed tomography showed the same lesion as an inhomogeneous calcified mass in the retroperitoneum below the lower pole of the left kidney.

^{131}I-MIBG scanning localizes pheochromocytomas[115] but adds little to the CT diagnosis of intra-adrenal lesions. Up to 15% of pheochromocytomas are ectopic, and under such circumstances both MRI and ^{131}I-MIBG scanning are helpful. ^{131}I-MIBG scintigraphy has the capability of scanning the entire body and detecting thoracic and abdominal paraspinal tumors, as well as intracranial, cervical (Fig. 125–30), and pelvic lesions. ^{123}I-MIBG is replacing ^{131}I-MIBG scanning because the shorter half-life allows a high dose of ^{123}I and permits single photon emission CT imaging.

ADRENAL MASSES

Incidentalomas, Metastases, and Other Masses

Endocrinologists are frequently consulted because a CT or MRI examination in a patient without evidence of adrenocortical or medullary dysfunction demonstrates an adrenal mass, commonly referred to as an "incidentaloma."[117, 118] They occur in about 3% of all patients undergoing abdominal CT, although the incidence of adrenal nodules in autopsy series is higher (10%–50%).[119, 120] Some masses (adrenal cyst, myelolipoma), by virtue of pathognomonic imaging characteristics, are diagnosed by CT findings alone (Fig. 125–31), but homogeneous unilateral or bilateral masses of soft tissue density in the 2- to 3-cm range require further workup. Even though most eventually prove to be nonhyperfunctioning adrenocortical adenomas, an endocrinologist is often called on to exclude more serious pathology. A careful history and physical examination with a few simple laboratory studies usually exclude adrenocortical hyperfunction or insufficiency, as well as pheochromocytoma.[118] Metastases from a known or an occult primary cancer are more difficult to exclude. Imaging can often provide clues that permit a fairly confident diagnosis of adenoma and a recommendation for a noninvasive follow-up study. Even in the presence of non–small cell lung cancer, more than 50% of adrenal lesions detected on CT are benign adenomas.[121]

Nonhyperfunctioning adrenocortical adenomas are homogeneous, smoothly outlined tumors up to 5 cm in diameter.[122, 123] Many appear radiolucent on CT.[124] Lee et al. reported that the differential diagnosis of adrenal masses may be based on their measured CT density.[125] Relatively lucent adrenal masses with Hounsfield values less than 0 are always nonhyperfunctioning adenomas, the less-than-water CT density reflecting a lipid content that is specific for adrenocortical tissue. When the adrenal mass is of soft tissue density (>10 HU), cortical adenomas, pheochromocytomas, and metastases cannot be distinguished. With a threshold of 0 HU, no malignant adrenal lesions were scored as benign (100% specificity), and these authors no longer recommend biopsy of adrenal masses with CT attenuation values less than 0 HU, even in patients with known cancer. With a threshold between 0 and 10 HU, specificity was also high (96%). With CT attenuation values greater than 10 HU, biopsy is necessary if discovery of a metastatic lesion would influence treatment. Other authors have confirmed the reliability of CT density measurements in distinguishing adrenocortical masses. Korobkin et al. used a CT threshold of 18 HU to distinguish adenomas with a positive predictive value of 100% and a negative predictive value of 77%.[16] Discriminations based on CT density measurements presuppose an unenhanced CT study, and many adrenal masses are discovered during contrast-enhanced studies for tumor staging. Rather than bring the patient back for an unenhanced scan, delayed images can be obtained at 1 hour: adenomas show rapid wash-out of contrast (11 HU) when compared with metastases (49 ± 8.3 HU).[18] At a threshold of 30 HU, the specificity and positive predictive value for the diagnosis of adenoma were 100% with a sensitivity of 95%. Other authors have confirmed the reliability of

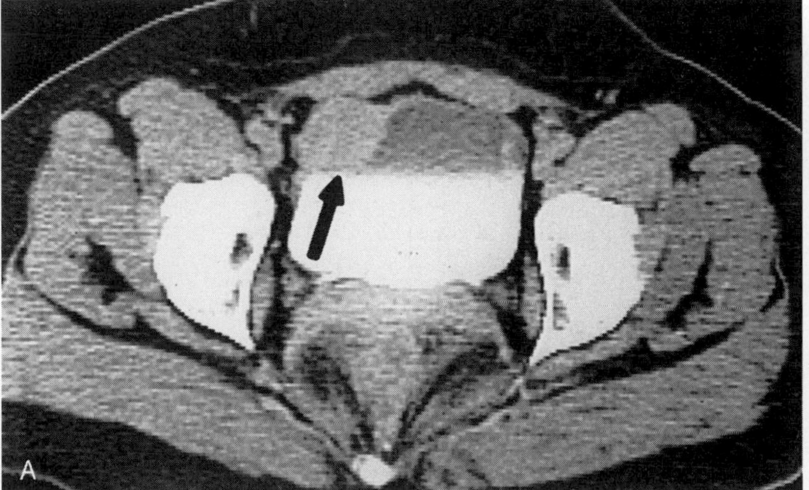

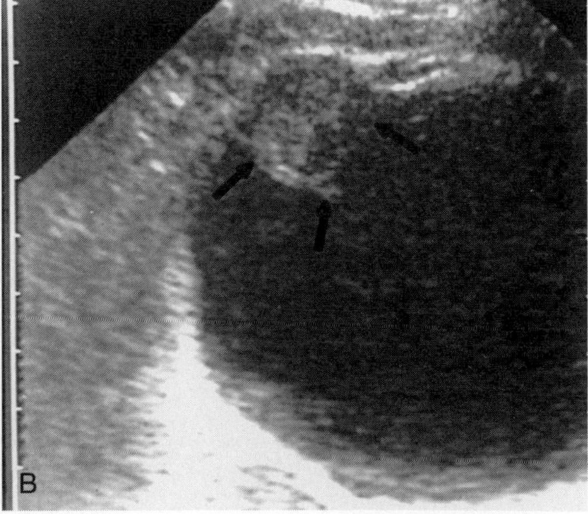

FIGURE 125–29. *A,* Pheochromocytoma in the right anterior wall of the bladder *(arrow)*. A bladder densely opacified with water-soluble contrast material, as occurs at the end of a bolus-enhanced abdominal computed tomographic study, might obscure a small tumor, but it is readily imaged by ultrasonography *(arrows, B)*.

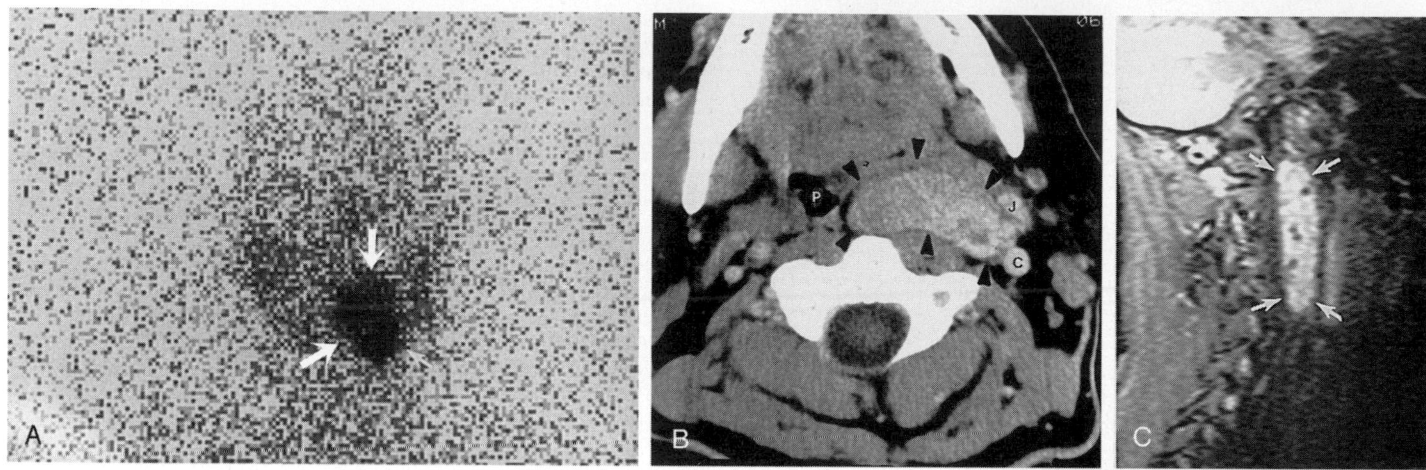

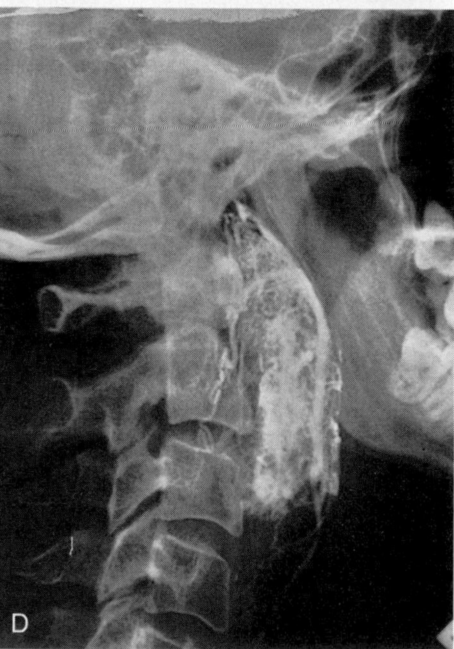

FIGURE 125–30. *A,* ^{131}I-meta-iodobenzylguanidine scan demonstrating high activity in the left cervical region *(arrows)* of a patient with clinical and biochemical findings of pheochromocytoma. *B,* Computed tomography demonstrating an enhancing mass *(arrowheads)* lying between the carotid artery and the jugular vein and growing medially to displace the air-filled nasopharynx. C, carotid artery; J, internal jugular vein; P, pharyngeal cavity. *C,* Sagittal magnetic resonance imaging demonstrating a high-intensity longitudinal mass *(arrows)* along the course of the vagus nerve. The low-signal foci represent flow-void phenomena in vessels within this hypervascular tumor. *D,* Left carotid arteriography revealing a hypervascular mass in the vicinity of the vagal body. A chemodectoma of the vagus nerve producing catecholamines was completely resected at surgery.

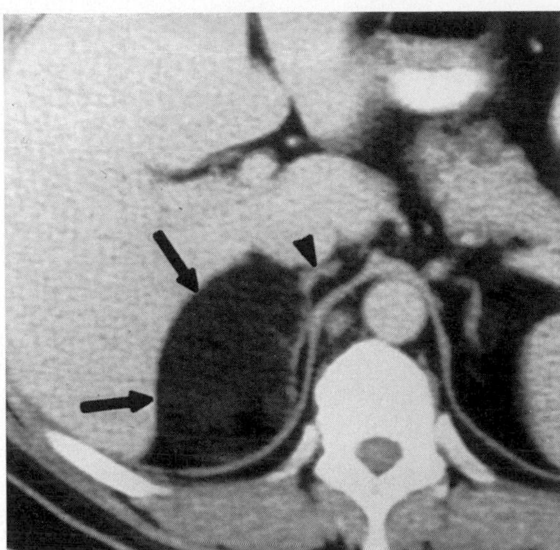

FIGURE 125–31. An adrenal mass of fat density *(arrows)* (computed tomographic density below 0 Hounsfield units) is diagnostic of myelolipoma. Note the normal right adrenal gland *(arrowhead)* from which it arises. Even minute amounts of fat in an otherwise water-density mass establish the diagnosis of myelolipoma, and biopsy is not indicated. On T1-weighted magnetic resonance imaging, myelolipomas are bright because of their fat content.

delayed contrast-enhanced CT to characterize adenoma.[19] A size threshold does not have the specificity of an attenuation threshold.

In addition to CT, MRI may help distinguish a nonhyperfunctioning adenoma from a small adrenocortical carcinoma, metastasis, or silent pheochromocytoma. Doppman et al.[20] originally reported that nonhyperfunctioning adenomas have low signal intensity similar to the liver on T2 weighted images. Mass-liver ratios less than 1:2 indicated adenoma, ratios greater than 1:4 indicated metastases (Fig. 125–32) or adrenal carcinomas (Fig. 125–33), and ratios greater than 3:1 indicated pheochromocytomas. With the use of T2 ratios investigators reported sensitivities between 75% and 85% with an indeterminate ratio range in 15% to 25% of patients. In-phase/out-of phase MRI has replaced T_2 ratios as the definitive MRI study for distinguishing incidentalomas from metastases. The lipid content of adrenocortical adenomas results in loss of signal when out-of-phase images are compared with conventional in-phase images. Mitchel et al. originally proposed the technique,[21] and multiple investigators have reported positive predictive values up to 95%.[22–25] A comparison of nonenhanced CT scans and chemical shift MRI found no clear evidence that either technique was more accurate in the characterization of adrenal masses.[126] Because CT is more readily available, we recommend that the initial study be nonenhanced CT. If the density of the adrenal mass is less than 0 HU, a confident diagnosis of adenoma can be made and no further studies are indicated. Lesions with a density greater than 20 HU are probably malignant and should undergo biopsy. For CT indeterminate lesions (HU $> 0 < 20$) chemical shift imaging should be performed. An adrenal-spleen ratio less than 70 indicates a benign lesion; adrenal-spleen ratios greater than 70 on in-phase/out-of-phase imaging are probably indicative of malignancy and biopsy should be performed.

Scintigraphy with NP-59 may also distinguish nonhyperfunctioning adenomas from metastases.[127] Although frequently described as "nonfunctioning adenomas," these lesions usually take up iodocholesterol, often with suppression of uptake in the contralateral gland, much like nontoxic functioning (hot) nodules in the thyroid gland. Cases of transient acute adrenal insufficiency after resection of nonhyperfunctioning adrenocortical adenomas have been described.[128, 129] The presence of iodocholesterol uptake in an adrenal mass excludes metastases. Such cases could be safely monitored by serial CT studies to exclude growth, although under conditions of stress, adrenocortical nodules have demonstrated enlargement.

Most adrenocortical carcinomas are larger than 6 cm and easily imaged by CT.[130–132] Staging rather than detection is the principal goal of imaging studies. Patients can have Cushing's syndrome as well as masculinization, but because the tumors are not as efficient in hormone production as benign adenomas, NP-59 scanning may be negative. Adrenocortical carcinomas invade the inferior vena cava with a frequency similar to that of renal tumors.[133] Caval involvement can usually be detected by coronal or sagittal MRI studies; only seldom is inferior venacavography required. Adrenocortical carcinomas have high signal intensity on T2-weighted images. Aggressive invasion into adjacent structures, as well as distant metastases along with failure to respond to chemotherapy or radiotherapy, results in a rather dismal prognosis (see Fig. 125–33).

In summary, CT, scintigraphy, and MRI are all useful in distinguishing an incidentally discovered nonhyperfunctioning adenoma from more serious pathology in patients without obvious endocrinologic abnormalities. The high incidence of adenomas among incidentally discovered adrenal masses, even in an oncologic population, emphasizes the need for a less invasive modality than fine-needle aspiration (Fig. 125–34). A reasonable approach in a patient with an incidentally discovered adrenal mass is as follows: functional adrenal endocrinopathy should first be excluded by physical examination and screening

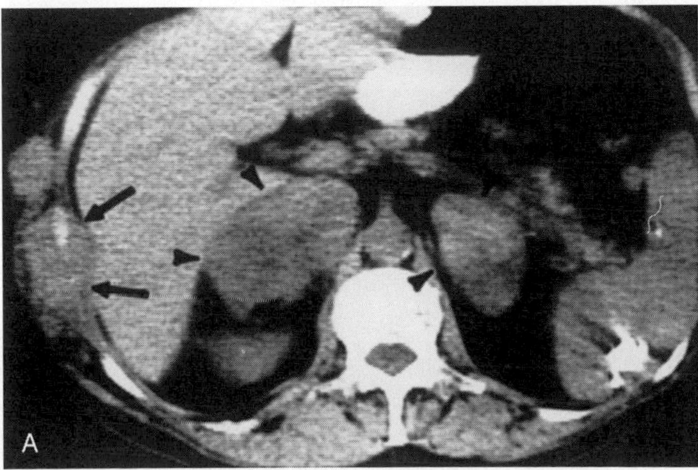

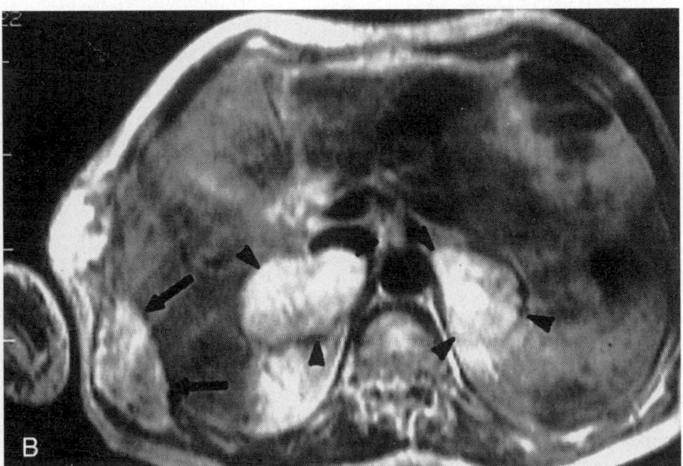

FIGURE 125–32. *A,* Computed tomography in a patient with renal cell carcinoma shows large bilateral adrenal masses *(arrowheads),* as well as evidence of metastatic disease involving the right ribs *(arrows). B,* On T2-weighted images, both the adrenal *(arrowheads)* and the costal *(arrows)* metastases have high signal intensity. Some metastases, particularly melanoma and colon cancer, may be of low signal intensity on T2-weighted images, and in critical cases with small masses, needle aspiration is required.

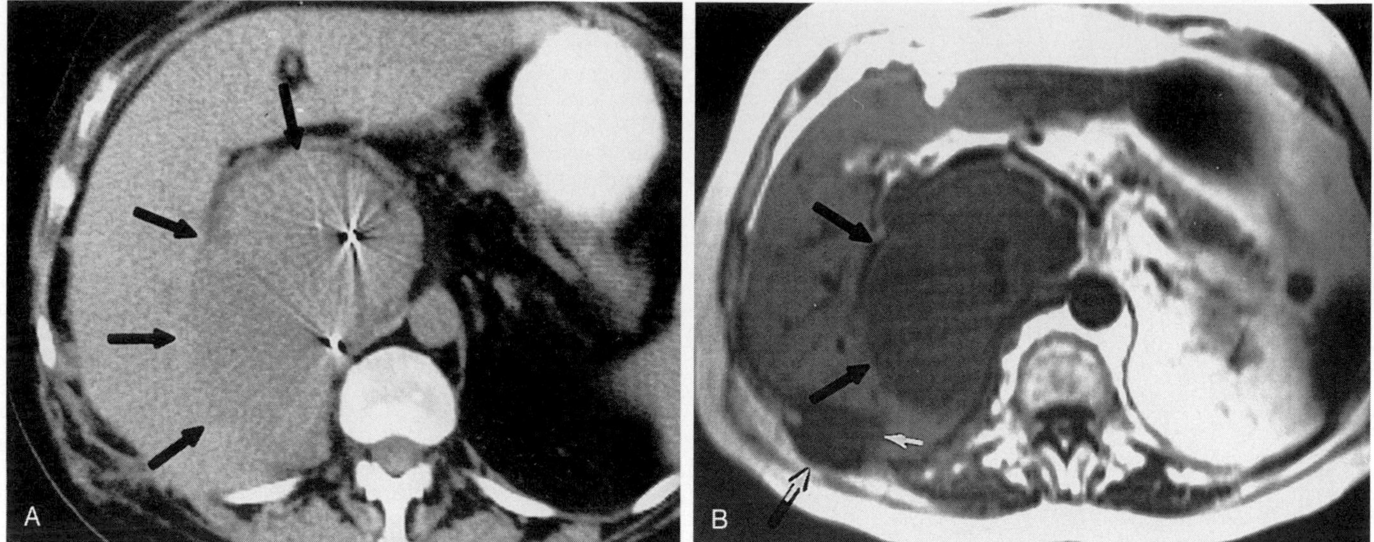

FIGURE 125–33. *A,* Computed tomography (CT) demonstrates a large carcinoma *(arrows)* arising from the right adrenal gland and containing clips from previous surgery. *B,* A T1-weighted image demonstrates a mass of low signal intensity *(black arrows)* more clearly separable from the liver than on the CT study. Note the metastatic lesion in the liver *(white arrows)*. On T2-weighted images, multiple small metastases were seen in the liver in addition to the primary tumor and the large hepatic metastases.

laboratory studies. In a patient without a known primary tumor, a mass smaller than 4 cm in diameter and of less-than-water density on CT can be presumed to be an adenoma, but a single follow-up CT at 3 to 6 months to demonstrate stability is recommended. When imaging characteristics on CT are not definitive, chemical shift (in-phase/out-of-phase) MRI is recommended. NP-59 scintigraphy can be used if CT and MRI are indeterminate and a diagnosis is essential for tumor staging. Fine-needle aspiration is not indicated when the CT, scintigraphic, or MRI characteristics suggest adenoma and the patient has no known primary tumor.

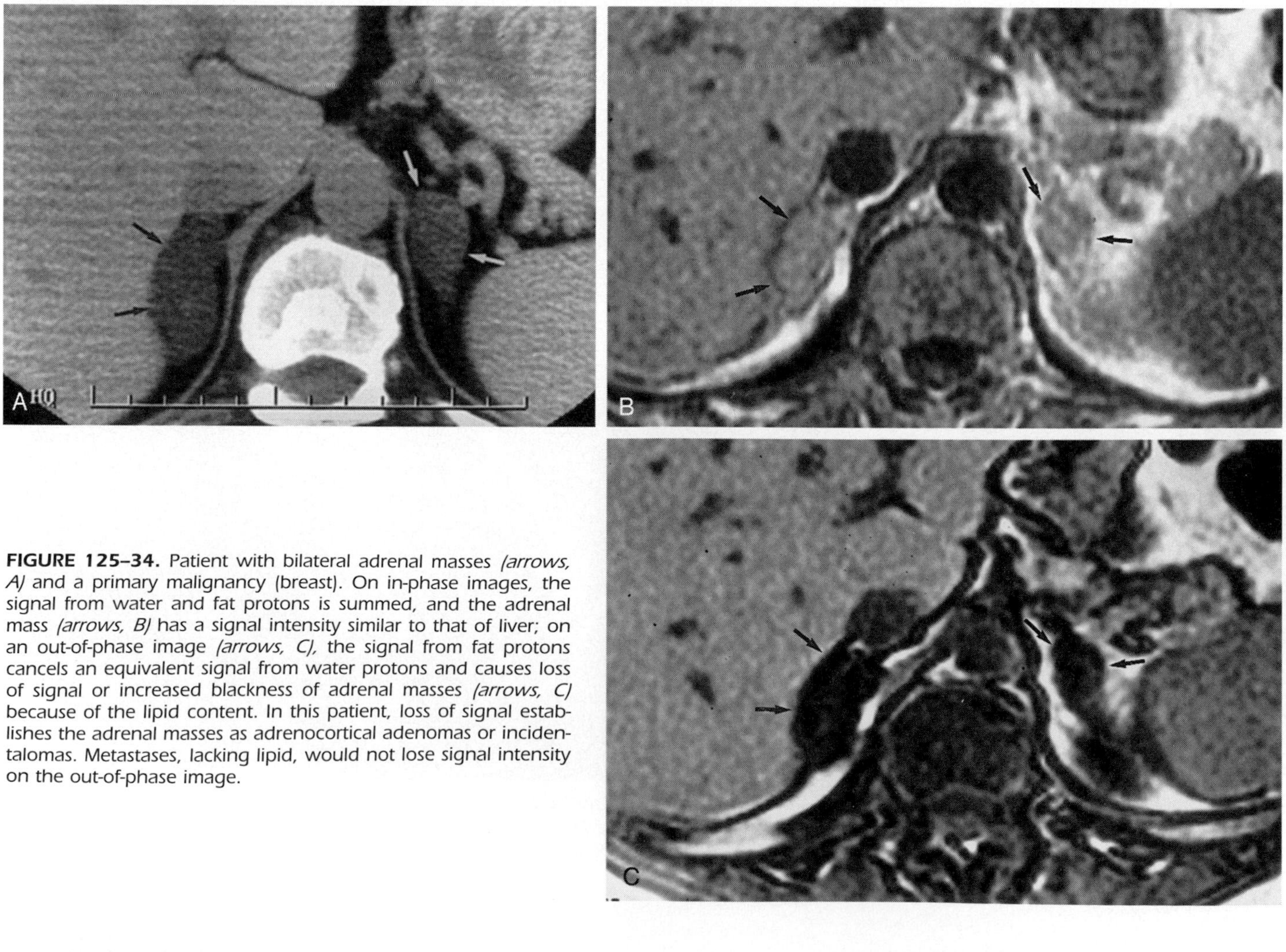

FIGURE 125–34. Patient with bilateral adrenal masses *(arrows, A)* and a primary malignancy (breast). On in-phase images, the signal from water and fat protons is summed, and the adrenal mass *(arrows, B)* has a signal intensity similar to that of liver; on an out-of-phase image *(arrows, C)*, the signal from fat protons cancels an equivalent signal from water protons and causes loss of signal or increased blackness of adrenal masses *(arrows, C)* because of the lipid content. In this patient, loss of signal establishes the adrenal masses as adrenocortical adenomas or incidentalomas. Metastases, lacking lipid, would not lose signal intensity on the out-of-phase image.

REFERENCES

1. Miller DL, Doppman JL: Diagnostic imaging of the adrenal gland. *In* Becker KL (ed): Principles and Practice of Endocrinology and Metabolism. Philadelphia, JB Lippincott, 1990, pp 684–689.
2. Korobkin M: Overview of adrenal imaging/adrenal CT. Urol Radiol 11:221–226, 1989.
3. Dunnick NR: Adrenal imaging. Current status. AJR 154:927–936, 1990.
4. Lack EE, Travis WD: Pathology of the Adrenal Glands. New York, Churchill Livingstone, 1990.
5. Wilms G, Baert A, Marchal G, et al: Computed tomography of the normal adrenal glands. Correlative study with autopsy specimens. J Comput Assist Tomogr 3:467–469, 1979.
6. El Shirf MA, Hemmingsson A: Computed tomography of the normal adrenal gland. Acta Radiol 23:433–442, 1982.
7. McCorkell SJ, Miles NL: Fine needle aspiration of catecholamine-producing adrenal masses, a possibly fatal mistake. AJR 145:113–114, 1985.
8. Casola G, Nicolet V, van Sonnenberg E, et al: Unsuspected pheochromocytomas; risk of blood pressure alterations during percutaneous adrenal biopsy. Radiology 159:733–735, 1986.
9. Montagne JP, Kressel HR, Korobkin M: Computed tomography of the normal adrenal glands. AJR 130:963–966, 1978.
10. Karstaedt N, Sagel S, Stanley R, et al: Computed tomography of the adrenal gland. Radiology 129:723–730, 1978.
11. Korobkin N, White EA, Kressel HY, et al: Computed tomography in the diagnosis of adrenal diseases. AJR 132:231–238, 1979.
12. Berliner L, Bosniak MA, Megibow A: Adrenal pseudotumors on computed tomography. J Comput Assist Tomogr 6:281–285, 1982.
13. Silverman PM: Gastric diverticulum mimicking adrenal gland. CT demonstration. J Comput Assist Tomogr 10:709–710, 1986.
14. Mitty HA, Cohen BA, Sprayregen S, et al: Adrenal pseudotumors on CT due to dilated portal systemic veins. AJR 141:727–730, 1983.
15. Korobkin M, Giordano TJ, Brodur FJ, et al: Adrenal adenomas; relationship between histologic lipid and CT and MR findings. Radiology 200:743–747, 1996.
16. Korobkin M, Brodur FJ, Yutzy GG, et al: Differentiation of adrenal adenomas from non-adenomas on CT attenuation values. AJR 166:531–536, 1996.
17. McNicholas MJ, Lee MJ, Mayo-Smith WW, et al: An imaging algorithm for the differential diagnosis of adrenal adenomas and metastases. AJR 165:1453–1459, 1995.
18. Korobkin M, Brodur FJ, Francis IR, et al: Delayed enhanced CT for differentiation of benign and malignant adrenal masses. Radiology 200:737–742, 1996.
19. Boland GW, Hahn PF, Pena C, et al: Adrenal masses: Characterization with delayed contrast enhanced CT. Radiology 202:693–696, 1997.
20. Doppman JL, Reinig JW, Dwyer AJ, et al: Differentiation of adrenal masses by magnetic resonance imaging. Surgery 102:1018–1026, 1987.
21. Mitchell DG, Crovello M, Mattucci T, et al: Benign adrenal cortical masses; diagnosis with chemical shift MR imaging. Radiology 185:345–351, 1992.
22. Mayo-Smith WW, Lee MJ, McNicholas MM, et al: Characterization of adrenal masses (<5cm) by use of chemical shift MR imaging; observer performance versus quantitative measures. AJR 165:91–95, 1995.
23. Outwater EK, Siegelman ES, Radecki PD, et al: Distinction between benign and malignant adrenal masses; value of T1-weighted chemical shift MR imaging. AJR 165:579–583, 1995.
24. Bilby JH, McLaughlin RF, Kurkjan PS, et al: MR imaging of adrenal masses; value of chemical-shift imaging for distinguishing adenomas from other tumors. AJR 164:637–642, 1995.
25. Korobkin M, Lombardi CJ, Aisen AM, et al: Characterization of adrenal masses with chemical shift and gadolinium-enhanced MR imaging. Radiology 197:411–418, 1995.
26. Kalmannskog F, Kolbenstvedt A, Brekke JB: CT and angiography in adrenocortical carcinoma. Acta Radiol 33:45–59, 1992.
27. Young WF Jr, Hogan MJ, Klee GG, et al: Primary aldosteronism diagnosis and treatment. Mayo Clin Proc 65:16–110, 1990.
28. Doppman JL, Gill JR Jr: Hyperaldosteronism: Sampling the adrenal veins. Radiology 198:309–312, 1996.
29. Eagan RT, Page MI: Adrenal insufficiency following bilateral adrenal venography. JAMA 215:115–116, 1971.
30. Doppman JL, Gill JG, Miller DL, et al: Distinction between hyperaldosteronism due to bilateral hyperplasia and unilateral aldosteronoma: Reliability of CT. Radiology 184:677–682, 1992.
31. Dunnick NR, Doppman JL, Mills SR, et al: Preoperative diagnosis and localization of aldosteronomas by measurement of corticosteroids in adrenal venous blood. Radiology 133:331–333, 1979.
32. Hessel SJ, Adams DF, Abrams HL: Complications of angiography. Radiology 138:273–281, 1981.
33. Boova R, Carabasi A, Scott I, et al: Transvenous adrenalectomy for advanced carcinoma of the breast. Surg Gynecol Obstet 152:627–629, 1981.
34. Jablonsky RD, Meaney TF, Schumacher OP: Transcatheter adrenal ablation for metastatic carcinoma of the breast. Cleve Clin Q 44:57–63, 1977.
35. Zimmerman CE, Eisenberg H, Spark R, et al: Transvenous adrenal destruction; clinical trials in patients with metastatic malignancies. Surgery 75:550–556, 1974.
36. Rosenstock J, Allison D, Joplin GF, et al: Therapeutic adrenal venous infarction in ACTH-dependent Cushing's syndrome. Br J Radiol 54:912–915, 1981.
37. Dunnick NR, Doppman JL, Gill JR Jr: Failure to ablate the adrenal gland by injection of contrast material. Radiology 142:67–69, 1982.
38. Fink IJ, Girton M, Doppman JL: Absolute ethanol injection of the adrenal artery: Hypertensive reaction. Radiology 154:357–358, 1985.
39. Doppman JL, Girton M: Adrenal ablation by retrograde venous ethanol injection: An ineffective and dangerous procedure. Radiology 150:667–672, 1984.
40. Takeda M, Go H, Imai T, et al: Laparoscopic adrenalectomy for primary aldosteronism. Report of initial ten cases. Surgery 115:621–625, 1994.
41. Gagner M, Pomp A, Meniford BT, et al: Laparoscopic adrenalectomy: Lessons learned from 100 consecutive procedures. Ann Surg 226:238–246, 1997.
42. Lieberman LM, Beierwaltes WH, Conn JW, et al: Diagnosis of adrenal disease by visualization of human adrenal glands with ^{131}I-19-iodocholesterol. N Engl J Med 285:1387–1393, 1971.
43. Mishkin F, Freeman L: Miscellaneous applications for radionuclide imaging. *In* Freeman L, Johnson PM (eds): Freeman and Johnson's Clinical Radionuclide Imaging. Orlando, FL, Grune & Stratton, 1984, p 1365.
44. Sisson JC, Frager MS, Valk TW, et al: Scintigraphic localization of pheochromocytoma. N Engl J Med 305:12–17, 1981.
45. Doppman JL, Frank JA, Dwyer AJ, et al: Gadolinium-DTPA enhanced MR imaging of ACTH-secreting microadenomas of the pituitary. J Comput Assist Tomogr 12:728–735, 1988.
46. Oldfield EH, Doppman JL, Nieman LK, et al: Petrosal sinus sampling with and without corticotropin-releasing hormone for the differential diagnosis of Cushing's syndrome. N Engl J Med 325:897–905, 1991.
47. Perry RR, Nieman LK, Cutler GB Jr, et al: Primary adrenal causes of Cushing's syndrome: Diagnosis and surgical management. Ann Surg 210:59–68, 1989.
48. Fig LM, Gross MD, Shapiro B, et al: Adrenal localization in the adrenocorticotropic hormone–independent Cushing syndrome. Ann Intern Med 109:547–553, 1988.
49. Doppman JL, Miller DL, Dwyer AJ, et al: Macronodular adrenal hyperplasia in Cushing disease. Radiology 166:347–352, 1988.
50. Aron DC, Findling JW, Fitzgerald PA, et al: Pituitary ACTH-dependency of nodular adrenal hyperplasia in Cushing's syndrome; report of two cases and review of the literature. Am J Med 71:302–306, 1981.
51. Smals AGH, Pieters GFFM, van Haelst UJG, et al: Macronodular adrenocortical hyperplasia in long-standing Cushing's disease. J Clin Endocrinol Metab 58:25–31, 1984.
52. Steingart DE, Tsao HA: Coexistence of pituitary adrenocorticotrophin-dependent Cushing's syndrome with a solitary adrenal adenoma. J Clin Endocrinol Metab 50:961–966, 1980.
53. Leiba S, Shindel B, Weinberger I, et al: Cushing's disease coexisting with a single macronodule simulating adenoma of the adrenal cortex. Acta Endocrinol 112:323–328, 1986.
54. Stratakis CA, Kirscher LS: Clinical and genetic analysis of primary bilateral adrenal diseases (micro- and macronodular disease) leading to Cushing syndrome. Horm Metab Res 30:456–463, 1998.
55. Bornstein SR, Stratakis CA, Chrousos GP: Adrenocortical tumors: Recent advances in basic concepts and clinical management. Ann Intern Med 130:759–771, 1999.
56. Ruder HJ, Loriaux DL, Lipsett MB: Severe osteopenia in young adults associated with Cushing's syndrome due to micronodular adrenal disease. J Clin Endocrinol Metab 39:1138–1147, 1974.
57. Larsen JL, Cathey WJ, O'Dell WD: Primary adrenocortical nodular dysplasia, a distinct subtype of Cushing's syndrome. Am J Med 80:976–984, 1986.
58. Carney JA, Gorden H, Carpenter PC, et al: The complex of myxomas, spotty pigmentation and endocrine overactivity. Medicine (Baltimore) 64:270–283, 1985.
59. Teding van Berkhout F, Croughs RJ, Wulffraat NM, et al: Familial Cushing's syndrome due to nodular adrenocortical dysplasia: An inherited disease of immunologic origin. Clin Endocrinol (Oxf) 31:185–191, 1989.
60. Carney JA, Young WF Jr: Primary pigmented nodular adrenocortical disease and its associated conditions. Endocrinologist 2:6–21, 1992.
61. Young WF Jr, Carney JA, Musa BU, et al: Familial Cushing's syndrome due to primary pigmented nodular adrenocortical disease. Reinvestigation 50 years later. N Engl J Med 321:1659–1664, 1989.
62. Stratakis CA, Carney CA, Lin JP, et al: Carney's complex: A familial multiple neoplasia and lentiginous syndrome. Analysis of 11 kindreds and linkage to the short arm of chromosome 2. J Clin Invest 97:699–705, 1996.
63. Travis WD, Tsokos M, Doppman JL, et al: Primary pigmented nodular adrenocortical disease. A light and electron microscopic study of eight cases. Am J Surg Pathol 13:921–930, 1989.
64. Doppman JL, Travis WD, Nieman L, et al: Cushing syndrome due to primary pigmented nodular adrenocortical disease: Findings at CT and MR imaging. Radiology 172:415–420, 1989.
65. Sarlis H, Chrousos GP, Doppman JL, et al: Primary pigmented nodular adrenocortical disease (PPHAD): Re-evaluation of a patient with Carney complex 27 years after unilateral adrenalectomy. J Clin Endocrinol Metab 82:2037–2043, 1997.
66. Grant CS, Carney JA, Carpenter PC, et al: Primary pigmented nodular adrenocortical disease; diagnosis and management. Surgery 100:1178–1183, 1986.
67. Doppman JL, Nieman LK, Travis WD, et al: CT and MR imaging of massive macronodular adrenocortical disease: A rare cause of autonomous primary adrenal hypercortisolism. J Comput Assist Tomogr 15:773–779, 1991.
68. Doppman JL, Chrousos GP, Papanicoloau D, et al: Adrenocorticotropic (ACTH)-independent macronodular adrenal hyperplasia; an uncommon cause of primary adrenal hypercortisolism. Radiology (in press).
69. Lieberman SA, Eccleshall TR, Feldman D: ACTH-independent massive bilateral adrenal disease (AIMBAD): A subtype of Cushing's syndrome with major diagnostic and therapeutic implications. Eur J Endocrinol 131:67–73, 1994.
70. Lack EE, Travis WD, Oertel JE: Adrenocortical nodules, hyperplasia and hyperfunction. *In* Lack EE (ed): Pathology of the Adrenal Glands. New York, Churchill Livingstone, 1990, pp 75–113.
71. Hermus AR, Pieters GF, Smals AG, et al: Transition from pituitary-dependent to adrenal-dependent Cushing's syndrome. N Engl J Med 318:966–970, 1988.
72. Kirschner MA, Powell RD Jr, Lipsett MB: Cushing's syndrome; nodular cortical hyperplasia of adrenal glands with clinical and pathologic features suggesting adrenocortical tumor. J Clin Endocrinol 24:947–955, 1964.
73. Lacroix A, Bolte EE, Tremblay J, et al: Gastric inhibitory polypeptide–dependent

cortisol dependent secretion—a new cause of Cushing's syndrome. N Engl J Med 327:974–980, 1992.
74. Lacroix A, Tremblay J, Touyz RM, et al: Abnormal adrenal and vascular responses to vasopressin mediated by a V1-vasopressin receptor in a patient with adrenocorticotropin-independent macronodular adrenal hyperplasia, Cushing's syndrome and orthostatic hypertension. J Clin Endocrinol Metab 82:2414–2422, 1987.
75. Lacroix A, Tremblay J, Rousseau G, et al: Propranolol therapy for ectopic beta-adrenogenic receptors in adrenal Cushing's syndrome. N Engl J Med 337:429–434, 1997.
76. Lacroix A, Mircescu H, Hamet P: Clinical evaluation with a presence of abnormal hormone receptors in adrenal Cushing's syndrome. Endocrinologist 9:9–15, 1999.
77. Swan JM, Grant CS, Schlinker TRT, et al: Corticotrophin independent macronodular adrenal hyperplasia. Arch Surg 133:541–546, 1998.
78. Bravo EL, Tarizi RC, Dustan HP, et al: The changing clinical spectrum of primary aldosteronism. Am J Med 74:641–651, 1983.
79. Weinberger MH, Grim CE, Hollifield JW, et al: Primary aldosteronism. Diagnosis, localization and treatment. Ann Intern Med 90:386–395, 1979.
80. Miyake H, Maeda H, Tishiro M, et al: CT of adrenal tumors; frequency and clinical significance of low attenuation lesions. AJR 152:1005–1007, 1989.
81. Young WF Jr, Klee GG: Primary aldosteronism; diagnostic evaluation. Endocrinol Metab Clin North Am 17:367–395, 1988.
82. Grant CS, Carpenter P, van Heerden JA, et al: Primary aldosteronism. Clinical management. Arch Surg 119:585–590, 1984.
83. Doppman JL: The dilemma of bilateral adrenal cortical nodularity in Conn's and Cushing's syndromes. Radiol Clin North Am 31:1039–1050, 1993.
84. Young WF Jr, Stanson AW, Grant CS, et al: Primary aldosteronism; adrenal venous sampling. Surgery 120:913–920, 1996.
85. Young WF Jr: Primary aldosteronism; update on diagnosis and treatment. Endocrinologist 7:213–221, 1997.
86. Sheaves R, Golden J, Resnick RH, et al: Larger value of computed tomography scanning and venous sampling in establishing the cause of primary hyperaldosteronism. Eur J Endocrinol 134:308–313, 1996.
87. Ikeda DM, Francis IR, Glazer GM, et al: The detection of adrenal tumors and hyperplasia in patients with primary aldosteronism; comparison of scintigraphy, CT and MR imaging. AJR 153:301–306, 1989.
88. Doppman JL, Gill JR Jr, Nienhuis AW, et al: CT findings in Addison's disease. J Comput Assist Tomogr 6:757–761, 1982.
89. McMurry JF Jr, Long D, McClure R, et al: Addison's disease with adrenal enlargement on computed tomographic scans. Report of two cases of tuberculosis and review of the literature. Am J Med 77:365–368, 1984.
90. Kung AWC, Pun KK, Lamb K, et al: Addisonian crisis as the presenting feature in malignancies. Cancer 65:177–179, 1990.
91. Sheeler LR, Myers JH, Eversman JJ, et al: Adrenal insufficiency secondary to carcinoma metastatic to the adrenal gland. Cancer 52:1312–1316, 1983.
92. Osa SR, Peterson RE, Roberts RB: Recovery of adrenal reserve following treatment of disseminated South American blastomycosis. Am J Med 71:298–301, 1981.
93. Washburn RG, Bennett JE: Reversal of adrenal glucocorticoid dysfunction of a patient with disseminated histoplasmosis. Ann Intern Med 110:86–87, 1989.
94. Long JA Jr, Doppman JL, Nienhuis AW, et al: Computed tomographic analysis of beta-thalassemic syndrome with hemochromatosis. Pathologic findings with clinical and laboratory correlations. J Comput Assist Tomogr 4:159–165, 1980.
95. Freda TU, Wardlaw SL, Burdney K, et al: Primary adrenal insufficiency in patients with acquired immune-deficiency syndrome; report of five cases. J Clin Endocrinol Metab 79:1540–1545, 1994.
96. Pedrola G, Casado JL, Lopez E, et al: Clinical features of adrenal insufficiency in patients with acquired immuno-deficiency syndrome. Clin Endocrinol (Oxf) 45:97–101, 1996.
97. Merenich JA, McDermott MT, Asp AA, et al: Evidence of endocrine involvement early in the course of human immunodeficiency by this infection. J Clin Endocrinol Metab 70:566–571, 1990.
98. Amason JA, Graziano FM: Adrenal insufficiency in the antiphospholipid antibody syndrome. Semin Arthritis Rheum 25:109–116, 1995.
99. Caron P, Shabbonier MH, Cambus J-P, et al: Definitive adrenal insufficiency due to bilateral adrenal hemorrhage and primary antiphospholipid syndrome. J Clin Endocrinol Metab 83:1437–1439, 1998.
100. Rao RH, Vagnucci AH, Amico JA: Bilateral massive adrenal hemorrhage. Early recognition and treatment. Ann Intern Med 110:227–235, 1989.
101. Cary RM: The changing clinical spectrum of adrenal insufficiency. Ann Intern Med 127:1103–1105, 1997.
102. Streeten DHP: Adrenal hemorrhage. Endocrinologist 6:277–284, 1996.
103. Harinariyana CV, Renu G, Ammini AC, et al: Computed tomography in untreated congenital adrenal hyperplasia. Pediatr Radiol 21:103–105, 1991.
104. Falke THM, van Seters AP, Schaberg AA, et al: Computed tomography in untreated adults with virilising congenital adrenal cortical hyperplasia. Clin Radiol 37:155–160, 1986.
105. Seidenwurm D, Hoffman A, Kan P, et al: Intratesticular adrenal rests diagnosed by ultrasound. Radiology 155:479–481, 1985.
106. Rutgers JL, Young RH, Scully RE: The testicular "tumor" of the adrenogenital syndrome. A report of six cases and review of the literature on testicular masses in patients with adrenocortical disorders. Am J Surg Pathol 12:503–513, 1988.
107. Shawker TH, Doppman JL, Choyke PL, et al: Intratesticular masses associated with abnormally functioning adrenal glands. J Clin Ultrasound 20:51–58, 1992.
108. Stewart BH, Bravo EL, Haaga J, et al: Localization of pheochromocytoma by computed tomography. N Engl J Med 299:460–461, 1978.
109. Welch TJ, Sheedy PF II, van Heerden JA, et al: Pheochromocytoma: Value of computed tomography. Radiology 148:501–503, 1983.
110. Thomas JL, Bernadino ME, Samaan NA, et al: CT of pheochromocytoma. AJR 135:477–482, 1980.
111. Stein PP, Black HR: A simplified diagnostic approach to pheochromocytoma. Medicine (Baltimore) 70:46–66, 1990.
112. Fink IJ, Reinig JW, Dwyer AJ, et al: MR imaging of pheochromocytomas. J Comput Assist Tomogr 9:454–458, 1985.
113. Shapiro B, Sisson JC, Lloyd R, et al: Malignant pheochromocytoma. Clinical, biochemical and scintigraphic characterization. Clin Endocrinol 20:189–203, 1984.
114. Lips KJM, van der Sluy S, Ver J, et al: Bilateral occurrence of pheochromocytoma in patients with multiple endocrine neoplasia syndrome IIA (Sipple syndrome). Am J Med 70:1051–1060, 1981.
115. Shapiro B, Copp JE, Sisson JC, et al: ^{131}Meta-iodobenzylguanidine for the locating of suspected pheochromocytoma. Experience in 400 cases. J Nucl Med 26:576–585, 1985.
116. Schmedtje JF, Sax S, Pool JL, et al: Localization of ectopic pheochromocytomas by magnetic resonance imaging. Am J Med 83:770–772, 1987.
117. Copeland PM: The incidentally discovered adrenal mass. Ann Intern Med 98:940–945, 1983.
118. Ross NS, Aron DC: Hormonal evaluation of the patient with an incidentally discovered adrenal mass. N Engl J Med 323:1401–1405, 1990.
119. Dobbie JW: Adrenocortical nodular hyperplasia; the aging adrenal. J Pathol 99:1–18, 1969.
120. Hedeland H, Ostberg G, Hokfelt B: On the prevalence of adrenocortical adenomas in an autopsy material in relation to hypertension and diabetes. Acta Med Scand 184:211–214, 1968.
121. Oliver EW Jr, Bernadino ME, Miller JI, et al: Isolated adrenal masses in nonsmall cell bronchogenic carcinoma. Radiology 153:217–218, 1984.
122. Glazer HS, Wyman PJ, Sagel SS, et al: Nonfunctioning adrenal masses; incidental discovery on computed tomography. AJR 139:81–85, 1982.
123. Mitnick JS, Bosniak MA, Megibow AJ, et al: Nonfunctioning adrenal adenomas discovered incidentally on computed tomography. Radiology 148:495–499, 1983.
124. Hussain S, Belldegrun A, Seltzer SP, et al: Differentiation of malignant from benign adrenal masses; predictive indices on computed tomography. AJR 144:61–65, 1985.
125. Lee MJ, Hahn PF, Papanicolaou N, et al: Benign and malignant adrenal masses. CT distinction with attenuation coefficient size and observer analysis. Radiology 179:415–418, 1991.
126. Outwater EK, Siegelman ES, Hwang AD, et al: Adrenal masses; correlation between CT attenuation value and chemical shift ratio at MR imaging with in-phase and opposed-phase sequences. Radiology 200:749–752, 1996.
127. Francis IR, Smid A, Gross MD, et al: Adrenal masses in oncologic patients. Functional and morphologic evaluation. Radiology 166:353–356, 1988.
128. Huiras CM, Pehling GB, Caplan RH: Adrenal insufficiency after operative removal of apparently non-functioning adrenal adenomas. JAMA 261:894–898, 1989.
129. McLeod MK, Thompson NW, Gross MD, et al: Subclinical Cushing's syndrome in patients with adrenal gland incidentalomas. Am Surg 56:398–403, 1990.
130. Cohn K, Gottesman L, Brennan M: Adrenocortical carcinoma. Surgery 100:1170–1177, 1986.
131. Luton JP, Cerdos S, Billaud L, et al: Clinical features of adrenocortical carcinoma, prognostic factors and the effect of mitotane therapy. N Engl J Med 322:1195–1201, 1990.
132. Fishman EK, Deutch BM, Hartman DS, et al: Primary adrenocortical carcinoma: CT evaluation with clinical correlation. AJR 148:531–535, 1987.
133. Dunnick NR, Doppman JL, Geelhoed GW: Intravenous extension of endocrine tumors. AJR 135:471–476, 1980.

Chapter 126

Adrenal Cancer

David E. Schteingart

INCIDENCE AND AGE AT DIAGNOSIS

Adrenal cortical carcinomas are rare, highly malignant tumors that account for only 0.2% of deaths caused by cancer. Their incidence has been estimated at 2 per million population per year. Occasional children have been found to have adrenal cortical carcinomas, but most cases occur between the ages of 30 and 50 years.[1] Although the etiology of adrenal cancer remains unknown, some cases have been described in families with a hereditary cancer syndrome in whom mutations in tumor suppressor genes are an important factor in adrenal tumorigenesis. One such syndrome is the Li-Fraumeni syndrome, which is characterized by sarcoma, breast cancer, brain tumors, lung cancer, laryngeal carcinoma, leukemia, and adrenal cortical carcinoma. In these cases, the deleterious genotype has been expressed through several generations and is found in both children and adults.[2, 3]

Several theories have been put forth to explain tumorigenesis in adrenal cortical carcinoma, including the development of chromosomal alterations leading to dysregulation of a gene product or chronic stimulation of the gland. Some data support the presence of changes in the p53 tumor suppressor gene located on chromosome 17p and its 53-kDa protein. A germline mutation of the p53 gene was found in a patient with an incidentally detected adrenal cortical carcinoma.[4] This mutation resulted in a premature stop codon. However, mutations at the p53 loci have also been found in adrenal adenomas and pheochromocytomas.[5] Others have shown allelic loss at the p53 gene locus on chromosome 17p.[6, 7] In a study of 11 adrenal cortical carcinomas, 5 showed positive immunohistochemical staining for the p53 protein,[8] but 3 of them had only a small percentage of cells staining positive. In 2 of the 11 carcinomas, point mutations were shown in the p53 gene in exons 5 through 8. These mutations resulted in a single amino acid change, presumably resulting in a protein with an altered half-life. A deletion rearrangement was also found in 1 adrenal cortical carcinoma. Another study reported positive immunostaining for the p53 gene product in 22 of 42 cases of adrenal cortical carcinoma but was unable to show that the p53 status had any effect on long-term survival.[9]

Changes in the RB gene have also been reported, but the nature of the changes in this gene and its regulation have not been completely worked out. As with the p53 gene, allelic loss at the RB gene locus on chromosome 13q has been described in adrenal cortical carcinoma.[6] Other genetic markers examined included the H19, the insulin-like growth factor type II (IGF-II), and the $p57^{kip2}$ genes. These genes have been mapped to chromosome 11p15.5[10] and appear to be important for fetal growth and development. The levels of H19 and IGF-II gene expression are very high in human fetal adrenal glands,[11] but they subsequently decrease by 50% in adults. The gene product for $p57^{kip2}$ is a member of the p21CIP1 cyclin-dependent kinase family and appears to regulate self-proliferation, exit from the cell cycle, and maintenance of differentiated cells. This gene product is usually found to be high in most normal human tissues. H19 and $p57^{kip2}$ gene expression is dependent on adrenocorticotropic hormone (ACTH), and regulation of the $p57^{kip2}$ gene appears to be related to the cyclic adenosine monophosphate–dependent protein kinase pathway.[10] H19 gene expression is markedly reduced in adrenal cortical carcinomas, both nonfunctioning and functioning, especially in tumors producing cortisol and aldosterone.[10] Loss of activity of the $p57^{kip2}$ gene product is also observed in virilizing adenomas and adrenal cortical carcinomas,[10] which suggests that this gene product plays a role in the normal maintenance of adrenal cortical differentiation and function. In contrast, IGF-II gene expression has been shown to be high in adrenal cortical carcinomas. Finally, the c-*myc* gene has been evaluated for a possible role in adrenal tumorigenesis. C-*myc* gene expression is relatively high in neoplasms, and it is often linked to a poor prognosis. However, in adrenal cortical carcinomas, expression of c-*myc* is approximately 10% of that found in normal adrenal tissue.[12] The c-*myc* gene is generally expressed in normal adrenal glands and usually localized to the zona fasciculata and zona reticularis. The significance of low c-*myc* gene expression in adrenal cortical carcinomas needs to be elucidated.

CLINICAL AND BIOCHEMICAL EVALUATION

Approximately 50% of adrenal cortical carcinomas are functioning and produce hormonal and metabolic syndromes leading to their discovery. The other 50% are silent and discovered only when they attain large size and produce localized abdominal symptoms or metastases.

Cushing's syndrome is the most common clinical manifestation in adult patients. Characteristically, these patients describe rapid development (3–6 months) of the clinical symptoms of cortisol excess, including weight gain, muscle weakness, easy bruising, irritability, and insomnia. In addition, manifestations of androgen excess are commonly seen, including hirsutism, acne, and irregular menses or amenorrhea in women. Although virilization frequently accompanies Cushing's syndrome, the predominant clinical manifestations may be those of androgen excess with only subtle evidence of hypercortisolism. The androgen excess may decrease the severity of the catabolic effect of hypercortisolemia such that skin and muscle atrophy may not be as readily apparent as in those with benign tumors. Patients with metastatic disease complain of anorexia and weight loss rather than weight gain. Adrenal cortical carcinomas causing Cushing's syndrome are large with an average weight of 800 g, but the clinical manifestations of hormone excess may lead to earlier diagnosis and the finding of smaller tumors.

Hormonal studies in patients with clinical manifestations of Cushing's syndrome include measurement of urinary free cortisol, serum cortisol, and dehydroepiandrosterone sulfate (DHEAS) at baseline and during dexamethasone suppression. Patients with cortisol-secreting adrenal cortical carcinomas exhibit elevated baseline cortisol and DHEAS levels and failure to suppress with a high (8 mg) dose of dexamethasone. ACTH levels are usually suppressed. The steroid profile in serum or urine can sometimes help distinguish between benign and malignant adrenal cortical tumors because of the presence of intermediary precursors in the steroid biosynthetic pathway or their metabolites in patients with malignant neoplasms.

Sex hormone–producing carcinomas lead to virilization in women and manifestations of feminization in men. Women with virilizing adrenal cortical carcinomas have marked androgen-type hirsutism, male pattern baldness, deepening voice, breast atrophy, clitoral hypertrophy, decreased libido, and oligomenorrhea or amenorrhea. In contrast, manifestations of androgen excess are less noticeable in men. In prepubertal boys with androgen excess, precocious puberty develops without concomitant testicular enlargement. Feminizing tumors in women cause breast tenderness and dysfunctional uterine bleeding. Estrogen-secreting tumors in men are associated with gynecomastia, breast tenderness, testicular atrophy, and decreased libido. Early breast and uterine development and early onset of menarche develop in prepubertal girls with feminizing tumors.

Patients with virilizing tumors demonstrate high serum levels of testosterone, androstenedione, and DHEAS, whereas patients with feminizing tumors have high serum estradiol levels. Total testosterone levels in virilized women are greater than 2.0 ng/mL (normal, 0.3–0.6 ng/mL).

Aldosterone-producing adrenal cortical carcinomas are extremely rare. They cause clinical manifestations of primary aldosteronism with hypertension and hypokalemia. When compared with patients with benign aldosterone-secreting adenomas, those with carcinoma have larger tumors, higher aldosterone levels, and more severe hypokalemia.[13, 14] Evaluation should include measurement of serum electrolyte, aldosterone, and plasma renin levels. Findings include severe hypokalemia with potassium levels below 2.5 mEq/L, hypernatremia, and metabolic alkalosis. Serum aldosterone levels are high whereas plasma renin levels are suppressed.

A hormonal profile should also be obtained in patients with apparently nonfunctioning adrenal tumors. Some of these tumors produce biosynthetic steroid pathway intermediates such as progesterone and 11-deoxycortisol.[15] It is important to determine the level of these steroids in patients with adrenal cortical cancer before surgery because these hormones can be used as biochemical markers in postoperative follow-up.

Silent adrenal cortical carcinomas do not cause recognizable symptoms of excessive hormone production and are detected when they attain large size and cause local symptoms. Some of these tumors, however, may be detected incidentally in the course of investigation for unrelated abdominal complaints. Incidentally discovered adrenal masses are found in 1% to 3% of computed tomographic (CT) scanning of the abdomen. Most of these masses are benign, and adrenal cortical adenomas are 60 times more common than primary carcinomas.[16] When these adrenal masses are malignant, they are frequently metastatic from extra-adrenal neoplasms.

In evaluating incidentally found adrenal masses, size is an important consideration in determining whether the mass is likely to be benign or malignant. Masses less than 3 cm are usually benign[17]; in contrast, the probability that a mass is malignant is greatly increased when it measures greater than 6 cm. The probability is uncertain that a mass measuring 3 to 6 cm is malignant, and it is of concern that adrenal cortical carcinomas larger than 6 cm would have been small early in their development. Because early resection of these tumors offers the best chance for cure or long survival, accurate diagnosis of a small tumor becomes very important.

RADIOGRAPHIC DETECTION OF ADRENAL MASSES; EVALUATION OF WHETHER THEY ARE BENIGN OR MALIGNANT

A variety of imaging procedures can be useful in the localization and evaluation of the benign or malignant character of an adrenal cortical neoplasm.

1. *Computed Axial Tomography.* Unenhanced and contrast-enhanced CT scans have been used to distinguish benign from malignant adrenal masses.[18, 19] The distinction is based on the lipid content of the mass. Lipid-rich masses are usually benign, whereas lipid-poor masses are frequently malignant. Enhancement is measured in Hounsfield units (HU). Low-attenuation lesions have low HU values. Unenhanced CT has been used to show that adenomas have values less than +10 HU whereas nonadenomas have values greater than +18 HU. These criteria give a sensitivity of 73% for distinguishing adenomas from nonadenomas and a specificity of 96%. CT images obtained 1 hour after the injection of contrast show enhancement of 11 ± 13 HU (<30 HU) for adenomas and a value of 49 ± 8.3 HU (>30 HU) for nonadenomas, with a sensitivity of 95% for distinguishing adenomas from malignant masses and a specificity of 100%. Adenomas also exhibit greater than 50% washout within 15 minutes of contrast injection, whereas nonadenomas exhibit greater retention of contrast. Malignant adrenal masses are usually larger than 5 cm, have an inhomogeneous pattern because of areas of necrosis within the tumor, and are frequently invasive of the upper pole of the adjoining kidney and the inferior vena cava. The CT procedure also helps determine the presence of involved lymph nodes and hepatic or pulmonary metastases. A definition of metastatic involvement is important when determining the stage of the disease and the treatment goals for a given patient.

2. *Ultrasonography.* Malignant lesions vary in echo texture and are heterogeneous in appearance, with focal or scattered echopenic or echogenic zones representing areas of tumor necrosis, hemorrhage, and/or calcification.[18, 20]

3. *Magnetic resonance imaging* (MRI). Tumors appear as hypointense masses when compared with the liver on T1-weighted images and hyperintense when compared with the liver on T2-weighted images. MRI also demonstrates displacement or invasion of adjacent organs, as well as liver metastases. Superior blood vessel identification and the multiplanar capabilities of MRI make it the imaging modality of choice for evaluating the extent of disease and planning surgical excision.[21] The distinction between benign and malignant masses based on the presence of lipid can also be determined by chemical shift MRI. Lipid-rich adenomas show a 34% change in relative signal intensity between in-phase and out-of-phase imaging, whereas nonadenomas do not change. This technique gives a specificity of 100% and a sensitivity of 81% in distinguishing between these two types of lesions.[22]

4. *^{131}I-6β-iodomethylnorcholesterol scintigraphy.* Most adrenal cortical carcinomas fail to image with this radionuclide. Because cortisol production suppresses ACTH secretion and the function of the contralateral adrenal gland, patients with cortisol-producing adrenal cortical carcinomas fail to show an image either at the site of the tumor or in the contralateral gland. Aldosterone-, androgen-, or estrogen-secreting tumors usually appear as an area of decreased uptake on the side of the tumor mass. The decreased or absent tracer uptake by adrenal cortical carcinomas is in contrast with the increased concentration of radionuclide by benign tumors.[14] This distinction is not absolute. Patients with adrenal cortical carcinoma may occasionally give positive nuclear scans. Based on these imaging characteristics, CT and iodocholesterol scintigraphy can be used together for the diagnosis of small (<4 cm) euadrenal masses. A study of 119 patients found that concordant images (CT image and increased uptake on the same side) were 100% benign whereas discordant images (a CT tumor image on one side and increased uptake on the contralateral side) were malignant in 73% of cases.[23]

CLINICAL ASSESSMENT OF EXTENT OF DISEASE

Staging of adrenal cortical carcinoma can be based on the size of the primary tumor and extent of regional or distant tumor involvement according to the MacFarlane classification[24] as modified by Sullivan[25] (Table 126–1). The sites of tumor spread in stage IV are summarized in Table 126–2. The most frequent sites of metastases are the lung, liver, lymph nodes, and bone. The stage at which an adrenal cortical carcinoma is defined determines its prognosis.[26, 27] Whereas 50% of patients in stages I, II, and III are alive 40 months after diagnosis, only 10% of patients in stage IV are alive at that time.

TABLE 126–1. MacFarlane Classification of Adrenal Cortical Carcinoma Based on Size and Extent of Disease

Stage	Size	Lymphadenopathy	Local Invasion	Metastases
I	<5 cm	–	–	–
II	>5 cm	–	–	–
III	Any size	+	+	–
IV	Any size	+	+	+

MANAGEMENT OF ADRENAL CORTICAL CARCINOMA

Therapeutic interventions used to treat patients with adrenal cancer include surgery, radiation therapy, nonspecific systemic chemotherapy, and mitotane.[28]

Surgical resection, even if incomplete, should be considered the initial step in therapy. Because most adrenal carcinomas are large, the surgical approach should be either transabdominal or thoracoabdominal, with an incision of sufficient length to allow adequate exploration and resection of contiguous organs if necessary to remove gross tumor. The surgical goal should be resection of the entire tumor mass whenever possible. Even if such resection is not possible because of local extension into other structures, tumor debulking should be carried out to the maximum degree possible. It is frequently necessary to remove the adjoining kidney en bloc with the tumor because of invasion of the upper pole. In cases of liver metastases, partial lobectomy with resection of the involved portion of the liver has led to long-term remission.[29] These aggressive efforts to excise all gross tumor are justified because chemotherapy appears to be most effective with minimal tumor burden.

Another approach to treatment is radiation therapy and nonspecific chemotherapy. Adrenal cortical carcinomas have been reported to be resistant to radiation therapy, which only causes a transient reduction in local disease.[30] However, these earlier reports were based on techniques and equipment much less powerful than currently available, and it is possible that better responses could be attained with newer methodology.

Nonspecific chemotherapy has resulted in only temporary improvement. Chemotherapeutic agents used in the treatment of metastatic adrenal carcinoma include doxorubicin (Adriamycin), cisplatin, etoposide, paclitaxel (Taxol), 5-fluorouracil, vincristine (Oncovin), cyclophosphamide, and suramin. Although the consensus from several series is that systemic chemotherapy is not very effective in this stage of the disease, difficulty interpreting the response to therapy is encountered for the following reasons: (1) the series reported usually involve small numbers of patients. (2) Great variability in treatment is seen between and within series. (3) The extent of disease when people are treated has been variable and not well defined. (4) The malignancy grade is variable and series include patients with low-grade as well as patients with high-grade malignancy. (5) A uniform definition of response is lacking. (6) The duration of response is not always clearly stated. (7) Patients within a series frequently receive multiple treatments in variable sequence, so treatments are difficult to compare. (8) Radiation therapy is sometimes combined with chemotherapy.

TABLE 126–2. Sites of Metastasis in Stage IV Adrenal Cortical Carcinoma

Organ	Percentage (n = 33)
Lung	45
Liver	42
Lymph nodes	24
Bone	15
Pancreas	12
Spleen	6
Diaphragm	12
Miscellaneous (brain, peritoneum skin, palate)	12

Mitotane has been used consistently in the treatment of patients with metastatic adrenal cortical carcinoma, but not everyone agrees on its efficacy.[31, 32] Mitotane is an adrenolytic drug with selective action on the adrenal cortex. When given to patients with pituitary ACTH-dependent adrenal cortical hyperfunction, mitotane induces suppression of cortisol secretion and selective chemical ablation of the fasciculata and reticularis zones of the adrenal cortex. Mitotane belongs to the class of drugs that require metabolic transformation into active metabolites for therapeutic action. The active metabolite either covalently combines to specific targets in the cells responsive to the drug and/or induces oxygen activation leading to toxicity. Some evidence indicates that mitotane is transformed to an acylchloride by mitochondrial cytochrome P-450–mediated hydroxylation and that the acylchloride covalently combines to specific bionucleophiles within the adrenal cortical cell for the adrenolytic effect to take place. It is possible that adrenal tumors vary in their ability to effect metabolic transformation or initiate free radical production and therefore express variable sensitivity to mitotane. In a series of reports over the past 30 years,[33] mitotane has been associated with partial or complete response in only 33% of patients with adrenal cancer. The timing of initiation of chemotherapy may influence patient survival. It has been reported that adjuvant therapy with mitotane is associated with prolonged survival when initiated shortly after the primary tumor has been surgically excised and before local extension or additional metastases develop.[34, 35] However, prospective studies in which patients were randomly assigned to either adjuvant therapy with mitotane or no therapy failed to show a beneficial effect of mitotane in extending life expectancy.[36]

Mitotane causes significant toxicity in therapeutically effective doses. The adverse effects of mitotane are dose dependent and usually intolerable when doses exceed 6 g daily, a dose that may be required to achieve therapeutic blood levels of at least 14 μg/dL.[37] Treatment begins with doses of 1 g twice daily and gradually increased to tolerance. The drug is best administered with fat containing foods because its absorption and transport appear to be coupled to lipoproteins. The cortisol response to mitotane should be followed by measurement of urinary free cortisol. Mitotane increases binding of cortisol to corticosteroid-binding globulin, and serum cortisol levels can be elevated even when circulating free cortisol is not.[38] Treatment with mitotane inhibits hormone production and eventually causes necrosis of the contralateral adrenal gland. Patients need cortisol replacement, 25 to 35 mg daily. Synthetic glucocorticoids such as prednisone and dexamethasone are less desirable because their metabolism may be enhanced by mitotane, thus making it difficult to determine the optimal replacement dose. In low doses (2 to 4 g daily), mitotane has less adrenolytic effects on the zona glomerulosa and is less likely to suppress aldosterone production. With larger doses, replacement with fludrocortisol may be necessary.

Suramin, a drug known for its antiparasitic effects, has previously been shown to have adrenocorticolytic effects in primates. Suramin may have some therapeutic efficacy as monotherapy in patients with metastatic adrenal cortical carcinoma.[39] When given to patients with adrenal carcinoma, a partial to minor response was observed in some patients. A greater response was obtained when suramin and mitotane were combined.

LONG-TERM TREATMENT OUTCOME

Medical therapy for adrenal cortical carcinoma is of limited effectiveness.[40, 47] However, in a significant number of patients, life expectancy has been extended with acceptable morbidity. Combined surgical and medical treatment appears to be more effective than medical treatment alone, especially for patients with localized or regional disease (stages I–III). In a comparison of 18 patients treated with mitotane alone and 15 treated with combined surgical resection and mitotane chemotherapy, those who underwent surgical treatment had a more favorable response, with 33% of patients living more than 5 years from the time of first recurrence.[48] In a study of 49 patients with adrenal carcinoma, surgical excision offered the best chance for prolonged survival. Forty-three percent of patients with a completely resectable tumor were alive with no evidence of disease an average of 7.3 years postoperatively.[49] In a comparison of various types of therapy in 110 patients with adrenal cortical carcinoma, it was noted that 56% of patients responded to surgery for localized and regional disease with a disease-free survival time of at least 2 years. In contrast, abdominal radiation therapy was effective in 15%, systemic chemotherapy in 9%, and mitotane in 29%.[50] In a review of 82 patients, it was noted that survival in patients with metastatic disease was poor and not improved by treatment with mitotane, cytotoxic chemotherapy, or radiation therapy.[51]

Thus survival of patients with adrenal carcinoma and recurrent or metastatic disease is better in patients receiving surgical than medical treatment. With surgical treatment, 50% of patients survive an average of 70 months, whereas with medical treatment alone, less than 10% of patients are alive for this length of time. Surgical treatment involves not only resection of the primary lesion but also repeated resection of metastases.

THE USE OF INHIBITORS OF ADRENAL FUNCTION IN PATIENTS WITH FUNCTIONING ADRENAL CORTICAL CARCINOMA

The metabolic changes associated with excessive hormonal production can cause significant morbidity and shortened life expectancy in patients with residual disease who do not respond to antitumor therapy. A variety of inhibitors of adrenal function have been used to suppress steroid hormone production and improve the clinical manifestations of the disease. The most commonly used inhibitors include ketoconazole, metyrapone, and aminoglutethimide.

Ketoconazole is an imidazole derivative that inhibits the synthesis of cortisol by inhibiting mitochondrial cytochrome P-450–dependent enzymes such as cholesterol side chain cleavage and 11-β-hydroxylase in rat and mouse adrenal preparations. It has been found to be an important inhibitor of gonadal and adrenal steroidogenesis in vivo when given in doses as low as 200 to 600 mg/day. Ketoconazole has been used to treat patients with Cushing's syndrome and virilization caused by adrenal tumors.[52] Clinical improvement occurs frequently, but regression of metastatic disease is rare.[53] When patients are treated with ketoconazole, adrenal insufficiency is avoided by decreasing the dose sufficiently to maintain normal cortisol levels. The most frequent adverse reactions with ketoconazole are nausea and vomiting, abdominal pain, and pruritus in 1% to 3% of patients. Hepatotoxicity, primarily of the hepatocellular type, has been associated with its use.[52]

Metyrapone is an 11-β-hydroxylase inhibitor. In doses of 250 to 1000 mg twice daily, patients experience biochemical and clinical improvement. Nausea, vomiting, and dizziness can occur in association with treatment. Because of the high cost and side effects, metyrapone should be used only as temporary therapy in patients with severe hypercortisolemia associated with adrenal cortical carcinomas.

Aminoglutethimide inhibits cholesterol side chain cleavage and the conversion of cholesterol to pregnenolone in the adrenal cortex. As a consequence, synthesis of cortisol, aldosterone, and androgens is suppressed. The drug has been used in both adults and children in doses of 500 to 2000 mg/day. Cortisol levels fall gradually with regression of the clinical manifestations of Cushing's syndrome.[54] Eventually, patients may need glucocorticoid replacement. The effect of aminoglutethimide is promptly reversed by interruption of therapy. Aminoglutethimide causes gastrointestinal (anorexia, nausea, vomiting) and neurologic (lethargy, sedation, blurred vision) side effect and can induce hypothyroidism in 5% of patients. A skin rash is frequently observed during the first 10 days of treatment, but it usually subsides with continuation of treatment. Headaches have also been observed with the larger doses.

REFERENCES

1. Brennan MF: Adrenocortical carcinoma. CA Cancer J Clin 37:348–365, 1987.
2. Lynch HT, Katz DA, Bogard PJ, et al: The sarcoma, breast cancer, lung cancer and adrenocortical carcinoma syndrome revisited. Childhood cancer. Am J Dis Child 139:134–136, 1985.
3. Hartley AL, Birch JM, Marsden HB, et al: Adrenal cortical tumors: Epidemiological and familial aspects. Arch Dis Child 62:683–689, 1987.
4. Grayson GH, Moore S, Schneider BG, et al: Novel germline mutation of the p53 tumor suppressor gene in a child with incidentally discovered adrenal cortical carcinoma. Am J Pediatr Hematol Oncol 16:341–347, 1994.
5. Lin SR, Lee YJ, Tsai JH: Mutations of the p53 gene in human functional adrenocortical neoplasms. J Clin Endocrinol Metab 78:483–491, 1994.
6. Miyamoto H, Kubota Y, Shuin T, et al: Bilateral adrenocortical carcinoma showing loss of heterozygosity at the p53 and RB gene loci. Cancer Genet Cytogenet 88:181–183, 1966.
7. Yano T, Linehan M, Anglard P, et al: Genetic changes in human adrenocortical carcinomas. J Natl Cancer Inst 81:518–523, 1989.
8. Reincke M, Karl M, Travis WH, et al: p53 mutations in human adrenocortical neoplasms; immunohistochemical and molecular studies. J Clin Endocrinol Metab 78:790–794, 1994.
9. McNicol AM, Nolan CE, Struthers AJ, et al: Expression of p53 in adrenocortical tumours: Clinicopathological correlations. J Pathol 181:146–152, 1997.
10. Liu J, Kahri AI, Heikkilä P, et al: Ribonucleic acid expression of the clustered imprinted genes $p57^{kip2}$ insulin-like growth factor-II and H19 in adrenal tumors and cultured adrenal cells. J Clin Endocrinol Metab 82:1766–1771, 1997.
11. Liu J, Kahri AI, Heikkilä P, et al: H19 and insulin-like growth factor-II gene expression in adrenal tumors and cultured adrenal cells. J Clin Endocrinol Metab 80:492–496, 1995.
12. Liu J, Voutilainen R, Kahri AI, et al: Expression patterns of the c-*myc* gene in adrenocortical tumors and pheochromocytomas. J Endocrinol 152:175–181, 1997.
13. Farge D, Chatellier G, Pagny JY, et al: Isolated clinical syndrome of primary aldosteronism in four patients with adrenocortical carcinoma. Am J Med 83:635–640, 1987.
14. Arteaga E, Biglieri EG, Kater CE, et al: Aldosterone-producing adrenocortical carcinoma. Preoperative recognition and course in three cases. Ann Intern Med 101:316–321, 1984.
15. Grondal S, Curstedt T: Steroid profile in serum: Increased levels of sulphated pregnenolone and pregn-5-ene-3 beta, 20 alpha-diol in patients with adrenocortical carcinoma. Acta Endocrinol 124:381–385, 1991.
16. Copeland PM: The incidentally discovered adrenal masses. Ann Surg 199:116–122, 1984.
17. Bencsik Z, Szaboles I, Goth M, et al: Incidentally detected adrenal tumors (incidentalomas): Histological heterogeneity and differentiated therapeutic approach. J Intern Med 237:585–589, 1995.
18. Korobkin M, Francis IR, Kloos RT, et al: The incidental adrenal mass. Radiol Clin North Am 34:1037–1054, 1996.
19. Korobkin M, Brodeur FJ, Francis IR, et al: Delayed enhanced CT for differentiation of benign from malignant adrenal masses. Radiology 200:737–742, 1996.
20. Hamper UM, Fishman EK, Hartman DS, et al: Primary adrenocortical carcinoma: Sonographic evaluation with clinical and pathologic correlation in 26 patients. AJR 148:915–919, 1987.
21. Smith SM, Patel SK, Turner DA, et al: Magnetic resonance imaging of adrenal cortical carcinoma. Urol Radiol 11:1–6, 1989.
22. Korobkin M, Lombardi TJ, Aisen AM, et al: Characterization of adrenal masses with chemical shift and gadolinium enhanced imaging. Radiology 197:414–418, 1995.
23. Gross MD, Shapiro B, Bouffard J, et al: Distinguishing benign and malignant euadrenal masses. Ann Intern Med 109:613–618, 1988.
24. MacFarlane DA: Cancer of the adrenal cortex: The natural history, prognosis and treatment in the study of fifty five cases. Ann R Coll Surg Engl 23:155–186, 1958.
25. Sullivan M: Adrenal cortical carcinoma. Urology 120:660, 1978.
26. Hogan T: A clinical and pathological study of adrenocortical carcinoma; therapeutic implications. Cancer 45:2880, 1980.
27. Bradley E: Primary and adjunctive therapy in carcinoma of the adrenal cortex. Surg Gynecol Obstet 141:507, 1975.
28. Schteingart DE: Treating adrenal cancer. Endocrinologist 2:149–157, 1992.
29. Thompson NW: Adrenocortical carcinoma. *In* Thompson NW, Knowlton AH (eds): Endocrine Surgery Update. New York, Grune & Stratton, 1983, pp 119–128.
30. Percarpio B, Knowlton AH: Radiation therapy of adrenal cortical carcinoma. Acta Radiol Ther 15:288–292, 1976.
31. Hogan TF, Citrin DL, Johnson BM, et al: *o,p'*-DDD (mitotane) therapy of adrenal cortical carcinoma: Observations on drug dosage, toxicity and steroid replacement. Cancer 42:2177–2181, 1978.
32. Luton JP, Cerdas S, Billaud L, et al: Clinical features of adrenocortical carcinoma, prognostic factors, and the effect of mitotane therapy. N Engl J Med 322:1195–1201, 1990.
33. Wooten MD, King DK: Adrenal cortical carcinoma. Epidemiology and treatment with mitotane and a review of the literature. Cancer 72:3145–3155, 1993.
34. Schteingart DE, Motazedi A, Noonan RA, et al: The treatment of adrenal carcinoma. Arch Surg 117:1142, 1982.
35. Kasperlik-Zaluska A: Impact of adjuvant mitotane on the clinical course of patients with adrenocortical carcinoma. Cancer 73:1533–1534, 1994.
36. Vassilopoulou-Sellin R, Guinee VF, Klein MJ, et al: Impact of adjuvant mitotane on the clinical course of patients with adrenocortical cancer. Cancer 71:3119–3123, 1993.
37. Haak HR, Hermans J, VandeVelde CJH, et al: Optimal treatment of adrenal cortical carcinoma with mitotane: Results in a consecutive series of 96 patients. Br J Cancer 69:947–951, 1994.
38. VanSeters AP, Moolenaar AJ: Mitotane increases the blood levels of hormone-binding proteins. Acta Endocrinol 124:526–533, 1991.
39. La Rocca RV, Stein CA, Danesi R, et al: Suramin in adrenal cancer: Modulation of steroid hormone production, cytotoxicity in vitro, and clinical antitumor effect. J Clin Endocrinol Metab 71:497–504, 1990.
40. Venkatesh S, Hickey RC, Sellin RV, et al: Adrenal cortical carcinoma. Cancer 64:765–769, 1989.

41. Kasperlik-Zaluska A, Migdalska BM, Zgliczynski S, et al: Adrenocortical carcinoma: A clinical study and treatment results of 52 patients. Cancer 75:2587–2591, 1995.
42. Magee BJ, Gattamaneni HR, Pearson D: Adrenal cortical carcinoma: Survival after radiotherapy. Clin Radiol 38:587–588, 1987.
43. Teinturier C, Brugières L, Lemerle J, et al: Corticosurrénalomes de l'enfant: Analyse rétrospective de 54 cas. Arch Pediatr 3:235–240, 1996.
44. Didolkar MS, Bescher RA, Elias EG, et al: Natural history of adrenal cortical carcinoma: A clinicopathologic study of 42 patients. Cancer 47:2153–2161, 1981.
45. Nader S, Hickey RC, Sellin RV, et al: Adrenal cortical carcinoma: A study of 77 cases. Cancer 52:707–711, 1983.
46. Schlumberger M, Brugieres L, Gicquel C, et al: 5-Fluorouracil, doxorubicin and cisplatin as treatment for adrenal cortical carcinoma. Cancer 67:2997–3000, 1991.
47. Bukowski RM, Montie J, Crawford D, et al: Cisplatin (CDDP) and mitotane in metastatic adrenal carcinoma: A Southwest Oncology Group Study. Proc Am Soc Clin Oncol 9:296, 1990.
48. Jensen JC, Pass HI, Sindelar WF, et al: Recurrent or metastatic disease in select patients with adrenocortical carcinoma: Aggressive resection vs. chemotherapy. Arch Surg 126:457–461, 1991.
49. King D, Lack E: Adrenal cortical carcinoma; a clinical and pathological study of 49 cases. Cancer 44:239, 1979.
50. Bodie B, Novick AC, Pontes JE, et al: The Cleveland Clinic experience with adrenal cortical carcinoma. J Urol 141:257–260, 1989.
51. Bradley EL: Primary and adjunctive therapy in carcinoma of the adrenal cortex. Surg Gynecol Obstet 141:507–516, 1975.
52. Kruimel JW, Smals AG, Beex LU, et al: Favourable response of a virilizing adrenocortical carcinoma to preoperative treatment with ketoconazole and postoperative chemotherapy. Acta Endocrinol 124:492–496, 1991.
53. Contreras P, Rojas A, Biagini L, et al: Regression of metastatic adrenal carcinoma during palliative ketoconazole treatment. Lancet 2:151, 1985.
54. Schteingart DE, Cash R, Conn JW: Aminoglutethimide and metastatic adrenal cancer. Maintained reversal (six months) of Cushing's syndrome. JAMA 198:1007, 1966.

Chapter 127

Adrenal Surgery

Allan E. Siperstein ▪ Eren Berber

INDICATIONS
CONTRAINDICATIONS
PERIOPERATIVE MANAGEMENT
SURGICAL TECHNIQUE
RESULTS
CONCLUSION

Laparoscopic surgery has revolutionized adrenal surgery by decreasing morbidity and accelerating the return to full activity after operation. The first open adrenalectomies were performed by Roux and associates[1] and Mayo[2] via the anterior transabdominal approach in 1927. The posterior approach was described by Young in 1936; however, it was not until the late 1970s that the procedure was popularized.[3] Since then, the posterior approach has been the procedure of choice for most adrenal lesions including aldosterone-secreting tumors, benign adenomas measuring less than 6 cm, and relatively small pheochromocytomas. The transabdominal approach was commonly selected for patients with pheochromocytomas, for children, and also for some patients with adrenal carcinomas. The other conventional approaches include the flank and thoracoabdominal approaches. The flank approach is a variant of the posterior approach with the retroperitoneal space being entered after the 11th rib is resected. The thoracoabdominal approach was utilized for large adenomas, some large adrenal carcinomas, and pheochromocytomas.[4] The posterior or the flank approach avoids the peritoneal and thoracic cavities and minimizes the risk of mechanical ileus and pulmonary problems. The use of these direct approaches, however, was generally limited to the removal of smaller glands. These retroperitoneal approaches do not allow the intra-abdominal exploration, and bilateral incisions were required in patients with bilateral disease. The transabdominal approach provided access to the entire peritoneal cavity for exploration of the contralateral adrenal gland as well; however, it was associated with the morbidity of a major laparotomy. Although, the thoracoabdominal approach provided the widest exposure to the adrenal gland, it was accompanied by the morbidity of a thoracotomy. The morbidity associated with conventional techniques has been as high as 40%, and mortality has been 2% to 4%.[5, 6] Morbidity after an open adrenalectomy includes wound pain, intercostal neuralgia, pneumonia, wound infection, pulmonary atelectasis, and incisional hernia.[7]

In the past decade, however, there have been dramatic changes in adrenal surgery with the introduction of laparoscopic adrenalectomy techniques by Gagner and associates[8] in 1992 and by Mercan and colleagues in 1993.[9] The small size of the adrenal gland, the benign nature of most adrenal tumors, and the difficulty of exposure with open methods have made this gland particularly amenable to laparoscopic surgery. Laparoscopy provides a magnified view of the operative field allowing the precise identification of small vessels and more precise dissection with less blood loss, so that transfusion is rare. Through late 1997, almost 600 cases had been reported in the literature. These studies have established the safety, efficacy, and cost-effectiveness of laparoscopic adrenalectomy.[10–12] Because the incision rather than internal dissection affects the pain and recovery after surgery, laparoscopic adrenal surgery has resulted in a decrease in wound complications, lesser postoperative pain, shorter hospital stay, and rapid return to normal activity.[12–15] Laparoscopic surgery is regarded as the "gold standard" for the removal of benign adrenal lesions.[16]

INDICATIONS

The current indications for laparoscopic adrenalectomy include[17–19]:

1. Aldosterone-secreting adenoma
2. Glucocorticoid-secreting adenoma
3. Androgen-secreting adenoma
4. Pheochromocytoma (small to moderate-sized)
5. Bilateral macronodular adrenal hyperplasia
6. Selected cases of bilateral adrenal hyperlasia (if ectopic adrenocorticotropic hormone [ACTH]–producing tumors cannot be located or pituitary tumor is unsuccessfully removed by transsphenoidal hypophysectomy)
7. Hormonally inactive tumors larger than 3 to 5 cm
8. Nonfunctioning adrenal tumors less than 3 cm that have shown progressive growth on serial imaging studies
9. Solitary adrenal metastases

The discovery of an incidental adrenal mass has become more frequent with widespread use of sensitive radiologic studies including ultrasound, computed tomography (CT), and magnetic resonance imaging (MRI). The incidence of incidentalomas varies from 0.35% to 1.3%, whereas the incidence of adrenal tumors in autopsy series is between 1.4% and 8.7%. The management of an incidentaloma is guided by two principles: whether the tumor has hormonal activity or a potential for malignancy. Once clinically significant hormonal activity is ruled out with biochemical and hormonal studies, the possibility of malignancy must be excluded. The appropriate use of fine-needle aspiration in this workup is also very important. It is crucial that the diagnosis of pheochromocytoma is definitely ruled out biochemically before attempting a needle biopsy, because the procedure can provoke a hypertensive crisis in a patient with pheochromocytoma. Fine-needle aspiration cytology may be able to distinguish primary from metastatic carcinoma, but may not help distinguish a benign adenoma from a low-grade carcinoma. The diameter of adrenal carcinomas is generally greater than 5 cm, although there are increasing reports of adrenal carcinomas as small as 3 cm. The advent of the minimally invasive approach to adrenal surgery has resulted in the decrease in size of the incidentalomas referred to surgery. The referral of patients to surgical removal based on the size of the tumor on radiologic studies is also controversial, because the transverse size on a CT scan often underestimates the longitudinal axis dimension. Many authors advocate surgical resection on lesions greater than 4 cm.[20, 21]

CONTRAINDICATIONS

There are a few absolute contraindications to laparoscopic adrenalectomy. Although there have been some reports on the feasibility and safety of laparoscopic adrenalectomy for cancer in the literature,[11, 22] invasive adrenal carcinoma is currently considered to be a contraindication to the laparoscopic approach owing to the need for en bloc excision of the adrenal cancer and surrounding tissues and organs.[12] Open surgery also seems to be indicated for patients with malignant pheochromocytoma, especially those with preoperative demonstration of metastatic nodes in the periaortic area or close to the bladder.

Coagulation parameters should be fully investigated preoperatively and should be corrected if possible before surgery. Multiple previous abdominal procedures were initially considered to be a contraindication for laparoscopic surgery owing to the presence of adhesions in the abdominal cavity. Nevertheless, the abdominal cavity can be entered under direct view; these adhesions can be taken down with laparoscopic dissection or they can be totally avoided with use of the posterior retroperitoneal technique. A history of previous operations is no longer considered to be a contraindication for laparoscopic adrenalectomy. Morbid obesity is often listed as a relative contraindication. However, the open approach probably carries a higher relative risk. Also, in these patients with Cushing's syndrome, the obesity is less on the back, making this a relatively straightforward approach laparoscopically.[18]

Although the indication for the laparoscopic resection of pheochromocytoma was initially considered to be less definite, the advances in diagnosing, localizing, and blocking these patients preoperatively as well as in controlling their intraoperative hemodynamics have permitted the laparoscopic resection of most patients with pheochromocytoma.[10, 13, 18, 23] The fact that there is an ever-present risk of a life-threatening hypertensive crisis during manipulation of the adrenal gland during surgery in these patients has caused many surgeons to approach pheochromocytoma with caution. Furthermore, concerns have been raised that laparoscopy may increase the risk of such crises. However, it was shown that the amount of catecholamine excretion during laparoscopic surgery for pheochromocytoma is lower than that with open surgery.[24] Hypertension is triggered with direct manipulation of the adrenal gland and is not affected by pneumoperitoneum. Another important issue in the management of patients with pheochromocytoma is prompt surgical referral, because these patients are at significant risk of hypertensive crisis and adrenal hemorrhage in the preoperative period.

There is no consensus in the literature regarding the upper limit of tumor size that can be resected laparoscopically. The size limit for laparoscopic resection varies between 6 cm and 15 cm.[12, 13, 25, 26]

PERIOPERATIVE MANAGEMENT

Appropriate preoperative preparation of patients is essential to prevent complications. Preoperative preparation is similar with Cushing's and Conn's syndromes, addressing primarily the hypertension and electrolyte disturbances. Patients with primary aldosteronism and hypokalemic hypertension should be treated with spironolactone 100 to 300 mg/day for 4 to 6 weeks before surgery. This treatment safely reduces blood pressure and restores normal electrolytes in most cases.[27] Hypertension and hypokalemia in patients with Cushing's syndrome should also be treated with potassium-sparing diuretics, either spironolactone or amiloride, and potassium supplements are used when necessary. Of patients with Cushing's syndrome, 10% to 15% become diabetic and require insulin treatment. Thus, blood glucose levels should be closely observed, especially in the postoperative period when hypoglycemia may develop. These patients should also receive steroid supplementation for the perioperative period of stress and also to prevent withdrawal syndrome after resection of the gland. Several suitable regimens are available. The equivalent of 200 to 300 mg/day of cortisol is recommended for the high-stress period of 24 to 72 hours. An appropriate tapering regimen then follows. When cortisol is reduced below 75 mg/day, the addition of 0.1 to 0.2 mg of fludrocortisone may be necessary in patients who have undergone bilateral adrenalectomy.[28, 29]

In patients with pheochromocytoma, emphasis is placed on controlling hypertension and associated hypovolemia. α-Blockade should be started at least 10 to 14 days preoperatively. This normalizes blood pressure, controls paroxysms, and allows for volume expansion. Phenoxybenzamide is the drug of choice. The patients should be conditioned with the drug to the point of orthostatic hypotension to minimize perioperative fluctuations in blood pressure. β-Blockers may be added once adequate α-blockade is established and if tachycardia develops. If β-blockade is begun prematurely, unopposed α action may paradoxically worsen hypertension. Preoperative α-blockade, in conjunction with aggressive fluid intake and institution of a high-salt diet, minimizes intraoperative risk by decreasing the frequency of shifts in blood pressure during resection and eliminates the profound hypotension that occurred in unprepared patients in the past.[30] In patients whose blood pressure and symptoms are not adequately controlled with α-blockade, consideration should be directed at administrating metyrosine (Demser), a tyrosine hydroxylase inhibitor, 1 to 4 g/day for at least 2 weeks before surgery. The patients undergoing resection of pheochromocytoma also need rigorous intraoperative and postoperative anesthetic monitoring.

Pheochromocytoma in pregnancy presents a special challenge. A maternal and fetal mortality rate of 40% to 56% has been reported if the diagnosis is not made during pregnancy, whereas correct antenatal diagnosis reduces the maternal and fetal mortality rates to 0% and 15%, respectively.[31] If the diagnosis is made before 23 weeks of gestation, the tumor should be resected after α-blockade is established. After 23 weeks, the gravid uterus usually makes surgery technically dangerous. Surgery, in this case, should be postponed until fetal maturity, when simultaneous cesarean section and tumor resection can be performed.[32] Janetschek and associates[31] have successfully treated two pregnant patients with pheochromocytoma with laparoscopic adrenalectomy before 20 weeks of gestation.

Most patients without associated comorbid pathology can be admitted to the hospital on the morning of surgery. Patients with pheochromocytoma are best admitted during the evening before surgery to ensure intravenous volume expansion. Owing to chronic vasoconstriction, patients with pheochromocytoma have greatly reduced blood volume. It is essential that blood volume is repleted preoperatively, because profound hypotension may develop with induction of anesthesia owing to the vasodilatory effects of many of these agents. The anesthesiologist may then need to administer agents to acutely correct the hypotension that may result in overshoot and hypertension crisis in these patients. The collaboration of the endocrine surgeon, endocrinologist, and anesthesiologist is essential for the appropriate management of these patients with adrenal pathologies.

SURGICAL TECHNIQUE

Laparoscopic adrenal surgery is performed under endotracheal general anesthesia. In the lateral transabdominal approach, the patient is placed on the lateral decubitus position on a beanbag; the operating table is flexed at the waist; and the kidney rest is elevated (Fig. 127 1). The surgeon stands facing the back of the patient, and the assistant faces the front of the patient. Four 10-mm trocars are placed at the midclavicular, anterior axillary, midaxillary, and posterior axillary lines, 1 to 2 fingerbreadths below the costal margin. A fan retractor is inserted through the midclavicular cannula and a 30 degree laparoscope through the anterior axillary cannula. An atraumatic grasper and a pair of dissecting scissors are inserted through the midaxillary and posterior axillary cannulas. On the right, the liver is detached from the triangular ligament and rotated medially. The right kidney is identified; the Gerota fascia is incised; and the adrenal is identified. The anterior, lateral, and posterior surfaces of the adrenal are avascular and should be dissected first. The gland is not directly handled during dissection but is retracted by grasping the periadrenal tissue. We routinely use laparoscopic ultrasound to localize and guide dissection of the adrenal tumor. The adrenal vein is secured with laparoscopic clips. The right adrenal vein, which is medial to the right adrenal gland, drains directly into the inferior vena cava. On the left, three trocars are used. The spleen, pancreas, and splenic flexure of the colon are dissected from their retroperitoneal attachments. They are rotated medially and retracted by gravity, and a fan retractor is placed on the spleen or the posterior surface of the pancreas. The left adrenal vein is found medioinferiorly to the adrenal gland and drains into the left renal vein.

The excised lesion is removed in an endoscopic retrieval bag through the most anterior trocar site, where the subcutaneous tissue is thinnest. Small tumors (<2 cm) are removed intact after dilating the trocar site. Larger tumors are fractured in the specimen bag with ring forceps and then removed piecemeal.

In the posterior approach, the patient is taken to the operating room and endotracheal anesthesia is induced while the patient is on the gurney. The patient is then turned to the prone position on the operating table with the chest and abdomen supported laterally by a Wilson frame or parallel bolsters. This allows the abdominal contents to fall anteriorly so that during the procedure a minimum of CO_2

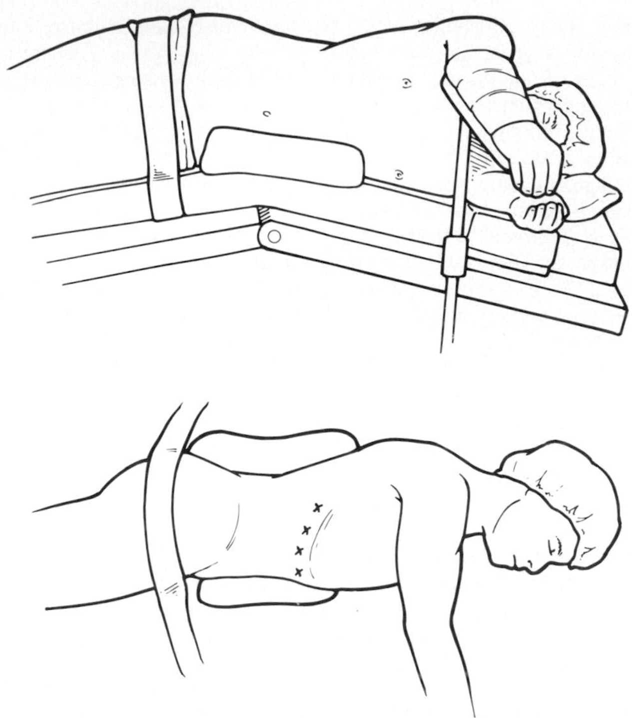

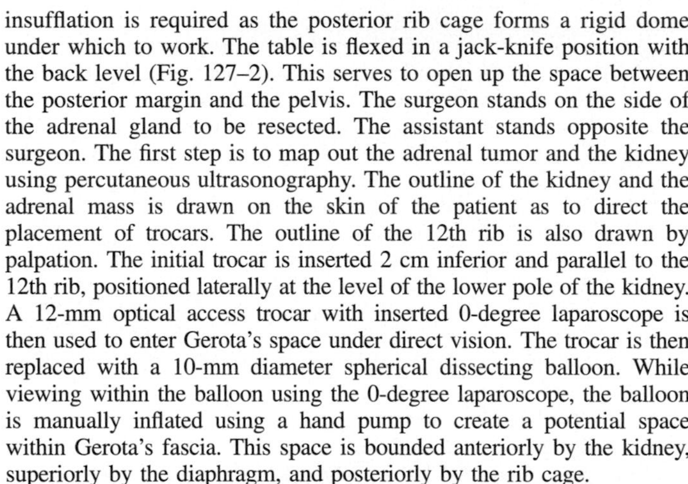

FIGURE 127–1. Patient positioning and trocar sites for a lateral transabdominal adrenalectomy.

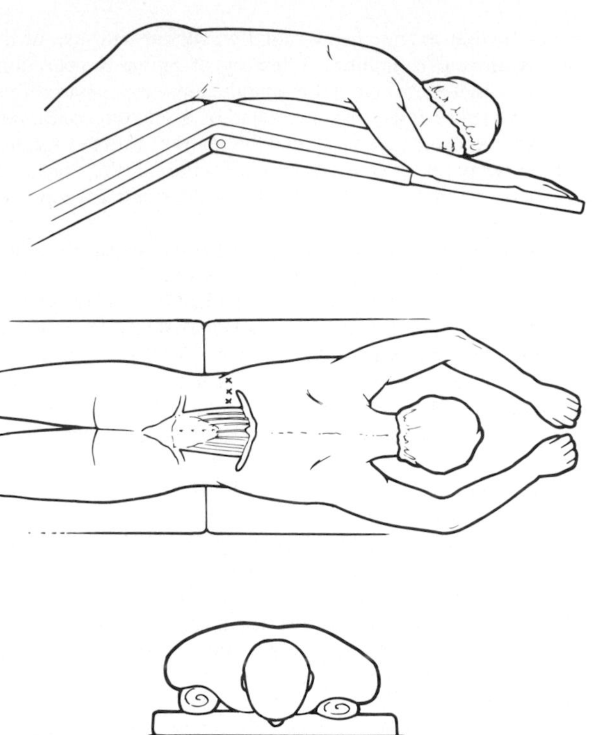

FIGURE 127–2. Positioning of the patient and the trocars for the posterior retroperitoneal adrenalectomy.

insufflation is required as the posterior rib cage forms a rigid dome under which to work. The table is flexed in a jack-knife position with the back level (Fig. 127–2). This serves to open up the space between the posterior margin and the pelvis. The surgeon stands on the side of the adrenal gland to be resected. The assistant stands opposite the surgeon. The first step is to map out the adrenal tumor and the kidney using percutaneous ultrasonography. The outline of the kidney and the adrenal mass is drawn on the skin of the patient as to direct the placement of trocars. The outline of the 12th rib is also drawn by palpation. The initial trocar is inserted 2 cm inferior and parallel to the 12th rib, positioned laterally at the level of the lower pole of the kidney. A 12-mm optical access trocar with inserted 0-degree laparoscope is then used to enter Gerota's space under direct vision. The trocar is then replaced with a 10-mm diameter spherical dissecting balloon. While viewing within the balloon using the 0-degree laparoscope, the balloon is manually inflated using a hand pump to create a potential space within Gerota's fascia. This space is bounded anteriorly by the kidney, superiorly by the diaphragm, and posteriorly by the rib cage.

The 12-mm trocar is then reinserted into this space, and 10 to 15 mm of CO_2 insufflation is applied. The procedure is performed with a 45-degree laparoscope. The adrenal is directly visible at this point. Two additional 12-mm optical access trocars are placed under direct vision, one on either side of the initial port. Laparoscopic ultrasonography is then performed to confirm the location and extent of the adrenal mass. Most adrenal neoplasms appear as a hypoechoic mass, and the normal adrenal tissue may be difficult to distinguish from the surrounding fat. This information regarding the relationship of the adrenal to the surrounding vessels and other structures is useful to guide dissection. Ultrasonic dissecting shears are used to perform essentially all the dissection, and an atraumatic grasper is used for countertraction. The dissection begins at the superior margin of the adrenal, separating it from the diaphragm. With division of the superior vessels, the gland may then be displaced inferiorly to facilitate mobilization. The lateral side is dissected next, followed by the inferior border with the kidney. The medial side is dissected last, and the adrenal veins are controlled with clips (Fig. 127–3). The gland is then placed in a specimen bag and withdrawn through the abdominal wall with morcellation if needed. Fascial and skin closure is done in the usual manner.

The average operating time is 225 minutes in the lateral approach and 176 minutes in the posterior approach in our series. Although technically more demanding, the posterior technique provides a more direct access to the adrenal gland by minimizing intra-abdominal dissection. Our current indications for the posterior technique include tumors less than 6 cm in size, bilateral tumors, and patients with a history of multiple previous abdominal surgeries. The lateral transabdominal approach is more suitable for larger tumors.

RESULTS

The mortality rate with laparoscopic adrenalectomy has been reported to be 0% and morbidity has been between 0% and 12%.[11–13, 16] Prinz[33] compared patients who underwent laparoscopic (n = 10), transabdominal (n = 11), and posterior (n = 13) adrenalectomy. There was no significant difference in the operative time for laparo-

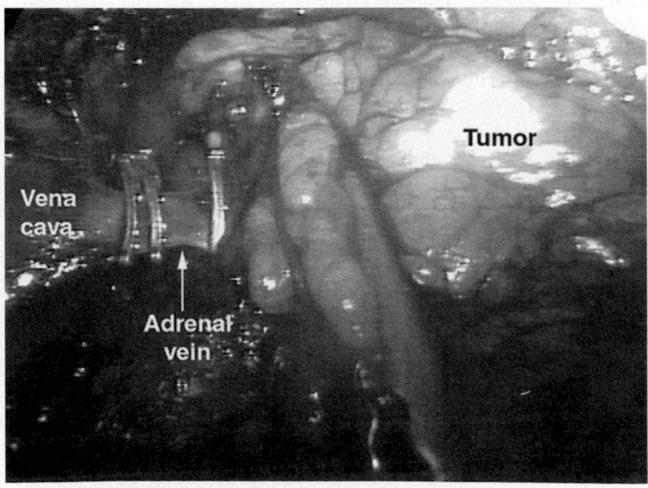

FIGURE 127–3. The adrenal vein is clipped in a 45-year-old male patient with a right-sided aldosteronoma during laparoscopic posterior adrenalectomy.

scopic and anterior adrenalectomy (212 ± 77 minutes versus 174 ± 41 minutes), but the time for posterior adrenalectomy was shorter (139 ± 36 minutes). The mean hospital stay after laparoscopic removal (2.1 ± 0.9 days) was significantly shorter than the stay after anterior (6.4 ± 1.5 days) and posterior (5.5 ± 2.9 days) adrenalectomy. The postoperative need for parenteral pain medication was significantly less with laparoscopic adrenalectomy compared with either open procedure.

The small size of the aldosterone-secreting adenomas has made them particularly amenable to laparoscopic treatment.[11–13, 18] We[34] have retrospectively compared our experience with 38 patients who underwent open adrenalectomy and 42 patients who underwent laparoscopic adrenalectomy for hyperaldosteronism. Patients who were treated with laparoscopic surgery were being referred with less severe hypertension and hypokalemia than were patients who were formerly treated with open adrenalectomy. Patients treated laparoscopically had fewer postoperative complications and were equally likely to improve in blood pressure and hypokalemia. Postoperatively, 81% of patients in the open surgery group and 88% of patients treated laparoscopically were normotensive.

Although patients with endogenous hypercortisolism have been traditionally thought to be at high risk for adrenalectomy with significant postoperative surgical morbidity and mortality, a report by van Heerden and associates[35] documented a 4.4% morbidity and 2.6% mortality in 91 patients with endogenous hypercortisolism who underwent open adrenalectomy. Laparoscopic surgery has been able to challenge these excellent results. In the 21 laparoscopic adrenalectomies performed for Cushing's adenoma in nine patients and Cushing's disease in six patients, Fernandez-Cruz and associates[36] reported no mortality and two cases of urinary infection. There was no recurrence of hypercortisolism in these patients with a mean follow-up of 9.2 months.

Although it was initially suggested that the pressure exerted by pneumoperitoneum would make the laparoscopic management of pheochromocytomas dangerous, studies have documented the safety and feasibility of laparoscopic excision of pheochromocytomas.[10–12, 31] In the 19 patients undergoing laparoscopic surgery for pheochromocytoma, Janetschek and associates[31] reported 11% minor intraoperative and 16% postoperative complications. In all patients, the catecholamine levels returned to normal, and no residual tumors were found at follow-up.

Although controversial at the moment, laparoscopic adrenalectomy for cancer has been reported by various groups[11, 12, 22] with no port site or local recurrences in follow-up.

CONCLUSION

Laparoscopic adrenalectomy has become the procedure of choice for the surgical management of most adrenal tumors. This revolution in technology has resulted in decreased morbidity and increased patient comfort compared with the traditional open adrenalectomy. Understanding the requirements for preoperative preparation for each adrenal pathology as well as the anesthetic management and postoperative care are essential for the safe management of these patients with potentially unstable physiologies.

REFERENCES

1. Roux C, Cited in Barbeau A, Marc-Aurello J et al: Le pheochromocytome bilateral: Presentation d'un cas et revue de la literature. Unin Med Can 87:165, 1928.
2. Mayo C: Paroxysmal hypertension with tumor of the retroperitoneal nerve. JAMA 89:1047, 1927.
3. Linos DA, Stylopoulos N, Boukis M et al: Anterior, posterior, or laparoscopic approach for the management of adrenal diseases? Am J Surg 173:120–125, 1997.
4. Vaughan ED Jr: Surgical options for open adrenalectomy. World J Urol 17:40–47, 1999.
5. McLeod MK: Complications following adrenal surgery. J Natl Med Assoc 83:161–164, 1991.
6. Sarkar R, Thompson NW, McLeod MK: The role of adrenalectomy in Cushing's syndrome. Surgery 108:1079–1084, 1990.
7. Bruining HA, Lamberts SW, Ong EG, van Seyen AJ: Results of adrenalectomy with various surgical approaches in the treatment of different diseases of the adrenal glands. Surg Gynecol Obstet 158:367–369, 1984.
8. Gagner M, Lacroix A, Bolte E: Laparoscopic adrenalectomy in Cushing's syndrome and pheochromocytoma (letter). N Engl J Med 327:1033, 1992.
9. Mercan S, Seven R, Ozarmagan S, Tezelman S: Endoscopic retroperitoneal adrenalectomy. Surgery 118:1071–1076, 1995.
10. Duh QY, Siperstein AE, Clark OH, et al: Laparoscopic adrenalectomy: Comparison of the lateral and posterior approaches. Arch Surg 131:870–876, 1996.
11. Siperstein A, Berber E, Engle KL et al: Laparoscopic posterior adrenalectomy: Technical considerations. Arch Surg (in press).
12. Gagner M, Pomp A, Heniford BT et al: Laparoscopic adrenalectomy: Lessons learned from 100 consecutive procedures. Ann Surg 226:238–247, 1997.
13. Jacobs JK, Goldstein RE, Geer RJ: Laparoscopic adrenalectomy: A new standard of care. Ann Surg 225:495–502, 1997.
14. Gagner M, Lacroix A, Prinz RA et al: Early experience with laparoscopic approach for adrenalectomy. Surgery 114:1120–1125, 1993.
15. Imai T, Kikumori T, Ohiwa M et al: A case-controlled study of laparoscopic compared with open lateral adrenalectomy. Am J Surg 178:50–54, 1999.
16. Smith CD, Weber CJ, Amerson JR: Laparoscopic adrenalectomy: New gold standard. World J Surg 23:389–396, 1999.
17. Winfield HN, Hamilton BD, Bravo EL: Technique of laparoscopic adrenalectomy. Urol Clin North Am 24:459–465, 1997.
18. Schell S, Talamini MA, Udelsman R: Laparoscopic adrenalectomy. Adv Surg 31:333–350, 1998.
19. Shichman SJ, Herndon CD, Sosa RE et al: Lateral transperitoneal laparoscopic adrenalectomy. World J Urol 17:48–53, 1999.
20. McGrath PC, Sloan DA, Schwartz RW, Kenady DE: Advances in the diagnosis and therapy of adrenal tumors. Curr Opin Oncol 10:52–57, 1998.
21. Bornstein SR, Stratakis CA, Chrousos GP: Adrenocortical tumors: Recent advances in basic concepts and clinical management. Ann Intern Med 130:759–771, 1999.
22. Heniford BT, Arca MJ, Walsh RM, Gill IS: Laparoscopic adrenalectomy for cancer. Semin Surg Oncol 16:293–306, 1999.
23. Orchard T, Grant CS, van Heerden JA, Weaver A: Pheochromocytoma—continuing evolution of surgical therapy. Surgery 114:1153–1159, 1993.
24. Fernandez-Cruz L, Taura P, Saenz A et al: Laparoscopic approach to pheochromocytoma: Hemodynamic changes and catecholamine secretion. World J Surg 20:762–768, 1996.
25. Fernandez-Cruz L: Laparoscopic adrenal surgery. Br J Surg 83:721–723, 1996.
26. Gagner M: Laparoscopic adrenalectomy. Surg Clin North Am 76:523–537, 1996.
27. Sergev OWM: Primary aldosteronism. *In* Cerny JC (ed): Medical and Surgical Management of Adrenal Diseases. Philadelphia, Lippincott Williams & Wilkins, 1999, pp 75–82.
28. Nelson D: Cushing's syndrome. *In* DeBroot L, Beser GM, Cahill GF et al (eds): Endocrinology. Philadelphia, WB Saunders, 1989, pp 1660–1675.
29. Marsh H, Kim JG: Anesthesia for adrenal surgery. *In* Cerny J (ed): Medical and Surgical Management of Adrenal Diseases. Philadelphia, Lippincott Williams & Wilkins, 1999, pp 131–139.
30. Bonzani RA, Thompson NW: Pheochromocytoma. *In* Cerny JC (ed): Medical and Surgical Management of Adrenal Diseases. Philadelphia, Lippincott Williams & Wilkins, 1999, pp 141–163.
31. Janetschek G, Finkenstedt G, Gasser R et al: Laparoscopic surgery for pheochromocytoma: Adrenalectomy, partial resection, excision of paragangliomas. J Urol 160:330–334, 1998.
32. Hadden DR: Adrenal disorders of pregnancy. Endocrinol Metab Clin North Am 24:139–151, 1995.
33. Prinz RA: A comparison of laparoscopic and open adrenalectomies. Arch Surg 130:489–494, 1995.
34. Shen WT, Lim RC, Siperstein AE et al: Laparoscopic vs open adrenalectomy for the treatment of primary hyperaldosteronism. Arch Surg 134:628–632, 1999.
35. van Heerden JA, Young WF Jr, Grant CS, Carpenter PC: Adrenal surgery for hypercortisolism—surgical aspects. Surgery 117:466–472, 1995.
36. Fernandez-Cruz L, Saenz A, Benarroch G et al: Laparoscopic unilateral and bilateral adrenalectomy for Cushing's syndrome: Transperitoneal and retroperitoneal approaches. Ann Surg 224:727–736, 1996.

Index

Note: Page numbers in *italics* refer to illustrations; page numbers followed by t refer to tables.

A

B

C

D

E

F

G

H

I

L

N

O

P

S

U

V

W

X

Y

Z

Set ISBN 0-7216-7840-8
Volume 2 ISBN 0-7216-7